drug listing. **If the drug is a combination drug** (containing two or more medications), then you might have to look for each of the components in separate listings.

For more information

For more information about how to use this book, see *To the Reader* (page vi), which discusses content in depth. In addition to the drug listings, this book contains general information about the use of your medications, a medication-identification chart, a pregnancy-precaution listing, a list of Canadian trade names, and a form to record all of your medications (My Medication Record).

What special dietary instructions should I follow? Lists any foods or beverages that should not be taken with the medication or any other dietary changes that you need to make while taking this medication.

What should I do if I forget to take a dose? Gives you specific instructions to follow if you forget to take your medication.

What side effects can this medicine cause? Lists both common and serious side effects and what to do if they happen to you.

---

2 Sertraline

ments, and herbal products you are taking or plan to take. Be sure to mention any of the following: anticoagulants ('blood thinners') such as warfarin (Coumadin); antidepressants (mood elevators) such as amitriptyline (Elavil), amoxapine (Asendin), clomipramine (Anafranil), desipramine (Norpramin), doxepin (Adapin, Sinequan), imipramine (Tofranil), nortriptyline (Aventyl, Pamelor), protriptyline (Vivactil), and trimipramine (Surmontil); aspirin and other nonsteroidal anti-inflammatory medications (NSAIDs) such as ibuprofen (Advil, Motrin) and naproxen (Aleve, Naprosyn); cimetidine (Tagamet); diazepam (Valium); digoxin (Lanoxin); lithium (Eskalith, Lithobid); medications for anxiety, mental illness, Parkinson's disease, and seizures; medications for irregular heartbeat such as flecainide (Tambocor) and propafenone (Rythmol); oral medications for diabetes such as tolbutamide (Orinase); medications for migraine headaches such as almotriptan (Axert), eletriptan (Relpax), frovatriptan (Frova), naratriptan (Amerge), rizatriptan (Maxalt), sumatriptan (Imitrex), and zolmitriptan (Zomig); sedatives; sleeping pills; and tranquilizers. Your doctor may need to change the doses of your medications or monitor you carefully for side effects.

- tell your doctor if you have recently had a heart attack and if you have or have ever had seizures or liver or heart disease.
- tell your doctor if you are pregnant, plan to become pregnant, or are breast-feeding. If you become pregnant while taking sertraline, call your doctor.
- you should know that sertraline may make you drowsy. Do not drive a car or operate machinery until you know how this medication affects you.
- ask your doctor about the safe use of alcoholic beverages while you are taking sertraline.

What special dietary instructions should I follow?
Unless your doctor tells you otherwise, continue your normal diet.

What should I do if I forget to take a dose?
Take the missed dose as soon as you remember it. However, if it is almost time for the next dose, skip the missed dose and continue your regular dosing schedule. Do not take a double dose to make up for a missed one.

What side effects can this medicine cause?
Sertraline may cause side effects. Tell your doctor if any of these symptoms are severe or do not go away:
- nausea
- diarrhea
- constipation
- vomiting
- dry mouth
- gas or bloating
- loss of appetite
- weight changes
- drowsiness
- dizziness
- excessive tiredness
- headache
- pain, burning, or tingling in the hands or feet
- nervousness
- uncontrollable shaking of a part of the body
- sore throat

Consumer Reports® Consumer Drug Reference

- changes in sex drive or ability
- excessive sweating

Some side effects can be serious. If you experience any of the following symptoms or those listed in the IMPORTANT WARNING section, call your doctor immediately:
- blurred vision
- seizures
- abnormal bleeding or bruising
- hallucinating (seeing things or hearing voices that do not exist)

Sertraline may cause other side effects. Call your doctor if you have any unusual problems while taking this medication.

What storage conditions are needed for this medicine?
Keep this medication in the container it came in, tightly closed, and out of reach of children. Store it at room temperature and away from excess heat and moisture (not in the bathroom). Throw away any medication that is outdated or no longer needed. Talk to your pharmacist about the proper disposal of your medication.

What should I do in case of overdose?
In case of overdose, call your local poison control center at 1-800-222-1222. If the victim has collapsed or is not breathing, call local emergency services at 911.

Symptoms of overdose may include:
- hair loss
- changes in sex drive or ability
- drowsiness
- excessive tiredness
- difficulty falling asleep or staying asleep
- diarrhea
- vomiting
- rapid, pounding or irregular heartbeat
- nausea
- dizziness
- excitement
- uncontrollable shaking of a part of the body
- seizures
- hallucinating (hearing voices or seeing things that do not exist)
- unconsciousness
- fainting

What other information should I know?
Keep all appointments with your doctor.
Do not let anyone else take your medication. Ask your pharmacist any questions you have about refilling your prescription.

Dosage Facts
For Informational Purposes

Caution: Do not change your dose, how often you take your medication, or the length of time you are to take it without first talking to your health-care provider.

The following dosage information was written using medical language for doctors and other healthcare professionals and is provided here for you to check your dosage. The dosage of this drug may differ for different patients. Therefore, always follow your doctor's instruc-

Access FREE updates online @ www.consumerdrugreference.org   © Copyright 2008 American Society of Health-System Pharmacists

---

What storage conditions are needed for this medicine? Tells you how to store the medication and what to do when it is outdated or no longer needed.

What should I do in case of overdose? Gives you the phone number to contact your local poison control center and lists effects that might occur if you take too much of the medication.

What other information should I know? Tells you any additional information that might be important when you take or use this medication.

Dosage Facts. Provides dosing information written for doctors and other health-care professionals and is provided here for you to check your dosage. **Do not change your dose, how often you take your medication, or the length of time you are to take it without first talking to your health-care provider.**

What's New in This Edition?

New for 2008

The 2008 Consumer Drug Reference was developed by pharmacists as a guide to help you and your family make safe and effective use of your medications. The easy-to-use format presents the critical drug information facts you need, drawing on current clinical research. New sections and expanded content have been added to help you continue to take an informed and active role in managing your medication use. The new and updated information includes:

- A "Guide to Over-the-Counter (OTC) Medicines" to help you choose and safely use many of the non-prescription products that you can buy at your pharmacy or other retail store. This section will also explain how to understand the information on each product's label. A summary of medications used for certain symptoms and conditions is included in the last part of this guide to help you select the most appropriate product for your needs.

- A section explaining the prescribing of medications for off-labeled uses and how to find out if the medication you are taking is being used for an FDA-approved indication.

- Information about Consumer Reports Best Buy Drugs, a public education initiative that provides free guidance (including cost information) about prescription medicines for consumers.

- An expanded Drug Identification section with over 1000 photographs of the most commonly used medications, with even more generic products now included, for you to verify that you are taking the right medication.

- Over 60 new drug listings, including many of the latest drugs approved by the FDA, detailed information about specific vaccines, chemotherapy agents (drugs used for the treatment of cancer), and medications that are used to help you stop smoking.

- Important safety warnings from the Food and Drug Administration (FDA) and drug manufacturers to keep you up to date about the risks and benefits of the medications that you are taking.

- An updated schedule of immunization information with the most current vaccination recommendations for children, teenagers, and adults.

- Newly approved uses for currently available medications.

- An updated pregnancy precaution section with classifications for new drugs.

How to Find More Drug Information Online

It is important for consumers to have access to the most current information about their medications. Go to our website, 24 hours a day, seven days a week to learn about new drugs and updated safety information.

Website address

Go to **www.consumerdrugreference.org**.

Access

You will need to enter the following name and password:

User name: crcdr

Password: moredrugs

Consumer Drug Reference

2008 Edition

American Society of Health-System Pharmacists®

Bethesda, Maryland

Consumer Reports
A Division of Consumers Union
Yonkers, New York

The *Consumer Drug Reference 2008*, is published by Consumer Reports, a division of Consumers Union of U.S., Inc. Consumers Union is an independent, nonprofit testing organization serving only consumers. Since 1936, it has been a comprehensive source for unbiased reporting about products and services, personal finance, health and nutrition, and other consumer concerns. It is chartered under the Not-For-Profit Corporation Law of the State of New York. Consumers Union derives its income mainly from the sale of *Consumer Reports*® magazine and other publications and services, such as Consumer Reports® Online, Consumer Reports® on Health, Consumer Reports® Medical Guide, and Consumer Reports® Money Adviser. Income is also derived from nonrestrictive, noncommercial contributions, grants, and fees. You may review our complete privacy policy for Consumer Reports information products, services, and programs at *www.ConsumerReports.org/privacy*.

NOTICE AND WARNING

Concerning US Patent or Trademark Rights

The inclusion in *Consumer Drug Reference* of entry on any drug in respect to which patent or trademark rights may exist shall not be deemed, and is not intended as, a grant of, or authority to exercise, any right or privilege protected by such patent or trademark. All such rights and privileges are vested in the patent or trademark owner, and no other person may exercise the same without express permission, authority, or license secured from such patent or trademark owner.

The listing of selected brand names is intended only for ease of reference. The inclusion of a brand name does not mean the American Society of Health-System Pharmacists or Consumers Union has any particular knowledge that the brand listed has properties different from other brands of the same drug, nor should it be interpreted as an endorsement by the American Society of Health-System Pharmacists or by Consumers Union. Similarly, the fact that a particular brand has not been included does not indicate that the product has been judged to be unsatisfactory or unacceptable.

Contents

Consumer Drug Reference

American Society of Health-System Pharmacists

Editorial Staff

Gerald K. McEvoy, Pharm.D.
Assistant Vice President, Drug Information Systems and Editor-in-Chief, *AHFS Drug Information*

Carol Wolfe
Vice President, Publications and Drug Information Systems Office

Barbara F. Young, Pharm.D., MHA
Project Editor

Michelle Schuchman, Pharm.D.
Jennifer Meyer Harris, Pharm.D.
Tzipora R. Lieder, R.Ph.
Theresa Lower, B.A., RN, CDE
Shana S. Mauer, Pharm.D.
Writers

Lisa Shannon
Project Manager

Johnna Hershey
Director, Publications Production Center

David Wade
Publishing Design Manager

Terry L. Griggs
Editorial Assistant

Silvia France
Office Manager

Jeffery Shick, B.S.
Director, eHealth Solutions

Edward D. Millikan, Pharm.D.
Assistant Director, eHealth Solutions Division

Kendra J. Grande, B.S., Pharm.
Laura Brady Sullivan, Pharm.D.
Contributors

Foreword

This reference book is designed to help make the challenging task of taking medications as simple, as effective, and as safe as possible. Taking a prescription or over-the-counter medication—and especially if you take more than one—is no simple matter. To work well, with a minimum of side effects, medications need to be taken according to directions. Taking them any other way is at best a waste of money and at worst a threat to your life. Over the last few years, roughly 500,000 adverse drug events have been reported annually to the US Food and Drug Administration; about 1 in 5 of those have been classified by the FDA as "serious." Recent studies also suggest that the total number of adverse drug events reported is just the tip of the iceberg—the vast majority of events that occur never get reported.

The Consumer Drug Reference (CDR), published annually since 1989 by Consumers Union, the not-for-profit publisher of Consumer Reports and the monthly newsletter, Consumer Reports on Health, is designed specifically for you, the healthcare consumer.

Good directions about medications can be hard to come by. Those distributed by your pharmacist may supply too little information, or even too much. If there's too little, you may overlook a possible problem. But if there's too much, the information can be so overwhelming and frightening that you may be tempted to shun a needed medication.

Other sources of drug information, such as drug ads on TV and radio, and in print, may misinform rather than inform. Ads spend considerably more time or space extolling the drug's benefits than warning about its limitations and side effects. In 2006, pharmaceutical companies spent over $5.5 billion advertising medications directly to the consumer. And many Web sites that also contain drug information often focus on selling the product.

All of the medicines on the market (except those that existed prior to the 1938 drug laws), have been approved by the Food and Drug Administration (FDA) for safety and efficacy when used as intended. However rigorous that approval process may be, it cannot guarantee that every drug on the market is always safe or is always effective. Even when drugs are taken as directed, side effects can be expected. Most of those are known from clinical trials done before the drug hits the market, but others that are less common only become evident after the drug has been in widespread use for a while.

This danger of side effects is magnified by the misuse of drugs by patient and doctor, who may take or prescribe too much or too little, for too long or too short a length of time. And if more than one medication is being taken, the risk of side effects is increased by drug-drug interactions. According to a report released by the Institute of Medicine in July 2006, this is especially a concern for roughly one-third of adults, who take five or more medications.

All New for 2008

The expanded 2008 edition of the Consumer Drug Reference contains an easy-to-use design that calls your attention to the most important information up front. It is the second edition published with our partner, the American Society of Health-System Pharmacists (ASHP). The mission of this not-for-profit organization is simply "to help people make the best use of medications." Founded in 1942, ASHP has grown to include over 30,000 practicing pharmacists, pharmacy students, and pharmacy technicians. The content of the CDR has been developed by pharmacists and other medical experts without industry influence or funding.

This volume, written for laypersons in understandable language, contains information on more than 12,000 drugs. The drugs are arranged alphabetically by their generic names with cross-references from many brand names in the easily accessible index. Important warnings head up the entries, followed by approved indications, how to use the medicine, and off-label uses (evidence-supported additional uses of a drug other than the FDA-approved indication). For more information about off-label use of medications, see page G-8. Special precautions, such as warnings for pregnant or nursing women, side effects (organized by degree of seriousness), and possible interactions with other drugs are also included.

A special full-color section includes photographs of more than 1000 commonly prescribed tablets, capsules, and other drug products. This section is included so that you can see what the medication looks like and be certain that it's the drug in your medication container.

A new detailed section on over-the-counter drugs, as well as an illustration and explanation of the over-the-counter "Drug Facts" label, are also included in this 2008 edition. And we've once again included a tear-out Medication Record form at the back of the book to help you keep track of your medications.

Online Updates Available

The CDR is a work in progress that is continually updated as new drugs come along and as old drugs get new safety warnings or new indications. For readers of this book, free access to the Web site www.consumerdrugreference.org is also available for up-to-the-minute drug listings and safety alerts.

You can access Consumer Reports drug information through www.ConsumerReportsHealth.org. That Web site also provides our Best Buy Drug Reports, which rate the efficacy, safety, and cost-effectiveness of many drugs. For more information about our Best Buy Drug project, see page BB-1. The above site also includes access to the Consumer Reports Medical Guide, which provides ratings of treatment options for more than 200 conditions and diseases. You can also access current information on thousands of natural medicines and dietary supplements.

We hope this book serves you well and enables you and the ones you care about to use medications safely and wisely.

Marvin M. Lipman, MD, FACP

To The Reader

When you receive a prescription medication or purchase an over-the-counter (nonprescription) product, you may have questions about your medicine such as:

- Why is this medication prescribed?
- How should this medication be used?
- What side effects can this medication cause?
- What storage conditions are needed for this medication?

You also may need to know specific instructions about how you are to use the medication, including whether you should take it with food or on an empty stomach or which other drugs and/or food may interact with the medication you are taking. It is important for you to know when it is necessary to talk to your doctor, pharmacist, or other healthcare provider to discuss how the medication is affecting you and your disease or condition.

Today's medicines are more complex and powerful than ever before. *Consumer Drug Reference 2008* can help you find the important information you need to use medications safely and effectively. This information is provided as a supplement to any specific instructions that your doctor, pharmacist, or other healthcare professional has given to you. Because everyone is unique in his or her experience when taking medicines, always talk to your pharmacist or doctor if you have specific questions about your medications.

Notice:

The information provided in the Drug Information section is not intended as individual advice, but should be used in addition to the information and instructions that your doctor, pharmacist, or other healthcare provider has discussed with you. These drug listings are summaries of the available information and do not contain all of the warnings, precautions, side effects, drug interactions, or other information that may be related to the use of the drug. While the listings address the manufacturer's information that accompanies the product, not all of the content is exactly the same, and there may be some additional information from other sources. It is not intended for the information contained in these monographs to provide a complete background for you to evaluate all of the risks and benefits of using this medication for your medical condition or disease. Instead, you should review this information and that from other sources with your doctor, pharmacist, or other healthcare professional if you have questions about your medication and/or how it may affect your medical condition. Always talk to your pharmacist or doctor if you need additional information about your medications.

The nature of drug information is that it is constantly changing because of new research and emerging knowledge from the ongoing use of the drug in patients. The information about medications is often subject to interpretation and the uniqueness of each patient and his or her medical condition. While care has been taken to ensure the accuracy of the information presented, the reader is advised that the authors, editors, reviewers, contributors, and publishers cannot be responsible that the information remains up-to-date or for any errors or omissions in this book or for any associated consequences. Newly recognized precautions, previously unreported side effects, and other new information may emerge at any time for any given drug and new drugs constantly are entering the marketplace. Because of the ever-changing nature of drug information, you should know that decisions regarding your medications and medical care must be based on your doctor's judgment, changing information about a drug (e.g., as reflected in the medical literature), and changing medical practices.

It is important for consumers to have access to the most current information about their medications. To find out about new drugs and safety information that has been reported after the *Consumer Drug Reference 2008* was published, you can visit several websites that contain updated information. The U.S. Food and Drug Administration (FDA) has a website (*www.fda.gov/cder/index.html*) that contains reports of new side effects, warnings, precautions, and other information about drug safety. To find new drug listings, safety alerts, and updated information for the Consumer Drug Reference, you can visit the website *www.consumerdrugreference.org* to easily find and print this information for your use.

However, if after reading and reviewing any information in this book or from other sources, you have special concerns about the medication(s) that you have been prescribed, you should first talk to your doctor before you make any changes in the way you take or use your medication. Do not stop taking your medication without talking to your doctor, pharmacist, or other healthcare provider.

Drugs are available under many brand (trade) names. The inclusion of various brand names in the text of the *Consumer Drug Reference 2008* is intended only to make it easier to reference a specific product. The inclusion of these brands does not mean that the publishers have any knowledge that any given brand has properties that differ from other brands of the same medicine nor does it represent an endorsement of a particular brand. Instead, this information is provided only for informational purposes to help the reader identify specific familiar products. For some drugs, there are too many brands available to list them all, and new brands and changes in formulations are introduced constantly. Therefore, missing specific brands of a medicine should not be interpreted to represent any judgment. In many cases, your doctor may prescribe a medicine by its generic (common) name or you may purchase over-the-counter (nonprescription) medicines by their generic name (e.g., acetaminophen for Tylenol®). If you have questions about the name of a medicine, especially if you wonder whether it is the same as another more familiar product, ask your pharmacist or doctor.

How to Use This Book

Consumer Drug Reference 2008 contains general information about how you should use your medications as well as a section of drug information about specific medicines. The General Section in the front of this reference (G-1) explains important considerations about taking your medicine, how to manage your medications, off-label use of medications, information about generic and brand-name drugs, safety issues, and how to store your medications. It is important to review the information in both of these sections to make the best use of your medications.

All drug products have a generic (common) name and many products also have a brand (trade) name. The generic name of the drug is determined when it is first brought to the market and is approved by the U.S. Adopted Name (USAN) Council and the World Health Organization (WHO). Many medicines also have brand names, which are created by manufacturers to promote recognition of their products on packaging and in advertising. Often, brand-name products may be available as less expensive generic medicines. In many cases, brand names are protected by patents for several years. Once the patent of a medicine expires, other manufacturers are allowed to manufacture it and call it by a generic name or other brand name. A generic drug is a copy that usually is the same as the brand-name medicine in dosage, safety, and strength, how it is taken, and in its quality, performance, and intended use. Since generic drugs use the same active ingredients and are shown to work the same way in the body, they have the same risks and benefits as their brand-name counterparts. For more information about generic drugs, see the General Information section titled "Generic and Brand-Name Drugs."

Each medication in *Consumer Drug Reference 2008* is listed alphabetically by the generic name of the drug in the Drug Information section. If you only know the brand name of your medicine, you can look in the index to find the generic name and the page number where the drug is listed in this reference. If the drug is a combination drug (containing two or more medications in the same product), you may have to look for each of the individual drugs in order to find information about the combination medicine.

Some generic names may be listed more than once with a description of how the drug is to be used in the body. For example, ciprofloxacin is listed as ciprofloxacin oral (for the tablets and liquid that are taken by mouth), ciprofloxacin injection (for the solution that is injected into a vein), and ciprofloxacin ophthalmic (for the solution and ointment that are used in the eye). Many drugs listed in this book are used in different ways in the body and the definitions for the manner in which the drugs are used are given below.

- Buccal—medication is placed in the mouth between the cheeks or lips and gum
- Nasal inhalation—medication is taken into the nose
- Oral inhalation—medication is taken into the lungs through the mouth
- Injection—medication that is injected into a vein or muscle or under the skin
- Nasal spray—medication is sprayed into the nose
- Ophthalmic—medication is placed into the eye
- Oral—medication is taken by mouth to be absorbed into the body

- Otic—medication is placed into the ear
- Rectal—medication is inserted into the rectum
- Subcutaneous injection—medication is given by syringe into the tissue just under the skin
- Sublingual—medication is placed under the tongue
- Topical—medication is applied directly on the skin
- Transdermal—a patch containing the medication is placed on the skin and the medication is slowly released
- Transmucosal—medication is placed in the mouth between the cheek and gum and allowed to dissolve slowly
- Vaginal—medication is inserted into the vagina

About AHFS MedMaster® Consumer Medication Information Database and AHFS DI Essentials® Dosing Information

Consumer Drug Reference 2008 contains the AHFS MedMaster® Consumer Medication Information database, which features more than 1000 drug listings about generic and brand-name medications that are written in easy to understand language for the consumer. This information is designed to supplement information about medications provided by doctors, pharmacists, and other healthcare professionals.

MedMaster® is based on the American Society of Health-System Pharmacists' (ASHP's) premier, unbiased drug information resources, which are developed independently by pharmacists and other medication experts. The mission is to provide a foundation for safe and effective drug therapy based on scientific evidence. Widely trusted for its established record in refuting unfounded claims, its rigorous science-based editorial process, and its independence from the influence of pharmaceutical manufacturers, these references have remained true to this mission for almost 50 years.

The **Dosage Facts** section is included for the consumer's informational purposes. The dosing section is derived from the *AHFS DI Essentials®* database, which is designed to offer healthcare professionals easy access to knowledge that is critical at the time they are providing care to patients. When you review this dosing information for the medications that you take or use, always contact your doctor, pharmacist, or other healthcare professional if you have any questions about the specific dosage of your medication. **You should never change the dosage of your prescription medicine, how often you take your medicine, or the length of time you are to take this medicine unless directed by your doctor or other healthcare professional.** For over-the-counter (nonprescription) medicines, consult the product labeling and follow the dosages listed there or take the medicine as directed by your healthcare professional. Never exceed recommended dosages unless specifically directed by your doctor.

About ASHP

The American Society of Health-System Pharmacists (ASHP) is the 30,000-member national professional association comprised of pharmacists who work with doctors and other health professionals in:

- Hospitals
- Ambulatory care clinics (e.g., HMOs)

- Long-term care facilities (e.g., nursing homes)
- Home care services

Since 1942, ASHP's mission has been to support pharmacists in helping people use medications safely and effectively. ASHP is widely recognized as a leader in promoting medication safety, and was one of the first publishers to produce drug information specifically directed at consumers almost 30 years ago. ASHP is a past recipient of an award of excellence for consumer education materials from FDA and the National Coalition for Consumer Education (NCCE). Staff members from ASHP serve on FDA's Drug Safety and Risk Management Committee and as experts for various drug safety and quality organizations (e.g., Institute of Medicine [IOM], National Quality Forum [NQF]). ASHP also serves on the Board of the National Council on Patient Information and Education (NCPIE).

Hospital and health-system pharmacists are licensed medication experts with at least five years of highly specialized pharmacy education. They often have completed doctoral degrees in pharmacy (Pharm.D.) and postgraduate residency programs. Health-system pharmacists:

- Evaluate new medications and advise doctors and other healthcare professionals about the safest and most effective drug therapies for individual patients
- Monitor every stage of medication therapy to improve drug effectiveness
- Provide critical safety and drug quality checks to prevent harmful drug interactions or reactions and potential mistakes
- Work under sterile conditions to create compounds that patients receive intravenously
- Supervise the dispensing and distribution of medications
- Counsel patients on the appropriate use of medicines

General Information

General Information about the Use of Medications

The following general information is provided to help you make safe use of your medications. You should always read the specific information in the Drug Listing section for each of your prescription medicines and also any medications that you buy without a prescription.

If you have any questions about your medication or how to use it, you should always talk to your doctor, pharmacist, or other healthcare professional.

What should I tell my doctor before taking or using this medication?

Before taking or using any medication:

- Tell your doctor if you are allergic to any medications, dyes, or other substances, including any foods.
- Tell your doctor or pharmacist what prescription and over-the-counter (nonprescription) medications, vitamins, nutritional supplements, and herbal products you are taking or plan to take. Remember, even occasional use of some nonprescription medications such as pain relievers, antacids, cold products, and laxatives could have effects on other medications you are taking.
- Tell your doctor if you have or ever have had a disease or condition such as diabetes or kidney or liver disease. Sometimes your doctor may want to know if anyone in your family has or has had a particular disease or disorder.
- Tell your doctor if you are pregnant or plan to become pregnant because some drugs may harm your unborn child. This is especially important during the first few weeks when fetal organs are forming. For other medications, their safety during pregnancy may not be known. If you become pregnant while taking any medication, call your doctor. For your convenience, a listing of drugs with FDA's rating for pregnancy risks is included in an appendix at the end of this book.
- Tell your doctor if you are breastfeeding or intend to breastfeed. Many medications get into your breast milk and can cause unwanted effects in your baby.
- Tell your doctor if you smoke or drink alcohol-containing beverages since some medications can be affected by chemicals in tobacco smoke and changes in your liver caused by alcohol. Alcohol also can increase drowsiness and confusion.
- If you are having surgery, including dental surgery, tell the doctor or dentist if you are taking any medications, vitamins, nutritional supplements, or herbal products since some can affect blood clotting and others can interact with anesthetic agents.
- Ask your pharmacist or doctor for a copy of the manufacturer's information for the patient or access it from the Food and Drug Administration website (*www.FDA.gov*).

Be sure to read this information carefully and discuss any questions you may have with your pharmacist or doctor.

- Tell your doctor if you have trouble with reading, opening medicine containers, or remembering to take your medicine.

How should I take or use this medication?

- Follow the directions on the prescription label carefully, and ask your doctor or pharmacist to explain any part you do not understand.
- For over-the-counter (nonprescription) medicines, follow the directions on the manufacturer's labeling carefully and ask your pharmacist or doctor to explain any part you do not understand.
- Read the label carefully each time and check the medication you are taking.
- Take or use your medication at about the same time(s) every day. If necessary, use calendars, timers, or pillboxes that remind you which drugs to take and when. Occasionally, some medicines are only taken as needed (e.g., analgesics), but do not exceed recommended dosages.
- If you take a drug several times each day and have trouble remembering to take it, ask your doctor if the drug is available in a dosage form, such as a long-acting tablet or capsule, that can be taken less often.
- Take your medication exactly as directed. Do not take more or less of it or take it more often than prescribed by your doctor.
- Take your medicine for as long as your doctor has told you. Do not stop taking your medication just because your symptoms disappear or you begin to feel better unless specifically told to do so.
- Bring all the medications and supplements (even those prescribed by other doctors) to your primary care doctor for review at least every six months.
- If you take certain medications regularly, be sure to allow enough time to order refills before you run out so that you won't miss any doses.
- Tell your doctor or pharmacist if you notice a change in the appearance (e.g., color, shape, size) of a medication that was refilled, unless an explanation has been given by your doctor or pharmacist.
- Do not take medications in the dark or without enough light to read the label. If you can't see well, you could take the wrong medication or dose.
- Medications that you take by mouth generally should be swallowed with a full glass (8 oz) of water unless your doctor or pharmacist has told you to take them with other liquids or food.
- You may need to take some medications with food to get the best effect or to reduce side effects in your stomach. Other medications may need to be taken on an empty stomach to get the best effect.
- Be sure to ask your pharmacist or doctor if you can safely split, chew, or crush the tablets or capsules that you are taking. Some long-acting medications should only be swallowed whole.

- Shake the liquids or suspension containers well before each use to mix the contents evenly.
- Always use the measuring device provided with liquid medications or ask your pharmacist to provide you with one. You should not use kitchen spoons because they can vary in size and may provide too much or too little medication.
- If you are having trouble taking one form of medication such as a large capsule, ask your pharmacist or doctor if it is available in another form that you can swallow more easily.
- Ask your doctor about the safe use of alcoholic beverages while you are taking your medication. Alcohol can make the side effects (e.g., drowsiness) from some medicines worse.
- Ask your doctor about the use of caffeinated beverages while you are taking your medication.

How to Use Special Dosage Forms

Provided here are instructions with pictures illustrating the best way to use several types of medication that are placed into your eye(s), nose, ear(s), or rectum. These descriptions are for general information only; you should always follow the specific instructions that come with your medication.

How to Use Eye Ointments and Gels Properly

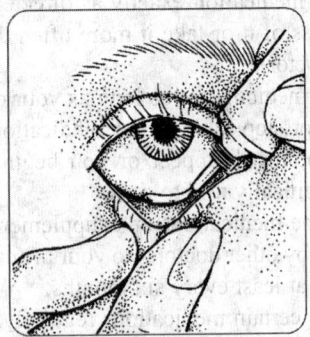

Adapted, with permission, from the Michigan Pharmacists Association's *Patient Education Program*. Illustration reproduced, with permission, from the *Atlas of Primary Eyecare Procedures*, Appleton Lange, Norwalk, CT, 1997.

(Using a mirror or having someone else apply the ointment or gel may make this procedure easier.)

1. Wash your hands thoroughly with soap and water.
2. Avoid touching the tip of the tube against your eye or anything else—the medication and its container must be kept clean.
3. Holding the tube between your thumb and forefinger, place it as near to your eyelid as possible without touching it.
4. Brace the remaining fingers of that hand against your face.

5. Tilt your head forward slightly.
6. With your index finger, pull the lower eyelid down to form a pocket.
7. Squeeze a ribbon of ointment or gel into the pocket made by the lower eyelid.
8. Blink your eye gently; then close your eye for 1 to 2 minutes.
9. With a tissue, wipe any excess ointment or gel from the eyelids and lashes. With another clean tissue, wipe the tip of the tube clean.
10. Repeat steps 3-9 if the ointment is also to be placed in the other eye.

How to Use Eyedrops Properly

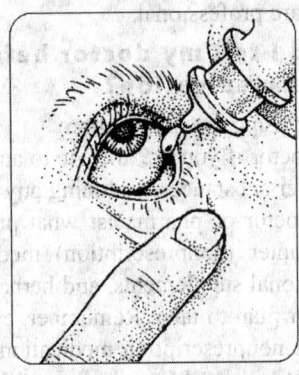

Adapted, with permission, from the Michigan Pharmacists Association's *Patient Education Program*. Illustration reproduced, with permission, from the *Atlas of Primary Eyecare Procedures*, Appleton Lange, Norwalk, CT, 1997.

(Using a mirror or having someone else give you the eyedrops may make this procedure easier.)

1. Wash your hands thoroughly with soap and water.
2. Check the dropper tip to make sure that it is not chipped or cracked.
3. Avoid touching the dropper tip against your eye or anything else—eyedrops and droppers must be kept clean.
4. While tilting your head back, pull down the lower lid of your eye with your index finger to form a pocket (see figure).
5. Hold the dropper (tip down) with the other hand, as close to the eye as possible without touching it.
6. Brace the remaining fingers of that hand against your face.
7. Gently squeeze the dropper so that the correct number of drops falls into the pocket made by the lower eyelid.
8. Close your eye for 2 to 3 minutes. Wipe any excess liquid from your face with a tissue.
9. Repeat steps 4-8 if the drops are also to be placed in the other eye.
10. Replace and tighten the cap right away. Do not wipe or rinse the dropper tip.
11. Wash your hands to remove any medication.

How to Use Ear Drops Properly

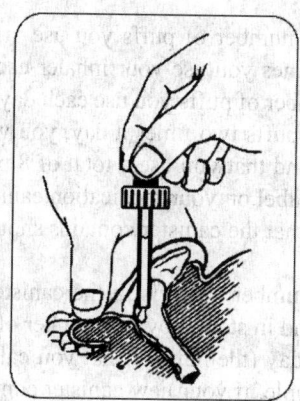

Adapted, with permission, from the Michigan Pharmacists Association's Patient Education Program.

(Having someone else give you the ear drops may make this procedure easier.)

1. Gently clean your ear with a damp facecloth and then dry your ear.
2. Wash your hands thoroughly with soap and water.
3. Warm the drops to near body temperature by holding the container in your hand for a few minutes.
4. If the drops are a cloudy suspension, shake the bottle well for 10 seconds.
5. Check the dropper tip to make sure that it is not chipped or cracked.
6. If the dropper is attached to the cap of your ear drop bottle, turn the bottle upside down to allow the drops to drip into the dropper.
7. If your ear drop bottle came with a regular cap, and you are using a separate dropper, place the tip of the dropper inside the bottle and squeeze the bulb gently to fill the dropper with drops.
8. Tilt the affected ear up or lie on your side.
9. Avoid touching the dropper tip against your ear or anything else—ear drops and the dropper must be kept clean.
10. Place the correct amount in your ear. Then tug gently on your ear to allow the drops to run in.
11. Keep your ear tilted up for a few minutes or insert a soft cotton plug in your ear, whichever method has been recommended by your pharmacist or doctor.

12. Replace and tighten the cap or dropper right away.
13. Wash your hands to remove any medication.

How to Use Metered-Dose Inhalers

Using Your Inhaler: You can use these general instructions to help you remember the right way to use your inhaler. However, your doctor or pharmacist should also give you specific directions for using the type of inhaler that was prescribed for you. Ask your doctor or pharmacist to show you how to use your inhaler and to watch you as you use it for the first time. Also ask your doctor or pharmacist for a copy of the manufacturer's information for the patient that comes with your inhaler and read this information carefully.

These directions explain how to use metered-dose inhalers. If you are using a different type of inhaler such as a dry powder inhaler, you will need to follow different directions. Ask your doctor or pharmacist if you need more information or if you do not know what type of inhaler you are using.

Most inhalers can be used alone or with a spacer (plastic tube that attaches to an inhaler and helps the medication to reach the lungs). Spacers are useful for all patients, especially children, older adults, and patients who are using inhaled corticosteroids (a type of medication used to prevent swelling of the airways in patients who have asthma). Ask your doctor if you should use your inhaler with a spacer. If you will be using a spacer, be sure you understand how to use and clean it. Ask your doctor or pharmacist if you have any questions.

1. Remove the cap and hold the inhaler upright.
2. Shake the inhaler.
3. Tilt your head back slightly and breathe out slowly.
4. Hold your inhaler in one of the following ways. (See Figure 1.) Methods A and B are best, but C is acceptable if you have trouble with A and B. Method C must be used for breath-activated inhalers.
5. If you are not using a spacer, press down on your inhaler **one** time to release medication and breathe in slowly through your mouth at the same time. If you are using a spacer, first press down on the inhaler, then within 5 seconds, begin to breathe in slowly through your mouth.

Figure 1.

A. Hold inhaler 1 to 2 inches in front of your mouth (about the width of your fingers).

B. Use a spacer/holding chamber. These come in many shapes and can be useful to any patient.

C. Put the inhaler in your mouth. Do not use for steroids.

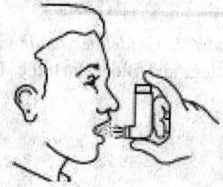
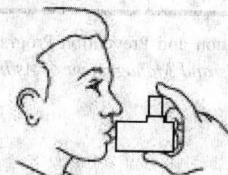
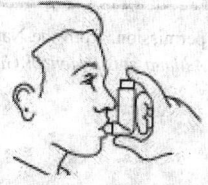

6. Continue to breathe in slowly for 3 to 5 seconds.

7. Hold your breath for 10 seconds if you can to allow the medication to reach deeply into your lungs.

8. Repeat steps 3-7 until you have inhaled the number of puffs that your doctor prescribed. If you are using a quick-relief medication (short-acting beta$_2$ agonists), wait about 1 minute between puffs. There is no need to wait between puffs for other types of medication. Ask your doctor or pharmacist if you need to wait between puffs of your medication.

Cleaning Your Inhaler:

1. Look at the hole where the medication sprays out of the inhaler.

2. If you see powder in or around the hole, then you need to clean the inhaler.

3. Remove the metal canister from the L-shaped plastic mouthpiece.

4. Rinse only the mouthpiece and cap in warm water.

5. Let the mouthpiece and cap dry overnight.

6. In the morning, put the canister back inside the mouthpiece and put the cap on the inhaler.

Knowing When to Replace Your Inhaler: You cannot see the medication in your inhaler, so it is hard to tell when it is empty. Some people think they can tell when their inhalers are empty by floating the canisters in water, spraying the medication into the air, or tasting the medication. However, studies show that none of these methods really work, and people who use these methods may continue to rely on their inhalers after the inhalers are empty. Follow the directions below as a guide to know when to replace your inhaler. However, because each inhaler device may vary, it is important to read and follow the package instructions or ask your pharmacist or doctor when to replace your inhaler so that you always receive your full dose of medication.

For long-term control medications that you take regularly each day:

1. Multiply the number of puffs you use at a time by the number of times you use your inhaler each day. This is the total number of puffs you use each day. For example, if you use 4 puffs two times a day, you would multiply 4 by 2 and find that you use a total of 8 puffs each day.

2. Look at the label on your medication canister. The number of puffs that the canister contains should be listed on the label.

3. Divide the number of puffs in the canister (the number that you found in step 2) by the number of puffs that you inhale each day (the number that you calculated in step 1). For example, if your new canister contains 200 puffs and you inhale 8 puffs per day, you would divide 200 by 8 and find that your canister would last 25 days.

4. Instead of following the steps above, you can use Table 1 to estimate how long your canister will last.

5. You should note the date that you begin using the canister and count ahead by the number of days you expect the canister to last. This will give you the date that you can expect your canister to be empty. For example, if you started using the new canister on May 1st, and the canister contains enough medication for 25 days, it should last until May 26th. Plan to refill you prescription before this date so that you will not run out of medication.

6. You can write the date on your canister to help you remember when you will need to refill your prescription.

For quick-relief medications that you use as needed:

1. You will need to count each puff that you use.

2. When the number of puffs used is near the total number of puffs in the canister, you will need to get a new canister.

Table 1:

How Often To Change Long-Term-Control Canisters

# Sprays	2 Sprays/Day	4 Sprays/Day	6 Sprays/Day	8 Sprays/Day	9 Sprays/Day	12 Sprays/Day	16 Sprays/Day
60	30 days	15 days	n/a	n/a	n/a	n/a	n/a
100	n/a	25 days	16 days	12 days	n/a	n/a	n/a
104	n/a	26 days	17 days	13 days	n/a	n/a	n/a
112	n/a	28 days	18 days	14 days	n/a	n/a	n/a
120	60 days	30 days	20 days	15 days	n/a	n/a	n/a
200	n/a	50 days	33 days	25 days	22 days	16 days	12 days
240	n/a	60 days	40 days	30 days	26 days	20 days	15 days

Reprinted, with permission, from the National Asthma Education and Prevention Program's *Expert Panel Report 2: Guidelines for the Diagnosis and Management of Asthma* and *Practical Guide for the Diagnosis and Management of Asthma*, National Heart, Lung, and Blood Institute, Bethesda, MD, 1997.

How to Use Nose Drops Properly

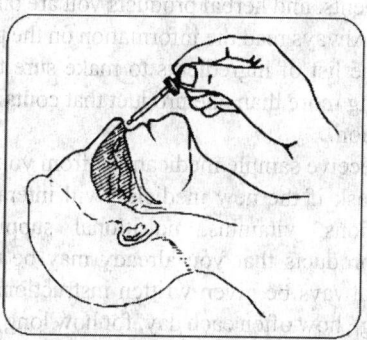

Adapted, with permission, from the Michigan Pharmacists Association's *Patient Education Program*.

(Having someone else give you the nose drops may make this procedure easier.)

1. Blow your nose gently.
2. Wash your hands thoroughly with soap and water
3. Check the dropper tip to make sure that it is not chipped or cracked.
4. Avoid touching the dropper tip against your nose or anything else—nose drops and the dropper must be kept clean.
5. Tilt your head as far back as possible, or lie down on your back on a flat surface (such as a bed) and hang your head over the edge.
6. Place the drops into your nose.
7. Bend your head forward toward your knees and move it left and right.
8. Remain in this position for a few minutes.
9. Clean the dropper tip with warm water. Cap the bottle right away.
10. Wash your hands to remove any medication.

How to Use Rectal Suppositories Properly

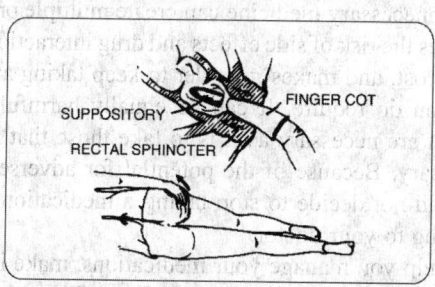

Adapted, with permission, from the Michigan Pharmacists Association's *Patient Education Program*.

1. Wash your hands thoroughly with soap and water.
2. If the suppository is soft, hold it under cool water to harden it before removing the wrapper.
3. Remove the wrapper, if present.
4. If you were told to use half of the suppository, cut it lengthwise with a clean, single-edge razor blade.
5. Put on a finger cot or disposable glove, if desired (available at a pharmacy).
6. Lubricate the suppository tip with a water-soluble lubricant such as K-Y Jelly, not petroleum jelly (such as

Vaseline). If you do not have this lubricant, moisten your rectal area with cool tap water.

7. Lie on your side with your lower leg straightened out and your upper leg bent forward toward your stomach.
8. Lift upper buttock to expose the rectal area.
9. Insert the suppository, pointed end first, with your finger until it passes the muscular sphincter of the rectum, about 1/2 to 1 inch in infants and young children and 1 inch in adults. If not inserted past this sphincter, the suppository may pop out.
10. Hold buttocks together for a few seconds.
11. Remain lying down for about 15 minutes to avoid having the suppository come out.
12. Discard used materials and wash your hands thoroughly.

What special dietary instructions should I follow?

- Unless your doctor tells you otherwise, continue your normal diet. Be sure to tell your doctor if you are following a special diet because some medications may contain other ingredients such as salt, sugar, or alcohol that could affect your diet.
- Some medications should not be taken with certain foods or beverages, such as grapefruit or grapefruit juice. Be sure to ask your pharmacist or doctor if there are certain foods or beverages that should not be taken with your medication.

What should I do if I forget to take a dose?

- You should review the specific information for the medication that you are taking. Generally, you should take the missed dose as soon as you remember it. However, if it is almost time for the next dose, skip the missed dose and continue your regular dosing schedule. Do not take a double dose to make up for a missed one.
- If you are using a cream, lotion, ointment, or gel, apply the missed dose as soon as you remember it. However, if it is almost time for the next dose, skip the missed dose and continue your regular dosing schedule. Do not apply extra cream, lotion, ointment, or gel to make up for a missed dose.

What side effects can my medication cause?

- Medications may cause side effects, and some can be serious. You should learn about those side effects and what you should do about them before you start taking your medication. If you experience any serious side effects, call your doctor immediately.
- Some medications may cause long-term risks. Talk to your doctor or pharmacist about all the risks and benefits of taking any medication.
- If you experience a serious side effect, you or your doctor may send a report to the Food and Drug Administration's (FDA) MedWatch Adverse Event Reporting program online [*www.fda.gov/MedWatch/index.html*] or by phone [1-800-332-1088].

How should I store my medication?

- Keep your medication in the container it came in, tightly closed, and out of reach of children and pets.
- Store it at room temperature and away from excess heat and moisture (not in the bathroom) unless your pharmacist or doctor told you to store it another way.
- Some medications may need to be stored under special conditions such as in a refrigerator or freezer. In general, you should avoid freezing liquid medications that you are told to store in a refrigerator. Check with your pharmacist or doctor to find out how you should store your medication.
- Keep each family member's medications separate from the others so that you do not mistakenly take someone else's medicine.
- Remove the cotton plug if there is one in the container when you open it. The cotton will attract moisture into the container if left in place after opening.
- Do not leave your medication in a car for long periods of time. It may be exposed to temperatures that are too high or too low.
- Throw away any medication that is outdated or no longer needed. However, be sure to talk to your doctor or pharmacist about the proper disposal of your medication.

What should I do if I take too much medication?

- In case of overdose, call your local poison control center at 800-222-1222. If the victim has collapsed or is not breathing, immediately call local emergency services at 911.

What other information should I know about my medication?

- Always know the generic and/or brand (trade) name of your medication. Ask your pharmacist or doctor if you are unsure which is the generic or brand name.
- Keep a list of all the medications that you are taking, including the name, dose, how often you take this medication, and the doctor who prescribed the medication. See "*My Medication Record*" section in the back of this book for a form that you can use to write down this information.
- Keep all appointments with your doctor and the laboratory. Your doctor sometimes may order certain lab tests to check your body's response to your medication.
- Before having any laboratory test, tell your doctor and the laboratory personnel what medications or supplements you are taking.
- Do not let anyone else take your medication.
- Ask your pharmacist any questions you have about refilling your prescription. Some prescriptions may not be refillable and your doctor will need to write another prescription if you are to continue using this medication.
- Ask your pharmacist any questions you have about over-the-counter medications (medications that you can buy without a prescription). Be sure to tell your pharmacist what other medications, vitamins, nutritional supplements, and herbal products you are taking or plan to take. Always read the information on the package and check the list of ingredients to make sure that you are not taking more than one product that contains the same medication.
- If you receive sample medications from your doctor, be sure to ask if the new medicine will interact with any medications, vitamins, nutritional supplements, or herbal products that you already may be taking. You should always be given written instructions on how to take (e.g., how often each day, for how long) any sample medication that you receive. Never rely just on your memory of what your doctor or his or her staff told you.

Managing Your Medications
Are you taking more prescription drugs than you need?

Prescription drugs have become the mainstay of modern medicine. Roughly half of people age 65 and over take five or more drugs, and 12 percent take ten or more. In many cases, such multiple medications are necessary. People with high blood pressure and increased cholesterol levels, for example, often require two drugs each, those with diabetes three, and people with heart failure or heart disease often demand five. Unfortunately, the more drugs you take, the more likely you are to get one you don't need. Indeed, research suggests that 20 to 60 percent of hospitalized Americans over the age of 65 take at least one unnecessary prescription drug, for these possible reasons: the medicine was improperly prescribed; it duplicates another drug being taken; the disorder has resolved; or the evidence no longer supports the drug's use. Many other people take medication that may be appropriate for most people in their condition but isn't essential for them based on their particular situation. Taking unnecessary medicine can create multiple problems. It increases the risk of side effects and drug interactions, adds needless cost, and makes it harder to keep taking any medication you do require. It can be equally harmful to skip drugs that are necessary as it is to take those that may not be necessary. Because of the potential for adverse effects, you should not decide to stop taking a medication without first talking to your doctor.

To help you manage your medications, make it a point to bring a list of your medications (see "My Medication Record" in the back of the book) to your primary doctor for review at each visit. You should also review your medication list with your physician or doctor if you:

- Take five or more drugs.
- Take drugs for three or more health problems.
- Get prescriptions from two or more healthcare providers.
- Have not reviewed all of your drugs and supplements with your primary-care doctor in the past six months.
- Have recently been discharged from a hospital.
- Have been taking a drug for more than a month that's known to cause addiction or rebound symptoms.

Be sure to include medications prescribed by each of your doctors, over-the-counter (nonprescription) drugs, and vitamin, mineral, or herbal supplements. For each of those items, as well as any new one a doctor prescribes, ask these questions:

Why do I need this medication?

A recent study found that some 20 percent of older people received prescriptions that weren't indicated or effective for their health problem. For example, a doctor may give antibiotics to someone with a viral infection, which won't respond to such drugs, or iron supplements to a woman who consumes an adequate diet and doesn't menstruate heavily. Or a doctor may prescribe a medication even after new evidence disproves the drug's presumed benefit, such as estrogen therapy for supposed heart protection in postmenopausal women. If you have any doubt about the appropriateness of your doctor's prescription, do your own research. Two good websites are Consumer Reports Medical Guide (*www.ConsumerReportsHealth.org*) and the National Library of Medicine's MedLine Plus (*www.medlineplus.gov*). Or ask your pharmacist if the drug seems right for your situation. If you still have concerns, talk with your doctor again or consider getting a second opinion.

Does this drug duplicate any other medication I'm taking?

That's especially likely if you get prescriptions from more than one doctor, as 40 percent of Americans do. Duplication sometimes occurs when multiple doctors treat the same disorder, a problem you may not notice if the drugs prescribed are either different drugs or the generic and brand-name versions of the same drug. In other cases, doctors may use related medications to treat different problems. For example, a primary-care doctor may prescribe a diuretic (water pill) to treat hypertension, while a neurologist may prescribe a beta-blocker, which also lowers blood pressure, to prevent migraines. Similarly, someone with both depression and diabetes-related nerve damage may be prescribed an antidepressant such as fluoxetine (Prozac®) by one doctor and a tricyclic antidepressant, which can relieve chronic pain, by another. In each of those cases, you may be able to keep taking the medication that treats both problems and stop the other drug.

Is this drug meant for short- or long-term use?

Doctors often intend to stop a medication after awhile but end up prescribing it indefinitely. Individuals taking a proton-pump inhibitor such as omeprazole (Prilosec®, Prilosec® OTC) for frequent heartburn or an antidepressant for mild to moderate depression should generally take a break after six months or a year, respectively, to see if the problem has eased. Other drugs, such as sleep aids or opiate pain relievers, should be used for even briefer periods but are often continued when patients become dependent on them. And many medications, including heartburn drugs as well as certain allergy or osteoarthritis drugs, can be used only when needed rather than continuously. However, you should not stop taking any medicine abruptly on your own since certain drugs should only be discontinued slowly over a period of time. You should always ask your doctor or pharmacist before stopping any medication. It's also especially important to review all medications that you are taking with your doctor when you check out of a hospital. Discharge plans often include medications started while you were there, though many, such as laxatives, sedatives, pain relievers, and stomach protectors, can usually be eliminated when you leave.

Can nondrug measures reduce or eliminate my need for this drug?

Doctors and patients often turn to medications before giving lifestyle changes or nondrug treatments a chance because they assume that medications work better. But that's not true in many cases. Studies show that spending just 10 to 15 minutes a day on exercises that strengthen the pelvic muscles, for example, is safer and at least as effective at treating urinary incontinence and possibly erectile dysfunction as common medications are.

Similarly, acupuncture, exercise, massage, spinal manipulation, and relaxation training may be better first choices for back pain than muscle relaxants or prescription painkillers. Changes in sleep, eating, or exercise patterns can often help relieve heartburn or insomnia. Headaches and allergies can be eased by identifying and avoiding the triggers. And people with only moderately elevated blood pressure, blood sugar (glucose), or cholesterol levels who start exercising, lose weight, and improve their diet may be able to reduce or even eliminate their need for drugs.

How important is this drug given my finances and overall health?

If you know that you can't afford all the drugs your doctor recommends, you should discuss this with your doctor or pharmacist. You can ask if lower-cost generic versions are available for the medications that you take. In some cases, programs sponsored by drug manufacturers may be available to pay for high-cost medications for patients who cannot afford them; ask your doctor or pharmacist if you have such a need and cannot afford a prescribed drug on your own. You and your doctor also can identify your most pressing health concerns and, if necessary, reduce or eliminate medications for less serious problems. It's also worth prioritizing medications when you or someone you're caring for has a terminal illness. In general, the shorter the expected life span, the wiser it is to choose drugs that ease symptoms, manage acute problems, or fight the current disease over those that help prevent future diseases. For example, someone with terminal cancer may not need to start or continue alendronate (Fosamax®) to prevent a first fracture caused by osteoporosis since that benefit typically won't appear until at least a year or so has passed.

Can I try a lower dose?

Even if you can't eliminate a drug, you can often get by with lower doses. Many studies have now identified effective, below-standard doses for numerous medications, including those for arthritis, high cholesterol, depression, hypertension, insomnia, and ulcers. However, you should not lower your dosage without first discussing it with your doctor or pharmacist.

Doctors may not try the low-dose approach because it requires extra monitoring at first to check how the drug is working for you. However, it can eventually yield more efficient care as side effects decline and patient compliance improves.

It's particularly worth considering a lower dose if you're older, female, thin, or small; have had reactions to medication; or are unusually sensitive to caffeine or alcohol because those characteristics may indicate a greater sensitivity to drugs in general. If your doctor is willing to try a low dose, be sure he or she monitors your progress especially during the first weeks or months.

Does this drug interact with any other medication or supplement I take?

When some drugs are used in combination, a decrease in the effectiveness of one or both medications may occur, while other combinations increase the risk of side effects. Some can even be life-threatening. Adding certain antibiotics or antifungals to cholesterol-lowering statin drugs, for example, increases the risk of potentially deadly kidney damage. Taking certain drugs and herbal products together can also have side effects. Echinacea may interact with immunosuppressants such as cyclosporine (Sandimmune®), saw palmetto with the prostate and hair-growth drug finasteride (Propecia®, Proscar®), and St. John's wort with dozens of medications. Even vitamins and minerals can complicate the use of medications. Calcium and iron can impair the absorption of drugs, and potassium supplements can lead to dangerously high levels of potassium in people who take ACE inhibitors or angiotensin-receptor blockers (ARBs).

Does my health or age make this drug unsafe for me?

Medications pose particular risks to older people, in part because changes in kidney function slow the elimination of many drugs from their body. Researchers have identified medicines that older people should always or almost always avoid, including some sedatives, pain relievers, antidepressant and antianxiety medications, antihistamines, and muscle relaxants. Many drugs and supplements also pose special risks to people with certain health problems, notably impaired kidney or liver function. Many other diseases can also make drugs more dangerous, including some that your doctor may overlook. For example, certain eye drops for treating glaucoma can potentially worsen asthma and heart failure.

Off-label Medication Use

When your doctor prescribes a medication for you, you assume that the US Food and Drug Administration (FDA) has found it to be safe and effective for the disorder being treated. However, that's not always the case. More than 20 percent of the prescriptions written are for "off-label" use — that is, for conditions other than the ones for which they received FDA approval. Sometimes these uses are called "unlabeled." In some cases, such as in children or people with cancer, off-label use is very common. The range of drugs used off label is far wider than thought, a federally funded study published in May 2006 shows. They include medications for allergies, convulsions, heart conditions, indigestion, ulcers, and asthma.

Before a drug can be marketed in the United States, the manufacturer must provide evidence to the FDA showing the safety and efficacy of a given drug in the treatment of a specific disease or disorder. A written summary of this information (also known as the label, prescribing information, or package insert) is subject to FDA approval. Under the Federal regulations, a drug approved for marketing in the US may be labeled, promoted, and advertised by the manufacturer only for those uses that were in the information submitted by the manufacturer to the FDA and that were reviewed and approved by the FDA. However, once the drug has been approved and is being marketed, those regulations do not restrict the doctor or other health professionals from prescribing that drug for disorders, in dosages, or in different groups of people (such as children or older adults) that are not included in the current FDA approved labeling.

Valid new uses for drugs often are first discovered after the drug has been in general use, by unexpected findings or successful use in disorders or diseases other than the condition for which the drug was intended. Further scientific studies may confirm the successful and appropriate prescribing for off-label uses of that medication. Because the submission of evidence and information of such new uses to the FDA may take considerable time and money, updating of the labeling with these new uses may never occur. Therefore, accepted medical practice (state-of-the-art) often includes the use of medications for disorders that are not included in the FDA-approved labeling. Off-label use does not mean that the use is improper or illegal. In fact, in many real-life medical situations, off-label use represents the most optimal therapy for patients. However off-label use of drugs is only as good as the evidence that backs up that use.

Not all off-label use has the evidence to support its use, and there can be concerns about the lack of supporting evidence for efficacy and safety in some cases. In the study cited above for example, doctors had little or no scientific evidence to back up their choices in 73 percent of the off-label cases. Therefore, it is important that you know whether there is well founded scientific evidence to support the off-label use of a medication for your particular condition. You should also know the expected benefits and potential risks of any off-label treatment for your disease or condition and discuss them with your doctor.

What can you do?

How can you find out if your medication is being used for an approved indication? Or how can you determine if there are safety issues associated with off-label use of a medication for your condition? The following suggestions may be helpful to find answers to these questions.

- Ask your doctor if your medication is approved by the FDA for use in your condition. Discuss any risks that may be associated with the use of the medication based on your health and any other medications or treatments that you may be receiving.

- Off-label uses are included for many medications in the Drug Listing portion of this book. Review the information in the section titled "Other Uses for This Medicine." Off-label uses included in the Consumer Drug Reference are based on ASHP's federally recognized drug reference, AHFS Drug Information, which carefully weighs the supporting evidence in coming to its conclusions.
- Check the FDA's Web site (*www.fda.gov*) to find the approved labeling in the Drugs@FDA link or on DailyMed on the US National Library of Medicine's Web site (*www.dailymed.nlm.nih.gov*). Look for your disease or condition under the section of the manufacturers labeling called "Indications and Usage."
- Access the drug reviews and review the information in the section "Other Uses for This Medicine" at *www.ConsumerReportsHealth.org*.
- Visit the Drug Safety section of the FDA's Web site *www.fda.gov*, to find if there are any specific warnings about the medication you are receiving for your condition in the section, "Safety Information for Specific Drugs."
- Always talk to your doctor if you have any concerns about using a medication for an off-label use.

Generic and Brand-name Drugs

What is the difference between generic and brand-name drugs?

Prescription drugs come in two basic forms—brand-name and generic drugs. Generic drugs are copies of brand-name products whose patents have expired. A generic drug has *exactly* the same active ingredient(s) as the brand-name drug it copies. The main differences between these products are price and how the medications look. Generics are much less expensive and by law are not allowed to look exactly like the brands they copy such as a certain color or shaped tablet. Certain inactive ingredients, colors, or flavors may also be different in the generic drug than the brand-name drug.

Are generic drugs as strong as brand-name drugs?

Many people believe that established generic medications are not as potent or effective as newer competing brand-name drugs. The truth is that the vast majority of generics continue to be useful medicines even years after their approval, and many remain the preferred first-line treatment even after newer brand-name competitor medicines emerge. Currently, over 50 percent of all prescriptions written in the U.S. are for generic drugs.

Are generic drugs as safe as brand-name drugs?

The Food and Drug Administration (FDA) requires that generic drugs be every bit as safe as brand-name drugs. The

FDA applies the same set of strict rules to generics as to brand-name drugs. Both must meet the same specifications for their ingredients and manufacturing process. The FDA requires generics to have the same quality, strength, purity, and chemical stability and to work the same way in the body. Both types of medications are tracked for their safety over time.

Because of US patent laws, generic drugs usually come on the market about 12 to 15 years after the brand-name drugs they copy were first approved. It is not uncommon for doctors and drug companies to find problems with new brand-name drugs that come to light only after they are approved. That's because even though new drugs undergo years of study to prove they are safe and effective, those studies may have involved only several thousand people; once a drug is used by millions of people, new problems can and sometimes do become known. Therefore, because they have been used for a longer period of time in many more people, generics drugs may actually be safer than newer brand-name drugs.

Why do I hear and read more about brand-name drugs — are they better?

In some cases, new brand-name drugs may be better for some conditions than older generics in terms of both safety and effectiveness. That is to be expected, and it reflects medical innovation and progress. But such advances are not as prevalent as you might believe. In fact, a growing number of experts, doctors, medical and health groups, and pharmacists believe that some newer and more expensive brand-name drugs are overused, while many generic drugs are underused. The reasons for this occurrence are complex, but the main ones are:

- brand-name drugs are widely promoted and advertised to doctors, while generic drugs are only minimally promoted, if at all. Brand marketing includes one-on-one sales pitches from drug representatives.
- brand-name drug manufacturers give doctors millions of doses of the newest drugs to hand out to patients as samples. This practice gets people to take the newest medicines, which can be the most costly. Some of these products will be better than available generics, but many will not.
- brand-name drug companies pay thousands of doctors every year to either give lectures on the newest drugs or use them as part of clinical studies. Both can be useful enterprises, but doctors often get used to prescribing the new drug instead of older, reliable drugs.
- brand-name drug companies spend tens (or even hundreds) of millions of dollars advertising their drugs directly to the public. Generic firms rarely advertise their drugs to the public.

How do I know if a generic drug is available for the brand-name drug that I take?

Not all medications have a generic counterpart because brand-name drugs are generally protected by a patent for more than a decade. When the patent expires, other drug companies can manufacture generic versions of the drugs, but these generic versions first must be tested and approved by the FDA prior to becoming available to patients.

You should ask your pharmacist or doctor if there are generic drugs available for the medication(s) that you are currently taking. Most states allow pharmacists to substitute the generic version of a drug when a doctor has written a prescription for the brand-name drug. But in many states, the pharmacist must ask the consumer's permission to make the switch. Sometimes consumers may be uncertain about making this change because they are afraid that they will get a drug their trusted doctor did not intend. If a pharmacist suggests substituting a generic drug at the time that your prescription is being filled, you can call your doctor if you are concerned about this switch. For new medications, you should talk to your doctor about your prescription when it is being written in his or her office. You should ask whether the prescription is for a brand or generic drug, and learn why your doctor has prescribed one or the other. If you pay for your medicines out-of-pocket because you lack insurance coverage for drugs, you should ask your doctor if there is a less expensive generic drug that would work for you. Even if you have insurance that covers your prescription medicines, the amount of your out-of-pocket co-pay may be much higher than you would pay with a less expensive generic.

Pharmacist Q & A

What basic items should be stored in a medicine cabinet?

- Antiseptics, first-aid ointments, hydrogen peroxide, and various sizes of bandages to treat cuts and scrapes. Gauze, adhesive tape, elastic bandages, and round-tipped scissors should also be included.
- Calamine lotion and hydrocortisone cream.
- Acetaminophen, aspirin, ibuprofen, or naproxen for aches and pain. Aspirin should not be used to treat flu symptoms or be given to children or teenagers.
- Oral hydration solution (such as Pedialyte) for children with severe diarrhea and/or vomiting.
- An oral syringe or measuring device to give medications to children.
- Thermometer (rectal thermometer for babies under 1 year).
- Your doctor or pharmacist may also recommend that you keep activated charcoal (an antidote for certain poisonings) on hand.
- Ipecac syrup is *not* recommended any longer for your medicine cabinet; discard any that you may have.

I've heard that you should pay attention to the expiration date on your prescription medication. Is that true?

Yes. Expired medicines often don't work as well, and they can even be harmful. To make sure that you don't accidentally take an out-of-date medication, you should clean out your medicine cabinet every year and properly dispose of:

- Any medication that is past the expiration date on the label.
- Any medication that has changed color, smells, or has formed a residue.
- Any liquid that looks cloudy or has thickened.
- Any container with cracks or leaks.
- Aspirin or acetaminophen that is crumbly or smells strange.
- Hydrogen peroxide that no longer bubbles when applied to the skin.

How should I dispose of my medications that I no longer need or are expired?

The disposal of medication is a complex issue. Throwing the medication into the trash can be risky if found and eaten by children or pets. The trash will most likely be taken to a landfill which will place the medication into the soil and water supply of our environment. Flushing unwanted medication down a toilet or rinsing it into a sink can also cause environmental concerns because the medication is put into the water supply. A better solution for the disposal of unwanted medications is to return the unwanted medication to your pharmacist or physician for disposal as hazardous waste material.

Does it make a difference where medicines are stored in my house?

Yes, it does. For instance, prescription medications should never be stored in a bathroom because heat and humidity can change the drug's chemical stability. Most medicines should be stored in a childproof area and kept at room temperature and away from sunlight. Some medications, however, must be refrigerated. Check with your pharmacist or doctor if you are not sure how to properly store a medication.

Can I split my medication in half?

Maybe. You should always check with your doctor or pharmacist before splitting any medication. Certain types of medication generally should *not* be split such as:

- Chemotherapy drugs.
- Medications to control seizures.
- Birth control pills.
- Blood thinners such as Coumadin® (warfarin).
- Capsules that contain powders or gel.
- Tablets with a hard outside coating.
- Long-acting tablets (designed to release medication slowly over time in your body).
- Tablets that are coated to protect your stomach.
- Tablets that crumble easily, irritate your mouth, taste bitter, or contain strong dyes that could stain your teeth and mouth.

Some medications can be safely split in half but should never be cut into smaller portions, such as thirds or quarters. Do not use a knife to split your tablet because it can be dangerous and often can result in unequal halves of the tablet. A pill splitter (relatively inexpensive and available from most pharmacies) should be used to split your tablets safely and accurately. Dividing your medication in half can be useful to get the correct dose of medication that is not commercially available or to save money. However, splitting your medication should only be done if your doctor thinks that it is a good idea for you, you learn how to do it properly, and you split only medications that should be split. If you split your medicine in half, use the other half as your next dose.

Medication Safety
Poison Prevention
Seniors

Seniors who take multiple medications are at increased risk for accidental poisonings. Older patients have complex medication regimens, often involving multiple medications prescribed by several doctors, which make older patients vulnerable to accidental poisonings.

Patients should:

- **Keep a list of your medications.** A written record of the medications you are taking, including drug name, dose, and frequency, is an important tool to have during doctor visits and in case of an emergency.
- **Communicate.** Inform your doctor and pharmacist of all the medications you are taking, including over-the-counter (nonprescription) medications and dietary supplements; this information will help reduce the chances of an interaction.
- **Learn about your medications.** Ask your doctor or pharmacist to explain why you are taking the medication you have been prescribed, the food and medicines you should avoid, and possible reactions and side effects.
- **Use one pharmacy.** Many seniors receive prescriptions from more than one doctor, making drug interactions more likely. By using one pharmacy, all of your prescriptions are consolidated and your pharmacist can check for possible interactions between medications.
- **Keep a journal.** Make note of all symptoms, especially after taking your medications. Painful or unexpected side effects may signal a need for adjusting your medication regimen.
- **Maintain a schedule.** Holding to a routine can decrease your chances of missing doses or taking more than needed.

Patients should immediately contact their doctor if they experience an adverse reaction to their medicines. If the doctor is not available, contact the local poison center using the toll free number **(800) 222-1222**. Eighty percent of directors and half of all staff members at poison control centers are pharmacists, healthcare professionals who are trained and highly educated on the complexities of today's medications.

Children

Did you know that many of the creative methods parents and caregivers use to get children to take their medicine can actually contribute to accidental poisonings? A recent consumer survey found that almost half of parents and caregivers said they have pretended to take their child's medication or called it candy to convince the child to take

the medicine. These methods are extremely dangerous and could lead to an overdose.

The Centers for Disease Control and Prevention (CDC) reports that approximately **9 of 10 accidental poisonings occur in the home**. Sixty percent of these victims are children younger than age six, and close to half of poisonings in children of this age group involve a misuse of medicines.

Every parent, caregiver, and grandparent should use these safety tips to prevent accidental poisonings:

- Avoid taking medications in the presence of children, as they often try to imitate adults.
- Don't call medicine candy.
- Use child-resistant closures on medicine and other products. Use of these closures has greatly decreased accidental poisonings by children. If you find it hard to open such closures, you may ask your pharmacist for an easier-to-open cap. You should take special precautions to keep such containers securely stored in a place that a child cannot access.
- Keep all medications (both prescription and nonprescription) in their original child-resistant containers.
- Always turn on the light when giving or taking medicine.
- Check your medications periodically for expiration dates. If the medication is not dated, consider it expired six months after purchase.
- Avoid putting medications in open trash containers in the kitchen or bathroom because many adult medications can be deadly to small children and pets.
- Be aware that multivitamins, particularly those containing iron, can be poisonous if taken in large doses. Children are especially susceptible to adverse effects from vitamin overdosing.
- Be aware the medication (transdermal) patches that you apply to your skin may be poisonous if chewed or swallowed by children or pets.
- **In case of overdose, call your local poison control center at 800-222-1222. If the child has collapsed or is not breathing, immediately call local emergency services at 911.**

Traveling Safely with Medications

Whether you are traveling domestically or internationally, you won't want an illness to disrupt either your vacation or business plans. This means planning well, managing your medications wisely, and consulting your doctor or pharmacist about proper precautions to take before you leave home.

- **Many medications can cause photosensitivity, or increased sensitivity to sunlight.** Even if you don't usually sunburn, taking medications that cause this reaction could greatly increase your chances of getting a bad burn. Your pharmacist can advise you about whether your medication can cause photosensitivity and recommend the right SPF (sun protection factor) for your skin type.
- **If you are flying, if possible, keep your medications in your carry-on luggage so that you have access to**

them during your flight and will not lose them in the event that your luggage gets lost. Plus, keeping your medications with you helps prevent exposure to extreme temperatures in the baggage compartment, which can alter the drug's effectiveness. Keep in mind that airport security requires that your medications be transported in their original, labeled containers. Some medications may not be placed in your carry-on luggage. For details, see the Transportation Security Administration website (*www.tsa.gov*).

- **If your medication requires you to use a syringe—insulin, for instance—you may need to carry your prescription label with you to ensure that you can pass through airport security.** The American Diabetes Association recommends that people with diabetes be prepared to provide airport security personnel with the prescription label for diabetes medications and supplies as well as complete contact information for the doctor.

- **Make sure that you carry your doctor's and your pharmacy's phone numbers with you when you are away from home.** In case you lose your medications, you may need a new prescription. You should also keep on hand a list of all your prescriptions.

- **If you are traveling through several time zones, consult with your doctor or pharmacist to work out a specific plan for adjusting the timing and dosage of your medications.** This will prevent you from taking too much or too little.

- **If you are visiting a foreign country, beware of buying over-the-counter (non-prescription) medications.** Many medicines that are available only by prescription in the United States are available over-the-counter in other countries. Some of these medications could have different ingredients and may not undergo comparable quality control. Buying these medications could put you at risk for allergic reactions, drug interactions, or other problems.

- **If you are visiting a hot, humid climate, be sure to keep your medications in a cool, dry place out of direct sunlight.** Never store medications in the glove compartment of your car. Also, because of the heat and humidity that build up in a bathroom, it is the worst place to store medication whether you are at home or on the road.

- **Take along more medication than the number of days you've planned to be away.** This precaution will allow you to be prepared for unexpected delays.

Emergency Preparedness and Medications

Consumers should be aware of their medication needs as they prepare for any emergency, including weather-related emergencies such as flooding and hurricanes. Following these tips can help you be ready:

- keep a list of all your medications in your wallet (include lists for your immediate family members, and drug name, strength, dosage form, and regimen).
- wear your medical-alert bracelet or necklace.

- store 3–5 days of medications that are important to your health.
- include any medications used to stabilize an existing medical condition or keep a condition from worsening or resulting in hospitalization, such as medications for asthma, seizures, cardiovascular disorders, diabetes, psychiatric conditions, HIV, and thyroid disorders. Carry these with you, if possible, in a purse or briefcase in labeled containers.
- don't store your medications in areas that are susceptible to extremes in heat, cold, and humidity (e.g., car or bathroom). This could decrease the effectiveness of the medication.
- use child-resistant containers and keep your purse or briefcase secure.
- rotate these medications whenever you get your prescriptions refilled to make sure they are used before their expiration date.
- refill your prescriptions while you still have at least a 5–7 day supply of medications left. Keep in mind that some sources, such as mail-order pharmacies, have a longer lead time to refill.
- if your child takes medications, talk to your school system to find out their emergency preparedness plans.
- if you are being treated with a complex medication regimen, talk to your doctor or pharmacist to create appropriate emergency preparation plans. Such regimens include injectable medications, including those delivered by pumps (e.g., insulin, analgesics, chemotherapy, parenteral nutrition); medications delivered by a nebulizer (e.g., antibiotics, bronchodilators); and dialysis.

Counterfeit Medications

While the U.S. drug supply is still the safest in the world, consumers should be particularly cautious about their medications given the recent rise in counterfeiting (fake products).

According to the U.S. Food and Drug Administration (FDA), counterfeit drug investigations have quadrupled since 2000. Additionally, the World Health Organization (WHO) estimates that up to 10 percent of the world market currently may be fake medications. These products may be expired, contain incorrect ingredients or the wrong amounts of active ingredients, or be enclosed in packaging that doesn't match the product inside.

It may be very difficult for patients to tell just by looking at a medication or its packaging if it is a counterfeit product. International counterfeiters are increasingly sophisticated, but that does not mean that you are helpless in the face of this new threat. You can do a lot by staying alert and following a few simple tips. And, when in doubt, always talk to your pharmacist, doctor, or other healthcare provider.

Consumers should follow a few simple safety tips when taking medication:

1. **Pay attention to your medicine**, particularly the instructions on how you should take it, the correct dosage, and warnings about interactions with other medications.

2. **Talk to your pharmacist or doctor if your medication:**

- Is different than you've experienced before in shape, color, taste, smell, or feel.
- Is packaged differently or if the container is altered or unsealed.
- Does not produce the expected results or if you are experiencing new side effects.

3. **Be extremely careful when ordering medications on the Internet**. To stay safe, only buy medications from pharmacy websites that post the National Association of Boards of Pharmacy's (NABP's) VIPPS (Verified Internet Pharmacy Practice Sites) symbol. For more information see the NABP website (*www.nabp.net/vipps/intro.asp*).

Consumer Reports®
BEST BUY DRUGS®

PROVEN • EFFECTIVE • AFFORDABLE

Free Guidance for Consumers on Prescription Medicines

Consumer Reports Best Buy Drugs is another resource to help you have an informed discussion with your doctor so that together you can find prescription medicines that offer the best value for your money.

At its Web site, *www.ConsumerReportsHealth.org,* you'll find free detailed evaluations of prescription drugs. These evaluations compare the drugs in a class or category (similar drugs that are used to treat a specific condition or illness)—based on their effectiveness, safety, side effects, and cost. CR Best Buy Drugs is a public education project grounded in the fact that for most conditions and diseases the drugs that your doctor has at his or her disposal are *not* equal. Each has strengths and weaknesses. A choice will have to be made, and you can and should take part in that choice.

For example, there are at present six drugs in the category of medicines called statins, the most widely used medicines to treat elevated cholesterol. Among these are generic lovastatin, pravastatin, and simvastatin, and the brand-name drugs Crestor, Lipitor, and Vytorin. In the *CR Best Buy Drugs* report on these medicines, you'll learn how effective each is, on average, at lowering "bad" (LDL) cholesterol, how strong the evidence is for each when it comes to reducing your risk of heart disease, and how much each drug costs.

Similarly, in the *CR Best Buy Drugs* report on sleeping pills, you can find out how each of four drugs in a class called the "newer sedatives" stacks up against the others when it comes to helping you fall asleep and stay asleep. You'll also learn that older, less expensive sleeping pills work just as well in most cases where people have only occasional problems falling asleep.

CR Best Buy Drugs has evaluated to date 20 categories of drugs used to treat almost every major ailment and disease. These include allergies, Alzheimer's disease, asthma, attention deficit hyperactivity disorder (ADHD), depression, diabetes, heartburn, heart disease, high blood pressure, schizophrenia, and stroke.

The *CR Best Buy Drugs* project is among the first attempts in the United States to translate for consumers the detailed findings of what doctors call "a systematic review of the scientific evidence." In this case, the reviews were conducted by the Drug Effectiveness Review Project, or DERP, which is currently funded by 15 states. Teams of researchers at academic medical centers spend up to a year pouring over the studies on a class of drugs. They then distill their findings in a way that highlights how the drugs compare when all the studies and data are taken into account.

Consumer Reports adds pricing data to the DERP reviews, and considers other factors, such as convenience of use and dosing. Based on all the factors and criteria, *CR Best Buy Drugs* chooses which drugs in a category it considers to be the *Best Buys*. Just as with other products and services that *Consumer Reports* evaluates and rates, a *Best Buy* drug is one that will—for most people—be as good or better than any other competing product in its class and offer you the best value for your money.

Many *CR Best Buy Drugs* are low-cost generics, but not all. In some cases, the evidence from the DERP indicates that a more expensive brand-name drug is clearly more effective for most people or a select group of patients with a certain condition.

Of course, no review or report can substitute for a doctor's close assessment of you and your medical problem, and the doctor's judgment about what treatment is best. Your unique medical history and circumstances may rule out a drug chosen as a *Best Buy*.

Just as *Consumer Drug Reference* will do, *CR Best Buy Drugs* will help you talk to your doctor about your prescription drugs choices. This will improve your chances of being prescribed a drug that not only will be best for your medical condition but also affordable. Since *CR Best Buy Drugs* was launched in December 2004, more than 2.5 million people have downloaded a drug report.

CR Best Buy Drugs is funded in part through generous grants from the Engelberg Foundation, a private philanthropy, and the National Library of Medicine of the National Institutes of Health.

As noted above, you can access the *CR Best Buy Drugs* Web site at *www.ConsumerReportsHealth.org* to view and print all its reports and other publications that will help you further understand prescription drugs and how to take them safely and wisely. New evaluations of classes of drugs, and updates of existing reports, are continuously being added.

Guide to Over-the-Counter (OTC) Medicines

General Information

In 2006, Americans spent over $15 billion dollars on OTC medications. The US Food and Drug Administration (FDA) has determined that OTC products are safe and effective for use without a doctor's prescription. But when these medications are used incorrectly, they can cause serious illness or even death. So what do you need to know about OTC products for you and your family to use them safely and effectively?

Over-the-counter or nonprescription products are most often used to treat common illnesses and complaints such as headaches, back pain, cough, colds, allergies, and constipation. OTC medications may contain a single active ingredient or several different active ingredients in the same product to treat your illness or condition. These medications primarily are used only for short periods of time. The instructions on the package tell you how long you should use the product. You should only use these medications for a longer period of time if your doctor or pharmacist has told you to do so.

It is important to know about the medication that you are taking and how to use it properly. It is always important to ask your doctor or pharmacist for information about OTC products that may be useful for you and your family. They will review your symptoms or complaint, general health, and other medications (both prescription and nonprescription) that you are taking to help you to select the right OTC product. You should not rely on television ads, coupons, or advice from friends and family to select an OTC product for your condition or illness.

Here are some important things for you to know or to ask your doctor or pharmacist about OTC medications:
- What does this medication do?
- When and how should I take this medication?
- What are the possible side effects?
- Will this medication interact with other medications or dietary supplements, food, or beverages?
- Are there any activities that I should avoid while taking the medication?
- How will I know that this medication is working?
- What should I do if my symptoms don't improve?

In recent years, some medications that used to be available only by prescription were reviewed by the FDA and now are allowed to be sold without a prescription. In fact, more than 700 nonprescription products currently available today use ingredients or dosages that were available only by prescription just 25 years ago. Because these medications are available without a prescription does not mean that they or other OTC medications are without side effects or risks, even when taken as instructed.

Herbal products and vitamins (dietary supplements) are not considered over-the-counter medications and are not regulated as such by the FDA. These products are considered to be 'foods' and the FDA and manufacturers do not need approval or review of safety and efficacy by the FDA before they are marketed. Always ask your doctor or pharmacist if you have any questions about dietary supplements. You should also ask for more information about the advertised benefits of these products because there may be little evidence to support some claims. However, you should treat these products like medications since they also can cause serious side effects just like drugs. If you take any of these products, always include them when you tell your doctor or pharmacist which medications you are taking. For more information about dietary supplements and natural medicines, go to *www.ConsumerReportsHealth.org*.

Just like prescription medications, OTC medications may be available in both brand and generic products. The generic products generally are less expensive, but you should always check to make sure that the type and amounts of the main ingredient(s) are the same. Ask your pharmacist if you need help to find the generic name of an OTC product that you are taking.

Important Things to Know About OTC Medications
Before You Buy an OTC Product

- Read the label carefully and completely before you buy the medication.
- Note what symptoms the medication should be used to treat. Do not buy a medication that is meant to treat more or different symptoms than you are experiencing.
- The product may not be right for you if you have certain medical condition such as diabetes, congestive heart failure, or high blood pressure. For example, certain pain relievers should not be used in people with liver or kidney disease.
- Be sure the medication is the right one for the age of the person that is to take the medication. Some products should not be used at all in young children or in older adults.
- Some products come in different strengths (amount of medication in the tablet or liquid). This will affect how much of the medication you will need to take.
- Check to see if the product should not be given with any of the prescription or other OTC medications, herbal products, or vitamins that you are currently taking.
- Choose OTC medications by their active ingredients, not by brand name. Drug manufacturers often use well-established brand names to launch a series of related— but different—products. For example, the manufacturer of the brand name cough product Robitussin (that contains only guaifenesin) also markets others labeled as Robitussin. These cough and cold products include

guaifenesin combined with one or more additional ingredients such as an antihistamine, a cough suppressant, another expectorant, a pain reliever, a decongestant, or even products that do not contain guaifenesin at all.

- Each time you buy a product, look for 'banners' or information on the package telling you about changes to the product or labeling such as new ingredients, dosages, or warnings.

Before You Take the OTC Medication

- Check the dosage carefully and be sure to give the right amount of medication based on your age or weight. Be sure to check exactly how many tablets or how much liquid you should take.
- Always check the label carefully to see how often you should take the medication.
- Review the warning section to see what side effects or events may happen after taking or using the medication and what you should do if they occur.
- Check the label to see if there are any foods or beverages that you should avoid when taking the medication.

Taking OTC Medication

- Only take or use the medication for the period of time that is recommended on the label unless your doctor has advised you differently. If you do not get better or if your condition or symptoms get worse, call your doctor or pharmacist.
- Always keep the medication in the original container to make sure that you don't mistakenly take the wrong medication.
- Do not take more than the recommended dose on the label. Taking more medicine or taking it more often will not make you feel better and can often cause harm. If you do not get relief from the medication, talk to your doctor about your symptoms or condition.
- Always use the measuring device (calibrated spoon, cup, or dropper) that comes with liquid medication. Ask the pharmacist for a measuring device if one is not provided with the product.
- Keep a record when you use OTC medications to help you take them at the recommended times. Do not take OTC products more often than is recommended on the label or as instructed by your doctor.
- Read the labels carefully to make sure that you are not taking two different brand name products that contain the same active ingredient. This is especially important if you are taking medications that contain more than one ingredient.
- If you have any side effects after taking or using the product, follow the instructions on the label or call your doctor.

Combination OTC Products

Many OTC products are referred to as "shot-gun" remedies since they can contain more than one ingredient to treat several symptoms. You should use these products only if you have all of the symptoms, otherwise you may be taking more medication than you need. Taking additional medications that you do not need increases the chance of side effects and/or interactions with other medications that you may be taking.

You should always check the label to see if the combination product contains a medication that you already may be taking. This is especially important with the use of the pain reliever and fever reducer acetaminophen. If you are taking acetaminophen (APAP, Genapap, paracetamol, Tylenol, others) and then begin to take a cough and cold medication that contains acetaminophen as one of the ingredients in the product, you will receive a double dose of acetaminophen. Some prescription medications also contain acetaminophen. In some cases, the label on the prescription bottle may not tell you all of the ingredients or may abbreviate acetaminophen as APAP. In countries outside of the US, acetaminophen is called paracetamol. Be sure to read all labels carefully. Taking too much of any one medication will increase the chance of side effects or injury.

OTC Safety — Protect Yourself Against Tampering

Companies that make OTC medicines seal most products in tamper-evident packaging to help make sure that no one has altered the medication that you have purchased. This packaging works by providing evidence to show you that the package has been disturbed. But OTC packaging cannot be 100 percent tamper-proof. Here's how to help protect you and your family:

- Look at the tamper-evident features on the package before you open it. These features are described on the label.
- Look at the outer packaging before you buy it. When you get home, check the medicine inside.
- Don't buy an OTC product if the packaging is damaged.
- Don't use any medicine that looks discolored or different in any way.
- If anything looks suspicious, be suspicious. Contact the store where you bought the product and take it back.

OTC Medication Considerations for Special Groups
Children

All medications, including OTC products, affect children differently than adults. It is very important to use these medications exactly as described on the label or as instructed by your child's doctor. Here are some other things to consider when giving OTC medications to children:

- Always purchase and store the medication in the original child-proof container.
- Give the appropriate product for your child. Pain relievers and fever reducers come in many different types of products, such as drops, liquid, and dissolvable or chewable tablets, to allow you to give the medication to the child in the easiest manner and at the correct dose. For instance, because it is difficult to get liquid medications into an infant's mouth, the concentrated infant

drops are made so that a smaller amount of liquid is needed for each dose.

- Follow the directions on the manufacturer's labeling carefully and ask your pharmacist or child's doctor to explain any part you do not understand.
- Always use the proper measuring device that comes with a specific liquid product. For instance, use only the dropper provided with the concentrated infant drops and do not use any other measuring device such as a household spoon or cup to measure the dose for your baby. Household spoons can measure too much or too little medicine. Ask the pharmacist for a measuring device if one does not come with the product.
- Check the dosage carefully. If there is a dosage range based on weight that is the best way to select the dose for your child. If you don't know your child's weight then the age range can be used to get the dose. Try to check your child's weight every so often as it can change between well-child visits to the doctor.
- Be sure to carefully follow the age and weight limit recommendations for dosage that are provided on the package. If the label states not to give to children under a certain age, check with your doctor or pharmacist before giving the medication. In some cases, they may be able to recommend an appropriate dose for your child. In other cases, they may tell you that the product should not be used for safety reasons. If you are not sure about what dosage to give, always ask your doctor or pharmacist.
- If your child is taking a medication that is only given when needed (e.g., fever-reducing medications), do not exceed recommended amounts for each dose or for the total number of doses for each day.
- Do not give aspirin to children and teenagers, especially if they have a viral illness such as a cold, flu, or chickenpox, because of the risk of Reye's syndrome (a serious condition affecting body organs, especially the liver and kidney).

Women Who Are Pregnant or Breast-feeding

There are special considerations for selecting and using OTC medications in pregnant and nursing women. Some OTC medications can cause problems with your baby or with your delivery. These medications can get into your breast milk and may be passed along to your baby if you are nursing. *Always* check with your doctor or pharmacist before taking any over-the-counter medication and follow the general information listed below.

- Talk to your doctor or pharmacist to find out about any non-medication treatment that can relieve your symptoms instead of taking or using an OTC product. For instance, a humidifier may help to relieve the congestion of a cold without taking a medication to treat your symptoms.
- Avoid taking OTC medications during the first trimester of pregnancy, unless your doctor or pharmacist tells you that you may do so.

- Avoid combination products, especially if they contain medications for symptoms that you may not need to treat.
- Avoid OTC products that stay in your body for longer periods of time such as 'extended-release' or '12-hour' products.
- Don't take aspirin or other non-steroidal anti-inflammatory medications (NSAIDs) such as ibuprofen (Advil, Motrin IB) or naproxen (Aleve) during the last trimester of pregnancy, unless instructed by your doctor to do so.
- Acetaminophen is generally safe for women who are pregnant or breast feeding to take occasionally, but you should check with your doctor or pharmacist before taking any acetaminophen product.
- Some antihistamines and nasal decongestants may interfere with the production of milk in the nursing mother and possibly cause side effects in the baby.
- If you are nursing, you may need to take oral medications just after feeding your baby or before your baby's longest time of sleep to minimize the amount of medication that gets into your breast milk.

Older Adults

Older adults are the biggest users of over-the-counter products. Seniors should use caution in selecting OTCs to avoid side effects and possible drug interactions with the other medications that they are taking. Older individuals often have changes in their bodies due to aging that may alter how drugs work and are removed from the body. It is important for older adults to realize that many OTC medications, such as pain relievers, laxatives, cough and cold products, antacids, and sleep medications, should only be used for a short period of time. If the symptoms continue, then you should talk to your doctor about your condition. Some specific advice for seniors who take OTC medications is listed below.

- Older adults should always tell their doctors and pharmacists all of the over-the-counter medications when they list their prescription medications. It is important not to take the same medications that you may already be taking or similar drugs for the same medical problem.
- Check cough and cold medications carefully for warnings about use in people with high blood pressure. Pseudoephedrine can increase blood pressure and the pressure in your eye so it should not be used in certain people with high blood pressure or glaucoma. Pseudoephedrine should also not be used in men with an enlarged prostate gland.
- Adults over 60 years of age who take OTC medications for pain such as ibuprofen (Advil, Motrin IB, others including generic versions) and naproxen (Aleve, others including generic versions) may have an increased chance of stomach ulcers or bleeding. This medication should also be used with caution if you have kidney or heart disease.
- If your doctor has told you to take a low dose of aspirin (such as 81-325 mg) each day to protect your heart or

prevent a stroke you should not use aspirin as a pain reliever or fever reducer because the benefits to your heart or brain may be lost when higher doses are used. The only exception is that a regular dose of aspirin (325 mg) should be taken if you suspect you may be having a heart attack. You should take the aspirin and then call 911 for help.

- If you are taking aspirin on a regular basis to prevent heart attack or stroke, do not take ibuprofen (Advil, Motrin IB, others including generic versions) to treat pain or fever without talking to your doctor or pharmacist. They will probably tell you to allow some time to pass between taking your daily dose of aspirin and taking a dose of ibuprofen.
- Older adults should be aware that some OTC sleeping aids such as diphenhydramine (which is also the active ingredient in the allergy medication Benadryl Allergy) may cause daytime sedation or confusion due to their effect on an aging central nervous system.
- Antacids, especially those containing calcium carbonate, may interfere with how other drugs are absorbed into the body. Older adults should check with their pharmacists or doctors before taking antacids together with their medications. Often antacids can be taken at separate times without affecting the other medication.
- Some antihistamines may affect medical conditions that are common in older adults such as angina, constipation, diabetes, glaucoma, sleep problems, or trouble urinating due to an enlarged prostate gland.
- Always start with the lowest dose of a medication to see how it will affect you. With aging, the normal drug doses may be too high for most seniors. For pain relievers, it may be best to follow the longer recommended time between doses to avoid having too much medication in the body.
- If you have trouble swallowing a tablet or capsule, ask your pharmacist if a liquid or chewable OTC product is available.
- If you have trouble opening OTC containers, look for an "easy open" or non-child proof packaging. Just be sure to keep these medications away from young children.

How to Read an OTC Label

Reading the product label is the most important part of taking care of you or your family when choosing and using an over-the-counter medication. It is important to take the time to read the label completely when deciding which product is best for you. The label tells you what your medication is for, how to use the product, and if a medication is right for your symptoms. Even if your doctor or pharmacist tells you which product to use, it is important to read the label completely so that you understand the instructions for use and any warnings about using the medication.

The Food and Drug Administration (FDA) has developed a Drug Facts label that has easy to read information displayed in the same sections for each product. You should read this information carefully each time you use this medication and ask your doctor or pharmacist if you have any questions.

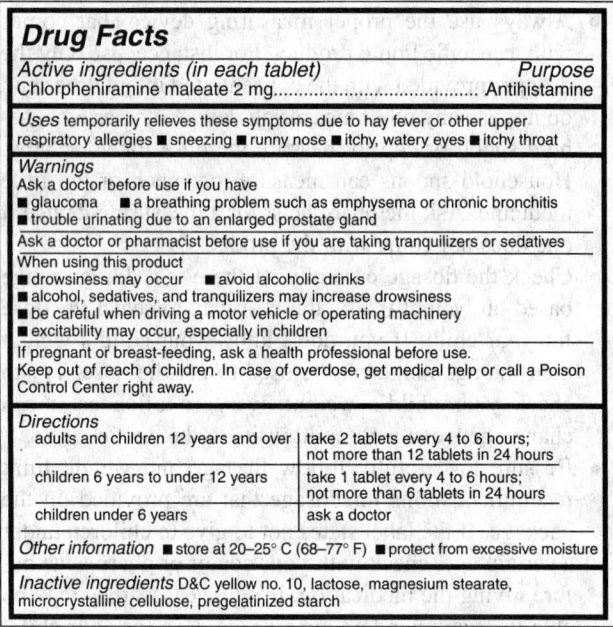

Some information may be on the container bottle and some on the box. It is best to keep all of the packaging to have this information available to you while you use the medication. For some products, you may need to peel back the container label to read all of the information.

These sections are on every OTC product label:

Active Ingredient. This is the name of the main medication or part of the product that works to relieve or treat your symptoms. This section also tells you how much medication is in each pill or specific amount of the liquid. Some products contain more than one active ingredient.

Uses. This section describes the symptoms or conditions that you can use the product to treat or prevent.

Warnings. This section lists the safety information and will tell you:

- when not to use the product
- what conditions may require advice from a doctor or pharmacist before taking the product
- things you shouldn't do while taking the medication
- when to stop using or taking the product and when to contact a doctor
- if you can take the product when you are pregnant or breastfeeding
- when to talk to a doctor or pharmacist
- always to keep the medication out of children's reach

Inactive Ingredients. This section lists the other parts or chemicals in the product such as coloring, flavoring, preservatives, or fillers. If you are allergic to certain dyes or chemicals, this is an important section to check for each OTC medication.

Purpose. This section tells you what the medication does in the body.

Directions. For specific age categories, this section tells you how and how much medication to take as well as how often and how long to take the product.

Other Information. This section includes how to properly store the product. It may also have information about how much sodium, calcium, or potassium is in the medication.

Additional sections may also be listed on the product or outside packaging such as:

Expiration date: tells you when the product should be properly thrown away

Lot or batch code: manufacturer information in case of a recall or to help identify the product

Name and address of manufacturer, packer, or distributor

Quantity: tells you how much product is in each container

Types of OTC Medications

Below is a summary of OTC medications used for certain conditions and symptoms. In addition, there is a table listing specific medications and brand name products for each type of OTC medication. For most of these medications, greater detail is provided in the Drug Listing section (indicated by a "*"). Be sure to read the information in the Drug Listing section and all of the information on the OTC product labeling before using any OTC product. Always talk to your doctor or pharmacist if you have any questions in choosing these medications for your specific needs. If your symptoms do not improve or if they get worse after using the product according to instructions on the medication label, talk to your doctor or pharmacist.

Pain and Fever Relievers

There are several types of OTC medications that are used to treat fever, pain, and muscle aches.

Nonsteroidal antiinflammatory drugs (NSAIDs) are used to reduce fever and to relieve mild pain from headaches, muscle aches, arthritis, menstrual periods, the common cold, toothaches, and backaches. They work by stopping the body's production of a substance (prostaglandins) that causes pain, fever, and inflammation. Be sure to read all of the 'warnings' information on the labels of these medications. Some of these warnings are listed below.

There is a risk of stomach problems or bleeding, especially if you:

- are age 60 or older
- have had stomach ulcers or bleeding problems
- take a blood thinning (anticoagulant) or steroid drug
- take other drugs containing an NSAID (aspirin, ibuprofen, naproxen, or others)
- have 3 or more alcoholic drinks every day while using this product
- take more or for a longer time than directed

Ask a doctor before using these products if you have:

- problems or serious side effects from taking pain relievers or fever reducers
- stomach pain
- ulcers
- bleeding problems
- high blood pressure
- heart or kidney disease
- taken a diuretic
- reached age 60 or older

Ask a doctor or pharmacist before use if you are:

- taking aspirin to prevent heart attack or stroke, because ibuprofen may decrease this benefit of aspirin
- taking any other drug containing an NSAID (prescription or nonprescription)
- taking a blood thinning (anticoagulant) or steroid drug
- under a doctor's care for any serious condition
- taking any other drug

NSAIDs	Brand name products
Ibuprofen *	Advil, Motrin IB
Naproxen *	Aleve

Acetaminophen is used to relieve mild to moderate pain from headaches, muscle aches, menstrual periods, colds and sore throats, toothaches, backaches, reactions to vaccinations (shots), and to reduce fever. Acetaminophen may also be used to relieve the pain of osteoarthritis (arthritis caused by the breakdown of the lining of the joints). Acetaminophen works by changing the way the body senses pain and by cooling the body.

Do not use acetaminophen with any other product containing acetaminophen. It is important to read labels carefully to see if they contain acetaminophen, especially combination products for cough and cold. If you use products from outside the US, you should be aware that in other countries acetaminophen is called paracetamol and should not be taken in addition to other acetaminophen products. Many prescription pain relievers, such as Percocet or Vicodin, also contain acetaminophen. Sometimes, the label on your prescription container may not mention that acetaminophen is one of the ingredients or may abbreviate it as APAP. Always ask your pharmacist if a prescription pain reliever that you are taking has acetaminophen as one of the ingredients.

If you are taking acetaminophen you should stop use and ask a doctor if:

- new symptoms occur
- redness or swelling is present
- pain gets worse or lasts for more than 10 days
- fever gets worse or lasts for more than 3 days
  These could be signs of a serious condition.

If you drink 3 or more alcoholic beverages every day, ask your doctor whether it is safe for you to take acetaminophen or other pain relievers/fever reducers.

Acetaminophen may cause liver damage, especially

when taken in higher doses or for longer periods of time than are recommended.

	Brand name products
Acetaminophen *	Feverall, Genapap, Tylenol

Aspirin is used to reduce fever and to relieve mild to moderate pain from headaches, menstrual periods, arthritis, colds, toothaches, and muscle aches. It is also used to prevent heart attacks in people who have had a heart attack in the past or who have angina (chest pain that occurs when the heart does not get enough oxygen). Aspirin is also used to reduce the risk of death in people who are experiencing or who have recently experienced a heart attack. It is also used to prevent ischemic strokes (strokes that occur when a blood clot blocks the flow of blood to the brain) or mini-strokes (strokes that occur when the flow of blood to the brain is blocked for a short time) in people who have had this type of stroke or mini-stroke in the past. Aspirin works by stopping the production of certain natural substances (prostaglandins) that cause fever, pain, swelling, and blood clots.

Aspirin is a NSAID like ibuprofen and naproxen, but it also has some special effects. Unlike the other NSAIDs, it does not increase the risk of heart attack or stroke. Instead, proper doses of aspirin may have life-saving effects on the heart.

	Brand name products
Aspirin *	Anacin, Bayer, Bufferin, Ecotrin, Excedrin, in Alka-Seltzer

Cold, Cough, and Allergy

Many OTC medications are available as single ingredient products or in combination to treat the symptoms of cold, cough, and allergies. Cough and cold medications that contain nasal decongestants, antihistamines, cough suppressants, and expectorants should be used with caution and only under the guidance of your child's doctor in children younger than 2 years of age. Improper use of these medications in young children can cause serious and life-threatening effects or death. The FDA is currently evaluating the safety and efficacy of the ingredients in cough and cold products used in children.

Oral Decongestants

Oral decongestants are used to relieve nasal discomfort or stuffiness caused by colds, allergies, and hay fever. They work by causing narrowing of the blood vessels of swollen nasal mucous membranes to reduce nasal congestion. These medications may provide short-term relief of nasal congestions in adults.

In the US, pseudoephedrine-containing medications are now only available as behind-the-counter medications as regulated by the Federal Government. Consumers can not select products containing this medication directly from the shelf in the OTC section, but must ask for it at the prescription counter or other space designated by the retail store. The reason pseudoephedrine is no longer available in the OTC section of the store is because it is used as an ingredient to make an illegal drug. This dangerous drug is called methamphetamine or "crystal meth" and is powerful and highly addictive when used or abused.

To purchase pseudoephedrine products, you must show a photo identification card issued by the State or the Federal Government (such as a driver's license) and provide your name, address, date, and signature in a log book. There is restriction on the amount of pseudoephedrine-containing medications that you can purchase in a single day or month. Ask your pharmacist or visit the FDA website at www.fda.gov if you have questions about buying pseudoephedrine-containing medications.

In response to these restrictions for the purchase and sale of pseudoephedrine products, some manufacturers have begun to sell oral decongestant products which substitute phenylephrine in place of pseudoephedrine. However, some experts have questioned the effectiveness of these phenylephrine products to reduce nasal congestion at the dose that is currently recommended and have suggested that further testing is needed.

Oral decongestant	Brand name products
Phenylephrine *	Sudafed PE
Pseudoephedrine *	Sudafed

Nasal Decongestants

Nasal decongestants are used to relieve nasal discomfort or stuffiness caused by colds, allergies, and hay fever. Nasal decongestants are given as sprays or drops directly into the nostrils. They work by causing narrowing of the blood vessels of swollen nasal mucous membranes to reduce nasal congestion. These products should only be used for the period of time stated on the label (usually about 3 days) to avoid the return of nasal congestion ('rebound' congestion). Your symptoms may actually get worse if these products are used for a longer time.

Nasal Decongestants	Brand name products
Naphazoline	Privine
Oxymetazoline	Afrin, Dristan
Phenylephrine	Neo Synephrine

Antihistamines

Antihistamines are used to relieve red, irritated, itchy, watery eyes; sneezing; and runny nose caused by hay fever, allergies, and the common cold. They work by blocking the action of histamine, a substance in the body that causes allergic symptoms. There are two types of antihistamines—sedating and non-sedating. The sedating type of antihistamine may give relief for the symptoms of sneezing and runny nose when used in combination with decongestants. However, the drowsiness caused by sedating antihistamines must be balanced against the relief provided by these medications. Sedating antihistamines also can be used to treat insomnia or difficulty in falling asleep (see Sleep Aids). Nonsedating antihistamines are used for the relief of allergies.

Antihistamines	Brand name products
Sedating antihistamines	
Brompheniramine *	In Bromfed, in Dimetapp, in Lodrane
Chlorpheniramine *	Chlor-Trimeton, Teldrin
Clemastine *	Tavist
Diphenhydramine *	Benadryl
Triprolidine *	In Actifed
Nonsedating antihistamines	
Loratadine *	Alavert, Claritin

Antitussives

Antitussives are used to relieve a nonproductive (dry or 'hacking') cough caused by a cold, the flu, or other conditions. They work to stop the cough reflex by affecting the area in the brain that causes you to cough. Codeine is available in some states as an OTC product, but in other states is only available with a prescription from a doctor. Some experts suggest that there is limited evidence based on available scientific studies that OTC cough medications are effective when used in children and adults for the relief of cough.

The FDA has warned that products that contain dextromethorphan have the potential for abuse. When taken in higher than recommended doses, dextromethorphan can cause serious conditions such as brain damage, seizures, loss of consciousness, changes in heartbeat, or even death. This is a particular concern for teenagers, as dextromethorphan is readily available as an OTC product. There has been a recent increase in the abuse of dextromethorphan by teenagers to get "high."

Antitussives	Brand name products
Codeine *	Robitussin AC
Dextromethorphan *	Delsym, Robitussin DM

Expectorants

Expectorants are used to relieve a productive ('wet' or a cough that brings up mucous) cough caused by colds, bronchitis, and other lung infections. They work by thinning the mucus in the air passages and making it easier to cough up the mucus and clear the airways, allowing you to breathe more easily.

Expectorant	Brand name products
Guaifenesin *	Robitussin

Gastrointestinal Disorders
Heartburn

Antacids are used to relieve the burning feeling in the stomach and throat. They work by reducing the amount of acid in the stomach.

Antacid	Brand name products
Aluminum hydroxide *	Alternagel, in Gelusil, in Mylanta, in Maalox
Bismuth subsalicylate *	Pepto Bismol
Calcium carbonate *	Alka mints, Tums, in Rolaids
Magnesium hydroxide *	Milk of Magnesia, in Gelusil, in Mylanta, in Maalox
Sodium bicarbonate *	In Alka Seltzer

Histamine$_2$-receptor antagonists are used to relieve the burning feeling in the stomach and throat. They work by reducing the amount of acid that is made by the stomach.

Histamine$_2$-receptor antagonists	Brand name products
Cimetidine *	Tagamet HB
Famotidine *	Pepcid AC, in Pepcid Complete
Nizatidine *	Axid AR
Ranitidine *	Zantac 75, Zantac 150

Proton pump inhibitors are used to relieve the burning feeling in the stomach and throat. They work by reducing the amount of acid that is made by the stomach.

Proton pump inhibitors	Brand name products
Omeprazole *	Prilosec OTC

Note: Both proton pump inhibitors and histamine$_2$-receptor antagonists usually last longer, provide more acid relief, and are taken less often than antacids. But they may take longer to work and may not provide relief for certain symptoms such as pain.

Gas

Antiflatulents are used to treat the symptoms of gas such as uncomfortable or painful pressure, fullness, and bloating.

They work by breaking up the gas bubbles that have formed in the stomach.

Antiflatulents	Brand name products
Simethicone *	Gas-X, Mylanta Gas, Mylicon, Phazyme

Constipation

Laxatives are used to treat symptoms of constipation such as hard stools, infrequent passing of stool, and bloating. There are several different types of laxatives which work in different ways to treat the symptoms of constipation. You should talk to your doctor or pharmacist before using OTC products to treat constipation, if you also have:

- abdominal pain, considerable bloating, or cramping
- considerable or unexplained gas
- fever
- nausea and/or vomiting
- need to use a laxative daily (except for fiber or bulk forming products)
- unexplained changes in bowel habits, especially if weight loss also occurs
- bloody stools or black and tarry stools
- change in width of stool, such as becoming pencil-thin
- bowel symptoms that last for longer than 2 weeks or happen again within 3 months
- bowel symptoms that happen again after treatment with medications or lifestyle changes
- diseases of the bowel such as inflammatory bowel syndrome or Crohn's disease

Some people become dependent on laxatives or may abuse them to lose weight in some eating disorders. Abuse of laxatives in eating disorders can be deadly.

Over-the-counter laxatives are classified by how they work to relieve the symptoms of constipation. Always use these products according to the instructions on the package or as directed by your doctor or pharmacist. Using more than recommended of these products or taking them too often or for a long period of time can cause serious medical problems.

Bulk forming laxatives work by absorbing fluid into the bowel and add the necessary bulk to help form an easily eliminated stool. These laxatives will not work right away, but generally produce an effect in 12 to 72 hours.

Emollient laxatives work by softening stools, making them easier to pass. These laxatives generally work in 1-2 days, but may take up to 3-5 days to work for some people.

Lubricant laxatives work by coating the stools and making them softer and easier to pass. These laxatives generally work in 6-8 hours after taking them orally and in 5-15 minutes when used as an enema.

Saline laxatives work by drawing more water into the bowel and stimulating the bowel to allow the stool to pass. These laxatives generally work in about ½ hour or up to to 3 hours when taken orally and in 2-5 minutes when used as an enema.

Hyperosmotic laxatives work by drawing fluid into the bowel and also to stimulate the bowel to allow the stool to pass. These laxatives generally work in about ½ hour when used as a suppository.

Stimulant laxatives work by increasing the action of the bowel to allow the stool to pass. These laxatives generally work within a day when taken by mouth and within an hour when given as a suppository or enema.

Laxative	Type	Brand name products
Psyllium *	Bulk forming	Metamucil
Methylcellulose	Bulk forming	Citrucel
Stool softeners *	Emollient	Colace
Mineral oil	Lubricant	Fleet mineral oil enema, Kondremul
Magnesium hydroxide *	Saline	Philip's Milk of Magnesia
Sodium phosphates	Saline	Fleet Enema
Glycerin	Hyperosmotic	Fleet glycerin suppository
Bisacodyl *	Stimulant	Correctol, Dulcolax, Feen-A-Mint
Stimulant laxatives *	Stimulant	Ex-Lax, Senokot

Diarrhea

Antidiarrheal medications are used to control the symptoms of diarrhea such as watery bowel movements or frequent passing of stools. These products work by slowing the movement of stool through the intestine. You should talk to your doctor before using OTC products to treat your symptoms of diarrhea, if you also have:

- high fever
- symptoms getting worse
- stool that contains blood or mucous
- symptoms continuing for longer than 48 hours
- signs of dehydration such as increasing thirst, dry mouth, weakness or lightheadedness (particularly if worse on standing), and a darkening of the urine or a decrease in urination

You should also talk to your doctor before using these products for infants and young children, frail, older adults, or in people with ongoing health conditions such as cancer, AIDS, or diabetes.

Antidiarrheals	Brand name products
Bismuth Subsalicylate *	Kaopectate, Pepto-Bismol
Loperamide *	Imodium AD

Sleep Aids

Over-the-counter sleep products are used to treat insomnia. They contain antihistamines and work because of the side effect of drowsiness caused by these medications. These medications should only be used for short-term sleep difficulties. Talk to your doctor if your sleep problems:

- occur for a month or longer
- cause you to frequently wake up at night or early in the morning

Sleep aid	Brand name products
Diphenhydramine *	Compoz, Sominex, Tylenol PM, Unisom Sleepgels
Doxylamine *	Unisom Nighttime Sleep Aid

Smoking Cessation

Nicotine replacement products are used to help people stop smoking. These products should be used together with a smoking cessation program, which may include support groups, counseling, or specific behavior change techniques. They work by providing nicotine to your body to decrease the withdrawal symptoms experienced when smoking is stopped and to reduce the urge to smoke. Talk to your doctor or pharmacist to help you decide which of these products may be best for you to use to help you quit smoking. These products should only be used to help you stop smoking—never to boost the effect of cigarettes since the increased amount of nicotine could be harmful to your body.

Nicotine replacement	Brand name products
Nicotine gum *	Nicorette
Nicotine lozenge *	Commit
Nicotine patches *	Nicoderm CQ, Nicotrol

Abbreviations List

AAP	American Academy of Pediatrics
ACC	American College of Cardiology
ACE	angiotensin-converting enzyme
ACLS	advanced cardiovascular life support
AHA	American Heart Association
ALT	alanine aminotransferase
AMI	acute myocardial infarction
ANC	absolute neutrophil count
aPTT	activated partial thromboplastin time
ARDS	adult respiratory distress syndrome
ASBMT	American Society of Bone Marrow Transplantation
ASCO	American Society of Clinical Oncology
AST	aspartate aminotransferase
ATS	American Thoracic Society
AUC	area under the serum concentration–time curve
AV	atrioventricular
BP	blood pressure
bpm	beats per minute
BUN	blood urea nitrogen
CABG	coronary artery bypass grafting
CAD	coronary artery disease
CAPD	continuous ambulatory peritoneal dialysis
CBC	complete blood count
CDC	US Centers for Disease Control and Prevention
CHD	coronary heart disease
CHF	congestive heart failure
CK	creatine kinase
Cl_{cr}	creatinine clearance
CNS	central nervous system
COX-1	cyclooxygenase-1
COPD	chronic obstructive pulmonary disease
CPK	creatine phosphokinase

CPR	cardiopulmonary resuscitation
CSF	cerebrospinal fluid
CYP	cytochrome P-450
DBP	diastolic blood pressure
DVT	deep-vein thrombosis
FDA	US Food and Drug Administration
FSH	follicle-stimulating hormone
GABA	γ-amino butyric acid
GFR	glomerular filtration rate
GI	gastrointestinal
GU	genitourinary
HCTZ	hydrochlorothiazide
HDL	high-density lipoprotein
HIV	human immunodeficiency virus
IDSA	Infectious Diseases Society of America
INR	international normalized rate
IM	intramuscular
IV	intravenous
JNC 7	Joint National Committee on the Prevention, Detection, and Treatment of Hypertension
LDH	lactate dehydrogenase
LDL	low-density lipoprotein
LH	luteinizing hormone
MAO	monoamine oxidase
MI	myocardial infarction
MIC	minimum inhibitory concentration
NSAIA	nonsteroidal anti-inflammatory agents
NSAID	nonsteroidal anti-inflammatory drugs
NYHA	New York Heart Association
OTC	over-the-counter or nonprescription
PCI	percutaneous coronary intervention
PSA	prostate-specific antigen
PT	prothrombin time
PVC	polyvinyl chloride
SA	sinoatrial
SBP	systolic blood pressure
S_{cr}	serum creatinine concentration
SIADH	syndrome of inappropriate antidiuretic hormone secretion

SSRI	selective serotonin-reuptake inhibitor	**VPCs**	ventricular premature complexes
Sub-Q	subcutaneous	**VT**	ventricular tachycardia
TIA	transient ischemic attack	**WBC**	white blood cell
TSH	thyrotropin, thyroid-stimulating hormone	**WHO**	World Health Organization
ULN	upper limit of normal	**>**	greater than
USPHS	US Public Health Service	**<**	less than
VLDL	very low density lipoprotein	**≥**	greater than or equal to
VF	ventricular fibrillation	**≤**	less than or equal to

Drug Identification Section

This Drug Identification Section has two parts that are designed to help check that you are taking the medication that your doctor prescribed. The first part consists of full-color photographs* of the most commonly prescribed medications in the United States so that you can check that the drug in your hand matches the drug identified in a photo. The second part is the drug imprint index to over 1000 drugs. Use this index to look up the alphanumeric code printed on most tablets and capsules as another way of checking that a drug you are about to take is the one you think it is.

The photographs of the products are arranged alphabetically by generic name; however, in some instances not all dosage forms and strengths are pictured. If additional dosage forms and strengths are available, a "dagger" symbol (†) precedes the product's name. These photographs are intended to closely approximate the size and color of the actual product; however, size and color can vary due to photographic and printing processes. Also be aware that manufacturers occasionally make changes to a product's appearance, and if this happens, the product may no longer look like the photographs shown here.

Just because a brand name is pictured in this section does not mean that the authors or organizations represented have any particular knowledge that the brand listed has properties different from other brands of the same drug, nor is it intended as a recommendation of the drugs listed. Additionally, if a brand name product is not listed, it does not indicate that the product has been evaluated to be unsatisfactory or substandard.

In the drug imprint index, the letters and/or numbers representing the manufacturer's identification code are listed so that you can find the name of the medication. These identification codes are often imprinted on the tablet or capsule. Imprints beginning with a number are listed first, and then an alphabetical listing follows. For medications such as tablets where there is writing on both the front and back, this writing is represented with a vertical line separating the front and back text (for example, "992 | 23" represents a tablet imprinted with "992" on the front and "23" on the back). Also included in the index is the manufacturer of the drug, the form of the drug (tablet or capsule), the strength, and a description of the product's shape and color(s).

This section is intended only as an initial guide to identifying medications. You should verify your findings with your pharmacist or doctor to be sure your medicine has been correctly identified. If you cannot find the identification code of your medication in this section, you should contact your pharmacist or doctor to find the name and strength of your medication.

*Drug images and imprints are reprinted by permission of First DataBank, Inc. all rights reserved.

Consumer Drug Reference 2008

Imprint	Generic Name	Strength	Form	Description
018 I	fexofenadine hcl	180 mg	tablet	oblong, peach
027 I logo	alprazolam	0.25 mg	tablet	white, round
029 I logo	alprazolam	0.5 mg	tablet	peach, round
03 I	fexofenadine hcl	30 mg	tablet	pinkish-brown, round
031 I logo	alprazolam	1 mg	tablet	blue, round
06 logo I	fexofenadine hcl	60 mg	tablet	oval, peach
06/012D I	pseudoephedrine hcl/fexofenadine hcl	120 mg-60 mg	capsule	white, tan, oblong
0698 I	benzonatate	200 mg	capsule	yellow, oblong
0863 I 93	ciprofloxacin hcl	250 mg	tablet	round, white
1 I	metoprolol tartrate	25 mg	tablet	round, white
1 KLONOPIN I ROCHE	clonazepam	1 mg	tablet	blue, round
1/2 KLONOPIN I ROCHE	clonazepam	0.5 mg	tablet	round, orange
10 I	olanzapine	10 mg	tablet	round, yellow, blue
10 00 I BMS 6071	metformin hcl	1,000 mg	tablet	oval, white
10 VALIUM I ROCHE ROCHE	diazepam	10 mg	tablet	blue, round
10 mg and 3513 I 10 mg and SB	d-amphetamine sulfate	10 mg	capsule	brown, clear, oblong
100 ER I	tramadol hcl	100 mg	tablet	white, round
1111 I 93	lisinopril	2.5 mg	tablet	round, white
1114 I 93	lisinopril	20 mg	tablet	oblong, red
1115 I 93	lisinopril	40 mg	tablet	oblong, yellow
112 I	sitagliptin phosphate	50 mg	tablet	light beige, round
12.5 I AD	amphetamine aspartate/amphetamine sulfate/dextroamphetamine	12.5 mg	tablet	orange, round
120 mg I Andrx 597	diltiazem hcl	120 mg	capsule	oblong, white, orange
15 I	olanzapine	15 mg	tablet	round, yellow
15 mg and 3514 I 15 mg and SB	d-amphetamine sulfate	15 mg	capsule	clear, oblong, brown
150 I AXID logo and Reliant	nizatidine	150 mg	capsule	oblong, pale yellow, dark yellow
166 I	metoprolol tartrate	50 mg	tablet	oblong, white
167 I	metoprolol tartrate	100 mg	tablet	oblong, white
180 mg I Andrx 598	diltiazem hcl	180 mg	capsule	yellow, oblong, orange
2 93 50	acetaminophen with codeine phosphate	300 mg-15 mg	tablet	white, round
2 KLONOPIN I ROCHE	clonazepam	2 mg	tablet	round, white
2 VALIUM I ROCHE ROCHE	diazepam	2 mg	tablet	white, round
2 1/2 I WARFARIN TARO	warfarin sodium	2.5 mg	tablet	green, oblong
2.5 I PERCOCET	oxycodone hcl/acetaminophen	2.5 mg-325 mg	tablet	oval, pink
20 I	olanzapine	20 mg	tablet	round, yellow
20 MG I F P	citalopram hydrobromide	20 mg	tablet	pink, oval
200 ER I	tramadol hcl	200 mg	tablet	round, white
201 I U U	hydrocodone bit/acetaminophen	7.5 mg-650 mg	tablet	oblong, white
2101 V I	amitriptyline hcl	10 mg	tablet	blue, round
2102 V I	amitriptyline hcl	25 mg	tablet	yellow, round

Imprint	Drug	Strength	Form	Description
2103 V I	amitriptyline hcl	50 mg	tablet	beige, round
2104 V I	amitriptyline hcl	75 mg	tablet	orange, round
2105 V I	amitriptyline hcl	100 mg	tablet	mauve, round
2106 I V	amitriptyline hcl	150 mg	tablet	blue, oblong
221 I	sitagliptin phosphate	25 mg	tablet	pink, round
222 I logo	hydrochlorothiazide	50 mg	tablet	peach, round
240 mg I Andrx 599	diltiazem hcl	240 mg	capsule	light brown, oblong, orange
241 1 I WATSON	lorazepam	1 mg	tablet	round, white
242 2 I WATSON	lorazepam	2 mg	tablet	white, round
266 I MRK	rizatriptan benzoate	5 mg	tablet	oblong, pale pink
277 I	sitagliptin phosphate	100 mg	tablet	beige, round
2771 I a heart	irbesartan	75 mg	tablet	oval, white
2772 I a heart	irbesartan	150 mg	tablet	oval, white
2773 I a heart	irbesartan	300 mg	tablet	oval, white
2775 I a heart	irbesartan/hydrochlorothiazide	150 mg-12.5 mg	tablet	oval, peach
2776 I a heart	irbesartan/hydrochlorothiazide	300 mg-12.5 mg	tablet	oval, peach
2788 I a heart	irbesartan/hydrochlorothiazide	300 mg-25 mg	tablet	oval, pink
3 I 93 150	acetaminophen with codeine phosphate	300 mg-30 mg	tablet	round, white
30 I ACTOS	pioglitazone hcl	30 mg	tablet	round, white
30 mg I LILLY 3240	duloxetine hcl	30 mg	capsule	blue, oblong, white
300 I AXID logo and Reliant	nizatidine	300 mg	capsule	brown, oblong, pale yellow
300 mg I Andrx 600	diltiazem hcl	300 mg	capsule	orange, oblong
300ER I	tramadol hcl	300 mg	tablet	white, round
306 I PFIZER	azithromycin	250 mg	tablet	oblong, red
308 AV I	pseudoephedrine hcl/fexofenadine hcl	240 mg-180 mg	tablet	round, white
311 I	ezetimibe/simvastatin	10 mg-10 mg	tablet	oblong, white
312 I	ezetimibe/simvastatin	10 mg-20 mg	tablet	oblong, white
313 I	ezetimibe/simvastatin	10 mg-40 mg	tablet	oblong, white
315 I	ezetimibe/simvastatin	10 mg-80 mg	tablet	white, oblong
35 95 I V	hydrocodone bit/acetaminophen	7.5 mg-650 mg	tablet	white, oblong
35 91 I V	hydrocodone bit/acetaminophen	2.5 mg-500 mg	tablet	oblong, white
35 92 I V	hydrocodone bit/acetaminophen	5 mg-500 mg	tablet	oblong, white
35 94 V I	hydrocodone bit/acetaminophen	7.5 mg-500 mg	tablet	oblong, white
35 95 I V	hydrocodone bit/acetaminophen	7.5 mg-650 mg	tablet	white, oblong
35 96 I V	hydrocodone bit/acetaminophen	7.5 mg-750 mg	tablet	oblong, white
35 98 I V	hydrocodone bit/acetaminophen	10 mg-660 mg	tablet	oval, white
3571 V I	hydrochlorothiazide	25 mg	tablet	peach, round
3572 V I	hydrochlorothiazide	50 mg	tablet	peach, round
36 01 I V	hydrocodone bit/acetaminophen	10 mg-325 mg	tablet	light yellow, oblong
3604 V I	hydrocodone bit/acetaminophen	5 mg-325 mg	tablet	oblong, white
3605 V I	hydrocodone bit/acetaminophen	7.5 mg-325 mg	tablet	light orange, oval
41 93 350	acetaminophen with codeine phosphate	300 mg-60 mg	tablet	round, white
40 I PD 157	atorvastatin calcium	40 mg	tablet	white, elliptical
40 MG I F P	citalopram hydrobromide	40 mg	tablet	oval, white
400 I SL	imatinib mesylate	400 mg	tablet	oval, yellow-orange
414 I	ezetimibe	10 mg	tablet	oblong, white
421 dp	estrogens, conj., synthetic a	0.625 mg	tablet	round, red
44 dp	estrogens, conj., synthetic a	1.25 mg	tablet	round, blue
45 I ACTOS	pioglitazone hcl	45 mg	tablet	round, white
461 80 mg I	aprepitant	80 mg	capsule	oblong, white

Imprint	Drug	Strength	Form	Description
462 125 mg	aprepitant	125 mg	capsule	oblong, pink, white
477	metoprolol tartrate	50 mg	tablet	round, white
49 93	metformin hcl	850 mg	tablet	white, oval
5	lisinopril	5 mg	tablet	pink, round
5 VALIUM ROCHE / ROCHE	diazepam	5 mg	tablet	round, yellow
5 mg RSN	risedronate sodium	5 mg	tablet	oval, yellow
5 or 10 FL	memantine hcl	5 mg (28)/10 mg (21)	tablet	multi-color (2), oblong
5 12	levothyroxine sodium	50 mg	tablet	white, oblong
50 GG 332	metformin hcl	500 mg	tablet	round, white
500 BMS 6060	metformin hcl	500 mg	tablet	oblong, white
5046 SOLVAY	eprosartan mesylate	600 mg	tablet	oblong, orange
5111 V	propoxyphene napsyl/acetaminophen	50 mg-325 mg	tablet	oblong, orange
5112 V	propoxyphene napsyl/acetaminophen	100 mg-650 mg	tablet	oblong, white
5113 V	propoxyphene napsyl/acetaminophen	100 mg-650 mg	tablet	oblong, pink
5114 V	propoxyphene napsyl/acetaminophen	100 mg-650 mg	tablet	oblong, pink
512	oxycodone hcl/acetaminophen	5 mg-325 mg	tablet	round, white
5157 93	lisinopril	30 mg	tablet	white, round
54 092	prednisone	1 mg	tablet	round, white
54 339	prednisone	2.5 mg	tablet	round, white
54 343	prednisone	50 mg	tablet	white, round
54 582	oxycodone hcl	5 mg	tablet	white, round
54 612	prednisone	5 mg	tablet	round, white
54 760	prednisone	20 mg	tablet	oval, pink
54 899	prednisone	10 mg	tablet	oval, pink
5410 logo and 50	fluconazole	50 mg	tablet	pink, oval
5411 logo and 100	fluconazole	100 mg	tablet	oval, pink
5412 logo and 150	fluconazole	150 mg	tablet	pink, oval
5413 logo and 200	fluconazole	200 mg	tablet	oval, pink
5431	simvastatin	80 mg	tablet	brick red, oblong
5553 DAN	doxycycline hyclate	100 mg	capsule	light orange, round
575	sitagliptin phosphate/metformin hcl	50 mg-500 mg	tablet	light pink, oblong
577	sitagliptin phosphate/metformin hcl	50 mg-1000 mg	tablet	oblong, red
6 WARFARIN TARO	warfarin sodium	6 mg	tablet	oblong, teal
60 mg LILLY 3237	duloxetine hcl	60 mg	capsule	blue, green, oblong
606 mg PRILOSEC 10	omeprazole	10 mg	capsule	amethyst, apricot, oblong
7.5 AD	amphetamine aspartate/amphetamine sulfate/dextroamphetamine	7.5 mg	tablet	blue, oval
707 SP 7.5	moexipril hcl	7.5 mg	tablet	pink, round
712 S P	moexipril hcl/hydrochlorothiazide	7.5 mg-12.5 mg	tablet	oval, yellow
715 SP 15	moexipril hcl	15 mg	tablet	salmon, round
7152 93	simvastatin	5 mg	tablet	round, light yellow
7153 93	simvastatin	10 mg	tablet	light pink, round
7154 93	simvastatin	20 mg	tablet	round, tan
7155 93	simvastatin	40 mg	tablet	red, round
7156 93	simvastatin	80 mg	tablet	red, oblong
7173 93	gabapentin	600 mg	tablet	oval, white
7174 93	gabapentin	800 mg	tablet	oval, white
7188 9 3	fluoxetine hcl	10 mg	tablet	blue, oval
7251 S P	moexipril hcl/hydrochlorothiazide	15 mg-25 mg	tablet	oval, yellow
726	simvastatin	5 mg	tablet	shield, buff
735	simvastatin	10 mg	tablet	shield, peach
74 ZE	erythromycin ethylsuccinate	400 mg	tablet	oblong, pink
740	simvastatin	20 mg	tablet	shield, tan
742 PRILOSEC 20	omeprazole	20 mg	capsule	amethyst, oblong
743 PRILOSEC 40	omeprazole	40 mg	capsule	apricot, oblong, amethyst
745	losartan potassium/hydrochlorothiazide	100 mg-12.5 mg	tablet	white, oval

Imprint	Drug	Strength	Form	Description
749	simvastatin	40 mg	tablet	brick red, shield
75 11171	clopidogrel bisulfate	75 mg	tablet	pink, round
7767 100	celecoxib	100 mg	capsule	oblong, white
8 SB	rosiglitazone maleate	8 mg	tablet	pentagon, red-brown
831 1 barr	warfarin sodium	1 mg	tablet	pink, oval
832 2 1/2 barr	warfarin sodium	2.5 mg	tablet	green, oval
833 5 barr	warfarin sodium	5 mg	tablet	oval, peach
869 2 barr	warfarin sodium	2 mg	tablet	lavender, oval
874 4 barr	warfarin sodium	4 mg	tablet	blue, oval
9 3 1174	penicillin v potassium	500 mg	tablet	oval, light green
903 ucb	hydrocodone bit/acetaminophen	7.5 mg-500 mg	tablet	oblong, white
910 ucb	hydrocodone bit/acetaminophen	10 mg-500 mg	tablet	pink, oblong
925 3 barr	warfarin sodium	3 mg	tablet	oval, tan
926 6 barr	warfarin sodium	6 mg	tablet	oval, teal
93 0864	ciprofloxacin hcl	500 mg	tablet	oblong, white
93 088	sulfamethoxazole/trimethoprim	400 mg-80 mg	tablet	round, white
93 089	sulfamethoxazole/trimethoprim	800 mg-160 mg	tablet	oval, white
93 1112	lisinopril	5 mg	tablet	red, round
93 3107 93 3107	amoxicillin trihydrate	250 mg	capsule	buff, oblong, caramel
93 3109 93 3109	amoxicillin trihydrate	500 mg	capsule	buff, oblong
93 3145 93 3145	cephalexin monohydrate	250 mg	capsule	gray, oblong, swedish orange
93 3147 93 3147	cephalexin monohydrate	500 mg	capsule	oblong, swedish orange
93 38	gabapentin	100 mg	capsule	gray, oblong
93 39 93 39	gabapentin	300 mg	capsule	orange, oblong
93 40 93 40	gabapentin	400 mg	capsule	caramel, oblong
93 42 93 42	fluoxetine hcl	10 mg	capsule	oblong, powder blue
93 43 93 43	fluoxetine hcl	20 mg	capsule	blue, white
93 7198 93 7198	fluoxetine hcl	40 mg	capsule	blue, orange, oblong
93 733	metoprolol tartrate	50 mg	tablet	pink, round
93 734	metoprolol tartrate	100 mg	tablet	blue, round
93 832	clonazepam	0.5 mg	tablet	yellow, round
93 833	clonazepam	1 mg	tablet	green, round
93 834	clonazepam	2 mg	tablet	round, white
93 2264	amoxicillin trihydrate	875 mg	tablet	off-white, oblong
93-4990	propoxyphene napsyl/acetaminophen	100 mg-650 mg	tablet	white, oblong
93-5	naproxen	375 mg	tablet	oblong, white
936 MRK	alendronate sodium	10 mg	tablet	oval, white
93-6	naproxen	500 mg	tablet	oblong, white
960 MRK	losartan potassium	100 mg	tablet	teardrop, dark green
A	desloratadine	5 mg	tablet	light red, round
A B	metoprolol succinate	25 mg	tablet	oval, white
A CF 004	candesartan cilexetil	4 mg	tablet	round, white
A CG 008	candesartan cilexetil	8 mg	tablet	light pink, round
A CH 016	candesartan cilexetil	16 mg	tablet	pink, round
A CJ 322	candesartan cilexetil/hydrochlorothiazide	32 mg-12.5 mg	tablet	oval, yellow
A CL 032	candesartan cilexetil	32 mg	tablet	pink, round
A CS 162	candesartan cilexetil/hydrochlorothiazide	16 mg-12.5 mg	tablet	oval, peach
A mo	metoprolol succinate	50 mg	tablet	round, white
A ms	metoprolol succinate	100 mg	tablet	round, white
A my	metoprolol succinate	200 mg	tablet	white, oval
A 301	cyclobenzaprine hcl	5 mg	tablet	orange, round
A 640 10	aripiprazole	10 mg	tablet	pink, round

Imprint	Drug	Strength	Form	Description
A 641	15	aripiprazole	15 mg	tablet	round, yellow
a bone outline	31	alendronate sodium	70 mg	tablet	white, oval
a square	rizatriptan benzoate	10 mg	tablet	round, white
a symbol	2	tolterodine tartrate	2 mg	capsule	blue-green, oblong
a triangle	rizatriptan benzoate	5 mg	tablet	white, round
A~	zolpidem tartrate	6.25 mg	tablet	round, pink
A-006	2	aripiprazole	2 mg	tablet	green, rectangular
A-007 5	aripiprazole	5 mg	tablet	blue, rectangular
A-008 10	aripiprazole	10 mg	tablet	pink, rectangular
A-009 15	aripiprazole	15 mg	tablet	round, yellow
A-010 20	aripiprazole	20 mg	tablet	round, white
A-011 30	aripiprazole	30 mg	tablet	pink, round
A500	A500	propoxyphene napsyl/acetaminophen	100 mg-500 mg	tablet	dark orange, oval
ACCOLATE 10	ZENECA	zafirlukast	10 mg	tablet	round, white
ACCOLATE 20	ZENECA	zafirlukast	20 mg	tablet	round, white
ACIPHEX 20	rabeprazole sodium	20 mg	tablet	round, light yellow
ADALAT CC	30	nifedipine	30 mg	tablet	pink, round
ADDERALL XR	10mg	amphetamine aspartate/amphetamine sulfate/dextroamphetamine	10 mg	capsule	blue, oblong
ALDACTAZIDE 25	SEARLE 1011	spironolactone/hydrochlorothiazide	25 mg-25 mg	tablet	round, tan
ALEVE	naproxen sodium	220 mg	tablet	round, yellow
ALTACE	5 mg MP	ramipril	5 mg	capsule	oblong, red
ALTACE 1.25 mg	MP	ramipril	1.25 mg	capsule	oblong, yellow
ALTACE 10 mg	MP	ramipril	10 mg	capsule	oblong, process blue
ALTACE 2.5 mg	MP	ramipril	2.5 mg	capsule	orange, oblong
alza 18	methylphenidate hcl	18 mg	tablet	oblong, yellow
alza 27	methylphenidate hcl	27 mg	tablet	gray, oblong
alza 36	methylphenidate hcl	36 mg	tablet	oblong, white
alza 54	methylphenidate hcl	54 mg	tablet	brownish-red, oblong
AMA RYL	logo logo	glimepiride	2 mg	tablet	green, oblong
AMB 10	5421	zolpidem tartrate	10 mg	tablet	oblong, white
AMB 5	5401	zolpidem tartrate	5 mg	tablet	oblong, pink
AMC	500/125	amoxicillin trihydrate/potassium clavulanate	500 mg-125 mg	tablet	oblong, white
AMOX 250	GG 848	amoxicillin trihydrate	250 mg	capsule	oblong, yellow
AMOX 500	GG 849	amoxicillin trihydrate	500 mg	capsule	oblong, yellow
ANSAID 100mg	flurbiprofen	100 mg	tablet	blue, oval
ANTIVERT	210	meclizine hcl	12.5 mg	tablet	blue, oval
ANZEMET	100	dolasetron mesylate	100 mg	tablet	oval, pink
APO	083	paroxetine hcl	20 mg	tablet	oval, reddish-brown
ARICEPT	10	donepezil hcl	10 mg	tablet	round, yellow
AVINZA	120 mg 508	morphine sulfate	120 mg	capsule	blue violet, oblong, white
AXID AR	nizatidine	75 mg	tablet	oblong, beige
b	40	bisoprolol fumarate/hydrochlorothiazide	10 mg-6.25 mg	tablet	round, white
B 145	digoxin	125 mcg	tablet	round, white
B 146	digoxin	250 mcg	tablet	round, yellow
B L	136	cephalexin monohydrate	250 mg	capsule	oblong, white
B2	logo	buprenorphine hcl	2 mg	tablet	oval, white
B2C	B2C	digoxin	100 mcg	capsule	oval, white
B8	logo	buprenorphine hcl	8 mg	tablet	oval, white
bar	834 7 1/2	warfarin sodium	7.5 mg	tablet	yellow, oval, white
BAYER	10	vardenafil hcl	10 mg	tablet	orange, round

Imprint	Drug	Strength	Form	Description
Benadryl	PD	diphenhydramine hcl	25 mg	capsule	oblong, pink, white
BMS	6072	glyburide/metformin hcl	1.25 mg-250 mg	tablet	oblong, pale yellow
BMS 150mg	3624	atazanavir sulfate	150 mg	capsule	blue, oblong, powder blue
BMS 1964	15	stavudine	15 mg	capsule	dark red, oblong, light yellow
BMS 1965	20	stavudine	20 mg	capsule	light brown, oblong
BMS 1966	30	stavudine	30 mg	capsule	dark orange, light orange, oblong
BMS 1967	40	stavudine	40 mg	capsule	dark orange, oblong
BMS 200mg	3631	atazanavir sulfate	200 mg	capsule	blue, oblong
BMS 6070	850	metformin hcl	850 mg	tablet	white, round
BMS 100mg	3623	atazanavir sulfate	100 mg	capsule	blue, oblong, white
BMS 6063	500	metformin hcl	500 mg	tablet	oblong, white
BMS 6064	750	metformin hcl	750 mg	tablet	oblong, pale red
BUSPAR	MJ 10	buspirone hcl	10 mg	tablet	oval, white
C 10	tadalafil	10 mg	tablet	almond, yellow
C 20	tadalafil	20 mg	tablet	almond, yellow
C 5	tadalafil	5 mg	tablet	almond, yellow
C2C	digoxin	200 mcg	capsule	green, oval
C5	desloratadine	5 mg	tablet	round, light blue
CALAN	40	verapamil hcl	40 mg	tablet	pink, round
CALAN 120	verapamil hcl	120 mg	tablet	brown, oval
CD	129	ranitidine hcl	150 mg	capsule	light brown, oblong
CDT 251	pfizer	amlodipine besylate/atorvastatin calcium	2.5 mg-10 mg	tablet	white
CDT 252	amlodipine besylate/atorvastatin calcium	2.5 mg-20 mg	tablet	white
CDT 254	amlodipine besylate/atorvastatin calcium	2.5 mg-40 mg	tablet	oblong, light orange
CG	HGH	valsartan/hydrochlorothiazide	80 mg-12.5 mg	tablet	pale green, round
CIBA	3	methylphenidate hcl	10 mg	tablet	white, round
CIBA 16	methylphenidate hcl	20 mg	tablet	round, white
CIPRO	250	ciprofloxacin hcl	250 mg	tablet	round, slightly yellow
CLARITIN 10	458	loratadine	10 mg	tablet	white, round
CLARITIN D	pseudoephedrine sulfate/loratadine	120 mg-5 mg	tablet	round, white
CLARITIN-D 24 HOUR	pseudoephedrine sulfate/loratadine	240 mg-10 mg	tablet	oval, white
COGNEX 10	tacrine hcl	10 mg	capsule	dark green, oblong, yellow
COGNEX 20	tacrine hcl	20 mg	capsule	yellow, light blue, oblong
COGNEX 30	tacrine hcl	30 mg	capsule	yellow, swedish orange, oblong
COGNEX 40	tacrine hcl	40 mg	capsule	lavender, oblong, yellow
COPLEY 225	potassium chloride	8 mEq	tablet	orange, round
CORGARD 20	BL 232	nadolol	20 mg	tablet	blue, round
CORGARD 40	BL 207	nadolol	40 mg	tablet	blue, round
CORGARD 80	BL 241	nadolol	80 mg	tablet	round, blue
COUMADIN 1	warfarin sodium	1 mg	tablet	pink, round
COUMADIN 10	warfarin sodium	10 mg	tablet	round, white
COUMADIN 2	warfarin sodium	2 mg	tablet	lavender, round
COUMADIN 2 1/2	warfarin sodium	2.5 mg	tablet	green, round
COUMADIN 3	warfarin sodium	3 mg	tablet	round, tan
COUMADIN 4	warfarin sodium	4 mg	tablet	blue, round

Imprint	Drug	Strength	Form	Description
COUMADIN 5	warfarin sodium	5 mg	tablet	peach, round
COUMADIN 6	warfarin sodium	6 mg	tablet	round, teal
COUMADIN 7 1/2	warfarin sodium	7.5 mg	tablet	round, yellow
COVERA-HS 2011	verapamil hcl	180 mg	tablet	round, lavender
COVERA-HS 2021	verapamil hcl	240 mg	tablet	pale yellow, round
COZAAR | MRK 952	losartan potassium	50 mg	tablet	green, teardrop
CR 250 | symbol	ciprofloxacin hcl	250 mg	tablet	oval, white
CR 500 | logo	ciprofloxacin hcl	500 mg	tablet	white, oblong
CR 750 | symbol	ciprofloxacin hcl	750 mg	tablet	white, oblong
CRESTOR I 40	rosuvastatin calcium	40 mg	tablet	oval, pink
CRESTOR 10 I	rosuvastatin calcium	10 mg	tablet	pink, round
CRESTOR 20 I	rosuvastatin calcium	20 mg	tablet	pink, round
CRESTOR 5 I	rosuvastatin calcium	5 mg	tablet	yellow, round
CRIXIVAN I 100 mg	indinavir sulfate	100 mg	capsule	oblong, white
D 24 I	pseudoephedrine sulfate/desloratadine	240 mg-5 mg	tablet	oval, light blue
d p I 46	estrogens, conj., synthetic a	0.45 mg	tablet	round, orange
D12 I	pseudoephedrine sulfate/desloratadine	120 mg-2.5 mg	tablet	blue, oval, white
DAN 5440 | DAN 5440	doxycycline hyclate	100 mg	capsule	blue, oblong
DAN 5535 | DAN 5535	doxycycline hyclate	50 mg	capsule	white, blue, oblong
DAN DAN | 5052	prednisone	5 mg	tablet	round, white
DARVOCET-N 100 I	propoxyphene napsyl/acetaminophen	100 mg-650 mg	tablet	dark orange, oblong
Darvon I	propoxyphene hcl	65 mg	capsule	pink
DARVON-N 100 I	propoxyphene napsyl	100 mg	tablet	elliptical, buff
Dia B I HOECHST	glyburide	2.5 mg	tablet	oblong, pink
Dia B I HOECHST	glyburide	1.25 mg	tablet	oblong, peach
DIFLUCAN 100 I RO-ERIG	fluconazole	100 mg	tablet	trapezoidal, pink
DIFLUCAN 200 I RO-ERIG	fluconazole	200 mg	tablet	pink, trapezoidal
DIFLUCAN 50 I RO-ERIG	fluconazole	50 mg	tablet	pink, trapezoidal
DILANTIN I 100 mg	phenytoin sodium extended	100 mg	capsule	clear, oblong
DISTA 3104 I PRO-ZAC 10 mg	fluoxetine hcl	10 mg	capsule	green, oblong
DISTA 3105 I PRO-ZAC 20 mg	fluoxetine hcl	20 mg	capsule	off-white, oblong, green
DISTA 3107 I PRO-ZAC 40 mg	fluoxetine hcl	40 mg	capsule	oblong, orange, green
DISTA H69 I KEFLEX 250 mg	cephalexin monohydrate	250 mg	capsule	dark green, oblong, green
DISTA H71 I KEFLEX 500 mg	cephalexin monohydrate	500 mg	capsule	oblong, dark green, light green
DO or DP I	ethinyl estradiol/drospirenone	0.03 mg-3 mg	tablet	multi-color (2), round
dp I 41	estrogens, conj., synthetic a	0.3 mg	tablet	green, round
DV I NVR	valsartan	80 mg	tablet	almond, pale red
DX I NVR	valsartan	160 mg	tablet	almond, gray orange
DXL I NVR	valsartan	320 mg	tablet	almond, dark grayish violet
e I 018	fexofenadine hcl	180 mg	tablet	oblong, peach
E 101 I	lisinopril	10 mg	tablet	pink, oval
E 102 I	lisinopril	20 mg	tablet	peach, oval
E 103 I	lisinopril	30 mg	tablet	oval, red
E 104 I	lisinopril	40 mg	tablet	oval, yellow
E 25 I	lisinopril	2.5 mg	tablet	oval, white
E 30 I	isosorbide mononitrate	30 mg	tablet	reddish-pink, oval
E 54 I	lisinopril	5 mg	tablet	oval, pink

Imprint	Drug	Strength	Form	Description
E 60	isosorbide mononitrate	60 mg	tablet	oval, yellow
E120	isosorbide mononitrate	120 mg	tablet	oval, white
EA logo	erythromycin base	500 mg	tablet	oblong, pink
EC logo	erythromycin base	250 mg	tablet	oval, white
ETH I 2 0	potassium chloride	20 mEq	tablet	oblong, white
ETHEX I 001	potassium chloride	10 mEq	capsule	clear, oblong
EXELON 1.5 mg	rivastigmine tartrate	1.5 mg	capsule	oblong, yellow
EXELON 3 mg	rivastigmine tartrate	3 mg	capsule	oblong, orange
EXELON 4.5 mg	rivastigmine tartrate	4.5 mg	capsule	oblong, red
EXELON 6 mg	rivastigmine tartrate	6 mg	capsule	oblong, orange, red
FL L 10	escitalopram oxalate	10 mg	tablet	round, white
FAMVIR I 125	famciclovir	125 mg	tablet	round, white, oval
FL I 10	memantine hcl	10 mg	tablet	gray, oblong
FL 10 I G	fluoxetine hcl	10 mg	tablet	white, oval
FL 20 I G	fluoxetine hcl	20 mg	capsule	oval, white
FL10 I G	fluoxetine hcl	10 mg	capsule	light green, light violet, oblong
FLAGYL I 375 mg	metronidazole	375 mg	capsule	iron gray, light green, oblong
FLAGYL 250 | SEARLE 1831	metronidazole	250 mg	tablet	blue, round
FLAGYL ER | SEARLE 1961	metronidazole	750 mg	tablet	blue, oval
Flomax 0.4 mg | BI 58	tamsulosin hcl	0.4 mg	capsule	oblong, olive green, orange
FLUOXETINE 20 MG | R148	fluoxetine hcl	20 mg	capsule	light blue, light turquoise blue, oblong
FLUOXETINE 40mg | R149	fluoxetine hcl	40 mg	capsule	blue, oblong, white
FOR SLEEP | M RESTORIL 22.5MG	temazepam	22.5 mg	capsule	blue, oblong
FP I 10 MG	citalopram hydrobromide	10 mg	tablet	beige, oval
G I 0.5	alprazolam	0.5 mg	tablet	blue, round
G 020 I 20	quinapril hcl	20 mg	tablet	brown, round
G 372 2 I	alprazolam	2 mg	tablet	oblong, white
G G24 9 I	quinapril hcl	10 mg	tablet	rectangular, white
G 019 I 10	quinapril hcl	10 mg	tablet	brown, triangular
G 021 I 40	quinapril hcl	40 mg	tablet	brown, elliptical
G 022 I 5	quinapril hcl	5 mg	tablet	brown, elliptical
G 22 I	gabapentin	800 mg	tablet	white, elliptical
G 3719 I	alprazolam	0.25 mg	tablet	oval, white
G 3720 I	alprazolam	0.5 mg	tablet	oval, peach
G 3721 I	alprazolam	1 mg	tablet	blue, oval
G 4900 I 50 mg	sertraline hcl	50 mg	tablet	light blue, oblong
G 4910 I 100 mg	sertraline hcl	100 mg	tablet	light yellow, oblong
GEIGY I 51 51	metoprolol tartrate	25 mg	tablet	light green, oblong
GG I 91	metoprolol tartrate	50 mg	tablet	oblong, pink
GG 165 I	lorazepam	0.5 mg	tablet	round, white
GG 172 I	triamterene/hydrochlorothiazide	37.5 mg-25 mg	tablet	round, green
GG 201 I	triamterene/hydrochlorothiazide	75 mg-50 mg	tablet	round, yellow
GG 21 I	furosemide	40 mg	tablet	round, white
GG 225 I	furosemide	20 mg	tablet	round, white
GG 235 I	promethazine hcl	25 mg	tablet	white, round
GG 263 I	promethazine hcl	50 mg	tablet	round, pink
GG 264 I	atenolol	50 mg	tablet	round, white
GG 580 I GG 580	triamterene/hydrochlorothiazide	50 mg-25 mg	capsule	oblong, red
GG 606 I GG 606	triamterene/hydrochlorothiazide	37.5 mg-25 mg	capsule	white, oblong

Imprint	Drug	Strength	Form	Description
GG 80	furosemide	80 mg	tablet	round, white
GG 92	lorazepam	1 mg	tablet	round, white
GG 93	lorazepam	2 mg	tablet	round, white
GG L7	atenolol	25 mg	tablet	round, white
GG N4	amoxicillin trihydrate/potassium clavulanate	400 mg-57 mg	chewable tablet	pink, round
GG N7	amoxicillin trihydrate/potassium clavulanate	875 mg-125 mg	tablet	oblong, white
GG 256	alprazolam	0.25 mg	tablet	oval, white
GG 257	alprazolam	0.5 mg	tablet	oval, peach
GG 258	alprazolam	1 mg	tablet	blue, oval
GG 330 137	levothyroxine sodium	137 mcg	tablet	oblong, turquoise
GG 331 25	levothyroxine sodium	25 mcg	tablet	oblong, orange
GG 333 75	levothyroxine sodium	75 mcg	tablet	oblong, blue
GG 334 88	levothyroxine sodium	88 mcg	tablet	olive, oval
GG 335 100	levothyroxine sodium	100 mcg	tablet	oblong, yellow
GG 336 112	levothyroxine sodium	112 mcg	tablet	oblong, rose
GG 337 125	levothyroxine sodium	125 mcg	tablet	oblong, brown
GG 338 150	levothyroxine sodium	150 mcg	tablet	oblong, blue
GG 339 175	levothyroxine sodium	175 mcg	tablet	lilac, oblong
GG 340 200	levothyroxine sodium	200 mcg	tablet	oblong, pink
GG 341 300	levothyroxine sodium	300 mcg	tablet	green, oblong
GG N6	amoxicillin trihydrate/potassium clavulanate	500 mg-125 mg	tablet	white, oblong
GGN2	amoxicillin trihydrate/potassium clavulanate	200 mg-28.5 mg	chewable tablet	pink, round
GGN5	amoxicillin trihydrate/potassium clavulanate	250 mg-125 mg	tablet	oblong, white
GLUCOTROL XL 10	glipizide	10 mg	tablet	round, white
GLUCOTROL XL 2.5	glipizide	2.5 mg	tablet	blue, round
GLUCOTROL XL 5	glipizide	5 mg	tablet	white, round
GLYBUR 364 364	glyburide	5 mg	tablet	oblong, blue
GLYNASE 1.5 PT PT	glyburide, micronized	1.5 mg	tablet	oval, white
GLYNASE 3 PT PT	glyburide, micronized	3 mg	tablet	oval, blue
GLYNASE 6 PT PT	glyburide, micronized	6 mg	tablet	oval, yellow
GP 111	lisinopril	2.5 mg	tablet	round, white
GP 112	lisinopril	5 mg	tablet	pink, round
GP 113	lisinopril	10 mg	tablet	round, white
GP 114	lisinopril	20 mg	tablet	peach, round
GP 115	lisinopril	40 mg	tablet	rose, round
GP 150	lisinopril	30 mg	tablet	peach, round
gsk 2/1000 10mg	rosiglitazone maleate/metformin hcl	2 mg-1,000 mg	tablet	oval, yellow
GSK COREG CR 10mg	carvedilol phosphate	10 mg	capsule	green, oblong, white
GSK COREG CR 20 mg	carvedilol phosphate	20 mg	capsule	oblong, yellow, white
GSK COREG CR 40 mg	carvedilol phosphate	40 mg	capsule	green, oblong, yellow
GSK COREG CR 80 mg	carvedilol phosphate	80 mg	capsule	green, oblong, white
GX 623	abacavir sulfate	300 mg	tablet	oblong, yellow
GX CL5	lamotrigine	25 mg	tablet	square (rounded corners), white
GX CG5	lamivudine	100 mg	tablet	oblong, butterscotch
GX CJ7	lamivudine	150 mg	tablet	diamond, white
GX CL2	lamotrigine	5 mg	tablet	oblong, white
GX EJ7	lamivudine	300 mg	tablet	diamond, gray
HYZAAR MRK 717	losartan potassium/hydrochlorothiazide	50 mg-12.5 mg	tablet	yellow, teardrop

Imprint	Drug	Strength	Form	Description
I 25	sumatriptan succinate	25 mg	tablet	triangular, white
IA NVR	deferasirox	125 mg	tablet	off-white, round
IB NVR	deferasirox	250 mg	tablet	off-white, round
IBU 400	ibuprofen	400 mg	tablet	white, round
IBU 600	ibuprofen	600 mg	tablet	oblong, white
IBU 800	ibuprofen	800 mg	tablet	oblong, white
IC NVR	deferasirox	500 mg	tablet	off-white, round
IMITREX 100	sumatriptan succinate	100 mg	tablet	pink, triangular
IMITREX 100 logo	sumatriptan succinate	100 mg	tablet	pink, triangular
IMITREX 50 logo	sumatriptan succinate	50 mg	tablet	triangular, white
INDERAL 60	propranolol hcl	60 mg	tablet	hexagonal, pink
INDERAL LA 120	propranolol hcl	120 mg	capsule	dark blue, light blue, oblong
INDERAL LA 160	propranolol hcl	160 mg	capsule	dark blue, oblong
INDERAL LA 60	propranolol hcl	60 mg	capsule	oblong, white, light blue
INDERAL LA 80	propranolol hcl	80 mg	capsule	oblong, light blue
IP 137 800	ibuprofen	800 mg	tablet	oblong, white
IP 132 600	ibuprofen	600 mg	tablet	oblong, white,
IPI 131 400	ibuprofen	400 mg	tablet	round, white
IPI 132 600	ibuprofen	600 mg	tablet	white, oblong
JANSSEN R 1	risperidone	1 mg	tablet	white, oblong
JSP 513	levothyroxine sodium	25 mcg	tablet	peach, round
K	desloratadine	2.5 mg	tablet	light red, round
KADIAN 100 mg	morphine sulfate	100 mg	capsule	green, oblong
KC M20	potassium chloride	20 mEq	tablet	green, white
KEFLEX 500 mg	cephalexin monohydrate	500 mg	capsule	dark green, light green, oblong
KEFLEX 750	cephalexin monohydrate	750 mg	capsule	oblong, dark green
KPI 4	hydrocodone bit/acetaminophen	7.5 mg-650 mg	tablet	oblong, white
L 22 M	lisinopril	2.5 mg	tablet	blue, round
L 26 M	lisinopril	40 mg	tablet	green, round
L 27 M	lisinopril	30 mg	tablet	blue, round
LAMICTAL 100	lamotrigine	100 mg	tablet	shield, peach
LAMICTAL 150	lamotrigine	150 mg	tablet	shield, cream
LAMICTAL 200	lamotrigine	200 mg	tablet	blue, shield
LAMICTAL 25	lamotrigine	25 mg	tablet	shield, white
LAMICTAL 25 or LAMICTAL 100	lamotrigine	25 mg (42)-100 mg (7)	tablet	shield, multi-color (2)
LAMICTAL 25	lamotrigine	25 mg (35)	tablet	shield, white
LANOXIN X3A	digoxin	250 mcg	tablet	round, yellow
LANOXIN Y3B	digoxin	125 mcg	tablet	round, white
LASIX HOECHST	furosemide	20 mg	tablet	oval, white
LASIX 40 HOECHST	furosemide	40 mg	tablet	round, white
LASIX 80 HOECHST	furosemide	80 mg	tablet	round, white
LESCOL XL 80	fluvastatin sodium	80 mg	tablet	round, yellow
LEVAQUIN 250	levofloxacin	250 mg	tablet	round, terra cotta pink
LEVOXYL dp 100	levothyroxine sodium	100 mcg	tablet	oval, yellow
Lilly 3145 AXID 300mg	nizatidine	300 mg	capsule	brown, oblong, pale yellow
LILLY 4112	olanzapine	2.5 mg	tablet	round, white
LILLY 4115	olanzapine	5 mg	tablet	round, white
LILLY 4116	olanzapine	7.5 mg	tablet	white, round
LILLY 4117	olanzapine	10 mg	tablet	white, round
Lilly 4165	raloxifene hcl	60 mg	tablet	elliptical, white
LILLY 4415	olanzapine	15 mg	tablet	blue, elliptical
LILLY 4420	olanzapine	20 mg	tablet	elliptical, pink
logo 3757	lisinopril	2.5 mg	tablet	white, round
logo 0 3 9	alprazolam	2 mg	tablet	rectangular, yellow

Imprint	Drug	Strength	Form	Description
logo 195	alprazolam	0.5 mg	tablet	round, white
logo 196	alprazolam	1 mg	tablet	oblong, yellow
logo 197	alprazolam	2 mg	tablet	blue, oblong
logo 198	alprazolam	3 mg	tablet	green, round
logo 20 LESCOL	fluvastatin sodium	20 mg	capsule	brown, oblong, tan
logo				
logo 33	clonazepam	0.5 mg	tablet	pink, round
logo 34	clonazepam	1 mg	tablet	round, yellow
logo 35	clonazepam	2 mg	tablet	white, round
logo 40 LESCOL	fluvastatin sodium	40 mg	capsule	oblong, brown, gold
logo				
logo DILACOR XR 120 mg	diltiazem hcl	120 mg	capsule	oblong, peach, pink
logo DILACOR XR 180 mg	diltiazem hcl	180 mg	capsule	lavender, oblong, peach
logo DILACOR XR 240 mg	diltiazem hcl	240 mg	capsule	light blue, peach, oblong,
logo Wellcome ZO-VIRAX 200	acyclovir	200 mg	capsule	blue, oblong
logo 182	trandolapril/verapamil hcl	2 mg-180 mg	tablet	oval, pink
logo and 4435 500	metformin hcl	500 mg	tablet	oval, white
logo 5311 250	ciprofloxacin hcl	250 mg	tablet	oblong, white
logo 567	hydrocodone bit/acetaminophen	10 mg-660 mg	tablet	light blue, oblong
logo and 100 5674	sertraline hcl	100 mg	tablet	oval, white
logo and 241	trandolapril/verapamil hcl	1 mg-240 mg	tablet	gold, oval
logo and 242	trandolapril/verapamil hcl	2 mg-240 mg	tablet	oval, reddish-brown
logo and 244	trandolapril/verapamil hcl	4 mg-240 mg	tablet	
logo and 25 5672	sertraline hcl	25 mg	tablet	light blue, round
logo and 2908	furosemide	20 mg	tablet	round, white
logo and 4073 logo and 4073	cephalexin monohydrate	250 mg	capsule	gray, oblong, red
logo and 4074 logo and 4074	cephalexin monohydrate	500 mg	capsule	oblong, red
logo and 4330 850	metformin hcl	850 mg	tablet	white, oval
logo and 4331 500	metformin hcl	500 mg	tablet	oval, white
logo and 4346 40	fluoxetine hcl	40 mg	capsule	light blue, oblong
logo and 4356 20 mg	fluoxetine hcl	20 mg	capsule	aqua blue, oblong
logo and 4357 150	ranitidine hcl	150 mg	tablet	beige, round
logo and 4358 300	ranitidine hcl	300 mg	tablet	beige, oval
logo and 4363 10	fluoxetine hcl	10 mg	capsule	aqua blue, white, oblong
logo and 4381 100 mg	gabapentin	100 mg	capsule	oblong, white
logo and 4382 300 mg	gabapentin	300 mg	capsule	oblong, white, yellow
logo and 4383 400 mg	gabapentin	400 mg	capsule	white, oblong, orange
logo and 4432 10 00 mg	metformin hcl	1,000 mg	tablet	oval, white
logo and 4440 100	gabapentin	100 mg	tablet	round, white
logo and 4441 300	gabapentin	300 mg	tablet	round, white
logo and 4442 400	gabapentin	400 mg	tablet	oval, white
logo and 4443 600	gabapentin	600 mg	tablet	oval, white
logo and 4444 800	gabapentin	800 mg	tablet	oval, white
logo and 4510	fluoxetine hcl	10 mg	tablet	light green, oval
logo and 4980	propoxyphene napsyl/acetaminophen	100 mg-650 mg	tablet	oblong, pink
logo and 50 5673	sertraline hcl	50 mg	tablet	light blue, oval
logo 5312 500	ciprofloxacin hcl	500 mg	tablet	oval, white

Imprint	Drug	Strength	Form	Description
logo and 5313 750 logo	ciprofloxacin hcl	750 mg	tablet	oval, white
logo and HC	divalproex sodium	500 mg	tablet	oval, gray
logo and HF	divalproex sodium	250 mg	tablet	oval, white
logo and KA	ritonavir/lopinavir	50 mg-200 mg	tablet	oval, yellow
logo and KJ	clarithromycin	500 mg	tablet	oval, yellow
logo and KT	clarithromycin	250 mg	tablet	oval, yellow
logo and NR	divalproex sodium	250 mg	tablet	oval, peach
logo and NS	divalproex sodium	500 mg	tablet	lavender, oval
logo and NT	divalproex sodium	125 mg	tablet	oval, salmon pink
logo and PK	ritonavir/lopinavir	33.3 mg-133.3 mg	capsule	oblong, orange
Lopid P-D 737	gemfibrozil	600 mg	tablet	elliptical, white
LOTENSIN 10	benazepril hcl	10 mg	tablet	round, dark yellow
LOTENSIN HCT 57 57	benazepril hcl/hydrochlorothiazide	5 mg-6.25 mg	tablet	white, oblong
LOTREL 0364	amlodipine besylate/benazepril hcl	10 mg-20 mg	capsule	amethyst, oblong
LOTREL 0384	amlodipine besylate/benazepril hcl	5 mg-40 mg	capsule	oblong, light blue
LOTREL 2255	amlodipine besylate/benazepril hcl	2.5 mg-10 mg	capsule	oblong, white
LOTREL 2260	amlodipine besylate/benazepril hcl	5 mg-10 mg	capsule	light brown, oblong
LOTREL 2265	amlodipine besylate/benazepril hcl	5 mg-20 mg	capsule	oblong, pink
Lotrel 0379	amlodipine besylate/benazepril hcl	10 mg-40 mg	capsule	dark blue, oblong
LSP 10	lisinopril	10 mg	tablet	round, yellow
LSP 20	lisinopril	20 mg	tablet	light gray, round
LSP 2 1/2	lisinopril	2.5 mg	tablet	pale yellow, round
LSP 30	lisinopril	30 mg	tablet	light gray, round
LSP 40	lisinopril	40 mg	tablet	light gray, round
LSP 5	lisinopril	5 mg	tablet	green, round
LUPIN 10	lisinopril	10 mg	tablet	pink, round
M 15	meloxicam	15 mg	tablet	pastel yellow
M 15 P F	morphine sulfate	15 mg	tablet	blue, round
M 18 scored	metoprolol tartrate	25 mg	tablet	round, white
M 30 P F	morphine sulfate	30 mg	tablet	round, purple
M 31	allopurinol	100 mg	tablet	white, round
M 312	verapamil hcl	180 mg	tablet	pink, round
M 32	metoprolol tartrate	50 mg	tablet	oblong, white
M 357	hydrocodone bit/acetaminophen	5 mg-500 mg	tablet	round, brown
M 36	amitriptyline hcl	50 mg	tablet	blue, round
M 37	amitriptyline hcl	75 mg	tablet	orange, round
M 38	amitriptyline hcl	100 mg	tablet	blue, round
M 411	verapamil hcl	240 mg	tablet	light blue, round
M 47	metoprolol tartrate	100 mg	tablet	light green, round
M 51	amitriptyline hcl	25 mg	tablet	beige, red, oblong
M 532 M 532	oxycodone hcl/acetaminophen	5 mg-500 mg	capsule	orange, round
M 60 P F	morphine sulfate	60 mg	tablet	round, white
M 71	allopurinol	300 mg	tablet	white, round
M E15	enalapril maleate	2.5 mg	tablet	light blue, round
M E16	enalapril maleate	5 mg	tablet	medium blue, round
M E17	enalapril maleate	10 mg	tablet	
M E18	enalapril maleate	20 mg	tablet	
M L23	lisinopril	5 mg	tablet	peach, round
M 200 P F	morphine sulfate	200 mg	tablet	green, oblong
M 244	metformin hcl	1,000 mg	tablet	white, oval
M 350	metformin hcl	750 mg	tablet	tan, oval
M 352	metformin hcl	500 mg	tablet	oval, tan
M 39	amitriptyline hcl	150 mg	tablet	oblong, peach
M052	sulfamethoxazole/trimethoprim	400 mg-80 mg	tablet	pink, round
M2	furosemide	20 mg	tablet	white, round
M357	hydrocodone bit/acetaminophen	5 mg-500 mg	tablet	oblong, white
M358	hydrocodone bit/acetaminophen	7.5 mg-500 mg	tablet	oblong, white
M359	hydrocodone bit/acetaminophen	7.5 mg-650 mg	tablet	oblong, white

Imprint	Drug	Strength	Form	Description
M360		hydrocodone bit/acetaminophen	7.5 mg-750 mg	tablet	oblong, white
M361		hydrocodone bit/acetaminophen	10 mg-650 mg	tablet	blue, oblong
M362		hydrocodone bit/acetaminophen	10 mg-660 mg	tablet	oblong, white
M363		hydrocodone bit/acetaminophen	10 mg-500 mg	tablet	oval, white
M364		hydrocodone bit/acetaminophen	10 mg-750 mg	tablet	oblong, white
M365		hydrocodone bit/acetaminophen	5 mg-325 mg	tablet	oval, white,
M366		hydrocodone bit/acetaminophen	7.5 mg-325 mg	tablet	white, oblong
M367		hydrocodone bit/acetaminophen	10 mg-325 mg	tablet	oblong, white
M522	7.5/325	oxycodone hcl/acetaminophen	7.5 mg-325 mg	tablet	oblong, white
M523	10/325	oxycodone hcl/acetaminophen	10 mg-325 mg	tablet	oblong, white
M562		oxycodone hcl/acetaminophen	10 mg-650 mg	tablet	oblong, white
M582		oxycodone hcl/acetaminophen	7.5 mg-500 mg	tablet	white, oval
M77		amitriptyline hcl	10 mg	tablet	round, white
MAXALT	MRK 267	rizatriptan benzoate	10 mg	tablet	oblong, pale pink
MERIDIA	10 and 10	sibutramine hcl m-hydrate	10 mg	capsule	blue, oblong, white
MIA	116	hydrocodone bit/acetaminophen	7.5 mg-325 mg	tablet	oblong, yellow-orange
MICRONASE 1.25		glyburide	1.25 mg	tablet	round, white
MICRONASE 2.5		glyburide	2.5 mg	tablet	dark pink, round
MICRONASE 5		glyburide	5 mg	tablet	round, blue
MJ 755		estradiol	1 mg	tablet	round, lavender
MJ 822	5 5 5	buspirone hcl	15 mg	tablet	rectangular, white
MJ 824	10 10 10	buspirone hcl	30 mg	tablet	pink, rectangular
MP 81		sulfamethoxazole/trimethoprim	400 mg-80 mg	tablet	round, white
MP 85		sulfamethoxazole/trimethoprim	800 mg-160 mg	tablet	white, oval
MRK	951	losartan potassium	25 mg	tablet	light green, teardrop
MRK 212	FOSAMAX	alendronate sodium	40 mg	tablet	triangular, white
MRK 925	a bone outline	alendronate sodium	5 mg	tablet	round, white
MSD 140	PRINZIDE	lisinopril/hydrochlorothiazide	20 mg-12.5 mg	tablet	round fluted-edge, yellow
MSD 142	PRINZIDE	lisinopril/hydrochlorothiazide	20 mg-25 mg	tablet	round fluted-edge, peach
MSD 106		lisinopril	10 mg	tablet	oval, light yellow
MSD 19		lisinopril	5 mg	tablet	oval, white
MSD 207		lisinopril	20 mg	tablet	oval, peach
MYLAN 186		verapamil hcl	120 mg	tablet	blue, oval
MYLAN 199		clonidine hcl	0.1 mg	tablet	round, white
MYLAN 244		clonidine hcl	0.2 mg	tablet	round, white
MYLAN 152		clonidine hcl	0.3 mg	tablet	white, round
MYLAN 1560	MYLAN 1560	phenytoin sodium extended	100 mg	capsule	light lavender, oblong, white
MYLAN 216	40	furosemide	40 mg	tablet	round, white
MYLAN 232	80	furosemide	80 mg	tablet	orange, round
MYLAN 2537	MYLAN 2537	triamterene/hydrochlorothiazide	37.5 mg-25 mg	capsule	peach, oblong
MYLAN 271		diazepam	2 mg	tablet	round, white
MYLAN 345		diazepam	5 mg	tablet	orange, round
MYLAN 4010	MYLAN 4010	temazepam	15 mg	capsule	green, round
MYLAN 477		diazepam	10 mg	tablet	oblong, yellow
MYLAN 5050	MYLAN 5050	temazepam	30 mg	capsule	green, oblong
MYLAN 5211	MYLAN 5211	omeprazole	10 mg	capsule	green, oblong
MYLAN 6150	MYLAN 6150	omeprazole	20 mg	capsule	green, oblong, aqua
MYLAN 6320	MYLAN 6320	verapamil hcl	120 mg	capsule	bluish-green, oblong, white

Imprint	Drug	Strength	Form	Description
MYLAN 6380	MYLAN 6380	verapamil hcl	180 mg	capsule	bluish-green, light green, oblong
MYLAN 6440	MYLAN 6440	verapamil hcl	240 mg	capsule	bluish-green, oblong
MYLAN 810	MYLAN 810	hydrochlorothiazide	12.5 mg	capsule	oblong, white
MYLAN A1		alprazolam	0.25 mg	tablet	white, round
MYLAN A1		alprazolam	1 mg	tablet	blue, round
MYLAN A3		alprazolam	0.5 mg	tablet	peach, round
MYLAN A4		alprazolam	2 mg	tablet	white, round
N 342	1.25	glyburide	1.25 mg	tablet	round, peach
N 343	2.5	glyburide	2.5 mg	tablet	round, peach
N 344	5	glyburide	5 mg	tablet	light green, round
N 544	150	ranitidine hcl	150 mg	tablet	round, white
N 547	300	ranitidine hcl	300 mg	tablet	oblong, white
N 548	150	fluconazole	150 mg	tablet	round, peach
N 550	50	fluconazole	50 mg	tablet	peach, round
N 551	100	fluconazole	100 mg	tablet	peach, round
N 552	200	fluconazole	200 mg	tablet	peach, round
N2	logo	buprenorphine hcl/naloxone hcl	2 mg-0.5 mg	tablet	hexagonal, orange
N8	logo	buprenorphine hcl/naloxone hcl	8 mg-2 mg	tablet	hexagonal, orange
Neurontin 100 mg	PD	gabapentin	100 mg	capsule	oblong, white
Neurontin 300 mg	PD	gabapentin	300 mg	capsule	oblong, yellow
Neurontin 400 mg	PD	gabapentin	400 mg	capsule	oblong, orange
NEXIUM 20mg		esomeprazole mag trihydrate	20 mg	capsule	amethyst, oblong
NEXIUM 40mg		esomeprazole mag trihydrate	40 mg	capsule	amethyst, oblong
NORVASC 2.5		amlodipine besylate	2.5 mg	tablet	diamond, white
NORVASC 10		amlodipine besylate	10 mg	tablet	white, round
NORVASC 5		amlodipine besylate	5 mg	tablet	octagonal, white
NPS 550		naproxen sodium	550 mg	tablet	dark blue, oblong
NPS 275		naproxen sodium	275 mg	tablet	light blue, oval
NT 16		gabapentin	600 mg	tablet	white, elliptical
NT 26		gabapentin	800 mg	tablet	white, elliptical
NVR	CTI	valsartan/hydrochlorothiazide	320 mg-25 mg	tablet	oval, yellow
OC	10	oxycodone hcl	10 mg	tablet	round, white
O-IR	PF 5 mg	oxycodone hcl	5 mg	capsule	beige, oblong, orange
O-M 180 or O-M 215 or O-M 250	O-M 180 or O-M 215 or O-M 250	tramadol hcl/acetaminophen	37.5 mg-325 mg	tablet	light yellow, oblong
O-M 706	logo	norgestimate-ethinyl estradiol	0.18 mg-25 mcg (7)/0.215 mg-25 mcg (7)/0.25 mg-25 mcg (7)	tablet	multi-color (4), round
OMNICEF 300 mg	logo	cefdinir	300 mg	capsule	turquoise, oblong, lavender
OP 706		disulfiram	250 mg	tablet	white, round
OP 707		disulfiram	500 mg	tablet	round, white
P		famotidine/calcium carbonate/magnesium	10 mg-800 mg-165 mg	chewable tablet	rose, round
P 20		pantoprazole sodium	20 mg	tablet	yellow, oval
par	034	meclizine hcl	12.5 mg	tablet	blue, oval, yellow
par 216	800	ibuprofen	800 mg	tablet	oblong, white
par 544		ranitidine hcl	150 mg	tablet	peach, round
par 545		ranitidine hcl	300 mg	tablet	oval, peach
PAXIL	10	paroxetine hcl	10 mg	tablet	oval, yellow
PAXIL CR	12.5	paroxetine hcl	12.5 mg	tablet	yellow, round
P-D 007		phenytoin	50 mg	chewable tablet	triangular, yellow
PD 220		quinapril hcl/hydrochlorothiazide	20 mg-12.5 mg	tablet	triangular, pink

Imprint	Drug	Strength	Form	Description
PD 222	quinapril hcl/hydrochlorothiazide	10 mg-12.5 mg	tablet	pink, elliptical
PD 223	quinapril hcl/hydrochlorothiazide	20 mg-25 mg	tablet	pink, round
P-D 365 / P-D 365	phenytoin sodium extended	30 mg	capsule	clear, oblong
PD 527 / 5	quinapril hcl	5 mg	tablet	brown, elliptical
PD 530 / 10	quinapril hcl	10 mg	tablet	triangular, brown
PD 532 / 20	quinapril hcl	20 mg	tablet	brown, round
PD 155 / 10	atorvastatin calcium	10 mg	tablet	elliptical, white
PD 156 / 20	atorvastatin calcium	20 mg	tablet	elliptical, white
PD 158 / 80	atorvastatin calcium	80 mg	tablet	elliptical, white
PD 535 / 40	quinapril hcl	40 mg	tablet	brown, elliptical
PEPCID / MSD 963	famotidine	20 mg	tablet	beige
Pepcid AC	famotidine	10 mg	chewable tablet	diamond, rose
Pepcid AC	famotidine	10 mg	tablet	oblong, rose, white
PERCOCET / 10	oxycodone hcl/acetaminophen	10 mg-650 mg	tablet	yellow, oval
PERCOCET 5	oxycodone hcl/acetaminophen	5 mg-325 mg	tablet	blue, round
PERCODAN	oxycodone hcl/aspirin	4.8355 mg-325 mg	tablet	round, yellow
PERCOGESIC	acetaminophen/phenyltoloxamine cit	325 mg-30 mg	tablet	light orange, round
PF / 100	morphine sulfate	100 mg	tablet	gray, round
PFIZER / 308	azithromycin	600 mg	tablet	oval, white
PFIZER 411	glipizide	5 mg	tablet	diamond, white
PFIZER 412	glipizide	10 mg	tablet	diamond, white
PL 500	amoxicillin trihydrate/potassium clavulanate	500 mg-125 mg	tablet	oval, white
PL 875	amoxicillin trihydrate/potassium clavulanate	875 mg-125 mg	tablet	white, oblong,
PLIVA / 563	cyclobenzaprine hcl	10 mg	tablet	round, yellow
PLIVA 433	trazodone hcl	50 mg	tablet	round, white
PLIVA 434	trazodone hcl	100 mg	tablet	round, white
PLIVA 441 / 50 50 50	trazodone hcl	150 mg	tablet	trapezoidal; white
PRAVACHOL 10 logo	pravastatin sodium	10 mg	tablet	pink, rectangular (rounded end)
PRAVACHOL 20 logo	pravastatin sodium	20 mg	tablet	rectangular (rounded end), yellow
PRAVACHOL 40 logo	pravastatin sodium	40 mg	tablet	green, rectangular (rounded end)
PREMARIN 0.625	estrogens, conjugated	0.625 mg	tablet	maroon, oval
PREMARIN 0.3	estrogens, conjugated	0.3 mg	tablet	green, oval
PREMARIN 0.45	estrogens, conjugated	0.45 mg	tablet	blue, oval
PREMARIN 0.625	estrogens, conjugated	0.625 mg	tablet	oval, maroon
PREMARIN 0.625 or PREMPHASE	estrogens, conjugated/medroxyprogesterone acet	0.625 mg (14)/ 0.625 mg-5 mg (14)	tablet	multi-color (2), oval
PREMARIN 0.9	estrogens, conjugated	0.9 mg	tablet	oval, white
PREMARIN 1.25	estrogens, conjugated	1.25 mg	tablet	oval, yellow
PREMPRO	estrogens, conjugated/medroxyprogesterone acet	0.625 mg-2.5 mg	tablet	oval, peach
PRINZIDE / MSD 145	lisinopril/hydrochlorothiazide	10 mg-12.5 mg	tablet	blue, hexagonal
PROCARDIA PFIZER 260	nifedipine	10 mg	capsule	oblong, orange
PROCARDIA XL 30	nifedipine	30 mg	tablet	rose pink, round
PROCARDIA XL 60	nifedipine	60 mg	tablet	rose pink, round
PROCARDIA XL 90	nifedipine	90 mg	tablet	rose pink, round
PROSCAR / MSD 72	finasteride	5 mg	tablet	apple, blue
PROTONIX	pantoprazole sodium	40 mg	tablet	oval, yellow
R / 125	ciprofloxacin hcl	100 mg	tablet	white, oval
R 4 / JANSSEN	risperidone	4 mg	tablet	green, oblong
R0.5	risperidone	0.5 mg	tablet	light coral, round
R1	risperidone	1 mg	tablet	light coral, square
R2	risperidone	2 mg	tablet	light coral, round
R3	risperidone	3 mg	tablet	coral, round
R4	risperidone	4 mg	tablet	coral, round
RAPAMUNE 1 mg	sirolimus	1 mg	tablet	white, triangular
RAPAMUNE 2 mg	sirolimus	2 mg	tablet	triangular, yellow
RAPAMUNE 2 mg	sirolimus	2 mg	tablet	triangular, yellow
RDY / 198	simvastatin	10 mg	tablet	brown, round
RDY 343	citalopram hydrobromide	20 mg	tablet	pink, round
RDY 344	citalopram hydrobromide	40 mg	tablet	white, round
REGLAN / AHR 10	metoclopramide hcl	10 mg	tablet	oblong, white
REGLAN 5 / AHR	metoclopramide hcl	5 mg	tablet	elliptical, green
REL900	omega-3 acid ethyl esters	1 gram	capsule	light yellow, oblong
RESTORIL 15 mg FOR SLEEP	temazepam	15 mg	capsule	maroon, oblong, pink
RESTORIL 30 mg FOR SLEEP	temazepam	30 mg	capsule	blue
RESTORIL 7.5 mg FOR SLEEP	temazepam	7.5 mg	capsule	blue, oblong, pink
REV / 10 mg	lenalidomide	10 mg	capsule	bluish-green, oblong
REV 15mg	lenalidomide	15 mg	capsule	oblong, powder blue, white
REV 25mg	lenalidomide	25 mg	capsule	blue, white
RIFADIN 150 / RIFADIN 150	rifampin	150 mg	capsule	maroon, oblong, scarlet
RIFADIN 300 / RIFADIN 300	rifampin	300 mg	capsule	maroon, oblong, scarlet
Ris 0.25 / JANSSEN	risperidone	0.25 mg	tablet	dark yellow, oblong
Ris 0.5 / JANSSEN	risperidone	0.5 mg	tablet	oblong, red brown
RSN / 30 mg	risedronate sodium	30 mg	tablet	oval, white
RX 7	lorazepam	0.5 mg	tablet	round, white
RX 709	ciprofloxacin hcl	250 mg	tablet	round, white
RX 773	lorazepam	1 mg	tablet	pink, round
RX 515	amoxicillin trihydrate	250 mg	chewable tablet	oblong, pink
RX 763	amoxicillin trihydrate	875 mg	tablet	oblong, yellow
RX654 / RX654	amoxicillin trihydrate	250 mg	capsule	maroon, yellow, oblong
RX655 / RX655	amoxicillin trihydrate	500 mg	capsule	green, oblong, white
RX656 / RX656	cephalexin monohydrate	250 mg	capsule	dark green, light green, oblong
RX657 / RX657	cephalexin monohydrate	500 mg	capsule	white, oblong
RX710	ciprofloxacin hcl	500 mg	tablet	oblong, white
RX711	ciprofloxacin hcl	750 mg	tablet	light pink, round
RX760	amoxicillin trihydrate	200 mg	chewable tablet	light pink, round
RX761	amoxicillin trihydrate	400 mg	chewable tablet	oblong, pink
RX762	amoxicillin trihydrate	500 mg	tablet	round, white
RX774	lorazepam	2 mg	tablet	peach, round
S 820	hydrochlorothiazide	25 mg	tablet	peach, round
S 821	hydrochlorothiazide	50 mg	tablet	oval, white
S P / 720	moexipril hcl/hydrochlorothiazide	15 mg-12.5 mg	tablet	light blue, round
S190	eszopiclone	1 mg	tablet	round, white
S191	eszopiclone	2 mg	tablet	dark blue, round
S193	eszopiclone	3 mg	tablet	white, round
SANKYO / C 14	olmesartan medoxomil	20 mg	tablet	oval, white
SB / 39	carvedilol	3.125 mg	tablet	oval, white
SB 4140 / SB 4140	carvedilol	6.25 mg	tablet	oval, white
SB 4141 / SB 4141	carvedilol	12.5 mg	tablet	white, oval
SB 4142 / SB 4142	carvedilol	25 mg	tablet	white, oval

Imprint	Drug	Strength	Form	Description
SCHWARZ 2489 | VERELAN 180 mg	verapamil hcl	180 mg	capsule	yellow, light gray, oblong
SCHWARZ 2490 | VERELAN 120 mg	verapamil hcl	120 mg	capsule	oblong, yellow
SCHWARZ 2491 | VERELAN 240 mg	verapamil hcl	240 mg	capsule	dark blue, oblong, yellow
SCHWARZ 2495 | VERELAN 360 mg	verapamil hcl	360 mg	capsule	yellow, lavender, oblong
SEA RLE 10 21 | AL-DACTAZIDE 50	spironolactone/hydrochlorothiazide	50 mg-50 mg	tablet	tan, oblong
SEA RLE 10 41 | AL-DACTONE 50	spironolactone	50 mg	tablet	light orange, oval
SEARLE 1001 | AL-DACTONE 25	spironolactone	25 mg	tablet	light yellow, round
SEARLE 103 | AL-DACTONE 100	spironolactone	100 mg	tablet	peach, round
SEPTRA DS M053	sulfamethoxazole/trimethoprim	800 mg-160 mg	tablet	pink, oval
SEROQUEL 300	quetiapine fumarate	300 mg	tablet	oblong, white
SEROQUEL 100	quetiapine fumarate	100 mg	tablet	round, yellow
SEROQUEL 200	quetiapine fumarate	200 mg	tablet	round, white
SEROQUEL 25	quetiapine fumarate	25 mg	tablet	round, peach
SEROQUEL 50	quetiapine fumarate	50 mg	tablet	white, round
SINEMET 647	carbidopa/levodopa	10 mg-100 mg	tablet	dark blue, oval
SINEMET CR 521	carbidopa/levodopa	50 mg-200 mg	tablet	peach, oval
SINEMET CR 601	carbidopa/levodopa	25 mg-100 mg	tablet	oval, pink
SINGULAIR MRK 117	montelukast sodium	10 mg	tablet	beige, square (rounded corners)
SOLVAY 5044	eprosartan mesylate	400 mg	tablet	oval, pink
SOLVAY 1023	estrogens, esterified/methyltestosterone	0.625 mg-1.25 mg	tablet	light green, oblong
SOLVAY 1026	estrogens, esterified/methyltestosterone	1.25 mg-2.5 mg	tablet	dark green, oblong
SUSTIVA 100 mg	efavirenz	100 mg	capsule	oblong, white, gold
SYNTHROID 100	levothyroxine sodium	100 mcg	tablet	round, yellow
T	benzonatate	100 mg	capsule	yellow, round
TEGRETOL 27 27	carbamazepine	200 mg	tablet	pink, oblong
TENORETIC 115	atenolol/chlorthalidone	50 mg-25 mg	tablet	round, white
TENORMIN 101	atenolol	100 mg	tablet	round, white, round
TI 01 logo	tiotropium bromide	18 mcg	capsule	oblong, white
Tiazac 120 | Tiazac 120	diltiazem hcl	120 mg	capsule	light green, oblong
Tiazac 180 | Tiazac 180	diltiazem hcl	180 mg	capsule	lavender, oblong
Tiazac 240 | Tiazac 240	diltiazem hcl	240 mg	capsule	blue-green, oblong, white
Tiazac 300 | Tiazac 300	diltiazem hcl	300 mg	capsule	oblong, blue-green, white
Tiazac 360 | Tiazac 360	diltiazem hcl	360 mg	capsule	green, lavender, white, lavender, oblong
Tiazac 420 | Tiazac 420	diltiazem hcl	420 mg	capsule	blue-green, oblong
Ticlid logo | 250 logo	ticlopidine hcl	250 mg	tablet	oblong, white
TOP 15 mg	topiramate	15 mg	capsule	oblong, white, clear
TOPAMAX 100	topiramate	100 mg	tablet	round, yellow
UAD 63 50	hydrocodone bit/acetaminophen	10 mg-650 mg	tablet	oblong, light blue
ucb 250	levetiracetam	250 mg	tablet	oblong, blue
ucb 500	levetiracetam	500 mg	tablet	oblong, yellow
ucb 750	levetiracetam	750 mg	tablet	oblong, orange
ULTRAM 06 59	tramadol hcl	50 mg	tablet	white, oblong

Imprint	Drug	Strength	Form	Description
US 10	potassium chloride	10 mEq	tablet	oblong, white
US 20	potassium chloride	20 mEq	tablet	oblong, white
V 35 97	hydrocodone bit/acetaminophen	10 mg-650 mg	tablet	light blue, oblong
VALTREX 1 gram	valacyclovir hcl	1,000 mg	tablet	oblong, blue
VALTREX 500 mg	valacyclovir hcl	500 mg	tablet	blue, oblong
VGR 100 | Pfizer	sildenafil citrate	100 mg	tablet	blue, diamond
VGR 25 | Pfizer	sildenafil citrate	25 mg	tablet	blue, diamond
VGR 50 | Pfizer	sildenafil citrate	50 mg	tablet	blue, diamond
VICODIN	hydrocodone bit/acetaminophen	5 mg-500 mg	tablet	oblong, white
VICODIN ES	hydrocodone bit/acetaminophen	7.5 mg-750 mg	tablet	oblong, white
VP logo	hydrocodone/ibuprofen	7.5 mg-200 mg	tablet	round, white
W 0.625/5	estrogens, conjugated/medroxyprogesterone acet	0.625 mg-5 mg	tablet	light blue, oval
W 100 705	venlafaxine hcl	100 mg	tablet	shield, peach
W 25 701	venlafaxine hcl	25 mg	tablet	peach, shield
W 37.5 781	venlafaxine hcl	37.5 mg	tablet	peach, shield
W 50 703	venlafaxine hcl	50 mg	tablet	peach, shield
W 75 704	venlafaxine hcl	75 mg	tablet	peach, shield
W Effexor XR 150	venlafaxine hcl	150 mg	capsule	dark orange, oblong, gray
W1502	isosorbide mononitrate	30 mg	tablet	white, oval
W1549	isosorbide mononitrate	60 mg	tablet	oblong, white
W1587	isosorbide mononitrate	120 mg	tablet	oblong, white
WATSON 240 0.5	lorazepam	0.5 mg	tablet	oblong, white
WATSON 3203	hydrocodone bit/acetaminophen	7.5 mg-325 mg	tablet	light orange, oblong
WATSON 3228	hydrocodone bit/acetaminophen	10 mg-750 mg	tablet	light yellow, oblong
WATSON 349	hydrocodone bit/acetaminophen	5 mg-500 mg	tablet	oblong, white
WATSON 385	hydrocodone bit/acetaminophen	7.5 mg-500 mg	tablet	oblong, white
WATSON 387	hydrocodone bit/acetaminophen	7.5 mg-750 mg	tablet	oblong, white
WATSON 388	hydrocodone bit/acetaminophen	2.5 mg-500 mg	tablet	oblong, white
WATSON 502	hydrocodone bit/acetaminophen	7.5 mg-650 mg	tablet	oblong, pink
WATSON 503	hydrocodone bit/acetaminophen	10 mg-650 mg	tablet	oblong, light green
WATSON 540	hydrocodone bit/acetaminophen	10 mg-500 mg	tablet	blue, oblong
WATSON 853	hydrocodone bit/acetaminophen	10 mg-325 mg	tablet	oblong, yellow
WC 722 2	estradiol	2 mg	tablet	green, oval
WELLBUTRIN 100	bupropion hcl	100 mg	tablet	round, red
WELLBUTRIN 75	bupropion hcl	75 mg	tablet	yellow-gold, round
WELLBUTRIN SR 100	bupropion hcl	100 mg	tablet	blue, round
WELLBUTRIN SR 150	bupropion hcl	150 mg	tablet	purple, round
WELLBUTRIN SR 200	bupropion hcl	200 mg	tablet	light pink, round
WELLBUTRIN XL 150	bupropion hcl	150 mg	tablet	round, creamy white
WELLBUTRIN XL 300	bupropion hcl	300 mg	tablet	creamy white, round
WPI 844	glipizide	5 mg	tablet	orange, round
WPI 845	glipizide	10 mg	tablet	round
WPI 900	glipizide	2.5 mg	tablet	round
WPI 4011	ibuprofen	600 mg	tablet	oblong, white
X I 0.5	alprazolam	0.5 mg	tablet	white, pentagon
XANAX 2	alprazolam	2 mg	tablet	oblong, white
XANAX 0.25	alprazolam	0.25 mg	tablet	white, oval
XANAX 0.5	alprazolam	0.5 mg	tablet	oval, peach
XANAX 1.0	alprazolam	1 mg	tablet	blue, oval
Z I 75	ranitidine hcl	75 mg	tablet	five-sided, pink
Z 2083	hydrochlorothiazide	25 mg	tablet	light orange, round
Z 2089	hydrochlorothiazide	50 mg	tablet	light orange, round

Access FREE updates online @ www.consumerdrugreference.org

Imprint	Drug	Strength	Form	Description
ZOCOR	MSD 726	simvastatin	5 mg	tablet	shield, buff
ZOLOFT	100 MG	sertraline hcl	100 mg	tablet	light yellow, oblong
ZOMIG 2.5	zolmitriptan	2.5 mg	tablet	round, yellow
ZOMIG 5	zolmitriptan	5 mg	tablet	pink, round
ZOVIRAX	a triangle	acyclovir	400 mg	tablet	shield, white
ZOVIRAX 800	acyclovir	800 mg	tablet	light blue, oval
ZYBAN 150	bupropion hcl	150 mg	tablet	purple, round
ZYLOPRIM 100	allopurinol	100 mg	tablet	white, round
ZYLOPRIM 300	allopurinol	300 mg	tablet	peach, round
ZYRTEC C10	cetirizine hcl	10 mg	chewable tablet	purple, round
ZYRTEC C5	cetirizine hcl	5 mg	chewable tablet	purple, round
ZYVOX 600 mg	linezolid	600 mg	tablet	white, oblong

Imprint	Drug	Strength	Form	Description
Z 2907	furosemide	40 mg	tablet	round, white
Z 2908	furosemide	20 mg	tablet	oval, white
ZANTAC 150	Glaxo	ranitidine hcl	150 mg	tablet	five-sided, peach
ZANTAC 300	Glaxo	ranitidine hcl	300 mg	tablet	oblong, yellow
ZBN	leflunomide	10 mg	tablet	round, white
ZBO	leflunomide	20 mg	tablet	light yellow, triangular
ZESTORETIC	141	lisinopril/hydrochlorothiazide	10 mg-12.5 mg	tablet	round, peach
ZESTRIL	130	lisinopril	5 mg	tablet	oblong, pink
ZESTRIL 10	131	lisinopril	10 mg	tablet	round, pink
ZESTRIL 2 1/2	135	lisinopril	2.5 mg	tablet	white, round
ZESTRIL 20	132	lisinopril	20 mg	tablet	rose, round
ZESTRIL 40	134	lisinopril	40 mg	tablet	round, yellow
ZESTRIL 30	133	lisinopril	30 mg	tablet	pink, round

ABACAVIR SULFATE

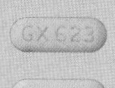

300 mg

†Ziagen®
GlaxoSmithKline

ACETAMINOPHEN/ CODEINE PHOSPHATE

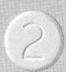

300 mg-15 mg

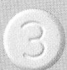

300 mg-30 mg

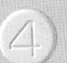

300 mg-60 mg

Acetaminophen/Codeine
Teva

ACETAMINOPHEN/ PHENYLTOLOXAMINE CITRATE

325 mg-30 mg

Percogesic®
Medtech Labs

ACYCLOVIR

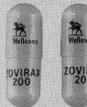

200 mg

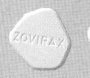

400 mg

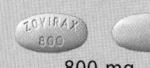

800 mg

†Zovirax®
GlaxoSmithKline

ALBUTEROL

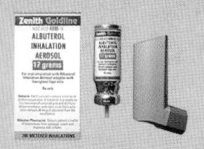

90 mcg

Albuterol
IVAX

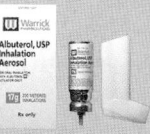

90 mcg

Albuterol
Warrick

ALBUTEROL SULFATE/ IPRATROPIUM BROMIDE

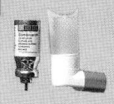

103 mcg (90 mcg)-18 mcg/ Actuation

Combivent®
Boehringer Ingelheim

ALENDRONATE SODIUM

5 mg

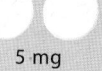

10 mg

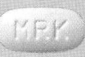

35 mg

40 mg

70 mg

†Fosamax®
Merck

ALLOPURINOL

100 mg

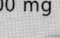 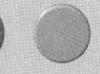

300 mg

Zyloprim®
Prometheus

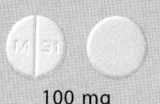

100 mg

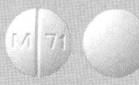

300 mg

Allopurinol
Mylan

ALPRAZOLAM

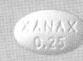

0.25 mg

0.5 mg

1 mg

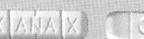

2 mg

Xanax®
Pfizer

0.5 mg

1 mg

2 mg

3 mg

Xanax XR®
Pfizer

 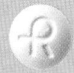

0.25 mg

0.5 mg

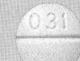

1 mg

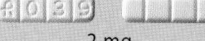

2 mg

Alprazolam
Actavis

0.5 mg

1 mg

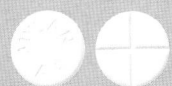

2 mg

†Alprazolam
Mylan

 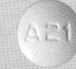

0.5 mg

 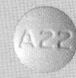

1 mg

2 mg

3 mg

Alprazolam ER
Mylan

0.25 mg

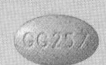 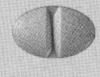

0.5 mg

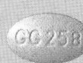

1 mg

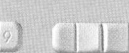

2 mg

Alprazolam
Sandoz

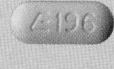

1 mg

2 mg

Alprazolam ER
Sandoz

---

†Additional dosage forms or strengths available.

AMITRIPTYLINE HCL

10 mg

25 mg

50 mg

75 mg

100 mg

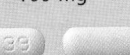

150 mg

Amitriptyline HCl
Mylan

AMLODIPINE BESYLATE

2.5 mg

5 mg

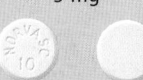

10 mg

Norvasc®
Pfizer

AMLODIPINE BESYLATE/ ATORVASTATIN CALCIUM

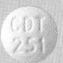

2.5 mg-10 mg

2.5 mg-20 mg

5 mg-10 mg

5 mg-20 mg

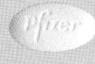

5 mg-40 mg

5 mg-80 mg

10 mg-10 mg

10 mg-20 mg

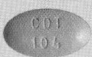

10 mg-40 mg

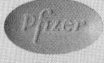

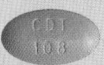

10 mg-80 mg

†Caduet®
Pfizer

AMLODIPINE BESYLATE/ BENAZEPRIL HCL

2.5 mg-10 mg

5 mg-10 mg

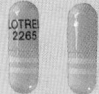

5 mg-20 mg

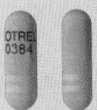

5 mg-40 mg

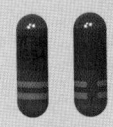

10 mg-20 mg

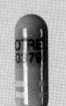

10 mg-40 mg

Lotrel®
Novartis

AMOXICILLIN TRIHYDRATE

200 mg

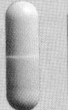

250 mg

250 mg

400 mg

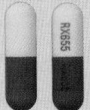

500 mg

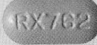

500 mg

875 mg

†Amoxicillin
Ranbaxy

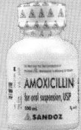

125 mg/5 mL

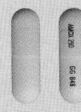

250 mg

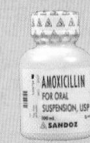

250 mg/5 mL

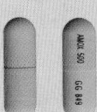

500 mg

†Amoxicillin
Sandoz

125 mg

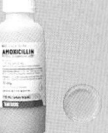

125 mg/5 mL

250 mg

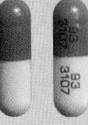

250 mg

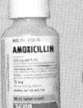

250 mg/5 mL

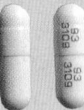

500 mg

500 mg

875 mg

†Amoxicillin
Teva

†Additional dosage forms or strengths available.

AMOXICILLIN/ CLAVULANATE POTASSIUM

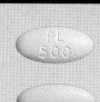

500 mg-125 mg

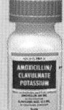

600 mg-42.9 mg/5 mL

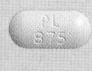

875 mg-125 mg

Amoxicillin/Clavulanate Potassium
IVAX

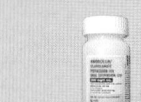

200 mg-28.5 mg/5 mL

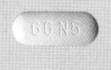

250 mg-125 mg

400 mg-57 mg

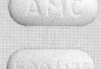

500 mg-125 mg

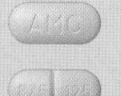

875 mg-125 mg

†Amoxicillin/Clavulanate Potassium
Sandoz

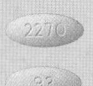

200 mg-28.5 mg

400 mg-57 mg

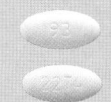

500 mg-125 mg

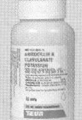

600 mg-42.9 mg/5 mL

875 mg-125 mg

†Amoxicillin/Clavulanate Potassium
Teva

AMPHETAMINE ASPARTATE/ AMPHETAMINE SULFATE/ DEXTROAMPHETAMINE

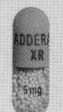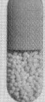

5 mg

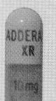

10 mg

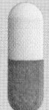

15 mg

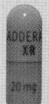

20 mg

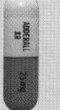

25 mg

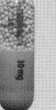

30 mg

Adderall XR®
Shire

ARIPIPRAZOLE

5 mg

10 mg

15 mg

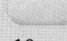

20 mg

30 mg

†Abilify®
Otsuka

ATAZANAVIR SULFATE

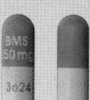

150 mg

200 mg

†Reyataz®
BMS

ATENOLOL

25 mg

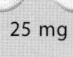

50 mg

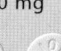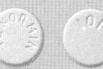

100 mg

Tenormin®
AstraZeneca

25 mg

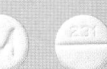

50 mg

100 mg

Atenolol
Mylan

25 mg

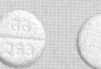

50 mg

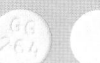

100 mg

Atenolol
Sandoz

ATENOLOL/ CHLORTHALIDONE

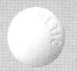

50 mg-25 mg

Tenoretic 50®
AstraZeneca

100 mg-25 mg

Tenoretic 100®
AstraZeneca

ATORVASTATIN CALCIUM

10 mg

20 mg

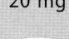

40 mg

80 mg

Lipitor®
Pfizer

†Additional dosage forms or strengths available.

Consumer Reports® Consumer Drug Reference 2008   DI-3

AZITHROMYCIN

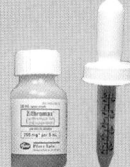

200 mg/5 mL

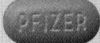

250 mg

500 mg

600 mg

†Zithromax®
Pfizer

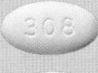

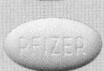

500 mg

Zithromax Tri-Pak®
Pfizer

250 mg

500 mg

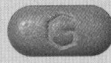

500 mg

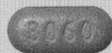

600 mg

†Azithromycin
Greenstone

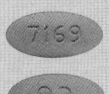

500 mg

Azithromycin
Teva

BENAZEPRIL HCL

5 mg

 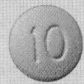

10 mg

 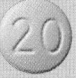

20 mg

 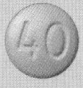

40 mg

Lotensin®
Novartis

BENAZEPRIL HCL/ HYDROCHLOROTHIAZIDE

 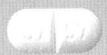

5 mg-6.25 mg

10 mg-12.5 mg

20 mg-12.5 mg

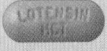 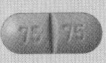

20 mg-25 mg

Lotensin HCT®
Novartis

BENZONATATE

100 mg

†Tessalon Perle®
Forest

BISOPROLOL/ HYDROCHLOROTHIAZIDE

5 mg-6.25 mg

 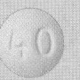

10 mg-6.25 mg

†Ziac®
Duramed/Barr

BUPRENORPHINE HCL

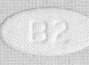

2 mg

8 mg

Subutex®
Reckitt Benckiser

BUPRENORPHINE HCL/ NALOXONE HCL

2 mg-0.5 mg

8 mg-2 mg

Suboxone®
Reckitt Benckiser

BUPROPION HCL

75 mg

100 mg

Wellbutrin®
GlaxoSmithKline

100 mg

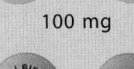

150 mg

 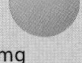

200 mg

Wellbutrin SR®
GlaxoSmithKline

150 mg

300 mg

Wellbutrin XL®
GlaxoSmithKline

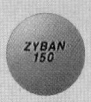 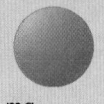

150 mg

Zyban®
GlaxoSmithKline

BUSPIRONE HCL

 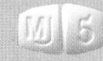

5 mg

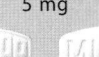 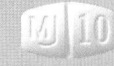

10 mg

15 mg

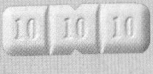

30 mg

Buspar®
BMS

CANDESARTAN CILEXETIL

4 mg

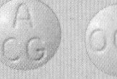 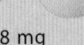

8 mg

 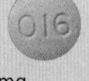

16 mg

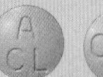

32 mg

Atacand®
AstraZeneca

†Additional dosage forms or strengths available.

CANDESARTAN CILEXETIL/ HYDROCHLOROTHIAZIDE

 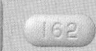

16 mg-12.5 mg

 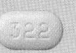

32 mg-12.5 mg

Atacand HCT®
AstraZeneca

CARBAMAZEPINE

100 mg

 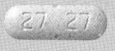

200 mg

†Tegretol®
Novartis

100 mg

200 mg

400 mg

Tegretol XR®
Novartis

CARBIDOPA/LEVODOPA

25 mg-100 mg

50 mg-200 mg

Sinemet CR®
BMS

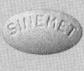

10 mg-100 mg

Sinemet-10/100®
BMS

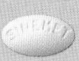

25 mg-100 mg

Sinemet-25/100®
BMS

†Additional dosage forms or strengths available.

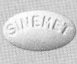

25 mg-250 mg

Sinemet-25/250®
BMS

CARVEDILOL

6.25 mg

12.5 mg

25 mg

†Coreg®
GlaxoSmithKline

CEFDINIR

250 mg/5 mL

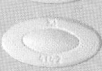

300 mg

†Omnicef®
Abbott

CELECOXIB

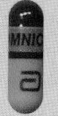 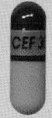

50 mg   100 mg

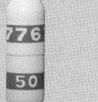

200 mg   400 mg

Celebrex®
Pfizer

CEPHALEXIN MONOHYDRATE

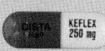

250 mg

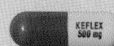

500 mg

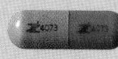...

750 mg

†Keflex®
Advancis Pharma

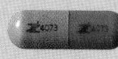

250 mg

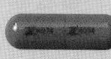

500 mg

Cephalexin
IVAX

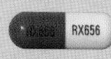

250 mg

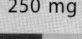

500 mg

†Cephalexin
Ranbaxy

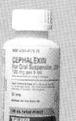

125 mg/5 mL

250 mg

250 mg

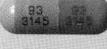

250 mg/5 mL

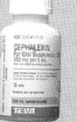

500 mg

500 mg

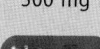

500 mg

Cephalexin
Teva

CETIRIZINE HCL

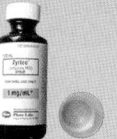

1 mg/mL

5 mg   10 mg

†Zyrtec®
Pfizer

CIPROFLOXACIN HCL

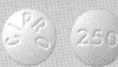

250 mg

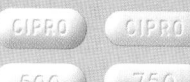

500 mg   750 mg

†Cipro®
Schering

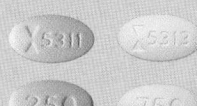

250 mg   750 mg

Ciprofloxacin HCl
IVAX

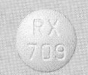

250 mg

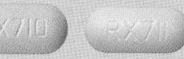

500 mg   750 mg

Ciprofloxacin HCl
Ranbaxy

250 mg

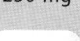

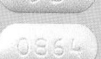

500 mg

750 mg

Ciprofloxacin HCl
Teva

CIPROFLOXACIN/ CIPROFLOXACIN HCL

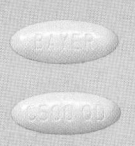

500 mg

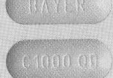

1,000 mg

Cipro XR®
Schering

CITALOPRAM HYDROBROMIDE

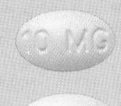

10 mg

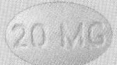

20 mg

40 mg

†Celexa®
Forest

CLARITHROMYCIN

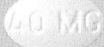

250 mg

500 mg

Biaxin®
Abbott

500 mg

Biaxin XL®
Abbott

CLONAZEPAM

0.5 mg

1 mg

2 mg

†Klonopin®
Roche

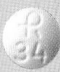 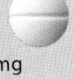

0.5 mg

1 mg

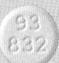

2 mg

Clonazepam
Actavis

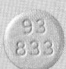

0.5 mg

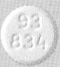

1 mg

2 mg

Clonazepam
Teva

CLONIDINE HCL

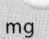

0.1 mg

0.2 mg

 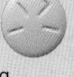

0.3 mg

Clonidine HCl
Mylan

CLOPIDOGREL BISULFATE

75 mg

Plavix®
BMS

CYCLOBENZAPRINE HCL

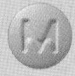 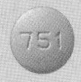

5 mg

10 mg

Cyclobenzaprine HCl
Mylan

10 mg

Cyclobenzaprine HCl
Pliva

DESLORATADINE

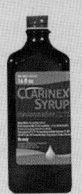

2.5 mg/5 mL

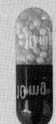 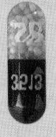

5 mg

Clarinex®
Schering

DEXTROAMPHETAMINE SULFATE

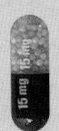 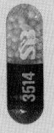

10 mg

 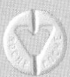

15 mg

†Dexedrine®
GlaxoSmithKline

DIAZEPAM

2 mg

5 mg

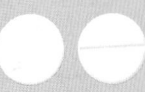

10 mg

Valium®
Roche

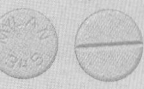

2 mg

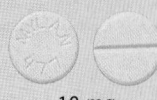

5 mg

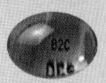

10 mg

Diazepam
Mylan

DIGOXIN

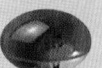

100 mcg

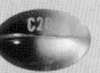

200 mcg

Lanoxicaps®
GlaxoSmithKline

125 mcg

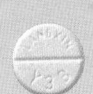

250 mcg

Lanoxin®
GlaxoSmithKline

125 mcg

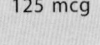 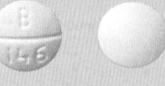

250 mcg

Digitek®
Bertek

†Additional dosage forms or strengths available.

DILTIAZEM HCL

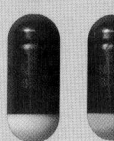

120 mg

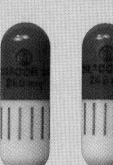

180 mg

240 mg

Dilacor XR®
Watson Pharma

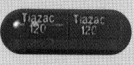

120 mg

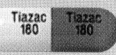

180 mg

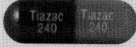

240 mg

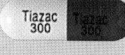

300 mg

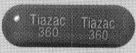

360 mg

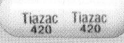

420 mg

Tiazac®
Forest

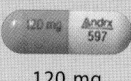

120 mg

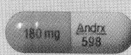

180 mg

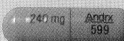

240 mg

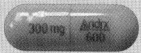

300 mg

Cartia XT®
Watson

DIPHENHYDRAMINE HCL

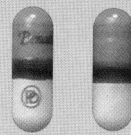

25 mg

†Benadryl®
Pfizer

DISULFIRAM

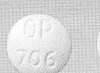

250 mg

†Antabuse®
Duramed/Barr

DIVALPROEX SODIUM

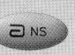

125 mg   250 mg   500 mg

Depakote®
Abbott

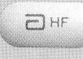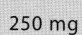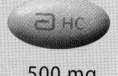

250 mg   500 mg

Depakote ER®
Abbott

DOLASETRON MESYLATE

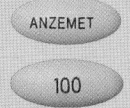

100 mg

Anzemet®
Aventis

DONEPEZIL HCL

5 mg

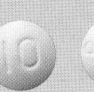

10 mg

Aricept®
Eisai

DOXYCYCLINE HYCLATE

50 mg

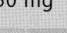

100 mg

100 mg

Doxycycline Hyclate
Watson

DULOXETINE HCL

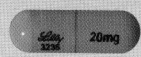

20 mg

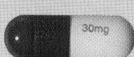

30 mg

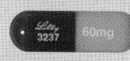

60 mg

Cymbalta®
Eli Lilly

EFAVIRENZ

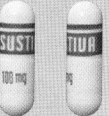

100 mg

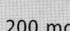

200 mg

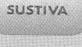

600 mg

†Sustiva®
BMS

ENALAPRIL MALEATE

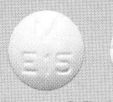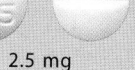

2.5 mg

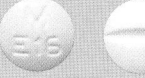

5 mg

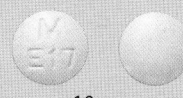

10 mg

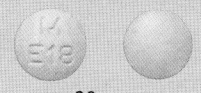

20 mg

Enalapril Maleate
Mylan

EPROSARTAN MESYLATE

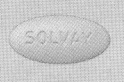

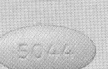

400 mg

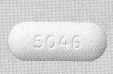

600 mg

Teveten®
Abbott

EPROSARTAN MESYLATE/ HYDROCHLOROTHIAZIDE

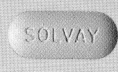

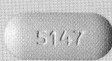

600 mg-12.5 mg

Teveten HCT®
Abbott

ERYTHROMYCIN BASE

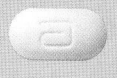

250 mg

333 mg

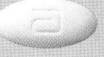

500 mg

Ery-Tab®
Abbott

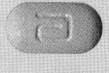

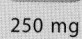

250 mg

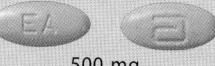

500 mg

Erythromycin Base®
Abbott

†Additional dosage forms or strengths available.

ERYTHROMYCIN ETHYLSUCCINATE

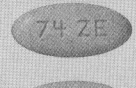

400 mg

†Erythromycin Ethylsuccinate®
Abbott

ERYTHROMYCIN STEARATE

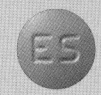

250 mg

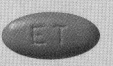 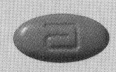

500 mg

Erythrocin Stearate®
Abbott

ESCITALOPRAM OXALATE

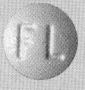

5 mg

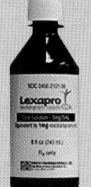

5 mg/5 mL

10 mg

20 mg

Lexapro®
Forest

ESOMEPRAZOLE

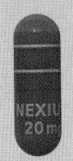 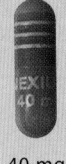

20 mg   40 mg

Nexium®
AstraZeneca

ESTRADIOL

1 mg

†Estrace®
WC Prof Prods

ESTROGENS, CONJUGATED, SYNTHETIC A

0.3 mg

0.45 mg

0.625 mg

 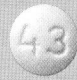

0.9 mg

1.25 mg

Cenestin®
Duramed/Barr

ESTROGENS,CONJUGATED

0.3 mg   0.45 mg   0.625 mg

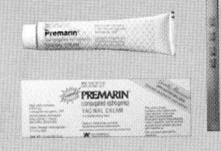

0.625 mg/gram

 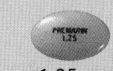

0.9 mg   1.25 mg

Premarin®
Wyeth

ESTROGENS,ESTERIFIED/ METHYLTESTOSTERONE

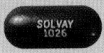 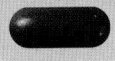

1.25 mg-2.5 mg

Estratest®
Solvay

0.625 mg-1.25 mg

Estratest H.S.®
Solvay

ESZOPICLONE

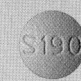 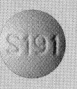

1 mg   2 mg   3 mg

Lunesta®
Sepracor

ETHINYL ESTRADIOL/ DROSPIRENONE

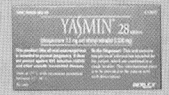 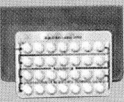

0.03 mg-3 mg

Yasmin 28®
Berlex

ETHINYL ESTRADIOL/ NORELGESTROMIN

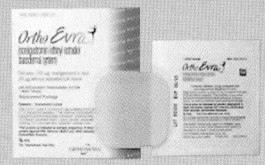

20 mcg-150 mcg/24 hour

Ortho Evra®
Ortho

EZETIMIBE

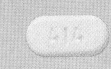

10 mg

Zetia®
Merck/Schering

EZETIMIBE/SIMVASTATIN

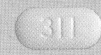

10 mg-10 mg   10 mg-20 mg

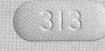

10 mg-40 mg

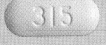

10 mg-80 mg

Vytorin®
Merck/Schering

FAMCICLOVIR

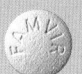

125 mg

 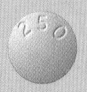

250 mg

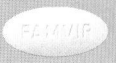

500 mg

Famvir®
Novartis

FAMOTIDINE

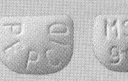

20 mg

†Pepcid®
Merck

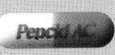

10 mg

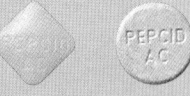

10 mg   10 mg

Pepcid AC®
Merck

FAMOTIDINE/CALCIUM CARBONATE/MAGNESIUM

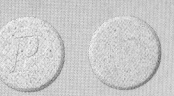

10 mg-800 mg-165 mg

Pepcid Complete®
Merck

FENOFIBRATE

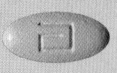

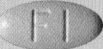

48 mg

145 mg

Tricor®
Abbott

†Additional dosage forms or strengths available.

FEXOFENADINE HCL

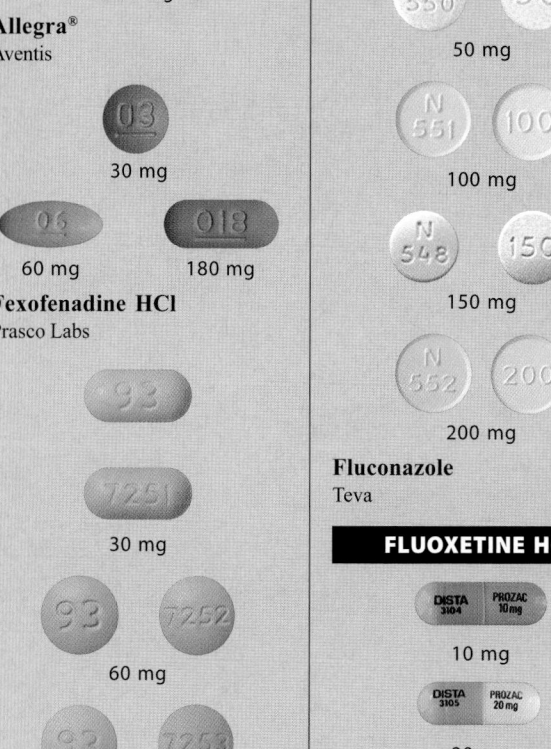

30 mg

60 mg

180 mg

Allegra®
Aventis

30 mg

60 mg   180 mg

Fexofenadine HCl
Prasco Labs

30 mg

60 mg

180 mg

Fexofenadine HCl
Teva

FINASTERIDE

1 mg

Propecia®
Merck

5 mg

Proscar®
Merck

FLUCONAZOLE

50 mg

100 mg

200 mg

†Diflucan®
Pfizer

50 mg

100 mg

150 mg

200 mg

Fluconazole
Teva

FLUOXETINE HCL

10 mg

20 mg

40 mg

†Prozac®
Dista

10 mg

10 mg

10 mg

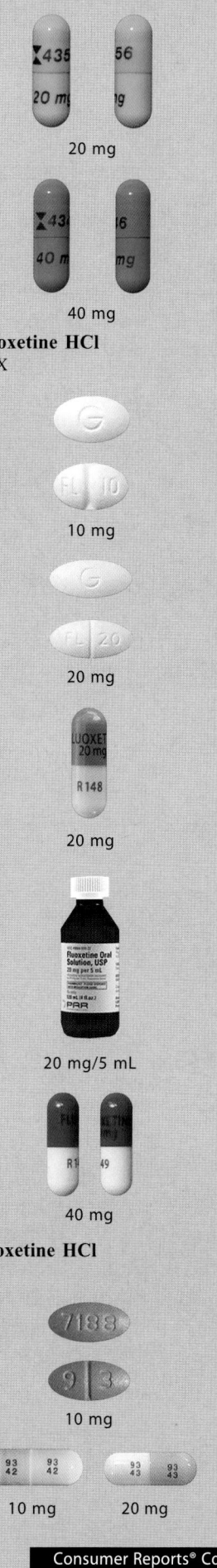

20 mg

40 mg

Fluoxetine HCl
IVAX

10 mg

20 mg

20 mg

20 mg/5 mL

40 mg

Fluoxetine HCl
Par

10 mg

10 mg   20 mg

20 mg/5 mL

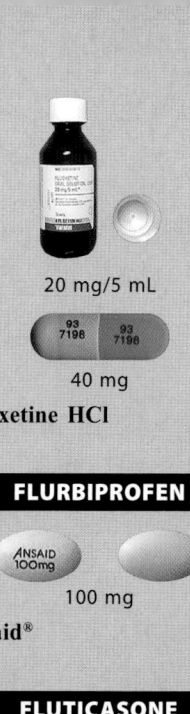

40 mg

Fluoxetine HCl
Teva

FLURBIPROFEN

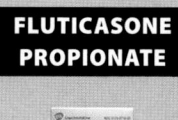

100 mg

Ansaid®
Pfizer

FLUTICASONE PROPIONATE

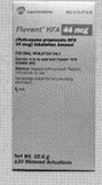

44 mcg

Flovent HFA®
GlaxoSmithKline

FLUTICASONE PROPIONATE/ SALMETEROL XINAFOATE

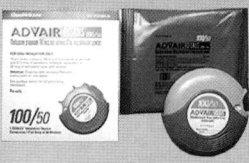

100 mcg-50 mcg/Dose

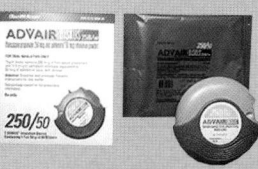

250 mcg-50 mcg/Dose

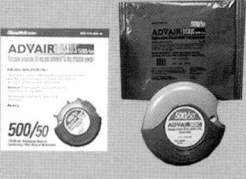

500 mcg-50 mcg/Dose

Advair Diskus®
GlaxoSmithKline

†Additional dosage forms or strengths available.

FLUVASTATIN SODIUM

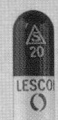 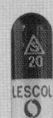

20 mg

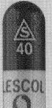 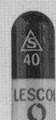

40 mg

Lescol®
Novartis

 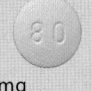

80 mg

Lescol XL®
Novartis

FOLIC ACID

 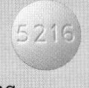

1 mg

Folic Acid
Watson

FUROSEMIDE

 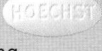 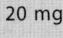

20 mg

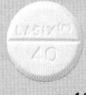 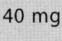

40 mg

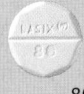 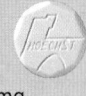

80 mg

Lasix®
Sanofi-Aventis

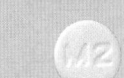

20 mg

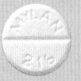 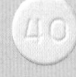

40 mg

80 mg

Furosemide
Mylan

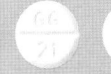

20 mg

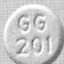

40 mg

80 mg

Furosemide
Sandoz

GABAPENTIN

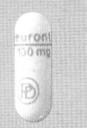 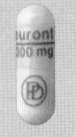 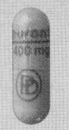

100 mg   300 mg   400 mg

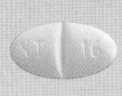

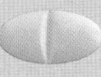

600 mg

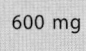

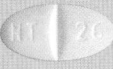

800 mg

†Neurontin®
Pfizer

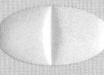

100 mg

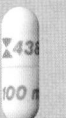 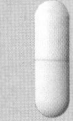

100 mg

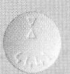 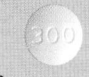

300 mg

Gabapentin
IVAX

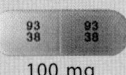

100 mg

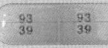

300 mg

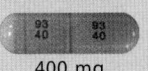

400 mg

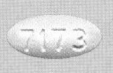

600 mg   800 mg

Gabapentin
Teva

GEMFIBROZIL

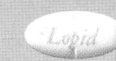 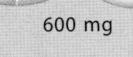

600 mg

Lopid®
Pfizer

GLIMEPIRIDE

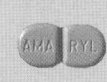 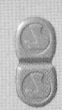

1 mg

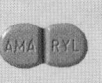

2 mg

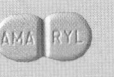 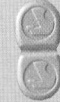

4 mg

Amaryl®
Sanofi-Aventis

GLIPIZIDE

5 mg

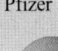

10 mg

Glucotrol®
Pfizer

2.5 mg   5 mg   10 mg

Glucotrol XL®
Pfizer

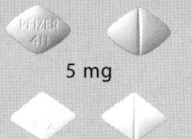

2.5 mg   5 mg   10 mg

Glipizide ER
Watson

GLYBURIDE

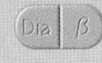 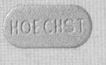

1.25 mg

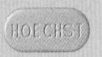

2.5 mg

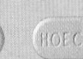

5 mg

Diabeta®
Sanofi-Aventis

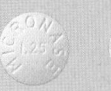

1.25 mg

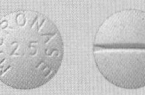

2.5 mg

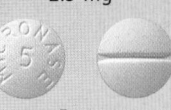

5 mg

Micronase®
Pfizer

GLYBURIDE, MICRONIZED

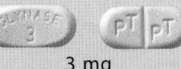

1.5 mg

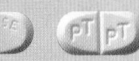

3 mg

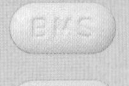

6 mg

Glynase®
Pfizer

GLYBURIDE/METFORMIN HCL

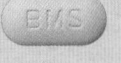

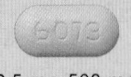

1.25 mg-250 mg

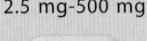

2.5 mg-500 mg

5 mg-500 mg

Glucovance®
BMS

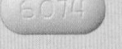

†Additional dosage forms or strengths available.

HYDROCHLOROTHIAZIDE

25 mg

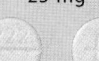

50 mg

Hydrochlorothiazide
Actavis

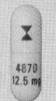

12.5 mg

25 mg   **50 mg**

Hydrochlorothiazide
Teva

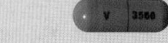

12.5 mg

25 mg   **50 mg**

Hydrochlorothiazide
Qualitest

HYDROCODONE/ ACETAMINOPHEN

10 mg-650 mg

Lorcet 10/650®
Forest

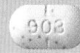

7.5 mg-650 mg

Lorcet Plus®
Forest

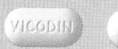

7.5 mg-500 mg

 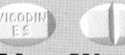

10 mg-500 mg

Lortab®
UCB Pharma

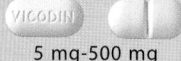

5 mg-500 mg

Vicodin®
Abbott

7.5 mg-750 mg

Vicodin ES®
Abbott

---

5 mg-400 mg

7.5 mg-400 mg

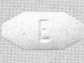

10 mg-400 mg

Zydone®
Endo

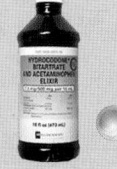

2.5 mg-167 mg/5 mL

5 mg-325 mg

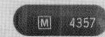

5 mg-500 mg

5 mg-500 mg

7.5 mg-325 mg

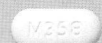

7.5 mg-500 mg

7.5 mg-650 mg

7.5 mg-750 mg

10 mg-325 mg

10 mg-500 mg

10 mg-650 mg

---

10 mg-660 mg

Hydrocodone/ Acetaminophen
Mallinckrodt

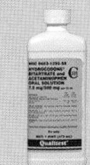

2.5 mg-167 mg/5 mL

5 mg-500 mg

7.5 mg-500 mg

7.5 mg-750 mg

10 mg-325 mg

10 mg-500 mg

10 mg-650 mg

Hydrocodone/ Acetaminophen
Qualitest

2.5 mg-500 mg

5 mg-325 mg

---

5 mg-500 mg

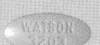

7.5 mg-325 mg

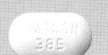

7.5 mg-500 mg

7.5 mg-650 mg

7.5 mg-750 mg

10 mg-325 mg

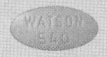

10 mg-500 mg

10 mg-650 mg

10 mg-750 mg

Hydrocodone/ Acetaminophen
Watson

HYDROCODONE/ IBUPROFEN

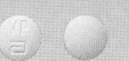

7.5 mg-200 mg

Vicoprofen®
Abbott

IBUPROFEN

400 mg

IBU 600

600 mg

IBU 800

800 mg

Ibuprofen
Par

600 mg

800 mg

†Ibuprofen
Watson

---

†Additional dosage forms or strengths available.

IMATINIB MESYLATE

100 mg

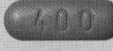

400 mg

Gleevec®
Novartis

INDINAVIR SULFATE

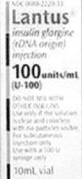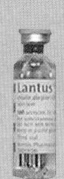

400 mg

†Crixivan®
Merck

INSULIN GLARGINE

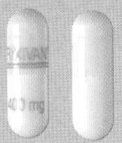

100 unit/mL

Lantus®
Aventis

IRBESARTAN

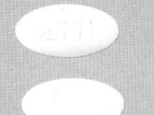

75 mg

150 mg

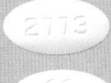

300 mg

Avapro®
BMS

IRBESARTAN/ HYDROCHLOROTHIAZIDE

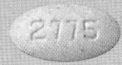

150 mg-12.5 mg

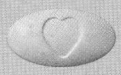

300 mg-12.5 mg

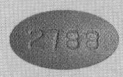

300 mg-25 mg

Avalide®
BMS

ISOSORBIDE MONONITRATE

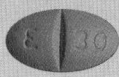

30 mg

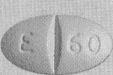

60 mg

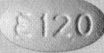

120 mg

Isosorbide Mononitrate
Ethex

60 mg

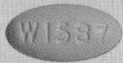

120 mg

Isosorbide Mononitrate
Warrick

ITRACONAZOLE

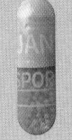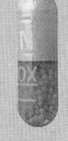

100 mg

Sporanox®
Janssen

LAMIVUDINE

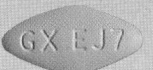

300 mg

†Epivir®
GlaxoSmithKline

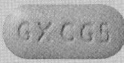

100 mg

†Epivir HBV®
GlaxoSmithKline

LAMOTRIGINE

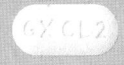

5 mg

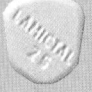

25 mg

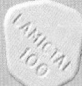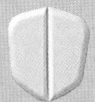

100 mg

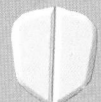

150 mg

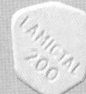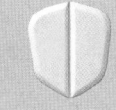

200 mg

Lamictal®
GlaxoSmithKline

LANSOPRAZOLE

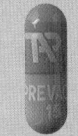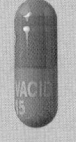

15 mg

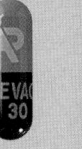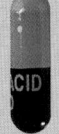

30 mg

Prevacid®
TAP

LATANOPROST

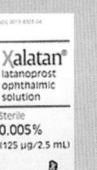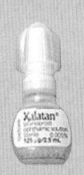

0.005 %

Xalatan®
Pfizer

LEFLUNOMIDE

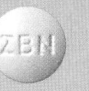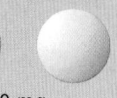

10 mg

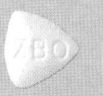

20 mg

Arava®
Sanofi-Aventis

LEVETIRACETAM

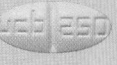

250 mg

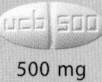

500 mg

750 mg

†Keppra®
UCB Pharma

LEVOFLOXACIN

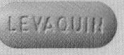

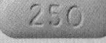

250 mg

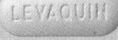

500 mg

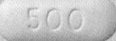

Levaquin®
Ortho

†Additional dosage forms or strengths available.

LEVOTHYROXINE SODIUM

  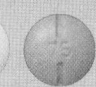

25 mcg | 50 mcg | 75 mcg

  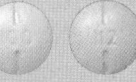

88 mcg | 100 mcg | 112 mcg

125 mcg | 137 mcg | 150 mcg

  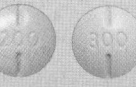

175 mcg | 200 mcg | 300 mcg

Synthroid®
Abbott

25 mcg

50 mcg

75 mcg

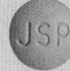

88 mcg

100 mcg

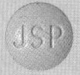

112 mcg

125 mcg

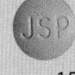

150 mcg

175 mcg

200 mcg

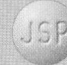

300 mcg

Levothyroxine Sodium
Lannett

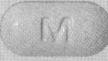

25 mcg

50 mcg

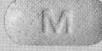

75 mcg

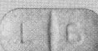

88 mcg

100 mcg

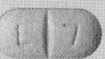

112 mcg

125 mcg

137 mcg

150 mcg

175 mcg

200 mcg

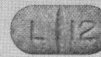

300 mcg

Levothyroxine Sodium
Mylan

25 mcg

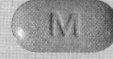

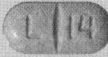

50 mcg

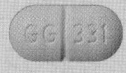

75 mcg

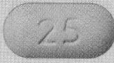

88 mcg

100 mcg

Levothyroxine Sodium
Sandoz

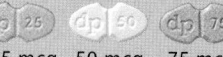

25 mcg | 50 mcg | 75 mcg

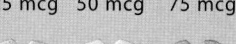

88 mcg | 100 mcg | 112 mcg

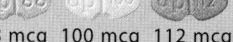

125 mcg | 137 mcg | 150 mcg

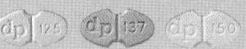

175 mcg | 200 mcg | 300 mcg

Levoxyl®
Monarch

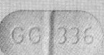

150 mcg

175 mcg

200 mcg

300 mcg

112 mcg

125 mcg

137 mcg

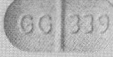

150 mcg

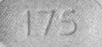

175 mcg

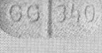

200 mcg

300 mcg

†Additional dosage forms or strengths available.

LINEZOLID

600 mg

Zyvox®
Pfizer

LISINOPRIL

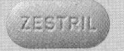 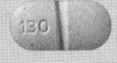

2.5 mg

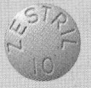 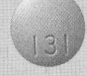

5 mg

10 mg

20 mg

 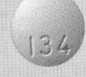

30 mg

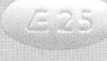

40 mg

Zestril®
AstraZeneca

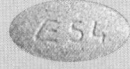

2.5 mg

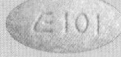

5 mg

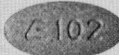

10 mg

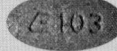

20 mg

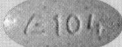

30 mg

40 mg

Lisinopril
Eon Labs

2.5 mg

10 mg

†Lisinopril
Lupin

2.5 mg

5 mg

10 mg

20 mg

30 mg

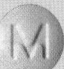 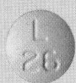

40 mg

Lisinopril
Mylan

 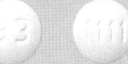

2.5 mg

5 mg

 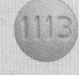

10 mg

20 mg

30 mg

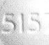

40 mg

Lisinopril
Teva

LISINOPRIL/HYDROCHLOROTHIAZIDE

10 mg-12.5 mg

20 mg-12.5 mg

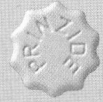 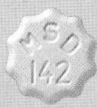

20 mg-25 mg

Prinzide®
Merck

 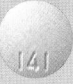

10 mg-12.5 mg

 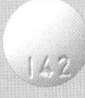

20 mg-12.5 mg

 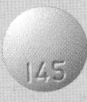

20 mg-25 mg

Zestoretic®
AstraZeneca

10 mg-12.5 mg

20 mg-12.5 mg

 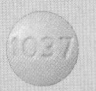

20 mg-25 mg

Lisinopril/HCTZ
Teva

LORATADINE

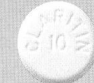 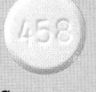

10 mg

Claritin®
S-P Healthcare

LORAZEPAM

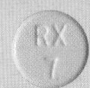 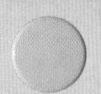

0.5 mg

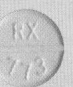

1 mg

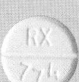 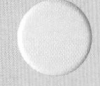

2 mg

Lorazepam
Ranbaxy

 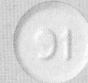

0.5 mg

1 mg

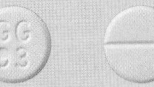

2 mg

Lorazepam
Sandoz

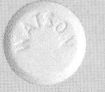 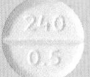

0.5 mg

1 mg

2 mg

Lorazepam
Watson

LOSARTAN POTASSIUM

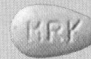

25 mg

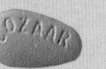 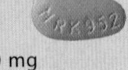

50 mg

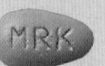 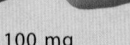

100 mg

Cozaar®
Merck

†Additional dosage forms or strengths available.

LOSARTAN POTASSIUM/ HYDROCHLOROTHIAZIDE

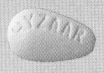

50 mg-12.5 mg

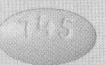 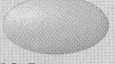

100 mg-12.5 mg

100 mg-25 mg

Hyzaar®
Merck

LOVASTATIN

 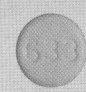

10 mg

20 mg

40 mg

Lovastatin
Actavis

MECLIZINE HCL

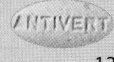

12.5 mg

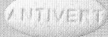

25 mg

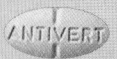 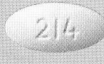

50 mg

Antivert®
Pfizer

MELOXICAM

 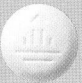

7.5 mg

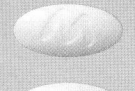

15 mg

Mobic®
Boehringer Ingelheim

MEMANTINE HCL

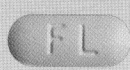

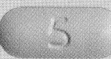

5 mg

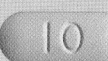

10 mg

†Namenda®
Forest

METFORMIN HCL

500 mg

850 mg

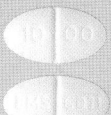

1,000 mg

Glucophage®
BMS

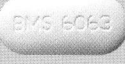

500 mg

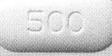

500 mg

750 mg

Glucophage XR®
BMS

 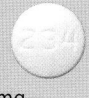

500 mg

850 mg

METFORMIN HCL
Mylan

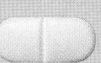

1,000 mg

Metformin HCl
Mylan

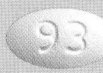

93

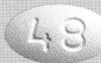

48

500 mg

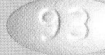

93

49

850 mg

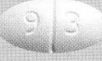

9 3

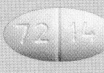

72 14

1,000 mg

Metformin HCl
Teva

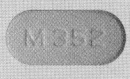

500 mg

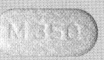

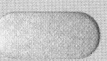

750 mg

Metformin HCl ER
Mylan

93

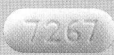

7267

500 mg

†Metformin HCl ER
Teva

METHYLPHENIDATE HCL

alza 18

18 mg

CONCERTA

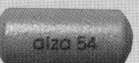

alza 27

27 mg

alza 36

36 mg

alza 54

54 mg

Concerta®
McNeil

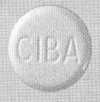 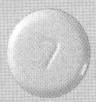

5 mg

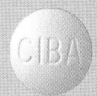 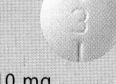

10 mg

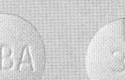

20 mg

Ritalin®
Novartis

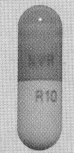 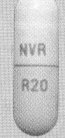

10 mg   20 mg

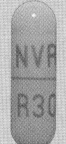 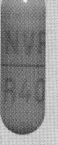

30 mg   40 mg

Ritalin LA®
Novartis

20 mg

Ritalin-SR®
Novartis

METOCLOPRAMIDE HCL

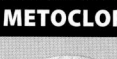

5 mg

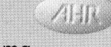 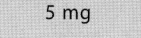

10 mg

Reglan®
Schwarz

---

†Additional dosage forms or strengths available.

METOPROLOL SUCCINATE

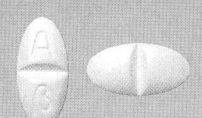
25 mg

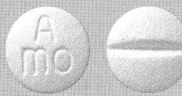
50 mg

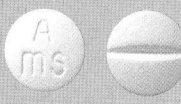
100 mg

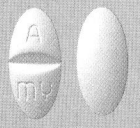
200 mg

Toprol XL®
AstraZeneca

METOPROLOL TARTRATE

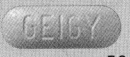 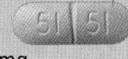
50 mg

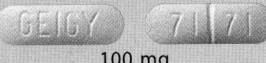
100 mg

Lopressor®
Novartis

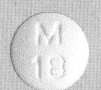 
25 mg

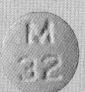
50 mg

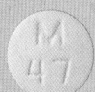
100 mg

Metoprolol Tartrate
Mylan

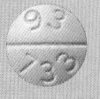
50 mg

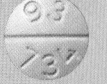 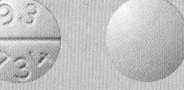
100 mg

Metoprolol Tartrate
Teva

METRONIDAZOLE

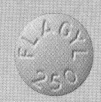 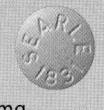
250 mg

 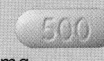
500 mg

Flagyl®
Pfizer

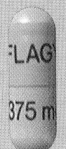 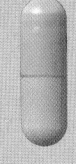
375 mg

Flagyl 375®
Pfizer

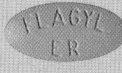
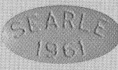
750 mg

Flagyl ER®
Pfizer

MOEXIPRIL HCL

 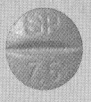
7.5 mg

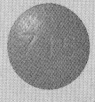 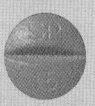
15 mg

Univasc®
Schwarz

MOEXIPRIL HCL/ HYDROCHLOROTHIAZIDE

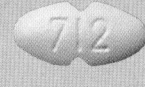
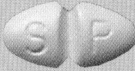
7.5 mg-12.5 mg

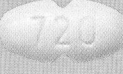
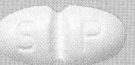
15 mg-12.5 mg

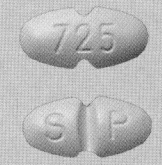
15 mg-25 mg

Uniretic®
Schwarz

MOMETASONE FUROATE

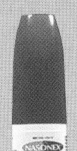
50 mcg

Nasonex®
Schering

MONTELUKAST SODIUM

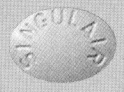
4 mg

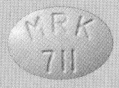
5 mg

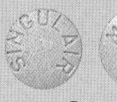
10 mg

†Singulair®
Merck

MORPHINE SULFATE

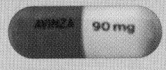

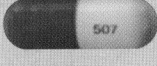
90 mg

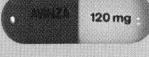

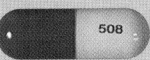
120 mg

†Avinza®
Monarch

 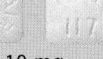

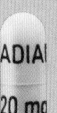 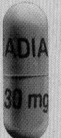
20 mg   30 mg

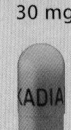
50 mg   60 mg

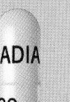 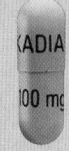
80 mg   100 mg

Kadian®
Alpharma BPD

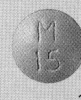 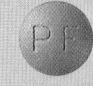
15 mg

30 mg

60 mg

100 mg

 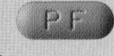
200 mg

MS Contin®
Purdue Pharma

NADOLOL

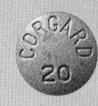 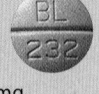
20 mg

40 mg

80 mg

Corgard®
Monarch

†Additional dosage forms or strengths available.

NAPROXEN

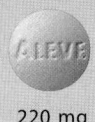

375 mg

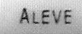

375 mg

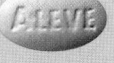

500 mg

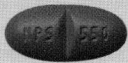

500 mg

†Naproxen
Teva

NAPROXEN SODIUM

220 mg

220 mg

220 mg

Aleve®
Bayer

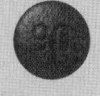

550 mg

Anaprox DS®
Roche

NIFEDIPINE

 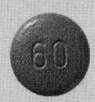

30 mg

60 mg

90 mg

Adalat CC®
Schering

10 mg

Procardia®
Pfizer

 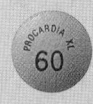

30 mg   60 mg   90 mg

Procardia XL®
Pfizer

NIZATIDINE

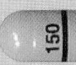

150 mg

300 mg

Axid®
Reliant

75 mg

Axid AR®
Wyeth

OLANZAPINE

2.5 mg   5 mg

7.5 mg   10 mg

15 mg

20 mg

Zyprexa®
Eli Lilly

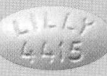

5 mg

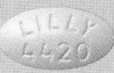

10 mg

†Zyprexa Zydis®
Eli Lilly

OLMESARTAN MEDOXOMIL

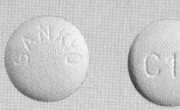

5 mg

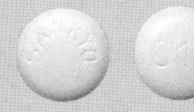

20 mg

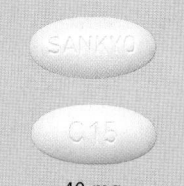

40 mg

Benicar®
Daiichi Sankyo

OLMESARTAN MEDOXOMIL/ HYDROCHLOROTHIAZIDE

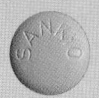 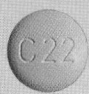

20 mg-12.5 mg

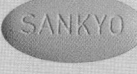

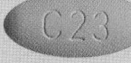

40 mg-12.5 mg

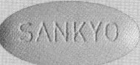

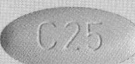

40 mg-25 mg

Benicar HCT®
Daiichi Sankyo

OMEPRAZOLE

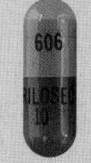 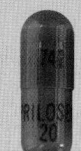 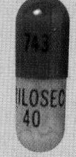

10 mg   20 mg   40 mg

Prilosec®
AstraZeneca

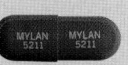

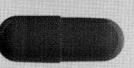

10 mg

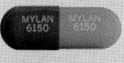

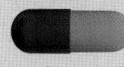

20 mg

Omeprazole
Mylan

OMEPRAZOLE MAGNESIUM

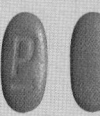

20 mg

Prilosec OTC®
Procter & Gamble

OXYCODONE HCL

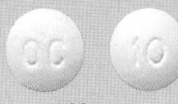

10 mg

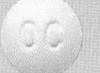

20 mg

40 mg

80 mg

†Oxycontin®
Purdue

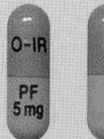

5 mg

OxyIR®
Purdue

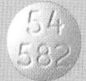 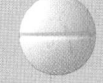

5 mg

Roxicodone®
Xanodyne

---

†Additional dosage forms or strengths available.

OXYCODONE HCL/ ACETAMINOPHEN

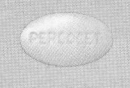

2.5 mg-325 mg

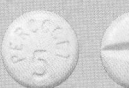

5 mg-325 mg

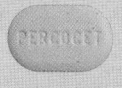

7.5 mg-325 mg

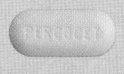

10 mg-325 mg

10 mg-650 mg

Percocet®
Endo

5 mg-325 mg

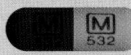

5 mg-500 mg

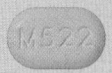

7.5 mg-325 mg

7.5 mg-325 mg

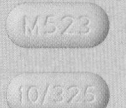

10 mg-325 mg

†Oxycodone/ Acetaminophen
Mallinckrodt

OXYCODONE HCL/ ASPIRIN

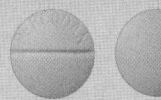

4.8355 mg-325 mg

Percodan®
Endo

PANTOPRAZOLE SODIUM

 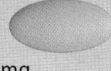

20 mg

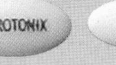

40 mg

Protonix®
Wyeth

PAROXETINE HCL

10 mg

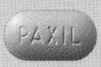 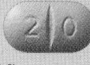

20 mg

30 mg

40 mg

†Paxil®
GlaxoSmithKline

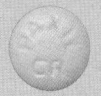

12.5 mg

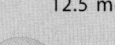

 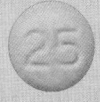

25 mg

 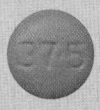

37.5 mg

Paxil CR®
GlaxoSmithKline

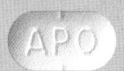

10 mg

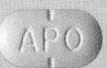 

20 mg

30 mg

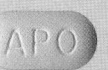

40 mg

Paroxetine HCl
Apotex

PENICILLIN V POTASSIUM

 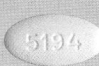

250 mg

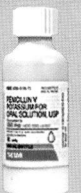

250 mg/5 mL

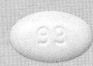 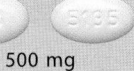

500 mg

Penicillin V Potassium
Teva

PHENYTOIN

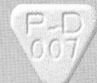 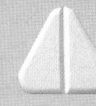

50 mg

Dilantin®
Pfizer

PHENYTOIN SODIUM EXTENDED

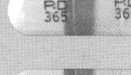

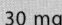

30 mg

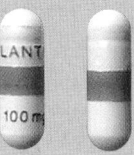

100 mg

Dilantin®
Pfizer

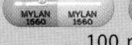 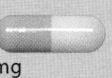

100 mg

Phenytoin Sodium, Extended
Mylan

PIOGLITAZONE HCL

 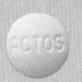

15 mg

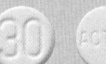

30 mg

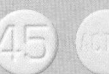

45 mg

Actos®
Takeda

POTASSIUM CHLORIDE

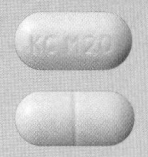

20 mEq

†Klor-Con M20
Upsher Smith

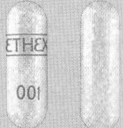

10 mEq

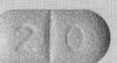

20 mEq

Potassium Chloride
Ethex

8 mEq

10 mEq

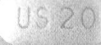

20 mEq

Potassium Chloride
Teva

†Additional dosage forms or strengths available.

PRAVASTATIN SODIUM

 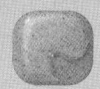

10 mg

20 mg

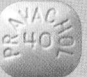

40 mg

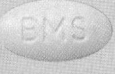

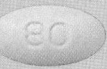

80 mg

Pravachol®
BMS

PREDNISONE

2.5 mg

5 mg

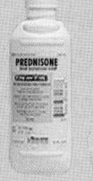

5 mg/5 mL

10 mg

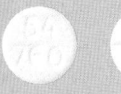

20 mg

†Prednisone
Roxane

5 mg

10 mg

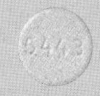

20 mg

Prednisone
Watson

PREGABALIN

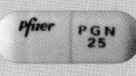

25 mg

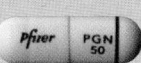

50 mg

75 mg

100 mg

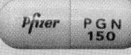

150 mg

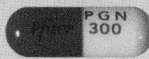

300 mg

†Lyrica®
Pfizer

PROMETHAZINE HCL

25 mg   50 mg

Promethazine HCl
Sandoz

PROPOXYPHENE NAPSYLATE

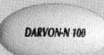

100 mg

Darvon-N®
Xanodyne Pharm

PROPOXYPHENE NAPSYLATE/ ACETAMINOPHEN

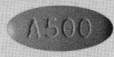

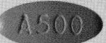

100 mg-500 mg

Darvocet A500®
Xanodyne Pharm

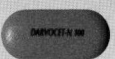

100 mg-650 mg

Darvocet-N 100®
Xanodyne Pharm

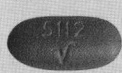

100 mg-650 mg

†Propoxyphene Napsylate/ APAP
Qualitest

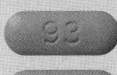

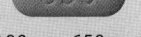

100 mg-650 mg

Propoxyphene Napsylate/ APAP
Teva

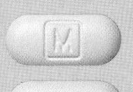

100 mg-650 mg

Propoxyphene Napsylate/ APAP
Mallinckrodt

PROPRANOLOL HCL

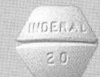

20 mg

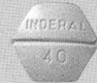

40 mg

 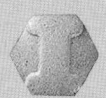

60 mg

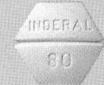

80 mg

†Inderal®
Wyeth

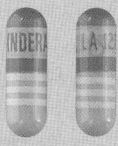

120 mg

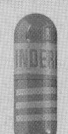 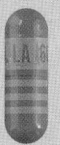

160 mg

†Inderal LA®
Wyeth

PSEUDOEPHEDRINE HCL/ FEXOFENADINE HCL

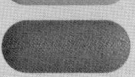

120 mg-60 mg

Allegra-D 12 Hour®
Aventis

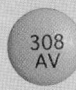

240 mg-180 mg

Allegra-D 24 Hour®
Sanofi

PSEUDOEPHEDRINE SULFATE/ DESLORATADINE

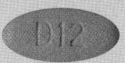

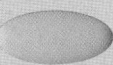

120 mg-2.5 mg

Clarinex-D 12 Hour®
Schering

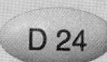

240 mg-5 mg

Clarinex-D 24 Hour®
Schering

PSEUDOEPHEDRINE SULFATE/LORATADINE

120 mg-5 mg

Claritin-D 12 Hour®
S-P Healthcare

240 mg-10 mg

Claritin-D 24 Hour®
S-P Healthcare

†Additional dosage forms or strengths available.

QUETIAPINE FUMARATE

25 mg   50 mg

100 mg   200 mg

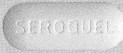

300 mg

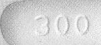

400 mg

Seroquel®
AstraZeneca

QUINAPRIL HCL

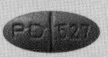 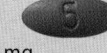

5 mg

10 mg

20 mg

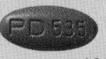 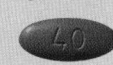

40 mg

Accupril®
Pfizer

QUINAPRIL HCL/ HYDROCHLOROTHIAZIDE

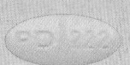

10 mg-12.5 mg

20 mg-12.5 mg

20 mg-25 mg

Accuretic®
Pfizer

RABEPRAZOLE SODIUM

20 mg

Aciphex®
Eisai

RALOXIFENE HCL

60 mg

Evista®
Eli Lilly

RAMIPRIL

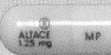

1.25 mg

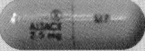

2.5 mg

5 mg

10 mg

Altace®
Monarch

RANITIDINE HCL

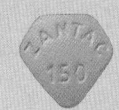 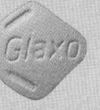

150 mg

 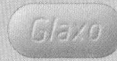

300 mg

Zantac®
GlaxoSmithKline

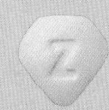

75 mg

Zantac 75®
Boehringer

150 mg

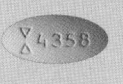

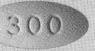

300 mg

Ranitidine HCl
IVAX

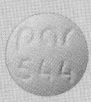

150 mg

300 mg

Ranitidine HCl
Par

150 mg

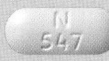

300 mg

Ranitidine HCl
Teva

RIFAMPIN

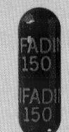 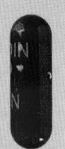

150 mg

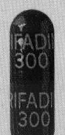 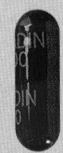

300 mg

Rifadin®
Sanofi-Aventis

RISEDRONATE SODIUM

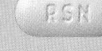

5 mg

 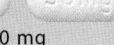

30 mg

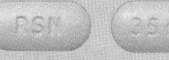

35 mg

Actonel®
Procter & Gamble

RISPERIDONE

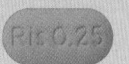

0.25 mg

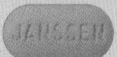

0.5 mg

1 mg

2 mg

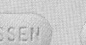 

3 mg

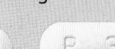

4 mg

Risperdal®
Janssen

RITONAVIR/LOPINAVIR

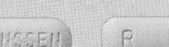

33.3 mg-133.3 mg

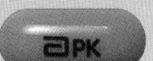

50 mg-200 mg

†Kaletra®
Abbott

RIVASTIGMINE TARTRATE

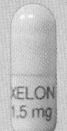 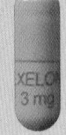

1.5 mg   3 mg

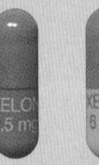 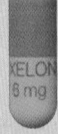

4.5 mg   6 mg

†Exelon®
Novartis

†Additional dosage forms or strengths available.

RIZATRIPTAN BENZOATE

5 mg

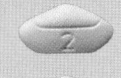

10 mg

Maxalt®
Merck

5 mg   10 mg

Maxalt MLT®
Merck

ROSIGLITAZONE MALEATE

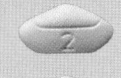
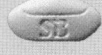

2 mg

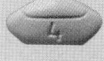

4 mg

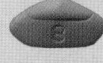

8 mg

Avandia®
GlaxoSmithKline

ROSIGLITAZONE MALEATE/GLIMEPIRIDE

4 mg-1 mg

4 mg-2 mg

4 mg-4 mg

Avandaryl®
GlaxoSmithKline

ROSIGLITAZONE MALEATE/METFORMIN HCL

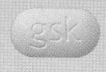

2 mg-500 mg

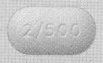

2 mg-1,000 mg

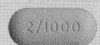

4 mg-500 mg

4 mg-1,000 mg

Avandamet®
GlaxoSmithKline

ROSUVASTATIN CALCIUM

5 mg   10 mg   20 mg

 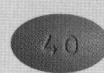

40 mg

Crestor®
AstraZeneca

SERTRALINE HCL

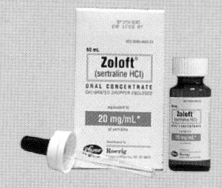

20 mg/mL

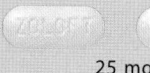

25 mg

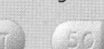

50 mg

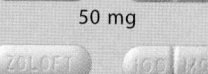

100 mg

Zoloft®
Pfizer

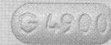

25 mg

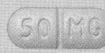

50 mg

100 mg

†Sertraline HCl
Greenstone

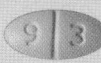

25 mg

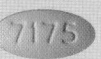

50 mg

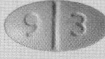

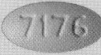

100 mg

Sertraline HCl
Teva

SIBUTRAMINE

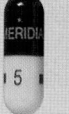

5 mg

10 mg

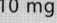 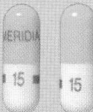

15 mg

Meridia®
Abbott

SILDENAFIL CITRATE

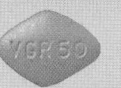

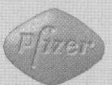

50 mg

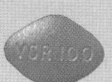

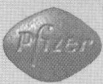

100 mg

†Viagra®
Pfizer

SIMVASTATIN

5 mg

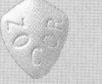

10 mg

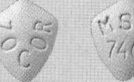

20 mg

 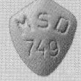

40 mg

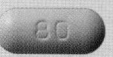

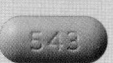

80 mg

Zocor®
Merck

5 mg   10 mg

20 mg   40 mg

†Simvastatin
Teva

---

†Additional dosage forms or strengths available.

SIROLIMUS

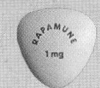 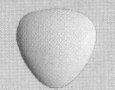

1 mg

†**Rapamune**®
Wyeth

SITAGLIPTIN PHOSPHATE

100 mg

†**Januvia**®
Merck

SPIRONOLACTONE

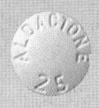

25 mg

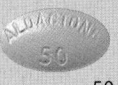 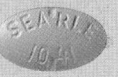

50 mg

100 mg

Aldactone®
Pfizer

SPIRONOLACTONE/ HYDROCHLOROTHIAZIDE

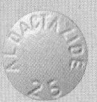 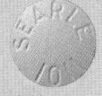

25 mg-25 mg

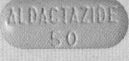

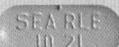

50 mg-50 mg

Aldactazide®
Pfizer

STAVUDINE

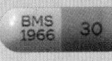

30 mg

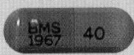

40 mg

†**Zerit**®
BMS

SULFAMETHOXAZOLE/ TRIMETHOPRIM

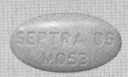

800 mg-160 mg

Septra DS®
Monarch

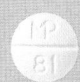

400 mg-80 mg

800 mg-160 mg

Sulfamethoxazole/ Trimethoprim
Mutual

400 mg-80 mg

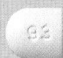

800 mg-160 mg

Sulfamethoxazole/ Trimethoprim
Teva

SUMATRIPTAN

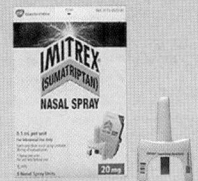

20 mg

Imitrex®
GlaxoSmithKline

SUMATRIPTAN SUCCINATE

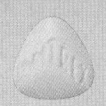 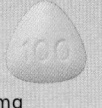

100 mg

†**Imitrex**®
GlaxoSmithKline

TACRINE HCL

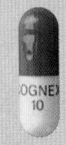 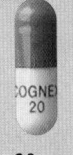

10 mg   20 mg

COGNEX

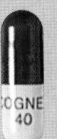

30 mg   40 mg

Cognex®
Sciele

TADALAFIL

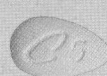

5 mg

10 mg

20 mg

Cialis®
Eli Lilly

TAMSULOSIN HCL

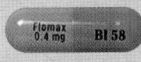

0.4 mg

Flomax®
Boehringer Ingelheim

TEMAZEPAM

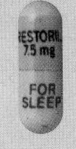 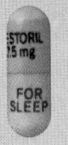

7.5 mg

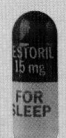 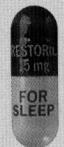

15 mg

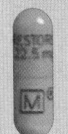 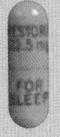

22.5 mg

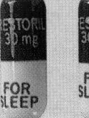

30 mg

Restoril®
Mallinckrodt

TEMAZEPAM

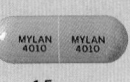

15 mg

30 mg

Temazepam
Mylan

TIAGABINE HCL

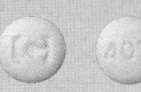

2 mg

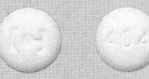

4 mg

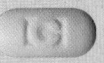

12 mg

16 mg

Gabitril®
Cephalon

TICLOPIDINE HCL

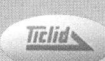 

250 mg

Ticlid®
Roche

TIOTROPIUM BROMIDE

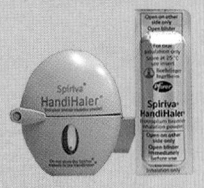

18 mcg

Spiriva®
Boehringer Ingelheim

TOLTERODINE TARTRATE

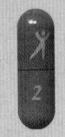 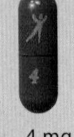

2 mg   4 mg

Detrol LA®
Pfizer

†Additional dosage forms or strengths available.

TOPIRAMATE

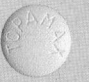

25 mg

50 mg

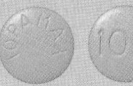

100 mg

200 mg

Topamax®
McNeil

TRAMADOL HCL

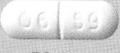

50 mg

Ultram®
McNeil

100 mg

200 mg

†Ultram ER®
McNeil

TRAMADOL HCL/ ACETAMINOPHEN

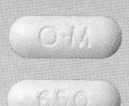

37.5 mg-325 mg

Ultracet®
McNeil

TRANDOLAPRIL

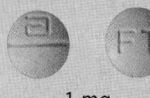

1 mg

2 mg

4 mg

Mavik®
Abbott

TRANDOLAPRIL/ VERAPAMIL HCL

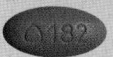

2 mg-180 mg

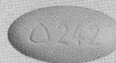

2 mg-240 mg

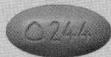

4 mg-240 mg

†Tarka®
Abbott

TRAZODONE HCL

 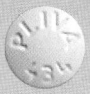

50 mg   100 mg

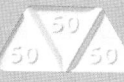

150 mg

Trazodone HCl
Pliva

TRIAMTERENE/ HYDROCHLOROTHIAZIDE

37.5 mg-25 mg

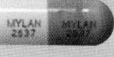

37.5 mg-25 mg

75 mg-50 mg

Triamterene/HCTZ
Mylan

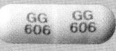

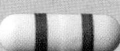

37.5 mg-25 mg

37.5 mg-25 mg

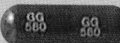

50 mg-25 mg

75 mg-50 mg

Triamterene/HCTZ
Sandoz

VALACYCLOVIR HCL

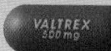

500 mg

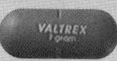

1,000 mg

Valtrex®
GlaxoSmithKline

VALSARTAN

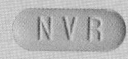

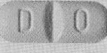

40 mg

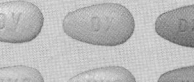

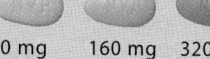

80 mg   160 mg   320 mg

Diovan®
Novartis

VALSARTAN/ HYDROCHLOROTHIAZIDE

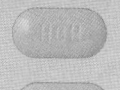

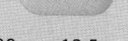

80 mg-12.5 mg

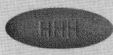

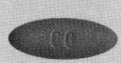

160 mg-12.5 mg

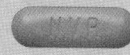

160 mg-25 mg

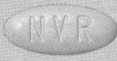

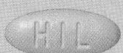

320 mg-12.5 mg

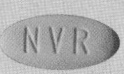

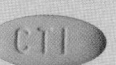

320 mg-25 mg

Diovan HCT®
Novartis

VARDENAFIL HCL

2.5 mg

5 mg

10 mg

20 mg

Levitra®
Schering

VENLAFAXINE HCL

25 mg

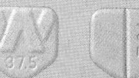

37.5 mg

50 mg

75 mg

100 mg

Effexor®
Wyeth

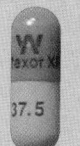 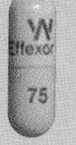 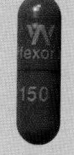

37.5 mg   75 mg   150 mg

Effexor XR®
Wyeth

VERAPAMIL HCL

 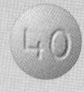

40 mg

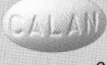 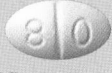

80 mg

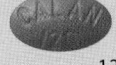 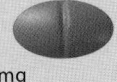

120 mg

Calan®
Pfizer

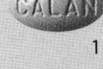 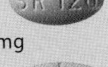

120 mg

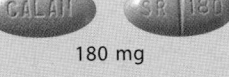

180 mg

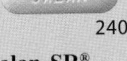

240 mg

Calan SR®
Pfizer

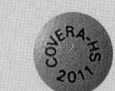

180 mg   240 mg

Covera-HS®
Pfizer

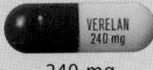

240 mg

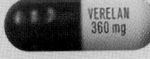

360 mg

†Verelan®
Schwarz

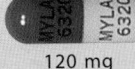

120 mg

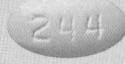

120 mg

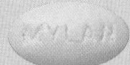

120 mg

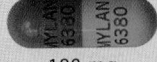

180 mg

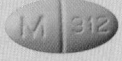

180 mg

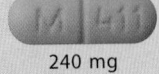

240 mg

240 mg

Verapamil HCl
Mylan

WARFARIN SODIUM

1 mg   2 mg   2.5 mg

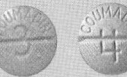 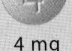 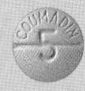

3 mg   4 mg   5 mg

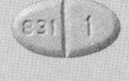 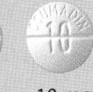

6 mg   7.5 mg   10 mg

Coumadin®
BMS

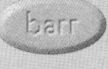

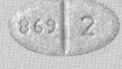

1 mg

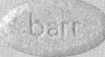

2 mg

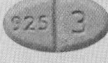

2.5 mg

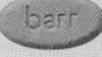

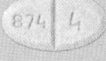

3 mg

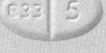

4 mg

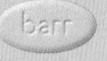

5 mg

Warfarin Sodium
Barr

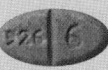

6 mg

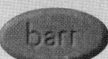

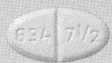

7.5 mg

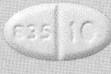

10 mg

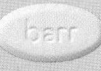

Warfarin Sodium
Barr

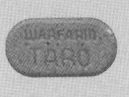 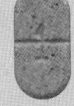

1 mg

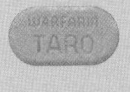 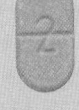

2 mg

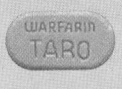 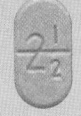

2.5 mg

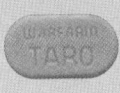 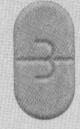

3 mg

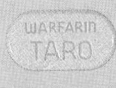 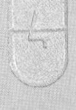

4 mg

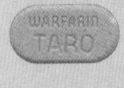 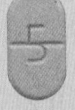

5 mg

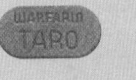

6 mg

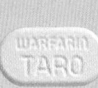 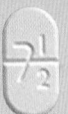

7.5 mg

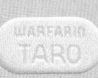 

10 mg

Warfarin Sodium
Taro

ZAFIRLUKAST

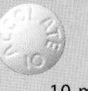

10 mg

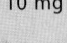 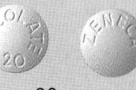

20 mg

Accolate®
AstraZeneca

ZOLMITRIPTAN

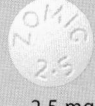 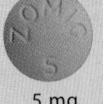

2.5 mg   5 mg

Zomig®
AstraZeneca

ZOLPIDEM TARTRATE

 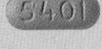

5 mg

 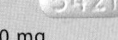

10 mg

Ambien®
Sanofi-Aventis

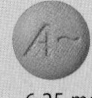 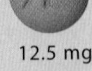

6.25 mg   12.5 mg

Ambien CR®
Sanofi-Aventis

ZONISAMIDE

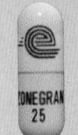 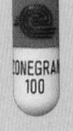

25 mg   100 mg

Zonegran®
Eisai

†Additional dosage forms or strengths available.

Index

The brand and generic drug names are listed in **boldface** type. When a brand name drug appears, the generic name of the drug will be provided and listed as "see (generic name)." The page number where the listing for that drug can be found is indicated after the generic name. The drug listings are arranged alphabetically by generic name in the Drug Information section. **If the drug is a combination drug** (containing two or more single medications in the product), then you may have to look for each of the individual drug components in separate drug listings if there is not a drug listing available for the combination drug.

There are many brands of drugs and the listing of selected brand names in this index are provided only for ease of reference. There are other brand name products that have not been included in the book. Because a brand name is listed in this index does not mean that the authors or organizations represented have any particular knowledge that the brand listed has properties different from other brands of the same drug, nor is it intended as a recommendation of the drugs listed. Additionally, if a brand name product is not listed it does not indicate that the product has been evaluated to be unsatisfactory or substandard.

§—Medications for which drug listings are not included in this published version of the Consumer Drug Reference due to space limitations. Copies of the drug listings are available on the website, *www.consumerdrugreference.org*. See "How to Find More Drug Information Online" in the introductory information, just inside the front cover, for details on accessing this site.

A

A-200° Lice Killing Shampoo— *See* Pyrethrin and Piperonyl Butoxide, 1479
Abacavir, 1
Abatacept Injection, 3
Abelcet°— *See* Amphotericin B Lipid Complex Injection, 101
Abilify°— *See* Aripiprazole, 129
Acamprosate, 4
Acarbose, 6
Accolate°— *See* Zafirlukast, 1787
Accuneb°— *See* Albuterol Inhalation, 41
Accupril°— *See* Quinapril, 1485
Accuretic°— *See* Hydrochlorothiazide, 829 *and See* Quinapril, 1485
Accutane°— *See* Isotretinoin, 943
Acebutolol, 8
Aceon°— *See* Perindopril, 1378
Acephen°— *See* Acetaminophen, 10
Acetaminophen, 10
Acetaminophen and Codeine, 13
Acetaminophen and Hydrocodone, 14
Acetaminophen and Oxycodone, 15
Acetaminophen and Propoxyphene, 16
Acetaminophen, Butalbital, and Caffeine, 17
Acetazolamide Oral, 18
AcipHex°— *See* Rabeprazole, 1492
Acitretin, 19
ACT°— *See* Fluoride, 720
ActHIB°— *See* Haemophilus influenzae type b Vaccine, 813
Actifed°— *See* Pseudoephedrine and Triprolidine, 1475
Actigall°— *See* Ursodiol, 1749
Actimmune°— *See* Interferon Gamma-1b Injection, 922
Actiq°— *See* Fentanyl Oral Transmucosal, 683
Activella°— *See* Estrogen and Progestin (Hormone Replacement Therapy), 631
Actonel°— *See* Risedronate, 1524
Actonel° with Calcium— *See* Risedronate, 1524
ActoPLUSMet°— *See* Pioglitazone, 1408
Actos°— *See* Pioglitazone, 1408
Actron°— *See* Ketoprofen, 959
Acular°— *See* Ketorolac Ophthalmic, 965
Acyclovir, 22
Acyclovir Injection, 26
Acyclovir Topical, 30
Adacel°— *See* Tetanus, Diphtheria, and Pertussis (Tdap) Vaccine, 1660

Adalat°— *See* Nifedipine, 1241
Adalat° CC— *See* Nifedipine, 1241
Adalimumab Injection, 32
Adapalene, 35
Adderall°— *See* Dextroamphetamine and Amphetamine, 473
Adefovir, 36
Adipex-P°— *See* Phentermine, 1391
Adprin B° Tri-Buffered Caplets°— *See* Aspirin, 132
Adrenalin° Chloride Solution— *See* Epinephrine Injection, 595
Advair°— *See* Fluticasone and Salmeterol Oral Inhalation, 734
Advicor°— *See* Lovastatin, 1052 *and See* Niacin, 1229
Advil° Caplets°— *See* Ibuprofen, 856
Advil° Children's— *See* Ibuprofen, 856
Advil° Cold & Sinus° Caplets°— *See* Ibuprofen, 856
Advil° Cold & Sinus Tablets— *See* Ibuprofen, 856
Advil° Flu & Body Ache Caplets°— *See* Ibuprofen, 856
Advil° Gel Caplets— *See* Ibuprofen, 856
Advil° Infants' Concentrated Drops— *See* Ibuprofen, 856
Advil° Junior Strength Chewable Tablets— *See* Ibuprofen, 856
Advil° Junior Strength Tablets— *See* Ibuprofen, 856
Advil° Liqui-Gels°— *See* Ibuprofen, 856
Advil° Migraine°— *See* Ibuprofen, 856
Advil° Tablets— *See* Ibuprofen, 856
AeroBid° Inhaler System— *See* Flunisolide Oral Inhalation, 715
AeroBid-M° Inhaler System— *See* Flunisolide Oral Inhalation, 715
Aftate° for Athlete's Foot Aerosol Spray Liquid— *See* Tolnaftate, 1703
Aftate° for Athlete's Foot Aerosol Spray Powder— *See* Tolnaftate, 1703
Aftate° for Jock Itch Aerosol Spray Powder— *See* Tolnaftate, 1703
Agenerase°— *See* Amprenavir, 112
Aggrenox°— *See* Aspirin, 132 *and See* Aspirin and Extended-Release Dipyridamole, 140
Agrylin°— *See* Anagrelide, 115
Ah-Chew°— *See* Chlorpheniramine, 318
A-hydroCort°— *See* Hydrocortisone Injection, 831
AKBeta°— *See* Levobunolol Ophthalmic, 1003

AK-Pred°— *See* Prednisolone Ophthalmic, 1437
AK-Sulf°— *See* Sulfacetamide Ophthalmic, 1607
AK-Tob°— *See* Tobramycin Ophthalmic, 1693
AK-Trol°— *See* Dexamethasone Ophthalmic, 461 *and See* Neomycin, Polymyxin, and Bacitracin Ophthalmic, 1220
Ala-Cort°— *See* Hydrocortisone Topical, 837
Alamag°— *See* Aluminum Hydroxide and Magnesium Hydroxide, 61
Ala-Scalpt°— *See* Hydrocortisone Topical, 837
Alavert° Allergy & Sinus D-12 Hour— *See* Loratadine, 1044
Alavert° Non-Drowsy Allergy Relief 24 Hour— *See* Loratadine, 1044
Albuterol, 39
Albuterol Inhalation, 41
Aldactazide°— *See* Hydrochlorothiazide, 829 *and See* Spironolactone and Hydrochlorothiazide, 1599
Aldactone°— *See* Spironolactone, 1596
Aldara°— *See* Imiquimod, 870
Aldochlor° 250— *See* Methyldopa, 1116
Aldoril°— *See* Hydrochlorothiazide, 829 *and See* Methyldopa, 1116 *and See* Methyldopa and Hydrochlorothiazide, 1118
Alefacept Injection, 45
Alendronate, 46
Alesse°— *See* Estrogen and Progestin (Oral Contraceptives), 633
Aleve°— *See* Naproxen, 1205
Alfuzosin, 49
Alglucerase Injection§
Alimta°— *See* Pemetrexed Injection, 1355
Alinia°— *See* Nitazoxanide, 1247
Aliskiren, 51
Alitretinoin, 52
Alka-Mints°— *See* Calcium Carbonate, 242
Alka-Seltzer° Effervescent Pain Reliever and Antacid— *See* Aspirin, 132
Alka-Seltzer° Extra Strength Effervescent Pain Reliever and Antacid— *See* Aspirin, 132
Alka-Seltzer° Flavored Effervescent Pain Reliever and Antacid— *See* Aspirin, 132
Alka-Seltzer° Gas Relief Maximum Strength Softgels°— *See* Simethicone, 1578
Alka-Seltzer Plus° Cold & Cough Medicine Liqui-Gels°— *See* Dextromethorphan, 477
Alka-Seltzer Plus° Cold Medicine Liqui-Gels°— *See* Chlorpheniramine, 318
Alka-Seltzer° Plus Cold & Sinus Medicine Effervescent— *See* Aspirin, 132

Cidofovir Injection, 334

Cilostazol, 336

Ciloxan®—*See* Ciprofloxacin Ophthalmic, 360

Cimetidine, 338

Cimetidine Hydrochloride Injection, 340

Cinacalcet, 343

Cipro®—*See* Ciprofloxacin, 345

Ciprodex®—*See* Ciprofloxacin and Dexamethasone Otic, 352

Ciprofloxacin, 345

Ciprofloxacin and Dexamethasone Otic, 352

Ciprofloxacin and Hydrocortisone Otic, 354

Ciprofloxacin Injection, 355

Ciprofloxacin Ophthalmic, 360

Cipro HC Otic—*See* Ciprofloxacin and Hydrocortisone Otic, 354

Cipro®I.V.—*See* Ciprofloxacin Injection, 355

Cipro® XR, Proquin®XR—*See* Ciprofloxacin, 345

Cisapride§

Citalopram, 363

Claforan®—*See* Cefotaxime Sodium Injection, 274

Claravis®—*See* Isotretinoin, 943

Clarinex®—*See* Desloratadine, 455

Clarinex® Reditabs®—*See* Desloratadine, 455

Clarithromycin, 366

Claritin-D® 12 Hour—*See* Loratadine, 1044

Claritin-D® 24 Hour—*See* Loratadine, 1044

Claritin® Hives Relief—*See* Loratadine, 1044

Claritin® 24 Hour—*See* Loratadine, 1044

Claritin® RediTabs® 24 Hour—*See* Loratadine, 1044

Clemastine, 370

Cleocin®—*See* Clindamycin, 371 *and See* Clindamycin Phosphate Injection, 374

Cleocin T®—*See* Clindamycin, 371

Cleocin T® Pledgets—*See* Clindamycin, 371

Cleocin® Vaginal Ovules—*See* Clindamycin, 371

Climara®—*See* Estradiol Transdermal, 621

Clinda-Derm®—*See* Clindamycin, 371

Clindagel®—*See* Clindamycin, 371

Clindamycin, 371

Clindamycin and Benzoyl Peroxide Topical, 373

Clindamycin Phosphate Injection, 374

Clindets® Pledgets—*See* Clindamycin, 371

Clindex®—*See* Chlordiazepoxide and Clidinium Bromide, 312

Clinoril®—*See* Sulindac, 1613

Clioquinol Topical, 377

Clobetasol, 378

Clobevate®—*See* Clobetasol, 378

Clofarabine Injection, 379

Clolar®—*See* Clofarabine Injection, 379

Clomid®—*See* Clomiphene, 381

Clomiphene, 381

Clomipramine, 382

Clonazepam, 385

Clonidine Tablets and Skin Patches, 387

Clopidogrel, 391

ClorazeCaps®—*See* Clorazepate, 393

Clorazepate, 393

ClorazeTabs®—*See* Clorazepate, 393

Clorpres®—*See* Chlorthalidone, 324 *and See* Clonidine Tablets and Skin Patches, 387

Clotrimazole, 394

Clozapine, 397

Clozaril®—*See* Clozapine, 397

Codal®-DM Syrup—*See* Dextromethorphan, 477

Codeine Oral, 400

Codimal® DM Syrup—*See* Dextromethorphan, 477

Codimal® PH Syrup—*See* Codeine Oral, 400

Cogentin®—*See* Benztropine Mesylate Oral, 187

Co-gesic®—*See* Acetaminophen and Hydrocodone, 14

Cognex®—*See* Tacrine, 1621

Colace®—*See* Stool Softeners, 1605

Colazal®—*See* Balsalazide, 172

Colchicine Oral, 403

Colesevelam, 405

Colestid®—*See* Colestipol, 406

Colestid® Flavored Granules—*See* Colestipol, 406

Colestid® Granules—*See* Colestipol, 406

Colestipol, 406

Colistimethate Injection, 408

Collyrium Fresh®—*See* Tetrahydrozoline Ophthalmic, 1666

Col-Probenecid®—*See* Probenecid, 1448

Colrex® Compound—*See* Codeine Oral, 400

Coly-Mycin® M Parenteral—*See* Colistimethate Injection, 408

CoLyte®—*See* Polyethylene glycol-electrolyte solution (PEG-ES), 1420

Combivent®—*See* Ipratropium and Albuterol Inhalation, 924

Combivir®—*See* Lamivudine and Zidovudine, 975

Comhist®—*See* Chlorpheniramine, 318

Commit® Lozenges—*See* Nicotine Lozenges, 1235

Compazine®—*See* Prochlorperazine, 1451

Compazine® Spansule®—*See* Prochlorperazine, 1451

Compazine® Syrup—*See* Prochlorperazine, 1451

Compoz® Nighttime Sleep Aid—*See* Diphenhydramine Oral, 515

Compoz® Nighttime Sleep Aid Gelcaps®—*See* Diphenhydramine Oral, 515

Compro®—*See* Prochlorperazine, 1451

Comtan®—*See* Entacapone, 590

Comtrex® Allergy-Sinus Maximum Strength Tablets®—*See* Chlorpheniramine, 318

Comtrex® Cold & Cough Multi-Symptom Relief Maximum Strength Caplets®—*See* Dextromethorphan, 477

Comtrex® Cold & Cough Multi-Symptom Relief Maximum Strength Tablets®—*See* Dextromethorphan, 477

Comtrex® Cough & Cold Day-Night Maximum Strength Caplets®—*See* Dextromethorphan, 477

Comtrex® Deep Chest Cold Multi-Symptom Softgels®—*See* Dextromethorphan, 477

Comtrex® Non-Drowsy Maximum Strength Caplets®—*See* Dextromethorphan, 477

Comvax®—*See* Haemophilus influenzae type b Vaccine, 813 *and See* Hepatitis B Vaccine, 824

Concerta®—*See* Methylphenidate, 1120

Congestac® Caplets—*See* Guaifenesin, 811

Constilac® Syrup—*See* Lactulose, 970

Constulose®—*See* Lactulose, 970

Contac® Day & Night Cold/Flu Caplets®—*See* Dextromethorphan, 477

Contac® Severe Cold and Flu Maximum Strength Caplets®—*See* Dextromethorphan, 477

Contac® Severe Cold and Flu Non-Drowsy Caplets®—*See* Dextromethorphan, 477

Control Rx®—*See* Fluoride, 720

Copaxone®—*See* Glatiramer Injection, 791

Cope®—*See* Aspirin, 132

Copegus®—*See* Ribavirin, 1514

Coppertone®—*See* Sunscreens, 1620

Cordarone®—*See* Amiodarone Oral, 75

Cordran®—*See* Flurandrenolide Topical, 729

Cordran® SP—*See* Flurandrenolide Topical, 729

Cordran® Tape—*See* Flurandrenolide Topical, 729

Coreg®—*See* Carvedilol, 256

Coreg CR®—*See* Carvedilol, 256

Corgard®—*See* Nadolol, 1194

Coricidin® HBP® Cold & Flu—*See* Chlorpheniramine, 318

Coricidin® HBP® Flu Maximum Strength—*See* Dextromethorphan, 477

Coricidin® HBP® Cough & Cold—*See* Dextromethorphan, 477

Cormax®—*See* Clobetasol, 378

Cormax® Scalp Application—*See* Clobetasol, 378

Correctol® Caplets—*See* Bisacodyl, 197

Correctol® Tablets—*See* Bisacodyl, 197

CortaGel® Extra Strength—*See* Hydrocortisone Topical, 837

Cortaid® FastStick® Maximum Strength—*See* Hydrocortisone Topical, 837

Cortaid® Intensive Therapy—*See* Hydrocortisone Topical, 837

Cortaid® Maximum Strength—*See* Hydrocortisone Topical, 837

Cortaid® Sensitive Skin Formula—*See* Hydrocortisone Topical, 837

Cortaid® Spray Maximum Strength—*See* Hydrocortisone Topical, 837

Cortef®—*See* Hydrocortisone Oral, 835

Cortenema®—*See* Hydrocortisone Topical, 837

Corticaine®—*See* Hydrocortisone Topical, 837

Cortifoam®—*See* Hydrocortisone Topical, 837

Cortisporin®—*See* Hydrocortisone Topical, 837

Cortisporin Ophthalmic®—*See* Hydrocortisone, Neomycin, and Polymyxin, 833

Cortisporin® Ophthalmic Ointment—*See* Neomycin, Polymyxin, and Bacitracin Ophthalmic, 1220

Cortisporin® Ophthalmic Suspension—*See* Neomycin, Polymyxin, and Bacitracin Ophthalmic, 1220

Cortizone®-5—*See* Hydrocortisone Topical, 837

Cortizone-10®—*See* Hydrocortisone Topical, 837

Cortizone-10® External Anal Itch Relief Creme—*See* Hydrocortisone Topical, 837

Cortizone-10® Scalp Itch Formula Liquid—*See* Hydrocortisone Topical, 837

Cortizone for Kids®—*See* Hydrocortisone Topical, 837

Corzide®—*See* Nadolol, 1194

Cosopt®—*See* Dorzolamide and Timolol Ophthalmic, 537

Co-trimoxazole Injection, 409

Co-trimoxazole Oral, 411

Cough-X®—*See* Dextromethorphan, 477

Coumadin®—*See* Warfarin, 1782

Covera-HS®—*See* Verapamil, 1773

Cozaar®—*See* Losartan, 1048

Creon® 5 Minimicrospheres®—*See* Pancrelipase, 1334

Creon® 10 Minimicrospheres®—*See* Pancrelipase, 1334

Creon® 20 Minimicrospheres®—*See* Pancrelipase, 1334

Crestor®—*See* Rosuvastatin, 1546

Crixivan®—*See* Indinavir, 875

Cromolyn Sodium Nasal Solution, 414

Cromolyn Sodium Oral Inhalation, 416

Cutivate®—*See* Fluticasone Topical, 745

Cyanocobalamin Injection, 418

Cyanocobalamin Nasal, 419

Cyclobenzaprine, 421

Dimetapp® Cold & Fever—*See* Brompheniramine, 215

Dimetapp® Decongestant Infant Drops—*See* Pseudoephedrine, 1473

Dimetapp® Decongestant Plus Cough Infant Drops—*See* Dextromethorphan, 477

Dimetapp® DM Cold & Cough Elixir—*See* Dextromethorphan, 477

Dimetapp® Elixir—*See* Brompheniramine, 215

Dimetapp® Nighttime Flu Children's—*See* Dextromethorphan, 477

Dimetapp® Non-Drowsy Flu Children's—*See* Dextromethorphan, 477

Dinoprostone, 514

Diovan®—*See* Valsartan, 1760

Diovan® HCT—*See* Hydrochlorothiazide, 829 *and See* Valsartan, 1760

Dipentum®—*See* Olsalazine, 1285

Diphen® AF Elixir—*See* Diphenhydramine Oral, 515

Diphenhist®—*See* Diphenhydramine Oral, 515

Diphenhist® Captabs®—*See* Diphenhydramine Oral, 515

Diphenhydramine Hydrochloride Caplets®—*See* Diphenhydramine Oral, 515

Diphenhydramine Oral, 515

Diphenhydramine Topical, 518

Diphenoxylate and Atropine, 519

Diphtheria, Tetanus, and Pertussis (DTaP) Vaccine, 520

Dipivefrin Ophthalmic, 522

Diprolene®—*See* Betamethasone Topical, 189

Diprolene® AF—*See* Betamethasone Topical, 189

Diprolene® Lotion—*See* Betamethasone Topical, 189

Dipyridamole, 523

Disalcid®—*See* Salsalate§

Disopyramide, 524

Disulfiram, 527

Ditropan®—*See* Oxybutynin, 1316

Ditropan XL®—*See* Oxybutynin, 1316

Diuril®—*See* Chlorothiazide, 315

Doan's® P.M. Extra Strength Caplets®—*See* Diphenhydramine Oral, 515

Dobutamine Hydrochloride Injection§

Dobutrex® Solution—*See* Dobutamine Hydrochloride Injection§

Docetaxel§

Docusate®—*See* Stool Softeners, 1605

Dofetilide, 528

Dolasetron, 530

Dolasetron Mesylate Injection, 532

Dolobid®—*See* Diflunisal, 501

Dolophine®—*See* Methadone, 1103

Donatussin® Pediatric Drops—*See* Guaifenesin, 811

Donatussin® Syrup—*See* Dextromethorphan, 477

Donepezil, 534

Donnatal®—*See* Belladonna Alkaloid Combinations and Phenobarbital§

Donnatal Extentabs®—*See* Belladonna Alkaloid Combinations and Phenobarbital§

Dornase Alfa, 536

Doryx®—*See* Doxycycline, 547

Dorzolamide and Timolol Ophthalmic, 537

Dorzolamide Ophthalmic, 539

DOS®—*See* Stool Softeners, 1605

Doxazosin, 541

Doxepin, 543

Doxepin Topical, 546

Doxinate®—*See* Stool Softeners, 1605

Doxy 100®—*See* Doxycycline Injection, 554

Doxy 200®—*See* Doxycycline Injection, 554

Doxycycline, 547

Doxycycline Injection, 554

Doxylamine, 558

Dramamine®—*See* Dimenhydrinate, 512

Dramamine® Chewable—*See* Dimenhydrinate, 512

Dramamine® Less Drowsy—*See* Meclizine, 1065

Dristan® Cold—*See* Chlorpheniramine, 318

Dristan® Cold No Drowsiness Formula Maximum Strength Caplets®—*See* Acetaminophen, 10

Dristan® Sinus Caplets®—*See* Ibuprofen, 856

Drixoral® Allergy/Sinus—*See* Brompheniramine, 215

Drixoral® Cold & Allergy—*See* Brompheniramine, 215

Drixoral® Cold & Flu—*See* Brompheniramine, 215

Drixoral® Nasal Decongestant—*See* Pseudoephedrine, 1473

Droxia®—*See* Hydroxyurea, 846

Duac®—*See* Clindamycin, 371

Duetact®—*See* Pioglitazone, 1408

Dulcolax®—*See* Bisacodyl, 197 *and See* Stimulant Laxatives, 1604

Dulcolax® Bowel Prep Kit—*See* Bisacodyl, 197

Duloxetine, 559

Duoneb®—*See* Ipratropium and Albuterol Inhalation, 924

Duraclon®—*See* Clonidine Tablets and Skin Patches, 387

Duradrin®—*See* Acetaminophen, 10

Duragesic®—*See* Fentanyl Skin Patches, 687

Duramorph®—*See* Morphine Sulfate Injection, 1178

Duratuss®—*See* Guaifenesin, 811

Duratuss® DM Elixir—*See* Dextromethorphan, 477

Duratuss® GP—*See* Guaifenesin, 811

Dura-Vent/®DA—*See* Chlorpheniramine, 318

Duricef®—*See* Cefadroxil, 261

Dutasteride, 562

Dyazide®—*See* Triamterene and Hydrochlorothiazide, 1735

Dyflex®-G—*See* Guaifenesin, 811

Dy-G®—*See* Guaifenesin, 811

Dynacin®—*See* Minocycline Oral, 1154

DynaCirc®—*See* Isradipine, 948

DynaCirc® CR®—*See* Isradipine, 948

Dyphylline GG®—*See* Guaifenesin, 811

Dyphylline GG® Elixir—*See* Guaifenesin, 811

Dyrenium®—*See* Triamterene, 1733

E

Easprin®—*See* Aspirin, 132

EC-Naprosyn®—*See* Naproxen, 1205

Econazole Topical, 564

Econopred® Plus—*See* Prednisolone Ophthalmic, 1437

Ecotrin®—*See* Aspirin, 132

Ecotrin® Adult Low Strength—*See* Aspirin, 132

Ecotrin® Maximum Strength—*See* Aspirin, 132

Edecrin®—*See* Ethacrynic Acid, 649

Edex®—*See* Alprostadil, 59

Efalizumab Injection, 565

Efavirenz, 568

Effexor®—*See* Venlafaxine, 1769

Effexor® XR—*See* Venlafaxine, 1769

Efidac 24® Chlorpheniramine—*See* Chlorpheniramine, 318

Efidac 24® Pseudoephedrine—*See* Pseudoephedrine, 1473

Eflornithine, 571

Efudex®—*See* Fluorouracil Topical, 721

Eldepryl®—*See* Selegiline, 1561

Elestat®—*See* Epinastine Ophthalmic, 593

Eletriptan, 573

Elidel®—*See* Pimecrolimus Topical, 1401

Eligard®—*See* Leuprolide, 995

Elimite®—*See* Permethrin, 1380

Elixophyllin®—*See* Theophylline§

Elixophyllin®-GG—*See* Guaifenesin, 811

Elmiron®—*See* Pentosan Polysulfate, 1376

Elocon®—*See* Mometasone Furoate, 1169

E-Lor®—*See* Acetaminophen and Propoxyphene, 16 *and See* Propoxyphene, 1464

Eloxatin®—*See* Oxaliplatin Injection, 1303

Embeline® E—*See* Clobetasol, 378

Emend®—*See* Aprepitant, 127

Empirin with Codeine®—*See* Aspirin and Codeine, 139

Emsam®—*See* Selegiline Transdermal, 1563

Emtricitabine, 575

Emtriva®—*See* Emtricitabine, 575

Enablex®—*See* Darifenacin, 444

Enalapril, 577

Enalapril and Felodipine, 580

Enalapril and Hydrochlorothiazide, 582

Enbrel®—*See* Etanercept Injection, 646

Endal®—*See* Guaifenesin, 811

Endocet®—*See* Acetaminophen and Oxycodone, 15

Endocodone®—*See* Oxycodone, 1321

Endodan®—*See* Oxycodone and Aspirin, 1323

Endolor®—*See* Acetaminophen, Butalbital, and Caffeine, 17

Enduron®—*See* Methyclothiazide, 1115

Enfuvirtide Injection, 584

Engerix-B®—*See* Hepatitis B Vaccine, 824

Enjuvia®—*See* Estrogen, 624

Enoxaparin Injection, 587

Entacapone, 590

Entecavir, 591

Entex® PSE—*See* Guaifenesin, 811

Enulose®—*See* Lactulose, 970

Enzone®—*See* Hydrocortisone Topical, 837

Epifoam®—*See* Hydrocortisone Topical, 837

Epinastine Ophthalmic, 593

Epinephrine Injection, 595

EpiPen® Auto-Injector—*See* Epinephrine Injection, 595

EpiPen® Jr. Auto-Injector—*See* Epinephrine Injection, 595

Epitol®—*See* Carbamazepine, 250

Epivir®—*See* Lamivudine, 972

Epivir-HBV®—*See* Lamivudine, 972

Eplerenone, 598

Epoetin Alfa Injection, 600

Epogen®—*See* Epoetin Alfa Injection, 600

Eprosartan, 604

Epzicom®—*See* Lamivudine, 972

Epzicon®—*See* Abacavir, 1

Equagesic®—*See* Aspirin, 132 *and See* Meprobamate, 1090

Equetro®—*See* Carbamazepine, 250

Erbitux®—*See* Cetuximab Injection, 306

Ercaf®—*See* Ergotamine and Caffeine§

Ergo-Caff®—*See* Ergotamine and Caffeine§

Ergoloid Mesylates§

Ergotamine and Caffeine§

Erlotinib, 606

ERYC®—*See* Erythromycin, 608

Fluvastatin, **746**

Fluvirin®—*See* Influenza Vaccine, Inactivated, 1731

Fluvoxamine, **748**

Fluzone®—*See* Influenza Vaccine, Inactivated, 1731

FML-S®—*See* Sulfacetamide Ophthalmic, 1607

Focalin®—*See* Dexmethylphenidate, 466

Folic Acid, **751**

Folvite®—*See* Folic Acid, 751

Foradil® Aerolizer® Inhaler—*See* Formoterol, 752

Formoterol, **752**

Fortabs®—*See* Aspirin, 132

Fortamet®—*See* Metformin, 1098

Fortaz®—*See* Ceftazidime Injection, 283

Forteo®—*See* Teriparatide (rDNA origin) Injection, 1649

Fortovase®—*See* Saquinavir, 1553

Fosamax®—*See* Alendronate, 46

Fosamax Plus D®—*See* Alendronate, 46

Fosamprenavir, **756**

Foscarnet Sodium Injection§

Foscavir®—*See* Foscarnet Sodium Injection§

Fosfomycin, **758**

Fosinopril, **759**

Fosrenol®—*See* Lanthanum, 986

Fostex®—*See* Benzoyl Peroxide, 186

Fragmin®—*See* Dalteparin Sodium Injection, 432

Frova®—*See* Frovatriptan, 762

Frovatriptan, **762**

Fulvestrant Injection, **763**

Fulvicin-U/F®—*See* Griseofulvin, 810

Fungizone® Intravenous—*See* Amphotericin B Injection, 96

Fungoid®—*See* Miconazole, 1149

Fungoid® Solution—*See* Clotrimazole, 394

Furadantin®—*See* Nitrofurantoin, 1248

Furosemide, **765**

Fuzeon®—*See* Enfuvirtide Injection, 584

G

Gabapentin, **767**

Gabarone®—*See* Gabapentin, 767

Gabitril®—*See* Tiagabine, 1675

Galantamine, **769**

Gammagard® S/D—*See* Immune Globulin Intravenous Injection, 872

Gamunex® 10%—*See* Immune Globulin Intravenous Injection, 872

Ganciclovir, **772**

Ganciclovir Injection, **775**

Ganidin® NR—*See* Guaifenesin, 811

Gani-Tuss® DM NR—*See* Dextromethorphan, 477

Gani-Tuss® NR—*See* Codeine Oral, 400 *and See* Guaifenesin, 811

Garamycin®—*See* Gentamicin Sulfate Injection, 788

Gardasil®—*See* Human Papillomavirus (HPV) Vaccine, 826

GasAid® Maximum Strength Softgels®—*See* Simethicone, 1578

Gas-X®—*See* Simethicone, 1578

Gas-X® Extra Strength—*See* Simethicone, 1578

Gas-X® Extra Strength Liquid—*See* Simethicone, 1578

Gas-X® Extra Strength Softgels®—*See* Simethicone, 1578

Gatifloxacin Ophthalmic, **779**

Gefitinib, **781**

Gel-Kam®—*See* Fluoride, 720

Gel-Kam® Oral Care Rinse—*See* Fluoride, 720

Gelpirin®—*See* Acetaminophen, 10 *and See* Aspirin, 132

Gel-Tin®—*See* Fluoride, 720

Gemfibrozil, **783**

Gemifloxacin, **784**

Genacote®—*See* Aspirin, 132

Genacote® Maximum Strength—*See* Aspirin, 132

Genagesic®—*See* Acetaminophen and Propoxyphene, 16

Genahist®—*See* Diphenhydramine Oral, 515

Genahist® Elixir—*See* Diphenhydramine Oral, 515

Genapap®—*See* Acetaminophen, 10

Genapap® Children's—*See* Acetaminophen, 10

Genapap® Drops Infant's—*See* Acetaminophen, 10

Genapap® Extra Strength Caplets®—*See* Acetaminophen, 10

Genapap® Extra Strength Tablets—*See* Acetaminophen, 10

Genapap® Gel-Coat Caplets®—*See* Acetaminophen, 10

Genaphed®—*See* Pseudoephedrine, 1473

Genasyme®—*See* Simethicone, 1578

Genasyme® Drops—*See* Simethicone, 1578

Genebs®—*See* Acetaminophen, 10

Genebs® Extra Strength Caplets®—*See* Acetaminophen, 10

Genebs® Extra Strength Tablets—*See* Acetaminophen, 10

Generlac®—*See* Lactulose, 970

Gengraf®—*See* Cyclosporine, 422

Genora®—*See* Estrogen and Progestin (Oral Contraceptives), 633

Genpril® Caplets®—*See* Ibuprofen, 856

Genpril® Tablets—*See* Ibuprofen, 856

Gentak®—*See* Gentamicin Ophthalmic, 786

Gentamicin Ophthalmic, **786**

Gentamicin Sulfate Injection, **788**

Gentasol®—*See* Gentamicin Ophthalmic, 786

Gentlax®—*See* Stimulant Laxatives, 1604

GenXene®—*See* Clorazepate, 393

Geodon®—*See* Ziprasidone, 1797

Gerimal®—*See* Ergoloid Mesylates§

Glatiramer Injection, **791**

Gleevec®—*See* Imatinib, 860

Glimepiride, **793**

Glipizide, **796**

GlucaGen Diagnostic Kit®—*See* Glucagon, 799

Glucagon, **799**

Glucophage®—*See* Metformin, 1098

Glucophage® XR—*See* Metformin, 1098

Glucotrol®—*See* Glipizide, 796

Glucovance®—*See* Glyburide and Metformin, 802

Glu-K®—*See* Potassium, 1422

Glyburide, **800**

Glyburide and Metformin, **802**

Glycopyrrolate, **805**

Glynase®—*See* Glyburide, 800

Glyset®—*See* Miglitol, 1152

GoLYTELY®—*See* Polyethylene glycol-electrolyte solution (PEG-ES), 1420

Goody's® Body Pain Powders—*See* Aspirin, 132

Goody's® Extra Strength Headache Powders—*See* Aspirin, 132

Goody's® Extra Strength Tablets—*See* Acetaminophen, 10 *and See* Aspirin, 132

Goody's® Fast Pain Relief Tablets—*See* Acetaminophen, 10

Goody's® Headache Powders—*See* Acetaminophen, 10

Goody's® PM Powder—*See* Diphenhydramine Oral, 515

Granisetron, **807**

Granisetron Hydrochloride Injection, **808**

Grifulvin V®—*See* Griseofulvin, 810

Griseofulvin, **810**

Gris-PEG®—*See* Griseofulvin, 810

Guaifed®-PD—*See* Guaifenesin, 811

Guaifed® Syrup—*See* Guaifenesin, 811

Guaifenesin, **811**

Guaifenesin AC® Liquid—*See* Guaifenesin, 811

Guaifenesin DAC®—*See* Codeine Oral, 400

Guaifenesin DM®—*See* Dextromethorphan, 477

Guaifenex® DM—*See* Dextromethorphan, 477

Guaifenex® PSE 120—*See* Guaifenesin, 811

Guaifenex® PSE 60—*See* Guaifenesin, 811

Guaifenex®-Rx 14-Day Treatment Regimen—*See* Guaifenesin, 811

Guaifenex®-Rx DM 14-Day Treatment Regimen—*See* Dextromethorphan, 477

GuaiMax-D®—*See* Guaifenesin, 811

Guanabenz§

Guanfacine§

Guiatuss AC® Syrup—*See* Codeine Oral, 400 *and See* Guaifenesin, 811

Guiatuss DAC® Syrup—*See* Codeine Oral, 400

Guiatuss DM®—*See* Dextromethorphan, 477

Guiatussin® DAC Syrup—*See* Codeine Oral, 400

Guiatussin® with Codeine—*See* Codeine Oral, 400

Guiatuss® Syrup—*See* Guaifenesin, 811

Gynazole-1®—*See* Butoconazole Vaginal Cream, 232

Gynecort® 10—*See* Hydrocortisone Topical, 837

Gyne-Lotrimin®—*See* Clotrimazole, 394

Gyne-Lotrimin®-3—*See* Clotrimazole, 394

Gyne-Lotrimin® 3 Combination Pack—*See* Clotrimazole, 394

Gynodiol®—*See* Estrogen, 624

H

Haemophilus influenzae type b Vaccine, **813**

Halcinonide Topical, **814**

Halcion®—*See* Triazolam, 1737

Haldol®—*See* Haloperidol Oral, 816

Haldol® Concentrate—*See* Haloperidol Oral, 816

Halfprin®—*See* Aspirin, 132

Halobetasol, **815**

Halog®—*See* Halcinonide Topical, 814

Halog®-E—*See* Halcinonide Topical, 814

Haloperidol Intensol®—*See* Haloperidol Oral, 816

Haloperidol Oral, **816**

Halotestin®—*See* Fluoxymesterone, 726

Halotussin® AC—*See* Guaifenesin, 811

Haltran®—*See* Ibuprofen, 856

HaNew Riversin® AC—*See* Codeine Oral, 400

HaNew Riversin® DAC—*See* Codeine Oral, 400

Haponal®—*See* Belladonna Alkaloid Combinations and Phenobarbital§

Havrix®—*See* Hepatitis A Vaccine, 823

Hawaiian Tropic®—*See* Sunscreens, 1620

Head and Shoulders Intensive Treatment Dandruff Shampoo®—*See* Selenium Sulfide, 1566

Helidac®—*See* Bismuth Subsalicylate, Metronidazole, and Tetracycline Combination, 201

Karigel® Maintenance-Neutral— *See* Fluoride, 720

Karigel® Professional APF Topical Gel with 0.1 M phosphate at pH 3.5— *See* Fluoride, 720

Kay Ciel®— *See* Potassium, 1422

Kayexalate®— *See* Sodium Polystyrene Sulfonate, 1590

K⁺ Care®— *See* Potassium, 1422

K⁺ Care® Effervescent Tablets— *See* Potassium, 1422

K-Dur® 10— *See* Potassium, 1422

K-Dur® 20— *See* Potassium, 1422

Keflex® Pulvules®— *See* Cephalexin, 301

Kemadrin®— *See* Procyclidine, 1453

Kenalog®— *See* Triamcinolone Topical, 1731

Kenalog® in Orabase®— *See* Triamcinolone Topical, 1731

Kenalog® Spray— *See* Triamcinolone Topical, 1731

Kepivance®— *See* Palifermin, 1327

Keppra®— *See* Levetiracetam, 1001

Ketek®— *See* Telithromycin, 1635

Ketoconazole, 954

Ketoconazole Topical, 957

Ketoprofen, 959

Ketorolac, 962

Ketorolac Ophthalmic, 965

Ketotifen Ophthalmic, 967

KG-Fed® Expectorant Syrup— *See* Codeine Oral, 400

KG-Fed® Pediatric Expectorant Syrup— *See* Codeine Oral, 400

KG-Fed® Syrup— *See* Codeine Oral, 400

Kidkare® Cough & Cold Liquid— *See* Dextromethorphan, 477

Kidkare® Decongestant Drops— *See* Pseudoephedrine, 1473

Kineret®— *See* Anakinra, 117

Kionex®— *See* Sodium Polystyrene Sulfonate, 1590

Klonopin®— *See* Clonazepam, 385

K-Lor®— *See* Potassium, 1422

Klor-Con® 8— *See* Potassium, 1422

Klor-Con® 10— *See* Potassium, 1422

Klor-Con®/EF— *See* Potassium, 1422

Klor-Con® Powder— *See* Potassium, 1422

Klor-Con®/25 Powder— *See* Potassium, 1422

Klotrix®— *See* Potassium, 1422

K-Lyte/CL® 50 Effervescent Tablets— *See* Potassium, 1422

K-Lyte/CL® Effervescent Tablets— *See* Potassium, 1422

K-Lyte® DS Effervescent Tablets— *See* Potassium, 1422

K-Lyte® Effervescent Tablets— *See* Potassium, 1422

Koate®-DVI— *See* Antihemophilic Factor (Human), 120

Kogenate® FS— *See* Antihemophilic Factor (Recombinant), 121

Kolephrin® Caplets®— *See* Chlorpheniramine, 318

Konsyl®— *See* Psyllium, 1476

Kristalose®— *See* Lactulose, 970

Kronofed-A-Jr.® Kronocaps®— *See* Chlorpheniramine, 318

Kronofed-A® Kronocaps®— *See* Chlorpheniramine, 318

K-Tab® Filmtab®— *See* Potassium, 1422

Ku-Zyme® HP— *See* Pancrelipase, 1334

Kytril®— *See* Granisetron, 807 *and See* Granisetron Hydrochloride Injection, 808

L

Labetalol Oral, 969

LactiCare®-HC— *See* Hydrocortisone Topical, 837

Lactulose, 970

Lamictal®— *See* Lamotrigine, 977

Lamisil®— *See* Terbinafine, 1645

Lamisil® AT— *See* Terbinafine, 1645

Lamivudine, 972

Lamivudine and Zidovudine, 975

Lamotrigine, 977

Lanacort® 10— *See* Hydrocortisone Topical, 837

Lanoxicaps®— *See* Digoxin Oral, 503

Lanoxin®— *See* Digoxin Oral, 503

Lanoxin® Elixir Pediatric— *See* Digoxin Oral, 503

Lansoprazole, 982

Lansoprazole/Clarithromycin/Amoxicillin, 984

Lanthanum, 986

Lantus®— *See* Insulin Glargine (rDNA origin) Injection, 894

Lariam®— *See* Mefloquine, 1074

Lasix®— *See* Furosemide, 765

Latanoprost, 987

Lazersporin-C®— *See* Hydrocortisone Topical, 837

Ledercillin VK®— *See* Penicillin V Potassium Oral, 1367

Leflunomide, 988

Legatrin PM® Caplets®— *See* Diphenhydramine Oral, 515

Lescol®— *See* Fluvastatin, 746

Lescol® XL— *See* Fluvastatin, 746

Letrozole, 990

Leucovorin Calcium, 992

Leukine®— *See* Sargramostim Injection, 1556

Leuprolide, 995

Levalbuterol Oral Inhalation, 999

Levaquin®— *See* Levofloxacin Oral, 1010

Levaquin® in Dextrose Injection Premix— *See* Levofloxacin Injection, 1007

Levatol®— *See* Penbutolol, 1357

Levbid®— *See* Hyoscyamine, 850

Levemir®— *See* Insulin Detemir (rDNA Origin) Injection, 891

Levetiracetam, 1001

Levitra®— *See* Vardenafil, 1764

Levlen®— *See* Estrogen and Progestin (Oral Contraceptives), 633

Levlite®— *See* Estrogen and Progestin (Oral Contraceptives), 633

Levobunolol Ophthalmic, 1003

Levocarnitine Injection§

Levodopa and Carbidopa, 1004

Levo-Dromoran®— *See* Levorphanol Oral, 1014

Levofloxacin Injection, 1007

Levofloxacin Oral, 1010

Levora®— *See* Estrogen and Progestin (Oral Contraceptives), 633

Levorphanol Oral, 1014

Levothroid®— *See* Levothyroxine, 1015

Levothyroxine, 1015

Levoxyl®— *See* Levothyroxine, 1015

Levsin®— *See* Hyoscyamine, 850

Levsin® Drops— *See* Hyoscyamine, 850

Levsinex® Timecaps®— *See* Hyoscyamine, 850

Levsin®/SL— *See* Hyoscyamine, 850

Lexapro®— *See* Escitalopram, 611

Lexiva— *See* Fosamprenavir, 756

Lexxel®— *See* Enalapril and Felodipine, 580

Librax®— *See* Chlordiazepoxide and Clidinium Bromide, 312

Librium®— *See* Chlordiazepoxide, 309

Lice Treatment® Maximum Strength Shampoo— *See* Pyrethrin and Piperonyl Butoxide, 1479

Licide®— *See* Pyrethrin and Piperonyl Butoxide, 1479

Lidex®— *See* Fluocinolone Topical, 716 *and See* Fluocinonide Topical, 718

Lidex-E®— *See* Fluocinonide Topical, 718

Lidex®-E Emollient Cream— *See* Fluocinolone Topical, 716

Lidex® Gel— *See* Fluocinolone Topical, 716

Lidocaine Transdermal, 1017

Lidocaine Viscous, 1019

Lidoderm®— *See* Lidocaine Transdermal, 1017

Limbitrol®— *See* Amitriptyline, 78 *and See* Chlordiazepoxide, 309

Limbitrol® DS— *See* Amitriptyline, 78 *and See* Chlordiazepoxide, 309

Lindane, 1020

Linezolid, 1023

Lioresal®— *See* Baclofen Oral, 170

Liothyronine, 1025

Lipitor®— *See* Atorvastatin, 151

Lipram® 4500— *See* Pancrelipase, 1334

Lipram®-CR5— *See* Pancrelipase, 1334

Lipram®-CR10— *See* Pancrelipase, 1334

Lipram®-CR20— *See* Pancrelipase, 1334

Lipram®-PN16— *See* Pancrelipase, 1334

Lipram®-PN10— *See* Pancrelipase, 1334

Lipram®-PN20— *See* Pancrelipase, 1334

Lipram®-UL12— *See* Pancrelipase, 1334

Lipram®-UL18— *See* Pancrelipase, 1334

Lipram®-UL20— *See* Pancrelipase, 1334

Liquid Pedvax HIB®— *See* Haemophilus influenzae type b Vaccine, 813

Liquiprin® Drops— *See* Acetaminophen, 10

Lisdexamfetamine, 1027

Lisinopril, 1029

Lisinopril and Hydrochlorothiazide, 1032

Lithium, 1034

Lithobid®— *See* Lithium, 1034

Locholest®— *See* Cholestyramine Resin, 327

Locholest® Light— *See* Cholestyramine Resin, 327

Locoid®— *See* Hydrocortisone Topical, 837

Lodine®— *See* Etodolac, 655

Lodine® XL— *See* Etodolac, 655

Lodoxamide Ophthalmic, 1037

Lodrane®— *See* Brompheniramine, 215

Lodrane® LD— *See* Brompheniramine, 215

Loestrin®— *See* Estrogen and Progestin (Oral Contraceptives), 633

Loestrin® Fe— *See* Estrogen and Progestin (Oral Contraceptives), 633

Lofibra®— *See* Fenofibrate, 678

Lomotil®— *See* Diphenoxylate and Atropine, 519

Lonide®— *See* Fluocinonide Topical, 718

Loniten®— *See* Minoxidil Oral, 1157

Lonox®— *See* Diphenoxylate and Atropine, 519

Lo/Ovral®— *See* Estrogen and Progestin (Oral Contraceptives), 633

Loperamide, 1039

Lopid®— *See* Gemfibrozil, 783

Lopinavir and Ritonavir, 1041

Lopressor®— *See* Metoprolol, 1139

Lopressor® HCT— *See* Hydrochlorothiazide, 829 *and See* Metoprolol, 1139

Loratadine, 1044

Lorazepam, 1046

Lorazepam Intensol®— *See* Lorazepam, 1046

Lorcet-HD®— *See* Acetaminophen and Hydrocodone, 14

Orphenadrine, 1296
Ortho-Cept®—*See* Estrogen and Progestin (Oral Contraceptives), 633
Ortho-Cyclen®—*See* Estrogen and Progestin (Oral Contraceptives), 633
Ortho Evra®—*See* Norelgestromin and Ethinyl Estradiol Transdermal System, 1258
Ortho-Novum®—*See* Estrogen and Progestin (Oral Contraceptives), 633
Ortho-Prefest®—*See* Estrogen and Progestin (Hormone Replacement Therapy), 631
Ortho Tri-Cyclen®—*See* Estrogen and Progestin (Oral Contraceptives), 633
Os-Cal 500®—*See* Calcium Carbonate, 242
Oseltamivir, 1298
Otocort Ear Solution®—*See* Hydrocortisone, Neomycin, and Polymyxin, 833
Otosporin®—*See* Hydrocortisone, Neomycin, and Polymyxin, 833
Ovcon®—*See* Estrogen and Progestin (Oral Contraceptives), 633
Ovral®—*See* Estrogen and Progestin (Oral Contraceptives), 633
Ovrette®—*See* Progestin-Only Oral Contraceptives, 1457
Oxacillin Sodium Injection, 1301
Oxaliplatin Injection, 1303
Oxandrin®—*See* Oxandrolone, 1305
Oxandrolone, 1305
Oxaprozin, 1307
Oxazepam, 1310
Oxcarbazepine, 1311
Oxiconazole, 1314
Oxistat®—*See* Oxiconazole, 1314
Oxy 10®—*See* Benzoyl Peroxide, 186
Oxybutynin, 1316
Oxybutynin Transdermal, 1318
Oxycodone, 1321
Oxycodone and Aspirin, 1323
OxyContin®—*See* Oxycodone, 1321
Oxydose®—*See* Oxycodone, 1321
OxyFast®—*See* Oxycodone, 1321
OxyIR®—*See* Oxycodone, 1321
Oxytocin Injection, 1325
Oxytrol®—*See* Oxybutynin Transdermal, 1318

P

P-A-C® Analgesic—*See* Aspirin, 132
Pacerone®—*See* Amiodarone Oral, 75
Palifermin, 1327
Paliperidone, 1328
Palivizumab Injection, 1330
Pamelor®—*See* Nortriptyline, 1264
Pamidronate Injection, 1331
Pamprin® Maximum Pain Relief Caplets®—*See* Acetaminophen, 10
Pamprin® Multi-Symptom—*See* Acetaminophen, 10
Panacet®—*See* Acetaminophen and Hydrocodone, 14
Pancrease®—*See* Pancrelipase, 1334
Pancrease® MT 16—*See* Pancrelipase, 1334
Pancrease® MT 4—*See* Pancrelipase, 1334
Pancrease® MT 10—*See* Pancrelipase, 1334
Pancrease® MT 20—*See* Pancrelipase, 1334
Pancrecarb® MS-16—*See* Pancrelipase, 1334
Pancrecarb® MS-4—*See* Pancrelipase, 1334
Pancrecarb® MS-8—*See* Pancrelipase, 1334
Pancrelipase, 1334
Pandel®—*See* Hydrocortisone Topical, 837
Pangestyme®—*See* Pancrelipase, 1334

Pangestyme® CN 10—*See* Pancrelipase, 1334
Pangestyme® CN 20—*See* Pancrelipase, 1334
Pangestyme® MT 16—*See* Pancrelipase, 1334
Pangestyme® UL 12—*See* Pancrelipase, 1334
Pangestyme® UL 18—*See* Pancrelipase, 1334
Pangestyme® UL 20—*See* Pancrelipase, 1334
Panokase®—*See* Pancrelipase, 1334
Panokase® 16—*See* Pancrelipase, 1334
PanOxyl®—*See* Benzoyl Peroxide, 186
Panretin®—*See* Alitretinoin, 52
Pantoprazole, 1335
Papaverine, 1337
Parafon Forte® DSC Caplets®—*See* Chlorzoxazone, 326
Para-Time® SR—*See* Papaverine, 1337
Parcopa®—*See* Levodopa and Carbidopa, 1004
Paregoric, 1338
Parlodel®—*See* Bromocriptine, 213
Parlodel® SnapTabs®—*See* Bromocriptine, 213
Parnate®—*See* Tranylcypromine, 1715
Paroxetine, 1339
Patanol®—*See* Olopatadine Ophthalmic, 1283
Paxil®—*See* Paroxetine, 1339
Paxil® CR—*See* Paroxetine, 1339
PC-CAP®—*See* Aspirin, 132 *and See* Propoxyphene, 1464
PCE® Dispertab®—*See* Erythromycin, 608
PediaCare® Cough-Cold Chewables—*See* Dextromethorphan, 477
Pediacare® Decongestant Plus Cough Infant Drops—*See* Dextromethorphan, 477
PediaCare® Decongestant Plus Cough Infant's Drops—*See* Guaifenesin, 811
PediaCare® Infants' Oral Decongestant Drops—*See* Pseudoephedrine, 1473
Pediacare® Long-Acting Cough Plus Cold—*See* Dextromethorphan, 477
PediaCare® Multisymptom Cold Liquid—*See* Dextromethorphan, 477
PediaCare® NightRest Cough-Cold Formula—*See* Dextromethorphan, 477
Pediacof® Cough Syrup—*See* Codeine Oral, 400
Pediaflor® Drops—*See* Fluoride, 720
Pedia Relief®—*See* Pseudoephedrine, 1473
Pediazole®—*See* Erythromycin and Sulfisoxazole, 610
Pedi-Dri®—*See* Nystatin, 1267
Pegasys®—*See* Peginterferon alfa-2a, 1343
Peginterferon Alfa-2a, 1343
Peginterferon Alfa-2b, 1349
PEG-Intron®—*See* Peginterferon Alfa-2b, 1349
Pemetrexed Injection, 1355
Penbutolol, 1357
Penciclovir Cream, 1358
Penecort®—*See* Hydrocortisone Topical, 837
Penicillin G Potassium or Sodium Injection, 1359
Penicillin V Potassium Oral, 1367
Penlac® Nail Lacquer—*See* Ciclopirox Topical Solution, 331
Pentacarinat®—*See* Pentamidine Inhalation, 1369
Pentam®—*See* Pentamidine Isethionate Injection, 1371
Pentam® 300—*See* Pentamidine Inhalation, 1369
Pentamidine Inhalation, 1369
Pentamidine Isethionate Injection, 1371
Pentasa®—*See* Mesalamine, 1091
Pentazocine and Naloxone, 1373
Pentobarbital Oral and Rectal, 1375
Pentosan Polysulfate, 1376
Pentoxifylline, 1377
Pentoxil®—*See* Pentoxifylline, 1377
Pen-Vee K®—*See* Penicillin V Potassium Oral, 1367

Pepcid®—*See* Famotidine, 669
Pepcid® AC—*See* Famotidine, 669
Pepcid® AC Gelcaps—*See* Famotidine, 669
Pepcid® AC Maximum Strength—*See* Famotidine, 669
Pepcid® Complete—*See* Famotidine, 669
Pepcid I.V.—*See* Famotidine Injection, 672
Pepcid Premixed in Iso-osmotic Sodium Chloride Injection—*See* Famotidine Injection, 672
Pepcid® RPD—*See* Famotidine, 669
Pepto-Bismol®—*See* Bismuth Subsalicylate, 669
Percocet®—*See* Acetaminophen and Oxycodone, 15
Percodan®—*See* Oxycodone and Aspirin, 1323
Percodan®-Demi—*See* Aspirin, 132
Percogesic®—*See* Acetaminophen, 10
Percogesic® Aspirin-Free Caplets® Extra Strength—*See* Diphenhydramine Oral, 515
Percogesic® Extra Strength Caplets®—*See* Acetaminophen, 10
Percolone®—*See* Oxycodone, 1321
Perdiem Fiber®—*See* Psyllium, 1476
Periactin®—*See* Cyproheptadine, 430
Perindopril, 1378
Permethrin, 1380
Perphenazine Oral, 1382
Persantine®—*See* Dipyridamole, 523
Pertussin® DM Extra Strength—*See* Dextromethorphan, 477
Pexeva®—*See* Paroxetine, 1339
Pfizerpen®—*See* Penicillin G Potassium or Sodium Injection, 1359
Phanasin® Diabetic Choice®—*See* Guaifenesin, 811
Phazyme® Infant Drops—*See* Simethicone, 1578
Phazyme®-166 Maximum Strength—*See* Simethicone, 1578
Phazyme®-166 Maximum Strength Softgels®—*See* Simethicone, 1578
Phazyme®-125 Softgels®—*See* Simethicone, 1578
Phenadoz®—*See* Promethazine, 1458
Phenaphen with Codeine (No.3 and No.4)®—*See* Acetaminophen and Codeine, 13
Phenazopyridine, 1383
Phenelzine, 1385
Phenergan®—*See* Promethazine, 1458
Phenergan® VC with Codeine Syrup—*See* Codeine Oral, 400
Phenergan® with Codeine Syrup—*See* Codeine Oral, 400
Phenergan® with Dextromethorphan Syrup—*See* Dextromethorphan, 477
Phenhist® DH with Codeine Modified Formula—*See* Codeine Oral, 400
Phenobarbital, 1388
Phenoxybenzamine, 1390
Phentermine, 1391
Phenylephrine, 1393
Phenytek®—*See* Phenytoin Oral, 1394
Phenytoin Oral, 1394
Phillips Milk of Magnesia®—*See* Magnesium Hydroxide, 1059
Phos-Flur® Gel—*See* Fluoride, 720
Phrenilin®—*See* Acetaminophen, 10
Phrenilin® Forte—*See* Acetaminophen, 10
Phytonadione, 1397
Pilocarpine Ophthalmic, 1399
Pilopine HS®—*See* Pilocarpine Ophthalmic, 1399
Pimecrolimus Topical, 1401
Pimozide, 1404

Readicat®—*See* Barium Sulfate, 173

Re-Azo®—*See* Phenazopyridine, 1383

Rebetol®—*See* Ribavirin, 1514

Rebif®—*See* Interferon Beta-1a Subcutaneous Injection, 917

Recombinate®—*See* Antihemophilic Factor (Recombinant), 121

Recombivax HB®—*See* Hepatitis B Vaccine, 824

Reese's® Pinworm Medicine—*See* Pyrantel, 1477

Reese's® Pinworm Medicine Caplets®—*See* Pyrantel, 1477

ReFacto®—*See* Antihemophilic Factor (Recombinant), 121

Reglan®—*See* Metoclopramide Hydrochloride Injection, 1134 *and See* Metoclopramide Oral, 1136

Reglan® Syrup—*See* Metoclopramide Oral, 1136

Regranex®—*See* Becaplermin, 175

Relafen®—*See* Nabumetone, 1191

Relenza®—*See* Zanamivir Inhalation, 1790

Relpax®—*See* Eletriptan, 573

Remeron®—*See* Mirtazapine, 1160

Remeron® SolTab®—*See* Mirtazapine, 1160

Remicade®—*See* Infliximab Injection, 881

Renagel®—*See* Sevelamer§

Renova® Emollient—*See* Tretinoin, 1723

Repaglinide, 1509

Repan®—*See* Acetaminophen, Butalbital, and Caffeine, 17

Requip®—*See* Ropinirole, 1540

Rescon®—*See* Chlorpheniramine, 318

Rescon®-DM—*See* Dextromethorphan, 477

Rescon®-ED—*See* Chlorpheniramine, 318

Rescon® GG—*See* Guaifenesin, 811

Rescon® JR—*See* Chlorpheniramine, 318

Rescriptor®—*See* Delavirdine, 449

Reserpine, 1511

Respahist®—*See* Brompheniramine, 215

Respaire®-120 SR—*See* Guaifenesin, 811

Respaire®-60 SR—*See* Guaifenesin, 811

Respa-1st®—*See* Guaifenesin, 811

Restasis®—*See* Cyclosporine Ophthalmic, 429

Restoril®—*See* Temazepam, 1639

Retapamulin, 1513

Retin-A®—*See* Tretinoin, 1723

Retin-A® Micro®—*See* Tretinoin, 1723

Retrovir®—*See* Zidovudine Injection§

Retrovir®—*See* Zidovudine Oral, 1793

Retrovir® I.V. Infusion—*See* Zidovudine Injection§

Retrovir® Syrup—*See* Zidovudine Oral, 1793

Rev-Eyes®—*See* Dapiprazole Ophthalmic, 438

ReVia®—*See* Naltrexone, 1202

Reyataz®—*See* Atazanavir, 142

Rheumatrex®—*See* Methotrexate, 1110

Rhinatate®—*See* Chlorpheniramine, 318

Rhinocort® Aqua Nasal Spray—*See* Budesonide, 216

Ribavirin, 1514

Ridaura®—*See* Auranofin, 155

RID® Maximum Strength Lice Killing Shampoo—*See* Pyrethrin and Piperonyl Butoxide, 1479

RID® Mousse—*See* Pyrethrin and Piperonyl Butoxide, 1479

Rifabutin, 1518

Rifadin®—*See* Rifampin, 1519

Rifamate®—*See* Isoniazid, 939 *and See* Rifampin, 1519

Rifampin, 1519

Rifater®—*See* Isoniazid, 939 *and See* Rifampin, 1519

Rifaximin, 1520

Rilutek®—*See* Riluzole, 1521

Riluzole, 1521

Rimactane®—*See* Rifampin, 1519

Rimantadine, 1523

Risedronate, 1524

Risperdal®—*See* Risperidone, 1527

Risperdal® M-TAB®—*See* Risperidone, 1527

Risperidone, 1527

Ritalin®—*See* Methylphenidate, 1120

Ritonavir, 1530

Rituxan®—*See* Rituximab Injection, 1533

Rituximab Injection, 1533

Rivastigmine, 1535

Rizatriptan, 1538

RMS®—*See* Morphine Rectal§

Robafen AC® Syrup—*See* Codeine Oral, 400

Robaxin®—*See* Methocarbamol Oral, 1109

Robicillin VK®—*See* Penicillin V Potassium Oral, 1367

Robinul®—*See* Glycopyrrolate, 805

Robinul® Forte—*See* Glycopyrrolate, 805

Robitussin®—*See* Guaifenesin, 811

Robitussin A-C® Syrup—*See* Codeine Oral, 400 *and See* Guaifenesin, 811

Robitussin® Allergy & Cough—*See* Dextromethorphan, 477

Robitussin®-CF®—*See* Dextromethorphan, 477

Robitussin® Cold & Congestion Caplets®—*See* Dextromethorphan, 477

Robitussin® Cold & Congestion Softgels®—*See* Dextromethorphan, 477

Robitussin® Cold Multi-Symptom Cold & Flu Softgels®—*See* Dextromethorphan, 477

Robitussin® Cold Severe Congestion Liqui-Gels®—*See* Guaifenesin, 811

Robitussin® Cough & Cold Infant Drops—*See* Dextromethorphan, 477

Robitussin® Cough & Cold Maximum Strength—*See* Dextromethorphan, 477

Robitussin® Cough & Cold Pediatric—*See* Dextromethorphan, 477

Robitussin® CoughGels®—*See* Dextromethorphan, 477

Robitussin®-DAC—*See* Codeine Oral, 400

Robitussin®-DM—*See* Dextromethorphan, 477

Robitussin® DM Infant Drops—*See* Dextromethorphan, 477

Robitussin® Flu—*See* Dextromethorphan, 477

Robitussin® Honey Cough Suppressant—*See* Dextromethorphan, 477

Robitussin® Maximum Strength Cough Suppressant—*See* Dextromethorphan, 477

Robitussin® Multi-Symptom Cold & Flu Caplets®—*See* Dextromethorphan, 477

Robitussin® Multi-Symptom Honey Flu—*See* Dextromethorphan, 477

Robitussin Night Relief®—*See* Dextromethorphan, 477

Robitussin® Nighttime Honey Flu—*See* Dextromethorphan, 477

Robitussin®-PE®—*See* Guaifenesin, 811

Robitussin® Pediatric Cough Suppressant—*See* Dextromethorphan, 477

Robitussin® PM Cough & Cold—*See* Dextromethorphan, 477

Robitussin® Sugar Free Cough—*See* Dextromethorphan, 477

Rocaltrol®—*See* Calcitriol, 240

Rocephin®—*See* Ceftriaxone Sodium Injection, 289

Roferon-A (alfa-2a)—*See* Interferon Alfa-2a and Alfa-2b Injection, 910

Rogaine®—*See* Minoxidil Topical, 1159

Rolaids Calcium Rich®—*See* Calcium Carbonate, 242

Rondec® DM—*See* Dextromethorphan, 477

Rondec® DM Drops—*See* Dextromethorphan, 477

Rondec® Syrup—*See* Brompheniramine, 215

Ropinirole, 1540

Rosiglitazone, 1543

Rosuvastatin, 1546

RotaTeq®—*See* Rotavirus Vaccine, 1548

Rotavirus Vaccine, 1548

Rowasa®—*See* Mesalamine, 1091

Roxanol®—*See* Morphine Oral, 1174

Roxanol®-T—*See* Morphine Oral, 1174

Roxicet®—*See* Acetaminophen and Oxycodone, 15

Roxicodone®—*See* Oxycodone, 1321

Roxicodone® Intensol®—*See* Oxycodone, 1321

Roxilox®—*See* Acetaminophen and Oxycodone, 15

Roxiprin®—*See* Oxycodone and Aspirin, 1323

Rozerem®—*See* Ramelteon, 1497

R-Tannate®—*See* Chlorpheniramine, 318

R-Tannate® Pediatric—*See* Chlorpheniramine, 318

Rulox®—*See* Aluminum Hydroxide and Magnesium Hydroxide, 61

Rum-K®—*See* Potassium, 1422

Ryna®—*See* Chlorpheniramine, 318

Ryna-C®—*See* Codeine Oral, 400

Ryna-CX®—*See* Codeine Oral, 400

Rynatan®—*See* Chlorpheniramine, 318

Rynatan® Pediatric—*See* Chlorpheniramine, 318

Rynatan®-S Pediatric—*See* Chlorpheniramine, 318

Rynatuss®—*See* Chlorpheniramine, 318

Rynatuss® Pediatric—*See* Chlorpheniramine, 318

Rythmol®—*See* Propafenone, 1461

Ry-Tuss®—*See* Chlorpheniramine, 318

Ry-Tuss® Pediatric—*See* Chlorpheniramine, 318

S

Safe Tussin®—*See* Dextromethorphan, 477

Safe Tussin® 30—*See* Dextromethorphan, 477

Salflex®—*See* Salsalate§

Salmeterol Oral Inhalation, 1550

Salsalate§

Salsitab®—*See* Salsalate§

Sanctura®—*See* Trospium, 1748

Sandimmune®—*See* Cyclosporine, 422

Sandimmune® I.V.—*See* Cyclosporine Injection, 427

Sandostatin®—*See* Octreotide Injection, 1269

Sandostatin LAR® Depot—*See* Octreotide Injection, 1269

Saquinavir, 1553

Sarafem®—*See* Fluoxetine, 722

Sargramostim Injection, 1556

Sarnol® HC—*See* Hydrocortisone Topical, 837

Scalp-Aid®—*See* Hydrocortisone Topical, 837

Scalpcort® Maximum Strength—*See* Hydrocortisone Topical, 837

Scopace®—*See* Scopolamine Patch, 1558

Scopolamine Patch, 1558

Seasonale®—*See* Estrogen and Progestin (Oral Contraceptives), 633

Seasonique®—*See* Estrogen and Progestin (Oral Contraceptives), 633

Secobarbital, 1560

U

Ultrabrom®— *See* Brompheniramine, 215
Ultrabrom® PD— *See* Brompheniramine, 215
Ultracet®— *See* Acetaminophen, 10 *and See* Tramadol, 1710
Ultram®— *See* Tramadol, 1710
Ultram® ER— *See* Tramadol, 1710
Ultrase®— *See* Pancrelipase, 1334
Ultrase® MT12— *See* Pancrelipase, 1334
Ultrase® MT18— *See* Pancrelipase, 1334
Ultrase® MT20— *See* Pancrelipase, 1334
Ultravate®— *See* Halobetasol, 815
Unasyn®— *See* Ampicillin Sodium and Sulbactam Sodium Injection, 107
Unipen®— *See* Nafcillin Sodium Injection, 1197
Uniphyl®— *See* Theophylline§
Uniretic®— *See* Hydrochlorothiazide, 829 *and See* Moexipril, 1166
Uniretic® HCT— *See* Hydrochlorothiazide, 829
Unisom® Nighttime Sleep Aid— *See* Doxylamine, 558
Unisom® SleepGels® Maximum Strength— *See* Diphenhydramine Oral, 515
Unithroid®— *See* Levothyroxine, 1015
Univasc®— *See* Moexipril, 1166
Urecholine®— *See* Bethanechol, 192
Urex®— *See* Methenamine, 1107
Urispas®— *See* Flavoxate, 703
Uro-Mag®— *See* Magnesium Oxide, 1059
Uroxatral®— *See* Alfuzosin, 49
Ursodiol, 1749
UTI Relief®— *See* Phenazopyridine, 1383

V

Vagifem®— *See* Estrogen Vaginal, 641
Valacyclovir, 1750
Valcyte®— *See* Valganciclovir, 1753
Valganciclovir, 1753
Valium®— *See* Diazepam, 478
Valproic Acid, 1756
Valsartan, 1760
Valtrex® Caplets— *See* Valacyclovir, 1750
Vanadom®— *See* Carisoprodol, 254
Vancocin®— *See* Vancomycin Hydrochloride Injection§
Vancocin®— *See* Vancomycin, 1762
Vancomycin, 1762
Vancomycin Hydrochloride Injection§
Vanex® Forte-R— *See* Chlorpheniramine, 318
Vaniqa®— *See* Eflornithine, 571
Vanquish® Caplets®— *See* Acetaminophen, 10 *and See* Aspirin, 132
Vantin®— *See* Cefpodoxime, 279
Vaqta®— *See* Hepatitis A Vaccine, 823
Vardenafil, 1764
Varenicline, 1766
Varicella (Chickenpox) Vaccine, 1767
Varivax®— *See* Varicella (Chickenpox) Vaccine, 1767
Vaseretic®— *See* Enalapril and Hydrochlorothiazide, 582
Vasocidin®— *See* Prednisolone Ophthalmic, 1437
Vasotec®— *See* Enalapril, 577
V-Cillin K®— *See* Penicillin V Potassium Oral, 1367
Veetids®— *See* Penicillin V Potassium Oral, 1367
Velcade®— *See* Bortezomib, 205

Venlafaxine, 1769
Ventolin HFA®— *See* Albuterol Inhalation, 41
Verapamil, 1773
Verapamil and Trandolapril, 1776
Verelan®— *See* Verapamil, 1773
Verelan® PM— *See* Verapamil, 1773
Vermox®— *See* Mebendazole, 1064
VESIcare®— *See* Solifenacin, 1591
Vfend®— *See* Voriconazole, 1777
Viadur®— *See* Leuprolide, 995
Viagra®— *See* Sildenafil, 1574
Vibramycin® Calcium Syrup— *See* Doxycycline, 547
Vibramycin® Hyclate— *See* Doxycycline, 547
Vibramycin® Hyclate Intravenous— *See* Doxycycline Injection, 554
Vibramycin® Monohydrate— *See* Doxycycline, 547
Vibra-Tabs®— *See* Doxycycline, 547
Vicks® 44 Cough Relief— *See* Dextromethorphan, 477
Vicks® DayQuil® Multi-Symptom Cold/Flu Relief— *See* Dextromethorphan, 477
Vicks® DayQuil® Multi-Symptom Cold/Flu Relief LiquiCaps®— *See* Dextromethorphan, 477
Vicks® 44D® Cough & Head Congestion Relief— *See* Dextromethorphan, 477
Vicks® 44E® Cough & Chest Congestion Relief— *See* Dextromethorphan, 477
Vicks® 44e® Pediatric Cough & Chest Congestion Relief— *See* Dextromethorphan, 477
Vicks® 44M® Cough Cold & Flu Relief— *See* Dextromethorphan, 477
Vicks® 44m® Cough & Cold Relief Pediatric— *See* Dextromethorphan, 477
Vicks® NyQuil® Cold/Cough Relief Children's— *See* Dextromethorphan, 477
Vicks® NyQuil® Cough— *See* Dextromethorphan, 477
Vicks® NyQuil® Multi-Symptom Cold/Flu Relief— *See* Dextromethorphan, 477
Vicks® NyQuil® Multi-Symptom Cold/Flu Relief LiquiCaps®— *See* Dextromethorphan, 477
Vicks® Vitamin C Drops— *See* Ascorbic Acid, 132
Vicodin®— *See* Acetaminophen and Hydrocodone, 14
Vicoprofen®— *See* Ibuprofen, 856
Videx®— *See* Didanosine, 495
Videx® EC— *See* Didanosine, 495
Videx® Pediatric— *See* Didanosine, 495
Vigamox®— *See* Moxifloxacin Ophthalmic, 1183
Vioform®— *See* Clioquinol Topical, 377
Viokase®— *See* Pancrelipase, 1334
Viokase® 16— *See* Pancrelipase, 1334
Viokase® 8— *See* Pancrelipase, 1334
Viracept®— *See* Nelfinavir, 1218
Viracept® Oral Powder— *See* Nelfinavir, 1218
Viramune®— *See* Nevirapine, 1226
Viread®— *See* Tenofovir, 1640
Visine®— *See* Tetrahydrozoline Ophthalmic, 1666
Visine® A.C.— *See* Tetrahydrozoline Ophthalmic, 1666
Visine® Moisturizing— *See* Tetrahydrozoline Ophthalmic, 1666
Visken®— *See* Pindolol, 1406
Vistaril®— *See* Hydroxyzine, 849
Vistide®— *See* Cidofovir Injection, 334
Vivactil®— *See* Protriptyline, 1470
Vivelle®— *See* Estradiol Transdermal, 621
Vivelle-Dot®— *See* Estradiol Transdermal, 621

Vivotif Berna®— *See* Typhoid Vaccine§
Voltaren®— *See* Diclofenac Ophthalmic, 489
Voltaren®-XR— *See* Diclofenac, 483
Voriconazole, 1777
Vorinostat, 1780
VoSpire ER®— *See* Albuterol, 39
Vytorin®— *See* Simvastatin, 1579
Vytorin®— *See* Ezetimibe, 664
Vyvanse®— *See* Lisdexamfetamine, 1027

W

Warfarin, 1782
WelChol®— *See* Colesevelam, 405
Wellbutrin®— *See* Bupropion, 225
Wellbutrin® SR— *See* Bupropion, 225
Wellbutrin® XL— *See* Bupropion, 225
Wellcovorin®— *See* Leucovorin Calcium, 992
Westcort®— *See* Hydrocortisone Topical, 837
Wigraine®— *See* Ergotamine and Caffeine§
Women's Tylenol® Menstrual Relief Caplets®— *See* Acetaminophen, 10
Wygesic®— *See* Acetaminophen and Propoxyphene, 16
Wytensin®— *See* Guanabenz§

X

Xalatan®— *See* Latanoprost, 987
Xanax®— *See* Alprazolam, 57
Xenical®— *See* Orlistat, 1295
Xifaxan®— *See* Rifaximin, 1520
Xolair®— *See* Omalizumab Injection, 1286
Xopenex®— *See* Levalbuterol Oral Inhalation, 999
X-Pect®— *See* Guaifenesin, 811
X-Prep® Bowel Evacuant Kit #1— *See* Bisacodyl, 197
Xylocaine Viscous®— *See* Lidocaine Viscous, 1019
Xyrem®— *See* Sodium Oxybate, 1587

Y

Yasmin®— *See* Estrogen and Progestin (Oral Contraceptives), 633
Yellow Fever Vaccine§
YF-VAX®— *See* Yellow Fever Vaccine§

Z

Zaditor®— *See* Ketotifen Ophthalmic, 967
Zafirlukast, 1787
Zaleplon, 1789
Zanaflex®— *See* Tizanidine, 1692
Zanamivir Inhalation, 1790
Zantac®— *See* Ranitidine, 1501 *and See* Ranitidine Hydrochloride Injection, 1504
Zantac® 75— *See* Ranitidine, 1501
Zantac® EFFERdose— *See* Ranitidine, 1501
Zantac® Premixed— *See* Ranitidine Hydrochloride Injection, 1504
Zantac® Syrup— *See* Ranitidine, 1501
Zarontin®— *See* Ethosuximide Oral, 651
Zarontin® Syrup— *See* Ethosuximide Oral, 651
Zaroxolyn®— *See* Metolazone, 1138
Zavesca®— *See* Miglustat§
Zeasorb®-AF— *See* Miconazole, 1149
Zeasorb®-AF Lotion— *See* Miconazole, 1149

Abacavir

(a ba ka' vir)

Brand Name: Epzicon® as a combination product containing Abacavir and Lamivudine, Trizivir® as a combination product containing Abacavir, Lamivudine, and Zidovudine, Ziagen®

Important Warning

Abacavir may cause severe allergic reactions that can lead to death. Stop taking abacavir and call your doctor immediately if you develop a rash or at least one symptom from two of the following groups:

- fever
- excessive tiredness
- upset stomach, vomiting, diarrhea, or stomach pain
- sore throat, shortness of breath, or cough

The Warning Card your pharmacist gives you will have a written list of these symptoms. Carry the card with you.

If you stop taking abacavir because you had an allergic reaction, never take abacavir again. If you stop taking abacavir for any other reason, do not start taking it again without talking to your doctor.

Abacavir may cause serious liver damage and a blood condition called lactic acidosis. Tell your doctor if you drink large amounts of alcohol and if you have or have ever had liver disease. If you experience any of the following symptoms, call your doctor immediately: unusual bleeding or bruising; loss of appetite; pain in the upper right part of the stomach; yellowing of the skin or eyes; or upset stomach and tiredness that do not get better.

Keep all appointments with your doctor and the laboratory. Your doctor will order certain lab tests to check your body's response to abacavir.

Why is this medicine prescribed?

Abacavir is used in combination with other medications to treat human immunodeficiency virus (HIV) infection in patients with or without acquired immunodeficiency syndrome (AIDS). Abacavir is in a class of antiviral medications called nucleoside reverse transcriptase inhibitors (NRTIs). It works by slowing the spread of HIV infection in the body. Abacavir is not a cure and may not decrease the number of HIV-related illnesses. Abacavir does not prevent the spread of HIV to other people.

How should this medicine be used?

Abacavir comes as a tablet and a solution (liquid) to take by mouth. It is usually taken twice a day with or without food.

To help you remember to take abacavir, take it around the same time every day. Follow the directions on your prescription label carefully, and ask your doctor or pharmacist to explain any part you do not understand. Take abacavir exactly as directed. Do not take more or less of it or take it more often than prescribed by your doctor.

Continue to take abacavir even if you feel well. Do not stop taking abacavir without talking to your doctor.

Before taking abacavir, carefully read the manufacturer's medication guide that comes with it.

Are there other uses for this medicine?

Abacavir is also used sometimes in combination with other antiviral medications to prevent HIV infection in people who have been exposed to it. Talk to your doctor about the possible risks of using this medication for your condition.

This medication may be prescribed for other uses; ask your doctor or pharmacist for more information.

What special precautions should I follow?

Before taking abacavir,

- tell your doctor and pharmacist if you are allergic to abacavir or any other medications.
- tell your doctor and pharmacist what prescription and nonprescription medications, vitamins, nutritional supplements, and herbal products you are taking. Be sure to mention the following: methadone. Your doctor may need to change the doses of your medications or monitor you carefully for side effects.
- in addition to the condition listed in the IMPORTANT WARNING section, tell your doctor if you have or have ever had kidney disease.
- tell your doctor if you are pregnant, plan to become pregnant, or are breast-feeding. If you become pregnant while taking abacavir, call your doctor. You should not breast-feed while taking abacavir.
- talk to your doctor about the safe use of alcohol while taking this medication.

What should I do if I forget to take a dose?

Take the missed dose as soon as you remember it. However, if it is almost time for the next dose, skip the missed dose and continue your regular dosing schedule. Do not take a double dose to make up for a missed one.

What side effects can this medicine cause?

Abacavir may cause side effects. Tell your doctor if any of these symptoms are severe or do not go away:

- upset stomach
- vomiting
- diarrhea
- loss of appetite
- tiredness
- difficulty falling asleep or staying asleep

Some side effects can be serious. The following symptoms are uncommon, but if you experience any of them or those listed in the IMPORTANT WARNING section, call your doctor immediately:

- muscle or joint pain
- headache
- pain, burning, or tingling in the hands or feet
- swelling of the hands, feet, ankles, or lower legs
- pink eye
- bruises in the mouth

Abacavir may cause other side effects. Call your doctor if you have any unusual problems while taking this medication.

If you experience a serious side effect, you or your doctor may send a report to the Food and Drug Administration's (FDA) MedWatch Adverse Event Reporting program online [at http://www.fda.gov/MedWatch/index.html] or by phone [1-800-332-1088].

What storage conditions are needed for this medicine?

Keep this medication in the container it came in, tightly closed, and out of reach of children. Store it at room temperature and away from excess heat and moisture (not in the bathroom). Store liquid medication at room temperature or in the refrigerator. Do not freeze. Throw away any medication that is outdated or no longer needed. Talk to your pharmacist about the proper disposal of your medication.

What should I do in case of overdose?

In case of overdose, call your local poison control center at 1-800-222-1222. If the victim has collapsed or is not breathing, call local emergency services at 911.

What other information should I know?

Do not let anyone else take your medication. Ask your pharmacist any questions you have about refilling your prescription.

Dosage Facts
For Informational Purposes

Caution: Do not change your dose, how often you take your medication, or the length of time you are to take it without first talking to your healthcare provider.

The following dosage information was written using medical language for doctors and other healthcare professionals and is provided here for you to check your dosage. The dosage of this drug may differ for different patients. Therefore, always follow your doctor's instructions or the directions on the label. Contact your healthcare provider or pharmacist if you have any questions about the specific dosage of your medication after reviewing this information.

General Dosage Information

Available as abacavir sulfate; dosage expressed in terms of abacavir.

Dosage of Epzicom® or Trizivir® expressed as number of tablets.

Abacavir must be used in conjunction with other antiretrovirals. The fixed-combination preparation containing abacavir and lamivudine (Epzicom®) is used with other antiretrovirals; the fixed-combination preparation containing abacavir, lamivudine, and zidovudine (Trizivir®) may be used alone or in conjunction with other antiretrovirals.

Pediatric Patients

Treatment of HIV Infection

ORAL:
- Children and adolescents 3 months to 16 years of age: 8 mg/kg (up to 300 mg) twice daily.
- Trizivir®: 1 tablet twice daily in adolescents weighing ≥40 kg.

Adult Patients

Treatment of HIV Infection

ORAL:
- 300 mg twice daily or 600 mg once daily.
- Epzicom®: 1 tablet once daily.
- Trizivir®: 1 tablet twice daily in adults weighing ≥40 kg.

Postexposure Prophylaxis of HIV†
Nonoccupational Exposure†

ORAL:
- 300 mg twice daily or 600 mg once daily.
- Used in an alternative nonnucleoside reverse transcriptase inhibitor-based (NNRTI-based) regimen in conjunction with efavirenz and (lamivudine or emtricitabine) and in various alternative HIV protease inhibitor-based (PI-based) regimens in conjunction with a PI (with or without low-dose ritonavir) and (lamivudine or emtricitabine).
- Initiate postexposure prophylaxis as soon as possible following exposure (preferably ≤72 hours after exposure) and continue for 28 days.

Special Populations

Hepatic Impairment

Treatment of HIV Infection

ORAL:
- Adults with mild hepatic impairment (Child-Pugh score 5–6): 200 mg twice daily (i.e., 10 mL of oral solution twice daily). Safety and efficacy not established in those with moderate to severe hepatic impairment.
- Epzicom® and Trizivir® not recommended in those with impaired hepatic function.

Renal Impairment

Treatment of HIV Infection

- No dosage recommendations available for patients with impaired renal function. Some experts state dosage adjustments not needed.
- Epzicom® and Trizivir® should not be used in those with Cl$_{cr}$ <50 mL/minute.

Abatacept Injection
(a ba ta′ sept)

Brand Name: Orencia®

Why is this medicine prescribed?

Abatacept is used alone or in combination with other medications to reduce the pain, swelling, difficulty with daily activities, and joint damage caused by rheumatoid arthritis (a condition in which the body attacks its own joints causing pain, swelling, and loss of function) in patients who have not been helped by other medications. Abatacept is in a class of medications called selective costimulation modulators (immunomodulators). It works by blocking the activity of T-cells, a type of immune cell in the body that causes swelling and joint damage in people who have arthritis.

How should this medicine be used?

Abatacept comes as a powder to be mixed with sterile water and infused (injected slowly) intravenously (into a vein) by a doctor or nurse. It is usually given in a doctor's office every 2 weeks for the first three doses and then every 4 weeks. It will take about 30 minutes for you to receive your entire dose of abatacept.

Your doctor will give you the manufacturer's patient information sheet to read before you receive each dose of abatacept. Read the information carefully and ask your doctor any questions you have.

Are there other uses for this medicine?

This medication may be prescribed for other uses; ask your doctor or pharmacist for more information.

What special precautions should I follow?

Before using abatacept,
- tell your doctor and pharmacist if you are allergic to abatacept or any other medications.
- tell your doctor and pharmacist what prescription and nonprescription medications, vitamins, nutritional supplements, and herbal products you are taking or plan to take. Be sure to mention any of the following: anakinra (Kineret), adalimumab (Humira), etanercept (Enbrel), and infliximab (Remicade). Your doctor may need to change the doses of your medications or monitor you carefully for side effects.
- tell your doctor if you have an infection anywhere in the body, including infections that come and go, such as cold sores, and chronic infections that do not go away, or if you often get any type of infection such as bladder infections. Also tell your doctor if you have or have ever had chronic obstructive pulmonary disease (COPD; a group of lung diseases that includes chronic bronchitis and emphysema); any disease that affects your nervous system, such as multiple sclerosis; any disease that affects your immune system, such as cancer, human immunodeficiency virus (HIV), acquired immunodeficiency syndrome (AIDS), or severe combined immunodeficiency syndrome (SCID). Also tell your doctor if you have or have ever had tuberculosis (TB; a lung infection that may not cause symptoms for many years and that may spread to other parts of the body) or if you have been around someone who has or has had tuberculosis. Your doctor may give you a skin test to see whether you are infected with tuberculosis. Tell your doctor if you have ever had a positive skin test for tuberculosis in the past.
- tell your doctor if you are pregnant, plan to become pregnant, or are breast-feeding. If you become pregnant while using abatacept, call your doctor.
- if you are having surgery, including dental surgery, tell the doctor or dentist that you are using abatacept.
- tell your doctor if you have recently received or are scheduled to receive any vaccines. You should not have any vaccinations while you are using abatacept or for 3 months after you stop using abatacept without talking to your doctor.

What special dietary instructions should I follow?

Unless your doctor tells you otherwise, continue your normal diet.

What should I do if I forget to take a dose?

If you miss an appointment to receive an abatacept infusion, call your doctor as soon as possible.

What side effects can this medicine cause?

Abatacept may cause side effects. Tell your doctor if any of these symptoms are severe or do not go away:
- headache
- runny nose
- sore throat
- nausea
- dizziness
- heartburn
- back pain
- arm or leg pain

Some side effects can be serious. If you experience any of these symptoms, call your doctor immediately:

- hives
- skin rash
- itching
- swelling of the eyes, face, lips, tongue, or throat
- difficulty breathing or swallowing
- shortness of breath
- fever, chills, and other signs of infection
- dry cough that doesn't go away
- weight loss
- night sweats
- frequent urination or sudden need to urinate right away
- burning during urination
- cellulitis (red, hot, swollen area on the skin)

Abatacept may increase the risk of developing certain types of cancer including lymphoma (cancer that begins in the cells that fight infection). People who have had severe rheumatoid arthritis for a long time may have a greater than normal risk of developing these cancers even if they do not use abatacept. Talk to your doctor about the risks of using this medication.

Abatacept may cause other side effects. Call your doctor if you have any unusual problems while using this medication.

What storage conditions are needed for this medicine?

Your doctor will store the medication in his or her office.

What should I do in case of overdose?

In case of overdose, call your local poison control center at 1-800-222-1222. If the victim has collapsed or is not breathing, call local emergency services at 911.

What other information should I know?

Be sure to schedule appointments with your doctor well in advance so that you will be able to receive abatacept on schedule and at times that are convenient for you.

Dosage Facts
For Informational Purposes

Caution: Do not change your dose, how often you take your medication, or the length of time you are to take it without first talking to your healthcare provider.

The following dosage information was written using medical language for doctors and other healthcare professionals and is provided here for you to check your dosage. The dosage of this drug may differ for different patients. Therefore, always follow your doctor's instructions or the directions on the label. Contact your healthcare provider or pharmacist if you have any questions about the specific dosage of your medication after reviewing this information.

Adult Patients

Rheumatoid Arthritis

IV:
- Adults weighing <60 kg: 500 mg at 0, 2, and 4 weeks, then every 4 weeks.
- Adults weighing 60–100 kg: 750 mg at 0, 2, and 4 weeks, then every 4 weeks.
- Adults weighing >100 kg: 1 g at 0, 2, and 4 weeks, then every 4 weeks.

Special Populations

No special population dosage recommendations at this time.

Acamprosate

(a kam′ pro sate)

Brand Name: Campral®

Why is this medicine prescribed?

Acamprosate is used along with counseling and social support to help people who have stopped drinking large amounts of alcohol to avoid drinking alcohol again. Drinking alcohol for a long time changes the way the brain works. Acamprosate works by helping the brains of people who have drunk large amounts of alcohol to work normally again. Acamprosate does not prevent the withdrawal symptoms that people may experience when they stop drinking alcohol. Acamprosate has not been shown to work in people who have not stopped drinking alcohol or in people who drink large amounts of alcohol and also overuse or abuse other substances such as street drugs or prescription medications.

How should this medicine be used?

Acamprosate comes as a delayed-release tablet to take by mouth. It is usually taken with or without food three times a day. To help you remember to take acamprosate, take it around the same times every day. Taking acamprosate with breakfast, lunch, and dinner may help you to remember all three doses. Follow the directions on your prescription label carefully, and ask your doctor or pharmacist to explain any part you do not understand. Take acamprosate exactly as directed. Do not take more or less of it or take it more often than prescribed by your doctor.

Swallow the tablets whole; do not split, chew, or crush them.

Acamprosate helps to prevent you from drinking alcohol only as long as you are taking it. Continue to take acamprosate even if you do not think you are likely to start drinking alcohol again. Do not stop taking acamprosate without talking to your doctor.

If you drink alcohol while you are taking acamprosate, continue to take the medication and call your doctor. Acamprosate will not cause you to have an unpleasant reaction if you drink alcohol during treatment.

Are there other uses for this medicine?

This medication may be prescribed for other uses; ask your doctor or pharmacist for more information.

What special precautions should I follow?

Before taking acamprosate,

- tell your doctor and pharmacist if you are allergic to acamprosate, any other medications, or sulfites.
- tell your doctor and pharmacist what prescription and nonprescription medications, vitamins, nutritional supplements, and herbal products you are taking. Be sure to mention antidepressants ('mood elevators'). Your doctor may need to change the doses of your medications or monitor you carefully for side effects.
- tell your doctor if you are thinking of, or have ever thought of, harming or killing yourself, if you have ever tried to do so, or if you use or have ever used street drugs or have overused prescription medications. Also tell your doctor if you have or have ever had depression or kidney disease.
- tell your doctor if you are pregnant, plan to become pregnant, or are breast-feeding. If you become pregnant while taking acamprosate, call your doctor.
- if you are having surgery, including dental surgery, tell the doctor or dentist that you are taking acamprosate.
- you should know that acamprosate may affect your thinking, ability to make decisions, and coordination. Do not drive a car or operate machinery until you know how this medication affects you.
- you should know that people who drink large amounts of alcohol often become depressed and sometimes try to harm or kill themselves. Taking acamprosate does not decrease and may increase the risk that you will try to harm yourself. You may develop depression while you are taking acamprosate even if you do not go back to drinking. You or your family should call the doctor right away if you experience symptoms of depression such as feelings of sadness, anxiousness, hopelessness, guilt, worthlessness, or helplessness; loss of interest or pleasure in activities you once enjoyed; lack of energy; difficulty concentrating, making decisions, or remembering; irritability; sleep problems; changes in appetite or weight; restlessness; or thinking about harming or killing yourself or planning or trying to do so. Be sure that your family knows which symptoms may be serious so they can call the doctor right away if you are unable to seek treatment on your own.

What special dietary instructions should I follow?

Unless your doctor tells you otherwise, continue your normal diet.

What should I do if I forget to take a dose?

Take the missed dose as soon as you remember it. However, if it is almost time for the next dose, skip the missed dose and continue your regular dosing schedule. Do not take a double dose to make up for a missed one.

What side effects can this medicine cause?

Acamprosate may cause side effects. Tell your doctor if any of these symptoms are severe or do not go away:

- diarrhea
- gas
- upset stomach
- loss of appetite
- dry mouth
- dizziness
- itching
- weakness

Some side effects can be serious. The following symptoms are uncommon, but if you experience either of them or those mentioned in the SPECIAL PRECAUTIONS section, call your doctor immediately:

- burning, tingling, or numbness in the hands, feet, arms, or legs
- rash

Acamprosate may cause other side effects. Call your doctor if you have any unusual problems while taking this medication.

If you experience a serious side effect, you or your doctor may send a report to the Food and Drug Administration's (FDA) MedWatch Adverse Event Reporting program online [at http://www.fda.gov/MedWatch/index.html] or by phone [1-800-332-1088].

What storage conditions are needed for this medicine?

Keep this medication in the container it came in, tightly closed, and out of reach of children. Store it at room temperature and away from excess heat and moisture (not in the bathroom). Throw away any medication that is outdated or no longer needed. Talk to your pharmacist about the proper disposal of your medication.

What should I do in case of overdose?

In case of overdose, call your local poison control center at 1-800-222-1222. If the victim has collapsed or is not breathing, call local emergency services at 911.

Symptoms of overdose may include:

- diarrhea

If you take too much acamprosate regularly for a long time, you may experience certain symptoms. Call your doctor if you experience any of these symptoms:

- loss of appetite
- upset stomach
- constipation

- extreme thirst
- tiredness
- muscle weakness
- restlessness
- confusion

What other information should I know?

Keep all appointments with your doctor and counselor or support group.

Do not let anyone else take your medication. Ask your pharmacist any questions you have about refilling your prescription.

Dosage Facts
For Informational Purposes

Caution: Do not change your dose, how often you take your medication, or the length of time you are to take it without first talking to your health-care provider.

The following dosage information was written using medical language for doctors and other healthcare professionals and is provided here for you to check your dosage. The dosage of this drug may differ for different patients. Therefore, always follow your doctor's instructions or the directions on the label. Contact your healthcare provider or pharmacist if you have any questions about the specific dosage of your medication after reviewing this information.

General Dosage Information

Available as acamprosate calcium; dosage expressed in terms of the salt.

Adult Patients

Alcohol Dependence
Maintenance of Abstinence of Alcohol Ingestion

ORAL:
- 666 mg 3 times daily.
- A lower dosage (1.3 grams daily given in 3 unequally divided doses of 666, 333, and 333 mg) also evaluated in clinical studies and may be effective in some patients.

Special Populations

Hepatic Impairment
- Dosage adjustment not required in patients with mild to moderate hepatic impairment.

Renal Impairment
- In patients with moderate renal impairment (Cl_{cr} 30–50 mL/minute), 333 mg 3 times daily.
- Do not use in patients with severe renal impairment (Cl_{cr}<30 mL/minute).

Geriatric Patients
- Select dosage carefully.

Acarbose
(ay′ car bose)

Brand Name: Prandase®, Precose®

Why is this medicine prescribed?

Acarbose is used (with diet only or diet and other medications) to treat type 2 diabetes (condition in which the body does not use insulin normally and therefore cannot control the amount of sugar in the blood). Acarbose works by slowing the action of certain chemicals that break down food to release glucose (sugar) into your blood. Slowing food digestion helps keep blood glucose from rising very high after meals.

This medication is sometimes prescribed for other uses; ask your doctor or pharmacist for more information.

How should this medicine be used?

Acarbose comes as a tablet to take by mouth. It is usually taken three times a day. It is very important to take each dose with the first bite of each main meal. Follow the directions on your prescription label carefully, and ask your doctor or pharmacist to explain any part you do not understand. Take acarbose exactly as directed. Do not take more or less of it or take it more often than prescribed by your doctor.

Continue to take acarbose even if you feel well. Do not stop taking acarbose without talking to your doctor.

What special precautions should I follow?

Before taking acarbose,
- tell your doctor and pharmacist if you are allergic to acarbose or any other drugs.
- tell your doctor and pharmacist what prescription and nonprescription medications you are taking, especially other medications for diabetes, digoxin (Lanoxin), diuretics ('water pills'), estrogens, isoniazid, medications for high blood pressure or colds, oral contraceptives, pancreatic enzymes, phenytoin (Dilantin), steroids, thyroid medications, and vitamins.
- tell your doctor if you have or have ever had ketoacidosis, cirrhosis, or intestinal disease such as inflammatory bowel disease or bowel obstruction.
- tell your doctor if you are pregnant, plan to become pregnant, or are breast-feeding. If you become pregnant while taking acarbose, call your doctor.
- if you are having surgery, including dental surgery, tell the doctor or dentist that you are taking acarbose.

What special dietary instructions should I follow?

Be sure to follow all exercise and dietary recommendations made by your doctor or dietitian. It is important to eat a healthful diet.

Alcohol may cause a decrease in blood sugar. Ask your doctor about the safe use of alcoholic beverages while you are taking acarbose.

What should I do if I forget to take a dose?

Take the missed dose as soon as you remember it. If you will be having a snack soon, take a dose with the snack. If it is almost time for the next dose, skip the missed dose and continue your regular dosing schedule. Do not take a double dose to make up for a missed one.

What side effects can this medicine cause?

When used in combination with insulin or other medications used to treat diabetes, acarbose may cause excessive lowering of blood sugar levels.

If you have any of these symptoms, glucose products (Insta-Glucose or B-D Glucose tablets) should be used and you should call your doctor. Because acarbose blocks the breakdown of table sugar and other complex sugars, fruit juice or other products containing these sugars will not help to increase blood sugar. It is important that you and other members of your household understand this difference between acarbose and other medications used to treat diabetes.

- shakiness
- dizziness or lightheadedness
- sweating
- nervousness or irritability
- sudden changes in behavior or mood
- headache
- numbness or tingling around the mouth
- weakness
- pale skin
- hunger
- clumsy or jerky movements

If hypoglycemia is not treated, severe symptoms may develop. Be sure that your family, friends, and other people who spend time with you know that if you have any of the following symptoms, they should get medical treatment for you immediately.

- confusion
- seizures
- loss of consciousness

Call your doctor immediately if you have any of the following symptoms of hyperglycemia (high blood sugar):

- extreme thirst
- frequent urination
- extreme hunger
- weakness
- blurred vision

If high blood sugar is not treated, a serious, life-threatening condition called diabetic ketoacidosis could develop. Call your doctor immediately if you have any of the these symptoms:

- dry mouth
- upset stomach and vomiting
- shortness of breath

- breath that smells fruity
- decreased consciousness

What storage conditions are needed for this medicine?

Keep this medication in the container it came in, tightly closed, and out of reach of children. Store it at room temperature and away from excess heat and moisture (not in the bathroom). Throw away any medication that is outdated or no longer needed. Talk to your pharmacist about the proper disposal of your medication.

What should I do in case of overdose?

In case of overdose, call your local poison control center at 1-800-222-1222. If the victim has collapsed or is not breathing, call local emergency services at 911.

What other information should I know?

Keep all appointments with your doctor and the laboratory. Your doctor will order certain lab tests to check your response to acarbose. Your doctor will also tell you how to check your response to this medication by measuring your blood or urine sugar levels at home. Follow these instructions carefully

You should always wear a diabetic identification bracelet to be sure you get proper treatment in an emergency.

Do not let anyone else take your medication. Ask your pharmacist any questions you have about refilling your prescription.

Dosage Facts
For Informational Purposes

Caution: Do not change your dose, how often you take your medication, or the length of time you are to take it without first talking to your healthcare provider.

The following dosage information was written using medical language for doctors and other healthcare professionals and is provided here for you to check your dosage. The dosage of this drug may differ for different patients. Therefore, always follow your doctor's instructions or the directions on the label. Contact your healthcare provider or pharmacist if you have any questions about the specific dosage of your medication after reviewing this information.

Adult Patients

Diabetes Mellitus

ORAL:
- Initially, 25 mg 3 times daily at the beginning of each main meal. In patients with adverse GI effects, initiate at 25 mg once daily and increase dosage gradually as necessary to 25 mg 3 times daily.
- Once dosage of 25 mg 3 times daily has been reached, in-

crease dosage at intervals of 4–8 weeks as tolerated to achieve the desired 1-hour postprandial glucose concentration (e.g., <180 mg/dL). Maintenance dosage ranges from 50–100 mg 3 times daily. Dosages higher than 100 mg 3 times daily are not recommended since such dosages have been associated with an increased risk of elevated serum aminotransferase concentrations. If no further therapeutic benefit occurs at the maximum recommended dosage, consider lowering the dosage.

Prescribing Limits

Adult Patients

Diabetes Mellitus

ORAL:
- Patients ≤60 kg: maximum 50 mg 3 times daily.
- Patients >60 kg: maximum 100 mg 3 times daily.

Acebutolol

(a se byoo' toe lole)

Brand Name: Sectral®
Also available generically.

Important Warning

Do not stop taking acebutolol without talking to your doctor first. If acebutolol is stopped suddenly, it may cause chest pain or heart attack in some people.

Why is this medicine prescribed?

Acebutolol is used to treat high blood pressure. It relaxes your blood vessels so your heart doesn't have to pump as hard. Acebutolol also is used to treat an irregular heartbeat.

This medication is sometimes prescribed for other uses; ask your doctor or pharmacist for more information.

How should this medicine be used?

Acebutolol comes as a capsule to take by mouth. It usually is taken once or twice a day. Follow the directions on your prescription label carefully, and ask your doctor or pharmacist to explain any part you do not understand. Take acebutolol exactly as directed. Do not take more or less of it or take it more often than prescribed by your doctor.

Acebutolol controls your condition but does not cure it. Continue to take acebutolol even if you feel well. Do not stop taking acebutolol without talking to your doctor.

Are there other uses for this medicine?

Acebutolol is also used sometimes to treat chest pain (angina). Talk to your doctor about the possible risks of using this drug for your condition.

What special precautions should I follow?

Before taking acebutolol,
- tell your doctor and pharmacist if you are allergic to acebutolol or any other drugs.
- tell your doctor and pharmacist what prescription and nonprescription medications you are taking, especially medications for migraine headaches, diabetes, asthma, allergies, colds, or pain; other medications for high blood pressure or heart disease; reserpine; and vitamins.
- tell your doctor if you have or have ever had heart, kidney, or liver disease; asthma or other lung diseases; diseases of the blood vessels; severe allergies; diabetes; or an overactive thyroid gland.
- tell your doctor if you are pregnant, plan to become pregnant, or are breast-feeding. If you become pregnant while taking acebutolol, call your doctor.
- if you are having surgery, including dental surgery, tell the doctor or dentist that you are taking acebutolol.
- you should know that this drug may make you drowsy. Do not drive a car or operate machinery until you know how this drug affects you.
- remember that alcohol can add to the drowsiness caused by this drug.

What special dietary instructions should I follow?

Talk to your doctor before using salt substitutes containing potassium. If your doctor prescribes a low-salt or low-sodium diet, follow these directions carefully.

What should I do if I forget to take a dose?

Take the missed dose as soon as you remember it. However, if it is almost time for the next dose, skip the missed dose and continue your regular dosing schedule. Do not take a double dose to make up for a missed one.

What side effects can this medicine cause?

Acebutolol may cause side effects. Tell your doctor if any of these symptoms are severe or do not go away:
- dizziness
- lightheadedness
- excessive tiredness
- headache
- constipation
- diarrhea
- upset stomach
- muscle aches

If you experience any of the following symptoms, call your doctor immediately:
- shortness of breath or wheezing
- swelling of the feet and lower legs
- chest pain

If you experience a serious side effect, you or your doctor may send a report to the Food and Drug Administration's (FDA) MedWatch Adverse Event Reporting program online

[at http://www.fda.gov/MedWatch/index.html] or by phone [1-800-332-1088].

What storage conditions are needed for this medicine?

Keep this medication in the container it came in, tightly closed, and out of reach of children. Store it at room temperature and away from excess heat and moisture (not in the bathroom). Throw away any medication that is outdated or no longer needed. Talk to your pharmacist about the proper disposal of your medication.

What should I do in case of overdose?

In case of overdose, call your local poison control center at 1-800-222-1222. If the victim has collapsed or is not breathing, call local emergency services at 911.

What other information should I know?

Keep all appointments with your doctor and the laboratory. Your blood pressure should be checked regularly to determine your response to acebutolol. Your doctor may ask you to check your pulse (heart rate). Ask your pharmacist or doctor to teach you how to take your pulse. If your pulse is faster or slower than it should be, call your doctor.

Do not let anyone else take your medication. Ask your pharmacist any questions you have about refilling your prescription.

Dosage Facts
For Informational Purposes

Caution: Do not change your dose, how often you take your medication, or the length of time you are to take it without first talking to your healthcare provider.

The following dosage information was written using medical language for doctors and other healthcare professionals and is provided here for you to check your dosage. The dosage of this drug may differ for different patients. Therefore, always follow your doctor's instructions or the directions on the label. Contact your healthcare provider or pharmacist if you have any questions about the specific dosage of your medication after reviewing this information.

General Dosage Information

Available as acebutolol hydrochloride; dosage expressed in terms of acebutolol.

Adult Patients

Hypertension

ORAL:
- Initially, 200–400 mg daily. Usual maintenance dosage is 200–800 mg daily, but some patients may achieve adequate BP control with dosages as low as 200 mg daily. Increase dosage up to 1.2 g daily in two divided doses in patients with

more severe hypertension or if adequate reduction of BP does not occur; alternatively, add another hypotensive agent (e.g., thiazide diuretic).

Ventricular Arrhythmias

ORAL:
- Initially, 200 mg twice daily. Increase gradually until optimum effect is achieved. Usual maintenance dosage is 600–1200 mg daily.

Angina

ORAL:
- Initially, 200 mg twice daily. Increase dosage gradually until optimum effect is achieved. Usual maintenance dosage is 800 mg or less daily, but patients with severe angina may require higher dosages.

Prescribing Limits

Adult Patients

Hypertension

ORAL:
- Maximum 1.2 g daily.

Special Populations

Renal Impairment

- Active metabolite (diacetolol) eliminated principally by the kidneys; dosage and/or frequency of administration must be modified in response to the degree of renal impairment.

Dosage Reductions in Patients with Renal Impairment

Reduction in Usual Daily Dosage	Cl_{cr} (mL/min)
50%	25–49 mL/minute
75%	<25 mL/minute

Acebutolol and diacetolol removed by hemodialysis; individualize dosage carefully in patients with severe renal impairment who undergo chronic intermittent hemodialysis.

Geriatric Patients

- Consider reduction in maintenance dosage. Avoid dosages >800 mg daily.

Acetaminophen

(a set a mee′ noe fen)

Brand Name: Acephen®, Anacin® Aspirin Free Maximum Strength Tablets®, FeverAll® Children's, FeverAll® Infants', FeverAll® Junior Strength, Gelpirin®, Genapap®, Genapap® Children's, Genapap® Drops Infant's, Genapap® Extra Strength Caplets®, Genapap® Extra Strength Tablets, Genapap® Gel-Coat Caplets®, Genebs®, Genebs® Extra Strength Caplets®, Genebs® Extra Strength Tablets, Liquiprin® Drops, Tylenol®, Tylenol® Arthritis Pain Extended Relief Caplets®, Tylenol® Meltaways Children's, Tylenol® Concentrated Drops Infant's, Tylenol® Extra Strength Adult, Tylenol® Extra Strength Caplets®, Tylenol® Extra Strength Gelcaps®, Tylenol® Extra Strength Geltabs®, Tylenol® Extra Strength Tablets, Tylenol® Meltaways Junior Strength, Tylenol® Suspension Children's
Also available generically.

Why is this medicine prescribed?

Acetaminophen is used to relieve mild to moderate pain from headaches, muscle aches, menstrual periods, colds and sore throats, toothaches, backaches, reactions to vaccinations (shots), and to reduce fever. Acetaminophen may also be used to relieve the pain of osteoarthritis (arthritis caused by the breakdown of the lining of the joints). Acetaminophen is in a class of medications called analgesics (pain relievers) and antipyretics (fever reducers). It works by changing the way the body senses pain and by cooling the body.

How should this medicine be used?

Acetaminophen comes as a tablet, chewable tablet, capsule, suspension or solution (liquid), drops (concentrated liquid), extended-release (long-acting) tablet, and orally disintegrating tablet (tablet that dissolves quickly in the mouth), to take by mouth, with or without food. Acetaminophen also comes as a suppository to use rectally. Acetaminophen is available without a prescription, but your doctor may prescribe acetaminophen to treat certain conditions. Follow the directions on the package or prescription label carefully, and ask your doctor or pharmacist to explain any part you do not understand. Take acetaminophen exactly as directed. Do not take more or less of it or take it more often than directed on the package label or prescribed by your doctor. Taking more than the recommended amount may cause damage to your liver.

If you are giving acetaminophen to your child, read the package label carefully to make sure that it is the right product for the age of the child. Do not give children acetaminophen products that are made for adults. Some products for adults and older children may contain too much acetaminophen for a younger child. Drops made for infants are more concentrated (much more medication in each drop) than liquids made for older children. Check the package label to find out how much medication the child needs. If you know how much your child weighs, give the dose that matches that weight on the chart. If you don't know your child's weight, give the dose that matches your child's age. Ask your child's doctor if you don't know how much medication to give your child.

Swallow the extended-release tablets whole; do not split, chew, crush, or dissolve them.

Place the orally disintegrating tablet ('Meltaways') in your mouth and allow to dissolve or chew it before swallowing.

Shake the suspension and drops well before each use to mix the medication evenly. Use the measuring cup provided by the manufacturer to measure each dose of the solution or suspension, and use the dosing device provided to measure each dose of the drops. Use the dosing device to slowly release the drops directly into the child's mouth near the inner cheek. Do not mix the drops with baby formula.

To insert an acetaminophen suppository into the rectum, follow these steps:
1. Remove the wrapper.
2. Dip the tip of the suppository in water.
3. Lie down on your left side and raise your right knee to your chest. (A left-handed person should lie on the right side and raise the left knee.)
4. Using your finger, insert the suppository into the rectum, about ½ to 1 inch in infants and children and 1 inch in adults. Hold it in place for a few moments.
5. Stand up after about 15 minutes. Wash your hands thoroughly and resume your normal activities.

Stop taking acetaminophen and call your doctor if your symptoms get worse, you develop new or unexpected symptoms, including redness or swelling, your pain lasts for more than 10 days, or your fever gets worse or lasts more than 3 days. Also stop giving acetaminophen to your child and call your child's doctor if your child develops new symptoms, including redness or swelling, or your child's pain lasts for longer than 5 days, or fever get worse or lasts longer than 3 days.

Do not give acetaminophen to a child who has a sore throat that is severe or does not go away, or that occurs along with fever, headache, rash, nausea, or vomiting. Call the child's doctor right away, because these symptoms may be signs of a more serious condition.

Are there other uses for this medicine?

Acetaminophen may also be used in combination with aspirin and caffeine to relieve the pain associated with migraine headache.

This medication is sometimes prescribed for other uses; ask your doctor or pharmacist for more information.

What special precautions should I follow?

Before taking acetaminophen,

- tell your doctor and pharmacist if you are allergic to acetaminophen, any other medications, or any of the ingredients in the product. Ask your pharmacist or check the label on the package for a list of ingredients.
- do not take two or more products that contain acetaminophen at the same time. Many prescription and non-prescription medications contain acetaminophen in combination with other medications. Read the package labels or ask your doctor or pharmacist to be sure that you do not take more than one product that contains acetaminophen at a time.
- tell your doctor and pharmacist what prescription and nonprescription medications, vitamins, nutritional supplements, or herbal products you are taking or plan to take. Be sure to mention anticoagulants ('blood thinners') such as warfarin (Coumadin); isoniazid (INH); certain medications for seizures including carbamazepine (Tegretol), phenobarbital, and phenytoin (Dilantin); medications for pain, fever, coughs, and colds; and phenothiazines (medications for mental illness and nausea). Your doctor may need to change the doses of your medications or monitor you carefully for side effects.
- tell your doctor if you have any serious medical condition.
- tell your doctor if you are pregnant, plan to become pregnant, or are breast-feeding. If you become pregnant while taking acetaminophen, call your doctor.
- if you drink three or more alcoholic beverages every day, ask your doctor if you should take acetaminophen. Ask your doctor or pharmacist about the safe use of alcoholic beverages while taking acetaminophen.
- you should know that combination acetaminophen products for cough and colds that contain nasal decongestants, antihistamines, cough suppressants, and expectorants should not be used in children less than 2 years of age without first talking to your child's doctor and following his or her instructions carefully. Improper use of these medications in young children can caused serious and life-threatening effects or death.
- if you have phenylketonuria (PKU, a inherited condition in which a special diet must be followed to prevent mental retardation), you should know that some brands of acetaminophen chewable tablets may be sweetened with aspartame that forms phenylalanine.

What special dietary instructions should I follow?

Unless your doctor tells you otherwise, continue your normal diet.

What should I do if I forget to take a dose?

This medication is usually taken as needed. If your doctor has told you to take acetaminophen regularly, take the missed dose as soon as you remember it. However, if it is almost time for the next dose, skip the missed dose and continue your regular dosing schedule. Do not take a double dose to make up for a missed one.

What side effects can this medicine cause?

Acetaminophen may cause side effects.

Some side effects can be serious. If you experience any of the following symptoms, call your doctor immediately:

- rash
- hives
- itching
- swelling of the face, throat, tongue, lips, eyes, hands, feet, ankles, or lower legs
- hoarseness
- difficulty breathing or swallowing

Acetaminophen may cause other side effects. Call your doctor if you have any unusual problems while you are taking this medication.

If you experience a serious side effect, you or your doctor may send a report to the Food and Drug Administration's (FDA) MedWatch Adverse Event Reporting program online [at http://www.fda.gov/MedWatch/index.html] or by phone [1-800-332-1088].

What storage conditions are needed for this medicine?

Keep this medication in the container it came in, tightly closed, and out of reach of children. Store it at room temperature and away from excess heat and moisture (not in the bathroom). Throw away any medication that is outdated or no longer needed. Talk to your pharmacist about the proper disposal of your medication.

What should I do in case of overdose?

In case of overdose, call your local poison control center at 1-800-222-1222. If the victim has collapsed or is not breathing, call local emergency services at 911.

If someone takes more than the recommended dose of acetaminophen, get medical help immediately, even if the person does not have any symptoms. Symptoms of overdose may include:

- nausea
- vomiting
- loss of appetite
- sweating
- extreme tiredness
- unusual bleeding or bruising
- pain in the upper right part of the stomach
- yellowing of the skin or eyes
- flu-like symptoms

What other information should I know?

Before having any laboratory test, tell your doctor and the laboratory personnel that you are taking acetaminophen.

Ask your pharmacist any questions you have about acetaminophen.

Dosage Facts
For Informational Purposes

Caution: Do not change your dose, how often you take your medication, or the length of time you are to take it without first talking to your healthcare provider.

The following dosage information was written using medical language for doctors and other healthcare professionals and is provided here for you to check your dosage. The dosage of this drug may differ for different patients. Therefore, always follow your doctor's instructions or the directions on the label. Contact your healthcare provider or pharmacist if you have any questions about the specific dosage of your medication after reviewing this information.

Pediatric Patients

Dosage in children should be guided by body weight.

Pain
ORAL:

Dosage for Self-medication of Pain in Children up to 11 Years of Age

Age	Weight	Oral Dose[a]
≤3 months	2.7–5 kg	40 mg
4–11 months	5–8 kg	80 mg
12–23 months	8–11 kg	120 mg
2–3 years	11–16 kg	160 mg
4–5 years	16–21.5 kg	240 mg
6–8 years	21.5–27 kg	320 mg
9–10 years	27–32.5 kg	400 mg
11 years	32.5–43 kg	480 mg

[a]Dose may be given every 4–6 hours as necessary (up to 5 times in 24 hours).

For *self-medication* in children ≥12 years of age, 650 mg or 1 g every 4–6 hours as necessary (maximum 4 g daily).
RECTAL:

Dosage for Self-medication of Pain in Children 2–12 Years of Age

Age	Rectal Dose[b]
2–4 years	160 mg
4–6 years	240 mg
6–9 years	320 mg
9–11 years	320–400 mg
11–12 years	320–480 mg

[b]Dose may be given every 4–6 hours as necessary (up to 5 times in 24 hours).

Individualize dosage in children <2 years of age.
For *self-medication* in children ≥12 years of age, 325–650 mg every 4 hours as necessary.

Fever
ORAL:

Dosage for Self-medication of Fever in Children up to 11 Years of Age

Age	Weight	Oral Dose[c]
≤3 months	2.7–5 kg	40 mg
4–11 months	5–8 kg	80 mg
12–23 months	8–11 kg	120 mg
2–3 years	11–16 kg	160 mg
4–5 years	16–21.5 kg	240 mg
6–8 years	21.5–27 kg	320 mg
9–10 years	27–32.5 kg	400 mg
11 years	32.5–43 kg	480 mg

[c]Dose may be given every 4–6 hours as necessary (up to 5 times in 24 hours).

For *self-medication* in children ≥12 years of age, 650 mg or 1 g every 4–6 hours as necessary (maximum 4 g daily).
RECTAL:

Dosage for Self-medication of Fever in Children 2–12 Years of Age

Age	Rectal Dose[d]
2–4 years	160 mg
4–6 years	240 mg
6–9 years	320 mg
9–11 years	320–400 mg
11–12 years	320–480 mg

[d]Dose may be given every 4 hours as necessary (up to 5 times in 24 hours).

Individualize dosage in children <2 years of age.
For *self-medication* in children ≥12 years of age, 325–650 mg every 4 hours as necessary.

Adult Patients

Pain

ORAL:
- For *self-medication*, 650 mg or 1 g every 4–6 hours as necessary (maximum 4 g daily). Alternatively, 1.3 g as extended-release tablets every 8 hours.

RECTAL:
- 325–650 mg every 4 hours as necessary.

Pain Associated with Migraine Headache

ORAL:
- For *self-medication*, 500 mg (combined with aspirin 500 mg and caffeine 130 mg) as a single dose.

Pain Associated with Osteoarthritis

ORAL:
- 1 g 4 times daily. Alternatively, 1.3 g as extended-release tablets every 8 hours.

Fever

ORAL:
- For *self-medication*, 650 mg or 1 g every 4–6 hours as necessary (maximum 4 g daily).

RECTAL:
- 325–650 mg every 4 hours as necessary.

Prescribing Limits

Pediatric Patients

Pain

ORAL:
- Do not exceed recommended daily dosage. *Self-medication* should not exceed 5 days.

Fever

ORAL:
- Do not exceed recommended daily dosage. *Self-medication* should not exceed 3 days.

Adult Patients

Pain

ORAL OR RECTAL:
- Maximum 4 g daily. *Self-medication* should not exceed 10 days.

Pain Associated with Migraine Headache

ORAL:
- For *self-medication*, maximum 500 mg (in combination with aspirin 500 mg and caffeine 130 mg) in 24 hours.

Pain Associated with Osteoarthritis

ORAL:
- Maximum 2.6 g daily for long-term (>10 days) use unless prescribed and monitored by a clinician.

Fever

ORAL OR RECTAL:
- Maximum 4 g daily. *Self-medication* should not exceed 3 days.

Acetaminophen and Codeine

(a set a mee′ noe fen) (koe′ deen)

Brand Name: Capital and Codeine®, Phenaphen with Codeine (No.3 and No.4)®, Tylenol with Codeine (No. 2, No. 3, No. 4)®

Why is this medicine prescribed?

This combination of drugs is used to relieve mild to moderate pain.

This medication is sometimes prescribed for other uses; ask your doctor or pharmacist for more information.

How should this medicine be used?

The combination of acetaminophen and codeine comes as a tablet, capsule, and liquid to take by mouth. It usually is taken every 6 hours as needed. Follow the directions on your prescription label carefully, and ask your doctor or phar-

macist to explain any part you do not understand. Take acetaminophen and codeine exactly as directed.

Codeine can be habit-forming. Do not take a larger dose, take it more often, or for a longer period than your doctor tells you to.

What special precautions should I follow?

Before taking acetaminophen and codeine,
- tell your doctor and pharmacist if you are allergic to acetaminophen, codeine, sulfite or any other drugs.
- tell your doctor and pharmacist what prescription and nonprescription medications you are taking, especially acetaminophen (Tylenol); antidepressants; medications for cough, cold, or allergies; other pain relievers; sedatives, sleeping pills, tranquilizers; and vitamins.
- tell your doctor if you have or have ever had liver or kidney disease, a history of alcoholism, lung or thyroid disease, prostatic hypertrophy, or urinary retention.
- tell your doctor if you are pregnant, plan to become pregnant, or are breast-feeding. If you become pregnant while taking acetaminophen and codeine, call your doctor.
- if you are having surgery, including dental surgery, tell the doctor or dentist that you are taking acetaminophen and codeine.
- you should know that this drug may make you drowsy. Do not drive a car or operate machinery until you know how this drug affects you.
- remember that alcohol can add to the drowsiness caused by this drug.

What should I do if I forget to take a dose?

This medication usually is taken as needed. If your doctor has told you to take acetaminophen and codeine regularly, take the missed dose as soon as you remember it. However, if it is almost time for the next dose, skip the missed dose and continue your regular dosing schedule. Do not take a double dose to make up for a missed one.

What side effects can this medicine cause?

Acetaminophen and codeine may cause side effects. Tell your doctor if any of these symptoms are severe or do not go away:
- dizziness
- lightheadedness
- drowsiness
- upset stomach
- vomiting
- constipation
- stomach pain
- rash
- difficulty urinating

If you experience either of the following symptoms, call your doctor immediately:
- difficulty breathing
- mood changes

If you experience a serious side effect, you or your doctor may send a report to the Food and Drug Administration's (FDA) MedWatch Adverse Event Reporting program online [at http://www.fda.gov/MedWatch/index.html] or by phone [1-800-332-1088].

What storage conditions are needed for this medicine?

Keep this medication in the container it came in, tightly closed, and out of reach of children. Store it at room temperature and away from excess heat and moisture (not in the bathroom). Throw away any medication that is outdated or no longer needed. Talk to your pharmacist about the proper disposal of your medication.

What should I do in case of overdose?

In case of overdose, call your local poison control center at 1-800-222-1222. If the victim has collapsed or is not breathing, call local emergency services at 911.

What other information should I know?

Keep all appointments with your doctor.

Too much acetaminophen may cause liver damage; do not take more than 4000 mg of acetaminophen per day.

Do not let anyone else take your medication. Ask your pharmacist any questions you have about refilling your prescription.

Talk to your doctor, pharmacist, or other healthcare professional if you have questions about dosing information for your medication.

Acetaminophen and Hydrocodone

(a set a mee′ noe fen) (hye droe koe′ done)

Brand Name: Anexsia®, Co-gesic®, Lorcet-HD®, Lortab®, Norco®, Panacet®, Vicodin®, Zydone®

Why is this medicine prescribed?

This combination of drugs is used to relieve moderate to moderately severe pain.

This medication is sometimes prescribed for other uses; ask your doctor or pharmacist for more information.

How should this medicine be used?

The combination of acetaminophen and hydrocodone comes as a tablet, capsule, and liquid to take by mouth. It usually is taken every 4-6 hours as needed. Follow the directions on your prescription label carefully, and ask your doctor or pharmacist to explain any part you do not understand. Take acetaminophen and hydrocodone exactly as directed.

Hydrocodone can be habit-forming. Do not take a larger dose, take it more often, or for a longer period than your doctor tells you to.

What special precautions should I follow?

Before taking acetaminophen and hydrocodone,

- tell your doctor and pharmacist if you are allergic to acetaminophen, codeine, hydrocodone, sulfite, or any other drugs.
- tell your doctor and pharmacist what prescription and nonprescription medications you are taking, especially acetaminophen (Tylenol); antidepressants; medications for cough, cold, or allergies; other pain relievers; sedatives; sleeping pills; tranquilizers; and vitamins.
- tell your doctor if you have or have ever had liver or kidney disease, a history of alcoholism, lung or thyroid disease, prostatic hypertrophy, or urinary retention.
- tell your doctor if you are pregnant, plan to become pregnant, or are breast-feeding. If you become pregnant while taking acetaminophen and hydrocodone, call your doctor.
- if you are having surgery, including dental surgery, tell the doctor or dentist that you are taking acetaminophen and hydrocodone.
- you should know that this drug may make you drowsy and dizzy; do not drive a car or operate heavy machinery until you know how acetaminophen and hydrocodone affects you.
- talk to your doctor about the safe use of alcohol. Alcohol may alter the effectiveness of acetaminophen and hydrocodone.

What should I do if I forget to take a dose?

This medication usually is taken as needed. If your doctor has told you to take acetaminophen and hydrocodone regularly, take the missed dose as soon as you remember it. However, if it is almost time for the next dose, skip the missed dose and continue your regular dosing schedule. Do not take a double dose to make up for a missed one.

What side effects can this medicine cause?

Acetaminophen and hydrocodone may cause side effects. Tell your doctor if any of these symptoms are severe or do not go away:

- lightheadedness
- dizziness
- drowsiness
- upset stomach
- vomiting
- constipation
- stomach pain
- rash
- difficulty urinating

If you experience either of the following symptoms, call your doctor immediately:

- difficulty breathing
- mood changes

If you experience a serious side effect, you or your doctor may send a report to the Food and Drug Administration's (FDA) MedWatch Adverse Event Reporting program online [at http://www.fda.gov/MedWatch/index.html] or by phone [1-800-332-1088].

What storage conditions are needed for this medicine?

Keep this medication in the container it came in, tightly closed, and out of reach of children. Store it at room temperature and away from excess heat and moisture (not in the bathroom). Throw away any medication that is outdated or no longer needed. Talk to your pharmacist about the proper disposal of your medication.

What should I do in case of overdose?

In case of overdose, call your local poison control center at 1-800-222-1222. If the victim has collapsed or is not breathing, call local emergency services at 911.

What other information should I know?

Keep all appointments with your doctor. If your pain is not controlled or continues, call your doctor.

Too much acetaminophen may cause liver damage; do not take more than 4000 mg of acetaminophen per day.

Do not let anyone else take your medication. Ask your pharmacist any questions you have about refilling your prescription.

Talk to your doctor, pharmacist, or other healthcare professional if you have questions about dosing information for your medication.

Acetaminophen and Oxycodone

(a set a mee' noe fen) (ox i koe' done)

Brand Name: Endocet®, Percocet®, Roxicet®, Roxilox®, Tylox®

Why is this medicine prescribed?

This combination of drugs is used to relieve moderate to moderately severe pain.

This medication is sometimes prescribed for other uses; ask your doctor or pharmacist for more information.

How should this medicine be used?

The combination of acetaminophen and oxycodone comes as a tablet, capsule, and liquid to take by mouth. It usually is taken every 6 hours as needed. Follow the directions on your prescription label carefully, and ask your doctor or pharmacist to explain any part you do not understand. Take acetaminophen and oxycodone exactly as directed.

Oxycodone can be habit-forming. Do not take a larger dose, take it more often, or for a longer period than your doctor tells you to.

What special precautions should I follow?

Before taking acetaminophen and oxycodone,

- tell your doctor and pharmacist if you are allergic to acetaminophen, codeine, oxycodone, sulfite, or any other drugs.
- tell your doctor and pharmacist what prescription and nonprescription medications you are taking, especially acetaminophen (Tylenol); antidepressants; medications for cough; cold; or allergies; other pain relievers; sedatives; sleeping pills; tranquilizers; and vitamins.
- tell your doctor if you have or have ever had liver or kidney disease, a history of alcoholism, lung or thyroid disease, prostatic hypertrophy, or urinary retention.
- tell your doctor if you are pregnant, plan to become pregnant, or are breast-feeding. If you become pregnant while taking acetaminophen and oxycodone, call your doctor.
- if you are having surgery, including dental surgery, tell the doctor or dentist that you are taking acetaminophen and oxycodone.
- you should know that this drug may make you drowsy. Do not drive a car or operate machinery until you know how this drug affects you.
- remember that alcohol can add to the drowsiness caused by this drug.

What should I do if I forget to take a dose?

This medication usually is taken as needed. If your doctor has told you to take acetaminophen and oxycodone regularly, take the missed dose as soon as you remember it. However, if it is almost time for the next dose, skip the missed dose and continue your regular dosing schedule. Do not take a double dose to make up for a missed one.

What side effects can this medicine cause?

Acetaminophen and oxycodone may cause side effects. Tell your doctor if any of these symptoms are severe or do not go away:

- dizziness
- lightheadedness
- drowsiness
- upset stomach
- vomiting
- constipation
- stomach pain
- rash
- difficulty urinating

If you experience either of the following symptoms, call your doctor immediately:

- difficulty breathing
- mood changes

If you experience a serious side effect, you or your doctor may send a report to the Food and Drug Administration's (FDA) MedWatch Adverse Event Reporting program online [at http://www.fda.gov/MedWatch/index.html] or by phone [1-800-332-1088].

What storage conditions are needed for this medicine?

Keep this medication in the container it came in, tightly closed, and out of reach of children. Store it at room temperature and away from excess heat and moisture (not in the bathroom). Throw away any medication that is outdated or no longer needed. Talk to your pharmacist about the proper disposal of your medication.

What should I do in case of overdose?

In case of overdose, call your local poison control center at 1-800-222-1222. If the victim has collapsed or is not breathing, call local emergency services at 911.

What other information should I know?

Keep all appointments with your doctor.

Too much acetaminophen may cause liver damage; do not take more than 4000 mg of acetaminophen per day.

Do not let anyone else take your medication. Ask your pharmacist any questions you have about refilling your prescription.

Talk to your doctor, pharmacist, or other healthcare professional if you have questions about dosing information for your medication.

Acetaminophen and Propoxyphene

(a set a mee′ noe fen) (proe pox′ i feen)

Brand Name: Darvocet-N®, E-Lor®, Genagesic®, Wygesic®

> ### Important Warning
>
> Propoxyphene in high doses, taken by itself or in combination with other drugs, has been associated with drug-related deaths. Do not take propoxyphene in combination with other drugs that cause drowsiness: alcohol, tranquilizers, sleep aids, antidepressant drugs, or antihistamines. Do not take a larger dose, take it more often, or for a longer period than your doctor tells you to.

Why is this medicine prescribed?

This combination of drugs is used to relieve mild to moderate pain. The drug also will help treat fever.

This medication is sometimes prescribed for other uses; ask your doctor or pharmacist for more information.

How should this medicine be used?

The combination of acetaminophen and propoxyphene comes as a tablet to take by mouth. It usually is taken every 4 hours as needed. Follow the directions on your prescription label carefully, and ask your doctor or pharmacist to explain any part you do not understand. Take acetaminophen and propoxyphene exactly as directed.

Propoxyphene can be habit-forming. Do not take a larger dose, take it more often, or for a longer period than your doctor tells you to.

What special precautions should I follow?

Before taking acetaminophen and propoxyphene,

- tell your doctor and pharmacist if you are allergic to acetaminophen, propoxyphene, sulfite, or any other drugs.
- tell your doctor and pharmacist what prescription and nonprescription medications you are taking, especially acetaminophen (Tylenol); anticoagulants ('blood thinners') such as warfarin (Coumadin); antidepressants; medications for cough, cold, or allergies; sedatives; seizure medications; sleeping pills; tranquilizers; and vitamins.
- tell your doctor if you have or have ever had liver or kidney disease, a history of alcoholism, lung or thyroid disease, prostatic hypertrophy, or urinary retention.
- tell your doctor if you are pregnant, plan to become pregnant, or are breast-feeding. If you become pregnant while taking acetaminophen and propoxyphene, call your doctor.
- if you are having surgery, including dental surgery, tell the doctor or dentist that you are taking acetaminophen and propoxyphene.
- you should know that this drug may make you drowsy. Do not drive a car or operate machinery until you know how this drug affects you.
- remember that alcohol can add to the drowsiness caused by this drug.

What should I do if I forget to take a dose?

This medication usually is taken as needed. If your doctor has told you to take acetaminophen and propoxyphene regularly, take the missed dose as soon as you remember it. However, if it is almost time for the next dose, skip the missed dose and continue your regular dosing schedule. Do not take a double dose to make up for a missed one.

What side effects can this medicine cause?

Acetaminophen and propoxyphene may cause side effects. Tell your doctor if any of these symptoms are severe or do not go away:

- dizziness
- lightheadedness

- drowsiness
- upset stomach
- vomiting
- constipation
- stomach pain
- rash
- difficulty urinating

If you experience either of the following symptoms, call your doctor immediately:

- difficulty breathing
- mood changes

If you experience a serious side effect, you or your doctor may send a report to the Food and Drug Administration's (FDA) MedWatch Adverse Event Reporting program online [at http://www.fda.gov/MedWatch/index.html] or by phone [1-800-332-1088].

What storage conditions are needed for this medicine?

Keep this medication in the container it came in, tightly closed, and out of reach of children. Store it at room temperature and away from excess heat and moisture (not in the bathroom). Throw away any medication that is outdated or no longer needed. Talk to your pharmacist about the proper disposal of your medication.

What should I do in case of overdose?

In case of overdose, call your local poison control center at 1-800-222-1222. If the victim has collapsed or is not breathing, call local emergency services at 911.

What other information should I know?

Keep all appointments with your doctor.

Too much acetaminophen may cause liver damage; do not take more than 4000 mg of acetaminophen per day.

Do not let anyone else take your medication. Ask your pharmacist any questions you have about refilling your prescription.

Talk to your doctor, pharmacist, or other healthcare professional if you have questions about dosing information for your medication.

Acetaminophen, Butalbital, and Caffeine

(a set a mee′ noe fen) (byoo tal′ bi tal) (kaf′ een)

Brand Name: Amaphen®, Anoquan®, Butace®, Endolor®, Esgic®, Fioricet®, Medigesic®, Repan®

Why is this medicine prescribed?

This combination of drugs is used to relieve tension headaches.

This medication is sometimes prescribed for other uses; ask your doctor or pharmacist for more information.

How should this medicine be used?

The combination of acetaminophen, butalbital, and caffeine comes as a capsule and tablet to take by mouth. It usually is taken every 4 hours as needed. Follow the directions on your prescription label carefully, and ask your doctor or pharmacist to explain any part you do not understand. Take acetaminophen, butalbital, and caffeine exactly as directed. Do not take more than six tablets or capsules in 1 day. If you think that you need more to relieve your symptoms, call your doctor.

This medication can be habit-forming. Do not take a larger dose, take it more often, or for a longer period than your doctor tells you to.

What special precautions should I follow?

Before taking acetaminophen, butalbital, and caffeine,

- tell your doctor and pharmacist if you are allergic to acetaminophen, butalbital, caffeine, or any other drugs.
- tell your doctor and pharmacist what prescription and nonprescription medications you are taking, especially anticoagulants ('blood thinners') such as warfarin (Coumadin), antidepressants, antihistamines, pain medications, sedatives, sleeping pills, tranquilizers, and vitamins. Many nonprescription pain relievers contain acetaminophen. Too much of this drug can be harmful.
- tell your doctor if you have or have ever had liver disease, porphyria, or depression.
- tell your doctor if you are pregnant, plan to become pregnant, or are breast-feeding. If you become pregnant while taking this medication, call your doctor.
- you should know that this drug may make you drowsy. Do not drive a car or operate machinery until you know how this drug affects you.
- remember that alcohol can add to the drowsiness caused by this drug.

What special dietary instructions should I follow?

Acetaminophen, butalbital, and caffeine may cause an upset stomach. Take this medicine with food or milk.

What should I do if I forget to take a dose?

Take the missed dose as soon as you remember it. However, if it is almost time for the next dose, skip the missed dose and continue your regular dosing schedule. Do not take a double dose to make up for a missed one.

What side effects can this medicine cause?

Acetaminophen, butalbital, and caffeine may cause side effects. Tell your doctor if any of these symptoms are severe or do not go away:

- drowsiness
- upset stomach
- vomiting
- stomach pain
- depression
- lightheadedness
- confusion

If you experience any of the following symptoms, call your doctor immediately:

- skin rash
- itching
- difficulty breathing

If you experience a serious side effect, you or your doctor may send a report to the Food and Drug Administration's (FDA) MedWatch Adverse Event Reporting program online [at http://www.fda.gov/MedWatch/index.html] or by phone [1-800-332-1088].

What storage conditions are needed for this medicine?

Keep this medication in the container it came in, tightly closed, and out of reach of children. Store it at room temperature, away from excess heat and moisture (not in the bathroom). Throw away any medication that is outdated or no longer needed. Talk to your pharmacist about the proper disposal of your medication.

What should I do in case of overdose?

In case of overdose, call your local poison control center at 1-800-222-1222. If the victim has collapsed or is not breathing, call local emergency services at 911.

What other information should I know?

Keep all appointments with your doctor.

Do not let anyone else take your medication. This medication is a controlled substance. Prescriptions may be refilled only a limited number of times; ask your pharmacist if you have any questions.

Talk to your doctor, pharmacist, or other healthcare professional if you have questions about dosing information for your medication.

Acetazolamide Oral

(a set a zole' a mide)

Brand Name: Diamox® Sequels®

Why is this medicine prescribed?

Acetazolamide is used to treat glaucoma, a condition in which increased pressure in the eye can lead to gradual loss of vision. Acetazolamide decreases the pressure in the eye. Acetazolamide is also used to reduce the severity and duration of symptoms (upset stomach, headache, shortness of breath, dizziness, drowsiness, and fatigue) of altitude (mountain) sickness. Acetazolamide is used with other medicines to reduce edema (excess water retention) and to help control seizures in certain types of epilepsy.

This medication is sometimes prescribed for other uses; ask your doctor or pharmacist for more information.

How should this medicine be used?

Acetazolamide comes as a tablet and capsule to take by mouth. Follow the directions on your prescription label carefully, and ask your doctor or pharmacist to explain any part you do not understand. Take acetazolamide exactly as directed. Do not take more or less of it or take it more often than prescribed by your doctor.

If you are taking the extended-release (long-acting) form of acetazolamide (Diamox Sequels), do not crush or chew the capsules.

What special precautions should I follow?

Before taking acetazolamide,

- tell your doctor and pharmacist if you are allergic to acetazolamide, sulfa drugs, diuretics ('water pills'), or any other drugs.
- tell your doctor and pharmacist what prescription and nonprescription medications you are taking, especially amphetamines, aspirin, cyclosporine (Neoral, Sandimmune), medications for depression or irregular heartbeat, diflunisal (Dolobid), digoxin (Lanoxin), diuretics ('water pills'), lithium (Eskalith, Lithobid), phenobarbital, primidone (Mysoline), and vitamins.
- tell your doctor if you have or have ever had heart, liver, or kidney disease; or diabetes.
- tell your doctor if you are pregnant, plan to become pregnant, or are breast-feeding. If you become pregnant while taking acetazolamide, call your doctor immediately.
- if you are having surgery, including dental surgery, tell the doctor or dentist that you are taking acetazolamide.
- you should know that this drug may make you drowsy. Do not drive a car or operate machinery until you know how this drug affects you.
- remember that alcohol can add to the drowsiness caused by this drug.

- plan to avoid unnecessary or prolonged exposure to sunlight and to wear protective clothing, sunglasses, and sunscreen. Acetazolamide may make your skin sensitive to sunlight.

What should I do if I forget to take a dose?

Take the missed dose as soon as you remember it. However, if it is almost time for the next dose, skip the missed dose and continue your regular dosing schedule. Do not take a double dose to make up for the missed one.

What side effects can this medicine cause?

Acetazolamide may cause side effects. Tell your doctor if any of these symptoms are severe or do not go away:

- upset stomach
- vomiting
- loss of appetite

If you experience any of the following symptoms, call your doctor immediately:

- numbness and tingling
- increased thirst and urination
- drowsiness
- headache
- confusion
- fever
- rash
- blood in urine
- painful urination
- yellowing of the skin or eyes
- seizures
- sore throat
- unusual bleeding or bruising

If you experience a serious side effect, you or your doctor may send a report to the Food and Drug Administration's (FDA) MedWatch Adverse Event Reporting program online [at http://www.fda.gov/MedWatch/index.html] or by phone [1-800-332-1088].

What storage conditions are needed for this medicine?

Keep this medication in the container it came in, tightly closed, and out of reach of children. Store it at room temperature and away from excess heat and moisture (not in the bathroom). Throw away any medication that is outdated or no longer needed. Talk to your pharmacist about the proper disposal of your medication.

What should I do in case of overdose?

In case of overdose, call your local poison control center at 1-800-222-1222. If the victim has collapsed or is not breathing, call local emergency services at 911.

What other information should I know?

Keep all appointments with your doctor and the laboratory. Your doctor will order certain tests to check your response to acetazolamide.

Do not let anyone else to take your medication. Ask your pharmacist any questions you have about refilling your prescription.

Talk to your doctor, pharmacist, or other healthcare professional if you have questions about dosing information for your medication.

Acitretin

(a si tre′ tin)

Brand Name: Soriatane®

Important Warning

For female patients:

Do not take acitretin if you are pregnant or plan to become pregnant within the next 3 years. Acitretin may harm the fetus. You should not begin taking acitretin until you have taken two pregnancy tests with negative results. You must use two acceptable forms of birth control for 1 month before you begin taking acitretin, during your treatment with acitretin, and for 3 years after treatment. Your doctor will tell you which methods of birth control are acceptable. You do not need to use two methods of birth control if you have had a hysterectomy (surgery to remove the womb), if your doctor tells you that you have finished menopause (change of life), or if you practice total sexual abstinence.

If you plan to use oral contraceptives (birth control pills) while taking acitretin, tell your doctor the name of the pill you will use. Acitretin interferes with the action of microdosed progestin ('minipill') oral contraceptives (Ovrette, Micronor, Nor-QD). Do not use this type of birth control while taking acitretin.

If you plan to use hormonal contraceptives (birth control pills, patches, implants, injections, and intrauterine devices), be sure to tell your doctor about all the medications, vitamins, and herbal supplements you are taking. Many medications interfere with the action of hormonal contraceptives. Do not take St. John's wort if you are using any type of hormonal contraceptive.

You will need to take pregnancy tests regularly while taking acitretin. Stop taking acitretin and call your doctor immediately if you become pregnant, miss a menstrual period, or have sex without using two forms of birth control. In some cases, your doctor can prescribe emergency contraception ('the morning after pill') to prevent pregnancy.

Do not consume foods, drinks, or prescription or nonprescription medications that contain alcohol while taking acitretin and for 2 months after treat-

continued on next page

Important Warning (cont'd)

ment. Alcohol and acitretin combine to form a substance that remains in the blood for a long time and can harm the fetus. Read medication and food labels carefully and ask your doctor or pharmacist if you are not sure whether a medication contains alcohol.

Your doctor will give you a Patient Agreement/ Informed Consent to read and sign before you begin treatment. Be sure to read this carefully and ask your doctor if you have any questions.

For male patients:

A small amount of acitretin is present in the semen of male patients who take this medication. It is not known whether this small amount of medication can harm the fetus. Talk to your doctor about the risks of taking this medication if your partner is pregnant or plans to become pregnant.

For male and female patients:

Do not donate blood while taking acitretin and for 3 years after treatment.

Acitretin may cause liver damage. Tell your doctor if you have or have ever had liver disease. If you experience any of the following symptoms, call your doctor immediately: upset stomach, extreme tiredness, unusual bruising or bleeding, lack of energy, loss of appetite, pain in the upper right part of the stomach, yellowing of the skin or eyes, dark urine, or flu-like symptoms.

Why is this medicine prescribed?

Actitretin is used to treat severe psoriasis (abnormal growth of skin cells that causes red, thickened, or scaly skin). Acitretin is in a class of medications called retinoids. The way acitretin works is not known.

How should this medicine be used?

Actitretin comes as a capsule to take by mouth. It is usually taken once a day with the main meal. Take acitretin at around the same time every day. Follow the directions on your prescription label carefully, and ask your doctor or pharmacist to explain any part you do not understand. Take acitretin exactly as directed. Do not take more or less of it or take it more often than prescribed by your doctor.

Your doctor may start you on a low dose of acitretin and gradually increase your dose.

Acitretin controls psoriasis but does not cure it. It may take 2-3 months or longer before you feel the full benefit of acitretin. Your psoriasis may get worse during the first few months of treatment. This does not mean that acitretin will not work for you, but tell your doctor if this happens. Continue to take acitretin even if you feel well. Do not stop taking acitretin without talking to your doctor.

After you stop taking acitretin, your symptoms may come back. Tell your doctor if this happens. Do not use leftover acitretin to treat a new flare-up of psoriasis. A different medication or dose may be needed.

Are there other uses for this medicine?

Acitretin is sometimes also used to treat Darier's disease (a type of skin disease); palmoplantar pustulosis (pus-filled blisters and red patches on the hands and feet); lichen sclerosus et atrophicus of the vulva (redness, scaling, and easy bleeding of the genital area in females); palmoplantar lichen nitidus (clusters of bumps on the hands and feet); and lichen planus (red, itchy bumps in various places on the body). It is also used to treat lamellar ichthyosis (scaly patches of skin that fall off the body); Sjogren-Larsson syndrome (dry, scaling skin, mental retardation, and trouble walking); and bullous and nonbullous ichthyosiform erythroderma (red, blistering, or peeling skin) in children. Talk to your doctor about the possible risks of using this drug for your condition.

This medication may be prescribed for other uses; ask your doctor or pharmacist for more information.

What special precautions should I follow?

Before taking acitretin,

- tell your doctor and pharmacist if you are allergic to acitretin, other retinoids such as adapalene (Differen), alitretinoin (Panretin), etretinate (Tegison), isotretinoin (Accutane), tazarotene (Tazorac), tretinoin (Renova, Retin-A, Vesanoid), Vitamin A, or any other medications.
- do not take methotrexate (Rheumatrex, Trexall) or tetracycline antibiotics such as demeclocycline (Declomycin), doxycycline (Doryx, Vibramycin), minocycline (Dynacin, Minocin), and tetracycline (Sumycin) while taking acitretin.
- tell your doctor and pharmacist what other prescription and nonprescription medications, vitamins, nutritional supplements, and herbal products you are taking. Be sure to mention the medications and herbs listed in the IMPORTANT WARNING section and any of the following: glyburide (Diabeta, Glynase, Micronase), other oral retinoids such as isotretinoin (Accutane) and tretinoin (Vesanoid), phenytoin (Dilantin, Phenytek), and vitamin A. Also tell your doctor if you have ever taken etretinate (Tegison). Your doctor may need to change the doses of your medications or monitor you carefully for side effects.
- tell your doctor if you have or have ever had the conditions mentioned in the IMPORTANT WARNING section; if you drink large amounts of alcohol; if you have a family history of high cholesterol or diabetes; if you have or have ever had diabetes, high cholesterol or triglycerides, spinal problems, depression, or stroke or mini-stroke; or if you have or have ever had joint, bone, kidney, or heart disease.
- do not breastfeed while taking acitretin or if you have recently stopped taking acitretin.
- you should know that acitretin may limit your ability to see at night. This problem may begin suddenly at any time during your treatment. Be very careful when driving at night.

- plan to avoid unnecessary or prolonged exposure to sunlight and to wear protective clothing, sunglasses, and sunscreen. Do not use sunlamps while taking acitretin. Acitretin may make your skin sensitive to sunlight.
- if you need to have phototherapy, tell your doctor that you are taking acitretin.
- you should know that acitretin may dry your eyes and make wearing contact lenses uncomfortable during or after treatment. Remove your contact lenses and call your doctor if this happens.

What special dietary instructions should I follow?

Unless your doctor tells you otherwise, continue your normal diet.

What should I do if I forget to take a dose?

Take the missed dose as soon as you remember it. However, if it is almost time for the next dose, skip the missed dose and continue your regular dosing schedule. Do not take a double dose to make up for a missed one.

What side effects can this medicine cause?

You may experience hypoglycemia (low blood sugar) while you are taking this medication. Your doctor will tell you what you should do if you develop hypoglycemia. He or she may tell you to check your blood sugar, eat or drink a food or beverage that contains sugar, such as hard candy or fruit juice, or get medical care. Follow these directions carefully if you have any of the following symptoms of hypoglycemia:

- shakiness
- dizziness or lightheadedness
- sweating
- nervousness or irritability
- sudden changes in behavior or mood
- headache
- numbness or tingling around the mouth
- weakness
- pale skin
- hunger
- clumsy or jerky movements

If hypoglycemia is not treated, severe symptoms may develop. Be sure that your family, friends, and other people who spend time with you know that if you have any of the following symptoms, they should get medical treatment for you immediately.

- confusion
- seizures
- loss of consciousness

Acitretin can also cause hyperglycemia (high blood sugar). Call your doctor immediately if you have any of the following symptoms of hyperglycemia:

- extreme thirst
- frequent urination
- extreme hunger

- weakness
- blurred vision

If high blood sugar is not treated, a serious, life-threatening condition called diabetic ketoacidosis could develop. Call your doctor immediately if you have any of the these symptoms:

- dry mouth
- upset stomach and vomiting
- shortness of breath
- breath that smells fruity
- decreased consciousness

Acitretin may cause other side effects. Tell your doctor if any of these symptoms are severe or do not go away:

- peeling, dry, itchy, scaling, cracked, blistered, sticky or infected skin
- brittle or weak fingernails and toenails
- dandruff
- sunburn
- abnormal skin odor
- excessive sweating
- hair loss
- changes in hair texture
- dry eyes
- loss of eyebrows or eyelashes
- hot flashes or flushing
- weak nails
- chapped or swollen lips
- swollen or bleeding gums
- excessive saliva
- tongue pain, swelling, or blistering
- mouth swelling or blisters
- stomach pain
- diarrhea
- increased appetite
- difficulty falling or staying asleep
- sinus infection
- runny nose
- dry nose
- nosebleed
- joint pain
- tight muscles

Some side effects can be serious. The following symptoms are uncommon, but if you experience any of them or those listed in the IMPORTANT WARNING section, call your doctor immediately:

- rash
- headache
- upset stomach
- vomiting
- blurred vision
- pain, swelling, or redness of eyes or eyelids
- eye pain
- eyes sensitive to light
- swelling of hands, feet, ankles, or lower legs
- redness or swelling in one leg only
- depression
- thoughts of hurting or killing yourself

- bone, muscle, or back pain
- difficulty moving any part of your body
- loss of feeling in hands or feet
- chest pain
- slow or difficult speech
- rash
- tingling in arms and legs
- loss of muscle tone
- weakness or heaviness in legs
- confusion
- cold, gray skin
- slow or irregular heartbeat
- pale skin
- dizziness
- fast heartbeat
- weakness
- shortness of breath

Acitretin may cause bone problems and slowing or stopping of growth in children. Talk to your child's doctor about the risks of giving this medication to your child.

Acitretin may cause other side effects. Call your doctor if you have any unusual problems while taking this medication.

If you experience a serious side effect, you or your doctor may send a report to the Food and Drug Administration's (FDA) MedWatch Adverse Event Reporting program online [at http://www.fda.gov/MedWatch/index.html] or by phone [1-800-332-1088].

What storage conditions are needed for this medicine?

Keep this medication in the container it came in, tightly closed, and out of reach of children. Store it at room temperature and away from excess heat and moisture (not in the bathroom). Throw away any medication that is outdated or no longer needed. Talk to your pharmacist about the proper disposal of your medication.

What should I do in case of overdose?

In case of overdose, call your local poison control center at 1-800-222-1222. If the victim has collapsed or is not breathing, call local emergency services at 911.

Symptoms of overdose may include:
- headache
- dizziness
- vomiting
- upset stomach
- dry, itchy skin
- loss of appetite
- bone or joint pain

If a female who could become pregnant takes an overdose of acitretin, she should take a pregnancy test after the overdose and use two forms of birth control for the next 3 years.

What other information should I know?

Keep all appointments with your doctor and the laboratory. Your doctor will order certain lab tests to check your body's response to acitretin.

Do not let anyone else take your medication. Ask your pharmacist any questions you have about refilling your prescription.

Talk to your doctor, pharmacist, or other healthcare professional if you have questions about dosing information for your medication.

Acyclovir
(ay sye' kloe veer)

Brand Name: Zovirax®
Also available generically.

Why is this medicine prescribed?

Acyclovir is used to decrease pain and speed the healing of sores or blisters in people who have varicella (chickenpox), herpes zoster (shingles; a rash that can occur in people who have had chickenpox in the past), and first-time or repeat outbreaks of genital herpes (a herpes virus infection that causes sores to form around the genitals and rectum from time to time). Acyclovir is also sometimes used to prevent outbreaks of genital herpes in people who are infected with the virus. Acyclovir is in a class of antiviral medications called synthetic nucleoside analogues. It works by stopping the spread of the herpes virus in the body. Acyclovir will not cure genital herpes and may not stop the spread of genital herpes to other people.

How should this medicine be used?

Acyclovir comes as a tablet, a capsule, and a suspension (liquid) to take by mouth. It is usually taken with or without food two to five times a day for 5 to 10 days, starting as soon as possible after your symptoms begin. When acyclovir is used to prevent outbreaks of genital herpes, it is usually taken two to five times a day for up to 12 months. Take acyclovir at around the same times every day. Follow the directions on your prescription label carefully, and ask your doctor or pharmacist to explain any part you do not understand. Take acyclovir exactly as directed. Do not take more or less of it or take it more often or for a longer time than prescribed by your doctor.

Shake the liquid well before each use to mix the medication evenly.

Your symptoms should improve during your treatment with acyclovir. Call your doctor if your symptoms do not improve or if they get worse.

Take acyclovir until you finish the prescription, even if you feel better. If you stop taking acyclovir too soon or skip doses, your infection may not be completely treated or may become more difficult to treat.

Are there other uses for this medicine?

Acyclovir is also sometimes used to treat eczema herpeticum (a skin infection caused by the herpes virus) to treat and prevent herpes infections of the skin, eyes, nose, and mouth in patients with human immunodeficiency virus (HIV), and to treat oral hairy leukoplakia (condition that causes hairy white or gray-colored patches on the tongue or inside of the cheek).

This medication may be prescribed for other uses; ask your doctor or pharmacist for more information.

What special precautions should I follow?

Before taking acyclovir,
- tell your doctor and pharmacist if you are allergic to acyclovir, valacyclovir (Valtrex), any other medications, or any of the ingredients in acyclovir. Ask your pharmacist for a list of the ingredients.
- tell your doctor and pharmacist what prescription and nonprescription medications, vitamins, nutritional supplements, and herbal products you are taking or plan to take. Be sure to mention any of the following: amphotericin B (Fungizone); aminoglycoside antibiotics such as amikacin (Amikin), gentamicin (Garamycin), kanamycin (Kantrex), neomycin (Nes-RX, Neo-Fradin), paramomycin (Humatin), streptomycin, and tobramycin (Tobi, Nebcin); aspirin and other nonsteroidal anti-inflammatory medications such as ibuprofen (Advil, Motrin), and naproxen (Aleve, Naprosyn); cyclosporine (Neoral, Sandimmune); medications to treat HIV or AIDS such as zidovudine (Retrovir, AZT); pentamidine (NebuPent); probenecid (Benemid); sulfonamides such as sulfamethoxazole and trimethoprim (Bactrim); tacrolimus (Prograf); and vancomycin. Many other medications may also interact with acyclovir, so be sure to tell your doctor about all the medications you are taking, even those that do not appear on this list. Your doctor may need to change the doses of your medications or monitor you carefully for side effects.
- tell your doctor if there is a possibility you may be dehydrated from a recent illness or activity, or if you have or have ever had problems with your immune system; human immunodeficiency virus infection (HIV); acquired immunodeficiency syndrome (AIDS); or kidney disease.
- tell your doctor if you are pregnant, plan to become pregnant, or are breast-feeding. If you become pregnant while taking acyclovir, call your doctor.
- if you are taking acyclovir to treat genital herpes, you should know that genital herpes can be spread through sexual contact even if you don't have blisters or other symptoms and possibly even if you are taking acyclovir. Talk to your doctor about ways to stop the spread of genital herpes and about whether your partner(s) should receive treatment.

What special dietary instructions should I follow?

Drink plenty of fluids while you are taking acyclovir.

What should I do if I forget to take a dose?

Take the missed dose as soon as you remember it and take any remaining doses for that day at evenly spaced intervals. However, if it is almost time for the next dose, skip the missed dose and continue your regular dosing schedule. Do not take a double dose to make up for a missed one.

What side effects can this medicine cause?

Acyclovir may cause side effects. Tell your doctor if any of these symptoms are severe or do not go away:
- upset stomach
- vomiting
- diarrhea
- dizziness
- tiredness
- agitation
- pain, especially in the joints
- hair loss
- changes in vision

Some side effects can be serious. If you experience any of the following symptoms, call your doctor immediately:
- hives
- rash or blisters
- itching
- difficulty breathing or swallowing
- swelling of the face, throat, tongue, lips, eyes, hands, feet, ankles, or lower legs
- hoarseness
- fast heartbeat
- weakness
- pale skin
- difficulty sleeping
- fever, sore throat, chills, cough, and other signs of infection
- unusual bruising or bleeding
- blood in the urine
- stomach pain or cramps
- bloody diarrhea
- decreased urination
- headache
- hallucinations (seeing things or hearing voices that do not exist)
- confusion
- aggressive behavior
- difficulty speaking
- numbness, burning, or tingling in the arms or legs
- temporary inability to move parts of your body
- shaking of a part of your body that you cannot control
- seizures
- loss of consciousness

Acyclovir may cause other side effects. Call your doctor

if you have any unusual problems while you are taking this medication.

If you experience a serious side effect, you or your doctor may send a report to the Food and Drug Administration's (FDA) MedWatch Adverse Event Reporting program online [at http://www.fda.gov/MedWatch/index.html] or by phone [1-800-332-1088].

What storage conditions are needed for this medicine?

Keep this medication in the container it came in, tightly closed, and out of reach of children. Store it at room temperature and away from excess heat and moisture (not in the bathroom). Throw away any medication that is outdated or no longer needed. Talk to your pharmacist about the proper disposal of your medication.

What should I do in case of overdose?

In case of overdose, call your local poison control center at 1-800-222-1222. If the victim has collapsed or is not breathing, call local emergency services at 911.

Symptoms of overdose may include:

- agitation
- seizures
- extreme tiredness
- loss of consciousness
- swelling of the hands, feet, ankles, or lower legs
- decreased urination

What other information should I know?

Keep all appointments with your doctor and the laboratory. Your doctor may order certain lab tests to check your response to acyclovir.

Do not let anyone else take your medication. Ask your pharmacist any questions you have about refilling your prescription.

Dosage Facts
For Informational Purposes

Caution: Do not change your dose, how often you take your medication, or the length of time you are to take it without first talking to your healthcare provider.

The following dosage information was written using medical language for doctors and other healthcare professionals and is provided here for you to check your dosage. The dosage of this drug may differ for different patients. Therefore, always follow your doctor's instructions or the directions on the label. Contact your healthcare provider or pharmacist if you have any questions about the specific dosage of your medication after reviewing this information.

General Dosage Information

Available as acyclovir and acyclovir sodium; dosage expressed in terms of acyclovir.

Pediatric Patients

Mucocutaneous, Ocular, and Systemic Herpes Simplex Virus (HSV) Infections
Treatment of Mucocutaneous HSV Infections

ORAL†:
- Immunocompromised children: 1 g daily given in 3–5 divided doses for 7–14 days.

HSV Gingivostomatitis

ORAL†:
- HIV-infected children with mild, symptomatic gingivostomatitis: CDC and others recommend 20 mg/kg (up to 400 mg) 3 times daily for 7–14 days.
- Immunocompetent children: 15 mg/kg (up to 200 mg) 5 times daily for 7 days has been used in a few children 1–6 years of age.

Chronic Suppressive or Maintenance Therapy (Secondary Prophylaxis) of HSV Infections†

ORAL:
- HIV-infected infants and children: 80 mg/kg daily (up to 1 g daily) in 3 or 4 divided doses.
- HIV-infected adolescents: 200 mg 3 times daily or 400 mg twice daily.

Prophylaxis Against Recurrent Ocular HSV Disease†

ORAL:
- Children ≥12 years of age: 400 mg twice daily. AAP recommends 80 mg/kg daily (up to 1 g daily) given in 3 divided doses.
- Optimum duration of prophylaxis unclear; has been continued for 12–18 months in clinical studies.

Prevention of HSV Recurrence in Hematopoietic Stem Cell Transplant (HSCT) Recipients†

ORAL:
- HSV-seropositive children: 0.6–1 g daily given in 3–5 divided doses.
- HSV-seropositive adolescents: 200 mg 3 times daily.
- Initiate prophylaxis at beginning of conditioning therapy and continue until engraftment or until mucositis resolves (approximately 30 days after allogeneic HSCT). Routine prophylaxis for >30 days after HSCT not recommended.

Genital Herpes
Treatment of First Episodes

ORAL:
- Children: AAP recommends 40–80 mg/kg daily (maximum 1 g daily) given in 3 or 4 divided doses for 5–10 days.
- Adolescents: CDC recommends 400 mg 3 times daily or 200 mg 5 times daily for 7–10 days; duration may be extended if healing is incomplete after 10 days.
- HIV-infected adolescents: CDC and others recommend 20 mg/kg (up to 400 mg) or 400 mg 3 times daily for 7–14 days.

Episodic Treatment of Recurrent Episodes

ORAL:
- Adolescents: CDC recommends 400 mg 3 times daily for 5 days, 800 mg twice daily for 5 days, or 800 mg 3 times daily for 2 days.
- HIV-infected adolescents: CDC recommends 400 mg 3 times daily for 5–10 days. Alternatively, acyclovir can be given for 7–14 days.
- Initiate episodic therapy at the earliest prodromal sign or symptom of recurrence or within 1 day of the onset of lesions.

Chronic Suppression of Recurrent Episodes

ORAL:

- Adolescents: CDC recommends 400 mg twice daily.
- HIV-infected adolescents: CDC recommends 400–800 mg 2 or 3 times daily.
- Discontinue periodically (e.g., after 12 months or once yearly) to reassess need for continued therapy.

Varicella-Zoster Infections
Treatment of Varicella (Chickenpox)

ORAL:

- Immunocompetent children ≥2 years of age: Manufacturer recommends 20 mg/kg 4 times daily (maximum 80 mg/kg daily) for 5 days in those weighing ≤40 kg and 800 mg 4 times daily for 5 days in those weighing >40 kg. Alternatively, some clinicians recommend 20 mg/kg (up to 800 mg) 4 times daily for 5 days.
- HIV-infected children with mild immunosuppression and mild varicella: CDC and others recommend 20 mg/kg (up to 800 mg) 4 times daily for 7 days or until no new lesions have appeared for 48 hours.
- Initiate therapy at the earliest sign or symptom of infection (within 24 hours of onset of rash).

Treatment of Herpes Zoster (Shingles, Zoster)

ORAL:

- Immunocompetent children ≥12 years of age: 800 mg every 4 hours 5 times daily (4 g daily) for 5–10 days.
- HIV-infected children with mild immunosuppression and mild varicella: CDC and others recommend 20 mg/kg (up to 800 mg) 4 times daily for 7–10 days.
- Initiate therapy preferably within 48 hours of onset of rash.

Adult Patients

Mucocutaneous, Ocular, and Systemic Herpes Simplex Virus (HSV) Infections
Treatment of Mucocutaneous HSV Infections

ORAL†:

- Immunocompromised or HIV-infected adults: 400 mg every 4 hours while awake (5 times daily) for 7–14 days.

Chronic Suppressive or Maintenance Therapy (Secondary Prophylaxis) of HSV Infections†

ORAL:

- HIV-infected adults: 200 mg 3 times daily or 400 mg twice daily.

Treatment of Orolabial HSV Infections

ORAL:

- 400 mg 5 times daily for 5 days.
- HIV-infected adults: CDC and others recommend 400 mg 3 times daily for 7–14 days.

Treatment of HSV Keratitis†

ORAL:

- HIV-infected adults: 400 mg 5 times daily. Long-term therapy may be required to prevent recurrence.

Prophylaxis Against Recurrent Ocular HSV Disease†

ORAL:

- Immunocompetent adults: 400 mg twice daily. Optimum duration of prophylaxis unclear; has been continued for 12–18 months in clinical studies.

Prevention of HSV Recurrence in Hematopoietic Stem Cell Transplant (HSCT) Recipients†

ORAL:

- HSV-seropositive adults: 200 mg 3 times daily initiated at beginning of conditioning therapy and continued until engraftment or until mucositis resolves (i.e., approximately 30 days after allogeneic HSCT). Routine prophylaxis for >30 days after HSCT not recommended.

Genital Herpes
Treatment of First Episodes

ORAL:

- Manufacturer recommends 200 mg every 4 hours while awake (5 times daily) for 10 days.
- CDC and others recommend 400 mg 3 times daily or 200 mg 5 times daily for 7–10 days; duration may be extended if healing is incomplete after 10 days.
- HIV-infected adults: CDC and others recommend 400 mg 3 times daily for 7–14 days.

Treatment of First Episode of Herpes Proctitis†

ORAL:

- 400 mg 5 times daily for 10 days or until clinical resolution occurs.

Episodic Treatment of Recurrent Episodes of Genital Herpes

ORAL:

- Manufacturer recommends 200 mg every 4 hours while awake (5 times daily) for 5 days.
- CDC recommends 400 mg 3 times daily for 5 days, 800 mg twice daily for 5 days, or 800 mg 3 times daily for 2 days.
- HIV-infected adults: CDC recommends 400 mg 3 times daily for 5–10 days. Alternatively, acyclovir can be given for 7–14 days.
- Initiate episodic therapy at the earliest prodromal sign or symptom of recurrence or within 1 day of the onset of lesions.

Chronic Suppression of Recurrent Episodes of Genital Herpes

ORAL:

- 400 mg twice daily; alternatively, 200 mg 3–5 times daily.
- HIV-infected adults: 400–800 mg 2 or 3 times daily.
- Discontinue periodically (e.g., after 12 months or once yearly) to reassess need for continued therapy.

Varicella-Zoster Infections
Treatment of Varicella (Chickenpox)

ORAL:

- 20 mg/kg (up to 800 mg) 4 times daily for 5 days.
- Initiate therapy at the earliest sign or symptom of infection (within 24 hours of onset of rash).

Treatment of Herpes Zoster (Shingles, Zoster)

ORAL:

- 800 mg every 4 hours (5 times daily) for 7–10 days.
- Initiate therapy preferably within 48 hours of onset of rash.

Treatment of Herpes Zoster Ophthalmicus†

ORAL:

- Immunocompetent adults: 600 mg every 4 hours 5 times daily (3 g daily) for 10 days.
- Initiate therapy within 72 hours (but no later than 7 days) after rash onset.

Treatment of Dermatomal Herpes Zoster†

ORAL:
- Immunocompromised adults: 800 mg 5 times daily for 10 days has been used, but CDC and others recommend oral famciclovir or valacyclovir for localized dermal infections in HIV-infected individuals.

Prescribing Limits

Pediatric Patients

ORAL:
- Maximum 20 mg/kg 4 times daily (1 g daily) in children ≥ 2 years of age weighing ≤ 40 kg.

Adult Patients

ORAL:
- 800 mg per dose.

Special Populations

Renal Impairment

Adjustment of Usual Oral Dosage

Oral Dosage in Renal Impairment

Usual Dosage Regimen	Cl_{cr} (mL/min per 1.73 m²)	Adjusted Dosage Regimen
200 mg every 4 h 5 times daily	>10	No adjustment necessary
	0–10	200 mg every 12 h
400 mg every 12 h	>10	No adjustment necessary
	0–10	200 mg every 12 h
800 mg every 4 h 5 times daily	>25	No adjustment necessary
	10–25	800 mg every 8 h
	0–10	800 mg every 12 h

Hemodialysis

Give supplemental oral dose immediately after each dialysis period.

Peritoneal Dialysis

Supplemental doses do not appear necessary.

HIV-infected Patients with Impaired Renal Function (Oral Administration)

Oral Dosage for HIV-infected Patients with Impaired Renal Function (Based on Usual Dosage of 200–800 mg Every 4–6 Hours)

Cl_{cr} (mL/min per 1.73 m²)	Adjusted Dosage Regimen
>80	No adjustment necessary
50–80	200–800 mg every 6–8 h
25–50	200–800 mg every 8–12 h
10–25	200–800 mg every 12–24 h
<10	200–400 mg every 24 h

Hemodialysis

Give supplemental usual oral dose after each dialysis period.

Geriatric Patients
- Cautious dosage selection; reduced dosage may be needed because of age-related decreases in renal function.

† Use is not currently included in the labeling approved by the US Food and Drug Administration.

Acyclovir Injection

(ay sye′ kloe ver)

Brand Name: Zovirax®
Also available generically.

About Your Treatment

Your doctor has ordered acyclovir, an antiviral agent, to help treat your infection. The medication will be added to an intravenous fluid that will drip through a needle or catheter placed in your vein for at least 60 minutes every 8 hours for 5 to 10 days.

Acyclovir is used to treat
- herpes infections of the skin, nose, and mouth in people with weak immune systems
- herpes infections in newborn infants
- herpes simplex encephalitis (brain infection with swelling caused by the herpes virus)
- varicella-zoster (shingles; a rash that can occur in people who have had chickenpox in the past) in people with weak immune systems
- the first outbreak of a genital herpes infection (a herpes virus infection that causes sores to form around the genitals and rectum from time to time)

Acyclovir is in a class of antiviral medications known as synthetic nucleoside analogues. It works by stopping the spread of the herpes virus in the body. Acyclovir will not cure genital herpes and may not stop the spread of genital herpes to other people. This medication may be prescribed for other uses; ask your doctor or pharmacist for more information.

This medication is most effective if started soon after the first signs of infection appear.

Your symptoms should improve during your treatment with acyclovir. Call your doctor if your symptoms do not improve or if they get worse.

Your health care provider (doctor, nurse, or pharmacist) may measure the effectiveness and side effects of your treatment using laboratory tests and physical examinations. It is important to keep all appointments with your doctor and the laboratory. The length of treatment depends on how your infection and symptoms respond to the medication.

Precautions

Before using acyclovir,
- tell your doctor and pharmacist if you are allergic to

acyclovir, valacyclovir (Valtrex), or any other medications.

- tell your doctor and pharmacist what prescription and nonprescription medications, vitamins, nutritional supplements, and herbal products you are taking or plan to take. Be sure to mention any of the following: amphotericin B (Fungizone); aminoglycoside antibiotics such as amikacin (Amikin), gentamicin (Garamycin), kanamycin (Kantrex), neomycin (Nes-RX, Neo-Fradin), paramomycin (Humatin), streptomycin, and tobramycin (Tobi, Nebcin); aspirin and other nonsteroidal anti-inflammatory medications such as ibuprofen (Advil, Motrin), and naproxen (Aleve, Naprosyn); cyclosporine (Neoral, Sandimmune); interferon; medications to treat HIV or AIDS such as zidovudine (Retrovir); methotrexate, pentamidine (NebuPent); probenecid (Benemid); sulfonamides such as sulfamethoxazole and trimethoprin (Bactrim); tacrolimus (Prograf); and vancomycin (Vancocin). Many other medications may also interact with acyclovir, so be sure to tell your doctor about all the medications you are taking, even those that do not appear on this list. Your doctor may need to change the doses of your medications or monitor you carefully for side effects.
- tell your doctor if there is a possibility that you may be dehydrated from a recent illness or activity, or if you have or have ever had problems with your immune system; human immunodeficiency virus infection (HIV); acquired immunodeficiency syndrome (AIDS); or kidney, liver, or nervous system disease.
- tell your doctor if you are pregnant, plan to become pregnant, or are breast-feeding. If you become pregnant while taking acyclovir, call your doctor.
- if you are using acyclovir to treat genital herpes, you should know that genital herpes can be spread through sexual contact even if you don't have blisters or other symptoms and possibly even if you are using acyclovir. Talk to your doctor about ways to stop the spread of genital herpes and about whether your partner(s) should receive treatment.
- be sure to drink plenty of fluids during your treatment with acyclovir.

Administering Your Medication

Before you use acyclovir, look at the solution closely. It should be clear and free of floating material. Gently squeeze the bag or observe the solution container to make sure there are no leaks. Do not use the solution if it is discolored, if it contains particles, or if the bag or container leaks. Use a new solution, but show the damaged one to your health care provider.

It is important that you use your medication exactly as directed. Do not stop your therapy on your own or skip doses for any reason because your infection could worsen and result in hospitalization or could become more difficult to treat. Do not change your dosing schedule without talking to your health care provider. Your health care provider may tell you

to stop your infusion if you have a mechanical problem (such as a blockage in the tubing, needle, or catheter). If you have to stop an infusion, call your health care provider immediately so your therapy can continue.

Side Effects

Acyclovir may cause side effects. Tell your health care provider if any of these symptoms are severe or do not go away:

- headache
- upset stomach
- vomiting
- diarrhea
- loss of appetite
- dizziness
- hair loss
- muscle or joint pain
- vision problems

Some side effects can be serious. If you experience any of the following symptoms, call your health care provider immediately:

- rash or blisters
- itching
- hives
- difficulty breathing or swallowing
- swelling of the face, throat, tongue, lips, eyes, hands, feet, ankles, or lower legs
- extreme tiredness
- confusion
- hallucinations (seeing things or hearing voices that are not really there)
- agitation
- shaking of a part of your body that you cannot control
- seizures
- unusual bleeding or bruising
- difficulty speaking
- numbness or tingling in the hands, arms, feet, or legs
- temporary inability to move part of your body
- stomach pain or cramps
- bloody diarrhea
- bloody urine
- fever

Acyclovir may cause other side effects. Call your doctor if you have any unusual problems while using this medication.

If you experience a serious side effect, you or your doctor may send a report to the Food and Drug Administration's (FDA) MedWatch Adverse Event Reporting program online [at http://www.fda.gov/MedWatch/index.html] or by phone [1-800-332-1088].

Storage Conditions

Your health care provider will probably tell you to store your medication at room temperature. Store your medication only as directed. Make sure you understand how to store your medication properly. Throw away any medication that is expired or no longer needed. Talk to your health care provider about the proper disposal of your medication.

Keep your supplies in a clean, dry place when you are not using them, and keep all medications and supplies out of reach of children. Your health care provider will tell you how to throw away used needles, syringes, tubing, and containers to avoid accidental injury.

Overdose

In case of overdose, call your local poison control center at 1-800-222-1222. If the victim has collapsed or is not breathing, call local emergency services at 911.

Symptoms of overdose may include:

- agitation
- seizures
- extreme tiredness
- loss of consciousness
- swelling of the hands, feet, ankles, or lower legs
- decrease in urination

Signs of Infection

If you are receiving acyclovir in your vein, you need to know the symptoms of a catheter-related infection (an infection where the needle enters your vein). If you experience any of these symptoms near your intravenous catheter, tell your health care provider as soon as possible:

- tenderness
- warmth
- irritation
- drainage
- redness
- swelling
- pain

Dosage Facts
For Informational Purposes

Caution: Do not change your dose, how often you take your medication, or the length of time you are to take it without first talking to your healthcare provider.

The following dosage information was written using medical language for doctors and other healthcare professionals and is provided here for you to check your dosage. The dosage of this drug may differ for different patients. Therefore, always follow your doctor's instructions or the directions on the label. Contact your healthcare provider or pharmacist if you have any questions about the specific dosage of your medication after reviewing this information.

General Dosage Information

Available as acyclovir and acyclovir sodium; dosage expressed in terms of acyclovir.

Pediatric Patients

Mucocutaneous, Ocular, and Systemic Herpes Simplex Virus (HSV) Infections
Treatment of Mucocutaneous HSV Infections

IV:

- Immunocompromised children <12 years of age: 10 mg/kg every 8 hours for 7–14 days.
- HIV-infected or immunocompromised adolescents and children ≥12 years of age: 5 mg/kg every 8 hours for 7–14 days. Alternatively, after lesions begin to regress, consider switching to oral acyclovir in a dosage of 400 mg 3 times daily and continue until lesions are completely healed.

HSV Gingivostomatitis

IV:

- HIV-infected children with moderate to severe gingivostomatitis: CDC and others recommend 5–10 mg/kg 3 times daily for 7–14 days. Consider chronic oral suppressive or maintenance therapy (secondary prophylaxis) in those with frequent or severe recurrences of gingivostomatitis.

Treatment of HSV Encephalitis or Disseminated Disease

IV:

- Immunocompromised children: 20 mg/kg every 8 hours in those 3 months to 12 years of age and 10–15 mg/kg every 8 hours in those ≥12 years of age. Manufacturer recommends a treatment duration of 10 days, but AAP and others recommend 14–21 days for disseminated or CNS infections.
- HIV-infected children: CDC and others recommend 10 mg/kg or 500 mg/m² 3 times daily for 21 days.
- HIV-infected adolescents: CDC and others recommend 10 mg/kg 3 times daily for 14–21 days.

Treatment of Neonatal HSV Infections

IV:

- Neonates and children ≤3 months of age: Manufacturer recommends 10 mg/kg every 8 hours for 10 days.
- Neonates and children ≤3 months of age: AAP recommends 20 mg/kg every 8 hours given for 14 days for infections of skin, eyes, or mouth or 21 days for disseminated or CNS infections.
- HIV-infected or -exposed neonates: CDC and others recommend 20 mg/kg 3 times daily given for 14 days for infections of skin, eyes, or mouth or 21 days for disseminated or CNS infections.

Prevention of HSV Recurrence in Hematopoietic Stem Cell Transplant (HSCT) Recipients†

IV:

- HSV-seropositive children: 250 mg/m² every 8 hours or 125 mg/m² every 6 hours.
- HSV-seropositive adolescents: 250 mg/m² every 12 hours.
- Initiate prophylaxis at beginning of conditioning therapy and continue until engraftment or until mucositis resolves (approximately 30 days after allogeneic HSCT). Routine prophylaxis for >30 days after HSCT not recommended.

Genital Herpes
Treatment of First Episodes

IV:

- Adolescents and children ≥12 years of age with severe initial episodes: 5–10 mg/kg every 8 hours.
- Manufacturer and some clinicians recommend 5–7 days of

IV acyclovir; CDC states IV acyclovir should be given for 2–7 days or until clinical improvement occurs, followed by an oral antiviral to complete at least 10 days of treatment.

Varicella-Zoster Infections
Treatment of Varicella (Chickenpox)

IV:

- Immunocompromised children: AAP recommends 10 mg/kg 3 times daily for 7–10 days for those <1 year of age and 500 mg/m² 3 times daily for 7–10 days in those ≥1 year of age.
- Immunocompromised adolescents and children: Some clinicians recommend 20 mg/kg every 8 hours for 7–10 days in those ≤12 years of age and 10 mg/kg every 8 hours for 7 days in those >12 years of age.
- HIV-infected children with moderate or severe immunosuppression and varicella associated with high fever or necrotic lesions: CDC and others recommend 10 mg/kg 3 times daily for 7 days or until no new lesions have appeared for 48 hours. Alternatively, a dosage of 500 mg/m² every 8 hours has been suggested for those ≥1 year of age.
- HIV-infected adolescents: CDC and others recommend 10 mg/kg every 8 hours for 7–10 days. After defervescence and if there is no evidence of visceral involvement, switch to oral acyclovir in a dosage of 800 mg 4 times daily.

Treatment of Herpes Zoster (Shingles, Zoster)

IV:

- Immunocompetent children: AAP recommends 10 mg/kg 3 times daily for 7–10 days for those <1 year of age and 500 mg/m² 3 times daily for 7–10 days in those ≥1 year of age.
- Immunocompromised children: 20 mg/kg every 8 hours for 7–10 days in those <12 years of age and 10 mg/kg every 8 hours for 7 days in those ≥12 years of age.
- HIV-infected children with severe immunosuppression and extensive multidermatomal zoster or zoster with trigeminal nerve involvement: CDC and others recommend 10 mg/kg 3 times daily for 7–10 days.
- HIV-infected adolescents: CDC and others recommend 10 mg/kg every 8 hours until cutaneous and visceral disease resolves.

Adult Patients

Mucocutaneous, Ocular, and Systemic Herpes Simplex Virus (HSV) Infections
Treatment of Mucocutaneous HSV Infections

IV:

- Immunocompromised or HIV-infected adults: CDC and others recommend 5 mg/kg every 8 hours for 7–14 days. Alternatively, after lesions begin to regress, consider switching to oral acyclovir in a dosage of 400 mg 3 times daily and continue until lesions are completely healed.

Treatment of HSV Encephalitis or Disseminated Disease

IV:

- 10–15 mg/kg every 8 hours. Manufacturer recommends a treatment duration of 10 days, but CDC and others recommend 14–21 days for disseminated or CNS infections.
- HIV-infected adults: CDC and others recommend 10 mg/kg 3 times daily for 14–21 days.

Prevention of HSV Recurrence in Hematopoietic Stem Cell Transplant (HSCT) Recipients†

IV:

- HSV-seropositive adults: 250 mg/m² every 12 hours initiated at beginning of conditioning therapy and continued until engraftment or until mucositis resolves (i.e., approximately 30 days after allogeneic HSCT). Routine prophylaxis for >30 days after HSCT not recommended.

Genital Herpes
Treatment of First Episodes

IV:

- Adults with severe initial episodes: 5–10 mg/kg every 8 hours.
- Manufacturer and some clinicians recommend 5–7 days of IV acyclovir; CDC states IV acyclovir should be given for 2–7 days or until clinical improvement occurs, followed by an oral antiviral to complete at least 10 days of therapy.

Varicella-Zoster Infections
Treatment of Varicella (Chickenpox)

IV, THEN ORAL:

- HIV-infected or immunocompromised adults: CDC and others recommend 10 mg/kg every 8 hours for 7–10 days. After defervescence and if there is no evidence of visceral involvement, switch to oral acyclovir in a dosage of 800 mg 4 times daily.

Treatment of Herpes Zoster (Shingles, Zoster)

IV:

- HIV-infected or immunocompromised adults: CDC and others recommend 10 mg/kg every 8 hours for 7 days or until cutaneous and visceral disease resolves.

Treatment of Herpes Zoster Ophthalmicus†

IV, THEN ORAL:

- HIV-infected adults: 10 mg/kg IV 3 times daily for 7 days followed by 800 mg orally 3–5 times daily has been used.

Treatment of Dermatomal Herpes Zoster†

Prescribing Limits
Pediatric Patients

IV:

- Maximum 20 mg/kg every 8 hours.

Adult Patients

IV:

- Maximum 20 mg/kg every 8 hours.

Special Populations

Renal Impairment

Adjustment of Usual IV Dosage

IV Dosage in Renal Impairment

Cl_{cr} (mL/min per 1.73 m²)	Percent of Recommended Dose	Dosing Interval (hours)
>50	100%	8
25–50	100%	12
10–25	100%	24
0–10	50%	24

Hemodialysis

Adjust dosing schedule so that a supplemental IV dose is administered immediately after each dialysis period.

CAPD

Supplemental doses do not appear necessary.

Alternative IV Dosage Regimens for End-Stage Renal Disease

93–185 mg/m² as a loading dose, followed by a maintenance dosage of 35–70 mg/m² every 8 hours, and 56–185 mg/m² immediately after dialysis.

250–500 mg/m² as a loading dose, followed by a maintenance dosage of 250–500 mg/m² every 48 hours, and 150–500 mg/m² immediately after dialysis.

2.5 mg/kg every 24 hours and 2.5 mg/kg after each dialysis period.

HIV-infected Patients with Impaired Renal Function (IV Administration)

IV Dosage for HIV-infected Patients with Impaired Renal Function (Based on Usual Dosage of 5 mg/kg Every 8 hours)

Cl_{cr} (mL/min per 1.73 m²)	Adjusted Dosage Regimen
>80	No adjustment necessary
50–80	No adjustment necessary
25–50	5 mg/kg every 12–24 hours
10–25	5 mg/kg every 12–24 hours
<10	2.5 mg/kg every 24 hours

Hemodialysis

Adjust dosing schedule so that daily IV dose is given after hemodialysis on dialysis days.

Geriatric Patients
- Cautious dosage selection; reduced dosage may be needed because of age-related decreases in renal function.

Obese Patients
- Use ideal body weight to determine IV dosage.

† *Use is not currently included in the labeling approved by the US Food and Drug Administration.*

Acyclovir Topical

(ay sye′ kloe veer)

Brand Name: Zovirax® Cream, Zovirax® Ointment

Why is this medicine prescribed?

Acyclovir cream is used to treat cold sores (fever blisters; blisters that are caused by a virus called herpes simplex) on the face or lips. Acyclovir ointment is used to treat first outbreaks of genital herpes (a herpes virus infection that causes sores to form around the genitals and rectum from time to time) and to treat certain types of sores caused by the herpes simplex virus in people with weak immune systems. Acyclovir is in a class of antiviral medications called synthetic nucleoside analogues. It works by stopping the spread of the herpes virus in the body. Acyclovir does not cure cold sores or genital herpes, does not prevent outbreaks of these conditions, and does not stop the spread of these conditions to other people.

How should this medicine be used?

Topical acyclovir comes as a cream and an ointment to apply to the skin. Acyclovir cream is usually applied five times a day for 4 days. Acyclovir cream may be applied at any time during a cold sore outbreak, but it works best when it is applied at the very beginning of a cold sore outbreak, when there is tingling, redness, itching, or a bump but the cold sore has not yet formed. Acyclovir ointment is usually applied six times a day (usually 3 hours apart) for 7 days. It is best to begin using acyclovir ointment as soon as possible after you experience the first symptoms of infection. Follow the directions on your prescription label carefully, and ask your doctor or pharmacist to explain any part you do not understand. Use topical acyclovir exactly as directed. Do not use more or less of it or use it more often than prescribed by your doctor.

Your symptoms should improve during your treatment with topical acyclovir. If your symptoms do not improve or if they get worse, call your doctor.

Acyclovir cream and ointment are for use only on the skin. Do not let acyclovir cream or ointment get into your eyes, or inside your mouth or nose, and do not swallow the medication.

Acyclovir cream should only be applied to skin where a cold sore has formed or seems likely to form. Do not apply acyclovir cream to any unaffected skin, or to genital herpes sores.

Do not apply other skin medications or other types of skin products such as cosmetics, sun screen, or lip balm to the cold sore area while using acyclovir cream unless your doctor tells you that you should.

To use acyclovir cream, follow these steps:
1. Wash your hands.
2. Clean and dry the area of skin where you will be applying the cream.
3. Apply a layer of cream to cover the skin where the cold sore has formed or seems likely to form.
4. Rub the cream into the skin until it disappears.
5. Leave the skin where you applied the medication uncovered. Do not apply a bandage or dressing unless your doctor tells you that you should.
6. Wash your hands with soap and water to remove any cream left on your hands.
7. Be careful not to wash the cream off of your skin. Do not bathe, shower, or swim right after applying acyclovir cream.

8. Avoid irritation of the cold sore area while using acyclovir cream.

To use acyclovir ointment, follow these steps:

1. Put on a clean finger cot or rubber glove.
2. Apply enough ointment to cover all of your sores.
3. Take off the finger cot or rubber glove and throw it away in a trash can that is out of reach of children.
4. Keep the affected area(s) clean and dry, and avoid wearing tight-fitting clothing over the affected area.

Ask your pharmacist or doctor for a copy of the manufacturer's information for the patient. Read this information before you start using acyclovir and each time you refill your prescription.

Are there other uses for this medicine?

This medication may be prescribed for other uses; ask your doctor or pharmacist for more information.

What special precautions should I follow?

Before using topical acyclovir,

- tell your doctor and pharmacist if you are allergic to acyclovir, valacyclovir (Valtrex), any other medications, or any of the ingredients in acyclovir cream or ointment. Ask your pharmacist for a list of the ingredients.
- tell your doctor and pharmacist what other prescription and nonprescription medications, vitamins, nutritional supplements, and herbal products you are taking or plan to take. Your doctor may need to change the doses of your medications or monitor you carefully for side effects.
- tell your doctor if you have or have ever had any condition that affects your immune system such as human immunodeficiency virus (HIV) or acquired immunodeficiency syndrome (AIDS).
- tell your doctor if you are pregnant, plan to become pregnant, or are breast-feeding. If you become pregnant while using acyclovir, call your doctor.

What special dietary instructions should I follow?

Unless your doctor tells you otherwise, continue your normal diet.

What should I do if I forget to take a dose?

Apply the missed dose as soon as you remember it. However, if it is almost time for the next dose, skip the missed dose and continue your regular dosing schedule. Do not apply extra cream or ointment to make up for a missed dose.

What side effects can this medicine cause?

Topical acyclovir may cause side effects. Tell your doctor if any of these symptoms are severe or do not go away:

- dry or cracked lips

- flaky, peeling, or dry skin
- burning or stinging skin
- redness, swelling, or irritation in the place where you applied the medication

Some side effects can be serious. If you experience any of these symptoms, call your doctor immediately:

- hives
- rash
- itching
- difficulty breathing or swallowing
- swelling of the face, throat, lips, eyes, hands, feet, ankles, or lower legs
- hoarseness

Topical acyclovir may cause other side effects. Call your doctor if you have any unusual problems while using this medication.

If you experience a serious side effect, you or your doctor may send a report to the Food and Drug Administration's (FDA) MedWatch Adverse Event Reporting program online [at http://www.fda.gov/MedWatch/index.html] or by phone [1-800-332-1088].

What storage conditions are needed for this medicine?

Keep this medication in the container it came in, with the cap on and tightly closed, and out of reach of children. Store it at room temperature and away from excess heat and moisture (not in the bathroom). Never leave this medication in your car in cold or hot weather. Throw away any medication that is outdated or no longer needed. Talk to your pharmacist about the proper disposal of your medication.

What should I do in case of overdose?

If someone swallows topical acyclovir, call your local poison control center at 1-800-222-1222. If the victim has collapsed or is not breathing, call local emergency services at 911.

What other information should I know?

Keep all appointments with your doctor.

Do not let anyone else use your medication. Ask your pharmacist any questions you have about refilling your prescription.

Dosage Facts
For Informational Purposes

Caution: Do not change your dose, how often you take your medication, or the length of time you are to take it without first talking to your healthcare provider.

The following dosage information was written using medical language for doctors and other healthcare professionals and is provided here for you to check your dosage. The dosage of this drug may differ for different

patients. Therefore, always follow your doctor's instructions or the directions on the label. Contact your healthcare provider or pharmacist if you have any questions about the specific dosage of your medication after reviewing this information.

Pediatric Patients

Herpes Labialis

TOPICAL:
- Children ≥12 years of age: Apply 5% cream to affected area 5 times daily for 4 days. Use sufficient quantity to adequately cover lesions or symptomatic area (e.g., area with tingling).
- Initiate at the earliest sign or symptom of herpes labialis (i.e., during the prodrome or when lesions appear).
- Do not exceed recommended dosage, frequency, and duration of therapy.

Adult Patients

Herpes Labialis

TOPICAL:
- Apply 5% cream to affected area times 5 times daily for 4 days. Use sufficient quantity to adequately cover lesions or symptomatic area (e.g., area with tingling).
- Initiate at the earliest sign or symptom of herpes labialis (i.e., during the prodrome or when lesions appear).
- Do not exceed recommended dosage, frequency, and duration of therapy.

Genital Herpes
Treatment of First Episodes

TOPICAL:
- Rub 5% ointment gently into the affected area every 3 hours 6 times daily for 7 days. Use sufficient quantity to adequately cover all lesions; usual dose varies according to total lesion area but should approximate a 1.25-cm (0.5-inch) ribbon of ointment for a skin surface area of 2.5 cm² (4 inch²).
- Initiate at the earliest sign or symptom of genital herpes (i.e., during the prodrome or when lesions appear).
- Do not exceed recommended dosage, frequency, and duration of therapy.

Mucocutaneous Herpes Simplex Virus (HSV) Infections
Non-life-threatening, Nongenital, Mucocutaneous HSV Infections

TOPICAL:
- Immunocompromised adults: Rub 5% ointment gently into the affected area every 3 hours 6 times daily for 7 days. Use sufficient quantity to adequately cover all lesions; usual dose varies according to total lesion area but should approximate a 1.25-cm (0.5-inch) ribbon of ointment for a skin surface area of 2.5 cm² (4 inch²).
- Do not exceed recommended dosage, frequency, and duration of therapy.

Adalimumab Injection

(a dal aye′ mu mab)

Brand Name: Humira®

Important Warning

Using adalimumab may decrease your ability to fight infection and increase the chance that you will develop a serious or life-threatening infection. Tell your doctor if you have any type of infection now, including minor infections (such as open cuts or sores), or if you have any signs of infection such as fever, cough, or flu-like symptoms. Also tell your doctor if you have or have ever had infections that come and go (such as cold sores) or chronic infections that do not go away, or if you often get any type of infection such as bladder infections. Also tell your doctor if you have or have ever had hepatitis B (a viral infection that affects the liver). Tell your doctor if you have any condition that affects your immune system or if you are taking medications that suppress the immune system such as azathioprine (Imuran), cyclosporine (Neoral, Sandimmune), sirolimus (Rapamune), and tacrolimus (Prograf). If you experience any of the following symptoms during or shortly after your treatment with adalimumab, call your doctor immediately: sore throat; cough; fever; weight loss; extreme tiredness; flu-like symptoms; warm, red, or painful skin; painful, difficult, or frequent urination; or other signs of infection.

Adalimumab may increase the risk that you will get some types of infections that are most common in certain parts of the United States and the world. Tell your doctor all the places you previously lived and all the places you recently visited or plan to visit while using adalimumab.

You may already be infected with tuberculosis but not have any symptoms of the disease. In this case, adalimumab may make your infection more serious and cause you to develop symptoms. Tell your doctor if you have or have ever had tuberculosis or have been around someone who has or has ever had tuberculosis. Before you begin your treatment, your doctor will perform a skin test to see if you have tuberculosis. If you do have tuberculosis, your doctor will treat this infection with antibiotics before you begin using adalimumab.

Talk to your doctor about the risks of using adalimumab.

Why is this medicine prescribed?

Adalimumab is used alone or with other medications to relieve the symptoms of certain autoimmune disorders (conditions in which the immune system attacks healthy parts of the body and causes pain, swelling, and damage) including:

- rheumatoid arthritis (a condition in which the body attacks its own joints, causing pain, swelling, and loss of function)
- Crohn's disease (a condition in which the body attacks the lining of the digestive tract, causing pain, diarrhea, weight loss, and fever) that has not improved when treated with other medications,
- ankylosing spondylitis (a condition in which the body attacks the joints of the spine and other areas causing pain and joint damage),
- psoriatic arthritis (a condition that causes joint pain and swelling and scales on the skin).

Adalimumab is in a class of medications called tumor necrosis factor (TNF) inhibitors. It works by blocking the action of TNF, a substance in the body that causes inflammation.

How should this medicine be used?

Adalimumab comes as a solution (liquid) to inject subcutaneously (under the skin). It is usually injected once every other week. If you are using adalimumab to treat Crohn's disease, your doctor may tell you to inject the medication more often at the beginning of your treatment. If you are using adalimumab to treat rheumatoid arthritis, your doctor may tell you to inject the medication once a week. To help you remember to inject adalimumab, mark the days you are scheduled to inject it on your calendar. Follow the directions on your prescription label carefully, and ask your doctor or pharmacist to explain any part you do not understand. Use adalimumab exactly as directed. Do not use more or less of it or use it more often than prescribed by your doctor.

You will receive your first dose of adalimumab in your doctor's office. After that, you can inject adalimumab yourself or have a friend or relative perform the injections. Before you use adalimumab yourself the first time, read the written instructions that come with it. Ask your doctor or pharmacist to show you or the person who will be injecting the medication how to inject it.

Adalimumab comes in prefilled syringes and dosing pens. Use each syringe or pen only once and inject all the solution in the syringe or pen. Even if there is still some solution left in the syringe or pen after you inject, do not inject again. Dispose of used syringes and pens in a puncture-resistant container. Talk to your doctor or pharmacist about how to dispose of the puncture-resistant container.

Be careful not to drop or crush the prefilled syringes or dosing pens. These devices are made of glass or contain glass and may break if they are dropped.

You can inject adalimumab anywhere on the front of your thighs or stomach except your navel and the area 2 inches around it. To reduce the chances of soreness or redness, use a different site for each injection. Give each injection at least 1 inch away from a spot that you have already used. Keep a list of the places where you have given injections so that you will not inject in these places again. Do not

inject into an area where the skin is tender, bruised, red, or hard or where you have scars or stretch marks.

Always look at adalimumab solution before injecting it. Check that the expiration date has not passed, that the syringe or dosing pen contains the correct amount of liquid, and that the liquid is clear and colorless. Do not use a syringe or dosing pen if it is expired, if it does not contain the correct amount of liquid, or if the liquid is cloudy or contains flakes.

Adalimumab may help control your condition but will not cure it. Continue to use adalimumab even if you feel well. Do not stop using adalimumab without talking to your doctor.

Are there other uses for this medicine?

This medication may be prescribed for other uses; ask your doctor or pharmacist for more information.

What special precautions should I follow?

Before using adalimumab,

- tell your doctor and pharmacist if you are allergic to adalimumab, mannitol, or any other medications. If you will be using the prefilled syringe, also tell your doctor if you or the person who will be helping you inject adalimumab are allergic to latex or rubber.
- tell your doctor and pharmacist what prescription and nonprescription medications, vitamins, nutritional supplements, and herbal products you are taking. Be sure to mention the medications listed in the IMPORTANT WARNING section, abatacept (Orencia) and anakinra (Kineret). Your doctor may need to change the doses of your medications or monitor you carefully for side effects.
- in addition to the conditions mentioned in the IMPORTANT WARNING section, tell your doctor if you have or have ever had numbness or tingling in any part of your body, any disease that affects your nervous system, such as multiple sclerosis (a disease in which the nerves do not function properly and patients may experience weakness, numbness, loss of muscle coordination and problems with vision, speech, and bladder control), or heart disease.
- tell your doctor if you are pregnant, plan to become pregnant, or are breast-feeding If you become pregnant while using adalimumab, call your doctor.
- if you are having surgery, including dental surgery, tell the doctor or dentist that you are using adalimumab.
- do not have any vaccinations without talking to your doctor.

What special dietary instructions should I follow?

Unless your doctor tells you otherwise, continue your normal diet.

What should I do if I forget to take a dose?

Inject the missed dose as soon as you remember it. Then inject the next dose on your regularly scheduled day. However, if it is almost time for the next dose, skip the missed dose and continue your regular dosing schedule. Do not use a double dose to make up for a missed one.

What side effects can this medicine cause?

Adalimumab may cause side effects. Tell your doctor if any of these symptoms are severe or do not go away:

- redness, itching, bruising, pain, or swelling in the place you injected adalimumab
- stomach pain
- nausea
- headache
- back pain

Some side effects can be serious. The following symptoms are uncommon, but if you experience any of them or those listed in the IMPORTANT WARNING section, call your doctor immediately:

- numbness or tingling
- problems with vision
- weakness in legs
- chest pain
- shortness of breath
- rash, especially a rash on the cheeks or arms that is sensitive to sunlight
- new joint pain
- hives
- itching
- swelling of the face, feet, ankles, or lower legs
- difficulty breathing or swallowing
- fever, sore throat, chills, and other signs of infection
- unusual bruising or bleeding
- pale skin
- dizziness

Using adalimumab may increase the risk of developing certain types of cancers including lymphoma (a cancer of the lymph system). People who have had severe rheumatoid arthritis for a long time may have a greater than normal chance of developing these cancers even if they do not use adalimumab. Talk to your doctor about the risks of using this medication.

Adalimumab may cause other side effects. Call your doctor if you have any unusual problems while using this medication.

If you experience a serious side effect, you or your doctor may send a report to the Food and Drug Administration's (FDA) MedWatch Adverse Event Reporting program online [at http://www.fda.gov/MedWatch/index.html] or by phone [1-800-332-1088].

What storage conditions are needed for this medicine?

Keep this medication in the container it came in, tightly closed, and out of reach of children. Store it in the refrigerator and protect it from light. Do not freeze it. If you are traveling and need to take adalimumab with you, keep it in a cooler with an ice pack and do not expose it to light. Throw away any medication that is outdated or no longer needed or that has been frozen. Talk to your pharmacist about the proper disposal of your medication.

What should I do in case of overdose?

In case of overdose, call your local poison control center at 1-800-222-1222. If the victim has collapsed or is not breathing, call local emergency services at 911.

What other information should I know?

Keep all appointments with your doctor.

Do not let anyone else use your medication. Ask your pharmacist any questions you have about refilling your prescription.

Dosage Facts
For Informational Purposes

Caution: Do not change your dose, how often you take your medication, or the length of time you are to take it without first talking to your healthcare provider.

The following dosage information was written using medical language for doctors and other healthcare professionals and is provided here for you to check your dosage. The dosage of this drug may differ for different patients. Therefore, always follow your doctor's instructions or the directions on the label. Contact your healthcare provider or pharmacist if you have any questions about the specific dosage of your medication after reviewing this information.

Adult Patients

Rheumatoid Arthritis

SUB-Q:
- 40 mg once every other week.
- Patients *not* receiving methotrexate may obtain additional benefit from once weekly doses of 40 mg.

Psoriatic Arthritis

SUB-Q:
- 40 mg once every other week.

Ankylosing Spondylitis

SUB-Q:
- 40 mg once every other week.

Adapalene

(a-dap′-a-leen)

Brand Name: Differin®

Why is this medicine prescribed?

Adapalene is used to treat acne. Adapalene is in a class of medications called retinoid-like compounds. It works by stopping pimples from forming under the surface of the skin.

How should this medicine be used?

Adapalene comes as a gel, a solution (liquid), and a cream to apply to the skin. The solution comes in a glass bottle with an applicator and as individual pledgets (medicated wipes for one time use). It is usually applied once a day at bedtime. Follow the directions on your prescription label carefully, and ask your doctor or pharmacist to explain any part you do not understand. Apply adapalene exactly as directed. Do not apply more or less of it or apply it more often than prescribed by your doctor. Applying more adapalene or applying adaplene more often than recommended will not speed up or improve results, but it may irritate your skin.

Adapalene controls acne but does not cure it. Your acne may get worse during the first few weeks of treatment, and it may take 8-12 weeks or longer before you feel the full benefit of adapalene. Pimples can take 6-8 weeks to form under the skin, and during the first weeks of your treatment, adapalene may bring these pimples to the skin surface. Continue to use adapalene even if your acne worsens or you do not see much improvement at first. Do not stop using adapalene without talking to your doctor.

Do not apply adapalene to skin that is sunburned, broken, or covered with eczema (a skin disease). If you have any of these conditions, do not apply adapalene until your skin has healed.

Be careful not to get adapalene in your eyes, nose, or mouth. If you do get adapalene in your eyes, wash them with plenty of water and call your doctor. Your eyes may become irritated, swollen, or infected.

To use the cream, gel, or solution, follow these steps:

1. Gently wash the affected skin with a mild soap or soapless cleanser and pat dry with a soft towel. Do not use harsh or abrasive cleansers, and do not scrub your skin vigorously. Ask your doctor or pharmacist to recommend a gentle cleanser.
2. If you are using the gel or cream, use your fingers to spread a thin film of medication over the affected area. If you are using a pledget, remove it from the foil pouch and gently wipe the entire affected area. If you are using the glass bottle of solution, apply a thin layer to the affected area using the applicator provided.
3. You may feel a slight warmth or stinging in the place where you applied adapalene. This feeling is normal and should go away by itself in a short time.
4. If you used a pledget, throw it away after use. Do not save it to use again.

Are there other uses for this medicine?

This medication may be prescribed for other uses; ask your doctor or pharmacist for more information.

What special precautions should I follow?

Before taking adapalene,

- tell your doctor and pharmacist if you are allergic to adapalene or any other medications.
- tell your doctor and pharmacist what prescription and nonprescription medications, vitamins, nutritional supplements, and herbal products you are taking or using. Be sure to mention all skin care products including soaps, cleansers, moisturizers, and cosmetics. Many skin care products can irritate your skin if you use them with adapalene. This is especially likely if you use products that are harsh, dry out the skin, or contain alcohol, spices, lime rind, sulfur, resorcinol, salicylic acid, or alpha hydroxy acid. If you have been using these products, your doctor may want you to wait for your skin to return to normal before you begin using adapalene.
- tell your doctor if you have or have ever had eczema or cancer.
- tell your doctor if you are pregnant, plan to become pregnant, or are breast-feeding. If you become pregnant while using adapalene, call your doctor.
- plan to avoid unnecessary or prolonged exposure to real and artificial sunlight and to wear protective clothing, sunglasses, and sunscreen with an SPF of 15 or higher, especially if you sunburn easily. Also avoid prolonged exposure to cold or wind. Adapalene may make your skin sensitive to sunlight or extreme weather.
- do not use hot wax to remove unwanted hair during your treatment with adapalene.

What special dietary instructions should I follow?

Unless your doctor tells you otherwise, continue your normal diet.

What should I do if I forget to take a dose?

Apply the missed dose as soon as you remember it. However, if it is almost time for the next dose, skip the missed dose and continue your regular dosing schedule. Do not apply a double dose to make up for a missed one.

What side effects can this medicine cause?

Adapalene may cause side effects. The following symptoms are likely to affect your skin during the first 2-4 weeks of treatment. Tell your doctor if any of these symptoms are severe or do not go away:

- redness
- scaling

- dryness
- burning or stinging
- itching

Medications that are similar to adapalene have caused tumors in laboratory animals who were given the medications and exposed to real or artificial sunlight. It is not known whether adapalene increases the risk of tumors in humans. Protect yourself from sunlight and sunlamps while taking adapalene, and talk to your doctor about the risks of taking this medication.

Adapalene may cause other side effects. Call your doctor if you have any unusual problems while taking this medication.

If you experience a serious side effect, you or your doctor may send a report to the Food and Drug Administration's (FDA) MedWatch Adverse Event Reporting program online [at http://www.fda.gov/MedWatch/index.html] or by phone [1-800-332-1088].

What storage conditions are needed for this medicine?

Keep this medication in the container it came in, tightly closed, and out of reach of children. Store it at room temperature and away from excess heat and moisture (not in the bathroom). If you are using a bottle of adapalene solution, be sure to store it upright. Throw away any medication that is outdated or no longer needed. Talk to your pharmacist about the proper disposal of your medication.

What should I do in case of overdose?

You should not swallow adapalene. If you regularly take adapalene by mouth, you may experience an overdose. If you swallow adapalene, call your local poison control center at 1-800-222-1222.

What other information should I know?

Keep all appointments with your doctor.

Do not let anyone else use your medication. Ask your pharmacist any questions you have about refilling your prescription.

Dosage Facts
For Informational Purposes

Caution: Do not change your dose, how often you take your medication, or the length of time you are to take it without first talking to your health-care provider.

The following dosage information was written using medical language for doctors and other healthcare professionals and is provided here for you to check your dosage. The dosage of this drug may differ for different patients. Therefore, always follow your doctor's instructions or the directions on the label. Contact your healthcare provider or pharmacist if you have any questions about the specific dosage of your medication after reviewing this information.

Pediatric Patients
Acne Vulgaris

TOPICAL:
- Children and adolescents ≥12 years of age: Apply once daily in the evening at bedtime.
- Improvement usually detectable within 8–12 weeks.

Adult Patients
Acne Vulgaris

TOPICAL:
- Apply once daily in the evening at bedtime.
- Improvement usually detectable within 8–12 weeks.

Prescribing Limits
Pediatric Patients
Acne Vulgaris

TOPICAL:
- Children and adolescents ≥12 years of age: most reported experience to date has been for treatment periods that did not exceed 12 weeks.

Adult Patients
Acne Vulgaris

TOPICAL:
- Most reported experience to date has been for treatment periods that did not exceed 12 weeks.

Adefovir
(a def′ o veer)

Brand Name: Hepsera®

Important Warning

Do not stop taking adefovir without talking to your doctor. When you stop taking adefovir your hepatitis may get worse. This is most likely to happen during the first 3 months after you stop taking adefovir. Be careful not to miss doses or run out of adefovir. Refill your prescription at least 5 days before you expect that you will need the new supply of medication. Tell your doctor if you have or have ever had liver disease other than hepatitis B or cirrhosis (scarring of the liver). If you experience any of the following symptoms after you stop taking adefovir, call your doctor immediately: extreme tiredness, weakness, upset stomach, vomiting, loss of appetite, yellowing of the skin or eyes, dark-colored urine, light-colored bowel movements, and muscle or joint pain.

Adefovir may cause kidney damage. Tell your

doctor if you have or have ever had kidney disease, high blood pressure, or diabetes. Tell your doctor and pharmacist if you are taking or have ever taken any of the following medications: aminoglycoside antibiotics such as amikacin (Amikin), gentamicin (Garamycin), kanamycin (Kantrex), neomycin (Neo-Rx, NeoFradin), paramomycin (Humatin), streptomycin, and tobramycin (Tobi, Nebcin); amphotericin B (Fungizone); aspirin and other non-steroidal antiinflammatory medications (NSAIDS) such as ibuprofen (Advil, Motrin) and naproxen (Aleve, Naprosyn); cyclosporine (Neoral, Samdimmune); tacrolimus (Prograf); or vancomycin. If you experience any of the following symptoms, call your doctor immediately: confusion; decreased urination; or swelling of the hands, feet, ankles, or lower legs.

If you have HIV or AIDS that is not being treated with medications and you take adefovir, your HIV infection may become difficult to treat. Tell your doctor if you have HIV or AIDS or if you have unprotected sex with more than one partner or use injectable street drugs. Your doctor may test you for HIV infection before you begin treatment with adefovir and at any time during your treatment when there is a chance that you were exposed to HIV.

Adefovir, when used alone or in combination with other antiviral medications, can cause serious or life-threatening damage to the liver and a condition called lactic acidosis (a build-up of acid in the blood). Tell your doctor if you drink or have ever drunk large amounts of alcohol, if you use or have ever used injectable street drugs, and if you have or have ever had any liver disease other than hepatitis B. Tell your doctor and pharmacist if you are taking or have ever taken the following medications: acetaminophen (Tylenol, others); cholesterol-lowering medications (statins); iron products; isoniazid (INH, Nydrazid); medications to treat HIV or AIDS; methotrexate (Rhuematrex); niacin (nicotinic acid); or rifampin (Rifadin, Rimactane). If you experience any of the following symptoms, call your doctor immediately: confusion; unusual bleeding or bruising; yellowing of the skin or eyes; dark-colored urine; light-colored bowel movements; difficulty breathing; stomach pain or swelling; upset stomach; vomiting; unusual muscle pain; loss of appetite for at least a few days; lack of energy; flu-like symptoms; itching; feeling cold, especially in the arms or legs; dizziness or lightheadedness; fast or irregular heart beat; or extreme weakness or tiredness.

Keep all appointments with your doctor and the laboratory before, during, and for a few months after your treatment with adefovir. Your doctor will order certain lab tests to check your body's response to adefovir during this time.

Talk to your doctor about the risks of taking adefovir.

Why is this medicine prescribed?

Adefovir is used to treat chronic (long-term) hepatitis B infection (swelling of the liver caused by a virus) in patients who have symptoms of the disease. Adefovir is in a class of medications called nucleotide analogs. It works by decreasing the amount of hepatitis B virus (HBV) in the body. Adefovir will not cure hepatitis B and may not prevent complications of chronic hepatitis B such as cirrhosis of the liver or liver cancer. Adefovir may not prevent the spread of hepatitis B to other people.

How should this medicine be used?

Adefovir comes as a tablet to take by mouth. It is usually taken once a day with or without food. Take adefovir at around the same time every day. Follow the directions on your prescription label carefully, and ask your doctor or pharmacist to explain any part you do not understand. Take adefovir exactly as directed. Do not take more or less of it or take it more often than prescribed by your doctor.

Are there other uses for this medicine?

This medication may be prescribed for other uses; ask your doctor or pharmacist for more information.

What special precautions should I follow?

Before taking adefovir,

- tell your doctor and pharmacist if you are allergic to adefovir or any other medications.
- tell your doctor and pharmacist what other prescription and nonprescription medications, vitamins, nutritional supplements, and herbal products you are taking or plan to take. Be sure to mention the medications listed in the IMPORTANT WARNING section and probenecid. Your doctor may need to change the doses of your medications or monitor you carefully for side effects. Do not take any other medications while you are taking adefovir unless your doctor has told you that you should.
- do not take adefovir if you are pregnant or plan to become pregnant. If you become pregnant while taking adefovir, call your doctor. Do not breast-feed while taking adefovir.
- if you are having surgery, including dental surgery, tell the doctor or dentist that you are taking adefovir.

What special dietary instructions should I follow?

Unless your doctor tells you otherwise, continue your normal diet.

What should I do if I forget to take a dose?

If you remember the missed dose on the day that you were supposed to take it, take the missed dose as soon as you remember it. However, if you do not remember the missed dose until the next day, skip the missed dose and continue your regular dosing schedule. Do not take more than one dose of adefovir on the same day. Do not take a double dose to make up for a missed one.

What side effects can this medicine cause?

Adefovir may cause side effects. Tell your doctor if any of these symptoms are severe or do not go away:

- weakness
- headache
- diarrhea
- gas
- indigestion
- cough
- sore throat
- runny nose

Some side effects can be serious. If you experience this symptom or any of those listed in the IMPORTANT WARNING section, call your doctor immediately:

- rash

Adefovir may cause other side effects. Call your doctor if you have any unusual problems while taking this medication.

If you experience a serious side effect, you or your doctor may send a report to the Food and Drug Administration's (FDA) MedWatch Adverse Event Reporting program online [at http://www.fda.gov/MedWatch/index.html] or by phone [1-800-332-1088].

What storage conditions are needed for this medicine?

Keep this medication in the container it came in, tightly closed, and out of reach of children. Store it at room temperature and away from excess heat and moisture (not in the bathroom). Throw away any medication that is outdated or no longer needed. Talk to your pharmacist about the proper disposal of your medication.

What should I do in case of overdose?

In case of overdose, call your local poison control center at 1-800-222-1222. If the victim has collapsed or is not breathing, call local emergency services at 911.

Symptoms of overdose may include:

- upset stomach
- stomach discomfort
- vomiting
- gas
- loose bowel movements
- loss of appetite

What other information should I know?

Do not let anyone else take your medication. Ask your pharmacist any questions you have about refilling your prescription.

Dosage Facts
For Informational Purposes

Caution: Do not change your dose, how often you take your medication, or the length of time you are to take it without first talking to your healthcare provider.

The following dosage information was written using medical language for doctors and other healthcare professionals and is provided here for you to check your dosage. The dosage of this drug may differ for different patients. Therefore, always follow your doctor's instructions or the directions on the label. Contact your healthcare provider or pharmacist if you have any questions about the specific dosage of your medication after reviewing this information.

General Dosage Information

Available as adefovir dipivoxil; dosage expressed in terms adefovir dipivoxil.

Adult Patients

Chronic Hepatitis B Virus (HBV) Infection

ORAL:
- 10 mg once daily.
- Optimal duration of treatment unknown.

Special Populations

Hepatic Impairment
- No dosage adjustments necessary in hepatic impairment.

Renal Impairment
- Decrease dosage in those with baseline Cl_{cr} <50 mL/minute.

Dosage for Adults with Renal Impairment

Cl_{cr} (mL/min)	Dosage
20–49	10 mg once every 48 hours
10–19	10 mg once every 72 hours
<10 (not undergoing hemodialysis)	Dosage recommendations not available
Hemodialysis patients	10 mg once every 7 days following dialysis

These dosage guidelines for adults with renal impairment have not been clinically evaluated. In addition, these dosages were derived from data involving patients with preexisting renal impairment and may not be appropriate for those in whom renal impairment evolves during adefovir therapy.

Albuterol

(al byoo′ ter ole)

Brand Name: VoSpire ER®
Also available generically.

Why is this medicine prescribed?

Albuterol is used to prevent and treat wheezing, difficulty breathing and chest tightness caused by lung diseases such as asthma and chronic obstructive pulmonary disease (COPD; a group of diseases that affect the lungs and airways). Albuterol is in a class of medications called bronchodilators. It works by relaxing and opening the air passages to the lungs to make breathing easier.

How should this medicine be used?

Albuterol comes as a tablet, a syrup, and an extended-release (long-acting) tablet to take by mouth. The tablets and syrup are usually taken three or four times a day. The extended-release tablets are usually taken once every 12 hours. Take albuterol at around the same times every day. Follow the directions on your prescription label carefully, and ask your doctor or pharmacist to explain any part you do not understand. Take albuterol exactly as directed. Do not take more or less of it or take it more often than prescribed by your doctor.

Swallow the extended-release tablets whole with plenty of water or other liquid. Do not split, chew, or crush them.

Your doctor may start you on a low dose of albuterol and gradually increase your dose.

Albuterol may help control your symptoms but will not cure your condition. Continue to take albuterol even if you feel well. Do not stop taking albuterol without talking to your doctor.

Call your doctor if your symptoms worsen or if you feel that albuterol no longer controls your symptoms.

Are there other uses for this medicine?

This medication may be prescribed for other uses; ask your doctor or pharmacist for more information.

What special precautions should I follow?

Before taking albuterol,

- tell your doctor and pharmacist if you are allergic to albuterol, any other medications, or any of the ingredients in albuterol tablets, extended-release tablets, or capsules. Ask your pharmacist for a list of the ingredients.
- tell your doctor and pharmacist what prescription and nonprescription medications, vitamins, nutritional supplements, and herbal products you are taking or plan to take. Be sure to mention any of the following: beta blockers such as atenolol (Tenormin), labetalol (Normodyne), metoprolol (Lopressor, Toprol XL), nadolol (Corgard), and propranolol (Inderal); digoxin (Lan-

oxin); diuretics ('water pills'); epinephrine (Epipen, Primatene Mist); other oral and inhaled medications for asthma and medications for colds. Also tell your doctor or pharmacist if you are taking the following medications or have stopped taking them within the past two weeks: antidepressants such as amitriptyline (Elavil), amoxapine (Asendin), clomipramine (Anafranil), desipramine (Norpramin), doxepin (Adapin, Sinequan), imipramine (Tofranil), nortriptyline (Aventyl, Pamelor), protriptyline (Vivactil), and trimipramine (Surmontil); and monoamine oxidase (MAO) inhibitors, including isocarboxazid (Marplan), phenelzine (Nardil), selegiline (Eldepryl, Emsam, Zelapar), and tranylcypromine (Parnate). Your doctor may need to change the doses of your medications or monitor you carefully for side effects.

- tell your doctor if you have or have ever had an irregular heartbeat, heart disease, high blood pressure, hyperthyroidism (condition in which there is too much thyroid hormone in the body), diabetes, or seizures.
- tell your doctor if you are pregnant, plan to become pregnant, or are breast-feeding. If you become pregnant while taking albuterol, call your doctor.
- you should know that albuterol sometimes causes wheezing and difficulty breathing. If this happens, call your doctor right away. Do not use albuterol again unless your doctor tells you that you should.

What special dietary instructions should I follow?

Unless your doctor tells you otherwise, continue your normal diet.

What should I do if I forget to take a dose?

Take the missed dose as soon as you remember it. However, if it is almost time for the next dose, skip the missed dose and continue your regular dosing schedule. Do not take a double dose to make up for a missed one.

What side effects can this medicine cause?

Albuterol may cause side effects. Tell your doctor if any of these symptoms are severe or do not go away:

- nervousness
- shakiness
- dizziness
- headache
- uncontrollable shaking of a part of the body
- muscle cramps
- excessive motion or activity
- sudden changes in mood
- nosebleed
- nausea
- increased or decreased appetite
- difficulty falling asleep or staying asleep
- pale skin

Some side effects can be serious. If you experience any of these symptoms, call your doctor immediately:

- fast, pounding, or irregular heartbeat
- chest pain
- fever
- blisters or rash
- hives
- itching
- swelling of the face, throat, tongue, lips, eyes, hands, feet, ankles, or lower legs
- increased difficulty breathing
- difficulty swallowing
- hoarseness

Albuterol may cause other side effects. Call your doctor if you have any unusual problems while taking this medication.

What storage conditions are needed for this medicine?

Keep this medication in the container it came in, tightly closed, and out of reach of children. Store it at room temperature and away from excess heat and moisture (not in the bathroom). Throw away any medication that is outdated or no longer needed. Talk to your pharmacist about the proper disposal of your medication.

What should I do in case of overdose?

In case of overdose, call your local poison control center at 1-800-222-1222. If the victim has collapsed or is not breathing, call local emergency services at 911.

Symptoms of overdose may include:

- seizures
- chest pain
- fast, irregular or pounding heartbeat
- nervousness
- headache
- uncontrollable shaking of a part of the body
- dry mouth
- nausea
- dizziness
- excessive tiredness
- lack of energy
- difficulty falling asleep or staying asleep

What other information should I know?

Keep all appointments with your doctor.

Do not let anyone else take your medication. Ask your pharmacist any questions you have about refilling your prescription.

Dosage Facts
For Informational Purposes

Caution: Do not change your dose, how often you take your medication, or the length of time you are to take it without first talking to your healthcare provider.

The following dosage information was written using medical language for doctors and other healthcare professionals and is provided here for you to check your dosage. The dosage of this drug may differ for different patients. Therefore, always follow your doctor's instructions or the directions on the label. Contact your healthcare provider or pharmacist if you have any questions about the specific dosage of your medication after reviewing this information.

General Dosage Information

Available as albuterol or albuterol sulfate; dosage expressed in terms of albuterol.

Pediatric Patients

Bronchospasm
Asthma

ORAL:

- Conventional tablets in children 6–12 years of age: Initially, 2 mg 3 or 4 times daily. If necessary, increase dosage cautiously and gradually as tolerated to a maximum of 6 mg 4 times daily (maximum 24 mg total daily dosage).
- Conventional tablets in adolescents ≥12 years of age: Initially, 2 or 4 mg 3 or 4 times daily. If necessary, increase dosage cautiously and gradually as tolerated to a maximum of 8 mg 4 times daily (maximum 32 mg total daily dosage).
- Extended-release tablets in children 6–12 years of age: Initially, 4 mg every 12 hours (VoSpire® ER). If necessary, increase dosage cautiously and gradually as tolerated to a maximum of 12 mg twice daily (maximum 24 mg total daily dosage).
- Extended-release tablets in adolescents ≥12 years of age: Initially, 8 mg every 12 hours. In some patients, 4 mg every 12 hours may be sufficient (e.g., low body weight). If necessary, increase dosage cautiously and gradually as tolerated to a maximum of 16 mg twice daily (maximum 32 mg total daily dosage). When transferring from conventional tablets to extended-release tablets, each 2 mg administered every 6 hours as conventional tablets is approximately equivalent to 4 mg every 12 hours as extended-release tablets.
- Oral solution in children 2–6 years of age: Initially, 0.1 mg/kg (up to 2 mg) 3 times daily. If necessary, increase dosage cautiously and gradually as tolerated to 0.2 mg/kg (up to 4 mg) 3 times daily (maximum 12 mg total daily dosage).
- Oral solution in children or adolescents >6–14 years of age: Initially, 2 mg 3 or 4 times daily. If necessary increase dosage cautiously and gradually as tolerated to a maximum of 24 mg daily in divided doses.
- Oral solution in adolescents >14 years of age: 2 or 4 mg 3–4 times daily. If necessary, increase dosage cautiously and gradually to a maximum of 8 mg 4 times daily.

Adult Patients

Bronchospasm
Asthma

ORAL:

- Conventional tablets or oral solution: Initially, 2 or 4 mg 3 or 4 times daily. If necessary, increase dosage cautiously and gradually as tolerated to a maximum of 8 mg 4 times daily.
- Extended-release tablets: Initially, 4 or 8 mg every 12 hours. In some patients (e.g., low body weight), 4 mg every 12 hours

may be sufficient. If necessary, increase dosage cautiously and gradually as tolerated to maximum of 16 mg twice daily.

Prescribing Limits

Pediatric Patients

Bronchospasm
Asthma

ORAL:
- Conventional tablets in children 6–12 years of age: Maximum 24 mg daily (in divided doses).
- Conventional tablets in adolescents 12 years of age: Maximum 8 mg 4 times daily.
- Extended-release tablets in children 6–12 years of age: Maximum 12 mg twice daily.
- Extended-release tablets in adolescents >12 years of age: Maximum 16 mg twice daily.
- Oral solution in children 2–6 years of age: Maximum 4 mg 3 times daily.
- Oral solution in children or adolescents >6 to 14 years of age: Maximum 24 mg daily in divided doses.
- Oral solution in adolescents >14 years of age: Maximum 8 mg 4 times daily.

Adult Patients

Bronchospasm
Asthma

ORAL:
- Conventional tablets or oral solution: Maximum 8 mg 4 times daily.
- Extended-release tablets: Maximum 16 mg twice daily.

Special Populations

Geriatric Patients
- Conventional tablets or oral solution: Initially, 2 mg 3 or 4 times daily. May increase gradually as tolerated up to a maximum of 8 mg 3 or 4 times daily (conventional tablets).
- Inhalation aerosol: Initiate therapy with dosages at the lower end of the usual range.

Patients Sensitive to Sympathomimetic Amines
- Conventional tablets or oral solution: Initially, 2 mg 3 or 4 times daily. May increase gradually as tolerated up to 8 mg 3 or 4 times daily.

Albuterol Inhalation

(al byoo′ ter ole)

Brand Name: Accuneb®, Proair HFA®, Proventil® HFA, Ventolin HFA®
Also available generically.

Why is this medicine prescribed?

Albuterol is used to prevent and treat wheezing, difficulty breathing and chest tightness caused by lung diseases such as asthma and chronic obstructive pulmonary disease (COPD; a group of diseases that affect the lungs and airways). Albuterol inhalation aerosol is also used to prevent breathing difficulties during exercise. Albuterol is in a class of medications called bronchodilators. It works by relaxing and opening air passages to the lungs to make breathing easier.

How should this medicine be used?

Albuterol comes as a solution (liquid) to inhale by mouth using a nebulizer (machine that turns medication into a mist that can be inhaled) and as an aerosol to inhale by mouth using an inhaler. When the inhalation aerosol is used to treat or prevent symptoms of lung disease, it is usually used every 4 to 6 hours as needed. When the inhalation aerosol is used to prevent breathing difficulty during exercise, it is usually used 15 to 30 minutes before exercise. The nebulizer solution is usually used three or four times a day. Follow the directions on your prescription label carefully, and ask your doctor or pharmacist to explain any part you do not understand. Use albuterol exactly as directed. Do not use more or less of it or use it more often than prescribed by your doctor.

Call your doctor if your symptoms worsen or if you feel that albuterol inhalation no longer controls your symptoms. If you were told to use albuterol as needed to treat your symptoms and you find that you need to use the medication more often than usual, call your doctor.

Albuterol controls symptoms of asthma and other lung diseases but does not cure them. Do not stop using albuterol without talking to your doctor.

If you are using the inhaler, your medication will come in canisters. Each canister of albuterol aerosol is designed to provide 200 inhalations. After the labeled number of inhalations has been used, later inhalations may not contain the correct amount of medication. Throw away the canister after you have used the labeled number of inhalations even if it still contains some liquid and continues to release a spray when it is pressed.

Your inhaler may come with an attached counter that keeps track of the number of sprays you have used. If you have this type of inhaler, you should not try to change the numbers or remove the counter from the canister. When the number that shows on the counter is 020, you should call your doctor or pharmacist to refill your prescription. When the number that shows on the counter is 000, you should not use that canister anymore. Throw away the empty canister.

If your inhaler does not come with an attached counter, you will need to keep track of the number of inhalations you have used. You can divide the number of inhalations in your inhaler by the number of inhalations you use each day to find out how many days your inhaler will last. Do not float the canister in water to see if it still contains medication.

The inhaler that comes with albuterol aerosol is designed for use only with a canister of albuterol. Never use it to inhale any other medication, and do not use any other inhaler to inhale albuterol.

Be careful not to get albuterol inhalation into your eyes.

Do not use your albuterol inhaler when you are near a flame or source of heat. The inhaler may explode if it is exposed to very high temperatures.

Before you use albuterol for the first time, read the written instructions that come with the inhaler or nebulizer. Ask your doctor, pharmacist, or respiratory therapist to show you how to use it. Practice using the inhaler or nebulizer while he or she watches.

If your child will be using the inhaler, be sure that he or she knows how to use it. Watch your child each time he or she uses the inhaler to be sure that he or she is using it correctly.

To use the aerosol inhaler, follow these steps:

1. Remove the protective dust cap from the end of the mouthpiece. If the dust cap was not placed on the mouthpiece, check the mouthpiece for dirt or other objects. Be sure that the canister is fully and firmly inserted in the mouthpiece.
2. If you are using the inhaler for the first time or if you have not used the inhaler in more than 14 days, you will need to prime it. You may also need to prime the inhaler if it has been dropped. Ask your pharmacist or check the manufacturer's information if this happens. To prime the inhaler, shake it well and then press down on the canister 4 times to release 4 sprays into the air, away from your face. Be careful not to get albuterol in your eyes.
3. Shake the inhaler well.
4. Breathe out as completely as possible through your mouth.
5. Hold the canister with the mouthpiece on the bottom, facing you and the canister pointing upward. Place the open end of the mouthpiece into your mouth. Close your lips tightly around the mouthpiece.
6. Breathe in slowly and deeply through the mouthpiece.At the same time, press down once on the container to spray the medication into your mouth.
7. Try to hold your breath for 10 seconds. remove the inhaler, and breathe out slowly.
8. If you were told to use 2 puffs, wait 1 minute and then repeat steps 3-7.
9. Replace the protective cap on the inhaler.

To inhale the solution using a nebulizer, follow these steps;

1. Remove one vial of albuterol solution from the foil pouch. Leave the rest of the vials in the pouch until you are ready to use them.
2. Look at the liquid in the vial. It should be clear and colorless. Do not use the vial if the liquid is cloudy or discolored.
3. Twist off the top of the vial and squeeze all of the liquid into the nebulizer reservoir. If you are using your nebulizer to inhale other medications, ask your doctor or pharmacist if you can place the other medications in the reservoir along with albuterol.
4. Connect the nebulizer reservoir to the mouthpiece or face mask.
5. Connect the nebulizer to the compressor.
6. Place the mouthpiece in your mouth or put on the face mask. Sit in an upright, comfortable position and turn on the compressor.
7. Breathe in calmly, deeply, and evenly for about 5-15 minutes until mist stops forming in the nebulizer chamber.

Clean your inhaler or nebulizer regularly. Follow the manufacturer's directions carefully and ask your doctor or pharmacist if you have any questions about cleaning your inhaler or nebulizer. If you do not clean your inhaler properly, the inhaler may become blocked and may not spray medication. If this happens, follow the manufacturer's directions for cleaning the inhaler and removing the blockage.

Are there other uses for this medicine?

Inhaled albuterol is also sometimes used to treat or improve muscle paralysis (inability to move parts of the body) in patients with a condition that causes attacks of paralysis. Talk to your doctor about the possible risks of using this medication for your condition.

This medication may be prescribed for other uses; ask your doctor or pharmacist for more information.

What special precautions should I follow?

Before using albuterol inhalation,
- tell your doctor and pharmacist if you are allergic to albuterol (Vospire ER, in Combivent, in Duoneb), levalbuterol (Xoponex), or any other medications.
- tell your doctor and pharmacist what prescription medications, vitamins, nutritional supplements, and herbal products you are taking or plan to take. Be sure to mention any of the following: beta blockers such as atenolol (Tenormin), labetalol (Normodyne), metoprolol (Lopressor, Toprol XL), nadolol (Corgard), and propranolol (Inderal); digoxin (Lanoxin); diuretics ('water pills'); epinephrine (Epipen, Primatene Mist); other inhaled medications used to relax the air passages such as metaproterenol (Alupent) and levalbuterol (Xoponex); and medications for colds. Also tell your doctor or pharmacist if you are taking the following medications or have stopped taking them within the past 2 weeks: antidepressants such as amitriptyline (Elavil), amoxapine (Asendin), clomipramine (Anafranil), desipramine (Norpramin), doxepin (Adapin, Sinequan), imipramine (Tofranil), nortriptyline (Aventyl, Pamelor), protriptyline (Vivactil), and trimipramine (Surmontil); and monoamine oxidase (MAO) inhibitors, including isocarboxazid (Marplan), phenelzine (Nardil), selegiline (Eldepryl, Emsam), and tranylcypromine (Parnate). Your doctor may need to change the doses of your medications or monitor you carefully for side effects.
- tell your doctor if you have or have ever had an irregular heartbeat, heart disease, high blood pressure, hyperthyroidism (condition in which there is too much thyroid hormone in the body), diabetes, or seizures.

- tell your doctor if you are pregnant, plan to become pregnant, or are breast-feeding. If you become pregnant while using albuterol, call your doctor.
- you should know that albuterol inhalation sometimes causes wheezing and difficulty breathing immediately after it is inhaled. If this happens, call your doctor right away. Do not use albuterol inhalation again unless your doctor tells you that you should.

What should I do if I forget to take a dose?

If you have been told to use albuterol inhalation on a regular schedule, use the missed dose as soon as you remember it. However, if it is almost time for the next dose, skip the missed dose and continue your regular dosing schedule. Do not use a double dose to make up for a missed one.

What side effects can this medicine cause?

Albuterol may cause side effects. Tell your doctor if any of these symptoms are severe or do not go away:
- uncontrollable shaking of a part of the body
- nervousness
- headache
- nausea
- vomiting
- cough
- throat irritation
- muscle, bone, or back pain

Some side effects can be serious. If you experience any of the following symptoms, call your doctor immediately:
- fast, pounding, or irregular heartbeat
- chest pain
- rash
- hives
- itching
- swelling of the face, throat, tongue, lips, eyes, hands, feet, ankles, or lower legs
- increased difficulty breathing
- difficulty swallowing
- hoarseness

Albuterol may cause other side effects. Call your doctor if you have any unusual problems while using this medication.

If you experience a serious side effect, you or your doctor may send a report to the Food and Drug Administration's (FDA) MedWatch Adverse Event Reporting program online [at http://www.fda.gov/MedWatch/index.html] or by phone [1-800-332-1088].

What storage conditions are needed for this medicine?

Keep this medication in the container it came in, tightly closed, and out of reach of children. Keep unused vials of nebulizer solution in the foil pouch until you are ready to use them. Store the medication at room temperature and away from excess heat and moisture (not in the bathroom).

Throw away any medication that is outdated or no longer needed. If you are using the nebulizer solution, throw away vials one week after you remove them from the foil pouch. If you are using the inhaler with an attached counter, throw away the inhaler 2 months after you remove it from the foil pouch. Talk to your pharmacist about the proper disposal of your medication. Do not puncture the aerosol canister, and do not discard it in an incinerator or fire.

What should I do in case of overdose?

In case of overdose, call your local poison control center at 1-800-222-1222. If the victim has collapsed or is not breathing, call local emergency services at 911.

Symptoms of overdose may include:
- seizures
- chest pain
- fast, irregular or pounding heartbeat
- nervousness
- headache
- uncontrollable shaking of a part of the body
- dry mouth
- nausea
- dizziness
- excessive tiredness
- lack of energy
- difficulty falling asleep or staying asleep

What other information should I know?

Keep all appointments with your doctor.

Do not let anyone else use your medication. Ask your pharmacist any questions you have about refilling your prescription.

Dosage Facts
For Informational Purposes

Caution: Do not change your dose, how often you take your medication, or the length of time you are to take it without first talking to your healthcare provider.

The following dosage information was written using medical language for doctors and other healthcare professionals and is provided here for you to check your dosage. The dosage of this drug may differ for different patients. Therefore, always follow your doctor's instructions or the directions on the label. Contact your healthcare provider or pharmacist if you have any questions about the specific dosage of your medication after reviewing this information.

General Dosage Information

Available as albuterol or albuterol sulfate; dosage expressed in terms of albuterol.

Pediatric Patients

Bronchospasm
Asthma

ORAL INHALATION:

- Inhalation aerosol without chlorofluorocarbons in children ≥4 years of age: 180 mcg (2 inhalations) every 4–6 hours (Ventolin® HFA, Proventil® HFA). Do not increase dosage or dosage frequency. Alternatively, 90 mcg (1 inhalation) every 4 hours may be sufficient.
- Inhalation aerosol with chlorofluorocarbons in adolescents ≥12 years of age: 180 mcg (2 inhalations) every 4–6 hours (Proventil®).
- Inhalation aerosol without chlorofluorocarbons in adolescents ≥12 years of age: 180 mcg (2 inhalations) every 4–6 hours (Proair® HFA).
- 0.042% Inhalation solution for nebulization in children 2–12 years of age: 0.63 or 1.25 mg 3 or 4 times daily. Dosage of 1.25 mg 3 or 4 times daily may improve initial response in children 6–12 years of age with more severe asthma (baseline FEV_1 <60% of predicted), patients weighing >40 kg, or children 11–12 years of age. For acute exacerbations, a 0.083% solution containing 2.5 mg of albuterol per 3 mL may be more appropriate, particularly in children ≥6 years of age.
- 0.083% Inhalation solution for nebulization in children 2–12 years of age: 2.5 mg 3 or 4 times daily in children weighing ≥15 kg. Do not increase dosage or dosage frequency. In children 2–12 years of age weighing<15 kg who require <2.5 mg per dose, the 0.5% inhalation solution should be used to prepare the appropriate dose for nebulization.
- 0.083% Inhalation solution for nebulization in adolescents ≥12 years of age: 2.5 mg 3 or 4 times daily (Proventil® single-use inhalation solution).
- 0.5% Inhalation solution for nebulization in adolescents ≥12 years of age: 2.5 mg 3–4 times daily.

Exercise-induced Bronchospasm
Prevention

ORAL INHALATION:

- Inhalation aerosol with chlorofluorocarbons in children ≥12 years of age: 180 mcg (2 inhalations) administered 15 minutes before exercise via metered-dose inhaler (Proventil®).
- Inhalation aerosol without chlorofluorocarbons in children ≥4 years of age: 180 mcg (2 inhalations) administered 15–30 minutes before exercise via metered-dose inhaler (Ventolin® HFA, Proventil® HFA).
- Inhalation aerosol without chlorofluorocarbons in children ≥12 years of age: 180 mcg (2 inhalations) administered 15–30 minutes before exercise via metered-dose inhaler (ProAir® HFA).

Adult Patients

Bronchospasm
Asthma

ORAL INHALATION:

- Inhalation aerosol: 180 mcg (2 inhalations) every 4–6 hours. Do not increase dosage or dosage frequency of orally inhaled albuterol aerosol. Alternatively, 90 mcg (1 inhalation) every 4 hours.
- Inhalation solution for nebulization: 2.5 mg 3 or 4 times daily. Do not increase dosage or dosage frequency.

Exercise-induced Bronchospasm
Prevention

ORAL INHALATION:

- Inhalation aerosol with chlorofluorocarbons: 180 mcg (2 inhalations) administered 15 minutes before exercise (Proventil®).
- Inhalation aerosol without chlorofluorocarbons: 180 mcg (2 inhalations) administered 15–30 minutes before exercise via the metered-dose inhaler (Ventolin® HFA, Proair® HFA, Proventil® HFA).

Bronchospasm
COPD

ORAL INHALATION:

- Inhalation aerosol: Initially, 180 mcg (2 inhalations) 4 times daily in fixed combination with ipratropium bromide (18 mcg per inhalation). If necessary, additional inhalations may be used, with dosage not exceeding 12 inhalations in 24 hours.
- Inhalation solution for nebulization: Initially, 2.5 mg 4 times daily in fixed combination with ipratropium bromide (0.5 mg per dose) (DuoNeb®). If necessary, may administer 2.5 mg in fixed combination with ipratropium bromide (0.5 mg per dose) up to 6 times daily.

Prescribing Limits

Pediatric Patients

Bronchospasm
Asthma

ORAL INHALATION:

- Inhalation aerosol with chlorofluorocarbons in adolescents ≥12 years of age: Maximum 180 mcg (2 inhalations) 4 times daily (Proventil®).
- Inhalation aerosol without chlorofluorocarbons in children ≥4 years of age: Maximum 180 mcg (2 inhalations) 4 times daily (Ventolin® HFA, Proventil® HFA).
- Inhalation solution for nebulization in children 2–12 years of age: Maximum 2.5 mg 4 times daily in children weighing at least 15 kg.
- Inhalation solution for nebulization in adolescents ≥12 years of age: Maximum 2.5 mg 4 times daily.

Exercise-induced Bronchospasm
Prevention

ORAL INHALATION:

- Inhalation aerosol: Maximum 12 inhalations in 24 hours in children ≥4 years of age (Ventolin® HFA, Proventil® HFA) or adolescents ≥12 years of age (Proventil®, ProAir® HFA).

Adult Patients

Bronchospasm
Asthma

ORAL INHALATION:

- Inhalation aerosol: Maximum 180 mcg (2 inhalations) 4 times daily.
- Inhalation solution for nebulization: Maximum 2.5 mg 4 times daily.

Exercise-induced Bronchospasm
Prevention

ORAL INHALATION:
- Inhalation aerosol: Maximum 12 inhalations in 24 hours.

Bronchospasm
COPD

ORAL INHALATION:
- Inhalation aerosol: Maximum 180 mcg (2 inhalations) 4 times daily in fixed combination with ipratropium bromide (18 mcg per inhalation).
- Inhalation solution for nebulization: Maximum 2.5 mg 6 times daily in fixed combination with ipratropium bromide (0.5 mg per dose).

Special Populations

Geriatric Patients
- Inhalation aerosol: Initiate therapy with dosages at the lower end of the usual range.

Alefacept Injection

(a la fa' cept)

Brand Name: Amevive®

Why is this medicine prescribed?

Alefacept is used to treat moderate to severe chronic plaque psoriasis (a skin disease in which red, scaly patches form on some areas of the body). Alefacept is in a class of medications called immunosuppressants. It works by stopping the action of certain cells in the body that cause the symptoms of psoriasis.

How should this medicine be used?

Alefacept comes as a solution to inject into a muscle or intravenously (into a vein). It is usually injected in a doctor's office once a week for 12 weeks. Sometimes a second 12-week cycle is given, but it is always separated from the first cycle by a period of at least 12 weeks without the medication.

Are there other uses for this medicine?

This medication may be prescribed for other uses; ask your doctor or pharmacist for more information.

What special precautions should I follow?

Before using alefacept,
- tell your doctor and pharmacist if you are allergic to alefacept or any other medications.
- tell your doctor and pharmacist what prescription and nonprescription medications, vitamins, nutritional supplements, and herbal products you are taking or plan to take. Be sure to mention medications that suppress the immune system such as azathioprine (Imuran); cancer chemotherapy; cyclosporine (Neoral, Sandimmune); methotrexate (Rheumatrex); oral steroids such as dexamethasone (Decadron, Dexone), methylprednisolone (Medrol), and prednisone (Deltasone); sirolimus (Rapamune); and tacrolimus (Prograf). Your doctor may need to change the doses of your medications or monitor you carefully for side effects.
- tell your doctor if you or any of your close relatives have or have ever had cancer and if you have or have ever had any disease that affects your immune system such as human immunodeficiency virus (HIV), acquired immunodeficiency syndrome (AIDS), or severe combined immunodeficiency syndrome (SCID); or kidney or liver disease. Also tell your doctor if you have any type of infection, including infections that come and go (such as cold sores), and chronic infections that do not go away such as tuberculosis (TB), varicella (chickenpox or shingles), or hepatitis, or if you frequently get any type of infection such as urinary tract or bladder infections.
- tell your doctor if your psoriasis is being treated with phototherapy (a treatment for psoriasis that involves exposing the skin to ultraviolet light).
- tell your doctor if you are pregnant, plan to become pregnant, or are breast-feeding. If you become pregnant while using alefacept or within 8 weeks of stopping alefacept, call your doctor.
- if you are having surgery, including dental surgery, tell the doctor or dentist that you are using alefacept.
- do not have any vaccinations (shots to prevent diseases) without talking to your doctor.
- you should know that alefacept may decrease your ability to fight infection and increase the risk that you will develop a serious infection. Stay away from people who are sick and wash your hands often while you are using this medication.

What special dietary instructions should I follow?

Unless your doctor tells you otherwise, continue your normal diet.

What should I do if I forget to take a dose?

If you miss an appointment to receive an alefacept injection, call your doctor as soon as possible.

What side effects can this medicine cause?

Alefacept may cause side effects. Tell your doctor if any of these symptoms are severe or do not go away:
- dizziness
- muscle pain
- pain, redness, swelling, or bleeding in the place where alefacept was injected

Some side effects can be serious. If you experience any of the following symptoms, call your doctor immediately:

- hives
- rash
- itching
- swelling of the face, throat, tongue, lips, eyes, hands, feet, ankles, or lower legs
- difficulty breathing or swallowing
- hoarseness
- fever, sore throat, chills, and other signs of infection
- cough
- changes in skin such as new or changed sores, spots, lumps or moles
- lumps or masses in any part of the body
- upset stomach
- vomiting
- loss of appetite
- extreme tiredness
- stomach pain
- yellowing of the skin or eyes
- easy bruising
- dark urine
- pale stools

Alefacept may increase the risk that you will develop cancer. Talk to your doctor about the risks of using this medication.

Alefacept may cause other side effects. Call your doctor if you have any unusual problems while using this medication.

If you experience a serious side effect, you or your doctor may send a report to the Food and Drug Administration's (FDA) MedWatch Adverse Event Reporting program online [at http://www.fda.gov/MedWatch/index.html] or by phone [1-800-332-1088].

What storage conditions are needed for this medicine?

Your doctor will store the medication in his office and give it to you each week.

What should I do in case of overdose?

In case of overdose, call your local poison control center at 1-800-222-1222. If the victim has collapsed or is not breathing, call local emergency services at 911.

Symptoms of overdose may include:

- chills
- headache
- joint pain
- sinus pain

What other information should I know?

Keep all appointments with your doctor and the laboratory. Your doctor will order certain lab tests before and during treatment to check your body's response to alefacept.

Dosage Facts
For Informational Purposes

Caution: Do not change your dose, how often you take your medication, or the length of time you are to take it without first talking to your healthcare provider.

The following dosage information was written using medical language for doctors and other healthcare professionals and is provided here for you to check your dosage. The dosage of this drug may differ for different patients. Therefore, always follow your doctor's instructions or the directions on the label. Contact your healthcare provider or pharmacist if you have any questions about the specific dosage of your medication after reviewing this information.

General Dosage Information

Monitor $CD4^+$ T-cell counts before initiation of therapy and every 2 weeks throughout the 12-week course of therapy. Do not initiate if $CD4^+$ T-cell counts are below normal range. If $CD4^+$ T-cell counts are $<250/mm^3$, withhold therapy and monitor $CD4^+$ T-cell counts *weekly*. Discontinue if $CD4^+$ T-cell counts remain $<250/mm^3$ for 1 month.

Adult Patients
Psoriasis

IV:
- 7.5 mg once weekly for 12 weeks. Monitor $CD4^+$ T-cell counts and adjust dosage accordingly.
- May initiate retreatment with additional 12-week course if $CD4^+$ T-cell counts are within normal range and ≥12 weeks have elapsed since previous course.

IM:
- 15 mg once weekly for 12 weeks. Monitor $CD4^+$ T-cell counts and adjust dosage accordingly.
- May initiate retreatment with additional 12-week course if $CD4^+$ T-cell counts are within normal range and ≥12 weeks have elapsed since previous course.

Alendronate

(a len' droe nate)

Brand Name: Fosamax®, Fosamax Plus D®

Why is this medicine prescribed?

Alendronate is used to treat and prevent osteoporosis (a condition in which the bones become thin and weak and break easily) in women who have undergone menopause (change of life; end of menstrual periods). Alendronate is also used to treat osteoporosis in men and women, who are taking corticosteroids (a type of medication that may cause osteoporosis in some patients). Alendronate is also used to treat Paget's disease of bone (a condition in which the bones are soft and weak and may be deformed, painful, or easily broken). Alendronate is in a class of medications called bisphosphonates. It works by preventing bone breakdown and increasing bone density thickness.

How should this medicine be used?

Alendronate comes as a tablet and a solution (liquid) to take by mouth. The solution is usually taken on an empty stomach once a week in the morning. The 5-mg and 10-mg tablets are usually taken on an empty stomach once a day in the morning, and the 30-mg and 70-mg tablets are usually taken on an empty stomach once a week in the morning. The 40-mg tablets are usually taken once a day in the morning for six months to treat Paget's disease of bone. Follow the directions on your prescription label carefully, and ask your doctor or pharmacist to explain any part you do not understand. Take alendronate exactly as directed. Do not take more or less of it or take it more often than prescribed by your doctor.

Alendronate may not work properly and may damage the esophagus (tube between the mouth and stomach) or cause sores in the mouth if it is not taken according to the following instructions. Tell your doctor if you do not understand, you do not think you will remember, or you are unable to follow these instructions:

- You must take alendronate just after you get out of bed in the morning, before you eat or drink anything. Never take alendronate at bedtime or before you wake up and get out of bed for the day.
- Swallow alendronate tablets with a full glass (6 to 8 ounces, about 1 cup) of plain water. Drink at least a quarter of a cup (2 ounces) of plain water after you drink alendronate liquid. Never take alendronate with tea, coffee, juice, milk, mineral water, sparkling water, or any liquid other than plain water.
- Swallow the tablets whole; do not split, chew or crush them. Do not suck on the tablets.
- After you take alendronate, do not eat, drink, or take any other medications (including vitamins or antacids) for at least 30 minutes. Do not lie down for at least 30 minutes after you take alendronate. Sit upright or stand upright until at least 30 minutes have passed and you have eaten your first food of the day.

Alendronate controls osteoporosis and Paget's disease of bone but does not cure these conditions. It may take 3 months or longer before your bone density begins to increase. Alendronate helps to treat and prevent osteoporosis only as long as it is taken regularly. Continue to take alendronate even if you feel well. Do not stop taking alendronate without talking to your doctor.

Ask your pharmacist or doctor for a copy of the manufacturer's information for the patient.

Are there other uses for this medicine?

This medication may be prescribed for other uses; ask your doctor or pharmacist for more information.

What special precautions should I follow?

Before taking alendronate,

- tell your doctor and pharmacist if you are allergic to alendronate, any other medications, or any of the ingredients in alendronate tablets or liquid. Ask your pharmacist for a list of the ingredients.
- tell your doctor and pharmacist what prescription and nonprescription medications, vitamins, nutritional supplements, and herbal products you are taking or plan to take. Be sure to mention any of the following: aspirin and other nonsteroidal anti-inflammatory medications (NSAIDs) such as ibuprofen (Advil, Motrin) and naproxen (Naprosyn, Aleve); cancer chemotherapy; or oral steroids such as dexamethasone (Decadron, Dexone), methylprednisolone (Medrol), and prednisone (Deltasone). Your doctor may need to change the doses of your medications or monitor you carefully for side effects.
- if you are taking any other medications including supplements, vitamins, or antacids by mouth, take them at least 30 minutes after you take alendronate.
- tell your doctor if you are unable to sit upright or stand upright for at least 30 minutes and if you have or have ever had a low level of calcium in your blood or any problems with your esophagus. Your doctor may tell you that you should not take alendronate.
- tell your doctor if are undergoing radiation therapy and if you have or have ever had anemia (condition in which the red blood cells do not bring enough oxygen to all the parts of the body); difficulty swallowing; heartburn; ulcers or other stomach problems; cancer; any type of infection, especially in your mouth; problems with your mouth, teeth, or gums; any condition that stops your blood from clotting normally; or dental or kidney disease.
- tell your doctor if you are pregnant or are breast-feeding. Also tell your doctor if you plan to become pregnant at any time in the future, because alendronate may remain in your body for many years after you stop taking it. Call your doctor if you become pregnant during or after your treatment.
- you should know that alendronate may cause serious problems with your jaw, especially if you have dental surgery or treatment while you are taking the medication. A dentist should examine your teeth and perform any needed treatments before you start to take alendronate. Be sure to brush your teeth and clean your mouth properly while you are taking alendronate. Talk to your doctor before having any dental treatments while you are taking this medication.
- you should know that alendronate may cause serious damage to the lining of your mouth, esophagus, or stom-

ach, especially if you do not take it according to the directions listed in the HOW section above. If you experience any of the following symptoms, stop taking alendronate, and call your doctor immediately: new or worsening heartburn, difficulty swallowing, pain on swallowing, or chest pain.

- talk to your doctor about other things you can do to prevent osteoporosis from developing or worsening. Your doctor will probably tell you to avoid smoking and drinking large amounts of alcohol and to follow a regular program of weight-bearing exercise.

What special dietary instructions should I follow?

You should eat and drink plenty of foods and drinks that are rich in calcium and vitamin D while you are taking alendronate. Your doctor will tell you which foods and drinks are good sources of these nutrients and how many servings you need each day. If you find it difficult to eat enough of these foods, tell your doctor. In that case, your doctor can prescribe or recommend a supplement.

What should I do if I forget to take a dose?

If you miss a dose of once-daily alendronate, do not take it later in the day. Skip the missed dose and take one dose the next morning as usual. If you miss a dose of once-weekly alendronate, take one dose the morning after you remember. Then return to taking one dose once each week on your regularly scheduled day. Never take a double dose to make up for a missed one, and never take more than one dose in 1 day.

What side effects can this medicine cause?

Alendronate may cause side effects. Tell your doctor if any of these symptoms are severe or do not go away:

- nausea
- stomach pain
- constipation
- diarrhea
- gas
- bloating or fullness in the stomach
- change in ability to taste food
- bone, muscle, or joint pain
- headache
- dizziness
- flu-like symptoms

Some side effects can be serious. If you experience any of the following symptoms, call your doctor immediately before you take any more alendronate:

- new or worsening heartburn
- difficulty swallowing
- pain on swallowing
- chest pain
- bloody vomit or vomit that looks like coffee grounds
- black, tarry, or bloody stools
- fever

- blisters or peeling skin
- rash (may be made worse by sunlight)
- itching
- hives
- swelling of eyes, face, lips, tongue, or throat
- difficulty breathing
- hoarseness
- painful or swollen gums
- loosening of the teeth
- numbness or heavy feeling in the jaw
- poor healing of the jaw
- eye pain

Alendronate may cause other side effects. Call your doctor if you have any unusual problems while taking this medication.

What storage conditions are needed for this medicine?

Keep this medication in the container it came in, tightly closed, and out of reach of children. Store it at room temperature and away from excess heat and moisture (not in the bathroom). Do not freeze alendronate solution. Throw away any medication that is outdated or no longer needed. Talk to your pharmacist about the proper disposal of your medication.

What should I do in case of overdose?

In case of overdose, give the victim a full glass of milk and call your local poison control center at 1-800-222-1222. If the victim has collapsed or is not breathing, call local emergency services at 911. Do not allow the victim to lie down and do not try to make the victim vomit.

Symptoms of overdose may include:

- heartburn
- nausea
- stomach pain
- bloody vomit or vomit that looks like coffee grounds
- difficulty swallowing or pain when swallowing
- bloody or black and tarry stool

What other information should I know?

Keep all appointments with your doctor and the laboratory. Your doctor may order certain lab tests to check your body's response to alendronate.

Do not let anyone else take your medication. Ask your pharmacist any questions you have about refilling your prescription.

Dosage Facts
For Informational Purposes

Caution: Do not change your dose, how often you take your medication, or the length of time you are to take it without first talking to your healthcare provider.

The following dosage information was written using medical language for doctors and other healthcare professionals and is provided here for you to check your dosage. The dosage of this drug may differ for different patients. Therefore, always follow your doctor's instructions or the directions on the label. Contact your healthcare provider or pharmacist if you have any questions about the specific dosage of your medication after reviewing this information.

General Dosage Information

Available as alendronate sodium; dosage expressed in terms of alendronate.

Adult Patients

Osteoporosis
Prevention of Postmenopausal Osteoporosis

ORAL:
• 5 mg once *daily* or 35 mg once *weekly*.

Treatment of Osteoporosis

ORAL:
• 10 mg once *daily* or 70 mg once *weekly* in men and postmenopausal women.

Corticosteroid-induced Osteoporosis
Prevention of Corticosteroid-induced Osteoporosis†

ORAL:
• 5 mg once *daily* in postmenopausal women receiving hormone replacement therapy (HRT), premenopausal women, and men.
• 10 mg once *daily* in postmenopausal women *not* receiving HRT.
• Continue alendronate as long as patient continues to receive corticosteroid therapy.

Treatment of Corticosteroid-induced Osteoporosis

ORAL:
• 5 mg once *daily* in postmenopausal women receiving HRT, premenopausal women, and men.
• 10 mg once *daily* in postmenopausal women *not* receiving HRT.
• Continue alendronate as long as patient continues to receive corticosteroid therapy.

Paget's Disease of Bone

ORAL:
• 40 mg once daily for 6 months.
• Consider retreatment after a 6-month posttreatment evaluation period if relapse occurs (i.e., increased serum alkaline phosphatase concentration) or if initial treatment failed to normalize serum alkaline phosphatase concentrations.

Special Populations

Renal Impairment
• No dosage adjustment required in patients with mild to moderate impairment (Cl_{cr} 35–60 mL/minute); not recommended in patients with severe impairment (Cl_{cr} <35 mL/minute).

† *Use is not currently included in the labeling approved by the US Food and Drug Administration.*

Alfuzosin
(al fyoo′ zoe sin)

Brand Name: Uroxatral®

Why is this medicine prescribed?

Alfuzosin is used in men to treat symptoms of an enlarged prostate (benign prostatic hyperplasia or BPH), which include difficulty urinating (hesitation, dribbling, weak stream, and incomplete bladder emptying), painful urination, and urinary frequency and urgency. Alfuzosin is in a class of medications called alpha blockers. It works by relaxing the muscles in the prostate and bladder to allow urine to flow more easily.

How should this medicine be used?

Alfuzosin comes as an extended-release (long-acting) tablet to take by mouth. It is usually taken once a day, immediately after a meal. Do not take alfuzosin on an empty stomach. To help you remember to take alfuzosin, take it after the same meal every day. Follow the directions on your prescription label carefully, and ask your doctor or pharmacist to explain any part you do not understand. Take alfuzosin exactly as directed. Do not take more or less of it or take it more often than prescribed by your doctor.

Swallow the tablets whole; do not split, chew, or crush them.

Alfuzosin controls BPH but does not cure it. Continue to take alfuzosin even if you feel well. Do not stop taking alfuzosin without talking to your doctor.

Are there other uses for this medicine?

This medication may be prescribed for other uses; ask your doctor or pharmacist for more information.

What special precautions should I follow?

Before taking alfuzosin,
• tell your doctor and pharmacist if you are allergic to alfuzosin, any other medications, or any of the ingredients in alfuzosin. Ask your pharmacist for a list of the ingredients.
• tell your doctor if you are taking itraconazole (Sporanox), ketoconazole (Nizoral), or ritonavir (Norvir, in Kaletra). Your doctor will probably tell you not to take alfuzosin.
• tell your doctor if you have liver disease. Your doctor may tell you not to take alfuzosin.
• tell your doctor and pharmacist what other prescription and nonprescription medications, vitamins, nutritional supplements, and herbal products you are taking or plan to take. Be sure to mention any of the following: amiodarone (Cordarone); aprepitant (Emend); atenolol (Tenormin); cimetidine (Tagamet); cisapride (not available in the U.S.); clarithormycin (Biaxin, in Prevpac);

cyclosporine (Neoral, Sandimmune); danazol (Danocrine); delavirdine (Rescriptor); diltiazem (Cardizem, Dilacor, Tiazac, others); disopyramide (Norpace); dofetilide (Tikosyn); efavirenz (Sustiva); erythromycin (E.E.S., E-Mycin, Erythrocin); fluconazole (Diflucan); fluoxetine (Prozac, Sarafem); fluvoxamine (Luvox); HIV protease inhibitors such as atazanavir (Reyataz), indinavir (Crixivan), lopinavir (in Kaletra), nelfinavir (Viracept), and saquinavir (Fortovase, Invirase); hormonal contraceptives (birth control pills, rings, and patches); isoniazid (INH, Nydrazid); lovastatin (Advicor, Altocor, Mevacor); medications for high blood pressure; medications for erectile dysfunction (ED) such as sildenafil (Viagra), tadalafil (Cialis), or vardenafil (Levitra); metronidazole (Flagyl); moxifloxacin (Avelox); nefazodone; other alpha blockers such as doxazosin (Cardura), prazosin (Minipress), terazosin (Hytrin), and tamsulosin (Flomax); pimozide (Orap); procainamide (Procanbid, Pronestyl); quinidine (Quinidex); sertraline (Zoloft); sotalol (Betapace,); sparfloxacin (Zagam); thioridazine (Mellaril); troleandomycin (TAO); verapamil (Calan, Covera, Isoptin, Verelan); and zafirlukast (Accolate). Your doctor may need to change the doses of your medications or monitor you carefully for side effects.

- tell your doctor if you or any member of your family have an irregular heartbeat; or if you have or have ever had prostate cancer; angina (chest pain); low blood pressure; or heart or kidney disease; and if you have ever become dizzy, fainted, or had low blood pressure after taking any medication.
- you should know that alfuzosin is only for use in men. Women should not take alfuzosin, especially if they are or could become pregnant or are breast-feeding. If a pregnant woman takes alfuzosin, she should call her doctor.
- if you are having surgery, including dental surgery, tell the doctor or dentist that you are taking alfuzosin. If you need to have eye surgery at any time during or after your treatment, be sure to tell your doctor that you are taking or have taken alfuzosin.
- you should know that alfuzosin may cause dizziness, lightheadedness, and fainting, especially when you get up too quickly from a lying position. This is more common when you first start taking alfuzosin. To avoid this problem, get out of bed slowly, resting your feet on the floor for a few minutes before standing up. If these symptoms do not improve, call your doctor. Avoid driving, operating machinery, or performing dangerous tasks until you know how this medication affects you.

What special dietary instructions should I follow?

Talk to your doctor about eating grapefruit or drinking grapefruit juice while taking this medication.

What should I do if I forget to take a dose?

Take the missed dose as soon as you remember it. However, if it is almost time for the next dose, skip the missed dose and continue your regular dosing schedule. Do not take a double dose to make up for a missed one.

What side effects can this medicine cause?

Alfuzosin may cause side effects. Tell your doctor if any of these symptoms or those listed in the SPECIAL PRECAUTIONS section are severe or do not go away:

- tiredness
- headache
- runny or stuffy nose
- pain
- stomach pain
- heartburn
- constipation
- nausea
- decrease in sexual ability
- sore throat, fever, chills, cough and other signs of infection.

Some side effects can be serious. If you experience any of these symptoms, call your doctor immediately:

- rash
- swelling of the face, throat, tongue, lips, eyes, hands, feet, ankles, or lower legs
- hoarseness
- difficulty swallowing or breathing
- chest pain
- fainting

Alfuzosin may cause other side effects. Call your doctor if you have any unusual problems while taking this medication.

What storage conditions are needed for this medicine?

Keep this medication in the container it came in, tightly closed, and out of reach of children. Store it at room temperature and away from light and excess heat and moisture (not in the bathroom). Throw away any medication that is outdated or no longer needed. Talk to your pharmacist about the proper disposal of your medication.

What should I do in case of overdose?

In case of overdose, call your local poison control center at 1-800-222-1222. If the victim has collapsed or is not breathing, call local emergency services at 911.

Symptoms of overdose may include:
- dizziness
- fainting
- lightheadedness
- blurred vision
- nausea

What other information should I know?

Keep all appointments with your doctor.

Do not let anyone else take your medication. Ask your pharmacist any questions you have about refilling your prescription.

Dosage Facts
For Informational Purposes

Caution: Do not change your dose, how often you take your medication, or the length of time you are to take it without first talking to your healthcare provider.

The following dosage information was written using medical language for doctors and other healthcare professionals and is provided here for you to check your dosage. The dosage of this drug may differ for different patients. Therefore, always follow your doctor's instructions or the directions on the label. Contact your healthcare provider or pharmacist if you have any questions about the specific dosage of your medication after reviewing this information.

General Dosage Information

Available as alfuzosin hydrochloride; dosage is expressed in terms of the salt.

Adult Patients

BPH

ORAL:
• 10 mg daily.

Aliskiren
(a lis kye′ ren)

Brand Name: Tekturna®

> ### Important Warning
>
> Do not take aliskiren if you are pregnant. If you become pregnant while taking aliskiren, call your doctor immediately. Aliskiren may harm the fetus.

Why is this medicine prescribed?

Aliskiren is used alone or in combination with other medications to treat high blood pressure. Aliskiren is in a class of medications called direct renin inhibitors. It works by decreasing certain natural chemicals that tighten the blood vessels, so blood vessels relax and the heart can pump blood more efficiently.

How should this medicine be used?

Aliskiren comes as a tablet to take by mouth. It is usually taken once a day. Aliskiren should be taken the same way each time, either always with food or always without food. Take aliskiren at around the same time every day. Follow the directions on your prescription label carefully, and ask your doctor or pharmacist to explain any part you do not understand. Take aliskiren exactly as directed. Do not take more or less of it or take it more often than prescribed by your doctor.

Your doctor will probably start you on an low dose of aliskiren and may increase your dose after you have been taking this medication for at least two weeks.

Aliskiren controls high blood pressure but does not cure it. Continue to take aliskiren even if you feel well. Do not stop taking aliskiren without talking to your doctor.

Ask your pharmacist or doctor for a copy of the manufacturer's information for the patient.

Are there other uses for this medicine?

This medication may be prescribed for other uses; ask your doctor or pharmacist for more information.

What special precautions should I follow?

Before taking aliskiren,
• tell your doctor and pharmacist if you are allergic to aliskiren or any other medications.
• tell your doctor and pharmacist what other prescription and nonprescription medications, vitamins, nutritional supplements, and herbal products you are taking or plan to take. Be sure to mention any of the following: angiotensin-converting enzyme (ACE) inhibitors such as benazepril (Lotensin), captopril (Capoten), enalapril (Vasotec), fosinopril (Monopril), lisinopril (Prinivil, Zestril), moexipril (Univasc), perindopril (Aceon), quinapril (Accupril), ramipril (Altace), and trandolapril (Mavik); antifungals such as ketoconazole (Nizoral); atorvastatin (Lipitor); diuretics ('water pills') such as hydrochlorothiazide (HCTZ) and furosemide (Lasix); irbesartan (Avapro); and other medications for heart disease or high blood pressure. Your doctor may need to change the doses of your medications or monitor you carefully for side effects.
• tell your doctor if you have or have ever had diabetes, seizures, or kidney disease.
• tell your doctor if you plan to become pregnant or are breast-feeding. Do not breastfeed while taking aliskiren.
• you should know that aliskiren may cause dizziness, lightheadedness, and fainting. Lie down if you feel faint or dizzy, and call your doctor right away.

What special dietary instructions should I follow?

Unless your doctor tells you otherwise, continue your normal diet.

What should I do if I forget to take a dose?

Take the missed dose as soon as you remember it. However, if it is almost time for the next dose, skip the missed dose and continue your regular dosing schedule. Do not take a double dose to make up for a missed one.

What side effects can this medicine cause?

Aliskiren may cause side effects. Tell your doctor if any of these symptoms are severe or do not go away:

- diarrhea
- stomach pain
- heartburn
- cough
- rash

Some side effects can be serious. If you experience any of these symptoms, call your doctor immediately:

- swelling of the face, throat, tongue, lips, eyes, hands, feet, ankles, or lower legs
- hoarseness
- difficulty swallowing or breathing
- lightheadedness
- fainting

Aliskiren may cause other side effects. Call your doctor if you have any unusual problems while taking this medication.

What storage conditions are needed for this medicine?

Keep this medication in the container it came in, tightly closed, and out of reach of children. Store it at room temperature and away from excess heat and moisture (not in the bathroom). Do not remove the desiccant (drying agent) from the bottle, if one has been provided. Throw away any medication that is outdated or no longer needed. Talk to your pharmacist about the proper disposal of your medication.

What should I do in case of overdose?

In case of overdose, call your local poison control center at 1-800-222-1222. If the victim has collapsed or is not breathing, call local emergency services at 911.

Symptoms of overdose may include:

- fainting
- dizziness
- blurred vision
- nausea

What other information should I know?

Keep all appointments with your doctor.

Do not let anyone else take your medication. Ask your pharmacist any questions you have about refilling your prescription.

Talk to your doctor, pharmacist, or other healthcare professional if you have questions about dosing information for your medication.

Alitretinoin

(a li tre′ ti noyn)

Brand Name: Panretin®

Why is this medicine prescribed?

Alitretinoin is used to treat skin lesions associated with Kaposi's sarcoma. It helps stop the growth of Kaposi's sarcoma cells.

This medication is sometimes prescribed for other uses; ask your doctor or pharmacist for more information.

How should this medicine be used?

Alitretinoin comes in topical gel. Alitretinoin is usually used twice a day. Your doctor may tell you to use alitretinoin more or less frequently depending on your response to it. Follow the directions on your prescription label carefully, and ask your doctor or pharmacist to explain any part you do not understand. Use alitretinoin exactly as directed. Do not use more or less of it or use it more often than prescribed by your doctor.

Alitretinoin controls Kaposi's sarcoma lesions but does not cure them. It will take at least 2 weeks of using alitretinoin before a benefit can be seen. For some patients, it may take 8-14 weeks to see results. Do not stop using alitretinoin without talking to your doctor. To apply alitretinoin, follow these steps:

1. Wash your hands and affected skin area thoroughly with mild soap (not medicated or abrasive soap or soap that dries the skin) and water.
2. Use clean fingertips, a gauze pad, or a cotton swab to apply the medication.
3. Apply enough gel to cover the lesion with a generous coating.
4. Apply the medication to the affected skin area only. Do not apply to unaffected areas; do not apply on or near mucus membranes.
5. Allow the gel to dry for 3-5 minutes before covering with clothing.

What special precautions should I follow?

Before using alitretinoin,

- tell your doctor and pharmacist if you are allergic to alitretinoin, etretinate, isotretinoin, tazarotene, tretinoin, or any other drugs.
- tell your doctor what other medications you are taking, including vitamins or herbal products. Do not use insect repellants that contain DEET while using alitretinoin.
- tell your doctor if you have or have ever had a type of skin cancer known as T-cell lymphoma.
- tell your doctor if you are pregnant, plan to become pregnant, or are breast-feeding. If you become pregnant while using alitretinoin, call your doctor immediately. You should not plan to become pregnant while using alitretinoin.

- plan to avoid unnecessary or prolonged exposure to sunlight and to wear protective clothing, sunglasses, and sunscreen. Alitretinoin may make your skin sensitive to sunlight.

What should I do if I forget to take a dose?

Apply the missed dose as soon as you remember. However, if it is almost time to apply the next dose, skip the missed dose and continue your regular application schedule.

What side effects can this medicine cause?

Alitretinoin may cause side effects. Tell your doctor if any of these symptoms are severe or do not go away:

- warmth or slight stinging of the skin
- lightening or darkening of the skin
- red, scaling skin
- rash
- swelling, blistering, or crusting of the skin
- pain at site of application
- itching

What storage conditions are needed for this medicine?

Keep this medication in the container it came in, tightly closed, and out of reach of children. Store it at room temperature and away from excess heat and moisture (not in the bathroom). Throw away any medication that is outdated or no longer needed. Talk to your pharmacist about the proper disposal of your medication.

What other information should I know?

Keep all appointments with your doctor. Alitretinoin is for external use only. Do not let alitretinoin get into your eyes, your nostrils, mouth, or any broken skin, and do not swallow it.

Do not apply dressings, bandages, cosmetics, lotions, or other skin medications to the area being treated unless your doctor tells you.

Do not let anyone else use your medication. Ask your pharmacist any questions you have about refilling your prescription. Tell your doctor if your skin condition gets worse or does not improve.

Dosage Facts
For Informational Purposes

Caution: Do not change your dose, how often you take your medication, or the length of time you are to take it without first talking to your healthcare provider.

The following dosage information was written using medical language for doctors and other healthcare professionals and is provided here for you to check your dosage. The dosage of this drug may differ for different

patients. Therefore, always follow your doctor's instructions or the directions on the label. Contact your healthcare provider or pharmacist if you have any questions about the specific dosage of your medication after reviewing this information.

Adult Patients

AIDS-related Kaposi's Sarcoma
TOPICAL:

- Initially, apply twice daily in sufficient amounts (to cover only affected areas). May increase application frequency gradually to 3 and then 4 times daily, according to individual lesion tolerance.
- In some patients, appreciable response occurred only after ≥14 weeks of therapy.
- Continue therapy as long as the patient derives benefit (has been applied for up to 175 weeks in clinical trials).

Allopurinol

(al oh pure′ i nole)

Brand Name: Aloprim®, Zyloprim®
Also available generically.

Why is this medicine prescribed?

Allopurinol is used to treat gout, high levels of uric acid in the body caused by certain cancer medications, and kidney stones. Allopurinol is in a class of medications called xanthine oxidase inhibitors. It works by reducing the production of uric acid in the body. High levels of uric acid may cause gout attacks or kidney stones. Allopurinol is used to prevent gout attacks, not to treat them once they occur.

How should this medicine be used?

Allopurinol comes as a tablet to take by mouth. It is usually taken once or twice a day, preferably after a meal. To help you remember to take allopurinol, take it around the same time every day. Follow the directions on your prescription label carefully, and ask your doctor or pharmacist to explain any part you do not understand. Take allopurinol exactly as directed. Do not take more or less of it or take it more often than prescribed by your doctor.

Your doctor will probably start you on a low dose of allopurinol and gradually increase your dose, not more than once a week.

It may take several months or longer before you feel the full benefit of allopurinol. Allopurinol may increase the number of gout attacks during the first few months that you take it, although it will eventually prevent attacks. Your doctor may prescribe another medication such as colchicine to prevent gout attacks for the first few months you take allopurinol. Continue to take allopurinol even if you feel well.

Do not stop taking allopurinol without talking to your doctor.

Are there other uses for this medicine?

Allopurinol is also sometimes used to treat seizures, pain caused by pancreas disease, and certain infections. It is also sometimes used to improve survival after bypass surgery, to reduce ulcer relapses, and to prevent rejection of kidney transplants. Talk to your doctor about the possible risks of using this medication for your condition.

This medication may be prescribed for other uses; ask your doctor or pharmacist for more information.

What special precautions should I follow?

Before taking allopurinol,

- tell your doctor and pharmacist if you are allergic to allopurinol or any other medications.
- tell your doctor and pharmacist what prescription and nonprescription medications, vitamins, nutritional supplements, and herbal products you are taking. Be sure to mention any of the following: amoxicillin (Amoxil, Trimox); ampicillin (Polycillin, Principen); anticoagulants ('blood thinners') such as warfarin (Coumadin); cancer chemotherapy drugs such as cyclophosphamide (Cytoxan) and mercaptopurine (Purinethol); chlorpropamide (Diabinese); diuretics ('water pills'); medications that suppress the immune system such as azathioprine (Imuran) and cyclosporine (Neoral, Sandimmune); other medications for gout such as probenecid (Benemid) and sulfinpyrazone (Anturane); and tolbutamide (Orinase). Your doctor may need to change the doses of your medications or monitor you carefully for side effects.
- tell your doctor if you have or have ever had kidney or liver disease or heart failure.
- tell your doctor if you are pregnant, plan to become pregnant, or are breast-feeding. If you become pregnant while taking allopurinol, call your doctor.
- you should know that allopurinol may make you drowsy. Do not drive a car or operate machinery until you know how this medication affects you.
- ask your doctor about the safe use of alcoholic beverages while you are taking allopurinol. Alcohol may decrease the effectiveness of allopurinol.

What special dietary instructions should I follow?

Drink at least eight glasses of water or other fluids each day while taking allopurinol unless directed to do otherwise by your doctor.

What should I do if I forget to take a dose?

Take the missed dose as soon as you remember it. However, if it is almost time for the next dose, skip the missed dose and continue your regular dosing schedule. Do not take a double dose to make up for a missed one.

What side effects can this medicine cause?

Allopurinol may cause side effects. Tell your doctor if any of these symptoms are severe or do not go away:

- upset stomach
- diarrhea
- drowsiness

Some side effects can be serious. The following symptoms are uncommon, but if you experience any of them, call your doctor immediately:

- skin rash
- painful urination
- blood in the urine
- irritation of the eyes
- swelling of the lips or mouth
- fever, sore throat, chills, and other signs of infection
- loss of appetite
- unexpected weight loss
- itching

Allopurinol may cause other side effects. Call your doctor if you have any unusual problems while taking this medication.

If you experience a serious side effect, you or your doctor may send a report to the Food and Drug Administration's (FDA) MedWatch Adverse Event Reporting program online [at http://www.fda.gov/MedWatch/index.html] or by phone [1-800-332-1088].

What storage conditions are needed for this medicine?

Keep this medication in the container it came in, tightly closed, and out of reach of children. Store it at room temperature and away from excess heat and moisture (not in the bathroom). Throw away any medication that is outdated or no longer needed. Talk to your pharmacist about the proper disposal of your medication.

What other information should I know?

Keep all appointments with your doctor and the laboratory. Your doctor will order certain lab tests to check your body's response to allopurinol.

Do not let anyone else take your medication. Ask your pharmacist any questions you have about refilling your prescription.

Dosage Facts
For Informational Purposes

Caution: Do not change your dose, how often you take your medication, or the length of time you are to take it without first talking to your healthcare provider.

The following dosage information was written using medical language for doctors and other healthcare professionals and is provided here for you to check your

dosage. The dosage of this drug may differ for different patients. Therefore, always follow your doctor's instructions or the directions on the label. Contact your healthcare provider or pharmacist if you have any questions about the specific dosage of your medication after reviewing this information.

General Dosage Information

Available as allopurinol (oral) or allopurinol sodium (for IV use); dosage is expressed in terms of allopurinol.

Pediatric Patients

Chemotherapy-induced Hyperuricemia

ORAL:

- Children <6 years of age: Initially, 150 mg daily.
- Children 6–10 years of age: Initially, 300 mg daily.
- Adjust dosage after about 48 hours according to patient response.

Adult Patients

Gout

ORAL:

- Initially, 100 mg daily. May increase dosage by 100 mg weekly until serum urate concentration falls to ≤6 mg/dL or until maximum recommended dosage of 800 mg daily is reached. Usual dosage is 200–300 mg daily in patients with mild gout and 400–600 mg daily in those with moderately severe tophaceous gout.
- After serum urate concentrations are controlled, dosage reduction may be possible; average maintenance dosage is 300 mg daily, and minimum effective dosage is 100–200 mg daily.

Chemotherapy-induced Hyperuricemia

ORAL:

- 600–800 mg daily for 2–3 days.

Recurrent Calcium Oxalate Renal Calculi

ORAL:

- Initially, 200–300 mg daily. Titrate dosage based on 24-hour urinary urate determinations.

Prescribing Limits

Adult Patients

ORAL:

- Maximum 800 mg daily.

Special Populations

Renal Impairment

ORAL:

Initial Oral Dosage in Patients with Renal Impairment

Cl_{cr} (mL/min)	Initial Dosage
10–20	200 mg daily
<10	≤100 mg daily
<3	Increase dosage interval (e.g., 300 mg twice weekly)

Maintenance Oral Dosage in Patients with Renal Impairment

Cl_{cr} (mL/min)	Maintenance Dosage
80	250 mg daily
60	200 mg daily
40	150 mg daily
20	100 mg daily
10	100 mg every 2 days
0	100 mg every 3 days

Almotriptan

(al moh trip′ tan)

Brand Name: Axert®

Why is this medicine prescribed?

Almotriptan is used to treat the symptoms of migraine headaches (severe, throbbing headaches that sometimes are accompanied by nausea and sensitivity to sound and light). Almotriptan is in a class of medications called selective serotonin receptor agonists. It works by narrowing blood vessels in the brain, stopping pain signals from being sent to the brain, and stopping the release of certain natural substances that cause pain, nausea, and other symptoms of migraine. Almotriptan does not prevent migraine attacks.

How should this medicine be used?

Almotriptan comes as a tablet to take by mouth. It is usually taken at the first sign of a migraine attack. If your symptoms improve after you take almotriptan but return after 2 hours or longer, you may take a second tablet. However, if your symptoms do not improve after you take almotriptan, do not take a second tablet before calling your doctor. Do not take more than two almotriptan tablets in any 24-hour period. Call your doctor if you need to take almotriptan more than four times a month. Follow the directions on your prescription label carefully, and ask your doctor or pharmacist to explain any part you do not understand. Take almotriptan exactly as directed. Do not take more or less of it or take it more often than prescribed by your doctor.

You may take your first dose of almotriptan in a doctor's office or other medical facility where you can be monitored for serious reactions.

Are there other uses for this medicine?

This medication may be prescribed for other uses; ask your doctor or pharmacist for more information.

What special precautions should I follow?

Before taking almotriptan,

- tell your doctor and pharmacist if you are allergic to almotriptan or any other medications.

- do not take almotriptan within 24 hours of another selective serotonin receptor agonist such as eletriptan (Relpax), frovatriptan (Frova), naratriptan (Amerge), rizatriptan (Maxalt), sumatriptan (Imitrex), or zolmitriptan (Zomig); or ergot-type medications such as bromocriptine (Parlodel), cabergoline (Dostinex), dihydroergotamine (D.H.E. 45, Migranal), ergoloid mesylates (Germinal, Hydergine), ergonovine (Ergotrate), ergotamine (Bellergal-S, Cafergot, Ergomar, Wigraine), methylergonovine (Methergine), methysergide (Sansert), and pergolide (Permax).
- tell your doctor and pharmacist what other prescription and nonprescription medications, vitamins, nutritional supplements, and herbal products you are taking, have recently stopped taking, or plan to take. Be sure to mention any of the following: antifungals such as fluconazole (Diflucan), itraconazole (Sporanox), and ketoconazole (Nizoral); cimetidine (Tagamet); clarithromycin (Biaxin); cyclosporine (Neoral, Sandimmune); danazol (Danocrine); delavirdine (Rescriptor); diltiazem (Cardizem, Dilacor, Tiazac); erythromycin (E.E.S., E-Mycin, Erythrocin); HIV protease inhibitors such as indinavir (Crixivan) and ritonavir (Norvir); isoniazid (INH, Nydrazid); metronidazole (Flagyl); nefazodone (Serzone); selective serotonin reuptake inhibitors (SSRIs) such as citalopram (Celexa), escitalopram (Lexapro), fluoxetine (Prozac, Sarafem, in Symbyax), fluvoxamine, paroxetine (Paxil), and sertraline (Zoloft); selective serotonin/norepinephrine reuptake inhibitors (SNRIs) such as duloxetine (Cymbalta) and venlafaxine (Effexor); troleandomycin (TAO); and zafirlukast (Accolate). Also tell your doctor or pharmacist if you are taking the following medications or if you have stopped taking them within the past two weeks: monoamine oxidase (MAO) inhibitors, including isocarboxazid (Marplan), phenelzine (Nardil), selegiline (Eldepryl), and tranylcypromine (Parnate). Your doctor may need to change the doses of your medications or monitor you carefully for side effects.
- tell your doctor if you smoke, if you or any family members have or have ever had heart disease, if you have gone through menopause (change of life), and if you have or have ever had a heart attack; angina (chest pain); high blood pressure; high cholesterol; diabetes; circulation problems; or kidney or liver disease.
- tell your doctor if you are pregnant, plan to become pregnant, or are breast-feeding. If you become pregnant while taking almotriptan, call your doctor.
- you should know that almotriptan may make you drowsy. Do not drive a car or operate machinery until you know how this medication affects you.
- talk to your doctor about your headache symptoms to make sure they are caused by migraine. Almotriptan should not be used to treat hemiplegic or basilar migraine or headaches caused by other conditions (such as cluster headaches).

What special dietary instructions should I follow?

Talk to your doctor about drinking grapefruit juice while taking this medicine.

What side effects can this medicine cause?

Almotriptan may cause side effects. Tell your doctor if any of these symptoms are severe or do not go away:

- upset stomach
- drowsiness
- headache
- dry mouth

Some side effects can be serious. The following symptoms are uncommon, but if you experience any of them, call your doctor immediately:

- rash or itching
- tightness, pain, pressure, or heaviness in the chest, throat, neck, and/or jaw
- slow or difficult speech
- dizziness or faintness
- weakness or numbness of an arm or leg
- severe stomach pain
- bloody diarrhea
- rapid, pounding, or irregular heartbeat
- difficulty breathing
- paleness or blue color of the fingers and toes
- pain, burning, or tingling in the hands or feet

Almotriptan may cause other side effects. Call your doctor if you have any unusual problems while taking this medication.

What storage conditions are needed for this medicine?

Keep this medication in the container it came in, tightly closed, and out of reach of children. Store it at room temperature and away from excess heat and moisture (not in the bathroom). Throw away any medication that is outdated or no longer needed. Talk to your pharmacist about the proper disposal of your medication.

What should I do in case of overdose?

In case of overdose, call your local poison control center at 1-800-222-1222. If the victim has collapsed or is not breathing, call local emergency services at 911.

Symptoms of overdose may include:

- tightness, pain, pressure, or heaviness in the chest, throat, neck, and/or jaw
- slow or difficult speech
- dizziness or faintness
- weakness or numbness of an arm or leg
- rapid, pounding, or irregular heart beat
- difficulty breathing
- headache

What other information should I know?

Keep all appointments with your doctor.

Do not let anyone else take your medication. Ask your pharmacist any questions you have about refilling your prescription.

Dosage Facts
For Informational Purposes

Caution: Do not change your dose, how often you take your medication, or the length of time you are to take it without first talking to your healthcare provider.

The following dosage information was written using medical language for doctors and other healthcare professionals and is provided here for you to check your dosage. The dosage of this drug may differ for different patients. Therefore, always follow your doctor's instructions or the directions on the label. Contact your healthcare provider or pharmacist if you have any questions about the specific dosage of your medication after reviewing this information.

General Dosage Information

Available as almotriptan malate; dosage is expressed in terms of almotriptan.

Adult Patients

Vascular Headaches
Migraine

ORAL:
- 6.25 or 12.5 mg as a single dose; individualize dosage selection, weighing the possible benefit (greater effectiveness) and risks (increased adverse effects) of the 12.5-mg dose. In clinical studies, doses >12.5 mg did not lead to substantially greater response.
- If headache recurs, dose may be repeated after 2 hours.
- Following failure to respond to first dose, reconsider diagnosis of migraine prior to administration of a second dose.

Prescribing Limits

Adult Patients

Vascular Headaches
Migraine

ORAL:
- Maximum 12.5 mg as a single dose; do not exceed 2 doses in any 24-hour period.
- Safety of treating an average of >4 headaches per 30-day period has not been established.

Special Populations

Hepatic Impairment
- Initial dose of 6.25 mg; maximum dosage of 12.5 mg over a 24-hour period.

Renal Impairment
- Initial dose of 6.25 mg; maximum dosage of 12.5 mg over a 24-hour period.

Geriatric Patients
- Cautious dosage selection recommended; generally start at low end of dosing range due to greater frequency of decreased hepatic, renal, or cardiac function and of concomitant illnesses or other drug therapy in geriatric population.
- In geriatric patients with normal renal function for their age, dosage is the same as that recommended for younger adults.

Alprazolam

(al pray′ zoe lam)

Brand Name: Alprazolam Intensol®, Xanax® Also available generically.

Why is this medicine prescribed?

Alprazolam is used to treat anxiety disorders and panic attacks. Alprazolam is in a class of medications called benzodiazepines. It works by decreasing abnormal excitement in the brain.

How should this medicine be used?

Alprazolam comes as a tablet and a concentrated solution (liquid) to take by mouth. It usually is taken two to four times a day. Follow the directions on your prescription label carefully, and ask your doctor or pharmacist to explain any part you do not understand. Take alprazolam exactly as directed.

To take the concentrated liquid, use only the dropper that came with your prescription. Draw into the dropper the amount prescribed for one dose. Squeeze the dropper contents into a liquid or semi-solid food such as water, juice, soda, applesauce, or pudding. Stir the liquid or food gently for a few seconds. The concentrated liquid will blend completely with the food. Drink or eat the entire mixture immediately. Do not store for future use.

Your doctor will probably start you on a low dose of alprazolam and gradually increase your dose, not more than once every 3 or 4 days.

Alprazolam can be habit-forming. Do not take a larger dose or take it more often or for a longer time than your doctor tells you to. Do not stop taking alprazolam without talking to your doctor. Suddenly stopping to take alprazolam may worsen your condition and cause withdrawal symptoms (anxiousness, sleeplessness, irritability, and seizures). Withdrawal symptoms may be worse if you take more than 4 mg of alprazolam every day. Your doctor will decrease your dose gradually.

Are there other uses for this medicine?

Alprazolam also is used sometimes to treat depression, fear of open spaces (agoraphobia), and premenstrual syndrome.

Talk to your doctor about the possible risks of using this medication for your condition.

This medication may be prescribed for other uses; ask your doctor or pharmacist for more information.

What special precautions should I follow?

Before taking alprazolam,

- tell your doctor and pharmacist if you are allergic to alprazolam, chlordiazepoxide (Librium, Librax), clonazepam (Klonopin), clorazepate (Tranxene), diazepam (Valium), estazolam (ProSom), flurazepam (Dalmane), halazepam (Paxipam), lorazepam (Ativan), oxazepam (Serax), prazepam (Centrax), quazepam (Doral), temazepam (Restoril), triazolam (Halcion), or any other medications.
- do not take alprazolam if you are taking itraconazole (Sporanox) or ketoconazole (Nizoral).
- tell your doctor and pharmacist what other prescription and nonprescription medications, vitamins, nutritional supplements, and herbal products you are taking. Be sure to mention any of the following: amiodarone (Cordarone, Pacerone); antidepressants ('mood elevators') such as desipramine (Norpramin), imipramine (Tofranil), and nefazodone (Serzone); antifungals such as fluconazole (Diflucan); antihistamines; cimetidine (Tagamet); clarithromycin (Biaxin); cyclosporine (Neoral, Sandimmune); diltiazem (Cardizem, Dilacor, Tiazac); ergotamine (Cafatine, Cafergot, Wigraine, others); erythromycin (E.E.S., E-Mycin, Erythrocin); isoniazid (INH, Nydrazid); medications for mental illness and seizures; nicardipine (Cardene); nifedipine (Adalat, Procardia); oral contraceptives (birth control pills); propoxyphene (Darvon); selective serotonin reuptake inhibitors (SSRIs) such as fluoxetine (Prozac, Sarafem), fluvoxamine (Luvox), paroxetine (Paxil), and sertraline (Zoloft); sedatives; sleeping pills; and tranquilizers. Your doctor may need to change the doses of your medications or monitor you carefully for side effects.
- tell your doctor if you have or have ever had glaucoma; depression; or lung, kidney, or liver disease.
- tell your doctor if you are pregnant, plan to become pregnant, or are breast-feeding. If you become pregnant while taking alprazolam, call your doctor immediately.
- if you are having surgery, including dental surgery, tell the doctor or dentist that you are taking alprazolam.
- you should know that alprazolam may make you drowsy. Do not drive a car or operate machinery until you know how this medication affects you.
- remember that alcohol can add to the drowsiness caused by this medication.

What special dietary instructions should I follow?

Talk to your doctor about drinking grapefruit juice while taking this medicine.

What should I do if I forget to take a dose?

Take the missed dose as soon as you remember it. However, if it is almost time for the next dose, skip the missed dose and continue your regular dosing schedule. Do not take a double dose to make up for a missed one.

What side effects can this medicine cause?

Alprazolam may cause side effects. Tell your doctor if any of these symptoms are severe or do not go away:

- drowsiness
- light-headedness
- tiredness
- dizziness
- irritability
- talkativeness
- dry mouth
- increased salivation
- changes in sex drive or ability
- changes in appetite
- weight changes
- difficulty urinating

Some side effects can be serious. The following symptoms are uncommon, but if you experience any of them, call your doctor immediately:

- seizures
- seeing things or hearing voices that do not exist (hallucinating)
- severe skin rash
- yellowing of the skin or eyes
- memory problems
- confusion
- problems with coordination

Alprazolam may cause other side effects. Call your doctor if you have any unusual problems while taking this medication.

If you experience a serious side effect, you or your doctor may send a report to the Food and Drug Administration's (FDA) MedWatch Adverse Event Reporting program online [at http://www.fda.gov/MedWatch/index.html] or by phone [1-800-332-1088].

What storage conditions are needed for this medicine?

Keep this medication in the container it came in, tightly closed, and out of reach of children. Store it at room temperature and away from excess heat and moisture (not in the bathroom). Throw away any medication that is outdated or no longer needed. Talk to your pharmacist about the proper disposal of your medication.

What should I do in case of overdose?

In case of overdose, call your local poison control center at 1-800-222-1222. If the victim has collapsed or is not breathing, call local emergency services at 911.

Symptoms of overdose may include:
- drowsiness
- confusion
- problems with coordination
- coma

What other information should I know?

Keep all appointments with your doctor.

Do not let anyone else take your medication. Ask your pharmacist any questions you have about refilling your prescription.

Dosage Facts

For Informational Purposes

Caution: Do not change your dose, how often you take your medication, or the length of time you are to take it without first talking to your healthcare provider.

The following dosage information was written using medical language for doctors and other healthcare professionals and is provided here for you to check your dosage. The dosage of this drug may differ for different patients. Therefore, always follow your doctor's instructions or the directions on the label. Contact your healthcare provider or pharmacist if you have any questions about the specific dosage of your medication after reviewing this information.

Adult Patients

Anxiety Disorders
Therapy with Conventional or Orally Disintegrating Tablets or Oral Concentrate

ORAL:
- Initially, 0.25–0.5 mg 3 times daily. Increase dosage gradually at intervals of 3 or 4 days according to individual requirements and response; maximum dosage of 4 mg daily given in divided doses.

Panic Disorder
Therapy with Conventional or Orally Disintegrating Tablets

ORAL:
- Dosages >4 mg daily have been required; dosage generally has averaged 5–6 mg daily but has ranged from 1–10 mg daily.
- Initiate at low dosage; increase dosage gradually until an acceptable therapeutic response is achieved, intolerable adverse effects occur, or a maximum dosage of 10 mg daily is achieved.
- Initially, 0.5 mg 3 times daily. Increase dosage as necessary at 3- or 4-day intervals in increments of ≤1 mg daily; slower titration to dosages ≥4 mg daily may be advisable so that full effects of a given dosage can be expressed.
- Periodic reassessment and consideration of dosage reduction recommended in patients receiving dosages >4 mg daily.
- To minimize risk of symptom emergence between doses, distribute doses evenly 3–4 times daily (while awake).

Therapy with Extended-release Tablets

ORAL:
- Dosage of 3–6 mg daily recommended, but dosage has ranged from 1–10 mg daily.
- Initiate at low dosage; increase dosage gradually until an acceptable therapeutic response is achieved, intolerable adverse effects occur, or a maximum dosage of 10 mg daily is achieved.
- Initially, 0.5–1 mg daily. Increase dosage as necessary (based on response) at 3- or 4-day intervals in increments of ≤1 mg daily; slower titration may be advisable so that full effects of a given dosage can be expressed.

Prescribing Limits

Adult Patients

Anxiety Disorders
ORAL:
- Maximum 4 mg daily.

Panic Disorder
ORAL:
- Maximum 10 mg daily.

Special Populations

Hepatic Impairment
- Prolonged elimination. Use the smallest effective dosage.
- Initially, 0.25 mg (as an immediate-release preparation) given 2 or 3 times daily or 0.5 mg (as extended-release tablets) once daily; adjust dosage according to individual tolerance and response.

Geriatric or Debilitated Patients
- Possible increased sensitivity to benzodiazepines. Use the smallest effective dosage.
- Initially, 0.25 mg (as an immediate-release preparation) given 2 or 3 times daily or 0.5 mg (as extended-release tablets) once daily; adjust dosage according to individual tolerance and response.

Alprostadil

(al pros' ta dil)

Brand Name: Caverject®, Caverject® Impulse®, Edex®, Muse®

Why is this medicine prescribed?

Alprostadil is used to produce a sexually functional erection in males with impotence (erectile dysfunction).

How should this medicine be used?

Alprostadil comes as a shot to inject into the penis. You must be trained by your doctor before using alprostadil at home. Use alprostadil before sex. It produces an erect penis within 5-20 minutes of injection (into the side of the upper third of the penis, as directed by your doctor). Generally, alprostadil should not be used more than three times a week or more than once every 24 hours. Follow the directions on your prescription label carefully, and ask your doctor or pharmacist to explain any part you do not understand. Use alprostadil exactly as directed. Do not use more or less of it or use it more often than prescribed by your doctor.

Your doctor will administer the first dose in his or her office to determine the appropriate dose you should receive.

Carefully read the patient directions that come with alprostadil vials. If you have questions about the volume of alprostadil to inject, ask your doctor or pharmacist.

Each needle, syringe with fluid, and vial with powder can be used only once.

The effects of alprostadil should last no longer than 1 hour. Call your doctor immediately if your erection lasts longer than 4 hours. Erections lasting more than 6 hours may result in permanent damage. If you use too much alprostadil by mistake, call your doctor immediately. Remember to wash your hands completely before using alprostadil and to clean the area of the penis that will be injected before the needle is inserted.

What special precautions should I follow?

Before using alprostadil,
- tell your doctor and pharmacist if you are allergic to alprostadil or any other drugs.
- tell your doctor and pharmacist what prescription and nonprescription medications you are taking, especially anticoagulants ('blood thinners') such as warfarin (Coumadin), and vitamins.
- tell your doctor if you have or have ever had anemia, bleeding disorders, sickle cell disease, leukemia, cancer, or kidney or liver disease. Alprostadil should not be used in patients with penile implants.

What side effects can this medicine cause?

Alprostadil may cause side effects. If you experience any of the following symptoms, call your doctor immediately:
- erection lasting more than 4 hours
- redness, swelling, tenderness, or unusual curving of the erect penis
- nodules or hard areas on the penis
- pain on injection
- bleeding

If you experience a serious side effect, you or your doctor may send a report to the Food and Drug Administration's (FDA) MedWatch Adverse Event Reporting program online [at http://www.fda.gov/MedWatch/index.html] or by phone [1-800-332-1088].

What storage conditions are needed for this medicine?

Keep this medication in the container it came in, tightly closed, and out of reach of children. Store it at room temperature and away from excess heat and moisture (not in the bathroom). Throw away any medication that is outdated or no longer needed. Talk to your pharmacist about the proper disposal of your medication.

What other information should I know?

Keep all appointments with your doctor.

Use precautions (such as condoms) to reduce the risk of spreading sexually transmitted diseases and human immunodeficiency virus (HIV) infection.

Do not let anyone else use your medication. Ask your pharmacist any questions you have about refilling your prescription.

Talk to your doctor, pharmacist, or other healthcare professional if you have questions about dosing information for your medication.

Aluminum Hydroxide
(a loo′ mi num) (hye drox′ ide)

Brand Name: AlternaGEL®, Alu-Cap®, Alu-Tab®, Amphojel®

Why is this medicine prescribed?

Aluminum hydroxide is used for the relief of heartburn, sour stomach, and peptic ulcer pain and to promote the healing of peptic ulcers.

This medication is sometimes prescribed for other uses; ask your doctor or pharmacist for more information.

How should this medicine be used?

Aluminum hydroxide comes as a capsule, a tablet, and an oral liquid and suspension. The dose and frequency of use depend on the condition being treated. The suspension needs to be shaken well before administration. Follow the directions on the package or prescription label carefully, and ask your doctor or pharmacist to explain any part you do not understand.

Are there other uses for this medicine?

Aluminum hydroxide is also used sometimes to decrease the amount of phosphate in the blood of patients with kidney disease. Talk to your doctor about the possible risks of using this drug for your condition.

What special precautions should I follow?

Before taking aluminum hydroxide,
- tell your doctor and pharmacist if you are allergic to aluminum hydroxide or any other drugs.
- tell your doctor and pharmacist what prescription and nonprescription medications you are taking, especially allopurinol (Lopurin, Zyloprim), alprazolam (Xanax), chlordiazepoxide (Librium, Mitran, and others), chloroquine (Aralen), cimetidine (Tagamet), clonazepam (Klonopin),

clorazepate, dexamethasone (Decadron and others), diazepam (Valium, Valrelease, and Zetran), diflunisal (Dolobid), digoxin (Lanoxin), ethambutol (Myambutol), famotidine (Pepcid), halazepam (Paxipam), hydrocortisone (Cortone, Hydrocortone), isoniazid (Laniazid, Nydrazid), levothyroxine (Levothroid, Levoxyl, Synthroid, and others), lorazepam (Ativan), methylprednisolone (Medrol), oxazepam (Serax), penicillamine (Cuprimine, Depen), prednisone (Deltasone, Orasone), products containing iron, tetracycline (Sumycin, Tetracap, and others), ticlopidine (Ticlid), and vitamins.

- be aware that aluminum hydroxide may interfere with other medicines, making them less effective. Take your other medications 1 hour before or 2 hours after aluminum hydroxide.
- tell your doctor if you have or have ever had hypertension, heart or kidney disease, or gastrointestinal bleeding.
- tell your doctor if you are pregnant, plan to become pregnant, or are breast-feeding. If you become pregnant while taking aluminum hydroxide, call your doctor.

What should I do if I forget to take a dose?

Take the missed dose as soon as you remember it. However, if it is almost time for the next dose, skip the missed dose and continue your regular dosing schedule. Do not take a double dose to make up for a missed one.

What side effects can this medicine cause?

Aluminum hydroxide may cause side effects. Tell your doctor if these symptoms are severe or do not go away:
- constipation
- loss of appetite

If you experience any of the following symptoms, call your doctor immediately:
- confusion
- unusual tiredness or discomfort
- muscle weakness

If you experience a serious side effect, you or your doctor may send a report to the Food and Drug Administration's (FDA) MedWatch Adverse Event Reporting program online [at http://www.fda.gov/MedWatch/index.html] or by phone [1-800-332-1088].

What storage conditions are needed for this medicine?

Keep this medication in the container it came in, tightly closed, and out of reach of children. Store it at room temperature and away from excess heat and moisture (not in the bathroom). Throw away any medication that is outdated or no longer needed. Talk to your pharmacist about the proper disposal of your medication.

What other information should I know?

Do not use aluminum hydroxide for more than 2 weeks unless your doctor tells you to do so.

Do not let anyone else take your medication. Ask your pharmacist any questions you have about refilling your prescription.

Talk to your doctor, pharmacist, or other healthcare professional if you have questions about dosing information for your medication.

Aluminum Hydroxide and Magnesium Hydroxide

(a loo′ mi num hye drox′ ide) (mag nee′ zhum hye drox′ ide)

Brand Name: Alamag®, Maalox®, Mag-Al®, Mylanta®, Rulox®

Why is this medicine prescribed?

Aluminum hydroxide and magnesium hydroxide are antacids used together to relieve heartburn, acid indigestion, and stomach upset. They may be used to treat these symptoms in patients with peptic ulcer, gastritis, esophagitis, hiatal hernia, or too much acid in the stomach (gastric hyperacidity). They combine with stomach acid and neutralize it. Aluminum hydroxide and magnesium hydroxide are available without a prescription.

This medication is sometimes prescribed for other uses; ask your doctor or pharmacist for more information.

How should this medicine be used?

This medication comes as a chewable tablet and liquid to take by mouth. Chew tablets thoroughly; do not swallow them whole. Drink a full glass of water after taking the tablets. Shake the oral liquid well before each use to mix the medicine evenly. The liquid may be mixed with water or milk.

Follow the directions on the package label or on your prescription label carefully, and ask your doctor or pharmacist to explain any part you do not understand. Take aluminum hydroxide and magnesium hydroxide antacids exactly as directed. Do not take more or less of it or take it more often than prescribed by your doctor. Do not take antacids for more than 1-2 weeks unless prescribed by your doctor.

What special precautions should I follow?

Before taking aluminum hydroxide and magnesium hydroxide antacids,
- tell your doctor and pharmacist if you are allergic to aluminum hydroxide and magnesium hydroxide antacids or any other drugs.
- tell your doctor and pharmacist what prescription and nonprescription medications you are taking, especially

aspirin, cinoxacin (Cinobac), ciprofloxacin (Cipro), digoxin (Lanoxin), diazepam (Valium), enoxacin (Penetrex), ferrous sulfate (iron), fluconazole (Diflucan), indomethacin, isoniazid (INH), itraconazole (Sporanox), ketoconazole (Nizoral), levofloxacin (Levaquin), lomefloxacin (Maxaquin), nalidixic acid (NegGram), norfloxacin (Noroxin), ofloxacin (Floxin), sparfloxacin (Zagam), tetracycline (Achromycin, Sumycin), and vitamins. If your doctor tells you to take antacids while taking these medications, do not take them within 2 hours of taking an antacid.

- tell your doctor if you have or have ever had kidney disease.
- tell your doctor if you are pregnant, plan to become pregnant, or are breast-feeding. If you become pregnant while taking aluminum hydroxide and magnesium hydroxide antacids, call your doctor.

What special dietary instructions should I follow?

If you are taking this medication for an ulcer, follow the diet prescribed by your doctor carefully.

What should I do if I forget to take a dose?

If you are taking scheduled doses of aluminum hydroxide and magnesium hydroxide, take the missed dose as soon as you remember it. However, if it is almost time for the next dose, skip the missed dose and continue your regular dosing schedule. Do not take a double dose to make up for a missed one.

What side effects can this medicine cause?

Side effects from aluminum hydroxide and magnesium hydroxide are not common. To avoid the chalky taste, take with water or milk. Tell your doctor if any of these symptoms are severe or do not go away:

- diarrhea
- constipation
- loss of appetite
- unusual tiredness
- muscle weakness

What storage conditions are needed for this medicine?

Keep this medication in the container it came in, tightly closed, and out of reach of children. Store it at room temperature and away from excess heat and moisture (not in the bathroom). Throw away any medication that is outdated or no longer needed. Talk to your pharmacist about the proper disposal of your medication.

What other information should I know?

If you are taking this medication under a doctor's care, keep all appointments with your doctor.

Do not let anyone else take your medication.

Talk to your doctor, pharmacist, or other healthcare professional if you have questions about dosing information for your medication.

Amantadine

(a man' ta deen)

Brand Name: Symmetrel®, Symmetrel® Syrup
Also available generically.

Why is this medicine prescribed?

Amantadine is used to treat Parkinson's disease and conditions similar to those of Parkinson's disease. It also is used to prevent and treat respiratory infections caused by influenza A virus.

This medication is sometimes prescribed for other uses; ask your doctor or pharmacist for more information.

How should this medicine be used?

Amantadine comes as a capsule and liquid to take by mouth. It is usually taken once or twice a day. Follow the directions on your prescription label carefully, and ask your doctor or pharmacist to explain any part you do not understand. Take amantadine exactly as directed. Do not take more or less of it or take it more often than prescribed by your doctor. Do not stop taking amantadine without talking to your doctor.

If this medication causes insomnia (difficulty sleeping), take the last dose several hours before bedtime.

What special precautions should I follow?

Before taking amantadine,

- tell your doctor and pharmacist if you are allergic to amantadine or any other drugs.
- tell your doctor and pharmacist what prescription and nonprescription medications you are taking, especially benztropine (Cogentin), hydrochlorothiazide with triamterene (Maxzide, Dyazide), medication for depression, other medication for Parkinson's disease, medication for spasms of the stomach or intestines, stimulants, trihexyphenidyl (Artane), and vitamins.
- tell your doctor if you have epilepsy or any other type of seizures, or have ever had heart, kidney, or liver disease, heart failure, low blood pressure, recurring skin rash, or mental illness.
- tell your doctor if you are pregnant, plan to become pregnant, or are breast-feeding. If you become pregnant while taking amantadine, call your doctor immediately. Amantadine may cause harm to the fetus.
- this medicine may cause blurred vision; be careful when driving or doing things requiring alertness.

What special dietary instructions should I follow?

Amantadine may cause an upset stomach. Take amantadine with food or milk.

What should I do if I forget to take a dose?

Take the missed dose as soon as you remember it. However, if it is almost time for the next dose, skip the missed dose and continue your regular dosing schedule. Do not take a double dose to make up for a missed one.

What side effects can this medicine cause?

Amantadine may cause side effects. Tell your doctor if any of these symptoms are severe or do not go away:

- blurred vision
- dizziness
- lightheadedness
- faintness
- trouble sleeping

If you experience any of the following side effects, call your doctor immediately:

- depression or anxiety
- swelling of the hands, legs, or feet
- difficulty urinating
- shortness of breath
- rash

If you experience a serious side effect, you or your doctor may send a report to the Food and Drug Administration's (FDA) MedWatch Adverse Event Reporting program online [at http://www.fda.gov/MedWatch/index.html] or by phone [1-800-332-1088].

What storage conditions are needed for this medicine?

Keep this medication in the container it came in, tightly closed, and out of reach of children. Store it at room temperature and away from excess heat and moisture (not in the bathroom). Do not freeze. Throw away any medication that is outdated or no longer needed. Talk to your pharmacist about the proper disposal of your medication.

What should I do in case of overdose?

In case of overdose, call your local poison control center at 1-800-222-1222. If the victim has collapsed or is not breathing, call local emergency services at 911.

What other information should I know?

Keep all appointments with your doctor and the laboratory. Your doctor may order certain lab tests to check your response to amantadine.

Do not let anyone else take your medication. Ask your pharmacist any questions you have about refilling your prescription. If you still have symptoms of infection after you finish the amantadine, call your doctor.

Dosage Facts
For Informational Purposes

Caution: Do not change your dose, how often you take your medication, or the length of time you are to take it without first talking to your healthcare provider.

The following dosage information was written using medical language for doctors and other healthcare professionals and is provided here for you to check your dosage. The dosage of this drug may differ for different patients. Therefore, always follow your doctor's instructions or the directions on the label. Contact your healthcare provider or pharmacist if you have any questions about the specific dosage of your medication after reviewing this information.

General Dosage Information

Available as amantadine hydrochloride; dosage expressed in terms of amantadine hydrochloride.

Usual dosage may need to be reduced in patients with congestive heart failure, peripheral edema, orthostatic hypotension, or impaired renal function.

Pediatric Patients

Treatment of Influenza A Virus Infections

ORAL:

- Children 1–9 years of age: 4.4–8.8 mg/kg (maximum 150 mg) daily recommended by manufacturer. AAP recommends 5 mg/kg (maximum 150 mg) daily in 2 divided doses.
- Children 9–12 years of age: 100 mg twice daily recommended by manufacturer.
- Children ≥10 years of age: AAP recommends 5 mg/kg daily in 2 divided doses in those weighing <40 kg or 200 mg daily in 2 divided doses in those weighing ≥40 kg.
- Children ≥12 years of age: 200 mg once daily or 100 mg twice daily recommended by manufacturer.
- Initiate amantadine treatment as soon as possible, preferably within 24–48 hours after onset of symptoms, and continue for up to 5 days or 24–48 hours after symptoms disappear.

Prevention of Influenza A Virus Infections

ORAL:

- Children 1–9 years of age: 4.4–8.8 mg/kg (maximum 150 mg) daily recommended by manufacturer. AAP recommends 5 mg/kg (maximum 150 mg) daily in 2 divided doses.
- Children 9–12 years of age: 100 mg twice daily recommended by manufacturer.
- Children ≥10 years of age: AAP recommends 5 mg/kg daily in 2 divided doses in those weighing <40 kg or 200 mg daily in 2 divided doses in those weighing ≥40 kg.
- Children ≥12 years of age: 200 mg once daily or 100 mg twice daily recommended by manufacturer.
- Alternatively, AAP states children weighing >20 kg can receive 100 mg daily.
- For prophylaxis of influenza A when influenza virus vaccine is contraindicated or unavailable or when a poor antibody

response to the vaccine is expected (e.g., severe immunodeficiency, HIV infection), amantadine can be started in anticipation of an influenza A outbreak and before or after contact with individuals with influenza A virus infection. Usually continue for ≥10 days following known exposure. Can be given for the duration of an influenza A outbreak in the community, which may be as long as 6–12 weeks.

- For prophylaxis in conjunction with influenza virus vaccine, amantadine should be administered for 2–4 weeks after vaccine administration. Children <9 years of age receiving influenza virus vaccine for the first time may require amantadine prophylaxis for up to 6 weeks following vaccination or until 2 weeks after the second dose of vaccine.

Adult Patients

Treatment of Influenza A Virus Infections

ORAL:
- 200 mg once daily or 100 mg twice daily.
- Dosage may be decreased to 100 mg daily in those who experience CNS or other toxicities with 200 mg daily; relative efficacy of lower dosage not elucidated.
- Initiate amantadine treatment as soon as possible, preferably within 24–48 hours after onset of symptoms, and continue for up to 5 days or 24–48 hours after symptoms disappear.

Prevention of Influenza A Virus Infections

ORAL:
- 200 mg once daily or 100 mg twice daily.
- Dosage may be decreased to 100 mg daily in those who experience CNS or other toxicities with 200 mg daily; relative efficacy of lower dosage not elucidated.
- For prophylaxis of influenza A when influenza virus vaccine is contraindicated or unavailable or when a poor antibody response to the vaccine is expected (e.g., severe immunodeficiency, HIV infection), amantadine can be started in anticipation of an influenza A outbreak and before or after contact with individuals with influenza A virus infection. Usually continue for ≥10 days following known exposure. Can be given for the duration of an influenza A outbreak in the community, which may be as long as 6–12 weeks.
- For prophylaxis in conjunction with influenza virus vaccine, amantadine should be administered for 2–4 weeks after vaccine administration.

Parkinsonian Syndrome and Drug-induced Extrapyramidal Effects

ORAL:
- 100 mg twice daily.
- Patients with serious illness or receiving other antiparkinsonian drugs: 100 mg once daily for ≥1 week, then increase to 100 mg twice daily if necessary.
- Dosage can be increased to 400 mg daily in divided doses in patients with parkinsonian syndrome.
- Dosage can be increased to 300 mg daily in divided doses in patients with drug-induced extrapyramidal reactions.

Prescribing Limits
Pediatric Patients
Treatment or Prevention of Influenza A Virus Infections

ORAL:
- Children 1–9 years of age: Maximum 150 mg daily.

Special Populations
Renal Impairment

Dosage in Adults with Renal Impairment

Cl$_{cr}$ (mL/minute)	Dosage
30–50	200 mg on first day, then 100 mg daily
15–29	200 mg on first day, then 100 mg every other day
<15	200 mg every 7 days
Hemodialysis patients	200 mg every 7 days

Geriatric Patients
- 100 mg daily for treatment or prophylaxis of influenza A virus infection in those ≥65 years of age. Dosage may need to be further reduced in some patients.

Amifostine Injection
(am i fos′ teen)

Brand Name: Ethyol®

About Your Treatment

Your doctor has ordered the drug amifostine to help treat your illness. The drug is given by injection into a vein.
This medication is used to:
- protect the kidneys against the harmful effects of the cancer-fighting drug cisplatin in patients with ovarian cancer or lung cancer
- reduce the severe dry mouth caused by radiation treatment after surgery for head and neck cancer

Amifostine is in a class of drugs known as chemoprotectants; it protects against the harmful effects of cisplatin and radiation treatment. The length of treatment depends on the types of drugs you are taking, how well your body responds to them, and the type of cancer you have.

This medication may be prescribed for other uses; ask your doctor or pharmacist for more information.

Precautions

Before taking amifostine,
- tell your doctor and pharmacist if you are allergic to amifostine or any other drugs.

- tell your doctor and pharmacist what prescription and nonprescription medications, vitamins, nutritional supplements, and herbal products you are taking. Be sure to mention medications for high blood pressure. Your doctor may need to change the doses of your medications or monitor you carefully for side effects.
- tell your doctor if you have or have ever had kidney disease, chest pain (angina), irregular heartbeats, heart failure, a stroke, or a mini-stroke.
- women who are pregnant or breast-feeding should tell their doctors before they begin taking this drug. You should not plan to have children while receiving chemotherapy or for a while after treatments. (Talk to your doctor for further details.) Use a reliable method of birth control to prevent pregnancy.
- you should know that the most common side effect of amifostine is a decrease in blood pressure, which may start while the drug is being given and lasts about 6 minutes. You will be told to lie on your back and your blood pressure will be checked regularly during your treatment. Your doctor may order fluids to be given by injection into a vein to help improve your blood pressure.

Side Effects

Amifostine may cause side effects. Tell your doctor if any of these symptoms are severe or do not go away:
- nausea
- vomiting
- flushing (feeling of warmth)
- chills (feeling of coldness)
- fever
- dizziness or lightheadedness
- drowsiness
- sneezing
- hiccups

Some side effects can be serious. The following symptoms are uncommon, but if you experience any of them, call your doctor immediately:
- shortness of breath
- fainting
- seizures
- chest tightness
- skin rash
- hives
- swelling of the throat

Amifostine may cause other side effects. Call your doctor if you have any unusual problems while taking this drug.

If you experience a serious side effect, you or your doctor may send a report to the Food and Drug Administration's (FDA) MedWatch Adverse Event Reporting program online [at http://www.fda.gov/MedWatch/index.html] or by phone [1-800-332-1088].

Overdose

In case of overdose, call your local poison control center at 1-800-222-1222. If the victim has collapsed or is not breathing, call local emergency services at 911.

Symptoms of overdose may include:
- dizziness
- lightheadedness
- fainting

Special Instructions

- You will probably be given anti-nausea medication before and during amifostine administration.
- Keep all appointments with your doctor and the laboratory. Your doctor may order certain lab tests to check your body's response to amifostine.

Dosage Facts
For Informational Purposes

Caution: Do not change your dose, how often you take your medication, or the length of time you are to take it without first talking to your healthcare provider.

The following dosage information was written using medical language for doctors and other healthcare professionals and is provided here for you to check your dosage. The dosage of this drug may differ for different patients. Therefore, always follow your doctor's instructions or the directions on the label. Contact your healthcare provider or pharmacist if you have any questions about the specific dosage of your medication after reviewing this information.

General Dosage Information

Available as the trihydrate form of amifostine; dosage expressed in terms of amifostine.

Adult Patients

Prophylaxis of Cisplatin-induced Nephrotoxicity

IV:
- Initially, 910 mg/m^2 once daily over 15 minutes, starting 30 minutes prior to cisplatin administration.
- If full initial dose is tolerated, repeat the full dose during subsequent courses of chemotherapy as tolerated.
- If the full dose cannot be administered, reduce dosage to 740 mg/m^2 during subsequent chemotherapy cycles.

Prophylaxis of Radiation Therapy-induced Xerostomia

IV:
- 200 mg/m^2 once daily over 3 minutes; initiate infusion 15–30 minutes prior to standard fractionated radiation therapy (1.8–2 Gy).

Special Populations

Hepatic Impairment
- No specific dosage recommendations at this time.

Renal Impairment
- No specific dosage recommendations at this time.

Geriatric Patients
- Careful dosage selection recommended due to possible age-related decreases in hepatic, renal, or cardiac function and concomitant diseases or drug therapies.

Amikacin Sulfate Injection

(am i kay′ sin)

Brand Name: Amikin®
Also available generically.

Important Warning

Amikacin can cause severe hearing and kidney problems. Before administering amikacin, tell your doctor and pharmacist what prescription and nonprescription medications you are taking, especially diuretics ('water pills'), cisplatin (Platinol), amphotericin (Amphotec, Fungizone), other antibiotics, and vitamins.

If you experience any of the following symptoms, call your health care provider immediately: dizziness, vertigo, ringing in the ears, hearing loss, numbness, muscle twitching or weakness, difficulty breathing, decreased urination, rash, itching, or sore throat.

About Your Treatment

Your doctor has ordered amikacin, an antibiotic, to help treat your infection. The drug will be either injected into a large muscle (such as your buttock or hip) or added to intravenous fluid that will drip through a needle or catheter placed in your vein for at least 30 minutes, one to three times a day.

Amikacin eliminates bacteria that cause many kinds of infections, including lung, skin, bone, joint, stomach, blood, and urinary tract infections. This medication is sometimes prescribed for other uses; ask your doctor or pharmacist for more information.

Your health care provider (doctor, nurse, or pharmacist) may measure the effectiveness and side effects of your treatment using laboratory tests and physical examinations. It is important to keep all appointments with your doctor and the laboratory. The length of treatment depends on how your infection and symptoms respond to the medication.

Precautions

Before administering amikacin,
- tell your doctor and pharmacist if you are allergic to amikacin, gentamicin (Garamycin), kanamycin (Kantrex), neomycin, netilmicin (Netromycin), streptomycin, tobramycin (Nebcin), or any other drugs.
- tell your doctor and pharmacist what prescription and nonprescription medications you are taking, especially diuretics ('water pills'), cisplatin (Platinol), amphotericin (Amphotec, Fungizone), other antibiotics, and vitamins.
- tell your doctor if you have or have ever had kidney disease, vertigo, hearing loss, ringing in the ears, myasthenia gravis, or Parkinson's disease.
- tell your doctor if you are pregnant, plan to become pregnant, or are breast-feeding. If you become pregnant while taking amikacin, call your doctor immediately. Amikacin can harm the fetus.

Administering Your Medication

Before you administer amikacin, look at the solution closely. It should be clear and free of floating material. Gently squeeze the bag or observe the solution container to make sure there are no leaks. Do not use the solution if it is discolored, if it contains particles, or if the bag or container leaks. Use a new solution, but show the damaged one to your health care provider.

It is important that you use your medication exactly as directed. Do not stop your therapy on your own for any reason because your infection could worsen and result in hospitalization. Do not change your dosing schedule without talking to your health care provider. Your health care provider may tell you to stop your infusion if you have a mechanical problem (such as a blockage in the tubing, needle, or catheter); if you have to stop an infusion, call your health care provider immediately so your therapy can continue.

Side Effects

Amikacin occasionally causes side effects. To reduce this risk, your health care provider may adjust your dose based on your blood test results. Follow the directions in the IMPORTANT WARNING section for symptoms listed there and tell your health care provider if any of the following symptoms are severe or do not go away:
- upset stomach
- vomiting
- fatigue
- pale skin

Storage Conditions

- Your health care provider probably will give you a several-day supply of amikacin at a time. If you are receiving amikacin intravenously (in your vein), you probably will be told to store it in the refrigerator or freezer.
- Take your next dose from the refrigerator 1 hour before using it; place it in a clean, dry area to allow it to warm to room temperature.
- If you are told to store additional amikacin in the freezer, always move a 24-hour supply to the refrigerator for the next day's use.
- Do not refreeze medications.

If you are receiving amikacin intramuscularly (in your muscle), your health care provider will tell you how to store it properly.

Store your medication only as directed. Make sure you understand what you need to store your medication properly.

Keep your supplies in a clean, dry place when you are not using them, and keep all medications and supplies out of reach of children. Your health care provider will tell you how to throw away used needles, syringes, tubing, and containers to avoid accidental injury.

Signs of Infection

If you are receiving amikacin in your vein or under your skin, you need to know the symptoms of a catheter-related infection (an infection where the needle enters your vein or skin). If you experience any of these effects near your intravenous catheter, tell your health care provider as soon as possible:

- tenderness
- warmth
- irritation
- drainage
- redness
- swelling
- pain

Dosage Facts
For Informational Purposes

Caution: Do not change your dose, how often you take your medication, or the length of time you are to take it without first talking to your healthcare provider.

The following dosage information was written using medical language for doctors and other healthcare professionals and is provided here for you to check your dosage. The dosage of this drug may differ for different patients. Therefore, always follow your doctor's instructions or the directions on the label. Contact your healthcare provider or pharmacist if you have any questions about the specific dosage of your medication after reviewing this information.

General Dosage Information

Available as amikacin sulfate; dosage expressed in terms of amikacin.

Dosage is identical for either IV or IM administration.

Dosage should be based on patient's pretreatment body weight and renal status.

Many clinicians recommend that dosage be determined using appropriate pharmacokinetic methods for calculating dosage requirements and patient-specific pharmacokinetic parameters (e.g., elimination rate constant, volume of distribution) derived from serum concentration-time data; in determining dosage, the susceptibility of the causative organism, the severity of infection, and the patient's immune and clinical status also must be considered.

Peak and trough serum amikacin concentrations should be determined periodically and dosage adjusted to maintain desired serum concentrations whenever possible, especially in patients with life-threatening infections, suspected toxicity or nonresponse to treatment, decreased or varying renal function, and/or when increased aminoglycoside clearance (e.g., patients with cystic fibrosis, burns) or prolonged therapy is likely.

Many clinicians recommend that dosage be adjusted to maintain peak and trough serum concentrations of 15–40 and <5–10 mcg/mL, respectively. The manufacturers state that peak serum concentrations (obtained 30–90 minutes after administration) of >35 mcg/mL and trough serum concentrations (obtained just before the next dose) of >10 mcg/mL should be avoided.

Once-daily administration† of aminoglycosides is at least as effective as, and may be less toxic than, conventional dosage regimens employing multiple daily doses.

Usual duration of treatment is 7–10 days. Safety of aminoglycoside treatment for >14 days *not* established. If clinical response does not occur within 3–5 days, in vitro susceptibility should be reassessed. In difficult and complicated infections, use of amikacin should be re-evaluated if treatment >10 days is being considered. If the drug is continued, serum amikacin concentrations and renal, auditory, and vestibular functions should be monitored closely.

Pediatric Patients

General Dosage for Neonates

IV OR IM:
- Manufacturer recommends an initial loading dose of 10 mg/kg followed by 7.5 mg/kg every 12 hours.
- Neonates <1 week of age: AAP recommends 7.5 mg/kg every 18–24 hours for those weighing <1.2 kg, 7.5 mg/kg every 12 hours for those weighing 1.2–2 kg, and 7.5–10 mg/kg every 12 hours in those weighing >2 kg.
- Neonates 1–4 weeks of age: AAP recommends 7.5 mg/kg every 18–24 hours for those weighing <1.2 kg, 7.5–10 mg/kg every 8 or 12 hours for those weighing 1.2–2 kg, and 10 mg/kg every 8 hours for those weighing >2 kg.

General Dosage for Infants and Children

IV OR IM:
- Older infants and children: manufacturer recommends 15 mg/kg daily given in equally divided doses at 8- or 12-hour intervals.
- Children ≥1 month of age: AAP recommends 15–22 mg/kg given in 3 divided doses.

Mycobacterial Infections
Active Tuberculosis

IV OR IM:
- Children <15 years of age: 15–30 mg/kg (up to 1 g) once daily or twice weekly.
- Children ≥15 years of age: 15 mg/kg daily (up to 1 g) as a single daily dose (usually 750–1000 mg daily) 5–7 times weekly for the first 2–4 months or until culture conversion; dosage can then be reduced to 15 mg/kg daily (up to 1 g) given 2 or 3 times weekly, depending on efficacy of the other drugs in the regimen.
- Must be used in conjunction with other antituberculosis agents. Multiple-drug regimen usually given for 12–18 months when rifampin-resistant *M. tuberculosis* are involved; for 18–24 months when isoniazid- and rifampin-resistant

strains are involved; or for 24 months when the strain is resistant to isoniazid, rifampin, ethambutol, and/or pyrazinamide.

Adult Patients

General Adult Dosage

IV OR IM:
- 15 mg/kg daily given in equally divided doses every 8–12 hours.

Urinary Tract Infections (UTIs)
Uncomplicated Infections

IV OR IM:
- 250 mg twice daily.

Mycobacterial Infections
Active Tuberculosis

IV OR IM:
- 15 mg/kg daily (up to 1 g) as a single daily dose (usually 750–1000 mg daily) 5–7 times weekly for the first 2–4 months or until culture conversion; dosage can then be reduced to 15 mg/kg daily (up to 1 g) given 2 or 3 times weekly, depending on efficacy of the other drugs in the regimen.
- Adults >59 years of age: 10 mg/kg (up to 750 mg) daily.
- Must be used in conjunction with other antituberculosis agents. Multiple-drug regimen usually given for 12–18 months when rifampin-resistant *M. tuberculosis* are involved; for 18–24 months when isoniazid- and rifampin-resistant strains are involved; or for 24 months when the strain is resistant to isoniazid, rifampin, ethambutol, and/or pyrazinamide.

Prescribing Limits

Pediatric Patients

IV OR IM:
- Daily dosage should not exceed 15 mg/kg or 1.5 g.

Adult Patients

IV OR IM:
- Daily dosage should not exceed 15 mg/kg or 1.5 g.

Special Populations

Renal Impairment
- Dosage adjustments necessary in patients with renal impairment.
- One method suggested by manufacturer is an initial loading dose of 7.5 mg/kg followed by 7.5 mg/kg given at intervals (in hours) calculated by multiplying the patient's steady-state serum creatinine (in mg/dL) by 9. The dosing method of Sarubbi and Hull, which is based on corrected creatinine clearance, also has been recommended.
- The above dosage calculation methods should *not* be used in patients undergoing hemodialysis or peritoneal dialysis. In adults with renal failure undergoing hemodialysis, some clinicians recommend supplemental doses of 50–75% of the initial loading dose at the end of each dialysis period. Serum concentrations of the drug should be monitored in dialysis patients and dosage adjusted to maintain desired serum concentrations.

Geriatric Patients
- Select dosage with caution and closely monitor renal function because of age-related decreases in renal function.

- No dosage adjustments except those related to renal impairment.

† Use is not currently included in the labeling approved by the US Food and Drug Administration.

Amiloride and Hydrochlorothiazide

(a mil′ oh ride) (hye droe klor oh thye′ a zide)

Brand Name: Moduretic®

Why is this medicine prescribed?

The combination of amiloride and hydrochlorothiazide, a 'water pill,' is used to treat high blood pressure and fluid retention caused by various conditions, including heart disease. It causes the kidneys to eliminate unneeded water and salt from the body into the urine.

This medicine is sometimes prescribed for other uses; ask your doctor or pharmacist for more information.

How should this medicine be used?

The combination of amiloride and hydrochlorothiazide comes as a tablet to take by mouth. It usually is taken once a day in the morning with food. Follow the directions on your prescription label carefully, and ask your doctor or pharmacist to explain any part you do not understand. Take amiloride and hydrochlorothiazide exactly as directed. Do not take more or less of it or take it more often than prescribed by your doctor.

This medication controls high blood pressure but does not cure it. Continue to take amiloride and hydrochlorothiazide even if you feel well. Do not stop taking amiloride and hydrochlorothiazide without talking to your doctor.

What special precautions should I follow?

Before taking amiloride and hydrochlorothiazide,
- tell your doctor and pharmacist if you are allergic to amiloride, hydrochlorothiazide, sulfa drugs, or any other drugs.
- tell your doctor and pharmacist what prescription and nonprescription medications you are taking, especially captopril (Capoten); digoxin (Lanoxin); enalapril (Vasotec); indomethacin (Indocin); lisinopril (Prinivil, Zestril); lithium (Eskalith, Lithobid); medications for arthritis, diabetes, or high blood pressure; potassium supplements; and vitamins. Do not take this medicine if you are taking spironolactone or triamterene.
- tell your doctor if you have or have ever had diabetes, gout, or kidney or liver disease.
- tell your doctor if you are pregnant, plan to become

pregnant, or are breast-feeding. If you become pregnant while taking amiloride and hydrochlorothiazide, call your doctor immediately.

- if you are having surgery, including dental surgery, tell the doctor or dentist that you are taking amiloride and hydrochlorothiazide.
- you should know that this drug may make you drowsy. Do not drive a car or operate machinery until you know how this drug affects you.
- remember that alcohol can add to the drowsiness caused by this drug.

What special dietary instructions should I follow?

Follow your doctor's directions for a low-salt or low-sodium diet and daily exercise program. Avoid potassium-containing salt substitutes. Limit your intake of potassium-rich foods (e.g., bananas, prunes, raisins, and orange juice). Ask your doctor for advice on how much of these foods you may have.

What should I do if I forget to take a dose?

Take the missed dose as soon as you remember it. However, if it is almost time for the next dose, skip the missed dose and continue your regular dosing schedule. Do not take a double dose to make up for a missed one.

What side effects can this medicine cause?

Amiloride and hydrochlorothiazide may cause side effects. Tell your doctor if any of these symptoms are severe or do not go away:

- upset stomach
- vomiting
- diarrhea
- loss of appetite
- stomach pain
- gas
- frequent urination
- dizziness
- headache

If you experience any of the following symptoms, call your doctor immediately:

- muscle weakness or cramps
- fatigue
- slow or irregular heartbeat
- sore throat
- unusual bleeding or bruising
- yellowing of the skin or eyes
- skin rash
- difficulty breathing or swallowing

If you experience a serious side effect, you or your doctor may send a report to the Food and Drug Administration's (FDA) MedWatch Adverse Event Reporting program online [at http://www.fda.gov/MedWatch/index.html] or by phone [1-800-332-1088].

What storage conditions are needed for this medicine?

Keep this medicine in the container it came in, tightly closed, and out of reach of children. Store it at room temperature and away from excess heat and moisture (not in the bathroom). Throw away any medicine that is outdated or no longer needed. Talk to your pharmacist about the proper disposal of your medicine.

What should I do in case of overdose?

In case of overdose, call your local poison control center at 1-800-222-1222. If the victim has collapsed or is not breathing, call local emergency services at 911.

What other information should I know?

Keep all appointments with your doctor and the laboratory. Your blood pressure should be checked regularly, and blood tests should be done occasionally.

Do not let anyone else take your medicine. Ask your pharmacist any questions you have about refilling your prescription.

Talk to your doctor, pharmacist, or other healthcare professional if you have questions about dosing information for your medication.

Aminophylline

(am in off″ i lin)

Why is this medicine prescribed?

Aminophylline is used to prevent and treat wheezing, shortness of breath, and difficulty breathing caused by asthma, chronic bronchitis, emphysema, and other lung diseases. It relaxes and opens air passages in the lungs, making it easier to breathe.

This medication is sometimes prescribed for other uses; ask your doctor or pharmacist for more information.

How should this medicine be used?

Aminophylline comes as a tablet and syrup to take by mouth. It usually is taken every 6, 8, or 12 hours. Follow the directions on your prescription label carefully, and ask your doctor or pharmacist to explain any part you do not understand. Take aminophylline exactly as directed. Do not take more or less of it or take it more often than prescribed by your doctor.

Take the tablets or oral liquid with a full glass of water on an empty stomach, at least 1 hour before or 2 hours after a meal. Do not chew or crush the long-acting tablets; swallow them whole.

Aminophylline controls symptoms of asthma and other lung diseases but does not cure them. Continue to take aminophylline even if you feel well. Do not stop taking aminophylline without talking to your doctor.

Are there other uses for this medicine?

Aminophylline is sometimes used to treat breathing problems in premature infants. Talk to your doctor about the possible risks of using this drug for your baby's condition.

What special precautions should I follow?

Before taking aminophylline,

- tell your doctor and pharmacist if you are allergic to aminophylline or any other drugs.
- tell your doctor and pharmacist what prescription medications you are taking, especially allopurinol (Zyloprim), azithromycin (Zithromax) carbamazepine (Tegretol), cimetidine (Tagamet), ciprofloxacin (Cipro), clarithromycin (Biaxin), diuretics ('water pills'), erythromycin, lithium (Eskalith, Lithobid), oral contraceptives, phenytoin (Dilantin), prednisone (Deltasone), propranolol (Inderal), rifampin (Rifadin), tetracycline (Sumycin), and other medications for infections or heart disease.
- tell your doctor and pharmacist what nonprescription medications and vitamins you are taking, especially nonprescription medications containing ephedrine, epinephrine, phenylephrine, phenylpropanolamine, or pseudoephedrine. Many nonprescription products contain these drugs (e.g., diet pills and medications for colds and asthma), so check labels carefully. Do not take these medications without talking to your doctor; they can increase the side effects of aminophylline.
- tell your doctor if you have or have ever had seizures, heart disease, an overactive or underactive thyroid gland, high blood pressure, or liver disease or if you have a history of alcohol abuse.
- tell your doctor if you are pregnant, plan to become pregnant, or are breast-feeding. If you become pregnant while taking aminophylline, call your doctor.
- tell your doctor if you use tobacco products. Cigarette smoking may affect the effectiveness of aminophylline.

What special dietary instructions should I follow?

Drinking or eating foods high in caffeine, like coffee, tea, cocoa, and chocolate, may increase the side effects caused by aminophylline. Avoid large amounts of these substances while you are taking aminophylline.

What should I do if I forget to take a dose?

Take the missed dose as soon as you remember it. However, if it is almost time for the next dose, skip the missed dose and continue your regular dosing schedule. Do not take a double dose to make up for a missed one. If you become severely short of breath, call your doctor.

What side effects can this medicine cause?

Aminophylline may cause side effects. Tell your doctor if any of these symptoms are severe or do not go away.

- upset stomach
- stomach pain
- diarrhea
- headache
- restlessness
- insomnia
- irritability

If you experience any of the following symptoms, call your doctor immediately:

- vomiting
- increased or rapid heart rate
- irregular heartbeat
- seizures
- skin rash

If you experience a serious side effect, you or your doctor may send a report to the Food and Drug Administration's (FDA) MedWatch Adverse Event Reporting program online [at http://www.fda.gov/MedWatch/index.html] or by phone [1-800-332-1088].

What storage conditions are needed for this medicine?

Keep this medication in the container it came in, tightly closed, and out of reach of children. Store it at room temperature and away from excess heat and moisture (not in the bathroom). Throw away any medication that is outdated or no longer needed. Talk to your pharmacist about the proper disposal of your medication.

What should I do in case of overdose?

In case of overdose, call your local poison control center at 1-800-222-1222. If the victim has collapsed or is not breathing, call local emergency services at 911.

What other information should I know?

Keep all appointments with your doctor and the laboratory. Your doctor will order certain lab tests to check your response to aminophylline.

Do not change from one brand of aminophylline to another without talking to your doctor.

Do not let anyone else take your medication. Ask your pharmacist any questions you have about refilling your prescription.

Dosage Facts
For Informational Purposes

Caution: Do not change your dose, how often you take your medication, or the length of time you are to take it without first talking to your health-care provider.

The following dosage information was written using medical language for doctors and other healthcare professionals and is provided here for you to check your dosage. The dosage of this drug may differ for different patients. Therefore, always follow your doctor's instructions or the directions on the label. Contact your healthcare provider or pharmacist if you have any questions about the specific dosage of your medication after reviewing this information.

General Dosage Information

Available as aminophylline anhydrous, aminophylline hydrous, and theophylline monohydrate; dosage expressed in terms of anhydrous theophylline. Also available as dyphylline; dosage expressed in terms of dyphylline.

Anhydrous Theophylline Content in Theophylline Derivatives

Drug	Anhydrous Theophylline Content
Aminophylline anhydrous	85.7% (±1.7%)
Aminophylline hydrous	78.9% (±1.6%)
Theophylline monohydrate	90.7% (±1.1%)

Theophylline has a low therapeutic index; cautious dosage determination is essential.

Individualize dosage carefully according to individual requirements and response, pulmonary function, and serum theophylline concentrations.

Calculate dosage on the basis of ideal body weight. Adjust dosage based on peak serum theophylline concentration.

In general, recommended dosage adjustments (see Adults: Dosage Adjustment, under Dosage and Administration) should not be exceeded in order to decrease the risk of potentially serious adverse effects associated with unexpected large increases in serum theophylline concentration.

Pediatric Patients

Bronchospasm
Dosage Initiation and Titration for Acute and Chronic Bronchospasm

Smaller and more frequently administered doses may be required to prevent breakthrough symptoms in patients who metabolize theophylline rapidly.

ORAL (IMMEDIATE-RELEASE PREPARATIONS):

Recommended Dosage Titration for Children <1 Year of Age

Age	Dosage Titration
Premature neonates <24 days postnatal	Initially, 1 mg/kg every 12 hours Adjust dosage to maintain a peak steady-state serum concentration of 5–10 mcg/mL (see Adults: Dosage Adjustment, under Dosage and Administration)
Premature neonates ≥24 days postnatal	Initially, 1.5 mg/kg every 12 hours Adjust dosage to maintain a peak steady-state serum concentration of 5–10 mcg/mL (see Adults: Dosage Adjustment, under Dosage and Administration)
Full-term infants <26 weeks of age	[(0.2 x age in weeks) + 5] x body weight (kg) = total daily dosage (mg); administer in 3 equally divided doses every 8 hours Adjust dose to maintain a peak steady-state serum concentration of 5–10 mcg/mL in neonates or 10–15 mcg/mL in older infants (see Adults: Dosage Adjustment, under Dosage and Administration)
Infants 26–52 weeks of age	[(0.2 x age in weeks) + 5] x body weight (kg) = total daily dosage (mg); administer in 4 equally divided doses every 6 hours Adjust dosage to maintain a peak steady-state serum concentration of 10–15 mcg/mL (see Adults: Dosage Adjustment, under Dosage and Administration)

Recommended Dosage Titration for Children ≥1 Year of Age

Age	Dosage Titration
Children ≥1 year of age (weighing <45 kg)	Initially, 12–14 mg/kg daily (maximum 300 mg daily); after 3 days, *if tolerated*, increase dosage to 16 mg/kg daily (maximum 400 mg daily); after 3 more days, *if tolerated and needed*, increase dosage to 20 mg/kg daily (maximum 600 mg daily) Administer in divided doses every 4–6 hours
Children ≥1 year of age (weighing >45 kg)	Initially, 300 mg daily; after 3 days, *if tolerated*, increase dosage to 400 mg daily; after 3 more days, *if tolerated and needed*, increase dosage to 600 mg daily Administer in divided doses every 6–8 hours

Children 1–15 years of age with risk factors for reduced theophylline clearance or for whom serum concentrations cannot be monitored	Initially 12–14 mg/kg daily (maximum 300 mg daily); after 3 days, *if tolerated*, increase dosage to maximum 16 mg/kg or 400 mg daily (whichever is less) Administer in divided doses every 4–6 hours
Adolescents >16 years of age with risk factors for reduced theophylline clearance or for whom serum concentrations cannot be monitored	Initially, 300 mg daily; after 3 days, *if tolerated*, increase dosage to maximum 400 mg daily Administer in divided doses every 6–8 hours

Switching to Extended-Release Preparations

ORAL:
- Twelve-hour preparations: Administer one-half the total daily dosage every 12 hours in children ≥6 years of age.
- Uniphyl®: Administer mg-for-mg total daily dosage once daily in appropriately selected children ≥12 years of age.

Chronic Bronchospasm

ORAL (12-HOUR EXTENDED-RELEASE PREPARATIONS):

Dosage Titration for Children ≥6 Years of Age

Age	Daily Dosage[a]
Children 6–15 years of age (weighing <45 kg)	Initially, 12–14 mg/kg daily (maximum 300 mg daily); after 3 days, *if tolerated*, increase dosage to 16 mg/kg daily (maximum 400 mg daily); after 3 more days, *if tolerated and needed*, increase dosage to 20 mg/kg daily (maximum 600 mg daily)
Children 6–15 years of age (weighing >45 kg) and adolescents ≥16 years of age	Initially, 300 mg daily; after 3 days, *if tolerated*, increase dose to 400 mg daily; after 3 more days, *if tolerated and needed*, increase dosage to 600 mg daily
Children 6–15 years of age with risk factors for reduced theophylline clearance or for whom serum concentrations cannot be monitored	Initially, 12–14 mg/kg daily (maximum 300 mg daily); after 3 days, *if tolerated*, increase dosage to maximum 16 mg/kg or 400 mg daily (whichever is less)
Adolescents ≥16 years of age with risk factors for reduced theophylline clearance or for whom serum concentrations cannot be monitored	Initially, 300 mg daily; after 3 days, *if tolerated*, increase dosage to maximum 400 mg daily

[a]Dosage given as total daily dosage; administer in divided doses every 12 hours.

ORAL (THEO-24® CAPSULES AND UNIPHYL® TABLETS):

Recommended Dosage Titration for Children ≥12 Years of Age

Age	Daily Dosage[b]
Children 12–15 years of age (weighing <45 kg) and adolescents ≥16 years of age	Initially, 12–14 mg/kg once daily (maximum 300 mg daily); after 3 days, *if tolerated*, increase dosage to 16 mg/kg once daily (maximum 400 mg daily); after 3 more days, *if tolerated and needed*, increase dosage to 20 mg/kg once daily (maximum 600 mg daily)
Children 12–15 years of age (weighing >45 kg)	Initially, 300–400 mg once daily; after 3 days, *if tolerated*, increase dosage to 400–600 mg once daily[c] Titrate doses >600 mg daily according to serum theophylline concentration (see Adults: Dosage Adjustment, under Dosage and Administration)
Children 12–15 years of age with risk factors for reduced theophylline clearance or for whom serum concentrations cannot be monitored	Initially, 12–14 mg/kg once daily (maximum 300 mg daily); after 3 days, *if tolerated*, increase dosage to 16 mg/kg or 400 mg once daily (whichever is less)
Adolescents ≥16 years of age with risk factors for reduced theophylline clearance or for whom serum concentrations cannot be monitored	Maximum 400 mg once daily

[b]Dosage given as total daily dosage; administer once daily every 24 hours.
[c]If caffeine-like adverse affects occur, consider decreasing dosage and slowing dosage titration.

Acute Bronchospasm in Patients Who Have Not Received Theophylline in the Previous 24 Hours

ORAL (IMMEDIATE-RELEASE PREPARATIONS):
- Loading dose: 5 mg/kg as a single dose in infants and children >1 year of age.

Dosing Guidelines in Infants and Children If Therapy Is Continued after Loading Dose

Age	Dosage (mg/kg)
Full-term infants <26 weeks of age	[(0.2 x age in weeks) + 5] x body weight (kg) = total daily dosage (mg); administer in 3 equally divided doses every 8 hours
Infants 26–52 weeks of age	[(0.2 x age in weeks) + 5] x body weight (kg) = total daily dosage (mg); administer in 4 equally divided doses every 6 hours
Children ≥1 year of age (weighing <45 kg)	20 mg/kg daily or 600 mg daily (whichever is less) in divided doses every 4–6 hours
Children ≥1 year of age (weighing >45 kg)	600 mg daily in divided doses every 6–8 hours
Children 1–15 years of age (weighing <45 kg) with risk factors for reduced theophylline clearance or for whom serum concentrations cannot be monitored	Maximum 16 mg/kg or 400 mg daily (whichever is less)
Children ≥16 years of age (weighing >45 kg) with risk factors for reduced theophylline clearance or for whom serum concentrations cannot be monitored	Maximum 400 mg daily in divided doses every 6–8 hours

Monitor serum theophylline concentration at 24-hour intervals to adjust final dosage. (See Adults: Dosage Adjustment, under Dosage and Administration.)

Adult Patients

Bronchospasm
Dosage Initiation and Titration for Acute and Chronic Bronchospasm

Smaller and more frequently administered doses may be required to prevent breakthrough symptoms in patients who metabolize theophylline rapidly.

ORAL (IMMEDIATE-RELEASE PREPARATIONS):
- Initially, 300 mg daily in divided doses every 6–8 hours. After 3 days, *if tolerated*, increase dosage to 400 mg daily in divided doses every 6–8 hours. After 3 more days, *if tolerated and needed*, increase dosage to 600 mg daily in divided doses every 6–8 hours.

- Patients with risk factors for reduced theophylline clearance or for whom serum concentrations cannot be monitored: Initially, 300 mg daily in divided doses every 6–8 hours. After 3 days, *if tolerated*, increase dosage to a maximum 400 mg daily in divided doses every 6–8 hours.

Switching to Extended-release Preparations

ORAL:
- Twelve-hour preparations: Administer one-half the total daily dosage every 12 hours.
- Uniphyl®: Administer mg-for-mg total daily dosage once daily.

Chronic Bronchospasm

ORAL (12-HOUR EXTENDED-RELEASE PREPARATIONS):
- Initially, 300 mg daily in 2 divided doses every 12 hours. After 3 days, *if tolerated*, increase dosage to 400 mg daily in 2 divided doses every 12 hours. After 3 more days, *if tolerated and needed*, increase dosage to 600 mg daily in 2 divided doses every 12 hours.

ORAL (THEO-24® CAPSULES AND UNIPHYL® TABLETS):
- Initially, 300–400 mg daily once daily. After 3 days, *if tolerated*, increase dosage to 400–600 mg once daily. After 3 more days, *if tolerated and needed*, titrate doses >600 mg according to serum theophylline concentration. (See Dosage Adjustment under Dosage and Administration.)

Acute Bronchospasm in Patients Who Have Not Received Theophylline in the Previous 24 Hours

ORAL (IMMEDIATE-RELEASE PREPARATIONS):
- Loading dose: 5 mg/kg as a single dose.
- Subsequently, 600 mg daily in divided doses every 6–8 hours in patients without risk factors for reduced theophylline clearance.
- Subsequently, 400 mg daily in divided doses every 6–8 hours in patients with risk factors for reduced theophylline clearance or for whom serum concentrations cannot be monitored.
- Monitor serum theophylline concentration at 24-hour intervals to adjust final dosage. (See Adults: Dosage Adjustment, under Dosage and Administration.)

Acute Bronchospasm

ORAL (DYPHYLLINE):
- Tablets: ≤15 mg/kg every 6 hours.
- Elixir: 200–400 mg every 6 hours.

Dosage Adjustment

Dosage adjustments should be based on peak serum theophylline concentration and patient's clinical response and tolerance. In general, the following recommended dosage adjustments should not be exceeded.

ORAL:

Oral Dosage Adjustment Based on Serum Theophylline Concentration

Serum Theophylline Concentration (mcg/mL)	Dosage Adjustment
<9.9	Increase dosage by 25% if symptoms are *not* controlled and current dosage is tolerated; recheck serum concentration after 3 days
10–14.9	Maintain dosage if symptoms are controlled and current dosage is tolerated; recheck serum concentration at 6- to 12-month intervals
	Consider adding additional agents if symptoms are not controlled and current dosage is tolerated
	Reduce dosage and/or measure serum theophylline concentration when adverse effects are present, physiologic abnormalities that reduce theophylline clearance (e.g., sustained fever) occur, or a drug that interacts is added or discontinued
15–19.9	Consider decreasing dosage by about 10% to provide greater margin of safety even if current dosage is tolerated
	Reduce dosage and/or measure serum theophylline concentration when adverse effects are present, physiologic abnormalities that reduce theophylline clearance (e.g., sustained fever) occur, or a drug that interacts is added or discontinued
20–24.9	Decrease dosage by 25% even if no adverse effects are present; recheck serum concentration after 3 days
25–30	Skip next dose and decrease subsequent doses by at least 25% even if no adverse effects are present
	Recheck serum concentration after 3 days; if symptomatic, consider whether treatment for overdose is indicated
>30	Treat overdose as indicated. If therapy is resumed, decrease subsequent doses by at least 50% and recheck serum concentration after 3 days

Prescribing Limits

Pediatric Patients

Bronchospasm
Dosage Initiation and Titration for Acute and Chronic Bronchospasm

ORAL:
- Children 1–15 years of age: Initially, maximum 300 mg daily; after 3 days, increase to maximum 400 mg daily; after 3 more days, increase to maximum 600 mg daily.
- Children 1–15 years of age with risk factors for reduced theophylline clearance or for whom serum concentrations cannot be monitored: Initially, maximum 300 mg daily; after 3 days, increase to maximum 400 mg daily or 16 mg/kg daily (whichever is less).

Acute Bronchospasm in Patients Who Have Not Received Theophylline in the Previous 24 Hours

ORAL (IMMEDIATE-RELEASE PREPARATIONS):
- Maximum 600 mg daily following administration of a loading dose.
- Children 1–15 years of age with risk factors for reduced theophylline clearance or for whom serum concentrations cannot be monitored: Maximum 16 mg/kg daily or 400 mg daily (whichever is less) following administration of a loading dose.

Adult Patients

Bronchospasm
Dosage Initiation and Titration for Acute and Chronic Bronchospasm

ORAL:
- Maximum 600 mg daily.
- Patients with risk factors for reduced theophylline clearance or for whom serum concentrations cannot be monitored: Maximum 400 mg daily.

Special Populations

Hepatic Impairment
- Decreased clearance; dosage reduction and frequent monitoring of serum theophylline concentrations recommended.

ORAL:
- Dyphylline: No dosage adjustment required.

Renal Impairment
- Dosage adjustment not required in adults and children >3 months of age.
- Dyphylline: Consider dosage reduction.

Geriatric Patients (>60 years)
- Select dosage with caution because of age-related decreases in hepatic, renal, and/or cardiac function and concomitant disease and drug therapy.

Oral
- Maximum 400 mg daily unless serum theophylline concentrations are monitored at 24-hour intervals, patient continues to be symptomatic, and serum concentration indicates need for larger dosage. Administer dosages >400 mg daily with caution.

† *Use is not currently included in the labeling approved by the US Food and Drug Administration.*

Amiodarone Oral

(a mee′ oh da rone)

Brand Name: Cordarone®, Pacerone®
Also available generically.

Important Warning

Amiodarone may cause lung disease that can be serious or life-threatening. Tell your doctor if you have or have ever had any type of lung disease. If you experience any of the following symptoms, call your doctor immediately: fever, shortness of breath, wheezing, cough, coughing up blood, and any other breathing problems.

Amiodarone also may cause liver disease. Tell your doctor if you have or have ever had liver disease. If your experience any of the following symptoms, call your doctor immediately: upset stomach, vomiting, dark colored urine, excessive tiredness, yellowing of the skin or eyes, itching, or pain in the upper right part of the stomach.

Amiodarone may cause your irregular heart rhythm (arrhythmia) to worsen or may cause you to develop new arrhythmias. Tell your doctor if you have ever been dizzy or lightheaded or have fainted because your heartbeat was too slow and if you have or have ever had low levels of potassium in your blood; heart or thyroid disease; or any problems with your heart rhythm other than the irregular heartbeat being treated. Tell your doctor and pharmacist if you are taking any of the following medications: antifungals such as fluconazole (Diflucan), ketoconazole (Nizoral), and itraconazole (Sporanox); azithromycin (Zithromax); beta blockers such as atenolol (Tenormin), labetalol (Normodyne), metoprolol (Lopressor, Toprol XL), nadolol (Corgard), and propranolol (Inderal); calcium channel blockers such as amlodipine (Norvasc), diltiazem (Cardizem, Dilacor, Tiazac, others), felodipine (Plendil), isradipine (DynaCirc), nicardipine (Cardene), nifedipine (Adalat, Procardia), nimodipine (Nimotop), nisoldipine (Sular), and verapamil (Calan, Covera, Isoptin, Verelan); cisapride (Propulsid); clarithromycin (Biaxin); diuretics ('water pills'); dofetilide (Tikosyn); erythromycin (E.E.S., E-Mycin, Erythrocin); fluoroquinolone antibiotics such as ciprofloxacin (Cipro), gatifloxacin (Tequin), levofloxacin (Levaquin), lomefloxacin (Maxaquin), moxifloxacin (Avelox), norfloxacin (Noroxin), ofloxacin (Floxin), and sparfloxacin (Zagam); other medications for irregular heartbeat such as digoxin (Lanoxin), disopyramide (Norpace), flecainide (Tambocor), phenytoin (Dilantin), procainamide (Procanbid, Pronestyl), quinidine (Quinidex) and sotalol (Betapace); and thioridazine (Mellaril). If you have any of the following symptoms, call your doctor immediately: lightheadedness; fainting; fast, slow, or pounding heartbeat; or feeling that your heart has skipped a beat.

You will probably be hospitalized for one week or longer when you begin your treatment with amiodarone. Your doctor will monitor you carefully during this time and for as long as you continue to take amiodarone. Your doctor will probably start you on a high dose of amiodarone and gradually decrease your dose as the medication begins to work. Your doctor may decrease your dose during your treatment if you develop side effects. Follow your doctor's directions carefully.

Keep all appointments with your doctor and the laboratory. Your doctor will order certain tests, such as blood tests, X-rays, and electrocardiograms (EKGs, tests that record the electrical activity of the heart) before and during your treatment to be sure that it is safe for you to take amiodarone and to check your body's response to the medication.

Your doctor or pharmacist will give you the manufacturer's patient information sheet (Medication Guide) when you begin treatment with amiodarone and each time you refill your prescription. Read the information carefully and ask your doctor or pharmacist if you have any questions. You also can obtain the Medication Guide from the FDA website: http://www.fda.gov/medwatch/SAFETY/2005/Cordarone_Med_Guide.pdf.

Talk to your doctor about the risks of taking amiodarone.

Why is this medicine prescribed?

Amiodarone is used to treat and prevent certain types of ventricular arrhythmias (abnormal heart rhythm). Amiodarone is in a class of medications called antiarrhythmics. It works by relaxing overactive heart muscles.

How should this medicine be used?

Amiodarone comes as a tablet to take by mouth. It is usually taken once or twice a day. Your doctor will tell you to take amiodarone with or without food; be sure to take it the same way each time. Follow the directions on your prescription label carefully, and ask your doctor or pharmacist to explain any part you do not understand. Take amiodarone exactly as directed. Do not take more or less of it or take it more often than prescribed by your doctor.

Amiodarone controls arrhythmias but does not cure them. Continue to take amiodarone even if you feel well. Do not stop taking amiodarone without talking to your doctor. If you suddenly stop taking amiodarone, your condition may get worse.

Are there other uses for this medicine?

This medication may be prescribed for other uses; ask your doctor or pharmacist for more information.

What special precautions should I follow?

Before taking amiodarone,

- tell your doctor and pharmacist if you are allergic to amiodarone, iodine, any other drugs, or corn.
- tell your doctor and pharmacist what prescription and nonprescription medications, vitamins, and nutritional supplements you are taking. Be sure to mention the medications listed in the IMPORTANT WARNING and any of the following: antidepressants ('mood elevators') such as fluoxetine (Prozac, Sarafem), fluvoxamine (Luvox), nefazodone (Serzone); anticoagulants ('blood thinners') such as warfarin (coumadin); cholesterol lowering medications such as atorvastatin (Lipitor), cholestyramine (Questran), lovastatin (Mevacor), simvastatin (Zocor); cimetidine (Tagamet); cyclosporine (Neoral, Sandimmune); danazol (Danocrine); delavirdine (Rescriptor); dextromethorphan (a medication in many cough preparations); dexamethasone (Decadron); fentanyl (Actiq, Duragesic); HIV protease inhibitors such as indinavir (Crixivan), and ritonavir (Norvir); isoniazid (INH, Nydrazid); medications for diabetes; medications for pain; medications for seizures such as carbamazepine (Tegretol), ethosuximide (Zarontin), phenobarbital (Luminal, Solfoton), phenytoin (Dilantin); metronidazole (Flagyl); methotrexate (Rheumatrex); oral contraceptives (birth control pills); rifabutin (Mycobutin); rifampin (Rifadin, Rimactane); troglitazone (Rezulin); troleandomycin (TAO); and zafirlukast (Accolate). Your doctor may have to change the doses of your medications or monitor you carefully for side effects.
- tell your doctor what herbal products you are taking, especially St. John's wort.
- tell your doctor if you have or have ever had problems with your blood pressure.
- tell your doctor if you are pregnant, plan to become pregnant, or are breast-feeding. You should use a reliable method of birth control to prevent pregnancy while you are taking amiodarone. If you become pregnant while taking amiodarone, call your doctor immediately. You should not breastfeed while you are taking amiodarone. Talk to your doctor if you plan to become pregnant or breastfeed during the first several months after your treatment because amiordarone may remain in your body for some time after you stop taking it.
- if you are having surgery, including dental surgery, tell your doctor or dentist that you are taking amiodarone.
- plan to avoid unnecessary or prolonged exposure to sunlight or sunlamps and to wear protective clothing, sunglasses, and sunscreen. Amiodarone may make your skin sensitive to sunlight. Exposed skin may turn blue-

gray and may not return to normal even after you stop using this medication.
- you should know that amiodarone may cause vision problems including permanent blindness. Be sure to have regular eye exams during your treatment and call your doctor if you have any changes with your eyes or notice any changes in your vision.
- you should know that amiodarone may remain in your body for several months after your stop taking it. You may continue to experience side effects of amiodarone during this time. Be sure to tell your health care provider who treats you or prescribes any medication for you during this time that you have recently stopped taking amiodarone.

What special dietary instructions should I follow?

Do not drink grapefruit juice while taking this medication.

What should I do if I forget to take a dose?

Take the missed dose as soon as you remember it. However, if it is almost time for the next dose, skip the missed dose and continue your regular dosing schedule. Do not take a double dose to make up for a missed one.

What side effects can this medicine cause?

Amiodarone may cause side effects. Tell your doctor if any of these symptoms are severe or do not go away:
- vomiting
- constipation
- headache
- decreased sex drive
- difficulty falling asleep or staying asleep
- flushing
- dry eyes
- changes in ability to taste and smell
- changes in amount of saliva

Some side effects can be serious. If you experience any of the following symptoms, or those listed in the IMPORTANT WARNING section, call your doctor immediately:
- rash
- weight loss or gain
- restlessness
- intolerance to heat or cold
- thinning hair
- excessive sweating
- changes in menstrual cycle
- swelling in the front of the neck (goiter)
- decreased vision or changes in your ability to see such as blurred vision or seeing halos
- eyes are sensitive to light
- eye pain
- swelling of the hands, feet, ankles, or lower legs
- shaking hands that you can not control
- movements that you can not control
- poor coordination or trouble walking

- numbness or tingling in the hands, legs, and feet
- muscle weakness

Laboratory animals who were given amiodarone developed thyroid tumors. It is not known if amiodarone increases the risk of developing thyroid tumors in humans.

Talk to your doctor about the risk of taking amiodarone.

Amiodarone may cause other side effects. Call your doctor if you have any unusual problems while taking this medication.

If you experience a serious side effect, you or your doctor may send a report to the Food and Drug Administration's (FDA) MedWatch Adverse Event Reporting program online [at http://www.fda.gov/MedWatch/index.html] or by phone [1-800-332-1088].

What storage conditions are needed for this medicine?

Keep this medication in the container it came in, tightly closed, and out of reach of children. Store it at room temperature and away from excess heat and moisture (not in the bathroom). Protect this medication from light. Throw away any medication that is outdated or no longer needed. Talk to your pharmacist about the proper disposal of your medication.

What should I do in case of overdose?

In case of overdose, call your local poison control center at 1-800-222-1222. If the victim has collapsed or is not breathing, call local emergency services at 911.

Symptoms of overdose may include:

- slow heartbeat
- upset stomach
- blurred vision
- lightheadedness
- fainting

What other information should I know?

Do not let anyone else take your medication. Ask your pharmacist any questions you have about refilling your prescription.

Dosage Facts
For Informational Purposes

Caution: Do not change your dose, how often you take your medication, or the length of time you are to take it without first talking to your healthcare provider.

The following dosage information was written using medical language for doctors and other healthcare professionals and is provided here for you to check your dosage. The dosage of this drug may differ for different patients. Therefore, always follow your doctor's instructions or the directions on the label. Contact your healthcare provider or pharmacist if you have any questions about the specific dosage of your medication after reviewing this information.

General Dosage Information

Available as amiodarone hydrochloride; dosage expressed in terms of the salt.

Pediatric Patients

Ventricular Arrhythmias†

ORAL:

- Initially (as loading dose), 10–15 mg/kg daily or 600–800 mg/1.73 m^2 daily for approximately 4–14 days and/or until adequate control of cardiac arrhythmias is achieved or adverse effects become prominent. Subsequently, reduce dosage to 5 mg/kg daily or 200–400 mg/1.73 m^2 daily for several weeks; if possible, reduce dosage to the lowest effective level.
- Children <1 year of age may require higher oral loading and maintenance dosages than older children when dosage is calculated on the basis of body weight, but not on the basis of body surface area†.

Supraventricular Arrhythmias†

ORAL:

- Initially (as loading dose), 10–15 mg/kg daily or 600–800 mg/1.73m^2 daily for approximately 4–14 days and/or until adequate control of cardiac arrhythmias is achieved or adverse effects become prominent. Subsequently, reduce dosage to 5 mg/kg daily or 200–400 mg/1.73 m^2 daily for several weeks; if possible, reduce dosage to the lowest effective level.
- Children <1 year of age may require higher oral loading and maintenance dosages than older children when dosage is calculated on the basis of body weight, but not on the basis of body surface area.†

Adult Patients

Ventricular Arrhythmias

ORAL:

Oral Loading and Maintenance Dosages

Loading Dose	800–1600 mg daily for 1–3 weeks or until initial therapeutic response occurs
Dosage Adjustment	When adequate control of ventricular arrhythmias is achieved or adverse effects become prominent, decrease dosage to 600–800 mg daily for about 1 month
Maintenance Dosage	400–600 mg daily; if possible, cautiously reduce dosage to 200 mg daily

Consult published protocols for specific information about oral loading doses >1600 mg daily or IV loading-dose regimens† followed by oral therapy. If an IV loading-dose regimen is used, initiate oral therapy as soon as possible after an adequate response is obtained and gradually eliminate IV amiodarone.

Supraventricular Arrhythmias†

ORAL:
- Initially (as loading dose), 600–800 mg daily for approximately 1–4 weeks and/or until adequate control of supraventricular arrhythmias is achieved or adverse effects become prominent. Gradually reduce dosage to the lowest effective maintenance dosage, usually 100–400 mg daily.
- Consult published protocols for specific information about oral loading-dose regimens using higher dosages.

Long-term Management of Recurrent Atrial Fibrillation†

ORAL:
- Initially, 10 mg/kg daily for 14 days, followed by 300 mg daily for 4 weeks, and then 200 mg daily.

Special Populations

Hepatic Impairment
- Dosage reduction recommended in patients with substantial hepatic impairment.

Renal Impairment
- Routine dosage reduction not required.

Geriatric Patients
- Careful dosage selection recommended due to possible age-related decrease in hepatic, renal, and/or cardiac function and concomitant disease and drug therapy; however, dosage requirements generally similar in geriatric and younger adults.
- Use caution with high dosages due to increased susceptibility to drug-induced bradycardia and conduction disturbances.

† Use is not currently included in the labeling approved by the US Food and Drug Administration.

Amitriptyline

(a mee trip′ ti leen)

Brand Name: Limbitrol® as a combination product containing amitriptyline and chlordiazepoxide, Limbitrol® DS as a combination product containing amitriptyline and chlordiazepoxide Also available generically.

Important Warning

A small number of children, teenagers, and young adults (up to 24 years of age) who took antidepressants ('mood elevators') such as amitriptyline during clinical studies became suicidal (thinking about harming or killing oneself or planning or trying to do so). Children, teenagers, and young adults who take antidepressants to treat depression or other mental illnesses may be more likely to become suicidal than children, teenagers, and young adults who do not take antidepressants to treat these conditions. However, experts are not sure about how great this risk is and how much it should be considered in deciding whether a child or teenager should take an antidepressant. Children younger than 18 years of age should not normally take amitriptyline, but in some cases, a doctor may decide that amitriptyline is the best medication to treat a child's condition.

You should know that your mental health may change in unexpected ways when you take amitriptyline or other antidepressants even if you are an adult over age 24. You may become suicidal, especially at the beginning of your treatment and any time that your dose is increased or decreased. You, your family, or your caregiver should call your doctor right away if you experience any of the following symptoms: new or worsening depression; thinking about harming or killing yourself, or planning or trying to do so; extreme worry; agitation; panic attacks; difficulty falling asleep or staying asleep; aggressive behavior; irritability; acting without thinking; severe restlessness; and frenzied abnormal excitement. Be sure that your family or caregiver knows which symptoms may be serious so they can call the doctor when you are unable to seek treatment on your own.

Your healthcare provider will want to see you often while you are taking amitriptyline, especially at the beginning of your treatment. Be sure to keep all appointments for office visits with your doctor.

The doctor or pharmacist will give you the manufacturer's patient information sheet (Medication Guide) when you begin treatment with amitriptyline. Read the information carefully and ask your doctor or pharmacist if you have any questions. You also can obtain the Medication Guide from the FDA website: http://www.fda.gov/cder/drug/antidepressants/antidepressants_MG_2007.pdf.

No matter your age, before you take an antidepressant, you, your parent, or your caregiver should talk to your doctor about the risks and benefits of treating your condition with an antidepressant or with other treatments. You should also talk about the risks and benefits of not treating your condition. You should know that having depression or another mental illness greatly increases the risk that you will become suicidal. This risk is higher if you or anyone in your family has or has ever had bipolar disorder (mood that changes from depressed to abnormally excited) or mania (frenzied, abnormally excited mood) or has thought about or attempted suicide. Talk to your doctor about your condition, symptoms, and personal and family medical history. You and your doctor will decide what type of treatment is right for you.

Why is this medicine prescribed?

Amitriptyline is used to treat symptoms of depression. Amitriptyline is in a class of medications called tricyclic antidepressants. It works by increasing the amounts of certain natural substances in the brain that are needed to maintain mental balance.

How should this medicine be used?

Amitriptyline comes as a tablet to take by mouth. It is usually taken one to four times a day. Take amitriptyline at around the same time(s) every day. Follow the directions on your prescription label carefully, and ask your doctor or pharmacist to explain any part you do not understand. Take amitriptyline exactly as directed. Do not take more or less of it or take it more often than prescribed by your doctor.

Your doctor will probably start you on a low dose of amitriptyline and gradually increase your dose.

It may take a few weeks or longer before you feel the full benefit of amitriptyline. Continue to take amitriptyline even if you feel well. Do not stop taking amitriptyline without talking to your doctor. If you suddenly stop taking amitriptyline, you may experience withdrawal symptoms such as nausea, headache, and lack of energy. Your doctor will probably decrease your dose gradually.

Are there other uses for this medicine?

Amitriptyline is also sometimes used to treat eating disorders and post-herpetic neuralgia (the burning, stabbing pains, or aches that may last for months or years after a shingles infection). Talk to your doctor about the possible risks of using this medication for your condition.

This medication may be prescribed for other uses; ask your doctor or pharmacist for more information.

What special precautions should I follow?

Before taking amitriptyline,
- tell your doctor and pharmacist if you are allergic to amitriptyline or any other medications.
- tell your doctor if you are taking cisapride (Propulsid) (not available in the U.S.) or monoamine oxidase (MAO) inhibitors such as isocarboxazid (Marplan), phenelzine (Nardil), selegiline (Eldepryl, Emsam, Zelapar), and tranylcypromine (Parnate), or if you have taken an MAO inhibitor during the past 14 days. Your doctor will probably tell you that you should not take amitriptyline.
- tell your doctor and pharmacist what other prescription and nonprescription medications, vitamins, nutritional supplements, and herbal products you are taking. Be sure to mention any of the following: antihistamines; cimetidine (Tagamet); diet pills; disulfiram (Antabuse); guanethidine (Ismelin); ipratropium (Atrovent); quinidine (Quinidex); medications for irregular heartbeats such as flecainide (Tambocor) and propafenone (Rythmol); medications for anxiety, asthma, colds, irritable

bowel disease, mental illness, nausea, Parkinson's disease, seizures, ulcers, or urinary problems; other antidepressants; phenobarbital (Bellatal, Solfoton); sedatives; selective serotonin reuptake inhibitors (SSRIs) such as citalopram (Celexa), fluoxetine (Prozac, Sarafem), fluvoxamine (Luvox), paroxetine (Paxil), and sertraline (Zoloft); sleeping pills; thyroid medications; and tranquilizers. Tell your doctor or pharmacist if you have stopped taking fluoxetine (Prozac, Sarafem) in the past 5 weeks. Your doctor may need to change the doses of your medications or monitor you carefully for side effects.
- tell your doctor if you have recently had a heart attack. Your doctor will probably tell you not to take amitriptyline.
- tell your doctor if you drink large amounts of alcohol and if you have or have ever had glaucoma (an eye condition); an enlarged prostate (a male reproductive gland); difficulty urinating; seizures; an overactive thyroid gland (hyperthyroidism); diabetes; schizophrenia (a mental illness that causes disturbed or unusual thinking, loss of interest in life, and strong or inappropriate emotions); or liver, kidney, or heart disease.
- tell your doctor if you are pregnant or plan to become pregnant. If you become pregnant while taking amitriptyline, call your doctor. Do not breast-feed while you are taking amitriptyline.
- if you are having surgery, including dental surgery, tell the doctor or dentist that you are taking amitriptyline.
- you should know that amitriptyline may make you drowsy. Do not drive a car or operate machinery until you know how this medication affects you.
- remember that alcohol can add to the drowsiness caused by this medication.

What special dietary instructions should I follow?

Unless your doctor tells you otherwise, continue your normal diet.

What should I do if I forget to take a dose?

Take the missed dose as soon as you remember it. However, if it is almost time for the next dose, skip the missed dose and continue your regular dosing schedule. Do not take a double dose to make up for a missed one.

What side effects can this medicine cause?

Amitriptyline may cause side effects. Tell your doctor if any of these symptoms are severe or do not go away:
- nausea
- vomiting
- drowsiness
- weakness or tiredness
- nightmares
- headaches
- dry mouth

- constipation
- difficulty urinating
- blurred vision
- pain, burning, or tingling in the hands or feet
- changes in sex drive or ability
- excessive sweating
- changes in appetite or weight
- confusion
- unsteadiness

Some side effects can be serious. If you experience any of the following symptoms or those listed in the IMPORTANT WARNING section, call your doctor immediately:

- slow or difficult speech
- dizziness or faintness
- weakness or numbness of an arm or a leg
- crushing chest pain
- rapid, pounding, or irregular heartbeat
- severe skin rash or hives
- swelling of the face and tongue
- yellowing of the skin or eyes
- jaw, neck, and back muscle spasms
- uncontrollable shaking of a part of the body
- fainting
- unusual bleeding or bruising
- seizures
- hallucinating (seeing things or hearing voices that do not exist)

Amitriptyline may cause other side effects. Call your doctor if you have any unusual problems while taking this medication.

If you experience a serious side effect, you or your doctor may send a report to the Food and Drug Administration's (FDA) MedWatch Adverse Event Reporting program online [at http://www.fda.gov/MedWatch/index.html] or by phone [1-800-332-1088].

What storage conditions are needed for this medicine?

Keep this medication in the container it came in, tightly closed, and out of reach of children. Store it at room temperature and away from excess heat and moisture (not in the bathroom). Throw away any medication that is outdated or no longer needed. Talk to your pharmacist about the proper disposal of your medication.

What should I do in case of overdose?

In case of overdose, call your local poison control center at 1-800-222-1222. If the victim has collapsed or is not breathing, call local emergency services at 911.

Symptoms of overdose may include:

- irregular heartbeat
- seizures
- coma (loss of consciousness for a period of time)
- confusion
- problems concentrating

- hallucinating (seeing things or hearing voices that do not exist)
- agitation
- drowsiness
- rigid muscles
- vomiting
- fever
- cold body temperature

What other information should I know?

Keep all appointments with your doctor and the laboratory. Your doctor may order certain lab tests to check your body's response to amitriptyline.

Do not let anyone else take your medication. Ask your pharmacist any questions you have about refilling your prescription.

Dosage Facts
For Informational Purposes

Caution: Do not change your dose, how often you take your medication, or the length of time you are to take it without first talking to your healthcare provider.

The following dosage information was written using medical language for doctors and other healthcare professionals and is provided here for you to check your dosage. The dosage of this drug may differ for different patients. Therefore, always follow your doctor's instructions or the directions on the label. Contact your healthcare provider or pharmacist if you have any questions about the specific dosage of your medication after reviewing this information.

General Dosage Information

Available as amitriptyline hydrochloride; dosage is expressed in terms of the salt.

Pediatric Patients

Major Depressive Disorder

ORAL:
- Adolescents ≥12 years of age: 10 mg 3 times daily plus 20 mg at bedtime.

Adult Patients

Major Depressive Disorder
Outpatients

ORAL:
- Initially, 75 mg daily in divided doses or 50–100 mg once daily at bedtime. Increase dosages in 25- or 50-mg increments until maximal therapeutic effect with minimal toxicity is achieved or up to a maximum dosage of 150 mg daily.
- Usual maintenance dosage: 50–100 mg daily, administered as a single daily dose, preferably at bedtime. For some, 25–40 mg daily may be sufficient. Continue therapy for at least 3 months to prevent relapse.

Hospitalized Patients

ORAL:
- Initially, 100 mg daily; dosage may be increased gradually to 200–300 mg daily as needed.

Prescribing Limits

Adult Patients

Major Depressive Disorder

Outpatients

ORAL:
- Maximum 150 mg daily.

Hospitalized Patients

ORAL:
- Maximum 300 mg daily.

Special Populations

Geriatric Patients
- 10 mg 3 times daily plus 20 mg at bedtime.

Amlexanox

(am lex′ an ox)

Brand Name: Aphthasol®

Why is this medicine prescribed?

Amlexanox is used to treat ulcers of the mouth called aphthous ulcers or canker sores. It decreases the time ulcers take to heal. Because amlexanox decreases the healing time, it also decreases the pain you feel.

This medication is sometimes prescribed for other uses; ask your doctor, dentist, or pharmacist for more information.

How should this medicine be used?

Amlexanox comes as a beige-colored paste. Amlexanox should be used as soon as possible after noticing symptoms of an ulcer. Amlexanox is usually applied four times a day, following brushing and flossing after breakfast, lunch, dinner, and at bedtime. Squeeze 1/4 inch of the paste on your finger. With gentle pressure, dab amlexanox onto each ulcer in the mouth. Wash hands immediately after using amlexanox. Amlexanox is only used until the ulcer has healed, usually within 10 days. Contact your physician or dentist if significant healing has not occurred within 10 days.

Follow the directions on your prescription label carefully, and ask your doctor, dentist, or pharmacist to explain any part you do not understand. Use amlexanox exactly as directed. Do not use more or less of it or use it more often than prescribed by your doctor or dentist.

What special precautions should I follow?

Before using amlexanox,
- tell your doctor or dentist and pharmacist if you are allergic to amlexanox or any other drugs.
- tell your doctor and pharmacist what prescription and nonprescription medications you are taking, including vitamins and herbal products.
- tell your doctor or dentist if you are pregnant, plan to become pregnant, or are breast-feeding. If you become pregnant while using amlexanox, call your doctor or dentist.

What should I do if I forget to take a dose?

Apply the missed dose as soon as you remember it. However, if it is almost time for the next dose, skip the missed dose and continue your regular dosing schedule. Do not apply a double dose to make up for a missed one.

What side effects can this medicine cause?

Amlexanox may cause side effects. Tell your doctor or dentist if any of these symptoms are severe or do not go away:
- slight pain, stinging, or burning of the skin that comes and goes
- nausea
- diarrhea

If you experience the following symptom, call your doctor or dentist immediately:
- rash

If you experience a serious side effect, you or your doctor may send a report to the Food and Drug Administration's (FDA) MedWatch Adverse Event Reporting program online [at http://www.fda.gov/MedWatch/index.html] or by phone [1-800-332-1088].

What storage conditions are needed for this medicine?

Keep this medication in the container it came in, tightly closed, and out of reach of children. Store it at room temperature and away from excess heat and moisture (not in the bathroom). Throw away any medication that is outdated or no longer needed. Talk to your pharmacist about the proper disposal of your medication.

What other information should I know?

Keep all appointments with your doctor or dentist. Amlexanox is for external use only. Do not let amlexanox get into your eyes. If it does get into your eyes, rinse them promptly.

Do not let anyone else use your medication. Ask your pharmacist any questions you have about refilling your prescription. Tell your doctor or dentist if your ulcers get worse or do not get better within 10 days.

Talk to your doctor, pharmacist, or other healthcare professional if you have questions about dosing information for your medication.

Amlodipine

(am loe' di peen)

Brand Name: Caduet® as a combination product containing Amlodipine and Atorvastatin, Norvasc®

Why is this medicine prescribed?

Amlodipine is used alone or in combination with other medications to treat high blood pressure and chest pain (angina). Amlodipine is in a class of medications called calcium channel blockers. It lowers blood pressure by relaxing the blood vessels so the heart does not have to pump as hard. It controls chest pain by increasing the supply of blood to the heart. If taken regularly, amlodipine controls chest pain, but it does not stop chest pain once it starts. Your doctor may prescribe a different medication to take when you have chest pain.

How should this medicine be used?

Amlodipine comes as a tablet to take by mouth. It is usually taken once a day. To help you remember to take amlodipine, take it around the same time every day. Follow the directions on your prescription label carefully, and ask your doctor or pharmacist to explain any part you do not understand. Take amlodipine exactly as directed. Do not take more or less of it or take it more often than prescribed by your doctor.

Your doctor will probably start you on a low dose of amlodipine and gradually increase your dose.

Amlodipine controls high blood pressure and chest pain (angina) but does not cure them. Continue to take amlodipine even if you feel well. Do not stop taking amlodipine without talking to your doctor.

Are there other uses for this medicine?

This medication may be prescribed for other uses; ask your doctor or pharmacist for more information.

What special precautions should I follow?

Before taking amlodipine,

- tell your doctor and pharmacist if you are allergic to amlodipine or any other medications.
- tell your doctor and pharmacist what prescription and nonprescription medications, vitamins, nutritional supplements, and herbal products you are taking.
- tell your doctor if you have or have ever had heart failure or liver disease.
- tell your doctor if you are pregnant, plan to become pregnant, or are breast-feeding. If you become pregnant while taking amlodipine, call your doctor.

What special dietary instructions should I follow?

If your doctor prescribes a low-salt or low-sodium diet, follow these directions carefully.

What should I do if I forget to take a dose?

Take the missed dose as soon as you remember it. However, if it is almost time for the next dose, skip the missed dose and continue your regular dosing schedule. Do not take a double dose to make up for a missed one.

What side effects can this medicine cause?

Amlodipine may cause side effects. Tell your doctor if any of these symptoms are severe or do not go away:

- swelling of the hands, feet, ankles, or lower legs
- headache
- upset stomach
- stomach pain
- dizziness or lightheadedness
- drowsiness
- excessive tiredness
- flushing (feeling of warmth)

Some side effects can be serious. The following symptoms are uncommon, but if you experience any of them, call your doctor immediately:

- more frequent or more severe chest pain
- rapid, pounding, or irregular heartbeat
- fainting

If you experience a serious side effect, you or your doctor may send a report to the Food and Drug Administration's (FDA) MedWatch Adverse Event Reporting program online [at http://www.fda.gov/MedWatch/index.html] or by phone [1-800-332-1088].

What storage conditions are needed for this medicine?

Keep this medication in the container it came in, tightly closed, and out of reach of children. Store it at room temperature and away from excess heat and moisture (not in the bathroom). Throw away any medication that is outdated or no longer needed. Talk to your pharmacist about the proper disposal of your medication.

What should I do in case of overdose?

In case of overdose, call your local poison control center at 1-800-222-1222. If the victim has collapsed or is not breathing, call local emergency services at 911.

Symptoms of overdose may include:

- dizziness
- fainting
- rapid heartbeat

What other information should I know?

Keep all appointments with your doctor. Your blood pressure should be checked regularly to determine your response to amlodipine.

Do not let anyone else take your medication. Ask your pharmacist any questions you have about refilling your prescription.

Dosage Facts
For Informational Purposes

Caution: Do not change your dose, how often you take your medication, or the length of time you are to take it without first talking to your healthcare provider.

The following dosage information was written using medical language for doctors and other healthcare professionals and is provided here for you to check your dosage. The dosage of this drug may differ for different patients. Therefore, always follow your doctor's instructions or the directions on the label. Contact your healthcare provider or pharmacist if you have any questions about the specific dosage of your medication after reviewing this information.

General Dosage Information

Available as amlodipine besylate; dosage is expressed in terms of amlodipine.

Pediatric Patients

Hypertension

ORAL:
- Children ≥6 years of age: Usual effective dosage is 2.5–5 mg once daily.

Adult Patients

Hypertension
Monotherapy

ORAL:
- Initially as monotherapy, 2.5–5 mg once daily.
- When adding to existing antihypertensive regimen, initially 2.5 mg once daily.
- Increase dosage gradually over 7–14 days until optimum control of BP is obtained. May increase more rapidly if symptoms so warrant and patient's tolerance and response are frequently assessed.
- Usual maintenance dosage is 5–10 mg once daily.

Amlodipine/Benazepril Combination Therapy

If BP is not adequately controlled by monotherapy with amlodipine or benazepril, can switch to the fixed-combination preparation containing amlodipine 2.5 mg and benazepril 10 mg, or amlodipine 5 mg and benazepril 10 or 20 mg, or, alternatively, amlodipine 10 mg and benazepril 20 mg.

If BP is adequately controlled by monotherapy with amlodipine, but edema has developed, can switch to the fixed-combination preparation containing amlodipine 2.5 mg and

benazepril 10 mg, or amlodipine 5 mg and benazepril 10 or 20 mg, or, alternatively, amlodipine 10 mg and benazepril 20 mg.

If BP is controlled with amlodipine and benazepril (administered separately), can switch to the fixed-combination preparation containing the corresponding individual doses for convenience.

Reduce amlodipine dosage in nonblack patients when benazepril is initiated to avoid excessive antihypertensive response.

Adjust dosage of amlodipine/benazepril fixed combination to patient's response; consider that steady-state plasma concentrations of amlodipine and benazepril are reached after 7 and 2 days, respectively.

Amlodipine/Atorvastatin Combination Therapy

Use as a *substitute* for individually titrated drugs; to provide *additional therapy* for patients currently receiving one component of the preparation; or to *initiate treatment* in patients requiring therapy for hypertension *and* dyslipidemias.

CAD
Angina

ORAL:
- Usual dosage is 5–10 mg once daily; adequate control usually requires a maintenance dosage of 10 mg daily.
- Amlodipine/Atorvastatin combination therapy: use as a *substitute* for individually titrated drugs; to provide *additional therapy* for patients currently receiving one component of the preparation; or to *initiate treatment* in patients requiring therapy for angina *and* dyslipidemias.

Angiographically Documented CAD

ORAL:
- Recommended dosage is 5–10 mg once daily.
- Amlodipine/Atorvastatin combination therapy: use as a *substitute* for individually titrated drugs; to provide *additional therapy* for patients currently receiving one component of the preparation; or to *initiate treatment* in patients requiring therapy for angiographically documented CAD *and* dyslipidemias.

Prescribing Limits

Pediatric Patients

Hypertension

ORAL:
- Children ≥6 years of age: Safety and efficacy of dosages >5 mg daily not established.

Special Populations

Hepatic Impairment

Hypertension

- Initially, 2.5 mg daily alone or in fixed combination with benazepril.

Angina

- Initially, 5 mg daily.

Renal Impairment

- Dosage modification not necessary.

Geriatric Patients
- Hypertension: Initially, 2.5 mg daily alone or in fixed combination with benazepril. Adjust subsequent dosage based on patient response and tolerance.
- Angina: Initially, 5 mg daily.

Amlodipine and Benazepril

(am loe′ di peen) (ben ay′ ze pril)

Brand Name: Lotrel®

Important Warning

Do not take amlodipine and benazepril if you are pregnant. If you become pregnant while taking amlodipine and benazepril, call your doctor immediately. Amlodipine and benazepril may harm the fetus.

Why is this medicine prescribed?

The combination of amlodipine and benazepril is used to treat high blood pressure. Amlodipine is in a class of medications called calcium channel blockers. It works by relaxing the blood vessels so the heart does not have to pump as hard. Benazepril is in a class of medications called angiotensin-converting enzyme (ACE) inhibitors. It works by decreasing certain chemicals that tighten the blood vessels, so blood flows more smoothly.

How should this medicine be used?

The combination of amlodipine and benazepril comes as a capsule to take by mouth. It is usually taken once a day. To help you remember to take amlodipine and benazepril, take it around the same time every day. Follow the directions on your prescription label carefully, and ask your doctor or pharmacist to explain any part you do not understand. Take amlodipine and benazepril exactly as directed. Do not take more or less of it or take it more often than prescribed by your doctor.

Amlodipine and benazepril controls high blood pressure but does not cure it. Continue to take amlodipine and benazepril even if you feel well. Do not stop taking amlodipine and benazepril without talking to your doctor.

Are there other uses for this medicine?

This medication may be prescribed for other uses; ask your doctor or pharmacist for more information.

What special precautions should I follow?

Before taking amlodipine and benazepril,
- tell your doctor and pharmacist if you are allergic to amlodipine (Norvasc), benazepril (Lotensin), captopril (Capoten), enalapril (Vasotec), fosinopril (Monopril), lisinopril (Prinivil, Zestril), moexipril (Univasc), perindopril (Aceon), quinapril (Accupril), ramipril (Altace), trandolapril (Mavik), or any other medications.
- tell your doctor and pharmacist what prescription and nonprescription medications, vitamins, nutritional supplements, and herbal products you are taking. Be sure to mention any of the following: diuretics ('water pills'), lithium (Eskalith, Lithobid), and potassium supplements. Your doctor may need to change the doses of your medications or monitor you carefully for side effects.
- tell your doctor if you have recently had severe diarrhea or vomiting and if you have or have ever had heart failure; lupus; scleroderma; heart, liver, or kidney disease; or diabetes.
- tell your doctor if you plan to become pregnant or are breast-feeding.
- if you are having surgery, including dental surgery, tell the doctor or dentist that you are taking amlodipine and benazepril.

What special dietary instructions should I follow?

Talk to your doctor before using salt substitutes containing potassium. If your doctor prescribes a low-salt or low-sodium diet, follow these directions carefully.

What should I do if I forget to take a dose?

Take the missed dose as soon as you remember it. However, if it is almost time for the next dose, skip the missed dose and continue your regular dosing schedule. Do not take a double dose to make up for a missed one.

What side effects can this medicine cause?

Amlodipine and benazepril may cause side effects. Tell your doctor if any of these symptoms are severe or do not go away:
- cough
- headache
- dizziness
- swelling of the hands, feet, ankles, or lower legs

Some side effects can be serious. The following symptoms are uncommon, but if you experience any of them, call your doctor immediately:
- swelling of the face, throat, tongue, lips, or eyes
- hoarseness
- difficulty swallowing or breathing
- fainting
- severe skin rash

     © Copyright 2008 American Society of Health-System Pharmacists

- yellowing of the skin or eyes
- more frequent or more severe chest pain

Amlodipine and benazepril may cause other side effects. Call your doctor if you have any unusual problems while taking this medication.

If you experience a serious side effect, you or your doctor may send a report to the Food and Drug Administration's (FDA) MedWatch Adverse Event Reporting program online [at http://www.fda.gov/MedWatch/index.html] or by phone [1-800-332-1088].

What storage conditions are needed for this medicine?

Keep this medication in the container it came in, tightly closed, and out of reach of children. Store it at room temperature and away from excess heat and moisture (not in the bathroom). Throw away any medication that is outdated or no longer needed. Talk to your pharmacist about the proper disposal of your medication.

What should I do in case of overdose?

In case of overdose, call your local poison control center at 1-800-222-1222. If the victim has collapsed or is not breathing, call local emergency services at 911.

What other information should I know?

Keep all appointments with your doctor and the laboratory. Your blood pressure should be checked regularly to determine your response to amlopidine and benazepril. Your doctor may order certain lab tests to check your body's response to amlodipine and benazepril.

Do not let anyone else take your medication. Ask your pharmacist any questions you have about refilling your prescription.

Dosage Facts
For Informational Purposes

Caution: Do not change your dose, how often you take your medication, or the length of time you are to take it without first talking to your healthcare provider.

The following dosage information was written using medical language for doctors and other healthcare professionals and is provided here for you to check your dosage. The dosage of this drug may differ for different patients. Therefore, always follow your doctor's instructions or the directions on the label. Contact your healthcare provider or pharmacist if you have any questions about the specific dosage of your medication after reviewing this information.

General Dosage Information

Available as amlodipine besylate; dosage is expressed in terms of amlodipine.

Adult Patients

Hypertension
Amlodipine/Benazepril Combination Therapy

If BP is not adequately controlled by monotherapy with amlodipine or benazepril, can switch to the fixed-combination preparation containing amlodipine 2.5 mg and benazepril 10 mg, or amlodipine 5 mg and benazepril 10 or 20 mg, or, alternatively, amlodipine 10 mg and benazepril 20 mg.

If BP is adequately controlled by monotherapy with amlodipine, but edema has developed, can switch to the fixed-combination preparation containing amlodipine 2.5 mg and benazepril 10 mg, or amlodipine 5 mg and benazepril 10 or 20 mg, or, alternatively, amlodipine 10 mg and benazepril 20 mg.

If BP is controlled with amlodipine and benazepril (administered separately), can switch to the fixed-combination preparation containing the corresponding individual doses for convenience.

Reduce amlodipine dosage in nonblack patients when benazepril is initiated to avoid excessive antihypertensive response.

Adjust dosage of amlodipine/benazepril fixed combination to patient's response; consider that steady-state plasma concentrations of amlodipine and benazepril are reached after 7 and 2 days, respectively.

Amoxapine

(a mox′ a peen)

Important Warning

A small number of children, teenagers, and young adults (up to 24 years of age) who took antidepressants ('mood elevators') such as amoxapine during clinical studies became suicidal (thinking about harming or killing oneself or planning or trying to do so). Children, teenagers, and young adults who take antidepressants to treat depression or other mental illnesses may be more likely to become suicidal than children, teenagers, and young adults who do not take antidepressants to treat these conditions. However, experts are not sure about how great this risk is and how much it should be considered in deciding whether a child or teenager should take an antidepressant. Children younger than 18 years of age should not normally take amoxapine, but in some cases, a doctor may decide that amoxapine is the best medication to treat a child's condition.

You should know that your mental health may change in unexpected ways when you take amox-

continued on next page

Important Warning (cont'd)

apine or other antidepressants even if you are an adult over age 24. You may become suicidal, especially at the beginning of your treatment and any time that your dose is increased or decreased. You, your family, or your caregiver should call your doctor right away if you experience any of the following symptoms: new or worsening depression; thinking about harming or killing yourself, or planning or trying to do so; extreme worry; agitation; panic attacks; difficulty falling asleep or staying asleep; aggressive behavior; irritability; acting without thinking; severe restlessness; and frenzied abnormal excitement. Be sure that your family or caregiver knows which symptoms may be serious so they can call the doctor when you are unable to seek treatment on your own.

Your healthcare provider will want to see you often while you are taking amoxapine, especially at the beginning of your treatment. Be sure to keep all appointments for office visits with your doctor.

The doctor or pharmacist will give you the manufacturer's patient information sheet (Medication Guide) when you begin treatment with amoxapine. Read the information carefully and ask your doctor or pharmacist if you have any questions. You also can obtain the Medication Guide from the FDA website: http://www.fda.gov/cder/drug/antidepressants/antidepressants_MG_2007.pdf.

No matter your age, before you take an antidepressant, you, your parent, or your caregiver should talk to your doctor about the risks and benefits of treating your condition with an antidepressant or with other treatments. You should also talk about the risks and benefits of not treating your condition. You should know that having depression or another mental illness greatly increases the risk that you will become suicidal. This risk is higher if you or anyone in your family has or has ever had bipolar disorder (mood that changes from depressed to abnormally excited) or mania (frenzied, abnormally excited mood) or has thought about or attempted suicide. Talk to your doctor about your condition, symptoms, and personal and family medical history. You and your doctor will decide what type of treatment is right for you.

Why is this medicine prescribed?

Amoxapine is used to treat depression. Amoxapine is in a class of medications called tricyclic antidepressants (TCAs). It works by increasing the amounts of certain natural substances in the brain that are needed to maintain mental balance.

How should this medicine be used?

Amoxapine comes as a tablet to take by mouth. It is usually taken one or more times a day. If you take amoxapine once a day, you should take it at bedtime. Try to take amoxapine at around the same time(s) every day. Follow the directions on your prescription label carefully, and ask your doctor or pharmacist to explain any part you do not understand. Take amoxapine exactly as directed. Do not take more or less of it or take it more often than prescribed by your doctor.

It may take several weeks or longer for you to feel the full effect of amoxapine. Continue to take amoxapine even if you feel well. Do not stop taking amoxapine without talking to your doctor. Your doctor probably will want to decrease your dose gradually.

Are there other uses for this medicine?

This medication may be prescribed for other uses; ask your doctor or pharmacist for more information.

What special precautions should I follow?

Before taking amoxapine,

- tell your doctor and pharmacist if you are allergic to amoxapine, doxepin (Sinequan), any other medications, or any of the inactive ingredients in amoxapine tablets. Ask your doctor or pharmacist for a list of the inactive ingredients.
- tell your doctor if you are taking a monoamine oxidase (MAO) inhibitor such as isocarboxazid (Marplan), phenelzine (Nardil), selegiline (Eldepryl, Emsam, Zelapar), and tranylcypromine (Parnate), or if you have stopped taking an MAO inhibitor within the past 14 days. Your doctor will probably tell you not to take amoxapine. If you stop taking amoxapine, you should wait at least 14 days before you start to take an MAO inhibitor.
- tell your doctor and pharmacist what prescription and nonprescription medications, vitamins, nutritional supplements, and herbal products you are taking or plan to take. Be sure to mention any of the following: anticoagulants (blood thinners) such as warfarin (Coumadin); antihistamines; cimetidine (Tagamet); flecainide (Tambocor); levodopa (Sinemet, Larodopa); lithium (Eskalith, Lithobid); medications for high blood pressure, seizures, Parkinson's disease, asthma, colds, or allergies; methylphenidate (Ritalin); muscle relaxants; propafenone (Rhythmol); quinidine; sedatives; selective serotonin reuptake inhibitors (SSRIs) such as citalopram (Celexa), escitalopram (Lexapro), fluoxetine (Prozac, Sarafem), fluvoxamine (Luvox), paroxetine (Paxil), and sertraline (Zoloft); sleeping pills; thyroid medications; and tranquilizers. Your doctor may need to change the doses of your medications or monitor you more carefully for side effects.
- tell your doctor if you are being treated with electroshock therapy (procedure in which small electric shocks are administered to the brain to treat certain mental illnesses) and if you have or have ever had a heart attack, glaucoma (an eye disease), an enlarged prostate (a male reproductive organ), difficulty urinating, seizures, an overactive thyroid gland, or liver, kidney, or heart disease.
- tell your doctor if you are pregnant, plan to become

pregnant, or are breast-feeding. If you become pregnant while taking amoxapine, call your doctor immediately.

- if you are having surgery, including dental surgery, tell the doctor or dentist that you are taking amoxapine.
- you should know that this medication may make you drowsy. Do not drive a car or operate machinery until you know how this medication affects you.
- remember that alcohol can add to the drowsiness caused by this medication.

What special dietary instructions should I follow?

Unless your doctor tells you otherwise, continue your normal diet.

What should I do if I forget to take a dose?

Take the missed dose as soon as you remember it. However, if it is almost time for the next dose, skip the missed dose and continue your regular dosing schedule. Do not take a double dose to make up for a missed one.

What side effects can this medicine cause?

Amoxapine may cause side effects. Tell your doctor if any of the following symptoms are severe or do not go away:

- nausea
- drowsiness
- weakness or tiredness
- nightmares
- dry mouth
- skin more sensitive to sunlight than usual
- changes in appetite or weight
- constipation
- difficulty urinating
- frequent urination
- blurred vision
- excessive sweating

Some side effects can be serious. If you experience any of the following symptoms or those listed in the IMPORTANT WARNING section, call your doctor immediately:

- muscle stiffness
- confusion
- fast or irregular heartbeat
- slow or difficult speech
- shuffling walk
- uncontrollable shaking or moving of a part of the body
- fever
- rash

If you experience a serious side effect, you or your doctor may send a report to the Food and Drug Administration's (FDA) MedWatch Adverse Event Reporting program online [at http://www.fda.gov/MedWatch/index.html] or by phone [1-800-332-1088].

Amoxapine may cause other side effects. Call your doctor if you have any unusual problems while you are taking this medication.

What storage conditions are needed for this medicine?

Keep this medication in the container it came in, tightly closed, and out of reach of children. Store it at room temperature and away from excess heat and moisture (not in the bathroom). Throw away any medication that is outdated or no longer needed. Talk to your pharmacist about the proper disposal of your medication.

What should I do in case of overdose?

In case of overdose, call your local poison control center at 1-800-222-1222. If the victim has collapsed or is not breathing, call local emergency services at 911.

Symptoms of overdose may include:

- seizures
- coma (loss of consciousness for a period of time)

What other information should I know?

Keep all appointments with your doctor.

Do not let anyone else take your medication. Ask your pharmacist any questions you have about refilling your prescription.

Dosage Facts
For Informational Purposes

Caution: Do not change your dose, how often you take your medication, or the length of time you are to take it without first talking to your healthcare provider.

The following dosage information was written using medical language for doctors and other healthcare professionals and is provided here for you to check your dosage. The dosage of this drug may differ for different patients. Therefore, always follow your doctor's instructions or the directions on the label. Contact your healthcare provider or pharmacist if you have any questions about the specific dosage of your medication after reviewing this information.

Adult Patients

Major Depressive Disorder

ORAL:

- Initially, 100–150 mg daily in 2–3 divided doses.At the end of the first week, if tolerated, may increase to 200–300 mg daily. If no response occurs after ≥2 weeks at 300 mg daily, increase to a maximum of 400 mg daily, as tolerated.
- Usual effective dosage: 200–300 mg daily.
- After symptoms are controlled, dosage should be gradually reduced to the lowest level that will maintain relief of symptoms.
- Hospitalized patients with no history of seizures, refractory to antidepressant therapy, and under close supervision may be increased cautiously up to 600 mg daily in divided doses.

Prescribing Limits

Adult Patients

Major Depressive Disorder

ORAL:
- Outpatients: Maximum 400 mg daily.
- Hospitalized patients: Maximum 600 mg daily.

Special Populations

Hepatic Impairment
- Clearance may be reduced; select dosage with caution in patients with hepatic disease.

Renal Impairment
- No specific dosage recommendations at this time.

Geriatric Patients
- Select dosage with caution, usually starting at a lower dose, because of age-related decreases in hepatic, renal, and/or cardiac function and concomitant disease and drug therapy.
- Initially, 50–75 mg daily in 2–3 divided doses. At the end of the first week, if tolerated, may increase to 100–150 mg daily in 2–3 divided doses. If required, dosage may be increased to a maximum 300 mg daily.

Amoxicillin

(a mox i sil′ in)

Brand Name: Amoxil®, Amoxil® Pediatric Drops, Trimox®, Trimox® Pediatric Drops
Also available generically.

Why is this medicine prescribed?

Amoxicillin is used to treat certain infections caused by bacteria, such as pneumonia; bronchitis; gonorrhea; and infections of the ears, nose, throat, urinary tract, and skin. It is also used in combination with other medications to eliminate *H. pylori*, a bacteria that causes ulcers. Amoxicillin is in a class of medications called penicillin-like antibiotics. It works by stopping the growth of bacteria. Antibiotics will not work for colds, flu, and other viral infections.

How should this medicine be used?

Amoxicillin comes as a capsule, a tablet, a chewable tablet, a suspension (liquid), and pediatric drops to take by mouth. It is usually taken every 12 hours (twice a day) or every 8 hours (three times a day) with or without food. To help you remember to take amoxicillin, take it around the same time every day. Follow the directions on your prescription label carefully, and ask your doctor or pharmacist to explain any part you do not understand. Take amoxicillin exactly as directed. Do not take more or less of it or take it more often than prescribed by your doctor.

Shake the liquid and pediatric drops well before each use to mix the medication evenly. Use the bottle dropper to measure the dose of pediatric drops. The pediatric drops and liquid may be placed on a child's tongue or added to formula, milk, fruit juice, water, ginger ale, or other cold liquid and taken immediately.

The chewable tablets should be crushed or chewed thoroughly before they are swallowed. The tablets and capsules should be swallowed whole and taken with a full glass of water.

Take amoxicillin until you finish the prescription, even if you feel better. Stopping amoxicillin too soon may cause bacteria to become resistant to antibiotics.

Are there other uses for this medicine?

Amoxicillin also is used sometimes to prevent anthrax infection after exposure and to treat anthrax infection of the skin and chlamydia infections during pregnancy. Talk with your doctor about the possible risks of using this medication for your condition.

This medication may be prescribed for other uses; ask your doctor or pharmacist for more information.

What special precautions should I follow?

Before taking amoxicillin,
- tell your doctor and pharmacist if you are allergic to amoxicillin, penicillin, cephalosporins, or any other medications.
- tell your doctor and pharmacist what prescription and nonprescription medications, vitamins, nutritional supplements, and herbal products you are taking. Be sure to mention any of the following: chloramphenicol (Chlormycetin), other antibiotics, and probenecid (Benemid). Your doctor may need to change the doses of your medications or monitor you carefully for side effects.
- tell your doctor if you have or have ever had kidney disease, allergies, asthma, hay fever, hives, or phenylketonuria.
- tell your doctor if you are pregnant, plan to become pregnant, or are breast-feeding. If you become pregnant while taking amoxicillin, call your doctor.

What special dietary instructions should I follow?

Unless your doctor tells you otherwise, continue your normal diet.

What should I do if I forget to take a dose?

Take the missed dose as soon as you remember it. However, if it is almost time for the next dose, skip the missed dose and continue your regular dosing schedule. Do not take a double dose to make up for a missed one.

What side effects can this medicine cause?

Amoxicillin may cause side effects. Tell your doctor if any of these symptoms are severe or do not go away:

- upset stomach
- vomiting
- diarrhea

Some side effects can be serious. The following symptoms are uncommon, but if you experience any of them, call your doctor immediately:

- severe skin rash
- hives
- seizures
- yellowing of the skin or eyes
- unusual bleeding or bruising
- pale skin
- excessive tiredness
- lack of energy

Amoxicillin may cause other side effects. Call your doctor if you have any unusual problems while taking this medication.

If you experience a serious side effect, you or your doctor may send a report to the Food and Drug Administration's (FDA) MedWatch Adverse Event Reporting program online [at http://www.fda.gov/MedWatch/index.html] or by phone [1-800-332-1088].

What storage conditions are needed for this medicine?

Keep this medication in the container it came in, tightly closed, and out of reach of children. Store the capsules and tablets at room temperature and away from excess heat and moisture (not in the bathroom). Throw away any medication that is outdated or no longer needed. The liquid medication preferably should be kept in the refrigerator, but it may be stored at room temperature. Throw away any unused medication after 14 days. Do not freeze. Talk to your pharmacist about the proper disposal of your medication.

What should I do in case of overdose?

In case of overdose, call your local poison control center at 1-800-222-1222. If the victim has collapsed or is not breathing, call local emergency services at 911.

What other information should I know?

Keep all appointments with your doctor and the laboratory. Your doctor may order certain lab tests to check your body's response to amoxicillin.

If you are diabetic, use Clinistix or TesTape (not Clinitest) to test your urine for sugar while taking this medication.

Do not let anyone else take your medication. Your prescription is probably not refillable. If you still have symptoms of infection after you finish the amoxicillin, call your doctor.

Dosage Facts
For Informational Purposes

Caution: Do not change your dose, how often you take your medication, or the length of time you are to take it without first talking to your healthcare provider.

The following dosage information was written using medical language for doctors and other healthcare professionals and is provided here for you to check your dosage. The dosage of this drug may differ for different patients. Therefore, always follow your doctor's instructions or the directions on the label. Contact your healthcare provider or pharmacist if you have any questions about the specific dosage of your medication after reviewing this information.

General Dosage Information

Available as the trihydrate; dosage expressed in terms of anhydrous amoxicillin.

Pediatric Patients

Neonates and infants ≤12 weeks (3 months) of age can receive amoxicillin in a dosage up to 30 mg/kg daily given in divided doses every 12 hours.

Pediatric dosage specified below is for those >3 months of age weighing <40 kg.

Children weighing ≥40 kg should receive usual adult dosage.

Otitis Media
Treatment of Acute Otitis Media (AOM)

ORAL:

- 80–90 mg/kg daily given in 2 or 3 divided doses† recommended by AAP, AAFP, CDC, and others.
- Usual duration is 10 days; optimal duration is uncertain. AAP and AAFP recommend 10 days in those <6 years of age and in those with severe disease and state 5–7 days may be appropriate in those ≥6 years of age with mild to moderate AOM.

Prevention of Recurrent AOM†

ORAL:

- 20 mg/kg daily given in 1 or 2 divided doses has been used.

Pharyngitis and Tonsillitis

ORAL:

- 45 mg/kg daily in 2 divided doses or 40 mg/kg daily in 3 divided doses for 10 days.
- 50 mg/kg once daily or 750 mg once daily for 10 days†.
- Follow-up throat cultures after treatment of pharyngitis and tonsillitis not indicated in asymptomatic patients, but recommended 2–7 days after treatment in those who remain symptomatic, develop recurring symptoms, or have a history of rheumatic fever and are at unusually high risk for recurrence.

Ear, Nose, and Throat Infections

ORAL:

- 25 mg/kg daily in divided doses every 12 hours or 20 mg/kg daily in divided doses every 8 hours for mild to moderate infections per manufacturer.
- 45 mg/kg daily in divided doses every 12 hours or 40 mg/kg in divided doses every 8 hours for severe infections per manufacturer.

Respiratory Tract Infections

ORAL:

- 45 mg/kg daily in divided doses every 12 hours or 40 mg/kg daily in divided doses every 8 hours for mild, moderate, or severe lower respiratory tract infections.

Skin and Skin Structure Infections

ORAL:

- 25 mg/kg daily in divided doses every 12 hours or 20 mg/kg daily in divided doses every 8 hours for mild to moderate infections.
- 45 mg/kg daily in divided doses every 12 hours or 40 mg/kg daily in divided doses every 8 hours for severe infections or those caused by less susceptible bacteria.

Urinary Tract Infections (UTIs)

ORAL:

- 25 mg/kg daily in divided doses every 12 hours or 20 mg/kg daily in divided doses every 8 hours for mild to moderate infections.
- 45 mg/kg daily in divided doses every 12 hours or 40 mg/kg daily in divided doses every 8 hours for severe infections or those caused by less susceptible bacteria.

Gonorrhea

ORAL:

- Prepubertal children ≥2 years of age: 50 mg/kg as a single dose given with a single dose of probenecid (25 mg/kg).
- No longer recommended for gonorrhea by the CDC or other experts.

Lyme Disease

ORAL:

- 25–50 mg/kg daily (up to 2 g daily) in 2–3 divided doses for 14–21 days for treatment of early localized or early disseminated Lyme disease†.
- 50 mg/kg daily in 3 divided doses for 14–28 days for mild Lyme carditis or for 28 days for Lyme arthritis (without associated neurologic disease).

Prevention of Bacterial Endocarditis

Patients Undergoing Certain Dental, Oral, Respiratory Tract, or Esophageal Procedures

ORAL:

- 50 mg/kg given 1 hour prior to the procedure.

Patients Undergoing Certain GU or GI (except Esophageal) Procedures

ORAL:

- 50 mg/kg as a single dose given 1 hour prior to the procedure for moderate-risk patients.
- For high-risk patients, give an initial IM or IV dose of ampicillin with IM or IV gentamicin within 30 minutes of starting the procedure followed by 25 mg/kg of amoxicillin 6 hours later.

Prevention of S. pneumoniae Infections in Asplenic Individuals†

ORAL:

- 20 mg/kg daily in children with anatomic or functional asplenia.
- In infants with sickle cell anemia, initiate prophylaxis as soon as diagnosis is established (preferably by 2 months of age); continue until approximately 5 years of age. Appropriate duration in children with asplenia from other causes unknown; some experts recommend that asplenic children at high risk receive prophylaxis throughout childhood and into adulthood.

Anthrax
Postexposure Prophylaxis

ORAL:

- 80 mg/kg daily (maximum 1.5 g daily) given in divided doses every 8 hours for 60 days for postexposure prophylaxis following exposure to *B. anthracis* spores (inhalational anthrax)†.
- 500 mg every 8 hours for 60 days in those weighing ≥20 kg.
- Use only if penicillin susceptibility is confirmed.

Inhalational Anthrax

ORAL:

- 80 mg/kg daily (maximum 1.5 g daily) given in divided doses every 8 hours for 60 days for treatment of inhalational anthrax in a mass-casualty setting†.
- 500 mg every 8 hours for 60 days for those weighing ≥20 kg.

Cutaneous Anthrax

ORAL:

- 80 mg/kg daily (maximum 1.5 g daily) given in divided doses every 8 hours for treatment of uncomplicated cutaneous anthrax†.
- Treat for 60 days if cutaneous anthrax occurred as the result of exposure to aerosolized anthrax spores; 7–10 days may be adequate if it occurred as the result of natural or endemic exposure to anthrax.

Adult Patients

Pharyngitis and Tonsillitis

ORAL:

- 500 mg 3 times daily or 750 mg once daily† for 10 days.
- Follow-up throat cultures after treatment of pharyngitis and tonsillitis not indicated in asymptomatic patients, but recommended 2–7 days after treatment in those who remain symptomatic, develop recurring symptoms, or have a history of rheumatic fever and are at unusually high risk for recurrence.

Ear, Nose, and Throat Infections

ORAL:

- 500 mg every 12 hours or 250 mg every 8 hours for mild to moderate infections per manufacturer.
- 875 mg every 12 hours or 500 mg every 8 hours for severe infections or those caused by less susceptible bacteria per manufacturer.

Respiratory Tract Infections

ORAL:

- 875 mg every 12 hours or 500 mg every 8 hours for mild, moderate, or severe lower respiratory tract infections.

Skin and Skin Structure Infections

ORAL:

- 500 mg every 12 hours or 250 mg every 8 hours for mild to moderate infections.
- 875 mg every 12 hours or 500 mg every 8 hours for severe infections or those caused by less susceptible bacteria.

Urinary Tract Infections (UTIs)

ORAL:

- 500 mg every 12 hours or 250 mg every 8 hours for mild to moderate infections.
- 875 mg every 12 hours or 500 mg every 8 hours for severe infections or those caused by less susceptible bacteria.

Gonorrhea

ORAL:

- 3 g as a single dose.
- No longer recommended for gonorrhea by the CDC or other experts.

Typhoid Fever

ORAL:

- 100 mg/kg daily or 1–1.5 g every 6 hours for 14 days.

Helicobacter pylori Infection and Duodenal Ulcer Disease

ORAL:

- 1 g 2 times daily for 10 or 14 days given in conjunction with clarithromycin and either lansoprazole or omeprazole (triple therapy).
- 1 g 3 times daily for 14 days given in conjunction with lansoprazole (dual therapy).

Lyme Disease

ORAL:

- 500 mg 3 times daily for 14–21 days for treatment of early localized or early disseminated Lyme disease†.
- 500 mg 3 times daily for 14–28 days for mild Lyme carditis or for 28 days for Lyme arthritis (without associated neurologic disease).

Chlamydial Infections

ORAL:

- 500 mg 3 times daily for 7 days for treatment of chlamydial infections in pregnant women†.
- Repeat testing (preferably by culture) recommended 3 weeks after completion of treatment.

Prevention of Bacterial Endocarditis
Patients Undergoing Certain Dental, Oral, Respiratory Tract, or Esophageal Procedures

ORAL:

- 2 g given 1 hour prior to the procedure.

Patients Undergoing Certain GU or GI (except Esophageal) Procedures

ORAL:

- 2 g given 1 hour prior to the procedure in moderate-risk patients.
- For high-risk patients, give an initial IM or IV dose of ampicillin with IM or IV gentamicin within 30 minutes of starting the procedure followed by 1 g of amoxicillin 6 hours later.

Anthrax
Postexposure Prophylaxis

ORAL:

- 500 mg every 8 hours for 60 days for postexposure prophylaxis following exposure to *B. anthracis* spores†; use only if penicillin susceptibility confirmed.

Inhalational Anthrax

ORAL:

- 500 mg every 8 hours for 60 days for treatment of inhalational anthrax†.

Cutaneous Anthrax

ORAL:

- 500 mg every 8 hours for treatment of inhalational anthrax†.
- Treat for 60 days if cutaneous anthrax occurred as the result of exposure to aerosolized anthrax spores; 7–10 days may be adequate if it occurred as the result of natural or endemic exposure to anthrax.

Prescribing Limits

Pediatric Patients

Neonates and Infants ≤12 weeks (3 Months) of Age

ORAL:

- Maximum 30 mg/kg daily in divided doses every 12 hours.

Prevention of Bacterial Endocarditis

ORAL:

- Dosage should not exceed adult dosage for prevention of bacterial endocarditis.

Special Populations

Renal Impairment

- Dosage adjustment necessary in severe renal impairment.
- Do not use 875-mg tablets in those with severe renal impairment and GFR <30 mL/minute.
- Dosage recommendations not available for pediatric patients with renal impairment.

Dosage for Adults with Renal Impairment

GFR (mL/min)	Daily Dosage
10–30	250 or 500 mg every 12 hours depending on infection severity
<10	250 or 500 mg every 24 hours depending on infection severity
Hemodialysis Patients	250 or 500 mg every 24 hours depending on infection severity; with an additional dose both during and at the end of dialysis

† Use is not currently included in the labeling approved by the US Food and Drug Administration.

Amoxicillin and Clavulanic Acid

(a mox i sil′ in) (klav′ yoo lan ic)

Brand Name: Augmentin ES-600®, Augmentin®, Augmentin® XR
Also available generically.

Why is this medicine prescribed?

The combination of amoxicillin and clavulanic acid is used to treat certain infections caused by bacteria, including infections of the ears, lungs, sinus, skin, and urinary tract. Amoxicillin is in a class of medications called penicillin-like antibiotics. It works by stopping the growth of bacteria. Clavulanic acid is in a class of medications called beta-lactamase inhibitors. It works by preventing bacteria from destroying amoxicillin. Antibiotics will not work for colds, flu, or other viral infections.

How should this medicine be used?

The combination of amoxicillin and clavulanic acid comes as a tablet, a chewable tablet, and a suspension (liquid) to take by mouth. It is usually taken with a meal or a snack every 8 hours (three times a day) or every 12 hours (twice a day). To help you remember to take amoxicillin and clavulanate, take it around the same time every day. Follow the directions on your prescription label carefully, and ask your doctor or pharmacist to explain any part you do not understand. Take amoxicillin and clavulanic acid exactly as directed. Do not take more or less of it or take it more often than prescribed by your doctor.

Shake the liquid well before each use to mix the medication evenly.

The chewable tablets should be chewed thoroughly before they are swallowed. The other tablets should be taken with a full glass of water.

The 250 mg and 500 mg tablets of amoxicillin and clavulanic acid contain the same amount of clavulanic acid. Do not substitute two 250 mg tablets for one 500 mg tablet. The 250 mg regular tablet and the 250 mg chewable tablet contain different amounts of clavulanic acid. They also should not be substituted.

Take amoxicillin and clavulanic acid until you finish the prescription, even if you feel better. Stopping amoxicillin and clavulanic acid too soon may cause bacteria to become resistant to antibiotics.

Are there other uses for this medicine?

Amoxicillin and clavulanic acid also is used sometimes to treat certain sexually transmitted diseases (STD). Talk to your doctor about the possible risks of using this medication for your condition.

This medication may be prescribed for other uses; ask your doctor or pharmacist for more information.

What special precautions should I follow?

Before taking amoxicillin and clavulanic acid,
- tell your doctor and pharmacist if you are allergic to amoxicillin (Amoxil, Trimox, Wymox), clavulanic acid, penicillin, cephalosporins, or any other medications.
- tell your doctor and pharmacist what prescription and nonprescription medications, vitamins, nutritional supplements, and herbal products you are taking. Be sure to mention either of the following: allopurinol (Lopurin, Zyloprim) and probenecid (Benemid). Your doctor may need to change the doses of your medications or monitor you carefully for side effects.
- tell your doctor if you have or have ever had kidney or liver disease, allergies, asthma, hay fever, hives, or mononucleosis.
- you should know that amoxicillin and clavulanic acid may decrease the effectiveness of oral contraceptives (birth control pills). Plan to use another form of birth control while taking amoxicillin and clavulanic acid.
- tell your doctor if you are pregnant, plan to become pregnant, or are breast-feeding. If you become pregnant while taking amoxicillin and clavulanic acid, call your doctor.

What special dietary instructions should I follow?

Unless your doctor tells you otherwise, continue your normal diet.

What should I do if I forget to take a dose?

Take the missed dose as soon as you remember it. However, if it is almost time for the next dose, skip the missed dose and continue your regular dosing schedule. Do not take a double dose to make up for a missed one.

What side effects can this medicine cause?

Amoxicillin and clavulanic acid may cause side effects. Tell your doctor if any of these symptoms are severe or do not go away:
- diarrhea
- upset stomach
- vomiting
- mild skin rash

If you experience any of the following symptoms, call your doctor immediately:
- severe skin rash
- itching
- hives
- difficulty breathing or swallowing
- wheezing
- vaginal itching and discharge
- yellowing of the skin or eyes

Amoxicillin and clavulanic acid may cause other side effects. Call your doctor if you have any unusual problems while taking this medication.

If you experience a serious side effect, you or your doctor may send a report to the Food and Drug Administration's (FDA) MedWatch Adverse Event Reporting program online [at http://www.fda.gov/MedWatch/index.html] or by phone [1-800-332-1088].

What storage conditions are needed for this medicine?

Keep this medication in the container it came in, tightly closed, and out of reach of children. Store the tablets at room temperature and away from excess heat and moisture (not in the bathroom). Throw away any medication that is outdated or no longer needed. Keep liquid medication in the refrigerator, tightly closed, and throw away any unused medication after 10 days. Do not freeze. Talk to your pharmacist about the proper disposal of your medication.

What should I do in case of overdose?

In case of overdose, call your local poison control center at 1-800-222-1222. If the victim has collapsed or is not breathing, call local emergency services at 911.

Symptoms of overdose may include:
- stomach pain
- vomiting
- diarrhea
- rash
- hyperactivity
- drowsiness

What other information should I know?

Keep all appointments with your doctor and the laboratory. Your doctor may order certain lab tests to check your body's response to amoxicillin and clavulanic acid.

If you are diabetic, use Clinistix or TesTape (not Clinitest) to test your urine for sugar while taking this medication.

Do not let anyone else take your medication. Your prescription is probably not refillable. If you still have symptoms of infection after you finish the amoxicillin and clavulanic acid, call your doctor.

Dosage Facts
For Informational Purposes

Caution: Do not change your dose, how often you take your medication, or the length of time you are to take it without first talking to your healthcare provider.

The following dosage information was written using medical language for doctors and other healthcare professionals and is provided here for you to check your dosage. The dosage of this drug may differ for different patients. Therefore, always follow your doctor's instructions or the directions on the label. Contact your healthcare provider or pharmacist if you have any questions about the specific dosage of your medication after reviewing this information.

General Dosage Information

Available as fixed combination containing amoxicillin and clavulanate potassium; dosage expressed in terms of amoxicillin.

Not all preparations of amoxicillin and clavulanate are interchangeable since they contain different amounts of clavulanic acid.

Powders for oral suspension contain a 4:1, 7:1, or 14:1 ratio of amoxicillin to clavulanic acid; chewable tablets contain a 4:1 or 7:1 ratio of the drugs; film-coated tablets contain a 2:1 or 4:1 ratio of the drugs; scored tablets contain a 7:1 ratio of the drugs; and extended-release tablets contain a 16:1 ratio of the drugs.

Pediatric Patients

Children weighing <40 kg should *not* receive film-coated tablets containing 250 mg of amoxicillin since this preparation contains a high dose of clavulanic acid.

The oral suspension containing 125 mg of amoxicillin/5 mL is the only preparation recommended for use in neonates and infants <12 weeks (3 months) of age.

Acute Otitis Media (AOM)
AOM in Neonates and Infants <12 Weeks (3 Months) of Age

ORAL:
- Oral suspension: Manufacturer recommends 30 mg/kg daily given in divided doses every 12 hours for 10 days using the oral suspension containing 125 mg/5 mL.

AOM in Children ≥12 Weeks of Age Weighing <40 kg

ORAL:
- Oral suspension: Manufacturer recommends 45 mg/kg daily given in divided doses every 12 hours for 10 days using the suspension containing 200 or 400 mg/5 mL; alternatively, 40 mg/kg daily given in divided doses every 8 hours using the suspension containing 125 or 250 mg/5 mL.
- Chewable tablets: Manufacturer recommends 45 mg/kg daily given in divided doses every 12 hours for 10 days using the chewable tablets containing 200 or 400 mg; alternatively, 40 mg/kg daily given in divided doses every 8 hours using chewable tablets containing 125 or 250 mg.

AOM in Children Weighing ≥40 kg

ORAL:
- Film-coated tablets: Manufacturer recommends one 250-mg tablet every 8 hours or one 500-mg tablet every 12 hours for 10 days.
- Oral suspension: Manufacturer recommends 500 mg every 12 hours for 10 days using the suspension containing 125 or 250 mg/5 mL.

AOM with Severe Illness or When β-Lactamase-producing Strains are Suspected

ORAL:
- 90 mg/kg daily given in divided doses every 12 hours recommended by AAP and AAFP.

- Usual duration is 10 days; optimal duration is uncertain. AAP and AAFP recommend 10 days in those <6 years of age and in those with severe disease and state 5–7 days may be appropriate in those ≥6 years of age with mild to moderate AOM.

AOM that Failed to Respond to Amoxicillin

ORAL:

- 90 mg/kg daily given in divided doses every 12 hours recommended by AAP and AAFP.
- Usual duration is 10 days; optimal duration is uncertain. AAP and AAFP recommend 10 days in those <6 years of age and in those with severe disease and state 5–7 days may be appropriate in those ≥6 years of age with mild to moderate AOM.

Persistent or Recurrent AOM
Infections in Children ≥3 Months of Age Weighing <40 kg

ORAL:

- Oral suspension: Manufacturer recommends 90 mg/kg daily given in divided doses every 12 hours for 10 days using the suspension containing 600 mg/5 mL.

Pediatric Dosage of Oral Suspension Containing 600 mg/5 mL (Augmentin ES-600®) for Persistent or Recurrent AOM

Weight (kg)	Volume of Suspension to Provide 90 mg/kg daily
8	3 mL twice daily
12	4.5 mL twice daily
16	6 mL twice daily
20	7.5 mL twice daily
24	9 mL twice daily
28	10.5 mL twice daily
32	12 mL twice daily
36	13.5 mL twice daily

Pharyngitis and Tonsillitis

ORAL:

- 40 mg/kg daily (up to 750 mg daily) in 3 divided doses for 10 days for treatment of multiple, recurrent episodes of pharyngitis known to be caused by *S. pyogenes*†.

Respiratory Tract Infections
Infections in Neonates and Infants <12 weeks (3 months) of Age

ORAL:

- Oral suspension: 30 mg/kg daily given in divided doses every 12 hours using the suspension containing 125 mg/5 mL.

Infections in Children ≥12 Weeks of Age Weighing <40 kg

ORAL:

- Oral suspension: 45 mg/kg daily given in divided doses every 12 hours using the suspension containing 200 or 400 mg/5 mL; alternatively, 40 mg/kg daily given in divided doses every 8 hours using the suspension containing 125 or 250 mg/5 mL.

- Chewable tablets: 45 mg/kg daily given in divided doses every 12 hours using chewable tablets containing 200 or 400 mg; alternatively, 40 mg/kg daily given in divided doses every 8 hours using chewable tablets containing 125 or 250 mg.

Infections in Children Weighing ≥40 kg

ORAL:

- Film-coated or scored tablets: One 500-mg tablet every 8 hours or one 875-mg tablet every 12 hours.
- Oral suspension: 500 mg every 8 hours using the suspension containing 125 or 250 mg/5 mL or 875 mg every 12 hours using the suspension containing 200 or 400 mg/5 mL.

Skin and Skin Structure Infections
Infections in Neonates and Infants <12 Weeks (3 Months) of Age

ORAL:

- Oral suspension: 30 mg/kg daily in divided doses every 12 hours using the suspension containing 125 mg/5 mL.

Infections in Children ≥12 Weeks of Age Weighing <40 kg

ORAL:

- Oral suspension: 25 mg/kg daily in divided doses every 12 hours using the suspension containing 200 or 400 mg/5 mL; alternatively, 20 mg/kg daily in divided doses every 8 hours using the suspension containing 125 or 250 mg/5 mL. For severe infections, 45 mg/kg daily in divided doses every 12 hours using the suspension containing 200 or 400 mg/5 mL; alternatively, 40 mg/kg daily in divided doses every 8 hours using the suspension containing 125 or 250 mg/5 mL.
- Chewable tablets: 25 mg/kg daily in divided doses every 12 hours using chewable tablets containing 200 or 400 mg. For severe infections, 45 mg/kg daily given in divided doses every 12 hours using chewable tablets containing 200 or 400 mg.

Infections in Children Weighing ≥40 kg

ORAL:

- Film-coated or scored tablets: One 250-mg tablet every 8 hours or one 500-mg tablet every 12 hours. For severe infections, one 500-mg tablet every 8 hours or one 875-mg tablet every 12 hours.
- Oral suspension: 500 mg every 12 hours using the suspension containing 125 or 250 mg/5 mL.

Urinary Tract Infections (UTIs)
Infections in Neonates and Infants <12 Weeks (3 Months) of Age

ORAL:

- Oral suspension: 30 mg/kg daily in divided doses every 12 hours using the suspension containing 125 mg/5 mL.

Infections in Children ≥12 Weeks of Age Weighing <40 kg

ORAL:

- Oral suspension: 25 mg/kg daily in divided doses every 12 hours using the suspension containing 200 or 400 mg/5 mL; alternatively, 20 mg/kg daily in divided doses every 8 hours using the suspension containing 125 or 250 mg/5 mL. For severe infections, 45 mg/kg daily in divided doses every 12 hours using the suspension containing 200 or 400 mg/5 mL;

alternatively, 40 mg/kg daily in divided doses every 8 hours using the suspension containing 125 or 250 mg/5 mL.
- Chewable tablets: 25 mg/kg daily in divided doses every 12 hours using chewable tablets containing 200 or 400 mg. For severe infections, 45 mg/kg daily given in divided doses every 12 hours using chewable tablets containing 200 or 400 mg.

Infections in Children Weighing ≥40 kg

ORAL:
- Film-coated or scored tablets: One 250-mg tablet every 8 hours or one 500-mg tablet every 12 hours. For severe infections, one 500-mg tablet every 8 hours or one 875-mg tablet every 12 hours.
- Oral suspension: 500 mg every 12 hours using the suspension containing 125 or 250 mg/5 mL.

Adult Patients

Respiratory Tract Infections

ORAL:
- Scored tablets: one 875-mg-tablet every 12 hours.
- Oral suspension: 875 mg every 12 hours using the suspension containing 200 or 400 mg/5 mL.

Community-acquired Pneumonia

ORAL:
- Extended-release tablets: Two 1-g tablets every 12 hours for 7–10 days.

Sinusitis

ORAL:
- Extended-release tablets: Two 1-g tablets every 12 hours for 10 days.

Acute Otitis Media (AOM)

ORAL:
- Film-coated tablets: One 500-mg tablet every 12 hours or one 250-mg tablet every 8 hours. For severe infections, one 875-mg tablet every 12 hours or one 500-mg tablet every 8 hours.
- Oral suspension: 500 mg every 12 hours using the suspension containing 125 or 250 mg/5 mL. For severe infections, 875 mg every 12 hours using the suspension containing 200 or 400 mg/5 mL.

Pharyngitis and Tonsillitis

ORAL:
- 500 mg twice daily for 10 days for treatment of multiple, recurrent episodes of pharyngitis known to be caused by *S. pyogenes*†. Adult dosage was extrapolated from pediatric dosage and has not been evaluated in clinical studies.

Skin and Skin Structure Infections

ORAL:
- Film-coated or scored tablets: One 500-mg tablet every 12 hours or one 250-mg tablet every 8 hours. For severe infections, one 875 mg-tablet every 12 hours or one 500-mg tablet every 8 hours.
- Oral suspension: 500 mg every 12 hours using the suspension containing 125 or 250 mg/5 mL. For severe infections, 875 mg every 12 hours using the suspension containing 200 or 400 mg/5 mL.

Urinary Tract Infections (UTIs)

ORAL:
- Film-coated or scored tablets: One 500-mg tablet every 12 hours or one 250-mg tablet every 8 hours. For severe infections, one 875-mg tablet every 12 hours or one 500-mg tablet every 8 hours.
- Oral suspension: 500 mg every 12 hours using the suspension containing 125 or 250 mg/5 mL. For severe infections, 875 mg every 12 hours using the suspension containing 200 or 400 mg/5 mL.

Special Populations

Hepatic Impairment
- Select dosage with caution and monitor hepatic function.

Renal Impairment
- Dosage adjustment necessary in patients with moderate to severe renal impairment.
- Do *not* use scored tablets containing 875 mg of amoxicillin in those with severe renal impairment and GFR <30 mL/ minute.
- Do *not* use extended-release tablets containing 1 g of amoxicillin in those with Cl_{cr} <30 mL/minute or in hemodialysis patients.

Dosage of Film-coated Tablets for Adults with Renal Impairment

GFR (mL/min)	Daily Dosage
10–30	250 or 500 mg every 12 hours depending on infection severity
<10	250 or 500 mg every 24 hours depending on infection severity
Hemodialysis Patients	250 or 500 mg every 24 hours depending on infection severity; with an additional dose both during and at the end of dialysis

Geriatric Patients
- No dosage adjustments except those related to renal impairment.

† *Use is not currently included in the labeling approved by the US Food and Drug Administration.*

Amphotericin B Injection

(am foe ter′ i sin)

Brand Name: Amphocin®, Fungizone® Intravenous

Also available generically.

Important Warning

Amphotericin B can cause serious side effects. This medication should only be used for the treatment of potentially life-threatening fungal infections and not to treat less serious fungal infections of the mouth, throat, or vagina in patients with a normal immune system (body's natural protection against infection).

About Your Treatment

Your doctor has ordered amphotericin B, an antifungal medication, to help treat your infection. It will be added to an intravenous fluid that will drip for about 2-6 hours through a needle or catheter placed in your vein once a day or once every other day.

Amphotericin B is used to kill fungus that can cause serious or life-threatening infections. Amphotericin B is not effective against bacterial infections or viruses. This medication is sometimes prescribed for other uses; ask your doctor or pharmacist for more information.

Your health care provider (doctor, nurse, or pharmacist) may measure the effectiveness and side effects of your treatment using laboratory tests and physical examinations. It is important to keep all appointments with your doctor and the laboratory. The length of treatment depends on how your infection and symptoms respond to the medication.

Precautions

Before administering amphotericin B,

- tell your doctor and pharmacist if you are allergic to amphotericin B, any other medications, or any of the ingredients in amphotericin B. Ask your health care provider for a list of the ingredients.
- tell your doctor and pharmacist what prescription and nonprescription medications, vitamins, nutritional supplements, and herbal products you are taking or plan to take. Be sure to mention any of the following: aminoglycoside antibiotics such as amikacin (Amikin), gentamicin (Garamycin), kanamycin (Kantrex), neomycin (Nes-RX, Neo-Fradin), paromomycin (Humatin), streptomycin, and tobramycin (Tobi, Nebcin); certain antifungals such as clotrimazole, fluconazole, itraconazole (Sporanox), ketoconazole, and miconazole; corticotropin (ACTH, H.P., Acthar Gel); cyclosporine (Neoral,

Sandimmune); digoxin (Digitek, Lanoxicaps, Lanoxin); flucytosine (Ancobon); medications for the treatment of cancer, such as nitrogen mustard; oral steroids such as dexamethasone (Decadron, Dexone), methylprednisolone (Medrol), and prednisone (Deltasone); and pentamidine (NebuPent, Pentam 300).
- tell your doctor if you are receiving transfusions or having radiation treatments. Also tell your doctor if you have or have ever had diabetes, or heart or kidney disease.
- tell your doctor if you are pregnant, or plan to become pregnant. If you become pregnant while taking amphotericin B, call your doctor.
- Do not breastfeed if you are taking amphotericin B.
- if you are having surgery, including dental surgery, tell the doctor or dentist that you are taking amphotericin B.

Administering Your Medication

Before you administer amphotericin B, look at the solution closely. It should be clear and free of floating material. Gently squeeze the bag or observe the solution container to make sure there are no leaks. Do not use the solution if it is discolored, if it contains particles, or if the bag or container leaks. Use a new solution, but show the damaged one to your health care provider. Protect the solution from light during administration.

It is important that you use amphotericin B exactly as directed. Do not stop your therapy on your own for any reason because your infection could worsen and result in hospitalization. Do not change your dosing schedule without talking to your health care provider. If your therapy is stopped for longer than one week for any reason, call your health care provider. If your infusion is restarted, it probably will be restarted at a lower dose. Your health care provider may tell you to stop your infusion if you have a mechanical problem (such as a blockage in the tubing, needle, or catheter); if you have to stop an infusion, call your health care provider immediately so your therapy can continue.

Side Effects

Amphotericin B may cause side effects. Some side effects are more severe and more common with the first few doses of amphotericin B. Your health care provider may prescribe other medications to decrease these side effects, or tell you to administer amphotericin B every other day. If you have never experienced any of the following side effects from previous doses and suddenly have symptoms, stop your infusion and call your health care provider immediately.

- fever
- chills
- fast breathing
- headache
- changes in heart beat
- dizziness
- fainting

- blurred vision
- nausea
- vomiting
- loss of appetite

Tell your health care provider if any of these symptoms are severe or do not go away:

- pale skin
- flushing
- tiredness
- diarrhea
- stomach cramping
- heartburn
- muscle or joint pain
- weight loss
- ringing in the ears
- hearing loss
- pain, burning, numbness, or tingling in the hands or feet

If you experience any of the following symptoms, call your health care provider immediately:

- rash
- itching
- hives
- difficulty breathing or swallowing
- wheezing
- confusion
- loss of responsiveness or consciousness
- seizures
- decreased urination
- change in heartbeat
- pain in the upper right part of the stomach
- extreme tiredness
- unusual bleeding or bruising
- black and tarry stools
- red blood in stools
- bloody vomit
- vomiting material that looks like coffee grounds
- lack of energy
- yellowing of the skin or eyes
- changes in vision
- flu-like symptoms
- sore throat, chills, cough, and other signs of infection

If you experience a serious side effect, you or your doctor may send a report to the Food and Drug Administration's (FDA) MedWatch Adverse Event Reporting program online [at http://www.fda.gov/MedWatch/index.html] or by phone [1-800-332-1088].

Storage Conditions

Talk to your health care provider about how you should store your medication. Your health care provider will probably tell you to store your medication in the refrigerator and to protect this solution from light. Your health care provider will tell you when and how you should throw away any unused medication and will probably mark this date on the medication container. Ask your health care provider if you do not understand the directions or you have any questions.

Keep your supplies in a clean, dry place when you are not using them, and keep all medications and supplies out of reach of children. Your health care provider will tell you how to throw away used needles, syringes, tubing, and containers to avoid accidental injury and to properly dispose of medical waste.

Overdose

In case of overdose, call your local poison control center at 1-800-222-1222. If the victim has collapsed or is not breathing, call local emergency services at 911.

Signs of Infection

If you are receiving amphotericin B in your vein or under your skin, you need to know the symptoms of a catheter-related infection (an infection where the needle enters your vein or skin). If you experience any of these effects near your intravenous catheter, tell your health care provider as soon as possible:

- tenderness
- warmth
- irritation
- drainage
- redness
- swelling
- pain

Dosage Facts
For Informational Purposes

Caution: Do not change your dose, how often you take your medication, or the length of time you are to take it without first talking to your healthcare provider.

The following dosage information was written using medical language for doctors and other healthcare professionals and is provided here for you to check your dosage. The dosage of this drug may differ for different patients. Therefore, always follow your doctor's instructions or the directions on the label. Contact your healthcare provider or pharmacist if you have any questions about the specific dosage of your medication after reviewing this information.

General Dosage Information

Available as conventional amphotericin B (formulated with sodium deoxycholate), amphotericin B cholesteryl sulfate complex, amphotericin B lipid complex, or amphotericin B liposomal; dosage is expressed as amphotericin B.

Dosage varies depending on whether the drug is administered as conventional amphotericin B or as amphotericin B cholesteryl sulfate complex, amphotericin B lipid complex, or amphotericin B liposomal. Dosage recommendations for the specific formulation being administered should be followed.

Prior to initiation of conventional IV amphotericin B therapy, a single test dose of the drug (1 mg in 20 mL of 5% dextrose injection) should be administered IV over 20–30 minutes and the patient carefully monitored (i.e., pulse and respiration rate, temperature, blood pressure) every 30 minutes for 2 hours. In patients with good cardiorenal function who tolerate the test dose, therapy may be initiated with a daily dosage of 0.25 mg/kg (0.3 mg/kg in those with severe or rapidly progressing fungal infections) given as a single daily dose. In patients with impaired cardiorenal function and in patients who have severe reactions to the test dose, therapy should be initiated with a smaller daily dosage (i.e., 5–10 mg). Depending on patient's cardiorenal status, dosage may gradually be increased by 5–10 mg daily to a final daily dosage of 0.5–0.7 mg/kg. Some clinicians suggest that higher initial IV dosages of conventional amphotericin B can be used and generally are necessary when initiating therapy in patients with severe, life-threatening infections.

Pediatric Patients

General Pediatric Dosage
Treatment of Invasive Fungal Infections

IV:
- Amphotericin B lipid complex: 5 mg/kg once daily.

Aspergillosis
Treatment of Aspergillosis

IV:
- Amphotericin B cholesteryl sulfate complex: 3–4 mg/kg once daily.
- Amphotericin B lipid complex: 5 mg/kg once daily. Median duration has been 25 days.
- Amphotericin B liposomal: 3–5 mg/kg once daily in children ≥1 month of age. Median duration has been 15–29 days.

Candida Infections
Treatment of Disseminated or Invasive Candida Infections

IV:
- Conventional amphotericin B: 0.4–0.6 mg/kg daily; higher dosage (i.e., 1 mg/kg daily or, rarely, 1.5 mg/kg daily) has been used for treatment of candidemia or rapidly progressing, potentially fatal infections. While 7–14 days may be adequate for non-life-threatening candidiasis in low-risk patients, more prolonged therapy (i.e., 6 weeks or longer) may be necessary in those at high-risk for morbidity and mortality.
- Amphotericin B lipid complex: 5 mg/kg once daily.
- Amphotericin B liposomal: 3–5 mg/kg once daily in children ≥1 month of age. Median duration has been 15–29 days; some candidal infections have been effectively treated with a median duration of 5–7 days.

Coccidioidomycosis
Prevention of Recurrence (Secondary Prophylaxis) of Coccidioidomycosis†

IV:
- Conventional amphotericin B: 1 mg/kg once weekly in HIV-infected infants, children, and adolescents. Initiate secondary prophylaxis after primary infection has been adequately treated.
- HIV-infected infants, children, and adolescents with a history of coccidioidomycosis should receive life-long suppressive therapy to prevent recurrence. The safety of discontinuing secondary prophylaxis in those receiving potent antiretroviral therapy has not been extensively studied.

Cryptococcosis
Treatment of Cryptococcosis

IV:
- Amphotericin B lipid complex: 5 mg/kg once daily.
- Amphotericin B liposomal: 3–5 mg/kg once daily in children ≥ 1 month of age.

Treatment of Cryptococcal Meningitis

IV:
- Amphotericin B liposomal: 6 mg/kg once daily in children ≥1 month of age.

Prevention of Recurrence (Secondary Prophylaxis) of Cryptococcosis†

IV:
- Conventional amphotericin B: 0.5–1 mg/kg 1–3 times weekly in HIV-infected infants, children, and adolescents. Initiate secondary prophylaxis after primary infection has been adequately treated.
- HIV-infected infants and children with a history of cryptococcosis should receive life-long suppressive therapy to prevent recurrence. The safety of discontinuing secondary prophylaxis in those receiving potent antiretroviral therapy has not been extensively studied. Consideration can be given to discontinuing secondary prophylaxis in HIV-infected adolescents according to recommendations in adults.

Histoplasmosis
Prevention of Recurrence (Secondary Prophylaxis) of Histoplasmosis†

IV:
- Conventional amphotericin B: 1 mg/kg once weekly in HIV-infected infants, children, and adolescents. Initiate secondary prophylaxis after primary infection has been adequately treated.
- HIV-infected infants, children, or adolescents with a history of histoplasmosis should receive life-long suppressive therapy to prevent recurrence. The safety of discontinuing secondary prophylaxis in those receiving potent antiretroviral therapy has not been extensively studied.

Leishmaniasis
Treatment of Cutaneous and Mucocutaneous Leishmaniasis

IV:
- Conventional amphotericin B: 0.25–0.5 mg/kg daily initially. Gradually increase dosage until 0.5–1 mg/kg daily is reached, at which time the drug usually is given on alternate days.
- Duration of therapy depends on severity of disease and response to the drug, but generally is 3–12 weeks. Total dose generally ranges from 1–3 g; mucocutaneous disease usually requires a higher total dose than cutaneous disease.

Treatment of Visceral Leishmaniasis (Kala-Azar)†

IV:
- Conventional amphotericin B†: 0.5–1 mg/kg administered on alternate days for 14–20 doses.
- Amphotericin B liposomal: 3 mg/kg once daily on days 1–5 and on days 14 and 21 in children ≥1 month of age; a second course of the drug may be useful if the infection is not completely cleared with a single course. For treatment of visceral leishmaniasis in immunocompromised children ≥1 month of age, dosage is 4 mg/kg once daily on days 1–5 and on days 10, 17, 24, 31, and 38; if the parasitic infection is not com-

pletely cleared after the first course or if relapses occur, an expert should be consulted regarding further treatment.

Primary Amebic Meningoencephalitis†
Treatment of Naegleria Infections†

IV:

• Conventional amphotericin B: 1 mg/kg daily. Optimal duration not determined.

Adult Patients

Aspergillosis
Treatment of Aspergillosis

IV:

• Conventional amphotericin B: 0.5–0.6 mg/kg daily. Higher dosage (i.e., 1 mg/kg daily or, rarely, 1.5 mg/kg daily) may be necessary in neutropenic patients or for treatment of rapidly progressing, potentially fatal infections. Optimal duration of therapy is uncertain; total doses of 1.5–4 g have been given over an 11-month period.
• Amphotericin B cholesteryl sulfate complex: 3–4 mg/kg once daily.
• Amphotericin B lipid complex: 5 mg/kg once daily. Median duration has been 25 days.
• Amphotericin B liposomal: 3–5 mg/kg once daily. Median duration has been 15–29 days.

Blastomycosis
Treatment of Blastomycosis

IV:

• Conventional amphotericin B: 0.5–1 mg/kg daily.

Candida Infections
Treatment of Disseminated or Invasive Candida Infections

IV:

• Conventional amphotericin B: 0.4–0.6 mg/kg daily; higher dosage (i.e., 1 mg/kg daily or, rarely, 1.5 mg/kg daily) has been used for treatment of candidemia or rapidly progressing, potentially fatal infections. While 7–14 days may be adequate for non-life-threatening candidiasis in low-risk patients, more prolonged therapy (i.e., 6 weeks or longer) may be necessary in those at high-risk for morbidity and mortality.
• Amphotericin B cholesteryl sulfate complex†: 3–6 mg/kg once daily. Dosages up to 7.5 mg/kg have been used in BMT patients.
• Amphotericin B lipid complex: 5 mg/kg once daily.
• Amphotericin B liposomal: 3–5 mg/kg once daily. Median duration has been 15–29 days; some candidal infections were effectively treated with a median duration of 5–7 days.

Treatment of Chronic Disseminated (Heptatosplenic) Candida Infections

IV:

• Conventional amphotericin B: 1 mg/kg daily in conjunction with oral flucytosine (100 mg/kg daily) has been used.

Treatment of Severe or Refractory Esophageal Candidiasis

IV:

• Conventional amphotericin B: 0.3 mg/kg daily for at least 5–7 days has been recommended for HIV-infected patients.

Treatment of Candiduria

IV:

• Conventional amphotericin B: 0.3 mg/kg daily given for 3–5 days.

Coccidioidomycosis
Treatment of Coccidioidomycosis

IV:

• Conventional amphotericin B: 0.5–1 mg/kg daily. Higher dosage (i.e., up to 1.5 mg/kg daily) has been used for treatment of rapidly progressing, potentially fatal infections. Duration depends on clinical response, but usually ranges from 4–12 weeks.

Prevention of Recurrence (Secondary Prophylaxis) of Coccidioidomycosis†

IV:

• Conventional amphotericin B: 1 mg/kg once weekly. Initiate secondary prophylaxis after primary infection has been adequately treated.
• HIV-infected adults with a history of coccidioidomycosis should receive life-long suppressive therapy to prevent recurrence. Although those who respond to potent antiretroviral therapy with increases in CD4+ T-cell counts to >100/mm³ may be at low risk for recurrence of fungal infections, data are insufficient to date to warrant a recommendation regarding discontinuance of secondary prophylaxis against coccidioidomycosis.

Cryptococcosis
Treatment of Cryptococcosis

IV:

• Conventional amphotericin B: 0.3–1 mg/kg daily (with or without oral flucytosine). Duration is determined by clinical response, but usually ranges from a minimum of 2–4 weeks up to several months.
• Amphotericin B cholesteryl sulfate complex†: 3–6 mg/kg once daily. Dosages up to 7.5 mg/kg have been used in BMT patients.
• Amphotericin B lipid complex: 5 mg/kg once daily.
• Amphotericin B liposomal: 3–5 mg/kg once daily.

Treatment of Cryptococcal Meningitis

IV:

• Conventional amphotericin B: 0.7 mg/kg daily for 4 weeks followed by 0.7 mg/kg given on alternate days for an additional 4 weeks has been used in HIV-infected patients. Alternatively, many clinicians recommend 0.7 mg/kg daily given in conjunction with oral flucytosine (100 mg/kg daily) for at least 2 weeks (or until the patient has stabilized) followed by 8–10 weeks of oral fluconazole (400 mg daily) or oral itraconazole (400 mg daily).
• Amphotericin B lipid complex: 5 mg/kg once daily for 6 weeks followed by 12 weeks of oral fluconazole.
• Amphotericin B liposomal: 6 mg/kg once daily.

Prevention of Recurrence (Secondary Prophylaxis) of Cryptococcosis†

IV:

• Conventional amphotericin B: 0.6–1 mg/kg 1–3 times weekly. Initiate secondary prophylaxis after the primary infection has been adequately treated.
• Consideration can be given to discontinuing secondary prophylaxis in HIV-infected adults who have successfully completed initial therapy for cryptococcosis, remain asymptomatic with respect to cryptococcosis, and have sustained (e.g., for ≥6 months) increases in CD4+ T-cell counts to >100–200/mm³ in response to potent antiretroviral therapy.

- Reinitiate secondary prophylaxis against cryptococcosis if CD4+ T-cell count decreases to <100–200/mm³.

Histoplasmosis
Treatment of Histoplasmosis

IV:
- Conventional amphotericin B: 0.5–0.6 mg/kg daily given for ≥4–8 weeks. Higher dosage (i.e., 0.7–1 mg/kg daily or, rarely, 1.5 mg/kg daily) has been recommended and may be necessary for treatment of rapidly progressing, potentially fatal infections. For HIV-infected patients, some clinicians recommend a dosage of 50 mg daily (1 mg/kg in individuals weighing less than 50 kg) for 2 weeks followed by the same dosage given on alternate days until a cumulative dose of 15 mg/kg is reached.

Prevention of Recurrence (Secondary Prophylaxis) of Histoplasmosis†

IV:
- Conventional amphotericin B: 1 mg/kg once weekly. Initiate after primary infection has been adequately treated.
- HIV-infected adults with a history of histoplasmosis should receive life-long suppressive therapy to prevent recurrence. Although those who respond to potent antiretroviral therapy with increases in CD4+ T-cell counts to >100/mm³ may be at low risk for recurrence of fungal infections, data are insufficient to date to warrant a recommendation regarding discontinuance of secondary prophylaxis against histoplasmosis.

Paracoccidioidomycosis†
Treatment of Paracoccidioidomycosis†

IV:
- Conventional amphotericin B: 0.4–0.5 mg/kg daily, although higher dosage (i.e., 1 mg/kg daily or, rarely, 1.5 mg/kg daily) has been used for treatment of rapidly progressing, potentially fatal infections. Prolonged therapy usually is required.

Sporotrichosis
Treatment of Sporotrichosis

IV:
- Conventional amphotericin B: 0.4–0.5 mg/kg daily for 2–3 months. Has been given for up to 9 months to provide a total dose of up to 2.5 g.
- Prolonged therapy with total IV doses of at least 2 g (alone or combined with intrathecal† therapy) have been given for the treatment of meningeal sporotrichosis in a limited number of patients.

Zygomycosis
Treatment of Zygomycosis

IV:
- Conventional amphotericin B: 1–1.5 mg/kg daily for 2–3 months. A total IV dose of 3–4 g is recommended for treatment of rhinocerebral phycomycosis; concomitant therapy has included irrigation† of the sinus cavities with a suspension of 1 mg/mL.
- Amphotericin B lipid complex: 5 mg/kg once daily.

Empiric Therapy in Febrile Neutropenic Patients

IV:
- Amphotericin B liposomal: 3 mg/kg once daily.

Prevention of Fungal Infections in Transplant or Cancer Patients†

IV:
- Conventional amphotericin B: 0.1–0.25 mg/kg daily.
- Amphotericin B liposomal: 2 mg/kg 3 times weekly.

Leishmaniasis
Cutaneous and Mucocutaneous Leishmaniasis

IV:
- Conventional amphotericin B: 0.25–0.5 mg/kg daily initially. Gradually increase dosage until 0.5–1 mg/kg daily is reached, at which time the drug usually is given on alternate days.
- Duration depends on the severity of disease and response to the drug, but generally is 3–12 weeks. Total dose generally ranges from 1–3 g; mucocutaneous disease usually requires a higher total dose than cutaneous disease.

Visceral Leishmaniasis (Kala-Azar)†

IV:
- Conventional amphotericin B†: 0.5–1 mg/kg administered on alternate days for 14–20 doses.
- Amphotericin B cholesteryl sulfate complex†: 2 mg/kg once daily for 7–10 days.
- Amphotericin B lipid complex†: 1–3 mg/kg once daily for 5 days has been used in patients who failed to respond to or relapsed after treatment with an antimony compound.
- Amphotericin B liposomal: 3 mg/kg once daily on days 1–5 and on days 14 and 21; a second course of the drug may be useful if the infection is not completely cleared with a single course. For treatment of visceral leishmaniasis in immunocompromised patients, 4 mg/kg once daily on days 1–5 and on days 10, 17, 24, 31, and 38; if the parasitic infection is not completely cleared after the first course or if relapses occur, an expert should be consulted regarding further treatment.

Primary Amebic Meningoencephalitis†
Naegleria Infections†

IV:
- Conventional amphotericin B: 1 mg/kg daily. Optimal duration not determined.

Prescribing Limits

Pediatric Patients

IV:
- Conventional amphotericin B: use lowest effective dose.

Adult Patients

IV:
- Conventional amphotericin B: daily dosage should not exceed 1.5 mg/kg.

† Use is not currently included in the labeling approved by the US Food and Drug Administration.

Amphotericin B Lipid Complex Injection

(am foe ter' I sin)

Brand Name: Abelcet®
Also available generically.

About Your Treatment

Your doctor has ordered amphotericin B lipid complex, an antifungal medication, to help treat your infection. It will be added to an intravenous fluid that will drip through a needle or catheter placed in your vein for several hours, once a day.

Amphotericin B lipid complex is used to kill some types of fungus that can cause serious and life-threatening infections. Amphotericin B lipid complex is not effective against bacterial infections or viruses. This medication is sometimes prescribed for other uses; ask your doctor or pharmacist for more information.

Your health care provider (doctor, nurse, or pharmacist) may measure the effectiveness and side effects of your treatment using laboratory tests and physical examinations. It is important to keep all appointments with your doctor and the laboratory. The length of treatment depends on how your infection and symptoms respond to the medication.

Precautions

Before administering amphotericin B lipid complex,

- tell your doctor and pharmacist if you are allergic to amphotericin B lipid complex or any other medications.
- tell your doctor and pharmacist what prescription and nonprescription medications, vitamins, nutritional supplements, and herbal products you are taking or plan to take. Be sure to mention any of the following: aminoglycoside antibiotics such as amikacin (Amikin), gentamicin (Garamycin), kanamycin (Kantrex), neomycin (Nes-RX, Neo-Fradin), paramomycin (Humatin), streptomycin, and tobramycin (Tobi, Nebcin); certain antifungals such as clotrimazole (Lotrimin, Mycelex, others), fluconazole (Diflucan), itraconazole (Sporanox), ketoconazole (Nizoral), and miconazole (Desenex, Lotrimin, Monistat, others); corticotropin (ACTH, H.P., Acthar Gel); cyclosporine (Neoral, Sandimmune); digoxin (Digitek, Lanoxicaps, Lanoxin); flucytosine (Ancobon); medications for the treatment of cancer; oral steroids such as dexamethasone (Decadron, Dexone), methylprednisolone (Medrol), and prednisone (Deltasone); pentamidine (NebuPent, Pentam 300); and zidovudine (AZT, Retrovir, in Combivir, Trizivir).
- tell your doctor if you are receiving transfusions, or have or have ever had diabetes or kidney disease.
- tell your doctor if you are pregnant or plan to become pregnant. If you become pregnant while taking amphotericin B lipid complex, call your doctor.
- Do not breastfeed if you are taking amphotericin B lipid complex.
- if you are having surgery, including dental surgery, tell the doctor or dentist that you are taking amphotericin B lipid complex.

Administering Your Medication

Before you administer amphotericin B lipid complex, look at the solution closely. It should be clear and free of floating material. Gently squeeze the bag or check the solution container to make sure there are no leaks. Do not use the solution if it is discolored, if it contains particles, or if the bag or container leaks. Use a new solution, but show the damaged one to your health care provider.

It is important that you use your medication exactly as directed. Do not stop your therapy on your own for any reason because your infection could worsen and result in hospitalization. Do not change your dosing schedule without talking to your health care provider. Your health care provider may tell you to stop your infusion if you have a mechanical problem (such as a blockage in the tubing, needle, or catheter); if you have to stop an infusion, call your health care provider immediately so your therapy can continue.

Side Effects

Amphotericin B lipid complex may cause side effects. Some side effects are usually more common and more severe with the first few doses of amphotericin B lipid complex. Your health care provider may prescribe other medications to decrease these side effects. If you have never experienced any of the following side effects from previous doses and suddenly have symptoms, stop your infusion and call your health care provider immediately.

- fever
- chills
- difficult or rapid breathing
- changes in heartbeat
- fainting
- dizziness
- blurred vision
- nausea
- vomiting
- cold clammy skin

Tell your health care provider if any of these symptoms are severe or do not go away:

- diarrhea
- stomach cramping or pain
- excessive tiredness
- pale skin
- headache
- difficulty sleeping
- weakness
- confusion
- fever, sore throat, cough, chills, and other signs of infection

If you experience any of the following symptoms, call your health care provider immediately:

- hives
- rash
- blisters on the palms or skin
- itching
- difficulty breathing or swallowing
- swelling of the face, throat, tongue, lips, eyes, hands, feet, ankles, or lower legs
- hoarseness
- chest pain
- unusual bleeding or bruising
- black and tarry stools
- red blood in stools
- bloody vomit
- vomiting material that looks like coffee grounds
- yellowing of the skin or eyes
- decreased urination

If you experience a serious side effect, you or your doctor may send a report to the Food and Drug Administration's (FDA) MedWatch Adverse Event Reporting program online [at http://www.fda.gov/MedWatch/index.html] or by phone [1-800-332-1088].

Storage Conditions

Talk to your health care provider about how you should store your medication. Your health care provider will probably tell you to store your medication in the refrigerator and to protect it from light. Do not allow this medication to freeze. Your health care provider will tell you when and how you should throw away any unused medication and will probably mark this date on the medication container. Ask your health care provider if you do not understand the directions or if you have any questions.

Keep your supplies in a clean, dry place when you are not using them, and keep all medications and supplies out of reach of children. Your health care provider will tell you how to throw away used needles, syringes, tubing, and containers to avoid accidental injury.

Overdose

In case of overdose, call your local poison control center at 1-800-222-1222. If the victim has collapsed or is not breathing, call local emergency services at 911.

Signs of Infection

If you are receiving amphotericin B lipid complex in your vein or under your skin, you need to know the symptoms of a catheter-related infection (an infection where the needle enters your vein or skin). If you experience any of these effects near your intravenous catheter, tell your health care provider as soon as possible:

- tenderness
- warmth
- irritation
- drainage
- redness
- swelling
- pain

Dosage Facts
For Informational Purposes

Caution: Do not change your dose, how often you take your medication, or the length of time you are to take it without first talking to your healthcare provider.

The following dosage information was written using medical language for doctors and other healthcare professionals and is provided here for you to check your dosage. The dosage of this drug may differ for different patients. Therefore, always follow your doctor's instructions or the directions on the label. Contact your healthcare provider or pharmacist if you have any questions about the specific dosage of your medication after reviewing this information.

General Dosage Information

Available as conventional amphotericin B (formulated with sodium deoxycholate), amphotericin B cholesteryl sulfate complex, amphotericin B lipid complex, or amphotericin B liposomal; dosage is expressed as amphotericin B.

Dosage varies depending on whether the drug is administered as conventional amphotericin B or as amphotericin B cholesteryl sulfate complex, amphotericin B lipid complex, or amphotericin B liposomal. Dosage recommendations for the specific formulation being administered should be followed.

Prior to initiation of conventional IV amphotericin B therapy, a single test dose of the drug (1 mg in 20 mL of 5% dextrose injection) should be administered IV over 20–30 minutes and the patient carefully monitored (i.e., pulse and respiration rate, temperature, blood pressure) every 30 minutes for 2 hours. In patients with good cardiorenal function who tolerate the test dose, therapy may be initiated with a daily dosage of 0.25 mg/kg (0.3 mg/kg in those with severe or rapidly progressing fungal infections) given as a single daily dose. In patients with impaired cardiorenal function and in patients who have severe reactions to the test dose, therapy should be initiated with a smaller daily dosage (i.e., 5–10 mg). Depending on patient's cardiorenal status, dosage may gradually be increased by 5–10 mg daily to a final daily dosage of 0.5–0.7 mg/kg. Some clinicians suggest that higher initial IV dosages of conventional amphotericin B can be used and generally are necessary when initiating therapy in patients with severe, life-threatening infections.

Pediatric Patients

General Pediatric Dosage
Treatment of Invasive Fungal Infections

IV:
- Amphotericin B lipid complex: 5 mg/kg once daily.

Aspergillosis
Treatment of Aspergillosis

IV:

- Amphotericin B cholesteryl sulfate complex: 3–4 mg/kg once daily.
- Amphotericin B lipid complex: 5 mg/kg once daily. Median duration has been 25 days.
- Amphotericin B liposomal: 3–5 mg/kg once daily in children ≥1 month of age. Median duration has been 15–29 days.

Candida Infections
Treatment of Disseminated or Invasive Candida Infections

IV:

- Conventional amphotericin B: 0.4–0.6 mg/kg daily; higher dosage (i.e., 1 mg/kg daily or, rarely, 1.5 mg/kg daily) has been used for treatment of candidemia or rapidly progressing, potentially fatal infections. While 7–14 days may be adequate for non-life-threatening candidiasis in low-risk patients, more prolonged therapy (i.e., 6 weeks or longer) may be necessary in those at high-risk for morbidity and mortality.
- Amphotericin B lipid complex: 5 mg/kg once daily.
- Amphotericin B liposomal: 3–5 mg/kg once daily in children ≥1 month of age. Median duration has been 15–29 days; some candidal infections have been effectively treated with a median duration of 5–7 days.

Coccidioidomycosis
Prevention of Recurrence (Secondary Prophylaxis) of Coccidioidomycosis†

IV:

- Conventional amphotericin B: 1 mg/kg once weekly in HIV-infected infants, children, and adolescents. Initiate secondary prophylaxis after primary infection has been adequately treated.
- HIV-infected infants, children, and adolescents with a history of coccidioidomycosis should receive life-long suppressive therapy to prevent recurrence. The safety of discontinuing secondary prophylaxis in those receiving potent antiretroviral therapy has not been extensively studied.

Cryptococcosis
Treatment of Cryptococcosis

IV:

- Amphotericin B lipid complex: 5 mg/kg once daily.
- Amphotericin B liposomal: 3–5 mg/kg once daily in children ≥1 month of age.

Treatment of Cryptococcal Meningitis

IV:

- Amphotericin B liposomal: 6 mg/kg once daily in children ≥1 month of age.

Prevention of Recurrence (Secondary Prophylaxis) of Cryptococcosis†

IV:

- Conventional amphotericin B: 0.5–1 mg/kg 1–3 times weekly in HIV-infected infants, children, and adolescents. Initiate secondary prophylaxis after primary infection has been adequately treated.
- HIV-infected infants and children with a history of cryptococcosis should receive life-long suppressive therapy to prevent recurrence. The safety of discontinuing secondary prophylaxis in those receiving potent antiretroviral therapy has

not been extensively studied. Consideration can be given to discontinuing secondary prophylaxis in HIV-infected adolescents according to recommendations in adults.

Histoplasmosis
Prevention of Recurrence (Secondary Prophylaxis) of Histoplasmosis†

IV:

- Conventional amphotericin B: 1 mg/kg once weekly in HIV-infected infants, children, and adolescents. Initiate secondary prophylaxis after primary infection has been adequately treated.
- HIV-infected infants, children, or adolescents with a history of histoplasmosis should receive life-long suppressive therapy to prevent recurrence. The safety of discontinuing secondary prophylaxis in those receiving potent antiretroviral therapy has not been extensively studied.

Leishmaniasis
Treatment of Cutaneous and Mucocutaneous Leishmaniasis

IV:

- Conventional amphotericin B: 0.25–0.5 mg/kg daily initially. Gradually increase dosage until 0.5–1 mg/kg daily is reached, at which time the drug usually is given on alternate days.
- Duration of therapy depends on severity of disease and response to the drug, but generally is 3–12 weeks. Total dose generally ranges from 1–3 g; mucocutaneous disease usually requires a higher total dose than cutaneous disease.

Treatment of Visceral Leishmaniasis (Kala-Azar)†

IV:

- Conventional amphotericin B†: 0.5–1 mg/kg administered on alternate days for 14–20 doses.
- Amphotericin B liposomal: 3 mg/kg once daily on days 1–5 and on days 14 and 21 in children ≥1 month of age; a second course of the drug may be useful if the infection is not completely cleared with a single course. For treatment of visceral leishmaniasis in immunocompromised children ≥1 month of age, dosage is 4 mg/kg once daily on days 1–5 and on days 10, 17, 24, 31, and 38; if the parasitic infection is not completely cleared after the first course or if relapses occur, an expert should be consulted regarding further treatment.

Primary Amebic Meningoencephalitis†
Treatment of Naegleria Infections†

IV:

- Conventional amphotericin B: 1 mg/kg daily. Optimal duration not determined.

Adult Patients

Aspergillosis
Treatment of Aspergillosis

IV:

- Conventional amphotericin B: 0.5–0.6 mg/kg daily. Higher dosage (i.e., 1 mg/kg daily or, rarely, 1.5 mg/kg daily) may be necessary in neutropenic patients or for treatment of rapidly progressing, potentially fatal infections. Optimal duration of therapy is uncertain; total doses of 1.5–4 g have been given over an 11-month period.
- Amphotericin B cholesteryl sulfate complex: 3–4 mg/kg once daily.
- Amphotericin B lipid complex: 5 mg/kg once daily. Median duration has been 25 days.

- Amphotericin B liposomal: 3–5 mg/kg once daily. Median duration has been 15–29 days.

Blastomycosis
Treatment of Blastomycosis

IV:
- Conventional amphotericin B: 0.5–1 mg/kg daily.

Candida Infections
Treatment of Disseminated or Invasive Candida Infections

IV:
- Conventional amphotericin B: 0.4–0.6 mg/kg daily; higher dosage (i.e., 1 mg/kg daily or, rarely, 1.5 mg/kg daily) has been used for treatment of candidemia or rapidly progressing, potentially fatal infections. While 7–14 days may be adequate for non-life-threatening candidiasis in low-risk patients, more prolonged therapy (i.e., 6 weeks or longer) may be necessary in those at high-risk for morbidity and mortality.
- Amphotericin B cholesteryl sulfate complex†: 3–6 mg/kg once daily. Dosages up to 7.5 mg/kg have been used in BMT patients.
- Amphotericin B lipid complex: 5 mg/kg once daily.
- Amphotericin B liposomal: 3–5 mg/kg once daily. Median duration has been 15–29 days; some candidal infections were effectively treated with a median duration of 5–7 days.

Treatment of Chronic Disseminated (Heptatosplenic) Candida Infections

IV:
- Conventional amphotericin B: 1 mg/kg daily in conjunction with oral flucytosine (100 mg/kg daily) has been used.

Treatment of Severe or Refractory Esophageal Candidiasis

IV:
- Conventional amphotericin B: 0.3 mg/kg daily for at least 5–7 days has been recommended for HIV-infected patients.

Treatment of Candiduria

IV:
- Conventional amphotericin B: 0.3 mg/kg daily given for 3–5 days.

Coccidioidomycosis
Treatment of Coccidioidomycosis

IV:
- Conventional amphotericin B: 0.5–1 mg/kg daily. Higher dosage (i.e., up to 1.5 mg/kg daily) has been used for treatment of rapidly progressing, potentially fatal infections. Duration depends on clinical response, but usually ranges from 4–12 weeks.

Prevention of Recurrence (Secondary Prophylaxis) of Coccidioidomycosis†

IV:
- Conventional amphotericin B: 1 mg/kg once weekly. Initiate secondary prophylaxis after primary infection has been adequately treated.
- HIV-infected adults with a history of coccidioidomycosis should receive life-long suppressive therapy to prevent recurrence. Although those who respond to potent antiretroviral therapy with increases in CD4+ T-cell counts to >100/mm³ may be at low risk for recurrence of fungal infections, data are insufficient to date to warrant a recommendation regard-

ing discontinuance of secondary prophylaxis against coccidioidomycosis.

Cryptococcosis
Treatment of Cryptococcosis

IV:
- Conventional amphotericin B: 0.3–1 mg/kg daily (with or without oral flucytosine). Duration is determined by clinical response, but usually ranges from a minimum of 2–4 weeks up to several months.
- Amphotericin B cholesteryl sulfate complex†: 3–6 mg/kg once daily. Dosages up to 7.5 mg/kg have been used in BMT patients.
- Amphotericin B lipid complex: 5 mg/kg once daily.
- Amphotericin B liposomal: 3–5 mg/kg once daily.

Treatment of Cryptococcal Meningitis

IV:
- Conventional amphotericin B: 0.7 mg/kg daily for 4 weeks followed by 0.7 mg/kg given on alternate days for an additional 4 weeks has been used in HIV-infected patients. Alternatively, many clinicians recommend 0.7 mg/kg daily given in conjunction with oral flucytosine (100 mg/kg daily) for at least 2 weeks (or until the patient has stabilized) followed by 8–10 weeks of oral fluconazole (400 mg daily) or oral itraconazole (400 mg daily).
- Amphotericin B lipid complex: 5 mg/kg once daily for 6 weeks followed by 12 weeks of oral fluconazole.
- Amphotericin B liposomal: 6 mg/kg once daily.

Prevention of Recurrence (Secondary Prophylaxis) of Cryptococcosis†

IV:
- Conventional amphotericin B: 0.6–1 mg/kg 1–3 times weekly. Initiate secondary prophylaxis after the primary infection has been adequately treated.
- Consideration can be given to discontinuing secondary prophylaxis in HIV-infected adults who have successfully completed initial therapy for cryptococcosis, remain asymptomatic with respect to cryptococcosis, and have sustained (e.g., for ≥6 months) increases in CD4+ T-cell counts to >100–200/mm³ in response to potent antiretroviral therapy.
- Reinitiate secondary prophylaxis against cryptococcosis if CD4+ T-cell count decreases to <100–200/mm³.

Histoplasmosis
Treatment of Histoplasmosis

IV:
- Conventional amphotericin B: 0.5–0.6 mg/kg daily given for ≥4–8 weeks. Higher dosage (i.e., 0.7–1 mg/kg daily or, rarely, 1.5 mg/kg daily) has been recommended and may be necessary for treatment of rapidly progressing, potentially fatal infections. For HIV-infected patients, some clinicians recommend a dosage of 50 mg daily (1 mg/kg in individuals weighing less than 50 kg) for 2 weeks followed by the same dosage given on alternate days until a cumulative dose of 15 mg/kg is reached.

Prevention of Recurrence (Secondary Prophylaxis) of Histoplasmosis†

IV:
- Conventional amphotericin B: 1 mg/kg once weekly. Initiate after primary infection has been adequately treated.
- HIV-infected adults with a history of histoplasmosis should

receive life-long suppressive therapy to prevent recurrence. Although those who respond to potent antiretroviral therapy with increases in CD4$^+$ T-cell counts to >100/mm^3 may be at low risk for recurrence of fungal infections, data are insufficient to date to warrant a recommendation regarding discontinuance of secondary prophylaxis against histoplasmosis.

Paracoccidioidomycosis†
Treatment of Paracoccidioidomycosis†

IV:
- Conventional amphotericin B: 0.4–0.5 mg/kg daily, although higher dosage (i.e., 1 mg/kg daily or, rarely, 1.5 mg/kg daily) has been used for treatment of rapidly progressing, potentially fatal infections. Prolonged therapy usually is required.

Sporotrichosis
Treatment of Sporotrichosis

IV:
- Conventional amphotericin B: 0.4–0.5 mg/kg daily for 2–3 months. Has been given for up to 9 months to provide a total dose of up to 2.5 g.
- Prolonged therapy with total IV doses of at least 2 g (alone or combined with intrathecal† therapy) have been given for the treatment of meningeal sporotrichosis in a limited number of patients.

Zygomycosis
Treatment of Zygomycosis

IV:
- Conventional amphotericin B: 1–1.5 mg/kg daily for 2–3 months. A total IV dose of 3–4 g is recommended for treatment of rhinocerebral phycomycosis; concomitant therapy has included irrigation† of the sinus cavities with a suspension of 1 mg/mL.
- Amphotericin B lipid complex: 5 mg/kg once daily.

Empiric Therapy in Febrile Neutropenic Patients

IV:
- Amphotericin B liposomal: 3 mg/kg once daily.

Prevention of Fungal Infections in Transplant or Cancer Patients†

IV:
- Conventional amphotericin B: 0.1–0.25 mg/kg daily.
- Amphotericin B liposomal: 2 mg/kg 3 times weekly.

Leishmaniasis
Cutaneous and Mucocutaneous Leishmaniasis

IV:
- Conventional amphotericin B: 0.25–0.5 mg/kg daily initially. Gradually increase dosage until 0.5–1 mg/kg daily is reached, at which time the drug usually is given on alternate days.
- Duration depends on the severity of disease and response to the drug, but generally is 3–12 weeks. Total dose generally ranges from 1–3 g; mucocutaneous disease usually requires a higher total dose than cutaneous disease.

Visceral Leishmaniasis (Kala-Azar)†

IV:
- Conventional amphotericin B†: 0.5–1 mg/kg administered on alternate days for 14–20 doses.
- Amphotericin B cholesteryl sulfate complex†: 2 mg/kg once daily for 7–10 days.
- Amphotericin B lipid complex†: 1–3 mg/kg once daily for 5

days has been used in patients who failed to respond to or relapsed after treatment with an antimony compound.
- Amphotericin B liposomal: 3 mg/kg once daily on days 1–5 and on days 14 and 21; a second course of the drug may be useful if the infection is not completely cleared with a single course. For treatment of visceral leishmaniasis in immuno-compromised patients, 4 mg/kg once daily on days 1–5 and on days 10, 17, 24, 31, and 38; if the parasitic infection is not completely cleared after the first course or if relapses occur, an expert should be consulted regarding further treatment.

Primary Amebic Meningoencephalitis†
Naegleria Infections†

IV:
- Conventional amphotericin B: 1 mg/kg daily. Optimal duration not determined.

Prescribing Limits
Pediatric Patients

IV:
- Conventional amphotericin B: use lowest effective dose.

Adult Patients

IV:
- Conventional amphotericin B: daily dosage should not exceed 1.5 mg/kg.

† Use is not currently included in the labeling approved by the US Food and Drug Administration.

Ampicillin Oral

(am pi sil′ in)

Brand Name: Principen®
Also available generically.

Why is this medicine prescribed?

Ampicillin is a penicillin-like antibiotic used to treat certain infections caused by bacteria such as pneumonia; bronchitis; and ear, lung, skin, and urinary tract infections. Antibiotics will not work for colds, flu, or other viral infections.

This medication is sometimes prescribed for other uses; ask your doctor or pharmacist for more information.

How should this medicine be used?

Ampicillin comes as a capsule, liquid, and pediatric drops to take by mouth. It is usually taken every 6 hours (four times a day). Follow the directions on your prescription label carefully, and ask your doctor or pharmacist to explain any part you do not understand. Take ampicillin exactly as directed. Do not take more or less of it or take it more often than prescribed by your doctor.

Shake the liquid and pediatric drops well before each

use to mix the medication evenly. Use the bottle dropper to measure the dose of pediatric drops. The pediatric drops and liquid may be placed on a child's tongue or added to formula, milk, fruit juice, water, ginger ale, or other cold liquid and taken immediately.

The capsules should be swallowed whole and taken with a full glass of water.

Continue to take ampicillin even if you feel well. Do not stop taking ampicillin without talking to your doctor.

What special precautions should I follow?

Before taking ampicillin,

- tell your doctor and pharmacist if you are allergic to ampicillin, penicillin, or any other drugs.
- tell your doctor and pharmacist what prescription and nonprescription medications you are taking, especially other antibiotics, allopurinol (Lopurin), anticoagulants ('blood thinners') such as warfarin (Coumadin), atenolol (Tenormin), oral contraceptives, probenecid (Benemid), rifampin, sulfasalazine, and vitamins.
- tell your doctor if you have or have ever had kidney or liver disease, allergies, asthma, blood disease, colitis, stomach problems, or hay fever.
- tell your doctor if you are pregnant, plan to become pregnant, or are breast-feeding. If you become pregnant while taking ampicillin, call your doctor.
- if you are having surgery, including dental surgery, tell the doctor or dentist that you are taking ampicillin.

What special dietary instructions should I follow?

Take ampicillin at least 1 hour before or 2 hours after meals.

What should I do if I forget to take a dose?

Take the missed dose as soon as you remember it. However, if it is almost time for the next dose, skip the missed dose and continue your regular dosing schedule. Do not take a double dose to make up for a missed one.

What side effects can this medicine cause?

Ampicillin may cause side effects. Tell your doctor if any of these symptoms are severe or do not go away:

- upset stomach
- diarrhea
- vomiting
- mild skin rash

If you experience any of the following symptoms, call your doctor immediately:

- severe skin rash
- itching
- hives
- difficulty breathing or swallowing
- wheezing
- vaginal infection

If you experience a serious side effect, you or your doc-

tor may send a report to the Food and Drug Administration's (FDA) MedWatch Adverse Event Reporting program online [at http://www.fda.gov/MedWatch/index.html] or by phone [1-800-332-1088].

What storage conditions are needed for this medicine?

Keep this medication in the container it came in, tightly closed, and out of reach of children. Store the capsules at room temperature and away from excess heat and moisture (not in the bathroom). Throw away any medication that is outdated or no longer needed. Keep liquid medicine in the refrigerator, tightly closed, and throw away any unused medication after 14 days. Do not freeze. The liquid is good for 7 days at room temperature. Talk to your pharmacist about the proper disposal of your medication.

What should I do in case of overdose?

In case of overdose, call your local poison control center at 1-800-222-1222. If the victim has collapsed or is not breathing, call local emergency services at 911.

What other information should I know?

Keep all appointments with your doctor and the laboratory. Your doctor may order certain lab tests to check your response to ampicillin.

If you are diabetic, use Clinistix or TesTape (not Clinitest) to test your urine for sugar while taking this drug.

Do not let anyone else take your medication. Your prescription is probably not refillable. If you still have symptoms of infection after you finish the ampicillin, call your doctor.

Dosage Facts
For Informational Purposes

Caution: Do not change your dose, how often you take your medication, or the length of time you are to take it without first talking to your healthcare provider.

The following dosage information was written using medical language for doctors and other healthcare professionals and is provided here for you to check your dosage. The dosage of this drug may differ for different patients. Therefore, always follow your doctor's instructions or the directions on the label. Contact your healthcare provider or pharmacist if you have any questions about the specific dosage of your medication after reviewing this information.

General Dosage Information

Available as ampicillin trihydrate and ampicillin sodium; dosage expressed in terms of ampicillin.

Duration of therapy depends on type and severity of infection and should be determined by clinical and bacteriologic response of the patient. For most infections, therapy should be continued for ≥48–72 hours after patient becomes asymptomatic or evidence of eradication of the infection has been obtained. More prolonged therapy may be necessary for some infections.

Pediatric Patients

General Pediatric Dosage

ORAL:
- Children ≥1 month of age: AAP recommends 50–100 mg/kg daily given in 4 divided doses for mild to moderate infections.
- AAP states oral route is inappropriate for severe infections.

GI Infections

ORAL:
- Children weighing ≤20 kg: 100 mg/kg daily in 4 divided doses.
- Children weighing >20 kg: 500 mg 4 times daily. Severe or chronic infections may require higher dosage.

Respiratory Tract Infections

ORAL:
- Children weighing ≤20 kg: 50 mg/kg daily in 3 or 4 divided doses.
- Children weighing >20 kg: 250 mg 4 times daily.

Urinary Tract Infections (UTIs)

ORAL:
- Children weighing ≤20 kg: 100 mg/kg daily in 4 divided doses.
- Children weighing >20 kg: 500 mg 4 times daily. Severe or chronic infections may require higher dosage.

Adult Patients

GI Infections

ORAL:
- 500 mg 4 times daily.

Respiratory Tract Infections

ORAL:
- 250 mg 4 times daily.

Urinary Tract Infections (UTIs)

ORAL:
- 500 mg 4 times daily.

Gonorrhea and Associated Infections
Uncomplicated Gonorrhea

ORAL:
- 3.5 g as a single dose (with 1 g of oral probenecid). No longer recommended for gonorrhea by CDC or other experts.

Prescribing Limits

Pediatric Patients

Pediatric dosage should not exceed adult dosage.

Special Populations

Renal Impairment
- Dosage adjustments necessary in patients with renal impairment.
- Some clinicians suggest that adults with GFR 10–50 mL/minute receive the usual dose every 6–12 hours and that adults with GFR <10 mL/minute receive the usual dose every

12–16 hours. Alternatively, some clinicians suggest that modification of usual dosage is unnecessary in adults with $Cl_{cr} \geq 30$ mL/minute, but that adults with $Cl_{cr} \leq 10$ mL/minute should receive the usual dose every 8 hours.
- Patients undergoing hemodialysis should receive a supplemental dose after each dialysis period.

Geriatric Patients
- No dosage adjustments except those related to renal impairment.

† Use is not currently included in the labeling approved by the US Food and Drug Administration.

Ampicillin Sodium and Sulbactam Sodium Injection

(am pi sill′ in) (sul bak′ tam)

Brand Name: Unasyn®
Also available generically.

About Your Treatment

Your doctor has ordered ampicillin and sulbactam, an antibiotic, to help treat your infection. The drug will be either injected into a large muscle (such as your buttock or hip) or added to an intravenous fluid that will drip through a needle or catheter placed in your vein for about 30 minutes, two to four times a day.

The combination of ampicillin and sulbactam eliminates bacteria that cause many kinds of infections, including gynecological, skin, and stomach infections. This medication is sometimes prescribed for other uses; ask your doctor or pharmacist for more information.

Your health care provider (doctor, nurse, or pharmacist) may measure the effectiveness and side effects of your treatment using laboratory tests and physical examinations. It is important to keep all appointments with your doctor and the laboratory. The length of treatment depends on how your infection and symptoms respond to the medication.

Precautions

Before administering ampicillin and sulbactam,
- tell your doctor and pharmacist if you are allergic to ampicillin, penicillin, cephalosporins [e.g., cefaclor (Ceclor), cefadroxil (Duricef), or cephalexin (Keflex)], or any other drugs.
- tell your doctor and pharmacist what prescription and nonprescription medications you are taking, especially other antibiotics, allopurinol (Lopurin), anticoagulants ('blood thinners') such as warfarin (Coumadin), atenolol (Tenormin), oral contraceptives, probenecid (Benemid), rifampin (Rifadin), sulfasalazine, and vitamins.

- tell your doctor if you have or have ever had asthma, hay fever, or kidney or gastrointestinal disease (especially colitis).
- tell your doctor if you are pregnant, plan to become pregnant, or are breast-feeding. If you become pregnant while taking ampicillin and sulbactam, call your doctor.
- if you have diabetes and regularly check your urine for sugar, use Clinistix or TesTape. Do not use Clinitest tablets because ampicillin and sulbactam may cause false positive results.

Administering Your Medication

Before you administer ampicillin and sulbactam, look at the solution closely. It should be clear and free of floating material. Gently squeeze the bag or observe the solution container to make sure there are no leaks. Do not use the solution if it is discolored, if it contains particles, or if the bag or container leaks. Use a new solution, but show the damaged one to your health care provider.

It is important that you use your medication exactly as directed. Do not stop your therapy on your own for any reason because your infection could worsen and result in hospitalization. Do not change your dosing schedule without talking to your health care provider. Your health care provider may tell you to stop your infusion if you have a mechanical problem (such as a blockage in the tubing, needle, or catheter); if you have to stop an infusion, call your health care provider immediately so your therapy can continue.

Side Effects

Ampicillin and sulbactam may cause side effects. If you are administering ampicillin and sulbactam into a muscle, it may be mixed with lidocaine (Xylocaine) to reduce pain at the injection site. Tell your health care provider if either of these symptoms is severe or does not go away:

- upset stomach
- diarrhea

If you experience any of the following symptoms, call your health care provider immediately:

- rash
- itching
- fever
- chills
- facial swelling
- wheezing
- difficulty breathing
- unusual bleeding or bruising
- dizziness
- seizures
- sore mouth or throat

If you experience a serious side effect, you or your doctor may send a report to the Food and Drug Administration's (FDA) MedWatch Adverse Event Reporting program online [at http://www.fda.gov/MedWatch/index.html] or by phone [1-800-332-1088].

Storage Conditions

- Your health care provider probably will give you a several-day supply of ampicillin and sulbactam at a time. If you are receiving ampicillin and sulbactam intravenously (in your vein), you probably will be told to store it in the refrigerator or freezer.
- Take your next dose from the refrigerator 1 hour before using it; place it in a clean, dry area to allow it to warm to room temperature.
- If you are told to store additional ampicillin and sulbactam in the freezer, always move a 24-hour supply to the refrigerator for the next day's use.
- Do not refreeze medications.

If you are receiving ampicillin and sulbactam intramuscularly (in your muscle), your health care provider will tell you how to store it properly.

Store your medication only as directed. Make sure you understand what you need to store your medication properly.

Keep your supplies in a clean, dry place when you are not using them, and keep all medications and supplies out of reach of children. Your health care provider will tell you how to throw away used needles, syringes, tubing, and containers to avoid accidental injury.

Overdose

In case of overdose, call your local poison control center at 1-800-222-1222. If the victim has collapsed or is not breathing, call local emergency services at 911.

Signs of Infection

If you are receiving ampicillin and sulbactam in your vein or under your skin, you need to know the symptoms of a catheter-related infection (an infection where the needle enters your vein or skin). If you experience any of these effects near your intravenous catheter, tell your health care provider as soon as possible:

- tenderness
- warmth
- irritation
- drainage
- redness
- swelling
- pain

Dosage Facts
For Informational Purposes

Caution: Do not change your dose, how often you take your medication, or the length of time you are to take it without first talking to your health-care provider.

The following dosage information was written using medical language for doctors and other healthcare professionals and is provided here for you to check your dosage. The dosage of this drug may differ for different

patients. Therefore, always follow your doctor's instructions or the directions on the label. Contact your health-care provider or pharmacist if you have any questions about the specific dosage of your medication after reviewing this information.

General Dosage Information

Available as fixed combination containing ampicillin sodium and sulbactam sodium; dosage generally expressed in terms of the total of the ampicillin and sulbactam content of the fixed combination. Potency of both ampicillin sodium and sulbactam sodium are expressed in terms of the bases.

Pediatric Patients

General Pediatric Dosage

IV:
- Children ≥1 month of age†: AAP recommends 100–150 mg/kg of ampicillin daily in 4 divided doses for treatment of mild to moderate infections or 200–400 mg/kg of ampicillin daily in 4 divided doses for treatment of severe infections.

Skin and Skin Structure Infections

IV:
- Children ≥1 year of age: 300 mg/kg daily (200 mg of ampicillin and 100 mg of sulbactam) in equally divided doses every 6 hours.
- Manufacturer recommends that IV treatment in pediatric patients not exceed 14 days; in clinical studies, most children received an appropriate oral anti-infective after an initial IV regimen of ampicillin and sulbactam.

Acute Pelvic Inflammatory Disease

IV:
- Adolescents: 3 g (2 g of ampicillin and 1 g of sulbactam) every 6 hours in conjunction with doxycycline (100 mg orally or IV every 12 hours). Parenteral regimen may be discontinued 24 hours after clinical improvement; oral doxycycline (100 mg twice daily) should be continued to complete 14 days of therapy.

Adult Patients

General Adult Dosage
Intra-abdominal, Gynecologic, or Skin and Skin Structure Infections

IV OR IM:
- 1.5 g (1 g of ampicillin and 0.5 g of sulbactam) to 3 g (2 g of ampicillin and 1 g of sulbactam) every 6 hours.

Acute Pelvic Inflammatory Disease

IV:
- 3 g (2 g of ampicillin and 1 g of sulbactam) every 6 hours in conjunction with doxycycline (100 mg orally or IV every 12 hours). Parenteral regimen may be discontinued 24 hours after clinical improvement; oral doxycycline (100 mg twice daily) should be continued to complete 14 days of therapy.

Prescribing Limits

Pediatric Patients

IV:
- Maximum sulbactam dosage is 4 g (i.e., 8 g of ampicillin and 4 g of sulbactam in fixed combination) daily.
- Duration of therapy should be ≤14 days.

Adult Patients

IV OR IM:
- Maximum sulbactam dosage is 4 g (i.e., 8 g of ampicillin and 4 g of sulbactam in fixed combination) daily.

Special Populations

Renal Impairment
- Dosage adjustments necessary in patients with renal impairment.
- Patients with renal impairment should receive the usually recommended dose but these doses should be given less frequently than usual; dosing intervals are based on the patient's Cl_{cr}. The manufacturer recommends that patients with Cl_{cr} ≥30 mL/minute per 1.73 m^2 should receive 1.5 g (1 g of ampicillin and 0.5 g of sulbactam) to 3 g (2 g of ampicillin and 1 g of sulbactam) every 6–8 hours and patients with Cl_{cr} 15–29 or 5–14 mL/minute per 1.73 m^2 receive these doses every 12 or 24 hours, respectively.
- Some clinicians suggest that patients undergoing hemodialysis receive 1.5 g (1 g of ampicillin and 0.5 g of sulbactam) to 3 g (2 g of ampicillin and 1 g of sulbactam) once every 24 hours and that the dose should preferably be given immediately after dialysis.

Geriatric Patients
- No dosage adjustments except those related to renal impairment.

† Use is not currently included in the labeling approved by the US Food and Drug Administration.

Ampicillin Sodium Injection

(am pi sill′ in)

Brand Name: Principen®
Also available generically.

About Your Treatment

Your doctor has ordered ampicillin, an antibiotic, to help treat your infection. The drug will be either injected into a large muscle (such as your buttock or hip) or added to an intravenous fluid that will drip through a needle or catheter placed in your vein for about 30 minutes, four to six times a day.

Ampicillin eliminates bacteria that cause many kinds of infection, including pneumonia; meningitis; and urinary tract, gastrointestinal tract, skin, bone, joint, blood, and heart valve infections. This medication is sometimes prescribed for other uses; ask your doctor or pharmacist for more information.

Your health care provider (doctor, nurse, or pharmacist) may measure the effectiveness and side effects of your treatment using laboratory tests and physical examinations. It is important to keep all appointments with your doctor and the laboratory. The length of treatment depends on how your infection and symptoms respond to the medication.

Precautions

Before administering ampicillin,

- tell your doctor and pharmacist if you are allergic to ampicillin, penicillin, cephalosporins [e.g., cefaclor (Ceclor), cefadroxil (Duricef), or cephalexin (Keflex)], or any other drugs.
- tell your doctor and pharmacist what prescription and nonprescription medications you are taking, especially other antibiotics, allopurinol (Lopurin), anticoagulants ('blood thinners') such as warfarin (Coumadin), atenolol (Tenormin), oral contraceptives, probenecid (Benemid), rifampin (Rifadin), sulfasalazine, and vitamins.
- tell your doctor if you have or have ever had kidney or liver disease, allergies, asthma, blood disease, colitis, stomach problems, or hay fever.
- tell your doctor if you are pregnant, plan to become pregnant, or are breast-feeding. If you become pregnant while taking ampicillin, call your doctor.
- if you have diabetes and regularly check your urine for sugar, use Clinistix or TesTape. Do not use Clinitest tablets because ampicillin may cause false positive results.

Administering Your Medication

Before you administer ampicillin, look at the solution closely. It should be clear and free of floating material. Gently squeeze the bag or observe the solution container to make sure there are no leaks. Do not use the solution if it is discolored, if it contains particles, or if the bag or container leaks. Use a new solution, but show the damaged one to your health care provider.

It is important that you use your medication exactly as directed. Do not stop your therapy on your own for any reason because your infection could worsen and result in hospitalization. Do not change your dosing schedule without talking to your health care provider. Your health care provider may tell you to stop your infusion if you have a mechanical problem (such as a blockage in the tubing, needle, or catheter); if you have to stop an infusion, call your health care provider immediately so your therapy can continue.

Side Effects

Ampicillin may cause side effects. Tell your doctor if any of these symptoms are severe or do not go away:

- upset stomach
- diarrhea
- vomiting
- mild skin rash

If you experience any of the following symptoms, call your health care provider immediately:

- severe skin rash

- itching
- hives
- difficulty breathing or swallowing
- wheezing
- unusual bleeding or bruising
- headache
- dizziness
- seizures
- sore mouth or throat

Storage Conditions

- Your health care provider probably will give you a several-day supply of ampicillin at a time. If you are receiving ampicillin intravenously (in your vein), you probably will be told to store it in the refrigerator or freezer.
- Take your next dose from the refrigerator 1 hour before using it; place it in a clean, dry area to allow it to warm to room temperature.
- If you are told to store additional ampicillin in the freezer, always move a 24-hour supply to the refrigerator for the next day's use.
- Do not refreeze medications.

If you are receiving ampicillin intramuscularly (in your muscle), your health care provider will tell you how to store it properly.

Store your medication only as directed. Make sure you understand what you need to store your medication properly.

Keep your supplies in a clean, dry place when you are not using them, and keep all medications and supplies out of reach of children. Your health care provider will tell you how to throw away used needles, syringes, tubing, and containers to avoid accidental injury.

Overdose

In case of overdose, call your local poison control center at 1-800-222-1222. If the victim has collapsed or is not breathing, call local emergency services at 911.

Signs of Infection

If you are receiving ampicillin in your vein or under your skin, you need to know the symptoms of a catheter-related infection (an infection where the needle enters your vein or skin). If you experience any of these effects near your intravenous catheter, tell your health care provider as soon as possible:

- tenderness
- warmth
- irritation
- drainage
- redness
- swelling
- pain

Dosage Facts
For Informational Purposes

Caution: Do not change your dose, how often you take your medication, or the length of time you are to take it without first talking to your health-care provider.

The following dosage information was written using medical language for doctors and other healthcare professionals and is provided here for you to check your dosage. The dosage of this drug may differ for different patients. Therefore, always follow your doctor's instructions or the directions on the label. Contact your health-care provider or pharmacist if you have any questions about the specific dosage of your medication after reviewing this information.

General Dosage Information

Available as ampicillin trihydrate and ampicillin sodium; dosage expressed in terms of ampicillin.

Duration of therapy depends on type and severity of infection and should be determined by clinical and bacteriologic response of the patient. For most infections, therapy should be continued for ≥48–72 hours after patient becomes asymptomatic or evidence of eradication of the infection has been obtained. More prolonged therapy may be necessary for some infections.

Pediatric Patients

General Pediatric Dosage

IV OR IM:
- Neonates <1 week of age: AAP recommends 25–50 mg/kg every 12 hours in those weighing ≤2 kg or 25–50 mg/kg every 8 hours in those weighing >2 kg.
- Neonates 1–4 weeks of age: AAP recommends 25–50 mg/kg every 12 hours for those weighing <1.2 kg, 25–50 mg/kg every 8 hours for those weighing 1.2–2 kg, or 25–50 mg/kg every 6 hours for those weighing >2 kg.
- Children ≥1 month of age: AAP recommends 100–150 mg/kg daily given in 4 divided doses for mild to moderate infections or 200–400 mg/kg daily given in 4 divided doses for severe infections.

Endocarditis
Treatment of Endocarditis Caused by Viridans Streptococci or S. bovis

IV:
- 300 mg/kg daily given in 4–6 divided doses for 4 weeks. Used in conjunction with IM or IV gentamicin (3 mg daily given during the first 2 weeks).

Treatment of Enterococcal Endocarditis

IV:
- 300 mg/kg daily given in 4–6 divided doses for 4–6 weeks. Used in conjunction with IM or IV gentamicin (3 mg daily given for 4–6 weeks).

Prevention of Bacterial Endocarditis in Patients Undergoing Certain Dental, Oral, Respiratory Tract, or Esophageal Procedures†

IV OR IM:
- 50 mg/kg given 30 minutes prior to the procedure.

Prevention of Enterococcal Endocarditis in Patients Undergoing Certain Genitourinary or GI (except Esophageal) Procedures†

IV OR IM:
- For moderate-risk patients, 50 mg/kg given 30 minutes prior to the procedure.
- For high-risk patients, 50 mg/kg (up to 2 g) as a single dose in conjunction with a single dose of gentamicin (1.5 mg/kg) given 30 minutes prior to the procedure followed a dose of IM or IV ampicillin (25 mg/kg) given 6 hours later or, alternatively, oral amoxicillin (25 mg/kg) given 6 hours later.

GI Infections

IV OR IM:
- Children weighing <40 kg: 50 mg/kg daily in divided doses every 6–8 hours.
- Children weighing ≥40 kg: 500 mg every 6 hours. Severe or chronic infections may require higher dosage.

Meningitis and Other CNS Infections
Empiric Treatment of Meningitis

IV:
- Neonates and children <2 months of age: 100–300 mg/kg daily given in divided doses; used in conjunction with IM gentamicin pending results of in vitro susceptibility tests.
- Children 2 months to 12 years of age: 200–400 mg/kg daily given in divided doses every 4–6 hours; used in conjunction with IV chloramphenicol.

Treatment of Meningitis Caused by S. agalactiae

IV:
- AAP recommends 200–300 mg/kg daily given in 3 divided for neonates ≤7 days of age or 300 mg/kg daily given in 4–6 divided doses for neonates >7 days of age.

Respiratory Tract Infections

IV OR IM:
- Children weighing <40 kg: 25–50 mg/kg daily in divided doses every 6–8 hours.
- Children weighing ≥40 kg: 250–500 mg every 6 hours.

Septicemia

IV OR IM:
- 150–200 mg/kg daily.

Skin and Skin Structure Infections

IV OR IM:
- Children weighing <40 kg: 25–50 mg/kg daily in divided doses every 6–8 hours.
- Children weighing ≥40 kg: 250–500 mg every 6 hours.

Urinary Tract Infections (UTIs)

IV OR IM:
- Children weighing <40 kg: 50 mg/kg daily in divided doses every 6–8 hours.
- Children weighing ≥40 kg: 500 mg every 6 hours. Severe or chronic infections may require higher dosage.

Adult Patients

Endocarditis
Treatment of Enterococcal Endocarditis

IV:
- 12 g daily (by continuous IV infusion or in 6 equally divided IV doses) in conjunction with IM or IV gentamicin (1 mg/kg every 8 hours). Treatment with both drugs generally should

be continued for 4–6 weeks, but patients who had symptoms of infection for >3 months before treatment was initiated and patients with prosthetic heart valves require ≥6 weeks of therapy with both drugs.

Treatment of Endocarditis Caused by HACEK group (i.e., H. parainfluenzae, H. aphrophilus, A. actinomycetemcomitans, C. hominis, E. corrodens, K. kingae)†

IV:
- 12 g daily (by continuous IV infusion or in 6 equally divided IV doses) in conjunction with IM or IV gentamicin (1 mg/kg every 8 hours). Treatment with both drugs generally should be continued for 4 weeks.

Prevention of Bacterial Endocarditis in Patients Undergoing Certain Dental, Oral, Respiratory Tract, or Esophageal Procedures†

IV OR IM:
- 2 g as a single dose given 30 minutes prior to the procedure.

Prevention of Enterococcal Endocarditis in Patients Undergoing Certain GU or GI (except Esophageal) Procedures†

IV OR IM:
- For moderate-risk patients, 2 g given 30 minutes prior to the procedure.
- For high-risk patients, 2 g as a single dose in conjunction with a single dose of gentamicin (1.5 mg/kg) given 30 minutes prior to the procedure followed by a dose of IM or IV ampicillin (1 g) given 6 hours later or, alternatively, a dose of oral amoxicillin (1 g) given 6 hours later.

GI Infections

IV OR IM:
- Adults weighing <40 kg: 50 mg/kg daily in divided doses every 6–8 hours.
- Adults weighing ≥40 kg: 500 mg every 6 hours.

Meningitis and Other CNS Infections

IV, THEN IM:
- 150–200 mg/kg daily in divided doses every 3–4 hours. Use IV initially, may switch to IM after 3 days.

Respiratory Tract Infections

IV OR IM:
- Adults weighing <40 kg: 25–50 mg/kg daily in divided doses every 6–8 hours.
- Adults weighing ≥40 kg: 250–500 mg every 6 hours.

Septicemia

IV OR IM:
- 150–200 mg/kg daily.

Skin and Skin Structure Infections

IV OR IM:
- Adults weighing <40 kg: 25–50 mg/kg daily in divided doses every 6–8 hours.
- Adults weighing ≥40 kg: 250–500 mg every 6 hours.

Urinary Tract Infections (UTIs)

IV OR IM:
- Adults weighing <40 kg: 50 mg/kg daily in divided doses every 6–8 hours.
- Adults weighing ≥40 kg: 500 mg every 6 hours.

Gonorrhea and Associated Infections
Gonococcal Urethritis

IV OR IM:
- 500 mg initially followed by 500 mg 8–12 hours later. No longer recommended by CDC or other experts.

Prevention of Perinatal Group B Streptococcal (GBS) Disease†

IV:
- An initial 2-g dose (at time of labor or rupture of membranes) followed by 1 g every 4 hours until delivery.

Prescribing Limits

Pediatric Patients

Pediatric dosage should not exceed adult dosage.

Special Populations

Renal Impairment
- Dosage adjustments necessary in patients with renal impairment.
- Some clinicians suggest that adults with GFR 10–50 mL/minute receive the usual dose every 6–12 hours and that adults with GFR <10 mL/minute receive the usual dose every 12–16 hours. Alternatively, some clinicians suggest that modification of usual dosage is unnecessary in adults with $Cl_{cr} \geq 30$ mL/minute, but that adults with $Cl_{cr} \leq 10$ mL/minute should receive the usual dose every 8 hours.
- Patients undergoing hemodialysis should receive a supplemental dose after each dialysis period.

Geriatric Patients
- No dosage adjustments except those related to renal impairment.

† Use is not currently included in the labeling approved by the US Food and Drug Administration.

Amprenavir

(am pren′ a veer)

Brand Name: Agenerase®

Important Warning

Amprenavir liquid should not be used by infants or children younger than 4 years of age, pregnant women, patients with liver or kidney failure, or patients taking disulfiram (Antabuse) or metronidazole (Flagyl). Amprenavir liquid should only be used when you cannot take amprenavir capsules or other antiretroviral agents. If you are using the liquid, but believe you could take capsules, you should speak to your doctor.

Why is this medicine prescribed?

Amprenavir is used in combination with other antiretroviral medications to treat human immunodeficiency virus (HIV). Amprenavir belongs to a class of drugs called protease inhibitors, which slow the spread of HIV infection in the body.

This medication is sometimes prescribed for other uses; ask your doctor or pharmacist for more information.

How should this medicine be used?

Amprenavir comes as a capsule and liquid to take by mouth. It is usually taken twice a day. Amprenavir may be taken with or without food. However, avoid taking amprenavir with high-fat foods or high-fat meals. The amount of drug in amprenavir capsules is not the same as the amount in amprenavir liquid. Do not switch between amprenavir capsules and amprenavir liquid unless your doctor tells you how many amprenavir capsules or how much amprenavir liquid you should take. Follow the directions on your prescription label carefully, and ask your doctor or pharmacist to explain any part you do not understand. Take amprenavir exactly as directed. Do not take more or less of it or take it more often than prescribed by your doctor.

Amprenavir is not a cure and may not decrease the number of HIV-related illnesses. Amprenavir does not prevent the spread of HIV to other people. Continue to take amprenavir even if you feel well. Do not stop taking amprenavir without talking to your doctor.

What special precautions should I follow?

Before taking amprenavir,

- tell your doctor and pharmacist if you are allergic to amprenavir, sulfa drugs, or any other drugs.
- tell your doctor and pharmacist what prescription and nonprescription medications you are taking in addition to those listed in the IMPORTANT WARNING section, especially alprazolam (Xanax); amiodarone (Cordarone); antacids; anticoagulants ('blood thinners') such as warfarin (Coumadin); astemizole (Hismanal); atorvastatin (Lipitor); bepridil (Vascor); betamethasone (Celestone); bepridil (Vascor); birth control pills; carbamazepine (Carbatrol, Epitol, Tegretol); cerivastatin (Baycol); cimetidine (Tagamet); cisapride (Propulsid); clorazepate (Tranxene); clozapine (Clozaril); cortisone acetate (Cortone); dapsone (Avlosulfon); delavirdine (Rescriptor); dexamethasone (Decadron, Hexadrol, others); diazepam (Valium); didanosine (Videx); dihydroergotamine (D.H.E. 45, Migranal); diltiazem (Cardizem, Dilacor); efavirenz (Sustiva); ergonovine (Ergotrate); ergotamine (Cafergot, Ercaf, others); erythromycin (E.E.S., E-Mycin, PCE, others); flurazepam (Dalmane); hydrocortisone (Cortef, Cortenema, Hydrocortone); itraconazole (Sporanox); lidocaine (Xylocaine, LidoPen Auto-Injector, others); loratadine (Claritin); lovastatin (Mevacor); medications for depression such as amitriptyline (Elavil), amoxapine (Asendin),

clomipramine (Anafranil), desipramine (Norpramin), doxepin (Adapin, Sinequan), imipramine (Tofranil), nortriptyline (Aventyl, Pamelor), protriptyline (Vivactil), and trimipramine (Surmontil); medications for diabetes; methylprednisolone (Depo-Medrol, others); midazolam (Versed); nevirapine (Viramune); nicardipine (Cardene); nifedipine (Adalat, Procardia); nimodipine (Nimotop); phenobarbital (Barbita); phenytoin (Dilantin, Diphenylan Sodium); pimozide (Orap); prednisolone (Delta-Cortef, Prelone); prednisone (Orasone, Deltasone, others); quinidine (Quinaglute, Cardioquin, Quinidex); rifabutin (Mycobutin); rifampin (Rifadin, Rifamate, Rifater, Rimactane); ritonavir (Norvir); sildenafil (Viagra); simvastatin (Zocor); steroid medications such as estrogen or progesterone; terfenadine (Seldane); triamcinolone (Aristocort, Kenacort); triazolam (Halcion); vitamin E and any other vitamins.
- take amprenavir 1 hour before or 1 hour after you take antacids or didanosine (Videx).
- tell your doctor and pharmacist what herbal products you are taking, especially St. John's wort or products containing St. John's wort.
- tell your doctor if you have or have ever had liver or kidney disease, diabetes, or hemophilia.
- tell your doctor if you are pregnant, plan to become pregnant, or are breast-feeding. Once you begin taking amprenavir, you should not plan to become pregnant or breast-feed. If you become pregnant while taking amprenavir capsules, call your doctor.
- if you are taking birth control pills, you should talk to your doctor about using another form of birth control because amprenavir may decrease the effectiveness of your birth control pills.
- if you are taking amprenavir liquid, you should avoid drinking alcohol.
- you should be aware that your body fat may increase or move to different areas of your body, such as your breasts and your upper back.

What special dietary instructions should I follow?

Do not take vitamin E supplements if you are taking amprenavir. Amprenavir capsules and solutions contain vitamin E and you do not need to take additional vitamin E to meet the daily requirement for this vitamin.

What should I do if I forget to take a dose?

If you miss a dose by less than 4 hours, take the missed dose as soon as you remember it. If you miss a dose by more than 4 hours, skip the missed dose and continue your regular dosing schedule. Do not take a double dose to make up for a missed one.

What side effects can this medicine cause?

Amprenavir may cause hyperglycemia (high blood sugar). Call your doctor immediately if you have any of the following symptoms:

- extreme thirst
- frequent urination
- extreme hunger
- weakness
- blurred vision

If high blood sugar is not treated, a serious, life-threatening condition called diabetic ketoacidosis could develop. Call your doctor immediately if you have any of the these symptoms:

- dry mouth
- upset stomach and vomiting
- shortness of breath
- breath that smells fruity
- decreased consciousness

Amprenavir may cause other side effects. Tell your doctor if any of these symptoms are severe or do not go away:

- upset stomach
- vomiting
- diarrhea or loose stools
- stomach pain
- change in taste
- tingling sensation around your mouth

If you experience any of the following symptoms, call your doctor immediately:

- rash
- seizures (if you are taking the liquid)
- confusion (if you are taking the liquid)
- rapid heart rate (if you are taking the liquid)

If you experience a serious side effect, you or your doctor may send a report to the Food and Drug Administration's (FDA) MedWatch Adverse Event Reporting program online [at http://www.fda.gov/MedWatch/index.html] or by phone [1-800-332-1088].

What storage conditions are needed for this medicine?

Keep this medication in the container it came in, tightly closed, and out of reach of children. Store it at room temperature and away from excess heat and moisture (not in the bathroom). Throw away any medication that is outdated or no longer needed. Talk to your pharmacist about the proper disposal of your medication.

What should I do in case of overdose?

In case of overdose, call your local poison control center at 1-800-222-1222. If the victim has collapsed or is not breathing, call local emergency services at 911.

What other information should I know?

It is important that you do not run out of your supply of amprenavir or other antiviral medications because the amount of HIV in your blood may increase if you stop taking them. When your supply of amprenavir is low, make sure you contact your doctor or pharmacist for a refill.

Keep all appointments with your doctor and the laboratory. Your doctor will order certain lab tests to check your response to amprenavir.

Do not let anyone else take your medication. Ask your pharmacist any questions you have about refilling your prescription.

Dosage Facts
For Informational Purposes

Caution: Do not change your dose, how often you take your medication, or the length of time you are to take it without first talking to your healthcare provider.

The following dosage information was written using medical language for doctors and other healthcare professionals and is provided here for you to check your dosage. The dosage of this drug may differ for different patients. Therefore, always follow your doctor's instructions or the directions on the label. Contact your healthcare provider or pharmacist if you have any questions about the specific dosage of your medication after reviewing this information.

General Dosage Information

Must be given in conjunction with other antiretrovirals. *If used with ritonavir capsules, dosage adjustment recommended and additional drug interactions must be considered.*

Pediatric Patients

Treatment of HIV Infection

ORAL:

Pediatric Dosage for Treatment of HIV

Age and Weight (kg)	Dosage for Liquid-filled Capsules	Dosage for Oral Solution
4–12 years of age weighing <50 kg	20 mg/kg twice daily or 15 mg/kg 3 times daily (maximum 2.4 g daily)	22.5 mg/kg (1.5 mL/kg) twice daily or 17 mg/kg (1.1 mL/kg) 3 times daily (maximum 2.8 g daily)
13–16 years of age weighing <50 kg	20 mg/kg twice daily or 15 mg/kg 3 times daily (maximum 2.4 g daily)	22.5 mg/kg (1.5 mL/kg) twice daily or 17 mg/kg (1.1 mL/kg) 3 times daily (maximum 2.8 g daily)
13–16 years of age weighing ≥50 kg	1.2 g twice daily	1.4 g twice daily
>16 years of age	1.2 g twice daily	1.4 g twice daily

Adult Patients

Treatment of HIV Infection

ORAL:
- Liquid-filled capsules: 1.2 g twice daily.
- If used in conjunction with low-dose ritonavir, manufacturer recommends amprenavir 1.2 g once daily with ritonavir 200 mg once daily or amprenavir 600 mg twice daily with ritonavir 100 mg twice daily.
- Oral solution: 1.4 g twice daily.

Special Populations

Hepatic Impairment
- Dosage recommendations not available for children with hepatic impairment since the drug has not been evaluated in these patients.
- Dosage adjustments necessary in adults with hepatic impairment based on Child-Pugh scores; oral solution contraindicated in those with hepatic failure.
- Liquid-filled capsules: 450 mg twice daily in adults with Child-Pugh scores 5–8 and 300 mg twice daily in those with Child-Pugh scores 9–12.
- Oral solution: 513 mg (34 mL) twice daily in adults with Child-Pugh scores 5–8 and 342 mg (23 mL) twice daily in those with Child-Pugh scores 9–12.

Renal Impairment
- Dosage adjustments not needed.
- Use oral solution with caution in patients with renal impairment; oral solution contraindicated in those with renal failure.

Geriatric Patients
- Cautious dosage selection; pharmacokinetics have not been studied in this age group.

Anagrelide

(an ag′ gre lide)

Brand Name: Agrylin®

Why is this medicine prescribed?

Anagrelide is used to decrease the number of platelets (a type of blood cell that is needed to control bleeding) in the blood of patients who have a myeloproliferative disorder (condition in which the body makes too many of one or more types of blood cells) such as essential thrombocythemia (condition in which the body makes too many platelets) or polycythemia vera (condition in which the body makes too many red blood cells and sometimes too many platelets). Anagrelide is in a class of medications called platelet-reducing agents. It works by slowing the production of platelets in the body.

How should this medicine be used?

Anagrelide comes as a capsule to take by mouth. It is usually taken with or without food two to four times a day. Take anagrelide at around the same times every day. Follow the directions on your prescription label carefully, and ask your doctor or pharmacist to explain any part you do not understand. Take anagrelide exactly as directed. Do not take more or less of it or take it more often than prescribed by your doctor.

Your doctor will probably start you on a low dose of anagrelide and gradually increase your dose, not more often than once a week. Your doctor may change your dose during your treatment based upon your body's response to the medication. Follow these directions carefully.

Anagrelide may help control your condition but will not cure it. Continue to take anagrelide even if you feel well. Do not stop taking anagrelide without talking to your doctor. If you suddenly stop taking anagrelide, the number of platelets in your blood will increase and you may experience symptoms.

Are there other uses for this medicine?

This medication may be prescribed for other uses; ask your doctor or pharmacist for more information.

What special precautions should I follow?

Before taking anagrelide,
- tell your doctor and pharmacist if you are allergic to anagrelide or any other medications.
- tell your doctor and pharmacist what other prescription and nonprescription medications, vitamins, nutritional supplements, and herbal products you are taking or plan to take. Be sure to mention any of the following: atazanavir (Reyataz); cilostazol (Pletal); cimetidine (Tagamet); clozapine (Clozaril); cyclobenzaprine (Flexeril); fluoroquinolone antibiotics including ciprofloxacin (Cipro), gatifloxacin (Tequin), levofloxacin (Levaquin), norfloxacin (Noroxin), ofloxacin (Floxin), others; fluvoxamine (Luvox); imipramine (Tofranil); inamrinone; mexiletine (Mexitil); milrinone (Primacor); naproxen (Aleve, Naprosyn, in Prevacid NapraPAC); riluzole (Rilutek); sucralfate (Carafate); tacrine (Cognex); theophylline (Elixophyllin, Theo-24, Theolair, others); and ticlopidine (Ticlid). Your doctor may need to change the doses of your medications or monitor you carefully for side effects.
- tell your doctor if you have or have ever had bleeding problems; high or low blood pressure; lactose intolerance (inability to digest dairy products) or heart, kidney, or liver disease.
- do not take anagrelide if you are pregnant or plan to become pregnant. You should use an effective form of birth control to prevent pregnancy during your treatment with anagrelide. Talk to your doctor about types of birth control that are right for you. If you become pregnant while taking anagrelide, call your doctor immediately. Do not breastfeed while you are taking anagrelide.
- if you are having surgery, including dental surgery, tell the doctor or dentist that you are taking anagrelide.

- you should know that anagrelide may make you dizzy, especially when you first start taking the medication. Do not drive a car or operate machinery until you know how this medication affects you.
- you should know that anagrelide may cause dizziness, lightheadedness, and fainting when you get up too quickly from a lying position. This is more common when you first start taking anagrelide. To avoid this problem, get out of bed slowly, resting your feet on the floor for a few minutes before standing up.
- plan to avoid unnecessary or prolonged exposure to sunlight and to wear protective clothing, sunglasses, and sunscreen. Anagrelide may make your skin sensitive to sunlight.

What special dietary instructions should I follow?

Talk to your doctor about eating grapefruit and drinking grapefruit juice while taking this medication.

What should I do if I forget to take a dose?

Take the missed dose as soon as you remember it. However, if it is almost time for the next dose, skip the missed dose and continue your regular dosing schedule. Do not take a double dose to make up for a missed one.

What side effects can this medicine cause?

Anagrelide may cause side effects. Tell your doctor if any of these symptoms are severe or do not go away:

- headache
- gas
- upset stomach
- vomiting
- diarrhea
- constipation
- stomach pain
- heartburn
- belching
- loss of appetite
- runny nose
- nosebleed
- sore throat
- mouth sores
- dizziness
- depression
- nervousness
- forgetfulness
- confusion
- difficulty falling asleep or staying asleep
- lack of energy or sleepiness
- weakness
- muscle, joint or back pain
- leg cramps
- hair loss
- fever
- flu-like symptoms

- painful urination
- ringing in the ears
- itching

If you experience any of the following symptoms, call your doctor immediately:

- rash
- hives
- unusual bleeding or bruising
- blood in urine or stool
- black or tarry stools
- chest pain
- fluttering sensation in the chest
- fast, forceful, or irregular heartbeats
- swelling of the arms, hands, feet, ankles or lower legs
- difficulty breathing
- cough
- slow or difficult speech
- fainting
- weakness or numbness of an arm or leg
- pain, burning, or tingling in the hands or feet
- seizure
- changes in vision

If you experience a serious side effect, you or your doctor may send a report to the Food and Drug Administration's (FDA) MedWatch Adverse Event Reporting program online [at http://www.fda.gov/MedWatch/index.html] or by phone [1-800-332-1088].

What storage conditions are needed for this medicine?

Keep this medication in the container it came in, tightly closed, and out of reach of children. Store it at room temperature and away from light or excess heat and moisture (not in the bathroom). Throw away any medication that is outdated or no longer needed. Talk to your pharmacist about the proper disposal of your medication.

What should I do in case of overdose?

In case of overdose, call your local poison control center at 1-800-222-1222. If the victim has collapsed or is not breathing, call local emergency services at 911.

Symptoms of overdose may include:

- unusual bleeding or bruising

What other information should I know?

Keep all appointments with your doctor and the laboratory. Your doctor will order certain lab tests to check your body's response to anagrelide.

Do not let anyone else take your medication. Ask your pharmacist any questions you have about refilling your prescription.

Talk to your doctor, pharmacist, or other healthcare professional if you have questions about dosing information for your medication.

Anakinra

(an a kin′ ra)

Brand Name: Kineret®

Why is this medicine prescribed?

Anakinra is used, alone or in combination with other medications, to reduce the pain and swelling associated with rheumatoid arthritis. Anakinra is in a class of medications called interleukin antagonists. It works by blocking the activity of interleukin, a protein in the body that causes joint damage.

How should this medicine be used?

Anakinra comes as a solution to inject subcutaneously (under the skin). It is usually injected once a day, at the same time every day. Follow the directions on your prescription label carefully, and ask your doctor or pharmacist to explain any part you do not understand. Take anakinra exactly as directed. Do not take more or less of it or take it more often than prescribed by your doctor.

Anakinra comes in prefilled glass syringes. There are seven syringes in each box, one for each day of the week. Use each syringe only once and inject all the solution in the syringe. Even if there is still some solution left in the syringe after you inject, do not inject again. Dispose of used syringes in a puncture-resistant container. Talk to your doctor or pharmacist about how to dispose of the puncture-resistant container.

Do not shake prefilled syringes. If the solution is foamy, allow the syringe to sit for a few minutes until it clears. Do not use a syringe if its contents look discolored or cloudy or if it has anything floating in it.

You can inject anakinra in the outer thigh or stomach. If someone else is giving you the injection, it can be injected in the back of the arms or buttocks. To reduce the chances of soreness or redness, use a different site for each injection. You do not have to change the part of the body every day, but the new injection should be given about 1 inch away from the previous injection. Do not inject close to a vein you can see under the skin.

Before you use anakinra for the first time, read the manufacturer's information for the patient that comes with it. Ask your doctor or pharmacist to show you how to inject anakinra.

To administer the injection, follow these steps:

1. Clean the injection site with an alcohol wipe using a circular motion, starting from the middle and moving outwards. Let the area dry completely.
2. Hold the syringe and pull the needle cover off by twisting the cover while pulling on it. Do not touch the needle.
3. Hold the syringe in the hand you use to inject yourself. If possible, use your other hand to pinch a fold of skin at the injection site. Do not lay the syringe down or allow the needle to touch anything.
4. Hold the syringe between your thumb and fingers so you have steady control. Insert the needle into the skin with a quick, short motion at a 45 to 90 degree angle. The needle should be inserted at least halfway.
5. Gently let go of the skin, but make sure the needle remains in your skin. Slowly push the plunger down into the syringe until it stops.
6. Remove the needle and do not recap it. Press dry gauze (NOT an alcohol wipe) over the injection site.
7. You may apply a small adhesive bandage over the injection site.
8. Place the entire used syringe in a puncture-resistant container.

It may take several weeks before you feel the full benefit of anakinra.

Are there other uses for this medicine?

This medication may be prescribed for other uses; ask your doctor or pharmacist for more information.

What special precautions should I follow?

Before taking anakinra,

- tell your doctor and pharmacist if you are allergic to anakinra, proteins made from bacterial cells (*E. coli*), latex, or any other medications.
- tell your doctor and pharmacist what prescription and nonprescription medications, vitamins, nutritional supplements, and herbal products you are taking. Be sure to mention any of the following: etanercept (Enbrel); infliximab (Remicade); and medications that suppress the immune system such as azathioprine (Imuran), cyclosporine (Neoral, Sandimmune), methotrexate (Rheumatrex), sirolimus (Rapamune), and tacrolimus (Prograf). Your doctor may need to change the doses of your medications or monitor you carefully for side effects.
- tell your doctor if you have an infection, asthma, HIV infection or AIDS, or kidney disease.
- tell your doctor if you are pregnant, plan to become pregnant, or are breast-feeding. If you become pregnant while taking anakinra, call your doctor.
- if you are having surgery, including dental surgery, tell the doctor or dentist that you are taking anakinra.
- do not have any vaccinations (e.g., measles or flu shots) without talking to your doctor.

What special dietary instructions should I follow?

Unless your doctor tells you otherwise, continue your normal diet.

What should I do if I forget to take a dose?

Take the missed dose as soon as you remember it. However, if it is almost time for the next dose, skip the missed dose and continue your regular dosing schedule. Do not take a double dose to make up for a missed one.

What side effects can this medicine cause?

Anakinra may cause side effects. Tell your doctor if any of these symptoms are severe or do not go away:

- redness, swelling, bruising, or pain at the site of injection
- headache
- upset stomach
- diarrhea
- runny nose
- stomach pain

Some side effects can be serious. The following symptoms are uncommon, but if you experience any of them, call your doctor immediately:

- rash
- flu-like symptoms
- fever, sore throat, chills, and other signs of infection
- coughing, wheezing, or chest pain
- hot, red, swollen area on the skin

Anakinra may cause other side effects. Call your doctor if you have any unusual problems while taking this medication.

If you experience a serious side effect, you or your doctor may send a report to the Food and Drug Administration's (FDA) MedWatch Adverse Event Reporting program online [at http://www.fda.gov/MedWatch/index.html] or by phone [1-800-332-1088].

What storage conditions are needed for this medicine?

Keep syringes and injection supplies out of the reach of children. Store anakinra syringes in the refrigerator. Do not freeze. Protect from light. Do not use a syringe that has been at room temperature for more than 24 hours. Throw away any medication left after the expiration date on the carton. Talk to your pharmacist about the proper disposal of your medication.

What should I do in case of overdose?

In case of overdose, call your local poison control center at 1-800-222-1222. If the victim has collapsed or is not breathing, call local emergency services at 911.

What other information should I know?

Keep all appointments with your doctor and the laboratory. Your doctor will order certain lab tests before and during treatment to check your body's response to anakinra.

Do not let anyone else take your medication. Ask your pharmacist any questions you have about refilling your prescription.

Dosage Facts
For Informational Purposes

Caution: Do not change your dose, how often you take your medication, or the length of time you are to take it without first talking to your healthcare provider.

The following dosage information was written using medical language for doctors and other healthcare professionals and is provided here for you to check your dosage. The dosage of this drug may differ for different patients. Therefore, always follow your doctor's instructions or the directions on the label. Contact your healthcare provider or pharmacist if you have any questions about the specific dosage of your medication after reviewing this information.

Adult Patients
Rheumatoid Arthritis

SUB-Q:
- 100 mg (entire contents [0.67 mL] of one prefilled syringe) daily.

Prescribing Limits
Adult Patients
Rheumatoid Arthritis

SUB-Q:
- Dosages >100 mg daily do not appear to provide additional benefit.

Special Populations
Renal Impairment
Rheumatoid Arthritis

SUB-Q:
- Consider decreasing dosage to 100 mg every *other* day in patients with severe renal insufficiency or end-stage renal disease (Cl_{cr} <30 mL/minute, as estimated from S_{cr}).

Anastrozole

(an as' troe zole)

Brand Name: Arimidex

About Your Treatment

Your doctor has ordered anastrozole to help treat your illness. Anastrozole comes as a tablet to take by mouth.

This medication is used alone or with other treatments such as surgery or radiation to treat:

- breast cancer in postmenopausal women (women who no longer get their periods).

Anastrozole is in a class of drugs known as non-steroidal aromatase inhibitors. It decreases the amount of estrogen the body makes. This can slow or stop the growth of many types of breast cancer cells that need estrogen to grow. The length of treatment depends on the types of drugs you are taking, how well your body responds to them, and the type of cancer you have.

Anastrozole is usually taken once a day with or without food. Take anastrozole at around the same time every day.

Follow the directions on your prescription label carefully and ask your doctor or pharmacist to explain anything you do not understand. Take anastrozole exactly as directed. Do not take more or less of it or take it more often than prescribed by your doctor. Continue to take anastrozole even if you feel well. Do not stop taking anastrozole without talking to your doctor.

Anastrozole is also sometimes used to prevent breast cancer in women who are at high risk of developing the disease. Talk to your doctor about the risks of using this medication for your condition.

This medication may be prescribed for other uses; ask your doctor or pharmacist for more information.

Precautions

Before taking anastrozole,

- tell your doctor and pharmacist if you are allergic to anastrozole or any other drugs.
- tell your doctor and pharmacist what prescription and nonprescription medications, vitamins, nutritional supplements, and herbal products you are taking or plan to take. Be sure to mention any of the following: medications containing estrogen such as hormone replacement therapy (HRT) or oral contraceptives (birth control pills); and tamoxifen (Nolvadex). Your doctor may need to change the doses of your medications or monitor you carefully for side effects.
- tell your doctor if you have or have ever had any medical condition, especially high cholesterol, liver disease, osteoporosis (a condition in which the bones are thin and fragile), abnormal vaginal bleeding, cancer of the uterus (womb), and blood clots.
- Anastrozole should only be taken by women who have undergone menopause and cannot become pregnant. However, if you are pregnant or breastfeeding, you should tell your doctor before you begin taking this drug. You should not plan to have children while receiving chemotherapy or for a while after treatments. Use a reliable method of birth control to prevent pregnancy. Talk to your doctor for further details. Anastrozole may harm the fetus.
- If you are having surgery, including dental surgery, tell the doctor or dentist that you are taking anastrozole.

Side Effects

Anastrozole may cause side effects. Tell your doctor if any of these symptoms are severe or do not go away:

- flu-like symptoms
- weakness
- headache
- flushing
- sweating
- nausea
- vomiting
- loss of appetite
- constipation
- diarrhea
- heartburn
- weight gain
- joint, bone, or muscle pain
- mood changes
- depression
- difficulty falling asleep or staying asleep
- nervousness
- dizziness
- vaginal bleeding
- vaginal dryness or irritation
- cough
- burning or tingling feeling
- dry mouth
- hair thinning

Some side effects can be serious. If you experience any of the following symptoms, call your doctor immediately:

- chest pain
- sore throat, fever, chills, swollen glands, and other signs of infection
- difficult, painful, or urgent urination
- blurred vision or vision changes
- pain, swelling, redness, warmth, or tenderness in 1 leg only
- pale skin
- fast heartbeat
- breast pain
- new lumps or masses in the breasts or other parts of the body
- blisters or peeling skin
- rash
- hives
- swelling of the eyes, face, lips, tongue, throat, arms, hands, feet, ankles, or lower legs

Anastrozole may cause or worsen osteoporosis. It can decrease the density of your bones and increase the chance of broken bones and fractures. Talk to your doctor about the risks of taking this medication and to find out what you can do to decrease these risks.

Anastrozole may cause other side effects. Call your doctor if you have any unusual problems while taking this drug.

If you experience a serious side effect, you or your doctor may send a report to the Food and Drug Administration's (FDA) MedWatch Adverse Event Reporting program online [at http://www.fda.gov/MedWatch/index.html] or by phone [1-800-332-1088].

Storage Conditions

Keep anastrozole in the container it came in, tightly closed, and out of reach of children. Store it at room temperature and away from excess heat and moisture (not in the bathroom). Throw away any medication that is outdated or no longer needed. Talk to your pharmacist about the proper disposal of your medication.

Overdose

In case of overdose, call your local poison control center at 1-800-222-1222. If the victim has collapsed or is not breathing, call local emergency services at 911.

Special Instructions

- Keep all appointments with your doctor.
- Do not let anyone else take your medication. Ask your pharmacist any questions you have about refilling your prescription.

Dosage Facts
For Informational Purposes

Caution: Do not change your dose, how often you take your medication, or the length of time you are to take it without first talking to your health-care provider.

The following dosage information was written using medical language for doctors and other healthcare professionals and is provided here for you to check your dosage. The dosage of this drug may differ for different patients. Therefore, always follow your doctor's instructions or the directions on the label. Contact your health-care provider or pharmacist if you have any questions about the specific dosage of your medication after reviewing this information.

Adult Patients

Breast Cancer
First-line Treatment of Locally Advanced or Metastatic Breast Cancer

ORAL:
- 1 mg once daily. Continue therapy until tumor progresses.

Second-line Treatment of Advanced Breast Cancer

ORAL:
- 1 mg once daily. Continue therapy until tumor progresses.

Adjuvant Treatment of Early Breast Cancer

ORAL:
- 1 mg once daily. Optimum duration unknown; ongoing clinical study designed for 5 year treatment period.

Antihemophilic Factor (Human)

(an tee hee moe fil′ ik) (fak tir)

Brand Name: Alphanate®, Hemofil® M Method M Monoclonal Purified, Humate-P®, Koate®-DVI, Monarc-M® Method M Monoclonal Purified, Monoclate-P®

About Your Treatment

Your doctor has ordered antihemophilic factor (human), an antihemophilic factor, to help your blood to clot. The drug will be either injected directly into your vein or added to an intravenous fluid that will drip through a needle or catheter placed in your vein for approximately 5-10 minutes. It will be given as often as your doctor determines you need it, possibly as often as every other day.

Antihemophilic factor (human), a substance naturally produced in your body, activates substances in your blood to form clots and decrease bleeding episodes. This medication is sometimes prescribed for other uses; ask your doctor or pharmacist for more information.

Your health care provider (doctor, nurse, or pharmacist) may measure the effectiveness and side effects of your treatment using laboratory tests and physical examinations. It is important to keep all appointments with your doctor and the laboratory. The length of treatment depends on how your symptoms respond to the medication.

Precautions

Before administering antihemophilic factor (human),
- tell your doctor and pharmacist if you have ever had a reaction to an antihemophilic factor or if you are allergic to any drugs.
- tell your doctor and pharmacist what prescription and nonprescription medications you are taking, especially aminocaproic acid (Amicar), anticoagulants ('blood thinners') such as warfarin (Coumadin), corticosteroids (e.g., prednisone), cyclophosphamide (Cytoxan), cyclosporine (Neoral, Sandimmune), heparin or low-molecular-weight heparin (Lovenox, Normiflo), interferon alfa (Roferon-A, Intron), vincristine (Oncovin), vitamin K, and other vitamins.
- tell your doctor if you are pregnant, plan to become pregnant, or are breast-feeding. If you become pregnant while taking antihemophilic factor (human), call your doctor.
- if you are having surgery, including dental surgery, tell the doctor or dentist that you are taking antihemophilic factor (human), before any surgeries or procedures.
- you should know antihemophilic factor (human) is prepared from human plasma. There is a risk that antihemophilic factor (human) may contain the human immunodeficiency virus (HIV) or viruses that may cause

hepatitis. Talk with your doctor about the potential risks of taking this medication.

Administering Your Medication

Before you administer antihemophilic factor (human), look at the solution closely. It should be clear and free of floating material. Gently squeeze the bag or observe the solution container to make sure there are no leaks. Do not use the solution if it is discolored, if it contains particles, or if the bag or container leaks. Use a new solution, but show the damaged one to your health care provider.

It is important that you use your medication exactly as directed. Do not stop your therapy on your own for any reason. Do not change your dosing schedule without talking to your health care provider. Your health care provider may tell you to stop your infusion if you have a mechanical problem (such as a blockage in the tubing, needle, or catheter); if you have to stop an infusion, call your health care provider immediately so your therapy can continue.

Side Effects

Antihemophilic factor (human) may cause side effects. Tell your health care provider if any of these symptoms are severe or do not go away:

- dizziness
- headache
- sore throat
- itching
- upset stomach
- vomiting
- tiredness

If you experience any of the following symptoms, stop your infusion and call your health care provider immediately:

- increased pulse rate
- hives
- unusual bleeding or bruising
- difficulty breathing
- chest discomfort or tightness
- chill
- fever

If you experience a serious side effect, you or your doctor may send a report to the Food and Drug Administration's (FDA) MedWatch Adverse Event Reporting program online [at http://www.fda.gov/MedWatch/index.html] or by phone [1-800-332-1088].

Storage Conditions

- Your health care provider will probably give you a several-day supply of antihemophilic factor (human) at a time. You will be told how to prepare each dose.

Store your medication only as directed. Make sure you understand what you need to store your medication properly.

Keep your supplies in a clean, dry place when you are not using them, and keep all medications and supplies out of reach of children. Your health care provider will tell you how to throw away used needles, syringes, tubing, and containers to avoid accidental injury.

Overdose

In case of overdose, call your local poison control center at 1-800-222-1222. If the victim has collapsed or is not breathing, call local emergency services at 911.

Signs of Infection

If you are receiving antihemophilic factor (human) in your vein or under your skin, you need to know the symptoms of a catheter-related infection (an infection where the needle enters your vein or skin). If you experience any of these effects near your intravenous catheter, tell your health care provider as soon as possible:

- tenderness
- warmth
- irritation
- drainage
- redness
- swelling
- pain

Talk to your doctor, pharmacist, or other healthcare professional if you have questions about dosing information for your medication.

Antihemophilic Factor (Recombinant)

(an tee hee moe fil' ik) (fak tir) (ree kom bi nant)

Brand Name: Helixate® FS, Kogenate® FS, Recombinate®, ReFacto®

About Your Treatment

Your doctor has ordered antihemophilic factor (recombinant) to help your blood to clot. The drug will be either injected directly into your vein or added to an intravenous fluid that will drip through a needle or catheter placed in your vein for approximately 5-10 minutes. It may be given as often as two or three times daily or only occasionally, such as once every two or more weeks.

Antihemophilic factor (recombinant), a synthetic version of substances naturally produced by the body, activates substances in your blood to form clots and decrease bleeding episodes. This medication is sometimes prescribed for other uses; ask your doctor or pharmacist for more information.

Your health care provider (doctor, nurse, or pharmacist) may measure the effectiveness and side effects of your treatment using laboratory tests and physical examinations. It is important to keep all appointments with your doctor and the laboratory. The length of treatment depends on how your symptoms respond to the medication.

Precautions

Before administering antihemophilic factor (recombinant),

- tell your doctor and pharmacist if you have ever had a reaction to an antihemophilic factor or if you are allergic to any drugs.
- tell your doctor and pharmacist what prescription and nonprescription medications you are taking, especially aminocaproic acid (Amicar), anticoagulants ('blood thinners') such as warfarin (Coumadin), corticosteroids (e.g., prednisone), cyclophosphamide (Cytoxan), cyclosporine (Neoral, Sandimmune), heparin or low-molecular-weight heparin (Lovenox, Normiflo), interferon alfa (Roferon-A, Intron), vincristine (Oncovin), vitamin K, and other vitamins.
- tell your doctor if you are pregnant, plan to become pregnant, or are breast-feeding. If you become pregnant while taking antihemophilic factor (recombinant), call your doctor.
- if you are having surgery, including dental surgery, tell the doctor or dentist that you are taking antihemophilic factor (recombinant), before any surgeries or procedures.

Administering Your Medication

Before you administer antihemophilic factor (recombinant), look at the solution closely. It should be clear and free of floating material. Gently squeeze the bag or observe the solution container to make sure there are no leaks. Do not use the solution if it is discolored, if it contains particles, or if the bag or container leaks. Use a new solution, but show the damaged one to your health care provider.

It is important that you use your medication exactly as directed. Do not stop your therapy on your own for any reason. Do not change your dosing schedule without talking to your health care provider. Your health care provider may tell you to stop your infusion if you have a mechanical problem (such as a blockage in the tubing, needle, or catheter); if you have to stop an infusion, call your health care provider immediately so your therapy can continue.

Side Effects

Antihemophilic factor (recombinant) may cause side effects. Tell your health care provider if any of these symptoms are severe or do not go away:

- dizziness
- headache
- sore throat
- itching
- upset stomach
- vomiting
- tiredness

If you experience any of the following symptoms, stop your infusion and call your health care provider immediately:

- increased pulse rate
- hives
- unusual bleeding or bruising
- difficulty breathing
- chest discomfort or tightness
- chills
- fever

If you experience a serious side effect, you or your doctor may send a report to the Food and Drug Administration's (FDA) MedWatch Adverse Event Reporting program online [at http://www.fda.gov/MedWatch/index.html] or by phone [1-800-332-1088].

Storage Conditions

- Your health care provider will probably give you a several-day supply of antihemophilic factor (recombinant) at a time. You will be told how to prepare each dose.

Store your medication only as directed. Make sure you understand what you need to store your medication properly.

Keep your supplies in a clean, dry place when you are not using them, and keep all medications and supplies out of reach of children. Your health care provider will tell you how to throw away used needles, syringes, tubing, and containers to avoid accidental injury.

Overdose

In case of overdose, call your local poison control center at 1-800-222-1222. If the victim has collapsed or is not breathing, call local emergency services at 911.

Signs of Infection

If you are receiving antihemophilic factor (recombinant) in your vein or under your skin, you need to know the symptoms of a catheter-related infection (an infection where the needle enters your vein or skin). If you experience any of these effects near your intravenous catheter, tell your health care provider as soon as possible:

- tenderness
- warmth
- irritation
- drainage
- redness
- swelling
- pain

Talk to your doctor, pharmacist, or other healthcare professional if you have questions about dosing information for your medication.

Apomorphine

(a poe mor′ feen)

Brand Name: Apokyn®

Why is this medicine prescribed?

Apomorphine is used to treat "off" episodes (times of difficulty moving, walking, and speaking that may happen as medication wears off or at random) in patients with Parkinson's disease (PD; a disorder of the nervous system that causes difficulties with movement, muscle control, and balance) who are taking other medications for their disorder. Apomorphine will not work to prevent "off" episodes, but will help improve symptoms when an "off" episode has already begun. Apomorphine is in a class of medications called dopamine agonists. Apomorphine works by mimicking the action of dopamine, a natural substance in the brain that is lacking in patients with PD.

How should this medicine be used?

Apomorphine comes as a solution to inject subcutaneously (just under the skin) and not into a vein. Apomorphine is usually injected when needed, according to your doctor's directions. Follow the directions on your prescription label carefully, and ask your doctor or pharmacist to explain any part you do not understand. Use apomorphine exactly as directed. Do not use more or less of it or use it more often than prescribed by your doctor.

Your doctor will give you another medication to take when you are using apomorphine. This medication will help decrease your chance of developing upset stomach and vomiting while you are using apomorphine, especially during the beginning of treatment. Your doctor will ask you to begin taking the other medication a few days before you begin to use apomorphine, and to continue taking the other medication for a few months. Do not stop taking the other medication until your doctor tells you to stop.

Your doctor will probably start you on a low dose of apomorphine and gradually increase your dose, not more than once every few days. Ask your doctor what to do if you do not use apomorphine for longer than 1 week. Your doctor will probably tell you to use a low dose and gradually increase your dose again.

Apomorphine solution comes in a glass cartridge to use with an injector pen. Some needles are provided with your pen and additional needles are sold separately. Ask your doctor or pharmacist if you have questions about the type of needle you need. Always use a new, sterile needle for each injection. Never reuse needles and never let a needle touch any surface except the place where you will inject the medicine. Throw away used needles in a puncture-resistant container kept out of reach of children. Talk to your doctor or pharmacist about how to throw away the puncture-resistant container.

You will receive your first dose of apomorphine in your doctor's office. After that, you can inject apomorphine yourself or have a friend or relative perform the injections. Your doctor will train the person who will be injecting the medication, and will test him to be sure he can give the injection correctly. Be sure that you and the person who will be giving the injections read the manufacturer's information for the patient that comes with apomorphine before you use it for the first time at home.

Be sure you know what numbers on the injector pen show your dose. Your doctor may have told you how many milligrams you need to use, but the pen is marked with milliliters. Ask your doctor or pharmacist if you are not sure how to find your dose on the injector pen.

The apomorphine injector pen is only for use by one person. Do not share your pen with anyone.

Be careful not to get apomorphine solution on your skin or in your eyes. If apomorphine does get on your skin or in your eyes, immediately wash your skin or flush your eyes with cold water.

You can inject apomorphine in your stomach area, upper arm, or upper leg. Do not inject into an area where the skin is sore, red, bruised, scarred, infected, or abnormal in any way. Use a different spot for each injection, choosing from among the spots you have been told to use. Keep a record of the date and spot of each injection. Do not use the same spot two times in a row.

To use the apomorphine injector pen, follow these steps:

1. Gather the supplies you will need to give the injection: alcohol swab, injector pen, apomorphine medication cartridge, and new, sterile needle unit. Wash your hands with soap and water.
2. If you already have a medication cartridge in the injector pen, go to step 7 below. To insert a new medication cartridge into the injector pen, follow steps 3-6.
3. Pull off the grey pen cap. Unscrew the cartridge holder from the body of the injector pen.
4. Look at the apomorphine medication cartridge you are going to put into the pen. Check the expiration date to make sure the medication is not expired. Only use a cartridge containing a clear and colorless solution. Do not use a cartridge containing a cloudy or green solution or a solution containing particles. If the apomorphine solution is not clear and colorless, if it contains particles, or if it is expired, do not use it and call your pharmacist.
5. Put the apomorphine cartridge into the cartridge holder. Put in the end with the metal cap first.
6. Lower the body of the pen onto the cartridge holder so that the rod presses against the cartridge plunger. Screw the cartridge holder onto the body of the injector pen. Tighten the pieces until no gap remains and one of the arrows lines up with the marker on the body of the pen.
7. Check the amount of solution in the cartridge through the window in the cartridge holder to be sure there is at least enough solution in the cartridge to give your dose. If the injector pen has been previously used, and the plunger has reached the red line on the cartridge, re-

move the cartridge and insert a new medication cartridge into the pen, beginning at step 3 above.

8. Remove the paper tab from the back of the needle unit.

9. Hold the injector pen by the cartridge holder and push the needle unit onto the pen. Turn the needle counterclockwise (to the left) to attach it to the cartridge holder.

10. Remove the outer needle shield with a gentle pull. Save the outer shield. Do not remove the inner needle shield yet. It is still needed to protect the needle.

11. Prime the injector pen to remove air bubbles. To prime, turn the dose knob to 0.1 mL. Carefully remove the inner needle shield and hold the injector pen with the needle pointing up. Hold the needle over a sink or surface that can be wiped easily and firmly push the injection button in as far as it will go and hold for at least 5 seconds. A small stream of medicine should come out of the end of the needle. If a medicine stream does not come out of the needle, repeat this step until a small stream of medicine comes out the end of the needle. Do this step three to four times when you begin to use a new cartridge and once each time you use the cartridge again. If the needle touches anything during the priming process, attach a new sterile needle unit to the injector pen.

12. Set your injection dose by turning the dose knob at the end of the pen until the correct dose (number of mL) is shown in the pen window. The dose will appear as a red number between black lines that line up next to the letters "mL" on the pen. Make sure the correct number appears in the window. Remember that you are setting your dose in mL (milliliters) and not mg (milligrams). If you are not sure how to set your dose, call your doctor or pharmacist. Never dial the dose or attempt to correct a dialing error while the pen needle is in the skin.

13. If you turn the dose knob past your dose by mistake, do not dial backwards. If you dial backwards, medication will be lost through the needle. To set the correct dose, continue to turn the dial until it is completely turned out. Press the injection button located on the end of the pen. This will reset the dial to zero without pushing medicine out of the needle. Repeat step 12 to set your correct dose.

14. Clean the skin in the area you chose to inject apomorphine with an alcohol swab and allow the skin to air dry.

15. With one hand pinch up about an inch of skin and fat tissue between your thumb and forefinger at the injection spot. With your other hand, insert the needle all the way into your pinched skin.

16. Push the injection button on the end of the injector pen all the way in. You will hear a clicking sound while the dose is injected. Push the injection button firmly for 5 seconds. Carefully remove the needle from your skin. Be careful not to stick another part of your body when you do this. If medicine is dripping from the needle, do not reinsert the needle. Remember to keep the needle in the skin longer the next time you inject apo-

morphine. Replace the outer needle shield and go to step 19.

17. If you are unable to push in the injection button, the medication cartridge is empty and no medication is being injected. Remove the needle from your skin, attach the needle shield and throw the needle away. Put a new medication cartridge and needle on the injector pen, choose and prepare a new injection site, and complete your injection.

18. If the injection button stops before you receive a complete dose, look at the number in the pen window. Remove the needle from your skin, attach the needle shield and throw away the needle. Put a new medication cartridge and needle on the injector pen. Set the injection dose to the number that last appeared in the pen window. Choose and prepare a new injection site, and complete your injection. Try to keep track of the number of times you have used a cartridge so you will know if the cartridge does not contain a complete dose.

19. Place the outer needle shield in the notch on the far left side of your pen carrying case. The opening of the needle shield should be pointing up. Carefully push the injector pen, needle pointing down, into the opening of the outer needle shield.

20. Pick up the pen and hold it by the cartridge holder. Unscrew the pen needle unit from the cartridge holder by turning in a counter-clockwise (to the left) direction. Throw away the needle unit properly.

21. Recap the pen. Never recap the pen with a needle attached.

Are there other uses for this medicine?

This medication may be prescribed for other uses; ask your doctor or pharmacist for more information.

What special precautions should I follow?

Before using apomorphine,

- tell your doctor and pharmacist if you are allergic to apomorphine, sulfa medications, any other medications, or sulfites.

- do not use apomorphine if you are taking a 5HT3 (serotonin) blocker such as alosetron (Lotronex), dolasetron (Anzemet), granisetron (Kytril), ondansetron (Zofran), or palonosetron (Aloxi).

- tell your doctor and pharmacist what other prescription and nonprescription medications, vitamins, nutritional supplements, and herbal products you are taking. Be sure to mention any of the following: allergy, cough and cold medications; amiodarone (Cordarone); antidepressants; antihistamines; cisapride (Propulsid); disopyramide (Norpace); diuretics ('water pills'); dofetilide (Tikosyn); erythromycin (E.E.S., E-Mycin, Erythrocin); haloperidol (Haldol); medications to treat mental illness or upset stomach, heart disease, high blood pressure, pain, or seizures; metoclopramide (Reglan); moxifloxacin (Avelox); muscle relaxants; other medications for

Parkinson's disease; phosphodiesterase inhibitors such as sildenafil (Viagra), tadalafil (Cialis), or vardenafil (Levitra); pimozide (Orap); procainamide (Procanbid, Pronestyl); quinidine (Quinidex); sedatives; sleeping pills; sotalol (Betapace); sparfloxacin (Zagam); tranquilizers; or nitrates such as isosorbide dinitrate (Isordril, Sorbitrate), isosorbide mononitrate (Imdur, ISMO), or nitroglycerin (Nitro-BID, nitro-Dur, Nitroquick, Nitrostat, others). Nitrates come as tablets, sublingual (under the tongue) tablets, sprays, patches, pastes, and ointments. Ask your doctor if you are not sure if any of your medications contain nitrates. Your doctor may need to change the doses of your medications or monitor you carefully for side effects.

- tell your doctor if you drink alcohol or if you have or have ever had asthma; dizziness; eye disease; fainting spells; irregular heartbeat; low blood pressure; mental illness; a sleep disorder; a stroke or mini-stroke, or other brain problems; sudden uncontrolled movements and falls; or heart, kidney, liver, or lung disease.
- tell your doctor if you are pregnant, plan to become pregnant, or are breast-feeding. If you become pregnant while using apomorphine, call your doctor.
- if you are having surgery, including dental surgery, tell the doctor or dentist that you are using apomorphine.
- you should know that apomorphine may make you drowsy. Do not drive a car, operate machinery, or do anything that might put you at risk of getting hurt until you know how this medication affects you.
- you should know that you may suddenly fall asleep during your regular daily activities while you are taking apomorphine. You may not feel drowsy before you fall asleep. If you suddenly fall asleep while you are doing something such as eating, talking, or watching television, call your doctor. Do not drive a car or operate machinery until you talk to your doctor.
- You should not drink alcohol while you are using apomorphine. Alcohol can make the side effects from apomorphine worse.
- you should know that apomorphine may cause dizziness, lightheadedness, upset stomach, sweating, and fainting when you get up too quickly from a lying or sitting position. This is more common when you first start using apomorphine or following an increase in dose. To avoid this problem, get out of bed or get up from a seated position slowly, resting your feet on the floor for a few minutes before standing up.

What special dietary instructions should I follow?

Unless your doctor tells you otherwise, continue your normal diet.

What should I do if I forget to take a dose?

This medication is usually taken as needed.

What side effects can this medicine cause?

Apomorphine may cause side effects. Tell your doctor if any of these symptoms are severe or do not go away:

- upset stomach
- vomiting
- constipation
- diarrhea
- headache
- yawning
- runny nose
- weakness
- paleness
- flushing
- bone or joint pain
- pain or difficulty in urination
- soreness, redness, pain, bruising, swelling, or itching in the place where you injected apomorphine

Some side effects can be serious. The following symptoms are uncommon, but if you experience any of them, call your doctor immediately:

- shortness of breath
- cough
- fast or pounding heart beat
- chest pain
- swelling of the hands, feet, ankles, or lower legs
- bruising
- sudden uncontrollable movements
- falling down
- hallucinations (seeing things or hearing voices that do not exist)
- depression
- confusion
- abnormal behavior
- change in vision
- painful erection that does not go away

Some laboratory animals who were given apomorphine developed eye disease. It is not known if apomorphine increases the risk of eye disease in humans. Talk to your doctor about the risks of using this medication.

Apomorphine may cause other side effects. Call your doctor if you have any unusual problems while taking this medication.

If you experience a serious side effect, you or your doctor may send a report to the Food and Drug Administration's (FDA) MedWatch Adverse Event Reporting program online [at http://www.fda.gov/MedWatch/index.html] or by phone [1-800-332-1088].

What storage conditions are needed for this medicine?

Keep this medication in the cartridge it came in and out of reach of children. Store the cartridge and injector pen in the carrying case, at room temperature away from dust, moisture (not in the bathroom) and cold or hot temperatures. Never store the pen with a needle attached. Throw away any medication cartridge that is outdated or no longer needed. Talk to your pharmacist about the proper disposal of your medication.

What should I do in case of overdose?

In case of overdose, call your local poison control center at 1-800-222-1222. If the victim has collapsed or is not breathing, call local emergency services at 911.

Symptoms of overdose may include:

- upset stomach
- fainting
- dizziness
- blurred vision
- slow heart beat
- abnormal behavior
- hallucinations (seeing things or hearing voices that do not exist)
- sudden uncontrollable movements

What other information should I know?

Keep all appointments with your doctor.

Do not let anyone else use your medication or injector pen. Ask your pharmacist any questions you have about refilling your prescription.

Apomorphine solution may stain fabric and other surfaces. If you do spill or drip apomorphine solution on a surface, you may wash it with lemon juice to prevent a stain from forming. Bleach will remove apomorphine stains, but should not be used on upholstery.

You may clean your apomorphine pen with a damp cloth as needed. Never use strong disinfectants or wash your pen under running water.

Dosage Facts
For Informational Purposes

Caution: Do not change your dose, how often you take your medication, or the length of time you are to take it without first talking to your healthcare provider.

The following dosage information was written using medical language for doctors and other healthcare professionals and is provided here for you to check your dosage. The dosage of this drug may differ for different patients. Therefore, always follow your doctor's instructions or the directions on the label. Contact your healthcare provider or pharmacist if you have any questions about the specific dosage of your medication after reviewing this information.

General Dosage Information

Available as apomorphine hydrochloride; dosage expressed in terms of the salt.

Provide dosing instructions for the patient or their caregiver in mL; dose on the dosing pen device is expressed in terms of mL.

Titrate dose according to patient's response and tolerance.

Adult Patients

Hypomobility Episodes Associated with Parkinson's Disease

SUB-Q:

- Initial test dose is 0.2 mL (2 mg). If the 0.2-mL (2-mg) dose is effective and tolerated, this dose may be used on an as-needed, outpatient basis. If necessary, the dose may be increased in 0.1-mL (1-mg) increments every few days.
- Patient is not a candidate for apomorphine therapy if clinically significant orthostatic hypotension occurs in response to initial 0.2-mL (2-mg) test dose.
- For patients who tolerate, but do not respond to the initial 0.2-mL (2-mg) test dose, administer a second test dose of 0.4 mL (4 mg) at the next observed "off" period, no sooner than 2 hours after the initial test dose. If the 0.4-mL (4-mg) dose is effective and tolerated, a 0.3-mL (3-mg) dose may be used on an as-needed, outpatient basis. If necessary, the dose may be increased in 0.1-mL (1-mg) increments every few days.
- For patients who respond, but do not tolerate the 0.4-mL (4-mg) test dose, administer a third test dose of 0.3 mL (3 mg) at the next observed "off" period, but no sooner than 2 hours after the 0.4-mL (4-mg) test dose. If the 0.3-mL (3-mg) dose is effective and tolerated, a 0.2-mL (2-mg) dose may be used on an as-needed, outpatient basis. If the 0.2-mL (2-mg) dose is tolerated, the dose may be increased, if needed, to 0.3 mL (3 mg) after a few days. The dose should not usually be increased to 0.4 mL (4 mg) on an outpatient basis in these patients.
- In clinical studies, most patients responded to doses of 0.3–0.6 mL (3–6 mg); average frequency of dosing was 3 times daily.
- If therapy has been interrupted for >1 week, reinitiate at a dose of 0.2 mL (2 mg) and gradually titrate to effect.

Prescribing Limits

Adult Patients

Hypomobility Episodes Associated with Parkinson's Disease

SUB-Q:

- No more than one dose of apomorphine should be administered for treatment of a single "off" episode. Safety and efficacy of a second dose during the same hypomobility episode in patients not responding to the initial dose have not been established.
- Doses >0.6 mL (6 mg) not associated with additional therapeutic effect and are not recommended.
- Limited experience with >5 doses per day or daily dosages >2 mL (20 mg).

Special Populations

Hepatic Impairment

- No special recommendations for patients with hepatic impairment.

Renal Impairment

- In patients with mild or moderate renal impairment, initial test dose and subsequent starting dose is 0.1 mg (1 mg).

Aprepitant

(ap-re′-pi-tant)

Brand Name: Emend®

Why is this medicine prescribed?

Aprepitant is used with other medications to prevent upset stomach and vomiting caused by cancer chemotherapy treatment. Aprepitant is in a class of medications called antiemetics. It works by blocking the action of neurokinin, a natural substance in the brain that causes upset stomach and vomiting.

How should this medicine be used?

Aprepitant comes as a capsule to swallow with a drink. Aprepitant is usually taken once daily, with or without food, during the first few days of your cancer chemotherapy treatment. You will probably take aprepitant 1 hour before your first dose of chemotherapy, and then each morning for the next 2 days. Follow the directions on your prescription label carefully, and ask your doctor or pharmacist to explain any part you do not understand. Take aprepitant exactly as directed. Do not take more or less of it or take it more often than prescribed by your doctor.

Aprepitant capsules come in two different strengths. Your doctor may prescribe both of the strengths for you to take at different times. You should be careful to take the right strength at the right time as directed by your doctor.

Aprepitant only works to prevent upset stomach and vomiting. If you already have these symptoms, do not take aprepitant. Call your doctor instead.

Aprepitant is used only during the first 3 days of cancer chemotherapy treatment cycles. Do not continue taking aprepitant longer than instructed by your doctor.

Are there other uses for this medicine?

This medication may be prescribed for other uses; ask your doctor or pharmacist for more information.

What special precautions should I follow?

Before taking aprepitant,

- tell your doctor and pharmacist if you are allergic to aprepitant or any other medications.
- do not take aprepitant if you are taking astemizole (Hismanal), cisapride (Propulsid), pimozide (Orap), or terfenadine (Seldane).
- tell your doctor and pharmacist what other prescription and nonprescription medications, vitamins, and nutritional supplements you are taking. Be sure to mention any of the following: anticoagulants ('blood thinners') such as warfarin (Coumadin); antifungals such as fluconazole (Diflucan), itraconzaole (Sporanox), and ketoconazole (Nizoral); benzodiazepines such as alprazolam (Xanax), diazepam (Valium), and triazolam (Halcion); buspirone (BuSpar); calcium channel blockers such as amlodipine (Norvasc), diltiazem (Cardizem, Dilacor, Tiazac,), felodipine (Lexxel, Plendil), nifedipine (Adalat, Procardia), nisoldipine (Sular), and verapamil (Calan, Isoptin, Verelan); chlolesterol-lowering medications (statins) such as atorvastatin (Lipitor), fluvastatin (Lescol); lovastatin (Altocor, Mevacor), and simvastin (Zocor); cancer chemotherapy medications such as docetaxel (Taxotere), etoposide (Toposar, VePesid), ifosfamide (Ifex), imatinib (Gleevec), irinotecan (Camptosar), paclitaxel (Taxol), tamoxifen (Nolvadex), vinblastine, vincristine (Vincasar), and vinorelbine (Navelbine); carbamazepine (Tegretol); celecoxib (Celebrex); chlorpheniramine (Chlor-Trimeton, other cough, cold and sinus medications); cimetidine (Tagamet); clarithromycin (Biaxin); cyclosporine (Neoral, Sandimmune); danazol (Danocrine); delavirdine (Rescriptor); dexamethasone (Decadron); diclofenac (Arthrotec, Voltaren); efavirenz (Sustiva); erythromycin (E.E.S., E-Mycin, Erythrocin); ethosuximide (Zarontin); fluoxetine (Prozac, Sarafem); fluvoxamine (Luvox); glipizide (Glucotrol); haloperidol (Haldol); HIV protease inhibitors such as indinavir (Crixivan), nelfinavir (Viracept), ritonavir (Norvir), and saquinavir (Fortovase, Invirase); ibuprofen (Advil, Motrin); irbesartan (Avapro, Avalide); isoniazid (INH, Nydriazid); losartan (Cozaar, Hyzaar); methadone (Dolophine, Methadose); methylprednisolone (Medrol); metronidazole (Flagyl); naproxen (Naprosyn); nefazadone (Serzone); oral contraceptives (birth control pills); phenobarbital (Luminal, Solfoton); phenytoin (Dilantin); piroxicam (Feldene); quinidine (Cardioglute, Quinaglute); quinine; rifabutin (Mycobutin); rifampin (Rifadin, Rimactane); tacrolimus (Prograf); sildenafil (Viagra); sulfamethoxazole (Bactrim, Septra, Sulfatrim); tolbutamide (Orinase); torsemide (Demadex); trazodone; troleandomycin (TAO); and zafirlukast (Accolate). Your doctor may need to change the doses of your medications or monitor you carefully for side effects.
- tell your doctor what herbal products you are taking, especially St. John's Wort.
- tell your doctor if you have or have ever had liver disease.
- tell your doctor if you are pregnant, plan to become pregnant, or are breast-feeding. If you become pregnant while taking aprepitant, call your doctor.

What special dietary instructions should I follow?

Talk to your doctor about drinking grapefruit juice while taking this medicine.

What should I do if I forget to take a dose?

Take the missed dose as soon as you remember it. However, if it is almost time for the next dose, skip the missed dose and continue your regular dosing schedule. Do not take a double dose to make up for a missed one.

What side effects can this medicine cause?

Aprepitant may cause side effects. Tell your doctor if any of these symptoms are severe or do not go away:

- weakness
- extreme tiredness
- dizziness
- diarrhea
- constipation
- stomach pain
- upset stomach
- hiccups
- loss of appetite

Some side effects can be serious. The following symptoms are uncommon, but if you experience any of them, call your doctor immediately:

- hives
- skin rash
- difficulty breathing or swallowing
- swelling of the face, throat, tongue, lips, eyes, hands, feet, ankles, or lower legs
- hoarseness

Laboratory animals who were given aprepitant developed tumors. It is not known if aprepitant increases the risk of tumors in humans. Talk to your doctor about the risks of taking aprepitant.

Aprepitant may cause other side effects. Call your doctor if you have any unusual problems while taking this medication.

If you experience a serious side effect, you or your doctor may send a report to the Food and Drug Administration's (FDA) MedWatch Adverse Event Reporting program online [at http://www.fda.gov/MedWatch/index.html] or by phone [1-800-332-1088].

What storage conditions are needed for this medicine?

Keep this medication in the container it came in, tightly closed, and out of reach of children. Store it at room temperature and away from excess heat and moisture (not in the bathroom). Throw away any medication that is outdated or no longer needed. Talk to your pharmacist about the proper disposal of your medication.

What should I do in case of overdose?

In case of overdose, call your local poison control center at 1-800-222-1222. If the victim has collapsed or is not breathing, call local emergency services at 911.

Symptoms of overdose may include:

- drowsiness
- headache

What other information should I know?

Keep all appointments with your doctor.

Do not let anyone else take your medication. Ask your pharmacist any questions you have about refilling your prescription.

Dosage Facts
For Informational Purposes

Caution: Do not change your dose, how often you take your medication, or the length of time you are to take it without first talking to your healthcare provider.

The following dosage information was written using medical language for doctors and other healthcare professionals and is provided here for you to check your dosage. The dosage of this drug may differ for different patients. Therefore, always follow your doctor's instructions or the directions on the label. Contact your healthcare provider or pharmacist if you have any questions about the specific dosage of your medication after reviewing this information.

Adult Patients

Cancer Chemotherapy-induced Nausea and Vomiting

Administer as part of a regimen that includes a 5-HT$_3$ receptor antagonist and a corticosteroid.

Highly Emetogenic Cancer Chemotherapy

ORAL:
- 125 mg administered 1 hour before chemotherapy on day 1, followed by 80 mg once daily in the morning on days 2 and 3 of the treatment regimen.
- In clinical studies, aprepitant was administered with IV ondansetron (32 mg 30 minutes before chemotherapy on day 1) and oral dexamethasone (12 mg 30 minutes before chemotherapy on day 1, followed by 8 mg once daily in the morning on days 2–4).

Moderately Emetogenic Cancer Chemotherapy

ORAL:
- 125 mg administered 1 hour before chemotherapy on day 1, followed by 80 mg once daily in the morning on days 2 and 3 of the treatment regimen.
- In a clinical study, aprepitant was administered with oral ondansetron (8 mg 30–60 minutes before chemotherapy on day 1, then 8 mg 8 hours after the first dose) and oral dexamethasone (12 mg 30 minutes before chemotherapy on day 1).

Special Populations

Hepatic Impairment
- No dosage adjustments necessary in patients with mild to moderate hepatic impairment. Not adequately studied in patients with severe hepatic impairment (Child-Pugh score >9).

Renal Impairment
- No dosage adjustments necessary in patients with renal impairment or end-stage renal disease requiring hemodialysis.

Geriatric Patients
- No dosage adjustments necessary.

Aripiprazole

(ay ri pip′ ray zole)

Brand Name: Abilify®

Important Warning

Studies have shown that older adults with dementia (a brain disorder that affects the ability to remember, think clearly, communicate, and perform daily activities and that may cause changes in mood and personality) who take antipsychotics (medications for mental illness) such as aripiprazole have an increased chance of death during treatment. Older adults with dementia may also have a greater chance of having a stroke or mini-stroke or other severe side effects during treatment. If you experience any of the following symptoms, call your doctor immediately: slow or difficult speech, sudden dizziness or faintness, weakness or numbness of an arm or leg. drowsiness, or difficulty swallowing.

Aripiprazole is not approved by the Food and Drug Administration (FDA) for the treatment of behavior problems in older adults with dementia. Talk to the doctor who prescribed this medication if you, a family member, or someone you care for has dementia and is taking aripiprazole. For more information visit the FDA website: http://www.fda.gov/cder

Why is this medicine prescribed?

Aripiprazole is used to treat the symptoms of schizophrenia (a mental illness that causes disturbed or unusual thinking, loss of interest in life, and strong or inappropriate emotions). It is also used to treat episodes of mania (frenzied, abnormally excited, or irritated mood) or mixed episodes (symptoms of mania and depression that happen together) in patients with bipolar disorder (manic depressive disorder; a disease that causes episodes of depression, episodes of mania, and other abnormal moods). Aripiprazole is in a class of medications called atypical antipsychotics. It works by changing the activity of certain natural substances in the brain.

How should this medicine be used?

Aripiprazole comes as a tablet, a solution (liquid), and an orally disintegrating tablet (tablet that dissolves quickly in the mouth) to take by mouth. It is usually taken once a day with or without food. Take aripiprazole at around the same time every day. Follow the directions on your prescription label carefully, and ask your doctor or pharmacist to explain any part you do not understand. Take aripiprazole exactly as directed. Do not take more or less of it or take it more often than prescribed by your doctor.

Do not try to push the orally disintegrating tablet through the foil. Instead, use dry hands to peel back the foil packaging. Immediately take out the tablet and place it on your tongue. The tablet will quickly dissolve and can be swallowed without liquid. If necessary, liquid can be used to take the orally disintegrating tablet. Do not split, chew, or crush the tablet.

Your doctor may start you on a low dose of aripiprazole and increase your dose after at least 2 weeks.

Aripiprazole may help control your symptoms, but will not cure your condition. It may take 2 weeks or longer before you feel the full benefit of aripiprazole. Continue to take aripiprazole even if you feel well. Do not stop taking aripiprazole without talking to your doctor.

Are there other uses for this medicine?

This medication may be prescribed for other uses; ask your doctor or pharmacist for more information.

What special precautions should I follow?

Before taking aripiprazole,

- tell your doctor and pharmacist if you are allergic to aripiprazole or any other medications.
- tell your doctor and pharmacist what prescription and nonprescription medications, vitamins, nutritional supplements, and herbal products you are taking or plan to take. Be sure to mention any of the following: amiodarone (Cordarone, Pacerone); antidepressants (mood elevators); antifungals such as fluconazole (Diflucan), itraconazole (Sporanox), and ketoconazole (Nizoral); antihistamines; bupropion (Wellbutrin); carbamazepine (Tegretol); celecoxib (Celebrex); chlorpromazine (Thorazine); cimetidine (Tagamet); clarithromycin (Biaxin); clomipramine (Anafranil); cyclosporine (Neoral, Sandimmune); danazol (Danocrine); delavirdine (Rescriptor); dexamethasone (Decadron); diltiazem (Cardizem, Dilacor, Tiazac); doxorubicin (Adriamycin); erythromycin (E.E.S., E-Mycin, Erythrocin); ethosuximide (Zarontin); fluoxetine (Prozac, Sarafem); fluvoxamine (Luvox); HIV protease inhibitors such as indinavir (Crixivan) and ritonavir (Norvir); ipratropium (Atrovent); isoniazid (INH, Nydrazid); lorazepam (Ativan); medications for anxiety, blood pressure, irritable bowel disease, mental illness, motion sickness, Parkinson's disease, seizures, ulcers, or urinary problems; metoclopramide (Reglan); methadone (Dolophine); metronidazole (Flagyl); nefazodone; hormonal contraceptives (birth control pills, patches, implants, rings and injections); paroxetine (Paxil); phenobarbital (Luminal, Solfoton); phenytoin (Dilantin); primidone (Mysoline); quinidine (Cardioquin, Quinaglute, Quinidex); ranitidine (Zantac); rifabutin (Mycobutin); rifampin (Rifadin, Rimactane); sedatives; sertraline (Zoloft); sleeping pills; terbinafine (Lamisil); tranquilizers; troglitazone (Rezulin) (not available in the United States); troleandomycin (TAO) (not available in the United States); verapamil

(Calan, Covera, Isoptin, Verelan); and zafirlukast (Accolate). Your doctor may need to change the doses of your medications or monitor you carefully for side effects.

- tell your doctor if you use or have ever used street drugs or have overused prescription medication and if you have or have ever had heart disease, heart failure, a heart attack, high or low blood pressure, a stroke, a ministroke, seizures, or any condition that makes it difficult for you to swallow, or if you or anyone in your family has or has ever had diabetes. Also tell your doctor if you have ever had to stop taking a medication for mental illness because of severe side effects.
- tell your doctor if you are pregnant or plan to become pregnant. If you become pregnant while taking aripiprazole, call your doctor. Do not breast-feed while taking aripiprazole.
- if you are having surgery, including dental surgery, tell the doctor or dentist that you are taking aripiprazole.
- you should know that aripiprazole may make you drowsy. Do not drive a car or operate machinery until you know how this medication affects you.
- you should know that alcohol can add to the drowsiness caused by this medication. Do not drink alcohol while taking aripiprazole.
- you should know that you may experience hyperglycemia (increases in your blood sugar) while you are taking this medication, even if you do not already have diabetes. If you have schizophrenia, you are more likely to develop diabetes than people who do not have schizophrenia, and taking aripiprazole or similar medications may increase this risk. Tell your doctor immediately if you have any of the following symptoms while you are taking aripiprazole: extreme thirst, frequent urination, extreme hunger, blurred vision, or weakness. It is very important to call your doctor as soon as you have any of these symptoms, because high blood sugar that is not treated can cause a serious condition called ketoacidosis. Ketoacidosis may become life-threatening if it is not treated at an early stage. Symptoms of ketoacidosis include: dry mouth, nausea and vomiting, shortness of breath, breath that smells fruity, and decreased consciousness.
- you should know that aripiprazole may cause dizziness, lightheadedness, and fainting when you get up too quickly from a lying position. This is more common when you first start taking aripiprazole. To avoid this problem, get out of bed slowly, resting your feet on the floor for a few minutes before standing up.
- you should know that aripiprazole may make it harder for your body to cool down when it gets very hot. Tell your doctor if you plan to do vigorous exercise or be exposed to extreme heat.
- if you have phenylketonuria (PKU, an inherited condition in which a special diet must be followed to prevent mental retardation), you should know that the orally disintegrating tablets contain phenylalanine. If you have

diabetes, you should know that aripiprazole solution contains sugar.

What special dietary instructions should I follow?

Talk to your doctor about drinking grapefruit juice while taking this medicine.

Be sure to drink plenty of water every day while you are taking this medication.

What should I do if I forget to take a dose?

Take the missed dose as soon as you remember it. However, if it is almost time for the next dose, skip the missed dose and continue your regular dosing schedule. Do not take a double dose to make up for a missed one.

What side effects can this medicine cause?

Aripiprazole may cause side effects. Tell your doctor if any of these symptoms are severe or do not go away:

- headache
- nervousness
- difficulty falling asleep or staying asleep
- drowsiness
- lightheadedness
- restlessness
- nausea
- heartburn
- constipation
- stomach pain
- weight gain
- dry mouth
- loss of appetite
- increased salivation
- joint pain

Some side effects can be serious. If you experience any of the following symptoms or those listed in the IMPORTANT WARNING section or the SPECIAL PRECAUTIONS section, call your doctor immediately:

- seizures
- slow, fast, or irregular heartbeat
- chest pain
- swelling of the hands, feet, ankles, or lower legs
- changes in vision
- unusual movements of your body or face that you cannot control
- high fever
- muscle stiffness
- confusion
- sweating
- rash
- hives
- itching
- difficulty breathing or swallowing

Aripiprazole may cause other side effects. Call your doctor if you have any unusual problems while taking this medication.

If you experience a serious side effect, you or your doctor may send a report to the Food and Drug Administration's (FDA) MedWatch Adverse Event Reporting program online [at http://www.fda.gov/MedWatch/index.html] or by phone [1-800-332-1088].

What storage conditions are needed for this medicine?

Keep this medication in the container it came in, tightly closed, and out of reach of children. Store the tablets, the solution, and the orally disintegrating tablets at room temperature and away from excess heat and moisture (not in the bathroom). Always store the orally disintegrating tablets in their sealed package, and use them immediately after opening the package. Throw away any medication that is outdated or no longer needed. Throw away any unused aripiprazole solution 6 months after you open the bottle, even if the expiration date marked on the bottle has not passed. Talk to your pharmacist about the proper disposal of your medication.

What should I do in case of overdose?

In case of overdose, call your local poison control center at 1-800-222-1222. If the victim has collapsed or is not breathing, call local emergency services at 911.

Symptoms of overdose may include:

- drowsiness
- weakness
- widened pupils (black circles in the middle of the eyes)
- nausea
- vomiting
- changes in heartbeat
- movements that you can not control
- confusion
- seizures
- loss of consciousness

What other information should I know?

Keep all appointments with your doctor.

Do not let anyone else take your medication. Ask your pharmacist any questions you have about refilling your prescription.

Dosage Facts

For Informational Purposes

Caution: Do not change your dose, how often you take your medication, or the length of time you are to take it without first talking to your healthcare provider.

The following dosage information was written using medical language for doctors and other healthcare professionals and is provided here for you to check your dosage. The dosage of this drug may differ for different patients. Therefore, always follow your doctor's instruc-

tions or the directions on the label. Contact your healthcare provider or pharmacist if you have any questions about the specific dosage of your medication after reviewing this information.

General Dosage Information

Oral solution may be given at same dose on mg-per-mg basis as the 5-, 10-, 15-, or 20-mg tablet strengths of the drug up to a dose of 25 mg. However, if oral solution is used in patients receiving aripiprazole 30-mg tablets, use a dose of 25 mg of the oral solution.

Adult Patients

Schizophrenia

ORAL:

- Initial and target dosage is 10 or 15 mg once daily.
- Dosages ranging from 10–30 mg daily were effective in clinical trials; dosages exceeding 10–15 mg daily did not result in greater efficacy.
- Adjust dosage at intervals of not less than 2 weeks, the time needed to achieve steady-state concentrations.
- In patients responding to aripiprazole therapy, continue the drug as long as clinically necessary and tolerated, but at lowest possible effective dosage; periodically reassess need for continued therapy.
- Long-term efficacy of aripiprazole has not been established, and optimum duration of therapy currently is not known. However, aripiprazole has been used as maintenance therapy for up to 26 weeks in clinical trials, and maintenance therapy with antipsychotic agents is well established.

Bipolar Disorder
Acute Mania and Mixed Episodes

ORAL:

- Initial dosage of 30 mg once daily as tablets was used in clinical trials.
- Dosage was decreased to 15 mg once daily in clinical trials if initial 30-mg dosage was not well tolerated.
- Safety of dosages >30 mg daily has not been established.
- Long-term efficacy (i.e., >6 weeks) of aripiprazole has not been established, and optimum duration of therapy currently is not known. Periodically reevaluate the long-term risks and benefits of the drug for the individual patient.

Special Populations

Patients Receiving CYP3A4 or CYP2D6 Inhibitors
- Reduce aripiprazole dosage to one-half the usual dosage in patients receiving concomitant therapy with inhibitors of CYP3A4 (e.g., ketoconazole) or CYP2D6 (e.g., fluoxetine, paroxetine, quinidine); increase aripiprazole dosage to the usual dosage after discontinuance of the CYP3A4 or CYP2D6 inhibitor.

Patients Receiving CYP3A4 Inducers
- Increase aripiprazole dosage to 20–30 mg daily upon initiation of concomitant therapy with drugs that induce CYP3A4 (e.g., carbamazepine); additional dosage escalation should be based on clinical evaluation. Decrease aripiprazole dosage to 10–15 mg daily if the CYP3A4 inducer is discontinued.

Ascorbic Acid

(a skor' bik)

Brand Name: Cecon® Drops, Cenolate®, Cevi-Bid®, Vicks® Vitamin C Drops

Why is this medicine prescribed?

Ascorbic acid is used to prevent and treat scurvy, a disease caused by a lack of vitamin C in the body.

This medication is sometimes prescribed for other uses; ask your doctor or pharmacist for more information.

How should this medicine be used?

Ascorbic acid comes in extended-release (long-acting) capsules and tablets, lozenges, syrup, chewable tablets, and liquid drops to be given by mouth. It usually is taken once a day. Follow the directions on the package or on your prescription label carefully, and ask your doctor or pharmacist to explain any part you do not understand. Take ascorbic acid exactly as directed. Do not take more or less of it or take it more often than prescribed by your doctor.

Some tablets should be chewed; other tablets and capsules should be swallowed with a full glass of water.

It may take up to 3 weeks for symptoms of scurvy to improve.

What special precautions should I follow?

Before taking ascorbic acid,

- tell your doctor and pharmacist if you are allergic to ascorbic acid or any other drugs.
- tell your doctor and pharmacist what prescription and nonprescription medications you are taking, including other vitamins.
- tell your doctor if you have or have ever had kidney stones. Diabetics should talk to their doctor or pharmacist for the correct way to test their urine while taking large amounts of ascorbic acid.
- tell your doctor if you are pregnant, plan to become pregnant, or are breast-feeding. If you become pregnant while taking ascorbic acid, call your doctor.

What special dietary instructions should I follow?

Some forms of ascorbic acid contain sodium and should be avoided if you are on a sodium- or salt-restricted diet.

Your doctor may suggest changes in your diet to give you more vitamin C.

What should I do if I forget to take a dose?

Take the missed dose as soon as you remember it. However, if it is almost time for the next dose, skip the missed dose and continue your regular dosing schedule. Do not take a double dose to make up for a missed one.

What side effects can this medicine cause?

Ascorbic acid may cause side effects. Tell your doctor if either of these symptoms is severe or does not go away:

- diarrhea
- upset stomach

What storage conditions are needed for this medicine?

Keep this medication in the container it came in, tightly closed, and out of reach of children. Store it at room temperature and away from excess heat and moisture (not in the bathroom). Throw away any medication that is outdated or no longer needed. Talk to your pharmacist about the proper disposal of your medication.

What should I do in case of overdose?

In case of overdose, call your local poison control center at 1-800-222-1222. If the victim has collapsed or is not breathing, call local emergency services at 911.

What other information should I know?

Keep all appointments with your doctor.

Do not let anyone else take your medication. Ask your pharmacist any questions you have about refilling your prescription.

Talk to your doctor, pharmacist, or other healthcare professional if you have questions about dosing information for your medication.

Aspirin

(as' pir in)

Brand Name: Adprin B® Tri-Buffered Caplets®, Alka-Seltzer® Effervescent Pain Reliever and Antacid, Alka-Seltzer® Extra Strength Effervescent Pain Reliever and Antacid, Alka-Seltzer® Flavored Effervescent Pain Reliever and Antacid, Ascriptin® Arthritis Pain Caplets®, Ascriptin® Enteric Adult Low Strength, Ascriptin® Enteric Regular Strength, Ascriptin® Maximum Extra Strength Caplets®, Ascriptin® Regular Strength, Aspergum®, Bayer® Aspirin with Calcium Regimen Caplets®, Bayer® Aspirin Arthritis Pain Regimen Extra Strength Caplets®, Bayer® Aspirin Caplets®, Bayer® Aspirin Extra Strength Caplets®, Bayer® Aspirin Extra Strength Gelcaps®, Bayer® Aspirin Extra Strength Tablets, Bayer® Aspirin Gelcaps®, Bayer® Aspirin Plus Buffered Extra Strength Caplets®, Bayer® Aspirin Regimen Adult Low Strength, Bayer® Aspirin Regimen Children's

Chewable, Bayer® Aspirin Regimen Regular Strength Caplets®, Bayer® Aspirin Tablets, Bufferin® Arthritis Strength Caplets®, Bufferin® Enteric Low Dose Caplets®, Bufferin® Extra Strength, Bufferin® Tablets, Easprin®, Ecotrin®, Ecotrin® Adult Low Strength, Ecotrin® Maximum Strength, Excedrin® Extra-Strength Caplets®, Excedrin® Extra-Strength Geltabs, Excedrin® Extra-Strength Tablets, Excedrin® Migraine Tablets, Genacote®, Genacote® Maximum Strength, Goody's® Extra Strength Headache Powders, Halfprin®, Magnaprin® Arthritis Strength, Magnaprin® Improved, Norwich® Aspirin, Norwich® Aspirin Maximum Strength, St. Joseph® Aspirin Adult Chewable®, Sureprin®, ZORprin®

Also available generically.

Why is this medicine prescribed?

Prescription aspirin is used to relieve the symptoms of rheumatoid arthritis (arthritis caused by swelling of the lining of the joints), osteoarthritis (arthritis caused by breakdown of the lining of the joints), systemic lupus erythematosus (condition in which the immune system attacks the joints and organs and causes pain and swelling) and certain other rheumatologic conditions (conditions in which the immune system attacks parts of the body). Nonprescription aspirin is used to reduce fever and to relieve mild to moderate pain from headaches, menstrual periods, arthritis, colds, toothaches, and muscle aches. Nonprescription aspirin is also used to prevent heart attacks in people who have had a heart attack in the past or who have angina (chest pain that occurs when the heart does not get enough oxygen). Nonprescription aspirin is also used to reduce the risk of death in people who are experiencing or who have recently experienced a heart attack. Nonprescription aspirin is also used to prevent ischemic strokes (strokes that occur when a blood clot blocks the flow of blood to the brain) or mini-strokes (strokes that occur when the flow of blood to the brain is blocked for a short time) in people who have had this type of stroke or mini-stroke in the past. Aspirin will not prevent hemorrhagic strokes (strokes caused by bleeding in the brain). Aspirin is in a group of medications called salicylates. It works by stopping the production of certain natural substances that cause fever, pain, swelling, and blood clots.

Aspirin is also available in combination with other medications such as antacids, pain relievers, and cough and cold medications. This monograph only includes information about the use of aspirin alone. If you are taking a combination product, read the information on the package or prescription label or ask your doctor or pharmacist for more information.

How should this medicine be used?

Prescription aspirin comes as an extended-release tablet (tablet that releases medication slowly over a period of time). Nonprescription aspirin comes as a regular tablet, an enteric-coated, delayed-release tablet (tablet that first begins to release medication some time after it is taken), a chewable tablet, and a gum to take by mouth and a suppository to use rectally. Prescription aspirin is usually taken two or more times a day. Nonprescription aspirin is usually taken once a day to lower the risk of a heart attack or stroke. Nonprescription aspirin is usually taken every 4 to 6 hours as needed to treat fever or pain. Follow the directions on the package or prescription label carefully, and ask your doctor or pharmacist to explain any part you do not understand. Take aspirin exactly as directed. Do not take more or less of it or take it more often than directed by the package label or prescribed by your doctor.

Swallow the extended-release tablets whole with a full glass of water. Do not break, crush, or chew them.

Swallow the tablets with a full glass of water.

Chewable aspirin tablets may be chewed, crushed, or swallowed whole. Drink a full glass of water, immediately after taking these tablets.

Ask a doctor before you give aspirin to your child or teenager. Aspirin may cause Reye's syndrome (a serious condition in which fat builds up on the brain, liver, and other body organs) in children and teenagers, especially if they have a virus such as chicken pox or the flu.

If you have had oral surgery or surgery to remove your tonsils in the last 7 days, talk to your doctor about which types of aspirin are safe for you.

Delayed-release tablets begin to work some time after they are taken. Do not take delayed-release tablets for fever or pain that must be relieved quickly.

Stop taking aspirin and call your doctor if your fever lasts longer than 3 days, if your pain lasts longer than 10 days, or if the part of your body that was painful becomes red or swollen. You may have a condition that must be treated by a doctor.

To insert an aspirin suppository into the rectum, follow these steps:

1. Remove the wrapper.
2. Dip the tip of the suppository in water.
3. Lie down on your left side and raise your right knee to your chest. (If you are left-handed, lie on your right side and raise your left knee.)
4. Using your finger, insert the suppository into the rectum, about 1/2 to 1 inch in infants and children and 1 inch in adults. Hold it in place for a few moments..
5. Do not stand up for at least 15 minutes. Then wash your hands thoroughly and resume your normal activities.

Are there other uses for this medicine?

Aspirin is also sometimes used to treat rheumatic fever (a serious condition that may develop after a strep throat infection and may cause swelling of the heart valves) and Kawasaki disease (an illness that may cause heart problems in children). Aspirin is also sometimes used to lower the risk of blood clots in patients who have artificial heart valves or certain other heart conditions and to prevent certain complications of pregnancy.

What special precautions should I follow?

Before taking aspirin,

- tell your doctor and pharmacist if you are allergic to aspirin, other medications for pain or fever, tartrazine dye, or any other medications.
- tell your doctor and pharmacist what prescription and nonprescription medications, vitamins, nutritional supplements, and herbal products you are taking or plan to take. Be sure to mention any of the following: acetazolamide (Diamox); angiotensin-converting enzyme (ACE) inhibitors such as benazepril (Lotensin), captopril (Capoten), enalapril (Vasotec), fosinopril (Monopril), lisinopril (Prinivil, Zestril), moexipril (Univasc), perindopril, (Aceon), quinapril (Accupril), ramipril (Altace), and trandolapril (Mavik); anticoagulants ('blood thinners') such as warfarin (Coumadin) and heparin; beta blockers such as atenolol (Tenormin), labetalol (Normodyne), metoprolol (Lopressor, Toprol XL), nadolol (Corgard), and propranolol (Inderal); diuretics ('water pills'); medications for diabetes or arthritis; medications for gout such as probenecid and sulfinpyrazone (Anturane); methotrexate (Trexall); other non steroidal anti-inflammatory medications (NSAIDs) such as naproxen (Aleve, Naprosyn); phenytoin (Dilantin); and valproic acid (Depakene, Depakote). Your doctor may need to change the doses of your medications or monitor you more carefully for side effects.
- if you are taking aspirin on a regular basis to prevent heart attack or stroke, do not take ibuprofen (Advil, Motrin) to treat pain or fever without talking to your doctor. Your doctor will probably tell you to allow some time to pass between taking your daily dose of aspirin and taking a dose of ibuprofen.
- tell your doctor if you have or have ever had asthma, frequent stuffed or runny nose, or nasal polyps (growths on the linings of the nose). If you have these conditions, there is a risk that you will have an allergic reaction to aspirin. Your doctor may tell you that you should not take aspirin.
- tell your doctor if you often have heartburn, upset stomach, or stomach pain and if you have or have ever had ulcers, anemia, bleeding problems such as hemophilia, or kidney or liver disease.
- tell your doctor if you are pregnant, especially if you are in the last few months of your pregnancy, you plan to become pregnant, or you are breast-feeding. If you become pregnant while taking aspirin, call your doctor. Aspirin may harm the fetus and cause problems with delivery if it is taken during the last few months of pregnancy.
- if you are having surgery, including dental surgery, tell the doctor or dentist that you are taking aspirin.
- if you drink three or more alcoholic drinks every day, ask your doctor if you should take aspirin or other medications for pain and fever.

What special dietary instructions should I follow?

Unless your doctor tells you otherwise, continue your normal diet.

What should I do if I forget to take a dose?

If your doctor has told you to take aspirin on a regular basis and you miss a dose, take the missed dose as soon as you remember it. However, if it is almost time for the next dose, skip the missed dose and continue your regular dosing schedule. Do not take a double dose to make up for a missed one.

What side effects can this medicine cause?

Aspirin may cause side effects. Tell your doctor if any of these symptoms are severe or do not go away:

- nausea
- vomiting
- stomach pain
- heartburn

Some side effects can be serious. If you experience any of the following symptoms, call your doctor immediately:

- hives
- rash
- swelling of the eyes, face, lips, tongue, or throat
- wheezing or difficulty breathing
- hoarseness
- fast heartbeat
- fast breathing
- cold, clammy skin
- ringing in the ears
- loss of hearing
- bloody vomit
- vomiting material that looks like coffee grounds
- bright red blood in stools
- black or tarry stools

Aspirin may cause other side effects. Call your doctor if you experience any unusual problems while you are taking this medication.

If you experience a serious side effect, you or your doctor may send a report to the Food and Drug Administration's (FDA) MedWatch Adverse Event Reporting program online [at http://www.fda.gov/MedWatch/index.html] or by phone [1-800-332-1088].

What storage conditions are needed for this medicine?

Keep this medication in the container it came in, tightly closed, and out of reach of children. Store it at room temperature and away from excess heat and moisture (not in the bathroom). Store aspirin suppositories in a cool place or in a refrigerator. Throw away any medication that is outdated or no longer needed and any tablets that have a strong vinegar smell. Talk to your pharmacist about the proper disposal of your medication.

What should I do in case of overdose?

In case of overdose, call your local poison control center at 1-800-222-1222. If the victim has collapsed or is not breathing, call local emergency services at 911.

Symptoms of overdose may include:
- burning pain in the throat or stomach
- vomiting
- decreased urination
- fever
- restlessness
- irritability
- talking a lot and saying things that do not make sense
- fear or nervousness
- dizziness
- double vision
- uncontrollable shaking of a part of the body
- confusion
- abnormally excited mood
- hallucination (seeing things or hearing voices that are not there)
- seizures
- drowsiness
- loss of consciousness for a period of time

What other information should I know?

Keep all appointments with your doctor.

If you are taking prescription aspirin, do not let anyone else take your medication. Ask your pharmacist any questions you have about refilling your prescription.

Dosage Facts
For Informational Purposes

Caution: Do not change your dose, how often you take your medication, or the length of time you are to take it without first talking to your healthcare provider.

The following dosage information was written using medical language for doctors and other healthcare professionals and is provided here for you to check your dosage. The dosage of this drug may differ for different patients. Therefore, always follow your doctor's instructions or the directions on the label. Contact your healthcare provider or pharmacist if you have any questions about the specific dosage of your medication after reviewing this information.

General Dosage Information

When used for pain, fever, or inflammatory diseases, attempt to titrate to the lowest effective dosage.

When used in anti-inflammatory dosages, development of tinnitus can be used as a sign of elevated plasma salicylate concentrations (except in patients with high-frequency hearing impairment).

Pediatric Patients

Dosage in children should be guided by body weight or body surface area.

Do not use in children and teenagers with varicella or influenza, unless directed by a clinician.

Pain

ORAL:
- Children 2–11 years of age: 1.5 g/m^2 daily administered in 4–6 divided doses (maximum 2.5 g/m^2 daily).

Dosage for Self-medication of Pain in Children <12 Years of Age

Age	Weight	Oral Dose[a]
<3 years of age	<14.5 kg	Consult clinician
3–<4 years	14.5–16 kg	160 mg
4–<6 years	16–20.5 kg	240 mg
6–<9 years	20.5–30 kg	320 mg
9–<11 years	30–35 kg	320–400 mg
11 years	35–38 kg	320–480 mg

[a]Dose may be given every 4 hours as necessary (up to 5 times in 24 hours).

For *self-medication* in children ≥12 years of age, 325–650 mg every 4 hours (maximum 4 g daily) or 1 g every 6 hours as necessary.

For *self-medication* in children ≥12 years of age, 454 mg (as chewing gum pieces) every 4 hours as necessary (maximum 3.632 g daily).

For *self-medication* in children ≥12 years of age, 650 mg (as highly buffered effervescent solution [Alka-Seltzer® Original]) every 4 hours (maximum 2.6 g daily); alternatively, 1 g (Alka-Seltzer® Extra Strength) every 6 hours (maximum 3.5 g daily).

RECTAL:
- Children 2–11 years of age: 1.5 g/m^2 daily administered in 4–6 divided doses (maximum 2.5 g/m^2 daily).
- Children ≥12 years of age: 325–650 mg every 4 hours as necessary (maximum 4 g daily).

Fever

ORAL:
- Children 2–11 years of age: 1.5 g/m^2 daily administered in 4–6 divided doses (maximum 2.5 g/m^2 daily).

Dosage for Self-medication of Fever in Children <12 Years of Age

Age	Weight	Oral Dose[b]
<3 years of age	<14.5 kg	Consult physician
3–<4 years	14.5–16 kg	160 mg
4–<6 years	16–20.5 kg	240 mg
6–<9 years	20.5–30 kg	320 mg
9–<11 years	30–35 kg	320–400 mg
11 years	35–38 kg	320–480 mg

[b]Dose may be given every 4 hours as necessary (up to 5 times in 24 hours).

Children ≥12 years of age: 325–650 mg every 4 hours as necessary (maximum 4 g daily).

For *self-medication* in children ≥12 years of age, 454 mg (as chewing gum pieces) every 4 hours as necessary (maximum 3.632 g daily).

RECTAL:
- Children 2–11 years of age: 1.5 g/m² daily administered in 4–6 divided doses (maximum 2.5 g/m² daily).
- Children ≥12 years of age: 325–650 mg every 4 hours as necessary (maximum 4 g daily).

Inflammatory Diseases
Juvenile Rheumatoid Arthritis

ORAL:
- Initially, 90–130 mg/kg daily in divided doses. Increase dosage as necessary for anti-inflammatory efficacy; target plasma salicylate concentration is 150–300 mcg/mL. Plasma concentrations >200 mcg/mL associated with an increased incidence of toxicity.

Rheumatic Fever†

ORAL:
- Initially, 90–130 mg/kg daily given in divided doses every 4–6 hours for up to 1–2 weeks for maximal suppression of acute inflammation, followed by 60–70 mg/kg daily in divided doses for 1–6 weeks. Adjust dosage based on response, tolerance, and plasma salicylate concentrations. Gradually withdraw over 1–2 weeks.
- Various regimens suggested depending on severity of initial manifestations. Consult published protocols for more information on specific dosages and schedules.

Thrombosis
Acute Ischemic Stroke†

ORAL:
- 2–5 mg/kg daily suggested by ACCP following discontinuance of anticoagulant (e.g., unfractionated or LMW heparin, warfarin) therapy.

Blalock-Taussig Shunt†

ORAL:
- 5 mg/kg daily has been suggested following intraoperative heparin.

Fontan Procedure†

ORAL:
- 5 mg/kg daily has been suggested; optimal duration of therapy unknown.

Mechanical Prosthetic Heart Valves†

ORAL:
- 6–20 mg/kg daily in combination with oral anticoagulation for patients with lack of response to oral anticoagulation or contraindication to full-dose oral anticoagulation suggested by ACCP.

Bioprosthetic Heart Valves†

ORAL:
- ACCP suggests same treatment as for adults (75–100 mg daily long term in those in sinus rhythm).

Kawasaki Disease

ORAL:
- Initially, 80–100 mg/kg daily given in 4 equally divided doses (in combination with IVIG); initiate within 10 days of onset of fever. May be necessary to monitor plasma salicylate concentrations. When fever subsides, decrease dosage to 3–5 mg/kg once daily.

- Continue indefinitely in those with coronary artery abnormalities; in the absence of such abnormalities, continue for 6–8 weeks after initial onset of illness or until platelet count and erythrocyte sedimentation rate return to normal.

Adult Patients

Pain

ORAL:
- For *self-medication*, 325–650 mg every 4 hours (maximum 4 g daily) or 0.5–1 g every 6 hours as necessary.
- For *self-medication*, 454 mg (as chewing gum pieces) every 4 hours as necessary (maximum 3.632 g daily).
- Adults <60 years of age for *self-medication*: 650 mg (as a highly buffered effervescent solution [Alka-Seltzer® Lemon-Lime or Original]) every 4 hours (maximum 2.6 g daily); alternatively, 1 g (Alka-Seltzer® Extra Strength) every 6 hours (maximum 3.5 g daily).
- Adults ≥60 years of age for *self-medication*: 650 mg (as a highly buffered effervescent solution [Alka-Seltzer® Lemon-Lime or Original]) every 4 hours (maximum 1.3 g daily); alternatively, 1 g (Alka-Seltzer® Extra Strength) every 6 hours (maximum 1.5 g daily).

RECTAL:
- 325–650 mg every 4 hours as necessary (maximum 4 g daily).

Pain Associated with Migraine Headache

ORAL:
- For *self-medication*, 500 mg (combined with acetaminophen 500 mg and caffeine 130 mg) as a single dose.

Fever

ORAL:
- 325–650 mg every 4 hours as necessary (maximum 4 g daily).
- For *self-medication*, 454 mg (as chewing gum pieces) every 4 hours as necessary (maximum 3.632 g daily).

RECTAL:
- 325–650 mg every 4 hours as necessary (maximum 4 g daily).

Inflammatory Diseases
Rheumatoid Arthritis and Arthritis and Pleurisy of SLE

ORAL:
- Initially, 3 g daily in divided doses. Increase dosage as necessary for anti-inflammatory efficacy; target plasma salicylate concentration is 150–300 mcg/mL. Plasma concentrations >200 mcg/mL associated with an increased incidence of toxicity.

Osteoarthritis

ORAL:
- Up to 3 g daily in divided doses.

Spondyloarthropathies

ORAL:
- Up to 4 g daily in divided doses.

Rheumatic Fever†

ORAL:
- Initially, 4.9–7.8 g daily in divided doses given for maximal suppression of acute inflammation. Adjust dosage based on response, tolerance, and plasma salicylate concentrations.

- Various regimens suggested depending on severity of initial manifestations. Consult published protocols for more information on specific dosages and schedules.

TIAs and Acute Ischemic Stroke
Secondary Prevention
ORAL:

- 50–325 mg daily in patients who experienced a noncardioembolic stroke or TIA (i.e., atherothrombotic, lacunar, or cryptogenic stroke).
- Alternatively, 25 mg (in combination with dipyridamole 200 mg) twice daily (morning and evening) or clopidogrel (75 mg daily).
- 50–100 mg daily suggested by some clinicians for patients at moderate to high risk of bleeding complications.
- Continue secondary prevention indefinitely.

Acute Treatment† of Ischemic Stroke
ORAL:

- 160–325 mg daily, initiated within 48 hours of stroke onset in patients who are not receiving thrombolytic therapy and continued for up to 2–4 weeks; then aspirin, dipyridamole and aspirin, or clopidogrel for secondary prevention.

CAD and MI
Suspected AMI or ACS
ORAL:

- 160–325 mg as soon as AMI or ACS is suspected (no later than 24 hours after symptom onset), continued daily after MI.
- Consider adjunctive therapy with clopidogrel (e.g., 300-mg loading dose, then 75 mg daily) for acute ST-segment elevation MI, unless contraindicated.
- 75–325 mg daily initially for non-ST-segment elevation (NSTE) ACS also has been recommended.

RECTAL:

- 300 mg daily may be considered for patients with severe nausea, vomiting, or upper GI tract disorders.

Secondary Prevention
ORAL:

- 75–325 or 75–162 mg once daily, continued indefinitely, has been recommended; current evidence suggests 75–81 mg daily sufficient for long-term cardiovascular disease prevention and associated with less GI bleeding risk.
- 75–162 mg (possibly 75–81 mg) daily in combination with long-term (up to 4 years), moderate-intensity (target INR: 2–3) oral anticoagulation recommended in post-MI patients where meticulous INR monitoring standard and routinely accessible.
- ≤100 mg (possibly 75–81 mg) daily in combination with short-term (3 months), moderate-intensity (target INR: 2–3) oral anticoagulation suggested in high-risk post-MI patients.
- ≤100 mg (possibly 75–81 mg) daily recommended in patients with history of aspirin-induced bleeding or risk factors for bleeding.

Primary Prevention† of MI
ORAL:

- 75–162 mg once daily. Continue indefinitely, provided there are no contraindications to aspirin.

Chronic Stable CAD
ORAL:

- 75–162 mg daily; continue indefinitely.
- 75–162 mg daily in combination with long-term clopidogrel therapy in patients with high risk of MI.

Angina
ORAL:

- 75–325 mg once daily, continued indefinitely; 75–162 mg daily recommended by ACCP for patients with chronic stable angina.
- Unstable angina: 75–325 mg (possibly 75–81 mg) once daily, continued indefinitely.

PCI and Revascularization Procedures
ORAL:

- PCI in adults who are already receiving aspirin: 75–325 mg initiated ≥2 hours before the procedure (e.g., PTCA, stent placement) in conjunction with a thienopyridine derivative.
- PCI in patients not already receiving long-term aspirin therapy: 300–325 mg daily, initiated at least 2 hours, preferably 24 hours, prior to PCI in conjunction with a thienopyridine derivative.
- Following PCI and bare-metal stent placement: 325 mg daily for ≥1 month in conjunction with a thienopyridine derivative; ideally, continue for ≤1 year in patients who are not at high risk for bleeding.
- Following PCI and drug-eluting stent placement: 75–100 mg daily for ≥12 months in combination with a thienopyridine derivative (e.g., clopidogrel 75 mg daily).
- Following PCI for prevention of myocardial ischemic events in patients requiring other antithrombotic agents (e.g., clopidogrel, warfarin):<100 mg (possibly 75–81 mg) daily recommended.
- Brachytherapy for restenosis following PCI and stent implantation†: 75–325 mg daily in combination with clopidogrel (75 mg daily) suggested by ACC and AHA and other clinicians.
- Continue indefinitely for secondary prevention of cardiovascular events.
- CABG: Some manufacturers recommend 325 mg daily, initiated 6 hours after surgery. If bleeding precludes earlier use, initiate as soon as possible thereafter.
- Saphenous vein CABG: 100–325 mg daily initiated within 48 hours after saphenous vein CABG suggested by ACC and AHA. 75–325 mg daily initiated at 6 hours after surgery recommended by ACCP.
- Internal mammary artery CABG: 75–162 mg daily, continued indefinitely, recommended by ACCP.
- Following CABG: Manufacturer recommends 325 mg daily for 1 year after CABG. ACCP recommend 75–162 mg daily continued indefinitely. ACC and AHA recommend >162 mg daily for <1 year following saphenous vein CABG.
- Carotid endarterectomy: ACCP recommends 75–325 mg daily initiated preoperatively and continued indefinitely. Manufacturer recommends 80 mg daily to 650 mg twice daily initiated preoperatively and continued indefinitely.
- Lower-extremity balloon angioplasty with or without stenting: 75–162 mg daily continued indefinitely.

Atrial Fibrillation/Flutter
ORAL:

- Patients at high risk for stroke who decline or have contraindications to oral anticoagulation: 325 mg daily.
- Intermediate risk for stroke: 325 mg daily or warfarin.
- ≥60 years of age and no other risk factors: 325 mg daily.
- Low risk for stroke: 325 mg daily.

Mitral Valve Prolapse†

ORAL:
- 50–162 mg daily long-term in those with unexplained TIAs.

Thrombosis in Other Arteries and Arteriovenous Communications

Carotid Stenosis

ORAL:
- 75–162 mg daily indefinitely recommended by ACCP for patients who are not surgical candidates.

Ischemic Events in Peripheral Arterial Occlusive Disease

ORAL:
- 75–325 mg daily. Continue indefinitely.

Vascular Grafts

ORAL:
- 75–325 mg daily in patients undergoing prosthetic infrainguinal bypass; initiate preoperatively.
- Use in combination with oral anticoagulation in patients at high risk of bypass occlusion or limb loss.
- Continue life-long aspirin prophylaxis.

Prosthetic Heart Valves

Mechanical Prosthetic Heart Valves†

ORAL:
- Optimal regimen not established. Consider low dosages (75–100 mg daily) of aspirin in combination with oral anticoagulation for patients at increased risk of thromboembolism (e.g., those with history of embolic event, atrial fibrillation, CHD, large left atrium, endocardial damage, low ejection fraction, caged ball or caged disk valve, >1 mechanical heart valve, mechanical valve in mitral position).
- 75–100 mg daily in combination with oral anticoagulation for patients who develop systemic embolism with oral anticoagulation alone. Increase dosage to 325 mg daily and/or titrate warfarin anticoagulation to a higher INR in patients who develop systemic embolism despite receiving combined therapy with oral anticoagulation and low dosages of aspirin.
- 80–100 mg daily recommended for patients with prosthetic heart valves in whom oral anticoagulation must be discontinued.
- Consult specialized references for additional information.

Bioprosthetic Heart Valves†

ORAL:
- Bioprosthetic valve in the aortic position: 80–100 mg daily recommended for the first 3 months following valve insertion.
- 75–100 mg daily long term for those in sinus rhythm with no other risk factors for thromboembolism.

Pericarditis

Acute Pericarditis† Following MI

ORAL:
- 162–325 mg daily. Higher dosages (e.g., 650 mg every 4–6 hours) may be required.

Complications of Pregnancy†

ORAL:
- Congenital thrombophilic defect† and recurrent spontaneous abortions, second-trimester or later pregnancy loss, severe or recurrent preeclampsia, or abruption: 75–162 mg daily combined with heparin or a low molecular weight heparin followed by postpartum anticoagulation (e.g., with warfarin).

- Antiphospholipid syndrome† and a history of multiple pregnancy losses, preeclampsia, intrauterine growth retardation, or abruption: 75–162 mg daily in combination with unfractionated or low molecular weight heparin, followed by postpartum oral anticoagulation suggested.
- Presence of antiphospholipid antibodies and no prior venous thromboembolic events or pregnancy loss: 75–162 mg daily suggested.

Prescribing Limits

Pediatric Patients

Pain

ORAL:
- Children 2–11 years of age: Maximum 2.5 g/m^2 daily.
- Children ≥12 years of age: Maximum 4 g daily. Maximum 2.6 g as highly buffered effervescent solution (Alka-Seltzer® Original) or 3.5 g (Alka-Seltzer® Extra Strength) in 24 hours.
- For *self-medication*, do not exceed recommended daily dosage. Treatment duration for *self-medication* for pain: ≤ 5 days. Treatment duration for *self-medication* of sore throat pain using chewing gum: ≤2 days.

RECTAL:
- Children 2–11 years of age: Maximum 2.5 g/m^2 daily.
- Children ≥12 years of age: Maximum 4 g daily.

Fever

ORAL:
- Children 2–11 years of age: Maximum 2.5 g/m^2 daily.
- Children ≥12 years of age: Maximum 4 g daily.
- For *self-medication*, do not exceed recommended daily dosage. Treatment duration for *self-medication*: <3 days.

RECTAL:
- Children 2–11 years of age: Maximum 2.5 g/m^2 daily.
- Children ≥12 years of age: Maximum 4 g daily.

Adult Patients

Pain

ORAL:
- Maximum 4 g daily. Treatment duration for *self-medication* for pain: ≤10 days. Aspirin chewing gum should not be used for *self-medication* of sore throat pain for longer than 2 days.
- Adults <60 years of age taking highly buffered effervescent solutions: Maximum 2.6 g (Alka-Seltzer® Lemon-lime or Original) or 3.5 g (Alka-Seltzer® Extra Strength) in 24 hours.
- Adults ≥60 years of age taking highly buffered effervescent solutions: Maximum 1.3 g (Alka-Seltzer® Lemon-lime or Original) or 1.5 g (Alka-Seltzer® Extra Strength) in 24 hours.

RECTAL:
- Maximum 4 g daily.

Pain Associated with Migraine Headache

ORAL:
- For *self-medication*, maximum 500 mg (in combination with acetaminophen 500 mg and caffeine 130 mg) in 24 hours.

Fever

ORAL OR RECTAL:
- Maximum 4 g daily.

Geriatric Patients
- Highly buffered effervescent solution: Maximum 1.3 g (Alka-Seltzer®Lemon-Lime or Original) or 1.5 g (Alka-Seltzer® Extra Strength) in 24 hours.

† Use is not currently included in the labeling approved by the US Food and Drug Administration.

Aspirin and Codeine

(as′ pir in) (koe′ deen)

Brand Name: Empirin with Codeine®

Why is this medicine prescribed?

This combination of drugs is used to relieve mild to moderately severe pain.

This medication is sometimes prescribed for other uses; ask your doctor or pharmacist for more information.

How should this medicine be used?

The combination of aspirin and codeine comes as a tablet to take by mouth. It usually is taken every 4 hours as needed. Follow the directions on your prescription label carefully, and ask your doctor or pharmacist to explain any part you do not understand. Take aspirin and codeine exactly as directed.

Codeine can be habit-forming. Do not take a larger dose, take it more often, or for a longer period than your doctor tells you to.

What special precautions should I follow?

Before taking aspirin and codeine,
- tell your doctor and pharmacist if you are allergic to aspirin, codeine, sulfite, or any other drugs.
- tell your doctor and pharmacist what prescription and nonprescription medications you are taking, especially other pain relievers; anticoagulants ('blood thinners') such as warfarin (Coumadin); antidepressants; corticosteroids; MAO inhibitors [phenelzine (Nardil) or tranylcypromine (Parnate)]; medications for cough, cold, or allergies; medications for diabetes, arthritis, or gout; sedatives; sleeping pills; tranquilizers; and vitamins.
- tell your doctor if you have or have ever had a bleeding disorder (hemophilia, von Willebrand's disease), ulcer disease, liver or kidney disease, a history of alcoholism, anemia, lung or thyroid disease, prostatic hypertrophy, or urinary problems.
- tell your doctor if you are pregnant, plan to become pregnant, or are breast-feeding. If you become pregnant while taking aspirin and codeine, call your doctor.
- if you are having surgery, including dental surgery, tell the doctor or dentist that you are taking aspirin and codeine.
- you should know that this drug may make you drowsy. Do not drive a car or operate machinery until you know how this drug affects you.
- remember that alcohol can add to the drowsiness caused by this drug.

What special dietary instructions should I follow?

Aspirin and codeine may cause an upset stomach. Take aspirin and codeine with food or milk.

What should I do if I forget to take a dose?

This medication usually is taken as needed. If your doctor has told you to take aspirin and codeine regularly, take the missed dose as soon as you remember it. However, if it is almost time for the next dose, skip the missed dose and continue your regular dosing schedule. Do not take a double dose to make up for a missed one.

What side effects can this medicine cause?

Aspirin and codeine may cause side effects. Tell your doctor if any of these symptoms are severe or do not go away:
- dizziness
- lightheadedness
- drowsiness
- upset stomach
- vomiting
- constipation
- stomach pain
- difficulty urinating

If you experience any of the following symptoms, call your doctor immediately:
- difficulty breathing
- rash or itching
- ringing in the ears or decreased hearing
- abnormal bruising or bleeding

If you experience a serious side effect, you or your doctor may send a report to the Food and Drug Administration's (FDA) MedWatch Adverse Event Reporting program online [at http://www.fda.gov/MedWatch/index.html] or by phone [1-800-332-1088].

What storage conditions are needed for this medicine?

Keep this medication in the container it came in, tightly closed, and out of reach of children. Store it at room temperature and away from excess heat and moisture (not in the bathroom). Throw away any medication that is outdated or no longer needed. Talk to your pharmacist about the proper disposal of your medication.

What should I do in case of overdose?

In case of overdose, call your local poison control center at 1-800-222-1222. If the victim has collapsed or is not breathing, call local emergency services at 911.

What other information should I know?

Keep all appointments with your doctor.

Do not let anyone else take your medication. Ask your pharmacist any questions you have about refilling your prescription.

Talk to your doctor, pharmacist, or other healthcare professional if you have questions about dosing information for your medication.

Aspirin and Extended-Release Dipyridamole

(dye peer id′ a mole)

Brand Name: Aggrenox®

Why is this medicine prescribed?

The combination of aspirin and extended-release dipyridamole is in a class of drugs called antiplatelet agents. It works by preventing excessive blood clotting. It is used to reduce the risk of stroke in patients who have had or are at risk of stroke.

This medication is sometimes prescribed for other uses; ask your doctor or pharmacist for more information.

How should this medicine be used?

The combination of aspirin and extended-release dipyridamole comes as a capsule to take by mouth. It is usually taken twice a day, one capsule in the morning and one in the evening. Aspirin and extended-release dipyridamole should be swallowed whole. Do not open, crush, break, or chew the capsules.

Follow the directions on your prescription label carefully, and ask your doctor or pharmacist to explain any part you do not understand. Use aspirin and extended-release dipyridamole exactly as directed. Do not use more or less of it or use it more often than prescribed by your doctor.

The combination of aspirin and extended-release dipyridamole decreases the risk of having a stroke but does not eliminate that risk. Continue to take aspirin and extended-release dipyridamole even if you feel well. Do not stop taking aspirin and extended-release dipyridamole without talking to your doctor.

What special precautions should I follow?

Before using aspirin and extended-release dipyridamole,

- tell your doctor and pharmacist if you are allergic to aspirin, celecoxib (Celebrex), choline salicylate (Arthropan), diclofenac (Cataflam), diflunisal (Dolobid), dipyridamole (Persantine), etodolac (Lodine), fenoprofen (Nalfon), flurbiprofen (Ansaid), ibuprofen (Advil, Motrin, Nuprin), indomethacin (Indocin), ketoprofen (Orudis, Oruvail), ketorolac (Toradol), magnesium salicylate (Nuprin Backache, Doan's), meclofenamate, mefenamic acid (Ponstel), meloxicam (Mobic), nabumetone (Relafen), naproxen (Aleve, Naprosyn), oxaprozin (Daypro), piroxicam (Feldene), rofecoxib (Vioxx), sulindac (Clinoril), tolmetin (Tolectin), or any other drugs.
- tell your doctor and pharmacist what prescription and nonprescription medications you are taking, especially acetazolamide (Diamox); ambenonium (Mytelase); angiotensin- converting enzyme inhibitors such as benazepril (Lotensin), captopril (Capoten), enalapril (Vasotec), fosinopril (Monopril), lisinopril (Prinivil, Zestril), moexipril (Univasc), quinapril (Accupril), ramipril (Altace), and trandolapril (Mavik); anticoagulants ('blood thinners') such as warfarin (Coumadin) and heparin; betablockers such as acebutolol (Sectral), atenolol (Tenormin), betaxolol (Kerlone), bisoprolol (Zebeta), carteolol (Cartrol), carvedilol (Coreg), labetalol (Normodyne), metoprolol (Lopressor), nadolol (Corgard), penbutolol (Levatol), Pindolol (Visken), propranolol (Inderal), sotalol (Betapace), and timolol (Blocadren); diabetes medications such as acetohexamide (Dymelor), chlorpropamide (Diabinese), glimepiride (Amaryl), glipizide (Glucotrol), glyburide (DiaBeta, Micronase, Glynase), repaglinide (Prandin), tolazamide (Tolinase), and tolbutamide (Orinase); diuretics ('water pills') such as amiloride (Midamor), bumetanide (Bumex), chlorothiazide (Diuril), chlorthalidone (Hygroton), ethacrynic acid (Edecrin), furosemide (Lasix), hydrochlorothiazide (Hydrodiuril), indapamide (Lozol), metolazone (Zaroxolyn), spironolactone (Aldactone), torsemide (Demadex), and triamterene (Dyrenium); methotrexate (Folex, Mexate, Rheumatrex); neostigmine (Prostigmin); nonsteroidal anti-inflammatory drugs such as celecoxib (Celebrex), choline salicylate (Arthropan), diclofenac (Cataflam), diflunisal (Dolobid), etodolac (Lodine), fenoprofen (Nalfon), flurbiprofen (Ansaid), ibuprofen (Advil, Motrin, Nuprin, others), indomethacin (Indocin), ketoprofen (Orudis, Oruvail), ketorolac (Toradol), magnesium salicylate (Nuprin Backache, Doan's), meclofenamate, mefenamic acid (Ponstel), meloxicam (Mobic), nabumetone (Relafen), naproxen (Aleve, Naprosyn), oxaprozin (Daypro), piroxicam (Feldene), rofecoxib (Vioxx), sulindac (Clinoril), and tolmetin (Tolectin); phenytoin (Dilantin); probenecid (Benemid); pyridostigmine (Mestinon); sulfinpyrazone (Anturane); valproic acid and related drugs (Depakene, Depakote); and vitamins and herbal products.
- tell your doctor if you have or have ever had disease of the liver, kidneys, or heart; a recent heart attack; bleeding disorders; low blood pressure; vitamin K deficiency; ulcers; the syndrome of asthma, rhinitis, and nasal polyps; or if you drink three or more alcoholic drinks a day.
- tell your doctor if you are pregnant, plan to become pregnant, or are breast-feeding. If you become pregnant while using aspirin and extended-release dipyridamole, call your doctor immediately.
- if you are having surgery, including dental surgery, tell the doctor or dentist that you are taking aspirin and ex-

tended-release dipyridamole. Your doctor may tell you to stop taking aspirin and extended-release dipyridamole before surgery.

What special dietary instructions should I follow?

Unless your doctor tells you otherwise, continue your normal diet while taking aspirin and extended-release dipyridamole.

What should I do if I forget to take a dose?

Take the missed dose as soon as you remember it. However, if it is almost time for the next dose, skip the missed dose and continue your regular dosing schedule. Do not take a double dose to make up for a missed one.

What side effects can this medicine cause?

Side effects from aspirin and extended-release dipyridamole can occur. Tell your doctor if any of these symptoms are severe or do not go away:

- headache
- heartburn
- stomach pain
- upset stomach
- vomiting
- diarrhea
- muscle and joint pain
- tiredness

If you experience any of the following symptoms, call your doctor immediately:

- bleeding
- severe rash
- swelling of the lips, tongue, or mouth
- difficulty breathing
- warm feeling
- flushing
- sweating
- restlessness
- weakness
- dizziness
- chest pain
- rapid heartbeat
- ringing in the ears

If you experience a serious side effect, you or your doctor may send a report to the Food and Drug Administration's (FDA) MedWatch Adverse Event Reporting program online [at http://www.fda.gov/MedWatch/index.html] or by phone [1-800-332-1088].

What storage conditions are needed for this medicine?

Keep this medication in the container it came in, tightly closed, and out of reach of children. Store it at room temperature and away from excess heat and moisture (not in the bathroom). Throw away any medication that is outdated or no longer needed. Talk to your pharmacist about the proper disposal of your medication.

What should I do in case of overdose?

In case of overdose, call your local poison control center at 1-800-222-1222. If the victim has collapsed or is not breathing, call local emergency services at 911.

What other information should I know?

Do not substitute the individual components of aspirin and dipyridamole (Persantine) for the combination product of aspirin and extended-release dipyridamole.

Because the use of aspirin by children and teenagers during viral illnesses may result in a serious condition (Reye's syndrome), keep aspirin and extended-release dipyridamole out of the reach of children.

Keep all appointments with your doctor and the laboratory. Your doctor may order certain lab tests to check your response to aspirin and extended-release dipyridamole.

Do not let anyone else take your medication. Ask your pharmacist any questions you have about refilling your prescription.

Talk to your doctor, pharmacist, or other healthcare professional if you have questions about dosing information for your medication.

Aspirin, Butalbital, and Caffeine

(as' pir in) (byoo tal' bi tal) (kaf' een)

Brand Name: Fiorinal®

Why is this medicine prescribed?

This combination of drugs is used to relieve tension headaches.

This medication is sometimes prescribed for other uses; ask your doctor or pharmacist for more information.

How should this medicine be used?

The combination of aspirin, butalbital, and caffeine comes as a capsule and tablet to take by mouth. It usually is taken every 4 hours as needed. Follow the directions on your prescription label carefully, and ask your doctor or pharmacist to explain any part you do not understand. Take aspirin, butalbital, and caffeine exactly as directed. Do not take more than six tablets or capsules in 1 day. If you think that you need more to relieve your symptoms, call your doctor.

This medication can be habit-forming. Do not take a larger dose, take it more often, or for a longer time than your doctor tells you to.

What special precautions should I follow?

Before taking aspirin, butalbital, and caffeine,

- tell your doctor and pharmacist if you are allergic to aspirin, butalbital, caffeine, other pain relievers such as ibuprofen (Motrin), or any other drugs.
- tell your doctor and pharmacist what prescription and nonprescription medications you are taking, especially acetazolamide (Diamox); anticoagulants ('blood thinners') such as warfarin (Coumadin); antidepressants; antihistamines; corticosteroids such as prednisone; medications for arthritis, gout, diabetes, or pain; methotrexate; sedatives; sleeping pills; tranquilizers; and vitamins.
- tell your doctor if you have or have ever had kidney disease, porphyria, bleeding problems, nasal polyps, ulcers, or a history of depression.
- tell your doctor if you are pregnant, plan to become pregnant, or are breast-feeding. If you become pregnant while taking this medication, call your doctor.
- you should know that this drug may make you drowsy. Do not drive a car or operate machinery until you know how this drug affects you.
- remember that alcohol can add to the drowsiness caused by this drug.

What special dietary instructions should I follow?

Aspirin, butalbital, and caffeine may cause an upset stomach. Take this medicine with food or milk.

What should I do if I forget to take a dose?

Take the missed dose as soon as you remember it. However, if it is almost time for the next dose, skip the missed dose and continue your regular dosing schedule. Do not take a double dose to make up for a missed one.

What side effects can this medicine cause?

Aspirin, butalbital, and caffeine may cause side effects. Tell your doctor if any of these symptoms are severe or do not go away:

- drowsiness
- upset stomach
- vomiting
- stomach pain
- lightheadedness
- confusion

If you experience any of the following symptoms, call your doctor immediately:

- skin rash
- itching
- difficulty breathing
- ringing in the ears
- bloody or black stools

If you experience a serious side effect, you or your doctor may send a report to the Food and Drug Administration's (FDA) MedWatch Adverse Event Reporting program online [at http://www.fda.gov/MedWatch/index.html] or by phone [1-800-332-1088].

What storage conditions are needed for this medicine?

Keep this medication in the container it came in, tightly closed, and out of reach of children. Store it at room temperature, away from excess heat and moisture (not in the bathroom). Throw away any medication that is outdated or no longer needed. Talk to your pharmacist about the proper disposal of your medication.

What should I do in case of overdose?

In case of overdose, call your local poison control center at 1-800-222-1222. If the victim has collapsed or is not breathing, call local emergency services at 911.

What other information should I know?

Keep all appointments with your doctor.

Do not let anyone else take your medication. This medication is a controlled substance. Prescriptions may be refilled only a limited number of times; ask your pharmacist if you have any questions.

Talk to your doctor, pharmacist, or other healthcare professional if you have questions about dosing information for your medication.

Atazanavir

(at a za na' veer)

Brand Name: Reyataz®

Why is this medicine prescribed?

Atazanavir is used in combination with other medications to treat human immunodeficiency virus (HIV) in patients with or without acquired immunodeficiency syndrome (AIDS). Atazanavir is in a class of medications called HIV protease inhibitors. It works by preventing the spread of HIV in the body. Atazanavir does not cure HIV and may not prevent you from developing HIV related illnesses. Atazanavir does not prevent the spread of HIV to other people.

How should this medicine be used?

Atazanavir comes as a capsule to take by mouth. It is usually taken once a day with a meal or snack. To help you remember to take atazanavir, take it at around the same time every day. Follow the directions on your prescription label carefully, and ask your doctor or pharmacist to explain any part you do not understand. Take atazanavir exactly as directed. Do not take more or less of it or take it more often than prescribed by your doctor.

You will take other medications for HIV while you are taking atazanavir. Your doctor will tell you whether these medications should be taken at the same time as atazanavir, or several hours before or after you take atazanavir. Follow this schedule carefully, and ask your doctor or pharmacist if you have questions about the times you should take your medications.

Swallow the capsules whole; do not split, chew, or open them.

Atazanavir controls HIV but does not cure it. Continue to take atazanavir even if you feel well. Do not stop taking atazanavir without talking to your doctor. If you miss doses or stop taking atazanavir, your condition may become more difficult to treat.

Are there other uses for this medicine?

This medication may be prescribed for other uses; ask your doctor or pharmacist for more information.

What special precautions should I follow?

Before taking atazanavir,

- tell your doctor and pharmacist if you are allergic to atazanavir or any other medications.
- do not take atazanavir if you are taking cisapride (Propulsid), ergot alkaloids such as dihydroergotamine (Migranal, D.H.E. 45), ergonovine (Ergotrate), ergotamine (Cafergot, Ercaf, others), or methylergonovine (Methergine); midazolam (Versed); pimozide (Orap); and triazolam (Halcion).
- tell your doctor and pharmacist what other prescription and nonprescription medications, vitamins, and nutritional supplements you are taking. Be sure to mention amiodarone (Cordarone); anticoagulants ('blood thinners') such as warfarin (Coumadin); antidepressants (mood elevators) such as amitriptyline (Elavil), amoxapine (Asendin), clomipramine (Anafranil), desipramine (Norpramin), doxepin (Adapin, Sinequan), fluoxetine (Prozac, Sarafem), fluvoxamine (Luvox), imipramine (Tofranil), nefazodone (Serzone), nortriptyline (Aventyl, Pamelor), protriptyline (Vivactil), and trimipramine (Surmontil); antifungals such as fluconazole (Diflucan), itraconazole (Sporanox), and ketoconazole (Nizoral); beta blockers such as atenolol (Tenormin), labetalol (Normodyne), metoprolol (Lopressor, Toprol XL), nadolol (Corgard), and propranolol (Inderal); calcium channel blockers such as bepridil (Vascor), diltiazem (Cardizem, Dilacor, Tiazac, others), felodipine (Plendil), nicardipine (Cardene), nifedipine (Adalat, Procardia) and verapamil (Calan, Isoptin, Verelan); carbamazepine (Tegretol); celecoxib (Vioxx); cholesterol-lowering medications (statins) such as atorvastatin (Lipitor), lovastatin (Mevacor), or simvastatin (Zocor); cimetidine (Tagamet); clarithromycin (Biaxin);

clozapine (Olozaril); cyclobenzaprine (Flexeril); danazol (Danocrine); dexamethasone (Decadron); diclofenac (Voltaren); digoxin (Lanoxin); ethosuximide (Zarontin); famotidine (Pepcid); fluvastatin (Lescol); glipizide (Glucotrol); ibuprofen (Advil, Motrin); irbesartan (Avapro); irinotecan (Camptosar); isoniazid (INH, Nydrazid); medications for irregular heartbeat; medications that suppress the immune system such as cyclosporine (Neoral, Sandimmune), sirolimus (Rapamune), and tacrolimus (Prograf); metronidazole (Flagyl); mexiletine (Mexetil); naproxen (Aleve, Naprosyn); nizatidine (Axid); oral contraceptives (birth control pills); other medications for HIV or AIDS such as delavirdine (Rescriptor), efavirenz (Sustiva), indinavir (Crixivan), nelfinavir (Viracept); ritonavir (Norvir), saquinavir (Fortovase, Invirase) and tenofovir (Viread); phenobarbital (Luminal, Solfoton); phenytoin (Dilantin); piroxicam (Feldene); proton-pump inhibitors used for indigestion, heartburn, or ulcers such as esomeprazole (Nexium), lansoprazole (Prevacid), omeprazole (Prilosec), pantoprazole (Protonix), and rabeprazole (Aciphex); quinidine (Quinidex); ranitidine (Zantac); rifabutin (Mycobutin); rifampin (Rimactane, Rifadin, others); tacrine (Cognex); theophylline (Theo-Dur, others); tolbutamide (Orinase); torsemide (Demadex); troleandomycin (TAO); and zafirlukast (Accolate). Your doctor may need to change the doses of your medications or monitor you carefully for side effects.

- If you are taking antacids, didanosine chewable or dispersible buffered tablets (Videx), or any other buffered medication such as buffered aspirin (Bufferin), take atazanavir 2 hours before or 1 hour after you take these medications. Ask your doctor or pharmacist if you are not sure if any of the medications you are taking are buffered.
- tell your doctor what herbal products you are taking, especially St. John's wort.
- tell your doctor if you are taking medications for erectile dysfunction such as sildenafil (Viagra), tadalafil (Cialis), or vardenafil (Levitra). You should know that atazanavir may increase the chance that you will experience serious side effects from these medications. If you are taking any of these medications and you experience dizziness, fainting, upset stomach, changes in vision, or a painful erection that lasts for several hours, call your doctor right away.
- tell your doctor if you have or have ever had an irregular heartbeat, diabetes, hemophilia (a condition in which the blood does not clot normally), liver disease such as hepatitis (a viral infection of the liver), or kidney, or heart disease.
- tell your doctor if you are pregnant or plan to become pregnant. If you become pregnant while taking atazanavir, call your doctor. You should not breastfeed if you are infected with HIV or are taking atazanavir.
- if you are having surgery, including dental surgery, tell the doctor or dentist that you are taking atazanavir.

- you should know that your body fat may increase or move to different areas of your body such as your breasts, waist, and upper back.

What special dietary instructions should I follow?

Talk to your doctor about drinking grapefruit juice while taking this medicine.

What should I do if I forget to take a dose?

Take the missed dose as soon as you remember it. However, if you are scheduled to take your next dose within the next 6 hours, skip the missed dose and continue your regular dosing schedule. Do not take a double dose to make up for a missed one.

What side effects can this medicine cause?

Atazanavir can cause high blood sugar (hyperglycemia). If you have any of these symptoms of high blood sugar, call your doctor immediately:

- thirst
- dry mouth
- tiredness
- flushing
- dry skin
- frequent urination
- loss of appetite
- trouble breathing

Atazanavir may cause side effects. Tell your doctor if any of these symptoms are severe or do not go away:

- headache
- diarrhea
- depression
- cough
- difficulty falling asleep or staying asleep
- pain, especially in joints, back, or muscles

Some side effects can be serious. The following symptoms are uncommon, but if you experience any of them, call your doctor immediately:

- dizziness
- lightheadedness
- upset stomach
- vomiting
- stomach pain
- extreme weakness and tiredness
- trouble breathing
- numbness, pain, or tingling in arms and legs
- fever
- yellowing of skin or eyes
- rash
- hives
- itching
- swelling of the face, throat, tongue, lips, eyes, hands, feet, ankles, or lower legs

- difficulty swallowing
- hoarseness

Atazanavir may cause other side effects. Call your doctor if you have any unusual problems while taking this medication.

If you experience a serious side effect, you or your doctor may send a report to the Food and Drug Administration's (FDA) MedWatch Adverse Event Reporting program online [at http://www.fda.gov/MedWatch/index.html] or by phone [1-800-332-1088].

What storage conditions are needed for this medicine?

Keep this medication in the container it came in, tightly closed, and out of reach of children. Store it at room temperature and away from excess heat and moisture (not in the bathroom). Throw away any medication that is outdated or no longer needed. Talk to your pharmacist about the proper disposal of your medication.

What should I do in case of overdose?

In case of overdose, call your local poison control center at 1-800-222-1222. If the victim has collapsed or is not breathing, call local emergency services at 911.

Symptoms of overdose may include:

- dizziness
- lightheadedness
- yellowing of skin or eyes

What other information should I know?

Keep all appointments with your doctor and the laboratory. Your doctor may order certain lab tests to check your body's response to atazanavir.

Do not let anyone else take your medication. Ask your pharmacist any questions you have about refilling your prescription.

Dosage Facts
For Informational Purposes

Caution: Do not change your dose, how often you take your medication, or the length of time you are to take it without first talking to your healthcare provider.

The following dosage information was written using medical language for doctors and other healthcare professionals and is provided here for you to check your dosage. The dosage of this drug may differ for different patients. Therefore, always follow your doctor's instructions or the directions on the label. Contact your healthcare provider or pharmacist if you have any questions about the specific dosage of your medication after reviewing this information.

General Dosage Information

Available as atazanavir sulfate; dosage expressed in terms of atazanavir.

Must be given in conjunction with other antiretrovirals. *If used with efavirenz, ritonavir, tenofovir, or saquinavir, dosage adjustment may be necessary. If used with certain didanosine preparations, administer at separate times.*

Used with low-dose ritonavir (*ritonavir-boosted* atazanavir) in treatment-experienced (previously treated) adults; atazanavir without low-dose ritonavir is not recommended in these patients.

Pediatric Patients

Treatment of HIV Infection

ORAL:

- Children ≥3 months of age: Optimal dosage not established; dose-finding studies underway. Children may need higher dosage on a mg/kg basis than adults.

Adult Patients

Treatment of HIV Infection
Treatment-naive Adults

ORAL:

- 400 mg once daily.

Treatment-experienced Adults

ORAL:

- 300 mg once daily *boosted* with low-dose ritonavir (100 mg once daily).

Postexposure Prophylaxis of HIV†
Occupational Exposure†

ORAL:

- 400 mg once daily. If tenofovir included in the regimen, use 300 mg of atazanavir once daily *boosted* with low-dose ritonavir (100 mg once daily).
- Used in alternative expanded regimens that include atazanavir and 2 NRTIs.
- Initiate postexposure prophylaxis as soon as possible following exposure (within hours rather than days) and continue for 4 weeks, if tolerated.

Nonoccupational Exposure†

ORAL:

- 400 mg once daily. If tenofovir included in the regimen, use 300 mg of atazanavir once daily *boosted* with low-dose ritonavir.
- Used in alternative PI-based regimens that include atazanavir and (lamivudine or emtricitabine) and (zidovudine or stavudine or abacavir or didanosine) or include *ritonavir-boosted* atazanavir and (lamivudine or emtricitabine) and tenofovir.
- Initiate postexposure prophylaxis as soon as possible following exposure (preferably ≤72 hours after exposure) and continue for 28 days.

Special Populations

Hepatic Impairment

ORAL:

- 300 mg once daily (without ritonavir) in adults with moderate hepatic impairment (Child-Pugh class B). Do not use in those with severe hepatic impairment (Child-Pugh class C).

Renal Impairment

- Data insufficient to make dosage recommendations; some experts state dosage adjustment not necessary.

Geriatric Patients

- Dosage adjustments based solely on age not required in patients ≥65 years of age.

† *Use is not currently included in the labeling approved by the US Food and Drug Administration.*

Atenolol

(a ten′ oh lole)

Brand Name: Tenoretic® as a combination product containing Atenolol and Chlorthalidone, Tenormin®
Also available generically.

Important Warning

Do not stop taking atenolol without talking to your doctor. Suddenly stopping atenolol may cause chest pain, heart attack, or irregular heartbeat. Your doctor will probably decrease your dose gradually.

Why is this medicine prescribed?

Atenolol is used alone or in combination with other medications to treat high blood pressure. It also is used to prevent angina (chest pain) and treat heart attacks. Atenolol is in a class of medications called beta blockers. It works by slowing the heart rate and relaxing the blood vessels so the heart does not have to pump as hard.

How should this medicine be used?

Atenolol comes as a tablet to take by mouth. It is usually taken once or twice a day. To help you remember to take atenolol, take it around the same time every day. Follow the directions on your prescription label carefully, and ask your doctor or pharmacist to explain any part you do not understand. Take atenolol exactly as directed. Do not take more or less of it or take it more often than prescribed by your doctor.

Atenolol controls high blood pressure and angina but does not cure them. It may take 1-2 weeks before you feel the full benefit of atenolol. Continue to take atenolol even if you feel well. Do not stop taking atenolol without talking to your doctor.

Are there other uses for this medicine?

Atenolol is also used sometimes to prevent migraine headaches and to treat alcohol withdrawal, heart failure, and irregular heartbeat. Talk to your doctor about the possible risks of using this medication for your condition.

This medication may be prescribed for other uses; ask your doctor or pharmacist for more information.

What special precautions should I follow?

Before taking atenolol,
- tell your doctor and pharmacist if you are allergic to atenolol or any other medications.
- tell your doctor and pharmacist what prescription and nonprescription medications, vitamins, nutritional supplements, and herbal products you are taking. Be sure to mention any of the following: calcium channel blockers such as diltiazem (Cardizem, Dilacor, Tiazac, others) and verapamil (Calan, Isoptin, Verelan); clonidine (Catapres); nonsteroidal anti-inflammatory medications (NSAIDs) such as indomethacin (Indocin); and reserpine (Serpalan, Serpasil, Serpatabs). Your doctor may need to change the doses of your medications or monitor you carefully for side effects.
- tell your doctor if you have or have ever had asthma or other lung disease; diabetes; severe allergies; an overactive thyroid gland (hyperthyroidism); pheochromocytoma; heart failure; a slow heart rate; circulation problems; or heart or kidney disease.
- tell your doctor if you are pregnant, plan to become pregnant, or are breast-feeding. If you become pregnant while taking atenolol, call your doctor immediately.
- if you are having surgery, including dental surgery, tell the doctor or dentist that you are taking atenolol.
- you should know that if you have allergic reactions to different substances, your reactions may be worse while you are using atenolol, and your allergic reactions may not respond to the usual doses of injectable epinephrine.

What special dietary instructions should I follow?

If your doctor prescribes a low-salt or low-sodium diet, follow these directions carefully.

What should I do if I forget to take a dose?

Take the missed dose as soon as you remember it. However, if it is almost time for the next dose, skip the missed dose and continue your regular dosing schedule. Do not take a double dose to make up for a missed one.

What side effects can this medicine cause?

Atenolol may cause side effects. Tell your doctor if any of these symptoms are severe or do not go away:
- dizziness
- lightheadedness
- tiredness
- drowsiness
- depression
- upset stomach
- diarrhea

Some side effects can be serious. The following symptoms are uncommon, but if you experience any of them, call your doctor immediately:
- shortness of breath
- swelling of the hands, feet, ankles, or lower legs
- unusual weight gain
- fainting

Atenolol may cause other side effects. Call your doctor if you have any unusual problems while taking this medication.

If you experience a serious side effect, you or your doctor may send a report to the Food and Drug Administration's (FDA) MedWatch Adverse Event Reporting program online [at http://www.fda.gov/MedWatch/index.html] or by phone [1-800-332-1088].

What storage conditions are needed for this medicine?

Keep this medication in the container it came in, tightly closed, and out of reach of children. Store it at room temperature and away from excess heat and moisture (not in the bathroom). Throw away any medication that is outdated or no longer needed. Talk to your pharmacist about the proper disposal of your medication.

What should I do in case of overdose?

In case of overdose, call your local poison control center at 1-800-222-1222. If the victim has collapsed or is not breathing, call local emergency services at 911.

Symptoms of overdose may include:
- lack of energy
- difficulty breathing
- wheezing
- slow heartbeat
- fainting
- swelling of the hands, feet, ankles, or lower legs
- unusual weight gain
- shakiness
- dizziness
- rapid heartbeat
- sweating or confusion
- blurred vision
- headache
- numbness or tingling of the mouth
- weakness
- excessive tiredness
- pale color
- sudden hunger

What other information should I know?

Keep all appointments with your doctor. Your blood pressure should be checked regularly to determine your response to atenolol. Your doctor may ask you to check your pulse (heart rate). Ask your pharmacist or doctor to teach you how to take your pulse. If your pulse is faster or slower than it should be, call your doctor.

Do not let anyone else take your medication. Ask your

pharmacist any questions you have about refilling your prescription.

Dosage Facts
For Informational Purposes

Caution: Do not change your dose, how often you take your medication, or the length of time you are to take it without first talking to your healthcare provider.

The following dosage information was written using medical language for doctors and other healthcare professionals and is provided here for you to check your dosage. The dosage of this drug may differ for different patients. Therefore, always follow your doctor's instructions or the directions on the label. Contact your healthcare provider or pharmacist if you have any questions about the specific dosage of your medication after reviewing this information.

Pediatric Patients

Hypertension†

ORAL:
- Some experts recommend an initial dosage of 0.5–1 mg/kg daily given as a single dose or in 2 divided doses. Increase dosage as necessary up to a maximum dosage of 2 mg/kg (up to 100 mg) daily given as a single dose or in 2 divided doses.

Adult Patients

Hypertension
Monotherapy

ORAL:
- Initially, 25–50 mg once daily. Full hypotensive response may require 2 weeks.
- If necessary, increase to 100 mg once daily. Some patients may have improved BP control with twice-daily dosing.

Combination Therapy.

ORAL:
- Atenolol in fixed combination with chlorthalidone: initially, 50 mg of atenolol and 25 mg of chlorthalidone once daily. If response is not optimal, 100 mg of atenolol and 25 mg of chlorthalidone once daily.
- Initial use of fixed-combination preparations is not recommended; adjust by administering each drug separately, then use the fixed combination if the optimum maintenance dosage corresponds to the ratio of drugs in the combination preparation. Administer separately for subsequent dosage adjustment.
- May add another antihypertensive agent when necessary (gradually using half of the usual initial dosage to avoid an excessive decrease in BP).

Angina

ORAL:
- Initially, 50 mg once daily.
- If optimum response is not achieved within 1 week, increase to 100 mg once daily.
- Some patients may require 200 mg once daily for optimum effect.

AMI
Early Treatment

ORAL (FOLLOWING IV DOSAGE):
- If the total IV dose is tolerated, administer 50 mg orally 10 minutes later, then 50 mg orally 12 hours later.
- Continue 100 mg daily (as a single daily dose or in 2 equally divided doses) for 6–9 days (or until a contraindication [e.g., bradycardia or hypotension requiring treatment] develops or the patient is discharged).
- If necessary, may reduce to 50 mg daily.

ORAL ALTERNATIVE DOSAGE:
- May eliminate IV doses and administer orally when safety of IV use is questionable and oral therapy is not contraindicated.
- Administer 100 mg once daily or in 2 equally divided doses for at least 7 days

Late Treatment

ORAL:
- If not initiated acutely, initiate long-term therapy within a few days of an AMI.
- Optimum duration remains to be clearly established, but studies suggest optimum benefit with at least 1–3 years of therapy after infarction (if not contraindicated).
- *Indefinite* continuation of therapy (unless contraindicated) has been recommended.

Supraventricular Tachyarrhythmias†
Atrial Fibrillation†

ORAL (FOLLOWING IV DOSAGE):
- 50 mg every 12 hours.

Vascular Headache†
Prevention of Common Migraine†

ORAL:
- Dosage has not been established; in clinical studies 100 mg daily was usual effective dosage.

Prescribing Limits

Pediatric Patients

Hypertension†

ORAL:
- Maximum 2 mg/kg (up to 100 mg) daily.

Adult Patients

Hypertension
Monotherapy

ORAL:
- Increasing beyond 100 mg daily usually does not result in further improvement in blood pressure control.

Special Populations

Hepatic Impairment
- Minimal hepatic metabolism; no dosage adjustment recommended.

Renal Impairment

Hypertension

ORAL:
- Modify doses and/or frequency of administration in response to the degree of renal impairment.
- Initial dose of 25 mg daily may be necessary.
- Measure BP just prior to the dose to ensure persistence of adequate BP reduction.

Cl$_{cr}$ 15–35 mL/minute per 1.73 m²

> Maximum 50 daily.

Cl$_{cr}$ <15 mL/minute per 1.73 m²

> Maximum 25 mg daily or 50 mg every other day.

Hemodialysis

> May administer 25 or 50 mg after each dialysis.

> Marked reductions in BP may occur; give under careful supervision.

Geriatric Patients
Hypertension
Oral

- Modification of dosage may be necessary because of age-related decreases in renal function.
- Initially, 25 mg daily may be necessary.
- Measure BP just prior to a dose to ensure persistence of adequate BP reduction.

Bronchospastic Disease

Oral

- Initially, 50 mg daily and use lowest possible dosage. If dosage must be increased, consider administering in 2 divided doses daily to decrease peak blood levels. A β_2-adrenergic agonist bronchodilator should be available.

† Use is not currently included in the labeling approved by the US Food and Drug Administration.

Atomoxetine

(at′ oh mox e teen)

Brand Name: Strattera®

Important Warning

Studies have shown that children and teenagers with attention-deficit hyperactivity disorder (ADHD; more difficulty focusing, controlling actions, and remaining still or quiet than other people who are the same age) who take atomoxetine are more likely to think about killing themselves than children and teenagers with ADHD who do not take atomoxetine. While your child is taking atomoxetine, you should watch his or her behavior very carefully, especially at the beginning of treatment and any time his or her dose is increased or decreased. Your child may develop serious symptoms very suddenly, so it is important to pay attention to his or her behavior every day. Ask other people who spend a lot of time with your child, such as brothers, sisters, and teachers to tell you if they notice changes in your child's behavior. Call your child's doctor right away if your child experiences any of these symptoms: acting more subdued or withdrawn than usual; feeling helpless, hopeless, or worth-

less; new or worsening depression; thinking or talking about harming or killing him- or herself or planning or trying to do so; extreme worry; agitation; panic attacks; difficulty falling asleep or staying asleep; irritability; aggressive or violent behavior; acting without thinking; extreme increase in activity or talking; frenzied, abnormal excitement; or any other sudden or unusual changes in behavior.

Your child's doctor will want to see your child often while he or she is taking atomoxetine, especially at the beginning of his or her treatment. Your child's doctor may also want to speak with you or your child by telephone from time to time. Be sure that your child keeps all appointments for office visits or telephone conversations with his or her doctor.

Your doctor or pharmacist will give you the manufacturer's patient information sheet (Medication Guide) when you begin treatment with atomoxetine and each time you refill your prescription. Read the information carefully and ask your doctor or pharmacist if you have any questions. You can also visit the Food and Drug Administration (FDA) website (http://www.fda.gov/cder) or the manufacturer's website to obtain the Medication Guide.

Talk to your doctor about the risks of giving atomoxetine to your child, of using other treatments for your child's condition, and of not treating your child's condition.

Why is this medicine prescribed?

Atomoxetine is used as part of a total treatment program to increase the ability to pay attention and decrease impulsiveness and hyperactivity in children and adults with ADHD. Atomoxetine is in a class of medications called selective norepinephrine reuptake inhibitors. It works by increasing the levels of norepinephrine, a natural substance in the brain that is needed to control behavior.

How should this medicine be used?

Atomoxetine comes as a capsule to take by mouth. It is usually taken either once a day in the morning, or twice a day in the morning and late afternoon or early evening. Atomoxetine may be taken with or without food. However, taking atomoxetine with food may help prevent the medication from upsetting your stomach. Take atomoxetine at around the same time(s) every day. Follow the directions on your prescription label carefully, and ask your doctor or pharmacist to explain any part you do not understand. Take atomoxetine exactly as directed. Do not take more or less of it or take it more often than prescribed by your doctor.

Swallow atomoxetine capsules whole; do not open, chew, or crush them. If a capsule is accidentally broken or opened, wash away the loose powder with water right away. Try not to touch the powder and be especially careful not to get the powder in your eyes. If you do get powder in your eyes, rinse them with water right away and call your doctor.

Your doctor will probably start you on a low dose of atomoxetine and increase your dose after at least 3 days. Your doctor may increase your dose again after 2-4 weeks. You may notice improvement in your symptoms during the first week of your treatment, but it may take up to one month for you to feel the full benefit of atomoxetine.

Atomoxetine may help control the symptoms of ADHD but will not cure the condition. Continue to take atomoxetine even if you feel well. Do not stop taking atomoxetine without talking to your doctor.

Are there other uses for this medicine?

This medication may be prescribed for other uses; ask your doctor or pharmacist for more information.

What special precautions should I follow?

Before taking atomoxetine,

- tell your doctor and pharmacist if you are allergic to atomoxetine, any other medications, or any of the inactive ingredients in atomoxetine capsules.
- tell your doctor if you are taking monoamine oxidase (MAO) inhibitors, including isocaraboxazid (Marplan), phenelzine (Nardil), selegiline (Eldepryl, Emsam, Zelapar), and tranylcypromine (Parnate), or if you have stopped taking them within the past 2 weeks. Your doctor will probably tell you not to take atomoxetine. If you stop taking atomoxetine, you should wait at least 2 weeks before you start taking an MAO inhibitor.
- tell your doctor and pharmacist what other prescription and nonprescription medications, vitamins, nutritional supplements, and herbal products you are taking or plan to take. Be sure to mention any of the following: albuterol syrup or tablets (Proventil, Ventolin), amiodarone (Cordarone, Pacerone), bupropion (Wellbutrin), chlorpheniramine (antihistamine in cold medications), cimetidine (Tagamet), clomipramine (Anafranil), fluoxetine (Prozac, Sarafem), haloperidol (Haldol), metaproterenol syrup or tablets, medications for high blood pressure, methadone (Dolophine), metoclopramide (Reglan), nefazodone, paroxetine (Paxil), quinidine, ritonavir (Norvir), and sertraline (Zoloft). Your doctor may need to change the doses of your medications or monitor you carefully for side effects.
- tell your doctor if you have or have ever had glaucoma (an eye disease that may cause vision loss). Your doctor may tell you not to take atomoxetine.
- tell your doctor if anyone in your family has or has ever had an irregular heartbeat or has died suddenly. Also tell your doctor if you have recently had a heart attack and if you have or have ever had a heart defect, an irregular heartbeat, heart or blood vessel disease, or other heart problems. Your doctor will probably examine you to see if your heart and blood vessels are healthy. Your doctor may tell you not to take atomoxetine if you have a heart condition or if there is a high risk that you may develop a heart condition.
- tell your doctor if you or anyone in your family has or

has ever had depression or bipolar disorder (manic depressive disorder; a condition that causes episodes of depression, episodes of frenzied, abnormal excitement and other abnormal moods) or has ever thought about or attempted suicide. Also tell your doctor if you have or have ever had high or low blood pressure, seizures, or liver disease.

- tell your doctor if you are pregnant, plan to become pregnant, or are breast-feeding. If you become pregnant while taking atomoxetine, call your doctor.
- you should know that atomoxetine may make you drowsy. Do not drive a car or operate machinery until you know how this medication affects you.
- you should know that atomoxetine has caused severe liver damage in some patients. Call your doctor right away if you have any of the following symptoms: itchy skin, dark urine, yellowing of your skin or eyes, pain in the upper right part of your stomach, or flu-like symptoms.
- you should know that atomoxetine may cause dizziness, lightheadedness, and fainting when you get up too quickly from a lying position. To avoid this problem, get out of bed slowly, resting your feet on the floor for a few minutes before standing up.
- you should know that atomoxetine should be used as part of a total treatment program for ADHD, which may include counseling and special education. Make sure to follow all of your doctor's and/or therapist's instructions.

What special dietary instructions should I follow?

Unless your doctor tells you otherwise, continue your normal diet.

What should I do if I forget to take a dose?

Take the missed dose as soon as you remember it. However, if it is almost time for the next dose, skip the missed dose and continue your regular dosing schedule. Do not take a double dose to make up for a missed one. Do not take more than the prescribed daily amount of atomoxetine in 24 hours.

What side effects can this medicine cause?

Atomoxetine may cause side effects. Tell your doctor if any of these symptoms are severe or do not go away:

- heartburn
- nausea
- vomiting
- loss of appetite
- weight loss
- constipation
- stomach pain
- gas
- dry mouth
- excessive tiredness
- dizziness
- headache
- mood swings

- decreased sex drive or ability
- difficulty urinating
- painful or irregular menstrual periods
- muscle pain
- sweating
- hot flashes
- unusual dreams
- burning or tingling in the hands, arms, feet, or legs

Some side effects can be serious. If you experience any of the following symptoms, or those listed in the IMPORTANT WARNING or SPECIAL PRECAUTIONS section, call your doctor immediately:

- fast or pounding heartbeat
- chest pain
- shortness of breath
- slow or difficult speech
- dizziness or faintness
- weakness or numbness of an arm or leg
- swelling of the face, throat, tongue, lips, eyes, hands, feet, ankles, or lower legs
- hoarseness
- difficulty swallowing or breathing
- hives
- rash
- abnormal thoughts
- hallucinating (seeing things or hearing voices that do not exist)
- erection that lasts for several hours or longer
- seizures

Atomoxetine may cause sudden death in children and teenagers with heart defects or serious heart problems. This medication also may cause sudden death, heart attack or stroke in adults, especially adults with heart defects or serious heart problems. Talk to your doctor about the risks of taking this medication or of giving this medication to your child.

Atomoxetine may slow down children's growth or weight gain. Your child's doctor will probably monitor your child carefully during his or her treatment with atomoxetine. Talk to your child's doctor about the risks of giving this medication to your child.

Atomoxetine may cause other side effects. Call your doctor if you have any unusual problems while taking this medication.

If you experience a serious side effect, you or your doctor may send a report to the Food and Drug Administration's (FDA) MedWatch Adverse Event Reporting program online [at http://www.fda.gov/MedWatch/index.html] or by phone [1-800-332-1088].

What storage conditions are needed for this medicine?

Keep this medication in the container it came in, tightly closed, and out of reach of children. Store it at room temperature and away from excess heat and moisture (not in the bathroom). Throw away any medication that is outdated or no longer needed. Talk to your pharmacist about the proper disposal of your medication.

What should I do in case of overdose?

In case of overdose, call your local poison control center at 1-800-222-1222. If the victim has collapsed or is not breathing, call local emergency services at 911.

Symptoms of overdose may include:

- sleepiness
- agitation
- an increase in activity or talking
- abnormal behavior
- stomach problems
- wide pupils (black circles in the middle of the eyes)
- fast heartbeat
- dry mouth

What other information should I know?

Keep all appointments with your doctor and the laboratory. Your doctor may order certain lab tests to check your body's response to atomoxetine.

Do not let anyone else take your medication. Ask your pharmacist any questions you have about refilling your prescription.

Dosage Facts
For Informational Purposes

Caution: Do not change your dose, how often you take your medication, or the length of time you are to take it without first talking to your healthcare provider.

The following dosage information was written using medical language for doctors and other healthcare professionals and is provided here for you to check your dosage. The dosage of this drug may differ for different patients. Therefore, always follow your doctor's instructions or the directions on the label. Contact your healthcare provider or pharmacist if you have any questions about the specific dosage of your medication after reviewing this information.

General Dosage Information

Available as atomoxetine hydrochloride; dosage expressed in terms of atomoxetine.

Pediatric Patients

ADHD

ORAL:
- Children and adolescents weighing ≤70 kg: Initially, approximately 0.5 mg/kg daily. Increase dosage after ≥3 days to target dosage of approximately 1.2 mg/kg daily (do not exceed 100 mg daily).
- Children and adolescents weighing >70 kg: Initially, 40 mg daily. Increase dosage after ≥3 days to target dosage of approximately 80 mg daily. If optimum response has not been

achieved after 2–4 additional weeks of therapy, may increase dosage to maximum of 100 mg daily.

Adult Patients

ADHD

ORAL:

- Initially, 40 mg daily. Increase dosage after ≥3 days to target dosage of approximately 80 mg daily. If optimum response has not been achieved after 2–4 additional weeks of therapy, may increase dosage to maximum of 100 mg daily.

Prescribing Limits

Pediatric Patients

ADHD

ORAL:

- Children and adolescents weighing ≤70 kg: Maximum 100 mg or 1.4 mg/kg daily (whichever is less); dosages >1.2 mg/kg daily have not been shown in clinical trials to result in additional therapeutic benefit.
- Children and adolescents weighing >70 kg: Maximum 100 mg daily; dosages >100 mg daily have not been shown in clinical trials to result in additional therapeutic benefit. Safety of single doses >120 mg and total daily dosages >150 mg has not been established.

Adult Patients

ADHD

ORAL:

- Maximum 100 mg daily; dosages >100 mg daily have not been shown in clinical trials to result in additional therapeutic benefit. Safety of single doses >120 mg and total daily dosages >150 mg has not been established.

Special Populations

Hepatic Impairment

- Reduce initial and target dosages by 50% in patients with moderate hepatic impairment (Child-Pugh class B) and by 75% in those with severe hepatic impairment (Child-Pugh class C).

Atorvastatin

(a tore′ va sta tin)

Brand Name: Caduet® (combination with amlodipine), Lipitor®

Why is this medicine prescribed?

Atorvastatin is used together with lifestyle changes (diet, weight-loss, exercise) to reduce the amount of cholesterol (a fat-like substance) and other fatty substances in the blood. Atorvastatin is in a class of medications called HMG-CoA reductase inhibitors (statins). It works by slowing the production of cholesterol in the body.

Buildup of cholesterol and other fats along the walls of the blood vessels (a process known as atherosclerosis) decreases blood flow and, therefore, the oxygen supply to the heart, brain, and other parts of the body. Lowering blood levels of cholesterol and other fats may help to decrease your chances of getting heart disease, angina (chest pain), strokes, and heart attacks. In addition to taking a cholesterol-lowering medication, making certain changes in your daily habits can also lower your cholesterol blood levels. You should eat a diet that is low in saturated fat and cholesterol (see SPECIAL DIETARY), exercise 30 minutes on most, if not all days, and lose weight if you are overweight.

How should this medicine be used?

Atorvastatin comes as a tablet to take by mouth. It is usually taken once a day with or without food. Take atorvastatin at around the same time every day. Follow the directions on your prescription label carefully, and ask your doctor or pharmacist to explain any part you do not understand. Take atorvastatin exactly as directed. Do not take more or less of it or take it more often than prescribed by your doctor.

Your doctor may start you on a low dose of atorvastatin and gradually increase your dose, not more than once every 2-4 weeks.

Continue to take atorvastatin even if you feel well. Do not stop taking atorvastatin without talking to your doctor.

Are there other uses for this medicine?

This medication may be prescribed for other uses; ask your doctor or pharmacist for more information.

What special precautions should I follow?

Before taking atorvastatin,

- tell your doctor and pharmacist if you are allergic to atorvastatin or any other medications.
- tell your doctor and pharmacist what prescription and nonprescription medications, vitamins, nutritional supplements, and herbal products you are taking or plan to take. Be sure to mention any of the following: antifungal medications such as itraconazole (Sporanox) and ketoconazole (Nizoral); cimetidine (Tagamet); cyclosporine (Neoral, Sandimmune); digoxin (Lanoxin); erythromycin (E.E.S., E-Mycin, Erythrocin); oral contraceptives (birth control pills); other cholesterol-lowering medications such as fenofibrate (Tricor), gemfibrozil (Lopid), and niacin (nicotinic acid, Niacor, Niaspan); and spironolactone (Aldactone). Your doctor may need to change the doses of your medications or monitor you carefully for side effects.
- tell your doctor if you have liver disease. Your doctor will probably tell you not to take lovastatin.
- tell your doctor if you drink large amounts of alcohol and if you have ever had liver disease.
- tell your doctor if you are pregnant or plan to become pregnant. If you become pregnant while taking atorvastatin, stop taking atorvastatin and call your doctor immediately. Atorvastatin may harm the fetus.
- Do not breastfeed while you are taking this medication.
- if you are having surgery, including dental surgery, tell the doctor or dentist that you are taking atorvastatin.

- ask your doctor about the safe use of alcoholic beverages while you are taking atorvastatin. Alcohol can increase the risk of serious side effects.

What special dietary instructions should I follow?

Eat a low-cholesterol, low-fat diet. This kind of diet includes cottage cheese, fat-free milk, fish (not canned in oil), vegetables, poultry, egg whites, and polyunsaturated oils and margarines (corn, safflower, canola, and soybean oils). Avoid foods with excess fat in them such as meat (especially liver and fatty meat), egg yolks, whole milk, cream, butter, shortening, lard, pastries, cakes, cookies, gravy, peanut butter, chocolate, olives, potato chips, coconut, cheese (other than cottage cheese), coconut oil, palm oil, and fried foods.

Talk to your doctor about drinking grapefruit juice while taking this medication.

What should I do if I forget to take a dose?

Take the missed dose as soon as you remember it. However, if it is almost time for the next dose, skip the missed dose and continue your regular dosing schedule. Do not take a double dose to make up for a missed one.

What side effects can this medicine cause?

Atorvastatin may cause side effects. Tell your doctor if any of these symptoms are severe or do not go away:

- diarrhea
- headache
- difficulty falling asleep or staying asleep
- dizziness
- joint pain
- sore throat
- upper respiratory infection

Some side effects can be serious. The following symptoms are uncommon, but if you experience any of them, call your doctor immediately:

- muscle pain, tenderness, or weakness
- lack of energy
- fever
- chest pain
- swelling of the hands, feet, ankles, or lower legs
- nausea
- extreme tiredness
- unusual bleeding or bruising
- loss of appetite
- pain in the upper right part of the stomach
- flu-like symptoms
- yellowing of the skin or eyes
- rash
- hives
- itching
- difficulty breathing or swallowing
- swelling of the face, throat, tongue, lips, eyes, hands, feet, ankles, or lower legs
- hoarseness

- pain during urination
- frequent urge to urinate

Atorvastatin may cause other side effects. Call your doctor if you have any unusual problems while taking this medication.

If you experience a serious side effect, you or your doctor may send a report to the Food and Drug Administration's (FDA) MedWatch Adverse Event Reporting program online [at http://www.fda.gov/MedWatch/index.html] or by phone [1-800-332-1088].

What storage conditions are needed for this medicine?

Keep this medication in the container it came in, tightly closed, and out of reach of children. Store it at room temperature and away from excess heat and moisture (not in the bathroom). Throw away any medication that is outdated or no longer needed. Talk to your pharmacist about the proper disposal of your medication.

What should I do in case of overdose?

In case of overdose, call your local poison control center at 1-800-222-1222. If the victim has collapsed or is not breathing, call local emergency services at 911.

What other information should I know?

Keep all appointments with your doctor and the laboratory. Your doctor will order certain lab tests before and during treatment to check your body's response to atorvastatin.

Before having any laboratory test, tell your doctor and the laboratory personnel that you are taking atorvastatin.

Do not let anyone else take your medication. Ask your pharmacist any questions you have about refilling your prescription.

Dosage Facts
For Informational Purposes

Caution: Do not change your dose, how often you take your medication, or the length of time you are to take it without first talking to your healthcare provider.

The following dosage information was written using medical language for doctors and other healthcare professionals and is provided here for you to check your dosage. The dosage of this drug may differ for different patients. Therefore, always follow your doctor's instructions or the directions on the label. Contact your healthcare provider or pharmacist if you have any questions about the specific dosage of your medication after reviewing this information.

General Dosage Information

Available as atorvastatin calcium; dosage expressed in terms of atorvastatin. Also available in fixed combination with amlodipine besylate (Caduet®).

Pediatric Patients

Dyslipidemias

ORAL:
- Children ≥10 years of age: Initially, 10 mg once daily.
- Adjust dosage at intervals ≥4 weeks until the desired effect on lipoprotein concentrations is observed or a daily dosage of 20 mg is reached.

Adult Patients

Dyslipidemias and Prevention of Cardiovascular Events
Primary Hypercholesterolemia and Mixed Dyslipidemia

ORAL:
- Initially, 10 or 20 mg once daily; patients who require a large reduction in LDL-cholesterol concentration (>45%) may receive 40 mg once daily. Determine serum lipoprotein concentrations within 2–4 weeks after initiating and/or titrating therapy and adjust dosage accordingly. Usual maintenance dosage is 10–80 mg once daily.
- Atorvastatin/amlodipine fixed combination (Caduet®): Use as a *substitute* for individually titrated drugs; to provide *additional therapy* for patients currently receiving one component of the preparation; or to *initiate treatment* in patients with dyslipidemias who have hypertension and/or CAD.

Homozygous Familial Hypercholesterolemia

ORAL:
- 10–80 mg once daily.

Prescribing Limits

Pediatric Patients

ORAL:
- Children ≥10 years of age: Maximum 20 mg daily.

Special Populations

Renal Impairment
- Dosage modification not required.

Atovaquone

(a toe′ va kwone)

Brand Name: Mepron®

Why is this medicine prescribed?

Atovaquone is used to treat Pneumocystis carinii pneumonia (PCP).

This medication is sometimes prescribed for other uses; ask your doctor or pharmacist for more information.

How should this medicine be used?

Atovaquone comes as a liquid to take by mouth. It usually is taken with food every 8 hours for 21 days. Always take atovaquone with snacks or meals. Follow the directions on your prescription label carefully, and ask your doctor or pharmacist to explain any part you do not understand. Take atovaquone exactly as directed. Do not take more or less of it or take it more often than prescribed by your doctor.

What special precautions should I follow?

Before taking atovaquone,
- tell your doctor and pharmacist if you are allergic to atovaquone or any other drugs.
- tell your doctor and pharmacist what prescription and nonprescription medications you are taking, especially rifampin (Rifadin), sulfa drugs, zidovudine and vitamins.
- tell your doctor if you have or have ever had stomach or intestinal disorders or allergies.
- tell your doctor if you are pregnant, plan to become pregnant, or are breast-feeding. If you become pregnant while taking atovaquone, call your doctor.
- you should know that this drug may make you drowsy. Do not drive a car or operate machinery until you know how this drug affects you.
- remember that alcohol can add to the drowsiness caused by this drug.

What should I do if I forget to take a dose?

Take the missed dose as soon as you remember it. However, if it is almost time for the next dose, skip the missed dose and continue your regular dosing schedule. Do not take a double dose to make up for a missed one.

What side effects can this medicine cause?

Atovaquone may cause side effects. Tell your doctor if any of these symptoms are severe or do not go away:
- upset stomach
- diarrhea
- constipation
- headache
- difficulty sleeping
- sweating
- dizziness
- altered sense of taste

If you experience any of the following symptoms, call your doctor immediately:
- skin rash
- fever
- vomiting
- itching
- unusual weakness

If you experience a serious side effect, you or your doctor may send a report to the Food and Drug Administration's (FDA) MedWatch Adverse Event Reporting program online [at http://www.fda.gov/MedWatch/index.html] or by phone [1-800-332-1088].

What storage conditions are needed for this medicine?

Keep this medication in the container it came in, tightly closed, and out of reach of children. Store it at room temperature and away from excess heat and moisture (not in the bathroom). Throw away any medication that is outdated or no longer needed. Talk to your pharmacist about the proper disposal of your medication.

What should I do in case of overdose?

In case of overdose, call your local poison control center at 1-800-222-1222. If the victim has collapsed or is not breathing, call local emergency services at 911.

What other information should I know?

Keep all appointments with your doctor and the laboratory. Your doctor will order certain lab tests to check your response to atovaquone.

Do not let anyone else take your medication. Your prescription is probably not refillable. If you still have symptoms of infection after you finish the atovaquone, call your doctor.

Talk to your doctor, pharmacist, or other healthcare professional if you have questions about dosing information for your medication.

Atropine Ophthalmic

(a′ troe peen)

Brand Name: Atropine Care® 1%, Atropisol®, Isopto® Atropine, Ocu-Tropine®

Why is this medicine prescribed?

Atropine is used before eye examinations to dilate (open) the pupil, the black part of the eye through which you see. It is also used to relieve pain caused by swelling and inflammation of the eye.

This medication is sometimes prescribed for other uses; ask your doctor or pharmacist for more information.

How should this medicine be used?

Atropine comes as eyedrops and eye ointment. The drops are usually applied 2 to 4 times a day. the ointment usually is applied 1 to 3 times a day. Follow the directions on your prescription label carefully, and ask your doctor or pharmacist to explain any part you do not understand. Use atropine exactly as directed. Do not use more or less of it or use it more often than prescribed by your doctor.

To use the eyedrops, follow these instructions:
1. Wash your hands thoroughly with soap and water.
2. Use a mirror or have someone else put the drops in your eye.
3. Remove the protective cap. Make sure that the end of the dropper is not chipped or cracked and that the eyedrops are clear (not cloudy).
4. Avoid touching the dropper tip against your eye or anything else.
5. Hold the dropper tip down at all times to prevent drops from flowing back into the bottle and contaminating the remaining contents.
6. Lie down or tilt your head back.
7. Holding the bottle between your thumb and index finger, place the dropper tip as near as possible to your eyelid without touching it.
8. Brace the remaining fingers of that hand against your cheek or nose.
9. With the index finger of your other hand, pull the lower lid of the eye down to form a pocket.
10. Drop the prescribed number of drops into the pocket made by the lower lid and the eye. Placing drops on the surface of the eyeball can cause stinging.
11. Close your eye and press lightly against the lower lid with your finger for 2-3 minutes to keep the medication in the eye. Do not blink.
12. Replace and tighten the cap right away. Do not wipe or rinse it off.
13. Wipe off any excess liquid from your cheek with a clean tissue. Wash your hands again.

To use the eye ointment, follow these instructions:
1. Wash your hands thoroughly with soap and water.
2. Use a mirror or have someone else apply the ointment.
3. Avoid touching the tip of the tube against your eye or anything else. The ointment must be kept clean.
4. Tilt your head forward slightly.
5. Holding the tube between your thumb and index finger, place the tube as near as possible to your eyelid without touching it.
6. Brace the remaining fingers of that hand against your cheek or nose.
7. With the index finger of your other hand, pull the lower lid of your eye down to form a pocket.
8. Place a small amount of ointment into the pocket made by the lower lid and theeye. A 1/2-inch strip of ointment usually is enough unless otherwise directed by your doctor.
9. Gently close your eyes and keep them closed for 1-2 minutes to allow the medication to be absorbed.
10. Replace and tighten the cap right away.
11. Wipe off any excess ointment from your eyelids and lashes with a clean tissue. Wash your hands again.

What special precautions should I follow?

Before using atropine eyedrops or eye ointment,
- tell your doctor and pharmacist if you are allergic to atropine, belladonna, or any other drugs.
- tell your doctor and pharmacist what prescription and nonprescription medications you are taking, especially antihistamines, cough and cold medicines, and vitamins.
- tell your doctor if you have glaucoma.

- tell your doctor if you are pregnant, plan to become pregnant, or are breast-feeding. If you become pregnant while using atropine, call your doctor immediately.

What should I do if I forget to take a dose?

Apply the eyedrops or eye ointment as soon as you remember the missed dose. Use any remaining doses for that day at evenly spaced intervals. However, if you remember a missed dose at the time the next one is due, use only the regularly scheduled dose. Do not apply a double dose to make up for a missed one.

What side effects can this medicine cause?

Atropine may cause side effects. Tell your doctor if any of these symptoms are severe or do not go away:

- eye irritation and redness
- swelling of the eyelids
- sensitivity to bright light
- dry mouth
- red or dry skin
- blurred vision

If you experience any of the following symptoms, call your doctor immediately:

- fever
- irritability
- fast pulse
- irregular heartbeat
- mental confusion
- difficulty urinating

If you experience a serious side effect, you or your doctor may send a report to the Food and Drug Administration's (FDA) MedWatch Adverse Event Reporting program online [at http://www.fda.gov/MedWatch/index.html] or by phone [1-800-332-1088].

What storage conditions are needed for this medicine?

Keep this medication in the container it came in, tightly closed, and out of reach of children. Store it at room temperature and away from excess heat and moisture (not in the bathroom). Throw away any medication that is outdated or no longer needed. Talk to your pharmacist about the proper disposal of your medication.

What other information should I know?

Keep all appointments with your doctor. Your doctor will order certain eye tests to check your response to atropine.

Do not let anyone else use your medication. Ask your pharmacist any questions you have about refilling your prescription.

Talk to your doctor, pharmacist, or other healthcare professional if you have questions about dosing information for your medication.

Auranofin

(au rane' oh fin)

Brand Name: Ridaura®

Why is this medicine prescribed?

Auranofin is used, with rest and nondrug therapy, to treat rheumatoid arthritis. It improves arthritis symptoms including painful or tender and swollen joints and morning stiffness.

This medication is sometimes prescribed for other uses; ask your doctor or pharmacist for more information.

How should this medicine be used?

Auranofin comes as a capsule to take by mouth. It usually is taken once or twice a day. It must be taken on a regular schedule, as prescribed by your doctor, to be effective. The full effect of this drug usually is not felt for 3-4 months; in some people, it may take up to 6 months. Follow the directions on your prescription label carefully, and ask your doctor or pharmacist to explain any part you do not understand. Take auranofin exactly as directed. Do not take more or less of it or take it more often than prescribed by your doctor.

Are there other uses for this medicine?

Auranofin is also used sometimes for psoriatic arthritis. Talk to your doctor about the possible risks of using this drug for your condition.

What special precautions should I follow?

Before taking auranofin,

- tell your doctor and pharmacist if you are allergic to auranofin or any other drugs.
- tell your doctor and pharmacist what prescription and non-prescription medications you are taking, especially arthritis medications, phenytoin (Dilantin), and vitamins.
- tell your doctor if you have or have ever had heart, kidney, or liver disease; diabetes; bleeding problems; inflammatory bowel disease; colitis; rash; eczema; SLE (systemic lupus erythematosus); or a history of bone marrow depression.
- tell your doctor if you are pregnant, plan to become pregnant, or are breast-feeding. If you become pregnant while taking auranofin, call your doctor. You should not try to become pregnant while taking auranofin or for at least 6 months after discontinuing the drug because it stays in the body for a long time.
- if you are having surgery, including dental surgery, tell the doctor or dentist that you are taking auranofin.
- be aware that you should not drink alcohol while taking this medication.
- plan to avoid unneccessary or prolonged exposure to sunlight and to wear protective clothing and sunscreen. Auranofin may make your skin more sensitive to sunlight.

What special dietary instructions should I follow?

Auranofin may cause an upset stomach. Take auranofin after meals or a light snack.

What should I do if I forget to take a dose?

Take the missed dose as soon as you remember it, and take any remaining doses for that day at evenly spaced intervals. Do not take a double dose to make up for a missed one.

What side effects can this medicine cause?

Auranofin may cause side effects. Tell your doctor if any of these symptoms are severe or do not go away:

- metallic taste
- loose stools or diarrhea
- stomach pain
- upset stomach
- vomiting
- gas
- hair loss

If you experience any of the following symptoms, call your doctor immediately:

- bloody or tarry stools
- itching
- skin rash
- sore throat
- mouth sores
- fever
- chills
- unusual bruising or bleeding
- blood in the urine
- fatigue

If you experience a serious side effect, you or your doctor may send a report to the Food and Drug Administration's (FDA) MedWatch Adverse Event Reporting program online [at http://www.fda.gov/MedWatch/index.html] or by phone [1-800-332-1088].

What storage conditions are needed for this medicine?

Keep this medication in the container it came in, tightly closed, and out of reach of children. Store it at room temperature and away from excess heat and moisture (not in the bathroom). Throw away any medication that is outdated or no longer needed. Talk to your pharmacist about the proper disposal of your medication.

What should I do in case of overdose?

In case of overdose, call your local poison control center at 1-800-222-1222. If the victim has collapsed or is not breathing, call local emergency services at 911.

What other information should I know?

Keep all appointments with your doctor and the laboratory. Your doctor will order certain lab tests to check your response to auranofin.

If you have a tuberculin (TB) skin test, tell the person performing the test that you take auranofin.

Do not let anyone else take your medication. Ask your pharmacist any questions you have about refilling your prescription.

Talk to your doctor, pharmacist, or other healthcare professional if you have questions about dosing information for your medication.

Azathioprine

(ay za thye′ oh preen)

Brand Name: Azasan®, Imuran®

<table>
<tr><td>

Important Warning

Azathioprine can cause a decrease in the number of blood cells in your bone marrow. If you experience any of the following symptoms, call your doctor immediately: unusual bleeding or bruising; excessive tiredness; pale skin; headache; confusion; dizziness; fast heartbeat; difficulty sleeping; weakness; shortness of breath; and sore throat, fever, chills, and other signs of infection. Your doctor will order tests before, during, and after your treatment to see if your blood cells are affected by this drug.

Azathioprine may increase your risk of developing certain types of cancer, especially skin cancer and lymphoma. Tell your doctor if you have or have ever had cancer and if you are taking or have ever taken alkylating agents such as chlorambucil (Leukeran), cyclophosphamide (Cytoxan), or melphalan (Alkeran) for cancer. Tell your doctor immediately if you notice any changes in your skin or any lumps or masses anywhere in your body. Talk to your doctor about the risks of taking this medication.

</td></tr>
</table>

Why is this medicine prescribed?

Azathioprine is used with other medications to prevent rejection of kidney transplants. It is also used to treat severe rheumatoid arthritis (a condition in which the body attacks its own joints, causing pain and swelling) when other medications and treatments have not helped. Azathioprine is in a class of medications called immunosuppressants. It works by weakening the body's immune system so it will not attack the transplanted organ or the joints.

How should this medicine be used?

Azathioprine comes as a tablet to take by mouth. It is usually taken once or twice a day after meals. To help you remember to take azathioprine, take it around the same time(s) every day. Follow the directions on your prescription label carefully, and ask your doctor or pharmacist to explain any part you do not understand. Take azathioprine exactly as directed. Do not take more or less of it or take it more often than prescribed by your doctor.

If you are taking azathioprine to treat rheumatoid arthritis, your doctor may start you on a low dose and gradually increase your dose after 6-8 weeks and then not more than once every 4 weeks. If you are taking azathioprine to prevent kidney transplant rejection, your doctor may start you on a high dose and decrease your dose gradually as your body adjusts to the transplant.

Azathioprine controls rheumatoid arthritis but does not cure it. It may take some time before you feel the full benefit of azathioprine. Azathioprine prevents transplant rejection only as long as you are taking the medication. Continue to take azathioprine even if you feel well. Do not stop taking azathioprine without talking to your doctor.

Are there other uses for this medicine?

Azathioprine is also used to treat ulcerative colitis (a condition in which sores develop in the intestine causing pain and diarrhea). Talk to your doctor about the possible risks of using this drug for your condition.

This medication is sometimes prescribed for other uses; ask your doctor or pharmacist for more information.

What special precautions should I follow?

Before taking azathioprine,

- tell your doctor and pharmacist if you are allergic to azathioprine or any other medications.
- tell your doctor and pharmacist what prescription and nonprescription medications, vitamins, nutritional supplements, and herbal products you are taking. Be sure to mention any of the medications mentioned in the IMPORTANT WARNING section and the following: allopurinol (Zyloprim); angiotensin-converting enzyme (ACE) inhibitors such as benazepril (Lotensin), captopril (Capoten), enalapril (Lexxel, Vasotec), fosinopril (Monopril), lisinopril (Prinivil, Zestril), moexipril (Univasc), perindopril (Aceon), quinapril (Accupril), ramipril (Altace), and trandolapril (Mavik, Tarka); anticoagulants ('blood thinners') such as warfarin (Coumadin); antimalarials such as chloroquine (Aralen), hydroxychloroquine (Plaquenil), mefloquine (Lariam), primaquine, proguanil (Malarone), pyrimethamine (Daraprim), and quinine; cancer chemotherapy medications; co-trimoxazole (Bactrim, Septra, Sulfatrim); cyclosporine (Neoral, Sandimmune); gold compounds such as auranofin (Ridaura) and aurothioglucose (Aurolate, Solganal); methotrexate (Rheumatrex); penicillamine (Cuprimine, Depen); sirolimus (Rapamune); and tacrolimus (Prograf).
- tell your doctor if you have any type of infection, or if you have or have ever had kidney, liver, or pancreas disease.

- tell your doctor if you are pregnant, plan to become pregnant, or are breast-feeding. You should use birth control to be sure you or your partner will not become pregnant while you are taking this medication. Do not breastfeed while you are taking this medication.
- if you are having surgery, including dental surgery, tell the doctor or dentist that you are taking azathioprine.
- Do not have any vaccinations (e.g., measles or flu shots) during or after your treatment without talking to your doctor.
- you should know that azathioprine may decrease your ability to fight infection. Stay away from people who are sick, and wash your hands often.

What special dietary instructions should I follow?

Unless your doctor tells you otherwise, continue your normal diet.

What should I do if I forget to take a dose?

Take the missed dose as soon as you remember it. However, if it is almost time for the next dose, skip the missed dose and continue your regular dosing schedule. Do not take a double dose to make up for a missed one.

What side effects can this medicine cause?

Azathioprine may cause side effects. Tell your doctor if any of these symptoms are severe or do not go away:
- upset stomach
- vomiting
- diarrhea
- muscle aches

Some side effects can be serious. The following symptoms are uncommon, but if you experience any of them or those listed in the IMPORTANT WARNING section, call your doctor immediately.
- mouth sores
- cough
- lack of energy
- loss of appetite
- pain in the upper right part of the stomach
- yellowing of the skin or eyes
- flu-like symptoms
- rash
- blurred vision
- stomach pain

If you experience a serious side effect, you or your doctor may send a report to the Food and Drug Administration's (FDA) MedWatch Adverse Event Reporting program online [at http://www.fda.gov/MedWatch/index.html] or by phone [1-800-332-1088].

What storage conditions are needed for this medicine?

Keep this medication in the container it came in, tightly closed, and out of reach of children. Store it at room tem-

perature and away from excess heat and moisture (not in the bathroom). Throw away any medication that is outdated or no longer needed. Talk to your pharmacist about the proper disposal of your medication.

What should I do in case of overdose?

In case of overdose, call your local poison control center at 1-800-222-1222. If the victim has collapsed or is not breathing, call local emergency services at 911.

Symptoms of overdose may include:
- upset stomach
- vomiting
- diarrhea
- sore throat, fever, chills, and other signs of infection

What other information should I know?

Keep all appointments with your doctor and the laboratory. Your doctor will order certain lab tests to check your response to azathioprine.

Do not let anyone else take your medication. Ask your pharmacist any questions you have about refilling your prescription.

Dosage Facts
For Informational Purposes

Caution: Do not change your dose, how often you take your medication, or the length of time you are to take it without first talking to your healthcare provider.

The following dosage information was written using medical language for doctors and other healthcare professionals and is provided here for you to check your dosage. The dosage of this drug may differ for different patients. Therefore, always follow your doctor's instructions or the directions on the label. Contact your healthcare provider or pharmacist if you have any questions about the specific dosage of your medication after reviewing this information.

General Dosage Information

Available as azathioprine and azathioprine sodium; dosage expressed as azathioprine.

Consider determining thiopurine methyl transferase (TPMT) phenotype or genotype prior to initiation of therapy and using results to select dosage. and

If rapid fall in leukocyte count, persistent leukopenia, or other evidence of bone marrow suppression develops, temporarily discontinue or reduce dosage. Consider TPMT testing in patients with abnormal CBC results that persist despite dosage reduction. and

If used with allopurinol, adjustment in the treatment regimen recommended.

If severe, continuous rejection occurs, it is probably preferable to allow the allograft to be rejected than to increase the dosage of azathioprine to very toxic levels.

Pediatric Patients
Renal Allotransplantation

ORAL:
- Initially, 3–5 mg/kg as a single daily dose has been used beginning on the day of transplantation (and in some cases 1–3 days before transplantation). Reduction to maintenance dosage of 1–3 mg/kg daily usually possible.

Crohn's Disease†

ORAL:
- 1.5–2 mg/kg daily has been used.

Adult Patients
Renal Allotransplantation

ORAL:
- Initially, 3–5 mg/kg as a single daily dose beginning on the day of transplantation (and in some cases 1–3 days before transplantation). Reduction to maintenance dosage of 1–3 mg/kg daily usually possible.

Rheumatoid Arthritis

ORAL:
- Initially, 1 mg/kg (50–100 mg) daily in 1 or 2 doses.
- If initial response unsatisfactory and there are no serious adverse effects after 6–8 weeks, the daily dosage may be increased by 0.5 mg/kg. Thereafter, daily dosage may be increased, if needed, by 0.5 mg/kg every 4 weeks up to a maximum dosage of 2.5 mg/kg daily. Patients whose disease does not improve after 12 weeks of therapy are considered nonresponders.
- When used for maintenance dosage, use lowest effective dosage to reduce toxicities. Dosage can be reduced in increments of 0.5 mg/kg (approximately 25 mg) daily every 4 weeks while other therapy is kept constant.
- Optimum duration of therapy undetermined.

Crohn's Disease†

ORAL:
- 2–4 mg/kg daily has been used.

Prescribing Limits
Adult Patients
Rheumatoid Arthritis

ORAL:
- Maximum 2.5 mg/kg daily.

Special Populations

Renal Impairment
- Use low initial dosage in patients with renal impairment.

Renal Allotransplantation
- Lower dosage may be necessary in relatively oliguric patients, especially in those with tubular necrosis in the immediate posttransplant period.

† Use is not currently included in the labeling approved by the US Food and Drug Administration.

Azelaic Acid Topical

(ay ze lay′ ik)

Brand Name: Azelex®, Finacea®

Why is this medicine prescribed?

Azelaic acid gel is used to clear the bumps, lesions, and swelling caused by rosacea (a skin disease that causes redness, flushing, and pimples on the face). Azelaic acid cream is used to treat acne. Azelaic acid is in a class of medications called dicarboxylic acids. It works to treat acne by killing the bacteria that infect pores and by decreasing production of keratin, a natural substance that can lead to the development of acne. The way azelaic acid works to treat rosacea is not known.

How should this medicine be used?

Azelaic acid comes as a gel and a cream to apply to the skin. It is usually applied twice a day, in the morning and the evening. To help you remember to use azelaic acid, use it at around the same times every day. Follow the directions on your prescription label carefully, and ask your doctor or pharmacist to explain any part you do not understand. Use azelaic acid exactly as directed. Do not use more or less of it or use it more often than prescribed by your doctor.

Azelaic acid controls acne and rosacea but does not cure these conditions. It may take 4 weeks or longer before you feel the full benefit of azelaic acid. Continue to use azelaic acid exactly as directed even if you do not notice much improvement at first.

To use the cream or gel, follow these steps:

1. Wash the affected skin with water and a mild soap or soapless cleansing lotion and pat dry with a soft towel. Ask your doctor to recommend a cleanser, and avoid alcoholic cleansers, tinctures, abrasives, astringents, and peeling agents, especially if you have rosacea.
2. Apply a thin layer of cream or gel to the affected skin. Gently and thoroughly massage it into the skin. Be careful not to get the medication in your eyes or mouth. If you do get azelaic acid in your eyes, wash with plenty of water and call your doctor if your eyes are irritated.
3. Do not cover the affected area with any bandages, dressings, or wrappings. You may apply non-irritating make up over the medication after it is dry.
4. Wash your hands with soap and water after you finish handling the medication.

Are there other uses for this medicine?

This medication may be prescribed for other uses; ask your doctor or pharmacist for more information.

What special precautions should I follow?

Before taking azelaic acid,

- tell your doctor and pharmacist if you are allergic to azelaic acid or any other medications.
- tell your doctor and pharmacist what prescription and nonprescription medications, vitamins, nutritional supplements, and herbal products you are taking.
- tell your doctor if you have or have ever had any medical condition.
- tell your doctor if you are pregnant, plan to become pregnant, or are breast-feeding. If you become pregnant while taking azelaic acid, call your doctor.
- you should know that azelaic acid may cause changes in your skin color, especially if you have a dark complexion. Tell your doctor if you notice any changes in your skin color.

What special dietary instructions should I follow?

If you have rosacea, you should avoid foods and drinks that cause you to flush or blush. These may include alcoholic drinks, spicy foods, and hot drinks such as coffee and tea.

If you have acne, continue your normal diet unless your doctor tells you otherwise.

What should I do if I forget to take a dose?

Take the missed dose as soon as you remember it. However, if it is almost time for the next dose, skip the missed dose and continue your regular dosing schedule. Do not take a double dose to make up for a missed one.

What side effects can this medicine cause?

Azelaic acid may cause side effects. The following symptoms are likely to affect the skin you are treating with azelaic acid cream or gel. Tell your doctor if any of these symptoms are severe or do not go away:

- itching
- burning
- stinging
- tingling

Some side effects can be serious. The following symptom is uncommon, but if you experience it, call your doctor immediately:

- rash

Azelaic acid may cause other side effects. Call your doctor if you have any unusual problems while taking this medication.

If you experience a serious side effect, you or your doctor may send a report to the Food and Drug Administration's (FDA) MedWatch Adverse Event Reporting program online [at http://www.fda.gov/MedWatch/index.html] or by phone [1-800-332-1088].

What storage conditions are needed for this medicine?

Keep this medication in the container it came in, tightly closed, and out of reach of children. Store it at room temperature and away from excess heat and moisture (not in the bathroom). Throw away any medication that is outdated or

no longer needed. Talk to your pharmacist about the proper disposal of your medication.

What other information should I know?

Keep all appointments with your doctor.

Do not let anyone else take your medication. Ask your pharmacist any questions you have about refilling your prescription.

Dosage Facts
For Informational Purposes

Caution: Do not change your dose, how often you take your medication, or the length of time you are to take it without first talking to your healthcare provider.

The following dosage information was written using medical language for doctors and other healthcare professionals and is provided here for you to check your dosage. The dosage of this drug may differ for different patients. Therefore, always follow your doctor's instructions or the directions on the label. Contact your healthcare provider or pharmacist if you have any questions about the specific dosage of your medication after reviewing this information.

Pediatric Patients

Acne

TOPICAL:
- Adolescents ≥12 years of age: Apply 20% cream in a thin film to affected areas twice daily (morning and evening).
- Improvement usually is detectable within 1–2 months of initiating therapy; however, maximum benefit generally requires more prolonged treatment.
- Usual duration of therapy is ≤6 months; however, therapy for ≥1 year has been required for control of individual lesions and repeat courses have been used for recurrences.

Adult Patients

Acne

TOPICAL:
- Apply 20% cream in a thin film to affected areas twice daily (morning and evening).
- Improvement usually is detectable within 1–2 months of initiating therapy; however, maximum benefit generally requires more prolonged treatment.
- Usual duration of therapy is ≤6 months; however, therapy for ≥1 year has been required for control of individual lesions and repeat courses have been used for recurrences.

Rosacea

TOPICAL:
- Apply 15% gel in a thin film to affected area twice daily (morning and evening).
- Safety and efficacy of therapy with gel for >12 weeks not established.

Prescribing Limits
Pediatric Patients

Acne

TOPICAL:
- Adolescents ≥12 years of age: Some clinicians suggest maximum 6 months of therapy; however, ≥1 year of therapy has been used in for control of individual lesions.

Adult Patients

Acne

TOPICAL:
- Some clinicians suggest maximum 6 months of therapy; however, ≥1 year of therapy has been used in for control of individual lesions.

Rosacea

TOPICAL:
- Safety and efficacy of therapy with gel for >12 weeks not established.

Special Populations

No special population dosage recommendations at this time.

Azelastine Nasal Spray

(a zel′ as teen)

Brand Name: Astelin® Nasal Spray

Why is this medicine prescribed?

Azelastine, an antihistamine, is used to treat hay fever and allergy symptoms including runny nose, sneezing, and itchy nose.

This medication is sometimes prescribed for other uses; ask your doctor or pharmacist for more information.

How should this medicine be used?

Azelastine comes as a nasal spray. Azelastine usually is sprayed in each nostril two times a day. Follow the directions on your prescription label carefully, and ask your doctor or pharmacist to explain any part you do not understand. Use azelastine exactly as directed. Do not use more or less of it or use it more often than prescribed by your doctor.

Before using azelastine for the first time, remove the child-resistant screw cap and replace with the pump unit. Prime the delivery system (pump unit) with four sprays or until a fine mist appears. If 3 days or more have elapsed since your last use of the nasal spray, reprime the pump with two sprays or until a fine mist appears.

What special precautions should I follow?

Before using azelastine,
- tell your doctor and pharmacist if you are allergic to azelastine or any other drugs.

- tell your doctor and pharmacist what prescription and nonprescription medications you are taking, especially other cold and allergy products, antihistamines, and vitamins.
- tell your doctor if you are pregnant, plan to become pregnant, or are breast-feeding. If you become pregnant while using azelastine, call your doctor.
- if you are having surgery, including dental surgery, tell the doctor or dentist that you are using azelastine.
- you should know that this drug may make you drowsy. Do not drive a car or operate machinery until you know how this drug affects you.
- remember that alcohol can add to the drowsiness caused by this drug.

What should I do if I forget to take a dose?

Use the missed dose as soon as you remember it. However, if it is almost time for the next dose, skip the missed dose and continue your regular dosing schedule. Do not use a double dose to make up for a missed one.

What side effects can this medicine cause?

Azelastine may cause side effects. Tell your doctor if any of these symptoms are severe or do not go away:

- bitter taste
- tiredness
- weight increase
- muscle pain
- nasal burning

What storage conditions are needed for this medicine?

Keep this medication in the container it came in, tightly closed, and out of reach of children. Store it at room temperature and away from excess heat and moisture (not in the bathroom). Throw away any medication that is outdated or no longer needed. Talk to your pharmacist about the proper disposal of your medication.

What other information should I know?

If a young child accidentally eats azelastine, call a doctor or a poison control center immediately.

Keep all appointments with your doctor.

Do not let anyone else use your medication. Ask your pharmacist any questions you have about refilling your prescription.

Dosage Facts
For Informational Purposes

Caution: Do not change your dose, how often you take your medication, or the length of time you are to take it without first talking to your health-care provider.

The following dosage information was written using medical language for doctors and other healthcare professionals and is provided here for you to check your dosage. The dosage of this drug may differ for different patients. Therefore, always follow your doctor's instructions or the directions on the label. Contact your healthcare provider or pharmacist if you have any questions about the specific dosage of your medication after reviewing this information.

General Dosage Information

Available as azelastine hydrochloride; dosage expressed in terms of the salt.

When properly primed, the nasal spray pump delivers approximately 100 metered doses per bottle.

Pediatric Patients

Seasonal Allergic Rhinitis

INTRANASAL:
- Children ≥12 years of age: 2 sprays (274 mcg) in each nostril twice daily.
- Children 5–11 years of age: 1 spray (137 mcg) in each nostril twice daily.

Nonallergic Rhinitis

INTRANASAL:
- Children ≥12 years of age: 2 sprays (274 mcg) in each nostril twice daily.

Allergic Conjunctivitis

OPHTHALMIC:
- Children ≥3 years of age: 1 drop of a 0.05% solution in the affected eye(s) twice daily.

Adult Patients

Seasonal Allergic Rhinitis

INTRANASAL:
- 2 sprays (274 mcg) in each nostril twice daily.

Nonallergic Rhinitis

INTRANASAL:
- 2 sprays (274 mcg) in each nostril twice daily.

Allergic Conjunctivitis

OPHTHALMIC:
- 1 drop of a 0.05% solution in the affected eye(s) twice daily.

Special Populations

Geriatric Patients
- Cautious dosing of nasal solution recommended.

Azelastine Ophthalmic

(a zel′ as teen)

Brand Name: Optivar®

Why is this medicine prescribed?

Azelastine is used to relieve the itching of allergic pink eye. Azelastine is in a class of medications called antihistamines. It works by blocking histamine, a substance in the body that causes allergic symptoms.

How should this medicine be used?

Azelastine comes as an eyedrop to apply to the eye. It is usually applied to the affected eye(s) twice a day. To help you remember to use azelastine, use it around the same time every day. Follow the directions on your prescription label carefully, and ask your doctor or pharmacist to explain any part you do not understand. Use azelastine exactly as directed. Do not use more or less of it or use it more often than prescribed by your doctor.

To apply the eyedrops, follow these steps:

1. Wash your hands thoroughly with soap and water.
2. Use a mirror or have someone else put the drops in your eye.
3. Remove the protective cap. Make sure the end of the dropper is not chipped or cracked.
4. Avoid touching the dropper against your eye or anything else.
5. Hold the dropper tip down at all times to prevent drops from flowing back into the bottle and contaminating the remaining contents.
6. Lie down or tilt your head back.
7. Holding the bottle between your thumb and index finger, place the dropper as near as possible to your eyelid without touching it.
8. Brace the remaining fingers of that hand against your cheek or nose.
9. With the index finger of your other hand, pull the lower lid of the eye down to form a pocket.
10. Drop the prescribed number of drops into the pocket made by the lower lid and the eye. Placing the drops on the surface of the eyeball can cause stinging.
11. Close your eye and press lightly against the lower lid with your finger for 2-3 minutes to keep the medication in the eye. Do not blink.
12. Replace and tighten the cap right away. Do not wipe or rinse it off.
13. Wipe off any excess liquid from your cheek with a clean tissue. Wash your hands again.

Are there other uses for this medicine?

This medication may be prescribed for other uses; ask your doctor or pharmacist for more information.

What special precautions should I follow?

Before using azelastine,

- tell your doctor and pharmacist if you are allergic to azelastine or any other medications.
- tell your doctor and pharmacist what prescription and nonprescription medications, vitamins, nutritional supplements, and herbal products you are taking.
- tell your doctor if you are pregnant, plan to become pregnant, or are breast-feeding. If you become pregnant while using azelastine, call your doctor.
- you should know that you should not wear contact lenses if your eye(s) is/are red. If your eye is not red and you wear contact lenses, you should know that azelastine solution contains benzalkonium chloride, which can be absorbed by soft contact lenses. Remove your contact lenses before applying azelastine and put them back in 10 minutes later.

What special dietary instructions should I follow?

Unless your doctor tells you otherwise, continue your normal diet.

What should I do if I forget to take a dose?

Apply the missed dose as soon as you remember it. However, if it is almost time for the next dose, skip the missed dose and continue your regular dosing schedule. Do not apply a double dose to make up for a missed one.

What side effects can this medicine cause?

Azelastine may cause side effects. Tell your doctor if any of these symptoms are severe or do not go away:

- eye burning or stinging
- headaches
- bitter taste
- eye pain
- blurred vision
- excessive tiredness
- sore throat

Some side effects can be serious. The following symptom is uncommon, but if you experience it, call your doctor immediately:

- difficulty breathing

Azelastine may cause other side effects. Call your doctor if you have any unusual problems while using this medication.

If you experience a serious side effect, you or your doctor may send a report to the Food and Drug Administration's (FDA) MedWatch Adverse Event Reporting program online [at http://www.fda.gov/MedWatch/index.html] or by phone [1-800-332-1088].

What storage conditions are needed for this medicine?

Keep this medication in the container it came in, tightly closed, and out of reach of children. Store it at room tem-

perature and away from excess heat and moisture (not in the bathroom). Throw away any medication that is outdated or no longer needed. Talk to your pharmacist about the proper disposal of your medication.

What other information should I know?

Keep all appointments with your doctor.

Do not let anyone else use your medication. Ask your pharmacist any questions you have about refilling your prescription.

Dosage Facts
For Informational Purposes

Caution: Do not change your dose, how often you take your medication, or the length of time you are to take it without first talking to your healthcare provider.

The following dosage information was written using medical language for doctors and other healthcare professionals and is provided here for you to check your dosage. The dosage of this drug may differ for different patients. Therefore, always follow your doctor's instructions or the directions on the label. Contact your healthcare provider or pharmacist if you have any questions about the specific dosage of your medication after reviewing this information.

General Dosage Information

Available as azelastine hydrochloride; dosage expressed in terms of the salt.

Pediatric Patients
Allergic Conjunctivitis

OPHTHALMIC:
- Children ≥3 years of age: 1 drop of a 0.05% solution in the affected eye(s) twice daily.

Adult Patients
Allergic Conjunctivitis

OPHTHALMIC:
- 1 drop of a 0.05% solution in the affected eye(s) twice daily.

Azithromycin

(az ith roe mye′ sin)

Brand Name: Zithromax®, Zithromax® Single Dose Packets, Zithromax® Tri-Paks®, Zithromax® Z-Pak®
Also available generically.

Why is this medicine prescribed?

Azithromycin is used to treat certain infections caused by bacteria, such as bronchitis; pneumonia; sexually transmitted diseases (STD); and infections of the ears, lungs, skin, and throat. Azithromycin is in a class of medications called macrolide antibiotics. It works by stopping the growth of bacteria. Antibiotics will not work for colds, flu, or other viral infections.

How should this medicine be used?

Azithromycin comes as a tablet and oral suspension (liquid) to take by mouth. It is usually taken with or without food once a day for 1-5 days. To help you remember to take azithromycin, take it around the same time every day. Follow the directions on your prescription label carefully, and ask your doctor or pharmacist to explain any part you do not understand. Take azithromycin exactly as directed. Do not take more or less of it or take it more often than prescribed by your doctor.

Shake the liquid well before each use to mix the medication evenly. Use only the syringe provided to measure the correct amount of medication. Rinse the syringe with water after taking the full dose of medication.

The tablets should be taken with a full glass of water.

Take azithromycin until you finish the prescription, even if you feel better. Stopping azithromycin too soon may cause bacteria to become resistant to antibiotics.

Are there other uses for this medicine?

Azithromycin is also used sometimes to treat *H. pylori* infection, early Lyme disease, and other infections. It is also used sometimes to prevent heart infection in patients having dental or other procedures and to prevent STD in victims of sexual assault. Talk to your doctor about the possible risks of using this medication for your condition.

This medication may be prescribed for other uses; ask your doctor or pharmacist for more information.

What special precautions should I follow?

Before taking azithromycin,
- tell your doctor and pharmacist if you are allergic to azithromycin, clarithromycin (Biaxin), dirithromycin (Dynabac), erythromycin (E.E.S., E-Mycin, Erythrocin), or any other medications.
- tell your doctor and pharmacist what prescription and nonprescription medications, vitamins, nutritional sup-

plements, and herbal products you are taking. Be sure to mention any of the following: anticoagulants ('blood thinners') such as warfarin (Coumadin); cyclosporine (Neoral, Sandimmune); digoxin (Lanoxin); dihydroergotamine (D.H.E. 45, Migranal); ergotamine (Ergomar); medications that suppress the immune system; nelfinavir (Viracept); phenytoin (Dilantin); and terfenadine (Seldane). Your doctor may need to change the doses of your medications or monitor you carefully for side effects.

- if you take antacids (Mylanta, Maalox), take them 2 hours before or 4 hours after azithromycin.
- tell your doctor if you have or have ever had cystic fibrosis, human immunodeficiency virus (HIV), irregular heartbeat, or kidney or liver disease.
- tell your doctor if you are pregnant, plan to become pregnant, or are breast-feeding. If you become pregnant while taking azithromycin, call your doctor.

What special dietary instructions should I follow?

Unless your doctor tells you otherwise, continue your normal diet.

What should I do if I forget to take a dose?

Take the missed dose as soon as you remember it. However, if it is almost time for the next dose, skip the missed dose and continue your regular dosing schedule. Do not take a double dose to make up for a missed one.

What side effects can this medicine cause?

Azithromycin may cause side effects. Tell your doctor if any of these symptoms are severe or do not go away:

- upset stomach
- diarrhea
- vomiting
- stomach pain
- mild skin rash

Some side effects can be serious. The following symptoms are uncommon, but if you experience any of them, call your doctor immediately:

- severe skin rash
- hives
- itching
- difficulty breathing or swallowing
- swelling of the face, throat, tongue, lips, eyes, hands, feet, ankles, or lower legs
- hoarseness
- yellowing of the skin or eyes
- rapid, pounding, or irregular heartbeat

Azithromycin may cause other side effects. Call your doctor if you have any unusual problems while taking this medication.

If you experience a serious side effect, you or your doctor may send a report to the Food and Drug Administration's (FDA) MedWatch Adverse Event Reporting program online [at http://www.fda.gov/MedWatch/index.html] or by phone [1-800-332-1088].

What storage conditions are needed for this medicine?

Keep this medication in the container it came in, tightly closed, and out of reach of children. Store the tablets at room temperature and away from excess heat and moisture (not in the bathroom). Throw away any medication that is outdated or no longer needed. Keep liquid medicine tightly closed at room temperature or in the refrigerator, and throw away any unused medication after 10 days. Do not freeze. Talk to your pharmacist about the proper disposal of your medication.

What should I do in case of overdose?

In case of overdose, call your local poison control center at 1-800-222-1222. If the victim has collapsed or is not breathing, call local emergency services at 911.

What other information should I know?

Keep all appointments with your doctor and the laboratory. Your doctor may order certain lab tests to check your body's response to azithromycin.

Do not let anyone else take your medication. Your prescription is probably not refillable. If you still have symptoms of infection after you finish the azithromycin, call your doctor.

Dosage Facts
For Informational Purposes

Caution: Do not change your dose, how often you take your medication, or the length of time you are to take it without first talking to your healthcare provider.

The following dosage information was written using medical language for doctors and other healthcare professionals and is provided here for you to check your dosage. The dosage of this drug may differ for different patients. Therefore, always follow your doctor's instructions or the directions on the label. Contact your healthcare provider or pharmacist if you have any questions about the specific dosage of your medication after reviewing this information.

General Dosage Information

Available as azithromycin dihydrate; dosage expressed in terms of anhydrous azithromycin.

Pediatric Patients

Acute Otitis Media (AOM)

ORAL:
- Children ≥6 months of age: 30 mg/kg as a single dose or 10 mg/kg once daily for 3 days. Alternatively, 10 mg/kg as a

single dose on day 1, followed by 5 mg/kg once daily on days 2–5.

Pharyngitis and Tonsillitis

ORAL:
- Children ≥2 years of age: 12 mg/kg once daily for 5 days.

GI Infections†
Mild to Moderate Campylobacter jejuni Infections†

ORAL:
- Adolescents: 500 mg once daily for 7 days recommended by CDC, NIH, and IDSA. If bacteremia is present, continue treatment for ≥2 weeks and consider use of a second anti-infective (e.g., an aminoglycoside).

Cryptosporidiosis†

ORAL:
- 10 mg/kg on day 1 followed by 5 mg/kg once daily (up to 600 mg daily) on days 2–10. Optimum duration of treatment unknown.

Shigella Infections†

ORAL:
- 12 mg/kg (up to 500 mg) on day 1 followed by 6 mg/kg orally once daily (up to 250 mg daily) on days 2–5. If bacteremia is present, continue for 14 days depending on the severity of infection.

Treatment of Travelers' Diarrhea†

ORAL:
- 10 mg/kg once daily for 3 days.

Respiratory Tract Infections
Acute Bacterial Sinusitis

ORAL:
- Children ≥6 months of age: 10 mg/kg once daily for 3 days.

Community-acquired Pneumonia

ORAL:
- Children ≥6 months of age: 10 mg/kg as a single dose on day 1, followed by 5 mg/kg once daily on days 2–5.

Pertussis†

ORAL:
- 10–12 mg/kg once daily (up to 600 mg daily) for 5 days. Alternatively, 10 mg/kg (up to 500 mg) on day 1 followed by 5 mg/kg (up to 250 mg) once daily on days 2–5 has been recommended for children 2 months to 16 years of age.

Babesiosis†

ORAL:
- 12 mg/kg once daily for 7–10 days; given in conjunction with atovaquone (20 mg/kg twice daily for 7–10 days).

Bartonella Infections†
Cat Scratch Disease Caused by Bartonella henselae†

ORAL:
- 10 mg/kg on day 1 followed by 5 mg/kg once daily on days 2–5.

Bartonella Infections in HIV-infected Individuals†

ORAL:
- Adolescents: 600 mg once daily for ≥3 months recommended by CDC, NIH, and IDSA. If relapse occurs, consider life-long secondary prophylaxis (chronic maintenance therapy) with erythromycin or doxycycline.

Chancroid†

ORAL:
- 12–15 mg/kg (maximum 1 g) as a single dose.

Chlamydial Infections
Uncomplicated Urethritis and Cervicitis†

ORAL:
- Children <8 years of age weighing ≥45 kg: 1 g as a single dose.
- Children ≥8 years of age: 1 g as a single dose.

Ocular Trachoma†

ORAL:
- 20 mg/kg as a single dose; 20 mg/kg once weekly for 3 weeks; or 20 mg/kg once every 4 weeks for a total of 6 doses.

Pneumonia in Infants or Conjunctivitis in Neonates†

ORAL:
- 20 mg/kg once daily for 3 days.

Lyme Disease†

ORAL:
- 10 mg/kg (maximum 500 mg) once daily for 7–10 days.

Mycobacterium avium Complex (MAC) Infections†
Primary Prevention of MAC in Children <13 Years of Age with Advanced HIV Infection

ORAL:
- 20 mg/kg (up to 1.2 g) once weekly or 5 mg/kg (maximum 250 mg) once daily.
- USPHS/IDSA recommends initiation of primary prophylaxis if CD4+ T-cell count is <750/mm³ in those <1 year, <500/mm³ in those 1–2 years, <75/mm³ in those 2–6 years, or <50/mm³ in those ≥6 years of age.

Primary Prevention of MAC in Adolescents with Advanced HIV Infection

ORAL:
- 1.2 g once weekly given alone.
- USPHS/IDSA recommends initiation of primary prophylaxis if CD4+ T-cell count is <50/mm³. May be discontinued if there is immune recovery in response to antiretroviral therapy with an increase in CD4+ T-cell count to >100/mm³ sustained for ≥3 months. Reinitiate prophylaxis if CD4+ T-cell count decreases to <50–100/mm³.

Treatment of Disseminated MAC in HIV-infected Infants and Children†

ORAL:
- 10–12 mg/kg once daily (up to 500 mg daily) in conjunction with ethambutol (15–25 mg/kg once daily [up to 1 g daily]) with or without rifabutin (10–20 mg/kg once daily [up to 300 mg daily]) recommended by CDC, NIH, and IDSA.

Treatment of Disseminated MAC in HIV-infected Adolescents†

ORAL:
- 500–600 mg once daily in conjunction with ethambutol (15 mg/kg once daily) with or without rifabutin (300 mg once daily) recommended by CDC, NIH, and IDSA.

Prevention of MAC Recurrence in HIV-infected Children <13 Years of Age†

ORAL:
- 10–12 mg/kg once daily (up to 500 mg daily) in conjunction with ethambutol (15–25 mg/kg once daily [up to 1 g daily])

with or without rifabutin (10–20 mg/kg once daily [up to 300 mg daily]) recommended by CDC, NIH, and IDSA.

- 5 mg/kg (maximum 250 mg) once daily, given in conjunction with ethambutol (with or without rifabutin) recommended by USPHS/IDSA.
- Secondary prophylaxis to prevent MAC recurrence in HIV-infected children usually continued for life. The safety of discontinuing secondary MAC prophylaxis in children whose CD4⁺ T-cell count increases in response to antiretroviral therapy has not been studied.

Prevention of MAC Recurrence in HIV-infected Adolescents†

ORAL:
- 500 mg once daily in conjunction with ethambutol (15 mg/kg once daily) with or without rifabutin (300 mg once daily) recommended by USPHS/IDSA, CDC, NIH, and IDSA.
- Secondary prophylaxis to prevent MAC recurrence usually continued for life in HIV-infected adolescents. USPHS/IDSA states that consideration can be given to discontinuing such prophylaxis after ≥12 months in those who remain asymptomatic with respect to MAC and have an increase in CD4⁺ T-cell count to >100/mm³ sustained for ≥6 months.

Toxoplasmosis†

ORAL:
- Adolescents: 900–1200 mg once daily in conjunction with pyrimethamine and leucovorin recommended by CDC, NIH, and IDSA.
- Continue acute treatment for ≥6 weeks; longer duration may be appropriate if disease is extensive or response incomplete at 6 weeks.

Typhoid Fever and Other Salmonella Infections†

ORAL:
- Children 3–17 years of age: 20 mg/kg once daily (up to 1 g daily) for 5–7 days.

Prevention of Bacterial Endocarditis†
Patients Undergoing Certain Dental, Oral, Respiratory Tract, or Esophageal Procedures

ORAL:
- 15 mg/kg as a single dose given 1 hour prior to the procedure.

Prophylaxis in Sexual Assault Victims†

ORAL:
- Adolescents: 1 g as a single dose in conjunction with IM ceftriaxone and oral metronidazole.

Adult Patients

Pharyngitis and Tonsillitis

ORAL:
- 500 mg as a single dose on day 1, followed by 250 mg once daily on days 2–5.

GI Infections†
Mild to Moderate Campylobacter jejuni Infections†

ORAL:
- 500 mg once daily for 7 days recommended by CDC, NIH, and IDSA. If bacteremia is present, continue treatment for ≥2 weeks and consider use of a second anti-infective (e.g., an aminoglycoside).

Cryptosporidiosis†

ORAL:
- HIV-infected adults: 600 mg once daily for 4 weeks; given in conjunction with paromomycin (1 g twice daily for 12 weeks).

Shigella Infections†

ORAL:
- 500 mg on day 1 followed by 250 mg once daily on days 2–5. If bacteremia is present, continue for 14 days depending on the severity of infection.

Treatment of Travelers' Diarrhea†

ORAL:
- 1 g as a single dose. Alternatively, 500 mg once daily for 3 days.

Respiratory Tract Infections
Acute Bacterial Sinusitis

ORAL:
- Conventional tablets or oral suspension: 500 mg once daily for 3 days.
- Extended-release oral suspension: 2 g given as a single dose.

Acute Bacterial Exacerbations of Chronic Obstructive Pulmonary Disease

ORAL:
- 500 mg once daily for 3 days or, alternatively, 500 mg as a single dose on day 1, followed by 250 mg once daily on days 2–5.

Mild to Moderate Community-acquired Pneumonia

ORAL:
- Conventional tablets or oral suspension: 500 mg as a single dose on day 1, followed by 250 mg once daily on days 2–5.
- Extended-release oral suspension: 2 g given as a single dose.

Moderate to Severe Community-acquired Pneumonia When IV therapy is Necessary

IV, THEN ORAL:
- Initiate treatment with an IV regimen of 500 mg once daily given for ≥2 days; then switch to an oral regimen of 500 mg once daily to complete 7–10 days of treatment.

Legionnaires' Disease†

ORAL:
- 500 mg once daily. Usual duration is 3–5 days for mild to moderate infections in immunocompetent patients; longer duration of treatment (at least 7–10 days or 3 weeks) may be necessary to prevent relapse in those with more severe infections or with underlying comorbidity or immunodeficiency.

IV:
- 500 mg once daily. Usual duration is 3–5 days for mild to moderate infections in immunocompetent patients; longer duration of treatment (at least 7–10 days or 3 weeks) may be necessary to prevent relapse in those with more severe infections or with underlying comorbidity or immunodeficiency.

Pertussis†

ORAL:
- 10 mg/kg on day 1 followed by 5 mg/kg once daily on days 2–5.

Skin and Skin Structure Infections

ORAL:
- 500 mg as a single dose on day 1, followed by 250 mg once daily on days 2–5.

Babesiosis†

ORAL:

- 600 mg daily for 7–10 days; given in conjunction with ato-vaquone (750 mg twice daily for 7–10 days).

Bartonella Infections†

Cat Scratch Disease Caused by Bartonella henselae†

ORAL:

- 500 mg on day 1 followed by 250 mg once daily on days 2–5.

Bartonella Infections in HIV-infected Patients

ORAL:

- 600 mg once daily for ≥3 months recommended by CDC, NIH, and IDSA. If relapse occurs, consider life-long secondary prophylaxis (chronic maintenance therapy) with erythromycin or doxycycline.

Chancroid

ORAL:

- 1 g as a single dose.

Chlamydial Infections

Uncomplicated Urethritis and Cervicitis

ORAL:

- 1 g as a single dose.

Ocular Trachoma†

ORAL:

- 20 mg/kg as a single dose or 1 g once weekly for 3 weeks.

Gonorrhea

ORAL:

- 2 g as a single dose.

Granuloma Inguinale (Donovanosis)†

ORAL:

- 1 g once weekly for at least 3 weeks or until all lesions have healed completely; consider adding IV aminoglycoside (e.g., gentamicin) if improvement is not evident within the first few days of treatment.

Mycobacterium avium Complex (MAC) Infections

Primary Prevention of MAC in Adults with Advanced HIV Infection

ORAL:

- 1.2 g once weekly given alone or with rifabutin.
- USPHS/IDSA recommends initiation of primary prophylaxis if CD4+ T-cell count is <50/mm³. May be discontinued if there is immune recovery in response to antiretroviral therapy with an increase in CD4+ T-cell count to >100/mm³ sustained for ≥3 months. Reinitiate prophylaxis if CD4+ T-cell count decreases to <50–100/mm³.

Treatment of Disseminated MAC in HIV-infected Adults

ORAL:

- Manufacturer recommends 600 mg once daily in conjunction with ethambutol (15 mg/kg daily), with or without an additional antimycobacterial.
- CDC, NIH, and IDSA recommend 500–600 mg once daily in conjunction with ethambutol (15 mg/kg once daily) with or without rifabutin (300 mg once daily).

Prevention of MAC Recurrence in HIV-infected Adults†

ORAL:

- 500 mg once daily in conjunction with ethambutol (15 mg/kg once daily) with or without rifabutin (300 mg once daily) recommended by USPHS/IDSA, CDC, NIH, and IDSA.
- Secondary prophylaxis to prevent MAC recurrence usually continued for life in HIV-infected adults. USPHS/IDSA states that consideration can be given to discontinuing such prophylaxis after ≥12 months in those who remain asymptomatic with respect to MAC and have an increase in CD4+ T-cell count to >100/mm³ sustained for ≥6 months.

Treatment of MAC Infections in HIV-negative Adults†

ORAL:

- ATS has recommended 250 mg once daily or 500 mg 3 times weekly in conjunction with ethambutol and rifabutin or rifampin.

Pelvic Inflammatory Disease

IV, THEN ORAL:

- 500 mg IV once daily for 1–2 days, followed by 250 mg orally once daily to complete 7 days of therapy. If anaerobic bacteria are suspected, an anti-infective active against anaerobes should also be used.

Syphilis†

Treatment of Primary or Secondary Syphilis in Penicillin-allergic Patients†

ORAL:

- 2 g as a single dose; close follow-up is essential since efficacy not well documented.

Toxoplasmosis†

ORAL:

- 900–1200 mg once daily in conjunction with pyrimethamine and leucovorin recommended by CDC, NIH, and IDSA.
- Continue acute treatment for ≥6 weeks; longer duration may be appropriate if disease is extensive or response incomplete at 6 weeks.

Typhoid Fever and Other Salmonella Infections†

ORAL:

- 1 g once daily for 5 days. Alternatively, 8–10 mg/kg daily for 7 days.

Prevention of Bacterial Endocarditis†

Patients Undergoing Certain Dental, Oral, Respiratory Tract, or Esophageal Procedures†

ORAL:

- 500 mg as a single dose given 1 hour prior to the procedure.

Prophylaxis in Sexual Assault Victims†

ORAL:

- 1 g as a single dose in conjunction with IM ceftriaxone and oral metronidazole.

Special Populations

Hepatic Impairment

- Manufacturer states dosage recommendations not available. Some clinicians state dosage adjustments not necessary in patients with class A or B liver cirrhosis.
- Use with caution; pharmacokinetics in hepatic impairment not completely established.

Renal Impairment
- No dosage adjustments recommended in renal impairment.
- Use with caution in severe renal impairment (GFR <10 mL/ minute).

Geriatric Patients
- Dosage adjustments not usually necessary in geriatric patients with normal renal and hepatic function receiving conventional or extended-release formulations.

† *Use is not currently included in the labeling approved by the US Food and Drug Administration.*

Aztreonam Injection

(az′ tree oh nam)

Brand Name: Azactam®, Azactam® in Iso-osmotic Dextrose Injection

About Your Treatment

Your doctor has ordered aztreonam, an antibiotic, to help treat your infection. The drug will be either injected into a large muscle (such as your buttock or hip) or added to an intravenous fluid that will drip through a needle or catheter placed in your vein for 30-60 minutes, two to four times a day.

Aztreonam eliminates bacteria that cause many kinds of infection, including pneumonia and gynecological, urinary tract, skin, bone, joint, stomach, and blood infections. This medication is sometimes prescribed for other uses; ask your doctor or pharmacist for more information.

Your health care provider (doctor, nurse, or pharmacist) may measure the effectiveness and side effects of your treatment using laboratory tests and physical examinations. It is important to keep all appointments with your doctor and the laboratory. The length of treatment depends on how your infection and symptoms respond to the medication.

Precautions

Before administering aztreonam,
- tell your doctor and pharmacist if you are allergic to aztreonam, penicillin, cephalosporins [e.g., cefaclor (Ceclor), cefadroxil (Duricef), or cephalexin (Keflex)], or any other drugs.
- tell your doctor and pharmacist what prescription and nonprescription medications you are taking, especially antibiotics and vitamins.
- tell your doctor if you have or have ever had kidney, heart, or gastrointestinal disease (especially colitis).
- tell your doctor if you are pregnant, plan to become pregnant, or are breast-feeding. If you become pregnant while taking aztreonam, call your doctor.
- if you have diabetes and regularly check your urine for sugar, use Clinistix or TesTape. Do not use Clinitest tablets because aztreonam may cause false positive results.

Administering Your Medication

Before you administer aztreonam, look at the solution closely. It should be clear and free of floating material. Gently squeeze the bag or observe the solution container to make sure there are no leaks. Do not use the solution if it is discolored, if it contains particles, or if the bag or container leaks. Use a new solution, but show the damaged one to your health care provider.

It is important that you use your medication exactly as directed. Do not stop your therapy on your own for any reason because your infection could worsen and result in hospitalization. Do not change your dosing schedule without talking to your health care provider. Your health care provider may tell you to stop your infusion if you have a mechanical problem (such as a blockage in the tubing, needle, or catheter); if you have to stop an infusion, call your health care provider immediately so your therapy can continue.

Side Effects

Aztreonam may cause side effects. Tell your health care provider if any of these symptoms are severe or do not go away:
- diarrhea
- upset stomach
- vomiting
- cramps
- bloating
- changes in taste sensation

If you experience any of the following symptoms, call your health care provider immediately:
- rash
- itching
- fever
- chills
- facial swelling
- sneezing
- wheezing
- difficulty breathing
- unusual bleeding or bruising
- unusual tiredness
- confusion
- seizures
- sore mouth or throat

If you experience a serious side effect, you or your doctor may send a report to the Food and Drug Administration's (FDA) MedWatch Adverse Event Reporting program online [at http://www.fda.gov/MedWatch/index.html] or by phone [1-800-332-1088].

Storage Conditions

- Your health care provider probably will give you a several-day supply of aztreonam at a time. If you are receiving aztreonam intravenously (in your vein), you probably will be told to store it in the refrigerator or freezer.

- Take your next dose from the refrigerator 1 hour before using it; place it in a clean, dry area to allow it to warm to room temperature.
- If you are told to store additional aztreonam in the freezer, always move a 24-hour supply to the refrigerator for the next day's use.
- Do not refreeze medications.

If you are receiving aztreonam intramuscularly (in your muscle), your health care provider will tell you how to store it properly.

Store your medication only as directed. Make sure you understand what you need to store your medication properly.

Keep your supplies in a clean, dry place when you are not using them, and keep all medications and supplies out of reach of children. Your health care provider will tell you how to throw away used needles, syringes, tubing, and containers to avoid accidental injury.

Overdose

In case of overdose, call your local poison control center at 1-800-222-1222. If the victim has collapsed or is not breathing, call local emergency services at 911.

Signs of Infection

If you are receiving aztreonam in your vein or under your skin, you need to know the symptoms of a catheter-related infection (an infection where the needle enters your vein or skin). If you experience any of these effects near your intravenous catheter, tell your health care provider as soon as possible:

- tenderness
- warmth
- irritation
- drainage
- redness
- swelling
- pain

Dosage Facts
For Informational Purposes

Caution: Do not change your dose, how often you take your medication, or the length of time you are to take it without first talking to your healthcare provider.

The following dosage information was written using medical language for doctors and other healthcare professionals and is provided here for you to check your dosage. The dosage of this drug may differ for different patients. Therefore, always follow your doctor's instructions or the directions on the label. Contact your healthcare provider or pharmacist if you have any questions about the specific dosage of your medication after reviewing this information.

General Dosage Information

Dosage and route of administration should be determined by the type and severity of infection, susceptibility of the causative organism, and condition of the patient. Dosages lower than those usually recommended should not be used.

Pediatric Patients

General Dosage for Neonates†

IV OR IM:

- Neonates <1 week of age†: AAP recommends 30 mg/kg every 12 hours in those weighing ≤2 kg or 30 mg/kg every 8 hours in those weighing >2 kg.
- Neonates 1–4 weeks of age†: AAP recommends 30 mg/kg every 12 hours in those weighing <1.2 kg, 30 mg/kg every 8 hours in those weighing 1.2–2 kg, or 30 mg/kg every 6 hours in those weighing >2 kg.

General Pediatric Dosage

IV:

- Children ≥9 months of age: Manufacturer recommends 30 mg/kg every 8 hours for treatment of mild to moderate infections or 30 mg/kg every 6 or 8 hours for treatment of moderate to severe infections.
- Children >1 month of age†: AAP recommends 90 mg/kg daily given in 3 divided doses for mild to moderate infections or 120 mg/kg daily given in 4 divided doses for severe infections.
- Children with cystic fibrosis: A dosage of 50 mg/kg every 6 or 8 hours (i.e., 150–200 mg/kg daily) has been suggested.

IM:

- Children >1 month of age†: AAP recommends 90 mg/kg daily given in 3 divided doses for mild to moderate infections or 120 mg/kg daily given in 4 divided doses for severe infections.

Adult Patients

General Adult Dosage
Moderately Severe Systemic Infections

IV:

- 1 or 2 g every 8 or 12 hours.

IM:

- 1 g every 8 or 12 hours.

Severe Systemic or Life-threatening Infections

IV:

- 2 g every 6 or 8 hours.

Urinary Tract Infections (UTIs)

IV OR IM:

- 500 mg or 1 g every 8 or 12 hours.
- Uncomplicated UTIs usually treated for 5–10 days; complicated UTIs usually treated for ≥10–18 days.

Prescribing Limits

Pediatric Patients

Treatment of Infections

IV:

- Maximum recommended in pediatric patients ≥9 months of age is 120 mg/kg daily, but higher dosage may be warranted in those with cystic fibrosis.

Adult Patients

Treatment of Infections

IV OR IM:
- Maximum 8 g daily.

Special Populations

Hepatic Impairment

Treatment of Infections

IV OR IM:
- Only limited experience with use of aztreonam in patients with impaired hepatic function.
- Some clinicians recommend that dosage be decreased by 20–25% in patients with alcoholic cirrhosis, especially if long-term therapy with the drug is required; others suggest that this decrease in dosage is unnecessary unless renal function also is impaired.
- Modification of usual dosage probably unnecessary in patients with stable primary biliary cirrhosis or other chronic hepatic disease unless renal function also is impaired.

Renal Impairment

Treatment of Infections

IV OR IM:
- Doses and/or frequency of administration in adults with Cl_{cr} ≤30 mL/minute should be modified in response to the degree of renal impairment.
- Serum creatinine concentrations alone may not be sufficiently accurate to assess the degree of renal impairment, especially in geriatric adults; dosage preferably should be based on the patient's measured or estimated Cl_{cr}.
- Adults with Cl_{cr} 10–30 mL/minute per 1.73 m^2: 1- or 2-g loading dose followed by maintenance doses equal to one-half the usual dose (i.e., 250 mg, 500 mg, or 1 g) given at the usual dosage intervals.
- Adults with Cl_{cr} <10 mL/minute per 1.73 m^2: A loading dose equal to the usual dose (i.e., 500 mg, 1 g, or 2 g) followed by maintenance doses equal to one-fourth the usual dose (i.e., 125 mg, 250 mg, or 500 mg) given at the usual dosage intervals.
- Adults undergoing hemodialysis: A loading dose equal to the usual dose (i.e., 500 mg, 1 g, or 2 g) followed by maintenance doses equal to one-fourth the usual dose (i.e., 125 mg, 250 mg, or 500 mg) given at the usual dosage intervals. Those with serious or life-threatening infections also should receive a supplemental dose equal to one-eighth the initial dose (i.e., 62.5 mg, 125 mg, or 250 mg) given immediately after each dialysis period.
- Adults undergoing CAPD: Some clinicians suggest that those with systemic infections should receive a loading dose equal to the usual dose (i.e., 500 mg, 1 g, or 2 g) followed by maintenance doses equal to one-fourth the usual dose (i.e., 125 mg, 250 mg, or 500 mg) given at the usual dosage intervals. Some clinicians suggest that adults undergoing CAPD who have peritonitis caused by susceptible organisms may receive a 1-g IV loading dose followed by maintenance doses of 500 mg given intraperitoneally† in 2 L of dialysate every 6 hours.
- Data insufficient to date to make dosage recommendations for pediatric patients with impaired renal function.

Geriatric Patients
- Select dosage based on renal function.
- Select dosage with caution because of age-related decreases in renal impairment.

† *Use is not currently included in the labeling approved by the US Food and Drug Administration.*

Baclofen Oral

(bak′ loe fen)

Brand Name: Lioresal®
Also available generically.

Why is this medicine prescribed?

Baclofen acts on the spinal cord nerves and decreases the number and severity of muscle spasms caused by multiple sclerosis or spinal cord diseases. It also relieves pain and improves muscle movement.

This medication is sometimes prescribed for other uses; ask your doctor or pharmacist for more information.

How should this medicine be used?

Baclofen comes as a tablet to take by mouth. It usually is taken three times a day at evenly spaced intervals. Follow the directions on your prescription label carefully, and ask your doctor or pharmacist to explain any part you do not understand. Take baclofen exactly as directed. Do not take more or less of it or take it more often than prescribed by your doctor. This drug must be taken regularly for a few weeks before its full effect is felt.

Continue to take baclofen even if you feel well. Do not stop taking baclofen without talking to your doctor, especially if you have taken large doses for a long time. Your doctor probably will want to decrease your dose gradually.

What special precautions should I follow?

Before taking baclofen,
- tell your doctor and pharmacist if you are allergic to baclofen or any other drugs.
- tell your doctor and pharmacist what prescription and nonprescription medications you are taking, especially muscle relaxants, sleeping pills, tranquilizers, and vitamins.
- tell your doctor if you have or have ever had kidney disease, epilepsy, ulcers, a stroke, a rheumatic disease, cerebral palsy, Parkinson's disease, or a psychiatric condition.
- tell your doctor if you are pregnant, plan to become pregnant, or are breast-feeding. If you become pregnant while taking baclofen, call your doctor immediately.

- you should know that this drug may make you drowsy. Do not drive a car or operate machinery until you know how baclofen affects you.
- remember that alcohol can add to the drowsiness caused by this drug.

What should I do if I forget to take a dose?

Take the missed dose as soon as you remember it. However, if it is almost time for the next dose, skip the missed dose and continue your regular dosing schedule. Do not take a double dose to make up for a missed one.

What side effects can this medicine cause?

Baclofen may cause side effects. Tell your doctor if any of these symptoms are severe or do not go away:

- drowsiness
- dizziness
- weakness
- confusion
- upset stomach

If you experience either of the following symptoms, call your doctor immediately:

- difficulty breathing
- seizures

If you experience a serious side effect, you or your doctor may send a report to the Food and Drug Administration's (FDA) MedWatch Adverse Event Reporting program online [at http://www.fda.gov/MedWatch/index.html] or by phone [1-800-332-1088].

What storage conditions are needed for this medicine?

Keep this medication in the container it came in, tightly closed, and out of reach of children. Store it at room temperature and away from excess heat and moisture (not in the bathroom). Throw away any medication that is outdated or no longer needed. Talk to your pharmacist about the proper disposal of your medication.

What should I do in case of overdose?

In case of overdose, call your local poison control center at 1-800-222-1222. If the victim has collapsed or is not breathing, call local emergency services at 911.

What other information should I know?

Keep all appointments with your doctor.

Do not let anyone else take your medication. Ask your pharmacist any questions you have about refilling your prescription.

Dosage Facts
For Informational Purposes

Caution: Do not change your dose, how often you take your medication, or the length of time you are to take it without first talking to your health-care provider.

The following dosage information was written using medical language for doctors and other healthcare professionals and is provided here for you to check your dosage. The dosage of this drug may differ for different patients. Therefore, always follow your doctor's instructions or the directions on the label. Contact your healthcare provider or pharmacist if you have any questions about the specific dosage of your medication after reviewing this information.

Pediatric Patients

Spasticity

ORAL:
- Children ≥12 Years of Age: Initially, 5 mg 3 times daily. Increase daily dosage by 15 mg (in 3 divided doses) at 3-day intervals (i.e., 5 mg 3 times daily for 3 days, then 10 mg 3 times daily for 3 days, then 15 mg 3 times daily for 3 days, then 20 mg 3 times daily for 3 days) until optimum effect is achieved.
- Usual dosage in children ≥12 years of age is 40–80 mg daily.

Adult Patients

Spasticity

ORAL:
- Initially, 5 mg 3 times daily. Increase daily dosage by 15 mg (in 3 divided doses) at 3-day intervals (i.e., 5 mg 3 times daily for 3 days, then 10 mg 3 times daily for 3 days, then 15 mg 3 times daily for 3 days, then 20 mg 3 times daily for 3 days) until optimum effect is achieved.
- Usual dosage is 40–80 mg daily.

Prescribing Limits
Pediatric Patients

Spasticity

ORAL:
- Some clinicians suggest that daily dosages up to 150 mg are well tolerated and provide additional therapeutic benefit in some patients; however, one manufacturer states that dosage should not exceed 80 mg daily (20 mg 4 times daily).

Adult Patients

Spasticity

ORAL:
- Some clinicians suggest that daily dosages up to 150 mg are well tolerated and provide additional therapeutic benefit in some patients; however, one manufacturer states that dosage should not exceed 80 mg daily (20 mg 4 times daily).

Special Populations

Renal Impairment
- Reduction of oral dosage may be necessary.

Geriatric Patients
- Increase oral dosage more gradually.

Patients with Psychiatric or Brain Disorders
- Increase oral dosage more gradually.

Balsalazide

(bal sal′ a zide)

Brand Name: Colazal®

Why is this medicine prescribed?

Balsalazide is used to treat ulcerative colitis, a condition in which the bowel is inflamed. Balsalazide is an anti-inflammatory drug. It is converted in the body to mesalamine and works by reducing bowel inflammation, diarrhea, rectal bleeding, and stomach pain.

This medication is sometimes prescribed for other uses; ask your doctor or pharmacist for more information.

How should this medicine be used?

Balsalazide comes as a capsule to take by mouth. It is usually taken three times a day. Follow the directions on your prescription label carefully, and ask your doctor or pharmacist to explain any part you do not understand. Take balsalazide exactly as directed. Do not take more or less of it or take it more often than prescribed by your doctor.

Balsalazide is usually taken for 8 weeks, but it may be taken for up to 12 weeks. Continue to take balsalazide even if you feel well. Do not stop taking balsalazide without talking to your doctor.

What special precautions should I follow?

Before taking balsalazide,

- tell your doctor and pharmacist if you are allergic to balsalazide, aspirin, choline magnesium trisalicylate (Tricosal, Trilisate), choline salicylate (Arthropan), diflunisal (Dolobid), magnesium salicylate (Nuprin Backache, Mobidin, Extra Strength Doan's, others), mesalamine (Asacol, Pentasa, Rowasa), salsalate (Argesic-AS, Disalcid, others), sodium salicylate, sodium thiosalicylate (Rexolate), sulfasalzine (Azulfidine), or any other drugs.
- tell your doctor and pharmacist what prescription and nonprescription medications you are taking, especially oral antibiotics and vitamins and herbal products.
- tell your doctor if you have or have ever had liver or kidney disease or pyloric stenosis (a condition in which the stomach empties slowly).
- tell your doctor if you are pregnant, plan to become pregnant, or are breast-feeding. If you become pregnant while taking balsalazide, call your doctor.

What should I do if I forget to take a dose?

Take the missed dose as soon as you remember it. However, if it is almost time for the next dose, skip the missed dose and continue your regular dosing schedule. Do not take a double dose to make up for a missed one.

What side effects can this medicine cause?

Side effects from balsalazide can occur. Tell your doctor if any of these symptoms are severe or do not go away:

- headache
- abdominal pain
- upset stomach
- diarrhea
- vomiting
- joint pain
- difficulty falling or staying asleep
- tiredness
- gas
- runny nose
- muscle or back pain
- coughing
- loss of appetite
- urinary tract infection
- constipation
- dry mouth

If you experience any of the following symptoms, call your doctor immediately:

- yellowing of the skin or eyes
- dark urine
- bloating or swelling of the stomach
- increased diarrhea
- rectal bleeding
- fever, sore throat, or flu-like symptoms

If you experience a serious side effect, you or your doctor may send a report to the Food and Drug Administration's (FDA) MedWatch Adverse Event Reporting program online [at http://www.fda.gov/MedWatch/index.html] or by phone [1-800-332-1088].

What storage conditions are needed for this medicine?

Keep this medication in the container it came in, tightly closed, and out of reach of children. Store it at room temperature and away from excess heat and moisture (not in the bathroom). Throw away any medication that is outdated or no longer needed. Talk to your pharmacist about the proper disposal of your medication.

What should I do in case of overdose?

In case of overdose, call your local poison control center at 1-800-222-1222. If the victim has collapsed or is not breathing, call local emergency services at 911.

What other information should I know?

Keep all appointments with your doctor and the laboratory.

Do not let anyone else take your medication. Ask your pharmacist any questions you have about refilling your prescription.

Dosage Facts
For Informational Purposes

Caution: Do not change your dose, how often you take your medication, or the length of time you are to take it without first talking to your healthcare provider.

The following dosage information was written using medical language for doctors and other healthcare professionals and is provided here for you to check your dosage. The dosage of this drug may differ for different patients. Therefore, always follow your doctor's instructions or the directions on the label. Contact your healthcare provider or pharmacist if you have any questions about the specific dosage of your medication after reviewing this information.

General Dosage Information

Available as balsalazide disodium; dosage expressed in terms of the salt.

Daily dosage of 6.75 g is equivalent to mesalamine 2.4 g.

Adult Patients
Ulcerative Colitis

ORAL:
- 2.25 g (three 750-mg capsules) 3 times daily for 8 weeks. Some patients may require up to 12 weeks of therapy.

Crohn's Disease

ORAL:
- 2–6 g daily may be used.

Prescribing Limits
Adult Patients

Safety and efficacy not established beyond 12 weeks.

Barium Sulfate

(ba′ ree um)

Brand Name: Baro-cat®, Baricon®, Barobag®, E-Z-Disk®, Intropaste®, Prepcat®, Readicat®, Tomocat®

Why is this medicine prescribed?

Barium sulfate is used to help doctors examine the esophagus (tube that connects the mouth and stomach), stomach, and intestine using x-rays or computed tomography (CAT scan, CT scan; a type of body scan that uses a computer to put together x-ray images to create cross-sectional or three dimensional pictures of the inside of the body). Barium sulfate is in a class of medications called radiopaque contrast media. It works by coating the esophagus, stomach, or intestine with a material that is not absorbed into the body so that diseased or damaged areas can be clearly seen by x-ray examination or CT scan.

How should this medicine be used?

Barium sulfate comes as a powder to be mixed with water, a suspension (liquid), a paste, and a tablet. The powder and water mixture and the suspension may be taken by mouth or may be given as an enema (liquid that is instilled into the rectum), and the paste and tablet are taken by mouth. Barium sulfate is usually taken one or more times before an x-ray examination or CT scan.

If you are using a barium sulfate enema, the enema will be administered by medical staff at the testing center. If you are taking barium sulfate by mouth, you may be given the medication after you arrive at the testing center or you may be given the medication to take at home at specific times the night before and/or the day of your test. If you are taking barium sulfate at home, take it exactly as directed. Do not take more or less of it or take it more often or at different times than directed.

Swallow the tablets whole; do not split, chew, or crush them.

Shake the liquid well before each use to mix the medication evenly. If you are given a powder to mix with water and take at home, be sure that you are also given directions for mixing and that you understand these directions. Ask your doctor or the staff at the testing center if you have any questions about mixing your medication.

You will be given specific directions to follow before and after your test. You may be told to drink only clear liquids after a certain time the day before your test, not to eat or drink after a specific time, and/or to use laxatives or enemas before your test. You may also be told to use laxatives to clear the barium sulfate from your body after your test. Be sure that you understand these directions and follow them carefully. Ask your doctor or the staff at the testing center if you are not given directions or if you have any questions about the directions you are given.

Are there other uses for this medicine?

This medication may be prescribed for other uses; ask your doctor or pharmacist for more information.

What special precautions should I follow?

Before taking or using barium sulfate,
- tell your doctor and the staff at the testing center if you are allergic to barium sulfate, other radiopaque contrast media, simethicone (Gas-X, Phazyme, others), any other medications, any foods, latex, or any of the ingredients in the type of barium sulfate that you will be taking or using. Ask the staff at the testing center for a list of the ingredients.
- tell your doctor and the staff at the testing center what prescription and nonprescription medications, vitamins, nutritional supplements, and herbal products you are

taking or plan to take. Your doctor will tell you whether you should take your medications on the day of your test and whether you should wait a certain amount of time between taking your regular medications and taking barium sulfate.

- tell your doctor if you have recently had a rectal biopsy (removal of a small amount of tissue from the rectum for laboratory examination) and if you have any blockage, sores, or holes in the esophagus, stomach, or intestine; or swelling or cancer of the rectum; Also tell your doctor if your infant or young child has any condition that affects his or her esophagus, stomach, or intestine, or has had surgery involving the intestines.Your doctor may tell you or your child not to take barium sulfate.

- tell your doctor if you have recently had any type of surgery especially surgery involving the colon (large intestine) or rectum if you have had a colostomy (surgery to create an opening for waste to leave the body through the abdomen), intracranial hypertension (pseudotumor cerebri; high pressure in the skull that may cause headaches, vision loss, and other symptoms), or if you have ever aspirated food (inhaled food into the lungs). Also tell your doctor if you or anyone in your family has or has ever had allergies and if you have or have ever had asthma; hay fever (allergy to pollen, dust, or other substances in the air); hives; eczema (red, itchy skin rash caused by allergy or sensitivity to substances in the environment); constipation; cystic fibrosis (inherited condition in which the body produces thick, sticky mucus that can interfere with breathing and digestion); Hirschsprung's disease (inherited condition in which the intestines do not work normally); high blood pressure; or heart disease.

- tell your doctor if you there is any chance that you are pregnant, if you plan to become pregnant, or if you are breast-feeding. The radiation used in x-rays and CT scans may harm the fetus.

What special dietary instructions should I follow?

Your doctor or the staff at the testing center will tell you what you may eat and drink the day before your test. Follow these directions carefully.

Drink plenty of fluids after your test is completed.

What should I do if I forget to take a dose?

If you were given barium sulfate to take at home and you forgot to take a dose, take the missed dose as soon as you remember it. Tell the staff at the testing center if you did not take the barium sulfate at the scheduled time.

What side effects can this medicine cause?

Barium sulfate may cause side effects. Tell your doctor if any of these symptoms are severe or do not go away:
- stomach cramps
- diarrhea

- nausea
- vomiting
- constipation
- weakness
- pale skin
- sweating
- ringing in the ears

Some side effects can be serious. If you experience any of these symptoms tell the staff at the testing center or call your doctor immediately:
- hives
- itching
- red skin
- swelling or tightening of the throat
- difficulty breathing or swallowing
- hoarseness
- agitation
- confusion
- fast heartbeat
- bluish skin color

Barium sulfate may cause other side effects. Call your doctor if you have any unusual problems while taking or after receiving this medication.

If you experience a serious side effect, you or your doctor may send a report to the Food and Drug Administration's (FDA) MedWatch Adverse Event Reporting program online [at http://www.fda.gov/MedWatch/index.html] or by phone [1-800-332-1088].

What storage conditions are needed for this medicine?

If you are given barium sulfate to take at home, keep the medication in the container it came in, tightly closed, and out of reach of children. Store it at room temperature and away from excess heat and moisture (not in the bathroom). You may be told to refrigerate the medication to chill it before you take it. Throw away any medication that is outdated or no longer needed. Talk to your pharmacist about the proper disposal of your medication.

What should I do in case of overdose?

In case of overdose, call your local poison control center at 1-800-222-1222. If the victim has collapsed or is not breathing, call local emergency services at 911.

Symptoms of overdose may include:
- stomach cramps
- diarrhea
- nausea
- vomiting
- constipation

What other information should I know?

Keep all appointments with your doctor and the testing center.

Do not let anyone else take your medication.

Talk to your doctor, pharmacist, or other healthcare professional if you have questions about dosing information for your medication.

Becaplermin

(be kap′ ler min)

Brand Name: Regranex®

Why is this medicine prescribed?

Becaplermin is used to treat ulcers of the foot, ankle, or leg in patients with diabetes. Becaplermin is a human-platelet-derived growth factor, a substance naturally produced by the body that helps in wound healing. It works, in combination with good ulcer care (cleaning, pressure relief, and infection control), by bringing the cells that the body uses to repair wounds to the site of the ulcer.

This medication is sometimes prescribed for other uses; ask your doctor or pharmacist for more information.

How should this medicine be used?

Becaplermin comes as a gel to apply to the skin. It is usually applied once daily to the ulcer. Your doctor or wound care-giver will tell you how much becaplermin gel to apply. The amount of gel to apply depends on the size of the ulcer. The amount you apply may be changed every 1 or 2 weeks as your ulcer heals. Follow the directions on your prescription label carefully, and ask your doctor or pharmacist to explain any part you do not understand. Use becaplermin exactly as directed. Do not use more or less of it or use it more often than prescribed by your doctor. Using more gel than your doctor prescribes will not make your ulcer heal faster.

To apply becaplermin gel, follow these steps:
1. Wash your hands thoroughly.
2. Squeeze the amount of gel your doctor has told you to use onto a clean, non-absorbent surface such as wax paper. The tip of the tube should not come in contact with the ulcer or any other surface. Recap the tube tightly after use.
3. With a clean cotton swab, tongue depressor, or other applicator, spread the gel over the ulcer surface in an even layer about 1/16th of an inch thick.
4. Moisten a piece of gauze dressing with saline (salt water) and cover the ulcer with the dressing.
5. After about 12 hours, remove the gauze dressing and rinse the ulcer gently with saline or water to remove whatever gel is left.
6. Cover the ulcer with a gauze dressing moistened with saline.

This drug must be used for a few weeks before your ulcer begins to heal. You may need to use becaplermin for up to 20 weeks. This drug must be used in combination with a good ulcer care program, including a strict non-weight-bearing program and good cleaning practices.

What special precautions should I follow?

Before using becaplermin,
- tell your doctor and pharmacist if you are allergic to becaplermin, parabens, or any other drugs.
- tell your doctor and pharmacist what prescription and nonprescription medications you are taking, especially other topical medications applied to the ulcer and vitamins and herbal products.
- tell your doctor if you have or have ever had a cancerous growth at the site of the ulcer.
- tell your doctor if you are pregnant, plan to become pregnant, or are breast-feeding. If you become pregnant while using becaplermin, call your doctor.

What should I do if I forget to take a dose?

Apply the missed dose as soon as you remember it. However, if it is almost time for the next application, skip the missed application and continue your regular application schedule. Do not apply a double amount of gel to make up for a missed application.

What side effects can this medicine cause?

Side effects from becaplermin can occur. Tell your doctor if this symptom is severe or does not go away:
- rash

What storage conditions are needed for this medicine?

Keep this medication in the refrigerator, tightly closed, and out of reach of children. Do not freeze it. Do not use the gel after the expiration date at the bottom of the tube. Throw away any medication that is outdated or no longer needed. Talk to your pharmacist about the proper disposal of your medication.

What other information should I know?

Keep all appointments with your doctor and the laboratory.

Do not use becaplermin gel for other wounds or ulcers unless your doctor tells you to.

Do not let anyone else take your medication. Ask your pharmacist any questions you have about refilling your prescription.

Talk to your doctor, pharmacist, or other healthcare professional if you have questions about dosing information for your medication.

Beclomethasone Nasal Inhalation

(be kloe meth' a sone)

Brand Name: Beconase AQ® Nasal Spray

Why is this medicine prescribed?

Beclomethasone, a corticosteroid, is used to prevent allergy symptoms including sneezing, itching, and runny or stuffed nose. It is also used to shrink nasal polyps (lumps) and prevent them from returning after surgical removal.

This medication is sometimes prescribed for other uses; ask your doctor or pharmacist for more information.

How should this medicine be used?

Beclomethasone comes as an aerosol and a solution to inhale through the nose. It usually is inhaled two to four times a day at evenly spaced intervals. Follow the directions on your prescription label carefully, and ask your doctor or pharmacist to explain any part you do not understand. Use beclomethasone exactly as directed. Do not use more or less of it or use it more often than prescribed by your doctor.

Beclomethasone controls symptoms of asthma and other lung diseases but does not cure them. Do not stop using beclomethasone without talking to your doctor.

Before you use beclomethasone the first time, read the written instructions that come with it. Ask your doctor, pharmacist, or respiratory therapist to demonstrate the proper technique. Practice using the inhaler while in his or her presence.

Before using beclomethasone, gently blow your nose to clear your nasal passages.

Avoid blowing your nose for 15 minutes after inhaling the prescribed dose.

What special precautions should I follow?

Before taking beclomethasone,

- tell your doctor and pharmacist if you are allergic to beclomethasone or any other drugs.
- tell your doctor and pharmacist what prescription and nonprescription medications you are taking, especially anticoagulants ('blood thinners') such as warfarin (Coumadin), arthritis medication, aspirin, cyclosporine (Neoral, Sandimmune), digoxin (Lanoxin), diuretics ('water pills'), estrogen (Premarin), ketoconazole (Nizoral), oral contraceptives, phenobarbital, phenytoin (Dilantin), rifampin (Rifadin), theophylline (Theo-Dur), and vitamins.
- if you have a nose infection or a fungal infection (other than on your skin), do not use beclomethasone without talking to your doctor.

- tell your doctor if you have or have ever had tuberculosis (TB); liver, kidney, intestinal, or heart disease; diabetes; an underactive thyroid gland; high blood pressure; mental illness; myasthenia gravis; osteoporosis; herpes eye infection; seizures; or ulcers.
- tell your doctor if you are pregnant, plan to become pregnant, or are breast-feeding. If you become pregnant while using beclomethasone, call your doctor.

What should I do if I forget to take a dose?

Use the missed dose as soon as you remember it. However, if it is almost time for the next dose, skip the missed dose and continue your regular dosing schedule. Do not use a double dose to make up for a missed one.

What side effects can this medicine cause?

Beclomethasone may cause side effects. Tell your doctor if any of these symptoms are severe or do not go away:

- headache
- nasal irritation or dryness
- sore throat
- sneezing
- nosebleed

If you experience any of the following symptoms, call your doctor immediately:

- increased difficulty breathing
- swollen face, lower legs, or ankles
- vision problems
- cold or infection that lasts a long time
- muscle weakness

If you experience a serious side effect, you or your doctor may send a report to the Food and Drug Administration's (FDA) MedWatch Adverse Event Reporting program online [at http://www.fda.gov/MedWatch/index.html] or by phone [1-800-332-1088].

What storage conditions are needed for this medicine?

Keep this medication in the container it came in, tightly closed, and out of reach of children. Store it at room temperature and away from excess heat and moisture (not in the bathroom). Throw away any medication that is outdated or no longer needed. Talk to your pharmacist about the proper disposal of your medication. Avoid puncturing the aerosol container, and do not discard it in an incinerator or fire.

What other information should I know?

Keep all appointments with your doctor.

Your symptoms may improve after just a few days. If they do not improve within 3 weeks, call your doctor.

Avoid exposure to chicken pox and measles. This drug makes you more susceptible to these illnesses. If you are exposed to them while using beclomethasone, call your doctor. Do not have a vaccination or other immunization unless your doctor tells you that you may.

Report any injuries or signs of infection (fever, sore throat, pain during urination, and muscle aches) that occur during treatment.

If your sputum (the matter you cough up during an asthma attack) thickens or changes color from clear white to yellow, green, or gray, call your doctor; these changes may be signs of an infection.

Inhalation devices require regular cleaning, and some require periodic replacement. Follow the directions that come with your inhaler.

When corticosteroids are used by children or teenagers for a long time, they may slow down growth. If you notice that your child who is taking beclomethasone seems to be growing slowly, talk to your child's doctor.

Do not let anyone else use your medication. Ask your pharmacist any questions you have about refilling your prescription.

Dosage Facts
For Informational Purposes

Caution: Do not change your dose, how often you take your medication, or the length of time you are to take it without first talking to your healthcare provider.

The following dosage information was written using medical language for doctors and other healthcare professionals and is provided here for you to check your dosage. The dosage of this drug may differ for different patients. Therefore, always follow your doctor's instructions or the directions on the label. Contact your healthcare provider or pharmacist if you have any questions about the specific dosage of your medication after reviewing this information.

General Dosage Information

After initial priming, each actuation of the nasal aqueous suspension spray pump delivers a dose of beclomethasone dipropionate monohydrate equivalent to 42 mcg of anhydrous beclomethasone dipropionate. Each spray bottle delivers 180 metered doses, after which the correct amount of drug in each spray cannot be assured.

Adjust dosage according to individual requirements and response.

Therapeutic effects of intranasal corticosteroids, unlike those of decongestants, are not immediate. This should be explained to the patient in advance to ensure compliance and continuation of the prescribed treatment regimen.

Use of topical nasal decongestants or oral antihistamines may be necessary until the effects of intranasal beclomethasone dipropionate are fully manifested. Use nasal vasoconstrictor for the first 2–3 days of therapy if excessive mucous secretion or nasal mucosal edema is present.

Symptomatic relief is usually evident within several days of continuous therapy; however, up to 2 weeks may be required for relief in some patients.

Do not continue therapy beyond 3 weeks in the absence of substantial symptomatic improvement.

Pediatric Patients

Seasonal Rhinitis

INTRANASAL INHALATION:
- Children 6–12 years of age: Initially, 1 spray (42 mcg) in each nostril twice daily (total dosage: 168 mcg/day).
- Increase dosage to 2 sprays (84 mcg) in each nostril twice daily (total dosage: 336 mcg/day) if response is inadequate or symptoms are severe.
- Reduce dosage to 1 spray in each nostril twice daily (total dosage: 168 mcg/day) once adequate symptom control is achieved.
- Adolescents ≥12 years of age: 1 or 2 sprays (42–84 mcg) in each nostril twice daily (total dosage: 168–336 mcg/day).

Perennial Rhinitis

INTRANASAL INHALATION:
- Children 6–12 years of age: Initially, 1 spray (42 mcg) in each nostril twice daily (total dosage: 168 mcg/day).
- Increase dosage to 2 sprays (84 mcg) in each nostril twice daily (total dosage: 336 mcg/day) if response is inadequate or symptoms are severe.
- Reduce dosage to 1 spray in each nostril twice daily (total dosage: 168 mcg/day) once adequate symptom control is achieved.
- Adolescents ≥12 years of age: 1 or 2 sprays (42–84 mcg) in each nostril twice daily (total dosage: 168–336 mcg/day).

Nasal Polyposis

INTRANASAL INHALATION:
- Children 6–12 years of age: Initially, 1 spray (42 mcg) in each nostril twice daily (total dosage: 168 mcg/day).
- Increase dosage to 2 sprays (84 mcg) in each nostril twice daily (total dosage: 336 mcg/day) if response is inadequate or symptoms are severe.
- Reduce dosage to 1 spray in each nostril twice daily (total dosage: 168 mcg/day) once adequate symptom control is achieved.
- Adolescents ≥12 years of age: 1 or 2 sprays (42–84 mcg) in each nostril twice daily (total dosage: 168–336 mcg/day).

Adult Patients

Seasonal Rhinitis

INTRANASAL INHALATION:
- 1 or 2 sprays (42–84 mcg) in each nostril twice daily (total dosage: 168–336 mcg/day).

Perennial Rhinitis

INTRANASAL INHALATION:
- 1 or 2 sprays (42–84 mcg) in each nostril twice daily (total dosage: 168–336 mcg/day).

Nasal Polyposis

INTRANASAL INHALATION:
- 1 or 2 sprays (42–84 mcg) in each nostril twice daily (total dose: 168–336 mcg/day).

Prescribing Limits

No evidence that higher than recommended dosages or increased frequency of administration is beneficial.

Exceeding the maximum recommended daily dosage may only increase the risk of adverse systemic effects (e.g., HPA-axis suppression, Cushing's syndrome).

Pediatric Patients

Seasonal Rhinitis

INTRANASAL INHALATION:
- Children 6–12 years of age: Maximum 84 mcg (2 sprays) in each nostril twice daily (total dosage: 336 mcg/day).
- Adolescents ≥12 years of age: Maximum 84 mcg (2 sprays) in each nostril twice daily (total dosage: 336 mcg/day).

Perennial Rhinitis

INTRANASAL INHALATION:
- Children 6–12 years of age: Maximum 84 mcg (2 sprays) in each nostril twice daily (total dosage: 336 mcg/day).
- Adolescents ≥12 years of age: Maximum 84 mcg (2 sprays) in each nostril twice daily (total dosage: 336 mcg/day).

Nasal Polyposis

INTRANASAL INHALATION:
- Children 6–12 years of age: Maximum 84 mcg (2 sprays) in each nostril twice daily (total dosage: 336 mcg/day).
- Adolescents ≥12 years of age: Maximum 84 mcg (2 sprays) in each nostril twice daily (total dosage: 336 mcg/day).

Adult Patients

Seasonal Rhinitis

INTRANASAL INHALATION:
- Maximum 84 mcg (2 sprays) in each nostril twice daily (total dosage: 336 mcg/day).

Perennial Rhinitis

INTRANASAL INHALATION:
- Maximum 84 mcg (2 sprays) in each nostril twice daily (total dosage: 336 mcg/day).

Nasal Polyposis

INTRANASAL INHALATION:
- Maximum 84 mcg (2 sprays) in each nostril twice daily (total dosage: 336 mcg/day).

Beclomethasone Oral Inhalation

(be kloe meth′ a sone)

Brand Name: QVAR® Oral Inhaler

Important Warning

If you are switching (or have recently switched) to beclomethasone inhalation from an oral corticosteroid such as dexamethasone (Decadron, Dexone), methylprednisolone (Medrol), or prednisone (Deltasone) and have an injury, infection, severe asthma attack, or surgery, use a full dose of oral corticosteroid (even if you have been gradually decreasing your dose) and call your doctor for additional instructions.

Carry an identification card saying that you may need to use extra doses of the corticosteroid during times of stress (injuries, infections, and severe asthma attacks). Write down the name of the medication and the full dose you took before decreasing it. Ask your pharmacist or doctor how to get this card. List your name, medical problems, medications and dosages, and doctor's name and telephone number on the card.

Why is this medicine prescribed?

Beclomethasone is used to prevent wheezing, shortness of breath, and breathing difficulties caused by severe asthma and other lung diseases. Beclomethasone is in a class of medications called corticosteroids. It works by reducing swelling in the airways.

How should this medicine be used?

Beclomethasone comes as an aerosol to inhale by mouth. It usually is inhaled three or four times a day at evenly spaced intervals. Follow the directions on your prescription label carefully, and ask your doctor or pharmacist to explain any part you do not understand. Use beclomethasone exactly as directed. Do not use more or less of it or use it more often than prescribed by your doctor.

If your doctor has prescribed a bronchodilator (a drug to be inhaled for rapid relief of difficult breathing), use it several minutes before your beclomethasone inhaler so that beclomethasone reaches deep into your lungs.

Beclomethasone controls symptoms of asthma and other lung diseases but does not cure them. Continue to use beclomethasone even if you feel well. Do not stop using beclomethasone without talking to your doctor.

Before you use beclomethasone the first time, read the written instructions that come with it. Ask your doctor, pharmacist, or respiratory therapist to show you how to use it. Practice using the inhaler while he or she watches.

To use the inhaler, follow these steps:
1. Shake the inhaler well. (Note: If you are using QVAR, you do not need to shake the inhaler.)
2. Remove the protective cap.
3. Exhale (breathe out) as completely as possible through your nose while keeping your mouth shut.
4. *Open Mouth Technique:* Open your mouth wide, and place the open end of the mouthpiece about 1-2 inches from your mouth.
   Closed Mouth Technique: Place the open end of the mouthpiece well into your mouth, past your front teeth. Close your lips tightly around the mouthpiece.
5. Take a slow, deep breath through the mouthpiece and, at the same time, press down on the container to spray the medication into your mouth. Be sure that the mist goes into your throat and is not blocked by your teeth or tongue. Adults giving the treatment to young children may hold the child's nose closed to be sure that the medication goes into the child's throat.

6. Hold your breath for 5-10 seconds, remove the inhaler, and exhale slowly through your nose or mouth. If you take two puffs, wait 2 minutes and shake the inhaler well before taking the second puff.
7. Replace the protective cap on the inhaler.
8. After each treatment, rinse your mouth with water or mouthwash.

If you have difficulty getting the medication into your lungs, a spacer (a special device that attaches to the inhaler) may help; ask your doctor, pharmacist, or respiratory therapist.

Are there other uses for this medicine?

This medication is sometimes prescribed for other uses; ask your doctor or pharmacist for more information.

What special precautions should I follow?

Before using beclomethasone,
- tell your doctor and pharmacist if you are allergic to beclomethasone or any other drugs.
- tell your doctor and pharmacist what prescription and nonprescription medications you are taking, especially arthritis medications, aspirin, digoxin (Lanoxin), diuretics (water pills), estrogen (Premarin), ketoconazole (Nizoral), oral contraceptives, phenobarbital, phenytoin (Dilantin), rifampin (Rifadin), theophylline (Theo-Dur), and vitamins.
- if you have a fungal infection (other than on your skin), do not use beclomethasone without talking to your doctor.
- tell your doctor if you have or have ever had liver, kidney, intestinal, or heart disease; diabetes; an underactive thyroid gland; high blood pressure; mental illness; myasthenia gravis; osteoporosis; herpes eye infection; seizures; or ulcers.
- tell your doctor if you are pregnant, plan to become pregnant, or are breast-feeding. If you become pregnant while using beclomethasone, call your doctor.
- if you have a history of ulcers or use large doses of aspirin or other arthritis medication, limit your consumption of alcoholic beverages while using this drug. Beclomethasone makes your stomach and intestines more susceptible to the irritating effects of alcohol, aspirin, and certain arthritis medications; this effect increases your risk of getting ulcers.
- do not use beclomethasone during a sudden asthma attack. You should have a fast-acting inhaler such as albuterol (Proventil, Ventolin) to use during asthma attacks.
- avoid exposure to chicken pox and measles. This drug makes you more likely to catch these illnesses. If you are exposed to them while using beclomethasone, call your doctor. Do not have a vaccination or other immunization without your doctor's approval.

What special dietary instructions should I follow?

Your doctor may tell you to follow a low-sodium, low-salt, potassium-rich, or high-protein diet. Follow these directions.

What should I do if I forget to take a dose?

Take the missed dose as soon as you remember it. However, if it is almost time for the next dose, skip the missed dose and continue your regular dosing schedule. Do not use a double dose to make up for a missed one.

What side effects can this medicine cause?

Beclomethasone may cause side effects. Tell your doctor if any of these symptoms are severe or do not go away:
- dry or irritated throat and mouth
- cough
- difficult or painful speech

If you experience any of the following symptoms, call your doctor immediately:
- skin rash
- increased difficulty breathing
- white spots or sores in your mouth
- swollen face, lower legs, or ankles
- vision problems
- cold or infection that lasts a long time
- muscle weakness

If you experience a serious side effect, you or your doctor may send a report to the Food and Drug Administration's (FDA) MedWatch Adverse Event Reporting program online [at http://www.fda.gov/MedWatch/index.html] or by phone [1-800-332-1088].

What storage conditions are needed for this medicine?

Keep this medication in the container it came in, tightly closed, and out of reach of children. Store it at room temperature and away from excess heat and moisture (not in the bathroom). Throw away any medication that is outdated or no longer needed. Talk to your pharmacist about the proper disposal of your medication. Avoid puncturing the aerosol container, and do not discard it in an incinerator or fire.

What other information should I know?

Keep all appointments with your doctor and the laboratory.

Report any injuries or signs of infection (fever, sore throat, pain during urination, and muscle aches) that occur during treatment.

If the sputum (spit) you cough up during an asthma attack thickens or changes color from clear white to yellow, green, or gray, call your doctor; these changes may be signs of an infection.

Inhalation devices require regular cleaning. Once a week, remove the drug container from the plastic mouthpiece, wash the mouthpiece with warm tap water, and dry it thoroughly.

Do not let anyone else use your medication. Ask your pharmacist any questions you have about refilling your prescription.

Dosage Facts

For Informational Purposes

Caution: Do not change your dose, how often you take your medication, or the length of time you are to take it without first talking to your healthcare provider.

The following dosage information was written using medical language for doctors and other healthcare professionals and is provided here for you to check your dosage. The dosage of this drug may differ for different patients. Therefore, always follow your doctor's instructions or the directions on the label. Contact your healthcare provider or pharmacist if you have any questions about the specific dosage of your medication after reviewing this information.

General Dosage Information

Available as beclomethasone dipropionate; dosage expressed in terms of the salt.

Oral inhalation aerosol releases 50 or 100 mcg of beclomethasone dipropionate, and delivers 40 or 80 mcg, respectively, from the actuator (mouthpiece) per metered spray.

Pediatric Patients

Asthma

ORAL INHALATION:
- Children 5–11 years of age receiving bronchodilators alone or inhaled corticosteroids previously: Initially, 40 mcg twice daily. If required, dosage may be increased to a maximum 80 mcg twice daily.
- Children ≥12 years of age receiving bronchodilators alone previously: Initially, 40–80 mcg twice daily. If required, dosage may be increased to a maximum 320 mcg twice daily.
- Children ≥12 years of age receiving inhaled corticosteroids previously: Initially, 40–160 mcg twice daily. If required, dosage may be increased to a maximum 320 mcg twice daily.

Adult Patients

Asthma

ORAL INHALATION:
- In adults receiving bronchodilators alone previously: Initially, 40–80 mcg twice daily. If required, dosage may be increased to a maximum 320 mcg twice daily.
- Adults receiving inhaled corticosteroids: Initially, 40–160 mcg twice daily. If required, dosage may be increased to a maximum of 320 mcg twice daily.

Prescribing Limits

Pediatric Patients

Asthma

ORAL INHALATION:
- Children 5–11 years of age: Maximum 80 mcg twice daily.
- Children ≥12 years of age: Maximum 320 mcg twice daily.

Adult Patients

Asthma

ORAL INHALATION:
- Maximum 320 mcg twice daily.

Special Populations

Geriatric Patients
- Consider initial dosages at the lower end of the usual range due to possible age-related decrease in hepatic, renal, and/or cardiac function and concomitant disease and drug therapy.

Benazepril

(ben ay' ze pril)

Brand Name: Lotensin®, Lotrel® as a combination product containing Benazepril Hydrochloride and Amlodipine Besylate
Also available generically.

Important Warning

Do not take benazepril if you are pregnant. If you become pregnant while taking benazepril, call your doctor immediately. Benazepril may harm the fetus.

Why is this medicine prescribed?

Benazepril is used alone or in combination with other medications to treat high blood pressure. Benazepril is in a class of medications called angiotensin-converting enzyme (ACE) inhibitors. It works by decreasing certain chemicals that tighten the blood vessels, so blood flows more smoothly.

How should this medicine be used?

Benazepril comes as a tablet to take by mouth. It is usually taken once or twice a day with or without food. To help you remember to take benazepril, take it around the same time every day. Follow the directions on your prescription label carefully, and ask your doctor or pharmacist to explain any part you do not understand. Take benazepril exactly as directed. Do not take more or less of it or take it more often than prescribed by your doctor.

Your doctor will probably start you on a low dose of benazepril and gradually increase your dose.

Benazepril controls high blood pressure but does not cure it. Continue to take benazepril even if you feel well. Do not stop taking benazepril without talking to your doctor.

Are there other uses for this medicine?

This medication may be prescribed for other uses; ask your doctor or pharmacist for more information.

What special precautions should I follow?

Before taking benazepril,

- tell your doctor and pharmacist if you are allergic to benazepril, captopril (Capoten), enalapril (Vasotec), fosinopril (Monopril), lisinopril (Prinivil, Zestril), moexipril (Univasc), perindopril (Aceon), quinapril (Accupril), ramipril (Altace), trandolapril (Mavik), or any other medications.
- tell your doctor and pharmacist what prescription and nonprescription medications, vitamins, nutritional supplements, and herbal products you are taking. Be sure to mention any of the following: diuretics ('water pills'), lithium (Eskalith, Lithobid), and potassium supplements. Your doctor may need to change the doses of your medications or monitor you carefully for side effects.
- tell your doctor if you have recently had severe diarrhea or vomiting and if you have or have ever had heart failure, kidney disease, lupus, scleroderma, or diabetes.
- tell your doctor if you plan to become pregnant or are breast-feeding.
- if you are having surgery, including dental surgery, tell the doctor or dentist that you are taking benazepril.
- you should know that diarrhea, vomiting, not drinking enough fluids, and sweating a lot can cause a drop in blood pressure, which may cause lightheadedness and fainting.

What special dietary instructions should I follow?

Talk to your doctor before using salt substitutes containing potassium. If your doctor prescribes a low-salt or low-sodium diet, follow these directions carefully.

What should I do if I forget to take a dose?

Take the missed dose as soon as you remember it. However, if it is almost time for the next dose, skip the missed dose and continue your regular dosing schedule. Do not take a double dose to make up for a missed one.

What side effects can this medicine cause?

Benazepril may cause side effects. Tell your doctor if any of these symptoms are severe or do not go away:

- cough
- headache
- dizziness
- drowsiness

Some side effects can be serious. The following symptoms are uncommon, but if you experience any of them, call your doctor immediately:

- swelling of the face, throat, tongue, lips, eyes, hands, feet, ankles, or lower legs
- hoarseness
- difficulty breathing or swallowing
- lightheadedness
- fainting
- rash
- yellowing of the skin or eyes
- fever, sore throat, chills, and other signs of infection

Benazepril may cause other side effects. Call your doctor if you have any unusual problems while taking this medication.

If you experience a serious side effect, you or your doctor may send a report to the Food and Drug Administration's (FDA) MedWatch Adverse Event Reporting program online [at http://www.fda.gov/MedWatch/index.html] or by phone [1-800-332-1088].

What storage conditions are needed for this medicine?

Keep this medication in the container it came in, tightly closed, and out of reach of children. Store it at room temperature and away from excess heat and moisture (not in the bathroom). Throw away any medication that is outdated or no longer needed. Talk to your pharmacist about the proper disposal of your medication.

What should I do in case of overdose?

In case of overdose, call your local poison control center at 1-800-222-1222. If the victim has collapsed or is not breathing, call local emergency services at 911.

Symptoms of overdose may include:

- dizziness
- fainting

What other information should I know?

Keep all appointments with your doctor and the laboratory. Your blood pressure should be checked regularly to determine your response to benazepril. Your doctor may order certain lab tests to check your body's response to benazepril.

Do not let anyone else take your medication. Ask your pharmacist any questions you have about refilling your prescription.

Dosage Facts
For Informational Purposes

Caution: Do not change your dose, how often you take your medication, or the length of time you are to take it without first talking to your healthcare provider.

The following dosage information was written using medical language for doctors and other healthcare professionals and is provided here for you to check your dosage. The dosage of this drug may differ for different patients. Therefore, always follow your doctor's instructions or the directions on the label. Contact your health-

care provider or pharmacist if you have any questions about the specific dosage of your medication after reviewing this information.

General Dosage Information

Available as benazepril hydrochloride; dosage expressed in terms of benazepril.

Pediatric Patients

Hypertension

ORAL:
- Children ≥6 years of age: Initially, 0.2 mg/kg (up to 10 mg) once daily. Adjust dosage until the desired BP goal is achieved (up to maximum dosage of 0.6 mg/kg or 40 mg daily).

Adult Patients

Hypertension

ORAL:
- Initially, 10 mg once daily as monotherapy. Adjust dosage at approximately monthly intervals (more aggressively in high-risk patients) to achieve BP control.
- In patients currently receiving diuretic therapy, discontinue diuretic, if possible, 2–3 days before initiating benazepril. May cautiously resume diuretic therapy if BP not controlled adequately with benazepril alone. If diuretic cannot be discontinued, increase sodium intake and give lower initial benazepril dose (5 mg) under close medical supervision.
- Usual dosage: 20–40 mg daily, given in 1 dose or 2 divided doses.
- If effectiveness diminishes toward end of dosing interval in patients treated once daily, consider increasing dosage or administering drug in 2 divided doses.

Benazepril/Hydrochlorothiazide Combination Therapy

ORAL:
- If BP is not adequately controlled by monotherapy with benazepril, can switch to the fixed-combination preparation containing benazepril 10 mg and hydrochlorothiazide 12.5 mg or, alternatively, benazepril 20 mg and hydrochlorothiazide 12.5 mg. Adjust dosage of either or both drugs according to patient's response.
- If BP is controlled by monotherapy with hydrochlorothiazide 25 mg daily but potassium loss is problematic, can switch to fixed-combination preparation containing benazepril 5 mg and hydrochlorothiazide 6.25 mg.

Benazepril/Amlodipine Combination Therapy

ORAL:
- Reduce amlodipine dosage in nonblack patients when benazepril is initiated.
- Adjust dosage of benazepril/amlodipine fixed combination according to patient's response; consider that steady-state plasma concentrations of benazepril and amlodipine are reached after 2 and 7 days, respectively.

Prescribing Limits

Pediatric Patients

Hypertension

ORAL:
- Maximum 0.6 mg/kg or 40 mg daily.

Adult Patients

Hypertension

ORAL:
- Maximum 80 mg daily.

Special Populations

Renal Impairment
- Initially, 5 mg once daily in adults with severe renal impairment (Cl_{cr} <30 mL/minute or S_{cr} >3 mg/dL); titrate until BP is controlled or to maximum of 40 mg daily. Use not recommended in pediatric patients with Cl_{cr} <30 mL/minute per 1.73 m².
- Benazepril/hydrochlorothiazide and benazepril/amlodipine fixed combinations are not recommended in patients with severe renal impairment.

Volume- and/or Salt-depleted Patients
- Correct volume and/or salt depletion prior to initiation of therapy or initiate therapy under close medical supervision using lower initial dosage.

Benazepril and Hydrochlorothiazide

(ben ay′ ze pril) (hye droe klor oh thye′ a zide)

Brand Name: Lotensin HCT®

Important Warning

Do not take benazepril and hydrochlorothiazide if you are pregnant. If you become pregnant while taking benazepril and hydrochlorothiazide, call your doctor immediately. Benazepril and hydrochlorothiazide may harm the fetus.

Why is this medicine prescribed?

The combination of benazepril and hydrochlorothiazide is used to treat high blood pressure. Benazepril is in a class of medications called angiotensin-converting enzyme (ACE) inhibitors. It works by decreasing certain chemicals that tighten the blood vessels, so blood flows more smoothly. Hydrochlorothiazide is in a class of medications called diuretics ('water pills'). It works by causing the kidneys to get rid of unneeded water and salt from the body into the urine.

How should this medicine be used?

The combination of benazepril and hydrochlorothiazide comes as a tablet to take by mouth. It is usually taken once a day. To help you remember to take benazepril and hydrochlorothiazide, take it around the same time every day. Follow the directions on your prescription label carefully, and ask your doctor or pharmacist to explain any part you do not understand. Take benazepril and hydrochlorothiazide exactly as directed. Do not take more or less of it or take it more often than prescribed by your doctor.

Benazepril and hydrochlorothiazide controls high blood pressure but does not cure it. Continue to take benazepril and hydrochlorothiazide even if you feel well. Do not stop taking benazepril and hydrochlorothiazide without talking to your doctor.

Are there other uses for this medicine?

This medication may be prescribed for other uses; ask your doctor or pharmacist for more information.

What special precautions should I follow?

Before taking benazepril and hydrochlorothiazide,

- tell your doctor and pharmacist if you are allergic to benazepril (Lotensin), hydrochlorothiazide (HCTZ, Hydrodiuril, Microzide), captopril (Capoten), enalapril (Vasotec), fosinopril (Monopril), lisinopril (Prinivil, Zestril), moexipril (Univasc), perindopril (Aceon), quinapril (Accupril), ramipril (Altace), trandolapril (Mavik), sulfa drugs, or any other medications.
- tell your doctor and pharmacist what prescription and nonprescription medications, vitamins, nutritional supplements, and herbal products you are taking. Be sure to mention any of the following: aspirin and other nonsteroidal anti-inflammatory medications (NSAIDs) such as ibuprofen (Advil, Motrin) and naproxen (Aleve, Naprosyn); cholestyramine (Questran); colestipol (Colestid); insulin; lithium (Eskalith, Lithobid); oral steroids such as dexamethasone (Decadron, Dexone), methylprednisolone (Medrol), and prednisone (Deltasone); other diuretics ('water pills'); other medications for high blood pressure; and potassium supplements. Your doctor may need to change the doses of your medications or monitor you carefully for side effects.
- tell your doctor if you have recently had severe diarrhea or vomiting and if you have or have ever had allergies; asthma; heart failure; diabetes; gout; high cholesterol; lupus; scleroderma; or kidney or liver disease.
- tell your doctor if you plan to become pregnant or are breast-feeding.
- if you are having surgery, including dental surgery, tell the doctor or dentist that you are taking benazepril and hydrochlorothiazide.
- you should know that diarrhea, vomiting, not drinking enough fluids, and sweating a lot can cause a drop in blood pressure, which may cause lightheadedness and fainting.

What special dietary instructions should I follow?

Talk to your doctor before using salt substitutes containing potassium. If your doctor prescribes a low-salt or low-sodium diet, or an exercise program, follow these directions carefully.

What should I do if I forget to take a dose?

Take the missed dose as soon as you remember it. However, if it is almost time for the next dose, skip the missed dose and continue your regular dosing schedule. Do not take a double dose to make up for a missed one.

What side effects can this medicine cause?

Benazepril and hydrochlorothiazide may cause side effects. Tell your doctor if any of these symptoms are severe or do not go away:

- cough
- dizziness
- excessive tiredness
- drowsiness

Some side effects can be serious. The following symptoms are uncommon, but if you experience any of them, call your doctor immediately:

- swelling of the face, throat, tongue, lips, eyes, hands, feet, ankles, or lower legs
- hoarseness
- difficulty breathing or swallowing
- rash
- lightheadedness
- fainting
- fever, sore throat, chills, and other signs of infection
- yellowing of the skin or eyes
- dry mouth
- thirst
- weakness
- lack of energy
- restlessness
- muscle pains or cramps
- infrequent urination
- upset stomach
- vomiting
- rapid, pounding, or irregular heartbeat

Benazepril and hydrochlorothiazide may cause other side effects. Call your doctor if you have any unusual problems while taking this medication.

If you experience a serious side effect, you or your doctor may send a report to the Food and Drug Administration's (FDA) MedWatch Adverse Event Reporting program online [at http://www.fda.gov/MedWatch/index.html] or by phone [1-800-332-1088].

What storage conditions are needed for this medicine?

Keep this medication in the container it came in, tightly closed, and out of reach of children. Store it at room temperature and away from excess heat and moisture (not in the bathroom). Throw away any medication that is outdated or

no longer needed. Talk to your pharmacist about the proper disposal of your medication.

What should I do in case of overdose?

In case of overdose, call your local poison control center at 1-800-222-1222. If the victim has collapsed or is not breathing, call local emergency services at 911.

What other information should I know?

Keep all appointments with your doctor and the laboratory. Your blood pressure should be checked regularly to determine your response to benazepril and hydrochlorothiazide. Your doctor may order certain lab tests to check your body's response to benazepril and hydrochlorothiazide.

Before having any laboratory test, tell your doctor and the laboratory personnel that you are taking benazepril and hydrochlorothiazide.

Do not let anyone else take your medication. Ask your pharmacist any questions you have about refilling your prescription.

Dosage Facts
For Informational Purposes

Caution: Do not change your dose, how often you take your medication, or the length of time you are to take it without first talking to your healthcare provider.

The following dosage information was written using medical language for doctors and other healthcare professionals and is provided here for you to check your dosage. The dosage of this drug may differ for different patients. Therefore, always follow your doctor's instructions or the directions on the label. Contact your healthcare provider or pharmacist if you have any questions about the specific dosage of your medication after reviewing this information.

General Dosage Information

Available as benazepril hydrochloride; dosage expressed in terms of benazepril.

Adult Patients

Hypertension
Benazepril/Hydrochlorothiazide Combination Therapy
ORAL:
- If BP is not adequately controlled by monotherapy with benazepril, can switch to the fixed-combination preparation containing benazepril 10 mg and hydrochlorothiazide 12.5 mg or, alternatively, benazepril 20 mg and hydrochlorothiazide 12.5 mg. Adjust dosage of either or both drugs according to patient's response.
- If BP is controlled by monotherapy with hydrochlorothiazide 25 mg daily but potassium loss is problematic, can switch to fixed-combination preparation containing benazepril 5 mg and hydrochlorothiazide 6.25 mg.

Special Populations
Renal Impairment
- Benazepril/hydrochlorothiazide fixed combinations are not recommended in patients with severe renal impairment.

Benzonatate

(ben zoe' na tate)

Brand Name: Tessalon® Capsules, Tessalon® Perles

Why is this medicine prescribed?

Benzonatate is used to treat cough due to the common cold, bronchitis, pneumonia, or other lung infections. Benzonatate is in a class of medications called antitussives (cough suppressants). It works by reducing the cough reflex in the lungs and air passages.

How should this medicine be used?

Benzonatate comes as a liquid-filled capsule (perle) and a regular capsule to take by mouth. It is usually taken three times a day as needed. Follow the directions on your prescription label carefully, and ask your doctor or pharmacist to explain any part you do not understand. Take benzonatate exactly as directed. Do not take more or less of it or take it more often than prescribed by your doctor.

Swallow the capsules and liquid-filled capsules whole; do not suck or chew on them. If the medication is released in the mouth, it may make the mouth numb and cause choking.

Are there other uses for this medicine?

This medication may be prescribed for other uses; ask your doctor or pharmacist for more information.

What special precautions should I follow?

Before taking benzonatate,
- tell your doctor and pharmacist if you are allergic to benzonatate, procaine (Novocain), tetracaine (Pontocaine), or any other medications.
- tell your doctor and pharmacist what prescription and nonprescription medications, vitamins, nutritional supplements, and herbal products you are taking.
- tell your doctor if you are pregnant, plan to become pregnant, or are breast-feeding. If you become pregnant while taking benzonatate, call your doctor.
- if you are having surgery, including dental surgery, tell the doctor or dentist that you are taking benzonatate.
- you should know that benzonatate may make you

drowsy. Do not drive a car or operate machinery until you know how this medication affects you.
- remember that alcohol can add to the drowsiness caused by this medication.

What special dietary instructions should I follow?

Unless your doctor tells you otherwise, continue your normal diet.

What should I do if I forget to take a dose?

This medication is usually taken as needed. If your doctor has told you to take benzonatate regularly, take the missed dose as soon as you remember it. However, if it is almost time for the next dose, skip the missed dose and continue your regular dosing schedule. Do not take a double dose to make up for a missed one.

What side effects can this medicine cause?

Benzonatate may cause side effects. Tell your doctor if any of these symptoms are severe or do not go away:
- upset stomach
- constipation
- drowsiness
- headache
- dizziness
- stuffed nose
- burning in the eyes

Some side effects can be serious. The following symptoms are uncommon, but if you experience any of them, call your doctor immediately:
- rash or hives
- itching
- difficulty breathing or swallowing
- confusion
- seeing things that do not exist (hallucinating)

Benzonatate may cause other side effects. Call your doctor if you have any unusual problems while taking this medication.

If you experience a serious side effect, you or your doctor may send a report to the Food and Drug Administration's (FDA) MedWatch Adverse Event Reporting program online [at http://www.fda.gov/MedWatch/index.html] or by phone [1-800-332-1088].

What storage conditions are needed for this medicine?

Keep this medication in the container it came in, tightly closed, and out of reach of children. Store it at room temperature and away from excess heat and moisture (not in the bathroom). Throw away any medication that is outdated or no longer needed. Talk to your pharmacist about the proper disposal of your medication.

What should I do in case of overdose?

In case of overdose, call your local poison control center at 1-800-222-1222. If the victim has collapsed or is not breathing, call local emergency services at 911.

Symptoms of overdose may include:
- restlessness
- shaking hands that you cannot control
- seizures
- unconsciousness

What other information should I know?

Keep all appointments with your doctor.

Do not let anyone else take your medication. Ask your pharmacist any questions you have about refilling your prescription.

Dosage Facts
For Informational Purposes

Caution: Do not change your dose, how often you take your medication, or the length of time you are to take it without first talking to your healthcare provider.

The following dosage information was written using medical language for doctors and other healthcare professionals and is provided here for you to check your dosage. The dosage of this drug may differ for different patients. Therefore, always follow your doctor's instructions or the directions on the label. Contact your healthcare provider or pharmacist if you have any questions about the specific dosage of your medication after reviewing this information.

Pediatric Patients

Cough

ORAL:
- Children ≤10 Years of Age: 8 mg/kg daily in 3–6 divided doses†, although safety and efficacy have not been established in this age group.
- Children >10 Years of Age: 100 or 200 mg 3 times daily.

Adult Patients

Cough

ORAL:
- 100 or 200 mg 3 times daily; doses up to 600 mg daily may be given in divided doses if necessary.

Prescribing Limits

Pediatric Patients

Cough

ORAL:
- Children >10 Years of Age: Maximum 600 mg daily in divided doses.

Adult Patients

Cough

ORAL:
- Maximum 600 mg daily in divided doses.

Benzoyl Peroxide

(ben′ zoe il)

Brand Name: Benoxyl®, Benzac®, Desquam®, Fostex®, Oxy 10®, PanOxyl®

Why is this medicine prescribed?

Benzoyl peroxide is used to treat mild to moderate acne.

How should this medicine be used?

Benzoyl peroxide comes in cleansing liquid or bar, lotion, cream, and gel for use on the skin. Benzoyl peroxide usually is used one or two times daily. Start with once daily to see how your skin reacts to this medication. Follow the directions on the package or on your prescription label carefully, and ask your doctor or pharmacist to explain any part you do not understand. Use benzoyl peroxide exactly as directed. Do not use more or less of it or use it more often than directed by your doctor.

The cleansing liquid and bar are used to wash the affected area as directed.

To use the lotion, cream, or gel, first wash the affected skin areas and gently pat dry with a towel. Then apply a small amount of benzoyl peroxide and rub it in gently.

Avoid anything that may irritate your skin (e.g., abrasive soaps or cleansers, alcohol-containing products, cosmetics or soaps that dry the skin, medicated cosmetics, sunlight, and sunlamps) unless directed otherwise by your doctor.

It may take 4-6 weeks to see the effects of this medication. If your acne does not improve after this time, call your doctor.

Do not allow medication to get into your eyes, mouth, and nose.

Do not use benzoyl peroxide on children less than 12 years of age without talking to a doctor.

What special precautions should I follow?

Before using benzoyl peroxide,
- tell your doctor and pharmacist if you are allergic to benzoyl peroxide or any other drugs.
- tell your doctor and pharmacist what prescription and nonprescription medications you are taking, including vitamins.
- tell your doctor if you are pregnant, plan to become pregnant, or are breast-feeding. If you become pregnant while using benzoyl peroxide, call your doctor.

What should I do if I forget to take a dose?

Apply the missed dose as soon as you remember it. However, if it is almost time for the next dose, skip the missed dose and continue your regular dosing schedule. Do not apply a double dose to make up for a missed one.

What side effects can this medicine cause?

Benzoyl peroxide may cause side effects. Tell your doctor if any of these symptoms are severe or do not go away:
- dryness or peeling of skin
- feeling of warmth
- tingling
- slight stinging

If you experience any of the following symptoms, call your doctor immediately:
- burning
- blistering
- itching
- redness
- rash
- swelling

If you experience a serious side effect, you or your doctor may send a report to the Food and Drug Administration's (FDA) MedWatch Adverse Event Reporting program online [at http://www.fda.gov/MedWatch/index.html] or by phone [1-800-332-1088].

What storage conditions are needed for this medicine?

Keep this medication in the container it came in, tightly closed, and out of reach of children. Store it at room temperature and away from excess heat and moisture (not in the bathroom). Throw away any medication that is outdated or no longer needed. Talk to your pharmacist about the proper disposal of your medication.

What other information should I know?

Keep all appointments with your doctor. Benzoyl peroxide is for external use only. Do not let benzoyl peroxide get into your eyes, nose, or mouth, and do not swallow it. Do not apply dressings, bandages, cosmetics, lotions, or other skin medications to the area being treated unless your doctor tells you.

Keep benzoyl peroxide away from your hair and colored fabrics because it may bleach them.

Do not let anyone else use your medication. Tell your doctor if your skin condition gets worse or does not go away.

Talk to your doctor, pharmacist, or other healthcare professional if you have questions about dosing information for your medication.

Benztropine Mesylate Oral

(benz′ troe peen)

Brand Name: Cogentin®
Also available generically.

Why is this medicine prescribed?

Benztropine mesylate is used to treat the symptoms of Parkinson's disease and tremors caused by other medical problems or drugs.

This medication is sometimes prescribed for other uses; ask your doctor or pharmacist for more information.

How should this medicine be used?

Benztropine mesylate comes as a tablet to take by mouth. It usually is taken at bedtime. It may be taken two or three times a day to treat tremors caused by other medical problems or drugs. You may not notice any improvement in your condition for 1-2 days. You may have to take benztropine mesylate for a long time to treat Parkinson's disease. However, it may only be needed for 1-2 weeks if your tremors are caused by other medical problems or drugs.

Your doctor may start with a small dose and increase it slowly after seeing your response to benztropine mesylate. Follow the directions on your prescription label carefully, and ask your doctor or pharmacist to explain any part you do not understand. Take benztropine mesylate exactly as directed. Do not take more or less of it or take it more often than prescribed by your doctor.

Do not stop taking benztropine mesylate suddenly without talking with your doctor, especially if you are also taking other medications. Sudden stoppage can cause symptoms of Parkinson's disease to return.

Are there other uses for this medicine?

Benztropine mesylate is also used occasionally in geriatric patients who cannot take cerebral-stimulating medicine. Talk with your doctor about the possible risks of using this drug for your condition.

What special precautions should I follow?

Before taking benztropine mesylate,
- tell your doctor and pharmacist if you are allergic to benztropine mesylate or any other drugs.
- tell your doctor and pharmacist what prescription and nonprescription medications you are taking, especially amantadine (Symmetrel), digoxin (Lanoxin), haloperidol (Haldol), levodopa (Larodopa, Sinemet), tranquilizers such as chlorpromazine (Thorazine) or thioridazine (Mellaril), and vitamins.
- tell your doctor if you have or have ever had kidney or liver disease; glaucoma; heart or blood pressure problems; myasthenia gravis; or problems with your urinary system, prostate, or stomach.
- tell your doctor if you are pregnant, plan to become pregnant, or are breast-feeding. If you become pregnant while taking benztropine mesylate, call your doctor.
- if you are having surgery, including dental surgery, tell the doctor or dentist that you are taking benztropine mesylate.
- you should know that this drug may make you drowsy. Do not drive a car or operate machinery until you know how this drug affects you.
- remember that alcohol can add to the drowsiness caused by this drug.
- plan to avoid unnecessary or prolonged exposure to sunlight and to wear protective clothing, sunglasses, and sunscreen. Benztropine mesylate may make your skin sensitive to sunlight.

What special dietary instructions should I follow?

Benztropine mesylate may cause an upset stomach. Take benztropine mesylate with food or milk.

What should I do if I forget to take a dose?

Take the missed dose as soon as you remember it. However, if it is almost time for the next dose, skip the missed dose and continue your regular dosing schedule. Do not take a double dose to make up for a missed one.

If you take benztropine mesylate once a day at bedtime and do not remember it until the next morning, skip the missed dose. Do not take a double dose to make up for a missed one.

What side effects can this medicine cause?

Side effects from benztropine mesylate are common. Tell your doctor if any of these symptoms are severe or do not go away:
- drowsiness
- dry mouth
- difficulty urinating
- constipation

If you experience any of the following symptoms, call your doctor immediately:
- skin rash
- fast, irregular, or pounding heartbeat
- fever
- confusion
- depression
- delusions or hallucinations
- eye pain

If you experience a serious side effect, you or your doctor may send a report to the Food and Drug Administration's (FDA) MedWatch Adverse Event Reporting program online [at http://www.fda.gov/MedWatch/index.html] or by phone [1-800-332-1088].

What storage conditions are needed for this medicine?

Keep this medication in the container it came in, tightly closed, and out of reach of children. Store it at room temperature and away from excess heat and moisture (not in the bathroom). Throw away any medication that is outdated or no longer needed. Talk to your pharmacist about the proper disposal of your medication.

What should I do in case of overdose?

In case of overdose, call your local poison control center at 1-800-222-1222. If the victim has collapsed or is not breathing, call local emergency services at 911.

Symptoms of overdose may include:
- excitement
- confusion
- nervousness
- seeing things that do not exist (hallucinating)
- dizziness
- muscle weakness
- dry mouth
- blurred vision
- rapid or pounding heartbeat
- upset stomach
- vomiting
- painful urination
- difficulty swallowing
- skin rash
- headache
- hot, dry, flushed skin
- bloody vomit
- seizure
- coma
- heat stroke
- heartburn
- constipation

What other information should I know?

Keep all appointments with your doctor and the laboratory. Your doctor will order certain lab tests to check your response to benztropine mesylate.

Do not let anyone else take your medication. Ask your pharmacist any questions you have about refilling your prescription.

Dosage Facts
For Informational Purposes

Caution: Do not change your dose, how often you take your medication, or the length of time you are to take it without first talking to your healthcare provider.

The following dosage information was written using medical language for doctors and other healthcare professionals and is provided here for you to check your dosage. The dosage of this drug may differ for different patients. Therefore, always follow your doctor's instructions or the directions on the label. Contact your healthcare provider or pharmacist if you have any questions about the specific dosage of your medication after reviewing this information.

General Dosage Information

Available as benztropine mesylate; dosage is expressed in terms of the salt.

Geriatric patients or those with less than average body weight generally cannot tolerate high dosages of the drug.

Pediatric Patients

Manufacturers make no specific dosage recommendations for children ≥ 3 years of age.

Adult Patients

Parkinsonian Syndrome

May require periodic dosage adjustments to maintain optimum symptomatic relief in patients receiving concomitant levodopa or combination levodopa-carbidopa therapy.

If used to replace or supplement other antiparkinsonian drugs, change should be gradual, with dosage of previous medication reduced as benztropine dosage is increased.

Avoid abrupt discontinuance of concomitantly administered antiparkinsonian drugs.

Idiopathic Parkinsonian Syndrome

ORAL:
- Initially, 0.5–1 mg as a single dose at bedtime. Dosages may be increased by 0.5-mg increments at 5–6 day intervals up to a maximum of 6 mg daily.
- Usual dosage: 1–2 mg daily (range: 0.5–6 mg daily).

Postencephalitic Parkinsonian Syndrome

ORAL:
- Initially, 2 mg daily, given in 1 or more divided doses. In highly sensitive patients, may give instead as a single 0.5 mg dose at bedtime. Dosages may be increased by 0.5-mg increments at 5- to 6-day intervals up to a maximum of 6 mg daily.
- Usual dosage: 1–2 mg daily (range: 0.5–6 mg daily).

Drug-Induced Extrapyramidal Reactions

ORAL:
- 1–4 mg once or twice daily.
- For extrapyramidal disorders that develop shortly after initiation of antipsychotic therapy, 1–2 mg 2 or 3 times daily usually provides relief within 1 or 2 days. Evaluate need for continued therapy after 1–2 weeks.

Prescribing Limits

Adult Patients

Parkinsonian Syndrome

ORAL:
- Maximum 6 mg daily.

Betamethasone Topical

(bay ta meth′ a sone)

Brand Name: Alphatrex®, Betatrex®, Beta-Val®, Diprolene®, Diprolene® AF, Diprolene® Lotion, Lotrisone® as a combination product containing Betamethasone Dipropionate and Clotrimazole, Luxiq®, Maxivate®
Also available generically.

Why is this medicine prescribed?

Betamethasone is used to treat the itching, redness, dryness, crusting, scaling, inflammation, and discomfort of various skin conditions.

This medication is sometimes prescribed for other uses; ask your doctor or pharmacist for more information.

How should this medicine be used?

Betamethasone comes in ointment, cream, lotion, and aerosol (spray) in various strengths for use on the skin. It is usually applied one to four times a day. Follow the directions on your prescription label carefully, and ask your doctor or pharmacist to explain any part you do not understand. Use betamethasone exactly as directed. Do not use more or less of it or use it more often than prescribed by your doctor. Do not apply it to other areas of your body or wrap or bandage the treated area unless directed to do so by your doctor.

Wash or soak the affected area thoroughly before applying the medicine, unless it irritates your skin. Then apply the ointment or cream sparingly in a thin film and rub it in gently.

To use the lotion on your scalp, part your hair, apply a small amount of the medicine on the affected area, and rub it in gently. Protect the area from washing and rubbing until the lotion dries. You may wash your hair as usual but not right after applying the medicine.

To apply an aerosol, shake well and spray on the affected area holding the container about 3 to 6 inches away. Spray for about 2 seconds to cover an area the size of your hand. Take care not to inhale the vapors. If you are spraying near your face, cover your eyes.

Avoid prolonged use on the face, in the genital and rectal areas, and in skin creases and armpits unless directed by your doctor.

If you are using betamethasone on your face, keep it out of your eyes.

If you are using betamethasone on a child's diaper area, do not use tight-fitting diapers or plastic pants. Such use may increase side effects.

Do not apply cosmetics or other skin preparations on the treated area without talking with your doctor.

If your doctor tells you to wrap or bandage the treated area, follow these instructions:

1. Soak the area in water or wash it well.
2. While the skin is moist, gently rub the medication into the affected areas.
3. Cover the area with plastic wrap (such as Saran Wrap or Handi-Wrap.) The plastic may be held in place with a gauze or elastic bandage or adhesive tape on the normal skin beside the treated area. (Instead of using plastic wrap, plastic gloves may be used for the hands, plastic bags for the feet, or a shower cap for the scalp.)
4. Carefully seal the edges of the plastic to make sure the wrap adheres closely to the skin. If the affected area is moist, you can leave the edges of the plastic wrap partly unsealed or puncture the wrap to allow excess moisture to escape.
5. Leave the plastic wrapping in place as long as instructed by your doctor. Usually plastic wraps are left in place not more than 12 hours each day.
6. Cleanse the skin and reapply the medication each time a new plastic wrapping is applied.

Call your doctor if the treated area gets worse or if burning, swelling, redness, or oozing of pus develops.

What special precautions should I follow?

Before using betamethasone,

- tell your doctor and pharmacist if you are allergic to betamethasone or any other drugs.
- tell your doctor and pharmacist what prescription and nonprescription medications you are taking, especially cancer chemotherapy agents, other topical medications, and vitamins.
- tell your doctor if you have an infection or have ever had diabetes, glaucoma, cataracts, a circulation disorder, or an immune disorder.
- tell your doctor if you are pregnant, plan to become pregnant, or are breast-feeding. If you become pregnant while using betamethasone, call your doctor immediately.

What should I do if I forget to take a dose?

Apply the missed dose as soon as you remember it. However, if it is almost time for the next dose, skip the missed dose and continue your regular dosing schedule. Do not apply a double dose to make up for a missed one.

What side effects can this medicine cause?

Betamethasone may cause side effects. Tell your doctor if any of these symptoms are severe or do not go away:

- drying or cracking of the skin
- acne
- itching
- burning
- change in skin color

If you experience any of the following symptoms, call your doctor immediately:

- severe skin rash
- difficulty breathing or swallowing

- wheezing
- skin infection (redness, swelling, or oozing pus)

If you experience a serious side effect, you or your doctor may send a report to the Food and Drug Administration's (FDA) MedWatch Adverse Event Reporting program online [at http://www.fda.gov/MedWatch/index.html] or by phone [1-800-332-1088].

What storage conditions are needed for this medicine?

Keep this medication in the container it came in, tightly closed, and out of reach of children. Store it according to the package instructions. Throw away any medication that is outdated or no longer needed. Do not use it to treat other skin conditions. Talk to your pharmacist about the proper disposal of your medication.

What other information should I know?

Keep all appointments with your doctor.

Do not let anyone else use your medication. Ask your pharmacist any questions you have about refilling your prescription.

Dosage Facts
For Informational Purposes

Caution: Do not change your dose, how often you take your medication, or the length of time you are to take it without first talking to your healthcare provider.

The following dosage information was written using medical language for doctors and other healthcare professionals and is provided here for you to check your dosage. The dosage of this drug may differ for different patients. Therefore, always follow your doctor's instructions or the directions on the label. Contact your healthcare provider or pharmacist if you have any questions about the specific dosage of your medication after reviewing this information.

General Dosage Information

Available as betamethasone dipropionate and betamethasone valerate; dosage usually expressed in terms of betamethasone.

Foam available as betamethasone valerate; dosage expressed in terms of betamethasone valerate.

Pediatric Patients

Administer the least amount of topical preparations that provides effective therapy.

Corticosteroid-responsive Dermatoses

TOPICAL (BETAMETHASONE DIPROPIONATE):
- Children ≥13 years of age: Apply 0.05% cream in a thin film to affected area, usually once daily or, if necessary, twice daily.
- Children ≥13 years of age: Apply 0.05% cream in optimized

(augmented) vehicle or 0.05% ointment in a thin film to affected area once or twice daily.
- Children ≥13 years of age: Apply a few drops of 0.05% lotion to affected area once or twice daily.
- Children ≥12 years of age: Apply 0.05% gel in optimized (augmented) vehicle or 0.05% ointment in optimized (augmented) vehicle in a thin film to affected area once or twice daily.
- Children ≥12 years of age: Apply a few drops of 0.05% lotion in optimized (augmented) vehicle to affected area once or twice daily.

TOPICAL (BETAMETHASONE VALERATE):
- Apply 0.1% cream or ointment to affected area 1–3 times daily; once- or twice-daily application often is effective.
- Apply a few drops of 0.1% lotion to affected area twice daily, in the morning and evening. Dosage may be increased in patients with resistant dermatoses; decrease frequency to once daily following clinical improvement.

Adult Patients

Corticosteroid-responsive Dermatoses

TOPICAL (BETAMETHASONE DIPROPIONATE):
- Apply 0.05% cream in a thin film to affected area, usually once daily or, if necessary, twice daily.
- Apply 0.05% cream in optimized (augmented) vehicle, 0.05% gel in optimized (augmented) vehicle, 0.05% ointment or ointment in optimized (augmented) vehicle in a thin film to affected area once or twice daily.
- Apply a few drops of 0.05% lotion or 0.05% lotion in optimized (augmented) vehicle to affected area once or twice daily.

TOPICAL (BETAMETHASONE VALERATE):
- Apply 0.1% cream or ointment to affected area 1–3 times daily; once- or twice-daily application is often effective.
- Apply 0.12% foam twice daily in the morning and evening. Discontinue when control is achieved; if response is inadequate within a 2-week course of therapy, consider reevaluation of diagnosis.
- Apply a few drops of 0.1% lotion to affected area twice daily, in the morning and evening. Dosage may be increased in patients with resistant dermatoses; decrease frequency to once daily following clinical improvement.

Symptomatic Inflammatory Tinea Pedis, Tinea Cruris, or Tinea Corporis

TOPICAL (BETAMETHASONE DIPROPIONATE AND CLOTRIMAZOLE):
- Apply combination (betamethasone dipropionate 0.05% and clotrimazole 1%) cream or lotion twice daily in the morning and evening.
- If response is inadequate within a 1-week (tinea corporis or tinea cruris) or 2-week (tinea pedis) course of therapy with combination (betamethasone 0.05% and clotrimazole 1%) cream or lotion, reevaluate diagnosis or discontinue combination preparation and consider clotrimazole alone.

Prescribing Limits

Pediatric Patients

Corticosteroid-responsive Dermatoses

TOPICAL (BETAMETHASONE DIPROPIONATE):

- Maximum 45 g weekly with 0.05% cream in optimized (augmented) vehicle or with 0.05% ointment in optimized (augmented) vehicle.
- Maximum 50 g weekly with 0.05% gel in optimized (augmented) vehicle or 50 mL weekly with 0.05% lotion in optimized (augmented) vehicle; do not exceed 2 consecutive weeks of therapy.

Adult Patients

Corticosteroid-responsive Dermatoses

TOPICAL (BETAMETHASONE DIPROPIONATE):

- Maximum 45 g weekly with 0.05% cream in optimized (augmented) vehicle or with 0.05% ointment in optimized (augmented) vehicle.
- Maximum 50 g weekly with 0.05% gel in optimized (augmented) vehicle or 50 mL weekly with 0.05% lotion in optimized (augmented) vehicle; do not exceed 2 consecutive weeks of therapy.

Symptomatic Inflammatory Tinea Pedis, Tinea Cruris, or Tinea Corporis

TOPICAL (BETAMETHASONE DIPROPIONATE AND CLOTRIMAZOLE):

- Maximum 45 g (cream) or 45 mL (lotion) weekly with combination (betamethasone dipropionate 0.05% and clotrimazole 1%) preparation; do not exceed 2 consecutive weeks of therapy in the treatment of tinea cruris or tinea corporis or 4 weeks in the treatment of tinea pedis.

Betaxolol Ophthalmic

(be tax′ oh lol)

Brand Name: Betoptic®, Betoptic S®

Why is this medicine prescribed?

Betaxolol is used to treat glaucoma, a condition in which increased pressure in the eye can lead to gradual loss of vision. Betaxolol decreases the pressure in the eye.

This medication is sometimes prescribed for other uses; ask your doctor or pharmacist for more information.

How should this medicine be used?

Betaxolol comes as eyedrops. Betaxolol usually is used twice a day. Follow the directions on your prescription label carefully, and ask your doctor or pharmacist to explain any part you do not understand. Use betaxolol exactly as directed. Do not use more or less of it or use it more often than prescribed by your doctor.

If you are using the suspension form of betaxolol eyedrops (Betoptic S), shake the bottle well before each dose. It is not necessary to shake betaxolol eyedrop solution.

Betaxolol controls glaucoma but does not cure it. Continue to use betaxolol even if you feel well. Do not stop using betaxolol without talking to your doctor.

To use the eyedrops, follow these instructions:

1. Wash your hands thoroughly with soap and water.
2. Use a mirror or have someone else put the drops in your eye.
3. If using the betaxolol suspension eyedrops, shake the bottle well.
4. Remove the protective cap. Make sure that the end of the dropper is not chipped or cracked.
5. Avoid touching the dropper tip against your eye or anything else.
6. Hold the dropper tip down at all times to prevent drops from flowing back into the bottle and contaminating the remaining contents.
7. Lie down or tilt your head back.
8. Holding the bottle between your thumb and index finger, place the dropper tip as near as possible to your eyelid without touching it.
9. Brace the remaining fingers of that hand against your cheek or nose.
10. With the index finger of your other hand, pull the lower lid of the eye down to form a pocket.
11. Drop the prescribed number of drops into the pocket made by the lower lid and the eye. Placing drops on the surface of the eyeball can cause stinging.
12. Close your eye and press lightly against the lower lid with your finger for 2-3 minutes to keep the medication in the eye. Do not blink.
13. Replace and tighten the cap right away. Do not wipe or rinse it off.
14. Wipe off any excess liquid from your cheek with a clean tissue. Wash your hands again.

What special precautions should I follow?

Before using betaxolol eyedrops,

- tell your doctor and pharmacist if you are allergic to betaxolol or any other drugs.
- tell your doctor and pharmacist what prescription and nonprescription medications you are taking, especially other eye medications; beta blockers such as atenolol (Tenormin), carteolol (Cartrol), labetalol (Normodyne, Trandate), metoprolol (Lopressor), nadolol (Corgard), propranolol (Inderal), sotalol (Betapace), or timolol (Blocadren); quinidine (Quinidex, Quinaglute Dura-Tabs); verapamil (Calan, Isoptin); and vitamins.
- tell your doctor if you have or have ever had thyroid, heart, or lung disease, congestive heart failure, or diabetes.
- tell your doctor if you are pregnant, plan to become pregnant, or are breast-feeding. If you become pregnant while using betaxolol, call your doctor immediately.
- if you are having surgery, including dental surgery, tell the doctor or dentist that you are using betaxolol.

- if you are using another eyedrop medication, use the eye medications at least 10 minutes apart.

What should I do if I forget to take a dose?

Apply the missed dose as soon as you remember it. However, if it is almost time for the next dose, skip the missed dose and continue your regular dosing schedule. Do not apply a double dose to make up for a missed one.

What side effects can this medicine cause?

Betaxolol may cause side effects. Tell your doctor if any of these symptoms are severe or do not go away:

- eye irritation
- eye tearing
- headache
- dizziness
- insomnia

If you experience any of the following symptoms, call your doctor immediately:

- difficulty breathing
- change in vision
- eye pain

If you experience a serious side effect, you or your doctor may send a report to the Food and Drug Administration's (FDA) MedWatch Adverse Event Reporting program online [at http://www.fda.gov/MedWatch/index.html] or by phone [1-800-332-1088].

What storage conditions are needed for this medicine?

Keep this medication in the container it came in, tightly closed, and out of reach of children. Store it at room temperature and away from excess heat and moisture (not in the bathroom). Throw away any medication that is outdated or no longer needed. Talk to your pharmacist about the proper disposal of your medication.

What other information should I know?

Keep all appointments with your doctor. Your doctor will order certain eye tests to check your response to betaxolol.

Do not let anyone else use your medication. Ask your pharmacist any questions you have about refilling your prescription.

Dosage Facts
For Informational Purposes

Caution: Do not change your dose, how often you take your medication, or the length of time you are to take it without first talking to your healthcare provider.

The following dosage information was written using medical language for doctors and other healthcare professionals and is provided here for you to check your dosage. The dosage of this drug may differ for different patients. Therefore, always follow your doctor's instructions or the directions on the label. Contact your healthcare provider or pharmacist if you have any questions about the specific dosage of your medication after reviewing this information.

General Dosage Information

Available as betaxolol hydrochloride; dosage expressed in terms of betaxolol.

Suspension is therapeutically equivalent (in terms of magnitude and duration of hypotensive effect) to solution.

Each 2.8 or 5.6 mg of betaxolol hydrochloride is equivalent to about 2.5 or 5 mg of betaxolol, respectively.

Adult Patients

Ocular Hypertension and Glaucoma

OPHTHALMIC:

- Betaxolol solution: 1–2 drops of a 0.5% solution in affected eye(s) twice daily.
- Betaxolol suspension: 1–2 drops of a 0.25% suspension in affected eye(s) twice daily.
- If further reduction of IOP is required, a topical miotic, topical dipivefrin, topical epinephrine, and/or a carbonic anhydrase inhibitor may be added.

Bethanechol

(be than' e kole)

Brand Name: Urecholine®

Why is this medicine prescribed?

Bethanechol is used to relieve difficulties in urinating caused by surgery, drugs, or other factors.

This medication is sometimes prescribed for other uses; ask your doctor or pharmacist for more information.

How should this medicine be used?

Bethanechol comes as a tablet to take by mouth. Bethanechol usually is taken two to four times a day. Follow the directions on your prescription label carefully, and ask your doctor or pharmacist to explain any part you do not understand. Take bethanechol exactly as directed. Do not take more or less of it or take it more often than prescribed by your doctor.

Bethanechol usually is taken at evenly spaced intervals during the day.

Take this medication on an empty stomach (at least 1 hour before or 2 hours after meals) to prevent stomach upset.

What special precautions should I follow?

Before taking bethanechol,

- tell your doctor and pharmacist if you are allergic to bethanechol or any other drugs.

- tell your doctor and pharmacist what prescription and nonprescription medications you are taking, especially procainamide (Pronestyl), quinidine (Quinaglute), medications for colds or nasal congestion, and vitamins.
- tell your doctor if you have or have ever had asthma, a bladder infection, epilepsy, high blood pressure, heart disease, Parkinson's disease, an overactive thyroid gland, or ulcers.
- tell your doctor if you are pregnant, plan to become pregnant, or are breast-feeding. If you become pregnant while taking bethanechol, call your doctor.
- you should know that this drug may make you drowsy. Do not drive a car or operate machinery until you know how this drug affects you.
- remember that alcohol can add to the drowsiness caused by this drug.

What should I do if I forget to take a dose?

Take the missed dose as soon as you remember it. However, if it is almost time for the next dose, skip the missed dose and continue your regular dosing schedule. Do not take a double dose to make up for a missed one.

What side effects can this medicine cause?

Bethanechol may cause side effects. Tell your doctor if any of these symptoms are severe or do not go away:
- upset stomach
- vomiting
- dizziness
- sweating or flushing

If you experience any of the following symptoms, call your doctor immediately:
- shortness of breath
- fainting
- slow heart rate (pulse less than 50 beats per minute)

If you experience a serious side effect, you or your doctor may send a report to the Food and Drug Administration's (FDA) MedWatch Adverse Event Reporting program online [at http://www.fda.gov/MedWatch/index.html] or by phone [1-800-332-1088].

What storage conditions are needed for this medicine?

Keep this medication in the container it came in, tightly closed, and out of reach of children. Store it at room temperature and away from excess heat and moisture (not in the bathroom). Throw away any medication that is outdated or no longer needed. Talk to your pharmacist about the proper disposal of your medication.

What should I do in case of overdose?

In case of overdose, call your local poison control center at 1-800-222-1222. If the victim has collapsed or is not breathing, call local emergency services at 911.

What other information should I know?

Keep all appointments with your doctor.

Do not let anyone else take your medication. Ask your pharmacist any questions you have about refilling your prescription.

Talk to your doctor, pharmacist, or other healthcare professional if you have questions about dosing information for your medication.

Bevacizumab Injection

(be va siz′ yoo mab)

Brand Name: Avastin®

Important Warning

Bevacizumab may cause you to develop a hole in the wall of your stomach or intestine. This is a serious and possibly life-threatening condition. If you experience any of the following symptoms, call your doctor immediately: stomach pain, constipation, nausea, vomiting, or fever.

Bevacizumab may slow the healing of wounds, such as cuts made by a doctor during surgery. In some cases, bevacizumab may cause a wound that has closed to split open. This is a serious and possibly life-threatening condition. If you experience this problem, call your doctor immediately. Tell your doctor if you have recently had surgery or if you plan to have surgery. If you have recently had surgery, you should not use bevacizumab until at least 28 days have passed and until the area has completed healed. If you are scheduled to have surgery, your doctor will stop your treatment with bevacizumab at least several weeks before the surgery.

Bevacizumab may cause severe, life-threatening bleeding in the lungs of people who are using bevacizumab along with chemotherapy to treat lung cancer. Tell your doctor if you have recently coughed up blood or if you cough up blood at any time during your treatment.

Talk to your doctor about the risks of using bevacizumab.

Why is this medicine prescribed?

Bevacizumab is used with chemotherapy to treat cancer of the colon (large intestine) or rectum that has spread to other parts of the body. Bevacizumab is also used with chemotherapy to treat certain types of lung cancer. Bevacizumab is in a class of medications called antiangiogenic agents. It works by stopping the formation of blood vessels that bring oxygen and nutrients to tumors. This may slow the growth and spread of tumors.

How should this medicine be used?

Bevacizumab comes as a solution to administer slowly into a vein. Bevacizumab is administered by a doctor or nurse in a medical office, infusion center, or hospital. Bevacizumab is usually given once every 2 weeks to treat cancer of the colon or rectum and once every 3 weeks to treat lung cancer.

It should take 90 minutes for you to receive your first dose of bevacizumab. A doctor or nurse will watch you closely to see how your body reacts to bevacizumab. If you do not have any serious problems when you receive your first dose of bevacizumab, it will usually take 30 to 60 minutes for you to receive each of your remaining doses of the medication.

Are there other uses for this medicine?

Bevacizumab is also sometimes used to treat wet age-related macular degeneration (AMD; an ongoing disease of the eye that causes loss of the ability to see straight ahead and may make it more difficult to read, drive, or perform other daily activities) and other types of cancer. Talk to your doctor about the risks of using bevacizumab to treat your condition.

This medication may be prescribed for other uses; ask your doctor or pharmacist for more information.

What special precautions should I follow?

Before receiving bevacizumab,
- tell your doctor and pharmacist if you are allergic to bevacizumab or any other medications.
- tell your doctor and pharmacist what prescription and nonprescription medications, vitamins, nutritional supplements, and herbal products you are taking or plan to take. Be sure to mention anticoagulants (blood thinners) such as warfarin (Coumadin) and irinotecan (Camptosar). Also tell your doctor if you are taking or if you have ever taken an anthracycline (a type of chemotherapy used for breast cancer and some types of leukemia) such as daunorubicin (Cerubidine), doxorubicin (Adriamycin, Rubex), epirubicin (Ellence), or idarubicin (Idamycin). Your doctor may need to change the doses of your medications or monitor you carefully for side effects.
- tell your doctor if you have ever been treated with radiation therapy to the left side of your chest, and if you have or have ever had cancer that spread to your brain or spine, high blood pressure, or any condition that affects your heart or blood vessels (tubes that move blood between the heart and other parts of the body).
- tell your doctor if you are pregnant or plan to become pregnant. Bevacizumab may harm the fetus and increase the risk of a pregnancy loss. You should use birth control to prevent pregnancy during your treatment with bevacizumab and for some time after you stop using the medication. If you become pregnant while using bevacizumab, call your doctor.
- tell your doctor if you are breast-feeding. You should not breastfeed during your treatment with bevacizumab and for some time after you stop using the medication.

What special dietary instructions should I follow?

Unless your doctor tells you otherwise, continue your normal diet.

What should I do if I forget to take a dose?

If you miss an appointment to receive a dose of bevacizumab, call your doctor as soon as possible.

What side effects can this medicine cause?

Bevacizumab may cause side effects. Tell your doctor if any of these symptoms are severe or do not go away:
- dizziness
- fainting
- nosebleeds
- bleeding gums
- weakness
- loss of appetite
- heartburn
- change in ability to taste food
- diarrhea
- weight loss
- dry mouth
- sores on the skin or in the mouth
- voice changes

Some side effects can be serious. If you experience any of these symptoms or those listed in the IMPORTANT WARNING section, call your doctor immediately:
- nosebleeds that cause dizziness or fainting or that do not stop after 10 to 15 minutes
- unusual bruising or bleeding
- black or bloody stools
- bright red blood in stools
- vomit that is bloody or looks like coffee grounds
- severe vaginal bleeding
- headache
- neck pain
- slow or difficult speech
- dizziness or faintness
- weakness or numbness of an arm or leg
- chest pain
- pain in the arms, neck, or upper back
- shortness of breath
- seizures
- extreme tiredness
- confusion
- change in vision or loss of vision
- sore throat, fever, chills, and other signs of infection
- swelling of the face, eyes, stomach, hands, feet, ankles, or lower legs
- unexplained weight gain
- foamy urine

- dry, hacking cough
- pain, tenderness, warmth, redness, or swelling in one leg only
- redness, itching, or scaling of the skin

Bevacizumab may cause other side effects. Call your doctor if you have any unusual problems while receiving this medication.

What storage conditions are needed for this medicine?

Bevacizumab will be stored in the medical office, infusion center, or hospital.

What should I do in case of overdose?

In case of overdose, call your local poison control center at 1-800-222-1222. If the victim has collapsed or is not breathing, call local emergency services at 911.

Symptoms of overdose may include:
- headache

What other information should I know?

Keep all appointments with your doctor. Your doctor will check your blood pressure and test your urine regularly during your treatment with bevacizumab.

Dosage Facts
For Informational Purposes

Caution: Do not change your dose, how often you take your medication, or the length of time you are to take it without first talking to your healthcare provider.

The following dosage information was written using medical language for doctors and other healthcare professionals and is provided here for you to check your dosage. The dosage of this drug may differ for different patients. Therefore, always follow your doctor's instructions or the directions on the label. Contact your healthcare provider or pharmacist if you have any questions about the specific dosage of your medication after reviewing this information.

Adult Patients
Colorectal Cancer

IV:
- 5 mg/kg every 14 days until disease progression occurs.
- Use in combination with IV fluorouracil-based chemotherapy. Consult respective manufacturers for information on the dosage, method, and sequence of administration of these other antineoplastic agents. In clinical studies, bevacizumab was used in combination with the IFL regimen (irinotecan 125 mg/m² , fluorouracil 500 mg/m² , and leucovorin 20 mg/m² , administered by IV injection once weekly for 4 out of every 6 weeks) or the 5-FU/LV regimen (leucovorin 500 mg/m² by IV infusion over 2 hours, then fluorouracil 500 mg/m² by slow IV injection [1 hour after initiation of leucovorin]

given once weekly for the first 6 weeks out of every 8-week cycle).

Dosage Modification for Toxicity

Dosage reductions not recommended in any patient; instead, temporarily or permanently discontinue therapy based on causality.

Discontinue therapy *permanently* if GI perforation, wound dehiscence (requiring medical intervention), severe bleeding, severe arterial thromboembolic event, nephrotic syndrome, or hypertensive crisis occurs.

Discontinue therapy *temporarily* in patients with evidence of moderate to severe proteinuria pending further evaluation; in patients with severe hypertension not controlled by medical management; or in patients with severe infusion reactions.

Special Populations

No dosage adjustment required in geriatric patients.

Bimatoprost Ophthalmic

(bi ma′ toe prost)

Brand Name: Lumigan®

Why is this medicine prescribed?

Bimatoprost is used to treat eye conditions, including glaucoma and ocular hypertension, in which increased pressure can lead to a gradual loss of vision. Bimatoprost is used for patients who cannot use other eye medications for their condition or whose eye condition has not responded to another medication. Bimatoprost is in a class of medications called prostamides. It lowers pressure in the eye by increasing the flow of natural eye fluids out of the eye.

How should this medicine be used?

Bimatoprost comes as an eyedrop to apply to the eye. It is usually applied to the affected eye(s) once a day in the evening. To help you remember to use bimatoprost, use it around the same time every day. Follow the directions on your prescription label carefully, and ask your doctor or pharmacist to explain any part you do not understand. Use bimatoprost exactly as directed. Do not use more or less of it or use it more often than prescribed by your doctor.

Bimatoprost controls glaucoma and ocular hypertension but does not cure them. Continue to use bimatoprost even if you feel well. Do not stop using bimatoprost without talking to your doctor.

To apply the eyedrops, follow these steps:
1. Wash your hands thoroughly with soap and water.
2. Use a mirror or have someone else put the drops in your eye.

3. Make sure the end of the dropper is not chipped or cracked.
4. Avoid touching the dropper against your eye or anything else.
5. Hold the dropper tip down at all times to prevent drops from flowing back into the bottle and contaminating the remaining contents.
6. Lie down or tilt your head back.
7. Holding the bottle between your thumb and index finger, place the dropper as near as possible to your eyelid without touching it.
8. Brace the remaining fingers of that hand against your cheek or nose.
9. With the index finger of your other hand, pull the lower lid of the eye down to form a pocket.
10. Drop the prescribed number of drops into the pocket made by the lower lid and the eye. Placing the drops on the surface of the eyeball can cause stinging.
11. Close your eye and press lightly against the lower lid with your finger for 2-3 minutes to keep the medication in the eye. Do not blink.
12. Replace and tighten the cap right away. Do not wipe or rinse it off.
13. Wipe off any excess liquid from your cheek with a clean tissue. Wash your hands again.

Are there other uses for this medicine?

This medication may be prescribed for other uses; ask your doctor or pharmacist for more information.

What special precautions should I follow?

Before using bimatoprost,
- tell your doctor and pharmacist if you are allergic to bimatoprost or any other medications.
- tell your doctor and pharmacist what prescription and nonprescription medications, vitamins, nutritional supplements, and herbal products you are taking.
- if you are using another topical eye medication, apply it at least 5 minutes before or after bimatoprost.
- tell your doctor if you have inflammation (swelling) of the eye or a torn or missing lens and if you have or have ever had liver or kidney disease.
- tell your doctor if you are pregnant, plan to become pregnant, or are breast-feeding. If you become pregnant while using bimatoprost, call your doctor.
- you should know that bimatoprost solution contains benzalkonium chloride, which can be absorbed by soft contact lenses. If you wear contact lenses, remove them before applying bimatoprost and put them back in 15 minutes later.
- if you have an eye injury, infection, or surgery while using bimatoprost, ask your doctor if you should continue using the same eyedrops container.

What special dietary instructions should I follow?

Unless your doctor tells you otherwise, continue your normal diet.

What should I do if I forget to take a dose?

Apply the missed dose as soon as you remember it. However, if it is almost time for the next dose, skip the missed dose and continue your regular dosing schedule. Do not apply a double dose to make up for a missed one.

What side effects can this medicine cause?

Bimatoprost may cause side effects. Tell your doctor if any of these symptoms are severe or do not go away:
- itchy eyes
- dry eyes
- burning eyes
- eye pain or irritation
- eye tearing
- headaches

Some side effects can be serious. The following symptoms are uncommon, but if you experience any of them, call your doctor immediately:
- sensitivity to light
- pink eye
- redness or swelling of the eyelid

Bimatoprost may change the color of your eye (to brown) and darken the skin around the eye. It may also cause your eyelashes to grow longer and thicker and darken in color. These changes usually occur slowly, but they may be permanent. If you use bimatoprost in only one eye, you should know that there may be a difference between your eyes after taking bimatoprost. Call your doctor if you notice these changes.

Bimatoprost may cause other side effects. Call your doctor if you have any unusual problems while using this medication.

If you experience a serious side effect, you or your doctor may send a report to the Food and Drug Administration's (FDA) MedWatch Adverse Event Reporting program online [at http://www.fda.gov/MedWatch/index.html] or by phone [1-800-332-1088].

What storage conditions are needed for this medicine?

Keep this medication in the container it came in, tightly closed, and out of reach of children. Store it at room temperature and away from excess heat and moisture (not in the bathroom). Throw away any medication that is outdated or no longer needed. Talk to your pharmacist about the proper disposal of your medication.

What other information should I know?

Keep all appointments with your doctor.

Do not let anyone else use your medication. Ask your

pharmacist any questions you have about refilling your prescription.

Dosage Facts
For Informational Purposes

Caution: Do not change your dose, how often you take your medication, or the length of time you are to take it without first talking to your healthcare provider.

The following dosage information was written using medical language for doctors and other healthcare professionals and is provided here for you to check your dosage. The dosage of this drug may differ for different patients. Therefore, always follow your doctor's instructions or the directions on the label. Contact your healthcare provider or pharmacist if you have any questions about the specific dosage of your medication after reviewing this information.

Adult Patients

Ocular Hypertension and Glaucoma

OPHTHALMIC:
- One drop of a 0.03% solution in the affected eye(s) once daily in the evening. More frequent dosing may paradoxically diminish the IOP-lowering effect of the drug.

Bisacodyl

(bis a koe' dill)

Brand Name: Alophen® Pills, Bisac-Evac®, Bisacodyl Uniserts®, Carter's Little Pills®, Correctol® Caplets®, Correctol® Tablets, Dulcolax®, Dulcolax® Bowel Prep Kit, Evac-Q-Kwik® Kit, Feen-A-Mint®, Fleet® Bisacodyl, Fleet® Bisacodyl Enema, Fleet® Prep Kit No. 1, Fleet® Prep Kit No. 2, Fleet® Prep Kit No. 3, LoSo® Prep® Kit, Tridate® Bowel Cleansing Kit, Tridate® Dry Bowel Cleansing Kit, X-Prep® Bowel Evacuant Kit #1

Also available generically.

Why is this medicine prescribed?

Bisacodyl, a laxative, is used on a short-term basis to treat constipation. It also is used to empty the bowels before surgery and examinations such as X-ray procedures using barium enemas. Bisacodyl is available with or without a prescription.

This medication is sometimes prescribed for other uses; ask your doctor or pharmacist for more information.

How should this medicine be used?

Bisacodyl comes as a tablet to take by mouth and a suppository and enema to use rectally. It is usually taken the evening before (tablets) or at the time that (suppositories or enema) a bowel movement is desired. Follow the directions on the package or on your prescription label carefully, and ask your doctor or pharmacist to explain any part you do not understand.

To empty the bowels, bisacodyl usually is taken orally the night before and rectally the morning of surgery or an examination. The tablets normally cause a bowel movement in 6-8 hours, suppositories in 15-60 minutes, and the enema in 3-5 minutes. Do not take bisacodyl more than once a day or for more than 1 week without talking to your doctor.

Do not crush or chew bisacodyl tablets; swallow them whole. Do not take tablets within 1 hour of drinking milk or taking antacids. Do not eat after taking bisacodyl tablets in preparation for a barium enema.

Take bisacodyl exactly as directed. Do not take more or less of it or take it more often than prescribed by your doctor. Frequent or continued use of bisacodyl may make you dependent on laxatives and cause your bowels to lose their normal ability. If you do not have a regular bowel movement or you have rectal bleeding after taking this medication as directed for 1 week, call your doctor. Do not give bisacodyl to a child less than 10 years of age unless a doctor tells you to.

If you are to insert a bisacodyl suppository, follow these steps:
1. Remove the wrapper.
2. Dip the tip of the suppository in lukewarm water.
3. Lie down on your left side and raise your right knee to your chest. (A left-handed person should lie on the right side and raise the left knee.)
4. Using your finger, insert the suppository high into your rectum. Hold it in place for a few moments. Try to keep it there for as long as possible.
5. Wash your hands thoroughly.

If you are to use a bisacodyl enema, follow these steps:
1. Shake the enema bottle well.
2. Remove the protective shield from the tip.
3. Lie down on your left side and raise your right knee to your chest. (A left-handed person should lie on the right side and raise the left knee.)
4. Gently insert the enema bottle into the rectum with the tip pointing toward the navel.
5. Squeeze the bottle gently until nearly all the medicine is expelled.
6. Remove the enema bottle from the rectum. Hold the enema contents in place for as long as possible.
7. Wash your hands thoroughly.

What special precautions should I follow?

Before taking bisacodyl,
- tell your doctor and pharmacist if you are allergic to bisacodyl, aspirin, or any other medications, or any

of the ingredients in these products. Check the label or ask your pharmacist for a list of these ingredients.

- tell your doctor and pharmacist what prescription and nonprescription medications you are taking.
- tell your doctor if you are pregnant, plan to become pregnant, or are breast-feeding. If you become pregnant while taking bisacodyl, call your doctor.

What should I do if I forget to take a dose?

This medication usually is taken as needed. If your doctor has told you to take bisacodyl regularly, take the missed dose as soon as you remember it. However, if it is almost time for the next dose, skip the missed dose and continue your regular dosing schedule. Do not take a double dose to make up for a missed one.

What side effects can this medicine cause?

Bisacodyl may cause side effects. Tell your doctor if any of these symptoms are severe or do not go away:

- stomach cramps
- upset stomach
- diarrhea
- stomach and intestinal irritation
- faintness
- irritation or burning in the rectum (from suppositories)

What storage conditions are needed for this medicine?

Keep this medication in the container it came in, tightly closed, and out of reach of children. Store it at room temperature and away from excess heat and moisture (not in the bathroom). Throw away any medication that is outdated or no longer needed. Talk to your pharmacist about the proper disposal of your medication.

What other information should I know?

Keep all appointments with your doctor.

Do not let anyone else take your medication. Ask your pharmacist any questions you have about refilling your prescription.

Dosage Facts
For Informational Purposes

Caution: Do not change your dose, how often you take your medication, or the length of time you are to take it without first talking to your healthcare provider.

The following dosage information was written using medical language for doctors and other healthcare professionals and is provided here for you to check your dosage. The dosage of this drug may differ for different patients. Therefore, always follow your doctor's instructions or the directions on the label. Contact your health-

care provider or pharmacist if you have any questions about the specific dosage of your medication after reviewing this information.

Pediatric Patients

Constipation

Stimulant laxatives generally avoided in children <6 years of age for occasional constipation, unless otherwise directed by a clinician.

ORAL:
- Children 3–11 Years of Age: A single 5- to 10-mg (usually 5-mg) or 0.3-mg/kg dose daily.
- Children ≥12 Years of Age: A single 5- to 15-mg (usually 10-mg) dose daily.

RECTAL (ENEMA):
- Children ≥12 Years of Age: A single 10-mg (30-mL) dose daily.

RECTAL (SUPPOSITORIES):
- Children <2 Years of Age: A single 5-mg (½ suppository) dose daily.
- Children 2–11 Years of Age: A single 5- or 10-mg (½ or 1 suppository, respectively) dose daily.
- Children ≥12 Years of Age: A single 10-mg (1 suppository) dose daily.

Adult Patients

Constipation

ORAL:
- Usually, 5–15 mg daily given as a single dose; some patients may require single daily doses up to 30 mg.

RECTAL (ENEMA):
- A single 10-mg (30-mL) dose daily.

RECTAL (SUPPOSITORIES):
- A single 10-mg (1 suppository) dose daily.

Colonic Evacuation

Up to 30 mg may be given orally when complete evacuation of the colon is required for special procedures.

One of the following regimens can be used to clear the bowel prior to surgical, radiologic, or endoscopic procedures. When available, provide patients with a copy of the manufacturers' instructions, which detail the specific regimen to be employed.

Bisacodyl Preparation for Barium Sulfate Enemas

ORAL AND RECTAL:
- Give up to 30 mg of bisacodyl orally the night before the procedure, followed by a 10-mg bisacodyl rectal suppository 1–2 hours before the procedure. Do not eat following administration of the tablets.

Bisacodyl and Magnesium Citrate Preparatory Regimens

ORAL AND RECTAL:
- Preparatory regimens using magnesium citrate, which acts mainly on the small intestine, in addition to administration of the usual oral (up to 30 mg) and rectal (10 mg) dose of bisacodyl also have been used.

Bisacodyl Antepatum Preparation

RECTAL (SUPPOSITORIES):

- To cleanse the colon prior to delivery, a single 10-mg bisacodyl rectal suppository is administered at least 2 hours before onset of the second stage of labor.

Bisacodyl Tannex Preparatory Enema

ENEMA:

- Bisacodyl tannex may be used prior to radiologic examinations or sigmoidoscopic or proctoscopic procedures.
- Give a residue-free diet the day before the prcedure, followed by 30–60 mL of castor oil orally 16 hours before the examination or procedure.
- Prepare a cleansing enema by dissolving bisacodyl tannex equivalent to 1.5 mg of bisacodyl and 2.5 g of tannic acid (one packet of the commercially available bisacodyl tannex product) in 1 L of lukewarm water.
- When used as a radiopaque enema adjuvant, bisacodyl tannex equivalent to 1.5–3 mg of bisacodyl (1–2 packets of the commercially available product) is dissolved in 1 L of barium sulfate suspension. The concentration of bisacodyl tannex should not exceed 0.5% (2 packets of the commercially available product per L).
- Administer the cleansing enema containing bisacodyl tannex the day of the procedure.
- If necessary, repeat the cleansing enema, but total dosage for one entire colonic examination (including the cleansing enema) should not exceed 4.5 mg of bisacodyl and 7.5 g of tannic acid (3 packets of the commercially available preparation), and no more than 6 mg of bisacodyl and 10 g of tannic acid (4 packets of the commercially available product) should be administered during a 72-hour period.

Dulcolax® Prep Kit

ORAL AND RECTAL:

- The regimen begins with a liquid meal at a prescribed time, followed by periodic clear liquid intake throughout the day and scheduled administration of oral laxatives, and concluding with rectal administration of a bisacodyl suppository.
- In the usual regimen, 300 mL of magnesium citrate is administered orally at 4 p.m. the day before the procedure, followed by 20 mg of bisacodyl orally at 6 p.m. the day before the procedure, and concluding with a 10-mg bisacodyl rectal suppository at 5:30 a.m. the morning of the procedure.

Evac-Q-Kwik® Kit

ORAL AND RECTAL:

- Each regimen begins with a liquid meal at a prescribed time, followed by scheduled clear liquid intake at various times and scheduled administration of oral laxatives, and concluding with rectal administration of a bisacodyl suppository.
- In the usual regimen, 300 mL of magnesium citrate is administered orally at 4 p.m. the day before the procedure, followed by 15 mg of bisacodyl orally at 7 p.m. the day before the procedure, and concluding with a 10-mg bisacodyl rectal suppository at 10 p.m. the day before the procedure.
- In the alternative regimen, 300 mL of magnesium citrate is administered orally at 7 p.m. the day before the procedure, followed by 15 mg of bisacodyl orally at 10 p.m. the day before the procedure, and concluding with a 10-mg bisacodyl rectal suppository at 6 a.m. the morning of the procedure.

E-Z-EM® LoSo Prep Kit

ORAL AND RECTAL:

- The regimen begins with liquid meals at prescribed times, followed by scheduled clear liquid intake at various times and scheduled administration of oral laxatives, and concluding with rectal administration of a bisacodyl suppository.
- In the usual regimen, one packet of magnesium citrate is dissolved in 240 mL cold water (yeilding a 16.4-g magnesium citrate solution) and administered orally at 5:30 p.m. the day before the procedure, followed by 20 mg of bisacodyl orally at 7:30 p.m. the day before the procedure, and concluding with a 10-mg bisacodyl rectal suppository at least 2 hours before the procedure.

Fleet® Prep Kits

ORAL AND RECTAL:

- Available in 3 kit combinations containing bisacodyl tablets, sodium phosphate oral solution, and either a bisacodyl suppository (kit #1), a large-volume cleansing enema (kit #2), or a bisacodyl enema (kit #3).
- Each kit can be administered in regimens beginning 18, 24, or 48 hours before the procedure; in most cases, the 24-hour regimen is followed.
- Each regimen begins with a light meal at a prescribed time, followed by scheduled clear liquid intake at various times and scheduled administration of oral laxatives, and concluding with rectal administration of either a bisacodyl suppository, bisacodyl enema, or cleansing ("bag") enema 1 hour before leaving for the procedure.
- In the 24-hour regimen, 45 mL of sodium phosphate is mixed with ½ glass of cold clear liquid and administered orally at 4 p.m. the day before the procedure, followed by 20 mg (or alternative dose per clinician) of bisacodyl orally at 9 p.m. the day before the procedure, and then by either a 10-mg bisacodyl rectal suppository (kit #1), a cleansing enema (kit #2), or a 10-mg (30-mL) bisacodyl enema administered 1 hour before leaving for the procedure.

LiquiPrep® Kit

ORAL AND RECTAL:

- The regimen begins with liquid meals at prescribed times, followed by scheduled clear liquid intake at various times and scheduled administration of oral laxatives, and concluding with rectal administration of a bisacodyl suppository.
- In the usual regimen, 300 mL of magnesium citrate is administered orally at 5:30 p.m. the day before the procedure, followed by 20 mg of bisacodyl orally at 9:30 p.m. the day before the procedure, and concluding with a 10-mg bisacodyl rectal suppository 1 hour before leaving for the procedure.

Tridate® Kit

ORAL AND RECTAL:

- The regimen begins with liquid meals at prescribed times, followed by scheduled clear liquid intake at various times and scheduled administration of oral laxatives, and concluding with rectal administration of a bisacodyl suppository.
- In the usual regimen, 300 mL of magnesium citrate is administered orally at 8 p.m. the day before the procedure, followed by 15 mg of bisacodyl orally at 10 p.m. the day before the procedure, and concluding with a 10-mg bisacodyl rectal suppository at 7 a.m. the morning of the procedure.

Tridate® Dry Kit

ORAL AND RECTAL:

- The regimen begins with liquid meals at prescribed times, followed by scheduled clear liquid intake at various times and scheduled administration of oral laxatives, and concluding with rectal administration of a bisacodyl suppository.
- In the usual regimen, one packet of magnesium citrate is dissolved in 240 mL room-temperature water (yielding a 19-g magnesium citrate solution; allow to dissolve for 20 minutes before drinking) and is administered orally in 2 divided doses at 6 p.m. and 6:15 p.m. the day before the procedure, followed by 15 mg of bisacodyl orally at bedtime (between 9 p.m. and midnight) the day before the procedure, and concluding with a 10-mg bisacodyl rectal suppository at 7 a.m. the morning of (at least 2 hours before) the procedure.

X-Prep® Kit-1

ORAL AND RECTAL:

- There are 3 recommended regimens, depending on the time of day the procedure is scheduled and whether the patients is to be admitted; the sequence of laxative administration is the same for all 3 regimens, with only the scheduled times changing. The sequence of liquid meals and clear liquid intake differs, and the manufacturer's instructions should be consulted for details.
- The regimen begins with an oral laxative, followed by an additional oral laxative, and concluding with rectal administration of a bisacodyl suppository.
- For morning procedures, 2 tablets (Senokot® S) containing standardized senna concentrate (sennosides 8.6 mg) and docusate sodium (50 mg) are administered orally at 7:30 a.m. the day before the procedure, followed by 74 mL (X-Prep® Liquid) containing standardized senna concentrate (sennosides 130 mg) orally at 3 p.m. the day before the procedure, and concluding with a 10-mg bisacodyl rectal suppository at least 1 hour before leaving for the procedure.
- For afternoon procedures, 2 tablets (Senokot® S) containing standardized senna concentrate (sennosides 8.6 mg) and docusate sodium (50 mg) are administered orally at noon with a liquid lunch the day before the procedure, followed by 74 mL (X-Prep® Liquid) containing standardized senna concentrate (sennosides 130 mg) orally at 11 p.m. the day before the procedure, and concluding with a 10-mg bisacodyl rectal suppository at least 1 hour before leaving for the procedure.
- For hospitalized patients admitted the afternoon before the procedure and for late admissions, 2 tablets (Senokot® S) containing standardized senna concentrate (sennosides 8.6 mg) and docusate sodium (50 mg) upon admission the day before the procedure, followed by 74 mL (X-Prep® Liquid) containing standardized senna concentrate (sennosides 130 mg) orally at 6–7 p.m. the day before the procedure, and concluding with a 10-mg bisacodyl rectal suppository at least 1 hour before leaving for the procedure.

Special Populations

Hepatic Impairment

- No specific dosage recommendations for hepatic impairment. Minimally absorbed systemically following oral or rectal administration.

Renal Impairment

- No specific dosage recommendations for renal impairment. Minimally absorbed systemically following oral or rectal administration.

Geriatric Patients

- No specific geriatric dosage recommendations.

Bismuth Subsalicylate

(biz muth) (sub sa lis' i late)

Brand Name: Kaopectate®, Pepto-Bismol®

Why is this medicine prescribed?

Bismuth subsalicylate is used to treat diarrhea, heartburn, and upset stomach in adults and children 12 years of age and older. Bismuth subsalicylate is in a class of medications called antidiarrhea agents. It works by decreasing the flow of fluids and electrolytes into the bowel, reduces inflammation within the intestine, and may kill the organisms that can cause diarrhea.

How should this medicine be used?

Bismuth subsalicylate comes as a liquid, tablet, or chewable tablet to be taken by mouth, with or without food. Follow the directions on the package carefully, and ask your doctor or pharmacist to explain any part you do not understand. Take bismuth subsalicylate exactly as directed. Do not take more or less of it or take it more often than recommended by the manufacturer or your doctor.

Swallow the tablets whole; do not chew them.

Shake the liquid well before each use to mix the medication evenly.

If your symptoms get worse or if your diarrhea lasts longer than 48 hours, stop taking this medication and call your doctor.

What special precautions should I follow?

Before taking bismuth subsalicylate,

- Ask your doctor or pharmacist if you are allergic to salicylate pain relievers such as aspirin, choline magnesium trisalicylate, choline salicylate (Arthropan), diflunisal (Dolobid), magnesium salicylate (Doan's, others), and salsalate (Argesic, Disalcid, Salgesic); or any other medication.
- tell your doctor and pharmacist what prescription and nonprescription medications, vitamins, nutritional supplements, and herbal products you are taking or plan to take. Be sure to talk to your doctor or pharmacist about taking bismuth subsalicylate if you take: anticoagulants ('blood thinners') such as warfarin (Coumadin); a daily aspirin; or medication for diabetes, arthritis or gout.
- If you are taking tetracycline antibiotics such as demeclocyline (Declomycin), doxycycline (Doryx, Vibramycin), minocycline (Dynacin, Minocin), and tetracycline (Sumycin), take them at least 1 hour before or 3 hours after taking bismuth subsalcylate.

- ask your doctor before taking this medication if you have ever had an ulcer, bleeding problem, stools that are bloody or blackened, or kidney disease. Also ask your doctor before taking bismuth subsalcylate if you have a fever or mucus in your stool. If you will be giving bismuth subsalcylate to a child or teenager, tell the child's doctor if the child has any of the following symptoms before he or she receives the medication: vomiting, listlessness, drowsiness, confusion, aggression, seizures, yellowing of the skin or eyes, weakness, or flu-like symptoms. Also tell the child's doctor if the child has not been drinking normally, has had excessive vomiting or diarrhea, or appears dehydrated.
- ask your doctor about taking this medication if you are pregnant or are breast-feeding.

What special dietary instructions should I follow?

Drink plenty of water or other beverages to replace fluids that you may have lost while having diarrhea.

Unless your doctor tells you otherwise, continue your normal diet.

What should I do if I forget to take a dose?

This medication is usually taken as needed. If your doctor has told you to take bismuth subsalicylate regularly, take the missed dose as soon as you remember it. However, if it is almost time for the next dose, skip the missed dose and continue your regular dosing schedule. Do not take a double dose to make up for a missed one.

What side effects can this medicine cause?

Bismuth subsalcylate may cause side effects.

Some side effects can be serious. If you experience this symptom, stop taking this medication and call your doctor immediately:

- ringing or buzzing in your ear(s)

Bismuth subsalcylate may cause other side effects. Call your doctor if you have any unusual problems while taking this medication.

What storage conditions are needed for this medicine?

Keep this medication in the container it came in, tightly closed, and out of reach of children. Store it at room temperature and away from excess heat and moisture (not in the bathroom). Throw away any medication that is outdated or no longer needed. Talk to your pharmacist about the proper disposal of your medication.

What should I do in case of overdose?

In case of overdose, call your local poison control center at 1-800-222-1222. If the victim has collapsed or is not breathing, call local emergency services at 911.

What other information should I know?

Ask your pharmacist any questions you have about bismuth salicylate.

You may notice darkening of the stool and/or tongue while you are taking bismuth salicylate. This darkening is harmless and usually goes away in a few days after you stop taking this medication.

Talk to your doctor, pharmacist, or other healthcare professional if you have questions about dosing information for your medication.

Bismuth Subsalicylate, Metronidazole, and Tetracycline Combination

(biz′ muth sub sal i′ sil ate), (me troe ni′ da zole), (tet ra sye′ kleen)

Brand Name: Helidac®

Important Warning

Metronidazole can cause cancer in laboratory animals. However, it is very important to heal ulcers. Talk to your doctor about the risks and benefits of using this combination containing metronidazole in the treatment of your ulcers.

Why is this medicine prescribed?

Bismuth subsalicylate, metronidazole, and tetracycline combination is used to treat duodenal ulcers. It fights infection by Helicobacter pylori bacteria, which often occurs with ulcers. Treating this infection keeps ulcers from coming back. It usually is used in combination with other ulcer medicines.

This medication is sometimes prescribed for other uses; ask your doctor or pharmacist for more information.

How should this medicine be used?

Bismuth subsalicylate, metronidazole, and tetracycline combination comes as four pills: two pink, round, chewable tablets (bismuth subsalicylate), one white tablet (metronidazole), and one pale orange and white capsule (tetracycline). It usually is taken four times a day at meals and bedtime. Follow the directions on your prescription label carefully, and ask your doctor or pharmacist to explain any part you do not understand. Take this medication exactly as directed.

Do not take more or less of it or take it more often than prescribed by your doctor.

Chew and swallow the bismuth subsalicylate tablets. Swallow the metronidazole tablet and tetracycline capsule whole with a full glass of water (8 ounces). Avoid taking this medication with dairy products or milk. Take the bedtime dose with plenty of fluid to prevent irritation of your throat and stomach.

Continue to take this medication even if you feel well. Most people will take it for 14 days. Do not stop taking it without talking to your doctor.

What special precautions should I follow?

Before taking bismuth subsalicylate, metronidazole, and tetracycline combination,

- tell your doctor and pharmacist if you are allergic to bismuth subsalicylate, metronidazole (Flagyl), aspirin or salicylates, tetracycline, or any other drugs.
- tell your doctor and pharmacist what prescription and nonprescription medications you are taking, especially oral contraceptives and medications that contain aspirin, antibiotics, or anticoagulants ('blood thinners') such as warfarin (Coumadin), and vitamins.
- tell your doctor if you have or have ever had kidney, blood, liver, or Crohn's disease.
- tell your doctor if you are pregnant, plan to become pregnant, or are breast-feeding. This medication may make oral contraceptives less effective. Use a different form of birth control while taking it. If you become pregnant while taking this medication, call your doctor immediately. Tetracycline can cause birth defects and may harm nursing babies.
- remember not to drink alcoholic beverages while taking this medication and for at least 1 day after treatment is finished. Metronidazole causes severe vomiting and illness when taken before or after drinking alcohol.
- plan to avoid unnecessary or prolonged exposure to sunlight and to wear protective clothing, sunglasses, and sunscreen. This medication may make your skin sensitive to sunlight.

What should I do if I forget to take a dose?

Take the missed dose as soon as you remember it. However, if it is almost time for the next dose, skip the missed dose and continue your regular dosing schedule. Do not take a double dose to make up for a missed one. If you miss more than four doses, call your doctor.

What side effects can this medicine cause?

Bismuth subsalicylate, metronidazole, and tetracycline combination may cause side effects. Darkening of the tongue and stool is temporary and harmless. Tell your doctor if any of these symptoms are severe or do not go away:

- headache
- blurred vision
- dizziness

- upset stomach
- diarrhea
- constipation
- loss of appetite
- stomach discomfort

If you have any of the following symptoms, stop taking this medication and call your doctor immediately:

- numbness in your hands or feet
- seizures
- confusion or agitation
- ringing in the ears
- bloody, black, or tarry stools

If you experience a serious side effect, you or your doctor may send a report to the Food and Drug Administration's (FDA) MedWatch Adverse Event Reporting program online [at http://www.fda.gov/MedWatch/index.html] or by phone [1-800-332-1088].

What storage conditions are needed for this medicine?

Keep this medication in the container it came in, tightly closed, and out of reach of children. Store it at room temperature and away from excess heat and moisture (not in the bathroom). Throw away any medication that is outdated or no longer needed. Talk to your pharmacist about the proper disposal of your medication.

What should I do in case of overdose?

In case of overdose, call your local poison control center at 1-800-222-1222. If the victim has collapsed or is not breathing, call local emergency services at 911.

What other information should I know?

Keep all appointments with your doctor and the laboratory. Your doctor may order certain lab tests to check your response to this medication.

Do not let anyone else take your medicine. Ask your pharmacist any questions you have about refilling your prescription.

Talk to your doctor, pharmacist, or other healthcare professional if you have questions about dosing information for your medication.

Bisoprolol

(bis oh′ proe lol)

Brand Name: Zebeta®, Ziac® (as a combination product containing Bisoprolol Fumarate and Hydrochlorothiazide)

Also available generically.

Why is this medicine prescribed?

Bisoprolol is used alone or in combination with other medications to treat high blood pressure. Bisoprolol is in a class of medications called beta blockers. It works by slowing the heart rate and relaxing the blood vessels so the heart does not have to pump as hard.

How should this medicine be used?

Bisoprolol comes as a tablet to take by mouth. It is usually taken once a day. To help you remember to take bisoprolol, take it around the same time every day. Follow the directions on your prescription label carefully, and ask your doctor or pharmacist to explain any part you do not understand. Take bisoprolol exactly as directed. Do not take more or less of it or take it more often than prescribed by your doctor.

Your doctor will probably start you on a low dose of bisoprolol and gradually increase your dose.

Bisoprolol controls high blood pressure but does not cure it. It may take a few weeks before you feel the full benefit of bisoprolol. Continue to take bisoprolol even if you feel well. Do not stop taking bisoprolol without talking to your doctor. Suddenly stopping bisoprolol may cause angina (chest pain), heart attack, or irregular heartbeat. Your doctor will probably decrease your dose gradually.

Are there other uses for this medicine?

Bisoprolol also is used sometimes to treat heart failure. Talk to your doctor about the possible risks of using this medication for your condition.

This medication may be prescribed for other uses; ask your doctor or pharmacist for more information.

What special precautions should I follow?

Before taking bisoprolol,
- tell your doctor and pharmacist if you are allergic to bisoprolol or any other medications.
- tell your doctor and pharmacist what prescription and nonprescription medications, vitamins, nutritional supplements, and herbal products you are taking. Be sure to mention any of the following: calcium channel blockers such as diltiazem (Cardizem, Dilacor, Tiazac, others) and verapamil (Calan, Isoptin, Verelan); clonidine (Catapres); guanethidine (Ismelin); medications for irregular heartbeat such as disopyramide (Norpace); other beta blockers; reserpine (Serpalan, Serpasil, Serpatabs); and rifampin (Rifadin, Rimactane). Your doctor may

need to change the doses of your medications or monitor you carefully for side effects.
- tell your doctor if you have or have ever had asthma or other lung disease; a slow heart rate; heart failure; heart, liver, or kidney disease; diabetes; severe allergies; circulation problems; or an overactive thyroid gland (hyperthyroidism).
- tell your doctor if you are pregnant, plan to become pregnant, or are breast-feeding. If you become pregnant while taking bisoprolol, call your doctor.
- if you are having surgery, including dental surgery, tell the doctor or dentist that you are taking bisoprolol.
- you should know that bisoprolol may make you drowsy. Do not drive a car or operate machinery until you know how this medication affects you.
- remember that alcohol can add to the drowsiness caused by this medication.
- you should know that if you have allergic reactions to different substances, your reactions may be worse while you are using bisoprolol, and your allergic reactions may not respond to the usual doses of injectable epinephrine.

What special dietary instructions should I follow?

If your doctor prescribes a low-salt or low-sodium diet, follow these directions carefully.

What should I do if I forget to take a dose?

Take the missed dose as soon as you remember it. However, if it is almost time for the next dose, skip the missed dose and continue your regular dosing schedule. Do not take a double dose to make up for a missed one.

What side effects can this medicine cause?

Bisoprolol may cause side effects. Tell your doctor if any of these symptoms are severe or do not go away:
- excessive tiredness
- vomiting
- diarrhea
- muscle aches
- runny nose

Some side effects can be serious. The following symptoms are uncommon, but if you experience any of them, call your doctor immediately:
- shortness of breath
- swelling of the hands, feet, ankles, or lower legs
- unusual weight gain
- fainting

Bisoprolol may cause other side effects. Call your doctor if you have any unusual problems while taking this medication.

If you experience a serious side effect, you or your doctor may send a report to the Food and Drug Administration's (FDA) MedWatch Adverse Event Reporting program online

[at http://www.fda.gov/MedWatch/index.html] or by phone [1-800-332-1088].

What storage conditions are needed for this medicine?

Keep this medication in the container it came in, tightly closed, and out of reach of children. Store it at room temperature and away from excess heat and moisture (not in the bathroom). Throw away any medication that is outdated or no longer needed. Talk to your pharmacist about the proper disposal of your medication.

What should I do in case of overdose?

In case of overdose, call your local poison control center at 1-800-222-1222. If the victim has collapsed or is not breathing, call local emergency services at 911.

Symptoms of overdose may include:

- swelling of the hands, feet, ankles, or lower legs
- unusual weight gain
- difficulty breathing or swallowing
- dizziness
- fainting
- shakiness
- sweating
- confusion
- blurred vision
- headache
- numbness or tingling of the mouth
- weakness
- extreme tiredness
- sudden hunger
- pale color

What other information should I know?

Keep all appointments with your doctor. Your blood pressure should be checked regularly to determine your response to bisoprolol. Your doctor may ask you to check your pulse (heart rate). Ask your pharmacist or doctor to teach you how to take your pulse. If your pulse is faster or slower than it should be, call your doctor.

Do not let anyone else take your medication. Ask your pharmacist any questions you have about refilling your prescription.

Dosage Facts
For Informational Purposes

Caution: Do not change your dose, how often you take your medication, or the length of time you are to take it without first talking to your healthcare provider.

The following dosage information was written using medical language for doctors and other healthcare professionals and is provided here for you to check your dosage. The dosage of this drug may differ for different patients. Therefore, always follow your doctor's instructions or the directions on the label. Contact your healthcare provider or pharmacist if you have any questions about the specific dosage of your medication after reviewing this information.

General Dosage Information

Available as bisoprolol fumarate; dosage expressed in terms of the fumarate.

Pediatric Patients

Hypertension†
Combination Therapy

ORAL:

- Some experts state that the initial dosage of the commercially available fixed-combination tablets (containing 2.5 mg of bisoprolol fumarate and 6.25 mg of hydrochlorothiazide) is 1 tablet daily. If needed, dosage may be increased to the fixed-combination preparation containing 10 mg of bisoprolol fumarate and 6.25 mg of hydrochlorothiazide administered once daily.

Adult Patients

Hypertension
Monotherapy

ORAL:

- Initially, 2.5–5 mg once daily.
- Increase dosage gradually up to 20 mg daily.

Bisoprolol/Hydrochlorothiazide Combination Therapy

ORAL:

- Patients in whom BP is not adequately controlled by monotherapy with bisoprolol fumarate 2.5–20 mg daily or those who respond adequately to a hydrochlorothiazide dosage of 50 mg daily, but potassium loss is problematic, can switch to a fixed-combination preparation containing bisoprolol and hydrochlorothiazide.
- Initial use of fixed-combination preparations generally is not recommended, adjust by administering each drug separately, then use the fixed combination if optimum maintenance dosage corresponds to the drug dosages in the combination preparation.
- Alternatively, may initiate daily therapy with the fixed-combination preparation containing bisoprolol fumarate 2.5 mg and hydrochlorothiazide 6.25 mg daily.

CHF†

ORAL:

- Initially, 1.25 mg daily for 2–4 weeks or less in adults with mild to moderately severe heart failure.
- If tolerated, increase to 2.5 mg daily for 2–4 weeks; subsequent dosages can be doubled every 2–4 weeks.
- If deterioration (usually transient) occurs during titration, increase dosage of concurrent diuretic and decrease dosage of β-blocker or temporarily discontinue β-blocker. Do not continue dosage titration until symptoms of worsening heart failure have stabilized. Initial difficulty in dosage titration should not preclude subsequent attempts to successfully titrate the dosage.
- Reduce dosage in patients with CHF who experience symptomatic bradycardia (e.g., dizziness) or 2nd or 3rd degree heart block.

Prescribing Limits

Pediatric Patients

Hypertension†
Combination Therapy

ORAL:

- Some experts state that the maximum dosage of bisoprolol fumarate in fixed combination with hydrochlorothiazide is 10 mg of bisoprolol fumarate and 6.25 mg of hydrochlorothiazide (i.e., 1 tablet of the 10/6.25-mg fixed combination) daily.

Adult Patients

Hypertension
Monotherapy

ORAL:

- Maximum is 20 mg daily. However, JNC 7 currently recommends a lower maximum dosage of 10 mg daily.

Combination Therapy

ORAL:

- Dosage of bisoprolol/hydrochlorothiazide fixed combination generally should not exceed bisoprolol fumarate 20 mg and hydrochlorothiazide 12.5 mg (i.e., 2 tablets of the 10/6.25-mg fixed combination) daily.

CHF†

ORAL:

- Maximum recommended by ACC and AHA: 10 mg once daily.

Special Populations

Hepatic Impairment

HEPATITIS OR CIRRHOSIS:

- Initially 2.5 mg once daily.
- Increase dosage with caution.

Renal Impairment

CL_{CR} <40 ML/MINUTE:

- Initially 2.5 mg daily.
- Increase dosage with caution.
- Discontinue bisoprolol/hydrochlorothiazide fixed combination if progressive renal impairment develops.

CL_{CR} <20 ML/MINUTE PER 1.73 M²:

- Generally, maximum 10 mg once daily.

HEMODIALYSIS:

- Apparently not removed by dialysis; supplemental dose is not required after dialysis.

Geriatric Patients

- Dosage adjustment not required unless appreciable renal or hepatic impairment is present.

Bronchospastic Disease

- Initially, 2.5 mg daily; use the possible lowest dosage.

† Use is not currently included in the labeling approved by the US Food and Drug Administration.

Bortezomib

(bor tez′ oh mib)

Brand Name: Velcade®

Why is this medicine prescribed?

Bortezomib is used to treat people with multiple myeloma (a type of cancer of the bone marrow) who have already been treated with at least one other medication. Bortezomib is also used to treat people with mantle cell lymphoma (a fast-growing cancer that begins in the cells of the immune system) who have already treated with at least one other medication. Bortezomib is in a class of medications called antineoplastic agents. It works by killing cancer cells.

How should this medicine be used?

Bortezomib comes as a solution (liquid) to inject into a vein. Bortezomib is given by a doctor or nurse in a medical office or clinic. It is usually given on a rotating schedule that alternates 2 weeks when bortezomib is given twice a week with 10 days when the medication is not given. During the weeks that bortezomib is given, doses will always be at least 72 hours apart. The rotating schedule may be followed for up to eight cycles. After that, your doctor may decide to continue your treatment, but you will receive bortezomib less often.

Be sure to tell your doctor how you are feeling during your treatment. Your doctor may stop your treatment for a while or decrease your dose of bortezomib if you experience side effects of the medication.

Ask your pharmacist or doctor for a copy of the manufacturer's information for the patient.

Are there other uses for this medicine?

This medication may be prescribed for other uses; ask your doctor or pharmacist for more information.

What special precautions should I follow?

Before using bortezomib,

- tell your doctor and healthcare provider if you are allergic to bortezomib, mannitol, any other medications, or boron.
- tell your doctor and pharmacist what other prescription and nonprescription medications, vitamins, or nutritional supplements you are taking or plan to take. Be sure to mention any of the following: amiodarone (Cordarone, Pacerone); cimetidine (Tagamet); clarithromycin (Biaxin, Prevpac); diltiazem (Cardizem, Dilacor, Tiazac, others); erythromycin (E.E.S., E-Mycin, Erythrocin); fluvoxamine; certain antifungals such as itraconazole (Sporanox) or ketoconazole (Nizoral); medications to treat diabetes or high blood pressure; certain medications to treat human immunodeficiency virus (HIV) or acquired immunodeficiency syndrome (AIDS)

such as indinavir (Crixivan), nelfinavir (Viracept), or ritonavir (Norvir); certain medications to treat seizures such as carbamazepine (Carbatrol, Tegretol), phenobarbital (Luminal, Solfoton), or phenytoin (Dilantin, Phenytek); mibefradil (no longer available in the U.S.); nefazodone; rifabutin (Mycobutin); rifampin (Rifadin, Rifamate, Rimactane, others); troleandomycin (TAO) (no longer available in the U.S.); or verapamil (Calan, Covera, Isoptin, in Tarka, others). Your doctor may need to change the doses of your medications or monitor you carefully for side effects.

- tell your doctor what herbal products you are taking, especially St. John's wort.
- tell your doctor if you or anyone in your family has or has ever had heart disease and if you have or have ever had a herpes infection (cold sores, shingles, or genital sores); diabetes; fainting; high cholesterol (fats in the blood); low or high blood pressure; peripheral neuropathy (numbness, pain, tingling, or burning feeling in the feet or hands) or weakness or loss of feeling or reflexes in a part of your body; or kidney or liver disease. Also tell your doctor if you smoke or drink large amounts of alcohol.
- tell your doctor if you are pregnant or plan to become pregnant. Bortezomib may harm the fetus. Use birth control to prevent pregnancy during your treatment with bortezomib. Ask your doctor if you have questions about types of birth control that will work for you. If you become pregnant while using bortezomib, call your doctor immediately.
- do not breast-feed during your treatment with bortezomib. After your treatment has finished, talk to your doctor or nurse about when it is safe to restart breast-feeding.
- if you are having surgery, including dental surgery, tell the doctor or dentist that you are using bortezomib.
- you should know that bortezomib may make you drowsy, dizzy, or lightheaded, or cause fainting or blurred vision. Do not drive a car or operate machinery or dangerous tools until you know how this medication affects you.
- you should know that bortezomib may cause dizziness, lightheadedness, and fainting when you get up too quickly from a lying position. This is more common in people who have fainted in the past, people who are dehydrated, and people who are taking medications that lower blood pressure. To avoid this problem, get out of bed slowly, resting your feet on the floor for a few minutes before standing up.

What special dietary instructions should I follow?

Talk to your doctor about eating grapefruit and drinking grapefruit juice while taking this medicine.

Drink plenty of fluids every day during your treatment with bortezomib, especially if you vomit or have diarrhea.

What should I do if I forget to take a dose?

If you miss an appointment to receive a dose of bortezomib, call your doctor right away.

What side effects can this medicine cause?

Bortezomib may cause side effects. Tell your doctor if any of these symptoms, or those in the SPECIAL PRECAUTIONS section, are severe or do not go away:

- general weakness
- nausea
- vomiting
- diarrhea
- stomach pain
- anxiety
- back pain
- bone, joint, or muscle pain
- muscle cramps
- difficulty falling asleep or staying asleep

Some side effects can be serious. If you experience any of these symptoms, call your doctor immediately:

- pain, burning, numbness, or tingling in the hands or feet
- weakness in the arms or legs
- changes in the sense of touch
- shortness of breath
- cough
- swelling of the feet, ankles, or lower legs
- hives
- rash
- itching
- difficulty breathing or swallowing
- swelling of the face, throat, tongue, lips, eyes, or hands
- hoarseness
- fever, sore throat, chills, or other signs of infection
- unusual bruising or bleeding
- black and tarry stools
- red blood in stools
- bloody vomit
- vomiting material that looks like coffee grounds
- slurred speech or inability to speak or understand speech
- loss of balance or coordination
- loss of memory
- paralysis (loss of ability to move a part of the body
- vision changes or loss of vision
- loss of consciousness
- excessive tiredness
- pale skin
- fast heartbeat
- fainting
- headache
- thoughts of harming or killing yourself
- difficulty thinking clearly, using good judgment, or understanding reality
- hallucinating (seeing things or hearing voices that do not exist)
- confusion
- restlessness

- thirst
- decreased urination
- loss of appetite
- constipation
- seizures
- skin blisters that are itchy or painful

Bortezomib may cause other side effects. Call your doctor if you have any unusual problems while taking this medication.

What storage conditions are needed for this medicine?

Bevacizumab will be stored in the medical office or clinic.

What should I do in case of overdose?

In case of overdose, call your local poison control center at 1-800-222-1222. If the victim has collapsed or is not breathing, call local emergency services at 911.

Symptoms of overdose may include:
- fainting
- dizziness
- blurred vision
- unusual bruising or bleeding

What other information should I know?

Keep all appointments with your doctor and the laboratory. Your doctor will order certain lab tests to check your body's response to bortezomib.

Dosage Facts
For Informational Purposes

Caution: Do not change your dose, how often you take your medication, or the length of time you are to take it without first talking to your healthcare provider.

The following dosage information was written using medical language for doctors and other healthcare professionals and is provided here for you to check your dosage. The dosage of this drug may differ for different patients. Therefore, always follow your doctor's instructions or the directions on the label. Contact your healthcare provider or pharmacist if you have any questions about the specific dosage of your medication after reviewing this information.

Adult Patients

Multiple Myeloma

IV:
- Standard regimen: 1.3 mg/m² twice weekly for 2 weeks (days 1, 4, 8, and 11), followed by a 10-day rest period (days 12–21).
- For extended therapy of >8 treatment cycles, continue standard 21-day regimen or initiate 35-day maintenance regimen of 1.3 mg/m² once weekly for 4 weeks (days 1, 8, 15, and 22), followed by a 13-day rest period (days 23–35).

- At least 72 hours should elapse between consecutive doses.
- In clinical studies, patients expected to benefit from extended therapy received a median of 7 additional treatment cycles, for a total median of 14 treatment cycles.

Dosage Modification for Peripheral Neuropathy

Adjust dosage and/or frequency of administration if severe peripheral neuropathy occurs.

Administer the adjusted regimen for 2 weeks, followed by a 10-day rest period.

Dosage Modification for Neuropathic Pain and/or Peripheral Sensory Neuropathy

Severity of Neuropathy and Manifestations	Comments
Grade 1 (paresthesias and/or loss of reflexes) *without* pain or loss of function	No dose modification necessary
Grade 1 *with* pain	Reduce dosage to 1 mg/m² twice weekly
Grade 2 (interfering with function but not with activities of daily living)	Reduce dosage to 1 mg/m² twice weekly
Grade 2 *with* pain	Temporarily discontinue; after manifestations of toxicity resolve, reinitiate at dosage of 0.7 mg/m² *once* weekly
Grade 3 (interfering with activities of daily living)	Temporarily discontinue; after manifestations of toxicity resolve, reinitiate at dosage of 0.7 mg/m² *once* weekly
Grade 4 (disabling)	Discontinue therapy

Dosage Modification for Other Severe Nonhematologic or Hematologic Effects

Temporarily discontinue therapy if grade 3 nonhematologic (other than peripheral neuropathy) or grade 4 hematologic toxicities (e.g., grade 4 thrombocytopenia [platelet count <25,000/mm³]) occur.

Once manifestations of toxicity resolve, reinitiate but reduce bortezomib dosage by 25% (i.e., reduce from 1.3 mg/m² per dose to 1 mg/m² per dose; reduce from 1 mg/m² per dose to 0.7 mg/m² per dose).

Administer the adjusted regimen for 2 weeks, followed by a 10-day rest period.

Bosentan

(boe sen′ tan)

Brand Name: Tracleer®

Important Warning

For female patients:

Do not take bosentan if you are pregnant or plan to become pregnant. Bosentan may harm the fetus. If you are sexually active and able to become pregnant, you should not begin taking bosentan until a pregnancy test has shown that you are not pregnant. You must use a reliable method of birth control and be tested for pregnancy every month during your treatment. Hormonal contraceptives (birth control pills, patches, rings, shots, implants, and intrauterine devices) may not work well when used with bosentan and should not be used as your only method of birth control. Talk to your doctor about birth control methods that will work for you. Call your doctor immediately if you miss a period or think that you may be pregnant while you are taking bosentan.

For male and female patients:

Bosentan may cause liver damage. Tell your doctor if you have or have ever had liver disease. If you experience any of the following symptoms, call your doctor immediately: upset stomach, vomiting, fever, stomach pain, yellowing of the skin or eyes, or extreme tiredness.

Keep all appointments with your doctor and the laboratory. Your doctor will order a blood test to be sure your liver is working normally before you start taking bosentan and every month during your treatment. Bosentan may damage the liver without causing symptoms. Regular blood tests are the only way to find liver damage before it becomes permanent and severe.

Bosentan is not available at retail pharmacies. Your medication will be mailed to you from a central pharmacy. This program is required to be sure that all patients who receive the medication are tested for liver damage and pregnancy. Ask your doctor if you have any questions about how you will receive your medication.

You will receive the manfacturer's patient information sheet (Medication Guide) when you begin treatment with bosentan and each time you refill the prescription. Read the information carefully each time and ask your doctor or pharmacist if you have any questions. You also can obtain the Medication Guide from the FDA website: http://www.fda.gov/cder/foi/label/2001/21290MedGuide.pdf.

Talk to your doctor about the risks of taking bosentan.

Why is this medicine prescribed?

Bosentan is used to treat pulmonary arterial hypertension (PAH, high blood pressure in the vessels that carry blood to the lungs). Bosentan may improve the ability to exercise and slow the worsening of symptoms in patients with PAH. Bosentan is in a class of medications called endothelin receptor antagonists. It works by stopping the action of endothelin, a natural substance that causes blood vessels to narrow and prevents normal blood flow in people who have PAH.

How should this medicine be used?

Bosentan comes as a tablet to take by mouth. It is usually taken with or without food twice a day in the morning and evening. To help you remember to take bosentan, take it at around the same times every day. Follow the directions on your prescription label carefully, and ask your doctor or pharmacist to explain any part you do not understand. Take bosentan exactly as directed. Do not take more or less of it or take it more often than prescribed by your doctor.

Your doctor will probably start you on a low dose of bosentan and increase your dose after 4 weeks.

Bosentan controls the symptoms of PAH but does not cure it. It may take 1-2 months or longer before you feel the full benefit of bosentan. Continue to take bosentan even if you feel well. Do not stop taking bosentan without talking to your doctor. If you suddenly stop taking bosentan, your symptoms may get worse. Your doctor may decrease your dose gradually.

Are there other uses for this medicine?

This medication may be prescribed for other uses; ask your doctor or pharmacist for more information.

What special precautions should I follow?

Before taking bosentan,

- tell your doctor and pharmacist if you are allergic to bosentan, any other medications, or corn.
- do not take cyclosporine (Sandimmune, Neoral) or glyburide (DiaBeta, Glynase, Micronase, others) while taking bosentan.
- tell your doctor and pharmacist what other prescription and nonprescription medications, vitamins, nutritional supplements, and herbal products you are taking. Be sure to mention any of the following: anticoagulants ('blood thinners') such as warfarin; cholesterol-lowering medications (statins) such as atorvastatin (Lipitor), fluvastatin (Lescol), lovastatin (Mevacor), pravastatin (Pravachol), and simvastatin (Zocor); hormonal contraceptives (birth control pills patches, rings, shots, implants, and intrauterine devices); ketoconazole (Nizoral); and medications for diabetes. Many other medications may also interact with bosentan, so be sure to tell your doctor about all the medications you are taking, even those that do not appear on this list. Your doctor may need to change the doses of your medications or monitor you carefully for side effects.

- tell your doctor if you have or have ever had anemia (condition in which red blood cells do not bring enough oxygen to the organs) or heart disease.

What special dietary instructions should I follow?

Talk to your doctor about drinking grapefruit juice while taking this medication.

What should I do if I forget to take a dose?

Take the missed dose as soon as you remember it. However, if it is almost time for the next dose, skip the missed dose and continue your regular dosing schedule. Do not take a double dose to make up for a missed one.

What side effects can this medicine cause?

Bosentan may cause side effects. Tell your doctor if any of these symptoms are severe or do not go away:

- headache
- flushing
- itching
- runny nose, sore throat, and other cold symptoms
- heartburn

Some side effects can be serious. The following symptoms are uncommon, but if you experience any of them or those listed in the IMPORTANT WARNING section, call your doctor immediately:

- swelling of the arms, hands, feet, ankles, or lower legs
- sudden weight gain
- fast, pounding, or irregular heartbeat
- fainting
- dizziness
- blurred vision
- pale skin
- confusion
- shortness of breath
- weakness

Male laboratory animals who were given medications similar to bosentan developed problems with their testicles and produced fewer sperm (male reproductive cells) than normal. It is not known if bosentan will damage the testicles or decrease the number of sperm produced in men. Talk to your doctor about the risks of taking bosentan if you would like to have children in the future.

Bosentan may cause other side effects. Call your doctor if you have any unusual problems while taking this medication.

If you experience a serious side effect, you or your doctor may send a report to the Food and Drug Administration's (FDA) MedWatch Adverse Event Reporting program online [at http://www.fda.gov/MedWatch/index.html] or by phone [1-800-332-1088].

What storage conditions are needed for this medicine?

Keep this medication in the container it came in, tightly closed, and out of reach of children. Store it at room temperature and away from excess heat and moisture (not in the bathroom). Throw away any medication that is outdated or no longer needed. Talk to your pharmacist about the proper disposal of your medication.

What should I do in case of overdose?

In case of overdose, call your local poison control center at 1-800-222-1222. If the victim has collapsed or is not breathing, call local emergency services at 911.

Symptoms of overdose may include:

- headache
- upset stomach
- vomiting
- fast heartbeat
- fainting
- dizziness
- blurred vision

What other information should I know?

Do not let anyone else take your medication. Ask your doctor any questions you have about refilling your prescription.

Dosage Facts
For Informational Purposes

Caution: Do not change your dose, how often you take your medication, or the length of time you are to take it without first talking to your healthcare provider.

The following dosage information was written using medical language for doctors and other healthcare professionals and is provided here for you to check your dosage. The dosage of this drug may differ for different patients. Therefore, always follow your doctor's instructions or the directions on the label. Contact your healthcare provider or pharmacist if you have any questions about the specific dosage of your medication after reviewing this information.

Adult Patients
Pulmonary Arterial Hypertension

ORAL:
- Initially, 62.5 mg twice daily for 4 weeks, followed by maintenance dosage of 125 mg twice daily.

Special Populations

Patients with Adverse Hepatic Effects
- If elevations in AST and ALT concentrations are accompanied by manifestations of hepatic disease (e.g., nausea, vomiting, fever, abdominal pain, jaundice, lethargy, fatigue) or bilirubin concentrations are ≥2 × ULN, discontinue bosen-

tan by gradually reducing dosage (e.g., 62.5 mg twice daily for 3–7 days).

- If confirmed (i.e., upon a repeat test) AST or ALT elevations of >3 but ≤5 × ULN develop during bosentan therapy, reduce dosage or interrupt therapy.
- If confirmed AST or ALT concentrations of >5 but ≤8 × ULN, discontinue bosentan by gradually reducing dosage.
- Monitor serum AST/ALT concentrations at least every 2 weeks following dosage reduction or discontinuance.
- May consider reinitiation of bosentan therapy at starting dosage of 62.5 mg twice daily following return of AST/ALT concentrations to pretreatment levels if AST/ALT elevations did *not* exceed 8 × ULN; check serum AST/ALT concentrations within 3 days of reinitiating therapy and every 2 weeks thereafter.
- Manufacturer states that reinitiation of bosentan therapy should *not* be considered if AST/ALT concentrations exceeded 8 × ULN. Clinical experience with reinitiation of bosentan therapy is lacking in such patients, as well as in those with AST/ALT elevations accompanied by manifestations of hepatic disease or by increases in bilirubin concentrations of ≥2 × ULN.

Patients with Low Body Weight
- In patients >12 years of age who weigh <40 kg, recommended dosage for both initial and maintenance therapy is 62.5 mg twice daily.

Brimonidine Ophthalmic

(bri moe′ ni deen)

Brand Name: Alphagan P®
Also available generically.

Why is this medicine prescribed?

Ophthalmic brimonidine is used to lower pressure in the eyes in patients who have glaucoma (high pressure in the eyes that may damage nerves and cause vision loss) and ocular hypertension (pressure in the eyes that is higher than normal but not high enough to cause vision loss). Brimonidine is in a class of drugs called alpha adrenergic agonists. Brimonidine works by decreasing the amount of fluid in the eyes.

How should this medicine be used?

Brimonidine ophthalmic comes as a solution (liquid) to instill in the eyes. It is usually instilled in the affected eye(s) three times a day. Use brimonidine eye drops at around the same times every day, and try to space your three daily doses about 8 hours apart. Follow the directions on your prescription label carefully, and ask your doctor or pharmacist to explain any part you do not understand. Use brimonidine eye drops exactly as directed. Do not use more or less of them or use them more often than prescribed by your doctor.

Brimonidine eye drops may control your condition, but will not cure it. Continue to use brimonidine eye drops even if you feel well. Do not stop using brimonidine eye drops without talking to your doctor.

To use the eye drops, follow these steps:
1. Wash your hands thoroughly with soap and water.
2. Use a mirror or have someone else put the drops in your eye.
3. Remove the protective cap. Make sure that the end of the dropper is not chipped or cracked.
4. Avoid touching the dropper tip against your eye or anything else.
5. Hold the dropper tip down at all times to prevent drops from flowing back into the bottle and contaminating the remaining contents.
6. Lie down or tilt your head back.
7. Holding the bottle between your thumb and index finger, place the dropper tip as near as possible to your eyelid without touching it.
8. Brace the remaining fingers of that hand against your cheek or nose.
9. With the index finger of your other hand, pull the lower lid of the eye down to form a pocket.
10. Drop the prescribed number of drops into the pocket made by the lower lid and the eye. Placing drops on the surface of the eyeball can cause stinging.
11. Close your eye and keep it closed for a few minutes. Do not blink.
12. Replace and tighten the cap right away. Do not wipe or rinse it off.
13. Wipe off any excess liquid from your cheek with a clean tissue. Wash your hands again.

Are there other uses for this medicine?

This medication may be prescribed for other uses; ask your doctor or pharmacist for more information.

What special precautions should I follow?

Before using brimonidine eye drops,
- tell your doctor or pharmacist if you are allergic to brimonidine eye drops or any other medications.
- do not use brimonidine eye drops if you are taking a monoamine oxidase inhibitor such as isocarboxazid (Marplan), phenelzine (Nardil), selegiline (Eldepryl), or tranylcypromine (Parnate).
- tell your doctor and pharmacist what prescription and nonprescription medications, vitamins, nutritional supplements, and herbal products you are taking or plan to take. Be sure to mention any of the following: antidepressants such as amitriptyline (Elavil), amoxapine (Asendin), clomipramine (Anafranil), desipramine (Norpramin), doxepin (Adapin, Sinequan), imipramine (Tofranil), nortriptyline (Aventyl, Pamelor), protriptyline (Vivactil), and trimipramine (Surmontil); barbitu-

rates such as phenobarbital and secobarbital (Seconal); digoxin (Lanoxin); medications for anxiety, high blood pressure, mental illness, pain, or seizures; sedatives; sleeping pills; and tranquilizers. Your doctor may need to change the doses of your medications or monitor you carefully for side effects.

- if you are using any other eye drops, instill them 5 minutes before or 5 minutes after you instill brimonidine eye drops.
- tell your doctor if you often feel dizzy when you sit or stand from a lying position and if you have or have ever had depression; conditions that affect your blood circulation including Raynaud's disease (a condition that causes attacks of low blood circulation to the fingers and toes), thromboangiitis obliterans (a condition that causes poor blood circulation in the hands and feet), and problems with blood flow to your heart or brain; or heart, kidney, or liver disease.
- tell your doctor if you are pregnant or plan to become pregnant. If you become pregnant while you are using brimonidine eye drops, call your doctor. Do not breast-feed while you are using brimonidine eye drops.
- if you are having surgery, including dental surgery, tell your doctor or dentist that you are using brimonidine eye drops.
- you should know that brimonidine eye drops may make you drowsy. Your vision may be blurry for a few minutes after you instill the eye drops. Do not drive a car or operate machinery until you know how this medication affects you.
- ask your doctor about the safe use of alcohol while you are using brimonidine eye drops. Alcohol can make the drowsiness caused by brimonidine eye drops worse.
- tell your doctor if you wear soft contact lenses. Remove your soft contact lenses before instilling brimonidine eye drops and wait at least 15 minutes after using the medication to replace your lenses.

What should I do if I forget to take a dose?

Instill the missed dose as soon as you remember it. However, if is almost time for the next dose, skip the missed dose and continue your regular dosing schedule. Do not instill a double dose to make up for a missed one.

What side effects can this medicine cause?

Brimonidine eye drops may cause side effects. Tell your doctor if any of these symptoms are severe or do not go away:

- itchy, irritated, red, stinging, or burning eyes
- dry eyes
- watery or runny eyes
- red or swollen eyelids
- sensitivity to light
- blurred vision
- headache
- drowsiness
- difficulty falling asleep or staying asleep
- dry mouth
- runny nose and other cold symptoms
- cough
- sore throat
- flu-like symptoms
- pain or pressure in the face
- heartburn

Some side effects can be serious. If you experience any of the following symptoms, call your doctor immediately:

- rash
- difficulty breathing
- seeing specks or flashes of light
- blind spots
- fainting
- dizziness
- upset stomach

If you experience a serious side effect, you or your doctor may send a report to the Food and Drug Administration's (FDA) MedWatch Adverse Event Reporting program online [at http://www.fda.gov/MedWatch/index.html] or by phone [1-800-332-1088].

What storage conditions are needed for this medicine?

Keep this medication in the container it came in, tightly closed, and out of reach of children. Store it at room temperature and away from excess heat and moisture (not in the bathroom). Throw away any medication that is outdated or no longer needed. Talk to your pharmacist about the proper disposal of your medication.

What other information should I know?

Keep all appointments with your doctor.

Do not let anyone else use your medication. Ask your pharmacist any questions you have about refilling your prescription.

Dosage Facts
For Informational Purposes

Caution: Do not change your dose, how often you take your medication, or the length of time you are to take it without first talking to your healthcare provider.

The following dosage information was written using medical language for doctors and other healthcare professionals and is provided here for you to check your dosage. The dosage of this drug may differ for different patients. Therefore, always follow your doctor's instructions or the directions on the label. Contact your healthcare provider or pharmacist if you have any questions about the specific dosage of your medication after reviewing this information.

Pediatric Patients

Ocular Hypertension and Glaucoma

OPHTHALMIC:

- The manufacturer makes no specific dosage recommendations for children ≥2 years of age.

Adult Patients

Ocular Hypertension and Glaucoma

OPHTHALMIC:

- One drop in the affected eye(s) 3 times daily, approximately 8 hours apart.

Brinzolamide Ophthalmic

(bryn xoe′ la mide)

Brand Name: Azopt®

Why is this medicine prescribed?

Brinzolamide ophthalmic is used to treat glaucoma, a condition that increases pressure in the eye and leads to vision loss. Brinzolamide ophthalmic is in a class of drugs called carbonic anhydrase inhibitors. It decreases the pressure in the eye.

This medication is sometimes prescribed for other uses; ask your doctor or pharmacist for more information.

How should this medicine be used?

Brinzolamide ophthalmic comes as eyedrops. One drop is usually applied three times a day. Shake the bottle well before each dose. Follow the directions on your prescription label carefully, and ask your doctor or pharmacist to explain any part you do not understand. Use brinzolamide ophthalmic exactly as directed. Do not use more or less of it or use it more often than prescribed by your doctor.

Brinzolamide ophthalmic controls glaucoma but does not cure it. Continue to use brinzolamide ophthalmic even if you feel well. Do not stop using brinzolamide ophthalmic without talking to your doctor.

To use the eyedrops, follow these instructions:

1. Wash your hands thoroughly with soap and water.
2. Use a mirror or have someone else put the drops in your eye.
3. Shake the bottle well for 10 seconds.
4. Remove the protective cap. Make sure the end of the dropper is not chipped or cracked.
5. Avoid touching the dropper tip against your eye or anything else.
6. Hold the dropper tip down at all times to prevent drops from flowing back into the bottle and contaminating the remaining contents.
7. Lie down or tilt your head back.
8. Holding the bottle between your thumb and index finger, place the dropper tip as near as possible to your eyelid without touching it.
9. Brace the remaining fingers of that hand against your cheek or nose.
10. With the index finger of your other hand, pull the lower lid of the eye down to form a pocket.
11. Drop the prescribed number of drops into the pocket made by the lower lid and the eye. Placing drops on the surface of the eyeball can cause stinging.
12. Close your eye and press lightly against the lower lid with your finger for 2 - 3 minutes to keep the medication in the eye. Do not blink.
13. Replace and tighten the cap right away. Do not wipe or rinse it off.
14. Wipe off any excess liquid from your cheek with a clean tissue. Wash your hands again.

What special precautions should I follow?

Before using brinzolamide ophthalmic eyedrops,

- tell your doctor and pharmacist if you are allergic to brinzolamide ophthalmic, other antibiotics, sulfa drugs, or any other drugs.
- tell your doctor and pharmacist what prescription and nonprescription medications you are taking, especially acetazolamide (Diamox), dichlorphenamide (Daranide), eye medications, methazolamide (Neptazane), products that contain aspirin, and vitamins and herbal products.
- tell your doctor if you have or have ever had kidney or liver disease.
- tell your doctor if you are pregnant, plan to become pregnant, or are breast-feeding.
- if you are having surgery, including dental surgery, tell the doctor or dentist that you are using brinzolamide ophthalmic.
- if you are using another eyedrop medication, use the eye medications at least 10 minutes apart.
- if you get an eye injury or infection, call your doctor to see if you should still use the same eyedrop bottle.
- tell your doctor if you wear soft contact lenses. Wait at least 15 minutes after using the medicine to put in soft contact lenses.
- use caution when driving or operating machinery because vision may be blurred after inserting the drops.

What should I do if I forget to take a dose?

Apply the missed dose as soon as you remember it. However, if it is almost time for the next dose, skip the missed dose and continue your regular dosing schedule. Do not apply a double dose to make up for a missed one.

What side effects can this medicine cause?

Brinzolamide ophthalmic may cause side effects. Tell your doctor if any of these symptoms are severe or do not go away:

- blurred vision
- bitter, sour, or unusual taste after inserting the drops
- dry eyes
- feeling that something is in your eye
- headache
- runny nose

If you experience any of the following symptoms, stop using brinzolamide ophthalmic and call your doctor immediately:

- itching eyes or skin
- redness or swelling of eyes, lips, tongue, or skin
- watery eyes
- eye pain
- skin rash, hives, or skin changes
- difficulty breathing or swallowing
- sore throat
- fever
- chest pain

If you experience a serious side effect, you or your doctor may send a report to the Food and Drug Administration's (FDA) MedWatch Adverse Event Reporting program online [at http://www.fda.gov/MedWatch/index.html] or by phone [1-800-332-1088].

What storage conditions are needed for this medicine?

Keep this medication in the container it came in, tightly closed, and out of reach of children. Store it at room temperature and away from excess heat and moisture (not in the bathroom). Throw away any medication that is outdated or no longer needed. Talk to your pharmacist about the proper disposal of your medication.

What other information should I know?

Keep all appointments with your doctor. Your doctor will order certain eye tests to check your response to brinzolamide ophthalmic.

Do not let anyone else use your medication. Ask your pharmacist any questions you have about refilling your prescription.

Dosage Facts
For Informational Purposes

Caution: Do not change your dose, how often you take your medication, or the length of time you are to take it without first talking to your healthcare provider.

The following dosage information was written using medical language for doctors and other healthcare professionals and is provided here for you to check your dosage. The dosage of this drug may differ for different patients. Therefore, always follow your doctor's instructions or the directions on the label. Contact your healthcare provider or pharmacist if you have any questions about the specific dosage of your medication after reviewing this information.

Adult Patients

Ocular Hypertension and Glaucoma

OPHTHALMIC:

- One drop of a 1% suspension in the affected eye(s) 3 times daily.

Bromocriptine

(broe moe krip′ teen)

Brand Name: Parlodel®, Parlodel® SnapTabs®

Why is this medicine prescribed?

Bromocriptine is used to treat amenorrhea, a condition in which the menstrual period does not occur; infertility (inability to get pregnant) in women; abnormal discharge of milk from the breast; hypogonadism; Parkinson's disease; and acromegaly, a condition in which too much growth hormone is in the body.

This medication is sometimes prescribed for other uses; ask your doctor or pharmacist for more information.

How should this medicine be used?

Bromocriptine comes as a capsule and tablet to take by mouth. It usually is taken once or twice a day. It also may be taken several times a day to treat certain conditions. Follow the directions on your prescription label carefully, and ask your doctor or pharmacist to explain any part you do not understand. Take bromocriptine exactly as directed. Do not take more or less of it or take it more often than prescribed by your doctor. Do not stop taking bromocriptine suddenly without talking with your doctor. It could make your condition worse.

If you are taking bromocriptine for amenorrhea, it usually takes 6-8 weeks for a menstrual period to occur. If you are taking bromocriptine to become pregnant, use a method of birth control other than oral contraceptives (birth control pills) until you have regular menstrual periods; then stop using birth control. If your menstrual period is 3 days late, call your doctor for a pregnancy test. Women who become pregnant while taking this medication should stop taking it and call their doctors immediately. If you do not wish to become pregnant, use a method of birth control other than oral contraceptives while taking bromocriptine.

Are there other uses for this medicine?

Bromocriptine is also used to treat certain tumors in men and women, a condition called neuroleptic malignant syndrome; cocaine addiction; and a painful breast condition. Talk with your doctor about the possible risks of using this drug for your condition.

What special precautions should I follow?

Before taking bromocriptine,

- tell your doctor and pharmacist if you are allergic to bromocriptine, ergotamine, or any other drugs.
- tell your doctor and pharmacist what prescription and nonprescription medications you are taking, especially erythromycin (E-Mycin); levodopa (Sinemet, Larodopa); medications for high blood pressure, migraine headaches, or depression; oral contraceptives; tranquilizers; and vitamins.
- tell your doctor if you have or have ever had kidney, heart, or liver disease, a heart attack, angina (chest pain), mental illness, or circulation problems in your fingers in cold weather.
- tell your doctor if you are pregnant, plan to become pregnant, or are breast-feeding. If you become pregnant while taking bromocriptine, call your doctor.
- you should know that this drug may make you drowsy. Do not drive a car or operate machinery until you know how this drug affects you.
- remember that alcohol can add to the drowsiness caused by this drug.

What special dietary instructions should I follow?

Bromocriptine may cause an upset stomach. Take bromocriptine with food or milk.

What should I do if I forget to take a dose?

If you take bromocriptine several times a day, take the missed dose as soon as you remember it and take any remaining doses for that day at evenly spaced intervals. However, if you remember a missed dose when it is almost time for your next scheduled dose, skip the missed dose. Do not take a double dose to make up for a missed one.

If you take bromocriptine once a day at bedtime and do not remember it until the next morning, skip the missed dose. Do not take a double dose to make up for a missed one.

What side effects can this medicine cause?

Bromocriptine may cause side effects. Tell your doctor if any of these symptoms are severe or do not go away:

- dizziness
- upset stomach
- headache
- fatigue
- vomiting
- constipation

If you experience any of the following symptoms, call your doctor immediately:

- swelling of the feet or ankles
- fast, irregular, or pounding heartbeat
- confusion
- watery discharge from nose

If you experience a serious side effect, you or your doctor may send a report to the Food and Drug Administration's (FDA) MedWatch Adverse Event Reporting program online [at http://www.fda.gov/MedWatch/index.html] or by phone [1-800-332-1088].

What storage conditions are needed for this medicine?

Keep this medication in the container it came in, tightly closed, and out of reach of children. Store it at room temperature, away from light and excess heat and moisture (not in the bathroom). Throw away any medication that is outdated or no longer needed. Talk to your pharmacist about the proper disposal of your medication.

What should I do in case of overdose?

In case of overdose, call your local poison control center at 1-800-222-1222. If the victim has collapsed or is not breathing, call local emergency services at 911.

What other information should I know?

Keep all appointments with your doctor and the laboratory. Your doctor will order certain lab tests to check your response to bromocriptine.

Do not let anyone else take your medication. Ask your pharmacist any questions you have about refilling your prescription.

Talk to your doctor, pharmacist, or other healthcare professional if you have questions about dosing information for your medication.

Brompheniramine

(brome fen ir′ a meen)

Brand Name: Allent® as a combination product containing Brompheniramine Maleate and Pseudoephedrine Hydrochloride, Andehist® Syrup as a combination product containing Brompheniramine Maleate and Pseudoephedrine Hydrochloride, Bromadrine PD® as a combination product containing Brompheniramine Maleate and Pseudoephedrine Hydrochloride, Bromadrine® as a combination product containing Brompheniramine Maleate and Pseudoephedrine Hydrochloride, Bromfed® as a combination product containing Brompheniramine Maleate and Pseudoephedrine Hydrochloride, Bromfed-PD® as a combination product containing Brompheniramine Maleate and Pseudoephedrine Hydrochloride, Bromfenex® as a combination product containing Brompheniramine Maleate and Pseudoephedrine Hydrochloride, Bromfenex® PD as a combination product containing Brompheniramine Maleate and Pseudoephedrine Hydrochloride, Brompheniramine-PSE® as a combination product containing Brompheniramine Maleate and Pseudoephedrine Hydrochloride, Dallergy®-JR as a combination product containing Brompheniramine Maleate and Pseudoephedrine Hydrochloride, Dexaphen® SA as a combination product containing Dexbrompheniramine Maleate and Pseudoephedrine Sulfate, Dimetapp® Cold & Fever as a combination product containing Brompheniramine Maleate, Acetaminophen, and Pseudoephedrine Hydrochloride, Dimetapp® Elixir as a combination product containing Brompheniramine Maleate and Pseudoephedrine Hydrochloride, Drixoral® Allergy/Sinus as a combination product containing Dexbrompheniramine Maleate, Acetaminophen, and Pseudoephedrine Sulfate, Drixoral® Cold & Allergy as a combination product containing Dexbrompheniramine Maleate and Pseudoephedrine Sulfate, Drixoral® Cold & Flu as a combination product containing Dexbrompheniramine Maleate, Acetaminophen, and Pseudoephedrine Sulfate, Lodrane® as a combination product containing Brompheniramine Maleate and Pseudoephedrine Hydrochloride, Lodrane® LD as a combination product containing Brompheniramine Maleate and Pseudoephedrine Hydrochloride, Respahist® as a combination product containing Brompheniramine Maleate and Pseudoephedrine Hydrochloride, Rondec® Syrup as a combination product containing Brompheniramine Maleate and Pseudoephedrine Hydrochloride, Ultrabrom® as a combination product containing Brompheniramine Maleate and Pseudoephedrine Hydrochloride, Ultrabrom® PD as a combination product containing Brompheniramine Maleate and Pseudoephedrine Hydrochloride

Why is this medicine prescribed?

Brompheniramine, an antihistamine, relieves red, irritated, itchy, watery eyes; sneezing; and runny nose caused by allergies, hay fever, and the common cold. It also may relieve the itching of insect bites, bee stings, poison ivy, and poison oak.

This medication is sometimes prescribed for other uses; ask your doctor or pharmacist for more information.

How should this medicine be used?

Brompheniramine comes as a regular tablet, extended-release (long-acting) tablet, and liquid to be taken by mouth. It usually is taken every 4, 6, 8, or 12 hours as needed. Follow the directions on the package label or on your prescription label carefully, and ask your doctor or pharmacist to explain any part you do not understand. Take brompheniramine exactly as directed. Do not take more or less of it or take it more often than indicated by the package label or your doctor.

Do not crush, break, or chew extended-release tablets; swallow them whole.

Do not give extended-release tablets to a child younger than 12 years of age and do not give regular tablets or oral liquid to a child younger than 6 years of age unless directed to do so by a doctor.

What special precautions should I follow?

Before taking brompheniramine,
- tell your doctor and pharmacist if you are allergic to brompheniramine or any other drugs.
- tell your doctor and pharmacist what prescription and nonprescription medications you are taking, especially other medications for colds, hay fever, or allergies; medications for depression or seizures; muscle relaxants; narcotics (medications for pain); sedatives; sleeping pills; tranquilizers; and vitamins. Do not take brompheniramine if you have taken an MAO inhibitor [phenelzine (Nardil) or tranylcypromine (Parnate)] within the last 2 weeks.
- tell your doctor if you have or have ever had asthma, diabetes, glaucoma, ulcers, difficulty urinating (due to an enlarged prostate gland), heart disease, high blood pressure, seizures, or an overactive thyroid gland.
- tell your doctor if you are pregnant, plan to become pregnant, or are breast-feeding. If you become pregnant while taking brompheniramine, call your doctor.
- if you are having surgery, including dental surgery, tell the doctor or dentist that you are taking brompheniramine.
- you should know that this drug may make you drowsy.

Do not drive a car or operate machinery until you know how this drug affects you.
- remember that alcohol can add to the drowsiness caused by this drug.

What should I do if I forget to take a dose?

Take the missed dose as soon as you remember it. However, if it is almost time for the next dose, skip the missed dose and continue your regular dosing schedule. Do not take a double dose to make up for a missed one.

What side effects can this medicine cause?

Brompheniramine may cause side effects. Tell your doctor if any of these symptoms are severe or do not go away:
- drowsiness
- dry mouth, nose, and throat
- upset stomach
- headache
- chest congestion
- diarrhea

If you experience any of the following symptoms, call your doctor immediately:
- vision problems
- difficulty urinating
- muscle weakness
- excitement (especially in children)
- prolonged drowsiness
- dizziness
- skin rash

If you experience a serious side effect, you or your doctor may send a report to the Food and Drug Administration's (FDA) MedWatch Adverse Event Reporting program online [at http://www.fda.gov/MedWatch/index.html] or by phone [1-800-332-1088].

What storage conditions are needed for this medicine?

Keep this medication in the container it came in, tightly closed, and out of reach of children. Store it at room temperature and away from excess heat and moisture (not in the bathroom). Throw away any medication that is outdated or no longer needed. Talk to your pharmacist about the proper disposal of your medication.

What should I do in case of overdose?

In case of overdose, call your local poison control center at 1-800-222-1222. If the victim has collapsed or is not breathing, call local emergency services at 911.

What other information should I know?

Keep all appointments with your doctor.

Do not let anyone else take your medication. Ask your pharmacist any questions you have about refilling your prescription.

Talk to your doctor, pharmacist, or other healthcare professional if you have questions about dosing information for your medication.

Budesonide

(byoo des' oh nide)

Brand Name: Rhinocort® Aqua Nasal Spray

Why is this medicine prescribed?

Budesonide is used to treat symptoms of stuffiness and runny nose due to allergies. It is in a class of drugs called corticosteroids (cortisone-like drugs).

This medication is sometimes prescribed for other uses; ask your doctor or pharmacist for more information.

How should this medicine be used?

Budesonide comes as an aerosol nasal spray to be sprayed in the nose. Budesonide usually is used once or twice a day. Follow the directions on your prescription label carefully, and ask your doctor or pharmacist to explain any part you do not understand. Use budesonide exactly as directed. Do not use more or less of it or use it more often than prescribed by your doctor.

Budesonide treats symptoms in your nose; you may need other drugs if you have other allergy symptoms. Do not stop taking budesonide without talking to your doctor.

Do not use budesonide if you have recently had a sinus infection, nasal bleeding, or surgery inside your nose.

If you have recently stopped taking a corticosteroid drug by mouth, tell your doctor if you have joint pain, muscle pain, depression, or tiredness. These symptoms may mean that you have too little corticosteroid in your body.

Before you use budesonide for the first time, read the written directions that come with it. Ask your doctor, pharmacist, or respiratory therapist to show you how to use the nasal spray, and practice using it in front of them. Follow these steps:
1. Blow your nose.
2. Open the canister by turning the arrow.
3. Shake the canister well, both before and between sprays.
4. Plug one nostril and place the end of the inhaler in the other nostril. Hold your breath and squeeze down on the canister to release the drug into your nose. If your doctor prescribes a second spray, repeat these steps with the inhaler in the other nostril.
5. Close the canister.

What special precautions should I follow?

Before using budesonide,
- tell your doctor and pharmacist if you are allergic to budesonide or any other drugs.

- tell your doctor and pharmacist what prescription and nonprescription medications you are taking, especially allergy and asthma medications and vitamins.
- tell your doctor if you have or have ever had tuberculosis, herpes, or other infections. Avoid people with chicken pox or measles because you may be more sensitive to infection.
- tell your doctor if you are pregnant, plan to become pregnant, or are breast-feeding. If you become pregnant while using budesonide, call your doctor.
- if you are having surgery, including dental surgery, tell the doctor or dentist that you are using budesonide.

What should I do if I forget to take a dose?

Use the missed dose as soon as you remember it. However, if it is almost time for the next dose, skip the missed dose and continue your regular dosing schedule. Do not use a double dose to make up for a missed one.

What side effects can this medicine cause?

Budesonide may cause side effects. Tell your doctor if any of these symptoms are severe or do not go away:
- nose irritation or burning
- bleeding or sores in the nose
- lightheadedness
- upset stomach
- cough
- hoarseness
- dry mouth

If you experience any of the following symptoms, call your doctor immediately:
- difficulty breathing
- white patches in the throat, mouth, or nose
- irregular menstrual periods
- severe acne
- swelling of the face

If you experience a serious side effect, you or your doctor may send a report to the Food and Drug Administration's (FDA) MedWatch Adverse Event Reporting program online [at http://www.fda.gov/MedWatch/index.html] or by phone [1-800-332-1088].

What storage conditions are needed for this medicine?

Keep this medication in the container it came in, tightly closed, and out of reach of children. Shake well before each use. After opening the aluminum pouch, use budesonide within 6 months. Store it at room temperature and away from excess heat and moisture (not in the bathroom). Throw away any medication that is outdated or no longer needed. Talk to your pharmacist about the proper disposal of your medication. Do not throw the container into an incinerator or store near heat or an open flame.

What other information should I know?

Keep all appointments with your doctor and the laboratory. Your doctor will order certain lab tests to check your response to budesonide.

Clean the nasal spray container regularly. Wash the plastic parts in very warm water with a mild soap. The plastic part can be reused with refills of your medication.

Do not let anyone else use your medication. Ask your pharmacist any questions you have about refilling your prescription.

Dosage Facts
For Informational Purposes

Caution: Do not change your dose, how often you take your medication, or the length of time you are to take it without first talking to your healthcare provider.

The following dosage information was written using medical language for doctors and other healthcare professionals and is provided here for you to check your dosage. The dosage of this drug may differ for different patients. Therefore, always follow your doctor's instructions or the directions on the label. Contact your healthcare provider or pharmacist if you have any questions about the specific dosage of your medication after reviewing this information.

General Dosage Information

After priming, nasal spray pump delivers about 32 mcg of budesonide per metered spray and about 120 metered doses per 8.6-g container.

Pediatric Patients

Titrate dosage to the lowest possible effective level.

Seasonal Allergic Rhinitis
INTRANASAL INHALATION:
- Children 6–11 years of age: initially, 32 mcg (1 spray) in each nostril once daily (64 mcg total). May be increased to 64 mcg (2 sprays) in each nostril once daily (128 mcg total).
- Children ≥12 years of age: initially, 32 mcg (1 spray) in each nostril once daily (64 mcg total). May be increased to 128 mcg (4 sprays) in each nostril once daily (256 mcg total).

Perennial Allergic Rhinitis
INTRANASAL INHALATION:
- Children 6–11 years of age: initially, 32 mcg (1 spray) in each nostril once daily (64 mcg total). May be increased to 64 mcg (2 sprays) in each nostril once daily (128 mcg total).
- Children ≥12 years of age: initially, 32 mcg (1 spray) in each nostril once daily (64 mcg total). May be increased to 128 mcg (4 sprays) in each nostril once daily (256 mcg total).

Adult Patients

Seasonal Allergic Rhinitis
INTRANASAL INHALATION:
- Initially, 32 mcg (1 spray) in each nostril once daily (64 mcg total). May be increased to 128 mcg (4 sprays) in each nostril once daily (256 mcg total).

Perennial Allergic Rhinitis

INTRANASAL INHALATION:

- Initially, 32 mcg (1 spray) in each nostril once daily (64 mcg total). May be increased to 128 mcg (4 sprays) in each nostril once daily (256 mcg total).

Prescribing Limits

Pediatric Patients

Seasonal Allergic Rhinitis

INTRANASAL INHALATION:

- Children 6–11 years of age: maximum 128 mcg (2 sprays in each nostril) once daily.
- Children ≥12 years of age: maximum 256 mcg (4 sprays in each nostril) once daily.

Perennial Allergic Rhinitis

INTRANASAL INHALATION:

- Children 6–11 years of age: maximum 128 mcg (2 sprays in each nostril) once daily.
- Children ≥12 years of age: maximum 256 mcg (4 sprays in each nostril) once daily.

Adult Patients

Seasonal Allergic Rhinitis

INTRANASAL INHALATION:

- Maximum 256 mcg (4 sprays in each nostril) once daily.

Perennial Allergic Rhinitis

INTRANASAL INHALATION:

- Maximum 256 mcg (4 sprays in each nostril) once daily.

Special Populations

Hepatic Impairment

- No specific dosage recommendations at this time.

Renal Impairment

- No specific dosage recommendations at this time.

Geriatric Patients

- No specific dosage recommendations at this time.

Budesonide Inhalation Powder

(byoo des' oh nide)

Brand Name: Pulmicort® Turbuhaler®, Pulmicort®Respules®

Important Warning

If you are switching (or have recently switched) from an oral corticosteroid such as budesonide, betamethasone, dexamethasone, methylprednisolone, prednisolone, or prednisone to budesonide inhalation and

suffer an injury, infection, or a severe asthma attack, take a full dose of the oral corticosteroid (even if you have been gradually decreasing the dose) and call your doctor for more directions.

Always carry an identification card that says you may need supplementary doses of an oral corticosteroid during periods of stress (injuries, infections, and severe asthma attacks). Ask your pharmacist or doctor how to get this card. List your name, medical problems, drugs and dosages, and doctor's name and telephone number on the card. Include the name of the oral corticosteroid and the full dose you took before decreasing it.

Why is this medicine prescribed?

Budesonide is used to prevent wheezing, shortness of breath, and troubled breathing caused by severe asthma and other lung diseases. It belongs to a class of drugs called corticosteroids.

This medication is sometimes prescribed for other uses; ask your doctor or pharmacist for more information.

How should this medicine be used?

Budesonide comes as a powder to inhale by mouth. Budesonide is usually inhaled once or twice a day. Follow the directions on your prescription label carefully, and ask your doctor or pharmacist to explain any part you do not understand. Use budesonide exactly as directed. Do not use more or less of it or use it more often than prescribed by your doctor.

Budesonide controls symptoms of asthma and other lung diseases but does not cure them. Improvement in your asthma may occur as soon as 24 hours after taking the medication, but full effects may not be seen for 1 to 2 weeks after taking it regularly. Continue to use budesonide even if you feel well. Do not stop using budesonide without talking to your doctor. Call your doctor if your symptoms do not improve during the first 2 weeks or if they get worse.

Do not use budesonide for rapid relief of asthma attacks. If you do not have another inhaler for prompt relief of breathing difficulties, ask your doctor to prescribe one. If your doctor has prescribed a bronchodilator (a drug to be inhaled for rapid relief of difficult breathing such as albuterol [Proventil, Ventolin]), use it several minutes before you use your budesonide. This helps the budesonide get into the deeper parts of your lungs. Call your doctor immediately if your asthma is not responding to usual treatment.

Before you use budesonide the first time, read the written directions that come with it. Ask your doctor, pharmacist, or respiratory therapist to show you the right way to use the inhaler. Practice using the inhaler in front of him or her, so you are sure you are doing it the right way.

To use the inhaler, follow these steps:

1. Turn the protective cover and lift it off.
2. The first time you use a new budesonide inhaler you must prime it. To do this, hold the inhaler upright (with mouth-

piece up), then twist the brown grip fully to the right as far as it will go, then back again fully to the left. You will hear a click. Repeat. The unit is now primed and ready to load the first dose. You do not have to prime the inhaler again after this, even if you do not use it for a long time.

3. Holding the inhaler upright, load the first dose by turning the grip fully to the right and fully to the left until it clicks.

4. Turn your head away from the inhaler and breathe out. Do not blow or exhale into the inhaler. Do not shake the inhaler after loading it.

5. Hold the inhaler in the upright (mouthpiece up) or horizontal position. Place the mouthpiece between your lips well into your mouth, past your front teeth. Tilt your head slightly back. Close your lips tightly around the mouthpiece and inhale deeply and forcefully. Be sure that the mist goes into your throat and is not blocked by your teeth or tongue. Adults giving the treatment to young children may hold the child's nose closed to be sure that the medication goes into the child's throat.

6. Remove the inhaler from your mouth and hold your breath for about 10 seconds. Do not exhale through the inhaler.

7. If you take 2 puffs (inhalations), wait 2 minutes before taking the second puff.

8. For the next puff and all other puffs, you do not have to prime the inhaler. However, it must be loaded in the upright position right before its use. Turn the grip fully to the right and then fully to the left until it clicks.

9. Replace the protective cap on the inhaler. After each treatment, rinse your mouth with water, but do not swallow the water.

Keep the inhaler clean and dry at all times. Do not bite or chew the mouthpiece. Do not use Pulmicort Turbuhaler with a spacer.

What special precautions should I follow?

Before using budesonide inhalation powder,

- tell your doctor and pharmacist if you are allergic to budesonide or any other drugs.
- tell your doctor and pharmacist what prescription and non-prescription medications you are taking, especially arthritis medications; aspirin; cimetidine (Tagamet); digoxin (Lanoxin); diuretics ('water pills'); estrogen (Premarin); ketoconazole (Nizoral); oral contraceptives (birth control pills); oral corticosteroids; phenobarbital (Donnatal, others); phenytoin (Dilantin); rifampin (Rifadin); theophylline (Theo-Dur); and vitamins or herbal products.
- if you have a fungal infection (other than on your skin), or any other type of infection, do not use budesonide without talking to your doctor.
- tell your doctor if you have or have ever had diabetes; thyroid problems; high blood pressure; mental illness; myasthenia gravis; osteoporosis; herpes eye infection; seizures; tuberculosis; ulcers; or liver, kidney, intestinal, or heart disease.
- tell your doctor if you are pregnant, plan to become

pregnant, or are breast-feeding. If you become pregnant while using budesonide, call your doctor.

- if you are having surgery, including dental surgery, tell the doctor or dentist that you are taking budesonide.
- avoid exposure to chicken pox and measles. If you are exposed to them while using budesonide, call your doctor. Do not have a vaccination or other immunization unless directed to by your doctor.

What special dietary instructions should I follow?

Unless your doctor tells you otherwise, continue your normal diet.

What should I do if I forget to take a dose?

Take the missed dose as soon as you remember it. However, if it is almost time for the next dose, skip the missed dose and continue your regular dosing schedule. Do not take a double dose to make up for a missed one.

What side effects can this medicine cause?

Budesonide may cause side effects. Tell your doctor if any of these symptoms are severe or do not go away:

- dry or irritated mouth or throat
- cough
- difficult or painful speech
- dizziness
- difficulty falling asleep or staying asleep
- neck pain
- stomach pain

If you experience any of the following symptoms, call your doctor immediately:

- vision problems
- white spots or sores in your mouth
- swollen face, lower legs, or ankles
- cold or infection that lasts a long time
- muscle weakness
- increased difficulty in breathing
- skin rash
- unusual bleeding or bruising
- fever
- sore throat
- pain during urination
- muscle aches

If you have been switched from oral corticosteroids to budesonide and are slowly tapering off your dose of the oral medication and you experience any of the following symptoms, call your doctor immediately:

- joint or muscle pain
- increased difficulty in breathing
- tiredness

If you experience a serious side effect, you or your doctor may send a report to the Food and Drug Administration's (FDA) MedWatch Adverse Event Reporting program online [at http://www.fda.gov/MedWatch/index.html] or by phone [1-800-332-1088].

What storage conditions are needed for this medicine?

Keep this medication in the container it came in, tightly closed, and out of reach of children. Store it at room temperature and away from excess heat and moisture (not in the bathroom). Throw away any medication that is outdated or no longer needed. Talk to your pharmacist about the proper disposal of your medication.

What other information should I know?

Keep all appointments with your doctor and the laboratory.

If your sputum (the stuff that you cough up during an asthma attack) thickens or changes color from clear white to yellow, green, or gray, call your doctor; these may be signs of an infection.

Only a small amount of the budesonide powder is released into your lungs when you inhale. Therefore, you may not taste or sense the presence of any medication, but the medication will be working in your lungs.

When there are 20 doses left in the budesonide inhaler, a red mark will appear in the indicator window. This is the time to get your budesonide inhaler refilled. When the red mark reaches the bottom of the window, your inhaler is empty. Discard it. (You may still hear a sound if you shake it; this sound is not the medication. It is the drying agent inside the inhaler.)

Breathing or inhalation devices require regular cleaning. Follow the written directions for care and cleaning that comes with the inhaler.

Do not let anyone else take your medication. Ask your pharmacist any questions you have about refilling your prescription.

Dosage Facts
For Informational Purposes

Caution: Do not change your dose, how often you take your medication, or the length of time you are to take it without first talking to your healthcare provider.

The following dosage information was written using medical language for doctors and other healthcare professionals and is provided here for you to check your dosage. The dosage of this drug may differ for different patients. Therefore, always follow your doctor's instructions or the directions on the label. Contact your healthcare provider or pharmacist if you have any questions about the specific dosage of your medication after reviewing this information.

General Dosage Information

Dose of budesonide inhalation powder is expressed in mcg delivered from the mouthpiece. The amount of drug powder delivered to the lungs depends on factors such as the patient's inspiratory flow.

Each actuation of the Turbuhaler® inhaler contains 200 mcg of budesonide inhalation powder and delivers approximately 160 mcg of budesonide per activation from the mouthpiece.

Delivery of oral inhalation suspension (Pulmicort® Respules®) to the lungs depends on the type of jet nebulizers used, performance of the compressor, and on factors such the patient's inspiratory flow.

Pediatric Patients

Asthma

ORAL INHALATION POWDER:
- Children ≥6 years of age who previously were receiving bronchodilators alone: Initially, 160 mcg twice daily. If required, dosage may be increased to a maximum of 320 mcg twice daily.
- Children ≥6 years of age who previously were receiving inhaled corticosteroids: Initially, 160 mcg twice daily. If required, dosage may be increased to a maximum of 320 mcg twice daily. In patients with mild-to-moderate asthma whose asthma is adequately controlled with inhaled corticosteroids, consider 160 or 320 mcg once daily.

Adult Patients

Asthma

ORAL INHALATION POWDER:
- Initially, 160–320 mcg twice daily in adults previously receiving bronchodilators. If required, dosage may be increased to a maximum of 320 mcg twice daily.
- Initially, 160–320 mcg twice daily in adults previously receiving inhaled corticosteroids. If required, dosage may be increased to a maximum 640 mcg twice daily. In patients with mild-to-moderate asthma whose asthma is adequately controlled with inhaled corticosteroids, consider 160 or 320 mcg once daily.
- Initially, 320–640 mcg twice daily in adults previously receiving oral corticosteroids. If required, dosage may be increased to a maximum of 640 mcg twice daily.

Prescribing Limits

Pediatric Patients

Asthma

ORAL INHALATION POWDER:
- Children ≥6 years of age: Maximum 320 mcg twice daily.

Adult Patients

Asthma

ORAL INHALATION POWDER:
- Maximum 320 mcg twice daily in adults previously receiving bronchodilators alone.
- Maximum 640 mcg twice daily in adults previously receiving inhaled corticosteroids.
- Maximum 640 mcg twice daily in adults previously receiving oral corticosteroids.

Bumetanide

(byoo met′ a nide)

Brand Name: Bumex®
Also available generically.

Important Warning
Bumetanide is a strong diuretic ('water pill'). It is important that you take it exactly as prescribed by your doctor.

Why is this medicine prescribed?

Bumetanide, a 'water pill,' is used to reduce the swelling and fluid retention caused by various medical problems, including heart or liver disease. It also is used to treat high blood pressure. It causes the kidneys to get rid of unneeded water and salt from the body into the urine.

This medicine is sometimes prescribed for other uses; ask your doctor or pharmacist for more information.

How should this medicine be used?

Bumetanide comes as a tablet to take by mouth. It usually is taken once a day, in the morning. Follow the directions on your prescription label carefully, and ask your doctor or pharmacist to explain any part you do not understand. Take bumetanide exactly as directed. Do not take more or less of it or take it more often than prescribed by your doctor.

Bumetanide controls high blood pressure but does not cure it. Continue to take bumetanide even if you feel well. Do not stop taking bumetanide without talking to your doctor.

What special precautions should I follow?

Before taking bumetanide,
- tell your doctor and pharmacist if you are allergic to bumetanide, sulfa drugs, or any other drugs.
- tell your doctor and pharmacist what prescription and nonprescription medications you are taking, especially other medications for high blood pressure, corticosteroids (e.g., prednisone), digoxin (Lanoxin), indomethacin (Indocin), lithium (Eskalith, Lithobid), probenecid (Benemid), and vitamins.
- tell your doctor if you have or have ever had diabetes, gout, or kidney or liver problems.
- tell your doctor if you are pregnant, plan to become pregnant, or are breast-feeding. Do not breast-feed while taking this medicine. If you become pregnant while taking bumetanide, call your doctor.
- if you are having surgery, including dental surgery, tell the doctor or dentist that you are taking bumetanide.

What special dietary instructions should I follow?

Follow your doctor's directions. They may include a daily exercise program and a low-sodium or low-salt diet, potassium supplements, and increased amounts of potassium-rich foods (e.g., bananas, prunes, raisins, and orange juice) in your diet.

What should I do if I forget to take a dose?

Take the missed dose as soon as you remember it. However, if it is almost time for your next dose, skip the missed dose and continue your regular dosing schedule. Do not take a double dose to make up for a missed one.

What side effects can this medicine cause?

Frequent urination may last for up to 6 hours after a dose and should decrease after you take bumetanide for a few weeks. Tell your doctor if any of these symptoms are severe or do not go away:
- muscle cramps
- weakness
- dizziness
- faintness
- thirst
- upset stomach
- vomiting
- diarrhea

If you have any of the following symptoms, call your doctor immediately:
- rapid, excessive weight loss
- sore throat with fever
- ringing in ears
- loss of hearing
- unusual bleeding or bruising
- severe rash with peeling skin
- difficulty breathing or swallowing

If you experience a serious side effect, you or your doctor may send a report to the Food and Drug Administration's (FDA) MedWatch Adverse Event Reporting program online [at http://www.fda.gov/MedWatch/index.html] or by phone [1-800-332-1088].

What storage conditions are needed for this medicine?

Keep this medicine in the container it came in, tightly closed, and out of reach of children. Store it at room temperature and away from excess heat and moisture (not in the bathroom). Throw away any medicine that is outdated or no longer needed. Talk to your pharmacist about the proper disposal of your medicine.

What should I do in case of overdose?

In case of overdose, call your local poison control center at 1-800-222-1222. If the victim has collapsed or is not breathing, call local emergency services at 911.

What other information should I know?

Keep all appointments with your doctor and the laboratory. Your blood pressure should be checked regularly, and blood tests should be done occasionally.

Do not let anyone else take your medicine. Ask your pharmacist any questions you have about refilling your prescription.

Dosage Facts
For Informational Purposes

Caution: Do not change your dose, how often you take your medication, or the length of time you are to take it without first talking to your healthcare provider.

The following dosage information was written using medical language for doctors and other healthcare professionals and is provided here for you to check your dosage. The dosage of this drug may differ for different patients. Therefore, always follow your doctor's instructions or the directions on the label. Contact your healthcare provider or pharmacist if you have any questions about the specific dosage of your medication after reviewing this information.

General Dosage Information

Individualize dosage according to individual requirements and response.

Since the diuretic response following oral or parenteral administration is similar, dosage for oral, IV, or IM administration is identical.

Manufacturer states that bumetanide may be substituted for furosemide in furosemide-allergic patients at approximately a 1:40 ratio (cross-sensitivity between the drugs does not appear to occur).

Adult Patients

Edema

ORAL:
- Initially, 0.5–2 mg daily. Repeat dose at 4- to 5-hour intervals until desired response is obtained or maximum dosage of 10 mg daily is reached.
- For maintenance therapy, effective dose may be administered intermittently.

Hypertension†

ORAL:
- Initially, 0.5 mg daily. 0.5–2 mg daily administered in 2 divided doses is recommended by JNC 7.
- Maintenance dosages of 1–4 mg daily have been used. Higher dosages may be necessary in some patients (e.g., those with renal insufficiency).

Prescribing Limits

Adult Patients

Edema

ORAL:
- Maximum recommended by manufacturer: 10 mg daily.

Special Populations

Hepatic Impairment

Edema

- Use minimum effective dosage; titrate carefully.

Renal Impairment

Edema

ORAL:
- Up to 20 mg daily has been administered. High dosages may be needed to produce an adequate diuretic response in patients with severe renal impairment (i.e., GFR <10 mL/minute).

Hypertension†

ORAL:
- Dosages >1–2 mg daily may be necessary for the management of hypertension† in adults with renal insufficiency. Dosage may be increased until the desired therapeutic response is achieved, adverse effects become intolerable, or a maximum dosage of 10 mg daily, in 2 divided doses, is attained. If an adequate response is not achieved with this maximum dosage, another hypotensive agent (e.g., an adrenergic inhibitor that preserves glomerular filtration rate and renal blood flow) may be added or substituted. Risk of adverse effects (e.g., ototoxicity) at these high dosages should be considered.

Geriatric Patients

- Select dosage with caution because of age-related decreases in hepatic, renal, and/or cardiac function and concomitant disease and drug therapy.

† Use is not currently included in the labeling approved by the US Food and Drug Administration.

Buprenorphine Sublingual and Buprenorphine and Naloxone Sublingual

(byoo pre nor′ feen)

Brand Name: Suboxone®, Subutex®
Also available generically.

Why is this medicine prescribed?

Buprenorphine (Subutex) and buprenorphine and naloxone (Suboxone) are used to treat opioid dependence (addiction to opioid drugs, including heroin and narcotic painkillers). Buprenorphine is in a class of medications called opioid partial agonist-antagonists, and naloxone is in a class of medications called opioid antagonists. Buprenorphine alone and the combination of buprenorphine and naloxone prevent withdrawal symptoms when someone stops taking opioid drugs by producing similar effects to these drugs.

How should this medicine be used?

Buprenorphine and the combination of buprenorphine and naloxone come as sublingual tablets to taken under the tongue. They are usually taken once a day. To help you remember to take buprenorphine or buprenorphine and naloxone, take it around the same time every day. Follow the directions on your prescription label carefully, and ask your doctor or pharmacist to explain any part you do not understand. Take buprenorphine or buprenorphine and naloxone exactly as directed. Do not take more or less of it or take it more often than prescribed by your doctor.

You will start your treatment with buprenorphine, which you will take in the doctor's office. Your doctor will start you on a low dose of buprenorphine and will increase your dose for several days before switching you to buprenorphine and naloxone. Your doctor may increase or decrease your buprenorphine and naloxone dose until the medication works properly.

Place the tablets under your tongue until they melt. This should take 2 to 10 minutes. If you are taking more than two tablets, either place them all under your tongue at the same time or place them under your tongue 2 at a time. Do not chew the tablets or swallow them whole.

Do not stop taking buprenorphine and naloxone without talking to your doctor. Stopping buprenorphine and naloxone too quickly can cause withdrawal symptoms. Your doctor will tell you when and how to stop taking buprenorphine and naloxone.

Are there other uses for this medicine?

This medication may be prescribed for other uses; ask your doctor or pharmacist for more information.

What special precautions should I follow?

Before taking buprenorphine or buprenorphine and naloxone,
- tell your doctor and pharmacist if you are allergic to buprenorphine, naloxone, or any other medications.
- do not take antidepressants ('mood elevators'), narcotic pain killers, sedatives, sleeping pills, or tranquilizers while taking buprenorphine or buprenorphine and naloxone.
- tell your doctor and pharmacist what prescription and non-prescription medications, vitamins, nutritional supplements, and herbal products you are taking. Be sure to mention any of the following: acetaminophen (Tylenol, others); antifungals such as fluconazole (Diflucan), itraconazole (Sporanox), and ketoconazole (Nizoral); carbamazepine (Tegretol); cholesterol-lowering medications (statins); cimetidine (Tagamet); clarithromycin (Biaxin); cyclosporine (Neoral, Sandimmune); danazol (Danocrine); delavirdine (Rescriptor); dexamethasone (Decadron); diltiazem (Cardizem, Dilacor, Tiazac); erythromycin (E.E.S., E-Mycin, Erythrocin); ethosuximide (Zarontin); fluoxetine (Prozac, Sarafem); fluvoxamine (Luvox); HIV protease inhibitors such as indinavir (Crixivan), nelfinavir (Viracept), and ritonavir (Norvir); iron products; isoniazid (INH, Nydrazid); medications for anxiety, mental illness, and sei-

zures; methotrexate (Rheumatrex); metronidazole (Flagyl); nefazodone (Serzone); niacin (nicotinic acid); oral contraceptives (birth control pills); phenobarbital (Luminal, Solfoton); phenytoin (Dilantin); rifabutin (Mycobutin); rifampin (Rifadin, Rimactane); troglitazone (Rezulin); troleandomycin (TAO); verapamil (Calan, Covera, Isoptin, Verelan); and zafirlukast (Accolate). Your doctor may need to change the doses of your medications or monitor you carefully for side effects.
- tell your doctor if you drink large amounts of alcohol and if you have or have ever had adrenal problems such as Addison's disease; benign prostatic hypertrophy (BPH, enlargement of the prostate gland); difficulty urinating; head injury; hallucinations (seeing things or hearing voices that do not exist); a curve in the spine that makes it hard to breathe; gallbladder disease; stomach conditions; and thyroid, kidney, liver, or lung disease.
- tell your doctor if you are pregnant, plan to become pregnant, or are breast-feeding. If you become pregnant while taking buprenorphine or buprenorphine and naloxone, call your doctor.
- if you are having surgery, including dental surgery, tell the doctor or dentist that you are taking buprenorphine or buprenorphine and naloxone.
- you should know that buprenorphine or buprenorphine and naloxone may make you drowsy. Do not drive a car or operate machinery until you know how this medication affects you.
- remember that alcohol can add to the breathing difficulties that can be caused by this medication.
- you should know that buprenorphine or buprenorphine and naloxone may cause dizziness, lightheadedness, and fainting when you get up too quickly from a lying position. This is more common when you first start taking buprenorphine or buprenorphine and naloxone. To avoid this problem, get out of bed slowly, resting your feet on the floor for a few minutes before standing up.

What special dietary instructions should I follow?

Talk to your doctor about drinking grapefruit juice while taking this medicine.

What should I do if I forget to take a dose?

Take the missed dose as soon as you remember it. However, if it is almost time for the next dose, skip the missed dose and continue your regular dosing schedule. Do not take a double dose to make up for a missed one.

What side effects can this medicine cause?

Buprenorphine or buprenorphine and naloxone may cause side effects. Tell your doctor if any of these symptoms are severe or do not go away:
- headache
- stomach pain
- constipation

- vomiting
- difficulty falling asleep or staying asleep
- sweating

Some side effects can be serious. The following symptoms are uncommon, but if you experience any of them, call your doctor immediately:

- hives
- skin rash
- itching
- difficulty breathing or swallowing
- slowed breathing
- upset stomach
- extreme tiredness
- unusual bleeding or bruising
- lack of energy
- loss of appetite
- pain in the upper right part of the stomach
- yellowing of the skin or eyes
- flu-like symptoms

Buprenorphine or buprenorphine and naloxone may cause other side effects. Call your doctor if you have any unusual problems while taking this medication.

If you experience a serious side effect, you or your doctor may send a report to the Food and Drug Administration's (FDA) MedWatch Adverse Event Reporting program online [at http://www.fda.gov/MedWatch/index.html] or by phone [1-800-332-1088].

What storage conditions are needed for this medicine?

Keep this medication in the container it came in, tightly closed, and out of reach of children. Store it at room temperature and away from excess heat and moisture (not in the bathroom). Buprenorphine or buprenorphine and naloxone can be a target for people who abuse prescription medications or street drugs. Keep your medication in a safe place to protect from theft. Throw away any medication that is outdated or no longer needed. Talk to your pharmacist about the proper disposal of your medication.

What should I do in case of overdose?

In case of overdose, call your local poison control center at 1-800-222-1222. If the victim has collapsed or is not breathing, call local emergency services at 911.

Symptoms of overdose may include:

- pinpoint pupils
- extreme drowsiness
- dizziness
- blurred vision
- slowed breathing

What other information should I know?

Keep all appointments with your doctor and the laboratory. Your doctor will order certain lab tests to check your body's response to buprenorphine and naloxone.

In case of an emergency, you or a family member should tell the treating doctor or emergency room staff that you are taking buprenorphine or buprenorphine and naloxone.

Do not inject buprenorphine or buprenorphine and naloxone sublingual tablets. Severe reactions may happen, including withdrawal symptoms.

Do not let anyone else take your medication. Ask your pharmacist any questions you have about refilling your prescription.

Dosage Facts
For Informational Purposes

Caution: Do not change your dose, how often you take your medication, or the length of time you are to take it without first talking to your healthcare provider.

The following dosage information was written using medical language for doctors and other healthcare professionals and is provided here for you to check your dosage. The dosage of this drug may differ for different patients. Therefore, always follow your doctor's instructions or the directions on the label. Contact your healthcare provider or pharmacist if you have any questions about the specific dosage of your medication after reviewing this information.

General Dosage Information

Available as buprenorphine hydrochloride (injection and sublingual tablets); dosage expressed in terms of buprenorphine.

Also available as fixed combination of buprenorphine hydrochloride and naloxone hydrochloride (sublingual tablets); dosage generally expressed in terms of the buprenorphine content.

Adult Patients

Opiate Dependence
Induction

SUBLINGUAL:

- Initially, buprenorphine 8 mg on day 1 and 16 mg on day 2. From day 3 onward, administer buprenorphine in fixed combination with naloxone at the same buprenorphine dose as on day 2.
- To avoid precipitating withdrawal, give the first dose when objective and clear signs of opiate withdrawal are evident.
- Manufacturer recommends that an adequate maintenance dosage, titrated to clinical effectiveness, be achieved as rapidly as possible to prevent undue opiate withdrawal symptoms.

Maintenance

SUBLINGUAL:

- Target dosage of buprenorphine in fixed combination with naloxone is 16 mg daily; however, dosages as low as 12 mg daily may be effective in some patients. Adjust dosage in increments/decrements of 2 or 4 mg daily to a dosage that suppresses opiate withdrawal symptoms and ensures that the patient continues treatment.
- Usual dosage: 4–24 mg daily depending on the individual patient.

SUBLINGUAL:
- The decision to discontinue therapy after a period of maintenance or brief stabilization should be made as part of a comprehensive treatment plan. Both gradual and abrupt discontinuance have been used; the best method for tapering dosage at the end of treatment has not been established.

† *Use is not currently included in the labeling approved by the US Food and Drug Administration.*

Bupropion

(byoo proe' pee on)

Brand Name: Wellbutrin®, Wellbutrin® SR, Wellbutrin® XL, Zyban®
Also available generically.

Important Warning

A small number of children, teenagers, and young adults (up to 24 years of age) who took antidepressants ('mood elevators') such as bupropion during clinical studies became suicidal (thinking about harming or killing oneself or planning or trying to do so). Children, teenagers, and young adults who take antidepressants to treat depression or other mental illnesses may be more likely to become suicidal than children, teenagers, and young adults who do not take antidepressants to treat these conditions. However, experts are not sure about how great this risk is and how much it should be considered in deciding whether a child or teenager should take an antidepressant. Children younger than 18 years of age should not normally take bupropion, but in some cases, a doctor may decide that bupropion is the best medication to treat a child's condition.

You should know that your mental health may change in unexpected ways when you take bupropion or other antidepressants even if you are an adult over age 24 or if you do not have a mental illness and you are taking bupropion to treat a different type of condition. You may become suicidal, especially at the beginning of your treatment and any time that your dose is increased or decreased. You, your family, or your caregiver should call your doctor right away if you experience any of the following symptoms: new or worsening depression; thinking about harming or killing yourself, or planning or trying to do so; extreme worry; agitation; panic attacks; difficulty falling asleep or staying asleep; aggressive behavior; irritability; acting without thinking; severe restlessness; and frenzied abnormal excitement. Be sure that your family or caregiver knows which symptoms may be serious so they can call the doctor when you are unable to seek treatment on your own.

Your healthcare provider will want to see you often while you are taking bupropion, especially at the beginning of your treatment. Be sure to keep all appointments or office visits with your doctor.

The doctor or pharmacist will give you the manufacturer's patient information sheet (Medication Guide) when you begin treatment with bupropion. Read the information carefully and ask your doctor or pharmacist if you have any questions. You also can obtain the Medication Guide from the FDA website: http://www.fda.gov/cder/drug/antidepressants/antidepressants_MG_2007.pdf.

No matter what your age, before you take an antidepressant, you, your parent, or your caregiver should talk to your doctor about the risks and benefits of treating your condition with an antidepressant or with other treatments. You should also talk about the risks and benefits of not treating your condition. You should know that having depression or another mental illness greatly increases the risk that you will become suicidal. This risk is higher if you or anyone in your family has or has ever had bipolar disorder (mood that changes from depressed to abnormally excited) or mania (frenzied, abnormally excited mood) or has thought about or attempted suicide. Talk to your doctor about your condition, symptoms, and personal and family medical history. You and your doctor will decide what type of treatment is right for you.

Why is this medicine prescribed?

Bupropion (Wellbutrin, Wellbutrin SR, Wellbutrin XL) is used to treat depression. Bupropion (Wellbutrin XL) is also used to treat seasonal affective disorder (SAD; episodes of depression that occur in the fall and winter each year). Bupropion (Zyban) is used to help people stop smoking. Bupropion is in a class of medications called antidepressants. It works by increasing certain types of activity in the brain.

How should this medicine be used?

Bupropion comes as a tablet and a sustained-release or extended-release (long-acting) tablet to take by mouth. The regular tablet (Wellbutrin) is usually taken three or four times a day, with doses at least 6 hours apart. The sustained-release tablet (Wellbutrin SR, Zyban) is usually taken twice a day, with doses at least 8 hours apart. The extended-release tablet (Wellbutrin XL) is usually taken once daily in the morning.When bupropion is used to treat seasonal affective disorder, it is usually taken once a day in the morning beginning in the early fall, continuing through the winter, and stopping in the early spring. Sometimes a lower dose of bupropion is taken for 2 weeks before the medication is stopped. Take bupropion with food if the medication upsets your stomach. Take bupropion at around the same time(s) every day. Follow the directions on your prescription label carefully, and ask your doctor or pharmacist to explain any part you do not understand. Take bupropion exactly as directed. Do not take more or less of it or take it more often than prescribed by your doctor.

Swallow the sustained-release and extended-release tablets whole; do not split, chew, or crush them.

Your doctor will probably start you on a low dose of bupropion and gradually increase your dose.

It may take 4 weeks or longer before you feel the full benefit of bupropion. Continue to take bupropion even if you feel well. Do not stop taking bupropion without talking to your doctor. Your doctor will probably decrease your dose gradually.

Are there other uses for this medicine?

Bupropion is also sometimes used to treat episodes of depression in patients with bipolar disorder (manic depressive disorder; a disease that causes episodes of depression, episodes of mania, and other abnormal moods) and to treat attention deficit disorder (ADHD; more difficulty focusing, controlling actions, and remaining still or quiet than other people who are the same age). Talk to your doctor about the possible risks of using this medication for your condition.

This medication may be prescribed for other uses; ask your doctor or pharmacist for more information.

What special precautions should I follow?

Before taking bupropion,

- tell your doctor and pharmacist if you are allergic to bupropion or any other medications.
- tell your doctor if you are taking a monoamine oxidase (MAO) inhibitor such as isocarboxazid (Marplan), phenelzine (Nardil), selegiline (Eldepryl, Emsam, Zelapar), and tranylcypromine (Parnate), or if you have stopped taking an MAO inhibitor within the past 14 days. Your doctor will probably tell you not to take bupropion.
- do not take more than one product containing bupropion at a time. You could receive too much medication and experience severe side effects.
- tell your doctor and pharmacist what other prescription and nonprescription medications, vitamins, nutritional supplements, and herbal products you are taking or plan to take. Be sure to mention any of the following: amantadine (Symmetrel); beta blockers such as atenolol (Tenormin), labetalol (Normodyne), metoprolol (Lopressor, Toprol XL), nadolol (Corgard), and propranolol (Inderal); cyclophosphamide (Cytoxan, Neosar); diet pills; insulin or oral medications for diabetes; medications for irregular heartbeat such as flecainide (Tambocor) and propafenone (Rythmol); medications for mental illness such as haloperidol (Haldol), risperidone (Risperdal), and thioridazine (Mellaril); medications for

seizures such as carbamazepine (Tegretol), phenobarbital (Luminal, Solfoton), and phenytoin (Dilantin); levodopa (Sinemet, Larodopa); nicotine patch; oral steroids such as dexamethasone (Decadron, Dexone), methylprednisolone (Medrol), and prednisone (Deltasone); orphenadrine (Norflex); other antidepressants such as desipramine (Norpramin), fluoxetine (Prozac), imipramine (Tofranil), nortriptyline (Aventyl, Pamelor), paroxetine (Paxil) and sertraline (Zoloft); sedatives; sleeping pills; theophylline (Theobid, Theo-Dur, others) and thiotepa. Your doctor may need to change the doses of your medications or monitor you carefully for side effects.

- tell your doctor if you have or have ever had seizures, anorexia nervosa (an eating disorder) or bulimia (an eating disorder). Also tell your doctor if you drink large amounts of alcohol but expect to suddenly stop drinking or you take sedatives but expect to suddenly stop taking them. Your doctor will probably tell you not to take bupropion.
- tell your doctor if you drink large amounts of alcohol, use street drugs, or overuse prescription medications and if you have or have ever had a heart attack; a head injury; a tumor in your brain or spine; high blood pressure; diabetes; or liver, kidney, or heart disease.
- tell your doctor if you are pregnant, plan to become pregnant, or are breast-feeding. If you become pregnant while taking bupropion, call your doctor.
- you should know that bupropion may make you drowsy. Do not drive a car or operate machinery until you know how this medication affects you.
- talk to your doctor about the safe use of alcoholic beverages while you are taking bupropion. Alcohol can make the side effects from bupropion worse.

What special dietary instructions should I follow?

Unless your doctor tells you otherwise, continue your normal diet.

What should I do if I forget to take a dose?

Skip the missed dose and continue your regular dosing schedule. Always allow the full scheduled amount of time to pass between doses of bupropion. Do not take a double dose to make up for a missed one.

What side effects can this medicine cause?

Bupropion may cause side effects. Tell your doctor if any of these symptoms are severe or do not go away:

- drowsiness
- excitement
- dry mouth
- dizziness
- headache
- nausea
- vomiting
- uncontrollable shaking of a part of the body

- weight loss
- constipation
- excessive sweating

Some side effects can be serious. If you experience any of the following symptoms or those listed in the IMPORTANT WARNING section, call your doctor immediately:

- seizures
- confusion
- hallucinating (seeing things or hearing voices that do not exist)
- irrational fears
- fever
- rash or blisters
- itching
- hives
- swelling of the face, throat, tongue, lips, eyes, hands, feet, ankles, or lower legs
- hoarseness
- difficulty breathing or swallowing
- chest pain
- muscle or joint pain
- rapid, pounding, or irregular heartbeat

Bupropion may cause other side effects. Call your doctor if you have any unusual problems while taking this medication.

If you experience a serious side effect, you or your doctor may send a report to the Food and Drug Administration's (FDA) MedWatch Adverse Event Reporting program online [at http://www.fda.gov/MedWatch/index.html] or by phone [1-800-332-1088].

What storage conditions are needed for this medicine?

Keep this medication in the container it came in, tightly closed, and out of reach of children. Store it at room temperature and away from excess heat and moisture (not in the bathroom). Throw away any medication that is outdated or no longer needed. Talk to your pharmacist about the proper disposal of your medication.

What should I do in case of overdose?

In case of overdose, call your local poison control center at 1-800-222-1222. If the victim has collapsed or is not breathing, call local emergency services at 911.

Symptoms of overdose may include:

- difficulty breathing or swallowing
- dizziness
- fainting
- shakiness
- sweating
- confusion
- blurred vision
- seizure
- hallucinating (seeing things or hearing voices that do not exist)
- loss of consciousness

- rapid or pounding heartbeat
- blurred vision
- lightheadedness
- confusion
- lack of energy
- upset stomach
- jitteriness

What other information should I know?

Keep all appointments with your doctor.

Do not let anyone else take your medication. Ask your pharmacist any questions you have about refilling your prescription.

If you are taking the extended-release tablet, you may notice something that looks like a tablet in your stool. This is just the empty tablet shell and does not mean that you did not get your complete dose of medication.

Dosage Facts
For Informational Purposes

Caution: Do not change your dose, how often you take your medication, or the length of time you are to take it without first talking to your healthcare provider.

The following dosage information was written using medical language for doctors and other healthcare professionals and is provided here for you to check your dosage. The dosage of this drug may differ for different patients. Therefore, always follow your doctor's instructions or the directions on the label. Contact your healthcare provider or pharmacist if you have any questions about the specific dosage of your medication after reviewing this information.

General Dosage Information

Available as bupropion hydrochloride; dosage expressed in terms of the salt.

Pediatric Patients

ADHD†

ORAL:

- Children weighing ≥20 kg: Initially, 1 mg/kg daily in 2–3 divided doses. After 3 days, titrate up to 3 mg/kg daily in 2–3 divided doses by day 7, then up to 6 mg/kg daily in 2–3 divided doses or 300 mg (whichever is smaller) by third week of therapy.
- Alternatively, may give initial dose of 37.5 or 50 mg twice daily with titration over 2 weeks up to a maximum of 250 mg daily (300–400 mg daily in adolescents).
- Pediatric dosage for ADHD generally has ranged from 50–100 mg 3 times daily for conventional tablets or 100–150 mg twice daily for extended-release tablets.

Adult Patients

Major Depression
Therapy with Conventional Tablets

ORAL:
- Initially, 100 mg twice daily. Alternatively, dosage may be initiated at 75 mg 3 times daily.
- If clinical improvement not apparent after >3 days, may increase to 100 mg 3 times daily.
- Dosages >300 mg should not be considered until completion of several weeks of therapy; if no improvement is apparent, then the dosage may be increased to 150 mg 3 times daily. Dosage should not be increased by more than 100 mg every 3 days.
- If no improvement after appropriate trial at 450 mg daily, the drug should be discontinued.

Therapy with Extended-release Tablets

ORAL:
- Extended-release, film-coated tablets (e.g., Wellbutrin® SR): Initially, 150 mg once daily. If tolerated, may increase to 150 mg twice daily as early as fourth day of therapy. Dosages >300 mg daily should not be considered until completion of several weeks of therapy; then, if no apparent improvement, may increase dosage to 200 mg 2 times daily.
- Extended-release tablets (Wellbutrin® XL): Initially, 150 mg once daily. If tolerated, may increase to 300 mg once daily as early as fourth day of therapy. Dosages >300 mg should not be considered until completion of several weeks of therapy; then, if no apparent improvement, may increase dosage to 450 mg once daily.
- When switching from conventional or extended-release film-coated tablets (e.g., Wellbutrin® SR) to extended-release tablets (Wellbutrin® XL), administer same total daily dose when possible.

Smoking Cessation
Therapy with Extended-release, Film-coated Tablets

ORAL:
- Initially, 150 mg daily for the first 3 days of therapy. Initiate 1–2 weeks prior to discontinuance of cigarette smoking.
- Maintenance, 150 mg twice daily. Continue therapy for 7–12 weeks; evaluate need for prolonged therapy after that period based on individual patient assessment.
- Cessation of smoking is unlikely in patients who do not show substantial progress toward abstinence after 7 weeks of therapy, so such therapy should be discontinued at that time in these patients.

Combination Therapy with Extended-release Tablets and Transdermal Nicotine Patches

ORAL:
- Initially, 150 mg daily, and after 3 days increase to 150 mg twice daily while still smoking.
- After about 1 week of therapy, when the patient is scheduled to stop smoking, initiate transdermal nicotine therapy at a dosage of 21 mg/24 hours.
- Taper transdermal nicotine to 14, then to 7 mg/24 hours during the eighth and ninth weeks of therapy, respectively.

Depression Associated With Bipolar Disorder†

ORAL:
- Dosages generally range from 75–400 mg in conjunction with a mood-stabilizing agent (e.g., carbamazepine, lithium, valproate).

ADHD†
Therapy with Conventional Tablets

ORAL:
- Initially, 150 mg daily. May be titrated up to 450 mg daily.

Prescribing Limits

Adult Patients

Major Depression

ORAL:
- Conventional tablets: Maximum 450 mg daily (not >150 mg per dose).
- Extended-release, film-coated tablets (e.g., Wellbutrin® SR): Maximum 400 mg daily (not >200 mg per dose).
- Extended-release tablets (Wellbutrin® XL): Maximum 450 mg daily.

Smoking Cessation

ORAL:
- Extended-release, film-coated tablets (e.g., Zyban®): 300 mg daily (not >150 mg per dose).

Special Populations

Hepatic Impairment

Maximum Dosage for Major Depression in Severe Hepatic Cirrhosis

Dosage Form	Maximum Dosage
Conventional tablets	75 mg once daily
Extended-release, film-coated tablets (e.g., Wellbutrin® SR)	100 mg once daily or 150 mg every other day
Extended-release tablets (Wellbutrin® XL)	150 mg every other day

For management of smoking cessation in patients with severe hepatic cirrhosis, maximum dosage is 150 mg every other day as extended-release, film-coated tablets (e.g., Zyban®).

Use with caution for management of major depression or smoking cessation in patients with mild to moderate hepatic impairment (e.g., mild to moderate hepatic cirrhosis); reduce dosage or frequency of administration as required.

Renal Impairment
- Use with caution. Monitor closely for possible adverse effects (e.g., seizures); reduce dosage or frequency of administration as required.

† Use is not currently included in the labeling approved by the US Food and Drug Administration.

Buspirone

(byoo spye' rone)

Brand Name: BuSpar®, BuSpar® Dividose

Why is this medicine prescribed?

Buspirone is used to treat anxiety disorders or in the short-term treatment of symptoms of anxiety.

This medication is sometimes prescribed for other uses; ask your doctor or pharmacist for more information.

How should this medicine be used?

Buspirone comes as a tablet to take by mouth. It usually is taken two or three times a day. Follow the directions on your prescription label carefully, and ask your doctor or pharmacist to explain any part you do not understand. Take buspirone exactly as directed. Do not take more or less of it or take it more often than prescribed by your doctor.

Continue to take buspirone even if you feel well. Do not stop taking buspirone without talking to your doctor, especially if you have taken large doses for a long time. Your doctor probably will decrease your dose gradually. This drug must be taken regularly for a few weeks before its full effect is felt.

Are there other uses for this medicine?

Buspirone is also used sometimes to treat the symptoms of premenstrual syndrome. Talk to your doctor about the possible risks of using this drug for your condition.

What special precautions should I follow?

Before taking buspirone,

- tell your doctor and pharmacist if you are allergic to buspirone or any other drugs.
- tell your doctor and pharmacist what prescription and nonprescription medications you are taking, especially antihistamines; anticonvulsants such as carbamazepine (Tegretol), phenobarbital (Barbita, Luminal, Solfoton), and phenytoin (Dilantin); dexamethasone (Decadron, others); diazepam (Valium); diltiazem (Cardizem, Dilacor, Tiazac); erythromycin ((E.E.S., E-Mycin, Erythrocin, others); haloperidol (Haldol); ketoconazole (Nizoral); itraconazole (Sporanox); MAO inhibitors [phenelzine (Nardil) and tranylcypromine (Parnate)]; muscle relaxants; nefazodone (Serzone); pain medications or narcotics; rifampin (Rifadin, Rimactane); ritonavir (Norvir); sedatives; sleeping pills; tranquilizers; trazodone (Desyrel); verapamil (Calan, Covera, Verelan); and vitamins.
- tell your doctor if you have or have ever had kidney or liver disease or a history of alcohol or drug abuse.
- tell your doctor if you are pregnant, plan to become pregnant, or are breast-feeding. If you become pregnant while taking buspirone, call your doctor.

- if you are having surgery, including dental surgery, tell the doctor or dentist that you are taking buspirone.
- you should know that this drug may make you drowsy. Do not drive a car or operate machinery until you know how this drug affects you.
- remember that alcohol can add to the drowsiness caused by this drug.

What special dietary instructions should I follow?

You may take buspirone either with or without food, but take it consistently, either always with food or always without food.

Avoid drinking large amounts of grapefruit juice while taking buspirone.

What should I do if I forget to take a dose?

Take the missed dose as soon as you remember it. However, if it is within 4 hours of the next dose, skip the missed dose and continue your regular dosing schedule. Do not take a double dose to make up for a missed one.

What side effects can this medicine cause?

Buspirone may cause side effects. Tell your doctor if any of these symptoms are severe or do not go away:

- drowsiness
- upset stomach
- vomiting
- constipation
- diarrhea
- stomach pain
- headache
- dry mouth
- depression
- excitement
- fatigue
- nervousness
- difficulty sleeping
- lightheadedness
- weakness
- numbness

If you experience any of the following symptoms, call your doctor immediately:

- skin rash
- itching
- fast or irregular heartbeat
- blurred vision
- unusual movements or the head or neck muscles

If you experience a serious side effect, you or your doctor may send a report to the Food and Drug Administration's (FDA) MedWatch Adverse Event Reporting program online [at http://www.fda.gov/MedWatch/index.html] or by phone [1-800-332-1088].

What storage conditions are needed for this medicine?

Keep this medication in the container it came in, tightly closed, and out of reach of children. Store it at room temperature, away from light, excess heat, and moisture (not in the bathroom). Throw away any medication that is outdated or no longer needed. Talk to your pharmacist about the proper disposal of your medication.

What should I do in case of overdose?

In case of overdose, call your local poison control center at 1-800-222-1222. If the victim has collapsed or is not breathing, call local emergency services at 911.

Symptoms of overdose may include:
- upset stomach
- vomiting
- dizziness
- drowsiness
- blurred vision

What other information should I know?

Keep all appointments with your doctor and the laboratory. Your doctor will order certain lab tests to check your response to buspirone.

Do not let anyone else take your medication. Ask your pharmacist any questions you have about refilling your prescription.

Dosage Facts
For Informational Purposes

Caution: Do not change your dose, how often you take your medication, or the length of time you are to take it without first talking to your healthcare provider.

The following dosage information was written using medical language for doctors and other healthcare professionals and is provided here for you to check your dosage. The dosage of this drug may differ for different patients. Therefore, always follow your doctor's instructions or the directions on the label. Contact your healthcare provider or pharmacist if you have any questions about the specific dosage of your medication after reviewing this information.

General Dosage Information

Available as buspirone hydrochloride; dosage is expressed in terms of the salt.

Adult Patients
Anxiety Disorders
ORAL:
- Initially, 10–15 mg daily in 2 or 3 divided doses. Increase dosage in increments of 5 mg daily every 2–4 days according to individual response and tolerance. Maintenance, 15–30 mg daily in 2 or 3 divided doses.

- Reduced dosage recommended in patients receiving concomitant therapy with potent CYP3A4 inhibitor.

Prescribing Limits
Adult Patients
Maximum 60 mg daily.

Special Populations
Hepatic Impairment
- Prolonged elimination. Consider dosage reduction. Manufacturer states that use in patients with severe hepatic impairment is not recommended.

Renal Impairment
- Some clinicians recommend that dosage be reduced by 25–50% in anuric patients. However, other clinicians state that dosage recommendations cannot be made for patients with renal impairment due to variability in plasma buspirone concentrations. Manufacturer states that use in patients with severe renal impairment is not recommended.

Butabarbital
(byoo ta bar' bi tal)

Brand Name: Butisol Sodium®

Why is this medicine prescribed?

Butabarbital, a barbiturate, is used in the short-term treatment of insomnia to help you fall asleep and stay asleep through the night. It is also used as a sedative to relieve anxiety, including anxiety before surgery.

This medication is sometimes prescribed for other uses; ask your doctor or pharmacist for more information.

How should this medicine be used?

Butabarbital comes as a tablet and elixir (liquid) to take by mouth. It usually is taken one to four times a day with or without food. If you take butabarbital once a day, take it at bedtime. Do not mix butabarbital oral liquid with other liquids, especially fruit juice. Follow the directions on your prescription label carefully, and ask your doctor or pharmacist to explain any part you do not understand. Take butabarbital exactly as directed.

Butabarbital can be habit-forming. Do not use butabarbital for more than 2 weeks. Do not take a larger dose, take it more often, or for a longer time than your doctor tells you to. Tolerance may develop with long-term or excessive use, making the drug less effective. Do not stop taking this drug without talking to your doctor, especially if you have been taking it for a long time. Stopping the drug suddenly can cause withdrawal symptoms (anxiousness, sleeplessness, and irritability). Your doctor probably will decrease your dose gradually.

If your sleep problems continue, talk to your doctor, who will determine whether this drug is right for you.

What special precautions should I follow?

Before taking butabarbital,

- tell your doctor and pharmacist if you are allergic to butabarbital, tartrazine (a yellow dye in some butabarbital tablets), aspirin, or any other drugs.
- tell your doctor and pharmacist what prescription and nonprescription medications you are taking, especially acetaminophen (Tylenol); anticoagulants ('blood thinners') such as warfarin (Coumadin); antihistamines; carbamazepine (Tegretol); clonazepam (Klonopin); disulfiram (Antabuse); felodipine (Plendil); fenoprofen (Nalfon); MAO inhibitors [phenelzine (Nardil) or tranylcypromine (Parnate)]; medications for depression, seizures, pain, Parkinson's disease, asthma, colds, or allergies; metoprolol (Lopressor, Toprol XL); metronidazole (Flagyl); muscle relaxants; phenylbutazone (Azolid, Butazolidin); propranolol (Inderal); rifampin (Rifadin); sedatives; sleeping pills; steroids; theophylline (Theo-Dur); tranquilizers; valproic acid (Depakene); verapamil (Calan); and vitamins. These medications may add to the drowsiness caused by butabarbital.
- tell your doctor if you have or have ever had anemia; asthma; seizures; or lung, heart, or liver disease.
- you should know that butabarbital can decrease the effectiveness of oral contraceptives. Use a different method of birth control while taking this medication.
- tell your doctor if you are pregnant, plan to become pregnant, or are breast-feeding. If you become pregnant while taking butabarbital, call your doctor immediately.
- if you are having surgery, including dental surgery, tell the doctor or dentist that you are taking butabarbital.
- you should know that this drug may make you drowsy. Do not drive a car or operate machinery until you know how this drug affects you.
- remember that alcohol can add to the drowsiness caused by this drug.

What should I do if I forget to take a dose?

Do not take the missed dose when you remember it. Skip it completely; then take the next dose at the regularly scheduled time. Do not take a double dose to make up for a missed one.

What side effects can this medicine cause?

Side effects from butabarbital are common and include:

- drowsiness
- headache
- dizziness
- depression
- excitement (especially in children)
- upset stomach

Tell your doctor if any of these symptoms are severe or do not go away:

- nightmares
- increased dreaming
- vomiting
- constipation
- joint or muscle pain

If you experience any of the following symptoms, call your doctor immediately:

- mouth sores
- sore throat
- easy bruising
- bloody nose
- unusual bleeding
- fever
- difficulty breathing or swallowing
- severe skin rash

If you experience a serious side effect, you or your doctor may send a report to the Food and Drug Administration's (FDA) MedWatch Adverse Event Reporting program online [at http://www.fda.gov/MedWatch/index.html] or by phone [1-800-332-1088].

What storage conditions are needed for this medicine?

Keep this medication in the container it came in, tightly closed, and out of reach of children. Store it at room temperature and away from excess heat and moisture (not in the bathroom). Throw away any medication that is outdated or no longer needed. Talk to your pharmacist about the proper disposal of your medication.

What should I do in case of overdose?

In case of overdose, call your local poison control center at 1-800-222-1222. If the victim has collapsed or is not breathing, call local emergency services at 911.

What other information should I know?

Keep all appointments with your doctor.

Do not let anyone else take your medication.

Talk to your doctor, pharmacist, or other healthcare professional if you have questions about dosing information for your medication.

Butoconazole Vaginal Cream

(byoo toe koe′ na zole)

Brand Name: Gynazole-1®, Mycelex®-3

Why is this medicine prescribed?

Butoconazole is used to treat yeast infections of the vagina.

This medication is sometimes prescribed for other uses; ask your doctor or pharmacist for more information.

How should this medicine be used?

Butoconazole comes as a cream to insert into the vagina. It is usually used daily at bedtime. Follow the directions on your prescription label carefully, and ask your doctor or pharmacist to explain any part you do not understand. Use butoconazole exactly as directed. Do not use more or less of it or use it more often than prescribed by your doctor.

To use the vaginal cream, read the instructions provided with the medication and follow these steps:

1. Fill the special applicator that comes with the cream to the level indicated.
2. Lie on your back with your knees drawn upward and spread apart.
3. Insert the applicator high into your vagina (unless you are pregnant), and then push the plunger to release the medication. If you are pregnant, insert the applicator gently. If you feel resistance (hard to insert), do not try to insert it further; call your doctor.
4. Withdraw the applicator and discard.
5. Wash your hands promptly to avoid spreading the infection.

The dose should be applied when you lie down to go to bed. The drug works best if you do not get up again after applying it except to wash your hands. You may wish to wear a sanitary napkin to protect your clothing against stains. Do not use a tampon because it will absorb the drug. Do not douche unless your doctor tells you to do so.

Continue to use butoconazole even if you feel well. Do not stop using butoconazole without talking to your doctor. Continue using this medication during your menstrual period.

What special precautions should I follow?

Before using butoconazole,

- tell your doctor and pharmacist if you are allergic to butoconazole or any other drugs.
- tell your doctor and pharmacist what prescription and nonprescription drugs you are taking, especially antibiotic medications and vitamins.
- tell your doctor if you have or have ever had diabetes, problems with your immune system, human immuno-deficiency virus infection (HIV), or acquired immuno-deficiency syndrome (AIDS).
- tell your doctor if you are pregnant, plan to become pregnant, or are breast-feeding. If you become pregnant while using butoconazole, call your doctor.

What should I do if I forget to take a dose?

Insert the missed dose as soon as you remember it. However, if it is almost time for the next dose, skip the missed dose and continue your regular dosing schedule. Do not insert a double dose to make up for a missed one.

What side effects can this medicine cause?

Butoconazole may cause side effects. If you experience any of the following symptoms, call your doctor immediately:

- burning in vagina when cream is inserted
- irritation in vagina when cream is inserted
- stomach pain
- fever
- foul-smelling discharge

If you experience a serious side effect, you or your doctor may send a report to the Food and Drug Administration's (FDA) MedWatch Adverse Event Reporting program online [at http://www.fda.gov/MedWatch/index.html] or by phone [1-800-332-1088].

What storage conditions are needed for this medicine?

Keep this medication in the container it came in, tightly closed, and out of reach of children. Store it at room temperature and away from excess heat and moisture (not in the bathroom). Do not freeze. Throw away any medication that is outdated or no longer needed. Talk to your pharmacist about the proper disposal of your medication.

What other information should I know?

Keep all appointments with your doctor. Butoconazole is for external use only. Do not let cream get into your eyes or mouth, and do not swallow it.

Refrain from sexual intercourse. An ingredient in the cream may weaken certain latex products like condoms or diaphragms; do not use such products within 72 hours of using this medication. Wear clean cotton panties (or panties with cotton crotches), not panties made of nylon, rayon, or other synthetic fabrics.

Do not let anyone else use your medication. Ask your pharmacist any questions you have about refilling your prescription. If you still have symptoms of infection after you finish the butoconazole, call your doctor.

Dosage Facts
For Informational Purposes

Caution: Do not change your dose, how often you take your medication, or the length of time you

are to take it without first talking to your health-care provider.

The following dosage information was written using medical language for doctors and other healthcare professionals and is provided here for you to check your dosage. The dosage of this drug may differ for different patients. Therefore, always follow your doctor's instructions or the directions on the label. Contact your healthcare provider or pharmacist if you have any questions about the specific dosage of your medication after reviewing this information.

Pediatric Patients
Uncomplicated Vulvovaginal Candidiasis
INTRAVAGINAL:
- Mycelex®-3: Children ≥12 years of age: One applicatorful of 2% cream (approximately 100 mg of the drug) once daily at bedtime for 3 consecutive days. May be used for *self-medication*.

Adult Patients
Uncomplicated Vulvovaginal Candidiasis
INTRAVAGINAL:
- Gynazole-1®: One applicatorful of 2% cream (approximately 100 mg of the drug) as a single dose.
- Mycelex®-3: One applicatorful of 2% cream (approximately 100 mg of the drug) once daily at bedtime for 3 consecutive days. May be used for *self-medication*.
- If clinical symptoms persist, tests should be repeated to rule out other pathogens, to confirm the original diagnosis, and to rule out other conditions that may predispose a patient to recurrent vaginal fungal infections.

HIV Infected Patients
INTRAVAGINAL:
- Use same intravaginal regimen recommended for other patients. Some experts recommend a duration of 3–7 days. Maintenance regimen of an intravaginal azole can be considered for those with recurrent episodes; *routine* primary or secondary prophylaxis (long-term suppressive or chronic maintenance therapy) not recommended.

Complicated Vulvovaginal Candidiasis
Recurrent Vulvovaginal Infections Caused by Candida albicans
INTRAVAGINAL:
- CDC and others recommend an initial intensive regimen (7–14 days of an intravaginal azole or 3-dose regimen of oral fluconazole) to achieve mycologic remission, followed by an appropriate maintenance regimen (6-month regimen of once-weekly oral fluconazole or, alternatively, an intravaginal azole given intermittently).

Other Complicated Vulvovaginal Infections
INTRAVAGINAL:
- CDC and others recommend 7–14 days of an intravaginal azole for vulvovaginal candidasis that is severe, caused by *Candida* other than *C. albicans*, or occurring in women with underlying medical conditions.

Butorphanol Injection
(byoo tor′ fa nole)

Brand Name: Stadol®
Also available generically.

About Your Treatment
Your doctor has ordered butorphanol, an analgesic (painkiller), to relieve your pain. The drug will be injected into a large muscle (such as your buttock or hip) or a vein.

You will probably receive butorphanol every 3 to 4 hours as needed for pain. Your doctor may also order other pain medications to make you more comfortable. This medication is sometimes prescribed for other uses; ask your doctor or pharmacist for more information.

Your health care provider (doctor, nurse, or pharmacist) may measure the effectiveness and side effects of your treatment using laboratory tests and physical examinations. It is important to keep all appointments with your doctor and the laboratory. The length of treatment depends on how you respond to the medication.

Precautions
Before administering butorphanol,
- tell your doctor and pharmacist if you are allergic to butorphanol or any other drugs.
- tell your doctor and pharmacist what prescription and nonprescription medications you are taking, especially antidepressants; medications for cough, cold, or allergies; naloxone (Narcan); naltrexone (ReVia); other pain relievers; sedatives; sleeping pills; tranquilizers; and vitamins.
- tell your doctor if you have or have ever had breathing difficulties including asthma and other respiratory diseases, liver or kidney disease, severe inflammatory bowel disease, or a history of drug dependence.
- tell your doctor if you are pregnant, plan to become pregnant, or are breast-feeding. If you become pregnant while taking butorphanol, call your doctor.
- if you are having surgery, including dental surgery, tell the doctor or dentist that you are taking butorphanol.
- you should know that this drug may make you drowsy. Do not drive a car or operate machinery until you know how butorphanol will affect you.
- remember that alcohol can add to the drowsiness caused by this drug.

Administering Your Medication
Before you administer butorphanol, look at the solution closely. It should be clear and free of floating material. Observe the solution container to make sure there are no leaks. Do not use the solution if it is discolored, if it contains particles, or if the container leaks. Use a new solution, but show the damaged one to your health care provider.

It is important that you use your medication exactly as directed. Butorphanol can be habit forming. Do not administer it more often or for a longer period than your doctor tells you. Do not change your dosing schedule without talking to your health care provider.

Side Effects

Butorphanol may cause side effects. Tell your doctor if any of these symptoms are severe or do not go away:

- upset stomach
- vomiting
- dry mouth
- stomach pain
- dizziness
- lightheadedness
- drowsiness
- headache
- difficulty sleeping
- constipation
- itchy skin
- unpleasant taste
- confusion or hallucinations
- unusual weakness
- nervousness, anxiety, or agitation

If you experience either of the following symptoms, call your doctor immediately:

- difficulty breathing
- fainting

If you experience a serious side effect, you or your doctor may send a report to the Food and Drug Administration's (FDA) MedWatch Adverse Event Reporting program online [at http://www.fda.gov/MedWatch/index.html] or by phone [1-800-332-1088].

Storage Conditions

- Your health care provider will probably give you a several-day supply of butorphanol at a time and provide you with directions on how to prepare each dose. Store the vials at room temperature.

Store your medication only as directed. Make sure you understand what you need to store your medication properly.

Keep your supplies in a clean, dry place when you are not using them, and keep all medications and supplies out of the reach of children. Your health care provider will tell you how to throw away used needles, syringes, tubing, and containers to avoid accidental injury.

Signs of Infection

If you are receiving butorphanol in your vein or under your skin, you need to know the symptoms of a catheter-related infection (an infection where the needle enters your vein or skin). If you experience any of these effects near your intravenous catheter, tell your health care provider as soon as possible:

- tenderness

- warmth
- irritation
- drainage
- redness
- swelling
- pain

Dosage Facts
For Informational Purposes

Caution: Do not change your dose, how often you take your medication, or the length of time you are to take it without first talking to your healthcare provider.

The following dosage information was written using medical language for doctors and other healthcare professionals and is provided here for you to check your dosage. The dosage of this drug may differ for different patients. Therefore, always follow your doctor's instructions or the directions on the label. Contact your healthcare provider or pharmacist if you have any questions about the specific dosage of your medication after reviewing this information.

General Dosage Information

Available as butorphanol tartrate; dosage expressed in terms of the salt.

After initial priming, the nasal solution spray pump delivers about 14–15 metered doses containing 1 mg per spray. If repriming of the pump is necessary, the spray pump will deliver about 8–10 metered doses, depending on the extent of repriming.

Adult Patients

Pain

IV:
- Initially, 1 mg; may repeat dose every 3–4 hours as necessary. Usual effective dosage, depending on severity of pain, is 0.5–2 mg repeated every 3–4 hours.

IM:
- Initially, 2 mg in patients able to remain recumbent; may repeat dose every 3–4 hours as necessary. Usual effective dosage, depending on severity of pain, is 1–4 mg repeated every 3–4 hours.

Preoperative Sedation and Analgesia

IM:
- Usual dosage is 2 mg administered 60–90 minutes before surgery.

Supplement to Surgical Anesthesia

IV:
- 2 mg shortly before induction of anesthesia and/or 0.5–1 mg administered during anesthesia in increments up to 0.06 mg/kg (depending on previous administration of sedatives, analgesics, and hypnotic agents). Usual total dose is 4–12.5 mg (approximately 0.06–0.18 mg/kg).

Obstetric Analgesia

IV OR IM:

- 1–2 mg administered in patients at full term in early labor; may repeat after 4 hours. Use alternative analgesia if delivery expected within 4 hours.

Prescribing Limits

Adult Patients

Pain

IM:

- Maximum 4 mg as a single dose.

Special Populations

Hepatic Impairment

Pain

IV:

- Initially, 0.5 mg. If necessary, repeat dose at an interval of ≥6 hours.

IM:

- Initially, 1 mg. If necessary, repeat dose at an interval of ≥6 hours.

Renal Impairment

- Patients with renal impairment may receive the same IV or IM dosages as patients with hepatic impairment.

Geriatric Patients

- Geriatric patients may receive the same IV or IM dosages as patients with hepatic impairment.

Butorphanol Nasal Spray

(byoo tor′ fa nole)

Brand Name: Stadol® NS®
Also available generically.

Why is this medicine prescribed?

Butorphanol nasal spray is used to relieve moderate to severe pain. It also is used to manage migraine headaches.

This medication is sometimes prescribed for other uses; ask your doctor or pharmacist for more information.

How should this medicine be used?

Butorphanol nasal spray comes in a pump. It usually is used as one spray in one nostril. If pain relief does not occur within 60-90 minutes, another single spray may be used. This two-dose sequence usually is repeated every 3-4 hours as needed. Follow the directions on your prescription label carefully, and ask your doctor or pharmacist to explain any part you do not understand.

Before you use butorphanol for the first time, read the written directions provided by the manufacturer. The pump must be primed (made ready to work) if it is not used for 48 hours or longer. One bottle provides approximately 8-10 doses (if priming is needed) or 14 or 15 doses (if no priming is needed between any doses).

To use the pump, follow these directions:

1. Wash your hands.
2. Gently blow your nose to clear your nasal passages.
3. Remove the clear cover and protective clip from the bottle.
4. With the nasal sprayer aimed away from all people and animals, prime the pump if needed. To prime the pump, pump the spray bottle firmly and quickly (up to eight strokes) until a fine spray appears.
5. Insert the tip of the sprayer approximately 1/4 inch into one nostril, pointing the tip toward the back of your nose.
6. Close your other nostril with your finger and tilt your head slightly forward.
7. Pump the spray firmly and quickly one time and sniff gently with your mouth closed.
8. Remove the sprayer from your nose.
9. Replace the protective clip and cover on the spray bottle.

Use butorphanol nasal spray exactly as directed. There is a small chance that the drug can be habit-forming. Do not use a larger dose, use it more often, or for a longer period than your doctor tells you to.

What special precautions should I follow?

Before using butorphanol nasal spray,

- tell your doctor and pharmacist if you are allergic to butorphanol or any other drugs.
- tell your doctor and pharmacist what prescription and nonprescription medications you are taking, especially other pain relievers; antidepressants; medications for cough, cold, or allergies; nasal sprays; sedatives; sleeping pills; tranquilizers; and vitamins.
- tell your doctor if you have or have ever had liver, kidney, lung, or heart disease.
- tell your doctor if you are pregnant, plan to become pregnant, or are breast-feeding. If you become pregnant while taking butorphanol nasal spray, call your doctor.
- if you are having surgery, including dental surgery, tell the doctor or dentist that you are taking butorphanol nasal spray.
- you should know that this drug may make you drowsy or dizzy. Do not drive a car or operate machinery for at least one hour after using butorphanol and until you no longer feel drowsy or dizzy.
- remember that alcohol can add to the drowsiness caused by this drug. You should not drink alcohol while using butorphanol.

What should I do if I forget to take a dose?

Butorphanol nasal spray usually is used as needed. If your doctor has told you to use butorphanol nasal spray regularly, use the missed dose as soon as you remember it. However, if it is almost time for the next dose, skip the missed dose and continue your regular dosing schedule. Do not use a double dose to make up for a missed one.

What side effects can this medicine cause?

Butorphanol nasal spray may cause side effects. Tell your doctor if any of these symptoms are severe or do not go away:

- drowsiness
- lightheadedness
- dizziness
- upset stomach
- vomiting
- headache
- congestion
- runny nose
- sore throat
- ringing in the ears

If you experience any of the following symptoms, call your doctor immediately:

- difficulty breathing
- fainting
- irregular heartbeat

If you experience a serious side effect, you or your doctor may send a report to the Food and Drug Administration's (FDA) MedWatch Adverse Event Reporting program online [at http://www.fda.gov/MedWatch/index.html] or by phone [1-800-332-1088].

What storage conditions are needed for this medicine?

After each use, replace the protective clip and clear cover on the spray bottle and return it to its child-resistant container. Store it at room temperature and away from excess heat and moisture (not in the bathroom). Throw away any medication that is outdated or no longer needed. Talk to your pharmacist about the proper disposal of your medication.

What should I do in case of overdose?

In case of overdose, call your local poison control center at 1-800-222-1222. If the victim has collapsed or is not breathing, call local emergency services at 911.

What other information should I know?

Keep all appointments with your doctor.

Do not let anyone else use your medication. Ask your pharmacist any questions you have about refilling your prescription.

Dosage Facts
For Informational Purposes

Caution: Do not change your dose, how often you take your medication, or the length of time you

are to take it without first talking to your healthcare provider.

The following dosage information was written using medical language for doctors and other healthcare professionals and is provided here for you to check your dosage. The dosage of this drug may differ for different patients. Therefore, always follow your doctor's instructions or the directions on the label. Contact your healthcare provider or pharmacist if you have any questions about the specific dosage of your medication after reviewing this information.

General Dosage Information

Available as butorphanol tartrate; dosage expressed in terms of the salt.

After initial priming, the nasal solution spray pump delivers about 14–15 metered doses containing 1 mg per spray. If repriming of the pump is necessary, the spray pump will deliver about 8–10 metered doses, depending on the extent of repriming.

Adult Patients

Pain

INTRANASAL:
- Initially, 1 mg (1 spray in 1 nostril); if adequate analgesia is not achieved, may give an additional 1-mg dose within 60–90 minutes. May repeat this initial dose sequence in 3–4 hours, if needed.
- For management of severe pain: Initially, 2 mg (1 spray in each nostril) in patients who can remain recumbent if drowsiness or dizziness occurs. Do not administer additional 2-mg doses at intervals <3–4 hours, since the incidence of adverse effects may be increased.

Special Populations

Hepatic Impairment

Pain

INTRANASAL:
- Initially, 1 mg (1 spray in 1 nostril); may give an additional 1-mg dose within 90–120 minutes, if necessary. May repeat this initial dose sequence at an interval of ≥6 hours.

Renal Impairment
- Patients with renal impairment may receive the same intranasal dosages as patients with hepatic impairment.

Geriatric Patients
- Geriatric patients may receive the same as patients intranasal dosages with hepatic impairment.

Calcitonin Salmon Injection

(kal si toe′ nin)

Brand Name: Miacalcin®
Also available generically.

Why is this medicine prescribed?

Calcitonin salmon injection is used to treat osteoporosis in postmenopausal women. Osteoporosis is a disease that causes bones to weaken and break more easily. Calcitonin salmon injection is also used to treat Paget's disease of bone and to quickly reduce calcium levels in the blood when needed. Calcitonin is a human hormone that is also found in salmon. It works by preventing bone breakdown and increasing bone density (thickness).

How should this medicine be used?

Calcitonin salmon comes as a solution to be injected under the skin (subcutaneously) or into the muscle (intramuscularly). It is usually used once a day or once every other day. Follow the directions on your prescription label carefully, and ask your doctor or pharmacist to explain any part you do not understand. Use calcitonin salmon injection exactly as directed. Do not use more or less of it or use it more often than prescribed by your doctor.

Your doctor, nurse, or pharmacist will show you how to administer the medication. Follow all directions carefully. Throw away all empty syringes and vials as directed by your health care provider.

Before preparing a dose, look at the vial. If the solution is discolored or contains particles, do not use it, and call your pharmacist.

Calcitonin salmon helps treat osteoporosis and Paget's disease but does not cure them. Continue to use calcitonin salmon even if you feel well. Do not stop using calcitonin salmon without talking to your doctor.

Are there other uses for this medicine?

Calcitonin salmon injection is also used sometimes to treat osteogenesis imperfecta. Talk to your doctor about the possible risks of using this medication for your condition.

This medication may be prescribed for other uses; ask your doctor or pharmacist for more information.

What special precautions should I follow?

Before using calcitonin salmon injection,

- tell your doctor and pharmacist if you are allergic to calcitonin salmon or any other medications. Your doctor may do a skin test before you start calcitonin salmon to make sure you do not have an allergic reaction to it.
- tell your doctor and pharmacist what prescription and nonprescription medications, vitamins, nutritional supplements, and herbal products you are taking.
- tell your doctor if you are pregnant, plan to become pregnant, or are breast-feeding. If you become pregnant while using calcitonin salmon, call your doctor.

What special dietary instructions should I follow?

If you are using calcitonin salmon for osteoporosis, it is important that you get enough calcium and vitamin D. Your doctor may prescribe supplements if your dietary intake is not enough.

What should I do if I forget to take a dose?

Do not administer a double dose to make up for a missed one. Use the following dosage schedule guidelines:

If your usual dose is two doses per day, use the missed dose if you remember it within 2 hours of your regularly scheduled dose. Otherwise, skip the missed dose and then continue on the regular dosing schedule.

If your usual dose is one dose per day, use the missed dose if you remember it during the same day. Otherwise, skip the missed dose and continue the regular dosing schedule the next day.

If your usual dose is every other day, use the missed dose as soon as you remember it, either on the regularly scheduled day or the next day. Then, continue a regular dosing schedule of every other day from that point.

If your usual dose is three times a week, give the missed dose on the next day and continue every other day thereafter. Resume the regular dosing schedule at the beginning of the next week.

What side effects can this medicine cause?

Calcitonin salmon may cause side effects. Tell your doctor if any of these symptoms are severe or do not go away:

- upset stomach
- vomiting
- redness, swelling, or irritation at the site of injection
- flushing (feeling of warmth) of the face or hands
- increased urination at night
- itching of the ear lobes
- feverish feeling
- eye pain
- decreased appetite
- stomach pain
- swelling of the feet
- salty taste

Some side effects can be serious. The following symptoms are uncommon, but if you experience any of them, call your doctor immediately:

- hives
- skin rash
- itching
- difficulty breathing or swallowing
- swelling of the tongue or throat

Calcitonin salmon may cause other side effects. Call your doctor if you have any unusual problems while taking this medication.

If you experience a serious side effect, you or your doctor may send a report to the Food and Drug Administration's (FDA) MedWatch Adverse Event Reporting program online [at http://www.fda.gov/MedWatch/index.html] or by phone [1-800-332-1088].

What storage conditions are needed for this medicine?

Store calcitonin salmon injection in its original container in the refrigerator. Do not freeze this medicine or shake the vials. Let the solution warm to room temperature before administration. Do not use calcitonin salmon injection if it has been out of the refrigerator for more than 24 hours. Keep all supplies in a clean, dry place and out of reach of children. Talk to your pharmacist about the proper disposal of used, empty syringes and vials.

What should I do in case of overdose?

In case of overdose, call your local poison control center at 1-800-222-1222. If the victim has collapsed or is not breathing, call local emergency services at 911.

Symptoms of overdose may include:

- upset stomach
- vomiting

What other information should I know?

Keep all appointments with your doctor and laboratory. Your doctor may order certain lab tests to check your body's response to calcitonin salmon.

Do not let anyone else use your medication. Ask your pharmacist any questions you have about refilling your prescription.

Dosage Facts
For Informational Purposes

Caution: Do not change your dose, how often you take your medication, or the length of time you are to take it without first talking to your healthcare provider.

The following dosage information was written using medical language for doctors and other healthcare professionals and is provided here for you to check your dosage. The dosage of this drug may differ for different patients. Therefore, always follow your doctor's instructions or the directions on the label. Contact your healthcare provider or pharmacist if you have any questions about the specific dosage of your medication after reviewing this information.

General Dosage Information

Activity of calcitonin salmon expressed in terms of International Units (units).

Intranasal spray pumps deliver 0.09 mL of solution per actuation; each 0.09-mL spray delivers 200-unit dose.

Adult Patients
Paget's Disease of Bone

SUB-Q OR IM:
- Initial dosage: 100 units (0.5 mL) daily.
- Maintenance: 50 units (0.25 mL) daily or every other day; higher dosage (100 units daily) appropriate in patients with serious deformity or neurologic involvement.
- Dosage >100 units daily usually does not produce an improved response in patients who relapse while receiving calcitonin.

Hypercalcemia

SUB-Q OR IM:
- Initially, 4 units/kg every 12 hours; may increase dosage after 1 or 2 days (if response not adequate) to 8 units/kg every 12 hours; may further increase dosage after 2 days (if response not adequate) to 8 units/kg every 6 hours.

Postmenopausal Osteoporosis

SUB-Q OR IM:
- Minimum effective dosage not established; 100 units every other day may be effective in preserving vertebral BMD.

Prescribing Limits
Adult Patients
Hypercalcemia

SUB-Q OR IM:
- Maximum 8 units/kg every 6 hours.

Calcitonin Salmon Nasal Spray

(kal si toe' nin)

Brand Name: Miacalcin®
Also available generically.

Why is this medicine prescribed?

Calcitonin salmon is used to treat osteoporosis in women who are at least 5 years past menopause and cannot or do not want to take estrogen products. Osteoporosis is a disease that causes bones to weaken and break more easily. Calcitonin is a human hormone that is also found in salmon. It works by preventing bone breakdown and increasing bone density (thickness).

How should this medicine be used?

Calcitonin salmon comes as a spray to be used in the nose. It is usually used once a day, alternating nostrils every day. To help you remember to use calcitonin salmon, use it around the same time every day. Follow the directions on your prescription label carefully, and ask your doctor or pharmacist to explain any part you do not understand. Use calcitonin salmon exactly as directed. Do not use more or less of it or use it more often than prescribed by your doctor.

Calcitonin salmon helps treat osteoporosis but does not cure it. Continue to use calcitonin salmon even if you feel well. Do not stop using calcitonin salmon without talking to your doctor.

Before using calcitonin salmon nasal spray the first time, read the written instructions that come with it. Ask your doctor or pharmacist to show you how to use it. Practice using the nasal spray while he or she watches.

To put the pump and bottle together, remove the rubber stopper from the bottle, and then remove the plastic protective cap from the bottom of the spray unit. Put the spray pump into the bottle and turn to tighten. Then take the plastic cover off of the top of the spray unit.

Before the first time you use a new bottle, you need to prime (activate) the pump. To prime the pump, follow these steps:

1. Allow the bottle to reach room temperature.
2. Hold the bottle upright, and press down on the two white side arms of the pump until a full spray is produced. The pump is now primed.

To use the nasal spray, follow these steps:

1. Keep your head up and place the nozzle in one nostril.
2. Press down on the pump to release the calcitonin salmon.
3. Use the opposite nostril each day.
4. Each bottle has enough medication for 14 doses.

Are there other uses for this medicine?

This medication may be prescribed for other uses; ask your doctor or pharmacist for more information.

What special precautions should I follow?

Before using calcitonin salmon,

- tell your doctor and pharmacist if you are allergic to calcitonin salmon or any other medications. Your doctor may do a skin test before you start calcitonin salmon to make sure you do not have an allergic reaction to it.
- tell your doctor and pharmacist what prescription and nonprescription medications, vitamins, nutritional supplements, and herbal products you are taking.
- tell your doctor if you are pregnant, plan to become pregnant, or are breast-feeding. If you become pregnant while using calcitonin salmon, call your doctor.

What special dietary instructions should I follow?

It is important that you get enough calcium and vitamin D while you are using calcitonin salmon. Your doctor may prescribe supplements if your dietary intake is not enough.

What should I do if I forget to take a dose?

Apply the missed dose as soon as you remember it. However, if it is almost time for the next dose, skip the missed dose and continue your regular dosing schedule. Do not use a double dose to make up for a missed one.

What side effects can this medicine cause?

Calcitonin salmon may cause side effects. Tell your doctor if any of these symptoms are severe or do not go away:

- runny nose
- nosebleed
- sinus pain
- nose symptoms such as crusts, dryness, redness, or swelling
- back pain
- joint pain
- upset stomach
- flushing (feeling of warmth)

Some side effects can be serious. The following symptoms are uncommon, but if you experience any of them, call your doctor immediately:

- hives
- skin rash
- itching
- difficulty breathing or swallowing
- swelling of the tongue or throat

Calcitonin salmon may cause other side effects. Call your doctor if you have any unusual problems while using this medication.

If you experience a serious side effect, you or your doctor may send a report to the Food and Drug Administration's (FDA) MedWatch Adverse Event Reporting program online [at http://www.fda.gov/MedWatch/index.html] or by phone [1-800-332-1088].

What storage conditions are needed for this medicine?

Keep this medication in the container it came in, tightly closed, and out of reach of children. Store unopened calcitonin salmon nasal spray in the refrigerator; do not freeze. Store opened bottles at room temperature in an upright position. Replace the plastic cover to keep the nozzle clean. Opened calcitonin salmon stored at room temperature should be thrown away after 30 days. Talk to your pharmacist about the proper disposal of your medication.

What should I do in case of overdose?

In case of overdose, call your local poison control center at 1-800-222-1222. If the victim has collapsed or is not breathing, call local emergency services at 911.

What other information should I know?

Keep all appointments with your doctor and the laboratory. Your doctor may order certain lab tests to check your body's response to calcitonin salmon. You will also need occasional examinations of the nose to make sure calcitonin salmon nasal spray is not causing injury to the nose.

Do not let anyone else use your medication. Ask your

pharmacist any questions you have about refilling your prescription.

Dosage Facts
For Informational Purposes

Caution: Do not change your dose, how often you take your medication, or the length of time you are to take it without first talking to your healthcare provider.

The following dosage information was written using medical language for doctors and other healthcare professionals and is provided here for you to check your dosage. The dosage of this drug may differ for different patients. Therefore, always follow your doctor's instructions or the directions on the label. Contact your healthcare provider or pharmacist if you have any questions about the specific dosage of your medication after reviewing this information.

General Dosage Information

Activity of calcitonin salmon expressed in terms of International Units (units).

Intranasal spray pumps deliver 0.09 mL of solution per actuation; each 0.09-mL spray delivers 200-unit dose.

Adult Patients

Postmenopausal Osteoporosis

INTRANASAL:
- 200 units (1 spray) daily.

Calcitriol
(kal si trye' ole)

Brand Name: Rocaltrol®

Why is this medicine prescribed?

Calcitriol is a form of vitamin D that is used to treat and prevent low levels of calcium in the blood of patients whose kidneys or parathyroid glands (glands in the neck that release natural substances to control the amount of calcium in the blood) are not working normally. Low blood levels of calcium may cause bone disease. Calcitriol is in a class of medications called vitamins. It works by helping the body to use more of the calcium found in foods or supplements.

How should this medicine be used?

Calcitriol comes as a capsule and a solution (liquid) to take by mouth. It usually is taken once a day or once every other day in the morning with or without food. Follow the directions on your prescription label carefully, and ask your doc-

tor or pharmacist to explain any part you do not understand. Take calcitriol exactly as directed. Do not take more or less of it or take it more often than prescribed by your doctor.

Your doctor will probably start you on a low dose of calcitriol and may gradually increase your dose, not more than once every 2-8 weeks.

Calcitriol may help to control your condition but will not cure it. Continue to take calcitriol even if you feel well. Do not stop taking cacitriol without talking to your doctor.

Are there other uses for this medicine?

Calcitriol is also sometimes used to treat rickets (softening and weakening of bones in children caused by lack of vitamin D), osteomalacia (softening and weakening of bones in adults caused by lack of vitamin D), and familial hypophosphatemia (rickets or osteomalacia caused by decreased ability to break down vitamin D in the body). Calcitriol is also sometimes used to increase the amount of calcium in the blood of premature (born early) babies. Talk to your doctor about the risks of using this medication for your condition.

This medication may be prescribed for other uses; ask your doctor or pharmacist for more information.

What special precautions should I follow?

Before taking calcitriol,
- tell your doctor and pharmacist if you are allergic to calcitriol, other forms of vitamin D such as calcifediol (Calderol), dihydrotachysterol (Hytakerol, DHT), doxercalciferol (Hectorol), ergocalciferol (Drisdol, Calciferol), paricalcitol (Zemplar) or any other medications or vitamins.
- tell your doctor and pharmacist what prescription and nonprescription medications. vitamins, nutritional supplements, and herbal products you are taking, especially antacids; calcium supplements; cholestyramine (Questran); colestipol (Colestid); digoxin (Lanoxin); diuretics ('water pills') ketoconazole (Nizoral); lanthanum (Fosrenol); laxatives; oral steroids such as dexamethasone (Decadron, Dexone), methylprednisolone (Medrol), and prednisone (Deltasone); other forms of vitamin D; phenobarbital (Luminal, Solfoton); phenytoin (Dilantin); and sevelamer (Renagel). Also tell your doctor or pharmacist if you are taking ergocalciferol (Drisdol, Calciferol) or have stopped taking it in the past few months.Your doctor may need to change the doses of your medications or monitor you carefully for side effects.
- you should know that many non-prescription medications are not safe to take with calcitriol. Ask your doctor before you take any non-prescription medications while you are taking calcitriol
- tell your doctor if you have recently had surgery or are unable to move around for any reason and if you have or have ever had kidney or liver disease.
- tell your doctor if you are pregnant, plan to become pregnant, or are breast-feeding. If you become pregnant

while taking calcitriol, call your doctor. You should not breastfeed while you are taking calcitriol.
- if you are having surgery, including dental surgery, tell the doctor or dentist that you are taking calcitriol.

What special dietary instructions should I follow?

Calcitriol will work only if you get the right amount of calcium from the foods you eat. If you get too much calcium from foods, you may experience serious side effects of calcitriol, and if you do not get enough calcium from foods, calcitriol will not control your condition. Your doctor will tell you which foods are good sources of these nutrients and how many servings you need each day. If you find it difficult to eat enough of these foods, tell your doctor. In that case, your doctor can prescribe or recommend a supplement.

If you are being treated with dialysis (process of cleaning the blood by passing it through a machine), your doctor may also prescribe a low-phosphate diet. Follow these directions carefully.

If you do not have kidney disease, you should drink plenty of fluids while taking calcitriol. If you have kidney disease, talk to your doctor about how much fluid you should drink each day.

What should I do if I forget to take a dose?

Take the missed dose as soon as you remember it. However, if it is almost time for the next dose, skip the missed dose and continue your regular dosing schedule. Do not take a double dose to make up for a missed one.

What side effects can this medicine cause?

Some side effects can be serious. The following symptoms are uncommon, but if you experience any of them, call your doctor immediately:
- weakness
- headache
- sluggishness
- upset stomach
- vomiting
- dry mouth
- constipation
- muscle pain
- bone pain
- metallic taste in mouth
- increased thirst
- decreased appetite
- weight loss
- increased urination (especially at night)
- difficult or painful urination
- changes in vision
- lack of interest in the things around you
- hallucination (seeing things or hearing voices that do not exist)
- fever or chills
- stomach pain

- pale, fatty stools
- yellowing of the skin or eyes
- runny nose
- decreased sexual desire
- irregular heartbeat
- rash
- hives
- itching
- difficulty breathing or swallowing

If you experience a serious side effect, you or your doctor may send a report to the Food and Drug Administration's (FDA) MedWatch Adverse Event Reporting program online [at http://www.fda.gov/MedWatch/index.html] or by phone [1-800-332-1088].

What storage conditions are needed for this medicine?

Keep this medication in the container it came in, tightly closed, and out of reach of children. Store it at room temperature and away from excess heat and moisture (not in the bathroom). Protect this medication from light. Throw away any medication that is outdated or no longer needed. Talk to your pharmacist about the proper disposal of your medication.

What should I do in case of overdose?

In case of overdose, call your local poison control center at 1-800-222-1222. If the victim has collapsed or is not breathing, call local emergency services at 911.

Symptoms of overdose may include:
- weakness
- headache
- sluggishness
- upset stomach
- vomiting
- dry mouth
- constipation
- muscle pain
- bone pain
- metallic taste in mouth
- increased thirst
- decreased appetite
- weight loss
- increased urination (especially at night)
- difficult or painful urination
- changes in vision
- lack of interest in the things around you
- hallucination (seeing things or hearing voices that do not exist)
- fever or chills
- stomach pain
- pale, fatty stools
- yellowing of the skin or eyes
- runny nose
- decreased sexual desire
- irregular heartbeat

What other information should I know?

Keep all appointments with your doctor and the laboratory. Your doctor will order certain lab tests to check your response to calcitriol.

Do not let anyone else take your medication. Ask your pharmacist any questions you have about refilling your prescription.

Talk to your doctor, pharmacist, or other healthcare professional if you have questions about dosing information for your medication.

Calcium Carbonate

(kal' see um kar' bon ate)

Brand Name: Alka-Mints®, Calel-D®, Caltrate 600®, Chooz®, Os-Cal 500®, Rolaids Calcium Rich®, Titralac®, Tums®

Why is this medicine prescribed?

Calcium carbonate is a dietary supplement used when the amount of calcium taken in the diet is not enough. Calcium is needed by the body for healthy bones, muscles, nervous system, and heart. Calcium carbonate also is used as an antacid to relieve heartburn, acid indigestion, and stomach upset. It is available with or without a prescription.

This medication is sometimes prescribed for other uses; ask your doctor or pharmacist for more information.

How should this medicine be used?

Calcium carbonate comes as a tablet, chewable tablet, capsule, and liquid to take by mouth. It usually is taken three or four times a day. Follow the directions on your prescription or package label carefully, and ask your doctor or pharmacist to explain any part you do not understand. Take calcium carbonate exactly as directed. Do not take more or less of it or take it more often than prescribed by your doctor. When using this medicine as a dietary supplement, take it with food or following meals.

Chewable tablets should be chewed thoroughly before being swallowed; do not swallow them whole. Drink a full glass of water after taking either the regular or chewable tablets or capsules. Some liquid forms of calcium carbonate must be shaken well before use.

Do not take calcium carbonate as an antacid for more than 2 weeks unless your doctor tells you to.

What special precautions should I follow?

Before taking calcium carbonate,
- tell your doctor and pharmacist if you are allergic to calcium carbonate or any other drugs.
- tell your doctor and pharmacist what prescription and nonprescription medications you are taking, especially digoxin (Lanoxin), etidronate (Didronel), phenytoin (Dilantin), tetracycline (Sumycin), and vitamins. Do not take calcium carbonate within 1-2 hours of taking other medicines. Calcium may decrease the effectiveness of the other medicine.
- tell your doctor if you have or have ever had kidney disease or stomach conditions.
- tell your doctor if you are pregnant, plan to become pregnant, or are breast-feeding. If you become pregnant while taking calcium carbonate, call your doctor.

What should I do if I forget to take a dose?

If you are taking calcium carbonate on a regular schedule, take the missed dose as soon you remember it. However, if it is almost time for the next dose, skip the missed dose and continue your regular dosing schedule. Do not take a double dose to make up for a missed one.

What side effects can this medicine cause?

Calcium carbonate may cause side effects. Tell your doctor if any of these symptoms are severe or do not go away:
- upset stomach
- vomiting
- stomach pain
- belching
- constipation
- dry mouth
- increased urination
- loss of appetite
- metallic taste

What storage conditions are needed for this medicine?

Keep this medication in the container it came in, tightly closed, and out of reach of children. Store it at room temperature and away from excess heat and moisture (not in the bathroom). Throw away any medication that is outdated or no longer needed. Talk to your pharmacist about the proper disposal of your medication.

What should I do in case of overdose?

In case of overdose, call your local poison control center at 1-800-222-1222. If the victim has collapsed or is not breathing, call local emergency services at 911.

What other information should I know?

If this medicine has been prescribed for you, keep all appointments with your doctor so that your response to calcium carbonate can be checked. Do not let anyone else take your medicine.

Talk to your doctor, pharmacist, or other healthcare professional if you have questions about dosing information for your medication.

Candesartan

(kan des ar′ tan)

Brand Name: Atacand®

Important Warning

Do not take candesartan if you are pregnant or breast-feeding. If you become pregnant while taking candesartan, call your doctor immediately.

Why is this medicine prescribed?

Candesartan is used to treat high blood pressure. It blocks the action of certain chemicals that tighten the blood vessels, so blood flows more smoothly. This medication is sometimes prescribed for other uses; ask your doctor or pharmacist for more information.

How should this medicine be used?

Candesartan comes as a tablet to take by mouth. It is usually taken once or twice a day with or without food. Follow the directions on your prescription label carefully, and ask your doctor or pharmacist to explain any part you do not understand. Take candesartan exactly as directed. Do not take more or less of it or take it more often than prescribed by your doctor.

Candesartan controls high blood pressure but does not cure it. Continue to take candesartan even if you feel well. Do not stop taking candesartan without talking to your doctor.

Are there other uses for this medicine?

Candesartan is sometimes used to treat congestive heart failure. Talk to your doctor about the possible risks of using this drug for your condition.

What special precautions should I follow?

Before taking candesartan,
- tell your doctor and pharmacist if you are allergic to candesartan, benazepril (Lotensin), captopril (Capoten), enalapril (Vasotec), fosinopril (Monopril), hydrochlorothiazide (HydroDIURIL), irbesartan (Avapro), lisinopril (Prinivil, Zestril), losartan (Cozaar), moexipril (Univasc), quinapril (Accupril), ramipril (Altace), sulfas, telmisartan (Micardis), trandolapril (Mavik), valsartan (Diovan), or any other drugs.
- tell your doctor and pharmacist what prescription and non-prescription medications you are taking, especially barbiturates; diuretics ('water pills'); lithium (Eskalith, Lithobid); medications for diabetes; nonsteroidal anti-inflammatory medications (ibuprofen [Motrin, Advil], naproxen [Naprosyn, Aleve], and others); other medications for high blood pressure; potassium supplements; and vitamins.
- tell your doctor if you have or have ever had heart, kidney, or liver disease or diabetes.

- if you are having surgery, including dental surgery, tell the doctor or dentist that you are taking candesartan.

What special dietary instructions should I follow?

Talk to your doctor before using salt substitutes containing potassium. If your doctor prescribes a low-salt or low-sodium diet, follow these directions carefully.

What should I do if I forget to take a dose?

Take the missed dose as soon as you remember it. However, if it is almost time for the next dose, skip the missed dose and continue your regular dosing schedule. Do not take a double dose to make up for a missed one.

What side effects can this medicine cause?

Candesartan may cause side effects. Tell your doctor if any of these symptoms are severe or do not go away:
- dizziness
- lightheadedness
- congestion
- cough
- diarrhea
- headache
- muscle aches
- back pain
- fever
- sore throat
- runny nose

If you experience any of the following symptoms, call your doctor immediately:
- swelling of the face, eyes, lips, tongue, arms, or legs
- difficulty breathing or swallowing
- fainting
- rash

If you experience a serious side effect, you or your doctor may send a report to the Food and Drug Administration's (FDA) MedWatch Adverse Event Reporting program online [at http://www.fda.gov/MedWatch/index.html] or by phone [1-800-332-1088].

What storage conditions are needed for this medicine?

Keep this medication in the container it came in, tightly closed, and out of reach of children. Store it at room temperature and away from excess heat and moisture (not in the bathroom). Throw away any medication that is outdated or no longer needed. Talk to your pharmacist about the proper disposal of your medication.

What should I do in case of overdose?

In case of overdose, call your local poison control center at 1-800-222-1222. If the victim has collapsed or is not breathing, call local emergency services at 911.

What other information should I know?

Keep all appointments with your doctor and the laboratory. Your blood pressure should be checked regularly to determine your response to candesartan.

Do not let anyone else take your medication. Ask your pharmacist any questions you have about refilling your prescription.

Dosage Facts
For Informational Purposes

Caution: Do not change your dose, how often you take your medication, or the length of time you are to take it without first talking to your healthcare provider.

The following dosage information was written using medical language for doctors and other healthcare professionals and is provided here for you to check your dosage. The dosage of this drug may differ for different patients. Therefore, always follow your doctor's instructions or the directions on the label. Contact your healthcare provider or pharmacist if you have any questions about the specific dosage of your medication after reviewing this information.

General Dosage Information

Available as candesartan cilexetil; dosage expressed in terms of the salt.

Adult Patients

Hypertension
Monotherapy
ORAL:
- Initially, 16 mg once daily in adults without intravascular volume depletion. Adjust dosage at approximately monthly intervals (more aggressively in high-risk patients) to achieve BP control.
- Usual dosage: 8–32 mg daily, given in 1 dose or 2 divided doses; no additional therapeutic benefit with higher dosages.

Combination Therapy
ORAL:
- If BP is not adequately controlled by monotherapy with candesartan 32 mg daily, can switch to fixed-combination tablets (candesartan 32 mg and hydrochlorothiazide 12.5 mg; then candesartan 32 mg and hydrochlorothiazide 25 mg).
- If BP is not adequately controlled by monotherapy with 25 mg of hydrochlorothiazide or if BP is controlled but hypokalemia is problematic at this dosage, can use fixed-combination tablets containing candesartan 16 mg and hydrochlorothiazide 12.5 mg.

CHF
Monotherapy
ORAL:
- Initially, 4 mg once daily. Increase dosage (by doubling the dosage at approximately 2-week intervals) as tolerated to a target dosage of 32 mg once daily.

Special Populations

Hepatic Impairment
- No initial dosage adjustments necessary in patients with mild hepatic impairment.
- Manufacturer recommends considering initial dosage reduction in patients with moderate hepatic impairment.
- Some clinicians recommend initial dosage of 4 or 8 mg daily in patients with severe hepatic impairment.

Renal Impairment
- Manufacturer states that no initial dosage adjustments are necessary in patients with renal impairment. However, some clinicians recommend initial dosage of 4 or 8 mg daily in those with severe impairment.

Volume- and/or Salt-Depleted Patients
- Correct volume and/or salt depletion prior to initiation of therapy or initiate therapy under close medical supervision using lower initial dosage.

Candesartan and Hydrochlorothiazide
(kan de sar′ tan) (hye droe klor oh thye′ a zide)

Brand Name: Atacand HCT®

> ## Important Warning
>
> Do not take candesartan and hydrochlorothiazide if you are pregnant. If you become pregnant while taking candesartan and hydrochlorothiazide, call your doctor immediately. Candesartan and hydrochlorothiazide may harm the fetus.

Why is this medicine prescribed?

The combination of candesartan and hydrochlorothiazide is used alone or with other medications to treat high blood pressure. Candesartan is in a class of medications called angiotensin II antagonists. It makes blood flow more smoothly by blocking the action of certain natural chemicals that tighten the blood vessels. Hydrochlorothiazide is in a class of medications called diuretics ('water pills'). It works by causing the the kidneys to get rid of unneeded water and salt from the body into the urine.

How should this medicine be used?

The combination of candesartan and hydrochlorothiazide comes as a tablet to take by mouth. It is usually taken once or twice a day with or without food. Follow the directions on your prescription label carefully, and ask your doctor or pharmacist to explain any part you do not understand. Take candesartan and hydrochlorothiazide exactly as directed. Do not take more or less of it or take it more often than prescribed by your doctor.

Candesartan and hydrochlorothiazide controls high blood pressure but does not cure it. It may take up to 4 weeks before you feel the full benefit of candesartan and hydrochlorothiazide. Continue to take candesartan and hydrochlorothiazide even if you feel well. Do not stop taking candesartan and hydrochlorothiazide without talking to your doctor.

Are there other uses for this medicine?

This medication may be prescribed for other uses; ask your doctor or pharmacist for more information.

What special precautions should I follow?

Before taking candesartan and hydrochlorothiazide,

- tell your doctor and pharmacist if you are allergic to candesartan (Atacand), hydrochlorothiazide (Hydro-DIURIL, Microzide), sulfa drugs, or any other medications.
- tell your doctor and pharmacist what prescription and nonprescription medications, vitamins, nutritional supplements, and herbal products you are taking. Be sure to mention any of the following: aspirin and other nonsteroidal anti-inflammatory medications (NSAIDS) such as ibuprofen (Advil, Motrin) and naproxen (Aleve, Naprosyn); cholestyramine (Questran); colestipol (Colestid); lithium (Eskalith, Lithobid); medications for diabetes; narcotic pain relievers; oral steroids such as dexamethasone (Decadron, Dexone), methylprednisolone (Medrol), and prednisone (Deltasone); other medications for high blood pressure; phenobarbital (Barbita, Luminal, Solfoton), and potassium supplements (K-Dur, Klor-Con, others). Your doctor may need to change the doses of your medications or monitor you carefully for side effects.
- tell your doctor if you are on dialysis and if you have or have ever had allergies, asthma, lupus (SLE), diabetes, heart failure, gout, or kidney or liver disease.
- tell your doctor if you plan to become pregnant or are breast-feeding.
- if you are having surgery, including dental surgery, tell the doctor or dentist that you are taking candesartan and hydrochlorothiazine.
- ask your doctor about the safe use of alcoholic beverages while you are taking candesartan and hydrochlorothiazide. Alcohol can make the side effects from candesartan and hydrochlorothiazide worse.
- you should know that candesartan and hydrochlorothiazide may cause dizziness, lightheadedness, and fainting when you get up too quickly from a lying position. This is more common when you first start taking candesartan and hydrochlorothiazide. To avoid this problem, get out of bed slowly, resting your feet on the floor for a few minutes before standing up.
- you should know that diarrhea, vomiting, not drinking enough fluids, and sweating a lot can cause a drop in blood pressure, which may cause lightheadedness and fainting.

What special dietary instructions should I follow?

Talk to your doctor before using salt substitutes containing potassium. If your doctor prescribes a low-salt or low-sodium diet or an exercise program, follow these directions carefully.

What should I do if I forget to take a dose?

Take the missed dose as soon as you remember it. However, if it is almost time for the next dose, skip the missed dose and continue your regular dosing schedule. Do not take a double dose to make up for a missed one.

What side effects can this medicine cause?

Candesartan and hydrochlorothiazide may cause side effects. Tell your doctor if any of these symptoms are severe or do not go away:

- dizziness
- back pain

Some side effects can be serious. The following symptoms are uncommon, but if you experience any of them, call your doctor immediately:

- lightheadedness
- fainting
- dry mouth
- thirst
- weakness
- lack of energy
- drowsiness
- restlessness
- confusion
- seizures
- muscle pain or cramps
- infrequent urination
- rapid or pounding heartbeat
- upset stomach
- vomiting

Candesartan and hydrochlorothiazide may cause other side effects. Call your doctor if you have any unusual problems while taking this medication.

If you experience a serious side effect, you or your doctor may send a report to the Food and Drug Administration's (FDA) MedWatch Adverse Event Reporting program online [at http://www.fda.gov/MedWatch/index.html] or by phone [1-800-332-1088].

What storage conditions are needed for this medicine?

Keep this medication in the container it came in, tightly closed, and out of reach of children. Store it at room temperature and away from excess heat and moisture (not in the bathroom). Throw away any medication that is outdated or no longer needed. Talk to your pharmacist about the proper disposal of your medication.

What should I do in case of overdose?

In case of overdose, call your local poison control center at 1-800-222-1222. If the victim has collapsed or is not breathing, call local emergency services at 911.

What other information should I know?

Keep all appointments with your doctor and the laboratory. Your doctor may order certain lab tests to check your body's response to candesartan and hydrochlorothiazide.

Do not let anyone else take your medication. Ask your pharmacist any questions you have about refilling your prescription.

Dosage Facts
For Informational Purposes

Caution: Do not change your dose, how often you take your medication, or the length of time you are to take it without first talking to your healthcare provider.

The following dosage information was written using medical language for doctors and other healthcare professionals and is provided here for you to check your dosage. The dosage of this drug may differ for different patients. Therefore, always follow your doctor's instructions or the directions on the label. Contact your healthcare provider or pharmacist if you have any questions about the specific dosage of your medication after reviewing this information.

General Dosage Information

Available as candesartan cilexetil; dosage expressed in terms of the salt.

Adult Patients

Hypertension
Combination Therapy

ORAL:
- If BP is not adequately controlled by monotherapy with candesartan 32 mg daily, can switch to fixed-combination tablets (candesartan 32 mg and hydrochlorothiazide 12.5 mg; then candesartan 32 mg and hydrochlorothiazide 25 mg).
- If BP is not adequately controlled by monotherapy with 25 mg of hydrochlorothiazide or if BP is controlled but hypokalemia is problematic at this dosage, can use fixed-combination tablets containing candesartan 16 mg and hydrochlorothiazide 12.5 mg.

Captopril
(kap′ toe pril)

Brand Name: Capoten®
Also available generically.

Important Warning

Do not take captopril if you are pregnant or breast-feeding. If you become pregnant while taking captopril, call your doctor immediately.

Why is this medicine prescribed?

Captopril is used to treat high blood pressure and heart failure. It decreases certain chemicals that tighten the blood vessels, so blood flows more smoothly and the heart can pump blood more efficiently.

This medication is sometimes prescribed for other uses; ask your doctor or pharmacist for more information.

How should this medicine be used?

Captopril comes as a tablet to take by mouth. It is usually taken two or three times a day on an empty stomach, 1 hour before or 2 hours after a meal. Follow the directions on your prescription label carefully, and ask your doctor or pharmacist to explain any part you do not understand. Take captopril exactly as directed. Do not take more or less of it or take it more often than prescribed by your doctor.

Captopril controls high blood pressure and heart failure but does not cure them.

Continue to take captopril even if you feel well. Do not stop taking captopril without talking to your doctor.

What special precautions should I follow?

Before taking captopril,
- tell your doctor and pharmacist if you are allergic to captopril or any other drugs.
- tell your doctor and pharmacist what prescription and nonprescription medications you are taking, especially diuretics ('water pills'), lithium (Eskalith, Lithobid), other medications for high blood pressure, potassium supplements, and vitamins.
- tell your doctor if you have or have ever had heart or kidney disease or diabetes.
- if you are having surgery, including dental surgery, tell the doctor or dentist that you are taking captopril.

What special dietary instructions should I follow?

Talk to your doctor before using salt substitutes containing potassium. If your doctor prescribes a low-salt or low-sodium diet, follow these instructions carefully.

What should I do if I forget to take a dose?

Take the missed dose as soon as you remember it. However, if it is almost time for the next dose, skip the missed dose and continue your regular dosing schedule. Do not take a double dose to make up for a missed one.

What side effects can this medicine cause?

Captopril may cause side effects. Tell your doctor if any of these symptoms are severe or do not go away:
- dizziness or lightheadedness
- salty or metallic taste, or decreased ability to taste
- cough
- sore throat
- fever
- mouth sores
- unusual bruising
- fast heartbeat
- excessive tiredness

If you experience any of the following symptoms, call your doctor immediately:
- chest pain
- swelling of the face, eyes, lips, tongue, arms, or legs
- difficulty breathing or swallowing
- fainting
- rash

If you experience a serious side effect, you or your doctor may send a report to the Food and Drug Administration's (FDA) MedWatch Adverse Event Reporting program online [at http://www.fda.gov/MedWatch/index.html] or by phone [1-800-332-1088].

What storage conditions are needed for this medicine?

Keep this medication in the container it came in, tightly closed, and out of reach of children. Store it at room temperature and away from excess heat and moisture (not in the bathroom). Throw away any medication that is outdated or no longer needed. Talk to your pharmacist about the proper disposal of your medication.

What should I do in case of overdose?

In case of overdose, call your local poison control center at 1-800-222-1222. If the victim has collapsed or is not breathing, call local emergency services at 911.

What other information should I know?

Keep all appointments with your doctor and the laboratory. Your blood pressure should be checked regularly to determine your response to captopril.

Captopril tablets may have a slight sulfur odor (like rotten eggs).

Do not let anyone else take your medication. Ask your pharmacist any questions you have about refilling your prescription.

Dosage Facts
For Informational Purposes

Caution: Do not change your dose, how often you take your medication, or the length of time you are to take it without first talking to your healthcare provider.

The following dosage information was written using medical language for doctors and other healthcare professionals and is provided here for you to check your dosage. The dosage of this drug may differ for different patients. Therefore, always follow your doctor's instructions or the directions on the label. Contact your healthcare provider or pharmacist if you have any questions about the specific dosage of your medication after reviewing this information.

Pediatric Patients

Hypertension

ORAL:
- Dosage has been reduced in proportion to body weight; titrate carefully. Some experts recommend an initial dosage of 0.9–1.5 mg/kg daily (given as 0.3–0.5 mg/kg 3 times daily). Increase dosage as necessary to a maximum of 6 mg/kg daily.

Adult Patients

Hypertension

ORAL:
- Initially, 25 mg 2 or 3 times daily. If BP is not adequately controlled after 1–2 weeks, increase dosage to 50 mg 2 or 3 times daily.
- Lower initial dosages (e.g., 6.25 mg twice daily to 12.5 mg 3 times daily) may be effective in some patients, particularly those already receiving a diuretic.
- Usual dosage: Manufacturers recommend 25–150 mg 2 or 3 times daily (usually not necessary to exceed 450 mg daily). JNC 7 recommends 25–100 mg daily given in 2 divided doses; JNC 7 recommends adding another drug, if needed, rather than continuing to increase dosage.
- If combination therapy is initiated with captopril/hydrochlorothiazide fixed-combination preparation, captopril 25 mg and hydrochlorothiazide 15 mg daily initially; adjust dosage (generally at 6-week intervals) by administering each drug separately or by advancing the fixed-combination preparation.

Hypertensive Crises

ORAL:
- 25 mg 2 or 3 times daily, initiated promptly under close supervision with frequent monitoring of BP. May continue previous diuretic therapy, but discontinue other hypotensive agents. May increase dosage at intervals of ≤24 hours under continuous supervision until optimum BP response is attained or 450 mg daily is given. Adjunctive therapy with other hypotensive agents may be necessary.
- Acute therapy (e.g., 12.5–25 mg, repeated once or twice if necessary at intervals of 30–60 minutes or longer) has been effective in adults with hypertensive urgencies† and emergencies†.

Nephropathy
Diabetic Nephropathy

ORAL:
- 25 mg 3 times daily.

CHF

ORAL:
- Manufacturer recommends initial dosage of 25 mg 3 times daily; in patients with normal or low BP who may be volume- and/or salt-depleted, initial dosage of 6.25 or 12.5 mg 3 times daily. Increase dosage gradually to 50 mg 3 times daily; delay further dosage increases for ≥2 weeks to assess response.
- Some clinicians recommend initial dosage of 6.25 or 12.5 mg 3 times daily, with gradual titration over several weeks to 50 mg 3 times daily, regardless of BP, salt/volume status, or concomitant diuretic therapy. Generally titrate dosage to pre-specified target (i.e., ≥150 mg daily) or highest tolerated dosage rather than according to response.

Left Ventricular Dysfunction after AMI

ORAL:
- Manufacturer recommends initiation of therapy ≥3 days post-MI with single dose of 6.25 mg, followed by 12.5 mg 3 times daily. Increase dosage over next several days to 25 mg 3 times daily and then over next several weeks (as tolerated) to 50 mg 3 times daily.
- Some clinicians recommend initiation of therapy <24 hours post-MI with initial dose of 6.25 mg, followed by 12.5 mg 2 hours later, 25 mg 10–12 hours later, and then 50 mg twice daily as tolerated. Recommended maintenance dosage: 50 mg 3 times daily.

Prescribing Limits

Pediatric Patients

Hypertension

ORAL:
- Maximum 6 mg/kg daily.

Adult Patients

Hypertension

ORAL:
- Maximum 450 mg daily.
- Dosage of captopril/hydrochlorothiazide fixed-combination generally should not exceed captopril 150 mg and hydrochlorothiazide 50 mg daily.

CHF

ORAL:
- Maximum dosage recommended by manufacturer and some experts is 450 mg daily. Other experts suggest maximum dosage of 50 mg 3 times daily.

Special Populations

Renal Impairment
- Manufacturer recommends initial dosage of <75 mg daily; increase dosage in small increments at 1- to 2-week intervals. After desired therapeutic effect has been attained, slowly reduce dosage to minimum effective level.
- Patients with Cl_{cr} 10–50 mL/minute: 75% of usual captopril dosage or administration of usual dose every 12–18 hours suggested by some clinicians.
- Cl_{cr} <10 mL/minute: 50% of usual dosage or administration of usual dose every 24 hours suggested by some clinicians.

- Patients undergoing hemodialysis may require supplemental dose after dialysis.
- Fixed-combination captopril/hydrochlorothiazide tablets usually are not recommended for patients with severe renal impairment.

Geriatric Patients

Hypertension
- Usual adult dosages generally have been used; dosages of 6.25–12.5 mg 1–4 times daily used occasionally.

Volume-and/or Salt-Depleted Patients
- Correct volume and/or salt depletion prior to initiation of therapy or initiate therapy under close medical supervision using lower initial dosage.

† Use is not currently included in the labeling approved by the US Food and Drug Administration.

Captopril and Hydrochlorothiazide

(kap′ toe pril) (hye droe klor oh thye′ a zide)

Brand Name: Capozide®

Important Warning

Do not take captopril and hydrochlorothiazide if you are pregnant. If you become pregnant while taking captopril and hydrochlorothiazide, call your doctor immediately. Captopril and hydrochlorothiazide may harm the fetus.

Why is this medicine prescribed?

The combination of captopril and hydrochlorothiazide is used to treat high blood pressure. Captopril is in a class of medications called angiotensin-converting enzyme (ACE) inhibitors. It works by decreasing certain chemicals that tighten the blood vessels, so blood flows more smoothly. Hydrochlorothiazide is in a class of medications called diuretics ('water pills'). It works by causing the kidneys to get rid of unneeded water and salt from the body into the urine.

How should this medicine be used?

The combination of captopril and hydrochlorothiazide comes as a tablet to take by mouth. It is usually taken once or twice a day on an empty stomach, 1 hour before meals. To help you remember to take captopril and hydrochlorothiazide, take it around the same time every day. Follow the directions on your prescription label carefully, and ask your doctor or pharmacist to explain any part you do not understand. Take captopril and hydrochlorothiazide exactly as directed. Do not take more or less of it or take it more often than prescribed by your doctor.

Your doctor may start you on a low dose of captopril and hydrochlorothiazide and gradually increase your dose, not more than once every 6 to 8 weeks.

Captopril and hydrochlorothiazide controls high blood pressure but does not cure it. Continue to take captopril and hydrochlorothiazide even if you feel well. Do not stop taking captopril and hydrochlorothiazide without talking to your doctor.

Are there other uses for this medicine?

This medication may be prescribed for other uses; ask your doctor or pharmacist for more information.

What special precautions should I follow?

Before taking captopril and hydrochlorothiazide,

- tell your doctor and pharmacist if you are allergic to captopril (Capoten), hydrochlorothiazide (HCTZ, Hydrodiuril, Microzide), benazepril (Lotensin), enalapril (Vasotec), fosinopril (Monopril), lisinopril (Prinivil, Zestril), moexipril (Univasc), perindopril (Aceon), quinapril (Accupril), ramipril (Altace), trandolapril (Mavik), sulfa drugs, or any other medications.
- tell your doctor and pharmacist what prescription and nonprescription medications, vitamins, nutritional supplements, and herbal products you are taking. Be sure to mention any of the following: amphotericin B (Fungizone); anticoagulants ('blood thinners') such as warfarin (Coumadin); aspirin and other nonsteroidal anti-inflammatory medications (NSAIDs) such as indomethacin (Indocin); calcium supplements; cancer chemotherapy drugs; cholestyramine (Questran); colestipol (Colestid); digoxin (Lanoxin); insulin or oral medications for diabetes; lithium (Eskalith, Lithobid); medications for gout such as probenecid (Benemid) and sulfinpyrazone (Anturane); medications that suppress the immune system; methenamine (Mandelamine, Hiprex); monoamine oxidase (MAO) inhibitors, including phenelzine (Nardil) and tranylcypromine (Parnate); nitrates such as isosorbide dinitrate (Isordil), isosorbide mononitrate (Imdur, ISMO, Monoket), and nitroglycerin (Nitrogard, Nitrolingual, Nitrostat, others); oral steroids such as dexamethasone (Decadron, Dexone), methylprednisolone (Medrol), and prednisone (Deltasone); other diuretics; other medications for high blood pressure; pain medications; phenobarbital (Luminal, Solfoton); and potassium supplements. Your doctor may need to change the doses of your medications or monitor you carefully for side effects.
- tell your doctor if you have or have ever had lupus; scleroderma; heart failure; diabetes; allergy; asthma; or liver or kidney disease.
- tell your doctor if you plan to become pregnant or are breast-feeding.
- if you are having surgery, including dental surgery, tell the doctor or dentist that you are taking captopril and hydrochlorothiazide.
- ask your doctor about the safe use of alcoholic beverages while you are taking captopril and hydrochlorothiazide. Alcohol can worsen the side effects of captopril and hydrochlorothiazide.
- you should know that diarrhea, vomiting, not drinking enough fluids, and sweating a lot can cause a drop in blood pressure, which may cause lightheadedness and fainting.

What special dietary instructions should I follow?

Talk to your doctor before using salt substitutes containing potassium. If your doctor prescribes a low-sodium (low-salt) diet, follow those directions carefully.

What should I do if I forget to take a dose?

Take the missed dose as soon as you remember it. However, if it is almost time for the next dose, skip the missed dose and continue your regular dosing schedule. Do not take a double dose to make up for a missed one.

What side effects can this medicine cause?

Captopril and hydrochlorothiazide may cause side effects. Tell your doctor if any of these symptoms are severe or do not go away:

- cough
- dizziness or lightheadedness
- taste changes
- rash and/or itching

Some side effects can be serious. The following symptoms are uncommon, but if you experience any of them, call your doctor immediately:

- swelling of the face, throat, tongue, lips, eyes, hands, feet, ankles, or lower legs
- hoarseness
- difficulty breathing or swallowing
- fever, sore throat, chills, and other signs of infection
- yellowing of the skin or eyes
- dry mouth
- thirst
- weakness
- lack of energy
- restlessness
- muscle pains or cramps
- infrequent urination
- upset stomach
- vomiting
- fainting
- chest pain
- rapid, pounding, or irregular heartbeat

Captopril and hydrochlorothiazide may cause other side effects. Call your doctor if you have any unusual problems while taking this medication.

If you experience a serious side effect, you or your doctor may send a report to the Food and Drug Administration's (FDA) MedWatch Adverse Event Reporting program online [at http://www.fda.gov/MedWatch/index.html] or by phone [1-800-332-1088].

What storage conditions are needed for this medicine?

Keep this medication in the container it came in, tightly closed, and out of reach of children. Store it at room temperature and away from excess heat and moisture (not in the bathroom). Throw away any medication that is outdated or no longer needed. Talk to your pharmacist about the proper disposal of your medication.

What should I do in case of overdose?

In case of overdose, call your local poison control center at 1-800-222-1222. If the victim has collapsed or is not breathing, call local emergency services at 911.

Symptoms of overdose may include:
- drowsiness
- coma
- difficulty breathing
- stomach pain

What other information should I know?

Keep all appointments with your doctor and the laboratory. Your blood pressure should be checked regularly to determine your response to captopril and hydrochlorothiazide. Your doctor may order certain lab tests to check your body's response to captopril and hydrochlorothiazide.

Before having any laboratory test, tell your doctor and the laboratory personnel that you are taking captopril and hydrochlorothiazide.

Do not let anyone else take your medication. Ask your pharmacist any questions you have about refilling your prescription.

Dosage Facts
For Informational Purposes

Caution: Do not change your dose, how often you take your medication, or the length of time you are to take it without first talking to your healthcare provider.

The following dosage information was written using medical language for doctors and other healthcare professionals and is provided here for you to check your dosage. The dosage of this drug may differ for different patients. Therefore, always follow your doctor's instructions or the directions on the label. Contact your healthcare provider or pharmacist if you have any questions about the specific dosage of your medication after reviewing this information.

Adult Patients

Hypertension

ORAL:
- If combination therapy is initiated with captopril/hydrochlorothiazide fixed-combination preparation, captopril 25 mg and hydrochlorothiazide 15 mg daily initially; adjust dosage (generally

at 6-week intervals) by administering each drug separately or by advancing the fixed-combination preparation.

Prescribing Limits

Adult Patients

Hypertension

ORAL:
- Dosage of captopril/hydrochlorothiazide fixed-combination generally should not exceed captopril 150 mg and hydrochlorothiazide 50 mg daily.

Special Populations

Renal Impairment
- Fixed-combination captopril/hydrochlorothiazide tablets usually are not recommended for patients with severe renal impairment.

† Use is not currently included in the labeling approved by the US Food and Drug Administration.

Carbamazepine

(kar ba maz′ e peen)

Brand Name: Carbatrol®, Epitol®, Equetro®, Tegretol®, Tegretol®-XR
Also available generically.

Important Warning

Carbamazepine may decrease the number of blood cells produced by your body. In rare cases, the number of blood cells may decrease enough to cause serious or life-threatening health problems. Tell your doctor if you have ever had a decreased number of blood cells, especially if it was caused by another medication. If you experience any of the following symptoms, call your doctor immediately: sore throat, fever, chills or other signs of infection; unusual bleeding or bruising; tiny purple dots or spots on the skin; mouth sores; or rash.

Keep all appointments with your doctor and the laboratory. Your doctor will order certain lab tests before and during your treatment to check your body's response to carbamazepine.

Why is this medicine prescribed?

Carbamazepine is used alone or in combination with other medications to treat certain types of seizures in patients with epilepsy. It is also used to treat trigeminal neuralgia (a condition that causes facial nerve pain). Carbamazepine extended-release capsules (Equetro brand only) are used to treat episodes of mania (frenzied, abnormally excited or irritated mood) or mixed episodes (symptoms of mania and depression that happen at the same time) in patients with bipolar I disorder (manic depressive disorder; a disease that causes episodes of depression, episodes of mania, and other abnormal moods). Carbamazepine is in a class of medications called anticonvulsants. It works by reducing abnormal excitement in the brain.

How should this medicine be used?

Carbamazepine comes as a tablet, a chewable tablet, an extended-release (long-acting) tablet, an extended-release capsule, and a suspension (liquid) to take by mouth. The regular tablet, chewable tablet, and liquid are usually taken two to four times a day with meals. The extended-release tablet is usually taken twice a day with meals. The extended-release capsule is usually taken twice a day with or without meals. To help you remember to take carbamazepine, take it at around the same times every day. Follow the directions on your prescription label carefully, and ask your doctor or pharmacist to explain any part you do not understand. Take carbamazepine exactly as directed. Do not take more or less of it or take it more often than prescribed by your doctor.

Swallow the extended-release tablets whole; do not split, chew, or crush them. The extended-release capsules may be opened and the beads inside sprinkled over food, such as a teaspoon of applesauce or similar food. Do not crush or chew the extended-release capsules or the beads inside them.

Shake the liquid well before each use to mix the medication evenly.

Your doctor will start you on a low dose of carbamazepine and gradually increase your dose.

It may take a few weeks or longer before you feel the full benefit of carbamazepine. Continue to take carbamazepine even if you feel well. Do not stop taking carbamazepine without talking to your doctor. If you have a seizure disorder and you suddenly stop taking carbamazepine, your seizures may become worse. Your doctor will probably decrease your dose gradually.

Are there other uses for this medicine?

Carbamazepine is also sometimes used to treat mental illnesses, depression, posttraumatic stress disorder, drug and alcohol withdrawal, restless legs syndrome, diabetes insipidus, certain pain syndromes, and a disease in children called chorea. Talk to your doctor about the possible risks of using this medication for your condition.

This medication may be prescribed for other uses; ask your doctor or pharmacist for more information.

What special precautions should I follow?

Before taking carbamazepine,

- tell your doctor and pharmacist if you are allergic to carbamazepine, amitriptyline (Elavil), amoxapine (Asendin), clomipramine (Anafranil), desipramine (Norpramin), doxepin (Adapin, Sinequan), imipramine (Tofranil), nortriptyline (Aventyl, Pamelor), other medications for seizures such as phenobarbital (Luminal,

Solfoton) or phenytoin (Dilantin), protriptyline (Vivactil), trimipramine (Surmontil), or any other medications.
- you should know that carbamazepine is the active ingredient in several products that have different names and may be prescribed to treat different conditions. Check the list of brand names at the beginning of this document carefully. All of the products listed contain carbamazepine and you should not take more than one of them at the same time.
- do not take carbamazepine if you are taking monoamine oxidase (MAO) inhibitors, including isocarboxazid (Marplan), phenelzine (Nardil) selegiline (Eldepryl); and tranylcypromine (Parnate), or have stopped taking them within the past 2 weeks.
- tell your doctor and pharmacist what other prescription and nonprescription medications, vitamins, nutritional supplements, and herbal products you are taking. Be sure to mention any of the following: acetaminophen (Tylenol); acetazolamide (Diamox); alprazolam (Xanax); anticoagulants ('blood thinners') such as warfarin (Coumadin); antidepressants such as amitriptyline (Elavil), buproprion (Wellbutrin, Zyban), buspirone (BuSpar), citalopram (Celexa), clomipramine (Anafranil), desipramine (Norpramin), fluoxetine (Prozac, Sarafem), fluvoxamine (Luvox), mirtazapine (Remeron), nortriptyline (Pamelor); antifungals such as itraconazole (Sporanox) and ketoconazole (Nizoral); cimetidine (Tagamet); cisplatin (Platinol); clarithromycin (Biaxin); clonazepam (Klonopin); clozapine (Clozaril); cyclosporine (Neoral, Sandimmune); daltopristin and quinupristin (Synercid); danazol (Danocrine); delviradine (Rescriptor); diltiazem (Cardizem, Dilacor, Tiazac); doxorubicin (Adriamycin, Rubex); doxycycline (Vibramycin); erythromycin (E.E.S., E-Mycin, Erythrocin); felodipine (Plendil); haloperidol (Haldol); HIV protease inhibitors including atazanavir (Reyataz), indinavir (Crixivan), lopinavir (in Kaletra), nelfinavir (Viracept), ritonavir (Norvir, in Kaletra), and saquinavir (Fortovase, Invirase); isoniazid (INH, Nydrazid); levothyroxine (Levoxyl, Synthroid); lithium (Lithobid); loratadine (Claritin); lorazepam (Ativan); certain medications to treat malaria such as chloroquine (Aralen) and mefloquine (Lariam); medications for anxiety or mental illness; other medications for seizures such as ethosuximide (Zarontin), felbamate (Felbatol), lamotrigine (Lamictal), methsuximide (Celontin), oxcarbazepine (Trileptal), phenobarbital (Luminal, Solfoton), phensuximide (Milontin) (not available in the United States), phenytoin (Dilantin), primidone (Mysoline), tiagabine (Gabitril), topiramate (Topamax), and valproic acid (Depakene, Depakote); methadone (Dolophine); nefazodone; niacinamide (nicotinamide, Vitamin B3); propoxyphene (Darvon); praziquantel (Biltricide); quinine; rifampin (Rifadin, Rimactane); sedatives; sleeping pills; terfenadine (Seldane) (not available in the United States); theophylline (Theobid, Theo-Dur); tramadol (Ultram); tranquilizers; troleandomycin (TAO); vera-

pamil (Calan, Covera, Isoptin, Verelan); and zileuton (Zyflo). Many other medications may also interact with carbamazepine, so be sure to tell your doctor about all the medications you are taking, even those that do not appear on this list. Your doctor may need to change the doses of your medications or monitor you carefully for side effects.

- if you are taking any other liquid medications, do not take them at the same time as carbamazepine liquid.
- tell your doctor what herbal products you are taking, especially St. John's Wort.
- tell your doctor if you have or have ever had glaucoma; psychosis; or heart, kidney, thyroid, or liver disease.
- you should know that carbamazepine may decrease the effectiveness of hormonal contraceptives (birth control pills, patches, rings, injections, implants, or intrauterine devices). Use another form of birth control while taking carbamazepine. Tell your doctor if you have unexpected vaginal bleeding or think you may be pregnant while you are taking carbamazepine.
- tell your doctor if you are pregnant or plan to become pregnant. Carbamazepine may harm the fetus. If you become pregnant while taking carbamazepine, call your doctor immediately.
- do not breastfeed while you are taking carbamazepine.
- if you are having surgery, including dental surgery, tell the doctor or dentist that you are taking carbamazepine.
- you should know that carbamazepine may make you drowsy. Do not drive a car or operate machinery until you know how this medication affects you.
- remember that alcohol can add to the drowsiness caused by this medication.

What special dietary instructions should I follow?

Talk to your doctor about drinking grapefruit juice while taking this medicine.

What should I do if I forget to take a dose?

Take the missed dose as soon as you remember it. However, if it is almost time for the next dose, skip the missed dose and continue your regular dosing schedule. Do not take a double dose to make up for a missed one.

What side effects can this medicine cause?

Carbamazepine may cause side effects. Tell your doctor if any of these symptoms are severe or do not go away:

- drowsiness
- dizziness
- unsteadiness
- upset stomach
- vomiting
- headache
- anxiety
- memory problems
- diarrhea

- constipation
- heartburn
- dry mouth
- back pain

Some side effects can be serious. The following symptoms are uncommon, but if you experience any of them or those listed in the IMPORTANT WARNING section, call your doctor immediately:

- rash
- confusion
- loss of contact with reality
- depression
- thinking about killing yourself or planning or trying to do so
- chest pain
- yellowing of the skin or eyes
- vision problems

Carbamazepine may cause other side effects. Call your doctor if you have any unusual problems while taking this medication.

If you experience a serious side effect, you or your doctor may send a report to the Food and Drug Administration's (FDA) MedWatch Adverse Event Reporting program online [at http://www.fda.gov/MedWatch/index.html] or by phone [1-800-332-1088].

What storage conditions are needed for this medicine?

Keep this medication in the container it came in, tightly closed, and out of reach of children. Store it at room temperature, away from excess heat and moisture (not in the bathroom). Throw away any medication that is outdated or no longer needed. Talk to your pharmacist about the proper disposal of your medication.

What should I do in case of overdose?

In case of overdose, call your local poison control center at 1-800-222-1222. If the victim has collapsed or is not breathing, call local emergency services at 911.

Symptoms of overdose may include:

- unconsciousness
- seizures
- restlessness
- muscle twitching
- abnormal movements
- shaking of a part of your body that you cannot control
- unsteadiness
- drowsiness
- dizziness
- blurred vision
- irregular or slowed breathing
- rapid or pounding heartbeat
- upset stomach
- vomiting
- difficulty urinating

What other information should I know?

Before having any laboratory test, tell your doctor and the laboratory personnel that you are taking carbamazepine.

Carbamazepine can interfere with the results of home pregnancy tests. Talk to your doctor if you think you might be pregnant while you are taking carbamazepine. Do not try to test for pregnancy at home.

The extended-release tablet does not dissolve in the stomach after swallowing. It slowly releases the medicine as it passes through your digestive system. You may notice the tablet coating in the stool.

Do not let anyone else take your medication. Ask your pharmacist any questions you have about refilling your prescription.

Dosage Facts

For Informational Purposes

Caution: Do not change your dose, how often you take your medication, or the length of time you are to take it without first talking to your healthcare provider.

The following dosage information was written using medical language for doctors and other healthcare professionals and is provided here for you to check your dosage. The dosage of this drug may differ for different patients. Therefore, always follow your doctor's instructions or the directions on the label. Contact your healthcare provider or pharmacist if you have any questions about the specific dosage of your medication after reviewing this information.

General Dosage Information

Initiate with a low dosage; adjust dosage carefully and slowly according to individual requirements and response. Do not discontinue abruptly due to risk of increased seizure frequency.

When adding to an existing anticonvulsant regimen, add gradually while dosage of other anticonvulsant(s) is maintained or gradually adjusted.

A given dose administered as oral suspension will produce higher peak plasma concentrations than when administered as tablets; initiate therapy with oral suspension with low, frequent doses and increase slowly to reduce risk of adverse effects (e.g., sedation).

To achieve therapeutic serum carbamazepine concentrations more rapidly (in about 2 hours), some clinicians recommend a loading-dose regimen (as oral suspension), preferably in a setting where plasma concentrations and the patient can be monitored closely.

When converting patients from oral tablets to oral suspension, divide total daily dosage administered as tablets into smaller, more frequent doses of suspension (e.g., transfer from twice-daily divided dosing of tablets to 3-times-daily divided dosing of suspension).

When converting patients from conventional, immediate-release formulations to extended-release capsules or tablets, administer same total daily dosage in 2 divided doses.

Pediatric Patients

Seizure Disorders

ORAL:

- Children <6 years of age: Initially, 10–20 mg/kg daily in 2–3 divided doses as chewable or conventional tablets or 4 divided doses as suspension. Increase dosage at weekly intervals to achieve optimal clinical response, which is generally achieved at maintenance dosages <35 mg/kg daily in 3 or 4 divided doses. If clinical response not achieved, obtain plasma carbamazepine concentrations to determine if in therapeutic range. Safety of dosages >35 mg/kg in a 24-hour period not established.
- Children 6–12 years of age: Initially, 100 mg twice daily as tablets (chewable, conventional, or extended-release) or 50 mg 4 times daily as oral suspension. Increase dosage at weekly intervals by up to 100 mg daily using a twice daily divided dosage regimen as extended-release tablets or a 3 or 4 times daily divided dosage regimen as conventional or chewable tablets or oral suspension until optimal response obtained, up to a maximum dosage of 1 g daily. When adequate seizure control is achieved, adjust dosage to minimum effective level, usually 400–800 mg daily.
- Children <12 years of age taking a total daily dosage of an immediate release formulation ≥400 mg may be converted to the same total daily dosage of extended-release capsules using a twice daily regimen.
- If rapid attainment of therapeutic serum carbamazepine concentrations is desired, some clinicians recommend an initial loading dose (as oral suspension) of 10 mg/kg in children <12 years of age.
- Children >12 years of age: Initially, 200 mg twice daily as tablets (conventional, chewable, or extended-release) or extended-release capsules or 100 mg 4 times daily as oral suspension. Increase dosage at weekly intervals by up to 200 mg daily using a twice daily divided dosage regimen as extended-release tablets or a 3 or 4 times daily divided dosage regimen as conventional or chewable tablets or oral suspension until optimal response obtained, up to a maximum dosage of 1 or 1.2 g in children 12–15 or >15 years of age, respectively. When adequate seizure control is achieved, adjust dosage to minimum effective level, usually 800 mg to 1.2 g daily.
- If rapid attainment of therapeutic serum carbamazepine concentrations is desired, some clinicians recommend an initial loading dose (as oral suspension) of 8 mg/kg in children ≥12 years of age.

Bipolar Disorder†

ORAL:

- Although dosage not established, experts generally recommend administering at the same range in dosage and therapeutic plasma concentrations as in the management of seizure disorders.
- Children >12 years of age: Initially, 200–600 mg daily, given in 3–4 divided doses; titrate dosage upward according to patient response and tolerability.
- In hospitalized patients >12 years of age with acute mania, increase dosage as tolerated in 200-mg daily increments up to 800 mg to 1 g daily, with slower increases thereafter as indicated. Do not exceed 1.6 g daily.
- In less acutely ill outpatients >12 years of age, adjust dosage more slowly, since rapid increases may cause patients to develop adverse GI or nervous system effects. If such adverse

effects occur, consider temporary dosage reductions. Once adverse effects resolve, increase dosage again more slowly.
- Maintenance dosages average about 1 g daily, but may range from 200 mg to 1.6 g daily in routine clinical practice.

Adult Patients

Seizure Disorders

ORAL:
- Initially, 200 mg twice daily as tablets (chewable, conventional, or extended-release) or capsules or 100 mg 4 times daily as oral suspension.
- Increase dosage by up to 200 mg daily at weekly intervals using a twice daily divided dosage regimen as extended-release tablets or capsules or a 3 or 4 times daily divided dosage regimen as conventional tablets or oral suspension until optimal response obtained, up to a maximum dosage of 1.2 g. In rare instances, dosages up to 1.6 g have been used.
- When adequate seizure control is achieved, adjust dosage to minimum effective level, usually 800 mg to 1.2 g daily.

Neuropathic Pain
Trigeminal Neuralgia

ORAL:
- Initially, 100 mg twice daily as tablets (conventional or extended-release), 200 mg once daily as extended-release capsules, or 50 mg 4 times daily as suspension on the first day of therapy.
- Increase dosage gradually by up to 200 mg daily using 200-mg increments for capsules, 100-mg increments every 12 hours for conventional or extended-release tablets, or 50-mg increments 4 times daily for the suspension until pain is relieved up to a total dosage of 1.2 g daily. The dosage necessary to relieve pain may range from 200 mg to 1.2 g daily.
- After pain control is achieved, maintenance dosage of 400–800 mg daily is usually adequate; some patients may require as little as 200 mg daily while others may require 1.2 g daily.
- At least once every 3 months, make attempt to decrease dosage to minimum effective level or to discontinue.

Bipolar Disorder†

ORAL:
- Dosage not established. Experts generally recommend the same range in dosage and therapeutic plasma concentrations as in the management of seizure disorders.
- Initially, 200–600 mg daily, given in 3–4 divided doses.
- Titrate dosage upward according to patient response and tolerability.
- In hospitalized patients with acute mania, increase dosage as tolerated in 200-mg daily increments up to 800 mg to 1 g daily, with slower increases thereafter as indicated. Do not exceed 1.6 g daily.
- In less acutely ill outpatients, adjust dosage more slowly, since rapid increases may cause patients to develop adverse GI or nervous system effects. If such adverse effects occur, consider temporary dosage reductions. Once adverse effects resolve, increase dosage again more slowly.
- Maintenance dosages average about 1 g daily, but may range from 200 mg to 1.6 g daily in routine clinical practice.

Prescribing Limits
Pediatric Patients

Seizure Disorders

ORAL:
- Children <6 years of age: Safety of dosages exceeding 35 mg/kg in a 24-hour period not established.
- Children 6–15 years of age: Generally should not exceed 1 g daily.
- Children >15 years of age: Generally should not exceed 1.2 g daily.

Adult Patients

Seizure Disorders

ORAL:
- Generally should not exceed 1.2 g daily; however, some patients have required up to 1.6–2.4 g daily.

Neuropathic Pain
Trigeminal Neuralgia

ORAL:
- Maximum 1.2 g daily.

Bipolar Disorder†

ORAL:
- Maximum 1.6 g daily.

† Use is not currently included in the labeling approved by the US Food and Drug Administration.

Carisoprodol

(kar eye soe proe′ dole)

Brand Name: Soma®, Soma® Compound as a combination product containing Carisoprodol and Aspirin, Soma® Compound with Codeine as a combination product containing Carisoprodol, Aspirin, and Codeine Phosphate, Vanadom® Also available generically.

Why is this medicine prescribed?

Carisoprodol, a muscle relaxant, is used with rest, physical therapy, and other measures to relax muscles and relieve pain and discomfort caused by strains, sprains, and other muscle injuries.

This medication is sometimes prescribed for other uses; ask your doctor or pharmacist for more information.

How should this medicine be used?

Carisoprodol comes as a tablet to take by mouth. It usually is taken three times daily and at bedtime. It may be taken with or without food. Follow the directions on your prescription label carefully, and ask your doctor or pharmacist to explain any part you do not understand. Take carisoprodol exactly as directed. Do not take more or less of it or take it more often than prescribed by your doctor.

What special precautions should I follow?

Before taking carisoprodol,

- tell your doctor and pharmacist if you are allergic to carisoprodol, meprobamate (Equanil, Meprospan, Miltown, Neuramate), or any other drugs.
- tell your doctor and pharmacist what prescription and nonprescription medications you are taking, especially medications for allergies, coughs, or colds; muscle relaxants; sedatives; sleeping pills; tranquilizers; and vitamins.
- tell your doctor if you have or have ever had kidney or liver disease.
- tell your doctor if you are pregnant, plan to become pregnant, or are breast-feeding. If you become pregnant while taking carisoprodol, call your doctor.
- you should know that this drug may make you drowsy. Do not drive a car or operate machinery until you know how carisoprodol affects you.
- remember that alcohol can add to the drowsiness caused by this drug.

What special dietary instructions should I follow?

Carisoprodol may cause an upset stomach. Take carisoprodol with food or milk.

What should I do if I forget to take a dose?

Take the missed dose as soon as you remember it. However, if it is almost time for the next dose, skip the missed dose and continue your regular dosing schedule. Do not take a double dose to make up for a missed one.

What side effects can this medicine cause?

Carisoprodol may cause side effects. Tell your doctor if any of these symptoms are severe or do not go away:

- drowsiness
- dizziness
- clumsiness
- headache
- fast heart rate
- upset stomach
- vomiting
- skin rash

If you experience any of the following symptoms, call your doctor immediately:

- difficulty breathing
- fever
- weakness
- burning in the eyes

If you experience a serious side effect, you or your doctor may send a report to the Food and Drug Administration's (FDA) MedWatch Adverse Event Reporting program online

[at http://www.fda.gov/MedWatch/index.html] or by phone [1-800-332-1088].

What storage conditions are needed for this medicine?

Keep this medication in the container it came in, tightly closed, and out of reach of children. Store it at room temperature and away from moisture and heat (not in the bathroom). Throw away any medication that is outdated or no longer needed. Talk to your pharmacist about the proper disposal of your medication.

What should I do in case of overdose?

In case of overdose, call your local poison control center at 1-800-222-1222. If the victim has collapsed or is not breathing, call local emergency services at 911.

What other information should I know?

Keep all appointments with your doctor.

Do not let anyone else take your medication. Ask your pharmacist any questions you have about refilling your prescription.

Dosage Facts
For Informational Purposes

Caution: Do not change your dose, how often you take your medication, or the length of time you are to take it without first talking to your healthcare provider.

The following dosage information was written using medical language for doctors and other healthcare professionals and is provided here for you to check your dosage. The dosage of this drug may differ for different patients. Therefore, always follow your doctor's instructions or the directions on the label. Contact your healthcare provider or pharmacist if you have any questions about the specific dosage of your medication after reviewing this information.

Pediatric Patients

Muscular Conditions

ORAL:
- Children ≥5 years of age: 25 mg/kg or 750 mg/m² daily in 4 divided doses has been suggested by some clinicians, although manufacturers state that safety and efficacy are not established in children <12 years of age.

Adult Patients

Muscular Conditions

ORAL:
- 350 mg 3 times daily and at bedtime.
- Reduce dosage if severe adverse CNS effects occur.

Carvedilol

(kar′ ve dil ol)

Brand Name: Coreg®, Coreg CR®

Why is this medicine prescribed?

Carvedilol is used to treat heart failure (condition in which the heart cannot pump enough blood to all parts of the body) and high blood pressure. It also is used to treat people whose hearts cannot pump blood well as a result of a heart attack. Carvedilol is often used in combination with other medications. Carvedilol is in a class of medications called beta-blockers. It works by relaxing the blood vessels to allow blood to flow through the body more easily.

How should this medicine be used?

Carvedilol comes as a tablet and an extended-release (long-acting) capsule to take by mouth. The tablet is usually taken twice a day with food. The extended-release capsule is usually taken once a day in the morning with food. Try to take carvedilol at around the same time(s) every day. Follow the directions on your prescription label carefully, and ask your doctor or pharmacist to explain any part you do not understand. Take carvedilol exactly as directed. Do not take more or less of it or take it more often than prescribed by your doctor.

Swallow the extended-release capsules whole. Do not chew or crush the capsules, and do not divide the beads inside a capsule into more than one dose. If you are unable to swallow the capsules, you may carefully open a capsule and sprinkle all of the beads it contains over a spoonful of cool or room temperature applesauce. Swallow the entire mixture immediately without chewing.

Your doctor will probably start you on a low dose of carvedilol and gradually increase your dose to allow your body to adjust to the medication. Talk to your doctor about how you feel and about any symptoms you experience during this time.

Carvedilol may help to control your condition but will not cure it. Continue taking carvedilol even if you feel well. Do not stop taking carvedilol without talking to your doctor. If you suddenly stop taking carvedilol, you may experience serious heart problems such as severe chest pain, a heart attack, or an irregular heartbeat. Your doctor will probably want to decrease your dose gradually over 1 to 2 weeks. Your doctor will watch you carefully and will probably tell you to avoid physical activity during this time.

Are there other uses for this medicine?

This medication may be prescribed for other uses. Ask your doctor or pharmacist for more information.

What special precautions should I follow?

Before taking carvedilol,

- tell your doctor and pharmacist if you have are allergic to carvedilol or any other medications.
- tell your doctor and pharmacist what prescription and nonprescription medications, vitamins, herbal products, and nutritional supplements you are taking or plan to take. Be sure to mention any of the following: cimetidine (Tagamet); clonidine (Catapres), cyclosporine (Neoral, Sandimmune); digoxin (Lanoxicaps, Lanoxin); diltiazem (Cardizem, Tiazac); epinephrine (Epipen); fluoxetine (Prozac); insulin; oral medications for diabetes; monoamine oxidase inhibitors (MAOIs) such as isocarboxazid (Marplan), phenelzine (Nardil), tranylcypromine (Parnate), and selegiline (Eldepryl, Emsam, Zelapar); paroxetine (Paxil); propafenone (Rythmol); quinidine; reserpine (Serpalan,); rifampin (Rifadin, Rimactane); and verapamil (Calan, Covera-HS, Verelan). Your doctor may need to change the doses of your medications or monitor you carefully for side effects.
- tell your doctor if you have or have ever had asthma or other breathing problems, a slow or irregular heartbeat, or liver disease. Your doctor may tell you not to take carvedilol.
- tell your doctor if you have or have ever had problems with blood flow in your feet or legs, diabetes or any other condition that causes you to have low blood sugar, hyperthyroidism (condition in which there is too much thyroid hormone in the body), low blood pressure, Prinzmetal's angina (chest pain that comes at rest with no obvious cause), or pheochromocytoma (a tumor that develops on a gland near the kidneys and may cause high blood pressure and fast heartbeat). Also tell your doctor if you have ever had a serious allergic reaction to a food or any other substance.
- tell your doctor if you are pregnant, plan to become pregnant, or are breast-feeding. If you become pregnant while taking carvedilol, call your doctor.
- if you are having surgery, including dental surgery, tell the doctor or dentist that you are taking carvedilol.
- you should know that this medication may make you feel tired, dizzy, or lightheaded, especially when you start taking carvedilol and when your dose is increased. Do not drive a car or operate machinery until you know how this medication affects you. Be especially careful during the first hour after you take the medication.
- do not drink any alcoholic drinks or take any prescription or nonprescription medications that contain alcohol for 2 hours before and 2 hours after you take carvedilol extended-release capsules. Ask your doctor or pharmacist if you do not know if a medication that you plan to take contains alcohol.
- you should know that carvedilol may cause dizziness, lightheadedness, and fainting, especially when you get up too quickly from a lying position. This is more common when you first start taking carvedilol. To avoid this

problem, get out of bed slowly, resting your feet on the floor for a few minutes before standing up.

- if you wear contact lenses, your eyes may become dry during your treatment with carvedilol. Tell your doctor if this becomes bothersome.

What special dietary instructions should I follow?

Unless your doctor tells you otherwise, continue your normal diet.

What should I do if I forget to take a dose?

Take the missed dose as soon as you remember it. However, if it is almost time for the next dose, skip the missed dose and continue your regular dosing schedule. Do not take a double dose to make up for a missed one.

What side effects can this medicine cause?

Carvedilol may cause hyperglycemia (high blood sugar). Call your doctor immediately if you have any of the following symptoms of hyperglycemia:

- extreme thirst
- frequent urination
- extreme hunger
- weakness
- blurred vision

Carvedilol may cause side effects. Tell your doctor if any of these symptoms are severe or do not go away:

- tiredness
- weakness
- lightheadedness
- dizziness
- headache
- diarrhea
- nausea
- vomiting
- vision changes
- joint pain
- difficulty falling asleep or staying asleep
- cough
- dry eyes
- numbness, burning, or tingling in the arms or legs

Some side effects may be serious. If you experience any of the following symptoms, call your doctor immediately:

- fainting
- shortness of breath
- weight gain
- swelling of the arms, hands, feet, ankles, or lower legs
- chest pain
- slow or irregular heartbeat
- rash
- hives
- itching
- difficulty breathing and swallowing

Carvedilol may cause other side effects. Tell your doctor if you experience any unusual problems while you are taking this medication.

If you experience a serious side effect, you or your doctor may send a report to the Food and Drug Administration's (FDA) MedWatch Adverse Event Reporting program online [at http://www.fda.gov/MedWatch/index.html] or by phone [1-800-332-1088].

What storage conditions are needed for this medicine?

Keep this medication in the container it came in, tightly closed, and out of reach of children. Store it at room temperature and away from excess heat and moisture (not in the bathroom). Throw away any medication that is outdated or no longer needed. Talk to your pharmacist about the proper disposal of your medication.

What should I do in case of overdose?

In case of overdose, call your local poison control center at 1-800-222-1222. If the victim has collapsed or is not breathing, call local emergency services at 911.

Symptoms of overdose may include:
- slow heartbeat
- dizziness
- fainting
- difficulty breathing
- vomiting
- loss of consciousness
- seizures

What other information should I know?

Keep all appointments with your doctor and the laboratory. Your doctor may order certain laboratory tests to check your body's response to carvedilol.

Do not let anyone else take your medication. Ask your pharmacist any questions you have about refilling your prescription.

Dosage Facts
For Informational Purposes

Caution: Do not change your dose, how often you take your medication, or the length of time you are to take it without first talking to your healthcare provider.

The following dosage information was written using medical language for doctors and other healthcare professionals and is provided here for you to check your dosage. The dosage of this drug may differ for different patients. Therefore, always follow your doctor's instructions or the directions on the label. Contact your healthcare provider or pharmacist if you have any questions about the specific dosage of your medication after reviewing this information.

Adult Patients

Hypertension

In hypertensive patients with left ventricular dysfunction, follow the usual CHF dosages and instructions (instead of those for hypertension); includes patients with CHF who already are receiving a cardiac glycoside, diuretic, and/or an ACE inhibitor. Such patients generally depend (at least in part) on β-adrenergic stimulation to maintain cardiovascular compensation.

Additive effects (e.g., hypotensive response, including increased orthostatic hypotension) may occur with concomitant carvedilol and diuretic therapy. Alternatively, consider addition of a drug from another antihypertensive class.

Monotherapy

ORAL:
- Initially, 6.25 mg twice daily for 7–14 days. If required, increase to 12.5 mg twice daily for 7–14 days. Dosage may be increased as tolerated to a maximum of 25 mg twice daily.
- Maintain dosage for 7–14 days between increments; full antihypertensive effect of each dosage level occurs within 7–14 days.
- Evaluate response and tolerance to the initial dosage and subsequent dosage adjustments by measurement of standing systolic pressure 1 hour after administration (trough BP).

CHF

If deterioration of heart failure is evident during titration, increase dosage of the concurrent diuretic; do not escalate β-blocker dosage until symptoms (e.g., fluid retention) have stabilized.

If heart failure manifestations do not resolve in response to an increase in diuretic dosage, consider decreasing dosage or temporarily discontinuing carvedilol.

Occurrence of increased heart failure manifestations during initiation or dosage titration that require dosage decreases or discontinuance should not prevent future consideration of resuming therapy with or increasing dosage of carvedilol.

If vasodilation occurs, consider decreasing diuretic or ACE inhibitor dosage; if this does not improved circulatory status, decrease carvedilol dosage.

If worsening heart failure or vasodilation occurs, do not increase carvedilol dosage until cardiovascular status is stable.

If bradycardia (heart rate <55 bpm) occurs, reduce carvedilol dosage.

ORAL:
- Initiate at very low dosage, usually 3.125 mg twice daily for 2 weeks.
- If initial dosage is tolerated, increase dosage to 6.25 mg twice daily for 2 weeks.
- If necessary, dosage may then be doubled every 2 weeks (with strict adherence to the monitoring regimen) to highest tolerated dosage.
- Maximum 50 mg daily (in patients weighing <85 kg) and 100 mg daily (in those weighing >85 kg).

Left Ventricular Dysfunction After AMI

ORAL:
- Initially, usually 6.25 mg twice daily for 3–10 days. If tolerated, increase to 12.5 mg twice daily for 3–10 days, and then increase to 25 mg twice daily (target dose).
- Maintain dosage for 3–10 days between increments to assess tolerance.

- If higher dosage is not tolerated, maintain on lower dosage.
- In patients with low BP, heart rate, or fluid retention, initiate at 3.125 mg twice daily and/or slow the rate of titration.

Prescribing Limits

Adult Patients

Hypertension

Initial dosage: maximum 6.25 mg twice daily (to minimize hypotension, syncope).

Maximum 50 mg daily.

CHF

Initial dosage: maximum 3.125 mg twice daily (to minimize hypotension, syncope).

Patients weighing <85 kg: maximum 25 mg daily.

Patients weighing >85 kg: maximum 50 mg daily.

Left Ventricular Dysfunction Following MI

Initial dosage: maximum 6.25 mg twice daily (to minimize hypotension, syncope).

Maximum (target dose): 25 mg twice daily.

Special Populations

Hepatic Impairment
- Not recommended for use in patients with clinical manifestations of hepatic impairment or severe impairment.

Renal Impairment
- No specific dosage adjustment recommendations.
- If a deterioration in renal function is detected in heart failure patients, decrease dosage or discontinue carvedilol.

Geriatric Patients
- Reduced initial dosage may be necessary because of increased risk of orthostatic hypotension and limited experience in patients ≥75 years of age.

Cefaclor

(sef' a klor)

Brand Name: Ceclor®, Ceclor® Pulvules®
Also available generically.

Why is this medicine prescribed?

Cefaclor is used to treat certain infections caused by bacteria, such as pneumonia and infections of the ears, lungs, throat, urinary tract, and skin. Cefaclor is in a class of medications called cephalosporin antibiotics. It works by stopping the growth of bacteria. Antibiotics will not work for colds, flu, or other viral infections.

How should this medicine be used?

Cefaclor comes as a capsule, an extended-release (long-acting) tablet, and a suspension (liquid) to take by mouth. The capsule and liquid are usually taken every 8 hours (three times a day) or every 12 hours (twice a day). The long-acting tablet is usually taken every 12 hours (twice a day), within 1 hour of eating a meal. To help you remember to take cefaclor, take it around the same time every day. Follow the directions on your prescription label carefully, and ask your doctor or pharmacist to explain any part you do not understand. Take cefaclor exactly as directed. Do not take more or less of it or take it more often than prescribed by your doctor.

Shake the liquid well before each use to mix the medication evenly.

The capsules and tablets should be swallowed whole and taken with a full glass of water. Swallow the long-acting tablets whole; do not split, chew, or crush them.

Take cefaclor until you finish the prescription, even if you feel better. Stopping cefaclor too soon may cause bacteria to become resistant to antibiotics.

Are there other uses for this medicine?

This medication may be prescribed for other uses; ask your doctor or pharmacist for more information.

What special precautions should I follow?

Before taking cefaclor,
- tell your doctor and pharmacist if you are allergic to cefaclor, penicillin, cefadroxil (Duricef), cefamandole (Mandol), cefazolin (Ancef, Kefzol), cefdinir (Omnicef), cefditoren (Spectracef), cefepime (Maxipime), cefixime (Suprax), cefmetazole (Zefazone), cefonicid (Monocid), cefoperazone (Cefobid), cefotaxime (Claforan), cefoxitin (Mefoxin), cefpodoxime (Vantin), cefprozil (Cefzil), ceftazidime (Ceptaz, Fortaz, Tazicef), ceftibuten (Cedax), ceftizoxime (Cefizox), ceftriaxone (Rocephin), cefuroxime (Ceftin, Kefurox, Zinacef), cephalexin (Keflex), cephapirin (Cefadyl), cephradine (Velosef), loracarbef (Lorabid), or any other medications.
- tell your doctor and pharmacist what prescription and nonprescription medications, vitamins, nutritional supplements, and herbal products you are taking. Be sure to mention either of the following: anticoagulants ('blood thinners') such as warfarin (Coumadin), and probenecid (Benemid). Your doctor may need to change the doses of your medications or monitor you carefully for side effects.
- tell your doctor if you have or have ever had allergies, kidney disease, colitis, or stomach problems.
- tell your doctor if you are pregnant, plan to become pregnant, or are breast-feeding. If you become pregnant while taking cefaclor, call your doctor.

What special dietary instructions should I follow?

Unless your doctor tells you otherwise, continue your normal diet.

What should I do if I forget to take a dose?

Take the missed dose as soon as you remember it. However, if it is almost time for the next dose, skip the missed dose and continue your regular dosing schedule. Do not take a double dose to make up for a missed one.

What side effects can this medicine cause?

Cefaclor may cause side effects. Tell your doctor if this symptom is severe or does not go away:
- diarrhea

Some side effects can be serious. The following symptoms are uncommon, but if you experience any of them, call your doctor immediately:
- severe skin rash
- itching
- hives
- difficulty breathing or swallowing
- wheezing
- joint pain
- fever
- painful sores in the mouth or throat
- vaginal itching and discharge

Cefaclor may cause other side effects. Call your doctor if you have any unusual problems while taking this medication.

If you experience a serious side effect, you or your doctor may send a report to the Food and Drug Administration's (FDA) MedWatch Adverse Event Reporting program online [at http://www.fda.gov/MedWatch/index.html] or by phone [1-800-332-1088].

What storage conditions are needed for this medicine?

Keep this medication in the container it came in, tightly closed, and out of reach of children. Store the capsules and tablets at room temperature and away from excess heat and moisture (not in the bathroom). Throw away any medication that is outdated or no longer needed. Keep liquid medicine in the refrigerator, tightly closed, and throw away any unused medication after 14 days. Do not freeze. Talk to your pharmacist about the proper disposal of your medication.

What should I do in case of overdose?

In case of overdose, call your local poison control center at 1-800-222-1222. If the victim has collapsed or is not breathing, call local emergency services at 911.

Symptoms of overdose may include:
- upset stomach
- vomiting
- stomach pain
- diarrhea

What other information should I know?

Keep all appointments with your doctor and the laboratory. Your doctor may order certain lab tests to check your body's response to cefaclor.

If you are diabetic, use Clinistix or TesTape (not Clinitest) to test your urine for sugar while taking this medication.

Do not let anyone else take your medication. Your prescription is probably not refillable. If you still have symptoms of infection after you finish the cefaclor, call your doctor.

Dosage Facts

For Informational Purposes

Caution: Do not change your dose, how often you take your medication, or the length of time you are to take it without first talking to your healthcare provider.

The following dosage information was written using medical language for doctors and other healthcare professionals and is provided here for you to check your dosage. The dosage of this drug may differ for different patients. Therefore, always follow your doctor's instructions or the directions on the label. Contact your healthcare provider or pharmacist if you have any questions about the specific dosage of your medication after reviewing this information.

General Dosage Information

Available as cefaclor monohydrate; dosage expressed in terms of anhydrous cefaclor.

Pediatric Patients

Lower Respiratory Tract Infections

ORAL:
- Children ≥1 month of age: 20 mg/kg daily in divided doses every 8 hours (as capsules or oral suspension). For more severe infections or those caused by less-susceptible organisms, 40 mg/kg daily in divided doses every 8 hours (as capsules or oral suspension).

Acute Otitis Media (AOM)

ORAL:
- Children ≥1 month of age: 40 mg/kg daily in divided doses every 8 or 12 hours (as capsules or oral suspension).

Pharyngitis and Tonsillitis

ORAL:
- Children ≥1 month of age: 20 mg/kg daily in divided doses every 8 or 12 hours for 10 days (as capsules or oral suspension). For more severe infections or those caused by less-susceptible organisms, 40 mg/kg daily in divided doses every 8 hours (as capsules or oral suspension).

Skin and Skin Structure Infections

ORAL:
- Children ≥1 month of age: 20 mg/kg daily in divided doses every 8 hours (as capsules or oral suspension). For more severe infections or those caused by less susceptible organisms, 40 mg/kg daily in divided doses every 8 hours (as capsules or oral suspension).

Urinary Tract Infections (UTIs)

ORAL:
- Children ≥1 month of age: 20 mg/kg daily in divided doses every 8 hours (as capsules or oral suspension). For more severe infections or those caused by less susceptible organisms, 40 mg/kg daily in divided doses every 8 hours (as capsules or oral suspension).

Adult Patients

Respiratory Tract Infections
Pneumonia

ORAL:
- 500 mg every 8 hours (as capsules or oral suspension).

Acute Bacterial Exacerbations of Chronic Bronchitis

ORAL:
- 500 mg every 12 hours for 7 days (as extended-release tablets).

Secondary Bacterial Infections of Acute Bronchitis

ORAL:
- 500 mg every 12 hours for 7 days (as extended-release tablets).

Acute Otitis Media (AOM)

ORAL:
- 250 mg every 8 hours (as capsules or oral suspension). For more severe infections or those caused by less susceptible organisms, 500 mg every 8 hours (as capsules or oral suspension).

Pharyngitis and Tonsillitis

ORAL:
- 250 mg every 8 hours (as capsules or oral suspension). For more severe infections or those caused by less susceptible organisms, 500 mg every 8 hours (as capsules or oral suspension).
- 375 mg every 12 hours for 10 days (as extended-release tablets).

Skin and Skin Structure Infections

ORAL:
- 250 mg every 8 hours (as capsules or oral suspension). For more severe infections or those caused by less susceptible organisms, 500 mg every 8 hours (as capsules or oral suspension).
- 375 mg every 12 hours for 7–10 days (as extended-release tablets).

Urinary Tract Infections (UTIs)

ORAL:
- 250 mg every 8 hours (as capsules or suspension). For more severe infections or those caused by less susceptible organisms, 500 mg every 8 hours (as capsules or oral suspension).

Prescribing Limits

Pediatric Patients

Maximum 1 g daily.

Special Populations

Renal Impairment
- No dosage adjustments required.
- Close clinical observation and appropriate laboratory tests recommended in those with moderate or severe renal impair-

ment. Use with caution in patients with markedly impaired renal function.

Geriatric Patients
- No age-related dosage adjustments required.

Cefadroxil

(sef a drox' il)

Brand Name: Duricef®
Also available generically.

Why is this medicine prescribed?

Cefadroxil is a cephalosporin antibiotic used to treat certain infections caused by bacteria such as skin, throat, and urinary tract infections. Antibiotics will not work for colds, flu, or other viral infections.

This medication is sometimes prescribed for other uses; ask your doctor or pharmacist for more information.

How should this medicine be used?

Cefadroxil comes as a capsule, tablet, and liquid to take by mouth. It is usually taken once a day or every 12 hours (twice a day) for 7-10 days. Follow the directions on your prescription label carefully, and ask your doctor or pharmacist to explain any part you do not understand. Take cefadroxil exactly as directed. Do not take more or less of it or take it more often than prescribed by your doctor.

Shake the liquid well before each use to mix the medication evenly.

The capsules and tablets should be swallowed whole and taken with a full glass of water.

Continue to take cefadroxil even if you feel well. Do not stop taking cefadroxil without talking to your doctor.

What special precautions should I follow?

Before taking cefadroxil,
- tell your doctor and pharmacist if you are allergic to cefadroxil or any other cephalosporin antibiotic such as cefaclor (Ceclor) or cephalexin (Keflex), penicillin, or any other drugs.
- tell your doctor and pharmacist what prescription and nonprescription medications you are taking, especially other antibiotics, anticoagulants ('blood thinners') such as warfarin (Coumadin), probenecid (Benemid), and vitamins.
- tell your doctor if you have or have ever had kidney or liver disease, colitis, or stomach problems.
- tell your doctor if you are pregnant, plan to become pregnant, or are breast-feeding. If you become pregnant while taking cefadroxil, call your doctor.
- if you are having surgery, including dental surgery, tell the doctor or dentist that you are taking cefadroxil.

What special dietary instructions should I follow?

Cefadroxil may cause an upset stomach. Take cefadroxil with food or milk.

What should I do if I forget to take a dose?

Take the missed dose as soon as you remember it. However, if it is almost time for the next dose, skip the missed dose and continue your regular dosing schedule. Do not take a double dose to make up for a missed one.

What side effects can this medicine cause?

Cefadroxil may cause side effects. Tell your doctor if any of these symptoms are severe or do not go away:
- upset stomach
- diarrhea
- vomiting
- mild skin rash

If you experience any of the following symptoms, call your doctor immediately:
- severe skin rash
- itching
- hives
- difficulty breathing or swallowing
- wheezing
- unusual bleeding or bruising
- sore throat
- painful mouth or throat sores
- vaginal infection

If you experience a serious side effect, you or your doctor may send a report to the Food and Drug Administration's (FDA) MedWatch Adverse Event Reporting program online [at http://www.fda.gov/MedWatch/index.html] or by phone [1-800-332-1088].

What storage conditions are needed for this medicine?

Keep this medication in the container it came in, tightly closed, and out of reach of children. Store the capsules and tablets at room temperature and away from excess heat and moisture (not in the bathroom). Throw away any medication that is outdated or no longer needed. Keep liquid medicine in the refrigerator, tightly closed, and throw away any unused medication after 14 days. Do not freeze. Talk to your pharmacist about the proper disposal of your medication.

What should I do in case of overdose?

In case of overdose, call your local poison control center at 1-800-222-1222. If the victim has collapsed or is not breathing, call local emergency services at 911.

What other information should I know?

Keep all appointments with your doctor and the laboratory. Your doctor will order certain lab tests to check your response to cefadroxil.

If you are diabetic, use Clinistix or TesTape (not Clinitest) to test your urine for sugar while taking this drug.

Do not let anyone else take your medication. Your prescription is probably not refillable. If you still have symptoms of infection after you finish the cefadroxil, call your doctor.

Dosage Facts
For Informational Purposes

Caution: Do not change your dose, how often you take your medication, or the length of time you are to take it without first talking to your healthcare provider.

The following dosage information was written using medical language for doctors and other healthcare professionals and is provided here for you to check your dosage. The dosage of this drug may differ for different patients. Therefore, always follow your doctor's instructions or the directions on the label. Contact your healthcare provider or pharmacist if you have any questions about the specific dosage of your medication after reviewing this information.

General Dosage Information

Available as the monohydrate; dosage expressed as cefadroxil.

Pediatric Patients

Pharyngitis and Tonsillitis
ORAL:
- 30 mg/kg daily given as a single dose or in 2 equally divided doses for ≥10 days.

Skin and Skin Structure Infections
Impetigo
ORAL:
- 30 mg/kg daily given as a single dose or in 2 equally divided doses.

Other Skin and Skin Structure Infections
ORAL:
- 30 mg/kg daily given in 2 equally divided doses.

Urinary Tract Infections (UTIs)
ORAL:
- 30 mg/kg daily given in 2 equally divided doses.

Prevention of Bacterial Endocarditis†
Patients Undergoing Certain Dental, Oral, Respiratory Tract, or Esophageal Procedures†
ORAL:
- 50 mg/kg (up to 2 g) as a single dose given 1 hour prior to the procedure.

Adult Patients

Pharyngitis and Tonsillitis
ORAL:
- 1 g daily given as a single dose or in 2 divided doses for 10 days.

Skin and Skin Structure Infections
ORAL:
- 1 g daily given as a single dose or in 2 divided doses.

Urinary Tract Infections (UTIs)
Uncomplicated Lower UTIs (e.g., Cystitis)
ORAL:
- 1 or 2 g daily given as a single dose or in 2 divided doses.

Other UTIs
ORAL:
- 2 g daily given in 2 divided doses.

Prevention of Bacterial Endocarditis†
Patients Undergoing Certain Dental, Oral, Respiratory Tract, or Esophageal Procedures†
ORAL:
- 2 g as a single dose given 1 hour prior to the procedure.

Special Populations

Renal Impairment
- Dosage adjustments required if $Cl_{cr} \leq 50$ mL/minute per 1.73 m². Use an initial 1-g induction dose followed by 500-mg maintenance doses given at intervals based on the degree of renal impairment.

Adult Dosage in Renal Impairment

Cl_{cr} (mL/min per 1.73 m²)	Induction Dose	Maintenance Dosage
25–50	1 g	500 mg every 12 hours
10–25	1 g	500 mg every 24 hours
0–10	1 g	500 mg every 36 hours

Geriatric Patients
- No dosage adjustments except those related to renal impairment. Cautious dosage selection because of age-related decreases in renal function.

† Use is not currently included in the labeling approved by the US Food and Drug Administration.

Cefazolin Sodium Injection
(sef a′ zoe lin)

Brand Name: Ancef®
Also available generically.

About Your Treatment

Your doctor has ordered cefazolin, an antibiotic, to help treat your infection. The drug will be either injected into a large muscle (such as your buttock or hip) or added to an intravenous fluid that will drip through a needle or catheter placed in your vein for 30 minutes, two to four times a day.

Cefazolin eliminates bacteria that cause many kinds of infections, including lung, skin, bone, joint, stomach, blood, heart valve, and urinary tract infections. This medication is sometimes prescribed for other uses; ask your doctor or pharmacist for more information.

Your health care provider (doctor, nurse, or pharmacist) may measure the effectiveness and side effects of your treatment using laboratory tests and physical examinations. It is important to keep all appointments with your doctor and the laboratory. The length of treatment depends on how your infection and symptoms respond to the medication.

Precautions

Before administering cefazolin,

- tell your doctor and pharmacist if you are allergic to cefazolin, any other cephalosporin [e.g., cefaclor (Ceclor), cefadroxil (Duricef), or cephalexin (Keflex)], penicillins, or any other drugs.
- tell your doctor and pharmacist what prescription and nonprescription medications you are taking, especially other antibiotics, probenecid (Benemid), and vitamins.
- tell your doctor if you have or have ever had kidney, liver, or gastrointestinal disease (especially colitis).
- tell your doctor if you are pregnant, plan to become pregnant, or are breast-feeding. If you become pregnant while taking cefazolin, call your doctor.
- if you have diabetes and regularly check your urine for sugar, use Clinistix or TesTape. Do not use Clinitest tablets because cefazolin may cause false positive results.

Administering Your Medication

Before you administer cefazolin, look at the solution closely. It should be clear and free of floating material. Gently squeeze the bag or observe the solution container to make sure there are no leaks. Do not use the solution if it is discolored, if it contains particles, or if the bag or container leaks. Use a new solution, but show the damaged one to your health care provider.

It is important that you use your medication exactly as directed. Do not stop your therapy on your own for any reason because your infection could worsen and result in hospitalization. Do not change your dosing schedule without talking to your health care provider. Your health care provider may tell you to stop your infusion if you have a mechanical problem (such as a blockage in the tubing, needle, or catheter); if you have to stop an infusion, call your health care provider immediately so your therapy can continue.

Side Effects

Cefazolin may cause side effects. If you are administering cefazolin into a muscle, it may be mixed with lidocaine (Xylocaine) to reduce pain at the injection site. Tell your health

care provider if any of these symptoms are severe or do not go away:

- diarrhea
- stomach pain
- upset stomach
- vomiting

If you experience any of the following symptoms, call your health care provider immediately:

- skin rash
- itching
- hives
- unusual bleeding or bruising
- difficulty breathing
- sore mouth or throat

If you experience a serious side effect, you or your doctor may send a report to the Food and Drug Administration's (FDA) MedWatch Adverse Event Reporting program online [at http://www.fda.gov/MedWatch/index.html] or by phone [1-800-332-1088].

Storage Conditions

- Your health care provider probably will give you a several-day supply of cefazolin at a time. If you are receiving cefazolin intravenously (in your vein), you probably will be told to store it in the refrigerator or freezer.
- Take your next dose from the refrigerator 1 hour before using it; place it in a clean, dry area to allow it to warm to room temperature.
- If you are told to store additional cefazolin in the freezer, always move a 24-hour supply to the refrigerator for the next day's use.
- Do not refreeze medications.

If you are receiving cefazolin intramuscularly (in your muscle), your health care provider will tell you how to store it properly.

Store your medication only as directed. Make sure you understand what you need to store your medication properly.

Keep your supplies in a clean, dry place when you are not using them, and keep all medications and supplies out of reach of children. Your health care provider will tell you how to throw away used needles, syringes, tubing, and containers to avoid accidental injury.

Overdose

In case of overdose, call your local poison control center at 1-800-222-1222. If the victim has collapsed or is not breathing, call local emergency services at 911.

Signs of Infection

If you are receiving cefazolin in your vein or under your skin, you need to know the symptoms of a catheter-related infection (an infection where the needle enters your vein or skin). If you experience any of these effects near your intravenous catheter, tell your health care provider as soon as possible:

- tenderness
- warmth

- irritation
- drainage
- redness
- swelling
- pain

Dosage Facts
For Informational Purposes

Caution: Do not change your dose, how often you take your medication, or the length of time you are to take it without first talking to your healthcare provider.

The following dosage information was written using medical language for doctors and other healthcare professionals and is provided here for you to check your dosage. The dosage of this drug may differ for different patients. Therefore, always follow your doctor's instructions or the directions on the label. Contact your healthcare provider or pharmacist if you have any questions about the specific dosage of your medication after reviewing this information.

General Dosage Information

Available as cefazolin sodium; dosage expressed in terms of cefazolin.

Pediatric Patients

Mild to Moderately Severe Infections

IV OR IM:
- Children >1 month of age: 25–50 mg/kg daily in 3 or 4 equally divided doses.

Severe Infections

IV:
- Children >1 month of age: 50–100 mg/kg daily in 3 or 4 equally divided doses.

Endocarditis
Treatment of Staphylococcal Endocarditis

IV:
- 100 mg/kg daily in 3 or 4 equally divided doses.
- For native valve endocarditis, duration of treatment is 6 weeks (with or without gentamicin given during the first 3–5 days).
- For endocarditis involving prosthetic valves or other prosthetic materials, duration of treatment is ≥6 weeks (with or without rifampin given for ≥6 weeks).

Prevention of Endocarditis in Patients Undergoing Certain Dental, Oral, Respiratory Tract, or Esophageal Procedures†

IV OR IM:
- 25 mg/kg given within 30 minutes prior to the procedure.

Perioperative Prophylaxis
Cardiac or Cardiothoracic Surgery

IV:
- 20–30 mg/kg given at induction of anesthesia (within 0.5–1 hour prior to incision). Some experts suggest additional doses of 20–30 mg/kg every 8 hours for up to 48–72 hours; others state that prophylaxis for ≤24 hours is appropriate.

Neurosurgery or Head and Neck Surgery

IV:
- 20–30 mg/kg given at induction of anesthesia (within 0.5–1 hour prior to incision).

GI, Pancreatic, or Biliary Tract Surgery

IV:
- 20–30 mg/kg given at induction of anesthesia (within 0.5–1 hour prior to incision).

Vascular or Orthopedic Surgery

IV:
- 20–30 mg/kg given at induction of anesthesia (within 0.5–1 hour prior to incision). Some experts also suggest 20–30 mg/kg every 8 hours for 24 hours.

Adult Patients

Mild Infections Caused by Gram-positive Bacteria

IV OR IM:
- 250–500 mg every 8 hours.

Moderate to Severe Infections

IV OR IM:
- 500 mg–1 g every 6–8 hours.

Severe, Life-threatening Infections

IV OR IM:
- 1–1.5 g every 6 hours. Dosage up to 12 g daily has been used.

Endocarditis
Treatment of Endocarditis

IV OR IM:
- 1–1.5 g every 6 hours. Dosage up to 12 g daily has been used.
- AHA recommends 2 g IV every 8 hours for 4–6 weeks for native valve staphylococcal endocarditis (with or without gentamicin during the first 3–5 days).

Prevention of Endocarditis in Patients Undergoing Certain Dental, Oral, Respiratory Tract, or Esophageal Procedures†

IV OR IM:
- 1 g given within 30 minutes prior to the procedure.

Respiratory Tract Infections
Pneumococcal Pneumonia

IV OR IM:
- 500 mg every 12 hours.

Septicemia

IV OR IM:
- 1–1.5 g every 6 hours. Doses up to 12 g daily have been used.

Urinary Tract Infections (UTIs)
Acute Uncomplicated Infections

IV OR IM:
- 1 g every 12 hours.

Prevention of Perinatal Group B Streptococcal (GBS) Disease†

IV:

- An initial 2-g dose (at time of labor or rupture of membranes) followed by 1 g every 8 hours until delivery.

Perioperative Prophylaxis
General Adult Dosage

IV OR IM:

- Manufacturers recommend 1 g given 0.5–1 hour prior to surgery; 0.5–1 g during surgery for lengthy procedures (e.g., ≥2 hours); and 0.5–1 g every 6–8 hours for 24 hours postoperatively. Manufacturers also recommend that prophylaxis be continued for 3–5 days following surgery where the occurrence of infection may be particularly devastating (e.g., open-heart surgery, prosthetic arthroplasty).
- Most clinicians recommend 1–2 g given no more than 0.5–1 hour before the incision and additional doses during the procedure (e.g., every 4–8 hours) only if surgery is prolonged >4 hours or major blood loss occurs. In most cases, postoperative doses are unnecessary and may increase the risk of toxicity and bacterial superinfection.

Cardiac, Cardiothoracic, or Noncardiac Thoracic Surgery.

IV:

- 1–2 g given at induction of anesthesia (within 0.5–1 hour prior to incision).
- In patients undergoing open-heart surgery, some experts recommend an additional dose when the patient is removed from bypass.
- For cardiothoracic surgery and heart and/or lung transplantation, some experts suggest additional 1-g doses every 8 hours for up to 48–72 hours; others state that prophylaxis for ≤24 hours is appropriate. There is no evidence to support continuing prophylaxis until chest and mediastinal drainage tubes are removed.

Neurosurgery or Head and Neck Surgery

IV:

- 1–2 g given at induction of anesthesia (within 0.5–1 hour prior to incision).
- For clean, contaminated head and neck surgery, some experts suggest 2 g given at induction of anesthesia and every 8 hours for 24 hours.

GI, Gastroduodenal, Colorectal, Pancreatic, or Biliary Tract Surgery

IV:

- 1–2 g given at induction of anesthesia (within 0.5–1 hour prior to incision).
- For colorectal surgery, use in conjunction with IV metronidazole.

Vascular or Orthopedic Surgery

IV:

- 1–2 g given at induction of anesthesia (within 0.5–1 hour prior to incision).
- Some experts suggest additional 1-g doses every 8 hours for up to 24 hours.

Gynecologic and Obstetric Surgery

IV:

- 1–2 g given at induction of anesthesia (within 0.5–1 hour prior to incision) for hysterectomy or as soon as umbilical cord is clamped for cesarean section.

Contaminated or Dirty Surgery Involving a Traumatic Wound†

IV:

- 1–2 g every 8 hours; continue postoperatively for about 5 days.

Special Populations

Hepatic Impairment

- No dosage recommendations.

Renal Impairment

- Dosage adjustments recommended in patients with Cl_{cr} <55 mL/minute.
- Administer an initial loading dose appropriate for the severity of the infection, followed by dosage based on the degree of renal impairment.

Dosage for Adults with Renal Impairment

Cl_{cr} (mL/minute)	Dose	Frequency
35–54	Full dose	≥8-hour intervals
11–34	50% of usual dose	Every 12 hours
≤10	50% of usual dose	Every 18–24 hours

Dosage for Children >1 Month of Age with Renal Impairment

Cl_{cr} (mL/minute)	Dose	Frequency
40–70	60% of usual dose	Every 12 hours
20–40	25% of usual dose	Every 12 hours
5–20	10% of usual dose	Every 24 hours

† *Use is not currently included in the labeling approved by the US Food and Drug Administration.*

Cefdinir

(sef′ di ner)

Brand Name: Omnicef®

Why is this medicine prescribed?

Cefdinir is an antibiotic used to treat certain infections caused by bacteria, such as pneumonia, bronchitis, ear infections, sinusitis, pharyngitis, tonsillitis, and skin infections. Antibiotics will not work for colds, flu, or other viral infections.

This medication is sometimes prescribed for other uses; ask your doctor or pharmacist for more information.

How should this medicine be used?

Cefdinir comes as a capsule and as an oral suspension. It is usually taken once or twice a day. Shake the suspension well before each use to mix the medication evenly. Follow the directions on your prescription label carefully, and ask your doctor or pharmacist to explain any part you do not understand. Take cefdinir exactly as directed. Do not take more or less of it or take it more often than prescribed by your doctor.

Continue to take cefdinir even if you feel well. Do not stop taking cefdinir without talking to your doctor.

What special precautions should I follow?

Before taking cefdinir,

- tell your doctor and pharmacist if you are allergic to cefdinir or any other cephalosporin antibiotic such as cefaclor (Ceclor) or cephalexin (Keflex), penicillin, or any other drugs.
- tell your doctor and pharmacist what prescription and nonprescription medications you are taking, especially probenecid (Benemid, Probalan) and vitamins.
- be aware that antacids containing magnesium or aluminum and products containing iron interfere with cefdinir, making it less effective. Take cefdinir 2 hours before or 2 hours after antacids or iron products.
- tell your doctor if you have or have ever had colitis, diabetes, or kidney disease.
- tell your doctor if you are pregnant, plan to become pregnant, or are breast-feeding. If you become pregnant while taking cefdinir, call your doctor.

What special dietary instructions should I follow?

Cefdinir may cause an upset stomach. Take cefdinir with food or milk.

What should I do if I forget to take a dose?

Take the missed dose as soon as you remember it. However, if it is almost time for the next dose, skip the missed dose and continue your regular dosing schedule. Do not take a double dose to make up for a missed one.

What side effects can this medicine cause?

Cefdinir may cause side effects. Tell your doctor if any of these symptoms are severe or do not go away:

- upset stomach
- vomiting
- loss of appetite
- diarrhea
- headache
- dizziness
- fatigue

If you experience any of the following symptoms, call your doctor immediately:

- rash
- hives
- swelling of the face, eyes, lips, tongue, arms, or legs
- difficulty breathing or swallowing
- vaginal infection

If you experience a serious side effect, you or your doctor may send a report to the Food and Drug Administration's (FDA) MedWatch Adverse Event Reporting program online [at http://www.fda.gov/MedWatch/index.html] or by phone [1-800-332-1088].

What storage conditions are needed for this medicine?

Keep this medication in the container it came in, tightly closed, and out of reach of children. Store it at room temperature and away from excess heat and moisture (not in the bathroom). Throw away any medication that is outdated or no longer needed. Talk to your pharmacist about the proper disposal of your medication.

What should I do in case of overdose?

In case of overdose, call your local poison control center at 1-800-222-1222. If the victim has collapsed or is not breathing, call local emergency services at 911.

What other information should I know?

Keep all appointments with your doctor and laboratory. Your doctor may order certain lab tests to check your response to cefdinir.

If you are diabetic, use Clinistix or TesTape (but not Clinitest) to test your urine for sugar while taking this drug; cefdinir may cause false positive results.

Do not let anyone else take your medication. Your prescription is probably not refillable. If you still have symptoms of infection after you finish the cefdinir, call your doctor.

Dosage Facts
For Informational Purposes

Caution: Do not change your dose, how often you take your medication, or the length of time you are to take it without first talking to your healthcare provider.

The following dosage information was written using medical language for doctors and other healthcare professionals and is provided here for you to check your dosage. The dosage of this drug may differ for different patients. Therefore, always follow your doctor's instructions or the directions on the label. Contact your healthcare provider or pharmacist if you have any questions about the specific dosage of your medication after reviewing this information.

Pediatric Patients

Acute Otitis Media (AOM)

ORAL:
- Children 6 months to 12 years of age weighing <43 kg: 14 mg/kg once daily for 10 days or 7 mg/kg every 12 hours for 5–10 days.

Pharyngitis and Tonsillitis

ORAL:

- Children 6 months to 12 years of age weighing <43 kg: 14 mg/kg once daily for 10 days or 7 mg/kg every 12 hours for 5–10 days.
- Children ≥13 year of age or weighing ≥43 kg: 600 mg once daily for 10 days or 300 mg every 12 hours for 5–10 days.

Respiratory Tract Infections

Acute Sinusitis

ORAL:

- Children 6 months through 12 years of age weighing <43 kg: 14 mg/kg once daily for 10 days or 7 mg/kg every 12 hours for 10 days.
- Children ≥13 years of age or weighing ≥43 kg: 600 mg once daily for 10 days or 300 mg every 12 hours for 10 days.

Acute Exacerbations of Chronic Bronchitis

ORAL:

- Children ≥13 year of age: 600 mg once daily for 10 days or 300 mg every 12 hours for 5–10 days.

Community-acquired Pneumonia

ORAL:

- Children ≥13 year of age: 300 mg every 12 hours for 10 days.

Skin and Skin Structure Infections

ORAL:

- Children 6 months to 12 years of age weighing <43 kg: 7 mg/kg every 12 hours for 10 days.
- Children ≥13 year of age or weighing ≥43 kg: 300 mg every 12 hours for 10 days.

Adult Patients

Pharyngitis and Tonsillitis

ORAL:

- 600 mg once daily for 10 days or 300 mg every 12 hours for 5–10 days.

Respiratory Tract Infections

Acute Sinusitis

ORAL:

- 600 mg once daily for 10 days or 300 mg every 12 hours for 10 days.

Acute Exacerbations of Chronic Bronchitis

ORAL:

- 600 mg once daily for 10 days or 300 mg every 12 hours for 5–10 days.

Community-acquired Pneumonia

ORAL:

- 300 mg every 12 hours for 10 days.

Skin and Skin Structure Infections

ORAL:

- 300 mg every 12 hours for 10 days.

Special Populations

Hepatic Impairment

- No dosage adjustments required.

Renal Impairment

- Dosage adjustments recommended in patients with severe renal impairment (Cl_{cr} <30 mL/minute).

- Adults: 300 mg once daily if Cl_{cr} <30 mL/minute.
- Children: 7 mg/kg (maximum 300 mg) once daily if Cl_{cr} <30 mL/minute.
- Patients maintained on long-term hemodialysis: Recommended initial dosage is 300 mg every 48 hours in adults and 7 mg/kg (maximum 300 mg) every 48 hours in children. Administer a supplemental dose (300 mg in adults or 7 mg/kg in children) at the end of each dialysis period.

Geriatric Patients

- No dosage adjustments except those related to renal impairment.

Cefditoren

(sef dit′ or in)

Brand Name: Spectracef®

Why is this medicine prescribed?

Cefditoren is used to treat infections such as community acquired pneumonia (a lung infection that developed in a person who was not in the hospital), flare-ups of chronic bronchitis (infection of the tubes that lead to the lungs), strep throat (sore throat caused by bacteria), tonsillitis (infection of the glands in the back of the throat), and some types of skin infections. Cefditoren is in a class of antibiotics called cephalosporins. It works by killing bacteria. Antibiotics will not work for colds, flu, or other viral infections.

How should this medicine be used?

Cefditoren comes as a tablet to take by mouth. It is usually taken twice a day with the morning and evening meals for 10 to 14 days. To help you remember to take cefditoren, take it at around the same times every day. Follow the directions on your prescription label carefully, and ask your doctor or pharmacist to explain any part you do not understand. Take cefditoren exactly as directed. Do not take more or less of it or take it more often than prescribed by your doctor.

Swallow the tablets with a full glass of water.

You should begin to feel better during your first few days of treatment with cefditoren. If you do not, call your doctor.

Take cefditoren until you finish the prescription, even if you feel better. If you stop taking cefditoren too soon or skip doses, your infection may not be completely cured and bacteria may become resistant to antibiotics.

Are there other uses for this medicine?

This medication may be prescribed for other uses; ask your doctor or pharmacist for more information.

What special precautions should I follow?

Before taking cefditoren,

- tell your doctor and pharmacist if you are allergic to

cefditoren or any other medications. It is especially important to tell your doctor if you are allergic to any other antibiotics because this may increase the chance that you will have an allergic reaction to cefditoren. Also tell your doctor if you are allergic to milk protein.

- tell your doctor and pharmacist what prescription and nonprescription medications, vitamins, nutritional supplements, and herbal products you are taking. Be sure to mention any of the following: antacids (Maalox, Mylanta, Tums, others); anticoagulants ('blood thinners') such as warfarin (Coumadin); medications that block stomach acid such as cimetidine (Tagamet), famotidine (Pepcid), nizatidine (Axid) and ranitidine (Zantac); or probenecid (Probalan).Your doctor may need to change the doses of your medications or monitor you carefully for side effects.
- tell your doctor if you have or have ever had carnitine deficiency (a rare condition in which the body does not have enough of a certain substance that is needed for energy production), or kidney or liver disease.
- tell your doctor if you are pregnant, plan to become pregnant, or are breast-feeding. If you become pregnant while taking cefditoren, call your doctor.
- you should know that cefditoren may cause a serious type of diarrhea during or after your treatment. Call your doctor if you have diarrhea at these times. Do not treat this diarrhea with over the counter medications.

What special dietary instructions should I follow?

Unless your doctor tells you otherwise, continue your normal diet.

What should I do if I forget to take a dose?

Take the missed dose as soon as you remember it. However, if it is almost time for the next dose, skip the missed dose and continue your regular dosing schedule. Do not take a double dose to make up for a missed one.

What side effects can this medicine cause?

Cefditoren may cause side effects. Tell your doctor if any of these symptoms are severe or do not go away:
- upset stomach
- vomiting
- stomach pain
- heartburn
- headache
- swelling, redness, irritation, burning, or itching of the vagina
- white vaginal discharge

Some side effects can be serious. The following symptoms are uncommon, but if you experience any of them, call your doctor immediately:
- hives
- rash
- itching

- difficulty breathing or swallowing
- closing of the throat
- fever
- seizures

Cefditoren may cause other side effects. Call your doctor if you have any unusual problems while taking this medication.

If you experience a serious side effect, you or your doctor may send a report to the Food and Drug Administration's (FDA) MedWatch Adverse Event Reporting program online [at http://www.fda.gov/MedWatch/index.html] or by phone [1-800-332-1088].

What storage conditions are needed for this medicine?

Keep this medication in the container it came in, tightly closed, and out of reach of children. Store it at room temperature and away from excess heat and moisture (not in the bathroom). Protect this medication from light. Throw away any medication that is outdated or no longer needed. Talk to your pharmacist about the proper disposal of your medication.

What should I do in case of overdose?

In case of overdose, call your local poison control center at 1-800-222-1222. If the victim has collapsed or is not breathing, call local emergency services at 911.

Symptoms of overdose may include:
- upset stomach
- vomiting
- stomach pain
- diarrhea
- seizures

What other information should I know?

Keep all appointments with your doctor

Before having any laboratory test, tell your doctor and the laboratory personnel that you are taking cefditoren.

If you are diabetic, use Clinistix or TesTape (not Clinitest) to test your urine for sugar while taking this medication.

Do not let anyone else take your medication. Your prescription is probably not refillable. If you still have symptoms of infection after you finish the cefditoren, call your doctor.

Dosage Facts
For Informational Purposes

Caution: Do not change your dose, how often you take your medication, or the length of time you are to take it without first talking to your healthcare provider.

The following dosage information was written using medical language for doctors and other healthcare pro-

fessionals and is provided here for you to check your dosage. The dosage of this drug may differ for different patients. Therefore, always follow your doctor's instructions or the directions on the label. Contact your health-care provider or pharmacist if you have any questions about the specific dosage of your medication after reviewing this information.

General Dosage Information

Available as cefditoren pivoxil; dosage expressed in terms of cefditoren.

Pediatric Patients

Respiratory Tract Infections
Acute Bacterial Exacerbations of Chronic Bronchitis

ORAL:
• Children ≥12 years of age: 400 mg twice daily for 10 days.

Community-acquired Pneumonia

ORAL:
• Children ≥12 years of age: 400 mg twice daily for 14 days.

Pharyngitis and Tonsillitis

ORAL:
• Children ≥12 years of age: 200 mg twice daily for 10 days.

Skin and Skin Structure Infections

ORAL:
• Children ≥12 years of age: 200 mg twice daily for 10 days.

Adult Patients

Respiratory Tract Infections
Acute Bacterial Exacerbations of Chronic Bronchitis

ORAL:
• 400 mg twice daily for 10 days.

Community-acquired Pneumonia

ORAL:
• 400 mg twice daily for 14 days.

Pharyngitis and Tonsillitis

ORAL:
• 200 mg twice daily for 10 days.

Skin and Skin Structure Infections

ORAL:
• 200 mg twice daily for 10 days.

Special Populations

Hepatic Impairment
• No dosage adjustments required in patients with mild or moderate hepatic impairment (Child-Pugh class A or B).
• Pharmacokinetics have not been studied in patients with severe hepatic impairment (Child-Pugh class C).

Renal Impairment
• No dosage adjustments required in patients with mild renal impairment (Cl_{cr} 50–80 mL/min per 1.73 m²).
• Maximum dosage of 200 mg twice daily for those with moderate renal impairment (Cl_{cr} 30–49 mL/min per 1.73 m²).
• Maximum dosage of 200 mg once daily for those with severe renal impairment (Cl_{cr} <30 mL/min per 1.73 m²).
• The appropriate dosage for patients with end-stage renal disease has not been determined.

Geriatric Patients
• No dosage adjustments except those related to renal impairment. Cautious dosage selection because of age-related decreases in renal function.

Cefepime Injection

(sef′ e pim)

Brand Name: Maxipime®

About Your Treatment

Your doctor has ordered cefepime, an antibiotic, to help treat your infection. The drug will be either injected into a large muscle (such as your buttock or hip) or added to an intravenous fluid that will drip through a needle or catheter placed in your vein for 30 minutes, one or two times a day.

Cefepime eliminates bacteria that cause many infections, including pneumonia and skin and urinary tract infections. This medication is sometimes prescribed for other uses; ask your doctor or pharmacist for more information.

Your health care provider (doctor, nurse, or pharmacist) may measure the effectiveness and side effects of your treatment using laboratory tests and physical examinations. It is important to keep all appointments with your doctor and the laboratory. The length of treatment depends on how your infection and symptoms respond to the medication.

Precautions

Before administering cefepime,
• tell your doctor and pharmacist if you are allergic to cefepime, penicillin, cephalosporins [cefaclor (Ceclor), cefadroxil (Duricef), or cephalexin (Keflex)], or any other drugs.
• tell your doctor and pharmacist what prescription and nonprescription medications you are taking, including vitamins.
• tell your doctor if you have or have ever had kidney, liver, or gastrointestinal disease (especially colitis).
• tell your doctor if you are pregnant, plan to become pregnant, or are breast-feeding. If you become pregnant while taking cefepime, call your doctor.
• if you have diabetes and regularly check your urine for sugar, use Clinistix or Tes-Tape. Do not use Clinitest tablets, because cefepime may cause false positive results.

Administering Your Medication

Before you administer cefepime, look at the solution closely. It should be clear and free of floating material. Gently squeeze the bag or observe the solution container to make sure there are no leaks. Do not use the solution if it is discolored, if it contains particles, or if the bag or container leaks. Use a new solution, but show the damaged one to your health care provider.

It is important that you use your medication exactly as directed. Do not stop your therapy on your own for any reason because your infection could worsen and result in hospitalization. Do not change your dosing schedule without talking to your health care provider. Your health care provider may tell you to stop your infusion if you have a mechanical problem (such as a blockage in the tubing, needle, or catheter); if you have to stop an infusion, call your health care provider immediately so your therapy can continue.

Side Effects

Cefepime may cause side effects. If you are administering cefepime into a muscle, it may be mixed with lidocaine (Xylocaine) to reduce pain at the injection site. Tell your health care provider if any of these symptoms are severe or do not go away:

- diarrhea
- stomach pain
- upset stomach
- vomiting

If you experience any of the following symptoms, call your health care provider immediately:

- skin rash
- unusual bleeding or bruising
- difficulty breathing
- hives
- sore mouth or throat

If you experience a serious side effect, you or your doctor may send a report to the Food and Drug Administration's (FDA) MedWatch Adverse Event Reporting program online [at http://www.fda.gov/MedWatch/index.html] or by phone [1-800-332-1088].

Storage Conditions

- Your health care provider probably will give you a several-day supply of cefepime at a time. If you are receiving cefepime intravenously (in your vein), you probably will be told to store it in the refrigerator.
- Take your next dose from the refrigerator 1 hour before using it; place it in a clean, dry area to allow it to warm to room temperature.

If you are receiving cefepime intramuscularly (in your muscle), your health care provider will tell you how to store it properly.

Store your medication only as directed. Make sure you understand what you need to store your medication properly.

Keep your supplies in a clean, dry place when you are not using them, and keep all medications and supplies out of reach of children. Your health care provider will tell you how to throw away used needles, syringes, tubing, and containers to avoid accidental injury.

Overdose

In case of overdose, call your local poison control center at 1-800-222-1222. If the victim has collapsed or is not breathing, call local emergency services at 911.

Signs of Infection

If you are receiving cefepime in your vein or under your skin, you need to know the symptoms of a catheter-related infection (an infection where the needle enters your vein or skin). If you experience any of these effects near your intravenous catheter, tell your health care provider as soon as possible:

- tenderness
- warmth
- irritation
- drainage
- redness
- swelling
- pain

Dosage Facts
For Informational Purposes

Caution: Do not change your dose, how often you take your medication, or the length of time you are to take it without first talking to your healthcare provider.

The following dosage information was written using medical language for doctors and other healthcare professionals and is provided here for you to check your dosage. The dosage of this drug may differ for different patients. Therefore, always follow your doctor's instructions or the directions on the label. Contact your healthcare provider or pharmacist if you have any questions about the specific dosage of your medication after reviewing this information.

General Dosage Information

Available as cefepime hydrochloride; dosage expressed in terms of cefepime.

Pediatric Patients
General Pediatric Dosage

IV OR IM:

- Children 2 months to 16 years of age weighing <40 kg: 50 mg/kg every 12 hours.
- AAP recommends 100–150 mg/kg daily in 3 divided doses for treatment of mild to moderate infections and 150 mg/kg daily in 3 divided doses for treatment of severe infections in children >1 month of age.

Respiratory Tract Infections
Pneumonia

IV:

- Children 2 months to 16 years of age weighing <40 kg: 50 mg/kg every 12 hours for 10 days.

Skin and Skin Structure Infections
Uncomplicated Infections

IV:

- Children 2 months to 16 years of age weighing <40 kg: 50 mg/kg every 12 hours for 10 days.

Urinary Tract Infections (UTIs)
Uncomplicated or Complicated UTIs

IV OR IM:

- Children 2 months to 16 years of age weighing <40 kg: 50 mg/kg every 12 hours for 7–10 days.

Empiric Therapy in Febrile Neutropenic Patients

IV:

- Children 2 months to 16 years of age weighing <40 kg: 50 mg/kg every 8 hours for 7 days or until neutropenia resolves.
- Frequently reevaluate need for continued anti-infective therapy if fever resolves but neutropenia remains for >7 days.

Adult Patients

Intra-abdominal Infections
Complicated Infections

IV:

- 2 g every 12 hours for 7–10 days; use in conjunction with IV metronidazole.

Respiratory Tract Infections
Moderate to Severe Pneumonia

IV:

- 1–2 g every 12 hours for 10 days.

Skin and Skin Structure Infections
Moderate to Severe Uncomplicated Infections

IV:

- 2 g every 12 hours for 10 days.

Urinary Tract Infections (UTIs)
Mild to Moderate Uncomplicated or Complicated UTIs

IV OR IM:

- 0.5–1 g every 12 hours for 7–10 days.

Severe Uncomplicated or Complicated UTIs

IV:

- 2 g every 12 hours for 10 days.

Empiric Therapy in Febrile Neutropenic Patients

IV:

- 2 g every 8 hours for 7 days or until neutropenia resolves.
- Frequently reevaluate need for continued anti-infective therapy if fever resolves but neutropenia remains for >7 days.

Prescribing Limits

Pediatric Patients

Dosage should not exceed recommended adult dosage.

Special Populations

Hepatic Impairment

- Dosage adjustments not required.

Renal Impairment

- Dosage adjustments necessary in patients with $Cl_{cr} \leq 60$ mL/minute.

- Adults with $Cl_{cr} \leq 60$ mL/minute: give an initial loading dose using the usually recommended adult dosage followed by maintenance dosage based on Cl_{cr}. and

Maintenance Dosage for Treatment of Infections in Adults with Renal Impairment

Cl_{cr} (mL/minute)	Initial dose: 500 mg	Initial dose: 1 g	Initial dose: 2 g
30–60	500 mg every 24 h	1 g every 24 h	2 g every 24 h
11–29	500 mg every 24 h	500 mg every 24 h	1 g every 24 h
<11	250 mg every 24 h	250 mg every 24 h	500 mg every 24 h

Maintenance Dosage for Empiric Therapy in Febrile Neutropenic Adults with Renal Impairment

Cl_{cr} (mL/minute)	Initial Dose: 2 g
30–60	2 g every 12 h
11–29	2 g every 24 h
<11	1 g every 24 h

Adults undergoing hemodialysis: 1 g on the first day of treatment followed by 500 mg every 24 hours for treatment of infections or 1 g on the first day followed by 1 g every 24 hours for empiric therapy in febrile neutropenic patients. Administer the dose at the same time each day (given at completion of procedure on hemodialysis days).

Adults undergoing CAPD: give usually recommended dose once every 48 hours.

Pediatric patients with renal impairment: make dosage adjustments similar to those recommended for adults.

Cefixime

(sef ix' eem)

Brand Name: Suprax®

Why is this medicine prescribed?

Cefixime is a cephalosporin antibiotic used to treat infections caused by bacteria such as pneumonia; bronchitis; gonorrhea; and ear, lung, throat, and urinary tract infections. Antibiotics will not work for colds, flu, or other viral infections.

This medication is sometimes prescribed for other uses; ask your doctor or pharmacist for more information.

How should this medicine be used?

Cefixime comes as a tablet and liquid to take by mouth. It is usually taken once a day or every 12 hours (twice a day) for 5-14 days. Gonorrhea may be treated in 1-10 days. Follow the directions on your prescription label carefully, and ask your doctor or pharmacist to explain any part you do not understand. Take cefixime exactly as directed. Do not take more or less of it or take it more often than prescribed by your doctor.

Shake the liquid well before each use to mix the medication evenly.

The tablets should be swallowed whole and taken with a full glass of water.

Continue to take cefixime even if you feel well. Do not stop taking cefixime without talking to your doctor.

What special precautions should I follow?

Before taking cefixime,

- tell your doctor and pharmacist if you are allergic to cefixime or other any cephalosporin antibiotic such as cefaclor (Ceclor) or cephalexin (Keflex), penicillin, or any other drugs.
- tell your doctor and pharmacist what prescription and nonprescription medications you are taking, especially other antibiotics, anticoagulants ('blood thinners') such as warfarin (Coumadin), aspirin, carbamazepine (Tegretol), probenecid (Benemid), and vitamins.
- tell your doctor if you have or have ever had kidney or liver disease, colitis, or stomach problems.
- tell your doctor if you are pregnant, plan to become pregnant, or are breast-feeding. If you become pregnant while taking cefixime, call your doctor.
- if you are having surgery, including dental surgery, tell the doctor or dentist that you are taking cefixime.

What special dietary instructions should I follow?

Cefixime may cause an upset stomach. Take cefixime with food or milk.

What should I do if I forget to take a dose?

Take the missed dose as soon as you remember it. However, if it is almost time for the next dose, skip the missed dose and continue your regular dosing schedule. Do not take a double dose to make up for a missed one.

What side effects can this medicine cause?

Cefixime may cause side effects. Tell your doctor if any of these symptoms are severe or do not go away:

- upset stomach
- diarrhea
- vomiting
- mild skin rash
- headache

If you experience any of the following symptoms, call your doctor immediately:

- severe skin rash
- itching
- hives

- difficulty breathing or swallowing
- wheezing
- vaginal infection

If you experience a serious side effect, you or your doctor may send a report to the Food and Drug Administration's (FDA) MedWatch Adverse Event Reporting program online [at http://www.fda.gov/MedWatch/index.html] or by phone [1-800-332-1088].

What storage conditions are needed for this medicine?

Keep this medication in the container it came in, tightly closed, and out of reach of children. Store the tablets at room temperature and away from excess heat and moisture (not in the bathroom). Throw away any medication that is outdated or no longer needed. Keep liquid medicine in the refrigerator, closed tightly, and throw away any unused medication after 14 days. Do not freeze. Talk to your pharmacist about the proper disposal of your medication.

What should I do in case of overdose?

In case of overdose, call your local poison control center at 1-800-222-1222. If the victim has collapsed or is not breathing, call local emergency services at 911.

What other information should I know?

Keep all appointments with your doctor and the laboratory. Your doctor will order certain lab tests to check your response to cefixime.

If you are diabetic, use Clinistix or TesTape (not Clinitest) to test your urine for sugar while taking this drug.

Do not let anyone else take your medication. Your prescription is probably not refillable. If you still have symptoms of infection after you finish the cefixime, call your doctor.

Dosage Facts
For Informational Purposes

Caution: Do not change your dose, how often you take your medication, or the length of time you are to take it without first talking to your healthcare provider.

The following dosage information was written using medical language for doctors and other healthcare professionals and is provided here for you to check your dosage. The dosage of this drug may differ for different patients. Therefore, always follow your doctor's instructions or the directions on the label. Contact your healthcare provider or pharmacist if you have any questions about the specific dosage of your medication after reviewing this information.

General Dosage Information

Available as cefixime trihydrate; dosage expressed in terms of cefixime.

Pediatric Patients

Respiratory Tract Infections
Acute Bronchitis

ORAL:
- Children 6 months to 12 years of age: 8 mg/kg once daily or 4 mg/kg every 12 hours for 10–14 days.
- Children >12 years of age or weighing >50 kg: 400 mg daily for 10–14 days.

Acute Exacerbations of Chronic Bronchitis

ORAL:
- Children 6 months to 12 years of age: 8 mg/kg once daily or 4 mg/kg every 12 hours for 10–14 days.
- Children >12 years of age or weighing >50 kg: 400 mg daily for 10–14 days.

Acute Otitis Media (AOM)

ORAL:
- Children 6 months to 12 years of age: 8 mg/kg once daily or 4 mg/kg every 12 hours for 10–14 days.
- Children >12 years of age or weighing >50 kg: 400 mg daily for 10–14 days.

Pharyngitis and Tonsillitis

ORAL:
- Children 6 months to 12 years of age: 8 mg/kg once daily or 4 mg/kg every 12 hours for ≥10 days.
- Children >12 years of age or weighing >50 kg: 400 mg daily for ≥10 days.

Urinary Tract Infections (UTIs)
Uncomplicated UTIs

ORAL:
- Children 6 months to 12 years of age: 8 mg/kg once daily or 4 mg/kg every 12 hours for 5–10 days.
- Children >12 years of age or weighing >50 kg: 400 mg daily 5–10 days.

Gonorrhea and Associated Infections
Uncomplicated Urethral, Endocervical, or Rectal† Gonorrhea

ORAL:
- Adolescents: 400 mg as a single dose.

Salmonella and Shigella Infections†
Typhoid Fever†

ORAL:
- Children 6 months to 13 years of age: 10 mg/kg daily in 2 divided doses for 14 days.

Shigellosis†

ORAL:
- 8 mg/kg daily for 5 days.

Adult Patients

Respiratory Tract Infections
Acute Bronchitis

ORAL:
- 400 mg once daily or 200 mg every 12 hours for 10–14 days.

Acute Exacerbations of Chronic Bronchitis

ORAL:
- 400 mg once daily or 200 mg every 12 hours for 10–14 days.

Acute Otitis Media (AOM)

ORAL:
- 400 mg once daily or 200 mg every 12 hours for 10–14 days.

Pharyngitis and Tonsillitis

ORAL:
- 400 mg once daily or 200 mg every 12 hours for ≥10 days.

Urinary Tract Infections (UTIs)
Uncomplicated UTIs

ORAL:
- 400 mg once daily or 200 mg every 12 hours for 5–10 days.

Gonorrhea and Associated Infections
Uncomplicated Urethral, Endocervical, or Rectal† Gonorrhea

ORAL:
- 400 mg as a single dose.

Disseminated Gonococcal Infections†

ORAL:
- 400 mg twice daily recommended by CDC; given to complete ≥1 week of treatment after an initial parenteral regimen of ceftriaxone, cefotaxime, ceftizoxime, or spectinomycin.

Lyme Disease†

ORAL:
- 200 mg daily for 100 days (administered with oral probenecid).

Special Populations

Renal Impairment
- Dosage adjustments necessary in patients with Cl_{cr} <60 mL/minute.

Dosage in Adults with Renal Impairment

Cl_{cr} (mL/min)	Dosage
21–60	75% of the usual dose given at usual intervals
<20	50% of the usual dose given at the usual intervals
Hemodialysis Patients	75% of the usual dose given at usual intervals; supplemental doses not necessary during or after hemodialysis
CAPD Patients	50% of the usual dose given at the usual intervals or the usual dose given at twice the usual dosing interval; supplemental doses not necessary during or after CAPD

Geriatric Patients
- No dosage adjustments except those related to renal impairment.

† Use is not currently included in the labeling approved by the US Food and Drug Administration.

Cefotaxime Sodium Injection

(sef oh taks′ eem)

Brand Name: Claforan®
Also available generically.

About Your Treatment

Your doctor has ordered cefotaxime, an antibiotic, to help treat your infection. The drug will be either injected into a large muscle (such as your buttock or hip) or added to an intravenous fluid that will drip through a needle or catheter placed in your vein for 30 minutes, two to four times a day.

Cefotaxime eliminates bacteria that cause many kinds of infections, including lung, skin, bone, joint, stomach, blood, gynecological, and urinary tract infections. This medication is sometimes prescribed for other uses; ask your doctor or pharmacist for more information.

Your health care provider (doctor, nurse, or pharmacist) may measure the effectiveness and side effects of your treatment using laboratory tests and physical examinations. It is important to keep all appointments with your doctor and the laboratory. The length of treatment depends on how your infection and symptoms respond to the medication.

Precautions

Before administering cefotaxime,

- tell your doctor and pharmacist if you are allergic to cefotaxime, any other cephalosporin [e.g., cefaclor (Ceclor), cefadroxil (Duricef), or cephalexin (Keflex)], penicillins, or any other drugs.
- tell your doctor and pharmacist what prescription and nonprescription medications you are taking, especially other antibiotics, probenecid (Benemid), and vitamins.
- tell your doctor if you have or have ever had kidney, liver, or gastrointestinal disease (especially colitis).
- tell your doctor if you are pregnant, plan to become pregnant, or are breast-feeding. If you become pregnant while taking cefotaxime, call your doctor.

Administering Your Medication

Before you administer cefotaxime, look at the solution closely. It should be clear and free of floating material. Gently squeeze the bag or observe the solution container to make sure there are no leaks. Do not use the solution if it is discolored, if it contains particles, or if the bag or container leaks. Use a new solution, but show the damaged one to your health care provider.

It is important that you use your medication exactly as directed. Do not stop your therapy on your own for any reason because your infection could worsen and result in hospitalization. Do not change your dosing schedule without talking to your health care provider. Your health care provider may tell you to stop your infusion if you have a mechanical problem (such as a blockage in the tubing, needle, or catheter); if you have to stop an infusion, call your health care provider immediately so your therapy can continue.

Side Effects

Cefotaxime may cause side effects. If you are administering cefotaxime into a muscle, it may be mixed with lidocaine (Xylocaine) to reduce pain at the injection site. Tell your health care provider if any of these symptoms are severe or do not go away:

- diarrhea
- stomach pain
- upset stomach
- vomiting

If you experience any of the following symptoms, call your health care provider immediately:

- unusual bleeding or bruising
- difficulty breathing
- skin rash
- itching
- hives
- sore mouth or throat

If you experience a serious side effect, you or your doctor may send a report to the Food and Drug Administration's (FDA) MedWatch Adverse Event Reporting program online [at http://www.fda.gov/MedWatch/index.html] or by phone [1-800-332-1088].

Storage Conditions

- Your health care provider probably will give you a several-day supply of cefotaxime at a time. If you are receiving cefotaxime intravenously (in your vein), you probably will be told to store it in the refrigerator or freezer.
- Take your next dose from the refrigerator 1 hour before using it; place it in a clean, dry area to allow it to warm to room temperature.
- If you are told to store additional cefotaxime in the freezer, always move a 24-hour supply to the refrigerator for the next day's use.
- Do not refreeze medications.

If you are receiving cefotaxime intramuscularly (in your muscle), your health care provider will tell you how to store it properly.

Store your medication only as directed. Make sure you understand what you need to store your medication properly.

Keep your supplies in a clean, dry place when you are not using them, and keep all medications and supplies out of reach of children. Your health care provider will tell you how to throw away used needles, syringes, tubing, and containers to avoid accidental injury.

Overdose

In case of overdose, call your local poison control center at 1-800-222-1222. If the victim has collapsed or is not breathing, call local emergency services at 911.

Signs of Infection

If you are receiving cefotaxime in your vein or under your skin, you need to know the symptoms of a catheter-related infection (an infection where the needle enters your vein or skin). If you experience any of these effects near your intravenous catheter, tell your health care provider as soon as possible:

- tenderness
- warmth
- irritation
- drainage
- redness
- swelling
- pain

Dosage Facts
For Informational Purposes

Caution: Do not change your dose, how often you take your medication, or the length of time you are to take it without first talking to your healthcare provider.

The following dosage information was written using medical language for doctors and other healthcare professionals and is provided here for you to check your dosage. The dosage of this drug may differ for different patients. Therefore, always follow your doctor's instructions or the directions on the label. Contact your healthcare provider or pharmacist if you have any questions about the specific dosage of your medication after reviewing this information.

General Dosage Information

Available as cefotaxime sodium; dosage expressed in terms of cefotaxime.

Pediatric Patients

General Dosage in Neonates <1 Week of Age

IV:

- 50 mg/kg every 12 hours for premature or full-term neonates <1 week of age.
- AAP recommends 50 mg/kg every 12 hours for neonates <1 week of age weighing ≤2 kg and 50 mg/kg every 8 or 12 hours for those weighing >2 kg.

General Dosage in Neonates 1–4 Weeks of Age

IV:

- 50 mg/kg every 8 hours.
- AAP recommends 50 mg/kg every 12 hours for neonates 1–4 weeks of age weighing <1.2 kg; 50 mg/kg every 8 hours for those weighing 1.2–2 kg; and 50 mg/kg every 6 or 8 hours for those weighing >2 kg.

General Dosage in Children 1 Month to 12 Years of Age

IV OR IM:

- 50–180 mg/kg daily given in 4–6 equally divided doses in those weighing <50 kg. The higher dosage should be used for more severe or serious infections.
- AAP recommends 75–100 mg/kg daily given in 3 or 4 equally divided doses for mild to moderate infections and 150–200 mg/kg daily given in 3 or 4 equally divided doses for severe infections.
- Children weighing >50 kg should receive the usual adult dosage.

Meningitis and Other CNS Infections

IV:

- AAP recommends 225–300 mg/kg daily given in 3 or 4 equally divided doses for treatment of meningitis, including meningitis caused by *S. pneumoniae*.
- Duration of treatment is 7 days for uncomplicated meningitis caused by susceptible *H. influenzae* or *N. meningitidis*; ≥10–14 days for complicated cases or meningitis caused by *S. pneumoniae*; and ≥21 days for meningitis caused by susceptible Enterobacteriaceae.

Gonorrhea and Associated Infections
Disseminated Gonococcal Infection or Gonococcal Scalp Abscess in Neonates†

IV OR IM:

- 25 mg/kg every 12 hours for 7 days recommended by CDC and AAP; if meningitis is documented, continue for 10–14 days.

Parenteral Prophylaxis in Neonates Born to Mothers with Gonococcal Infections†

IV OR IM:

- 100 mg/kg given as a single dose recommended by AAP.

Gonococcal Ophthalmia Neonatorum†

IV OR IM:

- 100 mg/kg given as a single dose recommended by AAP.

Disseminated Gonorrhea in Children ≥8 Years of Age or Weighing ≥45 kg†

IV:

- 1 g every 8 hours recommended by CDC and AAP. Continue for 7 days or discontinue 24–48 hours after improvement occurs and switch to an oral regimen to complete ≥7 days of treatment.

Lyme Disease†
Late or Persistent Manifestations†

IV:

- 150 mg/kg daily given in divided doses every 6–8 hours (up to 6 g daily) for 14–28 days.

Adult Patients

General Adult Dosage
Uncomplicated Infections

IV OR IM:

- 1 g every 12 hours.

Moderate to Severe Infections

IV OR IM:

- 1–2 g every 8 hours.

Severe or Life-threatening Infections

IV:
- 2 g every 6–8 hours. For life-threatening infections, 2 g every 4 hours.

Meningitis and Other CNS Infections

IV:
- 2 g every 6–8 hours for 7–21 days.
- Duration of treatment is 7 days for uncomplicated meningitis caused by susceptible *H. influenzae* or *N. meningitidis*; ≥10–14 days for complicated cases or meningitis caused by *S. pneumoniae*; and ≥21 days for meningitis caused by susceptible Enterobacteriaceae.

Meningitis Caused by S. pneumoniae

IV:
- Initially, 350 mg/kg daily given in 4 divided doses; reduce dosage to 225 mg/kg daily given in 3 divided doses if organism is susceptible to penicillin.

Respiratory Tract Infections
Community-acquired Pneumonia

IV OR IM:
- 1 g every 6–8 hours.
- Duration of treatment depends on the causative pathogen, illness severity at the onset of anti-infective therapy, response to treatment, comorbid illness, and complications. CAP secondary to *S. pneumoniae* generally can be treated for 7–10 days or 72 hours after the patient becomes afebrile. CAP caused by bacteria that can necrose pulmonary parenchyma generally should be treated for ≥2 weeks. Patients chronically treated with corticosteroids also may require at least 2 weeks of therapy.

Gonorrhea and Associated Infections
Uncomplicated Urethral, Cervical, or Rectal Gonorrhea

IM:
- 500 mg as a single dose.
- Manufacturer recommends 1 mg as a single dose for treatment of rectal gonorrhea in males.

Disseminated Gonorrhea†

IV:
- CDC recommends 1 g every 8 hours; continue for 24–48 hours after improvement begins and switch to an oral regimen (e.g., cefixime, ciprofloxacin, ofloxacin, levofloxacin) to complete ≥1 week of treatment.

Lyme Disease†
Late or Persistent Manifestations†

IV:
- 2 g every 8 hours for 14–28 days.

Perioperative Prophylaxis
Contaminated or Potentially Contaminated Surgery

IV OR IM:
- 1 g 30–90 minutes prior to surgery.

Cesarean Section

IV OR IM:
- 1 g IV as soon as the umbilical cord is clamped, followed by additional 1-g IM or IV doses given 6 and 12 hours after the first dose.

Prescribing Limits
Pediatric Patients

Maximum 12 g daily for children weighing >50 kg.

Adult Patients

Maximum 12 g daily.

Special Populations

Hepatic Impairment
- No dosage adjustments required.

Renal Impairment
- Patients with Cl_{cr} <20 mL/minute per 1.73 m² should receive 50% of the usual dose given at the usual time intervals.
- Patients undergoing hemodialysis should receive 0.5–2 g as a single daily dose with a supplemental dose after each dialysis period.

† Use is not currently included in the labeling approved by the US Food and Drug Administration.

Cefoxitin Sodium Injection
(se fox′ i tin)

Brand Name: Mefoxin®
Also available generically.

About Your Treatment

Your doctor has ordered cefoxitin, an antibiotic, to help treat your infection. The drug will be either injected into a large muscle (such as your buttock or hip) or added to an intravenous fluid that will drip through a needle or catheter placed in your vein for 30 minutes, two to four times a day.

Cefoxitin eliminates bacteria that cause many kinds of infections, including lung, skin, bone, joint, stomach, blood, gynecological, and urinary tract infections. This medication is sometimes prescribed for other uses; ask your doctor or pharmacist for more information.

Your health care provider (doctor, nurse, or pharmacist) may measure the effectiveness and side effects of your treatment using laboratory tests and physical examinations. It is important to keep all appointments with your doctor and the laboratory. The length of treatment depends on how your infection and symptoms respond to the medication.

Precautions

Before administering cefoxitin,
- tell your doctor and pharmacist if you are allergic to cefoxitin, any other cephalosporin [e.g., cefaclor (Ceclor), cefadroxil (Duricef), or cephalexin (Keflex)], penicillins, or any other drugs.

- tell your doctor and pharmacist what prescription and nonprescription medications you are taking, especially other antibiotics, probenecid (Benemid), and vitamins.
- tell your doctor if you have or have ever had kidney, liver, or gastrointestinal disease (especially colitis).
- tell your doctor if you are pregnant, plan to become pregnant, or are breast-feeding. If you become pregnant while taking cefoxitin, call your doctor.
- if you have diabetes and regularly check your urine for sugar, use Clinistix or TesTape. Do not use Clinitest tablets because cefoxitin may cause false positive results.

Administering Your Medication

Before you administer cefoxitin, look at the solution closely. It should be clear and free of floating material. Gently squeeze the bag or observe the solution container to make sure there are no leaks. Do not use the solution if it is discolored, if it contains particles, or if the bag or container leaks. Use a new solution, but show the damaged one to your health care provider.

It is important that you use your medication exactly as directed. Do not stop your therapy on your own for any reason because your infection could worsen and result in hospitalization. Do not change your dosing schedule without talking to your health care provider. Your health care provider may tell you to stop your infusion if you have a mechanical problem (such as a blockage in the tubing, needle, or catheter); if you have to stop an infusion, call your health care provider immediately so your therapy can continue.

Side Effects

Cefoxitin may cause side effects. If you are administering cefoxitin into a muscle, it probably will be mixed with lidocaine (Xylocaine) to reduce pain at the injection site. Tell your health care provider if any of these symptoms are severe or do not go away:

- diarrhea
- stomach pain
- upset stomach
- vomiting

If you experience any of the following symptoms, call your health care provider immediately:

- unusual bleeding or bruising
- difficulty breathing
- skin rash
- itching
- hives
- sore mouth or throat

If you experience a serious side effect, you or your doctor may send a report to the Food and Drug Administration's (FDA) MedWatch Adverse Event Reporting program online [at http://www.fda.gov/MedWatch/index.html] or by phone [1-800-332-1088].

Storage Conditions

- Your health care provider probably will give you a several-day supply of cefoxitin at a time. If you are receiving cefoxitin intravenously (in your vein), you probably will be told to store it in the refrigerator or freezer.
- Take your next dose from the refrigerator 1 hour before using it; place it in a clean, dry area to allow it to warm to room temperature.
- If you are told to store additional cefoxitin in the freezer, always move a 24-hour supply to the refrigerator for the next day's use.
- Do not refreeze medications.

If you are receiving cefoxitin intramuscularly (in your muscle), your health care provider will tell you how to store it properly.

Store your medication only as directed. Make sure you understand what you need to store your medication properly.

Keep your supplies in a clean, dry place when you are not using them, and keep all medications and supplies out of reach of children. Your health care provider will tell you how to throw away used needles, syringes, tubing, and containers to avoid accidental injury.

Overdose

In case of overdose, call your local poison control center at 1-800-222-1222. If the victim has collapsed or is not breathing, call local emergency services at 911.

Signs of Infection

If you are receiving cefoxitin in your vein or under your skin, you need to know the symptoms of a catheter-related infection (an infection where the needle enters your vein or skin). If you experience any of these effects near your intravenous catheter, tell your health care provider as soon as possible:

- tenderness
- warmth
- irritation
- drainage
- redness
- swelling
- pain

Dosage Facts
For Informational Purposes

Caution: Do not change your dose, how often you take your medication, or the length of time you are to take it without first talking to your healthcare provider.

The following dosage information was written using medical language for doctors and other healthcare professionals and is provided here for you to check your dosage. The dosage of this drug may differ for different patients. Therefore, always follow your doctor's instruc-

tions or the directions on the label. Contact your health-care provider or pharmacist if you have any questions about the specific dosage of your medication after reviewing this information.

General Dosage Information

Available as cefoxitin sodium; dosage expressed in terms of cefoxitin.

Pediatric Patients

General Pediatric Dosage

IV:
- Children ≥3 months of age: 80–160 mg/kg daily given in 4–6 equally divided doses.
- AAP recommends 80–100 mg/kg daily given in 3–4 equally divided doses for mild to moderate infections or 80–160 mg/kg daily given in 4–6 equally divided doses for severe infections in children >1 month of age.

Perioperative Prophylaxis

IV:
- Children ≥3 months of age: Manufacturer recommends 30–40 mg/kg given at induction of anesthesia (within 0.5–1 hour prior to incision), followed by 30–40 mg/kg every 6 hours for up to 24 hours.
- Some clinicians recommend additional doses during the procedure (e.g., every 2–3 hours), especially if surgery is prolonged >4 hours or major blood loss occurs. In most cases, postoperative doses are unnecessary and may increase the risk of toxicity and bacterial superinfection.

Adult Patients

General Adult Dosage
Uncomplicated Infections (Bacteremia Absent or Unlikely)

IV:
- 1 g every 6–8 hours.

Moderately Severe or Severe Infections

IV:
- 1 g every 4 hours or 2 g every 6–8 hours.

Infections Requiring Higher Dosage (e.g., Gangrene)

IV:
- 2 g every 4 hours or 3 g every 6 hours.

Gonorrhea†

IM†:
- 2 g as a single dose given with oral probenecid (1 g).

Pelvic Inflammatory Disease

IV:
- 2 g every 6 hours; used in conjunction with IV or oral doxycycline (100 mg every 12 hours). Cefoxitin may be discontinued 24 hours after clinical improvement occurs and oral doxycycline (100 mg every 12 hours) continued to complete 14 days of treatment.

IM†:
- 2 g as a single dose given with oral probenecid (1 g); followed by a 14-day regimen of oral doxycycline (100 mg twice daily) with or without oral metronidazole (500 mg twice daily).

Perioperative Prophylaxis
Gynecologic and Obstetric Surgery

IV:
- 1 or 2 g given at induction of anesthesia (within 0.5–1 hour prior to incision) for hysterectomy or as soon as umbilical cord is clamped for cesarean section.
- Some clinicians recommend additional doses during the procedure (e.g., every 2–3 hours), especially if surgery is prolonged >4 hours or major blood loss occurs.
- Manufacturer states 2 g can be given every 6 hours after the procedure for up to 24 hours. In most cases, postoperative doses are unnecessary and may increase the risk of toxicity and bacterial superinfection.

GI Surgery

IV:
- 1–2 g given at induction of anesthesia (within 0.5–1 hour prior to incision).
- Some clinicians recommend additional doses during the procedure (e.g., every 2–3 hours), especially if surgery is prolonged >4 hours or major blood loss occurs.
- Manufacturer states 2 g can be given every 6 hours after the procedure for up to 24 hours. In most cases, postoperative doses are unnecessary and may increase the risk of toxicity and bacterial superinfection.

Contaminated or Dirty Surgery Involving Ruptured Abdominal Viscus†

IV:
- 1 or 2 g every 6 hours; used with or without IV gentamicin (1.5 mg/kg every 8 hours). Continue postoperatively for about 5 days.

Prescribing Limits
Pediatric Patients

Maximum 12 g daily.

Adult Patients

Maximum 12 g daily.

Special Populations

Renal Impairment
- Dosage adjustments necessary in those with Cl_{cr} ≤50 mL/minute.
- Adults with Cl_{cr} ≤50 mL/minute: Give an initial loading dose of 1–2 g followed by maintenance dosage based on Cl_{cr}.

Maintenance Dosage for Adults with Renal Impairment

Cl_{cr} (mL/min)	Dosage
30–50	1–2 g every 8–12 h
10–29	1–2 g every 12–24 h
5–9	0.5–1 g every 12–24 h
<5	0.5–1 g every 24–48 h

Adults undergoing hemodialysis: Give a loading dose of 1–2 g after each dialysis period followed by maintenance dosage based on Cl_{cr}.

Pediatric patients with renal impairment: Make dosage adjustments similar to those recommended for adults.

Geriatric Patients
- Cautious dosage selection because of age-related decreases in renal function.

† *Use is not currently included in the labeling approved by the US Food and Drug Administration.*

Cefpodoxime

(sef pode ox′ eem)

Brand Name: Vantin®

Why is this medicine prescribed?

Cefpodoxime is a cephalosporin antibiotic used to treat certain infections caused by bacteria such as pneumonia; bronchitis; gonorrhea; and ear, skin, throat, and urinary tract infections. Antibiotics will not work for colds, flu, or other viral infections.

This medication is sometimes prescribed for other uses; ask your doctor or pharmacist for more information.

How should this medicine be used?

Cefpodoxime comes as a tablet and liquid to take by mouth. It is usually taken every 12 hours (twice a day) for 7-14 days. A single dose is given to treat gonorrhea. Follow the directions on your prescription label carefully, and ask your doctor or pharmacist to explain any part you do not understand. Take cefpodoxime exactly as directed. Do not take more or less of it or take it more often than prescribed by your doctor.

Shake the liquid well before each use to mix the medication evenly.

The tablets should be swallowed whole and taken with a full glass of water.

Continue to take cefpodoxime even if you feel well. Do not stop taking cefpodoxime without talking to your doctor.

What special precautions should I follow?

Before taking cefpodoxime,
- tell your doctor and pharmacist if you are allergic to cefpodoxime or any other cephalosporin antibiotic such as cefadroxil (Duricef) or cephalexin (Keflex), penicillin, or any other drugs.
- tell your doctor and pharmacist what prescription and nonprescription medications you are taking, especially other antibiotics, anticoagulants ('blood thinners') such as warfarin (Coumadin), probenecid (Benemid), and vitamins.
- tell your doctor if you have or have ever had kidney or liver disease, colitis, or stomach problems.
- tell your doctor if you are pregnant, plan to become pregnant, or are breast-feeding. If you become pregnant while taking cefpodoxime, call your doctor.
- if you are having surgery, including dental surgery, tell the doctor or dentist that you are taking cefpodoxime.

What special dietary instructions should I follow?

Take cefpodoxime tablets with food. The liquid may be taken with or without food.

What should I do if I forget to take a dose?

Take the missed dose as soon as you remember it. However, if it is almost time for the next dose, skip the missed dose and continue your regular dosing schedule. Do not take a double dose to make up for a missed one.

What side effects can this medicine cause?

Cefpodoxime may cause side effects. Tell your doctor if any of these symptoms are severe or do not go away:
- upset stomach
- diarrhea
- vomiting
- mild skin rash

If you experience any of the following symptoms, call your doctor immediately:
- severe skin rash
- itching
- hives
- difficulty breathing or swallowing
- wheezing
- unusual bleeding or bruising
- sore throat
- painful mouth or throat sores
- vaginal infection

If you experience a serious side effect, you or your doctor may send a report to the Food and Drug Administration's (FDA) MedWatch Adverse Event Reporting program online [at http://www.fda.gov/MedWatch/index.html] or by phone [1-800-332-1088].

What storage conditions are needed for this medicine?

Keep this medication in the container it came in, tightly closed, and out of reach of children. Store the tablets at room temperature and away from excess heat and moisture (not in the bathroom). Throw away any medication that is outdated or no longer needed. Keep liquid medicine in the refrigerator, tightly closed, and throw away any unused medication after 14 days. Do not freeze. Talk to your pharmacist about the proper disposal of your medication.

What should I do in case of overdose?

In case of overdose, call your local poison control center at 1-800-222-1222. If the victim has collapsed or is not breathing, call local emergency services at 911.

What other information should I know?

Keep all appointments with your doctor and the laboratory. Your doctor will order certain lab tests to check your response to cefpodoxime.

If you are diabetic, call your doctor before changing diet or dosage of medicine. Use Clinistix or TesTape (not Clinitest) to test your urine for sugar while taking this drug.

Do not let anyone else take your medication. Your prescription is probably not refillable. If you still have symptoms of infection after you finish the cefpodoxime, call your doctor.

Dosage Facts

For Informational Purposes

Caution: Do not change your dose, how often you take your medication, or the length of time you are to take it without first talking to your healthcare provider.

The following dosage information was written using medical language for doctors and other healthcare professionals and is provided here for you to check your dosage. The dosage of this drug may differ for different patients. Therefore, always follow your doctor's instructions or the directions on the label. Contact your healthcare provider or pharmacist if you have any questions about the specific dosage of your medication after reviewing this information.

General Dosage Information

Available as cefpodoxime proxetil; dosage expressed in terms of cefpodoxime.

Pediatric Patients

Acute Otitis Media (AOM)

ORAL:
- Children 2 months to 12 years of age: 5 mg/kg every 12 hours for 5 days.

Pharyngitis and Tonsillitis

ORAL:
- Children 2 months to 12 years of age: 5 mg/kg every 12 hours for 5–10 days.
- Children ≥12 years of age: 100 mg every 12 hours for 5–10 days.

Respiratory Tract Infections

Acute Sinusitis

ORAL:
- Children 2 months to 12 years of age: 5 mg/kg every 12 hours for 10 days.
- Children ≥12 years of age: 200 mg every 12 hours for 10 days.

Acute Exacerbations of Chronic Bronchitis

ORAL:
- Children ≥12 years of age: 200 mg every 12 hours for 10 days.

Community-acquired Pneumonia

ORAL:
- Children ≥12 years of age: 200 mg every 12 hours for 14 days.

Uncomplicated Gonorrhea

Uncomplicated Urethral or Cervical Gonorrhea in Adolescent Boys or Girls ≥12 Years of Age

ORAL:
- 200 mg as a single dose.

Uncomplicated Anorectal Gonorrhea in Adolescent Girls ≥12 Years of Age

ORAL:
- 200 mg as a single dose.

Skin and Skin Structure Infections

ORAL:
- Children ≥12 years of age: 400 mg every 12 hours for 7–14 days.

Urinary Tract Infections (UTIs)

ORAL:
- Children ≥12 years of age: 100 mg every 12 hours for 7 days.

Adult Patients

Pharyngitis and Tonsillitis

ORAL:
- 100 mg every 12 hours for 5–10 days.

Respiratory Tract Infections

Acute Maxillary Sinusitis

ORAL:
- 200 mg every 12 hours for 10 days.

Acute Exacerbations of Chronic Bronchitis

ORAL:
- 200 mg every 12 hours for 10 days.

Community-acquired Pneumonia

ORAL:
- 200 mg every 12 hours for 14 days.

Uncomplicated Gonorrhea

Uncomplicated Urethral or Cervical Gonorrhea in Men or Women

ORAL:
- 200 mg as a single dose.

Uncomplicated Anorectal Gonorrhea in Women

ORAL:
- 200 mg as a single dose.

Skin and Skin Structure Infections

ORAL:
- 400 mg every 12 hours for 7–14 days.

Urinary Tract Infections (UTIs)

ORAL:
- 100 mg every 12 hours for 7 days.

Prescribing Limits

Pediatric Patients

Acute Otitis Media (AOM)

ORAL:
- Maximum 200 mg every 12 hours for children 2 months to 12 years of age.

Pharyngitis and Tonsillitis

ORAL:
- Maximum 100 mg every 12 hours for children 2 months to 12 years of age.

Acute Maxillary Sinusitis

ORAL:
- Maximum 200 mg every 12 hours for children 2 months to 12 years of age.

Special Populations

Hepatic Impairment
- No dosage adjustments required in patients with cirrhosis (with or without ascites).

Renal Impairment
- Patients with Cl_{cr} <30 mL/minute: Give usual dose once every 24 hours.
- Patients maintained on hemodialysis: Give usual dose 3 times weekly after dialysis.

Geriatric Patients
- No dosage adjustments except those related to renal impairment.

Cefprozil

(sef proe′ zil)

Brand Name: Cefzil®

Why is this medicine prescribed?

Cefprozil is used to treat certain infections caused by bacteria, such as bronchitis and infections of the ears, throat, sinuses, and skin. Cefprozil is in a class of medications called cephalosporin antibiotics. It works by stopping the growth of bacteria. Antibiotics will not work for colds, flu, or other viral infections.

How should this medicine be used?

Cefprozil comes as a tablet and a suspension (liquid) to take by mouth. It is usually taken every 24 hours (once a day) or every 12 hours (twice a day) for 10 days. To help you remember to take cefprozil, take it around the same time every day. Follow the directions on your prescription label carefully, and ask your doctor or pharmacist to explain any part you do not understand. Take cefprozil exactly as directed. Do not take more or less of it or take it more often than prescribed by your doctor.

Shake the liquid well before each use to mix the medication evenly.

The tablets should be swallowed whole and taken with a full glass of water.

Take cefprozil until you finish the prescription, even if you feel better. Stopping cefprozil too soon may cause bacteria to become resistant to antibiotics.

Are there other uses for this medicine?

This medication may be prescribed for other uses; ask your doctor or pharmacist for more information.

What special precautions should I follow?

Before taking cefprozil,
- tell your doctor and pharmacist if you are allergic to cefprozil, penicillin, cefaclor (Ceclor), cefadroxil (Duricef), cefamandole (Mandol), cefazolin (Ancef, Kefzol), cefdinir (Omnicef), cefditoren (Spectracef), cefepime (Maxipime), cefixime (Suprax), cefmetazole (Zefazone), cefonicid (Monocid), cefoperazone (Cefobid), cefotaxime (Claforan), cefoxitin (Mefoxin), cefpodoxime (Vantin), ceftazidime (Ceptaz, Fortaz, Tazicef), ceftibuten (Cedax), ceftizoxime (Cefizox), ceftriaxone (Rocephin), cefuroxime (Ceftin, Kefurox, Zinacef), cephalexin (Keflex), cephapirin (Cefadyl), cephradine (Velosef), loracarbef (Lorabid), or any other medications.
- tell your doctor and pharmacist what prescription and nonprescription medications, vitamins, nutritional supplements, and herbal products you are taking. Be sure to mention any of the following: anticoagulants ('blood thinners') such as warfarin (Coumadin), diuretics ('water pills'), other antibiotics, and probenecid (Benemid). Your doctor may need to change the doses of your medications or monitor you carefully for side effects.
- tell your doctor if you have or have ever had kidney disease, phenylketonuria, colitis, or stomach problems.
- tell your doctor if you are pregnant, plan to become pregnant, or are breast-feeding. If you become pregnant while taking cefprozil, call your doctor.

What special dietary instructions should I follow?

Unless your doctor tells you otherwise, continue your normal diet.

What should I do if I forget to take a dose?

Take the missed dose as soon as you remember it. However, if it is almost time for the next dose, skip the missed dose and continue your regular dosing schedule. Do not take a double dose to make up for a missed one.

What side effects can this medicine cause?

Cefprozil may cause side effects. Tell your doctor if any of these symptoms are severe or do not go away:
- upset stomach
- diarrhea
- vomiting
- stomach pain
- dizziness

Some side effects can be serious. The following symptoms are uncommon, but if you experience any of them, call your doctor immediately:

- severe skin rash
- itching
- hives
- difficulty breathing or swallowing
- wheezing
- yellowing of the skin and eyes
- painful sores in the mouth or throat
- vaginal discharge and itching
- diaper rash

Cefprozil may cause other side effects. Call your doctor if you have any unusual problems while taking this medication.

If you experience a serious side effect, you or your doctor may send a report to the Food and Drug Administration's (FDA) MedWatch Adverse Event Reporting program online [at http://www.fda.gov/MedWatch/index.html] or by phone [1-800-332-1088].

What storage conditions are needed for this medicine?

Keep this medication in the container it came in, tightly closed, and out of reach of children. Store the tablets at room temperature and away from excess heat and moisture (not in the bathroom). Throw away any medication that is outdated or no longer needed. Keep liquid medicine in the refrigerator, closed tightly, and throw away any unused medication after 14 days. Do not freeze. Talk to your pharmacist about the proper disposal of your medication.

What should I do in case of overdose?

In case of overdose, call your local poison control center at 1-800-222-1222. If the victim has collapsed or is not breathing, call local emergency services at 911.

What other information should I know?

Keep all appointments with your doctor and the laboratory. Your doctor may order certain lab tests to check your body's response to cefprozil.

If you are diabetic, use Clinistix or TesTape (not Clinitest) to test your urine for sugar while taking this medication.

Do not let anyone else take your medication. Your prescription is probably not refillable. If you still have symptoms of infection after you finish the cefprozil, call your doctor.

Dosage Facts
For Informational Purposes

Caution: Do not change your dose, how often you take your medication, or the length of time you are to take it without first talking to your healthcare provider.

The following dosage information was written using medical language for doctors and other healthcare professionals and is provided here for you to check your dosage. The dosage of this drug may differ for different patients. Therefore, always follow your doctor's instructions or the directions on the label. Contact your healthcare provider or pharmacist if you have any questions about the specific dosage of your medication after reviewing this information.

General Dosage Information

Available as cefprozil monohydrate; dosage expressed as anhydrous cefprozil.

Pediatric Patients

Respiratory Tract Infections
Acute Sinusitis

ORAL:
- Children 6 months to 12 years of age: 7.5 mg/kg every 12 hours for 10 days. For moderate to severe infections, 15 mg/kg every 12 hours for 10 days.
- Children ≥13 years of age: 250 mg every 12 hours for 10 days. For moderate to severe infections, 500 mg every 12 hours for 10 days.

Secondary Bacterial Infections of Acute Bronchitis

ORAL:
- Children ≥13 years of age: 500 mg every 12 hours for 10 days.

Acute Exacerbations of Chronic Bronchitis

ORAL:
- Children ≥13 years of age: 500 mg every 12 hours for 10 days.

Acute Otitis Media (AOM)

ORAL:
- Children 6 months to 12 years of age: 15 mg/kg every 12 hours for 10 days.

Pharyngitis or Tonsillitis

ORAL:
- Children 2–12 years of age: 7.5 mg/kg every 12 hours for 10 days.
- Children ≥13 years of age: 500 mg once daily for 10 days.

Skin and Skin Structure Infections

ORAL:
- Children 2–12 years of age: 20 mg/kg once every 24 hours for 10 days.
- Children ≥13 years of age: 250 or 500 mg every 12 hours for 10 days or 500 mg once daily for 10 days.

Adult Patients

Respiratory Tract Infections
Acute Sinusitis

ORAL:
- 250 mg every 12 hours for 10 days. For moderate to severe infections, 500 mg every 12 hours for 10 days.

Secondary Bacterial Infections of Acute Bronchitis

ORAL:
- 500 mg every 12 hours for 10 days.

Acute Exacerbations of Chronic Bronchitis

ORAL:
- 500 mg every 12 hours for 10 days.

Pharyngitis or Tonsillitis

ORAL:
- 500 mg once daily for 10 days.

Skin and Skin Structure Infections

ORAL:
- 250 or 500 mg every 12 hours for 10 days or 500 mg once daily for 10 days.

Special Populations

Hepatic Impairment
- No dosage adjustments required.

Renal Impairment
- No dosage adjustments required in patients with Cl_{cr} $\geq$30 mL/minute.
- Patients with Cl_{cr} <30 mL/minute: administer 50% of the usual dose using the usual dosing intervals.
- Hemodialysis patients: administer cefprozil doses after dialysis sessions.

Geriatric Patients
- No dosage adjustments required except those related to renal impairment. Cautious dosage selection because of age-related decreases in renal function.

Ceftazidime Injection

(sef′ tay zi deem)

Brand Name: Ceptaz®, Fortaz®, Tazicef®

About Your Treatment

Your doctor has ordered ceftazidime, an antibiotic, to help treat your infection. The drug will be either injected into a large muscle (such as your buttock or hip) or added to an intravenous fluid that will drip through a needle or catheter placed in your vein for 30 minutes, one to three times a day.

Ceftazidime eliminates bacteria that cause many kinds of infections, including lung, skin, bone, joint, stomach, blood, gynecological, and urinary tract infections. This medication is sometimes prescribed for other uses; ask your doctor or pharmacist for more information.

Your health care provider (doctor, nurse, or pharmacist) may measure the effectiveness and side effects of your treatment using laboratory tests and physical examinations. It is important to keep all appointments with your doctor and the laboratory. The length of treatment depends on how your infection and symptoms respond to the medication.

Precautions

Before administering ceftazidime,
- tell your doctor and pharmacist if you are allergic to ceftazidime, any other cephalosporin [e.g., cefaclor (Ceclor), cefadroxil (Duricef), or cephalexin (Keflex)], penicillins, or any other drugs.
- tell your doctor and pharmacist what prescription and nonprescription medications you are taking, especially other antibiotics, probenecid (Benemid), and vitamins.
- tell your doctor if you have or have ever had kidney, liver, or gastrointestinal disease (especially colitis).
- tell your doctor if you are pregnant, plan to become pregnant, or are breast-feeding. If you become pregnant while taking ceftazidime, call your doctor.
- if you have diabetes and regularly check your urine for sugar, use Clinistix or TesTape. Do not use Clinitest tablets because ceftazidime may cause false positive results.

Administering Your Medication

Before you administer ceftazidime, look at the solution closely. It should be clear and free of floating material. Gently squeeze the bag or observe the solution container to make sure there are no leaks. Do not use the solution if it is discolored, if it contains particles, or if the bag or container leaks. Use a new solution, but show the damaged one to your health care provider.

It is important that you use your medication exactly as directed. Do not stop your therapy on your own for any reason because your infection could worsen and result in hospitalization. Do not change your dosing schedule without talking to your health care provider. Your health care provider may tell you to stop your infusion if you have a mechanical problem (such as a blockage in the tubing, needle, or catheter); if you have to stop an infusion, call your health care provider immediately so your therapy can continue.

Side Effects

Ceftazidime may cause side effects. If you are administering ceftazidime into a muscle, it may be mixed with lidocaine (Xylocaine) to reduce pain at the injection site. Tell your health care provider if any of these symptoms are severe or do not go away:
- diarrhea
- stomach pain
- upset stomach
- vomiting

If you experience any of the following symptoms, call your health care provider immediately:
- unusual bleeding or bruising
- difficulty breathing
- itching
- rash
- hives
- sore mouth or throat

If you experience a serious side effect, you or your doctor may send a report to the Food and Drug Administration's (FDA) MedWatch Adverse Event Reporting program online [at http://www.fda.gov/MedWatch/index.html] or by phone [1-800-332-1088].

Storage Conditions

- Your health care provider probably will give you a several-day supply of ceftazidime at a time. If you are receiving ceftazidime intravenously (in your vein), you probably will be told to store it in the refrigerator or freezer.
- Take your next dose from the refrigerator 1 hour before using it; place it in a clean, dry area to allow it to warm to room temperature.
- If you are told to store additional ceftazidime in the freezer, always move a 24-hour supply to the refrigerator for the next day's use.
- Do not refreeze medications.

If you are receiving ceftazidime intramuscularly (in your muscle), your health care provider will tell you how to store it properly.

Store your medication only as directed. Make sure you understand what you need to store your medication properly.

Keep your supplies in a clean, dry place when you are not using them, and keep all medications and supplies out of reach of children. Your health care provider will tell you how to throw away used needles, syringes, tubing, and containers to avoid accidental injury.

Overdose

In case of overdose, call your local poison control center at 1-800-222-1222. If the victim has collapsed or is not breathing, call local emergency services at 911.

Signs of Infection

If you are receiving ceftazidime in your vein or under your skin, you need to know the symptoms of a catheter-related infection (an infection where the needle enters your vein or skin). If you experience any of these effects near your intravenous catheter, tell your health care provider as soon as possible:

- tenderness
- warmth
- irritation
- drainage
- redness
- swelling
- pain

Dosage Facts
For Informational Purposes

Caution: Do not change your dose, how often you take your medication, or the length of time you are to take it without first talking to your healthcare provider.

The following dosage information was written using medical language for doctors and other healthcare professionals and is provided here for you to check your dosage. The dosage of this drug may differ for different patients. Therefore, always follow your doctor's instructions or the directions on the label. Contact your healthcare provider or pharmacist if you have any questions about the specific dosage of your medication after reviewing this information.

General Dosage Information

Available as ceftazidime pentahydrate and as ceftazidime sodium; dosage expressed as anhydrous ceftazidime.

Pediatric Patients

General Pediatric Dosage in Neonates

IV:
- Neonates ≤4 weeks of age: manufacturer recommends 30 mg/kg every 12 hours.
- Neonates <1 week of age: AAP recommends 50 mg/kg every 12 hours in those weighing ≤2 kg and 50 mg/kg every 8 or 12 hours in those weighing >2 kg.
- Neonates 1–4 weeks of age: AAP recommends 50 mg/kg every 12 hours in those weighing <1.2 kg and 50 mg/kg every 8 hours in those weighing ≥1.2 kg.

General Pediatric Dosage in Children 1 Month to 12 Years of Age

IV:
- 25–50 mg/kg every 8 hours.
- 50 mg/kg every 8 hours in immunocompromised children or children with cystic fibrosis or meningitis.

General Pediatric Dosage in Children >12 Years of Age

IV:
- Use usual adult dosage.

Empiric Therapy in Febrile Neutropenic Children†

IV:
- 50 mg/kg (maximum 2 g) every 8 hours has been used in pediatric patients ≥2 years of age.

Adult Patients

General Adult Dosage
Less Severe Infections

IV OR IM:
- 1 g every 8–12 hours.

Severe or Life-threatening Infections

IV:
- 2 g every 8 hours, especially in immunocompromised patients.

Bone and Joint Infections

IV:
- 2 g every 12 hours.

Intra-abdominal and Gynecologic Infections
Serious Infections

IV:
- 2 g every 8 hours.

Meningitis

IV:
- 2 g every 8 hours. Duration of treatment is ≥3 weeks for meningitis caused by susceptible gram-negative bacilli.

Respiratory Tract Infections
Uncomplicated Pneumonia

IV OR IM:
- 0.5–1 g every 8 hours.

Pseudomonas Lung Infections in Cystic Fibrosis Patients

IV:
- 30–50 mg/kg every 8 hours (up to 6 g daily).
- Clinical improvement may occur, but bacteriologic cures should not be expected in patients with chronic respiratory disease and cystic fibrosis.

Skin and Skin Structure Infections
Mild Infections

IV OR IM:
- 0.5–1 g every 8 hours.

Urinary Tract Infections (UTIs)
Uncomplicated Infections

IV OR IM:
- 250 mg every 12 hours.

Complicated Infections

IV OR IM:
- 500 mg every 8–12 hours.

Prescribing Limits
Pediatric Patients

Maximum 6 g daily.

Adult Patients

Maximum 6 g daily.

Special Populations

Hepatic Impairment
- Dosage adjustments not required unless renal function also impaired.

Renal Impairment
- Reduce dosage in patients with Cl_{cr} ≤50 mL/minute.
- Manufacturers recommend that adults with Cl_{cr} ≤50 mL/minute receive an initial loading dose of 1 g and a maintenance dosage based on Cl_{cr}.

Maintenance Dosage for Adults with Renal Impairment

Cl_{cr} (mL/minute)	Dosage
31–50	1 g every 12 h
16–30	1 g every 24 h
6–15	500 mg every 24 h
<5	500 mg every 48 h

Patients with renal impairment and severe infections who would generally receive 6 g daily if renal function were normal: increase dosage in table by 50% or dosing interval may be increased appropriately.

Patients undergoing hemodialysis: given an initial loading dose of 1 g followed by 1 g after each hemodialysis period.

Patients undergoing intraperitoneal dialysis or CAPD: given an initial loading dose of 1 g followed by 500 mg every 24 hours.

Geriatric Patients
- Cautious dosage selection because of age-related decreases in renal function.

† Use is not currently included in the labeling approved by the US Food and Drug Administration.

Ceftibuten

(sef tye′ byoo ten)

Brand Name: Cedax®

Why is this medicine prescribed?

Ceftibuten is a cephalosporin antibiotic used to treat certain infections caused by bacteria such as bronchitis and ear and throat infections. Antibiotics will not work for colds, flu, or other viral infections.

This medication is sometimes prescribed for other uses; ask your doctor or pharmacist for more information.

How should this medicine be used?

Ceftibuten comes as a capsule and liquid to take by mouth. It is usually taken once a day for 10 days. Follow the directions on your prescription label carefully, and ask your doctor or pharmacist to explain any part you do not understand. Take ceftibuten exactly as directed. Do not take more or less of it or take it more often than prescribed by your doctor.

Shake the liquid well before each use to mix the medication evenly.

The tablets should be swallowed whole and taken with a full glass of water.

Continue to take ceftibuten even if you feel well. Do not stop taking ceftibuten without talking to your doctor.

What special precautions should I follow?

Before taking ceftibuten,
- tell your doctor and pharmacist if you are allergic to ceftibuten or any other cephalosporin antibiotic such as cefaclor (Ceclor) or cephalexin (Keflex), penicillin, or any other drugs.
- tell your doctor and pharmacist what prescription and nonprescription medications you are taking, especially other antibiotics, anticoagulants ('blood thinners') such as warfarin (Coumadin), probenecid (Benemid), and vitamins.
- tell your doctor if you have or have ever had kidney or liver disease, colitis, or stomach problems.
- tell your doctor if you are pregnant, plan to become pregnant, or are breast-feeding. If you become pregnant while taking ceftibuten, call your doctor.
- if you are having surgery, including dental surgery, tell the doctor or dentist that you are taking ceftibuten.

What special dietary instructions should I follow?

Take ceftibuten liquid at least 1 hour before or 2 hours after meals. Ceftibuten may cause an upset stomach. Take ceftibuten capsules with food or milk.

What should I do if I forget to take a dose?

Take the missed dose as soon as you remember it. However, if it is almost time for the next dose, skip the missed dose and continue your regular dosing schedule. Do not take a double dose to make up for a missed one.

What side effects can this medicine cause?

Ceftibuten may cause side effects. Tell your doctor if any of these symptoms are severe or do not go away:

- upset stomach
- diarrhea
- vomiting
- mild skin rash

If you experience any of the following symptoms, call your doctor immediately:

- severe skin rash
- itching
- hives
- difficulty breathing or swallowing
- wheezing
- unusual bleeding or bruising
- sore throat
- painful mouth or throat sores
- vaginal infection

If you experience a serious side effect, you or your doctor may send a report to the Food and Drug Administration's (FDA) MedWatch Adverse Event Reporting program online [at http://www.fda.gov/MedWatch/index.html] or by phone [1-800-332-1088].

What storage conditions are needed for this medicine?

Keep this medication in the container it came in, tightly closed, and out of reach of children. Store the capsules at room temperature and away from excess heat and moisture (not in the bathroom). Throw away any medication that is outdated or no longer needed. Keep liquid medicine in the refrigerator, closed tightly, and throw away any unused medication after 14 days. Do not freeze. Talk to your pharmacist about the proper disposal of your medication.

What should I do in case of overdose?

In case of overdose, call your local poison control center at 1-800-222-1222. If the victim has collapsed or is not breathing, call local emergency services at 911.

What other information should I know?

Keep all appointments with your doctor and the laboratory. Your doctor will order certain lab tests to check your response to ceftibuten.

If you are diabetic, use Clinistix or TesTape (not Clinitest) to test your urine for sugar while taking this drug.

Do not let anyone else take your medication. Your prescription is probably not refillable. If you still have symptoms of infection after you finish the ceftibuten, call your doctor.

Dosage Facts
For Informational Purposes

Caution: Do not change your dose, how often you take your medication, or the length of time you are to take it without first talking to your healthcare provider.

The following dosage information was written using medical language for doctors and other healthcare professionals and is provided here for you to check your dosage. The dosage of this drug may differ for different patients. Therefore, always follow your doctor's instructions or the directions on the label. Contact your healthcare provider or pharmacist if you have any questions about the specific dosage of your medication after reviewing this information.

General Dosage Information

Available as ceftibuten dihydrate; dosage expressed in terms of anhydrous ceftibuten.

Pediatric Patients

Respiratory Tract Infections
Acute Exacerbations of Chronic Bronchitis

ORAL:
- Children ≥12 years of age: 400 mg once daily for 10 days.

Otitis Media
Acute Otitis Media (AOM)

ORAL:
- Children 6 months through 11 years of age: 9 mg/kg (up to 400 mg) once daily for 10 days.
- Children ≥12 years of age: 400 mg once daily for 10 days.

Pediatric Dosage of Ceftibuten Oral Suspension for AOM

Weight (kg)	Daily Dosage
10	90 mg once daily
20	180 mg once daily
40	360 mg once daily
>45	400 mg once daily

Otitis Media with Effusion†

ORAL:
- Children 7 months to 12 years of age: 9 mg/kg (up to 400 mg) once daily for 14 days.

Pharyngitis and Tonsillitis

ORAL:
- Children 6 months through 11 years of age: 9 mg/kg (up to 400 mg) once daily for 10 days.
- Children ≥12 years of age: 400 mg once daily for 10 days.

Pediatric Dosage of Ceftibuten Oral Suspension for Pharyngitis and Tonsillitis

Weight (kg)	Daily Dosage
10	90 mg once daily
20	180 mg once daily
40	360 mg once daily
>45	400 mg once daily

Adult Patients

Respiratory Tract Infections
Acute Exacerbations of Chronic Bronchitis

ORAL:
- 400 mg once daily for 10 days.

Acute Otitis Media (AOM)

ORAL:
- 400 mg once daily for 10 days.

Pharyngitis and Tonsillitis

ORAL:
- 400 mg once daily for 10 days.

Uncomplicated UTIs†

ORAL:
- 400 mg once daily for 7 days.

Prescribing Limits
Pediatric Patients

ORAL:
- Maximum 400 mg once daily for children 6 months through 11 years of age.

Adult Patients

ORAL:
- Maximum 400 mg once daily.

Special Populations

Hepatic Impairment
- No dosage adjustments required.

Renal Impairment

Dosage for Renal Impairment

Cl_{cr} (mL/min)	Daily Dosage
>50	9 mg/kg or 400 mg once every 24 hours
30–49	4.5 mg/kg or 200 mg once every 24 hours
5–29	2.25 mg/kg or 100 mg once every 24 hours

For patients undergoing hemodialysis 2 or 3 times weekly, a single 400-mg dose (given as a capsule) or 9 mg/kg (up to 400 mg; given as the oral suspension) may be given at the end of each dialysis period.

Geriatric Patients
- No dosage adjustments required other than those related to renal impairment.

† Use is not currently included in the labeling approved by the US Food and Drug Administration.

Ceftizoxime Sodium Injection

(sef ti zox′ eem)

Brand Name: Cefizox®

About Your Treatment

Your doctor has ordered ceftizoxime, an antibiotic, to help treat your infection. The drug will be either injected into a large muscle (such as your buttock or hip) or added to an intravenous fluid that will drip through a needle or catheter placed in your vein for 30 minutes, two or three times a day.

Ceftizoxime eliminates bacteria that cause many kinds of infections, including lung, skin, bone, joint, stomach, blood, and urinary tract infections. This medication is sometimes prescribed for other uses; ask your doctor or pharmacist for more information.

Your health care provider (doctor, nurse, or pharmacist) may measure the effectiveness and side effects of your treatment using laboratory tests and physical examinations. It is important to keep all appointments with your doctor and the laboratory. The length of treatment depends on how your infection and symptoms respond to the medication.

Precautions

Before administering ceftizoxime,
- tell your doctor and pharmacist if you are allergic to ceftizoxime, any other cephalosporin [e.g., cefaclor (Ceclor), cefadroxil (Duricef), or cephalexin (Keflex)], penicillins, or any other drugs.
- tell your doctor and pharmacist what prescription and nonprescription medications you are taking, especially other antibiotics, probenecid (Benemid), and vitamins.
- tell your doctor if you have or have ever had kidney, liver, or gastrointestinal disease (especially colitis).
- tell your doctor if you are pregnant, plan to become pregnant, or are breast-feeding. If you become pregnant while taking ceftizoxime, call your doctor.
- if you have diabetes and regularly check your urine for sugar, use Clinistix or TesTape. Do not use Clinitest

tablets because ceftizoxime may cause false positive results.

Administering Your Medication

Before you administer ceftizoxime, look at the solution closely. It should be clear and free of floating material. Gently squeeze the bag or observe the solution container to make sure there are no leaks. Do not use the solution if it is discolored, if it contains particles, or if the bag or container leaks. Use a new solution, but show the damaged one to your health care provider.

It is important that you use your medication exactly as directed. Do not stop your therapy on your own for any reason because your infection could worsen and result in hospitalization. Do not change your dosing schedule without talking to your health care provider. Your health care provider may tell you to stop your infusion if you have a mechanical problem (such as a blockage in the tubing, needle, or catheter); if you have to stop an infusion, call your health care provider immediately so your therapy can continue.

Side Effects

Ceftizoxime may cause side effects. If you are administering ceftizoxime into a muscle, it may be mixed with lidocaine (Xylocaine) to reduce pain at the injection site. Tell your health care provider if any of these symptoms are severe or do not go away:

- diarrhea
- stomach pain
- upset stomach
- vomiting

If you experience any of the following symptoms, call your health care provider immediately:

- unusual bleeding or bruising
- difficulty breathing
- itching
- rash
- hives
- sore mouth or throat

If you experience a serious side effect, you or your doctor may send a report to the Food and Drug Administration's (FDA) MedWatch Adverse Event Reporting program online [at http://www.fda.gov/MedWatch/index.html] or by phone [1-800-332-1088].

Storage Conditions

- Your health care provider probably will give you a several-day supply of ceftizoxime at a time. If you are receiving ceftizoxime intravenously (in your vein), you probably will be told to store it in the refrigerator or freezer.
- Take your next dose from the refrigerator 1 hour before using it; place it in a clean, dry area to allow it to warm to room temperature.
- If you are told to store additional ceftizoxime in the freezer, always move a 24-hour supply to the refrigerator for the next day's use.
- Do not refreeze medications.

If you are receiving ceftizoxime intramuscularly (in your muscle), your health care provider will tell you how to store it properly.

Store your medication only as directed. Make sure you understand what you need to store your medication properly.

Keep your supplies in a clean, dry place when you are not using them, and keep all medications and supplies out of reach of children. Your health care provider will tell you how to throw away used needles, syringes, tubing, and containers to avoid accidental injury.

Overdose

In case of overdose, call your local poison control center at 1-800-222-1222. If the victim has collapsed or is not breathing, call local emergency services at 911.

Signs of Infection

If you are receiving ceftizoxime in your vein or under your skin, you need to know the symptoms of a catheter-related infection (an infection where the needle enters your vein or skin). If you experience any of these effects near your intravenous catheter, tell your health care provider as soon as possible:

- tenderness
- warmth
- irritation
- drainage
- redness
- swelling
- pain

Dosage Facts
For Informational Purposes

Caution: Do not change your dose, how often you take your medication, or the length of time you are to take it without first talking to your healthcare provider.

The following dosage information was written using medical language for doctors and other healthcare professionals and is provided here for you to check your dosage. The dosage of this drug may differ for different patients. Therefore, always follow your doctor's instructions or the directions on the label. Contact your healthcare provider or pharmacist if you have any questions about the specific dosage of your medication after reviewing this information.

General Dosage Information

Available as ceftizoxime sodium; dosage expressed in terms of ceftizoxime.

Pediatric Patients

General Pediatric Dosage

IV OR IM:

- Children ≥6 months of age: 50 mg/kg every 6–8 hours. For serious infections, dosage may be increased to 200 mg/kg daily given in divided doses.
- AAP recommends 100–150 mg/kg daily given in 3 divided doses for mild to moderate infections or 150–200 mg/kg daily given in 3 or 4 equally divided doses for severe infections in children >4 weeks of age.

Disseminated Gonorrhea in Adolescents

IV:

- CDC recommends 1 g every 8 hours; continue for 24–48 hours after improvement begins and switch to an oral regimen (e.g., cefixime, ciprofloxacin, ofloxacin, levofloxacin) to complete ≥1 week of treatment.

Adult Patients

General Adult Dosage

IV OR IM:

- Usual dosage is 1–2 g every 8 or 12 hours.

Uncomplicated Infections

IV OR IM:

- 1 g every 8–12 hours.

Severe or Refractory Infections

IV OR IM:

- 1 g every 8 hours or 2 g every 8–12 hours.

Life-threatening Infections

IV:

- 3–4 g every 8 hours. Dosages up to 2 g every 4 hours have been used.

Septicemia

IV:

- 6–12 g daily for the first few days, then gradually decrease dosage according to clinical response and bacteriologic assessments.

Urinary Tract Infections (UTIs)
Uncomplicated UTIs

IV OR IM:

- 500 mg every 12 hours.
- Higher dosage recommended in infections caused by susceptible Ps. aeruginosa. Other therapy should be initiated if a prompt response is not obtained.

Gonorrhea
Uncomplicated Gonorrhea

IM:

- 1 g as a single dose recommended by manufacturer. CDC recommends 500 mg as a single dose.

Disseminated Gonorrhea

IV:

- CDC recommends 1 g every 8 hours; continue for 24–48 hours after improvement begins and switch to an oral regimen (e.g., cefixime, ciprofloxacin, ofloxacin, levofloxacin) to complete ≥1 week of treatment.

Pelvic Inflammatory Disease (PID)

IV OR IM:

- 2 g every 8 hours.

Prescribing Limits
Pediatric Patients

Maximum 12 g daily.

Special Populations

Renal Impairment

- The manufacturer recommends that adults with impaired renal function receive an initial IV or IM loading dose of 0.5–1 g followed by maintenance dosage based on Cl_{cr}.

Maintenance Dosage for Adults with Renal Impairment

Cl_{cr} (mL/min)	Less Severe Infections	Life-threatening Infections
50–79	500 mg every 8 hours	750 mg to 1.5 g every 8 hours
5–49	250–500 mg every 12 hours	0.5–1 g every 12 hours
<5	500 mg every 48 hours or 250 mg every 24 hours	0.5–1 g every 48 hours or 0.5 g every 24 hours

Patients undergoing hemodialysis: supplemental doses are unnecessary following hemodialysis but dosing regimen should be timed so that a ceftizoxime dose is scheduled at the end of the dialysis period.

Ceftriaxone Sodium Injection

(sef try ax' one)

Brand Name: Rocephin®
Also available generically.

About Your Treatment

Your doctor has ordered ceftriaxone, an antibiotic, to help treat your infection. The drug will be either injected into a large muscle (such as your buttock or hip) or added to an intravenous fluid that will drip through a needle or catheter placed in your vein for 30 minutes, one or two times a day.

Ceftriaxone eliminates bacteria that cause many kinds of infections, including lung, skin, bone, joint, stomach, blood, and urinary tract infections. This medication is sometimes prescribed for other uses; ask your doctor or pharmacist for more information.

Your health care provider (doctor, nurse, or pharmacist) may measure the effectiveness and side effects of your treatment using laboratory tests and physical examinations. It is important to keep all appointments with your doctor and the laboratory. The length of treatment depends on how your infection and symptoms respond to the medication.

Precautions

Before administering ceftriaxone,

- tell your doctor and pharmacist if you are allergic to ceftriaxone, any other cephalosporin [e.g., cefaclor (Ceclor), cefadroxil (Duricef), or cephalexin (Keflex)], penicillins, or any other drugs.
- tell your doctor and pharmacist what prescription and nonprescription medications you are taking, especially other antibiotics, probenecid (Benemid), and vitamins.
- tell your doctor if you have or have ever had kidney, liver, gallbladder, or gastrointestinal disease (especially colitis).
- tell your doctor if you are pregnant, plan to become pregnant, or are breast-feeding. If you become pregnant while taking ceftriaxone, call your doctor.
- if you have diabetes and regularly check your urine for sugar, use Clinistix or TesTape. Do not use Clinitest tablets because ceftriaxone may cause false positive results.

Administering Your Medication

Before you administer ceftriaxone, look at the solution closely. It should be clear and free of floating material. Gently squeeze the bag or observe the solution container to make sure there are no leaks. Do not use the solution if it is discolored, if it contains particles, or if the bag or container leaks. Use a new solution, but show the damaged one to your health care provider.

It is important that you use your medication exactly as directed. Do not stop your therapy on your own for any reason because your infection could worsen and result in hospitalization. Do not change your dosing schedule without talking to your health care provider. Your health care provider may tell you to stop your infusion if you have a mechanical problem (such as a blockage in the tubing, needle, or catheter); if you have to stop an infusion, call your health care provider immediately so your therapy can continue.

Side Effects

Ceftriaxone may cause side effects. If you are administering ceftriaxone into a muscle, it may be mixed with lidocaine (Xylocaine) to reduce pain at the injection site. Tell your health care provider if any of these symptoms are severe or do not go away:

- diarrhea
- stomach pain
- upset stomach
- vomiting

If you experience any of the following symptoms, call your health care provider immediately:

- unusual bleeding or bruising
- difficulty breathing
- itching
- rash
- hives
- sore mouth or throat

If you experience a serious side effect, you or your doctor may send a report to the Food and Drug Administration's (FDA) MedWatch Adverse Event Reporting program online [at http://www.fda.gov/MedWatch/index.html] or by phone [1-800-332-1088].

Storage Conditions

- Your health care provider probably will give you a several-day supply of ceftriaxone at a time. If you are receiving ceftriaxone intravenously (in your vein), you probably will be told to store it in the refrigerator or freezer.
- Take your next dose from the refrigerator 1 hour before using it; place it in a clean, dry area to allow it to warm to room temperature.
- If you are told to store additional ceftriaxone in the freezer, always move a 24-hour supply to the refrigerator for the next day's use.
- Do not refreeze medications.

If you are receiving ceftriaxone intramuscularly (in your muscle), your health care provider will tell you how to store it properly.

Store your medication only as directed. Make sure you understand what you need to store your medication properly.

Keep your supplies in a clean, dry place when you are not using them, and keep all medications and supplies out of reach of children. Your health care provider will tell you how to throw away used needles, syringes, tubing, and containers to avoid accidental injury.

Overdose

In case of overdose, call your local poison control center at 1-800-222-1222. If the victim has collapsed or is not breathing, call local emergency services at 911.

Signs of Infection

If you are receiving ceftriaxone in your vein or under your skin, you need to know the symptoms of a catheter-related infection (an infection where the needle enters your vein or skin). If you experience any of these effects near your intravenous catheter, tell your health care provider as soon as possible:

- tenderness
- warmth
- irritation
- drainage
- redness
- swelling
- pain

Dosage Facts
For Informational Purposes

Caution: Do not change your dose, how often you take your medication, or the length of time you

are to take it without first talking to your health-care provider.

The following dosage information was written using medical language for doctors and other healthcare professionals and is provided here for you to check your dosage. The dosage of this drug may differ for different patients. Therefore, always follow your doctor's instructions or the directions on the label. Contact your healthcare provider or pharmacist if you have any questions about the specific dosage of your medication after reviewing this information.

General Dosage Information

Available as ceftriaxone sodium; dosage expressed in terms of ceftriaxone.

Pediatric Patients

General Pediatric Dosage
Infections in Neonates ≤4 Weeks of Age

IV OR IM:
- AAP recommends 50 mg/kg once daily in neonates <1 week of age; 50 mg/kg once daily in those 1–4 weeks of age weighing <2 kg; and 50–75 mg/kg once daily in those 1–4 weeks of age weighing >2 kg.

Mild to Moderate Infections in Children >4 Weeks of Age

IV OR IM:
- AAP recommends 50–75 mg/kg given in 1 or 2 divided doses.

Severe Infections in Children >4 Weeks of Age

IV OR IM:
- AAP recommends 80–100 mg/kg given in 1 or 2 divided doses.
- Manufacturer recommends 50–75 mg/kg daily (maximum 2 g daily) given in 2 equally divided doses every 12 hours.

Acute Otitis Media (AOM)

IM:
- A single dose of 50 mg/kg (maximum 1 g).

Endocarditis†
Treatment of Native Valve Endocarditis Caused by Penicillin-susceptible Viridans Streptococci or S. bovis†

IV:
- 100 mg/kg once every 24 hours for 4 weeks recommended by AHA.
- If the streptococci are relatively resistant to penicillin (MIC 0.1–0.5 mcg/mL), AHA recommends concomitant gentamicin during the first 2 weeks of treatment.

Meningitis

IV:
- An initial dose of 100 mg/kg (≤4 g) followed by 100 mg/kg daily given as a single daily dose or in equally divided doses every 12 hours. Usual duration is 7–14 days.

Skin and Skin Structure Infections

IV OR IM:
- 50–75 mg/kg once daily or in equally divided doses twice daily.

Chancroid†

IM:
- Adolescents: a single dose of 250 mg recommended by CDC.

Gonorrhea and Associated Infections
Disseminated Gonococcal Infection or Gonococcal Scalp Abscess in Neonates†

IV OR IM:
- 25–50 mg/kg once daily for 7 days recommended by CDC and AAP; if meningitis is documented, continue for 10–14 days.

Parenteral Prophylaxis in Neonates Born to Mothers with Gonococcal Infections†

IV OR IM:
- A single dose of 25–50 mg/kg (maximum 125 mg) recommended by CDC and AAP.

Gonococcal Ophthalmia Neonatorum†

IV OR IM:
- A single dose of 25–50 mg/kg (maximum 125 mg) recommended by CDC and AAP.

Uncomplicated Urethral, Cervical, Rectal, or Pharyngeal Gonorrhea in Children

IM:
- Prepubertal children weighing <45 kg: a single dose of 125 mg recommended by CDC and AAP.
- Children ≥8 years of age or weighing ≥45 kg: a single dose of 125 mg recommended by CDC and AAP. Manufacturer recommends a single dose of 250 mg.

Disseminated Gonorrhea in Prepubertal Children Weighing <45 kg†

IV OR IM:
- 50 mg/kg (maximum 1 g) once daily for 7 days for disseminated infections with bacteremia or arthritis.
- 50 mg/kg (maximum 2 g) daily in equally divided doses every 12 hours for disseminated infections with endocarditis or meningitis. Duration of treatment is 10–14 days for meningitis or ≥28 days for endocarditis.

Disseminated Gonorrhea in Children ≥8 Years of Age or Weighing ≥45 kg†

IV OR IM:
- 1 g once daily recommended by CDC and AAP. Continue for 7 days or discontinue 24–48 hours after improvement occurs and switch to an oral regimen to complete ≥7 days of treatment.

Lyme Disease†
Early Disseminated or Late Lyme Disease with Serious Neurologic, Cardiac, and/or Arthritic Manifestations†

IV OR IM:
- 75–100 mg/kg once daily for 14–28 days. Additional courses generally are not recommended unless relapse of neurologic disease is documented with reliable objective measures.

Neisseria meningitidis Infections
Meningitis

IV:
- An initial dose of 100 mg/kg (≤4 g) followed by 100 mg/kg daily given as a single daily dose or in equally divided doses every 12 hours. Usual duration is 7–14 days.

Elimination of Pharyngeal Carrier State†

IM:

- A single 125-mg dose for children ≤12 years of age or a single 250-mg dose for older children recommended by AAP.
- A single 125-mg dose in children <15 years of age recommended by CDC.

Prophylaxis in Household or Other Close Contacts†

IV OR IM:

- A single 125-mg dose for children ≤12 years of age or a single 250-mg dose for older children recommended by AAP.
- A single 125-mg dose in children <15 years of age recommended by CDC.

Shigella Infections†

IV OR IM:

- 50 mg/kg once daily for 2–5 days.

Typhoid Fever and Other Salmonella Infections†
Typhoid Fever or Septicemia caused by S. typhi or S. paratyphi†

IV OR IM:

- 50–75 mg/kg once daily.
- May be effective for treatment of typhoid fever when given for 3–7 days, but anti-infective treatment usually continued for ≥14 days to prevent relapse. A duration of ≥4–6 weeks may be necessary in immunocompromised individuals (including those with HIV infection) or for treatment of *Salmonella* meningitis.

Prophylaxis in Sexual Assault Victims†

IM:

- Prepubertal children: a single dose of 125 mg given in conjunction with doxycycline or a macrolide (azithromycin, erythromycin).
- Adolescents: A single dose of 125 mg given in conjunction with oral metronidazole and either oral azithromycin or oral doxycycline.

Adult Patients

General Adult Dosage

IV OR IM:

- 1–2 g once daily or in equally divided doses twice daily.

Endocarditis†
Treatment of Native Valve Endocarditis Caused by Penicillin-susceptible Viridans Streptococci or S. bovis†

IV OR IM:

- 2 g once daily for 4 weeks recommended by AHA.
- Alternatively, a regimen of 2 g once daily for 2 weeks (given in conjunction with gentamicin) can be used in those with uncomplicated endocarditis. The 2-week regimen is *not* recommended by AHA for patients with complications such as extracardiac foci of infection or intracardiac abscesses.

Endocarditis Caused by HACEK Group (i.e., H. parainfluenzae, H. aphrophilus, A. actinomycetemcomitans, C. hominis, E. corrodens, K. kingae)†

IV OR IM:

- 2 g once daily for 3–4 weeks for native valve endocarditis or for 6 weeks for prosthetic valve endocarditis recommended by AHA.

Meningitis

IV:

- 2 g every 12 hours.
- While 7 days may be adequate for uncomplicated meningitis caused by susceptible *H. influenzae* or *N. meningitidis*, ≥10–14 days is suggested for complicated cases or meningitis caused by *S. pneumoniae* and ≥21 days is suggested for meningitis caused by susceptible Enterobacteriaceae (e.g., *E. coli, Klebsiella*).

Respiratory Tract Infections
Community-acquired Pneumonia

IV OR IM:

- 1 g every 12 or 24 hours in conjunction with other anti-infectives. Twice daily regimen recommended for critically ill patients.

Chancroid†

IM:

- A single dose of 250 mg recommended by CDC.

Gonorrhea and Associated Infections
Uncomplicated Cervical, Urethral, Rectal, or Pharyngeal Gonorrhea

IM:

- A single dose of 125 mg recommended by CDC and others. Manufacturer recommends a 250-mg single dose.

Disseminated Gonococcal Infections†

IV OR IM:

- 1 g once daily recommended by CDC and others. Continue for 24–48 hours after improvement begins; therapy may then be switched to an oral regimen to complete ≥1 week of treatment.
- For gonococcal meningitis or endocarditis, 1–2 g IV every 12 hours. Continue for 10–14 days in those with meningitis and for ≥4 weeks in those with endocarditis.

Gonococcal Conjunctivitis†

IM:

- A single dose of 1 g recommended by CDC and others.

Epididymitis†

IM:

- A single dose of 250 mg given in conjunction with a 10-day regimen of oral doxycycline.

Proctitis†

IM:

- A single dose of 125 mg given in conjunction with a 7-day regimen of oral doxycycline.

Lyme Disease†
Early Disseminated or Late Lyme Disease with Serious Neurologic, Cardiac, and/or Arthritic Manifestations†

IV:

- 2 g IV once daily for 14–28 days. Additional courses of antibiotic therapy generally are not recommended unless relapse of neurologic disease is documented with reliable objective measures.

Neisseria meningitidis Infections
Meningitis

IV:

- 2 g every 12 hours.

Elimination of Pharyngeal Carrier State†

IM:

- A single dose of 250 mg recommended by CDC and others.

Prophylaxis in Household or Other Close Contacts†

IM:

- A single dose of 250 mg recommended by CDC and others.

Pelvic Inflammatory Disease

IM:

- A single dose of 250 mg; followed by a 14-day regimen of oral doxycycline (100 mg twice daily) with or without oral metronidazole (500 mg twice daily).

Syphilis†

Early Syphilis in Penicillin-hypersensitive Patients†

IV OR IM:

- 1 g daily for 8–10 days has been recommended. CDC cautions that the optimal dosage and duration of the drug for treatment of early syphilis have not been defined.

Neurosyphilis in Penicillin-hypersensitive Patients†

IV OR IM:

- 2 g daily for 10–14 days has been suggested. CDC cautions that the optimal dosage and duration of the drug for treatment of early syphilis have not been defined.

Typhoid Fever and Other Salmonella Infections†

Typhoid Fever or Septicemia caused by S. typhi or S. paratyphi†

IV OR IM:

- 2–4 g once daily.
- May be effective for treatment of typhoid fever when given for 3–7 days, but anti-infective treatment usually continued for ≥14 days to prevent relapse. A duration of ≥4–6 weeks may be necessary in immunocompromised individuals (including those with HIV infection) or for the treatment of *Salmonella* meningitis.

Empiric Therapy in Febrile Neutropenic Patients†

IV:

- 30 mg/kg (2 g) once daily in conjunction with IV amikacin.

Perioperative Prophylaxis

IV:

- 1 g given 0.5–2 hours prior to surgery.

Prophylaxis in Sexual Assault Victims†

IV:

- A single 125-mg dose recommended by CDC and AAP; given in conjunction with oral metronidazole and either oral azithromycin or oral doxycycline.

Prescribing Limits

Pediatric Patients

Maximum 2 g daily for treatment of most infections. Maximum 4 g daily for treatment of meningitis.

Adult Patients

Maximum 4 g daily.

Special Populations

Hepatic Impairment

- Dosage adjustments not usually necessary in patients with only impaired hepatic function.

- Dosage should not exceed 2 g daily in patients with both hepatic and renal impairment unless serum ceftriaxone concentrations are monitored closely.

Renal Impairment

- Dosage adjustments not usually necessary in patients with only impaired renal function. Closely monitor patients with severe renal impairment (e.g., dialysis patients) and patients with both renal and hepatic impairment. If evidence of drug accumulation occurs, dosage should be adjusted accordingly.
- Dosage should not exceed 2 g daily in patients with both hepatic and renal impairment unless serum ceftriaxone concentrations are monitored closely.

† Use is not currently included in the labeling approved by the US Food and Drug Administration.

Cefuroxime

(se fyoor ox′ eem)

Brand Name: Ceftin®
Also available generically.

Why is this medicine prescribed?

Cefuroxime is used to treat certain infections caused by bacteria, such as bronchitis; gonorrhea; Lyme disease; and infections of the ears, throat, sinuses, urinary tract, and skin. Cefuroxime is in a class of medications called cephalosporin antibiotics. It works by stopping the growth of bacteria. Antibiotics will not work for colds, flu, or other viral infections.

How should this medicine be used?

Cefuroxime comes as a tablet and a suspension (liquid) to take by mouth. It is usually taken every 12 hours (twice a day) for 7-10 days. To treat gonorrhea, cefuroxime is taken as a single dose, and to treat Lyme disease, cefuroxime is taken twice a day for 20 days. The tablet may be taken with or without food, and the liquid must be taken with food. To help you remember to take cefuroxime, take it around the same time every day. Follow the directions on your prescription label carefully, and ask your doctor or pharmacist to explain any part you do not understand. Take cefuroxime exactly as directed. Do not take more or less of it or take it more often than prescribed by your doctor.

Shake the liquid well before each use to mix the medication evenly.

The tablets should be swallowed whole and taken with a full glass of water. Because the crushed tablet has a strong bitter taste, the tablet should not be crushed. Children who cannot swallow the tablet whole should take the liquid instead.

Take cefuroxime until you finish the prescription, even if you feel better. Stopping cefuroxime too soon may cause bacteria to become resistant to antibiotics.

Are there other uses for this medicine?

This medication may be prescribed for other uses; ask your doctor or pharmacist for more information.

What special precautions should I follow?

Before taking cefuroxime,

- tell your doctor and pharmacist if you are allergic to cefuroxime, penicillin, cefaclor (Ceclor), cefadroxil (Duricef), cefamandole (Mandol), cefazolin (Ancef, Kefzol), cefdinir (Omnicef), cefditoren (Spectracef), cefepime (Maxipime), cefixime (Suprax), cefmetazole (Zefazone), cefonicid (Monocid), cefoperazone (Cefobid), cefotaxime (Claforan), cefoxitin (Mefoxin), cefpodoxime (Vantin), cefprozil (Cefzil), ceftazidime (Ceptaz, Fortaz, Tazicef), ceftibuten (Cedax), ceftizoxime (Cefizox), ceftriaxone (Rocephin), cephalexin (Keflex), cephapirin (Cefadyl), cephradine (Velosef), loracarbef (Lorabid), or any other medications.
- tell your doctor and pharmacist what prescription and nonprescription medications, vitamins, nutritional supplements, and herbal products you are taking. Be sure to mention any of the following: anticoagulants ('blood thinners') such as warfarin (Coumadin), diuretics ('water pills'), medications for heartburn or ulcers, other antibiotics, and probenecid (Benemid). Your doctor may need to change the doses of your medications or monitor you carefully for side effects.
- tell your doctor if you have or have ever had kidney or liver disease, colitis, or stomach problems.
- tell your doctor if you are pregnant, plan to become pregnant, or are breast-feeding. If you become pregnant while taking cefuroxime, call your doctor.

What special dietary instructions should I follow?

Unless your doctor tells you otherwise, continue your normal diet.

What should I do if I forget to take a dose?

Take the missed dose as soon as you remember it. However, if it is almost time for the next dose, skip the missed dose and continue your regular dosing schedule. Do not take a double dose to make up for a missed one.

What side effects can this medicine cause?

Cefuroxime may cause side effects. Tell your doctor if any of these symptoms are severe or do not go away:

- upset stomach
- vomiting
- diarrhea
- stomach pain

If you experience any of the following symptoms, call your doctor immediately:

- severe skin rash
- itching
- hives
- difficulty breathing or swallowing
- wheezing
- diaper rash
- painful sores in the mouth or throat
- vaginal itching and discharge

Cefuroxime may cause other side effects. Call your doctor if you have any unusual problems while taking this medication.

If you experience a serious side effect, you or your doctor may send a report to the Food and Drug Administration's (FDA) MedWatch Adverse Event Reporting program online [at http://www.fda.gov/MedWatch/index.html] or by phone [1-800-332-1088].

What storage conditions are needed for this medicine?

Keep this medication in the container it came in, tightly closed, and out of reach of children. Store the tablets at room temperature and away from excess heat and moisture (not in the bathroom). Throw away any medication that is outdated or no longer needed. Keep liquid medicine at room temperature or in the refrigerator, tightly closed, and throw away any unused medication after 10 days. Do not freeze. Talk to your pharmacist about the proper disposal of your medication.

What should I do in case of overdose?

In case of overdose, call your local poison control center at 1-800-222-1222. If the victim has collapsed or is not breathing, call local emergency services at 911.

Symptoms of overdose may include:

- seizures

What other information should I know?

Keep all appointments with your doctor and the laboratory. Your doctor may order certain lab tests to check your body's response to cefuroxime.

If you are diabetic, use Clinistix or TesTape (not Clinitest) to test your urine for sugar while taking this medication.

Do not let anyone else take your medication. Your prescription is probably not refillable. If you still have symptoms of infection after you finish the cefuroxime, call your doctor.

Dosage Facts
For Informational Purposes

Caution: Do not change your dose, how often you take your medication, or the length of time you are to take it without first talking to your health-care provider.

The following dosage information was written using

medical language for doctors and other healthcare professionals and is provided here for you to check your dosage. The dosage of this drug may differ for different patients. Therefore, always follow your doctor's instructions or the directions on the label. Contact your healthcare provider or pharmacist if you have any questions about the specific dosage of your medication after reviewing this information.

General Dosage Information

Available as cefuroxime axetil or cefuroxime sodium; dosage expressed in terms of cefuroxime.

Tablets and oral suspension are *not* bioequivalent and are *not* substitutable on a mg/mg basis.

Pediatric Patients

General Pediatric Dosage
Mild to Moderate Infections

ORAL:
- AAP recommends 20–30 mg/kg daily given in 2 divided doses in children >4 weeks of age.

Severe Infections

ORAL:
- Oral route inappropriate for severe infections per AAP.

Acute Otitis Media (AOM)
Children 3 Months to 12 Years of Age

ORAL:
- Tablets (for children able to swallow tablets whole): 250 mg twice daily for 10 days.
- Oral suspension: 30 mg/kg daily (maximum 1 g daily) given in 2 divided doses for 10 days.

Pharyngitis and Tonsillitis
Children 3 Months to 12 Years of Age

ORAL:
- Oral suspension: 20 mg/kg daily (maximum 500 mg daily) in 2 divided doses for 10 days.

Adolescents ≥13 Years of Age

ORAL:
- Tablets: 250 mg twice daily for 10 days.

Respiratory Tract Infections
Acute Sinusitis in Children 3 Months to 12 Years of Age

ORAL:
- Tablets (for children able to swallow tablets whole): 250 mg twice daily for 10 days.
- Oral suspension: 30 mg/kg daily (maximum 1 g daily) given in 2 divided doses for 10 days.

Acute Sinusitis in Adolescents ≥13 Years of Age

ORAL:
- Tablets: 250 mg twice daily for 10 days.

Secondary Bacterial Infections of Acute Bronchitis in Adolescents ≥13 Years of Age

ORAL:
- Tablets: 250 or 500 mg twice daily for 5–10 days.

Acute Exacerbations of Chronic Bronchitis in Adolescents ≥13 Years of Age

ORAL:
- Tablets: 250 or 500 mg twice daily for 10 days. Efficacy of regimens <10 days has not been established.

Skin and Skin Structure Infections
Impetigo in Children 3 Months to 12 Years of Age

ORAL:
- Oral suspension: 30 mg/kg daily (maximum 1 g daily) in 2 divided doses for 10 days.

Uncomplicated Infections in Adolescents ≥13 Years of Age

ORAL:
- Tablets: 250 or 500 mg twice daily for 10 days.

Urinary Tract Infections (UTIs)
Uncomplicated Infections in Adolescents ≥13 Years of Age

ORAL:
- Tablets: 250 mg twice daily for 7–10 days.

Gonorrhea and Associated Infections
Uncomplicated Urethral, Cervical, or Rectal Gonorrhea In Adolescents ≥13 Years of Age

ORAL:
- Tablets: 1 g as a single dose.

Lyme Disease
Early Localized or Early Disseminated Lyme Disease

ORAL:
- Tablets: 500 mg twice daily for 20 days in adolescents ≥13 years of age.
- AAP, IDSA, and others recommend 30 mg/kg (maximum 500 mg) administered in 2 divided doses for 14–28 days in children.

Adult Patients

Pharyngitis and Tonsillitis

ORAL:
- Tablets: 250 mg twice daily for 10 days.

Respiratory Tract Infections
Acute Sinusitis

ORAL:
- Tablets: 250 mg twice daily for 10 days.

Secondary Bacterial Infections of Acute Bronchitis

ORAL:
- Tablets: 250 or 500 mg twice daily for 5–10 days.

Acute Exacerbations of Chronic Bronchitis

ORAL:
- Tablets: 250 or 500 mg twice daily for 10 days. Efficacy of regimens <10 days has not been established.

Pneumonia

ORAL:
- 500 mg twice daily for outpatient treatment of acute community-acquired pneumonia† (CAP) in immunocompetent adults.

Skin and Skin Structure Infections
Uncomplicated Infections

ORAL:
- Tablets: 250 or 500 mg twice daily for 10 days.

Urinary Tract Infections (UTIs)
Uncomplicated Infections

ORAL:
- Tablets: 250 mg twice daily for 7–10 days.

Gonorrhea and Associated Infections
Uncomplicated Urethral, Cervical, or Rectal Gonorrhea

ORAL:
- Tablets: 1 g as a single dose.

Lyme Disease
Early Localized or Early Disseminated Lyme Disease

ORAL:
- Tablets: 500 mg twice daily for 20 days.
- IDSA and others recommend 500 mg twice daily for 14–28 days.

Special Populations

Renal Impairment
- Dosage adjustments necessary in patients with $Cl_{cr} \leq 20$ mL/minute.
- No specific recommendations for adjusting dosage of oral cefuroxime in adults or children with renal impairment.

Geriatric Patients
- Cautious dosage selection because of age-related decreases in renal function.

† Use is not currently included in the labeling approved by the US Food and Drug Administration.

Cefuroxime Sodium Injection

(se fyoor ox′ eem)

Brand Name: Zinacef®
Also available generically.

About Your Treatment

Your doctor has ordered cefuroxime, an antibiotic, to help treat your infection. The drug will be either injected into a large muscle (such as your buttock or hip) or added to an intravenous fluid that will drip through a needle or catheter placed in your vein for 30 minutes, two to four times a day.

Cefuroxime eliminates bacteria that cause many kinds of infections, including lung, skin, bone, joint, stomach, blood, and urinary tract infections. This medication is sometimes prescribed for other uses; ask your doctor or pharmacist for more information.

Your health care provider (doctor, nurse, or pharmacist) may measure the effectiveness and side effects of your treatment using laboratory tests and physical examinations. It is important to keep all appointments with your doctor and the laboratory. The length of treatment depends on how your infection and symptoms respond to the medication.

Precautions

Before administering cefuroxime,
- tell your doctor and pharmacist if you are allergic to cefuroxime, any other cephalosporin [e.g., cefaclor (Ceclor), cefadroxil (Duricef), or cephalexin (Keflex)], penicillins, or any other drugs.
- tell your doctor and pharmacist what prescription and nonprescription medications you are taking, especially other antibiotics, probenecid (Benemid), and vitamins.
- tell your doctor if you have or have ever had kidney, liver, or gastrointestinal disease (especially colitis).
- tell your doctor if you are pregnant, plan to become pregnant, or are breast-feeding. If you become pregnant while taking cefuroxime, call your doctor.
- if you have diabetes and regularly check your urine for sugar, use Clinistix or TesTape. Do not use Clinitest tablets because cefuroxime may cause false positive results.

Administering Your Medication

Before you administer cefuroxime, look at the solution closely. It should be clear and free of floating material. Gently squeeze the bag or observe the solution container to make sure there are no leaks. Do not use the solution if it is discolored, if it contains particles, or if the bag or container leaks. Use a new solution, but show the damaged one to your health care provider.

It is important that you use your medication exactly as directed. Do not stop your therapy on your own for any reason because your infection could worsen and result in hospitalization. Do not change your dosing schedule without talking to your health care provider. Your health care provider may tell you to stop your infusion if you have a mechanical problem (such as a blockage in the tubing, needle, or catheter); if you have to stop an infusion, call your health care provider immediately so your therapy can continue.

Side Effects

Cefuroxime may cause side effects. If you are administering cefuroxime into a muscle, it may be mixed with lidocaine (Xylocaine) to reduce pain at the injection site. Tell your health care provider if any of these symptoms are severe or do not go away:
- diarrhea
- stomach pain
- upset stomach
- vomiting

If you experience any of the following symptoms, call your health care provider immediately:
- unusual bleeding or bruising
- difficulty breathing
- itching
- rash

- hives
- sore mouth or throat

If you experience a serious side effect, you or your doctor may send a report to the Food and Drug Administration's (FDA) MedWatch Adverse Event Reporting program online [at http://www.fda.gov/MedWatch/index.html] or by phone [1-800-332-1088].

Storage Conditions

- Your health care provider probably will give you a several-day supply of cefuroxime at a time. If you are receiving cefuroxime intravenously (in your vein), you probably will be told to store it in the refrigerator or freezer.
- Take your next dose from the refrigerator 1 hour before using it; place it in a clean, dry area to allow it to warm to room temperature.
- If you are told to store additional cefuroxime in the freezer, always move a 24-hour supply to the refrigerator for the next day's use.
- Do not refreeze medications.

If you are receiving cefuroxime intramuscularly (in your muscle), your health care provider will tell you how to store it properly.

Store your medication only as directed. Make sure you understand what you need to store your medication properly.

Keep your supplies in a clean, dry place when you are not using them, and keep all medications and supplies out of reach of children. Your health care provider will tell you how to throw away used needles, syringes, tubing, and containers to avoid accidental injury.

Overdose

In case of overdose, call your local poison control center at 1-800-222-1222. If the victim has collapsed or is not breathing, call local emergency services at 911.

Signs of Infection

If you are receiving cefuroxime in your vein or under your skin, you need to know the symptoms of a catheter-related infection (an infection where the needle enters your vein or skin). If you experience any of these effects near your intravenous catheter, tell your health care provider as soon as possible:

- tenderness
- warmth
- irritation
- drainage
- redness
- swelling
- pain

Dosage Facts
For Informational Purposes

Caution: Do not change your dose, how often you take your medication, or the length of time you are to take it without first talking to your healthcare provider.

The following dosage information was written using medical language for doctors and other healthcare professionals and is provided here for you to check your dosage. The dosage of this drug may differ for different patients. Therefore, always follow your doctor's instructions or the directions on the label. Contact your healthcare provider or pharmacist if you have any questions about the specific dosage of your medication after reviewing this information.

General Dosage Information

Available as cefuroxime axetil or cefuroxime sodium; dosage expressed in terms of cefuroxime.

Tablets and oral suspension are *not* bioequivalent and are *not* substitutable on a mg/mg basis.

Pediatric Patients

General Pediatric Dosage
Mild to Moderate Infections

IV OR IM:
- AAP recommends 75–100 mg/kg daily given in 3 divided doses in children >4 weeks of age.
- Manufacturer states 50–100 mg/kg daily given in 3 or 4 equally divided doses has been effective for most infections in children ≥3 months of age.

Severe Infections

IV OR IM:
- AAP recommends 100–150 mg/kg daily given in 3 divided doses in children >4 weeks of age.
- Manufacturer recommends 100 mg/kg daily given in 3 or 4 equally divided doses for children ≥3 months of age.

Bone and Joint Infections
Children 3 Months to 12 Years of Age

IV OR IM:
- 150 mg/kg daily given in equally divided doses every 8 hours.

Meningitis
Children 3 Months to 12 Years of Age

IV OR IM:
- 200–240 mg/kg daily given in equally divided doses every 6–8 hours.

Perioperative Prophylaxis
Cardiac, Cardiothoracic, or Noncardiac Thoracic Surgery

IV:
- 50 mg/kg given at induction of anesthesia (within 0.5–1 hour prior to incision). Some experts suggest additional doses of 50 mg/kg every 8 hours for up to 48–72 hours; others state that prophylaxis for ≤24 hours is appropriate.

Adult Patients

General Adult Dosage

IV OR IM:
- 750–1.5 g every 8 hours for 5–10 days.

Life-threatening Infections or Those Caused by Less Susceptible Organisms

IV OR IM:
- 1.5 g every 6 hours.

Bone and Joint Infections

IV OR IM:

- 1.5 g every 8 hours.

Meningitis

IV OR IM:

- Up to 3 g every 8 hours.

Respiratory Tract Infections

Pneumonia

IV OR IM:

- 750 mg every 8 hours. For severe or complicated infections, 1.5 g every 8 hours.

Skin and Skin Structure Infections

Uncomplicated Infections

IV OR IM:

- 750 mg every 8 hours.

Severe or Complicated Infections

IV OR IM:

- 1.5 g every 8 hours.

Urinary Tract Infections (UTIs)

Uncomplicated Infections

IV OR IM:

- 750 mg every 8 hours.

Severe or Complicated Infections

IV OR IM:

- 1.5 g every 8 hours.

Gonorrhea and Associated Infections

Uncomplicated Urethral, Cervical, or Rectal Gonorrhea

IM:

- 1.5 g as a single dose; divide the dose, give at 2 different sites. Given in conjunction with 1 g of oral probenecid.

Disseminated Gonococcal Infections

IV OR IM:

- 750 mg every 8 hours.

Perioperative Prophylaxis

General Adult Dosage

IV OR IM:

- Manufacturer recommends 1.5 g given IV just prior to surgery (approximately 0.5–1 hour prior to initial incision) and, in lengthy operations, 750 mg given IV or IM every 8 hours.
- Most clinicians recommend 1.5 g given no more than 0.5–1 hour before the incision and additional doses during the procedure (e.g., every 4–8 hours) only if surgery is prolonged >4 hours or major blood loss occurs. In most cases, postoperative doses are unnecessary and may increase the risk of toxicity and bacterial superinfection.

Cardiac, Cardiothoracic, or Noncardiac Thoracic Surgery

IV:

- For open-heart surgery, manufacturer recommends 1.5 g given at the time of induction of anesthesia and 1.5 g every 12 hours thereafter for a total dosage of 6 g.
- In patients undergoing cardiac surgery (prosthetic valve, coronary artery bypass, other open-heart surgery, pacemaker or defibrillator implant) or noncardiac thoracic surgery, some experts recommend 1.5 g given at induction of anesthesia (within 0.5–1 hour prior to incision) with an additional dose when the patient is removed from bypass.
- For cardiothoracic surgery and heart and/or lung transplantation, some experts suggest additional 1.5-g doses every 12 hours for up to 48–72 hours; others state that prophylaxis for ≤24 hours is appropriate. There is no evidence to support continuing prophylaxis until chest and mediastinal drainage tubes are removed.

Special Populations

Renal Impairment

- Dosage adjustments necessary in patients with Cl_{cr} ≤20 mL/minute.
- Adults with impaired renal function: 750 mg IM or IV every 12 hours in those with Cl_{cr} 10–20 mL/minute or 750 mg IM or IV every 24 hours in those with Cl_{cr} <10 mL/minute.
- Children with impaired renal function: Make adjustments to dosing frequency for IM or IV cefuroxime similar to those recommended for adults with renal impairment.

Geriatric Patients

- Cautious dosage selection because of age-related decreases in renal function.

† Use is not currently included in the labeling approved by the US Food and Drug Administration.

Celecoxib

(sell a kox′ ib)

Brand Name: Celebrex®

Important Warning

People who take nonsteroidal anti-inflammatory medications (NSAIDs) (other than aspirin) such as celecoxib may have a higher risk of having a heart attack or a stroke than people who do not take these medications. These events may happen without warning and may cause death. This risk may be higher for people who take NSAIDs for a long time. Tell your doctor if you or anyone in your family has or has ever had heart disease, a heart attack, or a stroke, if you smoke, and if you have or have ever had high cholesterol, high blood pressure, or diabetes. Get emergency medical help right away if you experience any of the following symptoms: chest pain, shortness of breath, weakness in one part or side of the body, or slurred speech.

If you will be undergoing a coronary artery bypass graft (CABG; a type of heart surgery), you should not take celecoxib right before or right after the surgery.

NSAIDs such as celecoxib may cause ulcers, bleeding, or holes in the stomach or intestine. These problems may develop at any time during treatment, may happen without warning symptoms, and may cause death. The risk may be higher for people who take NSAIDs for a long time, are older in age, have poor health, or drink large amounts of alcohol while taking celecoxib. Tell your doctor if you drink large amounts of alcohol or if you take any of the following medications: anticoagulants ('blood thinners') such as warfarin (Coumadin); aspirin; other NSAIDs such as ibuprofen (Advil, Motrin) or naproxen (Aleve, Naprosyn); or oral steroids such as dexamethasone (Decadron, Dexone), methylprednisolone (Medrol), and prednisone (Deltasone). Also tell your doctor if you have or have ever had ulcers or bleeding in your stomach or intestines or other bleeding disorders. If you experience any of the following symptoms, stop taking celecoxib and call your doctor: stomach pain, heartburn, vomiting a substance that is bloody or looks like coffee grounds, blood in the stool, or black and tarry stools.

Keep all appointments with your doctor and the laboratory. Your doctor will monitor your symptoms carefully and will probably order certain tests to check your body's response to celecoxib. Be sure to tell your doctor how you are feeling so that your doctor can prescribe the right amount of medication to treat your condition with the lowest risk of serious side effects.

Your doctor or pharmacist will give you the manufacturer's patient information sheet (Medication Guide) when you begin treatment with celecoxib and each time you refill your prescription. Read the information carefully and ask your doctor or pharmacist if you have any questions. You can also visit the Food and Drug Administration (FDA) website (http://www.fda.gov/cder) or the manufacturer's website to obtain the Medication Guide.

Why is this medicine prescribed?

Celecoxib is used to relieve pain, tenderness, swelling and stiffness caused by osteoarthritis (arthritis caused by a breakdown of the lining of the joints), rheumatoid arthritis (arthritis caused by swelling of the lining of the joints), and ankylosing spondylitis (arthritis that mainly affects the spine). Celecoxib is also used to treat painful menstrual periods and pain from other causes. It is also used with surgery and other treatments to reduce the number of polyps (abnormal growths) in the colon (large intestine) and rectum in patients with familial adenomatous polyposis (a condition in which hundreds or thousands of polyps form in the colon and cancer may develop). Celecoxib is in a class of NSAIDs called COX-2 inhibitors. It works by stopping the body's production of a substance that causes pain and inflammation.

How should this medicine be used?

Celecoxib comes as a capsule to take by mouth. It is usually taken once or twice a day. If you are taking up to 200 mg of celecoxib at a time, you may take the medication with or without food. If you are taking more than 200 mg of celecoxib at a time, you should take the medication with food. Ask your doctor or pharmacist if you are not sure if you need to take your medication with food. To help you remember to take celecoxib, take it around the same time(s) every day. Follow the directions on your prescription label carefully, and ask your doctor or pharmacist to explain any part you do not understand. Take celecoxib exactly as directed. Do not take more or less of it or take it more often than prescribed by your doctor.

Are there other uses for this medicine?

This medication may be prescribed for other uses; ask your doctor or pharmacist for more information.

What special precautions should I follow?

Before taking celecoxib,

- tell your doctor and pharmacist if you are allergic to celecoxib, aspirin or other NSAIDs such as ibuprofen (Advil, Motrin) and naproxen (Aleve, Naprosyn), sulfa medications, any other medications, or any of the inactive ingredients in celecoxib capsules. Ask your pharmacist for a list of the inactive ingredients.
- tell your doctor and pharmacist what prescription and nonprescription medications, vitamins, nutritional supplements, and herbal products you are taking or plan to take. Be sure to mention the medications listed in the IMPORTANT WARNING section and any of the following: amiodarone (Cordarone, Pacerone); angiotensin-converting enzyme (ACE) inhibitors such as benazepril (Lotensin), captopril (Capoten), enalapril (Vasotec), fosinopril (Monopril), lisinopril (Prinivil, Zestril), moexipril (Univasc), perindopril (Aceon), quinapril (Accupril), ramipril (Altace), and trandolapril (Mavik); certain antidepressants (mood elevators); atazanavir (Reyataz); clopidogrel (Plavix); codeine (in some cough medications and some pain medications); dextromethorphan (in some cough medications); diuretics ('water pills'); efavirenz (Sustiva); fluconazole (Diflucan); fluvastatin (Lescol); lithium (Eskalith, Lithobid); certain medications for mental illness; metoprolol (Lopressor, Toprol XL); metronidazole (Flagyl); mexiletine (Mexitil); ondansetron (Zofran); propafenone (Rhythmol); ritonavir (Norvir, in Kaletra); sulfamethoxazole (Bactrim, Septra); sulfinpyrazone (Anturane); tamoxifen (Nolvadex) timolol (Blocadren, Timolide, in some eye drops); tramadol (Ultram); and zafirlukast (Accolate). Your doctor may need to change the doses of your medications or monitor you carefully for side effects.
- tell your doctor if you have or have ever had any of the conditions mentioned in the IMPORTANT WARNING

section or asthma, especially if you also have frequent stuffed or runny nose or nasal polyps (swelling of the lining of the nose); swelling of the hands, arms, feet, ankles, or lower legs; or liver or kidney disease.

- tell your doctor if you are pregnant, especially if you are in the last few months of your pregnancy, you plan to become pregnant, or you are breast-feeding. If you become pregnant while taking celecoxib, call your doctor.
- if you are having surgery, including dental surgery, tell the doctor or dentist that you are taking celecoxib.

What special dietary instructions should I follow?

Unless your doctor tells you otherwise, continue your normal diet.

What should I do if I forget to take a dose?

Take the missed dose as soon as you remember it. However, if it is almost time for the next dose, skip the missed dose and continue your regular dosing schedule. Do not take a double dose to make up for a missed one.

What side effects can this medicine cause?

Celecoxib may cause side effects. Tell your doctor if any of these symptoms are severe or do not go away:

- diarrhea
- gas or bloating
- sore throat
- cold symptoms

Some side effects can be serious. If you experience any of the following symptoms or those mentioned in the IMPORTANT WARNING section, call your doctor immediately. Do not take any more celecoxib until you speak to your doctor.

- unexplained weight gain
- upset stomach
- excessive tiredness
- unusual bleeding or bruising
- itching
- lack of energy
- loss of appetite
- pain in the upper right part of the stomach
- yellowing of the skin or eyes
- flu-like symptoms
- blisters
- fever
- rash
- hives
- swelling of the face, throat, tongue, lips, eyes, hands, feet, ankles, or lower legs
- hoarseness
- difficulty swallowing or breathing
- pale skin
- fast heartbeat
- cloudy, discolored, or bloody urine

- back pain
- difficult or painful urination
- frequent urination, especially at night

Celecoxib may cause other side effects. Call your doctor if you have any unusual problems while taking this medication.

If you experience a serious side effect, you or your doctor may send a report to the Food and Drug Administration's (FDA) MedWatch Adverse Event Reporting program online [at http://www.fda.gov/MedWatch/index.html] or by phone [1-800-332-1088].

What storage conditions are needed for this medicine?

Keep this medication in the container it came in, tightly closed, and out of reach of children. Store it at room temperature and away from excess heat and moisture (not in the bathroom). Throw away any medication that is outdated or no longer needed. Talk to your pharmacist about the proper disposal of your medication.

What should I do in case of overdose?

In case of overdose, call your local poison control center at 1-800-222-1222. If the victim has collapsed or is not breathing, call local emergency services at 911.

Symptoms of overdose may include:

- lack of energy
- drowsiness
- upset stomach
- vomiting
- stomach pain
- vomiting material that is bloody or looks like coffee grounds
- bloody or black, tarry stools
- loss of consciousness
- hives
- rash
- swelling of the eyes, face, tongue, lips, throat, arms, hands, feet, ankles, or lower legs
- difficulty breathing or swallowing

What other information should I know?

Do not let anyone else take your medication. Ask your pharmacist any questions you have about refilling your prescription.

Dosage Facts
For Informational Purposes

Caution: Do not change your dose, how often you take your medication, or the length of time you are to take it without first talking to your health-care provider.

The following dosage information was written using medical language for doctors and other healthcare pro-

fessionals and is provided here for you to check your dosage. The dosage of this drug may differ for different patients. Therefore, always follow your doctor's instructions or the directions on the label. Contact your healthcare provider or pharmacist if you have any questions about the specific dosage of your medication after reviewing this information.

General Dosage Information

To minimize the potential risk of adverse cardiovascular and/or GI events, use lowest effective dosage and shortest duration of therapy consistent with the patient's treatment goals.

Attempt to titrate to the lowest effective dosage in adults with arthritis.

Pediatric Patients

Juvenile Arthritis

ORAL:
- Children ≥2 years of age weighing 10–25 kg: 50 mg twice daily.
- Children ≥2 years of age weighing >25 kg: 100 mg twice daily.

Adult Patients

Osteoarthritis

ORAL:
- 200 mg daily as a single dose or in 2 equally divided doses.
- No additional benefit from dosages >200 mg daily.

Rheumatoid Arthritis in Adults

ORAL:
- 100–200 mg twice daily.
- No additional benefit from higher dosages (400 mg twice daily).

Ankylosing Spondylitis

ORAL:
- Initially, 200 mg daily as a single dose or in 2 equally divided doses. If no response observed after 6 weeks, increase to 400 mg daily. If no response observed after 400 mg daily for 6 weeks, response is unlikely; consider alternative therapies.

Colorectal Polyps

ORAL:
- 400 mg twice daily.

Pain

ORAL:
- 400 mg initially as a single dose, followed by an additional dose of 200 mg, if necessary, on the first day. For continued relief, 200 mg twice daily as needed.

Dysmenorrhea

ORAL:
- 400 mg initially as a single dose, followed by an additional dose of 200 mg, if necessary, on the first day. For continued relief, 200 mg twice daily as needed.

Special Populations

Hepatic Impairment
- Reduce dosage by 50% in patients with moderate hepatic impairment; not recommended in patients with severe impairment.

Geriatric Patients
- Dosage adjustment based solely on age is not necessary; initiate at lowest recommended dosage in geriatric patients weighing <50 kg.

Cephalexin

(sef a lex′ in)

Brand Name: Keflex® Pulvules®
Also available generically.

Why is this medicine prescribed?

Cephalexin is a cephalosporin antibiotic used to treat certain infections caused by bacteria such as pneumonia and bone, ear, skin, and urinary tract infections. Antibiotics will not work for colds, flu, or other viral infections.

This medication is sometimes prescribed for other uses; ask your doctor or pharmacist for more information.

How should this medicine be used?

Cephalexin comes as a capsule, tablet, and liquid to take by mouth. It is usually taken every 6 hours (four times a day) or every 12 hours (twice a day) for 7-10 days. Follow the directions on your prescription label carefully, and ask your doctor or pharmacist to explain any part you do not understand. Take cephalexin exactly as directed. Do not take more or less of it or take it more often than prescribed by your doctor.

Shake the liquid well before each use to mix the medication evenly.

The capsules and tablets should be swallowed whole and taken with a full glass of water.

Continue to take cephalexin even if you feel well. Do not stop taking cephalexin without talking to your doctor.

What special precautions should I follow?

Before taking cephalexin,
- tell your doctor and pharmacist if you are allergic to cephalexin or any other cephalosporin antibiotic such as cefadroxil (Duricef) or cephradine (Velosef), penicillin, or any other drugs.
- tell your doctor and pharmacist what prescription and nonprescription medications you are taking, especially other antibiotics, anticoagulants ('blood thinners') such as warfarin (Coumadin), probenecid (Benemid), and vitamins.
- tell your doctor if you have or have ever had kidney or liver disease, colitis, or stomach problems.
- tell your doctor if you are pregnant, plan to become pregnant, or are breast-feeding. If you become pregnant while taking cephalexin, call your doctor.

- if you are having surgery, including dental surgery, tell the doctor or dentist that you are taking cephalexin.

What special dietary instructions should I follow?

Cephalexin may cause an upset stomach. Take cephalexin with food or milk.

What should I do if I forget to take a dose?

Take the missed dose as soon as you remember it. However, if it is almost time for the next dose, skip the missed dose and continue your regular dosing schedule. Do not take a double dose to make up for a missed one.

What side effects can this medicine cause?

Cephalexin may cause side effects. Tell your doctor if any of these symptoms are severe or do not go away:

- upset stomach
- diarrhea
- vomiting
- mild skin rash

If you experience any of the following symptoms, call your doctor immediately:

- severe skin rash
- itching
- hives
- difficulty breathing or swallowing
- wheezing
- unusual bleeding or bruising
- sore throat
- painful mouth or throat sores
- vaginal infection

If you experience a serious side effect, you or your doctor may send a report to the Food and Drug Administration's (FDA) MedWatch Adverse Event Reporting program online [at http://www.fda.gov/MedWatch/index.html] or by phone [1-800-332-1088].

What storage conditions are needed for this medicine?

Keep this medication in the container it came in, tightly closed, and out of reach of children. Store the capsules and tablets at room temperature and away from excess heat and moisture (not in the bathroom). Throw away any medication that is outdated or no longer needed. Keep liquid medicine in the refrigerator, tightly closed, and throw away any unused medication after 14 days. Do not freeze. Talk to your pharmacist about the proper disposal of your medication.

What should I do in case of overdose?

In case of overdose, call your local poison control center at 1-800-222-1222. If the victim has collapsed or is not breathing, call local emergency services at 911.

What other information should I know?

Keep all appointments with your doctor and the laboratory. Your doctor will order certain lab tests to check your response to cephalexin.

If you are diabetic, use Clinistix or TesTape (not Clinitest) to test your urine for sugar while taking this drug.

Do not let anyone else take your medication. Your prescription is probably not refillable. If you still have symptoms of infection after you finish the cephalexin, call your doctor.

Dosage Facts
For Informational Purposes

Caution: Do not change your dose, how often you take your medication, or the length of time you are to take it without first talking to your healthcare provider.

The following dosage information was written using medical language for doctors and other healthcare professionals and is provided here for you to check your dosage. The dosage of this drug may differ for different patients. Therefore, always follow your doctor's instructions or the directions on the label. Contact your healthcare provider or pharmacist if you have any questions about the specific dosage of your medication after reviewing this information.

General Dosage Information

Available as cephalexin monohydrate; dosage expressed in terms of cephalexin.

Pediatric Patients

Respiratory Tract Infections

ORAL:
- 25–50 mg/kg daily in 3–4 equally divided doses for mild to moderate infections.
- Manufacturers state dosage may be doubled for severe infections; AAP states the drug is inappropriate for severe infections.

Acute Otitis Media (AOM)

ORAL:
- 75–100 mg/kg daily in 4 divided doses.

Pharyngitis and Tonsillitis

ORAL:
- 25–50 mg/kg daily in 3–4 equally divided doses for ≥10 days. Daily dosage may be given in divided doses every 12 hours in those >1 year of age.
- Children >15 years of age: 500 mg every 12 hours for ≥10 days.

Bone and Joint Infections

ORAL:
- 25–50 mg/kg daily in 3–4 equally divided doses for mild to moderate infections.
- Manufacturers state dosage may be doubled for severe infec-

given either as a 5-mg dose once daily (as chewable tablets or oral solution), or alternatively, as a 2.5 mg dose every 12 hours (as oral solution).

Children ≥6 years of age: 5 or 10 mg once daily (as chewable or conventional tablets or oral solution), depending on symptom severity. In clinical trials, most children ≥12 years of age received an initial dosage of 10 mg daily; no additional benefit observed with 20-mg daily dosage.

Children ≥12 years of age: 5 mg twice daily (every 12 hours) (as fixed combination with 120 mg pseudoephedrine hydrochloride).

Perennial

ORAL:

- Children 6 months to <2 years of age: 2.5 mg once daily (as oral solution). In children 12–23 months of age, may increase dosage to a maximum of 5 mg daily, given as 2.5 mg every 12 hours.
- Children 2–5 years of age: 2.5 mg once daily (as oral solution); may increase dosage to a maximum of 5 mg daily, given either as a 5-mg dose once daily (as chewable tablets or oral solution), or alternatively, as a 2.5 mg dose every 12 hours (as oral solution).
- Children ≥6 years of age: 5 or 10 mg once daily (as chewable or conventional tablets or oral solution), depending on symptom severity. In clinical trials, most children ≥12 years of age received an initial dosage of 10 mg daily; no additional benefit observed with 20-mg daily dosage.
- Children ≥12 years of age: 5 mg twice daily (every 12 hours) (as fixed combination with 120 mg pseudoephedrine hydrochloride).

Chronic Idiopathic Urticaria

ORAL:

- Children 6 months to <2 years of age: 2.5 mg once daily (as oral solution). In children 12–23 months of age, may increase dosage to a maximum of 5 mg daily, given as 2.5 mg every 12 hours.
- Children 2–5 years of age: 2.5 mg once daily (as oral solution); may increase dosage to a maximum of 5 mg daily, given either as a 5-mg dose once daily (as chewable tablets or oral solution), or alternatively, as a 2.5 mg dose every 12 hours (as oral solution).
- Children ≥ 6 years of age: 5 or 10 mg once daily (as chewable or conventional tablets or oral solution), depending on symptom severity. In clinical trials, most children ≥12 years of age received an initial dosage of 10 mg daily; no additional benefit observed with 20-mg daily dosage.

Adult Patients

Allergic Rhinitis

ORAL:

- 5 or 10 mg once daily (as chewable or conventional tablets or oral solution), depending on symptom severity. In clinical trials, most patients received an initial dosage of 10 mg daily; no additional benefit observed with 20-mg daily dosage.
- 5 mg twice daily (every 12 hours) (as fixed combination with 120 mg pseudoephedrine hydrochloride).

Chronic Idiopathic Urticaria

ORAL:

- 5 or 10 mg once daily (as chewable or conventional tablets or oral solution), depending on symptom severity. In clinical

trials, most patients received an initial dosage of 10 mg daily; no additional benefit observed with 20-mg daily dosage.

Prescribing Limits

Pediatric Patients

Allergic Rhinitis

ORAL:

- Children 12 months to 5 years of age: Maximum 5 mg daily.
- Children ≥12 years of age: In clinical trials, a 20-mg daily dosage did not provide additional clinical benefit.
- Fixed-combination cetirizine hydrochloride/pseudoephedrine hydrochloride not recommended for children <12 years of age; contains 120 mg pseudoephedrine hydrochloride, which exceeds recommended single dose in such patients.

Chronic Idiopathic Urticaria

ORAL:

- Children 12 months to 5 years of age: Maximum 5 mg daily.
- Children ≥12 years of age: In clinical trials, a 20-mg daily dosage did not provide additional clinical benefit.

Adult Patients

Allergic Rhinitis

ORAL:

- In clinical trials, a 20-mg daily dosage did not provide additional clinical benefit.

Chronic Idiopathic Urticaria

ORAL:

- In clinical trials, a 20-mg daily dosage did not provide additional clinical benefit.

Special Populations

Hepatic Impairment

- Children <6 years of age: use not recommended.
- Adults and children ≥6 years of age: 5 mg once daily (as chewable or conventional tablets or oral solution).
- Adults and children ≥12 years of age: 5 mg once daily (in fixed combination with 120 mg pseudoephedrine hydrochloride).

Renal Impairment

- Children <6 years of age: use not recommended.
- Adults and children ≥6 years of age: 5 mg once daily (as chewable or conventional tablets or oral solution) in patients with impaired renal function (e.g., Cl_{cr} of 11–31 mL/minute) or those on hemodialysis (e.g., Cl_{cr} <7 mL/minute).
- Adults and children ≥12 years of age: 5 mg once daily (in fixed combination with 120 mg pseudoephedrine hydrochloride) in patients with impaired renal function (e.g., Cl_{cr} of 11–31 mL/minute) or those on hemodialysis (e.g., Cl_{cr} <7 mL/minute).

Geriatric Patients

- Patients ≥77 years of age: 5 mg once daily (as chewable or conventional tablets or oral solution) recommended.

Cetuximab Injection

(se tux' i mab)

Brand Name: Erbitux®

Important Warning

Cetuximab may cause severe or life-threatening reactions while you receive the medication. These reactions are more common with the first dose of cetuximab, but may occur at any time during treatment. Your doctor will watch you carefully while you receive each dose of cetuximab and for at least one hour afterwards. Tell your doctor if you experience any of the following symptoms during or after your infusion: shortness of breath, wheezing or noisy breathing, hoarseness, hives, fainting, dizziness, blurred vision, nausea, or chest pain or pressure. If you experience a severe reaction, your doctor will stop your infusion and treat the symptoms of the reaction. You will not be able to receive treatment with cetuximab in the future.

People with a head and neck cancer who are treated with radiation therapy and cetuximab may have an increased risk of cardiopulmonary arrest (condition in which the heart stops beating and breathing stops) and/or sudden death during or after their treatment. Tell your doctor if you have or have ever had coronary artery disease (condition that occurs when the blood vessels of the heart are narrowed by fat or cholesterol deposits); angina (chest pain or pressure); a heart attack; congestive heart failure; irregular heartbeat; other heart disease; or lower than normal levels of magnesium, potassium, or calcium in your blood.

Keep all appointments with your doctor and the laboratory. Your doctor will order certain tests during and after your treatment to check your body's response to cetuximab.

Talk to your doctor about the risks of using cetuximab.

Why is this medicine prescribed?

Cetuximab is used with or without radiation therapy to treat a certain type of cancer of the head and neck. Cetuximab is also used alone or in combination with another medication to treat a certain type of cancer of the colon (large intestine) or rectum that has spread to other parts of the body. Cetuximab has been shown to slow the growth of tumors in people who have cancer of the colon or rectum. However, it has not been shown to help people who have cancer of the colon or rectum feel better or live longer. Cetuximab is in a class of medications called monoclonal antibodies. It works by slowing or stopping the growth of cancer cells.

How should this medicine be used?

Cetuximab comes as a solution (liquid) to be infused (injected slowly) into a vein. Cetuximab is given by a doctor or nurse in a medical office or infusion center. It is usually given once a week.

Are there other uses for this medicine?

This medication may be prescribed for other uses; ask your doctor or pharmacist for more information.

What special precautions should I follow?

Before receiving treatment with cetuximab,

- tell your doctor and pharmacist if you are allergic to cetuximab, any medications that are made from murine (mouse) proteins, or any other medications. Ask your doctor or pharmacist if you don't know whether a medication that you are allergic to is made from murine proteins.
- tell your doctor and pharmacist what other prescription and nonprescription medications, vitamins, nutritional supplements, and herbal products you are taking or plan to take. Be sure to mention if you are receiving treatment with cisplatin (Platinol). Your doctor may need to change the doses of your medications or monitor you carefully for side effects.
- tell your doctor if you have or have ever had lung disease.
- tell your doctor if you are pregnant or plan to become pregnant. Use effective birth control to prevent pregnancy during your treatment with cetuximab. If you become pregnant while using cetuximab, call your doctor.
- tell your doctor if you are breast-feeding. You should not breastfeed during your treatment with cetuximab or for 60 days after you stop using the medication.
- plan to avoid unnecessary or prolonged exposure to sunlight and to wear protective clothing, a hat, sunglasses, and sunscreen. Cetuximab may make your skin sensitive to sunlight.

What special dietary instructions should I follow?

Unless your doctor tells you otherwise, continue your normal diet.

What should I do if I forget to take a dose?

If you miss an appointment to receive a dose of cetuximab, call your doctor right away.

What side effects can this medicine cause?

Cetuximab may cause side effects. Tell your doctor if any of these symptoms are severe or do not go away:

- acne-like rash
- dry or cracking skin
- swelling or pain in the fingernails or toenails

- red, watery, or itchy eye(s)
- red or swollen eyelid(s)
- pain or burning sensation in eye(s)
- sensitivity of eyes to light
- hair loss
- dry mouth
- chapped lips
- mouth sores
- difficulty swallowing
- headache
- tiredness
- weakness
- difficulty falling asleep or staying asleep
- depression
- nausea
- vomiting
- constipation
- stomach pain
- heartburn
- loss of appetite
- weight loss
- pain, especially in the back
- pain, redness, or swelling at injection spot

Some side effects can be serious. If you experience any of these symptoms or those listed in the IMPORTANT WARNING section, call your doctor immediately:

- swelling of the hands, feet, ankles, or lower legs
- fast heartbeat
- coughing up blood or dry cough
- shortness of breath or unusual tiredness during exercise
- fainting
- decreased urination
- muscle cramps
- shaking of the hands that you cannot control
- sudden tightening of the hands or feet
- twitching of the body that you cannot control
- sore throat, fever, chills, and other signs of infection
- diarrhea
- confusion
- itching
- hives
- red, swollen, or infected skin

Cetuximab may cause other side effects. Call your doctor if you have any unusual problems while using this medication.

What should I do in case of overdose?

In case of overdose, call your local poison control center at 1-800-222-1222. If the victim has collapsed or is not breathing, call local emergency services at 911.

What other information should I know?

Ask your doctor if you have any questions about your treatment with cetuximab.

Dosage Facts
For Informational Purposes

Caution: Do not change your dose, how often you take your medication, or the length of time you are to take it without first talking to your healthcare provider.

The following dosage information was written using medical language for doctors and other healthcare professionals and is provided here for you to check your dosage. The dosage of this drug may differ for different patients. Therefore, always follow your doctor's instructions or the directions on the label. Contact your healthcare provider or pharmacist if you have any questions about the specific dosage of your medication after reviewing this information.

Adult Patients

Head and Neck Cancer
Cetuximab/Radiation Combination Therapy

IV:

- Initially, 400 mg/m^2 over 2 hours as loading dose, administered 1 week prior to initiation of first course of radiation therapy. Then, 250 mg/m^2 over 1 hour once weekly (maintenance dosage) for duration of radiation therapy (6–7 weeks); a median of 8 doses was administered in clinical studies. In clinical studies, cetuximab was administered 1 hour prior to radiation therapy, beginning week 2.

Monotherapy

IV:

- Initially, 400 mg/m^2 over 2 hours as loading dose, followed by maintenance doses of 250 mg/m^2 over 1 hour once weekly until disease progression or unacceptable toxicity occurs. In clinical studies, a median of 11 doses was administered.

Colorectal Cancer

IV:

- Initially, 400 mg/m^2 over 2 hours as loading dose, followed by maintenance doses of 250 mg/m^2 over 1 hour once weekly.
- When used in combination with irinotecan, consult manufacturer of that drug for information on dosage, method, and sequence of administration. Dosage of irinotecan used in clinical studies was 350 mg/m^2 every 3 weeks, 180 mg/m^2 every 2 weeks, or 125 mg/m^2 weekly for 4 doses every 6 weeks.
- In clinical studies, a median of 12 or 7 doses of cetuximab was administered in patients receiving the cetuximab-irinotecan combination regimen or cetuximab monotherapy, respectively.

Dosage Modification for Toxicity
Infusion-related Reactions

If mild or moderate (grade 1 or 2) infusion-related reactions occur, *permanently* reduce infusion rate by 50%.

If severe (grade 3 or 4) infusion-related reactions occur, discontinue therapy immediately and *permanently*.

Dermatologic Toxicity

Dosage modification not necessary in patients experiencing severe radiation dermatitis.

If severe acneiform rash occurs, temporarily delay therapy;

reduce subsequent doses or discontinue therapy depending on patient's response as follows:

Cetuximab Dosage Modification for Severe Acneiform Rash

Occurrence of Severe Acneiform Rash	Intervention	Outcome	Cetuximab Dosage
First occurrence	Delay infusion for 1–2 weeks	Improvement	Continue weekly maintenance dose of 250 mg/m²
		No improvement	Discontinue cetuximab
Second occurrence	Delay infusion for 1–2 weeks	Improvement	Reduce weekly maintenance dose to 200 mg/m²
		No improvement	Discontinue cetuximab
Third occurrence	Delay infusion for 1–2 weeks	Improvement	Reduce weekly maintenance dose to 150 mg/m²
		No improvement	Discontinue cetuximab
Fourth occurrence	Discontinue cetuximab		

Special Populations

No special population dosage recommendations at this time.

Chloral Hydrate

(klor al hi′ drate)

Brand Name: Aquachloral®, Aquachloral Supprettes®

Why is this medicine prescribed?

Chloral hydrate, a sedative, is used in the short-term treatment of insomnia (to help you fall asleep and stay asleep for a proper rest) and to relieve anxiety and induce sleep before surgery. It is also used after surgery for pain and to treat alcohol withdrawal.

This medication is sometimes prescribed for other uses; ask your doctor or pharmacist for more information.

How should this medicine be used?

Chloral hydrate comes as a capsule and liquid to take by mouth and as a suppository to insert rectally. Follow the directions on your prescription label carefully, and ask your doctor or pharmacist to explain any part you do not understand. Take chloral hydrate exactly as directed. Do not take more or less of it or take it more often than prescribed by your doctor.

The liquid should be added to a half glass of water, fruit juice, or ginger ale and you should drink it immediately.

Swallow the capsule whole with a full glass of water or fruit juice; do not chew the capsule.

To use the suppository, follow these steps:
1. Remove the wrapper.
2. Dip the tip of the suppository in water.
3. Lie down on your left side and raise your right knee to your chest. (A left-handed person should lie on the right side and raise the left knee.)
4. Using your finger, insert the suppository into the rectum, about 1/2 to 1 inch in infants and children and 1 inch in adults. Hold it in place for a few moments.
5. Stand up after about 15 minutes. Wash your hands thoroughly and resume your normal activities.

Chloral hydrate can be habit-forming; do not take a larger dose, take it more often, or for a longer period than your doctor tells you to. Continue to take chloral hydrate even if you feel well. Do not stop taking chloral hydrate without talking to your doctor, especially if you have taken large doses for a long time. Your doctor probably will decrease your dose gradually.

What special precautions should I follow?

Before taking chloral hydrate,
- tell your doctor and pharmacist if you are allergic to chloral hydrate, aspirin, tartrazine (a yellow dye in some processed foods and drugs), or any other drugs.
- tell your doctor and pharmacist what prescription and nonprescription medications you are taking, especially anticoagulants ('blood thinners') such as warfarin (Coumadin), antihistamines, furosemide (Lasix), medications for depression or seizures, sedatives, sleeping pills, tranquilizers, and vitamins.
- tell your doctor if you have or have ever had kidney or liver disease, heart or stomach problems, a history of alcohol or drug abuse, or asthma.
- tell your doctor if you are pregnant, plan to become pregnant, or are breast-feeding. If you become pregnant while taking chloral hydrate, call your doctor.
- if you are having surgery, including dental surgery, tell the doctor or dentist that you are taking chloral hydrate.
- you should know that this drug may make you drowsy. Do not drive a car or operate machinery until you know how this drug affects you.
- remember that alcohol can add to the drowsiness caused by this drug.

What special dietary instructions should I follow?

Chloral hydrate may cause an upset stomach. Take chloral hydrate with food or milk.

What should I do if I forget to take a dose?

Do not take a missed dose when you remember it. Skip it completely; then take the next dose at the regularly scheduled time.

What side effects can this medicine cause?

Chloral hydrate may cause side effects. Tell your doctor if any of these symptoms are severe or do not go away:

- drowsiness
- upset stomach
- vomiting
- diarrhea

If you experience any of the following symptoms, call your doctor immediately:

- skin rash
- itching
- confusion
- difficulty breathing
- slow heartbeat
- extreme tiredness

If you experience a serious side effect, you or your doctor may send a report to the Food and Drug Administration's (FDA) MedWatch Adverse Event Reporting program online [at http://www.fda.gov/MedWatch/index.html] or by phone [1-800-332-1088].

What storage conditions are needed for this medicine?

Keep this medication in the container it came in, tightly closed, and out of reach of children. Store it at room temperature, away from excess heat and moisture (not in the bathroom). Protect the liquid from light; do not freeze. Throw away any medication that is outdated or no longer needed. Talk to your pharmacist about the proper disposal of your medication.

What should I do in case of overdose?

In case of overdose, call your local poison control center at 1-800-222-1222. If the victim has collapsed or is not breathing, call local emergency services at 911.

What other information should I know?

Keep all appointments with your doctor.

If you have diabetes, use TesTape or Clinistix to test your urine for sugar. Do not use Clinitest because chloral hydrate can cause false results.

Do not let anyone else take your medication. Chloral hydrate is a controlled substance. Prescriptions may be re-filled only a limited number of times; ask your pharmacist if you have any questions.

Talk to your doctor, pharmacist, or other healthcare professional if you have questions about dosing information for your medication.

Chlordiazepoxide

(klor dye az e pox′ ide)

Brand Name: Librium®, Limbitrol®, Limbitrol® DS
Also available generically.

Why is this medicine prescribed?

Chlordiazepoxide is used to relieve anxiety and to control agitation caused by alcohol withdrawal.

This medication is sometimes prescribed for other uses; ask your doctor or pharmacist for more information.

How should this medicine be used?

Chlordiazepoxide comes as a tablet and capsule to take by mouth. It usually is taken one to four times a day with or without food. Follow the directions on your prescription label carefully, and ask your doctor or pharmacist to explain any part you do not understand. Take chlordiazepoxide exactly as directed.

Chlordiazepoxide can be habit-forming. Do not take a larger dose, take it more often, or for a longer time than your doctor tells you to. Tolerance may develop with long-term or excessive use, making the drug less effective. This medication must be taken regularly to be effective. Do not skip doses even if you feel that you do not need them. Do not take chlordiazepoxide for more than 4 months or stop taking this medication without talking to your doctor. Stopping the drug suddenly can worsen your condition and cause withdrawal symptoms (anxiousness, sleeplessness, and irritability). Your doctor probably will decrease your dose gradually.

Are there other uses for this medicine?

Chlordiazepoxide is also used to treat irritable bowel syndrome. Talk to your doctor about the possible risks of using this drug for your condition.

What special precautions should I follow?

Before taking chlordiazepoxide,

- tell your doctor and pharmacist if you are allergic to chlordiazepoxide, alprazolam (Xanax), clonazepam (Klonopin), clorazepate (Tranxene), diazepam (Valium), estazolam (ProSom), flurazepam (Dalmane), lorazepam (Ativan), oxazepam (Serax), prazepam (Centrax), temazepam (Restoril), triazolam (Halcion), or any other drugs.

- tell your doctor and pharmacist what prescription and nonprescription drugs you are taking, especially antihistamines; cimetidine (Tagamet); digoxin (Lanoxin); disulfiram (Antabuse); fluoxetine (Prozac); isoniazid (INH, Laniazid, Nydrazid); ketoconazole (Nizoral); levodopa (Larodopa, Sinemet); medications for depression, seizures, Parkinson's disease, pain, asthma, colds, or allergies; metoprolol (Lopressor, Toprol XL); muscle relaxants; oral contraceptives; probenecid (Benemid); propoxyphene (Darvon); propranolol (Inderal); rifampin (Rifadin); sedatives; sleeping pills; theophylline (Theo-Dur); tranquilizers; valproic acid (Depakene); and vitamins. These medications may add to the drowsiness caused by chlordiazepoxide.
- tell your doctor if you have or have ever had glaucoma; seizures; or lung, heart, or liver disease.
- tell your doctor if you are pregnant, plan to become pregnant, or are breast-feeding. If you become pregnant while taking chlordiazepoxide, call your doctor immediately.
- if you are having surgery, including dental surgery, tell the doctor or dentist that you are taking chlordiazepoxide.
- you should know that this drug may make you drowsy. Do not drive a car or operate machinery until you know how this drug affects you.
- remember that alcohol can add to the drowsiness caused by this drug.
- tell your doctor if you use tobacco products. Cigarette smoking may decrease the effectiveness of this drug.

What should I do if I forget to take a dose?

If you take several doses per day and miss a dose, skip the missed dose and continue your regular dosing schedule. Do not take a double dose to make up for a missed one.

What side effects can this medicine cause?

Side effects from chlordiazepoxide are common and include:
- drowsiness
- dizziness
- tiredness
- weakness
- dry mouth
- diarrhea
- upset stomach
- changes in appetite

Tell your doctor if any of these symptoms are severe or do not go away:
- restlessness or excitement
- constipation
- difficulty urinating
- frequent urination
- blurred vision
- changes in sex drive or ability

If you experience any of the following symptoms, call your doctor immediately:
- shuffling walk
- persistent, fine tremor or inability to sit still
- fever
- difficulty breathing or swallowing
- severe skin rash
- yellowing of the skin or eyes
- irregular heartbeat

If you experience a serious side effect, you or your doctor may send a report to the Food and Drug Administration's (FDA) MedWatch Adverse Event Reporting program online [at http://www.fda.gov/MedWatch/index.html] or by phone [1-800-332-1088].

What storage conditions are needed for this medicine?

Keep this medication in the container it came in, tightly closed, and out of reach of children. Store it at room temperature and away from excess heat and moisture (not in the bathroom). Throw away any medication that is outdated or no longer needed. Talk to your pharmacist about the proper disposal of your medication.

What should I do in case of overdose?

In case of overdose, call your local poison control center at 1-800-222-1222. If the victim has collapsed or is not breathing, call local emergency services at 911.

What other information should I know?

Keep all appointments with your doctor.

Chlordiazepoxide can cause false results when using the Gravindex pregnancy test.

Do not let anyone else take your medication. Ask your pharmacist any questions you have about refilling your prescription.

Dosage Facts
For Informational Purposes

Caution: Do not change your dose, how often you take your medication, or the length of time you are to take it without first talking to your healthcare provider.

The following dosage information was written using medical language for doctors and other healthcare professionals and is provided here for you to check your dosage. The dosage of this drug may differ for different patients. Therefore, always follow your doctor's instructions or the directions on the label. Contact your healthcare provider or pharmacist if you have any questions about the specific dosage of your medication after reviewing this information.

General Dosage Information

Available as chlordiazepoxide hydrochloride; dosage expressed in terms of the salt.

Available as fixed combinations containing chlordiazepoxide and amitriptyline hydrochloride or chlordiazepoxide and clidinium bromide; dosage expressed in terms of chlordiazepoxide.

Fixed-combination preparation containing amitriptyline hydrochloride is available as a regular tablet containing 5 mg chlordiazepoxide and 12.5 mg amitriptyline hydrochloride (Limbitrol®) and as a double-strength tablet containing 10 mg chlordiazepoxide and 25 mg amitriptyline hydrochloride (Limbitrol® DS). Regular tablet (Limbitrol®) may be administered to patients who do not tolerate higher dosages.

Pediatric Patients

Initiate therapy with the lowest effective dosage and increase slowly as required.

Anxiety Disorders

ORAL:
- Children ≥6 years of age: Usual dosage is 5 mg 2–4 times daily; initial dosage should not exceed 10 mg daily. If required, may increase to 10 mg 2 or 3 times daily. Alternatively, some clinicians have recommended 0.5 mg/kg daily or 15 mg/m² daily, in 3 or 4 divided doses.

Preoperative Anxiolysis

ORAL:
- Children ≥6 years of age: 5 mg 2–4 times daily for several days prior to surgery; initial dosage should not exceed 10 mg daily. If required, may increase to 10 mg 2 or 3 times daily. Alternatively, some clinicians have recommended 0.5 mg/kg daily or 15 mg/m² daily, in 3 or 4 divided doses.

Adult Patients

Anxiety Disorders
Mild to Moderate Anxiety

ORAL:
- 5–10 mg 3 or 4 times daily.

Severe Anxiety

ORAL:
- 20–25 mg 3 or 4 times daily.

Preoperative Anxiolysis

ORAL:
- 5–10 mg 3 or 4 times daily for several days prior to surgery.

Alcohol Withdrawal

ORAL:
- Initially, 50–100 mg. Repeat doses until agitation is controlled, up to 300 mg daily. Reduce dosage slowly to maintenance levels.

Peptic Ulcer Disease, Irritable Bowel Syndrome, Acute Enterocolitis
Fixed-combination Therapy with Clidinium Bromide

ORAL:
- Maintenance dosage: 5 or 10 mg 3 or 4 times daily, given before meals and at bedtime.

Major Depressive Disorder with Associated Anxiety
Fixed-combination Therapy With Amitriptyline Hydrochloride

ORAL (LIMIBITROL® DS [DOUBLE STRENGTH]):
- Initially, 3 or 4 tablets (30 or 40 mg chlordiazepoxide) daily in divided doses; may increase to 6 tablets (60 mg chlordi-

azepoxide) daily in divided doses. Some patients may respond to 2 tablets daily.

ORAL (LIMIBITROL®):
- Patients who don't tolerate higher doses: Initially, 3 or 4 tablets (15 or 20 mg chlordiazepoxide) daily in divided doses.

Prescribing Limits

Pediatric Patients

Anxiety Disorders

ORAL:
- Maximum initial dosage 10 mg daily in divided doses; subsequently, maximum 10 mg 2 to 3 times daily.

Preoperative Anxiolysis

ORAL:
- Maximum initial dosage 10 mg daily in divided doses; subsequently, maximum 10 mg 2 to 3 times daily.

Adult Patients

Alcohol Withdrawal

ORAL:
- The manufacturer states the maximum dose is 300 mg daily. Some clinicians have used 600–800 mg daily to control symptoms without adverse effects.

Major Depressive Disorder with Associated Anxiety
Fixed-combination Therapy with Amitriptyline Hydrochloride

ORAL (LIMIBITROL® DS [DOUBLE STRENGTH]):
- Maximum 6 tablets (60 mg chlordiazepoxide) daily in divided doses.

Special Populations

Hepatic Impairment
- Decreased clearance. Select dosage with caution; use lower initial doses and increase gradually.

Renal Impairment
- GFR ≥10 mL/min: Dosage adjustment not required.
- GFR <10 mL/min: Decrease dosage by 50%.

Geriatric or Debilitated Patients
- Individualize dosage; use smallest effective dosage.

Oral
- Initial dose should not exceed 10 mg daily in divided doses. Increase gradually as needed and tolerated. 5 mg 2–4 times daily recommended.
- Fixed combination with clidinium bromide: Initially, 10 mg daily; increase gradually as needed and tolerated.

Chlordiazepoxide and Clidinium Bromide

(klor dye az e pox′ ide) (kli di′ nee um)

Brand Name: Clindex®, Librax®

Why is this medicine prescribed?

The combination of chlordiazepoxide and clidinium bromide is used to treat ulcers and irritable bowel syndrome. It helps relieve stomach spasms and abdominal cramps.

This medication is sometimes prescribed for other uses; ask your doctor or pharmacist for more information.

How should this medicine be used?

The combination of chlordiazepoxide and clidinium bromide comes as a capsule to be taken by mouth. It usually is taken three or four times a day, before meals and at bedtime. Follow the directions on your prescription label carefully, and ask your doctor or pharmacist to explain any part you do not understand. Take chlordiazepoxide and clidinium bromide exactly as directed.

Chlordiazepoxide can be habit-forming. Therefore, when taking chlordiazepoxide and clidinium bromide, do not take a larger dose, take it more often, or for a longer time than your doctor tells you to. Tolerance may develop with long-term or excessive use, making this medication less effective. This medication must be taken regularly to be effective. Do not skip doses even if you feel that you do not need them. Do not take chlordiazepoxide and clidinium bromide for more than 4 months or stop taking this medication without talking to your doctor. Stopping the drug suddenly can worsen your condition and cause withdrawal symptoms (anxiousness, sleeplessness, and irritability). Your doctor probably will decrease your dose gradually.

What special precautions should I follow?

Before taking chlordiazepoxide and clidinium bromide,
- tell your doctor and pharmacist if you are allergic to chlordiazepoxide, clidinium, alprazolam (Xanax), clonazepam (Klonopin), clorazepate (Tranxene), diazepam (Valium), estazolam (ProSom), flurazepam (Dalmane), lorazepam (Ativan), oxazepam (Serax), prazepam (Centrax), temazepam (Restoril), triazolam (Halcion), or any other drugs.
- tell your doctor and pharmacist what prescription and nonprescription drugs you are taking, especially amantadine (Symadine, Symmetrel); antihistamines; atenolol (Tenormin); cimetidine (Tagamet); digoxin (Lanoxin); disulfiram (Antabuse); fluoxetine (Prozac); isoniazid (INH, Laniazid, Nydrazid); ketoconazole (Nizoral); levodopa (Larodopa, Sinemet); medications for depression, thyroid, high blood pressure, seizures, Parkinson's disease, asthma, colds, or allergies; oral contraceptives;

muscle relaxants; probenecid (Benemid, Probalan); propoxyphene (Darvon); propranolol (Inderal); rifampin (Rifadin); sedatives; theophylline (Theo-Dur); tranquilizers; sleeping pills; valproic acid (Depakene); or vitamins. These medications may add to the drowsiness caused by chlordiazepoxide and clidinium bromide.
- tell your doctor if you have or have ever had glaucoma; prostate problems; high blood pressure; seizures; or lung, thyroid, kidney, heart, or liver disease.
- tell your doctor if you are pregnant, plan to become pregnant, or are breast-feeding. If you become pregnant while taking this medication, call your doctor immediately.
- if you are having surgery, including dental surgery, tell the doctor or dentist that you are taking chlordiazepoxide and clidinium bromide.
- you should know that this medication may make you drowsy. Do not drive a car or operate machinery until you know how it affects you.
- remember that alcohol can add to the drowsiness caused by this medication.
- tell your doctor if you use tobacco products. Cigarette smoking may decrease the effectiveness of this medication.

What should I do if I forget to take a dose?

If you take several doses per day and miss a dose, skip the missed dose and continue your regular dosing schedule. Do not take a double dose to make up for a missed one.

What side effects can this medicine cause?

Side effects from chlordiazepoxide and clidinium bromide are common and include:
- upset stomach
- drowsiness
- weakness or tiredness
- excitement
- sleeplessness
- dry mouth
- heartburn
- bloated feeling
- eyes more sensitive to sunlight than usual
- taste changes
- changes in appetite

Tell your doctor if any of these symptoms are severe or do not go away:
- constipation
- difficulty urinating
- frequent urination
- blurred vision
- dilated pupils
- changes in sex drive or ability

If you experience any of the following symptoms, call your doctor immediately:
- jaw, neck, and back muscle spasms
- slow or difficult speech

- shuffling walk
- persistent, fine tremor or inability to sit still
- fever
- difficulty breathing or swallowing
- severe skin rash
- yellowing of the skin or eyes
- irregular heartbeat

If you experience a serious side effect, you or your doctor may send a report to the Food and Drug Administration's (FDA) MedWatch Adverse Event Reporting program online [at http://www.fda.gov/MedWatch/index.html] or by phone [1-800-332-1088].

What storage conditions are needed for this medicine?

Keep this medication in the container it came in, tightly closed, and out of reach of children. Store it at room temperature and away from excess heat and moisture (not in the bathroom). Throw away any medication that is outdated or no longer needed. Talk to your pharmacist about the proper disposal of your medication.

What should I do in case of overdose?

In case of overdose, call your local poison control center at 1-800-222-1222. If the victim has collapsed or is not breathing, call local emergency services at 911.

What other information should I know?

Keep all appointments with your doctor.

Do not let anyone else take your medication. Ask your pharmacist any questions you have about refilling your prescription.

Talk to your doctor, pharmacist, or other healthcare professional if you have questions about dosing information for your medication.

Chloroquine Phosphate Oral

(klor′ oh kwin)

Brand Name: Aralen® Phosphate
Also available generically.

Why is this medicine prescribed?

Chloroquine phosphate is in a class of drugs called antimalarials and amebicides. It is used to prevent and treat malaria. It is also used to treat amebiasis.

This medication is sometimes prescribed for other uses; ask your doctor or pharmacist for more information.

How should this medicine be used?

Chloroquine phosphate comes as tablet to take by mouth. For prevention of malaria in adults, one dose is usually taken once a week on exactly the same day of the week. Your doctor will tell you how many tablets to take for each dose. One dose is taken beginning 2 weeks before traveling to an area where malaria is common, while you are in the area, and then for 8 weeks after you return from the area. If you are unable to start 2 weeks before traveling, your doctor may tell you to take double the dose right away.

For treatment of acute attacks of malaria in adults, one dose is usually taken right away, followed by half the dose 6 to 8 hours later and then half the dose once a day for the next 2 days.

For prevention and treatment of malaria in infants and children, the amount of chloroquine phosphate is based on the child's weight. Your doctor will calculate this amount and tell you how much chloroquine phosphate your child should receive.

For treatment of amebiasis, one dose is usually taken for 2 days and then half the dose every day for 2 to 3 weeks. It is usually taken in combination with other amebicides.

Chloroquine phosphate may cause an upset stomach. Take chloroquine phosphate with food.

Follow the directions on your prescription label carefully, and ask your doctor or pharmacist to explain any part you do not understand. Use chloroquine phosphate exactly as directed. Do not use more or less of it or use it more often than prescribed by your doctor.

Are there other uses for this medicine?

Chloroquine phosphate is used occasionally to decrease the symptoms of rheumatoid arthritis and to treat systemic and discoid lupus erythematosus, scleroderma, pemphigus, lichen planus, polymyositis, sarcoidosis, and porphyria cutanea tarda. Talk to your doctor about the possible risks of using this drug for your condition.

What special precautions should I follow?

Before using chloroquine phosphate,

- tell your doctor and pharmacist if you are allergic to chloroquine phosphate, chloroquine hydrochloride (Aralen HCl), hydroxychloroquine (Plaquenil), or any other drugs.
- tell your doctor and pharmacist what prescription and nonprescription medications you are taking, especially acetaminophen (Tylenol, others), cimetidine (Tagamet), iron products, isoniazid (Nydrazid), kaolin, magnesium trisilicate (Gaviscon), methotrexate (Rheumatrex), niacin, rifampin (Rifadin, Rimactane), and vitamins and herbal products.
- tell your doctor if you have or have ever had liver disease, G-6-PD deficiency, hearing problems, porphyria or other blood disorders, psoriasis, vision changes, weakness in your knees and ankles, or if you drink large amounts of alcohol.

- tell your doctor if you have ever had vision changes while taking chloroquine phosphate, chloroquine hydrochloride (Aralen HCl), or hydroxychloroquine (Plaquenil).
- tell your doctor if you are pregnant or plan to become pregnant. If you become pregnant while using chloroquine phosphate, call your doctor.
- tell your doctor if you are breast-feeding or plan to breast-feed. Chloroquine phosphate can harm a nursing infant.

What special dietary instructions should I follow?

Unless your doctor instructs you otherwise, continue your normal diet while taking chloroquine phosphate.

What should I do if I forget to take a dose?

Take the missed dose as soon as you remember it. However, if it is almost time for the next dose, skip the missed dose and continue your regular dosing schedule. Do not take a double dose to make up for a missed one.

What side effects can this medicine cause?

Side effects from chloroquine phosphate can occur. Tell your doctor if any of these symptoms are severe or do not go away:

- headache
- loss of appetite
- diarrhea
- upset stomach
- stomach pain
- skin rash or itching
- hair loss
- mood or mental changes

If you experience any of the following symptoms, call your doctor immediately:

- seeing light flashes and streaks
- blurred vision
- reading or seeing difficulties (words disappear, seeing half an object, misty or foggy vision)
- difficulty hearing
- ringing in ears
- muscle weakness
- drowsiness
- upset stomach
- vomiting
- irregular heartbeats
- convulsions
- difficulty breathing

If you experience a serious side effect, you or your doctor may send a report to the Food and Drug Administration's (FDA) MedWatch Adverse Event Reporting program online [at http://www.fda.gov/MedWatch/index.html] or by phone [1-800-332-1088].

What storage conditions are needed for this medicine?

Keep this medication in the container it came in, tightly closed, and out of reach of children. Store it at room temperature and away from light and excess heat and moisture (not in the bathroom). Throw away any medication that is outdated or no longer needed. Talk to your pharmacist about the proper disposal of your medication.

What should I do in case of overdose?

In case of overdose, call your local poison control center at 1-800-222-1222. If the victim has collapsed or is not breathing, call local emergency services at 911.

What other information should I know?

Children are especially sensitive to an overdose, so keep the medication out of the reach of children.

Keep all appointments with your doctor and the laboratory. Your doctor may order certain lab tests to check your response to chloroquine phosphate. Your doctor will also test your reflexes to see if you have muscle weakness that may be caused by the drug.

If you are taking chloroquine phosphate for a long period of time, your doctor will recommend frequent eye exams. It is very important that you keep these appointments. Chloroquine phosphate can cause serious vision problems. If you experience any changes in vision, stop taking chloroquine phosphate and call your doctor immediately.

Do not let anyone else take your medication. Ask your pharmacist any questions you have about refilling your prescription.

Dosage Facts
For Informational Purposes

Caution: Do not change your dose, how often you take your medication, or the length of time you are to take it without first talking to your healthcare provider.

The following dosage information was written using medical language for doctors and other healthcare professionals and is provided here for you to check your dosage. The dosage of this drug may differ for different patients. Therefore, always follow your doctor's instructions or the directions on the label. Contact your healthcare provider or pharmacist if you have any questions about the specific dosage of your medication after reviewing this information.

General Dosage Information

Available as chloroquine phosphate; dosage usually expressed in terms of chloroquine. Each 100 mg of chloroquine phosphate is equivalent to 60 mg of chloroquine.

Dosage of chloroquine in children should be calculated in proportion to adult dosage based on body weight.

Pediatric Patients

Malaria

Prevention of Malaria in Areas without Chloroquine-resistant Plasmodium

ORAL:

- 5 mg/kg (8.3 mg/kg of chloroquine phosphate) once weekly on the same day each week.
- Initiate prophylaxis 1–2 weeks prior to entering a malarious area and continue for 4–8 weeks after leaving the area. CDC states it may be advisable to initiate prophylaxis 3–4 weeks prior to travel to ensure that the drug or combination of drugs (in individuals receiving other drugs) is well tolerated and to allow ample time if a switch to another antimalarial agent is required.
- Terminal prophylaxis with primaquine may be indicated during the final 2 weeks of chloroquine prophylaxis if exposure occurred in areas where *P. ovale* or *P. vivax* are endemic.

Treatment of Uncomplicated Chloroquine-susceptible Malaria

ORAL:

- An initial dose of 10 mg/kg of chloroquine (16.7 mg/kg of chloroquine phosphate) followed by 5-mg/kg doses (8.3 mg/kg of chloroquine phosphate) given at 6, 24, and 48 hours after the initial dose.

Adult Patients

Malaria

Prevention of Malaria in Areas without Chloroquine-resistant Plasmodium

ORAL:

- 300 mg (500 mg of chloroquine phosphate) once weekly.
- Initiate prophylaxis 1–2 weeks prior to entering a malarious area and continue for 4–8 weeks after leaving the area. CDC states it may be advisable to initiate prophylaxis 3–4 weeks prior to travel to ensure that the drug or combination of drugs (in individuals receiving other drugs) is well tolerated and to allow ample time if a switch to another antimalarial agent is required.
- Terminal prophylaxis with primaquine may be indicated during the final 2 weeks of chloroquine prophylaxis if exposure occurred in areas where *P. ovale* or *P. vivax* are endemic.

Treatment of Uncomplicated Chloroquine-susceptible Malaria

ORAL:

- An initial dose of 600 mg of chloroquine (1 g of chloroquine phosphate) followed by 300-mg doses (500 mg of chloroquine phosphate) given at 6–8, 24, and 48 hours after the initial dose. This represents a total chloroquine dose of 1.5 g (2.5 g of chloroquine phosphate) in 3 days.

Prophylaxis of P. ovale or P. vivax When Primaquine Is Deferred during Pregnancy

ORAL:

- 300 mg (500 mg of chloroquine phosphate) once weekly for the duration of the pregnancy. Given after the usual treatment regimen and continued until primaquine can be given to provide a radical cure after delivery.

Extraintestinal Amebiasis

ORAL:

- 600 mg of chloroquine (1 g of chloroquine phosphate) once daily for 2 days, followed by 300 mg (500 mg of chloroquine phosphate) once daily for at least 2–3 weeks; usually used in conjunction with an intestinal amebicide.

Rheumatoid Arthritis†

ORAL:

- 150 mg (250 mg of chloroquine phosphate) daily. After remission or maximum improvement occurs, dosage should be reduced.
- A response may not occur until after >4–6 weeks of therapy. Some clinicians recommend that the drug be continued for 4 months before being considered ineffective for treatment of rheumatoid arthritis.

Lupus Erythematosus†

ORAL:

- 150 mg (250 mg of chloroquine phosphate) daily.
- When used in conjunction with topical corticosteroids in treatment of discoid lupus erythematosus, skin lesions may regress within 3–4 weeks and new lesions may not appear. When systemic and cutaneous manifestations of lupus erythematosus subside, reduce chloroquine dosage gradually over several months, and discontinue as soon as possible.

Prescribing Limits

Pediatric Patients

Malaria

Prevention of Malaria in Areas Without Chloroquine-resistant Plasmodium

ORAL:

- Maximum dosage of 300 mg (500 mg of chloroquine phosphate) daily, regardless of weight.

† Use is not currently included in the labeling approved by the US Food and Drug Administration.

Chlorothiazide

(klor oh thye′ a zide)

Brand Name: Diuril®
Also available generically.

Why is this medicine prescribed?

Chlorothiazide, a 'water pill,' is used to treat high blood pressure and fluid retention caused by various conditions, including heart disease. It causes the kidneys to get rid of unneeded water and salt from the body into the urine.

This medicine is sometimes prescribed for other uses; ask your doctor or pharmacist for more information.

How should this medicine be used?

Chlorothiazide comes as a tablet and liquid to take by mouth. It usually is taken once or twice a day. If you are to take it once a day, take it in the morning; if you are to take it twice a day, take it in the morning and in the late afternoon to avoid going to the bathroom during the night. Take this medication with meals or a snack. Follow the directions on your prescription label carefully, and ask your doctor or pharmacist to explain any part you do not understand. Take chlorothiazide exactly as directed. Do not take more or less of it or take it more often than prescribed by your doctor.

Chlorothizide controls high blood pressure but does not cure it. Continue to take chlorothiazide even if you feel well. Do not stop taking chlorothiazide without talking to your doctor.

Are there other uses for this medicine?

Chlorothiazide may also be used to treat patients with diabetes insipidus and certain electrolyte disturbances and to prevent kidney stones in patients with high levels of calcium in their blood. Talk to your doctor about the possible risks of using this medicine for your condition.

What special precautions should I follow?

Before taking chlorothiazide,

- tell your doctor and pharmacist if you are allergic to chlorothiazide, sulfa drugs, or any other drugs.
- tell your doctor and pharmacist what prescription and nonprescription medications you are taking, especially other medications for high blood pressure, anti-inflammatory medications such as ibuprofen (Motrin, Nuprin) or naproxen (Aleve), corticosteroids (e.g., prednisone), lithium (Eskalith, Lithobid), medications for diabetes, probenecid (Benemid), and vitamins. If you also are taking cholestyramine or colestipol, take it at least 1 hour after chlorothiazide.
- tell your doctor if you have or have ever had diabetes, gout, or kidney, liver, thyroid, or parathyroid disease.
- tell your doctor if you are pregnant, plan to become pregnant, or are breast-feeding. If you become pregnant while taking chlorothiazide, call your doctor immediately.
- if you are having surgery, including dental surgery, tell the doctor or dentist that you are taking chlorothiazide.
- plan to avoid unnecessary or prolonged exposure to sunlight and to wear protective clothing, sunglasses, and sunscreen. Chlorothiazide may make your skin sensitive to sunlight.

What special dietary instructions should I follow?

Follow your doctor's directions. They may include following a daily exercise program or a low-salt or low-sodium diet, potassium supplements, and increased amounts of potassium-rich foods (e.g., bananas, prunes, raisins, and orange juice) in your diet.

What should I do if I forget to take a dose?

Take the missed dose as soon as you remember it. However, if it is almost time for your next dose, skip the missed dose and continue your regular dosing schedule. Do not take a double dose to make up for a missed one.

What side effects can this medicine cause?

Frequent urination should go away after you take chlorothiazide for a few weeks. If you are dizzy or lightheaded when getting up, rise slowly from a lying or sitting position.

Tell your doctor if any of these symptoms are severe or do not go away:

- muscle weakness
- dizziness
- cramps
- thirst
- stomach pain
- upset stomach
- vomiting
- diarrhea
- loss of appetite
- headache
- hair loss

If you experience any of the following symptoms, call your doctor immediately:

- sore throat with fever
- unusual bleeding or bruising
- severe skin rash with peeling skin
- difficulty breathing or swallowing

If you experience a serious side effect, you or your doctor may send a report to the Food and Drug Administration's (FDA) MedWatch Adverse Event Reporting program online [at http://www.fda.gov/MedWatch/index.html] or by phone [1-800-332-1088].

What storage conditions are needed for this medicine?

Keep this medicine in the container it came in, tightly closed, and out of reach of children. Store it at room temperature and away from excess heat and moisture (not in the bathroom). Do not let the oral liquid freeze. Throw away any medicine that is outdated or no longer needed. Talk to your pharmacist about the proper disposal of your medicine.

What should I do in case of overdose?

In case of overdose, call your local poison control center at 1-800-222-1222. If the victim has collapsed or is not breathing, call local emergency services at 911.

What other information should I know?

Keep all appointments with your doctor and the laboratory. Your blood pressure should be checked regularly, and blood tests should be done occasionally.

Do not let anyone else take your medicine. Ask your pharmacist any questions you have about refilling your prescription.

Dosage Facts
For Informational Purposes

Caution: Do not change your dose, how often you take your medication, or the length of time you are to take it without first talking to your healthcare provider.

The following dosage information was written using medical language for doctors and other healthcare professionals and is provided here for you to check your dosage. The dosage of this drug may differ for different patients. Therefore, always follow your doctor's instructions or the directions on the label. Contact your healthcare provider or pharmacist if you have any questions about the specific dosage of your medication after reviewing this information.

General Dosage Information

Dosage of chlorothiazide sodium is expressed in terms of chlorothiazide.

Individualize according to requirements and response.

If added to potent hypotensive agent regimen, initially reduce hypotensive dosage to avoid the possibility of severe hypotension.

Pediatric Patients
Usual Dosage

ORAL:
- Infants <6 Months of Age: Up to 30 mg/kg daily given in 2 divided doses.
- Children 6 Months to 12 Years of Age: 10–20 mg/kg daily in 1 or 2 divided doses.

Adult Patients
Hypertension
Blood Pressure Monitoring and Treatment Goals

Carefully monitor blood pressure during initial titration or subsequent upward adjustment in dosage.

Avoid large or abrupt reductions in blood pressure.

Adjusted dosage at approximately monthly intervals (more aggressively in high-risk patients [stage 2 hypertension, comorbid conditions]) if blood pressure control is inadequate at a given dosage; it may take months to control hypertension adequately while avoiding adverse effects of therapy.

Systolic blood pressure is the principal clinical end point, especially in middle-aged and geriatric patients. Once the goal systolic blood pressure is attained, the goal diastolic blood pressure usually is achieved.

The goal is to achieve and maintain a lifelong systolic blood pressure <140 mm Hg and a diastolic blood pressure<90 mm Hg if tolerated.

The goal in hypertensive patients with diabetes mellitus or renal impairment is to achieve and maintain a systolic blood pressure <130 mm Hg and a diastolic blood pressure <80 mm Hg.

Monotherapy

ORAL:
- Initially, 125–250 mg daily.
- Gradually increase until the desired therapeutic response is achieved or adverse effects become intolerable, up to 500 mg daily.
- If adequate response is not achieved at maximum dosage, add or substitute another hypotensive agent.

MAINTENANCE:
- Usually, 125–500 mg daily in 1 or 2 divided doses.

Edema

ORAL:
- Usually, 500 mg to 1 g daily in 1 or 2 doses. Occasionally, up to 2 g daily in 1 or 2 doses.
- After several days or when nonedematous weight is attained, dosage reduction to a lower maintenance level may be possible.
- With an intermittent schedule, excessive response and the resulting undesirable electrolyte imbalance are less likely to occur.

Prescribing Limits
Pediatric Patients

ORAL:
- Infants <2 Years of Age: Maximum of 375 mg daily.
- Children ≥2 Years of Age: 1 g daily.

Adult Patients

Hypertension

ORAL:
- Maximum before switching/adding alternative drug is 500 mg daily.
- Higher dosages had been used (up to 2 g daily in divided doses) but no longer are recommended. Instead, switch to or add alternative drug.

Edema

ORAL:
- Maximum of 2 daily in divided doses.

Special Populations

Hepatic Impairment
- No specific dosage recommendations for hepatic impairment; caution because of risk of precipitating hepatic coma.

Renal Impairment
- No specific dosage recommendations for renal impairment; caution because of risk of precipitating azotemia.

Geriatric Patients
- No specific geriatric dosage recommendations.

Chlorpheniramine

(klor fen ir′ a meen)

Brand Name: Aller-Chlor®, Aller-Chlor® Syrup, Chlo-Amine®, Chlor-Trimeton® 12 Hour Allergy, Chlor-Trimeton® 4 Hour Allergy, Chlor-Trimeton® 8 Hour Allergy, Chlor-Trimeton® Allergy Syrup, Efidac 24® Chlorpheniramine, Polaramine®, Polaramine® Repetabs®, Polaramine® Syrup, Teldrin® Allergy

Also available generically.

Why is this medicine prescribed?

Chlorpheniramine, an antihistamine, relieves red, itchy, watery eyes; sneezing; and runny nose caused by allergies, hay fever, and the common cold. It may also relieve the itching of insect bites, bee stings, poison ivy, and poison oak.

This medication is sometimes prescribed for other uses; ask your doctor or pharmacist for more information.

How should this medicine be used?

Chlorpheniramine comes as a extended-release (long-acting) tablet and capsule, a regular tablet and capsule, chewable tablet, liquid, and syrup to take by mouth. It usually is taken every 4-6 hours or twice a day, in the morning and evening, as needed. Follow the directions on your prescription label carefully, and ask your doctor or pharmacist to explain any part you do not understand. Take chlorpheniramine exactly as directed. Do not take more or less of it or take it more often than prescribed by your doctor.

Do not break, crush, or chew extended-release tablets and do not open extended-release capsules; swallow them whole.

Do not give extended-release tablets or capsules to a child less than 12 years of age and do not give regular or chewable tablets or liquid to a child less than 6 years of age unless directed to do so by a doctor.

What special precautions should I follow?

Before taking chlorpheniramine,

- tell your doctor and pharmacist if you are allergic to chlorpheniramine or any other drugs.
- tell your doctor and pharmacist what prescription and nonprescription medications you are taking, especially other medications for colds, hay fever, or allergies; medications for depression or seizures; muscle relaxants; narcotics (pain medications); sedatives; sleeping pills; tranquilizers; and vitamins. Do not take chlorpheniramine if you have taken an MAO inhibitor [phenelzine (Nardil) or tranylcypromine (Parnate)] in the last 2 weeks.
- tell your doctor if you have or have ever had asthma, glaucoma, ulcers, diabetes, difficulty urinating (due to an enlarged prostate gland), heart disease, high blood pressure, seizures, or an overactive thyroid gland.
- tell your doctor if you are pregnant, plan to become pregnant, or are breast-feeding. If you become pregnant while taking chlorpheniramine, call your doctor.
- if you are having surgery, including dental surgery, tell the doctor or dentist that you are taking chlorpheniramine.
- you should know that this drug may make you drowsy. Do not drive a car or operate machinery until you know how this drug affects you.
- remember that alcohol can add to the drowsiness caused by this drug.

What should I do if I forget to take a dose?

Take the missed dose as soon as you remember it. However, if it is almost time for the next dose, skip the missed dose and continue your regular dosing schedule. Do not take a double dose to make up for a missed one.

What side effects can this medicine cause?

Chlorpheniramine may cause side effects. Tell your doctor if any of these symptoms are severe or do not go away:

- dry mouth, nose, and throat
- upset stomach
- headache
- chest congestion
- diarrhea

If you experience any of the following symptoms, call your doctor immediately:

- vision problems
- difficulty urinating
- difficulty breathing
- muscle weakness
- prolonged drowsiness
- excitement (especially in children)
- dizziness
- skin rash

If you experience a serious side effect, you or your doctor may send a report to the Food and Drug Administration's (FDA) MedWatch Adverse Event Reporting program online [at http://www.fda.gov/MedWatch/index.html] or by phone [1-800-332-1088].

What storage conditions are needed for this medicine?

Keep this medication in the container it came in, tightly closed, and out of reach of children. Store it at room temperature and away from excess heat and moisture (not in the bathroom). Throw away any medication that is outdated or no longer needed. Talk to your pharmacist about the proper disposal of your medication.

What should I do in case of overdose?

In case of overdose, call your local poison control center at 1-800-222-1222. If the victim has collapsed or is not breathing, call local emergency services at 911.

What other information should I know?

Keep all appointments with your doctor.

Do not let anyone else take your medication. Ask your pharmacist any questions you have about refilling your prescription.

Dosage Facts
For Informational Purposes

Caution: Do not change your dose, how often you take your medication, or the length of time you are to take it without first talking to your healthcare provider.

The following dosage information was written using medical language for doctors and other healthcare professionals and is provided here for you to check your dosage. The dosage of this drug may differ for different patients. Therefore, always follow your doctor's instructions or the directions on the label. Contact your healthcare provider or pharmacist if you have any questions about the specific dosage of your medication after reviewing this information.

General Dosage Information

Individualize dosage according to patient's response and tolerance.

Pediatric Patients

Allergic Rhinitis

ORAL:
- Children 2 to <6 years of age: 1 mg every 4–6 hours (as conventional formulations).
- Children 6 to <12 years of age: 2 mg every 4–6 hours (as conventional formulations) or 8 mg (as extended-release tablets) once daily at bedtime or during the day, as indicated.
- Children ≥12 years of age: 4 mg every 4–6 hours (as conventional formulations) or 8 or 12 mg (as extended-release tablets) twice daily in the morning and evening or 16-mg (as extended-release core tablet) once daily.

Adult Patients

Allergic Rhinitis

ORAL:
- 4 mg every 4–6 hours (as conventional formulations) or 8 or 12 mg (as extended-release tablets) twice daily in the morning and evening or 16-mg (as extended-release core tablets) once daily.

Prescribing Limits

Pediatric Patients

Allergic Rhinitis

ORAL:
- Children 2 to <6 years of age: Maximum 6 mg daily (as conventional formulations).
- Children 6 to <12 years of age: Maximum 12 mg daily (as conventional formulations) or maximum 8 mg daily (as extended-release tablets).

- Children ≥12 years of age: Maximum 24 mg daily (as immediate-release formulations or extended-release tablets) or maximum 16-mg daily (as extended-release core tablet).

Adult Patients

Allergic Rhinitis

ORAL:
- Maximum 24 mg daily (as conventional formulations or extended-release tablets) or maximum 16 mg daily (extended-release core tablets).

Chlorpromazine

(klor proe′ ma zeen)

Brand Name: Chlorpromazine Hydrochloride Intensol®, Thorazine®, Thorazine® Spansule®, Thorazine® Syrup

Also available generically.

Why is this medicine prescribed?

Chlorpromazine is used to treat psychotic disorders and symptoms such as hallucinations, delusions, and hostility. It also is used to prevent and treat nausea and vomiting, to treat behavior problems in children, and to relieve severe hiccups.

This medication is sometimes prescribed for other uses; ask your doctor or pharmacist for more information.

How should this medicine be used?

Chlorpromazine comes as a tablet, extended-release (long-acting) capsule, oral liquid (syrup and concentrate), and rectal suppository. Chlorpromazine usually is taken two to four times a day. For nausea and vomiting, it is taken every 4-6 hours (by mouth) or every 6-8 hours (rectally) as needed. Follow the directions on your prescription label carefully, and ask your doctor or pharmacist to explain any part you do not understand. Take chlorpromazine exactly as directed. Do not take more or less of it or take it more often than prescribed by your doctor.

Although chlorpromazine is not habit-forming, do not stop taking it abruptly, especially if you have been taking it for a long time. Your doctor probably will decrease your dose gradually.

Do not open extended-release capsules; swallow them whole.

Do not allow the liquid to touch your skin or clothing; it can cause skin irritation. Dilute the concentrate in water, milk, soft drink, coffee, tea, tomato or fruit juice, soup, or pudding just before taking it.

If you are to insert a rectal suppository, follow these steps:
1. If the suppository feels soft, hold it under cold, running water for 1 minute. Then remove the wrapper.
2. Dip the tip of the suppository in water.

3. Lie down on your left side and raise your right knee to your chest. (A left-handed person should lie on the right side and raise the left knee.)
4. Using your finger, insert the suppository into the rectum, about 1/2 to 1 inch in children and 1 inch in adults. Hold the suppository in place for a few moments.
5. Stand up after about 15 minutes. Wash your hands thoroughly and resume your normal activities.

What special precautions should I follow?

Before taking chlorpromazine,
- tell your doctor and pharmacist if you are allergic to chlorpromazine, any other tranquilizer, or any other drugs, or have had a bad reaction to insulin.
- tell your doctor and pharmacist what prescription and non-prescription medications you are taking, especially antihistamines; lithium (Eskalith, Lithobid); medications for depression, Parkinson's disease, seizures, hay fever, allergies, or colds; muscle relaxants; narcotics (pain medication); sedatives; sleeping pills; and vitamins.
- tell your doctor if you have or have ever had heart, liver, lung, or kidney disease; shock therapy; glaucoma; an enlarged prostate; difficulty urinating; asthma, emphysema, or chronic bronchitis; or seizures.
- tell your doctor if you are pregnant, plan to become pregnant, or are breast-feeding. If you become pregnant while taking chlorpromazine, call your doctor.
- if you are having surgery, including dental surgery, tell the doctor or dentist that you are taking chlorpromazine.
- you should know that this drug may make you drowsy. Do not drive a car or operate machinery until you know how this drug affects you.
- remember that alcohol can add to the drowsiness caused by this drug.
- plan to avoid unnecessary or prolonged exposure to sunlight and to wear protective clothing, sunglasses, and sunscreen. Chlorpromazine may make your skin sensitive to sunlight.

What should I do if I forget to take a dose?

Take the missed dose as soon as you remember it. However, if it is almost time for the next dose, skip the missed dose and continue your regular dosing schedule. Do not take a double dose to make up for a missed one.

What side effects can this medicine cause?

Chlorpromazine may cause side effects. Tell your doctor if either of these symptoms is severe or does not go away:
- dry mouth
- drowsiness

If you experience any of the following symptoms, call your doctor immediately:
- skin discoloration (yellowish-brown to greyish-purple)
- jaw, neck, and back muscle spasms
- pacing
- fine worm-like tongue movements
- rhythmic face, mouth, or jaw movements
- slow or difficult speech
- difficulty swallowing
- shuffling walk
- skin rash

If you experience a serious side effect, you or your doctor may send a report to the Food and Drug Administration's (FDA) MedWatch Adverse Event Reporting program online [at http://www.fda.gov/MedWatch/index.html] or by phone [1-800-332-1088].

What storage conditions are needed for this medicine?

Keep this medication in the container it came in, tightly closed, and out of reach of children. Store it at room temperature and away from excess heat and moisture (not in the bathroom). Throw away any medication that is outdated or no longer needed. Talk to your pharmacist about the proper disposal of your medication.

What should I do in case of overdose?

In case of overdose, call your local poison control center at 1-800-222-1222. If the victim has collapsed or is not breathing, call local emergency services at 911.

What other information should I know?

Keep all appointments with your doctor.

Do not let anyone else take your medication. Ask your pharmacist any questions you have about refilling your prescription.

Dosage Facts
For Informational Purposes

Caution: Do not change your dose, how often you take your medication, or the length of time you are to take it without first talking to your healthcare provider.

The following dosage information was written using medical language for doctors and other healthcare professionals and is provided here for you to check your dosage. The dosage of this drug may differ for different patients. Therefore, always follow your doctor's instructions or the directions on the label. Contact your healthcare provider or pharmacist if you have any questions about the specific dosage of your medication after reviewing this information.

General Dosage Information

Available as chlorpromazine and chlorpromazine hydrochloride; dosage expressed in terms of chlorpromazine and the salt, respectively.

Total daily dose for conventional oral preparations (i.e., solutions, tablets) generally may be used as the total daily dose for extended-release capsules.

The manufacturers state that the 100- and 200-mg tablets are intended for use in patients with severe neuropsychiatric conditions.

Pediatric Patients

Use not recommended in children <6 months of age except where potentially lifesaving.

Select route of administration according to severity of condition, and increase dosage gradually as required.

Psychotic Disorders

ORAL:
- Children 6 months to 12 years of age: Initially, 0.55 mg/kg every 4–6 hours as necessary. Increase dosage gradually as required. 50–100 mg daily may be required in hospitalized children with severe behavior disorders or psychotic conditions; hospitalized older children may require 200 mg or more daily.

RECTAL:
- Children 6 months to 12 years of age: 1.1 mg/kg every 6–8 hours as necessary. Increase dosage gradually as required.

Nausea and Vomiting

Adjust dosage and frequency according to symptom severity and patient response.

ORAL:
- Children 6 months to 12 years of age: 0.55 mg/kg every 4–6 hours.

RECTAL:
- Children 6 months to 12 years of age: 1.1 mg/kg every 6–8 hours as needed.

Surgery

ORAL:
- Children 6 months to 12 years of age: 0.55 mg/kg given 2–3 hours before surgery. May repeat every 4–6 hours as needed after surgery.

Adult Patients

Psychotic Disorders
Nonhospitalized Patients

ORAL:
- Initially, 30–75 mg daily given in 2–4 divided doses in patients with relatively mild symptoms. 75 mg daily given in 3 divided doses is recommended in patients with moderate to severe symptoms. After 1 or 2 days, gradually increase dosage twice weekly by 20–50 mg until symptoms are controlled. Once optimal dosage is achieved, continue for 2 weeks, then gradually reduce to the lowest possible effective dosage.
- Usual maintenance dosage: 200 mg daily; however, some patients (e.g., discharged psychiatric patients) may require up to 800 mg daily.

Hospitalized Patients

ORAL:
- Less acute agitation: Initially, 25 mg 3 times daily. Gradually increase subsequent doses until optimum therapeutic response is obtained; 400 mg daily may be sufficient.

Nausea and Vomiting

ORAL:
- Initially, 10–25 mg every 4–6 hours as needed. Increase dosage if necessary.

RECTAL:
- 100 mg every 6–8 hours as needed; in some patients, 50 mg every 6–8 hours is sufficient.

Acute Intermittent Porphyria

ORAL:
- 25–50 mg 3 or 4 times daily.
- Therapy usually can be discontinued after several weeks; some patients require maintenance therapy.

Intractable Hiccups

Initially, administer orally. If symptoms persist for 2–3 days, administer IM; if hiccups continue, give by slow IV infusion.

ORAL:
- Usual dosage: 25–50 mg 3 or 4 times daily for no more than 2–3 days.

Surgery

ORAL:
- 25–50 mg given 2–3 hours before surgery.
- 10–25 mg every 4–6 hours as needed after surgery.

Prescribing Limits

Pediatric Patients

Psychotic Disorders
Hospitalized

ORAL:
- Severely disturbed developmentally disabled children: There is little evidence that behavior improvement is further enhanced by dosages over 500 mg daily.

Special Populations

Hepatic Impairment
- No specific dosage recommendations at this time.

Renal Impairment
- No specific dosage recommendations at this time.

Geriatric Patients
- Use dosages in lower range and increase slowly.

Chlorpropamide

(klor proe′ pa mide)

Brand Name: Diabinese®
Also available generically.

Important Warning

Oral hypoglycemic drugs, including chlorpropamide, have been associated with increased cardiovascular mortality. Talk to your doctor about the possible risks, benefits, and alternatives of using this drug for your condition.

Why is this medicine prescribed?

Chlorpropamide is used to treat type 2 diabetes (condition in which the body does not use insulin normally and therefore cannot control the amount of sugar in the blood), particularly in people whose diabetes cannot be controlled by diet alone. Chlorpropamide lowers blood sugar by stimulating the pancreas to secrete insulin and helping the body to use insulin efficiently. The pancreas must produce insulin for this medication to work. Chlorpropamide is not used to treat type 1 diabetes (condition in which the body does not produce insulin and therefore cannot control the amount of sugar in the blood).

This medication is sometimes prescribed for other uses; ask your doctor or pharmacist for more information.

How should this medicine be used?

Chlorpropamide comes in tablets to take by mouth. It is usually taken once a day with breakfast. Follow the directions on your prescription label carefully, and ask your doctor or pharmacist to explain any part you do not understand. Take chlorpropamide exactly as directed. Do not take more or less of it or take it more often than prescribed by your doctor.

Continue to take chlorpropamide even if you feel well. Do not stop taking chlorpropamide without talking to your doctor.

What special precautions should I follow?

Before taking chlorpropamide,

- tell your doctor and pharmacist if you are allergic to chlorpropamide or any other drugs.
- tell your doctor and pharmacist what prescription and nonprescription medications you are taking, including vitamins.
- tell your doctor if you have or have ever had heart, liver, kidney, thyroid, adrenal, or pituitary disease.
- tell your doctor if you are pregnant, plan to become pregnant, or are breast-feeding. If you become pregnant while taking chlorpropamide, call your doctor.
- if you are having surgery, including dental surgery, tell the doctor or dentist that you are taking chlorpropamide.
- you should know that this drug may make you drowsy. Do not drive a car or operate machinery until you know how this drug affects you.
- remember that alcohol can add to the drowsiness caused by this drug.
- tell your doctor if you use tobacco products. Cigarette smoking may decrease the effectiveness of chlorpropamide.
- plan to avoid unnecessary or prolonged exposure to sunlight and to wear protective clothing, sunglasses, and sunscreen. Chlorpropamide may make your skin sensitive to sunlight.

What special dietary instructions should I follow?

Be sure to follow all exercise and dietary recommendations made by your doctor or dietitian. It is important to eat a healthful diet.

Alcohol may cause a decrease in blood sugar. Ask your doctor about the safe use of alcoholic beverages while you are taking chlorpropamide.

What should I do if I forget to take a dose?

Before you start to take chlorpropamide, ask your doctor what you should do if you forget to take a dose. Write these directions down so you can refer to them later.

As a general rule, take the missed dose as soon as you remember it unless it is almost time for the next dose. Do not take a double dose to make up for a missed one.

What side effects can this medicine cause?

This medication may cause changes in your blood sugar. You should know the symptoms of low and high blood sugar and what to do if you have these symptoms.

You may experience hypoglycemia (low blood sugar) while you are taking this medication. Your doctor will tell you what you should do if you develop hypoglycemia. He or she may tell you to check your blood sugar, eat or drink a food or beverage that contains sugar, such as hard candy or fruit juice, or get medical care. Follow these directions carefully if you have any of the following symptoms of hypoglycemia:

- shakiness
- dizziness or lightheadedness
- sweating
- nervousness or irritability
- sudden changes in behavior or mood
- headache
- numbness or tingling around the mouth
- weakness
- pale skin
- hunger
- clumsy or jerky movements

If hypoglycemia is not treated, severe symptoms may develop. Be sure that your family, friends, and other people who spend time with you know that if you have any of the following symptoms, they should get medical treatment for you immediately.

- confusion
- seizures
- loss of consciousness

Call your doctor immediately if you have any of the following symptoms of hyperglycemia (high blood sugar):

- extreme thirst
- frequent urination
- extreme hunger
- weakness
- blurred vision

If high blood sugar is not treated, a serious, life-threatening condition called diabetic ketoacidosis could develop. Call your doctor immediately if you have any of these symptoms:

- dry mouth
- upset stomach and vomiting
- shortness of breath
- breath that smells fruity
- decreased consciousness

Chlorpropamide may cause side effects. If you experience any of the following symptoms, call your doctor immediately:

- skin rash
- itching or redness
- exaggerated sunburn
- yellowing of the skin or eyes
- light-colored stools
- dark urine
- unusual bleeding or bruising
- fever
- sore throat

If you experience a serious side effect, you or your doctor may send a report to the Food and Drug Administration's (FDA) MedWatch Adverse Event Reporting program online [at http://www.fda.gov/MedWatch/index.html] or by phone [1-800-332-1088].

What storage conditions are needed for this medicine?

Keep this medication in the container it came in, tightly closed, and out of reach of children. Store it at room temperature and away from excess heat and moisture (not in the bathroom). Throw away any medication that is outdated or no longer needed. Talk to your pharmacist about the proper disposal of your medication.

What should I do in case of overdose?

In case of overdose, call your local poison control center at 1-800-222-1222. If the victim has collapsed or is not breathing, call local emergency services at 911.

What other information should I know?

Keep all appointments with your doctor and the laboratory. Your doctor will order certain lab tests to check your response to chlorpropamide. Your doctor will also tell you how to check your response to this medication by measuring your blood or urine sugar levels at home. Follow these instructions carefully.

You should always wear a diabetic identification bracelet to be sure you get proper treatment in an emergency.

Do not let anyone else take your medication. Ask your pharmacist any questions you have about refilling your prescription.

Dosage Facts
For Informational Purposes

Caution: Do not change your dose, how often you take your medication, or the length of time you are to take it without first talking to your healthcare provider.

The following dosage information was written using medical language for doctors and other healthcare professionals and is provided here for you to check your dosage. The dosage of this drug may differ for different patients. Therefore, always follow your doctor's instructions or the directions on the label. Contact your healthcare provider or pharmacist if you have any questions about the specific dosage of your medication after reviewing this information.

General Dosage Information

Administration of a loading dose is *not* recommended when initiating therapy.

Adult Patients

Diabetes Mellitus
Initial Dosage in Previously Untreated Patients

ORAL:
- Initially, 250 mg daily for 5–7 days. Subsequently, increase or decrease dosage by 50–125 mg daily at 3- to 5-day intervals; more frequent adjustments usually are undesirable.

Initial Dosage in Patients Transferred from Other Oral Antidiabetic Agents

ORAL:
- Initially, 250 mg daily for 5–7 days. Subsequently, increase or decrease dosage by 50–125 mg daily at 3- to 5-day intervals; more frequent adjustments usually are undesirable.
- May discontinue other oral antidiabetic agents immediately. When initiating therapy in patients previously receiving other sulfonylurea antidiabetic agents, consider the increased potency of chlorpropamide.

Initial Dosage in Patients Transferred from Insulin

ORAL:
- Initially, 250 mg daily for 5–7 days if insulin requirements were ≤ 40 units daily. Abruptly discontinue insulin.
- Initially, 250 mg daily for 5–7 days if insulin requirements were >40 units daily, and reduce insulin dosage by 50% daily for the first few days; subsequently adjust insulin dosage according to the therapeutic response.
- Subsequently, increase or decrease dosage by 50–125 mg daily at 3- to 5-day intervals; more frequent adjustments usually are undesirable.

Maintenance Dosage

ORAL:
- Usual maintenance dosage: 250 mg daily. Mild diabetics may respond to ≤100 mg daily; severe diabetics may require 500 mg daily. Patients who do not respond to 500 mg daily usually will not respond to a higher dosage.

Adult Patients

Diabetes Mellitus

ORAL:
- Maximum 750 mg daily.

Special Populations

Hepatic Impairment
- Conservative initial and maintenance dosages recommended.

Renal Impairment
- GFR >50ml/min: Initially, 125 mg daily. Conservative initial and maintenance dosages recommended.
- GFR ≤50 ml/min: Use not recommended.

Geriatric Patients
- Initially, 100–125 mg daily is recommended. Conservative initial and maintenance dosages recommended because of increased sensitivity to hypoglycemic effect and age-related decreases in hepatic and/or renal function and concomitant disease and drug therapy.

Debilitated or Malnourished Patients
- Conservative initial and maintenance dosages recommended.

Chlorthalidone

(klor thal′ i done)

Brand Name: Clorpres®, Tenoretic®, Thalitone® Also available generically.

Why is this medicine prescribed?

Chlorthalidone, a 'water pill,' is used to treat high blood pressure and fluid retention caused by various conditions, including heart disease. It causes the kidneys to get rid of unneeded water and salt from the body into the urine.

This medicine is sometimes prescribed for other uses; ask your doctor or pharmacist for more information.

How should this medicine be used?

Chlorthalidone comes as a tablet to take by mouth. It usually is taken once a day or every other day after a meal, preferably breakfast. It is best to take this medicine in the morning to avoid going to the bathroom during the night. Follow the directions on your prescription label carefully, and ask your doctor or pharmacist to explain any part you do not understand. Take chlorthalidone exactly as directed. Do not take more or less of it or take it more often than prescribed by your doctor.

Chlorthalidone controls high blood pressure but does not cure it. Continue to take chlorthalidone even if you feel well. Do not stop taking chlorthalidone without talking to your doctor.

Are there other uses for this medicine?

Chlorthalidone may also be used to treat patients with diabetes insipidus and certain electrolyte disturbances and to prevent kidney stones in patients with high levels of calcium in their blood. Talk to your doctor about the possible risks of using this medicine for your condition.

What special precautions should I follow?

Before taking chlorthalidone,
- tell your doctor and pharmacist if you are allergic to chlorthalidone, sulfa drugs, or any other drugs.
- tell your doctor and pharmacist what prescription and nonprescription medications you are taking, especially other medicines for high blood pressure, anti-inflammatory medications such as ibuprofen (Motrin, Nuprin) or naproxen (Aleve), corticosteroids (e.g., prednisone), lithium (Eskalith, Lithobid), medications for diabetes, probenecid (Benemid), and vitamins. If you also are taking cholestyramine or colestipol, take it at least 1 hour after chlorthalidone.
- tell your doctor if you have or have ever had diabetes, gout, or kidney, liver, thyroid, or parathyroid disease.
- tell your doctor if you are pregnant, plan to become pregnant, or are breast-feeding. If you become pregnant while taking chlorthalidone, call your doctor immediately.
- if you are having surgery, including dental surgery, tell the doctor or dentist that you are taking chlorthalidone.
- you should know that this drug may make you drowsy. Do not drive a car or operate machinery until you know how this drug affects you.
- remember that alcohol can add to the drowsiness caused by this drug.
- plan to avoid unnecessary or prolonged exposure to sunlight and to wear protective clothing, sunglasses, and sunscreen. Chlorthalidone may make your skin sensitive to sunlight.

What special dietary instructions should I follow?

Follow your doctor's directions. They may include following a daily exercise program or a low-salt or low-sodium diet, potassium supplements, and increased amounts of potassium-rich foods (e.g., bananas, prunes, raisins, and orange juice) in your diet.

What should I do if I forget to take a dose?

Take the missed dose as soon as you remember it. However, if it is almost time for your next dose, skip the missed dose and continue your regular dosing schedule. Do not take a double dose to make up for a missed one.

What side effects can this medicine cause?

Frequent urination should go away after you take chlorthalidone for a few weeks.

Tell your doctor if any of these symptoms are severe or do not go away:

- muscle weakness
- dizziness
- cramps
- thirst
- stomach pain
- upset stomach
- vomiting
- diarrhea
- loss of appetite
- headache
- hair loss

If you experience any of the following symptoms, call your doctor immediately:

- sore throat with fever
- unusual bleeding or bruising
- severe skin rash with peeling skin
- difficulty breathing or swallowing

If you experience a serious side effect, you or your doctor may send a report to the Food and Drug Administration's (FDA) MedWatch Adverse Event Reporting program online [at http://www.fda.gov/MedWatch/index.html] or by phone [1-800-332-1088].

What storage conditions are needed for this medicine?

Keep this medicine in the container it came in, tightly closed, and out of reach of children. Store it at room temperature and away from excess heat and moisture (not in the bathroom). Throw away any medicine that is outdated or no longer needed. Talk to your pharmacist about the proper disposal of your medicine.

What should I do in case of overdose?

In case of overdose, call your local poison control center at 1-800-222-1222. If the victim has collapsed or is not breathing, call local emergency services at 911.

What other information should I know?

Keep all appointments with your doctor and the laboratory. Your blood pressure should be checked regularly, and blood tests should be done occasionally.

Do not let anyone else take your medicine. Ask your pharmacist any questions you have about refilling your prescription.

Dosage Facts
For Informational Purposes

Caution: Do not change your dose, how often you take your medication, or the length of time you are to take it without first talking to your healthcare provider.

The following dosage information was written using medical language for doctors and other healthcare professionals and is provided here for you to check your dosage. The dosage of this drug may differ for different patients. Therefore, always follow your doctor's instructions or the directions on the label. Contact your healthcare provider or pharmacist if you have any questions about the specific dosage of your medication after reviewing this information.

General Dosage Information

Individualize according to requirements and response.

If added to potent hypotensive agent regimen, initially reduce hypotensive dosage to avoid the possibility of severe hypotension.

Thalitone® tablets are formulated with povidone to enhance oral bioavailability of chlorthalidone; because of the enhanced bioavailability of this formulation, Thalitone® tablets are *not* bioequivalent with other formulations of the drug, and the tablets cannot be substituted for other preparations or vice versa on a mg-for-mg basis.

Pediatric Patients

Usual Dosage

ORAL (CONVENTIONAL TABLETS):
- Children†: Usually, 2 mg/kg or 60 mg/m² 3 times weekly.

ORAL (ENHANCED BIOAVAILABILITY TABLETS [THALITONE®]):
- Dosage not established.

Hypertension†

ORAL (CONVENTIONAL TABLETS):
- Initially, 0.3 mg/kg once daily. Increase dosage as necessary up to a maximum of 2 mg/kg (up to 50 mg) once daily.

Adult Patients

Hypertension
BP Monitoring and Treatment Goals

Carefully monitor BP during initial titration or subsequent upward adjustment in dosage.

Avoid large or abrupt reductions in BP.

Adjust dosage at approximately monthly intervals (more aggressively in high-risk patients [stage 2 hypertension, comorbid conditions]) if BP control is inadequate at a given dosage; it may take months to control hypertension adequately while avoiding adverse effects of therapy.

SBP is the principal clinical end point, especially in middle-aged and geriatric patients. Once the goal SBP is attained, the goal DBP usually is achieved.

The goal is to achieve and maintain a lifelong SBP <140 mm Hg and a DBP <90 mm Hg if tolerated.

The goal in hypertensive patients with diabetes mellitus or renal impairment is to achieve and maintain a SBP <130 mm Hg and a DBP <80 mm Hg.

Monotherapy

ORAL (CONVENTIONAL TABLETS):
- Initially, 12.5–25 mg daily.
- May gradually increase dosage until the desired therapeutic response is achieved, adverse effects become intolerable, or a usual maximum adult dosage of 25 mg daily is attained.

- If an adequate response is not achieved with this maximum dosage, another hypotensive agent may be added or substituted.
- Dosages >100 mg daily usually do not increase efficacy.

ORAL (ENHANCED BIOAVAILABILITY TABLETS [THALITONE®]):
- Initially, 15 mg once daily.
- May increase dosage to 30 mg once daily and, if necessary, to 45–50 mg daily if response is inadequate after a sufficient trial.
- If BP control still is inadequate at the upper dosage, a second antihypertensive drug should be added rather than increasing the dosage of Thalitone® further.

Combination Therapy

ORAL (CONVENTIONAL TABLETS):
- Initially, administer each drug separately to adjust dosage.
- May use fixed combination if optimum maintenance dosage corresponds to drug ratio in combination preparation. Combination preparations do *not* contain chlorthalidone in enhanced bioavailability formulations; therefore, combination dosing does *not* apply to dosages attained with Thalitone®.
- Administer each drug separately whenever dosage adjustment is necessary.
- Alternatively, may initially use certain (low-dose chlorthalidone/other antihypertensive) fixed combinations for potentiation of antihypertensive effect and minimization of potential dose-related adverse effects of each drug.

Edema

ORAL (CONVENTIONAL TABLETS):
- Usually, 50–100 mg daily in a single dose after breakfast.
- Alternatively, initiate 100 mg every other day or 3 times a week; some patients require dosages of 150–200 mg daily or every other day.
- Dosages >200 mg daily do not produce a greater response.
- Maintenance: Reduction of dosage to a lower level may be possible after several days or when nonedematous weight is attained.

ORAL (ENHANCED BIOAVAILABILITY TABLETS [THALITONE®]):
- Usual initial dosage: 30–60 mg daily or 60 mg on alternate days.
- Adjust dosage as necessary to 90–120 mg on alternate days or daily.
- Dosages >120 mg daily usually do not produce a greater response.
- Maintenance: May be lower than initial dosages and therefore should be adjusted according to individual response.

Prescribing Limits

Pediatric Patients

Hypertension†

ORAL (CONVENTIONAL TABLETS):
- Maximum 2 mg/kg (up to 50 mg) once daily.

Adult Patients

Hypertension

ORAL (CONVENTIONAL TABLETS):
- Maximum before switching/adding alternative drug is 25 mg daily.

- Higher dosages had been used (up to 100 mg daily) but no longer are recommended. Instead, switch to or add alternative drug.

ORAL (ENHANCED BIOAVAILABILITY TABLETS [THALITONE®]):
- Maximum before switching/adding alternative drug is 50 mg daily.

Edema

ORAL (CONVENTIONAL TABLETS):
- Dosages >200 mg daily do not produce a greater response.

ORAL (ENHANCED BIOAVAILABILITY TABLETS [THALITONE®]):
- Dosages >120 mg daily usually do not produce a greater response.

Special Populations

Hepatic Impairment
- No specific dosage recommendations for hepatic impairment; caution because of risk of precipitating hepatic coma.

Renal Impairment
- No specific dosage recommendations for renal impairment; caution because of risk of precipitating azotemia.

Geriatric Patients
- Select dosage with caution because of age-related decreases in hepatic, renal, and/or cardiac function and concomitant disease and drug therapy.

† *Use is not currently included in the labeling approved by the US Food and Drug Administration.*

Chlorzoxazone

(klor zox′ a zone)

Brand Name: Parafon Forte® DSC Caplets®

Why is this medicine prescribed?

Chlorzoxazone is used to relieve pain and stiffness caused by muscle strains and sprains. It is used in combination with physical therapy, analgesics (such as aspirin or acetaminophen), and rest.

This medication is sometimes prescribed for other uses; ask your doctor or pharmacist for more information.

How should this medicine be used?

Chlorzoxazone comes as a tablet to take by mouth. It usually is taken three or four times a day. Follow the directions on your prescription label carefully, and ask your doctor or pharmacist to explain any part you do not understand. Take chlorzoxazone exactly as directed. Do not take more or less of it or take it more often than prescribed by your doctor.

What special precautions should I follow?

Before taking chlorzoxazone,
- tell your doctor and pharmacist if you are allergic to chlorzoxazone or any other drugs.

- tell your doctor and pharmacist what prescription and nonprescription medications you are taking, especially sedatives, sleeping pills, tranquilizers, and vitamins.
- tell your doctor if you have or have ever had liver disease.
- tell your doctor if you are pregnant, plan to become pregnant, or are breast-feeding. If you become pregnant while taking chlorzoxazone, call your doctor.
- you should know that this drug may make you drowsy. Do not drive a car or operate machinery until you know how this drug affects you.
- remember that alcohol can add to the drowsiness caused by this drug.

What should I do if I forget to take a dose?

Take the missed dose as soon as you remember it. However, if it is almost time for the next dose, skip the missed dose and continue your regular dosing schedule. Do not take a double dose to make up for a missed one.

What side effects can this medicine cause?

Chlorzoxazone may cause side effects. Your urine may turn purple or red; this effect is not harmful. Tell your doctor if any of these symptoms are severe or do not go away:
- upset stomach
- drowsiness
- dizziness
- lightheadedness
- weakness

If you experience any of the following symptoms, call your doctor immediately:
- skin rash or itching
- yellowing of the skin or eyes
- stomach pain

If you experience a serious side effect, you or your doctor may send a report to the Food and Drug Administration's (FDA) MedWatch Adverse Event Reporting program online [at http://www.fda.gov/MedWatch/index.html] or by phone [1-800-332-1088].

What storage conditions are needed for this medicine?

Keep this medication in the container it came in, tightly closed, and out of reach of children. Store it at room temperature and away from excess heat and moisture (not in the bathroom). Throw away any medication that is outdated or no longer needed. Talk to your pharmacist about the proper disposal of your medication.

What should I do in case of overdose?

In case of overdose, call your local poison control center at 1-800-222-1222. If the victim has collapsed or is not breathing, call local emergency services at 911.

What other information should I know?

Keep all appointments with your doctor.

Do not let anyone else take your medication. Ask your pharmacist any questions you have about refilling your prescription.

Dosage Facts
For Informational Purposes

Caution: Do not change your dose, how often you take your medication, or the length of time you are to take it without first talking to your healthcare provider.

The following dosage information was written using medical language for doctors and other healthcare professionals and is provided here for you to check your dosage. The dosage of this drug may differ for different patients. Therefore, always follow your doctor's instructions or the directions on the label. Contact your healthcare provider or pharmacist if you have any questions about the specific dosage of your medication after reviewing this information.

Adult Patients
Muscular Conditions

ORAL:
- Initially, 500 mg 3–4 times daily; if response inadequate, increase dosage to 750 mg 3–4 times daily.
- When desired response is obtained, reduce dosage to lowest effective level.
- Usual adult dosage: 250 mg 3–4 times daily.

Cholestyramine Resin

(koe less′ tir a meen)

Brand Name: Locholest®, Locholest® Light, Questran®, Questran® Light
Also available generically.

Why is this medicine prescribed?

Cholestyramine is used with diet changes (restriction of cholesterol and fat intake) to reduce the amount of cholesterol and certain fatty substances in your blood. Accumulation of cholesterol and fats along the walls of your arteries (a process known as atherosclerosis) decreases blood flow and, therefore, the oxygen supply to your heart, brain, and other parts of your body. Lowering your blood level of cholesterol and fats may help to prevent heart disease, angina (chest pain), strokes, and heart attacks.

This medication is sometimes prescribed for other uses; ask your doctor or pharmacist for more information.

How should this medicine be used?

Cholestyramine comes in a chewable bar and in a powder that must be mixed with fluids or food. It usually is taken two to four times a day. Follow the directions on your prescription label carefully, and ask your doctor or pharmacist to explain any part you do not understand. Take cholestyramine exactly as directed. Do not take more or less of it or take it more often than prescribed by your doctor.

Take this medication before a meal and/or at bedtime, and try to take any other medications at least 1 hour before or 4 hours after you take cholestyramine because cholestyramine can interfere with their absorption.

Continue to take cholestyramine even if you feel well. Do not stop taking cholestyramine without talking to your doctor. This precaution is especially important if you also take other drugs; changing your cholestyramine dose may change their effects.

Do not take the powder alone. To take the powder, follow these steps:

1. Stir the powder into a glass of water, milk, heavy or pulpy fruit juices such as orange juice, or other beverage. If you use a carbonated beverage, mix the powder slowly in a large glass to avoid excessive foaming.
2. Drink the mixture slowly.
3. Rinse the drinking glass with more of the beverage and drink it to be sure that you get all of the powder.

The powder also may be mixed with applesauce, crushed pineapple, pureed fruit, and soup. Although the powder may be mixed in hot foods, do not heat the powder. To improve the taste and for convenience, you can prepare doses for an entire day on the previous evening and refrigerate them.

To take the chewable bars, chew each bite thoroughly before swallowing.

Drink plenty of liquids while you are taking this medication.

What special precautions should I follow?

Before taking cholestyramine,

- tell your doctor and pharmacist if you are allergic to cholestyramine or any other drugs.
- tell your doctor and pharmacist what prescription and nonprescription medications you are taking, especially amiodarone (Cordarone), antibiotics, anticoagulants ('blood thinners') such as warfarin (Coumadin), digitoxin, digoxin (Lanoxin), diuretics ('water pills'), iron, loperamide (Imodium), mycophenolate (Cellcept), oral diabetes medications, phenobarbital, phenylbutazone, propranolol (Inderal), thyroid medications, and vitamins.
- tell your doctor if you have or have ever had heart disease, especially angina (heart pain); stomach, intestinal, or gallbladder disease; or phenylketonuria.
- tell your doctor if you are pregnant, plan to become pregnant, or are breast-feeding. If you become pregnant while taking cholestyramine, call your doctor.

- if you are having surgery, including dental surgery, tell the doctor or dentist that you are taking cholestyramine.

What special dietary instructions should I follow?

Eat a low-cholesterol, low-fat diet. This kind of diet includes cottage cheese, fat-free milk, fish (not canned in oil), vegetables, poultry, egg whites, and polyunsaturated oils and margarines (corn, safflower, canola, and soybean oils). Avoid foods with excess fat in them such as meat (especially liver and fatty meat), egg yolks, whole milk, cream, butter, shortening, lard, pastries, cakes, cookies, gravy, peanut butter, chocolate, olives, potato chips, coconut, cheese (other than cottage cheese), coconut oil, palm oil, and fried foods.

What should I do if I forget to take a dose?

Take the missed dose as soon as you remember it. However, if it is almost time for the next dose, skip the missed dose and continue your regular dosing schedule. Do not take a double dose to make up for a missed one.

What side effects can this medicine cause?

Cholestyramine may cause side effects. Tell your doctor if any of these symptoms are severe or do not go away:

- constipation
- bloating
- stomach pain
- gas
- upset stomach
- vomiting
- diarrhea
- loss of appetite
- heartburn
- indigestion

If you experience the following symptom, call your doctor immediately:

- unusual bleeding (such as bleeding from the gums or rectum)

If you experience a serious side effect, you or your doctor may send a report to the Food and Drug Administration's (FDA) MedWatch Adverse Event Reporting program online [at http://www.fda.gov/MedWatch/index.html] or by phone [1-800-332-1088].

What storage conditions are needed for this medicine?

Keep this medication in the container it came in, tightly closed, and out of reach of children. Store it at room temperature and away from excess heat and moisture (not in the bathroom). Throw away any medication that is outdated or no longer needed. Talk to your pharmacist about the proper disposal of your medication.

What other information should I know?

Keep all appointments with your doctor and the laboratory. Your doctor will order certain lab tests to check your response to cholestyramine.

Do not let anyone else take your medication. Ask your pharmacist any questions you have about refilling your prescription.

Dosage Facts
For Informational Purposes

Caution: Do not change your dose, how often you take your medication, or the length of time you are to take it without first talking to your healthcare provider.

The following dosage information was written using medical language for doctors and other healthcare professionals and is provided here for you to check your dosage. The dosage of this drug may differ for different patients. Therefore, always follow your doctor's instructions or the directions on the label. Contact your healthcare provider or pharmacist if you have any questions about the specific dosage of your medication after reviewing this information.

General Dosage Information

Available as cholestyramine resin; dosage expressed in terms of anhydrous (i.e., dried) cholestyramine resin.

Each 9 g of Questran® or generic cholestyramine (1 dose, 1 packet, or 1 level scoop), 5.5 g of Prevalite® (1 dose, 1 packet, or 1 level scoop), or 5 g of Questran® Light or generic cholestyramine light (1 dose, 1 packet, or 1 level scoop) contains about 4 g of anhydrous cholestyramine resin.

In calculating pediatric dosages, each 100 mg of the commercially available powders contains either 44.4 mg (e.g., Questran®, generic cholestyramine), 72.7 mg (e.g., Prevalite®), or 80 mg (e.g., Questran® Light, generic cholestyramine light) of anhydrous cholestyramine resin.

Pediatric Patients
Dyslipidemias†

ORAL:
- 240 mg/kg daily in 2–3 divided doses suggested by manufacturers and some clinicians.

Adult Patients
Dyslipidemias or Pruritus Associated with Partial Cholestasis

ORAL:
- Initially, 4 g of anhydrous resin (1 packet or 1 level scoop) once or twice daily at mealtime.
- Increase dosage gradually to minimize adverse GI effects (e.g., fecal impaction).
- Usual maintenance dosage recommended by manufacturers is 8–16 g daily, given in 2 divided doses. Usual dosage range suggested by National Cholesterol Education Program (NCEP) expert panel is 4–16 g daily.

- Although the recommended dosing schedule is twice daily, may be administered in 1–6 doses per day.
- In patients with preexisting constipation: Initially, 4 g of anhydrous resin (1 packet or 1 level scoop) once daily for 5–7 days; then increase dosage to 4 g twice daily and monitor constipation and serum lipoprotein values, at least twice, 4–6 weeks apart. Thereafter, increase dosage as needed by 1 dose (i.e., 4 g) per day (at monthly intervals) with periodic monitoring of serum lipoprotein values.
- If constipation worsens or the desired effect is not achieved with acceptable adverse effects with the usual dosage of 1–6 doses (i.e., 4–24 g) per day, consider combined therapy or alternative treatment.

Prescribing Limits
Pediatric Patients

ORAL:
- Maximum 8 g daily.

Adult Patients

ORAL:
- Maximum 24 g (6 packets or 6 level scoops) daily.

† Use is not currently included in the labeling approved by the US Food and Drug Administration.

Ciclesonide Nasal Spray

(sye kles' oh nide)

Brand Name: Omnaris ® Nasal Spray

Why is this medicine prescribed?

Ciclesonide nasal spray is used to treat the symptoms of seasonal (occurs only at certain times of the year), and perennial (occurs all year round) allergic rhinitis. These symptoms include sneezing and stuffy, runny or itchy nose. Ciclesonide is in a class of medications called corticosteroids. It works by preventing and decreasing inflammation (swelling that can cause other symptoms) in the nose.

How should this medicine be used?

Ciclesonide comes as a solution (liquid) to spray in the nose. It is usually sprayed in each nostril once daily. Use ciclesonide at around the same time every day. Follow the directions on your prescription label carefully, and ask your doctor or pharmacist to explain any part you do not understand. Use ciclesonide exactly as directed. Do not take more or less of it or take it more often than prescribed by your doctor.

Ciclesonide nasal spray is only for use in the nose. Do not swallow the nasal spray and be careful not to spray it in your eyes or directly onto the nasal septum (the wall between the two nostrils).

Ciclesonide controls the symptoms of rhinitis but does not cure it. Your symptoms probably will not begin to improve for at least 24-48 hours after your first dose and it may be longer before you feel the full benefit of ciclesonide. Continue to use ciclesonide even if you feel well. Do not stop taking ciclesonide without talking to your doctor.

Each bottle of ciclesonide nasal spray is designed to provide 120 sprays after the bottle is primed initially. The bottle must be thrown away after 4 months of use. You should count 4 months from the date that the bottle is removed from the foil pouch and write it on the sticker that is provided in the carton. Place the sticker in the space provided on the bottle to remind you of this date. It is also important to keep track of the number of sprays you have used and throw away the bottle after you have used 120 sprays, even if the bottle still contains some liquid and it is before the 4 months have passed.

To use the nasal spray, follow these steps:

1. Shake the bottle gently and remove the dust cover.
2. If you are using the pump for the first time, point the bottle away from your body and press down and release the pump eight times. If you have used the pump before but not within the last 4 days, press down and release the pump one time or until you see a fine spray.
3. Blow your nose until your nostrils are clear.
4. Hold one nostril closed with your finger.
5. With your other hand, hold the bottle firmly with your forefinger and middle finger on either side of the spray tip while supporting the base of the bottle with your thumb.
6. Tilt your head slightly forward and carefully put the tip of the nasal applicator into your open nostril keeping the bottle upright. Begin to breathe through your nose.
7. While you are breathing in, use your forefinger and middle finger to press quickly and firmly down on the applicator and release a spray.
8. Repeat steps 4-7 in the other nostril, unless your doctor has told you otherwise.
9. Wipe the applicator tip with a clean tissue and replace the dust cover.

Are there other uses for this medicine?

This medication may be prescribed for other uses; ask your doctor or pharmacist for more information.

What special precautions should I follow?

Before using ciclesonide nasal spray,

- Tell your doctor and pharmacist if you are allergic to ciclesonide; any other nasal corticosteroid such as beclomethasone (Beconase AQ), budesonide (Rhinocort Aqua), fluticasone (Flonase), momentasone (Flonase), triamcinolone (Nasacort AQ); or any other medications.
- Tell your doctor and pharmacist what prescription and nonprescription medications, vitamins, nutritional supplements and herbal products you are taking or have recently taken. Be sure to mention ketoconazole (Nizoral) or oral steroids such as dexamethasone (Decad-

ron, Dexone), methylprednisolone (Medrol) and prednisone (Deltasone). Your doctor may need to change the doses of your medications or monitor you carefully for side effects.

- Tell your doctor if you have or have ever had tuberculosis (TB), cataracts (clouding of the lens in your eye), or glaucoma (an eye disease), and if you now have sores in your nose, any type of untreated infection, or a herpes infection of your eye (a type of infection that causes a sore on the eyelid or surface of your eye). Also tell your doctor if you have recently had surgery on your nose or injured your nose in any way.
- Tell your doctor if you are pregnant, plan to become pregnant, or are breast-feeding. If you become pregnant while taking ciclesonide, call your doctor.
- If you are having surgery, including dental surgery, tell the doctor or dentist that you are taking ciclesonide.
- If you have been taking oral steroids such as dexamethasone (Decadron, Dexone), methylprednisolone (Medrol), prednisolone (Pediapred, Prelone) or prednisone (Deltasone) your doctor may want to gradually decrease your steroid dose after you begin using ciclesonide. Special caution is needed for several months as your body adjusts to the change in medication.
- If you have any other medical conditions, such as asthma, arthritis, or eczema (a skin disease), they may worsen when your oral steroid dose is decreased. Tell your doctor if this happens or if you experience any of the following symptoms during this time: extreme tiredness, muscle weakness or pain; sudden pain in stomach, lower body or legs; loss of appetite; weight loss; upset stomach; vomiting; diarrhea; dizziness; fainting; depression; irritability; and darkening of skin. Your body may be less able to cope with stress such as surgery, illness, severe asthma attack, or injury during this time. Call your doctor right away if you get sick and be sure that all health care providers who treat you know that you recently replaced your oral steroid with ciclesonide inhalation. Carry a card or wear a medical identification bracelet to let emergency personnel know that you may need to be treated with steroids in an emergency.
- You should know that ciclesonide may decrease your ability to fight infection. Stay away from people who are sick and wash your hands often. Be especially careful to stay away from people who have chicken pox or measles. Tell your doctor right away if you find out that you have been around someone who has one of these viruses.

What special dietary instructions should I follow?

Unless your doctor tells you otherwise, continue your normal diet.

What should I do if I forget to take a dose?

Use the missed dose as soon as you remember it. However, if it is almost time for the next dose, skip the missed dose and continue your regular dosing schedule. Do not use a double dose to make up for a missed one.

What side effects can this medicine cause?

Ciclesonide may cause side effects. Tell your doctor if any of these symptoms are severe or do not go away:

- headache
- nosebleed
- burning or irritation in the nose
- earache

Some side effects can be serious. If you experience any of these symptoms call your doctor immediately:

- painful white patches in nose or throat
- flu-like symptoms
- vision problems
- injury to nose
- new or increased acne (pimples)
- easy bruising
- enlarged face and neck
- extreme tiredness
- muscle weakness
- irregular menstruation (periods)
- hives
- rash
- itching
- swelling of the face, throat, lips, eyes, hands, feet, ankles or lower legs
- hoarseness
- difficulty breathing or swallowing
- wheezing

Ciclesonide may cause children to grow more slowly. It is not known whether using ciclesonide decreases the final adult height that children will reach. Talk to your doctor about the risks of giving this medication to your child.

Ciclesonide may cause other side effects. Call your doctor if you have any unusual problems while taking this medication.

What storage conditions are needed for this medicine?

Keep this medication in the container it came in, tightly closed, and out of reach of children. Store it at room temperature and away from excess heat and moisture (not in the bathroom). Do not freeze. Throw away any medication that is outdated or no longer needed. Talk to your pharmacist about the proper disposal of your medication.

What should I do in case of overdose?

If someone swallows ciclesonide, call your local poison control center at 1-800-222-1222. If the victim has collapsed or is not breathing, call local emergency services at 911.

Using too much ciclesonide on a regular basis over a long period of time may cause the following symptoms:

- enlarged face and neck
- new or worsening acne

- easy bruising
- extreme tiredness
- muscle weakness
- irregular menstrual periods

What other information should I know?

Keep all appointments with your doctor.

If your applicator becomes clogged, remove the dust cap and gently pull upwards to free the nasal applicator. Wash the dust cap and applicator with warm water. Dry and replace the applicator and press down and release the pump one time or until you see a fine spray. Replace the dust cap. Do not use pins or other sharp objects in the tiny spray hole on the nasal applicator to remove the blockage.

Do not let anyone else take your medication. Ask your pharmacist any questions you have about refilling your prescription.

Talk to your doctor, pharmacist, or other healthcare professional if you have questions about dosing information for your medication.

Ciclopirox Topical Solution

(sye kloe peer' ox)

Brand Name: Penlac® Nail Lacquer

Why is this medicine prescribed?

Ciclopirox topical solution is used along with regular nail trimming to treat fungal infections of the fingernails and toenails (an infection that may cause nail discoloration, splitting and pain). Ciclopirox is in a class of medications called antifungals. It works by stopping the growth of nail fungus.

How should this medicine be used?

Ciclopirox comes as a solution to apply to nails and the skin immediately surrounding and under the nails. It is usually applied once a day. To help you remember to use ciclopirox, apply it around the same time every day, usually at bedtime. Follow the directions on your prescription label carefully, and ask your doctor or pharmacist to explain any part you do not understand. Use ciclopirox exactly as directed. Do not use more or less of it or use it more often than prescribed by your doctor.

Ciclopirox is used to improve the condition of nails, but may not completely cure nail fungus. It may take 6 months or longer before you notice that your nails are getting better. Continue to use ciclopirox daily as directed. Do not stop using ciclopirox without talking to your doctor.

Ciclopirox topical solution will work best if you trim your nails regularly during your treatment. You should remove all loose nail or nail material using a nail clipper or nail file before you begin treatment and every week during your treatment. Your doctor will show you how to do this. Your doctor will also trim your nails once each month during your treatment.

Only apply ciclopirox topical solution to your nails and the skin under and around your nails. Be careful not to get the solution on any other areas of the skin or parts of your body, especially in or near your eyes, nose, mouth, or vagina.

Do not use nail polish or other nail cosmetic products on nails treated with ciclopirox topical solution.

Do not take a bath, shower, or swim for at least 8 hours after applying ciclopirox topical solution.

Ciclopirox topical solution may catch fire. Do not use this medication near heat or an open flame, such as a cigarette.

To use ciclopirox topical solution, follow these steps:

1. Be sure that you have trimmed your nails properly before your first treatment.
2. Use the applicator brush attached to the bottle cap to apply ciclopirox topical solution evenly to all affected nails. Also apply the solution to the underside of the nail and the skin beneath it if you can reach these areas.
3. Wipe off the bottle cap and neck and replace the cap tightly on the bottle.
4. Let the solution dry for about 30 seconds before you put on socks or stockings.
5. When it is time for your next dose, apply ciclopirox topical solution over the medication that is already on your nails.
6. Once a week, remove all the ciclopirox from your nail(s) with a cotton square or tissue soaked with rubbing alcohol. Then, remove as much of the damaged nail as possible using scissors, nail clippers, or nail files.

Are there other uses for this medicine?

This medication may be prescribed for other uses; ask your doctor or pharmacist for more information.

What special precautions should I follow?

Before using ciclopirox topical solution,

- tell your doctor and pharmacist if you are allergic to ciclopirox or any other medications.
- tell your doctor and pharmacist what other prescription and nonprescription medications, vitamins, nutritional supplements, and herbal products you are taking. Be sure to mention any of the following: inhaled steroids such as beclomethasone (Beconase, Vancenase), budesonide (Pulmicort, Rhinocort), flunisolide (AeroBid); fluticasone (Advair, Flonase, Flovent), mometasone (Nasonex), and triamcinolone (Azmacort, Nasacort, Tri-Nasal); oral medications to treat fungal infections such as fluconazole (Diflucan), itraconazole (Sporanox), ketoconazole (Nizoral), terbinafine (Lamisil) and voriconazole (Vfend); medications for seizures; and steroid creams, lotions, or ointments such as alclometasone (Aclovate), betamethasone (Alphatrex, Betatrex, Diprolene, others), clobetasol (Cormax, Temovate), desonide (DesOwen, Tridesilon), desoximetasone (Topicort), diflorasone (Maxiflor, Psorcon), fluocinolone (DermaSmoothe, Synalar), fluocinonide (Lidex), flurandrenolide (Cordran), halcinonide (Halor), hydrocortisone (Cortizone, Westcort, others), mometasone (Elocon), prednicarbate (Dermatop), and triamcinolone (Aristocort, Kenalog, others). Your doctor may need to change the doses of your medications or monitor you carefully for side effects.

- tell your doctor if you have or have ever had an organ transplant, if you have recently had chicken pox, and if you have or have ever had any disease that affects your immune system, such as human immunodeficiency virus (HIV) or acquired immunodeficiency syndrome (AIDS) or severe combined immunodeficiency syndrome (SCID); cancer; cold sores; diabetes; flaky, itchy, or crusty skin; genital herpes (sexually transmitted disease that causes painful blisters on reproductive organs); shingles (painful blisters caused by the chicken pox virus); fungal infections on your skin such as athlete's foot and ringworm (ring-shaped discolored patches of scales and blisters on the skin, hair, or nails); peripheral vascular disease (narrowing of blood vessels in feet, legs, or arms causing numbness, pain, or coldness in that part of the body); or seizures.

- tell your doctor if you are pregnant, plan to become pregnant, or are breast-feeding. If you become pregnant while taking ciclopirox, call your doctor.

- you should know that you should keep your nails clean and dry during treatment with ciclopirox topical solution. Do not share nail care tools. Use different tools for infected and healthy nails. If your toenails are affected, wear well-fitting, low heeled shoes, and change them change frequently, and do not go barefoot in public areas. Wear protective shoes and gloves when playing sports, using strong cleaners, or during work that might injure or irritate fingernails and toenails.

What special dietary instructions should I follow?

Unless your doctor tells you otherwise, continue your normal diet.

What should I do if I forget to take a dose?

Apply the missed dose as soon as you remember it. However, if it is almost time for the next dose, skip the missed dose and continue your regular dosing schedule. Do not apply a double dose to make up for a missed one.

What side effects can this medicine cause?

Ciclopirox topical solution may cause side effects. Tell your doctor if the following symptom is severe or does not go away:

- redness at the place where you applied ciclopirox

Some side effects can be serious. The following symptoms are uncommon, but if you experience any of them, call your doctor immediately:

- irritation, itching, burning, blistering, swelling, or oozing at the place where you applied ciclopirox
- pain at the affected nail(s) or surrounding area
- discoloration or change in shape of nail(s)
- ingrown nail(s)

Ciclopirox topical solution may cause other side effects. Call your doctor if you have any unusual problems while taking this medication.

If you experience a serious side effect, you or your doctor may send a report to the Food and Drug Administration's (FDA) MedWatch Adverse Event Reporting program online [at http://www.fda.gov/MedWatch/index.html] or by phone [1-800-332-1088].

What storage conditions are needed for this medicine?

Keep this medication in the container it came in, tightly closed, and out of reach of children. Store it at room temperature and away from excess heat and moisture (not in the bathroom). Keep the bottle of ciclopirox topical solution in the package it came in, away from light. Throw away any medication that is outdated or no longer needed. Talk to your pharmacist about the proper disposal of your medication.

What other information should I know?

Keep all appointments with your doctor.

Do not let anyone else use your medication. Ask your pharmacist any questions you have about refilling your prescription.

Dosage Facts
For Informational Purposes

Caution: Do not change your dose, how often you take your medication, or the length of time you are to take it without first talking to your healthcare provider.

The following dosage information was written using medical language for doctors and other healthcare professionals and is provided here for you to check your dosage. The dosage of this drug may differ for different patients. Therefore, always follow your doctor's instructions or the directions on the label. Contact your healthcare provider or pharmacist if you have any questions about the specific dosage of your medication after reviewing this information.

General Dosage Information

Available as ciclopirox and ciclopirox olamine; dosage expressed in terms of ciclopirox.

Pediatric Patients

Dermatophytoses and Cutaneous Candidiasis

TOPICAL:
- Children ≥10 years of age: Apply 0.77% cream or lotion twice daily.
- If clinical improvement does not occur after 4 weeks of treatment, reevaluate the diagnosis.

Pityriasis (Tinea) Versicolor

TOPICAL:
- Children ≥10 years of age: Apply 0.77% cream or lotion twice daily.
- Clinical improvement usually occurs after 2 weeks of treatment.

Adult Patients

Dermatophytoses and Cutaneous Candidiasis

TOPICAL:
- Apply 0.77% cream or lotion twice daily. Alternatively, in the treatment of interdigital tinea pedis or tinea corporis, apply 0.77% gel twice daily.
- If clinical improvement does not occur after 4 weeks of treatment, reevaluate the diagnosis.

Pityriasis (Tinea) Versicolor

TOPICAL:
- Apply 0.77% cream or lotion twice daily.
- Clinical improvement usually occurs after 2 weeks of treatment.

Seborrheic Dermatitis

TOPICAL:
- Apply 0.77% gel to affected areas twice daily.
- Alternatively, apply approximately 5 mL (10 mL for long hair) of 1% shampoo to wet hair and scalp and lather. Allow drug to remain on the scalp for 3 minutes and then rinse. Repeat treatment twice weekly for 4 weeks, with a minimum of 3 days between applications.
- If clinical improvement does not occur after 4 weeks of treatment, reevaluate the diagnosis.

Onychomycosis

TOPICAL:
- Apply 8% topical solution (nail lacquer) once daily (preferably at bedtime). Remove accumulated applications of the drug with alcohol every 7 days; daily removal of solution is not recommended.
- Initial improvement of symptoms may require 6 months of therapy and up to 48 weeks of continuous comprehensive therapy to achieve clear or almost clear nail(s).

Cidofovir Injection

(si dof′ o veer)

Brand Name: Vistide®

Important Warning

Cidofovir can cause kidney damage. Some people have had kidney failure after taking only one or two doses of cidofovir. These people have needed dialysis or have died. Your doctor will order laboratory tests to check your kidney function within 48 hours before each infusion of cidofovir. Your doctor will adjust the dose of cidofovir according to your kidney function.

Tell your doctor if you are taking any other medications that cause kidney damage, some of which include amikacin (Amikin), amphoteracin B (Fungizone), foscarnet (Foscarvir), gentamicin (Garamycin), pentamidine (Pentam 300), tobramycin (Nebcin), vancomycin (Vancocin) and non-steroidal anti-inflammatory agents (Advil, Aleve, others). You must stop taking these medications at least 7 days before starting to take cidofovir. Be sure to tell your doctor about all drugs, over-the-counter medicines and herbal products you are taking.

Talk to your doctor about taking cidofovir with extra fluids and probenecid.

Cidofovir can cause a decrease in the number of a certain type of white blood cell. Keep all appointments with your doctor and the laboratory. Your doctor will order certain lab tests to check your response to cidofovir.

Cidofovir should be used only for the treatment of cytomegalovirus (CMV) retinitis in patients with acquired immunodeficiency syndrome (AIDS).

Cidofovir has been shown to cause cancer, birth defects, and problems with sperm production in animals.

Talk to your doctor about the possible risks of taking this drug.

About Your Treatment

Your doctor has ordered cidofovir, an antiviral agent, to help treat your infection. The drug will be added to an intravenous fluid that will drip through a needle or catheter placed in your vein for 1 hour, weekly, or every 2 weeks.

Cidofovir is used to treat CMV retinitis in patients with AIDS.

Your health care provider (doctor, nurse, or pharmacist) may measure the effectiveness and side effects of your treatment using laboratory tests and physical examinations. It is important to keep all appointments with your doctor and the laboratory. The length of treatment depends on how your infection and symptoms respond to the medication.

Precautions

Before administering cidofovir,

- tell your doctor and pharmacist if you are allergic to cidofovir or any other drugs.
- tell your doctor and pharmacist what prescription and nonprescription medications you are taking, especially those listed in the IMPORTANT WARNING section, antibiotics, zidovudine, and vitamins.
- tell your doctor if you have or have ever had kidney or liver disease or diabetes.
- tell your doctor if you are pregnant, plan to become pregnant, or are breast-feeding. If you become pregnant while taking cidofovir, call your doctor. Women of childbearing age should use an effective method of birth control during therapy and for 1 month following therapy.
- Men should continue using condoms as standard precaution against spreading HIV disease.
- Men should talk to their doctor about any attempt to conceive a child.

Administering Your Medication

Before you administer cidofovir, look at the solution closely. It should be clear and free of floating material. Gently squeeze the bag or observe the solution container to make sure there are no leaks. Do not use the solution if it is discolored, if it contains particles, or if the bag or container leaks. Use a new solution, but show the damaged one to your health care provider.

It is important that you use your medication exactly as directed. Do not stop your therapy on your own for any reason because your infection could worsen and result in hospitalization. Do not change your dosing schedule without talking to your health care provider. Your health care provider may tell you to stop your infusion if you have a mechanical problem (such as a blockage in the tubing, needle, or catheter); if you have to stop an infusion, call your health care provider immediately so your therapy can continue.

Side Effects

Cidofovir may cause side effects. Tell your health care provider if any of these symptoms are severe or do not go away:

- headache
- diarrhea
- stomach pain, upset or vomiting
- constipation
- sore mouth or tongue
- joint and muscle pain
- coughing
- fever and chills

If you experience either of the following symptoms, call your health care provider immediately:

- skin rashes and itching of the skin
- eye pain and redness, sensitivity to light, and decreased vision

If you experience a serious side effect, you or your doctor may send a report to the Food and Drug Administration's

(FDA) MedWatch Adverse Event Reporting program online [at http://www.fda.gov/MedWatch/index.html] or by phone [1-800-332-1088].

Storage Conditions

- Your health care provider may give you one dose at a time; store it as directed. You will be told to store the doses in the refrigerator or freezer.
- Take your next dose from the refrigerator 1 hour before using it; place it in a clean, dry area to allow it to warm to room temperature.
- If you are told to store additional cidofovir in the freezer, always move a 24-hour supply to the refrigerator for the next day's use.
- Do not refreeze medications.

Store your medication only as directed. Make sure you understand what you need to store your medication properly.

Keep your supplies in a clean, dry place when you are not using them, and keep all medications and supplies out of reach of children. Your health care provider will tell you how to throw away used needles, syringes, tubing, and containers to avoid accidental injury.

Overdose

In case of overdose, call your local poison control center at 1-800-222-1222. If the victim has collapsed or is not breathing, call local emergency services at 911.

Signs of Infection

If you are receiving cidofovir in your vein or under your skin, you need to know the symptoms of a catheter-related infection (an infection where the needle enters your vein or skin). If you experience any of these effects near your intravenous catheter, tell your health care provider as soon as possible:

- tenderness
- warmth
- irritation
- drainage
- redness
- swelling
- pain

Dosage Facts
For Informational Purposes

Caution: Do not change your dose, how often you take your medication, or the length of time you are to take it without first talking to your health-care provider.

The following dosage information was written using medical language for doctors and other healthcare professionals and is provided here for you to check your dosage. The dosage of this drug may differ for different patients. Therefore, always follow your doctor's instruc-

tions or the directions on the label. Contact your health-care provider or pharmacist if you have any questions about the specific dosage of your medication after reviewing this information.

General Dosage Information

Available as cidofovir dihydrate; dosage is expressed in terms of anhydrous drug.

Pediatric Patients

Cytomegalovirus (CMV) Infections
CMV Retinitis in HIV-infected Adolescents†

IV:
- Initial induction therapy: 5 mg/kg once weekly for 2 consecutive weeks.
- Maintenance therapy: 5 mg/kg once every 2 weeks (i.e., every other week).

Prevention of Recurrence (Secondary Prophylaxis) of CMV Disease in HIV-infected Adolescents†

IV:
- 5 mg/kg once every other week. Initiate secondary prophylaxis after initial induction treatment.
- Consideration can be given to discontinuing secondary CMV prophylaxis in adolescents with sustained (e.g., for ≥6 months) increase in CD4+ T-cell counts to >100–150/mm³ in response to potent antiretroviral therapy.
- This decision should be made in consultation with an ophthalmologist and factors such as the magnitude and duration of CD4+ T-cell increase, anatomic location of the retinal lesion, vision in the contralateral eye, and feasibility of regular ophthalmic monitoring should be considered.
- Relapse of CMV retinitis could occur following discontinuance of secondary prophylaxis, especially in those whose CD4+ T-cell count decreases to <50/mm³; relapse has been reported rarely in those with CD4+ T-cell counts >100/mm³.
- Reinitiate secondary CMV prophylaxis if CD4+ T-cell count decreases to <100–150/mm³.

Herpes Simplex Virus (HSV) Infections†
Acyclovir-resistant HSV Infections in immunocompromised Adolescents†

IV:
- 5 mg/kg once weekly for 2–4 weeks until a response is obtained.

Adult Patients

Cytomegalovirus (CMV) Infections
CMV Retinitis in HIV-infected Adults

IV:
- Initial induction therapy: 5 mg/kg once weekly for 2 consecutive weeks.
- Maintenance therapy: 5 mg/kg once every 2 weeks (i.e., every other week).

Prevention of Recurrence (Secondary Prophylaxis) of CMV Disease in HIV-infected Adults†

IV:
- 5 mg/kg once every other week. Initiate secondary prophylaxis after initial induction treatment.
- Consideration can be given to discontinuing secondary CMV prophylaxis in adults with sustained (e.g., for ≥6 months)

increase in CD4+ T-cell counts to >100–150/mm³ in response to potent antiretroviral therapy.

- This decision should be made in consultation with an ophthalmologist and factors such as the magnitude and duration of CD4+ T-cell increase, anatomic location of the retinal lesion, vision in the contralateral eye, and feasibility of regular ophthalmic monitoring should be considered.
- Relapse of CMV retinitis could occur following discontinuance of secondary prophylaxis, especially in those whose CD4+ T-cell count decreases to <50/mm³; relapse has been reported rarely in those with CD4+ T-cell counts >100/mm³.
- Reinitiate secondary CMV prophylaxis if CD4+ T-cell count decreases to <100–150/mm³.

Herpes Simplex Virus (HSV) Infections†
Acyclovir-resistant HSV Infections in immunocompromised Adults†

IV:
- 5 mg/kg once weekly for 2–4 weeks until a response is obtained.

Smallpox†
Smallpox Vaccination Complications†

IV:
- CDC has proposed a cidofovir dosage of 5 mg/kg administered once as an IV infusion over 1 hour. If there is no response to the initial dose, administration of a second dose 1 week later can be considered. If a second dose is needed, cidofovir dosage may need to be adjusted if renal function has deteriorated.
- Information on dosage and administration of cidofovir and IND materials will be provided by CDC if the drug is released for treatment of certain serious complications of smallpox vaccination†.

Monkeypox†

IV:
- No specific dosage recommendations available. Information on appropriate dosage for severe monkeypox infection should be obtained as part of clinical consultation services provided by state health departments or CDC (877-554-4625).

Special Populations

Renal Impairment
- Contraindicated in patients with serum creatinine >1.5 mg/dL, calculated Cl$_{cr}$ ≤55 mL/minute, or urine protein ≥100 mg/dL (equivalent to 2+ or greater).
- If serum creatinine increases by 0.5 mg/dL or more above baseline or urinary proteinuria of 3+ or greater develops, cidofovir must be discontinued.
- Patients who develop 2+ proteinuria in the face of a stable serum creatinine during cidofovir therapy should be observed carefully (including close monitoring of serum creatinine and urinary protein) to detect potential deterioration that would warrant dose reduction or temporary discontinuance of the drug.

Cytomegalovirus (CMV) Infections
CMV Retinitis in HIV-infected Adults

IV:
- If clinically important decreases in renal function (e.g., increase in serum creatinine to 0.3–0.4 mg/dL above baseline) occur in patients receiving cidofovir, maintenance dosage must be reduced to 3 mg/kg administered IV at the usual rate and frequency. Some clinicians suggest a cidofovir dosage of 2.5–4 mg/kg administered IV at the usual rate and frequency in HIV-infected patients with a Cl$_{cr}$ 50–80 mL/minute.

Geriatric Patients
- Select dosage with caution because of age-related decreases in renal function.

† *Use is not currently included in the labeling approved by the US Food and Drug Administration.*

Cilostazol

(sil oh′ sta zol)

Brand Name: Pletal®
Also available generically.

Important Warning
Cilostazol should not be used by patients with congestive heart failure. If you have a history of heart disease, talk to your doctor about the potential risks associated with cilostazol before taking it.

Why is this medicine prescribed?

Cilostazol is used to reduce the symptoms of intermittent claudication (pain in the legs that happens when walking and goes away with rest). Cilostazol helps people walk a longer distance before leg pain starts.

This medication is sometimes prescribed for other uses; ask your doctor or pharmacist for more information.

How should this medicine be used?

Cilostazol comes as a tablet to take by mouth. It is usually taken two times a day. It should be taken at least 30 minutes before or 2 hours after breakfast and dinner. Follow the directions on the prescription label carefully, and ask your doctor or pharmacist to explain any part you do not understand. Take cilostazol exactly as directed. Do not take more or less of it or take it more often than prescribed by your doctor.

Cilostazol controls the symptoms of intermittent claudication but does not cure it. It may take up to 12 weeks before you notice a benefit (increased walking distance) from cilostazol. Continue taking cilostazol even if you feel well. Do not stop taking cilostazol without talking to your doctor.

What special precautions should I follow?

Before taking cilostazol,
- tell your doctor and pharmacist if you are allergic to cilostazol or any other drugs.

- tell your doctor and pharmacist what prescription and nonprescription medications you are taking, especially aspirin, azithromycin (Zithromax), citalopram (Celexa), clarithromycin (Biaxin), clopidogrel (Plavix), diltiazem (Cardizem, Dilacor XR), erythromycin (E-mycin, Ery-Tab, others), fluconazole (Diflucan), fluoxetine (Prozac), fluvoxamine (Luvox), itraconazole (Sporanox), ketoconazole (Nizoral), nefazadone (Serzone), omeprazole (Prilosec), sertraline (Zoloft), warfarin (Coumadin), and vitamins.
- tell your doctor if you have or have ever had heart or liver disease.
- tell your doctor if you are pregnant, plan to become pregnant, or are breast-feeding. If you become pregnant while taking cilostazol, call your doctor.
- tell your doctor if you use tobacco products. Cigarette smoking may decrease the effectiveness of cilostazol.

What special dietary instructions should I follow?

You should not drink grapefruit juice while taking cilostazol.

What should I do if I forget to take a dose?

Take the missed dose as soon as you remember it. However, if it is almost time for the next dose, skip the missed dose and continue your regular dosing schedule. Do not take a double dose to make up for a missed one.

What side effects can this medicine cause?

Cilostazol may cause side effects. Tell your doctor if any of these symptoms are severe or do not go away:
- headache
- fast or irregular heartbeats
- diarrhea
- dizziness
- upset stomach
- stomach pain
- abnormal stools
- runny nose
- sore throat
- flu-like symptoms

If you experience any of the following symptoms, call your doctor immediately:
- rash
- swelling of the hands, feet, ankles, or lower legs
- shortness of breath

If you experience a serious side effect, you or your doctor may send a report to the Food and Drug Administration's (FDA) MedWatch Adverse Event Reporting program online [at http://www.fda.gov/MedWatch/index.html] or by phone [1-800-332-1088].

What storage conditions are needed for this medicine?

Keep this medication in the container it came in, tightly closed, and out of reach of children. Store it at room temperature and away from excess heat and moisture (not in the bathroom). Throw away any medication that is outdated or no longer needed. Talk to your pharmacist about the proper disposal of your medication.

What should I do in case of overdose?

In case of overdose, call your local poison control center at 1-800-222-1222. If the victim has collapsed or is not breathing, call local emergency services at 911.

What other information should I know?

Keep all appointments with your doctor. You should read the patient information that comes with your prescription before you begin to take cilostazol and read it again every time you have your prescription filled in case the patient information changes.

Do not let anyone else take your medication. Ask your pharmacist any questions you have about refilling your prescription.

Dosage Facts
For Informational Purposes

Caution: Do not change your dose, how often you take your medication, or the length of time you are to take it without first talking to your healthcare provider.

The following dosage information was written using medical language for doctors and other healthcare professionals and is provided here for you to check your dosage. The dosage of this drug may differ for different patients. Therefore, always follow your doctor's instructions or the directions on the label. Contact your healthcare provider or pharmacist if you have any questions about the specific dosage of your medication after reviewing this information.

Adult Patients

Intermittent Claudication

ORAL:
- 100 mg twice daily.
- Patients receiving concomitant therapy with CYP3A4 (e.g., diltiazem, erythromycin, itraconazole, ketoconazole) or CYP2C19 (e.g., omeprazole) inhibitors: Initially, 50 mg twice daily.

Thrombotic Complications of Coronary Angioplasty†

ORAL:
- 100 mg twice daily alone or in combination with aspirin (e.g., 81 mg daily) has been used in a limited number of patients.

Special Populations

Hepatic Impairment
- No specific dosage recommendations at this time.

Renal Impairment
- No specific dosage recommendations at this time.

† *Use is not currently included in the labeling approved by the US Food and Drug Administration.*

Cimetidine

(sye met′ i deen)

Brand Name: Tagamet®, Tagamet® HB, Tagamet® Tiltab®
Also available generically.

Why is this medicine prescribed?

Cimetidine is used to treat ulcers; gastroesophageal reflux disease (GERD), a condition in which backward flow of acid from the stomach causes heartburn and injury of the food pipe (esophagus); and conditions where the stomach produces too much acid, such as Zollinger-Ellison syndrome. Over-the-counter cimetidine is used to prevent and treat symptoms of heartburn associated with acid indigestion and sour stomach. Cimetidine is in a class of medications called H_2 blockers. It decreases the amount of acid made in the stomach.

How should this medicine be used?

Cimetidine comes as a tablet and a liquid to take by mouth. It is usually taken once a day at bedtime or two to four times a day with meals and at bedtime. Over-the-counter cimetidine is usually taken once or twice a day with a glass of water. To prevent symptoms, it is taken within 30 minutes before eating or drinking foods that cause heartburn. Follow the directions on your prescription or the package label carefully, and ask your doctor or pharmacist to explain any part you do not understand. Take cimetidine exactly as directed. Do not take more or less of it or take it more often than prescribed by your doctor.

Do not take over-the-counter cimetidine for longer than 2 weeks unless your doctor tells you to. If symptoms of heartburn, acid indigestion, or sour stomach last longer than 2 weeks, stop taking cimetidine and call your doctor.

Are there other uses for this medicine?

Cimetidine is also used sometimes to treat stress ulcers, hives and itching, and viral warts, and to prevent aspiration pneumonia during anesthesia. Talk to your doctor about the possible risks of using this medication for your condition.

This medication may be prescribed for other uses; ask your doctor or pharmacist for more information.

What special precautions should I follow?

Before taking cimetidine,
- tell your doctor and pharmacist if you are allergic to cimetidine or any other medications.
- tell your doctor and pharmacist what prescription and nonprescription medications, vitamins, nutritional supplements, and herbal products you are taking. Be sure to mention any of the following: anticoagulants ('blood thinners') such as warfarin (Coumadin); antidepressants (mood elevators) such as amitriptyline (Elavil), amoxapine (Asendin), clomipramine (Anafranil), desipramine (Norpramin), doxepin (Adapin, Sinequan), imipramine (Tofranil), nortriptyline (Aventyl, Pamelor), protriptyline (Vivactil), and trimipramine (Surmontil); chlordiazepoxide (Librium); diazepam (Valium); lidocaine (Xylocaine); metronidazole (Flagyl); nifedipine (Adalat, Procardia); phenytoin (Dilantin); propranolol (Inderal); and theopylline (Theobid, Theo-Dur). Your doctor may need to change the doses of your medications or monitor you carefully for side effects.
- if you are taking antacids (Maalox, Mylanta, Tums), digoxin (Lanoxin), ketoconazole (Nizoral), or iron salts, take them 2 hours before cimetidine.
- tell your doctor if you have or have ever had human immunodeficiency virus (HIV), acquired immunodeficiency syndrome (AIDS), or kidney or liver disease.
- tell your doctor if you are pregnant, plan to become pregnant, or are breast-feeding. If you become pregnant while taking cimetidine, call your doctor.

What special dietary instructions should I follow?

Unless your doctor tells you otherwise, continue your normal diet.

What should I do if I forget to take a dose?

Take the missed dose as soon as you remember it. However, if it is almost time for the next dose, skip the missed dose and continue your regular dosing schedule. Do not take a double dose to make up for a missed one.

What side effects can this medicine cause?

Cimeditine may cause side effects. Tell your doctor if any of these symptoms are severe or do not go away:
- headache
- diarrhea
- dizziness
- drowsiness
- breast enlargement

Some side effects can be serious. The following symptoms are uncommon, but if you experience any of them, call your doctor immediately:
- confusion
- excitement
- depression
- nervousness
- seeing things or hearing voices that do not exist (hallucinating)

Cimetidine may cause other side effects. Call your doctor if you have any unusual problems while taking this medication.

If you experience a serious side effect, you or your doctor may send a report to the Food and Drug Administration's (FDA) MedWatch Adverse Event Reporting program online [at http://www.fda.gov/MedWatch/index.html] or by phone [1-800-332-1088].

What storage conditions are needed for this medicine?

Keep this medication in the container it came in, tightly closed, and out of reach of children. Store it at room temperature and away from excess heat and moisture (not in the bathroom). Throw away any medication that is outdated or no longer needed. Talk to your pharmacist about the proper disposal of your medication.

What should I do in case of overdose?

In case of overdose, call your local poison control center at 1-800-222-1222. If the victim has collapsed or is not breathing, call local emergency services at 911.

What other information should I know?

Keep all appointments with your doctor.

Do not let anyone else take your medicine. Ask your pharmacist any questions you have about refilling your prescription.

Dosage Facts
For Informational Purposes

Caution: Do not change your dose, how often you take your medication, or the length of time you are to take it without first talking to your healthcare provider.

The following dosage information was written using medical language for doctors and other healthcare professionals and is provided here for you to check your dosage. The dosage of this drug may differ for different patients. Therefore, always follow your doctor's instructions or the directions on the label. Contact your healthcare provider or pharmacist if you have any questions about the specific dosage of your medication after reviewing this information.

General Dosage Information

Dosage of cimetidine hydrochloride expressed in terms of cimetidine.

Pediatric Patients

20–40 mg/kg daily in divided doses has been used in a limited number of children when potential benefits are thought to outweigh the possible risks.

Heartburn, Acid Indigestion, or Sour Stomach
Heartburn Relief (Self-medication)

ORAL:
- Adolescents ≥12 years of age: 200 mg once or twice daily, or as directed by a clinician.

Prevention of Heartburn (Self-medication)

ORAL:
- Adolescents ≥12 years of age: 200 mg once or twice daily or as directed by a clinician; administer immediately (or up to 30 minutes) before ingestion of causative food or beverage.

Adult Patients

Duodenal Ulcer
Treatment of Active Duodenal Ulcer

ORAL:
- Dosage of choice: 800 mg once daily at bedtime.
- Patients with ulcer >1 cm in diameter who are heavy smokers (i.e., ≥1 pack daily) when rapid healing (e.g., within 4 weeks) is considered important: 1.6 g daily at bedtime.
- Administer for 4–6 weeks unless healing is confirmed earlier. If not healed or symptoms continue after 4 weeks, additional 2–4 weeks of full dosage therapy may be beneficial. More than 6–8 weeks at full dosage is rarely needed.
- Healing of active duodenal ulcers may occur in 2 weeks in some, and occurs within 4 weeks in most patients.
- Other regimens (no apparent rationale for these other than familiarity of use) that have been used: 300 mg 4 times daily with meals and at bedtime; 200 mg 3 times daily and 400 mg at bedtime; 400 mg twice daily in the morning and at bedtime.

Maintenance of Healing of Duodenal Ulcer

ORAL:
- 400 mg daily at bedtime. Efficacy not increased by higher dosages or more frequent administration.

Pathologic GI Hypersecretory Conditions
Zollinger-Ellison Syndrome

ORAL:
- 300 mg 4 times daily with meals and at bedtime.
- Higher doses administered more frequently may be necessary; adjust dosage according to response and tolerance but in general, do not exceed 2400 mg daily.
- Continue as long as necessary.

Gastric Ulcer

ORAL:
- Preferred regimen: 800 mg once daily at bedtime.
- Alternative regimen: 300 mg 4 times daily, with meals and at bedtime.
- Monitor to ensure rapid progress to complete healing.
- Studies limited to 6 weeks, efficacy for >8 weeks not established.

GERD

Once daily (at bedtime) not considered appropriate therapy.

Treatment of Symptomatic GERD†

ORAL:
- 300 mg 4 times daily has been used.

Treatment of Erosive Esophagitis

ORAL:

- 800 mg twice daily or 400 mg 4 times daily (e.g., before meals and at bedtime) for up to 12 weeks.

Upper GI Bleeding

Treatment of Upper GI Bleeding†

ORAL:

- 1–2 g daily in 4 divided doses has been used.

Heartburn, Acid Indigestion, or Sour Stomach

Heartburn (Self-medication)

ORAL:

- 200 mg once or twice daily, or as directed by clinician.
- Maximum 400 mg in 24 hours, but not continuously for >2 weeks except under clinician supervision.

Prevention of Heartburn (Self-medication)

ORAL:

- 200 mg once or twice daily or as directed by a clinician; administer immediately (or up to 30 minutes) before ingestion of causative food or beverage.
- Maximum 400 mg in 24 hours, but not continuously for >2 weeks except under clinician supervision.

Prescribing Limits

Pediatric Patients

Heartburn, Acid Indigestion, or Sour Stomach

Heartburn (Self-Medication)

ORAL:

- Adolescents ≥12 years of age: Maximum 400 mg in 24 hours, but not continuously for >2 weeks except under clinician supervision.

Prevention of Heartburn (Self-medication)

ORAL:

- Adolescents ≥12 years of age: Maximum 400 mg in 24 hours, but not continuously for >2 weeks except under clinician supervision.

Adult Patients

GERD

Short-term Treatment of Erosive Esophagitis

ORAL:

- Safety and efficacy beyond 12 weeks of administration have not been established.

Heartburn, Acid Indigestion, or Sour Stomach

Heartburn Relief (Self-medication)

ORAL:

- Maximum 400 mg in 24 hours, but not continuously for >2 weeks except under clinician supervision.

Prevention of Heartburn (Self-medication)

ORAL:

- Maximum 400 mg in 24 hours, but not continuously for >2 weeks except under clinician supervision.

Gastric Ulcer

Short-term treatment of Active Benign Gastric Ulcer

ORAL:

- Safety and efficacy beyond 8 weeks have not been established.

Pathologic GI Hypersecretory Conditions (e.g., Zollinger-Ellison Syndrome)

ORAL:

- Maximum usually 2.4 g daily.

Special Populations

Renal Impairment

Severe (Cl$_{cr}$< 30 mL/minute)

ORAL:

- 300 mg every 12 hours.
- Accumulation may occur; use lowest frequency of dosing compatible with adequate response.
- Increase frequency to every 8 hours or more frequently (with caution) if required.
- Presence of hepatic impairment may require further dosage reduction.

Hemodialysis

Decreases blood levels; administer at the end of hemodialysis and every 12 hours during interdialysis.

Hepatic Impairment

- May require further dosage reduction in the presence of severe renal impairment.

† Use is not currently included in the labeling approved by the US Food and Drug Administration.

Cimetidine Hydrochloride Injection

(sye met' i deen)

Brand Name: Tagamet®
Also available generically.

About Your Treatment

Your doctor has ordered cimetidine to decrease the amount of acid your stomach makes. It is used to treat and prevent ulcers and to treat other conditions in which the stomach makes too much acid. The drug will be injected into a large muscle (such as your buttock or hip); added to an intravenous fluid that will drip through a needle or catheter placed in your vein for at least 15 minutes, three or four times a day; or administered by constant infusion over 24 hours. This medication is sometimes prescribed for other uses; ask your doctor or pharmacist for more information.

Your health care provider (doctor, nurse, or pharmacist) may measure the effectiveness and side effects of your treatment using laboratory tests and physical examinations. It is important to keep all appointments with your doctor and the laboratory. The length of treatment depends on how you respond to the medication.

Precautions

Before administering cimetidine,

- tell your doctor and pharmacist if you are allergic to cimetidine or any other drugs.
- tell your doctor and pharmacist what prescription and nonprescription medications you are taking, especially amitriptyline (Elavil), anticoagulants ('blood thinners') such as warfarin (Coumadin), chlordiazepoxide (Librium), desipramine (Norpramin), diazepam (Valium), diuretics ('water pills'), imipramine (Tofranil), metronidazole (Flagyl), nifedipine (Adalat, Procardia), phenytoin (Dilantin), propranolol (Inderal), theophylline (Theo-Dur), triamterene (Dyrenium), and vitamins.
- tell your doctor if you have or have ever had kidney or liver disease.
- tell your doctor if you are pregnant, plan to become pregnant, or are breast-feeding. If you become pregnant while taking cimetidine, call your doctor.
- remember to administer it slowly. If cimetidine is administered too rapidly, you may develop severe dizziness and faintness. Do not administer your cimetidine faster than directed. If you feel faint or dizzy, call your health care provider immediately.

Administering Your Medication

Before you administer cimetidine, look at the solution closely. It should be clear and free of floating material. Gently squeeze the bag or observe the solution container to make sure there are no leaks. Do not use the solution if it is discolored, if it contains particles, or if the bag or container leaks. Use a new solution, but show the damaged one to your health care provider.

It is important that you use your medication exactly as directed. Do not stop your therapy on your own for any reason. Do not change your dosing schedule without talking to your health care provider. Your health care provider may tell you to stop your infusion if you have a mechanical problem (such as a blockage in the tubing, needle, or catheter); if you have to stop an infusion, call your health care provider immediately so your therapy can continue.

Side Effects

Cimetidine may cause side effects. Tell your health care provider if any of these symptoms are severe or do not go away:

- headache
- dizziness
- constipation
- diarrhea
- muscle pain

- drowsiness
- breast enlargement and soreness

If you experience any of the following symptoms, call your health care provider immediately:

- mental confusion
- skin rash
- itching
- hives
- difficulty breathing

If you experience a serious side effect, you or your doctor may send a report to the Food and Drug Administration's (FDA) MedWatch Adverse Event Reporting program online [at http://www.fda.gov/MedWatch/index.html] or by phone [1-800-332-1088].

Storage Conditions

- Your health care provider probably will give you a several-day supply of cimetidine at a time. If you are receiving cimetidine intravenously (in your vein), you probably will be told to store it in the refrigerator or freezer.
- Take your next dose from the refrigerator 1 hour before using it; place it in a clean, dry area to allow it to warm to room temperature.
- If you are told to store additional cimetidine in the freezer, always move a 24-hour supply to the refrigerator for the next day's use.
- Do not refreeze medications.

If you are receiving cimetidine intramuscularly (in your muscle), your health care provider will tell you how to store it properly.

Store your medication only as directed. Make sure you understand what you need to store your medication properly.

Keep your supplies in a clean, dry place when you are not using them, and keep all medications and supplies out of reach of children. Your health care provider will tell you how to throw away used needles, syringes, tubing, and containers to avoid accidental injury.

Overdose

In case of overdose, call your local poison control center at 1-800-222-1222. If the victim has collapsed or is not breathing, call local emergency services at 911.

Signs of Infection

If you are receiving cimetidine in your vein or under your skin, you need to know the symptoms of a catheter-related infection (an infection where the needle enters your vein or skin). If you experience any of these effects near your intravenous catheter, tell your health care provider as soon as possible:

- tenderness
- warmth
- irritation
- drainage

- redness
- swelling
- pain

Dosage Facts
For Informational Purposes

Caution: Do not change your dose, how often you take your medication, or the length of time you are to take it without first talking to your healthcare provider.

The following dosage information was written using medical language for doctors and other healthcare professionals and is provided here for you to check your dosage. The dosage of this drug may differ for different patients. Therefore, always follow your doctor's instructions or the directions on the label. Contact your healthcare provider or pharmacist if you have any questions about the specific dosage of your medication after reviewing this information.

General Dosage Information

Dosage of cimetidine hydrochloride expressed in terms of cimetidine.

Pediatric Patients

20–40 mg/kg daily in divided doses has been used in a limited number of children when potential benefits are thought to outweigh the possible risks.

Adult Patients

General Parenteral Dosage

Parenteral dosage regimens for GERD have not been established.

General parenteral dosage (in hospitalized patients with pathologic hypersecretory conditions or intractable ulcer, or for short-term use when oral therapy is not feasible):

IM:
- 300 mg every 6–8 hours.

INTERMITTENT DIRECT IV INJECTION:
- 300 mg every 6–8 hours.
- 300 mg more frequently if increased daily dosage is necessary (i.e., single doses not >300 mg), up to 2400 mg daily.

INTERMITTENT IV INFUSION:
- 300 mg every 6–8 hours.
- 300 mg more frequently if increased daily dosage is necessary (i.e., single doses not >300 mg), up to 2400 mg daily.

CONTINUOUS IV INFUSION:
- 900 mg over 24 hours (37.5 mg/hour).
- For more rapid increase in gastric pH, a loading dose of 150 mg may be given as an intermittent infusion before continuous infusion.

Pathologic GI Hypersecretory Conditions
Zollinger-Ellison Syndrome

CONTINUOUS IV INFUSION:
- Mean infused dose of 160 mg/hour (range: 40-600 mg/hour) in one study.

Upper GI Bleeding
Prevention of Upper GI Bleeding

CONTINUOUS IV INFUSION:
- 50 mg/hour; loading dose not required.
- Safety and efficacy of therapy beyond 7 days has not been established.
- Alternative dosage: Some clinicians recommend 300-mg IV loading dose over 5–20 minutes, then continuous IV infusion at 37.5–50 mg/hour; titrate with 25-mg/hour increments up to 100 mg/hour based on gastric pH (e.g., to maintain a pH of *at least* 3.5–4).
- Intermittent IV doses may be less effective in preventing upper GI bleeding than continuous IV infusion.

Treatment of Upper GI Bleeding†

IV:
- 1–2 g daily in 4 divided doses has been used.

Prescribing Limits
Adult Patients
General Parenteral Dosage

General parenteral dosage (hospitalized patients with pathologic hypersecretory conditions or intractable duodenal ulcer, or short-term use when oral therapy is not feasible):

DIRECT IV INJECTION:
- Maximum 2.4 g daily.
- Maximum 300 mg per dose.
- Maximum concentration 300 mg/20 mL.
- Maximum injection rate: 20 mL over not less than 5 minutes (4 mL per minute).

INTERMITTENT IV INFUSION:
- Maximum 2.4 g daily.
- Maximum 300 mg per dose.
- Maximum concentration 300 mg/50 mL.
- Maximum infusion rate: 15–20 minutes.

Duodenal Ulcer

INTERMITTENT DIRECT IV INJECTON:
- Maximum 2.4 g daily.

INTERMITTENT IV INFUSION:
- Maximum 2.4 g daily.

Gastric Ulcer
Short-term treatment of Active Benign Gastric Ulcer

INTERMITTENT DIRECT IV INJECTION:
- Maximum 2.4 g daily.

INTERMITTENT IV INFUSION:
- Maximum 2.4 g daily.

Pathologic GI Hypersecretory Conditions (e.g., Zollinger-Ellison Syndrome)

INTERMITTENT DIRECT IV INJECTION:
- Maximum 2.4 g daily.

INTERMITTENT IV INFUSION:
- Maximum 2.4 g daily.

Upper GI Bleeding
Prevention of Upper GI Bleeding

CONTINUOUS IV INFUSION:
- Safety and efficacy beyond 7 days have not been established.

Special Populations

Renal Impairment

Severe (Cl$_{cr}$< 30 mL/minute)

DIRECT IV INJECTION:

- 300 mg every 12 hours.
- Accumulation may occur; use lowest frequency compatible with adequate response.
- Increase frequency to every 8 hours or more frequently (with caution) if required.
- Presence of hepatic impairment may require further dosage reduction.

CONTINUOUS IV INFUSION:

- *Prevention of Upper GI Bleeding*: One-half recommended dosage (i.e., 25 mg/hour).

Hemodialysis

Decreases blood levels; administer at the end of hemodialysis and every 12 hours during interdialysis.

Hepatic Impairment

- May require further dosage reduction in the presence of severe renal impairment.

† *Use is not currently included in the labeling approved by the US Food and Drug Administration.*

Cinacalcet

(sin a cal′ set)

Brand Name: Sensipar®

Why is this medicine prescribed?

Cinacalcet is used alone or with other medications to treat secondary hyperparathyroidism [a condition in which the body produces too much parathyroid hormone (a natural substance needed to control the amount of calcium in the blood) which can cause serious problems with the bones, heart, blood vessels, and lungs] in patients with chronic kidney disease (condition in which the kidneys stop working slowly and gradually) who are being treated with dialysis (medical treatment to clean the blood when the kidneys are not working properly). Cinacalcet is also used to treat high levels of calcium in the blood of patients who have parathyroid cancer (cancer of the glands in the neck that make parathyroid hormone). Cinacalcet is in a class of medications called calcimimetics. It works by signaling the body to produce less parathyroid hormone in order to decrease the amount of calcium in the blood.

How should this medicine be used?

Cinacalcet comes as a tablet to take by mouth. It is usually taken once a day with food or shortly after a meal. To help you remember to take cinacalcet, take it at around the same time every day. Follow the directions on your prescription label carefully, and ask your doctor or pharmacist to explain any part you do not understand. Take cinacalcet exactly as directed. Do not take more or less of it or take it more often than prescribed by your doctor.

Swallow the tablets whole; do not split, chew, or crush them.

Your doctor will probably start you on a low dose of cinacalcet and gradually increase your dose, not more than once every 2-4 weeks.

Cinacalcet may help control your condition but will not cure it. Continue to take cinacalcet even if you feel well. Do not stop taking cinacalcet without talking to your doctor.

Are there other uses for this medicine?

This medication may be prescribed for other uses; ask your doctor or pharmacist for more information.

What special precautions should I follow?

Before taking cinacalcet,

- tell your doctor and pharmacist if you are allergic to cinacalcet or any other medications.
- tell your doctor and pharmacist what prescription and nonprescription medications, vitamins, nutritional supplements, and herbal products you are taking. Be sure to mention any of the following: antidepressants (mood elevators) such as amitriptyline (Elavil), clomipramine (Anafranil), desipramine (Norpramin), fluoxetine (Prozac, Sarafem), imipramine (Tofranil), nefazodone, nortriptyline (Aventyl, Pamelor), paroxetine (Paxil), protriptyline (Vivactil) and trimipramine (Surmontil); antifungals such as fluconazole (Diflucan), itraconazole (Sporanox), and ketoconazole (Nizoral); cimetidine (Tagamet); cyclosporine (Neoral, Sandimmune); danazol (Danocrine); delavirdine (Rescriptor); diltiazem (Cardizem, Dilacor, Tiazac); erythromycin (E.E.S., E-Mycin, Erythrocin); flecainide (Tambocor); HIV protease inhibitors such as indinavir (Crixivan) and ritonavir (Norvir); isoniazid (INH, Nydrazid); metronidazole (Flagyl); oral contraceptives (birth control pills); thioridazine (Mellaril); troleandomycin (TAO); verapamil (Calan, Covera, Isoptin, Verelan); vinblastine (Velban); and zafirlukast (Accolate). Your doctor may need to change the doses of your medications or monitor you carefully for side effects.
- tell your doctor if you have or have ever had seizures or liver disease.
- tell your doctor if you are pregnant, plan to become pregnant, or are breast-feeding. If you become pregnant while taking cinacalcet, call your doctor.

What special dietary instructions should I follow?

Talk to your doctor about drinking grapefruit juice while taking this medication.

What should I do if I forget to take a dose?

Take the missed dose as soon as you remember it. However, if it is almost time for the next dose, skip the missed dose and continue your regular dosing schedule. Do not take a double dose to make up for a missed one.

What side effects can this medicine cause?

Cinacalcet may cause side effects. Tell your doctor if any of these symptoms are severe or do not go away:

- upset stomach
- vomiting
- diarrhea
- dizziness
- weakness
- chest pain

Some side effects can be serious. The following symptoms are uncommon, but if you experience any of them, call your doctor immediately:

- burning, tingling, or unusual feelings of the lips, tongue, fingers, or feet
- muscle aches or cramps
- sudden tightening of the muscles in the hands, feet, face, or throat
- seizures
- infection of dialysis access (surgically created blood vessel where blood leaves and enters the body during dialysis)

Cinacalcet may cause other side effects. Call your doctor if you have any unusual problems while taking this medication.

If you experience a serious side effect, you or your doctor may send a report to the Food and Drug Administration's (FDA) MedWatch Adverse Event Reporting program online [at http://www.fda.gov/MedWatch/index.html] or by phone [1-800-332-1088].

What storage conditions are needed for this medicine?

Keep this medication in the container it came in, tightly closed, and out of reach of children. Store it at room temperature and away from excess heat and moisture (not in the bathroom). Throw away any medication that is outdated or no longer needed. Talk to your pharmacist about the proper disposal of your medication.

What should I do in case of overdose?

In case of overdose, call your local poison control center at 1-800-222-1222. If the victim has collapsed or is not breathing, call local emergency services at 911.

Symptoms of overdose may include:

- burning, tingling, or unusual feelings of the lips, tongue, fingers, or feet
- muscle aches or cramps
- sudden tightening of the muscles in the hands, feet, face, or throat
- seizures

What other information should I know?

Keep all appointments with your doctor and the laboratory. Your doctor will order certain lab tests to check your body's response to cinacalcet.

Do not let anyone else take your medication. Ask your pharmacist any questions you have about refilling your prescription.

Dosage Facts
For Informational Purposes

Caution: Do not change your dose, how often you take your medication, or the length of time you are to take it without first talking to your healthcare provider.

The following dosage information was written using medical language for doctors and other healthcare professionals and is provided here for you to check your dosage. The dosage of this drug may differ for different patients. Therefore, always follow your doctor's instructions or the directions on the label. Contact your healthcare provider or pharmacist if you have any questions about the specific dosage of your medication after reviewing this information.

General Dosage Information

Available as cinacalcet hydrochloride; dosage expressed in terms of cinacalcet.

Individualize dosage.

Adult Patients

Secondary Hyperparathyroidism Associated with Chronic Renal Disease

ORAL:

- Usual initial dosage: 30 mg once daily.
- Increase dosage no more frequently than every 2–4 weeks through sequential adjustments to 60, 90, 120, and 180 mg once daily to achieve a target intact parathyroid hormone (iPTH) concentration of 150–300 pg/mL (consistent with National Kidney Foundation-Kidney Dialysis Outcomes Quality Initiative [NKF-K/DOQI] recommendations for patients with chronic renal disease who are undergoing dialysis).
- Median dosage was 90 mg daily in clinical studies; patients with milder disease generally required lower dosages.
- Do not initiate cinacalcet if baseline serum calcium concentration is <8.4 mg/dL.
- Measure serum calcium and phosphorus concentrations within 1 week and iPTH concentrations 1–4 weeks after initiation or subsequent dosage adjustment.
- If serum calcium concentrations fall to <8.4 mg/dL but remain >7.5 mg/dL, or if manifestations of hypocalcemia occur, may use calcium-containing phosphate binders and/or vitamin D analogs to increase serum calcium concentrations.
- If serum calcium concentrations fall to <7.5 mg/dL, or hypocalcemia manifestations persist and vitamin D dosage cannot be increased, withhold cinacalcet. When serum calcium concentrations reach 8 mg/dL and/or manifestations of hypocalcemia have resolved, may reinitiate cinacalcet using the next lowest dosage.

- Once maintenance dosage is established, measure serum calcium and phosphorus concentrations monthly and iPTH concentration every 1–3 months.

Hypercalcemia Associated with Parathyroid Carcinoma

ORAL:
- Usual initial dosage: 30 mg twice daily.
- Increase dosage every 2–4 weeks through sequential adjustments to 60 mg twice daily, 90 mg twice daily, and 90 mg 3 or 4 times daily as needed to normalize serum calcium concentrations.
- Measure serum calcium concentration within 1 week of cinacalcet initiation or dosage adjustment; measure every 2 months once an appropriate maintenance dosage has been established.

Special Populations

No special population dosage recommendations at this time.

Ciprofloxacin

(sip roe flox′ a sin)

Brand Name: Cipro®, Cipro® XR, Proquin®XR

Why is this medicine prescribed?

Ciprofloxacin is an antibiotic used to treat or prevent certain infections caused by bacteria. Ciprofloxacin is also used to treat or prevent anthrax in people who may have been exposed to anthrax germs in the air. Ciprofloxacin extended-release (long-acting) tablets are used only to treat certain types of urinary tract infections. Ciprofloxacin is in a class of antibiotics called fluoroquinolones. It works by killing bacteria.

Antibiotics will not work for colds, flu, or other viral infections.

How should this medicine be used?

Ciprofloxacin comes as a tablet, a suspension (liquid) and an extended-release tablet to take by mouth. The tablet and suspension are usually taken twice a day in the morning and evening with or without food. The extended-release tablets are usually taken once a day. Cipro XR brand extended-release tablets may be taken with or without food. Proquin XR brand extended-release tablets should be taken with a main meal of the day, preferably the evening meal. Take ciprofloxacin at around the same time(s) every day. The length of your treatment depends on the type of infection you have. Your doctor will tell you how long to take ciprofloxacin. Follow the directions on your prescription label carefully, and ask your doctor or pharmacist to explain any part you do not understand. Take ciprofloxacin exactly as directed. Do not take more or less of it or take it more often than prescribed by your doctor.

One brand or type of ciprofloxacin cannot be substituted for another. Be sure that you receive only the brand of ciprofloxacin that was prescribed by your doctor. Ask your pharmacist if you have any questions about the type of ciprofloxacin you were given.

Swallow the extended-release tablets whole; do not split, crush, or chew them. If you cannot swallow tablets whole, tell your doctor.

If you are taking the liquid, shake the bottle very well for 15 seconds before each use to mix the medication evenly. Swallow the correct dose without chewing the granules in the liquid. Close the liquid ciprofloxacin bottle completely after each use. Do not give the liquid to a patient through a feeding tube.

You should begin feeling better during the first few days of treatment with ciprofloxacin. If your symptoms do not improve, or if they get worse, call your doctor. Fever and back pain may be symptoms of a worsening urinary tract infection. If you are being treated for this type of infection, call your doctor if you develop these symptoms during or after your treatment

Take ciprofloxacin until you finish the prescription, even if you feel better. If you stop taking ciprofloxacin too soon or if you skip doses, your infection may not be completely treated and the bacteria may become resistant to antibiotics.

Ask your pharmacist or doctor for a copy of the manufacturer's information for the patient.

Are there other uses for this medicine?

In the event of biological warfare, ciprofloxacin may be used to treat and prevent dangerous illnesses that are deliberately spread such as plague, tularemia, and anthrax of the skin or mouth. Talk to your doctor about the possible risks of using this medication for your condition.

This medication may be prescribed for other uses; ask your doctor or pharmacist for more information.

What special precautions should I follow?

Before taking ciprofloxacin,
- tell your doctor and pharmacist if you are allergic or have had a severe reaction to ciprofloxacin; or any other quinolone or fluoroquinolone antibiotics such as gatifloxacin (Tequin, not available in the U.S.), gemifloxacin (Factive), levofloxacin (Levaquin), lomefloxacin (Maxaquin), moxifloxacin (Avelox), nalidixic acid (NegGram), norfloxacin (Noroxin), and ofloxacin (Floxin); if you are allergic to any other medications; or if you are allergic to any of the ingredients in ciprofloxacin tablets or liquid. Ask your pharmacist for a list of the ingredients.
- tell your doctor if you are taking tizanidine (Zanaflex). Your doctor will probably tell you not to take ciprofloxacin while you are taking this medication.
- tell your doctor and pharmacist what other prescription and nonprescription medications, vitamins, nutritional supple-

ments, and herbal products you are taking or plan to take. Be sure to mention any of the following: acetazolamide (Diamox); anticoagulants ('blood thinners') such as warfarin (Coumadin); brinzolamide (Azopt); caffeine (NoDoz, Vivarin, others); cyclosporine (Neoral, Sandimmune); dorzolamide (Trusopt); glyburide (DiaBeta, Glucovance, Micronase, others); medications for diarrhea such as dicyclomine (Bentyl), diphenoxylate (Lomotil), and loperamide (Imodium); methazolamide; methotrexate (Rheumatrex, Trexall); metoclopramide (Reglan); nonsteroidal anti-inflammatory medications (NSAIDs) such as ibuprofen (Advil, Motrin) and naproxen (Aleve, Naprosyn); oral steroids such as dexamethasone (Decadron, Dexone), methylprednisolone (Medrol), and prednisone (Deltasone); phenytoin (Dilantin, Phenytek); potassium citrate and citric acid (Cytra-K, Polycitra-K); probenecid (Benemid); sodium bicarbonate (Soda Mint, baking soda); sodium citrate and citric acid (Bicitra, Oracit, Shohl's Solution); sodium lactate; or theophylline (Theobid, Theo-Dur, Slo-bid, others). Your doctor may need to change the doses of your medications or monitor you carefully for side effects. Many other medications may also interact with ciprofloxacin, so be sure to tell your doctor about all the medications you are taking, even those that do not appear on this list.

- if you are taking antacids (Maalox, Mylanta, Tums, others) or didanosine (Videx) oral solution (liquid); calcium, iron, zinc, or vitamin supplements; or sucralfate (Carafate); you will need to allow some time to pass between when you take a dose of any of these medications and when you take a dose of ciprofloxacin. Ask your doctor or pharmacist how many hours before or after you take ciprofloxacin you may take these medications.
- tell your doctor if you have or have ever had arthritis; asthma; cerebral palsy (CP, a condition of abnormal muscle or motor function); dementia (a condition associated with memory loss and personality changes); recent head injury; seizures; stroke or ministroke; or kidney or liver disease.
- tell your doctor if you have ever had tendonitis (swelling or tearing of the fiber that connects a bone to a muscle) and if you participate in regular athletic activity. There is a risk that you will develop tendonitis while you are taking ciprofloxacin, especially if you are also taking oral steroid medications. If you experience symptoms of tendonitis, such as pain, swelling, tenderness, stiffness, or difficulty in moving a muscle stop taking ciprofloxacin, rest, and call your doctor immediately.
- tell your doctor if you are pregnant, plan to become pregnant, or are breast-feeding. If you become pregnant while taking ciprofloxacin, call your doctor.
- if you are having surgery, including dental surgery, tell the doctor or dentist that you are taking ciprofloxacin.
- if you are having a radiologic test (X-ray, CT scan) that involves dye, tell the doctor or health care professional that you are taking ciprofloxacin.

- you should know that ciprofloxacin may cause confusion, dizziness, lightheadedness, and tiredness. Do not drive a car or operate machinery or participate in activities requiring alertness or coordination until you know how this medication affects you.
- plan to avoid unnecessary or prolonged exposure to sunlight or ultraviolet light (tanning beds) and to wear protective clothing, sunglasses, and sunscreen. Ciprofloxacin may make your skin sensitive to sunlight or ultraviolet light. If your skin becomes reddened, like a bad sunburn, stop taking ciprofloxacin and call your doctor.
- you should know that ciprofloxacin may cause diarrhea during or after your treatment. You should not treat this diarrhea with over the counter medications. If diarrhea does not go away, call your doctor to find out what to do.

What special dietary instructions should I follow?

Do not take ciprofloxacin with dairy products (like milk, ice cream, cheese, or yogurt) or calcium-added juices alone. You may take ciprofloxacin with a meal that includes these foods.

Do not drink or eat a lot of caffeine-containing products such as coffee, tea, energy drinks, cola, or chocolate. Ciprofloxacin may increase nervousness, sleeplessness, heart pounding, and anxiety caused by caffeine.

Make sure you drink plenty of water or other fluids every day while you are taking ciprofloxacin.

What should I do if I forget to take a dose?

If you miss a dose of ciprofloxacin tablets or suspension, take the missed dose as soon as you remember it. However, if it is almost time for the next dose, skip the missed dose and continue your regular dosing schedule. Do not take a double dose to make up for a missed one.

If you miss a dose of the extended-release tablets and remember that same day, take the missed dose as soon as you remember it. However, if you do not remember until the next day, skip the missed dose and continue your regular dosing schedule. Do not take more than one ciprofloxacin extended-release tablet in one day.

What side effects can this medicine cause?

Ciprofloxacin may cause side effects. Tell your doctor if any of these symptoms are severe or do not go away:
- nausea
- vomiting
- stomach pain
- indigestion
- diarrhea
- headache
- nervousness
- agitation
- anxiety

- difficulty falling asleep or staying asleep
- nightmares or abnormal dreams
- feelings of not trusting others or feelings that others want to hurt you
- vaginal itching and/or discharge

Some side effects can be serious. If you experience any of these symptoms, stop taking ciprofloxacin, and call your doctor immediately:

- rash or blisters
- hives
- itching
- tingling or swelling of the face, neck, throat, tongue, lips, eyes, hands, feet, ankles, or lower legs
- difficulty breathing or swallowing
- hoarseness
- rapid, irregular, or pounding heartbeat
- fainting
- fever
- joint or muscle pain
- unusual bruising or bleeding
- extreme tiredness
- lack of energy
- loss of appetite
- pain in the upper right part of the stomach
- yellowing of the skin or eyes
- flu-like symptoms
- seizures
- dizziness
- double vision
- pulsing sounds in the head or ringing in the ears
- confusion
- uncontrollable shaking of a part of the body
- hallucinations (seeing things or hearing voices that do not exist)
- depression
- thoughts about dying or killing yourself
- pain, burning, tingling, numbness, and/or weakness in a part of the body
- loss of ability to feel light touch, pain, heat or coldness, or vibration in a part of the body
- loss of ability to know position of a part of the body
- loss of muscle strength in a part of the body

Ciprofloxacin may cause joint damage in children. Ciprofloxacin should not normally be given to children younger than 18 years old unless they have certain serious infections that cannot be treated with other antibiotics or they have been exposed to anthrax in the air. If your doctor prescribes ciprofloxacin for your child, be sure to tell the doctor if your child has a history of joint-related problems. Call your doctor if your child develops joint problems while taking ciprofloxacin or after treatment with ciprofloxacin. Talk to your child's doctor about the risks of giving ciprofloxacin to your child.

Ciprofloxacin may cause other side effects. Call your doctor if you have any unusual problems while taking this medication.

What storage conditions are needed for this medicine?

Keep this medication in the container it came in, tightly closed, and out of reach of children. Store it at room temperature and away from excess heat and moisture (not in the bathroom). Store the suspension in the refrigerator or at room temperature, closed tightly, for up to 14 days. Do not freeze ciprofloxacin suspension. Throw away any liquid that is left over after 14 days and any medication that is outdated or no longer needed. Talk to your pharmacist about the proper disposal of your medication.

What should I do in case of overdose?

In case of overdose, call your local poison control center at 1-800-222-1222. If the victim has collapsed or is not breathing, call local emergency services at 911.

What other information should I know?

Keep all appointments with your doctor and the laboratory. Your doctor may order certain lab tests to check your body's response to ciprofloxacin.

Do not let anyone else take your medication. Your prescription is probably not refillable. If you still have symptoms of infection after you finish the ciprofloxacin, call your doctor.

Keep a list of all the medications you are taking and show it to your doctor and pharmacist during each visit.

Dosage Facts
For Informational Purposes

Caution: Do not change your dose, how often you take your medication, or the length of time you are to take it without first talking to your healthcare provider.

The following dosage information was written using medical language for doctors and other healthcare professionals and is provided here for you to check your dosage. The dosage of this drug may differ for different patients. Therefore, always follow your doctor's instructions or the directions on the label. Contact your healthcare provider or pharmacist if you have any questions about the specific dosage of your medication after reviewing this information.

General Dosage Information

Available as ciprofloxacin, ciprofloxacin hydrochloride, a mixture of ciprofloxacin and ciprofloxacin hydrochloride, and as ciprofloxacin lactate; dosage expressed in terms of ciprofloxacin.

Extended-release tablet preparations (Cipro® XR, ProQuin® XR) are used *only* for the treatment of certain urinary tract infections (UTIs). These extended-release preparations are *not* interchangeable with each other and are *not* interchangeable with other oral ciprofloxacin preparations (conventional tablets, oral suspension).

Based on pharmacokinetic parameters (i.e., AUC), the following regimens are considered equivalent: ciprofloxacin conventional tablets 250 mg every 12 hours—ciprofloxacin 200 mg IV every 12 hours; ciprofloxacin conventional tablets 500 mg every 12 hours—ciprofloxacin 400 mg IV every 12 hours; ciprofloxacin conventional tablets 750 mg every 12 hours—ciprofloxacin 400 mg IV every 8 hours.

Pediatric Patients

Urinary Tract Infections (UTIs)
Complicated UTIs and Pyelonephritis

ORAL:
- Children 1–17 years of age: 10–20 mg/kg (up to 750 mg) every 12 hours for 10–21 days.

Endocarditis†
Endocarditis Caused by the HACEK Group†

ORAL:
- 20–30 mg/kg daily given in 2 equally divided doses recommended by AHA and IDSA. Duration of treatment is 4 weeks for native valve endocarditis or 6 weeks for endocarditis involving prosthetic cardiac valves or other prosthetic cardiac material.

Culture-negative Endocarditis†

ORAL:
- 20–30 mg/kg daily given in 2 equally divided doses in conjunction with vancomycin (40 mg/kg daily given IV in 2 equally divided doses) and gentamicin (3 mg/kg daily given IM or IV in 3 equally divided doses) recommended by AHA and IDSA. All 3 drugs should be given for 4–6 weeks.

Anthrax
Postexposure Prophylaxis Following Exposure in the Context of Biologic Warfare or Bioterrorism

ORAL:
- 15 mg/kg (up to 500 mg) every 12 hours ≥60 days. Because of concerns regarding long-term use of ciprofloxacin in infants and children, consider changing (after 10–14 days) to amoxicillin to complete the full duration of postexposure prophylaxis if the strain is found to be susceptible to penicillin.
- Optimum duration of postexposure prophylaxis after an inhalation exposure to *B. anthracis* spores is unclear, but prolonged postexposure prophylaxis usually required. A duration of 60 days may be adequate for a low-dose exposure, but a duration >4 months may be necessary to reduce the risk following a high-dose exposure. CDC, US Working Group on Civilian Biodefense, and US Army Medical Research Institute of Infectious Diseases (USAMRIID) recommend that postexposure prophylaxis in unvaccinated individuals be continued for ≥60 days following a confirmed exposure (including in laboratory workers with confirmed exposures to *B. anthracis* cultures). The USPHS Advisory Committee on Immunization Practices (ACIP) and USAMRIID recommend that individuals who are partially or fully vaccinated against anthrax receive postexposure prophylaxis for ≥30 days; if given in conjunction with anthrax vaccine, continue prophylaxis for at least 7–14 days after the third vaccine dose.

Treatment of Inhalational, GI, or Oropharyngeal Anthrax†

ORAL:
- 15 mg/kg (up to 500 mg) every 12 hours given for ≥60 days.
- Initial parenteral regimen preferred; use oral regimen for initial treatment only when a parenteral regimen is not available (e.g., supply or logistic problems because large numbers of individuals require treatment in a mass casualty setting). Continue for total duration of ≥60 days if inhalational anthrax occurred as the result of exposure to anthrax spores in the context of biologic warfare or bioterrorism. Because of concerns regarding long-term use of ciprofloxacin in infants and children, consider changing (after 10–14 days) to amoxicillin to complete the treatment regimen if penicillin susceptibility is confirmed.

Treatment of Cutaneous Anthrax†

ORAL:
- 15 mg/kg (up to 500 mg) every 12 hour.
- For mild, uncomplicated cutaneous anthrax that occurs following natural or endemic exposure (e.g., known exposure to infected livestock or their products), 5–10 days of treatment may be sufficient.
- For cutaneous anthrax that occurs following exposure in the context of biologic warfare or bioterrorism, duration of treatment is ≥60 days. Because of concerns regarding long-term use of ciprofloxacin in infants and children, consider changing (after 10–14 days) to amoxicillin to complete the treatment regimen if penicillin susceptibility is confirmed.
- Oral regimen should not be used for initial treatment of cutaneous anthrax if there are signs of systemic involvement, extensive edema, or head and neck lesions or in infants <2 years of age.

Gonorrhea and Associated Infections†
Uncomplicated Urethral, Endocervical, Rectal, or Pharyngeal Gonorrhea†

ORAL:
- Adolescents and children weighing >45 kg: 500 mg as a single dose has been used for infections caused by susceptible *Neisseria gonorrhoeae*.
- Because of increased prevalence of quinolone-resistant *N. gonorrhoeae* (QRNG), CDC no longer recommends ciprofloxacin or other fluoroquinolones for treatment of gonorrhea or any associated infections involving *N. gonorrhoeae* (e.g., pelvic inflammatory disease [PID], epididymitis).
- Unless the presence of coexisting chlamydial infection has been excluded by appropriate testing, patients being treated for gonorrhea also should receive an anti-infective regimen effective for presumptive treatment of chlamydia (e.g., a single dose of oral azithromycin or a 7-day regimen of oral doxycycline).

Plague†
Treatment of Pneumonic Plague Occurring in Context of Biologic Warfare or Bioterrorism†

ORAL:
- Conventional tablets or oral suspension: 20 mg/kg twice daily. Usual duration of treatment is 10 days; some experts recommend a duration of at least 10–14 days.
- Initial parenteral regimen preferred; use oral regimen for initial treatment only when a parenteral regimen is not available (e.g., supply or logistic problems because large numbers of individuals require treatment in a mass casualty setting).

Postexposure Prophylaxis Following High-risk Exposure†

ORAL:
- Conventional tablets or oral suspension: 20 mg/kg twice daily for 7 days.

Tularemia†
Treatment of Tularemia Occurring in the Context of Biologic Warfare or Bioterrorism†

ORAL:
- Conventional tablets or oral suspension: 15 mg/kg twice daily. Usual duration of treatment is 10 days; some experts recommend a duration of at least 10–14 days.
- Initial parenteral regimen preferred; use oral regimen for initial treatment only when a parenteral regimen is not available (e.g., supply or logistic problems because large numbers of individuals require treatment in a mass casualty setting).

Postexposure Prophylaxis Following High-risk Exposure†

ORAL:
- Conventional tablets or oral suspension: 15 mg/kg twice daily for 14 days.

Vibrio Infections†
Cholera†

ORAL:
- Children 2–12 years of age: A single dose of 20 mg/kg (up to 750 mg) has been used for treatment of cholera caused by *V. cholerae* 01 or 0139.

Adult Patients

Bone and Joint Infections
Mild to Moderate Infections

ORAL:
- Conventional tablets or oral suspension: 500 mg every 12 hours for 4–6 weeks.

Severe or Complicated Infections

ORAL:
- Conventional tablets or oral suspension: 750 mg every 12 hours for 4–6 weeks.

Endocarditis†
Endocarditis Caused by the HACEK Group†

ORAL:
- 1 g daily given in 2 equally divided doses recommended by AHA and IDSA. Duration of treatment is 4 weeks for native valve endocarditis or 6 weeks for endocarditis involving prosthetic cardiac valves or other prosthetic cardiac material.

Staphylococcal Endocarditis in the Absence of Prosthetic Materials†

ORAL:
- 750 mg twice daily in conjunction with rifampin (300 mg orally twice daily) given for 28 days has been used for uncomplicated right-sided *S. aureus* endocarditis in IV drug abusers who will not comply with usually recommended parenteral regimens.

Culture-negative Endocarditis†

ORAL:
- 1 g daily given in 2 equally divided doses in conjunction with vancomycin (30 mg/kg daily given IV in 2 equally divided doses) and gentamicin (3 mg/kg daily given IM or IV in 3 equally divided doses) recommended by AHA and IDSA. All 3 drugs should be given for 4–6 weeks.

GI Infections
Infectious Diarrhea

ORAL:
- Conventional tablets or oral suspension: 500 mg every 12 hours for 5–7 days.

Cyclospora or Isospora Infections†

ORAL:
- Conventional tablets or oral suspension: 500 mg every 12 hours for 7 days.

Treatment of Travelers' Diarrhea†

ORAL:
- Conventional tablets or oral suspension: 500 mg every 12 hours for 1–3 days. Duration of 3–7 days recommended for empiric treatment in HIV-infected adults.

Prevention of Travelers' Diarrhea†

ORAL:
- Conventional tablets or oral suspension: 500 mg once daily.
- Although anti-infective prophylaxis generally is discouraged, some clinicians state that it can be given during the period of risk (for ≤3 weeks) beginning the day of travel and continuing for 1 or 2 days after leaving the area of risk.

Otic Infections†
Malignant Otitis Externa†

ORAL:
- 750 mg twice daily has been used. Although rapid relief of symptoms (pain, otorrhea) may occur, continue treatment for 6–8 weeks.
- Because ciprofloxacin-resistant *Pseudomonas aeruginosa* have been isolated from patients with malignant otitis externa with increasing frequency, in vitro susceptibility testing is indicated, especially if there is an inadequate response to treatment.

Respiratory Tract Infections
Acute Sinusitis

ORAL:
- Conventional tablets or oral suspension: 500 mg every 12 hours for 10 days.

Mild to Moderate Infections

ORAL:
- Conventional tablets or oral suspension: 500 mg every 12 hours for 7–14 days.

Severe or Complicated Infections

ORAL:
- Conventional tablets or oral suspension: 750 mg every 12 hours for 7–14 days.

Skin and Skin Structure Infections
Mild to Moderate Infections

ORAL:
- Conventional tablets or oral suspension: 500 mg every 12 hours for 7–14 days.

Severe or Complicated Infections

ORAL:
- Conventional tablets or oral suspension: 750 mg every 12 hours for 7–14 days.

Urinary Tract Infections (UTIs) and Prostatitis
Uncomplicated UTIs (Acute Cystitis)

ORAL:
- Conventional tablets or oral suspension: 250 mg every 12 hours for 3 days.
- Extended-release tablets (Cipro® XR): 1 tablet (500 mg) once daily for 3 days, preferably given with the evening meal.

- Extended-release tablets (ProQuin® XR): 1 tablet (500 mg) once daily for 3 days.

Mild to Moderate UTIs

ORAL:
- Conventional tablets or oral suspension: 250 mg every 12 hours for 7–14 days.

Complicated UTIs

ORAL:
- Conventional tablets or oral suspension: 500 mg every 12 hours for 7–14 days.
- Extended-release tablets (Cipro® XR): 1 tablet (1 g) once every 24 hours for 7–14 days.

Acute Uncomplicated Pyelonephritis

ORAL:
- Extended-release tablets: 1 g once every 24 hours for 7–14 days.

Mild to Moderate Chronic Prostatitis

ORAL:
- Conventional tablets or oral suspension: 500 mg every 12 hours for 28 days.

Anthrax
Postexposure Prophylaxis Following Exposure in the Context of Biologic Warfare or Bioterrorism

ORAL:
- Conventional tablets or oral suspension: 500 mg every 12 hours for ≥60 days.
- Optimum duration of postexposure prophylaxis after an inhalation exposure to *B. anthracis* spores is unclear, but prolonged postexposure prophylaxis usually required. A duration of 60 days may be adequate for a low-dose exposure, but a duration >4 months may be necessary to reduce the risk following a high-dose exposure. CDC, US Working Group on Civilian Biodefense, and US Army Medical Research Institute of Infectious Diseases (USAMRIID) recommend that postexposure prophylaxis in unvaccinated individuals be continued for ≥60 days following a confirmed exposure (including in laboratory workers with confirmed exposures to *B. anthracis* cultures). The USPHS Advisory Committee on Immunization Practices (ACIP) and USAMRIID recommend that individuals who are partially or fully vaccinated against anthrax receive postexposure prophylaxis for ≥30 days; if given in conjunction with anthrax vaccine, continue prophylaxis for at least 7–14 days after the third vaccine dose.

Postexposure Prophylaxis Following Ingestion of Bacillus anthracis Spores in Contaminated Meat†

ORAL:
- Conventional tablets or oral suspension: 500 mg every 12 hours has been recommended.

Treatment of Inhalational, GI, or Oropharyngeal Anthrax†

ORAL:
- Conventional tablets or oral suspension: 500 mg every 12 hours given for ≥60 days.
- Initial parenteral regimen preferred; use oral regimen for initial treatment only when a parenteral regimen is not available (e.g., supply or logistic problems because large numbers of individuals require treatment in a mass casualty setting). Continue for total duration of ≥60 days if inhalational anthrax occurred as the result of exposure to anthrax spores in the context of biologic warfare or bioterrorism.

Treatment of Cutaneous Anthrax†

ORAL:
- Conventional tablets or oral suspension: 500 mg every 12 hours.
- For mild, uncomplicated cutaneous anthrax that occurs following natural or endemic exposure, 5–10 days of treatment has been recommended.
- For cutaneous anthrax that occurs following exposure in the context of biologic warfare or bioterrorism, duration of treatment is ≥60 days.
- Oral regimen should not be used for initial treatment of cutaneous anthrax if there are signs of systemic involvement, extensive edema, or head and neck lesions.

Bartonella Infections†
Cat Scratch Disease Caused by Bartonella henselae†

ORAL:
- Conventional tablets or oral suspension: 500 mg twice daily for 10–16 days has been used.

Brucella Infections†

ORAL:
- Conventional tablets or oral suspension: 500 mg twice daily in conjunction with oral rifampin (600 mg once daily). Alternatively, 500 mg 2 or 3 times daily for 6–12 weeks or 750 mg 3 times daily for 6–8 weeks has been used for brucellosis or acute brucella arthritis-diskitis. Monotherapy or treatment regimens <4–6 weeks not recommended.

Chancroid†

ORAL:
- Conventional tablets or oral suspension: 500 mg twice daily for 3 days recommended by CDC and others.

Crohn's Disease†

ORAL:
- Conventional tablets or oral suspension: 500 mg twice daily (with or without metronidazole) has been used as an adjunct to conventional therapies for induction of remission of mildly to moderately active disease.

Gonorrhea and Associated Infections
Uncomplicated Urethral, Endocervical, Rectal†, or Pharyngeal† Gonorrhea

ORAL:
- Conventional tablets or oral suspension: 500 mg as a single dose has been used for infections caused by susceptible *N. gonorrhoeae*. Lower doses not recommended.
- Conventional tablets or oral suspension: 250 mg as a single dose recommended by manufacturer.
- Because of increased prevalence of QRNG, CDC no longer recommends ciprofloxacin or other fluoroquinolones for treatment of gonorrhea or any associated infections involving *N. gonorrhoeae* (e.g., PID, epididymitis).
- Unless the presence of coexisting chlamydial infection has been excluded by appropriate testing, patients being treated for gonorrhea also should receive an anti-infective regimen effective for presumptive treatment of chlamydia (e.g., a single dose of oral azithromycin or a 7-day regimen of oral doxycycline).

Granuloma Inguinale (Donovanosis)†

ORAL:

- Conventional tablets or oral suspension: 750 mg twice daily for ≥3 weeks or until all lesions have healed completely; consider adding IV aminoglycoside (e.g., gentamicin) if improvement is not evident within the first few days of therapy and in HIV-infected patients.
- Relapse can occur 6–18 months after apparently effective treatment.

Legionnaires' Disease†

ORAL:

- Conventional tablets or oral suspension: 500 mg every 12 hours for 2–3 weeks.

Mycobacterial Infections†

ORAL:

- Conventional tablets or oral suspension: 750 mg twice daily has been used in treatment of active tuberculosis caused by *M. tuberculosis* or treatment of infections caused by *M. avium* complex.

Neisseria meningitidis Infections†
Elimination of Pharyngeal Carrier State†

ORAL:

- Conventional tablets or oral suspension: 500 or 750 mg as a single dose. Alternatively, 250 mg twice daily for 2 days or 500 mg twice daily for 5 days.

Prophylaxis in Household or Other Close Contacts†

ORAL:

- Conventional tablets or oral suspension: 500 mg as a single dose.

Plague†
Treatment of Pneumonic Plague Occurring in Context of Biologic Warfare or Bioterrorism†

ORAL:

- Conventional tablets or oral suspension: 500 mg twice daily. Usual duration of treatment is 10 days; some experts recommend a duration of at least 10–14 days.
- Initial parenteral regimen preferred; use oral regimen for initial treatment only when a parenteral regimen is not available (e.g., supply or logistic problems because large numbers of individuals require treatment in a mass casualty setting).

Postexposure Prophylaxis Following High-risk Exposure†

ORAL:

- Conventional tablets or oral suspension: 500 mg twice daily for 7 days.

Tularemia†
Treatment of Tularemia Occurring in the Context of Biologic Warfare or Bioterrorism†

ORAL:

- Conventional tablets or oral suspension: 500 mg twice daily. Usual duration of treatment is 10 days; some experts recommend a duration of at least 10–14 days.
- Initial parenteral regimen preferred; use oral regimen for initial treatment only when a parenteral regimen is not available (e.g., supply or logistic problems because large numbers of individuals require treatment in a mass casualty setting).

Postexposure Prophylaxis Following High-risk Exposure†

ORAL:

- Conventional tablets or oral suspension: 500 mg twice daily for 14 days.

Typhoid Fever and Other Salmonella Infections
Mild to Moderate Typhoid Fever

ORAL:

- Conventional tablets or oral suspension: 500 mg every 12 hours for 10 days.

Chronic Typhoid Carriers†

ORAL:

- Conventional tablets or oral suspension: 750 mg every 12 hours for 28 days.

Prevention of Recurrence (Secondary Prophylaxis) in HIV-infected Patients†

ORAL:

- Conventional tablets or oral suspension: 500 mg every 12 hours for several months.

Vibrio Infections†
Cholera†

ORAL:

- 1 g given as a single dose or in 2 divided doses 12 hours apart has been used for treatment of cholera caused by *V. cholerae* 01 or 0139.

Perioperative Prophylaxis†

ORAL:

- Single 500-mg dose given prior to the procedure.

Prescribing Limits

Pediatric Patients

Urinary Tract Infections (UTIs)
Complicated UTIs and Pyelonephritis

ORAL:

- Children 1–17 years of age: Maximum 750 mg every 12 hours, even in those weighing >51 kg.

Anthrax
Postexposure Prophylaxis Following Exposure in the Context of Biologic Warfare or Bioterrorism

ORAL:

- Maximum 500 mg every 12 hours.

Adult Patients

Do not exceed usual dosage because of risk of crystalluria.

Special Populations

Hepatic Impairment

- Dosage adjustments not required in patients with stable chronic cirrhosis; pharmacokinetics not fully studied in those with acute hepatic insufficiency.
- Monitor ciprofloxacin concentrations in patients with both hepatic and renal impairment.

Renal Impairment

- Dosage adjustments may be necessary in adults with renal impairment, especially those with severe impairment. Dosage recommendations not available for pediatric patients with moderate to severe renal impairment (Cl_{cr} <50 mL/minute per 1.73 m²).

- Dosage of conventional tablets or oral suspension should be decreased in adults with Cl_{cr} ≤50 mL/minute. (See Tables.)
- Dosage adjustment unnecessary when extended-release tablets (ProQuin® XR) are used for uncomplicated UTIs in adults with mild to moderate renal impairment; efficacy not studied in severe renal impairment.
- Dosage adjustment unnecessary when extended-release tablets (Cipro® XR) are used for uncomplicated UTIs (acute cystitis), but dosage of this preparation should be reduced when used for complicated UTIs or acute uncomplicated pyelonephritis in adults with Cl_{cr} <30 mL/minute. (See Table.)
- If available, measurement of serum ciprofloxacin concentrations is the most reliable method for determining dosage, especially in those with severe renal impairment, changing renal function, or both renal and hepatic impairment. Peak ciprofloxacin concentrations (1–2 hours after an oral dose) generally should range from 2–4 mcg/mL.

Dosage of Conventional Tablets or Oral Suspension in Adults with Renal Impairment

Cl_{cr} (mL/min)	Dosage
30–50	250–500 mg every 12 hours
30–50 (with severe infections)	750 mg every 12 hours
5–29	250–500 mg every 18 hours
5–29 (with severe infections)	750 mg every 18 hours
Hemodialysis or Peritoneal Dialysis Patients	250–500 mg once every 24 hours; give dose after dialysis

Dosage of Extended-release Tablets (Cipro® XR) in Adults with Renal Impairment

Cl_{cr} (mL/min)	Dosage
<30 (Uncomplicated UTI; Acute Cystitis)	No dosage adjustment needed
<30 (Complicated UTI or Acute Uncomplicated Pyelonephritis)	500 mg once daily
Hemodialysis or Peritoneal Dialysis Patients	Give dose after dialysis period

Geriatric Patients
- No dosage adjustments except those related to renal impairment.
- Select dosage with caution because of age-related decreases in renal impairment.

† *Use is not currently included in the labeling approved by the US Food and Drug Administration.*

Ciprofloxacin and Dexamethasone Otic

(sip roe flox′ a sin) and (dex a meth′ a sone)

Brand Name: Ciprodex®

Why is this medicine prescribed?

Ciprofloxacin and dexamethasone otic is used to treat outer ear infections in adults and children and acute (suddenly occurring) middle ear infections in children with ear tubes. Ciprofloxacin is in a class of medications called quinolone antibiotics. Dexamethasone is in a class of medications called corticosteroids. The combination of ciprofloxacin and dexamethasone works by killing the bacteria that cause infection and reducing swelling in the ear.

How should this medicine be used?

Ciprofloxacin and dexamethasone otic comes as a suspension (liquid) to place into the ear. It is usually used twice a day, in the morning and evening, for 7 days. Use ciprofloxacin and dexamethasone otic at around the same times every day. Follow the directions on your prescription label carefully, and ask your doctor or pharmacist to explain any part you do not understand. Use ciprofloxacin and dexamethasone otic exactly as directed. Do not use more or less of it or use it more often than prescribed by your doctor.

Ciprofloxacin and dexamethasone otic is only for use in the ears. Do not use in the eyes.

You should begin to feel better during the first few days of treatment with ciprofloxacin otic. If your symptoms do not improve after one week or get worse, call your doctor.

Use ciprofloxacin and dexamethasone otic until you finish the prescription, even if you feel better. If you stop using ciprofloxacin and dexamethasone otic too soon or skip doses, your infection may not be completely treated and the bacteria may become resistant to antibiotics.

To use the eardrops, follow these steps:
1. Hold the bottle in your hand for one or two minutes to warm the solution.
2. Shake the bottle well.
3. Lie down with the affected ear upward.
4. Place the prescribed number of drops into your ear.
5. Be careful not to touch the tip to your ear, fingers, or any other surface.
6. For middle ear infections, push the tragus (small flap of cartilage just in front of the ear canal near the face) of the ear inward four times so that the drops will enter the middle ear.
7. Remain lying down with the affected ear upward for 60 seconds.
8. Repeat steps 1-7 for the opposite ear if necessary.

What special precautions should I follow?

Before using ciprofloxacin and dexamethasone otic,

- tell your doctor and pharmacist if you are allergic to ciprofloxacin (Cipro), dexamethasone (Decadron), cinoxacin (Cinobac) (not available in the U.S.), enoxacin (Penetrex) (not available in the U.S.), gatifloxacin (Tequin) (not available in the U.S.), gemifloxacin (Factive), levofloxacin (Levaquin), lomefloxacin (Maxaquin), moxifloxacin (Avelox), nalidixic acid (NegGram), norfloxacin (Noroxin), ofloxacin (Floxin), sparfloxacin (Zagam) (not available in the U.S.), trovafloxacin and alatrofloxacin combination (Trovan) (not available in the U.S.), or any other medications.
- tell your doctor and pharmacist what prescription and nonprescription medications, vitamins, nutritional supplements, and herbal products you are taking or plan to take.
- tell your doctor if you are pregnant, plan to become pregnant, or are breast-feeding. If you become pregnant while using ciprofloxacin and dexamethasone otic, call your doctor.
- you should know that you must keep your infected ear(s) clean and dry while using ciprofloxacin and dexamethasone otic. Avoid getting the infected ear(s) wet while bathing, and avoid swimming unless your doctor has told you otherwise.

What special dietary instructions should I follow?

Unless your doctor tells you otherwise, continue your normal diet.

What should I do if I forget to take a dose?

Apply the missed dose as soon as you remember it. However, if it is almost time for the next dose, skip the missed dose and continue your regular dosing schedule. Do not use extra eardrops to make up for a missed dose.

What side effects can this medicine cause?

Ciprofloxacin and dexamethasone otic may cause side effects. Tell your doctor if any of these symptoms are severe or do not go away:

- ear discomfort, pain, or itching

Some side effects can be serious. If you experience any of these symptoms, stop using ciprofloxacin and dexamethasone otic and call your doctor immediately:

- rash
- hives
- swelling of the face, throat, tongue, lips, eyes, hands, feet, ankles, or lower legs
- hoarseness
- difficulty swallowing or breathing

Ciprofloxacin and dexamethasone otic may cause other side effects. Call your doctor if you have any unusual problems while taking this medication.

What storage conditions are needed for this medicine?

Keep this medication in the container it came in, tightly closed, and out of reach of children. Store it at room temperature and away from excess heat and moisture (not in the bathroom). Do not freeze and protect from light. Throw away any medication that is outdated or no longer needed. Talk to your pharmacist about the proper disposal of your medication.

What should I do in case of overdose?

If someone swallows ciprofloxacin and dexamethasone otic, call your local poison control center at 1-800-222-1222. If the victim has collapsed or is not breathing, call local emergency services at 911.

What other information should I know?

Keep all appointments with your doctor.

Do not let anyone else use your medication. Your prescription is probably not refillable.

Dosage Facts
For Informational Purposes

Caution: Do not change your dose, how often you take your medication, or the length of time you are to take it without first talking to your healthcare provider.

The following dosage information was written using medical language for doctors and other healthcare professionals and is provided here for you to check your dosage. The dosage of this drug may differ for different patients. Therefore, always follow your doctor's instructions or the directions on the label. Contact your healthcare provider or pharmacist if you have any questions about the specific dosage of your medication after reviewing this information.

General Dosage Information

Available as ciprofloxacin hydrochloride; dosage expressed in terms of ciprofloxacin.

Pediatric Patients

Otic Infections
Otitis Externa (*S. aureus* or *Ps. aeruginosa*)

OTIC:
- Ciprofloxacin-dexamethasone otic suspension: In children ≥6 months of age, 4 drops into canal of affected ear(s) twice daily for 7 days.

Otitis Media (Acute)

OTIC:
- Ciprofloxacin-dexamethasone otic suspension: In children ≥6 months of age, 4 drops into affected ear(s) twice daily through tympanostomy tube for 7 days.

Adult Patients

Otic Infections
Otitis Externa (S. aureus or Ps. aeruginosa)

OTIC:
- Ciprofloxacin-dexamethasone otic suspension: 4 drops into canal of affected ear(s) twice daily for 7 days.

Ciprofloxacin and Hydrocortisone Otic

(sip roe flox′ a sin and hye droe kor′ ti sone)

Brand Name: Cipro HC Otic®

Why is this medicine prescribed?

Ciprofloxacin and hydrocortisone otic is used to treat outer ear infections in adults and children. Ciprofloxacin is in a class of medications called quinolone antibiotics. Hydrocortisone is in a class of medications called corticosteroids. The combination of ciprofloxacin and hydrocortisone works by killing the bacteria that cause infection and reducing swelling in the ear.

How should this medicine be used?

Ciprofloxacin and hydrocortisone otic comes as a suspension (liquid) to place into the ear. It is usually used twice a day, in the morning and evening, for 7 days. Use ciprofloxacin and hydrocortisone otic at around the same times every day. Follow the directions on your prescription label carefully, and ask your doctor or pharmacist to explain any part you do not understand. Use ciprofloxacin and hydrocortisone otic exactly as directed. Do not use more or less of it or use it more often than prescribed by your doctor.

Ciprofloxacin and hydrocortisone otic is only for use in the ears. Do not use in the eyes.

You should begin to feel better during the first few days of treatment with ciprofloxacin and hydrocortisone otic. If your symptoms do not improve after one week or get worse, call your doctor.

Use ciprofloxacin and hydrocortisone otic until you finish the prescription, even if you feel better. If you stop using ciprofloxacin and hydrocortisone otic too soon or skip doses, your infection may not be completely treated and the bacteria may become resistant to antibiotics.

To use the eardrops, follow these steps:
1. Hold the bottle in your hand for 1 or 2 minutes to warm the solution.
2. Shake the bottle well.
3. Lie down with the affected ear upward.
4. Place the prescribed number of drops into your ear.
5. Be careful not to touch the tip to your ear, fingers, or any other surface.

6. Remain lying down with the affected ear upward for 30-60 seconds.
7. Repeat steps 1-6 for the opposite ear if necessary.

Are there other uses for this medicine?

This medication may be prescribed for other uses; ask your doctor or pharmacist for more information.

What special precautions should I follow?

Before using ciprofloxacin and hydrocortisone otic,
- tell your doctor and pharmacist if you are allergic to ciprofloxacin (Cipro), hydrocortisone (Cortaid, Cortef, Cortizone, Hytone), cinoxacin (Cinobac) (not available in the U.S.), enoxacin (Penetrex) (not available in the U.S.), gatifloxacin (Tequin) (not available in the U.S.), gemifloxacin (Factive), levofloxacin (Levaquin), lomefloxacin (Maxaquin), moxifloxacin (Avelox), nalidixic acid (NegGram), norfloxacin (Noroxin), ofloxacin (Floxin), sparfloxacin (Zagam) (not available in the U.S.), trovafloxacin and alatrofloxacin combination (Trovan) (not available in the U.S.), or any other medications.
- tell your doctor and pharmacist what prescription and nonprescription medications, vitamins, nutritional supplements, and herbal products you are taking or plan to take.
- tell your doctor if you have a hole in your ear drum(s) or ear tube(s). Your doctor will tell you not to use this medication.
- tell your doctor if you are pregnant, plan to become pregnant, or are breast-feeding. If you become pregnant while using ciprofloxacin and hydrocortisone otic, call your doctor.
- you should know that you must keep your infected ear(s) clean and dry while using ciprofloxacin and hydrocortisone otic. Avoid getting the infected ear(s) wet while bathing, and avoid swimming unless your doctor has told you otherwise.

What special dietary instructions should I follow?

Unless your doctor tells you otherwise, continue your normal diet.

What should I do if I forget to take a dose?

Apply the missed dose as soon as you remember it. However, if it is almost time for the next dose, skip the missed dose and continue your regular dosing schedule. Do not use extra eardrops to make up for a missed dose.

What side effects can this medicine cause?

Ciprofloxacin and hydrocortisone otic may cause side effects. Tell your doctor if the following symptom is severe or does not go away:
- headache

Some side effects can be serious. If you experience any of these symptoms, stop using ciprofloxacin and hydrocortisone otic and call your doctor immediately:

- rash
- hives
- swelling of the face, throat, tongue, lips, eyes, hands, feet, ankles, or lower legs
- hoarseness
- difficulty swallowing or breathing

Ciprofloxacin and hydrocortisone otic may cause other side effects. Call your doctor if you have any unusual problems while taking this medication.

What storage conditions are needed for this medicine?

Keep this medication in the container it came in, tightly closed, and out of reach of children. Store it at room temperature and away from excess heat and moisture (not in the bathroom). Avoid freezing and protect from light. Throw away any medication that is outdated or no longer needed. Talk to your pharmacist about the proper disposal of your medication.

What should I do in case of overdose?

If someone swallows ciprofloxacin and hydrocortisone otic, call your local poison control center at 1-800-222-1222. If the victim has collapsed or is not breathing, call local emergency services at 911.

What other information should I know?

Keep all appointments with your doctor.

Do not let anyone else use your medication. Your prescription is probably not refillable.

Dosage Facts

For Informational Purposes

Caution: Do not change your dose, how often you take your medication, or the length of time you are to take it without first talking to your healthcare provider.

The following dosage information was written using medical language for doctors and other healthcare professionals and is provided here for you to check your dosage. The dosage of this drug may differ for different patients. Therefore, always follow your doctor's instructions or the directions on the label. Contact your healthcare provider or pharmacist if you have any questions about the specific dosage of your medication after reviewing this information.

General Dosage Information

Available as ciprofloxacin hydrochloride; dosage expressed in terms of ciprofloxacin.

Pediatric Patients

Otic Infections

Otitis Externa (S. aureus, Ps. aeruginosa, or P. mirabilis)

OTIC:

- Ciprofloxacin-hydrocortisone otic suspension: In children ≥1 year of age, 3 drops into canal of affected ear(s) twice daily for 7 days.

Adult Patients

Otic Infections

Otitis Externa (S. aureus, Ps. aeruginosa, or P. mirabilis)

OTIC:

- Ciprofloxacin-hydrocortisone otic suspension: 3 drops into canal of affected ear(s) twice daily for 7 days.

Ciprofloxacin Injection

(sip roe flox′ a sin)

Brand Name: Cipro®I.V.

Why is this medicine prescribed?

Ciprofloxacin is an antibiotic used to treat certain infections caused by bacteria. Ciprofloxacin is also used to prevent or treat anthrax in people who may have been exposed to anthrax germs in the air. Ciprofloxacin is in a class of antibiotics called fluoroquinolones. It works by killing bacteria. Antibiotics will not work for colds, flu, or other viral infections.

How should this medicine be used?

Ciprofloxacin injection comes as a solution (liquid) to be given through a needle or catheter placed in your vein. It is usually infused (injected slowly) intravenously (into a vein) over a period of 60 minutes, usually every 8 to 12 hours. Ciprofloxacin injection should be infused at around the same times every day. Follow the directions on your prescription label carefully, and ask your doctor or other health care provider to explain any part you do not understand. Use ciprofloxacin injection exactly as directed. Do not infuse it more quickly than directed, and do not use more or less of it, or use it more often than prescribed by your doctor. If this medication is infused more quickly than directed, there may be damage to the vein or to the skin near the injection area.

If you will be administering ciprofloxacin injection at home, your health care provider will show you how to infuse the medication. Be sure that you understand these directions, and ask your health care provider if you have any questions. Ask your health care provider what to do if you have any problems administering ciprofloxacin injection.

Before you administer ciprofloxacin, look at the solution closely. It should be clear and free of floating material.

Gently squeeze the bag or observe the solution container to make sure there are no leaks. Do not use the solution if it is discolored, if it contains particles, or if the bag or container leaks. Use a new solution, but show the damaged one to your health care provider.

Do not infuse ciprofloxacin into a vein at the same time as you infuse any other medication.

You should begin feeling better during the first few days of your treatment with ciprofloxacin. If your symptoms do not improve, or if they get worse, call your doctor.

Use ciprofloxacin until you finish the prescription, even if you feel better. If you stop using ciprofloxacin too soon or if you skip doses, your infection may not be completely treated and the bacteria may become resistant to antibiotics.

After you use one or more doses of ciprofloxacin injection, your doctor may tell you to start taking ciprofloxacin tablets or liquid by mouth instead of using ciprofloxacin injection. Make sure you understand and follow your doctor's directions.

Are there other uses for this medicine?

In the event of biological warfare, ciprofloxacin may be used to treat and prevent dangerous illnesses that are deliberately spread such as plague, tularemia, and anthrax of the skin or mouth. Talk to your doctor about the risks of using this medication for your condition.

This medication may be prescribed for other uses; ask your doctor or pharmacist for more information.

What special precautions should I follow?

Before using ciprofloxacin injection,
- tell your doctor and pharmacist if you are allergic or have had a severe reaction to ciprofloxacin; or any other quinolone or fluoroquinolone antibiotics such as gatifloxacin (Tequin) (not available in the U.S.), gemifloxacin (Factive), levofloxacin (Levaquin), lomefloxacin (Maxaquin), moxifloxacin (Avelox), nalidixic acid (NegGram), norfloxacin (Noroxin), and ofloxacin (Floxin); or if you are allergic to any other medications.
- tell your doctor if you are taking tizanidine (Zanaflex). Your doctor will probably tell you not take ciprofloxacin while you are taking this medication.
- tell your doctor and pharmacist what other prescription and nonprescription medications, vitamins, nutritional supplements, and herbal products you are taking or plan to take. Be sure to mention any of the following: acetazolamide (Diamox); anticoagulants ('blood thinners') such as warfarin (Coumadin); brinzolamide (Azopt); caffeine or medications that contain caffeine (NoDoz, Vivarin, others); cyclosporine (Neoral, Sandimmune); dorzolamide (Trusopt); glyburide (DiaBeta, Glucovance, Micronase, others); medications for diarrhea, such as dicyclomine (Bentyl), diphenoxylate (Lomotil), and loperamide (Immodium); methazolamide; methotrexate (Rheumatrex, Trexall); nonsteroidal anti-inflammatory medications (NSAIDs) such as ibuprofen (Advil, Mo-

trin) and naproxen (Aleve, Naprosyn); oral steroids such as dexamethasone (Decadron, Dexone), methylprednisolone (Medrol), and prednisone (Deltasone); phenytoin (Dilantin, Phenytek); potassium citrate and citric acid (Cytra-K, Polycitra-K); probenecid (Benemid); sodium bicarbonate (Soda Mint, baking soda); sodium citrate and citric acid (Bicitra, Oracit, Shohl's Solution); or theophylline (Theobid, Theo-Dur), Slo-bid, others). Many other medications may also interact with ciprofloxacin, so be sure to tell your doctor about all the medications you are taking, even those that do not appear on this list. Your doctor may need to change the doses of your medications or monitor you carefully for side effects.
- tell your doctor if you have or have ever had arthritis or other joint disease, cerebral palsy (CP, a condition of abnormal muscle or motor function), dementia (a condition associated with memory loss and personality changes), recent head injury, seizures, stroke or ministroke, or kidney or liver disease.
- tell your doctor if you have ever had tendonitis (swelling or tearing of the fiber that connects a bone to a muscle) and if you participate in regular athletic activity. There is a risk that you will develop tendonitis while you are using ciprofloxacin, especially if you are also taking steroid medications. If you experience symptoms of tendonitis, such as pain, swelling, tenderness, stiffness, or difficulty in moving a muscle, stop taking ciprofloxacin, rest, and call your doctor immediately.
- tell your doctor if you are pregnant, plan to become pregnant, or are breast-feeding. If you become pregnant while using ciprofloxacin, call your doctor.
- if you are having surgery, including dental surgery, tell the doctor or dentist that you are being treated with ciprofloxacin.
- if you are having a radiologic test (X-ray, CT scan) that involves dye, tell the doctor or health care professional that you are using ciprofloxacin.
- you should know that ciprofloxacin may make cause confusion, dizziness, lightheadedness, and tiredness. Do not drive a car or operate machinery or participate in activities requiring alertness or coordination until you know how this medication affects you.
- plan to avoid unnecessary or prolonged exposure to sunlight or ultraviolet light (tanning beds) and to wear protective clothing, sunglasses, and sunscreen. Ciprofloxacin may make your skin sensitive to sunlight or ultraviolet light. If your skin becomes reddened, like a bad sunburn, stop using ciprofloxacin and call your doctor.

What special dietary instructions should I follow?

Do not drink or eat a lot of caffeine-containing products such as coffee, tea, energy drinks, cola, or chocolate. Ciprofloxacin may increase nervousness, sleeplessness, heart pounding, and anxiety caused by caffeine.

Make sure you drink plenty of water or other fluids every day while you are using ciprofloxacin.

What should I do if I forget to take a dose?

Infuse the missed dose as soon as you remember it. However, if it is almost time for the next dose, skip the missed dose and continue your regular dosing schedule. Do not infuse a double dose to make up for a missed one.

What side effects can this medicine cause?

Ciprofloxacin may cause side effects. Tell your doctor if any of these symptoms are severe or do not go away:

- nausea
- vomiting
- stomach pain
- indigestion
- diarrhea
- headache
- nervousness
- restlessness
- feelings of not trusting others or feeling that others want to hurt you
- difficulty falling asleep or staying asleep
- nightmares
- irritation, pain, tenderness, redness, warmth, or swelling at the injection spot

Some side effects can be serious. If you experience any of these symptoms, stop using ciprofloxacin, and call your doctor immediately:

- rash or blisters
- hives
- itching
- swelling of the face, neck, throat, tongue, lips, eyes, hands, feet, ankles, or lower legs
- difficulty breathing or swallowing
- hoarseness
- fast, irregular, or pounding heart beat
- fainting
- fever
- joint or muscle pain
- unusual bruising or bleeding
- extreme tiredness
- lack of energy
- loss of appetite
- pain in the upper right part of the stomach
- yellowing of the skin or eyes
- seizures
- dizziness
- double vision
- pulsing sounds in the head or ringing in the ears
- confusion
- uncontrollable shaking of a part of the body
- hallucinations (seeing things or hearing voices that do not exist)
- depression
- thoughts about killing yourself

- pain, burning, tingling, numbness, and/or weakness in a part of the body
- loss of muscle strength in a part of the body
- loss of ability to feel light touch, pain, hot or cold, or vibration in a part of the body
- loss of ability to know position of a part of the body

Ciprofloxacin should not normally be given to children younger than 18 years old unless they have certain serious infections that cannot be treated with other antibiotics or they have been exposed to anthrax in the air. If your doctor prescribes ciprofloxacin for your child, be sure to tell the doctor if your child has or has ever had joint-related problems. Call your doctor if your child develops joint problems while using ciprofloxacin or after treatment with ciprofloxacin. Talk to your child's doctor about the risks of giving ciprofloxacin to your child.

Ciprofloxacin may cause other side effects. Call your doctor if you have any unusual problems while using this medication.

What storage conditions are needed for this medicine?

Your health care provider will probably tell you to store your medication at room temperature. Store your medication only as directed. Make sure you understand how to store your medication properly. Throw away any medication that is expired or no longer needed. Talk to your health care provider about the proper disposal of your medication.

Keep your supplies in a clean, dry place out of the reach of children when you are not using them. Your health care provider will tell you how to throw away used needles, syringes, tubing, and containers to avoid accidental injury.

What should I do in case of overdose?

In case of overdose, call your local poison control center at 1-800-222-1222. If the victim has collapsed or is not breathing, call local emergency services at 911.

What other information should I know?

Keep all appointments with your doctor. Your doctor may order certain lab tests to check your body's response to ciprofloxacin.

Do not let anyone else use your medication. If you still have symptoms of infection after you finish the ciprofloxacin, call your doctor.

Dosage Facts
For Informational Purposes

Caution: Do not change your dose, how often you take your medication, or the length of time you are to take it without first talking to your healthcare provider.

The following dosage information was written using medical language for doctors and other healthcare pro-

fessionals and is provided here for you to check your dosage. The dosage of this drug may differ for different patients. Therefore, always follow your doctor's instructions or the directions on the label. Contact your healthcare provider or pharmacist if you have any questions about the specific dosage of your medication after reviewing this information.

General Dosage Information

Available as ciprofloxacin, ciprofloxacin hydrochloride, a mixture of ciprofloxacin and ciprofloxacin hydrochloride, and as ciprofloxacin lactate; dosage expressed in terms of ciprofloxacin.

Extended-release tablet preparations (Cipro® XR, ProQuin® XR) are used *only* for the treatment of certain urinary tract infections (UTIs). These extended-release preparations are *not* interchangeable with each other and are *not* interchangeable with other oral ciprofloxacin preparations (conventional tablets, oral suspension).

Based on pharmacokinetic parameters (i.e., AUC), the following regimens are considered equivalent: ciprofloxacin conventional tablets 250 mg every 12 hours—ciprofloxacin 200 mg IV every 12 hours; ciprofloxacin conventional tablets 500 mg every 12 hours—ciprofloxacin 400 mg IV every 12 hours; ciprofloxacin conventional tablets 750 mg every 12 hours—ciprofloxacin 400 mg IV every 8 hours.

Pediatric Patients

Urinary Tract Infections (UTIs)
Complicated UTIs and Pyelonephritis

IV:
- Children 1–17 years of age: 6–10 mg/kg (up to 400 mg) every 8 hours. Switch to oral route when clinically indicated; total duration of IV and oral therapy 10–21 days.

Endocarditis†
Endocarditis Caused by the HACEK Group†

IV:
- 20–30 mg/kg daily given in 2 equally divided doses recommended by AHA and IDSA. Duration of treatment is 4 weeks for native valve endocarditis or 6 weeks for endocarditis involving prosthetic cardiac valves or other prosthetic cardiac material.

Culture-negative Endocarditis†

IV:
- 20–30 mg/kg daily given in 2 equally divided doses in conjunction with vancomycin (40 mg/kg daily given IV in 2 equally divided doses) and gentamicin (3 mg/kg daily given IM or IV in 3 equally divided doses) recommended by AHA and IDSA. All 3 drugs should be given for 4–6 weeks.

Meningitis and CNS Infections†
Salmonella Meningitis†

IV:
- 10–30 mg/kg daily has been given alone or in conjunction with cefotaxmine.

Anthrax
Postexposure Prophylaxis Following Exposure in the Context of Biologic Warfare or Bioterrorism

IV:
- 10 mg/kg (up to 400 mg) every 12 hours for ≥60 days.

Treatment of Inhalational, GI, or Oropharyngeal Anthrax†

IV, THEN ORAL:
- 10 mg/kg (up to 400 mg) IV every 12 hours.
- Used in conjunction with 1 or 2 other anti-infectives predicted to be effective. When clinical improvement occurs, switch IV ciprofloxacin to oral ciprofloxacin in a dosage of 15 mg/kg (up to 500 mg) twice daily and continue for a total duration of ≥60 days. Because of concerns regarding long-term use of ciprofloxacin in infants and children, consider changing (after 10–14 days) to amoxicillin to complete the treatment regimen if penicillin susceptibility is confirmed.

Treatment of Cutaneous Anthrax†

IV, THEN ORAL:
- 10 mg/kg (up to 400 mg) IV every 12 hours.
- Used in conjunction with 1 or 2 other anti-infectives predicted to be effective. When clinical improvement occurs, switch IV ciprofloxacin to oral ciprofloxacin in a dosage of 500 mg twice daily and continue for a total duration of ≥60 days. Because of concerns regarding long-term use of ciprofloxacin in infants and children, consider changing (after 10–14 days) to amoxicillin to complete the treatment regimen if penicillin susceptibility is confirmed.

Gonorrhea and Associated Infections†
Disseminated Gonococcal Infection†

IV, THEN ORAL:
- Adolescents and children weighing >45 kg: 400 mg IV every 12 hours has been used for initial treatment. IV regimen is continued for 24–48 hours after improvement begins, then switched to 500 mg orally twice daily to complete ≥1 week of treatment.
- Because of increased prevalence of QRNG, CDC no longer recommends ciprofloxacin or other fluoroquinolones for treatment of gonorrhea or any associated infections involving *N. gonorrhoeae* (e.g., PID, epididymitis). Use as an alternative treatment option for disseminated infections *only* if in vitro susceptibility can be documented by culture.
- Unless the presence of coexisting chlamydial infection has been excluded by appropriate testing, patients being treated for gonorrhea also should receive an anti-infective regimen effective for presumptive treatment of chlamydia (e.g., a single dose of oral azithromycin or a 7-day regimen of oral doxycycline).

Plague†
Treatment of Pneumonic Plague Occurring in Context of Biologic Warfare or Bioterrorism†

IV, THEN ORAL:
- 15 mg/kg IV twice daily. When clinical improvement occurs, IV ciprofloxacin may be switched to oral ciprofloxacin in a dosage of 20 mg/kg twice daily.
- Usual duration of treatment is 10 days; some experts recommend a duration of at least 10–14 days.

Tularemia†
Treatment of Tularemia Occurring in the Context of Biologic Warfare or Bioterrorism†

IV, THEN ORAL:
- 15 mg/kg IV twice daily.
- When clinical improvement occurs, switch IV ciprofloxacin to oral ciprofloxacin in a dosage of 15 mg/kg twice daily.

Usual total duration of treatment is 10 days; some experts recommend a duration of at least 10–14 days.

Adult Patients

Bone and Joint Infections
Mild to Moderate Infections

IV:
- 400 mg every 12 hours for ≥4–6 weeks.

Severe or Complicated Infections

IV:
- 400 mg every 8 hours for ≥4–6 weeks.

Endocarditis†
Endocarditis Caused by the HACEK Group†

IV:
- 800 mg daily given in 2 equally divided doses recommended by AHA and IDSA. Duration of treatment is 4 weeks for native valve endocarditis or 6 weeks for endocarditis involving prosthetic cardiac valves or other prosthetic cardiac material.

Culture-negative Endocarditis†

IV:
- 800 mg daily given in 2 equally divided doses in conjunction with vancomycin (30 mg/kg daily given IV in 2 equally divided doses) and gentamicin (3 mg/kg daily given IM or IV in 3 equally divided doses) recommended by AHA and IDSA. All 3 drugs should be given for 4–6 weeks.

Intra-abdominal Infections
Complicated Infections

IV, THEN ORAL:
- Initiate therapy with 400 mg IV every 12 hours given in conjunction with IV metronidazole. When appropriate, switch to oral ciprofloxacin in a dosage of 500 mg every 12 hours in conjunction with oral metronidazole. Total duration of therapy is 7–14 days.

Meningitis and CNS Infections†
Gram-negative Meningitis†

IV:
- 400 mg every 8 hours has been used alone or in conjunction with an aminoglycoside. Alternatively, 800–1200 mg daily has been recommended.

Respiratory Tract Infections
Acute Sinusitis

IV:
- 400 mg every 12 hours for 10 days.

Mild to Moderate Infections

IV:
- 400 mg every 12 hours for 7–14 days.

Severe or Complicated Infections

IV:
- 400 mg every 8 hours for 7–14 days.

Mild, Moderate, or Severe Nosocomial Pneumonia

IV:
- 400 mg every 8 hours for 10–14 days.

Skin and Skin Structure Infections
Mild to Moderate Infections

IV:
- 400 mg every 12 hours for 7–14 days.

Severe or Complicated Infections

IV:
- 400 mg every 8 hours for 7–14 days.

Urinary Tract Infections (UTIs) and Prostatitis
Mild to Moderate UTIs

IV:
- 200 mg every 12 hours for 7–14 days.

Complicated UTIs

IV:
- 400 mg every 12 hours for 7–14 days.

Mild to Moderate Chronic Prostatitis

IV:
- 400 mg every 12 hours for 28 days.

Anthrax
Postexposure Prophylaxis Following Exposure in the Context of Biologic Warfare or Bioterrorism

IV:
- 400 mg every 12 hours for ≥60 days.

Treatment of Inhalational, GI, or Oropharyngeal Anthrax†

IV, THEN ORAL:
- 400 mg IV every 12 hours.
- Used in conjunction with 1 or 2 other anti-infectives predicted to be effective. When clinical improvement occurs, switch IV ciprofloxacin to oral ciprofloxacin in a dosage of 500 mg twice daily and continue for a total duration of ≥60 days.

Treatment of Cutaneous Anthrax†

IV, THEN ORAL:
- 400 mg IV every 12 hours.
- Used in conjunction with 1 or 2 other anti-infectives predicted to be effective. When clinical improvement occurs, switch IV ciprofloxacin to oral ciprofloxacin in a dosage of 500 mg twice daily and continue for a total duration of ≥60 days.

Gonorrhea and Associated Infections
Disseminated Gonococcal Infections†

IV, THEN ORAL:
- 400 mg IV every 12 hours has been used for initial treatment. IV regimen is continued for 24–48 hours after improvement begins, then switched to 500 mg orally twice daily to complete ≥1 week of treatment.
- Because of increased prevalence of QRNG, CDC no longer recommends ciprofloxacin or other fluoroquinolones for treatment of gonorrhea or any associated infections involving *N. gonorrhoeae* (e.g., pelvic inflammatory disease [PID], epididymitis). Use as an alternative treatment option for disseminated infections *only* if in vitro susceptibility can be documented by culture.
- Unless the presence of coexisting chlamydial infection has been excluded by appropriate testing, patients being treated for gonorrhea also should receive an anti-infective regimen effective for presumptive treatment of chlamydia (e.g., a single dose of oral azithromycin or a 7-day regimen of oral doxycycline).

Legionnaires' Disease†

IV:
- 400 mg every 12 hours for 2–3 weeks.

Plague†
Treatment of Pneumonic Plague Occurring in Context of Biologic Warfare or Bioterrorism†

IV, THEN ORAL;
- 400 mg twice daily. When clinical improvement occurs, IV ciprofloxacin may be switched to oral ciprofloxacin in a dosage of 500 mg twice daily.
- Usual duration of treatment is 10 days; some experts recommend a duration of at least 10–14 days.

Tularemia†
Treatment of Tularemia Occurring in the Context of Biologic Warfare or Bioterrorism†

IV, THEN ORAL:
- 400 mg IV twice daily.
- When clinical improvement occurs, switch IV ciprofloxacin to oral ciprofloxacin in a dosage of 500 mg twice daily. Usual total duration of treatment is 10 days; some experts recommend a duration of at least 10–14 days.

Perioperative Prophylaxis†

IV:
- Single 400-mg dose given prior to the procedure. Begin IV infusion 1–2 hours prior to time of incision.

Empiric Therapy in Febrile Neutropenic Patients

IV:
- 400 mg every 8 hours; used in conjunction with IV piperacillin (50 mg/kg every 4 hours, not to exceed 24 g/daily or 300 mg/kg daily).
- Usual duration of treatment is 7–14 days.

Prescribing Limits

Pediatric Patients

Urinary Tract Infections (UTIs)
Complicated UTIs and Pyelonephritis

IV:
- Children 1–17 years of age: Maximum 400 mg every 8 hours, even in those weighing >51 kg.

Anthrax
Postexposure Prophylaxis Following Exposure in the Context of Biologic Warfare or Bioterrorism

IV:
- Maximum 400 mg every 12 hours.

Adult Patients

Do not exceed usual dosage because of risk of crystalluria.

Special Populations

Hepatic Impairment
- Dosage adjustments not required in patients with stable chronic cirrhosis; pharmacokinetics not fully studied in those with acute hepatic insufficiency.
- Monitor ciprofloxacin concentrations in patients with both hepatic and renal impairment.

Renal Impairment
- Dosage adjustments may be necessary in adults with renal impairment, especially those with severe impairment. Dosage recommendations not available for pediatric patients with moderate to severe renal impairment (Cl_{cr} <50 mL/minute per 1.73 m²).

- If available, measurement of serum ciprofloxacin concentrations is the most reliable method for determining dosage, especially in those with severe renal impairment, changing renal function, or both renal and hepatic impairment. Peak ciprofloxacin concentrations (1–2 hours after an oral dose or immediately after completion of IV infusion) generally should range from 2–4 mcg/mL.

IV Dosage in Adults with Renal Impairment

Cl_{cr} (mL/min)	Dosage
5–29	200–400 mg every 18–24 hours

Geriatric Patients
- No dosage adjustments except those related to renal impairment.
- Select dosage with caution because of age-related decreases in renal impairment.

† *Use is not currently included in the labeling approved by the US Food and Drug Administration.*

Ciprofloxacin Ophthalmic

(sip roe flox′ a sin)

Brand Name: Ciloxan®
Also available generically.

Why is this medicine prescribed?

Ciprofloxacin ophthalmic solution is used to treat bacterial infections of the eye including conjunctivitis (pinkeye; infection of the membrane that covers the outside of the eyeball and the inside of the eyelid) and corneal ulcers (infection and loss of tissue in the clear front part of the eye). Ciprofloxacin ophthalmic ointment is used to treat conjunctivitis. Ciprofloxacin is in a class of antibiotics called fluoroquinolones. It works by killing the bacteria that cause infection.

How should this medicine be used?

Ophthalmic ciprofloxacin comes as a solution (eye drops) and an ointment to apply to the eyes. Ciprofloxacin ophthalmic solution is usually used often, between once every 15 minutes to once every 4 hours while awake for 7 to 14 days or longer. Ciprofloxacin ophthalmic ointment is usually applied 3 times a day for 2 days and then twice a day for 5 days. To help you remember to use ophthalmic ciprofloxacin, use it at around the same times every day. Follow the directions on your prescription label carefully, and ask your doctor or pharmacist to explain any part you do not understand. Use ophthalmic ciprofloxacin exactly as directed. Do not use more or less of it or use it more often than prescribed by your doctor.

You should expect your symptoms to improve during your treatment. Call your doctor if your symptoms do not go away or get worse, or if you develop other problems with your eyes during your treatment.

Use ophthalmic ciprofloxacin until you finish the prescription, even if you feel better. If you stop using ophthalmic ciprofloxacin too soon, your infection may not be completely cured and the bacteria may become resistant to antibiotics.

When you use ophthalmic ciprofloxacin, be careful not to let the tip of the bottle or tube touch your eye, fingers, face, or any surface. If the tip does touch another surface, bacteria may get into the eye ointment or drops. Using eye ointment or drops that are contaminated with bacteria may cause serious damage to the eye or loss of vision. If you think your eye ointment or drops have become contaminated, call your doctor or pharmacist.

To use the eye drops or ointment, follow these steps:

1. Wash your hands thoroughly with soap and water.
2. Use a mirror or have someone else put the drops or ointment in your eye(s).
3. Remove the protective cap from the bottle or tube. Make sure that the end of the dropper tip is not chipped or cracked.
4. If you are using eye drops, hold the bottle with the tip down at all times to prevent drops from flowing back into the bottle and contaminating the medication inside.
5. Lie down and gaze upward or tilt your head back.
6. Holding the bottle or tube between your thumb and index finger, place the dropper tip or end of the tube as near as possible to your eyelid without touching it.
7. Brace the remaining fingers of that hand against your cheek or nose.
8. With the index finger of your other hand, pull the lower lid of the eye down to form a pocket.
9. If you are using the eye drops, drop the prescribed number of drops into the pocket made by the lower lid and the eye. Placing drops on the surface of the eyeball can cause stinging. Then close your eye and press lightly against the lower lid with your finger for 2-3 minutes to keep the medication in the eye. Do not blink. Use a clean tissue to wipe any excess liquid from your cheek.
10. If you are using the ointment, squeeze a thin ribbon of ointment into the pocket. Blink gently and close your eye for 1-2 minutes. Use a clean tissue to wipe excess ointment from your eyelids or eyelashes.
11. If your doctor told you to use ciprofloxacin eye drops or ointment in both eyes, repeat steps 6-10 above for your other eye.
12. Replace the cap on the tube or bottle and tighten it right away.
13. Wash your hands again.

Are there other uses for this medicine?

This medication may be prescribed for other uses; ask your doctor or pharmacist for more information.

What special precautions should I follow?

Before using ophthalmic ciprofloxacin,

- tell your doctor and pharmacist if you are allergic to ciprofloxacin (Cipro, Ciloxan), other quinolone antibiotics such as cinoxacin (Cinobac) (not available in the United States), enoxacin (Penetrex) (not available in the United States), gatifloxacin (Tequin, Zymar), levofloxacin (Levaquin, Quixin, Iquix), lomefloxacin (Maxaquin), moxifloxacin (Avelox, Vigamox), nalidixic acid (NegGram) (not available in the United States), norfloxacin (Noroxin), ofloxacin (Floxin, Ocuflox), and sparfloxacin (Zagam), any other medications, or benzalkonium chloride.
- tell your doctor and pharmacist what prescription and nonprescription medications, vitamins, nutritional supplements, and herbal products you are taking. Be sure to mention any of the following: anticoagulants ('blood thinners') such as warfarin (Coumadin), cyclosporine (Neoral, Sandimmune), and theophylline (Theo-Dur). Your doctor may need to change the doses of your medications or monitor you carefully for side effects.
- tell your doctor if you have or have ever had any medical condition.
- tell your doctor if you are pregnant, plan to become pregnant, or are breast-feeding. If you become pregnant while using ophthalmic ciprofloxacin, call your doctor.
- you should know that your vision may be blurred during your treatment with ciprofloxacin ophthalmic ointment. Avoid rubbing your eyes even if your vision is blurred. Do not drive a car or operate machinery if you are unable to see clearly.
- tell your doctor if you wear contact lenses. You should not wear contact lenses while you have symptoms of bacterial conjunctivitis or while you are applying eye drops or ointment.
- you should know that bacterial conjunctivitis spreads easily. Wash your hands often, especially after you touch your eyes. When your infection goes away, you should wash or replace any eye makeup, contact lenses, or other objects that touched your infected eye(s).

What special dietary instructions should I follow?

Talk to your doctor about drinking coffee or other beverages containing caffeine while you are taking this medication.

What should I do if I forget to take a dose?

Place the missed dose in your eye(s) as soon as you remember it. However, if it is almost time for the next dose, skip the missed dose and continue your regular dosing schedule. Do not use a double dose to make up for a missed one.

What side effects can this medicine cause?

Ophthalmic ciprofloxacin may cause side effects. Tell your doctor if any of these symptoms are severe or do not go away:

- burning, red, itchy, crusty, or irritated eyes
- eye pain
- feeling that something is in your eye
- unpleasant taste

Some side effects can be serious. The following symptoms are uncommon, but if you experience any of them, call your doctor immediately:

- rash
- hives
- itching
- tingling
- swelling of the face, throat, tongue, lips, eyes, hands, feet, ankles, or lower legs
- difficulty breathing or swallowing
- hoarseness

Ophthalmic ciprofloxacin may cause other side effects. Call your doctor if you have any unusual problems while taking this medication.

If you experience a serious side effect, you or your doctor may send a report to the Food and Drug Administration's (FDA) MedWatch Adverse Event Reporting program online [at http://www.fda.gov/MedWatch/index.html] or by phone [1-800-332-1088].

What storage conditions are needed for this medicine?

Keep this medication in the container it came in, tightly closed, and out of reach of children. Store it at room temperature and away from excess heat and moisture (not in the bathroom). Throw away any medication that is outdated or no longer needed. Talk to your pharmacist about the proper disposal of your medication.

What should I do in case of overdose?

If you place too many drops of the ophthalmic solution in your eye, wash your eye with plenty of warm tap water.

What other information should I know?

Keep all appointments with your doctor

Do not let anyone else use your medication. Your prescription is probably not refillable. If you still have symptoms of infection after you finish the ciprofloxacin ophthalmic solution or ointment, call your doctor.

Dosage Facts
For Informational Purposes

Caution: Do not change your dose, how often you take your medication, or the length of time you are to take it without first talking to your healthcare provider.

The following dosage information was written using medical language for doctors and other healthcare professionals and is provided here for you to check your dosage. The dosage of this drug may differ for different patients. Therefore, always follow your doctor's instructions or the directions on the label. Contact your healthcare provider or pharmacist if you have any questions about the specific dosage of your medication after reviewing this information.

General Dosage Information

Available as ciprofloxacin hydrochloride; dosage expressed in terms of ciprofloxacin.

Pediatric Patients

Ophthalmic Infections
Conjunctivitis (*S. aureus, S. epidermidis, S. pneumoniae, H. influenzae,* or viridans streptococci)

OPHTHALMIC:
- Ointment: In children ≥2 years of age, apply approximately 1.27 cm (½ inch) ribbon into conjunctival sac of affected eye(s) 3 times daily for 2 days, then twice daily for next 5 days.

Conjunctivitis (*S. aureus, S. epidermidis, S. pneumoniae,* or *H. influenzae*)

OPHTHALMIC:
- Solution: In children ≥1 year of age, 1 or 2 drops of 0.3% solution into conjunctival sac of affected eye(s) every 2 hours while awake for 2 days, then 1–2 drops every 4 hours while awake for next 5 days.

Keratitis

OPHTHALMIC:
- Solution: In children ≥1 year of age, 2 drops of 0.3% solution into affected eye(s) every 15 minutes for 6 hours, followed by 2 drops every 30 minutes for remainder of first day. On the second day, instill 2 drops into affected eye(s) every hour, and on days 3–14, instill 2 drops every 4 hours. May continue longer than 14 days if corneal reepithelialization is not complete.

Adult Patients

Ophthalmic Infections
Conjunctivitis (*S. aureus, S. epidermidis, S. pneumoniae, H. influenzae,* or viridans streptococci)

OPHTHALMIC:
- Ointment: Apply approximately 1.27 cm (½ inch) ribbon into conjunctival sac of affected eye(s) 3 times daily for 2 days, then twice daily for next 5 days.

Conjunctivitis (*S. aureus, S. epidermidis, S. pneumoniae,* or *H. influenzae*)

OPHTHALMIC:
- Solution: 1 or 2 drops of 0.3% solution into conjunctival sac of affected eye(s) every 2 hours while awake for 2 days, then 1–2 drops every 4 hours while awake for next 5 days.

Keratitis

OPHTHALMIC:
- Solution: 2 drops of 0.3% solution into affected eye(s) every 15 minutes for 6 hours, followed by 2 drops every 30 minutes for remainder of first day. On the second day, instill 2 drops

into affected eye(s) every hour, and on days 3–14, instill 2 drops every 4 hours. May continue longer than 14 days if corneal reepithelialization is not complete.

Citalopram

(sye tal′ oh pram)

Brand Name: Celexa®
Also available generically.

Important Warning

A small number of children, teenagers, and young adults (up to 24 years of age) who took antidepressants ('mood elevators') such as citalopram during clinical studies became suicidal (thinking about harming or killing oneself or planning or trying to do so). Children, teenagers, and young adults who take antidepressants to treat depression or other mental illnesses may be more likely to become suicidal than children, teenagers, and young adults who do not take antidepressants to treat these conditions. However, experts are not sure about how great this risk is and how much it should be considered in deciding whether a child or teenager should take an antidepressant. Children younger than 18 years of age should not normally take citalopram, but in some cases, a doctor may decide that citalopram is the best medication to treat a child's condition.

You should know that your mental health may change in unexpected ways when you take citalopram or other antidepressants even if you are an adult over age 24. You may become suicidal, especially at the beginning of your treatment and any time that your dose is increased or decreased. You, your family, or your caregiver should call your doctor right away if you experience any of the following symptoms: new or worsening depression; thinking about harming or killing yourself, or planning or trying to do so; extreme worry; agitation; panic attacks; difficulty falling asleep or staying asleep; aggressive behavior; irritability; acting without thinking; severe restlessness; and frenzied abnormal excitement. Be sure that your family or caregiver knows which symptoms may be serious so they can call the doctor when you are unable to seek treatment on your own.

Your healthcare provider will want to see you often while you are taking citalopram, especially at the beginning of your treatment. Be sure to keep all appointments for office visits with your doctor.

The doctor or pharmacist will give you the manufacturer's patient information sheet (Medication Guide) when you begin treatment with citalopram. Read the information carefully and ask your doctor or pharmacist if you have any questions. You also can obtain the Medication Guide from the FDA website: http://www.fda.gov/cder/drug/antidepressants/antidepressants_MG_2007.pdf.

No matter your age, before you take an antidepressant, you, your parent, or your caregiver should talk to your doctor about the risks and benefits of treating your condition with an antidepressant or with other treatments. You should also talk about the risks and benefits of not treating your condition. You should know that having depression or another mental illness greatly increases the risk that you will become suicidal. This risk is higher if you or anyone in your family has or has ever had bipolar disorder (mood that changes from depressed to abnormally excited) or mania (frenzied, abnormally excited mood) or has thought about or attempted suicide. Talk to your doctor about your condition, symptoms, and personal and family medical history. You and your doctor will decide what type of treatment is right for you.

Why is this medicine prescribed?

Citalopram is used to treat depression. Citalopram is in a class of antidepressants called selective serotonin reuptake inhibitors (SSRIs). It works by increasing the amount of serotonin, a natural substance in the brain that helps maintain mental balance.

How should this medicine be used?

Citalopram comes as a tablet and a solution (liquid) to take by mouth. It is usually taken once a day with or without food. Take citalopram at around the same time every day. Follow the directions on your prescription label carefully, and ask your doctor or pharmacist to explain any part you do not understand. Take citalopram exactly as directed. Do not take more or less of it or take it more often than prescribed by your doctor.

Your doctor may start you on a low dose of citalopram and gradually increase your dose, not more often than once a week.

It may take 1 to 4 weeks before you feel the full benefit of citalopram. Continue to take citalopram even if you feel well. If you suddenly stop taking citalopram, you may experience withdrawal symptoms such as mood changes, irritability, agitation, dizziness, numbness or tingling in the hands or feet, anxiety, confusion, headache, tiredness, and difficulty falling asleep or staying asleep. Do not stop taking citalopram without talking to your doctor. Your doctor will probably decrease your dose gradually.

Are there other uses for this medicine?

Citalopram is also sometimes used to treat eating disorders, alcoholism, panic disorder (condition that causes sudden attacks of extreme fear with no apparent cause), premenstrual dysphoric disorder (a group of physical and emotional symptoms that occur before the menstrual period each month), and social phobia (excessive anxiety about interacting with others). Talk to your doctor about the possible risks of using this medication for your condition.

This medication may be prescribed for other uses; ask your doctor or pharmacist for more information.

What special precautions should I follow?

Before taking citalopram,

- tell your doctor and pharmacist if you are allergic to citalopram, escitalopram (Lexapro), or any other medications.
- tell your doctor if you are taking pimozide (Orap) or a monoamine oxidase (MAO) inhibitor such as isocarboxazid (Marplan), phenelzine (Nardil), selegiline (Eldepryl, Emsam, Zelapar), and tranylcypromine (Parnate), or if you have stopped taking an MAO inhibitor within the past 14 days. Your doctor will probably tell you not to take citalopram. If you stop taking citalopram, you should wait at least 14 days before you start to take an MAO inhibitor.
- you should know that citalopram is very similar to another SSRI, escitalopram (Lexapro). You should not take these two medications together.
- tell your doctor and pharmacist what other prescription and nonprescription medications, and vitamins you are taking or plan to take. Be sure to mention any of the following: anticoagulants (blood thinners) such as warfarin (Coumadin); other antidepressants such as amitriptyline (Elavil), amoxapine (Asendin), clomipramine (Anafranil), desipramine (Norpramin), doxepin (Adapin, Sinequan), imipramine (Tofranil), nortriptyline (Aventyl, Pamelor), protriptyline (Vivactil), and trimipramine (Surmontil); aspirin and other nonsteroidal anti-inflammatory medications (NSAIDs) such as ibuprofen (Advil, Motrin) and naproxen (Aleve, Naprosyn); carbamazepine (Tegretol); cimetidine (Tagamet); ketoconazole (Nizoral); linezolid (Zyvox); lithium (Eskalith, Lithobid); medications for anxiety, mental illness, Parkinson's disease, and seizures; medications for migraine headaches such as almotriptan (Axert), eletriptan (Relpax), frovatriptan (Frova), naratriptan (Amerge), rizatriptan (Maxalt), sumatriptan (Imitrex), and zolmitriptan (Zomig); metoprolol (Lopressor, Toprol XL); sedatives; sleeping pills; tramadol (Ultram); and tranquilizers. Your doctor may need to change the doses of your medications or monitor you carefully for side effects.
- tell your doctor what nutritional supplements and herbal products you are taking, especially products that contain St. John's wort or tryptophan.
- tell your doctor if you have recently had a heart attack and if you have or have ever had seizures; or liver, kidney, or heart disease.
- tell your doctor if you are pregnant, plan to become pregnant, or are breast-feeding. If you become pregnant while taking citalopram, call your doctor.
- you should know that citalopram may make you drowsy. Do not drive a car or operate machinery until you know how this medication affects you.
- remember that alcohol can add to the drowsiness caused by this medication.

What special dietary instructions should I follow?

Unless your doctor tells you otherwise, continue your normal diet.

What should I do if I forget to take a dose?

Take the missed dose as soon as you remember it. However, if it is almost time for the next dose, skip the missed dose and continue your regular dosing schedule. Do not take a double dose to make up for a missed one.

What side effects can this medicine cause?

Citalopram may cause side effects. Tell your doctor if any of these symptoms are severe or do not go away:

- nausea
- diarrhea
- vomiting
- stomach pain
- drowsiness
- excessive tiredness
- uncontrollable shaking of a part of the body
- excitement
- nervousness
- muscle or joint pain
- dry mouth
- excessive sweating
- changes in sex drive or ability
- loss of appetite

Some side effects can be serious. If you experience either of the following symptoms or those listed in the IMPORTANT WARNING section, call your doctor immediately:

- seeing things or hearing voices that do not exist (hallucinating)
- seizures

Citalopram may cause other side effects. Call your doctor if you have any unusual problems while taking this medication.

What storage conditions are needed for this medicine?

Keep this medication in the container it came in, tightly closed, and out of reach of children. Store it at room temperature and away from excess heat and moisture (not in the bathroom). Throw away any medication that is outdated or no longer needed. Talk to your pharmacist about the proper disposal of your medication.

What should I do in case of overdose?

In case of overdose, call your local poison control center at 1-800-222-1222. If the victim has collapsed or is not breathing, call local emergency services at 911.

Symptoms of overdose may include:

- dizziness
- sweating
- upset stomach
- vomiting
- uncontrollable shaking of a part of the body
- drowsiness
- rapid, irregular, or pounding heartbeat
- memory loss
- confusion
- seizures
- coma
- rapid breathing

What other information should I know?

Keep all appointments with your doctor.

Do not let anyone else take your medication. Ask your pharmacist any questions you have about refilling your prescription.

Dosage Facts
For Informational Purposes

Caution: Do not change your dose, how often you take your medication, or the length of time you are to take it without first talking to your health-care provider.

The following dosage information was written using medical language for doctors and other healthcare professionals and is provided here for you to check your dosage. The dosage of this drug may differ for different patients. Therefore, always follow your doctor's instructions or the directions on the label. Contact your health-care provider or pharmacist if you have any questions about the specific dosage of your medication after reviewing this information.

General Dosage Information

Available as citalopram hydrobromide; dosages expressed in terms of citalopram.

Adult Patients

Major Depressive Disorder

ORAL:
- Initially, 20 mg once daily. If no clinical improvement is apparent, increase in 20-mg increments at intervals of ≥1 week.
- Optimum duration not established; may require several months of therapy or longer.

Obsessive-Compulsive Disorder†

ORAL:
- Initially, 20 mg once daily. Gradually increase dosage according to clinical response.

- Usual maintenance dosage: 40–60 mg daily.

Panic Disorder†

Usual initial dosage: 10 mg daily. Increase dosage after ≥1 week in 10- or 20-mg increments up to a dosage of 20–60 mg daily, depending on individual patient response and tolerability.

Usual maintenance dosage: 20–30 mg daily.

Prescribing Limits

Adult Patients

Major Depressive Disorder

ORAL:
- Maximum of 40 mg daily usually recommended; some patients may require up to 60 mg daily.

Obsessive-Compulsive Disorder†

Maximum 60 mg daily.

Panic Disorder†

Maximum 60 mg daily.

Special Populations

Hepatic Impairment

Major Depressive Disorder

ORAL:
- Initially, 20 mg once daily; titrate to 40 mg once daily *only* in nonresponders.

Renal Impairment

Major Depressive Disorder

ORAL:
- No dosage adjustment necessary in patients with mild to moderate renal impairment. Dosage adjustment may not be necessary in patients with severe renal impairment, but caution is recommended.

Geriatric Patients
- Initially, 20 mg once daily; titrate to 40 mg once daily *only* in nonresponders.

† Use is not currently included in the labeling approved by the US Food and Drug Administration.

Clarithromycin

(kla rith′ roe mye sin)

Brand Name: Biaxin® Filmtab®, Biaxin® Granules, Biaxin® XL Filmtab, Biaxin® XL Pac
Also available generically.

Why is this medicine prescribed?

Clarithromycin is used to treat certain infections caused by bacteria, such as pneumonia (a lung infection), bronchitis (infection of the tubes leading to the lungs), and infections of the ears, sinuses, skin, and throat. It also is used to treat and prevent disseminated Mycobacterium avium complex (MAC) infection [a type of lung infection that often affects people with human immunodeficiency virus (HIV)]. It is used in combination with other medications to eliminate *H. pylori*, a bacteria that causes ulcers. Clarithromycin is in a class of medications called macrolide antibiotics. It works by stopping the growth of bacteria. Antibiotics will not work for colds, flu, or other viral infections.

How should this medicine be used?

Clarithromycin comes as a tablet, an extended-release (long-acting) tablet, and a suspension (liquid) to take by mouth. The regular tablet and liquid are usually taken with or without food every 12 hours (twice a day) for 7-14 days. The long-acting tablet is usually taken with food every 24 hours (once a day) for 7-14 days. Take clarithromycin at around the same time(s) every day. Follow the directions on your prescription label carefully, and ask your doctor or pharmacist to explain any part you do not understand. Take clarithromycin exactly as directed. Do not take more or less of it or take it more often than prescribed by your doctor.

Shake the liquid well before each use to mix the medication evenly.

The tablets should be taken with a full glass of water. Swallow the long-acting tablets whole; do not split, chew, or crush them.

Take clarithromycin until you finish the prescription, even if you feel better. If you stop taking clarithromycin too soon, your infection may not be completely treated and the bacteria may become resistant to antibiotics.

Are there other uses for this medicine?

Clarithromycin also is used sometimes to treat other types of infections including Lyme disease (an infection that may develop after a person is bitten by a tick), crypotosporidiosis (an infection that causes diarrhea), cat scratch disease (an infection that may develop after a person is bitten or scratched by a cat), Legionnaires' disease (a type of lung infection), and pertussis (whooping cough; a serious infection that can cause severe coughing). It is also sometimes used to prevent heart infection in patients having dental or

other procedures. Talk to your doctor about the possible risks of using this medication for your condition.

This medication may be prescribed for other uses; ask your doctor or pharmacist for more information.

What special precautions should I follow?

Before taking clarithromycin,

- tell your doctor and pharmacist if you are allergic to clarithromycin, azithromycin (Zithromax), dirithromycin (Dynabac) (not available in the U.S.), erythromycin (E.E.S., E-Mycin, Erythrocin), telithromycin (Ketek), or any other medications
- tell your doctor if you are taking astemizole (Hismanal) (not available in the U.S.), cisapride (Propulsid), dihydroergotamine (DHE 45, Migranal), ergotamine (Ergomar, in Cafergot, in Migergot), pimozide (Orap), or terfenadine (Seldane) (not available in the U.S.). Your doctor may tell you not to take clarithromycin if you are taking one or more of these medications.
- tell your doctor and pharmacist what other prescription and nonprescription medications, vitamins, nutritional supplements, and herbal products you are taking or plan to take. Be sure to mention any of the following: anticoagulants ('blood thinners') such as warfarin (Coumadin); alfentanil (Alfenta); alprazolam (Xanax); bromocriptine (Parlodel); carbamazepine (Tegretol); cholesterol-lowering medications such as lovastatin (Mevacor) and simvastatin (Zocor); cilostazol (Pletal); colchicine; cyclosporine (Neoral, Sandimmune); darifenacin (Enablex); digoxin (Lanoxin); erlotinib (Tarceva); eszopiclone (Lunesta); fluconazole (Diflucan); certain medications for HIV such as nelfinavir (Viracept), ritonavir (Norvir), and ziodvudine (AZT, Retrovir); certain medications for irregular heartbeat such as disopyramide (Norpace) and quinidine; methylprednisolone (Medrol), midazolam (Versed); omeprazole (Prilosec); phenytoin (Dilantin); ranitidine (Zantac); rifabutin (Mycobutin); rifampin (Rifadin, Rimactane); sildenafil (Viagra), tacrolimus (Prograf); theophylline (Theo-Dur); triazolam (Halcion); valproate (Depacon) and valproic acid (Depakote). Many other medications may also interact with clarithromycin, so tell your doctor about all the medications you are taking, even those that do not appear on this list. Your doctor may need to change the doses of your medications or monitor you carefully for side effects.
- tell your doctor if you have or have ever had kidney or liver disease.
- tell your doctor if you are pregnant, plan to become pregnant, or are breast-feeding. If you become pregnant while taking clarithromycin, call your doctor.

What special dietary instructions should I follow?

Unless your doctor tells you otherwise, continue your normal diet.

What should I do if I forget to take a dose?

Take the missed dose as soon as you remember it. However, if it is almost time for the next dose, skip the missed dose and continue your regular dosing schedule. Do not take a double dose to make up for a missed one.

What side effects can this medicine cause?

Clarithromycin may cause side effects. Tell your doctor if any of these symptoms are severe or do not go away:

- diarrhea
- nausea
- heartburn
- abnormal taste
- stomach pain
- headache

Some side effects can be serious. If you experience any of the following symptoms, call your doctor immediately:

- rash
- hives
- itching
- swelling of the face, throat, tongue, lips, eyes, hands, feet, ankles, or lower legs
- difficulty breathing or swallowing
- hoarseness
- blisters or red splotches on skin
- fever
- yellowing of the skin or eyes
- unusual bruising or bleeding
- pain in the upper right part of the stomach
- lack of energy
- flu-like symptoms
- fast, pounding, or irregular heartbeat

Clarithromycin may cause other side effects. Call your doctor if you have any unusual problems while taking this medication.

If you experience a serious side effect, you or your doctor may send a report to the Food and Drug Administration's (FDA) MedWatch Adverse Event Reporting program online [at http://www.fda.gov/MedWatch/index.html] or by phone [1-800-332-1088].

What storage conditions are needed for this medicine?

Keep this medication in the container it came in, tightly closed, and out of reach of children. Store the tablets at room temperature and away from excess heat and moisture (not in the bathroom). Keep away from light. Throw away any medication that is outdated or no longer needed. Do not refrigerate the oral solution. Keep it at room temperature and away from excess heat and moisture. Throw away any unused oral solution after 14 days. Talk to your pharmacist about the proper disposal of your medication.

What should I do in case of overdose?

In case of overdose, call your local poison control center at 1-800-222-1222. If the victim has collapsed or is not breathing, call local emergency services at 911.

Symptoms of overdose may include:

- stomach pain
- nausea
- vomiting
- diarrhea

What other information should I know?

Keep all appointments with your doctor.

The extended-release tablet does not dissolve in the stomach after swallowing. It slowly releases the medicine as it passes through your digestive system. You may notice the tablet coating in the stool. This is normal and does not mean that you did not get the full dose of medication.

Do not let anyone else take your medication. Your prescription is probably not refillable. If you still have symptoms of infection after you finish the clarithromycin, call your doctor.

Dosage Facts
For Informational Purposes

Caution: Do not change your dose, how often you take your medication, or the length of time you are to take it without first talking to your healthcare provider.

The following dosage information was written using medical language for doctors and other healthcare professionals and is provided here for you to check your dosage. The dosage of this drug may differ for different patients. Therefore, always follow your doctor's instructions or the directions on the label. Contact your healthcare provider or pharmacist if you have any questions about the specific dosage of your medication after reviewing this information.

General Dosage Information

Extended-release tablets may be used *only* for treatment of acute maxillary sinusitis, acute bacterial exacerbations of chronic bronchitis, and CAP in adults; safety and efficacy not established for treatment of other infections in adults or for use in pediatric patients.

Pediatric Patients

Acute Otitis Media (AOM)

ORAL:
- 7.5 mg/kg every 12 hours for 10 days.

Pharyngitis and Tonsillitis

ORAL:
- 7.5 mg/kg every 12 hours for 10 days.

Respiratory Tract Infections
Acute Bacterial Sinusitis

ORAL:
- 7.5 mg/kg every 12 hours for 10 days.

Community-acquired Pneumonia (CAP)

ORAL:
- 7.5 mg/kg every 12 hours for 10 days.

Pertussis†

ORAL:
- 15–20 mg/kg daily in 2 divided doses (up to 1 g daily) for 7 days. 7.5 mg/kg twice daily for 7 days has been used in children 1 month to 16 years of age.

Skin and Skin Structure Infections

ORAL:
- 7.5 mg/kg every 12 hours for 10 days.

Bartonella Infections†
Cat Scratch Disease Caused by Bartonella henselae†

ORAL:
- 500 mg daily for 4 weeks.

Bartonella Infections in HIV-infected Individuals†

ORAL:
- Adolescents: 500 mg twice daily for ≥3 months recommended by CDC, NIH, and IDSA. If relapse occurs, consider lifelong secondary prophylaxis (chronic maintenance therapy) with erythromycin or doxycycline.

Lyme Disease†

ORAL:
- 7.5 mg/kg (up to 500 mg) twice daily for 14–21 days for treatment of early localized or early disseminated disease.

Mycobacterium avium Complex (MAC) Infections
Primary Prevention of MAC in Children with Advanced HIV Infection

ORAL:
- 7.5 mg/kg (up to 500 mg) every 12 hours.
- USPHS/IDSA recommends initiation of primary prophylaxis if $CD4^+$ T-cell count is <750/mm³ in those <1 year, <500/mm³ in those 1–2 years, <75/mm³ in those 2–6 years, or <50/mm³ in those ≥6 years of age.

Primary Prevention of MAC in Adolescents with Advanced HIV Infection

ORAL:
- 500 mg every 12 hours.
- USPHS/IDSA recommends initiation of primary prophylaxis if $CD4^+$ T-cell count is <50/mm³. May be discontinued if there is immune recovery in response to antiretroviral therapy and an increase in $CD4^+$ T-cell count to >100/mm³ sustained for ≥3 months. Reinitiate prophylaxis if $CD4^+$ T-cell count decreases to <50–100/mm³.

Treatment of Disseminated MAC in HIV-infected Children

ORAL:
- Manufacturer recommends 7.5 mg/kg (up to 500 mg) every 12 hours.
- CDC, NIH, and IDSA recommend 7.5–15 mg/kg (maximum 500 mg) twice daily in conjunction with ethambutol (15–25 mg/kg once daily [up to 1 g daily]) with or without rifabutin (10–20 mg/kg once daily [up to 300 mg daily]).

Treatment of Disseminated MAC in HIV-infected Adolescents

ORAL:
- 500 mg every 12 hours in conjunction with ethambutol (15 mg/kg daily) with or without a third drug (e.g., rifabutin 300 mg once daily) recommended by CDC, NIH, and IDSA. Higher dosage not recommended since such dosage has been associated with reduced survival in clinical studies.

Prevention of MAC Recurrence in HIV-infected Children

ORAL:
- 7.5 mg/kg (maximum 500 mg) twice daily in conjunction with ethambutol (15 mg/kg [maximum 900 mg] once daily) with or without rifabutin (5 mg/kg [maximum 300 mg] once daily).
- Secondary prophylaxis to prevent MAC recurrence in HIV-infected children usually continued for life. The safety of discontinuing secondary MAC prophylaxis in children whose $CD4^+$ T-cell count increases in response to antiretroviral therapy has not been studied.

Prevention of MAC Recurrence in HIV-infected Adolescents

ORAL:
- 500 mg every 12 hours in conjunction with ethambutol (15 mg/kg once daily) with or without rifabutin (300 mg once daily).
- Secondary prophylaxis to prevent MAC recurrence usually continued for life in HIV-infected adolescents. USPHS/IDSA states that consideration can be given to discontinuing such prophylaxis after ≥12 months in those who remain asymptomatic with respect to MAC and have an increase in $CD4^+$ T-cell count to >100/mm³ sustained for ≥6 months.

Treatment of Cutaneous Mycobacterium abscessus Infections†

ORAL:
- 15 mg/kg daily (with or without incision and drainage of lesions) has been used in children 1–15 years of age.

Prevention of Bacterial Endocarditis†
Patients Undergoing Certain Dental, Oral, Respiratory Tract, or Esophageal Procedures

ORAL:
- 15 mg/kg as a single dose given 1 hour prior to the procedure.

Adult Patients

Pharyngitis and Tonsillitis

ORAL:
- 250 mg every 12 hours for 10 days.

Respiratory Tract Infections
Acute Bacterial Sinusitis

ORAL:
- Conventional tablets or oral suspension: 500 mg every 12 hours for 14 days.
- Extended-release tablets: 1 g (two 500-mg extended release tablets) once daily for 14 days.

Acute Exacerbations of Chronic Bronchitis

ORAL:
- Conventional tablets or oral suspension: 500 mg every 12 hours for 7–14 days for *H. influenzae*, 500 mg every 12 hours

for 7 days for *H. parainfluenzae*, or 250 mg every 12 hours for 7–14 days for *M. catarrhalis* or *S. pneumoniae*.
- Extended-release tablets: 1 g (two 500-mg extended-release tablets) once daily for 7 days.

Community-acquired Pneumonia (CAP)

ORAL:
- Conventional tablets or oral suspension: 250 mg every 12 hours for 7 days for *H. influenzae* or for 7–14 days for *S. pneumoniae*, *C. pneumoniae*, or *M. pneumoniae*.
- Extended-release tablets: 1 g (two 500-mg extended-release tablets) once daily for 7 days.

Legionnaires' Disease†

ORAL:
- Conventional tablets or oral suspension: 500 mg twice daily. Usual duration is 10 days for mild to moderate infections in immunocompetent patients; longer duration of treatment (3 weeks) may be necessary to prevent relapse, especially in those with more severe infections or with underlying comorbidity or immunodeficiency.

Skin and Skin Structure Infections

ORAL:
- Conventional tablets or oral suspension: 250 mg every 12 hours for 7–14 days.

Helicobacter pylori Infection and Duodenal Ulcer Disease

ORAL:
- Conventional tablets or oral suspension: 500 mg twice daily for 10 or 14 days given in conjunction with amoxicillin and lansoprazole (triple therapy); 500 mg twice daily for 10 days given in conjunction with amoxicillin and omeprazole (triple therapy); 500 mg 3 times daily for 14 days given in conjunction with omeprazole or ranitidine bismuth citrate (dual therapy).

Bartonella Infections†
Cat Scratch Disease Caused by Bartonella henselae†

ORAL:
- Conventional tablets or oral suspension: 500 mg daily for 4 weeks.

Bartonella Infections in HIV-infected Individuals†

ORAL:
- Conventional tablets or oral suspension: 500 mg twice daily for ≥3 months recommended by CDC, NIH, and IDSA. If relapse occurs, consider lifelong secondary prophylaxis (chronic maintenance therapy) with erythromycin or doxycycline.

Lyme Disease†

ORAL:
- Conventional tablets or oral suspension: 500 mg twice daily for 14–21 days for treatment of early localized or early disseminated disease.

Mycobacterial Infections
Primary Prevention of MAC in Adults with Advanced HIV Infection

ORAL:
- Conventional tablets or oral suspension: 500 mg every 12 hours.
- USPHS/IDSA recommends initiation of primary prophylaxis

if CD4+ T-cell count is <50/mm³. May be discontinued if there is immune recovery in response to antiretroviral therapy and an increase in CD4+ T-cell count to >100/mm³ sustained for ≥3 months. Reinitiate prophylaxis if CD4+ T-cell count decreases to <50–100/mm³.

Treatment of Disseminated MAC in HIV-infected Adults

ORAL:
- Conventional tablets or oral suspension: 500 mg every 12 hours in conjunction with ethambutol (15 mg/kg daily) with or without a third drug (e.g., rifabutin 300 mg once daily). Higher dosage not recommended since such dosage has been associated with reduced survival in clinical studies.

Prevention of MAC Recurrence in HIV-infected Adults

ORAL:
- Conventional tablets or oral suspension: 500 mg every 12 hours in conjunction with ethambutol (15 mg/kg once daily) with or without rifabutin (300 mg once daily).
- Secondary prophylaxis to prevent MAC recurrence usually continued for life in HIV-infected adults. USPHS/IDSA states that consideration can be given to discontinuing such prophylaxis after ≥12 months in those who remain asymptomatic with respect to MAC and have an increase in CD4+ T-cell count to >100/mm³ sustained for ≥6 months.

Treatment of MAC in HIV-negative Adults†

ORAL:
- Conventional tablets or oral suspension: 500 mg every 12 hours in conjunction with ethambutol and rifabutin or rifampin.

Mycobacterium abscessus or M. chelonae Infections†

ORAL:
- Conventional tablets or oral suspension: 0.5–1 g twice daily for 6 months.

M. marinum Infections†

ORAL:
- Conventional tablets or oral suspension: 500 mg twice daily for at least 3 months.

Prevention of Bacterial Endocarditis†
Patients Undergoing Certain Dental, Oral, Respiratory Tract, or Esophageal Procedures

ORAL:
- Conventional tablets or oral suspension: 500 mg as a single dose given 1 hour prior to the procedure.

Special Populations

Hepatic Impairment
- No dosage adjustment required.

Renal Impairment
- If Cl_{cr} <30 mL/minute, reduce dose by 50% or double dosing interval. Alternatively (for conventional tablets or oral suspension), 500 mg initially followed by 250 mg twice daily (if the usual dosage in adults with normal renal function is 500 mg twice daily) or 250 mg daily (if the usual dosage in adults with normal renal function is 250 mg twice daily).

Geriatric Patients
- No dosage adjustments except those related to renal impairment.

† *Use is not currently included in the labeling approved by the US Food and Drug Administration.*

Clemastine

(klem′ as teen)

Brand Name: Anti-Hist®-1, Dayhist®-1, Tavist®, Tavist® Allergy (formerly Tavist-1®), Tavist® Syrup

Why is this medicine prescribed?

Clemastine, an antihistamine, is used to relieve hay fever and allergy symptoms, including itchy skin; hives; sneezing; runny nose; and red, itchy, tearing eyes.

This medication is sometimes prescribed for other uses; ask your doctor or pharmacist for more information.

How should this medicine be used?

Clemastine comes in regular and extended-release tablets and liquid to take by mouth. It usually is taken twice a day. Follow the directions on your prescription label carefully, and ask your doctor or pharmacist to explain any part you do not understand. Take clemastine exactly as directed. Do not take more or less of it or take it more often than prescribed by your doctor.

Do not crush or chew extended-release tablets; swallow them whole.

Speak with your doctor before giving this medication to a child younger than 12 years of age.

What special precautions should I follow?

Before taking clemastine,
- tell your doctor and pharmacist if you are allergic to clemastine or any other drugs.
- tell your doctor and pharmacist what prescription and nonprescription medications you are taking, especially other medications for colds, hay fever, or allergies; medications for depression or seizures; muscle relaxants; narcotics (pain medications); sedatives; sleeping pills; tranquilizers; and vitamins. Do not take clemastine if you have taken an MAO inhibitor [phenelzine (Nardil) or tranylcypromine (Parnate)] in the last two weeks.
- tell your doctor if you have or have ever had asthma or lung disease, diabetes, glaucoma, ulcers, difficulty urinating (due to an enlarged prostate gland), heart disease, high blood pressure, seizures, or an overactive thyroid gland.

- tell your doctor if you are pregnant, plan to become pregnant, or are breast-feeding. If you become pregnant while taking clemastine, call your doctor.
- if you are having surgery, including dental surgery, tell the doctor or dentist that you are taking clemastine.
- you should know that this drug may make you drowsy. Do not drive a car or operate machinery until you know how this drug affects you.
- remember that alcohol can add to the drowsiness caused by this drug.

What should I do if I forget to take a dose?

Take the missed dose as soon as you remember it. However, if it is almost time for the next dose, skip the missed dose and continue your regular dosing schedule. Do not take a double dose to make up for a missed one.

What side effects can this medicine cause?

Clemastine may cause side effects. Tell your doctor if any of these symptoms are severe or do not go away:
- drowsiness
- dry mouth, nose, and throat
- dizziness
- upset stomach
- chest congestion
- headache

If you experience any of the following symptoms, call your doctor immediately:
- dry mouth
- excitement (especially in children)
- nervousness
- enlargement of pupils in the eye
- increased sensitivity to sunlight

If you experience a serious side effect, you or your doctor may send a report to the Food and Drug Administration's (FDA) MedWatch Adverse Event Reporting program online [at http://www.fda.gov/MedWatch/index.html] or by phone [1-800-332-1088].

What storage conditions are needed for this medicine?

Keep this medication in the container it came in, tightly closed, and out of reach of children. Store it at room temperature and away from excess heat and moisture (not in the bathroom). Throw away any medication that is outdated or no longer needed. Talk to your pharmacist about the proper disposal of your medication.

What should I do in case of overdose?

In case of overdose, call your local poison control center at 1-800-222-1222. If the victim has collapsed or is not breathing, call local emergency services at 911.

What other information should I know?

Keep all appointments with your doctor.

Do not let anyone else take your medication. Ask your pharmacist any questions you have about refilling your prescription.

Talk to your doctor, pharmacist, or other healthcare professional if you have questions about dosing information for your medication.

Clindamycin

(klin da mye′ sin)

Brand Name: Cleocin T®, Cleocin T® 1%, Cleocin T® Pledgets, Cleocin®, Cleocin® Vaginal Ovules, Clinda-Derm®, Clindagel®, Clindets® Pledgets, Duac® as a combination product containing Clindamycin Phosphate and Benzoyl Peroxide

Also available generically.

Important Warning

Clindamycin may cause colitis, an infection of the colon that can be dangerous and sometimes life-threatening. If you experience any of the following symptoms while taking clindamycin or within a few weeks of stopping clindamycin, call your doctor immediately: severe persistent diarrhea, severe stomach cramps, or bloody stool. Talk to your doctor about the risk of taking clindamycin.

Why is this medicine prescribed?

Clindamycin, an antibiotic, is used to treat infections of the respiratory tract, skin, pelvis, vagina, and abdomen. Antibiotics will not work for colds, flu, or other viral infections.

This medication is sometimes prescribed for other uses; ask your doctor or pharmacist for more information.

How should this medicine be used?

Clindamycin comes as a capsule and liquid to take by mouth; topical solution, lotion, and gel for skin infections; and vaginal cream. Clindamycin usually is taken every 6 hours for respiratory, pelvis, or abdomen infections or applied twice a day for acne. Shake the oral liquid well before each use to mix the medication evenly. Drink a full glass of water after each dose (capsules and oral liquid).

For acne, it may take up to 12 weeks for the full effect of the drug to be seen. Shake the topical lotion well before each use. Apply this liquid, the solution, or the gel in a thin film after washing and drying the skin thoroughly. Avoid getting the medication in your eyes and mouth or on broken skin; if you do, use plenty of water to wash the drug away.

Follow the directions on your prescription label carefully, and ask your doctor or pharmacist to explain any part you do not understand. Take clindamycin exactly as directed. Do not take more or less of it or take it more often than prescribed by your doctor.

For vaginal infections, clindamycin is used once a day, at bedtime, for 7 days. Clindamycin cream for the vagina comes with a special applicator. The dose should be applied when you lie down to go to bed. The medicine works best if you do not get up again after applying the drug except to wash your hands and the applicator. Read the directions provided with it and follow these steps:

1. Fill the special applicator that comes with the cream to the level indicated.
2. Lie on your back with your knees drawn upward and spread apart.
3. Gently insert the applicator into your vagina and push the plunger to release the medication.
4. Withdraw the applicator and wash it with soap and warm water.
5. Wash your hands promptly to avoid spreading the infection.

You may wish to wear a sanitary napkin while using the vaginal cream to protect your clothing against stains. Do not use a tampon because it will absorb the drug. Do not douche unless your doctor tells you to do so. Continue using clindamycin vaginal cream even if you get your period during treatment.

What special precautions should I follow?

Before taking clindamycin,

- tell your doctor and pharmacist if you are allergic to clindamycin, tartrazine (a yellow dye in some processed foods and drugs), or any other drugs.
- tell your doctor and pharmacist what prescription and nonprescription medications you are taking, including vitamins. If you are using topical clindamycin, ask your doctor for advice on using other acne medications (e.g., benzoyl peroxide) and cosmetics. Some cosmetics make acne worse and interfere with the effectiveness of this medication.
- tell your doctor if you have or have ever had gastrointestinal, liver, or kidney disease.
- tell your doctor if you are pregnant, plan to become pregnant, or are breast-feeding. If you become pregnant while using clindamycin, call your doctor.

What should I do if I forget to take a dose?

Take the missed dose as soon as you remember it. However, if it is almost time for the next dose, skip the missed dose and take any remaining doses for that day at evenly spaced intervals. Do not take a double dose to make up for a missed one. Do not apply a missed topical dose.

What side effects can this medicine cause?

Clindamycin may cause side effects. Tell your doctor if any of these symptoms are severe or do not go away:

- upset stomach
- vomiting
- gas
- diarrhea

Tell your doctor if any these symptoms are severe or do not go away while using clindamycin vaginally or on your skin:

- dry skin
- redness or irritation
- peeling
- oiliness
- itching or burning

If you experience the following symptom, or any of those listed in the IMPORTANT WARNING section, stop taking clindamycin and call your doctor immediately:

- skin rash

If you experience a serious side effect, you or your doctor may send a report to the Food and Drug Administration's (FDA) MedWatch Adverse Event Reporting program online [at http://www.fda.gov/MedWatch/index.html] or by phone [1-800-332-1088].

What storage conditions are needed for this medicine?

Keep this medication in the container it came in, tightly closed, and out of reach of children. Store it at room temperature and away from excess heat and moisture (not in the bathroom). Throw away any medication that is outdated or no longer needed. Talk to your pharmacist about the proper disposal of your medication.

What should I do in case of overdose?

In case of overdose, call your local poison control center at 1-800-222-1222. If the victim has collapsed or is not breathing, call local emergency services at 911.

What other information should I know?

Keep all appointments with your doctor and the laboratory. Your doctor will order certain lab tests to check your response to clindamycin.

Do not let anyone else take your medication. Your prescription is probably not refillable. If you still have symptoms of infection after you finish the clindamycin, call your doctor.

Dosage Facts
For Informational Purposes

Caution: Do not change your dose, how often you take your medication, or the length of time you are to take it without first talking to your healthcare provider.

The following dosage information was written using medical language for doctors and other healthcare professionals and is provided here for you to check your dosage. The dosage of this drug may differ for different patients. Therefore, always follow your doctor's instructions or the directions on the label. Contact your healthcare provider or pharmacist if you have any questions about the specific dosage of your medication after reviewing this information.

Pediatric Patients

Acne Vulgaris

Number of inflammatory lesions generally decreases after 2–6 weeks of topical therapy; maximum benefit may not be seen for up to 12 weeks. Prolonged therapy (several months or years) may be necessary.

Continue as long as response is satisfactory and no severe or intolerable toxicity occurs.

Treatment with Single-entity Clindamycin Preparations

TOPICAL:
- Children ≥ 12 years of age: apply a thin film of gel, lotion, or solution to the cleansed affected area twice daily.

Treatment with Clindamycin and Benzoyl Peroxide Combination Preparations

TOPICAL:
- Children ≥ 12 years of age: apply a thin film of BenzaClin® gel to the cleansed affected area twice daily (morning and evening) or as directed by clinician.
- Children ≥ 12 years of age: apply a thin film of Duac® gel to the cleansed affected areas once daily in the evening or as directed by clinician.

Bacterial Vaginosis
Treatment in Nonpregnant Postmenarchal Females

INTRAVAGINAL:
- Vaginal suppositories: 1 suppository daily (preferably at bedtime) for 3 days.

Adult Patients

Acne Vulgaris

Number of inflammatory lesions generally decreases after 2–6 weeks of topical therapy; maximum benefit may not be seen for up to 12 weeks. Prolonged therapy (several months or years) may be necessary.

Continue as long as response is satisfactory and no severe or intolerable toxicity occurs.

Treatment with Single-entity Clindamycin Preparations

TOPICAL:
- Apply a thin film of gel, lotion, or solution to the cleansed affected area twice daily.

Treatment with Clindamycin and Benzoyl Peroxide Combination Preparations

TOPICAL:
- BenzaClin® gel: apply a thin film to the cleansed affected area twice daily (morning and evening) or as directed by clinician.
- Duac® gel: apply a thin film to the cleansed affected areas once daily in the evening or as directed by clinician.

Bacterial Vaginosis
Treatment in Nonpregnant Women
INTRAVAGINAL:
- Vaginal cream: 1 applicatorful once daily (preferably at bedtime) for 3 or 7 consecutive days. CDC recommends a 7-day regimen.
- Vaginal suppositories: 1 suppository once daily (preferably at bedtime) for 3 consecutive days.

Treatment in Pregnant Women
INTRAVAGINAL:
- Vaginal cream: 1 applicatorful once daily (preferably at bedtime) for 7 consecutive days.

Clindamycin and Benzoyl Peroxide Topical

(klin da mye′ sin) (ben′ zoe ill per ox′ ide)

Brand Name: BenzaClin® , Duac®

Why is this medicine prescribed?

The combination of clindamycin and benzoyl peroxide is used to treat acne. Clindamycin and benzoyl peroxide are in a class of medications called topical antibiotics. The combination of clindamycin and benzoyl peroxide works by killing the bacteria that cause acne.

How should this medicine be used?

The combination of clindamycin and benzoyl peroxide comes as a gel to apply to the skin. It is usually applied twice a day, in the morning and evening. To help you remember to use clindamycin and benzoyl peroxide gel, apply it at around the same times every day. Follow the directions on your prescription label carefully, and ask your doctor or pharmacist to explain any part you do not understand. Use clindamycin and benzoyl peroxide gel exactly as directed. Do not use more or less of it or use it more often than prescribed by your doctor.

To use the gel, follow these steps:
1. Wash the affected area with warm water and gently pat dry with a clean towel.
2. Use you fingertips to spread a thin layer of gel evenly over the affected area. Avoid getting the gel in your eyes, nose, mouth, or other body openings. If you do get the gel in your eyes, wash with warm water.
3. Look in the mirror. If you see a white film on your skin, you have used too much medication.
4. Wash your hands.

Are there other uses for this medicine?

This medication may be prescribed for other uses; ask your doctor or pharmacist for more information.

What special precautions should I follow?

Before using clindamycin and benzoyl peroxide,
- tell your doctor and pharmacist if you are allergic to clindamycin (Cleocin, Clinda-Derm, C/D/S), benzoyl peroxide (Benzac, Desquam, PanOxyl, Triaz, others), lincomycin, or any other medications.
- tell your doctor and pharmacist what prescription and nonprescription medications, vitamins, nutritional supplements, and herbal products you are taking. Be sure to mention any of the following: erythromycin (E.E.S., E-Mycin, Erythrocin) and other topical medications for acne. Your doctor may need to change the doses of your medications or monitor you carefully for side effects.
- tell your doctor if you have or have ever had stomach problems, ulcerative colitis, or severe diarrhea caused by antibiotics.
- tell your doctor if you are pregnant, plan to become pregnant, or are breast-feeding. If you become pregnant while using clindamycin and benzoyl peroxide, call your doctor.
- plan to avoid unnecessary or prolonged exposure to sunlight and to wear protective clothing, sunglasses, and sunscreen. Clindamycin and benzoyl peroxide may make your skin sensitive to sunlight.
- ask your doctor or pharmacist to recommend a moisturizer to keep your skin soft during treatment.

What special dietary instructions should I follow?

Unless your doctor tells you otherwise, continue your normal diet.

What should I do if I forget to take a dose?

Apply the missed dose as soon as you remember it. However, if it is almost time for the next dose, skip the missed dose and continue your regular dosing schedule. Do not apply a double dose to make up for a missed one.

What side effects can this medicine cause?

Clindamycin and benzoyl peroxide may cause side effects. Tell your doctor if any of these symptoms are severe or do not go away:
- dry skin
- itching
- peeling skin
- red skin

Some side effects can be serious. The following symptoms are uncommon, but if you experience any of them, call your doctor immediately:
- severe diarrhea
- blood or mucus in the stool
- severe stomach pain or cramps
- changes in your skin or nails that may be signs of infection with a fungus

Clindamycin and benzoyl peroxide may cause other side

effects. Call your doctor if you have any unusual problems while using this medication.

If you experience a serious side effect, you or your doctor may send a report to the Food and Drug Administration's (FDA) MedWatch Adverse Event Reporting program online [at http://www.fda.gov/MedWatch/index.html] or by phone [1-800-332-1088].

What storage conditions are needed for this medicine?

Keep this medication in the container it came in, tightly closed, and out of reach of children. Store it at room temperature and away from excess heat and moisture (not in the bathroom). Throw away any unused medication after 10 weeks. Talk to your pharmacist about the proper disposal of your medication.

What other information should I know?

Keep all appointments with your doctor.

Avoid getting clindamycin and benzoyl peroxide gel on your hair or clothing. Clindamycin and benzoyl peroxide may bleach hair or colored fabric.

Do not let anyone else use your medication. Ask your pharmacist any questions you have about refilling your prescription.

Dosage Facts

For Informational Purposes

Caution: Do not change your dose, how often you take your medication, or the length of time you are to take it without first talking to your healthcare provider.

The following dosage information was written using medical language for doctors and other healthcare professionals and is provided here for you to check your dosage. The dosage of this drug may differ for different patients. Therefore, always follow your doctor's instructions or the directions on the label. Contact your healthcare provider or pharmacist if you have any questions about the specific dosage of your medication after reviewing this information.

Pediatric Patients

Acne Vulgaris

Number of inflammatory lesions generally decreases after 2–6 weeks of topical therapy; maximum benefit may not be seen for up to 12 weeks. Prolonged therapy (several months or years) may be necessary.

Continue as long as response is satisfactory and no severe or intolerable toxicity occurs.

Treatment with Clindamycin and Benzoyl Peroxide Combination Preparations

TOPICAL:
- Children ≥ 12 years of age: apply a thin film of BenzaClin® gel to the cleansed affected area twice daily (morning and evening) or as directed by clinician.

- Children ≥ 12 years of age: apply a thin film of Duac® gel to the cleansed affected areas once daily in the evening or as directed by clinician.

Adult Patients

Acne Vulgaris

Number of inflammatory lesions generally decreases after 2–6 weeks of topical therapy; maximum benefit may not be seen for up to 12 weeks. Prolonged therapy (several months or years) may be necessary.

Continue as long as response is satisfactory and no severe or intolerable toxicity occurs.

Treatment with Clindamycin and Benzoyl Peroxide Combination Preparations

TOPICAL:
- BenzaClin® gel: apply a thin film to the cleansed affected area twice daily (morning and evening) or as directed by clinician.
- Duac® gel: apply a thin film to the cleansed affected areas once daily in the evening or as directed by clinician.

Clindamycin Phosphate Injection

(klin da mye′ sin)

Brand Name: Cleocin®
Also available generically.

Important Warning

Clindamycin may cause colitis. If you experience any of the following symptoms, call your doctor immediately: severe persistent diarrhea, severe stomach cramps, or bloody stool.

About Your Treatment

Your doctor has ordered clindamycin, an antibiotic, to help treat your infection. The drug will be either injected into a large muscle (such as your buttock or hip) or added to an intravenous fluid that will drip through a needle or catheter placed in your vein for 30 minutes, two to four times a day.

Clindamycin eliminates bacteria that cause many kinds of infections, including pneumonia, and gynecological, skin, stomach, and blood infections. This medication is sometimes prescribed for other uses; ask your doctor or pharmacist for more information.

Your health care provider (doctor, nurse, or pharmacist) may measure the effectiveness and side effects of your treatment using laboratory tests and physical examinations. It is important to keep all appointments with your doctor and the laboratory. The length of treatment depends on how your infection and symptoms respond to the medication.

Precautions

Before administering clindamycin,

- tell your doctor and pharmacist if you are allergic to clindamycin, lincomycin (Lincocin), or any other drugs.
- tell your doctor and pharmacist what prescription and nonprescription medications you are taking, especially antibiotics and vitamins.
- tell your doctor if you have or have ever had asthma or gastrointestinal, liver, or kidney disease.
- tell your doctor if you are pregnant, plan to become pregnant, or are breast-feeding. If you become pregnant while taking clindamycin, call your doctor.

Administering Your Medication

Before you administer clindamycin, look at the solution closely. It should be clear and free of floating material. Gently squeeze the bag or observe the solution container to make sure there are no leaks. Do not use the solution if it is discolored, if it contains particles, or if the bag or container leaks. Use a new solution, but show the damaged one to your health care provider.

It is important that you use your medication exactly as directed. Do not stop your therapy on your own for any reason because your infection could worsen and result in hospitalization. Do not change your dosing schedule without talking to your health care provider. Your health care provider may tell you to stop your infusion if you have a mechanical problem (such as a blockage in the tubing, needle, or catheter); if you have to stop an infusion, call your health care provider immediately so your therapy can continue.

Side Effects

Clindamycin may cause side effects. Tell your health care provider if any of these symptoms are severe or do not go away:

- upset stomach
- vomiting
- gas
- diarrhea

If you experience any of the following symptoms in addition to the symptoms listed in the IMPORTANT WARNING section, call your health care provider immediately:

- skin rash
- itching
- fever

If you experience a serious side effect, you or your doctor may send a report to the Food and Drug Administration's (FDA) MedWatch Adverse Event Reporting program online [at http://www.fda.gov/MedWatch/index.html] or by phone [1-800-332-1088].

Storage Conditions

- Your health care provider probably will give you several days supply of clindamycin. If you are receiving clindamycin intravenously (in your vein), you probably will be told to store it in the refrigerator or freezer.
- Take your next dose from the refrigerator 1 hour before using it; place it in a clean, dry area to allow it to warm to room temperature.
- If you are told to store additional clindamycin in the freezer, always move a 24-hour supply to the refrigerator for the next day's use.
- Do not refreeze medications.

If you are receiving clindamycin intramuscularly (in your muscle), your health care provider will tell you how to store it properly.

Store your medication only as directed. Make sure you understand what you need to store your medication properly.

Keep your supplies in a clean, dry place when you are not using them, and keep all medications and supplies out of reach of children. Your health care provider will tell you how to throw away used needles, syringes, tubing, and containers to avoid accidental injury.

Overdose

In case of overdose, call your local poison control center at 1-800-222-1222. If the victim has collapsed or is not breathing, call local emergency services at 911.

Signs of Infection

If you are receiving clindamycin in your vein or under your skin, you need to know the symptoms of a catheter-related infection (an infection where the needle enters your vein or skin). If you experience any of these effects near your intravenous catheter, tell your health care provider as soon as possible:

- tenderness
- warmth
- irritation
- drainage
- redness
- swelling
- pain

Dosage Facts
For Informational Purposes

Caution: Do not change your dose, how often you take your medication, or the length of time you are to take it without first talking to your healthcare provider.

The following dosage information was written using medical language for doctors and other healthcare professionals and is provided here for you to check your dosage. The dosage of this drug may differ for different patients. Therefore, always follow your doctor's instructions or the directions on the label. Contact your healthcare provider or pharmacist if you have any questions about the specific dosage of your medication after reviewing this information.

General Dosage Information

Available as clindamycin hydrochloride, clindamycin palmitate hydrochloride, and clindamycin phosphate; dosage expressed in terms of clindamycin.

Pediatric Patients

General Dosage in Neonates

IV OR IM:

- Manufacturer recommends 15–20 mg/kg daily given in 3 or 4 equally divided doses. The lower dosage may be adequate for premature neonates.
- Neonates <1 week of age: AAP recommends 5 mg/kg every 12 hours in those weighing ≤2 kg or 5 mg/kg every 8 hours in those weighing >2 kg.
- Neonates 1–4 weeks of age: AAP recommends 5 mg/kg every 12 hours in those weighing <1.2 kg, 5 mg/kg every 8 hours in those weighing 1.2–2 kg, and 5–7.5 mg/kg every 6 hours in those weighing >2 kg.

General Dosage in Children 1 Month to 16 Years of Age

IV OR IM:

- Manufacturer recommends 20–40 mg/kg daily given in 3 or 4 equally divided doses. Alternatively, manufacturer recommends 350 mg/m² daily for serious infections or 450 mg/m² daily for more severe infections.
- AAP recommends 15–25 mg/kg daily for mild to moderate infections and 25–40 mg/kg daily for severe infections. Daily dosage is given in 3 or 4 equally divided doses.

Malaria†
Treatment of Severe P. falciparum Malaria†

IV, THEN ORAL:

- 10-mg/kg IV loading dose followed by 5 mg/kg IV every 8 hours; when oral therapy is tolerated, switch to oral clindamycin 20 mg/kg daily in 3 divided doses and continue for a total duration of 7 days.
- Used in conjunction with IV quinidine gluconate (followed by oral quinine sulfate) given for a total duration of 3–7 days.

Pneumocystis jiroveci (Pneumocystis carinii) Pneumonia†
Treatment of Mild to Moderate Infections†

IV:

- Adolescents: 600–900 mg every 6–8 hours given for 21 days; used in conjunction with oral primaquine (15–30 mg once daily for 21 days).

Toxoplasmosis†
Treatment in Infants and Children†

IV:

- 5–7.5 mg/kg (up to 600 mg) 4 times daily; used in conjunction with oral pyrimethamine (2 mg/kg once daily for 3 days then 1 mg/kg once daily) and oral leucovorin (≥10–25 mg once daily).
- Continue acute treatment for ≥6 weeks; a longer duration may be appropriate if disease is extensive or response incomplete at 6 weeks.

Treatment in Adolescents†

IV:

- 600 mg every 6 hours; used in conjunction with oral pyrimethamine (200-mg loading dose then 50–75 mg once daily) and oral leucovorin (at least 10–20 mg once daily).

- Continue acute treatment for ≥6 weeks; longer duration may be appropriate if disease is extensive or response incomplete at 6 weeks.

Perioperative Prophylaxis†
Head or Neck Surgery†

IV:

- 15 mg/kg given at induction of anesthesia (within 0.5–1 hour prior to incision); used with or without IV gentamicin.
- Although postoperative doses of prophylactic drugs generally are unnecessary, some clinicians suggest the dose may be repeated every 8 hours for 24 hours.

Adult Patients

General Adult Dosage
Serious Infections

IV OR IM:

- 600 mg to 1.2 g daily in 2–4 equally divided doses.

More Severe Infections

IV OR IM:

- 1.2–2.7 g daily in 2–4 equally divided doses.
- For life-threatening infections, dosage may be increased up 4.8 g daily.

Gynecologic Infections
Pelvic Inflammatory Disease

IV, THEN ORAL:

- Initially, 900 mg IV every 8 hours; used in conjunction with IV or IM gentamicin. After clinical improvement occurs, discontinue IV clindamycin and gentamicin and switch to oral clindamycin in a dosage of 450 mg 4 times daily to complete 14 days of therapy. Alternatively, oral doxycycline can be used to complete 14 days of therapy.

Anthrax†
Treatment of Inhalational Anthrax†

IV:

- 900 mg every 8 hours.
- Used in multiple-drug regimens that initially include IV ciprofloxacin or IV doxycycline and 1 or 2 other anti-infectives predicted to be effective.
- Duration of treatment is 60 days if anthrax occurred as the result of exposure to anthrax spores in the context of biologic warfare or bioterrorism.

Babesiosis†

IV:

- 1.2 g twice daily given for 7–10 days; used in conjunction with oral quinine sulfate (650 mg 3 times daily for 7–10 days).

Malaria†
Treatment of Severe P. falciparum Malaria†

IV, THEN ORAL:

- 10-mg/kg IV loading dose followed by 5 mg/kg IV every 8 hours; when oral therapy is tolerated, switch to oral clindamycin 20 mg/kg daily in 3 divided doses and continue for a total duration of 7 days.
- Used in conjunction with IV quinidine gluconate (followed by oral quinine sulfate) given for a total duration of 3–7 days.

Pneumocystis jiroveci (Pneumocystis carinii) Pneumonia†
Treatment of Mild to Moderate Infections†

IV:
- 600–900 mg every 6–8 hours given for 21 days; used in conjunction with oral primaquine (15–30 mg once daily for 21 days).

Toxoplasmosis†
Treatment†

IV:
- 600 mg every 6 hours; used in conjunction with oral pyrimethamine (200-mg loading dose then 50–75 mg once daily) and oral leucovorin (at least 10–20 mg once daily).
- Continue acute treatment for ≥6 weeks.

Prevention of Perinatal Group B Streptococcal Disease†
Women at Risk Who Should Not Receive β-lactam Anti-infectives†

IV:
- 900 mg every 8 hours; initiate at time of labor or rupture of membranes and continue until delivery.

Perioperative Prophylaxis†
Head or Neck Surgery†

IV:
- 600–900 mg given at induction of anesthesia (within 0.5–1 hour prior to incision); used with or without IV gentamicin.
- Although postoperative doses of prophylactic drugs generally are unnecessary, some clinicians suggest that the dose be repeated every 8 hours for 24 hours.

Contaminated or Dirty Surgery Involving Ruptured Abdominal Viscus†

IV:
- 600 mg every 8 hours; used in conjunction with IV gentamicin. Continue postoperatively for about 5 days

Special Populations

Hepatic Impairment
- Dosage adjustments not necessary in those with mild or moderate hepatic impairment.

Renal Impairment
- Dosage adjustments not necessary in those with mild or moderate renal impairment.

† Use is not currently included in the labeling approved by the US Food and Drug Administration.

Clioquinol Topical
(klye oh kwin′ ole)

Brand Name: Vioform®

Why is this medicine prescribed?

Clioquinol is used to treat skin infections such as eczema, athlete's foot, jock itch, and ringworm.

This medication is sometimes prescribed for other uses; ask your doctor or pharmacist for more information.

How should this medicine be used?

Clioquinol comes as a cream, lotion, and ointment to apply to the skin. Clioquinol is usually used two to four times a day for 4 weeks (2 weeks for jock itch). Follow the directions on the label carefully, and ask your doctor or pharmacist to explain any part you do not understand. Use clioquinol exactly as directed. Do not use more or less of it or use it more often than indicated on the product label.

Thoroughly clean the infected area, allow it to dry, and then gently rub the medication in until most of it disappears. Use just enough medication to cover the affected area. You should wash your hands after applying the medication.

What special precautions should I follow?

Before using clioquinol,
- tell your doctor and pharmacist if you are allergic to clioquinol or any other drugs.
- tell your doctor and pharmacist what prescription and non-prescription drugs you are taking, including vitamins.
- tell your doctor and pharmacist if you are about to take a thyroid function test.
- tell your doctor if you are pregnant, plan to become pregnant, or are breast-feeding. If you become pregnant while using clioquinol, call your doctor.

What should I do if I forget to take a dose?

Apply the missed dose as soon as you remember it. However, if it is almost time for the next dose, skip the missed dose and continue your regular dosing schedule. Do not apply a double dose to make up for a missed one.

What side effects can this medicine cause?

Clioquinol may cause side effects. If you experience any of the following symptoms, call your doctor immediately:
- itching
- burning
- irritation or stinging
- redness
- swelling

If you experience a serious side effect, you or your doctor may send a report to the Food and Drug Administration's (FDA) MedWatch Adverse Event Reporting program online

[at http://www.fda.gov/MedWatch/index.html] or by phone [1-800-332-1088].

What storage conditions are needed for this medicine?

Keep this medication in the container it came in, tightly closed, and out of reach of children. Store it at room temperature and away from excess heat and moisture (not in the bathroom). Do not freeze. Protect it from light. Throw away any medication that is outdated or no longer needed. Talk to your pharmacist about the proper disposal of your medication.

What other information should I know?

Keep all appointments with your doctor. Clioquinol is for external use only and may stain your clothes, hair, skin, and nails yellow. Do not let clioquinol get into your eyes or mouth, and do not swallow it. Do not apply cosmetics, lotions, or other skin products to the area being treated unless your doctor tells you.

Do not let anyone else use your medication. If you still have the symptoms of infection after you finish the clioquinol, call your doctor.

Talk to your doctor, pharmacist, or other healthcare professional if you have questions about dosing information for your medication.

Clobetasol

(kloe bay′ ta sol)

Brand Name: Clobevate®, Cormax®, Cormax® Scalp Application, Embeline® E, Olux®, Temovate®, Temovate® E, Temovate® Scalp Application
Also available generically.

Why is this medicine prescribed?

Clobetasol is used to treat the itching, redness, dryness, crusting, scaling, inflammation, and discomfort of various skin and scalp conditions.

This medication is sometimes prescribed for other uses; ask your doctor or pharmacist for more information.

How should this medicine be used?

Clobetasol comes in cream and ointment for use on the skin and in lotion to apply to the scalp. Clobetasol is used once or twice a day. Follow the directions on your prescription label carefully, and ask your doctor or pharmacist to explain any part you do not understand. Use clobetasol exactly as directed. Do not use more or less of it or use it more often than prescribed by your doctor. Do not use clobetasol for longer than 14 days without your doctor's approval.

Thoroughly clean the infected area, allow it to dry, and then gently rub the medication in until most of it disappears. Use just enough medication to cover the affected area. You should wash your hands after applying the medication. The scalp lotion should be applied directly from the squeeze bottle to the affected area.

Clobetasol can be absorbed into your body if used in large amounts and can cause harmful effects.

What special precautions should I follow?

Before using clobetasol,
- tell your doctor and pharmacist if you are allergic to clobetasol or any other drugs.
- tell your doctor and pharmacist what prescription and nonprescription medications you are using, including vitamins.
- tell your doctor if you are pregnant, plan to become pregnant, or are breast-feeding. If you become pregnant while using clobetasol, call your doctor.

What should I do if I forget to take a dose?

Apply the missed dose as soon as you remember it. However, if it is almost time for the next dose, skip the missed dose and continue your regular dosing schedule. Do not apply a double dose to make up for a missed one.

What side effects can this medicine cause?

Clobetasol may cause side effects. If you experience any of the following symptoms, call your doctor:
- itching, burning, or irritation on the area of skin where clobetasol is applied

If you experience a serious side effect, you or your doctor may send a report to the Food and Drug Administration's (FDA) MedWatch Adverse Event Reporting program online [at http://www.fda.gov/MedWatch/index.html] or by phone [1-800-332-1088].

What storage conditions are needed for this medicine?

Keep this medication in the container it came in, tightly closed, and out of reach of children. Store it at room temperature and away from excess heat and moisture (not in the bathroom). Throw away any medication that is outdated or no longer needed. Talk to your pharmacist about the proper disposal of your medication.

What other information should I know?

Keep all appointments with your doctor. Clobetasol is for external use only. Do not let clobetasol get into your eyes, nose, or mouth, and do not swallow it. Do not apply dressings, bandages, cosmetics, lotions, or other skin medications to the area being treated unless your doctor tells you.

Do not let anyone else use your medication. Ask your pharmacist any questions you have about refilling your prescription.

If you still have symptoms of infection after you finish the clobetasol, call your doctor.

Dosage Facts
For Informational Purposes

Caution: Do not change your dose, how often you take your medication, or the length of time you are to take it without first talking to your health-care provider.

The following dosage information was written using medical language for doctors and other healthcare professionals and is provided here for you to check your dosage. The dosage of this drug may differ for different patients. Therefore, always follow your doctor's instructions or the directions on the label. Contact your health-care provider or pharmacist if you have any questions about the specific dosage of your medication after reviewing this information.

General Dosage Information

Available as clobetasol propionate; dosage expressed in terms of the salt.

Intermittent maintenance therapy, such as administration of the drug once or twice weekly for up to 6 months, has resulted in prolonged periods of remission from corticosteroid-responsive dermatoses in some patients.

Pediatric Patients

Administer the least amount of topical preparations that provides effective therapy.

Corticosteroid-responsive Dermatoses
TOPICAL:
- Children ≥12 years of age: Apply cream, ointment, gel, foam, or solution sparingly to affected area twice daily, preferably in the morning and evening.
- Discontinue when control is achieved; if improvement does not occur within 2 weeks, consider reassessment of the diagnosis.

Adult Patients

Corticosteroid-responsive Dermatoses
TOPICAL:
- Apply cream, ointment, gel, lotion, foam, or solution sparingly to affected area twice daily, preferably in the morning and evening.
- Discontinue when control is achieved; if improvement does not occur within 2 weeks, consider reassessment of the diagnosis.
- Emollient cream or lotion (applied to no more than 10% of body surface area) may be used for up to 4 consecutive weeks in the management of plaque psoriasis; however, the manufacturers state that additional benefits of extended treatment (i.e., >2 weeks) should be weighed against the risk of HPA-axis suppression.
- Apply shampoo to scalp once daily. Discontinue when control is achieved. If improvement does not occur within 4 weeks, consider reassessment of the diagnosis and consider substituting a less potent topical corticosteroid preparation.

Prescribing Limits
Pediatric Patients

Corticosteroid-responsive Dermatoses
TOPICAL:
- Maximum 50 g of 0.05% cream, ointment, or gel per week for no more than 2 consecutive weeks.
- Maximum 1 1/2 capfuls of foam per application; maximum 50 g per week for no more than 2 consecutive weeks.
- Maximum 50 mL (50 g) of 0.05% solution per week for no more than 2 consecutive weeks.

Adult Patients

Corticosteroid-responsive Dermatoses
TOPICAL:
- Maximum 50 g of 0.05% cream, ointment, gel, or lotion per week for no more than 2 consecutive weeks.
- Maximum 1 1/2 capfuls of foam per application; maximum 50 g per week for no more than 2 consecutive weeks.
- Maximum 50 mL (50 g) of 0.05% solution per week for no more than 2 consecutive weeks.
- In patients with plaque psoriasis, maximum 50 g of 0.05% emollient cream, shampoo, or lotion per week for no more than 4 consecutive weeks.
- In patients with psoriasis of the scalp, maximum 4 consecutive weeks of therapy with shampoo.

Special Populations

Geriatric Patients
- No dosage adjustments with cream, ointment, gel, or solution. Titrate dosage carefully when using foam, lotion, or shampoo; initiate therapy at the low end of the dosage range.

Clofarabine Injection
(kloe far′ a been)

Brand Name: Clolar®

Why is this medicine prescribed?

Clofarabine is used to treat acute lymphoblastic leukemia (ALL; a type of cancer of the white blood cells) in children and young adults 1-21 years old who have already received at least two other treatments. Clofarabine is in a class of medications called purine nucleoside antimetabolites. It works by killing existing cancer cells and limiting the development of new cancer cells.

How should this medicine be used?

Clofarabine comes as a solution to be injected into a vein. Clofarabine is administered by a doctor or nurse. It is usually given once a day for 5 days in a row. This dosing cycle may be repeated once every 2-6 weeks, depending on your response to the medication.

It will take at least 2 hours for you to receive each dose

of clofarabine. Tell your doctor or other healthcare provider right away if you feel anxious or restless while you are receiving the medication.

Are there other uses for this medicine?

This medication may be prescribed for other uses; ask your doctor or pharmacist for more information.

What special precautions should I follow?

Before using clofarabine,
- tell your doctor and pharmacist if you are allergic to clofarabine or any other medications.
- tell your doctor and pharmacist what prescription and nonprescription medications, vitamins, nutritional supplements, and herbal products you are taking or plan to take. Be sure to mention medications for high blood pressure and heart disease. Your doctor may need to change the doses of your medications or monitor you carefully for side effects.
- tell your doctor if you have or have ever had kidney or liver disease.
- tell your doctor if you are pregnant or plan to become pregnant. Clofarabine may harm the fetus. You should use birth control to prevent pregnancy during your treatment with clofarabine. Talk to your doctor about types of birth control that will work for you. If you become pregnant while using clofarabine, call your doctor.
- tell your doctor if you are breast-feeding. You should not breastfeed during your treatment with clofarabine.
- if you are having surgery, including dental surgery, tell the doctor or dentist that you are receiving clofarabine.
- you should know that clofarabine may cause a skin condition called hand-foot syndrome. If you develop this condition, you may experience tingling of the hands and feet, and then reddening, dryness, and flaking of the skin on the hands and feet. If this happens, ask your doctor to recommend a lotion that you can apply to these areas. You will need to apply the lotion lightly and avoid rubbing the areas forcefully. Your doctor may also prescribe medication to relieve these symptoms.

What special dietary instructions should I follow?

Drink plenty of fluids every day during your treatment with clofarabine, especially if you vomit or have diarrhea.

What side effects can this medicine cause?

Clofarabine may cause side effects. Tell your doctor if any of these symptoms are severe or do not go away:
- nausea
- vomiting
- stomach pain
- diarrhea
- constipation
- loss of appetite
- weight loss
- swelling of the inside of the mouth and nose
- painful white patches in the mouth
- headache
- anxiety
- depression
- irritability
- pain in the back, joints, arms, or legs
- drowsiness
- dry, itchy, or irritated skin
- flushing

Some side effects can be serious. If you experience any of these symptoms, call your doctor immediately:
- fast heartbeat
- fast breathing
- shortness of breath
- dizziness
- lightheadedness
- fainting
- decreased urination
- sore throat, cough, fever, chills, and other signs of infection
- pale skin
- excessive tiredness
- weakness
- confusion
- unusual bruising or bleeding
- nosebleed
- bleeding gums
- blood in urine
- small red or purple spots under the skin
- yellowing of the skin or eyes
- itching
- red, warm, swollen, tender skin
- uncontrollable shaking of a part of the body

Clofarabine may cause other side effects. Call your doctor if you have any unusual problems while using this medication.

What storage conditions are needed for this medicine?

This medication will be stored in the hospital.

What should I do in case of overdose?

In case of overdose, call your local poison control center at 1-800-222-1222. If the victim has collapsed or is not breathing, call local emergency services at 911.

Symptoms of overdose may include:
- yellowing of the skin or eyes
- vomiting
- rash

What other information should I know?

Keep all appointments with your doctor and the laboratory. Your doctor will order certain lab tests to check your body's response to clofarabine.

Dosage Facts
For Informational Purposes

Caution: Do not change your dose, how often you take your medication, or the length of time you are to take it without first talking to your healthcare provider.

The following dosage information was written using medical language for doctors and other healthcare professionals and is provided here for you to check your dosage. The dosage of this drug may differ for different patients. Therefore, always follow your doctor's instructions or the directions on the label. Contact your healthcare provider or pharmacist if you have any questions about the specific dosage of your medication after reviewing this information.

General Dosage Information

Dosage is based on the patient's body surface area and is calculated using the actual body weight and height of the patient before starting each cycle.

Pediatric Patients

Acute Lymphocytic Leukemia

IV:
- 1–21 years of age: 52 mg/m² by IV infusion over 2 hours daily for 5 consecutive days.
- Repeat treatment cycle following recovery or return to baseline organ function, approximately every 2–6 weeks.
- Discontinue infusion immediately and initiate appropriate supportive measures if early manifestations of cytokine release or capillary leak syndrome occur. Consider reinstitution of therapy, generally at a lower dosage, if patient is stable and organ function has returned to baseline levels.
- Discontinue infusion immediately if substantial increases in serum creatinine or bilirubin concentrations occur. Consider reinstitution of therapy, generally at a lower dosage, once the patient is stable and organ function has returned to baseline levels.
- Discontinue infusion immediately if hypotension develops. Consider reinstitution of therapy at a lower dosage if hypotension was transient and resolved without pharmacologic intervention.

Special Populations

No special population dosage recommendations at this time.

Clomiphene
(kloe′ mi feen)

Brand Name: Clomid®, Serophene®

Why is this medicine prescribed?

Clomiphene is used to induce ovulation (egg production) in women who do not produce ova (eggs) but wish to become pregnant. Clomiphene is in a class of medications called ovulatory stimulants. It works similarly to estrogen, a female hormone that causes eggs to develop in the ovaries and be released.

How should this medicine be used?

Clomiphene comes as a tablet to take by mouth. It is usually taken once a day for 5 days, beginning on or about day 5 of the cycle. To help you remember to take clomiphene, take it around the same time every day. Follow the directions on your prescription label carefully, and ask your doctor or pharmacist to explain any part you do not understand. Take clomiphene exactly as directed. Do not take more or less of it or take it more often than prescribed by your doctor.

Are there other uses for this medicine?

Clomiphene is also sometimes used to treat male infertility, menstrual abnormalities, fibrocystic breasts, and persistent breast milk production. Talk to your doctor about the possible risks of using this medication for your condition.

This medication may be prescribed for other uses; ask your doctor or pharmacist for more information.

What special precautions should I follow?

Before taking clomiphene,
- tell your doctor and pharmacist if you are allergic to clomiphene or any other medications.
- tell your doctor and pharmacist what prescription and nonprescription medications, vitamins, nutritional supplements, and herbal products you are taking.
- tell your doctor if you have or have ever had liver disease, ovarian cysts (except those from polycystic ovary syndrome), uterine fibroids, abnormal vaginal bleeding, a pituitary tumor, or thyroid or adrenal disease.
- tell your doctor if you are pregnant or breast-feeding. If you become pregnant while taking clomiphene, call your doctor immediately.
- you should know that clomiphene may cause blurred vision. Do not drive a car or operate machinery, especially in poor lighting, until you know how this medication affects you.
- you should know that clomiphene increases the chance of multiple pregnancy (twins or more). Talk to your doctor about the risks of multiple pregnancy.

What special dietary instructions should I follow?

Unless your doctor tells you otherwise, continue your normal diet.

What should I do if I forget to take a dose?

Take the missed dose as soon as you remember it. However, if it is almost time for the next dose, call your doctor for additional directions. Do not take a double dose to make up for a missed one.

What side effects can this medicine cause?

Clomiphene may cause side effects. Tell your doctor if any of these symptoms are severe or do not go away:
- flushing (feeling of warmth)
- upset stomach
- vomiting
- breast discomfort
- headache
- abnormal vaginal bleeding

Some side effects can be serious. The following symptoms are uncommon, but if you experience any of them, call your doctor immediately:
- blurred vision
- visual spots or flashes
- double vision
- stomach or lower stomach pain
- stomach swelling
- weight gain
- shortness of breath

Long-term use of clomiphene may increase the risk of ovarian cancer. Clomiphene should not be used for more than about six cycles. Talk to your doctor about the risks of taking this medication.

Clomiphene may cause other side effects. Call your doctor if you have any unusual problems while taking this medication.

If you experience a serious side effect, you or your doctor may send a report to the Food and Drug Administration's (FDA) MedWatch Adverse Event Reporting program online [at http://www.fda.gov/MedWatch/index.html] or by phone [1-800-332-1088].

What storage conditions are needed for this medicine?

Keep this medication in the container it came in, tightly closed, and out of reach of children. Store it at room temperature and away from excess heat and moisture (not in the bathroom). Throw away any medication that is outdated or no longer needed. Talk to your pharmacist about the proper disposal of your medication.

What should I do in case of overdose?

In case of overdose, call your local poison control center at 1-800-222-1222. If the victim has collapsed or is not breathing, call local emergency services at 911.

Symptoms of overdose may include:
- upset stomach
- vomiting
- hot flashes
- blurred vision
- visual spots or flashes
- blind spots
- stomach swelling
- stomach or lower stomach pain

What other information should I know?

Keep all appointments with your doctor and laboratory. Your doctor may order certain lab tests to check your body's response to clomiphene.

Do not let anyone else take your medication. Ask your pharmacist any questions you have about refilling your prescription.

Talk to your doctor, pharmacist, or other healthcare professional if you have questions about dosing information for your medication.

Clomipramine

(kloe mi′ pra meen)

Brand Name: Anafranil®
Also available generically.

Important Warning

A small number of children, teenagers, and young adults (up to 24 years of age) who took antidepressants ('mood elevators') such as clomipramine during clinical studies became suicidal (thinking about harming or killing oneself or planning or trying to do so). Children, teenagers, and young adults who take antidepressants to treat depression or other mental illnesses may be more likely to become suicidal than children, teenagers, and young adults who do not take antidepressants to treat these conditions. However, experts are not sure about how great this risk is and how much it should be considered in deciding whether a child or teenager should take an antidepressant. Children younger than 18 years of age should not normally take clomipramine, but in some cases, a doctor may decide that clomipramine is the best medication to treat a child's condition.

You should know that your mental health may change in unexpected ways when you take clomipramine or other antidepressants even if you are an adult over age 24. You may become suicidal, especially at the beginning of your treatment and any time that your dose is increased or decreased. You, your family, or your caregiver should call your doctor right away if you experience any of the following symptoms: new or worsening depression; thinking about harming or killing yourself, or planning or trying to do so; extreme worry; agitation; panic attacks; difficulty falling asleep or staying asleep; aggressive behavior; irritability; acting without thinking; severe restlessness; and frenzied abnormal excitement. Be sure that your family or caregiver knows which symptoms may be serious so they can call the doctor when you are unable to seek treatment on your own.

Your healthcare provider will want to see you often while you are taking clomipramine, especially at the beginning of your treatment. Be sure to keep all appointments for office visits with your doctor.

The doctor or pharmacist will give you the manufacturer's patient information sheet (Medication Guide) when you begin treatment with clomipramine. Read the information carefully and ask your doctor or pharmacist if you have any questions. You also can obtain the Medication Guide from the FDA website: http://www.fda.gov/cder/drug/antidepressants/antidepressants _ MG _ 2007.pdf.

No matter your age, before you take an antidepressant, you, your parent, or your caregiver should talk to your doctor about the risks and benefits of treating your condition with an antidepressant or with other treatments. You should also talk about the risks and benefits of not treating your condition. You should know that having depression or another mental illness greatly increases the risk that you will become suicidal. This risk is higher if you or anyone in your family has or has ever had bipolar disorder (mood that changes from depressed to abnormally excited) or mania (frenzied, abnormally excited mood) or has thought about or attempted suicide. Talk to your doctor about your condition, symptoms, and personal and family medical history. You and your doctor will decide what type of treatment is right for you.

Why is this medicine prescribed?

Clomipramine is used to treat people with obsessive-compulsive disorder (a condition that causes repeated unwanted thoughts and the need to perform certain behaviors over and over). Clomipramine is in a group of medications called tricyclic antidepressants. It works by increasing the amount of serotonin, a natural substance in the brain that is needed to maintain mental balance.

How should this medicine be used?

Clomipramine comes as a capsule to take by mouth. At the beginning of treatment, clomipramine is usually taken three times a day with meals as the body adjusts to the medication. After several weeks of treatment, clomipramine is usually taken once a day at bedtime. Follow the directions on your prescription label carefully, and ask your doctor or phar-

macist to explain any part you do not understand. Take clomipramine exactly as directed. Do not take more or less of it or take it more often than prescribed by your doctor.

Your doctor may start you on a low dose of clomipramine and gradually increase your dose.

It may take several weeks or longer for you to feel the full benefit of clomipramine. Continue to take clomipramine even if you feel well. Do not stop taking clomipramine without talking to your doctor. If you suddenly stop taking clomipramine, you may experience withdrawal symptoms such as dizziness, nausea, vomiting, headache, weakness, sleep problems, fever, and irritability. Your doctor probably will decrease your dose gradually.

What special precautions should I follow?

Before taking clomipramine,

- tell your doctor and pharmacist if you are allergic to clomipramine, other tricyclic antidepressants such as amitriptyline (Elavil), amoxapine (Asendin), desipramine (Norpramin), doxepin (Adapin, Sinequan), imipramine (Tofranil), nortriptyline (Aventyl, Pamelor), protriptyline (Vivactil), and trimipramine (Surmontil); any other medications, or any of the inactive ingredients in clomipramine capsules. Ask your doctor or pharmacist for a list of the inactive ingredients.
- tell your doctor if you are taking a monoamine oxidase (MAO) inhibitor such as isocarboxazid (Marplan), phenelzine (Nardil), selegiline (Eldepryl, Emsam, Zelapar), and tranylcypromine (Parnate), or if you have stopped taking an MAO inhibitor within the past 14 days. Your doctor will probably tell you not to take clomipramine. If you stop taking clomipramine, you should wait at least 14 days before you start to take an MAO inhibitor.
- tell your doctor and pharmacist what prescription and nonprescription medications, vitamins, nutritional supplements and herbal products you are taking or plan to take. Be sure to mention any of the following: anticoagulants ('blood thinners') such as warfarin (Coumadin); benztropine (Cogentin); cimetidine (Tagamet); clonidine (Catapres); dicyclomine (Bentyl); digoxin (Lanoxin); disulfiram; flecainide (Tambocor); guanethidine (Ismelin); haloperidol (Haldol); levodopa (Sinemet, Dopar); medications for nausea, dizziness, or mental illness; methylphenidate (Concerta, Metadate, Ritalin); oral contraceptives; phenobarbital; phenytoin; propafenone (Rythmol); quinidine; secobarbital (Seconal); sedatives; selective serotonin reuptake inhibitors (SSRIs) such as fluoxetine (Prozac, Sarafem), sertraline (Zoloft), and paroxetine (Paxil); tranquilizers; and trihexyphenidyl (Artane); and vitamins. Your doctor may need to change the doses of your medication or monitor you more carefully for side effects. Your doctor may tell you not to take clomipramine if you have stopped taking fluoxetine during the past 5 weeks.
- tell your doctor if you have recently had a heart attack. Your doctor may tell you that you should not take clomipramine.

- tell your doctor if you are being treated with electroshock therapy (procedure in which small electric shocks are administered to the brain to treat certain mental illnesses), if you drink or have ever drunk large amounts of alcohol and if you have or have ever had seizures, brain damage, problems with your urinary system or prostate (a male reproductive organ), glaucoma (an eye condition), irregular heartbeat, problems with your blood pressure, thyroid problems, or heart, kidney, or liver disease.
- tell your doctor if you are pregnant, plan to become pregnant, or are breast-feeding. If you become pregnant while taking clomipramine, call your doctor.
- if you are having surgery, including dental surgery, tell the doctor or dentist that you are taking clomipramine.
- you should know that this medication may make you drowsy and may increase the risk that you will have a seizure. Do not drive a car, operate machinery, swim, or climb until you know how this medication affects you.
- remember that alcohol can add to the drowsiness caused by this medication.
- tell your doctor if you use tobacco products. Cigarette smoking may decrease the effectiveness of this medication.

What special dietary instructions should I follow?

Unless your doctor tells you otherwise, continue your usual diet.

What should I do if I forget to take a dose?

Take the missed dose as soon as you remember it. However, if it is almost time for your next dose, skip the missed dose and continue your regular dosing schedule. Do not take a double dose to make up for a missed one.

What side effects can this medicine cause?

Clomipramine may cause side effects. Tell your doctor if any of these symptoms are severe or do not go away:

- drowsiness
- dry mouth
- nausea
- vomiting
- diarrhea
- constipation
- nervousness
- decreased sexual ability
- decreased memory or concentration
- headache
- stuffy nose
- change in appetite or weight

Some side effects may be serious. If you experience any of the following symptoms or those listed in the IMPORTANT WARNING section, call your doctor immediately:

- uncontrollable shaking of a part of the body
- seizures
- fast, irregular, or pounding heartbeat

- difficulty urinating or loss of bladder control
- believing things that are not true
- hallucinations (seeing things or hearing voices that do not exist)
- eye pain
- shakiness
- difficulty breathing or fast breathing
- severe muscle stiffness
- unusual tiredness or weakness
- sore throat, fever, and other signs of infection

If you experience a serious side effect, you or your doctor may send a report to the Food and Drug Administration's (FDA) MedWatch Adverse Event Reporting program online [at http://www.fda.gov/MedWatch/index.html] or by phone [1-800-332-1088].

What storage conditions are needed for this medicine?

Keep this medication in the container it came in, tightly closed, and out of reach of children. Store it at room temperature and away from excess heat and moisture (not in the bathroom). Throw away any medication that is outdated or no longer needed. Talk to your pharmacist about the proper disposal of your medication.

What should I do in case of overdose?

In case of overdose, call your local poison control center at 1-800-222-1222. If the victim has collapsed or is not breathing, call local emergency services at 911.

Symptoms of overdose may include:

- seizures
- coma (loss of consciousness for a period of time)
- drowsiness
- restlessness
- loss of coordination
- sweating
- stiff muscles
- unusual movements
- fast heartbeat
- slowed breathing
- blue discoloration of the skin
- fever
- widened pupils (dark circles in the center of the eye)
- decreased urination

What other information should I know?

Keep all appointments with your doctor.

Do not let anyone else take your medication. Ask your pharmacist any questions you have about refilling your prescription.

Dosage Facts
For Informational Purposes

Caution: Do not change your dose, how often you take your medication, or the length of time you

are to take it without first talking to your health-care provider.

The following dosage information was written using medical language for doctors and other healthcare professionals and is provided here for you to check your dosage. The dosage of this drug may differ for different patients. Therefore, always follow your doctor's instructions or the directions on the label. Contact your healthcare provider or pharmacist if you have any questions about the specific dosage of your medication after reviewing this information.

General Dosage Information

Available as clomipramine hydrochloride; dosage is expressed in terms of the salt.

Individualize dosage carefully according to individual requirements and response.

Allow 2–3 weeks to elapse between any further dosage adjustments after the initial dosage titration period for achievement of steady-state plasma concentrations.

Pediatric Patients

OCD

ORAL:
- Children >10 years of age: initially, 25 mg daily. Gradually increase dosage, as tolerated, during the first 2 weeks of therapy up to a maximum of 3 mg/kg or 100 mg daily, whichever is lower. Titrate dosage carefully. If necessary, dosages may be increased gradually during the next several weeks up to a maximum of 3 mg/kg or 200 mg daily (whichever is lower).
- Optimum duration not established; some clinicians recommend that therapy be continued in responding patients at the minimally effective dosage for at least 18 months before attempting to discontinue.

Adult Patients

OCD

ORAL:
- Initially, 25 mg daily. Gradually increase dosage, as tolerated, during the first 2 weeks of therapy to approximately 100 mg daily. If necessary, dosages may be increased gradually during the next several weeks up to a maximum of 250 mg daily.
- Optimum duration not established; some clinicians recommend that therapy be continued in responding patients at the minimally effective dosage for at least 18 months before attempting to discontinue.

Panic Disorder†

ORAL:
- Usual dosage: ≤50 mg daily (range: 12.5–150 mg daily); patients with agoraphobia may require higher dosage.

Major Depressive Disorder†

ORAL:
- 100–250 mg daily.

Chronic Pain†

ORAL:
- 100–250 mg daily.

Cataplexy and Associated Narcolepsy†

ORAL:
- 25–200 mg daily.

Prescribing Limits

Pediatric Patients

OCD

ORAL:
- Maximum 3 mg/kg or 200 mg daily, whichever is lower.

Adult Patients

OCD

ORAL:
- Maximum 250 mg daily.

Panic Disorder†

ORAL:
- Maximum 200 mg daily.

Special Populations

Geriatric Patients
- Manufacturer makes no specific recommendation for dosage adjustment but lower clomipramine hydrochloride dosages are recommended by some clinicians at least during initial therapy.
- Select dosage with caution because of age-related decreases in hepatic, renal, and/or cardiac function and potential for concomitant disease and drug therapy.

† Use is not currently included in the labeling approved by the US Food and Drug Administration.

Clonazepam

(kloe na′ ze pam)

Brand Name: Klonopin®
Also available generically.

Why is this medicine prescribed?

Clonazepam is used to control seizures. It is also used to relieve anxiety.

This medication is sometimes prescribed for other uses; ask your doctor or pharmacist for more information.

How should this medicine be used?

Clonazepam comes as a tablet to take by mouth. It usually is taken three times a day and may be taken with or without food. Follow the directions on your prescription label carefully, and ask your doctor or pharmacist to explain any part you do not understand. Take clonazepam exactly as directed.

Clonazepam can be habit-forming. Do not take a larger dose, take it more often, or for a longer time than your doctor tells you to. Tolerance may develop with long-term or excessive use, making the drug less effective. This medication must be taken regularly to be effective. Do not skip doses even if you feel that you do not need them. Do not take clonazepam for more than 4 months or stop taking this medication without talking to your doctor. Stopping the drug suddenly can worsen your condition and cause withdrawal symptoms (anxiousness, sleeplessness, and irritability). Your doctor probably will decrease your dose gradually.

Are there other uses for this medicine?

Clonazepam is also used to treat symptoms of Parkinson's disease, twitching, schizophrenia, and for pain management. Talk to your doctor about the possible risks of using this drug for your condition.

What special precautions should I follow?

Before taking clonazepam,

- tell your doctor and pharmacist if you are allergic to clonazepam, alprazolam (Xanax), chlordiazepoxide (Librium, Librax), clorazepate (Tranxene), diazepam (Valium), estazolam (ProSom), flurazepam (Dalmane), lorazepam (Ativan), oxazepam (Serax), prazepam (Centrax), temazepam (Restoril), triazolam (Halcion), or any other drugs.
- tell your doctor and pharmacist what prescription and nonprescription medications you are taking, especially antihistamines; cimetadine (Tagamet); digoxin (Lanoxin); disulfiram (Antabuse); fluoxetine (Prozac); isoniazide (INH, Laniazid, Nydrazid); ketoconazole (Nizoral); levodopa (Larodopa, Sinemet); medications for depression, seizures, pain, Parkinson's disease, asthma, colds, or allergies; metoprolol (Lopressor, Toprol XL), muscle relaxants; oral contraceptives; oral antifungals, phenytoin (Dilantin); probenecid (Benemid); propoxyphene (Darvon); propranolol (Inderal); rifampin (Rifadin); sedatives; sleeping pills; theophylline (TheoDur); tranquilizers; valproic acid (Depakene); and vitamins. These medications may add to the drowsiness caused by clonazepam.
- tell your doctor if you have or have ever had glaucoma; seizures; or lung, heart, or liver disease.
- tell your doctor if you are pregnant, plan to become pregnant, or are breast-feeding. If you become pregnant while taking clonazepam, call your doctor immediately. You should not nurse a baby while taking clonazepam.
- if you are having surgery, including dental surgery, tell the doctor or dentist that you are taking clonazepam.
- you should know that this drug may make you drowsy. Do not drive a car or operate machinery until you know how this drug affects you.
- remember that alcohol can add to the drowsiness caused by this drug. You should avoid drinking alcohol while taking clonazepam.
- tell your doctor if you use tobacco products. Cigarette smoking may decrease the effectiveness of this drug.

What should I do if I forget to take a dose?

If you take several doses per day and miss a dose, skip the missed dose and continue your regular dosing schedule. Do not take a double dose to make up for a missed one.

What side effects can this medicine cause?

Side effects from clonazepam are common and include:
- drowsiness
- dizziness
- tiredness
- weakness
- dry mouth
- diarrhea
- upset stomach
- changes in appetite

Tell your doctor if any of these symptoms are severe or do not go away:
- restlessness or excitement
- constipation
- difficulty urinating
- frequent urination
- blurred vision
- changes in sex drive or ability

If you experience any of the following symptoms, call your doctor immediately:
- seizures
- shuffling walk
- persistent, fine tremor or inability to sit still
- fever
- difficulty breathing or swallowing
- severe skin rash
- yellowing of the skin or eyes
- irregular heartbeat

If you experience a serious side effect, you or your doctor may send a report to the Food and Drug Administration's (FDA) MedWatch Adverse Event Reporting program online [at http://www.fda.gov/MedWatch/index.html] or by phone [1-800-332-1088].

What storage conditions are needed for this medicine?

Keep this medication in the container it came in, tightly closed, and out of reach of children. Store it at room temperature and away from excess heat and moisture (not in the bathroom). Throw away any medication that is outdated or no longer needed. Talk to your pharmacist about the proper disposal of your medication.

What should I do in case of overdose?

In case of overdose, call your local poison control center at 1-800-222-1222. If the victim has collapsed or is not breathing, call local emergency services at 911.

What other information should I know?

Keep all appointments with your doctor and the laboratory. Your doctor will order certain lab tests to check your response to clonazepam.

If you are taking clonazepam to control seizures and have an increase in their frequency or severity, call your doctor. Your dose may need to be adjusted. If you use clonazepam for seizures, carry identification (Medic Alert) stating that you have epilepsy and that you are taking clonazepam.

Do not let anyone else take your medication. Ask your pharmacist any questions you have about refilling your prescription.

Dosage Facts
For Informational Purposes

Caution: Do not change your dose, how often you take your medication, or the length of time you are to take it without first talking to your healthcare provider.

The following dosage information was written using medical language for doctors and other healthcare professionals and is provided here for you to check your dosage. The dosage of this drug may differ for different patients. Therefore, always follow your doctor's instructions or the directions on the label. Contact your healthcare provider or pharmacist if you have any questions about the specific dosage of your medication after reviewing this information.

Pediatric Patients
Seizure Disorders
ORAL:
- Infants and children <10 years of age or weighing <30 kg: Initially, 0.01–0.03 mg/kg daily; initial dosage should not exceed 0.05 mg/kg daily given in 2 or 3 divided doses.
- Increase dosage by no more than 0.5 mg every third day until seizure control is achieved with minimal adverse effects. Maintenance dosage of 0.1–0.2 mg/kg daily.
- Children ≥10 years of age or weighing ≥30 kg: Initial dosage should not exceed 1.5 mg daily given in 3 divided doses.
- Increase dosage in increments of 0.5–1 mg every third day (up to a maximum dosage of 20 mg daily) until seizure control is achieved with minimal adverse effects.

Adult Patients
Seizure Disorders
ORAL:
- Initial dosage should not exceed 1.5 mg daily given in 3 divided doses. Increase dosage in increments of 0.5–1 mg every third day (up to a maximum dosage of 20 mg daily) until seizure control is achieved with minimal adverse effects.

Panic Disorder
ORAL:
- Initially, 0.25 mg twice daily. After 3 days, increase dosage to usual maintenance dosage of 1 mg daily.
- Some clinicians recommend dosages of 1–2 mg daily. Certain patients may benefit from dosages up to 4 mg daily. In such cases, increase dosage by 0.125–0.25 mg twice daily every 3 days until panic disorder is controlled with minimal adverse effects.
- Discontinue therapy gradually by decreasing the dosage in increments of 0.125 mg twice daily every 3 days until the drug is completely withdrawn.

Prescribing Limits
Pediatric Patients
Seizure Disorders
ORAL:
- Maximum 0.2 mg/kg daily.

Adult Patients
Seizure Disorders
ORAL:
- Maximum 20 mg daily.

Panic Disorder
ORAL:
- Maximum 4 mg daily.

Special Populations
Geriatric Patients
- Initiate therapy at low dosage and observe closely.

Clonidine Tablets and Skin Patches
(kloe′ ni deen)

Brand Name: Catapres®, Catapres-TTS®, Clorpres®, Duraclon®

Why is this medicine prescribed?

Clonidine is used to treat high blood pressure. It works by decreasing your heart rate and relaxing the blood vessels so that blood can flow more easily through the body.

This medication is sometimes prescribed for other uses; ask your doctor or pharmacist for more information.

How should this medicine be used?

Clonidine comes as a tablet to take by mouth and a patch to apply to the skin. The tablet usually is taken two or three times a day at evenly spaced intervals. The patch is applied to the skin every 7 days. Follow the directions on your prescription label carefully, and ask your doctor or pharmacist to explain any part you do not understand. Take clonidine exactly as directed. Do not take more or less of it or take it more often than prescribed by your doctor.

If you are using the clonidine patch, ask your doctor or pharmacist for the manufacturer's patient instructions and read them carefully. To apply the patch, follow these directions:
1. Clean a relatively hairless area of unbroken skin on your upper arm or chest with mild soap and water and dry it completely.
2. Peel the clear plastic strip from the adhesive side of a patch.

3. Attach the patch to your skin by placing the adhesive side against it and pressing firmly. Place an overlay patch provided with your prescription over the top of the patch to secure it.
4. If the patch loosens before replacement time, place adhesive tape or an overlay patch over the top of the patch to secure it.
5. If the skin under the patch becomes irritated, remove the patch and replace it with a new one in a different area.
6. Fold the used patch in half with the sticky sides together and dispose of it carefully. The patch still contains active medication that could be harmful to children or pets. Always be sure to remove the old patch before applying another one.

Clonidine controls high blood pressure but does not cure it. Continue to take clonidine even if you feel well. Do not stop taking clonidine without talking to your doctor. Do not stop taking clonidine suddenly, that can cause a rise in blood pressure and symptoms such as nervousness, headache, and confusion. Your doctor will probably decrease your dose gradually over a few days.

Are there other uses for this medicine?

Clonidine is also used in the treatment of Tourette's syndrome, migraine headaches, ulcerative colitis, menopausal hot flashes, alcohol withdrawal, and as an aid in smoking cessation therapy. Talk to your doctor about the possible risks of using this drug for your condition.

What special precautions should I follow?

Before taking clonidine,
- tell your doctor and pharmacist if you are allergic to clonidine or any other drugs.
- tell your doctor and pharmacist what prescription and nonprescription medications you are taking, especially amitriptyline (Elavil); beta blockers such as atenolol (Tenormin), carteolol (Cartrol), labetalol (Normodyne, Trandate), metoprolol (Lopressor), nadolol (Corgard), propranolol (Inderal), sotalol (Betapace), and timolol (Blocadren); clomipramine (Anafranil); desipramine (Norpramin); doxepin (Adepin, Sinequan); imipramine (Tofranil); nortriptyline (Aventyl, Pamelor); protriptyline (Vivactil); sleeping pills; trimipramine (Surmontil); and vitamins.
- tell your doctor if you have or have ever had coronary artery disease, kidney disease, or a heart attack.
- tell your doctor if you are pregnant, plan to become pregnant, or are breast-feeding. If you become pregnant while taking clonidine, call your doctor.
- if you are having surgery, including dental surgery, tell the doctor or dentist that you are taking clonidine.
- you should know that this drug may make you drowsy or dizzy. Do not drive a car or operate machinery until you know how this drug affects you.
- ask your doctor about the safe use of alcohol while you are using clonidine. Alcohol can make the side effects from clonidine worse.

What special dietary instructions should I follow?

Your doctor may prescribe a low-salt or low-sodium diet. Follow these directions carefully.

What should I do if I forget to take a dose?

Take the missed dose as soon as you remember it. However, if it is almost time for the next dose, skip the missed dose and continue your regular dosing schedule. Do not take a double dose to make up for a missed one.

What side effects can this medicine cause?

Clonidine may cause side effects. Tell your doctor if any of these symptoms are severe or do not go away:
- dry mouth
- drowsiness
- dizziness
- constipation
- tiredness
- headache
- nervousness
- decreased sexual ability
- upset stomach
- vomiting
- rash

If you experience any of the following symptoms, call your doctor immediately:
- fainting
- increased or decreased heartbeat
- irregular heartbeat
- swollen ankles or feet

If you experience a serious side effect, you or your doctor may send a report to the Food and Drug Administration's (FDA) MedWatch Adverse Event Reporting program online [at http://www.fda.gov/MedWatch/index.html] or by phone [1-800-332-1088].

What storage conditions are needed for this medicine?

Keep this medication in the container it came in, tightly closed, and out of reach of children. Store at room temperature and away from excess heat and moisture (not in the bathroom). Throw away any medication that is outdated or no longer needed. Talk to your pharmacist about the proper disposal of your medication.

What should I do in case of overdose?

In case of overdose, call your local poison control center at 1-800-222-1222. If the victim has collapsed or is not breathing, call local emergency services at 911.

What other information should I know?

Keep all appointments with your doctor and the laboratory. Your blood pressure should be checked regularly to determine your response to clonidine.

Your doctor may ask you to check your pulse (heart rate) daily and will tell you how rapid it should be. Ask your doctor or pharmacist to teach you how to take your pulse. If your pulse is slower or faster than it should be, call your doctor before taking the drug that day.

To avoid dizziness or faintness, get up slowly from a sitting or lying position. If you feel dizzy or faint at any time, you should lie or sit down.

To relieve dry mouth caused by clonidine, chew gum or suck sugarless hard candy.

Use of sleeping pills or other medications may increase the drowsiness caused by this drug.

Do not let anyone else take your medication. Ask your pharmacist any questions you have about refilling your prescription.

Dosage Facts
For Informational Purposes

Caution: Do not change your dose, how often you take your medication, or the length of time you are to take it without first talking to your healthcare provider.

The following dosage information was written using medical language for doctors and other healthcare professionals and is provided here for you to check your dosage. The dosage of this drug may differ for different patients. Therefore, always follow your doctor's instructions or the directions on the label. Contact your healthcare provider or pharmacist if you have any questions about the specific dosage of your medication after reviewing this information.

General Dosage Information

Tablets: Available as clonidine hydrochloride. Dosage expressed in terms of clonidine hydrochloride.

Transdermal: Available as clonidine. Dosage expressed in terms of clonidine.

Discontinuation of oral therapy requires slow dosage reduction over a period of 2–4 days to avoid the possible precipitation of the withdrawal syndrome.

Pediatric Patients

Hypertension

ORAL:
- Children ≥12 years of age: 0.1 mg twice daily. Increase dosage by 0.1 mg daily at weekly intervals until the desired response is achieved.
- Maintenance: 0.2–0.6 mg daily in divided doses. Manufacturers report 2.4 mg daily to be the maximum effective dosage.

TRANSDERMAL:
- Children ≥12 years of age: Initially, apply one system delivering 0.1 mg/24 hours once every 7 days.
- Increase initial dosage by using 2 systems delivering 0.1 mg/24 hours or a larger dosage system if the desired reduction in BP is not achieved after 1–2 weeks; subsequent dosage adjustments may be made at weekly intervals.

- Dosages exceeding 0.6 mg/24 hours (2 systems each delivering 0.3 mg/24 hours) usually are not associated with additional efficacy.
- Gradually reduce dosage of other hypotensive agents when transdermal therapy is initiated since the hypotensive effect of transdermal clonidine may not begin until 2–3 days after application of the initial system; the other hypotensive agents may have to be continued, particularly in patients with more severe hypertension.

Hypertensive Crises†
Hypertensive Emergencies†

ORAL:
- Children 1–17 years of age: Initially for some hypertensive emergencies: 0.05–0.1 mg, may repeat up to maximum of 0.8 mg.

Hypertensive Urgencies†

ORAL:
- Children 1–17 years of age: Initially, 0.05–0.1 mg, may repeat up to maximum of 0.8 mg.

Attention Deficit Hyperactivity Disorder†

ORAL:
- Initially, 0.05 mg daily given as a single dose at bedtime.
- Increase cautiously over a period of 2–4 weeks as needed, in order to minimize development of adverse effects (e.g., sedation).
- Maintenance: 0.05–0.4 mg daily (depending on tolerance and patient's weight). Usually, give the maximum tolerated dosage for 2–8 weeks in order to assess treatment response, although the onset of action of clonidine may be more variable than that associated with stimulants or antidepressants.
- According to the AHA, ECG monitoring is not required in pediatric patients receiving clonidine for ADHD; however, some experts recommend weekly office visits during clonidine titration period to monitor both erect and supine BP and heart rate.

Adult Patients

Hypertension

Adjust dosage according to the patient's BP response and tolerance.

Minimize adverse effects such as drowsiness and dry mouth by increasing dosage gradually and/or taking the larger portion of the daily dose at bedtime.

Tolerance to the antihypertensive effect may develop, necessitating increased dosage or concomitant use of a diuretic to enhance the hypotensive response to the drug.

BP Monitoring and Treatment Goals

Carefully monitor BP during initial titration or subsequent upward adjustment in dosage.

Avoid large or abrupt reductions in BP.

Adjust dosage at approximately monthly intervals (more aggressively in high-risk patients [stage 2 hypertension, comorbid conditions]) if BP control is inadequate at a given dosage; it may take months to control hypertension adequately while avoiding adverse effects of therapy.

SBP is the principal clinical end point, especially in middle-aged and geriatric patients. Once the goal SBP is attained, the goal DBP usually is achieved.

The goal is to achieve and maintain a lifelong SBP <140 mm Hg and a DBP <90 mm Hg if tolerated.

The goal in hypertensive patients with diabetes mellitus or renal impairment is to achieve and maintain a SBP <130 mm Hg and a DBP <80 mm Hg.

Monotherapy

ORAL:
- Initially, 0.1 mg twice daily. Geriatric patients may benefit from a lower initial dosage of 0.05 mg twice daily.
- Most clinicians have reported satisfactory results with administration of the drug in 2 or 3 divided doses daily.
- Increase dosage by 0.1 mg daily at weekly intervals until the desired response is achieved. Manufacturers report 2.4 mg daily to be the maximum effective dosage.
- Usual dosage, per JNC 7 guidelines: 0.05–0.4 mg twice daily.

TRANSDERMAL:
- Initiate with one system delivering 0.1 mg/24 hours applied once every 7 days.
- Initiate therapy with this initial dosage in all patients, including those who had been receiving oral therapy, due to interpatient variability; titrate initial dosage subsequently according to individual requirements;
- Increase initial dosage by using 2 systems delivering 0.1 mg/24 hours or a larger dosage system if the desired reduction in BP is not achieved after 1–2 weeks; subsequent dosage adjustments may be made at weekly intervals.
- Usual dosage, per JNC 7 guidelines: 0.1–0.3 mg/24 hours applied once every 7 days.
- Dosages exceeding 0.6 mg/24 hours (2 systems each delivering 0.3 mg/24 hours) usually are not associated with additional efficacy.
- Consider continuing the usual oral dosage the first day the initial transdermal system is applied when transdermal therapy is initiated in patients who have been receiving low dosages of oral clonidine.
- Gradually reduce dosage of other hypotensive agents when transdermal therapy is initiated since the hypotensive effect of transdermal clonidine may not begin until 2–3 days after application of the initial system; the other hypotensive agents may have to be continued, particularly in patients with more severe hypertension.

Combination Therapy

ORAL:
- Preparations containing clonidine hydrochloride in fixed combination with chlorthalidone should not be used initially.
- Adjust dosage initially by administering each drug separately.
- Fixed combination may be used if it is determined that the optimum maintenance dosage corresponds to the ratio in a commercial combination preparation; administer each drug separately whenever dosage adjustment is necessary.
- Smaller than usual dosages of clonidine hydrochloride may be adequate in patients who are also receiving diuretics or other hypotensive drugs.

Hypertensive Urgencies†

ORAL:
- Initial dose: 0.1–0.2 mg, followed by hourly doses of 0.05–0.2 mg until a total dose of 0.5–0.7 mg has been given or DBP is controlled.
- Avoid excessive falls in BP since they may precipitate renal, cerebral, or coronary ischemia.

- Observe patient for several hours after last dose and ensure follow-up within 1 to a few days.
- Maintenance dose: Adjust according to the patient's response and tolerance.

Opiate Dependence†

Various dosage regimens have been used.

Carefully individualize dosage according to patient response and tolerance, and closely monitor and supervise.

May be difficult or impossible to establish a dosage regimen that adequately suppresses withdrawal without producing intolerable adverse effects because of varying sensitivity to clonidine's sedative, hypotensive, and withdrawal-suppressing effects.

ORAL:
- Initial Test Dose: 0.005 or 0.006 mg/kg; if signs and symptoms of withdrawal are suppressed, then give an oral dosage of 0.017 mg/kg daily, in 3 or 4 divided doses, generally for about 10 days.
- Initial Oral Dosage, Alternatively: 0.1 mg 3 or 4 times daily, with dosage adjusted by 0.1–0.2 mg per day according to the patient's response and tolerance.
- Dosage usually ranges from 0.3–1.2 mg daily.
- Discontinuing Therapy: Dosage has been reduced by increments of 50% per day for 3 days and then discontinued, or reduced by 0.1–0.2 mg daily.

Alcohol Dependence†

Optimal dosages have not been established.

ORAL:
- 0.5 mg twice or 3 times daily has reduced tremor, heart rate, and BP in alcohol withdrawal.

Smoking Cessation†

Optimal dosages have not been established and various regimens have been employed.

ORAL:
- Initial dosage: Typically, 0.1 mg twice daily; initiate therapy on the day set as the date of cessation of smoking or shortly before this date (e.g., up to 3 days prior).
- May increase dosage each week by 0.1 mg daily, if needed.

TRANSDERMAL:
- Initial dosage: Typically, one system delivering 0.1 mg/24 hours applied once every 7 days; intiate therapy on the day set as the date of cessation of smoking or shortly before this date (e.g., up to 3 days prior).
- May increase dose at weekly intervals by 0.1 mg/24 hours, if needed.

Pheochromocytoma, Diagnostic Use†

ORAL:
- Administer a single 0.3-mg dose.

Interpretation

Patient rests in the supine position for 30 minutes, after which time, 2 blood samples for baseline determination of catecholamine concentrations are drawn at 5-minute intervals. Administer the 0.3-mg dose; blood samples for catecholamine determinations are drawn at hourly intervals for 3 hours.

Patients *with* Pheochromocytoma: Plasma norepinephrine concentrations generally remain unchanged following administration of clonidine.

Patients *without* Pheochromocytoma: plasma norepinephrine concentrations generally decrease.

Migraine Headache Prophylaxis†

ORAL:

- Usually, 0.025 mg 2–4 times daily or up to 0.15 mg daily in divided doses.

Dysmenorrhea†

ORAL:

- Usually, 0.025 mg twice daily for 14 days before and during menses.

Vasomotor Symptoms Associated with Menopause†

ORAL:

- Usually, 0.025–0.2 mg twice daily.

TRANSDERMAL:

- Apply one transdermal system delivering 0.1 mg/24 hours once every 7 days.

Special Populations

Renal Impairment

- Smaller than usual doses may be adequate in patients with renal impairment. Adjust dosage according to the degree of renal impairment.
- $Cl_{cr} \geq 10$ mL/minute: Dosage adjustment does not appear necessary.
- $Cl_{cr} < 10$ mL/minute: Give 50–75% of the usual dosage.
- Supplemental doses after hemodialysis are not necessary.

Geriatric Patients

- May benefit from lower initial dosages of 0.05 mg twice daily for the management of hypertension.

† Use is not currently included in the labeling approved by the US Food and Drug Administration.

Clopidogrel

(kloh pid' oh grel)

Brand Name: Plavix®

Why is this medicine prescribed?

Clopidogrel is used to prevent strokes and heart attacks in patients at risk for these problems. Clopidogrel is in a class of medications called antiplatelet drugs. It works by helping to prevent harmful blood clots.

How should this medicine be used?

Clopidogrel comes as a tablet to take by mouth. It is usually taken once a day with or without food. Try to take clopidogrel at around the same time every day. Follow the directions on your prescription label carefully, and ask your doctor or pharmacist to explain any part you do not understand. Take clopidogrel exactly as directed. Do not take more or less of it or take it more often than prescribed by your doctor.

Continue to take clopidogrel even if you feel well. Do not stop taking clopidogrel without talking to your doctor.

Are there other uses for this medicine?

Clopidogrel is also sometimes used to prevent blood clots in people with mitral valve disease (a condition that affects the valve that separates the left upper and lower chambers of the heart) and people undergoing certain heart procedures. Talk to your doctor about the possible risks of using this medication for your condition.

This medication may be prescribed for other uses; ask your doctor or pharmacist for more information.

What special precautions should I follow?

Before taking clopidogrel,

- tell your doctor and pharmacist if you are allergic to clopidogrel or any other medications.
- tell your doctor and pharmacist what prescription and nonprescription medications, vitamins, nutritional supplements, and herbal products you are taking or plan to take. Be sure to mention any of the following: anticoagulants ('blood thinners') such as warfarin (Coumadin); aspirin and other nonsteroidal anti-inflammatory medications (NSAIDs) such as ibuprofen (Advil, Motrin) and naproxen (Aleve, Naprosyn); fluvastatin (Lescol); phenytoin (Dilantin); tamoxifen (Nolvadex); tolbutamide; and torsemide (Demadex). Your doctor may need to change the doses of your medications or monitor you carefully for side effects.
- tell your doctor if you have bleeding ulcers (sores in the lining of the stomach or small intestine that are bleeding), bleeding in the brain, or any other condition that causes severe bleeding. Your doctor may tell you that you should not take clopidogrel.
- tell your doctor if you have recently been injured and if you have or have ever had liver or kidney disease; or any condition that may cause bleeding including stomach problems such as ulcers and eye problems.
- tell your doctor if you are pregnant, plan to become pregnant, or are breast-feeding. If you become pregnant while taking clopidogrel, call your doctor.
- if you are having surgery, including dental surgery, tell the doctor or dentist that you are taking clopidogrel.
- you should know that you may bleed more easily or for a longer time than usual while you are taking clopidogrel. Be careful not to cut or hurt yourself while you are taking clopidogrel.

What special dietary instructions should I follow?

Unless your doctor tells you otherwise, continue your normal diet.

What should I do if I forget to take a dose?

Take the missed dose as soon as you remember it. However, if it is almost time for the next dose, skip the missed dose

and continue your regular dosing schedule. Do not take a double dose to make up for a missed one.

What side effects can this medicine cause?

Clopidogrel may cause side effects. Tell your doctor if any of these symptoms are severe or do not go away:

- excessive tiredness
- headache
- dizziness
- upset stomach
- stomach pain
- diarrhea
- nosebleed

Some side effects can be serious. If you experience any of the following symptoms, call your doctor immediately:

- hives
- rash
- itching
- difficulty breathing or swallowing
- swelling of face, throat, tongue, lips, eyes, hands, feet, ankles, or lower legs
- hoarseness
- black and tarry stools
- red blood in stools
- bloody vomit
- vomiting material that looks like coffee grounds
- unusual bleeding or bruising
- slow or difficult speech
- weakness or numbness of an arm or a leg
- vision loss
- shortness of breath
- fast heartbeat
- pale skin
- purple patches or bleeding under the skin
- confusion
- yellowing of the skin or eyes

Clopidogrel may cause other side effects. Call your doctor if you have any unusual problems while taking this medication.

If you experience a serious side effect, you or your doctor may send a report to the Food and Drug Administration's (FDA) MedWatch Adverse Event Reporting program online [at http://www.fda.gov/MedWatch/index.html] or by phone [1-800-332-1088].

What storage conditions are needed for this medicine?

Keep this medication in the container it came in, tightly closed, and out of reach of children. Store it at room temperature and away from excess heat and moisture (not in the bathroom). Throw away any medication that is outdated or no longer needed. Talk to your pharmacist about the proper disposal of your medication.

What should I do in case of overdose?

In case of overdose, call your local poison control center at 1-800-222-1222. If the victim has collapsed or is not breathing, call local emergency services at 911.

Symptoms of overdose may include:

- unusual bruising or bleeding

What other information should I know?

Keep all appointments with your doctor and the laboratory. Your doctor may order certain lab tests to check your body's response to clopidogrel.

Do not let anyone else take your medication. Ask your pharmacist any questions you have about refilling your prescription.

Dosage Facts
For Informational Purposes

Caution: Do not change your dose, how often you take your medication, or the length of time you are to take it without first talking to your healthcare provider.

The following dosage information was written using medical language for doctors and other healthcare professionals and is provided here for you to check your dosage. The dosage of this drug may differ for different patients. Therefore, always follow your doctor's instructions or the directions on the label. Contact your healthcare provider or pharmacist if you have any questions about the specific dosage of your medication after reviewing this information.

General Dosage Information

Available as clopidogrel bisulfate; dosage expressed in terms of clopidogrel.

Adult Patients

Prevention of Cardiovascular or Cerebrovascular Events
Recent MI, Recent Stroke, or Established Peripheral Arterial Disease

ORAL:
- 75 mg once daily.

Acute Coronary Syndrome

ORAL:
- 300 mg initial loading dose, then 75 mg daily given with aspirin (75–325 mg initially, then 75–162 mg daily).
- Discontinue before elective surgery (e.g., at least 5–7 days prior to CABG) if antiplatelet effect is not desired. In patients undergoing CABG who are allergic to aspirin, ACCP recommends initiation of the loading dose 6 hours after the procedure.
- Most patients in study also received heparin acutely.

Special Populations

No specific dosage recommendations at this time.

Clorazepate

(klor az' e pate)

Brand Name: ClorazeCaps®, ClorazeTabs®, GenXene®, Tranxene® T-TAB®, Tranxene®-SD, Tranxene®-SD Half Strength

Why is this medicine prescribed?

Clorazepate is used to relieve anxiety. It also is used to control agitation caused by alcohol withdrawal as well as seizures.

This medication is sometimes prescribed for other uses; ask your doctor or pharmacist for more information.

How should this medicine be used?

Clorazepate comes as a tablet and capsule to take by mouth. It usually is taken one to four times a day and may be taken with or without food. Follow the directions on your prescription label carefully, and ask your doctor or pharmacist to explain any part you do not understand. Take clorazepate exactly as directed.

Clorazepate can be habit-forming. Do not take a larger dose, take it more often, or for a longer time than your doctor tells you to. Tolerance may develop with long-term or excessive use, making the drug less effective. This medication must be taken regularly to be effective. Do not skip doses even if you feel that you do not need them. Do not take clorazepate for more than 4 months or stop taking this medication without talking to your doctor. Stopping the drug suddenly can worsen your condition and cause withdrawal symptoms (anxiousness, sleeplessness, and irritability). Your doctor probably will decrease your dose gradually.

Are there other uses for this medicine?

Clorazepate is also used to treat irritable bowel syndrome. Talk to your doctor about the possible risks of using this drug for your condition.

What special precautions should I follow?

Before taking clorazepate,

- tell your doctor and pharmacist if you are allergic to clorazepate, alprazolam (Xanax), chlordiazepoxide (Librium, Librax), clonazepam (Klonopin), diazepam (Valium), estazolam (ProSom), flurazepam (Dalmane), lorazepam (Ativan), oxazepam (Serax), prazepam (Centrax), temazepam (Restoril), triazolam (Halcion), or any other drugs.
- tell your doctor and pharmacist what prescription and nonprescription medications you are taking, especially antihistamines; cimetidine (Tagamet); digoxin (Lanoxin); disulfiram (Antabuse); fluoxetine (Prozac); isoniazid (INH, Laniazid, Nydrazid); ketoconazole (Nizoral); levodopa (Larodopa, Sinemet); medications for depression, seizures, Parkinson's disease, pain, asthma, colds, or allergies; metoprolol (Lopressor, Toprol XL); muscle relaxants; oral contraceptives; probenecid (Benemid); propoxyphene (Darvon); propranolol (Inderal); rifampin (Rifadin); sedatives; sleeping pills; theophylline (Theo-Dur); tranquilizers; valproic acid (Depakene); or vitamins. These medications may add to the drowsiness caused by clorazepate.
- tell your doctor if you have or have ever had glaucoma; seizures; or lung, heart, or liver disease.
- tell your doctor if you are pregnant, plan to become pregnant, or are breast-feeding. If you become pregnant while taking clorazepate, call your doctor immediately.
- if you are having surgery, including dental surgery, tell the doctor or dentist that you are taking clorazepate.
- you should know that this drug may make you drowsy. Do not drive a car or operate machinery until you know how this drug affects you.
- remember that alcohol can add to the drowsiness caused by this drug.
- tell your doctor if you use tobacco products. Cigarette smoking may decrease the effectiveness of this drug.

What should I do if I forget to take a dose?

If you take several doses per day and miss a dose, skip the missed dose and continue your regular dosing schedule. Do not take a double dose to make up for a missed one.

What side effects can this medicine cause?

Side effects from clorazepate are common and include:

- drowsiness
- dizziness
- tiredness
- weakness
- dry mouth
- diarrhea
- upset stomach
- changes in appetite

Tell your doctor if any of these symptoms are severe or do not go away:

- restlessness or excitement
- constipation
- difficulty urinating
- frequent urination
- blurred vision
- changes in sex drive or ability

If you experience any of the following symptoms, call your doctor immediately:

- seizures
- shuffling walk
- persistent, fine tremor or inability to sit still
- fever
- difficulty breathing or swallowing
- severe skin rash
- yellowing of the skin or eyes
- irregular heartbeat

If you experience a serious side effect, you or your doctor may send a report to the Food and Drug Administration's (FDA) MedWatch Adverse Event Reporting program online [at http://www.fda.gov/MedWatch/index.html] or by phone [1-800-332-1088].

What storage conditions are needed for this medicine?

Keep this medication in the container it came in, tightly closed, and out of reach of children. Store it at room temperature and away from excess heat and moisture (not in the bathroom). Throw away any medication that is outdated or no longer needed. Talk to your pharmacist about the proper disposal of your medication.

What should I do in case of overdose?

In case of overdose, call your local poison control center at 1-800-222-1222. If the victim has collapsed or is not breathing, call local emergency services at 911.

What other information should I know?

Keep all appointments with your doctor and the laboratory. Your doctor will order certain lab tests to check your response to clorazepate.

If you are taking clorazepate to control seizures and have an increase in their frequency or severity, call your doctor. Your dose may need to be adjusted. If you use clorazepate for seizures, carry identification (Medic Alert) stating that you have epilepsy and that you are taking clorazepate.

Do not let anyone else take your medication. Ask your pharmacist any questions you have about refilling your prescription.

Talk to your doctor, pharmacist, or other healthcare professional if you have questions about dosing information for your medication.

Clotrimazole

(kloe trim′ a zole)

Brand Name: Fungoid® Solution, Gyne-Lotrimin®, GyneLotrimin® 3, Gyne-Lotrimin® 3 Combination Pack, Gyne-Lotrimin®-3, Lotrim® AF Jock Itch Cream, Lotrimin®, Lotrimin® AF, Lotrisone® as a combination product containing Clotrimazole and Betamethasone Dipropionate, Mycelex® Troche, Mycelex®-7

Also available generically.

Why is this medicine prescribed?

Clotrimazole is used to treat yeast infections of the vagina, mouth, and skin such as athlete's foot, jock itch, and body ringworm. It can also be used to prevent oral thrush in certain patients.

This medication is sometimes prescribed for other uses; ask your doctor or pharmacist for more information.

How should this medicine be used?

Clotrimazole comes as a cream, lotion, and solution to apply to the skin; lozenges (called troches) to dissolve in the mouth; and vaginal tablets and vaginal cream to be inserted into the vagina. Clotrimazole is usually used five times a day for 14 days for oral thrush, twice a day (in the morning and evening) for 2 to 8 weeks for skin infections, and once a day at bedtime for 3 or 7 days for vaginal infections. Follow the directions on the package or your prescription label carefully, and ask your doctor or pharmacist to explain any part you do not understand. Use clotrimazole exactly as directed. Do not use more or less of it or use it more often than prescribed by your doctor.

To use the topical cream, lotion, or solution, thoroughly clean the infected area, allow it to dry, and then gently rub the medication in until most of it disappears. Use just enough medication to cover the affected area. You should wash your hands after applying the medication.

The lozenges should be placed in the mouth and dissolved slowly over about 15 to 30 minutes. Do not chew or swallow the lozenges whole.

To use clotrimazole vaginal cream or vaginal tablets, read the instructions provided with the medication and follow these steps:

1. Fill the special applicator that comes with the cream to the level indicated or unwrap a tablet, wet it with lukewarm water, and place it on the applicator as shown in the instructions that come with the product.
2. Lie on your back with your knees drawn upward and spread apart.
3. Insert the applicator high into your vagina (unless you are pregnant), and then push the plunger to release the medication. If you are pregnant, insert the applicator gently. If you feel resistance (hard to insert), do not try to insert it further; call your doctor.
4. Withdraw the applicator.
5. Discard the applicator if it is disposable. If the applicator is reusable, pull it apart and clean it with soap and warm water after each use.
6. Wash your hands promptly to avoid spreading the infection.

The vaginal cream or tablets should be applied when you lie down to go to bed. The drug works best if you do not get up again after applying it except to wash your hands. You may wish to wear a sanitary napkin while using the vaginal cream or tablets to protect your clothing against stains. Do not use a tampon because it will absorb the drug. Do not douche unless your doctor tells you to do so.

Continue to use clotrimazole even if you feel well. Do not stop using clotrimazole without talking to your doctor. Continue using this medication during your menstrual period.

If you obtained the clotrimazole skin cream, lotion, or solution without a prescription, use it for 4 weeks for athlete's foot and 2 weeks for jock itch or body ringworm. If your symptoms do not improve by that time, stop using the medication and consult either a pharmacist or doctor.

If you obtained clotrimazole vaginal cream or tablets without a prescription and this is the first time you have had vaginal itching and discomfort, talk with a physician before using clotrimazole. However, if a doctor previously told you that you had a yeast infection and if you have the same symptoms again, use the vaginal cream or tablets as directed on the package 3 or 7 consecutive days, preferably at night. If your symptoms do not improve within 3 or 7 days, call your doctor. If your symptoms return in less than 2 months, also call your doctor.

What special precautions should I follow?

Before using clotrimazole,

- tell your doctor and pharmacist if you are allergic to clotrimazole or any other drugs.
- tell your doctor and pharmacist what prescription and nonprescription drugs you are taking, especially antibiotic medications and vitamins.
- tell your doctor if you have or have ever had liver disease, problems with your immune system, human immunodeficiency virus infection (HIV), acquired immunodeficiency syndrome (AIDS), diabetes, or a history of alcohol abuse.
- tell your doctor if you are pregnant, plan to become pregnant, or are breast-feeding. If you become pregnant while using clotrimazole, call your doctor.
- tell your doctor if you drink alcohol.

What should I do if I forget to take a dose?

Take or insert the missed dose as soon as you remember it. However, if it is almost time for the next dose, skip the missed dose and continue your regular dosing schedule. Do not use a double dose to make up for a missed one.

What side effects can this medicine cause?

Clotrimazole may cause side effects. If you experience any of the following symptoms, call your doctor immediately:

- itching
- burning
- irritation
- redness
- swelling
- stomach pain
- fever
- foul-smelling discharge if using the vaginal product
- upset stomach or vomiting with the lozenges (troches)

If you experience a serious side effect, you or your doctor may send a report to the Food and Drug Administration's (FDA) MedWatch Adverse Event Reporting program online [at http://www.fda.gov/MedWatch/index.html] or by phone [1-800-332-1088].

What storage conditions are needed for this medicine?

Keep this medication in the container it came in, tightly closed, and out of reach of children. Store it at room temperature and away from excess heat and moisture (not in the bathroom). Do not freeze. Throw away any medication that is outdated or no longer needed. Talk to your pharmacist about the proper disposal of your medication.

What other information should I know?

Keep all appointments with your doctor. Clotrimazole cream, lotion, and solution are for external use only. Do not let clotrimazole get into your eyes. Do not swallow the topical cream, lotion, or solution. Do not swallow the vaginal tablets or vaginal cream.

If you have a vaginal infection, refrain from sexual intercourse. An ingredient in the cream may weaken certain latex products like condoms or diaphragms; do not use such products within 72 hours of using this medication. Wear clean cotton panties (or panties with cotton crotches), not panties made of nylon, rayon, or other synthetic fabrics.

Do not let anyone else use your medication. Ask your pharmacist any questions you have about refilling your prescription. If you still have symptoms of infection after you finish the clotrimazole, call your doctor.

Dosage Facts
For Informational Purposes

Caution: Do not change your dose, how often you take your medication, or the length of time you are to take it without first talking to your healthcare provider.

The following dosage information was written using medical language for doctors and other healthcare professionals and is provided here for you to check your dosage. The dosage of this drug may differ for different patients. Therefore, always follow your doctor's instructions or the directions on the label. Contact your healthcare provider or pharmacist if you have any questions about the specific dosage of your medication after reviewing this information.

Pediatric Patients

Dermatophytoses

TOPICAL:
- Apply 1% cream, lotion, or solution twice daily.
- If clinical improvement does not occur after 4 weeks of treatment, reevaluate the diagnosis. Some infections (especially tinea pedis) may require up to 8 weeks of therapy for mycological cure.

Self-medication of Tinea Corporis, Tinea Cruris, or Tinea Pedis

TOPICAL:
- Children ≥2 years of age: Apply topical cream or solution twice daily for 2 weeks (tinea cruris) or 4 weeks (tinea pedis or tinea corporis).

Pityriasis (Tinea) Versicolor

TOPICAL:
- Apply 1% cream, lotion, or solution twice daily.
- If clinical improvement does not occur after 4 weeks of treatment, reevaluate the diagnosis.

Cutaneous Candidiasis

TOPICAL:
- Apply 1% cream, lotion, or solution twice daily.
- If clinical improvement does not occur after 4 weeks of treatment, reevaluate the diagnosis. Some infections (especially tinea pedis) may require up to 8 weeks of therapy for mycological cure.

Oropharyngeal Candidiasis
Treatment

ORAL TOPICAL:
- Children ≥3 years of age: 10 mg (as lozenge) 5 times daily for 14 consecutive days.

Vulvovaginal Candidiasis

If response is inadequate following a course of therapy, reevaluate the diagnosis before instituting another course.

INTRAVAGINAL:
- Two 100-mg tablets or 1 applicatorful of 2% cream once daily for 3 consecutive days or one 100-mg tablet once daily for 7 consecutive days.
- Alternatively, 1 applicatorful of 1% cream once daily for 7–14 consecutive days.

Self-medication of Uncomplicated Vulvovaginal Candidiasis

INTRAVAGINAL:
- Children ≥12 years of age: One applicatorful of 1% cream once daily for 7 consecutive days; alternatively, 1 applicatorful of 2% cream once daily for 3 consecutive days.

TOPICAL:
- For adjunctive relief of external vulvar itching: Apply 1% topical vulvar cream 1 or 2 times daily for up to 7 days as needed.

Adult Patients

Dermatophytoses

TOPICAL:
- Apply 1% cream, lotion, or solution twice daily. If clinical improvement does not occur after 4 weeks of treatment, reevaluate the diagnosis. Some infections (especially tinea pedis) may require up to 8 weeks of therapy for mycological cure.
- If combination (clotrimazole 1% and betamethasone 0.05%) cream is used, apply twice daily for 2 weeks (tinea cruris or tinea corporis) or 4 weeks (tinea pedis); if infection persists beyond this period, discontinue combination preparation and initiate clotrimazole alone.

Self-medication of Tinea Corporis, Tinea Cruris, or Tinea Pedis

TOPICAL:
- Apply topical cream or solution twice daily for 2 weeks (tinea cruris) or 4 weeks (tinea pedis or tinea corporis).

Pityriasis (Tinea) Versicolor

TOPICAL:
- Apply 1% cream, lotion, or solution twice daily.
- If clinical improvement does not occur after 4 weeks of treatment, reevaluate the diagnosis.

Cutaneous Candidiasis

TOPICAL:
- Apply 1% cream, lotion, or solution twice daily.
- If clinical improvement does not occur after 4 weeks of treatment, reevaluate the diagnosis. Some infections (especially tinea pedis) may require up to 8 weeks of therapy for mycological cure.

Oropharyngeal Candidiasis
Treatment

ORAL TOPICAL:
- 10 mg (as lozenge) 5 times daily for 14 consecutive days.

Prophylaxis in Immunocompromised Patients

ORAL TOPICAL:
- 10 mg (as lozenge) 3 times daily for the duration of chemotherapy or until corticosteroid therapy is reduced to maintenance levels.

Vulvovaginal Candidiasis

If response is inadequate following a course of therapy, reevaluate the diagnosis before instituting another course.

INTRAVAGINAL:
- Two 100-mg tablets or 1 applicatorful of 2% cream once daily for 3 consecutive days or one 100-mg tablet once daily for 7 consecutive days.
- Alternatively, 1 applicatorful of 1% cream once daily for 7–14 consecutive days.

Self-medication of Uncomplicated Vulvovaginal Candidiasis

INTRAVAGINAL:
- One applicatorful of 1% cream once daily for 7 consecutive days; alternatively, 1 applicatorful of 2% cream once daily for 3 consecutive days.

TOPICAL:
- For adjunctive relief of external vulvar itching: Apply 1% topical vulvar cream 1 or 2 times daily for up to 7 days as needed.

Recurrent Vulvovaginal Infections Caused by Candida albicans

INTRAVAGINAL:
- CDC and others recommend an initial intensive regimen (7–14 days of an intravaginal azole or 3-dose regimen of oral fluconazole) to achieve mycologic remission, followed by a 6-month maintenance regimen of once-weekly oral fluconazole. If the oral maintenance regimen cannot be used, use intravaginal clotrimazole (200 mg twice weekly or 500 mg once weekly) or other intravaginal treatments intermittently.

Other Complicated Vulvovaginal Infections

INTRAVAGINAL:
- CDC and others recommend 7–14 days of an intravaginal azole for vulvovaginal candidiasis that is severe, caused by Candida other than C. albicans, or occurring in women with underlying medical conditions.

Vulvovaginal Candidiasis in HIV-infected Women

INTRAVAGINAL:

• CDC and other clinicians recommend same treatment as in women without HIV infection. Some experts recommend a duration of 3–7 days. Maintenance regimen of an intravaginal azole can be considered for those with recurrent episodes; *routine* primary or secondary prophylaxis (long-term suppressive or chronic maintenance therapy) not recommended.

Vulvovaginal Candidiasis in Pregnant Women

INTRAVAGINAL:

• CDC and others recommend a 7-day regimen of an intravaginal azole antifungal (e.g., clotrimazole).

Prescribing Limits

Pediatric Patients

Oropharyngeal Candidiasis

ORAL TOPICAL:

• Limit therapy to short-term use if possible; limited safety and efficacy data on prolonged therapy.

Adult Patients

Oropharyngeal Candidiasis

ORAL TOPICAL:

• Limit therapy to short-term use if possible; limited safety and efficacy data on prolonged therapy.

Clozapine

(kloe′ za peen)

Brand Name: Clozaril®, FazaClo®
Also available generically.

Important Warning

Clozapine can cause a serious blood condition. Your doctor will order certain lab tests before you start your treatment, during your treatment, and for at least 4 weeks after your treatment. Your doctor will order the lab tests once a week at first and may order the tests less often as your treatment continues. If you experience any of the following symptoms, call your doctor immediately: extreme tiredness; weakness; fever, sore throat, chills, or other signs of flu or infection; or sores in your mouth or throat.

A program has been set up by the manufacturers of clozapine to be sure that people do not take clozapine without the necessary monitoring. You, your doctor, and your pharmacist must be registered with the program, and your pharmacist will not dispense your medication unless he or she has received the results of your blood tests. Ask your doctor for more information about this program and how you will receive your medication.

Clozapine may cause seizures. Tell your doctor if you have or have ever had seizures. Do not drive a car, operate machinery, swim, or climb while taking clozapine, because if you suddenly lose consciousness, you could harm yourself or others.

Clozapine may cause myocarditis (swelling of the heart muscle that may be dangerous). If you experience any of the following symptoms, call your doctor immediately: extreme tiredness; difficulty breathing or fast breathing; fever; chest pain; or fast, irregular, or pounding heartbeat.

Clozapine may cause dizziness, lightheadedness, or fainting when you stand up, especially when you first start taking it or when your dose is increased. Tell your doctor if you are taking medications for anxiety such as diazepam (Valium), sleeping pills, or other medications for schizophrenia. Your doctor will probably start you on a low dose of clozapine and gradually increase your dose to give your body time to adjust to the medication and decrease the chance that you will experience this side effect. Talk to your doctor if you do not take clozapine for 2 days or longer. Your doctor will probably tell you to restart your treatment with a low dose of clozapine.

Use in Older Adults:

Studies have shown that older adults with dementia (a brain disorder that affects the ability to remember, think clearly, communicate, and perform daily activities and that may cause changes in mood and personality) who take antipsychotics (medications for mental illness) such as clozapine have an increased chance of death during treatment. If you experience any of the following symptoms, call your doctor immediately: slow or difficult speech, sudden dizziness or faintness, or weakness or numbness of an arm or leg.

Clozapine is not approved by the Food and Drug Administration (FDA) for the treatment of behavior problems in older adults with dementia. Talk to the doctor who prescribed clozapine if you, a family member, or someone you care for has dementia and is taking this medication. For more information visit the FDA website: http://www.fda.gov/cder

Why is this medicine prescribed?

Clozapine is used to treat the symptoms of schizophrenia (a mental illness that causes disturbed or unusual thinking, loss of interest in life, and strong or inappropriate emotions) in patients who have not been helped by other medications or who have tried to kill themselves and are likely to try to kill or harm themselves again. Clozapine is in a class of medications called atypical antipsychotics. It works by changing the activity of certain natural substances in the brain.

How should this medicine be used?

Clozapine comes as a tablet and an orally disintegrating tablet (tablet that dissolves quickly in the mouth) to take by mouth. It is usually taken one to three times a day. Take clozapine at around the same time(s) every day. Follow the directions on your prescription label carefully, and ask your doctor or pharmacist to explain any part you do not understand. Take clozapine exactly as directed. Do not take more or less of it or take it more often than prescribed by your doctor.

Do not try to push the orally disintegrating tablet through the foil packaging. Instead, use dry hands to peel back the foil. Immediately take out the tablet and place it on your tongue. The tablet will quickly dissolve and can be swallowed with saliva. No water is needed to swallow disintegrating tablets.

Clozapine controls schizophrenia but does not cure it. It may take several weeks or longer before you feel the full benefit of clozapine. Continue to take clozapine even if you feel well. Do not stop taking clozapine without talking to your doctor. Your doctor will probably want to decrease your dose gradually.

Are there other uses for this medicine?

This medication should not be prescribed for other uses; ask your doctor or pharmacist for more information.

What special precautions should I follow?

Before taking clozapine,

- tell your doctor and pharmacist if you are allergic to clozapine or any other medications.
- tell your doctor and pharmacist what prescription and nonprescription medications, vitamins, nutritional supplements, and herbal products you are taking or plan to take. Be sure to mention those listed in the IMPORTANT WARNING section and any of the following: antihistamines; benztropine (Cogentin); cimetidine (Tagamet); ciprofloxacin (Cipro); dicyclomine (Bentyl); epinephrine; erythromycin (E.E.S., E-Mycin, others); medications for high blood pressure, mental illness, or nausea; medications for irregular heartbeat such as encainide, flecainide (Tambocor), propafenone (Rythmol), and quinidine (Quinidex); medications for seizures such as carbamazepine (Tegretol) or phenytoin (Dilantin); rifampin (Rifadin, Rimactane); sedatives; selective serotonin reuptake inhibitors (SSRIs) such as citalopram (Celexa), fluoxetine (Prozac, Sarafem), fluvoxamine (Luvox), paroxetine (Paxil), and sertraline (Zoloft); sleeping pills; tranquilizers; and trihexyphenidyl (Artane). Your doctor may need to change the doses of your medications or monitor you carefully for side effects.
- in addition to the condition listed in the IMPORTANT WARNING section, tell your doctor if you have or have ever had problems with your urinary system or prostate (a male reproductive gland); paralytic ileus (condition in which food cannot move through the intestine); glaucoma; irregular heartbeat; high or low blood pressure; or heart, kidney, lung, or liver disease; or if you or anyone in your family has or has ever had diabetes. Also tell your doctor if you have ever had to stop taking a medication for mental illness because of severe side effects.
- tell your doctor if you are pregnant or plan to become pregnant. If you become pregnant while taking clozapine, call your doctor. Do not breast-feed while you are taking this medication.
- if you are having surgery, including dental surgery, tell the doctor or dentist that you are taking clozapine.
- you should know that alcohol can add to the drowsiness caused by this medication.
- tell your doctor if you use tobacco products. Cigarette smoking may decrease the effectiveness of this medication.
- you should know that you may experience hyperglycemia (increases in your blood sugar) while you are taking this medication, even if you do not already have diabetes. If you have schizophrenia, you are more likely to develop diabetes than people who do not have schizophrenia, and taking clozapine or similar medications may increase this risk. Tell your doctor immediately if you have any of the following symptoms while you are taking clozapine: extreme thirst, frequent urination, extreme hunger, blurred vision, or weakness. It is very important to call your doctor as soon as you have any of these symptoms, because high blood sugar can cause a serious condition called ketoacidosis. Ketoacidosis may become life-threatening if it is not treated at an early stage. Symptoms of ketoacidosis include: dry mouth, nausea and vomiting, shortness of breath, breath that smells fruity, and decreased consciousness.
- if you have phenylketonuria (PKU, an inherited condition in which a special diet must be followed to prevent mental retardation), you should know that the orally disintegrating tablets contain aspartame that forms phenylalanine.

What special dietary instructions should I follow?

Talk to your doctor about drinking caffeinated beverages while taking this medicine.

What should I do if I forget to take a dose?

Take the missed dose as soon as you remember it. However, if it is almost time for the next dose, skip the missed dose and continue your regular dosing schedule. Do not take a double dose to make up for a missed one.

If you miss taking clozapine for more than 2 days, you should call your doctor before taking any more medication. Your doctor may want to restart your medication at a lower dose.

What side effects can this medicine cause?

Clozapine may cause side effects. Tell your doctor if any of these symptoms are severe or do not go away:

- drowsiness
- dizziness

- increased salivation
- constipation
- dry mouth
- restlessness
- headache

Some side effects can be serious. If you experience any of the following symptoms or those listed in the IMPORTANT WARNINGS or SPECIAL PRECAUTIONS sections, call your doctor immediately:

- shaking hands that you cannot control
- seizures
- fainting
- difficulty urinating or loss of bladder control
- confusion
- changes in vision
- shakiness
- fever
- severe muscle stiffness
- sweating
- confusion
- changes in behavior
- sore throat
- unusual bleeding or bruising
- loss of appetite
- upset stomach
- yellowing of the skin or eyes
- pain in the upper right part of the stomach
- flu-like symptoms
- lack of energy

Clozapine may cause other side effects. Call your doctor if you have any unusual problems while taking this medication.

If you experience a serious side effect, you or your doctor may send a report to the Food and Drug Administration's (FDA) MedWatch Adverse Event Reporting program online [at http://www.fda.gov/MedWatch/index.html] or by phone [1-800-332-1088].

What storage conditions are needed for this medicine?

Keep this medication in the container it came in, tightly closed, and out of reach of children. Store it at room temperature and away from excess heat and moisture (not in the bathroom). Throw away any medication that is outdated or no longer needed and any orally disintegrating tablets that you removed from the blister pack but did not use immediately. Talk to your pharmacist about the proper disposal of your medication.

What should I do in case of overdose?

In case of overdose, call your local poison control center at 1-800-222-1222. If the victim has collapsed or is not breathing, call local emergency services at 911.

Symptoms of overdose may include:

- dizziness
- fainting
- slow breathing
- change in heartbeat
- loss of consciousness

What other information should I know?

Keep all appointments with your doctor and the laboratory. Your doctor will order certain lab tests to check your body's response to clozapine.

Do not let anyone else take your medication. Ask your pharmacist any questions you have about refilling your prescription.

Dosage Facts
For Informational Purposes

Caution: Do not change your dose, how often you take your medication, or the length of time you are to take it without first talking to your healthcare provider.

The following dosage information was written using medical language for doctors and other healthcare professionals and is provided here for you to check your dosage. The dosage of this drug may differ for different patients. Therefore, always follow your doctor's instructions or the directions on the label. Contact your healthcare provider or pharmacist if you have any questions about the specific dosage of your medication after reviewing this information.

General Dosage Information

Carefully adjust dosage according to individual requirements and response using lowest possible effective dosage. Avoid extended treatment in patients failing to show acceptable level of clinical response.

Due to possibility that high dosages may increase risk of adverse reactions, particularly seizures, allow adequate time to respond to a given dosage before dosage escalation is considered.

Pediatric Patients

Schizophrenia†

ORAL:
- Dosage not established in children <16 years of age.
- In a clinical study conducted by the National Institute of Mental Health (NIMH) in children (mean: 14 years of age), an initial dosage of 6.25–25 mg daily (depending on patient's weight) was used; dosages could be increased every 3–4 days by 1–2 times the initial dose on an individual basis up to a maximum of 525 mg daily.

Adult Patients

Schizophrenia

ORAL:
- Initially, 12.5 mg (one-half of a 25-mg tablet) once or twice daily. If therapy is initiated with orally disintegrating tablets, destroy the remaining half tablet. If well tolerated, increase by 25–50 mg daily over a 2-week period until dosage of 300–450 mg daily is achieved.

- Make subsequent dosage increases no more than once or twice weekly, in increments ≤50–100 mg.
- Continue daily administration in divided doses (e.g., 2–3 times daily) until effective and tolerable dosage reached, usually within 2–5 weeks, up to a maximum dosage of 900 mg daily.
- Many respond adequately to dosages between 200–600 mg daily, but 600–900 mg daily may be required in some.
- Optimum duration currently is not known, but maintenance therapy with antipsychotic agents is well established. In responsive patients, continue as long as clinically necessary and tolerated, but at lowest possible effective dosage; reassess need for continued therapy periodically.

Suicide Risk Reduction

ORAL:

- Initially, 12.5 mg once or twice daily. If therapy is initiated with orally disintegrating tablets, destroy the remaining half tablet. If well tolerated, increase by 25–50 mg daily over a 2-week period until a dosage of 300–450 mg daily is achieved.
- Make subsequent dosage increases no more than once or twice weekly, in increments ≤50–100 mg.
- In the principal supportive study, mean dosage was about 300 mg daily (range: 12.5–900 mg daily).
- Continue therapy for ≥2 years; after 2 years, reassess patient's risk of suicidal behavior. If clinician's assessment indicates that risk for suicidal behavior is still present, continue therapy. Thereafter, reevaluate need to continue therapy at regular intervals.
- If the clinician determines the patient is no longer at risk for suicidal behavior, discontinue gradually and resume treatment of underlying disorder with an antipsychotic agent to which patient has previously responded.

Discontinuance of Therapy
Oral

For planned termination of therapy, reduce dosage gradually over a 1- to 2-week period.

If abrupt discontinuance is required (e.g., due to leukopenia or agranulocytosis), observe carefully for recurrence of psychotic symptoms and symptoms related to cholinergic rebound (e.g., headache, nausea, vomiting, diarrhea). Sudden withdrawal can lead to rapid decompensation and rebound psychosis.

Reinitiation of Therapy
Oral

Do *not* reinitiate in patients in whom therapy was discontinued due to WBC count <2000/mm³ or an ANC <1000/mm³.

If restarted after brief interruption (i.e., ≥2 days) in therapy, reinitiate at dosage of 12.5 mg once or twice daily. If dosage well tolerated, it may be feasible to titrate back to therapeutic dosage more quickly than during initial treatment. However, reinitiate with extreme caution, even after brief interruptions of only 24 hours, in patients who have previously experienced respiratory or cardiac arrest during initial dosing but were subsequently titrated to therapeutic dosage.

Reexposure might enhance risk of an adverse effect and/or increase its severity (e.g., when immune-mediated mechanisms are involved); additional caution advised during reinitiation of treatment.

When reinitiating therapy, consider WBC count and ANC monitoring recommendations.

Prescribing Limits
Adult Patients
ORAL:
- Maximum 900 mg daily.

Special Populations

Geriatric Patients
- Select dosage with caution because of age-related decreases in hepatic, renal, and/or cardiac function and concomitant disease and drug therapy.

† Use is not currently included in the labeling approved by the US Food and Drug Administration.

Codeine Oral

(koe′ deen)

Brand Name: Ambenyl® Cough Syrup as a combination product containing Codeine Phosphate and Bromodiphenhydramine Hydrochloride, Bromanyl® Cough Syrup as a combination product containing Codeine Phosphate and Bromodiphenhydramine Hydrochloride, Brontex®, Cheracol® with Codeine Syrup, Codimal® PH Syrup as a combination product containing Codeine Phosphate, Phenylephrine Hydrochloride, and Pyrilamine Maleate, Colrex® Compound as a combination product containing Codeine Phosphate, Acetaminophen, Chlorpheniramine Maleate, and Phenylephrine Hydrochloride, Cycofed® Expectorant as a combination product containing Codeine Phosphate, Guaifenesin, and Pseudoephedrine Hydrochloride, Cycofed® Expectorant Pediatric as a combination product containing Codeine Phosphate, Guaifenesin, and Pseudoephedrine Hydrochloride, Decohistine® DH as a combination product containing Codeine Phosphate, Chlorpheniramine Maleate, and Pseudoephedrine Hydrochloride, Decohistine® Expectorant as a combination product containing Codeine Phosphate, Guaifenesin, and Pseudoephedrine Hydrochloride, Dihistine® DH Elixir as a combination product containing Codeine Phosphate, Chlorpheniramine Maleate, and Pseudoephedrine Hydrochloride, Dihistine® Expectorant as a combination product containing Codeine Phosphate, Guaifenesin, and Pseudoephedrine Hydrochloride, Gani-Tuss® NR, Guaifenesin DAC® as a combination product containing Codeine Phosphate, Guaifenesin, and Pseudoephedrine Hydrochloride, Guiatuss AC® Syrup, Guiatuss DAC® Syrup as a combination product containing Codeine Phosphate, Guaifenesin, and Pseudoephedrine Hydrochloride, Guiatussin® DAC Syrup as a combination product containing Codeine Phosphate, Guaifenesin, and Pseudoephedrine Hydrochloride, Guiatussin® with Codeine, HaNew Riversin® AC, HaNew Riversin® DAC as a combination product containing Codeine Phosphate, Guaifenesin, and Pseudoephedrine Hydrochloride, KG-Fed® Expectorant Syrup as a combination product containing Codeine Phosphate, Guaifenesin, and Pseudoephedrine Hydrochloride, KG-Fed® Pediatric Expectorant Syrup as a combination product containing Codeine Phosphate, Guaifenesin, and Pseudoephedrine Hydrochloride, KG-Fed® Syrup as a combination product containing Codeine Phosphate and Pseudoephedrine Hydrochloride, Mytussin® AC Cough Syrup, Mytussin® DAC as a combination product containing Codeine Phosphate, Guaifenesin, and Pseudoephedrine Hydrochloride, Novahistine® DH as a combination product containing Codeine Phosphate, Chlorpheniramine Maleate, and Pseudoephedrine Hydrochloride, Novahistine® Expectorant with Codeine as a combination product containing Codeine Phosphate, Guaifenesin, and Pseudoephedrine Hydrochloride, Nucofed® as a combination product containing Codeine Phosphate and Pseudoephedrine Hydrochloride, Nucofed® Expectorant as a combination product containing Codeine Phosphate, Guaifenesin, and Pseudoephedrine Hydrochloride, Nucofed® Pediatric Expectorant Syrup as a combination product containing Codeine Phosphate, Guaifenesin, and Pseudoephedrine Hydrochloride, Nucofed® Syrup as a combination product containing Codeine Phosphate and Pseudoephedrine Hydrochloride, Nucotuss® Expectorant as a combination product containing Codeine Phosphate, Guaifenesin, and Pseudoephedrine Hydrochloride, Nucotuss® Pediatric Expectorant as a combination product containing Codeine Phosphate, Guaifenesin, and Pseudoephedrine Hydrochloride, Pediacof® Cough Syrup as a combination product containing Codeine Phosphate, Chlorpheniramine Maleate, Phenylephrine Hydrochloride, and Potassium Iodide, Phenergan® VC with Codeine Syrup as a combination product containing Codeine Phosphate, Phenylephrine Hydrochloride, and Promethazine Hydrochloride, Phenergan® with Codeine Syrup as a combination product containing Codeine Phosphate and Promethazine Hydrochloride, Phenhist® DH with Codeine Modified Formula as a combination product containing Codeine Phosphate, Chlorpheniramine Maleate, and Pseudoephedrine Hydrochloride, Prometh® VC with Codeine Phos-

phate Cough Syrup as a combination product containing Codeine Phosphate, Phenylephrine Hydrochloride, and Promethazine Hydrochloride, Robafen AC® Syrup, Robitussin A-C® Syrup, Robitussin®-DAC as a combination product containing Codeine Phosphate, Guaifenesin, and Pseudoephedrine Hydrochloride, Ryna-C® as a combination product containing Codeine Phosphate, Chlorpheniramine Maleate, and Pseudoephedrine Hydrochloride, Ryna-CX® as a combination product containing Codeine Phosphate, Guaifenesin, and Pseudoephedrine Hydrochloride, Triacin-C® Cough Syrup as a combination product containing Codeine Phosphate, Pseudoephedrine Hydrochloride, and Triprolidine Hydrochloride, Tussar® SF Syrup as a combination product containing Codeine Phosphate, Guaifenesin, and Pseudoephedrine Hydrochloride, Tussar®-2 Syrup as a combination product containing Codeine Phosphate, Guaifenesin, and Pseudoephedrine Hydrochloride, Tussi-Organidin® NR, Tussi-Organidin®-S NR

Also available generically.

Why is this medicine prescribed?

Codeine is used, usually in combination with other medications, to reduce coughing. It also is used to relieve mild to moderate pain.

This medication is sometimes prescribed for other uses; ask your doctor or pharmacist for more information.

How should this medicine be used?

Codeine comes alone or in combination with other drugs as a tablet, capsule, and liquid to take by mouth. It usually is taken every 4-6 hours as needed. Follow the directions on your prescription label carefully, and ask your doctor or pharmacist to explain any part you do not understand. Take codeine exactly as directed.

Codeine can be habit-forming. Do not take a larger dose, take it more often, or for a longer period than your doctor tells you to.

Shake the liquid well before measuring a dose.

What special precautions should I follow?

Before taking codeine,

- tell your doctor and pharmacist if you are allergic to codeine or any other drugs.
- tell your doctor and pharmacist what prescription and nonprescription medications you are taking, especially other pain relievers; antidepressants; medications for cough, cold, or allergies; sedatives; sleeping pills; tranquilizers; and vitamins.
- tell your doctor if you have or have ever had liver, kidney, or lung disease.
- tell your doctor if you are pregnant, plan to become pregnant, or are breast-feeding. If you become pregnant while taking codeine, call your doctor.

- if you are having surgery, including dental surgery, tell the doctor or dentist that you are taking codeine.
- you should know that this drug may make you drowsy. Do not drive a car or operate machinery until you know how this drug affects you.
- remember that alcohol can add to the drowsiness caused by this drug.

What should I do if I forget to take a dose?

Codeine usually is taken as needed. If your doctor has told you to take codeine regularly, take the missed dose as soon as you remember it. However, if it is almost time for the next dose, skip the missed dose and continue your regular dosing schedule. Do not take a double dose to make up for a missed one.

What side effects can this medicine cause?

Codeine may cause side effects. Tell your doctor if any of these symptoms are severe or do not go away:
- dizziness
- lightheadedness
- drowsiness
- upset stomach
- vomiting
- constipation
- stomach pain
- rash
- difficulty urinating

If you experience either of the following symptoms, call your doctor immediately:
- difficulty breathing
- mood changes

If you experience a serious side effect, you or your doctor may send a report to the Food and Drug Administration's (FDA) MedWatch Adverse Event Reporting program online [at http://www.fda.gov/MedWatch/index.html] or by phone [1-800-332-1088].

What storage conditions are needed for this medicine?

Keep this medication in the container it came in, tightly closed, and out of reach of children. Store it at room temperature and away from excess heat and moisture (not in the bathroom). Throw away any medication that is outdated or no longer needed. Talk to your pharmacist about the proper disposal of your medication.

What should I do in case of overdose?

In case of overdose, call your local poison control center at 1-800-222-1222. If the victim has collapsed or is not breathing, call local emergency services at 911.

What other information should I know?

Keep all appointments with your doctor.

Do not let anyone else take your medication. Ask your pharmacist any questions you have about refilling your prescription.

Dosage Facts
For Informational Purposes

Caution: Do not change your dose, how often you take your medication, or the length of time you are to take it without first talking to your health-care provider.

The following dosage information was written using medical language for doctors and other healthcare professionals and is provided here for you to check your dosage. The dosage of this drug may differ for different patients. Therefore, always follow your doctor's instructions or the directions on the label. Contact your healthcare provider or pharmacist if you have any questions about the specific dosage of your medication after reviewing this information.

General Dosage Information

Available as codeine phosphate and codeine sulfate; dosage expressed in terms of the salt.

Pediatric Patients

Cough

ORAL:

Usual Pediatric Antitussive Dosages

Age	Daily Dosage
2–5 years	1 mg/kg daily in 4 equally divided doses every 4–6 hours
6–11 years	5–10 mg every 4–6 hours
≥12 years	10–20 mg every 4–6 hours

Alternatively, use the following dosages as a guide based on average body weight; reduce dosage for low-weight children.

Antitussive Dosages for Pediatric Patients Based on Weight

Age	Daily Dosage
2 years (averaging 12 kg)	3 mg every 4–6 hours (maximum 12 mg daily)
3 years (averaging 14 kg)	3.5 mg every 4–6 hours (maximum 14 mg daily)
4 years (averaging 16 kg)	4 mg every 4–6 hours (maximum 16 mg daily)
5 years (averaging 18 kg)	4.5 mg every 4–6 hours (maximum 18 mg daily)

Pain

ORAL:
- 3 mg/kg or 100 mg/m² daily in 6 divided doses. Alternatively, 0.5 mg/kg or 15 mg/m² every 4–6 hours.

Adult Patients

Cough

ORAL:
- 10–20 mg every 4–6 hours.

Pain

ORAL:
- 30 mg every 4 hours as needed; usual dosage range is 15–60 mg every 4 hours as needed.

Prescribing Limits

Pediatric Patients

Cough

ORAL:

Maximum Daily Antitussive Dosages for Pediatric Patients

Age	Maximum Daily Dosage
2 years (averaging 12 kg)	12 mg
3 years (averaging 14 kg)	14 mg
4 years (averaging 16 kg)	16 mg
5 years (averaging 18 kg)	18 mg
6–11 years	60 mg
≥12 years	120 mg

Adult Patients

Cough

ORAL:
- Maximum 120 mg daily.

Pain

ORAL:
- Maximum daily dosage in fixed combination with acetaminophen is 360 mg of codeine phosphate and 4 g of acetaminophen.

Special Populations

Geriatric Patients
- Reduce dosage in older patients.

Colchicine Oral

(kol' chi seen)

Why is this medicine prescribed?

Colchicine relieves swelling and pain caused by attacks of gout or gouty arthritis. It may also be taken regularly to prevent gout or gouty arthritis attacks.

This medication is sometimes prescribed for other uses; ask your doctor or pharmacist for more information.

How should this medicine be used?

Colchicine comes as a tablet to take by mouth. Follow the directions on your prescription label carefully, and ask your doctor or pharmacist to explain any part you do not understand. Take colchicine exactly as directed. Do not take more or less of it or take it more often than prescribed by your doctor.

If you are taking colchicine to relieve gout attack symptoms, start taking it at the first sign of pain. Relief usually begins within 12 hours, and symptoms disappear within 48–72 hours. This medicine will not be fully effective if you do not take it as soon as you feel pain.

What special precautions should I follow?

Before taking colchicine,
- tell your doctor and pharmacist if you are allergic to colchicine or any other drugs.
- tell your doctor and pharmacist what prescription and nonprescription medications you are taking, especially vitamin B_{12} and other vitamins.
- tell your doctor if you have or have ever had stomach, intestinal, blood disorder, kidney, liver, or heart problems.
- tell your doctor if you are pregnant, plan to become pregnant, or are breast-feeding. If you become pregnant while taking colchicine, call your doctor.
- if you are to have a urine test, tell your doctor and laboratory personnel that you are taking colchicine because it may affect the test results.

What should I do if I forget to take a dose?

Take the missed dose as soon as you remember it. However, if it is almost time for the next dose, skip the missed dose and continue your regular dosing schedule. Do not take a double dose to make up for a missed one.

What side effects can this medicine cause?

Colchicine may cause side effects. If you experience any of the following symptoms, call your doctor immediately:
- upset stomach
- vomiting
- diarrhea
- fever
- severe rash
- difficulty breathing
- seizures
- unusual bleeding or bruising
- blood in the urine or stool

If you experience a serious side effect, you or your doctor may send a report to the Food and Drug Administration's (FDA) MedWatch Adverse Event Reporting program online [at http://www.fda.gov/MedWatch/index.html] or by phone [1-800-332-1088].

What storage conditions are needed for this medicine?

Keep this medication in the container it came in, tightly closed, and out of reach of children. Store it at room tem-

perature and away from excess heat and moisture (not in the bathroom). Throw away medication that is outdated or no longer needed. Talk to your pharmacist about the proper disposal of your medication.

What should I do in case of overdose?

In case of overdose, call your local poison control center at 1-800-222-1222. If the victim has collapsed or is not breathing, call local emergency services at 911.

What other information should I know?

Keep all appointments with your doctor and the laboratory. Your doctor will order certain lab tests to check your response to colchicine.

Do not let anyone else take your medication. Ask your pharmacist any questions you have about refilling your prescription.

Dosage Facts
For Informational Purposes

Caution: Do not change your dose, how often you take your medication, or the length of time you are to take it without first talking to your healthcare provider.

The following dosage information was written using medical language for doctors and other healthcare professionals and is provided here for you to check your dosage. The dosage of this drug may differ for different patients. Therefore, always follow your doctor's instructions or the directions on the label. Contact your healthcare provider or pharmacist if you have any questions about the specific dosage of your medication after reviewing this information.

Adult Patients

Gouty Arthritis
Treatment to Relieve Pain in Acute Attacks

ORAL:
- Initially, 1–1.2 mg, followed by 0.5–0.6 mg every hour or 1–1.2 mg every 2 hours.
- Alternatively, 1–1.2 mg initially, then 0.5–0.6 mg every 2–3 hours may be sufficient.
- Continue course of therapy until pain is relieved; nausea, vomiting, or diarrhea occurs; or maximum recommended dosage is attained.
- Total amount usually required is 4–8 mg per course.
- Allow at least 3 days to elapse between oral courses of therapy to avoid toxicity from drug accumulation.
- Allow at least 7 days to elapse following a full **IV** course (i.e., total dose of 4 mg) before administering additional oral doses.
- When ACTH is used for acute attacks, administer at least 1 mg of colchicine daily during ACTH administration and for several days after ACTH is discontinued.

Prophylactic Therapy

Administer prophylactic doses *before* initiation of allopurinol or uricosurics.

ORAL:
- For ≤1 attack per year, usually 0.5–0.6 mg daily 3–4 times each week.
- For >1 attack per year, usually 0.5–0.6 mg daily; 1–1.8 mg daily may be required.
- Perioperative prophylaxis: 0.5–0.6 mg 3 times daily for 3 days before and 3 days after surgery.

Familial Mediterranean Fever†
Chronic Prophylactic Therapy

ORAL:
- 1–2 mg daily in divided doses.
- Reduce to 0.6 mg daily in patients who developed intolerable adverse GI effects at higher dosages.

Intermittent Use to Abort an Impending Acute Attack

ORAL:
- Initially, 0.6 mg when attack is first suspected, then 0.6 mg hourly for 3 doses, then 0.6 mg every 2 hours for 2 doses; may continue with 0.6 mg every 12 hours for 2 additional days.
- Relief may occur after the first 4 or 5 doses, and subsequent doses may not be necessary.

Prescribing Limits

Adult Patients

Gouty Arthritis
Treatment to Relieve Pain in Acute Attacks

ORAL:
- Maximum 8 mg per treatment course.

Special Populations

Renal Impairment

Prophylactic Treatment of Recurrent Gouty Arthritis

ORAL:
- Do not exceed 0.6 mg daily in patients with S_{cr} ≥1.6 mg/dL or Cl_{cr} ≤50 mL/minute; 0.6 mg every other day may be adequate. Generally do not administer to patients undergoing hemodialysis.

Geriatric Patients
- Select dosage with caution because of age-related decreases in hepatic, renal, and/or cardiac function and concomitant disease and drug therapy.
- For prophylactic therapy of recurrent gouty arthritis in patients with reduced muscle mass (e.g., geriatric or debilitated patients), initially 0.5 mg orally once daily (unless Cl_{cr} >50 mL/minute) has been recommended.

† Use is not currently included in the labeling approved by the US Food and Drug Administration.

Colesevelam

(koh le sev′ e lam)

Brand Name: WelChol®

Why is this medicine prescribed?

Colesevelam is used with exercise and diet changes (restriction of cholesterol and fat intake) to reduce the amount of cholesterol and certain fatty substances in your blood. It works by binding bile acids in your intestines. Bile acids are made when cholesterol is broken down in your body. Removing these bile acids helps to lower your blood cholesterol. Accumulation of cholesterol and fats along the walls of your arteries (a process known as atherosclerosis) decreases blood flow and, therefore, the oxygen supply to your heart, brain, and other parts of your body. Lowering your blood level of cholesterol and fats may help to prevent heart disease, angina (chest pain), strokes, and heart attacks. Colesevelam may be used alone or in combination with other lipid-lowering medications known as statins (atorvastatin [Lipitor], cerivastatin [Baycol], lovastatin [Mevacor], pravastatin [Pravachol], or simvastatin [Zocor]).

This medication is sometimes prescribed for other uses; ask your doctor or pharmacist for more information.

How should this medicine be used?

Colesevelam comes as a tablet to take by mouth. It is usually taken once or twice a day with meals and liquid. Your doctor will tell you how many tablets to take at each dose. Follow the directions on your prescription label carefully, and ask your doctor or pharmacist to explain any part you do not understand. Take colesevelam exactly as directed. Do not take more or less of it or take it more often than prescribed by your doctor.

Your lipid levels should lower within 2 weeks. Colesevelam lowers your lipid levels but does not cure high cholesterol. Continue to take colesevelam even if you feel well. Do not stop taking colesevelam without talking to your doctor.

What special precautions should I follow?

Before taking colesevelam,

- tell your doctor and pharmacist if you are allergic to colesevelam or any other drugs.
- tell your doctor and pharmacist what prescription and nonprescription medications you are taking, especially sustained-release formulations of verapamil (Calan SR) and vitamins and herbal products.
- tell your doctor if you have or have ever had gastrointestinal problems, especially bowel obstruction or difficulty swallowing foods, triglyceride levels greater than 300 mg/dl, bleeding problems, and low levels of fat-soluble vitamins (vitamins A, E, and K).
- tell your doctor if you are pregnant, plan to become pregnant, or are breast-feeding. If you become pregnant while taking colesevelam, call your doctor.

What special dietary instructions should I follow?

Eat a low-cholesterol, low-fat diet. This kind of diet includes cottage cheese, fat-free milk, fish (not canned in oil), vegetables, poultry, egg whites, and polyunsaturated oils and margarines (corn, safflower, canola, and soybean oils). Avoid foods with excess fat in them such as meat (especially liver and fatty meat), egg yolks, whole milk, cream, butter, shortening, lard, pastries, cakes, cookies, gravy, peanut butter, chocolate, olives, potato chips, coconut, cheese (other than cottage cheese), coconut oil, palm oil, and fried foods.

What should I do if I forget to take a dose?

Take the missed dose as soon as you remember it. However, if it is almost time for the next dose, skip the missed dose and continue your regular dosing schedule. Do not take a double dose to make up for a missed dose.

What side effects can this medicine cause?

Side effects from colesevelam can occur. Tell your doctor if any of these symptoms are severe or do not go away:

- gas
- constipation
- upset stomach
- headache
- weakness
- muscle pain
- throat infection

What storage conditions are needed for this medicine?

Keep this medication in the container it came in, tightly closed, and out of reach of children. Store it at room temperature and away from excess heat and moisture (not in the bathroom). Throw away any medication that is outdated or no longer needed. Talk to your pharmacist about the proper disposal of your medication.

What other information should I know?

Keep all appointments with your doctor and the laboratory. Your doctor will order certain lab tests to check your response to colesevelam.

Do not let anyone else take your medication. Ask your pharmacist any questions you have about refilling your prescription.

Dosage Facts
For Informational Purposes

Caution: Do not change your dose, how often you take your medication, or the length of time you

are to take it without first talking to your health-care provider.

The following dosage information was written using medical language for doctors and other healthcare professionals and is provided here for you to check your dosage. The dosage of this drug may differ for different patients. Therefore, always follow your doctor's instructions or the directions on the label. Contact your healthcare provider or pharmacist if you have any questions about the specific dosage of your medication after reviewing this information.

General Dosage Information

Available as colesevelam hydrochloride; dosage expressed in terms of colesevelam.

Adult Patients

Dyslipidemias
Primary Hypercholesterolemia

ORAL:
- Initially, 1.875 g (3 tablets) twice daily or 3.75 g (6 tablets) once daily. May increase dosage to 4.375 g (7 tablets) daily depending on desired therapeutic effect.

Colestipol

(koe les' ti pole)

Brand Name: Colestid®, Colestid® Flavored Granules, Colestid® Granules

Also available generically.

Why is this medicine prescribed?

Colestipol is used with diet changes (restriction of cholesterol and fat intake) to reduce the amount of cholesterol and certain fatty substances in your blood. Accumulation of cholesterol and fats along the walls of your arteries (a process known as atherosclerosis) decreases blood flow and, therefore, the oxygen supply to your heart, brain, and other parts of your body. Lowering your blood level of cholesterol and fats may help to prevent heart disease, angina (chest pain), strokes, and heart attacks.

This medication is sometimes prescribed for other uses; ask your doctor or pharmacist for more information.

How should this medicine be used?

Colestipol comes as granules to take by mouth. It usually is taken two to four times a day. Follow the directions on your prescription label carefully, and ask your doctor or pharmacist to explain any part you do not understand. Take colestipol exactly as directed. Do not take more or less of it or take it more often than prescribed by your doctor.

Take all other medications at least 1 hour before or 4 hours after you take colestipol because colestipol can interfere with their absorption.

Continue to take colestipol even if you feel well. Do not stop taking colestipol without talking to your doctor.

Do not take the granules dry. Add them to at least 3 ounces of a liquid (e.g., fruit juice, water, milk, or soft drink) and stir until completely mixed. If you use a carbonated beverage, mix it slowly in a large glass to minimize foaming. After taking the dose, rinse the glass with a small amount of additional liquid and drink it to be sure that you receive the entire dose.

For convenience and to improve taste, mix your entire next-day's dose in a liquid in the evening and refrigerate it. Colestipol also may be mixed with hot or regular breakfast cereals, thin soups (e.g., tomato and chicken noodle), or pulpy fruit (e.g., crushed pineapple, pears, peaches, and fruit cocktail).

What special precautions should I follow?

Before taking colestipol,
- tell your doctor and pharmacist if you are allergic to colestipol or any other drugs.
- tell your doctor and pharmacist what prescription and nonprescription medications you are taking, especially amiodarone (Cordarone), antibiotics, anticoagulants ('blood thinners') such as warfarin (Coumadin), digitoxin, digoxin (Lanoxin), diuretics ('water pills'), iron, loperamide (Imodium), mycophenolate (Cellcept), oral diabetes medications, phenobarbital, phenylbutazone, propranolol (Inderal), thyroid medications, and vitamins.
- tell your doctor if you have or have ever had unusual bleeding, an underactive thyroid gland, heart or intestinal disease, or if you have hemorrhoids.
- tell your doctor if you are pregnant, plan to become pregnant, or are breast-feeding. If you become pregnant while taking colestipol, call your doctor.

What special dietary instructions should I follow?

Eat a low-cholesterol, low-fat diet. This kind of diet includes cottage cheese, fat-free milk, fish (not canned in oil), vegetables, poultry, egg whites, and polyunsaturated oils and margarines (corn, safflower, canola, and soybean oils). Avoid foods with excess fat in them such as meat (especially liver and fatty meat), egg yolks, whole milk, cream, butter, shortening, lard, pastries, cakes, cookies, gravy, peanut butter, chocolate, olives, potato chips, coconut, cheese (other than cottage cheese), coconut oil, palm oil, and fried foods.

What should I do if I forget to take a dose?

Take the missed dose as soon as you remember it and take any remaining doses for that day at evenly spaced intervals. Do not take a double dose to make up for a missed one.

What side effects can this medicine cause?

Colestipol may cause side effects. Tell your doctor if any of these symptoms are severe or do not go away:

- constipation
- belching
- upset stomach
- vomiting
- gas

If you experience the following symptom, call your doctor immediately:

- unusual bleeding (such as bleeding from the gums or rectum)

If you experience a serious side effect, you or your doctor may send a report to the Food and Drug Administration's (FDA) MedWatch Adverse Event Reporting program online [at http://www.fda.gov/MedWatch/index.html] or by phone [1-800-332-1088].

What storage conditions are needed for this medicine?

Keep this medication in the container it came in, tightly closed, and out of reach of children. Store it at room temperature and away from excess heat and moisture (not in the bathroom). Throw away any medication that is outdated or no longer needed. Talk to your pharmacist about the proper disposal of your medication.

What other information should I know?

Keep all appointments with your doctor and the laboratory. Your doctor will order certain lab tests to check your response to colestipol.

Do not let anyone else take your medication. Ask your pharmacist any questions you have about refilling your prescription.

Dosage Facts
For Informational Purposes

Caution: Do not change your dose, how often you take your medication, or the length of time you are to take it without first talking to your healthcare provider.

The following dosage information was written using medical language for doctors and other healthcare professionals and is provided here for you to check your dosage. The dosage of this drug may differ for different patients. Therefore, always follow your doctor's instructions or the directions on the label. Contact your healthcare provider or pharmacist if you have any questions about the specific dosage of your medication after reviewing this information.

General Dosage Information

Available as colestipol hydrochloride; expressed in terms of the salt.

One dose (1 packet or 1 level teaspoon) of colestipol hydrochloride granules contains 5 g of colestipol hydrochloride. One dose (1 packet or 1 level scoop) of flavored colestipol hydrochloride granules contains 7.5 g of granules, which contains 5 g of colestipol hydrochloride.

Pediatric Patients

Dyslipidemias†

ORAL:

- Pediatric dosage has not been established; however, dosages of 10–20 g or 500 mg/kg daily in 2–4 divided doses have been used. Lower dosages (e.g., 125–250 mg/kg daily) have also been used in some children when serum cholesterol concentrations were only 15–20% above normal after dietary management alone.

Adult Patients

Dyslipidemias

ORAL (TABLETS):

- Initially, 2 g once or twice daily. Increase dosage by 2 g once or twice daily at intervals of 1 or 2 months. Usual daily dosage range is 2–16 g taken once or in divided doses.
- If the desired therapeutic effect is not achieved with the usual dosage of 2–16 g daily with good compliance and acceptable adverse effects, consider combined therapy or alternative treatment.
- If triglyceride concentrations increase markedly, consider reducing dosage, discontinuing therapy, or using combined or alternative treatment.

ORAL (GRANULES FOR ORAL SUSPENSION):

- Initially, 5 g (1 packet or 1 level scoop) once or twice daily. Titrate dose upward as necessary in 5-g increments at 1- or 2-month intervals. Usual daily dosage range is 5–30 g (1–6 packets or level scoops) taken once or in divided doses.
- If the desired therapeutic effect is not achieved with the usual dosage of 1–6 doses per day with good compliance and acceptable adverse effects, consider combined therapy or alternative treatment.
- If triglyceride concentrations increase markedly, consider reducing dosage, discontinuing therapy, or using combined or alternative treatment.
- Patients with preexisting constipation receiving granules for oral suspension: Initially, 5 g once daily for 5–7 days; then increase dosage to 5 g twice daily and monitor constipation and serum lipoprotein values, at least twice, 4–6 weeks apart. Thereafter, increase dosage as needed by 1 dose per day (at monthly intervals) with periodic monitoring of serum lipoprotein values; adjust dosage accordingly to achieve the desired effect while avoiding excessive dosage. If constipation worsens or the desired effect is not achieved with acceptable adverse effects with the usual dosage of 1–6 doses per day, consider combined therapy or alternative treatment.
- 30 g daily (as granules for oral suspension) has been used in combination with niacin in adults with heterozygous familial hypercholesterolemia.

† Use is not currently included in the labeling approved by the US Food and Drug Administration.

Colistimethate Injection

(koe lis ti meth′ ate)

Brand Name: Coly-Mycin® M Parenteral

About Your Treatment

Your doctor has ordered colistimethate, an antibiotic, to help treat your infection. The drug will be either injected directly into a vein through a needle or catheter or added to an intravenous fluid that will drip through a needle or catheter into a vein. You will either receive a continuous dose of this medication through your intravenous fluids or receive it two to four times a day.

Colistimethate eliminates bacteria that cause many kinds of infections. This medication is sometimes prescribed for other uses; ask your doctor or pharmacist for more information. Your health care provider (doctor, nurse, or pharmacist) may measure the effectiveness and side effects of your treatment using laboratory tests and physical examinations. It is important to keep all appointments with your doctor and the laboratory. The length of treatment depends on how you respond to the medication.

Precautions

Before administering colistimethate,

- tell your doctor and pharmacist if you are allergic to colistimethate or any other drugs.
- tell your doctor and pharmacist what prescription and nonprescription medications you are taking, especially antibiotics including amikacin (Amikin), cephalothin, gentamicin (Garamycin), netilmicin (Netromycin), tobramycin (Nebcin), amphotericin B (Fungizone), capreomycin (Capostat), polymixin B (Aerosporin); and vancomycin (Vancocin); succinylcholine; tubocurarine; and vitamins or herbal products.
- tell your doctor if you have or ever have had kidney disease or myasthenia gravis.
- tell your doctor if you are pregnant, plan to become pregnant, or are breast-feeding. If you become pregnant while taking colistimethate, call your doctor.
- you should know that this drug may make you drowsy. Do not drive a car or operate machinery until you know how colistimethate will affect you.
- you should know that this medication could cause severe muscle weakness and breathing difficulties if not used properly. Follow your health care provider's instructions to help avoid these effects.

Administering Your Medication

Before you administer colistimethate, look at the solution closely. It should be clear and free of floating material. Observe the solution container to make sure there are no leaks.

Do not use the solution if it is discolored or if it contains particles. Use a new solution, but show the damaged one to your health care provider.

It is important that you use your medication exactly as directed. Do not stop your therapy on your own for any reason because your infection could worsen and result in hospitalization. Do not administer it more often than or for longer periods than your doctor tells you. Do not change your dosing schedule without talking to your health care provider. Your health care provider may tell you to stop your infusion if you have a mechanical problem (such as blockage in the tubing, needle, or catheter); if you have to stop an infusion, call your health care provider immediately so your therapy can continue.

Side Effects

Colistimethate may cause side effects. Tell your doctor if any of these symptoms are severe or do not go away:

- dizziness
- itching
- hives
- rash
- fever
- muscle weakness
- upset stomach
- discomfort at injection site

If you experience any of the following symptoms, call your doctor immediately:

- diarrhea
- decreased urination
- numbness and tingling of the extremities and tongue
- change in urine color
- dizziness
- difficulty walking
- blurred vision
- slurred speech
- confusion
- difficulty breathing
- rash

If you experience a serious side effect, you or your doctor may send a report to the Food and Drug Administration's (FDA) MedWatch Adverse Event Reporting program online [at http://www.fda.gov/MedWatch/index.html] or by phone [1-800-332-1088].

Storage Conditions

Your health care provider will probably give you a several-day supply of colistimethate at a time. You will be told how to prepare each dose. Store your medication only as directed. Make sure you understand what you need to store your medication properly.

Keep your supplies in a clean, dry place when you are not using them, and keep all medications and supplies out of the reach of children. Your health care provider will tell you how to throw away used needles, syringes, tubing, and containers to avoid accidental injury..

Overdose

In case of overdose, call your local poison control center at 1-800-222-1222. If the victim has collapsed or is not breathing, call local emergency services at 911.

Signs of Infection

If you are receiving colistimethate in your vein or under your skin, you need to know the symptoms of a catheter-related infection (an infection where the needle enters your vein or skin). If you experience any of these effects near your intravenous catheter, tell your health care provider as soon as possible:

- tenderness
- warmth
- irritation
- drainage
- redness
- swelling
- pain

Talk to your doctor, pharmacist, or other healthcare professional if you have questions about dosing information for your medication.

Co-trimoxazole Injection

(coe try mox′ a zole)

Brand Name: Bactrim Injection®, Septra Injection ®

Also available generically.

About Your Treatment

Your doctor has ordered sulfamethoxazole and trimethoprim, an antibiotic, to help treat your infection. It will be added to an intravenous fluid that will drip through a needle or catheter placed in your vein for 60-90 or more minutes, two to four times a day.

The combination of sulfamethoxazole and trimethoprim eliminates bacteria that cause many kinds of infections, including pneumonia and urinary tract and intestinal infections. This medication is sometimes prescribed for other uses; ask your doctor or pharmacist for more information.

Your health care provider (doctor, nurse, or pharmacist) may measure the effectiveness and side effects of your treatment using laboratory tests and physical examinations. It is important to keep all appointments with your doctor and the laboratory. The length of treatment depends on how your infection and symptoms respond to the medication.

Precautions

Before administering sulfamethoxazole and trimethoprim,
- tell your doctor and pharmacist if you are allergic to sulfamethoxazole, trimethoprim, any other sulfa drug, diuretics ('water pills'), oral diabetes medications, or any other drugs.
- tell your doctor and pharmacist what prescription and nonprescription medications you are taking, particularly anticoagulants ('blood thinners') such as warfarin (Coumadin), cyclosporine (Neoral, Sandimmune), diabetes medications, diuretics ('water pills'), medications for seizures such as phenytoin (Dilantin), methotrexate (Folex, Rheumatrex), and vitamins.
- tell your doctor if you have a history of alcoholism and if you have or have ever had liver or kidney disease, asthma, severe allergies, anemia, or a glucose-6-phosphate dehydrogenase (G-6-PD) deficiency (an inherited blood disease).
- tell your doctor if you are pregnant, plan to become pregnant, or are breast-feeding. If you become pregnant while taking sulfamethoxazole and trimethoprim, call your doctor.

Administering Your Medication

Before you administer sulfamethoxazole and trimethoprim, look at the solution closely. It should be clear and free of floating material. Gently squeeze the bag or observe the solution container to make sure there are no leaks. Do not use the solution if it is discolored, if it contains particles, or if the bag or container leaks. Use a new solution, but show the damaged one to your health care provider.

It is important that you use your medication exactly as directed. Do not stop your therapy on your own for any reason because your infection could worsen and result in hospitalization. Do not change your dosing schedule without talking to your health care provider. Your health care provider may tell you to stop your infusion if you have a mechanical problem (such as a blockage in the tubing, needle, or catheter); if you have to stop an infusion, call your health care provider immediately so your therapy can continue.

Side Effects

Sulfamethoxazole and trimethoprim may cause side effects. Tell your health care provider if any of these symptoms are severe or do not go away:
- dizziness or loss of balance
- loss of appetite
- upset stomach

If you experience any of the following symptoms, call your health care provider immediately:
- sore throat
- difficulty breathing
- fever
- headache
- joint or muscle aches
- yellowing of the skin or eyes
- swelling of the lips or tongue
- swallowing problems
- skin rash or skin changes

- tiredness
- unusual bleeding or bruising
- weakness
- paleness
- cough
- diarrhea

If you experience a serious side effect, you or your doctor may send a report to the Food and Drug Administration's (FDA) MedWatch Adverse Event Reporting program online [at http://www.fda.gov/MedWatch/index.html] or by phone [1-800-332-1088].

Storage Conditions

- Your health care provider will probably teach you how to prepare each dose of sulfamethoxazole and trimethoprim. Since the medication is stable for only a short time after preparation, prepare your daily doses as directed by your health care provider.

  Store your medication only as directed. Make sure you understand what you need to store your medication properly.

  Keep your supplies in a clean, dry place when you are not using them, and keep all medications and supplies out of reach of children. Your health care provider will tell you how to throw away used needles, syringes, tubing, and containers to avoid accidental injury.

Overdose

In case of overdose, call your local poison control center at 1-800-222-1222. If the victim has collapsed or is not breathing, call local emergency services at 911.

Signs of Infection

If you are receiving sulfamethoxazole and trimethoprim in your vein or under your skin, you need to know the symptoms of a catheter-related infection (an infection where the needle enters your vein or skin). If you experience any of these effects near your intravenous catheter, tell your health care provider as soon as possible:

- tenderness
- warmth
- irritation
- drainage
- redness
- swelling
- pain

Dosage Facts
For Informational Purposes

Caution: Do not change your dose, how often you take your medication, or the length of time you are to take it without first talking to your healthcare provider.

The following dosage information was written using medical language for doctors and other healthcare pro-

fessionals and is provided here for you to check your dosage. The dosage of this drug may differ for different patients. Therefore, always follow your doctor's instructions or the directions on the label. Contact your healthcare provider or pharmacist if you have any questions about the specific dosage of your medication after reviewing this information.

General Dosage Information

Available as fixed combination containing sulfamethoxazole and trimethoprim; dosage expressed as both the sulfamethoxazole and trimethoprim content or as the trimethoprim content.

Pediatric Patients

GI Infections
Shigella Infections

IV:
- Children ≥2 months of age: 8–10 mg/kg of trimethoprim daily (as co-trimoxazole) in 2–4 equally divided doses given for 5 days.

Urinary Tract Infections (UTIs)
Severe UTIs

IV:
- Children ≥2 months of age: 8–10 mg/kg of trimethoprim daily (as co-trimoxazole) in 2–4 equally divided doses given for up to 14 days.

Pneumocystis jiroveci (Pneumocystis carinii) Pneumonia
Treatment

IV:
- Children ≥2 months of age: 15–20 mg/kg of trimethoprim daily (as co-trimoxazole) in 3 or 4 equally divided doses. Usual duration is 14–21 days.

Adult Patients

GI Infections
Shigella Infections

IV:
- 8–10 mg/kg of trimethoprim daily (as co-trimoxazole) in 2–4 equally divided doses given for 5 days.

Urinary Tract Infections (UTIs)
Severe UTIs

IV:
- 8–10 mg/kg of trimethoprim daily (as co-trimoxazole) in 2–4 equally divided doses given for up to 14 days.

Pneumocystis jiroveci (Pneumocystis carinii) Pneumonia
Treatment

IV:
- 15–20 mg/kg of trimethoprim daily in 3 or 4 equally divided doses every 6 or 8 hours given for up to 14 days. Some clinicians recommend 15 mg/kg of trimethoprim and 75 mg/kg of sulfamethoxazole daily in 3 or 4 divided doses for 14–21 days.

Special Populations

Renal Impairment
- In patients with Cl_{cr} 15–30 mL/minute, use 50% of usual dosage.

- Use not recommended in those with Cl_{cr} <15 mL/minute.

Geriatric Patients
- No dosage adjustments except those related to renal impairment.

† *Use is not currently included in the labeling approved by the US Food and Drug Administration.*

Co-trimoxazole Oral

(coe try mox′ a zole)

Brand Name: Bactrim®, Bactrim® DS, Septra®, Septra® DS, Septra® Grape Suspension, Septra® Suspension, Sulfatrim® Pediatric Suspension, Sulfatrim® Suspension
Also available generically.

Why is this medicine prescribed?

Co-trimoxazole is a combination of trimethoprim and sulfamethoxazole, a sulfa drug. It eliminates bacteria that cause various infections, including infections of the urinary tract, lungs (pneumonia), ears, and intestines. It also is used to treat 'travelers' diarrhea.' Antibiotics will not work for colds, flu, or other viral infections.

This medication is sometimes prescribed for other uses; ask your doctor or pharmacist for more information.

How should this medicine be used?

Co-trimoxazole comes as a tablet and a liquid to take by mouth. It usually is taken two times a day but may be taken up to four times a day for severe lung infections. Drink a full glass of water with each dose.

Shake the liquid well before each use to mix the medication evenly. Follow the directions on your prescription label carefully, and ask your doctor or pharmacist to explain any part you do not understand. Take co-trimoxazole exactly as directed. Do not take more or less of it or take it more often than prescribed by your doctor.

What special precautions should I follow?

Before taking co-trimoxazole,
- tell your doctor and pharmacist if you are allergic to co-trimoxazole, diuretics ('water pills'), oral diabetes medications, any sulfa drug, or any other drugs.
- tell your doctor and pharmacist what prescription and nonprescription medications you are taking, especially methotrexate, phenytoin (Dilantin), warfarin (Coumadin), and vitamins.
- tell your doctor if you have or have ever had liver or kidney disease, asthma, severe allergies, or glucose-6-phosphate dehydrogenase (G-6-PD) deficiency (an inherited blood disease).

- tell your doctor if you are pregnant, plan to become pregnant, or are breast-feeding. If you become pregnant while taking co-trimoxazole, call your doctor.
- plan to avoid unnecessary or prolonged exposure to sunlight and to wear protective clothing, sunglasses, and sunscreen. Co-trimoxazole may make your skin sensitive to sunlight.

What special dietary instructions should I follow?

Co-trimoxazole may cause an upset stomach. Take co-trimoxazole with food.

What should I do if I forget to take a dose?

Take the missed dose as soon as you remember it. However, if it is almost time for the next dose, skip the missed dose and continue your regular dosing schedule. Do not take a double dose to make up for a missed one.

What side effects can this medicine cause?

Co-trimoxazole may cause side effects. Tell your doctor if any of these symptoms are severe or do not go away:
- upset stomach
- vomiting
- loss of appetite

If you experience any of the following symptoms, call your doctor immediately:
- skin rash
- itching
- sore throat
- fever or chills
- mouth sores
- unusual bruising or bleeding
- yellowing of the skin or eyes
- paleness
- joint aches

If you experience a serious side effect, you or your doctor may send a report to the Food and Drug Administration's (FDA) MedWatch Adverse Event Reporting program online [at http://www.fda.gov/MedWatch/index.html] or by phone [1-800-332-1088].

What storage conditions are needed for this medicine?

Keep this medication in the container it came in, tightly closed, and out of reach of children. Store it at room temperature and away from excess heat and moisture (not in the bathroom). Throw away any medication that is outdated or no longer needed. Talk to your pharmacist about the proper disposal of your medication.

What should I do in case of overdose?

In case of overdose, call your local poison control center at 1-800-222-1222. If the victim has collapsed or is not breathing, call local emergency services at 911.

What other information should I know?

Keep all appointments with your doctor and the laboratory. Your doctor will order certain lab tests to check your response to co-trimoxazole.

Do not let anyone else take your medication. Your prescription is probably not refillable. If you still have symptoms of infection after you finish the co-trimoxazole, call your doctor.

Dosage Facts
For Informational Purposes

Caution: Do not change your dose, how often you take your medication, or the length of time you are to take it without first talking to your health-care provider.

The following dosage information was written using medical language for doctors and other healthcare professionals and is provided here for you to check your dosage. The dosage of this drug may differ for different patients. Therefore, always follow your doctor's instructions or the directions on the label. Contact your health-care provider or pharmacist if you have any questions about the specific dosage of your medication after reviewing this information.

General Dosage Information

Available as fixed combination containing sulfamethoxazole and trimethoprim; dosage expressed as both the sulfamethoxazole and trimethoprim content or as the trimethoprim content.

Pediatric Patients

Acute Otitis Media

ORAL:
- Children ≥2 months of age: 8 mg/kg of trimethoprim and 40 mg/kg of sulfamethoxazole daily in 2 divided doses every 12 hours. Usual duration is 10 days.

GI Infections
Shigella Infections

ORAL:
- Children ≥2 months of age: 8 mg/kg of trimethoprim and 40 mg/kg of sulfamethoxazole daily in 2 divided doses every 12 hours. Usual duration is 5 days.

Urinary Tract Infections (UTIs)

ORAL:
- Children ≥2 months of age: 8 mg/kg of trimethoprim and 40 mg/kg of sulfamethoxazole daily in 2 divided doses every 12 hours. Usual duration is 10 days.

Brucellosis†

ORAL:
- 10 mg/kg daily (up to 480 mg daily) of trimethoprim (as co-trimoxazole) in 2 divided doses for 4–6 weeks.

Cholera†

ORAL:
- 4–5 mg/kg of trimethoprim (as co-trimoxazole) twice daily given for 3 days.

Cyclospora Infections†

ORAL:
- 5 mg/kg of trimethoprim and 25 mg/kg of sulfamethoxazole twice daily given for 7–10 days. HIV-infected patients may require higher dosage and longer treatment.

Granuloma Inguinale (Donovanosis)†

ORAL:
- Adolescents: 160 mg of trimethoprim and 800 mg of sulfamethoxazole twice daily given for ≥3 weeks or until all lesions have healed completely; consider adding IV aminoglycoside (e.g., gentamicin) if improvement is not evident within the first few days of therapy and in HIV-infected patients.
- Relapse can occur 6–18 months after apparently effective treatment.

Isosporiasis†

ORAL:
- 5 mg/kg of trimethoprim and 25 mg/kg of sulfamethoxazole twice daily. Usual duration of treatment is 10 days; higher dosage or more prolonged treatment necessary in immunocompromised patients.

Pertussis†

ORAL:
- 8 mg/kg of trimethoprim and 40 mg/kg of sulfamethoxazole daily in 2 divided doses. Usual duration is 14 days for treatment or prevention.

Plague†
Postexposure Prophylaxis†

ORAL:
- Children ≥2 months of age: 320–640 mg of trimethoprim (as co-trimoxazole) daily in 2 divided doses given for 7 days. Alternatively, 8 mg/kg daily of trimethoprim (as co-trimoxazole) in 2 divided doses given for 7 days.

Pneumocystis jiroveci (Pneumocystis carinii) Pneumonia
Treatment

ORAL:
- Children ≥2 months of age: 15–20 mg/kg of trimethoprim and 75–100 mg/kg of sulfamethoxazole daily in 3 or 4 divided doses. Usual duration is 14–21 days.

Primary Prophylaxis in Infants and Children

ORAL:
- 150 mg/m² of trimethoprim and 750 mg/m² of sulfamethoxazole daily in 2 divided doses given on 3 consecutive days each week. Total daily dose should not exceed 320 mg of trimethoprim and 1.6 g of sulfamethoxazole.
- Alternatively, 150 mg/m² of trimethoprim and 750 mg/m² of sulfamethoxazole can be administered as a single dose 3 times each week on consecutive days, in 2 divided doses daily 7 days each week, or in 2 divided daily doses given 3 times each week on alternate days.
- CDC, USPHS/IDSA, AAP, and others recommend that primary prophylaxis be initiated in all infants born to HIV-infected women starting at 4–6 weeks of age, regardless of their CD4⁺ T-cell count. Infants who are first identified as being HIV-exposed after 6 weeks of age should receive primary prophylaxis beginning at the time of identification.
- Primary prophylaxis should be continued until 12 months of age in all HIV-infected infants and infants whose infection

status has not yet been determined; it can be discontinued in those found not to be HIV-infected.
- The need for subsequent prophylaxis should be based on age-specific CD4+ T-cell count thresholds. In HIV-infected children 1–5 years of age, primary prophylaxis should be initiated if CD4+ T-cell counts are <500/mm³ or CD4+ percentage is <15%. In HIV-infected children 6–12 years of age, primary prophylaxis should be initiated if CD4+ T-cell counts are <200/mm³ or CD4+ percentage is <15%.
- The safety of discontinuing prophylaxis in HIV-infected children receiving potent antiretroviral therapy has not been extensively studied.

Prevention of Recurrence (Secondary Prophylaxis) in Infants and Children
ORAL:
- 150 mg/m² of trimethoprim and 750 mg/m² of sulfamethoxazole daily in 2 divided doses given on 3 consecutive days each week. Total daily dose should not exceed 320 mg of trimethoprim and 1.6 g of sulfamethoxazole.
- Alternatively, 150 mg/m² of trimethoprim and 750 mg/m² of sulfamethoxazole can be administered as a single daily dose given for 3 consecutive days each week, in 2 divided doses daily, or in 2 divided daily doses given 3 times a week on alternate days.
- The safety of discontinuing secondary prophylaxis in HIV-infected children receiving potent antiretroviral therapy has not been extensively studied. Children who have a history of PCP should receive life-long suppressive therapy to prevent recurrence.

Primary and Secondary Prophylaxis in Adolescents
ORAL:
- Dosage for primary or secondary prophylaxis against *P. jiroveci* pneumonia in adolescents and criteria for initiation or discontinuance of such prophylaxis in this age group are the same as those recommended for adults.

Toxoplasmosis†
Primary Prophylaxis in Infants and Children†
ORAL:
- 150 mg/m² of trimethoprim and 750 mg/m² of sulfamethoxazole daily in 2 divided doses.
- The safety of discontinuing toxoplasmosis prophylaxis in HIV-infected children receiving potent antiretroviral therapy has not been extensively studied.

Primary Prophylaxis in Adolescents†
ORAL:
- Dosage for primary prophylaxis against toxoplasmosis in adolescents and criteria for initiation or discontinuance of such prophylaxis in this age group are the same as those recommended for adults.

Adult Patients

GI Infections
Treatment of Travelers' Diarrhea
ORAL:
- 160 mg of trimethoprim and 800 mg of sulfamethoxazole every 12 hours given for 3–5 days. A single 320-mg dose of trimethoprim (as co-trimoxazole) also has been used.

Prevention of Travelers' Diarrhea
ORAL:
- 160 mg of trimethoprim and 800 mg of sulfamethoxazole once daily during the period of risk. Use of anti-infectives for prevention of travelers' diarrhea generally is discouraged.

Shigella Infections
ORAL:
- 160 mg of trimethoprim and 800 mg of sulfamethoxazole every 12 hours given for 5 days.

Respiratory Tract Infections
Acute Exacerbations of Chronic Bronchitis
ORAL:
- 160 mg of trimethoprim and 800 mg of sulfamethoxazole every 12 hours given for 14 days.

Urinary Tract Infections (UTIs)
ORAL:
- 160 mg of trimethoprim and 800 mg of sulfamethoxazole every 12 hours.
- Usual duration of treatment is 10–14 days. A 3-day regimen may be effective for acute, uncomplicated cystitis in women.

Cholera†
ORAL:
- 160 mg of trimethoprim and 800 mg of sulfamethoxazole every 12 hours given for 3 days.

Cyclospora Infections†
ORAL:
- 160 mg of trimethoprim and 800 mg of sulfamethoxazole twice daily given for 7–10 days. HIV-infected patients may require higher dosage and longer-term treatment.

Granuloma Inguinale (Donovanosis)†
ORAL:
- 160 mg of trimethoprim and 800 mg of sulfamethoxazole twice daily given for ≥3 weeks or until all lesions have healed completely; consider adding IV aminoglycoside (e.g., gentamicin) if improvement is not evident within the first few days of therapy and in HIV-infected patients.
- Relapse can occur 6–18 months after apparently effective treatment.

Isosporiasis†
ORAL:
- 160 mg of trimethoprim and 800 mg of sulfamethoxazole twice daily. Usual duration of treatment is 10 days; higher dosage or more prolonged treatment necessary in immuno-compromised patients.

Mycobacterial Infections†
Mycobacterium marinum Infections
ORAL:
- 160 mg of trimethoprim and 800 mg of sulfamethoxazole twice daily given for ≥3 months recommended by ATS for treatment of cutaneous infections. A minimum of 4–6 weeks of treatment usually is necessary to determine whether the infection is responding.

Pertussis†
ORAL:
- 320 mg of trimethoprim (as co-trimoxazole) daily in 2 divided doses. Usual duration is 14 days for treatment or prevention.

Pneumocystis jiroveci (Pneumocystis carinii) Pneumonia

Treatment
ORAL:
- 15–20 mg/kg of trimethoprim and 75–100 mg/kg of sulfamethoxazole daily in 3 or 4 divided doses. Usual duration is 14–21 days.

Primary Prophylaxis
ORAL:
- 160 mg of trimethoprim and 800 mg of sulfamethoxazole once daily. Alternatively, 80 mg of trimethoprim and 400 mg of sulfamethoxazole can be given once daily.
- Initiate primary prophylaxis in patients with CD4+ T-cell counts <200/mm³ or a history of oropharyngeal candidiasis. Also consider primary prophylaxis if CD4+ T-cell percentage is <14% or there is a history of an AIDS-defining illness.
- Primary prophylaxis can be discontinued in adults and adolescents responding to potent antiretroviral therapy who have a sustained (≥3 months) increase in CD4+ T-cell counts from <200/mm³ to >200/mm³. However, it should be restarted if CD4+ T-cell count decreases to <200/mm³.

Prevention of Recurrence (Secondary Prophylaxis)
ORAL:
- 160 mg of trimethoprim and 800 mg of sulfamethoxazole once daily. Alternatively, 80 mg of trimethoprim and 400 mg of sulfamethoxazole can be given once daily.
- Initiate long-term suppressive therapy or chronic maintenance therapy (secondary prophylaxis) in those with a history of *P. jiroveci* pneumonia to prevent recurrence.
- Discontinuance of secondary prophylaxis is recommended in those who have a sustained (≥3 months) increase in CD4+ T-cell counts to >200/mm³ since such prophylaxis appears to add little benefit in terms of disease prevention and discontinuance reduces the medication burden, the potential for toxicity, drug interactions, selection of drug-resistant pathogens, and cost.
- Reinitiate secondary prophylaxis if CD4+ T-cell count decreases to <200/mm³ or if *P. jiroveci* pneumonia recurs at a CD4+ T-cell >200/mm³. It probably is prudent to continue secondary prophylaxis for life in those who had *P. jiroveci* episodes when they had CD4+ T-cell counts >200/mm³.

Toxoplasmosis†
Primary Prophylaxis
ORAL:
- 160 mg of trimethoprim and 800 mg of sulfamethoxazole once daily. Alternatively, 80 mg of trimethoprim and 400 mg of sulfamethoxazole may be used.
- Initiate primary prophylaxis against toxoplasmosis in HIV-infected adults and adolescents who are seropositive for *Toxoplasma* IgG antibody and have CD4+ T-cell counts <100/mm³.
- Consideration can be given to discontinuing primary prophylaxis in adults and adolescents who have a sustained (≥3 months) increase in CD4+ T-cell counts to >200/mm³ since such prophylaxis appears to add little benefit in terms of disease prevention for toxoplasmosis, and discontinuance reduces the pill burden, the potential for toxicity, drug interactions, selection of drug-resistant pathogens, and cost.
- Reinitiate primary prophylaxis against toxoplasmosis if CD4+ T-cell count decreases to <100–200/mm³.

Wegener's Granulomatosis†
ORAL:
- 160 mg of trimethoprim and 800 mg of sulfamethoxazole twice daily.

Special Populations
Renal Impairment
- In patients with Cl_{cr} 15–30 mL/minute, use 50% of usual dosage.
- Use not recommended in those with Cl_{cr} <15 mL/minute.

Geriatric Patients
- No dosage adjustments except those related to renal impairment.

† Use is not currently included in the labeling approved by the US Food and Drug Administration.

Cromolyn Sodium Nasal Solution

(kroe' moe lin)

Brand Name: Nasalcrom®
Also available generically.

Why is this medicine prescribed?

Cromolyn is used to prevent and treat stuffy nose, sneezing, runny nose, and other symptoms caused by allergies. It works by preventing the release of substances that cause inflammation (swelling) in the air passages of the lungs.

This medication is sometimes prescribed for other uses; ask your doctor or pharmacist for more information.

How should this medicine be used?

Cromolyn comes as a solution to use with a special nasal applicator. It usually is inhaled three to six times a day to prevent allergy symptoms. It is most effective when used before you come in contact with substances that cause allergies. If you have seasonal allergies, continue to use the drug until the season is over.

Follow the directions on the package or your prescription label carefully, and ask your doctor or pharmacist to explain any part you do not understand. Use cromolyn exactly as directed. Do not use more or less of it or use it more often than directed or prescribed by your doctor.

It may take up to 4 weeks for cromolyn to work. If your symptoms have not improved after 4 weeks, tell your doctor.

Cromolyn is used with a special applicator (Nasalmatic). Before you use cromolyn for the first time, read the instructions provided with the solution. Ask your doctor, pharmacist, or respiratory therapist to demonstrate the proper technique. Practice using the device while in his or her presence.

If you are to use the nasal spray, first blow your nose, and clear it as much as possible. Insert the applicator into a nostril. Sniff as you squeeze the sprayer once. To prevent mucous from entering the sprayer, do not release your grip until after you remove the sprayer from your nose. Repeat this process for your other nostril.

What special precautions should I follow?

Before using cromolyn,
- tell your doctor and pharmacist if you are allergic to cromolyn or any other drugs.
- tell your doctor and pharmacist what prescription and nonprescription medications you are taking, including vitamins.
- tell your doctor if you have or have ever had liver or kidney disease.
- tell your doctor if you are pregnant, plan to become pregnant, or are breast-feeding. If you become pregnant while using cromolyn, call your doctor.

What should I do if I forget to take a dose?

Use the missed dose as soon as you remember it. However, if it is almost time for the next dose, skip the missed dose and continue your regular dosing schedule. Do not use a double dose to make up for a missed one.

What side effects can this medicine cause?

Cromolyn may cause side effects. Tell your doctor if any of these symptoms are severe or do not go away:
- itching or burning nasal passages
- sneezing
- headache
- stomach pain

If you experience either of the following symptoms, call your doctor immediately:
- wheezing
- increased difficulty breathing

If you experience a serious side effect, you or your doctor may send a report to the Food and Drug Administration's (FDA) MedWatch Adverse Event Reporting program online [at http://www.fda.gov/MedWatch/index.html] or by phone [1-800-332-1088].

What storage conditions are needed for this medicine?

Keep this medication in the container it came in, tightly closed, and out of reach of children. Store it at room temperature and away from excess heat and moisture (not in the bathroom). Throw away any medication that is outdated or no longer needed. Talk to your pharmacist about the proper disposal of your medication.

What other information should I know?

Keep all appointments with your doctor.

Follow the written instructions for care and cleaning of the special nasal applicator. The applicator should be replaced every 6 months.

Do not let anyone else use your medication. Ask your pharmacist any questions you have about refilling your prescription.

Dosage Facts
For Informational Purposes

Caution: Do not change your dose, how often you take your medication, or the length of time you are to take it without first talking to your healthcare provider.

The following dosage information was written using medical language for doctors and other healthcare professionals and is provided here for you to check your dosage. The dosage of this drug may differ for different patients. Therefore, always follow your doctor's instructions or the directions on the label. Contact your healthcare provider or pharmacist if you have any questions about the specific dosage of your medication after reviewing this information.

General Dosage Information

Available as cromolyn sodium.

Pediatric Patients

Allergic Rhinitis

INTRANASAL:
- Children ≥2 years of age: 1 spray (5.2 mg) in each nostril 3 or 4 times daily given at regular intervals (morning, noon, dinner, bedtime) for ≤12 weeks. When necessary, may be used up to 6 times daily.

Adult Patients

Allergic Rhinitis

INTRANASAL:
- 1 spray (5.2 mg) in each nostril 3 or 4 times daily (morning, noon, dinner, bedtime) for ≤12 weeks. When necessary, may be used up to 6 times daily.

† Use is not currently included in the labeling approved by the US Food and Drug Administration.

Cromolyn Sodium Oral Inhalation

(kroe′ moe lin)

Brand Name: Intal®
Also available generically.

Why is this medicine prescribed?

Cromolyn is used to prevent the wheezing, shortness of breath, and troubled breathing caused by asthma. It also is used to prevent breathing difficulties (bronchospasm) during exercise. It works by preventing the release of substances that cause inflammation (swelling) in the air passages of the lungs.

This medication is sometimes prescribed for other uses; ask your doctor or pharmacist for more information.

How should this medicine be used?

Cromolyn comes as a solution and an aerosol to inhale by mouth. It is usually inhaled three or four times a day to prevent asthma attacks or within an hour before activities to prevent breathing difficulties caused by exercise.

Follow the directions on your prescription label carefully, and ask your doctor or pharmacist to explain any part you do not understand. Use cromolyn exactly as directed. Do not use more or less of it or use it more often than prescribed by your doctor.

It may take up to 4 weeks for cromolyn to work. You should use it regularly for it to be effective. If your symptoms have not improved after 4 weeks, tell your doctor.

Cromolyn is used with a special inhaler. Before you use cromolyn inhalation for the first time, read the instructions for your device. Ask your doctor, pharmacist, or respiratory therapist to demonstrate the proper technique. Practice using your inhalation device while in his or her presence.

To use the inhaler, follow these steps:

1. Shake the inhaler well.
2. Remove the protective cap.
3. Exhale (breathe out) as completely as possible through your nose while keeping your mouth shut.
4. *Open Mouth Technique:* Open your mouth wide, and place the open end of the mouthpiece about 1 or 2 inches from your mouth.
   Closed Mouth Technique: Place the open end of the mouthpiece well into your mouth, past your front teeth. Close your lips tightly around the mouthpiece.
5. Take a slow, deep breath through the mouthpiece and, at the same time, press down on the container to spray the medication into your mouth. Be sure that the mist goes into your throat and is not blocked by your teeth or tongue. Adults giving the treatment to young children

may hold the child's nose closed to be sure that the medication goes into the child's throat.
6. Hold your breath for 5 to 10 seconds, remove the inhaler, and exhale slowly through your nose or mouth. If you take two puffs, wait 2 minutes and shake the inhaler well before taking the second puff.
7. Replace the protective cap on the inhaler.

If you have difficulty getting the medication into your lungs, a spacer (a special device that attaches to the inhaler) may help; ask your doctor, pharmacist, or respiratory therapist.

What special precautions should I follow?

Before using cromolyn,

- tell your doctor and pharmacist if you are allergic to cromolyn or any other drugs.
- tell your doctor and pharmacist what prescription and nonprescription medications you are taking, especially isoproterenol (Aerolone, Isuprel, others) and vitamins.
- tell your doctor if you have or have ever had liver or kidney disease.
- tell your doctor if you are pregnant, plan to become pregnant, or are breast-feeding. If you become pregnant while using cromolyn, call your doctor.

What should I do if I forget to take a dose?

Use the missed dose as soon as you remember it. However, if it is almost time for the next dose, skip the missed dose and continue your regular dosing schedule. Do not use a double dose to make up for a missed one.

What side effects can this medicine cause?

Cromolyn may cause side effects. Tell your doctor if any of these symptoms are severe or do not go away:

- sore throat
- bad taste in the mouth
- stomach pain
- cough
- stuffy nose
- itching or burning nasal passages
- sneezing
- headache

If you experience any of the following symptoms, call your doctor immediately:

- wheezing
- increased difficulty breathing
- swelling of the tongue or throat

What storage conditions are needed for this medicine?

Keep this medication in the container it came in, tightly closed, and out of reach of children. Store it at room temperature and away from excess heat and moisture (not in the bathroom). Throw away any medication that is outdated or no longer needed. Talk to your pharmacist about the proper disposal of your medication. Avoid puncturing the aerosol container, and do not discard it in an incinerator or fire.

What other information should I know?

Keep all appointments with your doctor and the laboratory. Your doctor will order certain lab tests to check your response to cromolyn.

Do not use cromolyn to relieve an asthma attack that has already started; continue to use the medication prescribed for your acute attacks.

To relieve dry mouth or throat irritation caused by cromolyn inhalation, rinse your mouth with water, chew gum, or suck sugarless hard candy after each treatment.

Inhalation devices require regular cleaning. Once a week, remove the drug container from the plastic mouthpiece, wash the mouthpiece with warm tap water, and dry it thoroughly. Follow the written instructions for care of other inhalation devices.

Do not let anyone else use your medication. Ask your pharmacist any questions you have about refilling your prescription.

Dosage Facts
For Informational Purposes

Caution: Do not change your dose, how often you take your medication, or the length of time you are to take it without first talking to your healthcare provider.

The following dosage information was written using medical language for doctors and other healthcare professionals and is provided here for you to check your dosage. The dosage of this drug may differ for different patients. Therefore, always follow your doctor's instructions or the directions on the label. Contact your healthcare provider or pharmacist if you have any questions about the specific dosage of your medication after reviewing this information.

General Dosage Information

Available as cromolyn sodium.

Pediatric Patients

Asthma

ORAL INHALATION:
- Aerosol inhalation in children ≥5 years of age: 1.6 mg (2 inhalations) 4 times daily. Lower dosage may be effective, especially in younger patients. Following stabilization, gradually reduce the frequency of administration from 4 to 3 and then 3 to 2 times (2 inhalations per dose) daily.
- Inhalation solution for nebulization in children ≥2 years of age: 20 mg 4 times daily at regular intervals. Following stabilization, gradually reduce the frequency of administration from 4 to 3 times daily.
- If control deteriorates at a reduced dosage (< than 4 doses

daily), with or without concurrent agents at a reduced dosage, may need to increase the dosage of cromolyn sodium and reinitiate or increase the dosage of concurrent agent.

Prevention of Bronchospasm

ORAL INHALATION:
- Aerosol inhalation in children ≥5 years of age: 1.6 mg (2 inhalations) 10–15 minutes but ≤60 minutes before anticipated exercise or exposure to precipitating factor.
- Inhalation solution for nebulization in children ≥2 years of age: 20 mg 10–15 minutes before anticipated exercise or exposure to precipitating factor.

Adult Patients

Asthma

ORAL INHALATION:
- Aerosol inhalation: 1.6 mg (2 inhalations) 4 times daily. Following stabilization, gradually reduce the frequency of administration from 4 to 3 and then 3 to 2 times daily.
- Inhalation solution for nebulization: 20 mg 4 times daily. Following stabilization, gradually reduce the frequency of administration from 4 to 3 times daily.

Prevention of Bronchospasm

ORAL INHALATION:
- Aerosol inhalation: 1.6 mg (2 inhalations) 10–15 minutes but ≤60 minutes before anticipated exercise or exposure to precipitating factor.
- Inhalation solution for nebulization: 20 mg 10–15 minutes before anticipated exercise or exposure to precipitating factor.

Prescribing Limits

Pediatric Patients

Asthma

ORAL INHALATION:
- Children ≥5 years of age: Maximum 1.6 mg 4 times daily via metered-dose aerosol.

Adult Patients

Asthma

ORAL INHALATION:
- Maximum 1.6 mg 4 times daily via metered-dose aerosol.

Special Populations

Hepatic Impairment

Asthma/ Bronchospasm
- Reduce aerosol inhalation dosage.

Renal Impairment

Asthma/Bronchospasm
- Reduce aerosol inhalation dosage.

† Use is not currently included in the labeling approved by the US Food and Drug Administration.

Cyanocobalamin Injection

(sye an oh koe bal′ a min)

Why is this medicine prescribed?

Cyanocobalamin injection is used to treat and prevent a lack of vitamin B_{12} that may be caused by any of the following: pernicious anemia (lack of a natural substance needed to absorb vitamin B_{12} from the intestine); certain diseases, infections, or medications that decrease the amount of vitamin B_{12} absorbed from food; or a vegan diet (strict vegetarian diet that does not allow any animal products, including dairy products and eggs). Lack of vitamin B_{12} may cause anemia (condition in which the red blood cells do not bring enough oxygen to the organs) and permanent damage to the nerves. Cyanocobalamin injection also may be given as a test to see how well the body can absorb vitamin B_{12}. Cyanocobalamin injection is in a class of medications called vitamins. Because it is injected straight into the bloodstream, it can be used to supply vitamin B_{12} to people who cannot absorb this vitamin through the intestine.

How should this medicine be used?

Cyanocobalamin comes as a solution (liquid) to be injected into a muscle or just under the skin. It is usually injected by a health care provider in an office or clinic. You will probably receive cyanocobalamin injection once a day for the first 6-7 days of your treatment. As your red blood cells return to normal, you will probably receive the medication every other day for 2 weeks, and then every 3-4 days for 2-3 weeks. After your anemia has been treated, you will probably receive the medication once a month to prevent your symptoms from coming back.

Cyanocobalamin injection will supply you with enough vitamin B_{12} only as long as you receive injections regularly. You may receive cyanocobalamin injections every month for the rest of your life. Keep all appointments to receive cyanocobalamin injections even if you feel well. If you stop receiving cyanocobalamin injections, your anemia may return and your nerves may be damaged.

Are there other uses for this medicine?

Cyanocobalamin injection is also sometimes used to treat inherited conditions that decrease the absorption of vitamin B_{12} from the intestine. Cyanocobalamin injection is also sometimes used to treat methylmalonic aciduria (an inherited disease in which the body cannot break down protein) and is sometimes given to unborn babies to prevent methylmalonic aciduria after birth. Talk to your doctor about the possible risks of using this drug for your condition.

This medication may be prescribed for other uses; ask your doctor or pharmacist for more information.

What special precautions should I follow?

Before using cyanocobalamin injection,
- tell your doctor and pharmacist if you are allergic to cyanocobalamin injection, nasal gel, or tablets; hydroxycobalamin; multi-vitamins; any other medications or vitamins; or cobalt.
- tell your doctor and pharmacist what prescription and nonprescription medications, vitamins, nutritional supplements, and herbal products you are taking. Be sure to mention any of the following: antibiotics such as chloramphenicol; colchicine; folic acid; methotrexate (Rheumatrex, Trexall); para-aminosalicylic acid (Paser); and pyrimethamine (Daraprim). Your doctor may need to change the doses of your medications or monitor you carefully for side effects.
- tell your doctor if you drink or have ever drunk large amounts of alcohol and if you have or have ever had Leber's hereditary optic neuropathy (slow, painless loss of vision, first in one eye and then in the other) or kidney disease.
- tell your doctor if you are pregnant, plan to become pregnant, or are breast-feeding. If you become pregnant while using cyanocobalamin injection, call your doctor. Talk to your doctor about the amount of vitamin B_{12} you should get every day when you are pregnant or breastfeeding.

What special dietary instructions should I follow?

Unless your doctor tells you otherwise, continue your normal diet.

What should I do if I forget to take a dose?

If you miss an appointment to receive a cyanocobalamin injection, call your doctor as soon as possible.

What side effects can this medicine cause?

Cyanocobalamin injection may cause side effects. Tell your doctor if either of these symptoms is severe or does not go away:
- diarrhea
- feeling as if your entire body as swollen

Some side effects can be serious. The following symptoms are uncommon, but if you experience any of them, call your doctor immediately:
- muscle weakness, cramps, or pain
- leg pain
- extreme thirst
- frequent urination
- confusion
- shortness of breath, especially when you exercise or lie down
- coughing or wheezing
- fast heartbeat
- extreme tiredness

- swelling of the arms, hands, feet, ankles or lower legs
- pain, warmth, redness, swelling or tenderness in one leg
- headache
- dizziness
- red skin color, especially on the face
- hives
- rash
- itching
- difficulty breathing or swallowing

Cyanocobalamin injection may cause other side effects. Call your doctor if you have any unusual problems while taking this medication.

If you experience a serious side effect, you or your doctor may send a report to the Food and Drug Administration's (FDA) MedWatch Adverse Event Reporting program online [at http://www.fda.gov/MedWatch/index.html] or by phone [1-800-332-1088].

What storage conditions are needed for this medicine?

Your doctor will store this medication in his or her office.

What should I do in case of overdose?

In case of overdose, call your local poison control center at 1-800-222-1222. If the victim has collapsed or is not breathing, call local emergency services at 911.

What other information should I know?

Keep all appointments with your doctor and the laboratory. Your doctor will order certain lab tests to check your body's response to cyanocobalamin injection.

Talk to your doctor, pharmacist, or other healthcare professional if you have questions about dosing information for your medication.

Cyanocobalamin Nasal

(sye an oh koe bal' a min)

Brand Name: Nascobal®

Why is this medicine prescribed?

Cyanocobalamin nasal gel is used to prevent a lack of vitamin B_{12} that may be caused by any of the following: pernicious anemia (lack of a natural substance needed to absorb vitamin B_{12} from the intestine); certain diseases, infections or medications that decrease the amount of vitamin B_{12} absorbed from food; or a vegan diet (strict vegetarian diet that does not allow any animal products including eggs and dairy products). Lack of vitamin B_{12} can cause anemia (condition in which the red blood cells do not bring enough oxygen to the organs) and permanent damage to the nerves. This anemia must be treated with vitamin B_{12} injections. After the red blood cells have returned to normal, cyanocobalamin nasal gel can be used to stop anemia and other symptoms of lack of vitamin B_{12} from coming back. Cyanocobalamin nasal gel is also used to supply extra vitamin B_{12} to people who need unusually large amounts of this vitamin because they are pregnant or have certain diseases. Cyanocobalamin nasal gel is in a class of medications called vitamins. It enters the bloodstream through the nose, so it can be used to supply vitamin B_{12} to people who cannot take in this vitamin through the intestine.

How should this medicine be used?

Cyanocobalamin comes as a gel to apply to the inside of the nose. It is usually used once a week. To help you remember to use cyanocobalamin nasal gel, use it on the same day of the week every week. Follow the directions on your prescription label carefully, and ask your doctor or pharmacist to explain any part you do not understand. Use cyanocobalamin nasal gel exactly as directed. Do not use more or less of it or use it more often than prescribed by your doctor.

Cyanocobalamin nasal gel will supply you with enough vitamin B_{12} only as long as you use it regularly. You may need to use cyanocobalamin nasal gel every week for the rest of your life. Continue to use cyanocobalamin nasal gel even if you feel well. Do not stop using cyanocobalamin nasal gel without talking to your doctor. If you stop using cyanocobalamin nasal gel, your anemia may return and your nerves may be damaged.

Hot foods and drinks may cause your nose to produce mucus that can wash away cyanocobalamin nasal gel. Do not eat or drink hot foods or drinks for 1 hour before you plan to use cyanocobalamin nasal gel or for 1 hour after you use this medication.

Your doctor or pharmacist will show you how to use cyanocobalamin nasal gel. You will also be given the manufacturer's printed information on using this medication. Read the information carefully and ask your doctor or pharmacist if you have any questions.

To use the nasal gel, follow these steps:

1. Blow your nose gently to clear both nostrils.
2. Pull the clear cover off of the top of the pump.
3. If you are using the pump for the first time, press down on the finger grips of the pump firmly and quickly until you see a droplet of gel at the top of the pump. Then press down on the finger grips two more times.
4. Place the tip of the pump about halfway into one nostril. Be sure to point the tip toward the back of your nose.
5. Hold the pump in place with one hand. Press your other nostril closed with the forefinger of your other hand.
6. Press down firmly and quickly on the finger grips to release medication into your nostril.
7. Remove the pump from your nose.
8. Massage the nostril where you applied the medication for a few seconds.
9. Wipe the tip of the pump with a clean cloth or an alcohol swab and replace the clear cap on the tip of the pump.

Are there other uses for this medicine?

This medication may be prescribed for other uses; ask your doctor or pharmacist for more information.

What special precautions should I follow?

Before using cyanocobalamin nasal gel,

- tell your doctor and pharmacist if you are allergic to cyanocobalamin nasal gel, tablets, or injection; hydroxycobalamin; multi-vitamins; any other medications or vitamins; or cobalt.
- tell your doctor and pharmacist what prescription and non-prescription medications, vitamins, nutritional supplements, and herbal products you are taking. Be sure to mention any of the following: azathioprine; antibiotics such as chloramphenicol; cancer chemotherapy; colchicine; folic acid; iron supplements; medications for human immuno-deficiency virus (HIV) or acquired immunodeficiency syndrome (AIDS) such as lamivudine (Epivir) and zidovudine (Retrovir); methotrexate (Rheumatrex, Trexall), para-aminosalicylic acid (Paser), and pyrimethamine (Daraprim). Your doctor may need to change the doses of your medications or monitor you carefully for side effects.
- tell your doctor if you drink or have ever drunk large amounts of alcohol, if you have any type of infection, and if you have or have ever had Leber's hereditary optic neuropathy (slow, painless loss of vision, first in one eye and then in the other); allergies that often cause your nose to be stuffed, itchy, or runny; or kidney disease.
- tell your doctor if you get a cold or a runny or stuffy nose at any time during your treatment. You may have to use another form of vitamin B_{12} until your symptoms go away.
- tell your doctor if you are pregnant, plan to become pregnant, or are breast-feeding. If you become pregnant while using cyanocobalamin nasal gel, call your doctor. Talk to your doctor about the amount of vitamin B_{12} you should get every day when you are pregnant or breastfeeding.

What special dietary instructions should I follow?

Unless your doctor tells you otherwise, continue your normal diet.

What should I do if I forget to take a dose?

Use the missed dose as soon as you remember it. However, if it is almost time for the next dose, skip the missed dose and continue your regular dosing schedule. Do not use a double dose to make up for a missed one.

What side effects can this medicine cause?

Cyanocobalamin nasal gel may cause side effects. Tell your doctor if any of these symptoms are severe or do not go away:

- headache
- upset stomach
- stuffed or runny nose
- sore tongue
- weakness

Some side effects can be serious. The following symptoms are uncommon, but if you experience any of them, call your doctor immediately:

- unusual bruising or bleeding
- muscle weakness, cramps, or pain
- leg pain
- extreme thirst
- frequent urination
- confusion
- burning or tingling in the arms, legs, hands or feet
- sore throat, fever, chills, or other signs of infection
- rash
- hives
- itching
- difficulty breathing or swallowing

Cyanocobalamin nasal gel may cause other side effects. Call your doctor if you have any unusual problems while taking this medication.

If you experience a serious side effect, you or your doctor may send a report to the Food and Drug Administration's (FDA) MedWatch Adverse Event Reporting program online [at http://www.fda.gov/MedWatch/index.html] or by phone [1-800-332-1088].

What storage conditions are needed for this medicine?

Keep this medication upright in the carton it came in, tightly closed, and out of reach of children. Store it at room temperature and away from excess heat and moisture (not in the bathroom). Do not allow the medication to freeze. Throw away any medication that is outdated or no longer needed. Talk to your pharmacist about the proper disposal of your medication.

What should I do in case of overdose?

In case of overdose, call your local poison control center at 1-800-222-1222. If the victim has collapsed or is not breathing, call local emergency services at 911.

What other information should I know?

Keep all appointments with your doctor and the laboratory. Your doctor will order certain lab tests to check your body's response to cyanocobalamin nasal gel.

Do not let anyone else take your medication. Ask your pharmacist any questions you have about refilling your prescription.

Talk to your doctor, pharmacist, or other healthcare professional if you have questions about dosing information for your medication.

Cyclobenzaprine

(sye kloe ben′ za preen)

Brand Name: Flexeril®

Why is this medicine prescribed?

Cyclobenzaprine, a muscle relaxant, is used with rest, physical therapy, and other measures to relax muscles and relieve pain and discomfort caused by strains, sprains, and other muscle injuries.

This medication is sometimes prescribed for other uses; ask your doctor or pharmacist for more information.

How should this medicine be used?

Cyclobenzaprine comes as a tablet to take by mouth. It usually is taken two to four times a day. Do not take this drug for more than 3 weeks without talking to your doctor. Follow the directions on your prescription label carefully, and ask your doctor or pharmacist to explain any part you do not understand. Take cyclobenzaprine exactly as directed. Do not take more or less of it or take it more often than prescribed by your doctor.

What special precautions should I follow?

Before taking cyclobenzaprine,
- tell your doctor and pharmacist if you are allergic to cyclobenzaprine or any other drugs.
- tell your doctor and pharmacist what prescription and nonprescription drugs you are taking or have taken within the last 2 weeks, especially medications for depression, seizures, allergies, coughs, or colds; MAO inhibitors [phenelzine (Nardil), tranylcypromine (Parnate)]; sedatives; sleeping pills; tranquilizers; and vitamins.
- tell your doctor if you have an overactive thyroid gland, heart disease, glaucoma, or difficulty urinating.
- tell your doctor if you are pregnant, plan to become pregnant, or are breast-feeding. If you become pregnant while taking cyclobenzaprine, call your doctor immediately.
- you should know that this drug may make you drowsy. Do not drive a car or operate machinery until you know how cyclobenzaprine affects you.
- remember that alcohol can add to the drowsiness caused by this drug.

What should I do if I forget to take a dose?

Take the missed dose as soon as you remember it. However, if it is almost time for the next dose, skip the missed dose and continue your regular dosing schedule. Do not take a double dose to make up for the missed one.

What side effects can this medicine cause?

Cyclobenzaprine may cause side effects. Tell your doctor if any of these symptoms are severe or do not go away:
- drowsiness
- dry mouth
- dizziness
- upset stomach

If you experience any of the following symptoms, call your doctor immediately:
- severe skin rash
- swelling of the face or tongue
- difficulty breathing or swallowing
- irregular heart rate
- chest pain
- fever
- seizures

If you experience a serious side effect, you or your doctor may send a report to the Food and Drug Administration's (FDA) MedWatch Adverse Event Reporting program online [at http://www.fda.gov/MedWatch/index.html] or by phone [1-800-332-1088].

What storage conditions are needed for this medicine?

Keep this medication in the container it came in, tightly closed, and out of reach of children. Store it at room temperature and away from excess heat and moisture (not in the bathroom). Throw away any medication that is outdated or no longer needed. Talk to your pharmacist about the proper disposal of your medication.

What should I do in case of overdose?

In case of overdose, call your local poison control center at 1-800-222-1222. If the victim has collapsed or is not breathing, call local emergency services at 911.

What other information should I know?

Keep all appointments with your doctor.

Do not let anyone else take your medication. Ask your pharmacist any questions you have about refilling your prescription.

Dosage Facts
For Informational Purposes

Caution: Do not change your dose, how often you take your medication, or the length of time you are to take it without first talking to your healthcare provider.

The following dosage information was written using medical language for doctors and other healthcare professionals and is provided here for you to check your dosage. The dosage of this drug may differ for different patients. Therefore, always follow your doctor's instruc-

tions or the directions on the label. Contact your health-care provider or pharmacist if you have any questions about the specific dosage of your medication after reviewing this information.

General Dosage Information

Available as cyclobenzaprine hydrochloride; dosage expressed in terms of the salt.

Pediatric Patients

Muscular Conditions

ORAL:
- Adolescents ≥15 years of age: 5 mg 3 times daily; may increase dosage to 10 mg 3 times daily depending on response.

Adult Patients

Muscular Conditions

ORAL:
- 5 mg 3 times daily; may increase dosage to 10 mg 3 times daily depending on response.

Prescribing Limits

Pediatric Patients

Muscular Conditions

ORAL:
- Do not administer for more than 2–3 weeks.

Adult Patients

Muscular Conditions

ORAL:
- Do not administer for more than 2–3 weeks.

Special Populations

Hepatic Impairment
- Initiate with caution in patients with mild hepatic impairment. Consider less frequent dosing; start with 5-mg dose and increase slowly.
- Use not recommended in patients with moderate or severe hepatic impairment.

Geriatric Patients
- Consider less frequent dosing; start with 5-mg dose and increase slowly.

Cyclosporine
(sye′ kloe spor een)

Brand Name: Neoral®, Sandimmune®, Gengraf®

Important Warning

Cyclosporine is available in its original form and as another product that has been modified (changed) so that the medication can be better absorbed in the body. Original cyclosporine and cyclosporine (modified) are absorbed by the body in different amounts, so they cannot be substituted for one another. Take only the type of cyclosporine that was prescribed by your doctor. When your doctor gives you a written prescription, check to be sure that he or she has specified the type of cyclosporine you should receive. Each time you have your prescription filled, look at the brand name printed on your prescription label to be sure that you have received the same type of cyclosporine. Talk to your pharmacist if the brand name is unfamiliar or you are not sure you have received the right type of cyclosporine.

Taking cyclosporine or cyclosporine (modified) may increase the risk that you will develop an infection or cancer, especially lymphoma (cancer of a part of the immune system) or skin cancer. This risk may be higher if you take cyclosporine or cyclosporine (modified) with other medications that decrease the functioning of the immune system such as azathioprine (Imuran), cancer chemotherapy, methotrexate (Rheumatrex), sirolimus (Rapamune), and tacrolimus (Prograf). Tell your doctor if you are taking any of these medications, and if you have or have ever had any type of cancer. To reduce your risk of skin cancer, plan to avoid unnecessary or prolonged exposure to sunlight and to wear protective clothing, sunglasses, and sunscreen during your treatment. If you experience any of the following symptoms, call your doctor immediately: sore throat, fever, chills, and other signs of infection; flu-like symptoms; coughing; difficulty urinating; pain when urinating; a red, raised, or swollen area on the skin; new sores or discoloration on the skin; lumps or masses anywhere in your body; night sweats; swollen glands in the neck, armpits, or groin; trouble breathing; chest pain; weakness or tiredness that does not go away; or pain, swelling, or fullness in the stomach.

Cyclosporine and cyclosporine (modified) may cause high blood pressure and kidney damage. Tell your doctor if you have or have ever had high blood pressure or kidney disease. Also tell your doctor if you are taking any of the following medications: amphotericin B (Amphotec, Fungizone); cimetidine

(Tagamet); ciprofloxacin (Cipro); colchicine; fenofibrate (Lofibra); gemfibrozil (Lopid); gentamicin; ketoconazole (Nizoral); melphalan (Alkeran); non-steroidal anti-inflammatory medications such as diclofenac (Cataflam, Voltaren), naproxen (Aleve, Naprosyn), and sulindac (Clinoril); ranitidine (Zantac); tobramycin (Tobi); trimethoprim with sulfamethoxazole (Bactrim, Septra); and vancomycin (Vancocin). If you experience any of the following symptoms, call your doctor immediately: dizziness; swelling of the arms, hands, feet, ankles, or lower legs; fast, shallow breathing; upset stomach; or irregular heartbeat.

If you have psoriasis, tell your doctor about all the psoriasis treatments and medications you are using or have used in the past. The risk that you will develop skin cancer is greater if you have ever been treated with PUVA (psoralen and UVA; treatment for psoriasis that combines an oral or topical medication with exposure to ultraviolet A light), methotrexate (Rheumatrex) or other medications that suppress the immune system, UVB (exposure to ultraviolet B light to treat psoriasis), coal tar, or radiation therapy. You should not be treated with PUVA, UVB, or medications that suppress the immune system while you are taking cyclosporine (modified) to treat psoriasis.

Keep all appointments with your doctor and the laboratory. Your doctor will order certain lab tests to check your body's response to cyclosporine or cyclosporine (modified).

Why is this medicine prescribed?

Cyclosporine and cyclosporine (modified) are used with other medications to prevent transplant rejection (attack of the transplanted organ by the transplant recipient's immune system) in people who have received kidney, liver, and heart transplants. Cyclosporine (modified) is also used alone or with methotrexate (Rheumatrex) to treat the symptoms of rheumatoid arthritis (arthritis caused by swelling of the lining of the joints) in patients whose symptoms were not relieved by methotrexate alone. Cyclosporine (modified) is also used to treat psoriasis (a skin disease in which red, scaly patches form on some areas of the body) in certain patients who have not been helped by other treatments. Cyclosporine and cyclosporine (modified) are in a class of medications called immunosuppressants. They work by decreasing the activity of the immune system.

How should this medicine be used?

Cyclosporine and cyclosporine (modified) both come as a capsule and a solution (liquid) to take by mouth. Cyclosporine is usually taken once a day. Cyclosporine (modified) is usually taken twice a day. It is important to take both types of cyclosporine on a regular schedule. Take cyclosporine or cyclosporine (modified) at the same time(s) each day, and allow the same amount of time between doses and meals every day. Follow the directions on your prescription label carefully, and ask your doctor or pharmacist to explain any part you do not understand. Take cyclosporine or cyclosporine (modified) exactly as directed. Do not take more or less of the medication or take it more often than prescribed by your doctor.

Your doctor will probably adjust your dose of cyclosporine or cyclosporine (modified) during your treatment. If you are taking either type of cyclosporine to prevent transplant rejection, your doctor will probably start you on a high dose of the medication and gradually decrease your dose. If you are taking cyclosporine (modified) to treat rheumatoid arthritis or psoriasis, your doctor will probably start you on a low dose of the medication and gradually increase your dose. Your doctor may also decrease your dose if you experience side effects of the medication. Tell your doctor how you are feeling during your treatment.

Cyclosporine (modified) helps control the symptoms of psoriasis and rheumatoid arthritis, but does not cure these conditions. If you are taking cyclosporine (modified) to treat psoriasis, it may take 2 weeks or longer for your symptoms to begin to improve, and 12-16 weeks for you to feel the full benefit of the medication. If you are taking cyclosporine (modified) to treat rheumatoid arthritis, it may take 4-8 weeks for your symptoms to improve. Continue to take cyclosporine (modified) even if you feel well. Do not stop taking cyclosporine (modified) without talking to your doctor. Your doctor may decrease your dose gradually.

You may notice an unusual smell when you open a blister card of cyclosporine capsules. This is normal and does not mean that the medication is damaged or unsafe to use.

Cyclosporine (modified) oral solution may gel or become lumpy if it is exposed to temperatures below 68° F. You can use the solution even if it has gelled, or you can turn the solution back to a liquid by allowing it to warm to room temperature (77° F).

Cyclosporine and cyclosporine (modified) oral solution must be mixed with a liquid before use. Cyclosporine (modified) oral solution may be mixed with orange juice or apple juice but should not be mixed with milk. Cyclosporine oral solution may be mixed with milk, chocolate milk, or orange juice. You should choose one drink from the appropriate list and always mix your medication with that drink.

To take either type of oral solution, follow these steps:
- Fill a glass (not plastic) cup with the drink you have chosen.
- Remove the protective cover from the top of the dosing syringe that came with your medication.
- Place the tip of the syringe into the bottle of solution and pull back on the plunger to fill the syringe with the amount of solution your doctor has prescribed.
- Hold the syringe over the liquid in your glass and press down on the plunger to place the medication in the glass.
- Stir the mixture well.
- Drink all of the liquid in the glass right away.
- Pour a little more of the drink you have chosen into the glass, swirl the glass around to rinse, and drink the liquid.

- Dry the outside of the syringe with a clean towel and replace the protective cover. Do not wash the syringe with water. If you do need to wash the syringe, be sure that it is completely dry before you use it to measure another dose.

Are there other uses for this medicine?

Cyclosporine and cyclosporine (modified) are also sometimes used to treat Crohn's disease (a condition in which the body attacks the lining of the digestive tract, causing pain, diarrhea, weight loss, and fever) and to prevent rejection in patients who have received pancreas or cornea transplants. Cyclosporine and cyclosporine (modified) are also sometimes used to prevent graft-vs-host disease (attack on the recipient's body by transplanted bone marrow) in patients who have received a bone marrow transplant. Talk to your doctor about the possible risks of using this medication for your condition.

This medication may be prescribed for other uses. Ask your doctor or pharmacist for more information.

What special precautions should I follow?

Before taking cyclosporine or cyclosporine (modified),

- tell your doctor and pharmacist if you are allergic to cyclosporine, cyclosporine (modified), any other medications, or any of the inactive ingredients in cyclosporine or cyclosporine (modified) capsules or solution. Ask your pharmacist for a list of the inactive ingredients.
- tell your doctor and pharmacist what prescription and nonprescription medications, vitamins, and nutritional supplements you are taking, or plan to take. Be sure to mention the medications listed in the IMPORTANT WARNING section and any of the following: allopurinol (Zyloprim); amiodarone (Cordarone); angiotensin-converting enzyme (ACE) inhibitors such as benazepril (Lotensin), captopril (Capoten), enalapril (Vasotec), fosinopril (Monopril), lisinopril (Prinivil, Zestril), moexipril (Univasc), perindopril (Aceon), quinapril (Accupril), ramipril (Altace), and trandolapril (Mavik); angiotensin II receptor antagonists such as candesartan (Atacand), eprosartan (Teveten), irbesartan (Avapro), losartan (Cozaar), olmesartan (Benicar), telmisartan (Micardis), and valsartan (Diovan); certain antifungal medications such as fluconazole (Diflucan), and itraconazole (Sporanox); azithromycin (Zithromax); bromocriptine (Parlodel); calcium channel blockers such as diltiazem (Cardizem), nicardipine (Cardene), and verapamil (Calan); carbamazepine (Tegretol); cholesterol-lowering medications (statins) such as atorvastatin (Lipitor), fluvastatin (Lescol), lovastatin (Mevacor), pravastatin (Pravachol), and simvastatin (Zocor); clarithromycin (Biaxin); dalfopristin and quinapristin combination (Synercid); danazol; digoxin (Lanoxin); certain diuretics ('water pills') including amiloride (Midamor), spironolactone (Aldactone), and triamterene (Dyazide); erythromycin; HIV protease inhibitors such as indinavir (Crixivan), nelfinavir (Viracept), ritonavir (Norvir, in Kaletra), and saquinavir (Fortovase); imatinib (Gleevec); metoclopramide (Reglan); methylprednisolone (Medrol); nafcillin; octreotide (Sandostatin); oral contraceptives (birth control pills); orlistat (Xenical); potassium supplements; prednisolone (Pediapred); phenobarbital; phenytoin (Dilantin); rifabutin (Mycobutin); rifampin (Rifadin, Rimactane); sulfinpyrazone (Anturane); terbinafine (Lamisil); and ticlopidine (Ticlid). Your doctor may need to change the doses of your medications or monitor you more carefully for side effects.
- if you are taking sirolimus (Rapamune), take it 4 hours after you take cyclosporine or cyclosporine (modified).
- tell your doctor what herbal products you are taking, especially St. John's wort.
- tell your doctor if you have or have ever had any of the conditions mentioned in the IMPORTANT WARNING section or any of the following: high cholesterol, any condition that makes it difficult for your body to absorb nutrients, or liver disease.
- tell your doctor if you are pregnant or plan to become pregnant. If you become pregnant while taking either type of cyclosporine, call your doctor. Both types of cyclosporine may increase the risk that your baby will be born too early.
- do not breastfeed while you are taking either type of cyclosporine.
- do not have vaccinations (injections to prevent disease) without talking to your doctor.

What special dietary instructions should I follow?

Avoid drinking grapefruit juice or eating grapefruit while taking cyclosporine or cyclosporine (modified).

Your doctor may tell you to limit the amount of potassium in your diet. Follow these instructions carefully. Talk to your doctor about the amount of potassium-rich foods such as bananas, prunes, raisins, and orange juice you may have in your diet. Many salt substitutes contain potassium, so talk to your doctor about using them during your treatment.

What should I do if I forget to take a dose?

If you forget to take a dose, take the missed dose as soon as you remember it. However, if it is almost time for the next dose, skip the missed dose and continue your regular dosing schedule. Do not take a double dose to make up for a missed one.

What side effects can this medicine cause?

Cyclosporine and cyclosporine (modified) may cause side effects. Tell your doctor if any of these symptoms are severe or do not go away:

- headache
- diarrhea
- heartburn

- gas
- increased hair growth
- growth of extra tissue on the gums
- acne
- flushing
- shaking of a part of your body that you cannot control
- burning or tingling in the hands, arms, feet, or legs
- muscle or joint pain
- cramps
- pain or pressure in the face
- ear problems
- breast enlargement in men
- depression
- difficulty falling asleep or staying asleep

Some side effects can be serious. If you experience any of the following symptoms, or those listed in the IMPORTANT WARNING section, call your doctor immediately:

- unusual bleeding or bruising
- pale skin
- yellowing of the skin or eyes
- seizures
- loss of consciousness
- difficulty controlling body movements
- changes in vision
- confusion
- rash
- purple blotches on the skin

Cyclosporine and cyclosporine (modified) may cause other side effects. Talk to your doctor if you experience unusual problems while taking either medication.

If you experience a serious side effect, you or your doctor may send a report to the Food and Drug Administration's (FDA) MedWatch Adverse Event Reporting program online [at http://www.fda.gov/MedWatch/index.html] or by phone [1-800-332-1088].

What storage conditions are needed for this medicine?

Keep this medication in the container it came in, tightly closed and out of reach of children. Store it at room temperature and away from excess heat and moisture (not in the bathroom). Do not store this medicine in the refrigerator and do not freeze it. Throw away any medication that is outdated or no longer needed. Throw away any remaining solution 2 months after you first open the bottle. Talk to your pharmacist about the proper disposal of your medication.

What should I do in case of overdose?

In case of overdose, call your local poison control center at 1-800-222-1222. If the victim has collapsed or is not breathing, call local emergency services at 911.

Symptoms of overdose may include:

- yellowing of the skin or eyes
- swelling of the arms, hands, feet, ankles, or lower legs

What other information should I know?

Do not let anyone else take your medicine. Ask your pharmacist any questions you have about refilling your prescription.

Dosage Facts
For Informational Purposes

Caution: Do not change your dose, how often you take your medication, or the length of time you are to take it without first talking to your healthcare provider.

The following dosage information was written using medical language for doctors and other healthcare professionals and is provided here for you to check your dosage. The dosage of this drug may differ for different patients. Therefore, always follow your doctor's instructions or the directions on the label. Contact your healthcare provider or pharmacist if you have any questions about the specific dosage of your medication after reviewing this information.

General Dosage Information

Individualize dosage of cyclosporine.

Pediatric Patients

Transplant Recipients
Conventional Capsules and Oral Solution (Sandimmune®)

ORAL:

- Initially, 15 mg/kg administered as a single dose 4–12 hours before transplantation. Lower initial dosages (e.g., 10–14 mg/kg daily) may be preferred for renal allotransplantation.
- Postoperatively, continue initial dosage once daily for 1–2 weeks; then, taper by 5% per week (over about 6–8 weeks) to a maintenance dosage of 5–10 mg/kg daily. Maintenance dosages have been tapered to as low as 3 mg/kg daily in selected renal allograft recipients without an apparent increase in graft rejection rate.
- In several studies, pediatric patients have required and tolerated higher dosages.

Modified Capsules and Oral Solution (Gengraf® and Neoral®)

ORAL:

- Newly transplanted patients may receive the modified oral formulation at the same initial dose as for the conventional (nonmodified) oral formulation.
- Suggested initial dosages (based on a 1994 survey of average dosages of conventional formulations): 9 mg/kg for renal allograft recipients, 8 mg/kg for hepatic allograft recipients, and 7 mg/kg for cardiac allograft recipients administered in 2 equally divided doses daily. Give initial dose 4–12 hours before transplantation or postoperatively.
- Adjust dosage to attain a predefined blood cyclosporine concentration. Titrate dosage based on clinical evaluation of rejection and patient tolerability. Lower maintenance dosages may be possible with modified oral formulations compared with conventional (nonmodified) formulations.

Conversion from Conventional Oral Formulations (Sandimmune®) to Modified Oral Formulations (Gengraf®, Neoral®)

ORAL:

- Initial dosage of the modified formulation should be the same as the previous dosage of the conventional (nonmodified) oral formulation (1:1 conversion). Adjust dosage to attain trough blood concentrations that are similar to those achieved with the conventional oral formulation; however, attainment of therapeutic trough concentrations will result in greater exposure (AUC) to cyclosporine than would occur with the conventional oral formulation.
- Monitor trough blood cyclosporine concentrations every 4–7 days until they are the same as they were with the conventional (nonmodified) oral formulation. Monitor patient safety by determining S_{cr} and BP every 2 weeks for the first 2 months after the conversion. Adjust dosage if trough blood concentrations are outside of the desired range and/or measures of safety worsen. Dosage titration should be guided by trough blood concentrations, tolerability, and clinical response.
- Monitor trough blood concentrations closely following conversion from conventional (nonmodified) oral formulations to modified oral formulations in patients with suspected poor absorption of cyclosporine from the conventional formulations. Measure trough blood concentrations in these patients at least twice weekly (daily in patients receiving >10 mg/kg daily) until the trough blood cyclosporine concentration is maintained in the desired range, since higher bioavailability from the modified oral formulations may result in excessive trough concentrations after conversion to this formulation. Use caution with conversional dosages >10 mg/kg daily.

Adult Patients

Transplant Recipients
Conventional Capsules and Oral Solution (Sandimmune®)

ORAL:

- Initially, 15 mg/kg administered as a single dose 4–12 hours before transplantation. Lower initial dosages (e.g., 10–14 mg/kg daily) may be preferred for renal allotransplantation.
- Postoperatively, continue initial dosage once daily for 1–2 weeks; then, taper by 5% per week (over about 6–8 weeks) to a maintenance dosage of 5–10 mg/kg daily. Maintenance dosages have been tapered to as low as 3 mg/kg daily in selected renal allograft recipients without an apparent increase in graft rejection rate.

Modified Capsules and Oral Solution (Gengraf® and Neoral®)

ORAL:

- Newly transplanted patients may receive the modified oral formulation at the same initial dose as for the conventional (nonmodified) oral formulation.
- Suggested initial dosages (based on a 1994 survey of average dosages of conventional formulations): 9 mg/kg for renal allograft recipients, 8 mg/kg for hepatic allograft recipients, and 7 mg/kg for cardiac allograft recipients administered in 2 equally divided doses daily. Give initial dose 4–12 hours before transplantation or postoperatively.
- Adjust dosage to attain a predefined blood cyclosporine concentration. Titrate dosage based on clinical evaluation of rejection and patient tolerability. Lower maintenance dosages may be possible with modified oral formulations compared with conventional (nonmodified) formulations.

Conversion from Conventional Oral Formulations (Sandimmune®) to Modified Oral Formulations (Gengraf®, Neoral®)

ORAL:

- Initial dosage of the modified oral formulation should be the same as the previous dosage of the conventional (nonmodified) oral formulation (1:1 conversion). Adjust dosage to attain trough blood concentrations that are similar to those achieved with the conventional oral formulation; however, attainment of therapeutic trough concentrations will result in greater exposure (AUC) to cyclosporine than would occur with conventional oral formulation.
- Monitor trough blood cyclosporine concentrations every 4–7 days until they are the same as they were with the conventional (nonmodified) oral formulation. Monitor patient safety by determining S_{cr} and BP every 2 weeks for the first 2 months after the conversion. Adjust dosage if trough blood concentrations are outside of the desired range and/or measures of safety worsen. Dosage titration should be guided by trough blood concentrations, tolerability, and clinical response.
- Monitor trough blood concentrations closely following conversion from conventional (nonmodified) oral formulations to modified oral formulations in patients with suspected poor absorption of cyclosporine from the conventional formulations. Measure trough blood concentrations in these patients at least twice weekly (daily in patients receiving >10 mg/kg daily) until the trough blood cyclosporine concentration is maintained in the desired range, since higher bioavailability from the modified oral formulations may result in excessive trough concentrations after conversion to this formulation. Use caution with conversional dosages >10 mg/kg daily.

Rheumatoid Arthritis
Modified Capsules and Oral Solution (Gengraf® and Neoral®)

ORAL:

- Initially, 2.5 mg/kg daily in 2 divided doses. If response is insufficient but tolerance to the drug is good (including S_{cr} <30% above baseline), may increase dosage by 0.5–0.75 mg/kg daily after 8 weeks and, again, after 12 weeks (maximum 4 mg/kg daily).
- Reduce dosage by 25–50% to control adverse effects (e.g., hypertension, clinically important laboratory abnormalities) that occur. Manage persistent hypertension by further reduction of cyclosporine dosage or use of antihypertensive agents. Discontinue if adverse effects are severe or do not respond to dosage reduction.

Psoriasis
Modified Capsules and Oral Solution (Gengraf® and Neoral®)

ORAL:

- Initially, 1.25 mg/kg twice daily. Continue for ≥4 weeks unless prohibited by adverse effects. If initial dosage does not produce substantial clinical improvement within 4 weeks, increase dosage by approximately 0.5 mg/kg daily once every 2 weeks (maximum 4 mg/kg daily) based on the patient's tolerance and response.
- Use lowest dosage that maintains an adequate response (not necessarily total clearance of psoriasis). Dosages <2.5 mg/kg daily may be equally effective.
- Decrease dosage by 25–50% to control adverse effects (e.g.,

hypertension, clinically important laboratory test abnormalities) that occur. Discontinue if adverse effects are severe or do not respond to dosage reduction.

Crohn's Disease
Conventional (Nonmodified) Capsules (Sandimmune®)

ORAL:
- 3.8–8 mg/kg daily has been used.

Prescribing Limits
Adult Patients
Rheumatoid Arthritis
Modified Capsules and Oral Solution (Gengraf® and Neoral®)

ORAL:
- Maximum 4 mg/kg daily.

Psoriasis
Modified Capsules and Oral Solution (Gengraf® and Neoral®)

ORAL:
- Maximum 4 mg/kg daily.

Special Populations
Renal Impairment
- Monitor renal function closely; frequent dosage adjustments may be necessary.
- Contraindicated in rheumatoid arthritis or psoriasis patients with abnormal renal function.

Cyclosporine Injection
(sye′ kloe spor een)

Brand Name: Sandimmune® I.V.

Important Warning

Keep all appointments with your doctor and the laboratory while taking cyclosporine, especially if your doctor changes which type (capsules or liquid) or brand (Neoral or Sandimmune) of cyclosporine you are taking.

Cyclosporine makes you more susceptible to illnesses. If you are exposed to chicken pox, measles, or tuberculosis (TB) while taking cyclosporine, call your doctor. Do not have a vaccination, other immunization, or any skin test while you are taking cyclosporine unless your doctor tells you that you may. Call your doctor if you have any injuries or signs of infection (fever, sore throat, pain during urination, and muscle aches) that occur during treatment.

About Your Treatment

Your doctor has ordered cyclosporine, a drug used to reduce the body's natural immune system and to prevent rejection of organ transplants (heart, kidney, liver). The drug will be added to an intravenous fluid that will drip through a needle or catheter placed in your vein for 2-6 hours, once every day. This medication is sometimes prescribed for other uses; ask your doctor or pharmacist for more information.

Your health care provider (doctor, nurse, or pharmacist) may measure the effectiveness and side effects of your treatment using laboratory tests and physical examinations. It is important to keep all appointments with your doctor and the laboratory. The length of treatment depends on how you respond to the medication.

Precautions

Before administering cyclosporine,
- tell your doctor and pharmacist if you are allergic to cyclosporine or any other drugs.
- tell your doctor and pharmacist what prescription and nonprescription medications you are taking. While taking cyclosporine, do not take the following medications unless your doctor tells you to: allopurinol (Zyloprim), azithromycin (Zithromax), bromocriptine (Parlodel), carbamazepine (Tegretol), cimetidine (Tagamet), clarithromycin (Biaxin), danazol, diclofenac (Feldene), diltiazem (Cardizem), dirithromycin (Dynabac), erythromycin, fluconazole (Diflucan), itraconazole (Sporanox), ketoconazole (Nizoral), methotrexate, methylprednisolone (Medrol), metoclopramide (Reglan), octreotide (Sandostatin), phenobarbital, phenytoin (Dilantin), prednisolone, ranitidine (Zantac), rifabutin (Mycobutin), rifampin (Rifadin), spironolactone (Aldactone), tacrolimus (Prograf), ticlopidine (Ticlid), triamterene (Dyrenium), trimethoprim/sulfamethoxazole (Bactrim, Septra), verapamil (Calan), and vitamins.
- tell your doctor if you have or have ever had liver or kidney disease.
- tell your doctor if you are pregnant, plan to become pregnant, or are breast-feeding. If you become pregnant while taking cyclosporine, call your doctor.
- you should know that this drug may make you more likely to get infections. Avoid people with contagious diseases such as the flu. Keep cuts and scratches clean. Use good personal hygiene, particularly for your mouth, teeth, skin, hair, and hands. Call your doctor immediately if you have signs of an infection such as fever, sore throat, chills, and frequent and painful urination.

Administering Your Medication

Before you administer cyclosporine, look at the solution closely. It should be clear and free of floating material. Gently squeeze the bag or observe the solution container to make sure there are no leaks. Do not use the solution if it is discolored, if it contains particles, or if the bag or container leaks. Use a new solution, but show the damaged one to your health care provider.

It is important that you use your medication exactly as directed. Do not stop your therapy on your own for any reason. Do not change your dosing schedule without talking to your health care provider. Your health care provider may tell you to stop your infusion if you have a mechanical problem (such as a blockage in the tubing, needle, or catheter); if you have to stop an infusion, call your health care provider immediately so your therapy can continue.

Side Effects

Cyclosporine may cause side effects. Tell your health care provider if any of these symptoms are severe or do not go away:

- upset stomach
- vomiting
- diarrhea
- loss of appetite
- increased hair growth
- sinusitis
- breast enlargement

If you experience any of the following symptoms or those listed in the IMPORTANT WARNING section, call your health care provider immediately:

- tremors
- overgrowth of the gums
- unusual bleeding or bruising
- chills
- yellowing of the skin or eyes
- seizures
- decreased urination
- swelling (feet, ankles, lower legs, and hands)
- weight gain
- headache

If you experience a serious side effect, you or your doctor may send a report to the Food and Drug Administration's (FDA) MedWatch Adverse Event Reporting program online [at http://www.fda.gov/MedWatch/index.html] or by phone [1-800-332-1088].

Storage Conditions

- Your health care provider probably will give you a several-day supply of cyclosporine at a time. You may be told how to prepare each dose and how to store it properly.

Store your medication only as directed. Make sure you understand what you need to store your medication properly.

Keep your supplies in a clean, dry place when you are not using them, and keep all medications and supplies out of reach of children. Your health care provider will tell you how to throw away used needles, syringes, tubing, and containers to avoid accidental injury.

Overdose

In case of overdose, call your local poison control center at 1-800-222-1222. If the victim has collapsed or is not breathing, call local emergency services at 911.

Signs of Infection

If you are receiving cyclosporine in your vein or under your skin, you need to know the symptoms of a catheter-related infection (an infection where the needle enters your vein or skin). If you experience any of these effects near your intravenous catheter, tell your health care provider as soon as possible:

- tenderness
- warmth
- irritation
- drainage
- redness
- swelling
- pain

Dosage Facts
For Informational Purposes

Caution: Do not change your dose, how often you take your medication, or the length of time you are to take it without first talking to your healthcare provider.

The following dosage information was written using medical language for doctors and other healthcare professionals and is provided here for you to check your dosage. The dosage of this drug may differ for different patients. Therefore, always follow your doctor's instructions or the directions on the label. Contact your healthcare provider or pharmacist if you have any questions about the specific dosage of your medication after reviewing this information.

General Dosage Information

Individualize dosage of cyclosporine.

Pediatric Patients

Transplant Recipients
Concentrate for Injection

IV:
- Initially, 5–6 mg/kg as a single dose 4–12 hours before transplantation. Postoperatively, 5–6 mg/kg once daily until the patient is able to tolerate oral administration. Pediatric patients may require higher dosages.
- In patients unable to take cyclosporine orally, may administer the drug by IV infusion at about one-third the recommended oral dosage.

Adult Patients

Transplant Recipients
Concentrate for Injection

IV:
- Initially, 5–6 mg/kg as a single dose 4–12 hours before transplantation. Postoperatively, 5–6 mg/kg once daily until the patient is able to tolerate oral administration.
- In patients unable to take cyclosporine orally, may administer the drug by IV infusion at about one-third the recommended oral dosage.

Crohn's Disease
Concentrate for Injection

IV:
- Initially, 4 mg/kg daily for about 2–10 days has been used. Patients who respond to initial IV regimen may be switched to oral therapy.

Special Populations

Renal Impairment
- Monitor renal function closely; frequent dosage adjustments may be necessary.
- Contraindicated in rheumatoid arthritis or psoriasis patients with abnormal renal function.

Cyclosporine Ophthalmic

(sye′ kloe spor een)

Brand Name: Restasis®

Why is this medicine prescribed?

Cyclosporine ophthalmic is used to increase tear production in people with dry eye disease. Cyclosporine ophthalmic is in a class of medications called immunomodulators. It works by decreasing swelling in the eye to allow for tear production.

How should this medicine be used?

Cyclosporine ophthalmic comes as an emulsion (liquid) to apply to the eye. It is usually applied to each eye twice a day, about 12 hours apart. To help you remember to use cyclosporine eyedrops, apply them around the same times every day. Follow the directions on your prescription label carefully, and ask your doctor or pharmacist to explain any part you do not understand. Use cyclosporine eyedrops exactly as directed. Do not use more or less of them or use them more often than prescribed by your doctor.

Cyclosporine eyedrops are for use only in the eye(s). Do not swallow or apply cyclosporine eyedrops to the skin.

Cyclosporine eyedrops come in single-use vials (small bottles to be used for one dose). The liquid from one vial should be used immediately after opening for one or both eyes.

To apply the eyedrops, follow these steps:
1. Wash your hands thoroughly with soap and water.
2. Turn over the vial a few times until the liquid inside looks white and not see-through.
3. Open the vial.
4. Use a mirror or have someone else put the drops in your eye.
5. Avoid touching the dropper against your eye or anything else.
6. Hold the dropper tip down at all times to prevent drops from flowing back into the bottle and contaminating the remaining contents.
7. Lie down or tilt your head back.
8. Holding the bottle between your thumb and index finger, place the dropper as near as possible to your eyelid without touching it.
9. Brace the remaining fingers of that hand against your cheek or nose.
10. With the index finger of your other hand, pull the lower lid of the eye down to form a pocket.
11. Drop the prescribed number of drops into the pocket made by the lower lid and the eye. Placing the drops on the surface of the eyeball can cause stinging.
12. Close your eye and press lightly against the lower lid with your finger for 2-3 minutes to keep the medication in the eye. Do not blink.
13. If you are using the eyedrops for both eyes, repeat steps 7-11 for the other eye.
14. Wipe off any excess liquid from your cheek with a clean tissue.
15. Throw away the vial out of the reach of children even if it is not empty.
16. Wash your hands again.

Are there other uses for this medicine?

This medication may be prescribed for other uses; ask your doctor or pharmacist for more information.

What special precautions should I follow?

Before using cyclosporine eyedrops,
- tell your doctor and pharmacist if you are allergic to cyclosporine (Neoral, Sandimmune) or any other medications.
- tell your doctor and pharmacist what prescription and nonprescription medications, vitamins, nutritional supplements, and herbal products you are taking. Be sure to mention other eyedrops for dry eye disease.
- if you are using artificial tears, apply them at least 15 minutes before or after cyclosporine eyedrops.
- tell your doctor if you have an eye infection, if you have a punctal plug (stopper inserted by a doctor in a tear duct to keep tears in the eye), and if you have or have ever had a herpes infection of the eye.

- tell your doctor if you are pregnant, plan to become pregnant, or are breast-feeding. If you become pregnant while using cyclosporine eyedrops, call your doctor.
- you should know that cyclosporine eyedrops should not be applied while wearing contact lenses. If you wear contact lenses, remove them before applying cyclosporine eyedrops and put them back in 15 minutes later. Talk to your doctor about wearing contact lenses if you have dry eye disease.

What special dietary instructions should I follow?

Unless your doctor tells you otherwise, continue your normal diet.

What should I do if I forget to take a dose?

Apply the missed dose as soon as you remember it. However, if it is almost time for the next dose, skip the missed dose and continue your regular dosing schedule. Do not apply a double dose to make up for a missed one.

What side effects can this medicine cause?

Cyclosporine eyedrops may cause side effects. Tell your doctor if any of these symptoms are severe or do not go away:

- burning, itching, stinging, redness, or pain of the eyes
- overflow of tears
- red eyes
- eye discharge
- blurred vision or other vision changes
- feeling that something is in the eye

Cyclosporine eyedrops may cause other side effects. Call your doctor if you have any unusual problems while taking this medication.

What storage conditions are needed for this medicine?

Keep this medication in the container it came in, tightly closed, and out of reach of children. Store it at room temperature and away from excess heat and moisture (not in the bathroom). Throw away each vial after one use. Throw away any medication that is outdated or no longer needed. Talk to your pharmacist about the proper disposal of your medication.

What other information should I know?

Keep all appointments with your doctor.

Do not let anyone else take your medication. Ask your pharmacist any questions you have about refilling your prescription.

Dosage Facts
For Informational Purposes

Caution: Do not change your dose, how often you take your medication, or the length of time you

are to take it without first talking to your health-care provider.

The following dosage information was written using medical language for doctors and other healthcare professionals and is provided here for you to check your dosage. The dosage of this drug may differ for different patients. Therefore, always follow your doctor's instructions or the directions on the label. Contact your health-care provider or pharmacist if you have any questions about the specific dosage of your medication after reviewing this information.

Adult Patients
Keratoconjunctivitis Sicca

OPHTHALMIC:
- 1 drop of a 0.05% emulsion into each eye twice daily, approximately 12 hours apart.

Cyproheptadine

(si proe hep′ ta deen)

Brand Name: Periactin®
Also available generically.

Why is this medicine prescribed?

Cyproheptadine, an antihistamine, relieves red, irritated, itchy, watery eyes; sneezing; and runny nose caused by allergies, hay fever, and the common cold. It may also relieve the itching of insect bites, bee stings, poison ivy, and poison oak.

This medication is sometimes prescribed for other uses; ask your doctor or pharmacist for more information.

How should this medicine be used?

Cyproheptadine comes as tablets and a liquid to take by mouth. It usually is taken two or three times a day. Follow the directions on your prescription label carefully, and ask your doctor or pharmacist to explain any part you do not understand. Take cyproheptadine exactly as directed. Do not take more or less of it or take it more often than prescribed by your doctor.

Are there other uses for this medicine?

Cyproheptadine also is used to stimulate appetite and weight gain. Talk to your doctor about the possible risks of using this drug for your condition.

What special precautions should I follow?

Before taking cyproheptadine,
- tell your doctor and pharmacist if you are allergic to cyproheptadine or any other drugs.

- tell your doctor and pharmacist what prescription and nonprescription medications you are taking, especially other medications for allergies or colds, medications for depression or seizures, muscle relaxants, narcotics (pain medications), sedatives, sleeping pills, tranquilizers, and vitamins. Do not use cyproheptadine if you have taken an MAO inhibitor [phenelzine (Nardil) or tranylcypromine (Parnate)] in the last 2 weeks.
- tell your doctor if you have or have ever had asthma, diabetes, glaucoma, ulcers, difficulty urinating (due to an enlarged prostate gland), heart disease, high blood pressure, seizures, or an overactive thyroid gland.
- tell your doctor if you are pregnant, plan to become pregnant, or are breast-feeding. If you become pregnant while taking cyproheptadine, call your doctor.
- if you are having surgery, including dental surgery, tell the doctor or dentist that you are taking cyproheptadine.
- you should know that this drug may make you drowsy. Do not drive a car or operate machinery until you know how this drug affects you.
- remember that alcohol can add to the drowsiness caused by this drug.

What should I do if I forget to take a dose?

Take the missed dose as soon as you remember it. However, if it is almost time for the next dose, skip the missed dose and continue your regular dosing schedule. Do not take a double dose to make up for a missed one.

What side effects can this medicine cause?

Cyproheptadine may cause side effects. Tell your doctor if any of these symptoms are severe or do not go away:
- dry mouth, nose, and throat
- drowsiness
- dizziness
- upset stomach
- chest congestion
- headache
- diarrhea

If you experience any of the following symptoms, call your doctor immediately:
- excitement (especially in children)
- muscle weakness
- difficulty urinating
- vision problems
- skin rash

If you experience a serious side effect, you or your doctor may send a report to the Food and Drug Administration's (FDA) MedWatch Adverse Event Reporting program online [at http://www.fda.gov/MedWatch/index.html] or by phone [1-800-332-1088].

What storage conditions are needed for this medicine?

Keep this medication in the container it came in, tightly closed, and out of reach of children. Store it at room temperature and away from excess heat and moisture (not in the bathroom). Throw away any medication that is outdated or no longer needed. Talk to your pharmacist about the proper disposal of your medication.

What should I do in case of overdose?

In case of overdose, call your local poison control center at 1-800-222-1222. If the victim has collapsed or is not breathing, call local emergency services at 911.

What other information should I know?

Keep all appointments with your doctor.

Do not let anyone else take your medication. Ask your pharmacist any questions you have about refilling your prescription.

Dosage Facts
For Informational Purposes

Caution: Do not change your dose, how often you take your medication, or the length of time you are to take it without first talking to your healthcare provider.

The following dosage information was written using medical language for doctors and other healthcare professionals and is provided here for you to check your dosage. The dosage of this drug may differ for different patients. Therefore, always follow your doctor's instructions or the directions on the label. Contact your healthcare provider or pharmacist if you have any questions about the specific dosage of your medication after reviewing this information.

General Dosage Information

Available as cyproheptadine hydrochloride; dosage expressed in terms of the salt.

Pediatric Patients

Allergic Conditions

ORAL:
- Children 2–6 years of age: Usual dosage is 2 mg 2 or 3 times daily; adjust as needed based on the size and response of the patient, up to maximum of 12 mg daily.
- Children 7–14 years of age: Usual dosage is 4 mg 2 or 3 times daily; adjust as needed based on the size and response of the patient, up to maximum of 16 mg daily.
- Adolescents ≥15 years of age: Initially, 4 mg 3 times daily; adjust based on the size and response of the patient, up to 0.5 mg/kg daily. Dosage range: 4–20 mg daily; most patients require 12–16 mg daily.
- Alternatively, children ≥2 years of age may receive 0.25 mg/kg or 8 mg/m² daily in divided doses.

Anorexia Nervosa†

ORAL:
- Adolescents ≥13 years of age: Dosage of 2 mg 4 times daily, increased gradually over a 3-week period to up to 8 mg 4 times daily, has been used.

Adult Patients

Allergic Conditions

ORAL:
- Initially, 4 mg 3 times daily; adjust as needed based on the size and response of the patient, up to 0.5 mg/kg daily.
- Dosage range: 4–20 mg daily; most patients require 12–16 mg daily. Some patients may require up to 32 mg daily.

Cushing's Syndrome†

ORAL:
- Initially, 8 mg daily in divided doses; gradually increase dosage to up to 24 mg daily in divided doses.

Anorexia Nervosa†

ORAL:
- Dosage of 2 mg 4 times daily, increased gradually over a 3-week period to up to 8 mg 4 times daily, has been used.

Prescribing Limits

Pediatric Patients

Allergic Conditions

ORAL:
- Children 2–6 years of age: Maximum 12 mg daily.
- Children 7–14 years of age: Maximum 16 mg daily.
- Adolescents ≥15 years of age: Maximum 0.5 mg/kg daily.

Anorexia Nervosa†

ORAL:
- Adolescents ≥13 years of age: Maximum 32 mg daily.

Adult Patients

Allergic Conditions

ORAL:
- Maximum 0.5 mg/kg daily.

Cushing's Syndrome†

ORAL:
- Maximum 24 mg daily.

Anorexia Nervosa†

ORAL:
- Maximum 32 mg daily.

Special Populations

Geriatric Patients
- Select dosage with caution, starting at the lower end of the usual dosage range.

† Use is not currently included in the labeling approved by the US Food and Drug Administration.

Dalteparin Sodium Injection

(dal te pa′ rin)

Brand Name: Fragmin®

Important Warning

If you have epidural or spinal anesthesia or a spinal puncture while taking a 'blood thinner' such as dalteparin, you are at risk for internal bleeding that could cause you to become paralyzed.

Tell your doctor if you are taking abciximab (ReoPro); anagrelide (Agrylin); other anticoagulants ('blood thinners') such as warfarin (Coumadin); aspirin, ibuprofen (Advil, Motrin, or Nuprin), indomethacin (Indocin), ketoprofen (Actron, Orudis), naproxen (Aleve, Anaprox, Naprosyn), or other nonsteroidal anti-inflammatory drugs (NSAIDs); cilostazol (Pletal); clopidogrel (Plavix); dipyridamole (Persantine); eptifibatide (Integrilin); sulfinpyrazone (Anturane); ticlopidine (Ticlid); and tirofiban (Aggrastat).

If you experience any of the following symptoms, call your doctor immediately: numbness, tingling, leg weakness or paralysis, and loss of control over your bladder or bowels. Talk to your doctor about the risk of taking dalteparin.

About Your Treatment

Your doctor has ordered dalteparin sodium, an anticoagulant ('blood thinner'), to prevent harmful blood clots from forming. The drug will be injected under the skin (subcutaneously) once a day. This medication is sometimes prescribed for other uses; ask your doctor or pharmacist for more information.

Your health care provider (doctor, nurse, or pharmacist) may measure the effectiveness and side effects of your treatment using laboratory tests and physical examinations. It is important to keep all appointments with your doctor and the laboratory. The length of treatment depends on how you respond to the medication.

Precautions

Before administering dalteparin,
- tell your doctor and pharmacist if you are allergic to dalteparin, heparin, enoxaparin (Lovenox), any other drugs, or pork products.
- tell your doctor and pharmacist what prescription and nonprescription medications you are taking, especially those listed in the IMPORTANT WARNING section and vitamins.

- tell your doctor if you have or have ever had liver or kidney disease or diabetes.
- tell your doctor if you are pregnant, plan to become pregnant, or are breast-feeding. If you become pregnant while taking dalteparin, call your doctor.

Administering Your Medication

Before you administer dalteparin, look at the solution closely. It should be clear and free of floating material. Observe the solution container to make sure there are no leaks. Do not use the solution if it is discolored, if it contains particles, or if the container leaks. Use a new solution, but show the damaged one to your health care provider.

It is important that you use your medication exactly as directed. Do not change your dosing schedule without talking to your health care provider.

Side Effects

Dalteparin may cause side effects. Tell your health care provider if the following symptom is severe or does not go away:

- upset stomach

If you experience any of the following symptoms or those listed in the IMPORTANT WARNING section, call your doctor or health care provider immediately:

- unusual bleeding
- vomiting or spitting up blood or brown material that resembles coffee grounds
- bloody or black, tarry stools
- blood in urine
- red or dark-brown urine
- easy bruising
- excessive menstrual bleeding
- fever
- dizziness or lightheadedness

If you experience a serious side effect, you or your doctor may send a report to the Food and Drug Administration's (FDA) MedWatch Adverse Event Reporting program online [at http://www.fda.gov/MedWatch/index.html] or by phone [1-800-332-1088].

Storage Conditions

- Your health care provider will probably give you several days supply of dalteparin at a time. You will be told to store it at room temperature.

Store your medication only as directed. Make sure you understand what you need to store your medication properly.

Keep your supplies in a clean, dry place when you are not using them, and keep all medications and supplies out of reach of children. Your health care provider will tell you how to throw away used needles, syringes, tubing, and containers to avoid accidental injury.

Overdose

In case of overdose, call your local poison control center at 1-800-222-1222. If the victim has collapsed or is not breathing, call local emergency services at 911.

Signs of Infection

If you are receiving dalteparin under your skin, you need to know the symptoms of a catheter-related infection (an infection where the needle enters your skin). If you experience any of these effects near the infusion site, tell your health care provider as soon as possible:

- tenderness
- warmth
- irritation
- drainage
- redness
- swelling
- pain

Dosage Facts
For Informational Purposes

Caution: Do not change your dose, how often you take your medication, or the length of time you are to take it without first talking to your healthcare provider.

The following dosage information was written using medical language for doctors and other healthcare professionals and is provided here for you to check your dosage. The dosage of this drug may differ for different patients. Therefore, always follow your doctor's instructions or the directions on the label. Contact your healthcare provider or pharmacist if you have any questions about the specific dosage of your medication after reviewing this information.

General Dosage Information

Dosages for dalteparin sodium and regular (unfractionated heparin) or other low molecular weight (LMW) heparins cannot be used interchangeably on a unit-for-unit (or mg-for-mg) basis.

Available as dalteparin sodium; dosage expressed in anti-Factor Xa international units (IU, units).

Adult Patients

Unstable Angina and Non-ST-Segment Elevation/Non-Q-Wave MI

SUB-Q:
- 120 units/kg every 12 hours (up to a maximum of 10,000 units every 12 hours) until patient is clinically stabilized, generally for 5–8 days. Concurrent aspirin therapy is recommended in all patients unless contraindicated.

Prevention of Venous Thrombosis and Pulmonary Embolism
Hip-Replacement Surgery

SUB-Q:
- Initiate therapy either preoperatively or postoperatively; several regimens have been used. ACCP recommends initiation 12–24 hours postoperatively following achievement of hemostasis in patients at high risk for bleeding.
- Preoperative start, evening before surgery: 5000 units 10–14 hours before surgery, followed by 5000 units 4–8 hours after

surgery or later if hemostasis has not been achieved. Continue with 5000 units daily throughout the postoperative period (generally 5–10 days, but up to 14 days has been well tolerated).
- Preoperative start, day of surgery: 2500 units within 2 hours prior to surgery, followed by 2500 units 4–8 hours after surgery or later if hemostasis has not been achieved. Continue with 5000 units daily throughout the postoperative period (generally 5–10 days, but up to 14 days has been well tolerated).
- Alternative preoperative regimen recommended by ACCP: usual high-risk dosage (e.g., 5000 units) beginning 12 hours prior to surgery and continuing for ≥10 days postoperatively.
- Postoperative start: 2500 units 4–8 hours after surgery or later if hemostasis has not been achieved. Continue with 5000 units daily throughout the postoperative period (generally 5–10 days, but up to 14 days has been well tolerated).
- Alternative postoperative regimen recommended by ACCP: half the usual high-risk dosage (e.g., 2500 units) 4–6 hours after surgery, followed by the usual high-risk dosage (e.g., 5000 units daily) the next day for ≥10 days.
- Another alternative regimen recommended by ACCP: Usual high-risk dosage (e.g., 5000 units) 12–24 hours after surgery and continuing for ≥10 days.
- Extended prophylaxis: ACCP recommends continuation for ≤28–35 days postoperatively in patients considered at high risk for thromboembolism.

Hip-Fracture Surgery

SUB-Q:
- ACCP recommends the usual high-risk dosage (e.g., 5000 units daily) initiated either preoperatively or postoperatively. If surgery likely to be delayed, initiate preoperatively and reinstitute postoperatively after hemostasis achieved.
- Continue prophylaxis for ≥10 days (i.e., most patients will continue anticoagulation following hospital discharge).
- Extended prophylaxis: ACCP recommends continuation for ≤28–35 days postoperatively in patients considered at high risk for thromboembolism.

Knee-Replacement Surgery

SUB-Q:
- ACCP recommends the usual high-risk dosage (e.g., 5000 units daily) initiated either preoperatively or postoperatively.
- Continue prophylaxis for ≥10 days (i.e., most patients will continue anticoagulation following hospital discharge).

General Surgery

SUB-Q:
- Patients at moderate to high risk for thromboembolic complications: 2500 units initially, given 1–2 hours before surgery. Continue with 2500 units once daily throughout postoperative period, generally for 5–10 days, until the risk of DVT has diminished.
- Patients who are at high risk for thromboembolic complications: 5000 units on the evening prior to surgery (e.g., 8–12 hours prior to surgery). Such patients include those with malignant disease or a history of DVT or pulmonary embolism. Continue with 5000 units daily throughout the postoperative period, generally for 5–10 days.
- Patients with malignancy: 2500 units given 1–2 hours prior to surgery and repeated 12 hours later. Continue with 5000 units daily throughout the postoperative period, generally for 5–10 days.

- Extended prophylaxis: ACCP suggests continuation for 2–3 weeks after hospital discharge in patients at high risk for thromboembolism (e.g., major cancer surgery).

Medical Conditions Associated with Thromboembolism

SUB-Q:
- 5000 units once daily, generally for 12–14 days. Alternatively, ACCP recommends a dosage of 2500 units daily in general medical patients with high-risk factors for thromboembolism (e.g., cancer, CHF, severe lung disease, patients confined to bedrest).

Thromboembolism Occurring During Pregnancy

SUB-Q:
- *Treatment* of acute venous thromboembolism: 200 units/kg daily in 1 or 2 divided doses throughout pregnancy. Continue oral anticoagulation (e.g., with warfarin) for at least 6 weeks postpartum.
- *Primary prevention* in women with inherited causes of thrombophilia (e.g., antithrombin deficiency, heterozygous genetic mutation of both prothrombin G20210A and factor V Leiden, or homozygous genetic mutation for factor V Leiden or prothrombin G20210A): 5000 units once daily or every 12 hours throughout pregnancy suggested, followed by postpartum oral anticoagulation (e.g., with warfarin) for at least 4–6 weeks.
- *Primary prevention* in other patients with confirmed thrombophilia: 5000 units once daily throughout pregnancy suggested, followed by postpartum oral anticoagulation (e.g., with warfarin) for at least 4–6 weeks.
- *Secondary prevention* after a single episode of idiopathic venous thromboembolism in women not receiving long-term anticoagulation: 5000 units once daily throughout pregnancy suggested, followed by postpartum oral anticoagulation (e.g., with warfarin) for at least 4–6 weeks.
- *Secondary prevention* after a single episode of venous thromboembolism in women with risk factors (e.g., confirmed thrombophilia, strong family history of thrombosis) not receiving long-term anticoagulation: 5000 units once daily or every 12 hours throughout pregnancy suggested, followed by postpartum oral anticoagulation (e.g., with warfarin) for at least 4–6 weeks.
- *Secondary prevention* after >2 episodes of venous thromboembolism in women receiving long-term anticoagulation: 200 units/kg daily in 1 or 2 divided doses throughout pregnancy suggested, followed by postpartum resumption of long-term anticoagulation.
- Adjust dosage for extremes of body weight.
- Discontinue 24 hours prior to elective induction of labor.

Embolism Associated with Atrial Fibrillation/Flutter

SUB-Q:
- Patients with atrial fibrillation duration <48 hours undergoing cardioversion who have no contraindications to anticoagulation: 200 units/kg daily in 1 or 2 divided doses.
- ACCP suggests same regimen for anticoagulation in patients undergoing cardioversion for atrial flutter.

Treatment of DVT and Nonmassive Pulmonary Embolism

SUB-Q:

- 200 units/kg daily in 1 or 2 divided doses for at least 5 days has been recommended; administer on outpatient basis in selected patients with acute uncomplicated DVT.
- ACCP recommends *against* routine monitoring of anticoagulation (e.g., anti-factor X_a activity) with heparin treatment of acute venous thromboembolism.
- Initiate concurrently with oral anticoagulation (e.g., with warfarin) and overlap therapy until response to warfarin is adequate. Continue oral anticoagulation for at least 3 months.
- Patients with cancer or in whom oral anticoagulation contraindicated or inconvenient: 200 units/kg once daily for 1 month, followed by 150 units/kg once daily for at least 3–6 months. Continue anticoagulation indefinitely or until cancer is resolved.

Prescribing Limits

Adult Patients

Unstable Angina or Non-ST-Segment Elevation/Non-Q-Wave MI

SUB-Q:

- Maximum 10,000 units every 12 hours.

Danazol

(da′ na zole)

Brand Name: Danocrine®
Also available generically.

> ## Important Warning
>
> Do not take danazol if you are pregnant or breast-feeding. A method of birth control (contraception) other than oral contraceptives should be used while taking danazol. If you become pregnant, call your doctor immediately. Life-threatening strokes, increased pressure in the brain, and serious liver disease complicated by potentially life-threatening abdominal bleeding have been reported during therapy with danazol. Talk to your doctor about the potential risks associated with this medication.

Why is this medicine prescribed?

Danazol is used to treat endometriosis, a disease that causes infertility, pain before and during menstrual periods, pain during and after sexual activity, and heavy or irregular bleeding. Danazol is also used in fibrocystic breast disease to reduce breast pain, tenderness, and nodules (lumps). Danazol is also used to prevent attacks of angioedema in both males and females.

This medication is sometimes prescribed for other uses; ask your doctor or pharmacist for more information.

How should this medicine be used?

Danazol comes as a capsule to take by mouth. It usually is taken twice a day. Women should take the first dose during a menstrual period and take it continuously thereafter. Follow the directions on your prescription label carefully, and ask your doctor or pharmacist to explain any part you do not understand. Take danazol exactly as directed. Do not take more or less of it or take it more often than prescribed by your doctor.

Do not stop taking danazol without talking to your doctor. If you have fibrocystic breast disease, breast pain and tenderness usually improve during the first month that you take danazol and go away in 2-3 months; nodules should improve in 4-6 months.

What special precautions should I follow?

Before taking danzaol,

- tell your doctor and pharmacist if you are allergic to danazol or any other drugs.
- tell your doctor and pharmacist what prescription and nonprescription medications you are taking, especially anticoagulants ('blood thinners') such as warfarin (Coumadin); diabetes medications such as insulin; medications to prevent seizures, especially carbamazepine (Tegretol); and vitamins.
- tell your doctor if you have or have ever had migraine headaches; heart, liver, or kidney disease; seizures (epilepsy); or a history of stroke, blood clots, or breast cancer.

What should I do if I forget to take a dose?

Take the missed dose as soon as you remember it. However, if it is almost time for the next dose, skip the missed dose and continue your regular dosing schedule. Do not take a double dose to make up for a missed one.

What side effects can this medicine cause?

Danazol may cause side effects. Tell your doctor if any of these symptoms are severe or do not go away:

- acne
- decrease in breast size
- deepening of the voice, hoarseness, or sore throat
- weight gain
- swelling (water retention and bloating)
- oily skin or hair
- hair growth in unusual amounts and places
- flushing
- sweating
- vaginal dryness, burning, itching, or bleeding
- nervousness
- depression
- irritability

- absence of menstrual cycle, spotting, or change in menstrual cycle

If you experience any of the following symptoms, call your doctor immediately:

- skin rash
- yellowing of the skin or eyes
- persistent headache
- persistent upset stomach
- vomiting
- visual disturbances
- persistent abdominal pain
- for males, frequent, prolonged, or painful penile erections

If you experience a serious side effect, you or your doctor may send a report to the Food and Drug Administration's (FDA) MedWatch Adverse Event Reporting program online [at http://www.fda.gov/MedWatch/index.html] or by phone [1-800-332-1088].

What storage conditions are needed for this medicine?

Keep this medication in the container it came in, tightly closed, and out of reach of children. Store it at room temperature and away from excess heat and moisture (not in the bathroom). Throw away any medication that is outdated or no longer needed. Talk to your pharmacist about the proper disposal of your medication.

What should I do in case of overdose?

In case of overdose, call your local poison control center at 1-800-222-1222. If the victim has collapsed or is not breathing, call local emergency services at 911.

What other information should I know?

Keep all appointments with your doctor and the laboratory. You probably will have periodic blood tests; men also may have semen tests. Your doctor may change your dose, depending on your response to the medication.

Do not let anyone else take your medication. Ask your pharmacist any questions you have about refilling your prescription.

Dosage Facts
For Informational Purposes

Caution: Do not change your dose, how often you take your medication, or the length of time you are to take it without first talking to your healthcare provider.

The following dosage information was written using medical language for doctors and other healthcare professionals and is provided here for you to check your dosage. The dosage of this drug may differ for different patients. Therefore, always follow your doctor's instructions or the directions on the label. Contact your health-care provider or pharmacist if you have any questions about the specific dosage of your medication after reviewing this information.

Adult Patients

Endometriosis
Mild Endometriosis

ORAL:
- Initially, 200–400 mg daily in 2 divided doses. Adjust subsequent doses depending on patient tolerance and therapeutic response.
- Continue therapy *uninterrupted* for 3–6 months; may extend to 9 months if necessary. If symptoms recur after discontinuance, reinstitute therapy.

Moderate to Severe Endometriosis or Infertility due to Endometriosis

Initially, 800 mg daily in 2 divided doses; gradually reduce dosage, depending on therapeutic response, to a level sufficient to maintain amenorrhea.

Continue therapy *uninterrupted* for 3–6 months; may extend to 9 months if necessary. If symptoms recur after discontinuance, reinstitute therapy.

Fibrocystic Breast Disease

ORAL:
- Usual dose: 100–400 mg daily in 2 divided doses. Adjust therapy according to severity of disease and patient response.
- If symptoms recur after discontinuance, reinstitute therapy.

Hereditary Angioedema

ORAL:
- Initially, 200 mg given 2 or 3 times daily until a favorable response (i.e., prevention of episodes of edematous attacks) is attained.
- Determine subsequent maintenance dosage by decreasing dosage by ≤50% at intervals of 1–3 months or longer, based on frequency of attacks before therapy.
- Dosage may be increased by ≤200 mg daily if an attack occurs during therapy.
- If danazol was initiated during exacerbation of angioedema resulting from trauma, stress, or other cause, periodically attempt to reduce dosage or withdraw therapy.

Prescribing Limits

Adult Patients

Hereditary Angioedema

ORAL:
- Dosage may be increased by maximum of 200 mg daily if an attack occurs during therapy.

Special Populations

Hepatic Impairment
- No specific dosage recommendations at this time; contraindicated in patients with markedly impaired hepatic function.

Renal Impairment
- No specific dosage recommendations at this time; contraindicated in patients with markedly impaired renal function.

Dantrolene Oral

(dan' troe leen)

Brand Name: Dantrium®
Also available generically.

Important Warning

Dantrolene can cause severe liver damage. Do not use dantrolene for conditions other than those recommended by your doctor. Do not take more than the recommended amount prescribed by your doctor. Do not take dantrolene if you have active liver disease. If you experience any of the following symptoms, call your doctor immediately: yellowing of the skin or eyes, dark urine, black tarry stools, or severe nausea and vomiting.

Keep all appointments with your doctor and the laboratory. Your doctor will order certain lab tests to check your response to dantrolene.

Why is this medicine prescribed?

Dantrolene, a muscle relaxant, is used to treat spasticity or muscle spasms associated with spinal cord injuries, stroke, multiple sclerosis, cerebral palsy, or other conditions.

This medication is sometimes prescribed for other uses; ask your doctor or pharmacist for more information.

How should this medicine be used?

Dantrolene comes as a capsule to take by mouth. It usually is taken once a day at first and then increased gradually to two to four times a day. Follow the directions on your prescription label carefully, and ask your doctor or pharmacist to explain any part you do not understand. Take dantrolene exactly as directed. Do not take more or less of it or take it more often than prescribed by your doctor.

If you cannot swallow capsules, empty the contents into fruit juice and mix well just before taking the dose.

What special precautions should I follow?

Before taking dantrolene,
- tell your doctor and pharmacist if you are allergic to dantrolene or any other drugs.
- tell your doctor and pharmacist what prescription and nonprescription medications you are taking, especially diazepam (Valium); estrogen; medications for seizures, allergies, colds, or coughs; sedatives; sleeping pills; tranquilizers; and vitamins.
- tell your doctor if you have or have ever had liver, heart, rheumatic, or lung disease.
- tell your doctor if you are pregnant, plan to become pregnant, or are breast-feeding. If you become pregnant while taking dantrolene, call your doctor immediately.
- you should know that this drug may make you drowsy. Do not drive a car or operate machinery until you know how dantrolene affects you.
- remember that alcohol can add to the drowsiness caused by this drug.
- you should plan to avoid unnecessary or prolonged exposure to sunlight and to wear protective clothing, sunglasses, and sunscreen. Dantrolene may make your skin sensitive to sunlight.

What should I do if I forget to take a dose?

Take the missed dose as soon as you remember it. However, if it is almost time for the next dose, skip the missed dose and continue your regular dosing schedule. Do not take a double dose to make up for the missed one.

What side effects can this medicine cause?

Dantrolene may cause side effects. Tell your doctor if any of these symptoms are severe or do not go away:
- muscle weakness
- drowsiness
- dizziness
- diarrhea
- fatigue
- difficulty swallowing

In addition to the symptoms mentioned in the IMPORTANT WARNING section, if you experience the following symptom, call your doctor immediately:
- seizures

If you experience a serious side effect, you or your doctor may send a report to the Food and Drug Administration's (FDA) MedWatch Adverse Event Reporting program online [at http://www.fda.gov/MedWatch/index.html] or by phone [1-800-332-1088].

What storage conditions are needed for this medicine?

Keep this medication in the container it came in, tightly closed, and out of reach of children. Store it at room temperature and away from excess heat and moisture (not in the bathroom). Throw away any medication that is outdated or no longer needed. Talk to your pharmacist about the proper disposal of your medication.

What should I do in case of overdose?

In case of overdose, call your local poison control center at 1-800-222-1222. If the victim has collapsed or is not breathing, call local emergency services at 911.

What other information should I know?

Do not let anyone else take your medication. Ask your pharmacist any questions you have about refilling your prescription.

Dosage Facts
For Informational Purposes

Caution: Do not change your dose, how often you take your medication, or the length of time you are to take it without first talking to your healthcare provider.

The following dosage information was written using medical language for doctors and other healthcare professionals and is provided here for you to check your dosage. The dosage of this drug may differ for different patients. Therefore, always follow your doctor's instructions or the directions on the label. Contact your healthcare provider or pharmacist if you have any questions about the specific dosage of your medication after reviewing this information.

General Dosage Information

Available as dantrolene sodium; dosage expressed in terms of the salt.

Pediatric Patients
Spasticity

ORAL:
- Children ≥5 years of age: 0.5 mg/kg once daily for 7 days, followed by 0.5 mg/kg 3 times daily for 7 days, then 1 mg/kg 3 times daily for 7 days, and then 2 mg/kg 3 times daily, if necessary. Some patients may require doses 4 times daily.
- If no additional benefit is observed at the next higher dosage, decrease dosage to the previous (lower) dosage.

Malignant Hyperthermia Crisis
Preoperative Prophylaxis

ORAL:
- 4–8 mg/kg daily in 3 or 4 divided doses for 1–2 days prior to surgery; give the last dose approximately 3–4 hours before surgery with small amount of water.

Post-crisis Follow-up

ORAL:
- 4–8 mg/kg daily in 4 divided doses for up to 3 days after the crisis.

Adult Patients
Spasticity

ORAL:
- Initially, 25 mg once daily for 7 days, followed by 25 mg 3 times daily for 7 days, then 50 mg 3 times daily for 7 days, and then 100 mg 3 times daily, if necessary. Some patients may require doses 4 times daily.
- If no additional benefit is observed at the next higher dosage, decrease dosage to the previous (lower) dosage.

Malignant Hyperthermia Crisis
Preoperative Prophylaxis

ORAL:
- 4–8 mg/kg daily in 3 or 4 divided doses for 1–2 days prior to surgery; give the last dose approximately 3–4 hours before surgery with small amount of water.

Post-crisis Follow-up

ORAL:
- 4–8 mg/kg daily in 4 divided doses for up to 3 days after the crisis.

Prescribing Limits
Pediatric Patients
Spasticity

ORAL:
- Maximum 100 mg 4 times daily.

Adult Patients
Spasticity

ORAL:
- Maximum 100 mg 4 times daily.

Dapiprazole Ophthalmic

(da′ pi pray zole)

Brand Name: Rev-Eyes®

Why is this medicine prescribed?

Dapiprazole causes the pupil of the eye to constrict. It reverses pupil dilation caused by other drugs given during an eye examination.

This medication is sometimes prescribed for other uses; ask your doctor or pharmacist for more information.

How should this medicine be used?

Dapiprazole comes as eyedrops. Usually, 2 drops are applied following an eye examination, and 2 more drops are applied 5 minutes later. Follow the directions on your prescription label carefully, and ask your doctor or pharmacist to explain any part you do not understand. Use dapiprazole exactly as directed. Do not use more or less of it or use it more often than prescribed by your doctor.

To use the eyedrops, follow these instructions:
1. Wash your hands thoroughly with soap and water.
2. Use a mirror or have someone else put the drops in your eye.
3. Shake the container well.
4. Remove the protective cap. Make sure that the end of the dropper is not chipped or cracked.
5. Avoid touching the dropper tip against your eye or anything else.
6. Hold the dropper tip down at all times to prevent drops from flowing back into the bottle and contaminating the remaining contents.
7. Lie down or tilt your head back or lie down and gaze upward.

8. Holding the bottle between your thumb and index finger, place the dropper tip as near as possible to your eyelid without touching it.

9. Brace the remaining fingers of that hand against your cheek or nose.

10. With the index finger of your other hand, pull the lower lid of the eye down to form a pocket.

11. Drop the prescribed number of drops into the pocket made by the lower lid and the eye. Placing drops on the surface of the eyeball can cause stinging.

12. Close your eye and press lightly against the lower lid with your finger for 2-3 minutes to keep the medication in the eye. Do not blink.

13. Replace and tighten the cap right away. Do not wipe or rinse it off.

14. Wipe off any excess liquid from your cheek with a clean tissue. Wash your hands again.

What special precautions should I follow?

Before using dapiprazole eyedrops,

- tell your doctor and pharmacist if you are allergic to dapiprazole or any other drugs.
- tell your doctor and pharmacist what prescription and nonprescription medications you are taking, especially other eye medications, and vitamins.
- tell your doctor if you have eye problems or allergies.
- tell your doctor if you are pregnant, plan to become pregnant, or are breast-feeding. If you become pregnant while using dapiprazole, call your doctor immediately.
- if you are using another eyedrop medication, use the eye medications at least 10 minutes apart.

What should I do if I forget to take a dose?

Apply the missed dose as soon as you remember it. However, if it is almost time for the next dose, skip the missed dose and continue your regular dosing schedule. Do not apply a double dose to make up for a missed one.

What side effects can this medicine cause?

Dapiprazole may cause side effects. Tell your doctor if any of these symptoms are severe or do not go away:

- stinging, burning, or redness of the eye
- tearing

If you experience any of the following symptoms, stop using dapiprazole and call your doctor immediately:

- blurred or unstable vision, especially at night
- skin rash
- itching
- pain
- swelling around the eyes
- headache

If you experience a serious side effect, you or your doctor may send a report to the Food and Drug Administration's (FDA) MedWatch Adverse Event Reporting program online [at http://www.fda.gov/MedWatch/index.html] or by phone [1-800-332-1088].

What storage conditions are needed for this medicine?

Keep this medication in the container it came in, tightly closed, and out of reach of children. Store it at room temperature and away from excess heat and moisture (not in the bathroom). If the eyedrop solution becomes cloudy or contains particles, do not use it; obtain a fresh bottle. Throw away any medication that is outdated or no longer needed. Talk to your pharmacist about the proper disposal of your medication.

What other information should I know?

Keep all appointments with your doctor. Your doctor will order certain eye tests to check your response to dapiprazole.

Do not let anyone else use your medication. Ask your pharmacist any questions you have about refilling your prescription.

Talk to your doctor, pharmacist, or other healthcare professional if you have questions about dosing information for your medication.

Dapsone

(dap′ sone)

Why is this medicine prescribed?

Dapsone is used to treat leprosy and skin infections.

This medication is sometimes prescribed for other uses; ask your doctor or pharmacist for more information.

How should this medicine be used?

Dapsone comes as a tablet to take by mouth. Dapsone usually is taken either once a day or three times a week. Follow the directions on your prescription label carefully, and ask your doctor or pharmacist to explain any part you do not understand. Take dapsone exactly as directed. Do not take more or less of it or take it more often than prescribed by your doctor.

What special precautions should I follow?

Before taking dapsone,

- tell your doctor and pharmacist if you are allergic to dapsone, sulfa drugs, phenylhydrazine, naphthalene, niridazole, nitrofurantoin, primaquine, or any other drugs.
- tell your doctor and pharmacist what prescription and nonprescription medications you are taking, especially aminobenzoate potassium (Potaba), aminobenzoic acid, clofazimine (Lamprene), didanosine (Videx), probenecid (Benemid), pyrimethamine (Daraprim), rifampin (Rifadin), trimethoprim (Bactrim, Cotrim, Septra), or vitamins.

- tell your doctor if you have or have ever had anemia or liver disease.
- tell your doctor if you are pregnant, plan to become pregnant, or are breast-feeding. If you become pregnant while taking dapsone, call your doctor.
- plan to avoid unnecessary or prolonged exposure to sunlight and to wear protective clothing, sunglasses, and sunscreen. Dapsone may make your skin sensitive to sunlight.

What special dietary instructions should I follow?

Dapsone may cause an upset stomach. Take dapsone with food or milk.

What should I do if I forget to take a dose?

Take the missed dose as soon as you remember it. However, if it is almost time for the next dose, skip the missed dose and continue your regular dosing schedule. Do not take a double dose to make up for a missed one.

What side effects can this medicine cause?

Dapsone may cause side effects. Tell your doctor if any of these symptoms are severe or do not go away:
- upset stomach
- vomiting

If you experience any of the following symptoms, call your doctor immediately:
- sore throat
- fever
- rash
- yellowing of the skin or eyes
- unusual bruising

If you experience a serious side effect, you or your doctor may send a report to the Food and Drug Administration's (FDA) MedWatch Adverse Event Reporting program online [at http://www.fda.gov/MedWatch/index.html] or by phone [1-800-332-1088].

What storage conditions are needed for this medicine?

Keep this medication in the container it came in, tightly closed, and out of reach of children. Store it at room temperature and away from excess heat and moisture (not in the bathroom). Throw away any medication that is outdated or no longer needed. Talk to your pharmacist about the proper disposal of your medication.

What should I do in case of overdose?

In case of overdose, call your local poison control center at 1-800-222-1222. If the victim has collapsed or is not breathing, call local emergency services at 911.

What other information should I know?

Keep all appointments with your doctor and the laboratory. Your doctor will order certain lab tests to check your response to dapsone.

Do not let anyone else take your medication. Ask your pharmacist any questions you have about refilling your prescription.

Talk to your doctor, pharmacist, or other healthcare professional if you have questions about dosing information for your medication.

Darbepoetin Alfa Injection

(dar be poe' e tin)

Brand Name: Aranesp®

Important Warning

Darbepoetin alfa increases the risk of serious and life-threatening events, including heart attack, heart failure, stroke, TIA (ministroke) or cerebrovascular accident (blood clot to the brain), pulmonary embolus (blood clot to the lung), deep vein thrombosis (blood clot to the blood vessels), and death when treatment results in a higher than recommended amount of hemoglobin (red blood cells) in the blood. Call your doctor immediately if you experience any of the following symptoms: pain, tenderness, redness, warmth, and/or swelling in the legs; shortness of breath; cough that won't go away or coughing up blood; nausea; vomiting; chest pain, squeezing pressure, or tightness; discomfort or pain in the arms, shoulder, neck, jaw, or back; fast or irregular heartbeat; sweating; swelling of the hands, feet, or ankles; blue-grey coloring or darkening around mouth or nails; dizziness or lightheadedness; extreme tiredness or weakness; fainting or loss of consciousness; sudden trouble seeing in one or both eyes; sudden trouble speaking or understanding speech; sudden confusion; sudden weakness or numbness of an arm or leg (especially on one side of the body), or face; sudden trouble walking or loss of balance or coordination; sudden severe headache; seizure; increased blood pressure; or, if you are on hemodialysis and you notice blood clots in a vascular access port.

Darbepoetin alfa may increase the chance of death when used in people with cancer who are not receiving chemotherapy or radiation therapy at the same time they are using darbepoetin alfa. In people with cancer receiving chemotherapy, darbepoetin may cause a tumor to grow faster or shorten the time until death when the amount of hemoglobin (red blood cells) in the blood is higher than recommended.

Use of medications similar to darbepoetin in people a just before major surgery, increases the risk of blood clots. Call your doctor immediately if you experience any of the following symptoms: pain, tenderness, redness, warmth, and/or swelling in one or both legs.

Ask your pharmacist or doctor for a copy of the manufacturer's information for the patient.

Keep all appointments with your doctor and the laboratory. Your doctor will order certain lab tests to check your body's response to darbepoetin alfa.

Talk to your doctor about the risks of using darbepoetin alfa.

Why is this medicine prescribed?

Darbepoetin alfa is used to treat anemia (a lower than normal number of red blood cells) in people with chronic kidney failure (a condition where over a period of time there is a decrease in kidney function that is not reversible). Darbepoetin alfa is also used to treat anemia in people receiving chemotherapy (medications used to treat cancer). Darbepoetin alfa is in a class of medications called erythropoiesis-stimulating agents (ESAs). It works by causing the bone marrow (soft tissue inside the bones where blood is made) to make more red blood cells.

How should this medicine be used?

Darbepoetin alfa comes as a solution (liquid) to inject subcutaneously (just under the skin) or intravenously (into a vein). It is usually injected once a week every 1 to 3 weeks. Follow the directions on your prescription label carefully, and ask your doctor or pharmacist to explain any part you do not understand. Use darbepoetin alfa exactly as directed. Do not use more or less of it or use it more often than prescribed by your doctor.

Your doctor may start you on the lowest possible dose of darbepoetin alfa and gradually increase or decrease your dose, not more than once every month. Your doctor may also tell you to stop using darbepoetin alfa for a time. Follow these instructions carefully. If your doctor tells you to stop using darbepoetin alfa, do not begin using it again until your doctor tells you that you should. It is likely that your doctor will restart your treatment with a lower dose of darbepoetin alfa than you were using.

Darbepoetin alfa is used to reduce the need for red blood cell transfusions. Darbepoetin alfa controls anemia but does not cure it. It may take 2 to 6 weeks or longer before you feel the full benefit of darbepoetin alfa Continue to use darbepoetin alfa even if you feel well. Do not stop using darbepoetin alfa without talking to your doctor.

Darbepoetin alfa injections are usually given by a doctor or nurse. Your doctor may decide that you can inject darbepoetin alfa yourself, or that you may have a friend or relative give the injections.Your doctor will train the person who will be injecting the medication and will test him to be sure he can give the injection correctly. Be sure that you and the person who will be giving the injections know the correct dose, how to give the medication, and how often to give the medication. Be sure that you and the person who will be giving the injections read the manufacturer's information for the patient that comes with darbepoetin alfa before you use it for the first time at home.

Darbepoetin alfa comes in prefilled syringes and also in vials to use with disposable syringes. Use vials and prefilled or disposable syringes only once. Do not put a needle through the rubber stopper of a vial more than once. Throw away a vial, syringe, or prefilled syringe after one use, even if it is not empty. Throw away used syringes in a puncture-resistant container, out of the reach of children. Do not throw a filled container into the household trash or recycling. Talk to your doctor or pharmacist about how to throw away the puncture-resistant container. There may be special state and local laws for throwing away used needles and syringes.

If you are using vials of darbepoetin alfa, you will need to use disposable syringes to inject your medication. Your doctor or pharmacist will tell you what type of syringe you should use. Do not use any other type of syringe because you may not get the right amount of medication.

Always inject darbepoetin alfa solution in its own syringe; never mix it with any other medication.

If you are injecting darbepoetin alfa subcutaneously, you can inject it just under the skin anywhere on these parts of your body: the outer area of your upper arms, your stomach except for the two-inch area around your navel (belly button), the front of your middle thighs, and the upper outer areas of your buttocks.

Choose a new spot each time you inject darbepoetin alfa. Do not inject darbepoetin alfa into a spot that is tender, red, bruised, hard, lumpy, or swollen.

Carefully read the manufacturer's instructions that describe how to prepare and inject a dose of darbepoetin alpha. Be sure to ask your pharmacist or doctor if you have any questions about how to prepare or inject this medication.

Are there other uses for this medicine?

This medication may be prescribed for other uses; ask your doctor or pharmacist for more information.

What special precautions should I follow?

Before using darbepoetin alfa,

- tell your doctor and pharmacist if you are allergic to darbepoetin alfa, epoetin alfa (Epogen, Procrit), medications made from animal cells, albumin, any other medications, latex, or polysorbate 80. Ask your doctor or pharmacist if you don't know if a medication you are allergic to is made from animal cells.
- tell your doctor if you have or have had high blood pressure.Your doctor may tell you not to use darbepoetin alfa.

- tell your doctor and pharmacist what other prescription and nonprescription medications, vitamins, nutritional supplements, and herbal products you are taking or plan to take.
- tell your doctor if you have or have ever had bleeding or blood clotting problems; diseases that affect your blood such as hemolytic anemia (condition where a low number of red blood cells occurs because the cells are being destroyed in the body); sickle cell disease (an inherited blood disease that causes pain, anemia, and organ damage), thalassemia (an inherited blood disease that causes abnormal development and other problems), or porphyria (an inherited blood disease that may cause skin or nervous system problems); blood clots in your heart, legs, or lungs; a heart attack; high blood pressure; stroke or ministroke (TIA); tumors; heart disease, or any disease that affects your brain or nervous system.
- tell your doctor if you have used darbepoetin alfa or another erythropoietic protein such as epoetin alfa (Epogen, Procrit) in the past. Be sure to tell your doctor if your anemia worsened during your treatment with one of these medications, or if you were ever told to stop using one of these medications.
- tell your doctor if you are pregnant, plan to become pregnant, or are breast-feeding. If you become pregnant while using darbepoetin alfa, call your doctor.
- if you are having surgery, including dental surgery, tell the doctor or dentist that you are using darbepoetin alfa.
- you should know that your blood pressure may increase while you are using darbepoetin alfa. Your doctor may ask you to check your blood pressure often. Be sure to check your blood pressure as often as your doctor tells you that you should, to call your doctor if your blood pressure is higher than your doctor says it should be, and to take any medications your doctor prescribes to control your blood pressure exactly as directed.
- You should call your doctor if you are planning to travel or if your activity becomes limited, such as spending more time sitting or in bed.
- if you are on hemodialysis, you should know that blood clots may form in the tubing that goes into your vein. Call your doctor if you think there is a clot in your tubing.

What special dietary instructions should I follow?

If you are following a prescribed special diet because you have kidney disease or high blood pressure, follow it carefully, even if you feel better while using darbepoetin alfa. Darbepoetin alfa will not work unless your body has enough iron. Your doctor or dietician will probably tell you to eat foods that are rich in iron. If you cannot get enough iron from your diet, your doctor may prescribe an iron supplement. Take this supplement exactly as directed.

What should I do if I forget to take a dose?

Call your doctor to ask what to do if you miss a dose of darbepoetin alfa. Do not use a double dose to make up for a missed one.

What side effects can this medicine cause?

Darbepoetin alfa may cause side effects. Tell your doctor if any of these symptoms are severe or do not go away:

- headache
- nausea
- vomiting
- stomach pain
- diarrhea
- constipation
- body, joint, or muscle aches
- redness, swelling, bruising, itching, or a lump at the spot where you injected darbepoetin alfa

Some side effects can be serious. If you experience any of the following symptoms, or those listed in the IMPORTANT WARNING section, call your doctor immediately:

- rash over the whole body
- itching
- difficulty breathing or swallowing
- wheezing
- hoarseness
- swelling of the face, throat, tongue, lips, eyes, hands, feet, ankles, or lower legs
- dry mouth
- sunken eyes
- decreased urination
- fever, sore throat, chills, cough, and other signs of infection
- feeling cold most of the time
- pale skin

Darbepoetin alfa may cause other side effects. Call your doctor if you have any unusual problems or you do not feel well while taking this medication.

If you experience a serious side effect, you or your doctor may send a report to the Food and Drug Administration's (FDA) MedWatch Adverse Event Reporting program online [at http://www.fda.gov/MedWatch/index.html] or by phone [1-800-332-1088].

What storage conditions are needed for this medicine?

Keep this medication in the carton it came in, tightly closed, and out of reach of children. Once a vial or prefilled syringe has been taken out of its carton, keep it covered to protect it from room light until the dose is given. Store darbepoetin alfa in the refrigerator, but do not freeze it. Throw away any medication that has been frozen or is outdated or no longer needed. Talk to your pharmacist about the proper disposal of your medication.

When traveling, pack darbepoetin alfa in its original carton in an insulated container with a coolant such as blue ice.

To avoid freezing, make sure the darbepoetin alfa vial or prefilled syringe does not touch the coolant. Once you arrive, place darbepoetin alfa in a refrigerator as soon as possible.

What should I do in case of overdose?

In case of overdose, call your local poison control center at 1-800-222-1222. If the victim has collapsed or is not breathing, call local emergency services at 911.

Symptoms of overdose may include:

- unusual tiredness, weakness, or lack of energy
- shortness of breath
- cough that won't go away, or coughing up blood
- wheezing
- dizziness or lightheadedness
- swelling around the mouth or eyes
- blue-grey coloring or darkening around mouth or nails
- fast or irregular heartbeat
- sweating
- seizure
- fainting or loss of consciousness
- chest pain, squeezing pressure, or tightness
- discomfort or pain in the arms, shoulder, neck, jaw, or back
- nausea
- vomiting
- sudden weakness or numbness of an arm or leg (especially on one side of the body) or face
- sudden confusion
- sudden trouble speaking or understanding speech
- sudden trouble seeing in one or both eyes
- sudden trouble walking, or loss of balance or coordination
- sudden severe headache
- pain, tenderness, redness, warmth, and/or swelling in the legs
- swelling of the hands, feet, or ankles
- increased blood pressure
- blood clot in hemodialysis access port

What other information should I know?

Before having any laboratory test, tell your doctor and the laboratory personnel that you are using darbepoetin alfa.

Do not let anyone else use your medication. Ask your pharmacist any questions you have about refilling your prescription.

Dosage Facts
For Informational Purposes

Caution: Do not change your dose, how often you take your medication, or the length of time you are to take it without first talking to your healthcare provider.

The following dosage information was written using medical language for doctors and other healthcare professionals and is provided here for you to check your dosage. The dosage of this drug may differ for different patients. Therefore, always follow your doctor's instructions or the directions on the label. Contact your healthcare provider or pharmacist if you have any questions about the specific dosage of your medication after reviewing this information.

Pediatric Patients

Anemia of Chronic Renal Failure

IV OR SUB-Q:

- In pediatric patients >1 year of age currently receiving epoetin alfa, the manufacturer recommends the following initial dosage of darbepoetin alfa based on the weekly epoetin alfa dosage at the time of substitution:

Previous Weekly Epoetin Alfa Dosage (units/week)	Initial Weekly Darbepoetin Alfa Dosage (mcg/week)
<1500	*
1500–2499	6.25
2500–4999	10
5000–10,999	20
11,000–17,999	40
18,000–33,999	60
34,000–89,999	100
≥90,000	200

*For pediatric patients receiving a weekly epoetin alfa dosage of <1500 units/week, data are insufficient to determine initial darbepoetin alfa dosage.

Dosage adjustments should not be made more frequently than once a month.

If hemoglobin has increased by <1 g/dL during initial 4 weeks of therapy and iron stores are adequate, increase dosage by approximately 25% of the previous dosage. Dosage may be increased at intervals of ≥4 weeks until the lowest hemoglobin concentration that will avoid the need for blood transfusion (not to exceed 12 g/dL) is attained.

If hemoglobin concentration is increasing and approaching 12 g/dL, decrease dosage by approximately 25% of the previous dosage. If the hemoglobin concentration continues to increase, temporarily withhold therapy until hemoglobin concentration begins to decrease, at which point reinitiate therapy at a dosage approximately 25% below the previous dosage. If the hemoglobin concentration increases by >1 g/dL in any 2-week period, decrease dosage by approximately 25%.

Patients who fail to respond or maintain a response to dosages >1.5 mcg/kg per week may be resistant to the drug; failure or lack of response to darbepoetin alfa should be evaluated to determine causative factors.

Predialysis patients may require lower maintenance dosages compared with dialysis patients.

Adult Patients

Anemia of Chronic Renal Failure

IV OR SUB-Q:

- Initially, 0.45 mcg/kg administered as a single IV or sub-Q injection once weekly.
- In patients currently receiving epoetin alfa, the manufacturer recommends the following initial dosage of darbepoetin alfa based on the weekly epoetin alfa dosage at the time of substitution:

Previous Weekly Epoetin Alfa Dosage (units/week)	Initial Weekly Darbepoetin Alfa Dosage (mcg/week)
<1500	6.25
1500–2499	6.25
2500–4999	12.5
5000–10,999	25
11,000–17,999	40
18,000–33,999	60
34,000–89,999	100
≥90,000	200

Dosage adjustments should not be made more frequently than once a month.

If hemoglobin has increased by <1 g/dL during initial 4 weeks of therapy and iron stores are adequate, increase dosage by approximately 25% of the previous dosage. Dosage may be increased at intervals of ≥4 weeks until the lowest hemoglobin concentration that will avoid the need for blood transfusion (not to exceed 12 g/dL) is attained.

If hemoglobin concentration is increasing and approaching 12 g/dL, decrease dose by approximately 25% of the previous dosage. If the hemoglobin concentration continues to increase, temporarily withhold therapy until hemoglobin concentration begins to decrease, at which point reinitiate therapy at a dosage approximately 25% below the previous dosage. If the hemoglobin concentration increases by >1 g/dL in any 2-week period, decrease dosage by approximately 25% of the previous dosage.

Patients who fail to respond or maintain a response to dosages >1.5 mcg/kg per week may be resistant to the drug; failure or lack of response to darbepoetin alfa should be evaluated to determine causative factors.

Predialysis patients may require lower maintenance dosages compared with dialysis patients.

Anemia in Cancer Patients

SUB-Q:
- 2.25 mcg/kg once weekly.
- Alternatively, 500 mcg once every 3 weeks.
- Weekly dosage regimen: If hemoglobin concentration increases by <1 g/dL during the initial 6 weeks of therapy, increase dosage up to 4.5 mcg/kg weekly.
- Weekly or every 3 weeks dosage regimen: If hemoglobin concentration increases by >1 g/dL in any 2-week period or exceeds 11 g/dL, decrease dosage by approximately 40% of the previous dosage.
- Weekly or every 3 weeks dosage regimen: If hemoglobin concentration is >12 g/dL, withhold therapy until hemoglobin concentration decreases to 11 g/dL, at which point reinstitute at a dosage 40% below the previous dosage.

Darifenacin

(dar ee fen′ a sin)

Brand Name: Enablex®

Why is this medicine prescribed?

Darifenacin is used to treat an overactive bladder (a condition in which the bladder muscles contract uncontrollably and cause frequent urination, urgent need to urinate, and inability to control urination). Darifenacin is in a class of medications called antimuscarinics. It works by relaxing the bladder muscles to prevent urgent, frequent, or uncontrolled urination.

How should this medicine be used?

Darifenacin comes as an extended-release (long-acting) tablet to take by mouth. It is usually taken once a day with plenty of liquid. This medication may be taken with or without food. Take darifenacin at around the same time every day. Follow the directions on your prescription label carefully, and ask your doctor or pharmacist to explain any part you do not understand. Take darifenacin exactly as directed. Do not take more or less of it or take it more often than prescribed by your doctor.

Swallow the tablets whole; do not split, chew, or crush them.

Your doctor will start you on a low dose of darifenacin and may increase your dose after 2 weeks.

Ask your pharmacist or doctor for a copy of the manufacturer's information for the patient.

Are there other uses for this medicine?

This medication may be prescribed for other uses; ask your doctor or pharmacist for more information.

What special precautions should I follow?

Before taking darifenacin,
- tell your doctor and pharmacist if you are allergic to darifenacin or any other medications.
- tell your doctor and pharmacist what prescription and nonprescription medications, vitamins, nutritional supplements, and herbal products you are taking or plan to take. Be sure to mention any of the following: antidepressants such as amitriptyline (Elavil), amoxapine (Asendin), clomipramine (Anafranil), desipramine (Norpramin), doxepin (Adapin, Sinequan), imipramine (Tofranil), nortriptyline (Aventyl, Pamelor), protriptyline (Vivactil), and trimipramine (Surmontil); antihistamines; clarithromycin (Biaxin); flecainide (Tambocor); ipratropium (Atrovent); itraconazole (Sporanox); ketoconazole (Nizoral); medications for irritable bowel disease, motion sickness, Parkinson's disease, ulcers, or urinary problems; nefazodone (Serzone); nelfinavir (Viracept); ritonavir (Norvir); and thioridazine (Mel-

laril). Your doctor may need to change the doses of your medications or monitor you carefully for side effects.

- tell your doctor if you have or have ever had urinary obstruction (a blockage of urine flowing out of the bladder), any type of blockage in the digestive system, benign prostatic hypertrophy (enlargement of the prostate), severe constipation, ulcerative colitis (sores in the intestine that cause stomach pain and diarrhea), myasthenia gravis (a disorder of the nervous system that causes muscle weakness), glaucoma, or liver disease.
- tell your doctor if you are pregnant, plan to become pregnant, or are breast-feeding. If you become pregnant while taking darifenacin, call your doctor.
- if you are having surgery, including dental surgery, tell the doctor or dentist that you are taking darifenacin.
- you should know that darifenacin may cause blurred vision or make you dizzy. Do not drive a car or operate machinery until you know how this medication affects you.
- you should know that darifenacin causes decreased sweating, which may cause heat prostration (collapse because of high body temperature) in hot weather.

What special dietary instructions should I follow?

Unless your doctor tells you otherwise, continue your normal diet.

What should I do if I forget to take a dose?

Skip the missed dose and continue your regular dosing schedule. Do not take two doses in the same day or a double dose to make up for a missed one.

What side effects can this medicine cause?

Darifenacin may cause side effects. Tell your doctor if any of these symptoms are severe or do not go away:

- dry mouth
- constipation
- upset stomach
- stomach pain
- diarrhea
- weakness
- dry eyes

Some side effects can be serious. If you experience any of these symptoms, call your doctor immediately:

- difficulty urinating or being unable to urinate
- burning pain during urination
- rash
- itching

Darifenacin may cause other side effects. Call your doctor if you have any unusual problems while taking this medication.

If you experience a serious side effect, you or your doctor may send a report to the Food and Drug Administration's (FDA) MedWatch Adverse Event Reporting program online

[at http://www.fda.gov/MedWatch/index.html] or by phone [1-800-332-1088].

What storage conditions are needed for this medicine?

Keep this medication in the container it came in, tightly closed, and out of reach of children. Store it at room temperature and away from excess heat and moisture (not in the bathroom). Throw away any medication that is outdated or no longer needed. Talk to your pharmacist about the proper disposal of your medication.

What should I do in case of overdose?

In case of overdose, call your local poison control center at 1-800-222-1222. If the victim has collapsed or is not breathing, call local emergency services at 911.

Symptoms of overdose may include:

- vision problems

What other information should I know?

Keep all appointments with your doctor.

Do not let anyone else take your medication. Ask your pharmacist any questions you have about refilling your prescription.

Dosage Facts
For Informational Purposes

Caution: Do not change your dose, how often you take your medication, or the length of time you are to take it without first talking to your healthcare provider.

The following dosage information was written using medical language for doctors and other healthcare professionals and is provided here for you to check your dosage. The dosage of this drug may differ for different patients. Therefore, always follow your doctor's instructions or the directions on the label. Contact your healthcare provider or pharmacist if you have any questions about the specific dosage of your medication after reviewing this information.

General Dosage Information

Available as darifenacin hydrobromide; dosage expressed in terms of darifenacin.

Adult Patients

Overactive Bladder

ORAL:
- Initially, 7.5 mg once daily. May increase after 2 weeks to 15 mg once daily according to response.

Prescribing Limits

Adult Patients

Overactive Bladder

ORAL:
- Maximum 15 mg daily.

Special Populations

Hepatic Impairment

- No dosage adjustment required in patients with mild hepatic impairment (Child-Pugh class A).
- Maximum 7.5 mg daily in patients with moderate hepatic impairment (Child-Pugh class B).
- Use *not* recommended in patients with severe hepatic impairment (Child-Pugh class C).

Renal Impairment

- No dosage adjustment required.

Geriatric Patients

- No dosage adjustment required.

Darunavir

(da roon′ a veer)

Brand Name: Prezista®

Why is this medicine prescribed?

Darunavir is used with ritonavir (Norvir) and other medications to treat human immunodeficiency virus (HIV) in people who have already been treated for HIV. Darunavir is in a class of medications called protease inhibitors. It works by slowing the spread of HIV in the body. Darunavir does not cure HIV infection and may not prevent you from developing HIV-related illnesses. Darunavir does not prevent you from spreading HIV to other people.

How should this medicine be used?

Darunavir comes as a tablet to take by mouth. It is usually taken with food and with ritonavir twice a day. Take darunavir at around the same times every day. Follow the directions on your prescription label carefully, and ask your doctor or pharmacist to explain any part you do not understand. Take darunavir exactly as directed. Do not take more or less of it or take it more often than prescribed by your doctor.

Do not take darunavir without ritonavir.

Swallow the tablets whole with a drink such as water or milk. Do not chew the tablets.

Darunavir controls HIV but does not cure it. Continue to take darunavir even if you feel well. Do not stop taking darunavir without talking to your doctor. If you stop taking darunavir or skip doses, your condition may become more difficult to treat. When your supply of darunavir starts to run low, get more from your doctor or pharmacist.

Ask your pharmacist or doctor for a copy of the manufacturer's information for the patient.

Are there other uses for this medicine?

This medication may be prescribed for other uses; ask your doctor or pharmacist for more information.

What special precautions should I follow?

Before taking darunavir,

- tell your doctor and pharmacist if you are allergic to darunavir, ritonavir, sulfa medications, or any other medications. Ask your pharmacist if you are unsure if a medication you are allergic to is a sulfa medication.
- tell your doctor if you are taking any of the following medications: astemizole (Hismanal) (not available in the U.S.); cisapride (Propulsid); ergot-type medications such as dihydroergotamine (D.H.E. 45, Migranal), ergonovine (Ergotrate), ergotamine (Bellergal-S, Cafergot, Ergomar, Wigraine), and methylergonovine (Methergine); midazolam (Versed); pimozide (Orap); terfenadine (Seldane) (not available in the U.S.); or triazolam (Halcion). Your doctor will probably tell you not to take darunavir
- tell your doctor and pharmacist what other prescription and nonprescription medications, vitamins, and nutritional supplements you are taking or plan to take. Be sure to mention any of the following: anticoagulants ('blood thinners') such as warfarin (Coumadin); antifungals such as itraconazole (Sporanox), ketoconazole (Nizoral), and voriconazole (Vfend); calcium-channel blockers such as felodipine (in Lexxel, Plendil), nicardipine (Cardene), and nifedipine (Adalat, Procardia); cholesterol-lowering medications (statins) such as atorvastatin (in Caduet, Lipitor), lovastatin (Mevacor), pravastatin (Pravachol), and simvastatin (Zocor); dexamethasone (Decadron, Dexone); fluticasone (in Advair, Flonase, Flovent); certain phosphodiesterase inhibitors (PDE-5 inhibitors) such as sildenafil (Revatio, Viagra), tadalafil (Cialis), and vardenafil (Levitra); other medications for HIV including efavirenz (Sustiva), indinavir (Crixivan), lopinavir/ritonavir (Kaletra), and saquinavir (Invirase); medications for irregular heartbeat including amiodarone (Cordarone, Pacerone), bepridil (Vascor) (no longer available in the U.S.), and quinidine; certain medications for seizures such as carbamazepine (Equetro, Carbatrol, Tegretol), phenobarbital, and phenytoin (Dilantin, Phenytek); certain medications that suppress the immune system such as cyclosporine (Neoral, Sandimmune), sirolimus (Rapamune), and tacrolimus (Prograf); methadone (Dolophine, Methadose); rifabutin (Mycobutin); rifampin (Rimactane, Rifadin); certain selective serotonin reuptake inhibitors (SSRIs) such as paroxetine (Paxil) and sertraline (Zoloft); and trazodone. Many other medications may also interact with darunavir, so be sure to tell your doctor about all the medications you are taking, even those that do not appear on this list. Your doctor may need to change the doses of your medications or monitor you carefully for side effects.
- if you are taking didanosine (Videx), take it 1 hour before or 2 hours after you take darunavir.
- tell your doctor what herbal products you are taking, especially St. John's wort.

- tell your doctor if you have or have ever had diabetes or high blood sugar; hemophilia (bleeding disorder in which the blood does not clot properly); hepatitis (swelling of the liver caused by a virus) or any other liver disease; or an infection that does not go away or that comes and goes such as cytomegalovirus (CMV; a viral infection that may cause symptoms in patients with weak immune systems), mycobacterium avium complex disease (MAC; a bacterial infection that may cause serious symptoms in people with AIDS), pneumonia, or tuberculosis (TB; a type of lung infection).
- tell your doctor if you are pregnant, plan to become pregnant, or are breast-feeding. If you become pregnant while taking darunavir, call your doctor. Do not breast-feed if you are infected with HIV or are taking darunavir.
- you should know that darunavir may decrease the effectiveness of hormonal contraceptives (birth control pills, patches, rings, injections, or implants). Talk to your doctor about other ways to prevent pregnancy while you are taking this medication.
- you should know that your body fat may increase or move to different areas of your body such as your breasts, upper back, neck, chest, and stomach area. Loss of fat from the legs, arms, and face can also happen.

What special dietary instructions should I follow?

Talk to your doctor about eating grapefruit and drinking grapefruit juice while taking this medicine.

What should I do if I forget to take a dose?

If you miss a dose by less than 6 hours, take the missed dose as soon as you remember it and then take the next dose at the scheduled time. However, if you miss a dose by more than 6 hours, skip the missed dose and continue your regular dosing schedule. Do not take a double dose to make up for a missed one.

What side effects can this medicine cause?

Darunavir may cause hyperglycemia (high blood sugar). Call your doctor if you have any of the following symptoms of hyperglycemia:

- extreme thirst
- frequent urination
- extreme hunger
- weakness
- blurred vision

If high blood sugar is not treated, a serious, life-threatening condition called diabetic ketoacidosis could develop. Call your doctor immediately if you have any of these symptoms:

- dry mouth
- nausea and vomiting
- shortness of breath

- breath that smells fruity
- decreased consciousness

Darunavir may cause side effects. Tell your doctor if any of these symptoms are severe or do not go away:

- headache
- diarrhea
- nausea
- stomach pain
- constipation

Some side effects can be serious. If you experience any of these symptoms, call your doctor immediately:

- rash
- blisters
- fever
- swelling, tenderness, redness, or other signs of infection

Darunavir may cause other side effects. Call your doctor if you have any unusual problems while taking this medication.

What storage conditions are needed for this medicine?

Keep this medication in the container it came in, tightly closed, and out of reach of children. Store it at room temperature and away from excess heat and moisture (not in the bathroom). Throw away any medication that is outdated or no longer needed. Talk to your pharmacist about the proper disposal of your medication.

What should I do in case of overdose?

In case of overdose, call your local poison control center at 1-800-222-1222. If the victim has collapsed or is not breathing, call local emergency services at 911.

What other information should I know?

Keep all appointments with your doctor.

Do not let anyone else take your medication. Ask your pharmacist any questions you have about refilling your prescription.

Talk to your doctor, pharmacist, or other healthcare professional if you have questions about dosing information for your medication.

Deferasirox

(de fer′ a sir ox)

Brand Name: Exjade®

Why is this medicine prescribed?

Deferasirox is used to remove excess iron that is in the body because of blood transfusions. Deferasirox is in a class of medications called iron chelators. It works by attaching to iron molecules in the body so they can be excreted (removed from the body) in feces.

How should this medicine be used?

Deferasirox comes as a tablet for suspension (a tablet to dissolve in liquid) to take by mouth. It should be taken on an empty stomach once a day, at least 30 minutes before food. Take deferasirox at around the same time every day. Follow the directions on your prescription label carefully, and ask your doctor or pharmacist to explain any part you do not understand. Take deferasirox exactly as directed. Do not take more or less of it or take it more often than prescribed by your doctor.

Do not chew or swallow the tablets whole.

To take the tablets for suspension, follow these steps:

1. Place the number of tablets your doctor has told you to take in a cup.
2. If you are taking less than 1000 mg of deferasirox, fill the cup halfway (about 3.5 oz) with water, apple juice, or orange juice. If you are taking more than 1000 mg of deferasirox, fill the cup (about 7 oz) with water, apple juice, or orange juice. If you are not sure how much deferasirox you are to take, ask your doctor or pharmacist.
3. Stir the liquid until the tablet(s) is/are totally dissolved.
4. Drink the liquid immediately.
5. Add a small amount of liquid to the empty cup and stir.
6. Drink the rest of the liquid.

Are there other uses for this medicine?

This medication may be prescribed for other uses; ask your doctor or pharmacist for more information.

What special precautions should I follow?

Before taking deferasirox,

- tell your doctor and pharmacist if you are allergic to deferasirox or any other medications.
- tell your doctor and pharmacist what prescription and nonprescription medications, vitamins, nutritional supplements, you are taking or plan to take. Your doctor may need to change the doses of your medications or monitor you carefully for side effects.
- if you are taking aluminum-containing antacids such as Amphogel, Alternagel, Gaviscon, Maalox, or Mylanta, take them 2 hours before or after deferasirox.
- tell your doctor if you have or have ever had trouble hearing, ear problems, vision problems, or kidney or liver disease.
- tell your doctor if you are pregnant, plan to become pregnant, or are breast-feeding. If you become pregnant while taking deferasirox, call your doctor.
- you should know that deferasirox may make you dizzy. Do not drive a car or operate machinery until you know how this medication affects you.

What special dietary instructions should I follow?

Unless your doctor tells you otherwise, continue your normal diet.

What should I do if I forget to take a dose?

Take the missed dose later in the day, at least 2 hours after your last meal and 30 minutes before food. However, if it is almost time for the next dose or if you will not be able to take deferasirox on an empty stomach, skip the missed dose and continue your regular dosing schedule. Do not take a double dose to make up for a missed one.

What side effects can this medicine cause?

Deferasirox may cause side effects. Tell your doctor if any of these symptoms are severe or do not go away:

- headache
- stomach pain
- nausea
- vomiting
- diarrhea
- joint pain
- tiredness

Some side effects can be serious. If you experience any of these symptoms, call your doctor immediately:

- hearing loss
- vision problems
- decrease in urination
- fever
- unusual bleeding or bruising
- lack of energy
- loss of appetite
- pain in the upper right part of the stomach
- yellowing of the skin or eyes
- flu-like symptoms
- hives
- rash
- itching
- difficulty breathing or swallowing
- swelling of the face, throat, tongue, lips, eyes, hands, feet, ankles, or lower legs
- hoarseness

Deferasirox may cause other side effects. Call your doctor if you have any unusual problems while taking this medication.

If you experience a serious side effect, you or your doctor may send a report to the Food and Drug Administration's (FDA) MedWatch Adverse Event Reporting program online [at http://www.fda.gov/MedWatch/index.html] or by phone [1-800-332-1088].

What storage conditions are needed for this medicine?

Keep this medication in the container it came in, tightly closed, and out of reach of children. Store it at room temperature and away from excess heat and moisture (not in the bathroom). Throw away any medication that is outdated or no longer needed. Talk to your pharmacist about the proper disposal of your medication.

What should I do in case of overdose?

In case of overdose, call your local poison control center at 1-800-222-1222. If the victim has collapsed or is not breathing, call local emergency services at 911.

What other information should I know?

Keep all appointments with your doctor and the laboratory. Your doctor will order certain lab tests to check your body's response to deferasirox. Your doctor may adjust your dose of deferasirox every 3 to 6 months. You will need to have hearing and eye exams before starting deferasirox and once a year while taking this medication.

Do not let anyone else take your medication. Ask your pharmacist any questions you have about refilling your prescription.

Talk to your doctor, pharmacist, or other healthcare professional if you have questions about dosing information for your medication.

Delavirdine

(de la vir′ deen)

Brand Name: Rescriptor®

Important Warning

The benefit from using delavirdine may be limited. If disease progression occurs, a different therapy should be used. Delavirdine should always be used with another antiviral medication to avoid resistance to the HIV virus. If you experience the following symptom, call your doctor immediately: a severe skin rash. Keep all appointments with your doctor and the laboratory. Your doctor will order certain lab tests to check your response to delavirdine.

Why is this medicine prescribed?

Delavirdine is used to treat human immunodeficiency virus (HIV) infection in patients with or without acquired immunodeficiency syndrome (AIDS). Delavirdine is not a cure and may not decrease the number of HIV-related illnesses. Delavirdine does not prevent the spread of HIV to other people.

This medication is sometimes prescribed for other uses; ask your doctor or pharmacist for more information.

How should this medicine be used?

Delavirdine comes as a tablet to take by mouth. It usually is taken three times a day. Follow the directions on your prescription label carefully, and ask your doctor or pharmacist to explain any part you do not understand. Take delavirdine exactly as directed. Do not take more or less of it or take it more often than prescribed by your doctor.

If you have trouble swallowing the tablets, they may be dispersed in water. To prepare, add four tablets to at least 3 ounces of water, allow to stand for a few minutes, and then stir until a uniform dispersion occurs. Drink the delavirdine-water mixture right away. Rinse the glass and swallow the rinse to ensure that you have gotten the entire dose.

If you are taking antacids, wait at least 1 hour between taking the antacid and taking delavirdine.

What special precautions should I follow?

Before taking delavirdine,

- tell your doctor and pharmacist if you are allergic to delavirdine or any other drugs.
- tell your doctor and pharmacist what prescription and nonprescription medications you are taking, especially amprenavir (Agenerase); antacids; anticonvulsants such as carbamazepine (Tegretol), phenobarbital, phenytoin (Dilantin), andvalproic acid (Depakene); anticoagulants ('blood thinners') such as warfarin (Coumadin); antihistamines such as astemizole (Hismanal) and terfenadine (Seldane); benzodiazepines such as alprazolam (Xanax), midazolam (Versed), and triazolam (Halcion); calcium channel blockers such as amlodipine (Norvasc), felodipine (Plendil), isradipine (DynaCirc), nicardipine (Cardene), nifedipine (Adalat, Procardia), nimodipine (Nimotop), and nisoldipine (Sular); cisapride (Propulsid); clarithromycin (Biaxin); dapsone; ergot derivatives such as dihydroergotamine mesylate (DHE 45), ergotamine tartrate (Ergostat, Medihaler Ergotamine); fluoxetine (Prozac); medications for stomach acid such as cimetidine (Tagamet), famotidine (Pepcid), nizatidine (Axid), ranitidine (Zantac); quinidine (Quinaglute); rifabutin (Mycobutin); rifampin (Rifadin); sildenafil (Viagra); and vitamins.
- tell your doctor if you have or have ever had liver disease.
- tell your doctor if you are pregnant, plan to become pregnant, or are breast-feeding. If you become pregnant while taking delavirdine, call your doctor.
- if you are having surgery, including dental surgery, tell the doctor or dentist that you are taking delavirdine.

What special dietary instructions should I follow?

If your doctor has told you that you do have not enough stomach acid, you should take delavirdine with orange or cranberry juice. Delavirdine may be taken with or without food, although it may be best to take it the same way each day.

What should I do if I forget to take a dose?

Take the missed dose as soon as you remember it. However, if it is almost time for the next dose, skip the missed dose

and continue your regular dosing schedule. Do not take a double dose to make up for a missed one.

What side effects can this medicine cause?

Side effects from delavirdine are common. Tell your doctor if any of these symptoms are severe or do not go away:

- excessive tiredness
- headache
- upset stomach
- diarrhea
- vomiting
- hallucinations
- nightmares
- decreased libido (sex drive)
- rash

If you experience any of the following symptoms, or those listed in the IMPORTANT WARNING section, call your doctor immediately:

- chest pain
- irregular heartbeat
- hives
- itching
- difficulty breathing or swallowing
- wheezing
- fainting
- severe skin rash accompanied by fever, blistering, oral lesions, red eyes, swelling, or muscle or joint pain

If you experience a serious side effect, you or your doctor may send a report to the Food and Drug Administration's (FDA) MedWatch Adverse Event Reporting program online [at http://www.fda.gov/MedWatch/index.html] or by phone [1-800-332-1088].

What storage conditions are needed for this medicine?

Keep this medication in the container it came in, tightly closed, and out of reach of children. Store it at room temperature and away from excess heat and moisture (not in the bathroom). Throw away any medication that is outdated or no longer needed. Talk to your pharmacist about the proper disposal of your medication.

What should I do in case of overdose?

In case of overdose, call your local poison control center at 1-800-222-1222. If the victim has collapsed or is not breathing, call local emergency services at 911.

What other information should I know?

Keep all appointments with your doctor and the laboratory. Your doctor will order certain lab tests to check your response to delavirdine.

Do not let anyone else take your medication. Ask your pharmacist any questions you have about refilling your prescription.

Dosage Facts
For Informational Purposes

Caution: Do not change your dose, how often you take your medication, or the length of time you are to take it without first talking to your healthcare provider.

The following dosage information was written using medical language for doctors and other healthcare professionals and is provided here for you to check your dosage. The dosage of this drug may differ for different patients. Therefore, always follow your doctor's instructions or the directions on the label. Contact your healthcare provider or pharmacist if you have any questions about the specific dosage of your medication after reviewing this information.

General Dosage Information

Available as delavirdine mesylate; dosage expressed in terms of delavirdine mesylate.

Must be given in conjunction with other antiretrovirals. *If used with certain didanosine preparations, administer drugs at least 1 hour apart; if used with indinavir, adjustment in the treatment regimen necessary.*

Pediatric Patients
Treatment of HIV Infection

ORAL:
- Adolescents ≥16 years of age: 400 mg 3 times daily.

Adult Patients
Treatment of HIV Infection

ORAL:
- 400 mg 3 times daily.

Special Populations

Renal Impairment
- Dosage adjustments not necessary.

Geriatric Patients
- Select dosage with caution because of age-related decreases in hepatic, renal, and/or cardiac function and concomitant disease and drug therapy.

Demeclocycline

(dem e kloe sye' kleen)

Brand Name: Declomycin®
Also available generically.

Why is this medicine prescribed?

Demeclocycline is used to treat bacterial infections including pneumonia and other respiratory tract infections; acne; and infections of skin, genital, and urinary systems. Demeclocycline is in a class of medications called tetracycline antibiotics. It works by preventing the growth and spread of bacteria. Antibiotics will not work for colds, flu, or other viral infections.

How should this medicine be used?

Demeclocycline comes as a tablet to take by mouth. It usually is taken two to four times a day. Drink a full glass of water with each dose. Take demeclocycline on an empty stomach at least 1 hour before or 2 hours after meals. Do not take demeclocycline with food, especially dairy products such as milk, yogurt, cheese, and ice cream. Follow the directions on your prescription label carefully, and ask your doctor or pharmacist to explain any part you do not understand. Take demeclocycline exactly as directed. Do not take more or less of it or take it more often than prescribed by your doctor.

Are there other uses for this medicine?

This medication is sometimes prescribed for other uses; ask your doctor or pharmacist for more information.

What special precautions should I follow?

Before taking demeclocycline,
- tell your doctor and pharmacist if you are allergic to demeclocycline, tetracycline, minocycline, doxycycline, or any other medications.
- tell your doctor and pharmacist what prescription and nonprescription medications, vitamins, nutritional supplements, and herbal products you are taking or plan to take, especially antacids, anticoagulants ('blood thinners') such as warfarin (Coumadin), and penicillin. Demeclocycline decreases the effectiveness of some oral contraceptives; another form of birth control should be used while taking this drug.
- be aware that antacids, calcium supplements, iron products, and laxatives containing magnesium interfere with demeclocycline, making it less effective. Take demeclocycline 1 hour before or 2 hours after antacids (including sodium bicarbonate), calcium supplements, and laxatives containing magnesium. Take demeclocycline 2 hours before or 3 hours after iron preparations and vitamin products that contain iron.
- tell your doctor if you have or have ever had diabetes or kidney or liver disease.
- tell your doctor if you are pregnant, plan to become pregnant, or are breast-feeding. If you become pregnant while taking demeclocycline, call your doctor immediately. Demeclocycline can harm the fetus.
- if you are having surgery, including dental surgery, tell the doctor or dentist that you are taking demeclocycline.
- plan to avoid unnecessary or prolonged exposure to sunlight and to wear protective clothing, sunglasses, and sunscreen. Demeclocycline may make your skin sensitive to sunlight.

- you should know that when demeclocycline is used during pregnancy or in babies or children up to age 8, it can cause the teeth to become permanently stained. Demeclocycline should not be used in children under age 8 unless your doctor decides it is needed.

What special dietary instructions should I follow?

Unless your doctor tells you otherwise, continue your normal diet.

What should I do if I forget to take a dose?

Take the missed dose as soon as you remember it. However, if it is almost time for the next dose, skip the missed dose and continue your regular dosing schedule. Do not take a double dose to make up for a missed one.

What side effects can this medicine cause?

Demeclocycline may cause side effects. You may experience a darkened or discolored tongue. This effect will go away when you stop taking the medicine. Tell your doctor if any of these symptoms are severe or do not go away:
- diarrhea
- itching of the rectum or vagina
- sore mouth
- changes in skin color

Some side effects can be serious. If you experience any of these symptoms, call your doctor immediately:
- severe headache
- blurred vision
- skin rash
- redness of the skin (sunburn)
- hives
- difficulty breathing or swallowing
- yellowing of the skin or eyes
- itching
- dark-colored urine
- light-colored bowel movements
- loss of appetite
- upset stomach
- vomiting
- stomach pain
- extreme tiredness or weakness
- confusion
- decreased urination

If you experience a serious side effect, you or your doctor may send a report to the Food and Drug Administration's (FDA) MedWatch Adverse Event Reporting program online [at http://www.fda.gov/MedWatch/index.html] or by phone [1-800-332-1088].

What storage conditions are needed for this medicine?

Keep this medication in the container it came in, tightly closed, and out of reach of children. Store it at room tem-

perature and away from excess heat and moisture (not in the bathroom). Throw away any medication that is outdated or no longer needed. Talk to your pharmacist about the proper disposal of your medication.

What should I do in case of overdose?

In case of overdose, call your local poison control center at 1-800-222-1222. If the victim has collapsed or is not breathing, call local emergency services at 911.

What other information should I know?

Keep all appointments with your doctor and the laboratory. Your doctor will order certain lab tests to check your response to demeclocycline.

Before having any laboratory test, tell your doctor and the laboratory personnel that you are taking demeclocycline.

If you have diabetes, demeclocycline can cause false results in some tests for sugar in the urine. Check with your doctor before changing your diet or the dosage of your diabetes medicine.

Do not let anyone else take your medication. Your prescription is probably not refillable. If you still have symptoms of infection after you finish the demeclocycline, call your doctor.

Dosage Facts

For Informational Purposes

Caution: Do not change your dose, how often you take your medication, or the length of time you are to take it without first talking to your healthcare provider.

The following dosage information was written using medical language for doctors and other healthcare professionals and is provided here for you to check your dosage. The dosage of this drug may differ for different patients. Therefore, always follow your doctor's instructions or the directions on the label. Contact your healthcare provider or pharmacist if you have any questions about the specific dosage of your medication after reviewing this information.

Pediatric Patients

General Pediatric Dosage

ORAL:
• Children >8 years of age: 7–13 mg/kg daily given in 2–4 divided doses.

Adult Patients

General Adult Dosage

ORAL:
• 150 mg 4 times daily or 300 mg 2 times daily.

Gonorrhea and Associated Infections

ORAL:
• 600 mg initially followed by 300 mg every 12 hours for 4 days for a total of 3 g.

• No longer recommended for gonorrhea by CDC or other experts.

Syndrome of Inappropriate Antidiuretic Hormone Secretion†

ORAL:
• 600 mg to 1.2 g daily in 3 or 4 divided doses. Diuresis usually occurs within 5 days after initiation of therapy and reverses within 2–6 days after drug discontinued.

Prescribing Limits

Pediatric Patients

Maximum 600 mg daily.

Special Populations

Hepatic Impairment
• Adjust dosage by decreasing doses or increasing dosing interval.
• Use with caution.

Renal Impairment
• Adjust dosage by decreasing doses or increasing dosing interval.
• Use with caution.

† Use is not currently included in the labeling approved by the US Food and Drug Administration.

Desipramine

(des ip′ ra meen)

Brand Name: Norpramin®
Also available generically.

Important Warning

A small number of children, teenagers, and young adults (up to 24 years of age) who took antidepressants ('mood elevators') such as desipramine during clinical studies became suicidal (thinking about harming or killing oneself or planning or trying to do so). Children, teenagers, and young adults who take antidepressants to treat depression or other mental illnesses may be more likely to become suicidal than children, teenagers, and young adults who do not take antidepressants to treat these conditions. However, experts are not sure about how great this risk is and how much it should be considered in deciding whether a child or teenager should take an antidepressant. Children younger than 18 years of age should not normally take desipramine, but in some cases, a doctor may decide that desipramine is the best medication to treat a child's condition.

You should know that your mental health may

change in unexpected ways when you take desipramine or other antidepressants even if you are an adult over age 24. You may become suicidal, especially at the beginning of your treatment and any time that your dose is increased or decreased. You, your family, or your caregiver should call your doctor right away if you experience any of the following symptoms: new or worsening depression; thinking about harming or killing yourself, or planning or trying to do so; extreme worry; agitation; panic attacks; difficulty falling asleep or staying asleep; aggressive behavior; irritability; acting without thinking; severe restlessness; and frenzied abnormal excitement. Be sure that your family or caregiver knows which symptoms may be serious so they can call the doctor when you are unable to seek treatment on your own.

Your healthcare provider will want to see you often while you are taking desipramine, especially at the beginning of your treatment. Be sure to keep all appointments for office visits with your doctor.

The doctor or pharmacist will give you the manufacturer's patient information sheet (Medication Guide) when you begin treatment with desipramine. Read the information carefully and ask your doctor or pharmacist if you have any questions. You also can obtain the Medication Guide from the FDA website: http://www.fda.gov/cder/drug/antidepressants/antidepressants_MG_2007.pdf.

No matter your age, before you take an antidepressant, you, your parent, or your caregiver should talk to your doctor about the risks and benefits of treating your condition with an antidepressant or with other treatments. You should also talk about the risks and benefits of not treating your condition. You should know that having depression or another mental illness greatly increases the risk that you will become suicidal. This risk is higher if you or anyone in your family has or has ever had bipolar disorder (mood that changes from depressed to abnormally excited) or mania (frenzied, abnormally excited mood) or has thought about or attempted suicide. Talk to your doctor about your condition, symptoms, and personal and family medical history. You and your doctor will decide what type of treatment is right for you.

Why is this medicine prescribed?

Desipramine is used to treat depression. Desipramine is in a class of medications called tricyclic antidepressants. It works by increasing the amounts of certain natural substances in the brain that are needed for mental balance.

How should this medicine be used?

Desipramine comes as a tablet to take by mouth. It is usually taken one or more times a day and may be taken with or without food. Take desipramine at around the same time(s) every day. Follow the directions on your prescription label carefully, and ask your doctor or pharmacist to explain any part you do not understand. Take desipramine exactly as directed. Do not take more or less of it or take it more often than prescribed by your doctor.

Your doctor may start you on a low dose of desipramine and gradually increase your dose.

It may take 2-3 weeks for you to feel the full benefit of desipramine. Continue to take desipramine even if you feel well. Do not stop taking desipramine without talking to your doctor. If you suddenly stop taking desipramine, you may experience withdrawal symptoms such as nausea,, headache, and weakness. Your doctor will probably want to decrease your dose gradually.

Are there other uses for this medicine?

This medication is sometimes prescribed for other uses; ask your doctor or pharmacist for more information.

What special precautions should I follow?

Before taking desipramine,

- tell your doctor and pharmacist if you are allergic to desipramine, clomipramine (Anafranil), imipramine (Tofranil), trimipramine (Surmontil), any other medications, or any of the ingredients in desipramine tablets. Ask your doctor or pharmacist for a list of the ingredients.
- tell your doctor if you are taking a monoamine oxidase (MAO) inhibitor such as isocarboxazid (Marplan), phenelzine (Nardil), selegiline (Eldepryl, Emsam, Zelapar), and tranylcypromine (Parnate), or if you have stopped taking an MAO inhibitor within the past 14 days. Your doctor will probably tell you not to take desipramine. If you stop taking desipramine, you should wait at least 14 days before you start to take an MAO inhibitor.
- tell your doctor and pharmacist what prescription and nonprescription medications, vitamins, herbal products and nutritional supplements you are taking or plan to take. Be sure to mention any of the following: anticoagulants (blood thinners) such as warfarin (Coumadin); antihistamines; cimetidine (Tagamet); estrogens; flecainide (Tambocor); fluoxetine (Prozac); guanethedine (Ismelin); levodopa (Sinemet, Larodopa); lithium (Eskalith, Lithobid); medication for high blood pressure, seizures, Parkinson's disease, diabetes, mental illness, nausea, asthma, colds, or allergies; methylphenidate (Ritalin); muscle relaxants; oral contraceptives; phenobarbital; propafenone (Rhythmol); quinidine; sedatives; selective serotonin reuptake inhibitors (SSRIs) such as citalopram (Celexa), escitalopram (Lexapro), fluoxetine (Prozac, Sarafem), fluvoxamine (Luvox), paroxetine (Paxil), and sertraline (Zoloft); sleeping pills; thyroid medications; and tranquilizers. Your doctor may need to change the doses of your medications or monitor you carefully for side effects. Your doctor may tell you not to take desipramine if you have stopped taking fluoxetine during the past 5 weeks.

- tell your doctor if you have recently had a heart attack. Your doctor may tell you that you should not take desipramine.
- tell your doctor if you have or have ever had glaucoma, an enlarged prostate (a male reproductive gland), difficulty urinating, diabetes, seizures, an overactive thyroid gland, schizophrenia (a mental illness that causes disturbed or unusual thinking, loss of interest in life, and strong or inappropriate emotions), or liver, kidney, or heart disease.
- tell your doctor if you are pregnant, plan to become pregnant, or are breast-feeding. If you become pregnant while taking desipramine, call your doctor.
- if you are having surgery, including dental surgery, tell the doctor or dentist that you are taking desipramine.
- you should know that this medication may make you drowsy. Do not drive a car or operate machinery until you know how this medication affects you.
- ask your doctor about the safe use of alcohol while you are taking this medication.
- tell your doctor if you use tobacco products. Cigarette smoking may decrease the effectiveness of this medication.

What special dietary instructions should I follow?

Unless your doctor tells you otherwise, continue your normal diet.

What should I do if I forget to take a dose?

Take the missed dose as soon as you remember it. However, if it is almost time for the next dose, skip the missed dose and continue your regular dosing schedule. Do not take a double dose to make up for a missed one.

What side effects can this medicine cause?

Desipramine may cause side effects. Call your doctor if any of these symptoms become severe or do not go away:

- nausea
- drowsiness
- weakness or tiredness
- nightmares
- dry mouth
- skin more sensitive to sunlight than usual
- changes in appetite or weight
- constipation
- difficulty urinating
- frequent urination
- blurred vision
- changes in sex drive or ability
- excessive sweating

Some side effects can be serious. If you experience any of the following symptoms, or those listed in the IMPORTANT WARNING section, call your doctor immediately:

- jaw, neck, and back muscle spasms
- slow or difficult speech

- shuffling walk
- uncontrollable shaking or movement of a part of the body
- fever
- difficulty breathing or swallowing
- severe rash
- yellowing of the skin or eyes
- irregular heartbeat
- sore throat, fever, and other signs of infection

If you experience a serious side effect, you or your doctor may send a report to the Food and Drug Administration's (FDA) MedWatch Adverse Event Reporting program online [at http://www.fda.gov/MedWatch/index.html] or by phone [1-800-332-1088].

What storage conditions are needed for this medicine?

Keep this medication in the container it came in, tightly closed, and out of the reach of children. Store it at room temperature and away from excess heat and moisture (not in the bathroom). Throw away any medication that is outdated or no longer needed. Talk to your pharmacist about the proper disposal of your medication.

What should I do in case of overdose?

In case of overdose, call your local poison control center at 1-800-222-1222. If the victim has collapsed or is not breathing, call local emergency services at 911.

Symptoms of overdose may include

- irregular heartbeat
- seizures
- coma (loss of consciousness for a period of time)
- confusion
- hallucination (seeing things that do not exist)
- widened pupils (dark circles in the middle of the eyes)
- drowsiness
- agitation
- fever
- low body temperature
- stiff muscles
- vomiting

What other information should I know?

Keep all appointments with your doctor.

Do not allow anyone else to take your medication. Ask your pharmacist any questions you have about refilling your prescription.

Dosage Facts
For Informational Purposes

Caution: Do not change your dose, how often you take your medication, or the length of time you are to take it without first talking to your healthcare provider.

The following dosage information was written using medical language for doctors and other healthcare professionals and is provided here for you to check your dosage. The dosage of this drug may differ for different patients. Therefore, always follow your doctor's instructions or the directions on the label. Contact your healthcare provider or pharmacist if you have any questions about the specific dosage of your medication after reviewing this information.

General Dosage Information

Available as desipramine hydrochloride; dosage is expessed in terms of the salt.

Pediatric Patients

Major Depressive Disorder

ORAL:

- Adolescents ≥12 years of age: Initially, 25–50 mg daily. Increase dosage gradually until maximal therapeutic effect with minimal toxicity is achieved or up to a maximum dosage of 100 mg daily.
- Usual dosage: 25–100 mg daily. Dosage may be further increased to 150 mg daily, if necessary, in more seriously ill patients.
- After symptoms are controlled, gradually reduce dosage to the lowest level that will maintain relief of symptoms.

Adult Patients

Major Depressive Disorder

ORAL:

- Initially, 75–150 mg daily, depending on the severity of the condition being treated. Increase dosage gradually until maximal therapeutic effect with minimal toxicity is achieved.
- Usual dosage: 100–200 mg daily. Dosage may be further increased to 300 mg daily, if necessary, in more seriously ill patients.
- After symptoms are controlled, gradually reduce dosage to the lowest level that will maintain relief of symptoms.

Prescribing Limits

Pediatric Patients

Major Depressive Disorder

ORAL:

- Adolescents ≥12 years of age: Maximum 150 mg daily.

Adult Patients

Major Depressive Disorder

ORAL:

- Maximum 300 mg daily.

Special Populations

Geriatric Patients

- Initially, 25–50 mg daily. Increase dosage gradually until maximal therapeutic effect with minimal toxicity is achieved or up to a usual maximum dosage of 100 mg daily.
- Usual dosage: 25–100 mg daily. Dosage may be further increased to 150 mg daily, if necessary, in more seriously ill patients.

- After symptoms are controlled, gradually reduce dosage to the lowest level that will maintain relief of symptoms.

Desloratadine

(des lor at′ a deen)

Brand Name: Clarinex®, Clarinex® Reditabs®

Why is this medicine prescribed?

Desloratadine is used to relieve hay fever and allergy symptoms, including sneezing; runny nose; and red, itchy, tearing eyes. It is also used to treat hives. Desloratadine is in a class of medications called antihistamines. It works by blocking histamine, a substance in the body that causes allergic symptoms. Desloratadine may cause less drowsiness than other antihistamines.

How should this medicine be used?

Desloratadine comes as a tablet and an orally disintegrating tablet to take by mouth. It is usually taken once a day with or without food. Follow the directions on your prescription label carefully, and ask your doctor or pharmacist to explain any part you do not understand. Take desloratadine exactly as directed. Do not take more or less of it or take it more often than prescribed by your doctor.

To take the orally disintegrating tablet, use dry hands to peel back the foil packaging. Immediately take out the tablet and place it on your tongue. The tablet will quickly dissolve and can be swallowed with saliva. Orally disintegrating tablets may be taken with or without water.

Are there other uses for this medicine?

This medication may be prescribed for other uses; ask your doctor or pharmacist for more information.

What special precautions should I follow?

Before taking desloratadine,

- tell your doctor and pharmacist if you are allergic to desloratadine, loratadine (Claritin), or any other medications.
- tell your doctor and pharmacist what prescription and nonprescription medications, vitamins, nutritional supplements, and herbal products you are taking.
- tell your doctor if you have or have ever had kidney or liver disease or phenylketonuria (for orally disintegrating tablets).
- tell your doctor if you are pregnant, plan to become pregnant, or are breast-feeding. If you become pregnant while taking desloratadine, call your doctor.

What special dietary instructions should I follow?

Unless your doctor tells you otherwise, continue your normal diet.

What should I do if I forget to take a dose?

Take the missed dose as soon as you remember it. However, if it is almost time for the next dose, skip the missed dose and continue your regular dosing schedule. Do not take a double dose to make up for a missed one.

What side effects can this medicine cause?

Desloratadine may cause side effects. Tell your doctor if any of these symptoms are severe or do not go away:

- headache
- upset stomach
- dizziness
- sore throat
- dry mouth
- muscle pain
- extreme tiredness
- painful menstruation

Some side effects can be serious. The following symptom is uncommon, but if you experience it, call your doctor immediately:

- difficulty breathing

Desloratadine may cause other side effects. Call your doctor if you have any unusual problems while taking this medication.

If you experience a serious side effect, you or your doctor may send a report to the Food and Drug Administration's (FDA) MedWatch Adverse Event Reporting program online [at http://www.fda.gov/MedWatch/index.html] or by phone [1-800-332-1088].

What storage conditions are needed for this medicine?

Keep this medication in the container it came in, tightly closed, and out of reach of children. Store it at room temperature and away from excess heat and moisture (not in the bathroom). Throw away any medication that is outdated or no longer needed. Talk to your pharmacist about the proper disposal of your medication.

What should I do in case of overdose?

In case of overdose, call your local poison control center at 1-800-222-1222. If the victim has collapsed or is not breathing, call local emergency services at 911.

What other information should I know?

Keep all appointments with your doctor.

Do not let anyone else take your medication. Ask your pharmacist any questions you have about refilling your prescription.

Dosage Facts
For Informational Purposes

Caution: Do not change your dose, how often you take your medication, or the length of time you are to take it without first talking to your healthcare provider.

The following dosage information was written using medical language for doctors and other healthcare professionals and is provided here for you to check your dosage. The dosage of this drug may differ for different patients. Therefore, always follow your doctor's instructions or the directions on the label. Contact your healthcare provider or pharmacist if you have any questions about the specific dosage of your medication after reviewing this information.

General Dosage Information

Fixed-combination preparation contains 5 mg of desloratadine in an immediate-release outer shell and 240 mg of pseudoephedrine sulfate in an extended-release matrix core that slowly releases the drug.

Pediatric Patients

Allergic Rhinitis
Seasonal

ORAL:
- Children 2–5 years of age: 1.25 mg once daily (as oral solution).
- Children 6–11 years of age: 2.5 mg once daily (as oral solution or orally disintegrating tablets).
- Children ≥12 years of age: 5 mg once daily (as conventional tablets, oral solution, orally disintegrating tablets, or fixed-combination extended-release tablets with 240 mg pseudoephedrine sulfate).

Perennial

ORAL:
- Children 6–11 months of age: 1 mg once daily (as oral solution).
- Children 1–5 years of age: 1.25 mg once daily (as oral solution).
- Children 6–11 years of age: 2.5 mg once daily (as oral solution or orally disintegrating tablets).
- Children ≥12 years of age: 5 mg once daily (as conventional tablets, oral solution, or orally disintegrating tablets).

Chronic Idiopathic Urticaria

ORAL:
- Children 6–11 months of age: 1 mg once daily (as oral solution).
- Children 1–5 years of age: 1.25 mg once daily (as oral solution).
- Children 6–11 years of age: 2.5 mg once daily (as oral solution or orally disintegrating tablets).
- Children ≥12 years of age: 5 mg once daily (as conventional tablets, oral solution, or orally disintegrating tablets).

Adult Patients

Allergic Rhinitis
Seasonal

ORAL:
- 5 mg once daily (as conventional tablets, oral solution, orally disintegrating tablets, or fixed-combination extended-release tablets with pseudoephedrine sulfate).

Perennial

ORAL:
- 5 mg once daily (as conventional tablets, oral solution, or orally disintegrating tablets).

Chronic Idiopathic Urticaria

ORAL:
- 5 mg once daily (as conventional tablets, oral solution, or orally disintegrating tablets).

Prescribing Limits

Pediatric Patients

Allergic Rhinitis

ORAL:
- Children ≥12 years of age: Dosages >5 mg provide no additional benefit but may increase risk of adverse effects (e.g., somnolence).

Adult Patients

Allergic Rhinitis

ORAL:
- Dosages >5 mg provide no additional benefit but may increase risk of adverse effects (e.g., somnolence).

Special Populations

Dosage adjustment based on gender, race, or age generally not necessary.

Hepatic Impairment
- Pediatric patients: no specific dosage recommendations at this time because of lack of data.
- Adults: 5 mg every *other* day (as conventional tablets, oral solution, or orally disintegrating tablets). Avoid fixed-combination preparation.

Renal Impairment
- Pediatric patients: no specific dosage recommendations at this time because of lack of data.
- Adults: 5 mg every *other* day (as conventional tablets, oral solution, orally disintegrating tablets, or fixed-combination tablets).

Desmopressin

(des moe press′ in)

Brand Name: DDAVP®, DDAVP® Nasal Spray, DDAVP® Rhinal Tube, DDVP®, Stimate® Nasal Spray

Why is this medicine prescribed?

Desmopressin is a chemical that is similar to a hormone found naturally in your body. It increases urine concentration and decreases urine production. Desmopressin is used to prevent and control excessive thirst, urination, and dehydration caused by injury, surgery, and certain medical conditions, allowing you to sleep through the night without awakening to urinate. It is also used to treat specific types of diabetes insipidus and conditions after head injury or pituitary surgery.

How should this medicine be used?

Desmopressin comes in a liquid that is administered into the nose and as a nasal spray. It usually is used twice a day (every morning and evening). For bed wetting, it is used every evening at bedtime. Follow the directions on your prescription label carefully, and ask your doctor or pharmacist to explain any part you do not understand. Use desmopressin exactly as directed. Do not use more or less of it or use it more often than prescribed by your doctor.

Do not take the liquid by mouth. With the nasal liquid, you will receive a soft, flexible plastic tube with special markings for measuring the dose and instructions on how to measure and administer it. After drawing the dose into the tube, insert one end of the tube into your nose and the other end into your mouth. Blow on the tube to force the liquid high into your nose. Do not allow the liquid to run into your mouth. Follow the directions carefully; if you have difficulty using the drug or giving it to a child, ask your doctor or pharmacist for advice.

To use the nasal spray, first clear your nasal passages by gently blowing your nose. Insert the sprayer into a nostril. Sniff as you squeeze the sprayer once. To prevent mucus from entering the sprayer, release your grip after you remove the sprayer from your nose. Gently sniff two or three more times.

Are there other uses for this medicine?

Desmopressin nasal spray may be used to treat a condition called chronic autonomic failure (when the body is not able to control urine production).

Talk to your doctor about the possible risks of using this drug for your condition.

This medication is sometimes prescribed for other uses; ask your doctor or pharmacist for more information.

What special precautions should I follow?

Before using desmopressin,

- tell your doctor and pharmacist if you are allergic to desmopressin or any other drugs.
- tell your doctor and pharmacist what prescription and nonprescription medications you are taking, especially carbamazepine (Tegretol), chlorpropamide (Diabinese), clofibrate (Atromid-S), demeclocycline (Declomycin), epinephrine, lithium, and vitamins.
- tell your doctor if you have or have ever had heart disease, high blood pressure, coronary artery disease, nose or sinus problems or surgery, or cystic fibrosis.
- tell your doctor if you are pregnant, plan to become pregnant, or are breast-feeding. If you become pregnant while using desmopressin, call your doctor.
- you should know that this drug may make you drowsy. Do not drive a car or operate machinery until you know how this drug affects you.
- remember that alcohol can add to the drowsiness caused by this drug.

What special dietary instructions should I follow?

Your doctor may tell you to limit your intake of fluids. Follow your doctor's directions. Drinking too much may cause water retention (bloating and swelling of the feet, ankles, and lower legs).

What should I do if I forget to take a dose?

Use the missed dose as soon as you remember it. However, if it is almost time for the next dose, skip the missed dose and continue your regular dosing schedule. Do not use a double dose to make up for a missed one.

What side effects can this medicine cause?

Desmopressin may cause side effects. If you experience any of the following symptoms, call your doctor immediately:

- upset stomach
- headache
- stuffy or runny nose
- reddening of the skin
- stomach cramps
- pain in the external genital area (in women)

If you experience a serious side effect, you or your doctor may send a report to the Food and Drug Administration's (FDA) MedWatch Adverse Event Reporting program online [at http://www.fda.gov/MedWatch/index.html] or by phone [1-800-332-1088].

What storage conditions are needed for this medicine?

Keep this medication in the container it came in, tightly closed, and out of reach of children. Store it in the refrigerator; do not freeze. The nasal bottle contains 25 or 50 doses. Throw away any medication after that. Do not put any leftover medication into another bottle. Throw away any medication that is outdated or no longer needed. Talk to your pharmacist about the proper disposal of your medication.

What should I do in case of overdose?

In case of overdose, call your local poison control center at 1-800-222-1222. If the victim has collapsed or is not breathing, call local emergency services at 911.

What other information should I know?

Keep all appointments with your doctor and the laboratory. Your doctor will order certain lab tests to check your response to desmopressin.

If desmopressin loses its effectiveness (if urination increases or you wake up earlier than usual to urinate), call your doctor. Your dose may need to be changed.

Do not let anyone else use your medication. Ask your pharmacist any questions you have about refilling your prescription.

Talk to your doctor, pharmacist, or other healthcare professional if you have questions about dosing information for your medication.

Desonide Topical

(des' oh nide)

Brand Name: Tridesilon®, DesOwen®

Why is this medicine prescribed?

Desonide is used to treat the redness, swelling, itching, and discomfort of various skin conditions. Desonide is in a class of medications called topical corticosteroids. It works by activating natural substances in the skin to reduce swelling, redness, and itching.

How should this medicine be used?

Desonide comes as a cream, an ointment, and a lotion to apply to the skin. It is usually applied 2 or 3 times a day. Apply it at around the same times every day. Follow the directions on your prescription label carefully, and ask your doctor or pharmacist to explain any part you do not understand. Use desonide exactly as directed. Do not apply more or less of it or apply it more often than prescribed by your doctor. Do not apply it to other areas of your body or use it to treat other skin conditions unless directed to do so by your doctor.

Your skin condition should improve during the first 2 weeks of your treatment. Call your doctor if your symptoms do not improve during this time.

Shake the lotion well before each use to mix the medication evenly.

This medication is only for use on the skin. Do not let desonide get into your eyes, nose, or mouth and do not swallow it.

To use desonide, apply a small amount of ointment, cream, or lotion to cover the affected area of the skin with a thin even film and rub it in gently.

If you are applying desonide to a child's diaper area, do not cover the area with tight fitting diapers or plastic pants.

Do not wrap or bandage the treated area unless your doctor tells you that you should. If your doctor tells you to wrap or bandage the treated area, follow these instructions:

1. Soak the area in water or wash it well.
2. While the skin is moist, gently rub the medication into the affected areas.
3. Cover the area with plastic wrap (such as Saran Wrap® or Handi-Wrap®). The plastic may be held in place with a gauze or elastic bandage or adhesive tape on the normal skin beside the treated area. (Instead of using plastic wrap, plastic gloves may be used for the hands, plastic bags for the feet, or a shower cap for the scalp.)
4. Carefully seal the edges of the plastic to make sure the wrap adheres closely to the skin. If the affected area is moist, you can leave the edges of the plastic wrap partly unsealed or puncture the wrap to allow excess moisture to escape.
5. Leave the plastic wrap in place as long as directed by your doctor. Usually plastic wraps are left in place no more than 12 hours each day.
6. Cleanse the skin and reapply the medication each time a new plastic wrapping is applied. Do not discontinue treatment abruptly without talking to your doctor.

Are there other uses for this medicine?

This medication may be prescribed for other uses; ask your doctor or pharmacist for more information.

What special precautions should I follow?

Before using desonide,

- tell your doctor and pharmacist if you are allergic to desonide or any other medications.
- tell your doctor and pharmacist what other prescription and nonprescription medications, vitamins, nutritional supplements, and herbal products you are taking. Be sure to mention medications that suppress the immune system such as azathioprine (Imuran), cyclosporine (Neoral, Sandimmune), methotrexate (Rheumatrex), sirolimus (Rapamune), and tacrolimus (Prograf).Your doctor may need to change the doses of your medications or monitor you carefully for side effects.
- tell your doctor if you have or have ever had diabetes, Cushing's syndrome (an abnormal condition that is caused by excess hormones [corticosteroids]), problems with your circulation, or any condition that affects your immune system such as acquired immunodeficiency syndrome (AIDS) or severe combined immunodeficiency syndrome (SCID).

- tell your doctor if you are pregnant, plan to become pregnant, or are breast-feeding. If you become pregnant while taking desonide, call your doctor.

What special dietary instructions should I follow?

Unless your doctor tells you otherwise, continue your normal diet.

What should I do if I forget to take a dose?

Apply the missed dose as soon as you remember it. However, if it is almost time for the next dose, skip the missed dose and continue your regular dosing schedule. Do not apply a double amount to make up for a missed dose.

What side effects can this medicine cause?

Desonide may cause side effects. Tell your doctor if any of these symptoms are severe or do not go away:

- stinging, burning, irritation, peeling, dryness, and redness of the skin
- itching

Some side effects can be serious. The following symptoms are uncommon, but if you experience any of them, call your doctor immediately:

- redness, swelling, oozing pus or other signs of skin infection in the place where you applied desonide
- severe rash

Children who use desonide may have an increased risk of side effects including slowed growth and delayed weight gain. Talk to your child's doctor about the risks of applying this medication to your child's skin.

If you experience a serious side effect, you or your doctor may send a report to the Food and Drug Administration's (FDA) MedWatch Adverse Event Reporting program online [at http://www.fda.gov/MedWatch/index.html] or by phone [1-800-332-1088].

What storage conditions are needed for this medicine?

Keep this medication in the container it came in, tightly closed, and out of reach of children. Store it at room temperature and away from excess heat and moisture (not in the bathroom). Throw away any medication that is outdated or no longer needed. Talk to your pharmacist about the proper disposal of your medication.

What should I do in case of overdose?

If you apply more desonide or apply it for a longer time than prescribed by your doctor, you may receive an overdose of medication. This can affect your body in many ways. Call your doctor if you accidentally apply too much medication, especially if you experience unusual symptoms.

What other information should I know?

Keep all appointments with your doctor and the laboratory. Your doctor may order certain lab test to check your body's response to desonide.

Do not let anyone else use your medication. Ask your pharmacist any questions you have about refilling your prescription.

Talk to your doctor, pharmacist, or other healthcare professional if you have questions about dosing information for your medication.

Desoximetasone Topical

(des ox i met′ a sone)

Brand Name: Topicort®, Topicort LP®

Why is this medicine prescribed?

Desoximetasone is used to treat the redness, swelling, itching, and discomfort of various skin conditions. Desoximetasone is in a class of medications called topical corticosteroids. It works by activating natural substances in the skin to reduce swelling, redness, and itching.

How should this medicine be used?

Desoximetasone comes as a cream, an ointment, and a gel to apply to the skin. It is usually applied twice a day. Apply it at around the same times every day. Follow the directions on your prescription label carefully, and ask your doctor or pharmacist to explain any part you do not understand. Use desoximetasone exactly as directed. Do not apply more or less of it or apply it more often than prescribed by your doctor. Do not apply it to other areas of your body or use it to treat other skin conditions unless directed to do so by your doctor.

This medication is only for use on the skin. Do not let desoximetasone get into your eyes, nose, or mouth and do not swallow it.

To use desoximetasone, apply a small amount of ointment, cream, or gel to cover the affected area of skin with a thin even film and rub it in gently.

If you are applying desoximetasone to a child's diaper area, do not cover the area with tight fitting diapers or plastic pants.

Do not wrap or bandage the treated area unless your doctor tells you that you should. If your doctor tells you to wrap or bandage the treated area, follow these instructions:

1. Soak the area in water or wash it well.
2. While the skin is moist, gently rub the medication into the affected areas.
3. Cover the area with plastic wrap (such as Saran Wrap® or Handi-Wrap®). The plastic may be held in place with a gauze or elastic bandage or adhesive tape on the normal skin beside the treated area. (Instead of using plastic wrap, plastic gloves may be used for the hands, plastic bags for the feet, or a shower cap for the scalp.)
4. Carefully seal the edges of the plastic to make sure the wrap adheres closely to the skin. If the affected area is moist, you can leave the edges of the plastic wrap partly unsealed or puncture the wrap to allow excess moisture to escape.
5. Leave the plastic wrap in place as long as directed by your doctor. Usually plastic wraps are left in place no more than 12 hours each day.
6. Cleanse the skin and reapply the medication each time a new plastic wrapping is applied. Do not discontinue treatment abruptly without talking to your doctor.

Are there other uses for this medicine?

This medication may be prescribed for other uses; ask your doctor or pharmacist for more information.

What special precautions should I follow?

Before using desoximetasone,

- tell your doctor and pharmacist if you are allergic to desoximetasone or any other medications.
- tell your doctor and pharmacist what other prescription and nonprescription medications, vitamins, nutritional supplements, and herbal products you are taking. Be sure to mention medications that suppress the immune system such as azathioprine (Imuran), cyclosporine (Neoral, Sandimmune), methotrexate (Rheumatrex), sirolimus (Rapamune), and tacrolimus (Prograf). Your doctor may need to change the doses of your medications or monitor you carefully for side effects.
- tell your doctor if you have or have ever had diabetes, Cushing's syndrome (an abnormal condition that is caused by excess hormones [corticosteroids]), problems with your circulation, or any condition that affects your immune system such as acquired immunodeficiency syndrome (AIDS) or severe combined immunodeficiency syndrome (SCID).
- tell your doctor if you are pregnant, plan to become pregnant, or are breast-feeding. If you become pregnant while using desoximetasone, call your doctor.

What special dietary instructions should I follow?

Unless your doctor tells you otherwise, continue your normal diet.

What should I do if I forget to take a dose?

Apply the missed dose as soon as you remember it. However, if it is almost time for the next dose, skip the missed dose and continue your regular dosing schedule. Do not apply a double amount to make up for a missed dose.

What side effects can this medicine cause?

Desoximetasone may cause side effects. Tell your doctor if any of these symptoms are severe or do not go away:

- burning, itching, irritation, redness, or dryness of the skin
- swelling, redness, or pus filled blisters on the skin at the base of a hair
- tiny red bumps around the mouth
- unwanted hair growth
- pimples

Some side effects can be serious. The following symptoms are uncommon, but if you experience any of them, call your doctor immediately:

- severe rash
- redness, swelling, oozing pus, or other signs of skin infection in the place where you applied desoximetasone

Children who use desoximetasone have an increased risk of side effects including slowed growth and delayed weight gain. Talk to your child's doctor about the risks of applying this medication to your child's skin.

If you experience a serious side effect, you or your doctor may send a report to the Food and Drug Administration's (FDA) MedWatch Adverse Event Reporting program online [at http://www.fda.gov/MedWatch/index.html] or by phone [1-800-332-1088].

What storage conditions are needed for this medicine?

Keep this medication in the container it came in, tightly closed, and out of reach of children. Store it at room temperature and away from excess heat and moisture (not in the bathroom). Throw away any medication that is outdated or no longer needed. Talk to your pharmacist about the proper disposal of your medication.

What should I do in case of overdose?

If you apply more desoximetasone or apply it for a longer time than prescribed by your doctor, you may receive an overdose of medication. This can affect your body in many ways. Call your doctor if you accidentally apply too much medication, especially if you experience unusual symptoms.

What other information should I know?

Keep all appointments with your doctor and the laboratory. Your doctor may order certain lab tests to check your body's response to desoximetasone.

Do not let anyone else use your medication. Ask your pharmacist any questions you have about refilling your prescription.

Talk to your doctor, pharmacist, or other healthcare professional if you have questions about dosing information for your medication.

Dexamethasone Ophthalmic

(dex a meth′ a sone)

Brand Name: AK-Trol®, Dexasporin®, Maxidex®, Maxitrol®, Ocu-Trol®, TobraDex®
Also available generically.

Why is this medicine prescribed?

Dexamethasone reduces the irritation, redness, burning, and swelling of eye inflammation caused by chemicals, heat, radiation, infection, allergy, or foreign bodies in the eye. It is sometimes used after eye surgery.

How should this medicine be used?

Dexamethasone comes as eyedrops and eye ointment. Follow the directions on your prescription label carefully, and ask your doctor or pharmacist to explain any part you do not understand. Use dexamethasone exactly as directed. Do not use more or less of it or use it more often than prescribed by your doctor.

If you are using the suspension form of dexamethasone eyedrops (Maxidex), shake the bottle well before each dose. It is not necessary to shake dexamethasone eyedrop solution.

To use the eyedrops, follow these instructions:

1. Wash your hands thoroughly with soap and water.
2. Use a mirror or have someone else put the drops in your eye.
3. If using dexamethasone suspension eyedrops, shake the bottle well for 10 seconds.
4. Remove the protective cap. Avoid touching the dropper tip against your eye or anything else.
5. Make sure that the end of the dropper is not chipped or cracked.
6. Hold the dropper tip down at all times to prevent drops from flowing back into the bottle and contaminating the remaining contents.
7. Lie down or tilt your head back.
8. Holding the bottle between your thumb and index finger, place the dropper tip as near as possible to your eyelid without touching it.
9. Brace the remaining fingers of that hand against your cheek or nose.
10. With the index finger of your other hand, pull the lower lid of the eye down to form a pocket.
11. Drop the prescribed number of drops into the pocket made by the lower lid andthe eye. Placing drops on the surface of the eyeball can cause stinging.
12. Close your eye and press lightly against the lower lid with your finger for 2-3 minutes to keep the medication in the eye. Do not blink.

13. Replace and tighten the cap right away. Do not wipe or rinse it off.
14. Wipe off any excess liquid from your cheek with a clean tissue. Wash your hands again.

To use the eye ointment, follow these instructions:
1. Wash your hands thoroughly with soap and water.
2. Use a mirror or have someone else apply the ointment.
3. Avoid touching the tip of the tube against your eye or anything else. The ointment must be kept clean.
4. Tilt your head forward slightly.
5. Holding the tube between your thumb and index finger, place the tube as near as possible to your eyelid without touching it.
6. Brace the remaining fingers of that hand against your cheek or nose.
7. With the index finger of your other hand, pull the lower lid of your eye down to form a pocket.
8. Place a small amount of ointment into the pocket made by the lower lid and the eye. A 1/2-inch strip of ointment usually is enough unless otherwise directed by your doctor.
9. Gently close your eyes and keep them closed for 1-2 minutes to allow the medication to be absorbed.
10. Replace and tighten the cap right away.
11. Wipe off any excess ointment from your eyelids and lashes with a clean tissue. Wash your hands again.

Are there other uses for this medicine?

Dexamethasone eye drops may be used to reduce redness, burning, and swelling or inflammation in the ear. Talk to your doctor about the possible risks of using this drug for your condition.

This medication is sometimes prescribed for other uses; ask your doctor or pharmacist for more information.

What special precautions should I follow?

Before using dexamethasone eyedrops or eye ointment,
- tell your doctor and pharmacist if you are allergic to dexamethasone, sulfites, or any other drugs.
- tell your doctor and pharmacist what prescription and nonprescription medications you are taking, including vitamins.
- tell your doctor if you have or have ever had glaucoma or diabetes.
- tell your doctor if you are pregnant, plan to become pregnant, or are breast-feeding. If you become pregnant while using dexamethasone, call your doctor immediately. Talk to your doctor about stopping to breast-feed if you use dexamethasone eye drops.
- tell your doctor if you wear soft contact lenses. If the brand of dexamethasone you are using contains benzalkonium chloride, wait at least 15 minutes after using the medicine to put in soft contact lenses.

What should I do if I forget to take a dose?

Apply the missed drops or ointment as soon as you remember it. However, if it is almost time for the next dose, skip the missed dose and continue your regular dosing schedule. Do not apply a double dose to make up for a missed one.

What side effects can this medicine cause?

Dexamethasone may cause side effects. Tell your doctor if any of these symptoms are severe or do not go away:
- changes in vision, such as blurring and seeing halos around lights
- pressure and pain in the eye
- drooping of the eyelid

What storage conditions are needed for this medicine?

Keep this medication in the container it came in, tightly closed, and out of reach of children. Store it at room temperature and away from excess heat and moisture (not in the bathroom). Throw away any medication that is outdated or no longer needed. Talk to your pharmacist about the proper disposal of your medication.

What other information should I know?

Keep all appointments with your doctor.

Do not let anyone else use your medication. Ask your pharmacist any questions you have about refilling your prescription.

If you still have symptoms of eye irritation after you finish the dexamethasone, call your doctor.

Dosage Facts
For Informational Purposes

Caution: Do not change your dose, how often you take your medication, or the length of time you are to take it without first talking to your healthcare provider.

The following dosage information was written using medical language for doctors and other healthcare professionals and is provided here for you to check your dosage. The dosage of this drug may differ for different patients. Therefore, always follow your doctor's instructions or the directions on the label. Contact your healthcare provider or pharmacist if you have any questions about the specific dosage of your medication after reviewing this information.

Pediatric Patients

Ophthalmic Inflammation
Solution or Suspension

OPHTHALMIC:
- Severe inflammation: Initially, instill 1 or 2 drops of the suspension or solution into the conjunctival sac every hour during the day and every 2 hours during the night.

- Mild or moderate inflammation or when a favorable response is attained in severe cases: 1 drop every 4–8 hours.
- Also may use the ointment at night in conjunction with daytime use of a suspension or solution to reduce the frequent applications required with the liquid dosage forms.
- If improvement does not occur within several days, discontinue the drug and begin other therapy.
- Duration of treatment depends on the type and severity of the disease and may range from a few days to several weeks; avoid long-term therapy.
- Gradually taper the drug when it is discontinued to avoid exacerbation of the disease.

Ointment

OPHTHALMIC:

- Initially, apply 1.25–2.5 cm into the conjunctival sac 3 or 4 times daily; reduce frequency to once or twice daily when a favorable response is attained.
- Also may use the ointment at night in conjunction with daytime use of a suspension or solution to reduce the frequent applications required with the liquid dosage forms.
- If improvement does not occur within several days, discontinue the drug and begin other therapy.
- Duration of treatment depends on the type and severity of the disease and may range from a few days to several weeks; avoid long-term therapy.
- Gradually taper the drug when it is discontinued to avoid exacerbation of the disease.

Otic Inflammation

The ophthalmic solution is instilled into the ear (aural) canal.

Solution

OTIC:

- Instill 3 or 4 drops of the ophthalmic solution into the ear canal 2 or 3 times daily.
- Alternatively, a gauze wick saturated with the ophthalmic solution may be packed into the aural canal, kept moist with the solution, and allowed to remain in the canal for 12–24 hours; may be repeated as needed.

Adult Patients

Ophthalmic Inflammation
Solution or Suspension

OPHTHALMIC:

- Severe inflammation: Initially, instill 1 or 2 drops of the suspension or solution into the conjunctival sac every hour during the day and every 2 hours during the night.
- Mild or moderate inflammation or when a favorable response is attained in severe cases: 1 drop every 4–8 hours.
- Also may use ointment at night in conjunction with daytime use of a suspension or solution to reduce the frequent applications required with the liquid dosage forms.
- If improvement does not occur within several days, discontinue the drug and begin other therapy.
- Duration of treatment depends on the type and severity of the disease and may range from a few days to several weeks; avoid long-term therapy.
- Gradually taper the drug when it is discontinued to avoid exacerbation of the disease.

Ointment

OPHTHALMIC:

- Initially, apply 1.25–2.5 cm into the conjunctival sac 3 or 4 times daily; reduce frequency to once or twice daily when a favorable response is attained.
- Also may use the ointment at night in conjunction with daytime use of a suspension or solution to reduce the frequent applications required with the liquid dosage forms.
- If improvement does not occur within several days, discontinue the drug and begin other therapy.
- Duration of treatment depends on the type and severity of the disease and may range from a few days to several weeks; avoid long-term therapy.
- Gradually taper the drug when it is discontinued to avoid exacerbation of the disease.

Otic Inflammation

The ophthalmic solution is instilled into the ear (aural) canal.

Solution

OTIC:

- Instill 3 or 4 drops of the ophthalmic solution into the ear canal 2 or 3 times daily.
- Alternatively, a gauze wick saturated with the solution may be packed into the aural canal, kept moist with the solution, and allowed to remain in the canal for 12–24 hours; may be repeated as needed.

Special Populations

Hepatic Impairment
- No specific dosage recommendations for hepatic impairment.

Renal Impairment
- No specific dosage recommendations for renal impairment.

Geriatric Patients
- No specific geriatric dosage recommendations.

Dexamethasone Oral

(dex a meth′ a sone)

Brand Name: Decadron®, Dexamethasone Intensol®, Dexpak® Taperpak®
Also available generically.

Why is this medicine prescribed?

Dexamethasone, a corticosteroid, is similar to a natural hormone produced by your adrenal glands. It often is used to replace this chemical when your body does not make enough of it. It relieves inflammation (swelling, heat, redness, and pain) and is used to treat certain forms of arthritis; skin, blood, kidney, eye, thyroid, and intestinal disorders (e.g., colitis); severe allergies; and asthma. Dexamethasone is also used to treat certain types of cancer.

This medication is sometimes prescribed for other uses; ask your doctor or pharmacist for more information.

How should this medicine be used?

Dexamethasone comes as a tablet and a solution to take by mouth. Your doctor will prescribe a dosing schedule that is best for you. Follow the directions on your prescription label carefully, and ask your doctor or pharmacist to explain any part you do not understand. Take dexamethasone exactly as directed. Do not take more or less of it or take it more often than prescribed by your doctor.

Do not stop taking dexamethasone without talking to your doctor. Stopping the drug abruptly can cause loss of appetite, upset stomach, vomiting, drowsiness, confusion, headache, fever, joint and muscle pain, peeling skin, and weight loss. If you take large doses for a long time, your doctor probably will decrease your dose gradually to allow your body to adjust before stopping the drug completely. Watch for these side effects if you are gradually decreasing your dose and after you stop taking the tablets or oral liquid, even if you switch to an inhalation corticosteroid medication. If these problems occur, call your doctor immediately. You may need to increase your dose of tablets or liquid temporarily or start taking them again.

What special precautions should I follow?

Before taking dexamethasone,

- tell your doctor and pharmacist if you are allergic to dexamethasone, aspirin, tartrazine (a yellow dye in some processed foods and drugs), or any other drugs.
- tell your doctor and pharmacist what prescription and nonprescription medications you are taking especially anticoagulants ('blood thinners') such as warfarin (Coumadin), arthritis medications, aspirin, cyclosporine (Neoral, Sandimmune), digoxin (Lanoxin), diuretics ('water pills'), ephedrine, estrogen (Premarin), ketoconazole (Nizoral), oral contraceptives, phenobarbital, phenytoin (Dilantin), rifampin (Rifadin), theophylline (Theo-Dur), and vitamins.
- if you have a fungal infection (other than on your skin), do not take dexamethasone without talking to your doctor.
- tell your doctor if you have or have ever had liver, kidney, intestinal, or heart disease; diabetes; an underactive thyroid gland; high blood pressure; mental illness; myasthenia gravis; osteoporosis; herpes eye infection; seizures; tuberculosis (TB); or ulcers.
- tell your doctor if you are pregnant, plan to become pregnant, or are breast-feeding. If you become pregnant while taking dexamethasone, call your doctor.
- if you are having surgery, including dental surgery, tell the doctor or dentist that you are taking dexamethasone.
- if you have a history of ulcers or take large doses of aspirin or other arthritis medication, limit your consumption of alcoholic beverages while taking this drug. Dexamethasone makes your stomach and intestines more susceptible to the irritating effects of alcohol, aspirin, and certain arthritis medications: this effect increases your risk of ulcers.

What special dietary instructions should I follow?

Your doctor may instruct you to follow a low-sodium, low-salt, potassium-rich, or high-protein diet. Follow these directions.

Dexamethasone may cause an upset stomach. Take dexamethasone with food or milk.

What should I do if I forget to take a dose?

When you start to take dexamethasone, ask your doctor what to do if you forget a dose. Write down these instructions so that you can refer to them later.

If you take dexamethasone once a day, take the missed dose as soon as you remember it. However, if it is almost time for the next dose, skip the missed dose and continue your regular dosing schedule. Do not take a double dose to make up for a missed one.

What side effects can this medicine cause?

Dexamethasone may cause side effects. Tell your doctor if any of these symptoms are severe or do not go away:

- upset stomach
- stomach irritation
- vomiting
- headache
- dizziness
- insomnia
- restlessness
- depression
- anxiety
- acne
- increased hair growth
- easy bruising
- irregular or absent menstrual periods

If you experience any of the following symptoms, call your doctor immediately:

- skin rash
- swollen face, lower legs, or ankles
- vision problems
- cold or infection that lasts a long time
- muscle weakness
- black or tarry stool

If you experience a serious side effect, you or your doctor may send a report to the Food and Drug Administration's (FDA) MedWatch Adverse Event Reporting program online [at http://www.fda.gov/MedWatch/index.html] or by phone [1-800-332-1088].

What storage conditions are needed for this medicine?

Keep this medication in the container it came in, tightly closed, and out of reach of children. Store it at room temperature and away from excess heat and moisture (not in the bathroom). Throw away any medication that is outdated or

no longer needed. Talk to your pharmacist about the proper disposal of your medication.

What should I do in case of overdose?

In case of overdose, call your local poison control center at 1-800-222-1222. If the victim has collapsed or is not breathing, call local emergency services at 911.

What other information should I know?

Keep all appointments with your doctor and the laboratory. Your doctor will order certain lab tests to check your response to dexamethasone. Checkups are especially important for children because dexamethasone can slow bone growth.

If your condition worsens, call your doctor. Your dose may need to be adjusted.

Carry an identification card that indicates that you may need to take supplementary doses (write down the full dose you took before gradually decreasing it) of dexamethasone during periods of stress (injuries, infections, and severe asthma attacks). Ask your pharmacist or doctor how to obtain this card. List your name, medical problems, drugs and dosages, and doctor's name and telephone number on the card.

This drug makes you more susceptible to illnesses. If you are exposed to chicken pox, measles, or tuberculosis (TB) while taking dexamethasone, call your doctor. Do not have a vaccination, other immunization, or any skin test while you are taking dexamethasone unless your doctor tells you that you may.

Report any injuries or signs of infection (fever, sore throat, pain during urination, and muscle aches) that occur during treatment.

Your doctor may instruct you to weigh yourself every day. Report any unusual weight gain.

If your sputum (the matter you cough up during an asthma attack) thickens or changes color from clear white to yellow, green, or gray, call your doctor; these changes may be signs of an infection.

If you have diabetes, dexamethasone may increase your blood sugar level. If you monitor your blood sugar (glucose) at home, test your blood or urine more frequently than usual. Call your doctor if your blood sugar is high or if sugar is present in your urine; your dose of diabetes medication and your diet may need to be changed.

Do not let anyone else take your medication. Ask your pharmacist any questions you have about refilling your prescription.

Dosage Facts
For Informational Purposes

Caution: Do not change your dose, how often you take your medication, or the length of time you are to take it without first talking to your healthcare provider.

The following dosage information was written using medical language for doctors and other healthcare professionals and is provided here for you to check your dosage. The dosage of this drug may differ for different patients. Therefore, always follow your doctor's instructions or the directions on the label. Contact your healthcare provider or pharmacist if you have any questions about the specific dosage of your medication after reviewing this information.

General Dosage Information

Available as dexamethasone and dexamethasone sodium phosphate. Dosage of dexamethasone sodium phosphate is expressed in terms of dexamethasone phosphate.

After a satisfactory response is obtained, decrease dosage in small decrements to the lowest level that maintains an adequate clinical response, and discontinue the drug as soon as possible.

Monitor patients continually for signs that indicate dosage adjustment is necessary, such as remissions or exacerbations of the disease and stress (surgery, infection, trauma).

High dosages may be required for acute situations of certain rheumatic disorders and collagen diseases; after a response has been obtained, drug often must be continued for long periods at low dosage.

High or massive dosages may be required in the treatment of pemphigus, exfoliative dermatitis, bullous dermatitis herpetiformis, severe erythema multiforme, or mycosis fungoides. Early initiation of systemic glucocorticoid therapy may be lifesaving in pemphigus vulgaris. Reduce dosage gradually to the lowest effective level, but discontinuance may not be possible.

Massive dosages may be required for the treatment of shock.

Pediatric Patients

Base pediatric dosage on severity of the disease and patient response rather than on strict adherence to dosage indicated by age, body weight, or body surface area.

Usual Dosage
ORAL:
- 0.024–0.34 mg/kg daily or 0.66–10 mg/m^2 daily, administered in 4 divided doses.

Adult Patients

Usual Dosage
ORAL:
- Usually, 0.75–6 mg daily, depending on disease being treated, and usually divided into 2–4 doses.

Diagnostic Uses
Cushing's Syndrome
ORAL:
- Initially, 0.5 mg every 6 hours for 48 hours after baseline 24-hour urinary 17-hydroxycorticosteroid (17-OHCS) concentrations are determined.
- During the second 24 hours of administration, collect the urine and analyze for 17-OHCS.
- Alternatively, after a baseline plasma cortisol determination, administer 1-mg orally at 11 p.m., and determine plasma cortisol concentrations at 8 a.m. the following morning.
- Plasma cortisol and urinary output of 17-OHCS are depressed

following administration in healthy individuals but remain at basal levels in patients with Cushing's syndrome.

- To distinguish adrenal tumor from adrenal hyperplasia, 2 mg orally every 6 hours for 48 hours.
- During the second 24 hours of administration, collect the urine and analyze for 17-OHCS.
- In adrenal hyperplasia, urinary 17-OHCS levels are decreased and remain at basal levels in patients with adrenocortical tumors.

Depression†

ORAL:

- If used for dexamethasone suppression test (DST) for depression, 1 mg at 11 p.m.
- Following day, obtain venous blood samples at 8 a.m., 4 p.m. and 11 p.m; usually, only at 11 p.m. for outpatients.
- Depending on assay used, a serum cortisol concentration >4.5–5 mcg/dL for any blood sample is abnormal and represents a positive test.

† Use is not currently included in the labeling approved by the US Food and Drug Administration.

Dexmethylphenidate

(dex meth ill fen′ i date)

Brand Name: Focalin®

Important Warning

Dexmethylphenidate can be habit-forming. Do not take a larger dose, take it more often, take it for a longer time, or take it in a different way than prescribed by your doctor. If you take too much dexmethylphenidate, you may find that the medication no longer controls your symptoms, you may feel a need to take large amounts of the medication, and you may experience unusual changes in your behavior or a loss of contact with reality. Tell your doctor if you drink or have ever drunk large amounts of alcohol, use or have ever used street drugs, or have overused prescription medications.

Do not stop taking dexmethylphenidate without talking to your doctor, especially if you have overused the medication. Your doctor will probably decrease your dose gradually and monitor you carefully during this time. You may develop severe depression if you suddenly stop taking dexmethylphenidate after overusing it.

Your doctor or pharmacist will give you the manufacturer's patient information sheet (Medication Guide) when you begin treatment with dexmethylphenidate and each time you refill your prescription. Read the information carefully and ask your

doctor or pharmacist if you have any questions. You can also visit the Food and Drug Administration (FDA) website (http://www.fda.gov/cder) or the manufacturer's website to obtain the Medication Guide.

Why is this medicine prescribed?

Dexmethylphenidate is used as part of a treatment program to increase the ability to pay attention and to decrease impulsiveness and hyperactivity in people with Attention Deficit Hyperactivity Disorder (ADHD; more difficulty focusing, controlling actions, and remaining still or quiet than other people who are the same age). Dexmethylphenidate is in a class of medications called central nervous system (CNS) stimulants. It works by increasing the amounts of certain natural substances in the brain.

How should this medicine be used?

Dexmethylphenidate comes as a tablet and an extended-release (long-acting) capsule to take by mouth. The tablet is usually taken twice a day, at least 4 hours apart, with or without food. The extended-release capsule is usually taken once a day in the morning. The extended-release capsule can be taken with or without food but will start to work faster if it is taken without food. Take dexmethylphenidate at around the same time(s) every day. Follow the directions on your prescription label carefully, and ask your doctor or pharmacist to explain any part you do not understand.

Swallow the extended-release capsules whole; do not chew or crush them. If you are unable to swallow the extended-release capsule, you can carefully open the capsule and sprinkle the contents on a spoonful of applesauce. Swallow this mixture immediately, but do not chew it. Do not save this mixture to use at a later time.

Your doctor will probably start you on a low dose of dexmethylphenidate and gradually increase your dose, not more often than once a week.

Your condition should improve during your treatment. Call your doctor if your symptoms worsen at any time during your treatment or do not improve after one month.

Your doctor may tell you to stop taking dexmethylphenidate from time to time to see if the medication is still needed. Follow these directions carefully.

Before taking dexmethylphenidate, ask your pharmacist or doctor for a copy of the manufacturer's information for the patient and read it carefully.

Are there other uses for this medicine?

This medication may be prescribed for other uses; ask your doctor or pharmacist for more information.

What special precautions should I follow?

Before taking dexmethylphenidate,

- tell your doctor and pharmacist if you are allergic to dexmethylphenidate, methylphenidate (Concerta, Metadate, Methylin, Ritalin), or any other medications.

- tell your doctor if you are taking monoamine oxidase (MAO) inhibitors, including isocarboxazid (Marplan), phenelzine (Nardil), selegiline (Eldepryl), and tranylcypromine (Parnate), or if you have stopped taking them during the past 14 days. Your doctor will probably tell you not to take dexmethylphenidate until at least 14 days have passed since you last took an MAO inhibitor.

- tell your doctor and pharmacist what other prescription and nonprescription medications, vitamins, nutritional supplements, and herbal products you are taking or plan to take. Be sure to mention any of the following: anticoagulants ('blood thinners') such as warfarin (Coumadin); antidepressants (mood elevators) such as amitriptyline (Elavil), amoxapine (Asendin), clomipramine (Anafranil), desipramine (Norpramin), doxepin (Adapin, Sinequan), imipramine (Tofranil), nortriptyline (Aventyl, Pamelor), protriptyline (Vivactil), and trimipramine (Surmontil); clonidine (Catapres); medications for high blood pressure; medications for seizures such as phenobarbital phenytoin (Dilantin), and primidone (Mysoline); and selective serotonin reuptake inhibitors (SSRIs) such as citalopram (Celexa), fluoxetine (Prozac, Sarafem), fluvoxamine (Luvox), paroxetine (Paxil), and sertraline (Zoloft); and venlafaxine (Effexor). If you are taking the extended-release capsules, also tell your doctor if you are taking antacids or other medications for heartburn or ulcers. Your doctor may need to change the doses of your medications or monitor you carefully for side effects.

- tell your doctor if you or anyone in your family has or has ever had Tourette's syndrome (a condition characterized by the need to perform repeated motions or to repeat sounds or words), facial or motor tics (repeated uncontrollable movements), or verbal tics (repetition of sounds or words that is hard to control). Also tell your doctor if you have glaucoma, or feelings of anxiety, tension, or agitation. Your doctor will probably tell you not to take dexmethylphenidate.

- tell your doctor if anyone in your family has or has ever had an irregular heartbeat or has died suddenly. Also tell your doctor if you have recently had a heart attack and if you have or have ever had a heart defect, high blood pressure, an irregular heartbeat, heart or blood vessel disease, or other heart problems. Your doctor will probably examine you to see if your heart and blood vessels are healthy. Your doctor may tell you not to take dexmethylphenidate if you have a heart condition or if there is a high risk that you may develop a heart condition.

- tell your doctor if you or anyone in your family has or has ever had depression, bipolar disorder (mood that changes from depressed to abnormally excited), or mania (frenzied, abnormally excited mood), or has thought about or attempted suicide. Also tell your doctor if you ever have abnormal thoughts or visions or hear abnormal sounds.or if you have or have ever had depression; feelings of sadness, hopelessness, helplessness, or worthlessness; mental illness; seizures; an abnormal electroencephalogram (EEG; a test that measures electrical activity in the brain), or thyroid disease.

- tell your doctor if you are pregnant, plan to become pregnant, or are breast-feeding. If you become pregnant while taking dexmethylphenidate, call your doctor.

- you should know that dexmethylphenidate should be used as part of a total treatment program for ADHD, which may include counseling and special education. Make sure to follow all of your doctor's and/or therapist's instructions.

What special dietary instructions should I follow?

Unless your doctor tells you otherwise, continue your normal diet.

What should I do if I forget to take a dose?

Take the missed dose as soon as you remember it. However, if it is almost time for your next dose, skip the missed dose and continue your regular dosing schedule. Do not take a double dose to make up for a missed one.

What side effects can this medicine cause?

Dexmethylphenidate may cause side effects. Tell your doctor if any of these symptoms are severe or do not go away:

- stomach pain
- loss of appetite
- nausea
- vomiting
- heartburn
- weight loss
- dry mouth
- throat pain
- difficulty falling asleep or staying asleep
- dizziness
- drowsiness
- nervousness or jitteriness
- headache

Some side effects can be serious. If you experience any of the following symptoms, call your doctor immediately:

- fast, pounding, or irregular heartbeat
- chest pain
- shortness of breath
- excessive tiredness
- slow or difficult speech
- dizziness or faintness
- weakness or numbness of an arm or leg
- changes in vision or blurred vision
- seizures
- abnormal thinking
- aggressive behavior
- hallucinations (seeing things or hearing voices that do not exist)
- mood changes
- depression

- motor tics
- verbal tics
- rash
- hives
- itching
- purple blotches under the skin
- fever
- blisters
- joint pain

Dexmethylphenidate may cause sudden death in children and teenagers with heart defects or serious heart problems. This medication also may cause sudden death, heart attack or stroke in adults, especially adults with heart defects or serious heart problems. Talk to your doctor about the risks of taking this medication.

Dexmethylphenidate may slow children's growth or weight gain. Your child's doctor will watch his or her growth carefully. Talk to your child's doctor if you have concerns about your child's growth or weight gain while he or she is taking this medication. Talk to your child's doctor about the risks of giving dexmethylphenidate to your child.

Dexmethylphenidate may cause other side effects. Call your doctor if you have any unusual problems while taking this medication.

If you experience a serious side effect, you or your doctor may send a report to the Food and Drug Administration's (FDA) MedWatch Adverse Event Reporting program online [at http://www.fda.gov/MedWatch/index.html] or by phone [1-800-332-1088].

What storage conditions are needed for this medicine?

Keep this medication in the container it came in, tightly closed, and out of reach of children. Store it at room temperature and away from excess heat and moisture (not in the bathroom). Throw away any medication that is outdated or no longer needed. Talk to your pharmacist about the proper disposal of your medication.

Store dexmethylphenidate in a safe place so that no one else can take it accidentally or on purpose. Keep track of how many tablets or capsules are left so you will know if any are missing.

What should I do in case of overdose?

In case of overdose, call your local poison control center at 1-800-222-1222. If the victim has collapsed or is not breathing, call local emergency services at 911.

Symptoms of overdose may include:

- vomiting
- agitation
- uncontrollable shaking of a part of the body
- muscle twitching
- seizures
- unconsciousness
- inappropriate happiness
- confusion

- hallucinations (seeing things or hearing voices that do not exist)
- sweating
- flushing
- headache
- fever
- rapid, pounding, or irregular heartbeat
- blurred vision
- dry mouth

What other information should I know?

Keep all appointments with your doctor and the laboratory. Your doctor may order certain lab tests to check your body's response to dexmethylphenidate.

Do not let anyone else take your medication. This prescription is not refillable. Be sure to schedule appointments with your doctor on a regular basis so you do not run out of medication.

Dosage Facts
For Informational Purposes

Caution: Do not change your dose, how often you take your medication, or the length of time you are to take it without first talking to your healthcare provider.

The following dosage information was written using medical language for doctors and other healthcare professionals and is provided here for you to check your dosage. The dosage of this drug may differ for different patients. Therefore, always follow your doctor's instructions or the directions on the label. Contact your healthcare provider or pharmacist if you have any questions about the specific dosage of your medication after reviewing this information.

General Dosage Information

Available as dexmethylphenidate hydrochloride; dosage expressed in terms of the salt.

Pediatric Patients

ADHD
Conventional Tablets

ORAL:
- Children ≥6 years of age: Initially, 2.5 mg twice daily for children who currently are not receiving racemic methylphenidate or are receiving stimulants other than methylphenidate. Increase dosage by 2.5–5 mg daily at weekly intervals (up to maximum dosage of 20 mg daily).
- Children ≥6 years of age: Initially administer one-half the current methylphenidate hydrochloride dosage in children who are being transferred from racemic methylphenidate to dexmethylphenidate therapy.

Extended-release Capsules

ORAL:
- Children ≥6 years of age: Initially, 5 mg once daily for children who currently are not receiving dexmethylphenidate or

racemic methylphenidate or who are receiving stimulants other than methylphenidate. Increase dosage by 5 mg daily at weekly intervals (up to maximum dosage of 20 mg daily).
- Children ≥6 years of age: Substitute extended-release capsules for conventional tablets at same total daily dosage.
- Children ≥6 years of age: Initially administer one-half the current methylphenidate hydrochloride dosage in children who are being transferred from racemic methylphenidate to dexmethylphenidate therapy.

Adult Patients

ADHD
Extended-release Capsules

ORAL:
- Initially, 10 mg once daily for patients who currently are not receiving dexmethylphenidate or racemic methylphenidate or who are receiving stimulants other than methylphenidate. Increase dosage by 10 mg daily after 1 week (up to maximum dosage of 20 mg daily).
- Substitute extended-release capsules for conventional tablets at same total daily dosage.
- Initially administer one-half the current methylphenidate hydrochloride dosage in patients who are being transferred from racemic methylphenidate to dexmethylphenidate therapy.

Prescribing Limits

Pediatric Patients

ADHD
ORAL:
- Maximum 20 mg daily.
- Long-term use (>6 weeks for conventional tablets or >7 weeks for extended-release capsules) has not been studied systematically. If used for long-term therapy, periodically re-evaluate the usefulness of the drug.

Adult Patients

ADHD
ORAL:
- Maximum 20 mg daily.
- Long-term use (>6 weeks for conventional tablets or >7 weeks for extended-release capsules) has not been studied systematically. If used for long-term therapy, periodically re-evaluate the usefulness of the drug.

Special Populations

Hepatic Impairment
- No specific dosage recommendations.

Renal Impairment
- No specific dosage recommendations.

Dextroamphetamine
(dex troe am fet′ a meen)

Brand Name: Dexedrine®, DextroStat®
Also available generically.

Important Warning

Dextroamphetamine can be habit forming. Do not take a larger dose, take it more often, or take it for a longer time than prescribed by your doctor. If you take too much dextroamphetamine you may find that the medication no longer controls your symptoms, you may feel a need to take large amounts of the medication, and you may experience symptoms such as rash, difficulty falling asleep or staying asleep, irritability, hyperactivity, changes in your personality, and loss of contact with reality. Tell your doctor if you drink or have ever drunk large amounts of alcohol, use or have ever used street drugs, or have overused prescription medications.

Do not stop taking dextroamphetamine without talking to your doctor, especially if you have overused the medication. Your doctor will probably decrease your dose gradually and monitor you carefully during this time. You may experience depression and extreme tiredness if you suddenly stop taking dextroamphetamine after overusing it.

Do not let anyone else take your medication. Store dextroamphetamine in a safe place so that no one else can take it accidentally or on purpose. Keep track of how many tablets or capsules are left so you will know if any are missing.

Dextroamphetamine may cause sudden death or serious heart problems, especially if the medication is misused.

Your doctor or pharmacist will give you the manufacturer's patient information sheet (Medication Guide) when you begin treatment with dextroamphetamine and each time you refill your prescription. Read the information carefully and ask your doctor or pharmacist if you have any questions. You can also visit the Food and Drug Administration (FDA) website (http://www.fda.gov/cder) or the manufacturer's website to obtain the Medication Guide.

Why is this medicine prescribed?
Dextroamphetamine is used as part of a treatment program for attention deficit hyperactivity disorder (ADHD; more difficulty focusing, controlling actions, and remaining still or quiet than other people who are the same age). Dextroamphetamine is also used to treat narcolepsy (a sleep dis-

order that causes excessive daytime sleepiness and sudden attacks of sleep). Dextroamphetamine is in a class of medications called central nervous system stimulants. It works by changing the amounts of certain natural substances in the brain.

How should this medicine be used?

Dextroamphetamine comes as a tablet and an extended-release (long acting) capsule to take by mouth. The tablet is usually taken two to three times daily with or without food. The extended-release capsule is usually taken once a day with or without food. Take dextroamphetamine at around the same time(s) every day. If you are taking dextroamphetamine tablets, take your first dose as soon as you wake up in the morning, and space your doses by 4 to 6 hours. Do not take dextroamphetamine in the evening. Follow the directions on your prescription label carefully, and ask your doctor or pharmacist to explain any part you do not understand. Take dextroamphetamine exactly as directed.

Do not chew or crush the extended-release capsules.

Your doctor will probably start you on a low dose of dextroamphetamine and gradually increase your dose, not more often than once every week.

Your doctor may tell you to stop taking dextroamphetamine from time to time to see if the medication is still needed. Follow these directions carefully.

Are there other uses for this medicine?

Dextroamphetamine should not be used to treat excessive tiredness that is not caused by narcolepsy.

This medication may be prescribed for other uses; ask your doctor or pharmacist for more information.

What special precautions should I follow?

Before taking dextroamphetamine,

- tell your doctor and pharmacist if you are allergic to dextroamphetamine, any other medications, or any of the ingredients in dextroamphetamine tablets or capsules. If you are taking the tablets, tell your doctor if you are allergic to tartrazine (FD&C Yellow No. 5, a color additive) or aspirin.
- tell your doctor if you are taking monoamine oxidase (MAO) inhibitors, including isocarboxazid (Marplan), phenelzine (Nardil), selegiline (Eldepryl), and tranylcypromine (Parnate), or if you have stopped taking them within the past 2 weeks. Your doctor will probably tell you that you should not take dextroamphetamine until at least 14 days have passed since you last took an MAO inhibitor.
- tell your doctor and pharmacist what other prescription and nonprescription medications, vitamins, and herbal products you are taking. Be sure to mention any of the following: alpha blockers such as alfuzosin (Uroxatral), doxazosin (Cardura), prazosin (Minipress), tamsulosin (Flomax), and terazosin (Hytrin); antacids; antidepressants ('mood elevators') such as desipramine (Norpra-

min) and protriptyline (Vivactil), antihistamines; ascorbic acid (Vitamin C); beta blockers such as atenolol (Tenormin), labetalol (Normodyne), metoprolol (Lopressor, Toprol XL), nadolol (Corgard), and propranolol (Inderal); chlorpromazine (Thorazine); diuretics ('water pills') such as acetazolamide (Diamox); furazolidone (Furoxone); guanethidine (Ismelin); haloperidol (Haldol); lithium (Lithobid, Eskalith); medications for high blood pressure; medications for seizures such as ethosuximide (Zarontin), phenobarbital (Luminal, Solfoton), and phenytoin (Dilantin); meperidine (Demerol); methenamine (Hiprex, Urex); propoxyphene (Darvon, Darvon-N); reserpine (Serpalan); sodium bicarbonate (Arm and Hammer Baking Soda, Soda Mint); and sodium phosphate. Your doctor may need to change the doses of your medications or monitor you carefully for side effects.

- tell your doctor what nutritional supplements you are taking, especially glutamic acid (L-glutamine).
- tell your doctor if you have glaucoma (an eye disease), hyperthyroidism (a condition in which you have too much thyroid hormone in your body) or feelings of anxiety, tension, or agitation. Your doctor may tell you not to take dextroamphetamine.
- tell your doctor if anyone in your family has or has ever had an irregular heartbeat or has died suddenly. Also tell your doctor if you have recently had a heart attack and if you have or have ever had a heart defect, high blood pressure, an irregular heartbeat, heart or blood vessel disease, or other heart problems. Your doctor will probably examine you to see if your heart and blood vessels are healthy. Your doctor may tell you not to take dextroamphetamine and amphetamine if you have a heart condition or if there is a high risk that you may develop a heart condition.
- tell your doctor if you or anyone in your family has or has ever had depression, bipolar disorder (mood that changes from depressed to abnormally excited), or mania (frenzied, abnormally excited mood), facial or motor tics (repeated uncontrollable movements), verbal tics (repetition of sounds or words that is hard to control) or Tourette's syndrome (a condition characterized by the need to perform repeated motions or to repeat sounds or words), or has thought about or attempted suicide. Also tell your doctor if you have or have ever had mental illness or seizures. If your child is taking dextroamphetamine to treat ADHD, tell your child's doctor if your child has recently experienced unusual stress.
- tell your doctor if you are pregnant or plan to become pregnant. If you become pregnant while taking dextroamphetamine, call your doctor. Do not breastfeed while you are taking dextroamphetamine.
- you should know that dextroamphetamine may make it difficult for you to perform activities that require alertness or physical coordination. Do not drive a car or operate machinery until you know how this medication affects you.

- you should know that dextroamphetamine should be used as part of a total treatment program for ADHD, which may include counseling and special education. Make sure to follow all of your doctor's and/or therapist's instructions.

What special dietary instructions should I follow?

Talk to your doctor about drinking fruit juice while taking this medicine.

What should I do if I forget to take a dose?

Take the missed dose as soon as you remember it. However, if it is almost time for the next dose or if it is close to your bedtime, skip the missed dose and continue your regular dosing schedule. Do not take a double dose to make up for a missed one.

What side effects can this medicine cause?

Dextroamphetamine may cause side effects. Tell your doctor if any of these symptoms are severe or do not go away:

- restlessness
- difficulty falling asleep or staying asleep
- headache
- uncontrollable shaking of a part of your body
- dry mouth
- unpleasant taste
- diarrhea
- constipation
- loss of appetite
- weight loss
- changes in sex drive or ability

Some side effects can be serious. If you experience any of the following symptoms, call your doctor immediately:

- fast or pounding heartbeat
- shortness of breath
- chest pain
- excessive tiredness
- slow or difficult speech
- dizziness or faintness
- weakness or numbness of an arm or leg
- seizures
- mood changes
- psychosis (loss of contact with reality)
- hallucinating (seeing things or hearing voices that do not exist)
- mania (frenzied or abnormally excited mood)
- aggressive or hostile behavior
- abnormal movements
- verbal tics
- changes in vision or blurred vision
- hives

Dextroamphetamine may slow children's growth or weight gain. Your child's doctor will watch his or her growth carefully. Talk to your child's doctor if you have concerns about your child's growth or weight gain while he or she is taking this medication. Talk to your child's doctor about the risks of giving dextroamphetamine to your child.

Dextroamphetamine may cause sudden death in children and teenagers with heart defects or serious heart problems. Dextroamphetamine may cause sudden death, heart attack, or stroke in adults, especially adults who have heart defects or other serious heart problems. Talk to your doctor about the risks of taking dextroamphetamine.

Dextroamphetamine may cause other side effects. Call your doctor if you have any unusual problems while taking this medication.

If you experience a serious side effect, you or your doctor may send a report to the Food and Drug Administration's (FDA) MedWatch Adverse Event Reporting program online [at http://www.fda.gov/MedWatch/index.html] or by phone [1-800-332-1088].

What storage conditions are needed for this medicine?

Keep this medication in the container it came in, tightly closed, and out of reach of children. Store it at room temperature and away from excess heat and moisture (not in the bathroom). Throw away any medication that is outdated or no longer needed. Talk to your pharmacist about the proper disposal of your medication.

What should I do in case of overdose?

In case of overdose, call your local poison control center at 1-800-222-1222. If the victim has collapsed or is not breathing, call local emergency services at 911.

Symptoms of overdose may include:

- restlessness
- uncontrollable shaking of a part of your body
- dark red or cola colored urine
- muscle weakness or aching
- tiredness or weakness
- fast breathing
- fever
- confusion
- aggressive behavior
- hallucinations (seeing things or hearing voices that do not exist)
- panic
- depression
- irregular heartbeat
- dizziness
- fainting
- blurred vision
- upset stomach
- vomiting
- diarrhea
- stomach cramps
- seizures
- coma (loss of consciousness for a period of time)

What other information should I know?

Keep all appointments with your doctor.

Before having any laboratory test, tell your doctor and the laboratory personnel that you are taking dextroamphetamine.

This prescription is not refillable. Be sure to schedule appointments with your doctor on a regular basis so you do not run out of medication.

Dosage Facts
For Informational Purposes

Caution: Do not change your dose, how often you take your medication, or the length of time you are to take it without first talking to your healthcare provider.

The following dosage information was written using medical language for doctors and other healthcare professionals and is provided here for you to check your dosage. The dosage of this drug may differ for different patients. Therefore, always follow your doctor's instructions or the directions on the label. Contact your healthcare provider or pharmacist if you have any questions about the specific dosage of your medication after reviewing this information.

General Dosage Information

Dosages of dextroamphetamine sulfate alone and of total amphetamine base equivalence are the same.

Dextroamphetamine sulfate extended-release capsules can be substituted for their respective conventional short-acting preparations if less-frequent daily dosing is desirable.

Adjust dosage according to individual response and tolerance; the smallest dose required to produce the desired response should always be used.

When possible, therapy should be interrupted occasionally to determine if there is a recurrence of behavioral symptoms sufficient to require continued treatment.

Pediatric Patients

Attention Deficit Hyperactivity Disorder

Dosage titration usually requires 2–4 weeks.

Conventional Tablets (Dexedrine® and Generic Equivalents)

ORAL:
- Dosing in pediatric patients may begin with once-daily administration in the early morning, adding a noon dose if the effect does not last throughout the school day. Increasing the morning dose may extend its duration. A third dose may be added at around 4 p.m. if necessary.
- Children 3–5 years of age: Initially, 2.5 mg daily; the daily dosage is increased in 2.5-mg increments at weekly intervals until the optimum response is attained.
- Children ≥6 years of age: Initially, 5 mg once or twice daily; the daily dosage is increased in 5-mg increments at weekly intervals until the optimum response is attained. Total daily dosage rarely should exceed 40 mg.

Extended-release Capsules (Dexedrine® Spansules® and Generic Equivalents)

ORAL:
- Total daily dosage of dextroamphetamine sulfate is the same for extended-release capsules (Dexedrine® Spansules®) and conventional tablets (Dexedrine®).
- Although extended-release capsules usually are administered once daily, some patients may benefit from dividing the dosage into 2 doses daily.
- Children 3–5 years of age: Dosage must be initiated and titrated with conventional tablets in this age group. Can substitute with once-daily dosing *only* when the total daily dose is divisible by 5 mg.
- Children ≥6 years of age: Initially, 5 or 10 mg once daily; the daily dosage is increased in 5-mg increments at weekly intervals until the optimum response is attained. Total daily dosage rarely should exceed 40 mg.

Narcolepsy

When intolerable adverse effects occur (e.g., insomnia, anorexia), dosage should be reduced.

Conventional Tablets (Dexedrine and Generic Equivalents)

ORAL:
- Children 6–12 years of age: Initially, 5 mg daily; daily dosage is increased in 5-mg increments at weekly intervals until the optimum response is attained.
- Children ≥12 years of age: Initially, 10 mg daily; daily dosage is increased in 10-mg increments at weekly intervals until the optimum response is attained.
- Maintenance: Usually, 5–60 mg daily, depending on patient age and response, given in divided doses.

Extended-release Capsules (Dexedrine® Spansules® and Generic Equivalents)

ORAL:
- Total daily dosage of dextroamphetamine sulfate is the same for extended-release capsules (Dexedrine® Spansules®) and conventional tablets (Dexedrine®).
- Although extended-release capsules usually are administered once daily, some patients may benefit from dividing the dosage into 2 doses daily.
- Children 6–12 years of age: Initially, 5 mg once daily; daily dosage is increased in 5-mg increments at weekly intervals until the optimum response is attained.
- Children ≥12 years of age: Initially, 10 mg once daily; daily dosage is increased in 10-mg increments at weekly intervals until the optimum response is attained.
- Maintenance: Usually, 5–60 mg once daily, depending on patient age and response, given in divided doses.

Adult Patients

Attention Deficit Hyperactivity Disorder
Conventional Tablets (Dexedrine® and Generic Equivalents)

Dosage titration usually requires 2–4 weeks.

ORAL:
- Initially, 5 mg once or twice daily; the daily dosage is increased in 5- to 10-mg increments at weekly intervals until the optimum response is attained. Total daily dosage rarely should exceed 40 mg.

Extended-release Capsules (Dexedrine® Spansules® and Generic Equivalents)

ORAL:

- Total daily dosage of dextroamphetamine sulfate is the same for extended-release capsules (Dexedrine® Spansules®) and conventional tablets (Dexedrine®).
- Although extended-release capsules usually are administered once daily, some patients may benefit from dividing the dosage into 2 doses daily.
- Initially, 5 or 10 mg once daily; the daily dosage is increased in 5-mg increments at weekly intervals until the optimum response is attained. Total daily dosage rarely should exceed 40 mg.

Narcolepsy

When intolerable adverse effects occur (e.g., insomnia, anorexia), dosage should be reduced.

Conventional Tablets (Dexedrine® and Generic Equivalents)

ORAL:

- Initially, 10 mg daily; daily dosage is increased in 10-mg increments at weekly intervals until the optimum response is attained.
- Maintenance: Usually, 5–60 mg daily, depending on response, given in divided doses.

Prescribing Limits

Pediatric Patients

Attention Deficit Hyperactivity Disorder

Excessive dosage can cause pediatric patients to become overfocused on the medication or to appear dull or overly restricted. Rarely, psychotic reactions, mood disturbances, or hallucinations can occur.

Conventional Tablets (Dexedrine® and Generic Equivalents)

ORAL:

- Dosage rarely should exceed a total daily dosage of 40 mg. Individual doses rarely should exceed 10 mg each in children <25 kg.

Extended-release Capsules (Dexedrine® Spansules® and Generic Equivalents)

ORAL:

- Dosage rarely should exceed a total daily dosage of 40 mg. Individual doses rarely should exceed 10 mg each in children <25 kg.

Dextroamphetamine and Amphetamine

(dex troe am fet′ a meen) and (am fet′ a meen)

Brand Name: Adderall®

Important Warning

The combination of dextroamphetamine and amphetamine can be habit-forming. Do not take a larger dose, take it more often, or take it for a longer time than prescribed by your doctor. If you take too much dextroamphetamine and amphetamine you may find that the medication no longer controls your symptoms, you may feel a need to take large amounts of the medication, and you may experience symptoms such as rash, difficulty falling asleep or staying asleep, irritability, hyperactivity, and unusual changes in your personality or behavior. Tell your doctor if you drink or have ever drunk large amounts of alcohol, use or have ever used street drugs, or have overused prescription medications.

Do not stop taking dextroamphetamine and amphetamine without talking to your doctor, especially if you have overused the medication. Your doctor will probably decrease your dose gradually and monitor you carefully during this time. You may develop severe depression and extreme tiredness if you suddenly stop taking dextroamphetamine and amphetamine after overusing it.

Do not let anyone else take your medication. Store dextroamphetamine and amphetamine in a safe place so that no one else can take it accidentally or on purpose. Keep track of how many tablets or capsules are left so you will know if any are missing.

The combination of dextroamphetamine and amphetamine may cause sudden death or serious heart problems, especially if the medication is misused.

Your doctor or pharmacist will give you the manufacturer's patient information sheet (Medication Guide) when you begin treatment with dextroamphetamine and amphetamine and each time you refill your prescription. Read the information carefully and ask your doctor or pharmacist if you have any questions. You can also visit the Food and Drug Administration (FDA) website (http://www.fda.gov/cder) or the manufacturer's website to obtain the Medication Guide.

Why is this medicine prescribed?

The combination of dextroamphetamine and amphetamine is used as part of a treatment program for attention deficit hyperactivity disorder (ADHD; more difficulty focusing, controlling actions, and remaining still or quiet than other people who are the same age). Dextroamphetamine and amphetamine tablets are also used to treat narcolepsy (a sleep disorder that causes excessive daytime sleepiness and sudden attacks of sleep). The combination of dextroamphetamine and amphetamine is in a class of medications called central nervous system stimulants. It works by changing the amounts of certain natural substances in the brain.

How should this medicine be used?

The combination of dextroamphetamine and amphetamine comes as a tablet and an extended-release (long acting) capsule to take by mouth. The tablet is usually taken two to three times daily with or without food. The extended-release capsule is usually taken once daily in the morning with or without food. Dextroamphetamine and amphetamine combination should not be taken in the late afternoon or evening because it may cause difficulty falling asleep or staying asleep. Follow the directions on your prescription label carefully, and ask your doctor or pharmacist to explain any part you do not understand. Take dextroamphetamine and amphetamine exactly as directed.

You may swallow the extended-release capsule whole, or you may open the capsule and sprinkle the entire contents on a teaspoonful of applesauce. Swallow this mixture right away without chewing. Do not store the applesauce/medication mixture for future use, and do not divide the contents of one capsule into more than one dose.

Your doctor will probably start you on a low dose of dextroamphetamine and amphetamine and increase your dose gradually, not more often than once every week.

Your doctor may tell you to stop taking dextroamphetamine and amphetamine from time to time to see if the medication is still needed. Follow these directions carefully.

Are there other uses for this medicine?

The combination of dextroamphetamine and amphetamine should not be used to treat excessive tiredness that is not caused by narcolepsy.

This medication may be prescribed for other conditions; ask your doctor or pharmacist for more information.

What special precautions should I follow?

Before taking dextroamphetamine and amphetamine,
- tell your doctor and pharmacist if you are allergic to amphetamine, dextroamphetamine, or any other medications.
- tell your doctor if you are taking monoamine oxidase (MAO) inhibitors, including isocarboxazid (Marplan), phenelzine (Nardil), selegiline (Eldepryl), and tranylcypromine (Parnate), or if you have stopped taking them during the past 14 days. Your doctor will probably tell you not to take dextroamphetamine and amphetamine until at least 14 days have passed since you last took an MAO inhibitor.
- tell your doctor and pharmacist what other prescription and

nonprescription medications, vitamins, and herbal products you are taking. Be sure to mention any of the following: alpha blockers such as alfuzosin (Uroxatral), doxazosin (Cardura), prazosin (Minipress), tamsulosin (Flomax), and terazosin (Hytrin); antacids; antidepressants ('mood elevators'), antihistamines; ascorbic acid (Vitamin C); beta blockers such as atenolol (Tenormin), labetalol (Normodyne), metoprolol (Lopressor, Toprol XL), nadolol (Corgard), and propranolol (Inderal); chlorpromazine (Thorazine); diuretics ('water pills') such as acetazolamide (Diamox); guanethidine (Ismelin); haloperidol (Haldol); lithium (Lithobid, Eskalith); medications for high blood pressure; certain medications for seizures such as ethosuximide (Zarontin), phenobarbital (Luminal, Solfoton), and phenytoin (Dilantin); meperidine (Demerol); methenamine (Hiprex, Urex); propoxyphene (Darvon, Darvon-N); reserpine (Serpalan); sodium bicarbonate (Arm and Hammer Baking Soda, Soda Mint); and sodium phosphate. Your doctor may need to change the doses of your medications or monitor you carefully for side effects.
- tell your doctor what nutritional supplements you are taking, especially glutamic acid (L-glutamine).
- tell your doctor if you have glaucoma (an eye disease), hyperthyroidism (condition in which there is too much thyroid hormone in the body), or feelings of anxiety, tension, or agitation. Your doctor may tell you not to take dextroamphetamine and amphetamine.
- tell your doctor if anyone in your family has or has ever had an irregular heartbeat or has died suddenly. Also tell your doctor if you have recently had a heart attack and if you have or have ever had a heart defect, high blood pressure, an irregular heartbeat, heart or blood vessel disease, or other heart problems. Your doctor will probably examine you to see if your heart and blood vessels are healthy. Your doctor may tell you not to take dextroamphetamine and amphetamine if you have a heart condition or if there is a high risk that you may develop a heart condition.
- tell your doctor if you or anyone in your family has or has ever had depression, bipolar disorder (mood that changes from depressed to abnormally excited), or mania (frenzied, abnormally excited mood), motor tics (repeated uncontrollable movements), verbal tics (repetition of sounds or words that is hard to control), or Tourette's syndrome (a condition characterized by the need to perform repeated motions or to repeat sounds or words), or has thought about or attempted suicide. Also tell your doctor if you have or have ever had mental illness, seizures, or an abnormal electroencephalogram (EEG; a test that measures electrical activity in the brain).
- tell your doctor if you are pregnant, plan to become pregnant, or are breast-feeding. If you become pregnant while taking dextroamphetamine and amphetamine, call your doctor. You should not breastfeed while you are taking this medication.
- you should know that this medication may make it difficult for you to perform activities that require alertness

or physical coordination. Do not drive a car or operate machinery until you know how this medication affects you.

- you should know that dextroamphetamine and amphetamine should be used as part of a total treatment program for ADHD, which may include counseling and special education. Make sure to follow all of your doctor's and/or therapist's instructions.

What special dietary instructions should I follow?

Talk to your doctor about drinking fruit juice while taking this medicine.

What should I do if I forget to take a dose?

Take the missed dose as soon as you remember it. However, if it is almost time for the next dose, skip the missed dose and continue your regular dosing schedule. Do not take a double dose to make up for a missed one.

What side effects can this medicine cause?

Dextroamphetamine and amphetamine may cause side effects. Tell your doctor if any of these symptoms are severe or do not go away:

- nervousness
- restlessness
- difficulty falling asleep or staying asleep
- uncontrollable shaking of a part of the body
- headache
- changes in sex drive or ability
- dry mouth
- stomach pain
- nausea
- vomiting
- diarrhea
- constipation
- loss of appetite
- weight loss
- bad taste in mouth

Some side effects can be serious. If you experience any of the following symptoms, call your doctor immediately:

- fast or pounding heartbeat
- shortness of breath
- chest pain
- excessive tiredness
- slow or difficult speech
- dizziness or faintness
- weakness or numbness of an arm or leg
- seizures
- mood changes
- motor tics or verbal tics
- psychosis (loss of contact with reality)
- hallucinating (seeing things or hearing voices that do not exist)
- mania (frenzied or abnormally excited mood)
- aggressive or hostile behavior

- changes in vision or blurred vision
- fever
- blisters or rash
- hives
- itching
- swelling of the eyes, face, tongue, or throat
- difficulty breathing or swallowing
- hoarseness

Dextroamphetamine and amphetamine may cause sudden death in children and teenagers who have heart defects or serious heart problems. This medication also may cause sudden death, heart attack or stroke in adults, especially adults with heart defects or serious heart problems. Talk to your doctor about the risks of taking this medication.

Dextroamphetamine and amphetamine may slow children's growth or weight gain. Your child's doctor will watch his or her growth carefully. Talk to your child's doctor if you have concerns about your child's growth or weight gain while he or she is taking this medication. Talk to your child's doctor about the risks of giving dextroamphetamine and amphetamine to your child.

If you experience a serious side effect, you or your doctor may send a report to the Food and Drug Administration's (FDA) MedWatch Adverse Event Reporting program online [at http://www.fda.gov/MedWatch/index.html] or by phone [1-800-332-1088].

What storage conditions are needed for this medicine?

Keep this medication in the container it came in, tightly closed, and out of reach of children. Store it at room temperature, away from light and excess heat and moisture (not in the bathroom). Throw away any medication that is outdated or no longer needed. Talk to your pharmacist about the proper disposal of your medication.

What should I do in case of overdose?

In case of overdose, call your local poison control center at 1-800-222-1222. If the victim has collapsed or is not breathing, call local emergency services at 911.

Symptoms of overdose may include:

- restlessness
- confusion
- aggressive behavior
- feelings of panic
- hallucination (seeing things or hearing voices that do not exist)
- fast breathing
- shaking hands that you cannot control
- fever
- dark red or cola-colored urine
- muscle weakness or aching
- tirednessor weakness
- depression
- fast or irregular heartbeat
- fainting

- dizziness
- blurred vision
- upset stomach
- vomiting
- diarrhea
- seizures
- coma (loss of consciousness for a period of time)

What other information should I know?

Keep all your appointments with your doctor and the laboratory. Your doctor may order certain lab tests to determine your response to dextroamphetamine and amphetamine.

Before having any laboratory test, tell your doctor and the laboratory personnel that you are taking dextroamphetamine and amphetamine.

This prescription is not refillable. Be sure to schedule appointments with your doctor on a regular basis so that you do not run out of medication.

Dosage Facts

For Informational Purposes

Caution: Do not change your dose, how often you take your medication, or the length of time you are to take it without first talking to your healthcare provider.

The following dosage information was written using medical language for doctors and other healthcare professionals and is provided here for you to check your dosage. The dosage of this drug may differ for different patients. Therefore, always follow your doctor's instructions or the directions on the label. Contact your healthcare provider or pharmacist if you have any questions about the specific dosage of your medication after reviewing this information.

General Dosage Information

Fixed-combination extended-release capsules containing various salts of amphetamine and dextroamphetamine can be substituted for their respective conventional short-acting preparations if less-frequent daily dosing is desirable.

Dosage of fixed-combination preparations containing various salts of amphetamine and dextroamphetamine is expressed as total amphetamine base equivalence.

Adjust dosage according to individual response and tolerance; the smallest dose required to produce the desired response should always be used.

When possible, therapy should be interrupted occasionally to determine if there is a recurrence of behavioral symptoms sufficient to require continued treatment.

Pediatric Patients

Attention Deficit Hyperactivity Disorder

Dosage titration usually requires 2–4 weeks.

Extended-release Capsules (Adderall XR®)

ORAL:
- Children 6–12 years of age: Initially, 10 mg once daily; daily dosage may be increased in 5- or 10-mg increments at weekly

intervals to a maximum dosage of 30 mg daily. Alternatively, initiate with 5 mg once daily when lower initial dosage is appropriate.
- Adolescents 13–17 years of age: Initially, 10 mg once daily. Increase to 20 mg once daily after 1 week if symptoms not adequately controlled. No evidence that dosages >20 mg daily provide any additional benefit.
- When switching from conventional tablets to extended-release capsules, the total daily dosage may remain the same but may be given once daily.

Adult Patients

Attention Deficit Hyperactivity Disorder
Extended-release Capsules (Adderall XR®)

ORAL:
- 20 mg once daily as initial therapy or when switching from other drugs. No evidence that dosages >20 mg daily provide any additional benefit.
- When switching from conventional tablets to extended-release capsules, the total daily dosage may remain the same but may be given once daily.

Prescribing Limits

Pediatric Patients

Attention Deficit Hyperactivity Disorder

Excessive dosage can cause pediatric patients to become overfocused on the medication or to appear dull or overly restricted. Rarely, psychotic reactions, mood disturbances, or hallucinations can occur.

Extended-release Capsules (Adderall XR®)

ORAL:
- Children 6–12 years of age: Dosages >30 mg daily have not been studied systematically.
- Adolescents 13–17 years of age: Dosages up to 60 mg daily have been evaluated in clinical studies; however, no evidence that dosages >20 mg daily provide any additional benefit.
- Long-term use (>3 weeks in children or >4 weeks in adolescents) has not been studied systematically. If used for long-term therapy, periodically reevaluate the usefulness of the drug.

Adult Patients

Attention Deficit Hyperactivity Disorder
Extended-release Capsules (Adderall XR®)

ORAL:
- Dosages up to 60 mg daily have been evaluated in clinical studies; however, no evidence that dosages >20 mg daily provide any additional benefit.
- Long-term use (>4 weeks) has not been studied systematically. If used for long-term therapy, periodically reevaluate the usefulness of the drug.

Special Populations

Hepatic Impairment
- No specific hepatic dosage recommendations.
Renal Impairment
- No specific renal dosage recommendations.
Geriatric Patients
- No specific geriatric dosage recommendations.

Dextromethorphan

(dex troe meth or' fan)

Brand Name: Benylin® Adult Formula Cough Suppressant, Benylin® Pediatric Cough Suppressant, Codimal® DM Syrup as a combination product containing Dextromethorphan Hydrobromide, Phenylephrine Hydrochloride, and Pyrilamine Maleate, Cydec®-DM Drops as a combination product containing Dextromethorphan Hydrobromide, Carbinoxamine Maleate, and Pseudoephedrine Hydrochloride, Delsym®, Hold® DM, Pertussin® DM Extra Strength, Robitussin® CoughGels®, Robitussin® Honey Cough Suppressant, Robitussin® Maximum Strength Cough Suppressant, Robitussin® Pediatric Cough Suppressant, Simply Cough®, Sucrets® 8 Hour Cough Suppressant, Triaminic® Cough Softchews®, Vicks® 44 Cough Relief

Also available generically.

Why is this medicine prescribed?

Dextromethorphan, an antitussive, is used to relieve a nonproductive cough caused by a cold, the flu, or other conditions.

This medication is sometimes prescribed for other uses; ask your doctor or pharmacist for more information.

How should this medicine be used?

Dextromethorphan comes as a liquid or as a lozenge to take by mouth. It is usually taken every 4-8 hours as needed. Do not take more than 120 mg of dextromethorphan in a 24-hour period. Refer to the package or prescription label to determine the amount contained in each dose. The lozenge should dissolve slowly in your mouth. Drink plenty of water after taking a dose. Follow the directions on the package or prescription label carefully, and ask your doctor or pharmacist to explain any part you do not understand.

Take dextromethorphan exactly as directed. Do not take a larger dose, take it more often, or for a longer period than the label or your doctor tells you to.

What special precautions should I follow?

Before taking dextromethorphan,

- tell your doctor and pharmacist if you are allergic to dextromethorphan or any other drugs.
- tell your doctor and pharmacist what prescription and nonprescription medications you are taking, especially MAO inhibitors (Marplan [isocarboxazid]; Parnate [tranylcypromine]; Nardil [phenelzine]); other cough, cold, and allergy products; and vitamins.
- tell your doctor if you have or have ever had asthma, emphysema, or lung disease.
- tell your doctor if you are pregnant, plan to become

pregnant, or are breast-feeding. If you become pregnant while taking dextromethorphan, call your doctor.
- this medicine should not be used in children below the age of 2 years.

What should I do if I forget to take a dose?

Dextromethorphan is usually taken as needed. If your doctor has told you to take dextromethorphan regularly, take the missed dose as soon as you remember it. However, if it is almost time for the next dose, skip the missed dose and continue your regular dosing schedule. Do not take a double dose to make up for a missed one.

What side effects can this medicine cause?

Dextromethorphan may cause side effects. Tell your doctor if any of these symptoms are severe or do not go away:

- dizziness
- lightheadedness
- drowsiness
- nervousness
- restlessness
- upset stomach
- vomiting
- stomach pain

If you experience any of the following symptoms, call your doctor immediately:

- rash
- high fever
- persistent headache
- difficulty breathing
- mood changes
- slurred speech

If you experience a serious side effect, you or your doctor may send a report to the Food and Drug Administration's (FDA) MedWatch Adverse Event Reporting program online [at http://www.fda.gov/MedWatch/index.html] or by phone [1-800-332-1088].

What storage conditions are needed for this medicine?

Keep this medication in the container it came in, tightly closed, and out of reach of children. Store it at room temperature and away from excess heat and moisture (not in the bathroom). Throw away any medication that is outdated or no longer needed. Talk to your pharmacist about the proper disposal of your medication.

What should I do in case of overdose?

In case of overdose, call your local poison control center at 1-800-222-1222. If the victim has collapsed or is not breathing, call local emergency services at 911.

What other information should I know?

Keep all appointments with your doctor and the laboratory.

Do not let anyone else take your medication. Ask your

pharmacist any questions you have about refilling your prescription.

Dosage Facts
For Informational Purposes

Caution: Do not change your dose, how often you take your medication, or the length of time you are to take it without first talking to your healthcare provider.

The following dosage information was written using medical language for doctors and other healthcare professionals and is provided here for you to check your dosage. The dosage of this drug may differ for different patients. Therefore, always follow your doctor's instructions or the directions on the label. Contact your healthcare provider or pharmacist if you have any questions about the specific dosage of your medication after reviewing this information.

General Dosage Information

Dosage of dextromethorphan hydrobromide and dextromethorphan polistirex is expressed in terms of dextromethorphan hydrobromide.

Pediatric Patients

Cough
Immediate-release Preparations

ORAL:
- Children <2 years of age: dosage must be individualized.
- Children 2 to <6 years of age: 2.5–5 mg every 4 hours or 7.5 mg every 6–8 hours, not to exceed 30 mg daily, or as directed by a clinician.
- Children 6 to <12 years of age: 5–10 mg every 4 hours or 15 mg every 6–8 hours, not to exceed 60 mg daily, or as directed by a clinician.
- Children ≥12 years of age: 10–20 mg every 4 hours or 30 mg every 6–8 hours, not to exceed 120 mg daily, or as directed by a clinician.

Extended-release Oral Suspension (containing polistirex)

ORAL:
- Children 2 to <6 years of age: 15 mg twice daily.
- Children 6 to <12 years of age: 30 mg twice daily
- Children ≥12 years of age: 60 mg twice daily.

Adult Patients

Cough
Immediate-release Preparations

ORAL:
- 10–20 mg every 4 hours or 30 mg every 6–8 hours, not to exceed 120 mg daily, or as directed by a clinician.

Extended-release Oral Suspension (containing polistirex)

ORAL:
- 60 mg twice daily.

Prescribing Limits
Pediatric Patients

Cough

ORAL:
- Children 2 to <6 years of age: Maximum 30 mg daily, or as directed by a clinician.
- Children 6 to <12 years of age: Maximum 60 mg daily, or as directed by a clinician.
- Children ≥12 years of age: Maximum 120 mg daily, or as directed by a clinician.

Adult Patients

Cough

ORAL:
- Maximum 120 mg daily, or as directed by a clinician.

Special Populations

Hepatic Impairment
- No specific dosage recommendations for hepatic impairment.

Renal Impairment
- No specific dosage recommendations for renal impairment.

Geriatric Patients
- No specific geriatric dosage recommendations.

Diazepam

(dye az' e pam)

Brand Name: Diazepam Intensol®, Valium®
Also available generically.

Why is this medicine prescribed?

Diazepam is used to relieve anxiety, muscle spasms, and seizures and to control agitation caused by alcohol withdrawal.

How should this medicine be used?

Diazepam comes as a tablet, extended-release (long-acting) capsule, and concentrate (liquid) to take by mouth. Do not open, chew, or crush the extended-release capsules; swallow them whole. It usually is taken one to four times a day and may be taken with or without food. Follow the directions on your prescription label carefully, and ask your doctor or pharmacist to explain any part you do not understand. Take diazepam exactly as directed.

Diazepam concentrate (liquid) comes with a specially marked dropper for measuring the dose. Ask your pharmacist to show you how to use the dropper. Dilute the concentrate in water, juice, or carbonated beverages just before taking it. It also may be mixed with applesauce or pudding just before taking the dose.

Diazepam can be habit-forming. Do not take a larger

dose, take it more often, or for a longer time than your doctor tells you to. Tolerance may develop with long-term or excessive use, making the drug less effective. This medication must be taken regularly to be effective. Do not skip doses even if you feel that you do not need them. Do not take diazepam for more than 4 months or stop taking this medication without talking to your doctor. Stopping the drug suddenly can worsen your condition and cause withdrawal symptoms (anxiousness, sleeplessness, and irritability). Your doctor probably will decrease your dose gradually.

Are there other uses for this medicine?

Diazepam is also used to treat irritable bowel syndrome and panic attacks. Talk to your doctor about the possible risks of using this drug for your condition.

This medication is sometimes prescribed for other uses; ask your doctor or pharmacist for more information.

What special precautions should I follow?

Before taking diazepam,

- tell your doctor and pharmacist if you are allergic to diazepam, alprazolam (Xanax), chlordiazepoxide (Librium, Librax), clonazepam (Klonopin), clorazepate (Tranxene), estazolam (ProSom), flurazepam (Dalmane), lorazepam (Ativan), oxazepam (Serax), prazepam (Centrax), temazepam (Restoril), triazolam (Halcion), or any other drugs.
- tell your doctor and pharmacist what prescription and nonprescription medications you are taking, especially antihistamines; cimetadine (Tagamet); digoxin (Lanoxin); disulfiram (Antabuse); fluoxetine (Prozac); isoniazide (INH, Laniazid, Nydrazid); ketoconazole (Nizoral); levodopa (Larodopa, Sinemet); medications for depression, seizures, pain, Parkinson's disease, asthma, colds, or allergies; metoprolol (Lopressor, Toprol XL); muscle relaxants; oral contraceptives; probenecid (Benemid); propoxyphene (Darvon); propranolol (Inderal); ranitidine (Zantac); rifampin (Rifadin); sedatives; sleeping pills; theophylline (Theo-Dur); tranquilizers; valproic acid (Depakene); and vitamins. These medications may add to the drowsiness caused by diazepam.
- if you use antacids, take diazepam first, then wait 1 hour before taking the antacid.
- tell your doctor if you have or have ever had glaucoma; seizures; or lung, heart, or liver disease.
- tell your doctor if you are pregnant, plan to become pregnant, or are breast-feeding. If you become pregnant while taking diazepam, call your doctor immediately.
- if you are having surgery, including dental surgery, tell the doctor or dentist that you are taking diazepam.
- you should know that this drug may make you drowsy. Do not drive a car or operate machinery until you know how this drug affects you.
- remember that alcohol can add to the drowsiness caused by this drug.
- tell your doctor if you use tobacco products. Cigarette smoking may decrease the effectiveness of this drug.

What should I do if I forget to take a dose?

If you take several doses per day and miss a dose, skip the missed dose and continue your regular dosing schedule. Do not take a double dose to make up for a missed one.

What side effects can this medicine cause?

Side effects from diazepam are common and include:
- drowsiness
- dizziness
- tiredness
- weakness
- dry mouth
- diarrhea
- upset stomach
- changes in appetite

Tell your doctor if any of these symptoms are severe or do not go away:
- restlessness or excitement
- constipation
- difficulty urinating
- frequent urination
- blurred vision
- changes in sex drive or ability

If you experience any of the following symptoms, call your doctor immediately:
- seizures
- shuffling walk
- persistent, fine tremor or inability to sit still
- fever
- difficulty breathing or swallowing
- severe skin rash
- yellowing of the skin or eyes
- irregular heartbeat

If you experience a serious side effect, you or your doctor may send a report to the Food and Drug Administration's (FDA) MedWatch Adverse Event Reporting program online [at http://www.fda.gov/MedWatch/index.html] or by phone [1-800-332-1088].

What storage conditions are needed for this medicine?

Keep this medication in the container it came in, tightly closed, and out of reach of children. Store it at room temperature and away from excess heat and moisture (not in the bathroom). Throw away any medication that is outdated or no longer needed. Talk to your pharmacist about the proper disposal of your medication.

What should I do in case of overdose?

In case of overdose, call your local poison control center at 1-800-222-1222. If the victim has collapsed or is not breathing, call local emergency services at 911.

What other information should I know?

Keep all appointments with your doctor and the laboratory. Your doctor will order certain lab tests to check your response to diazepam.

Diazepam can cause false results in urine tests for sugar using Clinistix and Diastix. Diabetic patients should use TesTape to test their urine for sugar.

If you are taking diazepam to control seizures and have an increase in their frequency or severity, call your doctor. Your dose may need to be adjusted. If you use diazepam for seizures, carry identification (Medic Alert) stating that you have epilepsy and that you are taking diazepam.

Do not let anyone else take your medication. Ask your pharmacist any questions you have about refilling your prescription.

Dosage Facts
For Informational Purposes

Caution: Do not change your dose, how often you take your medication, or the length of time you are to take it without first talking to your healthcare provider.

The following dosage information was written using medical language for doctors and other healthcare professionals and is provided here for you to check your dosage. The dosage of this drug may differ for different patients. Therefore, always follow your doctor's instructions or the directions on the label. Contact your healthcare provider or pharmacist if you have any questions about the specific dosage of your medication after reviewing this information.

Pediatric Patients

Anxiety Disorders

ORAL:
- Children ≥6 months of age: Initially, 1–2.5 mg 3 or 4 times daily. Alternatively, 0.12–0.8 mg/kg or 3.5–24 mg/m² in 3 or 4 divided doses daily. Increase dosage gradually as needed and tolerated.

Seizure Disorders

ORAL:
- 6–15 mg daily (occasionally up to 30 mg daily) in divided doses has been used.

Skeletal Muscle Spasticity

ORAL:
- 0.12–0.8 mg/kg in 3 or 4 divided doses daily.

Adult Patients

Anxiety Disorders

ORAL:
- 2–10 mg 2–4 times daily, depending on the severity of the symptoms.

Alcohol Withdrawal

ORAL:
- 10 mg 3 or 4 times during the first 24 hours, followed by 5 mg 3 or 4 times daily as needed.

Seizure Disorders

ORAL:
- 2–10 mg 2–4 times daily.

Skeletal Muscle Spasticity

ORAL:
- 2–10 mg 2–4 times daily.

Night Terrors†

ORAL:
- Dosages of 5–20 mg at bedtime have been used.

Special Populations

Hepatic Impairment
- Reduce dosage; use the smallest effective dose to avoid oversedation.

Renal Impairment
- Use the smallest effective dose to avoid oversedation.

Geriatric Patients

Oral
- Initially, 2–2.5 mg once or twice daily. Increase dosage gradually as needed and tolerated.

Other Populations
- Use the smallest effective dosage in debilitated patient and patients with low serum albumin concentrations. In debilitated patients, observe maximum geriatric dosages.

† Use is not currently included in the labeling approved by the US Food and Drug Administration.

Diazepam Rectal

(dye az′ e pam)

Brand Name: Diastat®
Also available generically.

Why is this medicine prescribed?

Diazepam rectal is used in emergency situations to stop cluster seizures (episodes of increased seizure activity) in people who are taking other medications to treat epilepsy (seizures). Diazepam rectal is in a class of medications called benzodiazepines. It works by calming abnormal overactivity in the brain.

How should this medicine be used?

Diazepam comes as a gel to instill rectally using a prefilled syringe with a special plastic tip. Follow the directions on your prescription label carefully, and ask your doctor or pharmacist to explain any part you do not understand.

Before diazepam rectal gel is prescribed, the doctor will talk to your caregiver about how to recognize signs of the type of seizure activity that should be treated with this medication. Your caregiver will also be taught how to administer the rectal gel.

If used regularly, diazepam may be habit forming. Do not use a larger dose than your doctor tells you to. Diazepam rectal gel is not meant to be used on a daily basis. Diazepam rectal gel should not be used more than five times a month or more often than every 5 days. If you or your caregiver think that you need diazepam rectal more often than this, talk to your doctor.

Directions for the caregiver to administer the rectal gel:

1. Put the person having seizures on his/her side in a place where he/she cannot fall.
2. Remove the protective cover from the syringe by pushing it up with your thumb and then pulling it off.
3. Put lubricating jelly on the rectal tip.
4. Turn the person on his/her side facing you, bend his/her upper leg forward, and separate the his/her buttocks to expose the rectum.
5. Gently insert the syringe tip into the rectum until the rim is snug against the rectal opening.
6. Slowly count to 3 while pushing in the plunger until it stops.
7. Slowly count to 3 again, and then remove the syringe from the rectum.
8. Hold the buttocks together so the gel doesn't leak from the rectum, and slowly count to 3 before letting go.
9. Keep the person on his/her side. Take note of what time diazepam rectal gel was given, and continue to watch the person.

After administering the rectal gel, the caregiver should watch the person with seizures carefully. If any of the following occur, call 911:

- seizures continue for 15 minutes after diazepam rectal gel was given (or follow the doctor's instructions).
- the seizures seem different or worse than usual.
- you are worried about how often seizures are happening.
- you are worried about the skin color or breathing of the person with seizures.
- the person is having unusual or serious problems.

Ask your pharmacist or doctor for a copy of the manufacturer's administration instructions.

Are there other uses for this medicine?

This medication may be prescribed for other uses; ask your doctor or pharmacist for more information.

What special precautions should I follow?

Before using diazepam rectal gel,

- tell your doctor and pharmacist if you are allergic to diazepam (Valium) or any other medications.
- tell your doctor and pharmacist what prescription and non-prescription medications, vitamins, and nutritional supplements you are taking or plan to take. Be sure to mention any of the following: amiodarone (Cordarone, Pacerone); antidepressants ('mood elevators') including fluoxetine (Prozac, Sarafem), fluvoxamine (Luvox), imipramine (Tofranil), nefazodone, sertraline (Zoloft), and tranylcypromine (Parnate); antihistamines; aprepitant (Emend); carbamazepine (Carbatrol, Epitol, Tegretol); certain antifungals such as clotrimazole (Lotrimin), fluconazole (Diflucan), griseofulvin (Fulvicin, Grifulvin, Gris-PEG), itraconazole (Sporanox), ketoconazole (Nizoral), and voriconazole (Vfend); cimetidine (Tagamet); clarithromycin (Biaxin, in Prevpac); cyclosporine (Neoral, Sandimmune); delavirdine (Rescriptor); dexamethasone (Decadron, Dexpak); diltiazem (Cardizem, Dilacor, Tiazac, others); efavirenz (Sustiva); erythromycin (E.E.S., E-Mycin, Erythrocin); HIV protease inhibitors including atazanavir (Reyataz), indinavir (Crixivan), lopinavir (in Kaletra), nelfinavir (Viracept), ritonavir (Norvir, in Kaletra), and saquinavir (Fortovase, Invirase); hormonal contraceptives (birth control pills, rings, and patches); lansoprazole (Prevacid); lovastatin (Advicor, Altocor, Mevacor); modafinil (Provigil); medications for anxiety, mental illness, nausea, or pain; nevirapine (Viramune); omeprazole (Prilosec); paclitaxel (Taxol); phenobarbital; phenytoin (Dilantin, Phenytek); propranolol (Inderal); quinidine (Quinidex); rifabutin (Mycobutin); rifampin (Rifadin, Rimactane, in Rifamate); ritonavir (Norvir, in Kaletra); sedatives; sleeping pills; theophylline (Theo-Dur, Theo-24); ticlopidine (Ticlid); tranquilizers; troleandomycin (TAO); valproate (Depacon, Depakene, Depakote); verapamil (Calan, Covera, Isoptin, Verelan); warfarin (Coumadin); and zafirlukast (Accolate). Your doctor may need to change the doses of your medications or monitor you carefully for side effects.
- tell your doctor what herbal products you are taking, especially St. John's wort.
- tell your doctor if you drink large amounts of alcohol or use or have used street drugs and if you have or have ever had glaucoma, lung problems such as asthma or pneumonia, or liver or kidney disease.
- tell your doctor if you are pregnant, plan to become pregnant, or are breast-feeding. If you become pregnant while using diazepam rectal gel, call your doctor.
- you should know that diazepam rectal gel may make you drowsy. Do not drive a car, operate machinery, or ride a bicycle until the effects of diazepam rectal gel have passed.
- remember that alcohol can add to the drowsiness caused by this medication.

What special dietary instructions should I follow?

Talk to your doctor about eating grapefruit and drinking grapefruit juice while taking this medicine.

What side effects can this medicine cause?

Diazepam rectal gel may cause side effects. Tell your doctor if any of these symptoms are severe or do not go away:

- drowsiness
- dizziness
- headache
- pain

- stomach pain
- nervousness
- flushing
- diarrhea
- unsteadiness
- abnormal 'high' mood
- lack of coordination
- runny nose
- problems falling asleep or staying asleep

Some side effects can be serious. The following symptoms are uncommon, but if you experience any of them, call your doctor immediately:

- rash
- trouble breathing
- overexcitement
- hallucinating (seeing things or hearing voices that do not exist)
- rage

Diazepam rectal gel may cause other side effects. Call your doctor if you have any unusual problems while taking this medication.

If you experience a serious side effect, you or your doctor may send a report to the Food and Drug Administration's (FDA) MedWatch Adverse Event Reporting program online [at http://www.fda.gov/MedWatch/index.html] or by phone [1-800-332-1088].

What storage conditions are needed for this medicine?

Keep this medication in the container it came in, tightly closed, and out of reach of children. Store it at room temperature and away from excess heat and moisture (not in the bathroom). Throw away any medication that is outdated or no longer needed. Talk to your pharmacist about the proper disposal of your medication.

What should I do in case of overdose?

In case of overdose, call your local poison control center at 1-800-222-1222. If the victim has collapsed or is not breathing, call local emergency services at 911.

Symptoms of overdose may include:

- drowsiness
- confusion
- coma
- slow reflexes

What other information should I know?

Keep all appointments with your doctor. Your doctor will need to examine you about every 6 months to check if your dose of diazepam rectal should be changed.

If you have symptoms that are different from your usual seizures, you or your caregiver should call your doctor immediately.

Do not let anyone else take your medication. Ask your pharmacist any questions you have about refilling your prescription.

Dosage Facts
For Informational Purposes

Caution: Do not change your dose, how often you take your medication, or the length of time you are to take it without first talking to your healthcare provider.

The following dosage information was written using medical language for doctors and other healthcare professionals and is provided here for you to check your dosage. The dosage of this drug may differ for different patients. Therefore, always follow your doctor's instructions or the directions on the label. Contact your healthcare provider or pharmacist if you have any questions about the specific dosage of your medication after reviewing this information.

Pediatric Patients

Seizure Disorders

RECTAL:
- Children 2–5 years of age: Initially, 0.5 mg/kg as rectal gel, rounded up to the next available dose (i.e., the next multiple of 2.5 mg). If necessary, repeat initial dose in 4–12 hours. Administration of a third dose is not recommended by the manufacturer.

Recommended Doses of Diazepam Rectal Gel for Children 2–5 Years of Age

Weight (kg)	Rounded Dose (mg)
6–10	5
11–15	7.5
16–20	10
21–25	12.5
26–30	15
31–35	17.5
36–44	20

Children 6–11 years of age: Initially, 0.3 mg/kg as rectal gel, rounded up to the next available dose (i.e., the next multiple of 2.5 mg). If necessary, repeat initial dose in 4–12 hours. Administration of a third dose is not recommended by the manufacturer.

Recommended Doses of Diazepam Rectal Gel for Children 6–11 Years of Age

Weight (kg)	Rounded Dose (mg)
10–16	5
17–25	7.5
26–33	10
34–41	12.5
42–50	15
51–58	17.5
59–74	20

Children ≥12 years of age: Initially, 0.2 mg/kg as rectal gel, rounded up to the next available dose (i.e., the next multiple of 2.5 mg). If necessary, repeat initial dose in 4–12 hours. Administration of a third dose is not recommended by the manufacturer.

Recommended Doses of Diazepam Rectal Gel for Children ≥12 Years of Age

Weight (kg)	Rounded Dose (mg)
14–25	5
26–37	7.5
38–50	10
51–62	12.5
63–75	15
76–87	17.5
88–111	20

Usual dosage of parenteral solutions† administered rectally in children: 0.5 mg/kg (not to exceed 20 mg).

Adult Patients

Surgery

Seizure Disorders

RECTAL:
- Initially, 0.2 mg/kg as rectal gel, rounded up to next available dose (i.e., the next multiple of 2.5 mg). If necessary, repeat initial dose in 4–12 hours. Administration of a third dose is not recommended by the manufacturer.
- For rectal administration of parenteral solutions†, 0.5 mg/kg (not to exceed 20 mg).

Prescribing Limits

Pediatric Patients

Seizure Disorders

RECTAL:
- Maximum recommended frequency for administration by caregivers outside hospital is 1 treatment course every 5 days and 5 treatment courses per month.

Adult Patients

Seizure Disorders

RECTAL:
- Maximum recommended frequency for administration by caregivers outside hospital is 1 treatment course every 5 days and 5 treatment courses per month.

Special Populations

Hepatic Impairment
- Reduce dosage; use the smallest effective dose to avoid oversedation.

Renal Impairment
- Use the smallest effective dose to avoid oversedation.

Geriatric Patients

Rectal
- Dosage to be administered should be adjusted *downward* for the commercially available prefilled applicators of rectal gel.

Other Populations
- Use the smallest effective dosage in debilitated patient and patients with low serum albumin concentrations. In debilitated patients, observe maximum geriatric dosages.

† Use is not currently included in the labeling approved by the US Food and Drug Administration.

Diclofenac

(dye kloe′ fen ak)

Brand Name: Cataflam®, Voltaren®-XR
Also available generically.

Important Warning

People who take nonsteroidal anti-inflammatory medications (NSAIDs) (other than aspirin) such as diclofenac may have a higher risk of having a heart attack or a stroke than people who do not take these medications. These events may happen without warning and may cause death. This risk may be higher for people who take NSAIDs for a long time. Tell your doctor if you or anyone in your family has or has ever had heart disease, a heart attack, or a stroke, if you smoke, and if you have or have ever had high cholesterol, high blood pressure, or diabetes. Get emergency medical help right away if you experience any of the following symptoms: chest pain, shortness of breath, weakness in one part or side of the body, or slurred speech.

If you will be undergoing a coronary artery bypass graft (CABG; a type of heart surgery), you should not take diclofenac right before or right after the surgery.

NSAIDs such as diclofenac may cause ulcers, bleeding, or holes in the stomach or intestine. These problems may develop at any time during treatment, may happen without warning symptoms, and may cause death. The risk may be higher for people who take NSAIDs for a long time, are older in age, have poor health, or drink large amounts of alcohol while taking diclofenac. Tell your doctor if you take any of the following medications: anticoagulants ('blood thinners') such as warfarin (Coumadin); aspirin; other NSAIDS such as ibuprofen (Advil, Motrin) and naproxen (Aleve, Naprosyn); or oral steroids such as dexamethasone (Decadron, Dexone), methylprednisolone (Medrol), and prednisone (Deltasone). Also tell your doctor if you have or have ever had ulcers, bleeding in your stomach or intestines, or other bleeding disorders. If you experience any of the fol-

continued on next page

Important Warning (cont'd)

lowing symptoms, stop taking diclofenac and call your doctor: stomach pain, heartburn, vomiting a substance that is bloody or looks like coffee grounds, blood in the stool, or black and tarry stools.

Keep all appointments with your doctor and the laboratory. Your doctor will monitor your symptoms carefully and will probably order certain tests to check your body's response to diclofenac. Be sure to tell your doctor how you are feeling so that your doctor can prescribe the right amount of medication to treat your condition with the lowest risk of serious side effects.

Your doctor or pharmacist will give you the manufacturer's patient information sheet (Medication Guide) when you begin treatment with diclofenac and each time you refill your prescription. Read the information carefully and ask your doctor or pharmacist if you have any questions. You can also visit the Food and Drug Administration (FDA) website (http://www.fda.gov/cder) to obtain the Medication Guide.

Why is this medicine prescribed?

Diclofenac is used to relieve pain, tenderness, swelling, and stiffness caused by osteoarthritis (arthritis caused by a breakdown of the lining of the joints), rheumatoid arthritis (arthritis caused by swelling of the lining of the joints), and ankylosing spondylitis (arthritis that mainly affects the spine). Diclofenac immediate-release (short-acting) tablets are also used to treat painful menstrual periods and pain from other causes. Diclofenac is in a class of medications called NSAIDs. It works by stopping the body's production of a substance that causes pain, fever, and inflammation.

How should this medicine be used?

Diclofenac comes as an immediate-release tablet and an extended-release (long-acting) tablet to take by mouth. Diclofenac immediate-release tablets are usually taken two to four times a day. Diclofenac extended-release tablets are usually taken once a day, and in rare cases are taken twice a day. Take diclofenac at around the same time(s) every day. Follow the directions on your prescription label carefully, and ask your doctor or pharmacist to explain any part you do not understand. Take diclofenac exactly as directed. Do not take more or less of it or take it more often than prescribed by your doctor.

Are there other uses for this medicine?

Diclofenac is also used sometimes to treat pain caused by gout, painful shoulder and cancer. Talk to your doctor about the possible risks of using this medication for your condition.

This medication may be prescribed for other uses; ask your doctor or pharmacist for more information.

What special precautions should I follow?

Before taking diclofenac,

- tell your doctor and pharmacist if you are allergic to diclofenac (Cataflam, Voltaren XR, in Arthrotec), aspirin or other NSAIDs such as ibuprofen (Advil, Motrin) and naproxen (Aleve, Naprosyn), any other medications, or any of the inactive ingredients in diclofenac tablets or extended release tablets. Ask your pharmacist for a list of the inactive ingredients.
- tell your doctor and pharmacist what prescription and nonprescription medications, vitamins, nutritional supplements, and herbal products you are taking or plan to take. Be sure to mention the medications listed in the IMPORTANT WARNING section and any of the following: angiotensin-converting enzyme (ACE) inhibitors such as benazepril (Lotensin), captopril (Capoten), enalapril (Vasotec), fosinopril (Monopril), lisinopril (Prinivil, Zestril), moexipril (Univasc), perindopril (Aceon), quinapril (Accupril), ramipril (Altace), and trandolapril (Mavik); cyclosporine (Neoral, Sandimmune); digoxin (Lanoxin); diuretics ('water pills'); insulin and oral medication for diabetes; lithium (Eskalith, Lithobid); and methotrexate (Rheumatrex). Your doctor may need to change the doses of your medications or monitor you carefully for side effects.
- tell your doctor if you have or have ever had any of the conditions mentioned in the IMPORTANT WARNING section or asthma, especially if you also have frequent stuffed or runny nose or nasal polyps (swelling of the lining of the nose); lupus (a condition in which the body attacks many of its own tissues and organs, often including the skin, joints, blood, and kidneys); porphyria (an abnormal increase in the amount of certain natural substances made by the liver); liver, or kidney disease; or swelling of the hands, feet, ankles, or lower legs.
- tell your doctor if you are pregnant, especially if you are in the last few months of your pregnancy, you plan to become pregnant, or you are breast-feeding. If you become pregnant while taking diclofenac, call your doctor.
- if you are having surgery, including dental surgery, tell the doctor or dentist that you are taking diclofenac.

What special dietary instructions should I follow?

Unless your doctor tells you otherwise, continue your normal diet.

What should I do if I forget to take a dose?

Take the missed dose as soon as you remember it. However, if it is almost time for the next dose, skip the missed dose and continue your regular dosing schedule. Do not take a double dose to make up for a missed one.

What side effects can this medicine cause?

Diclofenac may cause side effects. Tell your doctor if any of these symptoms are severe or do not go away:

- diarrhea
- constipation
- gas or bloating
- headache
- dizziness
- ringing in the ears

Some side effects can be serious. If you experience any of the following symptoms or those mentioned in the IMPORTANT WARNING section, call your doctor immediately. Do not take any more diclofenac until you speak to your doctor.

- unexplained weight gain
- excessive tiredness
- lack of energy
- upset stomach
- loss of appetite
- itching
- pain in the upper right part of the stomach
- yellowing of the skin or eyes
- flu-like symptoms
- fever
- blisters
- rash
- hives
- swelling of the eyes, face, tongue, lips, throat, arms, hands, feet, ankles, or lower legs
- difficulty breathing or swallowing
- hoarseness
- pale skin
- fast heartbeat
- cloudy, discolored, or bloody urine
- back pain
- difficult or painful urination

Diclofenac may cause other side effects. Call your doctor if you have any unusual problems while taking this medication.

If you experience a serious side effect, you or your doctor may send a report to the Food and Drug Administration's (FDA) MedWatch Adverse Event Reporting program online [at http://www.fda.gov/MedWatch/index.html] or by phone [1-800-332-1088].

What storage conditions are needed for this medicine?

Keep this medication in the container it came in, tightly closed, and out of reach of children. Store it at room temperature and away from excess heat and moisture (not in the bathroom). Throw away any medication that is outdated or no longer needed. Talk to your pharmacist about the proper disposal of your medication.

What should I do in case of overdose?

In case of overdose, call your local poison control center at 1-800-222-1222. If the victim has collapsed or is not breathing, call local emergency services at 911.

Symptoms of overdose may include:

- upset stomach
- vomiting
- stomach pain
- bloody, black, or tarry stools
- vomiting a substance that is bloody or looks like coffee grounds
- drowsiness
- breathing
- loss of consciousness

What other information should I know?

Do not let anyone else take your medication. Ask your pharmacist any questions you have about refilling your prescription.

Dosage Facts
For Informational Purposes

Caution: Do not change your dose, how often you take your medication, or the length of time you are to take it without first talking to your healthcare provider.

The following dosage information was written using medical language for doctors and other healthcare professionals and is provided here for you to check your dosage. The dosage of this drug may differ for different patients. Therefore, always follow your doctor's instructions or the directions on the label. Contact your healthcare provider or pharmacist if you have any questions about the specific dosage of your medication after reviewing this information.

General Dosage Information

Available as diclofenac potassium or diclofenac sodium; dosage expressed in terms of the salt.

To minimize the potential risk of adverse cardiovascular and/or GI events, use lowest effective dosage and shortest duration of therapy consistent with the patient's treatment goals. Adjust dosage based on individual requirements and response; attempt to titrate to the lowest effective dosage.

Commercially available diclofenac sodium enteric-coated tablets (Voltaren®), diclofenac sodium extended-release tablets (Voltaren®-XR), and diclofenac potassium immediate-release tablets (Cataflam®) are not necessarily bioequivalent on a mg-per-mg basis.

Adult Patients

Inflammatory Diseases
Osteoarthritis

ORAL:

Preparation	Dosage
Diclofenac potassium conventional tablets	100–150 mg daily, given as 50 mg 2 or 3 times daily
Diclofenac sodium delayed-release tablets	100–150 mg daily, given as 50 mg 2 or 3 times daily or 75 mg twice daily
Diclofenac sodium extended-release tablets	100 mg once daily
Diclofenac sodium (in fixed combination with misoprostol)	50 mg 3 times daily[a]

[a]May change dosage to 50 or 75 mg twice daily in patients who do not tolerate usual dosage; however, these dosages may be less effective in preventing NSAIA-induced ulcers.

Rheumatoid Arthritis

ORAL:

Preparation	Dosage
Diclofenac potassium conventional tablets	150–200 mg daily, given as 50 mg 3 or 4 times daily
Diclofenac sodium delayed-release tablets	150–200 mg daily, given as 50 mg 3 or 4 times daily or 75 mg twice daily
Diclofenac sodium extended-release tablets	100 mg once daily; may increase to 100 mg twice daily
Diclofenac sodium (in fixed combination with misoprostol)	50 mg 3 or 4 times daily[b]

[b]May change dosage to 50 or 75 mg twice daily in patients who do not tolerate usual dosage; however, these dosages may be less effective in preventing NSAIA-induced ulcers.

Ankylosing Spondylitis

ORAL:

- 100–125 mg daily (as diclofenac sodium delayed-release tablets); administer as 25 mg 4 times daily, with 5th dose at bedtime as needed.

Pain

ORAL:

- 50 mg 3 times daily (as diclofenac potassium conventional tablets). Some patients may benefit from initial dose of 100 mg (followed by 50-mg doses).

Dysmenorrhea

ORAL:

- 50 mg 3 times daily (as diclofenac potassium conventional tablets). Some patients may benefit from initial dose of 100 mg (followed by 50-mg doses).

Special Populations

Renal Impairment

- Dosage adjustment not required.

Hepatic Impairment

- Dosage reductions may be necessary.

Diclofenac and Misoprostol

(dye kloe′ fen ak) and (mye soe prost′ ole)

Brand Name: Arthrotec® as a combination product containing diclofenac and misoprostol

Important Warning

For female patients:

Do not take diclofenac and misoprostol if you are pregnant or plan to become pregnant. If you become pregnant while taking diclofenac and misoprostol, stop taking the medication and call your doctor immediately. Diclofenac and misoprostol may cause miscarriage (pregnancy loss), serious bleeding, or premature birth (baby is born too early) if taken during pregnancy.

Women who can become pregnant generally should not take diclofenac and misoprostol. However, you and your doctor may decide that diclofenac and misoprostol combination is needed to treat your condition. In that case you must:

- agree to use a reliable method of birth control during your treatment and for at least 1 month or one menstrual cycle after your treatment;
- have a negative blood test for pregnancy no longer than 2 weeks before you start taking diclofenac and misoprostol;
- begin taking the medication only on the second or third day of the next normal menstrual period.

For all patients:

People who take nonsteroidal anti-inflammatory medications (NSAIDs) (other than aspirin) such as diclofenac and misoprostol combination may have a higher risk of having a heart attack or a stroke than people who do not take these medications. These events may happen without warning and may cause death. This risk may be higher for people who take NSAIDs for a long time. Tell your doctor if you or anyone in your family has or has ever had heart disease, a heart attack, or a stroke, if you smoke, and if you have or have ever had high cholesterol, high blood pressure, or diabetes. Get emergency medical help right away if you experience any of the following symptoms: chest pain, shortness of breath, weakness in one part or side of the body, or slurred speech.

If you will be undergoing a coronary artery bypass graft (CABG; a type of heart surgery), you should not take diclofenac and misoprostol right before or right after the surgery.

NSAIDs such as diclofenac may cause ulcers, bleeding, or holes in the stomach or intestine. Misoprostol is taken in combination with diclofenac to protect the stomach and intestine, but may not prevent all damage to these parts of the body. Problems with the stomach and intestine may develop at any time during treatment, may happen without warning symptoms, and may cause death. The risk may be higher for people who take NSAIDs for a long time, are older in age, have poor health, or drink large amounts of alcohol while taking diclofenac and misoprostol. Tell your doctor if you take any of the following medications: anticoagulants ('blood thinners') such as warfarin (Coumadin); aspirin; other NSAIDs such as ibuprofen (Advil, Motrin) and naproxen (Aleve, Naprosyn); or oral steroids such as dexamethasone (Decadron, Dexone), methylprednisolone (Medrol), and prednisone (Deltasone). Also tell your doctor if you have or have ever had ulcers, bleeding in your stomach or intestines, or other bleeding disorders. If you experience any of the following symptoms, stop taking diclofenac and misoprostol and call your doctor: stomach pain, heartburn, vomiting a substance that is bloody or looks like coffee grounds, blood in the stool, or black and tarry stools.

Keep all appointments with your doctor and the laboratory. Your doctor will monitor your symptoms carefully and will probably order certain tests to check your body's response to diclofenac and misoprostol. Be sure to tell your doctor how you are feeling so that your doctor can prescribe the right amount of medication to treat your condition with the lowest risk of serious side effects.

Do not give this medication to anyone else, especially a woman who is or could become pregnant.

Your doctor or pharmacist will give you the manufacturer's patient information sheet sheet for diclofenac and misoprostol and the general Medication Guide for NSAIDs when you begin your treatment and each time you refill your prescription. Read the information carefully and ask your doctor or pharmacist if you have any questions. You can also visit the Food and Drug Administration (FDA) website (http://www.fda.gov/cder) or the manufacturer's website to obtain the patient information sheet and Medication Guide.

Why is this medicine prescribed?

The combination of diclofenac and misoprostol is used to relieve the pain, tenderness, swelling, and stiffness caused by osteoarthritis (arthritis caused by a breakdown of the lining of the joints) and rheumatoid arthritis (arthritis caused by swelling of the lining of the joints) in patients who have a high risk of developing stomach ulcers. Diclofenac is in a class of medications called NSAIDs. It works by stopping the body's production of a substance that causes pain and inflammation. Misoprostol is in a class of medications called prostaglandins. It prevents ulcers caused by diclofenac by protecting the stomach lining and decreasing stomach acid production.

How should this medicine be used?

The combination of diclofenac and misoprostol comes as a tablet to take by mouth. It is usually taken with food two to four times a day. To help you remember to take diclofenac and misoprostol, take it at around the same times every day. Follow the directions on your prescription label carefully, and ask your doctor or pharmacist to explain any part you do not understand. Take diclofenac and misoprostol combination exactly as directed. Do not take more or less of it or take it more often than prescribed by your doctor.

Swallow the tablets whole; do not split, chew, or crush them.

Are there other uses for this medicine?

This medication may be prescribed for other uses; ask your doctor or pharmacist for more information.

What special precautions should I follow?

Before taking diclofenac and misoprostol,

- tell your doctor and pharmacist if you are allergic to diclofenac (Cataflam, Voltaren XR), misoprostol (Cytotec), aspirin or other NSAIDs such as ibuprofen (Advil, Motrin) and naproxen (Aleve, Naprosyn); prostaglandins such as alprostadil (Caverject, Muse), carboprost (Hemabate), dinoprostone (Cervidil, Prepidil, Prostin E2) and mifepristone (Mifeprex); any other medications, or any of the inactive ingredients in diclofenac and misoprostol tablets. Ask your pharmacist for a list of the inactive ingredients.
- tell your doctor and pharmacist what prescription and nonprescription medications, vitamins, nutritional supplements, and herbal products you are taking or plan to take. Be sure to mention any of the medications listed in the IMPORTANT WARNING section and any of the following: angiotensin-converting enzyme (ACE) inhibitors such as benazepril (Lotensin), captopril (Capoten), enalapril (Vasotec), fosinopril (Monopril), lisinopril (Prinivil, Zestril), moexipril (Univasc), perindopril (Aceon), quinapril (Accupril), ramipril (Altace), and trandolapril (Mavik); antacids containing magnesium (Mylanta, Maalox, others); cyclosporine (Neoral, Sandimmune); digoxin (Lanoxin); diuretics ('water pills'); insulin and oral medications for diabetes; methotrexate (Rheumatrex); lithium (Eskalith, Lithobid); and phenobarbital (Luminal, Solfoton). Your doctor may need to change the doses of your medications or monitor you carefully for side effects.

- tell your doctor if you have or have ever had any of the conditions mentioned in the IMPORTANT WARNING section or inflammatory bowel disease (swelling of the lining of the intestine that may cause painful or bloody diarrhea and cramping); asthma, especially if you also have frequent stuffed or runny nose or nasal polyps (swelling of the lining of the nose); lupus (a condition in which the body attacks many of its own tissues and organs, often including the skin, joints, blood, and kidneys); hepatic porphyria (an abnormal increase in the amount of certain natural substances made by the liver); liver or kidney disease; or swelling of the hands, feet, ankles, or lower legs.
- tell your doctor if you are breast-feeding. You should not breast-feed while you are taking this medication
- if you are having surgery, including dental surgery, tell the doctor or dentist that you are taking diclofenac and misoprostol.

What special dietary instructions should I follow?

Unless your doctor tells you otherwise, continue your normal diet.

What should I do if I forget to take a dose?

Take the missed dose as soon as you remember it. However, if it is almost time for the next dose, skip the missed dose and continue your regular dosing schedule. Do not take a double dose to make up for a missed one.

What side effects can this medicine cause?

Diclofenac and misoprostol may cause side effects. Tell your doctor if any of these symptoms are severe or do not go away:

- diarrhea
- gas or bloating

Some side effects can be serious. If you experience any of the following symptoms or those mentioned in the IMPORTANT WARNING section, call your doctor immediately. Do not take any more diclofenac and misoprostol until you speak to your doctor.

- unexplained weight gain
- excessive tiredness
- lack of energy
- itching
- upset stomach
- loss of appetite
- pain in the upper right part of the stomach
- yellowing of the skin or eyes
- flu-like symptoms
- pale skin
- fast heartbeat
- headache
- stiff neck
- sore throat
- muscle pain

- confusion
- sensitivity to light
- fever
- blisters
- rash
- hives
- swelling of the eyes, face, lips, tongue, throat, arms, hands, feet, ankles, or lower legs
- difficulty breathing or swallowing
- hoarseness
- unusual vaginal bleeding
- cloudy, discolored, or bloody urine
- back pain
- difficult or painful urination

Diclofenac and misoprostol may cause other side effects. Call your doctor if you have any unusual problems while taking this medication.

If you experience a serious side effect, you or your doctor may send a report to the Food and Drug Administration's (FDA) MedWatch Adverse Event Reporting program online [at http://www.fda.gov/MedWatch/index.html] or by phone [1-800-332-1088].

What storage conditions are needed for this medicine?

Keep this medication in the container it came in, tightly closed, and out of reach of children. Store it at room temperature and away from excess heat and moisture (not in the bathroom). Throw away any medication that is outdated or no longer needed. Talk to your pharmacist about the proper disposal of your medication.

What should I do in case of overdose?

In case of overdose, call your local poison control center at 1-800-222-1222. If the victim has collapsed or is not breathing, call local emergency services at 911.

Symptoms of overdose may include:
- stomach pain
- vomiting
- diarrhea
- confusion
- drowsiness
- low muscle tone
- shaking of a part of the body that you cannot control
- seizures
- shortness of breath
- fever
- fast, pounding, or slow heartbeat
- dizziness
- fainting

What other information should I know?

Before having any laboratory test, tell your doctor and the laboratory personnel that you are taking diclofenac and misoprostol.

Do not let anyone else take your medication. Ask your

pharmacist any questions you have about refilling your prescription.

Dosage Facts
For Informational Purposes

Caution: Do not change your dose, how often you take your medication, or the length of time you are to take it without first talking to your healthcare provider.

The following dosage information was written using medical language for doctors and other healthcare professionals and is provided here for you to check your dosage. The dosage of this drug may differ for different patients. Therefore, always follow your doctor's instructions or the directions on the label. Contact your healthcare provider or pharmacist if you have any questions about the specific dosage of your medication after reviewing this information.

General Dosage Information

Available as diclofenac potassium or diclofenac sodium; dosage expressed in terms of the salt.

To minimize the potential risk of adverse cardiovascular and/or GI events, use lowest effective dosage and shortest duration of therapy consistent with the patient's treatment goals. Adjust dosage based on individual requirements and response; attempt to titrate to the lowest effective dosage.

Adult Patients
Inflammatory Diseases
Osteoarthritis

ORAL:

Preparation	Dosage
Diclofenac potassium conventional tablets	100–150 mg daily, given as 50 mg 2 or 3 times daily
Diclofenac sodium delayed-release tablets	100–150 mg daily, given as 50 mg 2 or 3 times daily or 75 mg twice daily
Diclofenac sodium extended-release tablets	100 mg once daily
Diclofenac sodium (in fixed combination with misoprostol)	50 mg 3 times daily[a]

[a]May change dosage to 50 or 75 mg twice daily in patients who do not tolerate usual dosage; however, these dosages may be less effective in preventing NSAIA-induced ulcers.

Rheumatoid Arthritis

ORAL:

Preparation	Dosage
Diclofenac potassium conventional tablets	150–200 mg daily, given as 50 mg 3 or 4 times daily
Diclofenac sodium delayed-release tablets	150–200 mg daily, given as 50 mg 3 or 4 times daily or 75 mg twice daily
Diclofenac sodium extended-release tablets	100 mg once daily; may increase to 100 mg twice daily
Diclofenac sodium (in fixed combination with misoprostol)	50 mg 3 or 4 times daily[b]

[b]May change dosage to 50 or 75 mg twice daily in patients who do not tolerate usual dosage; however, these dosages may be less effective in preventing NSAIA-induced ulcers.

Special Populations

Renal Impairment
- Dosage adjustment not required.

Hepatic Impairment
- Dosage reductions may be necessary.

Diclofenac Ophthalmic
(dye kloe′ fen ak)

Brand Name: Voltaren®

Why is this medicine prescribed?

Diclofenac ophthalmic is used to treat eye pain, redness, and swelling in patients who are recovering from cataract surgery (procedure to treat clouding of the lens in the eye). Diclofenac ophthalmic is also used to temporarily relieve eye pain and sensitivity to light in patients who are recovering from corneal refractive surgery (surgery to improve vision). Diclofenac is in a class of medications called nonsteroidal anti-inflammatory medications. It works by stopping the production of certain natural substances that cause pain and swelling.

How should this medicine be used?

Diclofenac ophthalmic comes as a solution (liquid) to instill in the eyes. When diclofenac ophthalmic is used by patients recovering from cataract surgery, it is usually instilled 4 times a day beginning 24 hours after surgery and continuing for 2 weeks after surgery. When diclofenac ophthalmic is used by patients undergoing corneal refractive surgery, it is usually instilled one hour before the surgery, 15 minutes after the surgery, and then four times a day for up to 3 days. Use diclofenac eye drops at around the same times every day. Follow the directions on your prescription label carefully, and ask your doctor or pharmacist to explain any part you do not understand. Use diclofenac eye drops exactly as directed. Do not use more or less of them or use them more often than prescribed by your doctor.

To use the eye drops, follow these steps:

1. Use a mirror or have someone else put the drops in your eye.
2. Wash your hands thoroughly with soap and water.
3. Shake the container well.
4. Remove the protective cap. Make sure that the end of the dropper is not chipped or cracked.
5. Avoid touching the dropper tip against your eye or anything else.
6. Lie down or tilt your head back and look upward.
7. Hold the bottle between your thumb and index finger and place the dropper tip as near as possible to your eyelid without touching it.
8. Brace the remaining fingers of that hand against your cheek or nose.
9. Use the index finger of your other hand to gently press the skin just beneath the lower eyelid, then pull the lower eyelid down to form a pocket.
10. Drop the prescribed number of drops into the pocket made by the lower lid and the eye.
11. Close your eye gently.
12. Replace and tighten the cap right away. Do not rinse it off.
13. Wipe off any excess liquid from your cheek with a clean tissue. Wash your hands again.

Are there other uses for this medicine?

This medication may be prescribed for other uses; ask your doctor or pharmacist for more information.

What special precautions should I follow?

Before using diclofenac eye drops,

- tell your doctor and pharmacist if you are allergic to diclofenac; aspirin or other NSAIDs such as nepafenac (Nevanac), ibuprofen (Advil, Motrin), naproxen (Aleve, Naprosyn), or tolmetin (Tolectin); any other medications, or any of the ingredients in diclofenac eye drops. Ask your pharmacist for a list of the ingredients.
- tell your doctor and pharmacist what prescription and nonprescription medications, vitamins, nutritional supplements, and herbal products you are taking or plan to take. Be sure to mention any of the following: anticoagulants ('blood thinners') such as warfarin (Coumadin); aspirin and other NSAIDs such as ibuprofen (Advil, Motrin) and naproxen (Aleve, Naprosyn); and corticosteroid eye drops such as dexamethasone (Maxidex), fluorometholone (FML), hydrocortisone (in Cortisporin), loteprednol (Alrex, Lotemax), medrysone (HMS), prednisolone (Pred Mild), and rimexolone (Vexol). Your doctor may need to change the doses of your medications or monitor you carefully for side effects.

- tell your doctor if you have or have ever had diabetes, rheumatoid arthritis (arthritis caused by swelling of the lining of the joints), dry eye disease or any eye problem other than cataracts, or any condition that causes you to bleed easily.
- tell your doctor if you are pregnant, especially if you are in the last few months of your pregnancy, you plan to become pregnant, or you are breast-feeding. If you become pregnant while using diclofenac eye drops, call your doctor.
- tell your doctor if you wear soft contact lenses. Your doctor may tell you that you should not wear your contact lenses during your treatment with diclofenac eye drops.

What special dietary instructions should I follow?

Unless your doctor tells you otherwise, continue your normal diet.

What should I do if I forget to take a dose?

Instill the missed dose as soon as you remember it. However, if it is almost time for the next dose, skip the missed dose and continue your regular dosing schedule. Do not instill extra eye drops to make up for a missed dose.

What side effects can this medicine cause?

Diclofenac eye drops may cause side effects. Tell your doctor if any of these symptoms are severe or do not go away:

- burning or stinging in your eye just after you instill the drops
- itchy eyes
- stomach pain
- upset stomach
- vomiting
- difficulty falling asleep or staying asleep
- headache
- dizziness
- fever
- chills
- runny nose

Some side effects can be serious. If you experience any of these symptoms, call your doctor immediately:

- swelling of the eyes or face
- red or bloody eyes
- eye pain
- feeling that something is in the eye
- sensitivity to light
- blurred or decreased vision
- teary eyes
- eye discharge or crusting

Diclofenac eye drops may cause other side effects. Call your doctor if you have any unusual problems while using this medication.

If you experience a serious side effect, you or your doctor may send a report to the Food and Drug Administration's (FDA) MedWatch Adverse Event Reporting program online [at http://www.fda.gov/MedWatch/index.html] or by phone [1-800-332-1088].

What storage conditions are needed for this medicine?

Keep this medication in the container it came in, tightly closed, and out of reach of children. Store it at room temperature and away from excess heat and moisture (not in the bathroom). Throw away any medication that is outdated or no longer needed. Talk to your pharmacist about the proper disposal of your medication.

What should I do in case of overdose?

If someone swallows diclofenac eye drops, call your local poison control center at 1-800-222-1222. Give the victim plenty of liquids to drink. If the victim has collapsed or is not breathing, call local emergency services at 911.

What other information should I know?

Keep all appointments with your doctor.

Do not let anyone else use your medication. Ask your pharmacist any questions you have about refilling your prescription.

Talk to your doctor, pharmacist, or other healthcare professional if you have questions about dosing information for your medication.

Dicloxacillin

(dye klox a sill′ in)

Why is this medicine prescribed?

Dicloxacillin is a penicillin-like antibiotic used to treat certain infections caused by bacteria such as pneumonia and bone, ear, skin, and urinary tract infections. Antibiotics will not work for colds, flu, or other viral infections.

This medication is sometimes prescribed for other uses; ask your doctor or pharmacist for more information.

How should this medicine be used?

Dicloxacillin comes as a capsule and liquid to take by mouth. It is usually taken every 6 hours (four times a day). Follow the directions on your prescription label carefully, and ask your doctor or pharmacist to explain any part you do not understand. Take dicloxacillin exactly as directed. Do not take more or less of it or take it more often than prescribed by your doctor.

Shake the liquid well before each use to mix the medication evenly.

The capsules should be swallowed whole and taken with a full glass of water.

Continue to take dicloxacillin even if you feel well. Do not stop taking dicloxacillin without talking to your doctor.

What special precautions should I follow?

Before taking dicloxacillin,

- tell your doctor and pharmacist if you are allergic to dicloxacillin, penicillin, or any other drugs.
- tell your doctor and pharmacist what prescription and nonprescription medications you are taking, especially other antibiotics, anticoagulants ('blood thinners') such as warfarin (Coumadin), aspirin or other nonsteroidal anti-inflammatory medicine such as naproxen (Anaprox) or ibuprofen (Motrin), atenolol (Tenormin), oral contraceptives, probenecid (Benemid), and vitamins.
- tell your doctor if you have or have ever had kidney or liver disease, allergies, asthma, blood disease, colitis, stomach problems, or hay fever.
- tell your doctor if you are pregnant, plan to become pregnant, or are breast-feeding. If you become pregnant while taking dicloxacillin, call your doctor.
- if you are having surgery, including dental surgery, tell the doctor or dentist that you are taking dicloxacillin.

What special dietary instructions should I follow?

Take dicloxacillin at least 1 hour before or 2 hours after meals.

What should I do if I forget to take a dose?

Take the missed dose as soon as you remember it. However, if it is almost time for the next dose, skip the missed dose and continue your regular dosing schedule. Do not take a double dose to make up for a missed one.

What side effects can this medicine cause?

Dicloxacillin may cause side effects. Tell your doctor if any of these symptoms are severe or do not go away:

- upset stomach
- diarrhea
- vomiting
- mild skin rash

If you experience any of the following symptoms, call your doctor immediately:

- severe skin rash
- itching
- hives
- difficulty breathing or swallowing
- wheezing
- vaginal infection

If you experience a serious side effect, you or your doctor may send a report to the Food and Drug Administration's (FDA) MedWatch Adverse Event Reporting program online [at http://www.fda.gov/MedWatch/index.html] or by phone [1-800-332-1088].

What storage conditions are needed for this medicine?

Keep this medicine in the container it came in, tightly closed, and out of reach of children. Store the capsules at room temperature and away from excess heat and moisture (not in the bathroom). Throw away any medication that is outdated or no longer needed. Keep liquid medicine in the refrigerator, closed tightly, and throw away any unused medication after 14 days. Do not freeze. Talk to your pharmacist about the proper disposal of your medication.

What should I do in case of overdose?

In case of overdose, call your local poison control center at 1-800-222-1222. If the victim has collapsed or is not breathing, call local emergency services at 911.

What other information should I know?

Keep all appointments with your doctor and the laboratory. Your doctor will order certain lab tests to check your response to dicloxacillin.

If you are diabetic, use Clinistix or TesTape (not Clinitest) to test your urine for sugar while taking this drug.

Do not let anyone else take your medication. Your prescription is probably not refillable. If you still have symptoms of infection after you finish the dicloxacillin, call your doctor.

Dosage Facts
For Informational Purposes

Caution: Do not change your dose, how often you take your medication, or the length of time you are to take it without first talking to your healthcare provider.

The following dosage information was written using medical language for doctors and other healthcare professionals and is provided here for you to check your dosage. The dosage of this drug may differ for different patients. Therefore, always follow your doctor's instructions or the directions on the label. Contact your healthcare provider or pharmacist if you have any questions about the specific dosage of your medication after reviewing this information.

General Dosage Information

Available as dicloxacillin sodium; dosage expressed in terms of dicloxacillin.

Duration of treatment depends on type and severity of infection and should be determined by the clinical and bacteriologic response of the patient. Usually continued for ≥48 hours after cultures are negative and patient becomes afebrile and asymptomatic. For severe staphylococcal infections, continue therapy for ≥14 days; more prolonged therapy is necessary for treatment of osteomyelitis, endocarditis, or other metastatic infections.

Pediatric Patients

Staphylococcal Infections
Mild to Moderate Infections

ORAL:
- Children weighing <40 kg: 12.5 mg/kg daily given in divided doses every 6 hours.
- Children weighing ≥40 kg: 125 mg every 6 hours.
- Children ≥1 month of age: AAP recommends 25–50 mg/kg daily in 4 divided doses.

More Severe Infections

ORAL:
- Children weighing <40 kg: 25 mg/kg daily given in divided doses every 6 hours; higher dosage may be necessary depending on severity of infection.
- Children weighing ≥40 kg: 250 mg every 6 hours; higher dosage may be necessary depending on severity of infection.
- Inappropriate for severe infections per AAP.

Acute or Chronic Osteomyelitis

ORAL:
- 50–100 mg/kg daily given in divided doses every 6 hours as follow-up to initial parenteral therapy. If an oral regimen is used, compliance must be assured and some clinicians suggest that serum bactericidal titers (SBTs) be used to monitor adequacy of therapy and adjust dosage.
- When used as follow-up in treatment of acute osteomyelitis, oral regimen usually given for 3–6 weeks or until total duration of parenteral and oral therapy is ≥6 weeks; when used as follow-up in treatment of chronic osteomyelitis, oral regimen usually given for ≥1–2 months and has been given for as long as 1–2 years.

Adult Patients

Staphylococcal Infections
Mild to Moderate Infections

ORAL:
- 125 mg every 6 hours.

More Severe Infections

ORAL:
- 250 mg every 6 hours; higher dosage may be necessary depending on severity of infection.

Special Populations

Renal Impairment
- Dosage adjustment generally unnecessary in patients with renal impairment.

Dicyclomine

(dye sye' kloe meen)

Brand Name: Bentyl®, Bentyl® Syrup
Also available generically.

Why is this medicine prescribed?

Dicyclomine is used to treat the symptoms of irritable bowel syndrome. Dicyclomine is in a class of medications called anticholinergics. It relieves muscle spasms in the gastrointestinal tract by blocking the activity of a certain natural substance in the body.

How should this medicine be used?

Dicyclomine comes as a capsule, a tablet, and a syrup to take by mouth. It is usually taken four times a day. To help you remember to take dicyclomine, take it around the same time every day. Follow the directions on your prescription label carefully, and ask your doctor or pharmacist to explain any part you do not understand. Take dicyclomine exactly as directed. Do not take more or less of it or take it more often than prescribed by your doctor.

Your doctor will probably start you on a low dose of dicyclomine and gradually increase your dose.

Are there other uses for this medicine?

This medication may be prescribed for other uses; ask your doctor or pharmacist for more information.

What special precautions should I follow?

Before taking dicyclomine,

- tell your doctor and pharmacist if you are allergic to dicyclomine or any other medications.
- tell your doctor and pharmacist what prescription and nonprescription medications, vitamins, nutritional supplements, and herbal products you are taking. Be sure to mention any of the following: amantadine (Symmetrel); antacids; antidepressants such as amitriptyline (Elavil), amoxapine (Asendin), clomipramine (Anafranil), desipramine (Norpramin), doxepin (Adapin, Sinequan), imipramine (Tofranil), nortriptyline (Aventyl, Pamelor), protriptyline (Vivactil), and trimipramine (Surmontil); antihistamines; diet pills; digoxin (Lanoxin); ipratropium (Atrovent); isosorbide (Imdur, Ismo, Isordil, others); medications for anxiety, asthma, glaucoma, irregular heartbeat, mental illness, motion sickness, Parkinson's disease, seizures, ulcers, or urinary problems; metoclopramide (Reglan); monoamine oxidase (MAO) inhibitors, including phenelzine (Nardil) and tranylcypromine (Parnate); narcotic pain relievers such as meperidine (Demerol); nitroglycerin (Nitro-Bid, Nitrostat, others); sedatives; sleeping pills; and tranquilizers. Your doctor may need to change the doses of your medications or monitor you carefully for side effects.
- tell your doctor if you have or have ever had glaucoma; ulcerative colitis; an enlarged prostate (prostatic hyperplasia); difficulty urinating; esophageal reflux (heartburn); a blockage in the gastrointestinal tract; myasthenia gravis; high blood pressure; an overactive thyroid gland (hyperthyroidism); nerve disease (autonomic neuropathy); heart failure; rapid or pounding heartbeat; hiatal hernia; or liver, kidney, or heart disease.
- tell your doctor if you are pregnant, plan to become pregnant, or are breast-feeding. If you become pregnant while taking dicyclomine, call your doctor. Do not breast-feed while taking this medication.
- if you are having surgery, including dental surgery, tell the doctor or dentist that you are taking dicyclomine.
- you should know that dicyclomine may make you drowsy or cause blurred vision. Do not drive a car or operate machinery until you know how this medication affects you.
- remember that alcohol can add to the drowsiness caused by this medication.
- you should know that dicyclomine reduces the body's ability to cool off by sweating. In very high temperatures, dicyclomine can cause fever and heat stroke.

What special dietary instructions should I follow?

Unless your doctor tells you otherwise, continue your normal diet.

What should I do if I forget to take a dose?

Take the missed dose as soon as you remember it. However, if it is almost time for the next dose, skip the missed dose and continue your regular dosing schedule. Do not take a double dose to make up for a missed one.

What side effects can this medicine cause?

Dicyclomine may cause side effects. Tell your doctor if any of these symptoms are severe or do not go away:

- dry mouth
- upset stomach
- vomiting
- constipation
- stomach pain
- gas or bloating
- loss of appetite
- dizziness
- tingling
- headache
- drowsiness
- weakness
- blurred vision
- double vision
- difficulty urinating

Some side effects can be serious. The following symptoms are uncommon, but if you experience any of them, call your doctor immediately:

- hot, flushed, dry skin
- confusion
- forgetfulness
- seeing things or hearing voices that do not exist (hallucinating)
- unsteadiness
- coma
- anxiety
- excessive tiredness
- difficulty falling asleep or staying asleep
- excitement
- inappropriate mood
- muscle weakness
- rapid or pounding heartbeat
- fainting
- hives
- skin rash
- itching
- difficulty breathing or swallowing

Dicyclomine may cause other side effects. Call your doctor if you have any unusual problems while taking this medication.

If you experience a serious side effect, you or your doctor may send a report to the Food and Drug Administration's (FDA) MedWatch Adverse Event Reporting program online [at http://www.fda.gov/MedWatch/index.html] or by phone [1-800-332-1088].

What storage conditions are needed for this medicine?

Keep this medication in the container it came in, tightly closed, and out of reach of children. Store it at room temperature and away from excess heat and moisture (not in the bathroom). Throw away any medication that is outdated or no longer needed. Talk to your pharmacist about the proper disposal of your medication.

What should I do in case of overdose?

In case of overdose, call your local poison control center at 1-800-222-1222. If the victim has collapsed or is not breathing, call local emergency services at 911.

Symptoms of overdose may include:

- headache
- upset stomach
- vomiting
- blurred vision
- dilated pupils
- hot, dry skin
- dizziness
- dry mouth
- difficulty swallowing
- nervousness
- excitement

- seeing things or hearing voices that do not exist (hallucinating)

What other information should I know?

Keep all appointments with your doctor.

Do not let anyone else take your medication. Ask your pharmacist any questions you have about refilling your prescription.

Dosage Facts
For Informational Purposes

Caution: Do not change your dose, how often you take your medication, or the length of time you are to take it without first talking to your healthcare provider.

The following dosage information was written using medical language for doctors and other healthcare professionals and is provided here for you to check your dosage. The dosage of this drug may differ for different patients. Therefore, always follow your doctor's instructions or the directions on the label. Contact your healthcare provider or pharmacist if you have any questions about the specific dosage of your medication after reviewing this information.

General Dosage Information

Available as dicyclomine hydrochloride; dosage expressed in terms of the salt.

Pediatric Patients

GI Motility Disorders

ORAL:
- Infants >6 months of age†: 5 mg 3 or 4 times daily.
- Children†: 10 mg 3 or 4 times daily.

Adult Patients

GI Motility Disorders

ORAL:
- Usual initial dosage: 20 mg 4 times daily.
- Maintenance: Depending on response, increase dosage during the first week to 40 mg 4 times daily unless adverse effects limit upward titration.
- Only 40 mg 4 times daily has been shown clearly to be effective, but associated with a substantial incidence of adverse effects.
- Discontinue the drug if an adequate response is not obtained within 2 weeks or adverse effects limit dosage to <80 mg daily.

Prescribing Limits

Adult Patients

GI Motility Disorders

ORAL:
- Safety of 80–160 mg daily for longer than 2 weeks not established.

Special Populations

Hepatic Impairment
- No specific hepatic dosage recommendations; use with caution.

Renal Impairment
- No specific renal dosage recommendations; use with caution.

Geriatric Patients
- No specific geriatric dosage recommendations; use with caution since they may be more susceptible to adverse effects.

† Use is not currently included in the labeling approved by the US Food and Drug Administration.

Didanosine

(dye dan' oh seen)

Brand Name: Videx®, Videx® EC, Videx® Pediatric

Also available generically.

Important Warning

Didanosine, when used alone or in combination with other medications, can cause serious damage to the liver and pancreas and a condition called lactic acidosis. Tell your doctor if you drink or have ever drunk large amounts of alcohol; if you use or have used street drugs; or if you have or have ever had Crohn's disease, cystic fibrosis, diabetes, high cholesterol, or liver or pancreas disease. Tell your doctor and pharmacist if you are taking stavudine (Zerit), especially if you are pregnant. Tell your doctor and pharmacist if you are taking or have taken any of the following medications: acetaminophen (Tylenol, others); allopurinol (Zyloprim); amiodarone (Cordarone, Pacerone); azathioprine (Imuran); cholesterol-lowering medications (statins); dantrolene (Dantrium); furosemide (Lasix); hormone replacement therapy; iron products; isoniazid (INH, Nydrazid); ketoconazole (Nizoral); medications to treat HIV or AIDS; 6-mercaptopurine (Purinethol); methotrexate (Rheumatrex); methyldopa (Aldoril); niacin (nicotinic acid); oral contraceptives (birth control pills); oral steroids such as dexamethasone (Decadron, Dexone), methylprednisolone (Medrol), and prednisone (Deltasone); pentamidine (Nebupent, Pentam); piroxicam (Feldene); pyrazinamide (Rifater); ribavirin (Rebetron); rifampin (Rifadin, Rimactane); salicylate pain relievers such as aspirin, choline magnesium trisalicylate (Trisalate), choline salicylate (Arthropan), diflunisal (Dolobid), magnesium salicylate (Doan's, others), and salsalate (Argesic, Disalcid, Salgesic); sulfonamide antibiotics such as sulfadiazine, sulfamethizole (Urobiotic), sulfasalazine (Azulfidine), and sulfisoxazole (Eryzole, Gantrisin, Pediazole); sulindac (Clinoril); valproic acid (Depakene, Depakote); or products containing kava. If you experience any of the following symptoms, call your doctor immediately: upset stomach, vomiting, loss of appetite, stomach pain or swelling, severe back pain, extreme tiredness, weakness, dizziness, light-headedness, fast heart beat, sudden development of a slow or irregular heartbeat, deep or rapid breathing, shortness of breath, dark yellow or brown urine, unusual bleeding or bruising, yellowing of the skin or eyes, feeling cold, fever, or flu-like symptoms.

Ask your doctor about the safe use of alcohol while you are taking didanosine. Drinking alcohol can increase the risk that you will develop serious side effects of didanosine.

Keep all appointments with your doctor and the laboratory. Your doctor will order certain lab tests to check your body's response to didanosine. Talk to your doctor about the risks of taking didanosine.

Why is this medicine prescribed?

Didanosine is used with other medications to treat human immunodeficiency virus (HIV) infection in patients with or without acquired immunodeficiency syndrome (AIDS). Didanosine is in a class of medications called nucleoside reverse transcriptase inhibitors (NRTIs). Didanosine works by slowing the spread of HIV in the body. Didanosine does not cure HIV infection and may not prevent you from developing HIV-related illnesses. Didanosine does not prevent you from spreading HIV to other people.

How should this medicine be used?

Didanosine comes as extended-release (long-acting) capsules, tablets that can be chewed or mixed with water, a powder to be mixed with water, and a solution (liquid). All are taken by mouth. Didanosine is usually taken once or twice a day on an empty stomach, 30 minutes before or 2 hours after eating. To help you remember to take didanosine, take it around the same time(s) every day. Follow the directions on your prescription label carefully, and ask your doctor or pharmacist to explain any part you do not understand. Take didanosine exactly as directed. Do not take more or less of it, or take it more often than prescribed by your doctor.

If you are using the extended-release capsules, swallow them whole; do not split, chew, crush, or open them.

If you are using the tablets, do not swallow them whole. Chew the tablets well or mix them in at least 1 ounce of water and stir well to dissolve the tablets before swallowing. You may add one ounce (2 tablespoonfuls) of clear apple juice to the mixture for flavor, if needed. Do not use any other kind of juice. Drink all of the liquid right away.

If you are using the powder, you must mix it with water immediately before you take it. Open the packet and pour the powder into a glass with four ounces (1/2 cup) of water. Stir the mixture for 2 or 3 minutes until the powder is completely dissolved. Drink all of the liquid right away. Do not mix the powder with fruit juice or any other liquid.

If you are using the solution, you should shake it well before each use to mix the medication evenly. Use a dose-measuring spoon or cup to measure the correct dose, not a regular household spoon.

Didanosine controls HIV infection but does not cure it. Continue to take didanosine even if you feel well. Do not stop taking didanosine without talking to your doctor. If you miss doses or stop taking didanosine, your condition may become more difficult to treat.

Are there other uses for this medicine?

Didanosine is also used with another medication to help prevent infection in health care workers or other people who were accidentally exposed to HIV. Talk to your doctor about the possible risks of using this drug for your condition.

This medication may be prescribed for other uses; ask your doctor or pharmacist for more information.

What special precautions should I follow?

Before taking didanosine,
- tell your doctor and pharmacist if you are allergic to didanosine, aspartame (Nutrasweet), antacids, or any other medications.
- tell your doctor and pharmacist what other prescription and nonprescription medications, vitamins, and nutritional supplements you are taking. Be sure to mention any of the medications listed in the IMPORTANT WARNING section and the following: antacids; cancer chemotherapy medications; ganciclovir (Cytovene); methadone (Dolophine, Methadose); tenofovir (Viread); or zalcitabine (HIVID). Your doctor may need to change the doses of your medications or monitor you carefully for side effects.
- you should know that some medications must be taken several hours before or after you take didanosine. If you are taking any of the following medications, ask your doctor exactly when you should take them: anticoagulants ('blood thinners') such as warfarin (Coumadin); antifungals such as itraconazole (Sporanx) and ketoconazole (Nizoral); delavirdine (Rescriptor), digoxin (Lanoxin, Lanoxicaps); indinavir (Crixivan); nelfinavir (Viracept); quinolone antibiotics such as cinoxacin (Cinobac), ciprofloxacin (Cipro), enoxacin (Penetrex), gatifloxacin (Tequin), levofloxacin (Levaquin), lomefloxacin (Maxaquin), moxifloxacin (Avelox), nalidixic acid (NegGram), norfloxacin (Noroxin), ofloxacin (Floxin), sparfloxacin (Zagam), and trovafloxacin and alatrofloxacin combination (Trovan); tetracycline antibiotics such as demeclocycline

(Declomycin), doxycycline (Doryx, Vibramycin), minocycline (Dynacin, Minocin), and tetracycline (Sumycin); and zinc supplements.
- tell your doctor if you are on a low-salt diet and if you have or have ever had eye disease or problems with your vision, muscle problems, gout, peripheral neuropathy (numbness, tingling, burning, or pain sensation in your hands or feet, or decreased ability to feel temperature or touch in your hands or feet), radiation therapy, phenylketonuria (PKU, a disease in which you must avoid certain foods), or heart or kidney disease.
- tell your doctor if you are pregnant, plan to become pregnant, or are breast-feeding. If you become pregnant while taking didanosine, call your doctor. You should not breastfeed if you are infected with HIV or are taking didanosine.
- you should know that didanosine may cause side effects that must be treated right away before they become serious. Children who are taking didanosine may not be able to tell you about the side effects they are feeling. If you are giving didanosine to a child, ask the child's doctor how you can tell if the child is having these serious side effects.
- you should know that your body fat may increase or move to different areas of your body such as your breasts and upper back.

What special dietary instructions should I follow?

Unless your doctor tells you otherwise, continue your normal diet.

What should I do if I forget to take a dose?

Take the missed dose as soon as you remember it. However, if it is almost time for the next dose, skip the missed dose and continue your regular dosing schedule. Do not take a double dose to make up for a missed one.

What side effects can this medicine cause?

Didanosine may cause side effects. Tell your doctor if any of these symptoms are severe or do not go away:
- diarrhea
- headache
- muscle pain

Some side effects can be serious. The following symptoms are uncommon, but if you experience any of them, or those mentioned in the IMPORTANT WARNING section, call your doctor immediately:
- hives
- skin rash
- itching
- difficulty breathing or swallowing
- numbness, tingling, burning, or pain in hands or feet
- blurred vision
- difficulty in seeing colors clearly
- chills

Didanosine may cause other side effects. Call your doctor if you have any unusual problems while taking this medication.

If you experience a serious side effect, you or your doctor may send a report to the Food and Drug Administration's (FDA) MedWatch Adverse Event Reporting program online [at http://www.fda.gov/MedWatch/index.html] or by phone [1-800-332-1088].

What storage conditions are needed for this medicine?

Keep didanosine capsules, tablets, and powder in the containers they came in, tightly closed, and out of reach of children. Store them at room temperature and away from excess heat and moisture (not in the bathroom). Use mixtures of tablets and apple juice within 1 hour, and mixtures of powder and water within 4 hours. Keep didanosine liquid in the refrigerator, closed tightly, and throw away any unused medication after 30 days. Throw away any medication that is outdated or no longer needed. Talk to your pharmacist about the proper disposal of your medication.

What should I do in case of overdose?

In case of overdose, call your local poison control center at 1-800-222-1222. If the victim has collapsed or is not breathing, call local emergency services at 911.

Symptoms of overdose may include:

- diarrhea
- numbness, tingling, burning, or pain in hands or feet
- upset stomach
- vomiting
- loss of appetite
- stomach pain
- swelling of the stomach
- severe back pain
- extreme tiredness
- weakness
- dizziness
- light-headedness
- fast heart beat
- sudden development of a slow or irregular heartbeat
- deep or rapid breathing
- shortness of breath
- dark yellow or brown urine
- unusual bleeding or bruising
- yellowing of the skin or eyes
- feeling cold
- fever
- flu-like symptoms

What other information should I know?

Do not let anyone else take your medication. Ask your pharmacist any questions you have about refilling your prescription.

If you spill a packet of didanosine powder or didanosine liquid, clean the area of the spill with a wet mop or damp sponge using soap and water. Clean the area slowly so you do not make dust in the air. Try to keep all of the spill in one area. Wash your hands and the clean-up materials well after use.

Dosage Facts
For Informational Purposes

Caution: Do not change your dose, how often you take your medication, or the length of time you are to take it without first talking to your healthcare provider.

The following dosage information was written using medical language for doctors and other healthcare professionals and is provided here for you to check your dosage. The dosage of this drug may differ for different patients. Therefore, always follow your doctor's instructions or the directions on the label. Contact your healthcare provider or pharmacist if you have any questions about the specific dosage of your medication after reviewing this information.

General Dosage Information

Adult dosage is based on weight. Delayed-release capsules generally used for adults. Dosage in pediatric patients is based on body surface area. The pediatric oral solution generally used for children.

Must be given in conjunction with other antiretrovirals. *If used with amprenavir, atazanavir, darunavir, delavirdine, indinavir, lopinavir, nelfinavir, ritonavir, tenofovir, or tipranavir, adjustment in the treatment regimen necessary.*

Pediatric Patients

Treatment of HIV Infection

ORAL:

- Pediatric oral solution admixed with antacid: Neonates and children 2 weeks through 8 months of age: 100 mg/m² twice daily. Some experts suggest 50 mg/m² every 12 hours is more appropriate in those 2 weeks to 4 months of age.
- Pediatric oral solution admixed with antacid: Children >8 months of age: 120 mg/m² twice daily. Clinical studies have used 90–150 mg/m² every 12 hours.
- Adolescents: Use usual adult dosage based on weight.

Adult Patients

Treatment of HIV Infection
Treatment in Adults Weighing <60 kg

ORAL:

- Delayed-release capsules: 250 mg once daily.
- Pediatric oral solution admixed with antacid: 125 mg twice daily. If once-daily administration required, 250 mg once daily.

Treatment in Adults Weighing ≥60 kg

ORAL:

- Delayed-release capsules: 400 mg once daily.
- Pediatric oral solution admixed with antacid: 200 mg twice daily. If once-daily administration required, 400 mg once daily.

Postexposure Prophylaxis of HIV†

Occupational Exposure†

ORAL:

- Delayed-release capsules: Adults weighing <60 kg: 250 mg once daily.
- Delayed-release capsules: Adults weighing ≥60 kg: 400 mg once daily.
- Used in alternative basic regimens with lamivudine or emtricitabine.
- Initiate postexposure prophylaxis as soon as possible following exposure and continue for 4 weeks, if tolerated.

Nonoccupational Exposure†

ORAL:

- Delayed-release capsules: Adults weighing <60 kg: 250 mg once daily.
- Delayed-release capsules: Adults weighing ≥60 kg: 400 mg once daily.
- Used in an alternative NNRTI-based regimen in conjunction with efavirenz and (lamivudine or emtricitabine) and in various alternative HIV protease inhibitor-based (PI-based) regimens in conjunction with a PI (with or without low-dose ritonavir) and (lamivudine or emtricitabine).
- Initiate postexposure prophylaxis as soon as possible following exposure (preferably ≤72 hours after exposure) and continue for 28 days.

Special Populations

Renal Impairment

Treatment of HIV Infection

ORAL:

Dosage in Adults with Renal Impairment (Delayed-release Capsules)

Cl_{cr} (mL/minute)	Weighing <60 kg	Weighing ≥60 kg
≥60	250 mg once daily	400 mg once daily
30–59	125 mg once daily	200 mg once daily
10–29	125 mg once daily	125 mg once daily
<10	Not recommended; use alternative didanosine formulation	125 mg once daily
Hemodialysis or CAPD Patients	Not recommended; use alternative didanosine formulation	125 mg once daily; supplemental doses unnecessary after hemodialysis

Dosage in Adults with Renal Impairment (Pediatric Oral Solution Admixed with Antacid)

Cl_{cr} (mL/minute)	Weighing <60 kg	Weighing ≥60 kg
≥60	125 mg twice daily or 250 mg once daily	200 mg twice daily or 400 mg once daily
30–59	150 mg once daily or 75 mg twice daily	200 mg once daily or 100 mg twice daily
10–29	100 mg once daily	150 mg once daily
<10	75 mg once daily	100 mg once daily
Hemodialysis or CAPD Patients	75 mg once daily; supplemental doses unnecessary after hemodialysis	100 mg once daily; supplemental doses unnecessary after hemodialysis

† Use is not currently included in the labeling approved by the US Food and Drug Administration.

Diethylpropion

(dye eth il proe′ pee on)

Brand Name: Tenuate®, Tenuate Dospan®

Why is this medicine prescribed?

Diethylpropion decreases appetite. It is used on a short-term basis (a few weeks), in combination with diet, to help you lose weight.

This medication is sometimes prescribed for other uses; ask your doctor or pharmacist for more information.

How should this medicine be used?

Diethylpropion comes as a regular and extended-release (long-acting) tablet. Diethylpropion usually is taken three times a day, 1 hour before meals (regular tablets), or once a day in midmorning (extended-release tablets). Follow the directions on your prescription label carefully, and ask your doctor or pharmacist to explain any part you do not understand. Take diethylpropion exactly as directed.

Do not crush, chew, or cut extended-release tablets; swallow them whole.

Diethylpropion may be habit-forming. Do not take a larger dose, take it more often, or for a longer period than your doctor tells you to. Call your doctor if diethylpropion loses its effect.

What special precautions should I follow?

Before taking diethylpropion,

- tell your doctor and pharmacist if you are allergic to

diethylpropion; amphetamines; other diet pills; medications for allergies, hay fever, and colds; or any other drugs.

- tell your doctor and pharmacist what prescription and nonprescription medications you are taking, especially guanethidine, insulin, and MAO inhibitors [phenelzine (Nardil) or tranylcypromine (Parnate)] even if you stopped taking them in the last 2 weeks, herbal products, and vitamins. Tell your doctor if you have taken other diet pills in the past year.
- tell your doctor if you have or have ever had heart or blood vessel disease, high blood pressure, an overactive thyroid gland, diabetes, glaucoma, pulmonary hypertension, seizures, or a history of drug abuse.
- tell your doctor if you are pregnant, plan to become pregnant, or are breast-feeding. If you become pregnant while taking diethylpropion, call your doctor.
- if you are having surgery, including dental surgery, tell the doctor or dentist that you are taking diethylpropion.
- you should know that this drug may make you drowsy. Do not drive a car or operate machinery until you know how this drug affects you.
- remember that alcohol can add to the drowsiness caused by this drug.

What special dietary instructions should I follow?

Follow your doctor's directions. Eat a low-calorie, well-balanced diet.

What should I do if I forget to take a dose?

Take the missed dose as soon as you remember it. However, if it is almost time for the next dose, skip the missed dose and continue your regular dosing schedule. Do not take a double dose to make up for a missed one.

What side effects can this medicine cause?

Diethylpropion may cause side effects. Tell your doctor if any of these symptoms are severe or do not go away:

- dry mouth
- unpleasant taste
- restlessness
- anxiety
- dizziness
- depression
- tremors
- upset stomach
- vomiting
- increased urination

If you experience any of the following symptoms, call your doctor immediately:

- fast or irregular heartbeat
- heart palpitations
- blurred vision
- skin rash
- itching

- difficulty breathing
- chest pain
- fainting
- swelling of the ankles or feet
- fever
- sore throat
- chills
- painful urination

If you experience a serious side effect, you or your doctor may send a report to the Food and Drug Administration's (FDA) MedWatch Adverse Event Reporting program online [at http://www.fda.gov/MedWatch/index.html] or by phone [1-800-332-1088].

What storage conditions are needed for this medicine?

Keep this medication in the container it came in, tightly closed, and out of reach of children. Store it at room temperature and away from excess heat and moisture (not in the bathroom). Throw away any medication that is outdated or no longer needed. Talk to your pharmacist about the proper disposal of your medication.

What should I do in case of overdose?

In case of overdose, call your local poison control center at 1-800-222-1222. If the victim has collapsed or is not breathing, call local emergency services at 911.

What other information should I know?

Keep all appointments with your doctor. Your doctor may order certain tests to check your response to diethylpropion.

Diethylpropion may affect blood sugar levels of diabetic patients and may cover up some signs and symptoms of hypoglycemia (low blood sugar). If you notice a change in the results of your urine or blood sugar tests, check with your doctor.

Do not let anyone else take your medication. Ask your pharmacist any questions you have about refilling your prescription.

Talk to your doctor, pharmacist, or other healthcare professional if you have questions about dosing information for your medication.

Diflorasone Topical

(dye flor′ a sone)

Brand Name: Psorcon E® Emollient Cream, Psorcon®

Why is this medicine prescribed?

Diflorasone is used to treat the itching, redness, dryness, crusting, scaling, inflammation (swelling), and discomfort of various skin conditions. Diflorasone is in a class of medications called topical steroids. It works by reducing inflammation and itching.

How should this medicine be used?

Diflorasone comes as a cream and an ointment to apply to the skin. It is usually applied to the affected area one to three times a day. To help you remember to use diflorasone, apply it around the same time every day. Follow the directions on your prescription label carefully, and ask your doctor or pharmacist to explain any part you do not understand. Use diflorasone exactly as directed. Do not use more or less of it or use it more often than prescribed by your doctor.

Wash or soak the affected area thoroughly before applying the medicine, unless it irritates your skin. Then apply the ointment or cream sparingly in a thin film and rub it in gently.

If you are using diflorasone on your face, keep it out of your eyes.

If you are using diflorasone on a child's diaper area, do not use tight-fitting diapers or plastic pants. Such use may increase side effects.

Do not apply cosmetics or other skin preparations on the treated area without talking with your doctor.

Do not wrap or bandage the treated area unless your doctor tells you to. If your doctor tells you to wrap or bandage the treated area, follow these instructions:

1. Soak the area in water or wash it well.
2. While the skin is moist, gently rub the medication into the affected areas.
3. Cover the area with plastic wrap (such as Saran Wrap or Handi-Wrap). The plastic may be held in place with a gauze or elastic bandage or adhesive tape on the normal skin beside the treated area. (Instead of using plastic wrap, plastic gloves may be used for the hands, plastic bags for the feet, or a shower cap for the scalp.)
4. Carefully seal the edges of the plastic to make sure the wrap adheres closely to the skin. If the affected area is moist, you can leave the edges of the plastic wrap partly unsealed or puncture the wrap to allow excess moisture to escape.
5. Leave the plastic wrapping in place as long as instructed by your doctor. Usually plastic wraps are left in place not more than 12 hours each day.
6. Cleanse the skin and reapply the medication each time a new plastic wrapping is applied.

Are there other uses for this medicine?

This medication may be prescribed for other uses; ask your doctor or pharmacist for more information.

What special precautions should I follow?

Before using diflorasone,

- tell your doctor and pharmacist if you are allergic to diflorasone or any other medications.
- tell your doctor and pharmacist what prescription and nonprescription medications, vitamins, nutritional supplements, and herbal products you are taking.
- tell your doctor if you are pregnant, plan to become pregnant, or are breast-feeding. If you become pregnant while using diflorasone, call your doctor.

What special dietary instructions should I follow?

Unless your doctor tells you otherwise, continue your normal diet.

What should I do if I forget to take a dose?

Apply the missed dose as soon as you remember it. However, if it is almost time for the next dose, skip the missed dose and continue your regular dosing schedule. Do not apply a double dose to make up for a missed one.

What side effects can this medicine cause?

Diflorasone may cause side effects. If you experience any of the following symptoms, call your doctor immediately:

- skin burning, itching, or irritation
- dry skin
- rash
- increased hair growth
- skin discoloration

Long-term use of diflorasone may cause children to grow more slowly. Talk to your doctor about the risks of using this medication.

Diflorasone may cause other side effects. Call your doctor if you have any unusual problems while using this medication.

If you experience a serious side effect, you or your doctor may send a report to the Food and Drug Administration's (FDA) MedWatch Adverse Event Reporting program online [at http://www.fda.gov/MedWatch/index.html] or by phone [1-800-332-1088].

What storage conditions are needed for this medicine?

Keep this medication in the container it came in, tightly closed, and out of reach of children. Store it at room temperature and away from excess heat and moisture (not in the bathroom). Throw away any medication that is outdated or no longer needed. Talk to your pharmacist about the proper disposal of your medication.

What other information should I know?

Keep all appointments with your doctor and the laboratory. Your doctor may order certain lab tests to check your body's response to diflorasone.

Do not let anyone else use your medication. Do not use this medication for a skin condition other than the one for which it was prescribed. Ask your pharmacist any questions you have about refilling your prescription.

Talk to your doctor, pharmacist, or other healthcare professional if you have questions about dosing information for your medication.

Diflunisal

(dye floo′ ni sal)

Brand Name: Dolobid®
Also available generically.

Important Warning

People who take nonsteroidal anti-inflammatory medications (NSAIDs) (other than aspirin) such as diflunisal may have a higher risk of having a heart attack or a stroke than people who do not take these medications. These events may happen without warning and may cause death. This risk may be higher for people who take NSAIDs for a long time. Tell your doctor if you or anyone in your family has or has ever had heart disease, a heart attack, or a stroke, if you smoke, and if you have or have ever had high cholesterol, high blood pressure, or diabetes. Get emergency medical help right away if you experience any of the following symptoms: chest pain, shortness of breath, weakness in one part or side of the body, or slurred speech.

If you will be undergoing a coronary artery bypass graft (CABG; a type of heart surgery), you should not take diflunisal right before or right after the surgery.

NSAIDs such as diflunisal may cause ulcers, bleeding, or holes in the stomach or intestine. These problems may develop at any time during treatment, may happen without warning symptoms, and may cause death. The risk may be higher for people who take NSAIDs for a long time, are older in age, have poor health, or drink large amounts of alcohol while you are taking diflunisal. Tell your doctor if you take any of the following medications: anticoagulants ('blood thinners') such as warfarin (Coumadin); aspirin; other NSAIDs such as ibuprofen (Advil, Motrin) and naproxen (Aleve, Naprosyn); or oral steroids such as dexamethasone (Decadron, Dexone),

---

methylprednisolone (Medrol), and prednisone (Deltasone). Also tell your doctor if you have or have ever had ulcers, bleeding in your stomach or intestines, or other bleeding disorders. If you experience any of the following symptoms, stop taking diflunisal and call your doctor: stomach pain, heartburn, vomiting a substance that is bloody or looks like coffee grounds, blood in the stool, or black and tarry stools.

Keep all appointments with your doctor and the laboratory. Your doctor will monitor your symptoms carefully and will probably order certain tests to check your body's response to diflunisal. Be sure to tell your doctor how you are feeling so that your doctor can prescribe the right amount of medication to treat your condition with the lowest risk of serious side effects.

Your doctor or pharmacist will give you the manufacturer's patient information sheet (Medication Guide) when you begin treatment with diflunisal and each time you refill your prescription. Read the information carefully and ask your doctor or pharmacist if you have any questions. You can also visit the Food and Drug Administration (FDA) website (http://www.fda.gov/cder) or the manufacturer's website to obtain the Medication Guide.

Why is this medicine prescribed?

Diflunisal is used to relieve pain, tenderness, swelling and stiffness caused by osteoarthritis (arthritis caused by a breakdown of the lining of the joints) and rheumatoid arthritis (arthritis caused by swelling of the lining of the joints). Diflunisal is also used to relieve mild to moderate pain from other causes. Diflunisal is in a class of medications called NSAIDs. It works by stopping the body's production of a substance that causes pain, fever, and inflammation.

How should this medicine be used?

Diflunisal comes as a tablet to take by mouth. It usually is taken with water, milk, or food every 8-12 hours Take diflunisal at around the same times every day. Follow the directions on your prescription label carefully, and ask your doctor or pharmacist to explain any part you do not understand. Take diflunisal exactly as directed. Do not take more or less of it or take it more often than prescribed by your doctor.

Swallow the tablets whole; do not split, chew, or crush them.

It may take several days or longer for you to feel the full benefit of diflunisal. Continue to take diflunisal until your doctor tells you that you should stop taking the medication.

Are there other uses for this medicine?

This medication is sometimes prescribed for other uses; ask your doctor or pharmacist for more information.

What special precautions should I follow?

Before taking diflunisal,

- tell your doctor and pharmacist if you are allergic to diflunisal, aspirin or other NSAIDs such as ibuprofen (Advil, Motrin) and naproxen (Aleve, Naprosyn), or any other medications.
- tell your doctor and pharmacist what prescription and nonprescription medications, vitamins, nutritional supplements, and herbal products you are taking or plan to take. Be sure to mention the medications listed in the IMPORTANT WARNING section and any of the following: acetaminophen (Tylenol); angiotensin-converting enzyme (ACE) inhibitors such as benazepril (Lotensin), captopril (Capoten), enalapril (Vasotec), fosinopril (Monopril), lisinopril (Prinivil, Zestril), moexipril (Univasc), perindopril (Aceon), quinapril (Accupril), ramipril (Altace), and trandolapril (Mavik); angiotensin II receptor antagonists such as candesartan (Atacand), eprosartan (Teveten), irbesartan (Avapro), losartan (Cozaar), olmesartan (Benicar), telmisartan (Micardis), and valsartan (Diovan); antacids; cyclosporine (Neoral, Sandimmune); diuretics ('water pills'); indomethacin (Indocin); lithium (Eskalith, Lithobid); methotrexate (Rheumatrex); and sulindac (Clinoril). Your doctor may need to change the dose of your medications or monitor you carefully for side effects.
- tell your doctor if you have or have ever had any of the conditions mentioned in the IMPORTANT WARNING section or asthma, especially if you also have frequent stuffed or runny nose or nasal polyps (swelling of the lining of the nose); swelling of the hands, feet, ankles, or lower legs; or liver or kidney disease.
- tell your doctor if you are pregnant, especially if you are in the last few months of your pregnancy, you plan to become pregnant, or you are breast-feeding. If you become pregnant while taking diflunisal, call your doctor.
- if you are having surgery, including dental surgery, tell the doctor or dentist that you are taking diflunisal.
- call your doctor if you think you may have a virus, such as chicken pox or the flu. Do not take diflunisal if you have a virus, and do not give diflunisal to a child who has a virus.

What special dietary instructions should I follow?

Unless your doctor tells you otherwise, continue your normal diet.

What should I do if I forget to take a dose?

Take the missed dose as soon as you remember it. However, if it is almost time for the next dose, skip the missed dose and continue your regular dosing schedule. Do not take a double dose to make up for a missed one.

What side effects can this medicine cause?

Diflunisal may cause side effects. Tell your doctor if any of these symptoms are severe or do not go away:

- vomiting
- diarrhea
- constipation
- gas
- headache
- dizziness
- ringing in the ears
- problems with vision

Some side effects can be serious. If you experience any of the following symptoms or those mentioned in the IMPORTANT WARNING section, call your doctor immediately. Do not take any more diflunisal until you speak to your doctor.

- upset stomach
- excessive tiredness
- unusual bleeding or bruising
- itching
- lack of energy
- loss of appetite
- pain in the upper right part of the stomach
- yellowing of the skin or eyes
- flu-like symptoms
- rash
- blisters
- fever or chills
- pale skin
- fast heartbeat
- easy bruising or bleeding
- muscle or joint pain
- unexplained weight gain
- back pain
- cloudy, discolored, or bloody urine
- difficult or painful urination
- frequent urination, especially at night
- swelling of the face, throat, tongue, lips, eyes, hands, feet, ankles, or lower legs
- hoarseness
- difficulty swallowing or breathing

Diflunisal may cause other side effects. Call your doctor if you have any unusual problems while taking this medication.

If you experience a serious side effect, you or your doctor may send a report to the Food and Drug Administration's (FDA) MedWatch Adverse Event Reporting program online [at http://www.fda.gov/MedWatch/index.html] or by phone [1-800-332-1088].

What storage conditions are needed for this medicine?

Keep this medication in the container it came in, tightly closed, and out of reach of children. Store it at room temperature and away from excess heat and moisture (not in the bathroom). Throw away any medication that is outdated or

no longer needed. Talk to your pharmacist about the proper disposal of your medication.

What should I do in case of overdose?

In case of overdose, call your local poison control center at 1-800-222-1222. If the victim has collapsed or is not breathing, call local emergency services at 911.

Symptoms of overdose may include:

- drowsiness
- vomiting
- upset stomach
- diarrhea
- decreased urination
- fast breathing
- fast heartbeat
- sweating
- ringing in the ears
- confusion
- coma (loss of consciousness for a period of time)

What other information should I know?

Before having any laboratory test, tell your doctor and the laboratory personnel that you are taking diflunisal.

Do not let anyone else take your medication. Ask your pharmacist any questions you have about refilling your prescription.

Dosage Facts
For Informational Purposes

Caution: Do not change your dose, how often you take your medication, or the length of time you are to take it without first talking to your healthcare provider.

The following dosage information was written using medical language for doctors and other healthcare professionals and is provided here for you to check your dosage. The dosage of this drug may differ for different patients. Therefore, always follow your doctor's instructions or the directions on the label. Contact your healthcare provider or pharmacist if you have any questions about the specific dosage of your medication after reviewing this information.

General Dosage Information

To minimize the potential risk of adverse cardiovascular and/or GI events, use lowest effective dosage and shortest duration of therapy consistent with the patient's treatment goals. Adjust dosage based on individual requirements and response; attempt to titrate to the lowest effective dosage.

Exhibits concentration-dependent pharmacokinetics. Plasma diflunisal concentrations increase more than proportionally with increasing and/or multiple doses; use caution when adjusting doses.

Adult Patients
Pain

ORAL:
- Mild to moderate pain: Initially, 1 g, followed by 500 mg every 12 hours. Some patients may require 500 mg every 8 hours.
- Patients with lower dosage requirements (less severe pain, heightened response, low body weight): Initially, 500 mg, followed by 250 mg every 8–12 hours.

Inflammatory Diseases
Osteoarthritis or Rheumatoid Arthritis

ORAL:
- 500 mg–1 g daily in 2 divided doses.

Prescribing Limits
Adult Patients

ORAL:
- Maximum 1.5 g daily.

Special Populations

Geriatric Patients
- Select dosage with caution because of age-related decreases in renal function.
- Initially, 500 mg, followed by 250 mg every 8–12 hours.

Digoxin Oral
(di jox′ in)

Brand Name: Digitek®, Lanoxicaps®, Lanoxin®, Lanoxin® Elixir Pediatric
Also available generically.

Why is this medicine prescribed?

Digoxin is used to treat heart failure and abnormal heart rhythms (arrhythmias). It helps the heart work better and it helps control your heart rate.

This medication is sometimes prescribed for other uses; ask your doctor or pharmacist for more information.

How should this medicine be used?

Digoxin comes as a tablet, capsule, or pediatric elixir (liquid) to take by mouth. Digoxin is usually taken once a day. The pediatric elixir comes with a specially marked dropper for measuring the dose. If you have difficulty, ask your pharmacist to show you how to use it. It is important that you always take the same brand of digoxin. Different brands of digoxin have different amounts of active drug and your dose would need to be changed.

Follow the directions on your prescription label carefully, and ask your doctor or pharmacist to explain any part you do not understand. Take digoxin exactly as directed. Do not take more or less of it or take it more often than prescribed by your doctor.

Digoxin helps control your condition but will not cure it. Continue to take digoxin even if you feel well. Do not stop taking digoxin without talking to your doctor.

Are there other uses for this medicine?

Digoxin is also used to treat heart pain (angina) and may be used after a heart attack. Talk to your doctor about the possible risks of using this drug for your condition.

What special precautions should I follow?

Before taking digoxin,

- tell your doctor and pharmacist if you are allergic to digoxin, digitoxin, or any other drugs.
- tell your doctor and pharmacist what prescription and nonprescription medications you are taking, especially antacids, antibiotics, calcium, corticosteroids, diuretics ('water pills'), other medications for heart disease, thyroid medications, and vitamins.
- tell your doctor if you have or have ever had thyroid problems, heart arrhythmias, cancer, or kidney disease.
- tell your doctor if you are pregnant, plan to become pregnant, or are breast-feeding. If you become pregnant while taking digoxin, call your doctor.
- if you are having surgery, including dental surgery, tell the doctor or dentist that you are taking digoxin.
- you should know that this drug may make you drowsy. Do not drive a car or operate machinery until you know how this drug affects you.
- remember that alcohol can add to the drowsiness caused by this drug.

What special dietary instructions should I follow?

Your doctor may recommend a low-sodium (low-salt) diet and a potassium supplement. Ask your pharmacist or doctor for a list of foods that are low in sodium and high in potassium. Follow all diet directions carefully.

What should I do if I forget to take a dose?

Take the missed dose as soon as you remember it. However, if it is almost time for the next dose, skip the missed dose and continue your regular dosing schedule. Do not take a double dose to make up for a missed one.

What side effects can this medicine cause?

Digoxin may cause side effects. Tell your doctor if any of these symptoms are severe or do not go away:

- dizziness or lightheadedness
- drowsiness
- vision changes (blurred or yellow)
- rash
- irregular heartbeat

If you experience any of the following symptoms, call your doctor immediately:

- upset stomach
- vomiting
- diarrhea
- loss of appetite
- swelling of the feet or hands
- unusual weight gain
- difficulty breathing

If you experience a serious side effect, you or your doctor may send a report to the Food and Drug Administration's (FDA) MedWatch Adverse Event Reporting program online [at http://www.fda.gov/MedWatch/index.html] or by phone [1-800-332-1088].

What storage conditions are needed for this medicine?

Keep this medication in the container it came in, tightly closed, and out of reach of children. Store it at room temperature and away from excess heat and moisture (not in the bathroom). Throw away any medication that is outdated or no longer needed. Talk to your pharmacist about the proper disposal of your medication.

What should I do in case of overdose?

In case of overdose, call your local poison control center at 1-800-222-1222. If the victim has collapsed or is not breathing, call local emergency services at 911.

What other information should I know?

Keep all appointments with your doctor and the laboratory. Your doctor will need to determine your response to digoxin. You may have electrocardiograms (EKGs) and blood tests periodically, and your dose may need to be adjusted. Your doctor may ask you to check your pulse (heart rate). Ask your pharmacist or doctor to teach you how to take your pulse. If your pulse is faster or slower than it should be, call your doctor.

Do not let anyone else take your medication. Ask your pharmacist any questions you have about refilling your prescription.

Dosage Facts
For Informational Purposes

Caution: Do not change your dose, how often you take your medication, or the length of time you are to take it without first talking to your healthcare provider.

The following dosage information was written using medical language for doctors and other healthcare professionals and is provided here for you to check your dosage. The dosage of this drug may differ for different patients. Therefore, always follow your doctor's instructions or the directions on the label. Contact your health-

care provider or pharmacist if you have any questions about the specific dosage of your medication after reviewing this information.

General Dosage Information

Dosage guidelines provided are based upon average patient response and substantial patient variation can be expected. Ultimate dosage selection must be based upon clinical assessment of the patient.

Pediatric Patients

Titrate dosage carefully in neonates, especially premature infants, because renal clearance of digoxin is reduced.

Infants and young children (up to 10 years of age) generally require proportionally larger doses than children older than 10 years of age and adults when calculated on the basis of lean or ideal body weight or body surface area.

Children >10 years of age require adult dosages in proportion to the child's body weight.

Liquid-filled capsules may not be the formulation of choice in infants and young children (<10 years of age) where dosage adjustment is frequent and outside of the fixed dosages provided by the capsules.

CHF

Digitalization may be accomplished by one of two approaches (i.e., rapid digitalization or slow digitalization) that vary in dosage and frequency of administration, but achieve the same total amount of digoxin accumulated in the body.

Rapid digitalization (if considered medically appropriate): Administer a loading dose based upon projected peak digoxin body stores. Daily maintenance dose (calculated as a percentage of the loading dose) will follow loading dose.)

Peak body digoxin stores of 8–12 mcg/kg generally provide therapeutic effect with minimum risk of toxicity in most patients with CHF, normal sinus rhythm, and normal renal function.

Slow digitalization: Initiate therapy with an appropriate daily maintenance dose, which allows digoxin body stores to accumulate slowly. Steady-state serum digoxin concentrations will be achieved in about 5 half-lives of the drug for the individual patient; depending on the patient's renal function, this may take 1–3 weeks.

Digitalizing (i.e., Loading) and Maintenance Dosages

Total digitalizing (i.e., loading) doses and maintenance dosages in pediatric patients (depending on the dosage form administered) are given in the tables that follow, and should provide therapeutic effect with minimum risk of toxicity in most patients with CHF, normal sinus rhythm, and normal renal function.

Administer the loading dose in divided doses, with about 50% of the total dose given as the first (i.e., initial) dose; additional fractions (generally 25%) are administered at 4- to 8-hour intervals IV or 6- to 8-hour intervals orally or IM, *with careful assessment of the patient's clinical response before each additional dose is administered.* If the patient's clinical response requires a change from the calculated loading dose, then calculation of the maintenance dose is based upon the amount (i.e., total loading dose) actually administered.

ORAL:

Usual Pediatric Maintenance Dosages for Digoxin Tablets (normal renal function, based on lean body weight)

Age	Oral Maintenance Dosage† (mcg/kg daily)
2–5 years of age	10–15
5–10 years of age	7–10
>10 years of age	3–5

†Divided daily dosing is generally recommended in infants and young children (<10 years of age).

Usual Pediatric Digitalizing and Maintenance Dosages for Digoxin Elixir (normal renal function, based on lean body weight)

Age	Oral Digitalizing* (Loading) Dose (mcg/kg)	Oral Maintenance Dosage† (mcg/kg daily)
Premature neonates	20–30	20–30% of oral loading dose**
Full-term neonates	25–35	25–35% of oral loading dose**
1–24 months	35–60	25–35% of oral loading dose**
2–5 years of age	30–40	25–35% of oral loading dose**
5–10 years of age	20–35	25–35% of oral loading dose**
>10 years of age	10–15	25–35% of oral loading dose**

*IV digitalizing doses are 80% of oral digitalizing doses of digoxin tablets or elixir.
†Divided daily dosing is generally recommended in infants and young children (<10 years of age).
**Estimated or actual digitalizing dose that provides desired clinical response.

Usual Pediatric Digitalizing and Maintenance Dosages for Digoxin Liquid-Filled Capsules (normal renal function, based on lean body weight)

Age	Oral Digitalizing* (Loading) Dose (mcg/kg)	Oral Maintenance Dosage† (mcg/kg daily)
2–5 years of age	25–35	25–35% of oral or IV loading dose**
5–10 years of age	15–30	25–35% of oral or IV loading dose**
>10 years of age	8–12	25–35% of oral or IV loading dose**

*IV digitalizing doses are the same as oral digitalizing doses of liquid-filled capsules.
†Divided daily dosing is generally recommended in infants and young children (<10 years of age).
**Estimated or actual digitalizing dose that provides desired clinical response.

Atrial Fibrillation

Peak digoxin body stores exceeding the 8–12 mcg/kg required for most patients with CHF and normal sinus rhythm have been used for control of ventricular rate in patients with atrial fibrillation. In the treatment of chronic atrial fibrillation, titrate dosage to the minimum dosage that achieves the desired ventricular rate control without causing undesirable adverse effects. Appropriate target resting or exercising rates have not been established.

Adult Patients

CHF

Digitalization may be accomplished by one of two approaches (i.e., rapid digitalization or slow digitalization) that vary in dosage and frequency of administration, but achieve the same total amount of digoxin accumulated in the body.

Rapid digitalization (if considered medically appropriate): Administer a loading dose based upon projected peak digoxin body stores. Daily maintenance dose (calculated as a percentage of the loading dose) will follow loading dose. Peak digoxin body stores of 8–12 mcg/kg generally provide therapeutic effect with minimum risk of toxicity in most patients with CHF, normal sinus rhythm, and normal renal function.

Slow digitalization: Initiate therapy with an appropriate daily maintenance dose, which allows digoxin body stores to accumulate slowly. Steady-state serum digoxin concentrations will be achieved in about 5 half-lives of the drug for the individual patient; depending on the patient's renal function, this may take 1–3 weeks.

Loading Dose (for rapid digitalization)

Administer the loading dose in divided doses, with about 50% of the total dose given as the first (i.e., initial) dose; additional fractions (generally 25%) are administered at 6- to 8-hour intervals orally *with careful assessment of the patient's clinical response before each additional dose is administered.* If the patient's clinical response requires a change from the calculated loading dose, then calculation of the maintenance dose is based upon the amount (i.e., total loading dose) actually administered.

ORAL:
- Usually, a single initial dose of 500–750 mcg (0.5–0.75 mg) of digoxin tablets or 400–600 mcg (0.4–0.6 mg) of digoxin liquid-filled capsules produces a detectable effect in 0.5–2 hours that becomes maximal in 2–6 hours.
- Cautiously administer additional doses of 125–375 mcg (0.125–0.375 mg) of digoxin tablets or 100–300 mcg (0.1–0.3 mg) of digoxin liquid-filled capsules at 6- to 8-hour intervals until clinical evidence of an adequate response is achieved.
- Usual amount (i.e., total loading dose) of digoxin tablets or liquid-filled capsules that a 70-kg patient requires to achieve 8–12 mcg/kg peak body stores is 750–1250 mcg (0.75–1.25 mg) or 600–1000 mcg (0.6–1 mg), respectively.

Maintenance Dosage

Daily maintenance dosage is a replacement of daily digoxin loss from the body and can be *estimated* by multiplying the daily percentage loss by the peak body stores (i.e., loading dose).

About 30% of total digoxin in the body is eliminated daily in patients with normal renal function; anuric patients eliminate approximately 14% of the total digoxin stores daily. The % of digoxin eliminated from the body daily can be *estimated* by the following equation:

Use this method with caution, since Cl_{cr} does not accurately measure renal or total body clearance of digoxin.

ORAL:
- Tablets: Usually, 125–500 mcg (0.125–0.5 mg) once daily; titrate according to the patient's age, lean body weight, and renal function. Generally, initiate at 250 mcg (0.25 mg) once daily in patients <70 years of age with normal renal function; may increase dosage every 2 weeks according to clinical response.
- Capsules (liquid-filled): Usually, 150–350 mcg (0.15–0.35 mg) daily in patients with Cl_{cr} of ≥50 mL/minute.

Atrial Fibrillation

Peak digoxin body stores exceeding the 8–12 mcg/kg required for most patients with CHF and normal sinus rhythm have been used for control of ventricular rate in patients with atrial fibrillation.

In the treatment of chronic atrial fibrillation, titrate dosage to the minimum dosage that achieves the desired ventricular rate control without causing undesirable adverse effects. Appropriate target resting or exercising rates have not been established.

Special Populations

Hepatic Impairment
- No dosage adjustment is necessary in liver disease if renal function is normal.

Renal Impairment
- Loading doses (based upon projected peak digoxin body stores) in patients with renal insufficiency (particularly those with Cl_{cr} <10 mL/minute) should be conservative (i.e., based upon peak digoxin body stores of 6–10 mcg/kg) because of altered digoxin distribution and elimination.
- Pediatric Patients: Cautiously adjust dosage based on clinical response.
- Adults: For maintenance dosage, generally initiate at 125 mcg once daily orally (digoxin tablets) in patients with impaired renal function or at 62.5 mcg once daily orally (digoxin tablets) in patients with marked renal impairment; may increase dosage every 2 weeks according to clinical response.

Geriatric Patients
- Reduce dosage, especially in those with CAD.
- Advanced age may be an indicator of decreased renal function even in patients with normal S_{cr} (i.e., <1.5 mg/dL).
- Geriatric Patients ≥70 years of age: For maintenance dosage, generally initiate at 125 mcg once daily orally (digoxin tablets).

Dihydroergotamine Injection and Nasal Spray

(dye hye droe er got' a meen)

Brand Name: D.H.E. 45®, Migranal® Nasal Spray

Important Warning

Do not take dihydroergotamine if you are taking any of the following medications: antifungals such as itraconazole (Sporanox) and ketoconazole (Nizoral); HIV protease inhibitors such as indinavir (Crixivan), nelfinavir (Viracept), and ritonavir (Norvir); or macrolide antibiotics such as clarithromycin (Biaxin), erythromycin (E.E.S., E-Mycin, Erythrocin), and troleandomycin (TAO).

Why is this medicine prescribed?

Dihydroergotamine is used to treat migraine headaches. Dihydroergotamine is in a class of medications called ergot alkaloids. It works by tightening blood vessels in the brain and by stopping the release of natural substances in the brain that cause swelling.

How should this medicine be used?

Dihydroergotamine comes as a solution to inject subcutaneously (under the skin) and as a spray to be used in the nose. It is taken as needed for migraine headaches. Follow the directions on your prescription label carefully, and ask your doctor or pharmacist to explain any part you do not understand. Take dihydroergotamine exactly as directed. Do not take more or less of it or take it more often than prescribed by your doctor.

Dihydroergotamine can damage the heart and other organs if it is used too often. Dihydroergotamine should be used only to treat a migraine that is in progress. Do not use dihydroergotamine to prevent a migraine from beginning or to treat a headache that feels different than your usual migraine. Dihydroergotamine should not be used every day. Your doctor will tell you how many times you may use dihydroergotamine each week.

You may receive your first dose of dihydroergotamine in your doctor's office so that your doctor can monitor your reaction to the medication and be sure that you know how to use the nasal spray or administer the injection correctly. After that, you may spray or inject dihydroergotamine at home. Be sure that you and anyone who will be helping you inject the medication read the manufacturer's information for the patient that comes with dihydroergotamine before using it for the first time at home.

If you are using the solution for injection, you should never reuse syringes. Dispose of syringes in a puncture resistant container. Ask your doctor or pharmacist how to dispose of the puncture resistant container.

To use the solution for injection, follow these steps:

1. Check your ampule to be sure it is safe to use. Do not use the ampule if it is broken, cracked, labeled with an expiration date that has passed, or contains a colored, cloudy, or particle filled liquid. Return that ampule to the pharmacy and use a different ampule.
2. Wash your hands well with soap and water.
3. Check to be sure all the liquid is at the bottom of ampule. If any liquid is at the top of the ampule, gently flick it with your finger until it falls to the bottom.
4. Hold the bottom of the ampule in one hand. Hold the top of the ampule between the thumb and pointer of your other hand. Your thumb should be over the dot on the top of the ampule. Push the top of the ampule backward with your thumb until it breaks off.
5. Tilt the ampule at a 45 degree angle and insert the needle into the ampule.
6. Pull back the plunger slowly and steadily until the top of the plunger is even with the dose your doctor told you to inject.
7. Hold the syringe with the needle pointing upward and check if it contains air bubbles. If the syringe does contain air bubbles, tap it with your finger until the bubbles rise to the top. Then slowly push the plunger up until you see a drop of medication at the tip of the needle.
8. Check the syringe to be sure it contains the correct dose, especially if you had to remove air bubbles. If the syringe does not contain the correct dose, repeat steps 5-7.
9. Choose a spot to inject the medication on either thigh, well above the knee. Wipe the area with an alcohol swab using a firm, circular motion, and allow it to dry.
10. Hold the syringe with one hand and hold a fold of skin around the injection site with the other hand. Push the needle all the way into the skin at a 45-90 degree angle.
11. Keep the needle inside the skin, and pull back slightly on the plunger.
12. If blood appears in the syringe, pull the needle slightly out of the skin and repeat step 11.
13. Push the plunger all the way down to inject the medication.
14. Pull the needle quickly out of the skin at the same angle you inserted it.
15. Press a new alcohol pad on the injection site and rub it.

To use the nasal spray, follow these steps:

1. Check your ampule to be sure it is safe to use. Do not use the ampule if it is broken, cracked, labeled with an expiration date that has passed, or contains a colored, cloudy, or particle filled liquid. Return that ampule to the pharmacy and use a different ampule.
2. Check to be sure all the liquid is at the bottom of the ampule. If any liquid is at the top of the ampule, gently flick it with your finger until it falls to the bottom.

Access FREE updates online @ www.consumerdrugreference.org

3. Place the ampule straight and upright in the well of the assembly case. The breaker cap should still be on and should be pointing up.
4. Push down the lid of the assembly case slowly but firmly until you hear the ampule snap open.
5. Open the assembly case, but do not remove the ampule from the well.
6. Hold the nasal sprayer by the metal ring with the cap pointing up. Press it onto the ampule until it clicks. Check the bottom of the sprayer to be sure the ampule is straight. If it is not straight, push it gently with your finger.
7. Remove the nasal sprayer from the well and remove the cap from the sprayer. Be careful not to touch the tip of the sprayer.
8. To prime the pump, point the sprayer away from your face and pump it four times. Some medication will spray in the air, but a full dose of medication will remain in the sprayer.
9. Place the tip of the sprayer in each nostril and press down to release one full spray. Do not tilt your head back or sniff while you are spraying. The medication will work even if you have a stuffy nose, cold, or allergies.
10. Wait fifteen minutes and release one full spray in each nostril again.
11. Throw away the sprayer and ampule. Place a new unit dose spray in your assembly case so you will be ready for your next attack. Throw away the assembly case after you have used it to prepare four sprayers.

Are there other uses for this medicine?

This medication may be prescribed for other uses; ask your doctor or pharmacist for more information.

What special precautions should I follow?

Before using dihydroergotamine,

- tell your doctor and pharmacist if you are allergic to dihydroergotamine, other ergot alkaloids such as bromocriptine (Parlodel), ergonovine (Ergotrate), ergotamine (Cafergot, Ercaf, others), methylergonovine (Methergine), and methysergide (Sansert), or any other medications.
- do not take dihydroergotamine within 24 hours of taking ergot alkaloids such as bromocriptine (Parlodel), ergonovine (Ergotrate), ergotamine (Cafergot, Ercaf, others), methylergonovine (Methergine), and methysergide (Sansert); or other medications for migraine such as frovatriptan (Frova), naratriptan (Amerge), rizatriptan (Maxalt), sumatriptan (Imitrex), and zolmitriptan (Zomig).
- tell your doctor and pharmacist what other prescription and nonprescription medications, vitamins, nutritional supplements, and herbal products you are taking. Be sure to mention any of the following: beta blockers such as propranolol (Inderal); cimetidine (Tagamet); clotri-

mazole (Lotrimin); cyclosporine (Neoral, Sandimmune); danazol (Danocrine); delavirdine (Rescriptor); diltiazem (Cardizem, Dilacor, Tiazac); epinephrine (Epipen); fluconazole (Diflucan); isoniazid (INH, Nydrazid); medications for colds and asthma; metronidazole (Flagyl); nefazodone (Serzone); oral contraceptives (birth control pills); selective serotonin reuptake inhibitors (SSRIs) such as citalopram (Celexa), fluoxetine (Prozac, Sarafem), fluvoxamine (Luvox), paroxetine (Paxil), and sertraline (Zoloft); saquinavir (Fortovase, Invirase); verapamil (Calan, Covera, Isoptin, Verelan); zafirlukast (Accolate); and zileuton (Zyflo). Your doctor may need to change the doses of your medications or monitor you carefully for side effects.
- tell your doctor if you have a family history of heart disease and if you have or have ever had high blood pressure; high cholesterol; diabetes; Raynaud's disease (a condition that affects the fingers and toes); any disease that affects your circulation or arteries; sepsis (a severe infection of the blood); surgery on your heart or blood vessels; a heart attack; or kidney, liver, lung, or heart disease.
- tell your doctor if you are pregnant, plan to become pregnant, or are breast-feeding. If you become pregnant while taking dihydroergotamine, call your doctor immediately.
- if you are having surgery, including dental surgery, tell the doctor or dentist that you are taking dihydroergotamine.
- tell your doctor if you use tobacco products. Smoking cigarettes while taking this medication increases the risk of serious side effects.

What special dietary instructions should I follow?

Talk to your doctor about drinking grapefruit juice while taking this medicine.

What side effects can this medicine cause?

Dihydroergotamine may cause side effects. Tell your doctor if any of these symptoms are severe or do not go away. Most of these symptoms, especially those that affect the nose, are more likely to occur if you use the nasal spray:

- stuffy nose
- tingling or pain in the nose or throat
- dryness in the nose
- nosebleed
- taste changes
- upset stomach
- vomiting
- dizziness
- extreme tiredness
- weakness

Some side effects can be serious. If you experience any of the following symptoms, call your doctor immediately:
- color changes, numbness or tingling in fingers and toes

- muscle pain in arms and legs
- weakness in arms and legs
- chest pain
- speeding or slowing of heart rate
- swelling
- itching
- cold, pale skin
- slow or difficult speech
- dizziness
- faintness

Dihydroergotamine may cause other side effects. Call your doctor if you have any unusual problems while taking this medication.

If you experience a serious side effect, you or your doctor may send a report to the Food and Drug Administration's (FDA) MedWatch Adverse Event Reporting program online [at http://www.fda.gov/MedWatch/index.html] or by phone [1-800-332-1088].

What storage conditions are needed for this medicine?

Keep this medication in the container it came in, tightly closed, and out of reach of children. Store it at room temperature and away from excess heat and moisture (not in the bathroom). Do not refrigerate or freeze. Throw away unused medication for injection 1 hour after you open the ampule. Throw away unused nasal spray 8 hours after you open the ampule. Throw away any medication that is outdated or no longer needed. Talk to your pharmacist about the proper disposal of your medication.

What should I do in case of overdose?

In case of overdose, call your local poison control center at 1-800-222-1222. If the victim has collapsed or is not breathing, call local emergency services at 911.

Symptoms of overdose may include:
- numbness, tingling, and pain in fingers and toes
- blue color in fingers and toes
- slowed breathing
- upset stomach
- vomiting
- fainting
- blurred vision
- dizziness
- confusion
- seizures
- coma
- stomach pain

What other information should I know?

Keep all appointments with your doctor. Your doctor may order certain tests to check your body's response to dihydroergotamine.

Do not let anyone else take your medication. Ask your pharmacist any questions you have about refilling your prescription.

Dosage Facts
For Informational Purposes

Caution: Do not change your dose, how often you take your medication, or the length of time you are to take it without first talking to your healthcare provider.

The following dosage information was written using medical language for doctors and other healthcare professionals and is provided here for you to check your dosage. The dosage of this drug may differ for different patients. Therefore, always follow your doctor's instructions or the directions on the label. Contact your healthcare provider or pharmacist if you have any questions about the specific dosage of your medication after reviewing this information.

General Dosage Information

Available as dihydroergotamine mesylate; dosage expressed in terms of the salt.

Adult Patients

Vascular Headaches
Migraine

INTRANASAL:
- 0.5 mg (1 spray) in each nostril (1 mg total) initially; repeat 15 minutes later for a total dose of 2 mg. Higher dosages provide no additional benefit.

SUB-Q:
- 1 mg initially, followed by 1 mg at 1-hour intervals until the attack has abated or a total of 3 mg has been given in a 24-hour period.

Cluster Headaches

SUB-Q:
- 1 mg initially, followed by 1 mg at 1-hour intervals until the attack has abated or a total of 3 mg has been given in a 24-hour period.

Prescribing Limits

Adult Patients

Vascular Headaches

INTRANASAL:
- Safety of >3 mg in any 24-hour period and >4 mg in any 7-day period has not been established.

SUB-Q:
- Maximum 3 mg in any 24-hour period.
- Maximum total weekly dosage: 6 mg.

† Use is not currently included in the labeling approved by the US Food and Drug Administration.

Diltiazem

(dil tye′ a zem)

Brand Name: Cardizem®, Cardizem® CD, Cardizem® SR, Cartia XT®, Dilacor XR®, Diltia XT®, Tiazac®
Also available generically.

Why is this medicine prescribed?

Diltiazem is used to treat high blood pressure and to control chest pain (angina). Diltiazem is in a class of medications called calcium-channel blockers. It works by relaxing the blood vessels so the heart does not have to pump as hard. It also increases the supply of blood and oxygen to the heart.

How should this medicine be used?

Diltiazem comes as a tablet and an extended- or dual-release (long-acting) capsule to take by mouth. The tablet is usually taken three or four times a day with or without food. The capsule is usually taken one or two times a day. The extended-release capsule (Cardizem SR, Dilacor XR, Diltia XT) should be taken on an empty stomach, at least 1 hour before or 2 hours after a meal. The extended-release capsule (Tiazac) may be taken with or without food. The dual-release capsule (Cardizem CD) may be taken with food.

Follow the directions on your prescription label carefully, and ask your doctor or pharmacist to explain any part you do not understand. Take diltiazem exactly as directed. Do not take more or less of it or take it more often than prescribed by your doctor.

Swallow the capsules whole; do not split, chew, or crush them.

Your doctor will probably start you on a low dose of diltiazem and gradually increase your dose.

If taken regularly, diltiazem controls chest pain, but it does not stop chest pain once it starts. Your doctor may give you a different medication to take when you have chest pain.

Diltiazem controls high blood pressure and chest pain (angina) but does not cure them. It may take up to 2 weeks before you feel the full benefit of diltiazem. Continue to take diltiazem even if you feel well. Do not stop taking diltiazem without talking to your doctor.

Are there other uses for this medicine?

Diltiazem is also used sometimes to treat Raynaud's syndrome. Talk to your doctor about the possible risks of using this drug for your condition.

This medication may be prescribed for other uses; ask your doctor or pharmacist for more information.

What special precautions should I follow?

Before taking diltiazem,
- tell your doctor and pharmacist if you are allergic to diltiazem or any other drugs.
- tell your doctor and pharmacist what prescription and nonprescription medications you are taking, especially heart and blood pressure medications such as beta-blockers, digoxin (Lanoxin), quinidine (Quinaglute, Quinidex), and diuretics (water pills); carbamazepine (Tegretol); cimetidine (Tagamet); cyclosporine (Neoral, Sandimmune); fentanyl (Duragesic); medications to treat depression; medications to treat glaucoma (increased pressure in the eye); theophylline; and vitamins.
- tell your doctor if you have or have ever had heart, liver, or kidney disease.
- tell your doctor if you are pregnant, plan to become pregnant, or are breast-feeding. If you become pregnant while taking diltiazem, call your doctor.
- if you are having surgery, including dental surgery, tell your doctor or dentist that you are taking diltiazem.

What special dietary instructions should I follow?

Talk to your doctor before using salt substitutes containing potassium. If your doctor prescribes a low-salt or low-sodium diet, follow these directions carefully.

What should I do if I forget to take a dose?

Take the missed dose as soon as you remember it. However, if it is almost time for the next dose, skip the missed dose and continue your regular dosing schedule. Do not take a double dose to make up for a missed one.

What side effects can this medicine cause?

Diltiazem may cause side effects. Tell your doctor if any of these symptoms are severe or do not go away:
- dizziness or lightheadedness
- flushing (feeling of warmth)
- headache
- excessive tiredness
- slower heartbeat
- upset stomach
- loss of appetite
- vomiting
- diarrhea
- constipation
- stomach pain
- dry mouth
- difficulty falling asleep or staying asleep

If you experience any of the following symptoms, call your doctor immediately:
- swelling of the face, eyes, lips, tongue, arms, or legs
- difficulty breathing or swallowing
- fainting
- rash
- yellowing of the skin or eyes
- fever
- increase in frequency or severity of chest pain (angina)

If you experience a serious side effect, you or your doctor may send a report to the Food and Drug Administration's (FDA) MedWatch Adverse Event Reporting program online [at http://www.fda.gov/MedWatch/index.html] or by phone [1-800-332-1088].

What storage conditions are needed for this medicine?

Keep this medication in the container it came in, tightly closed, and out of reach of children. Store it at room temperature and away from excess heat and moisture (not in the bathroom). Throw away any medication that is outdated or no longer needed. Talk to your pharmacist about the proper disposal of your medication.

What should I do in case of overdose?

In case of overdose, call your local poison control center at 1-800-222-1222. If the victim has collapsed or is not breathing, call local emergency services at 911.

What other information should I know?

Keep all appointments with your doctor and the laboratory. Your blood pressure should be checked regularly to determine your response to diltiazem.

Your doctor may ask you to check your pulse (heart rate) daily and will tell you how fast it should be. If your pulse is slower than it should be, call your doctor for directions on taking diltiazem that day. Ask your doctor or pharmacist to teach you how to check your pulse.

The extended-release capsule does not dissolve in the stomach after swallowing. It slowly releases the medicine as it passes through your small intestines. It is not unusual to see the capsule shell in your stool.

Do not let anyone else take your medication. Ask your pharmacist any questions you have about refilling your prescription.

Dosage Facts
For Informational Purposes

Caution: Do not change your dose, how often you take your medication, or the length of time you are to take it without first talking to your healthcare provider.

The following dosage information was written using medical language for doctors and other healthcare professionals and is provided here for you to check your dosage. The dosage of this drug may differ for different patients. Therefore, always follow your doctor's instructions or the directions on the label. Contact your healthcare provider or pharmacist if you have any questions about the specific dosage of your medication after reviewing this information.

General Dosage Information

Available as diltiazem hydrochloride; dosage expressed in terms of the salt.

Adult Patients

Prinzmetal Variant Angina
Conventional Tablets

ORAL:
- Initially, 30 mg 4 times daily. Increase gradually at 1- to 2-day intervals until optimum control is obtained. Usual maintenance dosage is 180–360 mg daily. After manifestations are controlled, reduce dosage to lowest level that will maintain relief of systems.

Extended-release Capsules

ORAL:
- Initially, 120 or 180 mg once daily when administered as extended-release capsules (Cardizem® CD, Cartia XT®). Individualize dosage based on response; titrate dosage increases over 7–14 days. Some patients may respond to higher dosages of up to 480 mg once daily.

Chronic Stable Angina
Conventional Tablets

ORAL:
- Initially, 30 mg 4 times daily. Increase gradually at 1- to 2-day intervals until optimum control is obtained. Usual maintenance dosage is 180–360 mg daily. After manifestations are controlled, reduce dosage to lowest level that will maintain relief of symtoms.

Extended-release Capsules

ORAL:
- Initially, 120 (Dilacor XR®, Diltia XT®, Dilt-XR®) or 120–180 mg (Cardizem® CD, Cartia XT®, Tiazac®, Taztia XT®) once daily when administered as extended-release capsules. Individualize dosage based on response; titrate dosage increases over 7–14 days. Some patients may respond to higher dosages of up to 480 (Cardizem® CD, Cartia XT®, Dilacor XR®, Diltia XT®, Dilt-XR®) to 540 mg (Tiazac®, Taztia XT®) once daily.

Extended-release Tablets

ORAL:
- Initially, 180 mg once daily when administered as extended-release tablets (Cardizem® LA). Individualize dosage based on response; titrate dosage increases over 7–14 days. Some patients may respond to higher dosages of up to 360 mg once daily.

Hypertension
Extended-release Capsules

ORAL:
- Maximum hypotensive effect associated with a given dosage level usually is observed within 14 days.

Recommended Dosages for Management of Hypertension

Preparation	Initial Dosage	Usual Maintenance Dosage
Cardizem® LA	180–240 mg once daily	120–540 mg
Cardizem® CD	180–240 mg once daily	240–360 mg daily
Cartia XT®	180–240 mg once daily	240–360 mg daily
Dilacor XR®	180–240 mg once daily	180–480 mg* once daily
Diltia XT®	180–240 mg once daily	180–480 mg* once daily
Diltiazem hydro-chloride ex-tended-release capsules (12 hours)	60–120 mg twice daily	240–360 mg daily
Dilt-XR®	180–240 mg once daily	180–480 mg* once daily
Tiazac®	120–240 mg once daily	120–540 mg* once daily
Taztia XT®	120–240 mg once daily	120–540 mg* once daily

*JNC 7 recommends a usual maximum dosage of 420 mg daily for these preparations.

Switching to Cardizem® CD Extended-release Capsules

ORAL:
- Patients whose BP is adequately controlled with diltiazem therapy (as tablets or other extended-release capsules) alone or in combination with another antihypertensive agent may be safely switched to Cardizem® CD or Cartia XT® extended-release capsules or Cardizem® LA extended-release tablets at the nearest equivalent daily dosage. Subsequent titration of dosage is based on the clinical response of the patient.

Conventional Tablets†

ORAL:
- Initially, 30 mg 3 times daily; may be increased to a maximum dosage of 360 mg daily given in 3 or 4 divided doses.

Extended-release Tablets

ORAL:
- Initially, 180–240 mg daily; however, some patients may respond to a lower dosage. Individualize dosage based on response; maximum hypotensive effect associated with a given dosage level usually is observed within 14 days. Usual maintenance dosage is 120–540 mg daily; however, JNC 7 recommends a usual maximum dosage of 420 mg daily.

Prescribing Limits

Adult Patients

Angina

ORAL:
- Cardizem® LA extended-release tablets: Maximum 360 mg daily.
- Cardizem® CD, Dilacor XR®, Diltia XT®, Dilt-XR®, and Cartia XT® extended-release capsules: Maximum 480 mg daily.

- Tiazac® and Taztia XT® extended-release capsules: Maximum 540 mg daily.

Hypertension

ORAL:
- Cardizem® conventional tablets†: Maximum 360 mg daily.
- Cardizem® CD and Cartia XT® extended release capsules: Maximum 480 mg daily.
- Dilt-XR®, Dilacor XR®, Diltia XT®, Taztia XT®, and Tiazac® extended-release capsules and Cardizem® LA extended-release tablets: maximum 540 mg daily.
- However, JNC 7 recommends a usual maximum dosage of 420 mg daily for these preparations.

Special Populations

Geriatric Patients

Angina
- Select dosage cautiously; geriatric patients may respond to lower dosages.

Hypertension
- Select dosage cautiously. The manufacturers of Dilacor XR®, Dilt-XR®, and Diltia XT® state that patients 60 years of age or older may respond to an initial daily dosage of 120 mg.

† Use is not currently included in the labeling approved by the US Food and Drug Administration.

Dimenhydrinate

(dye men hye′ dri nate)

Brand Name: Dramamine®, Dramamine® Chewable, TripTone®
Also available generically.

Why is this medicine prescribed?

Dimenhydrinate is used to prevent and treat nausea, vomiting, and dizziness caused by motion sickness. Dimenhydrinate is in a class of medications called antihistamines. It works by preventing problems with body balance.

How should this medicine be used?

Dimenhydrinate comes as a tablet and chewable tablet to take by mouth with or without food. To prevent motion sickness, the first dose should be taken 30 minutes to 1 hour before you travel or begin motion activity. Adults and children older than age 12 may usually take dimenhydrinate every 4 to 6 hours as needed to prevent or treat motion sickness. Children under age 12 may usually be given dimenhydrinate every 6 to 8 hours as needed to prevent or treat motion sickness. Follow the directions on the package carefully, and ask your doctor or pharmacist to explain any part you do not understand. Take dimenhydrinate exactly as directed. Do not take more or less of it or take it more often than directed by the package label.

Do not give dimenhydrinate to children younger than 2 years of age unless your doctor has told you to do so.

Are there other uses for this medicine?

Dimenhydrinate is also sometimes used to treat Meniere's disease (condition of the inner ear which causes extreme dizziness, loss of balance, ringing in the ears, and hearing loss) and other inner ear problems. Talk to your doctor about the risks of using this medication for your condition.

This medication may be prescribed for other uses; ask your doctor or pharmacist for more information.

What special precautions should I follow?

Before taking dimenhydrinate,

- talk with your doctor and pharmacist if you are allergic to dimenhydrinate or any other medications. If you are taking dimenhydrinate chewable tablets, talk to your doctor if you are allergic to tartrazine (FD&C Yellow No. 5, a color additive) or aspirin.
- talk with your doctor and pharmacist about what prescription and nonprescription medications, vitamins, nutritional supplements, and herbal products you are taking or plan to take. Be sure to mention any of the following: aminoglycoside antibiotics such as such as amikacin (Amikin), gentamicin (Garamycin), kanamycin (Kantrex), neomycin (Neo-Rx, Neo-Fradin), netilmycin (Netromycin), paromomycin (Humatin), streptomycin, and tobramycin (Tobi, Nebcin); antidepressants such as amitriptyline (Elavil), amoxapine (Asendin), clomipramine (Anafranil), desipramine (Norpramin), doxepin (Adapin, Sinequan), imipramine (Tofranil), nortriptyline (Aventyl, Pamelor), protriptyline (Vivactil), and trimipramine (Surmontil); antihistamines, such as diphenhydramine; cough and cold medications; ipratropium (Atrovent); medications for anxiety, irritable bowel disease, mental illness, Parkinson's disease, seizures, ulcers, or urinary problems; narcotic or strong pain relievers or muscle relaxants; sedatives; sleeping pills; and tranquilizers. Your doctor may need to change the doses of your medications or monitor you carefully for side effects.
- talk with your doctor if you have or have ever had asthma; shortness of breath or difficulty breathing, including chronic bronchitis (swelling of the air passages that lead to the lungs) or emphysema (damage to air sacs in the lungs); difficulty urinating due to enlargement of the prostate (male reproductive organ); glaucoma (an eye disease that can cause vision loss); or seizures.
- talk with your doctor if you are pregnant, plan to become pregnant, or are breast-feeding. If you become pregnant while taking dimenhydrinate, call your doctor.
- if you are having surgery, including dental surgery, tell the doctor or dentist that you are taking dimenhydrinate.
- you should know that dimenhydrinate may make you drowsy. Do not drive a car, operate machinery, or participate in potentially dangerous activities until you know how this medication affects you.
- Avoid alcoholic beverages or products containing alcohol while taking dimenhydrinate. Alcohol can make the side effects from dimenhydrinate worse.
- if you have phenylketonuria (PKU, an inherited condition in which a special diet must be followed to prevent mental retardation), read the package label carefully before taking dimenhydrinate. Dimenhydrinate chewable tablets contain aspartame that forms phenylalanine.

What special dietary instructions should I follow?

Unless your doctor tells you otherwise, continue your normal diet.

What should I do if I forget to take a dose?

This medication is usually taken as needed. If your doctor has told you to take dimenhydrinate regularly, take the missed dose as soon as you remember it. However, if it is almost time for the next dose, skip the missed dose and continue your regular dosing schedule. Do not take a double dose to make up for a missed one.

What side effects can this medicine cause?

Dimenhydrinate may cause side effects. Talk to your doctor if any of these symptoms are severe or do not go away:

- drowsiness
- excitement or hyperactivity (especially in children)
- headache
- new or worsening dizziness
- blurred vision
- ringing in the ears
- dry mouth, nose, or throat
- problems with coordination
- fainting
- dizziness
- nausea

Some side effects can be serious. If you experience the following symptom, call your doctor immediately:

- fast, pounding, or irregular heartbeat

Dimenhydrinate may cause other side effects. Call your doctor if you have any unusual problems while taking this medication.

What storage conditions are needed for this medicine?

Keep this medication in the container it came in, tightly closed, and out of reach of children. Store it at room temperature and away from excess heat and moisture (not in the bathroom). Throw away any medication that is outdated or no longer needed. Talk to your pharmacist about the proper disposal of your medication.

What should I do in case of overdose?

In case of overdose, call your local poison control center at 1-800-222-1222. If the victim has collapsed or is not breathing, call local emergency services at 911.

Symptoms of overdose may include:

- large pupils (black circles in the centers of the eyes)
- flushed face
- drowsiness or sleepiness
- excitation or hyperactivity
- hallucinations (seeing things or hearing voices that do not exist)
- difficulty understanding reality
- confusion
- difficulty speaking or swallowing
- unsteadiness
- seizures
- unresponsiveness or coma (loss of consciousness for a period of time)

What other information should I know?

Ask your pharmacist any questions you have about dimenhydrinate.

Dosage Facts
For Informational Purposes

Caution: Do not change your dose, how often you take your medication, or the length of time you are to take it without first talking to your healthcare provider.

The following dosage information was written using medical language for doctors and other healthcare professionals and is provided here for you to check your dosage. The dosage of this drug may differ for different patients. Therefore, always follow your doctor's instructions or the directions on the label. Contact your healthcare provider or pharmacist if you have any questions about the specific dosage of your medication after reviewing this information.

Pediatric Patients
Motion Sickness

ORAL:

- For prevention, take 30 minutes before exposure to motion.
- Children <2 Years of Age: Give only under the direction of a clinician.
- Children 2 to <6 Years of Age: 12.5–25 mg every 6–8 hours, not to exceed 75 mg in 24 hours, or as directed by a clinician.
- Children 6 to <12 Years of Age: 25–50 mg every 6–8 hours, not to exceed 150 mg in 24 hours, or as directed by a clinician.
- Children ≥12 Years of Age: Usually, 50–100 mg every 4–6 hours, not to exceed 400 mg in 24 hours, or as directed by a clinician.
- Children: Alternatively, 1.25 mg/kg or 37.5 mg/m² 4 times daily, up to a maximum of 300 mg daily.

Adult Patients
Motion Sickness

ORAL:

- For prevention, take 30 minutes before exposure to motion.
- Usually 50–100 mg every 4–6 hours, not to exceed 400 mg in 24 hours, or as directed by a clinician.

Ménière's Disease and Other Vestibular Disturbances
Maintenance of Symptomatic Relief

ORAL:

- 25–50 mg has been given 3 times daily.

Prescribing Limits
Pediatric Patients
Motion Sickness

ORAL:

- Children 2 to <6 Years of Age: Maximum 75 mg in 24 hours, or as directed by a clinician.
- Children 6 to <12 Years of Age: Maximum 150 mg in 24 hours, or as directed by a clinician.
- Children ≥12 Years of Age: Maximum 400 mg in 24 hours, or as directed by a clinician.
- Children: Alternatively, maximum 300 mg daily when given as 1.25 mg/kg or 37.5 mg/m².

Adult Patients
Motion Sickness

ORAL:

- Maximum 400 mg in 24 hours, or as directed by a clinician.

Special Populations

Hepatic Impairment
- No specific dosage recommendations for hepatic impairment.

Renal Impairment
- No specific dosage recommendations for renal impairment.

Geriatric Patients
- No specific geriatric dosage recommendations.

Dinoprostone
(dye noe prost′ one)

Brand Name: Cervidil®, Prepidil®, Prostin E2®

Why is this medicine prescribed?

Dinoprostone is used to prepare the cervix for the induction of labor in pregnant women who are at or near term. This medication is sometimes prescribed for other uses; ask your doctor or pharmacist for more information.

How should this medicine be used?

Dinoprostone comes as a vaginal insert and as a gel that is inserted high into the vagina. It is administered using a syringe, by a health professional in a hospital or clinic setting. After the dose has been administered you should remain lying down for up to 2 hours as directed by your physician. A second dose of the gel may be administered in 6 hours if the first dose does not produce the desired response.

What special precautions should I follow?

Before taking dinoprostone,

- tell your doctor and pharmacist if you are allergic to dinoprostone or any other drugs.
- tell your doctor and pharmacist what prescription and nonprescription medications you are taking, including vitamins.
- tell your doctor if you have or have ever had asthma; anemia; a cesarean section or any other uterine surgery; diabetes; high or low blood pressure; placenta previa; a seizure disorder; six or more previous term pregnancies; glaucoma or increased pressure in the eye; cephalopelvic disproportion; previous difficult or traumatic deliveries; unexplained vaginal bleeding; or heart, liver, or kidney disease.

What side effects can this medicine cause?

Side effects from dinoprostone are not common, but they can occur. Tell your doctor if any of these symptoms are severe or do not go away:

- upset stomach
- vomiting
- diarrhea
- dizziness
- flushing of the skin
- headache
- fever

If you experience any of the following symptoms, call your doctor immediately:

- unpleasant vaginal discharge
- continued fever
- chills and shivering
- increase in vaginal bleeding several days after treatment
- chest pain or tightness
- skin rash
- hives
- difficulty breathing
- unusual swelling of the face

If you experience a serious side effect, you or your doctor may send a report to the Food and Drug Administration's (FDA) MedWatch Adverse Event Reporting program online [at http://www.fda.gov/MedWatch/index.html] or by phone [1-800-332-1088].

What storage conditions are needed for this medicine?

Dinoprostone gel should be stored in a refrigerator. The inserts should be stored in a freezer. Keep this medication in the container it came in, tightly closed, and out of reach of children.

What other information should I know?

Keep all appointments with your doctor. Do not let anyone else use your medication.

Talk to your doctor, pharmacist, or other healthcare professional if you have questions about dosing information for your medication.

Diphenhydramine Oral

(dye fen hye′ dra meen)

Brand Name: AllerMax®, AllerMax® Caplets®, Benadryl®, Benadryl® Allergy, Benadryl® Allergy Chewables Children's, Benadryl® Allergy Kapseals®, Benadryl® Allergy Ultratab®, Benadryl® Dye-Free Allergy Children's, Benadryl® Dye-Free Allergy Liqui-Gels®, Compoz® Nighttime Sleep Aid, Compoz® Nighttime Sleep Aid Gelcaps®, Diphen® AF Elixir, Diphenhist®, Diphenhist® Captabs®, Diphenhydramine Hydrochloride Caplets®, Excedrin P.M.® Geltabs®, Excedrin P.M.® Tablets, Genahist®, Genahist® Elixir, Goody's® PM Powder, Hydramine® Cough Syrup, Hydramine® Elixir, Miles® Nervine Nighttime Sleep-Aid, Nytol® QuickCaps® Caplets®, Nytol® Quickgels® Maximum Strength, Simply Sleep® Nighttime Sleep Aid Caplets®, Sleepinal® Night-time Sleep Aid Softgels®, Sominex® Caplets®Maximum Strength, Sominex® Nighttime Sleep Aid, Twilite® Caplets®, Unisom® SleepGels® Maximum Strength Also available generically.

Why is this medicine prescribed?

Diphenhydramine, an antihistamine, relieves red, irritated, itchy, watery eyes; sneezing; and runny nose caused by hay fever, allergies, and the common cold. It also may relieve the itching of insect bites, sunburns, bee stings, poison ivy, poison oak, and minor skin irritation. Diphenhydramine is also used to prevent and treat motion sickness, induce sleep, treat Parkinson's disease, and relieve cough caused by minor throat or airway irritation.

This medication is sometimes prescribed for other uses; ask your doctor or pharmacist for more information.

How should this medicine be used?

Diphenhydramine comes as a tablet, capsule, and liquid to take by mouth. It usually is taken three or four times a day. For motion sickness, diphenhydramine is taken 30 minutes before departure and, if needed, before meals and at bedtime. Diphenhydramine is taken at bedtime for sleep. Follow the directions on the package or on your prescription label carefully, and ask your doctor or pharmacist to explain any part you do not understand. Take diphenhydramine exactly as directed. Do not take more or less of it or take it more often than prescribed by your doctor.

Do not give diphenhydramine to a child younger than 6 years of age unless directed to do so by a doctor.

What special precautions should I follow?

Before taking diphenhydramine,

- tell your doctor and pharmacist if you are allergic to diphenhydramine or any other drugs.
- tell your doctor and pharmacist what prescription and nonprescription medications you are taking, especially other medications for colds, hay fever, or allergies; medications for depression or seizures; muscle relaxants; narcotics (pain medications); sedatives; sleeping pills; tranquilizers; and vitamins.
- tell your doctor if you have or have ever had asthma, lung disease, glaucoma, ulcers, difficulty urinating (due to an enlarged prostate gland), heart disease, high blood pressure, seizures, or an overactive thyroid gland.
- tell your doctor if you are pregnant, plan to become pregnant, or are breast-feeding. If you become pregnant while taking diphenhydramine, call your doctor.
- if you are having surgery, including dental surgery, tell the doctor or dentist that you are taking diphenhydramine.
- you should know that this drug may make you drowsy. Do not drive a car or operate machinery until you know how this drug affects you.
- remember that alcohol can add to the drowsiness caused by this drug.

What should I do if I forget to take a dose?

Take the missed dose as soon as you remember it. However, if it is almost time for the next dose, skip the missed dose and continue your regular dosing schedule. Do not take a double dose to make up for a missed one.

What side effects can this medicine cause?

Diphenhydramine may cause side effects. Tell your doctor if any of these symptoms are severe or do not go away:

- dry mouth, nose, and throat
- drowsiness
- upset stomach
- chest congestion
- headache

If you experience any of the following symptoms, call your doctor immediately:

- vision problems
- difficulty urinating
- muscle weakness
- excitement (especially in children)
- nervousness

If you experience a serious side effect, you or your doctor may send a report to the Food and Drug Administration's (FDA) MedWatch Adverse Event Reporting program online [at http://www.fda.gov/MedWatch/index.html] or by phone [1-800-332-1088].

What storage conditions are needed for this medicine?

Keep this medication in the container it came in, tightly closed, and out of reach of children. Store it at room temperature and away from excess heat and moisture (not in the bathroom). Throw away any medication that is outdated or no longer needed. Talk to your pharmacist about the proper disposal of your medication.

What should I do in case of overdose?

In case of overdose, call your local poison control center at 1-800-222-1222. If the victim has collapsed or is not breathing, call local emergency services at 911.

What other information should I know?

Keep all appointments with your doctor.

Do not let anyone else take your medication. Ask your pharmacist any questions you have about refilling your prescription.

Dosage Facts
For Informational Purposes

Caution: Do not change your dose, how often you take your medication, or the length of time you are to take it without first talking to your healthcare provider.

The following dosage information was written using medical language for doctors and other healthcare professionals and is provided here for you to check your dosage. The dosage of this drug may differ for different patients. Therefore, always follow your doctor's instructions or the directions on the label. Contact your healthcare provider or pharmacist if you have any questions about the specific dosage of your medication after reviewing this information.

General Dosage Information

Available as diphenhydramine hydrochloride and diphenhydramine citrate; dosage is expressed in terms of diphenhydramine hydrochloride or diphenhydramine citrate.

Diphenhydramine citrate available only in fixed-combination preparations.

12.5 mg diphenhydramine hydrochloride equivalent to 19 mg diphenhydramine citrate.

Pediatric Patients

Allergic Conditions and the Common Cold
Allergic Rhinitis and the Common Cold

ORAL:
- *Self-medication* in children 2–5 years of age: 6.25 mg every 4–6 hours (as diphenhydramine hydrochloride) or 9.5 mg

every 4 hours (as diphenhydramine citrate) when directed by a clinician; do not exceed 37.5 mg (as diphenhydramine hydrochloride) or 57 mg (as diphenhydramine citrate) in 24 hours.

- *Self-medication* in children 6–11 years of age: 12.5–25 mg every 4–6 hours (as diphenhydramine hydrochloride) or 19 mg every 4 hours (as diphenhydramine citrate); do not exceed 150 mg (as diphenhydramine hydrochloride) or 76 mg (as diphenhydramine citrate) in 24 hours.
- *Self-medication* in children ≥12 years of age: 25–50 mg every 4–6 hours (as diphenhydramine hydrochloride) or 38 mg every 4 hours (as diphenhydramine citrate); do not exceed 300 mg (as diphenhydramine hydrochloride) or 152 mg (as diphenhydramine citrate) in 24 hours.

Insomnia

ORAL:
- Children 2–11 years of age†: 1 mg/kg (as diphenhydramine hydrochloride) 30 minutes before retiring; do not exceed 50 mg.
- *Self-medication* in children ≥12 years of age: 50 mg (as diphenhydramine hydrochloride) or 76 mg (as diphenhydramine citrate) at bedtime as needed, or as directed by a clinician. Higher dosages do not produce substantially greater benefit but may be associated with a higher incidence of adverse (e.g., anticholinergic) effects.
- Use not recommended for ≥7–10 nights.

Motion Sickness

ORAL:
- Children 2–5 years of age†: 6.25 mg (as diphenhydramine hydrochloride) 30–60 minutes before travel and every 4–6 hours during travel; do not exceed 37.5 mg in 24 hours.
- *Self-medication* in children 6–11 years of age: 12.5–25 mg (as diphenhydramine hydrochloride) 30–60 minutes before travel and every 4–6 hours during travel; do not exceed 150 mg in 24 hours.
- *Self-medication* in children ≥12 years of age: 25–50 mg (as diphenhydramine hydrochloride) 30 minutes before exposure to motion and then every 4–6 hours (before meals and at bedtime) for duration of exposure; do not exceed 300 mg in 24 hours.

Adult Patients

Allergic Conditions and the Common Cold

Allergic Rhinitis and the Common Cold

ORAL:
- *Self-medication*: 25–50 mg every 4–6 hours (as diphenhydramine hydrochloride) or 38 mg every 4 hours (as diphenhydramine citrate); do not exceed 300 mg (as diphenhydramine hydrochloride) or 152 mg (as diphenhydramine citrate) in 24 hours.

Insomnia

ORAL:
- *Self-medication*: 50 mg (as diphenhydramine hydrochloride) or 76 mg (as diphenhydramine citrate) at bedtime as needed, or as directed by a clinician. Higher dosages do not produce substantially greater benefit but may be associated with a higher incidence of adverse (e.g., anticholinergic) effects.
- Use not recommended for ≥7–10 nights.

Motion Sickness

ORAL:
- *Self-medication*: 25–50 mg (as diphenhydramine hydrochloride) 30 minutes before exposure to motion and then every 4–6 hours (before meals and at bedtime) for duration of exposure; do not exceed 300 mg in 24 hours.

Parkinsonian Syndrome

ORAL:
- Initially, 25 mg 3 times daily (as diphenhydramine hydrochloride). If necessary, gradually increase dosage to 50 mg 4 times daily.

Prescribing Limits

Pediatric Patients

ORAL:
- Children 2–5 years of age: maximum 37.5 mg (as diphenhydramine hydrochloride) or 57 mg (as diphenhydramine citrate) in 24 hours.
- Children 6–11 years of age: maximum 150 mg (as diphenhydramine hydrochloride) or 76 mg (as diphenhydramine citrate) in 24 hours.
- Children ≥12 years of age: maximum 300 mg (as diphenhydramine hydrochloride) or 152 mg (as diphenhydramine citrate) in 24 hours.

Adult Patients

ORAL:
- Maximum 300 mg in 24 hours.

† Use is not currently included in the labeling approved by the US Food and Drug Administration.

Diphenhydramine Topical

(dye fen hye′ dra meen)

Brand Name: Benadryl® Itch Relief Stick Extra Strength, Benadryl® Itch Stopping Cream Extra Strength, Benadryl® Itch Stopping Cream Original Strength, Benadryl® Itch Stopping Extra Strength Spray, Benadryl® Itch Stopping Gel Extra Strength, Benadryl® Itch Stopping Gel Original Strength, Benadryl® Itch Stopping Original Strength Spray, Dermamycin®, Dermamycin® Spray as a combination product containing Diphenhydramine Hydrochloride and Menthol, Dermarest® Maximum Strength as a combination product containing Diphenhydramine Hydrochloride and Resorcinol, Dermarest® Plus as a combination product containing Diphenhydramine Hydrochloride and Menthol, Di-Delamine® as a combination product containing Diphenhydramine Hydrochloride and Tripelennamine

Why is this medicine prescribed?

Diphenhydramine, an antihistamine, is used to relieve the itching of insect bites, sunburns, bee stings, poison ivy, poison oak, and minor skin irritation.

This medication is sometimes prescribed for other uses; ask your doctor or pharmacist for more information.

How should this medicine be used?

Diphenhydramine topical comes in cream, lotion, gel, and spray to be applied to the skin. It is used three or four times a day. Follow the directions on the package or on your prescription label carefully, and ask your doctor or pharmacist to explain any part you do not understand. Use diphenhydramine exactly as directed. Do not use more or less of it or use it more often than directed by your doctor.

Thoroughly clean the infected area, allow it to dry, and then gently rub the medication in until most of it disappears. Use just enough medication to cover the affected area. You should wash your hands after applying the medication.

Do not apply diphenhydramine on chicken pox or measles, and do not use it on a child younger than 2 years of age unless directed to do so by a doctor.

What special precautions should I follow?

Before using diphenhydramine,
- tell your doctor and pharmacist if you are allergic to diphenhydramine or any other drugs.
- tell your doctor and pharmacist what prescription and nonprescription medications you are taking, including vitamins.
- tell your doctor if you are pregnant, plan to become pregnant, or are breast-feeding. If you become pregnant while using diphenhydramine, call your doctor.
- plan to avoid unnecessary or prolonged exposure to sunlight and to wear protective clothing, sunglasses, and sunscreen. Diphenhydramine may make your skin sensitive to sunlight.

What should I do if I forget to take a dose?

Apply the missed dose as soon as you remember it. However, if it is almost time for the next dose, skip the missed dose and continue your regular dosing schedule. Do not apply a double dose to make up for a missed one.

What side effects can this medicine cause?

Diphenhydramine may cause side effects. Tell your doctor if any of these symptoms are severe or do not go away:
- skin rash
- sunburn
- increased sensitivity to sunlamps and sunlight

What storage conditions are needed for this medicine?

Keep this medication in the container it came in, tightly closed, and out of reach of children. Store it at room temperature and away from excess heat and moisture (not in the bathroom). The spray is flammable. Keep it away from flames and extreme heat. Throw away any medication that is outdated or no longer needed. Talk to your pharmacist about the proper disposal of your medication.

What other information should I know?

Keep all appointments with your doctor. Diphenhydramine is for external use only. Do not let diphenhydramine get into your eyes, nose, or mouth, and do not swallow it. Do not apply dressings, bandages, cosmetics, lotions, or other skin medications to the area being treated unless your doctor tells you.

Do not let anyone else use your medication. Ask your pharmacist any questions you have about refilling your prescription.

Tell your doctor if your skin condition becomes severe or does not go away.

Talk to your doctor, pharmacist, or other healthcare professional if you have questions about dosing information for your medication.

Diphenoxylate and Atropine

(dye fen ox′ i late) (a′ troe peen)

Brand Name: Lomotil®, Lonox®
Also available generically.

Why is this medicine prescribed?

Diphenoxylate and atropine is used to control diarrhea.

This medication is sometimes prescribed for other uses; ask your doctor or pharmacist for more information.

How should this medicine be used?

Diphenoxylate and atropine comes as a tablet and liquid to take by mouth. It is usually taken as needed up to four times a day. Follow the directions on your prescription label carefully, and ask your doctor or pharmacist to explain any part you do not understand.

The liquid comes in a container with a special dropper. Use the dropper to measure the exact dose carefully. Ask your pharmacist if you have questions about how to measure a dose.

Diphenoxylate can be habit forming. Do not take a larger dose, take it more often, or for a longer period than your doctor tells you to. Stopping the medicine suddenly after taking it for a long time may cause withdrawal. Symptoms of withdrawal include muscle cramps, stomach cramps, unusual sweating, upset stomach and vomiting, and shaking or trembling.

What special precautions should I follow?

Before taking diphenoxylate and atropine,
- tell your doctor and pharmacist if you are allergic to diphenoxylate, atropine, or any other drugs.
- tell your doctor and pharmacist what prescription and nonprescription medications you are taking, especially MAO inhibitors [phenelzine (Nardil) and tranylcypromine (Parnate)], muscle relaxants, narcotic cough or pain relievers, sleeping pills, tranquilizers, and vitamins.
- tell your doctor if you have or have ever had chronic lung disease, ulcerative colitis, or liver disease or a history of alcohol abuse.
- tell your doctor if you are pregnant, plan to become pregnant, or are breast-feeding. If you become pregnant while taking diphenoxylate and atropine, call your doctor.
- before having surgery, including dental surgery, tell the doctor or dentist that you are taking this medicine.
- you should know that this drug may make you drowsy. Do not drive a car or operate machinery until you know how this drug affects you.

- remember that alcohol can add to the drowsiness caused by this drug.

What should I do if I forget to take a dose?

If you are taking scheduled doses of diphenoxylate and atropine, take the missed dose as soon you remember it. However, if it is almost time for the next dose, skip the missed dose and continue the regular dosing schedule. Do not take a double dose to make up for a missed one.

What side effects can this medicine cause?

Diphenoxylate and atropine may cause side effects. To avoid thirst and dry mouth, drink a lot of fluids, chew gum, or suck sugarless hard candies.

If you experience any of the following symptoms, call your doctor immediately:
- severe upset stomach and vomiting
- severe stomach pain
- bloating
- severe drowsiness
- palpitations
- swelling
- rash
- loss of appetite
- dryness of the skin, nose, or mouth,
- difficulty breathing
- convulsions

If you experience a serious side effect, you or your doctor may send a report to the Food and Drug Administration's (FDA) MedWatch Adverse Event Reporting program online [at http://www.fda.gov/MedWatch/index.html] or by phone [1-800-332-1088].

What storage conditions are needed for this medicine?

Keep this medication in the container it came in, tightly closed, and out of reach of children. Store it at room temperature and away from excess heat and moisture (not in the bathroom). Throw away any medication that is outdated or no longer needed. Talk to your pharmacist about the proper disposal of your medication.

What should I do in case of overdose?

In case of overdose, call your local poison control center at 1-800-222-1222. If the victim has collapsed or is not breathing, call local emergency services at 911.

What other information should I know?

Keep all appointments with your doctor so that your response to diphenoxylate and atropine can be checked. Do not give this medicine to children under 2 years of age.

Do not let anyone else take your medication. Ask your pharmacist any questions you have about refilling your prescription. If this medicine does not control your diarrhea within 2 days or your diarrhea gets worse, call your doctor.

Dosage Facts
For Informational Purposes

Caution: Do not change your dose, how often you take your medication, or the length of time you are to take it without first talking to your healthcare provider.

The following dosage information was written using medical language for doctors and other healthcare professionals and is provided here for you to check your dosage. The dosage of this drug may differ for different patients. Therefore, always follow your doctor's instructions or the directions on the label. Contact your healthcare provider or pharmacist if you have any questions about the specific dosage of your medication after reviewing this information.

General Dosage Information

Available as diphenoxylate hydrochloride; dosage expressed in terms of the salt. Commercially available only in combination with atropine sulfate (in subtherapeutic quantity to discourage deliberate overdosage).

Pediatric Patients

Diarrhea

ORAL:
- Children 2–12 years of age: Initially, 0.3–0.4 mg/kg daily, given in 4 divided doses.

Approximate Initial Dosage for Children 2–12 Years of Age

Age	Approximate Weight	Dosage in mg (mL of 2.5-mg/5-mL oral solution)
2 years	11–14 kg	0.75–1.5 mg (1.5–3 mL) 4 times daily
3 years	12–16 kg	1–1.5 mg (2–3 mL) 4 times daily
4 years	14–20 kg	1–2 mg (2–4 mL) 4 times daily
5 years	16–23 kg	1.25–2.25 mg (2.5–4.5 mL) 4 times daily
6–8 years	17–32 kg	1.25–2.5 mg (2.5–5 mL) 4 times daily
9–12 years	23–55 kg	1.75–2.5 mg (3.5–5 mL) 4 times daily

Children 13–16 years of age: Initially, 5 mg 3 times daily.
Pediatric dosage schedules are approximations of an average dosage recommendation; adjust dosage downward according to overall nutritional status and degree of dehydration.
Continue dosage at initial levels until symptoms are controlled and then reduce for maintenance as required; not likely to be effective if no response occurs within 48 hours.
Maintenance dosages may be as low as one-fourth the initial daily dosage.

Adult Patients

Diarrhea

ORAL:
- Initially, 5 mg 4 times daily.

- Continue dosage at initial level until symptoms are controlled and then reduce for maintenance as required; not likely to be effective for treatment of acute diarrhea if no response occurs within 48 hours.
- Maintenance dosage may be as low as one-fourth (e.g., 5 mg daily) the initial daily dosage.
- If clinical improvement of chronic diarrhea after treatment with a maximum daily dosage of 20 mg is not observed within 10 days, symptoms are unlikely to be controlled by further administration.

Prescribing Limits

Do not exceed recommended dosage.

Pediatric Patients

Diarrhea

ORAL:
- Children 2–12 years of age: 0.4 mg/kg daily in divided doses.
- Children 13–16 years of age: 5 mg 3 times daily.

Adult Patients

Diarrhea

ORAL:
- 20 mg daily in divided doses.

Diphtheria, Tetanus, and Pertussis (DTaP) Vaccine

Brand Name: Daptacel®, Infanrix®, Tripedia®

Why get vaccinated?

Diphtheria, tetanus, and pertussis are serious diseases caused by bacteria. Diphtheria and pertussis are spread from person to person. Tetanus enters the body through cuts or wounds.

DIPHTHERIA causes a thick covering in the back of the throat. It can lead to breathing problems, paralysis, heart failure, and even death.

TETANUS (Lockjaw) causes painful tightening of the muscles, usually all over the body. It can lead to "locking" of the jaw so the victim cannot open his mouth or swallow. Tetanus leads to death in about 1 out of 10 cases.

PERTUSSIS (Whooping Cough) causes coughing spells so bad that it is hard for infants to eat, drink, or breathe. These spells can last for weeks. It can lead to pneumonia, seizures (jerking and staring spells), brain damage, and death.

Diphtheria, tetanus, and pertussis vaccine (DTaP) can help prevent these diseases. Most children who are vaccinated with DTaP will be protected throughout childhood. Many more children would get these diseases if we stopped vaccinating.

DTaP is a safer version of an older vaccine called DTP. DTP is no longer used in the United States.

Who should get DTaP vaccine and when?

Children should get **5 doses** of DTaP vaccine, one dose at each of the following ages: 2 months, 4 months, 6 months, 15-18 months, 4-6 years.

DTaP may be given at the same time as other vaccines.

Who should *not* get DTaP vaccine or should wait?

- Children with minor illnesses, such as a cold, may be vaccinated. But children who are moderately or severely ill should usually wait until they recover before getting DTaP vaccine.
- Any child who had a life-threatening allergic reaction after a dose of DTaP should not get another dose.
- Any child who suffered a brain or nervous system disease within 7 days after a dose of DTaP should not get another dose.
- Talk with your doctor if your child: had a seizure or collapsed after a dose of DTaP, cried non-stop for 3 hours or more after a dose of DTaP, or had a fever over 105°F after a dose of DTaP.

Ask your health care provider for more information. Some of these children should not get another dose of pertussis vaccine, but may get a vaccine without pertussis, called DT.

Older children and adults

DTaP should not be given to anyone 7 years of age or older because pertussis vaccine is only licensed for children under 7.

But older children, adolescents, and adults still need protection from tetanus and diphtheria. A booster shot called Td is recommended at 11-12 years of age, and then every 10 years.

What are the risks from DTaP vaccine?

Getting diphtheria, tetanus, or pertussis disease is much riskier than getting DTaP vaccine.

However, a vaccine, like any medicine, is capable of causing serious problems, such as severe allergic reactions. The risk of DTaP vaccine causing serious harm, or death, is extremely small.

Mild Problems (Common):
- Fever (up to about 1 child in 4)
- Redness or swelling where the shot was given (up to about 1 child in 4)
- Soreness or tenderness where the shot was given (up to about 1 child in 4)
- These problems occur more often after the 4th and 5th doses of the DTaP series than after earlier doses. Sometimes the 4th or 5th dose of DTaP vaccine is followed by swelling of the entire arm or leg in which the shot was given, lasting 1-7 days (up to about 1 child in 30).
- **Other mild problems include:** fussiness (up to about 1 child in 3), tiredness or poor appetite (up to about 1 child in 10), vomiting (up to about 1 child in 50).

Moderate Problems (Uncommon):
- Seizure (jerking or staring) (about 1 child out of 14,000)
- Non-stop crying, for 3 hours or more (up to about 1 child out of 1,000)

- High fever, over 105°F (about 1 child out of 16,000)

Severe Problems (Very Rare):
- Serious allergic reaction (less than 1 out of a million doses)
- Several other severe problems have been reported after DTaP vaccine. These include: long-term seizures, coma, or lowered consciousness; permanent brain damage. These are so rare it is hard to tell if they are caused by the vaccine.

Controlling fever is especially important for children who have had seizures, for any reason. It is also important if another family member has had seizures. You can reduce fever and pain by giving your child an aspirin-free pain reliever (such as acetaminophen) when the shot is given, and for the next 24 hours, following the package instructions.

What if there is a moderate or severe reaction?

What should I look for?
- Any unusual conditions, such as a serious allergic reaction, high fever or unusual behavior. Serious allergic reactions are extremely rare with any vaccine. If one were to occur, it would most likely be within a few minutes to a few hours after the shot. Signs can include difficulty breathing, hoarseness or wheezing, hives, paleness, weakness, a fast heart beat or dizziness. If a high fever or seizure were to occur, it would usually be within a week after the shot.

What should I do?
- Call a doctor, or get the person to a doctor right away.
- Tell your doctor what happened, the date and time it happened, and when the vaccination was given.
- Ask your health care provider to file a Vaccine Adverse Event Reporting System (VAERS) form if you have any reaction to the vaccine. Or call VAERS yourself at 1-800-822-7967, or visit their website at http://vaers.hhs.gov.

The National Vaccine Injury Compensation Program

In the rare event that you or your child has a serious reaction to a vaccine, a federal program has been created to help pay for the care of those who have been harmed.

For details about the National Vaccine Injury Compensation Program, call 1-800-338-2382 or visit the program's website at http://www.hrsa.gov/vaccinecompensation.

How can I learn more?

- Ask your doctor or other health care provider. They can give you the vaccine package insert or suggest other sources of information.
- Call your local or state health department's immunization program.
- Contact the Centers for Disease Control and Prevention (CDC): call 1-800-232-4636 (1-800-CDC-INFO) or visit the National Immunization Program's website at http://www.cdc.gov/nip.

DTaP Vaccine Information Statement. U.S. Department of Health and Human Services/Centers for Disease Control and Prevention National Immunization Program. 7/30/2001.

Dipivefrin Ophthalmic

(dye pi′ ve frin)

Brand Name: Propine®
Also available generically.

Why is this medicine prescribed?

Dipivefrin is used to treat glaucoma, a condition in which increased pressure in the eye can lead to gradual loss of vision. Dipivefrin decreases the pressure in the eye.

This medication is sometimes prescribed for other uses; ask your doctor or pharmacist for more information.

How should this medicine be used?

Dipivefrin comes as eyedrops. Dipivefrin usually is applied every 12 hours. Follow the directions on your prescription label carefully, and ask your doctor or pharmacist to explain any part you do not understand. Use dipivefrin exactly as directed. Do not use more or less of it or use it more often than prescribed by your doctor.

Dipivefrin controls glaucoma but does not cure it. Continue to use dipivefrin even if you feel well. Do not stop using dipivefrin without talking to your doctor.

To use the eyedrops, follow these instructions:

1. Wash your hands thoroughly with soap and water.
2. Use a mirror or have someone else put the drops in your eye.
3. Remove the protective cap. Make sure that the end of the dropper is not chipped or cracked.
4. Avoid touching the dropper tip against your eye or anything else.
5. Hold the dropper tip down at all times to prevent drops from flowing back into the bottle and contaminating the remaining contents.
6. Lie down or tilt your head back.
7. Holding the bottle between your thumb and index finger, place the dropper tip as near as possible to your eyelid without touching it.
8. Brace the remaining fingers of that hand against your cheek or nose.
9. With the index finger of your other hand, pull the lower lid of the eye down to form a pocket.
10. Drop the prescribed number of drops into the pocket made by the lower lid and the eye. Placing drops on the surface of the eyeball can cause stinging.
11. Close your eye and press lightly against the lower lid with your finger for 2-3 minutes to keep the medication in the eye. Do not blink.
12. Replace and tighten the cap right away. Do not wipe or rinse it off.
13. Wipe off any excess liquid from your cheek with a clean tissue. Wash your hands again.

What special precautions should I follow?

Before using dipivefrin eyedrops,

- tell your doctor and pharmacist if you are allergic to dipivefrin, epinephrine, sulfites, or any other drugs.
- tell your doctor and pharmacist what prescription and nonprescription medications you are using, especially eye medications, and vitamins.
- tell your doctor if you have or have ever had high blood pressure, heart or blood vessel disease, irregular heartbeat, or asthma.
- tell your doctor if you are pregnant, plan to become pregnant, or are breast-feeding. If you become pregnant while using dipivefrin, call your doctor immediately.
- if you are having surgery, including dental surgery, tell the doctor or dentist that you are using dipivefrin.
- if you are using another eyedrop medication, use the eye medications at least 10 minutes apart.

What should I do if I forget to take a dose?

Apply the missed dose as soon as you remember it. However, if it is almost time for the next dose, skip the missed dose and continue your regular dosing schedule. Do not apply a double dose to make up for a missed one.

What side effects can this medicine cause?

Dipivefrin may cause side effects. Tell your doctor if any of these symptoms are severe or do not go away:

- eye irritation or discomfort
- swelling or pain of the eye
- blurred vision
- increased sensitivity to light and glare

If you experience any of the following symptoms, call your doctor immediately:

- fast or irregular heartbeat
- chest pain
- wheezing
- difficulty breathing

If you experience a serious side effect, you or your doctor may send a report to the Food and Drug Administration's (FDA) MedWatch Adverse Event Reporting program online [at http://www.fda.gov/MedWatch/index.html] or by phone [1-800-332-1088].

What storage conditions are needed for this medicine?

Keep this medication in the container it came in, tightly closed, and out of reach of children. Store it at room temperature in the dark and away from excess heat and moisture (not in the bathroom). Exposure to air and light causes the liquid to darken or become discolored and lose its effectiveness. If this happens, do not use the medication; obtain a new supply. Throw away any medication that is outdated or no longer needed. Talk to your pharmacist about the proper disposal of your medication.

What other information should I know?

Keep all appointments with your doctor. Your doctor will order certain eye tests to check your response to dipivefrin eyedrops.

Do not let anyone else use your medication. Ask your pharmacist any questions you have about refilling your prescription.

Dosage Facts
For Informational Purposes

Caution: Do not change your dose, how often you take your medication, or the length of time you are to take it without first talking to your healthcare provider.

The following dosage information was written using medical language for doctors and other healthcare professionals and is provided here for you to check your dosage. The dosage of this drug may differ for different patients. Therefore, always follow your doctor's instructions or the directions on the label. Contact your healthcare provider or pharmacist if you have any questions about the specific dosage of your medication after reviewing this information.

General Dosage Information

Available as dipivefrin hydrochloride; dosage expressed in terms of the salt.

Adult Patients

Ocular Hypertension and Glaucoma
Initial Therapy

OPHTHALMIC:
- 1 drop of a 0.1% solution in affected eye(s) every 12 hours.

Adjunctive Therapy

OPHTHALMIC:
- In patients receiving several drugs for the treatment of glaucoma, adjustments to the regimen should involve one drug at a time and should usually occur at intervals of at least 1 week.
- Initially, 1 drop of a 0.1% solution every 12 hours while therapy with other drugs is continued. Beginning on the following day and continuing at intervals of at least 1 week until optimum response is achieved, reduce dosage of one of the other drugs or discontinue one of the other drugs. Adjust remaining regimen according to the IOP response of the patient.

Conversion to Dipivefrin Therapy

OPHTHALMIC:
- Conversion from monotherapy with epinephrine: Discontinue epinephrine and initiate dipivefrin at 1 drop of a 0.1% solution into affected eye(s) every 12 hours at the time of the next scheduled dose of epinephrine.
- Conversion from monotherapy with antiglaucoma agents other than epinephrine: On day 1, continue other antiglaucoma agent and add 1 drop of a 0.1% dipivefrin solution every 12 hours. On day 2, discontinue the other drug and continue dipivefrin.

Dipyridamole
(dye peer id' a mole)

Brand Name: Persantine®

Why is this medicine prescribed?

Dipyridamole is used with other drugs to reduce the risk of blood clots after heart valve replacement. It works by preventing excessive blood clotting.

This medication is sometimes prescribed for other uses; ask your doctor or pharmacist for more information.

How should this medicine be used?

Dipyridamole comes as a tablet to take by mouth. It usually is taken four times a day. Follow the directions on your prescription label carefully, and ask your doctor or pharmacist to explain any part you do not understand. Take dipyridamole exactly as directed. Do not take more or less of it or take it more often than prescribed by your doctor.

Continue to take dipyridamole even if you feel well. Do not stop taking dipyridamole without talking to your doctor.

Are there other uses for this medicine?

Dipyridamole is also used with aspirin to reduce the risk of death after a heart attack and to prevent another heart attack. Talk to your doctor about the possible risks of using this drug for your condition.

What special precautions should I follow?

Before taking dipyridamole,
- tell your doctor and pharmacist if you are allergic to dipyridamole or any other drugs.
- tell your doctor and pharmacist what prescription and nonprescription medications you are taking, especially aspirin and vitamins.
- tell your doctor if you have or have ever had low blood pressure.
- tell your doctor if you are pregnant, plan to become pregnant, or are breast-feeding. If you become pregnant while taking dipyridamole, call your doctor.
- if you are having surgery, including dental surgery, tell the doctor or dentist that you are taking dipyridamole.

What should I do if I forget to take a dose?

Take the missed dose as soon as you remember it. However, if it is almost time for the next dose, skip the missed dose and continue your regular dosing schedule. Do not take a double dose to make up for a missed one.

What side effects can this medicine cause?

Dipyridamole may cause side effects. Tell your doctor if any of these symptoms are severe or do not go away:
- dizziness

- stomach pain
- headache
- rash
- diarrhea
- vomiting
- flushing (feeling of warmth)
- itching

If you experience any of the following symptoms, call your doctor immediately:

- unusual bleeding or bruising
- yellowing of the skin or eyes
- chest pain

If you experience a serious side effect, you or your doctor may send a report to the Food and Drug Administration's (FDA) MedWatch Adverse Event Reporting program online [at http://www.fda.gov/MedWatch/index.html] or by phone [1-800-332-1088].

What storage conditions are needed for this medicine?

Keep this medication in the container it came in, tightly closed, and out of reach of children. Store it at room temperature and away from excess heat and moisture (not in the bathroom). Throw away any medication that is outdated or no longer needed. Talk to your pharmacist about the proper disposal of your medication.

What should I do in case of overdose?

In case of overdose, call your local poison control center at 1-800-222-1222. If the victim has collapsed or is not breathing, call local emergency services at 911.

What other information should I know?

Keep all appointments with your doctor and the laboratory.

Do not let anyone else take your medication. Ask your pharmacist any questions you have about refilling your prescription.

Dosage Facts
For Informational Purposes

Caution: Do not change your dose, how often you take your medication, or the length of time you are to take it without first talking to your healthcare provider.

The following dosage information was written using medical language for doctors and other healthcare professionals and is provided here for you to check your dosage. The dosage of this drug may differ for different patients. Therefore, always follow your doctor's instructions or the directions on the label. Contact your healthcare provider or pharmacist if you have any questions about the specific dosage of your medication after reviewing this information.

Adult Patients

Thromboembolism Associated with Prosthetic Heart Valves
Prophylaxis

ORAL:
- Conventional tablets: 75–100 mg 4 times daily; use in conjunction with coumarin anticoagulant therapy.

Cerebral Thromboembolism
Secondary Prevention

ORAL:
- Fixed combination with aspirin: 200 mg of extended-release dipyridamole and 25 mg of aspirin (one capsule) twice daily in the morning and evening.
- Dose of aspirin in fixed-combination product may not be adequate to prevent recurrent MI or angina pectoris in patients with stroke or TIA.

Embolism Associated with Valvular Heart Disease

ORAL:
- Rheumatic mitral valve disease and a history of systemic embolism or atrial fibrillation† with aspirin intolerance: 400 mg daily.

† Use is not currently included in the labeling approved by the US Food and Drug Administration.

Disopyramide

(dye soe peer' a mide)

Brand Name: Norpace®, Norpace® CR
Also available generically.

Important Warning

Studies have shown that some antiarrhythmic drugs may increase the risk of death, especially if you have had a previous heart attack. This information also may apply to disopyramide. Disopyramide usually is used only to treat life-threatening arrhythmias.

Why is this medicine prescribed?

Disopyramide is used to treat abnormal heart rhythms (arrhythmias). It works by making your heart more resistant to abnormal activity.

This medication is sometimes prescribed for other uses; ask your doctor or pharmacist for more information.

How should this medicine be used?

Disopyramide comes as a capsule to take by mouth. Immediate-acting disopyramide may be taken three or four times a day. The long-acting product usually is taken twice a day. Do not cut, crush, or chew extended-release capsules; swallow them whole.

Follow the directions on your prescription label carefully, and ask your doctor or pharmacist to explain any part you do not understand. Take disopyramide exactly as directed. Do not take more or less of it or take it more often than prescribed by your doctor.

Disopyramide helps control your condition but will not cure it. Continue to take disopyramide even if you feel well. Do not stop taking disopyramide without talking to your doctor.

What special precautions should I follow?

Before taking disopyramide,

- tell your doctor and pharmacist if you are allergic to disopyramide or any other drugs.
- tell your doctor and pharmacist what prescription and nonprescription medications you are taking, especially clarithromycin (Biaxin), erythromycin (E.E.S., E-mycin, others), itraconazole (Sporanox), ketoconazole (Nizoral), other medications for arrhythmias such as quinidine (Quinidex) or procainamide (Pronestil, Rhythmin), phenytoin (Dilantin), potassium supplements (K-Dur, Klor-Con), propranolol (Inderal), verapamil (Calan, Covera, Verelan), and vitamins.
- tell your doctor if you have or have ever had congestive heart disease, high blood pressure, diabetes, kidney or liver disease, glaucoma, myasthenia gravis, urinary retention, or benign prostatic hypertrophy.
- tell your doctor if you are pregnant, plan to become pregnant, or are breast-feeding. If you become pregnant while taking disopyramide, call your doctor.
- if you are having surgery, including dental surgery, tell the doctor or dentist that you are taking disopyramide.
- you should know that this drug may make you drowsy. Do not drive a car or operate machinery until you know how this drug affects you.
- remember that alcohol can add to the drowsiness caused by this drug.
- talk to your doctor about the use of cigarettes and caffeine-containing beverages. These products may increase the irritability of your heart and interfere with the action of disopyramide.

What should I do if I forget to take a dose?

Take the missed dose as soon as you remember it. However, if it is almost time for the next dose, skip the missed dose and continue your regular dosing schedule. Do not take a double dose to make up for a missed one.

What side effects can this medicine cause?

Disopyramide may cause side effects. Tell your doctor if any of these symptoms are severe or do not go away:

- dizziness or lightheadedness
- difficult urination
- dry mouth
- constipation
- blurred vision
- stomach pain or bloating
- headache

If you experience any of the following symptoms, call your doctor immediately:

- chest pain
- swelling of the feet or hands
- unusual weight gain
- irregular heartbeat
- shortness of breath
- fever, chills, or sore throat
- skin rash or yellowing of the skin

If you experience a serious side effect, you or your doctor may send a report to the Food and Drug Administration's (FDA) MedWatch Adverse Event Reporting program online [at http://www.fda.gov/MedWatch/index.html] or by phone [1-800-332-1088].

What storage conditions are needed for this medicine?

Keep this medication in the container it came in, tightly closed, and out of reach of children. Store it at room temperature and away from excess heat and moisture (not in the bathroom). Throw away any medication that is outdated or no longer needed. Talk to your pharmacist about the proper disposal of your medication.

What should I do in case of overdose?

In case of overdose, call your local poison control center at 1-800-222-1222. If the victim has collapsed or is not breathing, call local emergency services at 911.

What other information should I know?

Keep all appointments with your doctor and the laboratory. Your doctor will need to determine your response to disopyramide.

Do not let anyone else take your medication. Ask your pharmacist any questions you have about refilling your prescription.

Dosage Facts
For Informational Purposes

Caution: Do not change your dose, how often you take your medication, or the length of time you are to take it without first talking to your healthcare provider.

The following dosage information was written using medical language for doctors and other healthcare professionals and is provided here for you to check your dosage. The dosage of this drug may differ for different patients. Therefore, always follow your doctor's instructions or the directions on the label. Contact your health-

care provider or pharmacist if you have any questions about the specific dosage of your medication after reviewing this information.

General Dosage Information

Available as disopyramide phosphate; dosage expressed in terms of disopyramide.

Reduce dosage in patients with moderate or severe renal insufficiency, hepatic insufficiency, cardiomyopathy, possible cardiac decompensation, AMI, and in patients weighing <50 kg.

Pediatric Patients

Ventricular Arrhythmias

ORAL:

- Optimum pediatric dosage has not been established; however, dosage recommendations have been made based on clinical experience.
- Initiate dose titration at the lower end of the recommended ranges; monitor plasma drug concentrations and therapeutic response carefully.
- For children unable to swallow the capsules, a suspension may be extemporaneously prepared by mixing the contents of disopyramide phosphate conventional capsules in cherry syrup to produce suspensions that contain 1–10 mg of disopyramide per mL. The extended-release capsules should *not* be used for the preparation of an extemporaneous suspension.
- Give total daily dose in equally divided doses every 6 hours or at intervals according to individual requirements.

Total Daily Pediatric Dosage Based on Age and Weight

Age	Total Daily Pediatric Dosage
<1 year of age	10–30 mg/kg
1–4 years of age	10–20 mg/kg
4–12 years of age	10–15 mg/kg
12–18 years of age	6–15 mg/kg

Adult Patients

Ventricular Arrhythmias

ORAL (CONVENTIONAL CAPSULES):

- Usual dosage: 400–800 mg daily, given in divided doses.
- Adults weighing ≥50 kg: Usually 150 mg every 6 hours.
- Adults weighing <50 kg: Usually 100 mg every 6 hours.

ORAL (EXTENDED-RELEASE CAPSULES):

- Usual dosage: 400–800 mg daily, given in divided doses.
- Adults weighing ≥50 kg: Usually 300 mg every 12 hours.
- Adults weighing <50 kg: Usually 200 mg every 12 hours.

Rapid Control

ORAL (CONVENTIONAL CAPSULES):

- Adults weighing ≥50 kg: Initially, 300 mg followed by 150 mg every 6 hours.
- Adults weighing <50 kg: Initially, 200 mg followed by 150 mg every 6 hours.
- If there is no therapeutic response and if no toxic effects occur within 6 hours after the initial 300-mg dose, 200-mg doses may be given every 6 hours. If there is no response to this dosage in 48 hours, discontinue disopyramide and initiate alternative therapy.

- Alternatively, the patient may be hospitalized, closely evaluated, and continuously monitored while the dosage is increased to 250 or 300 mg every 6 hours.

Severe Refractory VT

ORAL (CONVENTIONAL CAPSULES):

- Up to 400 mg every 6 hours may be required (resulting in plasma disopyramide concentrations up to 9 mcg/mL).
- Patients should be hospitalized, closely evaluated, and continuously monitored.

Rapid Control In Patients with Cardiomyopathy or Possible Cardiac Decompensation

ORAL (CONVENTIONAL CAPSULES):

- Do *not* administer an initial loading dose.
- Do *not* exceed an initial dosage of 100 mg every 6 hours.
- Carefully adjust dosage in these patients while closely monitoring for hypotension and/or CHF.

Switching from Another Class I Antiarrhythmic Agent

ORAL (CONVENTIONAL CAPSULES OR EXTENDED-RELEASE CAPSULES):

- Administer the usual dosage of disopyramide (without an initial loading dose) 6–12 hours after the last dose of quinidine sulfate or 3–6 hours after the last dose of procainamide.
- If withdrawal of quinidine or procainamide is likely to produce life-threatening arrhythmias, hospitalize and closely monitor patient.

Switching from Conventional to Extended-release Capsules

ORAL (EXTENDED-RELEASE):

- Initiate usual maintenance schedule (e.g., 300 mg every 12 hours) of extended-release capsules 6 hours after the last dose of the conventional capsules.

Dosage Modification for Toxicity

If increased anticholinergic adverse effects occur, monitor plasma concentrations of disopyramide and adjust dosage accordingly. Dosage may be reduced by one-third and the same dosing interval maintained (e.g., 600 mg daily reduced to 400 mg daily).

Prescribing Limits

Adult Patients

Ventricular Arrhythmias

Patients with Cardiomyopathy or Possible Cardiac Decompensation

ORAL (CONVENTIONAL CAPSULES):

- Maximum initial dosage: 100 mg every 6 hours.

Special Populations

Hepatic Impairment

ORAL:

- Usual dosage: 100 mg every 6 hours as conventional capsules or 200 mg every 12 hours as extended-release capsules.

Renal Impairment

ORAL:

- Do *not* use extended-release capsules in patients with a Cl_{cr} ≤40 mL/minute.
- Patients with moderately impaired renal function (Cl_{cr} >40 mL/minute): Usually, 100 mg every 6 hours as conventional capsules or 200 mg every 12 hours as extended-release capsules.

- In patients with severely impaired renal function ($Cl_{cr} \leq 40$ mL/minute), the usual dosage of conventional capsules is 100 mg (with or without an initial 150-mg dose) given at the following approximate intervals depending on the patient's Cl_{cr}:

Cl_{cr} (mL/minute)	Dosage Interval
30–40	every 8 h
15–30	every 12 h
<15	every 24 h

Geriatric Patients

- Select dosage with caution (generally starting at the low end of the dosing range) because of age-related decreases in hepatic, renal, and/or cardiac function, and concomitant disease and drug therapy.
- If adverse anticholinergic effects occur, monitor plasma disopyramide concentrations and adjust dosage as needed.

Disulfiram

(dye sul′ fi ram)

Brand Name: Antabuse®
Also available generically.

Important Warning

Never give disulfiram to a patient in a state of alcohol intoxication or without the patient's full knowledge. The patient should not take disulfiram for at least 12 hours after drinking. A reaction may occur for up to 2 weeks after disulfiram has been stopped.

Why is this medicine prescribed?

Disulfiram is used to treat chronic alcoholism. It causes unpleasant effects when even small amounts of alcohol are consumed. These effects include flushing of the face, headache, nausea, vomiting, chest pain, weakness, blurred vision, mental confusion, sweating, choking, breathing difficulty, and anxiety. These effects begin about 10 minutes after alcohol enters the body and last for 1 hour or more. Disulfiram is not a cure for alcoholism, but discourages drinking.

This medication is sometimes prescribed for other uses; ask your doctor or pharmacist for more information.

How should this medicine be used?

Disulfiram comes in tablets to take by mouth. It should be taken once a day. Follow the directions on your prescription label carefully, and ask your doctor or pharmacist to explain any part you do not understand. Take disulfiram exactly as

directed. Do not take more or less of it or take it more often than prescribed by your doctor.

If you cannot swallow the tablets, crush them and mix the medication with water, coffee, tea, milk, soft drink, or fruit juice.

What special precautions should I follow?

Before taking disulfiram,

- tell your doctor and pharmacist if you are allergic to disulfiram or any other drugs.
- tell your doctor and pharmacist what prescription and nonprescription medications you are taking, especially amitriptyline (Elavil), anticoagulants ('blood thinners') such as warfarin (Coumadin), isoniazid, metronidazole (Flagyl), phenytoin (Dilantin), any nonprescription drugs that might contain alcohol, and vitamins.
- tell your doctor if you have or have ever had diabetes, thyroid disease, epilepsy, brain damage, or kidney or liver disease.
- tell your doctor if you are pregnant, plan to become pregnant, or are breast-feeding. If you become pregnant while taking disulfiram, call your doctor.
- if you are having surgery, including dental surgery, tell the doctor or dentist that you are taking disulfiram.
- you should know that this drug may make you drowsy. Do not drive a car or operate machinery until you know how this drug affects you.

What special dietary instructions should I follow?

Do not drink any alcoholic beverages (including wine, beer, and medications that contain alcohol such as cough syrup) while taking disulfiram, during the 12-hour period before you take your first dose, and for several weeks after stopping the drug.

Avoid sauces, vinegars, and all foods and beverages containing alcohol.

What should I do if I forget to take a dose?

Take the missed dose as soon as you remember it. However, if it is almost time for the next dose, skip the missed dose and continue your regular dosing schedule. Do not take a double dose to make up for a missed one.

What side effects can this medicine cause?

Disulfiram may cause side effects. Tell your doctor if any of these symptoms are severe or do not go away:

- skin rash
- acne
- mild headache
- drowsiness
- tiredness
- impotence
- metallic taste or garlic-like taste in the mouth

If you experience any of the following symptoms, call your doctor immediately:

- excessive tiredness
- weakness
- lack of energy
- loss of appetite
- upset stomach
- vomiting
- yellowness of the skin or eyes
- dark urine

What storage conditions are needed for this medicine?

Keep this medication in the container it came in, tightly closed, and out of reach of children. Store it at room temperature and away from excess heat and moisture (not in the bathroom). Throw away any medication that is outdated or no longer needed. Talk to your pharmacist about the proper disposal of your medication.

What should I do in case of overdose?

In case of overdose, call your local poison control center at 1-800-222-1222. If the victim has collapsed or is not breathing, call local emergency services at 911.

What other information should I know?

Keep all appointments with your doctor and the laboratory. Your doctor will order certain lab tests to check your response to disulfiram.

Always carry an identification card stating that you are taking disulfiram and indicating the doctor or institution to be contacted in an emergency. If you need an identification card, ask your pharmacist or doctor how to get one.

Do not come in contact with or breathe the fumes of paint, paint thinner, varnish, shellac, and other products containing alcohol. Exercise caution when applying alcohol-containing products (e.g., aftershave lotions, colognes, and rubbing alcohol) to your skin. These products, in combination with disulfiram, may cause headache, nausea, local redness, or itching. Before using an alcohol-containing product, test it by applying some to a small area of your skin for 1-2 hours. If no redness, itching, or unwanted effects occur, you can use the product safely.

Do not let anyone else take your medication. Ask your pharmacist any questions you have about refilling your prescription.

Dosage Facts
For Informational Purposes

Caution: Do not change your dose, how often you take your medication, or the length of time you are to take it without first talking to your healthcare provider.

The following dosage information was written using medical language for doctors and other healthcare professionals and is provided here for you to check your dosage. The dosage of this drug may differ for different patients. Therefore, always follow your doctor's instructions or the directions on the label. Contact your healthcare provider or pharmacist if you have any questions about the specific dosage of your medication after reviewing this information.

General Dosage Information

Do not administer until patient has abstained from alcohol for ≥12 hours. Never administer without the patient's knowledge.

Adult Patients

Alcohol Dependence

ORAL:
- Initially, maximum 500 mg once daily for 1–2 weeks.
- Average maintenance dosage: 250 mg daily (range 125–500 mg daily) until a basis for permanent self-control is established. Treatment may be required for months or years.

Prescribing Limits

Adult Patients

Alcohol Dependence

ORAL:
- Maximum 500 mg daily.

Special Populations

Hepatic Impairment
- Use with extreme caution; however, no specific dosage recommendations at this time.

Renal Impairment
- Use with extreme caution; however, no specific dosage recommendations at this time.

Geriatric Patients
- Select dosage with caution and at the low end of the dosing range because of age-related decreases in hepatic, renal, and/or cardiac function, and concomitant disease and drug therapy.

Dofetilide
(doe fet′ il ide)

Brand Name: Tikosyn®

Important Warning

Tikosyn can cause your heart to beat irregularly. You will need to be in a hospital or another place where you can be monitored closely by your doctor for at least 3 days when you are started or restarted on dofetilide. It is important to read the patient information provided to you every time you begin therapy with dofetilide.

Why is this medicine prescribed?

Dofetilide is used to treat irregular heartbeats. It improves your heart rhythm by relaxing an overactive heart.

This medication is sometimes prescribed for other uses; ask your doctor or pharmacist for more information.

How should this medicine be used?

Dofetilide comes as a capsule to take by mouth. It is usually taken twice a day. Follow the directions on your prescription label carefully, and ask your doctor or pharmacist to explain any part you do not understand. Take dofetilide exactly as directed. Do not take more or less of it or take it more often than prescribed by your doctor. Do not take a double dose.

Dofetilide controls abnormal heart rhythms but does not cure them. Continue to take dofetilide even if you feel well. Do not stop taking dofetilide without talking to your doctor.

What special precautions should I follow?

Before taking dofetilide,

- tell your doctor and pharmacist if you are allergic to dofetilide or any other drugs.
- tell your doctor and pharmacist what prescription and nonprescription medications you are taking, especially antipsychotics, bepridil (Vascor), cimetidine (Tagamet), cisapride (Propulsid), clarithromycin (Biaxin), diltiazem (Cardizem), diuretics ('water pills'), erythromycin (E.E.S., E-Mycin, others), HIV protease inhibitors such as ritonavir (Norvir), itraconazole (Sporanox), ketoconazole (Nizoral), medications for dizziness or nausea, medications for depression such as amitriptyline (Elavil) or fluoxetine (Prozac), megestrol (Megace), metformin (Glucophage), other medications for irregular heart beats such as amiodarone (Cordarone), norfloxacin (Noroxin), prochlorperazine (Compazine), quinine (Formula Q), trimethoprim (Proloprim, Trimpex), trimethoprim and sulfamethoxazole (Bactrim, Septra), verapamil (Calan, Covera, Verelan), zafirlukast (Accolate), and vitamins.
- tell your doctor if you have or have ever had long QT syndrome (a type of heart problem), or kidney or liver disease.
- tell your doctor if you are pregnant, plan to become pregnant, or are breast-feeding. If you become pregnant while taking dofetilide, call your doctor.

What special dietary instructions should I follow?

Talk to your doctor before drinking grapefruit juice. It may be best to drink other fruit juices while taking dofetilide.

What should I do if I forget to take a dose?

Skip the missed dose and continue your regular dosing schedule. Do not take a double dose to make up for a missed one.

What side effects can this medicine cause?

Dofetilide may cause side effects. Tell your doctor if any of these symptoms are severe or do not go away:

- headache
- chest pain
- dizziness
- respiratory infection
- flu-like symptoms
- stomach pain
- back pain
- diarrhea
- difficulty sleeping

If you experience any of the following symptoms, call your doctor immediately:

- irregular heartbeat
- rash
- sweating
- upset stomach
- vomiting
- loss of appetite or thirst

If you experience a serious side effect, you or your doctor may send a report to the Food and Drug Administration's (FDA) MedWatch Adverse Event Reporting program online [at http://www.fda.gov/MedWatch/index.html] or by phone [1-800-332-1088].

What storage conditions are needed for this medicine?

Keep this medication in the container it came in, tightly closed, and out of reach of children. Store it at room temperature and away from excess heat and moisture (not in the bathroom). Throw away any medication that is outdated or no longer needed. Talk to your pharmacist about the proper disposal of your medication.

What should I do in case of overdose?

In case of overdose, call your local poison control center at 1-800-222-1222. If the victim has collapsed or is not breathing, call local emergency services at 911.

What other information should I know?

Keep all appointments with your doctor and the laboratory. Your heart rhythm should be checked regularly to determine your response to dofetilide. Your doctor will also want to follow your kidney function and blood level of potassium closely while you are taking dofetilide.

If you are ill for more than 24 hours with diarrhea, vomiting, or sweating and have not been able to take in much fluid or nutrition you should call your doctor before taking your next dose of dofetilide.

Do not let anyone else take your medication. Ask your pharmacist any questions you have about refilling your prescription.

Dosage Facts
For Informational Purposes

Caution: Do not change your dose, how often you take your medication, or the length of time you are to take it without first talking to your healthcare provider.

The following dosage information was written using medical language for doctors and other healthcare professionals and is provided here for you to check your dosage. The dosage of this drug may differ for different patients. Therefore, always follow your doctor's instructions or the directions on the label. Contact your healthcare provider or pharmacist if you have any questions about the specific dosage of your medication after reviewing this information.

Adult Patients

Supraventricular Tachyarrhythmias

ORAL:
- Initially, 500 mcg twice daily; modify dosage according to Cl_{cr} and QT_c interval. and

Table 1. Initial Dosage in Adults Based on Renal Function

Calculated Cl_{cr} (mL/minute)	Dosage
>60	500 mcg twice daily
40–60	250 mcg twice daily
20 to <40	125 mcg twice daily
<20	Dofetilide is contraindicated

Within 2–3 hours after administration of the first dose, determine the QT_c interval. If QT_c interval has increased by >15% or >500 msec (550 msec in patients with ventricular conduction abnormalities), adjust subsequent dosages as follows:

Table 2. Dosage Modification for QT_c Prolongation

Initial Dosage (Based on Cl_{cr})	Adjusted Dosage (for QT_c Prolongation)
500 mcg twice daily	250 mcg twice daily
250 mcg twice daily	125 mcg twice daily
125 mcg twice daily	125 mcg once daily

Therapy may be initiated at lower dosages due to the risk of torsades de pointes.

Prescribing Limits

Adult Patients

Supraventricular Tachyarrhythmias

ORAL:
- Dosages >500 mcg twice daily have been associated with an increased incidence of torsades de pointes.

Special Populations

Hepatic Impairment
- No dosage adjustment is required in patients with mild to moderate hepatic impairment (Child-Pugh class A or B). Use with particular caution in patients with severe hepatic insufficiency (Child-Pugh class C).

Renal Impairment
- Modify dosage according to the degree of renal impairment.
- Not studied in those undergoing dialysis; dosage recommendations are not known.

Geriatric Patients
- Select dosage with caution because of age-related decreases in renal function.

Dolasetron

(dol a' se tron)

Brand Name: Anzemet®

Why is this medicine prescribed?

Dolasetron is used to prevent nausea and vomiting caused by cancer chemotherapy, anesthesia, or surgery. Dolasetron is in a class of medications called serotonin 5-HT$_3$ receptor antagonists. It works by blocking the vomiting reflex in the brain.

How should this medicine be used?

Dolasetron comes as a tablet to take by mouth. It is usually taken within 1 hour before chemotherapy or within 2 hours before surgery. Follow the directions on your prescription label carefully, and ask your doctor or pharmacist to explain any part you do not understand. Take dolasetron exactly as directed. Do not take more or less of it or take it more often than prescribed by your doctor.

Are there other uses for this medicine?

This medication may be prescribed for other uses; ask your doctor or pharmacist for more information.

What special precautions should I follow?

Before taking dolasetron,
- tell your doctor and pharmacist if you are allergic to dolasetron, alosetron (Lotronex), granisetron (Kytril), ondansetron (Zofran), or any other medications.
- tell your doctor and pharmacist what prescription and nonprescription medications, vitamins, nutritional supplements, and herbal products you are taking. Be sure to mention any of the following: cimetidine (Tagamet); cisapride (Propulsid); diuretics ('water pills'); dofetilide (Tikosyn); erythromycin (E.E.S., E-Mycin, Erythrocin);

medications for irregular heartbeat such as amiodarone (Cordarone), disopyramide (Norpace), pimozide (Orap), procainamide (Procanbid, Pronestyl), quinidine (Quinidex), and sotalol (Betapace, Betapace AF); moxifloxacin (Avelox); rifampin (Rifadin, Rimactane); sparfloxacin (Zagam); and thioridazine (Mellaril). Your doctor may need to change the doses of your medications or monitor you carefully for side effects.

- tell your doctor if you have or have ever had low blood levels of magnesium or potassium, or heart disease.
- tell your doctor if you are pregnant, plan to become pregnant, or are breast-feeding. If you become pregnant while taking dolasetron, call your doctor.

What special dietary instructions should I follow?

Unless your doctor tells you otherwise, continue your normal diet.

What should I do if I forget to take a dose?

Take the missed dose as soon as you remember it. However, if it is almost time for the next dose, skip the missed dose and continue your regular dosing schedule. Do not take a double dose to make up for a missed one.

What side effects can this medicine cause?

Dolasetron may cause side effects. Tell your doctor if any of these symptoms are severe or do not go away:

- headache
- diarrhea
- excessive tiredness
- dizziness
- pain
- heartburn
- chills
- rash
- fever
- itching

Some side effects can be serious. The following symptom is uncommon, but if you experience it, call your doctor immediately:

- rapid, pounding, or irregular heartbeat

Dolasetron may cause other side effects. Call your doctor if you have any unusual problems while taking this medication.

If you experience a serious side effect, you or your doctor may send a report to the Food and Drug Administration's (FDA) MedWatch Adverse Event Reporting program online [at http://www.fda.gov/MedWatch/index.html] or by phone [1-800-332-1088].

What storage conditions are needed for this medicine?

Keep this medication in the container it came in, tightly closed, and out of reach of children. Store it at room temperature and away from excess heat and moisture (not in the bathroom). Throw away any medication that is outdated or no longer needed. Talk to your pharmacist about the proper disposal of your medication.

What should I do in case of overdose?

In case of overdose, call your local poison control center at 1-800-222-1222. If the victim has collapsed or is not breathing, call local emergency services at 911.

Symptoms of overdose may include:

- dizziness
- fainting

What other information should I know?

Keep all appointments with you doctor.

Do not let anyone else take your medication. Ask your pharmacist any questions you have about refilling your prescription.

Dosage Facts
For Informational Purposes

Caution: Do not change your dose, how often you take your medication, or the length of time you are to take it without first talking to your healthcare provider.

The following dosage information was written using medical language for doctors and other healthcare professionals and is provided here for you to check your dosage. The dosage of this drug may differ for different patients. Therefore, always follow your doctor's instructions or the directions on the label. Contact your healthcare provider or pharmacist if you have any questions about the specific dosage of your medication after reviewing this information.

General Dosage Information

Available as dolasetron mesylate; dosage expressed in terms of the salt.

Pediatric Patients

Cancer Chemotherapy-induced Nausea and Vomiting
Prevention

ORAL:
- Children 2–16 years of age: 1.8 mg/kg (maximum 100 mg) as a single dose within 1 hour before administration of chemotherapy.
- If dolasetron mesylate injection is administered *orally* in children, administer same dosage as for tablets.

Postoperative Nausea and Vomiting
Prevention

ORAL:
- Children 2–16 years of age: 1.2 mg/kg (maximum 100 mg) as a single dose within 2 hours before surgery.
- If dolasetron mesylate injection is administered *orally* in children, administer same dosage as for tablets.

Adult Patients

Cancer Chemotherapy-induced Nausea and Vomiting
Prevention

ORAL:
- 100 mg as a single dose within 1 hour before administration of chemotherapy.

Postoperative Nausea and Vomiting
Prevention

ORAL:
- 100 mg as a single dose within 2 hours before surgery. Higher dosages not associated with improved efficacy.

Prescribing Limits

Pediatric Patients

Cancer Chemotherapy-induced Nausea and Vomiting
Prevention

ORAL:
- Children 2–16 years of age: 1.8 mg/kg (100 mg maximum) as a single dose.

Postoperative Nausea and Vomiting
Prevention

ORAL:
- Children 2–16 years of age: 1.2 mg/kg (100 mg maximum) as a single dose.

Adult Patients

Cancer Chemotherapy-induced Nausea and Vomiting
Prevention

ORAL:
- 100 mg as a single dose.

Postoperative Nausea and Vomiting
Prevention

ORAL:
- 100 mg as a single dose.

Special Populations

Hepatic Impairment
- No dosage adjustments required.

Renal Impairment
- No dosage adjustments required.

Dolasetron Mesylate Injection

(dol a′ se tron)

Brand Name: Anzemet®

About Your Treatment

Your doctor has ordered dolasetron to prevent nausea and vomiting that may be caused by cancer chemotherapy or to treat nausea and vomiting caused by anesthesia. The drug will be either injected directly into your vein over 30 seconds or added to an intravenous fluid that will drip through a needle or catheter placed in your vein for at least 15 minutes. It is given about 30 minutes before chemotherapy or shortly before the end of your surgery. This medication is sometimes prescribed for other uses; ask your doctor or pharmacist for more information.

Your health care provider (doctor, nurse, or pharmacist) may measure the effectiveness and side effects of your treatment using laboratory tests and physical examinations. It is important to keep all appointments with your doctor and the laboratory. The length of treatment depends on how you respond to the medication.

Precautions

Before administering dolasetron,
- tell your doctor and pharmacist if you are allergic to dolasetron, granisetron (Kytril), odansetron (Zofran), or any other drugs.
- tell your doctor and pharmacist what prescription and nonprescription medications you are taking, especially amitriptyline (Elavil, Endep), astemizole (Hismanal), chlorpromazine (Thorazine), cimetidine (Tagamet, Tagamet HB), clomipramine (Anafranil), desipramine (Norpramin, Pertofrane), disopyramide (Norpace, Norpace CR), doxepin (Adapin, Sinequan), flecainide (Tambocor), fluphenazine (Permitil, Prolixin), imipramine (Tofranil), medications used to treat arrhythmias (especially amiodarone [Cordarone]), moricizine (Ethmozine), nortriptyline (Aventyl, Pamelor), perphenazine (Trilafon), procainamide (Procan SR, Pronestyl, and others), propafenone (Rythmol), protriptline (Vivactil), quinidine (Quinidex, Quinaglute, and others), rifampin (Rifadin, Rimactane), sotalol (Betapace)], thioridazine (Mellaril), trifluoperazine (Stelazine), trimipramine (Surmontil), and vitamins.
- tell your doctor if you have or ever had heart or liver disease, irregular heartbeats, low potassium levels, or low magnesium levels.
- tell your doctor if you are pregnant, plan to become pregnant, or are breast-feeding. If you become pregnant while taking dolasetron, call your doctor.

Administering Your Medication

Before you administer dolasetron, look at the solution closely. It should be clear and free of floating material. Gently squeeze the bag or observe the solution container to make sure there are no leaks. Do not use the solution if it is discolored, if it contains particles, or if the bag or container leaks. Use a new solution, but show the damaged one to your health care provider.

It is important that you use your medication exactly as directed. Do not change your dosing schedule without talking to your health care provider. Your health care provider may tell you to stop your infusion if you have a mechanical problem (such as a blockage in the tubing, needle, or catheter); if you have to stop an infusion, call your health care provider immediately so your therapy can continue.

Side Effects

Dolasetron may cause side effects. Tell your health care provider if any of these symptoms are severe or do not go away:
- headache
- diarrhea
- constipation
- dizziness
- drowsiness
- fever
- chills
- difficulty urinating

If you experience any of the following symptoms, call your health care provider immediately:
- chest pain
- irregular heartbeat
- fainting
- difficulty breathing
- rash

If you experience a serious side effect, you or your doctor may send a report to the Food and Drug Administration's (FDA) MedWatch Adverse Event Reporting program online [at http://www.fda.gov/MedWatch/index.html] or by phone [1-800-332-1088].

Storage Conditions

- Your health care provider will probably give you a 1- to 2-day supply of dolasetron at a time. Depending on the number of days supplied, you will be told to store it at room temperature or in the refrigerator.
- If you store your dolasetron in the refrigerator, take your next dose from the refrigerator 1 hour before using it; place it in a clean, dry area to allow it to warm to room temperature.

Store your medication only as directed. Make sure you understand what you need to store your medication properly. Keep your supplies in a clean, dry place when you are not using them, and keep all medications and supplies out of reach of children. Your health care provider will tell you how to throw away used needles, syringes, tubing, and containers to avoid accidental injury.

Overdose

In case of overdose, call your local poison control center at 1-800-222-1222. If the victim has collapsed or is not breathing, call local emergency services at 911.

Signs of Infection

If you are receiving dolasetron in your vein or under your skin, you need to know the symptoms of a catheter-related infection (an infection where the needle enters your vein or skin). If you experience any of these effects near your intravenous catheter, tell your health care provider as soon as possible:
- tenderness
- warmth
- irritation
- drainage
- redness
- swelling
- pain

Dosage Facts
For Informational Purposes

Caution: Do not change your dose, how often you take your medication, or the length of time you are to take it without first talking to your healthcare provider.

The following dosage information was written using medical language for doctors and other healthcare professionals and is provided here for you to check your dosage. The dosage of this drug may differ for different patients. Therefore, always follow your doctor's instructions or the directions on the label. Contact your healthcare provider or pharmacist if you have any questions about the specific dosage of your medication after reviewing this information.

General Dosage Information

Available as dolasetron mesylate; dosage expressed in terms of the salt.

Pediatric Patients

Cancer Chemotherapy-induced Nausea and Vomiting
Prevention

IV:
- Children 2–16 years of age: 1.8 mg/kg (maximum 100 mg) as a single dose approximately 30 minutes before administration of chemotherapy.

Postoperative Nausea and Vomiting
Prevention

IV:
- Children 2–16 years of age: 0.35 mg/kg (maximum 12.5 mg) as a single dose approximately 15 minutes before cessation of anesthesia.

Treatment

IV:

- Children 2–16 years of age: 0.35 mg/kg (maximum 12.5 mg) as a single dose as soon as nausea or vomiting develops.

Adult Patients

Cancer Chemotherapy-induced Nausea and Vomiting
Prevention

IV:

- 1.8 mg/kg as a single dose (given by IV infusion) approximately 30 minutes before administration of chemotherapy. Alternatively, a single 100-mg dose administered over 30 seconds.

Postoperative Nausea and Vomiting
Prevention

IV:

- 12.5 mg as a single dose administered approximately 15 minutes before cessation of anesthesia. Higher dosages not associated with improved efficacy.

Treatment

IV:

- 12.5 mg as a single dose administered as soon as nausea and/or vomiting develops. Higher dosages not associated with improved efficacy.

Prescribing Limits

Pediatric Patients

Cancer Chemotherapy-induced Nausea and Vomiting
Prevention

IV:

- Children 2–16 years of age: 1.8 mg/kg (100 mg maximum) as a single dose.

Postoperative Nausea and Vomiting
Prevention

IV:

- Children 2–16 years of age: 0.35 mg/kg (12.5 mg maximum) as single dose.

Treatment

IV:

- Children 2–16 years of age: 0.35 mg/kg (12.5 mg maximum) as a single dose.

Adult Patients

Cancer Chemotherapy-induced Nausea and Vomiting
Prevention

IV:

- 1.8 mg/kg or 100 mg as a single dose.

Postoperative Nausea and Vomiting
Prevention

IV:

- 12.5 mg as a single dose.

Treatment

IV:

- 12.5 mg as a single dose.

Special Populations

Hepatic Impairment

- No dosage adjustments required.

Renal Impairment

- No dosage adjustments required.

Donepezil

(doe nep′ e zil)

Brand Name: Aricept®, Aricept® ODT

Why is this medicine prescribed?

Donepezil is used to treat dementia (a brain disorder that affects the ability to remember, think clearly, communicate, and perform daily activities and may cause changes in mood and personality) associated with Alzheimer's disease (AD; a brain disease that slowly destroys the memory and the ability to think, learn, communicate and handle daily activities). Donepezil is in a class of medications called cholinesterase inhibitors. It improves mental function (such as memory, attention, social interaction, reasoning and language abilities, and ability to perform activities of daily living) by increasing the amount of a certain naturally occurring substance in the brain. Donepezil may improve the ability to think and remember or slow the loss of these abilities in people who have AD. However, donepezil will not cure AD or prevent the loss of mental abilities at some time in the future.

How should this medicine be used?

Donepezil comes as a tablet and an orally disintegrating tablet (tablet that dissolves quickly in the mouth) to take by mouth. It is usually taken once a day, in the evening at bedtime, with or without food. Take donepezil at around the same time every day. Follow the directions on your prescription label carefully, and ask your doctor or pharmacist to explain any part you do not understand. It may take awhile before you experience the full benefits of donepezil. Take donepezil exactly as directed. Do not take more or less of it or take it more often than prescribed by your doctor.

Donepezil helps control the symptoms of Alzheimer's disease but does not cure it. Continue to take donepezil even if you feel well. Do not stop taking donepezil without talking to your doctor.

Your doctor may start you on a low dose of donepezil and increase your dose after 4-6 weeks.

To take the orally disintegrating tablet, place the tablet on your tongue. The tablet will quickly dissolve and can be followed with a drink of water.

Are there other uses for this medicine?

This medication may be prescribed for other uses; ask your doctor or pharmacist for more information.

What special precautions should I follow?

Before taking donepezil,

- tell your doctor and pharmacist if you are allergic to donepezil or any other medications.
- tell your doctor and pharmacist what prescription and nonprescription medications, vitamins, nutritional supplements, and herbal products you are taking or plan to take. Be sure to mention any of the following: antihistamines; aspirin and other nonsteroidal anti-inflammatory medications (NSAIDs) such as ibuprofen (Advil, Motrin) and naproxen (Aleve, Naprosyn); bethanechol (Duvoid, Urabeth, Urecholine); carbamazepine (Tegretol); dexamethasone (Decadron, Dexone); ipratropium (Atrovent); ketoconazole (Nizoral); medications for glaucoma, irritable bowel disease, motion sickness, myasthenia gravis, Parkinson's disease, ulcers, or urinary problems; phenobarbital (Luminal, Solfoton); phenytoin (Dilantin); quinidine (Quinidex); and rifampin (Rifadin, Rimactane). Your doctor may need to change the doses of your medications or monitor you carefully for side effects.
- tell your doctor if you have or have ever had gastrointestinal (GI) bleeding; an ulcer, asthma, or obstructive pulmonary disease (chronic bronchitis or emphysema), or heart disease.
- tell your doctor if you are pregnant, plan to become pregnant, or are breast-feeding. If you become pregnant while taking donepezil, call your doctor.
- if you are having surgery, including dental surgery, tell the doctor or dentist that you are taking donepezil.

What special dietary instructions should I follow?

Unless your doctor tells you otherwise, continue your normal diet.

What should I do if I forget to take a dose?

If you forget to take a dose of donepezil, skip the missed dose and continue with your regular dosing schedule. Do not take a double dose to make up for a missed one. If you do not take donepezil, for 1 week or longer, you should call your doctor before starting to take this medication again.

What side effects can this medicine cause?

Donepezil may cause side effects. Tell your doctor if any of these symptoms are severe or do not go away:

- nausea
- vomiting
- diarrhea
- loss of appetite
- weight loss
- frequent urination
- muscle cramps
- joint pain, swelling, or stiffness
- pain

- excessive tiredness
- drowsiness
- headache
- dizziness
- nervousness
- depression
- confusion
- changes in behavior
- abnormal dreams
- difficulty falling asleep or staying asleep
- discoloration or bruising of the skin
- red, scaling, itchy skin

Some side effects can be serious. If you experience any of these symptoms, call your doctor immediately:

- fainting
- slow heartbeat
- chest pain
- black or tarry stools
- red blood in stools
- bloody vomit
- vomiting material that looks like coffee grounds
- inability to control urination
- difficulty urinating or pain when urinating
- lower back pain
- fever
- seizures

Donepezil may cause other side effects. Call your doctor if you have any unusual problems while taking this medication.

What storage conditions are needed for this medicine?

Keep this medication in the container it came in, tightly closed, and out of reach of children. Store it at room temperature and away from excess heat and moisture (not in the bathroom). Throw away any medication that is outdated or no longer needed. Talk to your pharmacist about the proper disposal of your medication.

What should I do in case of overdose?

In case of overdose, call your local poison control center at 1-800-222-1222. If the victim has collapsed or is not breathing, call local emergency services at 911.

Symptoms of overdose may include:

- nausea
- vomiting
- drooling
- sweating
- slow heartbeat
- difficulty breathing
- muscle weakness
- fainting
- seizures

What other information should I know?

Keep all appointments with your doctor.

Do not let anyone else take your medication. Ask your

pharmacist any questions you have about refilling your prescription.

Dosage Facts
For Informational Purposes

Caution: Do not change your dose, how often you take your medication, or the length of time you are to take it without first talking to your healthcare provider.

The following dosage information was written using medical language for doctors and other healthcare professionals and is provided here for you to check your dosage. The dosage of this drug may differ for different patients. Therefore, always follow your doctor's instructions or the directions on the label. Contact your healthcare provider or pharmacist if you have any questions about the specific dosage of your medication after reviewing this information.

General Dosage Information

Available as donepezil hydrochloride; dosage expressed in terms of the salt.

Adult Patients

Alzheimer's Disease

ORAL:
- Initially, 5 mg daily.
- Some data suggest the possibility of additional benefit with higher (10 mg daily) dosage in some patients; however, additional benefit with the 10-mg dosage has not been demonstrated in controlled clinical studies. Adverse cholinergic effects are more likely with the 10-mg dosage.
- Daily administration of 10 mg should not be considered until patient has received 5 mg daily for 4–6 weeks, since occurrence of adverse effects may be influenced by the rate of increase in dosage.

Special Populations

Hepatic Impairment
- No specific recommendation for dosage adjustment.

Dornase Alfa

(door′ nace)

Brand Name: Pulmozyme®

Why is this medicine prescribed?

Dornase alfa is used to reduce the number of lung infections and to improve lung function in patients with cystic fibrosis. It breaks down the thick secretions in the airways, allowing air to flow better and preventing bacteria from building up.

This medication is sometimes prescribed for other uses; ask your doctor or pharmacist for more information.

How should this medicine be used?

Dornase alfa comes as a solution to inhale by mouth. It usually is taken one or two times a day. Follow the directions on your prescription label carefully, and ask your doctor or pharmacist to explain any part you do not understand. Use dornase alfa exactly as directed. Do not use more or less of it or use it more often than prescribed by your doctor.

Dornase alfa is used to treat cystic fibrosis but does not cure it. Continue to use dornase alfa even if you feel well. Do not stop using dornase alfa without talking to your doctor.

Before you use dornase alfa the first time, read the written instructions that come with it. Ask your doctor, pharmacist, or respiratory therapist to demonstrate the proper technique. Practice using the nebulizer while in his or her presence. Only use a nebulizer that is recommended by your doctor.

What special precautions should I follow?

Before using dornase alfa,

- tell your doctor and pharmacist if you are allergic to dornase alfa or any other drugs.
- tell your doctor and pharmacist what prescription and nonprescription medications you are taking, including vitamins.
- tell your doctor if you are pregnant, plan to become pregnant, or are breast-feeding. If you become pregnant while using dornase alfa, call your doctor.

What should I do if I forget to take a dose?

Use the missed dose as soon as you remember it. However, if it is almost time for the next dose, skip the missed dose and continue your regular dosing schedule. Do not use a double dose to make up for a missed one.

What side effects can this medicine cause?

Dornase alfa may cause side effects. Tell your doctor if any of these symptoms are severe or do not go away.

- voice changes
- sore throat
- hoarseness
- eye irritation
- rash

If you experience either of the following symptoms, call your doctor immediately.

- increased difficulty breathing
- chest pain

If you experience a serious side effect, you or your doctor may send a report to the Food and Drug Administration's (FDA) MedWatch Adverse Event Reporting program online [at http://www.fda.gov/MedWatch/index.html] or by phone [1-800-332-1088].

What storage conditions are needed for this medicine?

Keep this medicine in the container it came in, tightly closed, and out of reach of children. Store it in the refrigerator and protect it from sunlight. Do not expose the drug to room temperature for more than 24 hours. Any ampule that has been open for more than 24 hours should be discarded. Discard ampules if the solution is cloudy or discolored. Talk to your pharmacist about the proper disposal of medicine that is outdated or no longer needed.

What other information should I know?

Keep all appointments with your doctor and the laboratory. Your doctor may order certain lab tests to check your response to dornase alfa.

Do not dilute or mix dornase alfa with other drugs in the nebulizer.

Inhalation devices require regular cleaning. Follow the manufacturer's written instructions for the care of the nebulizer.

Do not let anyone else use your medication. Ask your pharmacist any questions you have about refilling your prescription.

Dosage Facts
For Informational Purposes

Caution: Do not change your dose, how often you take your medication, or the length of time you are to take it without first talking to your healthcare provider.

The following dosage information was written using medical language for doctors and other healthcare professionals and is provided here for you to check your dosage. The dosage of this drug may differ for different patients. Therefore, always follow your doctor's instructions or the directions on the label. Contact your healthcare provider or pharmacist if you have any questions about the specific dosage of your medication after reviewing this information.

General Dosage Information

Each single-use ampul delivers 2.5 mg (2.5 mL of undiluted solution) to the nebulizer cup.

Pediatric Patients

Cystic Fibrosis

ORAL INHALATION:
- Children ≥5 years of age: 2.5 mg once daily. Some patients (e.g., those with FVC >85%) may benefit from 2.5 mg twice daily.

Adult Patients

Cystic Fibrosis

ORAL INHALATION:
- 2.5 mg once daily. Some patients (e.g., ≥21 years of age, those with FVC >85%) may benefit from 2.5 mg twice daily.

Prescribing Limits
Pediatric Patients

Cystic Fibrosis

ORAL INHALATION:
- In clinical studies, dosages >2.5 mg twice daily did not provide additional improvement in pulmonary function (e.g., FEV_1).
- Safety and efficacy of daily administration for >12 months of continuous therapy not established.

Adult Patients

Cystic Fibrosis

ORAL INHALATION:
- In clinical studies, dosages >2.5 mg twice daily did not provide additional improvement in pulmonary function (e.g., FEV_1).
- Safety and efficacy of daily administration for >12 months of continuous therapy not established.

Special Populations

No special population dosage recommendations at this time.

Dorzolamide and Timolol Ophthalmic

(dor zole' a mide) (tye' moe lole)

Brand Name: Cosopt®, Ocumeter® Plus

Why is this medicine prescribed?

The combination of dorzolamide and timolol is used to treat eye conditions, including glaucoma and ocular hypertension, in which increased pressure can lead to a gradual loss of vision. Dorzolamide and timolol is used for patients whose eye condition has not responded to another medication. Dorzolamide is in a class of medications called topical carbonic anhydrase inhibitors. Timolol is in a class of medications called topical beta blockers. Dorzolamide and timolol lowers pressure in the eye by decreasing the production of natural fluids in the eye.

How should this medicine be used?

The combination of dorzolamide and timolol comes as an eyedrop to apply to the eye. It is usually applied to the affected eye(s) twice a day. To help you remember to use dorzolamide and timolol, use it around the same time every day. Follow the directions on your prescription label carefully, and ask your doctor or pharmacist to explain any part you do not understand. Use dorzolamide and timolol exactly as directed. Do not use more or less of it or use it more often than prescribed by your doctor.

Dorzolamide and timolol controls glaucoma and ocular

hypertension but does not cure them. Continue to use dorzolamide and timolol even if you feel well. Do not stop using dorzolamide and timolol without talking to your doctor.

To apply the eyedrops, follow these steps:

1. Wash your hands thoroughly with soap and water.
2. Use a mirror or have someone else put the drops in your eye.
3. Before using the eyedrops bottle for the first time, make sure the safety strip on the front of the bottle is unbroken.
4. Tear off the safety strip to break the seal.
5. To open the bottle, unscrew the cap by turning as indicated by the arrows.
6. Avoid touching the dropper against your eye or anything else.
7. Lie down or tilt your head back.
8. Holding the bottle between your thumb and index finger, place the dropper as near as possible to your eyelid without touching it.
9. Brace the remaining fingers of that hand against your cheek or nose.
10. With the index finger of your other hand, pull the lower lid of the eye down to form a pocket.
11. Press lightly with the thumb or index finger over the Finger Push Area until a single drop is dispensed into the pocket made by the lower lid and the eye. Placing the drops on the surface of the eyeball can cause stinging.
12. Close your eye and press lightly against the lower lid with your finger for 2-3 minutes to keep the medication in the eye. Do not blink.
13. Replace and tighten the cap right away. Do not wipe or rinse it off.
14. Wipe off any excess liquid from your cheek with a clean tissue. Wash your hands again.

Are there other uses for this medicine?

This medication may be prescribed for other uses; ask your doctor or pharmacist for more information.

What special precautions should I follow?

Before using dorzolamide and timolol,

- tell your doctor and pharmacist if you are allergic to dorzolamide (Trusopt), timolol (Timoptic), sulfa drugs, or any other medications.
- tell your doctor and pharmacist what prescription and nonprescription medications, vitamins, nutritional supplements, and herbal products you are taking. Be sure to mention any of the following: beta blockers such as atenolol (Tenormin), labetalol (Normodyne), metoprolol (Lopressor, Toprol XL), nadolol (Corgard), and propranolol (Inderal); calcium channel blockers such as amlodipine (Norvasc), diltiazem (Cardizem, Dilacor, Tiazac, others), felodipine (Plendil), isradipine (DynaCirc), nicardipine (Cardene), nifedipine (Adalat, Procardia), nimodipine (Nimotop), nisoldipine (Sular),

and verapamil (Calan, Isoptin, Verelan); carbonic anhydrase inhibitors such as acetazolamide (Diamox), dichlorphenamide (Danaride), and methazolamide (GlaucTabs, Neptazane); clonidine (Catapres, Catapres-TTS); digoxin (Lanoxin); diuretics ('water pills'); quinidine (Quinidex); reserpine (Serpalan, Serpasil, Serpatabs); and salicylate pain relievers such as aspirin, choline magnesium trisalicylate, choline salicylate (Arthropan), diflunisal (Dolobid), magnesium salicylate (Doan's, others), and salsalate (Argesic, Disalcid, Salgesic). Your doctor may need to change the doses of your medications or monitor you carefully for side effects.

- if you are using another topical eye medication, apply it at least 10 minutes before or after dorzolamide and timolol.
- tell your doctor if you have or have ever had asthma, lung disease (including chronic bronchitis and emphysema), heart disease, diabetes, an overactive thyroid gland (hyperthyroidism), severe allergic reactions, myasthenia gravis, and kidney or liver disease.
- tell your doctor if you are pregnant, plan to become pregnant, or are breast-feeding. If you become pregnant while using dorzolamide and timolol, call your doctor.
- if you are having surgery, including dental surgery, tell the doctor or dentist that you are using dorzolamide and timolol.
- you should know that dorzolamide and timolol solution contains benzalkonium chloride, which can be absorbed by soft contact lenses. If you wear contact lenses, remove them before applying dorzolamide and timolol and put them back in 15 minutes later.
- if you have an eye injury, infection, or surgery while using dorzolamide and timolol, ask your doctor if you should continue using the same eyedrops container.
- you should know that if you have allergic reactions to different substances, your reactions may be worse while you are using dorzolamide and timolol, and your allergic reactions may not respond to the usual doses of injectable epinephrine.

What special dietary instructions should I follow?

Unless your doctor tells you otherwise, continue your normal diet.

What should I do if I forget to take a dose?

Take the missed dose as soon as you remember it. However, if it is almost time for the next dose, skip the missed dose and continue your regular dosing schedule. Do not take a double dose to make up for a missed one.

What side effects can this medicine cause?

Dorzolamide and timolol may cause side effects. Tell your doctor if any of these symptoms are severe or do not go away:

- taste changes (bitter, sour, or unusual taste)
- eye burning or stinging
- itchy eyes
- dry eyes
- eye tearing
- dizziness

Some side effects can be serious. The following symptoms are uncommon, but if you experience any of them, call your doctor immediately:

- blurred vision
- skin rash
- swelling of the hands, feet, ankles, or lower legs
- shortness of breath
- pink eye
- redness or swelling of the eyelid
- muscle weakness

Dorzolamide and timolol may cause other side effects. Call your doctor if you have any unusual problems while using this medication.

If you experience a serious side effect, you or your doctor may send a report to the Food and Drug Administration's (FDA) MedWatch Adverse Event Reporting program online [at http://www.fda.gov/MedWatch/index.html] or by phone [1-800-332-1088].

What storage conditions are needed for this medicine?

Keep this medication in the container it came in, tightly closed, and out of reach of children. Store it at room temperature and away from excess heat and moisture (not in the bathroom). Throw away any medication that is outdated or no longer needed. Talk to your pharmacist about the proper disposal of your medication.

What should I do in case of overdose?

In case of overdose, call your local poison control center at 1-800-222-1222. If the victim has collapsed or is not breathing, call local emergency services at 911.

Symptoms of overdose may include:

- dizziness
- headache
- shortness of breath
- difficulty breathing or swallowing
- chest pain
- confusion

What other information should I know?

Keep all appointments with your doctor.

Do not let anyone else use your medication. Ask your pharmacist any questions you have about refilling your prescription.

Dosage Facts
For Informational Purposes

Caution: Do not change your dose, how often you take your medication, or the length of time you

are to take it without first talking to your health-care provider.

The following dosage information was written using medical language for doctors and other healthcare professionals and is provided here for you to check your dosage. The dosage of this drug may differ for different patients. Therefore, always follow your doctor's instructions or the directions on the label. Contact your healthcare provider or pharmacist if you have any questions about the specific dosage of your medication after reviewing this information.

General Dosage Information

Available as dorzolamide hydrochloride; dosage expressed in terms of dorzolamide.

Adult Patients

Ocular Hypertension and Glaucoma
OPHTHALMIC:
- Dorzolamide in fixed-combination with timolol: 1 drop in the affected eye(s) twice daily.

Dorzolamide Ophthalmic
(dor zole′ a mide)

Brand Name: Trusopt® Ocumeter® Plus

Why is this medicine prescribed?

Dorzolamide is used to treat glaucoma, a condition in which increased pressure in the eye can lead to gradual loss of vision. Dorzolamide decreases the pressure in the eye.

This medication is sometimes prescribed for other uses; ask your doctor or pharmacist for more information.

How should this medicine be used?

Dorzolamide comes as eyedrops. Dorzolamide eyedrops usually are applied three times a day. Follow the directions on your prescription label carefully, and ask your doctor or pharmacist to explain any part you do not understand. Use dorzolamide exactly as directed. Do not use more or less of it or use it more often than prescribed by your doctor.

Dorzolamide controls glaucoma but does not cure it. Continue to use dorzolamide even if you feel well. Do not stop using dorzolamide without talking to your doctor.

To use the eyedrops, follow these instructions:
1. Wash your hands thoroughly with soap and water.

2. Use a mirror or have someone else put the drops in your eye.

3. Remove the protective cap. Make sure that the end of the dropper is not chipped or cracked.

4. Avoid touching the dropper tip against your eye or anything else.

5. Hold the dropper tip down at all times to prevent drops from flowing back into the bottle and contaminating the remaining contents.

6. Lie down or tilt your head back.

7. Holding the bottle between your thumb and index finger, place the dropper tip as near as possible to your eyelid without touching it.

8. Brace the remaining fingers of that hand against your cheek or nose.

9. With the index finger of your other hand, pull the lower lid of the eye down to form a pocket.

10. Drop the prescribed number of drops into the pocket made by the lower lid and the eye. Placing drops on the surface of the eyeball can cause stinging.

11. Close your eye and press lightly against the lower lid with your finger for 2-3 minutes to keep the medication in the eye. Do not blink.

12. Replace and tighten the cap right away. Do not wipe or rinse it off.

13. Wipe off any excess liquid from your cheek with a clean tissue. Wash your hands again.

What special precautions should I follow?

Before using dorzolamide eyedrops,

- tell your doctor and pharmacist if you are allergic to dorzolamide, other antibiotics, sulfa drugs, or any other drugs.
- tell your doctor and pharmacist what prescription and nonprescription medications you are taking, especially eye medications, products that contain aspirin, and vitamins.
- tell your doctor if you have or have ever had kidney disease.
- tell your doctor if you are pregnant, plan to become pregnant, or are breast-feeding. If you become pregnant while using dorzolamide, call your doctor immediately.
- if you are having surgery, including dental surgery, tell the doctor or dentist that you are using dorzolamide.
- if you are using another eyedrop medication, use the eye medications at least 10 minutes apart.
- tell your doctor if you wear soft contact lenses. Wait at least 15 minutes after using the medicine to put in soft contact lenses.

What should I do if I forget to take a dose?

Apply the missed dose as soon as you remember it. However, if it is almost time for the next dose, skip the missed dose and continue your regular dosing schedule. Do not apply a double dose to make up for a missed one.

What side effects can this medicine cause?

Dorzolamide may cause side effects. Tell your doctor if any of these symptoms are severe or do not go away:

- stinging, burning, or discomfort in the eye after inserting the drops
- bitter taste after inserting the drops
- sensitivity to light
- upset stomach
- vomiting

If you experience any of the following symptoms, stop using dorzolamide and call your doctor immediately:

- itching eyes
- redness or swelling eyes
- watery eyes
- dryness
- skin rash

If you experience a serious side effect, you or your doctor may send a report to the Food and Drug Administration's (FDA) MedWatch Adverse Event Reporting program online [at http://www.fda.gov/MedWatch/index.html] or by phone [1-800-332-1088].

What storage conditions are needed for this medicine?

Keep this medication in the container it came in, tightly closed, and out of reach of children. Store it at room temperature and away from excess heat and moisture (not in the bathroom). Throw away any medication that is outdated or no longer needed. Talk to your pharmacist about the proper disposal of your medication.

What other information should I know?

Keep all appointments with your doctor. Your doctor will order certain eye tests to check your response to dorzolamide.

Do not let anyone else use your medication. Ask your pharmacist any questions you have about refilling your prescription.

Dosage Facts
For Informational Purposes

Caution: Do not change your dose, how often you take your medication, or the length of time you are to take it without first talking to your health-care provider.

The following dosage information was written using medical language for doctors and other healthcare professionals and is provided here for you to check your dosage. The dosage of this drug may differ for different patients. Therefore, always follow your doctor's instructions or the directions on the label. Contact your health-care provider or pharmacist if you have any questions about the specific dosage of your medication after reviewing this information.

General Dosage Information

Available as dorzolamide hydrochloride; dosage expressed in terms of dorzolamide.

Adult Patients

Ocular Hypertension and Glaucoma

OPHTHALMIC:
- Dorzolamide 2% solution: 1 drop in the affected eye(s) 3 times daily.
- Fixed-combination with timolol: 1 drop in the affected eye(s) twice daily.

Doxazosin

(dox ay′ zoe sin)

Brand Name: Cardura®, Cardura ® XL
Also available generically.

Why is this medicine prescribed?

Doxazosin (Cardura, Cardura XL) is used in men to treat the symptoms of an enlarged prostate (benign prostatic hyperplasia or BPH), which include difficulty urinating (hesitation, dribbling, weak stream, and incomplete bladder emptying), painful urination, and urinary frequency and urgency. Doxazosin (Cardura) is also used alone or in combination with other medications to treat high blood pressure. Doxazosin is in a class of medications called alpha-blockers. It relieves the symptoms of BPH by relaxing the muscles of the bladder and prostate. It lowers blood pressure by relaxing the blood vessels so that blood can flow more easily through the body.

How should this medicine be used?

Doxazosin comes as a tablet and an extended-release tablet to take by mouth. The doxazosin tablet is usually taken with or without food once a day in the morning or in the evening. The doxazosin extended-release tablet is usually taken once a day with breakfast. To help you remember to take doxazosin, take it around the same time every day. Follow the directions on your prescription label carefully, and ask your doctor or pharmacist to explain any part you do not understand. Take doxazosin exactly as directed. Do not take more or less of it or take it more often than prescribed by your doctor.

Swallow the extended-release tablets whole; do not split, chew, or crush them.

Your doctor will start you on a low dose of doxazosin and gradually increase your dose, not more than once every 1 to 2 weeks. If you stop taking doxazosin for a few days or longer, call your doctor. Your doctor will have to start you again on the lowest dose of doxazosin and gradually increase your dose.

Doxazosin controls high blood pressure and the symptoms of BPH but does not cure them. It may take a few weeks before you feel the full benefit of doxazosin. Continue to take doxazosin even if you feel well. Do not stop taking doxazosin without talking to your doctor.

Are there other uses for this medicine?

This medication may be prescribed for other uses; ask your doctor or pharmacist for more information.

What special precautions should I follow?

Before taking doxazosin,
- tell your doctor and pharmacist if you are allergic to doxazosin, prazosin (Minipress), terazosin (Hytrin), or any other medications.
- tell your doctor and pharmacist what prescription and nonprescription medications, vitamins, nutritional supplements, and herbal products you are taking or plan to take. Be sure to mention any of the following: antihistamines; clarithromycin (Biaxin, in Prevpac); ipratropium (Atrovent); itraconazole (Sporanox); ketoconazole (Nizoral); medications for erectile dysfunction (ED) such as sildenafil (Viagra), tadalafil (Cialis), or vardenafil (Levitra); medications for high blood pressure; medications for HIV/AIDS including atazanavir (Reyataz), indinavir (Crixivan), nelfinavir (Viracept), ritonavir (Norvir, in Kaletra), or saquinavir (Fortovase, Invirase); medications for irritable bowel disease, motion sickness, Parkinson's disease, ulcers, or urinary problems; nefazodone; telithromycin (Ketek); and voriconazole (Vfend). Your doctor may need to change the doses of your medications or monitor you carefully for side effects.
- tell your doctor if you have angina (chest pain); low blood pressure; or if you have or have ever had prostate cancer or liver disease. If you are taking the extended-release tablet, tell you doctor if you have constipation, short bowel syndrome (a condition where more than half of the small intestine has been removed by surgery or damaged by disease), or narrowing or a blockage of the intestines.
- tell your doctor if you are pregnant, plan to become pregnant, or are breast-feeding. If you become pregnant while taking doxazosin, call your doctor.
- if you are having surgery, including dental surgery, tell the doctor or dentist that you are taking doxazosin. If you need to have eye surgery at any time during or after your treatment, be sure to tell your doctor that you are taking or have taken doxazosin.
- you should know that doxazosin may make you drowsy or dizzy. Do not drive a car, operate machinery, or perform dangerous tasks for 24 hours after the first time you take doxazosin or after your dose is increased.
- you should know that doxazosin may cause dizziness, lightheadedness, and fainting when you get up too quickly from a lying position. This is more common

when you first start taking doxazosin, when your dose is increased, or if your treatment has been stopped for more than a few days. To avoid this problem, get out of bed slowly, resting your feet on the floor for a few minutes before standing up. If you experience these symptoms, sit or lie down. If these symptoms do not improve, call your doctor.

What special dietary instructions should I follow?

Follow your doctor's directions for your meals, including advice for a reduced salt (sodium) diet.

What should I do if I forget to take a dose?

Take the missed dose as soon as you remember it. However, if it is almost time for the next dose, skip the missed dose and continue your regular dosing schedule. Do not take a double dose to make up for a missed one. Check with your doctor if you have missed two or more doses.

What side effects can this medicine cause?

Doxazosin may cause side effects. Tell your doctor if any of these symptoms or those listed in the SPECIAL PRECAUTIONS section are severe or do not go away:

- headache
- tiredness
- swelling of the hands, feet, ankles, or lower legs
- shortness of breath
- weight gain
- muscle or joint pain or weakness
- abnormal vision
- runny nose
- decreased sexual ability

Some side effects can be serious. If you experience any of these symptoms, call your doctor immediately:

- rapid, pounding, or irregular heartbeat
- chest pain
- shortness of breath
- hives
- painful erection of the penis that lasts for hours

Doxazosin may cause other side effects. Call your doctor if you have any unusual problems while taking this medication.

What storage conditions are needed for this medicine?

Keep this medication in the container it came in, tightly closed, and out of reach of children. Store it at room temperature and away from excess heat and moisture (not in the bathroom). Throw away any medication that is outdated or no longer needed. Talk to your pharmacist about the proper disposal of your medication.

What should I do in case of overdose?

In case of overdose, call your local poison control center at 1-800-222-1222. If the victim has collapsed or is not breathing, call local emergency services at 911.

Symptoms of overdose may include:

- drowsiness
- dizziness
- lightheadedness
- fainting
- seizure

What other information should I know?

If you are taking doxazosin extended-release tablets, you may notice something that looks like a tablet in your stool. This is just the empty tablet shell, and this does not mean that you did not get your complete dose of medication.

Keep all appointments with your doctor. If you are taking doxazosin to control high blood pressure, your blood pressure should be checked regularly to determine your response to doxazosin.

Do not let anyone else take your medication. Ask your pharmacist any questions you have about refilling your prescription.

Dosage Facts
For Informational Purposes

Caution: Do not change your dose, how often you take your medication, or the length of time you are to take it without first talking to your healthcare provider.

The following dosage information was written using medical language for doctors and other healthcare professionals and is provided here for you to check your dosage. The dosage of this drug may differ for different patients. Therefore, always follow your doctor's instructions or the directions on the label. Contact your healthcare provider or pharmacist if you have any questions about the specific dosage of your medication after reviewing this information.

General Dosage Information

Available as doxazosin mesylate; dosage expressed in terms of doxazosin.

Individualize dosage according to patient response and tolerance. Initiate at low dosage to minimize frequency of postural hypotension and syncope.

Postural effects are most likely to occur 2–6 hours after a dose; monitor BP during this period after first dose and with any dosage increases.

If therapy is interrupted for several days, restart using initial dosage regimen.

Pediatric Patients

Hypertension†

ORAL:
- Initially, 1 mg once daily. Increase dosage as necessary up to a maximum of 4 mg once daily.

Adult Patients

Hypertension

ORAL:

- Initially, 1 mg once daily. Do *not* initiate with higher dosages.
- Depending on patient response (standing BP 2–6 and 24 hours after initial dose), may increase dosage to 2 mg once daily; make subsequent dosage adjustments by doubling dose at intervals of 2 weeks–1 month until desired BP control is achieved, drug is not tolerated, or maximum daily dosage of 16 mg is reached.
- Increased likelihood of excessive postural effects (e.g., syncope, postural dizziness/vertigo, postural hypotension) with dosages >4 mg daily; substantial risk of postural effects with dosages >16 mg daily.
- Careful monitoring of BP is recommended during initial titration or subsequent upward dosage adjustment; avoid large or abrupt reductions in BP.

BPH

ORAL:

- Initially, 1 mg once daily in the morning or evening; some clinicians recommend administration at bedtime to minimize postural effects. Do *not* initiate with higher dosages.
- To achieve desired improvement in symptoms and urodynamics, may increase dosage in a stepwise manner to 2, 4, and 8 mg daily as necessary, at intervals ≥1–2 weeks. Do not exceed 8 mg daily.
- Evaluate BP routinely, particularly with initiation of therapy and subsequent dosage adjustment.

Prescribing Limits

Pediatric Patients

Hypertension†

ORAL:

- Maximum 4 mg daily.

Adult Patients

Hypertension

ORAL:

- Maximum 16 mg daily.

BPH

ORAL:

- Maximum 8 mg daily.

Special Populations

Geriatric Patients

Hypertension

- Select dosage carefully, usually initiating therapy at the low end of the dosage range, because of possible age-related decreases in hepatic, renal, and/or cardiac function and concomitant disease and drug therapy; generally, increase dosage more slowly in geriatric patients than in younger adults.

† Use is not currently included in the labeling approved by the US Food and Drug Administration.

Doxepin

(dox′ e pin)

Important Warning

A small number of children, teenagers, and young adults (up to 24 years of age) who took antidepressants ('mood elevators') such as doxepin during clinical studies became suicidal (thinking about harming or killing oneself or planning or trying to do so). Children, teenagers, and young adults who take antidepressants to treat depression or other mental illnesses may be more likely to become suicidal than children, teenagers, and young adults who do not take antidepressants to treat these conditions. However, experts are not sure about how great this risk is and how much it should be considered in deciding whether a child or teenager should take an antidepressant. Children younger than 18 years of age should not normally take doxepin, but in some cases, a doctor may decide that doxepin is the best medication to treat a child's condition.

You should know that your mental health may change in unexpected ways when you take doxepin or other antidepressants even if you are an adult over age 24. You may become suicidal, especially at the beginning of your treatment and any time that your dose is increased or decreased. You, your family, or your caregiver should call your doctor right away if you experience any of the following symptoms: new or worsening depression; thinking about harming or killing yourself, or planning or trying to do so; extreme worry; agitation; panic attacks; difficulty falling asleep or staying asleep; aggressive behavior; irritability; acting without thinking; severe restlessness; and frenzied abnormal excitement. Be sure that your family or caregiver knows which symptoms may be serious so they can call the doctor when you are unable to seek treatment on your own.

Your healthcare provider will want to see you often while you are taking doxepin, especially at the beginning of your treatment. Be sure to keep all appointments for office visits with your doctor.

The doctor or pharmacist will give you the manufacturer's patient information sheet (Medication Guide) when you begin treatment with doxepin. Read the information carefully and ask your doctor or pharmacist if you have any questions. You also can obtain the Medication Guide from the FDA website: http://www.fda.gov/cder/drug/antidepressants/antidepressants_MG_2007.pdf.

No matter your age, before you take an antidepressant, you, your parent, or your caregiver should talk to your doctor about the risks and benefits of

continued on next page

Important Warning (cont'd)

treating your condition with an antidepressant or with other treatments. You should also talk about the risks and benefits of not treating your condition. You should know that having depression or another mental illness greatly increases the risk that you will become suicidal. This risk is higher if you or anyone in your family has or has ever had bipolar disorder (mood that changes from depressed to abnormally excited) or mania (frenzied, abnormally excited mood) or has thought about or attempted suicide. Talk to your doctor about your condition, symptoms, and personal and family medical history. You and your doctor will decide what type of treatment is right for you.

Why is this medicine prescribed?

Doxepin is used to treat depression and anxiety. Doxepin is in a class of medications called tricyclic antidepressants. It works by increasing the amounts of certain natural substances in the brain that are needed for mental balance.

How should this medicine be used?

Doxepin comes as a capsule or concentrate (liquid) to take by mouth. It is usually taken one to three times a day and may be taken with or without food. Try to take doxepin at around the same time(s) every day. Follow the directions on your prescription label carefully, and ask your doctor or pharmacist to explain any part you do not understand. Take doxepin exactly as directed. Do not take more or less of it or take it more often than prescribed by your doctor.

Doxepin concentrate (oral liquid) comes with a specially marked dropper for measuring the dose. Ask your pharmacist to show you how to use the dropper. Dilute the concentrate in 4 ounces (120 mL) of water, whole or skim milk, or orange, grapefruit, tomato, prune, or pineapple juice just before taking it. Do not mix it with carbonated beverages (soft drinks).

It may take several weeks or longer for you to feel the full effect of doxepin. Continue to take doxepin even if you feel well. Do not stop taking doxepin without talking to your doctor. Your doctor will probably want to decrease your dose gradually.

Are there other uses for this medicine?

This medication may be prescribed for other uses. Ask your doctor or pharmacist for more information.

What special precautions should I follow?

Before taking doxepin,

- tell your doctor and pharmacist if you are allergic to doxepin, amoxapine, or any other medications.
- tell your doctor if you are taking a monoamine oxidase (MAO) inhibitor such as isocarboxazid (Marplan), phenelzine (Nardil), selegiline (Eldepryl, Emsam, Zelapar),

and tranylcypromine (Parnate), or if you have stopped taking an MAO inhibitor within the past 14 days. Your doctor will probably tell you not to take doxepin. If you stop taking doxepin, you should wait at least 14 days before you start to take an MAO inhibitor.

- tell your doctor and pharmacist what prescription and nonprescription medications, vitamins, nutritional supplements, and herbal products you are taking or plan to take. Be sure to mention any of the following: antihistamines; anticoagulants (blood thinners) such as warfarin (Coumadin); cimetidine (Tagamet); flecainide (Tambocor); levodopa (Sinemet, Larodopa); lithium (Eskalith, Lithobid); medication for high blood pressure, seizures, Parkinson's disease, diabetes, asthma, colds, or allergies; methylphenidate (Ritalin); muscle relaxants; propafenone (Rhythmol); quinidine; sedatives; selective serotonin reuptake inhibitors (SSRIs) such as citalopram (Celexa), escitalopram (Lexapro), fluoxetine (Prozac, Sarafem), fluvoxamine (Luvox), paroxetine (Paxil), and sertraline (Zoloft); sleeping pills; thyroid medications; tolazamide (Tolinase); and tranquilizers. Your doctor may need to change the doses of your medications or monitor you carefully for side effects. Your doctor may tell you not to take doxepin if you have taken fluoxetine in the past 5 weeks.
- tell your doctor if you have or have ever had glaucoma (an eye condition) or difficulty urinating. Your doctor will probably tell you not to take duloxetine.
- tell your doctor if you have or have ever had an enlarged prostate (a male reproductive gland), diabetes, seizures, an overactive thyroid gland, or liver, kidney, or heart disease.
- tell your doctor if you are pregnant, plan to become pregnant, or are breast-feeding. If you become pregnant while taking this medication, call your doctor.
- if you are having surgery, including dental surgery, tell the doctor or dentist that you are taking doxepin.
- you should know that this medication may make you drowsy. Do not drive a car or operate machinery until you know how this medication affects you.
- remember that alcohol can add to the drowsiness caused by this medication.

What special dietary instructions should I follow?

Unless your doctor tells you otherwise, continue your normal diet

What should I do if I forget to take a dose?

Take the missed dose as soon as you remember it. However, if it is almost time for your next dose, skip the missed dose and continue your regular dosing schedule. Do not take a double dose to make up for a missed one.

What side effects can this medicine cause?

Doxepin may cause side effects. Call your doctor if any of these symptoms are severe or do not go away:

- nausea
- drowsiness
- weakness or tiredness
- nightmares
- dry mouth
- skin more sensitive to sunlight than usual
- changes in appetite or weight
- constipation
- difficulty urinating
- frequent urination
- blurred vision
- changes in sex drive or ability
- excessive sweating

If you experience any of the following symptoms or those listed in the IMPORTANT WARNING section, call your doctor immediately:

- jaw, neck, and back muscle spasms
- slow or difficult speech
- shuffling walk
- uncontrollable shaking of a part of the body
- fever
- difficulty breathing or swallowing
- rash
- yellowing of the skin or eyes
- irregular heartbeat

If you experience a serious side effect, you or your doctor may send a report to the Food and Drug Administration's (FDA) MedWatch Adverse Event Reporting program online [at http://www.fda.gov/MedWatch/index.html] or by phone [1-800-332-1088].

Doxepin may cause other side effects. Call your doctor if you have any unusual problems while you are taking this medication.

What storage conditions are needed for this medicine?

Keep this medication in the container it came in, tightly closed, and out of reach of children. Store it at room temperature and away from excess heat and moisture (not in the bathroom). Throw away any medication that is outdated or no longer needed. Talk to your pharmacist about the proper disposal of your medication.

What should I do in case of overdose?

In case of overdose, call your local poison control center at 1-800-222-1222. If the victim has collapsed or is not breathing, call local emergency services at 911.

What other information should I know?

Keep all appointments with your doctor.

Do not let anyone else take your medication. Ask your pharmacist any questions you have about refilling your prescription.

Dosage Facts
For Informational Purposes

Caution: Do not change your dose, how often you take your medication, or the length of time you are to take it without first talking to your healthcare provider.

The following dosage information was written using medical language for doctors and other healthcare professionals and is provided here for you to check your dosage. The dosage of this drug may differ for different patients. Therefore, always follow your doctor's instructions or the directions on the label. Contact your healthcare provider or pharmacist if you have any questions about the specific dosage of your medication after reviewing this information.

General Dosage Information

Available as doxepin hydrochloride; dosage expressed in terms of doxepin.

Adult Patients

Major Depressive Disorder

ORAL:

- Mild to moderate symptoms: Initially, 75 mg daily in divided doses or as a single dose. Gradually adjust dosage to maximum therapeutic effect with minimal toxicity. After symptoms are controlled, dosage should be gradually reduced to the lowest level that will maintain relief of symptoms. Usual dose range is 75–150 mg daily.
- Very mild symptoms or emotional symptoms accompanying organic brain syndrome: Lower than average doses recommended; 25–50 mg daily may be sufficient.
- Severe symptoms: Higher than average doses may be required, with gradual increases to 300 mg daily in divided doses if necessary.
- Hospitalized patients under close supervision generally may be given higher dosages than outpatients.

Prescribing Limits

Adult Patients

Major Depressive Disorder

ORAL:

- Maximum 150 mg administered as single daily dose.
- Maximum 300 mg daily in divided doses. Manufacturer states that dosages >300 mg daily rarely produce additional therapeutic benefits.

Special Populations

Hepatic Impairment

- No specific dosage recommendations at this time.

Renal Impairment

- No specific dosage recommendations at this time.

Geriatric Patients

- Select dosage with caution, usually initiating therapy at the low end of the dosage range, and increase cautiously because of age-related decreases in hepatic, renal, and/or cardiac function and concomitant disease and drug therapy.

Doxepin Topical

(dox' e pin)

Brand Name: Zonalon®, Prudoxin®

Why is this medicine prescribed?

Doxepin topical is used to relieve itching of the skin caused by eczema. Doxepin is in a class of medications called topical antipruritics. It may work by blocking histamine, a substance in the body that causes certain symptoms, such as itching.

How should this medicine be used?

Doxepin comes as a cream to apply to the skin. It is usually applied four times a day, at least 3 to 4 hours apart, for up to 8 days. Use doxepin at around the same times every day. Follow the directions on your prescription label carefully, and ask your doctor or pharmacist to explain any part you do not understand. Use doxepin topical exactly as directed. Do not use more or less of it or use it more often than prescribed by your doctor.

To use the cream, follow these steps:

1. Wash the affected skin with water and a mild soap or soapless cleansing lotion and pat dry with a soft towel.
2. Apply a thin layer of cream to the affected skin. Gently and thoroughly massage it into the skin. Be careful not to get the medication in your eyes or mouth. If you do get doxepin in your eyes, wash with plenty of water and call your doctor if your eyes are irritated.
3. Do not cover the affected area with any bandages, dressings, or wrappings.
4. Wash your hands with soap and water after you finish handling the medication.

Are there other uses for this medicine?

This medication may be prescribed for other uses; ask your doctor or pharmacist for more information.

What special precautions should I follow?

Before using doxepin cream,

- tell your doctor and pharmacist if you are allergic to doxepin (Adapin, Sinequan) or any other medications.
- tell your doctor and pharmacist what prescription and nonprescription medications, vitamins, nutritional supplements, and herbal products you are taking or plan to take. Be sure to mention any of the following: antidepressants (mood elevators); antihistamines; carbamazepine (Tegretol); cimetidine (Tagamet); medications for irregular heart beat, including encainide (Enkaid), flecainide (Tambocor), propafenone (Rythmol), and quinidine (Quinaglute, Quinidex); and medications for mental illness and nausea. Also tell your doctor or pharmacist if you are taking the following medications or have stopped taking them within the past 2 weeks: monoamine oxidase (MAO) inhibitors, including isocarboxazid (Marplan), phenelzine (Nardil), and tranylcypromine (Parnate). Your doctor may need to change the doses of your medications or monitor you carefully for side effects.
- tell your doctor if you have or have ever had glaucoma, benign prostatic hypertrophy (enlargement of the prostate), or urinary retention (inability to empty your bladder completely or at all).
- tell your doctor if you are pregnant, plan to become pregnant, or are breast-feeding. If you become pregnant while using doxepin, call your doctor. You should not use doxepin if you are breast-feeding.
- if you are having surgery, including dental surgery, tell the doctor or dentist that you are using doxepin.
- you should know that doxepin may make you drowsy. Do not drive a car or operate machinery until you know how this medication affects you. If you become very drowsy from doxepin, talk to your doctor.
- remember that alcohol can add to the drowsiness caused by this medication.

What special dietary instructions should I follow?

Unless your doctor tells you otherwise, continue your normal diet.

What should I do if I forget to take a dose?

Apply the missed dose as soon as you remember it. However, if it is almost time for the next dose, skip the missed dose and continue your regular dosing schedule. Do not apply extra cream to make up for a missed dose.

What side effects can this medicine cause?

Doxepin may cause side effects. Tell your doctor if any of these symptoms are severe or do not go away:

- drowsiness
- dry mouth
- dry lips
- thirst
- headache
- extreme tiredness
- dizziness
- mood changes
- taste changes
- burning or stinging at affected area
- worsened itching
- dryness and tightness of skin at affected area
- tingling of the fingers or toes
- swelling of the affected area

Doxepin may cause other side effects. Call your doctor if you have any unusual problems while taking this medication.

What storage conditions are needed for this medicine?

Keep this medication in the container it came in, tightly closed, and out of reach of children. Store it at room temperature and away from excess heat and moisture (not in the bathroom). Throw away any medication that is outdated or no longer needed. Talk to your pharmacist about the proper disposal of your medication.

What should I do in case of overdose?

In case of overdose, call your local poison control center at 1-800-222-1222. If the victim has collapsed or is not breathing, call local emergency services at 911.

Symptoms of overdose may include:

- drowsiness
- unconsciousness
- blurred vision
- very dry mouth
- difficulty breathing
- dizziness
- fainting
- seizures
- change in body temperature
- fast or irregular heart beat
- urinary retention
- enlarged pupils (dark part of eye)

What other information should I know?

Keep all appointments with your doctor.

Do not let anyone else use your medication. Ask your pharmacist any questions you have about refilling your prescription.

Talk to your doctor, pharmacist, or other healthcare professional if you have questions about dosing information for your medication.

Doxycycline

(dox i sye′ kleen)

Brand Name: Doryx®, Monodox®, Vibramycin® Calcium Syrup, Vibramycin® Hyclate, Vibramycin® Monohydrate, Vibra-Tabs®
Also available generically.

Why is this medicine prescribed?

Doxycycline is used to treat bacterial infections, including pneumonia and other respiratory tract infections; Lyme disease; acne; infections of skin, genital, and urinary systems;

and anthrax (after inhalational exposure). It is also used to prevent malaria. Doxycycline is in a class of medications called tetracycline antibiotics. It works by preventing the growth and spread of bacteria. Antibiotics will not work for colds, flu, or other viral infections.

How should this medicine be used?

Doxycycline comes as a regular and a coated capsule, a tablet, a syrup, and a suspension (liquid), all to take by mouth. Doxycycline is usually taken once or twice a day. Drink a full glass of water with each dose of the capsule or tablet. If your stomach becomes upset when you take doxycycline, you may take it with food or milk. However, taking doxycycline with milk or food may decrease the amount of medication absorbed from your stomach. Talk with your doctor or pharmacist about the best way to take doxycycline if your stomach becomes upset. Follow the directions on your prescription label carefully, and ask your doctor or pharmacist to explain any part you do not understand. Take doxycycline exactly as directed. Do not take more or less of it or take it more often than prescribed by your doctor.

Shake the syrup or suspension well before each use to mix the medication evenly.

If you are taking doxycycline for the prevention of malaria, start taking it 1 or 2 days before traveling to an area where there is malaria. Continue taking doxycycline for 4 weeks after leaving the area where there is malaria. You should not take doxycycline for the prevention of malaria for more than 4 months.

Continue to take doxycycline even if you feel well. Take all the medication until you are finished, unless your doctor tells you otherwise.

Are there other uses for this medicine?

Doxycycline may also be used for the treatment of malaria. Talk to your doctor about the possible risks of using this medication for your condition.

This medication is sometimes prescribed for other uses; ask your doctor or pharmacist for more information.

What special precautions should I follow?

Before taking doxycycline,

- tell your doctor and pharmacist if you are allergic to doxycycline, minocycline, tetracycline, sulfites (for doxycycline syrup only), or any other medications.
- tell your doctor and pharmacist what prescription and nonprescription medications you are taking, especially antacids, anticoagulants ('blood thinners') such as warfarin (Coumadin), carbamazepine (Tegretol), penicillin, phenobarbital, phenytoin (Dilantin), and vitamins. Doxycycline decreases the effectiveness of some oral contraceptives; another form of birth control should be used while taking this drug.
- be aware that antacids, calcium supplements, iron products, and laxatives containing magnesium interfere with doxycycline, making it less effective. Take doxycycline

1 hour before or 2 hours after antacids (including sodium bicarbonate), calcium supplements, and laxatives containing magnesium. Take doxycycline 2 hours before or 3 hours after iron preparations and vitamin products that contain iron.

- tell your doctor if you have or have ever had diabetes or kidney or liver disease.
- tell your doctor if you are pregnant, plan to become pregnant, or are breast-feeding. If you become pregnant while taking doxycycline, call your doctor immediately. Doxycycline can harm the fetus.
- if you are having surgery, including dental surgery, tell the doctor or dentist that you are taking doxycycline.
- plan to avoid unnecessary or prolonged exposure to sunlight and to wear protective clothing, sunglasses, and sunscreen. Doxycycline may make your skin sensitive to sunlight.
- you should know that when you are receiving doxycycline for prevention of malaria, you should also use protective measures such as effective insert repellent, mosquito nets, clothing covering the whole body, and staying in well-screened areas, especially from early nighttime until dawn. Taking doxycycline does not give you full protection against malaria.
- you should know that when doxycycline is used during pregnancy or in babies or children up to age 8, it can cause the teeth to become permanently stained. Doxycycline should not be used in children under age 8 except for inhalational anthrax or if your doctor decides it is needed.

What special dietary instructions should I follow?

Unless your doctor tells you otherwise, continue your normal diet.

What should I do if I forget to take a dose?

Take the missed dose as soon as you remember it. However, if it is almost time for the next dose, skip the missed dose and continue your regular dosing schedule. Do not take a double dose to make up for a missed one.

What side effects can this medicine cause?

Doxycycline may cause side effects. Tell your doctor if any of these symptoms are severe or do not go away:

- diarrhea
- itching of the rectum or vagina
- sore mouth

Some side effects can be serious. If you experience any of these symptoms, call your doctor immediately:

- severe headache
- blurred vision
- skin rash
- hives
- difficulty breathing or swallowing

- redness of the skin (sunburn)
- yellowing of the skin or eyes
- itching
- dark-colored urine
- light-colored bowel movements
- loss of appetite
- upset stomach
- vomiting
- stomach pain
- extreme tiredness or weakness
- confusion
- decreased urination

What storage conditions are needed for this medicine?

Keep this medication in the container it came in, tightly closed, and out of reach of children. Store it at room temperature and away from excess heat and moisture (not in the bathroom). Throw away any medication that is outdated or no longer needed. Talk to your pharmacist about the proper disposal of your medication.

What should I do in case of overdose?

In case of overdose, call your local poison control center at 1-800-222-1222. If the victim has collapsed or is not breathing, call local emergency services at 911.

What other information should I know?

Keep all appointments with your doctor and laboratory. Your doctor will want to check your response to doxycycline.

Before having any laboratory test, tell your doctor and the laboratory personnel that you are taking doxycycline.

If you have diabetes, doxycycline can cause false results in some tests for sugar in the urine. Check with your doctor before changing your diet or the dosage of your diabetes medicine.

Do not let anyone else take your medication. Your prescription is probably not refillable. If you still have symptoms of infection after you finish the doxycycline, call your doctor.

Dosage Facts
For Informational Purposes

Caution: Do not change your dose, how often you take your medication, or the length of time you are to take it without first talking to your healthcare provider.

The following dosage information was written using medical language for doctors and other healthcare professionals and is provided here for you to check your dosage. The dosage of this drug may differ for different patients. Therefore, always follow your doctor's instructions or the directions on the label. Contact your health-

care provider or pharmacist if you have any questions about the specific dosage of your medication after reviewing this information.

General Dosage Information

Available as doxycycline calcium, doxycycline hyclate, and doxycycline monohydrate; dosage expressed in terms of doxycycline.

Pediatric Patients

General Pediatric Dosage

ORAL:
- Children >8 years of age weighing ≤45 kg: 4.4 mg/kg in 2 divided doses on day 1 followed by 2.2 mg/kg daily in 1 or 2 divided doses. For severe infections, up to 4.4 mg/kg daily.
- Children >8 years of age weighing >45 kg: 100 mg every 12 hours on day 1 followed by 100 mg daily in 1 or 2 divided doses. For more severe infections, 100 mg every 12 hours.

Anthrax

Postexposure Prophylaxis Following Exposure in the Context of Biologic Warfare or Bioterrorism

ORAL:
- Children ≤8 years of age† or weighing <45 kg: 2.2 mg/kg (up to 100 mg) twice daily given for ≥60 days. Because of concerns regarding long-term doxycycline use in infants and children, consider changing (after 10–14 days) to amoxicillin to complete the prophylaxis regimen if penicillin susceptibility is confirmed.
- Children >8 years of age weighing ≥45 kg: 100 mg twice daily given for ≥60 days.
- Optimum duration of postexposure prophylaxis after an inhalation exposure to *B. anthracis* spores is unclear, but prolonged postexposure prophylaxis usually required. A duration of 60 days may be adequate for a low-dose exposure, but a duration >4 months may be necessary to reduce the risk following a high-dose exposure. CDC and US Working Group on Civilian Biodefense recommend that postexposure prophylaxis following a confirmed exposure (including in laboratory workers with confirmed exposures to *B. anthracis* cultures) be continued for 60 days. The US Army Medical Research Institute of Infectious Diseases (USAMRIID) recommends that postexposure prophylaxis be continued for *at least* 60 days in individuals who are not fully immunized against anthrax and when anthrax vaccine is unavailable or cannot be used for postexposure vaccination.

Treatment of Inhalational, GI, or Oropharyngeal Anthrax

ORAL:
- Children ≤8 years of age† or weighing <45 kg: 2.2 mg/kg twice daily (up to 200 mg daily).
- Children >8 years of age weighing ≥45 kg: 100 mg twice daily. Some experts recommend an initial 200-mg dose, then 100 mg every 12 hours.
- Initial parenteral regimen preferred; use oral regimen for initial treatment only when a parenteral regimen is not available (e.g., when there are supply or logistic problems because large numbers of individuals require treatment in a mass casualty setting). Continue for total duration of ≥60 days if inhalational anthrax occurred as the result of exposure to anthrax spores in the context of biologic warfare or bioterror-

ism. Because of concerns regarding long-term doxycycline use in infants and children, consider changing (after 10–14 days) to amoxicillin to complete the treatment regimen in children <8 years of age if penicillin susceptibility is confirmed.

Treatment of Cutaneous Anthrax

ORAL:
- Children ≤8 years of age† or weighing <45 kg: 2.2 mg/kg (up to 100 mg) twice daily.
- Children >8 years of age weighing ≥45 kg: 100 mg twice daily.
- For mild, uncomplicated cutaneous anthrax that occurs following natural or endemic exposure, 5–10 days of treatment has been recommended.
- For cutaneous anthrax that occurs following exposure in the context of biologic warfare or bioterrorism, duration of treatment is ≥60 days. Because of concerns regarding long-term doxycycline use in infants and children, consider changing (after 10–14 days) to amoxicillin to complete the treatment regimen in children <8 years of age if penicillin susceptibility is confirmed.
- Oral regimen should not be used for initial treatment of cutaneous anthrax if there are signs of systemic involvement, extensive edema, or head and neck lesions and should not be used for initial treatment in infants and children <2 years of age.

Bartonella Infections

ORAL:
- Adolescents with HIV infection: 100 mg every 12 hours for ≥3 months for bartonellosis (including CNS infections). Also consider doxycycline long-term suppressive therapy† in those with relapse or reinfection.

Brucellosis

Treatment of Brucellosis

ORAL:
- Children ≥8 years of age: 2–4 mg/kg daily (up to 200 mg daily) in 2 divided doses. Some experts recommend 2.2 mg/kg twice daily (up to 200 mg daily).
- Usual duration of therapy is 4–6 weeks; more prolonged therapy may be required for complicated disease (e.g., hepatitis, splenitis, meningoencephalitis, endocarditis, osteomyelitis). Meningoencephalitis and endocarditis should be treated for ≥90 days and may require ≥6 months of treatment.
- Usually used in conjunction with rifampin or other anti-infectives to decrease risk of relapse. If infection is severe or if endocarditis, meningitis, or osteomyelitis is present, administer IM streptomycin or gentamicin during the first 1–3 weeks of doxycycline therapy.

Burkholderia Infections†

Follow-up Maintenance Regimen after Initial Treatment of Severe Disease†

ORAL:
- Children ≥8 years of age or weighing ≥45 kg: 100 mg twice daily given in conjunction with oral co-trimoxazole.
- Prolonged oral maintenance regimen recommended to reduce risk of relapse after initial treatment with IV ceftazidime, imipenem, or meropenem (with or without IV doxycycline). Maintenance regimen usually continued for ≥4–6 months; a duration of 6–12 months may be necessary depending on

response to therapy and severity of illness. Lifelong follow-up recommended for all patients to identify relapse.

Chlamydial Infections
Uncomplicated Urethral, Endocervical, or Rectal Infections

ORAL:
- Children >8 years of age: 100 mg twice daily given for 7 days.

Presumptive Treatment of Chlamydial Infection in Gonorrhea Patients

ORAL:
- Adolescents: 100 mg twice daily given for 7 days.

Lymphogranuloma Venereum

ORAL:
- Adolescents: 100 mg twice daily given for 21 days.

Ehrlichiosis†

ORAL:
- AAP and CDC recommend 2.2 mg/kg (up to 100 mg) twice daily. Initiate promptly since delay can result in severe disease and fatal outcome.
- Optimum duration of therapy not established. Usually continued ≥5–10 days and until patient is afebrile for ≥3 days and clinically improved. Severe illness may require longer duration of therapy. CDC recommends a duration of 10–14 days in those with HGA since this provides an appropriate duration of therapy for possible concurrent early Lyme disease.
- Oral therapy generally appropriate for patients with early disease, those treated as outpatients, or inpatients who are not vomiting or obtunded.

Gonorrhea and Associated Infections
Empiric Treatment of Epididymitis

ORAL:
- Children ≥8 years of age: 100 mg twice daily given for 10 days; as follow-up to single-dose IM ceftriaxone.

Granuloma Inguinale (Donovanosis)

ORAL:
- Adolescents: 100 mg twice daily given for ≥3 weeks or until all lesions have healed completely; consider adding IV aminoglycoside (e.g., gentamicin) if improvement is not evident within the first few days of therapy and in HIV-infected patients.
- Relapse can occur 6–18 months after apparently effective treatment.

Lyme Disease†
Early Localized or Early Disseminated Lyme Disease†

ORAL:
- Children ≥8 years of age: 1–2 mg/kg in 2 divided doses (up to 100 mg each dose).
- Duration of treatment is 14–21 days for most patients with early localized or early disseminated disease in the absence of neurologic involvement. Some experts recommend a duration of 21–28 days for early disseminated disease associated with mild carditis or isolated facial nerve palsy.

Lyme Arthritis†

ORAL:
- Children ≥8 years of age: 1–2 mg/kg twice daily (up to 100 mg each dose) for 28 days.

Malaria
Prevention of Malaria

ORAL:
- Children ≥8 years of age: 2 mg/kg (up to 100 mg) once daily.
- Initiate prophylaxis 1–2 days prior to entering malarious area; continue during the stay and for 4 weeks after leaving area. If there are concerns about tolerance or drug interactions, it may be advisable to initiate prophylaxis 3–4 weeks prior to travel in individuals receiving other drugs to ensure that the combination of drugs is well tolerated and to allow ample time if a switch to another antimalarial is required.
- Terminal prophylaxis with primaquine may be indicated during the final 2 weeks of doxycycline prophylaxis if exposure occurred in areas where *P. ovale* or *P. vivax* are endemic.

Treatment of Uncomplicated Chloroquine-resistant P. falciparum Malaria†

ORAL:
- Children ≥8 years of age: 4 mg/kg daily given in 2 equally divided doses (up to 200 mg daily) for 7 days; used in conjunction with oral quinine sulfate (10 mg/kg 3 times daily given for 3 days if infection was acquired in Africa or South America or for 7 days if acquired in Southeast Asia).

Treatment of Uncomplicated P. vivax Malaria†

ORAL:
- Children ≥8 years of age: 4 mg/kg daily in 2 equally divided doses (up to 200 mg daily) for 7 days; used in conjunction with oral quinine sulfate (10 mg/kg 3 times daily given for 3 days if infection was acquired in Africa or South America or for 7 days if acquired in Southeast Asia).
- In addition, a 14-day regimen of oral primaquine (0.6 mg/kg once daily) may be indicated to provide a radical cure and prevent delayed attacks or relapse of *P. vivax* malaria.

Treatment of Severe P. falciparum Malaria†

ORAL:
- Children ≥8 years of age: 4 mg/kg daily in 2 equally divided doses (up to 200 mg daily) given for 7 days; used in conjunction with IV quinidine gluconate (followed by oral quinine sulfate) given for a total duration of 3–7 days.

Presumptive Self-treatment of Malaria†

ORAL:
- Children ≥8 years of age: 4 mg/kg daily in 2 equally divided doses for 7 days; used in conjunction with oral quinine sulfate (10 mg/kg 3 times daily given for 3 days if infection was acquired in Africa or South America or for 7 days if acquired in Southeast Asia). Initiate presumptive self-treatment if malaria is suspected (fever, chills, or other influenza-like illness) and professional medical care will not be available within 24 hours.
- *Not* recommended for self-treatment of malaria in individuals currently taking the drug for prophylaxis.

Nongonococcal Urethritis

ORAL:
- Adolescents: 100 mg twice daily given for 7 days.

Pelvic Inflammatory Disease†

ORAL:
- Adolescents: 100 mg every 12 hours given for 14 days. Used in conjunction with and as follow-up to other anti-infectives.

Plague

Postexposure Prophylaxis Following High-risk Exposure†

ORAL:

- Children weighing <45 kg: 2.2 mg/kg twice daily (up to 200 mg daily).
- Children weighing ≥45 kg: 100 mg twice daily. Alternatively, 2–4 mg/kg daily in 2 equally divided doses.
- Duration of prophylaxis following exposure to plague aerosol or a patient with suspected pneumonic plague is 7 days or the duration of exposure risk plus 7 days.

Rickettsial Infections

ORAL:

- Children >8 years of age weighing ≤45 kg: 4.4 mg/kg in 2 divided doses on day 1 followed by 2.2 mg/kg daily in 1 or 2 divided doses. For severe infections, up to 4.4 mg/kg daily.
- Children >8 years of age weighing >45 kg: 100 mg every 12 hours on day 1 followed by 100 mg daily in 1 or 2 divided doses. For severe infections, 100 mg every 12 hours.
- Continue therapy for 3–10 days or until patient is afebrile for approximately 2–3 days. Alternatively, a single 50-mg dose may be effective for louse-borne (epidemic) typhus, Brill-Zinsser disease, or scrub typhus.

Rocky Mountain Spotted Fever (RMSF)

ORAL:

- CDC recommends 2.2 mg/kg (up to 100 mg) twice daily. Initiate promptly since delay can result in severe disease and fatal outcome.
- Usually continued ≥5–10 days and until patient is afebrile for ≥3 days and clinically improved. Severe illness may require longer duration of therapy.
- Oral therapy generally appropriate for patients with early disease, those treated as outpatients, or inpatients who are not vomiting or obtunded.

Q Fever

ORAL:

- CDC recommends 2.2 mg/kg every 12 hours for ≥14 days for treatment of acute Q fever.
- For prophylaxis against Q fever†, 2.2 mg/kg twice daily given for 5–7 days may prevent clinical disease if initiated 8–12 days after exposure; such prophylaxis is not effective and may only prolong the onset of disease if given immediately (1–7 days) after exposure.

Syphilis

Primary or Secondary Syphilis

ORAL:

- Children >8 years of age: 100 mg twice daily given for 14 days.

Latent Syphilis or Tertiary Syphilis (Except Neurosyphilis)

ORAL:

- Children >8 years of age: 100 mg twice daily given for 14 days for early latent syphilis (duration <1 year) or 100 mg twice daily given for 28 days for late latent syphilis (duration ≥1 year), latent syphilis of unknown duration, or tertiary syphilis.

Tularemia

Postexposure Prophylaxis Following High-risk Exposure†

ORAL:

- Children weighing <45 kg: 2.2 mg/kg (up to 100 mg) twice daily.
- Children weighing ≥45 kg: 100 mg twice daily.
- Initiate postexposure prophylaxis within 24 hours of exposure and continue for ≥14 days.

Vibrio Infections

Cholera

ORAL:

- Children ≥8 years of age: 6 mg/kg (maximum 300 mg) as a single dose.

Prophylaxis in Sexual Assault Victims†

ORAL:

- Adolescents: 100 mg twice daily given for 7 days; used in conjunction with single doses of IM ceftriaxone and oral metronidazole.

Adult Patients

General Adult Dosage

ORAL:

- 100 mg every 12 hours on day 1 followed by 100 mg daily in 1 or 2 divided doses.
- For more severe infections, 100 mg every 12 hours.

Respiratory Tract Infections

Legionella Infections†

ORAL:

- 100 mg every 12 hours on the first day followed by 100 mg daily in 1 or 2 divided doses.
- For severe infections, 100 mg every 12 hours.

Anthrax

Postexposure Prophylaxis Following Exposure in the Context of Biologic Warfare or Bioterrorism

ORAL:

- 100 mg twice daily given for ≥60 days. Some experts recommend an initial 200-mg dose, then 100 mg every 12 hours.
- Optimum duration of postexposure prophylaxis after an inhalation exposure to *B. anthracis* spores is unclear, but prolonged postexposure prophylaxis usually required. A duration of 60 days may be adequate for a low-dose exposure, but a duration >4 months may be necessary to reduce the risk following a high-dose exposure. CDC and US Working Group on Civilian Biodefense recommend that postexposure prophylaxis following a confirmed exposure (including in laboratory workers with confirmed exposures to *B. anthracis* cultures) be continued for 60 days. The US Army Medical Research Institute of Infectious Diseases (USAMRIID) recommends that postexposure prophylaxis be continued for *at least* 60 days in individuals who are not fully immunized against anthrax and when anthrax vaccine is unavailable or cannot be used for postexposure vaccination.

Treatment of Inhalational, GI, or Oropharyngeal Anthrax

ORAL:

- 100 mg twice daily. Some experts recommend an initial 200-mg dose, then 100 mg every 12 hours.
- Initial parenteral regimen preferred; use oral regimen for ini-

tial treatment only when a parenteral regimen is not available (e.g., when there are supply or logistic problems because large numbers of individuals require treatment in a mass casualty setting). Continue for total duration of ≥60 days if inhalational anthrax occurred as the result of exposure to anthrax spores in the context of biologic warfare or bioterrorism.

Treatment of Cutaneous Anthrax

ORAL:
- 100 mg twice daily.
- For mild, uncomplicated cutaneous anthrax that occurs following natural or endemic exposure, 5–10 days of treatment has been recommended.
- For cutaneous anthrax that occurs following exposure in the context of biologic warfare or bioterrorism, duration of treatment is ≥60 days.
- Oral regimen should not be used for initial treatment of cutaneous anthrax if there are signs of systemic involvement, extensive edema, or head and neck lesions.

Bartonella Infections

ORAL:
- HIV-infected adults: 100 mg every 12 hours for ≥3 months for bartonellosis (including CNS infections). Also consider doxycycline long-term suppressive therapy† in those with relapse or reinfection.

Burkholderia Infections†
Treatment of Localized Disease†

ORAL:
- Mild, localized disease without toxicity: 100 mg twice daily for 60–150 days may be effective.
- Localized disease without toxicity: 100 mg twice daily for 20 weeks given in conjunction with oral co-trimoxazole.

Follow-up Maintenance Regimen after Initial Treatment of Severe Disease†

ORAL:
- 100 mg twice daily given in conjunction with oral co-trimoxazole.
- Prolonged oral maintenance regimen recommended to reduce risk of relapse after initial treatment with IV ceftazidime, imipenem, or meropenem (with or without IV doxycycline). Maintenance regimen usually continued for ≥4–6 months; a duration of 6–12 months may be necessary depending on response to therapy and severity of illness. Lifelong follow-up recommended for all patients to identify relapse.

Postexposure Prophylaxis†

ORAL:
- 200 mg once daily in conjunction with oral rifampin. Optimum duration unknown; continue for ≥10 days.

Brucellosis
Treatment of Brucellosis

ORAL:
- Some experts recommend 100 mg twice daily.
- Usual duration is 4–6 weeks; more prolonged therapy may be required for complicated disease (e.g., hepatitis, splenitis, meningoencephalitis, endocarditis, osteomyelitis). Meningoencephalitis and endocarditis should be treated for ≥90 days and may require ≥6 months of treatment.
- Usually used in conjunction with rifampin or other anti-infectives to decrease risk of relapse. If infection is severe or if endocarditis, meningitis, or osteomyelitis is present, administer IM streptomycin or gentamicin during the first 1–3 weeks of doxycycline therapy.

Postexposure Prophylaxis following Exposure in the Context of Biologic Warfare or Bioterrorism

ORAL:
- 200 mg once daily given for 3–6 weeks.

Chlamydial Infections
Uncomplicated Urethral, Endocervical, or Rectal Infections

ORAL:
- 100 mg twice daily given for 7 days.

Presumptive Treatment of Chlamydial Infection in Gonorrhea Patients

ORAL:
- 100 mg twice daily given for 7 days.

Acute Epididymo-orchitis or Proctitis caused by C. trachomatis

ORAL:
- 100 mg twice daily given for ≥10 days.

Lymphogranuloma Venereum

ORAL:
- 100 mg twice daily given for 21 days.

Psittacosis (Ornithosis)

ORAL:
- 100 mg twice daily given for ≥10–14 days after defervescence.

Ehrlichiosis†

ORAL:
- CDC and others recommend 100 mg twice daily. Initiate promptly since delay can result in severe disease and fatal outcome.
- Optimum duration of therapy not established. Usually continued ≥5–10 days and until patient is afebrile for ≥3 days and clinically improved. Severe illness may require longer duration of therapy. CDC recommends a duration of 10–14 days in those with HGA since this provides an appropriate duration of therapy for possible concurrent early Lyme disease.
- Oral therapy generally appropriate for patients with early disease, not requiring hospitalization, or inpatients who are not vomiting or obtunded.

Gonorrhea and Associated Infections
Uncomplicated Gonorrhea

ORAL:
- 100 mg twice daily given for 7 days recommended by manufacturer. Alternatively, 300 mg followed by another 300-mg dose 1 hour later.
- No longer recommended for gonorrhea by CDC or other experts.

Empiric Treatment of Epididymitis

ORAL:
- 100 mg twice daily given for 10 days; as follow-up to a single dose of IM ceftriaxone.

Epididymo-orchitis or Proctitis

ORAL:
- 100 mg twice daily given for ≥10 days for acute epididymo-orchitis or for 7 days for proctitis.

Granuloma Inguinale (Donovanosis)

ORAL:

- 100 mg twice daily given for ≥3 weeks or until all lesions have healed completely; consider adding IV aminoglycoside (e.g., gentamicin) if improvement is not evident within the first few days of therapy and in HIV-infected patients.
- Relapse can occur 6–18 months after apparently effective treatment.

Leptospirosis†
Treatment†

ORAL:

- 100 mg twice daily given for 7 days.

Prevention†

ORAL:

- 200 mg once weekly beginning 1–2 days prior to and continuing throughout the period of exposure.

Lyme Disease†
Early Localized or Early Disseminated Lyme Disease†

ORAL:

- 100 mg twice daily.
- Duration of treatment is 14–21 days for most patients with early localized or early disseminated disease in the absence of neurologic involvement. Some experts recommend a duration of 21–28 days for early disseminated disease associated with mild carditis or isolated facial nerve palsy.

Lyme Arthritis†

ORAL:

- 100 mg twice daily given for 28 days.

Acute Neurologic Manifestations (e.g., Meningitis, Radiculopathy)†

ORAL:

- 100–200 mg twice daily given for 14–28 days for patients who are intolerant of cephalosporins and penicillin.

Malaria
Prevention of Malaria

ORAL:

- 100 mg once daily.
- Initiate prophylaxis 1–2 days prior to entering malarious area; continue during the stay and for 4 weeks after leaving area. If there are concerns about tolerance or drug interactions, it may be advisable to initiate prophylaxis 3–4 weeks prior to travel in individuals receiving other drugs to ensure that the combination of drugs is well tolerated and to allow ample time if a switch to another antimalarial is required.
- Terminal prophylaxis with primaquine may be indicated during the final 2 weeks of doxycycline prophylaxis if exposure occurred in areas where *P. ovale* or *P. vivax* are endemic.

Treatment of Uncomplicated Chloroquine-resistant P. falciparum Malaria†

ORAL:

- 100 mg twice daily for 7 days; used in conjunction with oral quinine sulfate (650 mg 3 times daily given for 3 days if infection was acquired in Africa or South America or for 7 days if acquired in Southeast Asia).

Treatment of Uncomplicated P. vivax Malaria†

ORAL:

- 100 mg twice daily for 7 days; used in conjunction with oral quinine sulfate (650 mg 3 times daily given for 3 days if malaria was acquired in Africa or South America or for 7 days if acquired in Southeast Asia).
- In addition, a 14-day regimen of oral primaquine (30 mg once daily) also may be indicated to provide a radical cure and prevent delayed attacks or relapse of *P. vivax* malaria.

Treatment of Severe P. falciparum Malaria†

ORAL:

- 100 mg twice daily given for 7 days; used in conjunction with IV quinidine gluconate (followed by oral quinine sulfate) given for a total duration of 3–7 days.

Presumptive Self-treatment of Malaria†

ORAL:

- 100 mg twice daily for 7 days; used in conjunction with oral quinine sulfate (650 mg 3 times daily given for 3 days if malaria was acquired in Africa or South America or for 7 days if acquired in Southeast Asia). Initiate presumptive self-treatment if malaria is suspected (fever, chills, or other influenza-like illness) and professional medical care will not be available within 24 hours.
- *Not* recommended for self-treatment of malaria in individuals currently taking the drug for prophylaxis.

Mycobacterial Infections†
Mycobacterium marinum Infections†

ORAL:

- 100 mg twice daily given for ≥3 months recommended by ATS for treatment of cutaneous infections. A minimum of 4–6 weeks of treatment usually is necessary to determine whether the infection is responding.

Nongonococcal Urethritis

ORAL:

- 100 mg twice daily given for 7 days.

Pelvic Inflammatory Disease†

ORAL:

- 100 mg every 12 hours given for 14 days. Used in conjunction with and as follow-up to other anti-infectives.

Plague
Postexposure Prophylaxis Following High-risk Exposure†

ORAL:

- 100 mg every 12 hours. Alternatively, 100–200 mg daily in 2 equally divided doses.
- Duration of prophylaxis following exposure to plague aerosol or a patient with suspected pneumonic plague is 7 days or the duration of exposure risk plus 7 days.

Rickettsial Infections

ORAL:

- 100 mg every 12 hours on day 1 followed by 100 mg daily in 1 or 2 divided doses. For more severe infections, 100 mg every 12 hours.
- Continue therapy for 3–10 days or until patient is afebrile for approximately 2–3 days. Alternatively, a single dose of 100–200 mg may be effective for louse-borne (epidemic) typhus, Brill-Zinsser disease, or scrub typhus.

Rocky Mountain Spotted Fever (RMSF)

ORAL:

- CDC and others recommend 100 mg twice daily. Initiate promptly since delay can result in severe disease and fatal outcome.

- Usually continued ≥5–10 days and until patient is afebrile for ≥3 days and clinically improved. Severe illness may require longer duration of therapy.
- Oral therapy generally appropriate for patients with early disease, not requiring hospitalization, or inpatients who are not vomiting or obtunded.

Q Fever

ORAL:
- 100 mg twice daily given for 2–3 weeks recommended by CDC and others for acute Q fever.
- For acute Q fever with preexisting valvular heart disease, CDC recommends 200 mg daily given in conjunction with hydroxychloroquine for 1 year to prevent progression of acute disease to endocarditis. Patients with chronic Q fever endocarditis should receive the doxycycline and hydroxychloroquine regimen for 1.5–3 years.
- For prophylaxis against Q fever†, 100 mg every 12 hours given for 5–7 days may prevent clinical disease if initiated 8–12 days after exposure; such prophylaxis is not effective and may only prolong the onset of disease if given immediately (1–7 days) after exposure.

Syphilis
Primary or Secondary Syphilis

ORAL:
- 100 mg twice daily given for 14 days.

Latent Syphilis or Tertiary Syphilis (Except Neurosyphilis)

ORAL:
- 100 mg twice daily given for 14 days for early latent syphilis (duration <1 year) or 100 mg twice daily given for 28 days for late latent syphilis (duration≥1 year), latent syphilis of unknown duration, or tertiary syphilis.

Tularemia
Postexposure Prophylaxis Following High-risk Exposure†

ORAL:
- 100 mg twice daily.
- Initiate postexposure prophylaxis within 24 hours of exposure and continue for ≥14 days.

Vibrio Infections
Cholera

ORAL:
- 100 mg every 12 hours on the first day followed by 100 mg daily in 1 or 2 divided doses for 2 days. For severe infections, 100 mg every 12 hours for 3 days.
- Alternatively, 300 mg as a single dose may be effective.

Prophylaxis in Sexual Assault Victims†

ORAL:
- 100 mg twice daily for 7 days; used in conjunction with single doses of IM ceftriaxone and oral metronidazole.

Prescribing Limits

Pediatric Patients

General Pediatric Dosage

ORAL:
- Maximum 4.4 mg/kg daily for severe infections in children >8 years of age weighing ≤45 kg.

Malaria
Treatment of Uncomplicated Chloroquine-resistant P. falciparum Malaria†

ORAL:
- Children ≥8 years of age: Maximum 200 mg daily.

Treatment of Uncomplicated P. vivax Malaria†

ORAL:
- Children ≥8 years of age: Maximum 200 mg daily.

Treatment of Severe P. falciparum Malaria†

ORAL:
- Children ≥8 years of age: Maximum 200 mg daily.

Special Populations

Renal Impairment
- Dosage adjustments not necessary.

† Use is not currently included in the labeling approved by the US Food and Drug Administration.

Doxycycline Injection

(dox i sye′ kleen)

Brand Name: Doxy 100®, Doxy 200®, Vibramycin® Hyclate Intravenous
Also available generically.

Important Warning

Doxycycline should not be taken by children under 8 years of age or women who are pregnant or breast-feeding.

About Your Treatment

Your doctor has ordered doxycycline, an antibiotic, to help treat your infection. The drug will be added to an intravenous fluid that will drip through a needle or catheter placed in your vein for 1-4 hours, one or two times a day.

Doxycycline eliminates bacteria that cause many kinds of infections including Lyme disease, pneumonia, and urinary tract, skin, bone, and rectal infections. This medication is sometimes prescribed for other uses; ask your doctor or pharmacist for more information.

Your health care provider (doctor, nurse, or pharmacist) may measure the effectiveness and side effects of your treatment using laboratory tests and physical examinations. It is important to keep all appointments with your doctor and the laboratory. The length of treatment depends on how your infection and symptoms respond to the medication.

Precautions

Before administering doxycycline,

- tell your doctor and pharmacist if you are allergic to doxycycline, tetracycline, minocycline, or any other drugs.
- tell your doctor and pharmacist what prescription and nonprescription medications you are taking, especially antacids, anticoagulants ('blood thinners') such as warfarin (Coumadin), barbiturates, carbamazepine (Tegretol), penicillin, phenytoin (Dilantin), and vitamins. Doxycycline decreases the effectiveness of some oral contraceptives; use another form of birth control while taking this drug.
- tell your doctor if you have or have ever had diabetes or kidney or liver disease.
- tell your doctor if you are pregnant, plan to become pregnant, or are breast-feeding. If you become pregnant while taking doxycycline, call your doctor immediately. Doxycycline can harm the fetus.
- you should plan to avoid unnecessary or prolonged exposure to sunlight and to wear protective clothing, sunglasses, and sunscreen. Doxycycline may make your skin sensitive to sunlight.
- you should know that this drug may cause a false positive with some tests that are used to measure sugar in your blood. Ask your doctor or pharmacist for a product that can be used safely.

Administering Your Medication

Before you administer doxycycline, look at the solution closely. It should be clear and free of floating material. Gently squeeze the bag or observe the solution container to make sure there are no leaks. Do not use the solution if it is discolored, if it contains particles, or if the bag or container leaks. Use a new solution, but show the damaged one to your health care provider.

It is important that you use your medication exactly as directed. Do not stop your therapy on your own for any reason because your infection could worsen and result in hospitalization. Do not change your dosing schedule without talking to your health care provider. Your health care provider may tell you to stop your infusion if you have a mechanical problem (such as a blockage in the tubing, needle, or catheter); if you have to stop an infusion, call your health care provider immediately so your therapy can continue.

Side Effects

Doxycycline may cause side effects. Tell your health care provider if any of these symptoms are severe or do not go away:

- upset stomach
- diarrhea
- stomach pain
- itching of the rectum or vagina
- sore mouth or tongue
- headache
- loss of appetite

If you experience either of the following symptoms, call your health care provider immediately:

- skin rash
- yellowing of the skin or eyes

If you experience a serious side effect, you or your doctor may send a report to the Food and Drug Administration's (FDA) MedWatch Adverse Event Reporting program online [at http://www.fda.gov/MedWatch/index.html] or by phone [1-800-332-1088].

Storage Conditions

- Your health care provider probably will give you a several-day supply of doxycycline at a time. You will be told to store it in the refrigerator or freezer.
- Take your next dose from the refrigerator 1 hour before using it; place it in a clean, dry area to allow it to warm to room temperature.
- If you are told to store additional doxycycline in the freezer, always move a 24-hour supply to the refrigerator for the next day's use.
- Do not refreeze medications.

Store your medication only as directed. Make sure you understand what you need to store your medication properly.

Keep your supplies in a clean, dry place when you are not using them, and keep all medications and supplies out of reach of children. Your health care provider will tell you how to throw away used needles, syringes, tubing, and containers to avoid accidental injury.

Overdose

In case of overdose, call your local poison control center at 1-800-222-1222. If the victim has collapsed or is not breathing, call local emergency services at 911.

Signs of Infection

If you are receiving doxycycline in your vein or under your skin, you need to know the symptoms of a catheter-related infection (an infection where the needle enters your vein or skin). If you experience any of these effects near your intravenous catheter, tell your health care provider as soon as possible:

- tenderness
- warmth
- irritation
- drainage
- redness
- swelling
- pain

Dosage Facts
For Informational Purposes

Caution: Do not change your dose, how often you take your medication, or the length of time you are to take it without first talking to your healthcare provider.

The following dosage information was written using medical language for doctors and other healthcare professionals and is provided here for you to check your dosage. The dosage of this drug may differ for different patients. Therefore, always follow your doctor's instructions or the directions on the label. Contact your healthcare provider or pharmacist if you have any questions about the specific dosage of your medication after reviewing this information.

General Dosage Information

Available as doxycycline calcium, doxycycline hyclate, and doxycycline monohydrate; dosage expressed in terms of doxycycline.

Pediatric Patients

General Pediatric Dosage

IV:
- Children >8 years of age weighing ≤45 kg: 4.4 mg/kg in 1 or 2 divided doses on day 1 followed by 2.2–4.4 mg/kg daily in 1 or 2 infusions.
- Children >8 years of age weighing >45 kg: 200 mg on day 1 in 1 or 2 infusions followed by 100–200 mg daily.

Anthrax
Treatment of Inhalational, GI, or Oropharyngeal Anthrax

IV, THEN ORAL:
- Children ≤8 years of age† or weighing <45 kg: 2.2 mg/kg (up to 100 mg) twice daily.
- Children >8 years of age weighing ≥45 kg: 100 mg twice daily.
- Used in conjunction with 1 or 2 other anti-infectives predicted to be effective. When clinical improvement occurs, switch IV doxycycline to oral doxycycline in the same dosage and continue for a total duration of ≥60 days. Because of concerns regarding long-term doxycycline use in infants and children, consider changing (after 10–14 days) to amoxicillin to complete the treatment regimen in children <8 years of age if penicillin susceptibility is confirmed.

Treatment of Cutaneous Anthrax

IV, THEN ORAL:
- Children ≤8 years of age† or weighing <45 kg: 2.2 mg/kg (up to 100 mg) twice daily.
- Children >8 years of age weighing ≥45 kg: 100 mg every 12 hours.
- Used in conjunction with 1 or 2 other anti-infectives predicted to be effective. When clinical improvement occurs, switch IV doxycycline to oral doxycycline in the same dosage and continue for a total duration of ≥60 days. Because of concerns regarding long-term doxycycline use in infants and children, consider changing (after 10–14 days) to amoxicillin to com-

plete the treatment regimen in children <8 years of age if penicillin susceptibility is confirmed.

Bartonella Infections

IV:
- Adolescents with HIV infection: 100 mg every 12 hours for ≥3 months for bartonellosis (including CNS infections). Also consider doxycycline long-term suppressive therapy† in those with relapse or reinfection.

Burkholderia Infections†
Initial Treatment of Severe Disease†

IV:
- Children <8 years of age† or weighing <45 kg: 2.2 mg/kg twice daily (up to 200 mg daily) given in conjunction with IV ceftazidime, imipenem, or meropenem.
- Children ≥8 years of age or weighing ≥45 kg: 100 mg twice daily given in conjunction with IV ceftazidime, imipenem, or meropenem.
- Initial IV regimen continued for ≥14 days and until clinical improvement occurs. When appropriate, switch to a prolonged oral maintenance regimen.

Ehrlichiosis†

IV:
- AAP and CDC recommend 2.2 mg/kg (up to 100 mg) twice daily. Initiate promptly since delay can result in severe disease and fatal outcome.
- Optimum duration of therapy not established. Usually continued ≥5–10 days and until patient is afebrile for ≥3 days and clinically improved. Severe illness may require longer duration of therapy. CDC recommends a duration of 10–14 days in those with HGA since this provides an appropriate duration of therapy for possible concurrent early Lyme disease.
- IV therapy generally indicated for hospitalized patients.

Malaria
Treatment of Severe P. falciparum Malaria†

IV, THEN ORAL:
- Children ≥8 years of age weighing <45 kg: Initially 4 mg/kg daily in 2 equally divided doses IV; when oral therapy can be tolerated, switch to oral doxycycline in a dosage of 4 mg/kg daily in 2 equally divided doses (up to 200 mg daily) for a total duration of IV and oral doxycycline of 7 days. Used in conjunction with IV quinidine gluconate (followed by oral quinine sulfate) given for a total duration of 3–7 days.
- Children ≥8 years of age weighing ≥45 kg: Initially 100 mg of doxycycline IV every 12 hours; when oral therapy can be tolerated, switch to oral doxycycline in a dosage of 100 mg every 12 hours for a total duration of IV and oral doxycycline of 7 days. Used in conjunction with IV quinidine gluconate (followed by oral quinine sulfate) given for a total duration of 3–7 days.

Pelvic Inflammatory Disease†

IV, THEN ORAL:
- Adolescents: 100 mg every 12 hours. Initially, IV doxycycline in conjunction with IV cefoxitin or cefotetan. Switch IV doxycycline to oral doxycycline in the same dosage as soon as possible and continue for a total duration of 14 days; continue IV cephamycin for ≥24 hours after clinical improvement occurs.

Plague
Treatment of Pneumonic Plague Occurring in Context of Biologic Warfare or Bioterrorism

IV, THEN ORAL:
- Children weighing <45 kg: 2.2 mg/kg twice daily (up to 200 mg daily).
- Children weighing ≥45 kg: 100 mg twice daily or 200 mg once daily.
- Prompt initiation of treatment (within 18–24 hours of symptom onset) is essential. Oral doxycycline may be substituted in the same dosage when the patient's condition improves or if parenteral doxycycline is unavailable. Total duration of treatment is ≥10–14 days.

Rickettsial Infections
Rocky Mountain Spotted Fever (RMSF)

IV:
- CDC recommends 2.2 mg/kg (up to 100 mg) twice daily. Initiate promptly since delay can result in severe disease and fatal outcome.
- Usually continued ≥5–10 days and until patient is afebrile for ≥3 days and clinically improved. Severe illness may require longer duration of therapy.
- IV therapy generally indicated for hospitalized patients.

Tularemia
Treatment

IV, THEN ORAL:
- Children weighing <45 kg: 2.2 mg/kg (up to 100 mg) twice daily.
- Children weighing ≥45 kg: 100 mg twice daily.
- Oral doxycycline may be substituted in the same dosage when the patient's condition improves or if parenteral doxycycline is unavailable. Total duration of treatment is ≥14–21 days.

Adult Patients

General Adult Dosage

IV:
- 200 mg on day 1 in 1 or 2 IV infusions followed by 100–200 mg daily.

Anthrax
Treatment of Inhalational, GI, or Oropharyngeal Anthrax

IV, THEN ORAL:
- 100 mg twice daily. Some experts recommend an initial 200-mg dose, then 100 mg every 12 hours.
- Used in conjunction with 1 or 2 other anti-infectives predicted to be effective. When clinical improvement occurs, switch IV doxycycline to oral doxycycline in the same dosage and continue for a total duration of ≥60 days.

Treatment of Cutaneous Anthrax

IV, THEN ORAL:
- 100 mg twice daily.
- Used in conjunction with 1 or 2 other anti-infectives predicted to be effective. When clinical improvement occurs, switch IV doxycycline to oral doxycycline in the same dosage and continue for a total duration of ≥60 days.

Bartonella Infections

IV:
- HIV-infected adults: 100 mg every 12 hours for ≥3 months for bartonellosis (including CNS infections). Also consider doxycycline long-term suppressive therapy† in those with relapse or reinfection.

Burkholderia Infections†
Initial Treatment of Severe Disease†

IV:
- 100 mg twice daily given in conjunction with IV ceftazidime, imipenem, or meropenem.
- Initial IV regimen continued for ≥14 days and until clinical improvement occurs. When appropriate, switch to a prolonged oral maintenance regimen.

Chlamydial Infections
Psittacosis (Ornithosis)

IV:
- 4.4 mg/kg daily in 2 divided doses for initial treatment of severely ill patients.

Ehrlichiosis†

IV:
- CDC and others recommend 100 mg twice daily. Initiate promptly since delay can result in severe disease and fatal outcome.
- Optimum duration of therapy not established. Usually continued ≥5–10 days and until patient is afebrile for ≥3 days and clinically improved. Severe illness may require longer duration of therapy. CDC recommends a duration of 10–14 days in those with HGA since this provides an appropriate duration of therapy for possible concurrent early Lyme disease.
- IV therapy generally indicated for hospitalized patients.

Lyme Disease†
Acute Neurologic Manifestations (e.g., Meningitis, Radiculopathy)†

IV:
- 100–200 mg twice daily given for 14–28 days for patients who are intolerant of cephalosporins and penicillin.

Malaria
Treatment of Severe P. falciparum Malaria†

IV, THEN ORAL:
- Initially, 100 mg of doxycycline IV every 12 hours; when oral therapy can be tolerated, switch to oral doxycycline in a dosage of 100 mg every 12 hours for a total duration of IV and oral doxycycline of 7 days.
- Used in conjunction with IV quinidine gluconate (followed by oral quinine sulfate) given for a total duration of 3–7 days.

Pelvic Inflammatory Disease†

IV, THEN ORAL:
- 100 mg every 12 hours. Initially, IV doxycycline in conjunction with IV cefoxitin or cefotetan. Switch IV doxycycline to oral doxycycline in the same dosage as soon as possible and continue for a total duration of 14 days; continue IV cefoxitin or cefotetan for ≥24 hours after clinical improvement occurs.

Plague
Treatment of Pneumonic Plague Occurring in Context of Biologic Warfare or Bioterrorism

IV, THEN ORAL:
- 100 mg every 12 hours or 200 mg once daily.
- Prompt initiation of treatment (within 18–24 hours of symptom onset) is essential. Oral doxycycline may be substituted in the same dosage when the patient's condition improves or

if parenteral doxycycline is unavailable. Total duration of treatment is ≥10–14 days.

Rickettsial Infections
Rocky Mountain Spotted Fever (RMSF)

IV:
- CDC and others recommend 100 mg twice daily. Initiate promptly since delay can result in severe disease and fatal outcome.
- Usually continued ≥5–10 days and until patient is afebrile for ≥3 days and clinically improved. Severe illness may require longer duration of therapy.
- IV therapy generally indicated for hospitalized patients.

Syphilis
Primary or Secondary Syphilis

IV:
- 300 mg daily given for ≥10 days.

Latent Syphilis or Tertiary Syphilis (Except Neurosyphilis)

Tularemia
Treatment

IV, THEN ORAL:
- 100 mg twice daily.
- Oral doxycycline may be substituted in the same dosage when the patient's condition improves or if parenteral doxycycline is unavailable. Total duration of treatment is ≥14–21 days.

Prescribing Limits

Pediatric Patients

Malaria
Treatment of Severe P. falciparum Malaria†

IV:
- Children ≥8 years of age: Maximum 200 mg daily.

Special Populations

Renal Impairment
- Dosage adjustments not necessary.

† Use is not currently included in the labeling approved by the US Food and Drug Administration.

Doxylamine

(dox il′ a meen)

Brand Name: Nighttime Sleep Aid®, Sleep Aid® Liqui-Gels® Maximum Strength, Unisom® Nighttime Sleep Aid

Why is this medicine prescribed?

Doxylamine, an antihistamine, causes drowsiness as a side effect and is used in the short-term treatment of insomnia. It is also used, in combination with decongestants, to relieve cough and cold symptoms.

This medication is sometimes prescribed for other uses; ask your doctor or pharmacist for more information.

How should this medicine be used?

Doxylamine comes as a tablet to take by mouth. It usually is taken 30 minutes before bedtime for sleep. For cold symptoms, doxylamine usually is taken every 4-6 hours. Follow the directions on the package label or on your prescription label carefully, and ask your doctor or pharmacist to explain any part you do not understand. Take doxylamine exactly as directed. Do not take more or less of it or take it more often than prescribed by your doctor.

Do not give doxylamine to a child younger than 12 years of age unless directed to do so by a doctor.

What special precautions should I follow?

Before taking doxylamine,
- tell your doctor and pharmacist if you are allergic to doxylamine or any other drugs.
- tell your doctor and pharmacist what prescription and non-prescription medications you are taking, especially medications for colds, hay fever, or allergies; muscle relaxants; pain medications; sedatives; sleep medications; tranquilizers; and vitamins. Do not take doxylamine if you have taken an MAO inhibitor [phenelzine (Nardil) or tranylcypromine (Parnate)] in the last 2 weeks.
- tell your doctor if you have or have ever had asthma, lung disease, glaucoma, ulcers, difficulty urinating (due to an enlarged prostate gland), heart disease, high blood pressure, seizures, or an overactive thyroid gland.
- tell your doctor if you are pregnant, plan to become pregnant, or are breast-feeding. If you become pregnant while taking doxylamine, call your doctor.
- if you are having surgery, including dental surgery, tell the doctor or dentist that you are taking doxylamine.
- you should know that this drug may make you drowsy. Do not drive a car or operate machinery until you know how this drug affects you.
- remember that alcohol can add to the drowsiness caused by this drug.

What special dietary instructions should I follow?

Doxylamine may cause an upset stomach. Take doxylamine with food or milk.

What should I do if I forget to take a dose?

Take the missed dose as soon as you remember it. However, if it is almost time for the next dose, skip the missed dose and continue your regular dosing schedule. Do not take a double dose to make up for a missed one.

What side effects can this medicine cause?

Doxylamine may cause side effects. Tell your doctor if this symptom is severe or does not go away:
- dry mouth, nose, and throat

If you experience any of the following symptoms, call your doctor immediately:

- vision problems
- difficulty urinating
- muscle weakness
- excitement
- nervousness

If you experience a serious side effect, you or your doctor may send a report to the Food and Drug Administration's (FDA) MedWatch Adverse Event Reporting program online [at http://www.fda.gov/MedWatch/index.html] or by phone [1-800-332-1088].

What storage conditions are needed for this medicine?

Keep this medication in the container it came in, tightly closed, and out of reach of children. Store it at room temperature and away from excess heat and moisture (not in the bathroom). Throw away any medication that is outdated or no longer needed. Talk to your pharmacist about the proper disposal of your medication.

What should I do in case of overdose?

In case of overdose, call your local poison control center at 1-800-222-1222. If the victim has collapsed or is not breathing, call local emergency services at 911.

What other information should I know?

Keep all appointments with your doctor.

Do not let anyone else take your medication. Ask your pharmacist any questions you have about refilling your prescription.

Talk to your doctor, pharmacist, or other healthcare professional if you have questions about dosing information for your medication.

Duloxetine
(doo lox′ e teen)

Brand Name: Cymbalta®

Important Warning

A small number of children, teenagers, and young adults (up to 24 years of age) who took antidepressants ('mood elevators') such as duloxetine during clinical studies became suicidal (thinking about harming or killing oneself or planning or trying to do so). Children, teenagers, and young adults who take antidepressants to treat depression or other mental illnesses may be more likely to become suicidal than children, teenagers, and young adults who do not take antidepressants to treat these conditions. However, experts are not sure about how great this risk is and how much it should be considered in deciding whether a child or teenager should take an antidepressant. Children younger than 18 years of age should not normally take duloxetine, but in some cases, a doctor may decide that duloxetine is the best medication to treat a child's condition.

You should know that your mental health may change in unexpected ways when you take duloxetine or other antidepressants even if you are an adult over age 24. These changes may occur even if you do not have a mental illness and you are taking duloxetine to treat a different type of condition. You may become suicidal, especially at the beginning of your treatment and any time that your dose is increased or decreased. You, your family, or caregiver should call your doctor right away if you experience any of the following symptoms: new or worsening depression; thinking about harming or killing yourself, or planning or trying to do so; extreme worry; agitation; panic attacks; difficulty falling asleep or staying asleep; aggressive behavior; irritability; acting without thinking; severe restlessness; and frenzied abnormal excitement. Be sure that your family or caregiver knows which symptoms may be serious so they can call the doctor when you are unable to seek treatment on your own.

Your healthcare provider will want to see you often while you are taking duloxetine, especially at the beginning of your treatment. Be sure to keep all appointments for office visits with your doctor.

The doctor or pharmacist will give you the manufacturer's patient information sheet (Medication Guide) when you begin treatment with duloxetine. Read the information carefully and ask your doctor or pharmacist if you have any questions. You also can obtain the Medication Guide from the FDA website: http://www.fda.gov/cder/drug/antidepressants/antidepressants _ MG _ 2007.pdf.

No matter your age, before you take an antidepressant, you, your parent, or your caregiver should talk to your doctor about the risks and benefits of treating your condition with an antidepressant or with other treatments. You should also talk about the risks and benefits of not treating your condition. You should know that having depression or another mental illness greatly increases the risk that you will become suicidal. This risk is higher if you or anyone in your family has or has ever had bipolar disorder (mood that changes from depressed to abnormally excited) or mania (frenzied, abnormally excited mood) or has thought about or attempted suicide. Talk to your doctor about your condition, symptoms, and personal and family medical history. You and your doctor will decide what type of treatment is right for you.

Why is this medicine prescribed?

Duloxetine is used to treat depression and generalized anxiety disorder (GAD; excessive worry and tension that disrupts daily life and lasts for 6 months or longer). Duloxetine is also used to treat pain and tingling caused by diabetic neuropathy (damage to nerves that can develop in people who have diabetes). Duloxetine is in a class of medications called selective serotonin and norepinephrine reuptake inhibitors (SSNRIs). It works by increasing the amounts of serotonin and norepinephrine, natural substances in the brain that help maintain mental balance and stop the movement of pain signals in the brain.

How should this medicine be used?

Duloxetine comes as a delayed release (long-acting) capsule to take by mouth. When duloxetine is used to treat depression, it is usually taken once or twice a day with or without food. When duloxetine is used to treat generalized anxiety disorder or the pain of diabetic neuropathy, it is usually taken once a day with or without food. Take duloxetine at around the same time(s) every day. Follow the directions on your prescription label carefully, and ask your doctor or pharmacist to explain any part you do not understand. Take duloxetine exactly as directed. Do not take more or less of it, take it more often, or take it for a longer time than prescribed by your doctor.

Swallow the capsules whole; do not split, chew, or crush them. Do not open the capsules and mix the contents with liquids or sprinkle the contents on food.

If you are taking duloxetine to treat generalized anxiety disorder or the pain of diabetic neuropathy, your doctor may start you on a low dose of medication and gradually increase your dose.

Duloxetine may help control your symptoms but will not cure your condition. It may take 1-4 weeks or longer before you feel the full benefit of duloxetine. Continue to take duloxetine even if you feel well. Do not stop taking duloxetine without talking to your doctor. Your doctor will probably decrease your dose gradually. If you suddenly stop taking duloxetine, you may experience withdrawal symptoms such as dizziness, nausea, vomiting, headache, pain, burning or tingling in the hands or feet, irritability, and nightmares. Tell your doctor if you experience any of these symptoms when your dose of duloxetine is decreased.

Are there other uses for this medicine?

Duloxetine is also sometimes used to treat stress urinary incontinence (leakage of urine during physical activity such as coughing, sneezing, laughing, and exercise) in women. Talk to your doctor about using this medication to treat your condition.

This medication may be prescribed for other uses; ask your doctor or pharmacist for more information.

What special precautions should I follow?

Before taking duloxetine,

- tell your doctor and pharmacist if you are allergic to duloxetine or any other medications.
- tell your doctor if you are taking thioridazine or a monoamine oxidase (MAO) inhibitor, such as isocarboxazid (Marplan), phenelzine (Nardil), selegiline (Eldepryl, Emsam, Zelapar), and tranylcypromine (Parnate), or if you have stopped taking an MAO inhibitor within the past 14 days. Your doctor will probably tell you not to take duloxetine. If you stop taking duloxetine, you should wait at least 5 days before you start to take an MAO inhibitor.
- tell your doctor and pharmacist what other prescription and nonprescription medications, vitamins, and nutritional supplements you are taking or plan to take. Be sure to mention any of the following: anticoagulants ('blood thinners') such as warfarin (Coumadin); antidepressants such as amitriptyline (Elavil), amoxapine (Asendin), clomipramine (Anafranil), desipramine (Norpramin), doxepin (Adapin, Sinequan), imipramine (Tofranil), nortriptyline (Aventyl, Pamelor), protriptyline (Vivactil), and trimipramine (Surmontil); antihistamines; cimetidine (Tagamet); diuretics ('water pills'); linezolid (Zyvox); medications for irregular heartbeat such as amiodarone (Cordarone), flecainide (Tambocor), moricizine (Ethmozine), quinidine (Quinidex) and propafenone (Rythmol); medications for anxiety, high blood pressure, mental illness, pain, and nausea; propranolol (Inderal); medications for migraine headaches such as almotriptan (Axert), eletriptan (Relpax), frovatriptan (Frova), naratriptan (Amerge), rizatriptan (Maxalt), sumatriptan (Imitrex), and zolmitriptan (Zomig); lithium (Eskalith, Lithobid); proton pump inhibitors such as lansoprazole (Prevacid), omeprazole (Prilosec), pantoprazole (Protonix), and rabeprazole (Aciphex); quinolone antibiotics such as ciprofloxacin (Cipro) and enoxacin (Penetrex); sedatives; certain selective serotonin reuptake inhibitors (SSRIs) such as fluoxetine (Prozac, Sarafem), fluvoxamine (Luvox) and paroxetine (Paxil); sleeping pills; theophylline (Theochron, Theolair); tramadol (Ultram); and tranquilizers. Many other medications may interact with duloxetine, so be sure to tell your doctor about all the medications you are taking, even those that do not appear on this list. Your doctor may need to change the doses of your medications or monitor you carefully for side effects.
- tell your doctor what herbal products you are taking, especially products containing St. John's wort or tryptophan.
- tell your doctor if you have or have ever had glaucoma (an eye condition). Your doctor may tell you that you should not take duloxetine.
- tell your doctor if you drink or have ever drunk large amounts of alcohol or if you use or have ever used street drugs or have ever overused prescription medications.

Also tell your doctor if you have or have ever had a heart attack; high blood pressure; seizures; coronary artery disease (blockage or narrowing of the blood vessels that lead to the heart; or heart, liver, or kidney disease. If you have diabetes, be sure to talk to your doctor about how serious your condition is so your doctor can decide if duloxetine is right for you.

- tell your doctor if you are pregnant, plan to become pregnant, or are breast-feeding. If you become pregnant while taking duloxetine, call your doctor.
- if you are having surgery, including dental surgery, tell the doctor or dentist that you are taking duloxetine.
- you should know that duloxetine may make you drowsy or dizzy. Do not drive a car or operate machinery until you know how this medication affects you.
- ask your doctor about the safe use of alcoholic beverages while you are taking duloxetine. Alcohol can increase the risk of serious side effects from duloxetine.
- you should know that duloxetine may cause dizziness, lightheadedness, and fainting when you get up too quickly from a lying position. This is more common when you first start taking duloxetine. To avoid this problem, get out of bed slowly, resting your feet on the floor for a few minutes before standing up.

What special dietary instructions should I follow?

Unless your doctor tells you otherwise, continue your normal diet.

What should I do if I forget to take a dose?

Take the missed dose as soon as you remember it. However, if it is almost time for the next dose, skip the missed dose and continue your regular dosing schedule. Do not take a double dose to make up for a missed one.

What side effects can this medicine cause?

Duloxetine may cause side effects. Tell your doctor if any of these symptoms are severe or do not go away:

- nausea
- vomiting
- constipation
- diarrhea
- heartburn
- stomach pain
- decreased appetite
- dry mouth
- increased urination
- difficulty urinating
- sweating or night sweats
- dizziness
- headache
- extreme tiredness
- weakness
- muscle pain or cramps

- changes in sexual desire or ability
- uncontrollable shaking of a part of the body

Some side effects can be serious. If you experience any of the following side effects, or those mentioned in the IMPORTANT WARNING section, call your doctor immediately:

- unusual bruising or bleeding
- pain in the upper right part of the stomach
- itching
- yellowing of the skin or eyes
- dark colored urine
- flu-like symptoms
- blurred vision
- fever
- blisters
- rash
- hives
- swelling of the eyes, face, lips, tongue, throat, hands, arms, feet, ankles, or lower legs
- difficulty breathing or swallowing

Duloxetine may cause other side effects. Call your doctor if you have any unusual problems while taking this medication.

What storage conditions are needed for this medicine?

Keep this medication in the container it came in, tightly closed, and out of reach of children. Store it at room temperature and away from excess heat and moisture (not in the bathroom). Throw away any medication that is outdated or no longer needed. Talk to your pharmacist about the proper disposal of your medication.

What should I do in case of overdose?

In case of overdose, call your local poison control center at 1-800-222-1222. If the victim has collapsed or is not breathing, call local emergency services at 911.

Symptoms of overdose may include:

- agitation
- hallucinating (seeing things or hearing voices that do not exist)
- fast heartbeat
- fever
- loss of coordination
- nausea
- vomiting
- diarrhea
- drowsiness
- seizures

What other information should I know?

Keep all appointments with your doctor.

Do not let anyone else take your medication. Ask your pharmacist any questions you have about refilling your prescription.

Dosage Facts
For Informational Purposes

Caution: Do not change your dose, how often you take your medication, or the length of time you are to take it without first talking to your healthcare provider.

The following dosage information was written using medical language for doctors and other healthcare professionals and is provided here for you to check your dosage. The dosage of this drug may differ for different patients. Therefore, always follow your doctor's instructions or the directions on the label. Contact your healthcare provider or pharmacist if you have any questions about the specific dosage of your medication after reviewing this information.

General Dosage Information

Available as duloxetine hydrochloride; dosage expressed in terms of duloxetine.

Adult Patients

Major Depressive Disorder

ORAL:
- 40-60 mg daily (as a single dose or in 2 equally divided doses).
- Optimum duration not established; may require several months of therapy or longer.
- Periodically reassess need for continued therapy and appropriateness of dosage.

Neuropathic Pain
Diabetic Neuropathy

ORAL:
- 60 mg once daily; consider lower initial dosage if suspect tolerability issues in patient.
- Assess efficacy individually; progression of diabetic peripheral neuropathy is highly variable, and pain management is empirical.
- Long-term efficacy not established in controlled studies.

Prescribing Limits

Adult Patients

Major Depressive Disorder

ORAL:
- Dosages >60 mg daily apparently do not provide additional benefit.

Neuropathic Pain
Diabetic Neuropathy

ORAL:
- Dosages >60 mg daily apparently do not substantially increase benefit and are less well tolerated.

Special Populations

Hepatic Impairment
- Use not recommended.

Renal Impairment
- Consider lower initial dosage in patients with mild to moderate renal impairment (Cl_{cr} 30–80 mL/minute), and increase gradually; do not administer if Cl_{cr} <30 mL/minute or if end-stage renal disease (requiring dialysis) present.

Geriatric Patients
- No dosage adjustment recommended, but use caution when increasing dosage.

Breastfeeding Patients
- No dosage adjustment recommended.

Dutasteride

(doo tas′ teer ide)

Brand Name: Avodart®

Why is this medicine prescribed?

Dutasteride is used to treat an enlarged prostate (benign prostatic hyperplasia, or BPH). Dutasteride is in a class of medications called 5-alpha reductase inhibitors. It works by blocking the production of a natural substance that enlarges the prostate. This shrinks the prostate, relieves symptoms of BPH, such as frequent and difficult urination, and decreases the chance that surgery will be needed to treat this condition.

How should this medicine be used?

Dutasteride comes as a capsule to take by mouth. It is usually taken once a day with or without food. To help you remember to take dutasteride, take it around the same time every day. Follow the directions on your prescription label carefully, and ask your doctor or pharmacist to explain any part you do not understand. Take dutasteride exactly as directed. Do not take more or less of it or take it more often than prescribed by your doctor.

Swallow the capsules whole; do not split, chew, or crush them.

Are there other uses for this medicine?

This medication may be prescribed for other uses; ask your doctor or pharmacist for more information.

What special precautions should I follow?

Before taking dutasteride,
- tell your doctor and pharmacist if you are allergic to dutasteride, finasteride (Propecia, Proscar), or any other medications.
- tell your doctor and pharmacist what prescription and nonprescription medications, vitamins, nutritional supplements, and herbal products you are taking. Be sure to mention any of the following: antifungals such as fluconazole, (Diflucan), itraconazole (Sporanox), and ketoconazole (Nizoral); cimetidine (Tagamet); ciprofloxacin (Cipro); clarithromycin (Biaxin); cyclosporine (Neoral, Sandimmune); danazol (Danocrine); delavir-

dine (Rescriptor); diltiazem (Cardizem, Dilacor, Tiazac); erythromycin (E.E.S., E-Mycin, Erythrocin); fluoxetine (Prozac, Sarafem); fluvoxamine (Luvox); HIV protease inhibitors such as indinavir (Crixivan) and ritonavir (Norvir); isoniazid (INH, Nydrazid); metronidazole (Flagyl); nefazodone (Serzone); troleandomycin (TAO); verapamil (Calan, Covera, Isoptin, Verelan); and zafirlukast (Accolate). Your doctor may need to change the doses of your medications or monitor you carefully for side effects.
- tell your doctor if you have or have ever had liver disease or prostate cancer.
- you should know that dutasteride is for use only in men. Women, especially those who are or may become pregnant, should not handle dutasteride capsules. Touching the contents of the capsules may harm the fetus. Women who accidentally touch leaking capsules should wash the area with soap and water immediately.
- you should know that you should not donate blood while you are taking dutasteride and for 6 months after you stop taking this medication.

What special dietary instructions should I follow?

Talk to your doctor about drinking grapefruit juice while taking this medicine.

What should I do if I forget to take a dose?

Take the missed dose as soon as you remember it. However, if it is almost time for the next dose, skip the missed dose and continue your regular dosing schedule. Do not take a double dose to make up for a missed one.

What side effects can this medicine cause?

Dutasteride may cause side effects. Tell your doctor if any of these symptoms are severe or do not go away:
- inability to have or maintain an erection
- decrease in sex drive
- difficulty ejaculating
- breast tenderness or enlargement

Dutasteride may cause other side effects. Call your doctor if you have any unusual problems while taking this medication.

What storage conditions are needed for this medicine?

Keep this medication in the container it came in, tightly closed, and out of reach of children. Store it at room temperature and away from excess heat and moisture (not in the bathroom). Throw away any medication that is outdated or no longer needed. Talk to your pharmacist about the proper disposal of your medication.

What should I do in case of overdose?

In case of overdose, call your local poison control center at 1-800-222-1222. If the victim has collapsed or is not breathing, call local emergency services at 911.

What other information should I know?

Keep all appointments with your doctor and the laboratory. Your doctor will order certain lab tests to check your body's response to dutasteride.

Before having any laboratory test, tell your doctor and the laboratory personnel that you are taking dutasteride.

Do not let anyone else take your medication. Ask your pharmacist any questions you have about refilling your prescription.

Dosage Facts
For Informational Purposes

Caution: Do not change your dose, how often you take your medication, or the length of time you are to take it without first talking to your healthcare provider.

The following dosage information was written using medical language for doctors and other healthcare professionals and is provided here for you to check your dosage. The dosage of this drug may differ for different patients. Therefore, always follow your doctor's instructions or the directions on the label. Contact your healthcare provider or pharmacist if you have any questions about the specific dosage of your medication after reviewing this information.

Adult Patients
Benign Prostatic Hyperplasia
ORAL:
- Initially and for maintenance therapy, 0.5 mg once daily.
- While early symptomatic improvement (e.g., within 3 months) may occur, a minimum of 6 months of therapy may be necessary to determine clinical benefit. Generally, therapy is continued for life.

Special Populations
Hepatic Impairment
- No specific dosage recommendations for hepatic impairment.
Renal Impairment
- Dosage adjustment not required.
Geriatric Patients
- Dosage adjustment not required.

Econazole Topical

(e kon′ na zole)

Brand Name: Spectazole®
Also available generically.

Why is this medicine prescribed?

Econazole is used to treat skin infections such as athlete's foot, jock itch, and ringworm.

This medication is sometimes prescribed for other uses; ask your doctor or pharmacist for more information.

How should this medicine be used?

Econazole comes as a cream to apply to the skin. Econazole is usually used once or twice a day, in the morning and evening, for 2 weeks. Some infections require up to 6 weeks of treatment. Follow the directions on your prescription label carefully, and ask your doctor or pharmacist to explain any part you do not understand. Use econazole exactly as directed. Do not use more or less of it or use it more often than prescribed by your doctor.

Thoroughly clean the infected area, allow it to dry, and then gently rub the medication in until most of it disappears. Use just enough medication to cover the affected area. You should wash your hands after applying the medication.

Continue to use econazole even if you feel well. Do not stop using econazole without talking to your doctor.

What special precautions should I follow?

Before using econazole,
- tell your doctor and pharmacist if you are allergic to econazole or any other drugs.
- tell your doctor and pharmacist what prescription and nonprescription drugs you are taking, including vitamins.
- tell your doctor if you are pregnant, plan to become pregnant, or are breast-feeding. If you become pregnant while using econazole, call your doctor.

What should I do if I forget to take a dose?

Apply the missed dose as soon as you remember it. However, if it is almost time for the next dose, skip the missed dose and continue your regular dosing schedule. Do not apply a double dose to make up for a missed one.

What side effects can this medicine cause?

Econazole may cause side effects. If you experience any of the following symptoms, call your doctor immediately:
- itching
- burning
- irritation
- stinging
- redness
- rash

If you experience a serious side effect, you or your doctor may send a report to the Food and Drug Administration's (FDA) MedWatch Adverse Event Reporting program online [at http://www.fda.gov/MedWatch/index.html] or by phone [1-800-332-1088].

What storage conditions are needed for this medicine?

Keep this medication in the container it came in, tightly closed, and out of reach of children. Store it at room temperature and away from excess heat and moisture (not in the bathroom). Throw away any medication that is outdated or no longer needed. Talk to your pharmacist about the proper disposal of your medication.

What other information should I know?

Keep all appointments with your doctor. Econazole is for external use only. Do not let econazole get into your eyes or mouth, and do not swallow it. Do not apply cosmetics, lotions, or other skin medications to the area being treated unless your doctor tells you.

Do not let anyone else use your medication. Ask your pharmacist any questions you have about refilling your prescription. If you still have symptoms of infection after you finish econazole, call your doctor.

Dosage Facts
For Informational Purposes

Caution: Do not change your dose, how often you take your medication, or the length of time you are to take it without first talking to your healthcare provider.

The following dosage information was written using medical language for doctors and other healthcare professionals and is provided here for you to check your dosage. The dosage of this drug may differ for different patients. Therefore, always follow your doctor's instructions or the directions on the label. Contact your healthcare provider or pharmacist if you have any questions about the specific dosage of your medication after reviewing this information.

Pediatric Patients

Dermatophytoses
Tinea Corporis or Tinea Cruris

TOPICAL:
- Apply once daily for 2 weeks.
- If clinical improvement does not occur after treatment, re-evaluate diagnosis. Occasionally, a treatment duration of ≥6 weeks may be necessary.

Tinea Pedis

TOPICAL:
- Apply once daily for 1 month.
- If clinical improvement does not occur after treatment, re-

evaluate diagnosis. Occasionally, a treatment duration of ≥6 weeks may be necessary.

Pityriasis (Tinea) Versicolor

TOPICAL:
- Apply once daily for 2 weeks.
- If clinical improvement does not occur after treatment, re-evaluate diagnosis.

Cutaneous Candidiasis

TOPICAL:
- Apply twice daily (morning and evening) for 2 weeks.
- If clinical improvement does not occur after treatment, re-evaluate diagnosis. Occasionally, a treatment duration of ≥6 weeks may be necessary.

Adult Patients

Dermatophytoses

Tinea Corporis or Tinea Cruris

TOPICAL:
- Apply once daily for 2 weeks.
- If clinical improvement does not occur after treatment, re-evaluate diagnosis. Occasionally, a treatment duration of ≥6 weeks may be necessary.

Tinea Pedis

TOPICAL:
- Apply once daily for 1 month.
- If clinical improvement does not occur after treatment, re-evaluate diagnosis. Occasionally, a treatment duration of ≥6 weeks may be necessary.

Pityriasis (Tinea) Versicolor

TOPICAL:
- Apply once daily for 2 weeks.
- If clinical improvement does not occur after treatment, re-evaluate diagnosis.

Cutaneous Candidiasis

TOPICAL:
- Apply twice daily (morning and evening) for 2 weeks.
- If clinical improvement does not occur after treatment, re-evaluate diagnosis. Occasionally, a treatment duration of ≥6 weeks may be necessary.

Special Populations

No special population dosage recommendations at this time.

Efalizumab Injection

(e fa li zoo′ mab)

Brand Name: Raptiva®

Why is this medicine prescribed?

Efalizumab is used to treat chronic (long-lasting) plaque psoriasis (a skin disease in which red scaly patches form on some areas of the body) in patients who cannot be treated with medications that are applied to the skin. Efalizumab is in a class of medications called immunosuppressants. It works by stopping the action of cells in the body that cause the symptoms of psoriasis.

How should this medicine be used?

Efalizumab comes as a powder to mix with sterile water and inject subcutaneously (under the skin). It is usually injected once a week. You should inject efalizumab on the same day every week. Follow the directions on your prescription label carefully, and ask your doctor or pharmacist to explain any part you do not understand. Use efalizumab exactly as directed. Do not use more or less of it or use it more often or for a longer period of time than prescribed by your doctor.

Your doctor will probably start you on a low dose of efalizumab and increase your dose after 1 week.

Efalizumab controls chronic plaque psoriasis but does not cure it. It may take several weeks before you feel the full benefit of efalizumab. Do not stop taking efalizumab without talking to your doctor.

You can inject efalizumab yourself or have a friend or relative give the injections. Your doctor will train the person who will be injecting the medication, and will test him to be sure he can give the injections correctly. Be sure that you and the person who will be giving the injections read the manufacturer's information for the patient that comes with efalizumab before you use it for the first time at home.

If you are injecting efalizumab yourself, you can inject it anywhere on your thighs or stomach. If someone else will be giving you your injections, he or she can also inject the medication anywhere on the back of your upper arms or buttocks. To reduce the chances of soreness or redness, choose a different area for each injection. If your doctor has told you to use two injections for each dose, choose two spots that are at least 1 inch apart. Do not inject efalizumab near a vein that you can see through the surface of the skin. Try to inject efalizumab in skin that is free of symptoms of psoriasis.

Never reuse needles, syringes, vials of efalizumab, or syringes of sterile water. You can throw away used alcohol pads, needle caps, and vials in the trash. Throw away used needles and syringes in a puncture-resistant container out of the reach of children. Talk to your doctor or pharmacist about what to do with the puncture-resistant container when it is full.

Never mix efalizumab powder with any liquid other than the sterile water provided. Never add any other medications to the syringe you will use to inject efalizumab.

To prepare and inject efalizumab, follow these steps:
1. Take one or two blister trays of efalizumab and supplies out of the refrigerator and place the tray(s) on a clean, well-lit, flat work surface. You will need one tray if your doctor has told you to inject 1.25 mL or less each week or two trays if your doctor has told you to inject more than 1.25 mL each week. You will also need to prepare sterile gauze and an adhesive bandage.
2. Wash your hands well with soap and warm water.
3. Open the blister tray(s) and place the contents on the

work surface. Each tray should contain one vial of efalizumab, one prefilled syringe of sterile water, two alcohol pads, and two needles. The vial(s) of efalizumab and syringe(s) of sterile water should be marked with expiration dates that have not passed. Call your pharmacist if your tray(s) do not contain all of these supplies or if your medication or water has expired.

4. Wait to allow the medication and water to warm to room temperature

      Steps 5-14 tell how to mix efalizumab with sterile water. If your dose is more than 1.25 mL, you will need to follow these directions twice to prepare two separate vials of efalizumab.

5. Remove the plastic cap from the vial of efalizumab and wipe the rubber stopper with an alcohol pad. When you handle the vial, be careful not to touch the rubber stopper with your fingers.

6. Remove one of the needles from its package, but do not remove the cap.

7. Remove the cap from the tip of the prefilled syringe, and place the capped needle onto the syringe tip. Twist the needle cap to secure it into place.

8. Remove the cap from the needle but be careful not to touch the needle with your fingers.

9. Place the vial of efalizumab upright on a firm surface and slowly push the needle through the rubber stopper.

10. Aim the tip of the needle toward the wall of the vial and slowly push down on the plunger to inject all of the sterile water into the vial. The powder in the vial may foam when you inject the water.

11. Leave the needle and syringe in the vial stopper. Pick up the vial and swirl it gently to mix the medication. Do not shake the vial.

12. Wait 5 minutes to allow the medication to dissolve.

13. Look at the vial to be sure it contains a clear or pale yellow liquid. Call your pharmacist and do not use the liquid if it is cloudy, contains particles, or is a different color.

      Steps 14-29 tell how to fill the syringe with the correct amount of medication and inject the medication. If your dose is more than 1.25 mL, you will need to follow these steps twice to fill and inject two syringes that each contain half of your dose.

14. Pick up the vial and turn it upside down without removing the needle. The entire tip of the needle should be covered by the liquid in the vial.

15. Pull back the plunger to fill the syringe with the amount of medication your doctor told you to use. (If your dose is more than 1.25 mL, you will fill the syringe with half the amount of medication your doctor told you to use and then prepare a second syringe containing the other half of your dose.) Line up the plunger with the right number on the side of the syringe to fill the syringe with the right amount of medication.

16. Remove the needle and syringe from the vial. Place the needle cap on a flat surface and slide the needle into the cap. Push the cap all the way down over the needle.

17. Hold the syringe upright and tap it to push any air bubbles to the top. Gently push in the plunger to push the air bubbles out.

18. Check that the syringe contains the right amount of medication. If the amount of liquid in the syringe goes past the line that matches your dose, push the plunger up slowly to release the extra medication.

19. Twist the capped needle off of the syringe and throw it away in a puncture-resistant container.

20. Hold the plastic cover of the second needle and remove the needle from the package. Be careful not to touch the uncovered end of the needle.

21. Place the capped needle on the syringe tip and twist it in place. Put the syringe and needle on a flat surface.

22. Wash your hands and the skin in the area where you plan to inject the medication with soap and warm water.

23. Let the skin in the area where you will inject efalizumab air dry, then clean it with an alcohol pad or alcohol-soaked cotton ball using a circular motion. Allow the skin to air dry again and do not touch it with your fingers until after you are finished injecting your medication.

24. Pick up the syringe and remove the needle cap by twisting and pulling it. Be careful not to touch the needle to your fingers or any surface.

25. Hold the syringe firmly between your thumb and fingers with one hand and use your other hand to pinch a fold of skin in the area where you will inject your medication.

26. Push the needle straight into your skin at a 90-degree angle.

27. Let go of the pinched fold of skin and use that hand to slowly push down on the plunger until it stops.

28. Remove the needle from your skin and throw it away in a puncture-resistant container. Do not recap the needle.

29. Use a dry sterile gauze pad to press down on the spot where you injected efalizumab. Do not use an alcohol wipe. You may cover the spot with a small bandage if needed.

Are there other uses for this medicine?

This medication may be prescribed for other uses; ask your doctor or pharmacist for more information.

What special precautions should I follow?

Before using efalizumab,

- tell your doctor and pharmacist if you are allergic to efalizumab or any other medications.
- tell your doctor and pharmacist what prescription and nonprescription medications, vitamins, nutritional supplements, and herbal products you are taking or plan to take. Be sure to mention any of the following: other medications for psoriasis; oral steroids such as dexamethasone (Decadron, Dexone), methylprednisolone (Medrol), and prednisone (Deltasone); and medications

that suppress the immune system such as azathioprine (Imuran), cancer chemotherapy medications, cyclosporine (Neoral, Sandimmune), methotrexate (Rheumatrex), sirolimus (Rapamune), and tacrolimus (Prograf). Your doctor may need to change the doses of your medications or monitor you carefully for side effects.

- tell your doctor if you or any of your close relatives have or have ever had cancer or if you have or have ever had any disease that affects your immune system such as human immunodeficiency virus (HIV), acquired immunodeficiency syndrome (AIDS), or severe combined immunodeficiency syndrome (SCID), or if you have liver or kidney disease. Also tell your doctor if you have any type of infection, including infections that come and go (such as cold sores) and chronic infections that never go away, or if you frequently get any type of infection (such as urinary tract or bladder infections).
- tell your doctor if your psoriasis is being treated with phototherapy (a treatment for psoriasis that involves exposing the skin to ultraviolet light).
- tell your doctor if you are pregnant, plan to become pregnant, or are breast-feeding. If you become pregnant while using efalizumab or within 6 weeks after you stop using efalizumab, call your doctor.
- if you are having surgery, including dental surgery, tell the doctor or dentist that you are using efalizumab.
- do not have any vaccinations (shots to prevent diseases) without talking to your doctor.
- you should know that efalizumab may decrease your ability to fight infection and increase the risk that you will develop a serious infection. Stay away from people who are sick and wash your hands often while you are using this medication.
- you should know that your psoriasis may worsen or you may develop a new type of psoriasis during or after your treatment with efalizumab. Call your doctor if you notice a new or worsening rash during or after your treatment.
- tell your doctor if you gain or lose weight while you are using efalizumab. Your doctor may have to change the dose of your medication if your weight changes. Do not change the dose of your medication without talking to your doctor.

What special dietary instructions should I follow?

Unless your doctor tells you otherwise, continue your normal diet.

What should I do if I forget to take a dose?

Call your doctor to find out when you should inject your next dose and what schedule you should follow after that. Never inject a double dose to make up for a missed one.

What side effects can this medicine cause?

Efalizumab may cause side effects. Tell your doctor if any of these symptoms are severe or do not go away:

- headache, fever, chills, upset stomach, vomiting, and muscle pain within 48 hours of injecting the first two doses.
- back pain
- acne

Some side effects can be serious. If you experience any of the following symptoms, call your doctor immediately:

- sore throat, fever, chills, cough, or other signs of infection
- flu-like symptoms
- easy bruising or bleeding
- bleeding gums
- tiny red spots under surface of skin
- weakness
- lightheadedness
- dark or red urine
- yellowing of the skin or eyes
- red, stiff, swollen, or painful joints
- hives
- itching
- difficulty breathing or swallowing
- wheezing
- swelling of the face, throat, tongue, lips, eyes, hands, feet, ankles, or lower legs
- hoarseness
- rash or blisters
- unusual skin changes or sores on the skin
- new lumps or masses anywhere in your body

Efalizumab may increase the risk that you will develop cancer. Talk to your doctor about the risks of using this medication.

Efalizumab may cause other side effects. Call your doctor if you have any unusual problems while using this medication.

If you experience a serious side effect, you or your doctor may send a report to the Food and Drug Administration's (FDA) MedWatch Adverse Event Reporting program online [at http://www.fda.gov/MedWatch/index.html] or by phone [1-800-332-1088].

What storage conditions are needed for this medicine?

Keep this medication in the carton it came in, tightly closed, away from light, and out of reach of children. Store unopened blister trays of efalizumab in the refrigerator, but do not freeze them. You may store mixtures of efalizumab and sterile water for up to 8 hours at room temperature. Throw away mixtures of efalizumab and sterile water after 8 hours have passed and throw away any medication that is outdated or no longer needed. Talk to your pharmacist about the proper disposal of your medication.

What should I do in case of overdose?

In case of overdose, call your local poison control center at 1-800-222-1222. If the victim has collapsed or is not breathing, call local emergency services at 911.

Symptoms of overdose may include:
- severe vomiting

What other information should I know?

Keep all appointments with your doctor and the laboratory. Your doctor will order certain lab tests to check your body's response to efalizumab.

Before having any laboratory tests, tell your doctor and the laboratory personnel that you are using efalizumab.

Do not let anyone else use your medication. Ask your pharmacist any questions you have about refilling your prescription.

Dosage Facts
For Informational Purposes

Caution: Do not change your dose, how often you take your medication, or the length of time you are to take it without first talking to your healthcare provider.

The following dosage information was written using medical language for doctors and other healthcare professionals and is provided here for you to check your dosage. The dosage of this drug may differ for different patients. Therefore, always follow your doctor's instructions or the directions on the label. Contact your healthcare provider or pharmacist if you have any questions about the specific dosage of your medication after reviewing this information.

Adult Patients
Psoriasis

SUB-Q:
- Initial dose of 0.7 mg/kg, followed by 1 mg/kg (maximum 200 mg) once weekly.

Prescribing Limits
Adult Patients
Psoriasis

SUB-Q:
- Maximum single dose: 200 mg.
- Safety and efficacy of efalizumab therapy beyond one year's duration not established.

Efavirenz
(e fa veer′ ens)

Brand Name: Atripla® as a combination product containing Efavirenz, Emtricitabine, and Tenofovir, Sustiva®

Why is this medicine prescribed?

Efavirenz is used with other medications to treat human immunodeficiency virus (HIV) infection in patients with or without acquired immunodeficiency syndrome (AIDS). Efavirenz is in a class of medications called nonnucleoside reverse transcriptase inhibitors (NNRTIs). It works by slowing the spread of HIV in the body. Efavirenz does not cure HIV infection and may not prevent you from developing HIV-related illnesses. Efavirenz does not prevent you from spreading HIV to other people.

How should this medicine be used?

Efavirenz comes as a capsule and as a tablet to take by mouth. It is usually taken once a day with plenty of water on an empty stomach. Take efavirenz at around the same time every day. Taking efavirenz at bedtime may make side effects less bothersome. Follow the directions on your prescription label carefully, and ask your doctor or pharmacist to explain any part you do not understand. Take efavirenz exactly as directed. Do not take more or less of it or take it more often than prescribed by your doctor.

Efavirenz controls HIV infection, but does not cure it. Continue to take efavirenz even if you feel well. Do not stop taking efavirenz without talking to your doctor. When your supply of efavirenz starts to run low, get more from your doctor or pharmacist. If you miss doses or stop taking efavirenz, your condition may become more difficult to treat.

Are there other uses for this medicine?

Efavirenz is also used with another medication to help prevent infection in health care workers or other people who were accidentally exposed to HIV. Talk to your doctor about the possible risks of using this medication for your condition.

This medication may be prescribed for other uses; ask your doctor or pharmacist for more information.

What special precautions should I follow?

Before taking efavirenz,
- tell your doctor and pharmacist if you are allergic to efavirenz or any other medications.
- do not take astemizole (Hismanal) (no longer available in the United States); cisapride (Propulsid) (no longer available in the United States); ergot-type medications such as bromocriptine (Parlodel), cabergoline (Dostinex), dihydroergotamine (D.H.E. 45, Migranal), ergoloid mesylates (Germinal, Hydergine), ergonovine (Ergotrate), ergotamine (Bellergal-S, Cafergot, Ergomar,

Wigraine), methylergonovine (Methergine), methysergide (Sansert), and pergolide (Permax); midazolam (Versed); triazolam (Halcion); or voriconazole (Vfend) while taking efavirenz.

- tell your doctor and pharmacist what other prescription and nonprescription medications, vitamins, and nutritional supplements you are taking or plan to take. Be sure to mention any of the following: acetaminophen (Tylenol, others); anticoagulants ('blood thinners') such as warfarin (Coumadin); antidepressants; antifungals such as itraconazole (Sporanox), and ketoconazole (Nizoral); calcium channel blockers such as amlodipine (Norvasc), diltiazem (Cardizem, Dilacor, Tiazac, others), felodipine (Lexxel, Plendil), nifedipine (Adalat, Procardia), nisoldipine (Sular), and verapamil (Calan, Covera, Isoptin, Verelan); chlorpheniramine in over-the-counter cold products; cholesterol-lowering medications (statins); cimetidine (Tagamet); clarithromycin (Biaxin, Prevpac); danazol (Danocrine); dexamethasone (Decadron); erythromycin (E.E.S., E-Mycin, Erythrocin); iron products; isoniazid (INH, Nydrazid); medications for anxiety, mental illness, or pain; medications for HIV or AIDS such as amprenavir (Agenerase), atazanavir (Reyataz); indinavir (Crixivan), lopinavir (in Kaletra); ritonavir (Norvir, in Kaletra) and saquinavir (Invirase); medications for seizures such as carbamazepine (Tegretol), phenobarbital, and phenytoin (Dilantin, Phenytek); methotrexate (Rheumatrex); methadone (Dolophine); metronidazole (Flagyl); niacin (nicotinic acid); nonsteroidal anti-inflammatory medications (NSAIDs) such as celecoxib (Celebrex), diclofenac (Voltaren), ibuprofen (Advil, Motrin), naproxen (Aleve, Anaprox, Naprosyn), and piroxicam (Feldene); oral medications for diabetes such as glipizide (Glucotrol, Metaglip) and tolbutamide (Orinase); proton pump inhibitors such as lansoprazole (Prevacid), omeprazole (Prilosec), and pantoprazole (Protonix); quinidine (Quinidex); quinine; rifabutin (Mycobutin); rifampin (Rifadin, Rimactane); sedatives; sertraline (Zoloft); sildenafil (Viagra); sleeping pills; sulfamethoxazole (Bactrim, Septra); tamoxifen (Nolvadex); torsemide (Demadex); tranquilizers; troleandomycin (TAO); or zafirlukast (Accolate). Your doctor may need to change the doses of your medications or monitor you carefully for side effects.
- tell your doctor what herbal products you are taking, especially products that contain kava or St. John's wort.
- tell your doctor if you drink or have ever drunk large amounts of alcohol; if you use or have ever used street drugs or have overused prescription medications; or if you have or have ever had seizures; high cholesterol; depression or other mental illness; or heart, liver, or pancreas disease.
- you should not become pregnant while taking efavirenz. You will have to have a negative pregnancy test before you begin taking this medication and use effective birth control during your treatment. Efavirenz may interfere

with the action of hormonal contraceptives (birth control pills, patches, rings, implants, or injections, so you should not use these as your only method of birth control during your treatment. You must use a barrier method of birth control (device that blocks sperm from entering the uterus such as a condom or a diaphragm) along with any other method of birth control you have chosen. Ask your doctor to help you choose a method of birth control that will work for you. If you become pregnant while taking efavirenz, call your doctor. Efavirenz may harm the fetus.

- you should not breastfeed if you are infected with HIV or are taking efavirenz.
- if you are having surgery, including dental surgery, tell the doctor or dentist that you are taking efavirenz.
- you should know that efavirenz may make you drowsy, dizzy, or unable to concentrate. Do not drive a car or operate machinery until you know how this medication affects you.
- ask your doctor about the safe use of alcoholic beverages while you are taking efavirenz. Alcohol can make the side effects from efavirenz worse.
- you should know that your body fat may increase or move to different areas of your body such as your breasts and upper back.
- you should know that efavirenz may cause changes in your thoughts, behavior, or mental health. Call your doctor immediately if you develop any of the following symptoms while you are taking efavirenz: depression, thinking about killing yourself or planning or trying to do so, angry or aggressive behavior, hallucinations (seeing things or hearing voices that do not exist), or loss of touch with reality. Be sure your family knows which symptoms may be serious so that they can call your doctor if you are unable to seek treatment on your own.

What special dietary instructions should I follow?

Talk to your doctor about eating grapefruit and drinking grapefruit juice while taking this medication.

What should I do if I forget to take a dose?

Take the missed dose as soon as you remember it. However, if it is almost time for the next dose, skip the missed dose and continue your regular dosing schedule. Do not take a double dose to make up for a missed one.

What side effects can this medicine cause?

Efavirenz may cause side effects. Tell your doctor if any of these symptoms are severe or do not go away:
- upset stomach
- vomiting
- stomach pain
- diarrhea
- indigestion
- drowsiness

- dizziness
- headache
- difficulty concentrating
- confusion
- forgetfulness
- nervousness
- strange thoughts
- abnormally happy mood
- difficulty falling asleep or staying asleep
- unusual dreams
- pain

Some side effects can be serious. If you experience any of the following symptoms or those mentioned in the SPECIAL PRECAUTIONS section, call your doctor immediately:

- sore throat, cough, fever, chills, or other signs of infection
- rash
- itching
- blisters or sores on skin
- peeling skin
- fainting
- extreme tiredness
- lack of energy
- loss of appetite
- pain in the upper right part of the stomach
- unusual bleeding or bruising
- yellowing of the skin or eyes
- flu-like symptoms
- seizures

Efavirenz may cause other side effects. Call your doctor if you have any unusual problems while taking this medication.

If you experience a serious side effect, you or your doctor may send a report to the Food and Drug Administration's (FDA) MedWatch Adverse Event Reporting program online [at http://www.fda.gov/MedWatch/index.html] or by phone [1-800-332-1088].

What storage conditions are needed for this medicine?

Keep this medication in the container it came in, tightly closed, and out of reach of children. Store it at room temperature and away from excess heat and moisture (not in the bathroom). Throw away any medication that is outdated or no longer needed. Talk to your pharmacist about the proper disposal of your medication.

What should I do in case of overdose?

In case of overdose, call your local poison control center at 1-800-222-1222. If the victim has collapsed or is not breathing, call local emergency services at 911.

Symptoms of overdose may include:
- movements of your body that you cannot control
- dizziness
- headache

- difficulty concentrating
- nervousness
- confusion
- forgetfulness
- difficulty falling asleep or staying asleep
- unusual dreams
- drowsiness
- hallucinations (seeing things or hearing voices that do not exist)
- abnormally happy mood
- strange thoughts

What other information should I know?

Keep all appointments with your doctor and the laboratory. Your doctor may order certain lab tests to check your body's response to efavirenz.

Before having any laboratory test, tell your doctor and the laboratory personnel that you are taking efavirenz.

Do not let anyone else take your medication. Ask your pharmacist any questions you have about refilling your prescription.

Dosage Facts
For Informational Purposes

Caution: Do not change your dose, how often you take your medication, or the length of time you are to take it without first talking to your healthcare provider.

The following dosage information was written using medical language for doctors and other healthcare professionals and is provided here for you to check your dosage. The dosage of this drug may differ for different patients. Therefore, always follow your doctor's instructions or the directions on the label. Contact your healthcare provider or pharmacist if you have any questions about the specific dosage of your medication after reviewing this information.

General Dosage Information

Administer single-entity preparation (Sustiva®) in conjunction with other antiretrovirals.

The fixed-combination preparation containing efavirenz, emtricitabine, and tenofovir (Atripla®) may be used alone or in conjunction with other antiretrovirals.

If used in conjunction with atazanavir, fosamprenavir, indinavir, or lopinavir, adjustment in the treatment regimen necessary.

Dosage of Atripla® expressed as number of tablets.

Pediatric Patients

Treatment of HIV Infection

ORAL:

Dosage in Children ≥3 Years of Age

Weight in kg	Dosage
10 to <15	200 mg once daily
15 to <20	250 mg once daily
20 to <25	300 mg once daily
25 to <32.5	350 mg once daily
32.5 to <40	400 mg once daily
≥40	600 mg once daily

Adult Patients

Treatment of HIV Infection

ORAL:
- 600 mg once daily.
- Atripla®: 1 tablet once daily.

Postexposure Prophylaxis of HIV†

Occupational Exposure†

ORAL:
- 600 mg once daily.
- Used in alternative expanded regimens that include efavirenz and 2 NRTIs.
- Initiate postexposure prophylaxis as soon as possible following exposure (within hours rather than days) and continue for 4 weeks, if tolerated.

Nonoccupational Exposure†

ORAL:
- 600 mg once daily.
- Used in a preferred NNRTI-based regimen that includes efavirenz and (lamivudine or emtricitabine) and (zidovudine or tenofovir) or an alternative NNRTI-based regimen that includes efavirenz and (lamivudine or emtricitabine) and (abacavir, didanosine, or stavudine).
- Initiate postexposure prophylaxis as soon as possible following exposure (preferably ≤72 hours after exposure) and continue for 28 days.

Special Populations

Renal Impairment
- Dosage adjustments not necessary.
- Atripla®: Dosage adjustment not necessary in patients with Cl_{cr} ≥50 mL/minute. Not recommended in patients with Cl_{cr} <50 mL/minute.

Geriatric Patients
- Select dosage with caution because of age-related decreases in hepatic, renal, and/or cardiac function and concomitant disease and drug therapy.

† *Use is not currently included in the labeling approved by the US Food and Drug Administration.*

Eflornithine

(ee flor′ ni theen)

Brand Name: Vaniqa®

Why is this medicine prescribed?

Eflornithine is used to slow the growth of unwanted hair on the face in women, usually around the lips or under the chin. Eflornithine works by blocking a natural substance that is needed for hair to grow and is located in your hair follicle (the sac where each hair grows).

How should this medicine be used?

Eflornithine comes as a cream to apply to the skin. It is usually applied twice a day. To help you remember to apply eflornithine cream, apply it around the same times every day, such as in the morning and in the evening. You should wait at least 8 hours between applications of eflornithine. Follow the directions on your prescription label carefully, and ask your doctor or pharmacist to explain any part you do not understand. Apply eflornithine cream exactly as directed. Do not apply more or less of it or apply it more often than prescribed by your doctor.

Eflornithine cream slows hair growth but does not prevent it. You should continue to use your current method of hair removal (e.g., shaving, plucking, cutting) or treatment while using eflornithine cream. It may take four weeks or longer before you see the full benefit of eflornithine cream. Do not stop applying eflornithine without talking to your doctor. Stopping use of eflornithine will cause hair to grow as it did before treatment. You should notice improvement (less time spent using your current method of hair removal) within 6 months of beginning treatment with eflornithine. If no improvement is seen, your doctor will likely ask you to stop using eflornithine.

To use eflornithine cream, follow these steps:
1. Wash and dry the affected area(s).
2. Apply a thin layer to affected area(s) and rub in until absorbed.

Apply eflornithine cream only to affected skin areas. Do not allow the cream to get into your eyes, mouth, or vagina.

You should wait at least 4 hours after applying eflornithine cream before washing the area where it was applied.

You should wait at least 5 minutes after using your current method of hair removal before applying eflornithine.

You may apply cosmetics or sunscreen after an application of eflornithine cream has dried.

You may feel temporary stinging or burning if you apply eflornithine to broken skin.

Are there other uses for this medicine?

This medication may be prescribed for other uses; ask your doctor or pharmacist for more information.

What special precautions should I follow?

Before using eflornithine,

- tell your doctor and pharmacist if you are allergic to eflornithine or any other medications.
- tell your doctor and pharmacist what other prescription and nonprescription medications, vitamins, nutritional supplements, and herbal products you are taking.
- tell your doctor if you have or have ever had severe acne.
- tell your doctor if you are pregnant, plan to become pregnant, or are breast-feeding. If you become pregnant while using eflornithine, call your doctor.

What special dietary instructions should I follow?

Unless your doctor tells you otherwise, continue your normal diet.

What should I do if I forget to take a dose?

Apply the missed dose as soon as you remember it, if at least 8 hours has passed since your previous application. However, if it is almost time for the next application, skip the missed dose and continue your regular application schedule. Do not apply extra cream to make up for a missed dose.

What side effects can this medicine cause?

Eflornithine may cause side effects. Tell your doctor if any of these symptoms are severe or do not go away:

- stinging, burning, or tingling of the skin
- redness of the skin
- skin rash
- acne
- swollen patches of skin that are reddened and contain a buried hair

Some side effects can be serious. The following symptom is uncommon, but if you experience it, stop using eflornithine and call your doctor immediately:

- severe irritation of the skin

Eflornithine may cause other side effects. Call your doctor if you have any unusual problems while using this medication.

If you experience a serious side effect, you or your doctor may send a report to the Food and Drug Administration's (FDA) MedWatch Adverse Event Reporting program online [at http://www.fda.gov/MedWatch/index.html] or by phone [1-800-332-1088].

What storage conditions are needed for this medicine?

Keep this medication in the container it came in, tightly closed, and out of reach of children. Store it at room temperature and away from excess heat and moisture (not in the bathroom). Do not freeze eflornithine. Throw away any medication that is outdated or no longer needed. Talk to your pharmacist about the proper disposal of your medication.

What should I do in case of overdose?

You should not swallow eflornithine. If you apply extremely high doses (several tubes daily) of eflornithine to your skin you also may experience an overdose. If you swallow adapalene or apply extremely large amounts to your skin, call your local poison control center at 1-800-222-1222.

What other information should I know?

Keep all appointments with your doctor.

Do not let anyone else use your medication. Ask your pharmacist any questions you have about refilling your prescription.

Dosage Facts
For Informational Purposes

Caution: Do not change your dose, how often you take your medication, or the length of time you are to take it without first talking to your healthcare provider.

The following dosage information was written using medical language for doctors and other healthcare professionals and is provided here for you to check your dosage. The dosage of this drug may differ for different patients. Therefore, always follow your doctor's instructions or the directions on the label. Contact your healthcare provider or pharmacist if you have any questions about the specific dosage of your medication after reviewing this information.

General Dosage Information

Available as eflornithine hydrochloride; dosage expressed in terms of the salt.

Adult Patients

Reduction of Unwanted Facial Hair

TOPICAL:
- Apply a thin film twice daily at least 8 hours apart (or as directed by clinician).
- If skin irritation or intolerance develops, reduce application frequency to once daily. If irritation continues, discontinue therapy.

Eletriptan

(el ih trip′ tan)

Brand Name: Relpax®

Why is this medicine prescribed?

Eletriptan is used to treat the symptoms of migraine headache (severe throbbing headache that sometimes comes along with nausea and sensitivity to sound and light). Eletriptan is in a class of medications called selective serotonin receptor agonists. It works by reducing swelling of blood vessels in the brain, stopping pain signals from being sent to the brain, and blocking the release of certain natural substances that cause pain, nausea, and other symptoms of migraine. Eletriptan does not prevent migraine attacks or reduce the number of headaches you have.

How should this medicine be used?

Eletriptan comes as a tablet to take by mouth. It is usually taken at the first sign of a migraine attack. If your symptoms improve after you take eletriptan but return after 2 hours or longer, you may take a second tablet. However, if your symptoms do not improve after you take eletriptan, do not take a second tablet before calling your doctor. Do not take more than two eletriptan tablets in any 24-hour period. Call your doctor if you need to take eletriptan more than three times a month. Follow the directions on your prescription label carefully, and ask your doctor or pharmacist to explain any part you do not understand. Take eletriptan exactly as directed. Do not take more or less of it or take it more often than prescribed by your doctor.

You may take your first dose of eletriptan in a doctor's office or other medical facility where you can be monitored for serious reactions.

Are there other uses for this medicine?

This medication may be prescribed for other uses; ask your doctor or pharmacist for more information.

What special precautions should I follow?

Before taking eletriptan,
- tell your doctor and pharmacist if you are allergic to eletriptan or any other medications.
- do not take eletriptan within 24 hours of another selective serotonin receptor agonist such as almotriptan (Axert), frovatriptan (Frova), naratriptan (Amerge), rizatriptan (Maxalt), sumatriptan (Imitrex), or zolmitriptan (Zomig); or ergot-type medications such as bromocriptine (Parlodel), cabergoline (Dostinex), dihydroergotamine (D.H.E. 45, Migranal), ergoloid mesylates (Germinal, Hydergine), ergonovine (Ergotrate), ergotamine (Bellergal-S, Cafergot, Ergomar, Wigraine), methylergonovine (Methergine), methysergide (Sansert), and pergolide (Permax). Do not take eletriptan within 72

hours of clarithromycin (Biaxin), itraconazole (Sporanox), ketoconazole (Nizoral), nefazodone (Serzone), nelfinavir (Viracept), ritonavir (Norvir), and troleandomycin (TAO).
- tell your doctor and pharmacist what other prescription and nonprescription medications, vitamins, nutritional supplements, and herbal products you are taking. Be sure to mention any of the following: cimetidine (Tagamet); cyclosporine (Neoral, Sandimmune); danazol (Danocrine); delavirdine (Rescriptor); diltiazem (Cardizem, Dilacor, Tiazac); erythromycin (E.E.S., E-Mycin, Erythrocin); fluconazole (Diflucan); indinavir (Crixivan); isoniazid (INH, Nydrazid); metronidazole (Flagyl); selective serotonin reuptake inhibitors (SSRIs) such as citalopram (Celexa), fluoxetine (Prozac, Sarafem), fluvoxamine (Luvox), paroxetine (Paxil), and sertraline (Zoloft); verapamil (Calan, Covera, Isoptin, Verelan); and zafirlukast (Accolate). Your doctor may need to change the doses of your medications or monitor you carefully for side effects.
- tell your doctor if you smoke, if you or any family members have or have ever had heart disease, if you have gone through menopause (change of life), and if you have or have ever had a heart attack; angina (chest pain); high blood pressure; stroke or 'mini-stroke'; high cholesterol; diabetes; circulation problems such as ischemic bowel disease; or kidney or liver disease.
- tell your doctor if you are pregnant, plan to become pregnant, or are breast-feeding. If you become pregnant while taking eletriptan, call your doctor.
- you should know that eletriptan may make you drowsy. Do not drive a car or operate machinery until you know how this medication affects you.
- talk to your doctor about your headache symptoms to make sure they are caused by migraine. Eletriptan should not be used to treat hemiplegic or basilar migraine or headaches caused by other conditions (such as cluster headaches).

What special dietary instructions should I follow?

Talk to your doctor about drinking grapefruit juice while taking this medicine.

What side effects can this medicine cause?

Eletriptan may cause side effects. Tell your doctor if any of these symptoms are severe or do not go away:
- weakness
- upset stomach
- heartburn
- dizziness
- drowsiness
- headache
- dry mouth
- stomach pain or cramps

Some side effects can be serious. The following symptoms are uncommon, but if you experience any of them, call your doctor immediately:

- tightness, pain, pressure, or heaviness in the chest, throat, neck, and/or jaw
- slow or difficult speech
- dizziness or faintness
- weakness or numbness of an arm or leg
- severe stomach pain
- bloody diarrhea
- rapid, pounding, or irregular heart beat
- difficulty breathing
- paleness or blue color of the fingers and toes
- pain, burning, or tingling in the hands or feet

Eletriptan may cause other side effects. Call your doctor if you have any unusual problems while taking this medication.

If you experience a serious side effect, you or your doctor may send a report to the Food and Drug Administration's (FDA) MedWatch Adverse Event Reporting program online [at http://www.fda.gov/MedWatch/index.html] or by phone [1-800-332-1088].

What storage conditions are needed for this medicine?

Keep this medication in the container it came in, tightly closed, and out of reach of children. Store it at room temperature and away from excess heat and moisture (not in the bathroom). Throw away any medication that is outdated or no longer needed. Talk to your pharmacist about the proper disposal of your medication.

What should I do in case of overdose?

In case of overdose, call your local poison control center at 1-800-222-1222. If the victim has collapsed or is not breathing, call local emergency services at 911.

Symptoms of overdose may include:

- tightness, pain, pressure, or heaviness in the chest, throat, neck, and/or jaw
- slow or difficult speech
- dizziness or faintness
- weakness or numbness of an arm or leg
- rapid, pounding, or irregular heart beat
- difficulty breathing
- headache

What other information should I know?

Keep all appointments with your doctor.

Do not let anyone else take your medication. Ask your pharmacist any questions you have about refilling your prescription.

Dosage Facts
For Informational Purposes

Caution: Do not change your dose, how often you take your medication, or the length of time you are to take it without first talking to your healthcare provider.

The following dosage information was written using medical language for doctors and other healthcare professionals and is provided here for you to check your dosage. The dosage of this drug may differ for different patients. Therefore, always follow your doctor's instructions or the directions on the label. Contact your healthcare provider or pharmacist if you have any questions about the specific dosage of your medication after reviewing this information.

General Dosage Information

Available as eletriptan hydrobromide; dosage expressed in terms of eletriptan.

Adult Patients

Vascular Headaches
Migraine

ORAL:
- 20 or 40 mg as a single dose; individualize dosage selection, weighing the possible benefit (greater effectiveness) and risks (increased adverse effects) of the 40-mg dose. In clinical studies, doses >40 mg were effective but were associated with increased risk of adverse effects.
- If headache recurs, additional doses may be administered at intervals of ≥2 hours, up to a maximum dosage of 80 mg in any 24-hour period.
- If patient does not respond to first dose, additional doses are unlikely to provide benefit for the same headache.

Prescribing Limits

Adult Patients

Vascular Headaches
Migraine

ORAL:
- Maximum 40 mg as a single dose; do not exceed 80 mg in any 24-hour period.
- Safety of treating an average of >3 headaches per 30-day period has not been established.

Special Populations

Hepatic Impairment
- Dosage adjustment not necessary in patients with mild to moderate hepatic impairment. Contraindicated in those with severe hepatic impairment.

Emtricitabine

(em tri sit′ uh bean)

Brand Name: Atripla® as a combination product containing Efavirenz, Emtricitabine, and Tenofovir, Emtriva®, Truvada® as a combination product containing Emtricitabine and Tenofovir Disoproxil Fumarate

Important Warning

Medications that are similar to emtricitabine have caused serious damage to the liver and a life-threatening condition called lactic acidosis (buildup of lactic acid in the blood) when they were used alone or in combination with other medications that treat human immunodeficiency virus (HIV) or acquired immunodeficiency syndrome (AIDS). Tell your doctor if you have or have ever had liver disease. If you experience any of the following symptoms, call your doctor immediately: upset stomach; vomiting; stomach pain; loss of appetite; extreme tiredness; weakness; dizziness; light-headedness; fast or irregular heartbeat; trouble breathing; dark yellow or brown urine; light-colored bowel movements; yellowing of the skin or eyes; feeling cold, especially in the arms or legs; or muscle pain that is different than any muscle pain you usually experience.

Emtricitabine should not be used to treat hepatitis B virus infection (HBV; an ongoing liver infection). Tell your doctor if you have or think you may have HBV. Your doctor may test you to see if you have HBV before you begin your treatment with emtricitabine. If you have HBV and you take emtricitabine, your condition may suddenly worsen when you stop taking emtricitabine. Your doctor will examine you and order lab tests regularly for several months after you stop taking emtricitabine to see if your HBV has worsened.

Keep all appointments with your doctor and the laboratory. Your doctor may order certain tests to check your body's response to emtricitabine. Talk to your doctor about the risks of taking emtricitabine.

Why is this medicine prescribed?

Emtricitabine is used with other medications to treat HIV infection in patients with or without AIDS. Emtricitabine is in a class of medications called nucleoside reverse transcriptase inhibitors (NRTIs). This medication works by slowing the spread of HIV in the body. Emtricitabine does not cure HIV infection and may not prevent you from developing HIV-related illnesses. Emtricitabine does not prevent you from spreading HIV to other people.

How should this medicine be used?

Emtricitabine comes as a capsule and a solution (liquid) to take by mouth. It is usually taken once a day with or without food. Take emtricitabine at around the same time every day. Follow the directions on your prescription label carefully, and ask your doctor or pharmacist to explain any part you do not understand. Take emtricitabine exactly as directed. Do not take more or less of it or take it more often than prescribed by your doctor.

Emtricitabine controls HIV infection but does not cure it. Continue to take emtricitabine even if you feel well. Do not stop taking emtricitabine without talking to your doctor. When your supply of emtricitabine starts to run low, get more from your doctor or pharmacist. If you miss doses or stop taking emtricitabine, your condition may become more difficult to treat.

Ask your doctor or pharmacist for a copy of the manufacturer's information for the patient.

Are there other uses for this medicine?

This medication may be prescribed for other uses; ask your doctor or pharmacist for more information.

What special precautions should I follow?

Before taking emtricitabine,

- tell your doctor and pharmacist if you are allergic to emtricitabine or any other medications.
- tell your doctor and pharmacist what other prescription and nonprescription medications, vitamins, nutritional supplements, and herbal products you are taking or plan to take. Your doctor may need to change the doses of your medications or monitor you more carefully for side effects.
- tell your doctor if you have or have ever had the conditions mentioned in the IMPORTANT WARNING section, any type of infection that does not go away or that comes and goes such as tuberculosis (TB; a type of lung infection) or cytomegalovirus (CMV; a viral infection that may cause symptoms in patients with weak immune systems) or kidney disease.
- tell your doctor if you are pregnant or plan to become pregnant. If you become pregnant while taking emtricitabine, call your doctor. Tell your doctor if you are breast-feeding. You should not breastfeed if you are infected with HIV or if you are taking emtricitabine.
- you should know that your body fat may increase or move to different areas of your body such as your breasts and upper back.

What special dietary instructions should I follow?

Unless your doctor tells you otherwise, continue your normal diet.

What should I do if I forget to take a dose?

Take the missed dose as soon as you remember it. However, if it is almost time for the next dose, skip the missed dose and continue your regular dosing schedule. Do not take more than one dose of emtricitabine in one day and do not take a double dose to make up for a missed one.

What side effects can this medicine cause?

Emtricitabine may cause side effects. Tell your doctor if any of these symptoms are severe or do not go away:

- headache
- diarrhea
- change in skin color, especially on the palms of the hands or the soles of the feet
- indigestion
- joint pain
- unusual dreams
- depression
- trouble falling asleep or staying asleep
- numbness, burning, or tingling in the hands, arms, feet, or legs
- runny nose

Some side effects can be serious. If you experience any of the following symptoms, or those mentioned in the IMPORTANT WARNING section, call your doctor immediately:

- fever, chills, sore throat, cough, or other signs of infection
- rash

Emtricitabine may cause other side effects. Call your doctor if you have any unusual problems while taking this medication.

If you experience a serious side effect, you or your doctor may send a report to the Food and Drug Administration's (FDA) MedWatch Adverse Event Reporting program online [at http://www.fda.gov/MedWatch/index.html] or by phone [1-800-332-1088].

What storage conditions are needed for this medicine?

Keep this medication in the container it came in, tightly closed, and out of reach of children. Store the capsules at room temperature and away from excess heat and moisture (not in the bathroom). Store the solution in the refrigerator, but do not freeze it. If you prefer not to refrigerate the solution, you may store it at room temperature for up to 3 months. Throw away any medication that is outdated or no longer needed, and any unused solution that has not been refrigerated after 3 months. Talk to your pharmacist about the proper disposal of your medication.

What should I do in case of overdose?

In case of overdose, call your local poison control center at 1-800-222-1222. If the victim has collapsed or is not breathing, call local emergency services at 911.

What other information should I know?

Do not let anyone else take your medication. Ask your pharmacist any questions you have about refilling your prescription.

Dosage Facts
For Informational Purposes

Caution: Do not change your dose, how often you take your medication, or the length of time you are to take it without first talking to your healthcare provider.

The following dosage information was written using medical language for doctors and other healthcare professionals and is provided here for you to check your dosage. The dosage of this drug may differ for different patients. Therefore, always follow your doctor's instructions or the directions on the label. Contact your healthcare provider or pharmacist if you have any questions about the specific dosage of your medication after reviewing this information.

General Dosage Information

Emtricitabine capsules and oral solution are not bioequivalent.

Emtriva® and Truvada® must be given in conjunction with other antiretrovirals. Atripla® may be used alone or in conjunction with other antiretrovirals.

Dosage of Truvada® and Atripla® expressed as number of tablets.

Pediatric Patients

Treatment of HIV Infection†

ORAL:

- Infants 0–3 months of age: 3 mg/kg (as the oral solution) once daily.
- Children 3 months to 17 years of age: 6 mg/kg (up to a maximum of 240 mg as the oral solution) once daily.
- Children weighing >33 kg who can swallow an intact capsule: 200 mg (as the capsule) once daily.

Adult Patients

Treatment of HIV Infection

ORAL:

- 200 mg (as the capsule) once daily. Alternatively, 240 mg (as the oral solution) once daily.
- Truvada®: 1 tablet once daily.
- Atripla®: 1 tablet once daily.

Postexposure Prophylaxis of HIV†
Occupational Exposure†

ORAL:

- 200 mg (as the capsule) once daily.
- Used in basic regimens with zidovudine or tenofovir; alternatively, used in alternative basic regimens with stavudine or didanosine.
- Initiate postexposure prophylaxis as soon as possible following exposure (within hours rather than days) and continue for 4 weeks, if tolerated.

Nonoccupational Exposure†

ORAL:

- 200 mg (as the capsule) once daily.
- Used in conjunction with another NRTI in preferred and alternative nonnucleoside reverse transcriptase inhibitor-based (NNRTI-based) or HIV protease inhibitor-based (PI-based) regimens. The preferred NNRTI-based regimen is efavirenz and (lamivudine or emtricitabine) and (zidovudine or tenofovir) and the preferred PI-based regimen is the fixed combination of lopinavir and ritonavir and (lamivudine or emtricitabine) and zidovudine.
- Initiate postexposure prophylaxis as soon as possible following exposure (preferably ≤72 hours after exposure) and continue for 28 days.

Prescribing Limits

Pediatric Patients

Treatment of HIV Infection

ORAL:

- Children 3 months to 17 years of age: Maximum 240 mg (as the oral solution) once daily.

Special Populations

Renal Impairment

Treatment of HIV Infection

ORAL:

- Reduce dosage in adults with Cl_{cr} <50 mL/minute (see tables).
- Data insufficient to make specific dosage recommendations for pediatric patients with renal impairment; consider reducing dose and/or increasing dosing interval.

Table 1. Emtriva® Dosage in Adults with Renal Impairment

Cl_{cr} (mL/minute)	Dosage of Capsules	Dosage of Oral Solution
≥50	200 mg every 24 hours	240 mg every 24 hours
30–49	200 mg every 48 hours	120 mg every 24 hours
15–29	200 mg every 72 hours	80 mg every 24 hours
<15	200 mg every 96 hours	60 mg every 24 hours
Hemodialysis patients	200 mg every 96 hours; on day of dialysis, give dose after the procedure	60 mg every 24 hours; give dose after hemodialysis

Table 2. Truvada® Dosage in Adults with Renal Impairment

Cl_{cr} (mL/minute)	Dose and Dosing Interval
≥50	One tablet every 24 hours
30–49	One tablet every 48 hours (monitor clinical response and renal function since dosage has not been evaluated clinically)
<30 (including hemodialysis patients)	Not recommended

Atripla®: Dosage adjustment not necessary in patients with Cl_{cr} ≥50 mL/minute. Not recommended in patients with Cl_{cr} < 50 mL/minute.

Geriatric Patients

- Select dosage with caution because of age-related decreases in hepatic, renal, and/or cardiac function and concomitant disease and drug therapy.

† Use is not currently included in the labeling approved by the US Food and Drug Administration.

Enalapril

(e nal′ a pril)

Brand Name: Lexxel® as a combination product containing Enalapril Maleate and Felodipine, Vaseretic®, Vasotec®

Also available generically.

Important Warning

Do not take enalapril if you are pregnant. If you become pregnant while taking enalapril, call your doctor immediately. Enalapril may harm the fetus.

Why is this medicine prescribed?

Enalapril is used alone or in combination with other medications to treat high blood pressure. It is also used in combination with other medications to treat heart failure. Enalapril is in a class of medications called angiotensin-converting enzyme (ACE) inhibitors. It works by decreasing certain chemicals that tighten the blood vessels, so blood flows more smoothly and the heart can pump blood more efficiently.

How should this medicine be used?

Enalapril comes as a tablet to take by mouth. It is usually taken once or twice a day with or without food. To help you remember to take enalapril, take it around the same time every day. Follow the directions on your prescription label carefully, and ask your doctor or pharmacist to explain any part you do not understand. Take enalapril exactly as directed. Do not take more or less of it or take it more often than prescribed by your doctor.

Your doctor will probably start you on a low dose of enalapril and gradually increase your dose.

Enalapril controls high blood pressure and heart failure but does not cure them. Continue to take enalapril even if you feel well. Do not stop taking enalapril without talking to your doctor.

Are there other uses for this medicine?

Enalapril is also sometimes used to treat kidney disease related to diabetes. Talk to your doctor about the possible risks of using this medication for your condition.

This medication may be prescribed for other uses; ask your doctor or pharmacist for more information.

What special precautions should I follow?

Before taking enalapril,

- tell your doctor and pharmacist if you are allergic to enalapril, benazepril (Lotensin), captopril (Capoten), fosinopril (Monopril), lisinopril (Prinivil, Zestril), moexipril (Univasc), perindopril (Aceon), quinapril (Accupril), ramipril (Altace), trandolapril (Mavik), or any other medications.
- tell your doctor and pharmacist what prescription and nonprescription medications, vitamins, nutritional supplements, and herbal products you are taking. Be sure to mention any of the following: aspirin and other non-steroidal anti-inflammatory medications (NSAIDs) such as indomethacin (Indocin); diuretics ('water pills'); lithium (Eskalith, Lithobid); and potassium supplements. Your doctor may need to change the doses of your medications or monitor you carefully for side effects.
- tell your doctor if you have or have ever had heart or kidney disease; lupus; scleroderma; diabetes; or angioedema, a condition that causes difficulty swallowing or breathing and painful swelling of the the face, throat, tongue, lips, eyes, hands, feet, ankles, or lower legs.
- tell your doctor if you plan to become pregnant or are breast-feeding.
- if you are having surgery, including dental surgery, tell the doctor or dentist that you are taking enalapril.
- you should know that diarrhea, vomiting, not drinking enough fluids, and sweating a lot can cause a drop in blood pressure, which may cause lightheadedness and fainting.

What special dietary instructions should I follow?

Talk to your doctor before using salt substitutes containing potassium. If your doctor prescribes a low-salt or low-sodium diet, follow these directions carefully.

What should I do if I forget to take a dose?

Take the missed dose as soon as you remember it. However, if it is almost time for the next dose, skip the missed dose and continue your regular dosing schedule. Do not take a double dose to make up for a missed one.

What side effects can this medicine cause?

Enalapril may cause side effects. Tell your doctor if any of these symptoms are severe or do not go away:

- cough
- dizziness
- rash
- weakness

Some side effects can be serious. The following symptoms are uncommon, but if you experience any of them, call your doctor immediately:

- swelling of the face, throat, tongue, lips, eyes, hands, feet, ankles, or lower legs
- hoarseness
- difficulty breathing or swallowing
- yellowing of the skin or eyes
- fever, sore throat, chills, and other signs of infection
- lightheadedness
- fainting

Enalapril may cause other side effects. Call your doctor if you have any unusual problems while taking this medication.

If you experience a serious side effect, you or your doctor may send a report to the Food and Drug Administration's (FDA) MedWatch Adverse Event Reporting program online [at http://www.fda.gov/MedWatch/index.html] or by phone [1-800-332-1088].

What storage conditions are needed for this medicine?

Keep this medication in the container it came in, tightly closed, and out of reach of children. Store it at room temperature and away from excess heat and moisture (not in the bathroom). Throw away any medication that is outdated or no longer needed. Talk to your pharmacist about the proper disposal of your medication.

What should I do in case of overdose?

In case of overdose, call your local poison control center at 1-800-222-1222. If the victim has collapsed or is not breathing, call local emergency services at 911.

Symptoms of overdose may include:

- lightheadedness
- fainting

What other information should I know?

Keep all appointments with your doctor and the laboratory. Your blood pressure should be checked regularly to determine your response to enalapril. Your doctor may order certain lab tests to check your body's response to enalapril.

Do not let anyone else take your medication. Ask your pharmacist any questions you have about refilling your prescription.

Dosage Facts
For Informational Purposes

Caution: Do not change your dose, how often you take your medication, or the length of time you are to take it without first talking to your health-care provider.

The following dosage information was written using medical language for doctors and other healthcare professionals and is provided here for you to check your dosage. The dosage of this drug may differ for different patients. Therefore, always follow your doctor's instructions or the directions on the label. Contact your healthcare provider or pharmacist if you have any questions about the specific dosage of your medication after reviewing this information.

General Dosage Information

Available as enalapril maleate (oral tablets); dosage expressed in terms of the salt. Also available as enalaprilat (IV injection); dosage expressed in terms of the base.

Dosage of enalapril and enalaprilat are not identical; caution when converting from oral to IV therapy or vice versa.

Pediatric Patients

Hypertension

ORAL:
- Children 1 month to 16 years of age: Enalapril 0.08 mg/kg (up to 5 mg) once daily.
- Adjust dosage until the desired BP goal is achieved (up to maximum dosage of 0.58 mg/kg or 40 mg).

Adult Patients

Hypertension

ORAL:
- Initially, enalapril 2.5–5 mg daily as monotherapy. Adjust dosage at 2- to 4-week intervals to achieve BP control.
- In patients currently receiving diuretic therapy, discontinue diuretic, if possible, 2–3 days before initiating enalapril. May cautiously resume diuretic therapy if BP not controlled adequately with enalapril alone. If diuretic cannot be discontinued, give initial enalapril dose of 2.5 mg under close medical supervision (observe patient for ≥2 hours and until BP has stabilized for at least an additional hour).
- When switching from IV enalaprilat to oral enalapril, initiate enalapril at 5 mg once daily as monotherapy. If used with a diuretic, 2.5 mg once daily (in patients who responded to enalaprilat 0.625 mg every 6 hours). Adjust dosage as necessary.
- Usual dosage: Enalapril 10–40 mg daily, given in 1 dose or 2 divided doses.
- If effectiveness diminishes toward end of dosing interval in patients treated once daily, consider increasing dosage or administering drug in 2 divided doses.

Enalapril/Hydrochlorothiazide Combination Therapy

ORAL:
- If BP is not adequately controlled by monotherapy with either enalapril or hydrochlorothiazide, or if stable dosages of these drugs have been achieved, can switch to the fixed-combination preparation containing enalapril 5 mg and hydrochlorothiazide 12.5 mg or, alternatively, enalapril 10 mg and hydrochlorothiazide 25 mg.
- Adjust dosage of either or both drugs according to patient's response.

Enalapril/Felodipine Combination Therapy

ORAL:
- If BP is not adequately controlled by monotherapy with either enalapril (or another ACE inhibitor) or felodipine (or another dihydropyridine-derivative calcium-channel blocking agent), can switch to the fixed-combination preparation containing enalapril 5 mg and felodipine 5 mg daily. If BP is not adequately controlled after 1 or 2 weeks, increase dosage to enalapril 10 mg and felodipine 10 mg once daily. If necessary, may increase dosage to enalapril 20 mg and felodipine 10 mg once daily.
- If control of BP is still inadequate, consider adding a thiazide diuretic.

CHF

ORAL:
- Manufacturer recommends initial enalapril dosage of 2.5 mg twice daily. Usual maintenance dosage: 2.5–20 mg twice daily.
- Some clinicians recommend initial enalapril dosage of 2.5 mg once or twice daily in patients with normal renal function and serum sodium concentration. Usual maintenance dosage: 2.5–20 mg daily, given in 2 divided doses.
- Following initial dose, monitor closely for ≥2 hours and until BP has stabilized for at least an additional hour. To minimize risk of hypotension, reduce diuretic dosage, if possible, prior to initiating therapy. Adjust dosage gradually over several weeks to prespecified target (≥20 mg daily) or maximum tolerated dosage.
- In patients with hyponatremia (serum sodium concentration <130 mEq/L), manufacturer recommends initial enalapril dosage of 2.5 mg daily under close monitoring. Increase dosage at intervals of ≥4 days, to 2.5 mg twice daily, then 5 mg twice daily, and then higher, provided excessive hypotension or deterioration of renal function is not present at the time of intended dosage adjustment; dosage should not exceed 40 mg daily.

Asymptomatic Left Ventricular Dysfunction

ORAL:
- Initially, enalapril 2.5 mg twice daily. Titrate upward as tolerated to target dosage of 20 mg daily, given in divided doses. Following initial dose, monitor closely for ≥2 hours and until BP has stabilized for at least an additional hour. To minimize risk of hypotension, reduce diuretic dosage, if possible, prior to initiating therapy.

Prescribing Limits

Pediatric Patients

Hypertension

ORAL:
- Maximum 0.58 mg/kg or 40 mg of enalapril daily.

Adult Patients

Hypertension

ORAL:
- Dosage of enalapril/hydrochlorothiazide fixed combination generally should not exceed enalapril 20 mg and hydrochlorothiazide 50 mg daily.

CHF

ORAL:
- Maximum 40 mg of enalapril daily, given in 2 divided doses.

Special Populations

Renal Impairment

Hypertension

ORAL:

- Patients with Cl_{cr} >30 mL/minute: Manufacturer states that no dosage adjustment is required.
- Adults with Cl_{cr} ≤30 mL/minute or S_{cr} ≥3 mg/dL: Manufacturer recommends initial enalapril dosage of 2.5 mg once daily; titrate until BP is controlled or to maximum of 40 mg daily. When switching from IV enalaprilat, initiate oral therapy at 2.5 mg once daily; adjust dosage according to patient's BP response. Manufacturer does not recommend use of enalapril in pediatric patients with Cl_{cr} <30 mL/minute per 1.73 m^2.
- Some clinicians recommend dosage of 75–100% of usual enalapril dosage in patients with Cl_{cr} of 10–50 mL/minute and dosage of 50% of usual enalapril dosage in those with Cl_{cr} <10 mL/minute.
- Hemodialysis patients: Enalapril 2.5 mg on dialysis days; on days between dialysis, adjust dosage according to BP response.

Enalapril/Hydrochlorothiazide Combination Therapy

ORAL:

- Not recommended in patients with severe renal impairment.

Enalapril/Felodipine Combination Therapy

ORAL:

- Adults with Cl_{cr} ≤30 mL/minute or S_{cr} >3 mg/dL: Enalapril 2.5 mg daily recommended by manufacturer.

CHF

ORAL:

- Patients with S_{cr} >1.6 mg/dL: Enalapril 2.5 mg daily initially under close monitoring. Increase dosage at intervals of ≥4 days, to 2.5 mg twice daily, then 5 mg twice daily, and then higher, provided excessive hypotension or deterioration of renal function is not present at the time of intended dosage adjustment; do not exceed 40 mg daily.

Geriatric Patients

Hypertension

- Initiate therapy with enalapril/hydrochlorothiazide fixed combination at lower end of usual range.
- Initiate therapy with enalapril/felodipine fixed combination with initial enalapril dosage of 2.5 mg daily.

† *Use is not currently included in the labeling approved by the US Food and Drug Administration.*

Enalapril and Felodipine

(e nal′ a pril) (fe loe′ di peen)

Brand Name: Lexxel®

Important Warning

Do not take enalapril and felodipine if you are pregnant. If you become pregnant while taking enalapril and felodipine, call your doctor immediately.

Why is this medicine prescribed?

The combination of enalapril and felodipine is used to treat high blood pressure. It decreases certain chemicals that tighten the blood vessels so blood flows more smoothly and the heart can pump blood more efficiently. It also relaxes your blood vessels so your heart does not have to pump as hard. This medication is sometimes prescribed for other uses; ask your doctor or pharmacist for more information.

How should this medicine be used?

The combination of enalapril and felodipine comes as a tablet to take by mouth. It is usually taken once or twice a day. Do not chew, divide, or crush the tablets. Follow the directions on your prescription label carefully, and ask your doctor or pharmacist to explain any part you do not understand. Take enalapril and felodipine exactly as directed. Do not take more or less of it or take it more often than prescribed by your doctor.

Enalapril and felodipine controls high blood pressure but does not cure it. Continue to take enalapril and felodipine even if you feel well. Do not stop taking enalapril and felodipine without talking to your doctor.

What special precautions should I follow?

Before taking enalapril and felodipine,

- tell your doctor and pharmacist if you are allergic to enalapril, felodipine (Plendil), benazepril (Lotensin), captopril (Capoten), fosinopril (Monopril), lisinopril (Prinivil, Zestril), moexipril (Univasc), quinapril (Accupril), ramipril (Altace), trandolapril (Mavik), or any other drugs.
- tell your doctor and pharmacist what prescription and nonprescription medications you are taking, especially antiseizure medications such as phenytoin (Dilantin), carbamazepine (Tegretol), and phenobarbital; aspirin or other non-steroidal antiinflammatory drugs such as ibuprofen (Advil, Motrin) or naproxen (Aleve, Naprosyn); cimetidine (Tagamet, Tagamet HB); diuretics ('water pills'); lithium (Eskalith, Lithobid); other medications

for high blood pressure; potassium supplements; ranitidine (Zantac, Zantac 24), and vitamins.

- tell your doctor if you have or have ever had heart, liver, or kidney disease; diabetes; or angioedema, a condition that causes hives, difficulty breathing, and painful swelling of the face, lips, throat, tongue, hands, or feet.
- tell your doctor if you are breast-feeding. Enalapril and felodipine may pass into breast milk and harm infants. Talk to your doctor about stopping to breast-feed if you take enalapril and felodipine.
- if you are having surgery, including dental surgery, tell the doctor or dentist that you are taking enalapril and felodipine.

What special dietary instructions should I follow?

Take enalapril and felodipine without food or with a light meal.

Talk to your doctor about drinking grapefruit juice or eating grapefruit while taking enalapril and felodipine.

Talk to your doctor before using salt substitutes containing potassium. If your doctor prescribes a low-salt or low-sodium diet, follow these directions carefully.

What should I do if I forget to take a dose?

Take the missed dose as soon as you remember it. However, if it is almost time for the next dose, skip the missed dose and continue your regular dosing schedule. Do not take a double dose to make up for a missed one.

What side effects can this medicine cause?

Enalapril and felodipine may cause side effects. Tell your doctor if any of these symptoms are severe or do not go away:

- headache
- dizziness or lightheadedness
- swelling
- cough
- excessive tiredness
- flushing (feeling of warmth)
- sore throat
- enlargement of gum tissue around teeth
- rapid heartbeat

If you experience any of the following symptoms, call your doctor immediately:

- swelling of the face, eyes, lips, tongue, arms, or legs
- difficulty breathing or swallowing
- fainting
- rash
- yellowing of the skin or eyes

If you experience a serious side effect, you or your doctor may send a report to the Food and Drug Administration's (FDA) MedWatch Adverse Event Reporting program online [at http://www.fda.gov/MedWatch/index.html] or by phone [1-800-332-1088].

What storage conditions are needed for this medicine?

Keep this medication in the container it came in, tightly closed, and out of reach of children. Store it at room temperature and away from excess heat and moisture (not in the bathroom). Throw away any medication that is outdated or no longer needed. Talk to your pharmacist about the proper disposal of your medication.

What should I do in case of overdose?

In case of overdose, call your local poison control center at 1-800-222-1222. If the victim has collapsed or is not breathing, call local emergency services at 911.

What other information should I know?

Keep all appointments with your doctor and the laboratory. Your blood pressure should be checked regularly to determine your response to enalapril and felodipine.

Good dental hygiene decreases the chance and severity of gum swelling. Brush your teeth regularly and schedule dental cleanings for every 6 months.

Do not let anyone else take your medication. Ask your pharmacist any questions you have about refilling your prescription.

Dosage Facts
For Informational Purposes

Caution: Do not change your dose, how often you take your medication, or the length of time you are to take it without first talking to your healthcare provider.

The following dosage information was written using medical language for doctors and other healthcare professionals and is provided here for you to check your dosage. The dosage of this drug may differ for different patients. Therefore, always follow your doctor's instructions or the directions on the label. Contact your healthcare provider or pharmacist if you have any questions about the specific dosage of your medication after reviewing this information.

General Dosage Information

Available as enalapril maleate (oral tablets); dosage expressed in terms of the salt.

Adult Patients

Hypertension
Enalapril/Felodipine Combination Therapy

ORAL:
- If BP is not adequately controlled by monotherapy with either enalapril (or another ACE inhibitor) or felodipine (or another dihydropylidine-derivative calcium-channel blocking agent), can switch to the fixed-combination preparation containing enalapril 5 mg and felodipine 5 mg daily. If BP is not ade-

quately controlled after 1 or 2 weeks, increase dosage to enalapril 10 mg and felodipine 10 mg once daily. If necessary, may increase dosage to enalapril 20 mg and felodipine 10 mg once daily.

- If control of BP is still inadequate, consider adding a thiazide diuretic.

Special Populations

Renal Impairment

Hypertension
Enalapril/Felodipine Combination Therapy

ORAL:

- Adults with Cl_{cr} ≤30 mL/minute or S_{cr} >3 mg/dL: Enalapril 2.5 mg daily recommended by manufacturer.

Geriatric Patients

Hypertension

- Initiate therapy with enalapril/felodipine fixed combination with initial enalapril dosage of 2.5 mg daily.

† Use is not currently included in the labeling approved by the US Food and Drug Administration.

Enalapril and Hydrochlorothiazide

(e nal′ a pril) (hye droe klor oh thye′ a zide)

Brand Name: Vaseretic®

Important Warning

Do not take enalapril and hydrochlorothiazide if you are pregnant. If you become pregnant while taking enalapril and hydrochlorothiazide, call your doctor immediately. Enalapril and hydrochlorothiazide may harm the fetus.

Why is this medicine prescribed?

The combination of enalapril and hydrochlorothiazide is used to treat high blood pressure. Enalapril is in a class of medications called angiotensin-converting enzyme (ACE) inhibitors. It works by decreasing certain chemicals that tighten the blood vessels, so blood flows more smoothly. Hydrochlorothiazide is in a class of medications called diuretics ('water pills'). It works by causing the kidneys to get rid of unneeded water and salt from the body into the urine.

How should this medicine be used?

The combination of enalapril and hydrochlorothiazide comes as a tablet to take by mouth. It is usually taken with or without food once or twice a day. To help you remember to take enalapril and hydrochlorothiazide, take it around the same times every day. Follow the directions on your prescription label carefully, and ask your doctor or pharmacist to explain any part you do not understand. Take enalapril and hydrochlorothiazide exactly as directed. Do not take more or less of it or take it more often than prescribed by your doctor.

Enalapril and hydrochlorothiazide controls high blood pressure but does not cure it. Continue to take enalapril and hydrochlorothiazide even if you feel well. Do not stop taking enalapril and hydrochlorothiazide without talking to your doctor.

Are there other uses for this medicine?

This medication may be prescribed for other uses; ask your doctor or pharmacist for more information.

What special precautions should I follow?

Before taking enalapril and hydrochlorothiazide,

- tell your doctor and pharmacist if you are allergic to enalapril (Vasotec), hydrochlorothiazide (HCTZ, Hydrodiuril, Microzide), benazepril (Lotensin), captopril (Capoten), fosinopril (Monopril), lisinopril (Prinivil, Zestril), moexipril (Univasc), perindopril (Aceon), quinapril (Accupril), ramipril (Altace), trandolapril (Mavik), sulfa drugs, or any other medications.
- tell your doctor and pharmacist what prescription and nonprescription medications, vitamins, nutritional supplements, and herbal products you are taking. Be sure to mention any of the following: aspirin and other nonsteroidal anti-inflammatory medications (NSAIDs) such as indomethacin (Indocin); cholestyramine (Questran); colestipol (Colestid); diuretics ('water pills'); insulin or oral medications for diabetes; lithium (Eskalith, Lithobid); oral steroids such as dexamethasone (Decadron, Dexone), methylprednisolone (Medrol), and prednisone (Deltasone); other medications for high blood pressure; pain medications; phenobarbital (Luminal, Solfoton); and potassium supplements. Your doctor may need to change the doses of your medications or monitor you carefully for side effects.
- tell your doctor if you have or have ever had heart, parathyroid, liver, or kidney disease; lupus; diabetes; allergies; asthma; gout; or angioedema, a condition that causes hives, difficulty breathing, and painful swelling of the face, lips, throat, tongue, hands, or feet.
- tell your doctor if you plan to become pregnant or are breast-feeding.
- if you are having surgery, including dental surgery, tell the doctor or dentist that you are taking enalapril and hydrochlorothiazide.
- ask your doctor about the safe use of alcoholic beverages while you are taking enalapril and hydrochlorothiazide. Alcohol can make the side effects from enalapril and hydrochlorothiazide worse.
- you should know that diarrhea, vomiting, not drinking

enough fluids, and sweating a lot can cause a drop in blood pressure, which may cause lightheadedness and fainting.

What special dietary instructions should I follow?

Talk to your doctor before using salt substitutes containing potassium. If your doctor prescribes a low-salt or low-sodium diet, follow these directions carefully.

What should I do if I forget to take a dose?

Take the missed dose as soon as you remember it. However, if it is almost time for the next dose, skip the missed dose and continue your regular dosing schedule. Do not take a double dose to make up for a missed one.

What side effects can this medicine cause?

Enalapril and hydrochlorothiazide may cause side effects. Tell your doctor if any of these symptoms are severe or do not go away:
- cough
- dizziness
- headache
- excessive tiredness
- muscle cramps
- decrease in sexual ability

Some side effects can be serious. The following symptoms are uncommon, but if you experience any of them, call your doctor immediately:
- lightheadedness
- swelling of the face, throat, tongue, lips, eyes, hands, feet, ankles, or lower legs
- hoarseness
- difficulty breathing or swallowing
- fever, sore throat, chills, and other signs of infection
- yellowing of the skin or eyes
- dry mouth
- thirst
- weakness
- infrequent urination
- upset stomach
- vomiting
- fainting
- chest pain
- fast or irregular heartbeat

Enalapril and hydrochlorothiazide may cause other side effects. Call your doctor if you have any unusual problems while taking this medication.

If you experience a serious side effect, you or your doctor may send a report to the Food and Drug Administration's (FDA) MedWatch Adverse Event Reporting program online [at http://www.fda.gov/MedWatch/index.html] or by phone [1-800-332-1088].

What storage conditions are needed for this medicine?

Keep this medication in the container it came in, tightly closed, and out of reach of children. Store it at room temperature and away from excess heat and moisture (not in the bathroom). Throw away any medication that is outdated or no longer needed. Talk to your pharmacist about the proper disposal of your medication.

What should I do in case of overdose?

In case of overdose, call your local poison control center at 1-800-222-1222. If the victim has collapsed or is not breathing, call local emergency services at 911.

What other information should I know?

Keep all appointments with your doctor and the laboratory. Your blood pressure should be checked regularly to determine your response to enalapril and hydrochlorothiazide. Your doctor may order certain lab tests to check your body's response to enalapril and hydrochlorothiazide.

Do not let anyone else take your medication. Ask your pharmacist any questions you have about refilling your prescription.

Dosage Facts
For Informational Purposes

Caution: Do not change your dose, how often you take your medication, or the length of time you are to take it without first talking to your healthcare provider.

The following dosage information was written using medical language for doctors and other healthcare professionals and is provided here for you to check your dosage. The dosage of this drug may differ for different patients. Therefore, always follow your doctor's instructions or the directions on the label. Contact your healthcare provider or pharmacist if you have any questions about the specific dosage of your medication after reviewing this information.

General Dosage Information

Available as enalapril maleate (oral tablets); dosage expressed in terms of the salt.

Adult Patients

Hypertension
Enalapril/Hydrochlorothiazide Combination Therapy

ORAL:
- If BP is not adequately controlled by monotherapy with either enalapril or hydrochlorothiazide, or if stable dosages of these drugs have been achieved, can switch to the fixed-combination preparation containing enalapril 5 mg and hydrochlorothiazide 12.5 mg or, alternatively, enalapril 10 mg and hydrochlorothiazide 25 mg.

- Adjust dosage of either or both drugs according to patient's response.

Prescribing Limits

Adult Patients

Hypertension

ORAL:
- Dosage of enalapril/hydrochlorothiazide fixed combination generally should not exceed enalapril 20 mg and hydrochlorothiazide 50 mg daily.

CHF

Special Populations

Renal Impairment

Hypertension
Enalapril/Hydrochlorothiazide Combination Therapy

ORAL:
- Not recommended in patients with severe renal impairment.

Geriatric Patients

Hypertension
- Initiate therapy with enalapril/hydrochlorothiazide fixed combination at lower end of usual range.

† *Use is not currently included in the labeling approved by the US Food and Drug Administration.*

Enfuvirtide Injection

(en fyoo′ vir tide)

Brand Name: Fuzeon®

Why is this medicine prescribed?

Enfuvirtide is used in combination with other medications to treat human immunodeficiency virus (HIV) infection in patients who have not responded well enough to other antiviral medications. Enfuvirtide is in a class of medications called HIV fusion inhibitors. It works by stopping HIV from entering healthy cells. Enfuvirtide does not cure HIV and may not prevent you from developing HIV related illnesses. Enfuvirtide does not prevent the spread of HIV to other people.

How should this medicine be used?

Enfuvirtide comes as a powder to be mixed with sterile water and injected subcutaneously (under the skin). It is usually injected twice a day. To help you remember to inject enfuvirtide, inject it at about the same times each day. Follow the directions on your prescription label carefully, and ask your doctor or pharmacist to explain any part you do not understand. Use enfuvirtide exactly as directed. Do not use more or less of it or use it more often than prescribed by your doctor.

Enfuvirtide controls HIV but does not cure it. Continue to use enfuvirtide even if you feel well. Do not stop using enfuvirtide without talking to your doctor. If you miss doses or stop using enfuvirtide, your condition may become more difficult to treat.

You will receive your first dose of enfuvirtide in your doctor's office. After that, you can inject enfuvirtide yourself or have a friend or relative perform the injections. Your doctor will train the person who will be injecting the medication, and will test him to be sure he can give the injection correctly. Be sure that you and the person who will be giving the injections read the manufacturer's information for the patient that comes with enfuvirtide before you use it for the first time at home.

You can inject enfuvirtide anywhere on your thighs, stomach, or upper arms except your navel (belly button) and any area directly under a belt or waistband. To reduce the chances of soreness or redness, choose a different area for each injection. Use your fingertips to check your chosen area for hard bumps under the skin. Never inject enfuvirtide into any skin that has a scar, bruise, mole, or reaction to a previous injection of enfuvirtide.

Never reuse needles, syringes, vials of enfuvirtide, or vials of sterile water. Dispose of used needles and syringes in a puncture-resistant container. You can dispose of used alcohol pads and vials in the trash, but if you see blood on an alcohol pad, put it in the puncture-resistant container. Talk to your doctor or pharmacist about how to dispose of the puncture-resistant container.

Before preparing an enfuvirtide dose, wash your hands with soap and water. After you wash your hands, do not touch anything except the medication, supplies, and the area where you will inject the medication.

To prepare and inject enfuvirtide, follow these steps:
1. Open the packages of one 3-mL (large) syringe and one 1-mL (small) syringe and remove the caps from one vial of enfuvirtide and one vial of sterile water. Throw away the packages and caps.
2. Wipe each vial top with a new alcohol pad and allow to air dry. Be careful not to touch the tops of the vials after you clean them. If you do touch the tops, clean them again with a new alcohol pad.
3. Gently tap the enfuvirtide vial to loosen the powder.
4. Slowly pull back the plunger of the 3-mL syringe to the 1.1 mL mark. Be careful not to push the plunger past the 0.2 mL mark.
5. Insert the needle into the sterile water vial and slowly inject the air into the vial. Do not remove the needle from the vial.
6. Turn the vial upside down and check to be sure the needle tip is below the surface of the water. Slowly pull the plunger back to the 1.1 mL mark. The syringe should fill with 1.1 mL of water.
7. Check the syringe for air bubbles. Gently tap the syringe and push and pull the plunger to remove air bubbles. You may need to pull the plunger back further to get the full amount of water.

8. When you are certain that the syringe contains 1.1 mL of water and no air bubbles, carefully remove the needle from the vial.

9. Insert the needle of the syringe you have just filled into the enfuvirtide vial at an angle.

10. Push down the plunger slowly to inject the sterile water into the vial. The water should drip down the side of the vial onto the powder.

11. Remove the needle from the vial and push the plunger all the way down with the tip of your thumb until you hear a snap. The needle will spring back into the syringe. Dispose of the syringe properly.

12. Tap the enfuvirtide vial gently with your fingertip for 10 seconds. Then roll it between your hands for a short while, but do not shake it. Be sure there is no powder stuck to the walls of the vial.

13. If you are not ready to inject the medication, you may write the date and time you mixed the medication on the vial and place the vial in the refrigerator at this point. You may store the mixed medication in the refrigerator for up to 24 hours. Allow the medication to warm to room temperature and be sure that it is clear before you use it.

14. If you are ready to inject the medication, leave the vial upright on a flat surface and wait for the powder to dissolve. This may take up to 45 minutes. You will know the powder has dissolved when the vial is clear and not foamy. If there are small bubbles in the vial, tap the vial gently until they disappear. If there are particles in the vial, do not use the vial, and call the pharmacy that provided it.

15. Rub a new alcohol pad over the place where you will inject enfuvirtide using pressure and a circular motion. Allow the area to air dry.

16. Clean the vial top again with a new alcohol pad and allow it to air dry.

17. Pull back the plunger on the 1-mL syringe to the 1-mL mark. Be careful not to push it past the 0.05 mL mark.

18. Insert the needle into the enfuvirtide vial and slowly push down the plunger to inject air. Do not remove the needle from the vial.

19. Turn the vial upside down and check to be sure the needle is below the surface of the liquid. Slowly pull back the plunger to the 1 mL mark. The syringe should fill with 1mL of liquid.

20. Check the syringe for air bubbles. Gently tap the syringe and push and pull the plunger to remove air bubbles. You may need to pull the plunger back further to get the full amount of liquid.

21. When you are certain that the syringe contains 1 mL of liquid and no air bubbles, carefully remove the needle and syringe from the vial.

22. Pinch and hold a fold of skin around the cleaned area where you will inject enfuvirtide. With your other hand, hold the needle like a pencil at a 45 degree angle.

23. Push the needle into your skin until 3/4 of the needle is under the skin.

24. Use your thumb to push the plunger down as far as it will go. The needle should pull out of your skin and spring back into the syringe when you do this. If it does not, pull the needle out of your skin and push the plunger down until the needle goes into the syringe.

25. Dispose of the needle properly and cover the spot where you injected enfuvirtide with a small bandage if you see any blood or medication on your skin.

Are there other uses for this medicine?

This medication may be prescribed for other uses; ask your doctor or pharmacist for more information.

What special precautions should I follow?

Before using enfuvirtide,

- tell your doctor and pharmacist if you are allergic to enfuvirtide or any other medications.
- tell your doctor and pharmacist what prescription and nonprescription medications, vitamins, nutritional supplements, and herbal products you are taking.
- tell your doctor if you smoke, if you use or have ever used intravenous (injected into the vein) street drugs and if you have or have ever had kidney or lung disease.
- tell your doctor if you are pregnant, plan to become pregnant, or are breast-feeding. If you become pregnant while taking enfuvirtide, call your doctor. You should not breastfeed if you are infected with HIV or if you are taking enfuvirtide.
- you should know that enfuvirtide may make you dizzy. Do not drive a car or operate machinery until you know how this medication affects you.

What special dietary instructions should I follow?

Unless your doctor tells you otherwise, continue your normal diet.

What should I do if I forget to take a dose?

Inject the missed dose as soon as you remember it. However, if it is almost time for the next dose, skip the missed dose and continue your regular dosing schedule. Do not inject a double dose to make up for a missed one.

What side effects can this medicine cause?

Enfuvirtide may cause side effects. Tell your doctor if any of these symptoms are severe or do not go away:

- itching, swelling, pain, tenderness, redness, purple patches, hard skin, or bumps in the place where you injected enfuvirtide
- itching anywhere on the body
- difficulty falling or staying asleep
- depression
- nervousness
- weakness
- muscle pain

- loss of appetite
- changes in ability to taste food
- weight loss
- constipation
- flu-like symptoms
- warts or cold sores
- swollen glands

Some side effects can be serious. The following symptoms are uncommon, but if you experience any of them, call your doctor immediately:

- severe pain, oozing, swelling, heat, or increasing redness in the place you injected enfuvirtide
- cough
- fever
- fast breathing
- shortness of breath
- vomiting
- rash
- blood in urine
- swollen feet
- pale or fatty stools
- yellowing of skin or eyes
- dizziness
- fainting
- blurred vision
- pain or tingling in toes that spreads to legs
- numbness in any part of the body
- pain in hands or arms
- painful, red, or teary eyes

Enfuvirtide may cause other side effects. Call your doctor if you have any unusual problems while taking this medication.

If you experience a serious side effect, you or your doctor may send a report to the Food and Drug Administration's (FDA) MedWatch Adverse Event Reporting program online [at http://www.fda.gov/MedWatch/index.html] or by phone [1-800-332-1088].

What storage conditions are needed for this medicine?

Keep this medication and the sterile water that comes with it in the containers they came in, tightly closed, and out of reach of children. Store them at room temperature and away from excess heat and moisture (not in the bathroom). If you mix the medication and sterile water in advance, store the mixture in the vial in the refrigerator for up to 24 hours. Never store mixed medication in the syringe. Throw away any medication that is outdated or no longer needed. Talk to your pharmacist about the proper disposal of your medication.

What should I do in case of overdose?

In case of overdose, call your local poison control center at 1-800-222-1222. If the victim has collapsed or is not breathing, call local emergency services at 911.

What other information should I know?

Keep all appointments with your doctor and the laboratory. Your doctor will order certain lab tests to check your body's response to enfuvirtide.

Do not let anyone else use your medication. Ask your pharmacist any questions you have about refilling your prescription.

Dosage Facts
For Informational Purposes

Caution: Do not change your dose, how often you take your medication, or the length of time you are to take it without first talking to your healthcare provider.

The following dosage information was written using medical language for doctors and other healthcare professionals and is provided here for you to check your dosage. The dosage of this drug may differ for different patients. Therefore, always follow your doctor's instructions or the directions on the label. Contact your healthcare provider or pharmacist if you have any questions about the specific dosage of your medication after reviewing this information.

General Dosage Information

Must be given in conjunction with other antiretrovirals.

Pediatric Patients

Treatment of HIV Infection

SUB-Q:
- Children 6–16 years of age: 2 mg/kg (maximum 90 mg) twice daily.
- Adolescents >16 years of age: 90 mg twice daily.

Adult Patients

Treatment of HIV Infection

SUB-Q:
- 90 mg twice daily.

Postexposure Prophylaxis of HIV†
Occupational Exposure†

SUB-Q:
- 90 mg twice daily.
- Used with expert consultation in alternative expanded regimen.
- Initiate postexposure prophylaxis as soon as possible (within hours rather than days) and continue for 4 weeks, if tolerated.

Prescribing Limits

Pediatric Patients

Treatment of HIV Infection

SUB-Q:
- Children 6–16 years of age: Maximum 90 mg twice daily.

Special Populations

Hepatic Impairment
- Dosage recommendations not available.

Renal Impairment

Treatment of HIV Infection

- Dosage adjustments not needed.

† Use is not currently included in the labeling approved by the US Food and Drug Administration.

Enoxaparin Injection

(ee nox a pa′ rin)

Brand Name: Lovenox®

Important Warning

If you have epidural or spinal anesthesia or a spinal puncture while taking a "blood thinner" such as enoxaparin, you are at risk for collection of blood in the spinal column that could cause you to become paralyzed. Tell your doctor if you are taking other anticoagulants ("blood thinners") such as warfarin (Coumadin), abciximab (ReoPro), anagrelide (Agrylin), aspirin or nonsteroidal anti-inflammatory drugs (ibuprofen, naproxen), cilostazol (Pletal), clopidogrel (Plavix), dipyridamole (Persantine), eptifibatide (Integrilin), sulfinpyrazone (Anturane), ticlopidine (Ticlid), and tirofiban (Aggrastat).

If you experience any of the following symptoms, call your doctor immediately: numbness, tingling, leg weakness or paralysis, and loss of control over your bladder or bowels.

Talk to your doctor about the risk of taking enoxaparin. Keep all appointments with your doctor.

Why is this medicine prescribed?

Enoxaparin is used to prevent blood clots in the leg in patients who are on bedrest or who are having hip replacement, knee replacement, or stomach surgery. It is used in combination with aspirin to prevent complications from angina (chest pain) and heart attacks. It is also used in combination with warfarin to treat blood clots in the leg. Enoxaparin is in a class of medications called low molecular weight heparins. It works by stopping the formation of substances that cause clots.

How should this medicine be used?

Enoxaparin comes as an injection in a syringe to be injected just under the skin (subcutaneously) but not into your muscle. It is usually given twice a day. You will probably begin using the drug while you are in the hospital and then use it for a total of 10-14 days. Follow the directions on your pre-

scription label carefully, and ask your doctor or pharmacist to explain any part you do not understand. Use enoxaparin exactly as directed. Do not inject more or less of it or inject it more often than prescribed by your doctor.

Continue to use enoxaparin even if you feel well. Do not stop taking enoxaparin without talking to your doctor.

Your health care provider will teach you how to give yourself the shot or arrangements will be made for someone else to give you the shot. Enoxaparin is usually injected in the stomach area. You must use a different area of the stomach each time you give the shot. If you have questions about where to give the shot, ask your health care provider. Each syringe has enough drug in it for one shot. Do not use the syringe and needle more than one time. Your doctor, pharmacist, or health care provider will tell you how to throw away used needles and syringes to avoid accidental injury. Keep syringes and needles out of reach of children.

To inject enoxaparin, follow these instructions:

1. Wash your hands and the area of skin where you will give the shot.
2. Look at the syringe to be sure the drug is clear and colorless or pale yellow.
3. Take the cap off the needle. Do not push any air or drug out of the syringe before giving the shot unless your health care provider tells you to.
4. Lie down and pinch a fold of skin between your finger and thumb. Push the entire needle into the skin and then press down on the syringe plunger to inject the drug. Hold onto the skin the entire time you give the shot. Do not rub the site after you give the shot.

Are there other uses for this medicine?

This medication may be prescribed for other uses; ask your doctor or pharmacist for more information.

What special precautions should I follow?

Before taking enoxaparin,

- tell your doctor and pharmacist if you are allergic to enoxaparin, heparin, any other drugs, or pork products.
- tell your doctor and pharmacist what prescription and nonprescription medications you are taking, especially those listed in the IMPORTANT WARNING section and vitamins.
- tell your doctor if you have an artificial heart valve and if you have or have ever had kidney disease, an infection in your heart, a stroke, a bleeding disorder, ulcers, or a low platelet count.
- tell your doctor if you are pregnant, plan to become pregnant, or are breast-feeding. If you become pregnant while taking enoxaparin, call your doctor.
- if you are having surgery, including dental surgery, tell the doctor or dentist that you are taking enoxaparin.

What should I do if I forget to take a dose?

Inject the missed dose as soon as you remember it. However, if it is almost time for the next dose, skip the missed dose and continue your regular dosing schedule. Do not inject a double dose to make up for a missed one.

What side effects can this medicine cause?

Enoxaparin may cause side effects. Tell your doctor if any of these symptoms are severe or do not go away:

- upset stomach
- fever
- irritation or burning at site of injection

If you experience any of the following symptoms or those listed in the IMPORTANT WARNING section, call your doctor immediately:

- unusual bleeding or bruising
- black or bloody stools
- blood in urine
- swollen ankles and/or feet

If you experience a serious side effect, you or your doctor may send a report to the Food and Drug Administration's (FDA) MedWatch Adverse Event Reporting program online [at http://www.fda.gov/MedWatch/index.html] or by phone [1-800-332-1088].

What storage conditions are needed for this medicine?

Keep this medication out of reach of children. Store the syringes at room temperature and away from excess heat and moisture (not in the bathroom). Do not use the syringe if it leaks or if the fluid is dark or contains particles. Throw away any medication that is outdated or no longer needed. Talk to your pharmacist about the proper disposal of your medication.

What should I do in case of overdose?

In case of overdose, call your local poison control center at 1-800-222-1222. If the victim has collapsed or is not breathing, call local emergency services at 911.

What other information should I know?

Keep all appointments with your doctor and the laboratory. Your doctor will order certain lab tests to monitor your enoxaparin therapy.

Enoxaparin prevents blood from clotting so it may take longer than usual for you to stop bleeding if you are cut or injured. Avoid activities that have a high risk of causing injury. Call your doctor if bleeding is unusual.

Do not let anyone else use your medication. Your prescription is probably not refillable.

Dosage Facts

For Informational Purposes

Caution: Do not change your dose, how often you take your medication, or the length of time you are to take it without first talking to your healthcare provider.

The following dosage information was written using medical language for doctors and other healthcare professionals and is provided here for you to check your dosage. The dosage of this drug may differ for different patients. Therefore, always follow your doctor's instructions or the directions on the label. Contact your healthcare provider or pharmacist if you have any questions about the specific dosage of your medication after reviewing this information.

General Dosage Information

Available as enoxaparin sodium; dosage expressed in terms of the salt.

Dosages for enoxaparin sodium and regular (unfractionated) heparin or other low molecular weight heparins cannot be used interchangeably on a unit-for-unit (or mg-for-mg) basis.

Enoxaparin has an approximate anti-factor Xa activity of 100 units/mg using the World Health Organization (WHO) First International Low Molecular Weight Heparin Reference Standard.

Adult Patients

Prevention of Venous Thrombosis and Pulmonary Embolism

General Surgery

SUB-Q:

- In patients undergoing general (e.g., abdominal, gynecologic, urologic) surgery who are at moderate to very high risk for thromboembolic complications (e.g., those with malignancy, history of deep-vein thrombosis or pulmonary embolism, or obesity, or patients >40 years of age or undergoing major surgery under general anesthesia lasting >30 minutes), 40 mg once daily with the initial dose given 2 hours prior to surgery.
- Usual duration of therapy is 7–10 days, although up to 12 days of treatment has been well tolerated in clinical trials.
- Extended prophylaxis: ACCP suggests continuation for 2–3 weeks after hospital discharge in patients at high risk for thromboembolism.

Hip-Replacement Surgery

SUB-Q:

- Initially, 30 mg every 12 hours for ≥10 days; begin 12–24 hours after surgery provided hemostasis has been established.
- Alternatively, consider 40 mg once daily, with the initial dose given approximately 12 hours prior to surgery.
- Extended prophylaxis: Following the initial phase of thromboprophylaxis, continue 40 mg once daily for 28–35 days.

Knee-Replacement Surgery

SUB-Q:

- Initially, 30 mg every 12 hours for >10 days; begin 12–24 hours after surgery provided hemostasis has been established.

Long-Distance Travel

Long-distance travelers at increased risk for thromboembolism: single dose of <34 mg prior to departure.

Medical Conditions Associated with Thromboembolism

SUB-Q:

- Acute illness with impaired mobility: 40 mg once daily. Usual duration of therapy is 6–11 days; well tolerated up to 14 days in clinical trials.

Thromboembolism During Pregnancy

SUB-Q:

- Primary prevention in women with inherited causes of thrombophilia (e.g., antithrombin deficiency, heterozygous genetic mutation of both prothrombin G20210A and factor V Leiden, or homozygous genetic mutation for factor V Leiden or prothrombin G20210A): 1 mg/kg every 12 hours suggested.
- Primary prevention in other patients with confirmed thrombophilia: 40 mg once daily, followed by postpartum oral anticoagulation (e.g., with warfarin) suggested.
- Secondary prevention after a single episode of idiopathic venous thromboembolism with no long-term anticoagulation: 40 mg once daily.
- Secondary prevention after a single episode of venous thromboembolism with risk factors (e.g., confirmed thrombophilia, strong family history of thrombosis) and no long-term anticoagulation: 40 mg once or twice daily, followed by postpartum oral anticoagulation.
- Secondary prevention after >2 episodes of venous thromboembolism: 1 mg/kg twice daily throughout pregnancy followed by postpartum resumption of long-term anticoagulation.
- Secondary prevention in women who require long-term anticoagulation: 1 mg/kg twice daily throughout pregnancy.

Treatment of Deep-Vein Thrombosis with or without Pulmonary Embolism

SUB-Q:

- *Outpatient* treatment at home in patients without pulmonary embolism: 1 mg/kg every 12 hours.
- Pregnant women: 1 mg/kg every 12 hours for remainder of pregnancy.
- *Inpatient* (hospital) treatment in patients with or without pulmonary embolism (not candidates for outpatient treatment): 1 mg/kg every 12 hours or 1.5 mg/kg once daily at the same time every day.
- Average duration of therapy is 7 days, although up to 17 days of treatment has been well tolerated in clinical trials.
- Initiate concurrent warfarin sodium therapy when appropriate, usually within 72 hours of enoxaparin injection.
- Continue enoxaparin for a minimum of 5 days, until a therapeutic oral anticoagulant effect is achieved.

Embolism Associated with Atrial Fibrillation

SUB-Q:

- Patients with atrial fibrillation duration <48 hours undergoing cardioversion who have no contraindications to anticoagulation: 1 mg/kg every 12 hours.
- ACCP suggests same regimen for anticoagulation in patients undergoing cardioversion for atrial flutter.

Unstable Angina and Non-ST-Segment Elevation MI

SUB-Q:

- 1 mg/kg every 12 hours in conjunction with aspirin therapy.
- Administer for a minimum of 2 days and continue until clinical stabilization.
- Usual duration of treatment is 2–8 days, although up to 12.5 days of treatment has been well tolerated in clinical trials.
- In patients with unstable angina or non-ST-segment elevation MI undergoing PCI, further anticoagulation suggested based on time of last dose of enoxaparin sodium.
- Last dose within 8 hours of PCI: No additional anticoagulation suggested during procedure.
- Last dose administered 8–12 hours before PCI: 0.3 mg/kg given by directIV injection suggested at initiation of PCI.
- Last dose administered >12 hours prior to PCI: Conventional anticoagulation with unfractionated heparin suggested during PCI.

Special Populations

Hepatic Impairment

- No dosage recommendations. No dosage adjustments necessary in patients with mild (Cl$_{cr}$ 50–80 mL/minute) or moderate (Cl$_{cr}$ 30–50 mL/minute) renal impairment.

Renal Impairment

- Use with caution in renally impaired patients. No dosage adjustments necessary in patients with mild (Cl$_{cr}$ 50–80 mL/minute) or moderate (Cl$_{cr}$ 30–50 mL/minute) renal impairment.

Venous Thrombosis and Pulmonary Embolism

Prophylaxis in General (e.g., Abdominal) Surgery

SUB-Q:

- In patients with severe renal impairment (Cl$_{cr}$ <30 mL/minute), 30 mg once daily.

Prophylaxis in Hip or Knee Replacement Surgery

SUB-Q:

- In patients with severe renal impairment (Cl$_{cr}$ <30 mL/minute), 30 mg once daily.

Prophylaxis in Medical Conditions Associated with Thromboembolism

SUB-Q:

- In patients with severe renal impairment (Cl$_{cr}$ <30 mL/minute), 30 mg once daily.

Treatment of Deep-Vein Thrombosis with or without Pulmonary Embolism

SUB-Q:

- In patients with severe renal impairment (Cl$_{cr}$ <30 mL/minute), 1 mg/kg once daily, in conjunction with warfarin therapy.

Unstable Angina and Non-ST Segment Elevation MI

SUB-Q:

- In patients with severe renal impairment (Cl$_{cr}$ <30 mL/minute), 1 mg/kg once daily, in conjunction with aspirin therapy.

Geriatric Patients

- Use with caution.

Low-Weight Patients
- Consider adjustment of dosage for low weight (women ≤45 kg or men <57 kg).

† *Use is not currently included in the labeling approved by the US Food and Drug Administration.*

Entacapone

(en ta′ ka pone)

Brand Name: Comtan®

Why is this medicine prescribed?

Entacapone is an inhibitor of catechol-O-methyltransferase (COMT). It is used in combination with levodopa and carbidopa (Sinemet) to treat the end-of-dose 'wearing-off' symptoms of Parkinson's disease. Entacapone helps the levodopa and carbidopa work better by allowing more of it to reach the brain, where it has its effects.

This medication is sometimes prescribed for other uses; ask your doctor or pharmacist for more information.

How should this medicine be used?

Entacapone comes as a tablet to take by mouth. It is taken with every dose of levodopa and carbidopa, up to 8 times a day. Entacapone may be taken with or without food. Read your prescription label carefully, and ask your doctor or pharmacist to explain any part you do not understand. Take entacapone exactly as directed. Do not take more or less of it or take it more often than prescribed by your doctor.

Entacapone helps control the symptoms of Parkinson's disease, but it does not cure it. Continue to take entacapone even if you feel well. Do not stop taking entacapone without talking to your doctor. Stopping entacapone suddenly may make your Parkinson's disease worse and could have other dangerous effects. Your doctor probably will decrease your dose gradually if necessary.

What special precautions should I follow?

Before taking entacapone,
- tell your doctor and pharmacist if you are allergic to entacapone or any other drugs.
- tell your doctor and pharmacist what prescription and nonprescription medications you are taking, especially ampicillin, apomorphine (Zydis), bitolterol (Tornalate), chloramphenicol (AK-Chlor, Chloromycetin), cholestyramine (Cholybar, Questran, Questran Light, others), medications that cause drowsiness (including medications for anxiety and sleeping pills), dobutamine (Dobutrex), epinephrine (AsthmaHaler, EpiPen Auto-Injector, Primatene Mist, others), erythromycin (E-Base, E.E.S., E-Mycin, others), isoetharine (Arm-a-Med Isoetharine, Beta-2, Bronkometer, others), isoproterenol (Dispos-a-Med Isoproterenol, Isuprel, Medihaler-Iso, others), methyldopa (Aldomet), phenelzine (Nardil), probenecid (Benemid), rifampin (Rifadin, Rimactane), tranylcypromine (Parnate), and vitamins and herbal products.
- tell your doctor if you have or have ever had liver disease or a history of alcoholism.
- tell your doctor if you are pregnant, plan to become pregnant, or are breast-feeding. If you become pregnant while taking entacapone, call your doctor.
- if you are having surgery, including dental surgery, tell the doctor or dentist that you are taking entacapone.
- you should know that this medication may make you drowsy. Do not drive a car or operate heavy machinery until you know how entacapone affects you.

What should I do if I forget to take a dose?

Take the missed dose as soon as you remember it. However, if it is almost time for your next dose, skip the missed dose and continue your regular dosing schedule. Do not take a double dose to make up for a missed dose.

What side effects can this medicine cause?

Entacapone may cause side effects. Tell your doctor if any of these symptoms are severe or do not go away:
- dizziness
- diarrhea
- upset stomach
- movements you cannot control
- stomach pain
- drowsiness

If you experience any of the following symptoms, call your doctor immediately:
- difficulty breathing
- hallucinations
- high fever
- confusion
- muscle stiffness
- weakness with or without a fever

If you experience a serious side effect, you or your doctor may send a report to the Food and Drug Administration's (FDA) MedWatch Adverse Event Reporting program online [at http://www.fda.gov/MedWatch/index.html] or by phone [1-800-332-1088].

What storage conditions are needed for this medicine?

Keep this medication in the container it came in, tightly closed, and out of reach of children. Store it at room temperature and away from excess heat and moisture (not in the bathroom). Throw away any medication that is outdated or no longer needed. Talk to your pharmacist about the proper disposal of your medication.

What should I do in case of overdose?

In case of overdose, call your local poison control center at 1-800-222-1222. If the victim has collapsed or is not breathing, call local emergency services at 911.

What other information should I know?

Keep all appointments with your doctor and the laboratory. You may become dizzy when you get up after sitting or lying down, especially when you begin taking entacapone. To avoid this problem, make sure to get up slowly, especially if you have been sitting or lying down for a long time.

Entacapone may cause your urine to change to a brownish-orange color. This effect is common and is not harmful.

Do not let anyone else take your medicine. Ask your pharmacist any questions you have about refilling your prescription.

Dosage Facts

For Informational Purposes

Caution: Do not change your dose, how often you take your medication, or the length of time you are to take it without first talking to your healthcare provider.

The following dosage information was written using medical language for doctors and other healthcare professionals and is provided here for you to check your dosage. The dosage of this drug may differ for different patients. Therefore, always follow your doctor's instructions or the directions on the label. Contact your healthcare provider or pharmacist if you have any questions about the specific dosage of your medication after reviewing this information.

Adult Patients

Parkinsonian Syndrome

ORAL:
- 200 mg with each levodopa-carbidopa dose.
- May need to reduce daily levodopa dosage or administration frequency to optimize patient response. In clinical studies, most patients receiving ≥800 mg of levodopa daily or experiencing moderate or severe dyskinesias before initiating entacapone therapy required a reduction (average 25%) in levodopa dosage.

Transferring to the Fixed-combination Preparation (Stalevo®)

ORAL:
- Patients receiving levodopa-carbidopa conventional tablets containing a 1:4 ratio of carbidopa to levodopa: Switch to the corresponding strength of Stalevo®.
- No information on transferring patients receiving extended-release levodopa-carbidopa preparation or levodopa-carbidopa preparations containing a 1:10 ratio of carbidopa to levodopa.

Initiating Entacapone Using the Fixed-combination Preparation (Stalevo®)

ORAL:
- Patients receiving levodopa >600 mg daily or with history of moderate or severe dyskinesias: Administer levodopa-carbidopa (1:4 ratio) and entacapone as separate preparations to determine optimum maintenance dosage and then switch to corresponding strength of Stalevo®.
- Patients receiving levodopa <600 mg daily (conventional tablet, 1:4 ratio) with no dyskinesias: Switch to the strength of Stalevo® that corresponds to the dosage of levodopa-carbidopa being taken. Further adjustment may be needed.

Prescribing Limits

Adult Patients

Parkinsonian Syndrome

ORAL:
- Maximum of 8 doses (1.6 g) daily; clinical experience with dosages >1.6 g daily is limited.

Entecavir

(en te′ ka veer)

Brand Name: Baraclude®

Important Warning

Entecavir can cause serious or life-threatening damage to the liver and a condition called lactic acidosis (a buildup of acid in the blood). Tell your doctor if you drink or have ever drunk large amounts of alcohol, if you use or have ever used injectable street drugs, and if you have or have ever had cirrhosis (scarring) of the liver or any liver disease other than hepatitis B. If you experience any of the following symptoms, call your doctor immediately: yellowing of the skin or eyes; dark-colored urine; light-colored bowel movements; difficulty breathing; stomach pain or swelling; nausea; vomiting; unusual muscle pain; loss of appetite for at least several days; lack of energy; extreme weakness or tiredness; feeling cold especially in the arms or legs; dizziness or lightheadedness; or fast or irregular heartbeat.

Do not stop taking entecavir without talking to your doctor. When you stop taking entecavir your hepatitis may get worse. This is most likely to happen during the first several months after you stop taking entecavir. Take entecavir exactly as directed. Be careful not to miss doses or run out of entecavir. Refill your prescription at least 5 days before you expect that you will need the new supply of medication. If you experience any of the following symp-

continued on next page

Important Warning (cont'd)

toms after you stop taking entecavir, call your doctor immediately: extreme tiredness, weakness, nausea, vomiting, loss of appetite, yellowing of the skin or eyes, dark-colored urine, light-colored bowel movements, or muscle or joint pain.

Keep all appointments with your doctor and the laboratory before, during, and for a few months after your treatment with entecavir. Your doctor will order certain tests to check your body's response to entecavir during this time.

Ask your pharmacist or doctor for a copy of the manufacturer's information for the patient.

Talk to your doctor about the risks of taking entecavir.

Why is this medicine prescribed?

Entecavir is used to treat chronic (long-term) hepatitis B infection (swelling of the liver caused by a virus) in people who have liver damage. Entecavir is in a class of medications called nucleoside analogs. It works by decreasing the amount of hepatitis B virus (HBV) in the body. Entecavir does not cure HBV and may not prevent complications of chronic hepatitis B such as cirrhosis of the liver or liver cancer. Entecavir does not prevent the spread of HBV to other people.

How should this medicine be used?

Entecavir comes as a tablet and solution (liquid) to take by mouth. It is usually taken once a day on an empty stomach, at least 2 hours after a meal and at least 2 hours before the next meal. Take entecavir at around the same time every day. Follow the directions on your prescription label carefully, and ask your doctor or pharmacist to explain any part you do not understand. Take entecavir exactly as directed. Do not take more or less of it or take it more often than prescribed by your doctor.

To use the entecavir solution, follow these steps:

1. Hold the spoon that came with your medication upright and slowly fill it with entecavir solution up to the mark that matches your dose.
2. Hold the spoon with the volume marks facing you and check to see that the top of the liquid is level with the mark that matches your dose.
3. Swallow the medication right from the measuring spoon. Do not mix the medication with water or any other liquid
4. Rinse the spoon with water after each use, and allow it to air dry.
5. Put the spoon in a safe place where it will not get lost, because you will need to use it every time you take your medication. If you do lose the dosing spoon, call your doctor or pharmacist.

Are there other uses for this medicine?

This medication may be prescribed for other uses; ask your doctor or pharmacist for more information.

What special precautions should I follow?

Before taking entecavir,

- tell your doctor and pharmacist if you are allergic to entecavir, or any other medications, or any of the ingredients in entecavir tablets or solution. Ask your pharmacist for a list of the ingredients..
- tell your doctor and pharmacist what other prescription and nonprescription medications, vitamins, nutritional supplements, and herbal products you are taking or plan to take. Be sure to mention the medications listed in the IMPORTANT WARNING section and any of the following: aminoglycoside antibiotics such as amikacin (Amikin), gentamicin (Garamycin), kanamycin (Kantrex), neomycin (Neo-Rx, NeoFradin), paromomycin (Humatin), streptomycin, and tobramycin (Tobi, Nebcin); amphotericin B (Fungizone); medications to prevent rejection of a transplanted organ such as cyclosporine (Neoral, Sandimmune) or tacrolimus (Prograf); probenecid; or vancomycin. Your doctor may need to change the doses of your medications or monitor you carefully for side effects.
- tell your doctor if you have had a liver transplant (surgery to replace a diseased liver), HIV and/or AIDS, or if you have or have ever had kidney disease.
- tell your doctor if you are pregnant, plan to become pregnant, or are breast-feeding. If you become pregnant while taking entecavir, call your doctor. Do not breast-feed while you are taking entecavir.
- if you are having surgery, including dental surgery, tell the doctor or dentist that you are taking entecavir.

What special dietary instructions should I follow?

Unless your doctor tells you otherwise, continue your normal diet.

What should I do if I forget to take a dose?

Take the missed dose as soon as you remember it. However, if it is almost time for the next dose, skip the missed dose and continue your regular dosing schedule. Do not take a double dose to make up for a missed one.

What side effects can this medicine cause?

Entecavir may cause side effects. Tell your doctor if any of these symptoms are severe or do not go away:

- headache

Some side effects can be serious. If you experience any of the symptoms listed in the IMPORTANT WARNING section, call your doctor immediately.

Entecavir may cause other side effects. Call your doctor if you have any unusual problems while using this medication.

If you experience a serious side effect, you or your doctor may send a report to the Food and Drug Administration's (FDA) MedWatch Adverse Event Reporting program online

[at http://www.fda.gov/MedWatch/index.html] or by phone [1-800-332-1088].

What storage conditions are needed for this medicine?

Keep this medication in the container it came in, tightly closed, and out of reach of children and pets. Store it at room temperature and away from excess heat, light, and moisture (not in the bathroom medicine cabinet or near the kitchen sink). Throw away any medication that is outdated or no longer needed. Talk to your pharmacist about the proper disposal of your medication.

What should I do in case of overdose?

In case of overdose, call your local poison control center at 1-800-222-1222. If the victim has collapsed or is not breathing, call local emergency services at 911.

What other information should I know?

Do not let anyone else take your medication. Ask your pharmacist any questions you have about refilling your prescription.

Dosage Facts
For Informational Purposes

Caution: Do not change your dose, how often you take your medication, or the length of time you are to take it without first talking to your healthcare provider.

The following dosage information was written using medical language for doctors and other healthcare professionals and is provided here for you to check your dosage. The dosage of this drug may differ for different patients. Therefore, always follow your doctor's instructions or the directions on the label. Contact your healthcare provider or pharmacist if you have any questions about the specific dosage of your medication after reviewing this information.

General Dosage Information

Optimal duration of treatment for chronic HBV infection unknown. Entecavir has been administered for 52 weeks in controlled clinical studies.

Pediatric Patients

Chronic Hepatitis B Virus (HBV) Infection
Nucleoside-naive Individuals

ORAL:
- Adolescents ≥16 years of age: 0.5 mg once daily.

Lamivudine-refractory HBV

ORAL:
- Adolescents ≥16 years of age: 1 mg once daily.

HBV and HIV Coinfection†

ORAL:
- Adolescents ≥16 years of age: 1 mg once daily.

Adult Patients

Chronic Hepatitis B Virus (HBV) Infection
Nucleoside-naive Individuals

ORAL:
- 0.5 mg once daily.

Lamivudine-refractory HBV

ORAL:
- 1 mg once daily.

HBV and HIV Coinfection†

ORAL:
- 1 mg once daily.

Special Populations

Hepatic Impairment
- Dosage adjustment not required.

Renal Impairment
- Decrease dosage in those with Cl_{cr} <50 mL/minute, including those undergoing hemodialysis or CAPD.

Dosage for Treatment of Chronic HBV Infection in Patients with Renal Impairment

Cl_{cr} (mL/min)	Nucleoside-naive Individuals	Lamivudine-refractory HBV
30–49	0.25 mg once daily	0.5 mg once daily
10–29	0.15 mg once daily	0.3 mg once daily
<10	0.05 mg once daily	0.1 mg once daily
Hemodialysis or CAPD Patients	0.05 mg once daily; give dose after hemodialysis	0.1 mg once daily; give dose after hemodialysis

† Use is not currently included in the labeling approved by the US Food and Drug Administration.

Epinastine Ophthalmic

(ep i nas' tine)

Brand Name: Elestat®

Why is this medicine prescribed?

Epinastine ophthalmic solution is used to prevent itching of the eyes caused by allergic conjunctivitis (a condition in which the eyes become itchy, swollen, red, and teary when they are exposed to certain substances in the air). Epinastine is in a class of medications called antihistamines. It works by preventing the release of natural substances which cause allergic reactions in the eyes.

How should this medicine be used?

Epinastine comes as an ophthalmic solution (eye drops) to apply to the eyes. It is usually applied twice a day. To help you remember to use epinastine eyedrops, use them around the same times every day, usually morning and evening. Follow the directions on your prescription label carefully, and ask your doctor or pharmacist to explain any part you do not understand. Use epinastine eyedrops exactly as directed. Do not use more or less of them or use them more often than prescribed by your doctor.

Epinastine eyedrops are only for use in the eyes. Do not swallow this medication.

Epinastine eyedrops control the itching of allergic conjunctivitis only when they are used regularly. Epinastine eyedrops will not work if you use them only when you experience symptoms. Continue to use epinastine eyedrops even if you feel well. Do not stop using epinastine eyedrops without talking to your doctor.

When you apply epinastine eye drops, be careful not to let the tip of the bottle touch your eye, fingers, face, or any surface. If the tip does touch another surface, bacteria may get into the eye drops. Using eye drops that are contaminated with bacteria may cause serious damage to the eye or loss of vision. If you think your eye drops have become contaminated, call your doctor or pharmacist.

To use the eye drops, follow these steps:

1. Wash your hands thoroughly with soap and water.
2. Use a mirror or have someone else put the drops in your eye.
3. Remove the protective cap. Make sure that the end of the dropper tip is not chipped or cracked.
4. Avoid touching the dropper tip against your eye, face, nose, fingers, or anything else.
5. Hold the bottle with the tip down at all times to prevent drops from flowing back into the bottle and contaminating the medication inside.
6. Lie down and gaze upward or tilt your head back.
7. Holding the bottle between your thumb and index finger, place the dropper tip as near as possible to your eyelid without touching it.
8. Brace the remaining fingers of that hand against your cheek or nose.
9. With the index finger of your other hand, pull the lower lid of the eye down to form a pocket.
10. Drop the prescribed number of drops into the pocket made by the lower lid and the eye. Placing drops on the surface of the eyeball can cause stinging.
11. Close your eye and press lightly against the lower lid with your finger for 2-3 minutes to keep the medication in the eye. Do not blink.
12. Repeat steps 7-11 above for your other eye.
13. Replace the cap on the bottle and tighten it right away. Do not wipe or rinse off the tip.

14. Wipe off any excess liquid from your cheek with a clean tissue. Wash your hands again.

Are there other uses for this medicine?

This medication may be prescribed for other uses; ask your doctor or pharmacist for more information.

What special precautions should I follow?

Before using epinastine eyedrops,

- tell your doctor and pharmacist if you are allergic to epinastine or any other medications.
- tell your doctor and pharmacist what other prescription and nonprescription medications, vitamins, nutritional supplements, and herbal products you are taking. Your doctor may need to adjust the doses of your medications or monitor you carefully for side effects.
- tell your doctor if you wear contact lenses. You should not wear contact lenses if your eyes are red or irritated, and you should not use epinastine to treat eye irritation that you think may be caused by contact lenses.
- tell your doctor if you are pregnant, plan to become pregnant, or are breast-feeding. If you become pregnant while taking epinastine, call your doctor.
- tell your doctor if you wear contact lenses. You should not wear contact lenses if your eyes are red or irritated, and you should not use epinastine eyedrops to treat irritation that you think may be caused by contact lenses. You should also not apply epinastine eyedrops while you are wearing contact lenses. Remove your contact lenses before you use epinastine eyedrops and do not replace them for at least 10 minutes afterward. You may find it convenient to apply the eye drops before you put your lenses on in the morning and after you take them out in the evening.

What special dietary instructions should I follow?

Unless your doctor tells you otherwise, continue your normal diet.

What should I do if I forget to take a dose?

Apply the missed dose as soon as you remember it. However, if it is almost time for the next dose, skip the missed dose and continue your regular dosing schedule. Do not apply a double dose to make up for a missed one.

What side effects can this medicine cause?

Epinastine eyedrops may cause side effects. It may be hard to tell if the symptoms you experience are side effects of epinastine eyedrops or are caused by allergies. Tell your doctor if any of these symptoms are severe or do not go away:

- burning or itchy eyes
- swollen eyelids
- eye redness

- headache
- runny nose
- cough

Some side effects can be serious. The following symptoms are uncommon, but if you experience either of them, call your doctor immediately:

- sore throat
- fever, chills, and other signs of infection

Epinastine eyedrops may cause other side effects. Call your doctor if you have any unusual problems while taking this medication.

If you experience a serious side effect, you or your doctor may send a report to the Food and Drug Administration's (FDA) MedWatch Adverse Event Reporting program online [at http://www.fda.gov/MedWatch/index.html] or by phone [1-800-332-1088].

What storage conditions are needed for this medicine?

Keep this medication in the container it came in, tightly closed, and out of reach of children. Store it at room temperature and away from excess heat and moisture (not in the bathroom). Throw away any medication that is outdated or no longer needed. Talk to your pharmacist about the proper disposal of your medication.

What should I do in case of overdose?

In case of overdose, call your local poison control center at 1-800-222-1222. If the victim has collapsed or is not breathing, call local emergency services at 911.

What other information should I know?

Keep all appointments with your doctor.

Do not let anyone else take your medication. Ask your pharmacist any questions you have about refilling your prescription.

Dosage Facts
For Informational Purposes

Caution: Do not change your dose, how often you take your medication, or the length of time you are to take it without first talking to your healthcare provider.

The following dosage information was written using medical language for doctors and other healthcare professionals and is provided here for you to check your dosage. The dosage of this drug may differ for different patients. Therefore, always follow your doctor's instructions or the directions on the label. Contact your healthcare provider or pharmacist if you have any questions about the specific dosage of your medication after reviewing this information.

General Dosage Information

Available as epinastine hydrochloride; dosage expressed in terms of the salt.

Pediatric Patients

Allergic Conjunctivitis

OPHTHALMIC:

- Children ≥3 years of age: 1 drop of a 0.05% solution in each eye twice daily for up to 8 weeks.
- Continue therapy throughout period of exposure (i.e., until pollen season is over or until exposure to offending allergen is terminated), even in absence of symptoms.

Adult Patients

Allergic Conjunctivitis

OPHTHALMIC:

- 1 drop of a 0.05% solution in each eye twice daily for up to 8 weeks.
- Continue therapy throughout period of exposure (i.e., until pollen season is over or until exposure to offending allergen is terminated), even in absence of symptoms.

Epinephrine Injection
(ep i nef' rin)

Brand Name: Adrenalin® Chloride Solution, EpiPen® Auto-Injector, EpiPen® Jr. Auto-Injector

Also available generically.

Why is this medicine prescribed?

Epinephrine injection is used to treat life-threatening allergic reactions caused by insect bites, foods, medications, latex, and other causes. Symptoms of allergic reaction include wheezing, shortness of breath, low blood pressure, hives, itching, swelling, stomach cramps, diarrhea, and loss of bladder control. Epinephrine is in a class of medications called sympathomimetic agents. It works by relaxing the muscles in the airways and tightening the blood vessels.

How should this medicine be used?

Epinephrine injection comes as a single-dose pre-filled automatic injection device to be injected into the thigh. You should only use it when you are experiencing or are likely to begin experiencing a serious allergic reaction. Talk to your doctor about substances that may cause serious allergic reactions and symptoms of these reactions.

Under certain conditions, you may need more than one epinephrine injection to treat an allergic reaction. Your doctor will tell you if and when you should use a second dose. Follow the directions on your prescription label carefully and ask your doctor or pharmacist to explain any part you do not understand. Use epinephrine injection exactly as directed. Do not use more or less of it or use it more often than prescribed by your doctor.

To use the automatic injection device, follow these steps:

1. Hold the device firmly in your fist with the black tip pointing down. Do not touch the black tip; hold only the cylinder.
2. Remove the gray activation cap.
3. Move your hand so the black tip is near your outer thigh.
4. Swing your hand away from your body, then jab the black tip firmly into your outer thigh at a 90-degree angle. You may inject the needle through clothing that is covering your thigh.
5. Keep the device firmly in this position for several seconds.
6. Remove the device from your thigh and rub the area with your fingers.
7. Look at the black tip to see if the needle is showing. If the needle is not showing, repeat steps 3-6.
8. If the needle is showing, you have received the full dose of epinephrine. You will notice that most of the liquid remains in the device. This is extra liquid that cannot be used.
9. Press the needle against a hard surface.
10. Replace the device in the carrying tube (without the activation cap) and cover with the cap.

After you use the automatic injection device, follow these steps:

1. If you were stung by an insect, try to remove the stinger with your fingernails. Be careful not to push the stinger deeper into the skin and not to pinch or squeeze the area. If you can, put ice and/or baking soda soaks on the area.
2. Go to the nearest hospital emergency room right away. Take the used injection device with you. Tell the doctor that you have used the device and give it to him for disposal.
3. Rest and avoid physical activity as directed by your doctor.

Handle the automatic injection device carefully to avoid accidentally injecting the epinephrine into your hands. If you do accidentally inject the epinephrine into any part of your body except your thigh, go to the nearest emergency room right away.

Are there other uses for this medicine?

This medication may be prescribed for other uses; ask your doctor or pharmacist for more information.

What special precautions should I follow?

Before using epinephrine injection:

- tell your doctor or pharmacist if you are allergic to epinephrine, sulfites, or any other medications. Your doctor may tell you to use epinephrine injection even if you are allergic to one of the ingredients because it is a life-saving medication. The epinephrine automatic injection

device does not contain latex and is safe to use if you have a latex allergy.

- tell your doctor or pharmacist what prescription and nonprescription medications, vitamins, nutritional supplements, and herbal products you are taking. Be sure to mention any of the following: antidepressants such as amitriptyline (Elavil), amoxapine (Asendin), clomipramine (Anafranil), desipramine (Norpramin), doxepin (Adapin, Sinequan), imipramine (Tofranil), nortriptyline (Aventyl, Pamelor), protriptyline (Vivactil), and trimipramine (Surmontil); digoxin (Digitek, Lanoxicaps, Lanoxin); and quinidine (Quinidex). Also tell your doctor if you are taking a monoamine oxidase inhibitor such as phenelzine (Nardil) or tranylcypromine (Parnate) or have stopped taking it within the past two weeks. Your doctor may need to change the doses of your medications or monitor you carefully for side effects.
- tell your doctor if you have or have ever had chest pain or a heart attack, irregular heart beat, diabetes, high blood pressure, or an overactive thyroid gland (hyperthyroidism).
- tell your doctor if you are pregnant, plan to become pregnant, or are breast-feeding. If you become pregnant while taking epinephrine injection, call your doctor.

What special dietary instructions should I follow?

Unless your doctor tells you otherwise, continue your normal diet.

What side effects can this medicine cause?

Epinephrine injection may cause side effects. Tell your doctor if any of these symptoms are severe or do not go away:

- upset stomach
- vomiting
- sweating
- dizziness
- nervousness
- weakness
- pale skin
- headache
- shaking hands that you cannot control

Some side effects can be serious. The following symptoms are uncommon, but if you experience any of them, call your doctor immediately:

- difficulty breathing
- pounding, fast, or irregular heartbeat

Epinephrine injection may cause other side effects. Call your doctor if you have any unusual problems while taking this medication.

If you experience a serious side effect, you or your doctor may send a report to the Food and Drug Administration's (FDA) MedWatch Adverse Event Reporting program online [at http://www.fda.gov/MedWatch/index.html] or by phone [1-800-332-1088].

What storage conditions are needed for this medicine?

Keep this medication in the plastic carrying tube it came in, tightly closed, and out of reach of children. Store it in a dark place at room temperature and away from excess heat and moisture (not in the bathroom). Pay attention to the expiration date of your automatic injection device, and be sure to always have an unexpired device available. Look at the liquid in the clear window of the device from time to time. Throw away the device if the liquid has changed color, is cloudy, or contains solid pieces, or if the expiration date has passed. Talk to your pharmacist about the proper disposal of your medication.

If you are experiencing an allergic emergency and the liquid in your device is discolored or otherwise appears abnormal, consult your doctor. He may tell you to use the device if you cannot get a fresh one quickly.

What should I do in case of overdose?

In case of overdose, call your local poison control center at 1-800-222-1222. If the victim has collapsed or is not breathing, call local emergency services at 911.

What other information should I know?

Keep all appointments with your doctor.

Do not let anyone else use your medication. Ask your pharmacist any questions you have about refilling your prescription.

Dosage Facts
For Informational Purposes

Caution: Do not change your dose, how often you take your medication, or the length of time you are to take it without first talking to your health-care provider.

The following dosage information was written using medical language for doctors and other healthcare professionals and is provided here for you to check your dosage. The dosage of this drug may differ for different patients. Therefore, always follow your doctor's instructions or the directions on the label. Contact your healthcare provider or pharmacist if you have any questions about the specific dosage of your medication after reviewing this information.

General Dosage Information

Available as epinephrine and epinephrine hydrochloride; dosage expressed in terms of epinephrine.

Pediatric Patients

Sensitivity Reactions
Anaphylaxis

IM:

- Inject 0.01 mg/kg (0.01 mL/kg of a 1:1000 injection) (up to 0.5 mg/dose), repeated every 10–20 minutes as needed for up to 3 consecutive doses.

- For *self-administration* using a prefilled auto-injector (e.g., EpiPen®), inject 0.15 or 0.3 mg, depending on body weight; a dose of 0.01 mg/kg generally is recommended. Clinicians may recommend higher or lower doses depending on individual patient needs and considering the life-threatening nature of anaphylaxis. The 0.15-mg dose may be more appropriate for children <30 kg. If doses <0.15 mg are considered more appropriate, alternative injectable forms of the drug should be used. For severe persistent anaphylaxis, repeated doses may be needed.

Adult Patients

Bronchospasm
Treatment of Acute Exacerbations of Asthma

IM:

- For severe asthma, the usual initial dose is 0.1–0.5 mg (0.1–0.5 mL of a 1:1000 injection). Initial doses should be small and may be increased if necessary, but single doses should not exceed 1 mg.

Sensitivity Reactions
Anaphylaxis

IM:

- The usual initial dose is 0.1–0.5 mg (0.1–0.5 mL of a 1:1000 injection).
- For the treatment of reactions caused by drugs that were given IM, epinephrine may be administered at the site of injection of the other drug to minimize further absorption.
- Initial doses should be small and may be increased if necessary, but single doses should not exceed 1 mg.
- Alternatively, inject 0.3–0.5 mg (0.3–0.5 mL of a 1:1000 injection), repeated every 15–20 minutes, as needed.
- For *self-administration* using a prefilled auto-injector (e.g., EpiPen®), inject 0.3 mg. Clinicians may recommend higher or lower doses depending on individual patient needs and considering the life-threatening nature of anaphylaxis.
- For severe persistent anaphylaxis, repeated doses may be needed.

Prescribing Limits
Pediatric Patients

Sensitivity Reactions
Anaphylaxis

IM:
- Maximum for pediatric patients: 0.5 mg repeated no more frequently than every 10 minutes up to 3 times.

Adult Patients

Sensitivity Reactions
Anaphylaxis

IM:
- Single doses should not exceed 1 mg.

† Use is not currently included in the labeling approved by the US Food and Drug Administration.

Eplerenone

(e pler′ en one)

Brand Name: Inspra®

Why is this medicine prescribed?

Eplerenone is used alone or in combination with other medications to treat high blood pressure. Eplerenone is in a class of medications called mineralocorticoid receptor antagonists. It works by blocking the action of aldosterone, a natural substance in the body that raises blood pressure.

How should this medicine be used?

Eplerenone comes as a tablet to take by mouth. It is usually taken once or twice a day, with or without food. To help you remember to take eplerenone, take it around the same time every day. Follow the directions on your prescription label carefully, and ask your doctor or pharmacist to explain any part you do not understand. Take eplerenone exactly as directed. Do not take more or less of it or take it more often than prescribed by your doctor.

Your doctor may start you on a low dose of eplerenone and increase your dose after 4 weeks.

Eplerenone controls high blood pressure but does not cure it. It may take 4 weeks or longer before you feel the full benefit of eplerenone. Continue to take eplerenone even if you feel well. Do not stop taking eplerenone without talking to your doctor.

Are there other uses for this medicine?

This medication may be prescribed for other uses; ask your doctor or pharmacist for more information.

What special precautions should I follow?

Before taking eplerenone,

- tell your doctor and pharmacist if you are allergic to eplerenone or any other medications.
- do not take eplerenone if you are taking amiloride (Midamor), amiloride and hydrochlorothiazide (Moduretic), itraconazole (Sporanox), ketoconazole (Nizoral), potassium supplements, spironolactone (Aldactone), spironolactone and hydrochlorothiazide (Aldactazide), triamterene (Dyrenium), or triamterene and hydrochlorothiazide (Dyazide, Maxzide).
- tell your doctor and pharmacist what other prescription and nonprescription medications, vitamins, and nutritional supplements you are taking. Be sure to mention any of the following: angiotensin converting enzyme (ACE) inhibitors such as benazepril (Lotensin), captopril (Capoten), enalapril (Vasotec), fosinopril (Monopril), lisinopril (Prinivil, Zestril), and quinapril (Accupril); angiotensin II receptor antagonists such as eprosartan (Teveten), irbesartan (Avapro), losartan (Cozaar), olmesartan (Benicar), and valsartan (Diovan); as-

pirin and other nonsteroidal anti-inflammatory medications (NSAIDS) such as ibuprofen (Advil, Motrin) and naproxen (Aleve, Naprosyn); cimetidine (Tagamet); clarithromycin (Biaxin); danazol (Danocrine); delavirdine (Rescriptor); diltiazem (Cardizem, Dilacor, Tiazac); erythromycin (E.E.S., E-Mycin, Erythrocin); fluconazole (Diflucan); fluoxetine (Prozac, Sarafem); fluvoxamine (Luvox); HIV protease inhibitors such as indinavir (Crixivan), ritonavir (Norvir), and saquinavir (Fortovase, Invirase); isoniazid (INH, Nydrazid); lithium (Eskalith, Lithobid), metronidazole (Flagyl); nefazodone (Serzone); troleandomycin (TAO); verapamil (Calan, Covera, Isoptin, Verelan); and zafirlukast (Accolate). Your doctor may need to change the doses of your medications or monitor you carefully for side effects.

- tell your doctor what herbal products you are taking, especially St. John's wort.
- tell your doctor if you have or have ever had high blood levels of potassium, diabetes, gout, or liver or kidney disease.
- tell your doctor if you are pregnant, plan to become pregnant, or are breast-feeding. If you become pregnant while taking eplerenone, call your doctor.

What special dietary instructions should I follow?

Talk to your doctor about drinking grapefruit juice while taking this medicine.

Do not use salt substitutes containing potassium while you are taking eplerenone. If your doctor prescribes a low-salt or low-sodium diet, follow these directions carefully.

What should I do if I forget to take a dose?

Take the missed dose as soon as you remember it. However, if it is almost time for the next dose, skip the missed dose and continue your regular dosing schedule. Do not take a double dose to make up for a missed one.

What side effects can this medicine cause?

Eplerenone may cause side effects. Tell your doctor if any of these symptoms are severe or do not go away:

- headache
- dizziness
- diarrhea
- stomach pain
- cough
- excessive tiredness
- flu-like symptoms
- breast enlargement or tenderness
- abnormal vaginal bleeding

Some side effects can be serious. The following symptoms are uncommon, but if you experience any of them, call your doctor immediately:

- chest pain
- tingling in arms and legs

- loss of muscle tone
- weakness or heaviness in legs
- confusion
- lack of energy
- cold, gray skin
- irregular heartbeat

Eplerenone may cause other side effects. Call your doctor if you have any unusual problems while taking this medication.

If you experience a serious side effect, you or your doctor may send a report to the Food and Drug Administration's (FDA) MedWatch Adverse Event Reporting program online [at http://www.fda.gov/MedWatch/index.html] or by phone [1-800-332-1088].

What storage conditions are needed for this medicine?

Keep this medication in the container it came in, tightly closed, and out of reach of children. Store it at room temperature and away from excess heat and moisture (not in the bathroom). Throw away any medication that is outdated or no longer needed. Talk to your pharmacist about the proper disposal of your medication.

What should I do in case of overdose?

In case of overdose, call your local poison control center at 1-800-222-1222. If the victim has collapsed or is not breathing, call local emergency services at 911.

Symptoms of overdose may include:

- fainting
- dizziness
- blurred vision
- upset stomach
- tingiling in arms and legs
- loss of muscle tone
- weakness or heaviness in legs
- confusion
- lack of energy
- cold, gray skin
- irregular or slow heartbeat

What other information should I know?

Keep all appointments with your doctor and the laboratory. Your doctor will check your blood pressure regularly and order certain lab tests to check your body's response to eplerenone.

Do not let anyone else take your medication. Ask your pharmacist any questions you have about refilling your prescription.

Dosage Facts
For Informational Purposes

Caution: Do not change your dose, how often you take your medication, or the length of time you are to take it without first talking to your healthcare provider.

The following dosage information was written using medical language for doctors and other healthcare professionals and is provided here for you to check your dosage. The dosage of this drug may differ for different patients. Therefore, always follow your doctor's instructions or the directions on the label. Contact your healthcare provider or pharmacist if you have any questions about the specific dosage of your medication after reviewing this information.

Adult Patients

CHF after AMI

ORAL:

- Initially, 25 mg once daily. Titrate dosage as tolerated to a target dosage of 50 mg once daily, preferably within 4 weeks of initiation of therapy in patients without hyperkalemia (defined as serum potassium concentrations $\geq$5.5 mEq/L).

Dosage Modification in CHF for Serum Potassium Concentrations

Serum Potassium (mEq/L)	Dosage Adjustment
<5	In those receiving 25 mg every other day, increase to 25 mg daily
	In those receiving 25 mg daily, increase to 50 mg daily
5–5.4	None
5.5–5.9	In those receiving 50 mg daily, decrease to 25 mg daily
	In those receiving 25 mg daily, decrease to 25 mg every other day
	In those receiving 25 mg every other day, withhold therapy
$\geq$6	Withhold

Hypertension

ORAL:

- Dosage must be individualized and adjusted according to the BP response.
- Initially, 50 mg once daily. If BP is not adequately controlled after 4 weeks, increase dosage to 50 mg twice daily.
- In hypertensive patients currently receiving therapy with weak inhibitors of the CYP3A4 isoenzyme (e.g., erythromycin, saquinavir, verapamil, fluconazole), reduce the initial dosage to 25 mg once daily.

Prescribing Limits

Adult Patients

Hypertension

ORAL:

- 50 mg twice daily. No additional benefit from higher dosages (>100 mg daily) and such dosages have been associated with increased risk of hyperkalemia.

Special Populations

Hepatic Impairment
- No adjustment in the initial dosage is necessary in those with mild-to-moderate hepatic impairment.

Geriatric Patients
- No adjustment in the initial dosage is necessary.

Epoetin Alfa Injection

(e poe′ e tin)

Brand Name: Epogen®, Procrit®

Important Warning

Epoetin alfa increases the risk of serious and life-threatening events, including heart attack, heart failure, stroke, TIA (ministroke) or cerebrovascular accident (blood clot to the brain), pulmonary embolus (blood clot to the lung), deep vein thrombosis (blood clot to the blood vessels), and death when treatment results in a higher than recommended amount of hemoglobin (red blood cells) in the blood. Call your doctor immediately if you experience any of the following symptoms: pain, tenderness, redness, warmth, and/or swelling in the legs; shortness of breath; cough that won't go away or coughing up blood; chest pain, squeezing pressure, or tightness; nausea; vomiting; discomfort or pain in the arms, shoulder, neck, jaw, or back; fast or irregular heartbeat; sweating; swelling of the hands, feet, or ankles; blue-grey coloring or darkening around mouth or nails; dizziness or lightheadedness; extreme tiredness or weakness; fainting or loss of consciousness; sudden trouble seeing in one or both eyes; sudden trouble speaking or understanding speech; sudden confusion; sudden weakness or numbness of an arm or leg (especially on one side of the body), or face; sudden trouble walking or loss of balance or coordination; sudden severe headache; seizure; increased blood pressure; or, if you are on hemodialysis and you notice blood clots in a vascular access port.

Epoetin alfa may increase the chance of death when used in people with cancer who are not receiving chemotherapy or radiation therapy at the same time they are using epoetin alfa. In people with cancer, epoetin alpha may cause a tumor to grow faster when the amount of hemoglobin (red blood cells) in the blood is higher than recommended.

Use of medications similar to epoetin alpha in people just before major surgery increases the risk of blood clots. Call your doctor immediately if you experience any of the following symptoms: pain, ten-derness, redness, warmth, and/or swelling in one or both legs. Your doctor may prescribe an anticoagulant ('blood thinner') prior to surgery to help prevent blood clots.

Ask your pharmacist or doctor for a copy of the manufacturer's information for the patient.

Keep all appointments with your doctor and the laboratory. Your doctor will order certain lab tests to check your body's response to epoetin alfa.

Talk to your doctor about the risks of using epoetin alfa.

Why is this medicine prescribed?

Epoetin alfa is used to treat anemia (a lower than normal number of red blood cells) in people with chronic kidney failure (a condition where over a period of time there is a decrease in kidney function that is not reversible). Epoetin alfa is also used to treat anemia in people receiving certain medications, such as chemotherapy (medications to treat cancer) and zidovudine (AZT, Retrovir, in Trizivir, in Combivir), a medication used to treat human immunodeficiency virus (HIV). Epoetin alfa is also used before and after certain types of surgery to decrease the number of blood transfusions (transfer of one person's blood to another person's body) needed for expected or actual blood loss during surgery. Epoetin alfa is in a class of medications called erythropoiesis-stimulating agents (ESAs). It works by causing the bone marrow (soft tissue inside the bones where blood is made) to make more red blood cells.

How should this medicine be used?

Epoetin alfa comes as a solution (liquid) to inject subcutaneously (just under the skin) or intravenously (into a vein). It is usually injected one to three times weekly. When epoetin alfa is used to prevent and treat anemia due to surgery, it is sometimes injected once daily for 10 days before surgery, on the day of surgery and for 4 days after surgery. Alternatively, epoetin alfa is sometimes injected once weekly, beginning 3 weeks before surgery, with a dose also on the day of surgery. To help you remember to use epoetin alfa, mark a calendar to keep track of when you are to receive a dose. Follow the directions on your prescription label carefully, and ask your doctor or pharmacist to explain any part you do not understand. Use epoetin alfa exactly as directed. Do not use more or less of it or use it more often than prescribed by your doctor.

Your doctor may start you on the lowest possible dose of epoetin alfa and gradually increase or decrease your dose, usually not more than once every month. Your doctor may also tell you to stop using epoetin alfa for a time. Follow these instructions carefully. If your doctor tells you to stop using epoetin alfa, do not begin using it again until your doctor tells you that you should. It is likely that your doctor will restart your treatment with a lower dose of epoetin alfa than you were using.

Epoetin alfa is used to reduce the need for red blood

cell transfusions. It does not cure anemia. It may take up to 2 to 6 weeks before there is an increase in the number of red blood cells. Do not stop using epoetin alfa without talking to your doctor.

Epoetin alfa injections are usually given by a doctor or nurse. Your doctor may decide that you can inject epoetin alfa yourself or that you may have a friend or relative give the injections. Your doctor will make sure the person who will be injecting the medication can give the injection correctly. Always follow the instructions of your doctor concerning the dose, how to give the medication, and how often to give the medication. Be sure that you and the person who will be giving the injections read the manufacturer's information for the patient that comes with epoetin alfa before you use it for the first time at home.

If you are using epoetin alfa at home, you will need to use disposable syringes and needles to inject your medication. Your doctor or pharmacist will tell you what type of syringe you should use. Do not use any other type of syringe because you may not get the right amount of medication. Always keep a spare syringe and needle on hand.

Use a disposable syringe or needle only one time. Throw away used syringes in a puncture-resistant container, out of the reach of children. Talk to your doctor or pharmacist about how to throw away the puncture-resistant container. Do not throw the container in your household trash. There may be special state and local laws for throwing away used needles and syringes.

If your doctor has prescribed epoetin alfa in a single use vial, the vial can be used only one time. Do not put a needle through the rubber stopper of the vial more than once. Throw away the vial after you have used it for one dose, even if it is not empty.

Always inject epoetin alfa in its own syringe; never mix it with any other medication.

If you are injecting epoetin alfa subcutaneously, you can inject it just under the skin anywhere on the outer area of your upper arms, middle of the front thighs, stomach (except for a 2-inch area around the navel), or outer area of the buttocks. Do not inject epoetin alfa into a spot that is tender, red, bruised, hard, or has scars or stretch marks. Choose a new spot each time you inject epoetin alfa, as directed by your doctor. Write down the date, time, dose of epoetin alfa, and the spot where you injected your dose in a record book.

Carefully read the manufacturer's instructions that describe how to prepare and inject a dose of epoetin alpha. Be sure to ask your pharmacist or doctor if you have any questions about how to prepare or inject this medication.

Are there other uses for this medicine?

This medication may be prescribed for other uses, including anemia in premature (born too early) babies; anemia from rheumatoid arthritis (condition in which the body attacks its own joints, causing pain, swelling, and loss of function); Castleman disease (spread of growths in certain parts of the body that can cause anemia); Gaucher's disease (buildup of a fatty substance in certain parts of the body that can cause

liver, spleen, bone, and blood problems); myelodysplastic syndrome (a disease that causes bone marrow to make unhealthy red blood cells); paroxysmal nocturnal hemoglobinuria (disease where red blood cells are destroyed and leave the body through the urine during sleep); and sickle cell anemia (a type of anemia in which red blood cells have an abnormal shape). Ask your doctor or pharmacist for more information.

What special precautions should I follow?

Before using epoetin alfa,

- tell your doctor and pharmacist if you are allergic to epoetin alfa, darbepoetin alfa (Aranesp), medications made from animal cells, albumin, or any other medications, or if you are allergic to benzyl alcohol. Ask your doctor or pharmacist if you don't know if a medication you are allergic to is made from animal cells.
- tell your doctor and pharmacist what other prescription and nonprescription medications, vitamins, nutritional supplements, and herbal products you are taking or plan to take. Your doctor may need to change the doses of your medications or monitor you carefully for side effects.
- tell your doctor if you have or have had high blood pressure. Your doctor may tell you not to use epoetin alfa.
- tell your doctor if you have or have ever had bleeding or blood clotting problems; cancer; diseases that affect your blood such as leukemia, myelodysplastic syndrome (condition in which the bone marrow can not produce enough blood cells), sickle cell disease (an inherited blood disease that causes pain, anemia, and organ damage), thalassemia (an inherited blood disease that causes abnormal development and other problems), or porphyria (an inherited blood disease that may cause skin or nervous system problems); blood clots in your heart, legs, or lungs; a heart attack; an infection; stroke or ministroke (TIA); tumors; heart disease, or any disease that affects your brain or nervous system.
- tell your doctor if you have used epoetin alfa or another erythropoiesis-stimulating agents, such as darbepoetin alfa (Aranesp), in the past. Be sure to tell your doctor if your anemia worsened during your treatment with one of these medications, or if you were ever told to stop using one of these medications.
- tell your doctor if you are pregnant, plan to become pregnant, or are breast-feeding. If you become pregnant while using epoetin alfa, call your doctor. If you stopped menstruating (getting your period) because of your anemia, you may begin to menstruate again while you are using epoetin alfa. This may increase the chance that you will become pregnant. Talk to your doctor about the type of birth control that is right for you.
- if you are having surgery, including dental surgery, tell the doctor or dentist that you are using epoetin alfa.
- you should know that epoetin alfa may cause seizures, usually during the first 3 months of treatment. Talk to

your doctor about driving a car, operating machinery, or participating in dangerous activities during this time.

- you should know that your blood pressure may increase while you are using epoetin alfa. Your doctor may ask you to monitor your blood pressure frequently. Be sure to check your blood pressure as often as your doctor tells you that you should, to call your doctor if your blood pressure is higher than your doctor says it should be, and to take any medications your doctor prescribes to control your blood pressure exactly as directed.
- you should call your doctor if you are planning to travel or if your activity becomes limited, such as spending more time sitting or in bed.
- if you are on hemodialysis, you should know that blood clots may form in the tubing that goes into your vein. Call your doctor if you think there is a clot in your tubing.

What special dietary instructions should I follow?

If you are following a prescribed special diet because you have kidney disease or high blood pressure, follow it carefully, even if you feel better while using epoetin alfa. Epoetin alfa will not work unless your body has enough iron. Your doctor or dietician will probably tell you to eat foods that are rich in iron. If you cannot get enough iron from your diet, your doctor may prescribe an iron supplement. Take this supplement exactly as directed.

What should I do if I forget to take a dose?

Call your doctor to ask what to do if you miss a dose of epoetin alfa. Do not use a double dose to make up for a missed one.

What side effects can this medicine cause?

Epoetin alfa may cause side effects. Tell your doctor if any of these symptoms are severe or do not go away:

- headache
- joint or muscle aches, pain, or soreness
- nausea
- vomiting
- indigestion
- stomach pain
- diarrhea
- constipation
- difficulty falling asleep or staying asleep
- rash
- itching
- pain, burning, numbness, or tingling in the hands or feet

Some side effects can be serious. If you experience any of the following symptoms, or those listed in the IMPORTANT WARNING section, call your doctor immediately.

- hallucinating (seeing things or hearing voices that do not exist)
- fever, sore throat, chills, cough, and other signs of infection

- redness, swelling, pain, or itching at the injection spot
- spreading rash over the whole body
- hives
- swelling of the face, throat, tongue, lips, eyes
- wheezing
- difficulty breathing or swallowing
- hoarseness
- lack of energy
- feeling cold most of the time

Epoetin alfa may cause other side effects. Call your doctor if you have any unusual problems while taking this medication.

If you experience a serious side effect, you or your doctor may send a report to the Food and Drug Administration's (FDA) MedWatch Adverse Event Reporting program online [at http://www.fda.gov/MedWatch/index.html] or by phone [1-800-332-1088].

What storage conditions are needed for this medicine?

Keep this medication in the container it came in, tightly closed, and out of reach of children. Store it in the refrigerator, but do not freeze it. Keep epoetin alfa away from excess heat and moisture (not in the bathroom) and sunlight. Throw away any medication that is outdated or no longer needed. Throw away a multidose vial of epoetin alfa 21 days after you first use it. Talk to your pharmacist about the proper disposal of your medication.

When traveling, place epoetin alfa in its original box in an insulated cooler with coolant such as blue ice. Do not place epoetin alfa vials directly on ice or coolants, and do not allow them to freeze. If a vial does freeze, do not use it. Once you arrive, place the medication in a refrigerator as soon as possible.

What should I do in case of overdose?

In case of overdose, call your local poison control center at 1-800-222-1222. If the victim has collapsed or is not breathing, call local emergency services at 911.

Symptoms of overdose may include:

- pain, tenderness, redness, warmth, and/or swelling in the legs
- chest pain, squeezing pressure, or tightness
- discomfort or pain in the arms, shoulder, neck, jaw, or back
- fast or irregular heartbeat
- shortness of breath
- cough that won't go away or coughing up blood
- swelling of the hands, feet, or ankles
- blue-grey color or darkening around mouth or nails
- excessive sweating
- dizziness or lightheadedness
- fainting or loss of consciousness
- sudden trouble seeing in one or both eyes
- sudden confusion
- sudden trouble speaking or understanding speech

- sudden weakness or numbness of an arm or leg, (especially on one side of the body) or face
- sudden trouble walking or loss of balance or coordination
- sudden severe headache
- extreme tiredness or weakness
- seizure
- increased blood pressure
- blood clot in hemodialysis port

What other information should I know?

Before having any laboratory test, tell your doctor and the laboratory personnel that you are using epoetin alfa.

Do not let anyone else use your medication. Ask your pharmacist any questions you have about refilling your prescription.

Dosage Facts
For Informational Purposes

Caution: Do not change your dose, how often you take your medication, or the length of time you are to take it without first talking to your healthcare provider.

The following dosage information was written using medical language for doctors and other healthcare professionals and is provided here for you to check your dosage. The dosage of this drug may differ for different patients. Therefore, always follow your doctor's instructions or the directions on the label. Contact your healthcare provider or pharmacist if you have any questions about the specific dosage of your medication after reviewing this information.

Pediatric Patients

Anemia of Chronic Renal Failure

IV OR SUB-Q:
- Children and infants ≥1 month of age on dialysis: 50 units/kg 3 times weekly; IV administration recommended in patients undergoing hemodialysis.
- Children ≥3 months of age who do not require dialysis†: 50–250 units/kg 1–3 times weekly has been used.
- If the hemoglobin has not increased by ≥1 g/dL within 4 weeks and iron stores are adequate, increase dosage by approximately 25%. Thereafter, dosage may be increased at 4-week intervals until the suggested target hemoglobin of 10–12 g/dL is attained.
- Dosage adjustments should not be made more frequently than once a month; 2–6 weeks are required to elicit a clinically important change in hemoglobin following dosage adjustment.
- If the hemoglobin approaches 12 g/dL or increases by >1 g/dL in any 2-week period, reduce dosage by approximately 25%. If the hemoglobin continues to increase, withhold therapy temporarily until the hemoglobin begins to fall, then resume at a dosage approximately 25% less than the previous dosage.
- Maintenance dosages subject to interindividual variation; ti-

trate according to patient response. Median dosage of 167 units/kg (range 49–447 units/kg) or 76 units/kg (range 24–323 units/kg) per week in 2 or 3 divided doses weekly used in pediatric hemodialysis or peritoneal dialysis patients, respectively, in clinical studies.

Anemia in HIV-infected Patients
Zidovudine-associated Anemia†

IV OR SUB-Q:
- Children 8 months to 17 years of age have received dosages of 50–400 units/kg 2 or 3 times weekly.

Anemia in Cancer Patients
Chemotherapy-induced Anemia

IV:
- Initially, 600 units/kg (maximum 40,000 units) once weekly.
- If the hemoglobin has not increased by ≥1 g/dL within 4 weeks (in the absence of RBC transfusion), increase weekly dosage to 900 units/kg (maximum 60,000 units). Suggested target hemoglobin is 10–12 g/dL.
- If epoetin alfa therapy produces a very rapid hemoglobin response (e.g., an increase of >1 g/dL in any 2-week period) or if hemoglobin is >12 g/dL, reduce dosage by 25%. If hemoglobin >13 g/dL, withhold therapy until the hemoglobin falls to 12 g/dL, then resume at a dosage 25% less than the previous dosage.

Adult Patients

Anemia of Chronic Renal Failure

IV OR SUB-Q:
- 50–100 units/kg 3 times weekly; IV administration recommended in patients undergoing hemodialysis.
- If the hemoglobin has not increased by ≥1 g/dL within 4 weeks and iron stores are adequate, increase dosage by approximately 25%. Thereafter, dosage may be increased at 4-week intervals until the suggested target hemoglobin of 10–12 g/dL is attained.
- Dosage adjustments should not be made more frequently than once a month; 2–6 weeks are required to elicit a clinically important change in hemoglobin following dosage adjustment.
- If the hemoglobin approaches 12 g/dL or increases by >1 g/dL in any 2-week period, reduce dosage by approximately 25%. If the hemoglobin continues to increase, withhold therapy temporarily until the hemoglobin begins to fall, then resume at a dosage approximately 25% less than the previous dosage.
- Maintenance dosages: subject to interindividual variation; titrate according to patient response. Median dosage of 75 units/kg (range: 12.5–525 units/kg) 3 times weekly used in clinical studies.

Anemia in HIV-infected Patients
Zidovudine-associated Anemia

IV OR SUB-Q:
- Initially, 100 units/kg 3 times weekly for 8–12 weeks.
- If the response is not satisfactory (transfusion requirements not reduced or hemoglobin not increased) after 8 weeks, increase each dose by 50–100 units/kg. Thereafter, adjust each dose every 4–8 weeks in increments of 50–100 units/kg as necessary.
- If the hemoglobin is >13 g/dL, withhold drug until the hemoglobin decreases to 12 g/dL. Reduce dosage by 25% upon reinitiation; titrate according to response.

- Maintenance dosages: titrate dosage to maintain response, taking into consideration other concurrent response factors (e.g., changes in zidovudine dosage, infectious or inflammatory processes).
- Patients who have not responded to dosages of 300 units/kg 3 times weekly are unlikely to respond to higher dosages; some patients with AIDS reportedly have required much higher dosages, and dosage should be individualized.

Anemia in Cancer Patients
Chemotherapy-induced Anemia

SUB-Q:
- Three-times-weekly regimen: 150 units/kg 3 times weekly for 8 weeks.
- If the response is not satisfactory (transfusion requirements not reduced or hemoglobin not increased) after 8 weeks, increase dosage to 300 units/kg 3 times weekly. Suggested target hemoglobin is 10–12 g/dL.
- If the hemoglobin approaches 12 g/dL or increases by >1 g/dL in any 2-week period, reduce dosage by 25%. If the hemoglobin is >13 g/dL, withhold therapy temporarily until the hemoglobin falls to 12 g/dL, at which point therapy may be resumed at a dosage 25% less than the previous dosage.
- Once-weekly regimen: initially, 40,000 units weekly.
- If the hemoglobin has not increased by ≥1 g/dL within 4 weeks (in the absence of RBC transfusion), increase dosage to 60,000 units weekly.
- If epoetin alfa therapy produces a very rapid hemoglobin response (e.g., an increase of >1 g/dL in any 2-week period) or if hemoglobin is >12 g/dL, reduce dosage by 25%. If hemoglobin >13 g/dL, withhold therapy temporarily until the hemoglobin falls to 12 g/dL, then resume at a dosage 25% less than the previous dosage.

Reduction of Allogeneic Blood Transfusion in Surgical Patients

SUB-Q:
- 300 units/kg once daily for 10 days prior to surgery, on the day of surgery, and for 4 days after surgery.
- Alternatively, 600 units/kg once weekly for 3 weeks prior to surgery (i.e., days 21, 14, and 7 before surgery), with an additional dose given on the day of surgery.

Prescribing Limits
Pediatric Patients
Chemotherapy-induced Anemia

IV:
- Maximum 60,000 units once weekly.

Adult Patients
Zidovudine-associated Anemia

IV OR SUB-Q:
- Patients not responding to 300 units/kg 3 times weekly are unlikely to respond to higher dosages.

Special Populations

Geriatric Patients
- Surgical patients receiving once-weekly regimen: Insufficient experience to determine whether dosing requirements differ from those in younger adults.
- Anemia of chronic renal failure in patients requiring dialysis:

Careful and individualized dosing recommended to maintain target hemoglobin concentration.

† Use is not currently included in the labeling approved by the US Food and Drug Administration.

Eprosartan

(ep roe sar' tan)

Brand Name: Teveten®, Teveten® HCT as a combination product containing Eprosartan Mesylate and Hydrochlorothiazide

Important Warning

Do not take eprosartan if you are pregnant. If you become pregnant while taking eprosartan, call your doctor immediately. Eprosartan may harm the fetus.

Why is this medicine prescribed?

Eprosartan is used alone or in combination with other medications to treat high blood pressure. Eprosartan is in a class of medications called angiotensin II receptor antagonists. It works by blocking the action of certain chemicals that tighten the blood vessels, so blood flows more smoothly.

How should this medicine be used?

Eprosartan comes as a tablet to take by mouth. It is usually taken once or twice a day with or without food. To help you remember to take eprosartan, take it around the same time every day. Follow the directions on your prescription label carefully, and ask your doctor or pharmacist to explain any part you do not understand. Take eprosartan exactly as directed. Do not take more or less of it or take it more often than prescribed by your doctor.

Eprosartan controls high blood pressure but does not cure it. Continue to take eprosartan even if you feel well. Do not stop taking eprosartan without talking to your doctor.

Are there other uses for this medicine?

Eprosartan is also used sometimes to treat heart failure. Talk to your doctor about the possible risks of using this drug for your condition.

This medication may be prescribed for other uses; ask your doctor or pharmacist for more information.

What special precautions should I follow?

Before taking eprosartan,
- tell your doctor and pharmacist if you are allergic to eprosartan or any other medications.

- tell your doctor and pharmacist what prescription and nonprescription medications, vitamins, nutritional supplements, and herbal products you are taking. Be sure to mention the following: diuretics ('water pills'). Your doctor may need to change the doses of your medications or monitor you carefully for side effects.
- tell your doctor if you have or have ever had heart failure or kidney disease.
- tell your doctor if you plan to become pregnant or are breast-feeding.

What special dietary instructions should I follow?

If your doctor prescribes a low-salt or low-sodium diet, follow these directions carefully.

What should I do if I forget to take a dose?

Take the missed dose as soon as you remember it. However, if it is almost time for the next dose, skip the missed dose and continue your regular dosing schedule. Do not take a double dose to make up for a missed one.

What side effects can this medicine cause?

Eprosartan may cause side effects. Tell your doctor if any of these symptoms are severe or do not go away:

- runny nose
- sore throat
- cough
- excessive tiredness
- stomach pain
- joint pain
- depression

Some side effects can be serious. The following symptoms are uncommon, but if you experience any of them, call your doctor immediately:

- swelling of the face, throat, tongue, lips, eyes, hands, feet, ankles, or lower legs
- hoarseness
- difficulty breathing or swallowing
- fainting

Eprosartan may cause other side effects. Call your doctor if you have any unusual problems while taking this medication.

If you experience a serious side effect, you or your doctor may send a report to the Food and Drug Administration's (FDA) MedWatch Adverse Event Reporting program online [at http://www.fda.gov/MedWatch/index.html] or by phone [1-800-332-1088].

What storage conditions are needed for this medicine?

Keep this medication in the container it came in, tightly closed, and out of reach of children. Store it at room temperature and away from excess heat and moisture (not in the bathroom). Throw away any medication that is outdated or no longer needed. Talk to your pharmacist about the proper disposal of your medication.

What should I do in case of overdose?

In case of overdose, call your local poison control center at 1-800-222-1222. If the victim has collapsed or is not breathing, call local emergency services at 911.

What other information should I know?

Keep all appointments with your doctor. Your blood pressure should be checked regularly to determine your response to eprosartan.

Do not let anyone else take your medication. Ask your pharmacist any questions you have about refilling your prescription.

Dosage Facts
For Informational Purposes

Caution: Do not change your dose, how often you take your medication, or the length of time you are to take it without first talking to your healthcare provider.

The following dosage information was written using medical language for doctors and other healthcare professionals and is provided here for you to check your dosage. The dosage of this drug may differ for different patients. Therefore, always follow your doctor's instructions or the directions on the label. Contact your healthcare provider or pharmacist if you have any questions about the specific dosage of your medication after reviewing this information.

General Dosage Information

Available as eprosartan mesylate; dosages expressed in terms of eprosartan.

Adult Patients

Hypertension
Monotherapy

ORAL:
- Initially, 600 mg once daily in adults without intravascular volume depletion. Adjust dosage at approximately monthly intervals (more aggressively in high-risk patients) to achieve BP control.
- Usual dosage: 400–800 mg daily, given in 1 dose or 2 divided doses; limited experience with higher dosages.
- If effectiveness diminishes toward end of dosing interval in patients treated once daily, consider increasing dosage or administering drug in 2 divided doses.

Combination Therapy

ORAL:
- If BP is not adequately controlled by monotherapy with eprosartan or hydrochlorothiazide, can switch to fixed-combination tablets (eprosartan 600 mg and hydrochlorothiazide 12.5 mg; then eprosartan 600 mg and hydrochlorothiazide 25 mg), administered once daily.

- If BP response diminishes toward the end of the dosing interval during once daily administration, increase dosage of the fixed-combination tablets to eprosartan 600 mg and hydrochlorothiazide 25 mg daily or add eprosartan 300 mg each evening.

Special Populations

Hepatic Impairment
- No initial dosage adjustments necessary.

Renal Impairment
- No initial dosage adjustment generally is necessary in patients with moderate or severe renal impairment; maximum 600 mg daily.
- Eprosartan/hydrochlorothiazide fixed combination not recommended in patients with anuria.

Geriatric Patients
- No initial dosage adjustments necessary.

Volume- and/or Salt-Depleted Patients
- Correct volume and/or salt depletion prior to initiation of therapy or initiate therapy under close medical supervision.

Erlotinib
(er loe′ tye nib)

Brand Name: Tarceva®

About Your Treatment

Your doctor has ordered erlotinib to help treat your illness. Erlotinib comes as a tablet to take by mouth. It is usually taken once a day on an empty stomach. Take erlotinib at least 1 hour before or 2 hours after you eat a meal or snack. To help you remember to take erlotinib, take it at around the same time every day.

Follow the directions on your prescription label carefully and ask your doctor or pharmacist to explain anything you do not understand. Take erlotinib exactly as directed. Do not take more or less of it or take it more often than prescribed by your doctor. Do not stop taking erlotinib without talking to your doctor.

This medication is used to treat non-small cell lung cancer (a type of cancer that begins in the lungs) in patients who have already been treated with at least one other chemotherapy medication and have not gotten better.

Erlotinib is in a class of drugs known as Human Epidermal Growth Factor Receptor Type 1/Epidermal Growth Factor Receptor (HER1/EGFR) tyrosine kinase inhibitors. It slows the growth of cancer cells. The length of your treatment depends on the types of drugs you are taking, how well your body responds to them, and the type of cancer you have. Be sure to tell your doctor how you are feeling during your treatment.

This medication may be prescribed for other uses; ask your doctor or pharmacist for more information.

Precautions

Before taking erlotinib,
- tell your doctor and pharmacist if you are allergic to erlotinib or any other drugs.
- tell your doctor and pharmacist what prescription and nonprescription medications, vitamins, and nutritional supplements you are taking. Be sure to mention any of the following: amiodarone (Cordarone, Pacerone); anticoagulants ('blood thinners') such as warfarin (Coumadin); antifungals such as fluconazole (Diflucan), itraconazole (Sporanox), and ketoconazole (Nizoral); aspirin and other non-steroidal anti-inflammatory medications (NSAIDS) such as ibuprofen (Advil, Motrin) and naproxen (Aleve, Naprosyn); carbamazepine (Tegretol); cimetidine (Tagamet); clarithromycin (Biaxin); cyclosporine (Neoral, Sandimmune); danazol (Danocrine); delavirdine (Rescriptor); dexamethasone (Decadron); diltiazem (Cardizem, Dilacor, Tiazac); erythromycin (E.E.S., E-Mycin, Erythrocin); ethosuximide (Zarontin); fluvoxamine (Luvox); HIV protease inhibitors such as atazanavir (Reyataz), indinavir (Crixivan), nelfinavir (Viracept), ritonavir (Norvir), and saquinavir (Fortovase, Invirase); isoniazid (INH, Nydrazid); metronidazole (Flagyl); nefazodone; oral contraceptives (birth control pills); other chemotherapy drugs, especially carboplatin (Paraplatin), cisplatin (Platinol-AQ), gemcitabine (Gemzar), and paclitaxel (Onxol, Taxol); phenobarbital (Luminal, Solfoton); phenytoin (Dilantin); rifabutin (Mycobutin); rifampin (Rifadin, Rimactane); telithromycin (Ketek); troglitazone (Rezulin); troleandomycin (TAO); voriconazole (Vfend); verapamil (Calan, Covera, Isoptin, Verelan); and zafirlukast (Accolate). Your doctor may need to change the doses of your medications or monitor you carefully for side effects.
- tell your doctor what herbal products you are taking, especially St. John's wort.
- tell your doctor if you have ever been treated with radiation therapy (treatment for cancer that uses waves of high energy particles to kill cancer cells) and if you have or have ever had any medical condition, especially any type of lung disease other than lung cancer, cancer that began in another part of your body but has spread to your lungs, and liver or kidney disease.
- tell your doctor if you are pregnant. You should not plan to have children while receiving chemotherapy or for a while after treatments. Use a reliable method of birth control to prevent pregnancy during your treatment and for at least 2 weeks after you stop taking erlotinib. Talk to your doctor for further details. Erlotinib may harm the fetus.
- tell your doctor if you are breastfeeding. You should not breastfeed while you are taking erlotinib.
- tell your doctor if you use tobacco products. Cigarette smoking may decrease the effectiveness of this medication.

Side Effects

Erlotinib may cause side effects. Tell your doctor if any of these symptoms are severe or do not go away:

- diarrhea
- nausea
- vomiting
- stomach pain
- loss of appetite
- mouth sores
- itching
- dry skin
- tiredness

Some side effects can be serious. If you experience any of the following symptoms, call your doctor immediately:

- rash
- new or worsening shortness of breath, cough, or fever
- sore throat, chills and other signs of infection
- unusual bruising or bleeding
- black and tarry stools
- red blood in stools
- bloody vomit
- vomiting material that looks like coffee grounds
- dry, red, or irritated eyes
- sunken eyes
- dry mouth
- decreased urination
- lack of energy

Erlotinib may cause other side effects. Call your doctor if you have any unusual problems while taking this drug.

If you experience a serious side effect, you or your doctor may send a report to the Food and Drug Administration's (FDA) MedWatch Adverse Event Reporting program online [at http://www.fda.gov/MedWatch/index.html] or by phone [1-800-332-1088].

Storage Conditions

Keep erlotinib in the container it came in, tightly closed, and out of reach of children. Store it at room temperature and away from excess heat and moisture (not in the bathroom). Throw away any medication that is outdated or no longer needed. Talk to your pharmacist about the proper disposal of your medication.

Overdose

In case of overdose, call your local poison control center at 1-800-222-1222. If the victim has collapsed or is not breathing, call local emergency services at 911.

Symptoms of overdose may include:

- diarrhea
- rash

Special Instructions

Keep all appointments with your doctor and the laboratory. Your doctor may order certain lab tests to check your body's response to erlotinib.

Do not let anyone else take your medication. Ask your pharmacist any questions you have about refilling your prescription.

Dosage Facts
For Informational Purposes

Caution: Do not change your dose, how often you take your medication, or the length of time you are to take it without first talking to your healthcare provider.

The following dosage information was written using medical language for doctors and other healthcare professionals and is provided here for you to check your dosage. The dosage of this drug may differ for different patients. Therefore, always follow your doctor's instructions or the directions on the label. Contact your healthcare provider or pharmacist if you have any questions about the specific dosage of your medication after reviewing this information.

General Dosage Information

Available as erlotinib hydrochloride; dosage expressed in terms of erlotinib.

Adult Patients

Non-small Cell Lung Cancer

ORAL:

- 150 mg once daily. Continue therapy until disease progression or unacceptable toxicity occurs; once disease progression occurs, there is no evidence that continued therapy is beneficial. In principal efficacy study, therapy was continued for a median of 9.6 weeks.

Dosage Modification for Toxicity
Rash or GI Toxicity

Consider dosage reduction or temporary interruption of therapy if severe skin reactions or severe diarrhea (unresponsive to loperamide or resulting in dehydration) occurs. When dosage reduction is required, reduce dosage in 50-mg decrements.

Hepatotoxicity

Consider reducing dosage or interrupting therapy if severe (grade 3 or 4) hepatotoxicity (e.g., liver function abnormality) develops.

Pulmonary Toxicity

Interrupt therapy pending diagnostic evaluation upon acute onset of new or progressive pulmonary manifestations.

Special Populations

Hepatic Impairment

- Consider reducing dosage or interrupting therapy if severe adverse effects occur.

Geriatric Patients

- No dosage adjustment required.

Erythromycin

(er ith roe mye′ sin)

Brand Name: ERYC®, Ery-Tab®, Erythromycin Base Filmtab®, PCE® Dispertab®

Why is this medicine prescribed?

Erythromycin is an antibiotic used to treat certain infections caused by bacteria, such as bronchitis; diphtheria; Legionnaires' disease; pertussis (whooping cough); pneumonia; rheumatic fever; venereal disease (VD); and ear, intestine, lung, urinary tract, and skin infections. It is also used before some surgery or dental work to prevent infection. Antibiotics will not work for colds, flu, or other viral infections.

This medication is sometimes prescribed for other uses; ask your doctor or pharmacist for more information.

How should this medicine be used?

Erythromycin comes as a capsule, tablet, long-acting capsule, long-acting tablet, chewable tablet, liquid, and pediatric drops to take by mouth. It usually is taken every 6 hours (four times a day) or every 8 hours (three times a day) for 7-21 days. Some infections may require a longer time. Follow the directions on your prescription label carefully, and ask your doctor or pharmacist to explain any part you do not understand. Take erythromycin exactly as directed. Do not take more or less of it or take it more often than prescribed by your doctor.

Shake the liquid and pediatric drops well before each use to mix the medication evenly. Use the bottle dropper to measure the dose of pediatric drops.

The chewable tablets should be crushed or chewed thoroughly before they are swallowed. The other capsules and tablets should be swallowed whole and taken with a full glass of water.

Continue to take erythromycin even if you feel well. Do not stop taking erythromycin without talking to your doctor.

What special precautions should I follow?

Before taking erythromycin,

- tell your doctor and pharmacist if you are allergic to erythromycin, azithromycin (Zithromax), clarithromycin (Biaxin), dirithromycin (Dynabac), or any other drugs.
- tell your doctor and pharmacist what prescription and nonprescription medications you are taking, especially other antibiotics, anticoagulants ('blood thinners'), astemizole (Hismanal), carbamazepine (Tegretol), cisapride (Propulsid), clozapine (clozaril), cyclosporine (Neoral, Sandimmune), digoxin (Lanoxin), disopyramide (Norpace), ergotamine, felodipine (Plendil), lovastatin (Mevacor), phenytoin (Dilantin), pimozide (Orap), terfenadine (Seldane), theophylline (Theo-Dur), triazolam (Halcion), and vitamins.

- tell your doctor if you have or have ever had liver disease, yellowing of the skin or eyes, colitis, or stomach problems.
- tell your doctor if you are pregnant, plan to become pregnant, or are breast-feeding. If you become pregnant while taking erythromycin, call your doctor.
- if you are having surgery, including dental surgery, tell the doctor or dentist that you are taking erythromycin.

What special dietary instructions should I follow?

Take erythromycin at least 1 hour before or 2 hours after meals. Do not take this medication with, or just after, fruit juices or carbonated drinks. Certain brands of erythromycin may be taken with meals; check with your doctor or pharmacist.

What should I do if I forget to take a dose?

Take the missed dose as soon as you remember it. However, if it is almost time for the next dose, skip the missed dose and continue your regular dosing schedule. Do not take a double dose to make up for a missed one.

What side effects can this medicine cause?

Erythromycin may cause side effects. Tell your doctor if any of these symptoms are severe or do not go away:

- upset stomach
- diarrhea
- vomiting
- stomach cramps
- mild skin rash
- stomach pain

If you experience any of the following symptoms, call your doctor immediately:

- severe skin rash
- itching
- hives
- difficulty breathing or swallowing
- wheezing
- yellowing of the skin or eyes
- dark urine
- pale stools
- unusual tiredness
- vaginal infection

If you experience a serious side effect, you or your doctor may send a report to the Food and Drug Administration's (FDA) MedWatch Adverse Event Reporting program online [at http://www.fda.gov/MedWatch/index.html] or by phone [1-800-332-1088].

What storage conditions are needed for this medicine?

Keep this medication in the container it came in, tightly closed, and out of reach of children. Store the capsules and tablets at room temperature and away from excess heat and moisture (not in the bathroom). Throw away any medication that is outdated or no longer needed. Keep liquid medicine in the refrigerator, closed tightly, and throw away any unused medication after 14 days. Do not freeze. Talk to your pharmacist about the proper disposal of your medication.

What should I do in case of overdose?

In case of overdose, call your local poison control center at 1-800-222-1222. If the victim has collapsed or is not breathing, call local emergency services at 911.

What other information should I know?

Keep all appointments with your doctor and the laboratory. Your doctor will order certain lab tests to check your response to erythromycin.

Do not let anyone else take your medication. Your prescription is probably not refillable. If you still have symptoms of infection after you finish the erythromycin, call your doctor.

Talk to your doctor, pharmacist, or other healthcare professional if you have questions about dosing information for your medication.

Erythromycin and Benzoyl Peroxide Topical

(er ith roe mye′ sin) (ben′ zoe ill per ox′ ide)

Brand Name: Benzamycin®, Benzamycin Pak®

Why is this medicine prescribed?

The combination of erythromycin and benzoyl peroxide is used to treat acne. Erythromycin and benzoyl peroxide are in a class of medications called topical antibiotics. The combination of erythromycin and benzoyl peroxide works by killing the bacteria that cause acne.

How should this medicine be used?

The combination of erythromycin and benzoyl peroxide comes as a gel to apply to the skin. It is usually applied twice a day, in the morning and evening. To help you remember to use erythromycin and benzoyl peroxide gel, apply it at around the same times every day. Follow the directions on your prescription label carefully, and ask your doctor or pharmacist to explain any part you do not understand. Use erythromycin and benzoyl peroxide gel exactly as directed. Do not use more or less of it or use it more often than prescribed by your doctor.

It may take several weeks or longer before you feel the full benefit of this medication. Continue to use this medication even if you do not see much improvement at first.

To use the gel, follow these steps:

1. Wash the affected areas with a mild soapless cleanser and gently pat dry with a clean towel.
2. If your medication comes in a large jar, remove a pea-sized dab with your finger and go on to step 5.
3. If your medication comes in small pouches, use scissors or your fingers to tear off the top at the notched tab. Do not open the pouch with your teeth.
4. Squeeze the contents of the pouch onto your palm. You will see a clear gel and a white gel. Use your fingertip to blend the gels with 5-10 circular motions.
5. Use your fingertips to spread a thin layer of gel evenly over the affected area. Avoid getting the gel in your eyes, nose, mouth, or other body openings. If you do get the gel in your eyes, wash with warm water.
6. Look in the mirror. If you see a white film on your skin, you have used too much medication.
7. Throw away the empty pouch and wash your hands.

Are there other uses for this medicine?

This medication may be prescribed for other uses; ask your doctor or pharmacist for more information.

What special precautions should I follow?

Before using erythromycin and benzoyl peroxide,

- tell your doctor and pharmacist if you are allergic to erythromycin (E.E.S., E-Mycin, Erythrocin), benzoyl peroxide (Benzac, Desquam, PanOxyl, Triaz, others), or any other medications.
- tell your doctor and pharmacist what prescription and nonprescription medications, vitamins, nutritional supplements, and herbal products you are taking. Be sure to mention other topical medications for acne. Your doctor may need to change the doses of your medications or monitor you carefully for side effects.
- tell your doctor if you have or have ever had any medical conditions.
- tell your doctor if you are pregnant, plan to become pregnant, or are breast-feeding. If you become pregnant while using erythromycin and benzoyl peroxide, call your doctor.
- plan to avoid unnecessary or prolonged exposure to sunlight and to wear protective clothing, sunglasses, and sunscreen. Erythromycin and benzoyl peroxide may make your skin sensitive to sunlight.
- ask your doctor or pharmacist to recommend a moisturizer to keep your skin soft during treatment.
- you should know that Benzamycin Pak is flammable. Do not mix, apply, or store it near an open flame.

What special dietary instructions should I follow?

Unless your doctor tells you otherwise, continue your normal diet.

What should I do if I forget to take a dose?

Apply the missed dose as soon as you remember it. However, if it is almost time for the next dose, skip the missed dose and continue your regular dosing schedule. Do not apply a double dose to make up for a missed one.

What side effects can this medicine cause?

Erythromycin and benzoyl peroxide may cause side effects. Tell your doctor if any of these symptoms are severe or do not go away:

- dry skin
- peeling, itching, stinging, burning, tingling, or redness of the skin
- oily, tender, or discolored skin

Some side effects can be serious. The following symptoms are uncommon, but if you experience any of them, call your doctor immediately:

- severe diarrhea
- blood or mucus in the stool
- severe stomach pain or cramps
- swelling of the face or nose
- eye or eyelid irritation and swelling
- hives
- changes in your skin or nails that may be signs of infection with a fungus

Erythromycin and benzoyl peroxide may cause other side effects. Call your doctor if you have any unusual problems while using this medication.

If you experience a serious side effect, you or your doctor may send a report to the Food and Drug Administration's (FDA) MedWatch Adverse Event Reporting program online [at http://www.fda.gov/MedWatch/index.html] or by phone [1-800-332-1088].

What storage conditions are needed for this medicine?

Keep this medication in the container it came in, tightly closed, and out of reach of children. Store Benzamycin Gel in the refrigerator but do not freeze it. If you forget to refrigerate the gel for 1 day, you may refrigerate it when you remember and continue to use it. Store Benzamycin Pak at room temperature and away from excess heat and moisture (not in the bathroom). Throw away any unused Benzamycin Gel after 3 months and any medication that is outdated or no longer needed. Talk to your pharmacist about the proper disposal of your medication.

What other information should I know?

Keep all appointments with your doctor.

Avoid getting erythromycin and benzoyl peroxide gel on your hair or clothing. Erythromycin and benzoyl peroxide may bleach hair or colored fabric.

Do not let anyone else use your medication. Ask your pharmacist any questions you have about refilling your prescription.

Talk to your doctor, pharmacist, or other healthcare professional if you have questions about dosing information for your medication.

Erythromycin and Sulfisoxazole

(er ith roe mye′ sin) (sul fi sox′ a zole)

Brand Name: Eryzole®, Pediazole®

Why is this medicine prescribed?

The combination of erythromycin and sulfisoxazole (a sulfa drug) is used to treat certain ear infections caused by bacteria. It usually is used in children.

This medication is sometimes prescribed for other uses; ask your doctor or pharmacist for more information.

How should this medicine be used?

Erythromycin and sulfisoxazole comes as a liquid to take by mouth. It usually is taken every 6 hours (four times a day) for 10 days. Follow the directions on your prescription label carefully, and ask your doctor or pharmacist to explain any part you do not understand. Take erythromycin and sulfisoxazole exactly as directed. Do not take more or less of it or take it more often than prescribed by your doctor.

Shake the liquid well before each use to mix the medication evenly.

Drink a full glass of water after each dose.

Continue to take erythromycin and sulfisoxazole even if you feel well. Do not stop taking erythromycin and sulfisoxazole without talking to your doctor.

What special precautions should I follow?

Before taking erythromycin and sulfisoxazole,

- tell your doctor and pharmacist if you are allergic to erythromycin and sulfisoxazole, azithromycin (Zithromax), clarithromycin (Biaxin), dirithromycin (Dynabac), medication for diabetes, diuretics ('water pills'), or any other drugs.
- tell your doctor and pharmacist what prescription and nonprescription medications you are taking, especially other antibiotics, anticoagulants ('blood thinners') such as warfarin (Coumadin), astemizole (Hismanal), carbamazepine (Tegretol), clozapine (clozaril), cyclosporine (Neoral, Sandimmune), digoxin (Lanoxin), disopyramide (Norpace), ergotamine, felodipine (Plendil), lovastatin (Mevacor), oral contraceptives, phenytoin (Dilantin), terfenadine (Seldane), theophylline (Theo-Dur), triazolam (Halcion), and vitamins.
- tell your doctor if you have or have ever had kidney or liver disease, allergies, anemia, asthma, glucose-6-phosphate dehydrogenase (G-6-PD) deficiency, yellowing of the skin or eyes, colitis, or stomach problems.

- tell your doctor if you are pregnant, plan to become pregnant, or are breast-feeding. If you become pregnant while taking erythromycin and sulfisoxazole, call your doctor.
- if you are having surgery, including dental surgery, tell the doctor or dentist that you are taking erythromycin and sulfisoxazole.

What special dietary instructions should I follow?

Do not take this medication with, or just after, fruit juices, carbonated drinks, or tea. It can be taken with or between meals.

What should I do if I forget to take a dose?

Take the missed dose as soon as you remember it. However, if it is almost time for the next dose, skip the missed dose and continue your regular dosing schedule. Do not take a double dose to make up for a missed one.

What side effects can this medicine cause?

Erythromycin and sulfisoxazole may cause side effects. Tell your doctor if any of these symptoms are severe or do not go away:
- upset stomach
- diarrhea
- vomiting
- stomach cramps
- mild skin rash

If you experience any of the following symptoms, call your doctor immediately:
- severe skin rash
- itching
- hives
- difficulty breathing or swallowing
- wheezing
- stomach pain
- yellowing of the skin or eyes
- dark urine
- pale stools
- unusual tiredness
- sore throat
- fever
- joint pain
- blood in urine
- unusual bleeding or bruising
- dark, tarry stools

If you experience a serious side effect, you or your doctor may send a report to the Food and Drug Administration's (FDA) MedWatch Adverse Event Reporting program online [at http://www.fda.gov/MedWatch/index.html] or by phone [1-800-332-1088].

What storage conditions are needed for this medicine?

Keep this medication in the container it came in, tightly closed, and out of reach of children. Keep it in the refrigerator, and throw away any unused medication after 14 days. Do not freeze. Talk to your pharmacist about the proper disposal of your medication.

What should I do in case of overdose?

In case of overdose, call your local poison control center at 1-800-222-1222. If the victim has collapsed or is not breathing, call local emergency services at 911.

What other information should I know?

Keep all appointments with your doctor and the laboratory. Your doctor will order certain lab tests to check your response to erythromycin and sulfisoxazole.

Do not let anyone else take your medication. Your prescription is probably not refillable. If you still have symptoms of infection after you finish the erythromycin and sulfisoxazole, call your doctor.

Talk to your doctor, pharmacist, or other healthcare professional if you have questions about dosing information for your medication.

Escitalopram

(es sye tal' oh pram)

Brand Name: Lexapro®

Important Warning

A small number of children, teenagers, and young adults (up to 24 years of age) who took antidepressants ('mood elevators') such as escitalopram during clinical studies became suicidal (thinking about harming or killing oneself or planning or trying to do so). Children, teenagers, and young adults who take antidepressants to treat depression or other mental illnesses may be more likely to become suicidal than children, teenagers, and young adults who do not take antidepressants to treat these conditions. However, experts are not sure about how great this risk is and how much it should be considered in deciding whether a child or teenager should take an antidepressant. Children younger than 18 years of age should not normally take escitalopram, but in some cases, a doctor may decide that escitalopram is the best medication to treat a child's condition.

continued on next page

Important Warning (cont'd)

You should know that your mental health may change in unexpected ways when you take escitalopram or other antidepressants even if you are an adult over age 24. You may become suicidal, especially at the beginning of your treatment and any time that your dose is increased or decreased. You, your family, or your caregiver should call your doctor right away if you experience any of the following symptoms: new or worsening depression; thinking about harming or killing yourself, or planning or trying to do so; extreme worry; agitation; panic attacks; difficulty falling asleep or staying asleep; aggressive behavior; irritability; acting without thinking; severe restlessness; and frenzied abnormal excitement. Be sure that your family or caregiver knows which symptoms may be serious so they can call the doctor when you are unable to seek treatment on your own.

Your healthcare provider will want to see you often while you are taking escitalopram, especially at the beginning of your treatment. Be sure to keep all appointments for office visits with your doctor.

The doctor or pharmacist will give you the manufacturer's patient information sheet (Medication Guide) when you begin treatment with escitalopram. Read the information carefully and ask your doctor or pharmacist if you have any questions. You also can obtain the Medication Guide from the FDA website: http://www.fda.gov/cder/drug/antidepressants/antidepressants_MG_2007.pdf.

No matter your age, before you take an antidepressant, you, your parent, or your caregiver should talk to your doctor about the risks and benefits of treating your condition with an antidepressant or with other treatments. You should also talk about the risks and benefits of not treating your condition. You should know that having depression or another mental illness greatly increases the risk that you will become suicidal. This risk is higher if you or anyone in your family has or has ever had bipolar disorder (mood that changes from depressed to abnormally excited) or mania (frenzied, abnormally excited mood) or has thought about or attempted suicide. Talk to your doctor about your condition, symptoms, and personal and family medical history. You and your doctor will decide what type of treatment is right for you.

Why is this medicine prescribed?

Escitalopram is used to treat depression and generalized anxiety disorder (GAD; excessive worry and tension that disrupts daily life and lasts for 6 months or longer). Escitalopram is in a class of antidepressants called selective serotonin reuptake inhibitors (SSRIs). It works by increasing the amount of serotonin, a natural substance in the brain that helps maintain mental balance.

How should this medicine be used?

Escitalopram comes as a tablet and a solution (liquid) to take by mouth. It is usually taken once a day with or without food. To help you remember to take escitalopram, take it at around the same time every day, in the morning or in the evening. Follow the directions on your prescription label carefully, and ask your doctor or pharmacist to explain any part you do not understand. Take escitalopram exactly as directed. Do not take more or less of it or take it more often than prescribed by your doctor.

Your doctor may start you on a low dose of escitalopram and increase your dose after 1 week.

It may take 1-4 weeks or longer before you feel the full benefit of escitalopram. Continue to take escitalopram even if you feel well. Do not stop taking escitalopram without talking to your doctor. If you suddenly stop taking escitalopram, you may experience withdrawal symptoms such as mood changes, irritability, agitation, dizziness, numbness or tingling in the hands or feet, anxiety, confusion, headache, tiredness, and difficulty falling asleep or staying asleep. Your doctor will probably decrease your dose gradually.

Are there other uses for this medicine?

This medication may be prescribed for other uses; ask your doctor or pharmacist for more information.

What special precautions should I follow?

Before taking escitalopram,

- tell your doctor or pharmacist if you are allergic to escitalopram, citalopram (Celexa), or any other medications.
- tell your doctor if you are taking pimozide (Orap) or a monoamine oxidase (MAO) inhibitor such as isocarboxazid (Marplan), phenelzine (Nardil), selegiline (Eldepryl, Emsam, Zelapar), and tranylcypromine (Parnate), or if you have stopped taking an MAO inhibitor within the past 14 days. Your doctor will probably tell you not to take escitalopram. If you stop taking escitalopram, you should wait at least 14 days before you start to take an MAO inhibitor.
- you should know that escitalopram is very similar to another SSRI, citalopram (Celexa). You should not take these two medications together.
- tell your doctor or pharmacist what prescription and nonprescription medications, and vitamins you are taking or plan to take. Be sure to mention any of the following: anticoagulants ('blood thinners') such as warfarin (Coumadin); antihistamines; aspirin and other nonsteroidal anti-inflammatory medications (NSAIDs) such as ibuprofen (Advil, Motrin) and naproxen (Aleve, Naprosyn); carbamazepine (Tegretol); cimetidine (Tagamet); ketoconazole (Sporanox); lithium (Eskalith, Lithobid, Lithotabs); linezolid (Zyvox); medications for anxiety, mental illness, or seizures; medications for migraine headaches such as almotriptan (Axert), eletriptan

(Relpax), frovatriptan (Frova), naratriptan (Amerge), rizatriptan (Maxalt), sumatriptan (Imitrex), and zolmitriptan (Zomig); metoprolol (Lopressor, Toprol XL); other antidepressants such as desipramine (Norpramin); sedatives; sleeping pills; tramadol; and tranquilizers. Your doctor may need to change the doses of your medications or monitor you carefully for side effects.

- tell your doctor what nutritional supplements and herbal products you are taking, especially products containing St. John's wort or tryptophan.
- tell your doctor if you have recently had a heart attack and if you have or have ever had seizures or liver, kidney, thyroid, or heart disease.
- tell your doctor if you are pregnant, plan to become pregnant, or are breast-feeding. If you become pregnant while taking escitalopram, call your doctor.
- if you are having surgery, including dental surgery, tell the doctor or dentist that you are taking escitalopram.
- you should know that escitalopram may make you drowsy. Do not drive a car or operate machinery until you know how this medication affects you.
- remember that alcohol can add to the drowsiness caused by this medication.

What special dietary instructions should I follow?

Unless your doctor tells you otherwise, continue your normal diet.

What should I do if I forget to take a dose?

Take the missed dose as soon as you remember it. However, if it is almost time for the next dose, skip the missed dose and continue your regular dosing schedule. Do not take a double dose to make up for a missed one.

What side effects can this medicine cause?

Escitalopram may cause side effects. Tell your doctor if any of these symptoms are severe or do not go away:
- nausea
- diarrhea
- constipation
- changes in sex drive or ability
- drowsiness
- increased sweating
- dizziness
- heartburn
- stomach pain
- excessive tiredness
- dry mouth
- increased appetite
- flu-like symptoms
- runny nose
- sneezing

Some side effects can be serious. If you experience either of the following symptoms or those listed in the IM-

PORTANT WARNING section, call your doctor immediately:
- unusual excitement
- seeing things or hearing voices that do not exist (hallucinating)

Escitalopram may cause other side effects. Call your doctor if you have any unusual problems while taking this medication.

What storage conditions are needed for this medicine?

Keep this medication in the container it came in, tightly closed, and out of reach of children. Store it at room temperature and away from excess heat and moisture (not in the bathroom). Throw away any medication that is outdated or no longer needed. Talk to your pharmacist about the proper disposal of your medication.

What should I do in case of overdose?

In case of overdose, call your local poison control center at 1-800-222-1222. If the victim has collapsed or is not breathing, call local emergency services at 911.

Symptoms of overdose may include:
- dizziness
- sweating
- nausea
- vomiting
- tremor
- drowsiness
- fast or pounding heartbeat
- seizures
- confusion
- forgetfulness
- fast breathing
- coma (loss of consciousness for a period of time)

What other information should I know?

Keep all appointments with your doctor.

Do not let anyone else take your medication. Ask your pharmacist any questions you have about refilling your prescription.

Dosage Facts
For Informational Purposes

Caution: Do not change your dose, how often you take your medication, or the length of time you are to take it without first talking to your healthcare provider.

The following dosage information was written using medical language for doctors and other healthcare professionals and is provided here for you to check your dosage. The dosage of this drug may differ for different patients. Therefore, always follow your doctor's instructions or the directions on the label. Contact your health-

care provider or pharmacist if you have any questions about the specific dosage of your medication after reviewing this information.

General Dosage Information

Available as escitalopram oxalate; dosage is expressed in terms of escitalopram.

Escitalopram dosages of 10 mg daily appear to be comparable to racemic citalopram dosages of 40 mg daily.

Adult Patients

Major Depressive Disorder

ORAL:
- Initially, 10 mg daily. May be increased to 20 mg daily after ≥1 week; no additional therapeutic benefit with higher dosages.
- Optimum duration not established; may require several months of therapy or longer.

Generalized Anxiety Disorder

ORAL:
- Initially, 10 mg daily. Dosage may be increased to 20 mg daily after ≥1 week.
- Not studied >8 weeks of therapy; periodically reevaluate need for therapy.

Special Populations

Hepatic Impairment
- 10 mg daily.

Renal Impairment
- No dosage adjustment required in patients with mild to moderate renal impairment; not studied in patients with severe renal impairment (Cl_{cr} <20 mL/minute).

Geriatric Patients
- 10 mg daily.

Esomeprazole

(es oh me′ pray zol)

Brand Name: Nexium®

Why is this medicine prescribed?

Esomeprazole is used to treat gastroesophageal reflux disease (GERD), a condition in which backward flow of acid from the stomach causes heartburn and injury of the esophagus (food pipe between the mouth and stomach). Esomeprazole is used to treat the symptoms of GERD, allow the esophagus to heal, and prevent further damage to the esophagus. Esomeprazole is also used to decrease the chance of getting an ulcer in people who are taking nonsteroidal anti-inflammatory medications (NSAIDs). It is also used with other medications to treat and prevent the return of stomach ulcers caused by a certain type of bacteria (H. pylori). Esomeprazole is also used for long-term treatment conditions

(such as Zollinger-Ellison Syndrome) in which the stomach makes too much acid. Esomeprazole is in a class of medications called proton pump inhibitors. It works by decreasing the amount of acid made in the stomach.

How should this medicine be used?

Esomeprazole comes as a delayed-release (long-acting) capsule to take by mouth and as granules to mix with water to take by mouth or give through a feeding tube. Esomeprazole is usually taken once a day at least 1 hour before a meal. To help you remember to take esomeprazole, take it around the same time every day. Follow the directions on your prescription label carefully, and ask your doctor or pharmacist to explain any part you do not understand. Take esomeprazole exactly as directed. Do not take more or less of it or take it more often than prescribed by your doctor.

Swallow the capsules whole; do not split, chew, or crush them. If you cannot swallow the capsule, put 1 tablespoon of cool, soft applesauce in an empty bowl. Open one esomeprazole capsule and carefully sprinkle the pellets onto the applesauce. Mix the pellets with the applesauce, and swallow the entire tablespoonful of the applesauce and pellet mixture immediately. Do not chew the pellets in the applesauce. Do not save the pellets and applesauce for later use.

To mix the granules, follow these steps:
1. Place 1 tablespoon (15 mL) of water into a cup.
2. Open the esomeprazole packet and empty the granules into the cup containing the water.
3. Stir the granules into the water and leave the mixture alone for 2 to 3 minutes so that it will thicken.
4. Stir the mixture again, and drink all the mixture within 30 minutes.
5. If any material remains in the cup after drinking, add some more water and stir. Drink all of the mixture immediately.

Your doctor will tell you how long you will need to take esomeprazole. If you are taking esomeprazole for GERD, you may take it for 4–8 weeks or longer. If you are taking esomeprazole to treat an ulcer, you may take it with other medications for 10 days. If you are taking esomeprazole to decrease the risk of getting an ulcer while taking NSAIDs, you may take it for up to 6 months.

Your doctor will tell you how long it will take to feel the full benefit of esomeprazole. Call your doctor if your symptoms worsen or do not improve during this time. Continue to take esomeprazole even if you feel well. Do not stop taking esomeprazole without talking to your doctor.

Are there other uses for this medicine?

This medication may be prescribed for other uses; ask your doctor or pharmacist for more information.

What special precautions should I follow?

Before taking esomeprazole,
- tell your doctor and pharmacist if you are allergic to esomeprazole, lansoprazole (Prevacid), omeprazole

(Prilosec, Zegerid), pantoprazole (Protonix), rabeprazole (AcipHex), or any other medications.

- tell your doctor and pharmacist what other prescription and nonprescription medications, vitamins, nutritional supplements, and herbal products you are taking or plan to take. Be sure to mention atazanavir (Reyataz); anticoagulants ('blood thinners') such as warfarin (Coumadin); voriconazole (Vfend). Your doctor may need to change the doses of your medications or monitor you carefully for side effects.
- if you are taking digoxin (Lanoxin, Lanoxicaps), iron supplements, vitamins that contain iron, or ketoconazole (Nizoral), you should take these medications at least 2 hours before taking esomeprazole.
- tell your doctor if you have or have ever had liver disease.
- tell your doctor if you are pregnant, plan to become pregnant, or are breast-feeding. If you become pregnant while taking esomeprazole, call your doctor.
- you may take antacids with esomeprazole. If you feel you need an antacid, ask your doctor to recommend one and to tell you when and how to take it.

What special dietary instructions should I follow?

Talk to your doctor about your diet. Some foods and drinks can make your symptoms worse. Your doctor can tell you which foods and drinks you should avoid or eat/drink only in small quantities.

What should I do if I forget to take a dose?

Take the missed dose as soon as you remember it. However, if it is almost time for the next dose, skip the missed dose and continue your regular dosing schedule. Do not take a double dose to make up for a missed one.

What side effects can this medicine cause?

Esomeprazole may cause side effects. Tell your doctor if any of these symptoms are severe or do not go away:

- headache
- diarrhea
- nausea
- gas
- stomach pain
- constipation
- dry mouth

Some side effects can be serious. If you experience any of these symptoms, call your doctor immediately:

- blisters or peeling skin
- hives
- rash
- itching
- difficulty breathing or swallowing
- swelling of the face, throat, tongue, lips, eyes, hands, feet, ankles, or lower legs
- hoarseness

Some people who took a medication similar to esomeprazole for a long time developed atrophic gastritis, a condition in which the stomach muscles weaken and shrink. It is not known if taking esomeprazole increases your risk of developing this condition. Talk to your doctor about the risks of taking esomeprazole.

Esomeprazole may cause other side effects. Call your doctor if you have any unusual problems while taking this medication.

If you experience a serious side effect, you or your doctor may send a report to the Food and Drug Administration's (FDA) MedWatch Adverse Event Reporting program online [at http://www.fda.gov/MedWatch/index.html] or by phone [1-800-332-1088].

What storage conditions are needed for this medicine?

Keep this medication in the container it came in, tightly closed, and out of reach of children. Store it at room temperature and away from excess heat and moisture (not in the bathroom). Throw away any medication that is outdated or no longer needed. Talk to your pharmacist about the proper disposal of your medication.

What should I do in case of overdose?

In case of overdose, call your local poison control center at 1-800-222-1222. If the victim has collapsed or is not breathing, call local emergency services at 911.

Symptoms of overdose may include:

- confusion
- drowsiness
- blurred vision
- fast heartbeat
- nausea
- sweating
- flushing
- headache
- dry mouth

What other information should I know?

Keep all appointments with your doctor.

Do not let anyone else take your medication. Ask your pharmacist any questions you have about refilling your prescription.

Dosage Facts
For Informational Purposes

Caution: Do not change your dose, how often you take your medication, or the length of time you are to take it without first talking to your healthcare provider.

The following dosage information was written using medical language for doctors and other healthcare professionals and is provided here for you to check your

dosage. The dosage of this drug may differ for different patients. Therefore, always follow your doctor's instructions or the directions on the label. Contact your healthcare provider or pharmacist if you have any questions about the specific dosage of your medication after reviewing this information.

General Dosage Information

Available as esomeprazole magnesium and esomeprazole sodium; dosage expressed in terms of esomeprazole.

Pediatric Patients

GERD

ORAL:
• Adolescents 12–17 years of age: 20 or 40 mg once daily for up to 8 weeks.

Adult Patients

GERD

GERD Without Erosive Esophagitis

ORAL:
• 20 mg once daily for 4 weeks; may give an additional 4 weeks of therapy. Chronic proton-pump inhibitor therapy may be appropriate.

Treatment of Erosive Esophagitis

ORAL:
• 20 or 40 mg once daily for 4–8 weeks; may give an additional 4–8 weeks of therapy.

Maintenance of Healing of Erosive Esophagitis

ORAL:
• 20 mg once daily; not studied >6 months.

Duodenal Ulcer

Helicobacter pylori Infection and Duodenal Ulcer

ORAL:
• Triple therapy: 40 mg once daily for 10 days in conjunction with amoxicillin and clarithromycin.

NSAIA-associated Ulcers

Prevention of Gastric Ulcers

ORAL:
• 20 or 40 mg once daily; not studied >6 months.

Special Populations

Hepatic Impairment
• Oral dosage should *not* exceed 20 mg once daily in patients with severe (Child-Pugh class C) hepatic impairment. No dosage adjustment required for mild or moderate (Child-Pugh class A or B, respectively) hepatic impairment.

Estazolam

(es ta′ zoe lam)

Why is this medicine prescribed?

Estazolam is used on a short-term basis to help you fall asleep and stay asleep through the night.

This medication is sometimes prescribed for other uses; ask your doctor or pharmacist for more information.

How should this medicine be used?

Estazolam comes as a tablet to take by mouth and may be taken with or without food. It usually is taken before bedtime when needed. Follow the directions on your prescription label carefully, and ask your doctor or pharmacist to explain any part you do not understand. Take estazolam exactly as directed.

Estazolam can be habit-forming. Do not take a larger dose, take it more often, or for a longer time than your doctor tells you to. Tolerance may develop with long-term or excessive use, making the drug less effective. Do not take estazolam for more than 12 weeks or stop taking this medication without talking to your doctor. Your doctor probably will decrease your dose gradually. You may experience sleeping difficulties the first one or two nights after stopping this medication. If your sleep problems continue, talk to your doctor who will determine whether this drug is right for you.

What special precautions should I follow?

Before taking estazolam,
• tell your doctor and pharmacist if you are allergic to estazolam, alprazolam (Xanax), chlordiazepoxide (Librium, Librax), clonazepam (Klonopin), clorazepate (Tranxene), diazepam (Valium), flurazepam (Dalmane), lorazepam (Ativan), oxazepam (Serax), prazepam (Centrax), temazepam (Restoril), triazolam (Halcion), or any other drugs.
• tell your doctor and pharmacist what prescription and nonprescription medications you are taking, especially antihistamines; cimetidine (Tagamet); digoxin (Lanoxin); disulfiram (Antabuse); medications for depression, seizures, Parkinson's disease, pain, asthma, colds, or allergies; muscle relaxants; isoniazid (INH, Laniazid, Nydrazid); oral contraceptives; probenecid (Benemid); rifampin (Rifadin); sedatives; sleeping pills; theophylline (Theo-Dur); tranquilizers; and vitamins. These medications may add to the drowsiness caused by estazolam.
• tell your doctor if you have or have ever had glaucoma; seizures; or lung, heart, or liver disease.
• tell your doctor if you are pregnant, plan to become pregnant, or are breast-feeding. If you become pregnant while taking estazolam, call your doctor immediately.
• if you are having surgery, including dental surgery, tell the doctor or dentist that you are taking estazolam.

- you should know that this drug may make you drowsy. Do not drive a car or operate machinery until you know how this drug affects you.
- remember that alcohol can add to the drowsiness caused by this drug.
- tell your doctor if you use tobacco products. Cigarette smoking may decrease the effectiveness of this drug.

What should I do if I forget to take a dose?

If you miss a dose, skip the missed dose and continue your regular dosing schedule. Do not take a double dose to make up for a missed one.

What side effects can this medicine cause?

Side effects from estazolam are common and include:
- headache
- heartburn
- diarrhea
- hangover effect (grogginess)
- drowsiness
- dizziness or lightheadedness
- weakness
- dry mouth

Tell your doctor if any of these symptoms are severe or do not go away:
- constipation
- difficulty urinating
- frequent urination
- blurred vision

If you experience any of the following symptoms, call your doctor immediately:
- jaw, neck, and back muscle spasms
- slow or difficult speech
- persistent, fine tremor or inability to sit still
- fever
- difficulty breathing or swallowing
- severe skin rash
- yellowing of the skin or eyes
- irregular heartbeat

If you experience a serious side effect, you or your doctor may send a report to the Food and Drug Administration's (FDA) MedWatch Adverse Event Reporting program online [at http://www.fda.gov/MedWatch/index.html] or by phone [1-800-332-1088].

What storage conditions are needed for this medicine?

Keep this medication in the container it came in, tightly closed, and out of reach of children. Store it at room temperature and away from excess heat and moisture (not in the bathroom). Throw away any medication that is outdated or no longer needed. Talk to your pharmacist about the proper disposal of your medication.

What should I do in case of overdose?

In case of overdose, call your local poison control center at 1-800-222-1222. If the victim has collapsed or is not breathing, call local emergency services at 911.

What other information should I know?

Keep all appointments with your doctor and the laboratory. Do not let anyone else take your medication.

Talk to your doctor, pharmacist, or other healthcare professional if you have questions about dosing information for your medication.

Estradiol Topical

(es tra dye' ole)

Brand Name: Estrasorb®, EstroGel®
Also available generically.

Important Warning

Estradiol increases the risk that you will develop endometrial cancer (cancer of the lining of the uterus [womb]). The longer you use estradiol, the greater the risk that you will develop endometrial cancer. If you have not had a hysterectomy (surgery to remove the uterus), you should be given another medication called a progestin to take with topical estradiol. This may decrease your risk of developing endometrial cancer but may increase your risk of developing certain other health problems, including breast cancer. Before you begin using topical estradiol, tell your doctor if you have or have ever had cancer and if you have abnormal or unusual vaginal bleeding. Call your doctor immediately if you have abnormal or unusual vaginal bleeding during your treatment with topical estradiol. Your doctor will watch you closely to help ensure you do not develop endometrial cancer during or after your treatment.

In a large study, women who took estrogens (a group of medications that includes estradiol) by mouth with progestins had a higher risk of heart attacks, strokes, blood clots in the lungs or legs, breast cancer, and dementia (loss of ability to think, learn, and understand). Women who use topical estradiol alone or with progestins may also have a higher risk of developing these conditions. Tell your doctor if you smoke, or use tobacco if you have had a heart attack or a stroke in the past year and if you or anyone in your family has or has ever had blood clots or breast cancer. Also tell your doctor if you have or

continued on next page

Important Warning (cont'd)

have ever had high blood pressure, high blood levels of cholesterol or fats, diabetes, heart disease, lupus (a condition in which the body attacks its own tissues causing damage and swelling), breast lumps, or an abnormal mammogram (x-ray of the breast used to find breast cancer).

The following symptoms can be signs of the serious health conditions listed above. Call your doctor immediately if you experience any of the following symptoms while you are using topical estradiol: sudden, severe headache; sudden, severe vomiting; speech problems; dizziness or faintness; sudden complete or partial loss of vision; double vision; weakness or numbness of an arm or a leg; crushing chest pain or chest heaviness; coughing up blood; sudden shortness of breath; breast lumps or other breast changes; discharge from nipples; difficulty thinking clearly, remembering, or learning new things, or pain, tenderness, or redness in one leg.

You can take steps to decrease the risk that you will develop a serious health problem while you are using topical estradiol. Do not use topical estradiol alone or with a progestin to prevent heart disease, heart attacks, or strokes. Use the lowest dose of topical estradiol that controls your symptoms and only use topical estradiol as long as needed. Talk to your doctor every 3-6 months to decide if you should use a lower dose of topical estradiol or should stop using the medication.

You should examine your breasts every month and have a mammogram and a breast exam performed by a doctor every year to help detect breast cancer as early as possible. Your doctor will tell you how to properly examine your breasts and whether you should have these exams more often than once a year because of your personal or family medical history.

Tell your doctor if you are having surgery or will be on bedrest. Your doctor may tell you to stop using topical estradiol 4-6 weeks before the surgery or bedrest to decrease the risk that you will develop blood clots.

Talk to your doctor regularly about the risks and benefits of using topical estradiol.

Why is this medicine prescribed?

Estradiol topical gel and emulsion (lotion type mixture) are used to treat and prevent hot flushes (hot flashes; sudden strong feelings of heat and sweating) in women who are experiencing menopause (change of life; the end of monthly menstrual periods). Estradiol topical gel is also used to treat vaginal dryness, itching, and burning in women who are experiencing menopause. However, women whose only bothersome symptoms are vaginal burning, itching, and dryness may benefit more from a medication that is applied topically to the vagina. Estradiol is in a class of medications called estrogen hormones. It works by replacing estrogen that is normally produced by the body.

How should this medicine be used?

Topical estradiol comes as a gel and an emulsion to apply to the skin. It is usually applied once a day. Estradiol emulsion should be applied in the morning. Estradiol gel may be applied at any time of day, but should be applied at around the same time of day every day. Follow the directions on your prescription label carefully, and ask your doctor or pharmacist to explain any part you do not understand. Use topical estradiol exactly as directed. Do not use more or less of it or use it more often than prescribed by your doctor.

If you are using estradiol gel, you should apply it in a thin layer to one arm, from the wrist to the shoulder. If you are using estradiol emulsion, you should apply it to both thighs and calves (lower legs). Do not apply estradiol gel or emulsion to your breasts. Be sure that the skin where you will apply topical estradiol is clean and completely dry, and is not red, irritated, or broken.

If you take a bath or a shower or use a sauna, apply topical estradiol after you have finished bathing, showering or using the sauna and have dried your skin completely. If you plan to swim, allow as much time as possible between applying estradiol gel and swimming. Do not apply sunscreen shortly before, at the same time, or soon after you apply topical estradiol.

Estradiol gel may catch fire. When you apply estradiol gel, do not smoke or go near a fire or open flame until the gel dries.

Be careful not to get estradiol gel in your eyes. If you do get estradiol gel in your eyes, wash them with plenty of warm water right away. Call a doctor if your eyes become irritated.

You should apply estradiol gel yourself. Do not let anyone else rub the gel onto your skin.

To use estradiol gel, follow these steps:

1. Before you use your first dose of estradiol gel, remove the large cover of the pump and fully press down the pump twice. Wash the gel that comes out down the sink or throw it away in a trash can that is out of the reach of children and pets. This primes the pump so that it will dispense the same amount of medication each time it is pressed. Do not repeat this step after the first time you use the pump.
2. Hold the pump with one hand and cup your other hand below the nozzle of the pump. Press the pump firmly and fully to dispense one dose of gel onto your palm.
3. Use your hand to spread the gel as thinly as possible over your entire arm. Try to cover the inside and outside of your arm from your wrist to your shoulder with the gel.
4. Do not rub or massage the gel into your skin. Wait 5 minutes to allow the skin to dry before covering your arm with clothing.
5. Cover the pump with the small and large protective caps.
6. Wash your hands with soap and water.

To use estradiol emulsion, follow these steps:

1. Get two pouches of estradiol emulsion and sit in a comfortable position.
2. Open one pouch of estradiol emulsion by cutting or tearing across the notches near the top of the pouch.
3. Place the pouch flat on top of your left thigh with the open end facing your knee.
4. Hold the closed end of the pouch with one hand and use the forefinger of your other hand to push all of the emulsion in the pouch onto your thigh.
5. Use one or both hands to rub the emulsion into your entire thigh and calf for 3 minutes until completely absorbed.
6. Rub any emulsion that is left on your hands onto your buttocks.
7. Repeat steps 1-6 using a fresh pouch of estradiol emulsion and your right thigh so that you apply the contents of the second pouch to your right thigh and calf.
8. Wait until the skin where you applied estradiol emulsion is completely dry and cover it with clothing.
9. Wash your hands with soap and water.

Ask your pharmacist or doctor for a copy of the manufacturer's information for the patient.

Are there other uses for this medicine?

This medication may be prescribed for other uses; ask your doctor or pharmacist for more information.

What special precautions should I follow?

Before using topical estradiol,

- tell your doctor and pharmacist if you are allergic to estradiol gel or emulsion, any other estrogen products, any other medications, or any of the ingredients in estradiol gel or emulsion. Ask your pharmacist for a list of the ingredients in estradiol gel or emulsion or if you are not sure if a medication you are allergic to contains estrogen.
- tell your doctor and pharmacist what prescription and nonprescription medications, vitamins, and nutritional supplements, you are taking or plan to take. Be sure to mention any of the following: amiodarone (Cordarone, Pacerone); antifungals such as itraconazole (Sporanox) and ketoconazole (Nizoral); aprepitant (Emend); carbamazepine (Carbatrol, Epitol, Tegretol); cimetidine (Tagamet); clarithromycin (Biaxin); cyclosporine (Neoral, Sandimmune); dexamethasone (Decadron, Dexpak); diltiazem (Cardizem, Dilacor, Tiazac, others); erythromycin (E.E.S, Erythrocin); fluoxetine (Prozac, Sarafem); fluvoxamine (Luvox); griseofulvin (Fulvicin, Grifulvin, Gris-PEG); lovastatin (Altocor, Mevacor); certain medications for human immunodeficiency virus (HIV) or acquired immunodeficiency syndrome (AIDS) such as atazanavir (Reyataz), delaviridine (Rescriptor); efavirenz (Sustiva); indinavir (Crixivan), lopinavir (in Kaletra), nelfinavir (Viracept), nevirapine (Viramune); ritonavir (Norvir, in Kaletra), and saquinavir (Forto-

vase, Invirase); medications for thyroid disease; nefazodone; phenobarbital; phenytoin (Dilantin, Phenytek); rifabutin (Mycobutin); rifampin (Rifadin, Rimactane, in Rifamate); sertraline (Zoloft); troleandomycin (TAO); verapamil (Calan, Covera, Isoptin, Verelan); and zafirlukast (Accolate). Your doctor may need to change the doses of your medications or monitor you carefully for side effects.

- tell your doctor what herbal products you are taking, especially St. John's wort.
- tell your doctor if you have or have ever had asthma; seizures; migraine headaches; endometriosis (a condition in which the type of tissue that lines the uterus [womb] grows in other areas of the body); uterine fibroids (growths in the uterus that are not cancer); yellowing of the skin or eyes, especially during pregnancy or while you were using an estrogen product; very high or very low levels of calcium in your blood; porphyria (condition in which abnormal substances build up in the blood and cause problems with the skin or nervous system) or gallbladder, thyroid, liver, pancreas, or kidney disease.
- tell your doctor if you are pregnant, plan to become pregnant, or are breast-feeding. If you become pregnant while using topical estradiol, call your doctor.
- plan to avoid unnecessary or prolonged exposure to sunlight and to wear protective clothing, sunglasses, and sunscreen. Remember to allow some time between applying topical estradiol and applying sunscreen. Estradiol gel may make your skin sensitive to sunlight.
- you should know that topical estradiol may harm other people who touch the medication that is on your skin or in the container. It is most harmful to men and children. Do not let anyone else touch the skin where you applied topical estradiol for one hour after you apply the medication. If someone does touch topical estradiol, that person should wash his or her skin with soap and water as soon as possible.

What special dietary instructions should I follow?

Talk to your doctor about eating grapefruit and drinking grapefruit juice while taking this medicine.

What should I do if I forget to take a dose?

If you forget to apply a dose of estradiol gel but remember more than 12 hours before you are scheduled to apply your next dose, apply the missed dose right away. If you remember less than 12 hours before you are scheduled to apply your next dose, skip the missed dose and continue your regular dosing schedule the next day. Do not apply extra gel to make up for a missed dose.

If you forget to apply estradiol emulsion in the morning, apply it as soon as you remember. Do not apply extra emulsion to make up for a missed dose and do not apply estradiol emulsion more than once each day.

What side effects can this medicine cause?

Topical estradiol may cause side effects. Tell your doctor if any of these symptoms are severe or do not go away:

- headache
- breast pain or tenderness
- upset stomach
- diarrhea
- constipation
- gas
- heartburn
- weight gain or loss
- mood changes
- depression
- nervousness
- sleepiness
- difficulty falling asleep or staying asleep
- changes in sexual desire
- back pain
- runny nose
- cough
- flu-like symptoms
- hair loss
- unwanted hair growth
- darkening of the skin on the face
- difficulty wearing contact lenses
- irritation or redness of the skin where you applied topical estradiol
- swelling, redness, burning, irritation, or itching of the vagina
- vaginal discharge

Some side effects can be serious. If you experience any of these symptoms or those listed in the IMPORTANT WARNING section, call your doctor immediately:

- bulging eyes
- yellowing of the skin or eyes
- itching
- loss of appetite
- fever
- joint pain
- stomach tenderness, pain, or swelling
- movements that are difficult to control
- hives
- rash or blisters on the skin
- swelling, of the eyes, face, lips, tongue, throat, hands, feet, ankles, or lower legs
- hoarseness
- wheezing
- difficulty breathing or swallowing

Topical estradiol may increase your risk of developing cancer of the ovaries and gallbladder disease that may need to be treated with surgery. Talk to your doctor about the risks of using this medication.

Topical estradiol may cause other side effects. Call your doctor if you have any unusual problems while taking this medication.

If you experience a serious side effect, you or your doctor may send a report to the Food and Drug Administration's (FDA) MedWatch Adverse Event Reporting program online [at http://www.fda.gov/MedWatch/index.html] or by phone [1-800-332-1088].

What storage conditions are needed for this medicine?

Keep this medication in the container it came in, tightly closed, and out of reach of children. Store it at room temperature and away from excess heat and moisture (not in the bathroom). Do not freeze topical estradiol. Keep estradiol gel away from open flame. Throw away any medication that is outdated or no longer needed. Throw away your estradiol gel pump after you have used 64 doses even if it is not completely empty. Talk to your pharmacist about the proper disposal of your medication.

What should I do in case of overdose?

In case of overdose, call your local poison control center at 1-800-222-1222. If the victim has collapsed or is not breathing, call local emergency services at 911.

Symptoms of overdose may include:

- upset stomach
- vomiting
- vaginal bleeding

What other information should I know?

Keep all appointments with your doctor and the laboratory. Your doctor may order certain lab tests to check your body's response to topical estradiol.

Before having any laboratory test, tell your doctor and the laboratory personnel that you are using topical estradiol.

Do not let anyone else use your medication. Ask your pharmacist any questions you have about refilling your prescription.

Please see the Estrogen monograph to find dosing information for this medication.

Estradiol Transdermal

(es tra dye′ ole)

Brand Name: Alora®, Climara®, Estraderm®, Menostar®, Vivelle®, Vivelle-Dot®
Also available generically.

Important Warning

Estradiol increases the risk that you will develop endometrial cancer (cancer of the lining of the uterus [womb]). The longer you use estradiol, the greater the risk that you will develop endometrial cancer. If you have not had a hysterectomy (surgery to remove the uterus), you should be given another medication called a progestin to take with transdermal estradiol. This may decrease your risk of developing endometrial cancer but may increase your risk of developing certain other health problems, including breast cancer. Before you begin using transdermal estradiol, tell your doctor if you have or have ever had cancer and if you have unusual vaginal bleeding. Call your doctor immediately if you have abnormal or unusual vaginal bleeding during your treatment with transdermal estradiol. Your doctor will watch you closely to help ensure you do not develop endometrial cancer during or after your treatment.

In a large study, women who took estrogens (a group of medications that includes estradiol) by mouth with progestins had a higher risk of heart attacks, strokes, blood clots in the lungs or legs, breast cancer, and dementia (loss of ability to think, learn, and understand). Women who use transdermal estradiol alone or with progestins may also have a higher risk of developing these conditions. Tell your doctor if you smoke or use tobacco, if you have had a heart attack or a stroke in the past year, and if you or anyone in your family has or has ever had blood clots or breast cancer. Also tell your doctor if you have or have ever had high blood pressure, high blood levels of cholesterol or fats, diabetes, heart disease, lupus (a condition in which the body attacks its own tissues causing damage and swelling), breast lumps, or an abnormal mammogram (x-ray of the breast used to find breast cancer).

The following symptoms can be signs of the serious health conditions listed above. Call your doctor immediately if you experience any of the following symptoms while you are using transdermal estradiol: sudden, severe headache; sudden, severe vomiting; speech problems; dizziness or faintness; sudden complete or partial loss of vision; double vision; weakness or numbness of an arm or a leg; crushing chest pain or chest heaviness; coughing up blood; sudden shortness of breath; difficulty thinking clearly, remembering, or learning new things; breast lumps or other breast changes; discharge from nipples; or pain, tenderness, or redness in one leg.

You can take steps to decrease the risk that you will develop a serious health problem while you are using transdermal estradiol. Do not use transdermal estradiol alone or with a progestin to prevent heart disease, heart attacks, strokes, or dementia. Use the lowest dose of transdermal estradiol that controls your symptoms and only use transdermal estradiol as long as needed. Talk to your doctor every 3-6 months to decide if you should use a lower dose of transdermal estradiol or should stop using the medication.

You should examine your breasts every month and have a mammogram and a breast exam performed by a doctor every year to help detect breast cancer as early as possible. Your doctor will tell you how to properly examine your breasts and whether you should have these exams more often than once a year because of your personal or family medical history.

Tell your doctor if you are having surgery or will be on bedrest. Your doctor may tell you to stop using transdermal estradiol 4-6 weeks before the surgery or bedrest to decrease the risk that you will develop blood clots.

Talk to your doctor regularly about the risks and benefits of using transdermal estradiol.

Why is this medicine prescribed?

Most brands of estradiol transdermal patches are used to treat hot flushes (hot flashes; sudden strong feelings of heat and sweating) and/or vaginal dryness, itching, and burning in women who are experiencing menopause (change of life; the end of monthly menstrual periods). Transdermal estradiol is also used to prevent osteoporosis (a condition in which the bones become thin and weak and break easily) in women who are experiencing or have experienced menopause. Women who need to use transdermal estradiol for more than one of these reasons can benefit most from the medication. Women whose only bothersome symptoms are vaginal dryness, itching, or burning may benefit more from an estrogen product that is applied topically to the vagina. Women who only need a medication to prevent osteoporosis may benefit more from a different medication that does not contain estrogen. Most brands of estradiol transdermal patches are also sometimes used as a source of estrogen in young women who do not produce enough estrogen naturally. Estradiol is in a class of medications called estrogen hormones. It works by replacing estrogen that is normally produced by the body.

Menostar® brand patches contain less estrogen than other brands of estradiol transdermal patches. Menostar® patches are used only to prevent osteoporosis in women who are experiencing or have experienced menopause.

How should this medicine be used?

Transdermal estradiol comes as a patch to apply to the skin. Transdermal estradiol is usually applied once or twice a week, depending on the brand of patch that is used. Some women wear a patch all the time, and other women wear a patch according to a rotating schedule that alternates 3 weeks when the patch is worn followed by 1 week when the patch is not worn. Always apply your transdermal patch on the same day(s) of the week every week. There may be a calendar on the inner flap of your medication carton where you can keep track of your patch change schedule. Follow the directions on your prescription label carefully, and ask your doctor or pharmacist to explain any part you do not understand. Use transdermal estradiol exactly as directed. Do not apply more or fewer patches or apply the patches more often than prescribed by your doctor.

Your doctor will start you on a low dose of transdermal estradiol and may increase your dose if your symptoms are still bothersome. If you are already taking or using an estrogen medication, your doctor will tell you how to switch from the estrogen medication you are taking or using to transdermal estradiol. Be sure you understand these instructions. Talk to your doctor about how well transdermal estradiol works for you.

You should apply estradiol patches to clean, dry, cool skin in the lower stomach area, below your waistline. Some brands of patches may also be applied to the upper buttocks or the hips. Ask your doctor or pharmacist or read the manufacturer's information that comes with your patches to find the best place(s) to apply the brand of patches you have received. Do not apply any brand of estradiol patches to the breasts or to skin that is oily, damaged, cut, or irritated. Do not apply estradiol patches to the waistline where they may be rubbed off by tight clothing or to the lower buttocks where they may be rubbed off by sitting. Be sure that the skin in the area where you plan to apply an estradiol patch is free of lotion, powders, or creams. After you apply a patch to a particular area, wait at least 1 week before applying another patch to that spot. Some brands of patches should not be applied to an area of the skin that is exposed to sunlight. Talk to your doctor or pharmacist to find out whether your patch should be applied to an area that will not be exposed to sunlight.

Talk to your doctor or pharmacist or read the manufacturer's information that came with your medication to find out if you need to be careful when you swim, bathe, shower, or use a sauna while wearing an estradiol transdermal patch. Some brands of patches are not likely to be affected by these activities, but some brands of patches may loosen. Some types of patches may also be pulled and loosened by your clothes or towel when you change clothes or dry your body. You may need to check that your patch is still firmly attached after these activities.

If the patch loosens or falls off before it is time to replace it, try to press it back in place with your fingers. Be careful not to touch the sticky side of the patch with your fingers while you are doing this. If the patch cannot be pressed back on, fold it in half so it sticks to itself, throw it away in a trash can that is out of the reach of children and pets, and apply a fresh patch to a different area. Replace the fresh patch on your next scheduled patch change day.

Each brand of estradiol transdermal patches should be applied following the specific directions given in the manufacturer's information for the patient. Read this information carefully before you start using estradiol transdermal and each time you refill your prescription. Ask your doctor or pharmacist if you have any questions. The following general directions can help you remember some important things to do when you apply any type of estradiol transdermal patch.

1. Tear open the pouch with your fingers. Do not use scissors because they may damage the patch. Do not open the pouch until you are ready to apply the patch.
2. Remove the patch from the pouch. There may be a silver foil sticker used to protect the patch from moisture inside the pouch. Do not remove this sticker from the pouch.
3. Remove the protective liner from the patch and press the sticky side of the patch against your skin in the area you have chosen to wear your patch. Some patches have a liner that is made to peel off in two pieces. If your patch has that type of liner, you should peel off one part of the liner and press that side of the patch against your skin. Then fold back the patch, peel off the other part of the liner and press the second side of the patch against your skin. Always be careful not to touch the sticky side of the patch with your fingers.
4. Press down on the patch with your fingers or palm for 10 seconds. Be sure that the patch is firmly attached to your skin, especially around its edges.
5. Wear the patch all the time until it is time to remove it. When it is time to remove the patch, slowly peel it off of your skin. Fold the patch in half so that the sticky sides are pressed together and throw it away in a trash can that is out of reach of children and pets.
6. Some brands of patches may leave a sticky substance on your skin. In some cases, this can be rubbed off easily. In other cases, you should wait 15 minutes and then remove the substance using an oil or lotion. Read the information that came with your patches to find out what to do if a substance is left on your skin after you remove your patch.

Ask your pharmacist or doctor for a copy of the manufacturer's information for the patient.

Are there other uses for this medicine?

This medication may be prescribed for other uses; ask your doctor or pharmacist for more information.

What special precautions should I follow?

Before using transdermal estradiol,

- tell your doctor and pharmacist if you are allergic to any brand of transdermal estradiol, any other estrogen products, any other medications, or any adhesives. Ask your doctor or pharmacist if you are not sure if a medication you are allergic to contains estrogen.

- tell your doctor and pharmacist what prescription and nonprescription medications, vitamins, and nutritional supplements you are taking or plan to take. Be sure to mention any of the following: amiodarone (Cordarone, Pacerone); antifungals such as itraconazole (Sporanox) and ketoconazole (Nizoral); aprepitant (Emend); carbamazepine (Carbatrol, Epitol, Tegretol); cimetidine (Tagamet); clarithromycin (Biaxin); cyclosporine (Neoral, Sandimmune); dexamethasone (Decadron, Dexpak); diltiazem (Cardizem, Dilacor, Tiazac, others); erythromycin (E.E.S, Erythrocin); fluoxetine (Prozac, Sarafem); fluvoxamine (Luvox); griseofulvin (Fulvicin, Grifulvin, Gris-PEG); lovastatin (Altocor, Mevacor); medications for human immunodeficiency virus (HIV) or acquired immunodeficiency syndrome (AIDS) such as atazanavir (Reyataz), delaviridine (Rescriptor); efavirenz (Sustiva); indinavir (Crixivan), lopinavir (in Kaletra), nelfinavir (Viracept), nevirapine (Viramune); ritonavir (Norvir, in Kaletra), and saquinavir (Fortovase, Invirase); medications for thyroid disease; nefazodone; other medications that contain estrogen; phenobarbital; phenytoin (Dilantin, Phenytek); rifabutin (Mycobutin); rifampin (Rifadin, Rimactane, in Rifamate); sertraline (Zoloft); troleandomycin (TAO); verapamil (Calan, Covera, Isoptin, Verelan); and zafirlukast (Accolate). Your doctor may need to change the doses of your medications or monitor you carefully for side effects.
- tell your doctor what herbal products you are taking, especially St. John's wort.
- tell your doctor if you have or have ever had asthma; seizures; migraine headaches; endometriosis (a condition in which the type of tissue that lines the uterus [womb] grows in other areas of the body); uterine fibroids (growths in the uterus that are not cancer); yellowing of the skin or eyes, especially during pregnancy or while you were using an estrogen product; very high or very low levels of calcium in your blood; porphyria (condition in which abnormal substances build up in the blood and cause problems with the skin or nervous system)or gallbladder, thyroid, pancreas, liver or kidney disease.
- tell your doctor if you are pregnant or plan to become pregnant, or are breastfeeding. If you become pregnant while using transdermal estradiol, call your doctor.
- if you are using transdermal estradiol to prevent osteoporosis, talk to your doctor about additional ways to prevent the disease such as exercising and taking vitamin D and/or calcium supplements.

What special dietary instructions should I follow?

Talk to your doctor about eating grapefruit and drinking grapefruit juice while using this medication.

Talk to your doctor about ways to increase the amount of calcium and vitamin D in your diet.

What should I do if I forget to take a dose?

Apply the missed patch as soon as you remember. Then apply the next patch according to your regular schedule.Do not apply extra patches to make up for a missed patch.

What side effects can this medicine cause?

Transdermal estradiol may cause side effects. Tell your doctor if any of these symptoms are severe or do not go away:

- headache
- breast pain or tenderness
- upset stomach
- vomiting
- constipation
- gas
- heartburn
- weight gain or loss
- hair loss
- redness or irritation of the skin that was covered by the estradiol patch
- swelling, redness, burning, irritation or itching of the vagina
- vaginal discharge
- painful menstrual periods
- anxiety
- depression
- changes in mood
- change in sexual desire
- back, neck, or muscle pain
- runny nose or congestion
- cough
- darkening of skin on face (may not go away even after you stop using transdermal estradiol)
- unwanted hair growth
- difficulty wearing contact lenses

Some side effects can be serious. If you experience any of these symptoms or those listed in the IMPORTANT WARNING section, call your doctor immediately:

- bulging eyes
- yellowing of the skin or eyes
- loss of appetite
- fever
- joint pain
- stomach tenderness, pain, or swelling
- movements that are difficult to control
- itching
- hives
- rash, blisters on skin, or other skin changes
- swelling, of the eyes, face, lips, tongue, throat, hands, feet, ankles, or lower legs
- hoarseness
- difficulty breathing or swallowing

Transdermal estradiol may increase your risk of developing cancer of the ovaries and gallbladder disease that may need to be treated with surgery. Talk to your doctor about the risks of using transdermal estradiol.

Transdermal estradiol may cause growth to slow or stop

early in children who use large doses for a long time. Your child's doctor will monitor her carefully during her treatment with transdermal estradiol. Talk to your child's doctor about the risks of giving this medication to your child.

Transdermal estradiol may cause other side effects. Call your doctor if you have any unusual problems while using this medication.

If you experience a serious side effect, you or your doctor may send a report to the Food and Drug Administration's (FDA) MedWatch Adverse Event Reporting program online [at http://www.fda.gov/MedWatch/index.html] or by phone [1-800-332-1088].

What storage conditions are needed for this medicine?

Keep estradiol patches sealed in their original pouches and out of reach of children. Store the patches at room temperature and away from excess heat and moisture (not in the bathroom). Throw away any medication that is outdated or no longer needed. Talk to your pharmacist about the proper disposal of your medication.

What should I do in case of overdose?

In case of overdose, call your local poison control center at 1-800-222-1222. If the victim has collapsed or is not breathing, call local emergency services at 911.

Symptoms of overdose may include:
- upset stomach
- vomiting
- vaginal bleeding

What other information should I know?

Keep all appointments with your doctor and the laboratory. Your doctor may order certain lab tests to check your body's response to transdermal estradiol.

Before having any laboratory test, tell your doctor and the laboratory personnel that you are using transdermal estradiol.

Do not let anyone else use your medication. Ask your pharmacist any questions you have about refilling your prescription.

Please see the Estrogen monograph to find dosing information for this medication.

Estrogen

(ess' troe jen)

Brand Name: Cenestin®, Enjuvia®, Estrace®, Femtrace®, Gynodiol®, Menest®, Ogen®, Premarin®

Also available generically.

Important Warning

Estrogen increases the risk that you will develop endometrial cancer (cancer of the lining of the uterus [womb]). The longer you take estrogen, the greater the risk that you will develop endometrial cancer. If you have not had a hysterectomy (surgery to remove the uterus), you should be given another medication called a progestin to take with estrogen. This may decrease your risk of developing endometrial cancer, but may increase your risk of developing certain other health problems, including breast cancer. Before you begin taking estrogen, tell your doctor if you have or have ever had cancer and if you have unusual vaginal bleeding. Call your doctor immediately if you have abnormal or unusual vaginal bleeding during your treatment with estrogen. Your doctor will watch you closely to help ensure you do not develop endometrial cancer during or after your treatment.

In a large study, women who took estrogen with progestins had a higher risk of heart attacks, strokes, blood clots in the lungs or legs, breast cancer, and dementia (loss of ability to think, learn, and understand). Women who take estrogen alone may also have a higher risk of developing these conditions. Tell your doctor if you smoke or use tobacco, if you have had a heart attack or a stroke in the past year, and if you or anyone in your family has or has ever had blood clots or breast cancer. Also tell your doctor if you have or have ever had high blood pressure, high blood levels of cholesterol or fats, diabetes, heart disease, lupus (a condition in which the body attacks its own tissues causing damage and swelling), breast lumps, or an abnormal mammogram (x-ray of the breast used to find breast cancer).

The following symptoms can be signs of the serious health conditions listed above. Call your doctor immediately if you experience any of the following symptoms while you are taking estrogen: sudden, severe headache; sudden, severe vomiting; speech problems; dizziness or faintness; sudden complete or partial loss of vision; double vision; weakness or numbness of an arm or a leg; crushing chest pain or chest heaviness; coughing up blood; sudden shortness of breath; difficulty thinking clearly, remembering, or learning new things; breast lumps or other breast changes; discharge from nipples; or pain, tenderness, or redness in one leg.

You can take steps to decrease the risk that you will develop a serious health problem while you are taking estrogen. Do not take estrogen alone or with a progestin to prevent heart disease, heart attacks, strokes, or dementia. Take the lowest dose of estrogen that controls your symptoms and only take estrogen as long as needed. Talk to your doctor every 3-6 months to decide if you should take a lower dose of estrogen or should stop taking the medication.

You should examine your breasts every month and have a mammogram and a breast exam performed by a doctor every year to help detect breast cancer as early as possible. Your doctor will tell you how to properly examine your breasts and whether you should have these exams more often than once a year because of your personal or family medical history.

Tell your doctor if you are having surgery or will be on bedrest. Your doctor may tell you to stop taking estrogen 4-6 weeks before the surgery or bedrest to decrease the risk that you will develop blood clots.

Talk to your doctor regularly about the risks and benefits of taking estrogen.

Why is this medicine prescribed?

Estrogen is used to treat hot flushes ('hot flashes'; sudden strong feelings of heat and sweating) in women who are experiencing menopause ('change of life', the end of monthly menstrual periods). Some brands of estrogen are also used to treat vaginal dryness, itching, or burning, or to prevent osteoporosis (a condition in which the bones become thin and weak and break easily) in women who are experiencing or have experienced menopause. However, women who need a medication only to treat vaginal dryness or only to prevent osteoporosis should consider a different treatment. Some brands of estrogen are also to relieve symptoms of low estrogen in young women who do not produce enough estrogen naturally. Some brands of estrogen are also used to relieve the symptoms of certain types of breast and prostate (a male reproductive gland) cancer. Estrogen is in a class of medications called hormones. It works by replacing estrogen that is normally produced by the body.

How should this medicine be used?

Estrogen comes as a tablet to take by mouth. It is usually taken with or without food once a day. Estrogen is sometimes taken every day and sometimes taken according to a rotating schedule that alternates a period of time when estrogen is taken every day with a period of time when estrogen is not taken. When estrogen is used to relieve the symptoms of cancer, it is usually taken three times a day. Take estrogen at around the same time(s) every day. Follow the directions on your prescription label carefully, and ask your

doctor or pharmacist to explain any part you do not understand. Take estrogen exactly as directed. Do not take more or less of it or take it more often than prescribed by your doctor.

Your doctor may start you on a low dose of estrogen and gradually increase your dose if your symptoms are still bothersome, or decrease your dose if your symptoms are well-controlled. Talk to your doctor about how well estrogen works for you.

Ask your pharmacist or doctor for a copy of the manufacturer's information for the patient.

Are there other uses for this medicine?

This medication may be prescribed for other uses; ask your doctor or pharmacist for more information.

What special precautions should I follow?

Before taking estrogen,

- tell your doctor and pharmacist if you are allergic to any brand of oral estrogen, any other estrogen products, any other medications, or any of the ingredients in estrogen tablets. If you will be taking Estrace® brand tablets, tell your doctor and pharmacist if you are allergic to aspirin or tartrazine (a food color additive). Ask your pharmacist or check the manufacturer's patient information for a list of the inactive ingredients in the brand of estrogen tablets you plan to take.

- tell your doctor and pharmacist what prescription and nonprescription medications, vitamins, and nutritional supplements you are taking or plan to take. Be sure to mention any of the following: amiodarone (Cordarone, Pacerone); certain antifungals such as itraconazole (Sporanox) and ketoconazole (Nizoral); aprepitant (Emend); carbamazepine (Carbatrol, Epitol, Tegretol); cimetidine (Tagamet); clarithromycin (Biaxin); cyclosporine (Neoral, Sandimmune); dexamethasone (Decadron, Dexpak); diltiazem (Cardizem, Dilacor, Tiazac, others); erythromycin (E.E.S, Erythrocin); fluoxetine (Prozac, Sarafem); fluvoxamine (Luvox); griseofulvin (Fulvicin, Grifulvin, Gris-PEG); lovastatin (Altocor, Mevacor); medications for human immunodeficiency virus (HIV) or acquired immunodeficiency syndrome (AIDS) such as atazanavir (Reyataz), delavirdine (Rescriptor), efavirenz (Sustiva), indinavir (Crixivan), lopinavir (in Kaletra), nelfinavir (Viracept), nevirapine (Viramune), ritonavir (Norvir, in Kaletra), and saquinavir (Fortovase, Invirase); medications for thyroid disease; nefazodone; phenobarbital; phenytoin (Dilantin, Phenytek); rifabutin (Mycobutin); rifampin (Rifadin, Rimactane, in Rifamate); sertraline (Zoloft); troleandomycin (TAO); verapamil (Calan, Covera, Isoptin, Verelan); and zafirlukast (Accolate). Your doctor may need to change the doses of your medications or monitor you carefully for side effects.

- tell your doctor what herbal products you are taking, especially St. John's wort.

- tell your doctor if you have or have ever had yellowing of the skin or eyes during pregnancy or during your treatment with an estrogen product, endometriosis (a condition in which the type of tissue that lines the uterus [womb] grows in other areas of the body), uterine fibroids (growths in the uterus that are not cancer), asthma, migraine headaches, seizures, porphyria (condition in which abnormal substances build up in the blood and cause problems with the skin or nervous system), very high or very low levels of calcium in your blood, or thyroid, liver, kidney, gallbladder, or pancreatic disease.
- tell your doctor if you are pregnant, plan to become pregnant, or are breast-feeding. If you become pregnant while taking estrogen, call your doctor immediately.
- if you are taking estrogen to prevent osteoporosis, talk to your doctor about other ways to prevent the disease such as exercising and taking vitamin D and/or calcium supplements.

What special dietary instructions should I follow?

Talk to your doctor about eating grapefruit and drinking grapefruit juice while taking this medicine.

Talk to your doctor about ways to increase the amount of calcium and vitamin D in your diet, especially if you are taking estrogen to prevent osteoporosis.

What should I do if I forget to take a dose?

Take the missed dose as soon as you remember it. However, if it is almost time for the next dose, skip the missed dose and continue your regular dosing schedule. Do not take a double dose to make up for a missed one.

What side effects can this medicine cause?

Estrogen may cause side effects. Tell your doctor if any of these symptoms are severe or do not go away:

- breast pain or tenderness
- upset stomach
- vomiting
- heartburn
- constipation
- diarrhea
- gas
- weight gain or loss
- leg cramps
- nervousness
- depression
- dizziness
- burning or tingling in the arms or legs
- tight muscles
- hair loss
- unwanted hair growth
- spotty darkening of the skin on the face
- difficulty wearing contact lenses

- swelling, redness, burning, itching, or irritation of the vagina
- vaginal discharge
- change in sexual desire
- cold symptoms

Some side effects can be serious. If you experience any of these symptoms or those listed in the IMPORTANT WARNING section, call your doctor immediately:

- bulging eyes
- sore throat, fever, chills, cough, and other signs of infection
- pain, swelling, or tenderness in the stomach
- loss of appetite
- weakness
- yellowing of the skin or eyes
- joint pain
- movements that are difficult to control
- rash or blisters
- hives
- itching
- swelling of the eyes, face, tongue, throat, hands, arms, feet, ankles, or lower legs
- hoarseness
- difficulty breathing or swallowing

Estrogen may increase your risk of developing cancer of the ovaries or gallbladder disease that may need to be treated with surgery. Talk to your doctor about the risks of taking estrogen.

Estrogen may cause growth to slow or stop early in children who take large doses for a long time. Estrogen may also affect the timing and speed of sexual development in children. Your child's doctor will monitor him or her carefully during his or her treatment with estrogen. Talk to your child's doctor about the risks of giving this medication to your child.

Estrogen may cause other side effects. Call your doctor if you have any unusual problems while taking this medication.

If you experience a serious side effect, you or your doctor may send a report to the Food and Drug Administration's (FDA) MedWatch Adverse Event Reporting program online [at http://www.fda.gov/MedWatch/index.html] or by phone [1-800-332-1088].

What storage conditions are needed for this medicine?

Keep this medication in the container it came in, tightly closed, and out of reach of children. Store it at room temperature and away from excess heat and moisture (not in the bathroom). Throw away any medication that is outdated or no longer needed. Talk to your pharmacist about the proper disposal of your medication.

What should I do in case of overdose?

In case of overdose, call your local poison control center at 1-800-222-1222. If the victim has collapsed or is not breathing, call local emergency services at 911.

Symptoms of overdose may include:
- upset stomach
- vomiting
- vaginal bleeding

What other information should I know?

Keep all appointments with your doctor.

Before having any laboratory test, tell your doctor and the laboratory personnel that you are taking estrogen.

Do not let anyone else take your medication. Ask your pharmacist any questions you have about refilling your prescription.

Dosage Facts
For Informational Purposes

Caution: Do not change your dose, how often you take your medication, or the length of time you are to take it without first talking to your healthcare provider.

The following dosage information was written using medical language for doctors and other healthcare professionals and is provided here for you to check your dosage. The dosage of this drug may differ for different patients. Therefore, always follow your doctor's instructions or the directions on the label. Contact your healthcare provider or pharmacist if you have any questions about the specific dosage of your medication after reviewing this information.

Estrogens, Conjugated

General Dosage Information

Individualize dosage according to the condition being treated and the tolerance and therapeutic response of the patient.

To minimize risk of adverse effects, use the lowest possible effective dosage. Because of the potential increased risk of cardiovascular events, breast cancer, and venous thromboembolic events, limit estrogen and estrogen/progestin therapy to the lowest effective doses and shortest duration of therapy consistent with treatment goals and risks for the individual woman.

Periodically reevaluate estrogen and estrogen/progestin therapy (i.e., at 3- to 6-month intervals).

Pediatric Patients

Hypoestrogenism

ORAL:
- Conjugated estrogens USP: 0.15 mg daily may induce breast development. Increase dosage at 6- to 12-month intervals to achieve appropriate bone age advancement and epiphyseal closure.
- Conjugated estrogens USP: 0.625 mg daily (with progestins) sufficient to induce artificial cyclic menses and to maintain bone mineral density (BMD) after skeletal maturity.

Adult Patients

Estrogen Replacement Therapy
Vasomotor Symptoms

ORAL:
- Conjugated estrogens USP: Initially, 0.3 mg daily continuously or in cyclic regimen (25 days on, 5 days off). Adjust dosage based on patient response.
- Synthetic conjugated estrogens A: Initially, 0.45 mg daily. May increase dosage up to 1.25 mg daily.
- Conjugated estrogens USP in fixed combination with medroxyprogesterone acetate (Prempro®), monophasic regimen: Initially, conjugated estrogens USP 0.3 mg with medroxyprogesterone acetate 1.5 mg daily. Alternatively, conjugated estrogens USP 0.45 mg with medroxyprogesterone acetate 1.5 mg daily, conjugated estrogens USP 0.625 mg with medroxyprogesterone acetate 2.5 mg daily, or conjugated estrogens USP 0.625 mg with medroxyprogesterone acetate 5 mg daily.
- Conjugated estrogens USP with medroxyprogesterone acetate (Premphase®), biphasic regimen: Conjugated estrogens USP 0.625 mg daily; medroxyprogesterone acetate 5 mg daily on days 15–28 of the cycle.

Vulvar and Vaginal Atrophy

ORAL:
- Conjugated estrogens USP: Initially, 0.3 mg daily continuously or in cyclic regimen (25 days on, 5 days off). Adjust dosage based on patient response.
- Synthetic conjugated estrogens A: 0.3 mg daily.
- Conjugated estrogens USP in fixed combination with medroxyprogesterone acetate (Prempro®), monophasic regimen: Initially, conjugated estrogens USP 0.3 mg with medroxyprogesterone acetate 1.5 mg daily. Alternatively, conjugated estrogens USP 0.45 mg with medroxyprogesterone acetate 1.5 mg daily, conjugated estrogens USP 0.625 mg with medroxyprogesterone acetate 2.5 mg daily, or conjugated estrogens USP 0.625 mg with medroxyprogesterone acetate 5 mg daily.
- Conjugated estrogens USP with medroxyprogesterone acetate (Premphase®), biphasic regimen: Conjugated estrogens USP 0.625 mg daily; medroxyprogesterone acetate 5 mg daily on days 15–28 of the cycle.

Osteoporosis
Prevention in Postmenopausal Women

ORAL:
- Conjugated estrogens USP: Initially, 0.3 mg daily continuously or in cyclic regimen (25 days on, 5 days off). Adjust dosage based on clinical and BMD response.
- Conjugated estrogens USP in fixed combination with medroxyprogesterone acetate (Prempro®), monophasic regimen: Initially, conjugated estrogens USP 0.3 mg with medroxyprogesterone acetate 1.5 mg daily. Alternatively, conjugated estrogens USP 0.45 mg with medroxyprogesterone acetate 1.5 mg daily, conjugated estrogens USP 0.625 mg with medroxyprogesterone acetate 2.5 mg daily, or conjugated estrogens USP 0.625 mg with medroxyprogesterone acetate 5 mg daily. Adjust dosage based on clinical and BMD response.
- Conjugated estrogens USP with medroxyprogesterone acetate (Premphase®), biphasic regimen: Conjugated estrogens USP 0.625 mg daily; medroxyprogesterone acetate 5 mg daily on days 15–28 of the cycle.

Hypoestrogenism
Female Hypogonadism

ORAL:
- Conjugated estrogens USP: 0.3–0.625 mg daily in a cyclic regimen (3 weeks on, 1 week off). Adjust dosage based on symptom severity and endometrial responsiveness.

Female Castration or Primary Ovarian Failure

ORAL:
- Conjugated estrogens USP: 1.25 mg daily in a cyclic regimen. Adjust dosage based on symptom severity and clinical response.

Metastatic Breast Carcinoma

ORAL:
- Conjugated estrogens USP: 10 mg 3 times daily for ≥3 months.

Prostate Carcinoma

ORAL:
- Conjugated estrogens USP: 1.25–2.5 mg 3 times daily.

Individualize dosage according to the condition being treated and the tolerance and therapeutic response of the patient.

Estrone, Estropipate, Esterified Estrogens

General Dosage Information

To minimize risk of adverse effects, use the lowest possible effective dosage. Because of the potential increased risk of cardiovascular events, breast cancer, and venous thromboembolic events, limit estrogen and estrogen/progestin therapy to the lowest effective doses and shortest duration of therapy consistent with treatment goals and risks for the individual woman.

Periodically reevaluate estrogen and estrogen/progestin therapy (i.e., at 3- to 6-month intervals).

Adult Patients

Estrogen Replacement Therapy
Vasomotor Symptoms

ORAL:
- Estropipate: 0.75–6 mg daily in a cyclic regimen.
- Esterified estrogens: 1.25 mg daily in a cyclic regimen (3 weeks on, 1 week off).
- Esterified estrogens in fixed combination with methyltestosterone: Esterified estrogens 0.625 mg with methyltestosterone 1.25 mg daily in a cyclic regimen (3 weeks on, 1 week off). Alternatively, esterified estrogens 1.25 mg with methyltestosterone 2.5 mg daily in a cyclic regimen.

IM:
- Estrone: 0.1–1 mg weekly in single or divided doses. Some patients may require 0.5–2 mg weekly. Administer in a cyclic regimen (3 weeks on, 1 week off).

Vulvar and Vaginal Atrophy

ORAL:
- Estropipate: 0.75–6 mg daily in a cyclic regimen.
- Esterified estrogens: 0.3–≥1.25 mg daily in a cyclic regimen (3 weeks on, 1 week off).

IM:
- Estrone: 0.1–0.5 mg 2 or 3 times weekly in a cyclic regimen (3 weeks on, 1 week off).

Osteoporosis
Prevention in Postmenopausal Women

ORAL:
- Estropipate: 0.75 mg daily in a cyclic regimen (25 days on, 6 days off).

Hypoestrogenism
Female Hypogonadism

ORAL:
- Estropipate: 1.5–9 mg daily for 3 weeks followed by 8–10 days without the drug; if menstruation does not occur by the end of the 8- to 10-day drug-free period, repeat the same dosage schedule. Number of courses required to induce menstruation varies depending on endometrial responsiveness. If satisfactory withdrawal bleeding does not occur, may administer an oral progestin concomitantly during the third week of the cycle.
- Esterified estrogens: 2.5–7.5 mg daily in divided doses for 20 days, followed by 10 days without the drug. Number of courses required to induce menstruation varies depending on endometrial responsiveness. If menstruation does not occur by the end of the first complete cycle, repeat the same dosage schedule. If menstruation occurs before the end of the 10-day drug-free period, initiate estrogen-progestin regimen with esterified estrogens 2.5–7.5 mg given daily in divided doses for 20 days; administer oral progestin during the last 5 days of esterified estrogens administration. If menstruation begins before the estrogen-progestin regimen is completed, discontinue therapy and then reinstitute on the fifth day of menstruation.

Female Castration or Primary Ovarian Failure

ORAL:
- Estropipate: 1.5–9 mg daily for 3 weeks, followed by 8–10 days without the drug. Adjust dosage according to severity of symptoms and therapeutic response.
- Esterified estrogens: 1.25 mg daily in a cyclic regimen. Adjust dosage according to severity of symptoms and therapeutic response.

Metastatic Breast Carcinoma

ORAL:
- Esterified estrogens: 10 mg 3 times daily for ≥3 months.

IM:
- Estrone: 5 mg ≥3 times weekly according to severity of pain.

Prostate Carcinoma

ORAL:
- Esterified estrogens: 1.25–2.5 mg 3 times daily.

IM:
- Estrone: 2–4 mg 2 or 3 times weekly.

Abnormal Uterine Bleeding

IM:
- Estrone: 2–5 mg daily for several days.

Individualize dosage according to the condition being treated and the tolerance and therapeutic response of the patient.

Estradiol

General Dosage Information

To minimize risk of adverse effects, use the lowest possible effective dosage. Because of the potential increased risk of cardiovascular events, breast cancer, and venous thromboembolic events, limit estrogen and estrogen/progestin therapy to the lowest effective doses and shortest duration of therapy consistent with treatment goals and risks for the individual woman.

Periodically reevaluate estrogen and estrogen/progestin therapy (i.e., at 3- to 6-month intervals).

Estradiol 0.06% topical gel (EstroGel®): Each depression of the pump delivers 1.25 g of gel (0.75 mg of estradiol). Pump delivers 64 metered doses.

Estradiol topical emulsion (Estrasorb®): Each pouch contains 1.74 g of emulsion (4.35 mg of estradiol hemihydrate).

Adult Patients

ERT
Vasomotor Symptoms

ORAL:
- Estradiol: 1–2 mg daily in a cyclic regimen (3 weeks on, 1 week off).
- Estradiol in fixed combination with norethindrone acetate (Activella®): Estradiol 1 mg with norethindrone acetate 0.5 mg daily.
- Estradiol in fixed combination with drospirenone (Angeliq®): Estradiol 1 mg with drospirenone 0.5 mg daily.
- Estradiol with norgestimate (Prefest®): Estradiol 1 mg daily on days 1–3, then estradiol 1 mg with norgestimate 0.09 mg daily on days 4–6; repeat the pattern continuously.
- Ethinyl estradiol in fixed combination with norethindrone acetate (FemHRT®): Ethinyl estradiol 5 mcg with norethindrone acetate 1 mg daily.

IM:
- Estradiol cypionate: 1–5 mg every 3–4 weeks.
- Estradiol valerate: 10–20 mg every 4 weeks.
- Estradiol cypionate in fixed combination with testosterone cypionate: Estradiol cypionate 2 mg with testosterone cypionate 50 mg every 4 weeks.

TOPICAL (ESTRADIOL TRANSDERMAL SYSTEM):
- Estradiol (Esclim®): Initially, 1 system delivering 0.025 mg/24 hours twice weekly in a continuous regimen (women without a uterus) or cyclic regimen (women with a uterus).
- Estradiol (Vivelle®, Vivelle-Dot®): Initially, 1 system delivering 0.0375 mg/24 hours twice weekly in a continuous regimen (women without a uterus) or cyclic regimen (women with a uterus).
- Estradiol (Climara®): Initially, 1 system delivering 0.025 mg/24 hours once weekly in a continuous regimen.
- Estradiol (Alora®, Estraderm®): Initially, 1 system delivering 0.05 mg/24 hours twice weekly in a continuous regimen (women without a uterus) or cyclic regimen (women with a uterus).

TOPICAL (ESTRADIOL/PROGESTIN TRANSDERMAL SYSTEM):
- Estradiol in fixed combination with norethindrone acetate (CombiPatch®) continuous combined regimen: 1 system delivering 0.05 mg/24 hours of estradiol and 0.14 mg/24 hours of norethindrone acetate twice weekly in a continuous regimen. If necessary, increase dosage of norethindrone acetate by using dosage system that delivers 0.25 mg/24 hours of norethindrone acetate.
- Estradiol in fixed combination with norethindrone acetate (CombiPatch®) continuous sequential regimen: 1 system of transdermal estradiol delivering 0.05 mg/24 hours (i.e., Vivelle®) twice weekly for the first 14 days of a 28-day cycle, then 1 estradiol/norethindrone acetate (CombiPatch®) system delivering 0.05 mg/24 hours of estradiol and 0.14 mg/24 hours of norethindrone acetate twice weekly for the remaining 14 days of the cycle. If necessary, increase dosage of norethindrone acetate by using dosage system that delivers 0.25 mg/24 hours of norethindrone acetate.
- Estradiol in fixed combination with levonorgestrel (Climara Pro®) continuous combined regimen: 1 system delivering 0.045 mg/24 hours of estradiol and 0.015 mg/24 hours of levonorgestrel once weekly in a continuous regimen.

TOPICAL (GEL):
- Estradiol 0.06% (EstroGel®): Apply 1.25 g of gel (0.75 mg of estradiol) once daily. Lowest effective dose not determined.

TOPICAL (EMULSION):
- Estradiol (Estrasorb®): Apply contents of 2 pouches (3.48 g of emulsion delivering 0.05 mg/24 hours) once daily. Lowest effective dose not determined.

VAGINAL:
- Estradiol acetate vaginal ring (Femring®): Initially, 1 ring delivering estradiol 0.05 mg/24 hours inserted into the vaginal vault; ring should remain in place for 3 months. After 3 months, remove the ring and, if appropriate, replace with a new ring.

Vulvar and Vaginal Atrophy

ORAL:
- Estradiol: 1–2 mg daily in a cyclic regimen (3 weeks on, 1 week off).
- Estradiol in fixed combination with norethindrone acetate (Activella®): Estradiol 1 mg with norethindrone acetate 0.5 mg daily.
- Estradiol in fixed combination with drospirenone (Angeliq®): Estradiol 1 mg with drospirenone 0.5 mg daily.
- Estradiol with norgestimate (Prefest®): Estradiol 1 mg daily on days 1–3, then estradiol 1 mg with norgestimate 0.09 mg daily on days 4–6; repeat the pattern continuously. This may not be the lowest effective dosage for this indication.

IM:
- Estradiol valerate: 10–20 mg every 4 weeks.

TOPICAL (ESTRADIOL TRANSDERMAL SYSTEM):
- Estradiol (Esclim®): Initially, 1 system delivering 0.025 mg/24 hours twice weekly in a continuous regimen (women without a uterus) or cyclic regimen (women with a uterus).
- Estradiol (Vivelle®, Vivelle-Dot®): Initially, 1 system delivering 0.0375 mg/24 hours twice weekly in a continuous regimen (women without a uterus) or cyclic regimen (women with a uterus).
- Estradiol (Alora®, Estraderm®): Initially, 1 system delivering 0.05 mg/24 hours twice weekly in a continuous regimen (women without a uterus) or cyclic regimen (women with a uterus).

TOPICAL (ESTRADIOL/PROGESTIN TRANSDERMAL SYSTEM):
- Estradiol in fixed combination with norethindrone acetate (CombiPatch®) continuous combined regimen: 1 system delivering 0.05 mg/24 hours of estradiol and 0.14 mg/24 hours of norethindrone acetate twice weekly in a continuous regimen. If necessary, increase dosage of norethindrone acetate by using dosage system that delivers 0.25 mg/24 hours of norethindrone acetate.

- Estradiol in fixed combination with norethindrone acetate (CombiPatch®) continuous sequential regimen: 1 system of transdermal estradiol delivering 0.05 mg/24 hours (i.e., Vivelle®) twice weekly for the first 14 days of a 28-day cycle, then 1 estradiol/norethindrone acetate (CombiPatch®) system delivering 0.05 mg/24 hours of estradiol and 0.14 mg/24 hours of norethindrone acetate twice weekly for the remaining 14 days of the cycle. If necessary, increase dosage of norethindrone acetate by using dosage system that delivers 0.25 mg/24 hours of norethindrone acetate.

TOPICAL (GEL):
- Estradiol 0.06% (EstroGel®): Apply 1.25 g of gel (0.75 mg of estradiol) once daily. Lowest effective dose not determined.

VAGINAL:
- Estradiol vaginal ring (Estring®): 1 ring delivering estradiol 0.0075 mg/24 hours inserted into the upper third of the vaginal vault; ring should remain in place for 3 months. After 3 months, remove the ring and, if appropriate, replace with a new ring.
- Estradiol acetate vaginal ring (Femring®): Initially, 1 ring delivering estradiol 0.05 mg/24 hours inserted into the vaginal vault; ring should remain in place for 3 months. After 3 months, remove the ring and, if appropriate, replace with a new ring.
- Estradiol vaginal tablet (Vagifem®): Initially, 25 mcg once daily for 2 weeks; maintenance, 25 mcg twice weekly.
- Estradiol vaginal cream (Estrace®): Initially, 2–4 g of 0.01% cream daily for 1–2 weeks; reduce to one-half the initial dosage for 2 weeks. Maintenance, 1 g 1 to 3 times weekly.

Osteoporosis
Prevention in Postmenopausal Women

ORAL:
- Estradiol: 0.5 mg daily in a cyclic regimen (23 days on, 5 days off). Adjust dosage if necessary to control concurrent menopausal symptoms.
- Estradiol in fixed combination with norethindrone acetate (Activella®): Estradiol 1 mg with norethindrone acetate 0.5 mg daily. This may not be the lowest effective dosage.
- Estradiol with norgestimate (Prefest®): Estradiol 1 mg daily on days 1–3, then estradiol 1 mg with norgestimate 0.09 mg daily on days 4–6; repeat the pattern continuously. This may not be the lowest effective dosage.
- Ethinyl estradiol in fixed combination with norethindrone acetate (FemHRT®): Ethinyl estradiol 5 mcg with norethindrone acetate 1 mg daily.

TOPICAL (ESTRADIOL TRANSDERMAL SYSTEM):
- Estradiol (Alora®, Vivelle®, Vivelle-Dot®): Initially, 1 system delivering 0.025 mg/24 hours twice weekly in a continuous regimen (women without a uterus) or cyclic regimen (women with a uterus). Adjust dosage as necessary.
- Estradiol (Climara®): Initially, 1 system delivering 0.025 mg/24 hours once weekly in a continuous regimen. Adjust dosage based on biochemical markers and BMD.
- Estradiol (Estraderm®): Initially, 1 system delivering 0.05 mg/24 hours twice weekly in a continuous regimen (women without a uterus) or cyclic regimen (women with a uterus). Adjust dosage as necessary.
- Estradiol (Menostar®): 1 system delivering 0.014 mg/24 hours once weekly in a continuous regimen.

TOPICAL (ESTRADIOL/PROGESTIN TRANSDERMAL SYSTEM):
- Estradiol in fixed combination with levonorgestrel (Climara Pro®) continuous combined regimen: 1 system delivering 0.045 mg/24 hours of estradiol and 0.015 mg/24 hours of levonorgestrel once weekly in a continuous regimen.

Hypoestrogenism

ORAL:
- Estradiol: 1–2 mg daily; adjust dosage as necessary to control symptoms.

IM:
- Estradiol cypionate: 1.5–2 mg every month.
- Estradiol valerate: 10–20 mg every 4 weeks.

TOPICAL (ESTRADIOL TRANSDERMAL SYSTEM):
- Estradiol (Esclim®): Initially, 1 system delivering 0.025 mg/24 hours twice weekly in a continuous regimen (women without a uterus) or cyclic regimen (women with a uterus).
- Estradiol (Alora®): Initially, 1 system delivering 0.05 mg/24 hours twice weekly in a continuous regimen (women without a uterus) or cyclic regimen (women with a uterus).

Metastatic Breast Carcinoma

ORAL:
- Estradiol: 10 mg 3 times daily for ≥3 months.

Prostate Carcinoma

ORAL:
- Estradiol: 1–2 mg 3 times daily.

IM:
- Estradiol valerate: ≥30 mg every 1–2 weeks.

Estrogen and Progestin (Hormone Replacement Therapy)

(ess′ troe jen) (pro jes′ tin)

Brand Name: Activella®, FemHrt®, Ortho-Prefest®, Premphase®, Prempro®

Important Warning

Hormone replacement therapy may increase the risk of heart attack, stroke, breast cancer, and blood clots in the lungs and legs. Tell your doctor if you smoke and if you have or have ever had breast lumps or cancer; a heart attack; a stroke; blood clots; high blood pressure; high blood levels of cholesterol or fats; or diabetes. If you are having surgery or will be on bedrest, talk to your doctor about stopping estrogen and progestin at least 4-6 weeks before the surgery or bedrest.

If you experience any of the following side effects, call your doctor immediately: sudden, severe headache; sudden, severe vomiting; sudden partial or complete loss of vision; speech problems; dizziness or faintness; weakness or numbness of an arm or a leg; crushing chest pain or chest heaviness; coughing up blood; sudden shortness of breath; or calf pain.

Talk to your doctor about the risks and benefits of taking estrogen and progestin.

Why is this medicine prescribed?

Combinations of estrogen and progestin are used to treat certain symptoms of menopause. Estrogen and progestin are two female sex hormones. Hormone replacement therapy works by replacing estrogen hormone that is no longer being made by the body. Estrogen reduces feelings of warmth in the upper body and periods of sweating and heat (hot flashes), vaginal symptoms (itching, burning, and dryness) and difficulty with urination, but it does not relieve other symptoms of menopause such as nervousness or depression. Estrogen also prevents thinning of the bones (osteoporosis) in menopausal women. Progestin is added to estrogen in hormone replacement therapy to reduce the risk of uterine cancer in women who still have their uterus.

How should this medicine be used?

Hormone replacement therapy comes as a tablet to take by mouth. It is usually taken once a day. To help you remember to take hormone replacement therapy, take it around the same time every day. Follow the directions on your prescription label carefully, and ask your doctor or pharmacist to explain any part you do not understand. Take this medication exactly as directed. Do not take more or less of it or take it more often than prescribed by your doctor. Do not stop taking this medication without talking to your doctor.

Activella, FemHrt, and Prempro come as tablets containing estrogen and progestin. Take one tablet every day.

Ortho-Prefest comes in a blister card containing 30 tablets. Take one pink tablet (containing only estrogen) once daily for 3 days, then take one white tablet (containing estrogen and progestin) once daily for 3 days. Repeat this process until you finish all the tablets on the card. Begin a new blister card the day after you finish the last one.

Premphase comes in a dispenser containing 28 tablets. Take one maroon tablet (containing only estrogen) once daily on days 1 to 14, and take one light-blue tablet (containing estrogen and progestin) once daily on days 15 to 28. Begin a new dispenser the day after you finish the last one.

Before taking hormone replacement therapy, ask your pharmacist or doctor for a copy of the manufacturer's information for the patient and read it carefully.

Are there other uses for this medicine?

This medication may be prescribed for other uses; ask your doctor or pharmacist for more information.

What special precautions should I follow?

Before taking hormone replacement therapy,

- tell your doctor and pharmacist if you are allergic to estrogen, progestin, or any other medications.
- tell your doctor and pharmacist what prescription and nonprescription medications, vitamins, nutritional supplements, and herbal products you are taking. Be sure to mention any of the following: acetaminophen (Tylenol); anticoagulants ('blood thinners') such as warfarin (Coumadin); cyclosporine (Neoral, Sandimmune); medications for seizures such as carbamazepine (Tegretol), phenobarbital (Luminal, Solfoton), and phenytoin (Dilantin); morphine (Kadian, MS Contin, MSIR, others); oral steroids such as dexamethasone (Decadron, Dexone), methylprednisolone (Medrol), prednisone (Deltasone) and prednisolone (Prelone); rifampin (Rifadin, Rimactane); salicylic acid; temazepam (Restoril); theophylline (Theobid, Theo-Dur); and thyroid medication such as levothyroxine (Levothroid, Levoxyl, Synthroid). Your doctor may need to change the doses of your medications or monitor you carefully for side effects.
- in addition to the conditions listed in the IMPORTANT WARNING section, tell your doctor if you have had a hysterectomy and if you have or have ever had asthma; toxemia (high blood pressure during pregnancy); depression; epilepsy (seizures); migraine headaches; liver, heart, gallbladder, or kidney disease; jaundice (yellowing of the skin or eyes); vaginal bleeding between menstrual periods; and excessive weight gain and fluid retention (bloating) during the menstrual cycle.

- tell your doctor if you are pregnant, plan to become pregnant, or are breast-feeding. If you become pregnant while taking this medication, call your doctor immediately. Estrogen and progestin may harm the fetus.
- if you are having surgery, including dental surgery, tell the doctor or dentist you are taking hormone replacement therapy.
- tell your doctor if you smoke cigarettes. Smoking while taking this medication may increase your risk of serious side effects such as blood clots and stroke. Smoking also may decrease the effectiveness of this medication.
- tell your doctor and pharmacist if you wear contact lenses. If you notice changes in vision or ability to wear your lenses while taking hormone replacement therapy, see an eye doctor.

What special dietary instructions should I follow?

Ask your doctor about taking calcium supplements if you are taking this medication for prevention of osteoporosis. Follow all dietary and exercise recommendations, as both can help prevent bone disease.

What should I do if I forget to take a dose?

Take the missed dose as soon as you remember it. However, if it is almost time for the next dose, skip the missed dose and continue your regular dosing schedule. Do not take a double dose to make up for a missed one.

What side effects can this medicine cause?

Hormone replacement therapy may cause side effects. Tell your doctor if any of these symptoms are severe or do not go away:

- headache
- upset stomach
- vomiting
- stomach cramps or bloating
- diarrhea
- appetite and weight changes
- changes in sex drive or ability
- nervousness
- brown or black skin patches
- acne
- swelling of hands, feet, or lower legs (fluid retention)
- bleeding or spotting between menstrual periods
- changes in menstrual flow
- breast tenderness, enlargement, or discharge
- difficulty wearing contact lenses

Some side effects can be serious. The following symptoms are uncommon, but if you experience any of them or those listed in the IMPORTANT WARNING section, call your doctor immediately:

- double vision
- severe abdominal pain
- yellowing of the skin or eyes
- severe mental depression

- unusual bleeding
- loss of appetite
- rash
- extreme tiredness, weakness, or lack of energy
- fever
- dark-colored urine
- light-colored stool

Hormone replacement therapy may increase the risk of developing endometrial cancer and gallbladder disease. Talk to your doctor about the risks of taking this medication.

Hormone replacement therapy may cause other side effects. Call your doctor if you have any unusual problems while taking this medication.

If you experience a serious side effect, you or your doctor may send a report to the Food and Drug Administration's (FDA) MedWatch Adverse Event Reporting program online [at http://www.fda.gov/MedWatch/index.html] or by phone [1-800-332-1088].

What storage conditions are needed for this medicine?

Keep this medication in the container it came in, tightly closed, and out of reach of children. Store it at room temperature and away from heat and moisture (not in the bathroom). Throw way any medication that is outdated or no longer needed. Talk to your pharmacist about the proper disposal of your medication.

What should I do in case of overdose?

In case of overdose, call your local poison control center at 1-800-222-1222. If the victim has collapsed or is not breathing, call local emergency services at 911.

Symptoms of overdose may include:
- upset stomach
- vomiting

What other information should I know?

Keep all appointments with your doctor and the laboratory. You should have a complete physical exam, including blood pressure measurements, breast and pelvic exams, and a Pap test at least yearly. Follow your doctor's directions for examining your breasts; report any lumps immediately.

If you are taking hormone replacement therapy to treat symptoms of menopause, your doctor will check every 3 to 6 months to see if you still need this medication. If you are taking this medication to prevent thinning of the bones (osteoporosis), you will take it for a longer period of time.

Before you have any laboratory tests, tell the laboratory personnel that you take hormone replacement therapy, because this medication may interfere with some laboratory tests.

Do not let anyone else take your medication. Ask your pharmacist any questions you have about refilling your prescription.

Please see the Estrogen monograph to find dosing information for this medication.

Estrogen and Progestin (Oral Contraceptives)

(ess′ troe jen) (proe jes tin)

Brand Name: Alesse®, Apri®, Aviane®, Brevicon®, Demulen®, Desogen®, Estrostep®, Estrostep® Fe, Genora®, Jenest®, Levlen®, Levlite®, Levora®, Lo/Ovral®, Loestrin®, Loestrin® Fe, Low-Ogestrel®, Lybrel®, Microgestin®, Microgestin® Fe, Mircette®, Modicon®, Necon®, Norinyl®, Nordette®, Nortrel®, Ogestrel®, Ortho-Cept®, Ortho-Cyclen®, Ortho-Novum®, Ortho Tri-Cyclen®, Ovcon®, Ovral®, Seasonale®, Seasonique®, Tri-Levlen®, Tri-Norinyl®, Triphasil®, Trivora®, Yasmin®, Zovia®

Also available generically.

Important Warning

Cigarette smoking increases the risk of serious side effects from oral contraceptives, including heart attacks, blood clots, and strokes. This risk is higher for women over 35 years old and heavy smokers (15 or more cigarettes per day). If you take oral contraceptives, you should not smoke.

Why is this medicine prescribed?

Oral contraceptives (birth-control pills) are used to prevent pregnancy. Estrogen and progestin are two female sex hormones. Combinations of estrogen and progestin work by preventing ovulation (the release of eggs from the ovaries). They also change the lining of the uterus (womb) to prevent pregnancy from developing and change the mucus at the cervix (opening of the uterus) to prevent sperm (male reproductive cells) from entering. Oral contraceptives are a very effective method of birth control, but they do not prevent the spread of human immunodeficiency virus [HIV, the virus that causes acquired immunodeficiency syndrome (AIDS)] and other sexually transmitted diseases.

Some brands of oral contraceptives are also used to treat acne in certain patients. Oral contraceptives work to treat acne by decreasing the amounts of certain natural substances that can cause acne.

How should this medicine be used?

Oral contraceptives come in packets of 21, 28, or 91 tablets to take by mouth once a day, every day or almost every day of a regular cycle. To avoid nausea, take oral contraceptives with food or milk. Take your oral contraceptive at the same time every day. Follow the directions on your prescription label carefully, and ask your doctor or pharmacist to explain any part you do not understand. Take your oral contraceptive exactly as directed. Do not take more or less of it, take it more often, or take it for a longer time than prescribed by your doctor.

Oral contraceptives come in many different brands. Different brands of oral contraceptives contain slightly different medications or doses, are taken in slightly different ways, and have different risks and benefits. Be sure that you know which brand of oral contraceptives you are using and exactly how you should use it. Ask your doctor or pharmacist for a copy of the manufacturer's information for the patient and read it carefully.

If you have a 21-tablet packet, take one tablet daily for 21 days and then none for 7 days. Then start a new packet.

If you have a 28-tablet packet, take one tablet daily for 28 days. The last set of tablets in most 28 day packets are a different color. These tablets are reminder tablets. They do not contain any active ingredients but may contain iron. Taking one of these tablets every day will help you remember to start your next packet of birth control pills on time. One type of 28-tablet packet contains tablets that are all the same color. All of the tablets in this type of packet contain active ingredients. Whether your packet includes reminder tablets or only active tablets, you should take one tablet daily continuously for 28 days in the order specified in your packet. Start a new packet the day after you take your 28th tablet.

If you have a 91-day tablet packet, take one tablet daily for 91 days. Your packet will contain three trays of tablets. Start with the first tablet on the first tray and continue taking one tablet every day in the order specified on the packet until you have taken all of the tablets on all of the trays. The last days' tablets are a different color. These tablets may contain an inactive ingredient, or they may contain a very low dose of estrogen. Start your new packet the day after you take your 91st tablet.

Your doctor will tell you when you should start taking your oral contraceptive. Oral contraceptives are usually started on the first or fifth day of your menstrual period or on the first Sunday after or on which bleeding begins. Your doctor will also tell you whether you need to use another method of birth control during the first 7 days that you take your oral contraceptive and will help you choose a method. Follow these directions carefully.

You will probably experience withdrawal bleeding similar to a menstrual period while you are taking the inactive tablets or the low dose estrogen tablets or during the week that you do not take your oral contraceptive. If you are taking the type of packet that only contains active tablets, you will not experience any scheduled bleeding, but you may experience unexpected bleeding and spotting, especially at the beginning of your treatment. Be sure to start taking your new packet on schedule even if you are still bleeding.

You may need to use a backup method of birth control if you vomit or have diarrhea while you are taking an oral contraceptive. Talk to your doctor about this before you begin to take your oral contraceptive so that you can prepare a backup method of birth control in case it is needed. If you vomit or have diarrhea while you are taking an oral contraceptive, call your doctor to find out how long you should use the backup method.

If you have recently given birth, wait until 4 weeks after delivering to begin taking oral contraceptives. If you have had an abortion or miscarriage, talk to your doctor about when you should begin taking oral contraceptives.

Oral contraceptives will work to prevent pregnancy or treat acne only as long as they are taken regularly. Continue to take oral contraceptives every day even if you are spotting or bleeding, have an upset stomach, or do not think that you are likely to become pregnant. Do not stop taking oral contraceptives without talking to your doctor.

Are there other uses for this medicine?

Oral contraceptives are also sometimes used to treat heavy or irregular menstruation and endometriosis (a condition in which the type of tissue that lines the uterus [womb] grows in other areas of the body and causes pain, heavy or irregular menstruation [periods], and other symptoms). Talk to your doctor about the risks of using this medication for your condition.

This medication may be prescribed for other uses; ask your doctor or pharmacist for more information.

What special precautions should I follow?

Before taking oral contraceptives,
- tell your doctor and pharmacist if you are allergic to estrogen, progestin, or any other medications.
- tell your doctor and pharmacist what prescription and nonprescription medications, vitamins, and nutritional supplements you are taking. Be sure to mention any of the following: acetaminophen (APAP, Tylenol); antibiotics such as ampicillin (Principen), clarithromycin (Biaxin), erythromycin (E.E.S., E-Mycin, Erythrocin), isoniazid (INH, Nydrazid), metronidazole (Flagyl), rifabutin (Mycobutin), rifampin (Rifadin, Rimactane), tetracycline (Sumycin), and troleandomycin (TAO) (not available in the U.S.); anticoagulants ('blood thinners') such as warfarin (Coumadin); antifungals such as griseofulvin (Fulvicin, Grifulvin, Grisactin), fluconazole (Diflucan), itraconazole (Sporanox), and ketoconazole (Nizoral); atorvastatin (Lipitor); clofibrate (Atromid-S); cyclosporine (Neoral, Sandimmune); danazol (Danocrine); delavirdine (Rescriptor); diltiazem (Cardizem, Dilacor, Tiazac); fluoxetine (Prozac, Sarafem, in Symbyax); HIV protease inhibitors such as indinavir (Crixivan) and ritonavir (Norvir); medications for seizures such as carbamazepine (Tegretol), felbamate (Felbatol), lamotrigine (Lamictal), oxcarbazepine (Trileptal), phenobarbital (Luminal, Solfoton), phenytoin (Dilantin), primidone (Mysoline), and topiramate (Topamax); modafinil (Provigil); morphine (Kadian, MS Contin, MSIR, others); nefazodone; oral steroids such as dexamethasone (Decadron, Dexone), methylprednisolone (Medrol), prednisone (Deltasone), and prednisolone (Prelone); temazepam (Restoril); theophylline (Theobid, Theo-Dur); thyroid medication such as levothyroxine (Levothroid, Levoxyl, Synthroid); verapamil (Calan, Covera, Isoptin, Verelan); vitamin C; and zafirlukast (Accolate). Before taking Yasmin, also tell your doctor and pharmacist if you are taking angiotensin-converting enzyme (ACE) inhibitors such as benazepril (Lotensin), enalapril (Vasotec), and lisinopril (Prinivil, Zestril); angiotensin II antagonists such as irbesartan (Avapro), losartan (Cozaar), and valsartan (Diovan); aspirin and other nonsteroidal anti-inflammatory medications (NSAIDs) such as ibuprofen (Advil, Motrin) and naproxen (Aleve, Naprosyn); diuretics ('water pills') such as amiloride (Midamor), spironolactone (Aldactone), and triamterene (Dyrenium); or heparin. Your doctor may need to change the doses of your medications or monitor you carefully for side effects.
- tell your doctor what herbal products you are taking, especially St. John's wort.
- tell your doctor if you have or have ever had blood clots in your legs, lungs, or eyes; thrombophilia (condition in which the blood clots easily); coronary artery disease (clogged blood vessels leading to the heart); cerebrovascular disease (clogging or weakening of the blood vessels within the brain or leading to the brain); stroke or stroke; an irregular heartbeat; heart disease; a heart attack; chest pain; diabetes that has affected your circulation; headaches that come along with other symptoms such as vision changes, weakness, and dizziness; high blood pressure; breast cancer; cancer of the lining of the uterus, cervix, or vagina; liver cancer; liver tumors; yellowing of the skin or eyes during pregnancy or while you were using hormonal contraceptives (birth control pills, patches, rings, implants, or injections); or unexplained abnormal vaginal bleeding. Also tell your doctor if you have recently had surgery or have been unable to move around for any reason. Your doctor may tell you that you should not take oral contraceptives if you have or have had any of these conditions.
- Also tell your doctor if anyone in your family has had breast cancer and if you have or have ever had problems with your breasts such as lumps, an abnormal mammogram (breast x-ray), or fibrocystic breast disease (swollen, tender breasts and/or breast lumps that are not cancer); high blood cholesterol or fats; diabetes; asthma; toxemia (high blood pressure during pregnancy); heart attack; chest pain; seizures; migraine headaches; depression; gallbladder or kidney disease; adrenal insufficiency (for Yasmin); jaundice (yellowing of the skin or eyes); and excessive weight gain and fluid retention (bloating) during the menstrual cycle.
- do not take oral contraceptives if you are pregnant, plan to become pregnant, or are breast-feeding. If you become pregnant while taking oral contraceptives, call your doctor immediately.

- if you miss periods while you are taking oral contraceptives, you may be pregnant. If you are using a 91-tablet packet and you miss one period, call your doctor. If you are using another type of packet according to the directions and you miss one period, you may continue to take your tablets. However, if you have not taken your tablets as directed and you miss one period or if you have taken your tablets as directed and you miss two periods, call your doctor and use another method of birth control until you have a pregnancy test. If you are using a 28-tablet packet that contains only active tablets, you will not expect to have periods on a regular basis, so it may be hard to tell if you are pregnant. If you are using this type of oral contraceptive, call your doctor and have a pregnancy test if you experience symptoms of pregnancy such as nausea, vomiting, and breast tenderness, or if you suspect you may be pregnant.
- if you are having surgery, including dental surgery, tell the doctor or dentist that you are taking oral contraceptives.
- tell your doctor and pharmacist if you wear contact lenses. If you notice changes in vision or ability to wear your lenses while taking oral contraceptives, see an eye doctor.

What special dietary instructions should I follow?

Unless your doctor tells you otherwise, continue your normal diet.

What should I do if I forget to take a dose?

If you miss doses of your oral contraceptive, you may not be protected from pregnancy. You may need to use a backup method of birth control for 7 days or until the end of the cycle. Every brand of oral contraceptives comes with specific directions to follow if you miss one or more doses. Carefully read the directions in the manufacturer's information for the patient that came with your oral contraceptive. If you have any questions, call your doctor or pharmacist. Continue to take your tablets as scheduled and use a backup method of birth control until your questions are answered.

What side effects can this medicine cause?

Oral contraceptives may cause side effects. Tell your doctor if any of these symptoms are severe or do not go away:
- nausea
- vomiting
- stomach cramps or bloating
- diarrhea
- constipation
- gingivitis (swelling of the gum tissue)
- increased or decreased appetite
- weight gain or weight loss
- brown or black skin patches
- acne
- hair growth in unusual places

- bleeding or spotting between menstrual periods
- changes in menstrual flow
- painful or missed periods
- breast tenderness, enlargement, or discharge
- difficulty wearing contact lenses
- swelling, redness, irritation, burning, or itching of the vagina
- white vaginal discharge

Some side effects can be serious. The following symptoms are uncommon, but if you experience any of them, call your doctor immediately:
- severe headache
- severe vomiting
- speech problems
- dizziness or faintness
- weakness or numbness of an arm or leg
- crushing chest pain or chest heaviness
- coughing up blood
- shortness of breath
- pain, warmth, or heaviness in the back of the lower leg
- partial or complete loss of vision
- double vision
- bulging eyes
- severe stomach pain
- yellowing of the skin or eyes
- loss of appetite
- extreme tiredness, weakness, or lack of energy
- fever
- dark-colored urine
- light-colored stool
- swelling of the hands, feet, ankles or lower legs
- depression, especially if you also have trouble sleeping, tiredness, loss of energy, or other mood changes
- unusual bleeding
- rash
- menstrual bleeding that is unusually heavy or that lasts for longer than 7 days in a row

Oral contraceptives may increase the chance that you will develop liver tumors. These tumors are not a form of cancer, but they can break and cause serious bleeding inside the body. Oral contraceptives may also increase the chance that you will develop breast or liver cancer, or have a heart attack, a stroke, or a serious blood clot. Talk to your doctor about the risks of using oral contraceptives.

Oral contraceptives may cause other side effects. Call your doctor if you have any unusual problems while taking this medication.

If you experience a serious side effect, you or your doctor may send a report to the Food and Drug Administration's (FDA) MedWatch Adverse Event Reporting program online [at http://www.fda.gov/MedWatch/index.html] or by phone [1-800-332-1088].

What storage conditions are needed for this medicine?

Keep this medication in the packet it came in, tightly closed, and out of reach of children. Store it at room temperature and away from excess heat and moisture (not in the bathroom). Throw away any medication that is outdated or no longer needed. Talk to your pharmacist about the proper disposal of your medication.

What should I do in case of overdose?

In case of overdose, call your local poison control center at 1-800-222-1222. If the victim has collapsed or is not breathing, call local emergency services at 911.

Symptoms of overdose may include:

- nausea
- vaginal bleeding

What other information should I know?

Keep all appointments with your doctor and the laboratory. You should have a complete physical examination every year, including blood pressure measurements, breast and pelvic exams, and a Pap test. Follow your doctor's directions for examining your breasts; report any lumps immediately.

Before you have any laboratory tests, tell the laboratory personnel that you take oral contraceptives.

If you wish to stop taking oral contraceptives and become pregnant, your doctor may tell you to use another method of birth control until you begin to menstruate regularly again. It may take a long time for you to become pregnant after you stop taking oral contraceptives, especially if you have never had a baby or if you had irregular, infrequent, or complete absence of menstrual periods before taking oral contraceptives. However, it is possible to become pregnant within days of stopping certain oral contraceptives. If you want to stop taking oral contraceptives but do not want to become pregnant, you should begin using another type of birth control as soon as you stop taking oral contraceptives. Discuss any questions that you may have with your doctor.

Oral contraceptives may decrease the amount of folate in your body. Folate is important for the development of a healthy baby, so you should talk to your doctor if you want to become pregnant soon after you stop taking oral contraceptives.

Do not let anyone else take your medication. Ask your pharmacist any questions you have about refilling your prescription.

Dosage Facts
For Informational Purposes

Caution: Do not change your dose, how often you take your medication, or the length of time you are to take it without first talking to your healthcare provider.

The following dosage information was written using medical language for doctors and other healthcare professionals and is provided here for you to check your dosage. The dosage of this drug may differ for different patients. Therefore, always follow your doctor's instructions or the directions on the label. Contact your health-care provider or pharmacist if you have any questions about the specific dosage of your medication after reviewing this information.

General Dosage Information

The smallest dosage of estrogen and progestin compatible with a low failure rate and the individual needs of the woman should be used.

In establishing an oral contraceptive dosage cycle, the menstrual cycle is usually considered to be 28 days. The first day of bleeding is counted as the first day of the cycle.

Estrogen-progestin oral contraceptives are usually classified according to their formulation:

- those **monophasic** preparations containing 50 mcg of estrogen,
- those **monophasic** preparations containing <50 mcg of estrogen (usually 20–35 mcg),
- those containing <50 mcg of estrogen with 2 sequences of progestin doses (**biphasic**),
- those containing <50 mcg of estrogen with 3 sequences of progestin doses (**triphasic**), and
- those containing 3 sequences of estrogen (e.g., 20, 30, 35 mcg) with a fixed dose of progestin (**estrophasic**).

Oral contraceptives usually are described in terms of their estrogen content, although the progestin content of the formulations also varies. The estrogenic and progestinic dominance of oral contraceptives depends mainly on the amount of estrogen and the amount and specific progestin contained in the formulation. The estrogenic or progestinic dominance of an oral contraceptive may contribute to hormone-related adverse effects and may be useful in selecting an alternate formulation when unacceptable adverse effects occur with a given formulation.

Biphasic oral contraceptives contain 2 sequentially administered, fixed combinations of hormones per dosage cycle. The first sequence consists of tablets containing a fixed combination of low-dose estrogen and low-dose progestin, and the second sequence consists of tablets containing a fixed combination of low-dose estrogen and higher-dose progestin. Biphasic oral contraceptives are *not* the same as previously available "sequential" oral contraceptives, which consisted of an estrogen alone for the first sequence.

Triphasic oral contraceptives contain graduated sequences of progestin or estrogen per dosage cycle. With most commercially available triphasic oral contraceptives, each dosage cycle consists of 3 sequentially administered fixed combinations of the hormones in which the ratio of progestin to estrogen progressively increases with each sequence. The first sequence consists of tablets containing a fixed combination of low-dose estrogen and low-dose progestin, the second sequence consists of tablets containing a fixed combination of low-dose or low but slightly higher-dose estrogen and higher-dose progestin, and the third sequence consists of tablets containing low-dose estrogen and either an even higher-dose progestin or low-dose progestin.

Estrophasic oral contraceptives are triphasic preparations in which the estrogen component progressively increases with each sequence.

Fixed-combination, conventional-cycle oral contraceptives are available as 21- or 28-day dosage preparations. Some 28-day preparations contain 21 hormonally active tablets and 7 inert or ferrous fumarate-containing tablets. Other 28-day preparations contain 24 hormonally active tablets and 4 inert or ferrous fumarate-containing tablets.

One monophasic, fixed-combination, **extended-cycle** oral contraceptive (e.g., Seasonale®) is available as a 91-day dosage preparation containing 84 hormonally active tablets and 7 inert tablets. Another extended-cycle oral contraceptive (e.g., Seasonique®) is available as a 91-day preparation with 84 hormonally active tablets containing estrogen/progestin and 7 tablets containing low-dose estrogen.

The transdermal system (Ortho Evra®) is applied topically in a cyclic regimen using a 28-day cycle.

The vaginal contraceptive ring (NuvaRing®) is intended to be used for 1 cycle, which consists of a 3-week period of continuous use of the ring followed by a 1-week ring-free period.

Adult Patients

Contraception

ORAL (21- OR 28-DAY CONVENTIONAL-CYCLE PREPARATIONS):

- Start on the first Sunday after or on which menstrual bleeding begins or on the first day of the menstrual cycle.
- If the first dose is on the first Sunday on or after menstrual bleeding starts, use a back-up method of contraception (e.g., condoms, foam, sponge) for 7 days following initiation of oral contraceptive therapy. If the first dose is on the first day of the menstrual cycle, a back-up method of contraception is not necessary.
- With **21-day conventional-cycle preparations**, take 1 estrogen/progestin tablet once daily for 21 consecutive days, followed by 7 days without tablets. Begin repeat dosage cycles on the eighth day after the last hormonally active tablet (i.e., on the same day of the week as the initial cycle).
- With **28-day conventional-cycle preparations containing 21 hormonally active tablets**, take 1 estrogen/progestin tablet once daily for 21 consecutive days, followed by inert tablets or ferrous fumarate tablets for 7 days. Begin repeat dosage cycles on the eighth day after the last hormonally active tablet (i.e., on the same day of the week as the initial cycle).
- With **28-day conventional-cycle preparations containing 24 hormonally active tablets**, take 1 estrogen/progestin tablet once daily for 24 consecutive days, followed by inert tablets or ferrous fumarate tablets for 4 days. Begin repeat dosage cycles on the fifth day after the last hormonally active tablet (i.e., on the same day of the week as the initial cycle).
- When 1 estrogen/progestin tablet of a conventional-cycle oral contraceptive is missed, take the missed tablet as soon as it is remembered, followed by resumption of the regular schedule. Additional contraceptive methods are not necessary if only 1 tablet is missed.
- When 2 estrogen/progestin tablets are missed during the first 1 or 2 weeks of the cycle, take the 2 missed tablets as soon as they are remembered, take 2 tablets the next day, then resume the regular schedule. If 2 consecutive estrogen/progestin tablets are missed during the third or fourth week of a dosage cycle that was initiated on the first day of the menstrual cycle, discard the remainder of the tablets in the pack for that cycle and start a new dosage cycle the same day. If 2 consecutive estrogen/progestin tablets are missed during the third or fourth week of a dosage cycle that was initiated on the first Sunday on or after menstruation started, continue to take 1 tablet daily until Sunday, then discard the remainder of the tablets for that cycle and start a new dosage cycle that same day. When 2 or more estrogen/progestin tablets are missed on consecutive days, a back-up method of contracep-

tion should be used for each sexual encounter until a hormonally active tablet has been taken for 7 consecutive days.

- If 3 or more consecutive estrogen/progestin tablets are missed during a dosage cycle that was initiated on the first day of the menstrual cycle, discard the remainder of the tablets in that cycle and start a new dosage cycle the same day. If 3 or more consecutive estrogen/progestin tablets are missed during a dosage cycle that was initiated on the first Sunday on or after menstruation started, take 1 tablet daily until Sunday, then discard the remainder of the tablets for that cycle and start a new dosage cycle that same day. A back-up method of contraception should be used for each sexual encounter until a hormonally active tablet has been taken for 7 consecutive days.
- During week 4 of a 28-day dosage cycle, any inactive or ferrous fumarate tablets that are missed should be discarded; continue to take the remaining tablets until the cycle is finished. A back-up contraceptive method is not required during the fourth week as a result of missed inactive or ferrous fumarate tablets.
- With 28-day contraceptive cycles, a new cycle of tablets should be started the day after taking the last tablet of the previous 28-day dosage cycle (i.e., no days without tablets).
- If unsure of what drug regimen to take as a result of missed tablets, use a back-up method of contraception for each sexual encounter and take 1 estrogen/progestin tablet daily until the next clinician contact.
- **Oral (91-day extended-cycle preparations):** Start on the first Sunday after or on which bleeding begins. Use a back-up method of contraception (e.g., condom, spermicide) for 7 days following initiation of therapy.
- Take 1 estrogen/progestin tablet daily for 84 days, followed by inert tablets or tablets containing 10 mcg of estrogen for 7 days. Repeat dosage cycles begin on the same day of the week (Sunday) as the initial cycle. If a repeat cycle is started later than the scheduled day, use a back-up method of contraception until an estrogen/progestin tablet has been taken for 7 consecutive days.
- When 1 estrogen/progestin tablet is missed, take the missed tablet as soon as it is remembered, followed by resumption of the regular schedule. Additional contraceptive measures are not necessary if only one tablet is missed.
- When 2 estrogen/progestin tablets are missed, take the 2 missed tablets as soon as they are remembered, 2 tablets the next day, then resume the regular cycle. Use a back-up method of contraception until an estrogen/progestin tablet has been taken for 7 consecutive days.
- When 3 or more consecutive estrogen/progestin tablets are missed, continue to take 1 tablet daily; the missed tablets should be discarded. Use a back-up method of contraception until an estrogen/progestin tablet has been taken for 7 consecutive days.
- If unsure of what drug regimen to take as a result of missed tablets, use a back-up method of contraception for each sexual encounter, and take 1 tablet daily until the next clinician contact.
- Discard inert tablets or estrogen-containing tablets that are missed; continue to take the remainingtablets until the cycle is finished. If inert tablets or estrogen-containing tablets are missed, a back-up contraceptive method is not required.

Postcoital Contraception

ORAL:
- Preven® Emergency Contraceptive Kit: Take 2 tablets (total dose: ethinyl estradiol 100 mcg and levonorgestrel 0.5 mg) within 72 hours after unprotected intercourse, repeating the dose 12 hours later.
- "Yuzpe" regimen†: Take 100 mcg of ethinyl estradiol and 1 mg of norgestrel within 72 hours after unprotected intercourse, repeating the dose 12 hours later.
- Other regimens†: Take 120 mcg of ethinyl estradiol and 1.2 mg of norgestrel or 0.5–0.6 mg of levonorgestrel within 72 hours after intercourse, repeating the dose 12 hours later.

Dosage of Estrogen-progestin Combinations for Postcoital Contraception

Estrogen-progestin Combination Formulation [Brand Name]	Number and Color of Tablets per Dose*
Ethinyl estradiol (50 mcg) with levonorgestrel (0.25 mg) [Preven® Emergency Contraceptive Kit]	2 light-blue tablets
Ethinyl estradiol (50 mcg) with norgestrel (0.5 mg) [Ovral®]	2 white tablets (any of 21 tablets)
Ethinyl estradiol (50 mcg) with norgestrel (0.5 mg) [Ovral®-28]	2 white tablets (any of *first* 21 tablets)
Ethinyl estradiol (30 mcg) with norgestrel (0.3 mg) [Lo-Ovral®]	4 white tablets (any of 21 tablets)
Ethinyl estradiol (30 mcg) with norgestrel (0.3 mg) [Lo-Ovral®-28]	4 white tablets (any of *first* 21 tablets)
Ethinyl estradiol (30 mcg) with levonorgestrel (0.15 mg) [Nordette®]	4 light-orange tablets (any of 21 tablets)
Ethinyl estradiol (30 mcg) with levonorgestrel (0.15 mg) [Nordette®-28]	4 light-orange tablets (any of *first* 21 tablets)
Ethinyl estradiol (30 mcg) with levonorgestrel (0.15 mg) [Levlen® 21]	4 light-orange tablets (any of 21 tablets)
Ethinyl estradiol (30 mcg) with levonorgestrel (0.15 mg) [Levlen® 28]	4 light-orange tablets (any of *first* 21 tablets)
Ethinyl estradiol (30 mcg) with levonorgestrel (0.125 mg) [Tri-Levlen® 21]	4 yellow tablets (any of *last* 10 tablets)
Ethinyl estradiol (30 mcg) with levonorgestrel (0.125 mg) [Tri-Levlen® 28]	4 yellow tablets (any of tablets 12–21)
Ethinyl estradiol (30 mcg) with levonorgestrel (0.125 mg) [Tri-Phasil® 21]	4 yellow tablets (any of *last* 10 tablets)
Ethinyl estradiol (30 mcg) with levonorgestrel (0.125 mg) [Tri-Levlen® 28]	4 yellow tablets (any of tablets 12–21)

* Dose is administered initially and then repeated 12 hours later

Acne Vulgaris

ORAL:
- Ortho Tri-Cyclen® or Estrostep® is used in the same dosage and administration (i.e., timing of initiation of therapy) as used in contraception.

Premenstrual Dysphoric Disorder

ORAL:
- Yaz® is used in the same dosage and administration (i.e., timing of initiation of therapy) as used in contraception.

† Use is not currently included in the labeling approved by the US Food and Drug Administration.

Estrogen Injection

(ess′ troe jen)

Brand Name: Delestrogen®, DEPO-Estradiol®, Premarin Intravenous®

Important Warning

Estrogen increases the risk that you will develop endometrial cancer (cancer of the lining of the uterus [womb]). The longer you use estrogen, the greater the risk that you will develop endometrial cancer. If you have not had a hysterectomy (surgery to remove the uterus), you should be given another medication called a progestin to take with estrogen injection. This may decrease your risk of developing endometrial cancer, but may increase your risk of developing certain other health problems, including breast cancer. Before you begin using estrogen injection, tell your doctor if you have or have ever had cancer and if you have unusual vaginal bleeding. Call your doctor immediately if you have abnormal or unusual vaginal bleeding during your treatment with estrogen injection. Your doctor will watch you closely to help ensure you do not develop endometrial cancer during or after your treatment.

In a large study, women who took estrogen with progestins by mouth had a higher risk of heart attacks, strokes, blood clots in the lungs or legs, breast cancer, and dementia (loss of ability to think, learn, and understand). Women who use estrogen injection alone or with progestins may also have a higher risk of developing these conditions. Tell your doctor if you smoke or use tobacco, if you have had a heart attack or a stroke in the past year, and if you or anyone in your family has or has ever had blood clots or breast cancer. Also tell your doctor if you have or have ever had high blood pressure, high blood levels of cholesterol or fats, diabetes, heart disease, lupus (a condition in which the body attacks its own tissues causing damage and swelling), breast lumps, or an abnormal mammogram (x-ray of the breast used to find breast cancer).

The following symptoms can be signs of the serious health conditions listed above. Call your doctor immediately if you experience any of the following symptoms while you are using estrogen injection: sudden, severe headache; sudden, severe vomiting; speech problems; dizziness or faintness; sudden complete or partial loss of vision; double vision; weakness or numbness of an arm or a leg; crushing chest pain or chest heaviness; coughing up blood; sudden shortness of breath; difficulty thinking clearly, remembering, or learning new things; breast lumps or other breast changes; discharge from nipples; or pain, tenderness, or redness in one leg.

You can take steps to decrease the risk that you will develop a serious health problem while you are using estrogen injection. Do not use estrogen injection alone or with a progestin to prevent heart disease, heart attacks, strokes, or dementia. Use the lowest dose of estrogen that controls your symptoms and only use estrogen injection as long as needed. Talk to your doctor every 3-6 months to decide if you should use a lower dose of estrogen or should stop using the medication.

You should examine your breasts every month and have a mammogram and a breast exam performed by a doctor every year to help detect breast cancer as early as possible. Your doctor will tell you how to properly examine your breasts and whether you should have these exams more often than once a year because of your personal or family medical history.

Tell your doctor if you are having surgery or will be on bedrest. Your doctor may tell you to stop using estrogen injection 4-6 weeks before the surgery or bedrest to decrease the risk that you will develop blood clots.

Talk to your doctor regularly about the risks and benefits of using estrogen injection.

Why is this medicine prescribed?

The estradiol cypionate and estradiol valerate forms of estrogen injection are used to treat hot flushes (hot flashes; sudden strong feelings of heat and sweating) and/or vaginal dryness, itching, and burning in women who are experiencing menopause (change of life; the end of monthly menstrual periods). However, women who need a medication only to treat vaginal dryness, itching, or burning should consider a different treatment. These forms of estrogen injection are also sometimes used to treat the symptoms of low estrogen in young women who do not produce enough estrogen naturally. The estradiol valerate form of estrogen injection is also sometimes used to relieve the symptoms of certain types of prostate (a male reproductive organ) cancer. The conjugated estrogens form of estrogen injection is used to treat abnormal vaginal bleeding that a doctor has decided is caused only by a problem with the amounts of certain hormones in the body. Estrogen injection is in a class of medications called hormones. It works by replacing estrogen that is normally produced by the body.

How should this medicine be used?

The estradiol cypionate and estradiol valerate forms of long acting estrogen injection come as a liquid to inject into a muscle. These medications are usually injected by a health care professional once every 3-4 weeks. When the estradiol valerate form of estrogen injection is used to treat the symptoms of prostate cancer, it is usually injected by a health care professional once every 1-2 weeks.

The conjugated estrogens form of estrogen injection comes as a powder to mix with sterile water and inject into a muscle or vein. It is usually injected by a health care professional as a single dose. A second dose may be injected 6-12 hours after the first dose if it is needed to control vaginal bleeding.

If you are using estrogen injection to treat hot flushes, your symptoms should improve within 1-5 days after you receive the injection. Tell your doctor if your symptoms do not improve during this time.

Ask your pharmacist or doctor for a copy of the manufacturer's information for the patient.

Are there other uses for this medicine?

This medication may be prescribed for other uses; ask your doctor or pharmacist for more information.

What special precautions should I follow?

Before using estrogen injection,

- tell your doctor and pharmacist if you are allergic to estrogen injection, any other estrogen products, any other medications, or any of the ingredients in estrogen injection. Ask your pharmacist or check the manufacturer's patient information for a list of the ingredients in the brand of estrogen injection you plan to use.
- tell your doctor and pharmacist what prescription and nonprescription medications, vitamins, and nutritional supplements you are taking or plan to take. Be sure to mention any of the following: amiodarone (Cordarone, Pacerone); certain antifungals such as itraconazole (Sporanox) and ketoconazole (Nizoral); aprepitant (Emend); carbamazepine (Carbatrol, Epitol, Tegretol); cimetidine (Tagamet); clarithromycin (Biaxin); cyclosporine (Neoral, Sandimmune); dexamethasone (Decadron, Dexpak); diltiazem (Cardizem, Dilacor, Tiazac, others); erythromycin (E.E.S, Erythrocin); fluoxetine (Prozac, Sarafem); fluvoxamine (Luvox); griseofulvin (Fulvicin, Grifulvin, Gris-PEG); lovastatin (Altocor, Mevacor); medications for human immunodeficiency virus (HIV) or acquired immunodeficiency syndrome

(AIDS) such as atazanavir (Reyataz), delavirdine (Rescriptor), efavirenz (Sustiva), indinavir (Crixivan), lopinavir (in Kaletra), nelfinavir (Viracept), nevirapine (Viramune), ritonavir (Norvir, in Kaletra), and saquinavir (Fortovase, Invirase); medications for thyroid disease; nefazodone; phenobarbital; phenytoin (Dilantin, Phenytek); rifabutin (Mycobutin); rifampin (Rifadin, Rimactane, in Rifamate); sertraline (Zoloft); troleandomycin (TAO); verapamil (Calan, Covera, Isoptin, Verelan); and zafirlukast (Accolate). Your doctor may need to change the doses of your medications or monitor you carefully for side effects.

- tell your doctor what herbal products you are taking, especially St. John's wort.
- tell your doctor if you have or have ever had yellowing of the skin or eyes during pregnancy or during your treatment with an estrogen product, endometriosis (a condition in which the type of tissue that lines the uterus [womb] grows in other areas of the body), uterine fibroids (growths in the uterus that are not cancer), asthma, migraine headaches, seizures, porphyria (condition in which abnormal substances build up in the blood and cause problems with the skin or nervous system), very high or very low levels of calcium in your blood, or thyroid, liver, kidney, gallbladder, or pancreatic disease.
- tell your doctor if you are pregnant, plan to become pregnant, or are breast-feeding. If you become pregnant while using estrogen injection, call your doctor.

What special dietary instructions should I follow?

Talk to your doctor about eating grapefruit and drinking grapefruit juice while using this medicine.

What should I do if I forget to take a dose?

If you miss an appointment to receive a dose of estrogen injection, call your doctor as soon as possible.

What side effects can this medicine cause?

Estrogen injection may cause side effects. Tell your doctor if any of these symptoms are severe or do not go away:

- breast pain or tenderness
- upset stomach
- vomiting
- weight gain or loss
- dizziness
- nervousness
- depression
- irritability
- changes in sexual desire
- hair loss
- unwanted hair growth
- spotty darkening of the skin on the face
- difficulty wearing contact lenses
- leg cramps

- swelling, redness, burning, itching, or irritation of the vagina
- vaginal discharge

Some side effects can be serious. If you experience any of these symptoms or those listed in the IMPORTANT WARNING section, call your doctor immediately:

- bulging eyes
- pain, swelling, or tenderness in the stomach
- loss of appetite
- weakness
- yellowing of the skin or eyes
- joint pain
- movements that are difficult to control
- rash or blisters
- hives
- itching
- swelling of the eyes, face, tongue, throat, hands, arms, feet, ankles, or lower legs
- hoarseness
- difficulty breathing or swallowing

Estrogen may increase your risk of developing cancer of the ovaries or gallbladder disease that may need to be treated with surgery. Talk to your doctor about the risks of using estrogen injection.

Estrogen may cause growth to slow or stop early in children who receive large doses for a long time. Estrogen injection may also affect the timing and speed of sexual development in children. Your child's doctor will monitor him or her carefully during his or her treatment with estrogen. Talk to your child's doctor about the risks of giving this medication to your child.

Estrogen injection may cause other side effects. Call your doctor if you have any unusual problems while taking this medication.

If you experience a serious side effect, you or your doctor may send a report to the Food and Drug Administration's (FDA) MedWatch Adverse Event Reporting program online [at http://www.fda.gov/MedWatch/index.html] or by phone [1-800-332-1088].

What storage conditions are needed for this medicine?

Your doctor will store the medication in his or her office.

What should I do in case of overdose?

In case of overdose, call your local poison control center at 1-800-222-1222. If the victim has collapsed or is not breathing, call local emergency services at 911.

Symptoms of overdose may include:

- upset stomach
- vomiting
- vaginal bleeding

What other information should I know?

Keep all appointments with your doctor.

Before having any laboratory test, tell your doctor and

the laboratory personnel that you are using estrogen injection.

Please see the Estrogen monograph to find dosing information for this medication.

Estrogen Vaginal

(ess' troe jen)

Brand Name: Estrace®, Estring®, Femring®, Premarin®, Vagifem®

Important Warning

Estrogen increases the risk that you will develop endometrial cancer (cancer of the lining of the uterus [womb]). The longer you use estrogen, the greater the risk that you will develop endometrial cancer. If you have not had a hysterectomy (surgery to remove the uterus), you may be given another medication called a progestin to take with vaginal estrogen. This may decrease your risk of developing endometrial cancer, but may increase your risk of developing certain other health problems, including breast cancer. Before you begin using vaginal estrogen, tell your doctor if you have or have ever had cancer and if you have unusual vaginal bleeding. Call your doctor immediately if you have abnormal or unusual vaginal bleeding during your treatment with vaginal estrogen. Your doctor will watch you closely to help ensure you do not develop endometrial cancer during or after your treatment.

In a large study, women who took estrogen with progestins by mouth had a higher risk of heart attacks, strokes, blood clots in the lungs or legs, breast cancer, and dementia (loss of ability to think, learn, and understand). Women who use vaginal estrogen alone or with progestins may also have a higher risk of developing these conditions. Tell your doctor if you smoke or use tobacco, if you have had a heart attack or a stroke in the past year, and if you or anyone in your family has or has ever had blood clots or breast cancer. Also tell your doctor if you have or have ever had high blood pressure, high blood levels of cholesterol or fats, diabetes, heart disease, lupus (a condition in which the body attacks its own tissues causing damage and swelling), breast lumps, or an abnormal mammogram (x-ray of the breasts used to find breast cancer).

The following symptoms can be signs of the serious health conditions listed above. Call your doctor immediately if you experience any of the following symptoms while you are using vaginal estrogen: sud-
den, severe headache; sudden, severe vomiting; speech problems; dizziness or faintness; sudden complete or partial loss of vision; double vision; weakness or numbness of an arm or a leg; crushing chest pain or chest heaviness; coughing up blood; sudden shortness of breath; difficulty thinking clearly, remembering, or learning new things; breast lumps or other breast changes; discharge from nipples; or pain, tenderness, or redness in one leg.

You can take steps to decrease the risk that you will develop a serious health problem while you are using vaginal estrogen. Do not use vaginal estrogen alone or with a progestin to prevent heart disease, heart attacks, strokes, or dementia. Use the lowest dose of estrogen that controls your symptoms and only use vaginal estrogen as long as needed. Talk to your doctor every 3-6 months to decide if you should use a lower dose of estrogen or should stop using the medication.

You should examine your breasts every month and have a mammogram and a breast exam performed by a doctor every year to help detect breast cancer as early as possible. Your doctor will tell you how to properly examine your breasts and whether you should have these exams more often than once a year because of your personal or family medical history.

Tell your doctor if you are having surgery or will be on bed rest. Your doctor may tell you to stop using vaginal estrogen 4-6 weeks before the surgery or bed rest to decrease the risk that you will develop blood clots.

Talk to your doctor regularly about the risks and benefits of using vaginal estrogen.

Why is this medicine prescribed?

Vaginal estrogen is used to treat vaginal dryness, itching, and burning; painful or difficult urination; and sudden need to urinate immediately in women who are experiencing or have experienced menopause (change of life; the end of monthly menstrual periods). Femring® brand estradiol vaginal ring is also used to treat hot flushes ('hot flashes'; sudden strong feelings of heat and sweating) in women who are experiencing menopause. Premarin® brand vaginal cream is also used to treat kraurosis vulvae (a condition that may cause vaginal dryness and discomfort in women or girls of any age). Vaginal estrogen is in a class of medications called hormones. It works by replacing estrogen that is normally produced by the body.

How should this medicine be used?

Vaginal estrogen comes as a flexible ring and a tablet to insert in the vagina, and as a cream to apply to the inside of the vagina. Estrogen vaginal rings are usually inserted in the vagina and left in place for 3 months. After 3 months, the ring is removed, and a new ring may be inserted if treatment is still needed. Estrogen vaginal tablets are usually inserted once a day for the first 2 weeks of treatment and then are inserted twice a week as long as treatment is needed. Estrace® brand vaginal cream is usually applied once daily for 2-4 weeks, and then applied one to three times a week. Premarin® brand vaginal cream product is usually applied according to a rotating schedule that alternates several weeks when the cream is applied every day with one week when the cream is not applied. Use vaginal estrogen at around the same time of day every time you use it. Follow the directions on your prescription label carefully, and ask your doctor or pharmacist to explain any part you do not understand. Use vaginal estrogen exactly as directed. Do not use more or less of it or use it more often than prescribed by your doctor.

To use the vaginal ring, follow these steps:

1. Wash and dry your hands
2. Remove the vaginal ring from its pouch.
3. Stand with one leg up on a chair, step or other object, squat, or lie down. Choose the position that is most comfortable for you.
4. Hold the vaginal ring between your thumb and index finger and press the sides of the ring together. You may want to twist the ring into a figure-of-eight shape.
5. Hold open the folds of skin around your vagina with your other hand.
6. Place the tip of the ring into your vagina and then use your index finger to gently push the ring inside your vagina as far as you can.
7. The vaginal ring does not have to be positioned a certain way inside your vagina, but it will be more comfortable and less likely to fall out when it is placed as far back in your vagina as possible. The ring cannot go past your cervix, so it will not go too far in your vagina or get lost when you push it in. If you feel discomfort, use your index finger to push the ring further into your vagina.
8. Wash your hands again.
9. Leave the ring in place for 3 months. The ring may fall out if you have not inserted it deeply in your vagina, if your vaginal muscles are weak, or if you are straining to have a bowel movement. If the ring falls out, wash it with warm water and replace it in your vagina following the directions above. If the ring falls out and is lost, insert a new ring and leave the new ring in place for up to 3 months. Call your doctor if your ring falls out often.
10. You can leave the ring in place when you have sex. If you choose to remove it or if it falls out, wash it with warm water and replace it in your vagina as soon as possible.
11. When you are ready to remove the ring, wash your hands and stand or lie in a comfortable position.
12. Put a finger into your vagina and hook it through the ring. Gently pull downward and forward to remove the ring.
13. Wrap the ring in a tissue or a piece of toilet paper and throw it away in a trash can. Do not flush the ring in a toilet.

14. Wash your hands again.

To use the vaginal tablet, follow these steps:

1. Tear off one applicator from the strip of applicators in your carton.
2. Open the plastic wrap and remove the applicator.
3. Stand with one leg up on a chair, step, or other object, or lie down. Choose the position that is most comfortable for you.
4. Hold the applicator in one hand with a finger on the end of the plunger.
5. Use the other hand to gently guide the applicator into the vaginal opening. If the tablet falls out of the applicator, do not try to replace it. Throw away that applicator and tablet and use a fresh applicator.
6. Insert the applicator into your vagina as far as is comfortable. Do not force the applicator into your vagina or insert more than half of the applicator into your vagina.
7. Gently press the plunger until you hear a click.
8. Remove the empty applicator from your vagina and throw it away as you would a plastic tampon applicator. Do not save or reuse the applicator.

To use the vaginal cream, follow these steps:

1. Remove the cap from the tube of cream.
2. Screw the nozzle end of the applicator onto the open end of the tube.
3. Gently squeeze the tube from the bottom to fill the applicator with the amount of cream that your doctor has told you to use. Look at the markings on the side of the applicator to help measure your dose.
4. Unscrew the applicator from the tube.
5. Lie on your back and pull your knees up toward your chest.
6. Gently insert the applicator into your vagina and press the plunger downward to release the cream.
7. Remove the applicator from your vagina.
8. To clean the applicator, pull the plunger to remove it from the barrel. Wash the applicator and plunger with mild soap and warm water. Do not use hot water or boil the applicator.

Ask your pharmacist or doctor for a copy of the manufacturer's information for the patient.

Are there other uses for this medicine?

This medication may be prescribed for other uses; ask your doctor or pharmacist for more information.

What special precautions should I follow?

Before using vaginal estrogen,

- tell your doctor and pharmacist if you are allergic to vaginal estrogen, any other estrogen products, any other medications, or any of the ingredients in the type of vaginal estrogen you plan to use. Ask your pharmacist or check the manufacturer's patient information for a list of the ingredients.
- tell your doctor and pharmacist what prescription and nonprescription medications, vitamins, and nutritional

supplements, you are taking or plan to take. Be sure to mention any of the following: amiodarone (Cordarone, Pacerone); certain antifungals such as itraconazole (Sporanox) and ketoconazole (Nizoral); aprepitant (Emend); carbamazepine (Carbatrol, Epitol, Tegretol); cimetidine (Tagamet); clarithromycin (Biaxin); cyclosporine (Neoral, Sandimmune); dexamethasone (Decadron, Dexpak); diltiazem (Cardizem, Dilacor, Tiazac, others); erythromycin (E.E.S, Erythrocin); fluoxetine (Prozac, Sarafem); fluvoxamine (Luvox); griseofulvin (Fulvicin, Grifulvin, Gris-PEG); lovastatin (Altocor, Mevacor); medications for human immunodeficiency virus (HIV) or acquired immunodeficiency syndrome (AIDS) such as atazanavir (Reyataz), delavirdine (Rescriptor), efavirenz (Sustiva), indinavir (Crixivan), lopinavir (in Kaletra), nelfinavir (Viracept), nevirapine (Viramune), ritonavir (Norvir, in Kaletra), and saquinavir (Fortovase, Invirase); medications for thyroid disease; other medications that are used vaginally; nefazodone; phenobarbital; phenytoin (Dilantin, Phenytek); rifabutin (Mycobutin); rifampin (Rifadin, Rimactane, in Rifamate); sertraline (Zoloft); troleandomycin (TAO); verapamil (Calan, Covera, Isoptin, Verelan); and zafirlukast (Accolate). Your doctor may need to change the doses of your medications or monitor you carefully for side effects.
- tell your doctor what herbal products you are taking, especially St. John's wort.
- tell your doctor if you have or have ever had yellowing of the skin or eyes during pregnancy or during your treatment with an estrogen product, endometriosis (a condition in which the type of tissue that lines the uterus [womb] grows in other areas of the body), uterine fibroids (growths in the uterus that are not cancer), asthma, migraine headaches, seizures, porphyria (condition in which abnormal substances build up in the blood and cause problems with the skin or nervous system), very high or very low levels of calcium in your blood, or thyroid, liver, kidney, gallbladder, or pancreatic disease. If you will be using the vaginal ring, also tell your doctor if you have a vaginal infection; any condition that makes your vagina more likely to become irritated; a narrow vagina; or a condition where the rectum, bladder, or uterus has bulged or dropped into the vagina.
- tell your doctor if you are pregnant, plan to become pregnant, or are breast-feeding. If you become pregnant while using vaginal estrogen, call your doctor immediately.
- you should know that the manufacturer of one brand of estrogen vaginal cream states that use of the cream may weaken latex or rubber birth control devices such as condoms or diaphragms. These devices may not be effective if you use them during your treatment with estrogen vaginal cream. Talk to your doctor about methods of birth control that will work for you.

What special dietary instructions should I follow?

Talk to your doctor about eating grapefruit and drinking grapefruit juice while using this medicine.

What should I do if I forget to take a dose?

Apply or insert the missed dose as soon as you remember it. However, if it is almost time for the next dose, skip the missed dose and continue your regular dosing schedule. Do not use a double dose or apply extra cream to make up for a missed dose.

What side effects can this medicine cause?

Vaginal estrogen may cause side effects. Tell your doctor if any of these symptoms are severe or do not go away:
- breast pain or tenderness
- upset stomach
- heartburn
- vomiting
- dizziness
- nervousness
- depression
- irritability
- difficulty falling asleep or staying asleep
- changes in sexual desire
- hair loss
- unwanted hair growth
- spotty darkening of the skin on the face
- sudden feelings of heat or sweating
- difficulty wearing contact lenses
- leg cramps
- swelling, redness, burning, itching, or irritation of the vagina
- vaginal discharge
- painful or difficult urination
- back pain
- cold symptoms
- flu symptoms

Some side effects can be serious. If you experience any of these symptoms, call your doctor immediately:
- bulging eyes
- pain, swelling, or tenderness in the stomach
- loss of appetite
- weakness
- yellowing of the skin or eyes
- joint pain
- movements that are difficult to control
- rash or blisters
- hives
- itching
- swelling of the eyes, face, tongue, throat, hands, arms, feet, ankles, or lower legs
- hoarseness
- difficulty breathing or swallowing

Estrogen may increase your risk of developing cancer of the ovaries or gallbladder disease that may need to be treated with surgery. Talk to your doctor about the risks of using vaginal estrogen.

Estrogen may cause growth to slow or stop early in children who receive large doses for a long time. Vaginal estrogen may also affect the timing and speed of sexual development in children. Your child's doctor will monitor her carefully during her treatment with estrogen. Talk to your child's doctor about the risks of giving this medication to your child.

Vaginal estrogen may cause other side effects. Call your doctor if you have any unusual problems while taking this medication.

If you experience a serious side effect, you or your doctor may send a report to the Food and Drug Administration's (FDA) MedWatch Adverse Event Reporting program online [at http://www.fda.gov/MedWatch/index.html] or by phone [1-800-332-1088].

What storage conditions are needed for this medicine?

Keep this medication in the container it came in, tightly closed, and out of reach of children. Store it at room temperature and away from excess heat and moisture (not in the bathroom). Throw away any medication that is outdated or no longer needed. Talk to your pharmacist about the proper disposal of your medication.

What should I do in case of overdose?

If someone swallows vaginal estrogen, uses extra tablets or rings, or applies extra cream, call your local poison control center at 1-800-222-1222. If the victim has collapsed or is not breathing, call local emergency services at 911.

Symptoms of overdose may include:
- upset stomach
- vomiting
- vaginal bleeding

What other information should I know?

Keep all appointments with your doctor.

Before having any laboratory test, tell your doctor and the laboratory personnel that you are using vaginal estrogen.

Do not let anyone else use your medication. Ask your pharmacist any questions you have about refilling your prescription.

Please see the Estrogen monograph to find dosing information for this medication.

Eszopiclone

(es zoe′ pi clone)

Brand Name: Lunesta®

Why is this medicine prescribed?

Eszopiclone is used to treat insomnia (difficulty falling asleep or staying asleep). Eszopiclone is in a class of medications called hypnotics. It works by slowing activity in the brain.

How should this medicine be used?

Eszopiclone comes as a tablet to take by mouth. It is usually taken once a day at bedtime. Follow the directions on your prescription label carefully, and ask your doctor or pharmacist to explain any part you do not understand. Take eszopiclone exactly as directed. Do not take more or less of it or take it more often than prescribed by your doctor.

Do not take eszopiclone with or shortly after a heavy, high-fat meal. Eszopiclone may not work well if it is taken with high fat foods.

You will probably become very sleepy soon after you take eszopiclone and will remain sleepy for some time after you take the medication. Plan to go to bed right after you take eszopiclone, and to stay in bed for at least 8 hours. If you do not go to bed right after you take eszopiclone or if you get up too soon after taking eszopiclone, you may experience dizziness, lightheadedness, hallucinations (seeing things or hearing voices that do not exist), and problems with coordination and memory.

Swallow the tablets whole; do not split, chew, or crush them.

Your doctor may start you on a low dose of eszopiclone and gradually increase your dose. Your doctor may also decrease your dose if you are too drowsy during the daytime.

You should be sleeping well within 7 to 10 days after you start taking eszopiclone. Call you doctor if your sleep problems do not improve during this time or if they get worse at any time during your treatment.

Do not stop taking eszopiclone without talking to your doctor, especially if you have taken it for longer than 1-2 weeks. Your doctor will probably decrease your dose gradually. If you suddenly stop taking eszopiclone you may experience withdrawal symptoms such as anxiety, unusual dreams, stomach and muscle cramps, upset stomach, vomiting, sweating, shakiness, and, rarely, seizures.

After you stop taking eszopiclone, you may have more difficulty falling asleep and staying asleep than you did before you took the medication. These sleep problems are normal and usually get better without treatment after one or two nights.

Are there other uses for this medicine?

This medication may be prescribed for other uses; ask your doctor or pharmacist for more information.

What special precautions should I follow?

Before taking eszopiclone,

- tell your doctor and pharmacist if you are allergic to eszopiclone or any other medications.
- tell your doctor and pharmacist what prescription and nonprescription medications, vitamins, and nutritional supplements you are taking. Be sure to mention any of the following: amiodarone (Cordarone, Pacerone); antidepressants ('mood elevators'); antifungals such as fluconazole (Diflucan), itraconazole (Sporanox), and ketoconazole (Nizoral); antihistamines; carbamazepine (Tegretol); cimetidine (Tagamet); clarithromycin (Biaxin); cyclosporine (Neoral, Sandimmune); danazol (Danocrine); delavirdine (Rescriptor); dexamethasone (Decadron); diltiazem (Cardizem, Dilacor, Tiazac); ethosuximide (Zarontin); erythromycin (E.E.S., E-Mycin, Erythrocin); fluoxetine (Prozac, Sarafem); fluvoxamine (Luvox); HIV protease inhibitors such as indinavir (Crixivan) nelfinavir (Viracept), and ritonavir (Norvir); isoniazid (INH, Nydrazid); medications for anxiety, mental illness, or seizures; metronidazole (Flagyl); nefazodone; olanzapine (Zyprexa); oral contraceptives (birth control pills); phenobarbital (Luminal, Solfoton); phenytoin (Dilantin); rifabutin (Mycobutin); rifampin (Rifadin, Rimactane); sedatives; sleeping pills; tranquilizers; troglitazone (Rezulin); troleandomycin (TAO); verapamil (Calan, Covera, Isoptin, Verelan); and zafirlukast (Accolate). Your doctor may need to change the doses of your medications or monitor you carefully for side effects.
- tell your doctor what herbal products you are taking, especially St. John's wort.
- tell your doctor if you drink or have ever drunk large amounts of alcohol and if you use or have ever used street drugs or have overused prescription medications. Also tell your doctor if you have ever thought about killing yourself or tried to do so and if you have or have ever had any medical condition especially depression, mental illness, asthma, chronic obstructive pulmonary disease (COPD, a group of diseases that affect the lungs and airways), any other condition that affects your breathing, or liver disease.
- tell your doctor if you are pregnant, plan to become pregnant, or are breast-feeding. If you become pregnant while taking eszopiclone, call your doctor.
- if you are having surgery, including dental surgery, tell the doctor or dentist that you are taking eszopiclone.
- you should know that eszopiclone may make you drowsy during the daytime. Do not drive a car or operate machinery until you know how this medication affects you.
- do not drink alcoholic beverages while you are taking eszopiclone. Alcohol can make the side effects from eszopiclone worse.
- you should know that your mental health may change in unexpected ways while you are taking this medica-

tion. These changes may be caused by eszopiclone or if they may be caused by physical or mental illnesses that you already have or that you develop during your treatment. Tell your doctor right away if you experience any of the following symptoms: aggressiveness, strange or unusually outgoing behavior, hallucinations (seeing things or hearing voices that do not exist), feeling as if you are outside of your body, memory problems, new or worsening depression, thinking about killing yourself, confusion, and any other changes in your usual thoughts or behavior. Be sure that your family knows which symptoms may be serious so that they can call the doctor if you are unable to seek treatment on your own.

What special dietary instructions should I follow?

Talk to your doctor about drinking grapefruit juice while taking this medication

What should I do if I forget to take a dose?

Eszopiclone should only be taken at bedtime. If you did not take eszopiclone before you went to bed and you are unable to fall asleep, you may take eszopiclone if you will be able to stay in bed for at least 8 hours afterward. Do not take eszopiclone if you are not ready to go to sleep right away and stay asleep for at least 8 hours. Do not take a double dose of eszopiclone to make up for a missed dose.

What side effects can this medicine cause?

Eszopiclone may cause side effects. Tell your doctor if any of these symptoms are severe or do not go away:

- unpleasant taste
- headache
- cold-like symptoms
- pain
- daytime drowsiness
- lightheadedness
- dizziness
- loss of coordination
- upset stomach
- vomiting
- heartburn
- unusual dreams
- decreased sexual desire
- painful menstruation (periods)
- breast enlargement in males

Some side effects can be serious. The following symptoms are uncommon, but if you experience any of them, call your doctor immediately:

- rash
- itching
- chest pain
- swelling of the hands, feet, ankles, or lower legs
- painful or frequent urination

- bloody or cloudy urine
- back pain

Eszopiclone may cause other side effects. Call your doctor if you have any unusual problems while taking this medication.

If you experience a serious side effect, you or your doctor may send a report to the Food and Drug Administration's (FDA) MedWatch Adverse Event Reporting program online [at http://www.fda.gov/MedWatch/index.html] or by phone [1-800-332-1088].

What storage conditions are needed for this medicine?

Keep this medication in the container it came in, tightly closed, and out of reach of children. Store it at room temperature and away from excess heat and moisture (not in the bathroom). Throw away any medication that is outdated or no longer needed. Talk to your pharmacist about the proper disposal of your medication.

What should I do in case of overdose?

In case of overdose, call your local poison control center at 1-800-222-1222. If the victim has collapsed or is not breathing, call local emergency services at 911.

Symptoms of overdose may include:

- drowsiness
- loss of consciousness
- coma

What other information should I know?

Keep all appointments with your doctor.

Do not let anyone else take your medication. Ask your pharmacist any questions you have about refilling your prescription.

Dosage Facts
For Informational Purposes

Caution: Do not change your dose, how often you take your medication, or the length of time you are to take it without first talking to your healthcare provider.

The following dosage information was written using medical language for doctors and other healthcare professionals and is provided here for you to check your dosage. The dosage of this drug may differ for different patients. Therefore, always follow your doctor's instructions or the directions on the label. Contact your healthcare provider or pharmacist if you have any questions about the specific dosage of your medication after reviewing this information.

General Dosage Information

Individualize dosage; use smallest effective dosage to minimize adverse effects.

If used concomitantly with a potent CYP3A4 inhibitor, adjustment of eszopiclone dosage is recommended.

Adult Patients

Insomnia

ORAL:

- Adults <65 years of age: Initially, 2 mg. May consider an initial dosage of 3 mg or an increase in dosage to 3 mg if clinically indicated; 3-mg dosage is more effective than 2-mg dosage for sleep maintenance.

Special Populations

Hepatic Impairment

- In patients with severe hepatic impairment, 1 mg initially; doses >2 mg not recommended.
- No dosage adjustment required in patients with mild to moderate hepatic impairment.

Renal Impairment

- No dosage adjustment required.

Geriatric Patients

- In adults ≥65 years of age experiencing difficulty falling asleep, 1 mg initially. May increase dosage to 2 mg if clinically indicated.
- In adults ≥65 years of age experiencing difficulty staying asleep, 2 mg.
- Do not exceed 2 mg daily in adults ≥65 years of age.

Debilitated Patients

- Do not exceed 1 mg.

Etanercept Injection

(et a ner' set)

Brand Name: Enbrel®

Why is this medicine prescribed?

Etanercept is used alone or in combination with other medications to reduce the pain and swelling associated with rheumatoid arthritis, juvenile rheumatoid arthritis, and psoriatic arthritis. Etanercept is in a class of medications called tumor-necrosis factor (TNF) inhibitors. It works by blocking the activity of TNF, a substance in the body that causes swelling and joint damage in arthritis.

How should this medicine be used?

Etanercept comes as a solution to inject subcutaneously (under the skin). It is usually injected twice a week. Follow the directions on your prescription label carefully, and ask your doctor or pharmacist to explain any part you do not understand. Use etanercept exactly as directed. Do not use more or less of it or use it more often than prescribed by your doctor.

You can inject etanercept in the thigh, stomach, or upper arm. To reduce the chances of soreness or redness, use a different site for each injection. The new injection should be given at least 1 inch away from the previous injection. Do not inject into an area where the skin is tender, bruised, red, or hard.

Dispose of used needles and syringes in a puncture-resistant container. Talk to your doctor or pharmacist about how to dispose of the puncture-resistant container.

Before you use etanercept for the first time, read the manufacturer's information for the patient that comes with it. Ask your doctor or pharmacist to show you how to inject etanercept.

Before preparing an etanercept dose, wash your hands with soap and water. To prepare the area of the skin where you will inject etanercept, wipe it with an alcohol swab.

To prepare and inject etanercept, follow these steps:

1. Remove the pink plastic cap from the etanercept vial. Do not remove the gray stopper or silver metal ring.
2. Clean the gray stopper on the vial with an alcohol swab. Place the vial on a flat surface. Do not touch the stopper.
3. Slide the plunger into the syringe and turn it clockwise until it becomes more difficult to turn.
4. Pull the needle cover straight off the syringe. Do not touch the needle or allow it to touch anything, and do not push the plunger.
5. Insert the needle straight down through the center ring of the gray stopper of the etanercept vial. You will hear a pop as the needle goes through the stopper. You should see the needle tip in the stopper window.
6. Push the plunger down very slowly until all the liquid from the syringe is in the vial. Leave the syringe in place, and gently swirl the vial between your fingers in a circular motion to dissolve the powder. Do not shake.
7. The powder should dissolve in less than 10 minutes. The solution should be clear and colorless. There may be some bubbles in the solution. Do not inject the solution if it contains lumps, flakes, or particles.
8. To withdraw the solution from the vial, turn the vial upside down and hold it at eye level. Slowly pull the plunger down to the marking on the side of the syringe that corresponds to the correct dose. Make sure to keep the tip of the needle in the solution.
9. With the needle still inserted in the vial, check for air bubbles in the syringe. Gently tap the syringe to make any air bubbles rise to the top of the syringe. Then slowly push the plunger up to remove the air bubbles. If any solution is pushed back into the vial, slowly pull back on the plunger to draw the solution back into the syringe.
10. Remove the syringe and needle from the vial. Be careful not to touch the needle or touch it to any surface.
11. Gently pinch the cleaned area of skin with one hand and hold it firmly. With the other hand, hold the syringe like a pencil at a 45 degree angle to the skin.
12. Push the needle into the skin, and let go of the skin with the other hand.
13. Use the other hand to slowly push the plunger down to inject etanercept.

14. When the syringe is empty, pull the needle out of the skin, being careful to keep it at the same angle as when it was inserted.

If it is hard for you to prepare a dose because of arthritis of the hand, you may use another method to prepare etanercept. Speak to your health care provider and refer to the manufacturer's information.

Some children may use one vial of etanercept solution for more than one dose. Do not mix the contents of one etanercept vial with the contents of another vial. Ask your health care provider for directions on how to prepare a dose from a vial that was already used.

Are there other uses for this medicine?

Etanercept is also used sometimes to treat psoriasis and ankylosing spondylitis. Talk to your doctor about the possible risks of using this medication for your condition.

This medication may be prescribed for other uses; ask your doctor or pharmacist for more information.

What special precautions should I follow?

Before taking etanercept,

- tell your doctor and pharmacist if you are allergic to etanercept, latex, or any other medications.
- tell your doctor and pharmacist what prescription and nonprescription medications, vitamins, nutritional supplements, and herbal products you are taking. Be sure to mention any of the following: medications that suppress the immune system such as azathioprine (Imuran), cyclosporine (Neoral, Sandimmune), methotrexate (Rheumatrex), sirolimus (Rapamune), and tacrolimus (Prograf). Your doctor may need to change the doses of your medications or monitor you carefully for side effects.
- tell your doctor if you have an infection anywhere in the body and if you have or have ever had seizures, multiple sclerosis, inflammation of the optic nerve (optic neuritis), blood abnormalities, human immunodeficiency virus (HIV) or acquired immunodeficiency syndrome (AIDS), diabetes, or heart failure.
- tell your doctor if you are pregnant, plan to become pregnant, or are breast-feeding. If you become pregnant while taking etanercept, call your doctor.
- if you are having surgery, including dental surgery, tell the doctor or dentist that you are taking etanercept.
- do not have any vaccinations (e.g., measles or flu shots) without talking to your doctor.
- if you are exposed to chickenpox while taking etanercept, call your doctor immediately.

What special dietary instructions should I follow?

Unless your doctor tells you otherwise, continue your normal diet.

What should I do if I forget to take a dose?

Take the missed dose as soon as you remember it. However, if it is almost time for the next dose, skip the missed dose and continue your regular dosing schedule. Do not take a double dose to make up for a missed one.

What side effects can this medicine cause?

Etanercept may cause side effects. Tell your doctor if any of these symptoms are severe or do not go away:

- redness, itching, pain, or swelling at the site of injection
- bleeding or bruising at the site of injection
- runny nose
- sneezing
- headache
- dizziness
- upset stomach
- vomiting
- stomach pain
- weakness
- cough

Some side effects can be serious. The following symptoms are uncommon, but if you experience any of them, call your doctor immediately:

- fever, sore throat, chills, and other signs of infection
- coughing, wheezing, or chest pain
- hot, red, swollen area on the skin
- seizures
- bruising
- bleeding
- pale skin
- hives
- itching
- difficulty breathing or swallowing
- severe rash

Etanercept may cause other side effects. Call your doctor if you have any unusual problems while taking this medication.

If you experience a serious side effect, you or your doctor may send a report to the Food and Drug Administration's (FDA) MedWatch Adverse Event Reporting program online [at http://www.fda.gov/MedWatch/index.html] or by phone [1-800-332-1088].

What storage conditions are needed for this medicine?

Keep this medication in the container it came in, tightly closed, and out of reach of children. Store the tray containing etanercept powder in the refrigerator. Do not freeze. Once water is added to the powder, the solution may be stored in the refrigerator for up to 14 days. Throw away any medication that is outdated or no longer needed. Talk to your pharmacist about the proper disposal of your medication.

What should I do in case of overdose?

In case of overdose, call your local poison control center at 1-800-222-1222. If the victim has collapsed or is not breathing, call local emergency services at 911.

What other information should I know?

Keep all appointments with your doctor and the laboratory. Your doctor may order certain lab tests to check your body's response to etanercept.

Do not let anyone else take your medication. Ask your pharmacist any questions you have about refilling your prescription.

Dosage Facts
For Informational Purposes

Caution: Do not change your dose, how often you take your medication, or the length of time you are to take it without first talking to your healthcare provider.

The following dosage information was written using medical language for doctors and other healthcare professionals and is provided here for you to check your dosage. The dosage of this drug may differ for different patients. Therefore, always follow your doctor's instructions or the directions on the label. Contact your healthcare provider or pharmacist if you have any questions about the specific dosage of your medication after reviewing this information.

Pediatric Patients

Juvenile Arthritis

SUB-Q:
- Children 4–17 years of age: 0.8 mg/kg per week (up to a dosage of 50 mg per week).

Adult Patients

Rheumatoid Arthritis

SUB-Q:
- 50 mg weekly.

Psoriatic Arthritis

SUB-Q:
- 50 mg weekly.

Ankylosing Spondylitis

SUB-Q:
- 50 mg weekly.

Psoriasis

SUB-Q:
- Initially, 50 mg twice weekly for 3 months. Initial dosages of 25 mg once or twice weekly also have been effective; proportion of responders related to etanercept dosage.
- Maintenance dosage: 50 mg weekly.

Prescribing Limits

Pediatric Patients

Juvenile Arthritis

SUB-Q:
- Maximum 50 mg weekly.

Adult Patients

Rheumatoid Arthritis

SUB-Q:
- Maximum 50 mg weekly.

Psoriatic Arthritis

SUB-Q:
- Maximum 50 mg weekly.

Ankylosing Spondylitis

SUB-Q:
- Maximum 50 mg weekly.

Special Populations

Renal Impairment
- Limited data indicate that dosage adjustment is not necessary in patients with renal failure.

Ethacrynic Acid

(eth a krin' ik)

Brand Name: Edecrin®

Why is this medicine prescribed?

Ethacrynic acid, a 'water pill,' is used to treat high blood pressure and fluid retention caused by various medical problems. It causes the kidneys to get rid of unneeded water and salt from the body into the urine.

This medicine is sometimes prescribed for other uses; ask your doctor or pharmacist for more information.

How should this medicine be used?

Ethacrynic acid comes as a tablet to take by mouth. It usually is taken once or twice a day with food. If you take ethacrynic acid once a day, take it with breakfast in the morning. If you take it twice a day, take it in the morning and in the afternoon to avoid going to the bathroom during the night. Follow the directions on your prescription label carefully, and ask your doctor or pharmacist to explain any part you do not understand. Take ethacrynic acid exactly as directed. Do not take more or less of it or take it more often than prescribed by your doctor.

Ethacrynic acid controls high blood pressure but does not cure it. Continue to take ethacrynic acid even if you feel well. Do not stop taking ethacrynic acid without talking to your doctor.

Are there other uses for this medicine?

Ethacrynic acid is also used to treat high blood pressure and a certain type of diabetes insipidus that does not respond to other medicines. Talk to your doctor about the possible risks of using this medicine for your condition.

What special precautions should I follow?

Before taking ethacrynic acid,
- tell your doctor and pharmacist if you are allergic to ethacrynic acid or any other drugs.
- tell your doctor and pharmacist what prescription and nonprescription medications you are taking, especially other blood pressure medications, anticoagulants ('blood thinners') such as warfarin (Coumadin), corticosteroids (e.g., prednisone), digoxin (Lanoxin), heart medications, lithium (Eskalith, Lithobid), medications for diabetes, probenecid (Benemid), and vitamins.
- tell your doctor if you have or have ever had diabetes, gout, or liver disease.
- tell your doctor if you are pregnant, plan to become pregnant, or are breast-feeding. If you are pregnant or breast-feeding, do not take ethacrynic acid. If you become pregnant while taking ethacrynic acid, call your doctor immediately.
- if you are having surgery, including dental surgery, tell the doctor or dentist that you are taking ethacrynic acid.
- you should know that this drug may make you drowsy. Do not drive a car or operate machinery until you know how this drug affects you.
- remember that alcohol can add to the drowsiness caused by this drug.

What special dietary instructions should I follow?

Follow your doctor's directions. They may include a daily exercise program, a low-salt or low-sodium diet, potassium supplements, and increased amounts of potassium-rich foods (e.g., bananas, prunes, raisins, and orange juice) in your diet.

What should I do if I forget to take a dose?

Take the missed dose as soon as you remember it. However, if it is almost time for your next dose, skip the missed dose and continue your regular dosing schedule. Do not take a double dose to make up for a missed one.

What side effects can this medicine cause?

Frequent urination should go away after you take ethacrynic acid for a few weeks. Tell your doctor if any of these symptoms are severe or do not go away:
- upset stomach
- vomiting
- loss of appetite
- stomach pain
- thirst
- muscle cramps

- weakness
- headache
- diarrhea

If you experience any of the following symptoms, call your doctor immediately:

- loss of hearing
- confusion
- loss of balance
- ringing or fullness in the ears
- chills
- confusion
- sore throat
- unusual bleeding or bruising
- rash
- difficulty breathing or swallowing

If you experience a serious side effect, you or your doctor may send a report to the Food and Drug Administration's (FDA) MedWatch Adverse Event Reporting program online [at http://www.fda.gov/MedWatch/index.html] or by phone [1-800-332-1088].

What storage conditions are needed for this medicine?

Keep this medicine in the container it came in, tightly closed, and out of reach of children. Store it at room temperature and away from excess heat and moisture (not in the bathroom). Throw away any medicine that is outdated or no longer needed. Talk to your pharmacist about the proper disposal of your medicine.

What should I do in case of overdose?

In case of overdose, call your local poison control center at 1-800-222-1222. If the victim has collapsed or is not breathing, call local emergency services at 911.

What other information should I know?

Keep all appointments with your doctor and the laboratory. Your blood pressure should be checked regularly, and blood tests should be done occasionally.

Do not let anyone else take your medicine. Ask your pharmacist any questions you have about refilling your prescription.

Talk to your doctor, pharmacist, or other healthcare professional if you have questions about dosing information for your medication.

Ethambutol

(e tham′ byoo tole)

Brand Name: Myambutol®

Why is this medicine prescribed?

Ethambutol eliminates certain bacteria that cause tuberculosis (TB). It is used with other medicines to treat tuberculosis and to prevent you from giving the infection to others.

This medication is sometimes prescribed for other uses; ask your doctor or pharmacist for more information.

How should this medicine be used?

Ethambutol comes as a tablet to take by mouth. It usually is taken once a day in the morning. Follow the directions on your prescription label carefully, and ask your doctor or pharmacist to explain any part you do not understand. Take ethambutol exactly as directed. Do not take more or less of it or take it more often than prescribed by your doctor.

What special precautions should I follow?

Before taking ethambutol,

- tell your doctor and pharmacist if you are allergic to ethambutol or any other drugs.
- tell your doctor and pharmacist what prescription and nonprescription medications you are taking, especially antacids and vitamins. Antacids interfere with ethambutol, making it less effective. Take ethambutol 1 hour before or 2 hours after antacids.
- tell your doctor if you have or have ever had kidney disease, gout, or eye disorders such as cataracts.
- tell your doctor if you are pregnant, plan to become pregnant, or are breast-feeding. If you become pregnant while taking ethambutol, call your doctor.

What special dietary instructions should I follow?

Ethambutol may cause upset stomach. Take ethambutol with food.

What should I do if I forget to take a dose?

Take the missed dose as soon as you remember it. However, if it is almost time for the next dose, skip the missed dose and continue your regular dosing schedule. Do not take a double dose to make up for a missed one.

What side effects can this medicine cause?

Ethambutol may cause side effects. Tell your doctor if any of these symptoms are severe or do not go away:

- loss of appetite
- upset stomach
- vomiting
- numbness and tingling in the hands or feet

If you experience any of the following symptoms, call your doctor immediately:

- blurred vision
- inability to see the colors red and green
- sudden changes in vision
- skin rash
- itching

If you experience a serious side effect, you or your doctor may send a report to the Food and Drug Administration's (FDA) MedWatch Adverse Event Reporting program online [at http://www.fda.gov/MedWatch/index.html] or by phone [1-800-332-1088].

What storage conditions are needed for this medicine?

Keep this medication in the container it came in, tightly closed, and out of reach of children. Store it at room temperature and away from excess heat and moisture (not in the bathroom). Throw away any medication that is outdated or no longer needed. Talk to your pharmacist about the proper disposal of your medication.

What should I do in case of overdose?

In case of overdose, call your local poison control center at 1-800-222-1222. If the victim has collapsed or is not breathing, call local emergency services at 911.

What other information should I know?

Keep all appointments with your doctor and the laboratory. Your doctor will want to check your response to ethambutol. Blood, kidney, and liver tests may be done also. While you are taking ethambutol, your doctor will want to examine your eyes at least every 3-6 months.

Do not let anyone else take your medication. Ask your pharmacist any questions you have about refilling your prescription.

Talk to your doctor, pharmacist, or other healthcare professional if you have questions about dosing information for your medication.

Ethosuximide Oral

(eth oh sux' i mide)

Brand Name: Zarontin®, Zarontin® Syrup

Why is this medicine prescribed?

Ethosuximide is used to treat a type of seizure called absence (petit mal). Ethosuximide acts on the brain and nervous system in the treatment of epilepsy.

This medication is sometimes prescribed for other uses; ask your doctor or pharmacist for more information.

How should this medicine be used?

Ethosuximide comes as a capsule and liquid to take by mouth. It is taken one, two, or three times a day. Follow the directions on your prescription label carefully, and ask your doctor or pharmacist to explain any part you do not understand. Take ethosuximide exactly as directed. Do not take more or less of it or take it more often than prescribed by your doctor.

Continue to take ethosuximide even if you feel well. Do not stop taking ethosuximide without talking to your doctor, especially if you have taken large doses for a long time. Abruptly stopping the drug can cause seizures. Your doctor probably will decrease your dose gradually.

What special precautions should I follow?

Before taking ethosuximide,

- tell your doctor and pharmacist if you are allergic to ethosuximide or any other drugs.
- tell your doctor and pharmacist what prescription and nonprescription medications you are taking, especially other seizure medications, doxycycline (Vibramycin), Isoniazid (INH), medications for colds or allergies such as chlorpheniramine (Chlor-Trimeton), medications for depression such as amitriptyline (Elavil), oral contraceptives, and vitamins. Ethosuximide affects the action of other medications, and many medications can affect the action of ethosuximide. Tell your doctor and pharmacist everything you are taking.
- tell your doctor if you have or have ever had kidney or liver disease or a blood disorder.
- tell your doctor if you are pregnant, plan to become pregnant, or are breast-feeding. If you become pregnant while taking ethosuximide, call your doctor.
- if you are having surgery, including dental surgery, tell the doctor or dentist that you are taking ethosuximide.
- you should know that this drug may make you drowsy. Do not drive a car or operate machinery until you know how this drug affects you.
- remember that alcohol can add to the drowsiness caused by this drug.
- plan to protect your eyes in the sun. Ethosuximide may make your eyes more sensitive to light. Wear dark glasses in bright light.

What special dietary instructions should I follow?

Ethosuximide may cause an upset stomach. Take ethosuximide with food. Drink plenty of water.

What should I do if I forget to take a dose?

Take the missed dose as soon as you remember it. However, if it is within 4 hours of the next dose, skip the missed dose and continue your regular dosing schedule. Do not take a double dose to make up for a missed one.

What side effects can this medicine cause?

Ethosuximide may cause side effects. Tell your doctor if any of these symptoms are severe or do not go away:

- drowsiness
- upset stomach
- vomiting
- constipation
- diarrhea
- stomach pain
- loss of taste and appetite
- weight loss
- irritability
- mental confusion
- depression
- insomnia
- nervousness
- headache

If you experience any of the following symptoms, call your doctor immediately:

- difficulty coordinating movements
- joint pain
- red, itchy skin rash
- easy bruising
- tiny purple-colored skin spots
- bloody nose
- unusual bleeding
- yellowing of the skin or eyes
- dark urine
- fever
- sore throat

If you experience a serious side effect, you or your doctor may send a report to the Food and Drug Administration's (FDA) MedWatch Adverse Event Reporting program online [at http://www.fda.gov/MedWatch/index.html] or by phone [1-800-332-1088].

What storage conditions are needed for this medicine?

Keep this medication in the container it came in, tightly closed, and out of reach of children. Store it at room temperature, away from light, excess heat, and moisture (not in the bathroom). Throw away any medication that is outdated or no longer needed. Talk to your pharmacist about the proper disposal of your medication.

What should I do in case of overdose?

In case of overdose, call your local poison control center at 1-800-222-1222. If the victim has collapsed or is not breathing, call local emergency services at 911.

What other information should I know?

Keep all appointments with your doctor and the laboratory. Your doctor will order certain lab tests to check your response to ethosuximide.

Call your doctor if you continue to have seizures or convulsions while taking this medication.

If you give this drug to a child, observe and keep a record of the child's moods, behavior, attention span, hand-eye coordination, and ability to solve problems and perform tasks requiring thought. Ask the child's teacher to keep a similar record. This information can help the child's doctor determine whether to continue the drug or to change the dose or drug.

Wear identification (Medic Alert) indicating medication use and epilepsy.

Do not let anyone else take your medication. Ask your pharmacist any questions you have about refilling your prescription.

Talk to your doctor, pharmacist, or other healthcare professional if you have questions about dosing information for your medication.

Etidronate

(e ti droe′ nate)

Brand Name: Didronel®

Why is this medicine prescribed?

Etidronate is used to treat Paget's disease of bone (a condition in which the bones are soft and weak and may be deformed, painful, or easily broken) and to prevent and treat heterotopic ossification (growth of bone tissue in an area of the body other than the skeleton) in people who have had total hip replacement surgery (surgery to replace the hip joint with an artificial joint) or in people who have had an injury to the spinal cord. Etidronate is in a class of medications called bisphosphonates. It works by slowing the breakdown of old bone and the formation of new bone.

How should this medicine be used?

Etidronate comes as a tablet to take by mouth. It is usually taken once or twice a day on an empty stomach. To help you remember to take etidronate, take it at around the same time(s) every day. Follow the directions on your prescription label carefully, and ask your doctor or pharmacist to explain any part you do not understand. Take etidronate exactly as directed. Do not take more or less of it or take it more often or for a longer period of time than prescribed by your doctor.

You may swallow etidronate tablets with water or plain fruit juice. Do not swallow the tablets with milk, calcium fortified juice, or other drinks that contain calcium.

Do not eat for 2 hours before and 2 hours after you take etidronate. It is especially important not to eat or drink foods or drinks that are high in calcium such as milk for 2 hours before and after you take etidronate.

If you are taking etidronate to treat Paget's disease of bone, it may take some time for your condition to improve. You may experience new or worsening bone pain, especially at the beginning of your treatment. Tell your doctor about any new or worsening symptoms you experience, but do not stop taking etidronate without talking to your doctor.

Are there other uses for this medicine?

Etidronate is also used sometimes to treat and prevent osteoporosis caused by corticosteroids (a type of medication that may cause osteoporosis) treatment. Talk to your doctor about the possible risks of using this medication for your condition.

This medication may be prescribed for other uses; ask your doctor or pharmacist for more information.

What special precautions should I follow?

Before taking etidronate,

- tell your doctor and pharmacist if you are allergic to etidronate or any other medications.
- tell your doctor and pharmacist what prescription and nonprescription medications, vitamins, nutritional supplements, and herbal products you are taking or plan to take. Be sure to mention anticoagulants ('blood thinners') such as warfarin (Coumadin); cancer chemotherapy; and oral steroids such as dexamethasone (Decadron, Dexone), methylprednisolone (Medrol), and prednisone (Deltasone). Your doctor may need to change the doses of your medications or monitor you carefully for side effects.
- if you are taking vitamin and mineral supplements such as iron, or if you are taking antacids containing calcium, magnesium, or aluminum (Maalox, Mylanta, Tums, others), take them 2 hours before or 2 hours after you take etidronate.
- tell your doctor if you have or have ever had osteomalacia (softening of bones due to a lack of minerals). Your doctor may tell you not to take etidronate.
- tell your doctor if you have or have ever had anemia (condition in which the red blood cells so not bring enough oxygen to all the parts of the body); difficulty swallowing, heartburn, ulcers, or other stomach problems; cancer; enterocolitis (swelling in the intestines), any type of infection, especially in your mouth; problems with your mouth, teeth, or gums; any condition that stops your blood from clotting normally; dental or kidney disease. Tell the doctor who prescribed etidronate if you break a bone at any time during your treatment.
- tell your doctor if you are pregnant, plan to become pregnant, or are breast-feeding. Also tell your doctor if you plan to become pregnant at any time in the future because etidronate may remain in your body for years after you stop taking it. Call your doctor if you become pregnant during or after your treatment with etidronate.
- you should know that etidronate may cause serious problems with your jaw, especially if you have dental surgery or treatment while you are taking the medication. A dentist should examine your teeth and perform any needed treatments before you start to take etidron-

ate. Be sure to brush your teeth and clean your mouth properly while you are taking etidronate. Talk to your doctor before having any dental treatments while you are taking this medication.

What special dietary instructions should I follow?

It is important you get enough calcium and vitamin D and eat a balanced diet while you are taking etidronate. Your doctor will tell you which foods are good sources of these nutrients and how many servings you need each day. If you find it difficult to eat enough of these foods, tell your doctor. In that case, your doctor may prescribe or recommend a supplement.

What should I do if I forget to take a dose?

If you have not already eaten, take the missed dose as soon as you remember it. If you have already eaten, take the missed dose 2 hours after you last ate. However, if it is almost time for the next dose, skip the missed dose and continue your regular dosing schedule. Do not take a double dose to make up for a missed one.

What side effects can this medicine cause?

Etidronate may cause side effects. Tell your doctor if any of these symptoms are severe or do not go away:

- nausea
- diarrhea
- bone, joint, and/or muscle pain

Some side effects can be serious. If you experience any of the following symptoms, call your doctor immediately:

- swelling of the face, throat, tongue, lips, eyes, hands, feet, ankles, or lower legs
- hoarseness
- difficulty swallowing or breathing
- blisters on the skin
- fever

Etidronate may cause other side effects. Call your doctor if you have any unusual problems while taking this medication.

What storage conditions are needed for this medicine?

Keep this medication in the container it came in, tightly closed, and out of reach of children. Store it at room temperature and away from excess heat and moisture (not in the bathroom). Throw away any medication that is outdated or no longer needed. Talk to your pharmacist about the proper disposal of your medication.

What should I do in case of overdose?

In case of overdose, call your local poison control center at 1-800-222-1222. If the victim has collapsed or is not breathing, call local emergency services at 911.

Symptoms of overdose may include:
- vomiting
- stomach cramps
- diarrhea
- pain, burning, numbness, or tingling in the hands or feet
- muscle spasms and cramps

What other information should I know?

Keep all appointments with your doctor and the laboratory. Your doctor may order certain lab tests to check your body's response to etidronate.

Do not let anyone else take your medication. Ask your pharmacist any questions you have about refilling your prescription.

Dosage Facts
For Informational Purposes

Caution: Do not change your dose, how often you take your medication, or the length of time you are to take it without first talking to your healthcare provider.

The following dosage information was written using medical language for doctors and other healthcare professionals and is provided here for you to check your dosage. The dosage of this drug may differ for different patients. Therefore, always follow your doctor's instructions or the directions on the label. Contact your healthcare provider or pharmacist if you have any questions about the specific dosage of your medication after reviewing this information.

General Dosage Information

Available as etidronate disodium; dosage expressed in terms of the salt.

Adult Patients

Paget's Disease of Bone

ORAL:
- Initially, 5–10 mg/kg daily for ≤6 months, or 11–20 mg/kg daily for ≤3 months, have been used. Recommended initial dosage is 5 mg/kg daily for ≤6 months.
- Onset of therapeutic response may be delayed, and therapeutic effects may persist for months following a course of therapy. Avoid premature increases in dosage since increased dosage may cause mineralization defects.
- Patients who require immediate suppression of Paget's disease or in whom lower dosages are ineffective: >10 mg/kg daily for ≤3 months. Use with caution.
- Dosages >20 mg/kg daily not recommended.
- Retreatment: Dosage usually the same as initial treatment. Consider increasing dosage within the recommended range if inadequate response with original dosage.

Heterotopic Ossification
Prevention and Treatment

ORAL:
- Spinal cord injury: Initially, 20 mg/kg daily for 2 weeks followed by 10 mg/kg daily for an additional 10 weeks (12 weeks total).
- Total hip arthroplasty: Initially, 20 mg/kg daily administered preoperatively for 1 month and postoperatively for an additional 3 months (4 months total).

Corticosteroid-Induced Osteoporosis†
Prevention and Treatment

ORAL:
- 400 mg daily for 2 weeks every 3 months has been used, usually in conjunction with calcium (e.g., 500 mg daily) and vitamin D supplementation during the remaining 10–11 weeks of each cycle or continuously.
- Administer for as long as corticosteroid therapy continues.

Postmenopausal Osteoporosis†
Treatment

ORAL:
- 400 mg daily for 14 days every 3 months has been used, in conjunction with calcium supplementation during the last 10 weeks of each cycle.

Prescribing Limits

Adult Patients

Paget's Disease of Bone

ORAL:
- Maximum 20 mg/kg daily.
- Treatment duration: ≤6 months; continuous therapy for >6 months may increase the risk of fracture and osteomalacia.

Special Populations

Renal Impairment
- Reduce dosage in patients with reduced glomerular filtration; monitor such patients closely.

Geriatric Patients
- Select dosage with caution because of age-related decreases in hepatic, renal, and/or cardiac function and concomitant disease and drug therapy.

† Use is not currently included in the labeling approved by the US Food and Drug Administration.

Etodolac

(ee toe doe' lak)

Brand Name: Lodine®, Lodine® XL

Important Warning

People who take nonsteroidal anti-inflammatory medications (NSAIDs) (other than aspirin) such as etodolac may have a higher risk of having a heart attack or a stroke than people who do not take these medications. These events may happen without warning and may cause death. This risk may be higher for people who take NSAIDs for a long time. Tell your doctor if you or anyone in your family has or has ever had heart disease, a heart attack, or a stroke, if you smoke, and if you have or have ever had high cholesterol, high blood pressure, or diabetes. Get emergency medical help right away if you experience any of the following symptoms: chest pain, shortness of breath, weakness in one part or side of the body, or slurred speech.

If you will be undergoing a coronary artery bypass graft (CABG; a type of heart surgery), you should not take etodolac right before or right after the surgery.

NSAIDs such as etodolac may cause ulcers, bleeding, or holes in the stomach or intestine. These problems may develop at any time during treatment, may happen without warning symptoms, and may cause death. The risk may be higher for people who take NSAIDs for a long time, are older in age, have poor health, or drink large amounts of alcohol while you are taking etodolac. Tell your doctor if you take any of the following medications: anticoagulants ('blood thinners') such as warfarin (Coumadin); aspirin; other NSAIDs such as ibuprofen (Advil, Motrin) and naproxen (Aleve, Naprosyn); or oral steroids such as dexamethasone (Decadron, Dexone), methylprednisolone (Medrol), and prednisone (Deltasone). Also tell your doctor if you have or have ever had ulcers or bleeding in your stomach or intestines or other bleeding disorders. If you experience any of the following symptoms, stop taking etodolac and call your doctor: stomach pain, heartburn, vomiting a substance that is bloody or looks like coffee grounds, blood in the stool, or black and tarry stools.

Keep all appointments with your doctor and the laboratory. Your doctor will monitor your symptoms carefully and will probably order certain tests to check your body's response to etodolac. Be sure to tell your doctor how you are feeling so that your doctor can prescribe the right amount of medication to treat your condition with the lowest risk of serious side effects.

Your doctor or pharmacist will give you the manufacturer's patient information sheet (Medication Guide) when you begin treatment with etodolac and each time you refill your prescription. Read the information carefully and ask your doctor or pharmacist if you have any questions. You can also visit the Food and Drug Administration (FDA) website (http://www.fda.gov/cder) or the manufacturer's website to obtain the Medication Guide.

Why is this medicine prescribed?

Etodolac tablets, capsules, and extended-release (long-acting) tablets are used to relieve pain, tenderness, swelling, and stiffness caused by osteoarthritis (arthritis caused by a breakdown of the lining of the joints) and rheumatoid arthritis (arthritis caused by swelling of the lining of the joints). Etodolac tablets and capsules are also used to relieve pain from other causes. Etodolac is in a class of medications called NSAIDs. It works by stopping the body's production of a substance that causes pain, fever, and inflammation.

How should this medicine be used?

Etodolac comes as a tablet, a capsule, and an extended-release tablet to take by mouth. To treat arthritis, the tablet and capsule are usually taken two to three times a day and the extended-release tablet is usually taken once a day. To relieve pain from other causes, the tablets and capsules are usually taken every 6 to 8 hours. Take etodolac at around the same time(s) every day. Follow the directions on your prescription label carefully, and ask your doctor or pharmacist to explain any part you do not understand. Take etodolac exactly as directed. Do not take more or less of it or take it more often than prescribed by your doctor.

Swallow the extended-release tablets whole; do not split, chew, or crush them.

If you are taking etodolac for arthritis, your doctor may start you on a high dose and decrease your dose once your symptoms are controlled. It may take 1-2 weeks for you to feel the full benefit of this medication.

Are there other uses for this medicine?

This medication may be prescribed for other uses; ask your doctor or pharmacist for more information.

What special precautions should I follow?

Before taking etodolac,
- tell your doctor and pharmacist if you are allergic to etodolac, aspirin or other NSAIDs such as ibuprofen (Advil, Motrin) and naproxen (Aleve, Naprosyn), any other medications, or any of the inactive ingredients in etodolac tablets, capsules, or extended-release tablets. Ask your pharmacist for a list of inactive ingredients.
- tell your doctor and pharmacist what prescription and

nonprescription medications, vitamins, nutritional supplements, and herbal products you are taking or plan to take. Be sure to mention the medications listed in the IMPORTANT WARNING section and any of the following: angiotensin-converting enzyme (ACE) inhibitors such as benazepril (Lotensin), captopril (Capoten), enalapril (Vasotec), fosinopril (Monopril), lisinopril (Prinivil, Zestril), moexipril (Univasc), perindopril (Aceon), quinapril (Accupril), ramipril (Altace), and trandolapril (Mavik); cyclosporine (Neoral, Sandimmune); digoxin (Lanoxin); diuretics ('water pills'); lithium (Eskalith, Lithobid); and methotrexate (Rheumatrex). Your doctor may need to change the doses of your medications or monitor you carefully for side effects.

- tell your doctor if you have or have ever had asthma, especially if you also have frequent stuffed or runny nose or nasal polyps (swelling of the lining of the nose); swelling of the hands, feet, ankles, or lower legs; or kidney or liver disease.
- tell your doctor if you are pregnant, especially if you are in the last few months of your pregnancy, you plan to become pregnant, or you are breast-feeding. If you become pregnant while taking etodolac, call your doctor.
- if you are having surgery, including dental surgery, tell the doctor or dentist that you are taking etodolac.

What special dietary instructions should I follow?

Unless your doctor tells you otherwise, continue your normal diet.

What should I do if I forget to take a dose?

Take the missed dose as soon as you remember it. However, if it is almost time for the next dose, skip the missed dose and continue your regular dosing schedule. Do not take a double dose to make up for a missed one.

What side effects can this medicine cause?

Etodolac may cause side effects. Tell your doctor if any of these symptoms are severe or do not go away:

- constipation
- diarrhea
- gas or bloating
- vomiting
- headache
- dizziness
- ringing in the ears
- runny nose
- sore throat
- blurred vision

Some side effects can be serious. If you experience any of the following symptoms, or those mentioned in the IMPORTANT WARNING section, call your doctor immediately. Do not take any more etodolac until you speak to your doctor.

- unexplained weight gain
- swelling of the eyes, face, lips, tongue, throat, hands, feet, ankles, or lower legs
- fever or chills
- blisters
- rash
- itching
- hives
- hoarseness
- difficulty breathing or swallowing
- yellowing of the skin or eyes
- excessive tiredness
- unusual bleeding or bruising
- lack of energy
- loss of appetite
- pain in the upper right part of the stomach
- flu-like symptoms
- pale skin
- fast heartbeat
- cloudy, discolored, or bloody urine
- difficult or painful urination
- back pain

Etodolac may cause other side effects. Call your doctor if you have any unusual problems while taking this medication.

If you experience a serious side effect, you or your doctor may send a report to the Food and Drug Administration's (FDA) MedWatch Adverse Event Reporting program online [at http://www.fda.gov/MedWatch/index.html] or by phone [1-800-332-1088].

What storage conditions are needed for this medicine?

Keep this medication in the container it came in, tightly closed, and out of reach of children. Do not prepare doses of etodolac tablets in advance; keep the tablets in the original container until you are ready to take them. Store etodolac at room temperature and away from excess heat and moisture (not in the bathroom). Throw away any medication that is outdated or no longer needed. Talk to your pharmacist about the proper disposal of your medication.

What should I do in case of overdose?

In case of overdose, call your local poison control center at 1-800-222-1222. If the victim has collapsed or is not breathing, call local emergency services at 911.

Symptoms of overdose may include:

- lack of energy
- drowsiness
- upset stomach
- vomiting
- stomach pain
- bloody, black or tarry stool

- vomit that is bloody or looks like coffee grounds
- coma (loss of consciousness for a period of time)

What other information should I know?

Before having any laboratory test, tell your doctor and the laboratory personnel that you are taking etodolac.

If you have diabetes and you test your urine for ketones, you should know that etodolac may interfere with the results of this type of test. Talk to your doctor about how you should monitor your diabetes while you are taking etodolac.

Do not let anyone else take your medication. Ask your pharmacist any questions you have about refilling your prescription.

Dosage Facts
For Informational Purposes

Caution: Do not change your dose, how often you take your medication, or the length of time you are to take it without first talking to your healthcare provider.

The following dosage information was written using medical language for doctors and other healthcare professionals and is provided here for you to check your dosage. The dosage of this drug may differ for different patients. Therefore, always follow your doctor's instructions or the directions on the label. Contact your healthcare provider or pharmacist if you have any questions about the specific dosage of your medication after reviewing this information.

General Dosage Information

To minimize the potential risk of adverse cardiovascular and/or GI events, use lowest effective dosage and shortest duration of therapy consistent with the patient's treatment goals. Adjust dosage based on individual requirements and response; attempt to titrate to the lowest effective dosage.

Pediatric Patients

Inflammatory Diseases
Juvenile Rheumatoid Arthritis

ORAL:

Dosage Based on Child's Body Weight

Weight (kg)	Dosage (as extended-release tablets)
20–30	400 mg once daily
31–45	600 mg once daily
46–60	800 mg once daily
>60	1 g once daily

Adult Patients

Inflammatory Diseases
Osteoarthritis or Rheumatoid Arthritis

ORAL:
- Initially, 300 mg 2 or 3 times daily, 400 mg twice daily, or 500 mg twice daily as conventional capsules or tablets. Base subsequent dosage on clinical response and tolerance.
- Alternatively, initial dosage of 400–1000 mg once daily as extended-release tablets. Base subsequent dosage on clinical response and tolerance.

Pain

ORAL:
- 1 g daily as conventional capsules or tablets given in divided doses of 200–400 mg every 6–8 hours.

Prescribing Limits

Adult Patients

Inflammatory Diseases
Osteoarthritis or Rheumatoid Arthritis

ORAL:
- Maximum 1.2 g daily.

Pain

ORAL:
- Maximum 1 g daily.

Etonogestrel and Ethinyl Estradiol Vaginal Ring

(et oh noe jes′ trel)

(eth′ in il es tra dye′ ol)

Brand Name: NuvaRing®

Important Warning

Cigarette smoking increases the risk of serious side effects from etonogestrel and ethinyl estradiol vaginal ring, including heart attacks, blood clots, and strokes. This risk is higher for women over 35 years old and heavy smokers (15 or more cigarettes per day). If you use etonogestrel and ethinyl estradiol ring, you should not smoke.

Why is this medicine prescribed?

Etonogestrel and ethinyl estradiol vaginal ring is used to prevent pregnancy. Etonogestrel and ethinyl estradiol vaginal ring is in a class of medications called combination hormonal contraceptives (birth control medications). Etonogestrel is a progestin and ethinyl estradiol is an estrogen. Etonogestrel and ethinyl estradiol vaginal ring works by preventing ovulation (the release of an egg from the ovaries). It also changes the lining of the uterus (womb) to prevent pregnancy from developing and changes the mucus at the cervix (opening of the uterus) to prevent sperm (male reproductive cells) from entering. The contraceptive ring is a very effective method of birth control but does not prevent the spread of human immunodeficiency virus [HIV, the virus that causes acquired immunodeficiency syndrome (AIDS)] or other sexually transmitted diseases.

How should this medicine be used?

Etonogestrel and ethinyl estradiol combination comes as a flexible ring to place in the vagina. It is usually placed in the vagina and left in place for 3 weeks. After 3 weeks, it is removed for a 1-week break; then a new ring is inserted. Follow the directions on your prescription label carefully, and ask your doctor or pharmacist to explain any part you do not understand. Use the contraceptive ring exactly as directed. Never use more than one contraceptive ring at a time and always insert and remove the ring according to the schedule your doctor gives you.

You should always insert and remove the contraceptive ring on the same day of the week and at about the same time of day. Your menstrual period will probably start 2-3 days after you remove the contraceptive ring and may continue through that week. Be sure to insert your new ring at the end of the week on the same day and at the same time that you usually insert or remove the ring even if you have not stopped bleeding.

Your doctor will tell you when you should insert your first contraceptive ring. This depends on whether you were using a different type of birth control in the past month, were not using birth control, or have recently given birth or had an abortion or miscarriage. In some cases, you may need to use an additional method of birth control for the first seven days that you use the contraceptive ring. Your doctor will tell you whether you need to use backup birth control and will help you choose a method, such as male condoms and/ or spermicides. You should not use a diaphragm when a contraceptive ring is in place.

You do not need to position the contraceptive ring a certain way inside your vagina. The ring will work no matter how it is positioned, but will be more comfortable and less likely to fall out when it is placed as far back in your vagina as possible. The ring cannot get past the cervix, so it will not go too far into the vagina or get lost when you push it in.

The contraceptive ring will usually stay in your vagina until you remove it. It may sometimes slip out when you are removing a tampon or having a bowel movement, or if you are very constipated or have not placed it properly in your vagina. Call your doctor if your contraceptive ring slips out often.

If your contraceptive ring slips out, you should rinse it with cool or lukewarm (not hot) water and replace it in your vagina as soon as possible. If your ring falls out and gets lost, you should replace it with a new ring and remove the new ring at the same time you were scheduled to remove the ring that was lost. Try to replace your ring within 3 hours after it falls out. If you do not replace your ring within 3 hours, you must use a backup method of birth control until you have had the ring in place for 7 days in a row.

To use the contraceptive ring, follow these steps:
1. Wash and dry your hands.
2. Remove one contraceptive ring from its foil pouch, but do not throw away the pouch. Put the pouch in a safe place so you can use it to properly throw away the contraceptive ring after you remove it.
3. Lie down on your back with your knees bent, squat, or stand with one leg up on a chair, step, or other object. Choose the position that is most comfortable for you.
4. Hold the contraceptive ring between your thumb and index finger and press the opposite sides of the ring together.
5. Gently push the folded ring into your vagina.
6. If you feel discomfort, push the ring further back into your vagina with your index finger.
7. Wash your hands again.
8. When it is time to remove the contraceptive ring, hook your index finger under the front rim or hold the rim between your index and middle fingers and pull it out.
9. Put the used ring into the foil pouch and throw it away in a trash can that is out of the reach of children and pets. Do not throw the used ring in the toilet.
10. Wash your hands.
11. Wait one week, then insert a new ring following the directions above.

Are there other uses for this medicine?

This medication may be prescribed for other uses; ask your doctor or pharmacist for more information.

What special precautions should I follow?

Before using etonogestrel and ethinyl estradiol vaginal ring,
- tell your doctor and pharmacist if you are allergic to etonogestrel, ethinyl estradiol or any other medications.
- tell your doctor and pharmacist what other prescription and nonprescription medications, vitamins, nutritional supplements, you are taking. Be sure to mention any of the following: acetaminophen (Tylenol, others); antibiotics such as ampicillin (Omnipen, Principen others), clarithromycin (Biaxin), demeclocycline (Declomycin), doxycycline (Vibramycin, Doryx, others), erythromycin (E.E.S., E-Mycin, Erythrocin), minocycline (Vectrin, Minocin), rifampin (Rifadin, Rimactane), rifabutin (Mycobutin); tetracycline (Sumycin), and troleandomycin (TAO); antifungals such as fluconazole (Diflucan), griseofulvin (Grifulvin V, Fulvicin, others), itraconazole (Sporanox), and ketoconazole (Nizoral); ascorbic acid (Vitamin C); atorvastatin (Lipitor); ci-

metidine (Tagamet); clofibrate (Abitrate, Atromid-S); cyclosporine (Neoral, Sandimmune); danazol (Danocrine); dexamethasone (Decadron); diltiazem (Cardizem, Dilacor, Tiazac); ethosuxamide (Zarontin); fluoxetine (Prozac, Sarafem); fluvoxamine (Luvox); isoniazid (INH, Nydrazid); medications for HIV or AIDS such as delavirdine (Rescriptor), indinavir (Crixivan), nelfinavir (Viracept), Saquinavir (Fortovase, Invirase), and ritonavir (Norvir); medications for seizures such as carbamazepine (Tegretol), felbamate (Felbatol), oxcarbazepine (Trileptal), phenobarbital (Luminal, Solfoton), phenytoin (Dilantin), and topiramate (Topamax); metronidazole (Flagyl); morphine (MSIR, Oramorph, others); nefazodone; prednisolone (Prelone); primidone; theophylline (TheoDur, others); temazepam (Restoril); verapamil (Calan, Covera, Isoptin, Verelan); zafirlukast (Accolate) and any medication that is placed in the vagina. Your doctor may need to change the doses of your medications or monitor you carefully for side effects. You may need to use an extra method of birth control if you take some of these medications while you are using the contraceptive ring.

- tell your doctor what herbal products you are taking, especially products containing St. John's wort.
- tell your doctor if you have or have ever had, or anyone in your family has or has ever had, breast cancer, if you have ever had yellowing of the skin or eyes during pregnancy or while you were using another type of hormonal contraceptive (birth control pills, patches, rings, or injections), if you are on bed rest or are unable to walk around for any reason, or if you have or have ever had breast lumps; an abnormal mammogram (breast x-ray); fibrocystic breast disease (swollen, tender breasts and/or breast lumps that are not cancer); any type of cancer, especially cancer of the endometrium (lining of the uterus), cervix, or vagina; blood clots in your legs, lungs, or eyes; stroke or mini-stroke; coronary artery disease (clogged blood vessels leading to the heart); chest pain; a heart attack; any condition that affects your heart valves (flaps of tissue that open and close to control blood flow in the heart); high cholesterol or triglycerides; high blood pressure; diabetes; headaches; seizures; depression; unexplained vaginal bleeding; any condition that makes your vagina more likely to become irritated; bladder, uterus or rectum that has dropped or bulged into the vagina; constipation; or liver, kidney, thyroid, or gallbladder disease.
- tell your doctor if you are pregnant or plan to become pregnant. If you become pregnant while using etonogestrel and ethinyl estradiol vaginal ring, call your doctor immediately. You should suspect that you are pregnant and call your doctor if you have used the contraceptive ring correctly and you miss two periods in a row, or if you have not used the contraceptive ring according to the directions and you miss one period. You should not breastfeed while you are using the contraceptive ring.

- if you are having surgery, including dental surgery, tell the doctor or dentist that you are using etonogestrel and ethinyl estradiol vaginal ring.
- tell your doctor if you wear contact lenses. If you notice changes in your vision or your ability to wear your lenses while using etonogestrel and ethinyl estradiol vaginal ring, see an eye doctor.

What special dietary instructions should I follow?

Talk to your doctor about drinking grapefruit juice while using this medication.

What should I do if I forget to take a dose?

If you forget to insert a new contraceptive ring 1 week after you removed the old ring, you may not be protected from pregnancy. Check to be sure that you are not pregnant. If you are not pregnant, insert a new ring as soon as you remember and use a backup method of birth control until the new ring has been in place for 7 days in a row.

If you forget to remove the contraceptive ring on time but remember before 1 week has passed, remove the ring as soon as you remember. Wait 1 week and then insert a new ring. If you forget to remove the contraceptive ring and remember after more than 1 week has passed, you may not be protected from pregnancy. Check to be sure that you are not pregnant. If you are not pregnant, remove the ring as soon as you remember, wait 1 week and insert a new ring. Use a backup method of birth control until the new ring has been in place for 7 days in a row.

What side effects can this medicine cause?

Etonogestrel and ethinyl estradiol vaginal ring may cause side effects. Tell your doctor if any of these symptoms are severe or do not go away:

- swelling, redness, irritation, burning, itching, or infection of the vagina
- white or yellow vaginal discharge
- vaginal bleeding or spotting when it is not time for your period. (Call your doctor if the bleeding lasts longer than a few days or happens in more than one cycle.)
- headache
- runny nose
- upset stomach
- vomiting
- changes in appetite
- weight gain or loss
- stomach cramps or bloating
- nervousness
- breasts that are large, tender, or produce a liquid
- growth of hair on face
- loss of hair on scalp
- acne
- changes in sexual desire

Some side effects can be serious. The following symptoms are uncommon, but if you experience any of them call your doctor immediately:

- pain in the back of the lower leg
- sharp, sudden, or crushing chest pain
- heaviness in chest
- coughing up blood
- sudden shortness of breath
- sudden severe headache, vomiting, dizziness, or fainting
- sudden problems with speech
- weakness or numbness of an arm or leg
- sudden loss of vision
- double vision, blurred vision, or other changes in vision
- bulging eyes
- yellowing of the skin or eyes, especially if you also have fever, tiredness, loss of appetite, dark urine, and/or light-colored bowel movements
- depression, especially if you also have trouble sleeping, tiredness, loss of energy, or other mood changes
- pain, tenderness, or swelling of the abdomen (area between the chest and the waist)
- stomach pain that worsens after eating
- swelling of the hands, feet, ankles, or lower legs
- diarrhea
- painful, difficult, or frequent urination
- brown patches on the skin, especially the face
- rash

Etonogestrel and ethinyl estradiol vaginal ring may increase the chance that you will develop liver tumors. These tumors are not a form of cancer, but they can break and cause serious bleeding inside the body. The contraceptive ring may also increase the chance that you will develop breast or liver cancer, or have a heart attack, a stroke, or a serious blood clot. Talk to your doctor about the risks of using the contraceptive ring.

Etonogestrel and ethinyl estradiol vaginal ring may cause other side effects. Call your doctor if you have any unusual problems while taking this medication.

If you experience a serious side effect, you or your doctor may send a report to the Food and Drug Administration's (FDA) MedWatch Adverse Event Reporting program online [at http://www.fda.gov/MedWatch/index.html] or by phone [1-800-332-1088].

What storage conditions are needed for this medicine?

Keep this medication in the packet it came in, tightly closed, and out of reach of children. Store it at room temperature and away from excess heat and moisture (not in the bathroom). Throw away any medication that is outdated or no longer needed. Talk to your pharmacist about the proper disposal of your medication.

What should I do in case of overdose?

In case of overdose, call your local poison control center at 1-800-222-1222. If the victim has collapsed or is not breathing, call local emergency services at 911.

Etonogestrel and ethinyl estradiol vaginal ring is unlikely to cause an overdose. You will not receive too much medication if the ring breaks inside your vagina or if it is left in your vagina for too long.

Symptoms of overdose may include:

- upset stomach
- vomiting
- vaginal bleeding
- irregular period

What other information should I know?

Keep all appointments with your doctor and the laboratory. You should have a complete physical examination every year, including blood pressure measurements, breast and pelvic exams, and a Pap test. Follow your doctor's directions for examining your breasts; report any lumps immediately.

Before having any laboratory test, tell your doctor and the laboratory personnel that you are using etonogestrel and ethinyl estradiol vaginal ring.

Do not let anyone else use your medication. Ask your pharmacist any questions you have about refilling your prescription.

Please see the Estrogen and Progestin monograph to find dosing information for this medication.

Exemestane

(ex e mes' tane)

Brand Name: Aromasin®

Why is this medicine prescribed?

Exemestane is used to treat early breast cancer in women who have experienced menopause (change of life; end of monthly menstrual periods) and who have already been treated with a medication called tamoxifen (Nolvadex) for 2-3 years. This medication is also used to treat breast cancer in women whose breast cancer has worsened while they were taking tamoxifen. Exemestane is in a class of medications called aromatase inhibitors. It works by decreasing the amount of estrogen produced by the body. This can slow or stop the growth of some breast tumors that need estrogen to grow.

How should this medicine be used?

Exemestane comes as a tablet to take by mouth. It is usually taken once a day after a meal. Take exemestane at around the same time every day. Follow the directions on your prescription label carefully, and ask your doctor or pharmacist to explain any part you do not understand. Take exemestane exactly as directed. Do not take more or less of it or take it more often than prescribed by your doctor.

You may need to take exemestane for several years or

longer. Continue to take exemestane even if you feel well. Do not stop taking exemestane without talking to your doctor.

Are there other uses for this medicine?

This medication may be prescribed for other uses; ask your doctor or pharmacist for more information.

What special precautions should I follow?

Before taking exemestane,

- tell your doctor and pharmacist if you are allergic to exemestane or any other medications.
- tell your doctor and pharmacist what other prescription and nonprescription medications, vitamins, and nutritional supplements you are taking or plan to take. Be sure to mention any of the following: carbamazepine (Carbatrol, Epitol, Tegretol); medications that contain estrogen such as hormone replacement therapy and hormonal contraceptives (birth control pills, patches, rings, and injections); phenobarbital; phenytoin (Dilantin); and rifampin (Rifadin, in Rifater, in Rifamate). Your doctor may need to change the doses of your medications or monitor you carefully for side effects.
- tell your doctor what herbal products you are taking, especially St John's wort.
- tell your doctor if you have or have ever had liver or kidney disease.
- you should know that exemestane should only be used by women who have experienced menopause and cannot become pregnant. However, if you are pregnant or breastfeeding, you should tell your doctor before you begin taking this medication. Exemestane may harm the fetus.

What special dietary instructions should I follow?

Unless your doctor tells you otherwise, continue your normal diet.

What should I do if I forget to take a dose?

Take the missed dose as soon as you remember it. However, if it is almost time for the next dose, skip the missed dose and continue your regular dosing schedule. Do not take a double dose to make up for a missed one.

What side effects can this medicine cause?

Exemestane may cause side effects. Tell your doctor if any of these symptoms are severe or do not go away:

- hot flushes
- sweating
- muscle or joint pain
- tiredness
- headache
- dizziness
- nervousness
- depression

- difficulty falling asleep or staying asleep
- diarrhea
- hair loss
- red, itchy skin
- changes in vision

Some side effects can be serious. If you experience any of these symptoms, call your doctor immediately:

- shortness of breath
- chest pain

Your bone mineral density (BMD; a measure of the strength of the bones) may decrease while you are taking exemestane. This may increase the chance that you will develop osteoporosis (condition in which the bones are fragile and break easily). Talk to your doctor about the risks of taking exemestane.

Exemestane may cause other side effects. Call your doctor if you have any unusual problems while taking this medication.

What storage conditions are needed for this medicine?

Keep this medication in the container it came in, tightly closed, and out of reach of children. Store it at room temperature and away from excess heat and moisture (not in the bathroom). Throw away any medication that is outdated or no longer needed. Talk to your pharmacist about the proper disposal of your medication.

What should I do in case of overdose?

In case of overdose, call your local poison control center at 1-800-222-1222. If the victim has collapsed or is not breathing, call local emergency services at 911.

What other information should I know?

Keep all appointments with your doctor and the laboratory. Your doctor may order certain lab tests to check your body's response to exemestane.

Do not let anyone else take your medication. Ask your pharmacist any questions you have about refilling your prescription.

Dosage Facts
For Informational Purposes

Caution: Do not change your dose, how often you take your medication, or the length of time you are to take it without first talking to your healthcare provider.

The following dosage information was written using medical language for doctors and other healthcare professionals and is provided here for you to check your dosage. The dosage of this drug may differ for different patients. Therefore, always follow your doctor's instructions or the directions on the label. Contact your healthcare provider or pharmacist if you have any questions

about the specific dosage of your medication after reviewing this information.

Adult Patients

Breast Cancer

ORAL:
- 25 mg once daily; continue until tumor progression is evident.

Prescribing Limits

Adult Patients

Dosages >25 mg daily not shown to provide substantially greater suppression of plasma estrogens but may increase adverse effects.

Special Populations

Hepatic Impairment
- Dosage adjustment does not appear to be necessary.

Renal Impairment
- Dosage adjustment does not appear to be necessary.

Exenatide Injection

(ex en′ a tide)

Brand Name: Byetta®

Why is this medicine prescribed?

Exenatide is used in combination with metformin, a sulfonylurea, or a thiazolidinedione medication to treat type 2 diabetes (condition in which the body does not use insulin normally and, therefore, cannot control the amount of sugar in the blood). Exenatide is in a class of medications called incretin mimetics. It works by stimulating the pancreas to secrete insulin when blood sugar levels are high. Insulin helps move sugar from the blood into other body tissues where it is used for energy. Exenatide also slows the emptying of the stomach and causes a decrease in appetite. Exenatide is not used to treat type 1 diabetes (condition in which the body does not produce insulin and, therefore, cannot control the amount of sugar in the blood). Exenatide is not used instead of insulin to treat people with diabetes who need insulin.

How should this medicine be used?

Exenatide comes as a solution (liquid) in a prefilled dosing pen to inject subcutaneously (under the skin). It is usually injected twice a day within 60 minutes before the morning and evening meals. Exenatide should not be injected after meals. Your doctor will probably start you on a low dose of exenatide and may switch you to a pen with a higher dose of medication if your blood sugar control has not improved after you have used exenatide for 1 month. Follow the directions on your prescription label carefully, and ask your

doctor or pharmacist to explain any part you do not understand. Use exenatide injection exactly as directed. Do not use more or less of it or use it more often than prescribed by your doctor.

Exenatide controls diabetes but does not cure it. Continue to use exenatide even if you feel well. Do not stop using exenatide without talking to your doctor.

Exenatide comes in prefilled dosing pens that contain enough medication for 60 doses (two doses a day for 1 month). You will need to buy needles separately. Ask your doctor or pharmacist what type of needles you will need to inject your medication. Be sure to read and understand the manufacturer's instructions for injecting exenatide using the pen. Also make sure you know how and when to set up a new pen. Ask your doctor or pharmacist to show you how to use the pen. Follow the directions carefully. Never remove the cartridge from the pen or attempt to add any other type of medication to the cartridge.

Always look at your exenatide solution before you inject it. It should be as clear, colorless, and fluid as water. Do not use exenatide if it is colored, cloudy, thickened, or contains solid particles, or if the expiration date on the bottle has passed.

Never reuse needles and never share needles or pens. Always remove the needle right after you inject your dose. Throw away needles in a puncture-resistant container. Ask your doctor or pharmacist how to dispose of the puncture resistant container.

Exenatide can be administered in the thigh (upper leg), abdomen (stomach), or upper arm. Use a different site for each injection, about 1 inch away from the previous injection but in the same general area (for example, the thigh). Use all available sites in the same general area before switching to a different area (for example, the upper arm). Do not use the same injection site more often than once every month.

Are there other uses for this medicine?

This medication may be prescribed for other uses; ask your doctor or pharmacist for more information.

What special precautions should I follow?

Before using exenatide injection,
- tell your doctor and pharmacist if you are allergic to exenatide or any other medications.
- tell your doctor and pharmacist what prescription and nonprescription medications, vitamins, nutritional supplements, and herbal products you are taking or plan to take. Be sure to mention warfarin (Coumadin).
- if you are taking oral contraceptives (birth control pills) or antibiotics, take them at least 1 hour before exenatide injection. If you have been told to take these medications with food, take them with a meal or snack at a time when you do not use exenatide.
- tell your doctor if you have or have ever had severe stomach problems or kidney disease.
- tell your doctor if you are pregnant, plan to become

pregnant, or are breast-feeding. If you become pregnant while using exenatide, call your doctor.

- you should know that when exenatide is used in combination with a sulfonylurea medication, it may increase the risk of hypoglycemia (low blood sugar). Ask your doctor or pharmacist if you are not sure if the antidiabetic medication that you are taking is a sulfonylurea. Your doctor may lower your dose of sulfonylurea while you are using exenatide.
- you should know that exenatide may cause weight loss and a decrease in appetite.

What special dietary instructions should I follow?

Be sure to follow all exercise and dietary recommendations made by your doctor or dietitian. It is important to eat a healthy diet.

Alcohol may cause a decrease in blood sugar. Ask your doctor about the safe use of alcoholic beverages while you are using exenatide.

What should I do if I forget to take a dose?

Skip the missed dose and continue your regular dosing schedule. Do not inject a double dose to make up for a missed one.

What side effects can this medicine cause?

This medication may cause changes in your blood sugar. You should know the symptoms of low and high blood sugar and what to do if you have these symptoms.

You may experience hypoglycemia (low blood sugar) while you are taking this medication. Your doctor will tell you what you should do if you develop hypoglycemia. He or she may tell you to check your blood sugar, eat or drink a food or beverage that contains sugar, such as hard candy or fruit juice, or get medical care. Follow these directions carefully if you have any of the following symptoms of hypoglycemia:

- shakiness
- dizziness or lightheadedness
- sweating
- nervousness or irritability
- sudden changes in behavior or mood
- headache
- numbness or tingling around the mouth
- weakness
- pale skin
- hunger
- clumsy or jerky movements

If hypoglycemia is not treated, severe symptoms may develop. Be sure that your family, friends, and other people who spend time with you know that if you have any of the following symptoms, they should get medical treatment for you immediately.

- confusion

- seizures
- loss of consciousness

Call your doctor immediately if you have any of the following symptoms of hyperglycemia (high blood sugar) :

- extreme thirst
- frequent urination
- extreme hunger
- weakness
- blurred vision

If high blood sugar is not treated, a serious, life-threatening condition called diabetic ketoacidosis could develop. Call your doctor immediately if you have any of the these symptoms:

- dry mouth
- upset stomach and vomiting
- shortness of breath
- breath that smells fruity
- decreased consciousness

Exenatide injection may cause side effects. Tell your doctor if any of these symptoms are severe or do not go away:

- upset stomach
- vomiting
- diarrhea
- jittery feeling
- dizziness
- headache
- weakness
- acid stomach

Some side effects can be serious. If you experience any of the following symptoms, call your doctor immediately:

- severe stomach pain
- hives
- skin rash
- itching
- difficulty breathing or swallowing
- swelling of the face, throat, tongue, lips, eyes, hands, feet, ankles, or lower legs
- hoarseness

Exenatide may cause other side effects. Call your doctor if you have any unusual problems while taking this medication.

If you experience a serious side effect, you or your doctor may send a report to the Food and Drug Administration's (FDA) MedWatch Adverse Event Reporting program online [at http://www.fda.gov/MedWatch/index.html] or by phone [1-800-332-1088].

What storage conditions are needed for this medicine?

Store unused exenatide pens in their original carton in the refrigerator protected from light. Once in use, store exenatide pens at room temperature (up to 77° F) protected from light. Do not freeze. Do not use exenatide if it has been frozen. Do not store exenatide pens with the needle attached. Keep exenatide pens out of the reach of children.

When traveling, be sure to keep exenatide pens dry. Unused pens should be refrigerated or at a cold temperature between 36 to 46°F; pens that are in use can be stored at room temperature up to 77°F (not in a car glove compartment or other hot place).

Make a note of the date you first use an exenatide pen, and throw away the pen after 30 days, even if there is some solution left in the pen. Throw away any exenatide pens that are outdated or no longer needed. Talk to your pharmacist about the proper disposal of your medication.

What should I do in case of overdose?

In case of overdose, call your local poison control center at 1-800-222-1222. If the victim has collapsed or is not breathing, call local emergency services at 911.

Symptoms of overdose may include:

- severe upset stomach
- severe vomiting
- dizziness
- symptoms of hypoglycemia (See "What Side Effects can this medication cause?")

What other information should I know?

Keep all appointments with your doctor and the laboratory. Your blood sugar and glycosylated hemoglobin (HbA1c) should be checked regularly to determine your response to exenatide. Your doctor will also tell you how to check your response to this medication by measuring your blood or urine sugar levels at home. Follow these instructions carefully.

See your dentist twice yearly; see your eye doctor regularly; get your blood pressure checked regularly.

Keep yourself and your clothes clean. Wash cuts, scrapes, and other wounds quickly, and do not let them get infected. Wear medical alert identification (a bracelet or tag) that says you have diabetes.

Do not let anyone else use your medication. Ask your pharmacist any questions you have about refilling your prescription.

Dosage Facts
For Informational Purposes

Caution: Do not change your dose, how often you take your medication, or the length of time you are to take it without first talking to your healthcare provider.

The following dosage information was written using medical language for doctors and other healthcare professionals and is provided here for you to check your dosage. The dosage of this drug may differ for different patients. Therefore, always follow your doctor's instructions or the directions on the label. Contact your healthcare provider or pharmacist if you have any questions about the specific dosage of your medication after reviewing this information.

General Dosage Information

Give in combination with metformin and/or sulfonylurea therapy. If used in combination with a sulfonylurea, adjustment of sulfonylurea dosage may be necessary. No dosage adjustment is required when used in combination with metformin.(See Specific Drugs under Interactions.)

Adult Patients
Diabetes Mellitus

SUB-Q:
- Initially, 5 mcg twice daily. If needed, may increase to 10 mcg twice daily after 1 month.

Special Populations

Hepatic Impairment
- Dosage adjustment not required.

Renal Impairment
- No dosage adjustment required in mild to moderate impairment (Cl_{cr} 30–80 mL/min); use not recommended in end-stage renal disease or severe renal impairment (Cl_{cr} <30mL/min).

Geriatric Patients
- Careful dosage selection recommended due to possible age-related decrease in renal function and concomitant disease and drug therapy; however, dosage requirements generally similar in geriatric patients and younger adults.

Obese Patients
- Dosage adjustment not required.

Ezetimibe
(ez et′ i mibe)

Brand Name: Vytorin® (combination with simvastatin), Zetia®

Why is this medicine prescribed?

Ezetimibe is used together with lifestyle changes (diet, weight-loss, exercise) to reduce the amount of cholesterol (a fat-like substance) and other fatty substances in the blood. It may be used alone or in combination with a HMG-CoA reductase inhibitor (statin). Ezetimibe is in a class of medications called cholesterol-lowering medications. It works by preventing the absorption of cholesterol in the intestine.

Buildup of cholesterol and fats along the walls of the blood vessels (a process known as atherosclerosis) decreases blood flow and, therefore, the oxygen supply to the heart, brain, and other parts of the body. Lowering blood levels of cholesterol and fats may help to decrease your chances of getting heart disease, angina (chest pain), strokes, and heart attacks. In addition to taking a cholesterol-lowering medication, making certain changes in your daily habits can also lower your cholesterol blood levels. You should eat a diet that is low in saturated fat and cholesterol (see SPECIAL

DIETARY), exercise 30 minutes on most, if not all days, and lose weight if you are overweight.

How should this medicine be used?

Ezetimibe comes as a tablet to take by mouth. It is usually taken once a day with or without food. To help you remember to take ezetimibe, take it around the same time every day. Follow the directions on your prescription label carefully, and ask your doctor or pharmacist to explain any part you do not understand. Take ezetimibe exactly as directed. Do not take more or less of it or take it more often than prescribed by your doctor.

Continue to take ezetimibe even if you feel well. Do not stop taking ezetimibe without talking to your doctor.

Are there other uses for this medicine?

This medication may be prescribed for other uses; ask your doctor or pharmacist for more information.

What special precautions should I follow?

Before taking ezetimibe,
- tell your doctor and pharmacist if you are allergic to ezetimibe or any other medications.
- tell your doctor and pharmacist what prescription and nonprescription medications, vitamins, nutritional supplements, and herbal products you are taking. Be sure to mention any of the following: anticoagulants ('blood thinners') such as warfarin (Coumadin), cyclosporine (Neoral, Sandimmune), fenofibrate (TriCor), and gemfibrozil (Lopid). Your doctor may need to change the doses of your medications or monitor you carefully for side effects.
- if you are taking cholestyramine (Questran), colesevelam (WellChol), or colestipol (Colestid), take it 4 hours before or 2 hours after ezetimibe.
- tell your doctor if you have or have ever had liver disease.
- tell your doctor if you are pregnant, plan to become pregnant, or are breast-feeding. If you become pregnant while taking ezetimibe, call your doctor.

What special dietary instructions should I follow?

Eat a low-cholesterol, low-fat diet. This kind of diet includes cottage cheese, fat-free milk, fish (not canned in oil), vegetables, poultry, egg whites, and polyunsaturated oils and margarines (corn, safflower, canola, and soybean oils). Avoid foods with excess fat in them such as meat (especially liver and fatty meat), egg yolks, whole milk, cream, butter, shortening, lard, pastries, cakes, cookies, gravy, peanut butter, chocolate, olives, potato chips, coconut, cheese (other than cottage cheese), coconut oil, palm oil, and fried foods.

What should I do if I forget to take a dose?

Take the missed dose as soon as you remember it. However, if it is almost time for the next dose, skip the missed dose and continue your regular dosing schedule. Do not take a double dose to make up for a missed one.

What side effects can this medicine cause?

Ezetimibe may cause side effects. Tell your doctor if any of these symptoms are severe or do not go away:
- headache
- dizziness
- diarrhea
- sore throat
- runny nose
- sneezing
- joint pain

Some side effects can be serious. The following symptoms are uncommon, but if you experience any of them, call your doctor immediately:
- hives
- rash
- itching
- difficulty breathing or swallowing
- swelling of the face, throat, tongue, lips, eyes, hands, feet, ankles, or lower legs
- hoarseness
- upset stomach
- extreme tiredness
- unusual bleeding or bruising
- lack of energy
- loss of appetite
- pain in the upper right part of the stomach
- yellowing of the skin or eyes
- flu-like symptoms
- muscle pain or weakness
- fever
- chills
- pale or fatty stools
- chest pain

Ezetimibe may cause other side effects. Call your doctor if you have any unusual problems while taking this medication.

What storage conditions are needed for this medicine?

Keep this medication in the container it came in, tightly closed, and out of reach of children. Store it at room temperature and away from excess heat and moisture (not in the bathroom). Throw away any medication that is outdated or no longer needed. Talk to your pharmacist about the proper disposal of your medication.

What should I do in case of overdose?

In case of overdose, call your local poison control center at 1-800-222-1222. If the victim has collapsed or is not breathing, call local emergency services at 911.

What other information should I know?

Keep all appointments with your doctor and the laboratory. Your doctor will order certain lab tests before and during treatment to check your body's response to ezetimibe.

Do not let anyone else take your medication. Ask your pharmacist any questions you have about refilling your prescription.

Dosage Facts
For Informational Purposes

Caution: Do not change your dose, how often you take your medication, or the length of time you are to take it without first talking to your healthcare provider.

The following dosage information was written using medical language for doctors and other healthcare professionals and is provided here for you to check your dosage. The dosage of this drug may differ for different patients. Therefore, always follow your doctor's instructions or the directions on the label. Contact your healthcare provider or pharmacist if you have any questions about the specific dosage of your medication after reviewing this information.

Pediatric Patients

Dyslipidemias
Primary Hypercholesterolemia and Mixed Dyslipidemia

ORAL:
- Children ≥10 years of age: 10 mg once daily.

Homozygous Familial Hypercholesterolemia

ORAL:
- Children ≥10 years of age: 10 mg once daily.

Homozygous Familial Sitosterolemia

ORAL:
- Children ≥10 years of age: 10 mg once daily.

Adult Patients

Dyslipidemias
Primary Hypercholesterolemia and Mixed Dyslipidemia

ORAL:
- 10 mg once daily.
- Ezetimibe/simvastatin fixed combination (Vytorin®): Initially, ezetimibe 10 mg/simvastatin 20 mg once daily in the evening. In patients requiring less aggressive LDL-cholesterol lowering, consider dosage of ezetimibe 10 mg/simvastatin 10 mg once daily. In patients requiring LDL-cholesterol reductions ≥55%, may initiate therapy with ezetimibe 10 mg/simvastatin 40 mg once daily. Determine serum cholesterol concen-

trations ≥2 weeks after initiation of therapy and adjust dosage as needed. Usual maintenance dosage range is ezetimibe 10 mg and simvastatin 10–80 mg once daily.

Homozygous Familial Hypercholesterolemia

ORAL:
- 10 mg once daily.
- Ezetimibe/simvastatin fixed combination (Vytorin®): Ezetimibe 10 mg/simvastatin 40 mg or ezetimibe 10 mg/simvastatin 80 mg once daily in the evening. Use as adjunct to other lipid-lowering treatments (e.g., LDL apheresis) or if such treatments are unavailable.

Homozygous Familial Sitosterolemia

ORAL:
- 10 mg once daily.

Special Populations

Hepatic Impairment

Ezetimibe
- No dosage adjustment needed in patients with mild hepatic impairment. Do not use in patients with moderate or severe hepatic impairment.

Ezetimibe/Simvastatin Fixed Combination
- No dosage adjustment needed in patients with mild hepatic impairment. Do not use in patients with moderate or severe hepatic impairment.

Renal Impairment

Ezetimibe
- No dosage adjustment needed in patients with renal impairment.

Ezetimibe/Simvastatin Fixed Combination
- No dosage adjustment needed in patients with mild to moderate renal impairment. Do not use in patients with severe renal impairment unless patient has already tolerated treatment with a simvastatin dosage ≥5 mg daily; in such patients, exercise caution and monitor closely.

Geriatric Patients

Ezetimibe
- No dosage adjustment needed in geriatric patients (≥65 years of age).

Ezetimibe/Simvastatin Fixed Combination
- No dosage adjustment needed in geriatric patients (≥65 years of age).

Famciclovir

(fam sye′ kloe veer)

Brand Name: Famvir®

Why is this medicine prescribed?

Famciclovir is used to treat herpes zoster (shingles) and genital herpes. It does not cure herpes infections but decreases pain and itching, helps sores to heal, and prevents new ones from forming.

This medication is sometimes prescribed for other uses; ask your doctor or pharmacist for more information.

How should this medicine be used?

Famciclovir comes as a tablet to take by mouth. It is usually taken every 8 hours (three times a day) for 7 days to treat shingles. To treat genital herpes it is usually taken twice a day for 5 days. Follow the directions on your prescription label carefully, and ask your doctor or pharmacist to explain any part you do not understand. Take famciclovir exactly as directed. Do not take more or less of it or take it more often than prescribed by your doctor. Use this medication as soon as possible after symptoms appear.

Continue to take famciclovir even if you feel well. Do not stop taking famciclovir without talking to your doctor.

What special precautions should I follow?

Before taking famciclovir,

- tell your doctor and pharmacist if you are allergic to famciclovir, acyclovir (Zovirax), or any other drugs.
- tell your doctor and pharmacist what prescription and nonprescription medications you are taking, especially digoxin (Lanoxin), probenecid (Benemid), and vitamins.
- tell your doctor if you have or have ever had kidney or liver disease, problems with your immune system, human immunodeficiency virus infection (HIV), or acquired immunodeficiency syndrome (AIDS).
- tell your doctor if you are pregnant, plan to become pregnant, or are breast-feeding. If you become pregnant while taking famciclovir, call your doctor.

What special dietary instructions should I follow?

Famciclovir may cause an upset stomach. Take famciclovir with food or milk.

What should I do if I forget to take a dose?

Take the missed dose as soon as you remember it, and take any remaining doses for that day at evenly spaced intervals. However, if it is almost time for the next dose, skip the missed dose and continue your regular dosing schedule. Do not take a double dose to make up for a missed one.

What side effects can this medicine cause?

Famciclovir may cause side effects. Tell your doctor if any of these symptoms are severe or do not go away:

- headache
- upset stomach
- vomiting
- diarrhea or loose stools

If you experience any of the following side effects, call your doctor immediately:

- rash
- itching

If you experience a serious side effect, you or your doctor may send a report to the Food and Drug Administration's (FDA) MedWatch Adverse Event Reporting program online [at http://www.fda.gov/MedWatch/index.html] or by phone [1-800-332-1088].

What storage conditions are needed for this medicine?

Keep this medication in the container it came in, tightly closed, and out of reach of children. Store it at room temperature and away from excess heat and moisture (not in the bathroom). Throw away any medication that is outdated or no longer needed. Talk to your pharmacist about the proper disposal of your medication.

What should I do in case of overdose?

In case of overdose, call your local poison control center at 1-800-222-1222. If the victim has collapsed or is not breathing, call local emergency services at 911.

What other information should I know?

Keep all appointments with your doctor and the laboratory. Your doctor will order certain lab tests to check your response to famciclovir.

Do not have sexual intercourse when you can see the genital herpes lesions. However, genital herpes can be spread even when there are no symptoms.

Do not let anyone else take your medication. Ask your pharmacist any questions you have about refilling your prescription. If you still have symptoms of infection after you finish the famciclovir, call your doctor.

Dosage Facts

For Informational Purposes

Caution: Do not change your dose, how often you take your medication, or the length of time you are to take it without first talking to your health-care provider.

The following dosage information was written using medical language for doctors and other healthcare professionals and is provided here for you to check your dosage. The dosage of this drug may differ for different

patients. Therefore, always follow your doctor's instructions or the directions on the label. Contact your healthcare provider or pharmacist if you have any questions about the specific dosage of your medication after reviewing this information.

Pediatric Patients

Genital Herpes

ORAL:
- Postpubertal adolescents should receive dosage recommended for adults with genital herpes.

Mucocutaneous Herpes Simplex Virus (HSV) Infections

ORAL:
- 250 mg twice daily for chronic suppressive or maintenance therapy (secondary prophylaxis) of HSV infections in HIV-infected adolescents who have frequent or severe recurrences.

Adult Patients

Genital Herpes
Treatment of Initial Episodes

ORAL:
- 250 mg 3 times daily for 5–10 days for initial episodes of genital herpes†.
- CDC suggests duration of treatment may be extended if healing is incomplete after 10 days.

Episodic Treatment of Recurrent Episodes

ORAL:
- 125 mg twice daily for 5 days in immunocompetent adults; 500 mg twice daily for 5–10 days in HIV-infected adults.
- Initiate therapy at first sign or symptom of an episode; efficacy not established if initiated >6 hours after onset of signs or symptoms.

Chronic Suppression of Recurrent Episodes

ORAL:
- 250 mg twice daily in immunocompetent adults; 500 mg twice daily in HIV-infected adults.
- May be given for up to 1 year.

Mucocutaneous Herpes Simplex Virus (HSV) Infections
Episodic Treatment of Recurrent Episodes

ORAL:
- 500 mg every 12 hours for 7 days for treatment of recurrent infections (orolabial or genital herpes) in HIV-infected adults.

Chronic Suppression of Recurrent Episodes

ORAL:
- 250 mg twice daily forchronic suppressive or maintenance therapy (secondary prophylaxis) of HSV infections in HIV-infected adults who have frequent or severe recurrences.

Herpes Zoster

ORAL:
- 500 mg every 8 hours for 7 days.
- Initiate therapy promptly as soon as diagnosed; efficacy not established if initiated >72 hours after rash onset.

Special Populations

Renal Impairment

Genital Herpes

Dosage for Episodic Treatment of Recurrent Genital Herpes in Renal Impairment

Cl_{cr} (mL/min)	Daily Dosage
≥40	125 mg every 12 hours
20–39	125 mg once every 24 hours
<20	125 mg once every 24 hours
Hemodialysis Patients	125 mg following each dialysis

Dosage for Chronic Suppression of Recurrent Genital Herpes in Renal Impairment

Cl_{cr} (mL/min)	Daily Dosage
≥40	250 mg every 12 hours
20–39	125 mg every 12 hours
<20	125 mg once every 24 hours
Hemodialysis Patients	125 mg following each dialysis

Mucocutaneous Herpes Simplex Virus (HSV) Infections

Dosage for Episodic Treatment of Recurrent HSV (Orolabial or Genital Herpes) in HIV-infected Individuals with Renal Impairment

Cl_{cr} (mL/min)	Daily Dosage
≥40	500 mg every 12 hours
20–39	500 mg once every 24 hours
<20	250 mg once every 24 hours
Hemodialysis Patients	250 mg following each dialysis

Herpes Zoster

Dosage for Treatment of Herpes Zoster in Renal Impairment

Cl_{cr} (mL/min)	Daily Dosage
40–59	500 mg every 12 hours
20–39	500 mg once every 24 hours
<20	250 mg once every 24 hours
Hemodialysis Patients	250 mg following each dialysis

† *Use is not currently included in the labeling approved by the US Food and Drug Administration.*

Famotidine

(fa moe′ ti deen)

Brand Name: Pepcid®, Pepcid® AC, Pepcid® AC Gelcaps, Pepcid® AC Maximum Strength, Pepcid® Complete, Pepcid® RPD

Why is this medicine prescribed?

Prescription famotidine is used to to treat ulcers (sores on the lining of the stomach or small intestine); gastroesophageal reflux disease [GERD, a condition in which backward flow of acid from the stomach causes heartburn and injury of the esophagus (tube that connects the mouth and stomach)]; and conditions where the stomach produces too much acid, such as Zollinger-Ellison syndrome (tumors in the pancreas or small intestine that cause increased production of stomach acid). Over-the-counter famotidine is used to prevent and treat heartburn due to acid indigestion and sour stomach caused by eating or drinking certain foods or drinks. Famotidine is in a class of medications called H_2 blockers. It works by decreasing the amount of acid made in the stomach.

How should this medicine be used?

Prescription famotidine comes as a tablet and a suspension (liquid) to take by mouth. It is usually taken once daily at bedtime or two to four times a day. Over-the-counter famotidine comes as a tablet, a chewable tablet, and a capsule to take by mouth. It is usually taken once or twice a day. To prevent symptoms, it is taken 15 to 60 minutes before eating foods or drinking drinks that may cause heartburn. Follow the directions on your prescription or the package label carefully, and ask your doctor or pharmacist to explain any part you do not understand. Take famotidine exactly as directed. Do not take more or less of it or take it more often or for a longer time than prescribed by your doctor.

Shake the liquid well for 5 to 10 seconds before each use to mix the medicine evenly.

Swallow the tablets and capsules with a full glass of water.

Thoroughly chew the chewable tablets before swallowing them. Swallow the chewed tablet with a full glass of water.

Do not take more than two tablets, capsules, or chewable tablets of over-the -counter famotidine in 24 hours and do not take over-the-counter famotidine for longer than 2 weeks unless your doctor tells you that you should. If symptoms of heartburn, acid indigestion, or sour stomach last longer than 2 weeks, stop taking over-the-counter famotidine and call your doctor.

Are there other uses for this medicine?

This medication may be prescribed for other uses; ask your doctor or pharmacist for more information.

What special precautions should I follow?

Before taking famotidine,
- tell your doctor and pharmacist if you are allergic to famotidine, cimetidine (Tagamet), nizatidine (Axid), ranitidine (Zantac), or any other medications.
- tell your doctor and pharmacist what prescription and nonprescription medications, vitamins, nutritional supplements, and herbal products you are taking. Be sure to mention any other medications for heartburn. Do not take over-the-counter famotidine with any other prescription or nonprescription medications for heartburn unless a doctor tells you that you should.
- tell your doctor if you have phenylketonuria (PKU, an inborn disease in which mental retardation develops if a specific diet is not followed), and if you have or have ever had trouble swallowing or kidney disease.
- tell your doctor if you are pregnant, plan to become pregnant, or are breast-feeding. If you become pregnant while taking famotidine, call your doctor.

What special dietary instructions should I follow?

Unless your doctor tells you otherwise, continue your normal diet.

What should I do if I forget to take a dose?

If you forget a dose of prescription famotidine, take the missed dose as soon as you remember it. However, if it is almost time for the next dose, skip the missed dose and continue your regular dosing schedule. Do not take a double dose to make up for a missed one.

Over-the-counter famotidine is usually taken as needed. If your doctor has told you to take over-the-counter famotidine regularly, take the missed dose as soon as you remember it. However, if it is almost time for the next dose, skip the missed dose and continue your regular dosing schedule. Do not take a double dose to make up for a missed one.

What side effects can this medicine cause?

Famotidine may cause side effects. Tell your doctor if any of these symptoms are severe or do not go away:
- headache
- dizziness
- constipation
- diarrhea
- fussiness (in babies who take famotidine)

Some side effects can be serious. The following symptoms are uncommon, but if you experience any of them call your doctor immediately:
- hives
- skin rash
- itching
- swelling of the face, throat, tongue, lips, eyes, hands, feet, ankles, or lower legs

- hoarseness
- difficulty breathing or swallowing

Famotidine may cause other side effects. Call your doctor if you have any unusual problems while taking this medication.

If you experience a serious side effect, you or your doctor may send a report to the Food and Drug Administration's (FDA) MedWatch Adverse Event Reporting program online [at http://www.fda.gov/MedWatch/index.html] or by phone [1-800-332-1088].

What storage conditions are needed for this medicine?

Keep this medication in the container it came in, tightly closed, and out of reach of children. Store it at room temperature and away from excess heat and moisture (not in the bathroom). Do not allow the liquid to freeze. Throw away any medication that is outdated or no longer needed, and throw away unused famotidine liquid after 30 days. Talk to your pharmacist about the proper disposal of your medication.

What should I do in case of overdose?

In case of overdose, call your local poison control center at 1-800-222-1222. If the victim has collapsed or is not breathing, call local emergency services at 911.

What other information should I know?

Keep all appointments with your doctor.

Do not let anyone else take your medicine. Ask your pharmacist any questions you have about refilling your prescription.

Dosage Facts
For Informational Purposes

Caution: Do not change your dose, how often you take your medication, or the length of time you are to take it without first talking to your healthcare provider.

The following dosage information was written using medical language for doctors and other healthcare professionals and is provided here for you to check your dosage. The dosage of this drug may differ for different patients. Therefore, always follow your doctor's instructions or the directions on the label. Contact your healthcare provider or pharmacist if you have any questions about the specific dosage of your medication after reviewing this information.

Pediatric Patients

Gastroesophageal Reflux
Treatment of GERD in Infants <3 Months of Age

ORAL:
- 0.5 mg/kg once daily for up to 4 weeks.

- Infants should also be receiving conservative measures (e.g., thickened feedings).

Treatment of GERD in Infants 3 Months to <1 Year of Age

ORAL:
- 0.5 mg/kg twice daily for up to 4 weeks.
- Infants should also be receiving conservative measures (e.g., thickened feedings).

Treatment of GERD in Children 1–16 Years of Age

ORAL:
- 1 mg/kg daily in 2 divided doses (maximum 40 mg twice daily); up to 2 mg/kg daily has been used.
- Individualize duration and dosage based on clinical response and/or gastric or esophageal pH determination and endoscopy.

Treatment of Esophagitis in Children 1- 16 Years of Age

ORAL:
- 1 mg/kg daily in 2 divided doses (maximum 40 mg twice daily); up to 2 mg/kg daily has been used.
- Individualize duration and dosage based on clinical response and/or gastric or esophageal pH determination and endoscopy.

Self-medication for Heartburn in Adolescents ≥12 Years of Age

ORAL:
- 10-mg tablets: 10 mg once or twice daily (maximum 20 mg in 24 hours continuously for 2 weeks) or as directed by clinician.
- Chewable tablets: 10 mg once or twice daily (maximum 20 mg in 24 hours continuously for 2 weeks) or as directed by clinician. Do not swallow whole; chew completely before swallowing.
- 20-mg tablets: 20 mg once or twice daily (maximum 40 mg in 24 hours continuously for 2 weeks) or as directed by clinician.
- Fixed combination of famotidine, calcium carbonate, and magnesium hydroxide (Pepcid® Complete): 1 tablet (10 mg of famotidine) once or twice daily (maximum 2 tablets in 24 hours continuously for 2 weeks). Do not swallow whole; chew completely before swallowing.

Self-medication for Prevention of Heartburn In Adolescents ≥12 Years of Age

ORAL:
- 10-mg tablets: 10 mg once or twice daily (15–60 minutes before ingestion of causative food or beverage); maximum 20 mg in 24 hours continuously for 2 weeks or as directed by clinician.
- 10-mg chewable tablets: 10 mg once or twice daily (15–60 minutes before ingestion of causative food or beverage); maximum 20 mg in 24 hours continuously for 2 weeks or as directed by clinician. Do not swallow whole; chew completely before swallowing.
- 20-mg tablets: 20 mg once or twice daily (10–60 minutes before ingestion of causative food or beverage); maximum 40 mg in 24 hours continuously for 2 weeks or as directed by clinician.

Duodenal Ulcer
Treatment of Duodenal Ulcer in Children 1–16 Years of Age
ORAL:
- 0.5 mg/kg once daily at bedtime or in 2 divided doses daily (maximum 40 mg daily); up to 1 mg/kg daily has been used.
- Individualize duration and dosage based on clinical response and/or gastric or esophageal pH determination and endoscopy.

Gastric Ulcer
Treatment of Gastric Ulcer in Children 1–16 Years of Age
ORAL:
- 0.5 mg/kg once daily at bedtime or in 2 divided doses daily (maximum 40 mg daily); up to 1 mg/kg daily has been used.
- Individualize duration and dosage based on clinical response and/or gastric or esophageal pH determination and endoscopy.

Adult Patients

Gastroesophageal Reflux
Treatment of GERD
ORAL:
- 20 mg twice daily for up to 6 weeks.
- 40 mg once daily at bedtime also has been used, but is less effective and not considered appropriate therapy.

Treatment of Esophagitis
ORAL:
- 20 or 40 mg twice daily for up to 12 weeks.

Self-medication for Heartburn
ORAL:
- 10-mg tablets: 10 mg once or twice daily (maximum 20 mg in 24 hours continuously for 2 weeks) or as directed by clinician.
- Chewable tablets: 10 mg once or twice daily (maximum 20 mg in 24 hours continuously for 2 weeks) or as directed by clinician. Do not swallow whole; chew completely before swallowing.
- Fixed combination of famotidine, calcium carbonate, and magnesium hydroxide (Pepcid® Complete): 1 tablet (10 mg of famotidine) once or twice daily (maximum 2 tablets in 24 hours continuously for 2 weeks). Do not swallow whole; chew completely before swallowing.
- 20-mg tablets: 20 mg once or twice daily (maximum 40 mg in 24 hours continuously for 2 weeks) or as directed by clinician.

Self-medication for Prevention of Heartburn
ORAL:
- 10-mg tablets: 10 mg once or twice daily (15–60 minutes before ingestion of causative food or beverage); maximum 20 mg in 24 hours continuously for 2 weeks or as directed by clinician.
- Chewable tablets: 10 mg once or twice daily (15–60 minutes before ingestion of causative food or beverage); maximum 20 mg in 24 hours continuously for 2 weeks or as directed by clinician. Do not swallow whole; chew completely before swallowing.
- 20-mg tablets: 20 mg once or twice daily (10–60 minutes before ingestion of causative food or beverage); maximum 40 mg in 24 hours continuously for 2 weeks or as directed by clinician.

Duodenal Ulcer
Treatment of Active Duodenal Ulcer
ORAL:
- 40 mg once daily at bedtime, or 20 mg twice daily.
- Healing may occur within 2 weeks in some, and within 4 weeks in most patients; some patients may benefit from an additional 4 weeks of therapy.
- Occasionally may be necessary to continue full-dose therapy for >6–8 weeks.
- Safety and efficacy of continuing full-dose therapy for >8 weeks have not been established.

Maintenance of Healing of Duodenal Ulcer
ORAL:
- 20 mg once daily at bedtime.

Gastric Ulcer
ORAL:
- 40 mg daily at bedtime for up to 8 weeks.
- Complete healing of gastric ulcers usually occurs within 8 weeks.
- Safety and efficacy of therapy for >8 weeks have not been established.

Pathologic GI Hypersecretory Conditions
Zollinger-Ellison Syndrome
ORAL:
- 20 mg every 6 hours. Higher doses administered more frequently may be necessary; adjust dosage according to response and tolerance and continue as long as necessary.
- 20–160 mg every 6 hours generally has been necessary to maintain basal gastric acid secretion at <10 mEq/hour.
- Up to 160 mg every 6 hours, or 800 mg daily in divided doses, has been used in severe disease.

Prescribing Limits

Pediatric Patients

Gastroesophageal Reflux
Treatment of GERD in Infants <1 Year of Age
ORAL:
- Safety and efficacy for >4 weeks not established.

Treatment of GERD without Esophagitis in Children 1–16 Years of Age
ORAL:
- Maximum 40 mg twice daily.

Treatment of Esophagitis (including Erosions, Ulcerations) in Children 1- 16 Years of Age
ORAL:
- Maximum 40 mg twice daily.

Self-Medication For Heartburn in Adolescents ≥12 Years of Age
ORAL:
- Maximum 20 or 40 mg in 24 hours continuously for 2 weeks.

Self-medication for Prevention of Heartburn in Adolescents ≥12 Years of Age
ORAL:
- Maximum 20 or 40 mg in 24 hours continuously for 2 weeks.

Duodenal Ulcer

Treatment of Active Duodenal Ulcer in Children 1–16 Years of Age

ORAL:
• Maximum 40 mg daily.

Gastric Ulcer

Treatment of Gastric Ulcer in Children 1–16 Years of Age

ORAL:
• Maximum 40 mg daily.

Adult Patients

Gastroesophageal Reflux

Treatment of Symptomatic GERD

ORAL:
• Safety and efficacy for >6 weeks not established.

Treatment of Esophagitis

ORAL:
• Safety and efficacy for >12 weeks not established.

Self-medication for Heartburn

ORAL:
• Maximum 20 or 40 mg in 24 hours continuously for 2 weeks.

Self-medication for Prevention of Heartburn

Maximum 20 or 40 mg in 24 hours continuously for 2 weeks.

Duodenal Ulcer

Treatment of Active Duodenal Ulcer

ORAL:
• Safety for >8 weeks not established.

Gastric Ulcer

Short-term Treatment of Active Benign Gastric Ulcer

ORAL:
• Safety and efficacy for >8 weeks not established.

Pathologic GI Hypersecretory Conditions (e.g., Zollinger-Ellison Syndrome)

ORAL:
• Up to 160 mg every 6 hours, or 800 mg daily in divided doses.

Special Populations

Renal Impairment

Pediatric Patients

• Consider dosage adjustment in children with moderate or severe renal impairment.

Adults

• In adults, modify dose and/or frequency of administration to the degree of renal impairment; adverse CNS effects have been reported.

Moderate (Cl_{cr}<50 mL/minute) or Severe (Cl_{cr}< 10 mL/minute)

ORAL:
• Decrease to 50% of usual dosage.
• Alternatively, increase dosing interval to 36–48 hours according to response.

Cl_{cr} of 30–60 mL/minute per 1.48 m²

50% of usual adult dosage has been recommended.

Cl_{cr} < 30 mL/minute per 1.48 m²

25% of usual adult dosage has been recommended.

Famotidine Injection

(fa moe′ ti deen)

Brand Name: Pepcid I.V., Pepcid Premixed in Iso-osmotic Sodium Chloride Injection

About Your Treatment

Your doctor has ordered famotidine to decrease the amount of acid your stomach makes. It is used to treat and prevent ulcers and to treat other conditions in which the stomach makes too much acid. The drug will be either added to an intravenous fluid that will drip through a needle or catheter placed in your vein for at least 15 minutes, once or twice a day, or administered by constant infusion over 24 hours. This medication is sometimes prescribed for other uses; ask your doctor or pharmacist for more information.

Your health care provider (doctor, nurse, or pharmacist) may measure the effectiveness and side effects of your treatment using laboratory tests and physical examinations. It is important to keep all appointments with your doctor and the laboratory. The length of treatment depends on how you respond to the medication.

Precautions

Before administering famotidine,
• tell your doctor and pharmacist if you are allergic to famotidine, cimetidine (Tagamet), nizatidine (Axid), ranitidine (Zantac), or any other drugs.
• tell your doctor and pharmacist what prescription and nonprescription medications you are taking, including vitamins.
• tell your doctor if you have or have ever had kidney or liver disease.
• tell your doctor if you are pregnant, plan to become pregnant, or are breast-feeding. If you become pregnant while taking famotidine, call your doctor.

Administering Your Medication

Before you administer famotidine, look at the solution closely. It should be clear and free of floating material. Gently squeeze the bag or observe the solution container to make sure there are no leaks. Do not use the solution if it is discolored, if it contains particles, or if the bag or container leaks. Use a new solution, but show the damaged one to your health care provider.

It is important that you use your medication exactly as directed. Do not change your dosing schedule without talking to your health care provider. Your health care provider may tell you to stop your infusion if you have a mechanical problem (such as a blockage in the tubing, needle, or catheter); if you have to stop an infusion, call your health care provider immediately so your therapy can continue.

Side Effects

Famotidine may cause side effects. Tell your health care provider if any of these symptoms are severe or do not go away:

- headache
- dizziness
- constipation
- diarrhea

Storage Conditions

- Your health care provider probably will give you a several-day supply of famotidine at a time. If you are receiving famotidine intravenously (in your vein), you probably will be told to store it in the refrigerator or freezer.
- Take your next dose from the refrigerator 1 hour before using it; place it in a clean, dry area to allow it to warm to room temperature.
- If you are told to store additional famotidine in the freezer, always move a 24-hour supply to the refrigerator for the next day's use.
- Do not refreeze medications.

Store your medication only as directed. Make sure you understand what you need to store your medication properly.

Keep your supplies in a clean, dry place when you are not using them, and keep all medications and supplies out of reach of children. Your health care provider will tell you how to throw away used needles, syringes, tubing, and containers to avoid accidental injury.

Overdose

In case of overdose, call your local poison control center at 1-800-222-1222. If the victim has collapsed or is not breathing, call local emergency services at 911.

Signs of Infection

If you are receiving famotidine in your vein or under your skin, you need to know the symptoms of a catheter-related infection (an infection where the needle enters your vein or skin). If you experience any of these effects near your intravenous catheter, tell your health care provider as soon as possible:

- tenderness
- warmth
- irritation
- drainage
- redness
- swelling
- pain

Dosage Facts
For Informational Purposes

Caution: Do not change your dose, how often you take your medication, or the length of time you are to take it without first talking to your healthcare provider.

The following dosage information was written using medical language for doctors and other healthcare professionals and is provided here for you to check your dosage. The dosage of this drug may differ for different patients. Therefore, always follow your doctor's instructions or the directions on the label. Contact your healthcare provider or pharmacist if you have any questions about the specific dosage of your medication after reviewing this information.

Pediatric Patients

General Parenteral Dosage

May administer IV in hospitalized pediatric patients with pathologic hypersecretory conditions, intractable ulcer, or for short-term use when oral therapy is not feasible.

Safety and efficacy have not been established in children <1 year of age.

Treatment of Children 1–16 Years of Age

Individualize duration and dosage based on clinical response and/or gastric or esophageal pH determination and endoscopy.

INTERMITTENT DIRECT IV INJECTION:
- Initially, 0.25 mg/kg (15-minute infusion) every 12 hours (maximum 40 mg daily). Up to 0.5 mg/kg every 12 hours has provided gastric acid suppression.

INTERMITTENT IV INFUSION:
- Initially, 0.25 mg/kg (over not less than 2 minutes) every 12 hours (maximum 40 mg daily). Up to 0.5 mg/kg every 12 hours has provided gastric acid suppression

Gastroesophageal Reflux
Treatment of GERD in Infants <3 Months of Age

IV:
- Safety and efficacy not established.

Treatment of GERD in Infants 3 Months to <1 Year of Age

IV:
- Safety and efficacy not established.

Treatment of GERD in Children 1–16 Years of Age

IV:
- Dosage not established.

Treatment of Esophagitis in Children 1-16 Years of Age

IV:
- Dosage not established.

Adult Patients

General Parenteral Dosage

May administer IV in hospitalized adults with pathologic hypersecretory conditions, intractable ulcer, or for short-term use when oral therapy is not feasible.

Dosage for parenteral administration in patients with GERD has not been established.

INTERMITTENT DIRECT IV INJECTION:
- 20 mg every 12 hours (maximum 40 mg daily).

INTERMITTENT IV INFUSION:
- 20 mg every 12 hours (maximum 40 mg daily).

Pathologic GI Hypersecretory Conditions
Zollinger-Ellison Syndrome

INTERMITTENT IV INFUSION:
- 20 mg every 12 hours. Higher initial dosage may be required; adjust to individual needs and continue as long as necessary.

Prescribing Limits

Pediatric Patients

General Parenteral Dosage
Treatment of Children 1–16 Years of Age

INTERMITTENT DIRECT IV INJECTION:
- Maximum 40 mg daily.

INTERMITTENT IV INFUSION:
- Maximum 40 mg daily.

Adult Patients

General Parenteral Dosage

INTERMITTENT DIRECT IV INJECTION:
- Maximum 40 mg daily.

INTERMITTENT IV INFUSION:
- Maximum 40 mg daily.

Special Populations
Renal Impairment

Pediatric Patients
- Consider dosage adjustment in children with moderate or severe renal impairment.

Adults
- In adults, modify dose and/or frequency of administration to the degree of renal impairment; adverse CNS effects have been reported.

Moderate ($Cl_{cr} < 50$ mL/minute) or Severe ($Cl_{cr} < 10$ mL/minute)

IV:
- Decrease to 50% of usual dosage.
- Alternatively, increase dosing interval to 36–48 hours according to response.

Cl_{cr} of 30–60 mL/minute per 1.48 m²
50% of usual adult dosage has been recommended.

$Cl_{cr} < 30$ mL/minute per 1.48 m²
25% of usual adult dosage has been recommended.

Felbamate
(fel bam′ ate)

Brand Name: Felbatol®

Important Warning

Felbamate may cause a serious blood condition called aplastic anemia. Symptoms of aplastic anemia can start any time you are taking felbamate or for a period of time after stopping to take felbamate. Tell your doctor if you have or have ever had blood problems. Your doctor will probably tell you not to take felbamate. If you experience any of the following symptoms while taking felbamate or after you stop taking felbamate, call your doctor immediately: fever, sore throat, chills, other signs of infection, bleeding, easy bruising, extreme tiredness, weakness, or lack of energy.

Felbamate may cause liver damage. Tell your doctor if you have or have ever had liver disease. Your doctor will probably tell you not to take felbamate. If you experience any of the following symptoms, call your doctor immediately: nausea, extreme tiredness, unusual bleeding or bruising, lack of energy, loss of appetite, pain in the upper right part of the stomach, yellowing of the skin or eyes, and flu-like symptoms.

Keep all appointments with your doctor and the laboratory. Your doctor will order certain tests before, during, and after treatment to check your body's response to felbamate.

Talk to your doctor about the risks of taking felbamate. You will have to sign an informed consent form before starting to take felbamate.

Why is this medicine prescribed?

Felbamate is used to treat certain seizures in adults and children with epilepsy whose seizures have not improved with other treatments. It is used alone or in combination with other medications to treat partial seizures in adults. It is used in combination with other medications to treat partial and generalized seizures in children with Lennox-Gastaut syndrome. Felbamate is in a class of medications called anticonvulsants. It works by decreasing abnormal activity in the brain.

How should this medicine be used?

Felbamate comes as a tablet and a suspension (liquid) to take by mouth. It is usually taken with or without food three or four times a day. Take felbamate at around the same times every day. Follow the directions on your prescription label carefully, and ask your doctor or pharmacist to explain any part you do not understand. Take felbamate exactly as directed. Do not take more or less of it or take it more often than prescribed by your doctor.

Shake the liquid well before each use to mix the medication evenly.

Your doctor will probably start you on a low dose of felbamate and gradually increase your dose every one or two weeks.

Felbamate controls seizures but does not cure them. Continue to take felbamate even if you feel well. Do not stop taking felbamate without talking to your doctor. If you suddenly stop taking felbamate, your seizures may become worse. Your doctor will probably decrease your dose gradually.

Are there other uses for this medicine?

This medication should not be prescribed for other uses; ask your doctor or pharmacist for more information.

What special precautions should I follow?

Before taking felbamate,

- tell your doctor and pharmacist if you are allergic to felbamate; carbamate medications such as rivastigmine (Exelon), methocarbamol (Robaxin), and meprobamate (Miltown); or any other medications.
- tell your doctor and pharmacist what prescription and nonprescription medications, vitamins, nutritional supplements, and herbal products you are taking or plan to take. Be sure to mention any of the following: carbamazepine (Tegretol), phenobarbital (Luminal, Solfoton), phenytoin (Dilantin), oral contraceptives (birth control pills), and valproate (Depacon). Your doctor may need to change the doses of your medications or monitor you carefully for side effects.
- tell your doctor if you have or have ever had any of the conditions listed in the IMPORTANT WARNINGS section or kidney disease.
- tell your doctor if you are pregnant, plan to become pregnant, or are breast-feeding. If you become pregnant while taking felbamate, call your doctor.
- you should know that felbamate may make you drowsy. Do not drive a car or operate machinery until you know how this medication affects you.
- remember that alcohol can add to the drowsiness caused by this medication.

What special dietary instructions should I follow?

Unless your doctor tells you otherwise, continue your normal diet.

What should I do if I forget to take a dose?

Take the missed dose as soon as you remember it. However, if it is almost time for the next dose, skip the missed dose and continue your regular dosing schedule. Do not take a double dose to make up for a missed one.

What side effects can this medicine cause?

Felbamate may cause side effects. Tell your doctor if any of these symptoms are severe or do not go away:

- heartburn
- vomiting
- constipation
- diarrhea
- weight loss
- difficulty falling asleep or staying asleep
- nervousness
- drowsiness
- swelling of the face
- runny nose
- differences in menstrual bleeding

Some side effects can be serious. If you experience any of these symptoms or those listed in the IMPORTANT WARNING section, call your doctor immediately:

- hives
- rash
- itching
- difficulty breathing or swallowing
- rapid or pounding heartbeat

Felbamate may cause other side effects. Call your doctor if you have any unusual problems while taking this medication.

If you experience a serious side effect, you or your doctor may send a report to the Food and Drug Administration's (FDA) MedWatch Adverse Event Reporting program online [at http://www.fda.gov/MedWatch/index.html] or by phone [1-800-332-1088].

What storage conditions are needed for this medicine?

Keep this medication in the container it came in, tightly closed, and out of reach of children. Store it at room temperature and away from excess heat and moisture (not in the bathroom). Throw away any medication that is outdated or no longer needed. Talk to your pharmacist about the proper disposal of your medication.

What should I do in case of overdose?

In case of overdose, call your local poison control center at 1-800-222-1222. If the victim has collapsed or is not breathing, call local emergency services at 911.

Symptoms of overdose may include:

- upset stomach
- rapid heartbeat

What other information should I know?

Do not let anyone else take your medication. Ask your pharmacist any questions you have about refilling your prescription.

Dosage Facts

For Informational Purposes

Caution: Do not change your dose, how often you take your medication, or the length of time you are to take it without first talking to your healthcare provider.

The following dosage information was written using medical language for doctors and other healthcare professionals and is provided here for you to check your dosage. The dosage of this drug may differ for different patients. Therefore, always follow your doctor's instructions or the directions on the label. Contact your healthcare provider or pharmacist if you have any questions about the specific dosage of your medication after reviewing this information.

General Dosage Information

When adding to an existing anticonvulsant regimen, add gradually while reducing the dosage(s) of other anticonvulsant(s).

Pediatric Patients

Lennox-Gastaut Syndrome
Adjunctive Therapy

ORAL:
- Children 2–14 years of age: Initially, 15 mg/kg daily administered in 3 or 4 divided doses. Dosage may be increased by 15 mg/kg daily at weekly intervals to a maximum dosage of 45 mg/kg daily administered in 3 or 4 divided doses.
- As felbamate is added to the anticonvulsant regimen, the dosage(s) of other anticonvulsant(s) must be gradually decreased, initially by at least 20%; further reductions in dosage(s) of concomitant anticonvulsant(s) may be necessary as felbamate dosage is increased.

Partial Seizures With or Without Secondary Generalization

ORAL:
- Adolescents ≥14 years of age should receive dosages recommended for adults.

Adult Patients

Partial Seizures With or Without Secondary Generalization
Monotherapy

ORAL:
- Initially, 1.2 g daily administered in 3 or 4 divided doses. Titrate previously untreated patients under close clinical supervision, increasing dosage in 600-mg daily increments every 2 weeks to 2.4 g daily based on clinical response and thereafter to 3.6 g daily if clinically indicated. Felbamate has not been evaluated systematically as initial monotherapy.

Conversion to Felbamate Monotherapy

ORAL:
- Initially, 1.2 g daily administered in 3 or 4 divided doses. At the same time, reduce the dosage(s) of concomitantly administered anticonvulsant(s) by 33%. At week 2, increase the felbamate dosage to 2.4 g daily while reducing the dosage(s) of other anticonvulsant(s) by up to an additional 33% of their baseline dosage(s). At week 3, increase the felbamate dosage to 3.6 g daily and continue to reduce the dosage(s) of other anticonvulsant(s) as clinically indicated.

Adjunctive Therapy

ORAL:
- Initially, 1.2 g daily administered in 3 or 4 divided doses. Dosage may be increased by 1.2-g daily increments at weekly intervals to a maximum of 3.6 g daily administered in 3 or 4 divided doses.
- As felbamate is added to the anticonvulsant regimen, the dosage(s) of other anticonvulsant(s) must be gradually decreased, initially by at least 20%; further reductions in dosage(s) of concomitant anticonvulsant(s) may be necessary as felbamate dosage is increased.
- More rapid titration of felbamate dosage (e.g., increasing dosage to 3.6 g daily over a 3-day period) occasionally has been employed.

Prescribing Limits

Pediatric Patients

Lennox-Gastaut Syndrome

ORAL:
- Children 2–14 years of age: Maximum 45 mg/kg daily.

Partial Seizures With or Without Secondary Generalization

ORAL:
- Adolescents ≥14 years of age: Maximum 3.6 g daily.

Adult Patients

Partial Seizures With or Without Secondary Generalization

ORAL:
- Maximum 3.6 g daily.

Special Populations

Renal Impairment
- Reduce initial and maintenance dosages by 50%. Adjunctive therapy with drugs that affect plasma felbamate concentrations, especially other anticonvulsants, may warrant further reductions in felbamate daily dosage in patients with renal dysfunction.

Felodipine

(fe loe′ di peen)

Brand Name: Lexxel as a combination product containing Felodipine and Enalapril Maleate, Plendil

Why is this medicine prescribed?

Felodipine is used to treat high blood pressure. It relaxes your blood vessels so your heart does not have to pump as hard.

This medication is sometimes prescribed for other uses; ask your doctor or pharmacist for more information.

How should this medicine be used?

Felodipine comes as a tablet to take by mouth. It is usually taken once a day. Do not crush, chew, or divide felodipine tablets. Follow the directions on your prescription label carefully, and ask your doctor or pharmacist to explain any part you do not understand. Take felodipine exactly as directed. Do not take more or less of it or take it more often than prescribed by your doctor.

Felodipine controls high blood pressure but does not cure it. Continue to take felodipine even if you feel well. Do not stop taking felodipine without talking to your doctor.

Are there other uses for this medicine?

Felodipine is also used sometimes to treat Raynaud's syndrome and congestive heart failure. Talk to your doctor about the possible risks of using this drug for your condition.

What special precautions should I follow?

Before taking felodipine,

- tell your doctor and pharmacist if you are allergic to felodipine or any other drugs.
- tell your doctor and pharmacist what prescription and nonprescription medications you are taking, especially antiseizure medicines such as carbamazepine (Tegretol), phenytoin (Dilantin), and phenobarbital; cimetidine (Tagamet); erythromycin (E.E.S., E-Mycin, others); itraconazole (Sporanox); ketoconazole (Nizoral); ranitidine (Zantac); and vitamins.
- tell your doctor if you have or have ever had heart, liver, or kidney disease.
- tell your doctor if you are pregnant, plan to become pregnant, or are breast-feeding. If you become pregnant while taking felodipine, call your doctor.
- if you are having surgery, including dental surgery, tell your doctor or dentist that you take felodipine.

What special dietary instructions should I follow?

Talk to your doctor about drinking grapefruit juice or eating grapefruit while taking felodipine.

Talk to your doctor before using salt substitutes containing potassium. If your doctor prescribes a low-salt or low-sodium diet, follow these directions carefully.

What should I do if I forget to take a dose?

Take the missed dose as soon as you remember it. However, if it is almost time for the next dose, skip the missed dose and continue your regular dosing schedule. Do not take a double dose to make up for a missed one.

What side effects can this medicine cause?

Felodipine may cause side effects. Tell your doctor if any of these symptoms are severe or do not go away:

- headache
- flushing (feeling of warmth)
- dizziness or lightheadedness
- weakness
- fast heartbeat
- heartburn
- constipation
- enlargement of gum tissue around teeth

If you experience any of the following symptoms, call your doctor immediately:

- swelling of the face, eyes, lips, tongue, arms, or legs
- difficulty breathing or swallowing
- fainting
- rash

If you experience a serious side effect, you or your doctor may send a report to the Food and Drug Administration's (FDA) MedWatch Adverse Event Reporting program online [at http://www.fda.gov/MedWatch/index.html] or by phone [1-800-332-1088].

What storage conditions are needed for this medicine?

Keep this medication in the container it came in, tightly closed, and out of reach of children. Store it at room temperature and away from excess heat and moisture (not in the bathroom). Throw away any medication that is outdated or no longer needed. Talk to your pharmacist about the proper disposal of your medication.

What should I do in case of overdose?

In case of overdose, call your local poison control center at 1-800-222-1222. If the victim has collapsed or is not breathing, call local emergency services at 911.

What other information should I know?

Keep all appointments with your doctor and the laboratory. Your blood pressure should be checked regularly to determine your response to felodipine.

Good dental hygiene decreases the chance and severity of gum swelling. Brush your teeth regularly and schedule dental cleanings every 6 months.

Do not let anyone else take your medication. Ask your pharmacist any questions you have about refilling your prescription.

Dosage Facts
For Informational Purposes

Caution: Do not change your dose, how often you take your medication, or the length of time you are to take it without first talking to your healthcare provider.

The following dosage information was written using medical language for doctors and other healthcare professionals and is provided here for you to check your

dosage. The dosage of this drug may differ for different patients. Therefore, always follow your doctor's instructions or the directions on the label. Contact your healthcare provider or pharmacist if you have any questions about the specific dosage of your medication after reviewing this information.

Pediatric Patients

Hypertension†
Monotherapy

ORAL:
- Initially, 2.5 mg once daily. Increase dosage as necessary up to a maximum dosage of 10 mg once daily.

Adult Patients

Hypertension
Monotherapy

ORAL:
- Initially, 2.5–5 mg once daily. Adjust dosage at approximately monthly intervals (more aggressively in high-risk patients) to achieve BP control.
- Usual dosage: 2.5–10 mg daily. Some experts (JNC 7) state that dosage can be increased to 20 mg daily if necessary and tolerated.

Combination Therapy

ORAL:
- If BP is not adequately controlled by monotherapy with felodipine or enalapril, can switch to fixed-combination tablets (felodipine 5 mg and enalapril 5 mg; felodipine 10 mg and enalapril 10 mg; then felodipine 10 mg and enalapril 20 mg).

Prescribing Limits

Pediatric Patients

Hypertension†

ORAL:
- Maximum 10 mg daily.

Adult Patients

Hypertension

ORAL:
- Maximum 20 mg daily.

Special Populations

Hepatic Impairment
- Usual initial dosage: 2.5 mg daily. Closely monitor BP response with each dosage adjustment.

Geriatric Patients
- Usual initial dosage: 2.5 mg daily. Closely monitor BP response with each dosage adjustment.
- Risk of peripheral edema increased substantially with felodipine dosages >10 mg daily.

† *Use is not currently included in the labeling approved by the US Food and Drug Administration.*

Fenofibrate

(fen oh fye′ brate)

Brand Name: Antara®, Lofibra®, TriCor®, Triglide®

Also available generically.

Why is this medicine prescribed?

Fenofibrate is used with diet changes (restriction of cholesterol and fat intake) to reduce the amount of cholesterol and triglycerides (fatty substances) in your blood. Accumulation of cholesterol and fats along the walls of your arteries (a process known as atherosclerosis) decreases blood flow and, therefore, the oxygen supply to your heart, brain, and other parts of your body. Lowering your blood level of cholesterol and fats may help to prevent heart disease, angina (chest pain), strokes, and heart attacks.

This medication is sometimes prescribed for other uses; ask your doctor or pharmacist for more information.

How should this medicine be used?

Fenofibrate comes as a capsule to take by mouth. It is usually taken once a day with a meal. Follow the directions on your prescription label carefully, and ask your doctor or pharmacist to explain any part you do not understand. Take fenofibrate exactly as directed. Do not take more or less of it or take it more often than prescribed by your doctor.

Continue to take fenofibrate even if you feel well. Do not stop taking fenofibrate without talking to your doctor.

What special precautions should I follow?

Before taking fenofibrate,
- tell your doctor and pharmacist if you are allergic to fenofibrate or any other drugs.
- tell your doctor and pharmacist what prescription and nonprescription medications you are taking, especially anticoagulants ('blood thinners') such as warfarin (Coumadin); HMG-CoA reductase inhibitors (cholesterol-lowering agents) such as lovastatin (Mevacor), pravastatin (Pravachol), and simvastatin (Zocor); cholestyramine (Questran); cyclosporine (Sandimmune, Neoral); and vitamins or herbal products.
- tell your doctor if you have or have ever had heart disease, gallbladder disease, or liver or kidney disease.
- tell your doctor if you are pregnant, plan to become pregnant, or are breast-feeding. If you become pregnant while taking fenofibrate, call your doctor.

What special dietary instructions should I follow?

Eat a low-cholesterol, low-fat diet, which includes cottage cheese, fat-free milk, fish, vegetables, poultry, egg whites, and polysaturated oils and margarines (such as corn, safflower, canola, and soybean oils). Avoid foods with excess fat in them, such as meat (especially liver and fatty meat), egg yolks, whole milk, cream, butter, shortening, pastries, cakes, cookies, gravy, peanut butter, chocolate, olives, potato chips, coconut, cheese (other than cottage cheese), coconut oil, palm oil, and fried foods.

What should I do if I forget to take a dose?

Take the missed dose as soon as you remember it. However, if it is almost time for the next dose, skip the missed dose and continue your regular dosing schedule. Do not take a double dose to make up for a missed one.

What side effects can this medicine cause?

Fenofibrate may cause side effects. Tell your doctor if any of these symptoms are severe or do not go away:

- gas
- headache
- stomach pain
- upset stomach
- dizziness or lightheadedness
- constipation
- fatigue
- runny nose

If you experience any of the following symptoms, call your doctor immediately:

- weakness
- muscle pain or tenderness
- joint pain
- rash
- infection
- flu-like symptoms

If you experience a serious side effect, you or your doctor may send a report to the Food and Drug Administration's (FDA) MedWatch Adverse Event Reporting program online [at http://www.fda.gov/MedWatch/index.html] or by phone [1-800-332-1088].

What storage conditions are needed for this medicine?

Keep this medication in the container it came in, tightly closed, and out of reach of children. Store it at room temperature and away from excess heat and moisture (not in the bathroom). Throw away any medication that is outdated or no longer needed. Talk to your pharmacist about the proper disposal of your medication.

What should I do in case of overdose?

In case of overdose, call your local poison control center at 1-800-222-1222. If the victim has collapsed or is not breathing, call local emergency services at 911.

What other information should I know?

Keep all appointments with your doctor and the laboratory. Your doctor will order certain laboratory tests to check your response to fenofibrate.

Do not let anyone else take your medication. Ask your pharmacist any questions you have about refilling your prescription.

Dosage Facts
For Informational Purposes

Caution: Do not change your dose, how often you take your medication, or the length of time you are to take it without first talking to your healthcare provider.

The following dosage information was written using medical language for doctors and other healthcare professionals and is provided here for you to check your dosage. The dosage of this drug may differ for different patients. Therefore, always follow your doctor's instructions or the directions on the label. Contact your healthcare provider or pharmacist if you have any questions about the specific dosage of your medication after reviewing this information.

General Dosage Information

Monitor lipoprotein concentrations periodically; consider reducing dosage in patients whose serum lipoprotein concentrations fall below the desired target range. Discontinue therapy in patients who fail to achieve an adequate response after 2 months of therapy with the maximum recommended dosage.

Adult Patients

Dyslipidemias
Primary Hypercholesterolemia and Mixed Dyslipidemia

ORAL:
- Antara® micronized capsules: 130 mg daily.
- Lofibra® micronized tablets (or generic equivalents): 160 mg daily.
- Lofibra® micronized capsules (or generic equivalents): 200 mg daily.
- TriCor® tablets: 145 mg daily.
- Triglide® tablets: 160 mg daily.

Hypertriglyceridemia

ORAL:
- Antara® micronized capsules: 43–130 mg daily.
- Lofibra® micronized tablets (or generic equivalents): 54–160 mg daily.
- Lofibra® micronized capsules (or generic equivalents): 67–200 mg daily.
- TriCor® tablets: 48–145 mg daily.
- Triglide® tablets: 50–160 mg daily.
- Adjust dosage at intervals of 4–8 weeks until the desired effect on lipoprotein concentrations is observed.

Prescribing Limits

Adult Patients

Dyslipidemias
Hypertriglyceridemia

ORAL:
- Antara® micronized capsules: Maximum 130 mg daily.
- Lofibra® micronized tablets (or generic equivalents): Maximum 160 mg daily.

- Lofibra® micronized capsules (or generic equivalents): Maximum 200 mg daily.
- TriCor® tablets: Maximum 145 mg daily.
- Triglide® tablets: Maximum 160 mg daily.

Special Populations

Renal Impairment

Dyslipidemias

ORAL:

- Antara® micronized capsules: Initially, 43 mg daily in patients with renal impairment (Cl_{cr} <50 mL/minute).
- Lofibra® micronized tablets (or generic equivalents): Initially, 54 mg daily in patients with renal impairment (Cl_{cr} <50 mL/minute).
- Lofibra® micronized capsules (or generic equivalents): Initially, 67 mg daily in patients with renal impairment (Cl_{cr} <50 mL/minute).
- TriCor® tablets: Initially, 48 mg daily in patients with renal impairment (Cl_{cr} <50 mL/minute).
- Triglide® tablets: Initially, 50 mg daily in patients with renal impairment (Cl_{cr} <50 mL/minute).
- Increase dosage only after evaluating therapeutic response and the effects of the drug on renal function.

Geriatric Patients

- Antara® micronized capsules: Initially, 43 mg daily.
- Lofibra® micronized tablets (or generic equivalents): Initially, 54 mg daily.
- Lofibra® micronized capsules (or generic equivalents): Initially, 67 mg daily.
- TriCor® tablets: Initially, 48 mg daily.
- Triglide® tablets: Initially, 50 mg daily.

Fenoprofen

(fen oh proe′ fen)

Brand Name: Nalfon
Also available generically.

Important Warning

People who take nonsteroidal anti-inflammatory medications (NSAIDs) (other than aspirin) such as fenoprofen may have a higher risk of having a heart attack or a stroke than people who do not take these medications. These events may happen without warning and may cause death. This risk may be higher for people who take NSAIDs for a long time. Tell your doctor if you or anyone in your family has or has ever had heart disease, a heart attack, or a stroke, if you smoke, and if you have or have ever had high cholesterol, high blood pressure, or diabetes. Get emergency medical help right away if you experience any of the following symptoms: chest pain, shortness of breath, weakness in one part or side of the body, or slurred speech.

If you will be undergoing a coronary artery bypass graft (CABG; a type of heart surgery), you should not take fenoprofen right before or right after the surgery.

NSAIDs such as fenoprofen may cause ulcers, bleeding, or holes in the stomach or intestine. These problems may develop at any time during treatment, may happen without warning symptoms, and may cause death. The risk may be higher for people who take NSAIDs for a long time, are older in age, have poor health, or drink large amounts of alcohol while taking fenoprofen. Tell your doctor if you take any of the following medications: anticoagulants ('blood thinners') such as warfarin (Coumadin); aspirin; other NSAIDs such as ibuprofen (Advil, Motrin) and naproxen (Aleve, Naprosyn); or oral steroids such as dexamethasone (Decadron, Dexone), methylprednisolone (Medrol), and prednisone (Deltasone). Also tell your doctor if you have or have ever had ulcers, bleeding in your stomach or intestines, or other bleeding disorders. If you experience any of the following symptoms, stop taking fenoprofen and call your doctor: stomach pain, heartburn, vomiting a substance that is bloody or looks like coffee grounds, blood in the stool, or black and tarry stools.

Keep all appointments with your doctor and the laboratory. Your doctor will monitor your symptoms carefully and will probably order certain tests to check your body's response to fenoprofen. Be sure to tell your doctor how you are feeling so that your doctor can prescribe the right amount of medication to treat your condition with the lowest risk of serious side effects.

Your doctor or pharmacist will give you the manufacturer's patient information sheet (Medication Guide) when you begin treatment with fenoprofen and each time you refill your prescription. Read the information carefully and ask your doctor or pharmacist if you have any questions. You can also visit the Food and Drug Administration (FDA) website (http://www.fda.gov/cder) or the manufacturer's website to obtain the Medication Guide.

Why is this medicine prescribed?

Fenoprofen is used to relieve pain, tenderness, swelling, and stiffness caused by osteoarthritis (arthritis caused by a breakdown of the lining of the joints) and rheumatoid arthritis (arthritis caused by swelling of the lining of the joints). Fenoprofen is also used to relieve mild to moderate pain from other causes. Fenoprofen is in a class of medications called NSAIDs. It works by stopping the body's production of a substance that causes pain, fever, and inflammation.

How should this medicine be used?

Fenoprofen comes as a capsule and a tablet to take by mouth. It is usually taken with a full glass of water three or four times a day for arthritis or every 4-6 hours as needed for pain. Fenoprofen can be taken with meals or milk to reduce stomach upset. Your doctor may also recommend that you take fenoprofen with an antacid to reduce stomach upset. If you take fenoprofen regularly, take it at around the same times every day. Follow the directions on your prescription label carefully, and ask your doctor or pharmacist to explain any part you do not understand. Take fenoprofen exactly as directed. Do not take more or less of it or take it more often than prescribed by your doctor.

If you are taking fenoprofen to relieve the symptoms of arthritis, your symptoms may begin to improve within a few days. It may take 2-3 weeks or longer for you to feel the full benefit of fenoprofen.

Are there other uses for this medicine?

Fenoprofen is also used to treat ankylosing spondylitis (arthritis that mainly affects the spine) and gouty arthritis (attacks of severe joint pain and swelling caused by a build-up of certain substances in the joints). It is also sometimes used to reduce fever. Talk to your doctor about the risks of using this medication to treat your condition.

This medication is sometimes prescribed for other uses; ask your doctor or pharmacist for more information.

What special precautions should I follow?

Before taking fenoprofen,

- tell your doctor and pharmacist if you are allergic to fenoprofen, aspirin or other NSAIDs such as ibuprofen (Advil, Motrin) and naproxen (Aleve, Naprosyn), any other medications, or any of the inactive ingredients in fenoprofen capsules. Ask your pharmacist for a list of the inactive ingredients.
- tell your doctor and pharmacist what prescription and nonprescription medications, vitamins, nutritional supplements, and herbal products you are taking or plan to take. Be sure to mention the medications listed in the IMPORTANT WARNING section and any of the following: angiotensin-converting enzyme (ACE) inhibitors such as benazepril (Lotensin), captopril (Capoten), enalapril (Vasotec), fosinopril (Monopril), lisinopril (Prinivil, Zestril), moexipril (Univasc), perindopril (Aceon), quinapril (Accupril), ramipril (Altace), and trandolapril (Mavik); diuretics ('water pills'); lithium (Eskalith, Lithobid); oral medications for diabetes; methotrexate (Rheumatrex); phenobarbital; phenytoin (Dilantin); and sulfa antibiotics such as sulfisoxazole (Gantrisin) and sulfamethoxazole (in Bactrim, in Septra). Your doctor may need to change the doses of your medications or monitor you carefully for side effects.
- tell your doctor if you have or have ever had the conditions mentioned in the IMPORTANT WARNING section or asthma, especially if you also have frequent stuffed or runny nose or nasal polyps (swelling of the lining of the nose); swelling of the hands, feet, ankles, or lower legs; a hearing impairment; anemia (blood cells do not bring enough oxygen to all parts of the body); or liver or kidney disease.
- tell your doctor if you are pregnant, especially if you are in the last few months of your pregnancy, you plan to become pregnant, or you are breast-feeding. If you become pregnant while taking fenoprofen, call your doctor.
- if you are having surgery, including dental surgery, tell the doctor or dentist that you are taking fenoprofen.
- you should know that this drug may make you drowsy. Do not drive a car or operate machinery until you know how this drug affects you.
- remember that alcohol can add to the drowsiness caused by this drug. Do not drink alcohol while taking this medication.

What special dietary instructions should I follow?

Unless your doctor tells you otherwise, continue your normal diet.

What should I do if I forget to take a dose?

Take the missed dose as soon as you remember it. However, if it is almost time for the next dose, skip the missed dose and continue your regular dosing schedule. Do not take a double dose to make up for a missed one.

What side effects can this medicine cause?

Fenoprofen may cause side effects. Tell your doctor if any of these symptoms are severe or do not go away:
- headache
- nervousness
- drowsiness
- sweating
- constipation
- ringing in the ears

Some side effects can be serious. If you experience any of the following symptoms, or those mentioned in the IMPORTANT WARNING section, call your doctor immediately. Do not take any more fenoprofen until you speak to your doctor.
- blurred vision
- shaking of a part of the body that you cannot control
- unexplained weight gain
- fever
- blisters
- rash
- itching
- hives
- swelling of the eyes, face, lips, tongue, throat, hands, arms, feet, ankles, or lower legs
- hoarseness
- difficulty breathing or swallowing
- yellowing of the skin or eyes

- excessive tiredness
- unusual bleeding or bruising
- lack of energy
- upset stomach
- loss of appetite
- pain in the upper right part of the stomach
- flu-like symptoms
- pale skin
- fast or pounding heartbeat
- cloudy, discolored, or bloody urine
- back pain
- difficult or painful urination

Fenoprofen may cause other side effects. Call your doctor if you have any unusual problems while taking this medication.

If you experience a serious side effect, you or your doctor may send a report to the Food and Drug Administration's (FDA) MedWatch Adverse Event Reporting program online [at http://www.fda.gov/MedWatch/index.html] or by phone [1-800-332-1088].

What storage conditions are needed for this medicine?

Keep this medication in the container it came in, tightly closed, and out of reach of children. Store it at room temperature and away from excess heat and moisture (not in the bathroom). Throw away any medication that is outdated or no longer needed. Talk to your pharmacist about the proper disposal of your medication.

What should I do in case of overdose?

In case of overdose, call your local poison control center at 1-800-222-1222. If the victim has collapsed or is not breathing, call local emergency services at 911.

Symptoms of overdose may include:

- heartburn
- upset stomach
- vomiting
- stomach pain
- dizziness
- unsteadiness or difficulty balancing
- headache
- ringing in the ears
- shaking of a part of the body that you cannot control
- drowsiness
- confusion

What other information should I know?

Do not let anyone else take your medication. Ask your pharmacist any questions you have about refilling your prescription.

Dosage Facts
For Informational Purposes

Caution: Do not change your dose, how often you take your medication, or the length of time you are to take it without first talking to your healthcare provider.

The following dosage information was written using medical language for doctors and other healthcare professionals and is provided here for you to check your dosage. The dosage of this drug may differ for different patients. Therefore, always follow your doctor's instructions or the directions on the label. Contact your healthcare provider or pharmacist if you have any questions about the specific dosage of your medication after reviewing this information.

General Dosage Information

Available as fenoprofen calcium; dosage expressed in terms of fenoprofen.

Attempt to titrate to the lowest effective dosage and shortest duration of therapy.

Pediatric Patients

Inflammatory Diseases
Juvenile Rheumatoid Arthritis†

ORAL:
- Initially, 900 mg/m² daily has been used; increase dosage over 4 weeks to 1.8 g/m² daily.

Adult Patients

Inflammatory Diseases
Rheumatoid Arthritis and Osteoarthritis

ORAL:
- 300–600 mg 3–4 times daily.
- Patients with rheumatoid arthritis may require larger doses than those with osteoarthritis.
- Symptomatic improvement usually begins in a few days, but an additional 2–3 weeks may be needed to determine response.

Acute Gouty Arthritis†

ORAL:
- 800 mg given every 6 hours. Reduce dosage rapidly, depending on patient response.

Pain

ORAL:
- For mild to moderate pain, 200 mg every 4–6 hours as needed.

Fever†

ORAL:
- ≤400 mg as single doses.

Prescribing Limits

Pediatric Patients

Inflammatory Diseases
Juvenile Rheumatoid Arthritis†

ORAL:
- Maximum 1.8 g/m² daily.

Adult Patients

Inflammatory Diseases
Rheumatoid Arthritis and Osteoarthritis

ORAL:
- Maximum 3.2 g daily.

Fever†

ORAL:

- Maximum 400 mg as a single dose.

Special Populations

Hepatic Impairment

- No specific dosage recommendations at this time.

Renal Impairment

- No specific dosage recommendations at this time; contraindicated in patients with significantly impaired renal function.

Geriatric Patients

- No specific dosage recommendations at this time.

† *Use is not currently included in the labeling approved by the US Food and Drug Administration.*

Fentanyl Oral Transmucosal

(fen′ ta nil)

Brand Name: Actiq
Also available generically.

Important Warning

Fentanyl oral transmucosal may cause serious or life-threatening breathing difficulties, which can cause death, especially if not used properly. Fentanyl oral transmucosal should be used only for breakthrough (flare-up) cancer pain that occurs during treatment with a regularly scheduled narcotic (opiate) analgesic for chronic cancer pain. Fentanyl oral transmucosal should not be used to treat short-term pain, including pain from an injury or pain after an operation or medical or dental procedure. Fentanyl oral transmucosal should be used only for people who have already received regularly scheduled narcotic pain medication for at least a week and are narcotic-tolerant. If you are unsure if you are narcotic-tolerant, ask your doctor. Tell your doctor if you have or have ever had breathing difficulties, chronic obstructive pulmonary disease (COPD), or other lung disease. Tell your doctor and pharmacist if you are taking or plan to take any of the following medications or those listed in the SPECIAL PRECAUTIONS section below: amiodarone (Cordarone, Pacerone); aprepitant (Emend); certain antifungals such as fluconazole (Diflucan), itraconazole (Sporanox), ketoconazole (Nizoral), or voriconazole (Vfend); chloral hydrate; cimetidine (Tagamet); clarithromycin (Biaxin, in Prevpac); cyclosporine (Neoral, Sandimmune); diltiazem (Cardi-

zem, Dilacor, Tiazac, others); erythromycin (E.E.S., E-Mycin, Erythrocin); general anesthetics; haloperidol (Haldol); hormonal contraceptives (birth control pills, rings, implants, injections, and patches); lovastatin (Advicor, Altocor, Mevacor); medications for anxiety, depression, or mental illness; medications to control cough, cold, or allergies; medications to control nausea or vomiting; medications to treat HIV/AIDS; muscle relaxants; other narcotic pain medications; nefazodone; phenobarbital; sedatives, sleeping pills, or tranquilizers; troleandomycin (TAO); verapamil (Calan, Covera, Isoptin, Verelan); or zafirlukast (Accolate). Alcohol will add to the drowsiness caused by fentanyl oral transmucosal. Talk to your doctor about drinking alcohol while using fentanyl oral transmucosal. If you have any of the following symptoms, stop using fentanyl oral transmucosal and call your doctor immediately: slow, shallow breathing; extreme drowsiness with slow breathing; difficulty thinking, talking, or walking normally; dizziness; confusion; extreme tiredness; fainting; difficulty awakening; or loss of consciousness.

Fentanyl oral transmucosal contains an amount of narcotic pain medication that can be harmful or fatal to a child. Keep fentanyl oral transmucosal out of the reach of children. Fentanyl oral transmucosal should not be used in children and adolescents younger than 16 years old. Fentanyl oral transmucosal must be stored in a locked storage space. Child-resistant cabinet locks, a temporary storage bottle, and a portable locking pouch (fanny pack) are available from the manufacturer. Ask your doctor to help you obtain these items. Never leave unused or partially used fentanyl oral transmucosal units where children or pets can get to them. Partially used fentanyl oral transmucosal medication units contain enough medication to be harmful or fatal to a child or other adults who have not been prescribed fentanyl. To keep this medication away from children and pets, used or unused medication units must be placed in a child-resistant storage bottle available from the manufacturer until it can be completely destroyed in the sink or toilet, as described below. Carefully read all the child safety warnings contained in the manufacturer's information for the patient.

Talk to your doctor about the risks using this medication.

Why is this medicine prescribed?

Fentanyl oral transmucosal is used to treat breakthrough pain (flare ups) that is uncontrolled by a regularly prescribed narcotic pain medication in people with chronic cancer pain. Fentanyl oral transmucosal is in a class of medications called narcotic (opioid) analgesics. It works to treat pain by changing the way the brain and nervous system respond to pain.

How should this medicine be used?

Fentanyl oral transmucosal comes as a solid dosage unit on a handle to place in the mouth between the cheek and gum. Let this medication dissolve over 15 minutes by sucking on the unit and moving it to each side of the mouth. Pain relief should begin to occur in about 15 minutes after using the medication unit. Finishing the medication too quickly or over a longer period of time will cause less pain relief. Do not eat or drink anything while using fentanyl oral transmucosal. Fentanyl oral transmucosal should be used in addition to a regularly prescribed cancer pain medication as directed by your doctor. Follow the directions on your prescription label carefully, and ask your doctor or pharmacist to explain any part you do not understand. Use fentanyl oral transmucosal exactly as directed. Do not use more of it or use it more often than prescribed by your doctor.

Do not bite or chew fentanyl oral transmucosal.

Your doctor will probably start you on a low dose of fentanyl oral transmucosal and gradually increase your dose to find the dose that will relieve your breakthrough pain. If pain is not relieved, your doctor may allow you to use a second medication unit during the same episode of breakthrough pain. Do not use a second fentanyl oral transmucosal unit unless your doctor tells you that you may. A second dose may be used 15 minutes after the previous dose has been completed (a total of at least 30 minutes from the time the previous dose was started). Call your doctor if two doses of fentanyl oral transmucosal do not control your breakthrough pain; do not use more than two doses in a single pain episode. Keep a record of fentanyl oral transmucosal use over several episodes of breakthrough pain, and tell the doctor how well this medication is relieving your pain. When you and your doctor find a dose that controls your pain, call your doctor if you need to use fentanyl oral transmucosal more than four times a day.

Fentanyl oral transmucosal is used on an as-needed basis to control breakthrough pain. It may take some time to find the appropriate dose and frequency of use for fentanyl oral transmucosal. Do not stop taking your regularly prescribed narcotic pain medication while using fentanyl oral transmucosal.

Fentanyl oral transmucosal may be habit-forming. Do not use a larger dose of fentanyl oral transmucosal, use it more often, or use it for a longer period of time than prescribed by your doctor. Tell your doctor if you or your family drink or have ever drunk large amounts of alcohol, have overused narcotic pain medications, have used street drugs, or have or have ever had depression or mental illness. Call your doctor if you begin to use more medication than you have been prescribed, or if you begin "craving" this medication.

If you suddenly stop using fentanyl oral transmucosal while taking doses on a regular basis, you may have symptoms of withdrawal. Call your doctor if you experience any of these symptoms of withdrawal: restlessness, tearing from your eyes, runny nose, yawning, sweating, chills, feeling that your hair stands on end, muscle aches, large pupils (black circles in the center of the eyes), irritability, anxiety, backache, pain in the joints, weakness, stomach cramps, difficulty falling asleep or staying asleep, upset stomach, loss of appetite, vomiting, diarrhea, fast heartbeat or rapid breathing.

To use fentanyl oral transmucosal:

1. Check the blister package and the handle of the fentanyl oral transmucosal unit to make sure the unit contains the dose of medication you have been prescribed.
2. Use scissors to cut open the blister package containing fentanyl oral transmucosal, and remove the medication unit. Do not use the medication unit if the blister package has been damaged or opened before you are ready to use it, or if the medication is expired. If the medication is expired or damaged, call your pharmacist.
3. Place fentanyl oral transmucosal in your mouth, between your cheek and lower gum, and actively suck on the medication unit. Move the unit around in your mouth, from one side to the other, using the handle. Twirl the handle often.
4. Finish the fentanyl oral transmucosal in about 15 minutes.
5. If you begin to feel dizzy or sick to your stomach before you have finished the medication, remove it from your mouth; dispose of it immediately (as described below) or put it in the temporary storage bottle for later disposal. If you are not finishing the entire medication unit each time you use it, call your doctor, to see if future doses may need to be decreased.

Follow these directions to dispose of fentanyl oral transmucosal:

1. If the medication is completely used (dissolved), throw the handle away in a place that is out of the reach of children or pets.
2. If the handle is not totally clean and there is some medication remaining, place the handle under hot running water until the medication is gone. Then throw away the handle as previously directed.
3. If the handle is not totally clean and you cannot immediately dissolve the medication as described in Step 2, put the medication unit in the temporary storage bottle you received from the manufacturer. Push the medication unit into the opening on top of the storage bottle until it falls completely into the bottle.
4. Empty the temporary storage bottle of any handles and partially used medication units at least once a day, following the steps above.
5. Do not flush entire unused medication units, handles, or blister packages down the toilet.

Ask your pharmacist or doctor for a copy of the manufacturer's information for the patient and ask them any questions you may have about the safe use of fentanyl oral transmucosal.

Are there other uses for this medicine?

This medication may be prescribed for other uses; ask your doctor or pharmacist for more information.

What special precautions should I follow?

Before using fentanyl oral transmucosal,

- tell your doctor and pharmacist if you are allergic to fentanyl, other narcotic pain medications, any other medications, or any of the ingredients in fentanyl oral transmucosal. Ask your pharmacist for a list of the ingredients.
- tell your doctor and pharmacist what other prescription and nonprescription medications, vitamins, and nutritional supplements you are taking or plan to take. Be sure to mention the medications listed in the IMPORTANT WARNING section and any of the following medications: buprenorphine (Buprenex, Subutex, Suboxone); butorphanol (Stadol); carbamazepine (Carbatrol, Epitol, Tegretol); dexamethasone (Decadron, Dexpak); griseofulvin (Fulvicin, Grifulvin, Gris-PEG); nalbuphine (Nubain); naloxone (Narcan); pentazocine (Talwin); phenytoin (Dilantin, Phenytek); rifabutin (Mycobutin); rifampin (Rifadin, Rimactane, in Rifamate). Also tell your doctor or pharmacist if you are taking the following medications or have stopped taking them within the past two weeks: monoamine oxidase (MAO) inhibitors including isocarboxazid (Marplan), phenelzine (Nardil), procarbazine (Matulane), selegiline (Carbex, Eldepryl), and tranylcypromine (Parnate). Your doctor may need to change the doses of your medications or monitor you carefully for side effects.
- tell your doctor what herbal products you are taking, especially St. John's wort.
- tell your doctor if you have or have ever had any of the conditions listed in the IMPORTANT WARNING section or a head injury, a brain tumor, a stroke, or any other condition that caused high pressure inside your skull; loss of consciousness; seizures; slowed heart beat; prostate problems or any other condition that causes difficulty urinating; or kidney or liver disease.
- do not use fentanyl oral transmucosal if you are pregnant or plan to become pregnant. If you become pregnant while using fentanyl oral transmucosal, call your doctor. Do not breast-feed while using fentanyl oral transmucosal.
- if you are having surgery, including dental surgery, tell the doctor or dentist that you are using fentanyl oral transmucosal.
- you should know that fentanyl oral transmucosal may make you drowsy or dizzy. Do not drive a car or operate machinery until you know how this medication affects you.
- you should know that fentanyl oral transmucosal may cause dizziness, lightheadedness, and fainting when you get up too quickly from a lying position. This is more common when you first start using this medication. To avoid this problem, get out of bed slowly, resting your feet on the floor for a few minutes before standing up.

What special dietary instructions should I follow?

Talk to your doctor about eating grapefruit and drinking grapefruit juice while using this medication.

What should I do if I forget to take a dose?

This medication is usually used as needed. If your doctor has told you to use fentanyl oral transmucosal regularly, and you have forgotten to use a dose, use the missed dose as soon as you remember it. However, if it is almost time for the next dose, skip the missed dose and continue your regular dosing schedule. Do not use a double dose to make up for a missed one.

What side effects can this medicine cause?

Fentanyl oral transmucosal may cause side effects, especially during the beginning of treatment. Tell your doctor if any of these symptoms are severe or do not go away:

- drowsiness
- upset stomach
- vomiting
- constipation
- difficulty urinating
- weakness
- headache
- dizziness
- changes in vision
- anxiety
- nervousness
- depression
- elevated mood
- seeing or hearing voices that do not really exist (hallucinating)
- difficulty falling asleep or staying asleep
- decreased alertness
- dry mouth
- dental cavities
- loss of teeth
- gum disease
- sweating
- shaking hands you cannot control
- abnormal muscle contractions

Fentanyl oral transmucosal contains sugar. Dry mouth is associated with the use of narcotic medications and may also add to the risk of dental cavities or tooth decay when using this medication. You should see your dentist regularly to ensure proper dental care while using fentanyl oral transmucosal.

Some side effects can be serious. If you experience any of these symptoms, or those listed in the IMPORTANT WARNING section, call your doctor immediately:

- heart beat that is slower or faster than normal
- fainting
- seizures
- hives
- rash

- itching
- swelling of the face, throat, tongue, lips, eyes, hands, feet, ankles, or lower legs
- hoarseness

Fentanyl oral transmucosal may cause other side effects. Call your doctor if you have any unusual problems while using this medication.

If you experience a serious side effect, you or your doctor may send a report to the Food and Drug Administration's (FDA) MedWatch Adverse Event Reporting program online [at http://www.fda.gov/MedWatch/index.html] or by phone [1-800-332-1088].

What storage conditions are needed for this medicine?

Keep this medication in the blister package it came in, tightly closed, and out of reach of children. Store fentanyl oral transmucosal in a place that is secured with the child-resistant lock provided by the manufacturer. You may keep a small supply of fentanyl oral transmucosal in the portable locking pouch (fanny pack) provided by the manufacturer so that it is nearby for your immediate use. Keep this pouch secured with its lock and out of the reach and sight of children. Store fentanyl oral transmucosal at room temperature and away from excess heat and moisture (not in the bathroom). Do not refrigerate or freeze fentanyl oral transmucosal, or store it inside a car.

If you are no longer using fentanyl oral transmucosal, if you have changed to a different dose unit, or if you have unused fentanyl oral transmucosal in your home, follow these steps to dispose of the medication as soon as possible:

1. Remove all unneeded fentanyl oral transmucosal from the locked storage space.
2. Using scissors, remove one fentanyl oral transmucosal unit from its blister package. Hold it by its handle over the toilet bowl.
3. Using wire-cutting pliers, cut the medicine end off the unit so that it falls into the toilet bowl.
4. Throw away the empty medication unit handle in a place that is out of the reach of children.
5. Repeat Steps 1- 4 for each fentanyl oral transmucosal unit. Flush the toilet twice after 5 medication units have been cut and dropped into the toilet bowl. Do not flush more than 5 medication units at a time.
6. If you need help disposing of fentanyl oral transmucosal that is no longer needed, call your pharmacist or your local Drug Enforcement Administration (DEA) office.

Store fentanyl oral transmucosal in a safe place so that no one else can take it accidentally or on purpose. Keep track of how many medication units are left so you will know if any are missing.

What should I do in case of overdose?

In case of overdose, call your local poison control center at 1-800-222-1222. If the victim has collapsed or is not breathing, call local emergency services at 911.

If an overdose is suspected, the medication unit should be removed from the person's mouth immediately and disposed of properly. If the person is asleep, call their name and shake their arm or shoulder to keep them awake. Contact the numbers listed above for emergency care. Once the emergency situation is taken care of, call the doctor to find out if future doses of fentanyl oral transmucosal should be at a lower dose.

Symptoms of overdose may include:
- drowsiness
- itching, especially around the nose and eyes
- dizziness
- upset stomach
- vomiting
- slowed breathing or stopped breathing

What other information should I know?

Keep all appointments with your doctor.

Fentanyl oral transmucosal contains narcotic pain medication. Do not let anyone else use your medication. Selling or giving away this medication is against the law.

This prescription is not refillable. Be sure to schedule appointments with your doctor on a regular basis so that you do not run out of medication.

Dosage Facts
For Informational Purposes

Caution: Do not change your dose, how often you take your medication, or the length of time you are to take it without first talking to your healthcare provider.

The following dosage information was written using medical language for doctors and other healthcare professionals and is provided here for you to check your dosage. The dosage of this drug may differ for different patients. Therefore, always follow your doctor's instructions or the directions on the label. Contact your healthcare provider or pharmacist if you have any questions about the specific dosage of your medication after reviewing this information.

General Dosage Information

Available as fentanyl and fentanyl citrate; dosage expressed in terms of fentanyl.

Give the smallest effective dose and as infrequently as possible to minimize the development of tolerance and physical dependence.

Reduced dosage is indicated initially in poor-risk patients, in geriatric patients, and in patients receiving other CNS depressants.

Individualize dosage of intrabuccal (transmucosal) lozenges according to the clinical status of the patient, desired therapeutic effect, and age.

Adult Patients

Breakthrough Malignant (Cancer) Pain

BUCCAL (TRANSMUCOSAL) (ACTIQ®):

- Adults who are already being treated with, and are tolerant of, opiates: Initially, 200 mcg for breakthrough episode.
- Prescribe 6 lozenges initially, all of which should be used for various breakthrough episodes before the dose is increased.
- May be necessary to use more than 1 lozenge per episode of breakthrough cancer pain until the appropriate dose is attained; an additional lozenge may be administered 15 minutes after the previous lozenge has been consumed (i.e., 30 minutes after the first lozenge initially was placed in the mouth).
- Maximum of 2 lozenges per breakthrough pain episode may be given, if necessary.
- Increase dose to the next higher available strength after several consecutive breakthrough cancer pain episodes require the use of more than 1 lozenge per episode; again, prescribe only 6 lozenges of the new strength.
- Titration phase: Each new dose should be evaluated over several breakthrough cancer pain episodes (generally 1–2 days) to determine efficacy and tolerability of the drug.
- Once titrated to an adequate dose (average breakthrough pain episode is treated with a single lozenge), the patient should limit consumption to a maximum of 4 lozenges daily.
- If patient requires >4 lozenges daily, reevaluate dosage of opiates used for chronic cancer pain.
- Discontinuance of opiates: Gradually downward taper the dose of the opiate to avoid manifestations associated with abrupt withdrawal.
- Geriatric (>65 years of age) patients have been titrated to an adequate lozenge dose that generally was about 200 mcg lower than the dose required in younger patients.
- Use caution when individually titrating transmucosal dosage in geriatric patients.

Special Populations

Hepatic Impairment

- Exercise caution and reduce initial dosage.

Renal Impairment

- Exercise caution and reduce initial dosage.

Geriatric Patients

- Initial doses should be reduced in geriatric patients; response to initial dosing should be considered in determining subsequent incremental doses.
- Buccal (transmucosal) dosage (Actiq®): Geriatric (>65 years of age) doses generally are about 200 mcg lower than those required in younger patients. Exercise caution during individual dosage titration.

Fentanyl Skin Patches

(fen′ ta nil)

Brand Name: Duragesic®
Also available generically.

Important Warning

Fentanyl skin patches may cause serious or life-threatening breathing difficulties, which can cause death, especially if not used properly. Fentanyl skin patches should be used only for chronic (around the clock, long-lasting) pain that cannot be controlled by the use of other shorter-acting pain medications that are not as strong. Fentanyl skin patches should not be used to treat short-term pain or pain after an operation or medical or dental procedure. Fentanyl is not for occasional (as needed) use. Fentanyl should be used only for people who have already received narcotic (opiate) pain medication for at least a week and are narcotic tolerant. If you are unsure if you are narcotic-tolerant, ask your doctor. Tell your doctor if you have or have ever had breathing difficulties, chronic obstructive pulmonary disease (COPD), or other lung disease. Tell your doctor and pharmacist if you are taking or plan to take any of the following medications or those listed in SPECIAL PRECAUTIONS: amiodarone (Cordarone, Pacerone); certain antifungals such as fluconazole (Diflucan), itraconazole (Sporanox), ketoconazole (Nizoral), and voriconazole (Vfend); aprepitant (Emend); cimetidine (Tagamet); clarithromycin (Biaxin, in Prevpac); cyclosporine (Neoral, Sandimmune); delavirdine (Rescriptor); diltiazem (Cardizem, Dilacor, Tiazac, others); efavirenz (Sustiva); erythromycin (E.E.S., E-Mycin, Erythrocin); fluoxetine (Prozac, Sarafem); fluvoxamine (Luvox); HIV protease inhibitors including atazanavir (Reyataz), indinavir (Crixivan), lopinavir (Kaletra), nelfinavir (Viracept), ritonavir (Norvir, in Kaletra), and saquinavir (Fortovase, Invirase); hormonal contraceptives (birth control pills, rings, and patches); lovastatin (Advicor, Altocor, Mevacor); nefazodone; sertraline (Zoloft); troleandomycin (TAO); verapamil (Calan, Covera, Isoptin, Verelan); and zafirlukast (Accolate). If you have any of the following symptoms, call your doctor immediately: difficulty breathing; extreme drowsiness with slow breathing; difficulty thinking, talking, or walking normally; dizziness; confusion; extreme tiredness; fainting; or loss of consciousness.

Fentanyl skin patches are for use only on skin that is not irritated, broken out, burned, cut, or damaged in any way. Do not use a fentanyl skin patch-

continued on next page

Important Warning (cont'd)

that is cut, damaged, or changed in any way, as this can cause you to receive too much medication, which could cause death.

Fentanyl skin patches can be habit-forming. Tell your doctor if you or your family drink or have ever drunk large amounts of alcohol; have overused opiate (narcotic) pain medications, have used street drugs, or have or have ever had depression or mental illness. Call your doctor if you begin to use more medication than you have been prescribed, or if you begin 'craving' this medication.

Fentanyl skin patches contain a large amount of opiate (narcotic) pain medication. Fentanyl may be used by people who misuse or abuse prescription medications or street drugs. Do not let anyone else use your medication. Keep this medication in a safe place to protect it from theft. Selling or giving away this medication is against the law.

Fentanyl skin patches should not be used in children less than 2 years of age and should be used for children only if they are narcotic-tolerant and 2 years of age or older.

Talk to your doctor about the risks of using this medication.

Why is this medicine prescribed?

Fentanyl skin patches are used to relieve moderate to severe pain that occurs constantly. Fentanyl skin patches contain fentanyl inside.The medication is released from the patch continuously over a period of time and is absorbed through the skin into the bloodstream. Fentanyl is in a class of medications called opiate (narcotic) analgesics. It works to treat pain by changing the way the brain and nervous system respond to pain.

How should this medicine be used?

Fentanyl skin patches are placed on the skin. The patch usually is changed every 3 days. Change your patch at about the same time of day on the days you are supposed to change the patch. Follow the directions on your prescription label carefully, and ask your doctor or pharmacist to explain any part you do not understand. Apply fentanyl patches exactly as directed. Read the patient information that is given to you with your prescription before you start using fentanyl skin patches.

Your doctor may start you on a low dose of fentanyl skin patches and gradually increase your dose, not more often than once every 3 days after the first patch and every 6 days thereafter, based upon your level of pain control. If your pain is not controlled by this medication, call your doctor.

Fentanyl skin patches should never be placed in the mouth, chewed, or swallowed, or used in any way other than directed by your doctor or pharmacist. Do not try to open the patch or allow someone to have your patch (new or used) for this purpose. If the fentanyl gel leaks from the patch at any time, try not to touch the gel as you remove and throw away the patch according to the directions below. If you or a caregiver touch the gel, immediately wash the area with only large amounts of water. Using soap, alcohol, or other cleansers to remove the gel may actually increase the amount of medication that goes through the skin.

Accidental exposure to the medication inside the fentanyl skin patch can cause serious harm. This may occur through transfer of a patch from an adult's body to a child while hugging, accidentally sitting on a patch, accidental exposure of a caregiver's skin to the medication in the patch when applying or removing a patch, or in other ways. If the patch comes off the person for whom it was prescribed and sticks to the skin of another person, take the patch off that person right away, wash the area with water only, and seek immediate medical attention by calling your doctor, emergency room, or the poison control center. Accidental exposure of children to fentanyl skin patches is a medical emergency. It is important to store and handle this medication carefully to prevent accidental exposure to fentanyl skin patches.

Do not apply more than one patch at a time unless your doctor tells you to, and do not apply fentanyl skin patches more often, or for a longer period of time than your doctor tells you to. Do not stop using fentanyl skin patches without talking to your doctor. Your doctor will probably decrease your dose gradually when you are to stop using this medication. If you suddenly stop using fentanyl skin patches or use the patches less often than your doctor told you to, you may have symptoms of withdrawal. Call your doctor if you experience any of these symptoms of withdrawal: restlessness, tearing from your eyes, runny nose, yawning, sweating, chills, feeling that your hair stands on end, muscle aches, large pupils (black circles in the center of the eyes), irritability, anxiety, backache, pain in the joints, weakness, stomach cramps, difficulty falling asleep or staying asleep, upset stomach, loss of appetite, vomiting, diarrhea, fast heartbeat or rapid breathing.

To apply the patch, follow the directions provided by the manufacturer and these steps:

1. Select a clean, dry area of skin on your chest, back, upper arm, or side above the waist. You should choose an area of your body which is flat and hairless. Avoid areas that move a lot, areas where the skin is sensitive, an area of the skin that has been exposed to radiation (x-ray treatment); or an area where you have recently applied a skin patch. If the area is hairy, clip hair as close to the skin as possible with scissors, but do not shave it.
2. Clean the skin area, using only clear water. Pat the skin completely dry. Do not put anything on the skin (including soap, lotion, alcohol, or oil) before applying the patch.
3. Tear open the pouch containing the fentanyl skin patch along the dotted line, starting at the slit. Remove the skin patch from the pouch and peel off the protective liner from the back of the patch exposing the adhesive (sticky) surface. Try not to touch the sticky side.

4. Immediately press the adhesive side of the patch onto the skin with the palm of your hand.

5. Press the patch firmly, for at least 30 seconds. Be sure that the patch sticks well to your skin, especially around the edges.

6. If the patch does not stick well or comes loose after it is applied, tape the edges down to your skin with first aid tape.

7. When you are finished applying the patch, wash your hands promptly with only clear water.

8. Apply each new patch to a different skin area to avoid irritation. Remove the old patch before applying another one.

9. Fold used patches in half with the sticky sides together and flush down a toilet. Used patches may still contain some medication and may be dangerous to children, pets, or adults who have not been prescribed fentanyl skin patches.

If a patch accidentally comes off or if the skin under the patch becomes irritated, remove the patch and replace it with a new one in a different area, following the steps above.

Do not remove a skin patch from its protective pouch or remove the protective backing until just before applying it. Do not use a patch if the pouch or backing has been broken or damaged.

If fentanyl has been prescribed for a person who is unable to think well or for a child, the patch should be placed on his or her upper back so it is less likely that the patch could be removed and put in their mouth.

Are there other uses for this medicine?

This medication is sometimes prescribed for other uses; ask your doctor or pharmacist for more information.

What special precautions should I follow?

Before using fentanyl skin patches,

- tell your doctor and pharmacist if you are allergic to fentanyl, other opiate (narcotic) pain medications, adhesives (glues), any other medications, or any of the ingredients in fentanyl skin patches. Ask your pharmacist for a list of the ingredients.

- tell your doctor and pharmacist what other prescription and nonprescription medications, vitamins, and nutritional supplements you are taking or plan to take. Be sure to mention the medications listed in the IMPORTANT WARNING and any of the following medications: antidepressants; antihistamines; carbamazepine (Carbatrol, Epitol, Tegretol); dexamethasone (Decadron, Dexpak); griseofulvin (Fulvicin, Grifulvin, Gris-PEG); medications for anxiety; medications for cough, cold, or allergies; medications for upset stomach; muscle relaxants; nevirapine (Viramune); other medications for pain; phenobarbital; sedatives; sleeping pills; phenytoin (Dilantin, Phenytek); rifabutin (Mycobutin); rifampin (Rifadin, Rimactane, in Rifamate); or tranquilizers. Also tell your doctor or pharmacist if you are taking the following medications or have stopped taking them within the past 2 weeks: monoamine oxidase (MAO) inhibitors including furazolidone (Furoxone), isocarboxazid (Marplan), phenelzine (Nardil), procarbazine (Matulane), selegiline (Carbex, Eldepryl), and tranylcypromine (Parnate). Your doctor may need to change the doses of your medications or monitor you carefully for side effects.

- tell your doctor what herbal products you are taking, especially St. John's wort.

- tell your doctor if you have or have ever had a head injury, a brain tumor, a stroke or any other condition that caused high pressure inside your skull; seizures; irregular heartbeat; prostate problems or any other condition that causes difficulty urinating; Addison's disease (a condition in which the adrenal gland does not make enough of certain natural substances); gallbladder disease; low blood pressure; paralytic ileus or any other problem which causes blockage of the intestines; or thyroid, heart, liver, or kidney disease.

- tell your doctor if you are pregnant, plan to become pregnant, or are breast-feeding. If you become pregnant while using a fentanyl skin patch, call your doctor. Do not use fentanyl skin patches if you are breast-feeding.

- if you are having surgery, including dental surgery, tell the doctor or dentist that you are using fentanyl skin patches.

- you should know that this drug may make you drowsy. Do not drive a car, operate machinery, or do other possibly dangerous activities until you know how this drug affects you.

- you should know that fentanyl skin patches may cause dizziness, lightheadedness, and fainting when you get up too quickly from a lying position. This is more common when you first start using fentanyl skin patches. To avoid this problem, get out of bed slowly, resting your feet on the floor for a few minutes before standing up.

- remember that alcohol can add to the drowsiness caused by this medication. Do not drink any alcohol while using fentanyl skin patches.

- you should know that fentanyl skin patches may cause constipation (less frequent than usual or hard bowel movements). Talk to your doctor about the use of laxatives or stool softeners to prevent or treat constipation while you are using fentanyl skin patches.

- keep in mind that you should not expose a fentanyl skin patch to direct heat or sunlight, heating pads, electric blankets, sun lamps or tanning beds, hot tubs, saunas, heated water beds, or other heat sources. Heat may increase the amount of fentanyl you receive from the skin patch.

- you should know that if you have a fever the amount of fentanyl that you receive from the skin patch may increase significantly and possibly result in an overdosage of medication. Call your doctor right away if you have a fever higher than 102 °F. Your doctor may need to adjust your dose.

What special dietary instructions should I follow?

Talk to your doctor about eating grapefruit and drinking grapefruit juice while using this medication.

What should I do if I forget to take a dose?

If you forget to apply or change a fentanyl skin patch, apply the patch as soon as you remember it. Be sure to remove a used patch before applying a new patch. Leave the new patch on for the regular period of time prescribed by your doctor (usually 3 days) and then replace it. Do not wear two patches at once unless your doctor has told you to.

What side effects can this medicine cause?

Fentanyl skin patches may cause side effects. Tell your doctor if any of these symptoms or those listed in SPECIAL PRECAUTIONS are severe or do not go away:

- headache
- mood changes
- nervousness
- depression
- difficulty falling asleep or staying asleep
- shaking hands that you cannot control
- pain, burning, tingling, or numbness in the hands or feet
- dry mouth
- hiccups
- stomach pain
- indigestion
- gas
- back pain
- difficulty urinating
- itching
- skin irritation, redness, itching, swelling, or blisters at the area where the patch is worn
- flu-like symptoms
- sore throat

If you experience any of these symptoms or those listed in the IMPORTANT WARNING section, call your doctor immediately:

- heartbeat that is slower or faster than normal
- chest pain
- rash
- seizure

If you experience a serious side effect, you or your doctor may send a report to the Food and Drug Administration's (FDA) MedWatch Adverse Event Reporting program online [at http://www.fda.gov/MedWatch/index.html] or by phone [1-800-332-1088].

What storage conditions are needed for this medicine?

Keep this medication in the protective pouch it came in, tightly closed, and out of reach of children and pets. Store it at room temperature and away from excess heat and mois-ture (not in the bathroom). Do not store fentanyl skin patches inside your car.

Throw away any medication that is outdated or no longer needed by carefully removing the adhesive backing, folding the sticky sides of the patch together (until it sticks to itself), and flushing the patch down the toilet. Throw away the pouch and protective liner in the trash. Wash your hands well with water after throwing away fentanyl patches. Do not put used fentanyl skin patches in a garbage can. Used fentanyl patches still contain some medication after they are removed from the skin.

Store fentanyl skin patches in a safe place so that no one can take it accidentally or on purpose. Keep track of how many patches are left so you will know if any are missing.

What should I do in case of overdose?

In case of overdose, call your local poison control center at 1-800-222-1222. If the victim has collapsed or is not breathing, call local emergency services at 911.

Symptoms of overdose may include:

- difficulty breathing
- extreme sleepiness or tiredness
- difficulty thinking, talking, or walking normally
- small, pinpoint pupils (black circles in the center of the eye)
- faintness
- dizziness
- confusion
- coma

What other information should I know?

Keep all appointments with your doctor.

You may bathe, shower, and swim while wearing a fentanyl skin patch.

This prescription is not refillable. Be sure to schedule appointments with your doctor on a regular basis so that you do not run out of medication if your doctor wants you to continue using fentanyl skin patches.

Dosage Facts
For Informational Purposes

Caution: Do not change your dose, how often you take your medication, or the length of time you are to take it without first talking to your health-care provider.

The following dosage information was written using medical language for doctors and other healthcare professionals and is provided here for you to check your dosage. The dosage of this drug may differ for different patients. Therefore, always follow your doctor's instructions or the directions on the label. Contact your health-care provider or pharmacist if you have any questions about the specific dosage of your medication after reviewing this information.

General Dosage Information

Available as fentanyl and fentanyl citrate; dosage expressed in terms of fentanyl.

Give the smallest effective dose and as infrequently as possible to minimize the development of tolerance and physical dependence.

Reduced dosage is indicated initially in poor-risk patients, in geriatric patients, and in patients receiving other CNS depressants.

When the transdermal system is used concomitantly with other CNS depressants, dosage of one or both drugs should be substantially reduced.

Individualize dosage of transdermal fentanyl according to the clinical status of the patient, desired therapeutic effect, and age and weight; assess dosage at periodic intervals. The most important factor in determining the appropriate dose is the degree of existing opiate tolerance.

Pediatric Patients

Chronic Malignant (Cancer) Pain and Other Chronic Pain

Initial Dose Selection in Patients Being Switched to Transdermal Fentanyl Therapy

TRANSDERMAL:

- Use transdermal system only in children ≥2 years of age who are opiate tolerant. Risk of fatal respiratory depression when administered to patients not already opiate tolerant.
- When selecting the initial transdermal dose, consider the daily dose, potency, and characteristics (e.g., pure or partial agonist activity) of the opiate the patient has been receiving and the reliability of potency estimates, which may vary by route, used to calculate an equivalent transdermal dose. Fatal overdose possible with the first transdermal dose if the dose is overestimated.
- The manufacturers provide specific dosage recommendations for switching opiate-tolerant children ≥2 years of age from certain oral or parenteral opiates to transdermal fentanyl (see Tables 1 and 2); the manufacturers consider these initial dosages of transdermal fentanyl to be conservative estimates. *Do not use the dosage conversion guidelines in Tables 1 and 2 to convert patients from transdermal fentanyl to oral or parenteral opiates, since dosage of oral or parenteral opiates may be overestimated.*
- Alternatively, to convert children ≥2 years of age who currently are receiving other opiate therapy or dosages that are not listed in Table 1 or 2, calculate the opiate analgesic requirements during the previous 24 hours. Then calculate an equianalgesic 24-hour dosage of oral morphine sulfate using Table 3. Finally, calculate the equivalent dose of transdermal fentanyl using Table 4. The manufacturers state that this calculated initial dose of transdermal fentanyl may underestimate dosage requirements in about 50% of patients. However, this conservative initial dosage is recommended to reduce the risk of overdosage with the first dose.
- Use the lowest possible dose providing acceptable analgesia.
- For transdermal doses >100 mcg/hour, apply multiple systems at different sites simultaneously.
- If severe adverse effects (including overdosage) occur, monitor and treat patient for ≥24 hours because of long elimination half-life (17 hours).
- Dosing intervals <72 hours have not been evaluated in chil-

dren and adolescents and cannot be recommended in this population.

- Postpone the initial evaluation of maximum analgesia for ≥24 hours after initiation of therapy because of gradual percutaneous absorption from the initially applied system.
- Many patients are likely to require upward dosage titration. If analgesia is inadequate, dosage may be titrated upward after 72 hours.
- Give supplemental doses of a short-acting opiate as needed during the initial application period and subsequently thereafter as necessary to relieve breakthrough pain.

Dosage Adjustment to Achieve Adequate Analgesia

TRANSDERMAL:

- If analgesia is inadequate after initial application of a transdermal system, dosage may be titrated upward after 72 hours. Initial transdermal dose may be increased after 72 hours based on the daily dose of supplemental opiates during the second and third day after initial application.
- Because subsequent equilibrium with an increased dose may require up to 6 days to achieve, make further upward dose titration based on supplemental opiate requirements no more frequently than every 6 days (i.e., after two 72-hour application periods with a given dose).
- Conversion of supplemental opiate requirements to transdermal dose should be based on a ratio of 45 mg of oral morphine sulfate (during a 24-hour period) to each 12.5-mcg/hour delivery from the fentanyl transdermal system.

Discontinuance of Transdermal Fentanyl Therapy

TRANSDERMAL:

- To convert to another opiate, remove the transdermal system and titrate the dosage of the other opiate according to patient toleration and response.
- It generally takes ≥17 hours for serum fentanyl concentrations to decline by 50% following removal of the system. Symptoms of withdrawal (e.g., nausea, vomiting, diarrhea, anxiety, shivering) may occur in some patients following conversion to another opiate agonist or discontinuance of the fentanyl transdermal system.

Adult Patients

Chronic Malignant (Cancer) Pain and Other Chronic Pain

Initial Dose Selection in Patients Being Switched to Transdermal Fentanyl Therapy

TRANSDERMAL:

- Use transdermal system only in patients who are opiate tolerant. Risk of fatal respiratory depression when administered to patients not already opiate tolerant.
- When selecting the initial transdermal dose, consider the daily dose, potency, and characteristics (e.g., pure or partial agonist activity) of the opiate the patient has been receiving and the reliability of potency estimates, which may vary by route, used to calculate an equivalent transdermal dose. Fatal overdose possible with the first transdermal dose if the dose is overestimated.
- Geriatric, cachectic, or debilitated patients should *not* receive initial transdermal doses >25 mcg/hour unless they currently are receiving a continuous daily opiate dose equivalent to 25 mcg/hour of transdermal fentanyl.
- The manufacturers provide specific dosage recommendations for switching opiate-tolerant patients from certain oral or par-

enteral opiates to transdermal fentanyl (see Tables 1 and 2); the manufacturers consider these initial dosages of transdermal fentanyl to be conservative estimates. *Do not use the dosage conversion guidelines in Tables 1 and 2 to convert patients from transdermal fentanyl to oral or parenteral opiates, since dosage of oral or parenteral opiates may be overestimated.*

Table 1. Transdermal Fentanyl Dose Based on Current Oral Opiate Dosage

Daily Dosage of Oral Opiate (in mg/day)	Transdermal Fentanyl (in mcg/hr)
Morphine sulfate	
60–134	25
135–224	50
225–314	75
315–404	100
Oxycodone hydrochloride	
30–67	25
67.5–112	50
112.5–157	75
157.5–202	100
Codeine phosphate	
150–447	25
448–747	50
748–1047	75
1048–1347	100
Hydromorphone hydrochloride	
8–17	25
17.1–28	50
28.1–39	75
39.1–51	100
Methadone hydrochloride	
20–44	25
45–74	50
75–104	75
105–134	100

Table 2. Transdermal Fentanyl Dose Based on Current Parenteral Opiate Dosage

Daily Dosage of Parenteral Opiate (in mg/day)	Transdermal Fentanyl (in mcg/hr)
Morphine sulfate IV/IM	
10–22	25
23–37	50
38–52	75
53–67	100
Oxycodone hydrochloride IV/IM	
15–33	25
33.1–56	50
56.1–78	75
78.1–101	100

Hydromorphone hydrochloride IV	
1.5–3.4	25
3.5–5.6	50
5.7–7.9	75
8–10	100
Meperidine hydrochloride IM	
75–165	25
166–278	50
279–390	75
391–503	100
Methadone hydrochloride IM	
10–22	25
23–37	50
38–52	75
53–67	100

Alternatively, to convert patients who currently are receiving other opiate therapy or dosages that are not listed in Table 1 or 2, calculate the opiate analgesic requirements during the previous 24 hours. Then calculate an equianalgesic 24-hour dosage of oral morphine sulfate using Table 3. Finally, calculate the equivalent dose of transdermal fentanyl using Table 4. The manufacturers state that this calculated initial dose of transdermal fentanyl may underestimate dosage requirements in about 50% of patients. However, this conservative initial dosage is recommended to reduce the risk of overdosage with the first dose.

Use the lowest possible dose providing acceptable analgesia.

For transdermal doses >100 mcg/hour, apply multiple systems at different sites simultaneously.

If severe adverse effects (including overdosage) occur, monitor and treat patient for ≥24 hours because of long elimination half-life (17 hours).

Table 3. Equianalgesic Potency Conversion

| Opiate Agonist | Equianalgesic Dose (in mg) | |
	IM	Oral
Morphine sulfate	10	30 (based on clinical experience with chronic pain) to 60 (based on potency study in acute pain)
Codeine phosphate	130	200
Hydromorphone hydrochloride	1.5	7.5
Levorphanol tartrate	2	4
Meperidine hydrochloride	75	–
Methadone hydrochloride	10	20
Oxycodone hydrochloride	15	30
Oxymorphone hydrochloride	1	10 (rectal)

Doses in Table 3 are considered equivalent to 10 mg of IM morphine sulfate.

Equivalencies were based on single-dose studies comparing IM doses of these drugs, and oral doses are those recommended when changing from IM to oral therapy with each drug.

Table 4. Transdermal Fentanyl Dose Based on Daily Morphine Equivalence

Oral 24-hr Morphine (in mg/day)	Transdermal Fentanyl (in mcg/hr)
60–134	25
135–224	50
225–314	75
315–404	100
405–494	125
495–584	150
585–674	175
675–764	200
765–854	225
855–944	250
945–1034	275
1035–1124	300

Postpone the initial evaluation of maximum analgesia for ≥24 hours because of gradual percutaneous absorption from the initially applied system.

Many patients are likely to require upward dosage titration. If analgesia is inadequate, dosage may be titrated upward after 72 hours.

Give supplemental doses of a short-acting opiate as needed during the initial application period and subsequently thereafter as necessary to relieve breakthrough pain.

Dosage Adjustment to Achieve Adequate Analgesia

TRANSDERMAL:

- If analgesia is inadequate after initial application of a transdermal system, dosage may be titrated upward after 72 hours. Initial transdermal dose may be increased after 72 hours based on the daily dose of supplemental opiates during the second and third day after initial application.
- Because subsequent equilibrium with an increased dose may require up to 6 days to achieve, make further upward dose titration based on supplemental opiate requirements no more frequently than every 6 days (i.e., after two 72-hour application periods with a given dose).
- Conversion of supplemental opiate requirements to transdermal dose should be based on a ratio of 45 mg of oral morphine sulfate (during a 24-hour period) to each 12.5-mcg/hour delivery from the fentanyl transdermal system.
- Most patients are maintained adequately with transdermal systems applied at 72-hour intervals; however, some may require application of the systems at 48-hour intervals to maintain adequate analgesia. Before shortening the dosing interval for inadequate response to a given dose, evaluate a dose increase so that patients can be maintained on a 72-hour regimen if possible.

Discontinuance of Transdermal Fentanyl Therapy

TRANSDERMAL:

- To convert to another opiate, remove the transdermal system and titrate the dosage of the other opiate according to patient toleration and response.
- It generally takes ≥17 hours for serum fentanyl concentrations to decline by 50% following removal of the system. Symptoms of withdrawal (e.g., nausea, vomiting, diarrhea, anxiety, shivering) may occur in some patients following conversion to another opiate agonist or discontinuance of the fentanyl transdermal system.

Special Populations

Hepatic Impairment

- Exercise caution and reduce initial dosage.

Renal Impairment

- Exercise caution and reduce initial dosage.

Geriatric Patients

- Initial doses should be reduced in geriatric patients; response to initial dosing should be considered in determining subsequent incremental doses.
- Geriatric, cachectic, or debilitated patients should *not* receive initial transdermal doses >25 mcg/hour unless they currently are receiving a continuous daily opiate dose equivalent to 25 mcg of transdermal fentanyl per hour.

Ferrous Sulfate (Iron)

(fer′ us)

Brand Name: Feosol®, Feosol® Caplets, Feostat®, Feratab®, Fer-Gen-Sol® Drops, Fergon®, Fer-In-Sol® Drops, Ferrex®-150, Fe-Tinic® 150, Hemocyte®, Hytinic®, Icar® Pediatric, Ircon®, Mol-Iron®, Nephro-Fer®, Niferex®, Niferex® Elixir, Niferex®-150, Slow FE®

Also available generically.

Important Warning

Accidental overdose of products containing iron is a leading cause of fatal poisoning in children under the age of 6. Keep this product out of the reach of children. In case of an accidental overdose, call your doctor or a poison control center immediately.

Why is this medicine prescribed?

Ferrous sulfate provides the iron needed by the body to produce red blood cells. It is used to treat or prevent iron-deficiency anemia, a condition that occurs when the body has too few red blood cells because of pregnancy, poor diet, excess bleeding, or other medical problems.

This medication is sometimes prescribed for other uses; ask your doctor or pharmacist for more information.

How should this medicine be used?

Ferrous sulfate comes in regular, coated, and extended-release (long-acting) tablets; regular and extended-release capsules; and oral liquid (syrup, drops, and elixir). Ferrous sulfate usually is taken three times a day between meals. Follow the directions on your prescription label carefully, and ask your doctor or pharmacist to explain any part you do not understand. Take ferrous sulfate exactly as directed. Do not take more or less of it or take it more often than prescribed by your doctor.

Although symptoms of iron deficiency usually improve within a few days, you may have to take ferrous sulfate for 6 months if you have severe iron deficiency.

This medication should be taken on an empty stomach, at least 1 hour before or 2 hours after eating.

Ferrous sulfate drops come with a special dropper for measuring the dose. Ask your pharmacist to show you how to use it. The drops may be placed directly in the mouth or mixed with water or fruit juice (not with milk).

Do not crush or chew regular, coated, or extended-release tablets, and do not open regular or extended-release capsules; swallow them whole.

What special precautions should I follow?

Before taking ferrous sulfate,
- tell your doctor and pharmacist if you are allergic to ferrous sulfate, tartrazine (a yellow dye in some processed foods and drugs), or any other drugs.
- tell your doctor and pharmacist what prescription and nonprescription medications you are taking, especially chloramphenicol, cimetidine (Tagamet), levodopa (Larodopa, Sinemet), methyldopa (Aldomet), penicillamine, and vitamins. If you also are taking cinoxacin (Cinobac), ciprofloxacin (Cipro), demeclocycline, doxycycline, enoxacin (Penetrex), levofloxacin (Levaquin), lomefloxacin (Maxaquin), methacycline, minocycline, nalidixic acid (NegGram), norfloxacin (Noroxin), ofloxacin (Floxin), oxytetracycline, sparfloxacin (Zagam), or tetracycline, take it 3 hours after or 2 hours before taking ferrous sulfate. Do not take antacids at the same time as ferrous sulfate; take them as far apart as possible.
- tell your doctor if you have or have ever had ulcers, colitis, or intestinal disease.
- tell your doctor if you are pregnant, plan to become pregnant, or are breast-feeding. If you become pregnant while taking ferrous sulfate, call your doctor.

What special dietary instructions should I follow?

Fish, meat (especially liver), and fortified cereals and breads are good dietary sources of iron; emphasize them in a well-balanced diet.

What should I do if I forget to take a dose?

Take the missed dose as soon as you remember it. However, if it is almost time for the next dose, skip the missed dose and continue your regular dosing schedule. Do not take a double dose to make up for a missed one.

What side effects can this medicine cause?

Ferrous sulfate may cause side effects. Your stools will turn dark; this effect is harmless. Your teeth may stain from the liquid; mix each dose with water or fruit juice. You may clean your teeth once a week by rubbing them with a small amount of baking soda.

Tell your doctor if either of these symptoms is severe or does not go away:
- constipation
- stomach upset

If you experience a serious side effect, you or your doctor may send a report to the Food and Drug Administration's (FDA) MedWatch Adverse Event Reporting program online [at http://www.fda.gov/MedWatch/index.html] or by phone [1-800-332-1088].

What storage conditions are needed for this medicine?

Keep this medication in the container it came in, tightly closed, and out of reach of children. Store it at room temperature and away from excess heat and moisture (not in the bathroom). Throw away any medication that is outdated or no longer needed. Talk to your pharmacist about the proper disposal of your medication.

What should I do in case of overdose?

In case of overdose, call your local poison control center at 1-800-222-1222. If the victim has collapsed or is not breathing, call local emergency services at 911.

What other information should I know?

Keep all appointments with your doctor and the laboratory. Your doctor will order certain lab tests to check your response to ferrous sulfate.

Do not let anyone else take your medication. Ask your pharmacist any questions you have about refilling your prescription.

Dosage Facts
For Informational Purposes

Caution: Do not change your dose, how often you take your medication, or the length of time you are to take it without first talking to your healthcare provider.

The following dosage information was written using medical language for doctors® and other healthcare pro-

fessionals and is provided here for you to check your dosage. The dosage of this drug may differ for different patients. Therefore, always follow your doctor's instructions or the directions on the label. Contact your healthcare provider or pharmacist if you have any questions about the specific dosage of your medication after reviewing this information.

General Dosage Information

Dosage expressed in terms of elemental iron.
Do not exceed recommended dosage.

Table 1. Approximate Elemental Iron Content of Various Oral Iron Preparations

Drug	Elemental Iron
Ferric pyrophosphate	120 mg/g
Ferrous gluconate	120 mg/g
Ferrous sulfate	200 mg/g
Ferrous sulfate, dried	300 mg/g
Ferrous fumarate	330 mg/g
Ferrous carbonate, anhydrous	480 mg/g
Carbonyl iron	1000 mg/g[a]

[a]Carbonyl iron is elemental iron, not an iron salt.

Pediatric Patients

Iron Deficiency Anemia
Prevention

ORAL:
- Premature or low-birthweight infants: 2–4 mg/kg daily starting preferably at 1 month, but at least by 2 months, of age. Do not exceed 15 mg daily.
- Normal full-term infants who are not breast-fed or are only partially breast-fed: 1 mg/kg daily, preferably as iron-fortified formula, starting at birth and continuing during the first year of life. Do not exceed 15 mg daily.
- Children ≥10 years of age who have begun their pubertal growth spurt may require daily iron supplementation of 2 or 5 mg daily in males or females, respectively.

Table 2. Recommended Dietary Allowance (RDA)/Adequate Intake (AI) of Iron for Pediatric Patients

Age	RDA[sect] (mg/day)	AI* (mg/day)
Infants 0–6 months of age		0.27
Infants 7–12 months of age	11	
Children 1–3 years of age	7	
Children 4–8 years of age	10	
Children 9–13 years of age	8	
Children 14–18 years of age	Boys: 11 Girls: 15	

§Based on the need to maintain a normal functional iron concentration but only minimal stores, RDA is the *goal* for dietary intake in individuals.
*Established for infants through 6 months of age based on the observed mean iron intake of infants fed principally human milk.

Treatment

ORAL:
- Children: 3–6 mg/kg daily in 3 divided doses.
- If a satisfactory response is not noted after 3 weeks of oral iron therapy, consideration should be given to the possibilities of patient noncompliance, simultaneous blood loss, additional complicating factors, or incorrect diagnosis.

Adult Patients

Iron Deficiency Anemia
Prevention

ORAL:
- RDA for healthy men of all ages (≥19 years of age) is 8 mg daily.
- RDA for healthy women 19–50 years of age is 18 mg daily, and RDA for healthy women ≥51 years of age is 8 mg daily.

Treatment

ORAL:
- Usual therapeutic dosage: 50–100 mg 3 times daily. Smaller dosages (e.g., 60–120 mg daily) also recommended if patients are intolerant of oral iron, but the possibility that iron stores will be replenished at a slower rate should be considered.
- If a satisfactory response is not noted after 3 weeks of oral iron therapy, consider possibility of patient noncompliance, simultaneous blood loss, additional complicating factors, or incorrect diagnosis.
- Normal hemoglobin values usually obtained in 2 months unless blood loss continues. In severe deficiencies, continue iron therapy for approximately 6 months.

Special Populations

Renal Impairment

Iron Deficiency Anemia
Anemia of Chronic Renal Failure in Hemodialysis Patients Receiving Epoetin Alfa

ORAL:
- Children: 2–3 mg/kg daily in 2 or 3 divided doses.
- Adults: ≥200 mg daily in 2 or 3 divided doses.

Pregnant Women
- RDA for pregnant women 14–50 years of age is 27 mg daily.

Lactating Women
- RDA for lactating women 14–18 or 19–50 years of age is 10 or 9 mg daily, respectively.

Fexofenadine

(fex oh fen′ a deen)

Brand Name: Allegra®

Why is this medicine prescribed?

Fexofenadine is used to relieve the allergy symptoms of seasonal allergic rhinitis ('hay fever'), including runny nose; sneezing; red, itchy, or watery eyes; or itching of the nose, throat, or roof of the mouth in adults and children 2 years of age and older. It is also used to relieve symptoms of urticaria (hives; red, itchy raised areas of the skin), including itching and rash in adults and children 6 months of age and older. Fexofenadine is in a class of medications called antihistamines. It works by blocking the effects of histamine, a substance in the body that causes allergy symptoms.

How should this medicine be used?

Fexofenadine comes as a tablet and a suspension (liquid) to take by mouth. It is usually taken with water once or twice a day. Fexofenadine will work better if it is not taken with fruit juices such as orange, grapefruit, or apple juice. Take fexofenadine at around the same time(s) every day. Follow the directions on your prescription label carefully, and ask your doctor or pharmacist to explain any part you do not understand. Take fexofenadine exactly as directed. Do not take more or less of it or take it more often than prescribed by your doctor.

Fexofenadine controls the symptoms of seasonal allergic rhinitis and urticaria but does not cure these conditions. Continue to take fexofenadine even if you feel well and are not experiencing these symptoms. If you wait too long between doses, your symptoms may become worse.

Shake the suspension well before each use to mix the medication evenly.

Are there other uses for this medicine?

This medication may be prescribed for other uses; ask your doctor or pharmacist for more information.

What special precautions should I follow?

Before taking fexofenadine,
- tell your doctor and pharmacist if you are allergic to fexofenadine, any other medications, or any of the ingredients in fexofenadine tablets or suspension. Ask your pharmacist for a list of the ingredients.
- tell your doctor and pharmacist what prescription and nonprescription medications, vitamins, nutritional supplements, and herbal products you are taking or plan to take. Be sure to mention either of the following: erythromycin (E.E.S., E-Mycin, Erythrocin) and ketoconazole (Nizoral). Your doctor may need to change the doses of your medications or monitor you carefully for side effects.
- if you are taking an antacid containing aluminum or magnesium (Maalox, Mylanta, others), take the antacid a few hours before or after fexofenadine.
- tell your doctor if you have or have ever had kidney disease.
- tell your doctor if you are pregnant, plan to become pregnant, or are breast-feeding. If you become pregnant while taking fexofenadine, call your doctor.

What special dietary instructions should I follow?

Unless your doctor tells you otherwise, continue your normal diet.

What should I do if I forget to take a dose?

Take the missed dose as soon as you remember it. However, if it is almost time for the next dose, skip the missed dose and continue your regular dosing schedule. Do not take a double dose to make up for a missed one.

What side effects can this medicine cause?

Fexofenadine may cause side effects. Tell your doctor if any of these symptoms are severe or do not go away:
- headache
- dizziness
- diarrhea
- vomiting
- pain in the arms, legs, or back
- pain
- pain during menstrual period
- cough

Some side effects can be serious. If you experience any of these symptoms, call your doctor immediately:
- hives
- rash
- itching
- difficulty breathing or swallowing
- swelling of the face, throat, tongue, lips, eyes, hands, feet, ankles, or lower legs
- hoarseness
- difficulty swallowing or breathing

Fexofenadine may cause other side effects. Call your doctor if you have any unusual problems while taking this medication.

What storage conditions are needed for this medicine?

Keep this medication in the container it came in, tightly closed, and out of reach of children. Store it at room temperature and away from excess heat and moisture (not in the bathroom). Throw away any medication that is outdated or no longer needed. Talk to your pharmacist about the proper disposal of your medication.

What should I do in case of overdose?

In case of overdose, call your local poison control center at 1-800-222-1222. If the victim has collapsed or is not breathing, call local emergency services at 911.

Symptoms of overdose may include:
- dizziness
- drowsiness
- dry mouth

What other information should I know?

Keep all appointments with your doctor.

Do not let anyone else take your medication. Ask your pharmacist any questions you have about refilling your prescription.

Dosage Facts

For Informational Purposes

Caution: Do not change your dose, how often you take your medication, or the length of time you are to take it without first talking to your healthcare provider.

The following dosage information was written using medical language for doctors and other healthcare professionals and is provided here for you to check your dosage. The dosage of this drug may differ for different patients. Therefore, always follow your doctor's instructions or the directions on the label. Contact your healthcare provider or pharmacist if you have any questions about the specific dosage of your medication after reviewing this information.

General Dosage Information

Available as fexofenadine hydrochloride; dosage expressed in terms of the salt.

Fixed-combination preparations available as Allegra-D® 12 Hour and Allegra-D® 24 Hour. Allegra-D® 12 Hour and Allegra-D® 24 Hour tablets contain 60 or 180 mg of fexofenadine hydrochloride, respectively, in an immediate-release layer and 120 or 240 mg of pseudoephedrine hydrochloride, respectively, in an extended-release matrix layer that slowly releases the drug.

Pediatric Patients

Allergic Rhinitis

ORAL:
- Children 6–11 years of age: 30 mg twice daily (as conventional tablets).
- Children ≥12 years of age: 60 mg twice daily or 180 mg once daily (as conventional capsules or tablets).
- Children ≥12 years of age: 60 mg twice daily (as Allegra-D® 12 Hour) or 180 mg once daily (as Allegra-D® 24 Hour).

Chronic Idiopathic Urticaria

ORAL:
- Children 6–11 years of age: 30 mg twice daily (as conventional tablets).
- Children ≥12 years of age: 60 mg twice daily (as conventional capsules or tablets).

Adult Patients

Allergic Rhinitis

ORAL:
- 60 mg twice daily or 180 mg once daily (as conventional capsules or tablets).
- 60 mg twice daily (as Allegra-D® 12 Hour) or 180 mg once daily (as Allegra-D® 24 Hour).

Chronic Idiopathic Urticaria

ORAL:
- 60 mg twice daily (as conventional capsules or tablets).

Special Populations

Hepatic Impairment
- Dosage adjustment not necessary.

Renal Impairment
- Children 6–11 years of age with decreased renal function: 30 mg once daily (as conventional tablets).
- Adults and children ≥12 years of age with decreased renal function: 60 mg once daily (as conventional capsules or tablets or in fixed combination with 120 mg of pseudoephedrine hydrochloride [Allegra-D® 12 Hour]). Avoid use of fixed-combination preparation containing 180 mg of fexofenadine hydrochloride and 240 mg of pseudoephedrine hydrochloride (Allegra-D® 24 Hour) in patients with renal impairment because of possible risk of pseudoephedrine accumulation.

Geriatric Patients
- Select dosage carefully.

Fexofenadine and Pseudoephedrine

(fex oh fen' a deen) (soo doe e fed' rin)

Brand Name: Allegra-D® 12 Hour, Allegra-D® 24 Hour

Why is this medicine prescribed?

The combination of fexofenadine and pseudoephedrine is used in adults and children 12 years of age and older to relieve the allergy symptoms of seasonal allergic rhinitis ('hay fever'), including runny nose; sneezing; congestion (stuffy nose); red, itchy, or watery eyes; or itching of the nose, throat, or roof of the mouth. Fexofenadine is in a class of medications called antihistamines. It works by blocking the effects of histamine, a substance in the body that causes allergy symptoms. Pseudoephedrine is in a class of medications called decongestants. It works by drying up the nasal passages.

How should this medicine be used?

The combination of fexofenadine and pseudoephedrine comes as an extended-release (long-acting) tablet to take by mouth. The fexofenadine and pseudoephedrine 12-hour tablet is usually taken once or twice a day on an empty stomach with water. The fexofenadine and pseudoephedrine 24-hour tablet is usually taken once a day on an empty stomach with water. Fexofenadine and pseudoephedrine will work better if it is not taken with fruit juices such as orange, grapefruit, or apple juice. Take fexofenadine and pseudoephedrine at around the same time(s) every day. Follow the directions on your prescription label carefully, and ask your doctor or pharmacist to explain any part you do not understand. Take fexofenadine and pseudoephedrine exactly as directed. Do not take more or less of it or take it more often than prescribed by your doctor.

Fexofenadine and pseudoephedrine controls the symptoms of seasonal allergic rhinitis but does not cure this condition. Continue to take fexofenadine and pseudoephedrine even if you feel well and are not experiencing these symptoms. If you wait too long between doses, your symptoms may become worse.

Swallow the tablets whole; do not split, chew, or crush them.

Are there other uses for this medicine?

This medication may be prescribed for other uses; ask your doctor or pharmacist for more information.

What special precautions should I follow?

Before taking fexofenadine and pseudoephedrine,

- tell your doctor and pharmacist if you are allergic to fexofenadine (Allegra), pseudoephedrine (Sudafed, in Dimetapp, in Drixoral, others), any other medications, or any of the ingredients in the tablets. Ask your pharmacist for a list of the ingredients.
- do not take fexofenadine and pseudoephedrine if you are taking monoamine oxidase (MAO) inhibitors, including isocarboxazid (Marplan), phenelzine (Nardil), selegiline (Eldepryl), and tranylcypromine (Parnate), or have taken them within the past 14 days.
- tell your doctor and pharmacist what prescription and nonprescription medications, vitamins, nutritional supplements, and herbal products you are taking or plan to take. Be sure to mention any of the following: asthma medications; diet pills; digoxin (Digitek, Lanoxin, Lanoxicaps); erythromycin (E.E.S., E-Mycin, Erythrocin); ketoconazole (Nizoral); medications for high blood pressure such as methyldopa (Aldomet) and reserpine (Serpalan, Serpasil, Serpatabs); and over-the-counter antihistamines, decongestants, or stimulants. Your doctor may need to change the doses of your medications or monitor you carefully for side effects.
- if you are taking an antacid containing aluminum or magnesium (Maalox, Mylanta, others), take the antacid a few hours before or after fexofenadine.
- tell your doctor if you have glaucoma, difficulty urinating, high blood pressure, or coronary artery disease (condition that occurs when the blood vessels of the heart are narrowed by fat or cholesterol deposits). Also tell your doctor if you have had symptoms such as insomnia, dizziness, weakness, shaking of a part of your body that you can not control, or a fast, pounding, or irregular heartbeat after taking adrenergic medications such as phenylephrine (Neo-Synephrine), or epinephrine (Primatene Mist, EpiPen). Your doctor may tell you not to take fexofenadine and pseudoephedrine.
- tell your doctor if you have or have ever had angina (chest pain or pressure), diabetes, a heart attack, hyperthyroidism (an overactive thyroid gland), prostatic hypertrophy (an enlarged prostate), or heart or kidney disease.

- tell your doctor if you are pregnant, plan to become pregnant, or are breast-feeding. If you become pregnant while taking fexofenadine and pseudoephedrine, call your doctor.

What special dietary instructions should I follow?

Caffeine-containing beverages (coffee, tea, sodas, and energy drinks) may increase the restlessness and insomnia caused by pseudoephedrine in sensitive individuals, so you may wish to drink less of these beverages. Talk to your doctor about drinking these beverages while taking this medication.

What should I do if I forget to take a dose?

Take the missed dose as soon as you remember it. However, if it is almost time for the next dose, skip the missed dose and continue your regular dosing schedule. Do not take a double dose to make up for a missed one.

What side effects can this medicine cause?

Fexofenadine and pseudoephedrine may cause side effects. Tell your doctor if any of these symptoms are severe or do not go away:

- headache
- nausea
- stomach pain
- heartburn
- dry mouth
- throat irritation
- back pain
- pale skin

Some side effects can be serious. The following symptoms are uncommon, but if you experience any of them, call your doctor immediately:

- nervousness
- dizziness
- difficulty falling asleep or staying asleep
- weakness
- fear, anxiety, or tenseness
- hallucinating (seeing things or hearing voices that do not exist)
- shaking of a part of your body that you cannot control
- seizure
- fainting
- blurred vision
- hives
- rash
- itching
- difficulty breathing or swallowing
- swelling of the face, throat, tongue, lips, eyes, hands, feet, ankles, or lower legs
- hoarseness
- fast pounding, or irregular heartbeat
- difficulty or pain when urinating

Fexofenadine and pseudoephedrine may cause other side effects. Call your doctor if you have any unusual problems while taking this medication.

What storage conditions are needed for this medicine?

Keep this medication in the container it came in, tightly closed, and out of reach of children. Store it at room temperature and away from excess heat and moisture (not in the bathroom). Throw away any medication that is outdated or no longer needed. Talk to your pharmacist about the proper disposal of your medication.

What should I do in case of overdose?

In case of overdose, call your local poison control center at 1-800-222-1222. If the victim has collapsed or is not breathing, call local emergency services at 911.

Symptoms of overdose may include:
- dizziness
- drowsiness
- dry mouth
- giddiness
- headache
- nausea
- vomiting
- sweating
- thirst
- fast or pounding heartbeat
- chest pain
- difficulty breathing
- difficulty urinating
- muscle weakness or tenseness
- nervousness
- restlessness
- difficulty falling asleep or staying asleep
- hallucinating (hearing voices or seeing things that do not exist)
- seizures
- coma

What other information should I know?

If you are taking fexofenadine and pseudoephedrine 12-hour tablets, you may notice something that looks like a tablet in your stool. This is just the empty tablet shell, and this does not mean that you did not get your complete dose of medication.

Keep all appointments with your doctor.

Do not let anyone else take your medication. Ask your pharmacist any questions you have about refilling your prescription.

Dosage Facts
For Informational Purposes

Caution: Do not change your dose, how often you take your medication, or the length of time you are to take it without first talking to your healthcare provider.

The following dosage information was written using medical language for doctors and other healthcare professionals and is provided here for you to check your dosage. The dosage of this drug may differ for different patients. Therefore, always follow your doctor's instructions or the directions on the label. Contact your healthcare provider or pharmacist if you have any questions about the specific dosage of your medication after reviewing this information.

General Dosage Information

Available as fexofenadine hydrochloride; dosage expressed in terms of the salt.

Fixed-combination preparations available as Allegra-D® 12 Hour and Allegra-D® 24 Hour. Allegra-D® 12 Hour and Allegra-D® 24 Hour tablets contain 60 or 180 mg of fexofenadine hydrochloride, respectively, in an immediate-release layer and 120 or 240 mg of pseudoephedrine hydrochloride, respectively, in an extended-release matrix layer that slowly releases the drug.

Pediatric Patients

Allergic Rhinitis

ORAL:
- Children ≥12 years of age: 60 mg twice daily (as Allegra-D® 12 Hour) or 180 mg once daily (as Allegra-D® 24 Hour).

Adult Patients

Allergic Rhinitis

ORAL:
- 60 mg twice daily (as Allegra-D® 12 Hour) or 180 mg once daily (as Allegra-D® 24 Hour).

Chronic Idiopathic Urticaria

ORAL:
- 60 mg twice daily (as conventional capsules or tablets).

Special Populations

Hepatic Impairment
- Dosage adjustment not necessary.

Renal Impairment
- Adults and children ≥12 years of age with decreased renal function: 60 mg once daily (as conventional capsules or tablets or in fixed combination with 120 mg of pseudoephedrine hydrochloride [Allegra-D® 12 Hour]). Avoid use of fixed-combination preparation containing 180 mg of fexofenadine hydrochloride and 240 mg of pseudoephedrine hydrochloride (Allegra-D® 24 Hour) in patients with renal impairment because of possible risk of pseudoephedrine accumulation.

Geriatric Patients
- Select dosage carefully.

Filgrastim

(fil gra' stim)

Brand Name: Neupogen®

About Your Treatment

Your doctor has ordered the drug filgrastim to help treat your illness. The drug will be infused into a vein or injected under your skin.

This medication is used to:

- decrease the chance of infection in patients with non-myeloid cancers who receive anticancer therapy that lowers white blood cell counts.
- reduce the amount of time the white blood cell counts are low and prevent the consequences of low white blood cell counts in patients with nonmyeloid cancer who receive chemotherapy that destroys bone marrow in preparation for bone marrow transplant.
- mobilize hematopoietic progenitor cells into peripheral blood for collection by leukapheresis.
- decrease the chance and the duration of problems due to low white blood cell counts in patients with congenital, cyclic, and idiopathic neutropenia (low white blood cell counts).

This medication is sometimes prescribed for other uses; ask your doctor or pharmacist for more information.

Filgrastim is in a class of drugs known as growth factors; it promotes the growth of white blood cells which help to fight infections. The length of treatment depends on the types of drugs you are taking, how well your body responds to them, and the type of cancer you have.

Filgrastim also is used to increase white blood cell counts in adults with myelodysplastic syndrome (MDS) and to treat low white blood cell counts in adults with acute leukemia who have received chemotherapy. In patients with human immunodeficiency virus (HIV) infection, filgrastim is used to increase white blood cell counts or to prevent the further lowering of white blood cell counts due to the virus and/or to medication. Filgrastim has been used to increase white blood cell counts in people who do not have cancer but take medications that lower white blood cell counts.

Precautions

Before taking filgrastim,

- tell your doctor and pharmacist if you are allergic to filgrastim or any other drugs.
- tell your doctor and pharmacist what prescription and nonprescription medications you are taking, including vitamins.
- tell your doctor if you have or have ever had heart disease.
- tell your doctor if you are pregnant or breast-feeding. You should not plan to have children while receiving therapy or for a while after treatments. (Talk to your doctor for further details.) Use a reliable method of birth control to prevent pregnancy. Filgrastim may harm the fetus.

Side Effects

Side effects from filgrastim are common and include:

- bone pain
- weakness
- muscle aches
- nausea
- vomiting
- stomach pain

Tell your doctor if the following symptom is severe or lasts for several hours:

- redness, pain, and burning at the injection site

If you experience any of the following symptoms, call your doctor immediately:

- skin rash
- fever
- chills, shaking, or nighttime sweating
- trouble breathing
- early fullness after eating
- drowsiness
- loss of appetite

If you experience a serious side effect, you or your doctor may send a report to the Food and Drug Administration's (FDA) MedWatch Adverse Event Reporting program online [at http://www.fda.gov/MedWatch/index.html] or by phone [1-800-332-1088].

Storage Conditions

Keep this medication in the container it came in, tightly closed, and out of reach of children. Store it in the refrigerator; do not freeze. Throw away any medication that is outdated or no longer needed. Talk to your pharmacist about the proper disposal of your medication.

Overdose

In case of overdose, call your local poison control center at 1-800-222-1222. If the victim has collapsed or is not breathing, call local emergency services at 911.

Special Instructions

- Filgrastim can be taken at home. In that case, your doctor or nurse will instruct you on how to use it. Store filgrastim in the refrigerator. One hour before your dose, remove the medication from the refrigerator to allow it to warm to room temperature. The vial is for one dose only; do not save unused medication for your next dose.

Dosage Facts
For Informational Purposes

Caution: Do not change your dose, how often you take your medication, or the length of time you

are to take it without first talking to your health-care provider.

The following dosage information was written using medical language for doctors and other healthcare professionals and is provided here for you to check your dosage. The dosage of this drug may differ for different patients. Therefore, always follow your doctor's instructions or the directions on the label. Contact your healthcare provider or pharmacist if you have any questions about the specific dosage of your medication after reviewing this information.

Pediatric Patients

Chemotherapy-induced Neutropenia

IV OR SUB-Q:

- Individualize dosage depending on type and dosage of myelosuppressive chemotherapy. Initially, 5 mcg/kg once daily, administered by sub-Q injection, short (15–30 minutes) IV infusion, or continuous sub-Q or IV infusion, for up to 2 weeks or until the ANC reaches 10,000/mm^3 following the expected chemotherapy-induced ANC nadir. Administer the first dose no earlier than 24 hours after administration of chemotherapy. Dosage may be increased in increments of 5 mcg/kg with each chemotherapy cycle, according to the duration and severity of the ANC nadir.

Congenital, Cyclic, and Idiopathic Neutropenias
Congenital Neutropenia

SUB-Q:

- Initially, 6 mcg/kg administered by sub-Q injection twice daily; individualize dosage according to clinical course and neutrophil count.

Cyclic or Idiopathic Neutropenia

SUB-Q:

- Initially, 5 mcg/kg administered by sub-Q injection once daily; individualize dosage according to clinical course and neutrophil count.

Neutropenia Associated with HIV Infection and Antiretroviral Therapy†

SUB-Q:

- Adolescents: 5–10 mcg/kg administered by sub-Q injection once daily for 2–4 weeks.

Adult Patients

Chemotherapy-induced Neutropenia

IV OR SUB-Q:

- Individualize dosage depending on type and dosage of myelosuppressive chemotherapy. Initially, 5 mcg/kg once daily, administered by sub-Q injection, short (15–30 minutes) IV infusion, or continuous sub-Q or IV infusion, for up to 2 weeks or until the ANC reaches 10,000/mm^3 following the expected chemotherapy-induced ANC nadir. Administer the first dose no earlier than 24 hours after administration of chemotherapy. Dosage may be increased in increments of 5 mcg/kg with each chemotherapy cycle, according to the duration and severity of the ANC nadir.

Bone Marrow Transplantation

IV OR SUB-Q:

- Initially, 10 mcg/kg daily, administered by IV infusion over 4 or 24 hours or by sub-Q infusion over 24 hours. Administer the first dose ≥24 hours after cytotoxic chemotherapy and ≥24 hours after BMT. Reduce dosage to 5 mcg/kg daily when the ANC is >1000/mm^3 for 3 consecutive days. Discontinue filgrastim if the ANC remains >1000/mm^3 for an additional 3 consecutive days. If ANC is <1000/mm^3 following discontinuance of filgrastim, reinitiate therapy at 5 mcg/kg daily. If ANC is <1000/mm^3 at any time when the 5-mcg/kg daily dosage is being used, increase dosage to 10 mcg/kg daily and repeat preceding steps.

Peripheral Blood Progenitor Cell Transplantation
Mobilization of Hematopoietic Progenitor Cells

SUB-Q:

- 10 mcg/kg once daily, administered by sub-Q injection or continuous sub-Q infusion, for 6–7 days. Manufacturer recommends that filgrastim be administered for ≥4 days prior to first leukapheresis and be continued until the last leukapheresis is performed. Modify dosage if the leukocyte count increases to >100,000/mm^3.

Administration Following Reinfusion of PBPC Collection

SUB-Q:

- 5–24 mcg/kg daily until a sustainable ANC (≥500/mm^3) is attained.

Congenital, Cyclic, and Idiopathic Neutropenias
Congenital Neutropenia

SUB-Q:

- Initially, 6 mcg/kg administered by sub-Q injection twice daily; individualize dosage according to clinical course and neutrophil count.

Cyclic or Idiopathic Neutropenia

SUB-Q:

- Initially, 5 mcg/kg administered by sub-Q injection once daily; individualize dosage according to clinical course and neutrophil count.

Myelodysplastic Syndromes† and Aplastic Anemia†
Myelodysplastic Syndromes†

IV:

- Dosages of 50–400 mcg/m^2 administered once daily by IV infusion over 30 minutes have been uesd.

SUB-Q:

- Dosages of 0.3–10 mcg/kg administered once daily by sub-Q injection have been used.

Neutropenia Associated with HIV Infection and Antiretroviral Therapy†

SUB-Q:

- 5–10 mcg/kg administered by sub-Q injection once daily for 2–4 weeks.

Prescribing Limits

Pediatric Patients

Chemotherapy-induced Neutropenia

Dosages that increase the ANC to >10,000/mm³ may not result in any additional clinical benefit and may increase the risk of excessive leukocytosis.

Adult Patients

Chemotherapy-induced Neutropenia

Dosages that increase the ANC to >10,000/mm³ may not result in any additional clinical benefit and may increase the risk of excessive leukocytosis.

† Use is not currently included in the labeling approved by the US Food and Drug Administration.

Finasteride

(fi nas′ teer ide)

Brand Name: Proscar®

Why is this medicine prescribed?

Finasteride is used alone or in combination with other medications to treat benign prostatic hypertrophy (BPH, enlargement of the prostate gland). Finasteride improves symptoms of BPH such as frequent and difficult urination and may reduce the chance of acute urinary retention (suddenly being unable to pass urine). It also may decrease the chance of needing prostate surgery. Finasteride is in a class of medications called 5-alpha reductase inhibitors. It works by blocking the body's production of a male hormone that causes the prostate to enlarge.

How should this medicine be used?

Finasteride comes as a tablet to take by mouth. It is usually taken once a day with or without food. Take finasteride at around the same time every day. Follow the directions on your prescription label carefully, and ask your doctor or pharmacist to explain any part you do not understand. Take finasteride exactly as directed. Do not take more or less of it or take it more often than prescribed by your doctor.

Continue to take finasteride even if you feel well. Do not stop taking finasteride without talking to your doctor.

Ask your pharmacist or doctor for a copy of the manufacturer's information for the patient.

Are there other uses for this medicine?

Finasteride is also sometimes used to treat male pattern baldness. Talk to your doctor about the risks of using this drug for your condition.

What special precautions should I follow?

Before taking finasteride,
- tell your doctor and pharmacist if you are allergic to finasteride or any other medications.
- tell your doctor and pharmacist what prescription and nonprescription medications, vitamins, nutritional supplements, and herbal products you are taking or plan to take.
- tell your doctor if you have or have ever had a blockage of urine flow or liver disease.
- you should know that finasteride is only for use in men. If taken by pregnant women, finasteride can cause abnormalities in the male fetus. Women who are or may be pregnant should not touch broken or crushed finasteride tablets.

What should I do if I forget to take a dose?

Take the missed dose as soon as you remember it. However, if it is almost time for the next dose, skip the missed dose and continue your regular dosing schedule. Do not take a double dose to make up for a missed one.

What side effects can this medicine cause?

Finasteride may cause side effects. Tell your doctor if any of these symptoms are severe or do not go away:
- impotence (inability to have or maintain an erection)
- decreased libido (interest in sex)
- decreased volume of ejaculate (amount of semen)

Some side effects can be serious. If you experience any of these symptoms, call your doctor immediately:
- changes in the breasts such as lumps, pain, or nipple discharge

Finasteride may cause other side effects. Call your doctor if you have any unusual problems while taking this medication.

If you experience a serious side effect, you or your doctor may send a report to the Food and Drug Administration's (FDA) MedWatch Adverse Event Reporting program online [at http://www.fda.gov/MedWatch/index.html] or by phone [1-800-332-1088].

What storage conditions are needed for this medicine?

Keep this medication in the container it came in, tightly closed, and out of reach of children. Store it at room temperature and away from excess heat and moisture (not in the bathroom). Throw away any medication that is outdated or no longer needed. Talk to your pharmacist about the proper disposal of your medication.

What should I do in case of overdose?

In case of overdose, call your local poison control center at 1-800-222-1222. If the victim has collapsed or is not breathing, call local emergency services at 911.

What other information should I know?

Keep all appointments with your doctor.

Before having any laboratory test, tell your doctor and the laboratory personnel that you are taking finasteride.

Do not let anyone else take your medication. Ask your pharmacist any questions you have about refilling your prescription.

Talk to your doctor, pharmacist, or other healthcare professional if you have questions about dosing information for your medication.

Flavoxate

(fla vox′ ate)

Brand Name: Urispas®

Why is this medicine prescribed?

Flavoxate is used to relieve painful, frequent, or nighttime urination and urgency that may occur with infections of the prostate, bladder, or kidneys. The drug works by relaxing the muscles involved with urination. However, flavoxate is not an antibiotic; it does not cure infections.

This medication is sometimes prescribed for other uses; ask your doctor or pharmacist for more information.

How should this medicine be used?

Flavoxate comes as a tablet. Flavoxate usually is taken three or four times a day. This drug may be taken with or without food. Follow the directions on your prescription label carefully, and ask your doctor or pharmacist to explain any part you do not understand. Take flavoxate exactly as directed. Do not take more or less of it or take it more often than prescribed by your doctor.

What special precautions should I follow?

Before taking flavoxate,

- tell your doctor and pharmacist if you are allergic to flavoxate or any other drugs.
- tell your doctor and pharmacist what prescription and nonprescription medications you are taking, including vitamins.
- tell your doctor if you have or have ever had glaucoma, ulcers, paralytic ileus, or obstructive disease (blockage) of the stomach, kidneys, or intestines.
- tell your doctor if you are pregnant, plan to become pregnant, or are breast-feeding. If you become pregnant while taking flavoxate, call your doctor.
- if you are having surgery, including dental surgery, tell the doctor or dentist that you are taking flavoxate.
- you should know that this drug may make you drowsy. Do not drive a car or operate machinery until you know how this drug affects you.

- remember that alcohol can add to the drowsiness caused by this drug.

What should I do if I forget to take a dose?

Take the missed dose as soon as you remember it. However, if it is almost time for the next dose, skip the missed dose and continue your regular dosing schedule. Do not take a double dose to make up for a missed one.

What side effects can this medicine cause?

Flavoxate may cause side effects. Tell your doctor if any of these symptoms are severe or do not go away:

- vomiting
- upset stomach
- dry mouth or throat
- blurred vision
- eye pain
- increased sensitivity of your eyes to light

If you experience any of the following symptoms, call your doctor immediately:

- confusion (especially in the elderly)
- skin rash
- fast or irregular heartbeat
- severe dizziness or drowsiness
- sore throat with fever

If you experience a serious side effect, you or your doctor may send a report to the Food and Drug Administration's (FDA) MedWatch Adverse Event Reporting program online [at http://www.fda.gov/MedWatch/index.html] or by phone [1-800-332-1088].

What storage conditions are needed for this medicine?

Keep this medication in the container it came in, tightly closed, and out of reach of children. Store it at room temperature and away from excess heat and moisture (not in the bathroom). Throw away any medication that is outdated or no longer needed. Talk to your pharmacist about the proper disposal of your medication.

What should I do in case of overdose?

In case of overdose, call your local poison control center at 1-800-222-1222. If the victim has collapsed or is not breathing, call local emergency services at 911.

What other information should I know?

Keep all appointments with your doctor.

Do not let anyone else take your medication. Ask your pharmacist any questions you have about refilling your prescription.

Talk to your doctor, pharmacist, or other healthcare professional if you have questions about dosing information for your medication.

Fluconazole

(floo kon' na zole)

Brand Name: Diflucan®

Why is this medicine prescribed?

Fluconazole is used to treat fungal infections, including yeast infections of the vagina, mouth, throat, esophagus (tube leading from the mouth to the stomach), abdomen (area between the chest and waist), lungs, blood, and other organs. Fluconazole is also used to treat meningitis (infection of the membranes covering the brain and spine) caused by fungus. Fluconazole is also used to prevent yeast infections in patients who are likely to become infected because they are being treated with chemotherapy or radiation therapy before a bone marrow transplant (replacement of unhealthy spongy tissue inside the bones with healthy tissue). Fluconazole is in a class of antifungals called triazoles. It works by slowing the growth of fungi that cause infection.

How should this medicine be used?

Fluconazole comes as a tablet and a suspension (liquid) to take by mouth. It is usually taken once a day. You may need to take only one dose of fluconazole, or you may need to take fluconazole for several weeks or longer. The length of your treatment depends on your condition and on how well you respond to fluconazole. Follow the directions on your prescription label carefully, and ask your doctor or pharmacist to explain any part you do not understand. Take fluconazole exactly as directed. Do not take more or less of it or take it more often than prescribed by your doctor.

Your doctor may tell you to take a double dose of fluconazole on the first day of your treatment. Follow these directions carefully.

Shake the liquid well before each use to mix the medication evenly.

Continue to take fluconazole until your doctor tells you that you should stop, even if you feel better. Do not stop taking fluconazole without talking to your doctor. If you stop taking fluconazole too soon, your infection may come back after a short time.

Are there other uses for this medicine?

Fluconazole is also sometimes used to treat serious fungal infections that begin in the lungs and can spread through the body and fungal infections of the eye, prostate (a male reproductive organ), skin and nails. Fluconazole is also sometimes used to prevent fungal infections in people who are likely to become infected because they have human immunodeficiency virus (HIV) or cancer or have had a transplant operation (surgery to remove an organ and replace it with a donor or artificial organ). Talk to your doctor about the possible risks of using this drug for your condition.

This medication may be prescribed for other uses; ask your doctor or pharmacist for more information.

What special precautions should I follow?

Before taking fluconazole,
- tell your doctor and pharmacist if you are allergic to fluconazole, other antifungal medications such as itraconazole (Sporanox), ketoconazole (Nizoral), or voriconazole (Vfend), or any other medications.
- do not take cisapride (Propulsid) while taking fluconazole.
- tell your doctor and pharmacist what prescription and nonprescription medications, vitamins, nutritional supplements, and herbal products you are taking, especially amiodarone (Cordarone); anticoagulants ('blood thinners') such as warfarin (Coumadin); astemizole (Hismanal) (not available in the United States); benzodiazepines such as midazolam (Versed); cyclosporine (Neoral, Sandimmune); disopyramide (Norpace); diuretics ('water pills') such as hydrochlorothiazide (HydroDIURIL, Microzide); dofetilide (Tikosyn); erythromycin (E.E.S, E-Mycin, Erythrocin); isoniazid (INH, Nydrazid); moxifloxacin (Avelox); oral contraceptives (birth control pills); oral medicine for diabetes such as glipizide (Glucotrol), glyburide (Diabeta, Micronase, Glycron, others), and tolbutamide (Orinase); phenytoin (Dilantin); pimozide (Orap); procainamide (Procanbid, Pronestyl); quinidine (Quinidex); rifabutin (Mycobutin); rifampin (Rifadin, Rimactane); sotalolol (Betapace); sparfloxacin (Zagam); tacrolimus (Prograf); terfenadine (Seldane) (not available in the United States); theophylline (TheoDur); thioridazine (Mellaril); valproic acid (Depakene, Depakote); and zidovudine (Retrovir).
- tell your doctor if you drink or have ever drunk large amounts of alcohol and if you have or have ever had cancer; acquired immunodeficiency syndrome (AIDS); an irregular heartbeat; or heart, kidney or liver disease.
- tell your doctor if you are pregnant, plan to become pregnant, or are breast-feeding. If you become pregnant while taking fluconazole, call your doctor.

What special dietary instructions should I follow?

Unless your doctor tells you otherwise, continue your normal diet.

What should I do if I forget to take a dose?

Take the missed dose as soon as you remember it. However, if it is almost time for the next dose, skip the missed dose and continue your regular dosing schedule. Do not take a double dose to make up for a missed one.

What side effects can this medicine cause?

Fluconazole may cause side effects. Tell your doctor if any of these symptoms are severe or do not go away:
- headache
- dizziness

- diarrhea
- stomach pain
- heartburn
- change in ability to taste food

Some side effects can be serious. If you experience any of the following symptoms, call your doctor immediately:

- upset stomach
- extreme tiredness
- unusual bruising or bleeding
- lack of energy
- loss of appetite
- pain in the upper right part of the stomach
- yellowing of the skin or eyes
- flu-like symptoms
- dark urine
- pale stools
- seizures
- rash
- hives
- itching
- swelling of the face, throat, tongue, lips, eyes, hands, feet, ankles, or lower legs
- difficulty breathing or swallowing

If you experience a serious side effect, you or your doctor may send a report to the Food and Drug Administration's (FDA) MedWatch Adverse Event Reporting program online [at http://www.fda.gov/MedWatch/index.html] or by phone [1-800-332-1088].

What storage conditions are needed for this medicine?

Keep this medication in the container it came in, tightly closed, and out of reach of children. Store it at room temperature and away from excess heat and moisture (not in the bathroom). Throw away any medication that is outdated or no longer needed. Throw away any unused liquid medication after 14 days. Talk to your pharmacist about the proper disposal of your medication.

What should I do in case of overdose?

In case of overdose, call your local poison control center at 1-800-222-1222. If the victim has collapsed or is not breathing, call local emergency services at 911.

Symptoms of overdose may include:

- hallucinations (seeing things or hearing voices that do not exist)
- extreme fear that others are trying to harm you

What other information should I know?

Keep all appointments with your doctor and the laboratory. Your doctor may order certain lab tests to check your response to fluconazole.

Do not let anyone else take your medication. Ask your pharmacist if you have questions about refilling your prescription. If you still have symptoms of infection after you finish taking the fluconazole, call your doctor.

Dosage Facts
For Informational Purposes

Caution: Do not change your dose, how often you take your medication, or the length of time you are to take it without first talking to your healthcare provider.

The following dosage information was written using medical language for doctors and other healthcare professionals and is provided here for you to check your dosage. The dosage of this drug may differ for different patients. Therefore, always follow your doctor's instructions or the directions on the label. Contact your healthcare provider or pharmacist if you have any questions about the specific dosage of your medication after reviewing this information.

Pediatric Patients

General Pediatric Dosage
Treatment of Fungal Infections

ORAL:
- 3–12 mg/kg once daily.
- Dosage of 3, 6, or 12 mg/kg daily in pediatric patients is equivalent to dosage of 100, 200, or 400 mg daily, respectively, in adults.
- Based on available pharmacokinetic data in premature neonates, manufacturer recommends that neonates ≤2 weeks of age receive the usual pediatric dosage once every 72 hours; after 2 weeks of age, neonates should receive the usual dosage once daily.

Candida Infections
Treatment of Oropharyngeal and Esophageal Candidiasis

ORAL:
- 6 mg/kg on the first day, followed by 3 mg/kg once daily. Dosage for esophageal candidiasis may be increased up to 12 mg/kg daily if necessary, based on the condition of the patient and the response to the drug.
- Treatment for oropharyngeal candidiasis should be continued for ≥2 weeks to decrease the likelihood of relapse. Treatment of esophageal candidiasis should be continued for ≥3 weeks and for ≥2 weeks after symptoms resolve.

Treatment of Disseminated or Invasive Candida Infections

ORAL:
- 6–12 mg/kg daily.
- Neonates and infants ≤3 months of age†: 5–6 mg/kg once daily has been used for candidal meningitis or septicemia. An initial loading dose of 10 mg/kg followed by 5 mg/kg once daily also has been used for candidal septicemia.

Prevention of Recurrence (Secondary Prophylaxis) of Mucocutaneous Candidiasis†

ORAL:
- HIV-infected infants and children: 3–6 mg/kg once daily recommended by USPHS/IDSA.
- HIV-infected adolescents: 100–200 mg once daily recommended by USPHS/IDSA.
- The safety of discontinuing secondary prophylaxis against

mucocutaneous candidiasis in those receiving potent anti-retroviral therapy has not been extensively studied.

Coccidioidomycosis†
Prevention of Recurrence (Secondary Prophylaxis) of Coccidioidomycosis†

ORAL:
- HIV-infected infants and children: 6 mg/kg once daily recommended by USPHS/IDSA.
- HIV-infected adolescents: 400 mg once daily recommended by USPHS/IDSA.
- Initiate secondary prophylaxis after primary infection has been adequately treated. HIV-infected children and adolescents with a history of coccidioidomycosis should receive life-long suppressive therapy to prevent recurrence; data insufficient to date to warrant a recommendation regarding discontinuance in these patients.

Cryptococcal Infections
Treatment of Cryptococcal Meningitis

ORAL:
- 12 mg/kg on the first day, followed by 6 mg/kg once daily. Dosage may be increased to 12 mg/kg daily if necessary based on condition of the patient and response to the drug. Continue for 10–12 weeks after CSF becomes culture negative.

Prevention (Primary Prophylaxis) of Cryptococcosis†

ORAL:
- HIV-infected infants and children with severe immunosuppression: 3–6 mg/kg once daily recommended by USPHS/IDSA.
- HIV-infected adolescents with CD4+ T-cell counts <50/mm³: 100–200 mg once daily recommended by USPHS/IDSA.

Prevention of Recurrence (Secondary Prophylaxis) of Cryptococcosis†

ORAL:
- HIV-infected infants and children: 3–6 mg/kg once daily recommended by USPHS/IDSA.
- HIV-infected adolescents: 200 mg once daily recommended by USPHS/IDSA.
- Initiate secondary prophylaxis after primary infection has been adequately treated.
- HIV-infected infants and children with a history of cryptococcosis should receive life-long suppressive therapy to prevent recurrence. Consideration can be given to discontinuing secondary prophylaxis in HIV-infected adolescents receiving potent antiretroviral therapy according to recommendations in adults.

Dermatophytoses†
Tinea capitis†

ORAL:
- 3–6 mg/kg daily for 2–6 weeks has been effective in children 1.5–16 years of age.

Adult Patients

Blastomycosis†
Treatment of Blastomycosis†

ORAL:
- 400–800 mg once daily.

Candida Infections
Treatment of Oropharyngeal and Esophageal Candidiasis

ORAL:
- 200 mg given as a single dose on the first day, followed by 100 or 200 mg once daily.
- Up to 400 mg once daily may be used depending on the patient's response.
- Clinical evidence of oropharyngeal candidiasis generally resolves within several days, but the drug usually is continued for ≥2 weeks to decrease the likelihood of relapse.
- Patients with esophageal candidiasis should receive fluconazole for ≥3 weeks and for ≥2 weeks after symptoms resolve.

Treatment of Vulvovaginal Candidiasis

ORAL:
- Uncomplicated infections in nonpregnant women: a single 150-mg dose.
- Severe vulvovaginal candidiasis† (extensive vulvar erythema, edema, excoriation, and fissure formation) in nonpregnant women: a 2-dose regimen (two 150-mg doses given 3 days apart).
- Recurrent vulvovaginal candidiasis† caused by *C. albicans* in nonpregnant women: a 100-, 150-, or 200-mg dose given every 3 days for 3 doses to achieve mycologic remission, then a maintenance regimen of 100, 150, or 200 mg once weekly for 6 months to prevent recurrence.

Treatment of Disseminated or Invasive Candida Infections

ORAL:
- 400 mg given as a single dose on the first day, followed by 200 mg once daily.
- Urinary tract infections or peritonitis: 50–200 mg daily has been used.
- Candidemia, disseminated candidiasis, or pneumonia: up to 400 mg daily has been used. For candidemia, 400–800 mg once daily IV initially, followed by oral fluconazole has been recommended.
- Therapy should be continued for ≥ 4 weeks and for ≥2 weeks after symptoms resolve. Some recommend therapy be continued for 2 weeks after patient becomes afebrile and blood cultures are negative.

Prevention of Recurrence (Secondary Prophylaxis) of Mucocutaneous Candidiasis†

ORAL:
- HIV-infected adults: 100–200 mg once daily recommended by USPHS/IDSA and others.
- While fluconazole has been given in a dosage of 200 mg once weekly for long-term suppressive therapy in HIV-infected women with a history of oropharyngeal or vaginal candidiasis, this regimen is not included in current USPHS/IDSA guidelines and there are concerns that such a regimen would promote emergence of fluconazole-resistant strains of *Candida*.

Coccidioidomycosis†
Coccidioidal meningitis†

ORAL:
- 200–800 mg once daily.
- HIV-infected adults: 400–800 mg daily.

• Concomitant intracisternal, intraventricular, or intrathecal amphotericin B therapy has been used in some patients.

Prevention of Recurrence (Secondary Prophylaxis) of Coccidioidomycosis†

ORAL:

• HIV-infected adults: 400 mg once daily recommended by USPHS/IDSA. Initiate secondary prophylaxis after primary infection has been adequately treated.

• HIV-infected adults with a history of coccidioidomycosis should receive life-long suppressive therapy to prevent recurrence. Although those who respond to potent antiretroviral therapy with increases in CD4+ T-cell counts to >100/mm³ may be at low risk for recurrence of fungal infections, data are insufficient to date to warrant a recommendation regarding discontinuance of secondary prophylaxis against coccidioidomycosis.

Cryptococcal Infections
Cryptococcal Meningitis

ORAL:

• 400 mg given as a single dose on the first day, followed by 200-400 mg once daily. Some evidence suggests that the 400-mg dosage is more effective than lower dosage.

• HIV-infected adults: Higher dosage (i.e., 800–1000 mg daily) has been used.

• Usually continued for 10–12 weeks after CSF is sterile.

Prevention (Primary Prophylaxis) of Cryptococcosis†

ORAL:

• HIV-infected adults with CD4+ T-cell counts <50/mm³: 100–200 mg once daily recommended by USPHS/IDSA.

• While there is some evidence that a dosage of 400 mg once weekly may be effective, this regimen is not included in current USPHS/IDSA guidelines, and further study is needed to evaluate efficacy of regimens other than daily administration for primary prophylaxis.

Prevention of Recurrence (Secondary Prophylaxis) of Cryptococcosis†

ORAL:

• HIV-infected adults: 200 mg once daily recommended by USPHS/IDSA and others. Some clinicians recommend a dosage of 400 mg daily for the first 4 weeks, followed by 200 mg daily.

• Consideration can be given to discontinuing secondary prophylaxis in HIV-infected adults who have successfully completed initial therapy for cryptococcosis, remain asymptomatic with respect to cryptococcosis, and have sustained (e.g., for ≥6 months) increases in CD4+ T-cell counts to >100–200/mm³ in response to potent antiretroviral therapy.

• Reinitiate secondary prophylaxis against cryptococcosis if CD4+ T-cell count decreases to <100–200/mm³.

Dermatophytoses†
Tinea corporis, Tinea cruris, or Tinea pedis†

ORAL:

• 150 mg once weekly for 2–6 weeks has been effective.

Onychomycosis†

ORAL:

• 150–450 mg once weekly for 3–12 months has been effective.

Histoplasmosis†
Treatment of Histoplasmosis†

ORAL:

• 400–800 mg once daily.

Prevention of Fungal Infections in Transplant or Cancer Patients

ORAL:

• 400 mg once daily.

• In patients in whom severe granulocytopenia (neutrophil count <500/mm³) is anticipated, initiate several days before expected onset of neutropenia and continue for 7 days after neutrophil count is >1000/mm³.

Prescribing Limits
Pediatric Patients
Treatment of Fungal Infections

ORAL:

• Maximum of 600 mg daily.

Special Populations

Renal Impairment

Treatment of Fungal Infections

ORAL:

• Dosage must be modified in response to the degree of impairment and should be based on the patient's measured or estimated Cl_{cr}.

• Manufacturer recommends that adults with impaired renal function receive an initial loading dose of 50–400 mg (based on the type of infection being treated), then patients with Cl_{cr} >50 mL/minute should receive 100% of the usual daily dose and those with Cl_{cr} ≤50 mL/minute should receive 50% of the usual daily dose.

• Patients who are undergoing regular dialysis should receive 100% of the usual daily dose after each dialysis period.

• These dosage recommendations are based on pharmacokinetics following multiple doses; further dosage adjustments may be necessary depending on patient condition.

• Modification of the single-dose regimen of oral fluconazole for treatment of vulvovaginal candidiasis is unnecessary in impaired renal function.

• Pharmacokinetics not studied in children with impaired renal function; recommendations for dosage reduction in such children should parallel those recommended for adults.

Geriatric Patients

• Adjust dosage based on Cl_{cr}.

† *Use is not currently included in the labeling approved by the US Food and Drug Administration.*

Fluconazole Injection

(floo koe′ na zole)

Brand Name: Diflucan®, Diflucan® in Iso-osmotic Dextrose Injection, Diflucan® in Iso-osmotic Sodium Chloride Injection

About Your Treatment

Your doctor has ordered fluconazole, an antifungal antibiotic, to help treat your infection. The drug will be added to an intravenous fluid that will drip through a needle or catheter placed in your vein for 1-2 hours once a day.

Fluconazole is used to treat many kinds of fungal infections, including blood, lung, and skin infections. This medication is sometimes prescribed for other uses; ask your doctor or pharmacist for more information.

Your health care provider (doctor, nurse, or pharmacist) may measure the effectiveness and side effects of your treatment using laboratory tests and physical examinations. It is important to keep all appointments with your doctor and the laboratory. The length of treatment depends on how your infection and symptoms respond to the medication.

Precautions

Before administering fluconazole,

- tell your doctor and pharmacist if you are allergic to fluconazole or any other drugs.
- tell your doctor and pharmacist what prescription and nonprescription medications you are taking, especially anticoagulants ('blood thinners') such as warfarin (Coumadin), antiviral agents such as zidovudine (AZT, Retrovir), astemizole (Hismanal), asthma medications, cisapride (Propulsid), cyclosporine (Neoral, Sandimmune), didanosine (DDI), hydrochlorothiazide, medications for stomach problems such as cimetidine (Tagamet), oral contraceptives, oral medicine for diabetes, phenytoin (Dilantin), rifabutin (Mycobutin), rifampin (Rifadin), tacrolimus (Prograf), terfenadine (Seldane), and vitamins.
- tell your doctor if you have or have ever had kidney or liver disease or a history of alcohol abuse.
- tell your doctor if you are pregnant, plan to become pregnant, or are breast-feeding. If you become pregnant while taking fluconazole, call your doctor.
- tell your doctor if you drink alcohol.

Administering Your Medication

Before you administer fluconazole, look at the solution closely. It should be clear and free of floating material. Gently squeeze the bag or observe the solution container to make sure there are no leaks. Do not use the solution if it is discolored, if it contains particles, or if the bag or container leaks. Use a new solution, but show the damaged one to your health care provider.

It is important that you use your medication exactly as directed. Do not stop your therapy on your own for any reason because your infection could worsen and result in hospitalization. Do not change your dosing schedule without talking to your health care provider. Your health care provider may tell you to stop your infusion if you have a mechanical problem (such as a blockage in the tubing, needle, or catheter); if you have to stop an infusion, call your health care provider immediately so your therapy can continue.

Side Effects

Fluconazole may cause side effects. Tell your health care provider if any of these symptoms are severe or do not go away:

- upset stomach
- loss of appetite
- altered sense of taste
- diarrhea or loose stools
- headache
- dizziness
- fatigue

If you experience any of the following symptoms, call your health care provider immediately:

- rash
- itching
- vomiting
- yellowing of the skin or eyes
- dark urine
- pale stools
- unusual bleeding or bruising

Storage Conditions

- Your health care provider will probably give you a 1- or 2-day supply of fluconazole at a time and tell you to store it at room temperature or in the refrigerator and avoid direct light.
- If you store it in the refrigerator, take your next dose from the refrigerator 1 hour before using it; place it in a clean, dry area to allow it to warm to room temperature.
- Do not allow fluconazole to freeze.

Store your medication only as directed. Make sure you understand what you need to store your medication properly.

Keep your supplies in a clean, dry place when you are not using them, and keep all medications and supplies out of reach of children. Your health care provider will tell you how to throw away used needles, syringes, tubing, and containers to avoid accidental injury.

Overdose

In case of overdose, call your local poison control center at 1-800-222-1222. If the victim has collapsed or is not breathing, call local emergency services at 911.

Signs of Infection

If you are receiving fluconazole in your vein or under your skin, you need to know the symptoms of a catheter-related infection (an infection where the needle enters your vein or skin). If you experience any of these effects near your intravenous catheter, tell your health care provider as soon as possible:

- tenderness
- warmth
- irritation
- drainage
- redness
- swelling
- pain

Dosage Facts
For Informational Purposes

Caution: Do not change your dose, how often you take your medication, or the length of time you are to take it without first talking to your healthcare provider.

The following dosage information was written using medical language for doctors and other healthcare professionals and is provided here for you to check your dosage. The dosage of this drug may differ for different patients. Therefore, always follow your doctor's instructions or the directions on the label. Contact your healthcare provider or pharmacist if you have any questions about the specific dosage of your medication after reviewing this information.

General Dosage Information

Oral and IV dosage are identical.

Pediatric Patients

General Pediatric Dosage
Treatment of Fungal Infections

IV:
- 3–12 mg/kg once daily.
- Dosage of 3, 6, or 12 mg/kg daily in pediatric patients is equivalent to dosage of 100, 200, or 400 mg daily, respectively, in adults.
- Based on available pharmacokinetic data in premature neonates, manufacturer recommends that neonates ≤2 weeks of age receive the usual pediatric dosage once every 72 hours; after 2 weeks of age, neonates should receive the usual dosage once daily.

Candida Infections
Treatment of Oropharyngeal and Esophageal Candidiasis

IV:
- 6 mg/kg on the first day, followed by 3 mg/kg once daily. Dosage for esophageal candidiasis may be increased up to 12 mg/kg daily if necessary, based on the condition of the patient and the response to the drug.
- Treatment for oropharyngeal candidiasis should be continued for ≥2 weeks to decrease the likelihood of relapse. Treatment of esophageal candidiasis should be continued for ≥3 weeks and for ≥2 weeks after symptoms resolve.

Treatment of Disseminated or Invasive Candida Infections

IV:
- 6–12 mg/kg daily.
- Neonates and infants ≤3 months of age†: 5–6 mg/kg once daily has been used for candidal meningitis or septicemia. An initial loading dose of 10 mg/kg followed by 5 mg/kg once daily also has been used for candidal septicemia.

Cryptococcal Infections
Treatment of Cryptococcal Meningitis

IV:
- 12 mg/kg on the first day, followed by 6 mg/kg once daily. Dosage may be increased to 12 mg/kg daily if necessary based on condition of the patient and response to the drug. Continue for 10–12 weeks after CSF becomes culture negative.

Adult Patients

Blastomycosis†
Treatment of Blastomycosis†

IV:
- 400–800 mg once daily.

Candida Infections
Treatment of Oropharyngeal and Esophageal Candidiasis

IV:
- 200 mg given as a single dose on the first day, followed by 100 or 200 mg once daily.
- Up to 400 mg once daily may be used depending on the patient's response.
- Clinical evidence of oropharyngeal candidiasis generally resolves within several days, but the drug usually is continued for ≥2 weeks to decrease the likelihood of relapse.
- Patients with esophageal candidiasis should receive fluconazole for ≥3 weeks and for ≥2 weeks after symptoms resolve.

Treatment of Disseminated or Invasive Candida Infections

IV:
- 400 mg given as a single dose on the first day, followed by 200 mg once daily.
- Urinary tract infections or peritonitis: 50–200 mg daily has been used.
- Candidemia, disseminated candidiasis, or pneumonia: up to 400 mg daily has been used. For candidemia, 400–800 mg once daily IV initially, followed by oral fluconazole has been recommended.
- Therapy should be continued for ≥4 weeks and for ≥2 weeks after symptoms resolve. Some recommend therapy be continued for 2 weeks after patient becomes afebrile and blood cultures are negative.

Cryptococcal Infections
Cryptococcal Meningitis

IV:
- 400 mg given as a single dose on the first day, followed by 200-400 mg once daily. Some evidence suggests that the 400-mg dosage is more effective than lower dosage.
- HIV-infected adults: Higher dosage (i.e., 800–1000 mg daily) has been used.
- Usually continued for 10–12 weeks after CSF is sterile.

Histoplasmosis†

Treatment of Histoplasmosis†

IV:
- 400–800 mg once daily.

Prevention of Fungal Infections in Transplant or Cancer Patients

IV:
- 400 mg once daily.
- In patients in whom severe granulocytopenia (neutrophil count $<500/mm^3$) is anticipated, initiate several days before expected onset of neutropenia and continue for 7 days after neutrophil count is $>1000/mm^3$.

Prescribing Limits

Pediatric Patients

Treatment of Fungal Infections

IV:
- Maximum of 600 mg daily.

Special Populations

Renal Impairment

Treatment of Fungal Infections

IV:
- Dosage must be modified in response to the degree of impairment and should be based on the patient's measured or estimated Cl_{cr}.
- Manufacturer recommends that adults with impaired renal function receive an initial loading dose of 50–400 mg (based on the type of infection being treated), then patients with Cl_{cr} >50 mL/minute should receive 100% of the usual daily dose and those with Cl_{cr} ≤50 mL/minute should receive 50% of the usual daily dose.
- Patients who are undergoing regular dialysis should receive 100% of the usual daily dose after each dialysis period.
- These dosage recommendations are based on pharmacokinetics following multiple doses; further dosage adjustments may be necessary depending on patient condition.
- Modification of the single-dose regimen of oral fluconazole for treatment of vulvovaginal candidiasis is unnecessary in impaired renal function.
- Pharmacokinetics not studied in children with impaired renal function; recommendations for dosage reduction in such children should parallel those recommended for adults.

Geriatric Patients
- Adjust dosage based on Cl_{cr}.

† Use is not currently included in the labeling approved by the US Food and Drug Administration.

Fludrocortisone Acetate

(floo droe kor′ ti sone)

Brand Name: Florinef® Acetate
Also available generically.

Why is this medicine prescribed?

Fludrocortisone, a corticosteroid, is used to help control the amount of sodium and fluids in your body. It is used to treat Addison's disease and syndromes where excessive amounts of sodium are lost in the urine. It works by decreasing the amount of sodium that is lost (excreted) in your urine.

This medication is sometimes prescribed for other uses; ask your doctor or pharmacist for more information.

How should this medicine be used?

Fludrocortisone comes as a tablet to be taken by mouth. Your doctor will prescribe a dosing schedule that is best for you. Follow the directions on your prescription label carefully, and ask your doctor or pharmacist to explain any part you do not understand. Take fludrocortisone exactly as directed. Do not take more or less of it or take it more often than prescribed by your doctor.

Do not stop taking fludrocortisone without talking to your doctor. Stopping the drug abruptly can cause loss of appetite, an upset stomach, vomiting, drowsiness, confusion, headache, fever, joint and muscle pain, peeling skin, and weight loss. If you take large doses for a long time, your doctor probably will decrease your dose gradually to allow your body to adjust before stopping the drug completely. Watch for these side effects if you are gradually decreasing your dose and after you stop taking the tablets. If these problems occur, call your doctor immediately. You may need to increase your dose temporarily or start taking the tablets again.

Are there other uses for this medicine?

Fludrocortisone is also used to increase blood pressure. Talk to your doctor about the possible risks of using this drug for your condition.

What special precautions should I follow?

Before taking fludrocortisone,
- tell your doctor and pharmacist if you are allergic to fludrocortisone, aspirin, tartrazine (a yellow dye in some processed foods and drugs), or any other drugs.
- tell your doctor and pharmacist what prescription and nonprescription medications you are taking, especially anticoagulants ('blood thinners') such as warfarin (Coumadin), arthritis medications, aspirin, cyclosporine (Neoral, Sandimmune), digoxin (Lanoxin), diuretics ('water pills'), estrogen (Premarin), ketoconazole (Ni-

zoral), oral contraceptives, phenobarbital, phenytoin (Dilantin), rifampin (Rifadin), theophylline (Theo-Dur), and vitamins.
- if you have a fungal infection (other than on your skin), do not take fludrocortisone without talking to your doctor.
- tell your doctor if you have or have ever had liver, kidney, intestinal, or heart disease; diabetes; an underactive thyroid gland; high blood pressure; mental illness; myasthenia gravis; osteoporosis; herpes eye infection; seizures; tuberculosis (TB); or ulcers.
- tell your doctor if you are pregnant, plan to become pregnant, or are breast-feeding. If you become pregnant while taking fludrocortisone, call your doctor.
- if you are having surgery, including dental surgery, tell the doctor or dentist that you are taking fludrocortisone.
- if you have a history of ulcers or take large doses of aspirin or other arthritis medication, limit your consumption of alcoholic beverages while taking this drug. Fludrocortisone makes your stomach and intestines more susceptible to the irritating effects of alcohol, aspirin, and certain arthritis medications. This effect increases your risk of ulcers.

What special dietary instructions should I follow?

Your doctor may instruct you to follow a low-sodium, low-salt, potassium-rich, or high-protein diet. Follow these directions.

Fludrocortisone may cause an upset stomach. Take fludrocortisone with food or milk.

What should I do if I forget to take a dose?

When you start to take fludrocortisone, ask your doctor what to do if you forget a dose. Write down these instructions so that you can refer to them later.

If you take fludrocortisone once a day, take the missed dose as soon as you remember it. However, if it is almost time for the next dose, skip the missed dose and continue your regular dosing schedule. Do not take a double dose to make up for a missed one.

What side effects can this medicine cause?

Fludrocortisone may cause side effects. Tell your doctor if any of these symptoms are severe or do not go away:
- upset stomach
- stomach irritation
- vomiting
- headache
- dizziness
- insomnia
- restlessness
- depression
- anxiety
- acne
- increased hair growth

- easy bruising
- irregular or absent menstrual periods

If you experience any of the following symptoms, call your doctor immediately:
- skin rash
- swollen face, lower legs, or ankles
- vision problems
- cold or infection that lasts a long time
- muscle weakness
- black or tarry stool

If you experience a serious side effect, you or your doctor may send a report to the Food and Drug Administration's (FDA) MedWatch Adverse Event Reporting program online [at http://www.fda.gov/MedWatch/index.html] or by phone [1-800-332-1088].

What storage conditions are needed for this medicine?

Keep this medication in the container it came in, tightly closed, and out of reach of children. Store it at room temperature and away from excess heat and moisture (not in the bathroom). Throw away any medication that is outdated or no longer needed. Talk to your pharmacist about the proper disposal of your medication.

What should I do in case of overdose?

In case of overdose, call your local poison control center at 1-800-222-1222. If the victim has collapsed or is not breathing, call local emergency services at 911.

What other information should I know?

Keep all appointments with your doctor and the laboratory. Your doctor may order certain lab tests to check your response to fludrocortisone. Your blood pressure should be checked regularly to determine your response to fludrocortisone.

If your condition worsens, call your doctor. Your dose may need to be adjusted.

Carry an identification card that indicates that you may need to take supplementary doses (write down the full dose you took before gradually decreasing it) of fludrocortisone during periods of stress (injuries, infections, and severe asthma attacks). Ask your pharmacist or doctor how to obtain this card. List your name, medical problems, drugs and dosages, and doctor's name and telephone number on the card.

This drug makes you more susceptible to illnesses. If you are exposed to chicken pox, measles, or tuberculosis (TB) while taking fludrocortisone, call your doctor. Do not have a vaccination, other immunization, or any skin test while you are taking fludrocortisone unless your doctor tells you that you may.

Report any injuries or signs of infection (fever, sore throat, pain during urination, and muscle aches) that occur during treatment.

Your doctor may instruct you to weigh yourself every day. Report any unusual weight gain.

If your sputum (the matter you cough up during an asthma attack) thickens or changes color from clear white to yellow, green, or gray, call your doctor; these changes may be signs of an infection.

If you have diabetes, fludrocortisone may increase your blood sugar level. If you monitor your blood sugar (glucose) at home, test your blood or urine more frequently than usual. Call your doctor if your blood sugar is high or if sugar is present in your urine; your dose of diabetes medication and your diet may need to be changed.

Do not let anyone else take your medication. Ask your pharmacist any questions you have about refilling your prescription.

Dosage Facts
For Informational Purposes

Caution: Do not change your dose, how often you take your medication, or the length of time you are to take it without first talking to your health-care provider.

The following dosage information was written using medical language for doctors and other healthcare professionals and is provided here for you to check your dosage. The dosage of this drug may differ for different patients. Therefore, always follow your doctor's instructions or the directions on the label. Contact your healthcare provider or pharmacist if you have any questions about the specific dosage of your medication after reviewing this information.

General Dosage Information

Available as fludrocortisone acetate; dosage expressed in terms of the salt.

Adult Patients

Adrenocortical Insufficiency

ORAL:
- Usually, 0.1 mg daily; dosage may range from 0.1 mg 3 times weekly to 0.2 mg daily.
- If hypertension occurs, reduce dosage to 0.05 mg daily.
- Administer concomitantly with cortisone (10–37.5 mg daily in divided doses) or hydrocortisone (10–30 mg daily in divided doses).

Adrenogenital Syndrome

ORAL:
- 0.1–0.2 mg daily.

Postural Hypotension†

ORAL:
- 0.1–0.4 mg daily has been given to diabetic patients with postural hypotension†.
- 0.05–0.2 mg daily has been given to patients with postural hypotension secondary to levodopa therapy†.

Prescribing Limits

Adult Patients

Adrenocortical Insufficiency

ORAL:
- Maximum 0.2 mg daily.

Adrenogenital Syndrome

ORAL:
- Maximum 0.2 mg daily.

Special Populations

Hepatic Impairment
- No special population dosage recommendations at this time.

Renal Impairment
- No special population dosage recommendations at this time.

Geriatric Patients
- Careful dosage selection recommended due to possible age-related decreases in hepatic, renal, and/or cardiac function and concomitant disease and drug therapy.

† Use is not currently included in the labeling approved by the US Food and Drug Administration.

Flunisolide Nasal Inhalation

(floo niss′ oh lide)

Brand Name: Nasalide®
Also available generically.

Why is this medicine prescribed?

Flunisolide, a corticosteroid, is used to prevent allergy symptoms including sneezing, itching, and runny or stuffed nose.

This medication is sometimes prescribed for other uses; ask your doctor or pharmacist for more information.

How should this medicine be used?

Flunisolide comes as an solution to inhale through the nose. It usually is inhaled one to four times a day at evenly spaced intervals. Follow the directions on your prescription label carefully, and ask your doctor or pharmacist to explain any part you do not understand. Use flunisolide exactly as directed. Do not use more or less of it or use it more often than prescribed by your doctor. Do not stop using flunisolide without talking to your doctor.

Before you use flunisolide the first time, read the written instructions that come with it. Ask your doctor, pharmacist, or respiratory therapist to demonstrate the proper technique. Practice using the inhaler while in his or her presence.

To use the inhaler, follow these steps:
1. Wash your hands.
2. Gently blow your nose to clear your nasal passages.
3. Remove the cap from the nasal inhaler.
4. Shake the inhaler.
5. With the nasal sprayer aimed away from all people and animals, prime the pump before each use. Hold the sprayer by placing two fingers on the 'shoulders' of the bottle and your thumb on the bottom. Use your thumb to push the spray bottle firmly and quickly until a fine spray appears.
6. Insert the tip of the nasal inhaler approximately 1/4 inch into one nostril, pointing the tip toward the outer side of your nose.
7. Close your other nostril with your finger and tilt your head back slightly.
8. Press down on the container to release the medication and sniff gently with your mouth closed.
9. Hold your breath for a few seconds.
10. Breathe out through your mouth.
11. Remove the nasal inhaler from your nose.
12. Clean the tip of the nasal inhaler with a tissue and replace the cap.
13. Repeat Steps 3 through 12 for your other nostril if directed to do so by your doctor.
14. Wash your hands again.

Avoid blowing your nose for 15 minutes after inhaling the prescribed dose.

What special precautions should I follow?

Before using flunisolide,
- tell your doctor and pharmacist if you are allergic to flunisolide or any other drugs.
- tell your doctor and pharmacist what prescription and nonprescription medications you are taking, especially anticoagulants ('blood thinners') such as warfarin (Coumadin), arthritis medications, aspirin, cyclosporine (Neoral, Sandimmune), digoxin (Lanoxin), diuretics ('water pills'), estrogen (Premarin), ketoconazole (Nizoral), oral contraceptives, phenobarbital, phenytoin (Dilantin), rifampin (Rifadin), theophylline (Theo-Dur), and vitamins.
- if you have a nose infection or a fungal infection (other than on your skin), do not use flunisolide without talking to your doctor.
- tell your doctor if you have or have ever had tuberculosis (TB); liver, kidney, intestinal, or heart disease; diabetes; an underactive thyroid gland; high blood pressure; mental illness; myasthenia gravis; osteoporosis; herpes eye infection; seizures; or ulcers.
- tell your doctor if you are pregnant, plan to become pregnant, or are breast-feeding. If you become pregnant while using flunisolide, call your doctor.

What should I do if I forget to take a dose?

Use the missed dose as soon as you remember it. However, if it is almost time for the next dose, skip the missed dose and continue your regular dosing schedule. Do not use a double dose to make up for a missed one.

What side effects can this medicine cause?

Flunisolide may cause side effects. Tell your doctor if any of these symptoms are severe or do not go away:
- headache
- nasal irritation or dryness
- sore throat
- sneezing
- nosebleed

If you experience any of the following symptoms, call your doctor immediately:
- increased difficulty breathing
- swollen face, lower legs, or ankles
- vision problems
- cold or infection that lasts a long time
- muscle weakness

If you experience a serious side effect, you or your doctor may send a report to the Food and Drug Administration's (FDA) MedWatch Adverse Event Reporting program online [at http://www.fda.gov/MedWatch/index.html] or by phone [1-800-332-1088].

What storage conditions are needed for this medicine?

Keep this medication in the container it came in, tightly closed, and out of reach of children. Store it at room temperature and away from excess heat and moisture (not in the bathroom). Throw away any medication that is outdated or no longer needed. Talk to your pharmacist about the proper disposal of your medication. Avoid puncturing the aerosol container, and do not discard it in an incinerator or fire.

What other information should I know?

Keep all appointments with your doctor.

Your symptoms may improve after just a few days. If they do not improve within 3 weeks, call your doctor.

Avoid exposure to chicken pox and measles. This drug makes you more susceptible to these illnesses. If you are exposed to them while using flunisolide, call your doctor. Do not have a vaccination or other immunization unless your doctor tells you that you may.

Report any injuries or signs of infection (fever, sore throat, pain during urination, and muscle aches) that occur during treatment.

If your sputum (the matter that you cough up during an asthma attack) thickens or changes color from clear white to yellow, green, or gray, call your doctor; these changes may be signs of an infection.

Inhalation devices require regular cleaning, and some require periodic replacement. Follow the directions that come with your inhaler.

Do not let anyone else use your medication. Ask your

pharmacist any questions you have about refilling your prescription.

Dosage Facts
For Informational Purposes

Caution: Do not change your dose, how often you take your medication, or the length of time you are to take it without first talking to your healthcare provider.

The following dosage information was written using medical language for doctors and other healthcare professionals and is provided here for you to check your dosage. The dosage of this drug may differ for different patients. Therefore, always follow your doctor's instructions or the directions on the label. Contact your healthcare provider or pharmacist if you have any questions about the specific dosage of your medication after reviewing this information.

General Dosage Information

After priming, nasal inhaler delivers about 25 mcg of flunisolide per metered spray and about 200 metered sprays per 25-mL container.

Adjust dosage according to individual requirements and response.

Therapeutic effects of intranasal corticosteroids, unlike those of decongestants, are not immediate. This should be explained to the patient in advance to ensure compliance and continuation of the prescribed treatment regimen.

Symptomatic relief is usually evident within 2–3 days of continuous therapy; however, occasionally, up to 2–3 weeks may be required for optimum effectiveness.

Generally assess response to the initial dosage 4–7 days after starting therapy; about two-thirds will experience some relief within this time period.

Once symptoms of seasonal or perennial rhinitis have been controlled, gradually reduce dosage to the lowest effective level.

Discontinue intranasal flunisolide in patients who do not experience clinically important benefit within 3 weeks of initiating therapy.

Pediatric Patients

Seasonal Rhinitis

INTRANASAL INHALATION:
- Children 6–14 years of age: 1 spray (25 mcg) in each nostril 3 times daily or 2 sprays (50 mcg) in each nostril twice daily (total dose: 150–200 mcg/day).

Perennial Rhinitis

INTRANASAL INHALATION:
- Children 6–14 years of age: 1 spray (25 mcg) in each nostril 3 times daily or 2 sprays (50 mcg) in each nostril twice daily (total dose 150–200 mcg/day).

Adult Patients

Seasonal Rhinitis

INTRANASAL INHALATION:
- Usual initial dose is 50 mcg (2 sprays) in each nostril twice daily. When necessary, increase to 50 mcg (2 sprays) in each nostril 3 times daily.
- Maintenance: 25 mcg (1 spray) in each nostril daily (50 mcg total) may be sufficient.

Perennial Rhinitis

INTRANASAL INHALATION:
- Usual initial dose is 50 mcg (2 sprays) in each nostril twice daily. When necessary, increase to 50 mcg (2 sprays) in each nostril 3 times daily.
- Maintenance: 25 mcg (1 spray) in each nostril daily (50 mcg total) may be sufficient.

Prescribing Limits

No evidence that higher than recommended dosages or increased frequency of administration is beneficial.

Exceeding the maximum recommended daily dosage may only increase the risk of adverse systemic effects (e.g., HPA-axis suppression, Cushing's syndrome).

Pediatric Patients

Seasonal Rhinitis

INTRANASAL INHALATION:
- Children 6-14 years of age: daily dosage should not exceed 100 mcg (4 sprays) in each nostril (200 mcg total).

Perennial Rhinitis

INTRANASAL INHALATION:
- Children 6-14 years of age: daily dosage should not exceed 100 mcg (4 sprays) in each nostril (200 mcg total).

Adult Patients

Seasonal Rhinitis

INTRANASAL INHALATION:
- Daily dosage should not exceed 200 mcg (8 sprays) in each nostril (400 mcg total).

Perennial Rhinitis

INTRANASAL INHALATION:
- Daily dosage should not exceed 200 mcg (8 sprays) in each nostril (400 mcg total).

Special Populations

Hepatic Impairment
- No specific dosage recommendations for hepatic impairment.

Renal Impairment
- No specific dosage recommendations for renal impairment.

Geriatric Patients
- No specific geriatric dosage recommendations.

Flunisolide Oral Inhalation

(floo niss' oh lide)

Brand Name: AeroBid® Inhaler System, AeroBid-M® Inhaler System

Important Warning

If you are switching (or have recently switched) from an oral corticosteroid such as betamethasone, dexamethasone, methylprednisolone, prednisolone, or prednisone to flunisolide inhalation and have an injury, infection, or severe asthma attack, use a full dose (even if you have been gradually decreasing your dose) of the oral corticosteroid and call your doctor for additional instructions.

Carry an identification card that indicates that you may need to take supplementary doses (write down the full dose you took before gradually decreasing it) of the corticosteroid during periods of stress (injuries, infections, and severe asthma attacks). Ask your pharmacist or doctor how to obtain this card. List your name, medical problems, drugs and dosages, and doctor's name and telephone number on the card.

Why is this medicine prescribed?

Flunisolide, a corticosteroid, is used to prevent wheezing, shortness of breath, and troubled breathing caused by severe asthma and other lung diseases.

This medication is sometimes prescribed for other uses; ask your doctor or pharmacist for more information.

How should this medicine be used?

Flunisolide comes as an aerosol to inhale by mouth. It usually is inhaled three or four times a day at evenly spaced intervals. Follow the directions on your prescription label carefully, and ask your doctor or pharmacist to explain any part you do not understand. Use flunisolide exactly as directed. Do not use more or less of it or use it more often than prescribed by your doctor.

Do not stop using flunisolide without talking to your doctor.

Before you use flunisolide the first time, read the written instructions that come with it. Ask your doctor, pharmacist, or respiratory therapist to demonstrate the proper technique. Practice using the inhaler while in his or her presence.

To use the inhaler, follow these steps:
1. Shake the inhaler well.
2. Remove the protective cap.
3. Exhale (breathe out) as completely as possible through your nose while keeping your mouth shut.
4. *Open Mouth Technique:* Open your mouth wide, and place the open end of the mouthpiece about 1-2 inches from your mouth.
   Closed Mouth Technique: Place the open end of the mouthpiece well into your mouth, past your front teeth. Close your lips tightly around the mouthpiece.
5. Take a slow, deep breath through the mouthpiece and, at the same time, press down on the container to spray the medication into your mouth. Be sure that the mist goes into your throat and is not blocked by your teeth or tongue. Adults giving the treatment to young children may hold the child's nose closed to be sure that the medication goes into the child's throat.
6. Hold your breath for 5-10 seconds, remove the inhaler, and exhale slowly through your nose or mouth. If you take 2 puffs, wait 2 minutes and shake the inhaler well before taking the second puff.
7. Replace the protective cap on the inhaler.
   After each treatment, rinse your mouth with water or mouthwash.

If you have difficulty getting the medication into your lungs, a spacer (a special device that attaches to the inhaler) may help; ask your doctor, pharmacist, or respiratory therapist.

What special precautions should I follow?

Before using flunisolide,
- tell your doctor and pharmacist if you are allergic to flunisolide or any other drugs.
- tell your doctor and pharmacist what prescription and nonprescription medications you are using, especially arthritis medications, aspirin, digoxin (Lanoxin), diuretics ('water pills'), estrogen (Premarin), ketoconazole (Nizoral), oral contraceptives, phenobarbital, phenytoin (Dilantin), rifampin (Rifadin), theophylline (Theo-Dur), and vitamins.
- if you have a fungal infection (other than on your skin), do not use flunisolide without talking to your doctor.
- tell your doctor if you have or have ever had liver, kidney, intestinal, or heart disease; diabetes; an underactive thyroid gland; high blood pressure; mental illness; myasthenia gravis; osteoporosis; herpes eye infection; seizures; or ulcers.
- tell your doctor if you are pregnant, plan to become pregnant, or are breast-feeding. If you become pregnant while using flunisolide, call your doctor.
- if you have a history of ulcers or take large doses of aspirin or other arthritis medication, limit your consumption of alcoholic beverages while using this drug. Flunisolide makes your stomach and intestines more susceptible to the irritating effects of alcohol, aspirin, and certain arthritis medications. This effect increases your risk of ulcers.

What special dietary instructions should I follow?

Your doctor may instruct you to follow a low-sodium, low-salt, potassium-rich, or high-protein diet. Follow these directions.

What should I do if I forget to take a dose?

Use the missed dose as soon as you remember it. However, if it is almost time for the next dose, skip the missed dose and continue your regular dosing schedule. Do not use a double dose to make up for a missed one.

What side effects can this medicine cause?

Flunisolide may cause side effects. Tell your doctor if any of these symptoms are severe or do not go away:

- dry or irritated throat and mouth
- cough
- difficult or painful speech

If you experience any of the following symptoms, call your doctor immediately:

- skin rash
- increased difficulty breathing
- white spots or sores in your mouth
- swollen face, lower legs, or ankles
- vision problems
- cold or infection that lasts a long time
- muscle weakness

If you experience a serious side effect, you or your doctor may send a report to the Food and Drug Administration's (FDA) MedWatch Adverse Event Reporting program online [at http://www.fda.gov/MedWatch/index.html] or by phone [1-800-332-1088].

What storage conditions are needed for this medicine?

Keep this medication in the container it came in, tightly closed, and out of reach of children. Store it at room temperature and away from excess heat and moisture (not in the bathroom). Throw away any medication that is outdated or no longer needed. Talk to your pharmacist about the proper disposal of your medication. Avoid puncturing the aerosol container, and do not discard it in an incinerator or fire.

What other information should I know?

Keep all appointments with your doctor and the laboratory. Your doctor will order certain lab tests to check your response to flunisolide.

Flunisolide is not used for rapid relief of breathing problems. If you do not have another inhaler for prompt relief of breathing difficulty, ask your doctor to prescribe one.

If your doctor has prescribed a bronchodilator (a drug to be inhaled for rapid relief of difficult breathing), use it several minutes before you use your flunisolide inhaler so that flunisolide can reach deep into your lungs.

Avoid exposure to chicken pox and measles. This drug makes you more susceptible to these illnesses. If you are exposed to them while using flunisolide, call your doctor. Do not have a vaccination or other immunization unless your doctor tells you that you may.

Report any injuries or signs of infection (fever, sore throat, pain during urination, and muscle aches) that occur during treatment.

If your sputum (the matter you cough up during an asthma attack) thickens or changes color from clear white to yellow, green, or gray, call your doctor; these changes may be signs of an infection.

Inhalation devices require regular cleaning. Once a week, remove the drug container from the plastic mouthpiece, wash the mouthpiece with warm tap water, and dry it thoroughly.

Do not let anyone else use your medication. Ask your pharmacist any questions you have about refilling your prescription.

Talk to your doctor, pharmacist, or other healthcare professional if you have questions about dosing information for your medication.

Fluocinolone Topical

(floo oh sin′ oh lone)

Brand Name: Capex® Shampoo, Derma-Smoothe/FS®, Lidex®, Lidex® Gel, Lidex®-E Emollient Cream, Synalar®, Synemol® Emollient Cream
Also available generically.

Why is this medicine prescribed?

Fluocinolone is used to treat the itching, redness, dryness, crusting, scaling, inflammation, and discomfort of various skin conditions.

This medication is sometimes prescribed for other uses; ask your doctor or pharmacist for more information.

How should this medicine be used?

Fluocinolone comes in ointment, cream, solution, shampoo, and oil in various strengths for use on the skin. It usually is applied two to four times a day. Follow the directions on your prescription label carefully, and ask your doctor or pharmacist to explain any part you do not understand. Use fluocinolone exactly as directed. Do not use more or less of it or use it more often than prescribed by your doctor. Do not apply it to other areas of your body or wrap or bandage the treated area unless directed to do so by your doctor.

Wash or soak the affected area thoroughly before applying the medicine, unless it irritates your skin. Then apply the ointment, cream, solution, or oil sparingly in a thin film and rub it in gently.

Use the shampoo as you would any normal shampoo. Wet your hair and scalp. Apply the shampoo and gently massage the scalp. Rinse with water.

To use a solution on your scalp, part your hair, apply a small amount of the medicine on the affected area, and rub it in gently. Protect the area from washing and rubbing until the solution dries. You may wash your hair as usual but not right after applying the medicine.

Avoid prolonged use on the face, in the genital and rectal areas, and in skin creases and armpits unless directed by your doctor.

If you are using fluocinolone on your face, keep it out of your eyes.

If you are using fluocinolone on a child's diaper area, do not use tight-fitting diapers or plastic pants. Such use may increase side effects.

Do not apply cosmetics or other skin preparations on the treated area without talking with your doctor.

If your doctor tells you to wrap or bandage the treated area, follow these instructions:

1. Soak the area in water or wash it well.
2. While the skin is moist, gently rub the medication into the affected areas.
3. Cover the area with plastic wrap (such as Saran Wrap or Handi-Wrap). The plastic may be held in place with a gauze or elastic bandage or adhesive tape on normal skin beside the treated area. (Instead of using plastic wrap, plastic gloves may be used for the hands, plastic bags for the feet, or a shower cap for the scalp.)
4. Carefully seal the edges of the plastic to make sure the wrap adheres closely to the skin. If the affected area is moist, you can leave the edges of the plastic wrap partly unsealed or puncture the wrap to allow excess moisture to escape.
5. Leave the plastic wrapping in place as long as directed by your doctor. Usually wraps are left in place no more than 12 hours each day.
6. Cleanse the skin and reapply the medication each time a new plastic wrapping is applied. Call your doctor if the treated area gets worse or if burning, swelling, redness, or oozing of pus develops.

Do not discontinue treatment abruptly without talking to your doctor.

What special precautions should I follow?

Before using fluocinolone,
- tell your doctor and pharmacist if you are allergic to fluocinolone or any other drugs.
- tell your doctor and pharmacist what prescription and nonprescription medications you are taking, especially cancer chemotherapy agents, other topical medications, and vitamins.
- tell your doctor if you have an infection or have ever had diabetes, glaucoma, cataracts, a circulation disorder, or an immune disorder.
- tell your doctor if you are pregnant, plan to become pregnant, or are breast-feeding. If you become pregnant while using fluocinolone, call your doctor immediately.

What should I do if I forget to take a dose?

Apply the missed dose as soon as you remember it. However, if it is almost time for the next dose, skip the missed dose and continue your regular dosing schedule. Do not apply a double dose to make up for a missed one.

What side effects can this medicine cause?

Fluocinolone may cause side effects. Tell your doctor if any of these symptoms are severe or do not go away:
- drying or cracking of the skin
- acne
- itching
- burning
- change in skin color

If you experience any of the following symptoms, call your doctor immediately:
- severe skin rash
- difficulty breathing or swallowing
- wheezing
- skin infection (redness, swelling, or oozing pus)

If you experience a serious side effect, you or your doctor may send a report to the Food and Drug Administration's (FDA) MedWatch Adverse Event Reporting program online [at http://www.fda.gov/MedWatch/index.html] or by phone [1-800-332-1088].

What storage conditions are needed for this medicine?

Keep this medication in the container it came in, tightly closed, and out of reach of children. Store it at room temperature and away from excess heat. Do not allow it to freeze. Throw away any medication that is outdated or no longer needed. Do not use it to treat other skin conditions. Talk to your pharmacist about the proper disposal of your medication.

What other information should I know?

Keep all appointments with your doctor.

Do not let anyone else use your medication. Ask your pharmacist any questions you have about refilling your prescription.

Dosage Facts
For Informational Purposes

Caution: Do not change your dose, how often you take your medication, or the length of time you are to take it without first talking to your healthcare provider.

The following dosage information was written using medical language for doctors and other healthcare pro-

fessionals and is provided here for you to check your dosage. The dosage of this drug may differ for different patients. Therefore, always follow your doctor's instructions or the directions on the label. Contact your healthcare provider or pharmacist if you have any questions about the specific dosage of your medication after reviewing this information.

General Dosage Information

Available as fluocinolone acetonide and fluocinonide; dosage expressed in terms of the salt and the base, respectively.

Pediatric Patients

Administer the least amount of topical preparations that provides effective therapy.

Corticosteroid-responsive Dermatoses

TOPICAL:
- Apply cream, gel, ointment, or solution sparingly 2–4 times daily depending on the severity of the condition.
- For the treatment of moderate to severe atopic dermatitis in children ≥2 years of age, apply a thin film of fluocinolone acetonide 0.01% topical oil twice daily to affected areas for no longer than 4 weeks.

Adult Patients

Corticosteroid-responsive Dermatoses

TOPICAL:
- Apply cream, gel, ointment, or solution sparingly 2–4 times daily depending upon severity of condition.
- For the treatment of atopic dermatitis, apply fluocinolone acetonide 0.01% topical oil as a thin film 3 times daily.
- For the treatment of psoriasis of the scalp, apply a thin film of fluocinolone acetonide 0.01% topical oil to wet or dampened hair and scalp, massage well, and cover with the manufacturer-supplied shower cap. Allow oil to remain on the scalp overnight or for a minimum of 4 hours following application before being washed off with regular shampoo and rinsed thoroughly with water.
- For the treatment of seborrheic dermatitis of the scalp, apply ≤30 mL of fluocinolone acetonide 0.01% shampoo to the scalp once daily.

Prescribing Limits

Pediatric Patients

Corticosteroid-responsive Dermatoses

TOPICAL:
- For the treatment of moderate to severe atopic dermatitis in children ≥2 years of age, maximum 4 weeks of therapy.

Adult Patients

Corticosteroid-responsive Dermatoses

TOPICAL:
- For the treatment of seborrheic dermatitis of the scalp, maximum 30 mL of fluocinolone acetonide 0.01% shampoo applied to the scalp once daily.

Fluocinonide Topical

(floo oh sin' oh nide)

Brand Name: Fluonex®, Lidex®, Lidex-E®, Lonide®
Also available generically.

Why is this medicine prescribed?

Fluocinonide is used to treat the itching, redness, dryness, crusting, scaling, inflammation, and discomfort of various skin conditions.

This medication is sometimes prescribed for other uses; ask your doctor or pharmacist for more information.

How should this medicine be used?

Fluocinonide comes in ointment, cream, solution, and gel in various strengths for use on the skin. It usually is applied two to four times a day. Follow the directions on your prescription label carefully, and ask your doctor or pharmacist to explain any part you do not understand. Use fluocinonide exactly as directed. Do not use more or less of it or use it more often than prescribed by your doctor. Do not apply it to other areas of your body or wrap or bandage the treated area unless directed to do so by your doctor.

Wash or soak the affected area thoroughly before applying the medicine, unless it irritates your skin. Then apply the ointment, cream, solution, or gel sparingly in a thin film and rub it in gently.

To use the solution or gel on your scalp, part your hair, apply a small amount of the medicine on the affected area, and rub it in gently. Protect the area from washing and rubbing until the solution or gel dries. You may wash your hair as usual but not right after applying the medicine.

Avoid prolonged use on the face, in the genital and rectal areas, and in skin creases and armpits unless directed by your doctor.

If you are using fluocinonide on your face, keep it out of your eyes.

If you are using fluocinonide on a child's diaper area, do not use tight-fitting diapers or plastic pants. Such use may increase side effects.

Do not apply cosmetics or other skin preparations on the treated area without talking with your doctor.

If your doctor tells you to wrap or bandage the treated area, follow these instructions:
1. Soak the area or wash it well.
2. While the skin is moist, gently rub the medication into the affected areas.
3. Cover the area with plastic wrap (such as Saran Wrap or Handi-Wrap). The plastic may be held in place with a gauze or elastic bandage or adhesive tape on the normal skin beside the treated area. (Instead of using plastic wrap, plastic gloves may be used for the hands, plastic bags for the feet, or a shower cap for the scalp.)

4. Carefully seal the edges of the plastic to make sure the wrap adheres closely to the skin. If the affected area is moist, you can leave the edges of the plastic wrap partly unsealed or puncture the wrap to allow excess moisture to escape.

5. Leave the plastic wrapping in place as long as instructed by your doctor. Usually wrappings are left in place no more than 12 hours each day.

6. Cleanse the skin and reapply the medication each time a new plastic wrapping is applied.

Call your doctor if the treated area gets worse or if burning, swelling, or oozing of pus develops.

Do not discontinue treatment abruptly without talking to your doctor.

What special precautions should I follow?

Before using fluocinonide,

- tell your doctor and pharmacist if you are allergic to fluocinonide or any other drugs.
- tell your doctor and pharmacist what prescription and nonprescription medications you are taking, especially cancer chemotherapy agents, other topical medications, and vitamins.
- tell your doctor if you have an infection or have ever had diabetes, glaucoma, cataracts, a circulation disorder, or an immune disorder.
- tell your doctor if you are pregnant, plan to become pregnant, or are breast-feeding. If you become pregnant while using fluocinonide, call your doctor immediately.

What should I do if I forget to take a dose?

Apply the missed dose as soon as you remember it. However, if it is almost time for the next dose, skip the missed dose and continue your regular dosing schedule. Do not apply a double dose to make up for a missed one.

What side effects can this medicine cause?

Fluocinonide may cause side effects. Tell your doctor if any of these symptoms are severe or do not go away:

- drying or cracking of the skin
- acne
- itching
- burning
- change in skin color

If you experience any of the following symptoms, call your doctor immediately:

- severe skin rash
- difficulty breathing or swallowing
- wheezing
- skin infection (redness, swelling, or oozing pus)

If you experience a serious side effect, you or your doctor may send a report to the Food and Drug Administration's (FDA) MedWatch Adverse Event Reporting program online [at http://www.fda.gov/MedWatch/index.html] or by phone [1-800-332-1088].

What storage conditions are needed for this medicine?

Keep this medication in the container it came in, tightly closed, and out of reach of children. Store it at room temperature and away from excess heat. Do not allow it to freeze. Throw away any medication that is outdated or no longer needed. Do not use it to treat other skin conditions. Talk to your pharmacist about the proper disposal of your medication.

What other information should I know?

Keep all appointments with your doctor.

Do not let anyone else use your medication. Ask your pharmacist any questions you have about refilling your prescription.

Dosage Facts
For Informational Purposes

Caution: Do not change your dose, how often you take your medication, or the length of time you are to take it without first talking to your healthcare provider.

The following dosage information was written using medical language for doctors and other healthcare professionals and is provided here for you to check your dosage. The dosage of this drug may differ for different patients. Therefore, always follow your doctor's instructions or the directions on the label. Contact your healthcare provider or pharmacist if you have any questions about the specific dosage of your medication after reviewing this information.

General Dosage Information

Available as fluocinolone acetonide and fluocinonide; dosage expressed in terms of the salt and the base, respectively.

Pediatric Patients

Administer the least amount of topical preparations that provides effective therapy.

Corticosteroid-responsive Dermatoses
TOPICAL:
- Apply cream, gel, ointment, or solution sparingly 2–4 times daily depending on the severity of the condition.
- For the treatment of moderate to severe atopic dermatitis in children ≥2 years of age, apply a thin film of fluocinolone acetonide 0.01% topical oil twice daily to affected areas for no longer than 4 weeks.

Adult Patients

Corticosteroid-responsive Dermatoses
TOPICAL:
- Apply cream, gel, ointment, or solution sparingly 2–4 times daily depending upon severity of condition.
- For the treatment of atopic dermatitis, apply fluocinolone acetonide 0.01% topical oil as a thin film 3 times daily.
- For the treatment of psoriasis of the scalp, apply a thin film

of fluocinolone acetonide 0.01% topical oil to wet or dampened hair and scalp, massage well, and cover with the manufacturer-supplied shower cap. Allow oil to remain on the scalp overnight or for a minimum of 4 hours following application before being washed off with regular shampoo and rinsed thoroughly with water.

- For the treatment of seborrheic dermatitis of the scalp, apply ≤30 mL of fluocinolone acetonide 0.01% shampoo to the scalp once daily.

Prescribing Limits

Pediatric Patients

Corticosteroid-responsive Dermatoses

TOPICAL:
- For the treatment of moderate to severe atopic dermatitis in children ≥2 years of age, maximum 4 weeks of therapy.

Adult Patients

Corticosteroid-responsive Dermatoses

TOPICAL:
- For the treatment of seborrheic dermatitis of the scalp, maximum 30 mL of fluocinolone acetonide 0.01% shampoo applied to the scalp once daily.

Fluoride

(floor′ ide)

Brand Name: ACT®, APF Gel®, Control Rx®, DentinBloc® Dentin Desensitizer as a combination product containing Sodium Fluoride, Hydrogen Fluoride, and Stannous Fluoride, Fluorigard® Anti-Cavity Dental Rinse, Fluorinse®, Fluoritab®, Fluoritab® Liquid, FluoroCare® Dual Rinse Kit, Fluorofoam® APF One-Minute Foam, Flura-Drops®, Flura-Loz®, Flura-Tab®, Gel-Kam®, Gel-Kam® Oral Care Rinse, Gel-Tin®, Karidium®, Karigel® Maintenance APF Gel, Karigel® Maintenance-Neutral, Karigel® Professional APF Topical Gel with 0.1 M phosphate at pH 3.5, Luride® Drops, Luride® F Lozi-Tabs® Full-Strength, Luride® F Lozi-Tabs® Half-Strength, Luride® F Lozi-Tabs® Quarter-Strength, Minute-Foam®, Minute-Gel® with phosphate at pH 3.5, My Gel®, NeutraCare®, Neutra-Foam®, Omnii-Gel®, Pediaflor® Drops, Phos-Flur® Gel, PreviDent 5000 Plus®, Previ-Dent® Brush-On Gel, PreviDent® Dental Rinse, SF 5000 Plus®, SF Gel®, Stanimax® Ortho Rinse, Stop® Home Treatment 0.4%, Thera-Flur®-N Gel-Drops

Why is this medicine prescribed?

Fluoride is used to prevent tooth decay. It is taken up by teeth and helps to strengthen teeth, resist acid, and block the cavity-forming action of bacteria. Fluoride usually is prescribed for children and adults whose homes have water that is not fluoridated (already has fluoride added).

This medication is sometimes prescribed for other uses; ask your doctor or pharmacist for more information.

How should this medicine be used?

Fluoride comes as a liquid, tablet, and chewable tablet to take by mouth. It usually is taken once daily. Follow the directions on your prescription label carefully, and ask your doctor or pharmacist to explain any part you do not understand. Take fluoride exactly as directed. Do not take more or less of it or take it more often than prescribed by your doctor.

The fluoride liquid may be taken straight from the bottle or mixed with cereal, fruit juice, or other foods. Use a dropper or an oral syringe to measure out your dose. Tablets may be dissolved in the mouth, chewed, or added to drinking water or fruit juice. Tablets also may be added to water for use in infant formulas or other food.

Fluoride helps to strengthen teeth and prevent cavities; it is not a substitute for brushing or flossing.

What special precautions should I follow?

Before taking fluoride,
- tell your doctor and pharmacist if you are allergic to fluoride, tartrazine (a yellow dye in some processed foods and drugs), or any other drugs.
- tell your doctor and pharmacist what prescription and nonprescription medications you are taking, especially vitamins. Do not take calcium, magnesium, or iron supplements while taking fluoride without checking with your doctor.
- tell your doctor if you are pregnant, plan to become pregnant, or are breast-feeding. If you become pregnant while taking fluoride, call your doctor.
- tell your doctor if you are on a low-sodium or sodium-free diet.

What special dietary instructions should I follow?

Do not eat or drink dairy products 1 hour before or 1 hour after taking fluoride.

What should I do if I forget to take a dose?

Take the missed dose as soon as you remember it. However, if it is almost time for the next dose, skip the missed dose and continue your regular dosing schedule. Do not take a double dose to make up for a missed one.

What side effects can this medicine cause?

Fluoride may cause side effects. Tell your doctor if this symptom is severe or does not go away:
- staining of teeth

If you experience any of the following symptoms, call your doctor immediately:

- unusual increase in saliva
- salty or soapy taste
- stomach pain
- upset stomach
- vomiting
- diarrhea
- rash
- weakness
- tremor
- seizures

If you experience a serious side effect, you or your doctor may send a report to the Food and Drug Administration's (FDA) MedWatch Adverse Event Reporting program online [at http://www.fda.gov/MedWatch/index.html] or by phone [1-800-332-1088].

What storage conditions are needed for this medicine?

Keep this medication in the container it came in, tightly closed, and out of reach of children. Store it at room temperature and away from excess heat and moisture (not in the bathroom). Throw away any medication that is outdated or no longer needed. Talk to your pharmacist about the proper disposal of your medication.

What should I do in case of overdose?

In case of overdose, call your local poison control center at 1-800-222-1222. If the victim has collapsed or is not breathing, call local emergency services at 911.

What other information should I know?

Keep all appointments with your doctor.

Do not let anyone else take your medication. Ask your pharmacist any questions you have about refilling your prescription.

Talk to your doctor, pharmacist, or other healthcare professional if you have questions about dosing information for your medication.

Fluorouracil Topical

(flure oh yoor′ a sil)

Brand Name: Efudex®

Why is this medicine prescribed?

Fluorouracil cream and topical solution are used to treat actinic or solar keratoses (scaly or crusted lesions [skin areas] caused by years of too much exposure to sunlight). Fluorouracil cream and topical solution are also used to treat a type of skin cancer called superficial basal cell carcinoma if usual types of treatment cannot be used. Fluorouracil is in a class of medications called antimetabolites. It works by killing fast-growing cells such as the abnormal cells in actinic keratoses and basal cell carcinoma.

How should this medicine be used?

Fluorouracil comes as a solution and a cream to apply to the skin. It is usually applied to the affected areas twice a day. To help you remember to use fluorouracil, apply it around the same time every day. Follow the directions on your prescription label carefully, and ask your doctor or pharmacist to explain any part you do not understand. Use fluorouracil exactly as directed. Do not apply more or less of it or apply it more often than prescribed by your doctor.

If you are using fluorouracil to treat actinic or solar keratoses, you should continue using it until the lesions start to peel off. This usually takes about 2 to 4 weeks. However, the lesions may not be completely healed until 1 or 2 months after you stop using fluorouracil.

If you are using fluorouracil to treat basal cell carcinoma, you should continue using it until the lesions are gone. This usually takes at least 3 to 6 weeks, but may take as long as 10 to 12 weeks.

During the first few weeks of treatment, the skin lesions and surrounding areas will feel irritated and look red, swollen, and scaly. This is a sign that fluorouracil is working. Do not stop using fluorouracil unless your doctor has told you to do so.

Apply fluorouracil cream with a nonmetal applicator, a glove, or your finger. If you apply fluorouracil cream with your finger, be sure to wash your hands well immediately afterwards. Do not cover the treated areas with a bandage or dressing unless your doctor tells you to.

Do not apply fluorouracil cream or topical solution to the eyelids or the eyes, nose, or mouth.

Are there other uses for this medicine?

This medication may be prescribed for other uses; ask your doctor or pharmacist for more information.

What special precautions should I follow?

Before using fluorouracil,

- tell your doctor and pharmacist if you are allergic to fluorouracil or any other medications.
- tell your doctor and pharmacist what prescription and nonprescription medications, vitamins, nutritional supplements, and herbal products you are taking, especially other topical medications. Your doctor may need to change the doses of your medications or monitor you carefully for side effects.
- tell your doctor if you have or have ever had dihydropyrimidine dehydrogenase (DPD) enzyme deficiency (a lack of a naturally occurring enzyme in your body).
- tell your doctor if you are pregnant, plan to become pregnant, or are breast-feeding. If you become pregnant while using fluorouracil, call your doctor immediately. Fluorouracil can harm the fetus.

- plan to avoid unnecessary or prolonged exposure to sunlight and UV light (such as tanning booths) and to wear protective clothing, sunglasses, and sunscreen. Fluorouracil may make your skin sensitive to sunlight.

What special dietary instructions should I follow?

Unless your doctor tells you otherwise, continue your normal diet.

What should I do if I forget to take a dose?

Apply the missed dose as soon as you remember it. However, if it is almost time for the next dose, skip the missed dose and continue your regular dosing schedule. Do not apply a double dose to make up for a missed one.

What side effects can this medicine cause?

Fluorouracil may cause side effects. Tell your doctor if any of these symptoms are severe or do not go away:

- burning, crusting, redness, discoloration, irritation, pain, itching, rash, or soreness at the site of application

Some side effects can be serious. The following symptoms are uncommon, but if you experience any of them, call your doctor immediately:

- severe stomach pain
- bloody diarrhea
- vomiting
- fever
- chills
- severe red skin rash

Fluorouracil may cause other side effects. Call your doctor if you have any unusual problems while taking this medication.

If you experience a serious side effect, you or your doctor may send a report to the Food and Drug Administration's (FDA) MedWatch Adverse Event Reporting program online [at http://www.fda.gov/MedWatch/index.html] or by phone [1-800-332-1088].

What storage conditions are needed for this medicine?

Keep this medication in the container it came in, tightly closed, and out of reach of children. Store it at room temperature and away from excess heat and moisture (not in the bathroom). Throw away any medication that is outdated or no longer needed. Talk to your pharmacist about the proper disposal of your medication.

What should I do in case of overdose?

In case of overdose, call your local poison control center at 1-800-222-1222. If the victim has collapsed or is not breathing, call local emergency services at 911.

What other information should I know?

Keep all appointments with your doctor.

Do not let anyone else use your medication. Ask your

pharmacist any questions you have about refilling your prescription.

Talk to your doctor, pharmacist, or other healthcare professional if you have questions about dosing information for your medication.

Fluoxetine

(floo ox′ e teen)

Brand Name: Prozac®, Prozac® Weekly, Sarafem®, Symbyax® (as a combination product containing Fluoxetine and Olanzapine)

Also available generically.

Important Warning

A small number of children, teenagers, and young adults (up to 24 years of age) who took antidepressants ('mood elevators') such as fluoxetine during clinical studies became suicidal (thinking about harming or killing oneself or planning or trying to do so). Children, teenagers, and young adults who take antidepressants to treat depression or other mental illnesses may be more likely to become suicidal than children, teenagers, and young adults who do not take antidepressants to treat these conditions. However, experts are not sure about how great this risk is and how much it should be considered in deciding whether a child or teenager should take an antidepressant.

You should know that your mental health may change in unexpected ways when you take fluoxetine or other antidepressants even if you are an adult over age 24. You may become suicidal, especially at the beginning of your treatment and any time that your dose is increased or decreased. You, your family, or your caregiver should call your doctor right away if you experience any of the following symptoms: new or worsening depression; thinking about harming or killing yourself, or planning or trying to do so; extreme worry; agitation; panic attacks; difficulty falling asleep or staying asleep; aggressive behavior; irritability; acting without thinking; severe restlessness; and frenzied abnormal excitement. Be sure that your family or caregiver knows which symptoms may be serious so they can call the doctor when you are unable to seek treatment on your own.

Your healthcare provider will want to see you often while you are taking fluoxetine, especially at the beginning of your treatment. Be sure to keep all appointments for office visits with your doctor.

The doctor or pharmacist will give you the manufacturer's patient information sheet (Medication Guide) when you begin treatment with fluoxetine. Read the information carefully and ask your doctor or pharmacist if you have any questions. You also can obtain the Medication Guide from the FDA website: http://www.fda.gov/cder/drug/antidepressants/antidepressants_MG_2007.pdf.

No matter your age, before you take an antidepressant, you, your parent, or your caregiver should talk to your doctor about the risks and benefits of treating your condition with an antidepressant or with other treatments. You should also talk about the risks and benefits of not treating your condition. You should know that having depression or another mental illness greatly increases the risk that you will become suicidal. This risk is higher if you or anyone in your family has or has ever had bipolar disorder (mood that changes from depressed to abnormally excited) or mania (frenzied, abnormally excited mood) or has thought about or attempted suicide. Talk to your doctor about your condition, symptoms, and personal and family medical history. You and your doctor will decide what type of treatment is right for you.

Why is this medicine prescribed?

Fluoxetine (Prozac) is used to treat depression, obsessive-compulsive disorder (bothersome thoughts that won't go away and the need to perform certain actions over and over), some eating disorders, and panic attacks (sudden, unexpected attacks of extreme fear and worry about these attacks). Fluoxetine (Sarafem) is used to relieve the symptoms of premenstrual dysphoric disorder, including mood swings, irritability, bloating, and breast tenderness. Fluoxetine is in a class of medications called selective serotonin reuptake inhibitors (SSRIs). It works by increasing the amount of serotonin, a natural substance in the brain that helps maintain mental balance.

How should this medicine be used?

Fluoxetine (Prozac) comes as a capsule, a tablet, a delayed-release (long-acting) capsule, and a solution (liquid) to take by mouth. Fluoxetine may be taken with or without food. Fluoxetine (Sarafem) comes as a capsule to take by mouth. Fluoxetine (Prozac) capsules, tablets, and liquid are usually taken once a day in the morning or twice a day, in the morning and at noon. Fluoxetine delayed-released capsules are usually taken once a week. Fluoxetine (Sarafem) is usually taken once a day, either every day of the month or on certain days of the month. Take fluoxetine at around the same time(s) every day. Follow the directions on your prescription label carefully, and ask your doctor or pharmacist to explain any part you do not understand. Take fluoxetine exactly as directed. Do not take more or less of it or take it more often than prescribed by your doctor.

Your doctor may start you on a low dose of fluoxetine and gradually increase your dose.

It may take 4 to 5 weeks or longer before you feel the full benefit of fluoxetine. Continue to take fluoxetine even if you feel well. Do not stop taking fluoxetine without talking to your doctor. If you suddenly stop taking fluoxetine, you may experience withdrawal symptoms such as mood changes, irritability, agitation, dizziness, numbness or tingling in the hands or feet, anxiety, confusion, headache, tiredness, and difficulty falling asleep or staying asleep. Your doctor will probably decrease your dose gradually.

Are there other uses for this medicine?

Fluoxetine is also sometimes used to treat alcoholism, attention-deficit disorder, borderline personality disorder, sleep disorders, headaches, mental illness, posttraumatic stress disorder, Tourette's syndrome, obesity, sexual problems, and phobias. Talk to your doctor about the possible risks of using this medication for your condition.

This medication may be prescribed for other uses; ask your doctor or pharmacist for more information.

What special precautions should I follow?

Before taking fluoxetine,

- tell your doctor and pharmacist if you are allergic to fluoxetine or any other medications.
- tell your doctor if you are taking pimozide (Orap), thioridazine or monoamine oxidase (MAO) inhibitors such as isocarboxazid (Marplan), phenelzine (Nardil), selegiline (Eldepryl, Emsam, Zelapar), and tranylcypromine (Parnate), or if you have stopped taking a monoamine oxidase inhibitor within the past 2 weeks. Your doctor will probably tell you that you should not take fluoxetine. If you stop taking fluoxetine, you should wait at least 5 weeks before you begin to take thioridazine or a monoamine oxidase inhibitor.
- tell your doctor and pharmacist what other prescription and nonprescription medications and vitamins you are taking or plan to take. Be sure to mention any of the following: alprazolam (Xanax); anticoagulants ('blood thinners') such as warfarin (Coumadin); antidepressants (mood elevators) such as amitriptyline (Elavil), amoxapine (Asendin), clomipramine (Anafranil), desipramine (Norpramin), doxepin, imipramine (Tofranil), nortriptyline (Aventyl, Pamelor), protriptyline (Vivactil), and trimipramine (Surmontil); aspirin and other nonsteroidal anti-inflammatory medications (NSAIDs) such as ibuprofen (Advil, Motrin), and naproxen (Aleve, Naprosyn); diazepam (Valium); digoxin (Lanoxin); diuretics (water pills), flecainide (Tambocor); insulin or oral medications for diabetes; lithium (Eskalith, Lithobid); medications for anxiety and Parkinson's disease; medications for mental illness such as clozapine (Clozaril), haloperidol (Haldol), and pimozide (Orap); medications for migraine headaches such as almotriptan (Axert), eletriptan (Relpax), frovatriptan (Frova), naratriptan (Amerge), rizatriptan (Maxalt), sumatriptan (Imitrex), and zolmitriptan (Zomig); medications for seizures such as carbamazepine (Tegretol) and phenytoin (Dilantin); sedatives; sleeping pills; tramadol (Ultram);

tranquilizers; and vinblastine (Velban). Your doctor may need to change the doses of your medications or monitor you carefully for side effects.

- tell your doctor what nutritional supplements you are taking, especially products that contain St. John's wort or tryptophan.
- tell your doctor if you are being treated with electro-shock therapy (procedure in which small electric shocks are administered to the brain to treat certain mental illnesses), if you have recently had a heart attack and if you have or have ever had diabetes, seizures, or liver or heart disease.
- tell your doctor if you are pregnant, plan to become pregnant, or are breast-feeding. If you become pregnant while taking fluoxetine, call your doctor.
- you should know that fluoxetine may make you drowsy. Do not drive a car or operate machinery until you know how this medication affects you.
- remember that alcohol can add to the drowsiness caused by this medication.

What should I do if I forget to take a dose?

Take the missed dose as soon as you remember it. However, if it is almost time for the next dose, skip the missed dose and continue your regular dosing schedule. Do not take a double dose to make up for a missed one.

What side effects can this medicine cause?

Fluoxetine may cause side effects. Tell your doctor if any of these symptoms are severe or do not go away:

- nervousness
- nausea
- dry mouth
- sore throat
- drowsiness
- weakness
- uncontrollable shaking of a part of the body
- loss of appetite
- weight loss
- changes in sex drive or ability
- excessive sweating

Some side effects can be serious. If you experience any of the following symptoms or those listed in the IMPORTANT WARNING section, call your doctor immediately:

- rash
- hives
- fever
- joint pain
- swelling of the face, throat, tongue, lips, eyes, hands, feet, ankles, or lower legs
- difficulty breathing or swallowing
- seeing things or hearing voices that do not exist (hallucinating)
- seizures

Fluoxetine may cause other side effects. Call your doctor if you have any unusual problems while taking this medication.

What storage conditions are needed for this medicine?

Keep this medication in the container it came in, tightly closed, and out of reach of children. Store it at room temperature and away from excess heat and moisture (not in the bathroom). Throw away any medication that is outdated or no longer needed. Talk to your pharmacist about the proper disposal of your medication.

What should I do in case of overdose?

In case of overdose, call your local poison control center at 1-800-222-1222. If the victim has collapsed or is not breathing, call local emergency services at 911.

Symptoms of overdose may include:

- unsteadiness
- confusion
- unresponsiveness
- nervousness
- uncontrollable shaking of a part of the body
- dizziness
- rapid, irregular, or pounding heartbeat
- seeing things or hearing voices that do not exist (hallucinating)
- fever
- fainting
- coma (loss of consciousness for a period of time)

What other information should I know?

Keep all appointments with your doctor.

Do not let anyone else take your medication. Ask your pharmacist any questions you have about refilling your prescription

Dosage Facts
For Informational Purposes

Caution: Do not change your dose, how often you take your medication, or the length of time you are to take it without first talking to your healthcare provider.

The following dosage information was written using medical language for doctors and other healthcare professionals and is provided here for you to check your dosage. The dosage of this drug may differ for different patients. Therefore, always follow your doctor's instructions or the directions on the label. Contact your healthcare provider or pharmacist if you have any questions about the specific dosage of your medication after reviewing this information.

General Dosage Information

Available as fluoxetine hydrochloride; dosage is expressed in terms of fluoxetine.

Consider prolonged elimination half-life of fluoxetine and norfluoxetine when titrating dosage or discontinuing therapy. Several weeks may be required before full effect of dosage alterations is realized.

Pediatric Patients

Major Depressive Disorder

ORAL:
- Children and adolescents ≥8 years of age: initially, 10 or 20 mg daily. If therapy is initiated at 10 mg daily, it can be increased after 1 week to 20 mg daily.
- Manufacturer states that both the initial and target dose in lower weight children may be 10 mg daily.
- An increase in dosage to 20 mg daily may be considered after several weeks in lower weight children if insufficient clinical improvement is observed.

Obsessive-Compulsive Disorder

ORAL:
- Children and adolescents ≥7 years of age: initially, 10 mg daily.
- In adolescents and higher weight children, the dosage should be increased to 20 mg daily after 2 weeks; additional dosage increases may be considered after several more weeks if insufficient clinical improvement is observed.
- In lower weight children, dosage increases may be considered after several weeks if insufficient clinical improvement is observed.
- Usual dosages: 20−60 mg daily for adolescents and higher weight children or 20−30 mg daily for lower weight children.

Adult Patients

Major Depressive Disorder

ORAL:
- As conventional capsules, tablets, or solution: Initially, 20 mg once daily (in the morning). May initiate with lower dosage (e.g., 5 mg daily, 20 mg every 2−3 days). If no improvement is apparent after several weeks of therapy with 20 mg daily, an increase in dosage may be considered.
- Usual dosage: 10−80 mg daily.
- Delayed-release capsules: 90 mg once weekly, beginning 7 days after the last 20 mg daily dose as conventional capsules, tablets, or solution.
- If a satisfactory response is not maintained, consider reestablishing daily dosage regimen with conventional capsules, tablets, or solution.
- Optimum duration not established; may require several months of therapy or longer.

Obsessive-Compulsive Disorder

ORAL:
- Initially, 20 mg once daily. If no improvement is apparent after several weeks, dosage may be increased.
- Usual dosage: 20−60 mg daily.

Premenstrual Dysphoric Disorder

ORAL:
- 20 mg once daily given continuously throughout the menstrual cycle or intermittently (i.e., only during the luteal phase, starting 14 days prior to the anticipated onset of menstruation and continuing through the first full day of menses).
- If the intermittent dosing regimen is used, it should be repeated with each new menstrual cycle.

Eating Disorders
Bulimia Nervosa

ORAL:
- 60 mg daily (in the morning); dosage may be decreased as necessary to minimize adverse effects. Alternatively, dosage may be titrated up to recommended initial dosage over several days.

Anorexia Nervosa†

ORAL:
- 40 mg daily in weight-restored patients.

Panic Disorder

ORAL:
- Initially, 10 mg daily. Increase dosage after 1 week to 20 mg daily. 10−60 mg is effective; 20 mg daily most frequently used. Dosages >60 mg daily not systematically evaluated.

Bipolar Disorder
Monotherapy†

ORAL:
- 20−60 mg daily in conjunction with a mood-stabilizing agent (e.g., lithium).

Combination Therapy

Initially, 25 mg of fluoxetine and 6 mg of olanzapine once daily in the evening as a fixed-combination capsule (Symbyax® 6/25).

This dosage generally should be used as initial and maintenance therapy in patients with a predisposition to hypotensive reactions, patients with hepatic impairment, or those with factors that may slow metabolism of the drugs(s) (e.g., female gender, geriatric age, nonsmoking status); when indicated, dosage should be escalated with caution.

In other patients, increase dosages according to patient response and tolerance as indicated. In clinical trials, antidepressive efficacy was demonstrated at olanzapine dosages ranging from 6−12 mg daily and fluoxetine dosages ranging from 25−50 mg daily. Dosages exceeding 18 mg of olanzapine and 75 mg of fluoxetine not evaluated in clinical studies.

Cataplexy†

ORAL:
- 20 mg once or twice daily in conjunction with CNS stimulant therapy (e.g., dextroamphetamine, methylphenidate).

Alcohol Dependence†

ORAL:
- 60 mg daily has been used.
- Higher than average antidepressant SSRI dosage apparently is required for reduced alcohol intake; fluoxetine 40 mg daily is comparable to placebo in efficacy.

Prescribing Limits
Adult Patients

ORAL:
- Conventional capsules, tablets, or solution: Maximum 80 mg daily.

Special Populations

Hepatic Impairment
- Reduce dose and/or frequency; some clinicians recommend a 50% reduction in initial dosage for patients with well-compensated cirrhosis.

- Carefully individualize dosage in substantial hepatic impairment; adjust based on tolerance and therapeutic response.

Renal Impairment
- Consider reduction in dosage and/or frequency particularly in severe renal impairment. Supplemental doses after hemodialysis not necessary.

Geriatric Patients
- Consider reducing dose and/or frequency.

† *Use is not currently included in the labeling approved by the US Food and Drug Administration.*

Fluoxymesterone

(floo ox i mes' te rone)

Brand Name: Halotestin®

Why is this medicine prescribed?

Fluoxymesterone, an androgenic hormone, is similar to the male hormone testosterone. It is prescribed for males when this hormone is absent or low or to treat delayed onset of puberty in males. It is also used in females with certain kinds of breast cancer.

This medication is sometimes prescribed for other uses; ask your doctor or pharmacist for more information.

How should this medicine be used?

Fluoxymesterone comes as a tablet to take by mouth. It usually is taken once a day or three or four times a day. Follow the directions on your prescription label carefully, and ask your doctor or pharmacist to explain any part you do not understand. Take fluoxymesterone exactly as directed. Do not take more or less of it or take it more often than prescribed by your doctor.

Continue to take fluoxymesterone even if you feel well. Do not stop taking fluoxymesterone without talking to your doctor.

What special precautions should I follow?

Before taking fluoxymesterone,
- tell your doctor and pharmacist if you are allergic to fluoxymesterone, tartrazine (a yellow dye in some processed foods and drugs), or any other drugs.
- tell your doctor and pharmacist what prescription and nonprescription medications you are taking, especially anticoagulants ('blood thinners') such as warfarin (Coumadin), diabetes medications such as insulin, and vitamins.
- tell your doctor if you have or have ever had diabetes; migraine headaches; heart, liver, or kidney disease; high blood cholesterol or fats; cancer of the breast; depres-

sion; enlarged prostate or prostate cancer; or any blood disorder.
- tell your doctor if you are pregnant, plan to become pregnant or are breast-feeding. If you become pregnant while taking fluoxymesterone, call your doctor.

What special dietary instructions should I follow?

Fluoxymesterone may cause an upset stomach. Take fluoxymesterone with food or milk.

What should I do if I forget to take a dose?

Take the missed dose as soon as you remember it. However, if it is almost time for the next dose, skip the missed dose and continue your regular dosing schedule. Do not take a double dose to make up for a missed one.

Call your doctor for directions if you miss more than one dose.

What side effects can this medicine cause?

Fluoxymesterone may cause side effects. Tell your doctor if any of these symptoms are severe or do not go away:
- acne
- enlargement of the breast
- swelling or fluid retention
- absence of menstrual periods
- deepening of the voice or hoarseness
- facial hair growth
- headache
- anxiety
- depression
- tingling, prickling, burning, or tight sensations
- upset stomach
- vomiting
- increased number and/or duration of penile erections
- decreased sperm production
- increased blood cholesterol
- increased blood calcium

If you experience any of the following symptoms, call your doctor immediately:
- skin rash, itching, or hives
- difficulty breathing
- yellowing of the skin or eyes
- unusual or excessive bleeding
- severe swelling or fluid retention
- difficulty urinating (males)

If you experience a serious side effect, you or your doctor may send a report to the Food and Drug Administration's (FDA) MedWatch Adverse Event Reporting program online [at http://www.fda.gov/MedWatch/index.html] or by phone [1-800-332-1088].

What storage conditions are needed for this medicine?

Keep this medication in the container it came in, tightly closed, and out of reach of children. Store it at room tem-

perature and away from excess heat and moisture (not in the bathroom). Throw away any medication that is outdated or no longer needed. Talk to your pharmacist about the proper disposal of your medication.

What other information should I know?

Keep all appointments with your doctor and the laboratory. Your doctor will order certain lab tests to check your response to fluoxymesterone.

Do not let anyone else take your medication. Ask your pharmacist any questions you have about refilling your prescription.

Talk to your doctor, pharmacist, or other healthcare professional if you have questions about dosing information for your medication.

Fluphenazine

(floo fen′ a zeen)

Brand Name: Prolixin Decanoate®
Also available generically.

Why is this medicine prescribed?

Fluphenazine is an antipsychotic medication used to treat schizophrenia and psychotic symptoms such as hallucinations, delusions, and hostility.

This medication is sometimes prescribed for other uses; ask your doctor or pharmacist for more information.

How should this medicine be used?

Fluphenazine comes as a tablet or oral liquid (elixir and concentrate) to take by mouth. It is usually taken two or three times a day and may be taken with or without food. Follow the directions on your prescription label carefully, and ask your doctor or pharmacist to explain any part you do not understand. Take fluphenazine exactly as directed. Do not take more or less of it or take it more often than prescribed by your doctor.

Fluphenazine oral liquid comes with a specially marked dropper for measuring the dose. Ask your pharmacist to show you how to use the dropper. Do not allow the liquid to touch your skin or clothing; it can cause skin irritation. Dilute the concentrate in water, Seven-Up, carbonated orange beverage, milk, or V-8, pineapple, apricot, prune, orange, tomato, or grapefruit juice just before taking it. Do not use beverages containing caffeine (coffee, tea, and cola) or apple juice.

Continue to take fluphenazine even if you feel well. Do not stop taking fluphenazine without talking to your doctor, especially if you have taken large doses for a long time. Your doctor probably will want to decrease your dose gradually. This drug must be taken regularly for a few weeks before its full effect is felt.

What special precautions should I follow?

Before taking fluphenazine,

- tell your doctor and pharmacist if you are allergic to fluphenazine or any other drugs.
- tell your doctor and pharmacist what prescription and nonprescription drugs you are taking or have taken within the last 2 weeks, especially antidepressants; antihistamines; bromocriptine (Parlodel); diet pills; lithium (Eskalith, Lithobid); medication for high blood pressure, seizures, Parkinson's disease, asthma, colds, or allergies; meperidine (Demerol); methyldopa (Aldomet); muscle relaxants; propranolol (Inderal); sedatives; sleeping pills; thyroid medications, tranquilizers; and vitamins.
- tell your doctor if you have or have ever had glaucoma, an enlarged prostate, difficulty urinating, seizures, an overactive thyroid gland, or liver, kidney, or heart disease.
- tell your doctor if you are pregnant, plan to become pregnant, or are breast-feeding. If you become pregnant while taking fluphenazine, call your doctor immediately.
- if you are having surgery, including dental surgery, tell the doctor or dentist that you are taking fluphenazine.
- you should know that this drug may make you drowsy. Do not drive a car or operate machinery until you know how this drug affects you.
- remember that alcohol can add to the drowsiness caused by this drug.
- tell your doctor if you use tobacco products. Cigarette smoking may decrease the effectiveness of this drug.

What should I do if I forget to take a dose?

Take the missed dose as soon as you remember it. However, if it is almost time for the next dose, skip the missed dose and continue your regular dosing schedule. Do not take a double dose to make up for a missed one.

What side effects can this medicine cause?

Side effects from fluphenazine are common:
- upset stomach
- drowsiness
- weakness or tiredness
- excitement or anxiety
- insomnia
- nightmares
- dry mouth
- skin more sensitive to sunlight than usual
- changes in appetite or weight

Tell your doctor if any of these symptoms are severe or do not go away:
- constipation
- difficulty urinating
- frequent urination
- blurred vision
- changes in sex drive or ability
- excessive sweating

If you experience any of the following symptoms, call your doctor immediately:

- jaw, neck, and back muscle spasms
- slow or difficult speech
- shuffling walk
- persistent fine tremor or inability to sit still
- fever, chills, sore throat, or flu-like symptoms
- difficulty breathing or swallowing
- severe skin rash
- yellowing of the skin or eyes
- irregular heartbeat

If you experience a serious side effect, you or your doctor may send a report to the Food and Drug Administration's (FDA) MedWatch Adverse Event Reporting program online [at http://www.fda.gov/MedWatch/index.html] or by phone [1-800-332-1088].

What storage conditions are needed for this medicine?

Keep this medication in the container it came in, tightly closed, and out of reach of children. Store it at room temperature and away from excess heat and moisture (not in the bathroom). Throw away any medication that is outdated or no longer needed. Talk to your pharmacist about the proper disposal of your medication.

What should I do in case of overdose?

In case of overdose, call your local poison control center at 1-800-222-1222. If the victim has collapsed or is not breathing, call local emergency services at 911.

What other information should I know?

Keep all appointments with your doctor and the laboratory. Your doctor will order certain lab tests to check your response to fluphenazine.

Do not let anyone else take your medication. Ask your pharmacist any questions you have about refilling your prescription.

Dosage Facts
For Informational Purposes

Caution: Do not change your dose, how often you take your medication, or the length of time you are to take it without first talking to your healthcare provider.

The following dosage information was written using medical language for doctors and other healthcare professionals and is provided here for you to check your dosage. The dosage of this drug may differ for different patients. Therefore, always follow your doctor's instructions or the directions on the label. Contact your healthcare provider or pharmacist if you have any questions about the specific dosage of your medication after reviewing this information.

General Dosage Information

Available as fluphenazine hydrochloride or fluphenazine decanoate; dosage expressed in terms of the salt.

Carefully adjust dosage according to individual requirements and response, using lowest possible effective dosage.

Because of risk of adverse reactions associated with cumulative effects of phenothiazines, periodically evaluate patients with a history of long-term therapy with fluphenazine and/or other antipsychotic agents to determine whether maintenance dosage may be decreased or drug therapy discontinued.

Conversion from oral fluphenazine hydrochloride to long-acting decanoate injection may be indicated for psychotic patients stabilized on a fixed daily oral dosage. In patients without a history of therapy with phenothiazines, administer shorter-acting form for several weeks prior to instituting therapy with fluphenazine decanoate in order to determine patient's approximate dosage requirements and susceptibility to adverse effects.

Precise formula for converting therapy from fluphenazine hydrochloride to fluphenazine decanoate not established. An approximate conversion ratio of 12.5 mg every 3 weeks of fluphenazine decanoate for every 10 mg daily of fluphenazine hydrochloride has been used.

Adult Patients

Psychotic Disorders

ORAL:

- Fluphenazine hydrochloride: Initially, 2.5–10 mg daily given in divided doses every 6–8 hours. Dosage may be gradually increased, if necessary, until desired clinical effects are obtained.
- Optimum therapeutic effect often occurs with oral fluphenazine hydrochloride dosages <20 mg daily. Dosages up to 40 mg may be required in severely disturbed patients, but safety of prolonged administration of such dosages not established. Use dosages >20 mg daily with caution.
- After maximum response attained, reduce fluphenazine hydrochloride dosage gradually to maintenance dosage of 1–5 mg daily, often as a single dose. To avoid recurrence of psychotic symptoms, continued therapy is required following optimum therapeutic response.

Prescribing Limits

Adult Patients

Psychotic Disorders

ORAL:

- Fluphenazine hydrochloride: Safety of prolonged administration of dosages up to 40 mg daily not established. Use dosages >20 mg daily with caution.

Special Populations

Geriatric Patients
- Fluphenazine hydrochloride: Initially 1–2.5 mg orally daily. Increase dosage more gradually in debilitated, emaciated, or geriatric patients.

Flurandrenolide Topical

(flure an dren' oh lide)

Brand Name: Cordran®, Cordran® SP, Cordran® Tape

Why is this medicine prescribed?

Flurandrenolide is used to treat the itching, redness, dryness, crusting, scaling, inflammation, and discomfort of various skin conditions.

This medication is sometimes prescribed for other uses; ask your doctor or pharmacist for more information.

How should this medicine be used?

Flurandrenolide comes in ointment, cream, and lotion in various strengths for use on the skin. It also comes in tape to be applied to the skin as a dressing. It usually is applied two or three times a day. Follow the directions on your prescription label carefully, and ask your doctor or pharmacist to explain any part you do not understand. Use flurandrenolide exactly as directed. Do not use more or less of it or use it more often than prescribed by your doctor. Do not apply it to other areas of your body or wrap or bandage the treated area unless directed to do so by your doctor.

Wash or soak the affected area thoroughly before applying the medicine, unless it irritates the skin. Then apply the ointment, cream, or lotion sparingly in a thin film and rub it in gently.

To use the lotion on your scalp, part your hair, apply a small amount of the medicine on the affected area and rub it in gently. Protect the area from washing and rubbing until the lotion dries. You may wash your hair as usual but not right after applying the medicine.

Avoid prolonged use on the face, in the genital and rectal areas, and in skin creases and armpits unless directed by your doctor.

If you are using flurandrenolide on your face, keep it out of your eyes.

If you are using flurandrenolide on a child's diaper area, do not use tight-fitting diapers or plastic pants. Such use may increase side effects.

Do not apply cosmetics or other skin preparations on the treated area without talking with your doctor.

If your doctor directs you to use flurandrenolide tape, follow these steps and the special instructions that accompany this medication:

1. Gently clean the affected area with germicidal soap (ask your pharmacist to recommend a soap) and water, removing any scales and crusts. Dry your skin thoroughly.
2. Shave or clip the hair in the area to allow the tape to adhere well to your skin and for comfortable removal.
3. Cut (do not tear) a piece of tape slightly larger than the treatment area and round off the corners. Remove the

white paper from the tape, exposing the medicated surface. Do not let the tape stick to itself. Keep your skin smooth, and press the tape in place.

4. Replace the tape as directed on your prescription label (usually every 12 hours). Remove the old tape, wash your skin, and allow the area to dry for 1 hour before applying fresh tape.
5. If the ends of the tape loosen before it is time to replace it, trim off the ends and replace them with new tape.

If your doctor tells you to wrap or bandage the treated area, follow these instructions:

1. Soak the area in water or wash it well.
2. While the skin is moist, gently rub the medication into the affected areas.
3. Cover the area with plastic wrap (such as Saran Wrap or Handi-Wrap). The plastic may be held in place with a gauze or elastic bandage or adhesive tape on the normal skin beside the treated area. (Instead of using plastic wrap, plastic gloves may be used for the hands, plastic bags for the feet, or a shower cap for the scalp.)
4. Carefully seal the edges of the plastic to make sure the wrap adheres closely to the skin. If the affected area is moist, you can leave the edges of the plastic wrap partly unsealed or puncture the wrap to allow excess moisture to escape.
5. Leave the plastic wrap in place as long as directed by your doctor. Usually plastic wraps are left in place no more than 12 hours each day.
6. Cleanse the skin and reapply the medication each time a new plastic wrapping is applied. Do not discontinue treatment abruptly without talking to your doctor.

What special precautions should I follow?

Before using flurandrenolide,

- tell your doctor and pharmacist if you are allergic to flurandrenolide or any other drugs.
- tell your doctor and pharmacist what prescription and nonprescription medications you are taking, especially cancer chemotherapy agents, other topical medications, and vitamins.
- tell your doctor if you have an infection or have ever had diabetes, glaucoma, cataracts, a circulation disorder, or an immune disorder.
- tell your doctor if you are pregnant, plan to become pregnant, or are breast-feeding. If you become pregnant while using flurandrenolide, call your doctor immediately.

What should I do if I forget to take a dose?

Apply the missed dose as soon as you remember it. However, if it is almost time for the next dose, skip the missed dose and continue your regular dosing schedule. Do not apply a double dose to make up for a missed one.

What side effects can this medicine cause?

Flurandrenolide may cause side effects. Tell your doctor if any of these symptoms are severe or do not go away:

- drying or cracking of the skin
- acne
- itching
- change in skin color

If you experience any of the following symptoms, call your doctor immediately:

- severe skin rash
- difficulty breathing or swallowing
- wheezing
- skin infection (redness, swelling, or oozing pus)

If you experience a serious side effect, you or your doctor may send a report to the Food and Drug Administration's (FDA) MedWatch Adverse Event Reporting program online [at http://www.fda.gov/MedWatch/index.html] or by phone [1-800-332-1088].

What storage conditions are needed for this medicine?

Keep this medication in the container it came in, tightly closed, and out of reach of children. Store it at room temperature. Do not allow it to freeze. Throw away any medication that is outdated or no longer needed. Do not use it to treat other skin conditions. Talk to your pharmacist about the proper disposal of your medication.

What other information should I know?

Keep all appointments with your doctor.

Do not let anyone else use your medication. Ask your pharmacist any questions you have about refilling your prescription.

Talk to your doctor, pharmacist, or other healthcare professional if you have questions about dosing information for your medication.

Flurazepam

(flure az′ e pam)

Brand Name: Dalmane®

Why is this medicine prescribed?

Flurazepam is used to treat insomnia (difficulty falling asleep and staying asleep). Flurazepam is in a class of medications called benzodiazepines. It works by slowing activity in the brain.

How should this medicine be used?

Flurazepam comes as a capsule to take by mouth. It usually is taken before bedtime when needed. Follow the directions on your prescription label carefully, and ask your doctor or pharmacist to explain any part you do not understand. Take flurazepam exactly as directed.

Flurazepam can be habit-forming. Do not take a larger dose, take it more often, or take it for a longer time than prescribed by your doctor.

Flurazepam starts working slowly and continues to work for a short time after you stop taking it. It may take two or three nights before you experience the full benefit of flurazepam. You may continue to feel the effects of flurazepam for one to two nights after you stop taking the medication.

Do not stop taking flurazepam without talking to your doctor. Your doctor will probably decrease your dose gradually. If you suddenly stop taking flurazepam, especially after taking it regularly, you may develop withdrawal symptoms such as sadness, difficulty sleeping, seizures, shaking of a part of your body that you cannot control, stomach and muscle cramps, vomiting, and sweating.

Are there other uses for this medicine?

This medication may be prescribed for other uses; ask your doctor or pharmacist for more information.

What special precautions should I follow?

Before taking flurazepam,

- tell your doctor and pharmacist if you are allergic to flurazepam, any other medications, or corn.
- tell your doctor and pharmacist what prescription and nonprescription medications, vitamins, nutritional supplements, and herbal products you are taking or plan to take during your treatment with flurazepam and for several days afterward. Be sure to mention any of the following: antihistamines; medications for anxiety, depression mental illness, or seizures; muscle relaxants; sedatives; sleeping pills; andtranquilizers. Your doctor may need to change the doses of your medications or monitor you carefully for side effects.
- tell your doctor if you drink or have ever drunk large amounts of alcohol, use or have ever used street drugs, or have overused prescription medications. Also tell your doctor if you have or have ever had depression; mental illness; glaucoma; or lung, kidney, or liver disease.
- tell your doctor if you are pregnant, plan to become pregnant, or are breast-feeding. If you become pregnant while taking flurazepam, call your doctor immediately.
- if you are having surgery, including dental surgery, tell the doctor or dentist that you are taking flurazepam.
- you should know that this medication may make you drowsy and may increase the risk that you could fall. Take extra care to be sure you do not fall, especially if you get out of bed in the middle of the night.Do not drive a car or operate machinery until you know how this medication affects you.
- remember that alcohol can add to the drowsiness caused by this medication. Do not drink alcohol while you are taking flurazepam and for several days after you stop taking the medication.

- tell your doctor if you use tobacco products. Cigarette smoking may decrease the effectiveness of this medication.
- you should know that your mental health may change in unexpected ways while you are taking this medication. It is hard to tell if these changes are caused by flurazepam or if they are caused by physical or mental illnesses that you already have or suddenly develop. Tell your doctor right away if you experience any of the following symptoms: aggressiveness, strange or unusually outgoing behavior, hallucinations (seeing things or hearing voices that do not exist), feeling as if you are outside of your body, memory problems, new or worsening depression, thinking about killing yourself, confusion, and any other changes in your usual thoughts or behavior. Be sure that your family knows which symptoms may be serious so that they can call the doctor if you are unable to seek treatment on your own.

What special dietary instructions should I follow?

Unless your doctor tells you otherwise, continue your normal diet.

What should I do if I forget to take a dose?

Flurazepam should only be taken at bedtime. If you forget to take flurazepam at bedtime, you are unable to fall asleep, and you will still be able to stay in bed for a full night's sleep, you may take flurazepam at that time. Do not take a double dose of flurazepam to make up for a missed dose.

What side effects can this medicine cause?

Flurazepam may cause side effects. Tell your doctor if any of these symptoms are severe or do not go away:

- drowsiness
- dizziness or lightheadness
- loss of coordination
- headache
- heartburn
- upset stomach
- vomiting
- stomach pain
- diarrhea
- constipation
- nervousness
- talking more than usual
- weakness
- difficulty urinating

Some side effects can be serious. The following symptoms are uncommon, but if you experience any of them, call your doctor immediately:

- pounding heartbeat
- chest pain
- confusion
- rash

If you experience a serious side effect, you or your doctor may send a report to the Food and Drug Administration's (FDA) MedWatch Adverse Event Reporting program online [at http://www.fda.gov/MedWatch/index.html] or by phone [1-800-332-1088].

What storage conditions are needed for this medicine?

Keep this medication in the container it came in, tightly closed, and out of reach of children. Store it at room temperature and away from excess heat and moisture (not in the bathroom). Throw away any medication that is outdated or no longer needed. Talk to your pharmacist about the proper disposal of your medication.

What should I do in case of overdose?

In case of overdose, call your local poison control center at 1-800-222-1222. If the victim has collapsed or is not breathing, call local emergency services at 911.

Symptoms of overdose may include:

- drowsiness
- confusion
- coma

What other information should I know?

Keep all appointments with your doctor.

Do not let anyone else take your medication. Ask your pharmacist any questions you have about refilling your prescription.

Talk to your doctor, pharmacist, or other healthcare professional if you have questions about dosing information for your medication.

Flurbiprofen

(flure bi′ proe fen)

Brand Name: Ansaid
Also available generically.

Important Warning

People who take nonsteroidal anti-inflammatory medications (NSAIDs) (other than aspirin) such as flurbiprofen may have a higher risk of having a heart attack or a stroke than people who do not take these medications. These events may happen without warning and may cause death. This risk may be higher for people who take NSAIDs for a long time. Tell your doctor if you or anyone in your family has or has ever had heart disease, a heart attack, or a stroke, if you smoke, and if you have or have ever-

continued on next page

Important Warning (cont'd)

had high cholesterol, high blood pressure, or diabetes. Get emergency medical help right away if you experience any of the following symptoms: chest pain, shortness of breath, weakness in one part or side of the body, or slurred speech.

If you will be undergoing a coronary artery bypass graft (CABG; a type of heart surgery), you should not take flurbiprofen right before or right after the surgery.

NSAIDs such as flurbiprofen may cause ulcers, bleeding, or holes in the stomach or intestine. These problems may develop at any time during treatment, may happen without warning symptoms, and may cause death. The risk may be higher for people who take NSAIDs for a long time, are older in age, have poor health, or drink large amounts of alcohol while you are taking flurbiprofen. Tell your doctor if you take any of the following medications: anticoagulants ('blood thinners') such as warfarin (Coumadin); aspirin; other NSAIDs such as ibuprofen (Advil, Motrin) and naproxen (Aleve, Naprosyn); or oral steroids such as dexamethasone (Decadron, Dexone), methylprednisolone (Medrol), and prednisone (Deltasone). Also tell your doctor if you have or have ever had ulcers or bleeding in your stomach or intestines or other bleeding disorders. If you experience any of the following symptoms, stop taking flurbiprofen and call your doctor: stomach pain, heartburn, vomiting a substance that is bloody or looks like coffee grounds, blood in the stool, or black and tarry stools.

Keep all appointments with your doctor and the laboratory. Your doctor will monitor your symptoms carefully and will probably order certain tests to check your body's response to flurbiprofen. Be sure to tell your doctor how you are feeling so that your doctor can prescribe the right amount of medication to treat your condition with the lowest risk of serious side effects.

Your doctor or pharmacist will give you the manufacturer's patient information sheet (Medication Guide) when you begin treatment with flurbiprofen and each time you refill your prescription. Read the information carefully and ask your doctor or pharmacist if you have any questions. You can also visit the Food and Drug Administration (FDA) website (http://www.fda.gov/cder) or the manufacturer's website to obtain the Medication Guide.

Why is this medicine prescribed?

Flurbiprofen is used to relieve pain, tenderness, swelling, and stiffness caused by osteoarthritis (arthritis caused by a breakdown of the lining of the joints) and rheumatoid arthritis (arthritis caused by swelling of the lining of the joints). Flurbiprofen is in a class of medications called NSAIDs. It works by stopping the body's production of a substance that causes pain, fever, and inflammation.

How should this medicine be used?

Flurbiprofen comes as a tablet to take by mouth. It usually is taken two to four times a day. Take flurbiprofen at around the same times every day. Follow the directions on your prescription label carefully, and ask your doctor or pharmacist to explain any part you do not understand. Take flurbiprofen exactly as directed. Do not take more or less of it or take it more often than prescribed by your doctor.

Are there other uses for this medicine?

Flurbiprofen is also used to treat ankylosing spondylitis (arthritis that mainly affects the spine).

This medication is sometimes prescribed for other uses; ask your doctor or pharmacist for more information.

What special precautions should I follow?

Before taking flurbiprofen,

- tell your doctor and pharmacist if you are allergic to flurbiprofen, aspirin or other NSAIDs such as ibuprofen (Advil, Motrin) and naproxen (Aleve, Naprosyn), or any other medications.
- tell your doctor and pharmacist what prescription and nonprescription medications, vitamins, nutritional supplements, and herbal products you are taking or plan to take. Be sure to mention the medications listed in the IMPORTANT WARNING section and any of the following: angiotensin-converting enzyme (ACE) inhibitors such as benazepril (Lotensin), captopril (Capoten), enalapril (Vasotec), fosinopril (Monopril), lisinopril (Prinivil, Zestril), moexipril (Univasc), perindopril (Aceon), quinapril (Accupril), ramipril (Altace), and trandolapril (Mavik); beta blockers such as atenolol (Tenormin), labetalol (Normodyne), metoprolol (Lopressor, Toprol XL), nadolol (Corgard), and propranolol (Inderal); diuretics ('water pills'); lithium (Eskalith, Lithobid); and methotrexate (Rheumatrex).
- tell your doctor if you have or have ever had asthma, especially if you also have frequent stuffed or runny nose or nasal polyps (swelling of the lining of the nose); swelling of the hands, feet, ankles, or lower legs; or liver or kidney disease.
- tell your doctor if you are pregnant, especially if you are in the last few months of your pregnancy, you plan to become pregnant, or you are breast-feeding. If you become pregnant while taking flurbiprofen, call your doctor.
- if you are having surgery, including dental surgery, tell the doctor or dentist that you are taking flurbiprofen.

What special dietary instructions should I follow?

Unless your doctor tells you otherwise, continue your normal diet.

What should I do if I forget to take a dose?

Take the missed dose as soon as you remember it. However, if it is almost time for the next dose, skip the missed dose and continue your regular dosing schedule. Do not take a double dose to make up for a missed one.

What side effects can this medicine cause?

Flurbiprofen may cause side effects. Tell your doctor if any of these symptoms are severe or do not go away:

- headache
- nervousness or anxiety
- depression
- memory problems
- shaking of a part of the body that you cannot control
- difficulty falling asleep or staying asleep
- vomiting
- gas
- constipation
- diarrhea
- runny nose
- ringing in the ears

Some side effects can be serious. If you experience any of the following symptoms, or those listed in the IMPORTANT WARNING section, call your doctor immediately. Do not take any more flurbiprofen until you speak to your doctor.

- changes in vision (blurriness, difficulty seeing)
- unexplained weight gain
- fever
- blisters
- rash
- itching
- hives
- swelling of the eyes, face, lips, tongue, throat, hands, feet, ankles, or lower legs
- difficulty breathing or swallowing
- pale skin
- fast heartbeat
- excessive tiredness
- unusual bleeding or bruising
- lack of energy
- upset stomach
- loss of appetite
- pain in the upper right part of the stomach
- flu-like symptoms
- yellowing of the skin or eyes
- cloudy, discolored, or bloody urine
- back pain
- difficult or painful urination

Flurbiprofen may cause other side effects. Call your doctor if you have any unusual problems while taking this medication.

If you experience a serious side effect, you or your doctor may send a report to the Food and Drug Administration's (FDA) MedWatch Adverse Event Reporting program online [at http://www.fda.gov/MedWatch/index.html] or by phone [1-800-332-1088].

What storage conditions are needed for this medicine?

Keep this medication in the container it came in, tightly closed, and out of reach of children. Store it at room temperature and away from excess heat and moisture (not in the bathroom). Throw away any medication that is outdated or no longer needed. Talk to your pharmacist about the proper disposal of your medication.

What should I do in case of overdose?

In case of overdose, call your local poison control center at 1-800-222-1222. If the victim has collapsed or is not breathing, call local emergency services at 911.

Symptoms of overdose may include:

- lack of energy
- drowsiness
- upset stomach
- vomiting
- stomach pain
- bloody, black, or tarry stools
- vomiting a substance that is bloody or looks like coffee grounds
- difficulty breathing
- coma (loss of consciousness for a period of time)

What other information should I know?

Do not let anyone else take your medication. Ask your pharmacist any questions you have about refilling your prescription.

Dosage Facts
For Informational Purposes

Caution: Do not change your dose, how often you take your medication, or the length of time you are to take it without first talking to your healthcare provider.

The following dosage information was written using medical language for doctors and other healthcare professionals and is provided here for you to check your dosage. The dosage of this drug may differ for different patients. Therefore, always follow your doctor's instructions or the directions on the label. Contact your healthcare provider or pharmacist if you have any questions about the specific dosage of your medication after reviewing this information.

General Dosage Information

Attempt to titrate to the lowest effective dosage and shortest duration of therapy.

Adult Patients

Inflammatory Diseases

Osteoarthritis or Rheumatoid Arthritis

ORAL:
- 200–300 mg daily in 2–4 divided doses; do not exceed 100 mg in a single dose.

Prescribing Limits

Adult Patients

ORAL:
- Maximum 100 mg in a single dose.

Special Populations

Hepatic Impairment
- Consider dosage reduction; metabolism may be decreased.

Renal Impairment
- Consider dosage reduction; clearance may be decreased.

Geriatric Patients
- Select dosage with caution because of age-related decreases in hepatic, renal, and/or cardiac function, and concomitant disease and drug therapy.
- Use the lowest effective dose for the shortest possible duration to minimize possible GI effects.

Fluticasone and Salmeterol Oral Inhalation

(floo tik' a sone and sal me' te role)

Brand Name: Advair ®

Important Warning

In a large clinical study more patients with asthma who used salmeterol died of asthma problems than patients with asthma who did not use salmeterol. If you have asthma, use of salmeterol may increase the risk that you will develop serious or fatal asthma problems. There is not enough information available to tell whether inhaling fluticasone with salmeterol increases, decreases, or does not change this risk. Your doctor will only prescribe fluticasone and salmeterol if other medications have not controlled your asthma or if your asthma is so severe that two medications are needed to control it.

Do not use fluticasone and salmeterol if you have asthma that is quickly getting worse. Tell your doctor if you have had many severe asthma attacks or if you have ever been hospitalized because of asthma symptoms. If you have any of the following signs of worsening asthma, call your doctor immediately:

- your short-acting inhaler [inhaled medication such as albuterol (Proventil, Ventolin) that is used to treat sudden attacks of asthma symptoms] does not work as well as it did in the past
- you need to use more puffs than usual of your short-acting inhaler or use it more often
- you need to use four or more puffs per day of your short acting inhaler for 2 or more days in a row
- you use one whole canister (200 inhalations) of your short acting inhaler during an 8-week period
- your peak-flow meter (home device used to test breathing) results show that your breathing problems are worsening
- you need to go to the emergency room for asthma treatment
- your asthma symptoms do not improve after you use fluticasone and salmeterol inhalation regularly for 1 week or your symptoms get worse at any time during your treatment

Talk to your doctor about the risks of using this medication.

Your doctor or pharmacist will give you the manufacturer's patient information sheet (Medication Guide) when you begin treatment with fluticasone and salmeterol and each time you refill your prescription. Read the information carefully and ask your doctor or pharmacist if you have any questions. You can also visit the Food and Drug Administration (FDA) website (http://www.fda.gov/cder) or the manufacturer's website to obtain the Medication Guide.

Why is this medicine prescribed?

The combination of fluticasone and salmeterol is used to prevent wheezing, shortness of breath, and breathing difficulties caused by asthma and chronic obstructive pulmonary disease (COPD; a group of lung diseases that includes chronic bronchitis and emphysema). Fluticasone is in a class of medications called steroids. It works by reducing swelling in the airways. Salmeterol is in a class of medications called long-acting beta-agonists (LABAs). It works by relaxing and opening air passages in the lungs, making it easier to breathe.

How should this medicine be used?

The combination of fluticasone and salmeterol comes as a powder to inhale by mouth using a specially designed inhaler. It is usually used twice a day, in the morning and evening, about 12 hours apart. Use fluticasone and salmeterol at around the same times every day. Follow the directions on your prescription label carefully, and ask your doctor or pharmacist to explain any part you do not understand.

Use fluticasone and salmeterol exactly as directed. Do not use more or less of it or use it more often than prescribed by your doctor.

Talk to your doctor about how you should take your other oral or inhaled medications for asthma during your treatment with salmeterol and fluticasone inhalation. If you were using a short-acting beta agonist inhaler such as albuterol (Proventil, Ventolin) on a regular basis, your doctor will probably tell you to stop using it regularly but to continue to use it to treat sudden attacks of asthma symptoms. Follow these directions carefully. Do not change the way you use any of your medications or stop taking any of your medications without talking to your doctor.

Do not use fluticasone and salmeterol during an attack of asthma or COPD. Your doctor will prescribe a short-acting inhaler to use during attacks.

Fluticasone and salmeterol inhalation controls asthma and COPD but does not cure these conditions. It may take a week or longer before you feel the full benefit of fluticasone and salmeterol. Continue to use fluticasone and salmeterol even if you feel well. Do not stop using fluticasone and salmeterol without talking to your doctor. If you stop using fluticasone and salmeterol inhalation, your symptoms may return.

Before you use fluticasone and salmeterol inhalation for the first time, ask your doctor, pharmacist, or respiratory therapist to show you how to use the inhaler. Practice using your inhaler while he or she watches.

To use the inhaler, follow these steps:

1. If you will be using a new inhaler for the first time, remove it from the box and the foil wrapper. Fill in the blanks on the inhaler label with the date that you opened the pouch and the date 1 month later when you must replace the inhaler.
2. Hold the inhaler in one hand, and put the thumb of your other hand on the thumbgrip. Push your thumb away from you as far as it will go until the mouthpiece appears and snaps into position.
3. Hold the inhaler in a level, horizontal position with the mouthpiece toward you. Slide the lever away from you as far as it will go until it clicks.
4. Every time the lever is pushed back, a dose is ready to inhale. You will see the number in the dose counter go down. Do not waste doses by closing or tilting the inhaler, playing with the lever, or advancing the lever more than once.
5. Hold the inhaler level and away from your mouth, and breathe out as far as you comfortably can.
6. Keep the inhaler in a level, flat position. Put the mouthpiece to your lips. Breathe in quickly and deeply though the inhaler, not through your nose.
7. Remove the inhaler from your mouth, and hold your breath for 10 seconds or as long as you comfortably can. Breathe out slowly.
8. You will probably taste or feel the salmeterol powder released by the inhaler. Even if you do not, do not inhale another dose. If you are not sure you are getting your dose of fluticasone and salmeterol, call your doctor or pharmacist.
9. Rinse your mouth with water, but do not swallow.
10. Put your thumb on the thumbgrip and slide it back toward you as far as it will go. The inhaler will click shut.

Never exhale into the inhaler, take the inhaler apart, or wash the mouthpiece or any part of the inhaler. Keep the inhaler dry. Do not use the inhaler with a spacer.

Are there other uses for this medicine?

This medication may be prescribed for other uses; ask your doctor or pharmacist for more information.

What special precautions should I follow?

Before using fluticasone and salmeterol,

- tell your doctor and pharmacist if you are allergic to fluticasone (Flonase, Flovent), salmeterol (Serevent), any other medications, milk protein, or any foods.
- tell your doctor if you use another LABA such as formoterol (Foradil) or salmeterol (Serevent). These medications should not be used with fluticasone and salmeterol inhalation. Your doctor will tell you which medication you should use and which medication you should stop using.
- tell your doctor and pharmacist what other prescription and nonprescription medications, vitamins, nutritional supplements, and herbal products you are taking. Be sure to mention any of the following: antifungals such as fluconazole (Diflucan), itraconazole (Sporanox), and ketoconazole (Nizoral); beta-blockers such as atenolol (Tenormin), labetalol (Normodyne), metoprolol (Lopressor, Toprol XL), nadolol (Corgard), and propranolol (Inderal); cimetidine (Tagamet); clarithromycin (Biaxin); cyclosporine (Neoral, Sandimmune); danazol (Danocrine); delavirdine (Rescriptor); diltiazem (Cardizem, Dilacor, Tiazac); diuretics ('water pills'); fluoxetine (Prozac, Sarafem); fluvoxamine (Luvox); HIV protease inhibitors such as indinavir (Crixivan), nelfinavir (Viracept), and ritonavir (Norvir); isoniazid (INH, Nydrazid); other medications for asthma or COPD; medications for seizures; metronidazole (Flagyl); nefazodone; oral contraceptives (birth control pills); troleandomycin (TAO); verapamil (Calan, Covera, Isoptin, Verelan); and zafirlukast (Accolate). Also tell your doctor and pharmacist if you are taking the following medications or have stopped taking them during the past 2 weeks: antidepressants such as amitriptyline (Elavil), amoxapine (Asendin), clomipramine (Anafranil), desipramine (Norpramin), doxepin (Adapin, Sinequan), imipramine (Tofranil), nortriptyline (Aventyl, Pamelor), protriptyline (Vivactil), and trimipramine (Surmontil); and monoamine oxidase (MAO) inhibitors, including isocarboxazid (Marplan), phenelzine (Nardil), selegiline (Eldepryl), and tranylcypromine (Parnate). Your doctor may need to change the doses of your medications or monitor you carefully for side effects.

- tell your doctor if you or anyone in your family has or has ever had osteoporosis (a condition in which the bones become weak and fragile), and if you have or have ever had high blood pressure, irregular heartbeat, seizures, hyperthyroidism (overactive thyroid), diabetes, tuberculosis (TB), glaucoma (an eye disease), any condition that affects your immune system, liver disease, or heart disease. Also tell your doctor if you have a herpes eye infection or any other type of infection and if you smoke or use tobacco products, if you do not eat a healthy diet, or if you do not exercise very often.
- tell your doctor if you are pregnant, plan to become pregnant, or are breast-feeding. If you become pregnant while using fluticasone and salmeterol, call your doctor.
- if you are having surgery, including dental surgery, tell your doctor or dentist that you are using fluticasone and salmeterol.
- tell your doctor if you have never had chickenpox or measles and have not been vaccinated against these infections. Stay away from people who are sick, especially people who have chickenpox or measles. If you are exposed to these infections or if you develop symptoms of these infections, call your doctor immediately. You may need to get a vaccine (shot) to protect you from these infections.

What special dietary instructions should I follow?

Talk to your doctor about eating grapefruit or drinking grapefruit juice while taking this medication.

What should I do if I forget to take a dose?

Skip the missed dose and continue your regular dosing schedule. Do not inhale a double dose to make up for a missed one.

What side effects can this medicine cause?

Fluticasone and salmeterol may cause side effects. Tell your doctor if any of these symptoms are severe or do not go away:
- runny nose
- sneezing
- sore throat
- throat irritation
- sinus pain
- headache
- upset stomach
- vomiting
- diarrhea
- stomach pain
- muscle and bone pain
- dizziness
- weakness
- tiredness
- sweating

- tooth pain
- red or dry eyes
- shaking of a part of your body that you cannot control
- sleep problems

Some side effects can be serious. If you experience any of the following side effects, call your doctor immediately:
- coughing, wheezing, or chest tightness that begins soon after you inhale fluticasone and salmeterol
- hives
- rash
- swelling of the face, throat, tongue, lips, hands, feet, ankles, or lower legs
- choking or difficulty swallowing
- hoarseness
- noisy, high-pitched breathing
- pounding fast, or irregular heartbeat
- fainting
- chest pain
- cough
- burning or tingling in the hands or feet
- blurred vision
- white patches in the mouth
- fever, chills, and other signs of infection

Fluticasone and salmeterol may cause children to grow more slowly. Your child's doctor will monitor your child's growth carefully. Talk to your child's doctor about the risks of giving this medication to your child.

Fluticasone and salmeterol may increase the risk that you will develop glaucoma, cataracts, or osteoporosis. You will probably need to have regular eye exams and bone tests during your treatment with fluticasone and salmeterol. Talk to your doctor about the risks of using this medication.

Fluticasone and salmeterol may cause other side effects. Call your doctor if you have any unusual problems while using this medication.

If you experience a serious side effect, you or your doctor may send a report to the Food and Drug Administration's (FDA) MedWatch Adverse Event Reporting program online [at http://www.fda.gov/MedWatch/index.html] or by phone [1-800-332-1088].

What storage conditions are needed for this medicine?

Keep this medication in the container it came in, tightly closed, and out of reach of children. Store it at room temperature and away from sunlight, excess heat and moisture (not in the bathroom). Throw away the inhaler 1 month after you remove it from the foil overwrap or after every blister has been used (when the dose indicator reads 0), whichever comes first. Talk to your pharmacist about the proper disposal of your medication.

What should I do in case of overdose?

In case of overdose, call your local poison control center at 1-800-222-1222. If the victim has collapsed or is not breathing, call local emergency services at 911.

Symptoms of overdose may include:
- seizures
- chest pain
- dizziness
- fainting
- blurred vision
- fast, pounding, or irregular heartbeat
- nervousness
- headache
- shaking of a part of your body that you cannot control
- muscle cramps or weakness
- dry mouth
- upset stomach
- dizziness
- excessive tiredness
- lack of energy
- difficulty falling asleep or staying asleep

What other information should I know?

Keep all appointments with your doctor and your eye doctor.

Do not let anyone else use your medication. Ask your pharmacist any questions you have about refilling your prescription.

Dosage Facts
For Informational Purposes

Caution: Do not change your dose, how often you take your medication, or the length of time you are to take it without first talking to your healthcare provider.

The following dosage information was written using medical language for doctors and other healthcare professionals and is provided here for you to check your dosage. The dosage of this drug may differ for different patients. Therefore, always follow your doctor's instructions or the directions on the label. Contact your healthcare provider or pharmacist if you have any questions about the specific dosage of your medication after reviewing this information.

General Dosage Information

Doses of fluticasone propionate and salmeterol in the combination preparation (Advair® inhalation powder) are expressed as the nominal (labeled) doses contained in each foil-wrapped blister. The amount of drug powder delivered to the lungs depends on factors such as the patient's inspiratory flow.

Pediatric Patients

Asthma

INHALATION POWDER:
- Fixed combination of fluticasone propionate and salmeterol in children 4–11 years of age inadequately controlled with an inhaled corticosteroid: Initial and maintenance dosage is 100 mcg of fluticasone propionate and 50 mcg of salmeterol (1 inhalation) twice daily.

- Fixed combination of fluticasone propionate and salmeterol in children ≥12 years of age *not* currently receiving an orally inhaled corticosteroid: Initially, 100 mcg of fluticasone propionate and 50 mcg of salmeterol (1 inhalation) twice daily.
- The dosage of fluticasone propionate and salmeterol in fixed combination in adolescents receiving inhaled corticosteroids depends on the dosage of the inhaled corticosteroid currently in use.

Recommended Dosage of Advair® Diskus® for Adolescents ≥12 Years of Age Taking Inhaled Corticosteroids

	Current Daily Dosage of Inhaled Corticosteroid (mcg)	Recommended Strength of Fluticasone Propionate Contained in Advair® Diskus® (with 50 mcg of Salmeterol) at Twice-Daily Dosage (mcg)
Beclomethasone Dipropionate HFA Inhalation Aerosol	≤160	100
	320	250
	640	500
Budesonide Inhalation Aerosol	≤400	100
	800–1200	250
	1600	500
Flunisolide Inhalation Aerosol	≤1000	100
	1250–2000	250
Flunisolide HFA Inhalation Aerosol	≤320	100
	640	250
Fluticasone Propionate HFA Inhalation Aerosol	≤176	100
	440	250
	660–880	500
Fluticasone Propionate Inhalation Powder	≤200	100
	500	250
	1000	500
Mometasone Furoate Inhalation Powder	220	100
	440	250
	880	500
Triamcinolone Acetonide Inhalation Aerosol	≤1000	100
	1100–1600	250
	1100–1600	250

Adult Patients

Asthma

INHALATION POWDER:
- Fixed combination of fluticasone propionate and salmeterol in patients *not* currently receiving an orally inhaled corticosteroid: Initially, 100 or 250 mcg of fluticasone propionate and 50 mcg of salmeterol (1 inhalation) twice daily.
- The dosage of fluticasone propionate and salmeterol in fixed combination in patients currently receiving inhaled corticosteroids depends on the dosage of the inhaled corticosteroid currently in use.

Recommended Dosage of Advair® Diskus® for Adults Taking Inhaled Corticosteroids

	Current Daily Dosage of Inhaled Corticosteroid (mcg)	Recommended Strength of Fluticasone Propionate Contained in Advair® Diskus® (with 50 mcg of Salmeterol) at Twice-Daily Dosage (mcg)
Beclomethasone Dipropionate HFA Inhalation Aerosol	≤160	100
	320	250
	640	500
Budesonide Inhalation Aerosol	≤400	100
	800–1200	250
	1600	500
Flunisolide Inhalation Aerosol	≤1000	100
	1250–2000	250
Flunisolide HFA Inhalation Aerosol	≤320	100
	640	250
Fluticasone Propionate HFA Inhalation Aerosol	≤176	100
	440	250
	660–880	500
Fluticasone Propionate Inhalation Powder	≤200	100
	500	250
	1000	500
Mometasone Furoate Inhalation Powder	220	100
	440	250
	880	500
Triamcinolone Acetonide Inhalation Aerosol	≤1000	100
	1100–1600	250

If control of asthma is inadequate 2 weeks after initiation of therapy at the initial dosage, a higher strength may provide additional asthma control.

COPD

ORAL INHALATION:
• Fixed combination of fluticasone propionate and salmeterol: Initial and maintenance dosage is 250 mcg of fluticasone propionate and 50 mcg of salmeterol (1 inhalation) twice daily given approximately every 12 hours (morning and evening).

Prescribing Limits

Pediatric Patients

Asthma

INHALATION POWDER:
• Fixed combination of fluticasone propionate and salmeterol in children 4–11 years of age: Maximum 100 mcg of fluticasone propionate and 50 mcg salmeterol (1 inhalation) twice daily.
• Fixed combination of fluticasone propionate and salmeterol in children ≥12 years of age: Maximum 500 mcg of fluticasone propionate and 50 mcg salmeterol (1 inhalation) twice daily.

Adult Patients

Asthma

INHALATION POWDER:
• Fixed combination of fluticasone propionate and salmeterol: Maximum 500 mcg of fluticasone propionate and 50 mcg salmeterol (1 inhalation) twice daily. Use of higher than recommended dosage (500 mcg of fluticasone propionate and 50 mcg of salmeterol twice daily) does not improve lung function compared with recommended dosages.

COPD

ORAL INHALATION:
• Fixed combination of fluticasone propionate and salmeterol: Maximum 250 mcg fluticasone propionate and 50 mcg salmeterol (1 inhalation) twice daily. Use of higher than recommended dosage (250 mcg of fluticasone propionate and 50 mcg of salmeterol twice daily) does not improve lung function compared with the recommended dosage.

Special Populations

Geriatric Patients
• Inhalation powder of fluticasone propionate in fixed combination with salmeterol: Dosage adjustments not recommended solely because of age.

Fluticasone Nasal Spray

(floo tik' a sone)

Brand Name: Flonase® Nasal Spray

Why is this medicine prescribed?

Fluticasone nasal spray is used to treat the symptoms of seasonal (occurs only at certain times of year), and perennial (occurs all year round) allergic rhinitis and perennial nonallergic rhinitis. These symptoms include sneezing and stuffy, runny, or itchy nose. Fluticasone is in a class of medications called corticosteroids. It works by preventing and decreasing inflammation (swelling that can cause other symptoms) in the nose.

How should this medicine be used?

Fluticasone comes as a liquid to spray in the nose. It is usually sprayed in each nostril once daily or twice daily in the morning and evening. It is sometimes used only as needed to treat symptoms. Follow the directions on your prescription label carefully, and ask your doctor or pharmacist to explain any part you do not understand. Use fluticasone exactly as directed. Do not use more or less of it or use it more often than prescribed by your doctor.

Fluticasone nasal spray is only for use in the nose. Do not swallow the nasal spray and be careful not to spray it in your eyes.

Your doctor will probably start you on a high dose of fluticasone nasal spray and may decrease your dose after your symptoms are controlled.

Fluticasone nasal spray controls the symptoms of rhinitis but does not cure the condition. Your symptoms will probably not begin to improve for at least 12 hours after you first use fluticasone, and it may take several days or longer before you feel the full benefit of fluticasone. Fluticasone works best when used regularly. Use fluticasone on a regular schedule unless your doctor has told you to use it as needed. Continue to use fluticasone even if you feel well. Do not stop using fluticasone without talking to your doctor.

Each bottle of fluticasone nasal spray is designed to provide 120 sprays. The bottle might not be empty after 120 sprays have been used, but each spray might not contain the correct amount of medication. You should keep track of the number of sprays you have used and throw away the bottle after you have used 120 sprays even if it still contains some liquid.

To use the nasal spray, follow these steps:
1. Shake the bottle gently.
2. Remove the dust cover.
3. If you are using the pump for the first time or have not used it for a week or more, you must prime it by following steps 4-5 below. If you have used the pump in the past week, skip to step 6.
4. Hold the pump with the applicator between your forefinger and middle finger and the bottom of the bottle resting on your thumb. Point the applicator away from your body.
5. If you are using the pump for the first time, press down and release the pump six times. If you have used the pump before, but not within the past week, press down and release the pump until you see a fine spray.
6. Blow your nose until your nostrils are clear.
7. Hold one nostril closed with your finger.
8. Tilt your head slightly forward and carefully put the nasal applicator into your other nostril. Be sure to keep the bottle upright.
9. Hold the pump with the applicator between your forefinger and middle finger and the bottom resting on your thumb.
10. Begin to breathe in through your nose.
11. While you are breathing in, use your forefinger and middle finger to press firmly down on the applicator and release a spray.
12. Breathe gently in through the nostril and breathe out through your mouth.
13. If your doctor told you to use two sprays in that nostril, repeat steps 6-12.
14. Repeat steps 6-13 in the other nostril.
15. Wipe the applicator with a clean tissue and cover it with the dust cover.

Are there other uses for this medicine?

This medication may be prescribed for other uses; ask your doctor or pharmacist for more information.

What special precautions should I follow?

Before using fluticasone nasal spray,
- tell your doctor and pharmacist if you are allergic to fluticasone, or any other medications.
- tell your doctor and pharmacist what prescription and nonprescription medications, vitamins, nutritional supplements, and herbal products you are taking or have recently taken. Be sure to mention any of the following: amiodarone (Cordarone); antifungals such as fluconazole (Diflucan), itraconazole (Sporanox), and ketoconazole (Nizoral); cimetidine (Tagamet); clarithromycin (Biaxin); cyclosporine (Neoral, Sandimmune); danazol (Danocrine); delavirdine (Rescriptor); diltiazem (Cardizem, Dilacor, Tiazac); fluoxetine (Prozac, Sarafem); fluvoxamine (Luvox); HIV protease inhibitors such as indinavir (Crixivan) nelfinavir (Viracept), ritonavir (Norvir) and saquinavir (Fortovase, Invirase); isoniazid (INH, Nydrazid); metronidazole (Flagyl); nefazodone (Serzone); oral contraceptives (birth control pills); oral steroids such as dexamethasone (Decadron, Dexone), methylprednisolone (Medrol), and prednisone (Deltasone); paroxetine (Paxil); steroids that are inhaled by mouth such as beclomethasone (QVAR), budesonide (Pulmicort), flunisolide (Aerobid), fluticasone (Flovent), and triamcinolone (Azmacort); troleandomycin (TAO); verapamil (Calan, Covera, Isoptin, Verelan); and zafirlukast (Accolate). Your doctor may need to change the doses of your medications or monitor you carefully for side effects.
- tell your doctor if you have or have ever had tuberculosis (a type of infection) in your lungs, cataracts (clouding of the lens of the eye), or glaucoma (an eye disease), and if you now have sores in your nose, any type of untreated infection, or a herpes infection (a type of infection that causes a sore on the eyelid or eye surface) in your eye. Also tell your doctor if you have recently had surgery on your nose or injured your nose in any way.
- tell your doctor if you are pregnant, plan to become pregnant, or are breast-feeding. If you become pregnant while taking fluticasone, call your doctor.
- if you are having surgery, including dental surgery, tell the doctor or dentist that you are taking fluticasone.
- if you have been taking oral steroids such as dexamethasone (Decadron, Dexone), methylprednisolone (Medrol), prednisolone (Pediapred, Prelone) or prednisone (Deltasone), your doctor may want to gradually decrease your steroid dose after you begin using fluticasone. Special caution is needed for several months as your body adjusts to the change in medication. If you have any other medical conditions, such as arthritis, or eczema (a skin disease), they may worsen when your oral steroid dose is decreased. Tell your doctor if this happens or if you experience any of the following symptoms during this time: extreme tiredness, muscle weakness or pain; sudden pain in stomach, lower body or legs; loss of appetite; weight loss; upset stomach; vom-

iting; diarrhea; dizziness; fainting; depression; irritability; and darkening of skin. Your body may be less able to cope with stress such as surgery, illness, severe asthma attack, or injury during this time. Call your doctor right away if you get sick and be sure that all health care providers who treat you know that you recently replaced your oral steroid with fluticasone inhalation. Carry a card or wear a medical identification bracelet to let emergency personnel know that you may need to be treated with steroids in an emergency.

- you should know that fluticasone may decrease your ability to fight infection. Stay away from people who are sick and wash your hands often. Be especially careful to stay away from people who have chicken pox or measles. Tell your doctor right away if you find out that you have been around someone who hads one of these viruses.

What special dietary instructions should I follow?

Talk to your doctor about drinking grapefruit juice while taking this medication.

What should I do if I forget to take a dose?

Use the missed dose as soon as you remember it. However, if it is almost time for the next dose, skip the missed dose and continue your regular dosing schedule. Do not use a double dose to make up for a missed one.

What side effects can this medicine cause?

Fluticasone may cause side effects. Tell your doctor if any of these symptoms are severe or do not go away:

- headache
- nosebleed
- burning or irritation in the nose
- runny nose
- bloody mucus in nose
- cough
- upset stomach
- vomiting
- stomach pain
- diarrhea
- dizziness

Some side effects can be serious. The following symptoms are uncommon, but if you experience any of them, call your doctor immediately:

- painful white patches in nose or throat
- flu-like symptoms
- sore throat
- vision problems
- injury to nose
- new or increased acne (pimples)
- easy bruising
- enlarged face and neck
- extreme tiredness
- muscle weakness
- irregular menstruation (periods)

- hives
- rash
- itching
- swelling of the face, throat, tongue, lips, eyes, hands, feet, ankles, or lower legs
- hoarseness
- difficulty breathing or swallowing
- wheezing

Fluticasone may cause children to grow more slowly. It is not known whether using fluticasone decreases the final adult height that children will reach. Talk to your child's doctor about the risks of giving this medication to your child.

Fluticasone may cause other side effects. Call your doctor if you have any unusual problems while using this medication.

If you experience a serious side effect, you or your doctor may send a report to the Food and Drug Administration's (FDA) MedWatch Adverse Event Reporting program online [at http://www.fda.gov/MedWatch/index.html] or by phone [1-800-332-1088].

What storage conditions are needed for this medicine?

Keep this medication in the container it came in, tightly closed, and out of reach of children. Store it at room temperature and away from excess heat and moisture (not in the bathroom). Throw away any medication that is outdated or no longer needed. Talk to your pharmacist about the proper disposal of your medication.

What should I do in case of overdose?

In case of overdose, call your local poison control center at 1-800-222-1222. If the victim has collapsed or is not breathing, call local emergency services at 911.

Using too much fluticasone on a regular basis over a long period of time may cause the following symptoms:

- enlarged face and neck
- new or worsening acne
- easy bruising
- extreme tiredness
- muscle weakness
- irregular menstrual periods
- loss of appetite
- weight loss
- irritability
- depression
- fainting or dizziness when standing up from a sitting or lying position
- darkening of skin

What other information should I know?

Keep all appointments with your doctor.

You should clean your nasal spray applicator once a week. You will need to remove the dust cap and then pull on the applicator to remove it from the bottle. Wash the dust cap and applicator in warm water, let them dry at room temperature, and then put them back on the bottle. If the applicator is clogged, soak it in warm water and then rinse it in cold water and dry it. Do not use pins or other sharp objects to remove the blockage.

Do not let anyone else take your medication. Ask your pharmacist any questions you have about refilling your prescription.

Dosage Facts
For Informational Purposes

Caution: Do not change your dose, how often you take your medication, or the length of time you are to take it without first talking to your healthcare provider.

The following dosage information was written using medical language for doctors and other healthcare professionals and is provided here for you to check your dosage. The dosage of this drug may differ for different patients. Therefore, always follow your doctor's instructions or the directions on the label. Contact your healthcare provider or pharmacist if you have any questions about the specific dosage of your medication after reviewing this information.

General Dosage Information

Nasal inhaler delivers about 50 mcg of fluticasone propionate per metered spray and about 120 metered sprays per 16-g container.

Adjust dosage according to individual requirements and response.

Therapeutic effects of intranasal corticosteroids, unlike those of decongestants, are not immediate. This should be explained to the patient in advance to ensure compliance and continuation of the prescribed treatment regimen.

Generally assess response to the initial dosage 4–7 days after starting therapy; a reduction in maintenance dosage may be possible at that time.

Pediatric Patients

Seasonal Rhinitis

INTRANASAL INHALATION:
- Adolescents and children ≥4 years of age: 1 spray (50 mcg) in each nostril once daily (total dose: 100 mcg/day). Increase dosage to 2 sprays (100 mcg) in each nostril daily (total dose: 200 mcg/day) if response is inadequate.
- Reduce dosage to 1 spray in each nostril (total dose: 100 mcg/day) once adequate symptom control is achieved.
- Some patients ≥12 years of age with seasonal allergic rhinitis may find as needed (prn) use of 200 mcg (100 mcg in each nostril) doses (no more frequently than once daily) to be effective in controlling symptoms. Greater symptom control may be achieved with regular dosing.

Perennial Rhinitis

INTRANASAL INHALATION:
- Adolescents and children ≥4 years of age: 1 spray (50 mcg) in each nostril daily (total dose: 100 mcg/day). Increase dosage to 2 sprays (100 mcg) in each nostril daily (total dose: 200 mcg/day) if response is inadequate.

- Maintenance dose is 1 spray in each nostril (total dose: 100 mcg/day) once adequate symptom control is achieved.

Adult Patients

Seasonal Rhinitis
Treatment

INTRANASAL INHALATION:
- Usual initial dose is 2 sprays (100 mcg) in each nostril once daily (total 200 mcg/day). Alternatively, 1 spray (50 mcg) in each nostril twice daily (total 200 mcg/day).
- Maintenance dose is 1 spray in each nostril (total dose: 100 mcg/day) once adequate symptom control is achieved.
- Some patients with seasonal allergic rhinitis may find as needed (prn) use of 200-mcg (100 mcg in each nostril) doses (no more frequently than once daily) to be effective in controlling symptoms. Greater symptom control may be achieved with regular dosing.

Prophylaxis†

INTRANASAL INHALATION:
- Maintenance dose is 2 sprays (100 mcg) in each nostril daily (200 mcg total).

Perennial Rhinitis

INTRANASAL INHALATION:
- Usual initial dose is 2 sprays (100 mcg) in each nostril once daily (total dose: 200 mcg/day). Alternatively, 1 spray (50 mcg) in each nostril twice daily (total 200 mcg/day).
- Maintenance dose is 1 spray in each nostril (total dose: 100 mcg/day) once adequate symptom control is achieved.

Prescribing Limits

No evidence that higher than recommended dosages or increased frequency of administration is beneficial.

Exceeding the maximum recommended daily dosage may only increase the risk of adverse systemic effects (e.g., HPA-axis suppression, Cushing's syndrome).

Pediatric Patients

Seasonal Rhinitis

INTRANASAL INHALATION:
- Adolescents and children ≥4 years of age: Maximum 100 mcg (2 sprays) in each nostril (200 mcg total) daily.

Perennial Rhinitis

INTRANASAL INHALATION:
- Adolescents and children ≥4 years of age: Maximum 100 mcg (2 sprays) in each nostril (200 mcg total) daily.

Adult Patients

Seasonal Rhinitis

INTRANASAL INHALATION:
- Maximum 100 mcg (2 sprays) in each nostril (200 mcg total) daily.

Perennial Rhinitis

INTRANASAL INHALATION:
- Maximum 100 mcg (2 sprays) in each nostril (200 mcg total) daily.

Special Populations

Hepatic Impairment
- No specific dosage recommendations for hepatic impairment.

Renal Impairment
• No specific dosage recommendations for renal impairment.

Geriatric Patients
• No specific geriatric dosage recommendations.

† Use is not currently included in the labeling approved by the US Food and Drug Administration.

Fluticasone Oral Inhalation

(floo tik′ a sone)

Brand Name: Flovent® HFA

Why is this medicine prescribed?

Fluticasone oral inhalation is used to prevent difficulty breathing, chest tightness, wheezing and coughing caused by asthma. Fluticasone is in a class of medications called corticosteroids. It works by decreasing swelling and irritation in the airways to allow for easier breathing.

How should this medicine be used?

Fluticasone comes as an aerosol to inhale by mouth. Fluticasone is usually inhaled twice a day. Try to use fluticasone at around the same times every day. Follow the directions on your prescription label carefully, and ask your doctor or pharmacist to explain any part you do not understand. Use fluticasone exactly as directed. Do not use more or less of it or use it more often than prescribed by your doctor.

Talk to your doctor about how you should use your other oral and inhaled medications for asthma during your treatment with fluticasone inhalation. If you were taking an oral steroid such as dexamethasone (Decadron, Dexone), methylprednisolone (Medrol), or prednisone (Deltasone), your doctor may want to gradually decrease your steroid dose starting at least 1 week after you begin to use fluticasone. Special care will be needed in certain situations for several months as your body adjusts to the change in medication. Ask your doctor for more information.

Fluticasone helps to prevent asthma attacks (sudden episodes of shortness of breath, wheezing, and coughing) but will not stop an asthma attack that has already started. Do not use fluticasone during an asthma attack. Your doctor will prescribe a short-acting inhaler to use during asthma attacks.

Your doctor will probably start you on an average dose of fluticasone. Your doctor may decrease your dose when your symptoms are controlled or increase it if your symptoms have not improved after at least 2 weeks.

Fluticasone controls asthma but does not cure it. Your symptoms may improve 24 hours after you begin using fluticasone, but it may take 2 weeks or longer before you feel the full benefit of the medication. Continue to use fluticasone even if you feel well. Do not stop using fluticasone without talking to your doctor.

Tell your doctor if your asthma worsens during your treatment. Call your doctor if you have an asthma attack that does not stop when you use your fast acting asthma medication, or if you need to use more of your fast acting medication than usual.

The inhaler that comes with fluticasone aerosol is designed for use only with a canister of fluticasone. Never use it to inhale any other medication, and never use any other inhaler to inhale fluticasone.

Each canister of fluticasone aerosol is designed to provide 60 or 120 inhalations, depending on its size. After the labeled number of inhalations has been used, later inhalations may not contain the correct amount of medication. You should keep track of the number of inhalations you have used. You can divide the number of inhalations in your inhaler by the number of inhalations you use each day to find out how many days your inhaler will last. Throw away the canister after you have used the labeled number of inhalations even if it still contains some liquid and continues to release a spray when it is pressed. Do not float the canister in water to see if it still contains medication.

Before you use your fluticasone aerosol inhaler the first time, read the written instructions that come with it. Look at the diagrams carefully and be sure that you recognize all the parts of the inhaler. Ask your doctor, pharmacist, or respiratory therapist to show you how to use it. Practice using the inhaler while he or she watches.

Do not use your fluticasone inhaler while you are near an open flame or a heat source. The inhaler may explode if it is exposed to very high temperatures.

To use the aerosol inhaler, follow these steps:

1. Before you use the inhaler for the first time, remove it from the overwrap. Throw away the overwrap and the drying packet that is inside the overwrap.
2. Be sure that the inhaler is at room temperature.
3. Remove the cap from the mouthpiece. The strap on the side of the cap will stay attached to the actuator to keep the cap from getting lost. Check the mouthpiece for dirt and other objects before each use, especially if the cap was not used to cover the mouthpiece.
4. Be sure the canister is fully and firmly inserted in the actuator. Shake the inhaler well for 5 seconds.
5. If you are using the inhaler for the first time, prime it by releasing 4 test sprays into the air, away from your face. Shake the inhaler for 5 seconds before each spray. If you have not used the inhaler in more than 7 days, or if you have dropped the inhaler, shake the inhaler for 5 seconds and release one spray into the air. Be careful not to spray the medication into your eyes.
6. Breathe out through your mouth.
7. Hold the inhaler facing you with the mouthpiece on the bottom. Place your thumb under the mouthpiece and your index finger on the top of the canister. Place the mouthpiece in your mouth and close your lips around it.

8. Breathe in deeply and slowly through your mouth. At the same time, press down firmly on the top of the canister with your index finger. Remove your index finger as soon as the spray is released.

9. When you have breathed in fully, remove the inhaler from your mouth and close your mouth.

10. Try to hold your breath for 10 seconds.

11. If your doctor told you to inhale more than one puff, wait 30 seconds, shake the canister again, and repeat steps 6-10 for each puff.

12. Put the cap back on the mouthpiece.

13. Rinse your mouth with water and spit the water out. Do not swallow the water.

Clean your inhaler once a week after an evening dose. To clean your inhaler, follow these steps:

1. Remove the mouthpiece cap, but leave the canister in the actuator.

2. Dampen the tip of a cotton swab with water. Use the damp swab to clean the small hole where the medication comes out. Twist the swab in a circular motion to remove any medication that is left in or near the hole.

3. Repeat step 2 with a second cotton swab.

4. Dampen a clean tissue with water. Wipe the inside of the mouthpiece with the damp tissue.

5. Leave the mouthpiece uncovered overnight to allow it to air dry.

6. Replace the mouthpiece cap when the actuator is dry.

Are there other uses for this medicine?

This medication may be prescribed for other uses; ask your doctor or pharmacist for more information.

What special precautions should I follow?

Before using fluticasone oral inhalation,

- tell your doctor and pharmacist if you are allergic to fluticasone or any other medications.
- tell your doctor and pharmacist what prescription and nonprescription medications, vitamins, nutritional supplements, and herbal products you are taking or have recently taken. Be sure to mention any of the following: amiodarone (Cordarone); antifungals such as fluconazole (Diflucan), itraconazole (Sporanox), and ketoconazole (Nizoral); cimetidine (Tagamet); clarithromycin (Biaxin); cyclosporine (Neoral, Sandimmune); danazol (Danocrine); delavirdine (Rescriptor); diltiazem (Cardizem, Dilacor, Tiazac); fluoxetine (Prozac, Sarafem); fluvoxamine (Luvox); HIV protease inhibitors such as indinavir (Crixivan), nelfinavir (Viracept), ritonavir (Norvir) and saquinavir (Invirase, Fortovase); isoniazid (INH, Nydrazid); metronidazole (Flagyl); nefazodone; hormonal contraceptives (birth control pills, patches, rings, injections, or implants); oral steroids such as dexamethasone (Decadron, Dexone), methylprednisolone (Medrol), and prednisone (Deltasone); paroxetine (Paxil); troleandomycin (TAO); verapamil (Calan, Covera, Isoptin, Verelan); and zafirlukast (Accolate). Your

doctor may need to change the doses of your medications or monitor you carefully for side effects.

- if you are using any other inhaled medications, ask your doctor if you should inhale these medications a certain amount of time before or after you inhale fluticasone inhalation.
- tell your doctor if you have or have ever had tuberculosis (a type of infection) in your lungs, cataracts (clouding of the lens of the eye), glaucoma (an eye disease), or liver disease. Also tell your doctor if you have any type of untreated infection anywhere in your body or a herpes infection (a type of infection that causes a sore on the eyelid or eye surface) in your eye.
- tell your doctor if you are pregnant, plan to become pregnant, or are breast-feeding. If you become pregnant while using fluticasone, call your doctor.
- if you are having surgery, including dental surgery, tell the doctor or dentist that you are using fluticasone.
- you should know that your body may be less able to cope with stress such as surgery, illness, severe asthma attack, or injury. Call your doctor right away if you get sick and be sure that all health care providers who treat you know that you are using fluticasone.
- tell your doctor if you have never had chicken pox or measles and you have not been vaccinated against these infections. Stay away from people who are sick, especially people who have chicken pox or measles. If you are exposed to one of these infections or if you develop symptoms of one of these infections, call your doctor right away. You may need treatment to protect you from these infections.
- you should know that fluticasone inhalation sometimes causes wheezing and difficulty breathing immediately after it is inhaled. If this happens, use your fast acting (rescue) asthma medication right away and call your doctor. Do not use fluticasone inhalation again unless your doctor tells you that you should.

What special dietary instructions should I follow?

Talk to your doctor about drinking grapefruit juice while taking this medication.

What should I do if I forget to take a dose?

Skip the missed dose and continue your regular dosing schedule. Do not use a double dose to make up for a missed one.

What side effects can this medicine cause?

Fluticasone may cause side effects. Tell your doctor if any of these symptoms are severe or do not go away:

- headache
- stuffy or runny nose
- difficulty speaking
- sore or irritated throat
- painful white patches in the mouth or throat

Some side effects can be serious. If you experience any of the following symptoms, call your doctor immediately:

- new or increased acne (pimples)
- easy bruising
- enlarged face and neck
- growth of hair on the face
- depression
- anxiety
- extreme tiredness
- muscle weakness
- irregular menstruation (periods)
- pink or purple stretch marks on the skin
- hives
- rash
- itching
- swelling of the face, throat, tongue, lips, eyes, hands, feet, ankles, or lower legs
- hoarseness
- difficulty breathing or swallowing
- chest pain or tightness
- cough
- shortness of breath
- red or fluid filled bumps on skin
- burning, tingling, numbness, or weakness in arms or legs

Fluticasone may cause children to grow more slowly. There is not enough information to tell whether using fluticasone decreases the final height that children will reach when they stop growing. Your child's doctor will watch your child's growth carefully while your child is using fluticasone. Talk to your child's doctor about the risks of giving this medication to your child.

In rare cases, people who used fluticasone for a long time developed glaucoma or cataracts. Talk to your doctor about the risks of using fluticasone and how often you should have your eyes examined during your treatment.

Fluticasone may increase your risk of developing osteoporosis (a condition in which the bones become thin and weak and break easily). Talk to your doctor about the risks of using this medication.

Fluticasone may cause other side effects. Call your doctor if you have any unusual problems while using this medication.

If you experience a serious side effect, you or your doctor may send a report to the Food and Drug Administration's (FDA) MedWatch Adverse Event Reporting program online [at http://www.fda.gov/MedWatch/index.html] or by phone [1-800-332-1088].

What storage conditions are needed for this medicine?

Store your fluticasone inhaler with the mouthpiece down. Store it out of reach of children, at room temperature and away from excess heat and moisture (not in the bathroom). Do not store the inhaler near a heat source or an open flame. Protect the inhaler from freezing and direct sunlight. Throw away any medication that is outdated or no longer needed.

Talk to your pharmacist about the proper disposal of your medication. Do not puncture the aerosol container and do not throw it away in an incinerator or fire.

What should I do in case of overdose?

In case of overdose, call your local poison control center at 1-800-222-1222. If the victim has collapsed or is not breathing, call local emergency services at 911.

Inhaling too much fluticasone on a regular basis over a long period of time may cause the following symptoms:

- enlarged face and neck
- new or worsening acne
- easy bruising
- extreme tiredness
- muscle weakness
- irregular menstrual periods
- loss of appetite
- weight loss
- irritability
- depression
- fainting or dizziness when standing up from a sitting or lying position
- darkening of skin

What other information should I know?

Keep all appointments with your doctor.

Do not let anyone else use your medication. Ask your pharmacist any questions you have about refilling your prescription.

Dosage Facts
For Informational Purposes

Caution: Do not change your dose, how often you take your medication, or the length of time you are to take it without first talking to your healthcare provider.

The following dosage information was written using medical language for doctors and other healthcare professionals and is provided here for you to check your dosage. The dosage of this drug may differ for different patients. Therefore, always follow your doctor's instructions or the directions on the label. Contact your healthcare provider or pharmacist if you have any questions about the specific dosage of your medication after reviewing this information.

General Dosage Information

Unless otherwise stated, the dose of fluticasone propionate administered as an aerosol via metered-dose inhaler is expressed as the amount delivered from the actuator of the inhaler per metered spray.

Oral inhalation aerosol delivers 50, 125, or 250 mcg from the valve, and 44, 110, or 220 mcg, respectively, from the actuator per metered spray. The 10.6- or 12-g canister (labeled as containing 44, 110, or 220 mcg of fluticasone propionate) delivers 120 metered sprays of fluticasone propionate.

Pediatric Patients

Asthma

INHALATION AEROSOL:
- Children 4–11 years of age: Initial and maximal dosage is 88 mcg twice daily.
- Children ≥12 years of age previously receiving bronchodilators alone: Initially, 88 mcg twice daily. If control of asthma is inadequate after 2 weeks of therapy at the initial dosage, a higher strength may provide additional asthma control. If required, dosage may be increased to a maximum of 440 mcg twice daily. Consider initial dosages >88 mcg twice daily in children with inadequate asthma control.
- Children ≥12 years of age previously receiving inhaled corticosteroids: Initially, 88–220 mcg twice daily. If required, dosage may be increased to a maximum of 440 mcg twice daily. Consider initial dosages >88 mcg twice daily in those who were receiving inhaled corticosteroids at the higher end of the dosage range.
- Children ≥12 years of age previously receiving oral corticosteroids: Initially, 440 mcg twice daily and maximum dosage is 880 mcg twice daily.

Adult Patients

Asthma

INHALATION AEROSOL:
- Previously receiving bronchodilators alone: Initially, 88 mcg twice daily. If required, dosage may be increased to a maximum of 440 mcg twice daily. Consider initial dosages >88 mcg twice daily in adults with inadequate asthma control.
- Previously receiving inhaled corticosteroids: Initially, 88–220 mcg twice daily. If required, dosage may be increased to a maximum of 440 mcg twice daily. Consider initial dosages >88 mcg twice daily in those who were receiving inhaled corticosteroids at the higher end of the dosage range.
- Previously receiving oral corticosteroids: Initial and maximum dosage is 880 mcg twice daily.
- If control of asthma is inadequate after 2 weeks of therapy at the initial dosage, a higher strength may provide additional asthma control.

Prescribing Limits

Pediatric Patients

Asthma

INHALATION AEROSOL:
- Children 4–11 years of age: Maximum 88 mcg twice daily.
- Children ≥12 years of age previously receiving bronchodilators alone or inhaled corticosteroids: Maximum 440 mcg twice daily.
- Children ≥12 years of age previously receiving oral corticosteroids: Maximum 880 mcg twice daily.

Adult Patients

Asthma

INHALATION AEROSOL:
- Previously receiving bronchodilators alone or inhaled corticosteroids: Maximum 440 mcg twice daily.
- Previously receiving oral corticosteroids: Maximum 880 mcg twice daily.

Special Populations

Geriatric Patients
- Inhalation aerosol: Select dosage with caution, reflecting the greater frequency of decreased hepatic function, presence of coexisting conditions, or other drug therapies.

Fluticasone Topical

(floo tik′ a sone)

Brand Name: Cutivate®

Why is this medicine prescribed?

Fluticasone, a corticosteroid, is used to reduce inflammation and relieve itching, redness, dryness, and scaling associated with various skin disorders.

This medication is sometimes prescribed for other uses; ask your doctor or pharmacist for more information.

How should this medicine be used?

Fluticasone comes as an ointment and cream to apply to the skin. It usually is applied two to four times a day at evenly spaced intervals. Follow the directions on your prescription label carefully, and ask your doctor or pharmacist to explain any part you do not understand. Use fluticasone exactly as directed. Do not use more or less of it or use it more often than prescribed by your doctor.

Do not stop using fluticasone without talking to your doctor.

Thoroughly clean the affected area, allow it to dry, and then gently rub the medication in until most of it disappears. Use just enough medication to cover the affected area. You should wash your hands after applying the medication. The scalp lotion should be applied directly from the squeeze bottle to the affected area.

What special precautions should I follow?

Before using fluticasone,
- tell your doctor and pharmacist if you are allergic to fluticasone or any other drugs.
- tell your doctor and pharmacist what prescription and nonprescription medications you are using, especially skin products containing hydrocortisone and vitamins.
- tell your doctor if you have any other illnesses, infections, or allergies.
- tell your doctor if you are pregnant, plan to become pregnant, or are breast-feeding. If you become pregnant while taking fluticasone, call your doctor.

What should I do if I forget to take a dose?

Apply the missed dose as soon as you remember it. However, if it is almost time for the next dose, skip the missed dose and continue your regular dosing schedule. Do not apply a double dose to make up for a missed one.

What side effects can this medicine cause?

Fluticasone may cause side effects. Tell your doctor if any of these symptoms are severe or do not go away:

- itching
- burning
- swelling
- redness
- skin rash
- numbness of the fingers

What storage conditions are needed for this medicine?

Keep this medication in the container it came in, tightly closed, and out of reach of children. Store it at room temperature and away from excess heat and moisture (not in the bathroom). Throw away any medication that is outdated or no longer needed. Talk to your pharmacist about the proper disposal of your medication.

What other information should I know?

Keep all appointments with your doctor. Fluticasone is for external use only. Do not let it get into your eyes, nose, or mouth, and do not swallow it. Do not apply dressings, bandages, cosmetics, lotions, or other skin medications to the area being treated unless your doctor tells you.

Do not let anyone else use your medication. Ask your pharmacist any questions you have about refilling your prescription.

Talk to your doctor, pharmacist, or other healthcare professional if you have questions about dosing information for your medication.

Fluvastatin

(floo' va sta tin)

Brand Name: Lescol®, Lescol® XL

Why is this medicine prescribed?

Fluvastatin is used together with lifestyle changes (diet, weight-loss, exercise) to reduce the amount of cholesterol (a fat-like substance) and certain other fatty substances in the blood. Fluvastatin is in a class of medications called HMG-CoA reductase inhibitors (statins). It works by slowing the production of cholesterol in the body.

Buildup of cholesterol and other fats along the walls of the arteries (a process known as atherosclerosis) decreases blood flow and, therefore, the oxygen supply to the heart, brain, and other parts of the body. Lowering blood levels of cholesterol and other fats may help to decrease your chances

of getting heart disease, angina (chest pain), strokes, and heart attacks. In addition to taking a cholesterol-lowering medication, making certain changes in your daily habits can also lower your cholesterol blood levels. You should eat a diet that is low in saturated fat and cholesterol (see SPECIAL DIETARY), exercise 30 minutes on most, if not all days, and lose weight if you are overweight.

How should this medicine be used?

Fluvastatin comes as a capsule and an extended-release (long-acting) tablet to take by mouth. The capsule is usually taken with or without food once a day at bedtime or twice a day. The extended-release tablet is usually taken once a day at bedtime with or without food. Take fluvastatin at around the same time(s) every day. Follow the directions on your prescription label carefully, and ask your doctor or pharmacist to explain any part you do not understand. Take fluvastatin exactly as directed. Do not take more or less of it or take it more often than prescribed by your doctor.

Swallow the extended-release tablets whole; do not split, chew, or crush them.

Your doctor may start you on a low dose of fluvastatin and gradually increase your dose, not more than once every 4 weeks.

Continue to take fluvastatin even if you feel well. Do not stop taking fluvastatin without talking to your doctor.

Are there other uses for this medicine?

This medication may be prescribed for other uses; ask your doctor or pharmacist for more information.

What special precautions should I follow?

Before taking fluvastatin,

- tell your doctor and pharmacist if you are allergic to fluvastatin or any other medications.
- tell your doctor and pharmacist what prescription and nonprescription medications, vitamins, nutritional supplements, and herbal products you are taking or plan to take. Be sure to mention any of the following: anticoagulants ('blood thinners') such as warfarin; cimetidine (Tagamet); cyclosporine (Neoral, Sandimmune); diclofenac (Cataflam, Voltaren); digoxin (Lanoxin); erythromycin (E.E.S., E-Mycin, Erythrocin); glyburide (DiaBeta, Glynase, Micronase); ketoconazole (Nizoral); omeprazole (Prilosec); other cholesterol-lowering medications such as fenofibrate (Tricor) and gemfibrozil (Lopid); phenytoin (Dilantin); ranitidine (Zantac); rifampin (Rifadin, Rimactane); and spironolactone (Aldactone). Your doctor may need to change the doses of your medications or monitor you carefully for side effects.
- if you are taking cholestyramine (Questran), take it at least 4 hours before fluvastatin.
- tell your doctor if you have liver disease. Your doctor will probably tell you not to take fluvastatin.
- tell your doctor if you drink large amounts of alcohol

and if you have ever had liver or have or ever had diabetes or thyroid or kidney disease.

- tell your doctor if you are pregnant, or plan to become pregnant. If you become pregnant while taking fluvastatin, stop taking fluvastatin and call your doctor immediately. Fluvastatin may harm the fetus.
- do not breastfeed while you are taking this medication.
- if you are having surgery, including dental surgery, tell the doctor or dentist that you are taking fluvastatin.
- ask your doctor about the safe use of alcoholic beverages while you are taking fluvastatin. Alcohol can increase the risk of serious side effects.

What special dietary instructions should I follow?

Eat a low-cholesterol, low-fat diet. This kind of diet includes cottage cheese, fat-free milk, fish (not canned in oil), vegetables, poultry, egg whites, and polyunsaturated oils and margarines (corn, safflower, canola, and soybean oils). Avoid foods with excess fat in them such as meat (especially liver and fatty meat), egg yolks, whole milk, cream, butter, shortening, lard, pastries, cakes, cookies, gravy, peanut butter, chocolate, olives, potato chips, coconut, cheese (other than cottage cheese), coconut oil, palm oil, and fried foods.

What should I do if I forget to take a dose?

Take the missed dose as soon as you remember it. However, if it has been more than 12 hours since your last dose, skip the missed dose and continue your regular dosing schedule. Do not take a double dose to make up for a missed one.

What side effects can this medicine cause?

Fluvastatin may cause side effects. Tell your doctor if any of these symptoms are severe or do not go away:

- headache
- heartburn
- difficulty falling asleep or staying asleep
- sinus pain
- cough

Some side effects can be serious. The following symptoms are uncommon, but if you experience any of them, call your doctor immediately:

- muscle pain, tenderness, or weakness
- lack of energy
- fever
- yellowing of the skin or eyes
- pain in the upper right part of the stomach
- nausea
- extreme tiredness
- unusual bleeding or bruising
- loss of appetite
- flu-like symptoms
- rash
- hives
- itching
- difficulty breathing or swallowing

- swelling of the face, throat, tongue, lips, eyes, hands, feet, ankles, or lower legs
- hoarseness
- pain during urination
- frequent urge to urinate

Fluvastatin may cause other side effects. Call your doctor if you have any unusual problems while taking this medication.

If you experience a serious side effect, you or your doctor may send a report to the Food and Drug Administration's (FDA) MedWatch Adverse Event Reporting program online [at http://www.fda.gov/MedWatch/index.html] or by phone [1-800-332-1088].

What storage conditions are needed for this medicine?

Keep this medication in the container it came in, tightly closed, and out of reach of children. Store it at room temperature and away from excess heat and moisture (not in the bathroom). Throw away any medication that is outdated or no longer needed. Talk to your pharmacist about the proper disposal of your medication.

What should I do in case of overdose?

In case of overdose, call your local poison control center at 1-800-222-1222. If the victim has collapsed or is not breathing, call local emergency services at 911.

What other information should I know?

Keep all appointments with your doctor and the laboratory. Your doctor will order certain lab tests before and during your treatment to check your body's response to fluvastatin.

Before having any laboratory test, tell your doctor and the laboratory personnel that you are taking fluvastatin.

Do not let anyone else take your medication. Ask your pharmacist any questions you have about refilling your prescription.

Dosage Facts
For Informational Purposes

Caution: Do not change your dose, how often you take your medication, or the length of time you are to take it without first talking to your healthcare provider.

The following dosage information was written using medical language for doctors and other healthcare professionals and is provided here for you to check your dosage. The dosage of this drug may differ for different patients. Therefore, always follow your doctor's instructions or the directions on the label. Contact your healthcare provider or pharmacist if you have any questions about the specific dosage of your medication after reviewing this information.

General Dosage Information

Available as fluvastatin sodium; dosage expressed in terms of fluvastatin.

Pediatric Patients

Dyslipidemias

ORAL:
- Children 10–16 years of age: Initially, 20 mg once daily.
- Adjust dosage at 6-week intervals until the desired effect on lipoprotein concentrations is observed or a daily dosage of 80 mg is reached.

Adult Patients

Prevention of Cardiovascular Events or Dyslipidemias

ORAL:
- Initially, 20 mg once daily in the evening in patients who require reductions in LDL-cholesterol concentrations of <25% to achieve their goal.
- In patients who require larger reductions in LDL-cholesterol concentrations (i.e., >25%), initiate therapy at a dosage of 40 mg (as conventional capsules) once daily in the evening, 80 mg (as extended-release tablets) once daily at any time of day, or 40 mg (as conventional capsules) twice daily.
- Adjust dosage at intervals of ≥4 weeks until the desired effect on lipoprotein concentrations is observed.
- Usual maintenance dosage is 20–80 mg daily.

Prescribing Limits

Pediatric Patients

ORAL:
- Children 10–16 years of age: Maximum 80 mg daily.

Special Populations

Hepatic Impairment
- Use with caution in patients who consume substantial amounts of alcohol and/or have a history of liver disease; monitor such patients closely.
- Contraindicated in patients with active liver disease or unexplained, persistent increases in serum aminotransferase concentrations.

Renal Impairment
- Dosage modification is not necessary in patients with mild to moderate renal impairment.
- Dosages >40 mg daily have not been studied in patients with severe renal impairment; caution is advised when administering higher dosages to such patients.

Fluvoxamine

(floo vox′ a meen)

Important Warning

A small number of children, teenagers, and young adults (up to 24 years of age) who took antidepressants ('mood elevators') such as fluvoxamine during clinical studies became suicidal (thinking about harming or killing oneself or planning or trying to do so). Children, teenagers, and young adults who take antidepressants to treat depression or other mental illnesses may be more likely to become suicidal than children, teenagers, and young adults who do not take antidepressants to treat these conditions. However, experts are not sure about how great this risk is and how much it should be considered in deciding whether a child or teenager should take an antidepressant.

You should know that your mental health may change in unexpected ways when you take fluvoxamine or other antidepressants even if you are an adult over age 24. You may become suicidal, especially at the beginning of your treatment and any time that your dose is increased or decreased. You, your family, or your caregiver should call your doctor right away if you experience any of the following symptoms: new or worsening depression; thinking about harming or killing yourself, or planning or trying to do so; extreme worry; agitation; panic attacks; difficulty falling asleep or staying asleep; aggressive behavior; irritability; acting without thinking; severe restlessness; and frenzied abnormal excitement. Be sure that your family or caregiver knows which symptoms may be serious so they can call the doctor when you are unable to seek treatment on your own.

Your healthcare provider will want to see you often while you are taking fluvoxamine, especially at the beginning of your treatment. Be sure to keep all appointments for office visits with your doctor.

The doctor or pharmacist will give you the manufacturer's patient information sheet (Medication Guide) when you begin treatment with fluvoxamine. Read the information carefully and ask your doctor or pharmacist if you have any questions. You also can obtain the Medication Guide from the FDA website: http://www.fda.gov/cder/drug/antidepressants/antidepressants_MG_2007.pdf.

No matter your age, before you take an antidepressant, you, your parent, or your caregiver should talk to your doctor about the risks and benefits of treating your condition with an antidepressant or with other treatments. You should also talk about the risks and benefits of not treating your condition. You should know that having depression or another mental illness greatly increases the risk that you will become suicidal. This risk is higher if you or anyone in your family has or has ever had bipolar disorder (mood that changes from depressed to abnormally excited) or mania (frenzied, abnormally excited mood) or has thought about or attempted suicide. Talk to your doctor about your condition, symptoms, and personal and family medical history. You and your doctor will decide what type of treatment is right for you.

Why is this medicine prescribed?

Fluvoxamine is used to treat obsessive-compulsive disorder (bothersome thoughts that won't go away and the need to perform certain actions over and over). Fluvoxamine is in a class of medications called selective serotonin reuptake inhibitors (SSRIs).

How should this medicine be used?

Fluvoxamine comes as a tablet to take by mouth. It usually is taken either once daily at bedtime or twice daily, once in the morning and once at bedtime. Follow the directions on your prescription label carefully, and ask your doctor or pharmacist to explain any part you do not understand. Take fluvoxamine exactly as directed. Do not take more or less of it or take it more often than prescribed by your doctor.

It may take several weeks or longer for you to feel the full benefit of fluvoxamine. Continue to take fluvoxamine even if you feel well. Do not stop taking fluvoxamine without talking to your doctor. Your doctor probably will decrease your dose gradually.

Are there other uses for this medicine?

Fluvoxamine is also used sometimes to treat depression. Talk with your doctor about the possible risks of using this medication for your condition.

This medication is sometimes prescribed for other uses; ask your doctor or pharmacist for more information.

What special precautions should I follow?

Before taking fluvoxamine,

- tell your doctor and pharmacist if you are allergic to fluvoxamine or any other medications.
- tell your doctor if you are taking alosetron (Lotronex), astemizole (Hismanal) (not available in the U.S.), cisapride (Propulsid) (not available in the U.S.), pimozide (Orap), terfenadine (Seldane) (not available in the U.S.); tizanidine (Zanaflex) or thioridazine. Your doctor will probably tell you not to take fluvoxamine.
- tell your doctor and pharmacist what prescription and nonprescription medications, vitamins, and herbal products you are taking or plan to take. Be sure to mention any of the following: alprazolam (Xanax); anticoagulants ('blood thinners') such as warfarin (Coumadin);

buspirone (Buspar); carbamazepine (Tegretol); clozapine (Clozaril); cyclosporine (Neoral, Sandimmune); dextromethorphan (in cough medications); diazepam (Valium); diltiazem (Cardizem); diuretics ('water pills'); haloperidol (Haldol); heart medications; lithium; medications for depression; medications for migraine headaches such as almotriptan (Axert), eletriptan (Relpax), frovatriptan (Frova), naratriptan (Amerge), rizatriptan (Maxalt), sumatriptan (Imitrex), and zolmitriptan (Zomig); methadone; midazolam (Versed); phenytoin (Dilantin); theophylline (TheoDur); and triazolam (Halcion). Also tell your doctor if you are taking the following medications or if you have stopped taking them within the past 2 weeks: monoamine oxidase inhibitors (MAO inhibitors) such as isocarboxazid (Marplan), phenelzine (Nardil), selegiline (Eldepryl, Emsam, Zelapar), and tranylcypromine (Parnate). Your doctor may need to change the doses of your medications or monitor you carefully for side effects.

- tell your doctor what nutritional supplements you are taking, especially products that contain St. John's wort and tryptophan.
- tell your doctor if you drink or have ever drunk large amounts of alcohol or have used street drugs or have overused prescription medications. Also tell your doctor if you have or have ever had seizures, or heart, kidney, adrenal, or liver disease.
- tell your doctor if you are pregnant, plan to become pregnant, or are breast-feeding. If you become pregnant while taking fluvoxamine, call your doctor.
- if you are having surgery, including dental surgery, tell the doctor or dentist that you are taking fluvoxamine.
- you should know that this medication may make you drowsy. Do not drive a car or operate machinery until you know how this medication affects you.
- remember that alcohol can add to the drowsiness caused by this medication.
- tell your doctor if you use tobacco products. Cigarette smoking may decrease the effectiveness of this medication.
- plan to avoid unnecessary or prolonged exposure to sunlight and to wear protective clothing, sunglasses, and sunscreen. Fluvoxamine may make your skin sensitive to sunlight.

What special dietary instructions should I follow?

Unless your doctor tells you otherwise, continue your normal diet.

What should I do if I forget to take a dose?

Take the missed dose as soon as you remember it. However, if it is almost time for your next dose, skip the missed dose and continue your regular dosing schedule. Do not take a double dose to make up for a missed one.

What side effects can this medicine cause?

Fluvoxamine may cause side effects. Tell your doctor if any of these symptoms are severe or do not go away:

- drowsiness
- dry mouth
- nausea
- headache
- diarrhea
- constipation
- indigestion
- nervousness
- uncontrollable shaking of a part of the body
- weakness
- abnormal ejaculation

Some side effects can be serious. If you experience any of the following symptoms or those listed in the IMPORTANT WARNING section, call your doctor immediately:

- rapid heartbeat
- sweating
- rash
- hives
- seizures

Fluvoxamine may cause other side effects. Call your doctor if you have any unusual problems while you are taking this medication.

What storage conditions are needed for this medicine?

Keep this medication in the container it came in, tightly closed, and out of reach of children. Store it at room temperature and away from excess heat and moisture (not in the bathroom). Throw away any medication that is outdated or no longer needed. Talk to your pharmacist about the proper disposal of your medication.

What should I do in case of overdose?

In case of overdose, call your local poison control center at 1-800-222-1222. If the victim has collapsed or is not breathing, call local emergency services at 911.

What other information should I know?

It is important to keep all appointments with your doctor and the laboratory. Your doctor will order certain lab tests to check your response to fluvoxamine.

Do not let anyone else take your medication. Ask your pharmacist any questions you have about refilling your prescription.

Dosage Facts
For Informational Purposes

Caution: Do not change your dose, how often you take your medication, or the length of time you are to take it without first talking to your healthcare provider.

The following dosage information was written using medical language for doctors and other healthcare professionals and is provided here for you to check your dosage. The dosage of this drug may differ for different patients. Therefore, always follow your doctor's instructions or the directions on the label. Contact your healthcare provider or pharmacist if you have any questions about the specific dosage of your medication after reviewing this information.

General Dosage Information

Available as fluvoxamine maleate; dosage is expressed in terms of the salt.

Pediatric Patients

OCD

ORAL:
- Children >8 years of age: Initially, 25 mg at bedtime. Increase dosages in 25-mg increments every 4–7 days, as tolerated, until maximum therapeutic benefit is achieved or up to a maximum dosage of 200 mg daily in children ≤11 years of age or 300 mg daily in adolescents ≥12 years of age. Girls ≤11 years of age may require lower dosages.
- Optimum duration of therapy not established; may require several months of sustained drug therapy. Use the lowest possible dosage and periodically reassess need for continued therapy.

Adult Patients

OCD

ORAL:
- Initially, 50 mg at bedtime. Increase dosages in 50-mg increments every 4–7 days, as tolerated, until maximum therapeutic benefit is achieved or up to a maximum dosage of 300 mg daily.
- Optimum duration of therapy not established; may require several months of sustained drug therapy. Use the lowest possible dosage and periodically reassess need for continued therapy.

Prescribing Limits

Pediatric Patients

OCD

ORAL:
- Children ≤11 years of age: Maximum 200 mg daily.
- Adolescents ≥12 years of age: Maximum 300 mg daily.

Adult Patients

OCD

ORAL:
- Maximum 300 mg daily.

Special Populations

Hepatic Impairment

OCD

ORAL:
- Use lower initial dosage and titrate dosage slowly.

Renal Impairment

OCD

ORAL:
- Limited evidence indicates that dosage modification is not necessary.

Geriatric Patients
- Initially, 25 mg daily; titrate dosage slowly.

Folic Acid

(foe′ lik)

Brand Name: Folvite®
Also available generically.

Why is this medicine prescribed?

Folic acid is used to treat or prevent folic acid deficiency. It is a B-complex vitamin needed by the body to manufacture red blood cells. A deficiency of this vitamin causes certain types of anemia (low red blood cell count).

How should this medicine be used?

Folic acid comes in tablets. It usually is taken once a day. Follow the directions on your prescription label carefully, and ask your doctor or pharmacist to explain any part you do not understand. Take folic acid exactly as directed. Do not take more or less of it or take it more often than prescribed by your doctor.

If you are taking folic acid to treat a deficiency, you probably will feel better quickly, often within 24 hours. However, do not stop taking this drug until your doctor tells you to do so.

Are there other uses for this medicine?

This medication is sometimes prescribed for other uses; ask your doctor or pharmacist for more information.

What special precautions should I follow?

Before taking folic acid,
- tell your doctor and pharmacist if you are allergic to folic acid or any other drugs.
- tell your doctor and pharmacist what prescription and nonprescription medications you are taking, especially phenytoin (Dilantin) and vitamins.

What special dietary instructions should I follow?

Your doctor may tell you to eat more liver, foods prepared from dried yeast, fruit, and fresh leafy green vegetables to increase the folic acid in your diet.

What should I do if I forget to take a dose?

Take the missed dose as soon as you remember it. However, if it is almost time for the next dose, skip the missed dose and continue your regular dosing schedule. Do not take a double dose to make up for a missed one.

What side effects can this medicine cause?

Folic acid may cause side effects. If you experience any of the following symptoms, call your doctor immediately:
- skin rash
- itching
- redness
- difficulty breathing

If you experience a serious side effect, you or your doctor may send a report to the Food and Drug Administration's (FDA) MedWatch Adverse Event Reporting program online [at http://www.fda.gov/MedWatch/index.html] or by phone [1-800-332-1088].

What storage conditions are needed for this medicine?

Keep this medication in the container it came in, tightly closed, and out of reach of children. Store it at room temperature and away from excess heat and moisture (not in the bathroom). Throw away any medication that is outdated or no longer needed. Talk to your pharmacist about the proper disposal of your medication.

What should I do in case of overdose?

In case of overdose, call your local poison control center at 1-800-222-1222. If the victim has collapsed or is not breathing, call local emergency services at 911.

What other information should I know?

Keep all appointments with your doctor and the laboratory. Your doctor will order certain lab tests to check your response to folic acid.

Do not let anyone else take your medication. Ask your pharmacist any questions you have about refilling your prescription.

Dosage Facts
For Informational Purposes

Caution: Do not change your dose, how often you take your medication, or the length of time you are to take it without first talking to your healthcare provider.

The following dosage information was written using medical language for doctors and other healthcare professionals and is provided here for you to check your dosage. The dosage of this drug may differ for different patients. Therefore, always follow your doctor's instructions or the directions on the label. Contact your health-

care provider or pharmacist if you have any questions about the specific dosage of your medication after reviewing this information.

General Dosage Information

Dosage of sodium folate injection is expressed in terms of folic acid.

The Recommended Dietary Allowance (RDA) is expressed in terms of dietary folate equivalents/day. Dietary food folate equivalents (DFE) are calculated as follows: 1 mcg of dietary folate equivalent = 1 mcg of food folate = 0.5 mcg of folic acid taken in the fasting state = 0.6 mcg of folic acid taken with food.

Pediatric Patients

Anemia

ORAL OR PARENTERAL:
- Up to 1 mg folic acid daily; some patients may require larger doses.
- Usual maintenance dosage: 0.1 mg daily for infants, 0.3 mg daily for children <4 years of age, 0.4 mg daily for children ≥4 years of age.
- Higher maintenance dosages may be required in patients with hemolytic anemia, chronic infections, and those receiving anticonvulsants.

Dietary Requirements

ORAL:
- The Adequate Intake (AI) of folate for healthy infants <6 months of age is 65 mcg daily and for those 6–12 months of age is 80 mcg daily.
- The RDA for healthy children 1–3, 4–8, 9–13, or 14–18 years of age is 0.15, 0.2, 0.3, or 0.4 mg of DFE daily, respectively.

Adult Patients

Anemia

ORAL OR PARENTERAL:
- Up to 1 mg folic acid daily; some patients may require larger doses.
- Usual maintenance dosage: 0.4 mg daily.
- Usual maintenance dosage for pregnant and lactating women: 0.8 mg daily.
- Higher maintenance dosages may be required in alcoholics, patients with hemolytic anemia, chronic infections, and patients receiving anticonvulsants.

Dietary Requirements

ORAL:
- RDA for healthy adults: 0.4 mg DFE daily.
- RDA for lactating women: 0.5 mg DFE daily. Folate intake exceeding this RDA may be needed by mothers nursing more than one infant.

Prevention of Neural Tube Defects

ORAL:
- 0.4 mg of folic acid daily through fortified foods and/or supplements in addition to food folate consumed from a varied diet recommended for women of childbearing potential.
- For women with a history of prior pregnancy complicated by neural tube defects: 4 mg folic acid daily initiated 1 month before and continued for 3 months after conception. Such women should maintain the lower level of folic acid intake (i.e., 0.4 mg daily) during other periods of continued childbearing potential.
- RDA for pregnant women: 0.6 mg DFE daily. Folate intake exceeding this RDA may be needed by women who are pregnant with more than one fetus.

Formoterol

(for moh′ te rol)

Brand Name: Foradil® Aerolizer® Inhaler

Important Warning

In a large clinical study, more patients who used an asthma medication similar to formoterol died of asthma problems than patients who did not use the medication. If you have asthma, use of formoterol may increase the chance that you will experience serious or fatal asthma problems. Your doctor will only prescribe formoterol if other medications have not controlled your asthma or if your asthma is so severe that two medications are needed to control it. Formoterol should not be the first or the only medication that you use to treat your asthma.

Do not use formoterol if you have asthma that is quickly getting worse. Tell your doctor if you have had many severe asthma attacks or if you have ever been hospitalized because of asthma symptoms. If you have any of the following signs of worsening asthma, call your doctor immediately:

- your short-acting inhaler [inhaled medication such as albuterol (Proventil, Ventolin) that is used to treat sudden attacks of asthma symptoms] does not work as well as it did in the past
- you need to use more puffs than usual of your short-acting inhaler or use it more often
- you need to use four or more puffs per day of your short-acting inhaler for 2 or more days in a row
- you use more than one canister (200 inhalations) of your short-acting inhaler during an 8-week period
- your peak-flow meter (home device used to test breathing) shows your breathing is worsening
- you need to go to the emergency room for asthma treatment
- your symptoms do not improve after you use formoterol regularly for one week or your symptoms get worse at any time during your treatment

Talk to your doctor about the risks of using this medication.

Your doctor or pharmacist will give you the manufacturer's patient information sheet (Medication Guide) when you begin treatment with formoterol and each time you refill your prescription. Read the information carefully and ask your doctor or pharmacist if you have any questions. You can also visit the Food and Drug Administration (FDA) website (http://www.fda.gov/cder) or the manufacturer's website to obtain the Medication Guide.

Why is this medicine prescribed?

Formoterol is used to treat wheezing, shortness of breath, and breathing difficulties caused by asthma and chronic obstructive pulmonary disease (COPD; a group of lung diseases, which includes chronic bronchitis and emphysema). It also is used to prevent breathing difficulties (bronchospasm) during exercise. Formoterol is in a class of medications called long-acting beta agonists (LABAs). It works by relaxing and opening air passages in the lungs, making it easier to breathe.

How should this medicine be used?

Formoterol comes as a powder-filled capsule to inhale by mouth using a special inhaler. If you are using formoterol to treat asthma and COPD, you will probably inhale it twice a day in the morning and the evening. Always inhale your next dose of formoterol 12 hours after you inhaled your last dose and try to inhale formoterol at about the same times every day. If you are using formoterol to prevent breathing difficulties during exercise, you will probably inhale it at least 15 minutes before exercise, but not more often than once in 12 hours. If you are using formoterol twice a day on a regular basis, do not use an additional dose before exercising. Follow the directions on your prescription label carefully, and ask your doctor or pharmacist to explain any part you do not understand. Use formoterol exactly as directed. Do not use more or less of it or use it more often than prescribed by your doctor.

Talk to your doctor about how you should take your other oral or inhaled medications for asthma during your treatment with formoterol. If you were taking a corticosteroid (a type of medication used to prevent airway swelling in patients with asthma), your doctor will probably tell you to continue taking it just as you did before you began using formoterol. If you were using a short acting beta agonist inhaler such as albuterol (Proventil, Ventolin) on a regular basis, your doctor will probably tell you to stop using it regularly, but to continue to use it to treat sudden attacks of asthma symptoms. Follow these directions carefully. Do not change the way you use any of your medications without talking to your doctor.

Formoterol helps to prevent asthma or COPD attacks but will not stop an attack that has already started. Do not use formoterol during an attack of asthma or COPD. Your doctor will prescribe a short-acting inhaler to use during attacks.

Formoterol controls the symptoms of asthma and other lung diseases but does not cure these conditions. Do not stop using formoterol without talking to your doctor. If you suddenly stop using formoterol, your symptoms may worsen.

Before you use the formoterol inhaler the first time, ask your doctor, pharmacist, or respiratory therapist to show you how to use it. Practice using the inhaler while he or she watches.

To use the inhaler, follow these steps:

1. Before you use a new inhaler for the first time, find the sticker on the box that says "Use by" and has been marked with a date by your pharmacist. Remove this sticker from the box and attach it to the cover of your inhaler to remind you to stop using the inhaler by this date. If the sticker on your box is blank, fill in the expiration date that is stamped on the box or the date that is 4 months after you purchased the inhaler, whichever comes sooner.
2. Open the foil pouch containing a blister card of formoterol and set it aside. Do not remove a capsule until you are ready to inhale your dose.
3. Pull off the inhaler cover and twist the mouthpiece open in the direction shown by the arrow on the mouthpiece. Push the buttons on each side to be sure you can see four pins in the capsule well of the inhaler.
4. Separate one blister from the blister card by tearing along the dotted lines. Remove the capsule from the blister by peeling back the paper backing and pushing the capsule through the foil.
5. Place the capsule in the chamber. Do not place it directly into the mouthpiece. Twist to close.
6. Hold the inhaler upright and press in both side buttons at the same time. Do not press the buttons more than once. You will hear a click as the capsule is punctured. Release the buttons. If the buttons do not pop out, pull the wings of the buttons to release them.
7. Exhale (breathe out) as completely as possible but not into the mouthpiece.
8. Turn the inhaler on its side so that the blue buttons are on the left and right (not the top and bottom) of the inhaler. Hold the inhaler so that it is level.
9. Tilt your head back slightly, place the mouthpiece in your mouth, and close your lips. Breathe in quickly and deeply. As the medicine is released from the capsule, you'll get a sweet taste and hear a whirring noise. (If you don't, the capsule may be stuck. Tap on the side of the inhaler to loosen the capsule and repeat steps 7 to 9. Do not press the side buttons again.)
10. Remove the inhaler from your mouth and hold your breath for as long as you comfortably can. Then exhale.
11. Open the inhaler to see if there is any powder left in the capsule. If there is, repeat steps 7 to 10.
12. Once the capsule is empty, remove it and throw it away. Do not leave it in the chamber. Close the mouthpiece and replace the cover.

The inhaler is made to pierce the capsule so that the powder can be released. However, it is possible that the capsule may break into small pieces inside the inhaler. If this happens, a screen in the inhaler should stop the pieces of capsule from reaching your mouth as you inhale the medication. Very tiny pieces of the capsule may reach your mouth or throat, but this will not hurt you. The capsule is less likely to break if you are careful to store the capsules properly, to keep the capsules in the foil package until you are ready to use them, and to press the buttons on the inhaler only once.

Formoterol capsules should only be used with the special inhaler and should not be taken by mouth. Store capsules in the package and remove them immediately before use. Avoid exposing the capsules to moisture, and handle them with dry hands.

Do not use the dry powder inhaler with a spacer. Do not exhale into the device. Keep the inhaler dry; do not wash it. Always use the new inhaler that comes with a refill of your medication. Do not use the inhaler to inhale any other type of capsules.

Are there other uses for this medicine?

This medication may be prescribed for other uses; ask your doctor or pharmacist for more information.

What special precautions should I follow?

Before using formoterol,

- tell your doctor and pharmacist if you are allergic to formoterol, any other medications, or milk proteins.
- tell your doctor if you use another LABA such as fluticasone and salmeterol combination (Advair) or salmeterol (Serevent). These medications should not be used with formoterol. Your doctor will tell you which medication you should use and which medication you should stop using.
- tell your doctor and pharmacist what prescription and nonprescription medications, vitamins, nutritional supplements, and herbal products you are taking or plan to take. Be sure to mention any of the following: aminophylline (Truphylline); amiodarone (Cordarone); antidepressants such as amitriptyline (Elavil), amoxapine (Asendin), clomipramine (Anafranil), desipramine (Norpramin), doxepin (Adapin, Sinequan), imipramine (Tofranil), nortriptyline (Aventyl, Pamelor), protriptyline (Vivactil), and trimipramine (Surmontil); beta blockers such as atenolol (Tenormin), labetalol (Normodyne), metoprolol (Lopressor, Toprol XL), nadolol (Corgard), propranolol (Inderal), and sotalol (Betapace, Betapace AF); cisapride (Propulsid) (not available in the United States); clonidine (Catapres); diet pills; disopyramide (Norpace); diuretics ('water pills'); dofetilide (Tikosyn); dyphylline (Dilor, Lufyllin); erythromycin (E.E.S., E-Mycin, Erythrocin); guanabenz; medications for colds; monoamine oxidase (MAO) inhibitors, including isocarboxazid (Marplan), phenelzine (Nardil), seligiline (Eldepryl), and tranylcypromine (Parnate); midodrine (Orvaten); moxifloxacin (Avelox); oral steroids such as dexamethasone (Decadron, Dexone), meth-

yldopa (Aldomet); methylprednisolone (Medrol), and prednisone (Deltasone); pimozide (Orap); procainamide (Procanbid, Pronestyl); quinidine (Quinidex); sparfloxacin (Zagam); theophylline (Theo-Chron, Theolair); and thioridazine (Mellaril). Your doctor may need to change the doses of your medications or monitor you carefully for side effects.

- tell your doctor if you have or have ever had an irregular heartbeat, high blood pressure, seizures, diabetes, or heart or thyroid disease.
- tell your doctor if you are pregnant, plan to become pregnant, or are breast-feeding. If you become pregnant while using formoterol, call your doctor.

What special dietary instructions should I follow?

Talk to your doctor about drinking beverages that contain caffeine while using this medicine.

What should I do if I forget to take a dose?

Skip the missed dose and continue your regular dosing schedule. Do not use a double dose to make up for a missed one.

What side effects can this medicine cause?

Formoterol may cause side effects. Tell your doctor if any of these symptoms are severe or do not go away:

- nervousness
- headache
- uncontrollable shaking of a part of the body
- dry mouth
- muscle cramps
- back pain
- nausea
- heartburn
- stomach pain
- extreme tiredness
- dizziness
- difficulty falling asleep or staying asleep
- stuffed or runny nose
- sore throat

Some side effects can be serious. If you experience any of the following symptoms, call your doctor immediately:

- swelling of the face, throat, tongue, lips, eyes, hands, feet, ankles, or lower legs
- hoarseness
- difficulty swallowing or breathing
- hives
- rash
- fast, pounding, or irregular heartbeat
- chest pain
- lightheadedness
- fainting

Formoterol may cause other side effects. Call your doctor if you have any unusual problems while taking this medication.

What storage conditions are needed for this medicine?

Keep sealed in their blister cards until you are ready to use them. Keep this medication out of reach of children. Store it at room temperature and away from excess heat and moisture (not in the bathroom). Throw away any medication that is outdated or no longer needed, and throw away your old inhaler each time you refill your prescription. Talk to your pharmacist about the proper disposal of your medication.

What should I do in case of overdose?

In case of overdose, call your local poison control center at 1-800-222-1222. If the victim has collapsed or is not breathing, call local emergency services at 911.

Symptoms of overdose may include:

- chest pain
- fainting
- fast, pounding, or irregular heartbeat
- nervousness
- headache
- uncontrollable shaking of a part of the body
- seizures
- muscle cramps
- dry mouth
- nausea
- dizziness
- excessive tiredness
- difficulty falling asleep or staying asleep
- thirst
- dry mouth
- trouble breathing

What other information should I know?

Keep all appointments with your doctor.

Do not let anyone else take your medication. Ask your pharmacist any questions you have about refilling your prescription.

Dosage Facts
For Informational Purposes

Caution: Do not change your dose, how often you take your medication, or the length of time you are to take it without first talking to your healthcare provider.

The following dosage information was written using medical language for doctors and other healthcare professionals and is provided here for you to check your dosage. The dosage of this drug may differ for different patients. Therefore, always follow your doctor's instructions or the directions on the label. Contact your healthcare provider or pharmacist if you have any questions about the specific dosage of your medication after reviewing this information.

Pediatric Patients

Asthma

ORAL INHALATION:
- 12 mcg (contents of one capsule) twice daily in patients ≥5 years of age.

Exercise-induced Bronchospasm

ORAL INHALATION:
- 12 mcg (contents of one capsule) administered at least 15 minutes before exercise in patients ≥5 years of age.

Adult Patients

Asthma

ORAL INHALATION:
- 12 mcg (contents of one capsule) twice daily.

Exercise-induced Bronchospasm

ORAL INHALATION:
- 12 mcg (contents of one capsule) administered at least 15 minutes before exercise.

Chronic Obstructive Pulmonary Disease

ORAL INHALATION:
- 12 mcg (contents of one capsule) twice daily.

Prescribing Limits

Pediatric Patients

Asthma

ORAL INHALATION:
- 24 mcg daily (12 mcg every 12 hours) in patients ≥5 years of age.

Exercise-induced Bronchospasm

ORAL INHALATION:
- 24 mcg daily (12 mcg every 12 hours) in patients ≥5 years of age.

Adult Patients

Asthma

ORAL INHALATION:
- 24 mcg daily (12 mcg every 12 hours).

Exercise-induced Bronchospasm

ORAL INHALATION:
- 24 mcg daily (12 mcg every 12 hours).

Chronic Obstructive Pulmonary Disease

ORAL INHALATION:
- 24 mcg daily (12 mcg every 12 hours).

Special Populations

No special population dosage recommendations at this time.

Fosamprenavir

(fos' am pren a veer)

Brand Name: Lexiva

Why is this medicine prescribed?

Fosamprenavir is used with other medications to treat human immunodeficiency virus (HIV) infection in patients with or without acquired immunodeficiency syndrome (AIDS). Fosamprenavir is in a class of medications called protease inhibitors. It works by slowing the spread of HIV in the body. Fosamprenavir does not cure HIV infection and may not prevent you from developing HIV-related illnesses. Fosamprenavir does not prevent you from spreading HIV to other people.

How should this medicine be used?

Fosamprenavir comes as a tablet to take by mouth. It is usually taken with or without food once or twice a day. To help you remember to take fosamprenavir, take it around the same time(s) every day. Follow the directions on your prescription label carefully, and ask your doctor or pharmacist to explain any part you do not understand. Take fosamprenavir exactly as directed. Do not take more or less of it or take it more often than prescribed by your doctor.

Fosamprenavir controls HIV infection but does not cure it. Continue to take fosamprenavir even if you feel well. Do not stop taking fosamprenavir without talking to your doctor. If you miss doses or stop taking fosamprenavir, your condition may become more difficult to treat.

Are there other uses for this medicine?

This medication may be prescribed for other uses; ask your doctor or pharmacist for more information.

What special precautions should I follow?

Before taking fosamprenavir,

- tell your doctor and pharmacist if you are allergic to fosamprenavir, amprenavir (Agenerase), sulfa medications, or any other medications.
- do not take fosamprenavir if you are taking cisapride (Propulsid); ergot medications such as dihydroergotamine (D.H.E. 45, Migranal), ergoloid mesylates (Hydergine, Gerimal), ergonovine (Ergotrate), ergotamine (Bellamine, Cafergot, Migergot), methylergonovine (Methergine), and methysergide (Sansert); midazolam (Versed); pimozide (Orap); or triazolam (Halcion).
- do not take flecainide (Tambocor) or propafenone (Rhythmol) if you are taking fosamprenavir and ritonavir (Norvir) together.
- tell your doctor and pharmacist what other prescription and nonprescription medications, vitamins, and nutritional supplements you are taking. Be sure to mention any of the following: anticoagulants ('blood thinners')

such as warfarin (Coumadin); antidepressants such as amitriptyline (Elavil), amoxapine (Asendin), clomipramine (Anafranil), desipramine (Norpramin), doxepin (Adapin, Sinequan), fluoxetine (Prozac), fluvoxamine (Luvox), imipramine (Tofranil), nefazodone (Serzone), nortriptyline (Aventyl, Pamelor), paroxetine (Paxil), protriptyline (Vivactil), trazodone, and trimipramine (Surmontil); benzodiazepines such as alprazolam (Xanax), clorazepate (ClorazeCaps, Tranxene), diazepam (Valium), and flurazepam (Dalmane); buspirone (BuSpar); calcium channel blockers such as amlodipine (Lotrel, Norvasc), diltiazem (Cardizem, Dilacor, Tizac), felodipine (Lexxel, Plendil), isradipine (DynaCirc), nicardipine (Cardene), nifedipine (Adalat, Nifedical, Procardia), nimodipine (Nimotop), nisoldipine (Sular), and verapamil (Calan, Covera, Isoptin, Verelan); chlorpheniramine (antihistamine in cough and cold medicines); cholesterol-lowering medications (statins) such as atorvastatin (Lipitor), fluvastatin (Lescol), lovastatin (Altocor, Mevacor), and simvastatin (Zocor); clarithromycin (Biaxin); danazol (Danocrine); dexamethasone (Decadron); erythromycin (E.E.S., E-mycin, Erythrocin); fluconazole (Diflucan); histamine H2-receptor blockers such as cimetidine (Tagamet), famotidine (Pepcid), nizatidine (Axid), and ranitidine (Zantac); isoniazid (INH, Nydrazid); itraconazole (Sporanox); ketoconazole (Nizoral); medications for irregular heartbeat such as amiodarone (Cordarone, Pacerone), bepridil (Vascor), flecainide (Tambocor), propafenone (Rhythmol), and quinidine (Quinidex); medications for seizures such as carbamazepine (Tegretol), ethosuximide (Zarontin), phenobarbital (Luminal, Solfoton), and phenytoin (Dilantin); medications that suppress the immune system such as cyclosporine (Neoral, Sandimmune), sirolimus (Rapamune), or tacrolimus (Prograf); methadone (Dolophine, Methadose); metronidazole (Flagyl); other medications to treat HIV including amprenavir (Agenerase), delavirdine (Rescriptor), efavirenz (Sustiva), indinavir (Crixivan), lopinavir (Kaletra), nelfinavir (Viracept), nevirapine (Viramune), saquinavir (Fortovase, Invirase), and ritonavir (Norvir); proton-pump inhibitors such as esomeprazole (Nexium), lansoprazole (Prevacid), omeprazole (Prilosec), pantoprazole (Protonix), and rabeprazole (AcipHex); quinine; rifabutin (Mycobutin); rifampin (Rifadin, Rimactane); tamoxifen (Nolvadex); terfenadine (Allegra); troleandomycin (TAO); vincristine (Vincasar); and zafirlukast (Accolate). Your doctor may need to change the doses of your medications or monitor you carefully for side effects.

- tell your doctor if you are taking medications for erectile dysfunction such as sildenafil (Viagra), tadalafil (Cialis), or vardenafil (Levitra). You should know that fosamprenavir may increase the chance that you will experience serious side effects from these medications. If you are taking any of these medications and you experience dizziness, fainting, upset stomach, changes in vision, or a painful erection that lasts for several hours, call your doctor right away.

- tell your doctor what herbal products you are taking, especially St. John's wort.
- tell your doctor if you have or have ever had diabetes, hemophilia (a disease in which the blood does not clot normally), high cholesterol or triglycerides, kidney or liver disease, or if you drink or have ever drunk large amounts of alcohol.
- tell your doctor if you are pregnant or plan to become pregnant. If you become pregnant while taking fosamprenavir, call your doctor. You should not breastfeed if you are infected with HIV or are taking fosamprenavir.
- if you are having surgery, including dental surgery, tell the doctor or dentist that you are taking fosamprenavir.
- you should know that fosamprenavir may decrease the effectiveness of oral contraceptives (birth control pills). Talk to your doctor about other ways to prevent pregnancy while you are taking this medication.
- you should know that your body fat may increase or move to different areas of your body such as your breasts and upper back.

What special dietary instructions should I follow?

Talk to your doctor about drinking grapefruit juice while taking this medicine.

What should I do if I forget to take a dose?

If you miss a dose and remember after less than 4 hours have passed, take the missed dose immediately. However, if you remember after more than 4 hours have passed, call your doctor to find out if you should skip the missed dose. Do not take a double dose to make up for a missed dose.

What side effects can this medicine cause?

Fosamprenavir may cause hyperglycemia (high blood sugar). Call your doctor immediately if you have any of the following symptoms of hyperglycemia:

- extreme thirst
- frequent urination
- extreme hunger
- weakness
- blurred vision

If high blood sugar is not treated, a serious, life-threatening condition called diabetic ketoacidosis could develop. Call your doctor immediately if you have any of the these symptoms:

- dry mouth
- upset stomach and vomiting
- shortness of breath
- breath that smells fruity
- decreased consciousness

Fosamprenavir may cause other side effects. Tell your doctor if any of these symptoms are severe or do not go away:

- diarrhea
- upset stomach
- vomiting
- headache
- extreme tiredness

Some side effects can be serious. The following symptoms are uncommon, but if you experience any of them, call your doctor immediately:

- skin rash
- itching
- hives
- difficulty breathing or swallowing
- sore throat, fever, chills, cough, and other signs of infection

Fosamprenavir may cause other side effects. Call your doctor if you have any unusual problems while taking this medication.

Laboratory animals who were given amprenavir (Agenerase), a medication similar to fosamprenavir, developed tumors. It is not known if fosamprenavir increases the risk of tumors in humans. Talk to your doctor about the risks of taking this medication.

If you experience a serious side effect, you or your doctor may send a report to the Food and Drug Administration's (FDA) MedWatch Adverse Event Reporting program online [at http://www.fda.gov/MedWatch/index.html] or by phone [1-800-332-1088].

What storage conditions are needed for this medicine?

Keep this medication in the container it came in, tightly closed, and out of reach of children. Store it at room temperature and away from excess heat and moisture (not in the bathroom). Throw away any medication that is outdated or no longer needed. Talk to your pharmacist about the proper disposal of your medication.

What should I do in case of overdose?

In case of overdose, call your local poison control center at 1-800-222-1222. If the victim has collapsed or is not breathing, call local emergency services at 911.

What other information should I know?

Keep all appointments with your doctor and the laboratory. Your doctor may order certain lab tests to check your body's response to fosamprenavir.

Do not let anyone else take your medication. Ask your pharmacist any questions you have about refilling your prescription.

Dosage Facts
For Informational Purposes

Caution: Do not change your dose, how often you take your medication, or the length of time you

are to take it without first talking to your healthcare provider.

The following dosage information was written using medical language for doctors and other healthcare professionals and is provided here for you to check your dosage. The dosage of this drug may differ for different patients. Therefore, always follow your doctor's instructions or the directions on the label. Contact your healthcare provider or pharmacist if you have any questions about the specific dosage of your medication after reviewing this information.

General Dosage Information

Available as fosamprenavir calcium; dosage expressed in terms of fosamprenavir.

Must be given in conjunction with other antiretrovirals. *If used with both ritonavir and efavirenz, dosage adjustment may be needed depending on frequency of administration.*

Adult Patients

Treatment of HIV Infection
Treatment-naive Adults

ORAL:
- 1.4 g twice daily (without ritonavir).
- 1.4 g once daily *boosted* with low-dose ritonavir (200 mg once daily) or 700 mg twice daily *boosted* with low-dose ritonavir (100 mg twice daily).

PI-experienced Adults

ORAL:
- 700 mg twice daily *boosted* with low-dose ritonavir (100 mg twice daily). A once-daily regimen of *ritonavir-boosted* fosamprenavir not recommended in treatment-experienced patients.

Postexposure Prophylaxis of HIV†
Occupational Exposure†

ORAL:
- 1.4 g twice daily (without ritonavir). Alternatively, 1.4 g once daily with low-dose ritonavir (200 mg once daily) or 700 mg twice daily with low-dose ritonavir (100 mg twice daily).
- Used in alternative expanded regimens that include fosamprenavir (with or without low-dose ritonavir) and 2 NRTIs.
- Initiate postexposure prophylaxis as soon as possible following exposure (within hours rather than days) and continue for 4 weeks, if tolerated.

Nonoccupational Exposure†

ORAL:
- 1.4 g twice daily (without ritonavir).
- Used in an alternative PI-based regimen that includes fosamprenavir (with or without low-dose ritonavir) and (lamivudine or emtricitabine) and (zidovudine or stavudine or abacavir or tenofovir or didanosine).
- Initiate postexposure prophylaxis as soon as possible following exposure (preferably ≤72 hours after exposure) and continue for 28 days.

Prescribing Limits
Adult Patients

Treatment of HIV Infection
Treatment-naive Adults

ORAL:
- Maximum 1.4 g once daily with ritonavir 200 mg once daily or 700 mg twice daily with ritonavir 100 mg twice daily. Higher than recommended dosages of fosamprenavir and/or ritonavir associated with increased serum transaminase concentrations; higher dosages not recommended.

PI-experienced Adults

ORAL:
- Maximum 700 mg twice daily with ritonavir 100 mg twice daily. Higher than recommended dosages of fosamprenavir and/or ritonavir associated with increased serum transaminase concentrations; higher dosages not recommended.

Special Populations

Hepatic Impairment
- 700 mg twice daily (without ritonavir) in adults with mild to moderate hepatic impairment (Child-Pugh scores 5–8). Should not be used in adults with severe hepatic impairment (Child-Pugh scores 9–12).
- Data not available on use of *ritonavir-boosted* fosamprenavir in those with hepatic impairment.

Renal Impairment
- Dosage adjustment not necessary.

Geriatric Patients
- Select dosage with caution because of age-related decreases in hepatic, renal, and/or cardiac function and concomitant disease and drug therapy.

† Use is not currently included in the labeling approved by the US Food and Drug Administration.

Fosfomycin

(fos foe mye′ sin)

Brand Name: Monurol® Sachet

Why is this medicine prescribed?

Fosfomycin is an antibiotic used to treat infections of the urinary tract.

This medication is sometimes prescribed for other uses; ask your doctor or pharmacist for more information.

How should this medicine be used?

Fosfomycin comes as granules to be mixed with water and then taken by mouth. Do not take the dry granules by mouth without first diluting them in water. Follow the directions on your prescription label carefully, and ask your doctor or pharmacist to explain any part you do not understand. Take fosfomycin exactly as directed. Do not take more or less of it or take it more often than prescribed by your doctor.

To prepare a dose, pour the entire contents of a single-dose packet into a glass and add 3-4 ounces of cold water. Stir to dissolve. Do not use hot water. The dose should be taken by mouth as soon as it is prepared.

What special precautions should I follow?

Before taking fosfomycin,
- tell your doctor and pharmacist if you are allergic to fosfomycin or any other drugs.
- tell your doctor and pharmacist what prescription and nonprescription medications you are taking, especially cisapride (Propulsid), metoclopramide (Reglan), and vitamins.
- tell your doctor if you have or have ever had asthma or liver disease.
- tell your doctor if you are pregnant, plan to become pregnant, or are breast-feeding. If you become pregnant while taking fosfomycin, call your doctor.

What should I do if I forget to take a dose?

Take the missed dose as soon as you remember it. However, if it is almost time for the next dose, skip the missed dose and continue your regular dosing schedule. Do not take a double dose to make up for a missed one.

What side effects can this medicine cause?

Fosfomycin may cause side effects. Tell your doctor if any of these symptoms are severe or do not go away:
- upset stomach
- diarrhea
- headache
- vaginal itching
- runny nose
- back pain

If you experience any of the following symptoms, call your doctor immediately:
- fever
- rash
- joint pain
- swelling of the mouth or tongue
- yellowing of the skin or eyes

If you experience a serious side effect, you or your doctor may send a report to the Food and Drug Administration's (FDA) MedWatch Adverse Event Reporting program online [at http://www.fda.gov/MedWatch/index.html] or by phone [1-800-332-1088].

What storage conditions are needed for this medicine?

Keep this medication in the container it came in, tightly closed, and out of reach of children. Store it at room temperature and away from excess heat and moisture (not in the bathroom). Throw away any medication that is outdated or no longer needed. Talk to your pharmacist about the proper disposal of your medication.

What should I do in case of overdose?

In case of overdose, call your local poison control center at 1-800-222-1222. If the victim has collapsed or is not breathing, call local emergency services at 911.

What other information should I know?

Keep all appointments with your doctor and the laboratory. Your doctor may order certain lab tests to check your response to fosfomycin

Do not let anyone else take your medication. Your prescription is probably not refillable. If you still have symptoms of infection after you finish the fosfomycin, call your doctor.

Talk to your doctor, pharmacist, or other healthcare professional if you have questions about dosing information for your medication.

Fosinopril

(foe sin' oh pril)

Brand Name: Monopril®, Monopril®-HCT as a combination product containing Fosinopril Sodium and Hydrochlorothiazide

> ## Important Warning
>
> Do not take fosinopril if you are pregnant. If you become pregnant while taking fosinopril, call your doctor immediately. Fosinopril may harm the fetus.

Why is this medicine prescribed?

Fosinopril is used alone or in combination with other medications to treat high blood pressure. It is also used in combination with other medications to treat heart failure. Fosinopril is in a class of medications called angiotensin-converting enzyme (ACE) inhibitors. It works by decreasing certain chemicals that tighten the blood vessels, so blood flows more smoothly and the heart can pump blood more efficiently.

How should this medicine be used?

Fosinopril comes as a tablet to take by mouth. It is usually taken once or twice a day. To help you remember to take fosinopril, take it around the same time every day. Follow the directions on your prescription label carefully, and ask your doctor or pharmacist to explain any part you do not understand. Take fosinopril exactly as directed. Do not take more or less of it or take it more often than prescribed by your doctor.

Your doctor will probably start you on a low dose of fosinopril and gradually increase your dose.

Fosinopril controls high blood pressure and heart failure but does not cure them. Continue to take fosinopril even if you feel well. Do not stop taking fosinopril without talking to your doctor.

Are there other uses for this medicine?

This medication may be prescribed for other uses; ask your doctor or pharmacist for more information.

What special precautions should I follow?

Before taking fosinopril,

- tell your doctor and pharmacist if you are allergic to fosinopril, benazepril (Lotensin), captopril (Capoten), enalapril (Vasotec), lisinopril (Prinivil, Zestril), moexipril (Univasc), perindopril (Aceon), quinapril (Accupril), ramipril (Altace), trandolapril (Mavik), or any other medications.
- tell your doctor and pharmacist what prescription and nonprescription medications, vitamins, nutritional supplements, and herbal products you are taking. Be sure to mention any of the following: diuretics ('water pills'); lithium (Eskalith, Lithobid); and potassium supplements. Your doctor may need to change the doses of your medications or monitor you carefully for side effects.
- if you are taking antacids (Maalox, Mylanta), take them 2 hours before or after fosinopril.
- tell your doctor if you are on dialysis and if you have or have ever had lupus; scleroderma; heart failure; high blood pressure; diabetes; or liver or kidney disease.
- tell your doctor if you plan to become pregnant or are breast-feeding.
- if you are having surgery, including dental surgery, tell the doctor or dentist that you are taking fosinopril.
- you should know that diarrhea, vomiting, not drinking enough fluids, and sweating a lot can cause a drop in blood pressure, which may cause lightheadedness and fainting.

What special dietary instructions should I follow?

Talk to your doctor before using salt substitutes containing potassium. If your doctor prescribes a low-salt or low-sodium diet, follow these instructions carefully.

What should I do if I forget to take a dose?

Take the missed dose as soon as you remember it. However, if it is almost time for the next dose, skip the missed dose and continue your regular dosing schedule. Do not take a double dose to make up for a missed one.

What side effects can this medicine cause?

Fosinopril may cause side effects. Tell your doctor if any of these symptoms are severe or do not go away:

- dizziness
- cough
- upset stomach
- vomiting
- diarrhea
- headache
- excessive tiredness
- weakness

Some side effects can be serious. The following symptoms are uncommon, but if you experience any of them, call your doctor immediately:

- swelling of the face, throat, tongue, lips, eyes, hands, feet, ankles, or lower legs
- hoarseness
- difficulty breathing or swallowing
- yellowing of the skin or eyes
- fever, sore throat, chills, and other signs of infection
- lightheadedness
- fainting

Fosinopril may cause other side effects. Call your doctor if you have any unusual problems while taking this medication.

If you experience a serious side effect, you or your doctor may send a report to the Food and Drug Administration's (FDA) MedWatch Adverse Event Reporting program online [at http://www.fda.gov/MedWatch/index.html] or by phone [1-800-332-1088].

What storage conditions are needed for this medicine?

Keep this medication in the container it came in, tightly closed, and out of reach of children. Store it at room temperature and away from excess heat and moisture (not in the bathroom). Throw away any medication that is outdated or no longer needed. Talk to your pharmacist about the proper disposal of your medication.

What should I do in case of overdose?

In case of overdose, call your local poison control center at 1-800-222-1222. If the victim has collapsed or is not breathing, call local emergency services at 911.

Symptoms of overdose may include:

- dizziness
- lightheadedness
- fainting

What other information should I know?

Keep all appointments with your doctor and the laboratory. Your blood pressure should be checked regularly to determine your response to fosinopril. Your doctor may order certain lab tests to check your body's response to fosinopril.

Before having any laboratory test, tell your doctor and the laboratory personnel that you are taking fosinopril.

Do not let anyone else take your medication. Ask your pharmacist any questions you have about refilling your prescription.

Dosage Facts
For Informational Purposes

Caution: Do not change your dose, how often you take your medication, or the length of time you are to take it without first talking to your healthcare provider.

The following dosage information was written using medical language for doctors and other healthcare professionals and is provided here for you to check your dosage. The dosage of this drug may differ for different patients. Therefore, always follow your doctor's instructions or the directions on the label. Contact your healthcare provider or pharmacist if you have any questions about the specific dosage of your medication after reviewing this information.

General Dosage Information

Available as fosinopril sodium; dosage expressed in terms of the salt.

Pediatric Patients

Hypertension

ORAL:
- Children ≥6 years of age and weighing >50 kg: 5–10 mg once daily. Increase dosage until desired BP goal is achieved (up to maximum dosage of 40 mg daily). A dosage form suitable for providing an appropriate dosage for children weighing <50 kg is not commercially available in the US.

Adult Patients

Hypertension

ORAL:
- Initially, 10 mg once daily as monotherapy. Adjust dosage at approximately monthly intervals (more aggressively in high-risk patients) to achieve BP control.
- In patients currently receiving diuretic therapy, discontinue diuretic, if possible, 2–3 days before initiating fosinopril. May cautiously resume diuretic therapy if BP not controlled adequately with fosinopril alone. If diuretic cannot be discontinued, can increase sodium intake prior to initiating fosinopril. Manufacturer states that fosinopril may be initiated at the usual dose of 10 mg under close medical supervision for several hours until BP has stabilized; however, consider the desirability of initiating therapy at reduced dosage to minimize risk of hypotension.
- Usual dosage: 20–40 mg daily, given in 1 dose or 2 divided doses daily. Increasing dosage to 80 mg daily occasionally may result in further BP response.
- If effectiveness diminishes toward end of dosing interval in patients treated once daily, consider increasing dosage or administering drug in divided doses.

Fosinopril/Hydrochlorothiazide Combination Therapy

ORAL:
- If BP is not adequately controlled by monotherapy with fosinopril, can switch to the fixed-combination preparation containing fosinopril 10 mg and hydrochlorothiazide 12.5 mg, or alternatively, fosinopril 20 mg and hydrochlorothiazide 12.5 mg.
- On average, antihypertensive effect of fosinopril 10 mg and hydrochlorothiazide 12.5 mg is similar to that of fosinopril 40 mg or hydrochlorothiazide 37.5 mg as monotherapy.

CHF

ORAL:
- Initially, 10 mg daily. If patient has been treated vigorously with diuretics, 5 mg initially. Monitor closely for ≥2 hours until BP has stabilized. To minimize risk of hypotension, reduce diuretic dosage, if possible.
- Adjust dosage gradually over several weeks to maximum tolerated dosage (up to 40 mg daily).
- Usual dosage: 20–40 mg once daily.

Prescribing Limits

Pediatric Patients

Hypertension

ORAL:
- Maximum 40 mg daily.

Adult Patients

CHF

ORAL:
- Maximum 40 mg daily.

Special Populations

Hepatic Impairment
- No specific dosage recommendations.

Renal Impairment

Hypertension

- Dosage adjustment not required.
- Fosinopril/hydrochlorothiazide fixed combinations are not recommended in patients with Cl_{cr} <30 mL/minute or S_{cr} ≥3 mg/dL.

CHF

- Initially, 5 mg in patients with moderate to severe renal impairment.

Geriatric Patients
- Select dosage carefully; monitoring renal function may be useful.

Frovatriptan

(froe va trip′ tan)

Brand Name: Frova®

Why is this medicine prescribed?

Frovatriptan is used to treat the symptoms of migraine headaches (severe throbbing headaches that sometimes are accompanied by nausea and sensitivity to sound and light). Frovatriptan is in a class of medications called selective serotonin receptor agonists. It works by narrowing blood vessels in the brain. Frovatriptan does not prevent migraine attacks.

How should this medicine be used?

Frovatriptan comes as a tablet to take by mouth. It is usually taken at the first sign of a migraine attack. If your symptoms improve after you take frovatriptan but return after 2 hours or longer, you may take a second tablet. However, if your symptoms do not improve after you take frovatriptan, do not take a second tablet before calling your doctor. Do not take more than three frovatriptan tablets in any 24-hour period. Call your doctor if you need to take frovatriptan more than four times a month. Follow the directions on your prescription label carefully, and ask your doctor or pharmacist to explain any part you do not understand. Take frovatriptan exactly as directed. Do not take more or less of it or take it more often than prescribed by your doctor.

You may take your first dose of frovatriptan in a doctor's office or other medical facility where you can be monitored for serious reactions.

Before taking frovatriptan, read the manufacturer's information for patients that comes with it.

Are there other uses for this medicine?

This medication may be prescribed for other uses; ask your doctor or pharmacist for more information.

What special precautions should I follow?

Before taking frovatriptan,

- tell your doctor and pharmacist if you are allergic to frovatriptan or any other medications.
- do not take frovatriptan within 24 hours of another selective serotonin receptor agonist such as almotriptan (Axert), eletriptan (Relpax), naratriptan (Amerge), rizatriptan (Maxalt), sumatriptan (Imitrex), or zolmitriptan (Zomig); or ergot-type medications such as bromocriptine (Parlodel), cabergoline (Dostinex), dihydroergotamine (D.H.E. 45, Migranal), ergoloid mesylates (Germinal, Hydergine), ergonovine (Ergotrate), ergotamine (Bellergal-S, Cafergot, Ergomar, Wigraine), methylergonovine (Methergine), methysergide (Sansert), and pergolide (Permax).

- tell your doctor and pharmacist what other prescription and nonprescription medications, vitamins, nutritional supplements, and herbal products you are taking or plan to take. Be sure to mention any of the following: propranolol (Inderal); selective serotonin reuptake inhibitors (SSRIs) such as citalopram (Celexa), escitalopram (Lexapro), fluoxetine (Prozac, Sarafem, in Symbyax), fluvoxamine, paroxetine (Paxil), and sertraline (Zoloft); selective serotonin/norepinephrine reuptake inhibitors (SNRIs) such as duloxetine (Cymbalta) and venlafaxine (Effexor); and oral contraceptives (birth control pills). Your doctor may need to change the doses of your medications or monitor you carefully for side effects.
- tell your doctor if you smoke, if you or any family members have or have ever had heart disease, if you have gone through menopause (change of life), and if you have or have ever had a heart attack; angina (chest pain); pounding heartbeat or shortness of breath; a stroke or 'mini-stroke'; high blood pressure; high cholesterol; diabetes; circulation problems such as varicose veins, blood clots in the legs, Raynaud's disease (problems with blood flow to the fingers, toes, ears, and nose) or ischemic bowel disease (bloody diarrhea and stomach pain caused by decreased blood flow to the intestines); or liver disease.
- tell your doctor if you are pregnant, plan to become pregnant, or are breast-feeding. If you become pregnant while taking frovatriptan, call your doctor.
- you should know that frovatriptan may make you drowsy or dizzy. Do not drive a car or operate machinery until you know how this medication affects you.
- talk to your doctor about your headache symptoms to make sure they are caused by migraine. Frovatriptan should not be used to treat hemiplegic or basilar migraine or headaches caused by other conditions (such as cluster headaches).

What special dietary instructions should I follow?

Unless your doctor tells you otherwise, continue your normal diet.

What side effects can this medicine cause?

Frovatriptan may cause side effects. Tell your doctor if any of these symptoms are severe or do not go away:

- dizziness
- headache
- dry mouth
- indigestion
- excessive tiredness
- flushing
- hot or cold feeling
- pain in joints or bones

Some side effects can be serious. The following symptoms are uncommon, but if you experience any of them, call your doctor immediately:

- tightness, pain, pressure, or heaviness in the chest, throat, neck, and/or jaw
- slow or difficult speech
- faintness
- weakness or numbness of an arm or leg
- severe stomach pain
- bloody diarrhea
- rapid, pounding, or irregular heartbeat
- difficulty breathing
- paleness or blue color of the fingers and toes
- pain, burning, or tingling in the hands or feet
- rash or itching

Frovatriptan may cause other side effects. Call your doctor if you have any unusual problems while taking this medication.

What storage conditions are needed for this medicine?

Keep this medication in the container it came in, tightly closed, and out of reach of children. Store it at room temperature and away from excess heat and moisture (not in the bathroom). Throw away any medication that is outdated or no longer needed. Talk to your pharmacist about the proper disposal of your medication.

What should I do in case of overdose?

In case of overdose, call your local poison control center at 1-800-222-1222. If the victim has collapsed or is not breathing, call local emergency services at 911.

What other information should I know?

Keep all appointments with your doctor.

Do not let anyone else take your medication. Ask your pharmacist any questions you have about refilling your prescription.

Dosage Facts
For Informational Purposes

Caution: Do not change your dose, how often you take your medication, or the length of time you are to take it without first talking to your healthcare provider.

The following dosage information was written using medical language for doctors and other healthcare professionals and is provided here for you to check your dosage. The dosage of this drug may differ for different patients. Therefore, always follow your doctor's instructions or the directions on the label. Contact your healthcare provider or pharmacist if you have any questions about the specific dosage of your medication after reviewing this information.

General Dosage Information

Available as frovatriptan succinate; dosage is expressed in terms of frovatriptan.

Adult Patients

Vascular Headaches
Migraine

ORAL:

- 2.5 mg as a single dose. Higher dosages provide no additional benefit but may increase risk of adverse effects.
- If headache recurs, additional doses may be administered at intervals of ≥2 hours, up to a maximum dosage of 7.5 mg in any 24-hour period.
- If patient does not respond to first dose, additional doses are unlikely to provide benefit for the same headache.

Prescribing Limits
Adult Patients

Vascular Headaches
Migraine

ORAL:

- Maximum 7.5 mg in any 24-hour period.
- Safety of treating an average of >4 headaches per 30-day period has not been established.

Special Populations

Hepatic Impairment

- No dosage adjustment required in patients with mild to moderate hepatic impairment; not studied in patients with severe hepatic impairment.

Fulvestrant Injection

(ful ves' trant)

Brand Name: Faslodex®

Why is this medicine prescribed?

Fulvestrant is used to treat hormone receptor positive breast cancer (breast cancer that depends on hormones such as estrogen to grow) in women who have experienced menopause (change of life; end of monthly menstrual periods) and whose breast cancer has worsened after they were treated with antiestrogen medications such as tamoxifen (Nolvadex). Fulvestrant is in a class of medications called estrogen receptor antagonists. It works by blocking the action of estrogen on cancer cells. This can slow or stop the growth of some breast tumors that need estrogen to grow.

How should this medicine be used?

Fulvestrant comes as a solution (liquid) to be injected into a muscle in the buttocks. Fulvestrant is administered by a doctor or nurse in a medical office. It is usually given once a month. You may receive your entire dose of medication as a single injection, or the dose may be divided into two injections that are given one after another.

Ask your doctor or pharmacist for a copy of the manufacturer's information for the patient.

Are there other uses for this medicine?

This medication may be prescribed for other uses; ask your doctor or pharmacist for more information.

What special precautions should I follow?

Before taking fulvestrant,

- tell your doctor and pharmacist if you are allergic to fulvestrant or any other medications.
- tell your doctor and pharmacist what prescription and nonprescription medications, vitamins, nutritional supplements, and herbal products you are taking or plan to take. Be sure to mention anticoagulants (blood thinners) such as warfarin (Coumadin). Your doctor may need to change the doses of your medications or monitor you carefully for side effects.
- tell your doctor if you have or have ever had any bleeding problems or liver disease.
- you should know that fulvestrant should only be taken by women who have undergone menopause and cannot become pregnant. However, if you are pregnant, you should tell your doctor before you begin treatment with this medication. Your doctor may also check to see if you are pregnant before you begin treatment. Tell your doctor if you become pregnant during your treatment with fulvestrant. Fulvestrant may harm the fetus.
- tell your doctor if you are breast-feeding. You should not breast-feed during your treatment with fulvestrant.

What special dietary instructions should I follow?

Unless your doctor tells you otherwise, continue your normal diet.

What should I do if I forget to take a dose?

If you miss an appointment to receive a dose of fulvestrant, call your doctor as soon as possible.

What side effects can this medicine cause?

Fulvestrant may cause side effects. Tell your doctor if any of these symptoms are severe or do not go away:

- nausea
- vomiting
- constipation
- diarrhea
- stomach pain
- loss of appetite
- sore throat
- weakness

- flushing
- headache
- pain in bones, joints, or back
- pain, redness, or swelling in the place where your medication was injected
- swelling of the hands, feet, ankles, or lower legs
- dizziness
- difficulty falling asleep or staying asleep
- depression
- nervousness
- feelings of numbness, tingling, pricking, or burning on the skin
- sweating

Some side effects can be serious. If you experience any of these symptoms, call your doctor immediately:

- shortness of breath
- chest pain
- hives
- rash
- itching
- difficulty breathing or swallowing
- swelling of the face, throat, tongue, lips, or eyes

Fulvestrant may cause other side effects. Call your doctor if you have any unusual problems while taking this medication.

What should I do in case of overdose?

In case of overdose, call your local poison control center at 1-800-222-1222. If the victim has collapsed or is not breathing, call local emergency services at 911.

What other information should I know?

Keep all appointments with your doctor.

Dosage Facts
For Informational Purposes

Caution: Do not change your dose, how often you take your medication, or the length of time you are to take it without first talking to your healthcare provider.

The following dosage information was written using medical language for doctors and other healthcare professionals and is provided here for you to check your dosage. The dosage of this drug may differ for different patients. Therefore, always follow your doctor's instructions or the directions on the label. Contact your healthcare provider or pharmacist if you have any questions about the specific dosage of your medication after reviewing this information.

Adult Patients

Breast Cancer

IM:
- 250 mg once monthly.

Furosemide

(fyoor oh′ se mide)

Brand Name: Lasix®

Why is this medicine prescribed?

Furosemide, a 'water pill,' is used to reduce the swelling and fluid retention caused by various medical problems, including heart or liver disease. It is also used to treat high blood pressure. It causes the kidneys to get rid of unneeded water and salt from the body into the urine.

This medicine is sometimes prescribed for other uses; ask your doctor or pharmacist for more information.

How should this medicine be used?

Furosemide comes as a tablet and liquid to take by mouth. It usually is taken once a day in the morning or twice a day in the morning and afternoon. Follow the directions on your prescription label carefully, and ask your doctor or pharmacist to explain any part you do not understand. Take furosemide exactly as directed. Do not take more or less of it or take it more often than prescribed by your doctor.

Furosemide controls high blood pressure but does not cure it. Continue to take furosemide even if you feel well. Do not stop taking furosemide without talking to your doctor.

What special precautions should I follow?

Before taking furosemide,

• tell your doctor and pharmacist if you are allergic to furosemide, sulfa drugs, or any other drugs.

• tell your doctor and pharmacist what prescription and nonprescription medications you are taking, especially other medications for high blood pressure, aspirin, corticosteroids (e.g., prednisone), digoxin (Lanoxin), indomethacin (Indocin), lithium (Eskalith, Lithobid), medications for diabetes, probenecid (Benemid), and vitamins. If you also are taking cholestyramine or colestipol, take it at least 1 hour after taking furosemide.

• tell your doctor if you have or have ever had diabetes, gout, or kidney or liver disease.

• tell your doctor if you are pregnant, plan to become pregnant, or are breast-feeding. Do not breast-feed while taking this medicine. If you become pregnant while taking furosemide, call your doctor.

• if you are having surgery, including dental surgery, tell the doctor or dentist that you are taking furosemide.

• plan to avoid unnecessary or prolonged exposure to sunlight and to wear protective clothing, sunglasses, and sunscreen. Furosemide may make your skin sensitive to sunlight.

What special dietary instructions should I follow?

Follow your doctor's directions. They may include a daily exercise program and a low-sodium or low-salt diet, potassium supplements, and increased amounts of potassium-rich foods (e.g., bananas, prunes, raisins, and orange juice) in your diet.

What should I do if I forget to take a dose?

Take the missed dose as soon as you remember it. However, if it is almost time for your next dose, skip the missed dose and continue your regular dosing schedule. Do not take a double dose to make up for a missed one.

What side effects can this medicine cause?

Frequent urination may last for up to 6 hours after a dose and should decrease after you take furosemide for a few weeks. Tell your doctor if any of these symptoms are severe or do not go away:

• muscle cramps
• weakness
• dizziness
• confusion
• thirst
• upset stomach
• vomiting
• blurred vision
• headache
• restlessness
• constipation

If you have any of the following symptoms, call your doctor immediately:

• fever
• sore throat
• ringing in the ears
• unusual bleeding or bruising
• loss of hearing
• severe rash with peeling skin
• difficulty breathing or swallowing
• rapid, excessive weight loss

If you experience a serious side effect, you or your doctor may send a report to the Food and Drug Administration's (FDA) MedWatch Adverse Event Reporting program online

[at http://www.fda.gov/MedWatch/index.html] or by phone [1-800-332-1088].

What storage conditions are needed for this medicine?

Keep this medicine in the container it came in, tightly closed, and out of reach of children. Store it at room temperature and away from excess heat and moisture (not in the bathroom). Throw away unused furosemide liquid after 60 days. Throw away any medicine that is outdated or no longer needed. Talk to your pharmacist about the proper disposal of your medicine.

What should I do in case of overdose?

In case of overdose, call your local poison control center at 1-800-222-1222. If the victim has collapsed or is not breathing, call local emergency services at 911.

What other information should I know?

Keep all appointments with your doctor and the laboratory. Your blood pressure should be checked regularly, and blood tests should be done occasionally.

Do not let anyone else take your medicine. Ask your pharmacist any questions you have about refilling your prescription.

Dosage Facts
For Informational Purposes

Caution: Do not change your dose, how often you take your medication, or the length of time you are to take it without first talking to your healthcare provider.

The following dosage information was written using medical language for doctors and other healthcare professionals and is provided here for you to check your dosage. The dosage of this drug may differ for different patients. Therefore, always follow your doctor's instructions or the directions on the label. Contact your healthcare provider or pharmacist if you have any questions about the specific dosage of your medication after reviewing this information.

General Dosage Information

Individualize dosage according to patient's requirements and response; titrate dosage to gain maximum therapeutic effect while using the lowest possible effective dosage.

Pediatric Patients

Edema

ORAL:
- 2 mg/kg administered as a single dose. If necessary, increase in increments of 1 or 2 mg/kg every 6–8 hours to a maximum of 6 mg/kg. Generally not necessary to exceed individual doses of 4 mg/kg or a dosing frequency of once or twice daily. Use minimum effective dosage for maintenance therapy.

Hypertension†

ORAL:
- Initially, 0.5–2 mg/kg given once or twice daily. Increase as necessary up to a maximum of 6 mg/kg daily.

Adult Patients

Edema

ORAL:
- 20–80 mg given as a single dose, preferably in the morning. If needed, repeat same dose 6–8 hours later or increase dose by 20- to 40-mg increments and give no sooner than 6–8 hours after last dose until desired diuretic response (including weight loss) is obtained. May titrate carefully up to 600 mg daily in severe cases.
- The effective dose may be given once or twice daily thereafter, or, in some cases, by intermittent administration on 2–4 consecutive days each week. Dosage may be reduced for maintenance therapy.

Hypertension

ORAL:
- 40 mg twice daily. If desired BP not attained, consider adding other antihypertensive agents.
- Usual dosage recommended by JNC 7: 10–40 mg twice daily.

Prescribing Limits
Pediatric Patients

Edema

ORAL:
- Maximum of 6 mg/kg.

Hypertension†

ORAL:
- Maximum 6 mg/kg daily.

Adult Patients

Edema

ORAL:
- Maximum of 600 mg daily.

Special Populations

Renal Impairment
- Higher doses may be required for patients with acute or chronic renal failure.

Hypertension
- Higher doses may be required for patients with acute or chronic renal failure.

ORAL:
- Use of ≥3 antihypertensive agents usually is required to achieve a target BP <130/80 mm Hg.

† Use is not currently included in the labeling approved by the US Food and Drug Administration.

Gabapentin

(ga′ ba pen tin)

Brand Name: Gabarone®, Neurontin®
Also available generically.

Why is this medicine prescribed?

Gabapentin is used to help control certain types of seizures in patients who have epilepsy. Gabapentin is also used to relieve the pain of postherpetic neuralgia (PHN; the burning, stabbing pain or aches that may last for months or years after an attack of shingles). Gabapentin is in a class of medications called anticonvulsants. Gabapentin treats seizures by decreasing abnormal excitement in the brain. Gabapentin relieves the pain of PHN by changing the way the body senses pain.

How should this medicine be used?

Gabapentin comes as a capsule, a tablet, and an oral solution (liquid) to take by mouth. It is usually taken with a full glass of water (8 oz) three times a day. Gabapentin may be taken with or without food. Take this medication at evenly spaced times throughout the day and night; do not let more than 12 hours pass between doses. Follow the directions on your prescription label carefully, and ask your doctor or pharmacist to explain any part you do not understand. Take gabapentin exactly as directed. Do not take more or less of it or take it more often than prescribed by your doctor.

If your doctor tells you to take one-half of a tablet as part of your dose, carefully split the tablet along the score mark. Use the other half-tablet as part of your next dose. Properly throw away any half-tablets that you have not used within several days of breaking them.

Your doctor will probably start you on a low dose of gabapentin and gradually increase your dose as needed to treat your condition. If you are taking gabapentin to treat PHN, tell your doctor if your symptoms do not improve during your treatment.

Gabapentin may help to control your condition but will not cure it. Continue to take gabapentin even if you feel well. Do not stop taking gabapentin without talking to your doctor. If you suddenly stop taking gabapentin, you may experience withdrawal symptoms such as anxiety, difficulty falling asleep or staying asleep, nausea, pain, and sweating. If you are taking gabapentin to treat seizures and you suddenly stop taking the medication, you may experience seizures more often. Your doctor probably will decrease your dose gradually over at least a week.

Are there other uses for this medicine?

Gabapentin is also sometimes used to relieve the pain of diabetic neuropathy (numbness or tingling due to nerve damage in people who have diabetes), and to treat and prevent hot flashes (sudden strong feelings of heat and sweating) in women who are being treated for breast cancer or who have experienced menopause ('change of life', the end of monthly menstrual periods). Talk to your doctor about the risks of using this medication for your condition.

This medication may be prescribed for other uses; ask your doctor or pharmacist for more information.

What special precautions should I follow?

Before taking gabapentin,

- tell your doctor and pharmacist if you are allergic to gabapentin, any other medications, or any of the inactive ingredients in the type of gabapentin you plan to take. Ask your pharmacist for a list of the inactive ingredients.
- tell your doctor and pharmacist what prescription and nonprescription medications, vitamins, nutritional supplements, and herbal products you are taking or plan to take. Be sure to mention any of the following: hydrocodone (in Hydrocet, in Vicodin, others), morphine (Avinza, Kadian, MSIR, others), and naproxen (Aleve, Anaprox, Naprosyn, others). Your doctor may need to change the doses of your medications or monitor you carefully for side effects.
- if you are taking antacids such as Maalox or Mylanta, take them at least 2 hours before you take gabapentin.
- tell your doctor if you have or have ever had kidney disease.
- tell your doctor if you are pregnant, plan to become pregnant, or are breast-feeding. If you become pregnant while taking gabapentin, call your doctor.
- if you are having surgery, including dental surgery, tell the doctor or dentist that you are taking gabapentin.
- you should know that this medication may make you drowsy or dizzy. Do not drive a car or operate machinery until you know how this medication affects you.
- if you are giving gabapentin to your child, you should know that your child's behavior and mental abilities may change while he or she is taking gabapentin. Your child may have sudden changes in mood, become hostile or hyperactive, have difficulty concentrating or paying attention, or be drowsy or clumsy. Have your child avoid activities that could be dangerous, such as riding a bicycle, until you know how gabapentin affects him or her.
- remember that alcohol can add to the drowsiness caused by this medication.

What special dietary instructions should I follow?

Unless your doctor tells you otherwise, continue your normal diet.

What should I do if I forget to take a dose?

Take the missed dose as soon as you remember it. However, if it is almost time for the next dose, skip the missed dose

and continue your regular dosing schedule. Do not take a double dose to make up for a missed one.

What side effects can this medicine cause?

Gabapentin may cause side effects. Tell your doctor if any of these symptoms are severe or do not go away:

- drowsiness
- tiredness or weakness
- dizziness
- headache
- shaking of a part of your body that you cannot control
- double or blurred vision
- unsteadiness
- anxiety
- memory problems
- strange or unusual thoughts
- unwanted eye movements
- nausea
- vomiting
- heartburn
- diarrhea
- dry mouth
- constipation
- weight gain
- swelling of the hands, feet, ankles, or lower legs
- back or joint pain
- fever
- runny nose, sneezing, cough, sore throat, or flu-like symptoms
- ear pain
- red, itchy eyes (sometimes with swelling or discharge)

Some side effects may be serious. If you experience any of the following symptoms, call your doctor immediately:

- rash
- itching
- swelling of the face, throat, tongue, lips, eyes, hands, feet, ankles, or lower legs
- hoarseness
- difficulty swallowing or breathing
- seizures

Gabapentin may cause other side effects. Call your doctor if you have any unusual problems while taking this medication.

If you experience a serious side effect, you or your doctor may send a report to the Food and Drug Administration's (FDA) MedWatch Adverse Event Reporting program online [at http://www.fda.gov/MedWatch/index.html] or by phone [1-800-332-1088].

What storage conditions are needed for this medicine?

Keep this medication in the container it came in, tightly closed, and out of reach of children. Store the tablets and capsules at room temperature, away from excess heat and moisture (not in the bathroom). Store the oral solution in the refrigerator. Throw away any medication that is outdated or no longer needed. Talk to your pharmacist about the proper disposal of your medication.

What should I do in case of overdose?

In case of overdose, call your local poison control center at 1-800-222-1222. If the victim has collapsed or is not breathing, call local emergency services at 911.

Symptoms of overdose may include:

- double vision
- slurred speech
- drowsiness
- diarrhea

What other information should I know?

Keep all appointments with your doctor.

Before having any laboratory test, tell your doctor and the laboratory personnel that you are taking gabapentin.

If you use a dipstick to test your urine for protein, ask your doctor which product you should use while taking this medication.

Do not let anyone else take your medication. Ask your pharmacist any questions you have about refilling your prescription.

Dosage Facts
For Informational Purposes

Caution: Do not change your dose, how often you take your medication, or the length of time you are to take it without first talking to your health-care provider.

The following dosage information was written using medical language for doctors and other healthcare professionals and is provided here for you to check your dosage. The dosage of this drug may differ for different patients. Therefore, always follow your doctor's instructions or the directions on the label. Contact your health-care provider or pharmacist if you have any questions about the specific dosage of your medication after reviewing this information.

Pediatric Patients

Seizure Disorders
Partial Seizures

ORAL:
- Children 3–12 years of age: Initially, 10–15 mg/kg daily in 3 divided doses. Maintenance dosage of 40 mg/kg daily in 3 divided doses for children 3 or 4 years of age and 25–35 mg/kg daily in 3 divided doses for children 5–12 years of age.
- Children >12 years of age: Initially, 300 mg 3 times daily. Maintenance dosage of 900 mg to 1.8 g daily in 3 divided doses.

Adult Patients

Seizure Disorders
Partial Seizures

ORAL:
- Initially, 300 mg 3 times daily. Maintenance dosage of 900 mg to 1.8 g daily in 3 divided doses.

Neuropathic Pain
Postherpetic Neuralgia

ORAL:

- 300 mg on the first day, 300 mg twice daily on the second day, and 300 mg 3 times daily on the third day. Increase dosage as needed for relief of pain up to a total daily dosage of 1.8 g in 3 divided doses. No evidence of additional benefit with dosages >1.8 g daily.

Diabetic Neuropathy

ORAL:

- Dosages of 900 mg to 3.6 g daily have been used; however, pain relief generally observed in patients receiving dosages >1.8 g daily.

Vasomotor Symptoms†

ORAL:

- 300 mg 3 times daily has been effective; higher dosages may provide additional benefit.

Prescribing Limits
Pediatric Patients

Children 3–12 years of age: Dosages up to 50 mg/kg daily in divided doses have been tolerated as adjunctive therapy in the management of partial seizures.

Children >12 years of age: Dosage of 3.6 g daily has been tolerated as adjunctive therapy in the management of partial seizures.

Adult Patients

Dosage of 3.6 g daily has been tolerated as adjunctive therapy in the management of partial seizures.

Special Populations

Renal Impairment

- Not studied in children <12 years of age with renal impairment.
- In adults and children ≥12 years of age, base dosage on measured or estimated Cl_{cr}:

Dosage for Adults and Children ≤12 Years of Age with Renal Impairment

Cl_{cr} (mL/min)	Total Daily Dosage (mg/day)	Dosage Regimen
≥60	900–3600	300–1200 mg 3 times daily
30–59	400–1400	200–700 mg twice daily
15–29	200–700	200–700 mg once daily
15[a]	100–300	100–300 mg once daily
ESRD patients undergoing hemodialysis	—	125–350 mg[b]

[a]In patients with Cl_{cr} <15 mL/min, reduce dosage proportionally (e.g., a patient with a Cl_{cr} of 7.5 mL/min should receive one-half the dosage that a patient with a Cl_{cr} of 15 mL/min should receive).
[b]Give maintenance doses based on Cl_{cr}, with supplemental doses (125–350 mg) given after each 4-hour hemodialysis session.

Geriatric Patients

- Select dosage carefully, usually initiating therapy at the low end of the dosage range. Adjust dosage based on Cl_{cr}.

† Use is not currently included in the labeling approved by the US Food and Drug Administration.

Galantamine

(ga lan′ ta meen)

Brand Name: Razadyne®(formerly available as Reminyl®), Razadyne ®ER

Why is this medicine prescribed?

Galantamine is used to treat the symptoms of Alzheimer's disease (AD; a brain disease that slowly destroys the memory and the ability to think, learn, communicate and handle daily activities). Galantamine is in a class of medications called acetylcholinesterase inhibitors. It works by increasing the amount of a certain natural substance in the brain that is needed for memory and thought. Galantamine may improve the ability to think and remember or slow the loss of these abilities in people who have AD. However, galantamine will not cure AD or prevent the loss of mental abilities at some time in the future.

How should this medicine be used?

Galantamine comes as a tablet, an extended-release (long-acting) capsule, and a solution (liquid) to take by mouth. The tablets and liquid are usually taken twice a day, preferably with the morning and evening meals. The extended-release capsules are usually taken once a day in the morning. Take galantamine at around the same time(s) every day. Follow the directions on your prescription label carefully, and ask your doctor or pharmacist to explain any part you do not understand. Take galantamine exactly as directed. Do not take more or less of it or take it more often than prescribed by your doctor. You are less likely to experience side effects of galantamine if you follow the exact dosing schedule prescribed by your doctor.

Galantamine may upset your stomach, especially at the beginning of your treatment. Take galantamine with food and drink 6-8 glasses of water every day. This may decrease the chance that you will have an upset stomach during your treatment.

Your doctor will probably start you on a low dose of galantamine and gradually increase your dose, not more often than once every 4 weeks.

Continue to take galantamine even if you feel well. Do not stop taking galantamine without talking to your doctor. If you do stop taking galantamine for a few days or longer, call your doctor before you start to take galantamine again.

Your doctor will probably tell you to start with the lowest dose of galantamine and gradually increase your dose to the dose you had been taking.

Before you take galantamine oral solution for the first time, read the written instructions that come with it. Ask your doctor or pharmacist to show you how to take the oral solution. To take the oral solution, follow these steps:

1. Open the child-proof cap by pushing the cap down while turning it to the left. Remove the cap.
2. Pull the pipette (the tube that you use to measure the dose of galantamine) out of its case.
3. Place the pipette fully into the bottle of galantamine.
4. While holding the bottom ring of the pipette, pull the pipette plunger up to the marking that shows the dose your doctor prescribed.
5. Hold the bottom ring of the pipette and remove the pipette from the bottle. Be careful not to push the plunger in.
6. Prepare 3-4 ounces (about 1/2 cup) of any non-alcoholic beverage. Empty all the medicine from the pipette into the beverage by pushing the plunger all the way in.
7. Stir the beverage well.
8. Drink all of the mixture right away.
9. Put the plastic cap back on the bottle of galantamine and turn the cap to the right to close the bottle.
10. Rinse the empty pipette by putting its open end into a glass of water, pulling the plunger out, and pushing the plunger in to remove the water.

Are there other uses for this medicine?

This medication may be prescribed for other uses; ask your doctor or pharmacist for more information.

What special precautions should I follow?

Before taking galantamine,

- tell your doctor and pharmacist if you are allergic to galantamine, any other medications, or any of the inactive ingredients in galantamine tablets, solution, or extended-release capsules. Ask your pharmacist for a list of the inactive ingredients.
- tell your doctor and pharmacist what prescription and nonprescription medications, vitamins, nutritional supplements, and herbal products you are taking or plan to take. Be sure to mention any of the following: ambenonium chloride (Mytelase); amitriptyline (Elavil); anticholinergic medications such as atropine (Atropen, Sal-Tropine), belladonna (in Donnatal, Bellamine, Bel-Tabs, others); benztropine (Cogentin), biperiden (Akineton); clidinium (in Librax), dicyclomine (Bentyl), glycopyrrolate (Robinul), hyoscyamine (Cytospaz-M, Levbid, Levsin), ipratropium (Atrovent, in Combivent), oxybutynin (Ditropan), procyclidine (Kemadrin), propantheline (Pro-Banthine), scopolamine (Scopace, Transderm-Scop), tiotropium (Spiriva), tolterodine (Detrol), and trihexyphenidyl; certain antifungals such as fluconazole (Diflucan), itraconazole (Sporanox), keto-

conazole (Nizoral), and voriconazole (Vfend); aspirin or other nonsteroidal anti-inflammatory drugs (NSAIDs) such as ibuprofen (Advil, Motrin) and naproxen (Aleve, Naprosyn); bethanechol (Urecholine); cevimeline (Evoxac); cimetidine (Tagamet); clarithromycin (Biaxin, in Prevpac); digoxin (Lanoxin); fluoxetine (Prozac, Sarafem); fluvoxamine (Luvox); heart medications; nefazodone; neostigmine (Prostigmin); other medications for Alzheimer's disease; medications for human immunodeficiency syndrome (HIV) or acquired immunodeficiency syndrome (AIDS); medications for high blood pressure; paroxetine (Paxil); pyridostigmine (Mestinon); and quinidine (Quinidex). Your doctor may need to change the doses of your medications or monitor you carefully for side effects.

- tell your doctor if you have or have ever had asthma or any other lung disease; an enlarged prostate; ulcers; seizures; irregular heartbeat; or heart, kidney, or liver disease.
- tell your doctor if you are pregnant, plan to become pregnant, or are breast-feeding. If you become pregnant while taking galantamine, call your doctor.
- if you are having surgery, including dental surgery, tell the doctor or dentist that you are taking galantamine.
- you should know that galantamine may make you drowsy. Do not drive a car or operate machinery until you know how this medication affects you.
- remember that alcohol can add to the drowsiness caused by this medication.

What special dietary instructions should I follow?

Unless your doctor tells you otherwise, continue your normal diet.

What should I do if I forget to take a dose?

Take the missed dose as soon as you remember it. However, if it is almost time for the next dose, skip the missed dose and continue your regular dosing schedule. Do not take a double dose to make up for a missed one.

What side effects can this medicine cause?

Galantamine may cause side effects. Tell your doctor if any of these symptoms are severe or do not go away:

- upset stomach
- vomiting
- diarrhea
- loss of appetite
- stomach pain
- heartburn
- weight loss
- extreme tiredness
- dizziness
- pale skin
- headache
- shaking of a part of your body that you cannot control

- depression
- difficulty falling asleep or staying asleep
- runny nose

Some side effects can be serious. The following symptoms are uncommon, but if you experience any of them, call your doctor immediately:

- difficulty urinating
- blood in the urine
- pain or burning while urinating
- seizures
- slowed heartbeat
- fainting
- shortness of breath
- black and tarry stools
- red blood in the stools
- bloody vomit
- vomiting material that looks like coffee grounds

Galantamine may cause other side effects. Call your doctor if you have any unusual problems while taking this medication.

If you experience a serious side effect, you or your doctor may send a report to the Food and Drug Administration's (FDA) MedWatch Adverse Event Reporting program online [at http://www.fda.gov/MedWatch/index.html] or by phone [1-800-332-1088].

What storage conditions are needed for this medicine?

Keep this medication in the container it came in, tightly closed, and out of reach of children. Store it at room temperature and away from excess heat and moisture (not in the bathroom). Do not freeze. Throw away any medication that is outdated or no longer needed. Talk to your pharmacist about the proper disposal of your medication.

What should I do in case of overdose?

In case of overdose, call your local poison control center at 1-800-222-1222. If the victim has collapsed or is not breathing, call local emergency services at 911.

Symptoms of overdose may include:

- muscle weakness or twitching
- upset stomach
- vomiting
- stomach cramps
- drooling
- teary eyes
- increased urination
- need to have a bowel movement
- sweating
- slowed, fast, or irregular heartbeat
- lightheadedness
- dizziness
- fainting
- slowed breathing
- collapse
- loss of conciousness

- seizures
- dry mouth
- chest pain
- hallucinations (seeing things or hearing voices that do not exist)

What other information should I know?

Keep all appointments with your doctor.

Do not let anyone else take your medication. Ask your pharmacist any questions you have about refilling your prescription.

Dosage Facts
For Informational Purposes

Caution: Do not change your dose, how often you take your medication, or the length of time you are to take it without first talking to your healthcare provider.

The following dosage information was written using medical language for doctors and other healthcare professionals and is provided here for you to check your dosage. The dosage of this drug may differ for different patients. Therefore, always follow your doctor's instructions or the directions on the label. Contact your healthcare provider or pharmacist if you have any questions about the specific dosage of your medication after reviewing this information.

General Dosage Information

Available as galantamine hydrobromide; dosage is expressed in terms of galantamine.

If galantamine therapy has been interrupted for more than a few days for any reason and reinitiation of the drug is not contraindicated, resume therapy using the lowest dosage and titrate upward to prior dosages.

Adult Patients

Alzheimer's Disease

ORAL:

- Initially, 4 mg twice daily (as conventional tablets or oral solution) or 8 mg once daily (as extended-release capsules). Dosage may be increased after a minimum of 4 weeks to 8 mg twice daily (as conventional tablets or oral solution) or 16 mg once daily (as extended-release capsules).
- Subsequent increases to 12 mg twice daily (as conventional tablets or oral solution) or 24 mg once daily (as extended-release capsules) should be attempted after a minimum of 4 weeks of treatment at the previous dosage.
- Maintenance dosage recommended by the manufacturer is 8–12 mg twice daily (as conventional tablets and oral solution) or 16–24 mg once daily (as extended-release capsules). Galantamine 16–24 mg once daily (as extended-release capsules) was as effective as galantamine 8–12 mg twice daily (as conventional tablets). Higher dosages (e.g., 16 mg twice daily) do not result in greater efficacy and are less well tolerated than lower dosages.

Hepatic Impairment

Alzheimer's Disease

ORAL:
- Dosage generally should not exceed 16 mg daily in patients with moderate hepatic impairment (Child-Pugh score of 7–9). Use not recommended in patients with severe hepatic impairment (Child-Pugh score of 10–15).

Renal Impairment

Alzheimer's Disease

ORAL:
- Dosage generally should not exceed 16 mg daily in patients with moderate renal impairment. Use not recommended in patients with severe renal impairment (Cl_{cr} <9 mL/minute).

Galantamine

(gan sye' kloe veer)

Brand Name: Cytovene®
Also available generically.

Important Warning

Ganciclovir may lower the number of all types of cells in your blood, causing serious and life-threatening problems. Tell your doctor if you have or have ever had anemia (red blood cells do not bring enough oxygen to all parts of the body); neutropenia (less than normal number of white blood cells); thrombocytopenia (less than normal number of platelets); or other blood or bleeding problems. Tell your doctor if you have ever developed blood problems as a side effect of any medication. Tell your doctor and pharmacist if you are taking or have taken any of the following medications: anticoagulants ('blood thinners') such as warfarin (Coumadin); cancer chemotherapy medications; dapsone; flucytosine (Ancobon); heparin; immunosuppressants such as azathioprine (Azasan, Imuran), cyclosporine (Neoral, Sandimmune), methotrexate (Rheumatrex), sirolimus (Rapamune), and tacrolimus (Prograf); interferons (Infergen, Intron A, PEGASYS, PEG-Intron, Roferon-A); medications to treat human immunodeficiency virus (HIV) and acquired immunodeficiency syndrome (AIDS) including didanosine (Videx), zalcitabine (HIVID), or zidovudine (Retrovir, AZT); nonsteroidal anti-inflammatory medications to treat pain and swelling such as aspirin, ibuprofen (Advil, Motrin), naproxen (Aleve, Naprosyn), and others; pentamidine (NebuPent, Pentam); pyrimethamine (Daraprim, in Fansidar); steroids such as dexamethasone (Decadron), prednisone (Deltasone), or others; trimethoprim/sulfamethoxazole (co-trimoxazole, Bactrim, Septra); or if you have received or are receiving radiation (X-ray) therapy. If you experience any of the following symptoms, call your doctor immediately: excessive tiredness; pale skin; headache; dizziness; confusion; fast heartbeat; difficulty falling asleep or staying asleep; weakness; shortness of breath; unusual bleeding or bruising; or sore throat, fever, chills, cough, or other signs of infection.

Keep all appointments with your doctor and the laboratory. Your doctor will order certain tests to check your body's response to ganciclovir.

Laboratory animals who were given ganciclovir developed birth defects. It is not known if ganciclovir causes birth defects in people. If you can become pregnant, you should use effective birth control while taking ganciclovir. If you are a man and your partner can become pregnant, you should use a condom while taking this medication, and for 90 days after your treatment. Talk to your doctor if you have questions about birth control. Do not use ganciclovir if you are pregnant or plan to become pregnant. If you become pregnant while taking ganciclovir, call your doctor immediately.

Laboratory animals who were given ganciclovir developed a lower sperm count (fewer male reproductive cells) and fertility problems. It is not known if ganciclovir causes lower sperm counts in men or problems with fertility in women.

Laboratory animals who were given ganciclovir developed cancer. It is not known if ganciclovir increases the risk of cancer in humans.

The manufacturer warns that ganciclovir should only be used for treatment of patients with certain diseases because the medication may cause severe side effects and there is currently not enough information to support safety and effectiveness in other groups of patients. (See the section, WHY is this medication is prescribed?)

Talk to your doctor about the risks of taking ganciclovir.

Why is this medicine prescribed?

Ganciclovir capsules are used to treat cytomegalovirus (CMV) retinitis (eye infection that can cause blindness) in people whose immune system is not working normally. Ganciclovir capsules are used to treat CMV retinitis after the condition has been controlled by intravenous (injected into a vein) ganciclovir. Ganciclovir is also used to prevent cytomegalovirus (CMV) disease in people who have acquired immunodeficiency syndrome (AIDS) or who have received an organ transplant and are at risk of CMV disease. Ganciclovir is in a class of medications called antivirals. It works by preventing the spread of CMV disease or slowing the growth of CMV.

How should this medicine be used?

Ganciclovir comes as a capsule to take by mouth. It is usually taken with food three to six times a day. To help you remember to take ganciclovir, take it at around the same times every day. Follow the directions on your prescription label carefully, and ask your doctor or pharmacist to explain any part you do not understand. Take ganciclovir exactly as directed. Do not take more or less of it or take it more often than prescribed by your doctor.

Swallow the capsules whole; do not open, split, chew, or crush them.

Be careful when handling ganciclovir capsules. Do not allow your skin, eyes, mouth, or nose to come into contact with broken or crushed ganciclovir capsules. If such contact occurs, wash your skin well with soap and water or rinse your eyes well with plain water.

You generally will receive intravenous (into a vein) ganciclovir for several weeks before you begin to take ganciclovir capsules. If your condition gets worse during your treatment, you may be given a second course of intravenous ganciclovir. Your doctor may decrease your dose of ganciclovir capsules if you experience side effects.

Ganciclovir controls CMV but does not cure it. It may take some time before you feel the full benefit of ganciclovir. Continue to take ganciclovir even if you feel well. Do not stop taking ganciclovir without talking to your doctor. Stopping to take ganciclovir too soon may cause the amount of CMV in your blood to increase or the virus to become resistant to this medication.

Are there other uses for this medicine?

The manufacturer states that this medication should not be prescribed for other uses; ask your doctor or pharmacist for more information.

What special precautions should I follow?

Before taking ganciclovir,
- tell your doctor and pharmacist if you are allergic to ganciclovir, acyclovir (Zovirax), valganciclovir (Valcyte), or any other medications.
- do not take ganciclovir if you are taking valganciclovir (Valcyte).
- tell your doctor and pharmacist what other prescription and nonprescription medications, vitamins, nutritional supplements, and herbal products you are taking. Be sure to mention the medications listed in the IMPORTANT WARNING section and any of the following: aminoglycoside antibiotics such as amikacin (Amikin), gentamicin (Garamycin), neomycin (New-Rx, New-Fradin), netilmycin (Netromycin), streptomycin, tobramycin (Nebcin, Tobi), and others; amphotericin B (Fungizone); captopril (Capoten, in Capozide); diuretics ('water pills'); foscarnet (Foscavir); gold compounds such as auranofin (Ridaura) or aurothioglucose (Solganal); imipenem-cilastatin (Primaxin); immune globulin (gamma globulin, BayGam, Carimmune, Gam-

magard, others); methicillin (Staphcillin); muromonab-CD3 (OKT3); mycophenolate mofetil (CellCept); nitrates such as isosorbide dinitrate (Isordil, Sorbitrate) or nitroglycerin products; penicillamine (Cuprimine, Depen); primaquine; probenecid; rifampin (Rifadin, Rimactane); or other nucleoside analogues such as acyclovir (Zovirax), famciclovir (Famvir), and ribavirin (Copegus, Rebetol, Virazole, in Rebetron). Your doctor may need to change the doses of your medications or monitor you carefully for side effects.
- tell your doctor if you have or have ever had any of the conditions mentioned in the IMPORTANT WARNING section or any of the following conditions: mental illness; seizures; eye problems other than CMV retinitis; kidney, or liver disease.
- tell your doctor if you are breast-feeding. You should not breast-feed while taking ganciclovir. Talk to your doctor about when you may safely begin breast-feeding after you stop taking ganciclovir.
- if you are having surgery, including dental surgery, tell the doctor or dentist that you are taking ganciclovir.
- you should know that ganciclovir may make you drowsy, dizzy, unsteady, confused or less alert, or may cause seizures. Do not drive a car or operate machinery until you know how this medication affects you.

What special dietary instructions should I follow?

Be sure to drink plenty of fluids while you are taking ganciclovir.

What should I do if I forget to take a dose?

Take the missed dose as soon as you remember it. However, if it is almost time for the next dose, skip the missed dose and continue your regular dosing schedule. Do not take a double dose to make up for a missed one.

What side effects can this medicine cause?

Ganciclovir may cause side effects. Tell your doctor if any of these symptoms are severe or do not go away:
- upset stomach
- vomiting
- diarrhea
- constipation
- stomach pain
- belching
- loss of appetite
- changes in ability to taste food
- dry mouth
- mouth sores
- unusual dreams
- nervousness
- depression
- sweating
- flushing
- joint or muscle pain or cramps

Some side effects can be serious. The following symptoms are uncommon, but if you experience any of them, or those listed in the IMPORTANT WARNING section, call your doctor immediately:

- seeing specks, flashes of light, or a dark curtain over everything
- decreased urination
- hives
- rash
- itching
- swelling of the hands, arms, feet, ankles, or lower legs
- numbness, pain, burning, or tingling in the hands or feet
- shaking hands that you cannot control
- difficulty breathing or swallowing
- chest pain
- mood changes
- seizures

Ganciclovir may cause other side effects. Call your doctor if you have any unusual problems while taking this medication.

If you experience a serious side effect, you or your doctor may send a report to the Food and Drug Administration's (FDA) MedWatch Adverse Event Reporting program online [at http://www.fda.gov/MedWatch/index.html] or by phone [1-800-332-1088].

What storage conditions are needed for this medicine?

Keep this medication in the container it came in, tightly closed, and out of reach of children. Store it at room temperature and away from excess heat and moisture (not in the bathroom). Throw away any medication that is outdated or no longer needed. Talk to your pharmacist about the proper disposal of your medication.

What should I do in case of overdose?

In case of overdose, call your local poison control center at 1-800-222-1222. If the victim has collapsed or is not breathing, call local emergency services at 911.

Symptoms of overdose may include:

- upset stomach
- vomiting
- diarrhea
- loss of appetite
- unusual bleeding or bruising
- excessive tiredness
- weakness
- pale skin
- headache
- dizziness
- confusion
- fast heartbeat
- difficulty sleeping
- shortness of breath
- sore throat, fever, chills, cough, or other signs of infection

- decreased urination
- swelling of the hands, arms, feet, ankles, or lower legs
- seizures
- yellowing of the skin or eyes
- flu-like symptoms
- pain in the upper right part of the stomach

What other information should I know?

Your doctor may order regular eye exams while you are taking this medication. Keep all appointments with the ophthalmologist (eye exams).

Before having any laboratory test, tell your doctor and the laboratory personnel that you are taking ganciclovir.

Do not let anyone else take your medication. Ask your pharmacist any questions you have about refilling your prescription. Do not let your supply of ganciclovir run out.

Dosage Facts
For Informational Purposes

Caution: Do not change your dose, how often you take your medication, or the length of time you are to take it without first talking to your healthcare provider.

The following dosage information was written using medical language for doctors and other healthcare professionals and is provided here for you to check your dosage. The dosage of this drug may differ for different patients. Therefore, always follow your doctor's instructions or the directions on the label. Contact your healthcare provider or pharmacist if you have any questions about the specific dosage of your medication after reviewing this information.

General Dosage Information

Available as ganciclovir and ganciclovir sodium; dosage expressed in terms of ganciclovir.

Because the risk of toxicity may be increased with higher doses and/or more rapid infusion, recommended doses, frequencies of administration, and rate of IV infusion should *not* be exceeded.

Pediatric Patients

Cytomegalovirus (CMV) Infections
Treatment of CMV Retinitis

ORAL:
- Maintenance therapy in children >3 months of age†: after an initial IV induction regimen, 1 g 3 times daily. Alternatively, 500 mg 6 times daily (every 3 hours while awake).

Primary Prevention (Primary Prophylaxis) of CMV in HIV-infected Children and Adolescents

ORAL:
- Infants and children†: 30 mg/kg 3 times daily.
- Adolescents: 1 g 3 times daily.

Prevention of Recurrence (Secondary Prophylaxis) of CMV in HIV-infected Children and Adolescents

ORAL:

• 1 g 3 times daily. Initiate secondary prophylaxis after initial induction treatment.

Adult Patients

Cytomegalovirus (CMV) Infections
Treatment of CMV Retinitis

ORAL:

• Maintenance therapy after an initial IV induction regimen: 1 g 3 times daily. Alternatively, 500 mg 6 times daily (every 3 hours while awake).

Primary Prevention (Primary Prophylaxis) of CMV in HIV-infected Adults

ORAL:

• 1 g 3 times daily.

Prevention of Recurrence (Secondary Prophylaxis) of CMV in HIV-infected Adults

ORAL:

• 1 g 3 times daily. Initiate secondary prophylaxis after initial induction treatment.

Prevention of CMV Disease in Transplant Recipients

ORAL:

• 1 g 3 times daily.

Special Populations

Renal Impairment

• In patients with impaired renal function, doses and/or frequency of administration of oral ganciclovir must be modified in response to the degree of impairment. Dosage should be based on the patient's measured or estimated Cl_{cr}.

Oral Dosage for Adults with Renal Impairment

Cl_{cr} (mL/min)	Dosage
50–69	1.5 g once daily or 500 mg 3 times daily
25–49	1 g once daily or 500 mg 2 times daily
10–24	500 mg once daily
<10	500 mg 3 times weekly, following hemodialysis

Geriatric Patients

• Select dosage with caution because of age-related decreases in renal function.

† *Use is not currently included in the labeling approved by the US Food and Drug Administration.*

Ganciclovir Injection

(gan sye′ kloe veer)

Brand Name: Cytovene®-IV
Also available generically.

Important Warning

Ganciclovir may lower the number of all types of cells in your blood, causing serious and life-threatening problems. Tell your doctor if you have or have ever had anemia (red blood cells do not bring enough oxygen to all parts of the body); neutropenia (less than normal number of white blood cells); thrombocytopenia (less than normal number of platelets); or other blood or bleeding problems. Tell your doctor if you have ever developed blood problems as a side effect of any medication. Tell your doctor and pharmacist if you are taking or have taken any of the following medications: anticoagulants ('blood thinners') such as warfarin (Coumadin); cancer chemotherapy medications; dapsone; flucytosine (Ancobon); heparin; immunosuppressants such as azathioprine (Azasan, Imuran), cyclosporine (Neoral, Sandimmune), methotrexate (Rheumatrex), sirolimus (Rapamune), and tacrolimus (Prograf); interferons (Infergen, Intron A, PEGASYS, PEG-Intron, Roferon-A); medications to treat human immunodeficiency virus (HIV) and acquired immunodeficiency syndrome (AIDS) including didanosine (Videx), zalcitabine (HIVID), or zidovudine (Retrovir, AZT); nonsteroidal anti-inflammatory medications to treat pain and swelling such as aspirin, ibuprofen (Advil, Motrin), naproxen (Aleve, Naprosyn), and others; pentamidine (NebuPent, Pentam); pyrimethamine (Daraprim, in Fansidar); steroids such as dexamethasone (Decadron), prednisone (Deltasone), or others; trimethoprim/sulfamethoxazole (co-trimoxazole, Bactrim, Septra); or if you have received or are receiving radiation (X-ray) therapy. If you experience any of the following symptoms, call your doctor immediately: excessive tiredness; pale skin; headache; dizziness; confusion; fast heartbeat; difficulty falling asleep or staying asleep; weakness; shortness of breath; unusual bleeding or bruising; sore throat, fever, chills, cough, or other signs of infection.

Keep all appointments with your doctor and the laboratory. Your doctor will order certain tests to check your body's response to ganciclovir.

Laboratory animals who were given ganciclovir developed birth defects. It is not known if ganciclovir causes birth defects in people. If you can become pregnant, you should use effective birth control while

continued on next page

Important Warning (cont'd)

using ganciclovir. If you are a man and your partner can become pregnant you should use a condom while taking this medication, and for 90 days after your treatment. Talk to your doctor if you have questions about birth control. Do not use ganciclovir if you are pregnant or plan to become pregnant. If you become pregnant while taking ganciclovir, call your doctor immediately.

Laboratory animals who were given ganciclovir developed a lower sperm count (fewer male reproductive cells) and fertility problems. It is not known if ganciclovir causes lower sperm counts in men or problems with fertility in women.

Laboratory animals who were given ganciclovir developed cancer. It is not known if ganciclovir increases the risk of cancer in humans.

The manufacturer warns that ganciclovir should only be used for treatment of patients with certain diseases because the medication may cause severe side effects and there currently is not enough information to support safety and effectiveness in other groups of patients. (See the section, About Your Treatment.)

Talk to your doctor about the risks of using ganciclovir.

About Your Treatment

Your doctor has ordered ganciclovir, an antiviral medication, to help treat or prevent an infection with cytomegalovirus (CMV). This medication will be added to an IV (intravenous) fluid that will drip through a needle (catheter) placed in your vein, and will be given to you two times a day for 2-3 weeks, and then once a day, 5-7 days of each week. Your dose of ganciclovir will be given at a constant rate over at least 60 minutes. Giving ganciclovir too quickly may increase the side effects of this medication. The manufacturer states that this medication should not be prescribed for other uses. Ask your doctor or pharmacist for more information.

Ganciclovir works by preventing the spread of CMV disease or slowing the growth of CMV. Ganciclovir injection is used to treat cytomegalovirus (CMV) retinitis (eye infection) that can cause blindness in people whose immune system is not working normally, including people with acquired immune deficiency syndrome (AIDS). Ganciclovir is also used to prevent cytomegalovirus (CMV) disease in people who have received an organ transplant and who are at risk of getting CMV disease.

Ganciclovir does not cure CMV retinitis. Your doctor may increase your dose if your condition gets worse, or decrease your dose if you develop side effects.

Ganciclovir injection is for intravenous (into a vein) use only. Giving ganciclovir through intramuscular (into a muscle) or subcutaneous (just under the skin) injection may cause severe skin and tissue irritation.

Your health care provider (doctor, nurse, or pharmacist) may measure the effectiveness and side effects of your treatment using laboratory tests and physical examinations, including eye exams. It is important to keep all appointments with your doctor, the laboratory, and the ophthalmologist (eye exams). The length of treatment depends on how your infection and symptoms respond to the medication.

Precautions

Before administering ganciclovir,

- tell your doctor and pharmacist if you are allergic to ganciclovir, acyclovir (Zovirax), valganciclovir (Valcyte), or any other medications.
- do not use ganciclovir if you are taking valganciclovir (Valcyte).
- tell your doctor and pharmacist what other prescription and nonprescription medications, vitamins, nutritional supplements, and herbal products you are taking. Be sure to mention the medications listed in the IMPORTANT WARNING section and any of the following: aminoglycoside antibiotics such as amikacin (Amikin), gentamicin (Garamycin), neomycin (Neo-Rx, Neo-Fradin), netilmycin (Netromycin), streptomycin, tobramycin (Nebcin, Tobi), and others; amphotericin B (Fungizone); captopril (Capoten, in Capozide); diuretics ('water pills'); foscarnet (Foscavir), gold compounds such as auranofin (Ridaura) or aurothioglucose (Solganal); imipenem-cilastatin (Primaxin); immune globulin (gamma globulin, BayGam, Carimmune, Gammagard, others); methicillin (Staphcillin); muromonab-CD3 (OKT3); mycophenolate mofetil (CellCept); nitrates such as isosorbide dinitrate (Isordil, Sorbitrate) or nitroglycerin products; penicillamine (Cuprimine, Depen); primaquine; probenecid; rifampin (Rifadin, Rimactane); or other nucleoside analogues such as acyclovir (Zovirax), famciclovir (Famvir), and ribavirin (Copegus, Rebetol, Virazole, in Rebetron). Your doctor may need to change the doses of your medications or monitor you carefully for side effects.
- tell your doctor if you have or have ever had any of the conditions mentioned in the IMPORTANT WARNING section or any of the following conditions: seizures; mental illness; eye problems other than CMV retinitis; kidney, or liver disease.
- tell your doctor if you are breast-feeding. You should not breastfeed while using ganciclovir. Talk with your doctor about when you may safely begin breast-feeding after you stop using ganciclovir.
- if you are having surgery, including dental surgery, tell the doctor or dentist that you are using ganciclovir.
- you should know that ganciclovir may make you drowsy, dizzy, unsteady, confused or less alert, or may cause seizures. Do not drive a car or operate machinery until you know how this medication affects you.
- you should drink plenty of fluids while using this medication.

Administering Your Medication

Before you administer ganciclovir, look at the solution closely. It should be clear and free of floating material. Gently squeeze the bag or observe the solution container to make sure there are no leaks. Do not use the solution if it is discolored, if it contains particles, or if the bag or container leaks. Use a new solution, but show the damaged one to your health care provider.

It is important that you use your medication exactly as directed. Do not stop your therapy on your own for any reason because your infection could worsen and result in hospitalization. Do not change your dosing schedule without talking to your health care provider. Your health care provider may tell you to stop your infusion if you have a mechanical problem (such as a blockage in the tubing, needle, or catheter); if you have to stop an infusion, call your health care provider immediately so your therapy can continue.

Be careful not to get the ganciclovir solution on your skin, eyes, mouth, or nose. If such contact occurs, wash your skin thoroughly with soap and water and rinse your eyes thoroughly with plain water.

Side Effects

Ganciclovir may cause side effects. Tell your doctor if any of these symptoms are severe or do not go away:

- upset stomach
- vomiting
- diarrhea
- constipation
- stomach pain
- belching
- loss of appetite
- changes in ability to taste food
- dry mouth
- mouth sores
- unusual dreams
- nervousness
- depression
- sweating
- flushing
- joint or muscle pain or cramps

Some side effects can be serious. The following symptoms are uncommon, but if you experience any of them, or those listed in the IMPORTANT WARNING section, call your doctor immediately:

- swelling of the hands, arms, feet, ankles, or lower legs
- numbness, pain, burning, or tingling in the hands or feet
  - chest pain
  - seeing specks, flashes of light, or a dark curtain over everything
- decreased urination
- pain at the injection site
- hives
- rash
- itching
- difficulty breathing or swallowing
- shaking hands that you cannot control
- mood changes
- seizures

Ganciclovir may cause other side effects. Call your doctor if you have any unusual problems while using this medication.

If you experience a serious side effect, you or your doctor may send a report to the Food and Drug Administration's (FDA) MedWatch Adverse Event Reporting program online [at http://www.fda.gov/MedWatch/index.html] or by phone [1-800-332-1088].

Storage Conditions

- Your health care provider may give you several doses (enough for a day's supply) of premixed ganciclovir injection solution at one time. You should store premixed ganciclovir solution in the refrigerator. Do not freeze ganciclovir. Use premixed ganciclovir solution within 24 hours. Throw away any ganciclovir solution that is not used within 24 hours of preparation. Ask your health care provider if you have any questions about the storage of ganciclovir solution.

Store your medication only as directed. Make sure you understand what you need to do to store your medication properly.

Keep your supplies in a clean, dry place when you are not using them, and keep all medications and supplies out of reach of children. Your health care provider will tell you how to throw away used needles, syringes, tubing, and containers to avoid accidental injury.

Overdose

In case of overdose, call your local poison control center at 1-800-222-1222. If the victim has collapsed or is not breathing, call local emergency services at 911.

Symptoms of overdose may include:

- upset stomach
- vomiting
- diarrhea
- loss of appetite
- unusual bleeding or bruising
- excessive tiredness
- weakness
- pale skin
- headache
- dizziness
- confusion
- fast heartbeat
- difficulty sleeping
- shortness of breath
- sore throat, fever, chills, cough, or other signs of infection
- decreased urination
- swelling of the hands, arms, feet, ankles, or lower legs
- seizures
- yellowing of the skin or eyes

- flu-like symptoms
- pain in the upper right part of the stomach

Signs of Infection

If you are receiving ganciclovir injection you need to know the symptoms of a catheter-related infection (an infection where the needle enters your vein). If you experience any of these effects near your intravenous catheter, tell your health care provider as soon as possible:

- tenderness
- warmth
- irritation
- drainage
- redness
- swelling
- pain

Dosage Facts

For Informational Purposes

Caution: Do not change your dose, how often you take your medication, or the length of time you are to take it without first talking to your health-care provider.

The following dosage information was written using medical language for doctors and other healthcare professionals and is provided here for you to check your dosage. The dosage of this drug may differ for different patients. Therefore, always follow your doctor's instructions or the directions on the label. Contact your health-care provider or pharmacist if you have any questions about the specific dosage of your medication after reviewing this information.

General Dosage Information

Available as ganciclovir and ganciclovir sodium; dosage expressed in terms of ganciclovir.

Because the risk of toxicity may be increased with higher doses and/or more rapid infusion, recommended doses, frequencies of administration, and rate of IV infusion should *not* be exceeded.

Pediatric Patients

Cytomegalovirus (CMV) Infections
Treatment of CMV Retinitis

IV:

- Initial induction therapy in children >3 months of age†: 5 mg/kg every 12 hours for 14–21 days.
- Maintenance treatment in children >3 months of age†: 5 mg/kg once daily. Alternatively, 6 mg/kg once daily 5 days weekly.

Prevention of Recurrence (Secondary Prophylaxis) of CMV in HIV-infected Children and Adolescents

IV:

- Infants and children†: 5 mg/kg daily.
- Adolescents: 5–6 mg/kg once daily 5–7 days each week.
- Consideration can be given to discontinuing secondary CMV

prophylaxis in adolescents with sustained (e.g., for ≥6 months) increase in CD4+ T-cell counts to >100–150/mm³ in response to potent antiretroviral therapy. This decision should be made in consultation with an ophthalmologist and factors such as the magnitude and duration of CD4+ T-cell increase, anatomic location of the retinal lesion, vision in the contralateral eye, and feasibility of regular ophthalmic monitoring should be considered. Relapse of CMV retinitis could occur following discontinuance of secondary prophylaxis, especially in whose CD4+ T-cell count decreases to <50/mm³; relapse has been reported rarely in those with CD4+ T-cell counts >100/mm³.

- Reinitiate secondary CMV prophylaxis if CD4+ T-cell count decreases to <100–150/mm³.

Adult Patients

Cytomegalovirus (CMV) Infections
Treatment of CMV Retinitis

IV:

- Initial induction therapy: 5 mg/kg every 12 hours for 14–21 days.
- Maintenance therapy: 5 mg/kg once daily. Alternatively, 6 mg/kg once daily 5 days weekly.

Prevention of Recurrence (Secondary Prophylaxis) of CMV in HIV-infected Adults

IV:

- 5–6 mg/kg once daily 5–7 days each week.
- Consideration can be given to discontinuing secondary CMV prophylaxis in adults with sustained (e.g., for ≥6 months) increase in CD4+ T-cell counts to >100–150/mm³ in response to potent antiretroviral therapy. This decision should be made in consultation with an ophthalmologist and factors such as the magnitude and duration of CD4+ T-cell increase, anatomic location of the retinal lesion, vision in the contralateral eye, and feasibility of regular ophthalmic monitoring should be considered. Relapse of CMV retinitis could occur following discontinuance of secondary prophylaxis, especially in those whose CD4+ T-cell count decreases to <50/mm³; relapse has been reported rarely in those with CD4+ T-cell counts >100/mm³.
- Reinitiate secondary CMV prophylaxis if CD4+ T-cell count decreases to <100–150/mm³.

Prevention of CMV Disease in Transplant Recipients

IV:

- Initially, 5 mg/kg every 12 hours for 7–14 days, then 5 mg/kg once daily 7 days per week or 6 mg/kg once daily 5 days per week.
- Duration of ganciclovir maintenance in organ transplant recipients depends on several factors including the duration and degree of immunosuppression. Bone marrow allograft recipients have received IV ganciclovir for up to 100–120 days following transplantation. In cardiac allograft recipients, ganciclovir should be continued for >28 days in patients to prevent late development of CMV disease. Liver transplant recipients have received oral ganciclovir for up to 98 days following transplantation.

Special Populations

Renal Impairment

- In patients with impaired renal function, doses and/or frequency of administration of oral or IV ganciclovir must be modified in response to the degree of impairment. Dosage should be based on the patient's measured or estimated Cl_{cr}.

IV Dosage for Adults with Renal Impairment

Cl_{cr} (mL/min)	Induction Dosage	Maintenance Dosage
50–69	2.5 mg/kg every 12 h	2.5 mg/kg every 24 h
25–49	2.5 mg/kg every 24 h	1.25 mg/kg every 24 h
10–24	1.25 mg/kg every 24 h	0.625 mg/kg every 24
<10	1.25 mg/kg 3 times weekly, following hemodialysis	0.625 mg/kg 3 times weekly, following hemodialysis

Geriatric Patients
- Select dosage with caution because of age-related decreases in renal function.

† *Use is not currently included in the labeling approved by the US Food and Drug Administration.*

Gatifloxacin Ophthalmic

(ga ti floks' a sin)

Brand Name: Zymar®

Why is this medicine prescribed?

Gatifloxacin ophthalmic solution is used to treat bacterial conjunctivitis (pinkeye; infection of the membrane that covers the outside of the eyeballs and the inside of the eyelids). Gatifloxacin is in a class of antibiotics called fluoroquinolones. It works by killing the bacteria that cause infection.

How should this medicine be used?

Gatifloxacin comes as an ophthalmic solution (eye drops) to be placed in the eyes. It is usually used every 2 hours while awake (up to eight times a day) for 2 days, and then four times a day for 5 days. To help you remember to use gatifloxacin ophthalmic solution, use it at around the same times every day. Follow the directions on your prescription label carefully, and ask your doctor or pharmacist to explain any part you do not understand. Use gatifloxacin ophthalmic solution exactly as directed. Do not use more or less of it or use it more often than prescribed by your doctor.

You should expect your symptoms to improve during your treatment. Call your doctor if your symptoms do not go away or get worse, or if you develop other problems with your eyes during your treatment.

Use gatifloxacin ophthalmic solution until you finish the prescription, even if you feel better. If you stop using gatifloxacin ophthalmic solution too soon, your infection may not be completely cured and the bacteria may become resistant to antibiotics.

When you use gatifloxacin ophthalmic solution, be careful not to let the tip of the bottle touch your eye, fingers, face, or any surface. If the tip does touch another surface, bacteria may get into the eye drops. Using eye drops that are contaminated with bacteria may cause serious damage to the eye or loss of vision. If you think your eye drops have become contaminated, call your doctor or pharmacist.

To use the eye drops, follow these steps:
1. Wash your hands thoroughly with soap and water.
2. Use a mirror or have someone else put the drops in your eye.
3. Remove the protective cap from the bottle. Make sure that the end of the dropper tip is not chipped or cracked.
4. Hold the bottle with the tip down at all times to prevent drops from flowing back into the bottle and contaminating the medication inside.
5. Lie down and gaze upward or tilt your head back.
6. Holding the bottle between your thumb and index finger, place the dropper tip as near as possible to your eyelid without touching it.
7. Brace the remaining fingers of that hand against your cheek or nose.
8. With the index finger of your other hand, pull the lower lid of the eye down to form a pocket.
9. Drop the prescribed number of drops into the pocket made by the lower lid and the eye. Placing drops on the surface of the eyeball can cause stinging.
10. Close your eye and press lightly against the lower lid with your finger for 2-3 minutes to keep the medication in the eye. Do not blink.
11. If your doctor told you to place gatifloxacin ophthalmic solution in both eyes, repeat steps 6-10 above for your other eye.
12. Replace the cap on the bottle and tighten it right away. Do not wipe or rinse off the tip.
13. Wipe off any excess liquid from your cheek with a clean tissue. Wash your hands again.

Are there other uses for this medicine?

This medication may be prescribed for other uses; ask your doctor or pharmacist for more information.

What special precautions should I follow?

Before using gatifloxacin ophthalmic solution,
- tell your doctor and pharmacist if you are allergic to gatifloxacin (Tequin, Zymar), other quinolone antibiotics such as cinoxacin (Cinobac) (not available in the United States), ciprofloxacin (Cipro, Ciloxan), enoxacin

(Penetrex) (not available in the United States), levofloxacin (Levaquin, Quixin, Iquix), lomefloxacin (Maxaquin), moxifloxacin (Avelox, Vigamox), nalidixic acid (NegGram) (not available in the United States); norfloxacin (Noroxin), ofloxacin (Floxin, Ocuflox), sparfloxacin (Zagam), and trovafloxacin and alatrofloxacin combination (Trovan) (not available in the United States), any other medications, or benzalkonium chloride.

- tell your doctor and pharmacist what prescription and nonprescription medications, vitamins, nutritional supplements, and herbal products you are taking. Be sure to mention any of the following: anticoagulants ('blood thinners') such as warfarin (Coumadin), cyclosporine (Neoral, Sandimmune) and theophylline (TheoDur). Your doctor may need to change the doses of your medications or monitor you carefully for side effects.
- tell your doctor if you have or have ever had any medical condition.
- tell your doctor if you are pregnant, plan to become pregnant, or are breast-feeding. If you become pregnant while using gatifloxacin ophthalmic solution, call your doctor.
- tell your doctor if you wear contact lenses. You should not wear contact lenses while you have symptoms of bacterial conjunctivitis or while you are applying eye drops.
- you should know that bacterial conjunctivitis spreads easily. Wash your hands often, especially after you touch your eyes. When your infection goes away, you should wash or replace any eye makeup, contact lenses, or other objects that touched your infected eye(s).

What special dietary instructions should I follow?

Talk to your doctor about drinking coffee or other beverages containing caffeine while you are taking this medication.

What should I do if I forget to take a dose?

Place the missed dose in your eye(s) as soon as you remember it. However, if it is almost time for the next dose, skip the missed dose and continue your regular dosing schedule. Do not use a double dose to make up for a missed one.

What side effects can this medicine cause?

Gatifloxacin ophthalmic solution may cause side effects. Tell your doctor if any of these symptoms are severe or do not go away:

- red, irritated, itchy, or teary eyes
- blurred vision
- eye pain
- eye discharge
- swollen eyelids
- broken blood vessels in the eyes

- headache
- unpleasant taste

Some side effects can be serious. The following symptoms are uncommon, but if you experience any of them, call your doctor immediately:

- rash
- hives
- itching
- difficulty breathing or swallowing
- swelling of the face, throat, tongue, lips, eyes, hands, feet, ankles, or lower legs
- hoarseness

Gatifloxacin ophthalmic solution may cause other side effects. Call your doctor if you have any unusual problems while taking this medication.

If you experience a serious side effect, you or your doctor may send a report to the Food and Drug Administration's (FDA) MedWatch Adverse Event Reporting program online [at http://www.fda.gov/MedWatch/index.html] or by phone [1-800-332-1088].

What storage conditions are needed for this medicine?

Keep this medication in the container it came in, tightly closed, and out of reach of children. Store it at room temperature and away from excess heat and moisture (not in the bathroom). Do not allow the medication to freeze. Throw away any medication that is outdated or no longer needed. Talk to your pharmacist about the proper disposal of your medication.

What other information should I know?

Keep all appointments with your doctor.

Do not let anyone else use your medication. Your prescription is probably not refillable. If you still have symptoms of infection after you finish the gatifloxacin ophthalmic solution, call your doctor.

Dosage Facts
For Informational Purposes

Caution: Do not change your dose, how often you take your medication, or the length of time you are to take it without first talking to your healthcare provider.

The following dosage information was written using medical language for doctors and other healthcare professionals and is provided here for you to check your dosage. The dosage of this drug may differ for different patients. Therefore, always follow your doctor's instructions or the directions on the label. Contact your healthcare provider or pharmacist if you have any questions about the specific dosage of your medication after reviewing this information.

Pediatric Patients

Bacterial Ophthalmic Infections
Conjunctivitis

OPHTHALMIC:

- Children ≥1 year of age: 1 drop of 0.3% solution in the affected eye(s) every 2 hours while awake (up to 8 times daily) for 2 days, then 1 drop up to 4 times daily while awake for the next 5 days.

Adult Patients

Bacterial Ophthalmic Infections
Conjunctivitis

OPHTHALMIC:

- 1 drop of 0.3% solution in the affected eye(s) every 2 hours while awake (up to 8 times daily) for 2 days, then 1 drop up to 4 times daily while awake for the next 5 days.

Gefitinib

(ge fi′ ti nib)

Brand Name: Iressa®

Why is this medicine prescribed?

Gefitinib is used to treat non-small cell lung cancer in people who have already been treated with certain other chemotherapy medications and have not improved or whose condition has worsened. Gefitinib has not been shown to help people who have non-small cell lung cancer live longer. There are other medications that may help people who have non-small cell lung cancer live longer. Therefore, only people who have already taken gefitinib and benefited from the medication should continue to take it. People who have never taken gefitinib should start their treatment with a medication that is known to help patients with lung cancer live longer. Gefitinib is in a class of anti-cancer medications called epidermal growth factor receptor (EGFR) tyrosine kinase inhibitors. It works by blocking the action of a certain naturally occurring substance that may be needed to help cancer cells multiply.

How should this medicine be used?

Gefitinib comes as a tablet to take by mouth. It is usually taken with or without food once a day. Take gefitinib at around the same time every day. Follow the directions on your prescription label carefully, and ask your doctor or pharmacist to explain any part you do not understand. Take gefitinib exactly as directed. Do not take more or less of it or take it more often than prescribed by your doctor.

If you are unable to swallow the tablets, you may dissolve them in water. Place one tablet in a half a glass of plain, non-carbonated drinking water. Stir with a spoon for about 10 minutes until the tablet is dissolved. Do not use the spoon to crush the tablet. Drink the mixture right away.

Rinse the glass with another half glass of water and drink the rinse water to be sure that you swallow all of the medication.

Gefitinib is not available in pharmacies. You can only get gefitinib through a distribution program that has been set up by the manufacturer for people who have taken gefitinib in the past. You will need to sign a consent form before you receive any medication. You will receive your medication by mail from a specific mail order pharmacy. Ask your doctor if you have any questions about receiving your medication.

Are there other uses for this medicine?

This medication may be prescribed for other uses; ask your doctor or pharmacist for more information.

What special precautions should I follow?

Before taking gefitinib,

- tell your doctor and pharmacist if you are allergic to gefitinib or any other medications.
- tell your doctor and pharmacist what prescription and nonprescription medications, vitamins, and nutritional supplements you are taking or plan to take. Be sure to mention any of the following: anticoagulants ('blood thinners') such as warfarin (Coumadin); antifungals such as itraconazole (Sporanox), ketoconazole (Nizoral), and voriconazole (Vfend); carbamazepine (Carbatrol, Equetro, Tegretol); amiodarone (Cordarone, Pacerone); clarithromycin (Biaxin); diltiazem (Cardizem, Dilacor, Tiazac); erythromycin (E.E.S, E-Mycin, Erythrocin); fluvoxamine (Luvox); medications for heartburn and ulcers such as cimetidine (Tagamet), famotidine (Pepcid), nizatidine (Axid), and ranitidine (Zantac); metoprolol (Lopressor, Toprol XL); rifabutin (Mycobutin); rifampin (Rifadin, Rimactane); medications for human immunodeficiency virus (HIV) such as indinavir (Crixivan), nelfinavir (Viracept), and ritonavir (Norvir, in Kaletra); nefazodone; phenobarbital; phenytoin (Dilantin); verapamil (Calan, Covera, Isoptin, Verelan); and vinorelbine (Navelbine). Many other medications may interact with gefitinib, so be sure to tell your doctor about all the medications you are taking, even those that do not appear on this list. Your doctor may need to change the doses of your medications or monitor you carefully for side effects.
- tell your doctor what herbal products you are taking, especially St. John's wort.
- tell your doctor if you have or have ever had pulmonary fibrosis (scarring of the lungs), or liver or kidney disease.
- tell your doctor if you are pregnant or plan to become pregnant. You should use birth control to prevent pregnancy during your treatment with gefitinib and for some time after you stop using the medication. If you become pregnant while taking gefitinib, call your doctor. Gefitinib may harm the fetus and increase the risk of pregnancy loss.

- tell your doctor if you are breast-feeding. You should not breast-feed while you are taking gefitinib.

What special dietary instructions should I follow?

Talk to your doctor about eating grapefruit and drinking grapefruit juice while you are taking this medicine.

What should I do if I forget to take a dose?

Take the missed dose as soon as you remember it. However, if it is almost time for the next dose, skip the missed dose and continue your regular dosing schedule. Do not take a double dose to make up for a missed one.

What side effects can this medicine cause?

Gefitinib may cause side effects. Tell your doctor if any of these symptoms are severe or do not go away:

- dry skin
- itching
- rash
- acne
- mouth sores
- weight loss
- weakness

Some side effects can be serious. If you experience any of these symptoms, call your doctor immediately:

- new or worsening shortness of breath, cough, or fever
- diarrhea
- nausea
- vomiting
- loss of appetite
- eye pain, redness, or irritation
- change in vision
- growth of eyelashes on the inside of the eyelid
- hives
- swelling of the eyes, face, lips, tongue, throat, hands, arms, feet, ankles or lower legs

Gefitinib may cause other side effects. Call your doctor if you have any unusual problems while taking this medication.

What storage conditions are needed for this medicine?

Keep this medication in the container it came in, tightly closed, and out of reach of children. Store it at room temperature and away from excess heat and moisture (not in the bathroom). Throw away any medication that is outdated or no longer needed. Talk to your pharmacist about the proper disposal of your medication.

What should I do in case of overdose?

In case of overdose, call your local poison control center at 1-800-222-1222. If the victim has collapsed or is not breathing, call local emergency services at 911.

Symptoms of overdose may include:

- diarrhea
- rash

What other information should I know?

Keep all appointments with your doctor and the laboratory. Your doctor will order certain lab tests to check your body's response to gefitinib.

Do not let anyone else take your medication. Ask your pharmacist any questions you have about refilling your prescription.

Dosage Facts
For Informational Purposes

Caution: Do not change your dose, how often you take your medication, or the length of time you are to take it without first talking to your healthcare provider.

The following dosage information was written using medical language for doctors and other healthcare professionals and is provided here for you to check your dosage. The dosage of this drug may differ for different patients. Therefore, always follow your doctor's instructions or the directions on the label. Contact your healthcare provider or pharmacist if you have any questions about the specific dosage of your medication after reviewing this information.

Adult Patients

NSCLC

ORAL:
- 250 mg once daily. Higher dosages do not increase response and may increase toxicity.
- If used with potent CYP3A4 inducer, consider dosage adjustment.
- Discontinue gefitinib if interstitial lung disease develops.
- May interrupt therapy briefly (up to 14 days) if adverse dermatologic reactions or poorly tolerated diarrhea (sometimes with dehydration) occurs. Reinitiate at dosage of 250 mg once daily.
- Interrupt therapy if adverse ocular manifestations (e.g., pain, aberrant eyelash) develop; following resolution, make decision regarding reinitiation at dosage of 250 mg once daily.

Special Populations

Hepatic Impairment
- No dosage adjustments necessary in patients with moderate to severe hepatic impairment and liver metastases.

Renal Impairment
- No dosage adjustments necessary.

Gemfibrozil

(jem fi′ broe zil)

Brand Name: Lopid®
Also available generically.

Why is this medicine prescribed?

Gemfibrozil is used with diet changes (restriction of cholesterol and fat intake) to reduce the amount of cholesterol and triglycerides (other fatty substances) in the blood in certain people with very high triglycerides who are at risk of pancreatic disease (conditions affecting the pancreas, a gland that produces fluid to break down food and hormones to control blood sugar). Gemfibrozil is also used in people with a combination of low high-density lipoprotein (HDL; "good cholesterol") levels and high low-density lipoprotein (LDL; "bad cholesterol") and triglyceride levels. Gemfibrozil is in a class of lipid-regulating medications called fibrates. It works be reducing the production of triglycerides in the liver.

Buildup of cholesterol and fats along the walls of your arteries (a process known as atherosclerosis) decreases blood flow and, therefore, the oxygen supply to your heart, brain, and other parts of your body. Lowering your blood level of cholesterol and fats may help to decrease your chances of getting heart disease, angina (chest pain), strokes, and heart attacks. In addition to taking a cholesterol-lowering medication, making certain changes in your daily habits can also lower your cholesterol blood levels. You should eat a diet that is low in saturated fat and cholesterol (see SPECIAL DIETARY), exercise 30 minutes on most, if not all days, and lose weight if you are overweight.

How should this medicine be used?

Gemfibrozil comes as a tablet to take by mouth. It is usually taken twice a day, 30 minutes before the morning and evening meals. Take gemfibrozil at around the same times every day. Follow the directions on your prescription label carefully, and ask your doctor or pharmacist to explain any part you do not understand. Take gemfibrozil exactly as directed. Do not take more or less of it or take it more often than prescribed by your doctor.

Gemfibrozil controls high cholesterol and triglycerides but does not cure them. Continue to take gemfibrozil even if you feel well. Do not stop taking gemfibrozil without talking to your doctor.

Are there other uses for this medicine?

This medication may be prescribed for other uses; ask your doctor or pharmacist for more information.

What special precautions should I follow?

Before taking gemfibrozil,
- tell your doctor and pharmacist if you are allergic to gemfibrozil or any other medications.
- tell your doctor if you are taking cerivastatin (Baycol, not on market in U.S.). Your doctor will tell you not to take gemfibrozil while taking cerivastatin.
- tell your doctor and pharmacist what prescription and nonprescription medications, vitamins, nutritional supplements, and herbal products you are taking or plan to take. Be sure to mention any of the following: anticoagulants ('blood thinners') such as warfarin (Coumadin); cholesterol-lowering medications (statins) such as atorvastatin (Lipitor), fluvastatin (Lescol), lovastatin (Mevacor), pravastatin (Pravachol), and simvastatin (Zocor); and repaglinide (Prandin). Your doctor may need to change the doses of your medications or monitor you carefully for side effects.
- tell your doctor if you have kidney, liver, or gallbladder disease. Your doctor may tell you not to take gemfibrozil.
- tell your doctor if you are pregnant, plan to become pregnant, or are breast-feeding. If you become pregnant while taking gemfibrozil, call your doctor.

What special dietary instructions should I follow?

Eat a low-cholesterol, low-fat diet. This kind of diet includes cottage cheese, fat-free milk, fish (not canned in oil), vegetables, poultry, egg whites, and polyunsaturated oils and margarines (corn, safflower, canola, and soybean oils). Avoid foods with excess fat in them such as meat (especially liver and fatty meat), egg yolks, whole milk, cream, butter, shortening, lard, pastries, cakes, cookies, gravy, peanut butter, chocolate, olives, potato chips, coconut, cheese (other than cottage cheese), coconut oil, palm oil, and fried foods.

What should I do if I forget to take a dose?

Take the missed dose as soon as you remember it. However, if it is almost time for the next dose, skip the missed dose and continue your regular dosing schedule. Do not take a double dose to make up for a missed one.

What side effects can this medicine cause?

Gemfibrozil may cause side effects. Tell your doctor if any of these symptoms are severe or do not go away:
- stomach pain
- heartburn

Some side effects can be serious. If you experience any of these symptoms, call your doctor immediately:
- muscle pain, tenderness, or weakness
- blurred vision

A medication similar to gemfibrozil has caused cancer, gallbladder disease, and stomach pain leading to appendectomy. Talk to your doctor about the risks of taking this medication.

Gemfibrozil may cause other side effects. Call your doctor if you have any unusual problems while taking this medication.

If you experience a serious side effect, you or your doctor may send a report to the Food and Drug Administration's (FDA) MedWatch Adverse Event Reporting program online [at http://www.fda.gov/MedWatch/index.html] or by phone [1-800-332-1088].

What storage conditions are needed for this medicine?

Keep this medication in the container it came in, tightly closed, and out of reach of children. Store it at room temperature and away from excess heat and moisture (not in the bathroom). Throw away any medication that is outdated or no longer needed. Talk to your pharmacist about the proper disposal of your medication.

What should I do in case of overdose?

In case of overdose, call your local poison control center at 1-800-222-1222. If the victim has collapsed or is not breathing, call local emergency services at 911.

Symptoms of overdose may include:

- stomach cramps
- diarrhea
- joint and muscle pain
- nausea
- vomiting

What other information should I know?

Keep all appointments with your doctor and the laboratory. Your doctor will order certain lab tests to check your body's response to gemfibrozil.

Do not let anyone else take your medication. Ask your pharmacist any questions you have about refilling your prescription.

Dosage Facts
For Informational Purposes

Caution: Do not change your dose, how often you take your medication, or the length of time you are to take it without first talking to your healthcare provider.

The following dosage information was written using medical language for doctors and other healthcare professionals and is provided here for you to check your dosage. The dosage of this drug may differ for different patients. Therefore, always follow your doctor's instructions or the directions on the label. Contact your healthcare provider or pharmacist if you have any questions about the specific dosage of your medication after reviewing this information.

Adult Patients
Prevention of Cardiovascular Events

ORAL:
- 600 mg twice daily.

- Monitor lipoprotein concentrations periodically. Discontinue therapy in patients who fail to achieve an adequate response after 3 months of therapy.

Dyslipidemias

ORAL:
- 600 mg twice daily.
- Monitor lipoprotein concentrations periodically. Discontinue therapy in patients who fail to achieve an adequate response after 3 months of therapy.

Gemifloxacin

(gem ah flox′ a sin)

Brand Name: Factive®

Why is this medicine prescribed?

Gemifloxacin is used to treat infections such as pneumonia (lung infections) or bronchitis (infection of the tubes moving air in and out of the lungs) caused by certain bacteria. Gemifloxacin is in a class of antibiotics called fluoroquinolones. It works by eliminating bacteria that cause infections. Antibiotics do not work for colds, flu, or other viral infections

How should this medicine be used?

Gemifloxacin comes as a tablet to take by mouth. It is usually taken with or without food once daily for 5 to 7 days. To help you remember to take gemifloxacin, take it around the same time every day. Follow the directions on your prescription label carefully, and ask your doctor or pharmacist to explain any part you do not understand. Take gemifloxacin exactly as directed. Do not take more or less of it or take it more often than prescribed by your doctor.

Swallow the tablets whole with plenty of water; do not split, chew, or crush them.

You should begin feeling better during the first few days of treatment with gemifloxacin. If you do not, call your doctor.

Take gemifloxacin until you finish the prescription, even if you feel better. If you stop taking gemifloxacin too soon, your infection may not be completely cured and the bacteria may become resistant to antibiotics.

Are there other uses for this medicine?

This medication may be prescribed for other uses; ask your doctor or pharmacist for more information.

What special precautions should I follow?

Before taking gemifloxacin,

- tell your doctor and pharmacist if you are allergic to gemifloxacin; other quinolone and fluoroquinolone antibiotics such as cinoxacin (Cinobac), ciprofloxacin (Cipro), enoxacin (Penetrex), gatifloxacin (Tequin), levofloxacin (Levaquin), lomefloxacin (Maxaquin), moxifloxacin (Avelox), nalidixic acid (NegGram), norfloxacin (Noroxin), ofloxacin (Floxin), sparfloxacin (Zagam), trovafloxacin and alatrofloxacin combination (Trovan); or any other medications.

- tell your doctor and pharmacist what other prescription and nonprescription medications, vitamins, nutritional supplements, and herbal products you are taking. Be sure to mention any of the following: anticoagulants ('blood thinners') such as warfarin (Coumadin); antidepressants such as amitriptyline (Elavil), amoxapine (Asendin), clomipramine (Anafranil), desipramine (Norpramin), doxepin (Adapin, Sinequan), imipramine (Tofranil), nortriptyline (Aventyl, Pamelor), protriptyline (Vivactil), and trimipramine (Surmontil); aspirin and other nonsteroidal anti-inflammatory medications (NSAIDs) such as ibuprofen (Advil, Motrin) and naproxen (Aleve, Naprosyn); cisapride (Propulsid); diuretics ('water pills'); erythromycin (E.E.S., E-mycin, Erythrocin); gatifloxacin (Tequin); hormone replacement therapy; levofloxacin (Levaquin); medications for irregular heartbeat such as amiodarone (Cordarone), dofetilide (Tikosyn), disopyramide (Norpace), procainamide (Procanbid, Pronestyl), quinidine (Quinidex), and sotalol (Betapace); medications for mental illness; moxifloxacin (Avelox); oral contraceptives (birth control pills); oral steroids such as dexamethasone (Decadron, Dexone), methylprednisolone (Medrol), and prednisone (Deltasone); pimozide (Orap); probenecid; sparfloxacin (Zagam); or thioridazine (Stelazine). Your doctor may need to change the doses of your medications or monitor you carefully for side effects.
- if you are taking magnesium- and/or aluminum-containing antacids (ALternaGEL, Amphojel, Basaljel, Gaviscon, Maalox, Mylanta); didanosine (Videx) chewable tablets or solution (liquid); or iron, magnesium, or zinc in supplements or multivitamins; take them 3 hours before or 2 hours after gemifloxacin.
- if you are taking sucralfate (Carafate), take it at least 2 hours after gemifloxacin.
- tell your doctor if you or any of your family members have or have ever had irregular, slow, or pounding heartbeat; if you have recently had a heart attack; and if you have or have ever had blood problems; low potassium or magnesium levels in your blood; mental illness; recent head injury; seizures; or heart, kidney, or liver disease.
- you should know that antibiotics similar to gemifloxacin have caused serious and occasionally fatal allergic reactions in some patients. If you develop hives; difficulty breathing or swallowing; rapid, irregular or pounding heartbeat; fainting; dizziness; blurred vision; or other symptoms of a severe allergic reaction, seek emergency medical care right away. If you develop a skin rash, stop taking gemifloxacin and call your doctor. Call your doctor if you experience other signs of an allergic reaction such as itching; swelling of the face, throat, tongue, lips, eyes, hands, feet, ankles, or lower legs; fever; sore throat, chills or other sign of infection; hoarseness; joint or muscle pain; decreased urination; unusual bruising or bleeding; lack of energy; weakness; yellowing of the skin or eyes; or upset stomach.

- you should know that gemifloxacin may cause tendonitis (swelling or tearing of the fiber that connects a bone to a muscle). Tell your doctor if you have ever had tendonitis, and if you participate in regular athletic activity. If you experience symptoms of tendonitis, such as pain, swelling, tenderness, or difficulty in moving a muscle, stop taking gemifloxacin, rest, and call your doctor immediately.
- tell your doctor if you are pregnant, plan to become pregnant, or are breast-feeding. If you become pregnant while taking gemifloxacin, call your doctor.
- if you are having surgery, including dental surgery, tell the doctor or dentist that you are taking gemifloxacin.
- you should know that gemifloxacin may make you dizzy. Do not drive a car or operate machinery until you know how this medication affects you.
- plan to avoid unnecessary or prolonged exposure to sunlight, sunlamps, or tanning beds and wear protective clothing, sunglasses, and sunscreen when outside in sunlight. Gemifloxacin may make your skin sensitive to sunlight.

What special dietary instructions should I follow?

Be sure to drink plenty of fluids while taking this medication.

What should I do if I forget to take a dose?

Take the missed dose as soon as you remember it. However, if it is almost time for the next dose, skip the missed dose and continue your regular dosing schedule. Do not take more than one dose of gemifloxacin in one day.

What side effects can this medicine cause?

Gemifloxacin may cause side effects. Tell your doctor if any of these symptoms are severe or do not go away:

- diarrhea
- stomach pain
- vomiting
- lightheadedness
- confusion
- restlessness
- nervousness
- change in ability to taste
- difficulty falling asleep or staying asleep

Some side effects can be serious. The following symptoms are uncommon, but if you experience any of them, or those mentioned in the SPECIAL PRECAUTIONS section, call your doctor immediately:

- hallucinations (seeing things or hearing voices that do not exist)
- depression
- abnormal fear

- thoughts of hurting yourself
- shaking hands that you cannot control
- seizures
- lower back pain

You should know that gemifloxacin has slowed the growth and damaged the joints of young laboratory animals. It is not known if gemifloxacin has these effects on children. Therefore, gemifloxacin should not be given to people younger than 18 years old. Talk to your child's doctor about the risks of giving gemifloxacin to your child.

Gemifloxacin may cause other side effects. Call your doctor if you have any unusual problems while taking this medication.

If you experience a serious side effect, you or your doctor may send a report to the Food and Drug Administration's (FDA) MedWatch Adverse Event Reporting program online [at http://www.fda.gov/MedWatch/index.html] or by phone [1-800-332-1088].

What storage conditions are needed for this medicine?

Keep this medication in the container it came in, tightly closed, and out of reach of children. Store it at room temperature and away from light, and excess heat and moisture (not in the bathroom). Throw away any medication that is outdated or no longer needed. Talk to your pharmacist about the proper disposal of your medication.

What should I do in case of overdose?

In case of overdose, call your local poison control center at 1-800-222-1222. If the victim has collapsed or is not breathing, call local emergency services at 911.

What other information should I know?

Keep all appointments with your doctor and the laboratory. Your doctor may order certain lab tests to check your body's response to gemifloxacin.

Do not let anyone else take your medication. Your prescription is probably not refillable. If you still have symptoms of infection after you finish the gemifloxacin, call your doctor.

Dosage Facts
For Informational Purposes

Caution: Do not change your dose, how often you take your medication, or the length of time you are to take it without first talking to your healthcare provider.

The following dosage information was written using medical language for doctors and other healthcare professionals and is provided here for you to check your dosage. The dosage of this drug may differ for different patients. Therefore, always follow your doctor's instructions or the directions on the label. Contact your health-care provider or pharmacist if you have any questions about the specific dosage of your medication after reviewing this information.

General Dosage Information

Available as gemifloxacin mesylate; dosage expressed in terms of gemifloxacin.

Adult Patients

Respiratory Tract Infections
Acute Exacerbations of Chronic Bronchitis

ORAL:
- 320 mg once daily for 5 days.

Community-acquired Pneumonia (CAP)

ORAL:
- 320 mg once daily for 7 days.

Prescribing Limits
Adult Patients

Do not exceed usual dosage or duration of therapy.

Special Populations

Hepatic Impairment
- Dosage adjustments not required in adults with mild, moderate, or severe hepatic impairment (Child Pugh class A, B, or C).

Renal Impairment
- Reduce dosage to 160 mg once daily in adults with $Cl_{cr} \leq 40$ mL/minute, including those on hemodialysis or CAPD.
- Gemifloxacin partially removed by hemodialysis; administer dose after hemodialysis.

Geriatric Patients
- No dosage adjustments except those related to renal impairment.

Gentamicin Ophthalmic

(jen ta mye' sin)

Brand Name: Gentak®, Gentasol®, Ocu-Mycin®, Pred-G® Liquifilm®, Pred-G® S.O.P.®
Also available generically.

Why is this medicine prescribed?

Gentamicin kills bacteria that cause certain eye infections.

This medication is sometimes prescribed for other uses; ask your doctor or pharmacist for more information.

How should this medicine be used?

Gentamicin comes as eyedrops and eye ointment. The eyedrops usually are applied every 4-8 hours; the eye ointment usually is applied two to four times a day. Follow the directions on your prescription label carefully, and ask your doctor or pharmacist to explain any part that you do not understand. Use gentamicin exactly as directed. Do not use more or less of it or use it more often than prescribed by your doctor.

To use the eyedrops, follow these instructions:

1. Wash your hands thoroughly with soap and water.
2. Use a mirror or have someone else put the drops in your eye.
3. Remove the protective cap. Make sure that the end of the dropper is not chipped or cracked and that the eyedrops are clear (not cloudy).
4. Avoid touching the dropper tip against your eye or anything else.
5. Hold the dropper tip down at all times to prevent drops from flowing back into the bottle and contaminating the remaining contents.
6. Lie down or tilt your head back.
7. Holding the bottle between your thumb and index finger, place the dropper tip as near as possible to your eyelid without touching it.
8. Brace the remaining fingers of that hand against your cheek or nose.
9. With the index finger of your other hand, pull the lower lid of the eye down to form a pocket.
10. Drop the prescribed number of drops into the pocket made by the lower lid and the eye. Placing drops on the surface of the eyeball can cause stinging.
11. Close your eye and press lightly against the lower lid with your finger for 2-3 minutes to keep the medication in the eye. Do not blink.
12. Replace and tighten the cap right away. Do not wipe or rinse it off.
13. Wipe off any excess liquid from your cheek with a clean tissue. Wash your hands again.

To use the eye ointment, follow these instructions:

1. Wash your hands thoroughly with soap and water.
2. Use a mirror or have someone else apply the ointment.
3. Avoid touching the tip of the tube against your eye or anything else. The ointment must be kept clean.
4. Tilt your head forward slightly.
5. Holding the tube between your thumb and index finger, place the tube as near as possible to your eyelid without touching it.
6. Brace the remaining fingers of that hand against your cheek or nose.
7. With the index finger of your other hand, pull the lower lid of your eye down to form a pocket.
8. Place a small amount of ointment into the pocket made by the lower lid and the eye. A 1/2-inch strip of ointment usually is enough unless otherwise directed by your doctor.
9. Gently close your eyes and keep them closed for 1-2 minutes to allow the medication to be absorbed.
10. Replace and tighten the cap right away.
11. Wipe off any excess ointment from your eyelids and lashes with a clean tissue. Wash your hands again.

What special precautions should I follow?

Before using gentamicin eyedrops or eye ointment,

- tell your doctor and pharmacist if you are allergic to gentamicin, other antibiotics, or any other drugs.
- tell your doctor and pharmacist what prescription and nonprescription medications you are taking, especially other eye medications, and vitamins.
- tell your doctor if you are pregnant, plan to become pregnant, or are breast-feeding. If you become pregnant while using gentamicin, call your doctor immediately.
- tell your doctor if you wear soft contact lenses. If the brand of gentamicin you are using contains benzalkonium chloride, wait at least 15 minutes after using the medicine to put in soft contact lenses.

What should I do if I forget to take a dose?

Apply the missed dose as soon as you remember it. However, if it is almost time for the next dose, skip the missed dose and continue your regular dosing schedule. Do not apply a double dose to make up for a missed one.

What side effects can this medicine cause?

Gentamicin may cause side effects. Tell your doctor if any of these symptoms are severe or do not go away:

- eye irritation, burning, or stinging
- swelling of the eye

What storage conditions are needed for this medicine?

Keep this medication in the container it came in, tightly closed, and out of reach of children. Store it at room temperature and away from excess heat and moisture (not in the bathroom). Throw away any medication that is outdated or no longer needed. Talk to your pharmacist about the proper disposal of your medication.

What other information should I know?

Keep all appointments with your doctor.

Do not let anyone else use your medication. Ask your pharmacist any questions you have about refilling your prescription.

If you still have symptoms of infection after you finish the gentamicin, call your doctor.

Dosage Facts
For Informational Purposes

Caution: Do not change your dose, how often you take your medication, or the length of time you are to take it without first talking to your healthcare provider.

The following dosage information was written using medical language for doctors and other healthcare professionals and is provided here for you to check your

dosage. The dosage of this drug may differ for different patients. Therefore, always follow your doctor's instructions or the directions on the label. Contact your health-care provider or pharmacist if you have any questions about the specific dosage of your medication after reviewing this information.

General Dosage Information

Available as gentamicin sulfate; dosage expressed in terms of gentamicin.

Pediatric Patients

Bacterial Ophthalmic Infections

OPHTHALMIC:
- 1 or 2 drops of 0.3% solution instilled into the infected eye(s) every 4 hours. In severe infections, up to 2 drops every hour may be used.
- Alternatively, place a small amount (approximately 1.3-cm ribbon) of 0.3% ointment into the conjunctival sac 2 or 3 times daily.

Adult Patients

Bacterial Ophthalmic Infections

OPHTHALMIC:
- 1 or 2 drops of 0.3% solution instilled into the infected eye(s) every 4 hours. In severe infections, up to 2 drops every hour may be used.
- Alternatively, place a small amount (approximately 1.3-cm ribbon) of 0.3% ointment into the conjunctival sac 2 or 3 times daily.

Gentamicin Sulfate Injection

(jen ta mye' sin)

Brand Name: Garamycin®
Also available generically.

Important Warning

Gentamicin can cause severe hearing and kidney problems. Before administering gentamicin, tell your doctor and pharmacist what prescription and non-prescription medications you are taking, especially diuretics ('water pills'), cisplatin (Platinol), amphotericin (Amphotec, Fungizone), other antibiotics, and vitamins.

If you experience any of the following symptoms, call your health care provider immediately: dizziness, vertigo, ringing in the ears, hearing loss, numbness, muscle twitching or weakness, difficulty breathing, decreased urination, rash, itching, or sore throat.

About Your Treatment

Your doctor has ordered gentamicin, an antibiotic, to help treat your infection. The drug will be either injected into a large muscle (such as your buttock or hip) or added to an intravenous fluid that will drip through a needle or catheter placed in your vein for at least 30 minutes, one to three times a day.

Gentamicin eliminates bacteria that cause many kinds of infections, including lung, skin, bone, joint, stomach, blood, and urinary tract infections. This medication is sometimes prescribed for other uses; ask your doctor or pharmacist for more information.

Your health care provider (doctor, nurse, or pharmacist) may measure the effectiveness and side effects of your treatment using laboratory tests and physical examinations. It is important to keep all appointments with your doctor and the laboratory. The length of treatment depends on how your infection and symptoms respond to the medication.

Precautions

Before administering gentamicin,
- tell your doctor and pharmacist if you are allergic to amikacin (Amikin), gentamicin, kanamycin (Kantrex), neomycin, netilmicin (Netromycin), streptomycin, tobramycin (Nebcin), or any other drugs.
- tell your doctor and pharmacist what prescription and nonprescription medications you are taking, especially diuretics ('water pills'), cisplatin (Platinol), amphotericin (Amphotec, Fungizone), other antibiotics, and vitamins.
- tell your doctor if you have or have ever had kidney disease, vertigo, hearing loss, ringing in the ears, myasthenia gravis, or Parkinson's disease.
- tell your doctor if you are pregnant, plan to become pregnant, or are breast-feeding. If you become pregnant while taking gentamicin, call your doctor immediately. Gentamicin can harm the fetus.

Administering Your Medication

Before you administer gentamicin, look at the solution closely. It should be clear and free of floating material. Gently squeeze the bag or observe the solution container to make sure there are no leaks. Do not use the solution if it is discolored, if it contains particles, or if the bag or container leaks. Use a new solution, but show the damaged one to your health care provider.

It is important that you use your medication exactly as directed. Do not stop your therapy on your own for any reason because your infection could worsen and result in hospitalization. Do not change your dosing schedule without talking to your health care provider. Your health care provider may tell you to stop your infusion if you have a mechanical problem (such as a blockage in the tubing, needle, or catheter); if you have to stop an infusion, call your health care provider immediately so your therapy can continue.

Side Effects

Gentamicin occasionally causes side effects. To reduce this risk, your health care provider may adjust your dose based on your blood test results. Follow the directions in the IMPORTANT WARNING section for the symptoms listed there and tell your health care provider if any of the following symptoms are severe or do not go away:

- upset stomach
- vomiting
- fatigue
- pale skin

Storage Conditions

- Your health care provider probably will give you a several-day supply of gentamicin at a time. If you are receiving gentamicin intravenously (in your vein), you probably will be told to store it in the refrigerator or freezer.
- Take your next dose from the refrigerator 1 hour before using it; place it in a clean, dry area to allow it to warm to room temperature.
- If you are told to store additional gentamicin in the freezer, always move a 24-hour supply to the refrigerator for the next day's use.
- Do not refreeze medications.

If you are receiving gentamicin intramuscularly (in your muscle), your health care provider will tell you how to store it properly.

Store your medication only as directed. Make sure you understand what you need to store your medication properly.

Keep your supplies in a clean, dry place when you are not using them, and keep all medications and supplies out of reach of children. Your health care provider will tell you how to throw away used needles, syringes, tubing, and containers to avoid accidental injury.

Overdose

In case of overdose, call your local poison control center at 1-800-222-1222. If the victim has collapsed or is not breathing, call local emergency services at 911.

Signs of Infection

If you are receiving gentamicin in your vein or under your skin, you need to know the symptoms of a catheter-related infection (an infection where the needle enters your vein or skin). If you experience any of these effects near your intravenous catheter, tell your health care provider as soon as possible:

- tenderness
- warmth
- irritation
- drainage
- redness
- swelling
- pain

Dosage Facts
For Informational Purposes

Caution: Do not change your dose, how often you take your medication, or the length of time you are to take it without first talking to your healthcare provider.

The following dosage information was written using medical language for doctors and other healthcare professionals and is provided here for you to check your dosage. The dosage of this drug may differ for different patients. Therefore, always follow your doctor's instructions or the directions on the label. Contact your healthcare provider or pharmacist if you have any questions about the specific dosage of your medication after reviewing this information.

General Dosage Information

Available as gentamicin sulfate; dosage is expressed in terms of gentamicin.

Dosage is identical for either IV or IM administration.

Dosage should be based on patient's pretreatment body weight.

Many clinicians recommend that dosage be determined using appropriate pharmacokinetic methods for calculating dosage requirements and patient-specific pharmacokinetic parameters (e.g., elimination rate constant, volume of distribution) derived from serum concentration-time data; in determining dosage, the susceptibility of the causative organism, the severity of infection, and the patient's immune and clinical status also must be considered.

Peak and trough serum gentamicin concentrations should be determined periodically and dosage adjusted to maintain desired serum concentrations whenever possible, especially in patients with life-threatening infections, suspected toxicity or nonresponse to treatment, decreased or varying renal function, and/or when increased aminoglycoside clearance (e.g., patients with cystic fibrosis, burns) or prolonged therapy is likely.

In general, desirable peak serum concentrations of gentamicin are 4–12 mcg/mL and trough concentrations of the drug should not exceed 1–2 mcg/mL. Some evidence suggests that an increased risk of toxicity may be associated with prolonged peak serum gentamicin concentrations >10–12 mcg/mL and/or trough concentrations >2 mcg/mL.

Once-daily administration† of aminoglycosides is at least as effective as, and may be less toxic than, conventional dosage regimens employing multiple daily doses.

Pediatric Patients
General Dosage for Neonates

IV OR IM:

- Manufacturer recommends 2.5 mg/kg every 12 hours in premature or full-term neonates ≤1 week of age and 2.5 mg/kg every 8 hours for older neonates.
- Neonates <1 week of age: AAP recommends 2.5 mg/kg every 18–24 hours for those weighing <1.2 kg and 2.5 mg/kg every 12 hours for those weighing ≥1.2 kg.

- Neonates 1–4 weeks of age: AAP recommends 2.5 mg/kg every 18–24 hours for those weighing <1.2 kg, 2.5 mg/kg every 8 or 12 hours for those weighing 1.2–2 kg, and 2.5 mg/kg every 8 hours for those weighing >2 kg.

General Dosage for Infants and Children

IV OR IM:
- Older infants and children: manufacturer recommends 2.5 mg/kg every 8 hours for older neonates.
- Children ≥1 month of age: AAP recommends 3–7.5 mg/kg given in 3 divided doses for treatment of severe infections. Inappropriate for mild to moderate infections according to AAP.

Endocarditis†
Treatment of Staphylococcal Endocarditis†

IV OR IM:
- 3 mg/kg daily in 3 divided doses; dosage adjusted to achieve peak serum gentamicin concentrations approximately 3 mcg/mL and trough concentrations <1 mcg/mL.
- Used in conjunction with nafcillin, oxacillin, cefazolin, or vancomycin; gentamicin used only during the first 3–5 days for native valve infections or during the first 2 weeks for prosthetic valve infections.

Treatment of Endocarditis Caused by Viridans Streptococci or S. bovis†

IV OR IM:
- 3 mg/kg daily in 3 divided doses; dosage adjusted to achieve peak serum gentamicin concentrations approximately 3 mcg/mL and trough concentrations <1 mcg/mL.
- Used in conjunction with penicillin G or ceftriaxone; usual duration is 2 weeks for penicillin-susceptible strains (MIC ≤0.1 mcg/mL), 2 weeks for relatively resistant strains (MIC >0.1–0.5 mcg/mL), or 4–6 weeks for strains with high level penicillin resistance (MIC >0.5 mcg/mL). If used with vancomycin in patients unable to receive a β-lactam, a 6-week regimen is recommended.

Treatment of Enterococcal Endocarditis†

IV OR IM:
- 3 mg/kg daily in 3 divided doses; dosage adjusted to achieve peak serum gentamicin concentrations approximately 3 mcg/mL and trough concentrations <1 mcg/mL.
- Used in conjunction with penicillin G or ceftriaxone; usual duration is 2 weeks for penicillin-susceptible strains (MIC ≤0.1 mcg/mL), 2 weeks for relatively resistant strains (MIC >0.1–0.5 mcg/mL), or 4–6 weeks for strains with high level penicillin resistance (MIC >0.5 mcg/mL). If used with vancomycin in patients unable to receive a β-lactam, a 6-week regimen is recommended.

Prevention of Endocarditis in Patients Undergoing Certain Genitourinary or GI (except Esophageal) Procedures†

IV OR IM:
- For high-risk patients: 1.5 mg/kg (up to 120 mg) given within 30 minutes prior to the procedure; used in conjunction with recommended regimens of ampicillin or vancomycin.

Plague†
Treatment of Plague†

IV OR IM:
- Premature neonates and neonates ≤1 week of age: 2.5 mg/kg twice daily.

- Infants and older children: 2.5 mg/kg 3 times daily.
- Usual duration is 10 days; some experts recommend 10–14 days.

Tularemia†
Treatment of Tularemia†

IV OR IM:
- 2.5 mg/kg 3 times daily for 10 days.

Adult Patients

General Adult Dosage
Treatment of Serious Infections

IV OR IM:
- 3 mg/kg daily given in 3 equally divided doses every 8 hours.

Treatment of Life-threatening Infections

IV OR IM:
- ≤5 mg/kg daily given in 3 or 4 equally divided doses. Dosage should be reduced to 3 mg/kg daily when clinically indicated.

Endocarditis†
Treatment of Staphylococcal Endocarditis†

IV OR IM:
- 1 mg/kg every 8 hours. Used in conjunction with nafcillin, oxacillin, cefazolin, or vancomycin; gentamicin used only during the first 3–5 days of therapy for native valve infections or during the first 2 weeks for prosthetic valve infections.

Treatment of Endocarditis Caused by Viridans Streptococci or S. bovis†

IV OR IM:
- 1 mg/kg every 8 hours. Used in conjunction with penicillin G, ceftriaxone, or vancomycin; gentamicin used only during the first 2 weeks of therapy.

Treatment of Enterococcal Endocarditis†

IV OR IM:
- 1 mg/kg every 8 hours. Used in conjunction with penicillin G, ampicillin, or vancomycin; usual duration is 4–6 weeks.

Treatment of Endocarditis Caused by HACEK group†

IV:
- 1 mg/kg every 8 hours. Used in conjunction with ampicillin; usual duration is 4 weeks. (HACEK: H. parainfluenzae, H. aphrophilus, A. actinomycetemcomitans, C. hominis, E. corrodens, K. kingae)

Prevention of Endocarditis in Patients Undergoing Certain Genitourinary or GI (except Esophageal) Procedures†

IV OR IM:
- For high-risk patients: 1.5 mg/kg (up to 120 mg) given within 30 minutes prior to the procedure; used in conjunction with recommended regimens of ampicillin or vancomycin.

Gynecologic Infections†
Pelvic Inflammatory Disease† (PID)

IV OR IM:
- Initially, 2 mg/kg followed by 1.5 mg/kg every 8 hours; used in conjunction with IV clindamycin (900 mg every 8 hours). After clinical improvement occurs, discontinue IV clindamycin and gentamicin and switch to oral clindamycin (450 mg 4 times daily) or oral doxycycline (100 mg twice daily) to complete 14 days of therapy.

Granuloma Inguinale (Donovanosis)†

IV:

- 1 mg/kg every 8 hours; added as an adjunct to the recommended or alternative drugs (doxycycline, co-trimoxazole, ciprofloxacin, erythromycin, azithromycin) if improvement is not evident within the first few days of therapy or in pregnant or HIV-infected patients.

Plague†

Treatment of Plague†

IV OR IM:

- 5 mg/kg once daily or, alternatively, a 2-mg/kg loading dose following by 1.7 mg/kg 3 times daily. Usual duration is 10 days; some experts recommend 10–14 days.

Tularemia†

Treatment of Tularemia†

IV OR IM:

- 5 mg/kg once daily for 10 days; some experts recommend 3–5 mg/kg daily for 10–14 days.

Special Populations

Renal Impairment

- Dosage adjustments necessary in patients with renal impairment. Whenever possible monitor serum gentamicin concentrations, especially in patients with changing renal function.
- Various methods have been used to determine aminoglycoside dosage for patients with renal impairment and there is wide variation in dosage recommendations for these patients. The manufacturers recommend an initial dose of 1–1.7 mg/kg, followed by 1-mg/kg doses given at intervals (in hours) calculated by multiplying the patient's steady-state serum creatinine (in mg/dL) by 8. The dosing method of Sarubbi and Hull, which is based on corrected Cl_{cr} also has been recommended. Specialized references should be consulted for specific information on dosage for patients with renal impairment.
- Dosage calculation methods should *not* be used in patients undergoing hemodialysis or peritoneal dialysis. In patients with renal failure undergoing hemodialysis, the manufacturers recommend supplemental doses of 1–1.7 mg/kg at the end of each dialysis period in adults and supplemental doses of 2–2.5 mg/kg at the end of each dialysis period in children.

Geriatric Patients

- Select dosage with caution and closely monitor renal function because of age-related decreases in renal function.
- No dosage adjustments except those related to renal impairment.

† Use is not currently included in the labeling approved by the US Food and Drug Administration.

Glatiramer Injection

(gla tir′ a mer)

Brand Name: Copaxone®

Why is this medicine prescribed?

Glatiramer is used to reduce episodes of symptoms in patients with relapsing-remitting multiple sclerosis. Glatiramer is in a class of medications called immunomodulators. It works by stopping the body from damaging its own nerve cells (myelin).

How should this medicine be used?

Glatiramer comes as a solution to inject in the fatty layer just under the skin (subcutaneously). It is usually injected once a day. To help you remember to inject glatiramer, inject it around the same time every day. Follow the directions on your prescription label carefully, and ask your doctor or pharmacist to explain any part you do not understand. Use glatiramer exactly as directed. Do not use more or less of it or use it more often than prescribed by your doctor.

You will receive your first dose of glatiramer in your doctor's office. After that, you can inject glatiramer yourself or have a friend or relative perform the injections. Before you use glatiramer yourself the first time, read the written instructions that come with it. Ask your doctor or pharmacist to show you or the person who will be injecting the medication how to inject it.

Glatiramer comes in prefilled syringes. Use each syringe only once and inject all the solution in the syringe. Even if there is still some solution left in the syringe after you inject, do not inject again. Dispose of used syringes in a puncture-resistant container. Talk to your doctor or pharmacist about how to dispose of the puncture-resistant container.

You can inject glatiramer into seven parts of your body: right and left arms, thighs, and hips; and lower stomach. There are specific spots on each of these body parts where you can inject glatiramer. Refer to the diagram in the manufacturer's patient information for the exact places you can inject. You should inject in each of the body parts once a week, and you should pick a different place on the body part each time. Keep a list of the places where you have given injections so that you will not inject in these places again until some time has passed.

To inject glatiramer, follow these steps:

1. Remove one blister pack from the carton of glatiramer syringes and place it on a clean flat surface. Wait 20 minutes to allow the medication to warm to room temperature.
2. Wash your hands thoroughly with soap and water and dry them with a clean towel.
3. Peel back the paper label and remove the syringe from

the blister pack. Check your pre-filled syringe to be sure it is safe to use. It should be labeled with the correct name of the medication and should contain a clear colorless solution. Do not use the syringe if it is expired, is cloudy, or contains any particles. Small air bubbles in the syringe will not cause any problems and you should not try to remove them.

4. Wipe the place on your skin where you will inject glatiramer with a fresh alcohol pad and wait several seconds to allow it to dry.
5. Pick up the syringe like a pencil and remove the needle cover.
6. Use your other hand to pinch a 2 inch fold of skin between your thumb and index finger.
7. Hold the syringe at a 90 degree angle to your body and push the needle straight into your skin. When the needle is all the way in, let go of the pinched fold of skin.
8. Hold the syringe steady while slowly pushing down the plunger until the syringe is empty.
9. Pull the needle straight out.
10. Press a dry cotton ball on the injection site for a few minutes, but do not rub it.

Glatiramer controls multiple sclerosis but does not cure it. Continue to use glatiramer even if you feel well. Do not stop using glatiramer without talking to your doctor.

Are there other uses for this medicine?

This medication may be prescribed for other uses; ask your doctor or pharmacist for more information.

What special precautions should I follow?

Before taking glatiramer,
- tell your doctor and pharmacist if you are allergic to glatiramer, mannitol, or any other medications.
- tell your doctor and pharmacist what prescription and nonprescription medications, vitamins, nutritional supplements, and herbal products you are taking. Your doctor may need to change the doses of your medications or monitor you carefully for side effects.
- tell your doctor if you have or have ever had kidney disease.
- tell your doctor if you are pregnant, plan to become pregnant, or are breast-feeding. If you become pregnant while taking glatiramer, call your doctor.
- you should know that you may have a reaction immediately after you inject glatiramer. You may experience the following symptoms: flushing, chest pain, pounding heartbeat, anxiety, trouble breathing, closing of the throat, and hives. This reaction is most likely to occur several months into your treatment, but may happen at any time. These symptoms will usually go away without treatment in a short time. Get emergency medical care if these symptoms become severe or last longer than a few minutes. It is important to tell your doctor if this happens.

What special dietary instructions should I follow?

Unless your doctor tells you otherwise, continue your normal diet.

What should I do if I forget to take a dose?

Take the missed dose as soon as you remember it. However, if it is almost time for the next dose, skip the missed dose and continue your regular dosing schedule. Do not take a double dose to make up for a missed one.

What side effects can this medicine cause?

Glatiramer may cause side effects. Tell your doctor if any of these symptoms are severe or do not go away:
- pain, redness, swelling, itching, or lump in the place where you injected glatiramer
- weakness
- flushing
- depression
- abnormal dreams
- pain in the back, neck, or any other part of the body
- severe headache
- loss of appetite
- diarrhea
- upset stomach
- vomiting
- weight gain
- swelling of the hands, feet, ankles, or lower legs
- purple patches on skin
- joint pain
- confusion
- nervousness
- crossed eyes
- difficulty speaking
- shaking hands that you cannot control
- sweating
- ear pain
- painful or changed menstrual periods
- vaginal itching and discharge
- urgent need to urinate or defecate
- tightness in muscles
- white patches in the mouth

Some side effects can be serious. The following symptoms are uncommon, but if you experience any of them, call your doctor immediately. In some cases, your doctor may tell you to stop using glatiramer:
- dizziness
- excessive sweating
- chest pain
- sore throat, fever, chills, and other signs of infection
- runny nose
- coughing
- fast heartbeat
- fainting
- skin rash

- hives
- itching
- difficulty breathing or swallowing
- very severe pain at the injection site

Glatiramer affects your immune system, so it may increase your risk of developing cancer or a serious infection. Talk to your doctor about the risks of taking this medication.

Glatiramer may cause other side effects. Call your doctor if you have any unusual problems while taking this medication.

If you experience a serious side effect, you or your doctor may send a report to the Food and Drug Administration's (FDA) MedWatch Adverse Event Reporting program online [at http://www.fda.gov/MedWatch/index.html] or by phone [1-800-332-1088].

What storage conditions are needed for this medicine?

Keep this medication in the container it came in, tightly closed, and out of reach of children. Store it in a refrigerator but do not freeze it. If you will not have access to a refrigerator, you can store glatiramer at room temperature for up to 7 days, but do not expose it to bright light. Throw away any medication that is outdated or no longer needed. Talk to your pharmacist about the proper disposal of your medication.

What should I do in case of overdose?

In case of overdose, call your local poison control center at 1-800-222-1222. If the victim has collapsed or is not breathing, call local emergency services at 911.

What other information should I know?

Keep all appointments with your doctor.

Do not let anyone else take your medication. Ask your pharmacist any questions you have about refilling your prescription.

Dosage Facts
For Informational Purposes

Caution: Do not change your dose, how often you take your medication, or the length of time you are to take it without first talking to your healthcare provider.

The following dosage information was written using medical language for doctors and other healthcare professionals and is provided here for you to check your dosage. The dosage of this drug may differ for different patients. Therefore, always follow your doctor's instructions or the directions on the label. Contact your healthcare provider or pharmacist if you have any questions about the specific dosage of your medication after reviewing this information.

General Dosage Information

Available as glatiramer acetate; dosage expressed in terms of the salt.

Adult Patients

Multiple Sclerosis

SUB-Q:
- 20 mg once daily.
- Therapy should be continued indefinitely except when there is a clear lack of benefit, intolerable adverse effects, or availability of better treatments.

Special Populations

No special population dosage recommendations at this time.

Glimepiride

(glye' me pye ride)

Brand Name: Amaryl®
Also available generically.

Important Warning

Oral hypoglycemic drugs, including glimepiride, have been associated with increased cardiovascular mortality. Talk to your doctor about the possible risks, benefits, and alternatives of using this drug for your condition.

Why is this medicine prescribed?

Glimepiride is used with diet and exercise to treat type 2 diabetes (condition in which the body does not use insulin normally and therefore cannot control the amount of sugar in the blood). Glimepiride stimulates your pancreas to make more insulin and also makes your body more sensitive to insulin. Glimepiride may be used with or without insulin.

This medication is sometimes prescribed for other uses; ask your doctor or pharmacist for more information.

How should this medicine be used?

Glimepiride comes as a tablet to take by mouth. It is usually taken once a day. The tablet should be taken with breakfast or the first big meal of the day. Follow the directions on your prescription label carefully, and ask your doctor or pharmacist to explain any part you do not understand. Take glimepiride exactly as directed. Do not take more or less of it or take it more often than prescribed by your doctor.

Continue to take glimepiride even if you feel well. Do not stop taking glimepiride without talking to your doctor.

What special precautions should I follow?

Before taking glimepiride,

- tell your doctor and pharmacist if you are allergic to glimepiride or any other drugs.
- tell your doctor and pharmacist what prescription and nonprescription medications you are taking, especially antibiotics, anticoagulants ('blood thinners') such as warfarin (Coumadin), dexamethasone (Decadron), diuretics ('water pills'), estrogens, isoniazid (INH), MAO inhibitors [phenelzine (Nardil) and tranylcypromine (Parnate)], medications for high blood pressure or heart disease, niacin, oral contraceptives, phenytoin (Dilantin), prednisone, probenecid (Benemid), and vitamins.
- tell your doctor if you have or have ever had kidney disease or ketoacidosis.
- tell your doctor if you are pregnant, plan to become pregnant, or are breast-feeding. If you become pregnant while taking glimepiride, call your doctor immediately.
- if you are having surgery, including dental surgery, tell the doctor or dentist that you are taking glimepiride.

What special dietary instructions should I follow?

Be sure to follow all exercise and dietary recommendations made by your doctor or dietitian. It is important to eat a healthful diet.

Alcohol may cause a decrease in blood sugar. Ask your doctor about the safe use of alcoholic beverages while you are taking glimepiride.

What should I do if I forget to take a dose?

Take the missed dose as soon as you remember it. If you will be having a snack soon, take a dose with the snack. If it is almost time for the next dose, skip the missed dose and continue your regular dosing schedule. Do not take a double dose to make up for a missed one.

What side effects can this medicine cause?

This medication may cause changes in your blood sugar. You should know the symptoms of low and high blood sugar and what to do if you have these symptoms.

You may experience hypoglycemia (low blood sugar) while you are taking this medication. Your doctor will tell you what you should do if you develop hypoglycemia. He or she may tell you to check your blood sugar, eat or drink a food or beverage that contains sugar, such as hard candy or fruit juice, or get medical care. Follow these directions carefully if you have any of the following symptoms of hypoglycemia:

- shakiness
- dizziness or lightheadedness
- sweating

- nervousness or irritability
- sudden changes in behavior or mood
- headache
- numbness or tingling around the mouth
- weakness
- pale skin
- hunger
- clumsy or jerky movements

If hypoglycemia is not treated, severe symptoms may develop. Be sure that your family, friends, and other people who spend time with you know that if you have any of the following symptoms, they should get medical treatment for you immediately.

- confusion
- seizures
- loss of consciousness

Call your doctor immediately if you have any of the following symptoms of hyperglycemia (high blood sugar):

- extreme thirst
- frequent urination
- extreme hunger
- weakness
- blurred vision

If high blood sugar is not treated, a serious, life-threatening condition called diabetic ketoacidosis could develop. Call your doctor immediately if you have any of the these symptoms:

- dry mouth
- upset stomach and vomiting
- shortness of breath
- breath that smells fruity
- decreased consciousness

Glimepiride may cause other side effects. Call your doctor if you have any unusual problems while taking this medication.

If you experience a serious side effect, you or your doctor may send a report to the Food and Drug Administration's (FDA) MedWatch Adverse Event Reporting program online [at http://www.fda.gov/MedWatch/index.html] or by phone [1-800-332-1088].

What storage conditions are needed for this medicine?

Keep this medication in the container it came in, tightly closed, and out of reach of children. Store it at room temperature and away from excess heat and moisture (not in the bathroom). Throw away any medication that is outdated or no longer needed. Talk to your pharmacist about the proper disposal of your medication.

What should I do in case of overdose?

In case of overdose, call your local poison control center at 1-800-222-1222. If the victim has collapsed or is not breathing, call local emergency services at 911.

What other information should I know?

Keep all appointments with your doctor and the laboratory. Your doctor will order certain lab tests to check your response to glimepiride. Your doctor will also tell you how to check your response to this medication by measuring your blood or urine sugar levels at home. Follow these instructions carefully.

You should always wear a diabetic identification bracelet to be sure you get proper treatment in an emergency.

Do not let anyone else take your medication. Ask your pharmacist any questions you have about refilling your prescription.

Dosage Facts
For Informational Purposes

Caution: Do not change your dose, how often you take your medication, or the length of time you are to take it without first talking to your healthcare provider.

The following dosage information was written using medical language for doctors and other healthcare professionals and is provided here for you to check your dosage. The dosage of this drug may differ for different patients. Therefore, always follow your doctor's instructions or the directions on the label. Contact your healthcare provider or pharmacist if you have any questions about the specific dosage of your medication after reviewing this information.

General Dosage Information

With the fixed combination of glimepiride and rosiglitazone maleate, dosage of rosiglitazone component expressed in terms of rosiglitazone.

Adult Patients

Diabetes Mellitus
Glimepiride Monotherapy

ORAL:

- Initially, 1–2 mg once daily for previously untreated patients or patients transferred from other antidiabetic agents. In patients receiving 1 mg daily, increase dosage to 2 mg daily after 1–2 weeks if adequate glycemic control has not been achieved. Increase dosage in increments of no more than 2 mg daily at 1- to 2-week intervals up to a maximum of 8 mg once daily. Usual maintenance dosage is 1–4 mg once daily.
- Maximum *initial* dosage should not exceed 2 mg once daily.

Glimepiride/Rosiglitazone Fixed-combination Therapy

ORAL:

- Patients inadequately controlled on sulfonylurea or rosiglitazone monotherapy: Initially, 1 or 2 mg of glimepiride and 4 mg of rosiglitazone once daily.
- In patients previously receiving thiazolidinedione monotherapy, allow approximately 1–2 weeks to assess therapeutic response before adjusting dosage of the fixed-combination preparation. If additional glycemic control is needed, increase dosage based on the glimepiride component in increments of

≤2 mg at 1–2 week intervals to a maximum total daily dosage of 4 mg of glimepiride and 8 mg of rosiglitazone.
- In patients previously receiving sulfonylurea monotherapy, allow 2 weeks to observe reduction in blood glucose concentrations and 2–3 months to observe full therapeutic response to newly initiated rosiglitazone component. If additional glycemic control is needed, increase dosage based on glimepiride component to a maximum total daily dosage of 4 mg of glimepiride and 8 mg of rosiglitazone.
- For patients switching from combined therapy with separate preparations, the initial dosage of the fixed-combination preparation should be the same as the daily dosage of glimepiride and rosiglitazone currently being taken.
- If hypoglycemia occurs, reduce dosage of glimepiride component.

Concomitant Glimepiride and Insulin Therapy

ORAL:

- Initially, 8 mg once daily and a low insulin dosage in patients whose fasting plasma or serum glucose concentration exceeds 150 mg/dL despite appropriate oral antidiabetic monotherapy, diet, and exercise.
- Adjust insulin dosage upward at approximately weekly intervals until adequate glycemic control is achieved. Periodic adjustments in insulin dosage may be necessary during continued combination therapy.

Initial Dosage in Patients Transferred from Other Sulfonylurea Agents

ORAL:

- Initially, 1–2 mg once daily. May discontinue other sulfonylurea agents immediately. During transfer from chlorpropamide (a sulfonylurea with a long elimination half-life), monitor closely for hypoglycemia during the initial 1–2 weeks of the transition period.
- The *initial* dosage of glimepiride during transfer from other therapy should not exceed 2 mg daily.

Prescribing Limits

Adult Patients

Diabetes Mellitus

ORAL:

- Monotherapy: Maximum 8 mg of glimepiride daily.
- Fixed combination: Maximum 4 mg of glimepiride and 8 mg of rosiglitazone daily.

Special Populations

Hepatic Impairment

- Initially, 1 mg of glimepiride alone or in fixed combination with rosiglitazone once daily. Titrate dosage of glimepiride alone or in fixed combination with rosiglitazone upward based on fasting glucose concentrations in order to avoid hypoglycemic reactions. Conservative initial and maintenance dosages recommended.
- Do not initiate therapy with fixed combination of glimepiride and rosiglitazone in patients with clinical evidence of active liver disease or elevated serum aminotransferase concentrations (ALT >2.5 times the upper limit of normal).

Renal Impairment

- Initially, 1 mg of glimepiride alone or in fixed combination with rosiglitazone once daily. Titrate dosage of glimepiride alone or in fixed combination with rosiglitazone upward based on fasting glucose concentrations. Conservative initial and maintenance dosages recommended. Dosages >1 mg daily (of glimepiride) may not be required if Cl_{cr} <22 mL/minute.

Adrenal Insufficiency
- Initially, 1 mg of glimepiride in fixed combination with 4 mg of rosiglitazone once daily. Titrate dosage of glimepiride component upward with care to avoid hypoglycemic reactions. Conservative initial and maintenance dosages recommended.

Geriatric Patients
- Initially, 1 mg of glimepiride alone or in fixed combination with rosiglitazone once daily. Titrate dosage of glimepiride alone or in fixed combination with rosiglitazone upward with care. Conservative initial and maintenance dosages recommended.

Debilitated or Malnourished Patients
- Initially, 1 mg of glimepiride alone or in fixed combination with rosiglitazone once daily. Titrate dosage of glimepiride alone or in fixed combination with rosiglitazone upward with care. Conservative initial and maintenance dosages recommended.

Glipizide

(glip′ i zide)

Brand Name: Glucotrol®
Also available generically.

Important Warning

Oral hypoglycemic drugs, including glipizide, have been associated with increased cardiovascular mortality. Talk to your doctor about the possible risks, benefits, and alternatives of using this drug for your condition.

Why is this medicine prescribed?

Glipizide is used to treat type 2 diabetes (condition in which the body does not use insulin normally and therefore cannot control the amount of sugar in the blood), particularly in people whose diabetes cannot be controlled by diet alone. Glipizide lowers blood sugar by stimulating the pancreas to secrete insulin and helping the body use insulin efficiently. The pancreas must be capable of producing insulin for this medication to work. Glipizide is not used to treat type 1 diabetes (condition in which the body does not produce insulin and therefore cannot control the amount of sugar in the blood).

This medication is sometimes prescribed for other uses; ask your doctor or pharmacist for more information.

How should this medicine be used?

Glipizide comes in tablets to take by mouth. It is usually taken once a day, 30 minutes before breakfast. Follow the directions on your prescription label carefully, and ask your doctor or pharmacist to explain any part you do not understand. Take glipizide exactly as directed. Do not take more or less of it or take it more often than prescribed by your doctor.

Continue to take glipizide even if you feel well. Do not stop taking glipizide without talking to your doctor.

What special precautions should I follow?

Before taking glipizide,
- tell your doctor and pharmacist if you are allergic to glipizide or any other drugs.
- tell your doctor and pharmacist what prescription and nonprescription medications you are taking, especially antibiotics, anticoagulants ('blood thinners') such as warfarin (Coumadin), dexamethasone (Decadron), diuretics ('water pills'), estrogens, isoniazid (INH), MAO inhibitors [phenelzine (Nardil) and tranylcypromine (Parnate)], medications for high blood pressure or heart disease, niacin, oral contraceptives, phenytoin (Dilantin), prednisone, probenecid (Benemid), and vitamins.
- tell your doctor if you have or have ever had kidney, liver, heart, or thyroid disease or a severe infection.
- tell your doctor if you are pregnant, plan to become pregnant, or are breast-feeding. If you become pregnant while taking glipizide, call your doctor.
- if you are having surgery, including dental surgery, tell the doctor or dentist that you are taking glipizide.
- plan to avoid unnecessary or prolonged exposure to sunlight and to wear protective clothing, sunglasses, and sunscreen. Glipizide may make your skin sensitive to sunlight.

What special dietary instructions should I follow?

Be sure to follow all exercise and dietary recommendations made by your doctor or dietitian. It is important to eat a healthy diet.

Alcohol may cause a decrease in blood sugar. Ask your doctor about the safe use of alcoholic beverages while you are taking glipizide.

What should I do if I forget to take a dose?

Before you start taking glipizide, ask your doctor what to do if you forget to take a dose. Write these directions down so you can refer to them later.

As a general rule, take the missed dose as soon as you remember it unless it is almost time for the next dose. Do not take a double dose to make up for a missed one.

What side effects can this medicine cause?

This medication may cause changes in your blood sugar. You should know the symptoms of low and high blood sugar and what to do if you have these symptoms.

You may experience hypoglycemia (low blood sugar) while you are taking this medication. Your doctor will tell you what you should do if you develop hypoglycemia. He or she may tell you to check your blood sugar, eat or drink a food or beverage that contains sugar, such as hard candy or fruit juice, or get medical care. Follow these directions carefully if you have any of the following symptoms of hypoglycemia:

- shakiness
- dizziness or lightheadedness
- sweating
- nervousness or irritability
- sudden changes in behavior or mood
- headache
- numbness or tingling around the mouth
- weakness
- pale skin
- hunger
- clumsy or jerky movements

If hypoglycemia is not treated, severe symptoms may develop. Be sure that your family, friends, and other people who spend time with you know that if you have any of the following symptoms, they should get medical treatment for you immediately.

- confusion
- seizures
- loss of consciousness

Call your doctor immediately if you have any of the following symptoms of hyperglycemia (high blood sugar):

- extreme thirst
- frequent urination
- extreme hunger
- weakness
- blurred vision

If high blood sugar is not treated, a serious, life-threatening condition called diabetic ketoacidosis could develop. Call your doctor immediately if you have any of the these symptoms:

- dry mouth
- upset stomach and vomiting
- shortness of breath
- breath that smells fruity
- decreased consciousness

Glipizide may cause side effects. If you experience any of the following symptoms, call your doctor immediately:

- skin rash
- itching or redness
- exaggerated sunburn
- yellowing of the skin or eyes
- light-colored stools
- dark urine
- unusual bleeding or bruising
- fever
- sore throat

If you experience a serious side effect, you or your doctor may send a report to the Food and Drug Administration's (FDA) MedWatch Adverse Event Reporting program online [at http://www.fda.gov/MedWatch/index.html] or by phone [1-800-332-1088].

What storage conditions are needed for this medicine?

Keep this medication in the container it came in, tightly closed, and out of reach of children. Store it at room temperature and away from excess heat and moisture (not in the bathroom). Throw away any medication that is outdated or no longer needed. Talk to your pharmacist about the proper disposal of your medication.

What should I do in case of overdose?

In case of overdose, call your local poison control center at 1-800-222-1222. If the victim has collapsed or is not breathing, call local emergency services at 911.

What other information should I know?

Keep all appointments with your doctor and the laboratory. Your doctor will order certain lab tests to check your response to glipizide. Your doctor will also tell you how to check your response to this medication by measuring your blood or urine sugar levels at home. Follow these instructions carefully.

You should always wear a diabetic identification bracelet to be sure you get proper treatment in an emergency.

Do not let anyone else take your medication. Ask your pharmacist any questions you have about refilling your prescription.

Dosage Facts
For Informational Purposes

Caution: Do not change your dose, how often you take your medication, or the length of time you are to take it without first talking to your healthcare provider.

The following dosage information was written using medical language for doctors and other healthcare professionals and is provided here for you to check your dosage. The dosage of this drug may differ for different patients. Therefore, always follow your doctor's instructions or the directions on the label. Contact your healthcare provider or pharmacist if you have any questions about the specific dosage of your medication after reviewing this information.

Adult Patients

Diabetes Mellitus
Initial Dosage in Previously Untreated Patients

ORAL:
- Conventional or extended-release tablets: Initially, 5 mg daily. Titrate dosage of conventional tablets in increments of 2.5–5 mg daily at intervals of at least several days (usually 3–7 days). Maximum once daily dosage, 15 mg.
- For extended-release tablets, dosage adjustment should be based on at least 2 similar consecutive fasting glucose concentrations obtained at least 7 days after the previous dose adjustment.

Initial Dosage in Patients Transferred from Conventional to Extended-release Tablets

ORAL:
- When transferring, administer the nearest equivalent total daily dosage once daily. Alternatively, 5 mg once daily as extended-release tablets and titrate dosage.

Initial Dosage in Patients Transferred from Other Oral Antidiabetic Agents

ORAL:
- Individualize initial dosage of glipizide; usually 5–10 mg daily. The other oral antidiabetic agent may be discontinued abruptly.
- Patients being transferred from a sulfonylurea agent with a longer half life (e.g., chlorpropamide) should be closely monitored for the occurrence of hypoglycemia during the initial 1–2 weeks. A drug-free interval of 2–3 days may be advisable before glipizide therapy is initiated as conventional tablets in patients being transferred from chlorpropamide, particularly if blood glucose concentration was adequately controlled with chlorpropamide.

Initial Dosage in Patients Transferred from Insulin

ORAL:
- Initially, 5 mg once daily, if insulin requirements were ≤20 units daily. Abruptly discontinue insulin.
- 5 mg once daily if insulin requirements were >20 units daily, and reduce insulin dosage by 50%. Withdraw insulin gradually and adjust glipizide dosage in increments of 2.5–5 mg daily at intervals of at least several days.

Maintenance Dosage

ORAL:
- Maintenance dosage varies considerably, ranging from 2.5–40 mg daily. Most patients require 5–25 mg daily as conventional tablets or 5–10 mg daily as extended-release tablets, but higher dosages may be necessary.

Combination Therapy with Other Oral Antidiabetic Agents

ORAL:
- When added to therapy with other antidiabetic agents, the glipizide extended-release tablets may be initiated at a dosage of 5 mg daily. Base titration on clinical judgment.
- Fixed combination: 2.5 mg of glipizide and 250 mg of metformin hydrochloride once daily with a meal in treatment-naive patients.
- For more severe hyperglycemia (i.e., fasting plasma glucose concentrations of 280–320 mg/dL), 2.5 mg of glipizide and 500 mg of metformin hydrochloride twice daily.

- Dosage may be increased in increments of one tablet (using the tablet strength at which therapy was initiated, either 2.5 mg glipizide/250 mg metformin hydrochloride or 2.5 mg glipizide/500 mg metformin hydrochloride) daily every 2 weeks until the minimum effective dosage required to achieve adequate glycemic control is reached.
- Maximum daily dosage, 10 mg of glipizide and 2 g of metformin hydrochloride.
- In previously treated patients with inadequate glycemic control with monotherapy, 2.5 or 5 mg of glipizide and 500 mg of metformin hydrochloride twice daily with the morning and evening meals.
- The initial dosage of the fixed combination should not exceed the daily dosage of glipizide or metformin hydrochloride previously received.
- Titrate upward in increments not exceeding 5 mg of glipizide and 500 mg of metformin hydrochloride until adequate glycemic control is reached.
- Maximum daily dosage, 20 mg of glipizide and 2 g of metformin hydrochloride in previously treated patients.
- For patients previouly receiving both glipizide (or another sulfonylurea antidiabetic agent) and metformin, the initial dosage of the fixed-combination preparation should not exceed the daily dosages of glipizide (or equivalent dosage of another sulfonylurea) and metformin hydrochloride currently being taken. Such patients should be monitored for signs and symptoms of hypoglycemia following the switch. In the transfer, the decision to switch to the nearest equivalent dosage or to titrate dosage is based on clinical judgment.

Prescribing Limits

Adult Patients

Diabetes Mellitus

ORAL:
- Maximum once-daily dose as conventional tablets is 15 mg.
- Maximum total daily dosage is 40 mg as divided doses of conventional tablets or 20 mg as extended-release tablets.
- Maximum daily dosage of the fixed combination, 10 mg of glipizide and 2 g of metformin hydrochloride.

Special Populations

Hepatic Impairment
- Conventional tablets: Initially, 2.5 mg daily; conservative maintenance dosage.
- Extended-release tablets: Use conservative initial and maintenance dosage.
- Adjust dosage carefully.
- Generally, do *not* use in patients with severe hepatic impairment.

Renal Impairment
- Use conservative initial and maintenance dosage.
- Use generally not recommended in patients with severe renal impairment.
- Cautious dosing recommended.

Geriatric Patients
- Conventional tablets: Initially, 2.5 mg daily.
- Initially, 5 mg (extended-release tablets) may be used.
- Use conservative initial and maintenance dosage of glipizide-containing formulations.

- Adjust dosage carefully. Any dosage adjustment of glipizide in fixed combination with metformin hydrochloride requires careful assessment of renal function.
- Dosage of glipizide and metformin hydrochloride in fixed combination should not be titrated to the maximum dosage.

Debilitated or Malnourished Patients

- Conservative initial and maintenance dosage of conventional and extended-release tablets.
- Dosage of glipizide and metformin hydrochloride in fixed combination should not be titrated to the maximum dosage.

Glucagon

(gloo′ ka gon)

Brand Name: GlucaGen Diagnostic Kit®

Why is this medicine prescribed?

Glucagon is a hormone produced in the pancreas. Glucagon is used to raise very low blood sugar. Glucagon is also used in diagnostic testing of the stomach and other digestive organs.

This medication is sometimes prescribed for other uses; ask your doctor or pharmacist for more information.

How should this medicine be used?

Glucagon is usually given by injection beneath the skin, in the muscle, or in the vein. It comes as a powder and liquid that will need to be mixed just before administering the dose. Instructions for mixing and giving the injection are in the package. Glucagon should be administered as soon as possible after discovering that the patient is unconscious from low blood sugar. After the injection, the patient should be turned onto the side to prevent choking if they vomit. Once the glucagon has been given, contact your doctor. It is very important that all patients have a household member who knows the symptoms of low blood sugar and how to administer glucagon.

If you have low blood sugar often, keep a glucagon kit with you at all times. You should be able to recognize some of the signs and symptoms of low blood sugar (i.e., shakiness, dizziness or lightheadedness, sweating, confusion, nervousness or irritability, sudden changes in behavior or mood, headache, numbness or tingling around the mouth, weakness, pale skin, sudden hunger, clumsy or jerky movments). Try to eat or drink a food or beverage with sugar in it, such as hard candy or fruit juice, before it is necessary to administer glucagon.

Follow the directions on your prescription label carefully, and ask your pharmacist or doctor to explain any part you or your household members do not understand. Use glucagon exactly as directed. Do not use more or less of it or take it more often than prescribed by your doctor.

What special precautions should I follow?

Before taking glucagon,

- tell your doctor and pharmacist if you are allergic to glucagon, any other drugs, or beef or pork products.
- tell your doctor and pharmacist what prescription and nonprescription medications you are taking, including vitamins.
- tell your doctor if you have ever had adrenal gland problems, blood vessel disease, malnutrition, pancreatic tumors, insulinoma, or pheochromocytoma.
- tell your doctor if you are pregnant, plan to become pregnant, or are breast-feeding.

What side effects can this medicine cause?

Glucagon may cause side effects. Tell your doctor if any of these symptoms are severe or do not go away:

- upset stomach
- vomiting
- rash
- itching

If you experience any of the following symptoms, call your doctor immediately:

- difficulty breathing
- loss of consciousness

If you experience a serious side effect, you or your doctor may send a report to the Food and Drug Administration's (FDA) MedWatch Adverse Event Reporting program online [at http://www.fda.gov/MedWatch/index.html] or by phone [1-800-332-1088].

What storage conditions are needed for this medicine?

Keep this medication in the container it came in, tightly closed, and out of reach of children. Store it at room temperature and away from excess heat and moisture (not in the bathroom). Once the injection dose has been mixed, discard any unused portion.

What should I do in case of overdose?

In case of overdose, call your local poison control center at 1-800-222-1222. If the victim has collapsed or is not breathing, call local emergency services at 911.

What other information should I know?

Keep all appointments with your doctor and the laboratory.

Do not let anyone else take your medication. Ask your pharmacist any questions you have about refilling your prescription.

Talk to your doctor, pharmacist, or other healthcare professional if you have questions about dosing information for your medication.

Glyburide

(glye′ byoor ide)

Brand Name: Diabeta®, Glynase®, Micronase®
Also available generically.

Why is this medicine prescribed?

Glyburide is used to treat type 2 diabetes (condition in which the body does not use insulin normally and therefore cannot control the amount of sugar in the blood), particularly in people whose diabetes cannot be controlled by diet alone. Glyburide lowers blood sugar by stimulating the pancreas to secrete insulin and helping the body use insulin efficiently. The pancreas must produce insulin for this medication to work. Glyburide is not used to treat type 1 diabetes (condition in which the body does not produce insulin and therefore cannot control the amount of sugar in the blood).

This medication is sometimes prescribed for other uses; ask your doctor or pharmacist for more information.

How should this medicine be used?

Glyburide comes in tablets to take by mouth. It is usually taken once a day with breakfast or twice a day (when a large daily dose is required). Follow the directions on your prescription label carefully, and ask your doctor or pharmacist to explain any part you do not understand. Take glyburide exactly as directed. Do not take more or less of it or take it more often than prescribed by your doctor.

Continue to take glyburide even if you feel well. Do not stop taking glyburide without talking to your doctor.

What special precautions should I follow?

Before taking glyburide,

- tell your doctor and pharmacist if you are allergic to glyburide or any other drugs.
- tell your doctor and pharmacist what prescription and nonprescription medications you are taking, especially antibiotics, anticoagulants ('blood thinners') such as warfarin (Coumadin), dexamethasone (Decadron), diuretics ('water pills'), estrogens, isoniazid (INH), MAO inhibitors [phenelzine (Nardil) and tranylcypromine (Parnate)], medications for high blood pressure or heart disease, metformin (Glucophage), niacin (nicotinic acid), oral contraceptives, phenytoin (Dilantin), prednisone, probenecid (Benemid), and vitamins.
- tell your doctor if you have or have ever had heart or kidney disease.
- tell your doctor if you are pregnant, plan to become pregnant, or are breast-feeding. If you become pregnant while taking glyburide, call your doctor.
- if you are having surgery, including dental surgery, tell the doctor or dentist that you are taking glyburide.

- you should know that this drug may make you drowsy. Do not drive a car or operate machinery until you know how this drug affects you.
- remember that alcohol can add to the drowsiness caused by this drug.
- tell your doctor if you use tobacco products. Cigarette smoking may decrease the effectiveness of glyburide.
- plan to avoid unnecessary or prolonged exposure to sunlight and to wear protective clothing, sunglasses, and sunscreen. Glyburide may make your skin sensitive to sunlight.

What special dietary instructions should I follow?

Be sure to follow all exercise and dietary recommendations made by your doctor or dietitian. It is important to eat a healthful diet.

Alcohol may cause a decrease in blood sugar. Ask your doctor about the safe use of alcoholic beverages while you are taking glyburide.

What should I do if I forget to take a dose?

Before you start taking glyburide, ask your doctor what to do if you forget to take a dose. Write these directions down so you can refer to them later.

As a general rule, take the missed dose as soon as you remember it unless it is almost time for the next dose. Do not take a double dose to make up for a missed one.

What side effects can this medicine cause?

This medication may cause changes in your blood sugar. You should know the symptoms of low and high blood sugar and what to do if you have these symptoms.

You may experience hypoglycemia (low blood sugar) while you are taking this medication. Your doctor will tell you what you should do if you develop hypoglycemia. He or she may tell you to check your blood sugar, eat or drink a food or beverage that contains sugar, such as hard candy or fruit juice, or get medical care. Follow these directions carefully if you have any of the following symptoms of hypoglycemia:

- shakiness
- dizziness or lightheadedness
- sweating
- nervousness or irritability
- sudden changes in behavior or mood
- headache
- numbness or tingling around the mouth
- weakness
- pale skin
- hunger
- clumsy or jerky movements

If hypoglycemia is not treated, severe symptoms may develop. Be sure that your family, friends, and other people who spend time with you know that if you have any of the following symptoms, they should get medical treatment for you immediately.

- confusion
- seizures
- loss of consciousness

Call your doctor immediately if you have any of the following symptoms of hyperglycemia (high blood sugar):

- extreme thirst
- frequent urination
- extreme hunger
- weakness
- blurred vision

If high blood sugar is not treated, a serious, life-threatening condition called diabetic ketoacidosis could develop. Call your doctor immediately if you have any of these symptoms:

- dry mouth
- upset stomach and vomiting
- shortness of breath
- breath that smells fruity
- decreased consciousness

Glyburide may cause side effects. If you experience any of the following symptoms, call your doctor immediately:

- skin rash
- itching or redness
- exaggerated sunburn
- yellowing of the skin or eyes
- light-colored stools
- dark urine
- unusual bleeding or bruising
- fever
- sore throat

If you experience a serious side effect, you or your doctor may send a report to the Food and Drug Administration's (FDA) MedWatch Adverse Event Reporting program online [at http://www.fda.gov/MedWatch/index.html] or by phone [1-800-332-1088].

What storage conditions are needed for this medicine?

Keep this medication in the container it came in, tightly closed, and out of reach of children. Store it at room temperature and away from excess heat and moisture (not in the bathroom). Throw away any medication that is outdated or no longer needed. Talk to your pharmacist about the proper disposal of your medication.

What should I do in case of overdose?

In case of overdose, call your local poison control center at 1-800-222-1222. If the victim has collapsed or is not breathing, call local emergency services at 911.

What other information should I know?

Studies have shown that people who take oral antidiabetic drugs have a higher rate of death caused by heart problems than people whose diabetes is treated with diet and insulin. Talk to your doctor about the possible risks, benefits, and alternatives of taking glyburide for your condition.

Keep all appointments with your doctor and the laboratory. Your blood sugar and glycosylated hemoglobin (HbA1c) should be checked regularly to determine your response to glyburide. Your doctor will also tell you how to check your response to this medication by measuring your blood or urine sugar levels at home. Follow these instructions carefully.

You should always wear a diabetic identification bracelet to be sure you get proper treatment in an emergency.

Do not let anyone else take your medication. Ask your pharmacist any questions you have about refilling your prescription.

Dosage Facts
For Informational Purposes

Caution: Do not change your dose, how often you take your medication, or the length of time you are to take it without first talking to your healthcare provider.

The following dosage information was written using medical language for doctors and other healthcare professionals and is provided here for you to check your dosage. The dosage of this drug may differ for different patients. Therefore, always follow your doctor's instructions or the directions on the label. Contact your healthcare provider or pharmacist if you have any questions about the specific dosage of your medication after reviewing this information.

Adult Patients

Diabetes Mellitus
Initial Dosage in Previously Untreated Patients

ORAL:
- Conventional formulations: Initially, 2.5–5 mg daily.
- Micronized formulations: Initially, 1.5 –3 mg daily.
- Fixed combination with metformin hydrochloride: Initially, 1.25 mg of glyburide and 250 mg of metformin hydrochloride once daily. For severe hyperglycemia (baseline HbA_{1c} >9% or fasting blood glucose >200 mg/dL), 1.25 mg of glyburide and 250 mg of metformin hydrochloride *twice* daily, given with the morning and evening meals.

Initial Dosage in Patients Transferred from Other Oral Antidiabetic Agents

ORAL:
- Conventional formulations: Initially, 2.5–5 mg daily.
- Micronized formulations: Initially, 1.5–3 mg daily.
- May discontinue most other oral hypoglycemic agents (except chlorpropamide) immediately. During transfer from chlorpropamide (a drug with a long elimination half-life),

monitor closely for hypoglycemia during initial 2 weeks of transition period.
- Fixed combination with metformin hydrochloride: Initially, 2.5 or 5 mg of glyburide and 500 mg of metformin hydrochloride twice daily with morning and evening meals in patients not adequately controlled by monotherapy with glyburide (or another sulfonylurea) or metformin. For patients previously receiving combination therapy with glyburide (or another sulfonylurea) and metformin, initial dosage should not exceed previous individual dosages of glyburide (or equivalent dosage of another sulfonylurea) and metformin. Titrate in increments ≤5 mg of glyburide and 500 mg of metformin hydrochloride to achieve adequate blood glucose control.

Initial Dosage in Patients Transferred from Insulin

ORAL:
- Conventional formulations: Initially, 2.5–5 mg once daily (if insulin dosage is <20 units daily) or 5 mg once daily (if insulin dosage is 20–40 units daily); may discontinue insulin immediately. If insulin dosage is >40 units daily, reduce insulin dosage by 50% and initiate glyburide at 5 mg daily; withdraw insulin gradually and increase glyburide dosage in increments of 1.25–2.5 mg daily every 2–10 days.
- Micronized formulations: Initially, 1.5–3 mg once daily (if insulin dosage is <20 units daily) or 3 mg once daily (if insulin dosage is 20–40 units daily); may discontinue insulin immediately. If insulin dosage is >40 units daily, reduce insulin dosage by 50% and initiate glyburide at 3 mg daily; withdraw insulin gradually and increase glyburide dosage in increments of 0.75–1.5 mg daily every 2–10 days.

Titration and Maintenance Dosage

ORAL:
- Conventional formulations: Increase dosage in increments of ≤2.5 mg daily at weekly intervals. Usual maintenance dosage is 1.25–20 mg daily.
- Micronized formulations: Increase dosage in increments of ≤1.5 mg daily at weekly intervals. Usual maintenance dosage is 0.75–12 mg daily.
- Fixed combination with metformin hydrochloride: Titrate in increments of 1.25 mg of glyburide and 250 mg of metformin hydrochloride daily at 2-week intervals to achieve adequate blood glucose control.

Prescribing Limits

Adult Patients

Conventional formulations: Maximum 20 mg daily.
Micronized formulations: Maximum 12 mg daily.
Fixed combination with metformin hydrochloride: Maximum 20 mg of glyburide and 2 g of metformin hydrochloride daily.

Special Populations

Hepatic Impairment
- Conventional formulations: Initially, 1.25 mg daily.
- Micronized formulations: Initially, 0.75 mg daily.

Renal Impairment
- Conventional formulations: Initially, 1.25 mg daily.
- Micronized formulations: Initially, 0.75 mg daily.

Geriatric Patients
- Conventional formulations: Initially, 1.25 mg daily
- Micronized formulations: Initially, 0.75 mg daily.
- Fixed combination with metformin hydrochloride: Do not titrate to maximum recommended dosage.

Other Populations
- Cautious dosing recommended in debilitated or malnourished patients or in patients with adrenal or pituitary insufficiency.
- Conventional formulations: Initially, 1.25 mg daily
- Micronized formulations: Initially, 0.75 mg daily.
- Fixed combination with metformin hydrochloride: Do not titrate to maximum recommended dosage.

Glyburide and Metformin

(glye′ byoor ide) (met for′ min)

Brand Name: Glucovance®

Important Warning

Metformin may cause a serious condition called lactic acidosis. Tell your doctor if you are over 80 years old and if you have ever had kidney or liver disease. Do not drink large amounts of alcohol while taking glyburide and metformin. If you are having a radiologic test with injectable contrast agents (for example, a CT scan, angiogram, urogram, or MRI), talk to your doctor about stopping glyburide and metformin a few days before the test. If you are having surgery, including dental surgery, tell the doctor or dentist that you are taking glyburide and metformin. If you experience any of the following symptoms, stop taking glyburide and metformin and call your doctor immediately: severe shortness of breath, excessive tiredness, muscle aches, stomach pain after the first few weeks of treatment, feeling cold, dizziness, or a slow or irregular heartbeat.

Why is this medicine prescribed?

The combination of glyburide and metformin is used to treat type 2 diabetes (condition in which the body does not use insulin normally and therefore cannot control the amount of sugar in the blood) in people whose diabetes cannot be controlled by diet and exercise alone. Glyburide belongs to a class of drugs called sulfonylureas, and metformin is in a class of drugs called biguanides. Glyburide lowers blood sugar by stimulating the pancreas, the organ that makes insulin. Insulin helps control blood sugar levels. The pancreas must produce insulin for this medication to work. Metformin helps your body regulate the amount of glucose (sugar) in your blood. It decreases the amount of glucose you get from your diet and the amount made by your liver. It also helps your body use its own insulin more effectively. Glyburide and metformin are not used to treat type 1 diabetes (condition in which the body does not produce insulin and therefore cannot control the amount of sugar in the blood).

How should this medicine be used?

Glyburide and metformin combination comes as a tablet to take by mouth. It is usually taken one to two times daily with meals. Your doctor may gradually increase your dose, depending on your response to glyburide and metformin. Monitor your blood glucose closely. Follow the directions on your prescription label carefully, and ask your doctor or pharmacist to explain any part you do not understand. Take glyburide and metformin exactly as directed. Do not take more or less of it or take it more often than prescribed by your doctor.

Glyburide and metformin combination controls diabetes but does not cure it. Continue to take glyburide and metformin even if you feel well. Do not stop taking glyburide and metformin without talking to your doctor.

Are there other uses for this medicine?

This medication is sometimes prescribed for other uses; ask your doctor or pharmacist for more information.

What special precautions should I follow?

Before taking glyburide and metformin,
- tell your doctor and pharmacist if you are allergic to glyburide, metformin, or any other drugs.
- tell your doctor and pharmacist what prescription and nonprescription medications you are taking, especially albuterol (Proventil, Ventolin); allergy or cold medications; anticoagulants ('blood thinners') such as warfarin (Coumadin); antipsychotics such as mesoridazine (Serentil) or thioridazine (Mellaril); aspirin or other nonsteroidal anti-inflammatory drugs (NSAIDs) such as ibuprofen (Advil, Motrin) or naproxen (Aleve, Naprosyn); beta-blockers such as propranolol (Inderal); calcium channel blockers such as diltiazem (Cardizem, Tiazac), nifedipine (Adalat, Procardia), or verapamil (Calan, Verelan); chloramphenicol (Chloromycetin); chlorpromazine (Thorazine); cimetidine (Tagamet); ciprofloxacin (Cipro); corticosteroids such as dexamethasone (Decadron), methylprednisolone (Medrol), or prednisone (Deltasone, Orasone); digoxin (Lanoxin); diuretics ('water pills'); epinephrine; estrogens; isoniazid (INH); medications that contain alcohol or sugar; miconazole (Lotrimin, others); morphine (MS Contin, others); niacin; oral contraceptives (birth control pills); phenelzine (Nardil); phenytoin (Dilantin); probenecid (Benemid); procainamide (Procanbid, Pronestyl); prochlorperazine (Compazine); promethazine

(Phenergan); quinidine (Quinalan, Quinidex); quinine (Quinamm); ranitidine (Zantac); salicylates such as diflunisal (Dolobid) or salsalate (Disalcid); terbutaline (Brethine, Bricanyl); thyroid medications; tranylcypromine (Parnate); trimethoprim (Proloprim, Trimpex); vancomycin (Vancocin, others); and vitamins or herbal products.
- in addition to the conditions listed in the IMPORTANT WARNING section, tell your doctor if you have or have ever had heart, pituitary, or thyroid disease; adrenal insufficiency; acute or chronic metabolic acidosis; diabetic ketoacidosis; hormone problems; or gastrointestinal absorption problems.
- tell your doctor if you are pregnant, plan to become pregnant, or are breast-feeding. If you become pregnant while taking glyburide and metformin, call your doctor immediately.
- you should know that this drug may make you drowsy. Do not drive a car or operate machinery until you know how this drug affects you.
- remember that alcohol can add to the drowsiness caused by this drug.
- tell your doctor if you use tobacco products. Cigarette smoking may decrease the effectiveness of glyburide and metformin.
- plan to avoid unnecessary or prolonged exposure to sunlight and to wear protective clothing, sunglasses, and sunscreen. Glyburide and metformin may make your skin sensitive to sunlight.
- tell your doctor if you have fever, infection, injury, or illness with vomiting or diarrhea. These may affect your blood sugar level.

What special dietary instructions should I follow?

Be sure to follow all exercise and dietary recommendations made by your doctor or dietitian. Calorie reduction, weight loss, and exercise will help control your diabetes and will also make glyburide and metformin work better. It is important to eat a healthy diet.

Alcohol may decrease blood sugar and can affect the amount of lactic acid made. Ask your doctor about the safe use of alcoholic beverages while you are taking glyburide and metformin.

What should I do if I forget to take a dose?

Before you start taking glyburide and metformin, ask your doctor what to do if you forget to take a dose or accidentally take an extra dose. Write these directions down so you can refer to them later.

As a general rule, take the missed dose as soon as you remember it. However, if it is almost time for the next dose, skip the missed dose and continue your regular dosing schedule. Do not take a double dose to make up for a missed one.

What side effects can this medicine cause?

This medication may cause changes in your blood sugar. You should know the symptoms of low and high blood sugar and what to do if you have these symptoms.

You may experience hypoglycemia (low blood sugar) while you are taking this medication. Your doctor will tell you what you should do if you develop hypoglycemia. He or she may tell you to check your blood sugar, eat or drink a food or beverage that contains sugar, such as hard candy or fruit juice, or get medical care. Follow these directions carefully if you have any of the following symptoms of hypoglycemia:

- shakiness
- dizziness or lightheadedness
- sweating
- nervousness or irritability
- sudden changes in behavior or mood
- headache
- numbness or tingling around the mouth
- weakness
- pale skin
- hunger
- clumsy or jerky movements

If hypoglycemia is not treated, severe symptoms may develop. Be sure that your family, friends, and other people who spend time with you know that if you have any of the following symptoms, they should get medical treatment for you immediately.

- confusion
- seizures
- loss of consciousness

Call your doctor immediately if you have any of the following symptoms of hyperglycemia (high blood sugar):

- extreme thirst
- frequent urination
- extreme hunger
- weakness
- blurred vision

If high blood sugar is not treated, a serious, life-threatening condition called diabetic ketoacidosis could develop. Call your doctor immediately if you have any of the these symptoms:

- dry mouth
- upset stomach and vomiting
- shortness of breath
- breath that smells fruity
- decreased consciousness

Glyburide and metformin may cause side effects. Tell your doctor if any of these symptoms are severe or do not go away:

- headache
- nasal congestion
- runny nose
- stomach pain
- cough
- diarrhea

If you experience any of the following symptoms or those listed in the IMPORTANT WARNING section, call your doctor immediately:

- skin rash or hives
- itching or redness
- exaggerated sunburn
- yellowing of the skin or eyes
- light-colored stools
- dark or clay-colored urine
- unusual bleeding or bruising
- fever
- sore throat

If you experience a serious side effect, you or your doctor may send a report to the Food and Drug Administration's (FDA) MedWatch Adverse Event Reporting program online [at http://www.fda.gov/MedWatch/index.html] or by phone [1-800-332-1088].

What storage conditions are needed for this medicine?

Keep this medication in the container it came in (which is light resistant), tightly closed, and out of reach of children. Store it at room temperature and away from excess heat and moisture (not in the bathroom). Throw away any medication that is outdated or no longer needed. Talk to your pharmacist about the proper disposal of your medication.

What should I do in case of overdose?

In case of overdose, call your local poison control center at 1-800-222-1222. If the victim has collapsed or is not breathing, call local emergency services at 911.

What other information should I know?

Keep all appointments with your doctor and the laboratory. Your blood sugar and glycosylated hemoglobin (HbA1c) should be checked regularly to determine your response to glyburide and metformin. Your doctor may order other lab tests to check your response to glyburide and metformin. Your doctor will also tell you how to check your response to this medication by measuring your blood or urine sugar levels at home. Follow these instructions carefully.

Keep yourself and your clothes clean. Wash cuts, scrapes, and other wounds quickly, and do not let them get infected.

You should always wear a diabetic identification bracelet to be sure you get proper treatment in an emergency.

Do not let anyone else take your medication. Ask your pharmacist any questions you have about refilling your prescription.

Dosage Facts
For Informational Purposes

Caution: Do not change your dose, how often you take your medication, or the length of time you

are to take it without first talking to your health-care provider.

The following dosage information was written using medical language for doctors and other healthcare professionals and is provided here for you to check your dosage. The dosage of this drug may differ for different patients. Therefore, always follow your doctor's instructions or the directions on the label. Contact your healthcare provider or pharmacist if you have any questions about the specific dosage of your medication after reviewing this information.

Adult Patients

Diabetes Mellitus
Initial Dosage in Previously Untreated Patients

ORAL:

- Fixed combination with metformin hydrochloride: Initially, 1.25 mg of glyburide and 250 mg of metformin hydrochloride once daily. For severe hyperglycemia (baseline HbA_{1c} >9% or fasting blood glucose >200 mg/dL), 1.25 mg of glyburide and 250 mg of metformin hydrochloride *twice* daily, given with the morning and evening meals.

Initial Dosage in Patients Transferred from Other Oral Antidiabetic Agents

ORAL:

- Fixed combination with metformin hydrochloride: Initially, 2.5 or 5 mg of glyburide and 500 mg of metformin hydrochloride twice daily with morning and evening meals in patients not adequately controlled by monotherapy with glyburide (or another sulfonylurea) or metformin. For patients previously receiving combination therapy with glyburide (or another sulfonylurea) and metformin, initial dosage should not exceed previous individual dosages of glyburide (or equivalent dosage of another sulfonylurea) and metformin. Titrate in increments ≤5 mg of glyburide and 500 mg of metformin hydrochloride to achieve adequate blood glucose control.

Titration and Maintenance Dosage

ORAL:

- Fixed combination with metformin hydrochloride: Titrate in increments of 1.25 mg of glyburide and 250 mg of metformin hydrochloride daily at 2-week intervals to achieve adequate blood glucose control.

Prescribing Limits

Adult Patients

Fixed combination with metformin hydrochloride: Maximum 20 mg of glyburide and 2 g of metformin hydrochloride daily.

Special Populations

Geriatric Patients
- Fixed combination with metformin hydrochloride: Do not titrate to maximum recommended dosage.

Other Populations
- Cautious dosing recommended in debilitated or malnourished patients or in patients with adrenal or pituitary insufficiency.
- Fixed combination with metformin hydrochloride: Do not titrate to maximum recommended dosage.

Glycopyrrolate
(glye koe pye′ roe late)

Brand Name: Robinul®, Robinul® Forte
Also available generically.

Why is this medicine prescribed?

Glycopyrrolate is used in combination with other medications to treat ulcers. Glycopyrrolate is in a class of medications called anticholinergics. It decreases stomach acid production by blocking the activity of a certain natural substance in the body.

How should this medicine be used?

Glycopyrrolate comes as a tablet to take by mouth. It is usually taken 2 or 3 times a day. Follow the directions on your prescription label carefully, and ask your doctor or pharmacist to explain any part you do not understand. Take glycopyrrolate exactly as directed. Do not take more or less of it or take it more often than prescribed by your doctor.

Are there other uses for this medicine?

This medication may be prescribed for other uses; ask your doctor or pharmacist for more information.

What special precautions should I follow?

Before taking glycopyrrolate,

- tell your doctor and pharmacist if you are allergic to glycopyrrolate or any other medications.
- tell your doctor and pharmacist what prescription and nonprescription medications, vitamins, nutritional supplements, and herbal products you are taking. Be sure to mention any of the following: anticholinergics; antidepressants; ipratropium (Atrovent); mediations for anxiety, irritable bowel disease, mental illness, motion sickness, Parkinson's disease, seizures, ulcers, or urinary problems; sedatives; sleeping pills; and tranquilizers. Your doctor may need to change the doses of your medications or monitor you carefully for side effects.
- tell your doctor if you have or have ever had glaucoma; enlargement of the prostate (benign prostatic hypertrophy), ulcerative colitis, myasthenia gravis, gastrointestinal disease, overactive thyoid (hyperthyroidism), high blood pressure, heart failure, irregular or rapid heartbeats, coronary artery disease, hiatal hernia with reflux, disorders of the nervous system, or kidney or liver disease.
- tell your doctor if you are pregnant, plan to become pregnant, or are breast-feeding. If you become pregnant while taking glycopyrrolate, call your doctor.
- if you are having surgery, including dental surgery, tell the doctor or dentist that you are taking glycopyrrolate.

- you should know that glycopyrrolate may make you drowsy or cause blurred vision. Do not drive a car or operate machinery until you know how this medication affects you.
- remember that alcohol can add to the drowsiness caused by this medication.
- you should know that glycopyrrolate reduces the body's ability to cool off by sweating. In very high temperatures, glycopyrrolate can cause fever and heat stroke.

What special dietary instructions should I follow?

Unless your doctor tells you otherwise, continue your normal diet.

What should I do if I forget to take a dose?

Take the missed dose as soon as you remember it. However, if it is almost time for the next dose, skip the missed dose and continue your regular dosing schedule. Do not take a double dose to make up for a missed one.

What side effects can this medicine cause?

Glycopyrrolate may cause side effects. Tell your doctor if any of these symptoms are severe or do not go away:

- dry mouth
- decreased sweating
- difficulty urinating
- blurred vision
- vision problems
- loss of taste
- headaches
- nervousness
- confusion
- drowsiness
- weakness
- dizziness
- difficulty falling asleep or staying asleep
- upset stomach
- vomiting
- constipation
- bloated feeling

Some side effects can be serious. The following symptoms are uncommon, but if you experience any of them, call your doctor immediately:

- diarrhea
- rash or hives
- difficulty breathing or swallowing

Glycopyrrolate may cause other side effects. Call your doctor if you have any unusual problems while taking this medication.

If you experience a serious side effect, you or your doctor may send a report to the Food and Drug Administration's (FDA) MedWatch Adverse Event Reporting program online [at http://www.fda.gov/MedWatch/index.html] or by phone [1-800-332-1088].

What storage conditions are needed for this medicine?

Keep this medication in the container it came in, tightly closed, and out of reach of children. Store it at room temperature and away from excess heat and moisture (not in the bathroom). Throw away any medication that is outdated or no longer needed. Talk to your pharmacist about the proper disposal of your medication.

What should I do in case of overdose?

In case of overdose, call your local poison control center at 1-800-222-1222. If the victim has collapsed or is not breathing, call local emergency services at 911.

What other information should I know?

Keep all appointments with your doctor.

Do not let anyone else take your medication. Ask your pharmacist any questions you have about refilling your prescription.

Dosage Facts
For Informational Purposes

Caution: Do not change your dose, how often you take your medication, or the length of time you are to take it without first talking to your healthcare provider.

The following dosage information was written using medical language for doctors and other healthcare professionals and is provided here for you to check your dosage. The dosage of this drug may differ for different patients. Therefore, always follow your doctor's instructions or the directions on the label. Contact your healthcare provider or pharmacist if you have any questions about the specific dosage of your medication after reviewing this information.

Adult Patients

Peptic Ulcer Disease

ORAL:
- Initially, 1 mg 3 times daily (morning, early afternoon, and bedtime); may increase bedtime dose to 2 mg if needed to control overnight symptoms.
- Alternatively, 2 mg given 2 or 3 times daily at equally spaced intervals.
- Maintenance dosage of 1 mg twice daily is adequate in most adults.

Prescribing Limits
Adult Patients

Peptic Ulcer Disease

ORAL:
- Maximum 8 mg daily.

Special Populations

Renal Impairment
- Dosage reduction may be necessary.

Geriatric Patients
- Select dosage with caution because of age-related decreases in hepatic, renal, and/or cardiac function and concomitant disease and drug therapy.

Granisetron

(gra ni′ se tron)

Brand Name: Kytril®

Why is this medicine prescribed?

Granisetron is used to prevent nausea and vomiting caused by cancer chemotherapy and radiation therapy. Granisetron is in a class of medications called 5-HT$_3$ antagonists. It works by blocking serotonin, a natural substance in the body that causes nausea and vomiting.

How should this medicine be used?

Granisetron comes as a tablet and a solution (liquid) to take by mouth. When taken to prevent nausea and vomiting caused by chemotherapy, granisetron is usually taken 1 hour before chemotherapy is begun. A second dose may be taken 12 hours after the first dose. When taken to prevent nausea and vomiting caused by radiation, granisetron is usually taken within 1 hour before treatment. Follow the directions on your prescription label carefully, and ask your doctor or pharmacist to explain any part you do not understand. Take granisetron exactly as directed. Do not take more or less of it or take it more often than prescribed by your doctor.

Are there other uses for this medicine?

This medication may be prescribed for other uses; ask your doctor or pharmacist for more information.

What special precautions should I follow?

Before taking granisetron,
- tell your doctor and pharmacist if you are allergic to granisetron, dolasetron (Anzemet), ondansetron, (Zofran), or any other medications.
- tell your doctor and pharmacist what prescription and nonprescription medications, vitamins, nutritional supplements, and herbal products you are taking. Be sure to mention ketoconazole (Nizoral). Your doctor may need to change the doses of your medications or monitor you carefully for side effects.
- tell your doctor if you are pregnant, plan to become pregnant, or are breast-feeding. If you become pregnant while taking granisetron, call your doctor.

What special dietary instructions should I follow?

Unless your doctor tells you otherwise, continue your normal diet.

What should I do if I forget to take a dose?

Granisetron should only be taken before chemotherapy or radiation therapy, as instructed by your doctor. It should not be taken on a regularly scheduled basis.

What side effects can this medicine cause?

Granisetron may cause side effects. Tell your doctor if any of these symptoms are severe or do not go away:
- headache
- weakness
- stomach pain
- heartburn
- constipation
- diarrhea
- pain
- dizziness
- drowsiness
- difficulty falling asleep or staying asleep
- nervousness
- cough
- fever

Some side effects can be serious. The following symptoms are uncommon, but if you experience any of them, call your doctor immediately:
- hives
- skin rash
- itching
- difficulty breathing or swallowing
- fainting
- blurred vision

Granisetron may cause other side effects. Call your doctor if you have any unusual problems while taking this medication.

If you experience a serious side effect, you or your doctor may send a report to the Food and Drug Administration's (FDA) MedWatch Adverse Event Reporting program online [at http://www.fda.gov/MedWatch/index.html] or by phone [1-800-332-1088].

What storage conditions are needed for this medicine?

Keep this medication in the container it came in, tightly closed, and out of reach of children. Store it at room temperature and away from excess heat and moisture (not in the bathroom). Throw away any medication that is outdated or no longer needed. Talk to your pharmacist about the proper disposal of your medication.

What should I do in case of overdose?

In case of overdose, call your local poison control center at 1-800-222-1222. If the victim has collapsed or is not breathing, call local emergency services at 911.

Symptoms of overdose may include:

- headache

What other information should I know?

Keep all appointments with your doctor.

Do not let anyone else take your medication. Ask your pharmacist any questions you have about refilling your prescription.

Dosage Facts
For Informational Purposes

Caution: Do not change your dose, how often you take your medication, or the length of time you are to take it without first talking to your healthcare provider.

The following dosage information was written using medical language for doctors and other healthcare professionals and is provided here for you to check your dosage. The dosage of this drug may differ for different patients. Therefore, always follow your doctor's instructions or the directions on the label. Contact your healthcare provider or pharmacist if you have any questions about the specific dosage of your medication after reviewing this information.

General Dosage Information

Available as granisetron hydrochloride; dosage expressed in terms of granisetron.

Adult Patients

Cancer Chemotherapy-induced Nausea and Vomiting
Prevention

ORAL:

- 2 mg once daily up to 1 hour before administration of chemotherapy.
- Alternatively, 1 mg twice daily (first dose up to 1 hour before chemotherapy and second dose 12 hours after first dose).

Radiation-induced Nausea and Vomiting
Prevention

ORAL:

- 2 mg once daily within 1 hour of radiation.

Special Populations

Hepatic Impairment
- No dosage adjustment required.

Geriatric Patients
- No dosage adjustment required.

Granisetron Hydrochloride Injection
(gra ni′ se tron)

Brand Name: Kytril®

About Your Treatment

Your doctor has ordered granisetron to prevent nausea and vomiting caused by cancer chemotherapy. The drug will be added to an intravenous fluid that will drip through a needle or catheter placed in your vein for at least 5 minutes, about a half-hour before chemotherapy administration. This medication is sometimes prescribed for other uses; ask your doctor or pharmacist for more information.

Your health care provider (doctor, nurse, or pharmacist) may measure the effectiveness and side effects of your treatment using laboratory tests and physical examinations. It is important to keep all appointments with your doctor and the laboratory. The length of treatment depends on how you respond to the medication.

Precautions

Before administering granisetron,

- tell your doctor and pharmacist if you are allergic to granisetron or any other drugs.
- tell your doctor and pharmacist what prescription and nonprescription medications you are taking, including vitamins.
- tell your doctor if you are pregnant, plan to become pregnant, or are breast-feeding. If you become pregnant while taking granisetron, call your doctor.

Administering Your Medication

Before you administer granisetron, look at the solution closely. It should be clear and free of floating material. Gently squeeze the bag or observe the solution container to make sure there are no leaks. Do not use the solution if it is discolored, if it contains particles, or if the bag or container leaks. Use a new solution, but show the damaged one to your health care provider.

It is important that you use your medication exactly as directed. Do not change your dosing schedule without talking to your health care provider. Your health care provider may tell you to stop your infusion if you have a mechanical problem (such as a blockage in the tubing, needle, or catheter); if you have to stop an infusion, call your health care provider immediately so your therapy can continue.

Side Effects

Granisetron may cause side effects. Tell your health care provider if any of these symptoms are severe or do not go away:

- headache
- dizziness
- weakness
- drowsiness
- stomach pain
- constipation
- diarrhea

If you experience any of the following symptoms, call your health care provider immediately:

- chest pain
- irregular heartbeat
- trouble breathing
- fainting spells
- rash

If you experience a serious side effect, you or your doctor may send a report to the Food and Drug Administration's (FDA) MedWatch Adverse Event Reporting program online [at http://www.fda.gov/MedWatch/index.html] or by phone [1-800-332-1088].

Storage Conditions

- Your health care provider probably will give you a several-day supply of granisetron at a time. You will be told to store it at room temperature.

Store your medication only as directed. Make sure you understand what you need to store your medication properly.

Keep your supplies in a clean, dry place when you are not using them, and keep all medications and supplies out of reach of children. Your health care provider will tell you how to throw away used needles, syringes, tubing, and containers to avoid accidental injury.

Overdose

In case of overdose, call your local poison control center at 1-800-222-1222. If the victim has collapsed or is not breathing, call local emergency services at 911.

Signs of Infection

If you are receiving granisetron in your vein or under your skin, you need to know the symptoms of a catheter-related infection (an infection where the needle enters your vein or skin). If you experience any of these effects near your intravenous catheter, tell your health care provider as soon as possible:

- tenderness
- warmth
- irritation
- drainage
- redness
- swelling

Dosage Facts
For Informational Purposes

Caution: Do not change your dose, how often you take your medication, or the length of time you are to take it without first talking to your healthcare provider.

The following dosage information was written using medical language for doctors and other healthcare professionals and is provided here for you to check your dosage. The dosage of this drug may differ for different patients. Therefore, always follow your doctor's instructions or the directions on the label. Contact your healthcare provider or pharmacist if you have any questions about the specific dosage of your medication after reviewing this information.

General Dosage Information

Available as granisetron hydrochloride; dosage expressed in terms of granisetron.

Pediatric Patients

Cancer Chemotherapy-induced Nausea and Vomiting
Prevention

IV:
- Children 2–16 years of age: 10 mcg/kg by IV infusion or direct IV injection within 30 minutes before administration of chemotherapy.

Adult Patients

Cancer Chemotherapy-induced Nausea and Vomiting
Prevention

IV:
- 10 mcg/kg by IV infusion or direct IV injection within 30 minutes before administration of chemotherapy.

Postoperative Nausea and Vomiting
Prevention

IV:
- 1 mg as a single dose by direct IV injection before induction of or immediately before reversal of anesthesia.

Treatment

IV:
- 1 mg as a single dose by direct IV injection.

Radiation-induced Nausea and Vomiting

Special Populations

Hepatic Impairment
- No dosage adjustment required.

Geriatric Patients
- No dosage adjustment required.

Griseofulvin

(gri see oh ful′ vin)

Brand Name: Fulvicin-U/F®, Grifulvin V®, Gris-PEG®

Why is this medicine prescribed?

Griseofulvin is used to treat skin infections such as jock itch, athlete's foot, and ringworm; and fungal infections of the scalp, fingernails, and toenails.

This medication is sometimes prescribed for other uses; ask your doctor or pharmacist for more information.

How should this medicine be used?

Griseofulvin comes as a tablet, capsule, and liquid to take by mouth. It is usually taken once a day or can be taken two to four times a day. Although your symptoms may get better in a few days, you will have to take griseofulvin for a long time before the infection is completely gone. It is usually taken for 2 to 4 weeks for skin infections, 4 to 6 weeks for hair and scalp infections, 4 to 8 weeks for foot infections, 3 to 4 months for fingernail infections, and at least 6 months for toenail infections. Follow the directions on your prescription label carefully, and ask your doctor or pharmacist to explain any part you do not understand. Take griseofulvin exactly as directed. Do not take more or less of it or take it more often than prescribed by your doctor.

Shake the liquid well before each use to mix the medication evenly.

Continue to take griseofulvin even if you feel well. Do not stop taking griseofulvin without talking to your doctor.

What special precautions should I follow?

Before taking griseofulvin,

- tell your doctor and pharmacist if you are allergic to griseofulvin, penicillin, or any other drugs.
- tell your doctor and pharmacist what prescription and nonprescription medications you are taking, especially anticoagulants ('blood thinners') such as warfarin (Coumadin), oral contraceptives, cyclosporine (Neoral, Sandimmune), phenobarbital (Luminal), and vitamins.
- tell your doctor if you have or have ever had liver disease, porphyria, lupus, or a history of alcohol abuse.
- tell your doctor if you are pregnant, plan to become pregnant, or are breast-feeding. If you become pregnant while taking griseofulvin, call your doctor.
- tell your doctor if you drink alcohol.
- you should plan to avoid unnecessary or prolonged exposure to sunlight and to wear protective clothing, sunglasses, and sunscreen. Griseofulvin may make your skin sensitive to sunlight.

What should I do if I forget to take a dose?

Take the missed dose as soon as you remember it. However, if it is almost time for the next dose, skip the missed dose and continue your regular dosing schedule. Do not take a double dose to make up for a missed one.

What side effects can this medicine cause?

Griseofulvin may cause side effects. Tell your doctor if any of these symptoms are severe or do not go away:

- headache
- upset stomach
- vomiting
- diarrhea or loose stools
- thirst
- fatigue
- dizziness
- faintness

If you experience any of the following symptoms, call your doctor immediately:

- fever
- sore throat
- skin rash
- mouth soreness or irritation

If you experience a serious side effect, you or your doctor may send a report to the Food and Drug Administration's (FDA) MedWatch Adverse Event Reporting program online [at http://www.fda.gov/MedWatch/index.html] or by phone [1-800-332-1088].

What storage conditions are needed for this medicine?

Keep this medication in the container it came in, tightly closed, and out of reach of children. Store it at room temperature and away from excess heat and moisture (not in the bathroom). Keep the liquid away from light. Do not freeze. Throw away any medication that is outdated or no longer needed. Talk to your pharmacist about the proper disposal of your medication.

What should I do in case of overdose?

In case of overdose, call your local poison control center at 1-800-222-1222. If the victim has collapsed or is not breathing, call local emergency services at 911.

What other information should I know?

Keep all appointments with your doctor and the laboratory. Your doctor will order certain lab tests to check your response to griseofulvin.

Do not let anyone else take your medication. Ask your pharmacist any questions you have about refilling your prescription. If you still have symptoms of infection after you finish the griseofulvin, call your doctor.

Dosage Facts
For Informational Purposes

Caution: Do not change your dose, how often you take your medication, or the length of time you are to take it without first talking to your healthcare provider.

The following dosage information was written using medical language for doctors and other healthcare professionals and is provided here for you to check your dosage. The dosage of this drug may differ for different patients. Therefore, always follow your doctor's instructions or the directions on the label. Contact your healthcare provider or pharmacist if you have any questions about the specific dosage of your medication after reviewing this information.

General Dosage Information

Dosage varies depending on whether the drug is administered as griseofulvin microsize (Grifulvin V®) or griseofulvin ultramicrosize (Gris-PEG®).

Dosage and duration of treatment should be individualized according to the requirements and response of the patient. Griseofulvin generally should be continued for ≥4–12 weeks for treatment of tinea capitis; ≥2–4 weeks for treatment of tinea corporis; ≥4–8 weeks for tinea pedis; and from 4–6 months to a year or longer for tinea unguium.

Pediatric Patients

Dermatophytoses
Microsize (Grifulvin V®)

ORAL:
- 10–11 mg/kg daily, although dosages up to 20–25 mg/kg daily have been used.
- Manufacturer suggests that those weighing approximately 14–23 kg may receive 125–250 mg daily and that those weighing >23 kg may receive 250–500 mg daily.
- AAP recommends 10–20 mg/kg (maximum 1 g) daily in 1 or 2 doses. For tinea capitis, AAP recommends 15–20 mg/kg once daily.

Ultramicrosize (Gris-PEG®)

ORAL:
- Children >2 years of age: Usually 7.3 mg/kg daily, although dosages up to 10–15 mg/kg daily have been used.
- Manufacturer suggests that those weighing approximately 16–27 kg may receive 125–187.5 mg daily and those weighing >27 kg may receive 187.5–375 mg daily.
- AAP recommends 5–10 mg/kg (maximum 750 mg) once daily.

Adult Patients

Dermatophytoses
Microsize (Grifulvin V®)

ORAL:
- 500 mg daily for treatment of tinea capitis, tinea corporis, or tinea cruris. For more difficult infections (e.g., tinea pedis, tinea unguium), 1 g daily.

Ultramicrosize (Gris-PEG®)

ORAL:
- 375 mg once daily or in divided doses for treatment of tinea capitis, tinea corporis, or tinea cruris. For more difficult infections (e.g., tinea pedis, tinea unguium), 750 mg daily given in divided doses.

Guaifenesin
(gwye fen′ e sin)

Brand Name: Diabetic Tussin® EX, Ganidin® NR, Gani-Tuss® NR, Guaifenesin AC® Liquid, Guiatuss® Syrup, Humibid® Pediatric, Hytuss®, Hytuss-2X®, Mucinex®, Naldecon® Senior EX, Organidin® NR, Phanasin® Diabetic Choice®, Robitussin®, X-Pect®
Also available generically.

Why is this medicine prescribed?

Guaifenesin thins the mucus in the air passages and makes it easier to cough up the mucus and clear the airways, allowing you to breathe more easily. It relieves the coughs of colds, bronchitis, and other lung infections.

This medication is sometimes prescribed for other uses; ask your doctor or pharmacist for more information.

How should this medicine be used?

Guaifenesin comes as a regular and extended-release (long-acting) tablet and capsule and liquid to take by mouth. Follow the directions on the package or on your prescription label carefully, and ask your doctor or pharmacist to explain any part you do not understand. Take guaifenesin exactly as directed. Do not take more or less of it or take it more often than prescribed by your doctor.

Do not break, crush, or chew extended-release tablets and do not open extended-release capsules; swallow them whole.

Drink plenty of fluid while taking this medication (unless your doctor has directed you to limit the amount of fluid you drink). Guaifenesin comes alone and in combination with antihistamines, cough suppressants, and decongestants. Ask your doctor or pharmacist for advice on which form is best for your symptoms.

If your symptoms do not improve within 7 days or if you have a high fever, rash, or persistent headache, call your doctor.

What special precautions should I follow?

Before taking guaifenesin,
- tell your doctor and pharmacist if you are allergic to guaifenesin or any other drugs.

- tell your doctor and pharmacist what prescription and nonprescription medications you are taking, including vitamins.
- tell your doctor if you have or have ever had high blood pressure, heart disease, thyroid disease, or diabetes.
- tell your doctor if you are pregnant, plan to become pregnant, or are breast-feeding. If you become pregnant while taking guaifenesin, call your doctor.

What should I do if I forget to take a dose?

Take the missed dose as soon as you remember it. However, if it is almost time for the next dose, skip the missed dose and continue your regular dosing schedule. Do not take a double dose to make up for a missed one.

What side effects can this medicine cause?

Guaifenesin may cause side effects. Tell your doctor if any of these symptoms are severe or do not go away:
- headache
- upset stomach
- vomiting

What storage conditions are needed for this medicine?

Keep this medication in the container it came in, tightly closed, and out of reach of children. Store it at room temperature and away from excess heat and moisture (not in the bathroom). Throw away any medication that is outdated or no longer needed. Talk to your pharmacist about the proper disposal of your medication.

What should I do in case of overdose?

In case of overdose, call your local poison control center at 1-800-222-1222. If the victim has collapsed or is not breathing, call local emergency services at 911.

What other information should I know?

Keep all appointments with your doctor.

Do not let anyone else take your medication. Ask your pharmacist any questions you have about refilling your prescription.

Dosage Facts
For Informational Purposes

Caution: Do not change your dose, how often you take your medication, or the length of time you are to take it without first talking to your healthcare provider.

The following dosage information was written using medical language for doctors and other healthcare professionals and is provided here for you to check your dosage. The dosage of this drug may differ for different patients. Therefore, always follow your doctor's instruc-

tions or the directions on the label. Contact your healthcare provider or pharmacist if you have any questions about the specific dosage of your medication after reviewing this information.

Pediatric Patients

Cough

ORAL:
- Children <2 years of age: Individualize dosage.
- Children 2 to <6 years of age, conventional preparations: 50–100 mg every 4 hours, up to 600 mg daily.
- Children 2–6 years of age, extended-release preparations: 300 mg every 12 hours, up to 600 mg daily.
- Children 6 to <12 years of age, conventional preparations: 100–200 mg every 4 hours, up to 1.2 g daily.
- Children 6–12 years of age, extended-release preparations: 600 mg every 12 hours, up to 1.2 g daily.
- Children ≥12 years of age, conventional preparations: 200–400 mg every 4 hours, up to 2.4 g daily.
- Children ≥12 years of age, 600-mg extended-release tablets: 600 mg or 1.2 g every 12 hours, up to 2.4 g daily.

Adult Patients

Cough

ORAL:
- Conventional preparations: 200–400 mg every 4 hours, up to 2.4 g daily.
- 600-mg extended-release tablets: 600 mg or 1.2 g every 12 hours, up to 2.4 g daily.

Prescribing Limits
Pediatric Patients

Cough

ORAL:
- Children 2 to <6 years of age, conventional preparations: Maximum 600 mg daily.
- Children 2–6 years of age, extended-release preparations: Maximum 600 mg daily.
- Children 6 to <12 years of age, conventional preparations: Maximum 1.2 g daily.
- Children 6–12 years of age, extended-release preparations: Maximum 1.2 g daily.
- Children ≥12 years of age, conventional preparations: Maximum 2.4 g daily.
- Children ≥12 years of age, extended-release preparations: Maximum 2.4 g daily.

Adult Patients

Cough

ORAL:
- Conventional preparations: Maximum 2.4 g daily.
- Extended-release preparations: Maximum 2.4 g daily.

Haemophilus influenzae type b Vaccine

Brand Name: Liquid Pedvax HIB®, TriHIBit®, Comvax®, ActHIB®, HibTITER®

What is Hib disease?

Haemophilus influenzae type b (Hib) disease is a serious disease caused by a bacteria. It usually strikes children under 5 years old.

Your child can get Hib disease by being around other children or adults who may have the bacteria and not know it. The germs spread from person to person. If the germs stay in the child's nose and throat, the child probably will not get sick. But sometimes the germs spread into the lungs or the bloodstream, and then Hib can cause serious problems.

Before Hib vaccine, Hib disease was the leading cause of bacterial meningitis among children under 5 years old in the United States. Meningitis is an infection of the brain and spinal cord coverings, which can lead to lasting brain damage and deafness. Hib disease can also cause:

- pneumonia
- severe swelling in the throat, making it hard to breathe
- infections of the blood, joints, bones, and covering of the heart
- death

Before Hib vaccine, about 20,000 children in the United States under 5 years old got severe Hib disease each year and nearly 1,000 people died. Hib vaccine can prevent Hib disease. Many more children would get Hib disease if we stopped vaccinating.

Who should get Hib vaccine and when?

Children should get Hib vaccine at: 2 months of age, 6 months of age (depending on what brand of Hib vaccine is used, your child might not need the dose at 6 months of age. Your doctor or nurse will tell you if this dose is needed), 4 months of age, and 12-15 months of age.

If you miss a dose or get behind schedule, get the next dose as soon as you can. There is no need to start over. Hib vaccine may be given at the same time as other vaccines.

Children over 5 years old usually do not need Hib vaccine. But some older children or adults with special health conditions should get it. These conditions include sickle cell disease, HIV/AIDS, removal of the spleen, bone marrow transplant, or cancer treatment with drugs. Ask your doctor or nurse for details.

Who should *not* get Hib vaccine or should wait?

- People who have ever had a life-threatening allergic reaction to a previous dose of Hib vaccine should not get another dose.
- Children less than 6 weeks of age should not get Hib vaccine.
- People who are moderately or severely ill at the time the shot is scheduled should usually wait until they recover before getting Hib vaccine.

Ask your doctor or nurse for more information.

What are the risks from Hib vaccine?

A vaccine, like any medicine, is capable of causing serious problems, such as severe allergic reactions. The risk of Hib vaccine causing serious harm or death is extremely small.

Most people who get Hib vaccine do not have any problems with it.

Mild Problems:

- Redness, warmth, or swelling where the shot was given (up to 1/4 of children)
- Fever over 101°F (up to 1 out of 20 children)
- If these problems happen, they usually start within a day of vaccination. They may last 2-3 days.

What if there is a moderate or severe reaction?

What should I look for?

- Any unusual condition, such as a serious allergic reaction, high fever or behavior changes. Signs of a serious allergic reaction can include difficulty breathing, hoarseness or wheezing, hives, paleness, weakness, a fast heart beat, or dizziness within a few minutes to a few hours after the shot.

What should I do?

- Call a doctor, or get the person to a doctor right away.
- Tell your doctor what happened, the date and time it happened, and when the vaccination was given.
- Ask your health care provider to file a Vaccine Adverse Event Reporting System (VAERS) form if you have any reaction to the vaccine. Or call VAERS yourself at 1-800-822-7967, or visit their website at http://vaers.hhs.gov.

The National Vaccine Injury Compensation Program

In the rare event that you or your child has a serious reaction to a vaccine, a federal program has been created to help pay for the care of those who have been harmed.

For details about the National Vaccine Injury Compensation Program, call 1-800-338-2382 or visit the program's website at http://www.hrsa.gov/vaccinecompensation.

How can I learn more?

- Ask your doctor or other health care provider. They can give you the vaccine package insert or suggest other sources of information.
- Call your local or state health department's immunization program.
- Contact the Centers for Disease Control and Prevention (CDC): call 1-800-232-4636 (1-800-CDC-INFO) or visit the National Immunization Program's website at http://www.cdc.gov/nip.

Haemophilus influenzae type b (Hib) Vaccine Information Statement. U.S. Department of Health and Human Services/Centers for Disease Control and Prevention National Immunization Program. 12/16/1998.

Halcinonide Topical

(hal sin′ oh nide)

Brand Name: Halog®, Halog®-E

Why is this medicine prescribed?

Halcinonide is used to treat the itching, redness, dryness, crusting, scaling, inflammation, and discomfort of various skin conditions.

This medication is sometimes prescribed for other uses; ask your doctor or pharmacist for more information.

How should this medicine be used?

Halcinonide comes in ointment, cream, and liquid in various strengths for use on the skin. It is usually applied two or three times a day. Follow the directions on your prescription label carefully, and ask your doctor or pharmacist to explain any part you do not understand. Use halcinonide exactly as directed. Do not use more or less of it or use it more often than prescribed by your doctor. Do not apply it to other areas of your body or wrap or bandage the treated area unless directed to do so by your doctor.

Wash or soak the affected area thoroughly before applying the medicine, unless it irritates your skin. Then apply the ointment, cream, or liquid sparingly in a thin film and rub it in gently.

To use the liquid on your scalp, part your hair, apply a small amount of the medicine on the affected area, and rub it in gently. Protect the area from washing and rubbing until the liquid dries. You may wash your hair as usual but not right after applying this medicine.

Avoid prolonged use on the face, in the genital or rectal areas, and in skin creases and armpits unless directed by your doctor.

If you are using halcinonide on your face, keep it out of your eyes.

If you are using halcinonide on a child's diaper area, do not use tight-fitting diapers or plastic pants. Such use may increase side effects.

Do not apply cosmetics or other skin preparations on the treated area without talking to your doctor.

If your doctor tells you to wrap or bandage the treated area, follow these instructions:

1. Soak the area in water or wash it well.
2. While the skin is moist, gently rub the medication into the affected areas.
3. Cover the area with plastic wrap (such as Saran Wrap or Handi-Wrap). The plastic may be held in place with a gauze or elastic bandage or adhesive tape on the normal skin beside the treated area. (Instead of using plastic wrap, plastic gloves may be used for the hands, plastic bags for the feet, or a shower cap for the scalp.)
4. Carefully seal the edges of the plastic to make sure the wrap adheres closely to the skin. If the affected area is moist, you can leave the edges of the plastic wrap partly unsealed or puncture the wrap to allow excess moisture to escape.
5. Leave the plastic wrap in place as long as instructed by your doctor. Usually plastic wraps are left in place no more than 12 hours each day.
6. Cleanse the skin and reapply the medication each time a new plastic wrapping is applied. Notify your doctor if the treated area gets worse or if burning, swelling, redness, or oozing of pus develops.

Do not discontinue treatment abruptly without talking to your doctor.

What special precautions should I follow?

Before using halcinonide,

- tell your doctor and pharmacist if you are allergic to halcinonide or any other drugs.
- tell your doctor and pharmacist what prescription and nonprescription medications you are taking, especially cancer chemotherapy agents, other topical medications, and vitamins.
- tell your doctor if you have an infection or have ever had diabetes, glaucoma, cataracts, a circulation disorder, or an immune disorder.
- tell your doctor if you are pregnant, plan to become pregnant, or are breast-feeding. If you become pregnant while using halcinonide, call your doctor immediately.

What should I do if I forget to take a dose?

Apply the missed dose as soon as you remember it. However, if it is almost time for the next dose, skip the missed dose and continue your regular dosing schedule. Do not apply a double dose to make up for a missed one.

What side effects can this medicine cause?

Halcinonide may cause side effects. Tell your doctor if any of these symptoms are severe or do not go away:

- drying or cracking of the skin
- acne
- itching
- burning
- change in skin color

If you experience any of the following symptoms, call your doctor immediately:

- severe skin rash
- difficulty breathing or swallowing
- wheezing
- skin infection (redness, swelling, or oozing pus)

If you experience a serious side effect, you or your doctor may send a report to the Food and Drug Administration's (FDA) MedWatch Adverse Event Reporting program online [at http://www.fda.gov/MedWatch/index.html] or by phone [1-800-332-1088].

What storage conditions are needed for this medicine?

Keep this medication in the container it came in, tightly closed, and out of reach of children. Store it at room temperature and away from excess heat. Do not allow it to freeze. Throw away any medication that is outdated or no longer needed. Do not use it to treat other skin conditions. Talk to your pharmacist about the proper disposal of your medication.

What other information should I know?

Keep all appointments with your doctor.

Do not let anyone else use your medication. Ask your pharmacist any questions you have about refilling your prescription.

Talk to your doctor, pharmacist, or other healthcare professional if you have questions about dosing information for your medication.

Halobetasol

(hal oh bay' ta sol)

Brand Name: Ultravate®

Why is this medicine prescribed?

Halobetasol is used to treat swelling, inflammation, and itching associated with skin conditions such as eczema, dermatitis, rashes, insect bites, poison ivy, and allergies.

This medication is sometimes prescribed for other uses; ask your doctor or pharmacist for more information.

How should this medicine be used?

Halobetasol comes in ointment and cream for use on the skin. Halobetasol usually is used two to four times a day. Halobetasol should not be used for longer than 2 weeks. Follow the directions on your prescription label carefully, and ask your doctor or pharmacist to explain any part you do not understand. Use halobetasol exactly as directed. Do not use more or less of it or use it more often than prescribed by your doctor.

Thoroughly clean the infected area, allow it to dry, and then gently rub the medication in until most of it disappears. Use just enough medication to cover the affected area. You should wash your hands after applying the medication.

Do not use halobetasol if you have an infection or sores on the area to be treated.

What special precautions should I follow?

Before using halobetasol,

- tell your doctor and pharmacist if you are allergic to halobetasol or any other drugs.

- tell your doctor and pharmacist what prescription and nonprescription medications you are taking, especially skin products containing hydrocortisone.
- tell your doctor if you are pregnant, plan to become pregnant, or are breast-feeding. If you become pregnant while using halobetasol, call your doctor.

What should I do if I forget to take a dose?

Apply the missed dose as soon as you remember it. However, if it is almost time for the next dose, skip the missed dose and continue your regular dosing schedule. Do not apply a double dose to make up for a missed one.

What side effects can this medicine cause?

Halobetasol may cause side effects. Tell your doctor if any of these symptoms are severe or do not go away:
- burning
- stinging
- itching
- redness

What storage conditions are needed for this medicine?

Keep this medication in the container it came in, tightly closed, and out of reach of children. Store it at room temperature and away from excess heat and moisture (not in the bathroom). Throw away any medication that is outdated or no longer needed. Talk to your pharmacist about the proper disposal of your medication.

What other information should I know?

Keep all appointments with your doctor. Halobetasol is for external use only. Do not let halobetasol get into your eyes, nose, or mouth, and do not swallow it. Do not apply dressings, bandages, cosmetics, lotions, or other skin medications to the area being treated unless your doctor tells you.

Do not let anyone else use your medication. Ask your pharmacist any questions you have about refilling your prescription.

Tell your doctor if your skin condition gets worse or does not go away.

Talk to your doctor, pharmacist, or other healthcare professional if you have questions about dosing information for your medication.

Haloperidol Oral

(ha loe per′ i dole)

Brand Name: Haldol®, Haldol® Concentrate, Haloperidol Intensol®
Also available generically.

Why is this medicine prescribed?

Haloperidol is used to treat psychotic disorders and symptoms such as hallucinations, delusions, and hostility and to control muscular tics of the face, neck, hands, and shoulders. It is also used to treat severe behavioral problems in children and in hyperactive children (short-term use).

This medication is sometimes prescribed for other uses; ask your doctor or pharmacist for more information.

How should this medicine be used?

Haloperidol comes as a tablet and liquid concentrate to take by mouth. It usually is taken two or three times a day. Follow the directions on your prescription label carefully, and ask your doctor or pharmacist to explain any part you do not understand. Take haloperidol exactly as directed. Do not take more or less of it or take it more often than prescribed by your doctor.

The liquid concentrate must be diluted before use. It comes with a specially marked dropper for measuring the dose. Ask your pharmacist to show you how to use the dropper if you have difficulty. To dilute the liquid concentrate, add it to at least 2 ounces of milk, water, orange juice, or grapefruit juice just before you take it. If any beverage gets on the dropper, rinse the dropper with tap water before replacing it in the bottle. Do not allow the liquid concentrate to touch your skin or clothing; it can irritate your skin. If you spill the liquid concentrate on your skin, wash it off immediately with soap and water.

Continue to take haloperidol even if you feel well. Do not stop taking haloperidol without talking to your doctor, especially if you have taken large doses for a long time. Your doctor probably will decrease your dose gradually. This drug must be taken regularly for a few weeks before its full effect is felt.

Are there other uses for this medicine?

Haloperidol is also used to prevent and control nausea and vomiting. Talk to your doctor about the possible risks of using this drug for your condition.

What special precautions should I follow?

Before taking haloperidol,

- tell your doctor and pharmacist if you are allergic to haloperidol, aspirin, tartrazine (a yellow dye in some processed foods and drugs), or any other drugs.
- tell your doctor and pharmacist what prescription and nonprescription medications you are taking, especially antacids (Amphogel, Maalox), antihistamines, appetite reducers (amphetamines), benztropine (Cogentin), bromocriptine (Parlodel), carbamazepine (Tegretol), dicyclomine (Bentyl), fluoxetine (Prozac), guanethidine (Ismelin), lithium, meperidine (Demerol), methyldopa (Aldomet), phenytoin (Dilantin), propranolol (Inderal), sedatives, trihexyphenidyl (Artane), valproic acid (Depakane), medication for colds or depression, and vitamins.
- tell your doctor if you have or have ever had depression; seizures; shock therapy; allergies; asthma; emphysema; chronic bronchitis; problems with your urinary system or prostate; glaucoma; history of alcohol abuse; thyroid problems; bad reaction to insulin; angina; irregular heartbeat; problems with your blood pressure; blood disorders; or blood vessel, heart, kidney, liver, or lung disease.
- tell your doctor if you are pregnant, plan to become pregnant, or are breast-feeding. If you become pregnant while taking haloperidol, call your doctor.
- if you are having surgery, including dental surgery, tell the doctor or dentist that you are taking haloperidol.
- you should know that this drug may make you drowsy. Do not drive a car or operate machinery until you know how this drug affects you.
- remember that alcohol can add to the drowsiness caused by this drug.
- plan to avoid unnecessary or prolonged exposure to sunlight and to wear protective clothing, sunglasses, and sunscreen. Haloperidol may make your skin sensitive to sunlight.

What should I do if I forget to take a dose?

Take the missed dose as soon as you remember it and take any remaining doses for that day at evenly spaced intervals. However, if you remember a missed dose when it is almost time for your next scheduled dose, skip the missed dose. Do not take a double dose to make up for a missed one.

What side effects can this medicine cause?

Side effects from haloperidol are common. Your urine may turn pink or reddish-brown; this effect is not harmful. Tell your doctor if any of these symptoms are severe or do not go away:

- drowsiness
- dry mouth
- constipation
- restlessness
- headache
- weight gain

If you experience any of the following symptoms, call your doctor immediately:

- tremor
- restlessness or pacing
- fine worm-like tongue movements
- unusual face, mouth, or jaw movements

- shuffling walk
- slow, jerky movements
- seizures or convulsions
- fast, irregular, or pounding heartbeat
- difficulty urinating or loss of bladder control
- confusion
- eye pain or discoloration
- difficulty breathing or fast breathing
- fever
- skin rash
- severe muscle stiffness
- unusual tiredness or weakness
- unusual bleeding or bruising
- yellowing of the skin or eyes

If you experience a serious side effect, you or your doctor may send a report to the Food and Drug Administration's (FDA) MedWatch Adverse Event Reporting program online [at http://www.fda.gov/MedWatch/index.html] or by phone [1-800-332-1088].

What storage conditions are needed for this medicine?

Keep this medication in the container it came in, tightly closed, and out of reach of children. Store it at room temperature and away from excess heat and moisture (not in the bathroom). Protect the liquid from light. Throw away any medication that is outdated or no longer needed. Talk to your pharmacist about the proper disposal of your medication.

What should I do in case of overdose?

In case of overdose, call your local poison control center at 1-800-222-1222. If the victim has collapsed or is not breathing, call local emergency services at 911.

What other information should I know?

Keep all appointments with your doctor and the laboratory. Your doctor will order certain lab tests to check your response to haloperidol.

Do not let anyone else take your medication. Ask your pharmacist any questions you have about refilling your prescription.

Dosage Facts
For Informational Purposes

Caution: Do not change your dose, how often you take your medication, or the length of time you are to take it without first talking to your healthcare provider.

The following dosage information was written using medical language for doctors and other healthcare professionals and is provided here for you to check your dosage. The dosage of this drug may differ for different patients. Therefore, always follow your doctor's instructions or the directions on the label. Contact your healthcare provider or pharmacist if you have any questions about the specific dosage of your medication after reviewing this information.

General Dosage Information

Available as the base, decanoate (decanoic acid ester), and lactate salt; dosage is expressed in terms of haloperidol.

There is considerable interindividual variation in optimum dosage requirements; carefully adjust dosage according to individual requirements and response, using the lowest possible effective dosage.

Because of risk of adverse reactions associated with cumulative effects of butyrophenones, periodically evaluate patients with a history of long-term therapy with haloperidol and/or other antipsychotic agents to determine whether maintenance dosage can be decreased or drug therapy discontinued.

Pediatric Patients
Psychotic Disorders

ORAL:
- Children 3–12 years of age (weighing 15–40 kg): Initially, 0.5 mg daily given in 2 or 3 divided doses. Subsequent dosage may be increased by 0.5 mg daily at 5- to 7-day intervals, depending on the patient's tolerance and therapeutic response; usual dosage range is 0.05–0.15 mg/kg daily given in 2 or 3 divided doses.
- Severely disturbed psychotic children may require higher dosages.
- During prolonged maintenance therapy, keep dosage at the lowest possible effective level; once an adequate response has been achieved, gradually reduce dosage and make subsequent adjustments according to patient response and tolerance.

Tourette's Disorder

ORAL:
- Children 3–12 years of age (weighing 15–40 kg): Initially, 0.5 mg daily given in 2 or 3 divided doses. Subsequent dosage may be increased by 0.5 mg daily at 5- to 7-day intervals, depending on the patient's tolerance and therapeutic response; usual dosage range is 0.05–0.075 mg/kg daily given in 2 or 3 divided doses.
- Once an adequate response is achieved, gradually reduce dosage and make subsequent adjustments according to patient response and tolerance.

Disruptive Behavior Disorder and ADHD

ORAL:
- Children 3–12 years of age (weighing 15–40 kg): Initially, 0.5 mg daily given in 2 or 3 divided doses. Subsequent dosage may be increased by 0.5 mg daily at 5- to 7-day intervals, depending on the patient's tolerance and therapeutic response; usual dosage range is 0.05–0.075 mg/kg daily given in 2 or 3 divided doses.
- Non-psychotic or hyperactive behavioral problems in children may be acute, and short-term administration may be adequate.
- Maximum effective dosage for management of behavioral problems in children not established, but there is little evidence that improvement in behavior is further enhanced at dosages >6 mg daily.

Adult Patients

Psychotic Disorders
Moderate Symptomatology

ORAL:
- Initially, 0.5–2 mg 2 or 3 times daily. Carefully adjust subsequent dosage according to the patient's tolerance and therapeutic response. During prolonged maintenance therapy, keep dosage at lowest effective level.

Severe Symptomatology

ORAL:
- Initially, 3–5 mg 2 or 3 times daily.
- To achieve prompt control, higher dosages may be required in some patients. Patients who remain severely disturbed or inadequately controlled may require dosage adjustment.
- Dosages up to 100 mg daily may be required in some severely psychotic patients. Occasionally, dosages >100 mg daily have been used for the management of severely resistant disorders in adults; however, safety of prolonged administration of such dosages has not been demonstrated.

Chronic/Resistant Disorders

ORAL:
- Initially, 3–5 mg 2 or 3 times daily.
- Patients who remain severely disturbed or inadequately controlled may require dosage adjustment.
- Dosages up to 100 mg daily may be required in some severely psychotic patients. Occasionally, dosages >100 mg daily have been used for the management of severely resistant disorders in adults; however, safety of prolonged administration of such dosages has not been demonstrated.

Tourette's Disorder
Moderate Symptomatology

ORAL:
- Initially, 0.5–2 mg 2 or 3 times daily. Carefully adjust subsequent dosage according to patient's tolerance and therapeutic response.
- During prolonged maintenance therapy, keep dosage at lowest effective level.

Severe Symptomatology and/or Chronic/Resistant Patients

ORAL:
- Initially, 3–5 mg 2 or 3 times daily.
- Patients who remain inadequately controlled may require dosage adjustment.
- Dosages up to 100 mg daily may be required in some patients to achieve optimal response. Occasionally, dosages >100 mg daily have been used for management of severely resistant disorders in adults; however, safety of prolonged administration of such dosages has not been demonstrated.

Prescribing Limits
Pediatric Patients

ORAL:
- Maximum effective dosage not established, but there is little evidence that improvement in behavior is further enhanced at dosages >6 mg daily.

Adult Patients

ORAL:
- Safety of prolonged administration of dosages >100 mg not demonstrated.

Special Populations

Geriatric/Debilitated Patients
- In geriatric or debilitated patients, lower dosages may be required than those in younger adults; optimal response is usually obtained with more gradual dosage adjustments.
- Initially, 0.5–2 mg orally 2 or 3 times daily; increase dosage more gradually in debilitated, emaciated, or geriatric patients than in younger adults.

† Use is not currently included in the labeling approved by the US Food and Drug Administration.

Heparin Flush Injection 10 units/mL, 100 units/mL

(hep′ a rin)

Brand Name: HepFlush®-10, Hep-Lock® U/P, Hep-Pak® Lock Flush
Also available generically.

About Your Treatment

Your doctor has ordered heparin flush, an anticoagulant ('blood thinner'), to prevent the formation of clots that could block your intravenous (IV) catheter.

You will probably use heparin flush several times a day. Your health care provider will determine the number of heparin flushes you will need a day.

Precautions

Before administering heparin flush,
- tell your doctor and pharmacist if you are allergic to heparin, any other drugs, or pork products.
- tell your doctor and pharmacist what prescription and nonprescription medications you are taking, especially other blood thinners such as warfarin (Coumadin) and vitamins.
- tell your doctor if you have or have ever had liver disease or a bleeding disorder.
- tell your doctor if you are pregnant, plan to become pregnant, or are breast-feeding. If you become pregnant while taking heparin flush, call your doctor.
- if you are having surgery, including dental surgery, tell the doctor or dentist that you are taking heparin flush.

Administering Your Medication

Before you administer heparin flush, look at the solution closely. It should be clear and free of floating material. Do not use the solution if it is discolored or if it contains particles. Use a new solution, but show the damaged one to your health care provider.

It is important that you use your medication exactly as directed. Do not administer it more often than or for longer periods than your doctor tells you. Do not change your dosing schedule without talking to your health care provider. Your health care provider may tell you to stop the infusion if you have a mechanical problem (such as blockage in the tubing, needle or catheter); if you have to stop an infusion, call your health care provider immediately so your therapy can continue.

Side Effects

Heparin flush may cause side effects. Tell your doctor if the following symptom is severe or does not go away:

- irritation at the injection site

If you experience any of the following symptoms, call your doctor immediately:

- skin rash or peeling
- unusual bleeding or bruising
- blood in urine or stools

If you experience a serious side effect, you or your doctor may send a report to the Food and Drug Administration's (FDA) MedWatch Adverse Event Reporting program online [at http://www.fda.gov/MedWatch/index.html] or by phone [1-800-332-1088].

Storage Conditions

- Your health care provider will probably give you several days supply of heparin. You will be told how to prepare each dose.

Store your medication only as directed. Make sure you understand what you need to store your medication properly.

Keep your supplies in a clean, dry place when you are not using them, and keep all medications and supplies out of the reach of children. Your health care provider will tell you how to throw away used needles, syringes, tubing, and containers to avoid accidental injury.

Overdose

In case of overdose, call your local poison control center at 1-800-222-1222. If the victim has collapsed or is not breathing, call local emergency services at 911.

Signs of Infection

You need to know the symptoms of a catheter-related infection (an infection where the needle enters your vein or skin). If you experience any of these effects near your intravenous catheter, tell your health care provider as soon as possible:

- tenderness
- warmth
- irritation
- drainage
- redness

- swelling
- pain

Dosage Facts
For Informational Purposes

Caution: Do not change your dose, how often you take your medication, or the length of time you are to take it without first talking to your health-care provider.

The following dosage information was written using medical language for doctors and other healthcare professionals and is provided here for you to check your dosage. The dosage of this drug may differ for different patients. Therefore, always follow your doctor's instructions or the directions on the label. Contact your health-care provider or pharmacist if you have any questions about the specific dosage of your medication after reviewing this information.

General Dosage Information

Available as heparin sodium; dosage is expressed in terms of heparin sodium in USP units.

Adult Patients

Thrombosis Associated with Indwelling Venipuncture Devices

INTRACATHETER INSTILLATION:
- Inject a quantity of heparin lock flush solution (e.g., containing 10 or 100 units/mL) sufficient to fill the device after each use.

† Use is not currently included in the labeling approved by the US Food and Drug Administration.

Heparin Injection

(hep' a rin)

About Your Treatment

Your doctor has ordered heparin, a medication to thin your blood, to help prevent blood clots from forming in your body. Heparin may also be given to prevent blood clots that have already formed from getting any bigger. Heparin will be injected into a vein (intravenously) or under the skin (subcutaneously). Your doctor will decide the best dosing schedule for you.

You may receive heparin intravenously for 1 or 2 weeks, while subcutaneous injections may continue for up to 6 weeks or 6 months. This medication is sometimes prescribed for other uses; ask your doctor or pharmacist for more information.

Your health care provider (doctor, nurse, or pharmacist)

may measure the effectiveness and side effects of your treatment using laboratory tests and physical examinations. It is important to keep all appointments with your doctor and the laboratory. The length of treatment depends on how you respond to the medication.

Precautions

Before administering heparin,

- tell your doctor and pharmacist if you are allergic to heparin, pork products, or any other drugs.
- tell your doctor and pharmacist what prescription and nonprescription medications you are taking, especially aspirin, ibuprofen (Motrin), medications for headaches or pain, naproxen (Anaprox, Aleve), and vitamins.
- tell your doctor if you have or have ever had kidney disease or diabetes.
- tell your doctor if you are pregnant, plan to become pregnant, or are breast-feeding. If you become pregnant while taking heparin, call your doctor.

Administering Your Medication

Before you administer heparin, look at the solution closely. It should be clear and free of floating material. Gently squeeze the bag or observe the solution container to make sure there are no leaks. Do not use the solution if it is discolored, if it contains particles, or if the bag or container leaks. Use a new solution, but show the damaged one to your health care provider.

It is important that you use your medication exactly as directed. Do not change your dosing schedule without talking to your health care provider. Your health care provider may tell you to stop your infusion if you have a mechanical problem (such as a blockage in the tubing, needle, or catheter); if you have to stop an infusion, call your health care provider immediately so your therapy can continue.

Side Effects

Heparin may cause side effects. The most common side effect of heparin therapy is excessive bleeding (hemorrhage). If you experience any of the following symptoms, call your health care provider immediately:

- bleeding from the gums or nose
- unusually heavy menstrual bleeding
- excessive bleeding from cuts or wounds
- easy bruising
- purplish areas on the skin
- blood in urine or stools
- vomiting or coughing up blood
- chills
- fever
- itching
- rash

If you experience a serious side effect, you or your doctor may send a report to the Food and Drug Administration's (FDA) MedWatch Adverse Event Reporting program online

[at http://www.fda.gov/MedWatch/index.html] or by phone [1-800-332-1088].

Storage Conditions

- Your health care provider probably will give you several days supply of heparin. You will be directed to store it in a cool, clean, dry area.
- Do not allow heparin to freeze.

Store your medication only as directed. Make sure you understand what you need to store your medication properly.

Keep your supplies in a clean, dry place when you are not using them, and keep all medications and supplies out of reach of children. Your health care provider will tell you how to throw away used needles, syringes, tubing, and containers to avoid accidental injury.

Overdose

In case of overdose, call your local poison control center at 1-800-222-1222. If the victim has collapsed or is not breathing, call local emergency services at 911.

Signs of Infection

If you are receiving heparin in your vein or under your skin, you need to know the symptoms of a catheter-related infection (an infection where the needle enters your vein or skin). If you experience any of these effects near your intravenous catheter, tell your health care provider as soon as possible:

- tenderness
- warmth
- irritation
- drainage
- redness
- swelling
- pain

Dosage Facts
For Informational Purposes

Caution: Do not change your dose, how often you take your medication, or the length of time you are to take it without first talking to your healthcare provider.

The following dosage information was written using medical language for doctors and other healthcare professionals and is provided here for you to check your dosage. The dosage of this drug may differ for different patients. Therefore, always follow your doctor's instructions or the directions on the label. Contact your healthcare provider or pharmacist if you have any questions about the specific dosage of your medication after reviewing this information.

General Dosage Information

Available as heparin sodium; dosage is expressed in terms of heparin sodium in USP units.

Dosage requirements for full-dose therapy vary greatly among individuals; carefully individualize dosage based on the patient's weight and clinical and laboratory findings.

Pediatric Patients

Treatment of Venous Thrombosis and Pulmonary Embolism

IV:

- Neonates: Weight-based dosage sufficient to prolong the aPTT to a range that corresponds to an anti-factor X_a concentration of 0.35–0.7 units/mL. Initial treatment with unfractionated heparin sodium or low molecular weight heparin may be continued for 5–10 days; ACCP states that data are insufficient to make strong recommendations and that treatment should be individualized considering risks versus benefits. Follow-up with low molecular weight heparin for 10 days to 3 months. Convert to oral anticoagulation or initiate or resume therapy with a low molecular weight heparin if thrombus extends following discontinuance of IV heparin sodium.
- Neonates with unilateral renal vein thrombosis that extends into the inferior vena cava: Adjust dosage adjusted to prolong the aPTT to a range corresponding to an anti-factor X_a concentration of 0.35–0.7 unit/mL for 6 weeks to 3 months.
- Children >2 months of age with a first thromboembolic event: Adjust maintenance dosage to prolong the aPTT to a range corresponding to an anti-factor X_a concentration of 0.35–0.7 units/mL for 5–10 days. Massive or extensive venous thromboembolism may require a longer initial treatment period. Convert to warfarin therapy for follow-up oral anticoagulation.
- For full-dose IV heparin sodium therapy in children, some manufacturers recommend an initial loading dose of 50 units/kg followed by 100 units/kg every 4 hours by intermittent infusion or 20,000 units/m² per 24 hours by continuous IV infusion.
- For full-dose IV heparin sodium therapy in children, ACCP recommends a loading dose of 75–100 units/kg given over 10 minutes.
- Infants <1 year of age: An initial maintenance dosage of 28 units/kg per hour recommended by ACCP, with dosage adjusted to maintain an aPTT of 60–85 seconds (assuming this corresponds to an anti-factor X_a concentration of 0.35–0.7 units/mL).
- Children >1 year of age: An initial maintenance dosage of 20 units/kg per hour recommended by ACCP, with dosage adjusted to maintain an aPTT of 60–85 seconds (assuming this corresponds to an anti-factor X_a concentration of 0.35–0.7 units/mL).
- Weight-adjusted dosage required for older children is similar to that for adults (18 units/kg per hour).

Arterial Thromboembolism

IV:

- For neonates and children requiring cardiac catheterization via an artery: 100–150 units/kg by direct injection suggested; multiple doses may be required in prolonged procedures (>60 minutes).
- Neonates or children with femoral artery thrombosis associated with cardiac catheterization: 75–100 units/kg by direct injection, then 20–28 units/kg per hour depending on age for 5–7 days suggested; optimal duration unknown.
- Neonates with aortic thrombosis associated with umbilical artery catheters: 75–100 units/kg by direct injection, then 28 units/kg per hour for 5–7 days suggested; optimal duration unknown.

Disseminated Intravascular Coagulation

IV:

- 25–50 units/kg given by IV infusion or IV injection every 4 hours. Discontinue after 4–8 hours if there is no improvement.

Adult Patients

Treatment of Venous Thrombosis and Pulmonary Embolism

IV, THEN SUB-Q:

- Full-dose intermittent therapy (68-kg adult): 5000 units *IV* then 10,000–20,000 units sub-Q initially, followed by 8000–10,000 units sub-Q every 8 hours or 15,000–20,000 units sub-Q every 12 hours.
- Adjusted-dose therapy: 5000 units IV initially as a loading dose followed by 17,500 units sub-Q twice daily, with dosage adjusted to prolong the aPTT to 1.5–2.5 times the control value at the mid-dose interval recommended by some clinicians.

IV:

- Full-dose continuous therapy (68-kg adult): 5000 units initial loading dose, then 20,000–40,000 units in 1 L of 0.9% sodium chloride injection or other compatible IV solution infused over 24 hours recommended by some manufacturers. ACCP recommends an initial loading dose of 5000 units, then ≥30,000 units infused over the first 24 hours.
- Full-dose intermittent therapy (68-kg adult): 10,000 units initial loading dose, then 5000–10,000 units every 4–6 hours recommended by some manufacturers. ACCP states that intermittent IV regimens are associated with a higher risk of bleeding than continuous IV infusion and are not recommended.
- Adjusted-dose continuous therapy: ACCP recommends 80 units/kg loading dose, then 18 units/kg per hour for 24 hours.
- After 24 hours, adjust dosage to prolong the aPTT to a level corresponding with a plasma heparin concentration of 0.3–0.7 units/mL (amidolytic anti-factor X_a assay) for ≥5 days.
- Pregnant women: 5000 units by direct injection followed by a continuous infusion to maintain aPTT in the therapeutic range) for ≥5 days.

General Surgery Thromboprophylaxis

SUB-Q:

- Moderate-risk general surgery patients: 5000 units 1–2 hours prior to surgery, then every 12 hours after surgery until patient is ambulatory or discharged from the hospital.
- *High-risk* general surgery patients: 5000 units administered 1–2 hours prior to surgery, then every 8 hours; for patients with multiple risk factors, combine pharmacologic therapy with intermittent pneumatic compression (IPC) or graduated-compression stockings.
- Gynecologic laparoscopic surgery patients with additional risk factors: 5000 units 2–3 times daily recommended by ACCP.
- Major gynecologic surgery for benign disease: 5000 units twice daily until hospital discharge.
- Major gynecologic surgery with additional risk factors: 5000 units 3 times daily until hospital discharge.

- Major gynecologic surgery for cancer: 5000 units 3 times daily until hospital discharge.
- Major gynecologic surgery at particularly high-risk patients (e.g., >60 years of age, cancer surgery, history of venous thromboembolism): Continue prophylaxis for 2–4 weeks after hospital discharge.
- Major open urologic surgery: 5000 units 2–3 times daily.
- Urologic surgical patients with multiple risk factors: 5000 units 2–3 times daily in combination with IPC or graduated-compression stockings.

Neurosurgery Thromboprophylaxis

SUB-Q:
- Intracranial neurosurgery†: 5000 units administered 1–2 hours preoperatively, then every 8–12 hours is recommended.
- Elective spinal surgery with additional risk factors: 5000 units 2–3 times daily initiated postoperatively alone or in combination with IPC or graded compression stockings.
- Hip-fracture surgery: 5000 units administered 1-2 hours preoperatively, then every 8–12 hours.

Thromboprophylaxis in Selected Medical Conditions

SUB-Q:
- Hospitalized patients with CHF, severe respiratory disease, or impaired mobility and additional risk factors: 5000 units twice daily.
- Critically ill patients at moderate risk: 5000 units twice daily.

Thromboembolism During Pregnancy

SUB-Q:
- *Primary prevention* in women with antithrombin deficiency, heterozygous genetic mutation for factor V Leiden and prothrombin G20210A or homozygous gene mutation for factor V Leiden or prothrombin G20210A : 5000 units every 12 hours with dosage adjusted to maintain an anti-factor X_a concentration of 0.1–0.3 units/mL, followed by postpartum oral anticoagulation (e.g., with warfarin).
- *Primary prevention* in women with confirmed thrombophilia: 5000 units every 12 hours suggested.
- *Secondary prevention* after a single episode of idiopathic venous thromboembolism with or without thrombophilia with no long-term anticoagulation: 5000 units every 12 hours with or without adjustment of dosage to maintain an anti-factor X_a concentration of 0.1–0.3 units/mL, followed by postpartum oral anticoagulation.
- *Secondary prevention* after a single episode of venous thromboembolism and confirmed thrombophilia or family history of thrombosis not receiving long-term anticoagulation: 5000 units every 12 hours with or without adjustment of dosage to maintain an anti-factor X_a concentration of 0.1–0.3 units/mL, followed by postpartum oral anticoagulation.
- *Secondary prevention* after ≥2 episodes of venous thromboembolism and/or who are receiving long-term anticoagulation: Administer every 12 hours with dosage adjusted to maintain the mid-interval aPTT in the therapeutic range, followed by resumption of postpartum long-term oral anticoagulation.
- *Primary or secondary prevention* in women with antiphospholipid syndrome and a history of multiple pregnancy losses, preeclampsia, intrauterine growth retardation, or abruption: 5000 units twice daily or moderate twice-daily

dosage adjusted to maintain an anti-factor X_a concentration of 0.1–0.3 units/mL and low-dose aspirin.
- Atrial fibrillation with risk factors: 10,000–20,000 units every 12 hours with dosage adjusted to maintain the mid-interval aPTT (6 hours after dose) at 1.5 times the control value during the first trimester and last month of pregnancy.

IV:
- Atrial fibrillation with risk factors: Adjusted dose continuous therapy suggested to maintain the aPTT ≥1.5–2 times control value during first trimester and last month of pregnancy.

Embolism Associated with Atrial Fibrillation/Flutter

IV:
- Atrial fibrillation with AMI: 60 units/kg loading dose followed by 12 units/kg per hour to maintain an aPTT of approximately 1.5–2 times the control value.

Thromboembolism Associated with Prosthetic Heart Valves

SUB-Q:
- Pregnant women: Initially, 17,500–20,000 units every 12 hours and adjusted to maintain the mid-interval aPTT at least twice the control value or anti-factor X_a concentration of 0.35–0.7 units/mL throughout pregnancy suggested.
- Alternatively, 17,500–20,000 units every 12 hours adjusted to maintain the mid-interval aPTT ≥twice the control value or an anti-factor X_a concentration of 0.35–0.7 units/mL until week 13 of pregnancy, then transfer to warfarin until the middle of the third trimester, followed by adjusted-dose heparin until close to term.

Disseminated Intravascular Coagulation

IV:
- 50–100 units/kg by IV infusion or IV injection every 4 hours. Discontinue after 4–8 hours if there is no improvement.

Acute Ischemic Complications of ST-Segment Elevation AMI

IV:
- Conjunctive therapy with fibrin-selective thrombolytic agents: Initially, 60 units/kg (maximum 4000 units) loading dose.
- Maintenance dosage: 12 units/kg per hour (maximum 1000 units/hour in patients weighing >70 kg), adjusted to maintain a therapeutic aPTT for 48 hours. Follow-up therapy with oral anticoagulation (e.g., warfarin).
- Conjunctive therapy with non-fibrin-selective thrombolytic agents in patients who are at high risk for thromboembolism: 5000 units by direct injection followed by 800 units/hr for patients weighing ≤80 kg or 1000 units/hr for patients weighing >80 kg for 48 hours. After 48 hours, change to sub-Q heparin.
- Discontinue after 48 hours in patients at low risk for thromboembolism, convert to sub-Q therapy in patients at high risk of systemic embolization, and continue IV therapy in patients at high risk for coronary reocclusion.

SUB-Q:
- Conjunctive therapy with non-fibrin-selective thrombolytic agents in patients who are at high risk for thromboembolism: 12,500 units every 12 hours for 48 hours.
- Patients who did not receive thrombolytic therapy: 7500–

12,500 units every 12 hours for 48 hours. Continue therapy until patient is ambulatory in patients with impaired mobility.

Cardiac and Vascular Surgery Thromboprophylaxis

IV:

- Total body perfusion for open-heart surgery: Initially, ≥150 units/kg. Administer 300 units/kg for procedures estimated to last <1 hour. Administer 400 units/kg for those procedures estimated to last >1 hour.
- Vascular surgery patients with additional risk factors: 5000 or 7500 units twice daily recommended by ACCP.

Acute Ischemic Complications of PCI

IV:

- PCI without concurrent antiplatelet therapy with a GP IIb/IIIa-receptor inhibitor: Dosage adjusted to maintain an activated clotting time (ACT) of 250–300 seconds with the HemoTec device or 300–350 seconds with the Hemochron device.
- PCI with concurrent GP IIb/IIIa-receptor inhibitors: A loading dose of 50–70 units/kg targeted to an ACT of ≥200 seconds (using either the HemoTec or Hemochron device) recommended. Discontinue therapy immediately upon completion of an uncomplicated procedure.

Acute Ischemic Complications of Unstable Angina and Non-ST-Segment Elevation MI

IV:

- Adjusted-dose continuous therapy:70–80 units/kg loading dose followed by continuous IV infusion to maintain the aPTT between 1.5–2 times the control value for ≥48 hours in addition to aspirin and/or clopidogrel. Continue for ≥48 hours or until anginal pain resolves with pharmacologic therapy or with cardiac intervention (e.g., revascularization). Early treatment initiation appears to be necessary for beneficial effects.

Prescribing Limits

Acute Ischemic Complications of ST-Segment Elevation AMI

IV:

- Conjunctive therapy with fibrin-selective thrombolytic agents: Maximum 4000 units loading dose.
- Maintenance dosage: Maximum 1000 units/hour in patients weighing >70 kg, adjusted to maintain a therapeutic aPTT for 48 hours.

Special Populations

Geriatric Patients

- Patients >60 years of age may require a lower dosage. Consider lower dosages in geriatric patients undergoing PCI, particularly when combined with GP IIb/IIIa-receptor inhibitors.

Women

- Consider lower dosages in women undergoing PCI, particularly when combined with GP IIb/IIIa-receptor inhibitors.

† Use is not currently included in the labeling approved by the US Food and Drug Administration.

Hepatitis A Vaccine

Brand Name: Havrix®, Vaqta®, Twinrix®

What is hepatitis A?

Hepatitis A is a serious liver disease caused by the hepatitis A virus (HAV). HAV is found in the stool of persons with hepatitis A. It is usually spread by close personal contact and sometimes by eating food or drinking water containing HAV.

Hepatitis A can cause:
- mild "flu-like" illness
- jaundice (yellow skin or eyes)
- severe stomach pains and diarrhea

People with hepatitis A often have to be hospitalized (up to about 1 person in 5). Sometimes, people die as a result of hepatitis A (about 3-5 deaths per 1,000 cases). A person who has hepatitis A can easily pass the disease to others within the same household. Hepatitis A vaccine can prevent hepatitis A.

Who should get hepatitis A vaccine?

Some people should be routinely vaccinated with hepatitis A vaccine:
- All children 1 year (12 through 23 months) of age.
- Persons 1 year of age and older traveling to or working in countries with high or intermediate prevalence of hepatitis A, such as those located in Central or South America, Mexico, Asia (except Japan), Africa, and eastern Europe. For more information see http://www.cdc.gov/travel.
- Children and adolescents through 18 years of age who live in states or communities where routine vaccination has been implemented because of high disease incidence.
- Men who have sex with men.
- Persons who use street drugs.
- Persons with chronic liver disease.
- Persons who are treated with clotting factor concentrates.
- Persons who work with HAV-infected primates or who work with HAV in research laboratories.

Hepatitis A vaccine is not licensed for children younger than 1 year of age.

When should someone receive hepatitis A vaccine?

For children, the first dose should be given at 12-23 months of age. Children who are not vaccinated by 2 years of age can be vaccinated at later visits.

For travelers, the vaccine series should be started at least one month before traveling to provide the best protection. Persons who get the vaccine less than one month before traveling can also get a shot called immune globulin (IG). IG gives immediate, temporary protection.

For others, the hepatitis A vaccine series may be started whenever a person is at risk of infection.

Two doses of the vaccine are needed for lasting protection. These doses should be given at least 6 months apart.

Hepatitis A vaccine may be given at the same time as other vaccines.

Who should *not* get hepatitis A vaccine or should wait?

- Anyone who has ever had a severe (lifethreatening) allergic reaction to a previous dose of hepatitis A vaccine should not get another dose.
- Anyone who has a severe (life threatening) allergy to any vaccine component should not get the vaccine. Tell your doctor if you have any severe allergies. All hepatitis A vaccines contain alum and some hepatitis A vaccines contain 2-phenoxyethanol.
- Anyone who is moderately or severely ill at the time the shot is scheduled should probably wait until they recover. Ask your doctor or nurse. People with a mild illness can usually get the vaccine.
- Tell your doctor if you are pregnant. The safety of hepatitis A vaccine for pregnant women has not been determined. But there is no evidence that it is harmful to either pregnant women or their unborn babies. The risk, if any, is thought to be very low.

What are the risks from hepatitis A vaccine?

A vaccine, like any medicine, could possibly cause serious problems, such as severe allergic reactions. The risk of hepatitis A vaccine causing serious harm, or death, is extremely small. Getting hepatitis A vaccine is much safer than getting the disease.

Mild Problems:
- soreness where the shot was given (about 1 out of 2 adults, and up to 1 out of 6 children)
- headache (about 1 out of 6 adults and 1 out of 25 children)
- loss of appetite (about 1 out of 12 children)
- tiredness (about 1 out of 14 adults)
- If these problems occur, they usually last 1 or 2 days.

Severe problems:
- serious allergic reaction, within a few minutes to a few hours of the shot (very rare)

What if there is a moderate or severe reaction?

What should I look for?
- Any unusual condition, such as a high fever or behavior changes. Signs of a serious allergic reaction can include difficulty breathing, hoarseness or wheezing, hives, paleness, weakness, a fast heart beat or dizziness.

What should I do?
- Call a doctor, or get the person to a doctor right away.
- Tell your doctor what happened, the date and time it happened, and when the vaccination was given.
- Ask your health care provider to file a Vaccine Adverse Event Reporting System (VAERS) form if you have any reaction to the vaccine. Or call VAERS yourself at 1-800-822-7967, or visit their website at http://vaers.hhs.gov.

The National Vaccine Injury Compensation Program

In the rare event that you or your child has a serious reaction to a vaccine, a federal program has been created to help pay for the care of those who have been harmed.

For details about the National Vaccine Injury Compensation Program, call 1-800-338-2382 or visit the program's website at http://www.hrsa.gov/vaccinecompensation.

How can I learn more?

- Ask your doctor or other health care provider. They can give you the vaccine package insert or suggest other sources of information.
- Call your local or state health department's immunization program.
- Contact the Centers for Disease Control and Prevention (CDC): call 1-800-232-4636 (1-800-CDC-INFO) or visit the National Immunization Program's website at http://www.cdc.gov/nip.

Hepatitis A Vaccine Information Statement. U.S. Department of Health and Human Services/Centers for Disease Control and Prevention National Immunization Program. 3/21/2006.

Hepatitis B Vaccine

Brand Name: Engerix-B®, Recombivax HB®, Comvax®, Twinrix®

What is hepatitis B?

Hepatitis B is a serious disease that affects the liver. It is caused by the hepatitis B virus (HBV). HBV can cause:

Acute (short-term) illness. This can lead to:
- loss of appetite
- tiredness
- pain in muscles, joints, and stomach
- diarrhea and vomiting
- jaundice (yellow skin or eyes)

Chronic (long-term) infection. Some people go on to develop chronic HBV infection. This can be very serious, and often leads to:
- liver damage (cirrhosis)
- liver cancer
- death

Chronic infection is more common among infants and children than among adults. People who are infected can spread HBV to others, even if they don't appear sick.

- In 2005, about 51,000 people became infected with hepatitis B.
- About 1.25 million people in the United States have chronic HBV infection.
- Each year about 3,000 to 5,000 people die from cirrhosis or liver cancer caused by HBV.

Hepatitis B virus is spread through contact with the blood or other body fluids of an infected person. A person can become infected by:

- contact with a mother's blood and body fluids at the time of birth;
- contact with blood and body fluids through breaks in the skin such as bites, cuts, or sores;
- contact with objects that could have blood or body fluids on them such as toothbrushes or razors;
- having unprotected sex with an infected person;
- sharing needles when injecting drugs;
- being stuck with a used needle on the job.

Why get vaccinated?

Hepatitis B vaccine can prevent hepatitis B, and the serious consequences of HBV infection, including liver cancer and cirrhosis. Routine hepatitis B vaccination of U.S. children began in 1991. Since then, the reported incidence of acute hepatitis B among children and adolescents has dropped by more than 95% – and by 75% in all age groups. Hepatitis B vaccine is made from a part of the hepatitis B virus. It cannot cause HBV infection.

Hepatitis B vaccine is usually given as a series of 3 or 4 shots. This vaccine series gives long-term protection from HBV infection, possibly lifelong.

Hepatitis B is a serious disease. The hepatitis B virus (HBV) can cause short-term (acute) illness that leads to: loss of appetite, diarrhea and vomiting, tiredness, jaundice (yellow skin or eyes), and pain in muscles, joints, and stomach. It can also cause long-term (chronic) illness that leads to: liver damage (cirrhosis), liver cancer, or death. About 1.25 million people in the U.S. have chronic HBV infection.

Who should get hepatitis B vaccine?

Children and Adolescents

- All children should get their first dose of hepatitis B vaccine at birth and should have completed the vaccine series by 6-18 months of age.
- Children and adolescents through 18 years of age who did not get the vaccine when they were younger should also be vaccinated.

Adults

- All unvaccinated adults at risk for HBV infection should be vaccinated. This includes:
- sex partners of people infected with HBV,
- men who have sex with men,
- people who inject street drugs,
- people with more than one sex partner,
- people with chronic liver or kidney disease,
- people with jobs that expose them to human blood,
- household contacts of people infected with HBV,
- residents and staff in institutions for the developmentally disabled,
- kidney dialysis patients,
- people who travel to countries where hepatitis B is common,
- people with HIV infection.

Anyone else who wants to be protected from HBV infection may be vaccinated.

Who should *not* get hepatitis B vaccine or should wait?

- Anyone with a life-threatening allergy to baker's yeast, or to any other component of the vaccine, should not get hepatitis B vaccine. Tell your provider if you have any severe allergies.
- Anyone who has had a life-threatening allergic reaction to a previous dose of hepatitis B vaccine should not get another dose.
- Anyone who is moderately or severely ill when a dose of vaccine is scheduled should probably wait until they recover before getting the vaccine.

Your provider can give you more information about these precautions. Pregnant women who need protection from HBV infection may be vaccinated.

Hepatitis B vaccine risks

Hepatitis B is a very safe vaccine. Most people do not have any problems with it.

Mild Problems:

- Soreness where the shot was given (up to about 1 person in 4).
- Temperature of 99.9°F or higher (up to about 1 person in 15).

Severe Problems:

- Serious allergic reaction (very rare; believed to occur about once in 1.1 million doses)

A vaccine, like any medicine, could cause a serious reaction. But the risk of a vaccine causing serious harm, or death, is extremely small. More than 100 million people have gotten hepatitis B vaccine in the United States.

What if there is a moderate or severe reaction?

What should I look for?

- Any unusual condition, such as a high fever or behavior changes. Signs of a serious allergic reaction can include difficulty breathing, hoarseness or wheezing, hives, paleness, weakness, a fast heart beat or dizziness.

What should I do?

- Call a doctor, or get the person to a doctor right away.
- Tell your doctor what happened, the date and time it happened, and when the vaccination was given.
- Ask your health care provider to file a Vaccine Adverse Event Reporting System (VAERS) form if you have any reaction to the vaccine. Or call VAERS yourself at 1-800-822-7967, or visit their website at http://vaers.hhs.gov.

The National Vaccine Injury Compensation Program

In the event that you or your child has a serious reaction to a vaccine, a federal program has been created to help pay for the care of those who have been harmed.

For details about the National Vaccine Injury Compensation Program, call 1-800-338-2382 or visit their website at http://www.hrsa.gov/vaccinecompensation.

How can I learn more?

- Ask your doctor or other health care provider. They can give you the vaccine package insert or suggest other sources of information.
- Call your local or state health department.
- Contact the Centers for Disease Control and Prevention (CDC): call 1-800-232-4636 (1-800-CDC-INFO) or visit the National Immunization Program's website at http://www.cdc.gov/vaccines.

Hepatitis B Vaccine Information Statement (Interim). U.S. Department of Health and Human Services/Centers for Disease Control and Prevention National Immunization Program. 7/18/2007.

Human Papillomavirus (HPV) Vaccine

Brand Name: Gardasil®

What is HPV?

Genital human papillomavirus (HPV) is the most common sexually transmitted virus in the United States.

There are about 40 types of HPV. About 20 million people in the U.S. are infected, and about 6.2 million more get infected each year. HPV is spread through sexual contact.

Most HPV infections don't cause any symptoms, and go away on their own. But HPV is important mainly because it can cause cervical cancer in women. Every year in the U.S. about 10,000 women get cervical cancer and 3,700 die from it. It is the 2nd leading cause of cancer deaths among women around the world.

HPV is also associated with several less common types of cancer in both men and women. It can also cause genital warts and warts in the upper respiratory tract.

More than 50% of sexually active men and women are infected with HPV at sometime in their lives.

There is no treatment for HPV infection, but the conditions it causes can be treated.

Why get vaccinated?

HPV vaccine is an inactivated (not live) vaccine which protects against 4 major types of HPV.

These include 2 types that cause about 70% of cervical cancer and 2 types that cause about 90% of genital warts. *HPV vaccine can prevent most genital warts and most cases of cervical cancer.*

Protection from HPV vaccine is expected to be long-lasting. But vaccinated women still need cervical cancer screening because the vaccine does not protect against all HPV types that cause cervical cancer.

Who should get HPV vaccine and when?

HPV vaccine is routinely recommended for girls 11-12 years of age. Doctors may give it to girls as young as 9 years.

It is important for girls to get HPV vaccine before their first sexual contact - because they have not been exposed to HPV. For these girls, the vaccine can prevent almost 100% of disease caused by the 4 types of HPV targeted by the vaccine. However, if a girl or woman is already infected with a type of HPV, the vaccine will not prevent disease from that type.

The vaccine is also recommended for girls and women 13-26 years of age who did not receive it when they were younger.

HPV vaccine is given as a 3-dose series:
- 1st Dose: Now
- 2nd Dose: 2 months after Dose 1
- 3rd Dose: 6 months after Dose 1

Additional (booster) doses are not recommended.

HPV vaccine may be given at the same time as other vaccines.

Which girls or women should *not* get HPV vaccine or should wait?

- Anyone who has ever had a life-threatening allergic reaction to yeast, to any other component of HPV vaccine, or to a previous dose of HPV vaccine should not get the vaccine. Tell your doctor if the person getting the vaccine has any severe allergies.
- Pregnant women should not get the vaccine. The vaccine appears to be safe for both the mother and the unborn baby, but it is still being studied. Receiving HPV vaccine when pregnant is not a reason to consider terminating the pregnancy. Women who are breast feeding may safely get the vaccine.
- **Any woman who learns that she was pregnant when she got HPV vaccine is encouraged to call the HPV vaccine in pregnancy registry at 800-986-8999. Information from this registry will help us learn how pregnant women respond to the vaccine.**
- People who are mildly ill when the shot is scheduled can still get HPV vaccine. People with moderate or severe illnesses should wait until they recover.

What are the risks from HPV vaccine?

HPV vaccine does not appear to cause any serious side effects.

However, a vaccine, like any medicine, could possibly cause serious problems, such as severe allergic reactions. The risk of any vaccine causing serious harm, or death, is extremely small.

Mild Problems:
- Pain at the injection site (about 8 people in 10)
- Redness or swelling at the injection site (about 1 person in 4)
- Mild fever (100°F) (about 1 person in 10)
- Itching at the injection site (about 1 person in 30)
- Moderate fever (102°F) (about 1 person in 65)
- These symptoms do not last long and go away on their own.

Life-threatening allergic reactions from vaccines are very rare. If they do occur, it would be within a few minutes to a few hours after the vaccination.

Like all vaccines, HPV vaccine will continue to be monitored for unusual or severe problems.

What if there is a severe reaction?

What should I look for?
- Any unusual condition, such as a high fever or behavior changes. Signs of a serious allergic reaction can include difficulty breathing, hoarseness or wheezing, hives, paleness, weakness, a fast heart beat or dizziness.

What should I do?
- Call a doctor, or get the person to a doctor right away.
- Tell your doctor what happened, the date and time it happened, and when the vaccination was given.
- Ask your health care provider to file a Vaccine Adverse Event Reporting System (VAERS) form if you have any reaction to the vaccine. Or call VAERS yourself

at 1-800-822-7967, or visit their website at http://vaers.hhs.gov.

The National Vaccine Injury Compensation Program

In the rare event that you or your child has a serious reaction to a vaccine, a federal program has been created to help pay for the care of those who have been harmed.

For details about the National Vaccine Injury Compensation Program, call 1-800-338-2382 or visit the program's website at http://www.hrsa.gov/vaccinecompensation.

How can I learn more?

- Ask your doctor or other health care provider. They can give you the vaccine package insert or suggest other sources of information.
- Call your local or state health department's immunization program.
- Contact the Centers for Disease Control and Prevention (CDC): call 1-800-232-4636 (1-800-CDC-INFO) or visit the National Immunization Program's website at http://www.cdc.gov/nip.

HPV Vaccine Information Statement. U.S. Department of Health and Human Services/Centers for Disease Control and Prevention National Immunization Program. 2/2/2007.

Hydralazine

(hye dral' a zeen)

Brand Name: Hydra-Zide® (as a combination product containing Hydralazine Hydrochloride and Hydrochlorothiazide)
Also available generically.

Why is this medicine prescribed?

Hydralazine is used to treat high blood pressure. It works by relaxing the blood vessels so that blood can flow more easily through the body.

This medication is sometimes prescribed for other uses; ask your doctor or pharmacist for more information.

How should this medicine be used?

Hydralazine comes as a tablet to take by mouth. It usually is taken two to four a day at evenly spaced intervals. Follow the directions on your prescription label carefully, and ask your doctor or pharmacist to explain any part you do not understand. Take hydralazine exactly as directed. Do not take more or less of it or take it more often than prescribed by your doctor.

Hydralazine controls high blood pressure but does not cure it. Continue to take hydralazine even if you feel well. Do not stop taking hydralazine without talking to your doctor.

Are there other uses for this medicine?

Hydralazine is also used after heart valve replacement and in the treatment of congestive heart failure. Talk to your doctor about the possible risks of using this drug for your condition.

What special precautions should I follow?

Before taking hydralazine,

- tell your doctor and pharmacist if you are allergic to hydralazine, aspirin, tartrazine (a yellow dye in some processed foods and medications), or any other drugs.
- tell your doctor and pharmacist what prescription and nonprescription medications you are taking, especially indomethacin (Indocin), metoprolol (Lopressor), propranolol (Inderal), and vitamins.
- tell your doctor if you have or have ever had coronary artery disease, rheumatic heart disease, kidney or liver disease, or a heart attack.
- tell your doctor if you are pregnant, plan to become pregnant, or are breast-feeding. If you become pregnant while taking hydralazine, call your doctor.
- if you are having surgery, including dental surgery, tell the doctor or dentist that you are taking hydralazine.
- ask your doctor about the safe use of alcohol while you are taking hydralazine. Alcohol can make the side effects from hydralazine worse.

What special dietary instructions should I follow?

Take hydralazine with meals or a snack.

Your doctor may prescribe a low-salt or low-sodium diet. Follow these directions carefully.

What should I do if I forget to take a dose?

Take the missed dose as soon as you remember it. However, if it is almost time for the next dose, skip the missed dose and continue your regular dosing schedule. Do not take a double dose to make up for a missed one.

What side effects can this medicine cause?

Hydralazine may cause side effects. Tell your doctor if any of these symptoms are severe or do not go away:
- flushing (feeling of warmth)
- headache
- upset stomach
- vomiting
- loss of appetite
- diarrhea
- constipation
- eye tearing
- stuffy nose
- rash

If you experience any of the following symptoms, call your doctor immediately:
- fainting
- joint or muscle pain
- unexplained fever
- rapid heartbeat

- chest pain
- swollen ankles or feet
- numbing or tingling in hands or feet

If you experience a serious side effect, you or your doctor may send a report to the Food and Drug Administration's (FDA) MedWatch Adverse Event Reporting program online [at http://www.fda.gov/MedWatch/index.html] or by phone [1-800-332-1088].

What storage conditions are needed for this medicine?

Keep this medication in the container it came in, tightly closed, and out of reach of children. Store at room temperature and away from excess heat and moisture (not in the bathroom). Throw away any medication that is outdated or no longer needed. Talk to your pharmacist about the proper disposal of your medication.

What should I do in case of overdose?

In case of overdose, call your local poison control center at 1-800-222-1222. If the victim has collapsed or is not breathing, call local emergency services at 911.

What other information should I know?

Keep all appointments with your doctor and the laboratory. Your blood pressure should be checked regularly to determine your response to hydralazine.

Your doctor may ask you to check your blood pressure daily. Ask your doctor or pharmacist to teach you how.

Do not let anyone else take your medication. Ask your pharmacist any questions you have about refilling your prescription.

Dosage Facts
For Informational Purposes

Caution: Do not change your dose, how often you take your medication, or the length of time you are to take it without first talking to your healthcare provider.

The following dosage information was written using medical language for doctors and other healthcare professionals and is provided here for you to check your dosage. The dosage of this drug may differ for different patients. Therefore, always follow your doctor's instructions or the directions on the label. Contact your healthcare provider or pharmacist if you have any questions about the specific dosage of your medication after reviewing this information.

General Dosage Information

Available as hydralazine hydrochloride; dosage expressed in terms of the salt.

20–25 mg of IV hydralazine hydrochloride was approximately equal to 75–100 mg of oral hydralazine hydrochloride in one study.

Pediatric Patients
Hypertension†

ORAL:
- Initially, 0.75 mg/kg daily (or 25 mg/m^2 daily) given in 4 divided doses; initial dose should not exceed 25 mg.
- Dosages may be increased gradually (over 3–4 weeks) up to a maximum of 7.5 mg/kg daily (or 200 mg daily).

Adult Patients
Hypertension
Monotherapy

ORAL:
- Initially, 10 mg 4 times daily for 2–4 days. Dosage then can be increased to 25 mg 4 times daily for the remainder of the week. If necessary, dosage can be increased for the second and subsequent weeks to 50 mg 4 times daily. Usual dosages of 12.5–50 mg twice daily recommended by JNC 7.

Combination Therapy

ORAL:
- If BP is not adequately controlled by monotherapy with hydalazine or hydrochlorothiazide, can switch to fixed-combination capsules containing hydralazine hydrochloride 25 mg and hydrochlorothiazide 25 mg; then hydralazine hydrochloride 50 mg and hydrochlorothiazide 50 mg, administered twice daily.

CHF
Fixed-combination Therapy with Isosorbide Dinitrate in Self-identified Black Patients

ORAL:
- Initially, hydralazine hydrochloride 37.5 mg and isosorbide dinitrate 20 mg (1 tablet of BiDil®) 3 times daily. May titrate dosage to a maximum tolerated dosage not to exceed 2 tablets (a total of 75 mg of hydralazine hydrochloride and 40 mg of isosorbide dinitrate) 3 times daily. Rapid titration (over 3–5 days) may be possible; however, slower titration may be needed due to adverse effects. May decrease dosage to as little as one-half of the fixed-combination tablet 3 times daily in patients who experience intolerable effects, but attempt to titrate dosage up once adverse effects subside.

Prescribing Limits
Pediatric Patients
Hypertension

ORAL:
- Maximum 7.5 mg/kg daily (or 200 mg daily).

Adult Patients
Hypertension
Maintenance Therapy

ORAL:
- Maximum 100 mg daily; addition of another antihypertensive agent is preferable to increasing dosage beyond 100 mg because of poor patient tolerance.

CHF
Fixed-combination Therapy with Isosorbide Dinitrate in Self-identified Black Patients

ORAL:
- Maximum 75 mg of hydralazine hydrochloride and 40 mg of isosorbide dinitrate (2 tablets of BiDil®) 3 times daily.

Hydrochlorothiazide

(hye droe klor oh thye′ a zide)

Brand Name: HydroDIURIL®, Microzide®
Also available generically.

Why is this medicine prescribed?

Hydrochlorothiazide, a 'water pill,' is used to treat high blood pressure and fluid retention caused by various conditions, including heart disease. It causes the kidneys to get rid of unneeded water and salt from the body into the urine.

This medicine is sometimes prescribed for other uses; ask your doctor or pharmacist for more information.

How should this medicine be used?

Hydrochlorothiazide comes as a tablet and liquid to take by mouth. It usually is taken once or twice a day. If you are to take it once a day, take it in the morning; if you are to take it twice a day, take it in the morning and in the late afternoon to avoid going to the bathroom during the night. Take this medication with meals or a snack. Follow the directions on your prescription label carefully, and ask your doctor or pharmacist to explain any part you do not understand. Take hydrochlorothiazide exactly as directed. Do not take more or less of it or take it more often than prescribed by your doctor.

Hydrochlorothiazide controls high blood pressure but does not cure it. Continue to take hydrochlorothiazide even if you feel well. Do not stop taking hydrochlorothiazide without talking to your doctor.

Are there other uses for this medicine?

Hydrochlorothiazide may also be used to treat patients with diabetes insipidus and certain electrolyte disturbances and to prevent kidney stones in patients with high levels of calcium in their blood. Talk to your doctor about the possible risks of using this medicine for your condition.

What special precautions should I follow?

Before taking hydrochlorothiazide,
- tell your doctor and pharmacist if you are allergic to hydrochlorothiazide, sulfa drugs, or any other drugs.
- tell your doctor and pharmacist what prescription and nonprescription medications you are taking, especially other medicines for high blood pressure, anti-inflammatory medications such as ibuprofen (Motrin, Nuprin) or naproxen (Aleve), corticosteroids (e.g., prednisone), lithium (Eskalith, Lithobid), medications for diabetes, probenecid (Benemid), and vitamins. If you also are taking cholestyramine or colestipol, take it at least 1 hour after hydrochlorothiazide.
- tell your doctor if you have or have ever had diabetes, gout, or kidney, liver, thyroid, or parathyroid disease.
- tell your doctor if you are pregnant, plan to become pregnant, or are breast-feeding. If you become pregnant while taking hydrochlorothiazide, call your doctor immediately.
- if you are having surgery, including dental surgery, tell the doctor or dentist that you are taking hydrochlorothiazide.
- you should know that this drug may make you drowsy. Do not drive a car or operate machinery until you know how this drug affects you.
- remember that alcohol can add to the drowsiness caused by this drug.
- plan to avoid unnecessary or prolonged exposure to sunlight and to wear protective clothing, sunglasses, and sunscreen. Hydrochlorothiazide may make your skin sensitive to sunlight.

What special dietary instructions should I follow?

Follow your doctor's directions. They may include following a daily exercise program or a low-salt or low-sodium diet, potassium supplements, and increased amounts of potassium-rich foods (e.g., bananas, prunes, raisins, and orange juice) in your diet.

What should I do if I forget to take a dose?

Take the missed dose as soon as you remember it. However, if it is almost time for your next dose, skip the missed dose and continue your regular dosing schedule. Do not take a double dose to make up for a missed one.

What side effects can this medicine cause?

Frequent urination should go away after you take hydrochlorothiazide for a few weeks. Tell your doctor if any of these symptoms are severe or do not go away:
- muscle weakness
- dizziness
- cramps
- thirst
- stomach pain
- upset stomach

- vomiting
- diarrhea
- loss of appetite
- headache
- hair loss

If you experience any of the following symptoms, call your doctor immediately:

- sore throat with fever
- unusual bleeding or bruising
- severe skin rash with peeling skin
- difficulty breathing or swallowing

If you experience a serious side effect, you or your doctor may send a report to the Food and Drug Administration's (FDA) MedWatch Adverse Event Reporting program online [at http://www.fda.gov/MedWatch/index.html] or by phone [1-800-332-1088].

What storage conditions are needed for this medicine?

Keep this medicine in the container it came in, tightly closed, and out of reach of children. Store it at room temperature and away from excess heat and moisture (not in the bathroom). Do not allow the oral liquid to freeze. Throw away any medicine that is outdated or no longer needed. Talk to your pharmacist about the proper disposal of your medicine.

What should I do in case of overdose?

In case of overdose, call your local poison control center at 1-800-222-1222. If the victim has collapsed or is not breathing, call local emergency services at 911.

What other information should I know?

Keep all appointments with your doctor and the laboratory. Your blood pressure should be checked regularly, and blood tests should be done occasionally.

Do not let anyone else take your medicine. Ask your pharmacist any questions you have about refilling your prescription.

Dosage Facts
For Informational Purposes

Caution: Do not change your dose, how often you take your medication, or the length of time you are to take it without first talking to your healthcare provider.

The following dosage information was written using medical language for doctors and other healthcare professionals and is provided here for you to check your dosage. The dosage of this drug may differ for different patients. Therefore, always follow your doctor's instructions or the directions on the label. Contact your healthcare provider or pharmacist if you have any questions about the specific dosage of your medication after reviewing this information.

General Dosage Information

Individualize according to requirements and response. Use lowest dosage necessary to produce desired clinical effect.

If added to potent hypotensive agent regimen, initially reduce hypotensive dosage to avoid the possibility of severe hypotension.

Pediatric Patients

Usual Dosage

ORAL:
- Infants <6 months of age: Up to 3 mg/kg daily, in 2 divided doses; up to 37.5 mg daily.
- Infants 6 months to 2 years of age: Usually, 1–2 mg/kg daily, in a single or 2 divided doses, up to 37.5 mg daily.
- Children 2–12 years of age: 1–2 mg/kg daily, in a single or 2 divided doses, up to 100 mg daily.

Hypertension

ORAL:
- Initially, 1 mg/kg once daily. Increase dosage as necessary up to a maximum of 3 mg/kg (up to 50 mg) once daily.

Adult Patients

Hypertension
BP Monitoring and Treatment Goals

Carefully monitor BP during initial titration or subsequent upward adjustment in dosage.

Avoid large or abrupt reductions in BP.

Adjust dosage at approximately monthly intervals (more aggressively in high-risk patients [stage 2 hypertension, comorbid conditions]) if BP control is inadequate at a given dosage; it may take months to control hypertension adequately while avoiding adverse effects of therapy.

SBP is the principal clinical end point, especially in middle-aged and geriatric patients. Once the goal SBP is attained, the goal DBP usually is achieved.

The goal is to achieve and maintain a lifelong SBP <140 mm Hg and a DBP <90 mm Hg if tolerated.

The goal in hypertensive patients with diabetes mellitus or renal impairment is to achieve and maintain a SBP <130 mm Hg and a DBP <80 mm Hg.

Monotherapy

ORAL:
- Initially, 12.5–25 mg daily.
- Gradually increase until the desired therapeutic response is achieved or adverse effects become intolerable, up to 50 mg daily.
- If adequate response is not achieved at maximum dosage, add or substitute another hypotensive agent.

MAINTENANCE:
- Usually, 12.5–50 mg once daily.

Combination Therapy

ORAL:
- Initially, administer each drug separately to adjust dosage.
- May use fixed combination if optimum maintenance dosage corresponds to drug ratio in combination preparation.
- Administer each drug separately whenever dosage adjustment is necessary.
- Alternatively, may initially use certain (low-dose hydrochlorothiazide/other antihypertensive) fixed combinations for

potentiation of antihypertensive effect and minimiziation of potential dose-related adverse effects of each drug.

Edema

ORAL:

- Usually, 25–100 mg daily in 1–3 divided doses.
- Many patients also may respond to intermittent therapy (e.g., alternate days, 3–5 days weekly); decreased risk of excessive diuretic response and resulting electrolyte imbalance.

Prescribing Limits

Pediatric Patients

Usual Dosage

ORAL:

- Infants <2 years of age: Maximum 37.5 mg daily.
- Children 2–12 years of age: Maximum 100 mg daily.

Hypertension

ORAL:

- Maximum 3 mg/kg (up to 50 mg) once daily.

Adult Patients

Hypertension

ORAL:

- Maximum before switching/adding alternative drug is 50 mg daily.
- Higher dosages had been used in the past (up to 200 mg daily) but no longer are recommended because of the risk of adverse effects (e.g., markedly decreased serum potassium). Instead, switch to or add alternative drug.

Special Populations

Hepatic Impairment

- No specific dosage recommendations for hepatic impairment; caution because of risk of precipitating hepatic coma.

Renal Impairment

- No specific dosage recommendations for renal impairment; caution because of risk of precipitating azotemia.

Geriatric Patients

- Initiate therapy at the lowest dosage (12.5 mg daily); may adjust dosage in increments of 12.5 mg if needed.

Hydrocortisone Injection

(hye droe kor′ ti sone)

Brand Name: A-hydroCort®, Hydrocortone® Acetate, Hydrocortone® Phosphate, Solu-Cortef® Also available generically.

About Your Treatment

Your doctor has ordered hydrocortisone, a corticosteroid, to relieve inflammation (swelling, heat, redness, and pain). The drug will be injected into a large muscle (such as your buttock or hip), into your vein, or added to an intravenous fluid that will drip through a needle or catheter placed in your vein.

Hydrocortisone is similar to a natural hormone produced by your adrenal glands. It is used to treat, but not cure, certain forms of arthritis; asthma; and skin, blood, kidney, eye, thyroid, and intestinal disorders. It is sometimes used to reduce side effects from other medications. This medication is sometimes prescribed for other uses; ask your doctor or pharmacist for more information.

Your health care provider (doctor, nurse, or pharmacist) may measure the effectiveness and side effects of your treatment using laboratory tests and physical examinations. It is important to keep all appointments with your doctor. The length of treatment depends on how you respond to the medication.

Precautions

Before administering hydrocortisone,

- tell your doctor and pharmacist if you are allergic to hydrocortisone, medications containing sulfites, or any other drugs.
- tell your doctor and pharmacist what prescription and nonprescription medications you are taking, especially anticoagulants ('blood thinners') such as warfarin (Coumadin), arthritis medications, aspirin, cyclosporine (Neoral, Sandimmune), digoxin (Lanoxin), diuretics ('water pills'), estrogens, ketoconazole (Nizoral), oral contraceptives, phenobarbital, phenytoin (Dilantin), rifampin (Rifadin), theophylline (Theo-Dur), and vitamins.
- tell your doctor if you have a fungal infection (other than on your skin); do not take hydrocortisone without talking to your doctor.
- tell your doctor if you have or have ever had liver, kidney, intestinal, or heart disease; diabetes; an underactive thyroid gland; high blood pressure; mental illness; myasthenia gravis; osteoporosis; herpes eye infection; seizures; tuberculosis (TB); AIDS; or ulcers.
- tell your doctor if you are pregnant, plan to become pregnant, or are breast-feeding. If you become pregnant while taking hydrocortisone, call your doctor.
- if you are having surgery, including dental surgery, tell the doctor or dentist that you are taking hydrocortisone.

Administering Your Medication

Before you administer hydrocortisone, look at the solution closely. It should be clear and free of floating material. Gently squeeze the bag or observe the solution container to make sure there are no leaks. Do not use the solution if it is discolored, if it contains particles, or if the bag or container leaks. Use a new solution, but show the damaged one to your health care provider.

It is important that you use your medication exactly as

directed. Do not administer it more often than or for longer periods than your doctor tells you. Do not change your dosing schedule without talking to your health care provider. Your health care provider may tell you to stop the infusion if you have a mechanical problem (such as blockage in the tubing, needle or catheter); if you have to stop an infusion, call your health care provider immediately so your therapy can continue.

Side Effects

Hydrocortisone may cause side effects. Tell your doctor if any of these symptoms are severe or do not go away:

- headache
- upset stomach
- vomiting
- dizziness
- insomnia
- restlessness
- depression
- anxiety
- unusual moods
- increased sweating
- increased hair growth
- reddened face
- acne
- thinned skin
- easy bruising
- tiny purple skin spots
- irregular or absent menstrual periods

If you experience any of the following symptoms, call your doctor immediately:

- skin rash
- swollen feet, ankles, and lower legs
- vision problems
- eye pain
- muscle pain and weakness
- black, tarry stool
- unusual bleeding

If you experience a serious side effect, you or your doctor may send a report to the Food and Drug Administration's (FDA) MedWatch Adverse Event Reporting program online [at http://www.fda.gov/MedWatch/index.html] or by phone [1-800-332-1088].

Storage Conditions

- Your health care provider will probably give you a several-day supply of hydrocortisone at a time. You will be told how to prepare each dose.

Store your medication only as directed. Make sure you understand what you need to store your medication properly.

Keep your supplies in a clean, dry place when you are not using them, and keep all medications and supplies out of the reach of children. Your health care provider will tell you how to throw away used needles, syringes, tubing, and containers to avoid accidental injury.

Overdose

In case of overdose, call your local poison control center at 1-800-222-1222. If the victim has collapsed or is not breathing, call local emergency services at 911.

Signs of Infection

If you are receiving hydrocortisone in your vein or under your skin, you need to know the symptoms of a catheter-related infection (an infection where the needle enters your vein or skin). If you experience any of these effects near your intravenous catheter, tell your health care provider as soon as possible:

- tenderness
- warmth
- irritation
- drainage
- redness
- swelling
- pain

Dosage Facts
For Informational Purposes

Caution: Do not change your dose, how often you take your medication, or the length of time you are to take it without first talking to your healthcare provider.

The following dosage information was written using medical language for doctors and other healthcare professionals and is provided here for you to check your dosage. The dosage of this drug may differ for different patients. Therefore, always follow your doctor's instructions or the directions on the label. Contact your healthcare provider or pharmacist if you have any questions about the specific dosage of your medication after reviewing this information.

General Dosage Information

Available as hydrocortisone, hydrocortisone acetate, hydrocortisone sodium phosphate, and hydrocortisone sodium succinate; dosage of hydrocortisone sodium phosphate and sodium succinate is expressed in terms of hydrocortisone and dosage of hydrocortisone acetate is expressed in terms of hydrocortisone acetate.

After a satisfactory response is obtained, dosage should be decreased in small decrements to the lowest level that maintains an adequate clinical response, and discontinue the drug as soon as possible.

Monitor patients continually for signs that indicate dosage adjustment is necessary, such as remissions or exacerbations of the disease and stress (surgery, infection, trauma).

High dosages may be required for acute situations of certain rheumatic disorders and collagen diseases; after a response has been obtained, drug often must be continued for long periods at low dosage.

High or massive dosages may be required in the treatment of pemphigus, exfoliative dermatitis, bullous dermatitis herpetiformis, severe erythema multiforme, or mycosis fungoides. Early initiation of systemic glucocorticoid therapy may be life-saving in pemphigus vulgaris. Reduce dosage gradually to the lowest effective level, but discontinuance may not be possible.

Massive dosages may be required for the treatment of shock.

If used orally for prolonged anti-inflammatory therapy, consider an alternate-day dosage regimen. Following long-term therapy, withdraw gradually.

Pediatric Patients

Base pediatric dosage on severity of the disease and the response of the patient rather than on strict adherence to dosage indicated by age, body weight, or body surface area.

Usual Dosage

IV:
- Hydrocortisone sodium succinate: 0.16–1 mg/kg or 6–30 mg/m² IV 1 or 2 times daily.

IM:
- Hydrocortisone sodium phosphate: 0.16–1 mg/kg or 6–30 mg/m² IM 1 or 2 times daily.
- Hydrocortisone sodium succinate: 0.16–1 mg/kg or 6–30 mg/m² IM 1 or 2 times daily.

Adult Patients

Usual Dosage

IV:
- Hydrocortisone sodium phosphate: Initially, 15–240 mg IV daily depending on the disease being treated. In life-threatening situations, extremely high parenteral dosage may be justified and may be a multiple of the usual oral dosage.
- Hydrocortisone sodium succinate: 100 mg to 8 g daily. 100–500 mg IV initially, and every 2–10 hours as needed.

IM:
- Hydrocortisone sodium phosphate: 15–240 mg IM daily, depending on the disease being treated. In life-threatening situations, extremely high parenteral dosage may be justified and may be a multiple of the usual oral dosage.
- Hydrocortisone sodium succinate: 100 mg to 8 g daily. 100–500 mg IM initially and every 2–10 hours as needed.

Shock†

IV:
- Life-threatening shock: Massive doses of hydrocortisone sodium succinate such as 50 mg/kg by direct IV injection (over a period of one to several minutes) initially and repeated in 4 hours and/or every 24 hours if needed.
- Alternatively, 0.5–2 g by direct IV injection (over a period of one to several minutes) initially and repeated at 2- to 6-hour intervals as required.
- In such cases, administer by direct IV injection over a period of one to several minutes.
- Continue high-dose therapy only until the patient's condition has stabilized and usually not beyond 48–72 hours.
- If massive corticosteroid therapy is needed beyond 72 hours, use a corticosteroid which causes less sodium retention (e.g., methylprednisolone sodium succinate or dexamethasone sodium phosphate) to minimize the risk of hypernatremia.

† Use is not currently included in the labeling approved by the US Food and Drug Administration.

Hydrocortisone, Neomycin, and Polymyxin

(hye droe kor′ ti sone) (nee oh mye′ sin)
(pol i mix′ in)

Brand Name: Bacticort®, Cortisporin Ophthalmic®, Otocort Ear Solution®, Otosporin®

Why is this medicine prescribed?

The combination of hydrocortisone, neomycin, and polymyxin eliminates bacteria that cause ear, eye, and skin infections and relieves pain, inflammation, redness, and itching.

This medication is sometimes prescribed for other uses; ask your doctor or pharmacist for more information.

How should this medicine be used?

This combination of drugs comes in eardrops, eyedrops, and a skin cream. For eye infections, this medication usually is used every 3 to 4 hours; for ear and skin infections, it usually is used two to four times a day. Follow the directions on your prescription label carefully, and ask your doctor or pharmacist to explain any part you do not understand. Use this combination exactly as directed. Do not use more or less of it or use it more often than prescribed by your doctor. Do not use this medication for more than 10 days. If your infection does not improve within 1 week or if it worsens, call your doctor.

To apply the eardrops, follow these directions (to make this procedure easier, have someone else insert the drops):

1. Gently clean and dry your ear with a sterile cotton swab.
2. Wash your hands thoroughly with soap and water.
3. Check the dropper to make sure it is not chipped or cracked.
4. The eardrops must be kept clean. Avoid touching the dropper against your ear, fingers, or any other source of contamination.
5. Warm the drops to near (but not higher than) body temperature by holding the container in your hand for a few minutes.
6. If the drops are a cloudy suspension (not a clear solution), shake the container well for 10 seconds.
7. Draw some medication into the dropper.
8. Tilt your head so that the affected ear is up, or lie on your side with the affected ear up.
9. To allow the drops to run in, hold the ear lobe up and back for an adult and hold the ear lobe down and back for a child.
10. Place the prescribed number of drops in your ear and keep your ear tilted up for 5 minutes. To avoid injury, do not insert the dropper into your ear.

11. If you prefer, insert a soft cotton gauze wick plug (ask your doctor or pharmacist to recommend a product) and saturate it with the eardrops. Keep the cotton moist by adding eardrops every 4 hours or as directed by your doctor, and replace the cotton every 24 hours.

12. Wash your hands to remove any medicine.

To apply the eyedrops, shake the bottle well and follow these directions:

1. Wash your hands thoroughly with soap and water.
2. Use a mirror or have someone else put the drops in your eye.
3. Make sure that the end of the dropper is not chipped or cracked.
4. Avoid touching the dropper against your eye or against anything else that may contaminate the remaining medication. Hold the dropper tip down at all times to prevent drops from flowing back into the bottle and contaminating the remaining contents. Damage to the eye may result from using contaminated eye medications.
5. Lie down or tilt your head back.
6. Holding the bottle between your thumb and index finger, place the dropper tip as near as possible to your eyelid without touching it.
7. Brace the remaining fingers of that hand against your cheek or nose.
8. With the index finger of your other hand, pull the lower lid of the eye down to form a pocket.
9. Drop the prescribed number of drops into the pocket made by the lower lid and the eye. Placing drops on the surface of the eyeball can cause stinging.
10. Close your eye for 2 to 3 minutes to keep the medication in the eye. Do not blink.
11. Replace and tighten the cap right away. Do not wipe or rinse it off.
12. Wipe off any excess liquid from your cheek with a clean tissue. Wash your hands again to remove any medication.

To use the skin cream, wash the affected skin area thoroughly. Then apply a small amount of cream and rub it in gently. If you use the cream on your face, keep it out of your eyes.

When using the cream, do not bandage or otherwise wrap your skin unless directed by your doctor. Do not apply this medication to other areas of the body unless directed by your doctor.

Do not apply cosmetics or other skin preparations to the treated skin area without talking with your doctor.

If you use this medication on a child's diaper area, do not use tight-fitting diapers or plastic pants. Such use may increase side effects.

What special precautions should I follow?

Before using hydrocortisone, neomycin, and polymyxin,

- tell your doctor and pharmacist if you are allergic to hydrocortisone, neomycin, polymixin, or any other drugs.
- tell your doctor what prescription and nonprescription medications you are taking, especially cancer chemotherapy agents, other topical medications, and vitamins.

- tell your doctor if you have or have ever had kidney disease, a heart attack, diabetes, glaucoma, cataracts, a perforated eardrum, a circulation disorder, or an immune disorder.
- tell your doctor if you are pregnant, plan to become pregnant, or are breast-feeding. If you become pregnant while using hydrocortisone, neomycin, and polymyxin, call your doctor immediately.

What should I do if I forget to take a dose?

Apply the missed dose as soon as you remember it. However, if it is almost time for the next dose, skip the missed dose and continue your regular dosing schedule. Do not apply a double dose to make up for a missed one.

What side effects can this medicine cause?

Hydrocortisone, neomycin, and polymyxin may cause side effects. Tell your doctor if any of these symptoms are severe or do not go away:

- itching
- burning
- pain
- swelling
- drying or cracking of the skin
- acne
- change in skin color
- blurred vision
- hearing difficulty

If you experience any of the following symptoms, call your doctor immediately:

- severe skin rash
- difficulty breathing or swallowing
- wheezing

If you experience a serious side effect, you or your doctor may send a report to the Food and Drug Administration's (FDA) MedWatch Adverse Event Reporting program online [at http://www.fda.gov/MedWatch/index.html] or by phone [1-800-332-1088].

What storage conditions are needed for this medicine?

Keep this medication in the container it came in, tightly closed, and out of reach of children. Store it according to the package instructions. Throw away any medication that is outdated or no longer needed. Talk to your pharmacist about the proper disposal of your medications.

What other information should I know?

Keep all appointments with your doctor.

Do not let anyone else use your medication. Ask your pharmacist any questions you have about refilling your prescription.

Talk to your doctor, pharmacist, or other healthcare professional if you have questions about dosing information for your medication.

Hydrocortisone Oral

(hye droe kor′ ti sone)

Brand Name: Cortef®, Hydrocortone®
Also available generically.

Why is this medicine prescribed?

Hydrocortisone, a corticosteroid, is similar to a natural hormone produced by your adrenal glands. It is often used to replace this chemical when your body does not make enough of it. It relieves inflammation (swelling, heat, redness, and pain) and is used to treat certain forms of arthritis; skin, blood, kidney, eye, thyroid, and intestinal disorders (e.g., colitis); severe allergies; and asthma. Hydrocortisone is also used to treat certain types of cancer.

This medication is sometimes prescribed for other uses; ask your doctor or pharmacist for more information.

How should this medicine be used?

Hydrocortisone comes as a tablet and suspension to be taken by mouth. Your doctor will prescribe a dosing schedule that is best for you. Follow the directions on your prescription label carefully, and ask your doctor or pharmacist to explain any part you do not understand. Take hydrocortisone exactly as directed. Do not take more or less of it or take it more often than prescribed by your doctor.

Do not stop taking hydrocortisone without talking to your doctor. Stopping the drug abruptly can cause loss of appetite, an upset stomach, vomiting, drowsiness, confusion, headache, fever, joint and muscle pain, peeling skin, and weight loss. If you take large doses for a long time, your doctor probably will decrease your dose gradually to allow your body to adjust before stopping the drug completely. Watch for these side effects if you are gradually decreasing your dose and after you stop taking the tablets or oral liquid, even if you switch to an inhalation. If these problems occur, call your doctor immediately. You may need to increase your dose of oral hydrocortisone temporarily or start taking it again.

What special precautions should I follow?

Before taking hydrocortisone,

- tell your doctor and pharmacist if you are allergic to hydrocortisone, aspirin, tartrazine (a yellow dye in some processed foods and drugs), or any other drugs.
- tell your doctor and pharmacist what prescription and nonprescription medications you are taking, especially anticoagulants ('blood thinners') such as warfarin (Coumadin), arthritis medication, aspirin, cyclosporine (Neoral, Sandimmune), digoxin (Lanoxin), diuretics ('water pills'), estrogen (Premarin), ketoconazole (Nizoral), oral contraceptives, phenobarbital, phenytoin (Dilantin), rifampin (Rifadin), theophylline (Theo-Dur), and vitamins.

- if you have a fungal infection (other than on your skin), do not take hydrocortisone without talking to your doctor.
- tell your doctor if you have or have ever had liver, kidney, intestinal, or heart disease; diabetes; an underactive thyroid gland; high blood pressure; mental illness; myasthenia gravis; osteoporosis; herpes eye infection; seizures; tuberculosis (TB); or ulcers.
- tell your doctor if you are pregnant, plan to become pregnant, or are breast-feeding. If you become pregnant while taking hydrocortisone, call your doctor.
- if you are having surgery, including dental surgery, tell the doctor or dentist that you are taking hydrocortisone.
- if you have a history of ulcers or take large doses of aspirin or other arthritis medication, limit your consumption of alcoholic beverages while taking this drug. Hydrocortisone makes your stomach and intestines more susceptible to the irritating effects of alcohol, aspirin, and certain arthritis medications. This effect increases your risk of ulcers.

What special dietary instructions should I follow?

Your doctor may instruct you to follow a low-sodium, low-salt, potassium-rich, or high-protein diet. Follow these directions.

Hydrocortisone may cause an upset stomach. Take hydrocortisone with food or milk.

What should I do if I forget to take a dose?

When you start to take hydrocortisone, ask your doctor what to do if you forget a dose. Write down these instructions so that you can refer to them later.

If you take hydrocortisone once a day, take the missed dose as soon as you remember it. If you do not remember a missed dose until it is time for the next dose, skip the missed dose completely and take only the regularly scheduled dose.

If you take more than one dose a day, take the missed dose as soon as you remember it. However, if it is almost time for the next dose, skip the missed dose and continue your regular dosing schedule. Do not take a double dose to make up for a missed one.

What side effects can this medicine cause?

Hydrocortisone may cause side effects. Tell your doctor if any of these symptoms are severe or do not go away:

- upset stomach
- stomach irritation
- vomiting
- headache
- dizziness
- insomnia
- restlessness
- depression
- anxiety
- acne
- increased hair growth

- easy bruising
- irregular or absent menstrual periods

If you experience any of the following symptoms, call your doctor immediately:

- skin rash
- swollen face, lower legs, or ankles
- vision problems
- cold or infection that lasts a long time
- muscle weakness
- black or tarry stool

If you experience a serious side effect, you or your doctor may send a report to the Food and Drug Administration's (FDA) MedWatch Adverse Event Reporting program online [at http://www.fda.gov/MedWatch/index.html] or by phone [1-800-332-1088].

What storage conditions are needed for this medicine?

Keep this medication in the container it came in, tightly closed, and out of reach of children. Store it at room temperature and away from excess heat and moisture (not in the bathroom). Throw away any medication that is outdated or no longer needed. Talk to your pharmacist about the proper disposal of your medication.

What should I do in case of overdose?

In case of overdose, call your local poison control center at 1-800-222-1222. If the victim has collapsed or is not breathing, call local emergency services at 911.

What other information should I know?

Keep all appointments with your doctor and the laboratory. Your doctor will order certain lab tests to check your response to hydrocortisone. Checkups are especially important for children because hydrocortisone can slow bone growth.

If your condition worsens, call your doctor. Your dose may need to be adjusted.

Carry an identification card that indicates that you may need to take supplementary doses (write down the full dose you took before gradually decreasing it) of hydrocortisone during periods of stress (injuries, infections, and severe asthma attacks). Ask your pharmacist or doctor how to obtain this card. List your name, medical problems, drugs and dosages, and doctor's name and telephone number on the card.

This drug makes you more susceptible to illnesses. If you are exposed to chicken pox, measles, or tuberculosis (TB) while using hydrocortisone, call your doctor. Do not have a vaccination, other immunization, or any skin test while you are taking hydrocortisone unless your doctor tells you that you may.

Report any injuries or signs of infection (fever, sore throat, pain during urination, and muscle aches) that occur during treatment.

Your doctor may instruct you to weigh yourself every day. Report any unusual weight gain.

If your sputum (the matter you cough up during an asthma attack) thickens or changes color from clear white to yellow, green, or gray, call your doctor; these changes may be signs of an infection.

If you have diabetes, hydrocortisone may increase your blood sugar level. If you monitor your blood sugar (glucose) at home, test your blood or urine more frequently than usual. Call your doctor if your blood sugar is high or if sugar is present in your urine; your dose of diabetes medication and your diet may need to be changed.

Do not let anyone else take your medication. Ask your pharmacist any questions you have about refilling your prescription.

Dosage Facts
For Informational Purposes

Caution: Do not change your dose, how often you take your medication, or the length of time you are to take it without first talking to your healthcare provider.

The following dosage information was written using medical language for doctors and other healthcare professionals and is provided here for you to check your dosage. The dosage of this drug may differ for different patients. Therefore, always follow your doctor's instructions or the directions on the label. Contact your healthcare provider or pharmacist if you have any questions about the specific dosage of your medication after reviewing this information.

General Dosage Information

Available as hydrocortisone, hydrocortisone acetate, hydrocortisone sodium phosphate, and hydrocortisone sodium succinate; dosage of hydrocortisone sodium phosphate and sodium succinate is expressed in terms of hydrocortisone and dosage of hydrocortisone acetate is expressed in terms of hydrocortisone acetate.

After a satisfactory response is obtained, dosage should be decreased in small decrements to the lowest level that maintains an adequate clinical response, and discontinue the drug as soon as possible.

Monitor patients continually for signs that indicate dosage adjustment is necessary, such as remissions or exacerbations of the disease and stress (surgery, infection, trauma).

High dosages may be required for acute situations of certain rheumatic disorders and collagen diseases; after a response has been obtained, drug often must be continued for long periods at low dosage.

High or massive dosages may be required in the treatment of pemphigus, exfoliative dermatitis, bullous dermatitis herpetiformis, severe erythema multiforme, or mycosis fungoides. Early initiation of systemic glucocorticoid therapy may be lifesaving in pemphigus vulgaris. Reduce dosage gradually to the lowest effective level, but discontinuance may not be possible.

Massive dosages may be required for the treatment of shock.

If used orally for prolonged anti-inflammatory therapy,

consider an alternate-day dosage regimen. Following long-term therapy, withdraw gradually.

Pediatric Patients

Base pediatric dosage on severity of the disease and the response of the patient rather than on strict adherence to dosage indicated by age, body weight, or body surface area.

Usual Dosage

ORAL:
- Hydrocortisone: 0.56–8 mg/kg daily or 16–240 mg/m² daily, administered in 3 or 4 divided doses.

Adult Patients

Usual Dosage

ORAL:
- Hydrocortisone: Initially, 10–320 mg daily (usually administered in 3 or 4 divided doses), depending on the disease being treated.

† Use is not currently included in the labeling approved by the US Food and Drug Administration.

Hydrocortisone Topical

(hye droe kor′ ti sone)

Brand Name: Ala-Cort®, Ala-Scalpt®, Anucort-HC®, Anu-Med® HC, Anusert® HC-1, Anusol-HC®, Anusol-HC®-1, Aquanil HC®, Caldecort® Anti-Itch, Cetacort®, CortaGel® Extra Strength, Cortaid® FastStick® Maximum Strength, Cortaid® Intensive Therapy, Cortaid® Maximum Strength, Cortaid® Sensitive Skin Formula, Cortaid® Spray Maximum Strength, Cortenema®, Corticaine®, Cortifoam®, Cortizone for Kids®, Cortizone®-5, Cortizone-10®, Cortizone-10® External Anal Itch Relief Creme®, Cortizone-10® Scalp Itch Formula Liquid, Dermacort®, Dermarest® DriCort®, DermiCort®, Dermtex® HC, Dermtex® HC Spray, Gynecort® 10, Hemorrhoidal®-HC, Hemril-HC® Uniserts®, HydroSKIN®, Hytone®, LactiCare®-HC, Lanacort® 10, Locoid®, Massengill® Medicated Soft Cloth Towelette®, Nupercainal® Hydrocortisone Anti-Itch Cream, Nutracort®, Orabase® HCA, Pandel®, Penecort®, Preparation H® Hydrocortisone, Proctocort®, ProctoCream®-HC, ProctoFoam®-HC as a combination product containing Hydrocortisone Acetate and Pramoxine Hydrochloride, Sarnol® HC, Scalp-Aid®, Scalpcort® Maximum Strength, Texacort®, Westcort®

Also available generically.

Why is this medicine prescribed?

Hydrocortisone is available with or without a prescription. Low-strength preparations (0.5% or 1%) are used without a prescription for the temporary relief of (1) minor skin irritations, itching, and rashes caused by eczema, insect bites, poison ivy, poison oak, poison sumac, soaps, detergents, cosmetics, and jewelry; (2) itchy anal and rectal areas; and (3) itching and irritation of the scalp. It is also used to relieve the discomfort of mouth sores.

Hydrocortisone may be prescribed by your doctor to relieve the itching, redness, dryness, crusting, scaling, inflammation, and discomfort of various skin conditions; the inflammation of ulcerative colitis or proctitis; or the swelling and discomfort of hemorrhoids and other rectal problems.

This medication is sometimes prescribed for other uses; ask your doctor or pharmacist for more information.

How should this medicine be used?

Hydrocortisone comes as ointment, cream, lotion, liquid, gel, medicated cloth towelette, and spray for use on the skin; foam, suppositories, cream, ointment, and enema for rectal use; and paste for use in the mouth.

Hydrocortisone is usually used one to four times a day for skin problems.

For mouth sores, it usually is applied two or three times a day after meals and at bedtime. If mouth sores do not begin to heal within 7 days, call your doctor.

For colitis, hydrocortisone usually is used every night or twice a day (every morning and night) for 2 or 3 weeks. Although colitis symptoms may improve within 3-5 days, 2-3 months of regular enema use may be required. Call your doctor if your colitis symptoms do not improve within 3 weeks.

For proctitis, hydrocortisone usually is used one or two times a day for 2-3 weeks, then if necessary every other day until your condition improves. Proctitis symptoms may improve within 5-7 days.

For hemorrhoids, hydrocortisone usually is used twice a day (every morning and night) for 2-6 days.

Follow the directions on the label carefully, and ask your doctor or pharmacist to explain any part that you do not understand. Use hydrocortisone exactly as directed. Do not use more or less of it or use it more often than prescribed by your doctor.

If you obtained hydrocortisone without a prescription and your condition does not improve within 7 days, stop using it and call your doctor.

Call your doctor if any area treated with hydrocortisone gets worse or if redness, swelling, or oozing of pus develops.

To use hydrocortisone ointment, cream, lotion, liquid, or gel on your skin, wash or soak the affected area thoroughly before applying the medication, unless it irritates your skin. Then apply sparingly in a thin film and rub it in gently.

To use the lotion, liquid, or gel on your scalp, part your hair, apply a small amount of the medicine on the affected area, and rub it in gently. Protect the area from washing and rubbing until the medication dries. You may wash your hair as usual but not right after applying the medicine.

To apply the aerosol spray, shake well and spray on the

affected area holding the container about 3-6 inches away. Spray for about 2 seconds to cover an area the size of your hand. Take care not to inhale the vapors. If you are spraying near your face, cover your eyes.

Avoid prolonged use on the face, in the genital and rectal areas, and in skin creases and armpits unless directed to do so by your doctor.

If you are using hydrocortisone on your face, keep it out of your eyes.

If you are using hydrocortisone on a child's diaper area, do not use tight-fitting diapers or plastic pants. Such use may increase side effects.

Do not apply cosmetics or other skin preparations on the treated area without talking to your doctor.

If your doctor tells you to wrap or bandage the treated area, follow these instructions:

1. Soak the area in water or wash it well.
2. While the skin is moist, gently rub the medication into the affected areas.
3. Cover the area with plastic wrap (such as Saran Wrap or Handi-Wrap). The plastic may be held in place with a gauze or elastic bandage or adhesive tape on the normal skin beside the treated area. (Instead of using plastic wrap, plastic gloves may be used for the hands, plastic bags for the feet, or a shower cap for the scalp.)
4. Carefully seal the edges of the plastic to make sure the wrap adheres closely to the skin. If the affected area is moist, you can leave the edges of the plastic wrap partly unsealed or puncture the wrap to allow excess moisture to escape.
5. Leave the plastic wrap in place as long as directed by your doctor. Usually plastic wraps are left in place no more than 12 hours each day.
6. Cleanse the skin and reapply the medication each time a new plastic wrapping is applied.

Apply the rectal cream or ointment externally to the anal area. Some nonprescription creams may be applied to the genital and anal areas; read the label of the product you are using carefully.

The hydrocortisone enema comes with directions that you should follow carefully. Lie on your left side while using the enema and for 30 minutes afterward. Try to hold the enema in for at least 1 hour and preferably all night.

The rectal foam also comes with directions that you should follow carefully. A special applicator is provided and always should be used to apply the foam. Do not insert any part of the container into your rectum. After using the applicator, take it apart and clean it thoroughly with warm water.

To insert a rectal suppository, follow these steps:

1. Remove the wrapper. If the suppository is too soft to insert, chill it in the refrigerator for 30 minutes or run cold water over it before removing the foil wrapper.
2. Dip the tip of the suppository in water.
3. Lie down on your left side and raise your right knee to your chest. (A left-handed person should lie on the right side and raise the left knee.)

4. Using your finger, insert the suppository into the rectum (about 1/2 to 1 inch in infants and children and 1 inch in adults). Hold it in place for a few moments.
5. Remain lying down for 15 minutes. Then, stand up, wash your hands thoroughly, and resume your normal activities.

Note that some hydrocortisone suppositories may stain fabric, so take any precautions needed.

What special precautions should I follow?

Before using hydrocortisone,

- tell your doctor and pharmacist if you are allergic to hydrocortisone or any other drugs.
- tell your doctor and pharmacist what prescription and nonprescription medications you are taking, especially cancer chemotherapy agents, other topical medications, and vitamins.
- tell your doctor if you have an infection or have ever had diabetes, glaucoma, a circulation disorder, or an immune disorder.
- tell your doctor if you are pregnant, plan to become pregnant, or are breast-feeding. If you become pregnant while using hydrocortisone, call your doctor immediately.
- remember not to use hydrocortisone on children less than 2 years of age without talking to a doctor.

What should I do if I forget to take a dose?

Apply the missed dose as soon as you remember it. However, if it is almost time for the next dose, skip the missed dose and continue your regular dosing schedule. Do not apply a double dose to make up for a missed one.

What side effects can this medicine cause?

Hydrocortisone may cause side effects. Tell your doctor if any of these symptoms are severe or do not go away:

- drying or cracking of the skin
- acne
- itching
- burning
- change in skin color

If you experience any of the following symptoms, call your doctor immediately:

- severe skin rash
- difficulty breathing or swallowing
- wheezing
- skin infection (redness, swelling, or oozing of pus)

If you experience a serious side effect, you or your doctor may send a report to the Food and Drug Administration's (FDA) MedWatch Adverse Event Reporting program online [at http://www.fda.gov/MedWatch/index.html] or by phone [1-800-332-1088].

What storage conditions are needed for this medicine?

Keep this medication in the container it came in, tightly closed, and out of reach of children. Store it according to the package instructions. Throw away any medication that is outdated or no longer needed. Talk to your pharmacist about the proper disposal of your medication.

What other information should I know?

Keep all appointments with your doctor.

Do not let anyone else use your medication. Ask your pharmacist any questions you have about refilling your prescription.

Dosage Facts
For Informational Purposes

Caution: Do not change your dose, how often you take your medication, or the length of time you are to take it without first talking to your healthcare provider.

The following dosage information was written using medical language for doctors and other healthcare professionals and is provided here for you to check your dosage. The dosage of this drug may differ for different patients. Therefore, always follow your doctor's instructions or the directions on the label. Contact your healthcare provider or pharmacist if you have any questions about the specific dosage of your medication after reviewing this information.

General Dosage Information

Available as hydrocortisone (dosage expressed in terms of the base) and as hydrocortisone acetate, buteprate, butyrate, and valerate (dosage expressed in terms of the salt).

Pediatric Patients

Administer the least amount of topical preparations that provides effective therapy.

Corticosteroid-responsive Dermatoses
TOPICAL:
- Nonprescription hydrocortisone preparations should not be used in children <2 years of age unless directed and supervised by a clinician.
- Children ≥2 years of age: Apply appropriate cream, lotion, ointment, or solution sparingly 1–4 times daily.

Adult Patients

Corticosteroid-responsive Dermatoses
TOPICAL:
- Apply appropriate cream, lotion, ointment, or solution sparingly 1–4 times daily.
- Apply aerosol foam to affected area 2–4 times daily.
- Nonprescription preparations should not be used for *self-medication* for >7 days.
- If the condition worsens or symptoms persist, discontinue and consult a clinician.

Oral Lesions
TOPICAL:
- Apply a small amount of paste to the lesion 2 or 3 times daily after meals and at bedtime.

- If substantial regeneration or repair of oral tissues does not occur after 7 days, further investigate etiology of the lesions.

Ulcerative Colitis and Anorectal Disorders
RECTAL (AS RETENTION ENEMA):
- Adjunctive treatment of ulcerative colitis: 100 mg nightly. Some clinicians recommend 100 mg twice daily followed by 100 mg nightly when improvement occurs.
- Usually given for 21 days or until clinical and proctologic remissions are achieved.
- Lay on left side during and for 30 minutes after administration to distribute drug throughout the left colon. Retain for ≥1 hour, preferably all night.
- Symptoms may improve in 3–5 days, followed by proctologic improvement. Discontinue if clinical or proctologic improvement does not occur within 2–3 weeks.
- Protologic remission may require 2–3 months of therapy.
- Following treatment for >21 days, gradually withdraw use; give every other night for 2–3 weeks, then discontinue.

RECTAL (AS FOAM):
- Ulcerative proctitis of the distal rectum: 90 mg (1 applicatorful of a 10% aerosol foam suspension) 1 or 2 times daily for 2–3 weeks. Then, if necessary, every other day until clinical and proctologic improvement.
- Symptoms may improve within 5–7 days.

RECTAL (AS SUPPOSITORY):
- Adjunctive treatment of ulcerative colitis of the rectum and other inflammatory conditions of the anorectum: 25 mg in the morning and at night for 2 weeks.
- Severe proctitis: 25 mg 3 times daily or 50 mg twice daily.
- Adjunctive treatment of postirradiation or factitial proctitis: 25 mg in the morning and at night for 6–8 weeks (or less if an adequate response is attained).
- For internal hemorrhoid symptoms and adjunctive treatment of other anorectal inflammatory conditions: 10 mg in the morning and at night for 2–6 days.

Prescribing Limits

Pediatric Patients

Corticosteroid-responsive Dermatoses
Self-medication
TOPICAL:
- Maximum 7 days.

Adult Patients

Corticosteroid-responsive Dermatoses
Self-medication
TOPICAL:
- Maximum 7 days.

Hydromorphone Hydrochloride Injection

(hye droe mor' fone)

Brand Name: Dilaudid®, Dilaudid-HP®
Also available generically.

About Your Treatment

Your doctor has ordered hydromorphone, a strong analgesic (painkiller), to relieve your pain. The drug will be either injected into a large muscle (such as your buttock or hip) or added to an intravenous fluid that will drip through a needle or catheter placed in your vein or under your skin.

You probably will receive hydromorphone continuously for around-the-clock pain relief. Your doctor also may order other pain medications to make you more comfortable. This medication is sometimes prescribed for other uses; ask your doctor or pharmacist for more information.

Your health care provider (doctor, nurse, or pharmacist) may measure the effectiveness and side effects of your treatment using laboratory tests and physical examinations. It is important to keep all appointments with your doctor and the laboratory. The length of treatment depends on how you respond to the medication.

Precautions

Before administering hydromorphone,

- tell your doctor and pharmacist if you are allergic to hydromorphone, codeine (or medications that contain codeine such as Tylenol with Codeine), hydrocodone (e.g., Vicodin), morphine (e.g., MS Contin), oxycodone (e.g., Percocet), oxymorphone (Numorphan), or any other drugs.
- tell your doctor and pharmacist what prescription and nonprescription medications you are taking, especially other pain relievers; antidepressants; cough, cold, and allergy medications; sedatives; sleeping pills; tranquilizers; and vitamins.
- tell your doctor if you have or have ever had kidney, liver, heart, or thyroid disease; seizures; asthma; bronchitis or any other respiratory diseases; prostatic hypertrophy; or urinary problems.
- tell your doctor if you are pregnant, plan to become pregnant, or are breast-feeding. If you become pregnant while taking hydromorphone, call your doctor.
- if you are having surgery, including dental surgery, tell the doctor or dentist that you are taking hydromorphone.
- you should know that this drug may make you drowsy. Do not drive a car or operate machinery until you know how this drug affects you.
- remember that alcohol can add to the drowsiness caused by this drug.

Administering Your Medication

Before you administer hydromorphone, look at the solution closely. It should be clear and free of floating material. Gently squeeze the bag or observe the solution container to make sure there are no leaks. Do not use the solution if it is discolored, if it contains particles, or if the bag or container leaks. Use a new solution, but show the damaged one to your health care provider.

It is important that you use your medication exactly as directed. Hydromorphone can be habit forming. Do not administer it more often or for a longer period than your doctor tells you. Do not change your dosing schedule without talking to your health care provider. Your health care provider may tell you to stop your infusion if you have a mechanical problem (such as a blockage in the tubing, needle, or catheter); if you have to stop an infusion, call your health care provider immediately so your therapy can continue.

Side Effects

Hydromorphone may cause side effects. Tell your health care provider if any of these symptoms are severe or do not go away:

- dizziness
- lightheadedness
- drowsiness
- upset stomach
- vomiting
- constipation
- stomach pain
- rash
- difficulty urinating

If you experience either of the following symptoms, call your health care provider immediately:

- difficulty breathing
- fainting

If you experience a serious side effect, you or your doctor may send a report to the Food and Drug Administration's (FDA) MedWatch Adverse Event Reporting program online [at http://www.fda.gov/MedWatch/index.html] or by phone [1-800-332-1088].

Storage Conditions

- Your health care provider probably will give you a several-day supply of hydromorphone at a time. If you are receiving hydromorphone intravenously (in your vein), you probably will be told to store it in the refrigerator.
- Take your next dose from the refrigerator 1 hour before using it; place it in a clean, dry area to allow it to warm to room temperature.

If you are receiving hydromorphone intramuscularly (in your muscle), your health care provider will tell you how to store it properly.

Store your medication only as directed. Make sure you understand what you need to store your medication properly.

Keep your supplies in a clean, dry place when you are not using them, and keep all medications and supplies out of reach of children. Your health care provider will tell you how to throw away used needles, syringes, tubing, and containers to avoid accidental injury.

Overdose

In case of overdose, call your local poison control center at 1-800-222-1222. If the victim has collapsed or is not breathing, call local emergency services at 911.

Signs of Infection

If you are receiving hydromorphone in your vein or under your skin, you need to know the symptoms of a catheter-related infection (an infection where the needle enters your vein or skin). If you experience any of these effects near your intravenous catheter, tell your health care provider as soon as possible:

- tenderness
- warmth
- irritation
- drainage
- redness
- swelling
- pain

Dosage Facts
For Informational Purposes

Caution: Do not change your dose, how often you take your medication, or the length of time you are to take it without first talking to your healthcare provider.

The following dosage information was written using medical language for doctors and other healthcare professionals and is provided here for you to check your dosage. The dosage of this drug may differ for different patients. Therefore, always follow your doctor's instructions or the directions on the label. Contact your healthcare provider or pharmacist if you have any questions about the specific dosage of your medication after reviewing this information.

General Dosage Information

Available as hydromorphone hydrochloride; dosage expressed in terms of the salt.

Give the smallest effective dose as infrequently as possible to minimize the development of tolerance and physical dependence.

Reduce dosage in poor-risk patients, in pediatric or geriatric patients, and in patients receiving other CNS depressants.

In patients who are tolerant to opiate agonists and who require high dosages (e.g., patients with severe chronic pain associated with cancer), individualize dosage of highly potent preparations based on response and tolerance.

Avoid abrupt withdrawal from relatively high dosages (e.g., in chronic pain patients) since precipitation of severe abstinence syndrome is likely.

Pediatric Patients
Pain†

IV, IM, OR SUB-Q:
- Children 6–12 years of age: 0.015 mg/kg every 4–6 hours as needed.
- Children >12 years of age: 1–4 mg every 4–6 hours as needed.

Adult Patients
Pain

IV OR IM:
- 1.5–2 mg every 3–6 hours as necessary.
- For severe pain, 3–4 mg every 4–6 hours may be given.
- Pain associated with terminal cancer: individual doses of 1–14 mg.

SUB-Q:
- 2 mg every 4–6 hours as necessary.
- For severe pain, 3–4 mg every 4–6 hours.
- Pain associated with terminal cancer: individual doses of 1–14 mg; occasionally, individual 30-mg doses (60 mg total) in opiate-tolerant patients.

Special Populations

Geriatric and Debilitated Patients
- Select dosage with caution, and use lower than usual initial dosages.

† Use is not currently included in the labeling approved by the US Food and Drug Administration.

Hydromorphone Oral and Rectal

(hye droe mor′ fone)

Brand Name: Dilaudid®
Also available generically.

Why is this medicine prescribed?

Hydromorphone is used to relieve moderate to severe pain. It also may be used to decrease coughing.

This medication is sometimes prescribed for other uses; ask your doctor or pharmacist for more information.

How should this medicine be used?

Hydromorphone comes as a tablet and liquid to take by mouth. It also comes as a rectal suppository. The oral forms usually are taken every 4-6 hours as needed. The suppository usually is used every 6-8 hours as needed. Follow the directions on your prescription label carefully, and ask your doctor or pharmacist to explain any part you do not understand.

Shake the liquid well before measuring a dose. Take hydromorphone exactly as directed. Hydromorphone can be habit-forming. Do not take a larger dose, take it more often, or for a longer period than your doctor tells you to.

To insert a hydromorphone suppository rectally, follow these steps:

1. Remove the wrapper.
2. Dip the tip of the suppository in water.
3. Lie down on your left side and raise your right knee to your chest. (A left-handed person should lie on the right side and raise the left knee.)
4. Using your finger, insert the suppository into the rectum, about 1/2 to 1 inch for infants and children and about 1 inch for an adult.
5. Hold it in place with your finger for a few moments.
6. Stand up after about 15 minutes. Wash your hands thoroughly and resume normal activities.

What special precautions should I follow?

Before taking hydromorphone,

- tell your doctor and pharmacist if you are allergic to hydromorphone, aspirin, sulfites, tartrazine (yellow dye), or any other drugs.
- tell your doctor and pharmacist what prescription and nonprescription medications you are taking, especially other pain relievers; antidepressants; medications for cough, cold, or allergies; sedatives; sleeping pills; tranquilizers; and vitamins.
- tell your doctor if you have or have ever had liver or kidney disease, a history of alcoholism, lung or thyroid disease, heart disease, prostatic hypertrophy, or urinary problems.
- tell your doctor if you are pregnant, plan to become pregnant, or are breast-feeding. If you become pregnant while taking hydromorphone, call your doctor.
- if you are having surgery, including dental surgery, tell the doctor or dentist that you are taking hydromorphone.
- you should know that this drug may make you drowsy. Do not drive a car or operate machinery until you know how this drug affects you.
- remember that alcohol can add to the drowsiness caused by this drug.

What special dietary instructions should I follow?

Hydromorphone may cause an upset stomach. Take hydromorphone with food or milk.

What should I do if I forget to take a dose?

Hydromorphone usually is taken as needed. If your doctor has told you to take hydromorphone regularly, take the missed dose as soon as you remember it. However, if it is almost time for the next dose, skip the missed dose and continue your regular dosing schedule. Do not take a double dose to make up for a missed one.

What side effects can this medicine cause?

Hydromorphone may cause side effects. Tell your doctor if any of these symptoms are severe or do not go away:

- dizziness
- lightheadedness
- drowsiness
- upset stomach
- vomiting
- constipation
- stomach pain
- rash
- difficulty urinating

If you experience either of the following symptoms, call your doctor immediately:

- difficulty breathing
- fainting

If you experience a serious side effect, you or your doctor may send a report to the Food and Drug Administration's (FDA) MedWatch Adverse Event Reporting program online [at http://www.fda.gov/MedWatch/index.html] or by phone [1-800-332-1088].

What storage conditions are needed for this medicine?

Keep this medication in the container it came in, tightly closed, and out of reach of children. Store it at room temperature and away from excess heat and moisture (not in the bathroom). Throw away any medication that is outdated or no longer needed. Talk to your pharmacist about the proper disposal of your medication.

What should I do in case of overdose?

In case of overdose, call your local poison control center at 1-800-222-1222. If the victim has collapsed or is not breathing, call local emergency services at 911.

What other information should I know?

Keep all appointments with your doctor.

Do not let anyone else take your medication. Ask your pharmacist any questions you have about refilling your prescription.

Dosage Facts
For Informational Purposes

Caution: Do not change your dose, how often you take your medication, or the length of time you are to take it without first talking to your healthcare provider.

The following dosage information was written using medical language for doctors and other healthcare professionals and is provided here for you to check your dosage. The dosage of this drug may differ for different patients. Therefore, always follow your doctor's instructions or the directions on the label. Contact your healthcare provider or pharmacist if you have any questions about the specific dosage of your medication after reviewing this information.

General Dosage Information

Available as hydromorphone hydrochloride; dosage expressed in terms of the salt.

Give the smallest effective dose as infrequently as possible to minimize the development of tolerance and physical dependence.

Reduce dosage in poor-risk patients, in pediatric or geriatric patients, and in patients receiving other CNS depressants.

In patients who are tolerant to opiate agonists and who require high dosages (e.g., patients with severe chronic pain associated with cancer), individualize dosage of highly potent preparations based on response and tolerance.

Avoid abrupt withdrawal from relatively high dosages (e.g., in chronic pain patients) since precipitation of severe abstinence syndrome is likely.

Pediatric Patients

Pain†
ORAL:
- Children 6–12 years of age: 0.03–0.08 mg/kg every 4–6 hours as needed.
- Children >12 years of age: 1–4 mg every 4–6 hours as needed.

Cough†
ORAL:
- Children 6–12 years of age: 0.5 mg every 3–4 hours.
- Children >12 years of age: 1 mg every 3–4 hours.

Adult Patients

Pain
ORAL:
- Usually, 2 mg every 4–6 hours as necessary.
- For severe pain, 4 mg (or more) every 3–6 hours as indicated and tolerated.

RECTAL:
- Suppository: 3 mg every 6–8 hours as necessary.

Cough
ORAL:
- Usually, 1 mg every 3–4 hours.

Special Populations

Geriatric and Debilitated Patients
- Select dosage with caution, and use lower than usual initial dosages.

† Use is not currently included in the labeling approved by the US Food and Drug Administration.

Hydroxychloroquine
(hye drox ee klor′ oh kwin)

Brand Name: Plaquenil®
Also available generically.

Why is this medicine prescribed?

Hydroxychloroquine is in a class of drugs called antimalarials. It is used to prevent and treat acute attacks of malaria. It is also used to treat discoid or systemic lupus erythematosus and rheumatoid arthritis in patients whose symptoms have not improved with other treatments.

This medication is sometimes prescribed for other uses; ask your doctor or pharmacist for more information.

How should this medicine be used?

Hydroxychloroquine comes as a tablet to take by mouth. For prevention of malaria in adults, two tablets are usually taken once a week on exactly the same day of each week. The first dose is taken 1-2 weeks before traveling to an area where malaria is common, and then doses are continued for 8 weeks after exposure. For treatment of acute attacks of malaria in adults, four tablets are usually taken right away, followed by two tablets 6-8 hours later and then two tablets on each of the next 2 days.

For prevention or treatment of malaria in infants and children, the amount of hydroxychloroquine is based on the child's weight. Your doctor will calculate this amount and tell you how much hydroxychloroquine your child should receive.

For lupus erythematosus, one or two tablets are usually taken once or twice daily. For rheumatoid arthritis, one to three tablets are usually taken once a day.

Hydroxychloroquine can be taken with a glass of milk or a meal to decrease stomach upset. Follow the directions on your prescription label carefully, and ask your doctor or pharmacist to explain any part you do not understand. Take hydroxychloroquine exactly as directed. Do not take more or less of it or take it more often than prescribed by your doctor.

If you are taking hydroxychloroquine for symptoms of rheumatoid arthritis, your symptoms should improve within 6 months. If your rheumatoid arthritis symptoms do not improve, or if they worsen, stop taking the drug and call your doctor. Once you and your doctor are sure the drug works for you, do not stop taking hydroxychloroquine without talking to your doctor. Symptoms of rheumatoid arthritis will return if you stop taking hydroxychloroquine.

Are there other uses for this medicine?

Hydroxychloroquine is used occasionally to treat porphyria cutanea tarda. Talk to your doctor about the possible risks of using this drug for your condition.

What special precautions should I follow?

Before taking hydroxychloroquine,

- tell your doctor and pharmacist if you are allergic to hydroxychloroquine, chloroquine (Aralen), primaquine, or any other drugs.
- tell your doctor and pharmacist what prescription and nonprescription drugs you are taking, especially acetaminophen (Tylenol, others), digoxin (Lanoxin), iron-containing medications (including multivitamins), isoniazid (Nydrazid), methotrexate (Rheumatrex), niacin, rifampin (Rifadin, Rimactane), and vitamins and herbal products.
- tell your doctor if you have or have ever had liver disease, psoriasis, porphyria or other blood disorders, G-6-PD deficiency, dermatitis (skin inflammations), or if you drink large amounts of alcohol.
- tell your doctor if you have ever had vision changes while taking hydroxychloroquine, chloroquine (Aralen), or primaquine.
- tell your doctor if you are pregnant, plan to become pregnant, or are breast-feeding. If you become pregnant while taking hydroxychloroquine, call your doctor.

What should I do if I forget to take a dose?

Take the missed dose as soon as you remember it. However, if it is almost time for the next dose, skip the missed dose and continue your regular dosing schedule. Do not take a double dose to make up for a missed one.

What side effects can this medicine cause?

Hydroxychloroquine may cause side effects. Tell your doctor if any of these symptoms are severe or do not go away:

- headache
- dizziness
- loss of appetite
- upset stomach
- diarrhea
- stomach pain
- vomiting
- skin rash

If you experience any of the following symptoms, call your doctor immediately:

- reading or seeing difficulties (words, letters, or parts of objects missing)
- sensitivity to light
- blurred distance vision
- seeing light flashes or streaks
- difficulty hearing
- ringing in ears
- muscle weakness
- bleeding or bruising of the skin
- bleaching or loss of hair
- mood or mental changes
- irregular heartbeat
- drowsiness
- convulsions

If you experience a serious side effect, you or your doctor may send a report to the Food and Drug Administration's (FDA) MedWatch Adverse Event Reporting program online [at http://www.fda.gov/MedWatch/index.html] or by phone [1-800-332-1088].

What storage conditions are needed for this medicine?

Keep this medication in the container it came in, tightly closed, and out of reach of children. Store it at room temperature and away from excess heat and moisture (not in the bathroom). Throw away any medication that is outdated or no longer needed. Talk to your pharmacist about the proper disposal of your medication.

What should I do in case of overdose?

In case of overdose, call your local poison control center at 1-800-222-1222. If the victim has collapsed or is not breathing, call local emergency services at 911.

What other information should I know?

Children can be especially sensitive to an overdose, so keep the medication out of the reach of children. Children should not take hydroxychloroquine for long-term therapy.

Keep all appointments with your doctor and the laboratory. Your doctor may order certain lab tests to check your response to hydroxychloroquine.

If you are taking hydroxychloroquine for a long period of time, your doctor will recommend frequent eye exams. It is very important that you keep these appointments. Hydroxychloroquine can cause serious vision problems. If you experience any changes in vision, stop taking hydroxychloroquine and call your doctor immediately.

Do not let anyone else take your medication. Ask your pharmacist any questions you have about refilling your prescription.

Dosage Facts

For Informational Purposes

Caution: Do not change your dose, how often you take your medication, or the length of time you are to take it without first talking to your healthcare provider.

The following dosage information was written using medical language for doctors and other healthcare professionals and is provided here for you to check your dosage. The dosage of this drug may differ for different patients. Therefore, always follow your doctor's instructions or the directions on the label. Contact your healthcare provider or pharmacist if you have any questions about the specific dosage of your medication after reviewing this information.

General Dosage Information

Available as hydroxychloroquine sulfate; dosage usually expressed as hydroxychloroquine.

Each 200 mg of hydroxychloroquine sulfate is equivalent to 155 mg of hydroxychloroquine.

Pediatric Patients

Malaria

Prevention of Malaria in Areas Without Chloroquine-resistant Plasmodium

ORAL:
- 5 mg/kg (6.5 mg/kg of hydroxychloroquine sulfate) once weekly on the same day each week.
- Initiate prophylaxis 1–2 weeks prior to entering a malarious area and continue for 4 weeks after leaving the area. CDC states it may be advisable to initiate prophylaxis 3–4 weeks prior to travel to ensure that the drug or combination of drugs (in individuals receiving other drugs) is well tolerated and to allow ample time if a switch to another antimalarial agent is required.
- If not initiated prior to entering a malarious area, manufacturer recommends a loading dose of 10 mg/kg (13 mg/kg of hydroxychloroquine sulfate) given in 2 equally divided doses 6 hours apart followed by the usual dosage.

Treatment of Uncomplicated Chloroquine-susceptible Malaria

ORAL:
- An initial dose of 10 mg/kg (13 mg/kg of hydroxychloroquine sulfate) followed by 5-mg/kg doses (6.5 mg/kg of hydroxychloroquine sulfate) given at 6, 24, and 48 hours after the initial dose.

Adult Patients

Malaria

Prevention of Malaria in Areas Without Chloroquine-resistant Plasmodium

ORAL:
- 310 mg (400 mg of hydroxychloroquine sulfate) once weekly on the same day each week.
- Initiate prophylaxis 1–2 weeks prior to entering a malarious area and continue for 4 weeks after leaving the area. CDC states it may be advisable to initiate prophylaxis 3–4 weeks prior to travel to ensure that the drug or combination of drugs (in individuals receiving other drugs) is well tolerated and to allow ample time if a switch to another antimalarial agent is required.
- If not initiated prior to entering a malarious area, the manufacturer recommends a loading dose of 620 mg (800 mg of hydroxychloroquine sulfate) followed by the usual dosage regimen.

Treatment of Uncomplicated Chloroquine-susceptible Malaria

ORAL:
- An initial dose of 620 mg (800 mg of hydroxychloroquine sulfate) followed by 310-mg doses (400 mg of hydroxychloroquine sulfate) given 6–8 hours, 24, and 48 hours after the initial dose. This represents a total hydroxychloroquine dose of 1.55 g (2 g of hydroxychloroquine sulfate) in 3 days. Alternatively, adults may receive a single 620-mg dose (800 mg of hydroxychloroquine sulfate).

Rheumatoid Arthritis

ORAL:
- Initiate treatment with 310–465 mg (400–600 mg of hydroxychloroquine sulfate) daily. If adverse effects occur, dosage may be temporarily reduced; after 5–10 days, increase dosage gradually until an optimum response occurs without recurrence of adverse effects.
- A response may not occur until after 4–12 weeks and several months of therapy may be required to attain optimum response. When a good response is obtained, decrease dosage by 50% and continue treatment with a maintenance dosage of 155–310 mg (200–400 mg of hydroxychloroquine sulfate) daily.
- If relapse occurs after hydroxychloroquine is discontinued, the drug can be reinitiated or continued on an intermittent schedule if there is no evidence of adverse ocular effects.
- If objective improvement of rheumatoid arthritis (e.g., reduced joint swelling, increased mobility) does not occur within 6 months, hydroxychloroquine should be discontinued.

Lupus Erythematosus

ORAL:
- 310 mg (400 mg of hydroxychloroquine sulfate) once or twice daily for several weeks or months depending on response of the patient. For prolonged maintenance therapy, 155–310 mg (200–400 mg of hydroxychloroquine sulfate) daily may be adequate.

Q Fever†

Acute Q Fever in Patients with Preexisting Valvular Heart Disease†

ORAL:
- CDC recommends 465 mg (600 mg of hydroxychloroquine sulfate) daily in conjunction with oral doxycycline (200 mg daily) for 1 year. Adjust hydroxychloroquine dosage to maintain plasma hydroxychloroquine concentrations at 1 ± 0.2 mcg/mL.

Chronic Q Fever†

ORAL:
- CDC recommends 465 mg (600 mg of hydroxychloroquine sulfate) daily in conjunction with oral doxycycline (200 mg daily) for 1.5–3 years.

Prescribing Limits

Pediatric Patients

Malaria
Prevention of Malaria in Areas Without Chloroquine-resistant Plasmodium

ORAL:
- Maximum of 310 mg (400 mg of hydroxychloroquine sulfate) daily, regardless of weight.

† Use is not currently included in the labeling approved by the US Food and Drug Administration.

Hydroxyurea

(hye drox ee yoor ee′ a)

Brand Name: Droxia®, Hydrea®
Also available generically.

Important Warning

Hydroxyurea may cause severe, life-threatening side effects, including a low blood count (decrease in the number of blood cells in your body) Tell your doctor if you have or have ever had a blood disease. Tell your doctor and pharmacist about all the medications you are taking. If you take hydroxyurea with other medications that may cause a low blood count, the side effects of the medications may be more severe. If you experience any of the following symptoms, call your doctor immediately: fever, sore throat, chills, cough, and other signs of infection; excessive tiredness; weakness; pale skin; dizziness; confusion; fast heartbeat, shortness of breath; difficulty falling asleep or staying asleep; or unusual bleeding or bruising.

Keep all appointments with your doctor and the laboratory. Your doctor will order certain tests on a regular basis to check your body's response to hydroxyurea and to see if your blood count has dropped. Your doctor may need to change your dose or tell you to stop taking hydroxyurea for a period of time to allow your blood count to return to normal if it has dropped too low. Follow your doctor's directions carefully and ask your doctor if you do not know how much hydroxyurea you should take.

Taking hydroxyurea may increase the risk that you will develop cancer. This risk may be greater if you take hydroxyurea for a long time.

Talk to your doctor about the risks of taking hydroxyurea.

Women who are taking hydroxyurea, or whose male partners are taking hydroxyurea, may be less likely to become pregnant than women who are not taking hydroxyurea or whose partners are not taking the medication. However, you should not assume that you or your partner cannot become pregnant during your treatment. Tell your doctor if you are pregnant or plan to become pregnant. Use a reliable method of birth control to prevent pregnancy while you are taking hydroxyurea. If you become pregnant while taking hydroxyurea, call your doctor immediately. Hydroxyurea may cause harm or death to the fetus.

About Your Treatment

Your doctor has ordered hydroxyurea to help treat your illness. Hydroxyurea comes as a capsule to take by mouth.
This medication is used:
- to treat melanoma (a type of skin cancer)
- to treat chronic myelocytic leukemia (CML; cancer of the white blood cells)
- to treat recurrent, metastatic, or inoperable ovarian cancer [cancer of the ovary (a female reproductive organ) that has returned after treatment, that has spread, or that cannot be treated with surgery]
- with radiation therapy to control primary squamous cell carcinoma (a type of skin cancer) that affects any part of the head or neck except the lips
- to prevent crises (episodes of severe pain) and decrease the need for blood transfusions (transfer of one person's blood to another person's body) in people who have sickle cell anemia (a blood disease that may cause painful crises, a low number of red blood cells, infection, and damage to the internal organs).

Hydroxyurea is in a class of medications known as antineoplastic agents. Hydroxyurea treats cancer by slowing or stopping the growth of cancer cells. Hydroxyurea treats sickle cell anemia by changing red blood cells so that they are less likely to bend in an abnormal shape. The length of treatment depends on the condition you have and how well your body responds to this medication.

Hydroxyurea is usually taken once a day. When hydroxyurea is used to treat certain types of cancer, it may be taken once every third day. Try to take hydroxyurea at about the same time of day on the days that you are scheduled to take the medication. Follow the directions on your prescription label carefully and ask your doctor or pharmacist to explain anything you do not understand. Take hydroxyurea exactly as directed. Do not take more or less of it or take it more often than prescribed by your doctor.

Your doctor may start you on a low dose of hydroxyurea and gradually increase your dose.

Hydroxyurea may help control the symptoms of sickle cell anemia but does not cure the condition. Continue to take hydroxyurea even if you feel well. Do not stop taking this medication without talking to your doctor.

If you forget to take a dose of hydroxyurea, take the missed dose as soon as you remember it. However, if it is almost time for your next dose, skip the missed dose and continue your regular dosing schedule. Do not take a double dose to make up for a missed dose and do not take more than one dose in one day. Call your doctor if you miss more than one dose of hydroxyurea.

Hydroxyurea is also sometimes used to treat polycythemia vera (a condition in which the body produces too many blood cells), psoriasis (a skin disease in which red, scaly patches form on some areas of the body), and hypereosinophilic syndrome (a condition in which the body produces too many of a certain type of white blood cell). Talk to your doctor about the possible risks of using this medication for your condition.

This medication may be prescribed for other uses; ask your doctor or pharmacist for more information.

Precautions

Before taking hydroxyurea,

- tell your doctor and pharmacist if you are allergic to hydroxyurea, any other medications, or any of the inactive ingredients in hydroxyurea capsules. Ask your pharmacist for a list of the ingredients.
- tell your doctor if you are taking or have ever taken an interferon. (Interferons are a group of medications similar to substances produced by the body. They are used to treat diseases that involve the immune system such as certain types of cancer, hepatitis, multiple sclerosis, and genital warts. Brand names include Actimmune, Avonex, Betaseron, Rebif and others.) If you are taking or have ever taken an interferon, there is a greater chance that you will develop severe skin problems during your treatment with hydroxyurea. Ask your doctor or pharmacist if you are not sure if you are taking or have ever taken an interferon.
- tell your doctor and pharmacist what prescription and nonprescription medications, vitamins, nutritional supplements, and herbal products you are taking or plan to take. Be sure to mention any of the following: medications to treat human immunodeficiency virus (HIV) or acquired immunodeficiency syndrome (AIDS), especially didanosine (Videx) and stavudine (Zerit); probenecid; or sulfinpyrazone (Anturane). Your doctor may need to change the doses of your medications or monitor you carefully for side effects.
- tell your doctor if you have human immunodeficiency virus (HIV) or acquired immunodeficiency syndrome (AIDS), if you are being treated with or have ever been treated with radiation therapy or cancer chemotherapy; if you have or have ever had kidney, or liver disease.

- tell your doctor if you are breast-feeding. You should not breastfeed during your treatment with hydroxyurea.
- your doctor may prescribe a folic acid supplement for you to take during your treatment with hydroxyurea. Take this medication exactly as directed.
- you should know that hydroxyurea may be harmful if it gets on the skin. People who are not taking hydroxyurea should avoid touching hydroxyurea capsules or the bottle that contains the capsules. Always wear disposable gloves when handling hydroxyurea capsules or bottles containing hydroxyurea capsules and wash your hands before and after you touch the bottle or capsules. If the powder from a capsule spills, wipe it up immediately with a damp disposable towel, place the towel in a closed container, such as a plastic bag and throw it away in a trash can that is out of the reach of children and pets.

Side Effects

Hydroxyurea may cause side effects. Tell your doctor if any of these symptoms are severe or do not go away:

- nausea
- vomiting
- diarrhea
- constipation
- drowsiness

Some side effects can be serious. If you experience any of the following symptoms, or those listed in the IMPORTANT WARNING section, call your doctor immediately.

- rash
- purple, blue, or black discoloration of the skin or nails
- loss of feeling in one area of the body
- sores on the skin or in the mouth
- foul-smelling substance oozing from the skin.
- swelling of the hands, feet, ankles, or lower legs

Hydroxyurea may cause other side effects. Call your doctor if you have any unusual problems while taking this medication.

If you experience a serious side effect, you or your doctor may send a report to the Food and Drug Administration's (FDA) MedWatch Adverse Event Reporting program online [at http://www.fda.gov/MedWatch/index.html] or by phone [1-800-332-1088].

Storage Conditions

Keep hydroxyurea in the container it came in, tightly closed and out of reach of children and pets. Store it at room temperature and away from excess heat and moisture (not in the bathroom). Throw away any medication that is outdated or no longer needed. Talk to your doctor or pharmacist about the proper disposal of your medication.

Overdose

In case of overdose, call your local poison control center at 1-800-222-1222. If the victim has collapsed or is not breathing, call local emergency services at 911.

Symptoms of overdose may include:

- violet discoloration, swelling, and soreness of the palms and soles
- scaling of the skin on the hands and feet
- darkening of the skin
- sores in the mouth

Special Instructions

- Do not let anyone else take your medication. Ask your pharmacist if you have any questions about refilling your prescription.

Dosage Facts
For Informational Purposes

Caution: Do not change your dose, how often you take your medication, or the length of time you are to take it without first talking to your healthcare provider.

The following dosage information was written using medical language for doctors and other healthcare professionals and is provided here for you to check your dosage. The dosage of this drug may differ for different patients. Therefore, always follow your doctor's instructions or the directions on the label. Contact your healthcare provider or pharmacist if you have any questions about the specific dosage of your medication after reviewing this information.

Adult Patients
Chronic Myelogenous Leukemia

ORAL:

- 20–30 mg/kg as a single dose daily.
- Continue therapy indefinitely in patients who show regression or arrest of tumor growth.

Solid Tumors

ORAL:

- 80 mg/kg as a single dose every third day. Alternatively, 20–30 mg/kg as a single dose daily.

Head and Neck Cancer

ORAL:

- 80 mg/kg as a single dose every third day.
- Administration should begin at least 7 days before initiation of radiation therapy; continue during irradiation as well as afterward provided patient is closely monitored and no unusual or severe reactions occur.

Sickle Cell Anemia

ORAL:

- Initially, 15 mg/kg as a single dose.
- Adjust dosage according to patient's blood cell count. If

blood cell count is in an acceptable range, dosage may be increased in increments of 5 mg/kg daily once every 12 weeks to a maximum tolerated dosage of up to 35 mg/kg daily. Dosage should not be increased if blood cell counts are between the acceptable range and the toxic range.

- If blood cell count is in the toxic range, discontinue hydroxyurea until hematologic recovery occurs; treatment may then be resumed at a reduced daily dose.

Polycythemia Vera†

ORAL:

- Initially, 15–20 mg/kg daily.
- Most adults respond adequately to dosages of 500 mg to 1 g daily; some patients may respond to as little as 1.5–2 g *weekly* (along with occasional phlebotomy), while others may require dosages as high as 1.5–2 g or more daily.

Dosage Modification for Toxicity
Hematologic Toxicity

In patients receiving hydroxyurea for antineoplastic therapy, withhold therapy when leukocyte count is <2500/mm³ or platelet count is <100,000/mm³. Reevaluate leukocyte and platelet counts after 3 days; therapy may be resumed when the counts return to acceptable levels. Severe anemia may be managed without interrupting hydroxyurea therapy.

If hematologic recovery does not occur promptly during combined hydroxyurea and radiation therapy, irradiation may be interrupted.

In patients receiving hydroxyurea for sickle cell anemia, withhold therapy when neutrophil count is <2000/mm³, the platelet count is <80,000/mm³, the hemoglobin concentration is <4.5 g/dL, or the reticulocyte count is <80,000/mm³ with a hemoglobin concentration of <9 g/dL. Following hematologic recovery, resume therapy at a reduced daily dose of 2.5 mg/kg less than the dose that resulted in toxicity. Resume titration of the dosage by increasing or decreasing the daily dose in increments of 2.5 mg/kg once every 12 weeks to a maximum tolerated dosage (up to 35 mg/kg daily) at which the patient does not experience hematologic toxicity during 24 consecutive weeks of therapy. Further attempts should not be made to titrate to a dosage level that resulted in hematologic toxicity during 2 separate periods of dosage adjustment.

GI Toxicity

Temporarily discontinue hydroxyurea if severe gastric distress (e.g., nausea, vomiting, anorexia) resulting from combined hydroxyurea and radiation therapy occurs.

Prescribing Limits
Adult Patients
Sickle Cell Anemia

ORAL:

- Maximum 35 mg/kg daily.

Special Populations

Hepatic Impairment

- No specific dosage adjustment recommended, however close monitoring of hematologic parameters is recommended.

Renal Impairment
- Dosage reduction may be necessary; close monitoring of hematologic parameters recommended.

Sickle Cell Anemia

ORAL:
- If Cl_{cr} ≥60 mL/min, reduce initial dosage to 15 mg/kg daily.
- If Cl_{cr} is <60 mL/min, reduce initial dosage to 7.5 mg/kg daily.
- For hemodialysis patients, administer 7.5 mg/kg following dialysis.

Geriatric Patients
- Careful dosage selection recommended due to possible age-related decrease in renal function; lower dosages may be required.

† Use is not currently included in the labeling approved by the US Food and Drug Administration.

Hydroxyzine

(hye drox′ i zeen)

Brand Name: Anx®, Atarax®, Atarax® Syrup, Vistaril®

Also available generically.

Why is this medicine prescribed?

Hydroxyzine is used to relieve the itching caused by allergies and to control the nausea and vomiting caused by various conditions, including motion sickness. It is also used for anxiety and to treat the symptoms of alcohol withdrawal.

This medication is sometimes prescribed for other uses; ask your doctor or pharmacist for more information.

How should this medicine be used?

Hydroxyzine comes in capsules, tablets, a syrup, and suspension to take by mouth. It usually is taken three or four times a day. Follow the directions on your prescription label carefully, and ask your doctor or pharmacist to explain any part you do not understand. Take hydroxyzine exactly as directed. Do not take more or less of it or take it more often than prescribed by your doctor.

Shake the suspension (Vistaril) well before each use to mix the medication evenly.

Do not give this medication to children less than 12 years of age unless a doctor directs you to do so.

What special precautions should I follow?

Before taking hydroxyzine,
- tell your doctor and pharmacist if you are allergic to hydroxyzine or any other drugs.
- tell your doctor and pharmacist what prescription and nonprescription medications you are taking, especially antihistamines; medications for colds, allergies, or hay fever; medications for depression or seizures; muscle relaxants; narcotics (pain medications); sedatives; sleeping pills; tranquilizers; and vitamins.
- tell your doctor if you have or have ever had asthma, glaucoma, ulcers, difficulty urinating (due to an enlarged prostate gland), heart disease, liver disease, high blood pressure, seizures, or an overactive thyroid gland.
- tell your doctor if you are pregnant, plan to become pregnant, or are breast-feeding. If you become pregnant while taking hydroxyzine, call your doctor.
- if you are having surgery, including dental surgery, tell the doctor or dentist that you are taking hydroxyzine.
- you should know that this drug may make you drowsy. Do not drive a car or operate machinery until you know how this drug affects you.
- remember that alcohol can add to the drowsiness caused by this drug.

What should I do if I forget to take a dose?

Take the missed dose as soon as you remember it. However, if it is almost time for the next dose, skip the missed dose and continue your regular dosing schedule. Do not take a double dose to make up for a missed one.

What side effects can this medicine cause?

Hydroxyzine may cause side effects. Tell your doctor if any of these symptoms are severe or do not go away:
- dry mouth, nose, and throat
- upset stomach
- drowsiness
- dizziness
- chest congestion
- headache
- reddening of skin

If you experience any of the following symptoms, call your doctor immediately:
- difficulty breathing
- muscle weakness
- increased anxiety

If you experience a serious side effect, you or your doctor may send a report to the Food and Drug Administration's (FDA) MedWatch Adverse Event Reporting program online [at http://www.fda.gov/MedWatch/index.html] or by phone [1-800-332-1088].

What storage conditions are needed for this medicine?

Keep this medication in the container it came in, tightly closed, and out of reach of children. Store it at room tem-

perature and away from excess heat and moisture (not in the bathroom). Throw away any medication that is outdated or no longer needed. Talk to your pharmacist about the proper disposal of your medication.

What should I do in case of overdose?

In case of overdose, call your local poison control center at 1-800-222-1222. If the victim has collapsed or is not breathing, call local emergency services at 911.

What other information should I know?

Keep all appointments with your doctor.

Do not let anyone else take your medication. Ask your pharmacist any questions you have about refilling your prescription.

Dosage Facts
For Informational Purposes

Caution: Do not change your dose, how often you take your medication, or the length of time you are to take it without first talking to your healthcare provider.

The following dosage information was written using medical language for doctors and other healthcare professionals and is provided here for you to check your dosage. The dosage of this drug may differ for different patients. Therefore, always follow your doctor's instructions or the directions on the label. Contact your healthcare provider or pharmacist if you have any questions about the specific dosage of your medication after reviewing this information.

General Dosage Information

Available as hydroxyzine pamoate and hydroxyzine hydrochloride; dosage expressed in terms of the hydrochloride.
Use the smallest possible effective dosage.

Pediatric Patients

Anxiety

ORAL:
• Children <6 years of age: 50 mg daily given in divided doses.
• Children ≥6 years of age: 50–100 mg daily given in divided doses.

Pruritus

ORAL:
• Children <6 years of age: 50 mg daily given in divided doses.
• Children ≥6 years of age: 50–100 mg daily given in divided doses.

Preoperative and Postoperative Adjunctive Therapy
Sedation

ORAL:
• 0.6 mg/kg administered before and following general anesthesia.

Adult Patients

Anxiety

ORAL:
• 50–100 mg 4 times daily.

Pruritus

ORAL:
• 25 mg 3 or 4 times daily.

Preoperative and Postoperative Adjunctive Therapy
Sedation

ORAL:
• 50–100 mg administered before and following general anesthesia.

Special Populations

Geriatric Patients
• Use initial dosage at low end of the recommended dosage range.

Hyoscyamine
(hye oh sye′ a meen)

Brand Name: Anaspaz®, Cystospaz®, Cystospaz-M®, Hyosol® SL, Hyospaz®, Levbid®, Levsin®, Levsin® Drops, Levsin®/SL, Levsinex® Timecaps®, NuLev®

Why is this medicine prescribed?

Hyoscyamine is used to control symptoms associated with disorders of the gastrointestinal (GI) tract. It works by decreasing the motion of the stomach and intestines and the secretion of stomach fluids, including acid. Hyoscyamine is also used in the treatment of bladder spasms, peptic ulcer disease, diverticulitis, colic, irritable bowel syndrome, cystitis, and pancreatitis. Hyoscyamine may also be used to treat certain heart conditions, to control the symptoms of Parkinson's disease and rhinitis (runny nose), and to reduce excess saliva production.

This medication is sometimes prescribed for other uses; ask your doctor or pharmacist for more information.

How should this medicine be used?

Hyoscyamine comes as a tablet, an extended-release (long-acting) capsule, a liquid to take by mouth, and in an injectable form. The tablets and liquid are usually taken three or four times a day. The extended-release capsules are usually taken twice a day. Do not crush, chew, or divide the extended-release capsules. Hyoscyamine injections are given by qualified health care professionals. Follow the directions on your prescription label carefully, and ask your doctor or pharmacist to explain any part you do not understand. Take hyoscyamine exactly as directed. Do not take more or less of it or take it more often than prescribed by your doctor.

Hyoscyamine controls symptoms associated with disorders of the GI tract, but it does not cure the disorders. Continue to take hyoscyamine even if you feel well. Do not stop taking hyoscyamine without talking to your doctor.

What special precautions should I follow?

Before taking hyoscyamine,

- tell your doctor and pharmacist if you are allergic to hyoscyamine or any other drugs.
- tell your doctor and pharmacist what prescription and nonprescription medications you are taking, especially amantadine (Symadine, Symmetrel), amitriptyline (Elavil), chlorpromazine (Thorazine), clomipramine (Anafranil), desipramine (Norpramin), doxepin (Sinequan), fluphenazine (Prolixin), haloperidol (Haldol), imipramine (Tofranil), medications containing belladonna (Donnatal), mesoridazine (Serentil), nortriptyline (Pamelor), perphenazine (Trilafon), phenelzine (Nardil), prochlorperazine (Compazine), promazine (Sparine), promethazine (Phenergan), protriptyline (Vivactil), thioridazine (Mellaril), tranylcypromine (Parnate), trifluoperazine (Stelazine), triflupromazine (Vesprin), trimeprazine (Temaril), trimipramine (Surmontil), and vitamins.
- be aware that antacids may interfere with hyoscyamine, making it less effective. Take hyoscyamine 1 hour before or 2 hours after antacids.
- tell your doctor if you have or have ever had glaucoma; heart, lung, liver, or kidney disease; a urinary tract or intestinal obstruction; an enlarged prostate; ulcerative colitis; or myasthenia gravis.
- tell your doctor if you are pregnant, plan to become pregnant, or are breast-feeding. If you become pregnant while taking hyoscyamine, call your doctor.
- if you are having surgery, including dental surgery, tell your doctor or dentist that you take hyoscyamine.
- you should know that this drug may make you drowsy. Do not drive a car or operate machinery until you know how hyoscyamine will affect you.
- remember that alcohol can add to the drowsiness caused by this drug.

What special dietary instructions should I follow?

Your doctor may instruct you to take hyoscyamine 30-60 minutes before meals. Check with your doctor or pharmacist about the best times to take your medication.

What should I do if I forget to take a dose?

Take the missed dose as soon as you remember it. However, if it is almost time for the next dose, skip the missed dose and continue your regular dosing schedule. Do not take a double dose to make up for a missed one.

What side effects can this medicine cause?

Hyoscyamine may cause side effects. Tell your doctor if any of these symptoms are severe or do not go away:

- drowsiness
- dizziness or lightheadedness
- headache
- blurred vision
- flushing (feeling of warmth)
- dry mouth
- constipation
- difficulty urinating
- increased sensitivity to light

If you experience any of the following symptoms, call your doctor immediately:

- diarrhea
- skin rash
- eye pain
- fast or irregular heartbeat

If you experience a serious side effect, you or your doctor may send a report to the Food and Drug Administration's (FDA) MedWatch Adverse Event Reporting program online [at http://www.fda.gov/MedWatch/index.html] or by phone [1-800-332-1088].

What storage conditions are needed for this medicine?

Keep this medication in the container it came in, tightly closed, and out of reach of children. Store it at room temperature and away from excess heat and moisture (not in the bathroom). Throw away any medication that is outdated or no longer needed. Talk to your pharmacist about the proper disposal of your medication.

What should I do in case of overdose?

In case of overdose, call your local poison control center at 1-800-222-1222. If the victim has collapsed or is not breathing, call local emergency services at 911.

What other information should I know?

Keep all appointments with your doctor and the laboratory.

Do not let anyone else take your medication. Ask your pharmacist any questions you have about refilling your prescription.

Talk to your doctor, pharmacist, or other healthcare professional if you have questions about dosing information for your medication.

Ibandronate

(i ban′ droh nate)

Brand Name: Boniva®

Why is this medicine prescribed?

Ibandronate is used to prevent and treat osteoporosis (a condition in which the bones become thin and weak and break easily) in women who have undergone menopause ('change of life,' end of menstrual periods). Ibandronate is in a class of medications called bisphosphonates. It works by preventing bone breakdown and increasing bone density (thickness).

How should this medicine be used?

Ibandronate comes as a tablet to take by mouth. The 2.5-mg tablet is usually taken once a day in the morning on an empty stomach and the 150-mg tablet is usually taken once a month in the morning on an empty stomach. The 150-mg tablet should be taken on the same date each month. Follow the directions on your prescription label carefully, and ask your doctor or pharmacist to explain any part you do not understand. Take ibandronate exactly as directed. Do not take more or less of it or take it more often than prescribed by your doctor.

Ibandronate may not work properly and may damage the esophagus (tube between the mouth and stomach) or cause sores in the mouth if it is not taken according to the following instructions. Tell your doctor if you do not understand, you do not think you will remember, or you are unable to follow these instructions:

- You must take ibandronate just after you get out of bed in the morning, before you eat or drink anything. Never take ibandronate at bedtime or before you wake up and get out of bed for the day.
- Swallow the tablets with a full glass (6 to 8 ounces, about 1 cup) of plain water. Never take ibandronate with tea, coffee, juice, milk, mineral water, sparkling water, or any liquid other than plain water.
- Swallow the tablets whole; do not split, chew, or crush them. Do not suck on the tablets.
- After you take ibandronate, do not eat, drink, or take any other medications (including vitamins or antacids) for at least 60 minutes. Do not lie down for at least 60 minutes after you take ibandronate. Sit upright or stand upright for at least 60 minutes.

Ibandronate controls osteoporosis but does not cure it. Ibandronate helps to treat and prevent osteoporosis only as long as it is taken regularly. Continue to take ibandronate even if you feel well. Do not stop taking ibandronate without talking to your doctor.

Ask your pharmacist or doctor for a copy of the manufacturer's information for the patient.

Are there other uses for this medicine?

This medication may be prescribed for other uses; ask your doctor or pharmacist for more information.

What special precautions should I follow?

Before taking ibandronate,

- tell your doctor and pharmacist if you are allergic to ibandronate or any other medications, or any of the ingredients in ibandronate tablets. Ask your pharmacist for a list of the ingredients.
- tell your doctor and pharmacist what prescription and nonprescription medications, vitamins, nutritional supplements, and herbal products you are taking or plan to take. Be sure to mention any of the following: aspirin and other nonsteroidal anti-inflammatory medications (NSAIDs) such as ibuprofen (Advil, Motrin) and naproxen (Naprosyn, Aleve) cancer chemotherapy; and oral steroids such as dexamethasone (Decadron, Dexone), methylprednisolone (Medrol), and prednisone (Deltasone). Your doctor may need to change the doses of your medications or monitor you carefully for side effects.
- if you are taking any oral medications, including supplements, vitamins, or antacids, take them at least 60 minutes after you take ibandronate.
- tell your doctor if you are unable to sit upright or stand upright for at least 60 minutes and if you have or have ever had a low level of calcium in your blood. Your doctor may tell you not to take ibandronate.
- tell your doctor if are undergoing radiation therapy and if you have or have ever had anemia (condition in which the red blood cells do not bring enough oxygen to all the parts of the body); difficulty swallowing; heartburn; ulcers or other problems with your stomach or esophagus; cancer; any type of infection, especially in your mouth; problems with your mouth, teeth, or gums; any condition that stops your blood from clotting normally; or dental or kidney disease.
- tell your doctor if you are pregnant, plan to become pregnant, or are breast-feeding. Also tell your doctor if you plan to become pregnant at any time in the future, because ibandronate may remain in your body for many years after you stop taking it. Call your doctor if you become pregnant during or after your treatment.
- you should know that ibandronate may cause serious problems with your jaw, especially if you have dental surgery or treatment while you are taking the medication. A dentist should examine your teeth and perform any needed treatments before you start to take ibandronate. Be sure to brush your teeth and clean your mouth properly while you are taking ibandronate. Talk to your doctor before having any dental treatments while you are taking this medication.
- talk to your doctor about other things you can do to prevent osteoporosis from developing or worsening. Your doctor will probably tell you to avoid smoking

and drinking large amounts of alcohol and to follow a regular program of weight-bearing exercise.

What special dietary instructions should I follow?

You should eat and drink plenty of foods and drinks that are rich in calcium and vitamin D while you are taking ibandronate. Your doctor will tell you which foods and drinks are good sources of these nutrients and how many servings you need each day. If you find it difficult to eat enough of these foods, tell your doctor. In that case, your doctor may prescribe or recommend a supplement.

What should I do if I forget to take a dose?

If you forget to take the daily 2.5-mg tablet, do not take it later in the day. Skip the missed dose and continue your regular dosing schedule the next morning. Do not take two tablets of ibandronate on the same day.

If you forget to take the once-monthly 150-mg tablet, and your next scheduled day to take ibandronate is more than 7 days away, take one tablet the morning after you remember. Then return to taking one tablet each month on the regularly scheduled date. If you forget to take the once-monthly 150-mg tablet and your next scheduled day to take ibandronate is 7 or fewer days away, skip the dose and wait for your next scheduled day. You should not take two 150-mg tablets of ibandronate within 1 week.

If you are not sure what to do if you miss a dose of ibandronate, call your doctor.

What side effects can this medicine cause?

Ibandronate may cause side effects. Tell your doctor if any of these symptoms are severe or do not go away:
- nausea
- stomach pain
- diarrhea
- constipation
- back pain
- bone, joint, or muscle pain
- pain in the arms or legs
- weakness
- dizziness
- headache
- flu-like symptoms
- fever, sore throat, chills, cough, and other signs of infection
- frequent or urgent need to urinate
- painful urination

Some side effects can be serious. If you experience any of the following symptoms, call your doctor immediately before you take any more ibandronate:
- new or worsening heartburn
- difficulty swallowing
- pain on swallowing
- chest pain
- rash

- painful or swollen gums
- loosening of the teeth
- numbness or heavy feeling in the jaw
- poor healing of the jaw
- eye pain

Ibandronate may cause other side effects. Call your doctor if you have any unusual problems while taking this medication.

What storage conditions are needed for this medicine?

Keep this medication in the container it came in, tightly closed, and out of reach of children. Store it at room temperature and away from excess heat and moisture (not in the bathroom). Throw away any medication that is outdated or no longer needed. Talk to your pharmacist about the proper disposal of your medication.

What should I do in case of overdose?

In case of overdose, give the victim a full glass of milk and call your local poison control center at 1-800-222-1222. If the victim has collapsed or is not breathing, call local emergency services at 911. Do not allow the victim to lie down and do not try to make the victim vomit. Do not lie down.

Symptoms of overdose may include:
- nausea
- stomach pain
- heartburn

What other information should I know?

Keep all appointments with your doctor. Your doctor may order certain tests to check your body's response to ibandronate.

Before having any bone imaging study, tell your doctor and health care personnel that you are taking ibandronate

Do not let anyone else take your medication. Ask your pharmacist any questions you have about refilling your prescription.

Dosage Facts
For Informational Purposes

Caution: Do not change your dose, how often you take your medication, or the length of time you are to take it without first talking to your healthcare provider.

The following dosage information was written using medical language for doctors and other healthcare professionals and is provided here for you to check your dosage. The dosage of this drug may differ for different patients. Therefore, always follow your doctor's instructions or the directions on the label. Contact your healthcare provider or pharmacist if you have any questions about the specific dosage of your medication after reviewing this information.

General Dosage Information

Available as ibandronate sodium (as the monosodium monohydrate); dosage expressed in terms of ibandronate.

Adult Patients

Osteoporosis
Prevention in Postmenopausal Women

ORAL:
- 2.5 mg once daily. Alternatively, a dosage of 150 mg once monthly may be considered.

Treatment in Postmenopausal Women

ORAL:
- 2.5 mg once daily or 150 mg once monthly.

Special Populations

Hepatic Impairment
- Dosage adjustments not necessary.

Renal Impairment

ORAL:
- Dosage adjustments not necessary in patients with mild to moderate renal impairment ($Cl_{cr} \geq 30$ mL/minute); use not recommended in patients with severe renal impairment ($Cl_{cr} < 30$ mL/minute).

Geriatric Patients
- Dosage adjustments not necessary.

Ibandronate Injection

(i ban' droh nate)

Brand Name: Boniva® Injection

Why is this medicine prescribed?

Ibandronate injection is used to treat osteoporosis (a condition in which the bones become thin and weak and break easily) in women who have undergone menopause ('change of life,' end of menstrual periods). Ibandronate is in a class of medications called bisphosphonates. It works by preventing bone breakdown and increasing bone density (thickness).

How should this medicine be used?

Ibandronate injection comes as a solution (liquid) to be injected into a vein. Ibandronate injection is given only by a health care provider usually once every 3 months. Do not give an ibandronate injection to yourself.

Ibandronate injection controls osteoporosis but does not cure it. Ibandronate injection helps to treat osteoporosis only as long as you receive regular injections. It is important that you receive your ibandronate injection once every 3 months for as long as your health care provider prescribes it.

Ask your pharmacist or doctor for a copy of the manufacturer's information for the patient.

Are there other uses for this medicine?

This medication may be prescribed for other uses; ask your doctor or pharmacist for more information.

What special precautions should I follow?

Before receiving ibandronate injection,
- tell your doctor and pharmacist if you are allergic to ibandronate, any other medications, or any of the ingredients in ibandronate injection. Ask your doctor for a list of the ingredients.
- tell your doctor and pharmacist what prescription and nonprescription medications, vitamins, nutritional supplements, and herbal products you are taking or plan to take. Your doctor may need to change the doses of your medications or monitor you carefully for side effects.
- tell your doctor if you have hypocalcemia (lower than normal level of calcium in your blood). Your doctor will probably tell you not to use ibandronate injection.
- tell your doctor if are undergoing radiation therapy and if you have or have ever had anemia (condition in which the red blood cells do not bring enough oxygen to all the parts of the body); cancer; diabetes; any type of infection, especially in your mouth; problems with your mouth, teeth, or gums; high blood pressure; any condition that stops your blood from clotting normally; lower than normal levels of Vitamin D; or heart, or kidney disease.
- tell your doctor if you are pregnant, plan to become pregnant, or are breast-feeding. Also tell your doctor if you plan to become pregnant at any time in the future, because ibandronate may remain in your body for many years after you stop taking it. Call your doctor if you become pregnant during or after your treatment.
- you should know that ibandronate injection may cause serious problems with your jaw, especially if you have dental surgery or treatment while you are being treated with ibandronate injection. A dentist should examine your teeth and perform any needed treatments before you start treatment with ibandronate injection. Be sure to brush your teeth and clean your mouth properly while you are being treated with ibandronate injection. Talk to your dentist before having any dental treatments while you are receiving this medication.
- you should know that ibandronate injection may cause flu-like symptoms including fever; chills; joint, bone and/or muscle pain; and excessive tiredness. These symptoms usually occur only after the first ibandronate injection and generally do not happen again during treatment. Your health care provider or pharmacist can suggest a mild pain reliever to make you more comfortable. Without treatment, these symptoms usually disappear within 24 to 48 hours. Call your doctor if these symptoms get worse or do not go away.
- talk to your doctor about other things you can do to prevent osteoporosis from developing or worsening. Your doctor will probably tell you to avoid smoking

and drinking large amounts of alcohol and to follow a regular program of weight-bearing exercise.

What special dietary instructions should I follow?

Your doctor will tell you to take supplements of calcium and vitamin D while you are being treated with ibandronate injection.

What should I do if I forget to take a dose?

If you miss an appointment to receive an injection of ibandronate, you should call your health care provider as soon as possible. The missed dose should be given as soon as it can be rescheduled. After you receive the missed dose, your next injection should be scheduled 3 months from the date of your last injection. You should not receive an ibandronate injection more often than once every 3 months.

What side effects can this medicine cause?

Ibandronate injection may cause side effects. Tell your doctor if any of these symptoms are severe or do not go away:
- stomach pain
- nausea
- constipation
- diarrhea
- heartburn
- back pain
- rash
- bone, joint, or muscle pain
- pain in the arms or legs
- weakness
- tiredness
- dizziness
- headache
- fever, sore throat, chills, cough, and other signs of infection
- frequent or urgent need to urinate
- painful urination
- redness, or swelling at injection spot

Some side effects can be serious. If you experience any of the following symptoms, call your doctor immediately before receiving any more ibandronate injection:
- painful or swollen gums
- loosening of the teeth
- numbness or heavy feeling in the jaw
- poor healing of the jaw
- eye pain or swelling
- vision changes
- sensitivity to light

Ibandronate injection may cause other side effects. Call your doctor if you have any unusual problems while taking this medication.

What should I do in case of overdose?

In case of overdose, call your local poison control center at 1-800-222-1222. If the victim has collapsed or is not breathing, call local emergency services at 911.

What other information should I know?

Keep all appointments with your doctor and the laboratory. Your doctor will order certain tests to check your body's response to ibandronate injection.

Before having any bone imaging study, tell your doctor and health care personnel that you are receiving ibandronate injection

Dosage Facts
For Informational Purposes

Caution: Do not change your dose, how often you take your medication, or the length of time you are to take it without first talking to your health-care provider.

The following dosage information was written using medical language for doctors and other healthcare professionals and is provided here for you to check your dosage. The dosage of this drug may differ for different patients. Therefore, always follow your doctor's instructions or the directions on the label. Contact your healthcare provider or pharmacist if you have any questions about the specific dosage of your medication after reviewing this information.

General Dosage Information

Available as ibandronate sodium (as the monosodium monohydrate); dosage expressed in terms of ibandronate.

Adult Patients

Osteoporosis
Treatment in Postmenopausal Women
IV:
- 3 mg once every 3 months.

Special Populations

Hepatic Impairment
- Dosage adjustments not necessary.

Renal Impairment
IV:
- Should not be administered to patients with severe renal impairment (Cl_{cr} <30 mL/minute, S_{cr} >2.3 mg/dL).

Geriatric Patients
- Dosage adjustments not necessary.

Ibuprofen

(eye byoo' proe fen)

Brand Name: Advil® Caplets®, Advil® Children's, Advil® Gel Caplets, Advil® Infants' Concentrated Drops, Advil® Junior Strength Chewable Tablets, Advil® Junior Strength Tablets, Advil® Liqui-Gels®, Advil® Migraine®, Advil® Tablets, Genpril® Caplets ®, Genpril® Tablets, Haltran®, IBU®, Ibu-Tab®, Menadol® Captabs®, Midol® Cramp, Motrin®, Motrin® Caplets®, Motrin® Children's, Motrin® Drops, Motrin® IB Caplets®, Motrin® IB Gelcaps®, Motrin® IB Tablets, Motrin® Infants' Concentrated Drops, Motrin® Junior Strength, Motrin® Junior Strength Caplets®, Motrin® Migraine Pain Caplets®

Also available generically.

Important Warning

People who take nonsteroidal anti-inflammatory medications (NSAIDs) (other than aspirin) such as ibuprofen may have a higher risk of having a heart attack or a stroke than people who do not take these medications. These events may happen without warning and may cause death. This risk may be higher for people who take NSAIDs for a long time. Tell your doctor if you or anyone in your family has or has ever had heart disease, a heart attack, or a stroke, if you smoke, and if you have or have ever had high cholesterol, high blood pressure, or diabetes. Get emergency medical help right away if you experience any of the following symptoms: chest pain, shortness of breath, weakness in one part or side of the body, or slurred speech.

If you will be undergoing a coronary artery bypass graft (CABG; a type of heart surgery), you should not take ibuprofen right before or right after the surgery.

NSAIDs such as ibuprofen may cause ulcers, bleeding, or holes in the stomach or intestine. These problems may develop at any time during treatment, may happen without warning symptoms, and may cause death. The risk may be higher for people who take NSAIDs for a long time, are older in age, have poor health, or who drink 3 or more alcoholic drinks per day while taking ibuprofen. Tell your doctor if you take any of the following medications: anticoagulants ('blood thinners') such as warfarin (Coumadin); aspirin; other NSAIDS such as ketoprofen (Orudis KT, Actron) and naproxen (Aleve, Naprosyn); or oral steroids such as dexamethasone (Decadron, Dexone), methylprednisolone (Medrol), and prednisone (Deltasone). Also tell your doctor if you have or have ever had ulcers, bleeding in your stomach or intestines, or other bleeding disorders. If you experience any of the following symptoms, stop taking ibuprofen and call your doctor: stomach pain, heartburn, vomiting a substance that is bloody or looks like coffee grounds, blood in the stool, or black and tarry stools.

Keep all appointments with your doctor and the laboratory. Your doctor will monitor your symptoms carefully and will probably order certain tests to check your body's response to ibuprofen. Be sure to tell your doctor how you are feeling so that your doctor can prescribe the right amount of medication to treat your condition with the lowest risk of serious side effects.

Your doctor or pharmacist will give you the manufacturer's patient information sheet (Medication Guide) when you begin treatment with prescription ibuprofen and each time you refill your prescription. Read the information carefully and ask your doctor or pharmacist if you have any questions. You can also visit the Food and Drug Administration (FDA) website (http://www.fda.gov/cder) or the manufacturer's website to obtain the Medication Guide.

Why is this medicine prescribed?

Prescription ibuprofen is used to relieve pain, tenderness, swelling, and stiffness caused by osteoarthritis (arthritis caused by a breakdown of the lining of the joints) and rheumatoid arthritis (arthritis caused by swelling of the lining of the joints). It is also used to relieve mild to moderate pain, including menstrual pain (pain that happens before or during a menstrual period). Nonprescription ibuprofen is used to reduce fever and to relieve mild pain from headaches, muscle aches, arthritis, menstrual periods, the common cold, toothaches, and backaches. Ibuprofen is in a class of medications called NSAIDs. It works by stopping the body's production of a substance that causes pain, fever, and inflammation.

How should this medicine be used?

Prescription ibuprofen comes as a tablet to take by mouth. It is usually taken three or four times a day for arthritis or every 4-6 hours as needed for pain. Nonprescription ibuprofen comes as a tablet, chewable tablet, suspension (liquid), and drops (concentrated liquid). Adults and children older than 12 years of age may usually take nonprescription ibuprofen every 4-6 hours as needed for pain or fever. Children and infants may usually be given nonprescription ibuprofen every 6-8 hours as needed for pain or fever, but should not be given more than four doses in 24 hours. Ibuprofen may be taken with food or milk to prevent stomach upset. If you are taking ibuprofen on a regular basis, you should take it at the same time(s) every day.

Follow the directions on the package or prescription label carefully, and ask your doctor or pharmacist to explain any part you do not understand. Take ibuprofen exactly as directed. Do not take more or less of it or take it more often than directed by the package label or prescribed by your doctor.

The chewable tablets may cause a burning feeling in the mouth or throat. Take the chewable tablets with food or water.

Shake the suspension and drops well before each use to mix the medication evenly. Use the measuring cup provided to measure each dose of the suspension, and use the dosing device provided to measure each dose of the drops.

Stop taking nonprescription ibuprofen and call your doctor if your symptoms get worse, you develop new or unexpected symptoms, the part of your body that was painful becomes red or swollen, your pain lasts for more than 10 days, or your fever lasts more than 3 days. Stop giving nonprescription ibuprofen to your child and call your child's doctor if your child does not start to feel better during the first 24 hours of treatment. Also stop giving nonprescription ibuprofen to your child and call your child's doctor if your child develops new symptoms, including redness or swelling on the painful part of his body, or your child's pain or fever get worse or last longer than 3 days.

Do not give nonprescription ibuprofen to a child who has a sore throat that is severe or does not go away, or that comes along with fever, headache, upset stomach, or vomiting. Call the child's doctor right away, because these symptoms may be signs of a more serious condition.

Are there other uses for this medicine?

Ibuprofen is also sometimes used to treat ankylosing spondylitis (arthritis that mainly affects the spine), gouty arthritis (joint pain caused by a build-up of certain substances in the joints), and psoriatic arthritis (arthritis that occurs with a long-lasting skin disease that causes scaling and swelling). Talk to your doctor about the risks of using this drug for your condition.

This medication is sometimes prescribed for other uses; ask your doctor or pharmacist for more information.

What special precautions should I follow?

Before taking ibuprofen,
- tell your doctor and pharmacist if you are allergic to ibuprofen, aspirin or other NSAIDs such as ketoprofen (Orudis KT, Actron) and naproxen (Aleve, Naprosyn), any other medications, or any of the inactive ingredients in the type of ibuprofen you plan to take. Ask your pharmacist or check the label on the package for a list of the inactive ingredients.
- tell your doctor and pharmacist what prescription and nonprescription medications, vitamins, nutritional supplements, and herbal products you are taking or plan

to take. Be sure to mention the medications listed in the IMPORTANT WARNING section and any of the following: angiotensin-converting enzyme (ACE) inhibitors such as benazepril (Lotensin), captopril (Capoten), enalapril (Vasotec), fosinopril (Monopril), lisinopril (Prinivil, Zestril), moexipril (Univasc), perindopril (Aceon), quinapril (Accupril), ramipril (Altace), and trandolapril (Mavik); diuretics ('water pills'); lithium (Eskalith, Lithobid), and methotrexate (Rheumatrex). Your doctor may need to change the doses of your medications or monitor you more carefully for side effects.
- do not take nonprescription ibuprofen with any other medication for pain unless your doctor tells you that you should.
- tell your doctor if you have or have ever had any of the conditions mentioned in the IMPORTANT WARNING section or asthma, especially if you also have frequent stuffed or runny nose or nasal polyps (swelling of the inside of the nose); swelling of the hands, arms, feet, ankles, or lower legs; lupus (a condition in which the body attacks many of its own tissues and organs, often including the skin, joints, blood, and kidneys) or liver or kidney disease. If you are giving ibuprofen to a child, tell the child's doctor if the child has not been drinking fluids or has lost a large amount of fluid from repeated vomiting or diarrhea.
- tell your doctor if you are pregnant, especially if you are in the last few months of your pregnancy, you plan to become pregnant, or you are breast-feeding. If you become pregnant while taking ibuprofen, call your doctor.
- if you are having surgery, including dental surgery, tell the doctor or dentist that you are taking ibuprofen.
- if you have phenylketonuria (an inborn disease in which mental retardation develops if a specific diet is not followed), read the package label carefully before taking nonprescription ibuprofen. Some types of nonprescription ibuprofen contain aspartame that forms phenylalanine.

What special dietary instructions should I follow?

Unless your doctor tells you otherwise, continue your normal diet.

What should I do if I forget to take a dose?

If you are taking ibuprofen on a regular basis, take the missed dose as soon as you remember it. However, if it is almost time for the next dose, skip the missed dose and continue your regular dosing schedule. Do not take a double dose to make up for a missed one.

What side effects can this medicine cause?

Ibuprofen may cause side effects. Tell your doctor if any of these symptoms are severe or do not go away:

- constipation
- diarrhea
- gas or bloating
- dizziness
- nervousness
- ringing in the ears

Some side effects can be serious. If you experience any of the following symptoms, or those mentioned in the IMPORTANT WARNING section, call your doctor immediately. Do not take any more ibuprofen until you speak to your doctor.

- unexplained weight gain
- fever
- blisters
- rash
- itching
- hives
- swelling of the eyes, face, throat, arms, hands, feet, ankles, or lower legs
- difficulty breathing or swallowing
- hoarseness
- excessive tiredness
- pain in the upper right part of the stomach
- upset stomach
- loss of appetite
- yellowing of the skin or eyes
- flu-like symptoms
- pale skin
- fast heartbeat
- cloudy, discolored, or bloody urine
- back pain
- difficult or painful urination
- blurred vision, changes in color vision, or other vision problems
- red or painful eyes
- stiff neck
- headache
- confusion
- aggression

Ibuprofen may cause other side effects. Call your doctor if you have any unusual problems while taking this medication.

If you experience a serious side effect, you or your doctor may send a report to the Food and Drug Administration's (FDA) MedWatch Adverse Event Reporting program online [at http://www.fda.gov/MedWatch/index.html] or by phone [1-800-332-1088].

What storage conditions are needed for this medicine?

Keep this medication in the container it came in, tightly closed, and out of reach of children. Store it at room temperature and away from excess heat and moisture (not in the bathroom). Throw away any medication that is outdated or no longer needed. Talk to your pharmacist about the proper disposal of your medication.

What should I do in case of overdose?

In case of overdose, call your local poison control center at 1-800-222-1222. If the victim has collapsed or is not breathing, call local emergency services at 911.

Symptoms of overdosage may include:

- dizziness
- fast eye movements that you cannot control
- slow breathing or short periods of time without breathing
- blue color around the lips, mouth, and nose

What other information should I know?

If you are taking prescription ibuprofen, do not let anyone else take your medication. Ask your pharmacist any questions you have about refilling your prescription.

Dosage Facts
For Informational Purposes

Caution: Do not change your dose, how often you take your medication, or the length of time you are to take it without first talking to your healthcare provider.

The following dosage information was written using medical language for doctors and other healthcare professionals and is provided here for you to check your dosage. The dosage of this drug may differ for different patients. Therefore, always follow your doctor's instructions or the directions on the label. Contact your healthcare provider or pharmacist if you have any questions about the specific dosage of your medication after reviewing this information.

General Dosage Information

Dosage of ibuprofen lysine expressed in terms of ibuprofen.

To minimize the potential risk of adverse cardiovascular and/or GI events, use lowest effective dosage and shortest duration of therapy consistent with the patient's treatment goals. Adjust dosage based on individual requirements and response; attempt to titrate to the lowest effective dosage.

Pediatric Patients

Dosage in children should be guided by body weight.

Inflammatory Diseases
Juvenile Rheumatoid Arthritis

ORAL:
- 30–40 mg/kg daily divided into 3 or 4 doses. 20 mg/kg daily in divided doses may be adequate for children with mild disease.

Pain

ORAL:
- For mild to moderate pain in children 6 months to 12 years of age, 10 mg/kg every 6–8 hours.

Age- or Weight-Based Dosage for Self-medication of Minor Aches and Pain in Children 6 Months to 11 Years of Age

Age	Weight	Dose[a]
6–11 months	12–17 pounds (approximately 5–8 kg)	50 mg
12–23 months	18–23 pounds (approximately 8–10 kg)	75 mg
2–3 years	24–35 pounds (approximately 11–16 kg)	100 mg
4–5 years	36–47 pounds (approximately 16–21 kg)	150 mg
6–8 years	48–59 pounds (approximately 22–27 kg)	200 mg
9–10 years	60–71 pounds (approximately 27–32 kg)	250 mg
11 years	72–95 pounds (approximately 33–43 kg)	300 mg

[a]Dose may be administered every 6–8 hours.

For *self-medication* of minor aches and pain in children ≥12 years of age, 200 mg every 4–6 hours; may increase dosage to 400 mg every 4–6 hours if needed.

Fever

ORAL:
- For children 6 months to 12 years of age: 5 mg/kg for temperatures <39°C; 10 mg/kg for temperatures >39°C.

Age- or Weight-Based Dosage for Self-medication of Fever in Children 6 Months to 11 Years of Age

Age	Weight	Dose[b]
6–11 months	12–17 pounds (approximately 5–8 kg)	50 mg
12–23 months	18–23 pounds (approximately 8–10 kg)	75 mg
2–3 years	24–35 pounds (approximately 11–16 kg)	100 mg
4–5 years	36–47 pounds (approximately 16–21 kg)	150 mg
6–8 years	48–59 pounds (approximately 22–27 kg)	200 mg
9–10 years	60–71 pounds (approximately 27–32 kg)	250 mg
11 years	72–95 pounds (approximately 33–43 kg)	300 mg

[a]Dose may be administered every 6–8 hours.

For *self-medication* of fever in children ≥12 years of age, 200 mg every 4–6 hours; may increase dosage to 400 mg every 4–6 hours if needed.

Adult Patients

Inflammatory Diseases
Osteoarthritis or Rheumatoid Arthritis

ORAL:
- 1.2–3.2 g daily, given as 300 mg 4 times daily, or 400, 600, or 800 mg 3 or 4 times daily.

Pain

ORAL:
- For mild to moderate pain, 400 mg every 4–6 hours as needed.
- For *self-medication* of minor aches and pain, 200 mg every 4–6 hours; may increase dosage to 400 mg every 4–6 hours if needed.
- For *self-medication* of migraine pain, 400 mg once in a 24-hour period.

Dysmenorrhea

ORAL:
- 400 mg every 4 hours as necessary; initiate at earliest onset of pain.
- For *self-medication*, 200 mg every 4–6 hours; may increase to 400 mg every 4–6 hours if necessary.

Fever

ORAL:
- For *self-medication*, 200 mg every 4–6 hours; may increase to 400 mg every 4–6 hours if needed.

Prescribing Limits

Pediatric Patients

Inflammatory Diseases
Juvenile Rheumatoid Arthritis

ORAL:
- Maximum 50 mg/kg daily.

Pain

ORAL:
- For mild to moderate pain in children 6 months to 12 years of age, maximum 40 mg/kg daily.
- For *self-medication* of minor aches and pain in children 6 months to 11 years of age, do not exceed recommended dosage; do not administer recommended dose more than 4 times daily. *Self-medication* should not exceed 3 days unless otherwise directed by a clinician.
- For *self-medication* of minor aches and pain in children ≥12 years of age, maximum 1.2 g daily. *Self-medication* should not exceed 10 days unless otherwise directed by a clinician.

Fever

ORAL:
- Maximum 40 mg/kg daily in children 6 months to 12 years of age.
- For *self-medication* in children 6 months to 11 years of age, do not exceed recommended dosage; do not administer recommended dose more than 4 times daily. *Self-medication* should not exceed 3 days unless otherwise directed by a clinician.

- For *self-medication* in children ≥12 years of age, maximum 1.2 g daily. *Self-medication* should not exceed 3 days unless otherwise directed by a clinician.

Adult Patients

Inflammatory Diseases
Osteoarthritis or Rheumatoid Arthritis

ORAL:
- Maximum 3.2 g daily.

Pain

ORAL:
- For mild to moderate pain, maximum 3.2 g daily.
- For *self-medication* of minor aches and pain, maximum 1.2 g daily. *Self-medication* should not exceed 10 days unless otherwise directed by a clinician.
- For *self-medication* of migraine pain, maximum 400 mg in a 24-hour period unless otherwise directed by a clinician.

Dysmenorrhea

ORAL:
- Maximum 3.2 g daily.
- For *self-medication*, maximum 1.2 g daily.

Fever

ORAL:
- For *self-medication*, maximum 1.2 g daily. *Self-medication* should not exceed 3 days unless otherwise directed by a clinician.

Special Populations

Renal Impairment
- Consider dosage reduction in patients with substantial renal impairment.

Imatinib

(i mat′ in ib)

Brand Name: Gleevec®

Why is this medicine prescribed?

Imatinib is used to treat certain types of leukemia (cancer that begins in the white blood cells) and other cancers of the blood cells. Imatinib is also used to treat gastrointestinal stromal tumors (GIST; a type of tumor that grows in the walls of the digestive passages and may spread to other parts of the body). Imatinib is also used to treat dermatofibrosarcoma protuberans (a tumor that forms under the top layer of skin) when the tumor cannot be removed surgically, has spread to other parts of the body, or has come back after surgery. Imatinib is in a class of medications called protein-tyrosine kinase inhibitors. It works by blocking the action of the abnormal protein that signals cancer cells to multiply. This helps stop the spread of cancer cells.

How should this medicine be used?

Imatinib comes as a tablet to take by mouth. It is usually taken with a meal and a large glass of water once or twice a day. Take imatinib at around the same time(s) every day. Follow the directions on your prescription label carefully, and ask your doctor or pharmacist to explain any part you do not understand. Take imatinib exactly as directed. Do not take more or less of it or take it more often than prescribed by your doctor.

If you are unable to swallow imatinib tablets, you may place all of the tablets that you need for one dose into a glass of water or apple juice. Use 50 mL (a little less than 2 ounces) of liquid for each 100 mg tablet and 100 mL (a little less than 4 ounces) of liquid for each 400 mg tablet. Stir with a spoon until the tablets crumble completely and drink the mixture immediately.

If your doctor has told you to take 800 mg of imatinib, you should take two of the 400 mg tablets. Do not take 8 of the 100 mg tablets. The tablet coating contains iron, and you will receive too much iron if you take 8 of the 100 mg tablets.

Your doctor may increase or decrease your dose of imatinib during your treatment. This depends on how well the medication works for you and on the side effects you experience. Talk to your doctor about how you are feeling during your treatment. Continue to take imatinib even if you feel well. Do not stop taking imatinib without talking to your doctor.

Are there other uses for this medicine?

This medication may be prescribed for other uses; ask your doctor or pharmacist for more information.

What special precautions should I follow?

Before taking imatinib,
- tell your doctor and pharmacist if you are allergic to imatinib or any other medications.
- tell your doctor and pharmacist what prescription and nonprescription medications, vitamins, and nutritional supplements you are taking or plan to take. Be sure to mention any of the following: acetaminophen (Tylenol); certain antibiotics including erythromycin (E.E.S., E-Mycin, Erythrocin), clarithromycin (Biaxin), and rifampin (Rifadin, in Rifamate); anticoagulants ('blood thinners') such as warfarin (Coumadin); antifungals such as ketoconazole (Nizoral) and itraconazole (Sporanox); calcium channel blockers such as amlodipine (Norvasc, in Caduet), diltiazem (Cardizem, Tiazac), felodipine (Plendil), isradipine (Dynacirc), nicardipine (Cardene), nifedipine (Adalat, Procardia, others), nimodipine (Nimotop), nisoldipine (Sular), or verapamil (Calan, Covera, Isoptin, Verelan); cholesterol-lowering medications (statins) such as atorvastatin (Lipitor), lovastatin (Mevacor), and simvastatin (Zocor); cyclospor-

ine (Neoral, Sandimmune); dexamethasone; hormonal contraceptives (birth control pills, patches, rings, injections or implants); pimozide (Orap); medications for anxiety; medications for seizures such as carbamazepine (Tegretol), phenobarbital, and phenytoin (Dilantin); sedatives; sleeping pills; and tranquilizers. Other medications may also interact with imatinib, so be sure to tell your doctor about all the medications you are taking, even those that do not appear on this list. Your doctor may need to change the doses of your medications or monitor you carefully for side effects.

- tell your doctor what herbal products you are taking, especially St. John's wort.
- tell your doctor if you have or have ever had high blood pressure a heart attack; an irregular heartbeat; diabetes; or heart, lung, thyroid, or liver disease. Also tell your doctor if you smoke, if you use street drugs, and if you drink or have ever drunk large amounts of alcohol.
- tell your doctor if you are pregnant or plan to become pregnant. You should not become pregnant while you are taking imatinib. Talk to your doctor about birth control methods that you can use during your treatment. If you become pregnant while taking imatinib, call your doctor. Imatinib may harm the fetus.
- tell your doctor if you are breast-feeding. You should not breast-feed while you are taking imatinib.
- talk to your doctor about what you should do if you develop diarrhea during your treatment. Do not take any medications to treat diarrhea without talking to your doctor.

What special dietary instructions should I follow?

Talk to your doctor about drinking grapefruit juice or eating grapefruit while taking this medication.

What should I do if I forget to take a dose?

Take the missed dose as soon as you remember it. However, if it is almost time for the next dose, skip the missed dose and continue your regular dosing schedule. Do not take a double dose to make up for a missed one.

What side effects can this medicine cause?

Imatinib may cause side effects. Tell your doctor if any of these symptoms are severe or do not go away:

- diarrhea
- constipation
- gas
- nausea
- vomiting
- loss of appetite
- indigestion
- joint pain
- muscle cramps

- depression
- anxiety
- night sweats
- teary eyes

Some side effects can be serious. If you experience any of these symptoms call your doctor immediately:

- puffiness under the eyes
- swelling of the hands, feet, ankles, or lower legs
- weight gain
- shortness of breath
- fast, irregular, or pounding heartbeat
- difficulty falling asleep or staying asleep
- fainting
- coughing up pink or bloody mucus
- increased urination, especially at night
- chest pain
- fever
- rash or blisters
- yellowing of the skin or eyes
- blood in the stool
- unusual bruising or bleeding
- sore throat, fever, chills, and other signs of infection
- excessive tiredness or weakness
- headache
- dizziness

Imatinib may cause other side effects. Call your doctor if you have any unusual problems while taking this medication.

What storage conditions are needed for this medicine?

Keep this medication in the container it came in, tightly closed, and out of reach of children. Store it at room temperature and away from excess heat and moisture (not in the bathroom). Throw away any medication that is outdated or no longer needed. Talk to your pharmacist about the proper disposal of your medication.

What should I do in case of overdose?

In case of overdose, call your local poison control center at 1-800-222-1222. If the victim has collapsed or is not breathing, call local emergency services at 911.

Symptoms of overdose may include:

- muscle cramps
- swollen or bloated stomach

What other information should I know?

Keep all appointments with your doctor and the laboratory. Your doctor will order certain lab tests to check your body's response to imatinib.

Do not let anyone else take your medication. Ask your pharmacist any questions you have about refilling your prescription.

Dosage Facts

For Informational Purposes

Caution: Do not change your dose, how often you take your medication, or the length of time you are to take it without first talking to your healthcare provider.

The following dosage information was written using medical language for doctors and other healthcare professionals and is provided here for you to check your dosage. The dosage of this drug may differ for different patients. Therefore, always follow your doctor's instructions or the directions on the label. Contact your healthcare provider or pharmacist if you have any questions about the specific dosage of your medication after reviewing this information.

General Dosage Information

Available as imatinib mesylate; dosage expressed in terms of imatinib.

Pediatric Patients

CML

ORAL:

- Children >3 years of age: 260 mg/m^2 given once daily or in 2 divided doses (once in the morning and once in the evening). If there is evidence of disease progression (at any time), inadequate hematologic response after at least 3 months of therapy, inadequate cytogenetic response after 6–12 months of therapy, or loss of a previously achieved hematologic or cytogenetic response, increase dosage (in the absence of severe adverse drug or hematologic effects) to 340 mg/m^2 daily.

Adult Patients

CML
Chronic Phase

ORAL:

- 400 mg daily. If there is evidence of disease progression (at any time), inadequate hematologic response after at least 3 months of therapy, inadequate cytogenetic response after 6–12 months of therapy, or loss of a previously achieved hematologic or cytogenetic response, increase dosage (in the absence of severe adverse drug or hematologic effects) to 600 mg daily.

Accelerated Phase or Blast Crisis

ORAL:

- 600 mg daily. If there is evidence of disease progression (at any time), inadequate hematologic response after at least 3 months of therapy, inadequate cytogenetic response after 6–12 months of therapy, or loss of a previously achieved hematologic or cytogenetic response, increase dosage (in the absence of severe adverse drug or hematologic effects) to 800 mg daily (administered as 400 mg twice daily).

GIST

ORAL:

- 400 or 600 mg once daily.

Dose Modification for Toxicity
Nonhematologic Adverse Effects

If a severe non-hematologic adverse reaction (e.g., severe hepatotoxicity, severe fluid retention) occurs, withhold imatinib until the event has resolved. Thereafter, resume therapy as appropriate, depending on the initial severity of the event.

If substantial increases in bilirubin (>3 times ULN) or hepatic transaminase concentrations (>5 times ULN) occur, withhold imatinib until bilirubin or transaminase concentrations decrease to <1.5 or <2.5 times ULN, respectively. Resume therapy at a reduced daily dosage. Adult patients previously receiving a dosage of 400 or 600 mg daily may resume therapy at a dosage of 300 or 400 mg daily, respectively; pediatric patients previously receiving a dosage of 260 or 340 mg/m^2 daily may resume therapy at a dosage of 200 or 260 mg/m^2 daily, respectively.

Adverse Hematologic Effects

Adjust dosage if neutropenia and/or thrombocytopenia occur.

Dose Adjustments for Neutropenia and Thrombocytopenia

Use (Initial Dosage)	Hematologic Measurements	Comments
Chronic Phase CML (initial dosage: 400 mg daily in adults, 260 mg/m^2 daily in pediatric patients) GIST (initial dosage: 400 or 600 mg daily)	ANC <1000/mm^3 and/or Platelets <50,000/mm^3	1. Discontinue imatinib until ANC ≥1500/mm^3 and platelets ≥75,000/mm^3 2. Resume imatinib at original dosage (400 or 600 mg once daily in adults; 260 mg/m^2 daily in pediatric patients) 3. If recurrence of ANC <1000/mm^3 and/or platelets <50,000/mm^3 occurs, repeat step 1 and resume therapy at a reduced dosage (reduce from 400 mg to 300 mg or from 600 mg to 400 mg once daily in adults; reduce from 260 mg/m^2 to 200 mg/m^2 daily in pediatric patients)

| Accelerated Phase CML and Blast Crisis (initial dosage: 600 mg daily in adults) | ANC <500/mm³ and/or Platelets <10,000/ mm³ occurring after at least 1 month of treatment | 1. If cytopenia is unrelated to CML (as determined by marrow aspirate or biopsy), reduce dosage to 400 mg once daily
2. If cytopenia persists for 2 weeks, further reduce dosage to 300 mg once daily
3. If cytopenia persists for 4 weeks and is still unrelated to CML, withhold therapy until ANC ≥1000/mm³ and platelets ≥20,000/mm³; then reinitiate therapy at 300 mg once daily |

Special Populations

Patients Receiving CYP3A4 Inducers
- Increase imatinib dosage by at least 50% and carefully monitor clinical response in patients receiving concomitant therapy with imatinib and CYP3A4 inducers (e.g., phenytoin, rifampin).

Imiglucerase Injection

(i mi gloo' ser ace)

Brand Name: Cerezyme®

About Your Treatment

Your doctor has ordered imiglucerase to help treat your illness. The drug will be added to an intravenous fluid that will drip through a needle or catheter into your vein for 1-2 hours. Your doctor will determine how often you will receive this medication. Imiglucerase is an enzyme used to help treat the signs and symptoms of Type 1 Gaucher's disease. This medication is sometimes prescribed for other uses; ask your doctor or pharmacist for more information.

Your health care provider (doctor, nurse, or pharmacist) may measure the effectiveness and side effects of your treatment using laboratory tests and physical examinations. It is important to keep all appointments with your doctor and the laboratory. The length of treatment depends on how you respond to the medication.

Precautions

Before administering imiglucerase,
- tell your doctor and pharmacist if you are allergic to imiglucerase, alglucerase (Ceredase), or any other drugs.
- tell your doctor and pharmacist what prescription and nonprescription medications you are taking, including vitamins.
- tell your doctor if you are pregnant, plan to become pregnant, or are breast-feeding. If you become pregnant while taking imiglucerase, call your doctor.
- if you are having surgery, including dental surgery, tell the doctor or dentist that you are taking imiglucerase.

Administering Your Medication

Before you administer imiglucerase, look at the solution closely. It should be clear and free of floating material. Gently squeeze the bag or observe the solution container to make sure there are no leaks. Do not use the solution if it is discolored or if it contains particles or the bag or container leaks. Use a new solution, but show the damaged one to your health care provider.

It is important that you use your medication exactly as directed. Do not stop your therapy on your own for any reason. Do not administer it more often or for longer periods than your doctor tells you. Do not change your dosing schedule without talking to your health care provider. Your health care provider may tell you to stop your infusion if you have a mechanical problem (such as a blockage in the tubing, needle, or catheter); if you have to stop an infusion, call your health care provider immediately so your therapy can continue.

Side Effects

Imiglucerase may cause side effects. Tell your health care provider if any of these symptoms are severe or do not go away:
- fever
- chills
- stomach pain
- upset stomach
- vomiting
- itching
- headache
- dizziness

Storage Conditions

- Your health care provider will probably give you a several-day supply of imiglucerase at a time. Discard any unused medication.
- Imiglucerase needs to be stored in the refrigerator. Take your dose from the refrigerator 1 hour before using it; place it in a clean, dry area to allow it to warm to room temperature.
- Do not allow imiglucerase to freeze.

Your health care provider may provide you with directions on how to prepare each dose.

Store your medication only as directed. Make sure you understand what you need to store your medication properly.

Keep your supplies in a clean, dry place when you are not using them, and keep all medications and supplies out of the reach of children. Your health care provider will tell you how to throw away used needles, syringes, tubing, and containers to avoid accidental injury.

Overdose

In case of overdose, call your local poison control center at 1-800-222-1222. If the victim has collapsed or is not breathing, call local emergency services at 911.

Signs of Infection

If you are receiving imiglucerase in your vein, you need to know the symptoms of a catheter-related infection (an infection where the needle enters your skin). If you experience any of these effects near your intravenous catheter, tell your health care provider as soon as possible:

- tenderness
- warmth
- irritation
- drainage
- redness
- swelling
- pain

Dosage Facts
For Informational Purposes

Caution: Do not change your dose, how often you take your medication, or the length of time you are to take it without first talking to your healthcare provider.

The following dosage information was written using medical language for doctors and other healthcare professionals and is provided here for you to check your dosage. The dosage of this drug may differ for different patients. Therefore, always follow your doctor's instructions or the directions on the label. Contact your healthcare provider or pharmacist if you have any questions about the specific dosage of your medication after reviewing this information.

Pediatric Patients
Gaucher's Disease

IV:
- Children and adolescents 2–16 years of age: Initially, dosage ranges from 2.5 units/kg 3 times weekly to 60 units/kg every 2 weeks.
- Increase or decrease dosage and/or frequency of administration according to disease severity and patient response and convenience.
- Individual doses occasionally may be increased or decreased

slightly to avoid wasting a partially used vial, as long as the total monthly dosage is not altered substantially.
- Clinical improvement in hematologic and visceral manifestations generally occurs within the first year of therapy; response to skeletal manifestations may require 2–3 years of therapy.
- Failure to respond within 6 months may indicate the need for increased dosages.

Adult Patients
Gaucher's Disease

IV:
- Adults >16 years of age: Initially, dosage ranges from 2.5 units/kg 3 times weekly to 60 units/kg every 2 weeks.
- Increase or decrease dosage and/or frequency of administration according to disease severity and patient response and convenience.
- Individual doses occasionally may be increased or decreased slightly to avoid wasting a partially used vial, as long as the total monthly dosage is not altered substantially.
- Clinical improvement in hematologic and visceral manifestations generally occurs within the first year of therapy; response to skeletal manifestations may require 2–3 years of therapy.
- Failure to respond within 6 months may indicate the need for increased dosages.

Imipenem and Cilastatin Sodium Injection

(i mi pen' em) (sye la stat' in)

Brand Name: Primaxin®

About Your Treatment

Your doctor has ordered imipenem and cilastatin, an antibiotic, to help treat your infection. The drug will be either injected into a large muscle (such as your buttock or thigh) or added to an intravenous fluid that will drip through a needle or catheter placed in your vein for about 30 minutes, two to four times a day.

The combination of imipenem and cilastatin eliminates bacteria that cause many kinds of infections, including pneumonia and gynecological, skin, stomach, blood, bone, joint, urinary tract, and heart valve infections. This medication is sometimes prescribed for other uses; ask your doctor or pharmacist for more information.

Your health care provider (doctor, nurse, or pharmacist) may measure the effectiveness and side effects of your treatment using laboratory tests and physical examinations. It is important to keep all appointments with your doctor and the laboratory. The length of treatment depends on how your infection and symptoms respond to the medication.

Precautions

Before administering imipenem and cilastatin,

- tell your doctor and pharmacist if you are allergic to imipenem, penicillin, cephalosporins [e.g., cefaclor (Ceclor), cefadroxil (Duricef), and cephalexin (Keflex)], or any other drugs.
- tell your doctor and pharmacist what prescription and nonprescription medications you are taking, especially antibiotics and vitamins.
- tell your doctor if you have or have ever had seizures; a brain injury; kidney, liver, or gastrointestinal disease (especially colitis); or asthma.
- tell your doctor if you are pregnant, plan to become pregnant, or are breast-feeding. If you become pregnant while taking imipenem and cilastatin, call your doctor.
- if you have diabetes and regularly check your urine for sugar, use Clinistix or TesTape. Do not use Clinitest tablets because this drug may cause false positive results.

Administering Your Medication

Before you administer imipenem and cilastatin, look at the solution closely. It should be clear and free of floating material. Gently squeeze the bag or observe the solution container to make sure there are no leaks. Do not use the solution if it is discolored, if it contains particles, or if the bag or container leaks. Use a new solution, but show the damaged one to your health care provider.

It is important that you use your medication exactly as directed. Do not stop your therapy on your own for any reason because your infection could worsen and result in hospitalization. Do not change your dosing schedule without talking to your health care provider. Your health care provider may tell you to stop your infusion if you have a mechanical problem (such as a blockage in the tubing, needle, or catheter); if you have to stop an infusion, call your health care provider immediately so your therapy can continue.

Side Effects

Imipenem and cilastatin may cause side effects. If you are administering imipenem and cilastatin into a muscle, it probably will be mixed with lidocaine (Xylocaine) to reduce pain at the injection site. Tell your health care provider if any of these symptoms are severe or do not go away:

- upset stomach
- vomiting
- stomach pain

If you experience any of the following symptoms, call your health care provider immediately:

- diarrhea
- rash
- itching
- fever
- chills
- facial swelling
- wheezing

- difficulty breathing
- unusual bleeding or bruising
- decreased urination
- dizziness
- confusion
- seizures
- sore mouth or throat

If you experience a serious side effect, you or your doctor may send a report to the Food and Drug Administration's (FDA) MedWatch Adverse Event Reporting program online [at http://www.fda.gov/MedWatch/index.html] or by phone [1-800-332-1088].

Storage Conditions

- Your health care provider probably will give you a several-day supply of imipenem and cilastatin at a time. If you are receiving imipenem and cilastatin intravenously (in your vein), you probably will be told to store it in the refrigerator.
- Take your next dose from the refrigerator 1 hour before using it; place it in a clean, dry area to allow it to warm to room temperature.

If you are receiving imipenem and cilastatin intramuscularly (in your muscle), your health care provider will tell you how to store it properly.

Store your medication only as directed. Make sure you understand what you need to store your medication properly.

Keep your supplies in a clean, dry place when you are not using them, and keep all medications and supplies out of reach of children. Your health care provider will tell you how to throw away used needles, syringes, tubing, and containers to avoid accidental injury.

Overdose

In case of overdose, call your local poison control center at 1-800-222-1222. If the victim has collapsed or is not breathing, call local emergency services at 911.

Signs of Infection

If you are receiving imipenem and cilastatin in your vein or under your skin, you need to know the symptoms of a catheter-related infection (an infection where the needle enters your vein or skin). If you experience any of these effects near your intravenous catheter, tell your health care provider as soon as possible:

- tenderness
- warmth
- irritation
- drainage
- redness
- swelling
- pain

Dosage Facts
For Informational Purposes

Caution: Do not change your dose, how often you take your medication, or the length of time you are to take it without first talking to your healthcare provider.

The following dosage information was written using medical language for doctors and other healthcare professionals and is provided here for you to check your dosage. The dosage of this drug may differ for different patients. Therefore, always follow your doctor's instructions or the directions on the label. Contact your healthcare provider or pharmacist if you have any questions about the specific dosage of your medication after reviewing this information.

General Dosage Information

Available as fixed-combination containing imipenem monohydrate and cilastatin sodium; dosage generally expressed in terms of the imipenem content (as anhydrous imipenem).

To minimize risk of seizures, closely adhere to dosage recommendations, especially in patients with factors known to predispose to seizure activity; dosage adjustment recommended for patients with advanced age and/or renal impairment. Anticonvulsant therapy should be continued in patients with existing seizure disorders.

Duration of therapy depends on type and severity of infection. Safety and efficacy of the IM route for >14 days have not been established.

Pediatric Patients

General Dosage for Neonates

IV:
- Neonates <1 week of age weighing ≥1.5 kg: 25 mg/kg every 12 hours.
- Neontes 1–4 weeks of age weighing ≥1.5 kg: 25 mg/kg every 8 hours.

General Dosage for Infants and Children

IV:
- Children 1–3 months of age weighing ≥1.5 kg: 25 mg every 6 hours.
- Children ≥3 months of age: 15–25 mg/kg every 6 hours.

Mild to Moderately Severe Infections
Gynecologic, Lower Respiratory Tract, or Skin and Skin Structure Infections

IM:
- Children ≥12 years of age: 500 or 750 mg every 12 hours.

Intra-abdominal Infections

IM:
- Children ≥12 years of age: 750 mg every 12 hours.

Adult Patients

Recommended IV adult dosages are for adults weighing ≥70 kg. Modification of dosage is recommended for patients weighing <70 kg.

Mild Infections
Fully Susceptible Aerobic or Anaerobic Bacteria

IV:
- Adults weighing ≥70 kg: 250 mg every 6 hours (1 g daily).

Moderately Susceptible Aerobic or Anaerobic Bacteria

IV:
- Adults weighing ≥70 kg: 500 mg every 6 hours (2 g daily).

Moderately Severe Infections
Fully Susceptible Aerobic or Anaerobic Bacteria

IV:
- Adults weighing ≥70 kg: 500 mg every 8 hours (1.5 g daily) or 500 mg every 6 hours (2 g daily).

Moderately Susceptible Aerobic or Anaerobic Bacteria

IV:
- Adults weighing ≥70 kg: 500 mg every 6 hours (2 g daily) or 1 g every 8 hours (3 g daily).

Severe, Life-threatening Infections
Fully Susceptible Aerobic or Anaerobic Bacteria

IV:
- Adults weighing ≥70 kg: 500 mg every 6 hours (2 g daily).

Moderately Susceptible Aerobic or Anaerobic Bacteria

IV:
- Adults weighing ≥70 kg: 1 g every 6 hours (4 g daily) or 1 g every 8 hours (3 g daily).

Urinary Tract Infections (UTIs)
Uncomplicate UTIs

IV:
- Adults weighing ≥70 kg: 250 mg every 6 hours (1 g daily).

Complicated UTIs

IV:
- Adults weighing ≥70 kg: 500 mg every 6 hours (2 g daily).

Mild to Moderately Severe Infections
Gynecologic, Lower Respiratory Tract, or Skin and Skin Structure Infections

IM:
- 500 or 750 mg every 12 hours.

Intra-abdominal Infections

IM:
- 750 mg every 12 hours.

Empiric Therapy in Febrile Neutropenic Patients†

IV:
- 500 mg every 6 hours (1 g daily).

Prescribing Limits

Pediatric Patients

IV:
- 2 g daily in those with infections caused by fully susceptible bacteria or 4 g daily in those with infections caused by moderately susceptible bacteria (e.g., some strains of *Ps. aeruginosa*). Higher dosage (up to 90 mg/kg daily in older children) has been used in some cystic fibrosis patients.

Adult Patients

IV:
- 50 mg/kg daily or 4 g daily, whichever is lower.

IM:
• 1.5 g daily.

Special Populations

Renal Impairment

Infections in Adults

IV:
• Dosage adjustments recommended in adults with Cl_{cr} <70 mL/minute per 1.73 m². Serum creatinine concentrations alone may not be sufficiently accurate to assess the degree of renal impairment; dosage preferably should be based on the patient's measured or estimated Cl_{cr}.
• Manufacturer makes the following recommendations for dosage in adults with Cl_{cr} <70 mL/minute per 1.73 m² and/or body weight <70 kg (see manufacturer's prescribing information).
• Impenem should be used in patients undergoing hemodialysis only when potential benefits outweigh the potential risk of drug-induced seizures. If used IV in hemodialysis patients, a supplemental dose of the drug should be given after each dialysis period and at 12-hour intervals thereafter. In addition, patients should be monitored closely for adverse CNS effects (e.g., confusion, myoclonic activity, seizures), especially those with CNS disease.
• Patients with Cl_{cr} ≤5 mL/minute per 1.73² should not receive imipenem and cilastatin sodium IV unless hemodialysis is instituted within 48 hours.

IM:
• IM route should not be used in patients with Cl_{cr} <20 mL/minute per 1.73 m².

Infections in Pediatric Patients

IV:
• Not recommended in pediatric patients weighing <30 kg with impaired renal function.

Adults with Low Body Weight
• Dosage adjustment recommended when IV imipenem used in adults with body weight <70 kg. IV dosage recommended for these adults is the same as that recommended for adults with renal impairment. (See Tables.)

Geriatric Patients
• No dosage adjustments except those related to renal impairment.

† *Use is not currently included in the labeling approved by the US Food and Drug Administration.*

Imipramine

(im ip′ ra meen)

Brand Name: Tofranil®, Tofranil® PM
Also available generically.

Important Warning

A small number of children, teenagers, and young adults (up to 24 years of age) who took antidepressants ('mood elevators') such as imipramine during clinical studies became suicidal (thinking about harming or killing oneself or planning or trying to do so). Children, teenagers, and young adults who take antidepressants to treat depression or other mental illnesses may be more likely to become suicidal than children, teenagers, and young adults who do not take antidepressants to treat these conditions. However, experts are not sure about how great this risk is and how much it should be considered in deciding whether a child or teenager should take an antidepressant. Children younger than 18 years of age should not normally take imipramine except to prevent bedwetting, but in some cases, a doctor may decide that imipramine is the best medication to treat a child's condition.

You should know that your mental health may change in unexpected ways when you take imipramine or other antidepressants even if you are an adult over age 24. You may become suicidal, especially at the beginning of your treatment and any time that your dose is increased or decreased. You, your family, or your caregiver should call your doctor right away if you experience any of the following symptoms: new or worsening depression; thinking about harming or killing yourself, or planning or trying to do so; extreme worry; agitation; panic attacks; difficulty falling asleep or staying asleep; aggressive behavior; irritability; acting without thinking; severe restlessness; and frenzied abnormal excitement. Be sure that your family or caregiver knows which symptoms may be serious so they can call the doctor when you are unable to seek treatment on your own.

Your healthcare provider will want to see you often while you are taking imipramine, especially at the beginning of your treatment. Be sure to keep all appointments for office visits with your doctor.

The doctor or pharmacist will give you the manufacturer's patient information sheet (Medication Guide) when you begin treatment with imipramine. Read the information carefully and ask your doctor or pharmacist if you have any questions. You also can obtain the Medication Guide from the FDA

continued on next page

Important Warning (cont'd)

website: http://www.fda.gov/cder/drug/antidepressants/antidepressants_MG_2007.pdf.

No matter your age, before you take an antidepressant, you, your parent, or your caregiver should talk to your doctor about the risks and benefits of treating your condition with an antidepressant or with other treatments. You should also talk about the risks and benefits of not treating your condition. You should know that having depression or another mental illness greatly increases the risk that you will become suicidal. This risk is higher if you or anyone in your family has or has ever had bipolar disorder (mood that changes from depressed to abnormally excited) or mania (frenzied, abnormally excited mood) or has thought about or attempted suicide. Talk to your doctor about your condition, symptoms, and personal and family medical history. You and your doctor will decide what type of treatment is right for you.

Why is this medicine prescribed?

Imipramine tablets and capsules are used to treat depression. Imipramine tablets are also used to prevent bedwetting in children. Imipramine is in a class of medications called tricyclic antidepressants. It treats depression by increasing the amounts of certain natural substances in the brain that are needed to maintain mental balance. There is not enough information to explain how imipramine prevents bedwetting.

How should this medicine be used?

Imipramine comes as a tablet and a capsule to take by mouth. When imipramine tablets or capsules are used to treat depression, they are usually taken one or more times a day and may be taken with or without food. When imipramine tablets are used to prevent bedwetting in children, they are usually taken one hour before bedtime. Children who wet the bed early in the evening may be given one dose in the midafternoon and another dose at bedtime. Try to take imipramine at around the same time(s) every day. Follow the directions on your prescription label carefully, and ask your doctor or pharmacist to explain any part you do not understand. Take imipramine exactly as directed. Do not take more or less of it or take it more often than prescribed by your doctor.

Your doctor may start you on a low dose of imipramine and gradually increase your dose.

It may take 1-3 weeks or longer for you to feel the full benefit of imipramine. Continue to take imipramine even if you feel well. Do not stop taking imipramine without talking to your doctor. Your doctor will probably want to decrease your dose gradually.

Are there other uses for this medicine?

Imipramine is also used occasionally to treat eating disorders and panic disorders. Talk to your doctor about the possible risks of using this medication for your condition.

This medication may be prescribed for other uses. Ask your doctor or pharmacist for more information.

What special precautions should I follow?

Before taking imipramine,

- tell your doctor and pharmacist if you are allergic to imipramine or any other medications.
- tell your doctor if you are taking a monoamine oxidase (MAO) inhibitor such as isocarboxazid (Marplan), phenelzine (Nardil), selegiline (Eldepryl, Emsam, Zelapar), and tranylcypromine (Parnate), or if you have stopped taking an MAO inhibitor within the past 14 days. Your doctor will probably tell you not to take imipramine. If you stop taking imipramine, you should wait at least 14 days before you start to take an MAO inhibitor.
- tell your doctor and pharmacist what prescription and nonprescription medications, vitamins, nutritional supplements, and herbal products you are taking or plan to take. Be sure to mention any of the following: anticoagulants (blood thinners) such as warfarin (Coumadin); antihistamines; cimetidine (Tagamet); flecainide (Tambocor); levodopa (Sinemet, Larodopa); lithium (Eskalith, Lithobid); medication for high blood pressure, mental illness, nausea, seizures, Parkinson's disease, asthma, colds, or allergies; methylphenidate (Ritalin); muscle relaxants; propafenone (Rhythmol); quinidine; sedatives; selective serotonin reuptake inhibitors (SSRIs) such as citalopram (Celexa), escitalopram (Lexapro), fluoxetine (Prozac, Sarafem), fluvoxamine (Luvox), paroxetine (Paxil), and sertraline (Zoloft); sleeping pills; thyroid medications; and tranquilizers. Your doctor may need to change the doses of your medications or monitor you carefully for side effects. Your doctor may tell you not to take imipramine if you have taken fluoxetine in the past 5 weeks.
- tell your doctor if you have recently had a heart attack. Your doctor may tell you not to take imipramine.
- tell your doctor if you are being treated with electroshock therapy (procedure in which small electric shocks are administered to the brain to treat certain mental illnesses), and if you have or have ever had glaucoma (an eye condition), an enlarged prostate (a male reproductive gland), difficulty urinating, seizures, an overactive thyroid gland, or liver, kidney, or heart disease.
- tell your doctor if you are pregnant, plan to become pregnant, or are breast-feeding. If you become pregnant while taking imipramine, call your doctor.
- if you are having surgery, including dental surgery, tell the doctor or dentist that you are taking imipramine.
- you should know that this medication may make you drowsy. Do not drive a car or operate machinery until you know how this medication affects you.

- remember that alcohol can add to the drowsiness caused by this medication.
- tell your doctor if you use tobacco products. Cigarette smoking may decrease the effectiveness of this medication.
- plan to avoid unnecessary or prolonged exposure to sunlight and to wear protective clothing, sunglasses, and sunscreen. Imipramine may make your skin sensitive to sunlight.

What special dietary instructions should I follow?

Unless your doctor tells you otherwise, continue your normal diet.

What should I do if I forget to take a dose?

Take the missed dose as soon as you remember it. However, if it is almost time for your next dose, skip the missed dose and continue your regular dosing schedule.

What side effects can this medicine cause?

Imipramine may cause side effects. Tell your doctor if any of these symptoms are severe or do not go away:

- nausea
- drowsiness
- weakness or tiredness
- excitement or anxiety
- nightmares
- dry mouth
- skin more sensitive to sunlight than usual
- changes in appetite or weight
- constipation
- difficulty urinating
- frequent urination
- blurred vision
- changes in sex drive or ability
- excessive sweating

Some side effects can be serious. If you experience any of the following symptoms or those listed in the IMPORTANT WARNING section, call your doctor immediately:

- jaw, neck, and back muscle spasms
- slow or difficult speech
- shuffling walk
- uncontrollable shaking of a part of the body
- fever, sore throat, or other signs of infection
- difficulty breathing or swallowing
- severe rash
- yellowing of the skin or eyes
- irregular heartbeat

If you experience a serious side effect, you or your doctor may send a report to the Food and Drug Administration's (FDA) MedWatch Adverse Event Reporting program online [at http://www.fda.gov/MedWatch/index.html] or by phone [1-800-332-1088].

Imipramine may cause other side effects. Tell you doctor if you have any unusual problems while you are taking this medication.

What storage conditions are needed for this medicine?

Keep this medication in the container it came in, tightly closed, and out of reach of children. Store it at room temperature and away from excess heat and moisture (not in the bathroom). Throw away any medication that is outdated or no longer needed. Talk to your pharmacist about the proper disposal of your medication.

What should I do in case of overdose?

In case of overdose, call your local poison control center at 1-800-222-1222. If the victim has collapsed or is not breathing, call local emergency services at 911.

What other information should I know?

Keep all appointments with your doctor.

Do not let anyone else take your medication. Ask your pharmacist any questions you have about refilling your prescription.

Dosage Facts
For Informational Purposes

Caution: Do not change your dose, how often you take your medication, or the length of time you are to take it without first talking to your healthcare provider.

The following dosage information was written using medical language for doctors and other healthcare professionals and is provided here for you to check your dosage. The dosage of this drug may differ for different patients. Therefore, always follow your doctor's instructions or the directions on the label. Contact your healthcare provider or pharmacist if you have any questions about the specific dosage of your medication after reviewing this information.

General Dosage Information

Available as imipramine hydrochloride or imipramine pamoate; dosage is expressed in terms of imipramine hydrochloride.

Individualize dosage carefully according to individual requirements and response.

Pediatric Patients

Enuresis

ORAL:
- Children ≥6 years of age: Initially, 25 mg daily, administered 1 hour prior to bedtime. If satisfactory response not obtained within 1 week, dosage may be increased to 50 mg nightly for children <12 years of age or 75 mg nightly for children ≥12 years of age. Higher dosages provide no additional therapeutic benefit but may increase risk of adverse effects. Maximum 2.5 mg/kg daily.

- For children who are early-night bedwetters, better results may be obtained by administering 25 mg in midafternoon and again at bedtime.

Adult Patients

Major Depressive Disorder
Outpatients

ORAL:
- Initially, 75 mg daily. May increase dosage to 150 mg daily and then if necessary to 200 mg daily.
- Maintenance dosages: 50–150 mg daily.

Hospitalized Patients

ORAL:
- Initially, 100–150 mg daily (administered in divided doses). May increase dosages to 200 mg daily and then if there is no response after 2 weeks to 250–300 mg daily.

Prescribing Limits

Pediatric Patients

Enuresis

ORAL:
- Maximum 2.5 mg/kg daily.

Adult Patients

Major Depressive Disorder
Outpatients

ORAL:
- Maximum 200 mg daily.

Hospitalized Patients

ORAL:
- Maximum 300 mg daily.

Special Populations

Geriatric Patients
- Initially, 25–50 mg daily as imipramine hydrochloride (Tofranil®). Increase dosage based on response and tolerance up to a maximum of 100 mg daily.

Imiquimod

(i mi kwi′ mod)

Brand Name: Aldara®

Why is this medicine prescribed?

Imiquimod is used topically to treat warts on the skin of the genital and anal areas. Imiquimod does not cure warts, and new warts may appear during treatment.

This medication is sometimes prescribed for other uses; ask your doctor or pharmacist for more information.

How should this medicine be used?

Imiquimod comes as a topical cream in unit-of-use packages. It is important to wash your hands before and after applying imiquimod to your skin. One packet of imiquimod is used to apply a thin layer of cream to the wart area three times per week, just before going to sleep. A schedule of Monday, Wednesday, Friday or Tuesday, Thursday, Saturday is suggested. Rub the cream into the skin until no more cream is visible. Do not put any covering on the area. Imiquimod should be left on the skin for 6 to 10 hours. Upon waking, wash the area with mild soap and water to remove excess cream. Follow the directions on your prescription label carefully, and ask your doctor or pharmacist to explain any part you do not understand. Use imiquimod exactly as directed. Do not use more or less of it or use it more often than prescribed by your doctor.

What special precautions should I follow?

Before using imiquimod,
- tell your doctor and pharmacist if you are allergic to imiquimod or any other drugs.
- tell your doctor and pharmacist what prescription and nonprescription medications you are taking, including vitamins.
- tell your doctor if you are pregnant, plan to become pregnant, or are breast-feeding. If you become pregnant while using imiquimod, call your doctor.

What should I do if I forget to take a dose?

Apply imiquimod just before going to bed on the day that you remember. Apply only the single dose, do not apply a double dose. Resume a Monday, Wednesday, Friday or Tuesday, Thursday, Saturday schedule, depending on what day you resume treatment.

What side effects can this medicine cause?

Imiquimod may cause side effects. Tell your doctor if any of these symptoms are severe or do not go away:
- redness, itching, or burning of the skin
- flaking of the skin
- swelling or pain in the area where imiquimod was applied
- blisters, scabs, or bumps on the skin
- change in skin color
- headache
- muscle weakness or pain
- fever
- flu-like symptoms
- fungal infection

What storage conditions are needed for this medicine?

Keep this medication in the container it came in, tightly closed, and out of reach of children. Store it at room temperature and away from excess heat and moisture (not in the bathroom). Throw away any medication that is outdated or no longer needed. Talk to your pharmacist about the proper disposal of your medication.

What other information should I know?

Keep all appointments with your doctor. Imiquimod is for external use only. Avoid sexual contact while the cream is on the skin. Imiquimod may also weaken condoms and vaginal diaphragms.

Do not apply dressings, bandages, cosmetics, lotions, or other skin medications to the area being treated unless your doctor tells you to.

Do not let anyone else use your medication. Ask your pharmacist any questions you have about refilling your prescription. Tell your doctor if your skin condition gets worse or does not go away.

Dosage Facts
For Informational Purposes

Caution: Do not change your dose, how often you take your medication, or the length of time you are to take it without first talking to your healthcare provider.

The following dosage information was written using medical language for doctors and other healthcare professionals and is provided here for you to check your dosage. The dosage of this drug may differ for different patients. Therefore, always follow your doctor's instructions or the directions on the label. Contact your healthcare provider or pharmacist if you have any questions about the specific dosage of your medication after reviewing this information.

Pediatric Patients

HPV Infections
External Genital and Perianal HPV Warts
TOPICAL:
- Children ≥12 years of age: Apply thin layer of 5% cream to HPV wart area at bedtime 3 times weekly (e.g., Monday, Wednesday, Friday or Tuesday, Thursday, Saturday) until warts have cleared completely or for a maximum of 16 weeks. Remove drug in the morning (6–10 hours after application) by washing with soap and water.
- HIV-infected children†: Apply thin layer of 5% cream to wart area at bedtime 3 times weekly (nonconsecutive days) for ≤16 weeks. Remove drug in the morning by washing with soap and water.
- Follow-up examinations not generally required for patients self-administering imiquimod, but may be useful several weeks after initiation of therapy to determine response to treatment, to monitor and treat complications of therapy, and provide additional patient education and counseling. A follow-up examination 3 months after completion of treatment may be beneficial since identification of external genital warts may be difficult.

Adult Patients

Actinic Keratosis
TOPICAL:
- Apply thin layer of 5% cream to affected area of face or scalp at bedtime twice weekly (e.g., Monday and Thursday or Tues-

day and Friday) for 16 weeks. Treatment area should be a single contiguous area approximately 25 cm² (e.g., 5 cm long and 5 cm wide) occurring on the face (e.g., forehead or one cheek) or on the scalp; both areas should not be treated concurrently. Remove drug in the morning (6–10 hours after application) by washing with soap and water.
- Assess response to treatment after local skin reactions and/or application site reactions have resolved. Lesions that do not respond to treatment should be carefully reevaluated and management reconsidered. Safety and efficacy of repeat courses of imiquimod not established.

Basal Cell Carcinoma
Biopsy-confirmed Superficial Basal Cell Carcinoma
TOPICAL:
- Apply thin layer of 5% cream to affected area at bedtime 5 times weekly (e.g., Monday through Friday) for 6 weeks. Treatment area should include the target tumor and a 1-cm margin of skin around the tumor. (See Table.) Remove drug in the morning (6–10 hours after application) by washing with soap and water.
- Assess response to treatment after local skin reactions and/or application site reactions have resolved and skin has regenerated (approximately 12 weeks after treatment ends). If there is clinical evidence of persistent tumor after treatment, a biopsy or other alternative intervention should be considered. Lesions that do not respond to treatment should be carefully reevaluated and management reconsidered. Safety and efficacy of repeat courses of imiquimod not established.

Dosage for Treatment of Superficial Basal Cell Carcinoma

Target Tumor Diameter (cm)	Cream Droplet Diameter (mm)	Approximate Dosage in Cream Droplet
0.5 to <1.0	4	10 mg 5 times weekly for 6 weeks
≥1.0 to <1.5	5	25 mg 5 times weekly for 6 weeks
≥1.5 to 2.0 cm	7	40 mg 5 times weekly for 6 weeks

HPV Infections
External Genital and Perianal HPV Warts
TOPICAL:
- Apply thin layer of 5% cream to HPV wart area at bedtime 3 times weekly (e.g., Monday, Wednesday, Friday or Tuesday, Thursday, Saturday) until warts have cleared completely or for a maximum of 16 weeks. Remove drug in the morning (6–10 hours after application) by washing with soap and water.
- HIV-infected adults†: Apply thin layer of 5% cream to wart area at bedtime 3 times weekly (nonconsecutive days) for ≤16 weeks. Remove drug in the morning by washing with soap and water.
- Follow-up examinations not generally required for patients self-administering imiquimod, but may be useful several weeks after initiation of therapy to determine response to treatment, to monitor and treat complications of therapy, and

provide additional patient education and counseling. A follow-up examination 3 months after completion of treatment may be beneficial since identification of external genital warts may be difficult.

Prescribing Limits

Pediatric Patients

HPV Infections
External Genital and Perianal HPV Warts

TOPICAL:
- Children ≥12 years of age: Maximum of 16 weeks of treatment (3 times weekly).

Adult Patients

Actinic Keratosis

TOPICAL:
- Maximum of 16 weeks of treatment (2 times weekly).
- Maximum treatment area is 25 cm².
- Safety and efficacy of repeated use (i.e., multiple courses of treatment) in the same area of actinic keratosis not established.

Superficial Basal Cell Carcinoma

TOPICAL:
- Maximum of 6 weeks of treatment (5 times weekly).
- Safety and efficacy of repeat courses of imiquimod not established.

HPV Infections
External Genital and Perianal HPV Warts

TOPICAL:
- Maximum of 16 weeks of treatment (3 times weekly).

Special Populations

No special population dosage recommendations.

† Use is not currently included in the labeling approved by the US Food and Drug Administration.

Immune Globulin Intravenous Injection

(glob' yoo lin)

Brand Name: Carimune® NF, Flebogamma® 5%, Gammagard® S/D, Gamunex® 10%, Iveegam® EN, Octagam® 5%, Polygam® S/D

Important Warning

Immune globulin intravenous (IGIV) may cause kidney failure. Tell your doctor if you are over 65 years old or if you have or have ever had kidney disease, diabetes, sepsis, plasma cell disease, or volume depletion. Tell your doctor if you are taking amikacin (Amikin), gentamicin (Garamycin), streptomycin, or other medications that can cause kidney damage. Keep all appointments with your doctor and the laboratory. Your doctor will order certain lab tests to check your response to IGIV. If you experience any of the following symptoms, call your doctor immediately: decreased urination, suden wight gain, swelling of the legs or ankles, or shortness of breath.

About Your Treatment

Your doctor has ordered IGIV. The drug may be given alone or added to an intravenous fluid that will drip through a needle or catheter placed in your vein for 2-4 hours, once a day for 2-7 days. You will receive another single dose every 10-21 days or every 3-4 weeks, depending on your condition.

IGIV boosts the body's natural response in patients with compromised immune systems [e.g., patients with human immunodeficiency virus (HIV) and premature babies]. It also increases the number of platelets (part of the blood) in patients with idiopathic thrombocytopenic purpura. This medication is sometimes prescribed for other uses; ask your doctor or pharmacist for more information.

Your health care provider (doctor, nurse, or pharmacist) may measure the effectiveness and side effects of your treatment using laboratory tests and physical examinations. It is important to keep all appointments with your doctor and the laboratory. The length of treatment depends on how you respond to the medication.

Precautions

Before administering IGIV,
- tell your doctor and pharmacist if you are allergic to any drugs.
- tell your doctor and pharmacist what prescription and nonprescription medications you are taking, especially those listed in the IMPORTANT WARNING section, antibiotics, and vitamins.
- tell your doctor if you are pregnant, plan to become pregnant, or are breast-feeding. If you become pregnant while taking IGIV, call your doctor.
- tell your doctor if you had a vaccine for measles, mumps, or rubella in the last 3 months.

Administering Your Medication

Before you administer IGIV, look at the solution closely. It should be clear and free of floating material. Gently squeeze the bag or observe the solution container to make sure there are no leaks. Do not use the solution if it is discolored, if it contains particles, or if the bag or container leaks. Use a new solution, but show the damaged one to your health care provider.

It is important that you use your medication exactly as

directed. Do not change your dosing schedule without talking to your health care provider. Your health care provider may tell you to stop your infusion if you have a mechanical problem (such as a blockage in the tubing, needle, or catheter); if you have to stop an infusion, call your health care provider immediately so your therapy can continue.

Side Effects

IGIV may cause side effects. Tell your health care provider if any of these symptoms are severe or do not go away:

- backache
- headache
- joint or muscle pain
- general feeling of discomfort
- leg cramps
- rash
- pain at the injection site

If you experience any of the following symptoms or those listed in the IMPORTANT WARNING section, call your health care provider immediately:

- hives
- chest tightness
- dizziness
- unusual tiredness or weakness
- chills
- fever
- sweating
- redness of the face
- upset stomach
- vomiting

If you experience a serious side effect, you or your doctor may send a report to the Food and Drug Administration's (FDA) MedWatch Adverse Event Reporting program online [at http://www.fda.gov/MedWatch/index.html] or by phone [1-800-332-1088].

Storage Conditions

- Your health care provider probably will give you a 1-day supply of IGIV at a time. Depending on the product you receive, you may be told to store it in the refrigerator.
- If you store IGIV in the refrigerator, take your next dose from the refrigerator 1 hour before using it; place it in a clean, dry area to allow it to warm to room temperature.
- Do not allow IGIV to freeze.

Your health care provider may provide you with directions on how to prepare each dose.

Store your medication only as directed. Make sure you understand what you need to store your medication properly.

Keep your supplies in a clean, dry place when you are not using them, and keep all medications and supplies out of reach of children. Your health care provider will tell you how to throw away used needles, syringes, tubing, and containers to avoid accidental injury.

Overdose

In case of overdose, call your local poison control center at 1-800-222-1222. If the victim has collapsed or is not breathing, call local emergency services at 911.

Signs of Infection

If you are receiving IGIV in your vein or under your skin, you need to know the symptoms of a catheter-related infection (an infection where the needle enters your vein or skin). If you experience any of these effects near your intravenous catheter, tell your health care provider as soon as possible:

- tenderness
- warmth
- irritation
- drainage
- redness
- swelling
- pain

Talk to your doctor, pharmacist, or other healthcare professional if you have questions about dosing information for your medication.

Indapamide

(in dap′ a mide)

Brand Name: Lozol®
Also available generically.

Why is this medicine prescribed?

Indapamide, a 'water pill,' is used to reduce the swelling and fluid retention caused by heart disease. It also is used to treat high blood pressure. It causes the kidneys to get rid of unneeded water and salt from the body into the urine.

This medicine is sometimes prescribed for other uses; ask your doctor or pharmacist for more information.

How should this medicine be used?

Indapamide comes as a tablet to take by mouth. It usually is taken once a day, in the morning. Follow the directions on your prescription label carefully, and ask your doctor or pharmacist to explain any part you do not understand. Take indapamide exactly as directed. Do not take more or less of it or take it more often than prescribed by your doctor.

Indapamide controls high blood pressure but does not cure it. Continue to take indapamide even if you feel well. Do not stop taking indapamide without talking to your doctor.

Are there other uses for this medicine?

Indapamide also is used to treat swelling and fluid retention caused by various medical conditions other than heart disease. Talk to your doctor about the possible risks of using this medicine for your condition.

What special precautions should I follow?

Before taking indapamide,

- tell your doctor and pharmacist if you are allergic to indapamide, sulfa drugs, or any other drugs.
- tell your doctor and pharmacist what prescription and nonprescription medications you are taking, especially other medications for high blood pressure, corticosteroids (e.g., prednisone), digoxin (Lanoxin), indomethacin (Indocin), lithium (Eskalith, Lithobid), probenecid (Benemid), and vitamins.
- tell your doctor if you have or have ever had heart rhythm problems, diabetes, gout, or kidney, liver, thyroid, or parathyroid disease.
- tell your doctor if you are pregnant, plan to become pregnant, or are breast-feeding. Do not breast-feed while taking this medicine. If you become pregnant while taking indapamide, call your doctor.
- if you are having surgery, including dental surgery, tell the doctor or dentist that you are taking indapamide.
- you should know that this drug may make you drowsy. Do not drive a car or operate machinery until you know how this drug affects you.
- remember that alcohol can add to the drowsiness caused by this drug.

What special dietary instructions should I follow?

Follow your doctor's directions. They may include a daily exercise program and a low-sodium or low-salt diet, potassium supplements, and increased amounts of potassium-rich foods (e.g., bananas, prunes, raisins, and orange juice) in your diet.

What should I do if I forget to take a dose?

Take the missed dose as soon as you remember it. However, if it is almost time for your next dose, skip the missed dose and continue your regular dosing schedule. Do not take a double dose to make up for a missed one.

What side effects can this medicine cause?

Frequent urination may last for up to 6 hours after a dose and should decrease after you take indapamide for a few weeks. Tell your doctor if any of these symptoms are severe or do not go away:

- muscle cramps
- drowsiness
- dizziness
- confusion
- thirst
- upset stomach
- vomiting
- stomach cramps
- decreased sexual ability
- blurred vision

If you have any of the following symptoms, call your doctor immediately:

- rapid, excessive weight loss
- severe skin rash with itching
- difficulty breathing or swallowing

If you experience a serious side effect, you or your doctor may send a report to the Food and Drug Administration's (FDA) MedWatch Adverse Event Reporting program online [at http://www.fda.gov/MedWatch/index.html] or by phone [1-800-332-1088].

What storage conditions are needed for this medicine?

Keep this medicine in the container it came in, tightly closed, and out of reach of children. Store it at room temperature and away from excess heat and moisture (not in the bathroom). Throw away any medicine that is outdated or no longer needed. Talk to your pharmacist about the proper disposal of your medicine.

What should I do in case of overdose?

In case of overdose, call your local poison control center at 1-800-222-1222. If the victim has collapsed or is not breathing, call local emergency services at 911.

What other information should I know?

Keep all appointments with your doctor and the laboratory. Your blood pressure should be checked regularly, and blood tests should be done occasionally.

Do not let anyone else take your medicine. Ask your pharmacist any questions you have about refilling your prescription.

Dosage Facts
For Informational Purposes

Caution: Do not change your dose, how often you take your medication, or the length of time you are to take it without first talking to your healthcare provider.

The following dosage information was written using medical language for doctors and other healthcare professionals and is provided here for you to check your dosage. The dosage of this drug may differ for different patients. Therefore, always follow your doctor's instructions or the directions on the label. Contact your healthcare provider or pharmacist if you have any questions about the specific dosage of your medication after reviewing this information.

General Dosage Information

Individualize dosage according to individual requirements and response.

Adult Patients

Hypertension
BP Monitoring and Treatment Goals

Carefully monitor BP during initial titration or subsequent upward adjustment in dosage.

Avoid large or abrupt reductions in BP.

Adjust dosage at approximately monthly intervals (more aggressively in high-risk patients [stage 2 hypertension, comorbid conditions]) if BP control is inadequate at a given dosage; it may take months to control hypertension adequately while avoiding adverse effects of therapy.

SBP is the principal clinical end point, especially in middle-aged and geriatric patients. Once the goal SBP is attained, the goal DBP usually is achieved.

The goal is to achieve and maintain a lifelong SBP <140 mm Hg and a DBP <90 mm Hg if tolerated.

The goal in hypertensive patients with diabetes mellitus or renal impairment is to achieve and maintain a SBP <130 mm Hg and a DBP <80 mm Hg.

Monotherapy
ORAL:
- Initially, 1.25 mg once daily in the morning.
- If response is inadequate, dosage may be increased at 4-week intervals to 2.5 mg daily and subsequently to 5 mg daily.
- Dosages >5 mg daily do not appear to result in further improvement in BP and increase the risk of hypokalemia.
- If adequate response is not achieved with the 5-mg daily dosage, add or substitute another antihypertensive agent.
- Although JNC previously recommended a usual dosage range of 1.25–5 mg daily, these experts currently (JNC 7) recommend a lower usual dosage range of 1.25–2.5 mg daily.

Maintenance
ORAL:
- In patients whose BP is controlled adequately with 2.5 or 5 mg daily, reduction in dosage, including alternate-day therapy, may be attempted.
- Dosage reduction should be gradual and deliberate and under close medical supervision.

Combination Therapy
ORAL:
- If concomitant therapy with other antihypertensive agents is required, the usual dose of the other agent may need to be reduced initially by up to 50%; subsequent dosage adjustments should be based on BP response. Dosage reduction of both drugs may be required.

Edema in CHF
ORAL:
- Initially, 2.5 mg once daily in the morning.
- If response is inadequate after 1 week, dosage may be increased to 5 mg daily given as a single dose in the morning.
- Dosages >5 mg daily do not appear to result in further improvement in heart failure and increase the risk of hypokalemia.

Edema (General)
ORAL:
- Similar dosages to those employed for the management of edema associated with CHF have been used in the management of edema from other causes†.

Prescribing Limits

Adult Patients

ORAL:
- Dosages >5 mg daily do not appear to result in further improvement in heart failure or BP and are associated with increased risk of hypokalemia; such dosages have been employed only in a limited number of clinical studies.

Special Populations

Hepatic Impairment
- No specific dosage recommendations.

Renal Impairment
- No specific dosage recommendations.

Geriatric Patients
- No specific dosage recommendations.

† Use is not currently included in the labeling approved by the US Food and Drug Administration.

Indinavir

(in din′ a veer)

Brand Name: Crixivan®

Why is this medicine prescribed?

Indinavir is used to treat human immunodeficiency virus (HIV) infection in adults. It belongs to a class of drugs called protease (pro′ tee ace) inhibitors, which slow the spread of HIV infection in the body. It is usually taken with other antiviral medications. Indinavir is not a cure and may not decrease the number of HIV-related illnesses. Indinavir does not prevent the spread of HIV to other people.

This medication is sometimes prescribed for other uses; ask your doctor or pharmacist for more information.

How should this medicine be used?

Indinavir comes as a capsule to take by mouth. It is usually taken every 8 hours (three times a day). Follow the directions on your prescription label carefully, and ask your doctor or pharmacist to explain any part you do not understand. Take indinavir exactly as directed. Do not take more or less of it or take it more often than prescribed by your doctor.

Continue to take indinavir even if you feel well. Do not stop taking indinavir without talking to your doctor.

Are there other uses for this medicine?

Indinavir is also used sometimes in combination with zidovudine (Retrovir, AZT) and lamivudine (Epivir) to treat health-care workers and other individuals exposed to HIV infection after accidental contact with HIV-contaminated blood, tissues, or other body fluids. Talk to your doctor about the possible risks of using this drug for your condition.

What special precautions should I follow?

Before taking indinavir,
- tell your doctor and pharmacist if you are allergic to indinavir or any other drugs.
- tell your doctor and pharmacist what prescription and nonprescription medications you are taking, especially astemizole (Hismanal), atorvastatin (Lipitor), cerivastatin (Baycol), cisapride (Propulsid), clarithromycin (Biaxin), delavirdine (Rescriptor), dexamethasone (Decadron), efavirenz (Sustiva), fluconazole (Diflucan), isoniazid (INH), itraconazole (Sporanox), ketoconazole (Nizoral), lovastatin (Mevacor), medications for seizures, midazolam (Versed), oral contraceptives, quinidine, rifabutin (Mycobutin), rifampin (Rifadin), sildenafil (Viagra), simvastatin (Zocor), terfenadine (Seldane), and triazolam (Halcion).
- tell your doctor what vitamins and herbal products you are taking, especially St. John's wort.
- if you are taking didanosine, take it at least one hour before or after indinavir.
- tell your doctor if you have or have ever had hemophilia or kidney or liver disease or a history of alcohol abuse.
- tell your doctor if you are pregnant, plan to become pregnant, or are breast-feeding. If you become pregnant while taking indinavir, call your doctor.
- tell your doctor if you drink alcohol.

What special dietary instructions should I follow?

Take indinavir on an empty stomach, 1 hour before meals or 2 hours after meals, with plenty of fluids (an 8-ounce glass of water). However, if indinavir upsets your stomach, it may be taken with a light meal, such as dry toast or cornflakes with skim milk. Do not take with grapefruit juice. If you are also taking didanosine (DDI), take 1 hour apart on an empty stomach.

Drink at least 48 ounces (six 8-ounce glasses) of water or other liquids every 24 hours.

What should I do if I forget to take a dose?

Take the missed dose as soon as you remember it. However, if it is almost time for the next dose, skip the missed dose and continue your regular dosing schedule. Do not take a double dose to make up for a missed one.

What side effects can this medicine cause?

Indinavir may cause side effects. Tell your doctor if any of these symptoms are severe or do not go away:
- headache
- stomach pain
- change in the distribution of body fat

If you experience any of the following symptoms, call your doctor immediately:
- rash
- back pain
- pain in the side of your body
- blood in urine
- muscle pain
- upset stomach
- excessive tiredness
- unusual bleeding or bruising
- loss of appetite
- pain in the upper right part of your stomach
- flu-like symptoms
- dark yellow or brown urine
- yellowing of the skin or eyes
- paleness

Indinavir may increase the sugar level in your blood. If you experience any of the following symptoms, call your doctor immediately:
- frequent urination
- increased thirst
- weakness
- dizziness
- headache

If you experience a serious side effect, you or your doctor may send a report to the Food and Drug Administration's (FDA) MedWatch Adverse Event Reporting program online [at http://www.fda.gov/MedWatch/index.html] or by phone [1-800-332-1088].

What storage conditions are needed for this medicine?

Keep this medication in the container it came in, tightly closed, and out of reach of children. A desiccant (drying agent) is included with your capsules; keep this in your medicine bottle at all times. Store it at room temperature and away from excess heat and moisture (not in the bathroom). Throw away any medication that is outdated or no longer needed. Talk to your pharmacist about the proper disposal of your medication.

What should I do in case of overdose?

In case of overdose, call your local poison control center at 1-800-222-1222. If the victim has collapsed or is not breathing, call local emergency services at 911.

What other information should I know?

Keep all appointments with your doctor and the laboratory. Your doctor will order certain lab tests to check your response to indinavir.

Do not let anyone else take your medication. Ask your pharmacist any questions you have about refilling your prescription.

Dosage Facts
For Informational Purposes

Caution: Do not change your dose, how often you take your medication, or the length of time you

are to take it without first talking to your health-care provider.

The following dosage information was written using medical language for doctors and other healthcare professionals and is provided here for you to check your dosage. The dosage of this drug may differ for different patients. Therefore, always follow your doctor's instructions or the directions on the label. Contact your healthcare provider or pharmacist if you have any questions about the specific dosage of your medication after reviewing this information.

General Dosage Information

Available as indinavir sulfate; dosage expressed as indinavir.

Must be given in conjunction with other antiretrovirals. *If used with delavirdine, certain didanosine preparations, efavirenz, lopinavir/ritonavir, nelfinavir, nevirapine, or ritonavir, adjustment in the treatment regimen recommended.*

Pediatric Patients

Treatment of HIV Infection

ORAL:
- Children 4–15 years of age†: 500 mg/m^2 every 8 hours under investigation.

Adult Patients

Treatment of HIV Infection

ORAL:
- 800 mg every 8 hours. If *ritonavir-boosted* indinavir is used, 800 mg twice daily with low-dose ritonavir (100 or 200 mg twice daily).

Postexposure Prophylaxis of HIV†
Occupational Exposure†

ORAL:
- 800 mg twice daily *boosted* with low-dose ritonavir (100 mg twice daily). Alternatively, 800 mg every 8 hours (without low-dose ritonavir).
- Used in alternative expanded regimens that include indinavir with low-dose ritonavir and 2 NRTIs.
- Initiate postexposure prophylaxis as soon as possible following exposure (within hours rather than days) and continue for 4 weeks, if tolerated.

Nonoccupational Exposure†

ORAL:
- 800 mg twice daily *boosted* with low-dose ritonavir (100 or 200 mg every 12 hours). Alternatively, 800 mg every 8 hours (without low-dose ritonavir).
- Used in an alternative PI-based regimen that includes indinavir (or *ritonavir-boosted* indinavir) and (lamivudine or emtricitabine) and (zidovudine or stavudine or abacavir or tenofovir or didanosine).
- Initiate postexposure prophylaxis as soon as possible following exposure (preferably ≤72 hours after exposure) and continue for 28 days.

Special Populations

Hepatic Impairment

Treatment of HIV Infection

ORAL:
- Adults with mild to moderate hepatic impairment due to cirrhosis: 600 mg every 8 hours.

Renal Impairment

Treatment of HIV Infection

ORAL:
- Dosage adjustment not needed.

Geriatric Patients
- Select dosage with caution.

† *Use is not currently included in the labeling approved by the US Food and Drug Administration.*

Indomethacin

(in doe meth′ a sin)

Brand Name: Indocin®
Also available generically.

Important Warning

People who take nonsteroidal anti-inflammatory medications (NSAIDs) (other than aspirin) such as indomethacin may have a higher risk of having a heart attack or a stroke than people who do not take these medications. These events may happen without warning and may cause death. This risk may be higher for people who take NSAIDs for a long time. Tell your doctor if you or anyone in your family has or has ever had heart disease, a heart attack, or a stroke, if you smoke, and if you have or have ever had high cholesterol, high blood pressure, or diabetes. Get emergency medical help right away if you experience any of the following symptoms: chest pain, shortness of breath, weakness in one part or side of the body, or slurred speech.

If you will be undergoing a coronary artery bypass graft (CABG; a type of heart surgery), you should not take indomethacin right before or right after the surgery.

NSAIDs such as indomethacin may cause ulcers, bleeding, or holes in the stomach or intestine. These problems may develop at any time during treatment, may happen without warning symptoms, and may cause death. The risk may be higher for people who take NSAIDs for a long time, are older in age, have poor health, or drink large amounts of

continued on next page

Important Warning (cont'd)

alcohol while you are taking indomethacin. Tell your doctor if you take any of the following medications: anticoagulants ('blood thinners') such as warfarin (Coumadin); aspirin; other NSAIDS such as diflunisal (Dolobid), ibuprofen (Advil, Motrin) and naproxen (Aleve, Naprosyn); or oral steroids such as dexamethasone (Decadron, Dexone), methylprednisolone (Medrol), and prednisone (Deltasone). Also tell your doctor if you have or have ever had ulcers or bleeding in your stomach or intestines or other bleeding disorders. If you experience any of the following symptoms, stop taking indomethacin and call your doctor: stomach pain, heartburn, vomiting a substance that is bloody or looks like coffee grounds, blood in the stool, or black and tarry stools.

Keep all appointments with your doctor and the laboratory. Your doctor will monitor your symptoms carefully and will probably order certain tests to check your body's response to indomethacin. Be sure to tell your doctor how you are feeling so that your doctor can prescribe the right amount of medication to treat your condition with the lowest risk of serious side effects.

Your doctor or pharmacist will give you the manufacturer's patient information sheet (Medication Guide) when you begin treatment with indomethacin and each time you refill your prescription. Read the information carefully and ask your doctor or pharmacist if you have any questions. You can also visit the Food and Drug Administration (FDA) website (http://www.fda.gov/cder) or the manufacturer's website to obtain the Medication Guide.

Why is this medicine prescribed?

Indomethacin is used to relieve moderate to severe pain, tenderness, swelling, and stiffness caused by osteoarthritis (arthritis caused by a breakdown of the lining of the joints), rheumatoid arthritis (arthritis caused by swelling of the lining of the joints), and ankylosing spondylitis (arthritis that mainly affects the spine). Indomethacin is also used to treat pain in the shoulder caused by bursitis (inflammation of a fluid-filled sac in the shoulder joint) and tendinitis (inflammation of the tissue that connects muscle to bone). Indomethacin immediate-release capsules, suspension (liquid) and suppositories are also used to treat acute gouty arthritis (attacks of severe joint pain and swelling caused by a build-up of certain substances in the joints). Indomethacin is in a class of medications called NSAIDs. It works by stopping the body's production of a substance that causes pain, fever, and inflammation.

How should this medicine be used?

Indomethacin comes as a capsule, an extended-release (long-acting) capsule, and a suspension to take by mouth and as a suppository to be used rectally. Indomethacin capsules, liq-

uid, and suppositories usually are taken two to four times a day. Extended-release capsules are usually taken one or two times a day. Indomethacin capsules, extended release capsules, and suspension should be taken with food, immediately after meals, or with antacids. Take indomethacin at around the same times every day. Follow the directions on your prescription label carefully, and ask your doctor or pharmacist to explain any part you do not understand. Take indomethacin exactly as directed. Do not take more or less of it or take it more often than prescribed by your doctor.

Swallow the extended-release capsules whole; do not split, chew, or crush them.

Shake the suspension well before each use to mix the medication evenly.

Your doctor may change the dose of your medication during your treatment. In some cases, your doctor may start you on a low dose of indomethacin and gradually increase your dose, not more often than once a week. In other cases, your doctor may start you on an average dose of indomethacin and decrease your dose once your symptoms are controlled. Follow these directions carefully and ask your doctor or pharmacist if you have any questions.

To use indomethacin suppositories, follow these steps:
1. Remove the wrapper.
2. Dip the tip of the suppository in water.
3. Lie down on your left side and raise your right knee to your chest. (A left-handed person should lie on the right side and raise the left knee.)
4. Using your finger, insert the suppository about 1 inch into the rectum. Hold it in place for a few moments.
5. Stand up after about 15 minutes. Wash your hands thoroughly and resume your normal activities.
6. You should try to keep the suppository in place and avoid having a bowel movement for 1 hour after you insert the suppository.

Are there other uses for this medicine?

Indomethacin is also sometimes used to relieve fever, pain, and inflammation caused by many types of conditions or injuries, to reduce the amount of calcium in the blood, and to treat a certain type of low blood pressure Talk to your doctor about the risks of using this medication for your condition.

This medication may be prescribed for other uses; ask your doctor or pharmacist for more information.

What special precautions should I follow?

Before taking indomethacin,
- tell your doctor and pharmacist if you are allergic to indomethacin, aspirin or other NSAIDs such as ibuprofen (Advil, Motrin) and naproxen (Aleve, Naprosyn), any other medications, or any of the inactive ingredients in indomethacin capsules, suspension, extended release capsules, or suppositories. Ask your pharmacist for a list of the inactive ingredients.
- tell your doctor and pharmacist what prescription and

nonprescription medications, vitamins, nutritional supplements, and herbal products you are taking or plan to take. Be sure to mention the medications listed in the IMPORTANT WARNING section and any of the following: angiotensin-converting enzyme (ACE) inhibitors such as benazepril (Lotensin), captopril (Capoten), enalapril (Vasotec), fosinopril (Monopril), lisinopril (Prinivil, Zestril), moexipril (Univasc), perindopril (Aceon), quinapril (Accupril), ramipril (Altace), and trandolapril (Mavik); angiotensin II receptor antagonists such as candesartan (Atacand), eprosartan (Teveten), irbesartan (Avapro), losartan (Cozaar), olmesartan (Benicar), telmisartan (Micardis), and valsartan (Diovan); beta blockers such as atenolol (Tenormin), labetalol (Normodyne), metoprolol (Lopressor, Toprol XL), nadolol (Corgard), and propranolol (Inderal); cyclosporine (Neoral, Sandimmune); digoxin (Lanoxin); diuretics ('water pills') such as triamterene (Dyrenium, in Dyazide); lithium (Eskalith, Lithobid); methotrexate (Rheumatrex); phenytoin (Dilantin); and probenecid (Benemid).

- tell your doctor if you have or have ever had asthma, especially if you also have frequent stuffed or runny nose or nasal polyps (swelling of the lining of the nose); seizures; Parkinson's disease; depression or mental illness; or liver or kidney disease. If you will be using indomethacin suppositories, also tell your doctor if you have or have ever had proctitis (inflammation of the rectum) or have or have recently had rectal bleeding.
- tell your doctor if you are pregnant especially if you are in the last few months of your pregnancy, you plan to become pregnant, or you are breast-feeding. If you become pregnant while taking indomethacin, call your doctor.
- if you are having surgery, including dental surgery, tell the doctor or dentist that you are taking indomethacin.
- you should know that this medication may make you drowsy. Do not drive a car or operate machinery until you know how this medication affects you.
- remember that alcohol can add to the drowsiness caused by this medication.

What special dietary instructions should I follow?

Unless your doctor tells you otherwise, continue your normal diet.

What should I do if I forget to take a dose?

Take the missed dose as soon as you remember it. However, if it is almost time for the next dose, skip the missed dose and continue your regular dosing schedule. Do not take a double dose to make up for a missed one.

What side effects can this medicine cause?

Indomethacin may cause side effects. Tell your doctor if any of these symptoms are severe or do not go away:

- headache
- dizziness
- vomiting
- diarrhea
- constipation
- irritation of the rectum
- constant feeling of the need to empty the bowel
- ringing in the ears

Some side effects can be serious. If you experience any of the following symptoms or those mentioned in the IMPORTANT WARNING section, call your doctor immediately. Do not take any more indomethacin until you speak to your doctor.

- unexplained weight gain
- fever
- blisters
- rash
- itching
- hives
- swelling of the eyes, face, tongue, lips, throat, hands, feet, ankles, or lower legs
- difficulty breathing or swallowing
- hoarseness
- pale skin
- fast heartbeat
- excessive tiredness
- unusual bleeding or bruising
- lack of energy
- upset stomach
- loss of appetite
- pain in the upper right part of the stomach
- flu-like symptoms
- yellowing of the skin or eyes
- cloudy, discolored, or bloody urine
- back pain
- difficult or painful urination
- blurred vision or other problems with sight

Indomethacin may cause other side effects. Call your doctor if you have any unusual problems while taking this medication.

If you experience a serious side effect, you or your doctor may send a report to the Food and Drug Administration's (FDA) MedWatch Adverse Event Reporting program online [at http://www.fda.gov/MedWatch/index.html] or by phone [1-800-332-1088].

What storage conditions are needed for this medicine?

Keep this medication in the container it came in, tightly closed, and out of reach of children. Store it at room temperature and away from excess heat and moisture (not in the bathroom). Throw away any medication that is outdated or no longer needed. Talk to your pharmacist about the proper disposal of your medication.

What should I do in case of overdose?

In case of overdose, call your local poison control center at 1-800-222-1222. If the victim has collapsed or is not breathing, call local emergency services at 911.

Symptoms of overdose may include:

- upset stomach
- vomiting
- headache
- dizziness
- confusion
- extreme tiredness
- feeling of numbness, pricking, burning, or creeping on the skin
- seizures

What other information should I know?

Before having any laboratory test, tell your doctor and the laboratory personnel that you are taking indomethacin.

Do not let anyone else take your medication. Ask your pharmacist any questions you have about refilling your prescription.

Dosage Facts
For Informational Purposes

Caution: Do not change your dose, how often you take your medication, or the length of time you are to take it without first talking to your healthcare provider.

The following dosage information was written using medical language for doctors and other healthcare professionals and is provided here for you to check your dosage. The dosage of this drug may differ for different patients. Therefore, always follow your doctor's instructions or the directions on the label. Contact your healthcare provider or pharmacist if you have any questions about the specific dosage of your medication after reviewing this information.

General Dosage Information

Available as indomethacin and indomethacin sodium; dosage expressed in terms of indomethacin.

To minimize the potential risk of adverse cardiovascular and/or GI events, use lowest effective dosage and shortest duration of therapy consistent with the patient's treatment goals. Adjust dosage based on individual requirements and response; attempt to titrate to the lowest effective dosage.

Pediatric Patients

Inflammatory Diseases
Juvenile Rheumatoid Arthritis†

ORAL:
- Children ≥2 years of age: Initially, 2 mg/kg daily in divided doses. Increase dosage until a satisfactory response is achieved, up to maximum dosage of 4 mg/kg daily or 150–200 mg daily (whichever is less) in divided doses. As symp-

toms subside, reduce dosage to the lowest effective level or discontinue the drug.

Pericarditis†

ORAL:
- 50–100 mg daily in 2–4 divided doses.

Adult Patients

Inflammatory Diseases
Osteoarthritis, Rheumatoid Arthritis, or Ankylosing Spondylitis

ORAL:
- Conventional capsules or oral suspension: Initially, 25 mg 2 or 3 times daily. If needed, increase dosage by 25 or 50 mg daily at weekly intervals until a satisfactory response is obtained up to a maximum dosage of 150–200 mg daily.
- Extended-release capsules: Initially, 75 mg once daily. May increase dosage to 75 mg twice daily.

RECTAL:
- 25 mg 2 or 3 times daily. If needed, increase dosage by 25 or 50 mg daily at weekly intervals until a satisfactory response is obtained up to a maximum dosage of 150–200 mg daily.

Gout

ORAL:
- Conventional capsules: 50 mg 3 times daily until pain is tolerable; then reduce dosage rapidly and discontinue.

Painful Shoulder

ORAL:
- Conventional capsules or oral suspension: 75–150 mg daily in 3 or 4 divided doses. Discontinue once symptoms have been controlled for several days; usual course of therapy is 7–14 days.
- Extended-release capsules: 75 mg once or twice daily. Discontinue once symptoms have been controlled for several days; usual course of therapy is 7–14 days.

RECTAL:
- 75–150 mg daily in 3 or 4 divided doses. Discontinue once symptoms have been controlled for several days; usual course of therapy is 7–14 days.

Pericarditis†

ORAL:
- 75–200 mg daily in 3 or 4 divided doses.

Prescribing Limits

Pediatric Patients

Juvenile Rheumatoid Arthritis

ORAL:
- Maximum 4 mg/kg or 150–200 mg daily, whichever is less.

Adult Patients

Inflammatory Diseases
Rheumatoid Arthritis, Osteoarthritis, or Ankylosing Spondylitis

ORAL:
- Maximum 200 mg daily.

RECTAL:
- Maximum 200 mg daily.

Special Populations

Geriatric Patients
- Careful dosage selection recommended due to possible age-related decreases in renal function.

† Use is not currently included in the labeling approved by the US Food and Drug Administration.

Infliximab Injection

(in flix′ i mab)

Brand Name: Remicade®

Important Warning

Infliximab may decrease your ability to fight infection and increase the risk that you will get a serious or life-threatening infection. Tell your doctor if you have any type of infection now, including minor infections (such as open cuts or sores), infections that come and go (such as cold sores) and chronic infections that do not go away, or if you often get any type of infection such as bladder infections. Also tell your doctor if you are taking medications that suppress the immune system such as azathioprine (Imuran), cancer chemotherapy medications, cyclosporine (Neoral, Sandimmune), oral corticosteroids; 6-mercaptopurine (Purinethol); methotrexate (Rheumatrex), sirolimus (Rapamune), and tacrolimus (Prograf). If you experience any of the following symptoms during or shortly after your treatment with infliximab, call your doctor immediately: sore throat; cough; fever; extreme tiredness; flu-like symptoms; warm, red, or painful skin; or other signs of infection.

Infliximab increases the risk that you will get some types of infections that are most common in certain parts of the United States and the world. Tell your doctor all the places you previously lived and all the places you recently visited or plan to visit while using infliximab.

You may be infected with tuberculosis (TB, a type of lung infection) but not have any symptoms of the disease. In this case, infliximab may increase the risk that your infection will become more serious and you will develop symptoms. Your doctor will perform a skin test to see if you have an inactive TB infection. If necessary, your doctor will give you medication to treat this infection before you start using infliximab. Tell your doctor if you have or have ever had TB, or if you have been around someone who has TB.

Keep all appointments with your doctor. Your doctor will monitor your health carefully to be sure you do not develop a serious infection.

Some children and young adults with Crohn's disease (a condition in which the body attacks the lining of the digestive tract, causing pain, diarrhea, weight loss, and fever) who used infliximab developed a rare type of cancer called hepatosplenic T-cell lymphoma. These patients were also taking azathioprine (Imuran) or 6-mercaptopurine (Purinethol) when they developed this cancer.

Your doctor or pharmacist will give you the manufacturer's patient information sheet (Medication Guide) when you begin treatment with infliximab and each time you receive the medication. Read the information carefully and ask your doctor or pharmacist if you have any questions. You can also visit the Food and Drug Administration (FDA) website (http://www.fda.gov/cder) or the manufacturer's website to obtain the Medication Guide.

Talk to your doctor about the risks of using infliximab.

Why is this medicine prescribed?

Infliximab is used to relieve the symptoms of certain autoimmune disorders (conditions in which the immune system attacks healthy parts of the body and causes pain, swelling, and damage) including:
- rheumatoid arthritis (a condition in which the body attacks its own joints, causing pain, swelling, and loss of function) that is also being treated with methotrexate (Rheumatrex, Trexall)
- Crohn's disease (a condition in which the body attacks the lining of the digestive tract, causing pain, diarrhea, weight loss, and fever) that has not improved when treated with other medications
- ulcerative colitis (condition that causes swelling and sores in the lining of the large intestine) that has not improved when treated with other medications,
- ankylosing spondylitis (a condition in which the body attacks the joints of the spine and other areas causing pain and joint damage),
- psoriasis (a skin disease in which red, scaly patches form on some areas of the body),
- psoriatic arthritis (joint pain and swelling and scales on the skin).

Infliximab is in a class of medications called tumor necrosis factor-alpha (TNF-alpha) inhibitors. It works by blocking the action of TNF-alpha, a substance in the body that causes inflammation.

How should this medicine be used?

Infliximab comes as a powder to be mixed with sterile water and administered intravenously (into a vein) by a doctor or nurse. It is usually given in a doctor's office every 2-8 weeks. It will take about 2 hours for you to receive your entire dose of infliximab.

Infliximab may cause serious allergic reactions during an infusion and for 2 hours afterward. A doctor or nurse will monitor you during this time to be sure you are not having a serious reaction to the medication. You may be given other medications to treat or prevent reactions to infliximab. Tell your doctor or nurse immediately if you experience any of the following symptoms during or shortly after your infusion: hives; rash; itching; swelling of the face, eyes, mouth, throat, tongue, lips, hands, feet, ankles, or lower legs; difficulty breathing or swallowing; flushing dizziness; fainting; fever; chills; seizures; and chest pain.

Infliximab may help control your symptoms, but it will not cure your condition. Your doctor will watch you carefully to see how well infliximab works for you. If you have rheumatoid arthritis or Crohn's disease, your doctor may increase the amount of medication you receive, if needed. If you have Crohn's disease and your condition has not improved after 14 weeks, your doctor may stop treating you with infliximab. It is important to tell your doctor how you are feeling during your treatment.

Are there other uses for this medicine?

Infliximab is also sometimes used to treat juvenile arthritis (joint pain and swelling that begins in childhood), and Behcet's syndrome (ulcers in the mouth and on the genitals and inflammation of various parts of the body). Talk to your doctor about the possible risks of using this medication for your condition.

This medication may be prescribed for other uses; ask your doctor or pharmacist for more information.

What special precautions should I follow?

Before using infliximab,

- tell your doctor and pharmacist if you are allergic to infliximab, any medications made from murine (mouse) proteins, or any other medications. Ask your doctor or pharmacist if you don't know whether a medication you are allergic to is made from murine proteins.
- tell your doctor and pharmacist what prescription and nonprescription medications, vitamins, nutritional supplements, and herbal products you are taking or plan to take. Be sure to mention the medications listed in the IMPORTANT WARNING section, anakinra (Kineret) and etanercept (Enbrel). Your doctor may need to change the doses of your medications or monitor you carefully for side effects.
- tell your doctor if you have or have ever had congestive heart failure (condition in which the heart cannot pump enough blood to other parts of the body). Your doctor may tell you not to use infliximab.
- tell your doctor if you have ever been treated with phototherapy (a treatment for psoriasis that involves exposing the skin to ultraviolet light) and if you have or have ever had a disease that affects your nervous system, such as multiple sclerosis (MS; loss of coordination, weakness, and numbness due to nerve damage), Guillain-

Barre syndrome (weakness, tingling, and possible paralysis due to sudden nerve damage) or optic neuritis (inflammation of the nerve that sends messages from the eye to the brain); numbness, burning or tingling in any part of your body; seizures; chronic obstructive pulmonary disease (COPD; a group of diseases that affect the lungs and airways); any type of cancer; bleeding problems or diseases that affect your blood; or heart disease.

- tell your doctor if you have or have ever had hepatitis B (a viral liver infection), have been told that you are a carrier (you are not sick, but the virus is still in your blood) of hepatitis B, or have been in close contact with someone who has hepatitis B. If you are a carrier of hepatitis B, your doctor will watch you carefully to be sure you do not develop an active infection while you are taking infliximab.
- tell your doctor if you are pregnant, plan to become pregnant, or are breast-feeding. If you become pregnant while using infliximab, call your doctor. You should not breast-feed while using infliximab.
- if you are having surgery, including dental surgery, tell the doctor or dentist that you are using infliximab.
- do not have any vaccinations without talking to your doctor. Tell your doctor if you have recently received a vaccine. If your child will be using infliximab, be sure that your child has received all the shots that are required for children of his or her age before he or she begins treatment with infliximab.
- if you were treated with infliximab in the past and you are now starting a second course of treatment, you may have a delayed allergic reaction 3-12 days after you receive infliximab. Tell your doctor if you experience any of the following symptoms several days or longer after your treatment: muscle or joint pain; fever; rash; hives; itching; swelling of the hands, face, or lips; difficulty swallowing; sore throat; and headache.

What special dietary instructions should I follow?

Unless your doctor tells you otherwise, continue your normal diet.

What should I do if I forget to take a dose?

If you miss an appointment to receive an infliximab infusion, call your doctor as soon as possible.

What side effects can this medicine cause?

Infliximab may cause side effects. Tell your doctor if any of these symptoms are severe or do not go away:

- stomach pain
- nausea
- heartburn
- headache
- runny nose
- back pain

- white patches in the mouth
- vaginal itching, burning, and pain or other signs of a yeast infection
- flushing

Some side effects can be serious. The following symptoms are uncommon, but if you experience any of them, or those listed in the IMPORTANT WARNING section, call your doctor immediately:

- any type of rash, including a rash on the cheeks or arms that gets worse in the sun
- chest pain
- swelling of the feet, ankles, stomach, or lower legs
- sudden weight gain
- shortness of breath
- blurred vision or vision changes
- weakness in arms or legs
- muscle or joint pain
- numbness or tingling in any part of the body
- seizures
- yellowing of the skin or eyes
- dark colored urine
- loss of appetite
- pain in the upper right part of the stomach
- unusual bruising or bleeding
- blood in stool
- pale skin

Studies have shown that people who use infliximab or similar medications may be more likely to develop lymphoma (cancer that begins in the cells that fight infection) than people who do not take these medications. Patients who have autoimmune diseases are more likely to develop certain types of cancer than people who do not have these conditions. This is especially true if their disease is very active. Using infliximab may increase this risk. People who have COPD may have a higher risk of developing cancer while they are using infliximab than people who do not have this condition. Talk to your doctor about the risk of using infliximab.

Infliximab may cause other side effects. Call your doctor if you have any unusual problems while taking this medication.

If you experience a serious side effect, you or your doctor may send a report to the Food and Drug Administration's (FDA) MedWatch Adverse Event Reporting program online [at http://www.fda.gov/MedWatch/index.html] or by phone [1-800-332-1088].

What storage conditions are needed for this medicine?

Your doctor will store the medication in his or her office.

What should I do in case of overdose?

In case of overdose, call your local poison control center at 1-800-222-1222. If the victim has collapsed or is not breathing, call local emergency services at 911.

What other information should I know?

Be sure to schedule appointments with your doctor well in advance so that you will be able to receive infliximab on schedule and at times that are convenient for you.

Dosage Facts
For Informational Purposes

Caution: Do not change your dose, how often you take your medication, or the length of time you are to take it without first talking to your healthcare provider.

The following dosage information was written using medical language for doctors and other healthcare professionals and is provided here for you to check your dosage. The dosage of this drug may differ for different patients. Therefore, always follow your doctor's instructions or the directions on the label. Contact your healthcare provider or pharmacist if you have any questions about the specific dosage of your medication after reviewing this information.

Pediatric Patients

Crohn's Disease†

IV:
- Children ≥ 6 years of age: 5 mg/kg. Pediatric patients have received 1–3 doses over a 12-week period.

Adult Patients

Crohn's Disease
Management of Moderate or Severe Active Crohn's Disease or Fistulizing Crohn's Disease

IV:
- 5 mg/kg at 0, 2, and 6 weeks (induction regimen), then every 8 weeks (maintenance regimen).
- Consider dose of 10 mg/kg for patients who respond initially but subsequently lose response.
- Patients who do not respond by week 14 are unlikely to respond with continued administration; consider discontinuing the drug.

Rheumatoid Arthritis
Moderate to Severe Active Rheumatoid Arthritis

IV:
- 3 mg/kg at 0, 2, and 6 weeks, then every 8 weeks.
- Increase dosage up to 10 mg/kg and/or administer as often as once every 4 weeks for patients who have an incomplete response to 3 mg/kg; consider that risk of serious infection is increased with higher dosages.

Ankylosing Spondylitis

IV:
- 5 mg/kg at 0, 2, and 6 weeks, then every 6 weeks.

Psoriatic Arthritis

IV:
- 5 mg/kg at 0, 2, and 6 weeks, then every 8 weeks.

Influenza Vaccine, Inactivated

Brand Name: Fluarix®, FluLaval®, Fluvirin®, Fluzone®

Why get vaccinated?

Influenza ("flu") is a contagious disease. It is caused by the influenza virus, which spreads from infected persons to the nose or throat of others. Other illnesses can have the same symptoms and are often mistaken for influenza. But only an illness caused by the influenza virus is really influenza.

Anyone can get influenza, but rates of infection are highest among children. For most people, it lasts only a few days. It can cause: fever, sore throat, chills, fatigue, cough, headache, and muscle aches.

Some people get much sicker. Influenza can lead to pneumonia and can be dangerous for people with heart or breathing conditions. It can cause high fever and seizures in children. On average, 226,000 people are hospitalized every year because of influenza and 36,000 die - mostly elderly.

Influenza vaccine can prevent influenza.

Inactivated Influenza vaccine

There are two types of influenza vaccine:
- An inactivated (killed) vaccine, or "flu shot," is given by injection into the muscle.
- Live, attenuated (weakened) influenza vaccine, called LAIV, is sprayed into the nostrils. This vaccine is described in a separate monograph.

For most people influenza vaccine prevents serious influenza-related illness. But it will not prevent "influenza-like" illnesses caused by other viruses.

Influenza viruses are always changing. Because of this, influenza vaccines are updated every year, and an annual vaccination is recommended. Protection lasts up to a year.

It takes about 2 weeks for protection to develop after the vaccination.

Some inactivated influenza vaccine contains thimerosal, a preservative that contains mercury. Some people believe thimerosal may be related to developmental problems in children. In 2004 the Institute of Medicine published a report concluding that, based on scientific studies, there is no evidence of such a relationship. If you are concerned about thimerosal, ask your doctor about thimerosal-free influenza vaccine.

Who should get inactivated influenza vaccine?

People 6 months of age and older can receive inactivated influenza vaccine. It is recommended for anyone who is at risk of complications from influenza or more likely to require medical care:
- All children from 6 months up to 5 years of age.
- Anyone 50 years of age or older.
- Anyone 6 months to 18 years of age on long-term aspirin treatment (they could develop Reye Syndrome if they got influenza).
- Women who will be pregnant during influenza season.
- Anyone with long-term health problems with heart disease; kidney disease; lung disease; metabolic disease, such as diabetes; asthma; anemia, and other blood disorders.
- Anyone with a weakened immune system due to HIV/AIDS or other diseases affecting the immune system; long-term treatment with drugs such as steroids; cancer treatment with x-rays or drugs.
- Anyone with certain muscle or nerve disorders (such as seizure disorders or severe cerebral palsy) that can lead to breathing or swallowing problems.
- Residents of nursing homes and other chronic-care facilities.

Influenza vaccine is also recommended for anyone who lives with or cares for people at high risk for influenza related complications:
- Health care providers.
- Household contacts and caregivers of children from birth up to 5 years of age.
- Household contacts and caregivers of people 50 years and older, and those with medical conditions that put them at higher risk for severe complications from influenza.

A yearly influenza vaccination should be *considered* for:
- People who provide essential community services.
- People living in dormitories or under other crowded conditions, to prevent outbreaks.
- People at high risk of influenza complications who travel to the Southern hemisphere between April and September, or to the tropics or in organized tourist groups at any time.

Influenza vaccine is also recommended for anyone who wants to reduce the likelihood of becoming ill with influenza or spreading influenza to others.

When should I get influenza vaccine?

Plan to get influenza vaccine in October or November if you can. But getting vaccinated in December, or even later, will still be beneficial in most years. You can get the vaccine as soon as it is available, and for as long as illness is occurring. Influenza illness can occur any time from November through May. Most cases usually occur in January or February.

Most people need one dose of influenza vaccine each year. Children younger than 9 years of age getting influenza vaccine for the first time should get 2 doses. For inactivated vaccine, these doses should be given at least 4 weeks apart.

Influenza vaccine may be given at the same time as other vaccines, including pneumococcal vaccine.

Some people should talk with a doctor before getting influenza vaccine

Some people should not get inactivated influenza vaccine or should wait before getting it.

- Tell your doctor if you have any severe (life-threatening) allergies. Allergic reactions to influenza vaccine are rare. Influenza vaccine virus is grown in eggs. People with a severe egg allergy should not get the vaccine. A severe allergy to any vaccine component is also a reason to not get the vaccine. If you have had a severe reaction after a previous dose of influenza vaccine, tell your doctor.
- Tell your doctor if you ever had Guillain-Barré Syndrome (a severe paralytic illness, also called GBS). You may be able to get the vaccine, but your doctor should help you make the decision.
- People who are moderately or severely ill should usually wait until they recover before getting flu vaccine. If you are ill, talk to your doctor or nurse about whether to reschedule the vaccination. People with a mild illness can usually get the vaccine.

What are the risks from inactivated influenza vaccine?

A vaccine, like any medicine, could possibly cause serious problems, such as severe allergic reactions. The risk of a vaccine causing serious harm, or death, is extremely small.

Serious problems from influenza vaccine are very rare. The viruses in inactivated influenza vaccine have been killed, so you cannot get influenza from the vaccine.

Mild Problems:
- soreness, redness, or swelling where the shot was given
- fever
- aches
- If these problems occur, they usually begin soon after the shot and last 1-2 days.

Severe Problems:
- Life-threatening allergic reactions from vaccines are very rare. If they do occur, it is within a few minutes to a few hours after the shot.
- In 1976, a certain type of influenza (swine flu) vaccine was associated with Guillain-Barré Syndrome (GBS). Since then, flu vaccines have not been clearly linked to GBS. However, if there is a risk of GBS from current

flu vaccines, it would be no more than 1 or 2 cases per million people vaccinated. This is much lower than the risk of severe influenza, which can be prevented by vaccination.

What if there is a severe reaction?
What should I look for?
- Any unusual condition, such as a high fever or behavior changes. Signs of a serious allergic reaction can include difficulty breathing, hoarseness or wheezing, hives, paleness, weakness, a fast heart beat or dizziness.

What should I do?
- Call a doctor, or get the person to a doctor right away.
- Tell your doctor what happened, the date and time it happened, and when the vaccination was given.
- Ask your health care provider to file a Vaccine Adverse Event Reporting System (VAERS) form if you have any reaction to the vaccine. Or call VAERS yourself at 1-800-822-7967, or visit their website at http://vaers.hhs.gov.

The National Vaccine Injury Compensation Program

In the rare event that you or your child has a serious reaction to a vaccine, a federal program has been created to help pay for the care of those who have been harmed.

For details about the National Vaccine Injury Compensation Program, call 1-800-338-2382 or visit the program's website at http://www.hrsa.gov/vaccinecompensation.

How can I learn more?
- Ask your doctor or other health care provider. They can give you the vaccine package insert or suggest other sources of information.
- Call your local or state health department's immunization program.
- Contact the Centers for Disease Control and Prevention (CDC): call 1-800-232-4636 (1-800-CDC-INFO) or visit the National Immunization Program's website at http://www.cdc.gov/vaccines.

Inactivated Influenza Vaccine Information Statement. U.S. Department of Health and Human Services/Centers for Disease Control and Prevention National Immunization Program. 7/16/2007.

Influenza Vaccine, Live Intranasal

Brand Name: FluMist®

Why get vaccinated?

Influenza ("flu") is a contagious disease. It is caused by the influenza virus, which spreads from infected persons to the nose or throat of others. Other illnesses can have the same symptoms and are often mistaken for influenza. But only an illness caused by the influenza virus is really influenza.

Anyone can get influenza, but rates of infection are highest among children. For most people, it lasts only a few days. It can cause: fever, sore throat, chills, fatigue, cough, headache, and muscle aches.

Some people get much sicker. Influenza can lead to pneumonia and can be dangerous for people with heart or breathing conditions. It can cause high fever and seizures in children. On average, 226,000 people are hospitalized every year because of influenza and 36,000 die - mostly elderly.

Influenza vaccine can prevent influenza.

Live, attenuated influenza vaccine (nasal spray)

There are two types of influenza vaccine:

- **Live, attenuated influenza vaccine (LAIV)** contains live but attenuated (weakened) influenza virus. It is sprayed into the nostrils rather than injected into the muscle.
- **Inactivated influenza vaccine**, sometimes called the "flu shot," is given by injection. This vaccine is described in a separate monograph.

For most people influenza vaccine prevents serious influenza-related illness. But it will not prevent "influenza-like" illnesses caused by other viruses.

Influenza viruses are always changing. Because of this, influenza vaccines are updated every year, and an annual vaccination is recommended. Protection lasts up to a year.

It takes about 2 weeks for protection to develop after the vaccination.

LAIV does not contain thimerosal or other preservatives.

Who can get LAIV?

Live, intranasal influenza vaccine is approved for healthy people from 2 through 49 years of age, who are not pregnant. This includes people who can spread influenza to others at high risk, such as:

- Household contacts and out-of-home caregivers of children from birth up to 5 years of age.
- Physicians and nurses, and family members or any one else in close contact with people at risk of serious influenza.

Influenza vaccine should be given to anyone who wants to reduce the likelihood of becoming ill with influenza or spreading influenza to others. LAIV may be considered for:

- People who provide essential community services.
- People living in dormitories or under other crowded conditions, to prevent outbreaks.

Who should *not* get LAIV?

LAIV is not licensed for everyone. The following people should check with their healthcare provider about getting the inactivated vaccine (flu shot).

- Adults 50 years of age and older or children 6 months up to 2 years of age. (Children younger than 6 months cannot get either influenza vaccine.)
- People who have long-term health problems with heart disease; kidney disease; lung disease; metabolic disease, such as diabetes; asthma; anemia, and other blood disorders.
- Anyone with a weakened immune system.
- Children or adolescents on long-term aspirin treatment.
- Pregnant women.
- Anyone with a history of Guillain-Barré syndrome (a severe paralytic illness, also called GBS).

Inactivated influenza vaccine is the preferred vaccine for people (including healthcare workers, and family members) coming in close contact with anyone who has a severely weakened immune system (that is, anyone who requires care in a protected environment).

Some people should talk with a doctor before getting either influenza vaccine:

- Anyone who has ever had a serious allergic reaction to eggs or another vaccine component, or to a previous dose of influenza vaccine.
- People who are moderately or severely ill should usually wait until they recover before getting flu vaccine. If you are ill, talk to your doctor or nurse about whether to reschedule the vaccination. People with a mild illness can usually get the vaccine.

When should I get influenza vaccine?

Plan to get influenza vaccine in October or November if you can. But getting vaccinated in December, or even later, will still be beneficial in most years. You can get the vaccine as soon as it is available, and for as long as illness is occurring. Influenza illness can occur any time from November through May. Most cases usually occur in January or February.

Most people need one dose of influenza vaccine each year. Children younger than 9 years of age getting influenza vaccine for the first time should get 2 doses For LAIV, these doses should be given 6-10 weeks apart.

LAIV may be given at the same time as other vaccines.

What are the risks from LAIV?

A vaccine, like any medicine, could possibly cause serious problems, such as severe allergic reactions. However, the risk of a vaccine causing serious harm, or death, is extremely small. Live influenza vaccine viruses rarely spread from person to person. Even if they do, they are not likely to cause illness. LAIV is made from weakened virus and does not cause influenza. The vaccine *can* cause mild symptoms in people who get it (see below).

Mild Problems (In children and adolescents 2-17 years of age):

- runny nose, nasal congestion or cough
- headache and muscle aches
- fever
- abdominal pain or occasional vomiting or diarrhea

Mild Problems (In adults 18-49 years of age):

- runny nose or nasal congestion
- cough, chills, tiredness/weakness
- sore throat
- headache

These symptoms did not last long and went away on their own. Although they can occur after vaccination, they may not have been caused by the vaccine.

Severe Problems:

- Life-threatening allergic reactions from vaccines are very rare. If they do occur, it is within a few minutes to a few hours after the vaccination.
- If rare reactions occur with any new product, they may not be identified until thousands, or millions, of people have used it. Over six million doses of LAIV have been distributed since it was licensed, and no serious problems have been identified. Like all vaccines, LAIV will continue to be monitored for unusual or severe problems.

What if there is a severe reaction?

What should I look for?

- Any unusual condition, such as a high fever or behavior changes. Signs of a serious allergic reaction can include difficulty breathing, hoarseness or wheezing, hives, paleness, weakness, a fast heart beat or dizziness.

What should I do?

- Call a doctor, or get the person to a doctor right away.
- Tell your doctor what happened, the date and time it happened, and when the vaccination was given.
- Ask your healthcare provider to file a Vaccine Adverse Event Reporting System (VAERS) form if you have any reaction to the vaccine. Or call VAERS yourself at 1-800-822-7967, or visit their website at http://vaers.hhs.gov.

The National Vaccine Injury Compensation Program

In the rare event that you or your child has a serious reaction to a vaccine, a federal program has been created to help pay for the care of those who have been harmed.

For details about the National Vaccine Injury Compensation Program, call 1-800-338-2382 or visit the program's website at http://www.hrsa.gov/vaccinecompensation.

How can I learn more?

- Ask your doctor or other health care provider. They can give you the vaccine package insert or suggest other sources of information.
- Call your local or state health department's immunization program.
- Contact the Centers for Disease Control and Prevention (CDC): call 1-800-232-4636 (1-800-CDC-INFO) or visit the National Immunization Program's website at http://www.cdc.gov/vaccines.

Live Attenuated Influenza Vaccine Information Statement. U.S. Department of Health and Human Services/Centers for Disease Control and Prevention National Immunization Program. 7/16/2007. (Rev 9/19/07)

Insulin Aspart (rDNA Origin) Injection

(in′ su lin as′ part)

Brand Name: NovoLog®

Why is this medicine prescribed?

Insulin aspart is used to treat type 1 diabetes (condition in which the body does not produce insulin and therefore cannot control the amount of sugar in the blood). It is also used to treat people with type 2 diabetes (condition in which the body does not use insulin normally and therefore cannot control the amount of sugar in the blood) who need insulin to control their diabetes. Insulin aspart is a short-acting, man-made version of human insulin. It works by helping move sugar from the blood into other body tissues where it is used for energy. It also stops the liver from producing more sugar.

How should this medicine be used?

Insulin aspart comes as a solution (liquid) to inject subcutaneously (under the skin). It is usually injected immediately before meals (5 to 10 minutes before eating). Insulin aspart can also be infused under the skin using an external insulin pump. Follow the directions on your prescription label carefully, and ask your doctor or pharmacist to explain any part you do not understand. Use insulin aspart injection exactly as directed. Do not use more or less of it or use it more often than prescribed by your doctor.

Because insulin aspart is a short-acting insulin, it may be used as an injection in combination with some other longer-acting insulins. If insulin aspart is mixed with NPH human insulin, insulin aspart should be drawn into the syringe first, and the solution should be injected immediately after mixing. When insulin aspart is used in an insulin pump, it should not be diluted or mixed with any other insulin or solution.

Insulin aspart controls diabetes but does not cure it. Continue to use insulin aspart even if you feel well. Do not stop using insulin aspart without talking to your doctor. Do not switch to another brand or type of insulin or change the dose of any type of insulin you are using without talking to your doctor.

Insulin aspart comes in vials, cartridges that contain medication and are to be placed in dosing pens, and dosing pens that contain cartridges of medication. Be sure you know what type of container your insulin aspart comes in and what other supplies, such as needles, syringes, or pens, you will need to inject your medication.

If your insulin aspart comes in vials, you will need to use syringes to inject your dose. Ask your doctor or pharmacist if you have questions about the type of syringe you should use.

If your insulin aspart comes in cartridges, you will need to buy an insulin pen separately. Check the manufacturer's information for the patient to see what type of pen is right for the cartridge size you are using. Carefully read the instructions that come with your pen, and ask your doctor or pharmacist to show you how to use it. Ask your doctor or pharmacist if you have questions about the type of pen you should use.

If your insulin aspart comes in pens, be sure to read and understand the manufacturer's instructions. Ask your doctor or pharmacist to show you how to use the pen. Follow the directions carefully. Never remove the cartridge from the pen or attempt to add any other type of insulin to the cartridge.

Never reuse needles or syringes and never share needles, syringes, cartridges, or pens. If you are using an insulin pen, always remove the needle right after you inject your dose. Throw away needles and syringes in a puncture-resistant container. Ask your doctor or pharmacist how to dispose of the puncture resistant container.

Always look at your insulin aspart before you inject it. It should be as clear, colorless, and fluid as water. Do not use your insulin aspart if it is colored, cloudy, thickened, or contains solid particles, or if the expiration date on the bottle has passed.

If your insulin aspart comes in vials, follow these steps to prepare your dose:

1. Wash your hands.
2. If you are using a new bottle, flip off the plastic cap, but do not remove the stopper.
3. Wipe the top of the bottle with an alcohol swab.
4. Pull back the plunger of the syringe until the top of the plunger is even with the dose your doctor told you to inject.
5. Push the needle through the rubber stopper on the bottle.
6. Push down on the plunger to inject the air into the bottle.

7. Turn the bottle upside down without removing the syringe.
8. Be sure the tip of the needle is under the liquid in the bottle. Slowly pull back on the plunger until the top of the plunger is even with the dose your doctor told you to inject.
9. While the needle is still in the bottle, check whether there are air bubbles in the syringe. If there are bubbles, hold the syringe upright and tap on it to push the bubbles to the top. Push the plunger up to move the bubbles out of the syringe, and then pull the plunger back down to the correct dose.
10. Remove the needle from the bottle and lay the syringe down so that the needle is not touching anything.

To inject a prepared dose of insulin aspart using a syringe or pen, follow these steps:

1. Use an alcohol pad to wipe the area where you plan to inject your medication.
2. Pinch up a large area of skin, or spread the skin flat with your hands.
3. Insert the needle into your skin. Your doctor will tell you exactly how to do this.
4. If you are using a syringe, push the plunger all the way down. If you are using a pen, follow the manufacturer's instructions for dispensing a dose.
5. Pull the needle out and press down on the spot for several seconds, but do not rub it.

Use a different site for each injection, about 1 inch away from the previous injection but in the same general area (for example, the thigh). Use all available sites in the same general area before switching to a different area (for example, the upper arm). Do not use the same injection site more often than once every month.

If you use insulin aspart in an insulin pump, change the tubing and needle and throw away any solution left in the reservoir at least every 48 hours. You should also change the injection site at least every 48 hours.

Are there other uses for this medicine?

This medication may be prescribed for other uses; ask your doctor or pharmacist for more information.

What special precautions should I follow?

Before using insulin aspart injection,

- tell your doctor and pharmacist if you are allergic to insulin (Humulin, Iletin, Novolin, Velosulin, others) or any other medications.
- tell your doctor and pharmacist what prescription and nonprescription medications, vitamins, nutritional supplements, and herbal products you are taking. Be sure to mention any of the following: angiotensin-converting enzyme (ACE) inhibitors such as benazepril (Lotensin), captopril (Capoten), enalapril (Vasotec), fosinopril (Monopril), lisinopril (Prinivil, Zestril), moexipril (Univasc), perindopril, (Aceon), quinapril (Accupril), ramipril (Altace), and trandolapril (Mavik); beta blockers

such as atenolol (Tenormin), labetalol (Normodyne), metoprolol (Lopressor, Toprol XL), nadolol (Corgard), and propranolol (Inderal); clonidine (Catapres, Catapres-TTS); danazol (Danocrine); disopyramide (Norpace, Norpace CR); diuretics ('water pills'); fenofibrate (Lofibra, TriCor); fluoxetine (Prozac, Sarafem); gemfibrozil (Lopid); guanethidine (Ismelin); hormone replacement therapy; isoniazid (INH, Laniazid, Nydrazid); lithium (Eskalith, Lithobid, Lithotabs); medications for asthma, colds, mental illness, and nausea; monoamine oxidase (MAO) inhibitors, including phenelzine (Nardil) and tranylcypromine (Parnate); niacin (nicotinic acid, Niaspan, Slo-Niacin); oral contraceptives (birth control pills); oral medications for diabetes; oral steroids such as dexamethasone (Decadron, Dexone), methylprednisolone (Medrol), and prednisone (Deltasone); pentamidine (NebuPent, Pentam 300); propoxyphene; reserpine (Serpalan, Serpasil); salicylate pain relievers such as aspirin, choline magnesium trisalicylate (Tricosal, Trilisate), choline salicylate (Arthropan), diflunisal (Dolobid), magnesium salicylate (Doan's, others), and salsalate (Argesic, Disalcid, Salgesic); sulfa antibiotics; and thyroid medications. Your doctor may need to change the doses of your medications or monitor you carefully for side effects.

- tell your doctor if you have or have ever had nerve damage caused by your diabetes or kidney or liver disease.
- tell your doctor if you are pregnant, plan to become pregnant, or are breast-feeding. If you become pregnant while using insulin aspart, call your doctor.

What special dietary instructions should I follow?

Be sure to follow all exercise and dietary recommendations made by your doctor or dietitian. It is important to eat a healthy diet.

Alcohol may cause a decrease in blood sugar. Ask your doctor about the safe use of alcoholic beverages while you are using insulin aspart.

What should I do if I forget to take a dose?

Insulin aspart must be injected shortly before or after a meal. If you remember your dose before or shortly after your meal, inject the missed dose right away. If some time has passed since your meal, call your doctor to find out whether you should inject the missed dose. Do not inject a double dose to make up for a missed one.

What side effects can this medicine cause?

This medication may cause changes in your blood sugar. You should know the symptoms of low and high blood sugar and what to do if you have these symptoms.

You may experience hypoglycemia (low blood sugar) while you are taking this medication. Your doctor will tell you what you should do if you develop hypoglycemia. He or she may tell you to check your blood sugar, eat or drink a food or beverage that contains sugar, such as hard candy or fruit juice, or get medical care. Follow these directions carefully if you have any of the following symptoms of hypoglycemia:

- shakiness
- dizziness or lightheadedness
- sweating
- nervousness or irritability
- sudden changes in behavior or mood
- headache
- numbness or tingling around the mouth
- weakness
- pale skin
- hunger
- clumsy or jerky movements

If hypoglycemia is not treated, severe symptoms may develop. Be sure that your family, friends, and other people who spend time with you know that if you have any of the following symptoms, they should get medical treatment for you immediately.

- confusion
- seizures
- loss of consciousness

Call your doctor immediately if you have any of the following symptoms of hyperglycemia (high blood sugar):

- extreme thirst
- frequent urination
- extreme hunger
- weakness
- blurred vision

If high blood sugar is not treated, a serious, life-threatening condition called diabetic ketoacidosis could develop. Call your doctor immediately if you have any of the these symptoms:

- dry mouth
- upset stomach and vomiting
- shortness of breath
- breath that smells fruity
- decreased consciousness

Insulin aspart injection may cause side effects. Tell your doctor if any of these symptoms are severe or do not go away:

- redness, swelling, or itching at the site of the injection
- changes in the feel of your skin, skin thickening (fat build-up), or a little depression in the skin (fat breakdown)

Some side effects can be serious. The following symptoms are uncommon, but if you experience any of them, call your doctor immediately:

- rash and/or itching over the whole body
- shortness of breath
- wheezing
- dizziness
- blurred vision
- fast heartbeat
- sweating

Insulin aspart may cause other side effects. Call your doctor if you have any unusual problems while taking this medication.

If you experience a serious side effect, you or your doctor may send a report to the Food and Drug Administration's (FDA) MedWatch Adverse Event Reporting program online [at http://www.fda.gov/MedWatch/index.html] or by phone [1-800-332-1088].

What storage conditions are needed for this medicine?

Store unopened insulin aspart vials, cartridges, and pens in the refrigerator. Do not freeze. Unopened refrigerated insulin aspart can be stored until the date shown on the company's label.

If no refrigerator is available (for example, when on vacation), store the vials or cartridges at room temperature and away from direct sunlight and extreme heat. Unrefrigerated vials, cartridges, and pens can be used within 28 days or they must be thrown away. Opened vials can be stored for 28 days at room temperature or in the refrigerator. Opened cartridges and pens may be stored at room temperature for up to 28 days; do not refrigerate them. Throw away any insulin aspart that has been exposed to extreme heat or cold.

Throw away any medication that is outdated or no longer needed. Talk to your pharmacist about the proper disposal of your medication.

What should I do in case of overdose?

In case of overdose, call your local poison control center at 1-800-222-1222. If the victim has collapsed or is not breathing, call local emergency services at 911.

Symptoms of overdose may include the symptoms of hypoglycemia listed above and the following:

- loss of consciousness
- confusion

What other information should I know?

Keep all appointments with your doctor and the laboratory. Your blood sugar and glycosylated hemoglobin (HbA1c) should be checked regularly to determine your response to insulin aspart. Your doctor will also tell you how to check your response to this medication by measuring your blood or urine sugar levels at home. Follow these instructions carefully.

Your dose of insulin aspart may need to be changed when you are ill (especially with fever, vomiting, or diarrhea), have emotional changes or stress, gain or lose weight, or change the amount of food you eat or amount of exercise you do. If any of these things happen, call your doctor.

See your dentist twice yearly; see your eye doctor regularly; get your blood pressure checked regularly.

If you travel across time zones, ask your doctor how to time your injections. When you travel, take extra insulin and supplies with you.

Keep yourself and your clothes clean. Wash cuts, scrapes, and other wounds quickly, and do not let them get infected. Wear medical alert identification (a bracelet or tag) that says you have diabetes.

Do not let anyone else use your medication. Ask your pharmacist any questions you have about refilling your prescription.

Dosage Facts
For Informational Purposes

Caution: Do not change your dose, how often you take your medication, or the length of time you are to take it without first talking to your healthcare provider.

The following dosage information was written using medical language for doctors and other healthcare professionals and is provided here for you to check your dosage. The dosage of this drug may differ for different patients. Therefore, always follow your doctor's instructions or the directions on the label. Contact your healthcare provider or pharmacist if you have any questions about the specific dosage of your medication after reviewing this information.

General Dosage Information

Patients previously receiving insulin may require a change in dosage if insulin therapy is changed to insulin aspart.

Adult Patients

Diabetes Mellitus

SUB-Q INJECTION:
- Individualize dosage; adjust dosage regularly based on blood glucose determinations.
- Usually, the total daily insulin requirement is 0.5–1 unit/kg. When used in a preprandial sub-Q injection treatment regimen, 50–70% of total insulin requirements may be provided by insulin aspart, with the remainder provided by an intermediate-acting or long-acting insulin.

SUB-Q INFUSION:
- Individualize dosage; adjust dosage regularly based on blood glucose determinations. Glucose monitoring is particularly important for patients receiving insulin via an external infusion pump.
- When used in external infusion pumps, initial programming of the pump is based on total daily insulin dosage previously used.
- Although there is substantial interpatient variability, preprandial administration of insulin aspart injection comprises approximately 50% of the total daily insulin dosage, with the remainder given as a basal infusion.
- Some patients may require more basal insulin and a greater total daily insulin dosage to prevent preprandial hyperglycemia when using insulin aspart than when using insulin human (regular).

SUB-Q INJECTION:

- Individualize dosage; adjust dosage regularly based on blood glucose determinations.
- When the fixed combination is used as monotherapy, initially, 0.4–0.6 units/kg daily given in 2 divided doses (before the morning and evening meal) has been recommended. Titrate subsequent dosage in increments of 2–4 units every 3–4 days to achieve the target fasting plasma glucose concentration.
- When used in combination with oral antidiabetic agents, initially, 0.2–0.3 unit/kg daily has been recommended. Titrate subsequent dosage to target glycemic goals.
- When used to replace isophane insulin alone or a biphasic insulin product (e.g., premixed isophane and regular insulin) in patients with adequate glycemic control, initial dosage of fixed-combination insulin aspart/insulin aspart protamine should be identical to previous insulin dosage, with subsequent dosage adjustment as required.
- Patients inadequately controlled on previous therapy with isophane insulin may require increases of 10–20% in the dosage of fixed-combination insulin aspart/insulin aspart protamine during the first week.
- In patients transferring from a multiple-daily-dose regimen consisting of an intermediate-acting (e.g., isophane) insulin and a rapid- or short-acting insulin at mealtimes, the initial dosage of the insulin aspart protamine component of the fixed combination should be same as the dosage of the previously used intermediate-acting insulin.

Special Populations

Hepatic Impairment

- Insulin aspart and/or insulin aspart protamine requirements may be reduced. Careful monitoring of blood glucose and adjustment of dosage may be necessary.

Renal Impairment

- Insulin aspart and/or insulin aspart protamine requirements may be reduced. Careful monitoring of blood glucose and adjustment of dosage may be necessary.

Geriatric Patients

- Careful dosage selection recommended due to possible age-related decrease in hepatic, renal, and/or cardiac function and concomitant disease and drug therapy. Initiate dosage at lower end of the usual range.

Insulin Detemir (rDNA Origin) Injection

(in′ su lin de′ te mir)

Brand Name: Levemir®

Why is this medicine prescribed?

Insulin detemir is used to treat type 1 diabetes (condition in which the body does not produce insulin and therefore cannot control the amount of sugar in the blood). It is also used to treat people with type 2 diabetes (condition in which the body does not use insulin normally and, therefore, cannot control the amount of sugar in the blood) who need insulin to control their diabetes. Insulin detemir is a long-acting, man-made version of human insulin. It works by helping move sugar from the blood into other body tissues where it is used for energy. It also stops the liver from producing more sugar.

How should this medicine be used?

Insulin detemir comes as a solution (liquid) to inject subcutaneously (under the skin). It is usually injected once a day, with the evening meal or at bedtime, or twice a day, in the morning and in the evening with the evening meal or at bedtime. Inject insulin detemir at around the same time(s) every day. Follow the directions on your prescription label carefully, and ask your doctor or pharmacist to explain any part you do not understand. Use insulin detemir exactly as directed. Do not use more or less of it or use it more often than prescribed by your doctor.

Insulin detemir should not be used in insulin infusion pumps.

Insulin detemir should not be mixed or diluted with other insulin products.

Insulin detemir controls diabetes but does not cure it. Continue to use insulin detemir even if you feel well. Do not stop using insulin detemir without talking to your doctor. Do not switch to another brand or type of insulin or change the dose of any type of insulin you are using without talking to your doctor.

Insulin detemir comes in vials, cartridges that contain medication and are to be placed in dosing pens, and dosing pens that contain cartridges of medication. Be sure you know what type of container your insulin detemir comes in and what other supplies, such as needles, syringes, or pens, you will need to inject your medication.

If your insulin detemir comes in vials, you will need to use syringes to inject your dose. Ask your doctor or pharmacist if you have questions about the type of syringe you should use.

If your insulin detemir comes in cartridges, you will need to buy an insulin pen separately. Check the manufacturer's information for the patient to see what type of pen is right for the cartridge size you are using. Carefully read the instructions that come with your pen, and ask your doctor or pharmacist to show you how to use it. Ask your doctor or pharmacist if you have questions about the type of pen you should use.

If your insulin detemir comes in pens, be sure to read and understand the manufacturer's instructions. Ask your doctor or pharmacist to show you how to use the pen. Follow the directions carefully. Never remove the cartridge from the pen or attempt to add any other type of insulin to the cartridge.

Never reuse needles or syringes and never share needles, syringes, cartridges, or pens. If you are using an insulin pen, always remove the needle right after you inject your dose. Throw away needles and syringes in a puncture-resistant container. Ask your doctor or pharmacist how to dispose of the puncture resistant container.

Always look at your insulin detemir before you inject it. It should be as clear, colorless, and fluid as water. Do not use your insulin detemir if it is colored, cloudy, thickened, or contains solid particles, or if the expiration date on the bottle has passed.

If your insulin detemir comes in vials, follow these steps to prepare your dose:

1. Wash your hands.
2. If you are using a new bottle, flip off the plastic cap, but do not remove the stopper.
3. Wipe the top of the bottle with an alcohol swab.
4. Pull back the plunger of the syringe until the top of the plunger is even with the dose your doctor told you to inject.
5. Push the needle through the rubber stopper on the bottle.
6. Push down on the plunger to inject the air into the bottle.
7. Turn the bottle upside down without removing the syringe.
8. Be sure the tip of the needle is under the liquid in the bottle. Slowly pull back on the plunger until the top of the plunger is even with the dose your doctor told you to inject.
9. While the needle is still in the bottle, check whether there are air bubbles in the syringe. If there are bubbles, hold the syringe upright and tap on it to push the bubbles to the top. Push the plunger up to move the bubbles out of the syringe, and then pull the plunger back down to the correct dose.
10. Remove the needle from the bottle and lay the syringe down so that the needle is not touching anything.

To inject a prepared dose of insulin detemir using a syringe or pen, follow these steps:

1. Use an alcohol pad to wipe the area where you plan to inject your medication.
2. Pinch up a large area of skin, or spread the skin flat with your hands.
3. Insert the needle into your skin. Your doctor will tell you exactly how to do this.
4. If you are using a syringe, push the plunger all the way down. If you are using a pen, follow the manufacturer's instructions for dispensing a dose.
5. Pull the needle out and press down on the spot for several seconds, but do not rub it.

Use a different site for each injection, about 1 inch away from the previous injection but in the same general area (for example, the thigh). Use all available sites in the same general area before switching to a different area (for example, the upper arm). Do not use the same injection site more often than once every month.

Are there other uses for this medicine?

This medication may be prescribed for other uses; ask your doctor or pharmacist for more information.

What special precautions should I follow?

Before using insulin detemir,

- tell your doctor and pharmacist if you are allergic to insulin (Humulin, Iletin, Novolin, Velosulin, others) or any other medications.
- tell your doctor and pharmacist what prescription and nonprescription medications, vitamins, nutritional supplements, and herbal products you are taking. Be sure to mention any of the following: angiotensin-converting enzyme (ACE) inhibitors such as benazepril (Lotensin), captopril (Capoten), enalapril (Vasotec), fosinopril (Monopril), lisinopril (Prinivil, Zestril), moexipril (Univasc), perindopril, (Aceon), quinapril (Accupril), ramipril (Altace), and trandolapril (Mavik); antihistamines; beta blockers such as atenolol (Tenormin), labetalol (Normodyne), metoprolol (Lopressor, Toprol XL), nadolol (Corgard), and propranolol (Inderal); clonidine (Catapres, Catapres-TTS); danazol (Danocrine); disopyramide (Norpace, Norpace CR); diuretics ('water pills'); fenofibrate (Lofibra, TriCor); fluoxetine (Prozac, Sarafem); gemfibrozil (Lopid); guanethidine (Ismelin); hormone replacement therapy; isoniazid (INH, Laniazid, Nydrazid); lithium (Eskalith, Lithobid, Lithotabs); medications for asthma, colds, mental illness, and nausea; monoamine oxidase (MAO) inhibitors, including isocarboxazid (Marplan), phenelzine (Nardil), selegiline (Eldepryl), and tranylcypromine (Parnate); oral contraceptives (birth control pills); oral medications for diabetes; oral steroids such as dexamethasone (Decadron, Dexone), methylprednisolone (Medrol), and prednisone (Deltasone); pentamidine (NebuPent, Pentam 300); propoxyphene (Darvon); reserpine (Serpalan, Serpasil); salicylate pain relievers such as aspirin, choline magnesium trisalicylate (Tricosal, Trilisate), choline salicylate (Arthropan), diflunisal (Dolobid), magnesium salicylate (Doan's, others), and salsalate (Argesic, Disalcid, Salgesic); sulfa antibiotics; and thyroid medications. Your doctor may need to change the doses of your medications or monitor you carefully for side effects.
- tell your doctor if you have or have ever had nerve damage caused by your diabetes or kidney or liver disease.
- tell your doctor if you are pregnant, plan to become pregnant, or are breast-feeding. If you become pregnant while using insulin detemir, call your doctor.
- if you are having surgery, including dental surgery, tell the doctor or dentist that you are using insulin detemir.
- ask your doctor what to do if you get sick, experience unusual stress, plan to travel across more than two time zones, or change your exercise or activity schedule. These changes can affect your dosing schedule and the amount of insulin you will need.

What special dietary instructions should I follow?

Be sure to follow all exercise and dietary recommendations made by your doctor or dietitian. It is important to eat a healthy diet.

Alcohol may cause a decrease in blood sugar. Ask your doctor about the safe use of alcoholic beverages while you are using insulin detemir.

What should I do if I forget to take a dose?

If you remember your dose shortly after the time you were supposed to take it, inject the missed dose as soon as you remember it. If some time has passed since your regular dosing time, call your doctor to find out whether you should inject the missed dose. Do not inject a double dose to make up for a missed one.

What side effects can this medicine cause?

This medication may cause changes in your blood sugar. You should know the symptoms of low and high blood sugar and what to do if you have these symptoms.

You may experience hypoglycemia (low blood sugar) while you are taking this medication. Your doctor will tell you what you should do if you develop hypoglycemia. He or she may tell you to check your blood sugar, eat or drink a food or beverage that contains sugar, such as hard candy or fruit juice, or get medical care. Follow these directions carefully if you have any of the following symptoms of hypoglycemia:

- shakiness
- dizziness or lightheadedness
- sweating
- nervousness or irritability
- sudden changes in behavior or mood
- headache
- numbness or tingling around the mouth
- weakness
- pale skin
- hunger
- clumsy or jerky movements

If hypoglycemia is not treated, severe symptoms may develop. Be sure that your family, friends, and other people who spend time with you know that if you have any of the following symptoms, they should get medical treatment for you immediately.

- confusion
- seizures
- loss of consciousness

Call your doctor immediately if you have any of the following symptoms of hyperglycemia (high blood sugar):

- extreme thirst
- frequent urination
- extreme hunger
- weakness
- blurred vision

If high blood sugar is not treated, a serious, life-threatening condition called diabetic ketoacidosis could develop. Call your doctor immediately if you have any of the these symptoms:

- dry mouth
- upset stomach and vomiting

- shortness of breath
- breath that smells fruity
- decreased consciousness

Insulin detemir injection may cause side effects. Tell your doctor if any of these symptoms are severe or do not go away:

- redness, swelling, or itching at the site of the injection
- changes in the feel of your skin, skin thickening (fat build-up), or a little depression in the skin (fat breakdown)

Some side effects can be serious. The following symptoms are uncommon, but if you experience any of them, call your doctor immediately:

- rash and/or itching over the whole body
- shortness of breath
- wheezing
- dizziness
- blurred vision
- fast heartbeat
- sweating
- swelling of the hands, feet, ankles, or lower legs

Insulin detemir may cause other side effects. Call your doctor if you have any unusual problems while taking this medication.

What storage conditions are needed for this medicine?

Store unopened insulin detemir vials, cartridges, and pens in the refrigerator. Do not freeze. Do not use insulin detemir if it has been frozen. Unopened refrigerated insulin detemir can be stored until the date shown on the company's label.

If no refrigerator is available (for example, when on vacation), store the vials or cartridges at room temperature and away from direct sunlight and extreme heat. Unrefrigerated vials, cartridges, and pens can be used within 42 days or they must be thrown away. Opened vials can be stored for 42 days at room temperature or in the refrigerator. Opened cartridges and pens may be stored at room temperature for up to 42 days; do not refrigerate them. Throw away any insulin detemir that has been exposed to extreme heat or cold.

When traveling, protect your insulin detemir vials, cartridges, and pens from bumps or other rough handling (wrap them in clothes in the middle of a suitcase). Do not keep insulin in hot areas of a car such as the glove compartment or trunk. When traveling by airplane, do not put insulin in checked luggage since the luggage may be lost. Always keep insulin with you or in carry-on luggage.

Throw away any medication that is outdated or no longer needed. Talk to your pharmacist about the proper disposal of your medication.

What should I do in case of overdose?

In case of overdose, call your local poison control center at 1-800-222-1222. If the victim has collapsed or is not breathing, call local emergency services at 911.

Symptoms of overdose may include the symptoms of hypoglycemia listed above and the following:

- seizure
- loss of consciousness
- confusion

What other information should I know?

Keep all appointments with your doctor and the laboratory. Your blood sugar and glycosylated hemoglobin (HbA1c) should be checked regularly to determine your response to insulin detemir. Your doctor will also tell you how to check your response to insulin by measuring your blood or urine sugar levels at home. Follow these instructions carefully.

You should always wear a diabetic identification bracelet to be sure you get proper treatment in an emergency.

Do not let anyone else use your medication. Ask your pharmacist any questions you have about refilling your prescription.

Dosage Facts
For Informational Purposes

Caution: Do not change your dose, how often you take your medication, or the length of time you are to take it without first talking to your healthcare provider.

The following dosage information was written using medical language for doctors and other healthcare professionals and is provided here for you to check your dosage. The dosage of this drug may differ for different patients. Therefore, always follow your doctor's instructions or the directions on the label. Contact your healthcare provider or pharmacist if you have any questions about the specific dosage of your medication after reviewing this information.

Pediatric Patients
Diabetes Mellitus

SUB-Q:
- Individualize dosage based on blood glucose determinations.
- When substituted for another intermediate- or long-acting insulin in patients with type 1 diabetes mellitus receiving combination therapy with a short- or rapid-acting insulin and a longer-acting insulin, initial dosage can be identical (on a unit-for-unit basis) to the dosage of the previous longer-acting insulin. Adjust subsequent dosage to achieve glycemic goals.
- In patients with type 1 diabetes mellitus currently receiving a basal insulin only, substitute insulin detemir on a unit-for-unit basis for the basal insulin currently in use.
- Closely monitor blood glucose concentrations during the transition and in the initial weeks thereafter. May need to adjust dosage and timing of the concurrent short- or rapid-acting insulin.

Adult Patients
Diabetes Mellitus

SUB-Q:
- Individualize dosage based on blood glucose determinations.
- In insulin-naive patients with type 2 diabetes mellitus who

are inadequately controlled on oral antidiabetic agents, recommended initial dosage is 0.1–0.2 units/kg given once daily in the evening or 10 units given once or twice daily; adjust subsequent dosage to achieve glycemic goals.
- When substituted for another intermediate- or long-acting insulin in patients with type 1 or 2 diabetes mellitus receiving combination therapy with a short- or rapid-acting insulin and a longer-acting insulin, initial dosage can be identical (on a unit-for-unit basis) to the dosage of the previous longer-acting insulin. Adjust subsequent dosage to achieve glycemic goals.
- Some patients with type 2 diabetes mellitus who are switched from isophane insulin human to insulin detemir may require an insulin detemir dosage that is higher than their previous dosage of isophane insulin human (0.77 versus 0.52 units/kg daily [in conjunction with one or more oral antidiabetic agents] in one study).
- In patients currently receiving a basal insulin only, substitute insulin detemir on a unit-for-unit basis for the basal insulin currently in use.
- Closely monitor blood glucose concentrations during the transition and in the initial weeks thereafter. May need to adjust dosage and timing of the concurrent short- or rapid-acting insulin or other concomitant antidiabetic agents.

Insulin Glargine (rDNA origin) Injection

(in′ su lin glar′ geen)

Brand Name: Lantus®

Why is this medicine prescribed?

Insulin glargine is used to treat type 1 diabetes (condition in which the body does not produce insulin and therefore cannot control the amount of sugar in the blood). It is also used to treat people with type 2 diabetes (condition in which the body does not use insulin normally and, therefore, cannot control the amount of sugar in the blood) who need long-acting insulin to control their diabetes. Insulin glargine is a long-acting, man-made version of human insulin. Insulin is a hormone made in the pancreas. Insulin helps move sugar from the blood into other body tissues where it is used for energy. It also helps the body break down carbohydrates, fats, and proteins from the diet. In a person with diabetes, the pancreas does not produce enough insulin for the body's needs, so additional insulin is required. People with diabetes may gradually develop serious nerve, blood vessel, kidney, and eye problems if the diabetes is not controlled properly.

This medication is sometimes prescribed for other uses; ask your doctor or pharmacist for more information.

How should this medicine be used?

Insulin glargine comes as an injection to inject subcutaneously (beneath the skin, not into a vein). It is injected once a day at bedtime. The medication comes in vials (bottles) and also prefilled containers called cartridges. The amount of insulin glargine you need depends on diet, other diseases, exercise, and other drugs you are taking and may change with time. Your doctor will tell you how much you should take. Follow the directions on your prescription label carefully, and ask your doctor or pharmacist to explain any part you do not understand. Take insulin glargine exactly as directed. Do not take more or less of it or take it more often than directed by the package label or prescribed by your doctor.

Insulin glargine controls diabetes but does not cure it. It must be taken regularly. Continue to take insulin glargine even if you feel well. Do not stop taking insulin glargine without talking to your doctor.

You do not have to shake the vial or cartridge of insulin glargine before use. Do not dilute or mix insulin glargine with any other insulin or solution. The syringe must not have any other medicine or residue in it.

If your insulin glargine comes in cartridges, the medication will already be inside. You must only use the OptiPen One Insulin Delivery Device with the cartridges. Before you use the device for the first time, read the written directions that come with it. Ask your doctor, pharmacist, or nurse to show you the right way to use this device. Practice while your health care provider watches.

If your insulin glargine comes in vials, you will have to withdraw (draw up) the medication into a syringe. Before you do this for the first time, read the written directions that come with it. Ask your doctor or pharmacist to show you the right way to withdraw the insulin glargine and to inject the medication subcutaneously. Practice while your health care provider watches.

If your insulin glargine comes in vials you will need to use syringes. Always use a syringe that is marked for U-100 insulin products. If you use the wrong syringe, you may get the wrong dose, and your blood glucose level may end up being too low or too high.

Plastic syringes are disposable; use a new one for each injection. Used needles will hurt more and may cause an infection. Never share needles and syringes. To withdraw insulin glargine into the syringe, follow these steps:

1. Wash your hands.
2. Hold the vial in your hands to warm the medicine. Look at the medicine in the vial. Make sure it is clear and colorless. If it is cloudy or has particles (specks) in it, throw the vial away and get a new one.
3. If you are using a new vial, remove the protective cap. Do not remove the stopper (the rubber inside the cap).
4. Wipe the top of the vial with an alcohol swab or cotton dipped in rubbing alcohol.
5. It is easier to withdraw insulin glargine if you first inject air into the vial. To do this, pull the plunger (the cylinder inside the syringe) back to the number of insulin glargine units you will have to take. Now your syringe is filled with the right amount of air. Insert the needle

through the rubber cap and push on the plunger to inject the air into the vial.
6. Keep the syringe in the vial and turn both upside down. Hold the syringe and vial firmly with one hand.
7. Make sure the tip of the needle is in the insulin. With your free hand, pull back on the plunger to withdraw insulin glargine into the syringe, and measure the correct number of units of insulin glargine.
8. Before you take the needle out of the vial, be sure that there are no bubbles in the syringe. If there are bubbles in the syringe, hold the syringe straight up and tap the side of the syringe until the bubbles float to the top. Push the bubbles out with the plunger and draw insulin glargine back in until you have the correct dose.
9. Remove the needle from the vial. Do not let the needle touch anything. You are now ready to inject.
10. If you have trouble seeing the small markings on the syringe, have someone help you. Also, let your doctor and pharmacist know about this problem. They can provide syringes that are easier to read, special tools to help you fill the syringe, or prefilled syringes.

To inject your insulin glargine dose, follow these steps:
1. Decide on an injection area—either your abdomen, buttocks, thighs, or arms.
2. Clean the skin at the injection site with an alcohol pad or cotton dipped in rubbing alcohol.
3. Pinch a fold of skin with your fingers at least 3 inches apart and insert the needle at a 45- to 90-degree angle.
4. Then slowly push the plunger of the syringe all the way, making sure you have injected all the insulin glargine. Leave the needle in the skin for several seconds.
5. Pull the needle straight out and press lightly on the spot where you injected yourself for several seconds. Do not rub the area.
6. Follow the directions given to you for throwing away the needle and syringe.

Use a different site for each injection, about 1 inch away from the previous injection but in the same general area (for example, the thigh). Use all available sites in the same general area before switching to a different area (for example, the upper arm). Do not use the same injection site more often than once every month.

What special precautions should I follow?

Before taking insulin glargine,
- tell your doctor and pharmacist if you are allergic to insulin or any other drugs.
- tell your doctor and pharmacist what prescription and nonprescription medications you are taking, especially acetazolamide (Diamox); AIDS antiviral medications; albuterol (Proventil, Ventolin); allergy or cold medications; angiotensin-converting enzyme inhibitors (ACE inhibitors) such as captopril (Capoten), enalapril (Vasotec), or lisinopril (Prinivil, Zestril); antibiotics; antipsychotics such as fluphenazine (Prolixin), mesoridazine (Serentil), or thioridazine (Mellaril); beta-blockers such

as propranolol (Inderal); calcitonin (Calcimar); chloroquine (Aralen); chlorpromazine (Thorazine); clofibrate (Atromid-S); clonidine (Catapres); corticosteroids such as dexamethasone (Decadron), methylprednisolone (Medrol), or prednisone (Deltasone, Orasone); danazol (Danocrine); disopyramide (Norpace); diuretics ('water pills'); epinephrine; estrogens; fenofibrate (TriCor); fluoxetine (Prozac, Sarafem); gemfibrozil (Lopid); guanethidine (Ismelin); isoniazid (INH); lithium (Eskalith, Lithobid); mebendazole (Vermox); medications that contain alcohol or sugar; morphine (MS Contin, others); niacin; nicotine; octreotide (Sandostatin); oral contraceptives (birth control pills); oral medications for diabetes; pentamidine (Pentam); phenelzine (Nardil); phenytoin (Dilantin); prochlorperazine (Compazine); promethazine (Phenergan); propoxyphene (Darvon); reserpine (Serpalan, others); salicylates such as aspirin, diflunisal (Dolobid), or salsalate (Disalcid); somatropin (human growth hormone); sulfa drugs; sulfinpyrazone (Anturane); terbutaline (Brethine, Bricanyl); thyroid medications; tranylcypromine (Parnate); trimeprazine (Temaril); and vitamins or herbal products.

- tell your doctor if you have or have ever had thyroid, liver, or kidney disease.
- tell your doctor if you are pregnant, plan to become pregnant, or are breast-feeding. If you become pregnant while taking insulin glargine, call your doctor.
- if you are having surgery, including dental surgery, tell the doctor or dentist that you are taking insulin glargine.
- tell your doctor if you have fever, infection, injury, or illness with vomiting or diarrhea. These may affect your blood sugar level.

What special dietary instructions should I follow?

Be sure to follow all exercise and dietary recommendations made by your doctor or dietitian. It is important to eat a healthful diet. Do not start a diet or an exercise program without talking to your doctor. Your insulin dose may need to be changed.

Alcohol may cause a decrease in blood sugar. Ask your doctor about the safe use of alcoholic beverages while you are using insulin glargine.

What should I do if I forget to take a dose?

Before you start taking insulin glargine, ask your doctor what to do if you forget to take a dose or if you accidentally take an extra dose. Write these directions down so you can refer to them later.

What side effects can this medicine cause?

This medication may cause changes in your blood sugar. You should know the symptoms of low and high blood sugar and what to do if you have these symptoms.

You may experience hypoglycemia (low blood sugar) while you are taking this medication. Your doctor will tell

you what you should do if you develop hypoglycemia. He or she may tell you to check your blood sugar, eat or drink a food or beverage that contains sugar, such as hard candy or fruit juice, or get medical care. Follow these directions carefully if you have any of the following symptoms of hypoglycemia:

- shakiness
- dizziness or lightheadedness
- sweating
- nervousness or irritability
- sudden changes in behavior or mood
- headache
- numbness or tingling around the mouth
- weakness
- pale skin
- hunger
- clumsy or jerky movements

If hypoglycemia is not treated, severe symptoms may develop. Be sure that your family, friends, and other people who spend time with you know that if you have any of the following symptoms, they should get medical treatment for you immediately.

- confusion
- seizures
- loss of consciousness

Call your doctor immediately if you have any of the following symptoms of hyperglycemia (high blood sugar):

- extreme thirst
- frequent urination
- extreme hunger
- weakness
- blurred vision

If high blood sugar is not treated, a serious, life-threatening condition called diabetic ketoacidosis could develop. Call your doctor immediately if you have any of the these symptoms:

- dry mouth
- upset stomach and vomiting
- shortness of breath
- breath that smells fruity
- decreased consciousness

Insulin glargine can cause side effects. Tell your doctor if any of these symptoms are severe or do not go away:

- redness, swelling, pain, and itching at the injection site
- changes in the feel of your skin, skin thickening (fat build-up), or a little depression in the skin (fat breakdown)

If you experience any of the following symptoms, call your doctor immediately:

- exaggerated sunburn
- difficulty speaking or moving
- skin rash or hives all over the body
- itching or redness
- swelling of hands or feet
- difficulty swallowing
- wheezing (trouble breathing)

- fast pulse
- low blood pressure

What storage conditions are needed for this medicine?

Store unopened insulin glargine vials and cartridges in the refrigerator. Never allow insulin glargine to freeze; do not use insulin glargine that has been frozen and thawed. Never heat insulin glargine to warm it. Unopened refrigerated insulin glargine can be stored until the date shown on the company's label.

If no refrigerator is available (for example, when on vacation), store the vials or cartridges at room temperature and away from direct sunlight and extreme heat. Unrefrigerated 10-mL vials or cartridges can be used within 28 days or they must be thrown away. Unrefrigerated 5-mL vials can be used for 14 days or they must be thrown away. Refrigerated 5-mL vials can be used for up to 28 days. Once the cartridge is placed in the OptiPen One Insulin Delivery Device, do not refrigerate. Throw away any insulin that has been exposed to extreme heat or cold.

Throw away any medication that is outdated or no longer needed. Talk to your pharmacist about the proper disposal of your medication.

What should I do in case of overdose?

In case of overdose, call your local poison control center at 1-800-222-1222. If the victim has collapsed or is not breathing, call local emergency services at 911.

What other information should I know?

Keep all appointments with your doctor and the laboratory. Your blood sugar and glycosylated hemoglobin (HbA1c) should be checked regularly to determine your response to insulin glargine. Your doctor will also tell you how to check your response to this medication by measuring your blood or urine sugar levels at home. Follow these instructions carefully.

Your dose of insulin glargine may need to be changed when you are ill (especially with fever, vomiting, or diarrhea), have emotional changes or stress, gain or lose weight, or change the amount of food you eat or amount of exercise you do. If any of these things happen, call your doctor.

See your dentist twice yearly; see your eye doctor regularly; get your blood pressure checked regularly.

If you travel across time zones, ask your doctor how to time your injections. When you travel, take extra insulin and supplies with you.

Keep yourself and your clothes clean. Wash cuts, scrapes, and other wounds quickly, and do not let them get infected. Wear medical alert identification (a bracelet or tag) that says you have diabetes.

Do not let anyone else take your medication. Ask your pharmacist any questions you have about refilling your prescription.

Dosage Facts
For Informational Purposes

Caution: Do not change your dose, how often you take your medication, or the length of time you are to take it without first talking to your healthcare provider.

The following dosage information was written using medical language for doctors and other healthcare professionals and is provided here for you to check your dosage. The dosage of this drug may differ for different patients. Therefore, always follow your doctor's instructions or the directions on the label. Contact your healthcare provider or pharmacist if you have any questions about the specific dosage of your medication after reviewing this information.

Pediatric Patients

Diabetes Mellitus

SUB-Q:
- Individualize dosage.
- In children ≥6 years of age with type 1 diabetes mellitus, recommendations for changing from another insulin to insulin glargine are the same as for adults.

Adult Patients

Diabetes Mellitus

SUB-Q:
- Individualize dosage.
- In a clinical study in patients with type 2 diabetes mellitus, the initial dosage of insulin glargine in insulin-naive patients receiving oral antidiabetic agents was 10 units once daily, with subsequent dosage adjustments based on blood glucose concentrations; total daily dosages ranged from 2–100 units.
- When patients were transferred from once-daily isophane insulin human or extended insulin human zinc to insulin glargine in clinical studies, the initial dosage generally was the same.
- When patients are transferred from twice-daily isophane insulin to insulin glargine once daily, the manufacturer recommends that the initial dosage be reduced by approximately 20% for the first week to reduce the risk of hypoglycemia; dosage should then be adjusted on the basis of blood glucose concentrations.

Special Populations

Hepatic Impairment
- Insulin glargine requirements may be reduced. Careful monitoring of blood glucose and adjustment of dosage may be necessary.

Renal Impairment
- Insulin glargine requirements may be reduced. Careful monitoring of blood glucose and adjustment of dosage may be necessary.

Geriatric Patients
- Conservative initial dosage, dose increments, and maintenance dosage recommended to avoid hypoglycemia.

Insulin Glulisine (rDNA origin) Injection

(in′ su lin gloo′ lis een)

Brand Name: Apidra®

Why is this medicine prescribed?

Insulin glulisine is used to treat type 1 diabetes (condition in which the body does not make insulin and therefore cannot control the amount of sugar in the blood). It is also used to treat people with type 2 diabetes (condition in which the blood sugar is too high because the body does not produce or use insulin normally) who need insulin to control their diabetes. Insulin glulisine is a man-made version of human insulin that begins working quickly and continues to work for a short time to control increases in blood sugar that may occur after meals. It is used together with a longer-acting insulin or an insulin pump (a device that delivers insulin to the body at all times through a small tube that is inserted under the skin) to control blood sugar. Insulin glulisine works by helping move sugar from the blood into other body tissues where it is used for energy. It also stops the liver from producing more sugar.

How should this medicine be used?

Insulin glulisine comes as a solution (liquid) to inject subcutaneously (under the skin). It is usually injected up to 15 minutes before a meal or within 20 minutes after starting a meal. Insulin glulisine can also be infused under the skin using an external insulin pump. Follow the directions on your prescription label carefully, and ask your doctor or pharmacist to explain any part you do not understand. Use insulin glulisine exactly as directed. Do not use more or less of it or use it more often than prescribed by your doctor.

Never use insulin glulisine when you have symptoms of hypoglycemia (low blood sugar) or if you have checked your blood sugar and found it to be low. Call your doctor in these cases.

Insulin glulisine controls diabetes but does not cure it. Continue to use insulin glulisine even if you feel well. Do not stop using insulin glulisine without talking to your doctor. Do not switch to another brand or type of insulin or change the dose of any type of insulin you are using without talking to your doctor.

Insulin glulisine comes in vials and in cartridges. The cartridges are designed to be placed in dosing pens. Be sure you know what type of container your insulin glulisine comes in and what other supplies, such as needles, syringes, or pens, you will need to inject your medication.

If your insulin glulisine comes in vials, you will need to use syringes or an insulin pump to inject your dose. Always use a syringe marked for U-100 insulin to be sure that you get the right dose. Ask your doctor or pharmacist if you have questions about the type of syringe you should use.

Carefully read the manufacturer's instructions to learn how to draw insulin glulisine into a syringe and inject your dose. Ask your doctor or pharmacist if you have questions about how to inject your dose.

If your insulin glulisine comes in cartridges, you will need to buy an insulin pen separately. Check the manufacturer's information to see what type of pen is right for insulin glulisine cartridges. Ask your doctor or pharmacist if you have any questions about the type of pen you should use. Carefully read the instructions that come with your pen, and ask your doctor or pharmacist to show you how to use it.

Never reuse needles or syringes and never share needles, syringes, cartridges, or pens. If you are using an insulin pen, always remove the needle right after you inject your dose. Throw away needles and syringes in a puncture-resistant container. Ask your doctor or pharmacist how to dispose of the puncture-resistant container.

Insulin glulisine may be mixed only with NPH insulin (Novolin N, Humulin N) to be injected using a syringe. Do not mix or dilute insulin glulisine with any other type of insulin. If you mix insulin glulisine with NPH insulin, draw insulin glulisine into the syringe first, then draw the NPH insulin into the syringe and inject the solution immediately after mixing. If you use insulin glulisine in an insulin pump, do not dilute insulin glulisine or mix it with any other insulin or solution.

Always look at your insulin glulisine before you inject it. It should be as clear, colorless, and fluid as water. Do not use your insulin glulisine if it is colored, cloudy, thickened, or contains solid particles, or if the expiration date on the bottle has passed.

If you use syringes or a pen, you may inject insulin glulisine into your upper arm; stomach area, except for a two inch circle around the navel (belly button); or upper leg. If you use an insulin pump, infuse insulin glulisine into your stomach area. Never inject insulin glulisine into muscles or veins, or in or near moles or scars. Use a different site for each injection, about 1 inch away from the previous injection site but in the same general area (for example, the thigh). Use all available sites in the same general area before switching to a different area (for example, the upper arm).

If you use insulin glulisine in an insulin pump, change the tubing and needle and throw away any solution left in the reservoir at least every 48 hours. You should also change the infusion site (spot where the pump is attached to the body) at least every 48 hours. You may need to change the needles, tubing, infusion site, and medication more often if the medication has been exposed to high temperatures or direct sunlight, if your blood sugar increases unexpectedly, if the skin around the infusion site becomes irritated, or if there are problems with your pump. Be sure that you know what to do if you have any problems with your pump. Your blood sugar may increase very quickly if your pump stops working, and you may need to inject insulin with a syringe. Read the manufacturer's information carefully and ask your doctor or pharmacist for more information.

Are there other uses for this medicine?

This medication may be prescribed for other uses; ask your doctor or pharmacist for more information.

What special precautions should I follow?

Before using insulin glulisine,

- tell your doctor and pharmacist if you are allergic to insulin (Humulin, Novolin, others) or any other medications.
- tell your doctor and pharmacist what prescription and nonprescription medications, vitamins, nutritional supplements, and herbal products you are taking or plan to take. Be sure to mention any of the following: angiotensin-converting enzyme (ACE) inhibitors such as benazepril (Lotensin), captopril (Capoten), enalapril (Vasotec), fosinopril (Monopril), lisinopril (Zestril), moexipril (Univasc), perindopril, (Aceon), quinapril (Accupril), ramipril (Altace), and trandolapril (Mavik); albuterol (Proventil, Ventolin, Vospire ER); antihistamines; beta blockers such as atenolol (Tenormin), labetalol (Normodyne), metoprolol (Lopressor, Toprol XL), nadolol (Corgard), and propranolol (Inderal); clonidine (Catapres, Catapres-TTS); danazol; diazoxide (Proglycem); disopyramide (Norpace); diuretics ('water pills'); epinephrine (Bronitin Mist, EpiPen, Primatene Mist); fenofibrate (Antara, Lipofen, Tricor); fluoxetine (Prozac, Sarafem); gemfibrozil (Lopid); glucagon (Glucagen); guanethidine (Ismelin); hormone replacement therapy; isoniazid (INH, Laniazid); lithium (Eskalith, Lithobid); medications for asthma, colds, irregular menstrual bleeding, and nausea; certain medications for human immunodeficiency virus (HIV) including amprenavir (Agenerase), atazanavir (Reyataz), fosamprenavir (Lexiva), indinavir (Crixivan), lopinavir (in Kaletra), nelfinavir (Viracept), ritonavir (in Kaletra, Norvir), saquinavir (Invirase), and tipranavir (Aptivus); certain antipsychotics (medications for mental illness) including clozapine (Clozaril, Fazaclo) and olanzapine (Zyprexa, in Symbyax); monoamine oxidase (MAO) inhibitors such as isocarboxazid (Marplan), phenelzine (Nardil), selegiline (Eldepryl, Emsam, Zelapar), and tranylcypromine (Parnate); hormonal contraceptives (birth control pills, patches, rings, injections, or implants); oral medications for diabetes; oral steroids such as dexamethasone (Decadron, Dexone), methylprednisolone (Medrol), and prednisone (Deltasone); pentoxifylline (Pentoxil, Trental); propoxyphene (Darvon, in Darvocet, in Wygesic); reserpine (Serpalan); salicylate pain relievers such as aspirin; somatropin (Humatrope, Norditropin, Nutropin); sulfa antibiotics; terbutaline (Brethine); and thyroid medications. Your doctor may need to change the doses of your medications or monitor you carefully for side effects.
- tell your doctor if you have or have ever had nerve damage caused by your diabetes or kidney or liver disease.
- tell your doctor if you are pregnant, plan to become pregnant, or are breast-feeding. If you become pregnant while using insulin glulisine, call your doctor.
- if you are having surgery, including dental surgery, tell the doctor or dentist that you are using insulin glulisine.
- ask your doctor what to do if you get sick, experience unusual stress, plan to travel across time zones, or change your exercise and activity level. These changes can affect your blood sugar and the amount of insulin you may need.

What special dietary instructions should I follow?

Be sure to follow all exercise and dietary recommendations made by your doctor or dietitian. It is important to eat a healthy diet and to eat about the same amounts of the same kinds of food at about the same times each day. Skipping or delaying meals or changing the amount or kind of food you eat can cause problems with your blood sugar control.

Alcohol may cause a decrease in blood sugar. Ask your doctor about the safe use of alcoholic beverages while you are using insulin glulisine.

What should I do if I forget to take a dose?

Insulin glulisine must be injected up to 15 minutes before or within 20 minutes after starting a meal. If some time has passed since your meal, check your blood sugar and call your doctor to find out whether you should inject the missed dose. Do not inject a double dose to make up for a missed one.

What side effects can this medicine cause?

Insulin glulisine may cause changes in your blood sugar. You should know the symptoms of low and high blood sugar and what to do if you have these symptoms.

You may experience hypoglycemia (low blood sugar) while you are taking this medication. Your doctor will tell you what you should do if you develop hypoglycemia. He or she may tell you to check your blood sugar, eat or drink a food or beverage that contains sugar, such as hard candy or fruit juice, or get medical care. Follow these directions carefully if you have any of the following symptoms of hypoglycemia:

- shakiness
- dizziness or lightheadedness
- sweating
- nervousness or irritability
- sudden changes in behavior or mood
- headache
- numbness or tingling around the mouth, hands, or feet
- weakness
- pale skin
- hunger
- clumsy or jerky movements
- nightmares
- difficulty falling asleep or staying asleep
- blurred vision

- slurred speech
- fast heartbeat

If hypoglycemia is not treated, severe symptoms may develop. Be sure that your family, friends, and other people who spend time with you know that if you have any of the following symptoms, they should get medical treatment for you immediately.

- confusion
- seizures
- loss of consciousness

Call your doctor immediately if you have any of the following symptoms of hyperglycemia (high blood sugar):

- extreme thirst
- frequent urination
- extreme hunger
- weakness
- blurred vision

If high blood sugar is not treated, a serious, life-threatening condition called diabetic ketoacidosis could develop. Get medical care immediately if you have any of these symptoms:

- dry mouth
- nausea and vomiting
- stomach pain
- shortness of breath
- breath that smells fruity
- decreased consciousness

Insulin glulisine may cause side effects. Tell your doctor if any of these symptoms are severe or do not go away:

- redness, swelling, or itching at the site of the injection
- changes in the feel of your skin, skin thickening (fat build-up), or a little indentation in the skin (fat breakdown)
- muscle pain

Some side effects can be serious. The following symptoms are uncommon, but if you experience any of them, call your doctor immediately:

- rash and/or itching over the whole body
- shortness of breath
- wheezing
- dizziness
- blurred vision
- fast heartbeat
- sweating
- difficulty breathing or swallowing

Insulin glulisine may cause other side effects. Call your doctor if you have any unusual problems while using this medication.

What storage conditions are needed for this medicine?

Store unopened insulin glulisine vials and cartridges in the refrigerator away from light. Do not freeze. Opened insulin glulisine vials may be refrigerated or may be stored at room temperature, away from direct sunlight and heat, for up to 28 days. Opened insulin glulisine cartridges that have not been inserted into a pen may be refrigerated or may be stored at room temperature, away from direct heat and sunlight, for up to 28 days. Opened insulin glulisine cartridges that have been inserted into a pen should not be refrigerated; they should be stored inside the pen at room temperature for up to 28 days after the first use. Throw away opened insulin glulisine cartridges and vials after 28 days. Throw away unopened, refrigerated insulin glulisine after the expiration date printed on the label has passed. Throw away any insulin glulisine that has been frozen or exposed to extreme heat.

Throw away any medication that is outdated or no longer needed. Talk to your pharmacist about the proper disposal of your medication.

What should I do in case of overdose?

In case of overdose, call your local poison control center at 1-800-222-1222. If the victim has collapsed or is not breathing, call local emergency services at 911.

Symptoms of overdose may include:

- loss of consciousness
- seizures
- confusion

What other information should I know?

Keep all appointments with your doctor and the laboratory. Your blood sugar and glycosylated hemoglobin (HbA1c) should be checked regularly to determine your response to insulin glulisine. Your doctor will also tell you how to check your response to insulin by measuring your blood or urine sugar levels at home. Follow these instructions carefully.

You should always wear a diabetic identification bracelet to be sure you get proper treatment in an emergency.

Do not let anyone else use your medication. Ask your pharmacist any questions you have about refilling your prescription.

Dosage Facts
For Informational Purposes

Caution: Do not change your dose, how often you take your medication, or the length of time you are to take it without first talking to your healthcare provider.

The following dosage information was written using medical language for doctors and other healthcare professionals and is provided here for you to check your dosage. The dosage of this drug may differ for different patients. Therefore, always follow your doctor's instructions or the directions on the label. Contact your healthcare provider or pharmacist if you have any questions about the specific dosage of your medication after reviewing this information.

Adult Patients

Diabetes Mellitus

Whenever possible, patients should self-monitor blood glucose concentrations.

SUB-Q INJECTION:

- Individualize dosage based on blood glucose determinations. No specific dosage recommendations by the manufacturer.
- When insulin glulisine is used as a mealtime insulin, a longer-acting insulin (e.g., insulin glargine, isophane insulin human) is used concomitantly to meet basal insulin needs and to provide more optimal glycemic control.

SUB-Q INFUSION:

- Individualize dosage based on blood glucose determinations. No specific dosage recommendations by the manufacturer.

Special Populations

Hepatic Impairment

- Dosage reduction may be necessary.

Renal Impairment

- Dosage reduction may be necessary.

Insulin Human (rDNA Origin) Inhalation

(in' su lin)

Brand Name: Exubera®

Why is this medicine prescribed?

Insulin inhalation is used in combination with a long-acting insulin to treat type 1 diabetes (condition in which the body does not produce insulin and therefore cannot control the amount of sugar in the blood). It is also used alone or in combination with other medications to treat people with type 2 diabetes (condition in which the body does not use insulin normally and, therefore, cannot control the amount of sugar in the blood) who need insulin to control their diabetes. Insulin inhalation is a short-acting, man-made version of human insulin that starts to work within 10 to 20 minutes after it is inhaled and continues to work for about 6 hours. It helps control blood sugar levels by moving sugar from the blood into other body tissues where it is used for energy. It also stops the liver from producing more sugar.

How should this medicine be used?

Insulin inhalation comes as a powder to inhale by mouth using a specially designed inhaler. It is usually taken immediately before meals (within 10 minutes before eating). Follow the directions on your prescription label carefully, and ask your doctor or pharmacist to explain any part you do not understand. Use insulin inhalation exactly as directed. Do not use more or less of it or use it more often than prescribed by your doctor.

Insulin inhalation controls diabetes but does not cure it. Continue to use insulin inhalation even if you feel well. Do not stop using insulin inhalation without talking to your doctor. Do not switch to another brand or type of insulin without talking to your doctor.

When you begin using insulin inhalation, your doctor may need to adjust the doses of your other diabetes medications, such as long-acting insulin and oral medications for diabetes. Your doctor may also need to adjust your dose of insulin inhalation during your treatment. Follow these directions carefully and ask your doctor if you have any questions. Do not change the dose of insulin inhalation or any other medication for diabetes without talking to your doctor.

Insulin inhalation powder comes in small foil dose packets called blisters. Do not open or puncture the blisters. The blisters will open after they are put in the inhaler. Do not swallow the contents of the blister or inhale them without the proper inhaler. After you use a blister, throw it away in a garbage can that is out of the reach of children and pets. Do not try to reuse a blister.

Do not use three 1-mg blisters in place of one 3-mg blister. You may get too much insulin. If needed, you can use two 1-mg blisters in place of one 3-mg blister. Then check your blood sugar level and get a new supply of 3-mg blisters as soon as possible.

Call your doctor if you develop a cold or a cough or if you become congested at any time during your treatment. You will still be able to use insulin inhalation, but your doctor may adjust your dose or tell you to check your blood sugar level more often.

Ask your pharmacist or doctor for a copy of the manufacturer's Medication Guide. Carefully read the instructions on how to use the insulin inhaler, how to clean the insulin inhaler, and how often to replace the parts of the inhaler.

Are there other uses for this medicine?

This medication may be prescribed for other uses; ask your doctor or pharmacist for more information.

What special precautions should I follow?

Before using insulin inhalation,

- tell your doctor and pharmacist if you are allergic to insulin (Humulin, Iletin, Novolin, Velosulin, others), any other medications, or any of the inactive ingredients in insulin inhalation. Ask your pharmacist or check the Medication Guide for a list of the ingredients.
- tell your doctor and pharmacist what prescription and nonprescription medications, vitamins, nutritional supplements, and herbal products you are taking or plan to take. Be sure to mention any of the following: albuterol (Proventil, Ventolin); angiotensin-converting enzyme (ACE) inhibitors such as benazepril (Lotensin), enalapril (Vasotec), fosinopril (Monopril), lisinopril (Prinivil, Zestril), quinapril (Accupril), and ramipril (Altace); an-

tihistamines; beta blockers such as atenolol (Tenormin), labetalol (Normodyne), metoprolol (Lopressor, Toprol XL), nadolol (Corgard), and propranolol (Inderal); clonidine (Catapres, Catapres-TTS); clozapine (Clozaril); danazol (Danocrine); diazoxide (Proglycem); disopyramide (Norpace, Norpace CR); diuretics ('water pills'); epinephrine; fenofibrate (Lofibra, TriCor); fluoxetine (Prozac, Sarafem); gemfibrozil (Lopid); guanethidine (Ismelin); HIV protease inhibitors including atazanavir (Reyataz), indinavir (Crixivan), lopinavir (in Kaletra), nelfinavir (Viracept), ritonavir (Norvir, in Kaletra), and saquinavir (Fortovase, Invirase); hormone replacement therapy; hormonal contraceptives (birth control pills, patches, rings, and injections); isoniazid (Laniazid, Nydrazid); lithium (Eskalith, Lithobid, Lithotabs); medications for asthma, colds, mental illness, and nausea; monoamine oxidase (MAO) inhibitors, including isocarboxazid (Marplan), phenelzine (Nardil), tranylcypromine (Parnate), and selegiline (Eldepryl); oral contraceptives (birth control pills); oral medications for diabetes; oral steroids such as dexamethasone (Decadron, Dexone), methylprednisolone (Medrol), and prednisone (Deltasone); other inhaled medications; olanzapine (Zyprexa); pentamidine (NebuPent, Pentam 300); pentoxifylline (Pentoxil, Trental); propoxyphene; reserpine (Serpalan, Serpasil); salicylate pain relievers such as aspirin; somatropin (Humatrope, Serostim, Zorbtive); sulfa antibiotics; terbutaline (Brethine); and thyroid medications. Your doctor may need to change the doses of your medications or monitor you carefully for side effects.

- tell your doctor if you smoke or have stopped smoking within the past 6 months, or if you have asthma, chronic obstructive pulmonary disease (COPD; a group of lung diseases including chronic bronchitis and emphysema), or other lung disease. Your doctor may tell you not to use insulin inhalation.
- do not smoke during your treatment with insulin inhalation. If you do start smoking, stop using insulin inhalation and call your doctor right away.
- tell your doctor if you have or have ever had nerve damage caused by your diabetes; or kidney or liver disease.
- tell your doctor if you are pregnant, plan to become pregnant, or are breast-feeding. If you become pregnant while using insulin inhalation, call your doctor.
- if you are having surgery, including dental surgery, tell the doctor or dentist that you are using insulin inhalation.
- ask your doctor what to do if you get sick, experience unusual stress, plan to travel across more than two time zones, or change your exercise or activity schedule. These changes can affect your dosing schedule and the amount of insulin you will need.
- ask your doctor how often you should check your blood sugar. Be aware that low blood sugar may affect your ability to perform tasks such as driving and ask your

doctor if you need to check your blood sugar before driving or operating machinery.
- you should know that insulin inhalation may decrease lung function. Your doctor will order certain tests to check how well your lungs are working before and during insulin inhalation treatment.

What special dietary instructions should I follow?

Be sure to follow all exercise and dietary recommendations made by your doctor or dietitian. It is important to eat a healthy diet and to eat about the same amounts of the same kinds of food at about the same times each day. Skipping or delaying meals or changing the amount or kind of food you eat can cause problems with your blood sugar control.

Alcohol may cause a decrease in blood sugar. Ask your doctor about the safe use of alcoholic beverages while you are using insulin inhalation.

What should I do if I forget to take a dose?

Skip the missed dose and continue your regular dosing schedule. Do not inhale a dose at a later time or inhale a double dose to make up for a missed one. When you realize that you have missed a dose, check your blood sugar and call your doctor if it is too high.

What side effects can this medicine cause?

This medication may cause changes in your blood sugar. You should know the symptoms of low and high blood sugar and what to do if you have these symptoms.

You may experience hypoglycemia (low blood sugar) while you are taking this medication. Your doctor will tell you what you should do if you develop hypoglycemia. He or she may tell you to check your blood sugar, eat or drink a food or beverage that contains sugar, such as hard candy or fruit juice, or get medical care. Follow these directions carefully if you have any of the following symptoms of hypoglycemia:

- shakiness
- dizziness or lightheadedness
- sweating
- nervousness or irritability
- sudden changes in behavior or mood
- headache
- numbness or tingling around the mouth
- weakness
- pale skin
- hunger
- clumsy or jerky movements
- nightmares
- difficulty falling asleep or staying asleep
- blurred vision
- slurred speech
- fast heartbeat

If hypoglycemia is not treated, severe symptoms may

develop. Be sure that your family, friends, and other people who spend time with you know that if you have any of the following symptoms, they should get medical treatment for you immediately.

- confusion
- seizures
- loss of consciousness

Call your doctor immediately if you have any of the following symptoms of hyperglycemia (high blood sugar):

- extreme thirst
- frequent urination
- extreme hunger
- weakness
- blurred vision

If high blood sugar is not treated, a serious, life-threatening condition called diabetic ketoacidosis could develop. Get medical care immediately if you have any of these symptoms:

- dry mouth
- nausea and vomiting
- loss of appetite
- pain in the stomach
- fast heartbeat
- fast, deep breathing
- breath that smells fruity
- decreased consciousness

Insulin inhalation may cause side effects. Tell your doctor if any of these symptoms are severe or do not go away:

- chest pain
- cough
- coughing up mucus
- mild shortness of breath
- sore throat
- hoarse, changed, or lost voice
- runny nose
- nosebleed

Some side effects can be serious. If you experience any of these symptoms, call your doctor immediately:

- rash and/or itching over the whole body
- hives
- wheezing

Insulin inhalation may cause other side effects. Call your doctor if you have any unusual problems while using this medication.

What storage conditions are needed for this medicine?

Keep this medication in the container it came in, tightly closed, and out of reach of children. Store it at room temperature and keep the unit dose blisters away from excess heat and moisture (not in the bathroom). Do not refrigerate. Do not freeze. Throw away any blister that has been exposed to moisture or excessive heat or that has been frozen. Throw away any medication that is outdated or no longer needed. Talk to your pharmacist about the proper disposal of your medication.

What should I do in case of overdose?

In case of overdose, call your local poison control center at 1-800-222-1222. If the victim has collapsed or is not breathing, call local emergency services at 911.

Insulin inhalation overdose can occur if you take too much insulin inhalation or if you take the right amount of insulin inhalation but eat or exercise less than usual. Insulin inhalation overdose can cause hypoglycemia. If you have any of the symptoms of hypoglycemia listed above, follow your doctor's instructions for what you should do if you develop hypoglycemia.

What other information should I know?

Keep all appointments with your doctor and the laboratory. Your blood sugar and glycosylated hemoglobin (HbA1c) should be checked regularly to determine your response to insulin inhalation. Your doctor will also tell you how to check your response to insulin by measuring your blood or urine sugar levels at home. Follow these instructions carefully.

You should always wear a diabetic identification bracelet to be sure you get proper treatment in an emergency.

Do not let anyone else use your medication. Ask your pharmacist any questions you have about refilling your prescription.

Dosage Facts
For Informational Purposes

Caution: Do not change your dose, how often you take your medication, or the length of time you are to take it without first talking to your healthcare provider.

The following dosage information was written using medical language for doctors and other healthcare professionals and is provided here for you to check your dosage. The dosage of this drug may differ for different patients. Therefore, always follow your doctor's instructions or the directions on the label. Contact your healthcare provider or pharmacist if you have any questions about the specific dosage of your medication after reviewing this information.

General Dosage Information

Patients receiving insulin should be monitored with regular laboratory evaluations, including blood glucose determinations and glycosylated hemoglobin (hemoglobin A_{1c} [HbA_{1c}]) concentrations, to determine the minimum effective dosage of insulin when used alone, with other insulins, or in combination with an oral antidiabetic agent.

Insulin Injection

(in' su lin)

Brand Name: Humulin R®, Humulin N®, Humulin 70/30®, Humulin 50/50®, Humulin R U-500®, Novolin R®, Novolin N®, Novolin 70/30®

Why is this medicine prescribed?

Insulin injection is used to control blood sugar in people who have type 1 diabetes (condition in which the body does not make insulin and therefore cannot control the amount of sugar in the blood) or in people who have type 2 diabetes (condition in which the blood sugar is too high because the body does not produce or use insulin normally) that cannot be controlled with oral medications alone. Insulin injection is in a class of medications called hormones. Insulin injection is used to take the place of insulin that is normally produced by the body. It works by helping move sugar from the blood into other body tissues where it is used for energy. It also stops the liver from producing more sugar. All of the types of insulin that are available work in this way. The types of insulin differ only in how quickly they begin to work and how long they continue to control blood sugar.

How should this medicine be used?

Insulin comes as a solution (liquid) and a suspension (liquid with particles that will settle on standing) to be injected subcutaneously (under the skin). Insulin is usually injected several times a day, and more than one type of insulin may be needed. Your doctor will tell you which type(s) of insulin to use, how much insulin to use, and how often to inject insulin. Follow these directions carefully. Do not use more or less insulin or use it more often than prescribed by your doctor.

Insulin controls high blood sugar but does not cure diabetes. Continue to use insulin even if you feel well. Do not stop using insulin without talking to your doctor. Do not switch to another brand or type of insulin or change the dose of any type of insulin you use without talking to your doctor.

Insulin comes in vials, pre-filled disposable dosing devices, and cartridges. The cartridges are designed to be placed in dosing pens. Be sure you know what type of container your insulin comes in and what other supplies, such as needles, syringes, or pens, you will need to inject your medication. Make sure that the name and letter on your insulin are exactly what your doctor prescribed.

If your insulin comes in vials, you will need to use syringes to inject your dose. Be sure that you know whether your insulin is U-100 or U-500 and always use a syringe marked for that type of insulin. Always use the same brand and model of needle and syringe. Ask your doctor or pharmacist if you have questions about the type of syringe you should use. Carefully read the manufacturer's instructions to learn how to draw insulin into a syringe and inject your dose.

Ask your doctor or pharmacist if you have questions about how to inject your dose.

If your insulin comes in cartridges, you may need to buy an insulin pen separately. Talk to your doctor or pharmacist about the type of pen you should use. Carefully read the instructions that come with your pen, and ask your doctor or pharmacist to show you how to use it.

If your insulin comes in a disposable dosing device, read the instructions that come with the device carefully. Ask your doctor or pharmacist to show you how to use the device.

Never reuse needles or syringes and never share needles, syringes, cartridges, or pens. If you are using an insulin pen, always remove the needle right after you inject your dose. Throw away needles and syringes in a puncture-resistant container. Ask your doctor or pharmacist how to dispose of the puncture-resistant container.

Your doctor may tell you to mix two types of insulin in the same syringe. Your doctor will tell you exactly how to draw both types of insulin into the syringe. Follow these directions carefully. Always draw the same type of insulin into the syringe first, and always use the same brand of needles. Never mix more than one type of insulin in a syringe unless you are told to do so by your doctor.

Always look at your insulin before you inject. If you are using a regular insulin (Humulin R, Novolin R), the insulin should be as clear, colorless, and fluid as water. Do not use this type of insulin if it appears cloudy, thickened, or colored, or if it has solid particles. If you are using an NPH insulin (Humulin N, Novolin N) or a pre-mixed insulin that contains NPH (Humulin 70/30, Humulin 50/50, Novolin 70/30), the insulin should appear cloudy or milky after you mix it. Do not use these types of insulin if there are clumps in the liquid or if there are solid white particles sticking to the bottom or walls of the bottle. Do not use any type of insulin after the expiration date printed on the bottle has passed.

Some types of insulin must be shaken or rotated to mix before use. Ask your doctor or pharmacist if the type of insulin you are using should be mixed and how you should mix it if necessary.

Talk to your doctor or pharmacist about where on your body you should inject insulin. Insulin is usually injected in the stomach (except for 2 inches around the belly button), upper arm, upper leg, or buttocks. Do not inject insulin into muscles, scars, or moles. Use a different site for each injection, at least 1/2 inch away from the previous injection site but in the same general area (for example, the thigh). Use all available sites in the same general area before switching to a different area (for example, the upper arm).

Are there other uses for this medicine?

This medication may be prescribed for other uses. Ask your doctor or pharmacist for more information.

What special precautions should I follow?

Before using insulin,

- tell your doctor and pharmacist if you are allergic to any type of insulin or any other medications.
- tell your doctor and pharmacist what prescription and nonprescription medications, vitamins, nutritional supplements, and herbal products you are taking or plan to take. Be sure to mention any of the following: alpha blockers such as doxazosin (Cardura), prazosin (Minipress), terazosin (Hytrin), tamsulosin (Flomax), and alfuzosin (Uroxatral); angiotensin-converting enzyme (ACE) inhibitors such as benazepril (Lotensin), captopril (Capoten), enalapril (Vasotec), fosinopril (Monopril), lisinopril (Zestril), moexipril (Univasc), perindopril, (Aceon), quinapril (Accupril), ramipril (Altace), and trandolapril (Mavik); antidepressants; asparaginase (Elspar); beta blockers such as atenolol (Tenormin), carvedilol (Coreg), labetalol (Normodyne), metoprolol (Lopressor, Toprol XL), nadolol (Corgard), pindolol, propranolol (Inderal), sotalol (Betapace, Sorine), and timolol (Blocadren); diazoxide (Proglycem); diuretics ('water pills'); medications for asthma and colds; monoamine oxidase (MAO) inhibitors such as isocarboxazid (Marplan), phenelzine (Nardil), selegiline (Eldepryl, Emsam, Zelapar), and tranylcypromine (Parnate); hormonal contraceptives (birth control pills, patches, rings, injections, or implants); niacin (Niacor, Niaspan, Slo-Niacin); octreotide (Sandostatin); oral medications for diabetes; oral steroids such as dexamethasone (Decadron, Dexone), methylprednisolone (Medrol), and prednisone (Deltasone); quinine; quinidine; salicylate pain relievers such as aspirin; sulfa antibiotics; and thyroid medications. Your doctor may need to change the doses of your medications or monitor you carefully for side effects.
- tell your doctor if you have or have ever had nerve damage caused by diabetes; or adrenal (a small gland near the kidneys), pituitary (a small gland in the brain), thyroid, liver, or kidney disease.
- tell your doctor if you are pregnant, plan to become pregnant, or are breast-feeding. If you become pregnant while using insulin, call your doctor.
- if you are having surgery, including dental surgery, tell the doctor or dentist that you are using insulin.
- ask your doctor what to do if you get sick, experience unusual stress, plan to travel across time zones, or change your exercise and activity level. These changes can affect your blood sugar and the amount of insulin you may need.

What special dietary instructions should I follow?

Be sure to follow all exercise and dietary recommendations made by your doctor or dietitian. It is important to eat a healthy diet and to eat about the same amounts of the same kinds of foods at about the same times every day. Skipping or delaying meals or changing the amount or kind of food you eat can cause problems with your blood sugar control.

Alcohol may cause a decrease in blood sugar. Ask your doctor about the safe use of alcoholic beverages while you are using insulin.

What should I do if I forget to take a dose?

When you first start using insulin, ask your doctor what to do if you forget to inject a dose at the correct time. Write down these directions so that you can refer to them later.

What side effects can this medicine cause?

This medication causes changes in your blood sugar. You should know the symptoms of low and high blood sugar and what to do if you have these symptoms.

You may experience hypoglycemia (low blood sugar) while you are using this medication. Your doctor will tell you what you should do if you develop hypoglycemia. He or she may tell you to check your blood sugar, eat or drink a food or beverage that contains sugar, such as hard candy or fruit juice, or get medical care. Follow these directions carefully if you have any of the following symptoms of hypoglycemia. You should be especially alert to these symptoms if you previously used an animal-source insulin and have switched to a human insulin. Your hypoglycemia symptoms may be different or less noticeable while you are using a human insulin. Symptoms of hypoglycemia include:

- shakiness
- dizziness or lightheadedness
- sweating
- nervousness or irritability
- sudden changes in behavior or mood
- headache
- numbness or tingling around the mouth
- weakness
- pale skin
- hunger
- clumsy or jerky movements

If hypoglycemia is not treated, severe symptoms may develop. Be sure that your family, friends, and other people who spend time with you know that if you have any of the following symptoms, they should get medical treatment for you immediately.

- confusion
- seizures
- loss of consciousness

Call your doctor immediately if you have any of the following symptoms of hyperglycemia (high blood sugar):

- extreme thirst
- frequent urination
- extreme hunger
- weakness
- blurred vision

If high blood sugar is not treated, a serious, life-threatening condition called diabetic ketoacidosis could develop.

Call your doctor immediately if you have any of the these symptoms:

- dry mouth
- upset stomach and vomiting
- shortness of breath
- breath that smells fruity
- decreased consciousness

Insulin may cause side effects. Tell your doctor if any of these symptoms are severe or do not go away:

- redness, swelling, and itching at the injection site
- changes in the feel of your skin, fat build-up, or fat breakdown

Some side effects can be serious. If you experience any of the following symptoms, call your doctor immediately:

- rash and/or itching over the whole body
- shortness of breath
- wheezing
- dizziness
- blurred vision
- fast heartbeat
- sweating
- difficulty breathing or swallowing

If you experience a serious side effect, you or your doctor may send a report to the Food and Drug Administration's (FDA) MedWatch Adverse Event Reporting program online [at http://www.fda.gov/MedWatch/index.html] or by phone [1-800-332-1088].

What storage conditions are needed for this medicine?

Store unopened vials of insulin, unopened disposable dosing devices and unopened insulin pens in the refrigerator. Do not freeze insulin and do not use insulin that has been frozen. Opened vials of insulin should be stored in the refrigerator but may also be stored at room temperature, in a cool place that is away from heat and direct sunlight. Store opened insulin pens and opened dosing devices at room temperature. Check the manufacturer's information to find out how long you may keep your pen or dosing device after the first use. Throw away any medication that is outdated or no longer needed. Talk to your doctor or pharmacist about the proper disposal of your medication.

What should I do in case of overdose?

In case of overdose, call your local poison control center at 1-800-222-1222. If the victim has collapsed or is not breathing, call local emergency services at 911.

Symptoms of overdose may include the hypoglycemia symptoms listed above as well as the following:

- loss of consciousness
- seizures
- confusion

What other information should I know?

Keep all appointments with your doctor and the laboratory. Your blood sugar and glycosylated hemoglobin (HbA1c)

should be checked regularly to determine your response to insulin. Your doctor will also tell you how to check your response to insulin by measuring your blood or urine sugar levels at home. Follow these directions carefully.

You should always wear a diabetic identification bracelet to be sure you get proper treatment in an emergency.

Do not let anyone else use your medication. Ask your pharmacist any questions you have about refilling your prescription.

Dosage Facts
For Informational Purposes

Caution: Do not change your dose, how often you take your medication, or the length of time you are to take it without first talking to your healthcare provider.

The following dosage information was written using medical language for doctors and other healthcare professionals and is provided here for you to check your dosage. The dosage of this drug may differ for different patients. Therefore, always follow your doctor's instructions or the directions on the label. Contact your healthcare provider or pharmacist if you have any questions about the specific dosage of your medication after reviewing this information.

General Dosage Information

Patients receiving insulin should be monitored with regular laboratory evaluations, including blood glucose determinations and glycosylated hemoglobin (hemoglobin A_{1c} [HbA_{1c}]) concentrations, to determine the minimum effective dosage of insulin when used alone, with other insulins, or in combination with an oral antidiabetic agent.

Pediatric Patients

Diabetes Mellitus

SUB-Q:
- Dosage must be individualized.
- In newly diagnosed children with severe diabetes mellitus, unstable diabetes mellitus, or diabetes mellitus with complications, *insulin (regular) (i.e., purified pork insulin)* generally is given sub-Q in a dosage of 2–4 units, 15–30 minutes before meals and at bedtime.
- In patients who are currently controlled on purified pork insulins, no change in dosage usually is required when transferring to insulin human, except routine dosage adjustments that are necessary to maintain stable glycemic control.

Adult Patients

Diabetes Mellitus

SUB-Q:
- Dosage must be individualized.
- In newly diagnosed patients with severe diabetes mellitus, unstable diabetes mellitus, or diabetes mellitus with complications, *insulin (regular) (i.e., purified pork insulin)* generally is given sub-Q in a dosage of 5–10 units, 15–30 minutes before meals and at bedtime.
- In patients who are currently controlled on purified pork in-

sulins, no change in dosage usually is required when transferring to insulin human, except routine dosage adjustments that are necessary to maintain stable glycemic control.

† Use is not currently included in the labeling approved by the US Food and Drug Administration.

Insulin Lispro Injection

(in′ su lin lye′ sproe)

Brand Name: Humalog®

Why is this medicine prescribed?

Insulin lispro is used to control blood sugar in people who have diabetes. Insulin lispro is in a class of medications called hormones. People who have diabetes do not produce enough natural insulin, a substance that is needed to break down carbohydrates, fats, and proteins from food and to move sugar from the blood to other parts of the body. Insulin lispro works by replacing the insulin that is normally produced by the body. Insulin lispro starts working more quickly but continues to work for a shorter time than regular insulin. Insulin lispro is always used with other medications for diabetes. You will need to use another type of insulin or take an oral medication, depending on the type of diabetes you have.

How should this medicine be used?

Insulin lispro comes as a solution (liquid) to inject subcutaneously (under the skin). It is usually injected 15 minutes before a meal or immediately after a meal. Your doctor will tell you how many times you should inject insulin lispro each day. Follow the directions on your prescription label carefully, and ask your doctor or pharmacist to explain any part you do not understand. Use insulin lispro exactly as directed. Do not use more or less of it or use it more often than prescribed by your doctor.

Never use insulin lispro when you have symptoms of hypoglycemia (low blood sugar) or if you have checked your blood sugar and found it to be low. Call your doctor in these cases.

Insulin lispro controls diabetes but does not cure it. Continue to use insulin lispro even if you feel well. Do not stop using insulin lispro without talking to your doctor. Do not switch to another brand or type of insulin or change the dose of any type of insulin you are using without talking to your doctor.

Insulin lispro comes in vials, cartridges that contain medication and are to be placed in dosing pens, and dosing pens that contain cartridges of medication. Be sure you know what type of container your insulin lispro comes in and what other supplies, such as needles, syringes, or pens you will need to inject your medication.

If your insulin lispro comes in vials, you will need to use syringes to inject your dose. Be sure to use syringes that are marked U-100. Ask your doctor or pharmacist if you have questions about the type of syringe you should use.

If your insulin lispro comes in cartridges, you will need to purchase an insulin pen separately. Check the manufacturer's information for the patient to see what type of pen is right for the cartridge size you are using. Carefully read the instructions that come with your pen, and ask your doctor or pharmacist to show you how to use it. Ask your doctor or pharmacist if you have questions about the type of pen you should use.

If your insulin lispro comes in pens, be sure to read and understand the manufacturer's instructions. Ask your doctor or pharmacist to show you how to use the pen. Follow the directions carefully, and always prime the pen before use. Never remove the cartridge from the pen or attempt to add any other type of insulin to the cartridge.

Never reuse needles or syringes and never share needles, syringes, cartridges, or pens. If you are using an insulin pen, always remove the needle right after you inject your dose. Throw away needles and syringes in a puncture-resistant container. Ask your doctor or pharmacist how to dispose of the puncture resistant container.

Your doctor may tell you to mix your insulin lispro with another type of insulin in the same syringe. Your doctor will tell you exactly how to do this. Always draw insulin lispro into the syringe first, always use the same brand of syringe, and always inject the insulin immediately after mixing.

You can inject your insulin lispro in your thighs, stomach, or upper arms. Each time you inject insulin lispro you should choose a spot that is at least 1/2 inch away from the spot where you gave your last injection.

Always look at your insulin lispro before you inject it. It should be as clear, colorless, and fluid as water. Do not use your insulin lispro if it is colored, cloudy, thickened, or contains solid particles, or if the expiration date on the bottle has passed.

If your insulin lispro comes in vials, follow these steps to prepare your dose:
1. Wash your hands.
2. If you are using a new bottle, flip off the plastic cap, but do not remove the stopper.
3. Wipe the top of the bottle with an alcohol swab.
4. Pull back the plunger of the syringe until the top of the plunger is even with the dose your doctor told you to inject.
5. Push the needle through the rubber stopper on the bottle.
6. Push down on the plunger to inject the air into the bottle.
7. Turn the bottle upside down without removing the syringe.
8. Be sure the tip of the needle is under the liquid in the bottle. Slowly pull back on the plunger until the top of the plunger is even with the dose your doctor told you to inject.
9. While the needle is still in the bottle, check whether there are air bubbles in the syringe. If there are bubbles,

hold the syringe upright and tap on it to push the bubbles to the top. Push the plunger up to move the bubbles out of the syringe, and then pull the plunger back down to the correct dose.

10. Remove the needle from the bottle and lay the syringe down so that the needle is not touching anything.

To inject a prepared dose of insulin lispro using a syringe or pen, follow these steps:

1. Use an alcohol pad to wipe the area where you plan to inject your medication.
2. Pinch up a large area of skin, or spread the skin flat with your hands.
3. Insert the needle into your skin. Your doctor will tell you exactly how to do this.
4. If you are using a syringe, push the plunger all the way down. If you are using a pen, follow the manufacturer's instructions for dispensing a dose.
5. Pull the needle out and press down on the spot for several seconds, but do not rub it.

Are there other uses for this medicine?

This medication may be prescribed for other uses; ask your doctor or pharmacist for more information.

What special precautions should I follow?

Before using insulin lispro,

- tell your doctor and pharmacist if you are allergic to insulin (Humulin, Iletin, Novolin, Velosulin, others) or any other medications.
- tell your doctor and pharmacist what prescription and nonprescription medications, vitamins, nutritional supplements, and herbal products you are taking. Be sure to mention any of the following: angiotensin converting enzyme (ACE) inhibitors such as benazepril (Lotensin), captopril (Capoten), enalapril (Vasotec), fosinopril (Monopril), lisinopril (Prinivil, Zestril), moexipril (Univasc), perindopril, (Aceon), quinapril (Accupril), ramipril (Altace), and trandolapril (Mavik); antacids; antihistamines; beta blockers such as atenolol (Tenormin), labetalol (Normodyne), metoprolol (Lopressor, Toprol XL), nadolol (Corgard), and propranolol (Inderal); digoxin (Digitek, Lanoxin); diuretics ('water pills'); cholesterol-lowering medications such as niacin (Niacor, Niaspan); hormone replacement therapy; isoniazid (INH, Nydrazid); laxatives; medications for mental illness and upset stomach; monoamine oxidase inhibitors including isocarboxazid (Marplan), phenelzine (Nardil), selegiline (Eldepryl) and tranylcypromine (Parnate); oral contraceptives (birth control pills); oral medications for diabetes; oral steroids such as dexamethasone (Decadron, Dexone), methylprednisolone (Medrol), and prednisone (Deltasone); salicylate pain relievers such as aspirin, choline magnesium trisalicylate (Trisalate), choline salicylate (Arthropan), diflunisal (Dolobid), magnesium salicylate (Doan's, others), and salsalate (Argesic, Disalcid, Salgesic); sodium polystyrene sulfonate (Kayexalate); sulfa antibiotics; theophylline (TheoDur) and thyroid medications. Your doctor may need to change the doses of your medications or monitor you carefully for side effects.

- tell your doctor if you have or have ever had nerve damage caused by your diabetes; any disease that affects your adrenal (a gland near the kidney that produces chemicals needed for fluid balance), pituitary (a gland in the head that produces many chemicals), or thyroid glands; or liver or kidney disease.
- tell your doctor if you are pregnant, plan to become pregnant, or are breast-feeding. If you become pregnant while using insulin lispro, call your doctor.
- if you are having surgery, including dental surgery, tell the doctor or dentist that you are using insulin lispro.
- ask your doctor what to do if you get sick, experience unusual stress, plan to travel across more than two time zones, or change your exercise or activity schedule. These changes can affect your dosing schedule and the amount of insulin you will need.
- ask your doctor how often you should check your blood sugar. Be aware that hypoglycemia may affect your ability to perform tasks such as driving and ask your doctor if you need to check your blood sugar before driving or operating machinery.

What special dietary instructions should I follow?

Be sure to follow all dietary recommendations made by your doctor or dietitian. It is important to eat a healthful diet, and to eat about the same amounts of the same kinds of food at about the same times each day. Skipping or delaying meals or changing the amount or kind of food you eat can cause problems with your blood sugar control.

Alcohol may cause a decrease in blood sugar. Ask your doctor about the safe use of alcoholic beverages while you are using insulin lispro.

What should I do if I forget to take a dose?

Insulin lispro must be injected shortly before or after a meal. If you remember your dose before or shortly after your meal, inject the missed dose right away. If some time has passed since your meal, call your doctor to find out whether you should inject the missed dose. Do not inject a double dose to make up for a missed one.

What side effects can this medicine cause?

This medication may cause changes in your blood sugar. You should know the symptoms of low and high blood sugar and what to do if you have these symptoms.

You may experience hypoglycemia (low blood sugar) while you are taking this medication. Your doctor will tell you what you should do if you develop hypoglycemia. He or she may tell you to check your blood sugar, eat or drink a food or beverage that contains sugar, such as hard candy or fruit juice, or get medical care. Follow these directions carefully if you have any of the following symptoms of hypoglycemia:

- shakiness
- dizziness or lightheadedness
- sweating
- nervousness or irritability
- sudden changes in behavior or mood
- headache
- numbness or tingling around the mouth
- weakness
- pale skin
- hunger
- clumsy or jerky movements

If hypoglycemia is not treated, severe symptoms may develop. Be sure that your family, friends, and other people who spend time with you know that if you have any of the following symptoms, they should get medical treatment for you immediately.

- confusion
- seizures
- loss of consciousness

Call your doctor immediately if you have any of the following symptoms of hyperglycemia (high blood sugar):

- extreme thirst
- frequent urination
- extreme hunger
- weakness
- blurred vision

If high blood sugar is not treated, a serious, life-threatening condition called diabetic ketoacidosis could develop. Call your doctor immediately if you have any of the these symptoms:

- dry mouth
- upset stomach and vomiting
- shortness of breath
- breath that smells fruity
- decreased consciousness

Insulin lispro may cause side effects. Tell your doctor if the following symptom is severe or does not go away:

- redness, swelling, or itching in the place where you injected insulin lispro

Some side effects can be serious. The following symptoms are uncommon, but if you experience any of them, call your doctor immediately:

- rash and itching
- difficulty breathing or swallowing
- hives
- wheezing
- fast heartbeat
- changes in the feel of your skin such as skin thickening or a little indentation in the skin
- muscle weakness
- tingling in arms or legs
- constipation
- stomach cramps
- depression

Insulin lispro may cause other side effects. Call your doctor if you have any unusual problems while taking this medication.

If you experience a serious side effect, you or your doctor may send a report to the Food and Drug Administration's (FDA) MedWatch Adverse Event Reporting program online [at http://www.fda.gov/MedWatch/index.html] or by phone [1-800-332-1088].

What storage conditions are needed for this medicine?

Keep this medication in the container it came in, tightly closed, and out of reach of children. Store vials of insulin lispro in the refrigerator but do not freeze them. If necessary, you may store the vial you are using outside the refrigerator in a cool dark place for up to 28 days. If your doctor tells you to dilute your insulin lispro, the vial of diluted medication can be stored for 28 days in the refrigerator or 14 days at room temperature. Store extra insulin lispro pens and cartridges that are not in use in the refrigerator but do not freeze them. Store the pen and cartridge you are using outside the refrigerator in a cool dark place for up to 28 days. Throw away any medication that is outdated or no longer needed. Talk to your pharmacist about the proper disposal of your medication.

What should I do in case of overdose?

In case of overdose, call your local poison control center at 1-800-222-1222. If the victim has collapsed or is not breathing, call local emergency services at 911.

Insulin lispro overdose can occur if you take too much insulin lispro or if you take the right amount of insulin lispro but eat or exercise less than usual. Insulin lispro overdose can cause hypoglycemia. If you have any of the symptoms of hypoglycemia listed above, follow your doctor's instructions for what you should do if you develop hypoglycemia. Other symptoms of overdose:

- coma
- seizures

What other information should I know?

Keep all appointments with your doctor and the laboratory. Your doctor will order certain lab tests to check your body's response to insulin lispro. Your doctor will also tell you how to check your response to insulin by measuring your blood or urine sugar levels at home. Follow these instructions carefully.

You should always wear a diabetic identification bracelet to be sure you get proper treatment in an emergency.

Do not let anyone else take your medication. Ask your pharmacist any questions you have about refilling your prescription.

Dosage Facts

For Informational Purposes

Caution: Do not change your dose, how often you take your medication, or the length of time you are to take it without first talking to your healthcare provider.

The following dosage information was written using medical language for doctors and other healthcare professionals and is provided here for you to check your dosage. The dosage of this drug may differ for different patients. Therefore, always follow your doctor's instructions or the directions on the label. Contact your healthcare provider or pharmacist if you have any questions about the specific dosage of your medication after reviewing this information.

General Dosage Information

Dosage of insulin lispro is always expressed in USP units.

Pediatric Patients

Diabetes Mellitus

SUB-Q INJECTION:
- Individualize dosage; adjust dosage regularly based on blood glucose determinations. Usually, the total daily insulin requirement in children with type 1 diabetes mellitus ranges from 0.2–1 units/kg (generally 0.5–0.8 units/kg daily). Adolescents in a growth phase may require an initial insulin dosage of 1–1.5 units/kg daily. No specific dosage recommendations by manufacturer. When used as a preprandial treatment regimen in clinical trials, 26–64% of total insulin requirements have been provided by insulin lispro, with the remainder provided by an intermediate-acting or long-acting insulin.

SUB-Q INFUSION:
- Individualize dosage; adjust dosage regularly based on blood glucose determinations. Glucose monitoring is particularly important for patients receiving insulin via an external infusion pump.
- No specific dosage recommendations by manufacturer. In a clinical trial, preprandial administration of insulin lispro injection comprised approximately 66% of the total daily insulin dosage, with the remainder given as a basal infusion.

Adult Patients

Diabetes Mellitus

SUB-Q INJECTION:
- Individualize dosage; adjust dosage regularly based on blood glucose determinations. Usually, the total daily insulin requirements in patients with type 1 diabetes mellitus is 0.5–1 unit/kg. No specific dosage recommendations by manufacturer. When used in a preprandial treatment regimen in clinical trials, 39–66% of total insulin requirements have been provided by insulin lispro, with the remainder provided by an intermediate-acting or long-acting insulin.
- In patients with type 2 diabetes mellitus who are not controlled on intermediate-acting or long-acting insulin, some clinicians suggest initiating preprandial therapy with a short-acting or rapid-acting insulin, with the preprandial injection comprising 40–50% of the total insulin dosage.

SUB-Q INFUSION:
- Individualize dosage; adjust dosage regularly based on blood glucose determinations. Glucose monitoring is particularly important for patients receiving insulin via an external infusion pump.
- No specific dosage recommendations by the manufacturer. In patients with type 1 diabetes mellitus, preprandial administration of insulin lispro injection has been used in clinical trials, comprising approximately 21–46% of the total daily insulin dosage, with the remainder given as a basal infusion.

Therapy with Fixed-Combination Insulin Lispro and Insulin Lispro Protamine

SUB-Q INJECTION:
- Individualize dosage; adjust dosage regularly based on blood glucose determinations.
- No specific dosage recommendations by the manufacturer. Initially, 0.3–0.5 units/kg daily given in 2 divided doses (before morning and evening meal) has been used in patients with type 2 diabetes mellitus. Subsequent dosage has been titrated in increments of 2–4 units per injection per day every 2–3 days to achieve the targeted fasting blood glucose concentration. Mean daily maintenance insulin dosage achieved was 0.46–0.66 units/kg.
- In patients with type 1 diabetes mellitus in a clinical trial, mean daily maintenance insulin dosage achieved was 0.64 units/kg.

Special Populations

Renal or Hepatic Impairment
- Careful monitoring of blood glucose and dosage adjustment may be necessary.

Interferon Alfa-2a and Alfa-2b Injection

(in ter feer' on)

Brand Name: Intron A (alfa-2b), Roferon-A (alfa-2a)

About Your Treatment

Your doctor has ordered interferon alfa-2a or alfa-2b to help treat your illness. This drug will be injected under the skin (subcutaneously) or into a muscle (intramuscularly).

This medication is given to prevent tumor cells or viruses from growing inside your body. It does not work for all patients, however, and some patients respond to the drug better than others. This medication is sometimes prescribed for other uses; ask your doctor or pharmacist for more information.

For the first 10-24 weeks, you will have a daily injection (the induction period). After that time, you will receive an injection three times a week (the maintenance period). Generally, therapy lasts for at least 6 months. This medication is sometimes prescribed for other uses; ask your doctor or pharmacist for more information.

Your health care provider (doctor, nurse, or pharmacist) may measure the effectiveness and side effects of your treatment using physical examinations and laboratory tests before and during your treatment. It is important to keep all appointments with your doctor and the laboratory. The length of treatment depends on how you respond to the medication.

Precautions

Before administering interferon alfa,

- tell your doctor and pharmacist if you are allergic to interferon alfa or any other drugs.
- tell your doctor and pharmacist what prescription and nonprescription medications you are taking, especially antibiotics and vitamins.
- tell your doctor if you have or have ever had heart, kidney or liver disease; asthma; depression; mental illness; or diabetes.
- tell your doctor if you are pregnant, plan to become pregnant, or are breast-feeding. If you become pregnant while taking interferon alfa, call your doctor.
- remember you should never change brands of interferon without telling your health care provider.

Administering Your Medication

Before you administer interferon alfa-2a or alfa-2b, look at the solution closely. It should be clear and free of floating material. Observe the solution container to make sure there are no leaks. Do not use the solution if it is discolored, if it contains particles, or if the container leaks. Use a new solution, but show the damaged one to your health care provider.

It is important that you use your medication exactly as directed. Do not change your dosing schedule without talking to your health care provider. Your health care provider may tell you to stop your infusion if you have a mechanical problem (such as a blockage in the tubing, needle, or catheter); if you have to stop an infusion, call your health care provider immediately so your therapy can continue.

Side Effects

The most common side effect of interferon alfa-2a or alfa-2b therapy is a flu-like reaction with fever, fatigue, irritability, chills, headaches, and muscle aches. These effects should become less severe and less frequent as you continue your therapy. Tell your health care provider if any of these problems continue or worsen.

Tell your health care provider if any of these symptoms are severe or do not go away:

- upset stomach
- loss of appetite
- stomach pain
- diarrhea
- skin rash
- dry skin
- itching

If you experience either of the following symptoms, call your health care provider immediately:

- dizziness
- numbness or tingling in the arms, hands, legs, or feet

If you experience a serious side effect, you or your doctor may send a report to the Food and Drug Administration's (FDA) MedWatch Adverse Event Reporting program online [at http://www.fda.gov/MedWatch/index.html] or by phone [1-800-332-1088].

Storage Conditions

- Your health care provider probably will give you several days supply of interferon alfa at a time. The drug comes either as a white to beige powder with a solution for mixing or as a colorless solution ready for use. All medications and solutions must be stored in the refrigerator.
- Take your next dose from the refrigerator 1 hour before using it; place it in a clean, dry area to allow it to warm to room temperature.
- Follow all directions provided by your health care provider for preparation of the drug. Let the solution warm to room temperature before administration. Do not use the medication if it has been out of the refrigerator for 24 hours or more or if it has been in the refrigerator longer than 30 days.
- Do not allow interferon alfa-2a or alfa 2b to freeze; do not shake the vials.

Store your medication only as directed. Make sure you understand what you need to store your medication properly.

Keep your supplies in a clean, dry place when you are not using them, and keep all medications and supplies out of reach of children. Your health care provider will tell you how to throw away used needles, syringes, tubing, and containers to avoid accidental injury.

Overdose

In case of overdose, call your local poison control center at 1-800-222-1222. If the victim has collapsed or is not breathing, call local emergency services at 911.

Signs of Infection

If you are receiving interferon alfa under your skin, you need to know the symptoms of a catheter-related infection (an infection where the needle enters your skin). If you experience any of these effects near the infusion site, tell your health care provider as soon as possible:

- tenderness
- warmth
- irritation
- drainage
- redness

- swelling
- pain

Talk to your doctor, pharmacist, or other healthcare professional if you have questions about dosing information for your medication.

Interferon Alfacon-1 Injection

(in ter feer′ on)

Brand Name: Infergen®

About Your Treatment

Your doctor has ordered interferon alfacon-1 to help treat your hepatitis C infection. The drug will be injected under your skin (subcutaneously) three times a week. Your health care provider will show you what to do.

Interferon alfacon-1 is a synthetic interferon that helps to prevent the hepatitis C virus from growing inside your body. This medication is sometimes prescribed for other uses; ask your doctor or pharmacist for more information.

Your health care provider (doctor, nurse, or pharmacist) may measure the effectiveness and side effects of your treatment using laboratory tests and physical examinations. It is important to keep all appointments with your doctor and the laboratory. The length of treatment depends on how you respond to the medication.

Precautions

Before administering interferon alfacon-1,

- tell your doctor and pharmacist if you are allergic to interferon alfacon-1, alfa interferons, E. coli-derived products, or any other drugs.
- tell your doctor and pharmacist what prescription and nonprescription medications you are taking, including carbamazepine (Tegretol); chloramphenicol (Chlormycetin); medications that contain gold (auranofin [Ridaura], aurothioglucose [(Solganol]); medications that suppress your immune system, such as chemotherapy agents; penicillamine (Cuprimine, Depen); phenylbutazone; phenytoin (Dilantin); sulfa drugs; thyroid medications; zidovudine (Retrovir); and vitamins or herbal products.
- tell your doctor if you have or have ever had heart, liver, or autoimmune disease; a recent organ transplant; depression or psychiatric illness; blood disorders; diabetes; thyroid problems; high blood pressure; or vision problems.
- tell your doctor if you are pregnant, plan to become pregnant, or are breast-feeding. If you become pregnant while taking interferon alfacon-1, call your doctor.
- if you are having surgery, including dental surgery, tell the doctor or dentist that you are taking interferon alfacon-1.

Administering Your Medication

Before you administer interferon alfacon-1, look at the solution closely. It should be clear and free of floating material. Observe the solution container to make sure there are no leaks. Do not use the solution if it is discolored or if it contains particles. Use a new solution, but show the damaged one to your health care provider.

It is important that you use your medication exactly as directed. Do not stop your therapy on your own for any reason because your infection may worsen and result in hospitalization. Do not administer it more often than or for longer periods than your doctor tells you. Do not change your dosing schedule without talking to your health care provider.

Side Effects

Interferon alfacon-1 may cause side effects. Interferon alfacon-1 sometimes causes a flu-like reaction, including chills, headache, fever, muscle pain, sweating, and joint pain. The effects should become less severe and less frequent as you continue your therapy.

Tell your health care provider if any of these symptoms are severe or do not go away:

- nervousness
- pain and irritation at site of injection
- difficulty sleeping
- tiredness
- dizziness
- stomach pain
- upset stomach
- diarrhea
- body aches
- headache

If you experience any of the following symptoms, call your doctor immediately:

- vision changes
- difficulty breathing
- swelling of the face, eyelids, lips, or neck
- hives or rash
- chest pain
- chest pressure or heaviness
- depression and thoughts of suicide
- unusual bleeding or bruising
- fast or irregular heartbeats

If you experience a serious side effect, you or your doctor may send a report to the Food and Drug Administration's (FDA) MedWatch Adverse Event Reporting program online [at http://www.fda.gov/MedWatch/index.html] or by phone [1-800-332-1088].

Storage Conditions

Your health care provider will probably give you a several-day supply of interferon alfacon-1 at a time. You will be told to store it in the refrigerator and to protect it from light.

Take your dose from the refrigerator 1 hour before using it; place it in a clean, dry area to allow it to warm to room temperature.

Do not allow interferon alfacon-1 to freeze; do not vigorosly shake the vials. Store your medication only as directed. Make sure you understand what you need to store your medication properly.

Keep your supplies in a clean, dry place when you are not using them, and keep all medications and supplies out of the reach of children. Your health care provider will tell you how to throw away used needles, syringes, tubing, and containers to avoid accidental injury.

Overdose

In case of overdose, call your local poison control center at 1-800-222-1222. If the victim has collapsed or is not breathing, call local emergency services at 911.

Signs of Infection

You should be aware of the symptoms of infection. If you experience any of these effects near the site where you administer your interferon alfacon-1, tell your health care provider as soon as possible:

- tenderness
- warmth
- irritation
- drainage
- redness
- swelling
- pain

Talk to your doctor, pharmacist, or other healthcare professional if you have questions about dosing information for your medication.

Interferon beta-1a Intramuscular Injection

(in-ter-feer′-on bay′-ta wun aye)

Brand Name: Avonex®

Why is this medicine prescribed?

Interferon beta-1a is used to decrease the number of episodes of symptoms and slow the development of disability in patients with relapsing-remitting (symptoms come and go) multiple sclerosis (MS, a disease in which the nerves do not function properly and patients may experience weakness, numbness, loss of muscle coordination and problems with vision, speech, and bladder control). Interferon beta-1a has not been shown to help patients with chronic progressive (symptoms are almost always present and worsen over time) MS. Interferon beta-1a is in a class of medications called immunomodulators. It is not known how interferon beta-1a works to treat MS.

How should this medicine be used?

Interferon beta-1a intramuscular injection comes as a powder to be mixed into a solution for injection, and also as a prefilled injection syringe. This medication is injected into a muscle, usually once a week, on the same day each week. It is best to inject the medication at around the same time of day on your injection days, usually in the late afternoon or evening. Follow the directions on your prescription label carefully, and ask your doctor or pharmacist to explain any part you do not understand. Use interferon beta-1a exactly as directed. Do not use more or less of it or use it more often than prescribed by your doctor.

Interferon beta-1a controls the symptoms of MS, but does not cure it. Continue to use interferon beta-1a even if you feel well. Do not stop using interferon beta-1a without talking to your doctor.

You will receive your first dose of interferon beta-1a in your doctor's office. After that, you can inject interferon beta-1a yourself or have a friend or relative perform the injections. Ask your doctor or pharmacist to show you or the person who will be injecting the medication how to inject it.

Your doctor or pharmacist will give you the manufacturer's patient information sheet (medication guide) when you begin treatment with interferon beta-1a and each time you refill your prescription. Read the information carefully and ask your doctor or pharmacist if you have any questions. You can also visit the Food and Drug Administration (FDA) website (http://www.fda.gov/cder) to obtain the interferon beta-1a Medication Guide.

Always use a new, unopened vial or prefilled syringe and needle for each injection. Never reuse vials, syringes, or needles. Throw away used syringes and needles in a puncture-resistant container, kept out of reach of children. Talk to your doctor or pharmacist about how to throw away the puncture-resistant container.

You can inject interferon beta-1a in your upper arms or thighs. Use a different spot for each injection. Keep a record of the date and spot of each injection. Do not use the same spot two times in a row. Do not inject into an area where the skin is sore, red, bruised, scarred, infected, irritated, or abnormal in any way.

To prepare interferon beta-1a powder for injection, follow these steps:

1. Wash your hands well with antibacterial soap.
2. Remove the interferon beta-1a vial from the refrigerator. Allow it to warm to room temperature for about 30 minutes before using. Do not use a heat source such as hot water or a microwave to warm the vial.
3. Set up a clean, well lit, flat work surface, like a table, to collect all the supplies you will need. Assemble these supplies: vial of interferon beta-1a, vial of sterile water, sterile syringe, sterile needle, blue MICRO PIN (vial access pin), alcohol wipes, and puncture-resistant container.

4. Check the expiration dates on the vials of interferon beta-1a powder and sterile water. If either vial is expired, do not use that vial and call your pharmacist.

5. Remove the caps from the vials of interferon beta-1a powder and sterile water. Clean the rubber stopper on the top of each vial with an alcohol wipe.

6. Remove the small light blue protective cover from the end of the syringe barrel with a counterclockwise (toward the left) turn.

7. Attach the blue MICRO PIN to the syringe by turning clockwise (toward the right) until it is tight. Do not overtighten.

8. Pull the MICRO PIN cover straight off, without twisting. Save the cover for later use.

9. Pull back the syringe plunger to the 1.1-mL mark on the syringe.

10. Firmly push the MICRO PIN on the syringe down through the center of the rubber stopper of the sterile water vial.

11. Push down on the plunger of the syringe until it cannot be pushed down any further.

12. Keep the MICRO PIN in the vial and turn the vial and syringe upside down.

13. Keep the MICRO PIN in the liquid while you slowly pull back on the syringe plunger to the 1.1 mL mark.

14. Gently tap the syringe with your finger to make any air bubbles rise to the top. If there are bubbles, slowly press the plunger in just enough to push the bubbles (but not liquid) out of the syringe. Make sure there is still 1.1 mL of sterile water in the syringe.

15. Slowly pull the MICRO PIN out of the sterile water vial.

16. Carefully push the MICRO PIN through the center of the rubber stopper of the interferon beta-1a powder vial. Pushing the MICRO PIN through the vial stopper off-center can cause the stopper to fall into the vial. If the stopper falls into the vial, do not use that vial. Get a new vial and continue to prepare your dose.

17. Slowly push down on the plunger until the syringe is empty. Do not aim the stream of water directly on the medication powder. A forceful or direct stream of liquid on the powder will cause foaming and make it difficult to withdraw the medication.

18. Without removing the syringe, gently swirl the vial until the interferon beta-1a powder is dissolved. Do not shake. The solution should be clear to slightly yellow and should not have any particles. Do not use the vial if the solution is cloudy, has particles in it, or is another color.

19. Turn the vial and syringe upside down. Slowly pull back on the plunger of the syringe until it is filled to the 1.0-mL mark. If bubbles appear, push the solution slowly back into the vial and try again.

20. Continue to hold the vial and syringe upside down. Tap the syringe gently to make any air bubbles rise to the top. Press the plunger in until the solution moves up to the top of the syringe and there is still 1.0 mL of solution left in the syringe. Pull the MICRO PIN out of the vial.

21. Hold the syringe upright and carefully replace the cover on the MICRO PIN. Then remove the MICRO PIN from the syringe with a counterclockwise (to the left) turn.

22. Attach the sterile needle for injection to the syringe by turning the needle clockwise (to the right) until it is tight.

23. Throw away the blue MICRO PIN in a puncture-resistant container. See below for injection instructions.

To prepare a prefilled syringe of interferon beta-1a intramuscular injection, follow these steps:

1. Wash your hands well with antibacterial soap. Set up a clean, well-lit, flat work surface, like a table, to collect all the supplies you will need. Remove the prefilled syringe from the refrigerator and allow it to warm to room temperature for about 30 minutes before using. Do not use a heat source such as hot water or a microwave to warm the syringe.

2. Check the syringe to be sure it is safe to use. The syringe should be labeled with the correct name of the medication and an expiration date that has not passed and should contain a clear, colorless solution filled to the 0.5-mL mark. Hold the syringe so that the rubber cap is facing down and the 0.5-mL mark on the syringe is at eye level. Check to make sure the lowest point of the curved surface of the liquid in the syringe is level with or very close to the 0.5-mL mark. If the syringe does not have the correct amount of liquid, the syringe is expired, or the solution is cloudy, discolored, or contains any particles, do not use the syringe and call your pharmacist.

3. Hold the prefilled syringe upright, with the rubber cap facing up.

4. Remove the rubber cap by turning and gently pulling the cap in a clockwise (toward the right) direction.

5. Open the needle package and attach the needle to the syringe by firmly pressing it onto the syringe and turning it a half-turn clockwise (toward the right). Be sure to attach the needle tightly so medication will not leak.

To inject an intramuscular dose of interferon beta-1a, follow these steps:

1. Use a new alcohol wipe to clean the skin in the spot where you will inject interferon beta-1a. Use a circular motion, starting at the injection spot and moving outward. Let the skin dry before you inject interferon beta-1a.

2. Pull the protective cover straight off the needle without twisting.

3. Use one hand to stretch the skin out around the spot where you will inject the medication. Use your other hand to hold the syringe like a pencil. Use a quick motion to stick the needle in the skin at a 90-degree angle (straight up and down) and push the needle through the skin and into your muscle.

4. If you are injecting your medication using a prefilled syringe, skip this step and go on to Step 5. If you are in-

jecting your medication using a syringe that you filled yourself, let go of the skin and use that hand to gently pull back slightly on the syringe plunger. If you see blood come into the syringe, pull the needle out of the injection spot and put pressure on the spot with a gauze pad. You will need to replace the needle with a new needle, choose a new spot for injection, and go back to Step 1.

5. Hold the syringe with one hand and use the other hand to slowly push the plunger down until the syringe is empty.

6. Hold a gauze pad near the needle at the injection spot and pull the needle straight out of the skin. Use the gauze pad to apply pressure to the spot for a few seconds or rub gently in a circular motion.

7. If there is slight bleeding at the spot, wipe it off with the gauze pad, and apply an adhesive bandage if necessary.

8. Throw away the used syringe and needle in a puncture-resistant container.

9. After 2 hours, check the injection site for redness, swelling, or tenderness. If you have redness, swelling, or tenderness that does not go away in a few days or is severe, call your doctor.

Are there other uses for this medicine?

This medication may be prescribed for other uses; ask your doctor or pharmacist for more information.

What special precautions should I follow?

Before using interferon beta-1a,

- tell your doctor and pharmacist if you are allergic to interferon beta-1a, any other interferon product, any other medications, human albumin, natural rubber, latex, or any of the ingredients in interferon beta-1a intramuscular injection. Ask your pharmacist for a list of the ingredients in interferon beta-1a.

- tell your doctor and pharmacist what other prescription and nonprescription medications, vitamins, nutritional supplements, and herbal products you are taking or plan to take. Be sure to mention any of the following: acetaminophen (Tylenol, others); antidepressants; azathioprine (Imuran); cancer chemotherapy medications; cholesterol-lowering medications (statins); cyclosporine (Neoral, Sandimmune); iron products; isoniazid (INH, Nydrazid); medications for acquired immunodeficiency syndrome (AIDS) or human immunodeficiency virus (HIV); methotrexate (Rheumatrex); niacin (nicotinic acid); rifampin (Rifadin, Rimactane); salicylate pain relievers such as aspirin, choline magnesium trisalicylate, choline salicylate (Arthropan), difunisal (Dolobid), magnesium salicylate (Doan's, others), and salsalate (Argesic, Disalcid, Salgesic); sirolimus (Rapamune); and tacrolimus (Prograf). Your doctor may need to change the doses of your medications or monitor you carefully for side effects.

- tell your doctor if you drink or have ever drunk large amounts of alcohol and if you have or have ever had

AIDS or HIV; an autoimmune disease other than MS (a disease in which the body attacks its own cells; ask your doctor if you are unsure if you have this type of disease); blood problems such as anemia (red blood cells that do not bring enough oxygen to all parts of the body), low white blood cells, or easy bruising or bleeding; cancer; anxiety, depression, other mood disorders, or mental illness; difficulty falling asleep or staying asleep; seizures; angina (recurring chest pain); or heart, liver, or thyroid disease.

- tell your doctor if you are pregnant, plan to become pregnant, or are breast-feeding. If you become pregnant while using interferon beta-1a, stop using the medication and call your doctor immediately. Interferon beta-1a may harm the fetus.

- if you are having surgery, including dental surgery, tell the doctor or dentist that you are using interferon beta-1a.

- ask your doctor about the safe use of alcoholic beverages while you are using interferon beta-1a. Alcohol can increase the risk that you will develop serious side effects from interferon beta-1a.

- you should know that you may have flu-like symptoms such as headache, fever, chills, sweating, muscle aches, upset stomach, vomiting, and tiredness that last for a day after your injection. Your doctor may tell you to inject your medication at bedtime and take an over-the-counter pain and fever medication to help with these symptoms. These symptoms usually lessen or go away over time. Talk to your doctor if these symptoms last longer than the first few months of therapy, or if they are difficult to manage or become severe.

What special dietary instructions should I follow?

Unless your doctor tells you otherwise, continue your normal diet.

What should I do if I forget to take a dose?

Inject the missed dose as soon as you remember it. Do not inject interferon beta-1a two days in a row. Do not inject a double dose to make up for a missed dose. Return to your regular dosing schedule the following week. Call your doctor if you miss a dose and have questions about what to do.

What side effects can this medicine cause?

Interferon beta-1a may cause side effects. Tell your doctor if any of these symptoms are severe or do not go away:

- tight muscles
- dizziness
- numbness, burning, tingling, or pain in hands or feet
- joint pain
- stomach pain
- eye problems
- runny nose
- toothache

- hair loss
- bruising, pain, redness, swelling, bleeding, or irritation at the injection spot

Some side effects can be serious. The following symptoms are uncommon, but if you experience any of them, call your doctor immediately:

- depression
- thoughts of hurting or killing yourself
- feeling very emotional
- hallucinating (seeing things or hearing voices that do not exist)
- seizures
- unexplained weight gain or loss
- feeling cold or hot all the time
- trouble breathing when lying flat in bed
- increased need to urinate during the night
- painful or difficult urination
- decreased ability to exercise
- chest pain or tightness
- fast or irregular heartbeat
- pale skin
- excessive tiredness
- lack of energy
- loss of appetite
- unusual bleeding or bruising
- pain or swelling in the upper right part of the stomach
- yellowing of the skin or eyes
- dark brown urine
- light-colored bowel movements
- sore throat, cough, or other signs of infection
- hives
- rash
- itching
- swelling of the face, throat, tongue, lips, eyes, hands, arms, feet, ankles, or lower legs
- difficulty breathing or swallowing
- hoarseness
- flushing

Interferon beta-1a may cause other side effects. Call your doctor if you have any unusual problems while taking this medication.

If you experience a serious side effect, you or your doctor may send a report to the Food and Drug Administration's (FDA) MedWatch Adverse Event Reporting program online [at http://www.fda.gov/MedWatch/index.html] or by phone [1-800-332-1088].

What storage conditions are needed for this medicine?

Keep this medication in the container it came in, tightly closed, and out of reach of children. Store interferon beta-1a prefilled syringes and vials in the refrigerator. Do not freeze interferon beta-1a, and do not expose the medication to high temperatures. If a refrigerator is not available, you can store the vials of interferon beta-1a at room temperature, away from heat and light, for up to 30 days. After you mix interferon beta-1a powder with sterile water, store it in the refrigerator and use it within 6 hours. Use prefilled syringes within 12 hours after you take them out of the refrigerator. Throw away mixed vials or syringes after this time has passed. Throw away any medication that is outdated or no longer needed. Talk to your pharmacist about the proper disposal of your medication.

What should I do in case of overdose?

In case of overdose, call your local poison control center at 1-800-222-1222. If the victim has collapsed or is not breathing, call local emergency services at 911.

What other information should I know?

Keep all appointments with your doctor and the laboratory. Your doctor will order certain lab tests to check your body's response to interferon beta-1a.

Do not let anyone else take your medication. Ask your pharmacist any questions you have about refilling your prescription.

Dosage Facts
For Informational Purposes

Caution: Do not change your dose, how often you take your medication, or the length of time you are to take it without first talking to your healthcare provider.

The following dosage information was written using medical language for doctors and other healthcare professionals and is provided here for you to check your dosage. The dosage of this drug may differ for different patients. Therefore, always follow your doctor's instructions or the directions on the label. Contact your healthcare provider or pharmacist if you have any questions about the specific dosage of your medication after reviewing this information.

General Dosage Information

Available as interferon beta-1a; dosage and potency expressed in terms of international units (IU, units) or mg.

Each mg of interferon beta-1a is approximately equivalent to 200 million units (for Avonex®).

Adult Patients

Relapsing-remitting MS
Interferon beta-1a (Avonex®)

IM:
- 6 million units (30 mcg) once weekly. Safety and efficacy of Avonex® given for >3 years not established.

Prescribing Limits

Adult Patients

IM:
- Safety of interferon beta-1a (Avonex®) dosages >12 million units (60 mcg) once weekly not established.

Special Populations

Hepatic Impairment

- Consider decreasing dosages if serum ALT concentrations >5 times ULN.
- Discontinue therapy if hepatic transaminase (AST, ALT) concentrations >10 times ULN (with or without jaundice or other clinical symptoms of liver dysfunction) or if the serum bilirubin >5 times ULN.
- When concentrations return to normal, interferon beta therapy may be restarted at a 50% dose reduction, if clinically appropriate.

Geriatric Patients

- Titrate dosage, usually initiating therapy at the low end of the dosage range due to possible age-related decreases in hepatic, renal, and/or cardiac function and of concomitant disease and drug therapy.

Interferon beta-1a Subcutaneous Injection

(in-ter-feer'-on bay'-ta wun aye)

Brand Name: Rebif®

Why is this medicine prescribed?

Interferon beta-1a is used to prevent episodes of symptoms and slow the development of disability in patients with relapsing-remitting multiple sclerosis (MS, a disease in which the nerves do not function properly and patients may experience weakness, numbness, loss of muscle coordination and problems with vision, speech, and bladder control). Interferon beta-1a has not been shown to help patients with chronic progressive MS. Interferon beta-1a is in a class of medications called immunomodulators. It is not known how interferon beta-1a works to treat MS.

How should this medicine be used?

Interferon beta-1a subcutaneous injection comes as a solution to inject subcutaneously (under the skin) three times a week. You should inject this medication on the same 3 days every week, for example, every Monday, Wednesday, and Friday. The injections should be spaced at least 48 hours apart, so it is best to inject your medication around the same time of day on each of your injection days. The best time to inject this medication is in the late afternoon or evening. Follow the directions on your prescription label carefully, and ask your doctor or pharmacist to explain any part you do not understand. Use interferon beta-1a exactly as directed. Do not use more or less of it or use it more often than prescribed by your doctor.

Your doctor may start you on a low dose of interferon beta-1a and gradually increase your dose, not more than once every 2 weeks.

Interferon beta-1a controls symptoms of MS, but does not cure it. Continue to take interferon beta-1a even if you feel well. Do not stop taking interferon beta-1a without talking to your doctor.

You will receive your first dose of interferon beta-1a in your doctor's office. After that, you can inject interferon beta-1a yourself or have a friend or relative perform the injections. Before you use interferon beta-1a yourself the first time, read the written instructions that come with it. Ask your doctor or pharmacist to show you or the person who will be injecting the medication how to inject it.

Interferon beta-1a comes in prefilled syringes. Use each syringe and needle only once and inject all the solution in the syringe. Even if there is still some solution left in the syringe after you inject, do not inject again. Throw away used syringes and needles in a puncture-resistant container kept out of reach of children. Talk to your doctor or pharmacist about how to throw away the puncture-resistant container.

You can inject interferon beta-1a in areas of your body with a layer of fat between the skin and muscle, such as your thigh, the outer surface of your upper arms, your stomach, or your buttocks. If you are very thin, only inject in your thigh or the outer surface of your arm for injection. Use a different spot for each injection. Keep a record of the date and spot of each injection. Do not use the same spot two times in a row. Do not inject near your navel (belly button) or waistline or into an area where the skin is sore, red, bruised, scarred, infected, or abnormal in any way.

To inject interferon beta-1a, follow these steps:

1. Remove the prefilled syringe from the refrigerator and allow it to warm to room temperature for about 30 minutes before using. Do not use a heat source such as hot water or a microwave to warm the syringe.
2. Check the syringe to be sure it is safe to use. The syringe should be labeled with the correct name of the medication and an expiration date that has not passed and should contain a clear to slightly yellow solution. If the syringe is expired, or the solution is cloudy, discolored, or contains particles, do not use it and call your pharmacist.
3. Set-up a clean, well-lit, flat work surface, like a table, to collect all the supplies you will need to inject interferon beta-1a. Assemble these supplies: alcohol wipes, gauze pad, small adhesive bandage, and puncture-resistant container for disposal of used syringes and needles.
4. Wash your hands well with antibacterial soap.
5. Choose a spot to inject interferon beta-1a and clean it with an alcohol wipe, using a circular motion. Let the skin air dry.
6. Remove the cap from the syringe needle.
7. The syringe should be filled with interferon beta-1a to the 0.5 mL mark. This is a full dose. If your doctor has told you to use less than the full dose, slowly push the

syringe plunger in until the amount of medication left in the syringe is the amount your doctor told you to use.

8. Use your thumb and forefinger to pinch up a pad of skin around the spot where you will inject interferon beta-1a. Hold the syringe like a pencil with your other hand.

9. Hold the syringe at a 90-degree angle (straight up and down), and push the needle straight into your skin, stopping just underneath the skin.

10. When the needle is in, let go of the pinched skin and slowly push down on the syringe plunger until the syringe is empty.

11. Hold a gauze pad near the needle and pull the needle straight out of the skin. Use the gauze pad to apply pressure to the spot for a few seconds. You may cover the spot with a bandage.

12. Throw away the used syringe, needle, and gauze pad properly.

13. Apply a cold compress or ice pack to the injection spot to help reduce redness, swelling, or tenderness that may occur.

14. After 2 hours, check the injection spot for redness, swelling, or tenderness. If you have redness, swelling, or tenderness that does not go away in a few days or is severe, call your doctor.

Are there other uses for this medicine?

This medication may be prescribed for other uses; ask your doctor or pharmacist for more information.

What special precautions should I follow?

Before using interferon beta-1a,

- tell your doctor and pharmacist if you are allergic to interferon beta-1a, any other interferon product, any other medications, or human albumin.

- tell your doctor and pharmacist what other prescription and nonprescription medications, vitamins, nutritional supplements, and herbal products you are taking. Be sure to mention any of the following: acetaminophen (Tylenol, others); antidepressants; azathioprine (Imuran); cancer chemotherapy medications; carbamazepine (Tegretol); chloramphenicol (Chloromycetin); cholesterol-lowering medications (statins); cyclosporine (Neoral, Sandimmune); gold compounds such as auranofin (Ridaura) and aurothioglucose (Solganol); heparin; iron products; isoniazid (INH, Nydrazid); medications for acquired immunodeficiency syndrome (AIDS) or human immunodeficiency virus (HIV); methotrexate (Rheumatrex); niacin (nicotinic acid); penicillamine (Cuprimine, Depen); phenytoin (Dilantin, Phenytek); rifampin (Rifadin, Rimactane); sirolimus (Rapamune); sulfa antibiotics such as sulfamethoxazole (Bactrim, Septra) and sulfisoxazole (Gantrisin); thyroid medications; and tacrolimus (Prograf). Your doctor may need to change the doses of your medications or monitor you carefully for side effects.

- tell your doctor if you drink or have ever drunk large

amounts of alcohol and if you have or have ever had AIDS or HIV; an autoimmune disease (a disease in which the body attacks its own cells; ask your doctor if you are not sure if you have this type of disease); blood problems such as anemia (low red blood cells) or easy bruising or bleeding; anxiety, depression, or mental illness; cancer; seizures; or kidney, liver, or thyroid disease.

- tell your doctor if you are pregnant, plan to become pregnant, or are breast-feeding. If you become pregnant while taking interferon beta-1a, call your doctor immediately.

- if you are having surgery, including dental surgery, tell the doctor or dentist you are using interferon beta-1a.

- ask your doctor about the safe use of alcoholic beverages while you are using interferon beta-1a. Alcohol can make the side effects of interferon beta-1a worse.

- you should know that you may have flu-like symptoms such as headache, fever, chills, sweating, muscle aches, back pain, and tiredness that last for a day after your injection. Your doctor may tell you to take an over-the-counter pain and fever medication to help with these symptoms. These symptoms usually improve or go away over time. Talk to your doctor if these symptoms last longer than the first few months of therapy, or if they are difficult to manage or become severe.

What special dietary instructions should I follow?

Unless your doctor tells you otherwise, continue your normal diet.

What should I do if I forget to take a dose?

Inject the missed dose as soon as you remember it. If you are scheduled for a dose the following day, skip that dose. Do not inject interferon beta-1a 2 days in a row. Do not inject a double dose to make up for a missed dose. You should return to your regular dosing schedule the following week. Call your doctor if you miss a dose and have questions about what to do.

What side effects can this medicine cause?

Interferon beta-1a may cause side effects. Tell your doctor if any of these symptoms are severe or do not go away:

- dry eyes
- dry mouth
- upset stomach
- vomiting
- stomach pain
- tight muscles
- bruising, pain, redness, swelling, or tenderness in the place where you injected interferon beta-1a

Some side effects can be serious. The following symptoms are uncommon, but if you experience any of them, call your doctor immediately:

- depression

- thoughts of hurting yourself or others
- anxiety
- hives
- skin rash
- itching
- flushing
- difficulty breathing or swallowing
- lightheadedness
- fainting
- seizures
- loss of coordination
- vision problems
- extreme tiredness
- lack of energy
- loss of appetite
- pain in the upper right part of the stomach
- yellowing of the skin or eyes
- pale skin
- chest pain
- fast heartbeat
- difficulty sleeping
- unusual bruising or bleeding
- swollen glands in your neck
- sore throat, cough, fever, chills, or other signs of infection
- unexplained weight gain or loss
- feeling cold or hot all the time
- blackening of skin or drainage in the place where you injected interferon beta-1a

Interferon beta-1a may cause other side effects. Call your doctor if you have any unusual problems while taking this medication.

If you experience a serious side effect, you or your doctor may send a report to the Food and Drug Administration's (FDA) MedWatch Adverse Event Reporting program online [at http://www.fda.gov/MedWatch/index.html] or by phone [1-800-332-1088].

What storage conditions are needed for this medicine?

Keep this medication in the container it came in, tightly closed, and out of reach of children. Store it in the refrigerator, but do not freeze it. If a refrigerator is not available, you can store the medication at room temperature away from heat and light for up to 30 days. Throw away any medication that is outdated or no longer needed. Talk to your pharmacist about the proper disposal of your medication.

What should I do in case of overdose?

In case of overdose, call your local poison control center at 1-800-222-1222. If the victim has collapsed or is not breathing, call local emergency services at 911.

What other information should I know?

Keep all appointments with your doctor and the laboratory. Your doctor will order certain lab tests to check your body's response to interferon beta-1a.

Do not let anyone else take your medication. Ask your pharmacist any questions you have about refilling your prescription.

Dosage Facts
For Informational Purposes

Caution: Do not change your dose, how often you take your medication, or the length of time you are to take it without first talking to your healthcare provider.

The following dosage information was written using medical language for doctors and other healthcare professionals and is provided here for you to check your dosage. The dosage of this drug may differ for different patients. Therefore, always follow your doctor's instructions or the directions on the label. Contact your healthcare provider or pharmacist if you have any questions about the specific dosage of your medication after reviewing this information.

General Dosage Information

Available as interferon beta-1a; dosage and potency expressed in terms of international units (IU, units) or mg.

Each mg of interferon beta-1a is approximately equivalent to 270 million units (for Rebif®).

Adult Patients

Relapsing-remitting MS
Interferon beta-1a (Rebif®)

SUB-Q:
- Gradually titrate dosage over a 4-week period to 6 million units (22 mcg) or 12 million units (44 mcg) 3 times weekly using the following schedule:

Rebif® Dosage Titration Schedule

	Recommended Titration (% of Final Target)	Rebif® 22 mcg Target Dose	Rebif® 44 mcg Target Dose
Weeks 1–2	20%	1.2 million units (4.4 mcg)	2.4 million units (8.8 mcg)
Weeks 3–4	50%	3 million units (11 mcg)	6 million units (22 mcg)
Weeks 5+	100%	6 million units (22 mcg)	12 million units (44 mcg)

Special Populations

Hepatic Impairment
- Consider decreasing dosages if serum ALT concentrations >5 times ULN.
- Discontinue therapy if hepatic transaminase (AST, ALT) concentrations >10 times ULN (with or without jaundice or other

clinical symptoms of liver dysfunction) or if the serum bilirubin >5 times ULN.

- When concentrations return to normal, interferon beta therapy may be restarted at a 50% dose reduction, if clinically appropriate.

Geriatric Patients

- Titrate dosage, usually initiating therapy at the low end of the dosage range due to possible age-related decreases in hepatic, renal, and/or cardiac function and of concomitant disease and drug therapy.

Interferon Beta-1b Injection

(in ter feer′ on)

Brand Name: Betaseron®

About Your Treatment

Your doctor has ordered interferon beta-1b, a biologic response modifier. This medication is used to treat patients with multiple sclerosis (MS), a disease in which the nerves do not function properly and patients may experience weakness; numbness; loss of muscle coordination; and problems with vision, speech, and bladder control. This medication will be injected subcutaneously (under the skin) every other day. Your health care provider will show you how to prepare and give the injection.

Interferon beta-1b is a man-made version of a naturally occuring protein. It is used to treat patients with relapsing forms of MS (course of disease where symptoms flare up for a short time, then go away). Interferon beta-1b does not cure MS but may reduce the number of disease flare-ups. Interferon beta-1b may be prescribed for other uses; ask your doctor or pharmacist for more information.

Your health care provider (doctor, nurse, or pharmacist) may measure the effectiveness and side effects of your treatment using laboratory tests and physical examinations. It is important to keep all appointments with your doctor and the laboratory. The length of treatment depends on how you respond to the medication.

Precautions

Before using interferon beta-1b,

- tell your doctor and pharmacist if you are allergic to interferon beta-1b, or any other medications, or human albumin.
- tell your doctor and pharmacist what other prescription and nonprescription medications, vitamins, nutritional supplements, and herbal products you are taking or plan to take. Your doctor may need to change the doses of your medications or monitor you carefully for side effects.

- tell your doctor if you drink or have ever drunk large amounts of alcohol, if you have or have ever had anemia (low red blood cells) or low white blood cells, blood problems such as bruising easily or bleeding, diabetes, anxiety, depression, mental illness, thoughts of hurting yourself, seizures, trouble falling asleep or staying asleep, or prostate, skin, thyroid, blood, heart, or liver disease.
- tell your doctor if you are pregnant, plan to become pregnant, or are breast-feeding. If you become pregnant while taking interferon beta-1b, stop using interferon beta-1b immediately and call your doctor.

Administering Your Medication

Before you administer interferon beta-1b, look at the solution closely. It should be clear and free of floating material. Observe the solution container to make sure there are no leaks and check the expiration date. Do not use the solution if it is discolored, if it contains particles, or if the container leaks or it is expired. Use a new solution, but show the damaged or expired one to your health care provider.

It is important that you use your medication exactly as directed. Your health care provider may start you on a low dose of interferon beta-1b and gradually increase your dose. Do not change your dosing schedule without talking to your health care provider. Your injections should be approximately 48 hours (2 days) apart, so it is best to give them at the same time, preferably in the evening just before bedtime.

Do not inject interferon beta-1b into an area of skin that is irritated, sore, red, bruised, infected, damaged, or abnormal in any way. It is important that you change your injection area each time interferon beta-1b is injected; keeping a record will help you to remember to rotate injection sites. Do not use the same injection area two times in a row. Do not inject interferon beta-1b near the navel (bellybutton) or waistline.

If you miss a dose of interferon beta-1b, inject your next dose as soon as you remember or are able to give it. Your next injection should then be given 48 hours (2 days) after that dose. Do not use interferon beta-1b on 2 days in a row. If you accidentally take more than your prescribed dose, or give it on 2 days in a row, call your health care provider right away.

Side Effects

Side effects from interferon beta-1b can occur. Interferon beta-1b sometimes causes a flu-like illness with headache, fever, chills, sweating, muscle aches, tiredness, and general discomfort. Tell your health care provider if any of these problems continue or worsen. You should talk with your health care provider about whether to take an over the counter medication for pain or fever before or after taking your dose of interferon beta-1b.

Tell your health care provider if any of these symptoms are severe or do not go away:

- upset stomach

- indigestion
- diarrhea
- constipation
- weight gain or weight loss
- feeling cold or hot much of the time
- dizziness
- increased urinary frequency
- incontinence
- flushing
- hair loss
- joint or muscle weakness or pain
- leg cramps
- difficulty falling asleep or staying asleep
- changes in sex drive or ability (in men)
- increased menstrual pain

If you experience any of the following symptoms, call your health care provider immediately:

- extreme tiredness
- lack of energy
- unusual bruising or bleeding
- loss of appetite
- pain in the upper right part of the stomach
- yellowing of the skin or eyes
- hives
- rash
- itching
- difficulty breathing or swallowing
- swelling of the face, throat, tongue, lips, eyes, hands, feet, ankles, abdomen (stomach), or lower legs
- hoarseness
- vaginal bleeding or spotting between menstrual periods
- change in coordination
- heart palpitations or rapid heart rate
- chest pain
- nervousness
- depression
- anxiety
- thoughts of hurting yourself
- swollen lymph nodes

Interferon beta-1b affects your immune system so it may increase your risk of developing a serious infection. Talk to your health care provider about the risks of using this medication.

Interferon beta-1b may cause other side effects. Call your health care provider if you have any unusual problems while taking this medication.

If you experience a serious side effect, you or your doctor may send a report to the Food and Drug Administration's (FDA) MedWatch Adverse Event Reporting program online [at http://www.fda.gov/MedWatch/index.html] or by phone [1-800-332-1088].

Storage Conditions

- Your health care provider probably will give you a several-day supply of interferon beta-1b at a time and provide you with directions on how to prepare each dose. Store the vials at room temperature.

- You should use a prepared dose immediately after mixing and allowing any foam in the solution to settle. If you must wait to give the injection, you may refrigerate the prepared dose and use it within 3 hours after bringing it to room temperature before injecting. Avoid shaking the vial. Use a vial and syringe only once, and do not reenter a needle into the vial. Throw away any unused portion of medication.
- Do not allow interferon beta-1b to freeze.

Store your medication only as directed. Make sure you understand what you need to store your medication properly.

Keep your supplies in a clean, dry place when you are not using them, and keep all medications and supplies out of reach of children. Do not throw needles or syringes in the household trash or recycle. Your health care provider will tell you how to throw away used needles and syringes in a puncture-proof container to avoid accidental injury.

Overdose

In case of overdose, call your local poison control center at 1-800-222-1222. If the victim has collapsed or is not breathing, call local emergency services at 911.

Signs of Infection

If you are receiving interferon beta-1b under your skin, you need to know the signs of an injection area infection (an infection at the area where you have given your medication subcutaneously). If you experience any of these signs near an injection area, call your health care provider as soon as possible:

- swelling
- lump
- pain
- irritation
- redness
- bruising
- drainage
- dark discoloration
- other skin problems

Dosage Facts
For Informational Purposes

Caution: Do not change your dose, how often you take your medication, or the length of time you are to take it without first talking to your health-care provider.

The following dosage information was written using medical language for doctors and other healthcare professionals and is provided here for you to check your dosage. The dosage of this drug may differ for different patients. Therefore, always follow your doctor's instructions or the directions on the label. Contact your health-care provider or pharmacist if you have any questions about the specific dosage of your medication after reviewing this information.

General Dosage Information

Available as interferon beta-1a or interferon beta-1b; dosage and potency expressed in terms of international units (IU, units) or mg.

Each mg of interferon beta-1a is approximately equivalent to 270 million units (for Rebif®).

Adult Patients

Relapsing-remitting MS
Interferon beta-1b (Betaseron®)

SUB-Q:
- Gradually titrate dosage over a 6-week period to 8 million units (0.25 mg) every other day using the following schedule:

Betaseron® Dosage Titration Schedule

	Betaseron® Dose
Weeks 1–2	2 million units (0.0625 mg)
Weeks 3–4	4 million units (0.125 mg)
Weeks 5–6	6 million units (0.1875 mg)
Weeks 7+	8 million units (0.25 mg)

Safety and efficacy of interferon beta-1b (Betaseron®) given for >3 years not established.

Special Populations

Hepatic Impairment
- Consider decreasing dosages if serum ALT concentrations >5 times ULN.
- Discontinue therapy if hepatic transaminase (AST, ALT) concentrations >10 times ULN (with or without jaundice or other clinical symptoms of liver dysfunction) or if the serum bilirubin >5 times ULN.
- When concentrations return to normal, interferon beta therapy may be restarted at a 50% dose reduction, if clinically appropriate.

Geriatric Patients
- Titrate dosage, usually initiating therapy at the low end of the dosage range due to possible age-related decreases in hepatic, renal, and/or cardiac function and of concomitant disease and drug therapy.

Interferon Gamma-1b Injection

(in ter feer′ on)

Brand Name: Actimmune®

About Your Treatment

Your doctor has ordered interferon gamma-1b. This drug is a manmade version of a substance normally produced by your body's cells to help fight infections, and it is used to treat patients with chronic granulomatous disease. The drug will be injected under your skin three times a week. This medication is sometimes prescribed for other uses; ask your doctor or pharmacist for more information.

Your health care provider (doctor, nurse, or pharmacist) may measure the effectiveness and side effects of your treatment using laboratory tests and physical examinations. It is important to keep all appointments with your doctor and the laboratory. The length of treatment depends on how you respond to the medication.

Precautions

Before administering interferon gamma-1b,
- tell your doctor and pharmacist if you are allergic to interferon gamma-1b or any other drugs.
- tell your doctor and pharmacist what prescription and nonprescription medications you are taking, including vitamins.
- tell your doctor if you have or have ever had heart disease or seizures.
- tell your doctor if you are pregnant, plan to become pregnant, or are breast-feeding. If you become pregnant while taking interferon gamma-1b, call your doctor.

Administering Your Medication

Before you administer interferon gamma-1b, look at the solution closely. It should be clear and free of floating material. Observe the solution container to make sure there are no leaks. Do not use the solution if it is discolored, if it contains particles, or if the container leaks. Use a new solution, but show the damaged one to your health care provider.

It is important that you use your medication exactly as directed. Do not stop your therapy on your own for any reason. Do not change your dosing schedule without talking to your health care provider.

Side Effects

The most common side effects from interferon gamma-1b are flu-like symptoms which include fever, headache, chills, muscle pain, and fatigue. Your health care provider may advise you to inject your dose of interferon gamma-1b at bedtime to lessen these effects.

If you experience any of the following symptoms, call your health care provider immediately:
- unusual bleeding or bruising
- pinpoint red spots on skin
- black, tarry stools
- blood in urine or stool

Storage Conditions

- Your health care provider probably will give you a several-day supply of interferon gamma-1b at a time. If you are receiving interferon gamma-1b, you probably will be told to store it in the refrigerator.

- Take your next dose from the refrigerator 1 hour before using it; place it in a clean, dry area to allow it to warm to room temperature. Do not let the vial remain out of the refrigerator for more than 12 hours.
- Do not allow interferon gamma-1b to freeze.

Store your medication only as directed. Make sure you understand what you need to store your medication properly.

Keep your supplies in a clean, dry place when you are not using them, and keep all medications and supplies out of reach of children. Your health care provider will tell you how to throw away used needles, syringes, and containers to avoid accidental injury.

Overdose

In case of overdose, call your local poison control center at 1-800-222-1222. If the victim has collapsed or is not breathing, call local emergency services at 911.

Signs of Infection

If you are receiving interferon gamma-1b under your skin, you need to know the symptoms of an infection where the needle enters your skin. If you experience any of these effects near your site of injection, tell your health care provider as soon as possible:

- tenderness
- warmth
- irritation
- drainage
- redness
- swelling
- pain

Dosage Facts
For Informational Purposes

Caution: Do not change your dose, how often you take your medication, or the length of time you are to take it without first talking to your health-care provider.

The following dosage information was written using medical language for doctors and other healthcare professionals and is provided here for you to check your dosage. The dosage of this drug may differ for different patients. Therefore, always follow your doctor's instructions or the directions on the label. Contact your healthcare provider or pharmacist if you have any questions about the specific dosage of your medication after reviewing this information.

General Dosage Information

Each mg of interferon gamma-1b is approximately equivalent to 20 million international units (equivalent to the amount that formerly was expressed as 30 million units).

Pediatric Patients

Chronic Granulomatous Disease

SUB-Q:
- 50 mcg/m^2 (1 million international units per m^2) 3 times weekly for patients with body surface area (BSA) >0.5 m^2 and 1.5 mcg/kg 3 times weekly for those with body surface area ≤0.5 m^2.
- If a severe adverse reaction (e.g., flu-like symptoms) occurs, reduce dosage by 50% or discontinue drug until adverse reaction abates.

Osteopetrosis

SUB-Q:
- 50 mcg/m^2 (1 million international units per m^2) 3 times weekly for patients with body surface area >0.5 m^2 and 1.5 mcg/kg 3 times weekly for those with body surface area ≤0.5 m^2.
- If a severe adverse reaction (e.g., flu-like symptoms) occurs, reduce dosage by 50% or discontinue drug until adverse reaction abates.

Adult Patients

Chronic Granulomatous Disease

SUB-Q:
- 50 mcg/m^2 (1 million international units per m^2) 3 times weekly.
- If a severe adverse reaction (e.g., flu-like symptoms) occurs, reduce dosage by 50% or discontinue drug until adverse reaction abates.

Osteopetrosis

SUB-Q:
- 50 mcg/m^2 (1 million international units per m^2) 3 times weekly.
- If a severe adverse reaction (e.g., flu-like symptoms) occurs, reduce dosage by 50% or discontinue drug until adverse reaction abates.

Prescribing Limits

Pediatric Patients

Chronic Granulomatous Disease

SUB-Q:
- Safety and efficacy of dosages >50 mcg/m^2 3 times weekly not established.

Osteopetrosis

SUB-Q:
- Safety and efficacy of dosages >50 mcg/m^2 3 times weekly not established.

Adult Patients

Chronic Granulomatous Disease

SUB-Q:
- Safety and efficacy of dosages >50 mcg/m^2 3 times weekly not established.

Osteopetrosis

SUB-Q:
- Safety and efficacy of dosages >50 mcg/m^2 3 times weekly not established.

Ipratropium and Albuterol Inhalation

(i pra troe′ pee um) (al byoo′ ter ole)

Brand Name: Combivent®, Duoneb®

Why is this medicine prescribed?

The combination of ipratropium and albuterol is used to prevent wheezing, difficulty breathing, chest tightness, and coughing in people with chronic obstructive pulmonary disease (COPD; a group of diseases that affect the lungs and airways) such as chronic bronchitis (swelling of the air passages that lead to the lungs) and emphysema (damage to the air sacs in the lungs). Ipratropium and albuterol combination is used by people whose symptoms have not been controlled by a single inhaled medication. Ipratropium and albuterol are in a class of medications called bronchodilators. Ipratropium and albuterol combination works by relaxing and opening the air passages to the lungs to make breathing easier.

How should this medicine be used?

The combination of ipratropium and albuterol comes as a solution (liquid) to inhale by mouth using a nebulizer (machine that turns medication into a mist that can be inhaled) and as an aerosol to inhale by mouth using an inhaler. It is usually inhaled four times a day. Follow the directions on your prescription label carefully, and ask your doctor or pharmacist to explain any part you do not understand. Use ipratropium and albuterol exactly as directed. Do not use more or less of it or use it more often than prescribed by your doctor.

Your doctor may tell you to use additional doses of ipratropium and albuterol combination if you experience symptoms such as wheezing, difficulty breathing, or chest tightness. Follow these directions carefully, and do not use extra doses of medication unless your doctor tells you that you should. Do not use more than two extra doses of the nebulizer solution per day. Do not use more than 12 puffs of the inhalation aerosol in 24 hours.

Call your doctor if your symptoms worsen or if you feel that ipratropium and albuterol inhalation no longer controls your symptoms. If you were told to use ipratropium and albuterol as needed to treat your symptoms and you find that you need to use the medication more often than usual, call your doctor.

If you are using the inhaler, your medication will come in canisters. Each canister of ipratropium and albuterol aerosol is designed to provide 200 inhalations. After the labeled number of inhalations has been used, later inhalations may not contain the correct amount of medication. You should keep track of the number of inhalations you have used. You can divide the number of inhalations in your inhaler by the number of inhalations you use each day to find out how many days your inhaler will last. Throw away the canister after you have used the labeled number of inhalations even if it still contains some liquid and continues to release a spray when it is pressed. Do not float the canister in water to see if it still contains medication.

Be careful not to get ipratropium and albuterol into your eyes. If you are using the inhaler, keep your eyes closed when you use the medication. If you get ipratropium and albuterol in your eyes, you may develop narrow angle glaucoma (a serious eye condition that may cause loss of vision). If you already have narrow angle glaucoma, your condition may worsen. You may experience widened pupils (black circles in the center of the eyes), eye pain or redness, blurred vision, and vision changes such as seeing halos around lights. Call your doctor if you get ipratropium and albuterol into your eyes or if you develop these symptoms.

The inhaler that comes with ipratropium and albuterol aerosol is designed for use only with a canister of ipratropium and albuterol. Never use it to inhale any other medication, and do not use any other inhaler to inhale ipratropium and albuterol.

Do not use your ipratropium and albuterol inhaler when you are near a flame or source of heat. The inhaler may explode if it is exposed to very high temperatures.

Before you use ipratropium and albuterol for the first time, read the written instructions that come with the inhaler or nebulizer. Ask your doctor, pharmacist, or respiratory therapist to show you how to use it. Practice using the inhaler or nebulizer while he or she watches.

To use the inhaler, follow these steps:

1. Hold the inhaler with the clear end pointing upward. Place the metal canister into the clear end of the inhaler. Be sure that the canister is fully and firmly in place.
2. Remove the protective dust cap from the end of the mouthpiece. If the dust cap was not placed on the mouthpiece, check the mouthpiece for dirt or other objects.
3. If you are using the inhaler for the first time or if you have not used the inhaler in more than 24 hours, you will need to prime it. Shake it well for at least 10 seconds and then press down on the canister three times to release three sprays into the air, away from your face. Be careful not to get ipratropium and albuterol in your eyes.
4. Hold the inhaler between your thumb and your next two fingers with the mouthpiece on the bottom, facing you. Shake the inhaler well for at least 10 seconds.
5. Immediately breathe out deeply through your mouth.
6. Hold the canister with the mouthpiece on the bottom and facing you and the canister pointing upward. Place the open end of the mouthpiece into your mouth. Close your lips tightly around the mouthpiece. Close your eyes.
7. Breathe in slowly and deeply through the mouthpiece. At the same time, press down once on the container to spray the medication into your mouth.

8. Hold your breath for 10 seconds. Then remove the inhaler, and breathe out slowly.
9. If you were told to use two puffs, wait about 2 minutes and then repeat steps 4 to 8.
10. Replace the protective cap on the inhaler.

To inhale the solution using a nebulizer, follow these steps:

1. Remove one vial of medication from the foil pouch. Put the rest of the vials back into the pouch until you are ready to use them.
2. Twist off the top of the vial and squeeze all of the liquid into the reservoir of the nebulizer.
3. Connect the nebulizer reservoir to the mouthpiece or face mask.
4. Connect the nebulizer reservoir to the compressor.
5. Put the mouthpiece in your mouth or put on the face mask. Sit in a comfortable, upright position and turn on the compressor.
6. Breathe in calmly, deeply, and evenly through your mouth for about 5 to 15 minutes until mist stops forming in the nebulizer chamber.

Clean your inhaler or nebulizer regularly. Follow the manufacturer's directions carefully and ask your doctor or pharmacist if you have any questions about cleaning your inhaler or nebulizer.

Are there other uses for this medicine?

This medication may be prescribed for other uses. Ask your doctor or pharmacist for more information.

What special precautions should I follow?

Before using ipratropium and albuterol,

- tell your doctor and pharmacist if you are allergic to ipratropium (Atrovent), atropine (Atropen), albuterol (Proventil HFA, Ventolin HFA, Vospire ER), levalbuterol (Xoponex), any other medications, or soya lecithin soybeans, or peanuts.
- tell your doctor and pharmacist what prescription and nonprescription medications, vitamins, nutritional supplements and herbal products you are taking or plan to take. Be sure to mention any of the following: beta blockers such as atenolol (Tenormin), labetalol (Normodyne), metoprolol (Lopressor, Toprol XL), nadolol (Corgard), and propranolol (Inderal); diuretics ('water pills'); epinephrine (Epipen, Primatene Mist); medications for colds; other inhaled medications, especially other medications for asthma such as formoterol (Foradil), metaproterenol (Alupent), levalbuterol (Xopenex), and salmeterol (Serevent); and terbutaline (Brethine). Also tell your doctor if you are taking any of the following medications or if you have stopped taking them within the past two weeks: antidepressants such as amitriptyline (Elavil), amoxapine (Asendin), clomipramine (Anafranil), desipramine (Norpramin), doxepin (Sinequan), imipramine (Tofranil), nortriptyline (Pamelor), protriptyline (Vivactil), and trimipramine (Sur-

montil); or monoamine oxidase inhibitors (MAOIs) such as isocarboxazid (Marplan), phenelzine (Nardil), tranylcypromine (Parnate), and selegiline (Eldepryl, Emsam). Your doctor may have to change the doses of your medications or monitor you carefully for side effects.
- tell your doctor if you have or have ever had glaucoma (an eye condition); difficulty urinating; a prostate (a male reproductive gland) condition; seizures; hyperthyroidism (condition in which there is too much thyroid hormone in the body); high blood pressure; an irregular heartbeat; diabetes; or heart, liver, or kidney disease.
- tell your doctor if you are pregnant, plan to become pregnant, or are breast-feeding. If you become pregnant while using ipratropium and albuterol, call your doctor.
- if you are having surgery, including dental surgery, tell the doctor or dentist that you are using ipratropium and albuterol.
- you should know that ipratropium and albuterol inhalation sometimes causes wheezing and difficulty breathing immediately after it is inhaled. If this happens, call your doctor right away. Do not use ipratropium and albuterol inhalation again unless your doctor tells you that you should.

What special dietary instructions should I follow?

Unless your doctor tells you otherwise, continue your normal diet.

What should I do if I forget to take a dose?

Use the missed dose as soon as you remember it. However, if it is almost time for the next dose, skip the missed dose and continue your regular dosing schedule. Do not use a double dose to make up for a missed one.

What side effects can this medicine cause?

This medication may cause side effects. Tell your doctor if any of these symptoms are severe or do not go away:

- cough
- headache
- nausea
- heartburn
- diarrhea
- constipation
- leg cramps
- pain
- difficulty urinating
- frequent urination
- pain when urinating
- voice changes

Some side effects can be serious. If you experience any of the following symptoms, call your doctor immediately:

- fast heartbeat
- chest pain
- hives

- rash
- itching
- swelling of the eyes, face, lips, tongue, throat, hands, feet, ankles, or lower legs
- difficulty breathing or swallowing
- sore throat, fever, chills, and other signs of infection

Ipratropium and albuterol may cause other side effects. Call your doctor if you have any unusual problems while you are using this medication.

What storage conditions are needed for this medicine?

Keep this medication in the container it came in, tightly closed, and out of reach of children. Keep unused vials of nebulizer solution in the foil pouch until you are ready to use them. Store the medication at room temperature and away from excess heat and moisture (not in the bathroom). Throw away any medication that is outdated or no longer needed. Talk to your pharmacist about the proper disposal of your medication. Do not puncture the aerosol canister, and do not discard it in an incinerator or fire.

What should I do in case of overdose?

In case of overdose, call your local poison control center at 1-800-222-1222. If the victim has collapsed or is not breathing, call local emergency services at 911.

Symptoms of overdose may include:
- chest pain
- fast heartbeat

What other information should I know?

Keep all appointments with your doctor.

Do not let anyone else use your medication. Ask your pharmacist any questions you have about refilling your prescription.

Dosage Facts
For Informational Purposes

Caution: Do not change your dose, how often you take your medication, or the length of time you are to take it without first talking to your health-care provider.

The following dosage information was written using medical language for doctors and other healthcare professionals and is provided here for you to check your dosage. The dosage of this drug may differ for different patients. Therefore, always follow your doctor's instructions or the directions on the label. Contact your healthcare provider or pharmacist if you have any questions about the specific dosage of your medication after reviewing this information.

Pediatric Patients

COPD

INHALATION:
- Patients ≥12 years of age: 36 mcg (2 inhalations) 4 times daily via a metered-dose aerosol, given in fixed combination with albuterol (90 mcg via the mouthpiece). Additional inhalations should not exceed 216 mcg (12 inhalations) of ipratropium bromide in 24 hours.

Adult Patients

COPD

INHALATION:
- Initially, 36 mcg (2 inhalations) 4 times daily via a metered-dose aerosol, given with the fixed combination of ipratropium with albuterol (90 mcg from the mouthpiece). Additional inhalations should not exceed 216 mcg (12 inhalations) in 24 hours.
- Via a nebulizer with the fixed combination of ipratropium bromide with albuterol sulfate (DuoNeb®), 500 mcg 4 times daily. Additional inhalations should not exceed 6 inhalations daily.

Prescribing Limits
Pediatric Patients

COPD

INHALATION:
- Maximum 12 inhalations via metered-dose inhaler in 24 hours with the fixed combination of ipratropium bromide and albuterol sulfate.

Adult Patients

COPD

INHALATION:
- Maximum 12 inhalations via metered-dose inhaler in 24 hours with the fixed combination of ipratropium bromide and albuterol sulfate.

Special Populations

Geriatric Patients
- Dosage adjustments based solely on age are not necessary.

Ipratropium Oral Inhalation

(i pra troe′ pee um)

Brand Name: Atrovent®
Also available generically.

Why is this medicine prescribed?

Ipratropium oral inhalation is used to prevent wheezing, difficulty breathing, chest tightness, and coughing in people with chronic obstructive pulmonary disease (COPD; a group of diseases that affect the lungs and airways) such as chronic bronchitis (swelling of the air passages that lead to the lungs) and emphysema (damage to the air sacs in the lungs). Ipratropium is in a class of medications called bronchodilators. It works by relaxing and opening the air passages to the lungs to make breathing easier.

How should this medicine be used?

Ipratropium comes as a solution (liquid) to inhale by mouth using a nebulizer (machine that turns medication into a mist that can be inhaled) and as an aerosol to inhale by mouth using an inhaler. The nebulizer solution is usually used three or four times a day, once every 6 to 8 hours. The aerosol is usually used four times a day. Follow the directions on your prescription label carefully, and ask your doctor or pharmacist to explain any part you do not understand. Use ipratropium exactly as directed. Do not use more or less of it or use it more often than prescribed by your doctor.

Talk to your doctor about what you should do if you experience symptoms such as wheezing, difficulty breathing, or chest tightness. Your doctor will probably give you a different inhaler that acts more quickly than ipratropium to relieve these symptoms. Your doctor may also tell you to use additional puffs of ipratropium along with other medications to treat these symptoms. Follow these directions carefully and be sure you know when you should use each of your inhalers. Do not use extra puffs of ipratropium unless your doctor tells you that you should. Never use more than 12 puffs of ipratropium inhalation aerosol in a 24-hour period.

Call your doctor if your symptoms worsen or if you feel that ipratropium inhalation no longer controls your symptoms. Also call your doctor if you were told to use extra doses of ipratropium and you find that you need to use more doses than usual.

If you are using the inhaler, your medication will come in canisters. Each canister of ipratropium aerosol is designed to provide 200 inhalations. After the labeled number of inhalations has been used, later inhalations may not contain the correct amount of medication. You should keep track of the number of inhalations you have used. You can divide the number of inhalations in your inhaler by the number of inhalations you use each day to find out how many days your inhaler will last. Throw away the canister after you have used the labeled number of inhalations even if it still contains some liquid and continues to release a spray when it is pressed. Do not float the canister in water to see if it still contains medication.

Be careful not to get ipratropium into your eyes. If you are using the inhaler, keep your eyes closed when you use the medication. If you are using the nebulizer solution, you should use a nebulizer with a mouthpiece instead of a face mask. If you must use a face mask, ask your doctor how you can prevent the medication from leaking. If you get ipratropium in your eyes, you may develop narrow angle glaucoma (a serious eye condition that may cause loss of vision). If you already have narrow angle glaucoma, your condition may worsen. You may experience widened pupils (black circles in the center of the eyes), eye pain or redness, blurred vision, and vision changes such as seeing halos around lights. Call your doctor if you get ipratropium into your eyes or if you develop these symptoms.

The inhaler that comes with ipratropium aerosol is designed for use only with a canister of ipratropium. Never use it to inhale any other medication, and do not use any other inhaler to inhale ipratropium.

Do not use your ipratropium inhaler when you are near a flame or source of heat. The inhaler may explode if it is exposed to very high temperatures.

Before you use ipratropium inhalation for the first time, read the written instructions that come with it. Ask your doctor, pharmacist, or respiratory therapist to show you how to use the inhaler or nebulizer. Practice using the inhaler or nebulizer while he or she watches.

To use the inhaler, follow these steps:
1. Hold the inhaler with the clear end pointing upward. Place the metal canister inside the clear end of the inhaler. Be sure that it is fully and firmly in place and that the canister is at room temperature.
2. Remove the protective dust cap from the end of the mouthpiece. If the dust cap was not placed on the mouthpiece, check the mouthpiece for dirt or other objects
3. If you are using the inhaler for the first time or if you have not used the inhaler in 3 days, prime it by pressing down on the canister to release two sprays into the air, away from your face. Be careful not to spray medication into your eyes while you are priming the inhaler.
4. Breathe out as completely as possible through your mouth.
5. Hold the inhaler between your thumb and your next two fingers with the mouthpiece on the bottom, facing you. Place the open end of the mouthpiece into your mouth. Close your lips tightly around the mouthpiece. Close your eyes.
6. Breathe in slowly and deeply through the mouthpiece. At the same time, press down firmly on the canister.
7. Hold your breath for 10 seconds. Then remove the inhaler, and breathe out slowly.
8. If you were told to use two puffs, wait at least 15 seconds and then repeat steps 4 to 7.
9. Replace the protective cap on the inhaler.

To inhale the solution using a nebulizer, follow these steps:
1. Twist off the top of one vial of ipratropium solution and squeeze all of the liquid into the nebulizer reservoir.
2. Connect the nebulizer reservoir to the mouthpiece or face mask.
3. Connect the nebulizer to the compressor.
4. Place the mouthpiece in your mouth or put on the face mask. Sit in an upright, comfortable position and turn on the compressor.
5. Breathe in calmly, deeply, and evenly for about 5 to 15 minutes until mist stops forming in the nebulizer chamber.

Clean your inhaler or nebulizer regularly. Follow the

manufacturer's directions carefully and ask your doctor or pharmacist if you have any questions about cleaning your inhaler or nebulizer.

Are there other uses for this medicine?

Ipratropium is also sometimes used to treat the symptoms of asthma. Talk to your doctor about the risks of using this medication for your condition

What special precautions should I follow?

Before using ipratropium inhalation,

- tell your doctor and pharmacist if you are allergic to ipratropium, atropine (Atropen), or any other medications.
- tell your doctor and pharmacist what prescription and nonprescription medications, vitamins, nutritional supplements, and herbal products you are taking or plan to take. Be sure to mention any of the following: antihistamines; or medications for irritable bowel disease, motion sickness, Parkinson's disease, ulcers, or urinary problems. Your doctor may need to change the doses of your medications or monitor you carefully for side effects.
- if you are using any other inhaled medications, ask your doctor if you should use these medications a certain amount of time before or after you use ipratropium inhalation. If you are using a nebulizer, ask your doctor if you can mix any of your other medications with ipratropium in the nebulizer.
- tell your doctor if you have or have ever had glaucoma, urinary problems or a prostate (a male reproductive organ) condition.
- tell your doctor if you are pregnant, plan to become pregnant, or are breast-feeding. If you become pregnant while using ipratropium, call your doctor.
- if you will be having surgery, including dental surgery, tell the doctor or dentist that you are using ipratropium.
- you should know that ipratropium inhalation sometimes causes wheezing and difficulty breathing immediately after it is inhaled. If this happens, call your doctor right away. Do not use ipratropium inhalation again unless your doctor tells you that you should.

What special dietary instructions should I follow?

Unless your doctor tells you otherwise, continue your normal diet.

What should I do if I forget to take a dose?

Use the missed dose as soon as you remember it. However, if it is almost time for the next dose, skip the missed dose and continue your regular dosing schedule. Do not use a double dose to make up for a missed one.

What side effects can this medicine cause?

Ipratropium may cause side effects. Tell your doctor if any of these symptoms are severe or do not go away:

- dizziness
- nausea
- heartburn
- constipation
- dry mouth
- difficulty urinating
- pain when urinating
- frequent need to urinate
- back pain

Some side effects can be serious. If you experience any of the following symptoms, call your doctor immediately:

- rash
- hives
- itching
- swelling of the eyes, face, lips, tongue, throat, hands, feet, ankles, or lower legs
- hoarseness
- difficulty breathing or swallowing
- fast or pounding heartbeat
- chest pain

Ipratropium may cause other side effects. Call your doctor if you have any unusual problems while using this medication.

What storage conditions are needed for this medicine?

Keep this medication in the container it came in, tightly closed, and out of reach of children. Store unused vials of the solution in the foil pack until you are ready to use them. Store the medication at room temperature and away from excess heat and moisture (not in the bathroom). Talk to your pharmacist about the proper disposal of medication that is outdated or no longer needed. Do not puncture the aerosol canister, and do not discard it in an incinerator or fire.

What should I do in case of overdose?

In case of overdose, call your local poison control center at 1-800-222-1222. If the victim has collapsed or is not breathing, call local emergency services at 911.

What other information should I know?

Keep all appointments with your doctor.

Do not let anyone else use your medication. Ask your pharmacist any questions you have about refilling your prescription.

Dosage Facts
For Informational Purposes

Caution: Do not change your dose, how often you take your medication, or the length of time you are to take it without first talking to your healthcare provider.

The following dosage information was written using medical language for doctors and other healthcare pro-

fessionals and is provided here for you to check your dosage. The dosage of this drug may differ for different patients. Therefore, always follow your doctor's instructions or the directions on the label. Contact your healthcare provider or pharmacist if you have any questions about the specific dosage of your medication after reviewing this information.

General Dosage Information

Available as ipratropium bromide.

Dosage of oral inhalation aerosol expressed in terms of the monohydrate.

Dosage of inhalation solution for nebulization expressed in terms of anhydrous drug.

Using in vitro testing at an average flow rate of 3.6 L per minute for an average of ≤15 minutes, the Pari-LC Plus® nebulizer delivered at the mouthpiece approximately 46 or 42% of the original dosage of albuterol or ipratropium bromide, respectively.

Pediatric Patients

COPD

INHALATION:
- Patients ≥12 years of age: 36 mcg (2 inhalations) 4 times daily via a metered-dose aerosol, given alone or in fixed combination with albuterol (90 mcg via the mouthpiece). Additional inhalations should not exceed 216 mcg (12 inhalations) of ipratropium bromide in 24 hours.
- Patients ≥12 years of age: 500 mcg (contents of 1 unit-dose vial) 3 or 4 times daily (i.e., every 6–8 hours) via a nebulizer.

Adult Patients

COPD

INHALATION:
- Initially, 36 mcg (2 inhalations) 4 times daily via a metered-dose aerosol, given alone or in fixed combination with albuterol (90 mcg from the mouthpiece). Additional inhalations should not exceed 216 mcg (12 inhalations) in 24 hours.
- Initially, 500 mcg 3 or 4 times daily (i.e., every 6–8 hours) via a nebulizer. With ipratropium bromide in fixed combination with albuterol sulfate (DuoNeb®), 500 mcg 4 times daily. Additional inhalations should not exceed 6 inhalations daily.

Prescribing Limits

Pediatric Patients

COPD

INHALATION:
- Maximum 216 mcg (12 inhalations via a metered-dose inhaler) in 24 hours.
- Maximum 12 inhalations via metered-dose inhaler in 24 hours with the fixed combination of ipratropium bromide and albuterol sulfate.
- 500 mcg 3–4 times daily via a nebulizer in patients ≥12 years of age.

Adult Patients

COPD

INHALATION:
- Maximum 216 mcg (12 inhalations via a metered-dose inhaler) in 24 hours; frequency of administration should not exceed 4 times daily.

- Maximum 12 inhalations via metered-dose inhaler in 24 hours with the fixed combination of ipratropium bromide and albuterol sulfate.
- 500 mcg 3–4 times daily via a nebulizer.

Special Populations

Geriatric Patients
- Dosage adjustments based solely on age are not necessary.

Irbesartan

(ir be sar′ tan)

Brand Name: Avapro®

Important Warning

Do not take irbesartan if you are pregnant. If you become pregnant while taking irbesartan, call your doctor immediately. Irbesartan may harm the fetus.

Why is this medicine prescribed?

Irbesartan is used alone or in combination with other medications to treat high blood pressure. It is also used to treat kidney disease caused by diabetes in patients with type 2 diabetes (condition in which the body does not use insulin normally and therefore cannot control the amount of sugar in the blood) and high blood pressure. Irbesartan is in a class of medications called angiotensin II receptor antagonists. It works by blocking the action of certain chemicals that tighten the blood vessels, so blood flows more smoothly.

How should this medicine be used?

Irbesartan comes as a tablet to take by mouth. It is usually taken once a day with or without food. To help you remember to take irbesartan, take it around the same time every day. Follow the directions on your prescription label carefully, and ask your doctor or pharmacist to explain any part you do not understand. Take irbesartan exactly as directed. Do not take more or less of it or take it more often than prescribed by your doctor.

Your doctor may start you on a low dose of irbesartan and gradually increase your dose.

Irbesartan controls high blood pressure but does not cure it. Continue to take irbesartan even if you feel well. Do not stop taking irbesartan without talking to your doctor.

Are there other uses for this medicine?

Irbesartan is also used sometimes to treat heart failure. Talk to your doctor about the possible risks of using this medication for your condition.

This medication may be prescribed for other uses; ask your doctor or pharmacist for more information.

What special precautions should I follow?

Before taking irbesartan,

- tell your doctor and pharmacist if you are allergic to irbesartan or any other medications.
- tell your doctor and pharmacist what prescription and nonprescription medications, vitamins, nutritional supplements, and herbal products you are taking. Be sure to mention any of the following: diuretics ('water pills'), nifedipine (Adalat, Procardia), and tolbutamide (Orinase). Your doctor may need to change the doses of your medications or monitor you carefully for side effects.
- tell your doctor if you are on dialysis and if you have or have ever had heart failure or kidney disease.
- tell your doctor if you plan to become pregnant or are breast-feeding.

What special dietary instructions should I follow?

If your doctor prescribes a low-salt or low-sodium diet, follow these directions carefully.

What should I do if I forget to take a dose?

Take the missed dose as soon as you remember it. However, if it is almost time for your next dose, skip the missed dose and continue your regular dosing schedule. Do not take a double dose to make up for a missed one.

What side effects can this medicine cause?

Irbesartan may cause side effects. Tell your doctor if any of these symptoms are severe or do not go away:

- runny nose
- sore throat
- diarrhea
- heartburn
- excessive tiredness

Some side effects can be serious. The following symptoms are uncommon, but if you experience any of them, call your doctor immediately:

- swelling of the face, throat, tongue, lips, eyes, hands, feet, ankles, or lower legs
- hoarseness
- difficulty breathing or swallowing
- hives
- fainting

Irbesartan may cause other side effects. Call your doctor if you have any unusual problems while taking this medication.

If you experience a serious side effect, you or your doctor may send a report to the Food and Drug Administration's (FDA) MedWatch Adverse Event Reporting program online [at http://www.fda.gov/MedWatch/index.html] or by phone [1-800-332-1088].

What storage conditions are needed for this medicine?

Keep this medication in the container it came in, tightly closed, and out of reach of children. Store it at room temperature and away from excess heat and moisture (not in the bathroom). Throw away any medication that is outdated or no longer needed. Talk to your pharmacist about the proper disposal of your medication.

What should I do in case of overdose?

In case of overdose, call your local poison control center at 1-800-222-1222. If the victim has collapsed or is not breathing, call local emergency services at 911.

Symptoms of overdose may include:

- dizziness
- fainting
- rapid or pounding heartbeat

What other information should I know?

Keep all appointments with your doctor. Your blood pressure should be checked regularly to determine your response to irbesartan.

Do not let anyone else take your medication. Ask your pharmacist any questions you have about refilling your prescription.

Dosage Facts
For Informational Purposes

Caution: Do not change your dose, how often you take your medication, or the length of time you are to take it without first talking to your healthcare provider.

The following dosage information was written using medical language for doctors and other healthcare professionals and is provided here for you to check your dosage. The dosage of this drug may differ for different patients. Therefore, always follow your doctor's instructions or the directions on the label. Contact your healthcare provider or pharmacist if you have any questions about the specific dosage of your medication after reviewing this information.

Pediatric Patients

Hypertension

ORAL:
- Children 6–12 years of age: Initially, 75 mg once daily. Dosage may be increased as tolerated up to 150 mg daily.
- Adolescents 13–16 years of age: Initially, 150 mg once daily. Dosage may be increased as tolerated up to 300 mg daily.

Adult Patients

Hypertension

Monotherapy

ORAL:
- Initially, 150 mg once daily in adults without intravascular volume depletion. Adjust dosage at approximately monthly intervals (more aggressively in high-risk patients) to achieve BP control.
- Usual dosage: 150–300 mg once daily; no additional therapeutic benefit with higher dosages or with twice-daily dosing.

Combination Therapy

ORAL:
- If BP is not adequately controlled by monotherapy with irbesartan or hydrochlorothiazide, can switch to fixed-combination tablets (irbesartan 150 mg and 12.5 mg hydrochlorothiazide; then irbesartan 300 mg and hydrochlorothiazide 12.5 mg), administered once daily. Can increase dosage to irbesartan 300 mg and hydrochlorothiazide 25 mg daily, if needed, to control BP.

Diabetic Nephropathy

ORAL:
- Initial dosage of 75 mg once daily used in clinical trial. Increase dosage to target maintenance dosage of 300 mg once daily. No data available on effects of lower dosages.

Prescribing Limits

Pediatric Patients

Hypertension

ORAL:
- Children 6–12 years of age: Maximum 150 mg daily.
- Adolescents 13–16 years of age: Maximum 300 mg daily.

Special Populations

Hepatic Impairment
- No initial dosage adjustments necessary.

Renal Impairment
- No initial dosage adjustments necessary.
- Irbesartan/hydrochlorothiazide fixed combination not recommended in patients with severe renal impairment.

Geriatric Patients
- No initial dosage adjustments necessary.

Volume- and/or Salt-depleted Patients
- Correct volume and/or salt depletion prior to initiation of therapy or initiate therapy under close medical supervision using lower initial dosage (75 mg once daily).

Irbesartan and Hydrochlorothiazide

(ir be sar′ tan) (hye dro klor oh thye′ a zide)

Brand Name: Avalide®

Important Warning

Do not take irbesartan and hydrochlorothiazide if you are pregnant. If you become pregnant while taking irbesartan and hydrochlorothiazide, call your doctor immediately. Irbesartan and hydrochlorothiazide may harm the fetus.

Why is this medicine prescribed?

The combination of irbesartan and hydrochlorothiazide is used to treat high blood pressure. Irbesartan is in a class of medications called angiotensin II antagonists. It works by blocking the action of certain natural chemicals that tighten the blood vessels, making blood flow more smoothly. Hydrochlorothiazide is in a class of medications called diuretics ('water pills'). It works by causing the the kidneys to get rid of unneeded water and salt from the body into the urine.

How should this medicine be used?

The combination of irbesartan and hydrochlorothiazide comes as a tablet to take by mouth. It is usually taken once a day with or without food. Follow the directions on your prescription label carefully, and ask your doctor or pharmacist to explain any part you do not understand. Take irbesartan and hydrochlorothiazide exactly as directed. Do not take more or less of it or take it more often than prescribed by your doctor.

Irbesartan and hydrochlorothiazide controls high blood pressure but does not cure it. It may take 2 to 4 weeks before you feel the full benefit of irbesartan and hydrochlorothiazide. Continue to take irbesartan and hydrochlorothiazide even if you feel well. Do not stop taking irbesartan and hydrochlorothiazide without talking to your doctor.

Are there other uses for this medicine?

This medication may be prescribed for other uses; ask your doctor or pharmacist for more information.

What special precautions should I follow?

Before taking irbesartan and hydrochlorothiazide,
- tell your doctor and pharmacist if you are allergic to irbesartan, hydrochlorothiazide, sulfa drugs, or any other medications.
- tell your doctor and pharmacist what prescription and nonprescription medication, vitamins, nutritional sup-

plements, and herbal products you are taking. Be sure to mention any of the following: aspirin and other non-steroidal anti-inflammatory medications (NSAIDS) such as ibuprofen (Advil, Motrin) and naproxen (Aleve, Naprosyn); cholestyramine (Questran); colestipol (Colestid); lithium (Eskalith, Lithobid); medications for diabetes; narcotic pain relievers; oral steroids such as dexamethasone (Decadron, Dexone), methylprednisolone (Medrol), and prednisone (Deltasone); other medications for high blood pressure; phenobarbital (Luminal, Solfoton); and tolbutamide (Orinase). Your doctor may need to change the doses of your medications or monitor you carefully for side effects.

- tell your doctor if you are on dialysis and if you have or have ever had asthma, lupus (SLE), diabetes, heart failure, gout, or kidney or liver disease.
- tell your doctor if you are breast-feeding.
- you should know that irbesartan and hydrochlorothiazide may make you drowsy. Do not drive a car or operate machinery until you know how this medication affects you.
- ask your doctor about the safe use of alcoholic beverages while you are taking irbesartan and hydrochlorothiazide. Alcohol can make the side effects from irbesartan and hydrochlorothiazide worse.
- you should know that irbesartan and hydrochlorothiazide may cause dizziness, lightheadedness, and fainting when you get up too quickly from a lying position. This is more common when you first start taking irbesartan and hydrochlorothiazide. To avoid this problem, get out of bed slowly, resting your feet on the floor for a few minutes before standing up.
- you should know that diarrhea, vomiting, not drinking enough fluids, and sweating a lot can cause a drop in blood pressure, which may cause lightheadedness and fainting.

What special dietary instructions should I follow?

Talk to your doctor before using salt substitutes containing potassium. If your doctor prescribes a low-salt or low-sodium diet or an exercise program, follow these directions carefully.

What should I do if I forget to take a dose?

Take the missed dose as soon as you remember it. However, if it is almost time for the next dose, skip the missed dose and continue your regular dosing schedule. Do not take a double dose to make up for a missed one.

What side effects can this medicine cause?

Irbesartan and hydrochlorothiazide may cause side effects. Tell your doctor if any of these symptoms are severe or do not go away:
- dizziness
- extreme tiredness
- upset stomach
- vomiting
- stomach pain
- heartburn
- chest pain
- flu-like symptoms

Some side effects can be serious. The following symptoms are uncommon, but if you experience any of them, call your doctor immediately:
- dry mouth
- thirst
- weakness
- lack of energy
- restlessness
- confusion
- seizures
- muscle pain or cramps
- infrequent urination
- rapid heartbeat
- lightheadedness
- fainting

Irbesartan and hydrochlorothiazide may cause other side effects. Call your doctor if you have any unusual problems while taking this medication.

If you experience a serious side effect, you or your doctor may send a report to the Food and Drug Administration's (FDA) MedWatch Adverse Event Reporting program online [at http://www.fda.gov/MedWatch/index.html] or by phone [1-800-332-1088].

What storage conditions are needed for this medicine?

Keep this medication in the container it came in, tightly closed, and out of reach of children. Store it at room temperature and away from excess heat and moisture (not in the bathroom). Throw away any medication that is outdated or no longer needed. Talk to your pharmacist about the proper disposal of your medication.

What should I do in case of overdose?

In case of overdose, call your local poison control center at 1-800-222-1222. If the victim has collapsed or is not breathing, call local emergency services at 911.

What other information should I know?

Keep all appointments with your doctor and the laboratory. Your doctor may order certain lab tests to check your body's response to irbesartan and hydrochlorothiazide.

Do not let anyone else take your medication. Ask your pharmacist any questions you have about refilling your prescription.

Dosage Facts
For Informational Purposes

Caution: Do not change your dose, how often you take your medication, or the length of time you

are to take it without first talking to your healthcare provider.

The following dosage information was written using medical language for doctors and other healthcare professionals and is provided here for you to check your dosage. The dosage of this drug may differ for different patients. Therefore, always follow your doctor's instructions or the directions on the label. Contact your healthcare provider or pharmacist if you have any questions about the specific dosage of your medication after reviewing this information.

Adult Patients

Hypertension
Combination Therapy

ORAL:
- If BP is not adequately controlled by monotherapy with irbesartan or hydrochlorothiazide, can switch to fixed-combination tablets (irbesartan 150 mg and 12.5 mg hydrochlorothiazide; then irbesartan 300 mg and hydrochlorothiazide 12.5 mg), administered once daily. Can increase dosage to irbesartan 300 mg and hydrochlorothiazide 25 mg daily, if needed, to control BP.

Isocarboxazid

(eye soe kar box' azid)

Brand Name: Marplan®

Important Warning

A small number of children, teenagers, and young adults (up to 24 years of age) who took antidepressants ('mood elevators') such as isocarboxazid during clinical studies became suicidal (thinking about harming or killing oneself or planning or trying to do so). Children, teenagers, and young adults who take antidepressants to treat depression or other mental illnesses may be more likely to become suicidal than children, teenagers, and young adults who do not take antidepressants to treat these conditions. However, experts are not sure about how great this risk is and how much it should be considered in deciding whether a child or teenager should take an antidepressant. Children younger than 18 years of age should not normally take isocarboxazid, but in some cases, a doctor may decide that isocarboxazid is the best medication to treat a child's condition.

You should know that your mental health may change in unexpected ways when you take isocarboxazid or other antidepressants even if you are an adult over age 24. You may become suicidal, especially at the beginning of your treatment and any time that your dose is increased or decreased. You, your family, or your caregiver should call your doctor right away if you experience any of the following symptoms: new or worsening depression; thinking about harming or killing yourself, or planning or trying to do so; extreme worry; agitation; panic attacks; difficulty falling asleep or staying asleep; aggressive behavior; irritability; acting without thinking; severe restlessness; and frenzied abnormal excitement. Be sure that your family or caregiver knows which symptoms may be serious so they can call the doctor when you are unable to seek treatment on your own.

Your healthcare provider will want to see you often while you are taking isocarboxazid, especially at the beginning of your treatment. Be sure to keep all appointments for office visits with your doctor.

The doctor or pharmacist will give you the manufacturer's patient information sheet (Medication Guide) when you begin treatment with isocarboxazid. Read the information carefully and ask your doctor or pharmacist if you have any questions. You also can obtain the Medication Guide from the FDA website: http://www.fda.gov/cder/drug/antidepressants/antidepressants_MG_2007.pdf.

No matter what your age, before you take an antidepressant, you, your parent, or your caregiver should talk to your doctor about the risks and benefits of treating your condition with an antidepressant or with other treatments. You should also talk about the risks and benefits of not treating your condition. You should know that having depression or another mental illness greatly increases the risk that you will become suicidal. This risk is higher if you or anyone in your family has or has ever had bipolar disorder (mood that changes from depressed to abnormally excited) or mania (frenzied, abnormally excited mood) or has thought about or attempted suicide. Talk to your doctor about your condition, symptoms, and personal and family medical history. You and your doctor will decide what type of treatment is right for you.

Why is this medicine prescribed?

Isocarboxazid is used to treat depression in people who have not been helped by other antidepressants. Isocarboxazid is in a class of medications called monoamine oxidase inhibitors (MAOIs). It works by increasing the amounts of certain natural substances in the brain that help maintain mental balance.

How should this medicine be used?

Isocarboxazid comes as a tablet to take by mouth. It is usually taken between two and four times a day. Take isocarboxazid at around the same times every day. Follow the directions on your prescription label carefully, and ask your doctor or pharmacist to explain any part you do not understand. Take isocarboxazid exactly as directed.

Swallow the tablets with water or another liquid. If you are unable to swallow the tablets, you can crumble them and swallow the crumbled tablets with food or liquid.

Isocarboxazid may be habit-forming. Do not take a larger dose, take it more often, or take it for a longer period of time than prescribed by your doctor.

Your doctor will probably start you on a low dose of isocarboxazid and gradually increase your dose, not more often than once every 2-4 days at first, and then not more often than once every week. After your symptoms improve, your doctor will probably gradually decrease your dose of isocarboxazid.

Isocarboxazid is used to treat depression but does not cure it. It may take 3-6 weeks or longer before you feel the full benefit of isocarboxazid. Tell your doctor if your symptoms do not improve during the first 6 weeks of your treatment with isocarboxazid. If your symptoms do improve during your treatment, continue to take isocarboxazid. Do not stop taking isocarboxazid without talking to your doctor.

Are there other uses for this medicine?

This medication may be prescribed for other uses; ask your doctor or pharmacist for more information.

What special precautions should I follow?

Before taking isocarboxazid,

- tell your doctor and pharmacist if you are allergic to isocarboxazid, any other medications, or any of the inactive ingredients in isocarboxazid tablets. Ask your pharmacist for a list of the inactive ingredients.
- do not take isocarboxazid if you are taking or plan to take any of the following prescription or nonprescription medications: certain other antidepressants such as amitriptyline (Elavil), amoxapine (Asendin), clomipramine (Anafranil), desipramine (Norpramin), doxepin (Sinequan), imipramine (Tofranil), maprotiline, nortriptyline (Aventyl, Pamelor), protriptyline (Vivactil), trimipramine (Surmontil), and selective serotonin reuptake inhibitors (SSRIs) such as fluoxetine (Prozac), fluvoxamine (Luvox), paroxetine (Paxil), and sertraline (Zoloft); amphetamines such as amphetamine (in Adderall), benzphetamine (Didrex), dextroamphetamine (Dexedrine, Dextrostat, in Adderall), and methamphetamine (Desoxyn); antihistamines; barbiturates such as pentobarbital (Nembutal), phenobarbital (Luminal), and secobarbital (Seconal); bupropion (Wellbutrin, Zyban); buspirone (BuSpar); caffeine (No-Doz, Quick-Pep, Vivarin); cyclobenzaprine (Flexeril); dextromethorphan (Robitussin, others); diuretics ('water pills'); duloxetine (Cymbalta), ephedrine (in cough and cold medications, formerly available in the United States as an ingredient in dietary supplements); epinephrine (Epipen); guanethidine (Ismelin; not commercially available in the United States); levodopa (Laradopa, in Sinemet); medications for allergies, asthma, cough, and cold symptoms, including nose drops; medications for high blood pressure, mental illness, anxiety, pain, or weight loss (diet pills); medications for seizures such as carbamazepine (Tegretol); methyldopa (Aldomet); methylphenidate (Concerta, Metadate, Ritalin, others); other MAOIs such as phenelzine (Nardil), procarbazine (Matulane), tranylcypromine (Parnate), and selegiline (Eldepryl, Emsam, Zelapar); reserpine (Serpalan); sedatives; sleeping pills; tranquilizers; and medications containing alcohol (Nyquil, elixirs, others). Tell your doctor if you have recently taken any of these medications.

- tell your doctor and pharmacist what other prescription and nonprescription medications, vitamins, and herbal products you are taking or plan to take. Be sure to mention any of the following: disulfiram (Antabuse), doxepin cream (Zonalon); insulin, oral medications for diabetes, and medications for upset stomach. Your doctor may need to change the doses of your medications or monitor you carefully for side effects.

- you should know that isocarboxazid may remain in your body for 2 weeks after you stop taking the medication. Tell your doctor and pharmacist that you have recently stopped taking isocarboxazid before you start taking any new medications during the first 2 weeks after you stop taking isocarboxazid.

- tell your doctor if you are taking any nutritional supplements, especially phenylalanine (DLPA; contained in aspartame sweetened products such as diet sodas and foods, over-the-counter medications, and some prescription medications), tyrosine, or tryptophan.

- tell your doctor if you or anyone in your family has or has ever had schizophrenia (a mental illness that causes disturbed thinking, loss of interest in life, and strong or unusual emotions). Also tell your doctor if you have ever used street drugs or overused prescription medications and if you have or have ever had a head injury; hyperactivity; headaches; high blood pressure; chest pain; a heart attack; a stroke or mini-stroke; pheochromocytoma (tumor on a small gland near the kidneys); seizures; diabetes; or liver, kidney, thyroid, or heart disease.

- tell your doctor if you are pregnant, plan to become pregnant, or are breast-feeding. If you become pregnant while taking isocarboxazid, call your doctor.

- if you are having surgery, including dental surgery, or any x-ray procedure, tell the doctor or dentist that you are taking isocarboxazid.

- you should know that isocarboxazid may make you drowsy. Do not drive a car, pilot an airplane, operate machinery, climb ladders, or work in high places until you know how this medication affects you.

- remember that alcohol can add to the drowsiness caused by this medication. Do not drink alcohol while you are taking isocarboxazid.

- you should know that isocarboxazid may cause dizziness, lightheadedness, and fainting when you get up too quickly from a lying position. This is more common when you first start taking isocarboxazid. To avoid this problem, get out of bed slowly, resting your feet on the floor for a few minutes before standing up.

What special dietary instructions should I follow?

You may experience a serious reaction if you eat foods that are high in tyramine during your treatment with isocarboxazid. Tyramine is found in many foods, including meat, poultry, fish, or cheese that has been smoked, aged, improperly stored, or spoiled; certain fruits, vegetables, and beans; alcoholic beverages; and yeast products that have fermented. Your doctor or dietitian will tell you which foods you must avoid completely, and which foods you may eat in small amounts. You should also avoid foods and drinks that contain caffeine during your treatment with isocarboxazid. Follow these directions carefully. Ask your doctor or dietitian if you have any questions about what you may eat and drink during your treatment.

What should I do if I forget to take a dose?

Take the missed dose as soon as you remember it. However, if it has been more than 2 hours since you were supposed to take the dose, skip the missed dose and continue your regular dosing schedule. Do not take a double dose to make up for a missed one.

What side effects can this medicine cause?

Isocarboxazid may cause side effects. Tell your doctor if any of these symptoms are severe or do not go away:
- dry mouth
- constipation
- diarrhea
- weakness
- extreme tiredness
- forgetfulness
- decreased sexual ability
- frequent, painful, or difficult urination

Some side effects can be serious. If you experience any of the following symptoms or those listed in the IMPORTANT WARNING section, call your doctor immediately:
- headaches
- fast or pounding heartbeat
- chest pain
- sweating
- fever
- chills
- cold, clammy skin
- dizziness
- tightness in the chest or throat
- stiff or sore neck
- upset stomach
- vomiting
- fainting
- blurred vision

- sensitivity to light
- wide pupils (black circle in the middle of the eye)
- yellowing of the skin or eyes
- uncontrollable shaking of a part of the body
- sudden jerking of a part of the body
- seizures
- numbness, burning, or tingling in the arms or legs

Isocarboxazid may cause other side effects. Call your doctor if you have any unusual problems while taking this medication.

If you experience a serious side effect, you or your doctor may send a report to the Food and Drug Administration's (FDA) MedWatch Adverse Event Reporting program online [at http://www.fda.gov/MedWatch/index.html] or by phone [1-800-332-1088].

What storage conditions are needed for this medicine?

Keep this medication in the container it came in, tightly closed, and out of reach of children. Store it at room temperature and away from excess heat and moisture (not in the bathroom). Throw away any medication that is outdated or no longer needed. Talk to your pharmacist about the proper disposal of your medication.

What should I do in case of overdose?

In case of overdose, call your local poison control center at 1-800-222-1222. If the victim has collapsed or is not breathing, call local emergency services at 911.

Symptoms of overdose may include:
- fast heartbeat
- dizziness
- fainting
- blurred vision
- upset stomach
- coma (loss of consciousness for a length of time)
- seizures
- slowed breathing
- slowed reflexes
- fever
- sweating

What other information should I know?

Keep all appointments with your doctor and the laboratory. Your doctor will check your blood pressure often and will order certain lab tests to check your body's response to isocarboxazid.

Do not let anyone else take your medication. Ask your pharmacist any questions you have about refilling your prescription.

Dosage Facts
For Informational Purposes

Caution: Do not change your dose, how often you take your medication, or the length of time you

are to take it without first talking to your health-care provider.

The following dosage information was written using medical language for doctors and other healthcare professionals and is provided here for you to check your dosage. The dosage of this drug may differ for different patients. Therefore, always follow your doctor's instructions or the directions on the label. Contact your healthcare provider or pharmacist if you have any questions about the specific dosage of your medication after reviewing this information.

Adult Patients

Major Depressive Disorder

ORAL:
- Initially, 10 mg twice daily. If tolerated, dosage may be increased every 2–4 days by 10 mg daily, up to 40 mg daily in divided doses by the end of the first week. If required, may increase dosage by increments of ≤20 mg weekly to a maximum 60 mg daily; however, dosages >40 mg daily should be administered with caution.
- After symptoms are controlled, gradually reduce dosage over several weeks to the lowest level that will maintain relief of symptoms.
- Transferring from another MAO inhibitor: Initially, 5 mg twice daily for at least 7 days.

Prescribing Limits

Adult Patients

ORAL:
- Maximum 60 mg daily.

Special Populations

Hepatic Impairment
- No specific dosage recommendations at this time; however, should not be used in patients with a history of liver disease or in those with abnormal liver function tests.

Renal Impairment
- No specific dosage recommendations at this time; however, should not be used in patients with severe renal function impairment.

Geriatric Patients
- Select dosage with caution, usually starting at a lower dose, because of age-related decreases in hepatic, renal, and/or cardiac function and concomitant disease and drug therapy.

Isoetharine Oral Inhalation

(eye soe eth′ a reen)

Brand Name: Beta-2®

Why is this medicine prescribed?

Isoetharine is used to prevent and treat wheezing, shortness of breath, and troubled breathing caused by asthma, chronic bronchitis, emphysema, and other lung diseases. It relaxes and opens air passages in the lungs, making it easier to breathe.

This medication is sometimes prescribed for other uses; ask your doctor or pharmacist for more information.

How should this medicine be used?

Isoetharine comes as an aerosol and a solution to inhale by mouth. It is used as needed to relieve symptoms but usually should not be used more than every 4 hours. Follow the directions on your prescription label carefully, and ask your doctor or pharmacist to explain any part you do not understand. Use isoetharine exactly as directed. Do not use more or less of it or use it more often than prescribed by your doctor.

Isoetharine controls symptoms of asthma and other lung diseases but does not cure them. Do not stop using isoetharine without talking to your doctor.

Before you use isoetharine the first time, read the written instructions that come with it. Ask your doctor, pharmacist, or respiratory therapist to demonstrate the proper technique. Practice using the inhaler while in his or her presence.

To use the inhaler, follow these steps:
1. Shake the inhaler well.
2. Remove the protective cap.
3. Exhale (breathe out) as completely as possible through your nose while keeping your mouth shut.
4. *Open Mouth Technique:* Open your mouth wide, and place the open end of the mouthpiece about 1-2 inches from your mouth.
   Closed Mouth Technique: Place the open end of the mouthpiece well into your mouth, past your front teeth. Close your lips tightly around the mouthpiece.
5. Take a slow, deep breath through the mouthpiece and, at the same time, press down on the container to spray the medication into your mouth. Be sure that the mist goes into your throat and is not blocked by your teeth or tongue. Adults giving the treatment to young children may hold the child's nose closed to be sure that the medication goes into the child's throat.
6. Hold your breath for 5-10 seconds, remove the inhaler, and exhale slowly through your nose or mouth. If you

take 2 puffs, wait 2 minutes and shake the inhaler well before taking the second puff.

7. Replace the protective cap on the inhaler.

If you have difficulty getting the medication into your lungs, a spacer (a special device that attaches to the inhaler) may help; ask your doctor, pharmacist, or respiratory therapist.

What special precautions should I follow?

Before using isoetharine,

- tell your doctor and pharmacist if you are allergic to isoetharine or any other drugs.
- tell your doctor and pharmacist what prescription medications you are taking, especially atenolol (Tenormin); carteolol (Cartrol); labetalol (Normodyne, Trandate); metoprolol (Lopressor); nadolol (Corgard); phenelzine (Nardil); propranolol (Inderal); sotalol (Betapace); theophylline (Theo-Dur); timolol (Blocadren); tranylcypromine (Parnate); and other medications for asthma, heart disease, or depression.
- tell your doctor and pharmacist what nonprescription medications and vitamins you are taking, including ephedrine, phenylephrine, phenylpropanolamine, or pseudoephedrine. Many nonprescription products contain these drugs (e.g., diet pills and medications for colds and asthma), so check labels carefully. Do not take any of these medications without talking to your doctor (even if you never had a problem taking them before).
- tell your doctor if you have or have ever had an irregular heartbeat, increased heart rate, glaucoma, heart disease, high blood pressure, an overactive thyroid gland, diabetes, or seizures.
- tell your doctor if you are pregnant, plan to become pregnant, or are breast-feeding. If you become pregnant while using isoetharine, call your doctor.
- if you are having surgery, including dental surgery, tell the doctor or dentist that you are using isoetharine.

What should I do if I forget to take a dose?

Use the missed dose as soon as you remember it. However, if it is almost time for the next dose, skip the missed dose and continue your regular dosing schedule. Do not use a double dose to make up for a missed one.

What side effects can this medicine cause?

Isoetharine may cause side effects. Tell your doctor if any of these symptoms are severe or do not go away:

- tremor
- nervousness
- headache
- upset stomach
- dry mouth
- throat irritation

If you experience any of the following symptoms, call your doctor immediately:

- increased difficulty breathing
- rapid or increased heart rate
- irregular heartbeat
- chest pain or discomfort

If you experience a serious side effect, you or your doctor may send a report to the Food and Drug Administration's (FDA) MedWatch Adverse Event Reporting program online [at http://www.fda.gov/MedWatch/index.html] or by phone [1-800-332-1088].

What storage conditions are needed for this medicine?

Keep this medication in the container it came in, tightly closed, and out of reach of children. Store it at room temperature and away from excess heat and moisture (not in the bathroom). Do not use the liquid if it is pink, yellow, or dark in color or if it contains floating particles. Throw away any medication that is outdated or no longer needed. Talk to your pharmacist about the proper disposal of your medication. Avoid puncturing the aerosol container, and do not discard it in an incinerator or fire.

What other information should I know?

Keep all appointments with your doctor and the laboratory. Your doctor will order certain lab tests to check your response to isoetharine.

To relieve dry mouth or throat irritation, rinse your mouth with water, chew gum, or suck sugarless hard candy after using isoetharine.

Inhalation devices require regular cleaning. Once a week, remove the drug container from the plastic mouthpiece, wash the mouthpiece with warm tap water, and dry it thoroughly.

Do not let any one else use your medication. Ask your pharmacist any questions you have about refilling your prescription.

Talk to your doctor, pharmacist, or other healthcare professional if you have questions about dosing information for your medication.

Isometheptene Mucate, Dichloralphenazone, and Acetaminophen

(eye soe me thep′ teen myoo kate)
(dye klor al phen′ a zone) (a seet a min′ oh fen)

Brand Name: Iso-Acetazone®, Isocom®, Isopap®, Midchlor®, Midrin®, Migratine®, Mitride®

Why is this medicine prescribed?

The combination of isometheptene mucate, dichloralphenazone, and acetaminophen is used to relieve migraine and tension headaches. It prevents blood vessels in your head from expanding and causing headaches.

This medication is sometimes prescribed for other uses; ask your doctor or pharmacist for more information.

How should this medicine be used?

The combination of isometheptene mucate, dichloralphenazone, and acetaminophen comes as a capsule to take by mouth. It usually is taken when a headache first begins and then as needed. Do not take more than five capsules in 12 hours or more than eight capsules per day. Follow the directions on your prescription label carefully, and ask your doctor or pharmacist to explain any part you do not understand. Take isometheptene mucate, dichloralphenazone, and acetaminophen exactly as directed. Do not take more or less of it or take it more often than prescribed by your doctor.

What special precautions should I follow?

Before taking isometheptene mucate, dichloralphenazone, and acetaminophen,

- tell your doctor and pharmacist if you are allergic to isometheptene mucate, dichloralphenazone, acetaminophen, or any other drugs.
- tell your doctor and pharmacist what prescription and nonprescription medications you are taking, especially antihistamines, MAO inhibitors [phenelzine (Nardil) and tranylcypromine (Parnate)], medications for depression such as chlorpromazine (Thorazine), sleeping pills, tranquilizers, and vitamins.
- tell your doctor if you have or have ever had heart, kidney, or liver disease; glaucoma; high blood pressure; or artery disease.
- tell your doctor if you are pregnant, plan to become pregnant, or are breast-feeding. If you become pregnant while taking this medication, call your doctor.
- you should know that this drug may make you drowsy. Do not drive a car or operate machinery until you know how this drug affects you.
- remember that alcohol can add to the drowsiness caused by this drug.

What should I do if I forget to take a dose?

This medication usually is taken as needed. If your doctor has told you to take isometheptene mucate, dichloralphenazone, and acetaminophen regularly, take the missed dose as soon as you remember it. However, if it is almost time for the next dose, skip the missed dose and continue your regular dosing schedule. Do not take a double dose to make up for a missed one.

What side effects can this medicine cause?

Isometheptene mucate, dichloralphenazone, and acetaminophen may cause side effects. Tell your doctor if this symptom is severe or does not go away:

- drowsiness

  If you experience the following symptom, call your doctor immediately:

- skin rash

  If you experience a serious side effect, you or your doctor may send a report to the Food and Drug Administration's (FDA) MedWatch Adverse Event Reporting program online [at http://www.fda.gov/MedWatch/index.html] or by phone [1-800-332-1088].

What storage conditions are needed for this medicine?

Keep this medication in the container it came in, tightly closed, and out of reach of children. Store it at room temperature, away from excess heat and moisture (not in the bathroom). Throw away any medication that is outdated or no longer needed. Talk to your pharmacist about the proper disposal of your medication.

What should I do in case of overdose?

In case of overdose, call your local poison control center at 1-800-222-1222. If the victim has collapsed or is not breathing, call local emergency services at 911.

What other information should I know?

Keep all appointments with your doctor.

Do not let anyone else take your medication. Ask your pharmacist any questions you have about refilling your prescription.

Talk to your doctor, pharmacist, or other healthcare professional if you have questions about dosing information for your medication.

Isoniazid

(eye soe nye′ a zid)

Brand Name: Nydrazid®, Rifamate® as a combination product containing Isoniazid and Rifampin, Rifater® as a combination product containing Isoniazid, Pyrazinamide, and Rifampin

Important Warning

Isoniazid may cause severe and sometimes fatal liver damage. Tell your doctor if you have or have ever had liver disease or a history of alcoholism or injection drug use. Keep all appointments with your doctor and the laboratory. Your doctor will order certain lab tests to check your response to isoniazid.

If you experience any of the following symptoms, call your doctor immediately: excessive tiredness, weakness, lack of energy, loss of appetite, upset stomach, vomiting, dark yellow or brown urine, and yellowing of the skin or eyes.

Why is this medicine prescribed?

Isoniazid is used alone or with other drugs to treat tuberculosis (TB) and to prevent it in people who have had contact with tuberculosis bacteria. It eliminates only active (growing) bacteria. Since the bacteria may exist in a resting (nongrowing) state for long periods, therapy with isoniazid (and other antituberculosis drugs) must be continued for a long time (usually 6-12 months).

This medication is sometimes prescribed for other uses; ask your doctor or pharmacist for more information.

How should this medicine be used?

Isoniazid comes as a tablet and a syrup to take by mouth. It usually is taken once a day, on an empty stomach, 1 hour before or 2 hours after meals. However, if isoniazid causes an upset stomach, it may be taken with food. Follow the directions on your prescription label carefully, and ask your doctor or pharmacist to explain any part you do not understand. Take isoniazid exactly as directed. Do not take more or less of it or take it more often than prescribed by your doctor.

What special precautions should I follow?

Before taking isoniazid,
- tell your doctor and pharmacist if you are allergic to isoniazid or any other drugs.
- tell your doctor and pharmacist what prescription and nonprescription medications you are taking, especially acetaminophen (Tylenol), antacids, carbamazepine (Tegretol), disulfiram (Antabuse), ketoconazole (Nizoral), phenytoin (Dilantin), theophylline (Theobid, Theo-Dur), valproic acid (Depakene, Depakote), and vitamins.
- in addition to the conditions listed in the IMPORTANT WARNING section, tell your doctor if you have or have ever had kidney disease; diabetes; tingling, burning, and pain in the fingers or toes (peripheral neuropathy); or human immunodeficiency virus (HIV).
- tell your doctor if you are pregnant or plan to become pregnant. If you become pregnant while taking isoniazid, call your doctor.
- be aware that you should not drink alcoholic beverages while taking this drug.

What special dietary instructions should I follow?

Unless your doctor tells you otherwise, continue your normal diet.

What should I do if I forget to take a dose?

Take the missed dose as soon as you remember it. However, if it is almost time for the next dose, skip the missed dose and continue your regular dosing schedule. Do not take a double dose to make up for a missed one.

What side effects can this medicine cause?

Isoniazid may cause side effects. Tell your doctor if any of these symptoms are severe or do not go away:
- diarrhea
- vision problems

If you experience any of the following symptoms or those listed in the IMPORTANT WARNING section, call your doctor immediately:
- eye pain
- numbness or tingling in the hands and feet
- skin rash
- fever
- swollen glands
- sore throat
- unusual bleeding or bruising
- stomach pains or tenderness

If you experience a serious side effect, you or your doctor may send a report to the Food and Drug Administration's (FDA) MedWatch Adverse Event Reporting program online [at http://www.fda.gov/MedWatch/index.html] or by phone [1-800-332-1088].

What storage conditions are needed for this medicine?

Keep this medication in the container it came in, tightly closed, and out of reach of children. Store it at room temperature and away from excess heat and moisture (not in the bathroom). Throw away any medication that is outdated or no longer needed. Talk to your pharmacist about the proper disposal of your medication.

What should I do in case of overdose?

In case of overdose, call your local poison control center at 1-800-222-1222. If the victim has collapsed or is not breathing, call local emergency services at 911.

What other information should I know?

If you have diabetes, do not use Clinitest to test your urine for sugar because isoniazid can cause false results in this test.

Do not let anyone else take your medication. Ask your pharmacist any questions you have about refilling your prescription.

Talk to your doctor, pharmacist, or other healthcare professional if you have questions about dosing information for your medication.

Isosorbide

(eye soe sor′ bide)

Brand Name: Dilatrate®-SR, Imdur®, Ismo®, Isordil®, Isordil® Titradose®, Monoket®

Why is this medicine prescribed?

Isosorbide is used to prevent or treat chest pain (angina). It works by relaxing the blood vessels to the heart, so the blood and oxygen supply to the heart is increased.

This medication is sometimes prescribed for other uses; ask your doctor or pharmacist for more information.

How should this medicine be used?

Isosorbide comes as a regular, sublingual, chewable, and extended-release (long-acting) tablet and extended-release (long-acting) capsule to be taken by mouth. The tablet usually is taken every 6 hours. The extended-release tablet usually is taken one or two times a day. The extended-release capsule usually is taken every 8-12 hours. Do not crush, chew, or divide the extended-release tablets or capsules. The sublingual or chewable tablet is used as needed to relieve chest pain that has already started or to prevent pain before activities known to provoke attacks (e.g., climbing stairs, sexual activity, heavy exercise, or being outside in cold weather). The chewable tablet also may be used every 2-3 hours to prevent chest pain. Follow the directions on your prescription label carefully, and ask your doctor or pharmacist to explain any part you do not understand. Take isosorbide exactly as directed. Do not take more or less of it or take it more often than prescribed by your doctor.

Isosorbide controls chest pain but does not cure it. Continue to take isosorbide even if you feel well. Do not stop taking isosorbide without talking to your doctor. Stopping the drug abruptly may cause chest pain.

Isosorbide can lose its effectiveness when used for a long time. This effect is called tolerance. If your angina attacks happen more often, last longer, or are more severe, call your doctor.

If you are using isosorbide sublingual or chewable tablets for acute chest pain, you should carry the tablets with you at all times. If you are taking isosorbide and your chest pain is not relieved within 5-10 minutes, take another dose. Call for emergency assistance or go to a hospital emergency department if pain persists after you have taken three tablets (at 5-10-minute intervals) and 15-30 minutes have passed.

When an attack occurs, sit down. If you use chewable tablets, chew a tablet thoroughly and swallow it. To use the sublingual tablets, place a tablet under your tongue or between your cheek and gum and allow it to dissolve. Do not swallow the tablet. Try not to swallow saliva too often until the tablet dissolves.

Are there other uses for this medicine?

Isosorbide tablets are also used with other drugs to treat congestive heart failure. Talk to your doctor about the possible risks of using this drug for your condition.

What special precautions should I follow?

Before taking isosorbide,

- tell your doctor and pharmacist if you are allergic to isosorbide; nitroglycerin tablets, patches, or ointment; or any other drugs.
- tell your doctor and pharmacist what prescription and nonprescription medications you are taking, especially aspirin; beta blockers such as atenolol (Tenormin), carteolol (Cartrol), labetalol (Trandate, Normodyne), metoprolol (Lopressor), nadolol (Corgard), propranolol (Inderal), sotalol (Betapace), and timolol (Blocadren); calcium channel blockers such as amlodipine (Norvasc), diltiazem (Cardizem), felodipine (Plendil), isradipine (DynaCirc), nifedipine (Procardia), and verapamil (Calan, Isoptin); dihydroergotamine (D.H.E. 45); sildenafil (Viagra); tadalafil (Cialis); vardenafil (Levitra); and vitamins.
- tell your doctor if you have or have ever had low red blood cell counts (anemia), glaucoma, or recent head trauma.
- tell your doctor if you are pregnant, plan to become pregnant, or are breast-feeding. If you become pregnant while taking isosorbide, call your doctor.
- if you are having surgery, including dental surgery, tell the doctor or dentist that you are taking isosorbide.
- you should know that this drug may make you drowsy or dizzy. Do not drive a car or operate machinery until you know how it affects you.
- tell your doctor if you consume large amounts of alcohol regularly and ask about the safe use of alcoholic beverages while you are taking isosorbide. Alcohol can make the side effects from isosorbide worse.

What special dietary instructions should I follow?

Take isosorbide tablets on an empty stomach (at least 1 hour before or 2 hours after meals) with a full glass of water.

What should I do if I forget to take a dose?

Take the missed dose as soon as you remember it. However, if it is almost time for the next dose, skip the missed dose and continue your regular dosing schedule. Do not take a double dose to make up for a missed one.

What side effects can this medicine cause?

Side effects from isosorbide are common. Tell your doctor if any of these symptoms are severe or do not go away:

- headache
- rash
- dizziness
- upset stomach
- headache
- flushing (feeling of warmth)

If you experience any of the following symptoms, call your doctor immediately:

- blurred vision
- dry mouth
- chest pain
- fainting

If you experience a serious side effect, you or your doctor may send a report to the Food and Drug Administration's (FDA) MedWatch Adverse Event Reporting program online [at http://www.fda.gov/MedWatch/index.html] or by phone [1-800-332-1088].

What storage conditions are needed for this medicine?

Keep this medication in the container it came in, tightly closed, and out of reach of children. Store it at room temperature and away from excess heat and moisture (not in the bathroom). Keep sublingual and chewable tablets in the original container. Do not open a container of sublingual or chewable isosorbide until you need a dose. Do not use tablets that are more than 12 months old. Throw away any medication that is outdated or no longer needed. Talk to your pharmacist about the proper disposal of your medication.

What should I do in case of overdose?

In case of overdose, call your local poison control center at 1-800-222-1222. If the victim has collapsed or is not breathing, call local emergency services at 911.

What other information should I know?

Keep all appointments with your doctor and the laboratory.

Isosorbide regular and extended-release tablets or capsules should not be used for acute angina attacks. Continue to use isosorbide sublingual or chewable tablets to relieve chest pain that has already started.

If headache continues, ask your doctor if you may take acetaminophen. Your isosorbide dose may need to be adjusted. Do not take aspirin or any other medication for headache while using isosorbide unless you doctor tells you to.

The tablets may cause a sweet, tingling sensation when placed under your tongue. This sensation is not an accurate indicator of drug strength; the absence of a tingling sensation does not mean that the drug is not working.

Do not let anyone else take your medication. Ask your pharmacist any questions you have about refilling your prescription.

Dosage Facts
For Informational Purposes

Caution: Do not change your dose, how often you take your medication, or the length of time you are to take it without first talking to your healthcare provider.

The following dosage information was written using medical language for doctors and other healthcare professionals and is provided here for you to check your dosage. The dosage of this drug may differ for different patients. Therefore, always follow your doctor's instructions or the directions on the label. Contact your healthcare provider or pharmacist if you have any questions about the specific dosage of your medication after reviewing this information.

General Dosage Information

Adjust dosage of isosorbide dinitrate and isosorbide mononitrate carefully according to the patient's requirements and response; use the smallest effective dosage.

Although many clinicians do not gradually reduce the dosage when discontinuance of oral nitrates is planned, it appears prudent that dosage be gradually reduced (e.g., over a period of about 1–2 weeks) to avoid withdrawal manifestations. Supplementary sublingual nitroglycerin doses should be given if necessary during dosage reduction.

Adult Patients

Angina
Acute Symptomatic Relief and Prophylactic Management

Do *not* use extended-release isosorbide dinitrate preparations or any isosorbide mononitrate preparation to abort an acute anginal episode or for acute relief of angina or in the prophylactic management in situations likely to provoke angina attacks; onset is not sufficiently rapid.

SUBLINGUAL:
- Patients who fail to respond to nitroglycerin lingual or sublingual: 2.5–5 mg of isosorbide dinitrate.
- If relief is not attained after a single dose during an acute attack, may give additional doses at 5- to 10-minute intervals; give no more than 3 doses in a 15- to 30-minute period.
- Prophylactic management in situations likely to provoke an-

gina attacks in patients who fail to respond to sublingual nitroglycerin: place 2.5–5 mg of isosorbide dinitrate under the tongue about 15 minutes prior to engaging in such activities.

INTRABUCCAL:

- Patients who fail to respond to nitroglycerin lingual or sublingual: 2.5–5 mg of isosorbide dinitrate.
- If relief is not attained after a single dose during an acute attack, may give additional doses at 5- to 10-minute intervals; no more than 3 doses should be given in a 15- to 30-minute period.
- Prophylactic management in situations likely to provoke angina attacks in patients who fail to respond to sublingual nitroglycerin: 2.5–5 mg of isosorbide dinitrate should be placed under the tongue approximately 15 minutes prior to engaging in such activities.

Long-term Prophylactic Management

ORAL (ISOSORBIDE DINITRATE CONVENTIONAL TABLETS):

- Initially, isosorbide dinitrate conventional tablets (e.g., Isordil® Titradose®) 5–20 mg administered 2–3 times daily, followed by maintenance dosage of 10–40 mg administered 2–3 times daily (some patients may require higher dosages).
- Suggested schedules: Usually, at 7 a.m., 12 p.m., and 5 p.m. in chronic stable angina or at 7 a.m. and 12 p.m. in less severely symptomatic angina in order to allow for a nitrate-free interval of 10–14 hours.
- May need to adjust schedule for those arising earlier than 7 a.m. since early morning angina is common.
- Less frequent administration of isosorbide dinitrate may reduce the development of tolerance to the drug's antianginal effects.)

ORAL (ISOSORBIDE DINITRATE EXTENDED-RELEASE CAPSULES):

- An interdosing interval sufficient to avoid tolerance to Dilatrate®-SR extended-release capsules is not known, but it must exceed 18 hours.
- Do not exceed daily Dilatrate®-SR dosages of 160 mg (4 capsules).

ORAL (ISOSORBIDE MONONITRATE CONVENTIONAL TABLETS):

- Usual initial dosage of conventional tablets (e.g., Monoket®): 20 mg twice daily, with the 2 doses administered 7 hours apart.
- Particularly small stature, initially: 5 mg (½ of a 10-mg tablet) twice daily, for no longer than initial 2 days.
- Particularly small stature, maintenance: Increased to at least 10 mg twice daily by the second or third day.

ORAL (ISOSORBIDE MONONITRATE EXTENDED-RELEASE TABLETS):

- Initially, (e.g., Imdur®): 30 mg (as a single 30-mg tablet or as ½ of a 60-mg tablet) or 60 mg (as a single 60-mg tablet) once daily.
- May increase dosage to 120 mg (as a single 120-mg tablet or as two 60-mg tablets) once daily after several days; 240-mg dosages rarely needed.

CHF
Fixed-combination Therapy with Hydralazine in Self-identified Black Patients

ORAL (ISOSORBIDE DINITRATE IN FIXED COMBINATION WITH HYDRALAZINE HYDROCHLORIDE TABLETS):

- Initially, isosorbide dinitrate 20 mg and hydralazine hydrochloride 37.5 mg (1 tablet of BiDil®) 3 times daily. May titrate dosage to a maximum tolerated dosage not to exceed 2 tablets (a total of 40 mg of isosorbide dinitrate and 75 mg of hydralazine hydrochloride) 3 times daily. Rapid titration (over 3–5 days) may be possible; however, slower titration may be needed due to adverse effects. May decrease dosage to as little as ½ of the fixed-combination tablet 3 times daily in patients who experience intolerable effects, but attempt to titrate dosage up once adverse effects subside.

Other Therapies in the General Population†

ORAL (ISOSORBIDE DINITRATE CONVENTIONAL TABLETS):

- Initially, 80 mg of isosorbide dinitrate (administered as ½ of a 40 mg conventional tablet 4 times daily) daily in combination with oral dosages of 150 mg of hydralazine hydrochloride (as a single 37.5 mg tablet 4 times daily) daily for 2 weeks.
- If initial dosages are tolerated, increase daily dosages to 160 mg of isosorbide dinitrate and 300 mg of hydralazine hydrochloride.

Diffuse Esophageal Spasm

ORAL (ISOSORBIDE DINITRATE CONVENTIONAL TABLETS):

- 10–30 mg 4 times daily.

Prescribing Limits

Adult Patients

Angina
Acute Symptomatic Relief and Prophylactic Management

SUBLINGUAL:

- No more than 3 doses in a 15- to 30-minute period.

INTRABUCCAL:

- No more than 3 doses in a 15- to 30-minute period.

Long-term Prophylactic Management

ORAL (ISOSORBIDE DINITRATE EXTENDED-RELEASE CAPSULES):

- Maximum daily dosage of Dilatrate®-SR: 160 mg (4 capsules).

ORAL (ISOSORBIDE MONONITRATE EXTENDED-RELEASE TABLETS):

- Dosages of 240 mg are rarely needed.

CHF
Fixed-combination Therapy with Hydralazine Hydrochloride in Self-identified Black Patients

ORAL (ISOSORBIDE DINITRATE IN FIXED COMBINATION WITH HYDRALAZINE HYDROCHLORIDE TABLETS):

- Maximum 40 mg of isosorbide dinitrate and 75 mg of hydralazine hydrochloride (2 tablets of BiDil®) 3 times daily.

Special Populations

Hepatic Impairment
- No specific dosage recommendations for hepatic impairment.

Renal Impairment
- No specific dosage recommendations for renal impairment.

Geriatric Patients
- One manufacturer of isosorbide mononitrate states that dosage should be selected with caution, usually initiating therapy at the low end of the range, although age, renal, hepatic, and cardiovascular dysfunction do not appear to have a significant effect on drug clearance.
- The manufacturer of the fixed combination of isosorbide dinitrate and hydralazine hydrochloride states that dosage should be selected with caution because of age-related decreases in hepatic, renal, and/or cardiac function and concomitant disease and drug therapy.

† Use is not currently included in the labeling approved by the US Food and Drug Administration.

Isotretinoin

(eye soe tret′ i noyn)

Brand Name: Accutane®, Amnesteem®, Claravis®, Sotret®

Important Warning

For all patients:

Isotretinoin must not be taken by patients who are pregnant or who may become pregnant. There is a high risk that isotretinoin will cause loss of the pregnancy, or will cause the baby to be born too early, to die shortly after birth, or to be born with birth defects (physical problems that are present at birth).

A program called iPLEDGE has been set up to make sure that pregnant women do not take isotretinoin and that women do not become pregnant while taking isotretinoin. All patients, including women who cannot become pregnant and men, can get isotretinoin only if they are registered with iPLEDGE, have a prescription from a doctor who is registered with iPLEDGE and fill the prescription at a pharmacy that is registered with iPLEDGE. Do not buy isotretinoin over the internet.

You will receive information about the risks of taking isotretinoin and must sign an informed consent sheet stating that you understand this information before you can receive the medication. You will need to see your doctor every month during your treatment to talk about your condition and the side effects you are experiencing. At each visit, your doctor may give you a prescription for up to a 30 day supply of medication with no refills. You must have this prescription filled within 7 days. If you do not have your prescription filled within 7 days and you are a woman who can become pregnant, you will not be able to get isotretinoin until it is time for your next office visit, 23 days after the 7 days have passed. If you are a man or if you are a woman who cannot become pregnant, you will need to visit your doctor again to talk about the safe use of isotretinoin and to get a new prescription. You may have the new prescription filled right away.

Tell your doctor if you do not understand everything you were told about isotretinoin and the iPLEDGE program or if you do not think you will be able to keep appointments or fill your prescription on schedule every month.

Your doctor will give you an identification number and card when you start your treatment. You will need this number to fill your prescriptions and to get information from the iPLEDGE website and phone line. Keep the card in a safe place where it will not get lost. If you do lose your card, you can ask for a replacement through the website or phone line.

Do not donate blood while you are taking isotretinoin and for 1 month after your treatment.

Do not share isotretinoin with anyone else, even someone who has the same symptoms that you have.

Your doctor or pharmacist will give you the manufacturer's patient information sheet (Medication Guide) when you begin treatment with isotretinoin and each time you refill your prescription. Read the information carefully and ask your doctor or pharmacist if you have any questions. You can also visit the Food and Drug Administration (FDA) website (http://www.fda.gov/cder), the manufacturer's website, or the iPLEDGE program website (http://www.ipledgeprogram.com) to obtain the Medication Guide.

Talk to your doctor about the risks of taking isotretinoin.

For female patients:

If you can become pregnant, you will need to meet certain requirements during your treatment with isotretinoin. You need to meet these requirements even if you have not started menstruating (having monthly periods) or have had a tubal ligation ('tubes tied'; surgery to prevent pregnancy). You may be excused from meeting these requirements only if you have not menstruated for 12 months in a row and your doctor says you have passed menopause (change of life) or you have had surgery to remove your uterus and/or both ovaries. If none of these are true for you, then you must meet the requirements below.

continued on next page

Important Warning (cont'd)

You must use two acceptable forms of birth control for 1 month before you begin to take isotretinoin, during your treatment, and for 1 month after your treatment. Your doctor will tell you which forms of birth control are acceptable, and will give you written information about birth control. You can also have a free visit with a doctor or family planning expert to talk about birth control that is right for you. You must use these two forms of birth control at all times unless you can promise that you will not have any sexual contact with a male for 1 month before your treatment, during your treatment, and for 1 month after your treatment.

If you choose to take isotretinoin, it is your responsibility to avoid pregnancy for 1 month before, during, and for 1 month after your treatment. You must understand that any form of birth control can fail. Therefore, it is very important to decrease the risk of accidental pregnancy by using two forms of birth control. Tell your doctor if you do not understand everything you were told about birth control or you do not think that you will be able to use two forms of birth control at all times.

If you plan to use oral contraceptives (birth control pills) while taking isotretinoin, tell your doctor the name of the pill you will use. Isotretinoin interferes with the action of microdosed progestin ('minipill') oral contraceptives (Ovrette, Micronor, Nor-QD). Do not use this type of birth control while taking isotretinoin.

If you plan to use hormonal contraceptives (birth control pills, patches, implants, injections, rings, or intrauterine devices), be sure to tell your doctor about all the medications, vitamins, and herbal supplements you are taking. Many medications interfere with the action of hormonal contraceptives. Do not take St. John's wort if you are using any type of hormonal contraceptive.

You must have two negative pregnancy tests before you can begin to take isotretinoin. Your doctor will tell you when and where to have these tests. You will also need to be tested for pregnancy in a laboratory each month during your treatment, when you take your last dose, and 30 days after you take your last dose.

You will need to contact the iPLEDGE system by phone or the internet every month to confirm the two forms of birth control you are using and to answer two questions about the iPLEDGE program. You will only be able to continue to get isotretinoin if you have done this, if you have visited your doctor to talk about how you are feeling and how you are using your birth control and if you have had a negative pregnancy test within the past 7 days.

Stop taking isotretinoin and call your doctor right away if you think you are pregnant, you miss a menstrual period, or you have sex without using two forms of birth control. If you become pregnant during your treatment or within 30 days after your treatment, your doctor will contact the iPLEDGE program, the manufacturer of isotretinoin, and the Food and Drug Administration (FDA). You will also talk with a doctor who specializes in problems during pregnancy who can help you make choices that are best for you and your baby. Information about your health and your baby's health will be used to help doctors learn more about the effects of isotretinoin on unborn babies.

For male patients:

A very small amount of isotretinoin will probably be present in your semen when you take prescribed doses of this medication. It is not known if this small amount of isotretinoin may harm the fetus if your partner is or becomes pregnant. Tell your doctor if your partner is pregnant, plans to become pregnant, or becomes pregnant during your treatment with isotretinoin.

Why is this medicine prescribed?

Isotretinoin is used to treat severe recalcitrant nodular acne (a certain type of severe acne) that has not been helped by other treatments, such as antibiotics. Isotretinoin is in a class of medications called retinoids. It works by slowing the production of certain natural substances that can cause pimples to form.

How should this medicine be used?

Isotretinoin comes as a capsule to take by mouth. Isotretinoin is usually taken twice a day with meals. Follow the directions on your prescription label carefully, and ask your doctor or pharmacist to explain any part you do not understand. Take isotretinoin exactly as directed. Do not take more or less of it or take it more often than prescribed by your doctor.

Swallow the capsules whole with a full glass of liquid. Do not chew or suck on the capsules.

Your doctor will probably start you on an average dose of isotretinoin and increase or decrease your dose depending on how well you respond to the medication and the side effects you experience. Follow these directions carefully and ask your doctor or pharmacist if you are not sure how much isotretinoin you should take.

It may take several weeks or longer for you to feel the full benefit of isotretinoin. Your acne may get worse during the beginning of your treatment with isotretinoin. This is normal and does not mean that the medication is not working.

Are there other uses for this medicine?

Isotretinoin has been used to treat certain other skin conditions and some types of cancer. Talk to your doctor about the possible risks of using this medication for your condition.

This medication may be prescribed for other uses. Ask your doctor or pharmacist for more information.

What special precautions should I follow?

Before taking isotretinoin,

- tell your doctor and pharmacist if you are allergic to isotretinoin, any other medications, parabens (a preservative), or any of the ingredients in isotretinoin capsules. Ask your pharmacist or check the Medication Guide for a list of the inactive ingredients.
- tell your doctor and pharmacist what prescription and nonprescription medications, vitamins, herbal products, and nutritional supplements you are taking or plan to take. Be sure to mention medications for seizures such as phenytoin (Dilantin); oral steroids such as dexamethasone (Decadron, Dexone), methylprednisolone (Medrol), and prednisone (Deltasone); tetracycline antibiotics such as demeclocycline (Declomycin), doxycycline (Monodox, Vibramycin, others), minocycline (Minocin, Vectrin), oxytetracycline (Terramycin), and tetracycline (Sumycin, Tetrex, others); and vitamin A supplements. Your doctor may need to change the doses of your medications or monitor you carefully for side effects.
- tell your doctor if you or anyone in your family has thought about or attempted suicide and if you or anyone in your family has or has ever had depression, mental illness, diabetes, asthma, osteoporosis (a condition in which the bones are fragile and break easily) or other conditions that cause weak bones, a high triglyceride (fats in the blood) level, anorexia nervosa (an eating disorder in which very little is eaten), or heart or liver disease.
- do not breastfeed while you are taking isotretinoin and for 1 month after you stop taking isotretinoin.
- plan to avoid unnecessary or prolonged exposure to sunlight and to wear protective clothing, sunglasses, and sunscreen. Isotretinoin may make your skin sensitive to sunlight.
- you should know that isotretinoin may cause changes in your thoughts, behavior, or mental health. Some patients who took isotretinoin have developed depression or psychosis (loss of contact with reality), have become violent, have thought about killing or hurting themselves, and have tried or succeeded in doing so. You or your family should call your doctor right away if you experience any of the following symptoms: anxiety, sadness, crying spells, loss of interest in activities you used to enjoy, poor performance at school or work, sleeping more than usual, difficulty falling asleep or staying asleep, irritability, anger, aggression, changes in appetite or weight, difficulty concentrating, withdrawing from friends or family, lack of energy, feelings of worthlessness or guilt, thinking about killing or hurting yourself, acting on dangerous thoughts, or hallucinations (seeing or hearing things that do not exist). Be sure that your family members know which symptoms are serious so that they can call the doctor if you are unable to seek treatment on your own.
- you should know that isotretinoin may cause your eyes to feel dry and make wearing contact lenses uncomfortable during and after your treatment.
- you should know that isotretinoin may limit your ability to see in the dark. This problem may begin suddenly at any time during your treatment and may continue after your treatment is stopped. Be very careful when you drive or operate machinery at night.
- plan to avoid hair removal by waxing, laser skin treatments, and dermabrasion (surgical smoothing of the skin) while you are taking isotretinoin and for 6 months after your treatment. Isotretinoin increases the risk that you will develop scars from these treatments. Ask your doctor when you can safely undergo these treatments.
- talk to your doctor before you participate in hard physical activity such as sports. Isotretinoin may cause the bones to weaken or thicken abnormally and may increase the risk of certain bone injuries in people who perform some types of physical activity. If you break a bone during your treatment, be sure to tell all your health care providers that you are taking isotretinoin.

What special dietary instructions should I follow?

Unless your doctor tells you otherwise, continue your normal diet.

What should I do if I forget to take a dose?

Skip the missed dose and continue your regular dosing schedule. Do not take a double dose to make up for a missed one.

What side effects can this medicine cause?

Isotretinoin may cause side effects. Tell your doctor if any of these symptoms are severe or do not go away:

- red, cracked, and sore lips
- dry skin, eyes, mouth, or nose
- nosebleeds
- changes in skin color
- peeling skin, especially on the palms and soles
- changes in the nails
- slowed healing of cuts or sores
- bleeding or swollen gums
- hair loss or unwanted hair growth
- sweating
- flushing
- voice changes
- tiredness
- cold symptoms

Some side effects can be serious. If you experience any of the following symptoms or those listed in the IMPORTANT WARNING section, call your doctor immediately:

- headache
- blurred vision

- dizziness
- upset stomach
- vomiting
- seizures
- slow or difficult speech
- weakness or numbness of one part or side of the body
- stomach pain
- chest pain
- difficulty swallowing or pain when swallowing
- new or worsening heartburn
- diarrhea
- rectal bleeding
- yellowing of the skin or eyes
- dark colored urine
- back, bone, joint or muscle pain
- muscle weakness
- difficulty hearing
- ringing in the ears
- vision problems
- painful or constant dryness of the eyes
- unusual thirst
- frequent urination
- trouble breathing
- fainting
- fast or pounding heartbeat
- fever
- rash
- red patches or bruises on the legs
- swelling of the eyes, face, lips, tongue, throat, arms, hands, feet, ankles, or lower legs

Isotretinoin may cause the bones to stop growing too soon in teenagers. Talk to your child's doctor about the risks of giving this medication to your child.

Isotretinoin may cause other side effects. Call your doctor if you have any unusual problems while taking this medication.

If you experience a serious side effect, you or your doctor may send a report to the Food and Drug Administration's (FDA) MedWatch Adverse Event Reporting program online [at http://www.fda.gov/MedWatch/index.html] or by phone [1-800-332-1088].

What storage conditions are needed for this medicine?

Keep this medication in the container it came in, tightly closed, and out of reach of children. Store it at room temperature and away from excess heat and moisture (not in the bathroom). Throw away any medication that is outdated or no longer needed. Talk to your pharmacist about the proper disposal of your medication.

What should I do in case of overdose?

In case of overdose, call your local poison control center at 1-800-222-1222. If the victim has collapsed or is not breathing, call local emergency services at 911.

Symptoms of overdose may include:

- vomiting
- flushing
- severe chapped lips
- stomach pain
- headache
- dizziness
- loss of coordination

Anyone who has taken an overdose of isotretinoin should know about the risk of birth defects caused by isotretinoin and should not donate blood for 1 month after the overdose. Pregnant woman should talk to their doctors about the risks of continuing the pregnancy after the overdose. Women who can become pregnant should use two forms of birth control for 1 month after the overdose. Men whose partners are or may become pregnant should use condoms or avoid sexual contact with that partner for 1 month after the overdose because isotretinoin may be present in the semen.

What other information should I know?

Keep all appointments with your doctor and the laboratory. Your doctor will order certain lab tests to check your response to isotretinoin.

Dosage Facts
For Informational Purposes

Caution: Do not change your dose, how often you take your medication, or the length of time you are to take it without first talking to your healthcare provider.

The following dosage information was written using medical language for doctors and other healthcare professionals and is provided here for you to check your dosage. The dosage of this drug may differ for different patients. Therefore, always follow your doctor's instructions or the directions on the label. Contact your healthcare provider or pharmacist if you have any questions about the specific dosage of your medication after reviewing this information.

Pediatric Patients

Severe Nodular Acne

ORAL:
- Adolescents ≥12 years of age: usual initial dosage is 0.5–1 mg/kg daily given in 2 divided doses with food. Adjust subsequent dosage after ≥2 weeks of treatment according to individual tolerance and response, using the lowest possible effective dosage.
- Usual duration of therapy: 15–20 weeks; discontinue therapy sooner if the total number of cysts has been reduced by more than 70%.
- A second course of therapy may be initiated if severe nodular acne persists and it is thought that the patient could benefit from further treatment; optimum interval between initial and subsequent courses of isotretinoin therapy has not been defined for adolescents who have not completed skeletal growth.

Adult Patients

Severe Nodular Acne

ORAL:

- Usual initial dosage: 0.5–1 mg/kg daily given in 2 divided doses with food. Adjust subsequent dosage after ≥2 weeks of treatment according to individual tolerance and response, using the lowest possible effective dosage. If disease is severe or is mainly evident on the chest and back, instead of the face, dosages up to 2 mg/kg daily may be required.
- Usual duration of therapy: 15–20 weeks; discontinue therapy sooner if the total number of cysts has been reduced by more than 70%.
- A second course of therapy may be initiated if severe nodular acne persists and it is thought that the patient could benefit from further treatment; however, at least 2 months should elapse between courses in adults to assess the degree of improvement and the need for further therapy.

Prescribing Limits

Pediatric Patients

Severe Nodular Acne

ORAL:

- Maximum 2 mg/kg daily.

Adult Patients

Severe Nodular Acne

ORAL:

- Maximum 2 mg/kg daily.

Isoxsuprine Oral

(eye sox′ syoo preen)

Available generically.

Why is this medicine prescribed?

Isoxsuprine is used to relieve the symptoms of central and peripheral vascular diseases such as arteriosclerosis, Buerger's disease, and Raynaud's disease.

This medication is sometimes prescribed for other uses; ask your doctor or pharmacist for more information.

How should this medicine be used?

Isoxsuprine comes as a tablet to take by mouth. It is usually taken three or four times a day. Follow the directions on your prescription label carefully, and ask your doctor or pharmacist to explain any part you do not understand. Take isoxsuprine exactly as directed. Do not take more or less of it or take it more often than prescribed by your doctor.

Are there other uses for this medicine?

Isoxsuprine is also used occasionally to treat menstrual pain or prevent premature labor. Talk to your doctor about the possible risks of using this drug for your condition.

What special precautions should I follow?

Before taking isoxsuprine,

- tell your doctor and pharmacist if you are allergic to isoxsuprine or any other drugs.
- tell your doctor and pharmacist what prescription and nonprescription medications and vitamins you are taking.
- tell your doctor if you are pregnant, plan to become pregnant, or are breast-feeding. If you become pregnant while taking isoxsuprine, call your doctor immediately.
- if you are having surgery, including dental surgery, tell your doctor or dentist that you are taking isoxsuprine.
- you should know that this drug may make you drowsy or dizzy. Do not drive a car or operate machinery until you know how isoxsuprine will affect you. Avoid sudden changes in posture and get up slowly when lying down.

What should I do if I forget to take a dose?

Take the missed dose as soon as you remember it. However, if it is almost time for the next dose, skip the missed dose and continue your regular dosing schedule. Do not take a double dose to make up for a missed one.

What side effects can this medicine cause?

Isoxsuprine may cause side effects. Tell your doctor if any of these symptoms are severe or do not go away:

- weakness
- dizziness
- flushing (feeling of warmth)
- upset stomach
- vomiting
- stomach pain

If you experience any of the following symptoms, call your doctor immediately:

- rash
- fast heartbeat
- chest pain

If you experience a serious side effect, you or your doctor may send a report to the Food and Drug Administration's (FDA) MedWatch Adverse Event Reporting program online [at http://www.fda.gov/MedWatch/index.html] or by phone [1-800-332-1088].

What storage conditions are needed for this medicine?

Keep this medication in the container it came in, tightly closed, and out of reach of children. Store it at room temperature and away from excess heat and moisture (not in the bathroom). Throw away any medication that is outdated or no longer needed. Talk to your pharmacist about the proper disposal of your medication.

What should I do in case of overdose?

In case of overdose, call your local poison control center at 1-800-222-1222. If the victim has collapsed or is not breathing, call local emergency services at 911.

What other information should I know?

Keep all appointments with your doctor and the laboratory.

Do not let anyone else take your medication. Ask your pharmacist any questions you have about refilling your prescription.

Talk to your doctor, pharmacist, or other healthcare professional if you have questions about dosing information for your medication.

Isradipine

(iz ra′ di peen)

Brand Name: DynaCirc®, DynaCirc® CR®

Why is this medicine prescribed?

Isradipine is used to treat high blood pressure. It relaxes your blood vessels so your heart does not have to pump as hard.

This medication is sometimes prescribed for other uses; ask your doctor or pharmacist for more information.

How should this medicine be used?

Isradipine comes as a regular capsule and an extended-release (long-acting) tablet to take by mouth. The capsule is usually taken two times a day, while the tablet is usually taken once a day. The tablet should be swallowed whole. Do not chew, divide, or crush the tablet. Follow the directions on your prescription label carefully, and ask your doctor or pharmacist to explain any part you do not understand. Take isradipine exactly as directed. Do not take more or less of it or take it more often than prescribed by your doctor.

Isradipine controls high blood pressure but does not cure it. Continue to take isradipine even if you feel well. Do not stop taking isradipine without talking to your doctor.

What special precautions should I follow?

Before taking isradipine,
- tell your doctor and pharmacist if you are allergic to isradipine or any other drugs.
- tell your doctor and pharmacist what prescription and nonprescription medications you are taking, especially cimetidine (Tagamet), fentanyl (Duragesic), heart and blood pressure medications such as beta-blockers and diuretics ('water pills'), medications to treat glaucoma (increased pressure in the eye), ranitidine (Zantac), rifampin (Rifadin, Rimactane), and vitamins.
- tell your doctor if you have or have ever had heart, liver, or kidney disease or a history of gastrointestinal obstruction (strictures).

- tell your doctor if you are pregnant, plan to become pregnant, or are breast-feeding. If you become pregnant while taking isradipine, call your doctor.
- if you are having surgery, including dental surgery, tell your doctor or dentist that you are taking isradipine.

What special dietary instructions should I follow?

Talk to your doctor about drinking grapefruit juice or eating grapefruit while taking isradipine.

Talk to your doctor before using salt substitutes containing potassium. If your doctor prescribes a low-salt or low-sodium diet, follow these directions carefully.

What should I do if I forget to take a dose?

Take the missed dose as soon as you remember it. However, if it is almost time for the next dose, skip the missed dose and continue your regular dosing schedule. Do not take a double dose to make up for a missed one.

What side effects can this medicine cause?

Isradipine may cause side effects. Tell your doctor if any of these symptoms are severe or do not go away:
- headache
- dizziness or lightheadedness
- flushing (feeling of warmth)
- fast heartbeat
- excessive tiredness
- upset stomach
- vomiting
- diarrhea

If you experience any of the following symptoms, call your doctor immediately:
- chest pain
- swelling of the face, eyes, lips, tongue, arms, or legs
- difficulty breathing or swallowing
- fainting
- rash

If you experience a serious side effect, you or your doctor may send a report to the Food and Drug Administration's (FDA) MedWatch Adverse Event Reporting program online [at http://www.fda.gov/MedWatch/index.html] or by phone [1-800-332-1088].

What storage conditions are needed for this medicine?

Keep this medication in the container it came in, tightly closed, and out of reach of children. Store it at room temperature and away from excess heat and moisture (not in the bathroom). Throw away any medication that is outdated or no longer needed. Talk to your pharmacist about the proper disposal of your medication.

What should I do in case of overdose?

In case of overdose, call your local poison control center at 1-800-222-1222. If the victim has collapsed or is not breathing, call local emergency services at 911.

What other information should I know?

Keep all appointments with your doctor and the laboratory. Your blood pressure should be checked regularly to determine your response to isradipine.

The extended-release tablet does not dissolve in the stomach after being swallowed. It slowly releases medicine as it passes through your small intestines. It is not unusual to see the tablet shell in the stool.

Do not let anyone else take your medication. Ask your pharmacist any questions you have about refilling your prescription.

Dosage Facts
For Informational Purposes

Caution: Do not change your dose, how often you take your medication, or the length of time you are to take it without first talking to your healthcare provider.

The following dosage information was written using medical language for doctors and other healthcare professionals and is provided here for you to check your dosage. The dosage of this drug may differ for different patients. Therefore, always follow your doctor's instructions or the directions on the label. Contact your healthcare provider or pharmacist if you have any questions about the specific dosage of your medication after reviewing this information.

Pediatric Patients

Hypertension†
Conventional Capsules

ORAL:
- Initially, 0.15–0.2 mg/kg daily given in 3–4 divided doses. Increase dosage as necessary up to a maximum dosage of 0.8 mg/kg (up to 20 mg) daily.

Extended-release Core Tablets

ORAL:
- Initially, 0.15–0.2 mg/kg daily given once daily or in 2 divided doses. Increase dosage as necessary up to a maximum dosage of 0.8 mg/kg (up to 20 mg) daily.

Hypertensive Urgencies or Emergencies†

ORAL CAPSULES, EXTENDED-RELEASE TABLETS, OR EXTEMPORANEOUS SUSPENSION:
- Children and adolescents 1–17 years of age: 0.05–0.1 mg/kg per dose.
- Prepare extemporaneous isradipine suspension containing 1 mg/mL for those unable to swallow capsules or extended-release tablets. Open twenty four 5-mg capsules and grind the contents to a fine powder with a mortar and pestle; levigate

with a small amount of glycerin to form a paste. Add simple syrup in increasing amounts while mixing thoroughly; transfer the suspension to a graduated cylinder. Add any remaining drug in the mortar to the graduated container; the final volume of the suspension should be 120 mL. Transfer contents of the graduated cylinder into an appropriate size amber bottle. The isradipine suspension is stable for 35 days when refrigerated. Shake well before each use.

Adult Patients

Hypertension
Conventional Capsules

ORAL:
- Initially, 1.25–2.5 mg twice daily as monotherapy or when added to thiazide diuretic therapy. However, a dosage form suitable for administering 1.25-mg doses is not commercially available in the US.
- Full hypotensive effect may not be seen for 2–4 weeks. If BP control is inadequate after this period, increase dosage in increments of 5 mg daily at intervals of 2–4 weeks, up to a maximum of 20 mg daily, according to patient's BP response.
- Dosages >10 mg daily usually do not result in further improvement in BP control and may increase risk of adverse effects. The JNC recommends a usual range of 2.5–10 mg daily.

Extended-release Core Tablets

ORAL:
- Initially, 5 mg once daily as monotherapy or when added to thiazide diuretic therapy.
- If necessary, increase dosage in increments of 5 mg daily at intervals of 2–4 weeks, up to a maximum of 20 mg daily, according to patient's BP response.
- Dosages >10 mg daily usually do not result in further improvement in BP control and may increase risk of adverse effects. The JNC recommends a usual range of 2.5–10 mg daily.

Prescribing Limits
Pediatric Patients

Hypertension†

ORAL:
- Conventional capsules: Maximum 0.8 mg/kg (up to 20 mg) daily.
- Extended-release core tablets: Maximum 0.8 mg/kg (up to 20 mg) daily.

Adult Patients

Hypertension

ORAL:
- Conventional capsules: Maximum 20 mg daily.
- Extended-release core tablets: Maximum 20 mg daily.

Special Populations

Hepatic Impairment
- Some clinicians recommend dosage modification (i.e., reduced dosage) and careful titration, but the manufacturer recommends usual initial adult dosage.

Renal Impairment
- Dosage modification not necessary.

Geriatric Patients
- Initial dosage modification not necessary, but slower dosage escalation recommended; BP may be adequately controlled with relatively low dosages and once-daily dosing.

† *Use is not currently included in the labeling approved by the US Food and Drug Administration.*

Itraconazole

(i tra ko′ na zole)

Brand Name: Sporanox®
Also available generically.

Important Warning

Itraconazole can cause congestive heart failure (condition in which the heart cannot pump enough blood through the body). Tell your doctor if you have or have ever had heart failure; a heart attack; an irregular heartbeat; any other type of heart disease; lung, liver, or kidney disease; or any other serious health problem. If you experience any of the following symptoms, stop taking itraconazole and call your doctor immediately: shortness of breath, coughing up white or pink phlegm, weakness, excessive tiredness, fast heartbeat, swelling of the feet, ankles, or legs; and sudden weight gain.

Do not take cisapride (Propulsid), dofetilide (Tikosyn), pimozide (Orap), or quinidine (Quinaglute, Quinidex, others), while taking itraconazole. Taking these medications with itraconazole can cause serious irregular hearbeats.

Talk to your doctor about the risks of taking itraconazole.

Why is this medicine prescribed?

Itraconazole capsules are used to treat fungal infections that begin in the lungs and can spread through the body. Itraconazole capsules are also used to treat fungal infections of the fingernails and/or toenails. Itraconazole oral solution is used to treat yeast infections of the mouth and throat and suspected fungal infections in patients with fever and certain other signs of infection. Itraconazole is in a class of antifungals called triazoles. It works by slowing the growth of fungi that cause infection.

How should this medicine be used?

Itraconazole comes as a capsule and a solution (liquid) to take by mouth. Itraconazole capsules are usually taken with a full meal one to three times a day for at least 3 months.

When itraconazole capsules are used to treat fungal infections of the fingernails, they are usually taken twice a day for one week, not taken at all for three weeks, and then taken twice a day for an additional week. Itraconazole solution is usually taken on an empty stomach once or twice a day for 1 to 4 weeks or longer. Follow the directions on your prescription label carefully, and ask your doctor or pharmacist to explain any part you do not understand. Take itraconazole exactly as directed. Do not take more or less of it or take it more often than prescribed by your doctor.

Your doctor may tell you to take itraconazole capsules with a cola soft drink if you have certain medical conditions or are taking any of the following medications: cimetidine (Tagamet); famotidine (Pepcid); nizatadine (Axid); proton-pump inhibitors such as esomeprazole (Nexium), lansoprazole (Prevacid), omeprazole (Prilosec), pantoprazole (Protonix), and rabeprazole (AcipHex); or ranitidine (Zantac) Follow these directions carefully.

To take itraconazole oral solution for fungal infections of the mouth or throat, swish 10 mL (about 2 teaspoons) of the solution in your mouth for a few seconds and swallow. Repeat if necessary until you have taken your entire dose.

Itraconazole capsules and oral solution are absorbed into the body in different ways and work to treat different conditions. Do not substitute the capsules for the liquid or the liquid for the capsules. Be sure that your pharmacist gives you the form of itraconazole that your doctor prescribed.

Your doctor may tell you to take higher doses of itraconazole or to take itraconazole more often at the beginning of your treatment. Follow these directions carefully.

If you are taking itraconazole to treat a nail infection, your nails will probably not look healthier until new nails grow. It can take up to 6 months to grow a new fingernail and up to 12 months to grow a new toenail, so you should not expect to see improvement during your treatment or for several months afterward. Continue to take itraconazole even if you do not see any improvement.

Continue to take itraconazole until your doctor tells you to stop even if you feel well. Do not stop taking itraconazole without talking to your doctor. If you stop taking itraconazole too soon, your infection may come back after a short time.

Are there other uses for this medicine?

Itraconazole is also sometimes used to treat other types of fungal infections and to prevent fungal infections in people who have human immunodeficiency virus (HIV) or acquired immunodeficiency syndrome (AIDS). Talk to your doctor about the possible risks of using this drug for your condition.

This medication may be prescribed for other uses; ask your doctor or pharmacist for more information.

What special precautions should I follow?

Before taking itraconazole,
- tell your doctor and pharmacist if you are allergic to

itraconazole; other antifungal medications such as fluconazole (Diflucan), ketoconazole (Nizoral), or voriconazole (Vfend); orany other medications. If you are taking itraconazole oral solution, tell your doctor if you are allergic to saccharin or sulfa medications.

- do not take itraconazole if you are taking any of the medications listed in the IMPORTANT WARNING section or any of the following medications: ergot-type medications such as dihydroergotamine (D.H.E. 45, Migranal), ergoloid mesylates (Germinal, Hydergine), ergonovine (Ergotrate), ergotamine (Bellergal-S, Cafergot, Ergomar, Wigraine), methylergonovine (Methergine), and methysergide (Sansert); lovastatin (Mevacor); simvastatin (Zocor); or triazolam (Halcion).
- tell your doctor and pharmacist what other prescription and nonprescription medications, vitamins, nutritional supplements and herbal products you are taking, especially alfentanil (Alfenta); alprazolam (Xanax); anticoagulants ('blood thinners') such as warfarin (Coumadin); atorvastatin (Lipitor); buspirone (BuSpar); busulfan (Myleran); calcium channel blockers such as amlodipine (Norvasc), felodipine (Plendil), isradipine (Dynacirc), nifedipine (Adalat, Procardia) nicardipine (Cardene) nimodipine (Nimotop), nisoldipine (Sular), and verapamil (Calan, Covera, Isoptin, Verelan); carbamazepine (Tegretol); cerivastatin (Baycol) (not available in the United States); cilostazol (Pletal); clarithromycin (Biaxin); cyclosporine (Neoral, Sandimmune); diazepam (Valium); digoxin (Lanoxin); disopyramide (Norpace); docetaxel (Taxotere); eletriptan (Relpax); erythromycin (E.E.S., Erythrocin, E-Mycin); halofantrine (Halfan); HIV protease inhibitors such as indinavir (Crixivan), ritonavir (Norvir), and saquinavir (Fortovase, Invirase); isoniazid (INH, Nydrazid); medications for erectile dysfunction such as sildenafil (Viagra), tadalafil (Cialis), and vardenafil (Levitra); midazolam (Versed); nevirapine (Viramune)' oral contraceptives (birth control pills); oral medicine for diabetes; phenobarbital (Luminal, Solfoton); phenytoin (Dilantin); rifabutin (Mycobutin); rifampin (Rifadin, Rimactane); sirolimus (Rapamune); steroids such as dexamethasone (Decadron), budesonide (Entocort EC), and methylprednisolone (Medrol); tacrolimus (Prograf); trimetrexate (Neutrexin); vinblastine (Velban); vincristine (Oncovin); and vinorelbine (Navelbine). Many other medications may also interact with itraconazole, so be sure to tell your doctor about all the medications you are taking, even those that do not appear on this list.
- you should know that itraconazole may remain in your body for several months after you stop taking it. Tell your doctor that you have recently stopped taking itraconazole before you start taking any other medications during the first few months after your treatment.
- if you are taking an antacid, take it 1 hour before or 2 hours after you take itraconazole.
- tell your doctor if you have or have ever had the conditions mentioned in the IMPORTANT WARNING section, AIDS, cystic fibrosis (an inborn disease that causes problems with breathing, digestion, and reproduction), or any condition that decreases the amount of acid in your stomach.
- tell your doctor if you are pregnant, plan to become pregnant, or are breast-feeding. You should not take itraconazole to treat nail fungus if you are pregnant or could become pregnant. You may start to take itraconazole to treat nail fungus only on the second or third day of your menstrual period when you are sure you are not pregnant. You must use effective birth control during your treatment and for 2 months afterward. If you become pregnant while taking itraconazole to treat any condition, call your doctor.

What special dietary instructions should I follow?

Talk to your doctor about drinking grapefruit juice while taking this medication.

What should I do if I forget to take a dose?

Take the missed dose as soon as you remember it. However, if it is almost time for the next dose, skip the missed dose and continue your regular dosing schedule. Do not take a double dose to make up for a missed one.

What side effects can this medicine cause?

Itraconazole may cause side effects. Tell your doctor if any of these symptoms are severe or do not go away:

- diarrhea or loose stools
- constipation
- gas
- stomach pain
- heartburn
- sore or bleeding gums
- sores in or around the mouth
- headache
- dizziness
- sweating
- muscle pain
- decreased sexual desire or ability
- nervousness
- depression
- runny nose and other cold symptoms
- unusual dreams

Some side effects can be serious. If you experience any of the following symptoms or those listed in the IMPORTANT WARNING section, call your doctor immediately:

- excessive tiredness
- loss of appetite
- upset stomach
- vomiting
- yellowing of the skin or eyes
- dark urine
- pale stools
- tingling or numbness of the hands or feet

- fever, chills, or other signs of infection
- frequent or painful urination
- shaking hands that you cannot control
- rash
- hives
- itching
- difficulty breathing or swallowing

One of the ingredients in itraconazole oral solution caused cancer in some types of laboratory animals. It is not known whether people who take itraconazole solution have an increased risk of developing cancer. Talk to your doctor about the risks of taking itraconazole solution.

If you experience a serious side effect, you or your doctor may send a report to the Food and Drug Administration's (FDA) MedWatch Adverse Event Reporting program online [at http://www.fda.gov/MedWatch/index.html] or by phone [1-800-332-1088].

What storage conditions are needed for this medicine?

Keep this medication in the container it came in, tightly closed, and out of reach of children. Store it at room temperature and away from excess heat and moisture (not in the bathroom). Throw away any medication that is outdated or no longer needed. Talk to your pharmacist about the proper disposal of your medication.

What should I do in case of overdose?

In case of overdose, call your local poison control center at 1-800-222-1222. If the victim has collapsed or is not breathing, call local emergency services at 911.

What other information should I know?

Keep all appointments with your doctor and the laboratory. Your doctor will order certain lab tests to check your response to itraconazole.

Do not let anyone else take your medication. Ask your pharmacist any questions you have about refilling your prescription. If you still have symptoms of infection after you finish the itraconazole, call your doctor.

Dosage Facts
For Informational Purposes

Caution: Do not change your dose, how often you take your medication, or the length of time you are to take it without first talking to your healthcare provider.

The following dosage information was written using medical language for doctors and other healthcare professionals and is provided here for you to check your dosage. The dosage of this drug may differ for different patients. Therefore, always follow your doctor's instructions or the directions on the label. Contact your healthcare provider or pharmacist if you have any questions

about the specific dosage of your medication after reviewing this information.

General Dosage Information

Because of differences in oral bioavailability, itraconazole capsules and oral solution should *not* be used interchangeably on a mg-for-mg basis.

Only the oral solution (not capsules) is indicated for treatment of oropharyngeal or esophageal candidiasis.

For treatment of life-threatening systemic fungal infections, IV itraconazole or oral itraconazole capsules should be initiated using a loading dosage given for the first 3–4 days.

For treatment of systemic fungal infections, itraconazole usually is continued for >3 months and until clinical parameters and laboratory tests indicate that the active fungal infection has subsided. Some clinicians state that while the optimal duration of therapy for serious fungal infections has not been established, itraconazole probably should be continued for 6–12 months for blastomycosis and for ≥12 months for disseminated or chronic pulmonary histoplasmosis. An inadequate period of treatment can result in recurrence of active infection.

Pediatric Patients

Candida Infections†
Prevention of Recurrence (Secondary Prophylaxis) of Mucocutaneous Candidiasis†

ORAL:
- HIV-infected infants and children with frequent or severe recurrences: 5 mg/kg (oral solution) once daily recommended by USPH/IDSA.
- HIV-infected adolescents with frequent or severe recurrences: 200 mg (oral solution) once daily recommended by USPHS/IDSA.
- The safety of discontinuing secondary prophylaxis against mucocutaneous candidiasis in those receiving potent antiretroviral therapy has not been extensively studied.

Coccidioidomycosis†
Prevention of Recurrence (Secondary Prophylaxis) of Coccidioidomycosis†

ORAL:
- HIV-infected infants and children: 2–5 mg/kg every 12–48 hours recommended by USPHS/IDSA.
- HIV-infected adolescents: 200 mg (capsule) twice daily recommended by USPHS/IDSA.
- Initiate secondary prophylaxis after primary infection has been adequately treated.
- HIV-infected children and adolescents with a history of coccidioidomycosis should receive life-long suppressive therapy to prevent recurrence; data insufficient to date to warrant a recommendation regarding discontinuance in patients receiving potent antiretroviral therapy.

Cryptococcosis†
Prevention (Primary Prophylaxis) of Cryptococcosis†

ORAL:
- HIV-infected infants and children with severe immunosuppression: 2–5 mg/kg every 12–24 hours recommended by USPHS/IDSA.
- HIV-infected adolescents with CD4+ T-cell counts <50/mm³: 200 mg (capsule) once daily recommended by USPHS/IDSA.

Prevention of Recurrence (Secondary Prophylaxis) of Cryptococcosis†

ORAL:

- HIV-infected infants and children: 2–5 mg/kg every 12–24 hours recommended by USPHS/IDSA.
- HIV-infected adolescents: 200 mg (capsule) once daily recommended by USPHS/IDSA.
- Initiate secondary prophylaxis after primary infection has been adequately treated.
- HIV-infected infants and children with a history of cryptococcosis should receive life-long suppressive therapy to prevent recurrence. Consideration can be given to discontinuing secondary prophylaxis in HIV-infected adolescents receiving potent antiretroviral therapy according to recommendations in adults.

Histoplasmosis†

Prevention (Primary Prophylaxis) of Histoplasmosis†

ORAL:

- HIV-infected infants and children with severe immunosuppression: 2–5 mg/kg every 12–24 hours recommended by USPHS/IDSA.
- HIV-infected adolescents with CD4$^+$ T-cell counts <100/mm^3: 200 mg (capsule) once daily recommended by USPHS/IDSA.

Prevention of Recurrence (Secondary Prophylaxis) of Histoplasmosis†

ORAL:

- HIV-infected infants and children: 2–5 mg/kg every 12–48 hours recommended by USPHS/IDSA.
- HIV-infected adolescents: 200 mg (capsule) twice daily recommended by USPHS/IDSA.
- Initiate secondary prophylaxis after primary infection has been adequately treated.
- HIV-infected infants, children, or adolescents with a history of histoplasmosis should receive life-long suppressive therapy to prevent recurrence; data insufficient to date to warrant a recommendation regarding discontinuance in patients receiving potent antiretroviral therapy.

Adult Patients

General Adult Dosage
Treatment of Serious, Life-threatening Systemic Fungal Infections

ORAL:

- Capsules: initial loading dosage of 200 mg 3 times daily (600 mg daily) for the first 3–4 days, then 200–400 mg daily thereafter.

Aspergillosis
Treatment of Pulmonary or Extrapulmonary Aspergillosis

ORAL:

- Capsules: 200–400 mg daily. Higher oral dosages (i.e., 600 mg daily) also have been used; some clinicians recommend dosages of at least 400 mg daily for treatment of invasive aspergillosis.

Blastomycosis
Treatment of Pulmonary or Extrapulmonary Blastomycosis

ORAL:

- Capsules: 200 mg once daily. If there is evidence of progression or no apparent improvement, increase dosage in 100-mg increments daily up to a maximum dosage of 400 mg daily. Usual duration is 6–12 months.
- Some clinicians suggest 200–400 mg daily for ≥6 months (12 months in those with bone disease).

Candida Infections
Treatment of Oropharyngeal Candidiasis

ORAL:

- Oral solution: 200 mg (20 mL) daily for 1–2 weeks. Clinical signs and symptoms generally resolve within several days.
- For retreatment in patients who failed to respond to or are refractory to oral fluconazole, the recommended itraconazole dosage is 100 mg (10 mL) twice daily. A response to itraconazole in these patients generally is evident within 2–4 weeks; however, relapse may be expected shortly after the drug is discontinued.

Treatment of Esophageal Candidiasis

ORAL:

- Oral solution: 100 mg (10 mL) daily. Depending on patient response, a dosage up to 200 mg (20 mL) daily may be given. Usual duration is ≥3 weeks; continue for 2 weeks after symptoms resolve.

Prevention of Recurrence (Secondary Prophylaxis) of Mucocutaneous Candidiasis†

ORAL:

- Oral solution: 200 mg once daily recommended by USPHS/IDSA in HIV-infected adults.
- The safety of discontinuing secondary prophylaxis against mucocutaneous candidiasis in those receiving potent antiretroviral therapy has not been extensively studied.

Coccidioidomycosis†
Prevention of Recurrence (Secondary Prophylaxis) of Coccidioidomycosis†

ORAL:

- Capsules: 200 mg twice daily recommended by USPHS/IDSA in HIV-infected adults. Initiate secondary prophylaxis after primary infection has been adequately treated.
- HIV-infected adults with a history of coccidioidomycosis should receive life-long suppressive therapy to prevent recurrence. Although those who respond to potent antiretroviral therapy with increases in CD4$^+$ T-cell counts to >100/mm^3 may be at low risk for recurrence of fungal infections, data are insufficient to date to warrant a recommendation regarding discontinuance of secondary prophylaxis against coccidioidomycosis.

Cryptococcosis†
Prevention (Primary Prophylaxis) of Cryptococcosis†

ORAL:

- Capsules: 200 mg once daily recommended by USPHS/IDSA in HIV-infected adults with CD4$^+$ T-cell counts <50/mm^3.

Prevention of Recurrence (Secondary Prophylaxis) of Cryptococcosis†

ORAL:

- Capsules: 200 mg once daily recommended by USPHS/IDSA in HIV-infected adults.
- Initiate secondary prophylaxis after primary infection has been adequately treated.
- Consideration can be given to discontinuing secondary prophylaxis in HIV-infected adults who have successfully completed initial therapy for cryptococcosis, remain asympto-

matic with respect to cryptococcosis, and have sustained (e.g., for ≥6 months) increases in CD4+ T-cell counts to >100–200/mm³ in response to potent antiretroviral therapy.

- Reinitiate secondary prophylaxis against cryptococcosis if CD4+ T-cell count decreases to <100–200/mm³.

Histoplasmosis
Treatment of Histoplasmosis (Nonmeningeal)

ORAL:
- Capsules: 200 mg once daily. If there is evidence of progression or no apparent improvement, increase dosage in 100-mg increments daily up to a maximum dosage of 400 mg daily. Usual duration is ≥12 months.
- Some clinicians recommend 200 mg once or twice daily for 12–24 months for treatment of chronic pulmonary histoplasmosis or for 6–18 months for treatment of mild to moderate, nonmeningeal, disseminated infections.

Prevention (Primary Prophylaxis) of Histoplasmosis†

ORAL:
- Capsules: 200 mg once daily recommended by USPHS/IDSA in HIV-infected adults with CD4+ T-cell counts <100/mm³.

Prevention of Recurrence (Secondary Prophylaxis) of Histoplasmosis†

ORAL:
- Capsules: 200 mg twice daily recommended by USPHS/IDSA in HIV-infected adults.
- Initiate secondary prophylaxis after primary infection has been adequately treated.
- HIV-infected adults with a history of histoplasmosis should receive life-long suppressive therapy to prevent recurrence. Although those who respond to potent antiretroviral therapy with increases in CD4+ T-cell counts to >100/mm³ may be at low risk for recurrence of fungal infections, data are insufficient to date to warrant a recommendation regarding discontinuance of secondary prophylaxis against histoplasmosis.

Onychomycosis
Onychomycosis of the Fingernails (Without Toenail Involvement)

ORAL:
- Capsules: pulse-dosing regimen of 200 mg twice daily during the first week, no itraconazole during weeks 2–4, and 200 mg twice daily during the fifth week.

Onychomycosis of the Toenails (With or Without Fingernail Involvement)

ORAL:
- Capsules: 200 mg once daily for 12 consecutive weeks.
- Capsules: a pulse-dosing regimen of 400 mg once daily for one week each month for 3 months† also has been effective.

Sporotrichosis†
Treatment of Sporotrichosis†

ORAL:
- Capsules: 100–200 mg once daily for 3–6 months for cutaneous or lymphocutaneous infections or 200 mg twice daily for 12 months for osteoarticular infections.

Special Populations
Renal Impairment
Treatment of Fungal Infections

ORAL:
- Adjustment of oral itraconazole dosage in patients with renal impairment does not appear to be necessary.

† Use is not currently included in the labeling approved by the US Food and Drug Administration.

Ketoconazole
(kee toe kon′ na zole)

Brand Name: Nizoral®
Also available generically.

Important Warning

Ketoconazole may cause liver damage. Tell your doctor if you drink or have ever drunk large amounts of alcohol and if you have or have ever had liver disease. Tell your doctor and pharmacist if you are taking acetaminophen (Tylenol, others); cholesterol-lowering medications (statins) such as atorvastatin (Lipitor), fluvastatin (Lescol), lovastatin (Mevacor), pravastatin (Pravachol), or simvastatin (Zocor); isoniazid (INH, Nydrazid); methotrexate (Rheumatrex); niacin (nicotinic acid); or rifampin. If you experience any of the following symptoms, call your doctor immediately: extreme tiredness, loss of appetite, upset stomach, vomiting, yellowing of the skin or eyes, dark yellow urine, pale stools, pain in the upper right part of the stomach, or flu-like symptoms.

Keep all appointments with your doctor and the laboratory. Your doctor will order certain tests to check your body's response to ketoconazole.

Do not take astemizole (Hismanal) (not available in the United States), cisapride (Propulsid), or terfenadine (Seldane) (not available in the United States) while you are taking ketoconazole.

Why is this medicine prescribed?

Ketoconazole is used to treat fungal infections. Ketoconazole is most often used to treat fungal infections that can spread to different parts of the body through the bloodstream such as yeast infections of the mouth, skin, urinary tract, and blood, and certain fungal infections that begin on the skin or in the lungs and can spread through the body. Ketoconazole is also used to treat fungal infections of the skin or nails that cannot be treated with other medications. Ketoconazole is in a class of antifungals called imidazoles. It works by slowing the growth of fungi that cause infection.

How should this medicine be used?

Ketoconazole comes as a tablet to take by mouth. It is usually taken once a day. To help you remember to take ketoconazole, take it at around the same time every day. Follow the directions on your prescription label carefully, and ask your doctor or pharmacist to explain any part you do not understand. Take ketoconazole exactly as directed. Do not take more or less of it or take it more often than prescribed by your doctor.

If you have certain medical conditions, your doctor will tell you to take ketoconazole tablets dissolved in an acid solution. Your doctor will tell you exactly how to do this. Follow these directions carefully.

Your doctor will probably start you on an average dose of ketoconazole. Your doctor may increase your dose if your infection is very serious or your condition does not improve.

You may need to take ketoconazole for several weeks or months to cure your infection completely. Your doctor will probably order laboratory tests to be sure your infection has been treated. Continue to take ketoconazole until your doctor tells you that you should stop, even if you feel better. Do not stop taking ketoconazole without talking to your doctor. If you stop taking ketoconazole too soon, your infection may come back after a short time.

Are there other uses for this medicine?

Ketoconazole is also sometimes used to treat vaginal yeast infections, tinea versicolor (spots on skin caused by yeast), eumycetoma (a severe fungal skin infection that often affects the foot), leishmaniasis (a disease caused by the bite of an infected sand fly), prostate cancer (cancer that begins in a male reproductive organ), high blood levels of calcium in patients with certain conditions, Cushing's syndrome (high blood levels of a natural substance called cortisol), and excessive hair growth in women. Talk to your doctor about the possible risks of using this drug for your condition.

This medication may be prescribed for other uses; ask your doctor or pharmacist for more information.

What special precautions should I follow?

Before taking ketoconazole,
- tell your doctor and pharmacist if you are allergic to ketoconazole, other antifungal medications such as fluconazole (Diflucan), itraconazole (Sporonox), or voriconazole (Vfend); any other medications; or corn.
- do not take ketoconazole if you are taking any of the medications listed in the IMPORTANT WARNING section or triazolam (Halcion).
- tell your doctor and pharmacist what other prescription and nonprescription medications, vitamins, nutritional supplements, and herbal products you are taking. Be sure to mention the medications listed in the IMPORTANT WARNING section and any of the following:

alprazolam (Xanax); anticoagulants ('blood thinners') such as warfarin (Coumadin); buspirone (Buspar); calcium channel blockers such as amlodipine (Norvasc), diltiazem (Cardizem, Dilacor, Tiazac), felodipine (Plendil), nifedipine (Adalat, Procardia), nisoldipine (Sular), and verapamil (Calan, Covera, Isoptin, Verelan); clarithromycin (Biaxin); cyclosporine (Neoral, Sandimmune); diazepam (Valium); digoxin (Lanoxin); erythromycin (E.E.S., E-Mycin, Erythrocin); HIV protease inhibitors such as indinavir (Crixivan), ritonavir (Norvir), and saquinavir (Invirase, Fortovase); loratadine (Claritin); medications for diabetes; medications for erectile dysfunction such as sildenafil (Viagra), tadalafil (Cialis) and vardenafil (Levitra); methadone (Dolophine); methylprednisolone (Medrol); midazolam (Versed); phenytoin (Dilantin); pimozide (Orap); quinidine (Quinidex, Quinaglute); quinine; tacrolimus (Prograf); tamoxifen (Nolvadex); telithromycin (Ketek); trazodone (Desyrel); and vincristine (Vincasar). Your doctor may need to change the doses of your medications or monitor you carefully for side effects.
- if you are taking antacids; antihistamines; medications for heartburn or ulcers such as cimetidine (Tagamet), famotidine (Pepcid), nizatadine (Axid), or ranitidine (Zantac); or medications for irritable bowel disease, motion sickness, Parkinson's disease, ulcers, or urinary problems, take them 2 hours after you take ketoconazole.
- tell your doctor if you have or have ever had the conditions mentioned in the IMPORTANT WARNING section or any condition that decreases the amount of acid in your stomach.
- tell your doctor if you are pregnant, plan to become pregnant, or are breast-feeding. If you become pregnant while taking ketoconazole, call your doctor. Do not breastfeed while you are taking ketoconazole.
- ask your doctor about the safe use of alcoholic beverages while you are taking ketoconazole. You may experience unpleasant symptoms such as flushing, rash, upset stomach, headache, and swelling of the hands, feet, ankles, or lower legs if you drink alcohol while you are taking ketoconazole.

What special dietary instructions should I follow?

Unless your doctor tells you otherwise, continue your normal diet.

What should I do if I forget to take a dose?

Take the missed dose as soon as you remember it. However, if it is almost time for the next dose, skip the missed dose and continue your regular dosing schedule. Do not take a double dose to make up for a missed one.

What side effects can this medicine cause?

Ketoconazole may cause side effects. Tell your doctor if either of these symptoms is severe or does not go away:

- stomach pain
- depression

Some side effects can be serious. The following symptoms are uncommon, but if you experience any of them or those listed in the IMPORTANT WARNING section, call your doctor immediately:

- rash
- hives
- itching
- difficulty breathing or swallowing
- thinking about harming or killing yourself or planning or trying to do so

A small number of patients who were taking high doses of ketoconazole for prostate cancer died soon after they began taking the medication. It is not known whether they died because of their disease or their treatment with ketoconazole or for other reasons. Talk to your doctor about the risks of taking ketoconazole.

Ketoconazole may cause a decrease in the number of sperm (male reproductive cells) produced, especially if it is taken at high doses. Talk to your doctor about the risks of taking this medication if you are a man and would like to have children.

Ketoconazole may cause other side effects. Call your doctor if you have any unusual problems while taking this medication.

If you experience a serious side effect, you or your doctor may send a report to the Food and Drug Administration's (FDA) MedWatch Adverse Event Reporting program online [at http://www.fda.gov/MedWatch/index.html] or by phone [1-800-332-1088].

What storage conditions are needed for this medicine?

Keep this medication in the container it came in, tightly closed, and out of reach of children. Store it at room temperature and away from excess heat and moisture (not in the bathroom). Throw away any medication that is outdated or no longer needed. Talk to your pharmacist about the proper disposal of your medication.

What should I do in case of overdose?

In case of overdose, call your local poison control center at 1-800-222-1222. If the victim has collapsed or is not breathing, call local emergency services at 911.

What other information should I know?

Before having any laboratory test, tell your doctor and the laboratory personnel that you are taking ketoconazole.

Do not let anyone else take your medication. Ask your pharmacist if you have any questions about refilling your prescription. If you still have symptoms of infection after you finish the ketoconazole, call your doctor.

Dosage Facts
For Informational Purposes

Caution: Do not change your dose, how often you take your medication, or the length of time you are to take it without first talking to your healthcare provider.

The following dosage information was written using medical language for doctors and other healthcare professionals and is provided here for you to check your dosage. The dosage of this drug may differ for different patients. Therefore, always follow your doctor's instructions or the directions on the label. Contact your healthcare provider or pharmacist if you have any questions about the specific dosage of your medication after reviewing this information.

Pediatric Patients

General Pediatric Dosage
Treatment of Fungal Infections

ORAL:
- Children >2 years of age: 3.3–6.6 mg/kg once daily has been used.

Adult Patients

General Adult Dosage
Treatment of Fungal Infections

ORAL:
- 200 mg once daily. Dosage may be increased to 400 mg once daily for severe infections or if the expected clinical response is not achieved.

Blastomycosis

ORAL:
- Some clinicians suggest 400 mg once or twice daily. Treatment usually continued for 6–12 months.

Candidiasis
Oropharyngeal and Esophageal Candidiasis

ORAL:
- 200–400 mg daily.

Vulvovaginal Candidiasis†

ORAL:
- Treatment of uncomplicated vulvovaginal candidiasis† in nonpregnant women: 200–400 mg twice daily for 5 days.
- When used as a maintenance regimen to reduce the frequency of recurrent episodes of vulvovaginal candidiasis† in women who have received an initial intensive antifungal regimen (i.e., 7–14 days of an intravaginal azole antifungal or a 2-dose fluconazole regimen), ketoconazole has been given in a dosage of 100 mg once daily for up to 6 months.

Chromomycosis

ORAL:
- 200–400 mg daily. Treatment usually continued for 6–12 months.

Coccidioidomycosis

ORAL:
- 400 mg once or twice daily. Treatment usually continued for 6–12 months.

Dermatophytoses

ORAL:

- 200–400 mg daily has been given for 1–2 months. Infections involving glabrous skin require a minimum of 4 weeks of treatment; palmar and plantar infections may respond more slowly. Tinea unguium (onychomycosis) may require ≥6–12 months of treatment.

Histoplasmosis

ORAL:

- 400 mg once or twice daily. A dosage of 200 mg once or twice daily also has been used.
- A minimum of 6 months of therapy usually required, but 2–6 months has been effective in some patients.

Paracocciodioidomycosis

ORAL:

- 200–400 mg daily.
- A minimum of 6 months of therapy usually required, but 2–6 months has been effective in some patients.

Leishmaniasis†

Cutaneous and Mucocutaneous Leishmaniasis†

ORAL:

- 400–600 mg daily for 4–8 weeks has been used.

Visceral Leishmaniasis (Kala-Azar)†

ORAL:

- 400–600 mg daily for 4–8 weeks has been used.

Prostate Cancer†

ORAL:

- 400 mg every 8 hours has been used for treatment of prostatic carcinoma† or as an adjunct in the management of disseminated intravascular coagulation (DIC) associated with prostatic carcinoma†. Risk of depressed adrenocortical function at this high dosage should be considered.

† Use is not currently included in the labeling approved by the US Food and Drug Administration.

Ketoconazole Topical

(kee toe kon′ na zole)

Brand Name: Nizoral®, Nizoral AD®
Also available generically.

Why is this medicine prescribed?

Ketoconazole cream is used to treat tinea corporis (ringworm; fungal skin infection that causes a red scaly rash on different parts of the body), tinea cruris (jock itch; fungal infection of the skin in the groin or buttocks), tinea pedis (athlete's foot; fungal infection of the skin on the feet and between the toes), tinea versicolor (fungal infection that causes brown or light colored spots on the chest, back, arms, legs, or neck), and yeast infections of the skin. Prescription ketoconazole shampoo is used to treat tinea versicolor. Over-the-counter ketoconazole shampoo is used to control flaking, scaling, and itching of the scalp caused by dandruff. Ketoconazole is in a class of antifungal medications called imidazoles. It works by slowing the growth of fungi that cause infection.

How should this medicine be used?

Prescription ketoconazole comes as a cream and a shampoo to apply to the skin. Over-the-counter ketoconazole comes as a shampoo to apply to the scalp. Ketoconazole cream is usually applied once a day for 2-6 weeks. Prescription ketoconazole shampoo is usually applied one time to treat the infection. Over-the-counter ketoconazole shampoo is usually used every 3-4 days for up to 8 weeks, and then used as needed to control dandruff. Follow the directions on your prescription label carefully, and ask your doctor or pharmacist to explain any part you do not understand. Use ketoconazole exactly as directed. Do not use more or less of it or use it more often than prescribed by your doctor.

One treatment with prescription ketoconazole shampoo may successfully treat your tinea versicolor infection. However, it may take several months for your skin color to return to normal, especially if your skin is exposed to sunlight. After your infection is treated, there is a chance that you will develop another tinea versicolor infection.

If you are using over-the-counter ketoconazole shampoo to treat dandruff, your symptoms should improve during the first 2-4 weeks of your treatment. Call your doctor if your symptoms do not improve during this time or if your symptoms get worse at any time during your treatment.

If you are using ketoconazole cream, your symptoms should improve at the beginning of your treatment. Continue to use ketoconazole cream even if you are feeling well. If you stop using ketoconazole cream too soon, your infection may not be completely cured and your symptoms may return.

Ketoconazole cream and shampoos are only for use on the skin or scalp. Do not let ketoconazole cream or shampoo get into your eyes or mouth, and do not swallow the medication. If you do get ketoconazole cream or shampoo in your eyes, wash them with plenty of water.

To use the cream, apply enough cream to cover the affected area and all of the skin around it.

To use the prescription shampoo, follow these steps:

1. Use a small amount of water to wet your skin in the area where you will apply ketoconazole shampoo.
2. Apply the shampoo to the affected skin and a large area around it.
3. Use your fingers to rub the shampoo until it forms a lather.
4. Leave the shampoo on your skin for 5 minutes.
5. Rinse the shampoo off of your skin with water.

To use the over-the-counter shampoo, follow these steps:

1. Be sure that your scalp is not broken, cut, or irritated. Do

not use ketoconazole shampoo if your scalp is broken or irritated.
2. Wet your hair thoroughly.
3. Apply the shampoo to your hair.
4. Use your fingers to rub the shampoo until it forms a lather.
5. Rinse all of the shampoo out of your hair with plenty of water.
6. Repeat steps 2-5.

Are there other uses for this medicine?

Ketoconazole cream and prescription shampoo are also sometimes used to treat dandruff and seborrheic dermatitis (condition that causes flaking of the skin). Ketoconazole cream is sometimes used to treat tinea manuum (fungal infection of the skin on the hands). Ketoconazole cream is also sometimes used with other medications to treat skin conditions that are often worsened by fungal infection such as diaper rash, eczema (skin irritation caused by allergies), impetigo (blisters caused by a bacterial infection), and psoriasis (a lifelong skin condition). Talk to your doctor about the possible risks of using this drug for your condition.

This medication may be prescribed for other uses; ask your doctor or pharmacist for more information.

What special precautions should I follow?

Before using ketoconazole,
- tell your doctor and pharmacist if you are allergic to ketoconazole or any other medications, creams, or shampoos. If you will be using the cream, tell your doctor if you are allergic to sulfites.
- tell your doctor and pharmacist what prescription and nonprescription medications, vitamins, nutritional supplements, and herbal products you are taking. Your doctor may need to change the doses of your medications or monitor you carefully for side effects.
- tell your doctor if you have or have ever had any medical condition. If you will be using the cream, tell your doctor if you have or have ever had asthma.
- tell your doctor if you are pregnant, plan to become pregnant, or are breast-feeding. If you become pregnant while using ketoconazole, call your doctor.

What special dietary instructions should I follow?

Unless your doctor tells you otherwise, continue your normal diet.

What should I do if I forget to take a dose?

Apply the missed dose as soon as you remember it. However, if it is almost time for the next dose, skip the missed dose and continue your regular dosing schedule. Do not apply a double dose to make up for a missed one.

What side effects can this medicine cause?

Ketoconazole may cause side effects. Tell your doctor if any of these symptoms are severe or do not go away:
- changes in hair texture
- blisters on scalp
- dry skin
- itching
- oily or dry hair or scalp
- irritation, itching, or stinging in the place where you applied the medication

Some side effects can be serious. The following symptoms are uncommon, but if you experience any of them, call your doctor immediately:
- rash
- hives
- difficulty breathing or swallowing
- redness, tenderness, swelling, pain, or warmth in the place where you applied the medication

Ketoconazole may cause other side effects. Call your doctor if you have any unusual problems while taking this medication.

If you experience a serious side effect, you or your doctor may send a report to the Food and Drug Administration's (FDA) MedWatch Adverse Event Reporting program online [at http://www.fda.gov/MedWatch/index.html] or by phone [1-800-332-1088].

What storage conditions are needed for this medicine?

Keep this medication in the container it came in, tightly closed, and out of reach of children. Store it at room temperature and away from excess heat and moisture (not in the bathroom). Protect the medication from light and do not allow it to freeze. Throw away any medication that is outdated or no longer needed. Talk to your pharmacist about the proper disposal of your medication.

What should I do in case of overdose?

If someone swallows ketoconazole cream or shampoo, call your local poison control center at 1-800-222-1222. If the victim has collapsed or is not breathing, call local emergency services at 911.

What other information should I know?

Keep all appointments with your doctor.

Ketoconazole shampoo may remove the curl from hair that has been permanently waved ('permed').

Do not let anyone else use your medication. Your prescription is probably not refillable. If you still have symptoms of infection after you finish the ketoconazole, call your doctor.

Dosage Facts
For Informational Purposes

Caution: Do not change your dose, how often you take your medication, or the length of time you are to take it without first talking to your healthcare provider.

The following dosage information was written using medical language for doctors and other healthcare professionals and is provided here for you to check your dosage. The dosage of this drug may differ for different patients. Therefore, always follow your doctor's instructions or the directions on the label. Contact your healthcare provider or pharmacist if you have any questions about the specific dosage of your medication after reviewing this information.

Pediatric Patients

Dandruff

TOPICAL:
- For *self-medication* in children >12 years of age: apply 1% shampoo to wet hair, lather, and rinse thoroughly; then repeat application, lathering, and rinsing. Use every 3 or 4 days for up to 8 weeks as needed or as directed by a clinician. Thereafter, use as needed to control dandruff.

Adult Patients

Dermatophytoses
Tinea Corporis or Tinea Cruris

TOPICAL:
- Apply 2% cream and rub gently into affected and surrounding areas of skin once or twice daily for 2 weeks.

Tinea Pedis

TOPICAL:
- Apply 2% cream and rub gently into affected and surrounding areas of skin once or twice daily for 6 weeks. Moccasin-type (dry-type) tinea pedis may require more prolonged therapy.

Cutaneous Candidiasis

TOPICAL:
- Apply 2% cream and rub gently into affected and surrounding areas of skin once or twice daily for 2 weeks.

Pityriasis (Tinea) Versicolor

TOPICAL:
- Topical cream: Apply 2% cream and rub gently into affected and surrounding areas once daily for 2 weeks.
- Shampoo: Apply 2% shampoo to the damp skin of the affected area and a wide margin surrounding this area and lather; after 5 minutes, rinse with water. A single application of 2% shampoo should be sufficient, although once-daily application for 3 days also has been used.
- Once-weekly application of the 2% shampoo has been used to prevent relapses.

Seborrheic Dermatitis and Dandruff
Dermatitis

TOPICAL:
- Apply 2% cream and rub gently into affected areas twice daily for 4 weeks or until clinical clearing.

Dandruff

TOPICAL:
- For *self-medication*, apply 1% shampoo to thoroughly wet hair, lather, rinse thoroughly, and then repeat application, lathering, and rinsing. Use every 3 or 4 days for up to 8 weeks as needed or as directed by a clinician. Thereafter, use as needed to control dandruff.

Ketoprofen
(kee toe proe′ fen)

Brand Name: Actron®
Also available generically.

Important Warning

People who take nonsteroidal anti-inflammatory medications (NSAIDs) other than aspirin, such as ketoprofen, may have a higher risk of having a heart attack or a stroke than people who do not take these medications. These events may happen without warning and may cause death. This risk may be higher for people who take NSAIDs for a long time. Tell your doctor if you or anyone in your family has or has ever had heart disease, a heart attack, or a stroke, if you smoke, and if you have or have ever had high cholesterol, high blood pressure, or diabetes. Get emergency medical help right away if you experience any of the following symptoms: chest pain, shortness of breath, weakness in one part or side of the body, or slurred speech.

If you will be undergoing a coronary artery bypass graft (CABG; a type of heart surgery), you should not take ketoprofen right before or right after the surgery.

NSAIDs such as ketoprofen may cause ulcers, bleeding, or holes in the stomach or intestine. These problems may develop at any time during treatment, may happen without warning symptoms, and may cause death. The risk may be higher for people who take NSAIDs for a long time, are older in age, have poor health, or drink more than three alcoholic drinks per day while taking ketoprofen. Tell your doctor if you drink large amounts of alcohol or if you take any of the following medications: anticoagulants ('blood thinners') such as warfarin (Coumadin); aspirin; other NSAIDs such as ibuprofen (Advil, Motrin) or naproxen (Aleve, Naprosyn); or oral steroids such as dexamethasone (Decadron, Dexone), methylprednisolone (Medrol), and prednisone (Deltasone). Also tell your doctor if you have or have ever had ulcers

continued on next page

Important Warning (cont'd)

or bleeding in your stomach or intestines or other bleeding disorders. If you experience any of the following symptoms, stop taking ketoprofen and call your doctor: stomach pain, heartburn, vomiting a substance that is bloody or looks like coffee grounds, blood in the stool, or black and tarry stools.

Keep all appointments with your doctor and the laboratory. Your doctor will monitor your symptoms carefully and will probably order certain tests to check your body's response to ketoprofen. Be sure to tell your doctor how you are feeling so that your doctor can prescribe the right amount of medication to treat your condition with the lowest risk of serious side effects.

Your doctor or pharmacist will give you the manufacturer's patient information sheet (Medication Guide) when you begin treatment with prescription ketoprofen and each time you refill your prescription. Read the information carefully and ask your doctor or pharmacist if you have any questions. You can also visit the Food and Drug Administration (FDA) website (http://www.fda.gov/cder) to obtain the Medication Guide.

Why is this medicine prescribed?

Prescription ketoprofen is used to relieve pain, tenderness, swelling, and stiffness caused by osteoarthritis (arthritis caused by a breakdown of the lining of the joints) and rheumatoid arthritis (arthritis caused by swelling of the lining of the joints). Prescription ketoprofen capsules are also used to relieve pain, including menstrual pain (pain that occurs before or during a menstrual period). Nonprescription ketoprofen is used to relieve minor aches and pain from headaches, menstrual periods, toothaches, the common cold, muscle aches, and backaches, and to reduce fever. Ketoprofen is in a class of medications called NSAIDs. It works by stopping the body's production of a substance that causes pain, fever, and inflammation.

How should this medicine be used?

Prescription ketoprofen comes as a capsule and extended-release (long-acting) capsule to take by mouth. The capsules are usually taken three or four times a day for arthritis or every 6-8 hours as needed for pain. The extended-release capsules are usually taken once daily. If you take ketoprofen regularly, take it at around the same times every day.

Nonprescription ketoprofen comes as a tablet to take by mouth. It is usually taken with a full glass of water or other liquid every 4-6 hours as needed.

Follow the directions on the package or prescription label carefully, and ask your doctor or pharmacist to explain any part you do not understand. Take ketoprofen exactly as directed. Do not take more or less of it or take it more often than prescribed by your doctor or written on the label.

Ketoprofen may be taken with food or milk to prevent upset stomach. Your doctor may also recommend that you take ketoprofen with an antacid to reduce stomach upset.

Your doctor may start you on an average dose of prescription ketoprofen and may increase or decrease on your dose depending on how well you respond to the medication and the side effects you experience. Follow these directions carefully.

Stop taking nonprescription ketoprofen and call your doctor if your symptoms get worse, you develop new or unexpected symptoms, the part of your body that was painful becomes red or swollen, your pain lasts for more than 10 days or your fever lasts for more than 3 days.

Are there other uses for this medicine?

Ketoprofen is also sometimes used to treat juvenile rheumatoid arthritis (a type of arthritis that affects children), ankylosing spondylitis (arthritis that mainly affects the spine), Reiter's syndrome (condition in which many parts of the body including the joints, eyes, genitals, bladder, and digestive system become swollen), shoulder pain caused by bursitis (inflammation of a fluid-filled sac in the shoulder joint) and tendinitis (inflammation of the tissue that connects muscle to bone), and gouty arthritis (attacks of joint pain caused by a build-up of certain substances in the joints). Talk to your doctor about the risks of using this medication for your condition.

This medication is sometimes prescribed for other uses; ask your doctor or pharmacist for more information.

What special precautions should I follow?

Before taking ketoprofen,

- tell your doctor and pharmacist if you are allergic to ketoprofen, aspirin or other NSAIDs such as ibuprofen (Advil, Motrin) and naproxen (Aleve, Naprosyn), any other medications, or any of the inactive ingredients in ketoprofen capsules or extended release capsules. Ask your pharmacist for a list of the inactive ingredients.
- tell your doctor and pharmacist what prescription and nonprescription medications, vitamins, nutritional supplements, and herbal products you are taking, or plan to take. Be sure to mention the medications listed in the IMPORTANT WARNING section and any of the following: angiotensin-converting enzyme (ACE) inhibitors such as benazepril (Lotensin), captopril (Capoten), enalapril (Vasotec), fosinopril (Monopril), lisinopril (Prinivil, Zestril), moexipril (Univasc), perindopril (Aceon), quinapril (Accupril), ramipril (Altace), and trandolapril (Mavik); diuretics ('water pills'); lithium (Eskalith, Lithobid); medications for diabetes; methotrexate (Rheumatrex); phenytoin (Dilantin); probenecid (Benemid); and sulfa antibiotics such as sulfisoxazole (Gantrisin) and sulfamethoxazole (in Bactrim, in Septra). Your doctor may need to change the doses of your medications or monitor you more carefully for side effects.

- tell your doctor if you have or have ever had any of the conditions mentioned in the IMPORTANT WARNING section or asthma, especially if you also have frequent stuffed or runny nose or nasal polyps (swelling of the lining of the nose); swelling of the hands, arms, feet, ankles, or lower legs; or liver or kidney disease.
- tell your doctor if you are pregnant especially if you are in the last few months of your pregnancy, you plan to become pregnant, or you are breast-feeding. If you become pregnant while taking ketoprofen, call your doctor.
- if you are having surgery, including dental surgery, tell the doctor or dentist that you are taking ketoprofen.

What special dietary instructions should I follow?

Unless your doctor tells you otherwise, continue your normal diet.

What should I do if I forget to take a dose?

Take the missed dose as soon as you remember it. However, if it is almost time for the next dose, skip the missed dose and continue your regular dosing schedule. Do not take a double dose to make up for a missed one.

What side effects can this medicine cause?

Ketoprofen may cause side effects. Tell your doctor if any of these symptoms are severe or do not go away:

- constipation
- diarrhea
- sores in the mouth
- headache
- dizziness
- nervousness
- drowsiness
- difficulty falling asleep or staying asleep
- ringing in the ears

Some side effects may be serious. If you experience any of the following symptoms or those mentioned in the IMPORTANT WARNING section, call your doctor immediately. Do not take any more ketoprofen until you speak to your doctor.

- changes in vision
- unexplained weight gain
- fever
- blisters
- rash
- itching
- hives
- swelling of the eyes, face, lips, tongue, throat, arms, hands, feet, ankles, or lower legs
- hoarseness
- difficulty breathing or swallowing

- excessive tiredness
- unusual bleeding or bruising
- lack of energy
- loss of appetite
- upset stomach
- pain in the upper right part of the stomach
- flu-like symptoms
- yellowing of the skin or eyes
- pale skin
- fast heartbeat
- cloudy, discolored, or bloody urine
- back pain
- difficult or painful urination

Ketoprofen may cause other side effects. Call your doctor if you have any unusual problems while taking this medication.

If you experience a serious side effect, you or your doctor may send a report to the Food and Drug Administration's (FDA) MedWatch Adverse Event Reporting program online [at http://www.fda.gov/MedWatch/index.html] or by phone [1-800-332-1088].

What storage conditions are needed for this medicine?

Keep this medication in the container it came in, tightly closed, and out of reach of children. Store it at room temperature and away from excess heat and moisture (not in the bathroom). Throw away any medication that is outdated or no longer needed. Talk to your pharmacist about the proper disposal of your medication.

What should I do in case of overdose?

In case of overdose, call your local poison control center at 1-800-222-1222. If the victim has collapsed or is not breathing, call local emergency services at 911.

Symptoms of overdose may include:

- lack of energy
- drowsiness
- upset stomach
- vomiting
- stomach pain
- shallow breathing
- seizures
- coma

What other information should I know?

Before having any laboratory test, tell your doctor and the laboratory personnel that you are taking ketoprofen.

Do not let anyone else take your medication. Ask your pharmacist any questions you have about refilling your prescription.

Dosage Facts
For Informational Purposes

Caution: Do not change your dose, how often you take your medication, or the length of time you are to take it without first talking to your healthcare provider.

The following dosage information was written using medical language for doctors and other healthcare professionals and is provided here for you to check your dosage. The dosage of this drug may differ for different patients. Therefore, always follow your doctor's instructions or the directions on the label. Contact your healthcare provider or pharmacist if you have any questions about the specific dosage of your medication after reviewing this information.

General Dosage Information

To minimize the potential risk of adverse cardiovascular and/or GI events, use lowest effective dosage and shortest duration of therapy consistent with the patient's treatment goals. Adjust dosage based on individual requirements and response; attempt to titrate to the lowest effective dosage.

Adult Patients

Inflammatory Diseases
Osteoarthritis or Rheumatoid Arthritis

ORAL:
- Conventional capsules: Initially, 75 mg 3 times daily or 50 mg 4 times daily. Base subsequent dosage on clinical response and tolerance.
- Extended-release capsules: Initially, 200 mg once daily. Base subsequent dosage on clinical response and tolerance.

Pain

ORAL:
- Conventional capsules: Usual dosage is 25–50 mg every 6–8 hours as needed.

Dysmenorrhea

ORAL:
- Conventional capsules: Usual dosage is 25–50 mg every 6–8 hours as needed.

Prescribing Limits

Adult Patients

Inflammatory Diseases
Osteoarthritis or Rheumatoid Arthritis

ORAL:
- Conventional capsules: Maximum 300 mg daily.
- Extended-release capsules: Maximum 200 mg daily.

Pain or Dysmenorrhea

ORAL:
- Conventional capsules: Maximum 300 mg daily.

Special Populations

Hepatic Impairment
- Maximum recommended initial total dosage is 100 mg daily in patients with hepatic impairment and serum albumin concentrations <3.5 g/dL.

Renal Impairment
- Mild renal impairment: Maximum recommended dosage is 150 mg daily.
- Severe renal impairment (GFR <25 mL/minute per 1.73 m² or end-stage renal impairment): Maximum recommended dosage is 100 mg daily. ()

Geriatric Patients
- Consider reduced initial dosage in patients >75 years of age.

Ketorolac
(kee toe role′ ak)

Brand Name: Toradol®

Important Warning

Ketorolac is used for the short-term relief of moderately severe pain and should not be used for longer than 5 days, for mild pain, or for pain from chronic (long-term) conditions. You will receive your first doses of ketorolac by intravenous (into a vein) or intramuscular (into a muscle) injection in a hospital or medical office. After that, your doctor may choose to continue your treatment with oral ketorolac. You must stop taking oral ketorolac on the fifth day after you received your first ketorolac injection. Talk to your doctor if you still have pain after 5 days or if your pain is not controlled with this medication. Ketorolac may cause serious side effects, especially when taken improperly. Take ketorolac exactly as directed. Do not take more of it or take it more often than prescribed by your doctor.

People who take nonsteroidal anti-inflammatory medications (NSAIDs) (other than aspirin) such as ketorolac may have a higher risk of having a heart attack or a stroke than people who do not take these medications. These events may happen without warning and may cause death. This risk may be higher for people who take NSAIDs for a long time. Tell your doctor if you or anyone in your family has or has ever had heart disease, a heart attack, or a stroke or 'mini-stroke' if you smoke, and if you have or have ever had high cholesterol, high blood pressure, bleeding or clotting problems, or diabetes. Get emergency medical help right away if you experience any of the following symptoms: chest pain, shortness of breath, weakness in one part or side of the body, or slurred speech.

If you are having surgery, including dental surgery, tell the doctor or dentist that you are taking ketorolac. If you will be undergoing a coronary artery bypass graft (CABG; a type of heart surgery), you should not take ketorolac right before or right after the surgery.

NSAIDs such as ketorolac may cause ulcers, bleeding, or holes in the stomach or intestine. These problems may develop at any time during treatment, may happen without warning symptoms, and may cause death. The risk may be higher for people who take NSAIDs for a long time, are older in age, have poor health, or drink large amounts of alcohol while taking ketorolac. Tell your doctor if you take any of the following medications: anticoagulants ('blood thinners') such as warfarin (Coumadin); aspirin; or oral steroids such as dexamethasone (Decadron, Dexone), methylprednisolone (Medrol), and prednisone (Deltasone). Do not take aspirin or other NSAIDs such as ibuprofen (Advil, Motrin) and naproxen (Aleve, Naprosyn) while you are taking ketorolac. Also tell your doctor if you have or have ever had ulcers or bleeding in your stomach or intestines. If you experience any of the following symptoms, stop taking ketorolac and call your doctor: stomach pain, heartburn, vomiting a substance that is bloody or looks like coffee grounds, blood in the stool, or black and tarry stools.

Ketorolac may cause kidney failure. Tell your doctor if you have kidney or liver disease, if you have had severe vomiting or diarrhea or think you may be dehydrated, and if you are taking angiotensin-converting enzyme (ACE) inhibitors such as benazepril (Lotensin), captopril (Capoten), enalapril (Vasotec), fosinopril (Monopril), lisinopril (Prinivil, Zestril), moexipril (Univasc), perindopril (Aceon), quinapril (Accupril), ramipril (Altace), and trandolapril (Mavik); or diuretics ('water pills'). If you experience any of the following symptoms, stop taking ketorolac and call your doctor: swelling of the hands, arms, feet, ankles, or lower legs; unexplained weight gain; confusion; or seizures.

Some people have severe allergic reactions to ketorolac. Tell your doctor if you are allergic to ketorolac, aspirin or other NSAIDs such as ibuprofen (Advil, Motrin) or naproxen (Aleve, Naprosyn), or any other medications. Also tell your doctor if you have or have ever had asthma, especially if you also have frequent stuffed or runny nose or nasal polyps (swelling of the lining of the nose). If you experience any of the following symptoms, stop taking ketorolac and call your doctor right away: rash; hives; itching; swelling of the eyes, face, throat, tongue, arms, hands, ankles, or lower legs; difficulty breathing or swallowing; or hoarseness.

Do not breastfeed while you are taking ketorolac.

Keep all appointments with your doctor and the laboratory. Your doctor will monitor your symptoms carefully and will probably order certain tests to check your body's response to ketorolac. Be sure to tell your doctor how you are feeling so that your doctor can prescribe the right amount of medication to treat your condition with the lowest risk of serious side effects.

Your doctor or pharmacist will give you the manufacturer's patient information sheet (Medication Guide) when you begin treatment with ketorolac and each time you refill your prescription. Read the information carefully and ask your doctor or pharmacist if you have any questions. You can also visit the Food and Drug Administration (FDA) website (http://www.fda.gov/cder) to obtain the Medication Guide.

Why is this medicine prescribed?

Ketorolac is used to relieve moderately severe pain, usually after surgery. Ketorolac is in a class of medications called NSAIDs. It works by stopping the body's production of a substance that causes pain, fever, and inflammation.

How should this medicine be used?

Ketorolac comes as a tablet to take by mouth. It is usually taken every 4-6 hours on a schedule or as needed for pain. If you are taking ketorolac on a schedule, take it at around the same times every day. Follow the directions on your prescription label carefully, and ask your doctor or pharmacist to explain any part you do not understand.

Are there other uses for this medicine?

This medication is sometimes prescribed for other uses; ask your doctor or pharmacist for more information.

What special precautions should I follow?

Before taking ketorolac,
- do not take ketorolac if you are taking probenecid.
- tell your doctor and pharmacist what prescription and nonprescription medications, vitamins, nutritional supplements, and herbal products you are taking or plan to take. Be sure to mention the medications listed in the IMPORTANT WARNING section and any of the following: antidepressants; medications for anxietyor mental illness; medications for seizures such as phenytoin (Dilantin) or carbamazepine (Tegretol); methotrexate (Rheumatrex); sedatives; sleeping pills; and tranquilizers. Your doctor may need to change the doses of your medications or monitor you more carefully for side effects.
- tell your doctor if you have or have ever had the con-

ditions mentioned in the IMPORTANT WARNING section or swelling of the hands, feet, ankles, or lower legs.

- tell your doctor if you are pregnant, especially if you are in the last few months of your pregnancy, or you plan to become pregnant. If you become pregnant while taking ketorolac, call your doctor.
- you should know that this medication may make you drowsy or dizzy. Do not drive a car or operate machinery until you know how this medication affects you.
- remember that alcohol can add to the drowsiness caused by this medication. Talk to your doctor about the safe use of alcohol while taking this medication.

What special dietary instructions should I follow?

Unless your doctor tells you otherwise, continue your normal diet.

What should I do if I forget to take a dose?

If your doctor has told you to take ketorolac regularly, take the missed dose as soon as you remember it. However, if it is almost time for the next dose, skip the missed dose and continue your regular dosing schedule. Do not take a double dose to make up for a missed one.

What side effects can this medicine cause?

Ketorolac may cause side effects. Tell your doctor if any of these symptoms are severe or do not go away:

- headache
- dizziness
- drowsiness
- diarrhea
- constipation
- gas
- sores in the mouth
- sweating

Some side effects can be serious. If you experience any of the following symptoms, or those mentioned in the IMPORTANT WARNING section, call your doctor immediately. Do not take any more ketorolac until you speak to your doctor.

- fever
- blisters
- yellowing of the skin or eyes
- excessive tiredness
- unusual bleeding or bruising
- lack of energy
- upset stomach
- loss of appetite
- pain in the upper right part of the stomach
- flu-like symptoms
- pale skin
- fast hearbeat

- cloudy, discolored, or bloody urine
- back pain
- difficult or painful urination

Ketorolac may cause other side effects. Call your doctor if you have any unusual problems while taking this medication.

If you experience a serious side effect, you or your doctor may send a report to the Food and Drug Administration's (FDA) MedWatch Adverse Event Reporting program online [at http://www.fda.gov/MedWatch/index.html] or by phone [1-800-332-1088].

What storage conditions are needed for this medicine?

Keep this medication in the container it came in, tightly closed, and out of reach of children. Store it at room temperature and away from excess heat and moisture (not in the bathroom). Throw away any medication that is outdated or no longer needed. Talk to your pharmacist about the proper disposal of your medication.

What should I do in case of overdose?

In case of overdose, call your local poison control center at 1-800-222-1222. If the victim has collapsed or is not breathing, call local emergency services at 911.

Symptoms of overdose may include:

- upset stomach
- vomiting
- stomach pain
- bloody, black, or tarry stools
- vomiting a substance that is bloody or looks like coffee grounds
- drowsiness
- slowed breathing or fast, shallow breathing
- coma (loss of consciousness for a period of time)

What other information should I know?

Do not let anyone else take your medication. Ask your pharmacist any questions you have about refilling your prescription.

Dosage Facts
For Informational Purposes

Caution: Do not change your dose, how often you take your medication, or the length of time you are to take it without first talking to your healthcare provider.

The following dosage information was written using medical language for doctors and other healthcare professionals and is provided here for you to check your dosage. The dosage of this drug may differ for different patients. Therefore, always follow your doctor's instructions or the directions on the label. Contact your healthcare provider or pharmacist if you have any questions

about the specific dosage of your medication after reviewing this information.

General Dosage Information

Available as ketorolac tromethamine; dosage expressed in terms of the salt.

To minimize the potential risk of adverse cardiovascular and/or GI events, use lowest effective dosage and shortest duration of therapy consistent with the patient's treatment goals. Adjust dosage based on individual requirements and response; attempt to titrate to the lowest effective dosage.

For breakthrough pain, supplement with low doses of opiate analgesics (unless contraindicated) as needed rather than higher or more frequent doses of ketorolac.

Adult Patients

Pain

ORAL:
- When switching from parenteral to oral therapy, the first oral dose is 20 mg, followed by 10 mg every 4–6 hours (maximum 40 mg in a 24-hour period).
- Weight <50 kg: When switching from parenteral to oral therapy, 10 mg every 4–6 hours (maximum 40 mg in a 24-hour period).

Prescribing Limits

Adult Patients

Pain

Total combined duration of parenteral and oral therapy should not exceed 5 days.

ORAL:
- All adults: Maximum 40 mg in a 24-hour period.

Special Populations

Hepatic Impairment
- Need for dosage adjustment not fully established; evidence in patients with cirrhosis suggests that dosage adjustment may not be necessary.

Renal Impairment

Pain

- Safety not established in patients with S_{cr} >5 mg/dL and/or those undergoing dialysis.

ORAL:
- When switching from parenteral to oral therapy, 10 mg every 4–6 hours (maximum 40 mg in a 24-hour period).

Geriatric Patients
- Dosage recommendations are the same as those for patients with moderately increased S_{cr} or for those weighing <50 kg.

Ketorolac Ophthalmic

(kee toe role′ ak)

Brand Name: Acular®

Why is this medicine prescribed?

Ketorolac ophthalmic is used to treat itchy eyes caused by allergies. It also is used to treat swelling and redness (inflammation) that can occur after cataract surgery. Ketorolac ophthalmic is in a class of drugs called nonsteroidal anti-inflammatory drugs. It works by stopping the release of substances that cause allergy symptoms and inflammation.

How should this medicine be used?

Ketorolac ophthalmic comes as eyedrops. For allergy symptoms, one drop is usually applied to the affected eyes four times a day. For inflammation after cataract surgery, one drop is usually applied to the affected eye four times a day for 2 weeks beginning 24 hours after surgery. Follow the directions on your prescription label carefully, and ask your doctor or pharmacist to explain any part you do not understand. Use ketorolac ophthalmic exactly as directed. Do not use more or less of it or use it more than prescribed by your doctor.

Your allergy symptom (itchy eyes) should improve when you apply the eyedrops. If your symptoms do not improve or they worsen, call your doctor.

For treatment of itchy eyes caused by allergies, continue to use ketorolac ophthalmic until you are no longer exposed to the substance that causes your symptom, allergy season is over, or your doctor tells you to stop using it.

To use the eyedrops, follow these instructions:
- Wash your hands thoroughly with soap and water.
- Use a mirror or have someone else put the drops in your eye.
- Remove the protective cap. Make sure the end of the dropper is not chipped or cracked.
- Avoid touching the dropper tip against your eye or anything else.
- Hold the dropper tip down at all times to prevent drops from flowing back into the bottle and contaminating the remaining contents.
- Lie down or tilt your head back.
- Holding the bottle between your thumb and index finger, place the dropper tip as near as possible to your eyelid without touching it.
- Brace the remaining fingers of that hand against your cheek or nose.
- With the index finger of your other hand, pull the lower lid of the eye down to form a pocket.
- Drop the prescribed number of drops into the pocket made by the lower lid and the eye. Placing drops on the surface of the eyeball can cause stinging.

- Close your eye and press lightly against the lower lid with your finger for 2-3 minutes to keep the medication in the eye. Do not blink.
- Replace and tighten the cap right away. Do not wipe or rinse it off.
- Wipe off any excess liquid from your cheek with a clean tissue. Wash your hands again.

What special precautions should I follow?

Before using ketorolac eyedrops,

- tell your doctor or pharmacist if you are allergic to ketorolac ophthalmic, aspirin, or any other drugs.
- tell your doctor and pharmacist what prescription and nonprescription medications you are taking, especially anticoagulants (''blood thinners'') such as warfarin (Coumadin); aspirin; nonsteroidal anti-inflammatory agents, such as celecoxib (Celebrex), diclofenec (Voltaren), etodolac (Lodine), fenoprofen (Nalfon), flurbiprofen (Ansaid), ibuprofen (Advil, Motrin, Midol), indomethacin (Indocin), ketoprofen (Orudis, Oruvail), ketorolac (Toradol), meclofenamate, mefenamic (Ponstel), nabumetone (Relafen), naproxen (Aleve, Naprosyn), oxaprozin (Daypro), Piroxicam (Feldene), refecoxib (Vioxx), sulindac (Clinoril), and tolmetin (Tolectin); and vitamins or herbal products.
- tell your doctor if you have or have ever had heart, kidney, or liver disease or bleeding problems.
- tell your doctor if you are pregnant, plan to become pregnant, or are breastfeeding.
- tell your doctor if you wear soft contact lenses. You should not use ketorolac ophthalmic while wearing your soft contact lenses.
- use caution when driving or operating machinery because your vision may be blurred after inserting the drops.

What should I do if I forget to take a dose?

Apply the missed dose as soon as you remember it. However, if is almost time for the next dose, skip the missed dose and continue your regular dosing schedule. Do not apply a double dose to make up for a missed one.

What side effects can this medicine cause?

Ketorolac ophthalmic may cause side effects. Tell your doctor if any of these symptoms are severe or do not go away:

- stinging and burning of the eyes
- blurry vision

If you experience any of the following symptoms, stop using ketorolac ophthalmic and call your doctor immediately:

- redness or swelling of eyes, lips, tongue, or skin
- infection in or around the eye
- skin rash, hives, or skin changes
- difficulty breathing or swallowing

If you experience a serious side effect, you or your doctor may send a report to the Food and Drug Administration's (FDA) MedWatch Adverse Event Reporting program online [at http://www.fda.gov/MedWatch/index.html] or by phone [1-800-332-1088].

What storage conditions are needed for this medicine?

Keep this medication in the container it came in, tightly closed, and out of reach of children. Store it at room temperature and away from excess heat and moisture (not in the bathroom). Throw away any medication that is outdated or no longer needed. Talk to your pharmacist about the proper disposal of your medication.

What other information should I know?

Keep all appointments with your doctor.

Do not let anyone else use your medication. Ask your pharmacist any questions you have about refilling your prescription.

Dosage Facts
For Informational Purposes

Caution: Do not change your dose, how often you take your medication, or the length of time you are to take it without first talking to your healthcare provider.

The following dosage information was written using medical language for doctors and other healthcare professionals and is provided here for you to check your dosage. The dosage of this drug may differ for different patients. Therefore, always follow your doctor's instructions or the directions on the label. Contact your healthcare provider or pharmacist if you have any questions about the specific dosage of your medication after reviewing this information.

General Dosage Information

Available as ketorolac tromethamine; dosage expressed in terms of the salt.

Pediatric Patients

Conjunctivitis

OPHTHALMIC:
- Children ≥3 years of age: 1 drop (250 mg) of a 0.5% solution in the affected eye(s) 4 times daily.

Postoperative Ocular Inflammation

OPHTHALMIC:
- Children ≥3 years of age: 1 drop (250 mcg) of a 0.5% solution in the eye(s) undergoing surgery 4 times daily beginning 24 hours after surgery and typically continuing for 2 weeks after surgery.

Postoperative Ocular Pain

OPHTHALMIC:

- Children ≥3 years of age undergoing ocular incisional refractive surgery: 1 drop (250 mcg) of a 0.5% preservative-free solution 4 times daily in the eye(s) that underwent surgery as needed for up to 3 days after surgery.
- Children ≥3 years of age undergoing corneal refractive surgery: 1 drop (200 mcg) of a 0.4% solution 4 times daily in the eye(s) that underwent surgery as needed for up to 4 days after surgery.

Adult Patients

Conjunctivitis

OPHTHALMIC:

- 1 drop (250 mg) of a 0.5% solution in the affected eye(s) 4 times daily.

Postoperative Ocular Inflammation

OPHTHALMIC:

- 1 drop (250 mcg) of a 0.5% solution in the eye(s) undergoing surgery 4 times daily beginning 24 hours after surgery and typically continuing for 2 weeks after surgery.

Postoperative Ocular Pain

OPHTHALMIC:

- Patients undergoing ocular incisional refractive surgery: 1 drop (250 mcg) of a 0.5% preservative-free solution 4 times daily in the eye(s) that underwent surgery as needed for up to 3 days after surgery.
- Patients undergoing corneal refractive surgery: 1 drop (200 mcg) of a 0.4% solution 4 times daily in the eye(s) that underwent surgery as needed for up to 4 days after surgery.

Cystoid Macular Edema
Postoperative Cystoid Macular Edema†

OPHTHALMIC:

- 1–2 drops (250–500 mcg) of a 0.5% solution in the eye(s) undergoing surgery every 6–8 hours beginning 24 hours prior to surgery and continuing for 3–4 weeks after surgery.

Chronic Aphakic or Pseudophakic Cystoid Macular Edema†

OPHTHALMIC:

- 1–2 drops (250–500 mcg) of a 0.5% solution in the affected eye(s) 4 times daily for 2–3 months.

† Use is not currently included in the labeling approved by the US Food and Drug Administration.

Ketotifen Ophthalmic
(kee toe tye′ fen)

Brand Name: Zaditor®

Why is this medicine prescribed?

Ketotifen is used to relieve the itching of allergic pink eye. Ketotifen is in a class of medications called antihistamines. It works by blocking histamine, a substance in the body that causes allergic symptoms.

How should this medicine be used?

Ketotifen comes as a solution to apply to the eye. It is usually applied to the affected eye(s) twice daily, 8 to 12 hours apart. To help you remember to use ketotifen, apply it around the same times every day. Follow the directions on your prescription label carefully, and ask your doctor or pharmacist to explain any part you do not understand. Use ketotifen exactly as directed. Do not use more or less of it or use it more often than prescribed by your doctor.

To apply the eyedrops, follow these steps:

1. Wash your hands thoroughly with soap and water.
2. Use a mirror or have someone else put the drops in your eye.
3. Remove the protective cap. Make sure the end of the dropper is not chipped or cracked.
4. Avoid touching the dropper against your eye or anything else.
5. Hold the dropper tip down at all times to prevent drops from flowing back into the bottle and contaminating the remaining contents.
6. Lie down or tilt your head back.
7. Holding the bottle between your thumb and index finger, place the dropper as near as possible to your eyelid without touching it.
8. Brace the remaining fingers of that hand against your cheek or nose.
9. With the index finger of your other hand, pull the lower lid of the eye down to form a pocket.
10. Drop the prescribed number of drops into the pocket made by the lower lid and the eye. Placing the drops on the surface of the eyeball can cause stinging.
11. Close your eye and press lightly against the lower lid with your finger for 2-3 minutes to keep the medication in the eye. Do not blink.
12. Replace and tighten the cap right away. Do not wipe or rinse it off.
13. Wipe off any excess liquid from your cheek with a clean tissue. Wash your hands again.

Are there other uses for this medicine?

This medication may be prescribed for other uses; ask your doctor or pharmacist for more information.

What special precautions should I follow?

Before using ketotifen,

- tell your doctor and pharmacist if you are allergic to ketotifen or any other medications.
- tell your doctor and pharmacist what prescription and nonprescription medications, vitamins, nutritional supplements, and herbal products you are taking.
- tell your doctor if you are pregnant, plan to become pregnant, or are breast-feeding. If you become pregnant while using ketotifen, call your doctor.
- you should know that you should not wear contact lenses if your eye(s) is/are red. If your eye is not red and you wear contact lenses, you should know that ketotifen solution contains benzalkonium chloride, which can be absorbed by soft contact lenses. Remove your contact lenses before applying azelastine and put them back in 10 minutes later.

What special dietary instructions should I follow?

Unless your doctor tells you otherwise, continue your normal diet.

What should I do if I forget to take a dose?

Apply the missed dose as soon as you remember it. However, if it is almost time for the next dose, skip the missed dose and continue your regular dosing schedule. Do not apply a double dose to make up for a missed one.

What side effects can this medicine cause?

Ketotifen may cause side effects. Tell your doctor if any of these symptoms are severe or do not go away:

- headache
- runny nose
- burning or stinging of the eye
- eye discharge
- dry eyes
- eye pain
- eyelid problems
- itching
- problem with tear production
- blurred vision
- sensitivity to light
- rash
- flu-like symptoms
- sore throat

Ketotifen may cause other side effects. Call your doctor if you have any unusual problems while using this medication.

What storage conditions are needed for this medicine?

Keep this medication in the container it came in, tightly closed, and out of reach of children. Store it at room temperature and away from excess heat and moisture (not in the bathroom). Throw away any medication that is outdated or no longer needed. Talk to your pharmacist about the proper disposal of your medication.

What other information should I know?

Keep all appointments with your doctor.

Do not let anyone else use your medication. Ask your pharmacist any questions you have about refilling your prescription.

Dosage Facts
For Informational Purposes

Caution: Do not change your dose, how often you take your medication, or the length of time you are to take it without first talking to your healthcare provider.

The following dosage information was written using medical language for doctors and other healthcare professionals and is provided here for you to check your dosage. The dosage of this drug may differ for different patients. Therefore, always follow your doctor's instructions or the directions on the label. Contact your healthcare provider or pharmacist if you have any questions about the specific dosage of your medication after reviewing this information.

General Dosage Information

Available as ketotifen fumarate; dosage is expressed in terms of ketotifen.

Pediatric Patients

Allergic Conjunctivitis

OPHTHALMIC:
- One drop of a 0.025% solution in the affected eye(s) twice daily (at an interval of 8–12 hours) for those ≥3 years of age.

Adult Patients

Allergic Conjunctivitis

OPHTHALMIC:
- One drop of a 0.025% solution in the affected eye(s) twice daily (at an interval of 8–12 hours).

Labetalol Oral

(la bet′ a lole)

Brand Name: Normodyne®, Trandate®
Also available generically.

Important Warning

Do not stop taking labetalol without talking to your doctor first. If labetalol is stopped suddenly, it may cause chest pain or heart attack in some people.

Why is this medicine prescribed?

Labetalol is used to treat high blood pressure. It relaxes your blood vessels so your heart doesn't have to pump as hard. This medication is sometimes prescribed for other uses; ask your doctor or pharmacist for more information.

How should this medicine be used?

Labetalol comes as a tablet to take by mouth. It usually is taken two or three times a day. Follow the directions on your prescription label carefully, and ask your doctor or pharmacist to explain any part you do not understand. Take labetalol exactly as directed. Do not take more or less of it or take it more often than prescribed by your doctor.

Labetalol controls high blood pressure but does not cure it. Continue to take labetalol even if you feel well. Do not stop taking labetalol without talking to your doctor.

Are there other uses for this medicine?

Labetalol is also used sometimes to treat chest pain (angina) and to treat patients with tetanus. Talk to your doctor about the possible risks of using this drug for your condition.

What special precautions should I follow?

Before taking labetalol,
- tell your doctor and pharmacist if you are allergic to labetalol or any other drugs.
- tell your doctor and pharmacist what prescription and nonprescription medications you are taking, especially other medications for high blood pressure or heart disease; cimetidine (Tagamet); nitroglycerin; medications for asthma, headaches, allergies, colds, or pain; and vitamins.
- tell your doctor if you have or have ever had heart, kidney, or liver disease; asthma or other lung disease; severe allergies; diabetes; or pheochromocytoma.
- tell your doctor if you are pregnant, plan to become pregnant, or are breast-feeding. If you become pregnant while taking labetalol, call your doctor.
- if you are having surgery, including dental surgery, tell the doctor or dentist that you are taking labetalol.
- you should know that this drug may make you drowsy. Do not drive a car or operate machinery until you know how this drug affects you.
- remember that alcohol can add to the drowsiness caused by this drug.

What special dietary instructions should I follow?

Talk to your doctor before using salt substitutes containing potassium. If your doctor prescribes a low-salt or low-sodium diet, follow these directions carefully.

Labetalol may be taken with or without food, but it should be taken the same way every day.

What should I do if I forget to take a dose?

Take the missed dose as soon as you remember it. However, if it is almost time for the next dose, skip the missed dose and continue your regular dosing schedule. Do not take a double dose to make up for a missed one.

What side effects can this medicine cause?

Labetalol may cause side effects. Tell your doctor if any of these symptoms are severe or do not go away:
- dizziness
- tingling scalp or skin
- lightheadedness
- excessive tiredness
- headache
- upset stomach
- stuffy nose

If you experience any of the following symptoms, call your doctor immediately:
- shortness of breath or wheezing
- swelling of the feet and lower legs
- sudden weight gain
- chest pain

If you experience a serious side effect, you or your doctor may send a report to the Food and Drug Administration's (FDA) MedWatch Adverse Event Reporting program online [at http://www.fda.gov/MedWatch/index.html] or by phone [1-800-332-1088].

What storage conditions are needed for this medicine?

Keep this medication in the container it came in, tightly closed, and out of reach of children. Store it at room temperature and away from excess heat and moisture (not in the bathroom). Throw away any medication that is outdated or no longer needed. Talk to your pharmacist about the proper disposal of your medication.

What should I do in case of overdose?

In case of overdose, call your local poison control center at 1-800-222-1222. If the victim has collapsed or is not breathing, call local emergency services at 911.

What other information should I know?

Keep all appointments with your doctor and the laboratory. Your blood pressure should be checked regularly to determine your response to labetalol. Your doctor may ask you to check your pulse (heart rate). Ask your pharmacist or doctor to teach you how to take your pulse. If your pulse is faster or slower than it should be, call your doctor.

Do not let anyone else take your medication. Ask your pharmacist any questions you have about refilling your prescription.

Dosage Facts
For Informational Purposes

Caution: Do not change your dose, how often you take your medication, or the length of time you are to take it without first talking to your healthcare provider.

The following dosage information was written using medical language for doctors and other healthcare professionals and is provided here for you to check your dosage. The dosage of this drug may differ for different patients. Therefore, always follow your doctor's instructions or the directions on the label. Contact your healthcare provider or pharmacist if you have any questions about the specific dosage of your medication after reviewing this information.

General Dosage Information

Available as labetalol hydrochloride; dosage expressed in terms of the salt.

Pediatric Patients

Hypertension†

ORAL:
- Initially, 1–3 mg/kg daily given in 2 divided doses. Increase dosage as necessary up to a maximum of 10–12 mg/kg or 1.2 g daily given in 2 divided doses.

Adult Patients

Hypertension
Monotherapy

ORAL:
- Initially, 100 mg twice daily.
- Adjust dosage in increments of 100 mg twice daily every 2 or 3 days until optimum BP response is achieved.
- For maintenance, manufacturer recommends a usual dosage of 200–400 mg twice daily. Manufacturer states that some adults with severe hypertension may require up to 1.2 g–2.4 g administered in 2 or 3 divided doses daily.
- JNC 7 recommends a usual range of 100–400 mg twice daily. JNC recommends adding another drug, if needed, rather than continuing to increase dosage.

Combination Therapy

ORAL:
- Initially, 100 mg twice daily, in combination with a diuretic.
- Adjustment of labetalol dosage may be necessary when di-

uretic is initiated in a patient already receiving labetalol; optimum maintenance dosage is usually lower.

Severe Hypertension and Hypertensive Crisis

ORAL (FOLLOWING IV DOSAGE):
- Discontinue IV therapy and initiate oral labetalol therapy when the DBP begins to increase.
- Initially 200 mg, followed in 6–12 hours by an additional dose of 200 or 400 mg, depending on the BP response.
- If necessary, oral dosage may be increased in usual increments at *1-day* intervals while the patient is hospitalized.
- Follow the usual oral dosage recommendations for subsequent outpatient dosage titration or maintenance dosing.

Prescribing Limits
Pediatric Patients

Hypertension

ORAL:
- Maximum 10–12 mg/kg or 1.2 g daily.

Adult Patients

Hypertension

ORAL:
- Maximum titration increment of 200 mg twice daily.

Special Populations

Hepatic Impairment
- Dosage reduction may be necessary, but specific data are currently not available.

Renal Impairment
- No dosage adjustment required in patients with mild to moderate renal impairment. In patients with severe renal impairment (i.e., Cl_{cr} <10 mL/minute) undergoing dialysis, once-daily dosing may be adequate.

Geriatric Patients

Oral
- Adjustment in initial dosage not required. Maintenance dosage requirements are lower in most geriatric patients; 100–200 mg twice daily usually required.

† Use is not currently included in the labeling approved by the US Food and Drug Administration.

Lactulose

(lak′ tyoo lose)

Brand Name: Cholac® Syrup, Constilac® Syrup, Constulose®, Enulose®, Evalose® Syrup, Generlac®, Heptalac®, Kristalose®
Also available generically.

Why is this medicine prescribed?

Lactulose is a synthetic sugar used to treat constipation. It is broken down in the colon into products that pull water out from the body and into the colon. This water softens stools. Lactulose is also used to reduce the amount of ammonia in the blood of patients with liver disease. It works by drawing ammonia from the blood into the colon where it is removed from the body.

This medication is sometimes prescribed for other uses; ask your doctor or pharmacist for more information.

How should this medicine be used?

Lactulose comes as liquid to take by mouth. It usually is taken once a day for treatment of constipation and three or four times a day for liver disease. Your prescription label tells you how much medicine to take at each dose. Follow the directions on your prescription label carefully, and ask your doctor or pharmacist to explain any part you do not understand. Take lactulose exactly as directed. Do not take more or less of it or take it more often than prescribed by your doctor.

What special precautions should I follow?

Before taking lactulose,
- tell your doctor and pharmacist if you are allergic to lactulose or any other drugs.
- tell your doctor and pharmacist what prescription and nonprescription medications you are taking, especially antacids, antibiotics including neomycin (Mycifradin), and other laxatives.
- tell your doctor if you have diabetes or require a low-lactose diet.
- tell your doctor if you are pregnant, plan to become pregnant, or are breast-feeding. If you become pregnant while taking lactulose, call your doctor.
- if you are having surgery or tests on your colon or rectum, tell the doctor or dentist that you are taking lactulose.

What should I do if I forget to take a dose?

Take the missed dose as soon as you remember it. However, if it is almost time for the next dose, skip the missed dose and continue your regular dosing schedule. Do not take a double dose to make up for a missed one.

What side effects can this medicine cause?

Lactulose may cause side effects. Tell your doctor if any of these symptoms are severe or do not go away:
- diarrhea
- gas
- upset stomach

If you have any of the following symptoms, stop taking lactulose and call your doctor immediately:
- stomach pain or cramps
- vomiting

If you experience a serious side effect, you or your doctor may send a report to the Food and Drug Administration's (FDA) MedWatch Adverse Event Reporting program online

[at http://www.fda.gov/MedWatch/index.html] or by phone [1-800-332-1088].

What storage conditions are needed for this medicine?

Keep this medication in the container it came in, tightly closed, and out of reach of children. Store it at room temperature and away from excess heat and moisture (not in the bathroom). Throw away any medication that is outdated or no longer needed. Talk to your pharmacist about the proper disposal of your medication.

What other information should I know?

Keep all appointments with your doctor.

To improve the taste of lactulose, mix your dose with one-half glass of water, milk, or fruit juice.

Do not let anyone else take your medicine. Ask your pharmacist any questions you have about refilling your prescription.

Dosage Facts
For Informational Purposes

Caution: Do not change your dose, how often you take your medication, or the length of time you are to take it without first talking to your healthcare provider.

The following dosage information was written using medical language for doctors and other healthcare professionals and is provided here for you to check your dosage. The dosage of this drug may differ for different patients. Therefore, always follow your doctor's instructions or the directions on the label. Contact your healthcare provider or pharmacist if you have any questions about the specific dosage of your medication after reviewing this information.

General Dosage Information

Each 15 mL of commercially available lactulose solution provides approximately 10 g of the drug; corresponding doses provided by 2.5, 5, 7.5, 10, 30, 40, 45, 90, 150, and 300 mL of the commercial solution are approximately 1.67, 3.3, 5, 6.67, 20, 27, 30, 60, 100, and 200 g, respectively. Following reconstitution of the oral powder as directed, a 10- or 20-g dose is provided by administering the total volume.

Pediatric Patients

Portal-Systemic Encephalopathy
ORAL:
- Infants (limited data): Initially, 1.67–6.67 g daily in divided doses.
- Older children and adolescents: Initially, 27–60 g daily recommended by manufacturer.
- Adjust dosage every 1–2 days as necessary to produce 2–3 soft stools daily.
- If the initial dose produces diarrhea, reduce dose immediately; if diarrhea persists, discontinue drug.

Chronic Constipation

At least 5 g daily, usually given as a single dose after breakfast, has been used.

Adult Patients

Portal-Systemic Encephalopathy

ORAL:

- 20–30 g 3 or 4 times daily.
- Adjust dosage every 1–2 days as necessary to produce 2 or 3 soft stools daily. Usually dosage is 60–100 g daily; some patients may require higher dosage.
- Some clinicians recommend dosage adjustment according to acidity of colonic contents by measuring stool pH (with indicator paper) at initiation of therapy and adjusting dosage until stool pH is about 5. This pH is usually achieved when the patient has 2 or 3 soft stools daily during therapy.
- In the management of acute PSE episodes, give 20–30 g orally at 1- to 2-hour intervals to induce rapid laxation. When the laxative effect has been achieved, reduce dosage to the amount required to produce 2 or 3 soft stools daily.
- During treatment, improvement in patient's clinical condition usually occurs within 1–3 days.
- Continuous long-term therapy with lactulose may decrease severity and prevent recurrence of PSE.

Chronic Constipation

ORAL:

- Usual initial dosage is 10–20 g daily. Dosage may be increased to 40 g daily if necessary.
- Following oral administration, 24–48 hours may be required to restore normal bowel movements.
- To facilitate bowel movements in patients undergoing hemorrhoidectomy†, administer 10 g twice daily on the day before surgery and twice daily for 5 days postoperatively.
- To induce bowel evacuation in geriatric patients with colonic retention of barium and severe constipation following barium meal examination†, 3.3–6.7 g twice daily for 1–4 weeks has been administered.

Special Populations

Hepatic Impairment

Hepatic Impairment

ORAL:

- No specific dosage recommendations for patients with hepatic impairment.

Renal Impairment

Renal Impairment

ORAL:

- No specific dosage recommendations for patients with renal impairment.

Geriatric Patients

- No specific dosage recommendations for geriatric patients.

† *Use is not currently included in the labeling approved by the US Food and Drug Administration.*

Lamivudine

(la mi′ vyoo deen)

Brand Name: Combivir® (as a combination product containing Lamivudine and Zidovudine), Epivir®, Epivir-HBV®, Epzicom® (as a combination product containing Lamivudine and Abacavir Sulfate), Trizivir® (as a combination product containing Lamivudine, Abacavir Sulfate, and Zidovudine)

Important Warning

Lamivudine, when used alone or in combination with other antiviral medications, can cause serious damage to the liver and a condition called lactic acidosis. If you experience any of the following symptoms, call your doctor immediately: upset stomach, loss of appetite, excessive tiredness, weakness, dark yellow or brown urine, unusual bleeding or bruising, flu-like symptoms, yellowing of the skin or eyes, and pain in the upper right part of your stomach. Keep all appointments with your doctor and the laboratory. Your doctor will order certain lab tests to check your response to lamivudine.

Epivir tablets and liquid (used to treat human immunodeficiency virus [HIV]) are not interchangeable with Epivir-HBV tablets and liquid (used to treat hepatitis B infection). Epivir contains a higher dose of lamivudine than Epivir-HBV. Treatment with Epivir-HBV in patients infected with HIV may cause the HIV virus to be less treatable with lamivudine and other medicines. If you have both HIV and hepatitis B, you should take only Epivir. If you are taking Epivir-HBV for hepatitis B infection, talk to your doctor about your risks for HIV infection.

Why is this medicine prescribed?

Lamivudine (Epivir) is used in combination with other medications to treat human immunodeficiency virus (HIV) infection in patients with acquired immunodeficiency syndrome (AIDS). Lamivudine is not a cure and may not decrease the number of HIV-related illnesses. Lamivudine does not prevent the spread of HIV to other people. Lamivudine (Epivir-HBV) is used to treat hepatitis B infection. Lamivudine is in a class of medications called nucleoside reverse transcriptase inhibitors. It works by stopping the spread of the HIV and hepatitis B viruses.

How should this medicine be used?

Lamivudine comes as a tablet and liquid to take by mouth. Lamivudine (Epivir) is usually taken every 12 hours (twice a day). Lamivudine (Epivir-HBV) is usually taken once a day. Follow the directions on your prescription label carefully, and ask your doctor or pharmacist to explain any part you do not understand. Take lamivudine exactly as directed. Do not take more or less of it or take it more often than prescribed by your doctor.

Continue to take lamivudine even if you feel well. Do not stop taking lamivudine without talking to your doctor.

Are there other uses for this medicine?

Lamivudine is also used sometimes in combination with zidovudine (Retrovir, AZT) to treat health-care workers or other individuals exposed to HIV infection after accidental contact with HIV-contaminated blood, tissues, or other body fluids. Talk to your doctor about the possible risks of using this drug for your condition.

This medication may be prescribed for other uses; ask your doctor or pharmacist for more information.

What special precautions should I follow?

Before taking lamivudine,

- tell your doctor and pharmacist if you are allergic to lamivudine or any other drugs.
- tell your doctor and pharmacist what prescription and nonprescription medications you are taking, especially trimethoprim/sulfamethoxazole (Bactrim, Septra), and vitamins.
- tell your doctor if you have or have ever had hepatitis B, kidney disease, or pancreas disease (in children only).
- tell your doctor if you are pregnant, plan to become pregnant, or are breast-feeding. If you become pregnant while taking lamivudine, call your doctor. You should not breast-feed while taking lamivudine.

What should I do if I forget to take a dose?

Take the missed dose as soon as you remember it. However, if it is almost time for the next dose, skip the missed dose and continue your regular dosing schedule. Do not take a double dose to make up for a missed one.

What side effects can this medicine cause?

Lamivudine may cause side effects. Tell your doctor if any of these symptoms are severe or do not go away:

- diarrhea
- headache
- fatigue
- chills
- upset stomach
- vomiting
- loss of appetite
- dizziness

- trouble sleeping
- depression
- stuffy nose
- cough

If you experience any of the following symptoms or those listed in the IMPORTANT WARNING section, call your doctor immediately:

- rash
- stomach pain
- vomiting (in children)
- upset stomach (in children)
- fever
- muscle pain
- numbness, tingling, or burning in the fingers or toes

If you experience a serious side effect, you or your doctor may send a report to the Food and Drug Administration's (FDA) MedWatch Adverse Event Reporting program online [at http://www.fda.gov/MedWatch/index.html] or by phone [1-800-332-1088].

What storage conditions are needed for this medicine?

Keep this medication in the container it came in, tightly closed, and out of reach of children. Store it at room temperature and away from excess heat and moisture (not in the bathroom). The liquid does not need to be refrigerated; however, it should be stored in a cool place. Throw away any medication that is outdated or no longer needed. Talk to your pharmacist about the proper disposal of your medication.

What should I do in case of overdose?

In case of overdose, call your local poison control center at 1-800-222-1222. If the victim has collapsed or is not breathing, call local emergency services at 911.

What other information should I know?

Do not let anyone else take your medication. Ask your pharmacist any questions you have about refilling your prescription.

Dosage Facts
For Informational Purposes

Caution: Do not change your dose, how often you take your medication, or the length of time you are to take it without first talking to your health-care provider.

The following dosage information was written using medical language for doctors and other healthcare professionals and is provided here for you to check your dosage. The dosage of this drug may differ for different patients. Therefore, always follow your doctor's instructions or the directions on the label. Contact your healthcare provider or pharmacist if you have any questions

about the specific dosage of your medication after reviewing this information.

General Dosage Information

Dosage of Combivir®, Epzicom®, and Trizivir® expressed as number of tablets.

Epivir®, Epzicom®, and Combivir® must be used in conjunction with other antiretrovirals; Trizivir® may be used alone or in conjunction with other antiretrovirals.

Pediatric Patients

Treatment of HIV Infection

ORAL:
- Infants <30 days of age†: 2 mg/kg twice daily (Epivir®) suggested by some experts.
- Children 3 months to 16 years of age: 4 mg/kg (maximum 150 mg) twice daily (Epivir®).
- Adolescents ≥16 years of age weighing ≥50 kg: 150 mg twice daily or 300 mg once daily (Epivir®).
- Adolescents ≥16 years of age weighing <50 kg: 4 mg/kg (maximum 150 mg) twice daily (Epivir®).
- Combivir®: 1 tablet twice daily in adolescents ≥12 years of age.
- Trizivir®: 1 tablet twice daily in adolescents weighing ≥40 kg.

Prevention of Maternal-fetal Transmission of HIV†
Zidovudine and Lamivudine Regimen

ORAL:
- Neonates born to women who received no antiretroviral therapy prior to labor: 2 mg/kg every 12 hours (Epivir®) given for 7 days in conjunction with a 7-day regimen of oral zidovudine (4 mg/kg every 12 hours).
- Used in conjunction with intrapartum regimen of oral zidovudine and lamivudine in the mother.

Chronic Hepatitis B Virus (HBV) Infection

ORAL:
- Children 2–17 years of age: 3 mg/kg once daily (maximum 100 mg) (Epivir-HBV®).
- Optimal duration of treatment unknown; safety and efficacy >1 year not established.

Adult Patients

Treatment of HIV Infection

ORAL:
- 150 mg twice daily or 300 mg once daily (Epivir®).
- Combivir®: 1 tablet twice daily.
- Epzicom®: 1 tablet once daily.
- Trizivir®: 1 tablet twice daily in adults weighing ≥40 kg.

Prevention of Maternal-fetal Transmission†
Zidovudine and Lamivudine Regimen

ORAL:
- Women in labor who have received no prior antiretroviral therapy: 150 mg at onset of labor, then 150 mg every 12 hours during labor. Given with oral zidovudine (600 mg at onset of labor, then 300 mg every 3 hours during labor).

- Used in conjunction with a 7-day regimen of oral zidovudine and lamivudine in the neonate.

Postexposure Prophylaxis of HIV†
Occupational Exposure†

ORAL:
- 300 mg once daily or 150 mg twice daily (Epivir®).
- Used in basic regimens with zidovudine or tenofovir; used in alternative basic regimens with stavudine or didanosine.
- Initiate postexposure prophylaxis as soon as possible following exposure (within hours rather than days) and continue for 4 weeks, if tolerated.

Nonoccupational Exposure†

ORAL:
- 300 mg once daily or 150 mg twice daily (Epivir®).
- Used in conjunction with another NRTI in preferred and alternative nonnucleoside reverse transcriptase inhibitor-based (NNRTI-based) or HIV protease inhibitor-based (PI-based) regimens.
- Initiate postexposure prophylaxis as soon as possible following exposure (preferably ≤72 hours after exposure) and continue for 28 days.

Chronic Hepatitis B Virus (HBV) Infection

ORAL:
- 100 mg once daily (Epivir-HBV®).
- Optimal duration of treatment unknown; safety and efficacy >1 year not established.

Prescribing Limits

Pediatric Patients

Treatment of HIV Infection

ORAL:
- Children 3 months to 16 years of age: Maximum 150 mg twice daily (Epivir®).

Chronic Hepatitis B Virus (HBV) Infection

ORAL:
- Children 2–17 years of age: Maximum 100 mg daily (Epivir-HBV®).

Special Populations

Hepatic Impairment

Treatment of HIV Infection

ORAL:
- Dosage adjustment not needed.

Chronic Hepatitis B Virus (HBV) Infection

ORAL:
- Dosage adjustment not needed.

Renal Impairment

Treatment of HIV Infection
Oral

- Consider reducing dose and/or increasing dosing interval in pediatric patients with renal impairment; data insufficient to make a specific recommendation.

Dosage in Adults and Adolescents with Renal Impairment (Epivir®)

Cl$_{cr}$ (mL/minute)	Dosage
≥50	150 mg twice daily or 300 mg once daily
30–49	150 mg once daily
15–29	150 mg first dose, then 100 mg once daily
5–14	150 mg first dose, then 50 mg once daily
<5	50 mg first dose, then 25 mg once daily
Hemodialysis Patients	Supplemental doses not necessary with routine (4-hour) hemodialysis
Peritoneal Dialysis Patients	Supplemental doses not necessary after peritoneal dialysis

Chronic Hepatitis B Virus (HBV) Infection

ORAL:
• Consider reducing dose in pediatric patients with renal impairment; data insufficient to make a specific recommendation.

Dosage in Adults with Renal Impairment (Epivir-HBV®)

Cl$_{cr}$ (mL/minute)	Dosage
≥50	100 mg once daily
30–49	100 mg first dose, then 50 mg once daily
15–29	100 mg first dose, then 25 mg once daily
5–14	35 mg first dose, then 15 mg once daily
<5	35 mg first dose, then 10 mg once daily
Hemodialysis Patients	Supplemental doses not necessary with routine (4-hour) hemodialysis
Peritoneal Dialysis Patients	Supplemental doses not necessary after peritoneal dialysis

Geriatric Patients
• Select dosage with caution because of age-related decreases in hepatic, renal, and/or cardiac function and concomitant disease and drug therapy.

† *Use is not currently included in the labeling approved by the US Food and Drug Administration.*

Lamivudine and Zidovudine

(la mi′ vyoo deen) (zye doe′ vyoo deen)

Brand Name: Combivir®

Important Warning

Lamivudine and zidovudine may stop your body from making enough blood cells. Tell your doctor if you have or have ever had any blood disorders such as anemia or bone marrow problems. If you experience any of the following symptoms, call your doctor immediately: unusual bleeding or bruising; shortness of breath; pale skin; fever, sore throat, chills, and other signs of infection; or unusual tiredness or weakness.

Lamivudine and zidovudine may cause muscle disorders. Tell your doctor if you have or have ever had any disease or swelling of the muscles. If you experience muscle pain or weakness, call your doctor immediately.

When used alone or in combination with other antiretroviral medication, lamivudine and zidovudine may also cause serious damage to the liver and a condition called lactic acidosis. Tell your doctor if you drink or have ever drunk large amounts of alcohol and if you have or have ever had liver disease. Tell your doctor and pharmacist if you are taking acetaminophen (Tylenol) and if you have been taking medication to treat HIV infection for a long time. If you experience any of the following symptoms, call your doctor immediately: fatty and foul-smelling stools, upset stomach, extreme tiredness, unusual bleeding or bruising, lack of energy, loss of appetite, pain in the upper right part of the stomach, yellowing of the skin or eyes, or flu-like symptoms.

Keep all appointments with your doctor and the laboratory. Your doctor will order certain lab tests to check your body's response to lamivudine and zidovudine.

Why is this medicine prescribed?

The combination of lamivudine and zidovudine is used to treat human immunodeficiency virus (HIV) in patients with or without acquired immunodeficiency syndrome (AIDS). Lamivudine and zidovudine are in a class of antiviral medications called synthetic nucleoside analogues. They work by slowing the spread of HIV infection in the body. Lamivudine and zidovudine is not a cure and may not decrease the number of HIV-related illnesses. Lamivudine and zidovudine does not prevent the spread of HIV to other people.

How should this medicine be used?

The combination of lamivudine and zidovudine comes as a tablet to take by mouth. It is usually taken twice a day with or without food. To help you remember to take this medication, take it around the same time every day. Follow the directions on your prescription label carefully and ask your doctor or pharmacist to explain any part you do not understand. Take this medication exactly as directed. Do not take more or less of it or take it more often than prescribed by your doctor.

Lamivudine and zidovudine controls HIV infection but does not cure it. Continue to take lamivudine and zidovudine even if you feel well. Do not stop taking lamivudine and zidovudine without talking to your doctor.

Are there other uses for this medicine?

This medication may be prescribed for other uses; ask your doctor or pharmacist for more information.

What special precautions should I follow?

Before taking lamivudine and zidovudine,

- tell your doctor or pharmacist if you are allergic to lamivudine (Epivir, Epivir HBV); zidovudine (Retrovir); lamivudine, zidovudine, and abacavir (Trizivir); or any other medications.
- you should know that lamivudine and zidovudine are also available individually with the brand names Epivir, Epivir HBV, and Retrovir, and in another combination as Trizivir. Tell your doctor if you are taking any of these medications, to be sure you do not receive the same medication twice.
- tell your doctor and pharmacist what prescription and nonprescription medications, vitamins, nutritional supplements and herbal products you are taking. Be sure to mention any of the following: acetaminophen (Tylenol), acyclovir (Zovirax), atovaquone (Mepron), cancer chemotherapy drugs, cidofovir (Vistide), dapsone (Avlosulfon), didanosine (ddI, Videx), doxorubicin (Adriamycin, Rubex), fluconazole (Diflucan), foscarnet (Foscavir), ganciclovir (Cytovene, Vitrasert), interferon alpha (Alferon N, Infergen, Intron A, Roferon A), interferon beta-1b (Betaseron), methadone, nelfinavir (Viracept), probenecid (Benemid, Probalan), ribavarin (Rebetol, Virazole), rifabutin (Mycobutin), rifampin (Rifadin, Rimactane), ritonavir (Norvir), stavudine (Zerit), trimethoprim (Trimpex, Proloprim), trimethoprim and sulfamethoxazole (Bactrim, Septra), valproic acid (Depakene, Depakote), and zalcitabine (ddC, Hivid). Your doctor may need to change the doses of your medications or monitor you carefully for side effects.
- in addition to the conditions listed in the IMPORTANT WARNING section, tell your doctor if you have or have ever had kidney disease.
- tell your doctor if you are pregnant, plan to become pregnant, or are breast-feeding. If you become pregnant while taking lamivudine and zidovudine, call your doctor. You should not breast-feed while taking lamivudine and zidovudine.
- you should be aware that your body fat may increase or move to different areas of your body, such as your breasts and your upper back.

What special dietary instructions should I follow?

Unless your doctor tells you otherwise, continue your normal diet.

What should I do if I forget to take a dose?

Take the missed dose as soon as you remember it. However, if it is almost time for the next dose, skip the missed dose and continue your regular dosing schedule. Do not take a double dose to make up for a missed one.

What side effects can this medicine cause?

Lamivudine and zidovudine may cause side effects. Tell your doctor if any of these symptoms are severe or do not go away:

- headache
- upset stomach
- diarrhea
- constipation
- loss of appetite
- dizziness
- difficulty falling asleep or staying asleep
- excessive tiredness
- depression
- stuffy nose
- cough
- hair loss

Some side effects can be serious. The following side effects are uncommon, but if you experience any of them, or any of those listed in the IMPORTANT WARNING section, call your doctor immediately:

- hives
- skin rash
- itching
- difficulty breathing or swallowing
- seizures
- numbness, tingling, or burning in your fingers or toes
- fever
- wheezing

Lamivudine and zidovudine may cause other side effects. Call your doctor if you have any unusual problems while taking lamivudine and zidovudine.

If you experience a serious side effect, you or your doctor may send a report to the Food and Drug Administration's (FDA) MedWatch Adverse Event Reporting program online [at http://www.fda.gov/MedWatch/index.html] or by phone [1-800-332-1088].

What storage conditions are needed for this medicine?

Keep this medication in the container it came in, tightly closed, and out of reach of children. Store it at room temperature and away from excess heat and moisture (not in the bathroom). Throw away any medication that is outdated or no longer needed. Talk to your pharmacist about the proper disposal of your medication.

What should I do in case of overdose?

In case of overdose, call your local poison control center at 1-800-222-1222. If the victim has collapsed or is not breathing, call local emergency services at 911.

What other information should I know?

Keep all appointments with your doctor and the laboratory.

Before having any laboratory test, tell your doctor and the laboratory personnel that you are taking lamivudine and zidovudine.

Do not let anyone else take your medication. Ask your pharmacist any questions you have about refilling your prescription.

Dosage Facts
For Informational Purposes

Caution: Do not change your dose, how often you take your medication, or the length of time you are to take it without first talking to your healthcare provider.

The following dosage information was written using medical language for doctors and other healthcare professionals and is provided here for you to check your dosage. The dosage of this drug may differ for different patients. Therefore, always follow your doctor's instructions or the directions on the label. Contact your healthcare provider or pharmacist if you have any questions about the specific dosage of your medication after reviewing this information.

General Dosage Information

Dosage of Combivir® expressed as number of tablets.

Combivir® must be used in conjunction with other antiretrovirals.

Pediatric Patients

Treatment of HIV Infection

ORAL:
- Combivir®: 1 tablet twice daily in adolescents ≥12 years of age.

Adult Patients

Treatment of HIV Infection

ORAL:
- Combivir®: 1 tablet twice daily.

† Use is not currently included in the labeling approved by the US Food and Drug Administration.

Lamotrigine

(la moe' tri jeen)

Brand Name: Lamictal®

Important Warning

Lamotrigine may cause serious rashes that may need to be treated in a hospital or cause permanent disability or death. Tell your doctor if you are taking valproic acid (Depakene) or divalproex (Depakote), because taking these medications with lamotrigine may increase your risk of developing a serious rash.

Your doctor will start you on low dose of lamotrigine and gradually increase your dose, not more than once every 1-2 weeks. You may be more likely to develop a serious rash if you take a higher starting dose or increase your dose faster than your doctor tells you that you should. Be sure to take lamotrigine exactly as directed. Do not take more or less of it or take it more often than prescribed by your doctor.

Serious rashes usually develop during the first 2-8 weeks of treatment with lamotrigine, but can develop at any time during treatment. If you develop any of the following symptoms while you are taking lamotrigine, call your doctor immediately: rash; fever; swelling of the face, throat, tongue, lips, eyes, hands, feet, ankles, or lower legs; hoarseness; difficulty breathing or swallowing; upset stomach; extreme tiredness; unusual bruising or bleeding; lack of energy; loss of appetite; pain in the upper right part of the stomach; yellowing of the skin or eyes; flu-like symptoms; pale skin; headache; dizziness; fast heartbeat; weakness;; shortness of breath; sore throat, fever, chills, and other signs of infection; dark red or cola-colored urine; muscle weakness or aching; or painful sores in your mouth or around your eyes.

Talk to your doctor about the risks of taking lamotrigine or of giving lamotrigine to your child. Children who take lamotrigine are more likely to develop serious rashes than adults who take the medication.

Why is this medicine prescribed?

Lamotrigine is used to treat certain types of seizures in patients who have epilepsy or Lennox-Gastaut syndrome (a disorder that causes seizures and often causes developmental delays). Lamotrigine is also used to increase the time between episodes of depression, mania (frenzied or abnormally excited mood), and other abnormal moods in patients with bipolar I disorder (manic depressive disorder; a disease that causes episodes of depression, episodes of mania, and other abnormal moods). Lamotrigine has not been shown to be effective when people experience the actual episodes of depression or mania, so other medications must be used to help people recover from these episodes. Lamotrigine is in a class of medications called anticonvulsants. It works by decreasing abnormal excitement in the brain.

How should this medicine be used?

Lamotrigine comes as a regular tablet and a chewable dispersible (can be chewed or dissolved in liquid) tablet to take by mouth. It is usually taken once or twice a day. It is sometimes taken once every other day at the beginning of treatment. Follow the directions on your prescription label carefully and ask your doctor or pharmacist to explain any part you do not understand.

There are other medications that have names similar to the brand name for lamotrigine. You should be sure that you receive lamotrigine and not one of the similar medications each time you fill your prescription. Be sure that the prescription your doctor gives you is clear and easy to read. Talk to your pharmacist to be sure that you are given lamotrigine. After you receive your medication, compare the tablets to the pictures in the manufacturer's patient information sheet. If you think you were given the wrong medication, talk to your pharmacist. Do not take any medication unless you are certain it is the medication that your doctor prescribed.

Swallow the regular tablets whole; do not split, chew, or crush them.

If you are taking the chewable dispersible tablets, you may swallow them whole, chew them, or dissolve them in liquid. If you chew the tablets, drink a small amount of water or diluted fruit juice afterward to wash down the medication. To dissolve the tablets in liquid, place 1 teaspoon of water or diluted fruit juice in a glass or on a spoon. Place the tablet in the liquid and wait 1 minute to allow it to dissolve. Then mix the liquid and drink all of it immediately.

If you were taking another medication to treat seizures and are switching to lamotrigine, your doctor will gradually decrease your dose of the other medication and gradually increase your dose of lamotrigine. Follow these directions carefully and ask your doctor or pharmacist if you have questions about how much of each medication you should take.

Lamotrigine may control your condition, but it will not cure it. Continue to take lamotrigine even if you feel well.

Do not stop taking lamotrigine without talking to your doctor. Your doctor will probably decrease your dose gradually. If you suddenly stop taking lamotrigine, you may experience seizures. If you do stop taking lamotrigine for any reason, do not start taking it again without talking to your doctor.

Your doctor or pharmacist will give you the manufacturer's patient information sheet. Read it carefully before you begin taking lamotrigine and each time you refill your prescription. Ask your doctor or pharmacist if you have any questions.

Are there other uses for this medicine?

This medication may be prescribed for other uses; ask your doctor or pharmacist for more information.

What special precautions should I follow?

Before taking lamotrigine,

- tell your doctor and pharmacist if you are allergic to lamotrigine, or any other medications. If you will be taking the chewable dispersible tablets, tell your doctor if you are allergic to sulfa medications or saccharin.
- tell your doctor and pharmacist what prescription and nonprescription medications, vitamins, nutritional supplements, and herbal products you are taking. Be sure to mention the medications listed in the IMPORTANT WARNING section and methotrexate (Rheumatrex, Trexall); other medications for seizures such as carbamazepine (Tegretol), oxcarbazepine (Trileptal), phenobarbital (Luminal, Solfoton), phenytoin (Dilantin), and primidone (Mysoline); rifampin (Rifadin, Rimactane); and trimethoprim (Proloprim). Your doctor may need to change the doses of your medications or monitor you carefully for side effects.
- tell your doctor if you are taking female hormonal medications such as hormonal contraceptives (birth control pills, patches, rings, injections, implants, or intrauterine devices), or hormone replacement therapy (HRT). Talk to your doctor before you start or stop taking any of these medications while you are taking lamotrigine. If you are taking a female hormonal medication, tell your doctor if you have any bleeding between expected menstrual periods.
- tell your doctor if you have or have ever had heart, kidney, or liver disease or a blood disorder.
- tell your doctor if you are pregnant, plan to become pregnant, or are breast-feeding. If you become pregnant while taking lamotrigine, call your doctor.
- if you are having surgery, including dental surgery, tell the doctor or dentist that you are taking lamotrigine.
- you should know that this medication may make you drowsy. Do not drive a car or operate machinery until you know how this medication affects you.
- remember that alcohol can add to the drowsiness caused by this medication.

What special dietary instructions should I follow?

Unless your doctor tells you otherwise, continue your normal diet.

What should I do if I forget to take a dose?

Take the missed dose as soon as you remember it. However, if it is almost time for the next dose, skip the missed dose and continue your regular dosing schedule. Do not take a double dose to make up for a missed one.

What side effects can this medicine cause?

Lamotrigine may cause side effects. Tell your doctor if any of these symptoms are severe or do not go away:

- loss of balance or coordination
- double vision
- blurred vision
- crossed eyes
- difficulty thinking or concentrating
- difficulty speaking
- drowsiness
- dizziness
- vomiting
- diarrhea
- constipation
- heartburn
- problems with ears or teeth
- irritability
- nervousness
- mood changes
- difficulty falling asleep or staying asleep
- stomach, back, or joint pain
- runny nose
- cough
- missed or painful menstrual periods
- swelling, itching, or irritation of the vagina
- dry mouth

Some side effects can be serious. If you experience any of the following symptoms or those described in the IMPORTANT WARNING section, call your doctor immediately:

- seizures that happen more often, last longer, or are different than the seizures you had in the past
- chest pain
- swelling of the hands, feet, ankles, or lower legs
- depression

If you experience a serious side effect, you or your doctor may send a report to the Food and Drug Administration's (FDA) MedWatch Adverse Event Reporting program online [at http://www.fda.gov/MedWatch/index.html] or by phone [1-800-332-1088].

What storage conditions are needed for this medicine?

Keep this medication in the container it came in, tightly closed, and out of reach of children. Store it at room temperature, away from excess heat and moisture (not in the bathroom). Throw away any medication that is outdated or no longer needed. Talk to your pharmacist about the proper disposal of your medication.

What should I do in case of overdose?

In case of overdose, call your local poison control center at 1-800-222-1222. If the victim has collapsed or is not breathing, call local emergency services at 911.

Symptoms of overdose may include:

- loss of balance or coordination
- crossed eyes
- increased seizures
- loss of consciousness
- coma

What other information should I know?

Keep all appointments with your doctor and the laboratory. Your doctor may order certain lab tests to check your response to lamotrigine.

Do not let anyone else take your medication. Ask your pharmacist any questions you have about refilling your prescription.

Dosage Facts
For Informational Purposes

Caution: Do not change your dose, how often you take your medication, or the length of time you are to take it without first talking to your healthcare provider.

The following dosage information was written using medical language for doctors and other healthcare professionals and is provided here for you to check your dosage. The dosage of this drug may differ for different patients. Therefore, always follow your doctor's instructions or the directions on the label. Contact your healthcare provider or pharmacist if you have any questions about the specific dosage of your medication after reviewing this information.

General Dosage Information

When adding lamotrigine to an existing anticonvulsant regimen, add gradually while maintaining or gradually adjusting dosage of the other anticonvulsant(s).

Addition of other anticonvulsants (e.g., carbamazepine, phenobarbital, phenytoin, primidone, valproic acid) to, or their discontinuance from, an anticonvulsant regimen including lamotrigine may require modification of the dosage of lamotrigine and/or the other anticonvulsant(s).

If lamotrigine therapy is interrupted for >5 half-lives for any reason and reinitiation of the drug is not contraindicated, resume therapy using recommended initial dosage and dosage escalation regimens.

Pediatric Patients

Seizure Disorders
Adjunctive Therapy

ORAL:

- Recommended initial dosages and dosage escalations for lamotrigine when added to an anticonvulsant regimen containing valproic acid or containing carbamazepine, phenobarbital, phenytoin, or primidone (without valproic acid) are summarized in Table 1 or 2, respectively.
- Manufacturer makes no specific dosage recommendations for adding lamotrigine to an anticonvulsant regimen containing oxcarbazepine or levetiracetam or anticonvulsants with unknown potential for interacting with lamotrigine. Conservative initial dosages and dosage escalations (as with concomitant valproic acid) are recommended; an appropriate maintenance dosage probably would be greater than the maintenance dosage with valproic acid and lower than the maintenance dosage with carbamazepine, phenobarbital, phenytoin, or primidone (without valproic acid).
- Maintenance dosages usually are achieved after several weeks to months of therapy and should be individualized. Maintenance dosages in patients weighing <30 kg, regardless of age or concomitant anticonvulsant(s), may need to be increased by as much as 50%, based on clinical response.

Table 1. Recommended Pediatric Dosages of Lamotrigine When Added to Anticonvulsant Regimens Containing Valproic Acid

	Children 2–12 Years of Age[a]	Children >12 Years of Age
Weeks 1 and 2	0.15 mg/kg daily in 1 dose or 2 divided doses	25 mg every other day
Weeks 3 and 4	0.3 mg/kg daily in 1 dose or 2 divided doses	25 mg daily
Week 5 onward	Increase dosage in increments of 0.3 mg/kg daily every 1–2 weeks until an effective maintenance dosage is reached	Increase dosage in increments of 25–50 mg daily every 1–2 weeks until an effective maintenance dosage is reached
Usual maintenance dosage[b]	1–5 mg/kg daily (maximum 200 mg daily in 1 dose or 2 divided doses) 1–3 mg/kg daily if added to anticonvulsant regimen containing valproic acid alone	100–400 mg daily in 1 dose or 2 divided doses 100–200 mg daily if added to anticonvulsant regimen containing valproic acid alone

[a]Round dosage down to the nearest whole tablet.
[b]Increase maintenance dosage by as much as 50%, based on clinical response, in patients weighing <30 kg, regardless of age or concomitant anticonvulsant(s).

Table 2. Recommended Pediatric Dosages of Lamotrigine When Added to Anticonvulsant Regimens Containing Carbamazepine, Phenobarbital, Phenytoin, or Primidone (without Valproic Acid)

	Children 2–12 Years of Age[a]	Children >12 Years of Age
Weeks 1 and 2	0.6 mg/kg daily in 2 divided doses	50 mg daily
Weeks 3 and 4	1.2 mg/kg daily in 2 divided doses	100 mg daily in 2 divided doses
Week 5 onward	Increase dosage in increments of 1.2 mg/kg daily every 1–2 weeks until an effective maintenance dosage is reached	Increase dosage in increments of 100 mg daily every 1–2 weeks until an effective maintenance dosage is reached
Usual maintenance dosage[b]	5–15 mg/kg daily (maximum 400 mg daily in 2 divided doses)	300–500 mg daily in 2 divided doses

[a]Round dosage down to the nearest whole tablet.
[b]Increase maintenance dosage by as much as 50%, based on clinical response, in patients weighing <30 kg, regardless of age or concomitant anticonvulsant(s).

Patients receiving rifampin but not receiving valproic acid should receive lamotrigine dosages recommended for individuals receiving carbamazepine, phenobarbital, phenytoin, or primidone (without valproic acid).

Conversion to Lamotrigine Monotherapy

Adolescents ≥16 years of age should receive dosage recommended for adults.

Adult Patients

Seizure Disorders
Adjunctive Therapy

ORAL:

- Recommended initial dosages and dosage escalations for lamotrigine when added to an anticonvulsant regimen containing valproic acid or containing carbamazepine, phenobarbital, phenytoin, or primidone (without valproic acid) are summarized in Table 3.
- Manufacturer makes no specific dosage recommendations for adding lamotrigine to an anticonvulsant regimen containing oxcarbazepine or levetiracetam or anticonvulsants with unknown potential for interacting with lamotrigine. Conservative initial dosages and dosage escalations (as with concomitant valproic acid) are recommended; an appropriate maintenance dosage probably would be greater than the maintenance dosage with valproic acid and lower than the maintenance dosage with carbamazepine, phenobarbital, phenytoin, or primidone (without valproic acid).
- Maintenance dosages usually are achieved after several weeks to months of therapy and should be individualized.

Table 3. Recommended Adult Dosage of Lamotrigine When Added to Existing Anticonvulsant Regimens

	Regimens Containing Valproic Acid	Regimens Containing Carbamazepine, Phenobarbital, Phenytoin, or Primidone (Without Valproic Acid)
Weeks 1 and 2	25 mg every other day	50 mg daily
Weeks 3 and 4	25 mg daily	100 mg daily in 2 divided doses
Week 5 onward	Increase dosage in increments of 25–50 mg daily every 1–2 weeks until an effective maintenance dosage is reached	Increase dosage in increments of 100 mg daily every 1–2 weeks until an effective maintenance dosage is reached
Usual maintenance dosage	100–400 mg daily in 1 dose or 2 divided doses 100–200 mg daily if added to anticonvulsant regimen containing valproic acid alone	300–500 mg daily in 2 divided doses

Patients receiving rifampin but not receiving valproic acid should receive lamotrigine dosages recommended for individuals receiving carbamazepine, phenobarbital, phenytoin, or primidone (without valproic acid).

Conversion to Lamotrigine Monotherapy
ORAL:
• Conversion from monotherapy with carbamazepine, phenobarbital, phenytoin, or primidone: Titrate dosage until a maintenance lamotrigine dosage of 500 mg daily is reached); then withdraw concomitant anticonvulsant by 20% decrements each week over a 4-week period.
• Conversion from monotherapy with valproic acid:

Table 4. Conversion from Monotherapy with Valproic Acid to Lamotrigine Monotherapy

	Lamotrigine	Valproic Acid
Step 1	Achieve a dosage of 200 mg daily according to guidelines in Table 3 (if not already receiving 200 mg daily)	Maintain previous stable dosage
Step 2	Maintain at 200 mg daily	Decrease to 500 mg daily in decrements no greater than 500 mg daily every week and then maintain dosage of 500 mg daily for 1 week
Step 3	Increase to 300 mg daily and maintain for 1 week	Simultaneously decrease to 250 mg daily and maintain for 1 week
Step 4	Increase in increments of 100 mg daily every week to achieve maintenance dosage of 500 mg daily	Discontinue

Manufacturer makes no specific dosage recommendations for conversion to lamotrigine monotherapy in patients receiving anticonvulsants other than carbamazepine, phenobarbital, phenytoin, primidone, or valproic acid.

Bipolar Disorder
Maintenance Therapy
ORAL:
• Recommended initial dosages and dosage escalations for lamotrigine in patients receiving valproic acid or receiving carbamazepine, phenobarbital, phenytoin, primidone, or rifampin (without valproic acid) are summarized in Table 5.
• Optimum duration of therapy has not been established; periodically reevaluate the usefulness of the drug during prolonged therapy (i.e., >18 months).

Table 5. Lamotrigine Dosage Titration Regimen for Patients with Bipolar Disorder

	For Patients *Not* Receiving Carbamazepine, Phenobarbital, Phenytoin, Primidone, Rifampin, or Valproic Acid	For Patients Receiving Valproic Acid	For Patients Receiving Carbamazepine, Phenobarbital, Phenytoin, Primidone, or Rifampin (without Valproic Acid)
Weeks 1 and 2	25 mg daily	25 mg every other day	50 mg daily
Weeks 3 and 4	50 mg daily	25 mg daily	100 mg daily in divided doses
Week 5	100 mg daily	50 mg daily	200 mg daily in divided doses
Week 6	200 mg daily	100 mg daily	300 mg daily in divided doses
Week 7 (target dosages)	200 mg daily	100 mg daily	Up to 400 mg daily in divided doses

Recommended adjustments to lamotrigine dosage following discontinuance of rifampin or concomitantly administered psychotropic agents are summarized in Table 6.

Table 6. Dosage Adjustments for Patients with Bipolar Disorder following Discontinuance of Rifampin or Concomitantly Administered Psychotropic Agents

	Lamotrigine Dosage after Discontinuance of Psychotropic Agents *Excluding* Carbamazepine, Phenobarbital, Phenytoin, Primidone, or Valproic Acid	Lamotrigine Dosage after Discontinuance of Valproic Acid (when current lamotrigine dosage = 100 mg daily)	Lamotrigine Dosage after Discontinuance of Carbamazepine, Phenobarbital, Phenytoin, Primidone, or Rifampin (when current lamotrigine dosage = 400 mg daily)
Week 1	Maintain current lamotrigine dosage	150 mg daily	400 mg daily
Week 2	Maintain current lamotrigine dosage	200 mg daily	300 mg daily
Week 3 onward	Maintain current lamotrigine dosage	200 mg daily	200 mg daily

Prescribing Limits

Pediatric Patients

Seizure Disorders
Adjunctive Therapy

ORAL:
- Children 2–12 years of age: Maximum 200 mg daily when added to an anticonvulsant regimen containing valproic acid. Maximum 400 mg daily when added to an anticonvulsant regimen containing carbamazepine, phenobarbital, phenytoin, or primidone (without valproic acid).

Adult Patients

Bipolar Disorder
Maintenance Therapy

ORAL:
- Maximum 200 mg daily in patients *not* receiving concomitant therapy with carbamazepine, phenobarbital, phenytoin, primidone, rifampin, or valproic acid.

Special Populations

Hepatic Impairment
- Manufacturer generally recommends reducing initial, escalation, and maintenance dosages by approximately 50% in patients with moderate (Child-Pugh class B) and 75% in patients with severe (Child-Pugh class C) hepatic impairment. Adjust dosage according to clinical response.

Renal Impairment
- A reduced maintenance dosage may be effective and generally should be used in patients with substantial renal impairment; however, manufacturer makes no specific recommendation for dosage adjustment in such patients.

Geriatric Patients
- Manufacturer suggests that geriatric patients receive initial dosage at the lower end of the usual range.

Lansoprazole

(lan soe′ pra zole)

Brand Name: Prevacid®, Prevacid® NapraPAC®, Prevacid® SoluTab®, Prevpac®

Why is this medicine prescribed?

Lansoprazole is used to treat ulcers; gastroesophageal reflux disease (GERD), a condition in which backward flow of acid from the stomach causes heartburn and injury of the food pipe (esophagus); and conditions where the stomach produces too much acid, such as Zollinger-Ellison syndrome. Lansoprazole is used in combination with other medications to eliminate *H. pylori*, a bacteria that causes ulcers. Lansoprazole is in a class of medications called proton-pump inhibitors. It works by decreasing the amount of acid made in the stomach.

How should this medicine be used?

Lansoprazole comes as a delayed-release (long-acting) capsule and granules to make a delayed-release solution (liquid) to take by mouth. Lansoprazole is usually taken once a day, before eating. When taken in combination with other medications to eliminate *H. pylori*, lansoprazole is taken twice a day (every 12 hours) or three times a day (every 8 hours) for 10 to 14 days. To help you remember to take lansoprazole, take it around the same time every day. Follow the directions on your prescription label carefully, and ask your doctor or pharmacist to explain any part you do not understand. Take lansoprazole exactly as directed. Do not take more or less of it or take it more often than prescribed by your doctor.

The capsule should be swallowed whole. If you have difficulty swallowing capsules, lansoprazole capsules can be opened, and the granules can be sprinkled on 1 tablespoon of applesauce, Ensure pudding, cottage cheese, yogurt, or strained pears and swallowed immediately. The granules should not be chewed or crushed. The capsules can also be emptied into 2 ounces of orange juice or tomato juice, mixed briefly, and swallowed immediately. Rinse the glass with some additional juice and drink immediately.

For patients who have a nasogastric tube, lansoprazole capsules can be opened and the granules mixed in 40 mL of apple juice. The mixture should be injected through the nasogastric tube into the stomach. Then the tube should be flushed with some more apple juice.

To use lansoprazole oral solution, empty the contents of a packet into a container containing 2 tablespoons of water. Stir well and drink immediately. If any granules remain, add more water, stir, and drink immediately. Do not use liquids or foods other than water. Do not crush or chew the granules.

Continue to take lansoprazole even if you feel well. Do not stop taking lansoprazole without talking to your doctor.

Are there other uses for this medicine?

This medication may be prescribed for other uses; ask your doctor or pharmacist for more information.

What special precautions should I follow?

Before taking lansoprazole,
- tell your doctor and pharmacist if you are allergic to lansoprazole or any other medications.
- tell your doctor and pharmacist what prescription and nonprescription medications, vitamins, nutritional supplements, and herbal products you are taking. Be sure to mention any of the following: ampicillin (Omnipen, Polycillin, Totacillin), digoxin (Lanoxin), ketoconazole (Nizoral), theophylline (Theo-bid, TheoDur), and vitamins containing iron. Your doctor may need to change the doses of your medications or monitor you carefully for side effects.
- if you are taking sucralfate (Carafate), take it at least 30 minutes after lansoprazole.

- tell your doctor if you have or have ever had liver or kidney disease.
- tell your doctor if you are pregnant, plan to become pregnant, or are breast-feeding. If you become pregnant while taking lansoprazole, call your doctor.

What special dietary instructions should I follow?

Unless your doctor tells you otherwise, continue your normal diet.

What should I do if I forget to take a dose?

Take the missed dose as soon as you remember it. However, if it is almost time for the next dose, skip the missed dose and continue your dosing schedule. Do not take a double dose to make up for a missed one.

What side effects can this medicine cause?

Lansoprazole may cause side effects. Tell your doctor if either of these symptoms is severe or does not go away:
- stomach pain
- diarrhea

Lansoprazole may cause other side effects. Call your doctor if you have any unusual problems while taking this medication.

What storage conditions are needed for this medicine?

Keep this medication in the container it came in, tightly closed, and out of reach of children. Store it at room temperature and away from excess heat and moisture (not in the bathroom). Throw away any medication that is outdated or no longer needed. Talk to your pharmacist about the proper disposal of your medication.

What should I do in case of overdose?

In case of overdose, call your local poison control center at 1-800-222-1222. If the victim has collapsed or is not breathing, call local emergency services at 911.

What other information should I know?

Keep all appointments with your doctor.

Do not let anyone else take your medicine. Ask your pharmacist any questions you have about refilling your prescription.

Dosage Facts
For Informational Purposes

Caution: Do not change your dose, how often you take your medication, or the length of time you are to take it without first talking to your health-care provider.

The following dosage information was written using medical language for doctors and other healthcare professionals and is provided here for you to check your dosage. The dosage of this drug may differ for different patients. Therefore, always follow your doctor's instructions or the directions on the label. Contact your healthcare provider or pharmacist if you have any questions about the specific dosage of your medication after reviewing this information.

Pediatric Patients

Gastroesophageal Reflux

GERD

ORAL:
- Children 1–11 years of age: Children weighing ≤30 kg: 15 mg once daily for up to 12 weeks. Those weighing >30 kg: 30 mg once daily for up to 12 weeks. Dosage has been increased up to 30 mg twice daily after ≥2 weeks in patients remaining symptomatic.
- Children 12–17 years of age: 15 mg daily for up to 8 weeks.

Treatment of Erosive Esophagitis

ORAL:
- Children 1–11 years of age. Children weighing ≤30 kg: 15 mg once daily for up to 12 weeks. Those weighing >30 kg: 30 mg once daily for up to 12 weeks. Dosage has been increased up to 30 mg twice daily after ≥2 weeks in patients remaining symptomatic.
- Children 12–17 years of age: 30 mg daily for up to 8 weeks.

Adult Patients

Gastroesophageal Reflux

Chronic, lifelong therapy with proton-pump inhibitor is appropriate for many GERD patients.

GERD

ORAL:
- 15 mg once daily for up to 8 weeks.

Treatment of Erosive Esophagitis

ORAL:
- 30 mg once daily for up to 8 weeks. May give additional 8 weeks of therapy (up to 16 weeks for a single course) if not healed. If recurs, consider additional 8 weeks of therapy.

Maintenance of Healing of Erosive Esophagitis

ORAL:
- 15 mg once daily. Not studied >1 year.

Duodenal Ulcer

Treatment of Active Duodenal Ulcer

ORAL:
- 15 mg once daily for 4 weeks.

Treatment of Helicobacter pylori Infection and Duodenal Ulcer

ORAL:
- Triple therapy: 30 mg every 12 hours for 10 or 14 days in conjunction with amoxicillin and clarithromycin.
- Dual therapy: 30 mg every 8 hours for 14 days in conjunction with amoxicillin.

Maintenance of Duodenal Ulcer Healing

ORAL:
- 15 mg daily. Safety and efficacy beyond 1 year not established.

Gastric Ulcer

Benign Gastric Ulcer

ORAL:
- 30 mg once daily for up to 8 weeks.

NSAIA-induced Gastric Ulcer

Treatment

ORAL:
- 30 mg once daily for 8 weeks.

Risk Reduction

ORAL:
- 15 mg once daily for up to 12 weeks.

Pathologic GI Hypersecretory Conditions (e.g., Zollinger-Ellison Syndrome)

ORAL:
- 60 mg once daily initially. Adjust dosage according to patient response and tolerance; continue therapy as long as necessary. May require dosages of up to 90 mg twice daily. Administer daily dosages >120 mg in divided doses. Patients with Zollinger-Ellison syndrome have been treated for up to 4 years.

Special Populations

Hepatic Impairment
- Consider dosage reduction in patients with severe hepatic impairment.

Lansoprazole/ clarithromycin/ amoxicillin

(lan soe' pra zole) (kla rith' roe mye sin)
(a mox i sil' in)

Brand Name: Prevpac®

Why is this medicine prescribed?

Prevpac (lansoprazole, clarithromycin, and amoxicillin) is used to treat Helicobacter pylori infections associated with ulcers. Each daily administration pack contains a single day's dose of lansoprazole, clarithromycin, and amoxicillin.

How should this medicine be used?

Prevpac comes as an individual card containing a single day's dose of lansoprazole (two capsules), clarithromycin (two tablets), and amoxicillin (four capsules). You should take one lansoprazole capsule, one clarithromycin tablet, and two amoxicillin capsules twice a day. The individual dosing cards are supplied in boxes of 14 cards, which will give you a 2-week supply of medication. The tablets and capsules should be taken by mouth. All three medications can be taken at the same time. Follow the directions on your prescription label carefully, and ask your doctor or pharmacist to explain any part you do not understand. Take the medication in Prevpac exactly as directed. Do not take more or less of it or take it more often than prescribed by your doctor.

What special precautions should I follow?

Before taking Prevpac,

- tell your doctor and pharmacist if you are allergic to amoxicillin, azithromycin (Zithromax), clarithromycin (Biaxin), dirithromycin (Dynabac), erythromycin, lansoprazole (Prevacid), penicillin, or any other drugs.
- tell your doctor and pharmacist what prescription and nonprescription medications you are taking, especially allopurinol (Lopurin, Zyloprim), other antibiotics, anticoagulants ('blood thinners') such as warfarin (Coumadin), astemizole (Hismanal), carbamazepine (Tegretol), cisapride (Propulsid), cyclosporine (Neoral, Sandimmune), digoxin (Lanoxin, Lanoxicaps), dihydroergotamine (D.H.E. 45, Migranol), disopyramide (Norpace), ergotamine, felodipine (Plendil), fluconazole (Diflucan), ketoconazole (Nizoral), lovastatin (Mevacor), oral contraceptives, phenytoin (Dilantin), pimozide (Orap), probenecid (Benemid), sucralfate (Carafate), tacrolimus (Prograf), theophylline (Theo-Dur, Slo-Bid, Slo-Phyllin, others), triazolam (Halcion), zidovudine (Retrovir, AZT), and vitamins.
- tell your doctor if you have or have ever had asthma; irregular heartbeats; jaundice or yellowing of the skin or eyes; colitis; stomach problems; or liver or kidney disease.
- tell your doctor if you are pregnant, plan to become pregnant or are breast-feeding. If you become pregnant while taking the medications in Prevpac, call your doctor.
- if you are having surgery, including dental surgery, tell your doctor or dentist that you take Prevpac.

What special dietary instructions should I follow?

Clarithromycin and amoxicillin may cause an upset stomach. Take your medication doses with food or milk.

What should I do if I forget to take a dose?

Take the missed dose (one lansoprazole capsule, one clarithromycin tablet, and 2 amoxicillin capsules) as soon as you remember it. However, if it is almost time for the next dose, skip the missed dose and continue your regular dosing schedule. Do not take a double dose to make up for a missed one.

What side effects can this medicine cause?

The medications in Prevpac may cause side effects. Tell your doctor if any of these symptoms are severe or do not go away:

- diarrhea
- stomach pain or cramps
- vomiting
- upset stomach
- altered taste sensation
- headache
- dizziness or lightheadedness
- sour stomach

If you experience any of the following symptoms, call your doctor immediately:

- swelling of the face, eyes, lips, tongue, arms, or legs
- difficulty breathing or swallowing
- rash
- hives
- unusual bleeding or bruising
- yellowing of the eyes of skin
- dark urine
- pale stools
- unusual tiredness
- vaginal infection

If you experience a serious side effect, you or your doctor may send a report to the Food and Drug Administration's (FDA) MedWatch Adverse Event Reporting program online [at http://www.fda.gov/MedWatch/index.html] or by phone [1-800-332-1088].

What storage conditions are needed for this medicine?

Keep this medication in the daily packets and storage box they came in, tightly closed, and out of reach of children. Store it at room temperature and away from excess heat and moisture (not in the bathroom). Throw away any medication that is outdated or no longer needed. Talk to your pharmacist about the proper disposal of your medication.

What should I do in case of overdose?

In case of overdose, call your local poison control center at 1-800-222-1222. If the victim has collapsed or is not breathing, call local emergency services at 911.

What other information should I know?

Keep all appointments with your doctor and the laboratory. Do not let anyone else take your medication. Your prescription is probably not refillable. If you still have symptoms after you finish your prescription, call your doctor.

Talk to your doctor, pharmacist, or other healthcare professional if you have questions about dosing information for your medication.

Lanthanum

(lan' tha num)

Brand Name: Fosrenol®

Why is this medicine prescribed?

Lanthanum is used to reduce blood levels of phosphate in patients with kidney disease. High levels of phosphate in the blood can cause bone problems. Lanthanum is in a class of medications called phosphate binders. It works by preventing absorption of phosphate from food in the stomach.

How should this medicine be used?

Lanthanum comes as a chewable tablet to take by mouth. It is usually taken three times a day with or immediately after meals. Follow the directions on your prescription label carefully, and ask your doctor or pharmacist to explain any part you do not understand. Take lanthanum exactly as directed. Do not take more or less of it or take it more often than prescribed by your doctor.

Chew the tablets completely before swallowing; do not swallow the tablets whole.

Your doctor will probably start you on a low dose of lanthanum and gradually increase your dose, not more than once every 2 to 3 weeks.

Are there other uses for this medicine?

This medication may be prescribed for other uses; ask your doctor or pharmacist for more information.

What special precautions should I follow?

Before taking lanthanum,

- tell your doctor and pharmacist if you are allergic to lanthanum or any other medications.
- tell your doctor and pharmacist what prescription and nonprescription medications, vitamins, nutritional supplements, and herbal products you are taking.
- if you are taking cinoxacin (Cinobac) (no longer available in the US); ciprofloxacin (Cipro); dicumarol; digoxin (Lanoxin); enoxacin (Penetrex) (no longer available in the US); gatifloxacin (Tequin); indomethacin (Indocin); iron salts; isoniazid (INH, Nydrazid); ketoconazole (Nizoral); lomefloxacin (Maxaquin); moxifloxacin (Avelox); nalidixic acid (NegGram) (no longer available in the US); norfloxacin (Noroxin); ofloxacin (Floxin); salicylate pain relievers such as aspirin, choline magnesium trisalicylate (Tricosal, Trilisate), choline salicylate (Arthropan), diflunisal (Dolobid), magnesium salicylate (Doan's, others), and salsalate (Argesic, Disalcid, Salgesic); sparfloxacin (Zagam); tetracycline antibiotics such as demeclocycline (Declomycin), doxycycline (Doryx, Vibramycin), minocycline (Dynacin, Minocin), and tetracycline (Sumycin); or trovafloxacin and alatrofloxacin combination (Trovan) (no

longer available in the US), take them 2 hours before or after lanthanum.
- tell your doctor if you have or have ever had an ulcer, ulcerative colitis, Crohn's disease, or bowel obstruction.
- tell your doctor if you are pregnant, plan to become pregnant, or are breast-feeding. If you become pregnant while taking lanthanum, call your doctor.

What special dietary instructions should I follow?

Unless your doctor tells you otherwise, continue your normal diet.

What should I do if I forget to take a dose?

Take the missed dose as soon as you remember it. However, if it is almost time for the next dose, skip the missed dose and continue your regular dosing schedule. Do not take a double dose to make up for a missed one.

What side effects can this medicine cause?

Lanthanum may cause side effects. Tell your doctor if any of these symptoms are severe or do not go away:

- upset stomach
- vomiting
- stomach pain
- diarrhea
- constipation
- problems with the dialysis graft
- headache
- dizziness
- blurred vision

Lanthanum may cause other side effects. Call your doctor if you have any unusual problems while taking this medication.

What storage conditions are needed for this medicine?

Keep this medication in the container it came in, tightly closed, and out of reach of children. Store it at room temperature and away from excess heat and moisture (not in the bathroom). Throw away any medication that is outdated or no longer needed. Talk to your pharmacist about the proper disposal of your medication.

What should I do in case of overdose?

In case of overdose, call your local poison control center at 1-800-222-1222. If the victim has collapsed or is not breathing, call local emergency services at 911.

What other information should I know?

Keep all appointments with your doctor and the laboratory. Your doctor will order certain lab tests to check your body's response to lanthanum.

Do not let anyone else take your medication. Ask your

pharmacist any questions you have about refilling your prescription.

Dosage Facts
For Informational Purposes

Caution: Do not change your dose, how often you take your medication, or the length of time you are to take it without first talking to your healthcare provider.

The following dosage information was written using medical language for doctors and other healthcare professionals and is provided here for you to check your dosage. The dosage of this drug may differ for different patients. Therefore, always follow your doctor's instructions or the directions on the label. Contact your healthcare provider or pharmacist if you have any questions about the specific dosage of your medication after reviewing this information.

General Dosage Information

Available as lanthanum carbonate; dosage expressed in terms of lanthanum.

Adult Patients

Hyperphosphatemia
ESRD

ORAL:
- Initially, 750 mg–1.5 g daily.
- Adjust dosage at 2- to 3-week intervals until serum phosphorus concentration is acceptable; generally titrated in increments of 750 mg daily in clinical studies.
- Dosage of 1.5–3 g daily usually is required to reduce serum phosphorus concentrations to <6 mg/dL; dosages up to 3.75 g daily have been studied.
- Monitor serum phosphorus concentrations as needed during titration and regularly thereafter.

Latanoprost

(la ta′ noe prost)

Brand Name: Xalatan®

Why is this medicine prescribed?

Latanoprost is a topical eye medication used to reduce pressure inside the eye. It is used to treat eye conditions, including glaucoma and ocular hypertension, in which increased pressure can lead to a gradual loss of vision.

This medication is sometimes prescribed for other uses; ask your doctor or pharmacist for more information.

How should this medicine be used?

Latanoprost comes as eyedrops. Usually, one drop is applied to the affected eye(s) once a day in the evening. If latanoprost is used with other topical eye medications, allow at least 5 minutes between each medication. Follow the directions on your prescription label carefully, and ask your doctor or pharmacist to explain any part you do not understand. Use latanoprost exactly as directed. Do not use more or less of it or use it more often than prescribed by your doctor.

Latanoprost controls glaucoma but does not cure it. Continue to use latanoprost even if you feel well. Do not stop using latanoprost without talking to your doctor.

To apply the eyedrops, follow these steps:
1. Wash your hands thoroughly with soap and water.
2. Use a mirror or have someone else put the drops in your eye.
3. Make sure the end of the dropper is not chipped or cracked.
4. Avoid touching the dropper against your eye or anything else.
5. Hold the dropper tip down at all times to prevent drops from flowing back into the bottle and contaminating the remaining contents.
6. Lie down or tilt your head back.
7. Holding the bottle between your thumb and index finger, place the dropper as near as possible to your eyelid without touching it.
8. Brace the remaining fingers of that hand against your cheek or nose.
9. With the index finger of your other hand, pull the lower lid of the eye down to form a pocket.
10. Drop the prescribed number of drops into the pocket made by the lower lid and the eye. Placing the drops on the surface of the eyeball can cause stinging.
11. Close your eye and press lightly against the lower lid with your finger for 2-3 minutes to keep the medication in the eye. Do not blink.
12. Replace and tighten the cap right away. Do not wipe or rinse it off.
13. Wipe off any excess liquid from your cheek with a clean tissue. Wash your hands again.

If you still have symptoms of glaucoma (eye pain or blurred vision) after using this medication for a couple of days, call your doctor.

What special precautions should I follow?

Before using latanoprost,
- tell your doctor and pharmacist if you are allergic to latanoprost or any other drugs.
- tell your doctor and pharmacist what prescription and nonprescription medications you are taking, including vitamins.
- tell your doctor if you have inflammation of the eye, and if you have or have ever had liver or kidney disease.
- tell your doctor if you are pregnant, plan to become pregnant, or are breast-feeding. If you become pregnant while using latanoprost, call your doctor.
- if you are having surgery, including dental surgery, tell the doctor or dentist that you are using latanoprost.

What should I do if I forget to take a dose?

Apply the missed dose as soon as you remember it. However, if it is almost time for the next dose, skip the missed dose and continue your regular dosing schedule. Do not apply a double dose to make up for a missed one.

What side effects can this medicine cause?

Latanoprost may cause side effects. Tell your doctor if any of these symptoms are severe or do not go away:

- stinging, burning, itching, watering, or swelling of the eye
- redness of the eyelids
- irritation
- dry eyes

Latanoprost may increase the brown pigmentation in your iris, changing your eye color to brown. The pigmentation changes may be more noticeable in patients who already have some brown eye coloring. Latanoprost may also cause your eyelashes to grow longer and thicker and darken in color. These changes usually occurs slowly, but they may be permanent. If you use latanoprost in only one eye, you should know that there may be a difference between your eyes after taking latanoprost. Call your doctor if you notice these changes.

What storage conditions are needed for this medicine?

Keep this medication in the container it came in, tightly closed, and out of reach of children. Store it at room temperature and away from excess heat and moisture (not in the bathroom). Throw away any medication that is outdated or no longer needed. Talk to your pharmacist about the proper disposal of your medication.

What other information should I know?

Keep all appointments with your doctor. Your doctor will order certain eye tests to check your response to latanoprost.

Remove contact lenses before using latanoprost. You may replace the lenses 15 minutes after applying latanoprost.

Do not let anyone else take your medication. Ask your pharmacist any questions you have about refilling your prescription.

Dosage Facts
For Informational Purposes

Caution: Do not change your dose, how often you take your medication, or the length of time you are to take it without first talking to your healthcare provider.

The following dosage information was written using medical language for doctors and other healthcare professionals and is provided here for you to check your dosage. The dosage of this drug may differ for different patients. Therefore, always follow your doctor's instructions or the directions on the label. Contact your healthcare provider or pharmacist if you have any questions about the specific dosage of your medication after reviewing this information.

Adult Patients

Ocular Hypertension and Glaucoma

OPHTHALMIC:
- One drop of a 0.005% solution (1.5 mcg) in the affected eye(s) once daily in the evening. More frequent dosing may paradoxically diminish the IOP-lowering effect of the drug. If a dose is missed, omit the dose and apply the next dose the following evening.

Leflunomide

(le floo′ na mide)

Brand Name: Arava®
Also available generically.

Important Warning

Pregnant women and women of childbearing age who are not using a reliable method of birth control should not take leflunomide. Pregnancy must be avoided during treatment and for 2 years after treatment with leflunomide. If your period is late or you miss a period during treatment with leflunomide, call your doctor immediately. Talk to your doctor if you plan to become pregnant after stopping treatment with leflunomide. Your doctor can prescribe a treatment that will decrease the risk of harm to the fetus.

Why is this medicine prescribed?

Leflunomide is used to treat rheumatoid arthritis. Leflunomide decreases the symptoms of rheumatoid arthritis and slows damage to joints caused by the disease.

This medication is sometimes prescribed for other uses; ask your doctor or pharmacist for more information.

How should this medicine be used?

Leflunomide comes as a tablet to take by mouth. It is usually taken once a day. You will need to take a larger dose for the first 3 days of treatment. Follow the directions on your prescription label carefully, and ask your doctor or pharmacist to explain any part you do not understand. Take leflunomide exactly as directed. Do not take more or less of it or take it more often than prescribed by your doctor.

What special precautions should I follow?

Before taking leflunomide,

- tell your doctor and pharmacist if you are allergic to leflunomide or any other drugs.
- tell your doctor and pharmacist what prescription and nonprescription medications you are taking, especially cholestyramine (Cholybar, Questran), colestipol (Colestid), felbamate (Felbatol), mercaptopurine (Purinethol), rifampin (Rifadin, Rimactane, Rifater), methotrexate (Rheumatrex), tolbutamide (Orinase), troglitazone (Rezulin), and vitamins.
- tell your doctor if you have or have ever had liver or kidney disease, hepatitis, severe infections, or conditions affecting the bone marrow or the immune system (including human immunodeficiency virus [HIV] and acquired immunodeficiency syndrome [AIDS]).
- tell your doctor if you are breast-feeding.
- if you are planning to father a child, you should talk to your doctor about stopping leflunomide prior to conception.
- you should not receive any vaccinations while taking leflunomide unless you have talked with your doctor.
- you should know that there is a special treatment for removing leflunomide from your body once you stop taking it. Ask your doctor or pharmacist for more information about this treatment.

What should I do if I forget to take a dose?

Take the missed dose as soon as you remember it. However, if it is almost time for your next dose, skip the missed dose and continue your regular dosing schedule. Do not take a double dose to make up for a missed one.

What side effects can this medicine cause?

Leflunomide may cause side effects. Tell your doctor if any of these symptoms are severe or do not go away:

- diarrhea
- hair loss
- headache
- dizziness
- upset stomach
- vomiting
- stomach pain
- loss of appetite
- weight loss
- mouth sores
- runny nose
- back pain
- dry or itchy skin
- muscle pain or weakness
- flu-like symptoms
- urinary tract infection

If you experience any of the following symptoms, call your doctor immediately:

- rash
- difficulty breathing
- chest pain
- increased heart rate

If you experience a serious side effect, you or your doctor may send a report to the Food and Drug Administration's (FDA) MedWatch Adverse Event Reporting program online [at http://www.fda.gov/MedWatch/index.html] or by phone [1-800-332-1088].

What storage conditions are needed for this medicine?

Keep this medication in the container it came in, tightly closed, and out of reach of children. Store it at room temperature and away from excess heat and moisture (not in the bathroom). Throw away any medication that is outdated or no longer needed. Talk to your pharmacist about the proper disposal of your medication.

What should I do in case of overdose?

In case of overdose, call your local poison control center at 1-800-222-1222. If the victim has collapsed or is not breathing, call local emergency services at 911.

What other information should I know?

Keep all appointments with your doctor. Your doctor will order certain laboratory tests to monitor your response to leflunomide.

Do not let anyone else take your medication. Ask your pharmacist any questions you have about refilling your prescription.

Dosage Facts
For Informational Purposes

Caution: Do not change your dose, how often you take your medication, or the length of time you are to take it without first talking to your healthcare provider.

The following dosage information was written using medical language for doctors and other healthcare professionals and is provided here for you to check your dosage. The dosage of this drug may differ for different patients. Therefore, always follow your doctor's instructions or the directions on the label. Contact your healthcare provider or pharmacist if you have any questions about the specific dosage of your medication after reviewing this information.

Adult Patients

Rheumatoid Arthritis in Adults

ORAL:

- 100 mg once daily for 3 days, then 20 mg once daily. If this dosage is not tolerated, decrease to 10 mg once daily. Dosage adjustment or discontinuance may be required in patients who experience hepatotoxicity.
- Eliminating the 3-day loading dose may decrease the risk of

adverse effects. Elimination of loading dose may be especially important for patients at increased risk of hematologic or hepatic toxicity.

Solid Organ Transplantation
Renal or Hepatic Transplant Recipients†

ORAL:
- Initial loading dosage of 1.2–1.4 g (administered in divided doses over 5–7 days), then 10–120 mg daily.

Prescribing Limits

Adult Patients

Rheumatoid Arthritis in Adults

ORAL:
- Maintenance therapy: Maximum 20 mg daily. Dosages of 25 mg daily associated with higher incidence of alopecia, weight loss, and increases in serum liver enzyme concentrations.

Special Populations

Hepatic Impairment
- Not recommended in patients with substantial hepatic impairment or those who are seropositive for hepatitis B or C.

† Use is not currently included in the labeling approved by the US Food and Drug Administration.

Letrozole
(let′ roe zole)

Brand Name: Femara®

About Your Treatment

Your doctor has prescribed letrozole for you. Letrozole comes as a tablet to take by mouth.

This medication is used in women who have experienced menopause (change of life; end of monthly menstrual periods) to:
- treat breast cancer that has spread within the breast or to other areas of the body.
- treat early breast cancer in women who have already been treated with surgery, radiation and/or chemotherapy. Letrozole is sometimes used right after these treatments and sometimes after 5 years of treatment with a medication called tamoxifen (Nolvadex). Letrozole is used to stop any cancer cells that remain after these treatments from spreading.

Letrozole is in a class of medications known as nonsteroidal aromatase inhibitors. It decreases the amount of estrogen produced by the body. This can slow or stop the growth of some breast tumors that need estrogen to grow.

Letrozole is usually taken once a day, with or without food. Try to take letrozole at around the same time every day. Follow the directions on your prescription label carefully and ask your doctor or pharmacist to explain anything you do not understand. Take letrozole exactly as directed. Do not take more or less of it or take it more often than prescribed by your doctor.

You may need to take letrozole for several years or longer. Continue to take letrozole even if you feel well. Do not stop taking letrozole without talking to your doctor.

If you forget to take a dose of letrozole, take the missed dose as soon as you remember it. However, if it is almost time for your next dose, skip the missed dose and continue your regular dosing schedule. Do not take a double dose to make up for a missed dose and do not take more than one dose of letrozole in one day.

This medication may be prescribed for other uses. Ask your doctor or pharmacist for more information.

Precautions

Before taking letrozole,
- tell your doctor and pharmacist if you are allergic to letrozole, any other medications, or any of the inactive ingredients in letrozole tablets. Ask your doctor or pharmacist for a list of the inactive ingredients.
- tell your doctor or pharmacist what prescription and nonprescription medications, vitamins, nutritional supplements and herbal products you are taking or plan to take. Be sure to mention any of the following: other medications to treat cancer, medications that contain estrogen such as hormone replacement therapy and hormonal contraceptives (birth control pills, patches, rings, and injections), tamoxifen (Nolvadex), and raloxifene (Evista). Your doctor may need to change the doses of your medications or monitor you carefully for side effects.
- tell your doctor if you have or have ever had any medical condition, especially liver disease and osteoporosis (condition in which the bones are weak and break easily).
- you should know that letrozole should only be used by women who have experienced menopause and cannot become pregnant. However, if you are pregnant or breastfeeding, you should tell your doctor before you begin taking this medication. Use a reliable method of birth control to prevent pregnancy during your treatment. Letrozole may harm the fetus.
- you should know that letrozole may make you drowsy. Do not drive a car or operate machinery until you know how this medication affects you.

Side Effects

Letrozole may cause side effects. Tell your doctor if any of these symptoms are severe or do not go away:
- hot flushes
- night sweats
- nausea
- vomiting

- muscle, joint, or bone pain
- excessive tiredness
- headache
- dizziness
- muscle weakness
- swelling of the hands, feet, ankles, or lower legs
- loss of appetite
- constipation
- diarrhea
- stomach pain
- difficulty falling asleep or staying asleep
- vaginal bleeding or irritation
- breast pain
- flu-like symptoms
- difficulty urinating
- pain on urination
- cough
- rash

Some side effects can be serious. If you experience any of the following symptoms, call your doctor immediately:

- chest pain
- difficulty breathing

Letrozole may cause or worsen osteoporosis. Talk to your doctor about the risk of taking this medication and to find out what you can do to decrease this risk.

Letrozole may cause other side effects. Call your doctor if you have any unusual problems while you are taking this medication.

Storage Conditions

Keep letrozole in the container it came in, tightly closed, and out of reach of children. Store it at room temperature and away from excess heat and moisture (not in the bathroom). Throw away any medication that is outdated or no longer needed. Talk to your pharmacist about the proper disposal of your medication.

Overdose

In case of overdose, call your local poison control center at 1-800-222-1222. If the victim has collapsed or is not breathing, call local emergency services at 911.

Special Instructions

- Keep all appointments with your doctor.
- Do not let anyone else take your medication. Ask your pharmacist if you have any questions about refilling your prescription.

Dosage Facts
For Informational Purposes

Caution: Do not change your dose, how often you take your medication, or the length of time you are to take it without first talking to your healthcare provider.

The following dosage information was written using medical language for doctors and other healthcare professionals and is provided here for you to check your dosage. The dosage of this drug may differ for different patients. Therefore, always follow your doctor's instructions or the directions on the label. Contact your healthcare provider or pharmacist if you have any questions about the specific dosage of your medication after reviewing this information.

Adult Patients

Breast Cancer
Adjuvant Treatment of Early-stage Breast Cancer

ORAL:
- 2.5 mg once daily. Optimal duration unknown. Planned duration of treatment in clinical study was 5 years; median duration of treatment at time of analysis was 24 months; median duration of follow-up was 26 months. Discontinue if relapse occurs.

Extended Adjuvant Treatment of Early-stage Breast Cancer

ORAL:
- 2.5 mg once daily. Optimal duration unknown. Planned duration of treatment in clinical study was 5 years; median duration of treatment at time of analysis was 24 months; median duration of follow-up was 28 months. Discontinue if relapse occurs.

First-line Treatment of Locally Advanced or Metastatic Breast Cancer

ORAL:
- 2.5 mg once daily. Continue therapy until tumor progresses.

Second-line Treatment of Advanced Breast Cancer

ORAL:
- 2.5 mg once daily. Continue therapy until tumor progresses.

Special Populations

Hepatic Impairment
- Cirrhosis and severe hepatic impairment (Child-Pugh class C): Decrease dosage to 2.5 mg every other day.
- Mild to moderate hepatic impairment: No dosage adjustment recommended.

Renal Impairment
- $Cl_{cr} \geq 10$ mL/minute: No dosage adjustment necessary.

Geriatric Patients
- No dosage adjustment necessary.

Leucovorin Calcium

(loo koe vor′ in)

Brand Name: Wellcovorin®

About Your Treatment

Your doctor has ordered the drug leucovorin to help treat your illness. The drug is given by injection into a vein, intramuscularly (into a muscle), or taken by mouth.

This medication is used:

- to prevent or treat the toxicities of medications known as folic acid antagonists such as methotrexate (MTX, Rheumatrex), trimetrexate (Neutrexin), trimethoprim (Proloprim, Trimpex), trimethoprim/sulfamethoxazole (Bactrim, Septra), pyrimethamine (Daraprim), and pyrimethamine/sulfadoxine (Fansider).
- to treat folate-deficient megaloblastic anemias.
- in combination with fluorouracil (Adrucil, 5-FU) for the treatment of advanced colorectal cancer.

This medication is sometimes prescribed for other uses; ask your doctor or pharmacist for more information.

Leucovorin is a vitamin derivative. When used in combination with fluorouracil, it enhances the ability of the chemotherapy to slow or stop the growth of cancer cells in your body. In diseases where the amount of folate is low, it can replace the body's supply of the vitamin. Leucovorin also can prevent or treat the toxicities associated with a group of drugs known as folate antagonists. The length of treatment depends on the types of drugs you are taking, how well your body responds to them, and the type of disease you have.

Leucovorin in combination with fluorouracil is also used to treat other types of gastrointestinal cancers. Talk to your doctor about the possible risks of using this drug for your condition.

Precautions

Before taking leucovorin,

- tell your doctor and pharmacist if you are allergic to leucovorin or any other drugs.
- tell your doctor and pharmacist what prescription and nonprescription medications you are taking, including vitamins.
- women who are pregnant or breast-feeding should tell their doctors before they begin taking this drug. You should not plan to have children while receiving chemotherapy or for a while after treatments. (Talk to your doctor for further details.) Use a reliable method of birth control to prevent pregnancy.

Side Effects

If you experience any of the following symptoms, call your doctor immediately:

- shortness of breath
- rash
- itching

If you experience a serious side effect, you or your doctor may send a report to the Food and Drug Administration's (FDA) MedWatch Adverse Event Reporting program online [at http://www.fda.gov/MedWatch/index.html] or by phone [1-800-332-1088].

Storage Conditions

Keep leucovorin in the container it came in, tightly closed, and out of reach of children. Store it at room temperature and away from excess heat and moisture (not in the bathroom). Throw away any medication that is outdated or no longer needed. Talk to your pharmacist about the proper disposal of your medication.

Overdose

In case of overdose, call your local poison control center at 1-800-222-1222. If the victim has collapsed or is not breathing, call local emergency services at 911.

Special Instructions

- Follow the directions on your prescription label carefully, and ask your doctor or pharmacist to explain any part you do not understand. Take leucovorin exactly as directed. Do not take more or less of it or take it more often than prescribed by your doctor. Continue to take leucovorin even if you feel well. Do not stop taking leucovorin without talking to your doctor.

Dosage Facts
For Informational Purposes

Caution: Do not change your dose, how often you take your medication, or the length of time you are to take it without first talking to your healthcare provider.

The following dosage information was written using medical language for doctors and other healthcare professionals and is provided here for you to check your dosage. The dosage of this drug may differ for different patients. Therefore, always follow your doctor's instructions or the directions on the label. Contact your healthcare provider or pharmacist if you have any questions about the specific dosage of your medication after reviewing this information.

General Dosage Information

Available as leucovorin calcium; dosage expressed in terms of leucovorin.

Pediatric Patients

Toxicity Associated with Folic Acid Antagonists
Prevention of Pyrimethamine Toxicity†

ORAL:
- For pyrimethamine dosages of 25–100 mg daily or 1–2 mg/

kg daily (for treatment of toxoplasmosis): 10–25 mg administered with each pyrimethamine dose.

- For pyrimethamine dosages of 25–50 mg once daily (given with clindamycin or sulfadiazine for secondary prophylaxis of toxoplasmosis in adolescents): 10–25 mg once daily.
- For pyrimethamine dosage of 1 mg/kg once daily (given with dapsone or clindamycin for primary or secondary prophylaxis of toxoplasmosis, respectively, in HIV-infected children): 5 mg once every 3 days.
- For pyrimethamine dosage of 25 mg once daily (given with atovaquone for primary or secondary prophylaxis against toxoplasmosis in HIV-infected adolescents): 10 mg daily, administered concomitantly with pyrimethamine.
- For pyrimethamine dosage of 50 or 75 mg once weekly (given with dapsone for primary prevention of *Pneumocystis jiroveci* [formerly *Pneumocystis carinii*] pneumonia or toxoplasmosis or for secondary prophylaxis of *P. jiroveci* pneumonia in HIV-infected adolescents): 25 mg once weekly, administered concomitantly with pyrimethamine.

Adult Patients

Toxicity Associated with Folic Acid Antagonists

Methotrexate Overdosage

ORAL, IV, OR IM:

- 15 mg (approximately 10 mg/m^2) every 6 hours until serum methotrexate concentration declines to <0.005 mcg/mL (0.01 μM); initiate administration as soon as possible after overdosage and within 24 hours following methotrexate administration if delayed elimination is detected.
- If 24-hour S_{cr} increases 50% over baseline, 24-hour methotrexate concentration is >2.27 mcg/mL (5 μM, or 48-hour methotrexate concentration is >0.409 mcg/mL (0.9 μM), increase dosage immediately to 150 mg (approximately 100 mg/m^2) IV every 3 hours until serum methotrexate concentration declines to <0.005 mcg/mL (0.01 μM).

Pyrimethamine or Trimethoprim Overdosage

ORAL:

- 5–15 mg daily is recommended by some clinicians.

Rescue after High-dose Methotrexate Therapy

ORAL, IV, OR IM:

- 15 mg (approximately 10 mg/m^2) every 6 hours for 10 doses, starting at 24 hours after initiation of methotrexate (12–15 g/m^2) infusion for patients with normal methotrexate elimination (i.e., serum methotrexate concentration approximately 4.54 mcg/mL [10 μM] at 24 hours after administration, 0.454 mcg/mL [1 μM] at 48 hours, and <0.091 mcg/mL [0.2 μM] at 72 hours).
- Continue therapy and maintain adequate hydration and urinary alkalization (pH $\geq$7) until methotrexate concentration declines to <0.023 mcg/mL (0.05 μM).
- If substantial clinical toxicity occurs in patients with mild abnormalities in methotrexate elimination or renal function, extend rescue therapy for an additional 24 hours (i.e., 14 doses over 84 hours) for subsequent methotrexate courses.
- Monitor S_{cr} and methotrexate concentration at least once daily. Adjust dosage and duration of therapy based on methotrexate elimination pattern and patient's renal function.

Table 1. Guidelines for Leucovorin Dosage Adjustment in Patients with Delayed Late Methotrexate Elimination

Serum Methotrexate Concentration	Leucovorin Dosage Adjustment
>0.091 mcg/mL (0.2 μM) at 72 hours and >0.023 mcg/mL (0.05 μM) at 96 hours following methotrexate administration	Continue leucovorin 15 mg every 6 hours until methotrexate concentration declines to <0.023 mcg/mL (0.05 μM)

Table 2. Guidelines for Leucovorin Dosage Adjustment in Patients with Delayed Early Methotrexate Elimination and/or Evidence of Acute Renal Injury

Serum Methotrexate and/or S_{cr} Concentration	Leucovorin Dosage Adjustment and Monitoring
$\geq$22.7 mcg/mL (50 μM) at 24 hours or $\geq$2.27 mcg/mL (5 μM) at 48 hours after methotrexate administration and/or $\geq$100% increase in S_{cr} at 24 hours after administration	Leucovorin 150 mg IV every 3 hours until methotrexate concentration declines to <0.454 mcg/mL (1 μM), then leucovorin 15 mg IV every 3 hours until methotrexate concentration declines to <0.023 mcg/mL (0.05 μM)
	If nonoliguric renal failure develops, monitor fluid and electrolyte status until methotrexate concentration declines to 0.023 mcg/mL (0.05 μM) and renal failure has resolved

Prevention of Pyrimethamine Toxicity†

ORAL:

- For pyrimethamine dosages of 25–100 mg daily or 1–2 mg/kg daily (for treatment of toxoplasmosis): 10–25 mg administered with each pyrimethamine dose.
- For pyrimethamine dosages of 25–50 mg once daily (given with clindamycin or sulfadiazine for secondary prophylaxis of toxoplasmosis): 10–25 mg once daily.
- For pyrimethamine dosage of 25 mg once daily (given with atovaquone for primary or secondary prophylaxis of toxoplasmosis in HIV-infected individuals): 10 mg daily, administered concomitantly with pyrimethamine.
- For pyrimethamine dosage of 50 or 75 mg once weekly (given with dapsone for primary prevention of *P. jiroveci* pneumonia or toxoplasmosis or for secondary prophylaxis of *P. jiroveci* pneumonia in HIV-infected individuals): 25 mg once weekly, administered concomitantly with pyrimethamine.

Prevention of Trimetrexate Toxicity†

ORAL OR IV:

- For trimetrexate dose of 45 mg/m^2: 20 mg/m^2 every 6 hours (total daily dose: 80 mg/m^2).
- Alternatively, dose may be based on body weight.

Table 3. Leucovorin Dosage Based on Body Weight

Body Weight (kg)	Trimetrexate Dosage (mg/kg/day)	Leucovorin Dosage (mg/kg Every 6 Hours)
<50	1.5	0.6
50–80	1.2	0.5
>80	1.0	0.5

Round calculated oral dose up to the next 25-mg increment. Continue leucovorin therapy for at least 72 hours after last trimetrexate dose (usual duration: 24 days).

Adjust dosage if hematologic toxicities occur, based on the worst of the two blood cell counts.

Table 4. Dosage Adjustments for Hematologic Toxicities[a]

Toxicity Grade	ANC (cells/mm^3)	Platelets (cells/mm^3)	Dosage Adjustments
1	>1000	>75,000	No adjustment in trimetrexate or leucovorin dosages
2	750–1000	50,000–75,000	No adjustment in trimetrexate dosage; increase leucovorin to 40 mg/m^2 every 6 hours
3	500–749	25,000–49,999	Decrease trimetrexate dose to 22 mg/m^2 once daily; increase leucovorin to 40 mg/m^2 every 6 hours
4	<500	<25,000	Day 1–9: Discontinue trimetrexate; increase leucovorin to 40 mg/m^2 every 6 hours for an additional 72 hours Day 10–21: Discontinue trimetrexate; increase leucovorin to 40 mg/m^2 every 6 hours for an additional 72 hours. If hematologic toxicity improves within 96 hours to grade 3 or grade 2, reinitiate trimetrexate at 22 mg/m^2 or 45 mg/m^2, respectively, once daily; continue leucovorin for 72 hours after the last trimetrexate dose

[a]Adjust dosage based on the worse of the two blood counts

Megaloblastic Anemia

IM:
- Up to 1 mg daily; no evidence that doses >1 mg daily are more effective.
- Duration of therapy depends on hematologic response. In general, improved sense of well-being occurs within first 24 hours; bone marrow begins to become normoblastic within 48 hours; and reticulocytosis begins within 2–5 days after initiation of therapy.

Colorectal Cancer

IV:
- Leucovorin 20 mg/m^2 followed by IV fluorouracil (425 mg/m^2) daily for 5 days or leucovorin 200 mg/m^2 by slow IV injection (over a minimum of 3 minutes) followed by IV fluorouracil (370 mg/m^2) daily for 5 days; no evidence of superiority of either regimen.
- Repeat either regimen at 4-week intervals for 2 additional courses, then at 4- to 5-week intervals provided toxicity from the previous course has subsided.
- Do not administer repeat courses until WBC >4000/mm^3 and platelet count >130,000/mm^3. If blood counts do not return to these levels within 2 weeks, discontinue therapy. Discontinue therapy when there is clear evidence of tumor progression.
- If WBC and platelet count return to >4000/mm^3 and >130,000/mm^3, respectively, within 2 weeks, adjust subsequent fluorouracil dosages based on severity of GI toxicity and nadir blood counts from previous course; leucovorin dosage generally not adjusted according to toxicity. If no toxicity occurred in the prior course, increase subsequent fluorouracil dosage by 10%.

Table 5. Fluorouracil Dosage Adjustments for Hematologic or GI Toxicities[a]

Toxicity after Prior Dose	Fluorouracil Daily Dosage for Subsequent Course
If moderate diarrhea and/or stomatitis or WBC nadir of 1000–1900/mm^3 or Platelet nadir of 25,000–75,000/mm^3 occurs	Reduce dosage by 20%
If severe diarrhea and/or stomatitis or WBC nadir of <1000/mm^3 or Platelet nadir of <25,000/mm^3 occurs	Reduce dosage by 30%

[a]Adjust dosage based on the most severe toxicity.

Prescribing Limits

Pediatric Patients

ORAL:
- Administration of doses >25 mg not recommended.

Adult Patients

ORAL:
- Administration of doses >25 mg not recommended.

Special Populations

Patients with Delayed Methotrexate Elimination
- Higher dosages and extended duration of therapy may be required if delayed methotrexate excretion is caused by third space fluid accumulation (i.e., ascites, pleural effusion), renal impairment, or inadequate hydration.

† *Use is not currently included in the labeling approved by the US Food and Drug Administration.*

Leuprolide

(loo proe′ lide)

Brand Name: Eligard®, Lupron®, Lupron Depot®, Lupron Depot®-3 Month, Lupron Depot®-4 Month, Lupron Depot-PED®, Viadur®
Also available generically.

About Your Treatment

Your doctor has ordered the drug leuprolide to help treat your illness. Leuprolide comes as a solution (Lupron) that is injected subcutaneously (just under the skin) and is usually given once daily. Leuprolide also comes as a long-acting suspension (Eligard) that is injected subcutaneously and is usually given every 1, 3, 4, or 6 months. This medication also comes as a long-acting suspension that is injected intramuscularly (into a muscle) and is usually given once a month (Lupron Depot, Lupron Depot-PED) or every few months (Lupron Depot-3 month, Lupron Depot-4 month). Leuprolide is also available as an implant (a small, thin metal tube containing medication) (Viadur) that is inserted under the skin and is usually given once a year.

Leuprolide is used to treat:
- symptoms of advanced prostate cancer in men
- endometriosis (condition in which cells normally found in the uterus become implanted in other areas of the body) in women
- uterine fibroids (noncancerous growths in the uterus) in women
- central precocious puberty (a condition causing children to enter puberty too soon, resulting in accelerated bone growth and the development of sexual characteristics) in girls usually younger than 8 years of age and in boys usually younger than 9 years of age

If you receive leuprolide long-acting suspension (Eligard) as a subcutaneous injection, you may notice a small bump when you first receive an injection. This bump should eventually go away.

If you receive leuprolide as an implant under the skin, keep the area where the implant was inserted clean and dry for 24 hours. Do not swim or bathe during this time. Cover the area with a bandage for a few days until the wound heals. Avoid heavy lifting and physical activity for 48 hours after receiving the implant and avoid bumping the area around the implant for a few days.

Leuprolide prescribed for children with precocious puberty will likely be discontinued by your child's doctor before age 11 for girls and age 12 for boys.

Leuprolide is in a class of drugs known as gonadotropin-releasing (GnRH or LH-RH) hormone agonists. It decreases the production of testosterone (male hormone) in men and estrogen (female hormone) in women. Decreasing the production of these hormones is desirable because they stimulate the growth of the diseased cells involved in prostate cancer and endometriosis, and they stimulate the development of sexual characteristics in children with early puberty.

Your doctor will tell you how long your treatment with leuprolide will last. When used to treat advanced prostate cancer, leuprolide controls the symptoms of prostate cancer but does not cure it. Continue to use leuprolide even if you feel well. Do not stop using leuprolide without talking to your doctor.

If your doctor has told you or your caregiver to give a subcutaneous injection of leuprolide, follow these steps:
1. Wash your hands well with soap and water.
2. Look at the liquid in the container. If the liquid is cloudy or contains particles, do not use it and call your pharmacist.
3. If using a new container of leuprolide, flip off the plastic cover to expose the gray rubber stopper. Wipe the metal ring and rubber stopper on the container with an alcohol wipe, just before each use.
4. Remove the outer wrapping from a new syringe. Pull the plunger back until the tip of the plunger is at the right mark for your dose. If you do not know the right mark for your dose, call your doctor or pharmacist.
5. Carefully pull the cover off the needle. Do not touch the needle. Place the container on a clean, flat surface and push the needle through the center of the rubber stopper of the container.
6. Push the plunger all the way down to inject air into the container.
7. Keep the needle in the container while turning the container straight upside down. Check to make sure the tip of the needle is in the liquid.
8. Slowly pull back on the syringe plunger until the syringe fills with liquid to the right mark for your dose.
9. While keeping the needle in the container and the container upside down, check for air bubbles in the syringe. If you see any, push the plunger in slowly to push the air bubbles out of the syringe. Keep the tip of the needle in the liquid and pull the plunger back again to fill the syringe to the mark for your dose.
10. Remove the needle from the container and lay the sy-

ringe down on a clean, flat surface without touching the needle or touching it to any surface. Carefully recap the syringe if it will be left for a period of time.

11. Choose an injection spot and clean it with a new alcohol wipe. Use a different injection spot each day.

12. Hold the syringe in one hand and pull up skin at the injection spot with the other hand.

13. While holding the syringe like a pencil, quickly insert the needle all the way into the skin at a 90 degree angle.

14. Push the plunger in to inject the complete dose of leuprolide.

15. Pull the needle out from the skin at the same angle it was inserted. Dab an alcohol wipe on the skin at the injection spot.

16. Throw the syringe and needle away in a puncture-resistant container out of the reach of children. Talk to your doctor or pharmacist about the proper way to throw away syringes and needles.

17. Do not try to get every last drop of medication out of the leuprolide container. There is extra medication in the container so that you can withdraw the recommended number of doses without drawing air into the syringe.

18. Ask your pharmacist or doctor for a copy of the manufacturer's information for the patient.

This medication is sometimes prescribed for other uses; ask your doctor or pharmacist for more information.

Precautions

Before taking leuprolide,

- tell your doctor and pharmacist if you are allergic to leuprolide; any of the ingredients in leuprolide injection or implant; other gonadotropin-releasing hormones including gonadorelin hydrochloride (Factrel), goserelin (Zoladex), or nafarelin (Synarel); any other medications; or benzyl alcohol. Ask your doctor or pharmacist if you are not sure if a medication you are allergic to is a gonadotropin-releasing hormone. Ask your pharmacist for a list of ingredients in leuprolide injection and leuprolide implant.

- tell your doctor and pharmacist what prescription and nonprescription medications, nutritional supplements, and herbal products you are taking or plan to take. Be sure to mention aluminum-containing antacids; cancer chemotherapy corticosteroids such as dexamethasone (Decadron, Dexone), methylprednisolone (Medrol), and prednisone (Deltasone); cyclosporine (Neoral, Restasis, Sandimmune); diuretics ('water pills'); heparin; lanthanum carbonate (Fosrenol); lithium; medications to control seizures; medications for thyroid disease; phenothiazines; sevelamer (Renagel); or tetracycline.

- tell your doctor if you have a history of drinking alcohol or using tobacco products for a long period of time; or if you have or have ever had anorexia nervosa (an eating disorder), cancer of the spine (backbone), Cushing's disease (condition where adrenal gland produces excess cortisol), diabetes, high cholesterol or lipids (fats in the blood), malabsorption disease (difficulty absorbing nutrients from food), osteoporosis (condition where bones are thin and more likely to break), rheumatoid arthritis, abnormal vaginal bleeding which has not been evaluated or diagnosed by a doctor, urinary obstruction in men (blockage that causes difficulty urinating), or heart, kidney, liver, parathyroid, or thyroid disease.

- you should know that leuprolide may interfere with the normal menstrual cycle (period) in women who have not been through menopause. However, if leuprolide causes amenorrhea (stopping of the menstrual cycle) while you are using it, you should not assume that you cannot get pregnant. Leuprolide should not be used by women who are pregnant or who may become pregnant. Use a reliable method of birth control to prevent pregnancy while using leuprolide. Ask your doctor what type of birth control is best for you. If you become pregnant while using leuprolide, call your doctor immediately. Leuprolide may harm the fetus. Leuprolide should not be used in women who are breast-feeding.

- you should know that medication may decrease sperm production in men. However, you should not assume that you cannot get a woman pregnant while using leuprolide.

Side Effects

Leuprolide may cause side effects. Tell your doctor if any of these symptoms are severe or do not go away:

- weakness
- headache
- dizziness
- hot flashes (a sudden wave of mild or intense body heat)
- sweating or night sweats
- tiredness
- nausea
- vomiting
- diarrhea
- constipation
- loss of appetite
- change in weight
- increased need to urinate, especially at night
- breast tenderness or change in breast size in both men and women
- decrease in sexual desire in men and women or ability to perform in men
- decrease in size of testicles
- vaginal discharge, dryness, or itching in women
- absence of menstrual periods in women
- spotting (light vaginal bleeding)
- swelling of the hands, feet, ankles, or lower legs
- depression
- difficulty concentrating
- anxiety or nervousness
- difficulty with memory
- difficulty falling asleep or staying asleep
- flu-like symptoms
- muscle aches

- itching, swelling, burning, stinging, pain, bruising, redness, or development of a sore at injection spot
- firmness or hardness at subcutaneous injection spot
- bleeding, bruising, burning, pain, pressure, itching, swelling, or redness at the place where the implant was inserted
- hair loss
- acne

Some side effects can be serious. If you experience any of the following symptoms, call your doctor immediately:

- hives
- rash
- itching
- difficulty breathing or swallowing
- numbness, tingling, weakness, or pain in the feet or lower legs
- painful or difficult urination
- blood in urine
- bone pain
- testicular or prostate pain
- inability to move arms or legs

There is an increased risk of osteoporosis (condition in which the bones become weak and fragile and can break easily) while using leuprolide. Talk with your doctor about the risks of using leuprolide.

In children receiving leuprolide for early puberty, signs of sexual development may not decrease or may increase during the first few weeks of treatment. In girls receiving leuprolide for early puberty, the onset of menstruation or spotting (light vaginal bleeding) may occur during the first two months of treatment. If bleeding continues beyond the second month, call your doctor.

Leuprolide may cause other side effects. Call your doctor if you have any unusual problems while using this medication.

If you experience a serious side effect, you or your doctor may send a report to the Food and Drug Administration's (FDA) MedWatch Adverse Event Reporting program online [at http://www.fda.gov/MedWatch/index.html] or by phone [1-800-332-1088].

Storage Conditions

If you are receiving leuprolide injections at home, keep leuprolide in the carton it came in and out of reach of children. Keep syringes and needles out of reach of children. Store leuprolide at room temperature and away from light, excess heat (such as a radiator) and moisture (not in the bathroom). Do not allow leuprolide to freeze. Throw away any medication that is outdated or no longer needed. Talk to your pharmacist about the proper disposal of your medication.

Overdose

In case of overdose, call your local poison control center at 1-800-222-1222. If the victim has collapsed or is not breathing, call local emergency services at 911.

Special Instructions

- Keep all appointments with your doctor and the laboratory. Your doctor will order certain lab tests to check your body's response to leuprolide.
- Before having any laboratory tests, tell your doctor and the laboratory personnel that you are using leuprolide.
- If you are receiving your leuprolide injections at home, do not run out of leuprolide. Tell your pharmacist when you will need more leuprolide so that it will be at the pharmacy when you need it.
- If you have a leuprolide implant and your doctor prescribes an X-ray or MRI, the implant will not be affected but will be seen on the films. Before having an X-ray or MRI, tell the medical personnel that you have a leuprolide implant.

Dosage Facts
For Informational Purposes

Caution: Do not change your dose, how often you take your medication, or the length of time you are to take it without first talking to your healthcare provider.

The following dosage information was written using medical language for doctors and other healthcare professionals and is provided here for you to check your dosage. The dosage of this drug may differ for different patients. Therefore, always follow your doctor's instructions or the directions on the label. Contact your healthcare provider or pharmacist if you have any questions about the specific dosage of your medication after reviewing this information.

General Dosage Information

Available as leuprolide acetate; dosage of injection and suspension expressed in terms of the salt, and dosage of implant expressed in terms of leuprolide.

Pediatric Patients

Central Precocious Puberty

Individualize dosage according to actual body weight; younger children (i.e., children weighing <25 kg) generally appear to require higher dosages on a mg/kg basis than older children (i.e., children weighing ≥25 kg).

Confirm inhibition of gonadotropin secretion and suppression of ovarian or testicular steroidogenesis after 1–2 months of initial therapy or when changing dosage by evaluation of GnRH stimulation test, Tanner staging, and sex steroid concentrations.

Prior to initiation of therapy, perform baseline evaluations.

In most children, the first dosage found to adequately inhibit gonadotropin secretion and suppress ovarian or testicular steroidogenesis can be maintained for the duration of therapy.

Data currently are insufficient for specific dosage recommendations in children in whom therapy was initiated at a low dosage and at a very young age and whose weight has changed such that the patient would be in a different weight range/dose category. The manufacturer recommends that inhibition of gonadotropin secretion and suppression of ovarian or testicular steroidogenesis be monitored closely in children whose weight has increased considerably while receiving therapy.

IM:
- Leuprolide acetate suspension (Lupron Depot-Ped®): Initially, 0.3-mg/kg (minimum 7.5 mg) every 4 weeks in girls <8 years of age or boys <9 years of age.

Initial Dosage for Children (Girls <8 Years of Age or Boys <9 Years of Age)

Weight	Dosage of leuprolide acetate suspension (Lupron Depot-Ped®)
≤25 kg	7.5 mg every 4 weeks
25–37.5 kg	11.25 mg every 4 weeks
>37.5 kg	15 mg every 4 weeks

Titrate dose upward in increments of 3.75 mg every 4 weeks until clinical or laboratory tests indicate no disease progression.

Therapy usually is continued until fusion of the epiphyses or attainment of appropriate chronologic pubertal age (e.g., consideration made at 11 and 12 years of age in girls and boys, respectively).

SUB-Q:
- Leuprolide acetate injection (Lupron® for Pediatric Use): Initially 50 mcg/kg once daily for girls <8 years of age or boys <9 years of age. If total suppression of ovarian or testicular steroidogenesis is not achieved, titrate dosage upward by 10 mcg/kg daily to establish maintenance dosage.

Adult Patients

Advanced Prostate Cancer
Daily Therapy with Leuprolide Acetate Injection

SUB-Q:
- Usually, 1 mg daily.
- Dosages up to 20 mg daily have been used by some clinicians; however, dosages >1 mg daily have not resulted in a greater incidence of remission.
- For patients at risk of serious adverse affects, consider initiating therapy with daily administration of leuprolide acetate injection for 2 weeks prior to IM administration of leuprolide acetate suspension (Lupron Depot®) to permit discontinuance of therapy if warranted.

Therapy with Extended-release Suspension

IM:
- 7.5 mg once monthly as the monthly formulation (Lupron Depot®), or 22.5 mg every 3 months (84 days) as the 3-month formulation (Lupron Depot®-3 month 22.5 mg), or 30 mg once every 4 months (16 weeks) as the 4-month formulation (Lupron Depot®-4 month 30 mg).
- If a monthly dose is missed, a delay of ≤12 days may or may not compromise the patient's treatment; however, if a monthly dose is missed by ≥2 weeks, serum testosterone concentrations will increase substantially.

SUB-Q:
- Eligard®: 7.5 mg once monthly as the monthly formulation, or 22.5 mg once every 3 months as the 3-month formulation,

or 30 mg once every 4 months as the 4-month formulation, or 45 mg once every 6 months as the 6-month formulation.

Therapy with Leuprolide Acetate (Viadur®) Implant

SUB-Q:
- One 65-mg implant every 12 months.
- One implant delivers 120 mcg of leuprolide acetate daily for 12 months.
- Remove implant 12 months after insertion. At time of implant removal, may insert another implant to continue therapy.

Endometriosis
Initial Treatment

IM:
- 3.75 mg once monthly as the monthly formulation (Lupron Depot®) for 6 consecutive months or 11.25 mg every 3 months as the 3-month formulation (Lupron Depot®-3 month 11.25 mg) for a total of 6 months. Administer with or without norethindrone acetate (5 mg daily).

Retreatment If Symptoms Recur after Initial Treatment

Retreatment with additional courses of leuprolide alone is *not* recommended; if retreatment is considered, administer a *single* 6-month course of leuprolide acetate suspension in conjunction with norethindrone acetate.

Assess BMD prior to therapy to ensure that values are within normal limits.

IM:
- 3.75 mg once monthly as the monthly formulation (Lupron Depot®) for a total of 6 months or 11.25 mg every 3 months as the 3-month formulation (Lupron Depot®-3 month 11.25 mg) for a total of 6 months. Administer in conjunction with oral norethindrone acetate (5 mg daily).
- Additional courses of treatment after a single 6-month retreatment course are not recommended.

Uterine Leiomyomata

IM:
- 3.75 mg once monthly as the monthly formulation (Lupron Depot®) for up to 3 consecutive months in conjunction with iron therapy.
- 11.25 mg of the 3-month formulation (Lupron Depot®-3 month 11.25 mg) as a single injection in conjunction with iron therapy. Use of the 3-month formulation recommended *only* when 3 months of hormonal suppression is necessary.
- If additional therapy is considered, assess BMD prior to therapy to ensure that values are within normal limits.

Prescribing Limits

Adult Patients

Endometriosis
Initial Treatment

IM:
- Limit initial course of therapy to 6 months.

Retreatment If Symptoms Recur after Initial Treatment

IM:
- Limit retreatment of symptom recurrence to 6 months.
- Additional courses of treatment after a single 6-month retreatment course are not recommended.

Uterine Leiomyomata

IM:

- Lupron Depot® 3.75 mg monthly formulation: Maximum 3 consecutive months of therapy recommended.
- Lupron Depot® 11.25 mg (3-month formulation): A single injection of 11.25 mg recommended.
- Safety and efficacy of >6 months of therapy not evaluated.

Levalbuterol Oral Inhalation

(lev al byoo′ ter ol)

Brand Name: Xopenex®

Why is this medicine prescribed?

Levalbuterol is used to prevent or relieve the wheezing, shortness of breath, and difficulty breathing caused by asthma. Levalbuterol is in a class of medications called beta agonists. It works by relaxing and opening air passages, making it easier to breathe.

How should this medicine be used?

Levalbuterol comes as a solution to inhale using a nebulizer. It is usually used three times a day. Follow the directions on your prescription label carefully, and ask your doctor or pharmacist to explain any part you do not understand. Use levalbuterol exactly as directed. Do not use more or less of it or use it more often than prescribed by your doctor.

Levalbuterol controls asthma but does not cure it. Continue to use levalbuterol even if you feel well. Do not stop using levalbuterol without talking to your doctor.

To use the solution for oral inhalation, follow these steps:

1. Tear the serrated edge on the foil pouch to open and remove one vial. Look at the solution in the vial to be sure it is colorless. If it is not colorless, call your doctor or pharmacist and do not use the solution.
2. Twist off the top of the vial and squeeze all of the liquid into the reservoir of your nebulizer. Do not add any other medications to the nebulizer because it may not be safe to mix them with levalbuterol. Use all nebulized medications separately unless your doctor specifically tells you to mix them.
3. Connect the nebulizer reservoir to your mouthpiece or facemask.
4. Connect the nebulizer to the compressor.
5. Sit upright and place the mouthpiece in your mouth or put on the facemask.
6. Turn on the compressor.
7. Breathe calmly, deeply, and evenly until mist stops forming in the nebulizer. This should take between 5 and 15 minutes.
8. Clean the nebulizer according to the manufacturer's instructions.

Are there other uses for this medicine?

This medication may be prescribed for other uses; ask your doctor or pharmacist for more information.

What special precautions should I follow?

Before using levalbuterol,

- tell your doctor and pharmacist if you are allergic to levalbuterol, albuterol (Proventil, Ventolin, others), or any other medications.
- tell your doctor and pharmacist what other prescription and nonprescription medications, vitamins, nutritional supplements, and herbal products you are taking. Be sure to mention any of the following: beta blockers such as atenolol (Tenormin), labetalol (Normodyne), metoprolol (Lopressor, Toprol XL), nadolol (Corgard), and propranolol (Inderal); digoxin (Digitek, Lanoxin); diuretics ('water pills') such as bumetanide (Bumex), chlorthalidone (Thalitone), ethacrynic acid (Edecrin), furosemide (Lasix), and hydrochlorthiazide (Hydro-DIURIL, Microzide); epinephrine (Epipen, Primatene Mist); medications for colds; and other inhaled medications for asthma such as metaproterenol (Alupent) and pirbuterol (Maxair). Also tell your doctor or pharmacist if you are taking the following medications or have stopped taking them within the past two weeks: antidepressants (mood elevators) such as amitriptyline (Elavil), amoxapine (Asendin), clomipramine (Anafranil), desipramine (Norpramin), doxepin (Asapin, Sinequan), imipramine (Tofranil), nortriptyline (Aventyl, Pamelor), protriptyline (Vivactil), and trimipramine (Surmontil); and monoamine oxidase inhibitors including phenelzine (Nardil) and tranylcypromine (Parnate). Your doctor may need to change the doses of your medications or monitor you carefully for side effects.
- tell your doctor if you have or have ever had high blood pressure, irregular heartbeat, any other type of heart disease, seizures, diabetes, or hyperthyroidism (overactive thyroid gland).
- tell your doctor if you are pregnant, plan to become pregnant, or are breast-feeding. If you become pregnant while taking levalbuterol, call your doctor.

What special dietary instructions should I follow?

Unless your doctor tells you otherwise, continue your normal diet.

What should I do if I forget to take a dose?

Take the missed dose as soon as you remember it. However, if it is almost time for the next dose, skip the missed dose and continue your regular dosing schedule. Do not take a double dose to make up for a missed one.

What side effects can this medicine cause?

Levalbuterol may cause side effects. Tell your doctor if any of these symptoms are severe or do not go away:

- headache
- dizziness
- nervousness
- shaking hands that you cannot control
- upset stomach
- vomiting
- flu-like symptoms
- cough
- runny nose
- weakness
- fever
- diarrhea
- constipation
- frequent urination

Some side effects can be serious. The following symptoms are uncommon, but if you experience any of them, call your doctor immediately:

- chest pain
- fast or pounding heartbeat
- hives
- skin rash
- itching
- increased difficulty breathing or difficulty swallowing
- hoarseness
- swelling of the face, throat, tongue, lips, eyes, hands, feet, ankles, or lower legs
- depression
- muscle pain, weakness, or cramping
- difficulty moving a part of the body

Levalbuterol may cause other side effects. Call your doctor if you have any unusual problems while taking this medication.

If you experience a serious side effect, you or your doctor may send a report to the Food and Drug Administration's (FDA) MedWatch Adverse Event Reporting program online [at http://www.fda.gov/MedWatch/index.html] or by phone [1-800-332-1088].

What storage conditions are needed for this medicine?

Keep this medication in the container it came in, tightly closed, and out of reach of children. Store it at room temperature and away from excess heat and moisture (not in the bathroom). Throw away any medication that is outdated or no longer needed. Talk to your pharmacist about the proper disposal of your medication.

Levalbuterol must be protected from light. Store unused vials in the foil pouch, and discard all unused vials 2 weeks after you opened the pouch. If you remove a vial from the pouch, you should protect it from light and use it within one week.

What should I do in case of overdose?

In case of overdose, call your local poison control center at 1-800-222-1222. If the victim has collapsed or is not breathing, call local emergency services at 911.

Symptoms of overdose may include:

- seizures
- chest pain
- fainting
- dizziness
- blurred vision
- upset stomach
- fast, pounding, or irregular heartbeat
- nervousness
- headache
- dry mouth
- shaking hands that you cannot control
- extreme tiredness
- weakness
- difficulty falling or staying asleep
- frequent urination
- depression
- muscle weakness or cramps
- constipation
- vomiting
- difficulty moving a part of the body

What other information should I know?

Keep all appointments with your doctor

If your asthma symptoms become worse, if levalbuterol inhalation becomes less effective, or if you need more doses than usual of the asthma medications you use as needed, your condition may be getting worse. Call your doctor.

Do not let anyone else take your medication. Ask your pharmacist any questions you have about refilling your prescription.

Dosage Facts
For Informational Purposes

Caution: Do not change your dose, how often you take your medication, or the length of time you are to take it without first talking to your healthcare provider.

The following dosage information was written using medical language for doctors and other healthcare professionals and is provided here for you to check your dosage. The dosage of this drug may differ for different patients. Therefore, always follow your doctor's instructions or the directions on the label. Contact your healthcare provider or pharmacist if you have any questions about the specific dosage of your medication after reviewing this information.

General Dosage Information

Available as levalbuterol hydrochloride and levalbuterol tartrate; dosages are expressed in terms of levalbuterol.

Pediatric Patients

Bronchospasm in Asthma

ORAL INHALATION AEROSOL:
- Children ≥4 years of age: Initially, 90 mcg every 4–6 hours. Some patients may find 45 mcg every 4 hours to be sufficient.

ORAL INHALATION SOLUTION:
- Children 6–11 years of age: Initially, 0.31 mg 3 times daily via nebulization. Children 6–11 years of age with more severe asthma or those not responding adequately to the 0.31-mg dose may benefit from a dosage of up to 0.63 mg 3 times daily. Some experts on asthma management recommend a dosage of 0.025 mg/kg (minimum 0.63 mg, maximum 1.25 mg) every 4-8 hours in children ≤12 years of age.
- Adolescents ≥12 years of age: Initially, 0.63 mg 3 times daily (every 6–8 hours) via nebulization. Adolescents ≥12 years of age with more severe asthma or those not responding adequately to the 0.63-mg dose may benefit from a dosage of 1.25 mg 3 times daily.
- Some experts on asthma management recommend a dosage of 0.63-2.5 mg/kg every 4-8 hours in adolescents >12 years of age.

Adult Patients

Bronchospasm in Asthma

ORAL INHALATION AEROSOL:
- Initially, 90 mcg every 4–6 hours. Some patients may find 45 mcg every 4 hours to be sufficient.

ORAL INHALATION SOLUTION:
- Initially, 0.63 mg of levalbuterol 3 times daily (every 6–8 hours) via nebulization. Patients with more severe asthma or those not responding adequately to the 0.63-mg dose may benefit from a dosage of 1.25 mg 3 times daily.
- Some experts on asthma management recommend a dosage of 0.63-2.5 mg/kg every 4-8 hours in adults.

Prescribing Limits

Pediatric Patients

Bronchospasm in Asthma

ORAL INHALATION AEROSOL:
- Children ≥4 years of age: Maximum 90 mcg every 4–6 hours.

ORAL INHALATION SOLUTION:
- Children 6-11 years of age: Maximum 0.63 mg 3 times daily.
- Adolescents ≥12 years of age: Maximum 1.25 mg 3 times daily.

Adult Patients

Bronchospasm in Asthma

ORAL INHALATION AEROSOL:
- Maximum 90 mcg every 4–6 hours.

ORAL INHALATION SOLUTION:
- Maximum 1.25 mg 3 times daily.

Special Populations

Renal Impairment
- Inhalation aerosol: Use caution when administering high dosages.

Geriatric Patients
- Inhalation aerosol: Use caution and select initial dosage at the lower end of dosing range because of age-related decreases in hepatic, renal, and/or cardiac function and concomitant disease and drug therapy.
- Inhalation solution: Increase dosage as tolerated with careful monitoring.

Levetiracetam

(lee ve tye ra′ se tam)

Brand Name: Keppra®

Why is this medicine prescribed?

Levetiracetam is used in combination with other medications to treat certain types of seizures in people with epilepsy. Levetiracetam is in a class of medications called anticonvulsants. It works by decreasing abnormal excitement in the brain.

How should this medicine be used?

Levetiracetam comes as a solution (liquid) and a tablet to take by mouth. It is usually taken twice a day, once in the morning and once at night, with or without food. Try to take levetiracetam at around the same times every day. Follow the directions on your prescription label carefully, and ask your doctor or pharmacist to explain any part you do not understand. Take levetiracetam exactly as directed. Do not take more or less of it or take it more often than prescribed by your doctor.

Swallow the tablets whole; do not split, chew, or crush them.

If you are taking the oral solution, do not use a household spoon to measure your dose. You might not get the right amount of medication. Ask your doctor or pharmacist to recommend a medicine dropper, spoon, cup, or syringe and to show you how to use it to measure your medication.

Your doctor may start you on a low dose of levetiracetam and gradually increase your dose, not more often than once every 2 weeks.

Levetiracetam controls epilepsy but does not cure it. Continue to take levetiracetam even if you feel well. Do not stop taking levetiracetam without talking to your doctor. If you suddenly stop taking levetiracetam, your seizures may become worse. Your doctor will probably decrease your dose gradually.

Are there other uses for this medicine?

This medication may be prescribed for other uses; ask your doctor or pharmacist for more information.

What special precautions should I follow?

Before taking levetiracetam,
- tell your doctor and pharmacist if you are allergic to levetiracetam or any other medications.

- tell your doctor and pharmacist what prescription and nonprescription medications, vitamins, nutritional supplements, and herbal products you are taking. Your doctor may need to change the doses of your medications or monitor you carefully for side effects.
- tell your doctor if you have or have ever had kidney disease.
- tell your doctor if you are pregnant or plan to become pregnant. If you become pregnant while taking levetiracetam, call your doctor. Do not breastfeed while you are taking levetiracetam
- you should know that levetiracetam may make you dizzy or drowsy. Do not drive a car or operate machinery until you know how this medication affects you.

What special dietary instructions should I follow?

Unless your doctor tells you otherwise, continue your normal diet.

What should I do if I forget to take a dose?

If it has only been a few hours since the time you were scheduled to take the dose, take the missed dose as soon as you remember it. However, if it is almost time for the next dose, skip the missed dose and continue your regular dosing schedule. Do not take a double dose to make up for a missed one.

What side effects can this medicine cause?

Levetiracetam may cause side effects. Tell your doctor if any of these symptoms are severe or do not go away:

- drowsiness
- weakness
- unsteady walking
- coordination problems
- headache
- pain
- forgetfulness
- anxiety
- agitation or hostility
- dizziness
- moodiness
- nervousness
- numbness, burning, or tingling in the hands or feet
- loss of appetite
- vomiting
- diarrhea
- constipation
- changes in skin color

Some side effects can be serious. If you experience any of the following symptoms, call your doctor immediately:

- depression
- hallucinating (hearing voices or seeing visions that do not exist)
- thoughts of killing yourself

- seizures that are worse or different than the seizures you had before
- fever, sore throat, and other signs of infection
- double vision
- itching
- rash
- swelling of the face

Levetiracetam may cause other side effects. Call your doctor if you have any unusual problems while taking this medication.

If you experience a serious side effect, you or your doctor may send a report to the Food and Drug Administration's (FDA) MedWatch Adverse Event Reporting program online [at http://www.fda.gov/MedWatch/index.html] or by phone [1-800-332-1088].

What storage conditions are needed for this medicine?

Keep this medication in the container it came in, tightly closed, and out of reach of children. Store it at room temperature and away from excess heat and moisture (not in the bathroom). Throw away any medication that is outdated or no longer needed. Talk to your pharmacist about the proper disposal of your medication.

What should I do in case of overdose?

In case of overdose, call your local poison control center at 1-800-222-1222. If the victim has collapsed or is not breathing, call local emergency services at 911.

Symptoms of overdose may include:

- drowsiness
- agitation
- aggression
- decreased consciousness or loss of consciousness
- difficulty breathing

What other information should I know?

Keep all appointments with your doctor.

Do not let anyone else take your medication. Ask your pharmacist any questions you have about refilling your prescription.

Dosage Facts
For Informational Purposes

Caution: Do not change your dose, how often you take your medication, or the length of time you are to take it without first talking to your healthcare provider.

The following dosage information was written using medical language for doctors and other healthcare professionals and is provided here for you to check your dosage. The dosage of this drug may differ for different patients. Therefore, always follow your doctor's instructions or the directions on the label. Contact your health-

care provider or pharmacist if you have any questions about the specific dosage of your medication after reviewing this information.

Adult Patients

Seizure Disorders
Partial Seizures

ORAL:
- Initially, 500 mg twice daily.
- If response is inadequate, dosage may be increased by 1 g daily at 2-week intervals.
- Some clinicians reportedly initiate therapy with dosages of 2–4 g daily.
- Dosages >3 g daily may not be associated with increased therapeutic benefit.
- Do not discontinue abruptly; withdraw gradually by reducing dosage by 1 g daily at 2-week intervals.

Prescribing Limits

Adult Patients

Seizure Disorders
Partial Seizures

ORAL:
- Maximum 3 g daily recommended by the manufacturer.

Special Populations

Renal Impairment
- Modify dosage according to the degree of impairment based on patient's measured or estimated Cl_{cr}.

Recommended Dosage Based on Cl_{cr}

Renal Function	Cl_{cr} (mL/minute)	Dosage
Normal	>80	500–1500 mg every 12 hours
Mild	50–80	500–1000 mg every 12 hours
Moderate	30–50	250–750 mg every 12 hours
Severe	<30	250–500 mg every 12 hours
ESRD patients using dialysis	–	500–1000 mg every 24 hours; following dialysis, a 250- to 500-mg supplemental dose is recommended

Geriatric Patients
- Select dosage carefully and consider monitoring renal function during therapy.

Levobunolol Ophthalmic

(lee voe byoo′ noe lole)

Brand Name: AKBeta®, Betagan®

Why is this medicine prescribed?

Levobunolol is used to treat glaucoma, a condition in which increased pressure in the eye can lead to gradual loss of vision. Levobunolol decreases the pressure in the eye.

This medication is sometimes prescribed for other uses; ask your doctor or pharmacist for more information.

How should this medicine be used?

Levobunolol comes as eyedrops. Levobunolol usually is applied once or twice a day. Follow the directions on your prescription label carefully, and ask your doctor or pharmacist to explain any part you do not understand. Use levobunolol exactly as directed. Do not use more or less of it or use it more often than prescribed by your doctor.

Levobunolol controls glaucoma but does not cure it. Continue to use levobunolol even if you feel well. Do not stop using levobunolol without talking to your doctor.

To use the eyedrops, follow these instructions:
1. Wash your hands thoroughly with soap and water.
2. Use a mirror or have someone else put the drops in your eye.
3. Remove the protective cap. Make sure that the end of the dropper is not chipped or cracked.
4. Avoid touching the dropper tip against your eye or anything else.
5. Hold the dropper tip down at all times to prevent drops from flowing back into the bottle and contaminating the remaining contents.
6. Lie down or tilt your head back.
7. Holding the bottle between your thumb and index finger, place the dropper tip as near as possible to your eyelid without touching it.
8. Brace the remaining fingers of that hand against your cheek or nose.
9. With the index finger of your other hand, pull the lower lid of the eye down to form a pocket.
10. Drop the prescribed number of drops into the pocket made by the lower lid and the eye. Placing drops on the surface of the eyeball can cause stinging.
11. Close your eye and press lightly against the lower lid with your finger for 2-3 minutes to keep the medication in the eye. Do not blink.
12. Replace and tighten the cap right away. Do not wipe or rinse it off.
13. Wipe off any excess liquid from your cheek with a clean tissue. Wash your hands again.

What special precautions should I follow?

Before using levobunolol eyedrops,

- tell your doctor and pharmacist if you are allergic to levobunolol, other beta blockers, sulfites, or any other drugs.
- tell your doctor and pharmacist what prescription and nonprescription medications you are taking, especially other eye medications, beta blockers, such as atenolol (Tenormin), carteolol (Cartrol), labetalol (Normodyne, Trandate), metoprolol (Lopressor), nadolol (Corgard), propranolol (Inderal), sotalol (Betapace), or timolol (Blocadren); quinidine (Quinidex, Quinaglute Dura-Tabs); verapamil (Calan, Isoptin); and vitamins.
- tell your doctor if you have or have ever had thyroid, heart, or lung disease; congestive heart failure; or diabetes.
- tell your doctor if you are pregnant, plan to become pregnant, or are breast-feeding. If you become pregnant while using levobunolol, call your doctor immediately.
- if you are having surgery, including dental surgery, tell the doctor or dentist that you are using levobunolol.
- if you are using another eyedrop medication, use the eye medications at least 10 minutes apart.

What should I do if I forget to take a dose?

Apply the missed dose as soon as you remember it. However, if it is almost time for the next dose, skip the missed dose and continue your regular dosing schedule. Do not apply a double dose to make up for a missed one.

What side effects can this medicine cause?

Levobunolol may cause side effects. Tell your doctor if any of these symptoms are severe or do not go away:

- eye stinging or burning
- discomfort, redness, or itching of the eye
- swelling of the eyelids
- decreased vision

If you experience any of the following symptoms, stop using the eyedrops and call your doctor immediately:

- difficulty breathing
- wheezing
- slow or irregular heartbeat
- faintness
- swelling of the feet and legs
- sudden weight gain

If you experience a serious side effect, you or your doctor may send a report to the Food and Drug Administration's (FDA) MedWatch Adverse Event Reporting program online [at http://www.fda.gov/MedWatch/index.html] or by phone [1-800-332-1088].

What storage conditions are needed for this medicine?

Keep this medication in the container it came in, tightly closed, and out of reach of children. Store it at room temperature and away from excess heat and moisture (not in the bathroom). Throw away any medication that is outdated or no longer needed. Talk to your pharmacist about the proper disposal of your medication.

What other information should I know?

Keep all appointments with your doctor. Your doctor will order certain eye tests to check your response to levobunolol.

Do not let anyone else use your medication. Ask your pharmacist any questions you have about refilling your prescription.

Talk to your doctor, pharmacist, or other healthcare professional if you have questions about dosing information for your medication.

Levodopa and Carbidopa

(lee voe doe′ pa) (kar bi doe′ pa)

Brand Name: Parcopa®, Sinemet®, Sinemet CR®, Stalevo® (Levodopa and Carbidopa in combination with Entacapone)
Also available generically.

Why is this medicine prescribed?

The combination of levodopa and carbidopa is used to treat the symptoms of Parkinson's disease and Parkinson's-like symptoms that may develop after encephalitis (swelling of the brain) or injury to the nervous system caused by carbon monoxide poisoning or manganese poisoning. Parkinson's symptoms, including tremors (shaking), stiffness, and slowness of movement, are caused by a lack of dopamine, a natural substance usually found in the brain. Levodopa is in a class of medications called central nervous system agents. It works by being converted to dopamine in the brain. Carbidopa is in a class of medications called decarboxylase inhibitors. It works by preventing levodopa from being broken down before it reaches the brain. This allows for a lower dose of levodopa, which causes less nausea and vomiting.

How should this medicine be used?

The combination of levodopa and carbidopa comes as a regular tablet, an orally disintegrating tablet, and an extended-release (long-acting) tablet to take by mouth. The regular and orally disintegrating tablets are usually taken three or four times a day. The extended-release tablet is usually taken two to four times a day. Take levodopa and carbidopa at around the same times every day. Follow the directions on your prescription label carefully, and ask your doctor or pharmacist to explain any part you do not understand. Take levodopa and carbidopa exactly as directed. Do not take more or less of it or take it more often than prescribed by your doctor.

Swallow the extended-release tablets whole; do not split, chew, or crush them.

To take the orally disintegrating tablet, remove the tablet from the bottle using dry hands and immediately place it in your mouth. The tablet will quickly dissolve and can be swallowed with saliva. No water is needed to swallow disintegrating tablets.

If you are switching from levodopa (Dopar or Larodopa; no longer available in the US) to the combination of levodopa and carbidopa, follow your doctor's instructions. You will probably be told to wait at least 12 hours after your last dose of levodopa to take your first dose of levodopa and carbidopa.

Your doctor may start you on a low dose of levodopa and carbidopa and gradually increase your dose of the regular or orally disintegrating tablet every day or every other day as needed. The dose of the extended-release tablet may be gradually increased after 3 days as needed.

Levodopa and carbidopa controls Parkinson's disease but does not cure it. It may take several months before you feel the full benefit of levodopa and carbidopa. Continue to take levodopa and carbidopa even if you feel well. Do not stop taking levodopa and carbidopa without talking to your doctor. If you suddenly stop taking levodopa and carbidopa, you could develop a serious syndrome that causes fever, rigid muscles, unusual body movements, and confusion. Your doctor will probably decrease your dose gradually.

Are there other uses for this medicine?

This medication may be prescribed for other uses; ask your doctor or pharmacist for more information.

What special precautions should I follow?

Before taking levodopa and carbidopa,

- tell your doctor and pharmacist if you are allergic to levodopa and carbidopa any other medications, or any of the ingredients in levodopa and carbidopa tablets. Ask your pharmacist for a list of the ingredients.
- tell your doctor if you are taking phenelzine (Nardil) or tranyllcypromine (Parnate) or if you have stopped taking them in the past 2 weeks. Your doctor will probably tell you not to take levodopa and carbidopa.
- tell your doctor and pharmacist what prescription and nonprescription medications, vitamins, nutritional supplements, and herbal products you are taking or plan to take. Be sure to mention any of the following: antidepressants ('mood elevators') such as amitriptyline (Elavil), amoxapine (Asendin), clomipramine (Anafranil), desipramine (Norpramin), doxepin (Adapin, Sinequan), imipramine (Tofranil), nortriptyline (Aventyl, Pamelor), protriptyline (Vivactil), and trimipramine (Surmontil); antihistamines; haloperidol (Haldol); ipratropium (Atrovent); iron pills and vitamins containing iron; isocarboxazid (Marplan); isoniazid (INH, Nydra-

zid); medications for high blood pressure, irritable bowel disease, mental illness, motion sickness, nausea, ulcers, or urinary problems; metoclopramide (Reglan); papaverine (Pavabid); phenytoin (Dilantin); rasagiline (Azilect); risperidone (Risperdal); and selegiline (Eldepryl).Your doctor may need to change the doses of your medications or monitor you carefully for side effects.

- tell your doctor if you have or have ever had glaucoma, melanoma (skin cancer), or a skin growth that has not been diagnosed. Your doctor may tell you not to take levodopa and carbidopa.
- tell your doctor if you have or have ever had hormone problems; asthma; emphysema; mental illness; diabetes; ulcers; heart attacks; irregular heartbeat; or blood vessel, heart, kidney, liver or lung disease.
- tell your doctor if you are pregnant, plan to become pregnant, or are breast-feeding. If you become pregnant while taking levodopa and carbidopa, call your doctor.
- if you are having surgery, including dental surgery, tell the doctor or dentist that you are taking levodopa and carbidopa.
- you should know that while taking levodopa and carbidopa, your saliva, urine, or sweat may become a dark color (red, brown, or black). This is harmless, but your clothing may become stained.
- if you have phenylketonuria (PKU, an inherited condition in which a special diet must be followed to prevent mental retardation), you should know that the orally disintegrating tablets contain aspartame that forms phenylalanine.

What special dietary instructions should I follow?

Talk to your doctor if you plan on changing your diet to foods that are high in protein, such as meat, poultry, and dairy products.

What should I do if I forget to take a dose?

Take the missed dose as soon as you remember it. However, if it is almost time for the next dose, skip the missed dose and continue your regular dosing schedule. Do not take a double dose to make up for a missed one.

What side effects can this medicine cause?

Levodopa and carbidopa may cause side effects. Tell your doctor if any of these symptoms are severe or do not go away:
- dizziness
- nausea
- vomiting
- loss of appetite
- diarrhea
- dry mouth
- constipation
- change in sense of taste
- forgetfulness or confusion

- nervousness
- nightmares
- difficulty falling asleep or staying asleep
- headaches
- weakness
- increased sweating
- drowsiness

Some side effects can be serious. If you experience any of the following symptoms, call your doctor immediately:

- unusual or uncontrolled movements of the mouth, tongue, face, head, neck, arms, and legs
- fast, irregular, or pounding heartbeat
- depression
- thoughts of death or killing oneself
- hallucinating (seeing things or hearing voices that do not exist)
- swelling of the face, throat, tongue, lips, eyes, hands, feet, ankles, or lower legs
- hoarseness
- difficulty swallowing or breathing
- hives
- black and tarry stools
- red blood in stools
- bloody vomit
- vomiting material that looks like coffee grounds

What storage conditions are needed for this medicine?

Keep this medication in the container it came in, tightly closed, and out of reach of children. Store it at room temperature and away from excess heat and moisture (not in the bathroom). Throw away any medication that is outdated or no longer needed. Talk to your pharmacist about the proper disposal of your medication.

What should I do in case of overdose?

In case of overdose, call your local poison control center at 1-800-222-1222. If the victim has collapsed or is not breathing, call local emergency services at 911.

What other information should I know?

Keep all appointments with your doctor and the laboratory. Your doctor will order certain lab tests to check your response to levodopa and carbidopa.

Before having any laboratory test, tell your doctor and the laboratory personnel that you are taking levodopa and carbidopa.

Levodopa and carbidopa can lose its effect completely over time or only at certain times during the day. Call your doctor if your Parkinson's disease symptoms (shaking, stiffness, and slowness of movement) worsen or vary in severity.

As your condition improves and it is easier for you to move, be careful not to overdo physical activities. Increase your activity gradually to avoid falls and injuries.

Levodopa and carbidopa can cause false results in urine tests for sugar (Clinistix, Clinitest, and TesTape) and ketones (Acetest, Ketostix, and Labstix). Diabetic patients should use TesTape to test urine for glucose (sugar); better results can be obtained by holding the tape vertically, inserting the lower portion of the tape into the urine sample, and reading the color at the top of the damp area.

Do not let anyone else take your medication. Ask your pharmacist any questions you have about refilling your prescription

Dosage Facts
For Informational Purposes

Caution: Do not change your dose, how often you take your medication, or the length of time you are to take it without first talking to your healthcare provider.

The following dosage information was written using medical language for doctors and other healthcare professionals and is provided here for you to check your dosage. The dosage of this drug may differ for different patients. Therefore, always follow your doctor's instructions or the directions on the label. Contact your healthcare provider or pharmacist if you have any questions about the specific dosage of your medication after reviewing this information.

General Dosage Information

Dosage expressed in terms of levodopa and carbidopa.

Available in combination products containing a 1:4 or 1:10 ratio of carbidopa to levodopa. Additional carbidopa can be administered separately if a higher carbidopa dosage than is available in the combination preparations is needed. The treatment regimen can include levodopa-carbidopa extended-release tablets, conventional tablets, and orally disintegrating tablets and carbidopa tablets based on individual requirements. Levodopa no longer is commercially available in the US as a single-entity preparation.

Also available as a fixed-combination preparation containing levodopa, carbidopa, and entacapone (Stalevo®); available in a 1:4 ratio of carbidopa to levodopa. Used if optimum maintenance dosage of the 3 drugs corresponds to the dosage in the combination preparation. No experience transferring patients receiving levodopa-carbidopa extended-release tablets or levodopa-carbidopa preparations containing the 1:10 ratio.

For some patients (maintenance levodopa dosage ≤600 mg daily, no dyskinesias), the fixed combination containing levodopa, carbidopa, and entacapone (Stalevo®) can be used when initiating entacapone therapy if optimum maintenance dosage of levodopa-carbidopa corresponds to dosage in the combination preparation.

Adjust levodopa-carbidopa dosage carefully according to individual requirements, response, and tolerance.

Dosage adjustment may be needed when other antiparkinsonian drugs are added to or discontinued from the regimen.

Daily dosage of carbidopa should be at least 70–100 mg daily; patients receiving <70–100 mg daily are likely to experience nausea and vomiting.

Observe patient closely if dosage is reduced abruptly or

the drug is discontinued; risk of precipitating a symptom complex resembling neuroleptic malignant syndrome (NMS).

If general anesthesia required, continue therapy as long as patient permitted to take oral medications; resume as soon as patient is able to take oral medication. If therapy interrupted, observe for NMS.

Adult Patients

Parkinsonian Syndrome
Levodopa-Carbidopa Conventional Tablets or Orally Disintegrating Tablets

ORAL:
- Initially, levodopa 100 mg/carbidopa 25 mg (as 1 tablet) 3 times daily.
- Increase dosage by levodopa 100 mg/carbidopa 25 mg (1 tablet) daily or every other day until a daily dosage of levodopa 800 mg/carbidopa 200 mg is reached or adverse effects prevent further increases or necessitate discontinuance.
- Alternatively, initiate with levodopa 100 mg/carbidopa 10 mg (as 1 tablet) 3 or 4 times daily; this dosage will not provide an adequate dose of carbidopa for most patients. Increase dosage by levodopa 100 mg/carbidopa 10 mg (1 tablet) daily or every other day until a daily dosage of levodopa 800 mg/ carbidopa 80 mg is reached.

Levodopa-Carbidopa Extended-release Tablets

ORAL:
- Initially, levodopa 200 mg/carbidopa 50 mg (as 1 extended-release tablet) twice daily; initial dosage should not be given at intervals <6 hours. Adjust dosage based on response and tolerance at intervals ≥3 days. Most patients are treated adequately with levodopa 400 mg to 1.6 g daily and carbidopa 100–400 mg daily, administered in divided doses at intervals ranging from 4–8 hours while awake. Higher dosages (levodopa 2.4 g/carbidopa 600 mg) and shorter intervals (<4 hours) have been used but usually are not recommended. If the dosing interval is <4 hours and/or the divided doses are not equal, the smaller doses can be given at the end of the day.
- Dosage may be initiated, titrated, and stabilized initially with conventional (immediate-release) tablets.
- Transfer to extended-release tablets: initial dosage should provide 10% more levodopa daily than dosage previously received as conventional tablets; levodopa dosage may need to be increased up to 30% more daily, depending on response.

Carbidopa

Carbidopa: 25 mg with first dose of levodopa/carbidopa each day for patients who need additional carbidopa; additional 12.5- or 25-mg doses may given during the day with each dose of levodopa/carbidopa.

Prescribing Limits

Adult Patients
Parkinsonian Syndrome

ORAL:
- Experience with carbidopa dosages >200 mg daily is limited.

Levofloxacin Injection

(lee voe flox′ a sin)

Brand Name: Levaquin® in Dextrose Injection Premix

About Your Treatment

Your doctor has ordered levofloxacin, an antibiotic, to help treat your infection. The drug will be added to an intravenous fluid that will drip through a needle or catheter placed in your vein for at least 60 minutes, once a day.

Levofloxacin eliminates bacteria that cause many infections, including skin, respiratory tract, and urinary tract infections. It also kills bacteria that cause many venereal diseases. This medication is sometimes prescribed for other uses; ask your doctor or pharmacist for more information.

Your health care provider (doctor, nurse, or pharmacist) may measure the effectiveness and side effects of your treatment using laboratory tests and physical examinations. It is important to keep all appointments with your doctor and the laboratory. Before having any laboratory test, tell your doctor and the laboratory personnel that you are taking levofloxacin. The length of treatment depends on how your infection and symptoms respond to the medication.

Precautions

Before administering levofloxacin,
- tell your doctor and pharmacist if you are allergic to cinoxacin (Cinobac), ciprofloxacin (Cipro), enoxacin (Penetrex), erythromycin, levofloxacin, lomefloxacin (Maxaquin), nalidixic acid (NegGram), norfloxacin (Noroxin), ofloxacin (Floxin), sparfloxacin (Zagam), or any other drugs.
- tell your doctor and pharmacist what prescription and nonprescription medications you are taking, especially other antibiotics; anticoagulants ('blood thinners') such as warfarin (Coumadin); aspirin and other nonsteroidal anti-inflammatory medications (NSAIDs) such as ibuprofen (Advil, Motrin) and naproxen (Aleve, Naprosyn); cancer chemotherapy agents; cimetidine (Tagamet); cisapride (Propulsid); cyclosporine (Neoral, Sandimmune); medications for irregular heartbeats such as amiodarone (Cordarone), disopyramide (Norpace), dofetilide (Tikosyn), procainamide (Procanbid, Pronestyl), quinidine (Quinidex), and sotalol (Betapace, Betapace AF); oral steroids such as dexamethasone (Decadron, Dexone), methylprednisolone (Medrol), and prednisone (Deltasone); phenytoin (Dilantin); pimozide (Orap); probenecid (Benemid); theophylline (Theo-Dur); thioridazine (Mellaril); and vitamins.
- tell your doctor if you have or have ever had kidney or liver disease, seizures, colitis, stomach problems, vision problems, heart disease, or a history of stroke.
- tell your doctor if you are pregnant, plan to become

pregnant, or are breast-feeding. If you become pregnant while taking levofloxacin, call your doctor immediately.

- you should know that this drug may cause dizziness, lightheadedness, and tiredness. Do not drive a car or operate machinery until you know how levofloxacin affects you.
- plan to avoid unnecessary or prolonged exposure to sunlight and to wear protective clothing, sunglasses, and sunscreen. Levofloxacin may make your skin sensitive to sunlight.
- keep in mind that it causes increased or decreased blood sugar in patients taking antidiabetes medications or insulin. Careful monitoring of blood glucose is advised. If you experience a significant drop in blood glucose, stop taking levofloxacin and call your doctor.

Administering Your Medication

Before you administer levofloxacin, look at the solution closely. It should be clear and free of floating material. Gently squeeze the bag or observe the solution container to make sure there are no leaks. Do not use the solution if it is discolored, if it contains particles, or if the bag or container leaks. Use a new solution, but show the damaged one to your health care provider.

It is important that you use your medication exactly as directed. Do not stop your therapy on your own for any reason because your infection could worsen and result in hospitalization. Do not change your dosing schedule without talking to your health care provider. Your health care provider may tell you to stop your infusion if you have a mechanical problem (such as a blockage in the tubing, needle, or catheter); if you have to stop an infusion, call your health care provider immediately so your therapy can continue.

Side Effects

Levofloxacin may cause side effects. Tell your health care provider if any of these symptoms are severe or do not go away:

- upset stomach
- diarrhea
- vomiting
- stomach pain
- headache
- restlessness

If you experience any of the following symptoms, call your health care provider immediately:

- skin rash
- itching
- hives
- difficulty breathing or swallowing
- swelling of the face or throat
- yellowing of the skin or eyes
- dark urine
- pale or dark stools
- blood in urine
- pain, inflammation, or rupture of a tendon

- seizures
- rapid, irregular, or pounding heartbeats

Storage Conditions

- Your health care provider probably will give you a several-day supply of levofloxacin at a time. If you are receiving levofloxacin intravenously (in your vein), you probably will be told to store it in the refrigerator or freezer.
- Take your next dose from the refrigerator 1 hour before using it; place it in a clean, dry area to allow it to warm to room temperature.
- If you are told to store additional levofloxacin in the freezer, always move a 24-hour supply to the refrigerator for the next day's use.
- Do not refreeze medications.

Store your medication only as directed. Make sure you understand what you need to store your medication properly.

Keep your supplies in a clean, dry place when you are not using them, and keep all medications and supplies out of reach of children. Your health care provider will tell you how to throw away used needles, syringes, tubing, and containers to avoid accidental injury.

Overdose

In case of overdose, call your local poison control center at 1-800-222-1222. If the victim has collapsed or is not breathing, call local emergency services at 911.

Signs of Infection

If you are receiving levofloxacin in your vein or under your skin, you need to know the symptoms of a catheter-related infection (an infection where the needle enters your vein or skin). If you experience any of these effects near your intravenous catheter, tell your health care provider as soon as possible:

- tenderness
- warmth
- irritation
- drainage
- redness
- swelling
- pain

Dosage Facts
For Informational Purposes

Caution: Do not change your dose, how often you take your medication, or the length of time you are to take it without first talking to your healthcare provider.

The following dosage information was written using medical language for doctors and other healthcare professionals and is provided here for you to check your dosage. The dosage of this drug may differ for different

patients. Therefore, always follow your doctor's instructions or the directions on the label. Contact your healthcare provider or pharmacist if you have any questions about the specific dosage of your medication after reviewing this information.

General Dosage Information

Dosage of oral and IV levofloxacin is identical. No dosage adjustment needed when switching from IV to oral administration, or vice versa.

Adult Patients

Respiratory Tract Infections
Acute Bacterial Sinusitis

IV:
- 500 mg once every 24 hours for 10–14 days.
- Alternatively, 750 mg once every 24 hours for 5 days.

Acute Exacerbations of Chronic Bronchitis

IV:
- 500 mg once every 24 hours for 7 days.

Community-acquired Pneumonia (CAP)

IV:
- 500 mg once every 24 hours for 7–14 days.
- Alternatively, 750 mg once every 24 hours for 5 days can be used for treatment of CAP caused by S. pneumoniae (penicillin-susceptible strains), H. influenzae, H. parainfluenzae, C. pneumoniae, or M. pneumoniae.
- For empiric treatment of CAP, the IDSA and ATS recommend 750 mg once daily.

Nosocomial Pneumonia

IV:
- 750 mg once every 24 hours for 7–14 days.

Skin and Skin Structure Infections
Uncomplicated Infections

IV:
- 500 mg once every 24 hours for 7–10 days.

Complicated Infections

IV:
- 750 mg once every 24 hours for 7–14 days.

Urinary Tract Infections (UTIs) and Prostatitis
Uncomplicated UTIs

IV:
- 250 mg once every 24 hours for 3 days.

Complicated UTIs

IV:
- 250 mg once every 24 hours for 10 days.

Acute Pyelonephritis

IV:
- 250 mg once every 24 hours for 10 days.

Chronic Prostatitis

IV:
- 500 mg once every 24 hours for 28 days.

Anthrax
Postexposure Prophylaxis Following Inhalational Exposure

IV:
- 500 mg once daily. Initiate as soon as possible following suspected or confirmed exposure to aerosolized B. anthracis.
- Optimum duration of postexposure prophylaxis after an inhalation exposure to B. anthracis spores is unclear, but prolonged postexposure prophylaxis usually required. A duration of 60 days may be adequate for a low-dose exposure, but a duration >4 months may be necessary to reduce the risk following a high-dose exposure. CDC, US Working Group on Civilian Biodefense, and US Army Medical Research Institute of Infectious Diseases (USAMRIID) recommend that postexposure prophylaxis in unvaccinated individuals be continued for ≥60 days following a confirmed exposure (including in laboratory workers with confirmed exposures to B. anthracis cultures). The US Public Health Service Advisory Committee on Immunization Practices (ACIP) and USAMRIID recommend that individuals who are partially or fully vaccinated against anthrax receive postexposure prophylaxis for ≥30 days; if given in conjunction with anthrax vaccine, continue prophylaxis for at least 7–14 days after the third vaccine dose.
- Safety of levofloxacin given for >28 days has not been evaluated. Manufacturer states prolonged therapy should be used only when potential benefits outweigh risks.

Treatment of Inhalational Anthrax†

IV:
- 500 mg once daily for ≥60 days.
- Initial parenteral regimen preferred; use oral regimen for initial treatment only when a parenteral regimen is not available (e.g., supply or logistic problems because large numbers of individuals require treatment in a mass casualty setting). Continue for total duration of ≥60 days if inhalational anthrax occurred as the result of exposure to anthrax spores in the context of biologic warfare or bioterrorism.

Disseminated Gonococcal Infections†

IV, THEN ORAL:
- 250 mg IV once daily has been used for initial treatment. IV regimen is continued for 24–48 hours after improvement begins, then switched to 500 mg orally once daily to complete ≥1 week of treatment.
- Because of increased prevalence of QRNG, CDC no longer recommends fluoroquinolones for treatment of gonorrhea or any associated infections involving N. gonorrhoeae (e.g., PID, epididymitis). Use as an alternative treatment option for disseminated infections only if in vitro susceptibility can be documented by culture.
- Unless the presence of coexisting chlamydial infection has been excluded by appropriate testing, patients being treated for gonorrhea should also receive an anti-infective regimen effective for presumptive treatment of chlamydia (e.g., a single dose of oral azithromycin or a 7-day regimen of oral doxycycline).

Mycobacterial Infections†
Active Tuberculosis†

IV:
- 0.5–1 g once daily. Must be used in conjunction with other antituberculosis agents.
- Multiple-drug regimen usually given for 12–18 months when rifampin-resistant *M. tuberculosis* are involved; for 18–24 months when isoniazid- and rifampin-resistant strains are involved; or for 24 months when the strain is resistant to isoniazid, rifampin, ethambutol, and/or pyrazinamide.

Pelvic Inflammatory Disease†

IV:
- 500 mg once daily; used with or without IV metronidazole (500 mg every 8 hours).
- Should be used for treatment of PID *only* when cephalosporins are not feasible, community prevalence and individual risk of gonorrhea is low, and in vitro susceptibility has been confirmed.

Prescribing Limits
Adult Patients

Do not exceed usual dosage or duration of therapy.

Special Populations
Hepatic Impairment
- Dosage adjustments not required.

Renal Impairment
- Dosage adjustment not needed for treatment of uncomplicated UTIs in adults with renal impairment.
- Dosage adjustment not needed for treatment of complicated UTIs or acute pyelonephritis in adults with $Cl_{cr} \geq 20$ mL/minute.
- For other indications, dosage adjustments required in adults with $Cl_{cr} < 50$ mL/minute.

Dosage for Treatment of Acute Bacterial Sinusitis, Acute Bacterial Exacerbations of Chronic Bronchitis, Community-acquired Pneumonia, Uncomplicated Skin and Skin Structure Infections, or Chronic Prostatitis in Adults with Renal Impairment

Cl_{cr} (mL/min)	Dosage
20–49	Initial 500-mg dose, then 250 mg once every 24 hours
10–19	Initial 500-mg dose, then 250 mg once every 48 hours
Hemodialysis or CAPD Patients	Initial 500-mg dose, then 250 mg once every 48 hours; supplemental doses not required after dialysis

Dosage for Treatment of Nosocomial Pneumonia or Complicated Skin and Skin Structure Infections in Adults with Renal Impairment

Cl_{cr} (mL/min)	Dosage
20–49	Initial 750-mg dose, then 750 mg once every 48 hours
10–19	Initial 750-mg dose, then 500 mg once every 48 hours
Hemodialysis or CAPD Patients	Initial 750-mg dose, then 500 mg once every 48 hours; supplemental doses not required after dialysis

Dosage for Treatment of Complicated UTIs or Acute Pyelonephritis in Adults with Renal Impairment

Cl_{cr} (mL/min)	Dosage
≥20	No dosage adjustment required
10–19	Initial 250-mg dose, then 250 mg once every 48 hours

Geriatric Patients
- No dosage adjustments except those related to renal impairment.

† Use is not currently included in the labeling approved by the US Food and Drug Administration.

Levofloxacin Oral

(lee voe flox′ a sin)

Brand Name: Levaquin®

Why is this medicine prescribed?

Levofloxacin is used treat infections such as pneumonia; chronic bronchitis; and sinus, urinary tract, kidney, and skin infections. Levofloxacin is in a class of antibiotics called fluoroquinolones. It works by eliminating bacteria that cause infections. Antibiotics will not work for colds, flu, or other viral infections.

How should this medicine be used?

Levofloxacin comes as a tablet to take by mouth. It is usually taken once daily for 7-14 days. Treatment for some infections may take 6 weeks or longer. Follow the directions on your prescription label carefully, and ask your doctor or pharmacist to explain any part you do not understand. Take levofloxacin exactly as directed. Do not take more or less of it or take it more often than prescribed by your doctor.

Tablets should be taken with a full glass of water.

Continue to take levofloxacin even if you feel well. Do not stop taking levofloxacin without talking to your doctor.

Are there other uses for this medicine?

This medication may be prescribed for other uses; ask your doctor or pharmacist for more information.

What special precautions should I follow?

Before taking levofloxacin,

- tell your doctor and pharmacist if you are allergic to levofloxacin, ciprofloxacin (Cipro), enoxacin (Penetrex), lomefloxacin (Maxaquin), norfloxacin (Noroxin), ofloxacin (Floxin), sparfloxacin (Zagam), cinoxacin (Cinobac), nalidixic acid (NegGram), or any other drugs.
- tell your doctor and pharmacist what prescription and nonprescription medications, vitamins, nutritional supplements, and herbal products you are taking or plan to take. Be sure to mention any of the following: other antibiotics; anticoagulants ('blood thinners') such as warfarin (Coumadin); cancer chemotherapy agents; cimetidine (Tagamet); cisapride (Propulsid); cyclosporine (Neoral, Sandimmune); medications for irregular heartbeats such as amiodarone (Cordarone), disopyramide (Norpace), dofetilide (Tikosyn), procainamide (Procanbid, Pronestyl), quinidine (Quinidex), and sotalol (Betapace, Betapace AF); oral steroids such as dexamethasone (Decadron, Dexone), methylprednisolone (Medrol), and prednisone (Deltasone); phenytoin (Dilantin); pimozide (Orap); probenecid (Benemid); sucralfate (Carafate); theophylline (Theo-Dur); and thioridazine (Mellaril). Your doctor may need to change the doses of your medications or monitor you carefully for side effects.
- do not take with antacids (Mylanta, Maalox), didanosine (Videx) chewable/buffered tablets or solution, iron or zinc supplements, sucralfate (Carafate), or vitamins that contain iron or zinc. Take these medications 2 hours before or after levofloxacin.
- tell your doctor if you have or have ever had kidney or liver disease, convulsions, colitis, stomach problems, vision problems, heart disease, or history of stroke.
- tell your doctor if you are pregnant, plan to become pregnant, or are breast-feeding. If you become pregnant while taking levofloxacin, call your doctor.
- if you are having surgery, including dental surgery, tell the doctor or dentist that you are taking levofloxacin.
- you should know that this medication may cause dizziness, lightheadedness, and tiredness. Do not drive a car or work on dangerous machines until you know how levofloxacin will affect you.
- plan to avoid unnecessary or prolonged exposure to sunlight and to wear protective clothing, sunglasses, and

sunscreen. Levofloxacin may make your skin sensitive to sunlight.
- keep in mind that it causes increased or decreased blood sugar in patients taking antidiabetes medications or insulin. Careful monitoring of blood glucose is advised. If you experience a significant drop in blood glucose, stop taking levofloxacin and call your doctor.

What special dietary instructions should I follow?

Levofloxacin can be taken with or without food. If an upset stomach occurs, take with food. Drink at least eight full glasses of water or other liquid every day.

What should I do if I forget to take a dose?

Take the missed dose as soon as you remember it. However, if it is almost time for the next dose, skip the missed dose and continue your regular dosing schedule. Do not take a double dose to make up for a missed one.

What side effects can this medicine cause?

Levofloxacin may cause side effects. Tell your doctor if any of these symptoms are severe or do not go away:
- upset stomach
- diarrhea
- vomiting
- stomach pain
- headache
- restlessness

Some side effects can be serious. If you experience any of these symptoms, call your doctor immediately:
- skin rash
- itching
- hives
- difficulty breathing or swallowing
- swelling of the face or throat
- yellowing of the skin or eyes
- dark urine
- pale or dark stools
- blood in urine
- pain, inflammation, or rupture of a tendon
- rapid, irregular, or pounding heartbeats

Levofloxacin may cause other side effects. Call your doctor if you have any unusual problems while taking this medication.

What storage conditions are needed for this medicine?

Keep this medication in the container it came in, tightly closed, and out of reach of children. Store the tablets at room temperature and away from excess heat and moisture (not in the bathroom). Keep away from light. Throw away any medication that is outdated or no longer needed. Talk to your pharmacist about the proper disposal of your medication.

What should I do in case of overdose?

In case of overdose, call your local poison control center at 1-800-222-1222. If the victim has collapsed or is not breathing, call local emergency services at 911.

What other information should I know?

Keep all appointments with your doctor and the laboratory. Your doctor will order certain lab tests to check your response to levofloxacin.

Before having any laboratory test, tell your doctor and the laboratory personnel that you are taking levofloxacin.

Do not let anyone else take your medication. Your prescription is probably not refillable. If you still have symptoms of infection after you finish the levofloxacin, call your doctor.

Dosage Facts
For Informational Purposes

Caution: Do not change your dose, how often you take your medication, or the length of time you are to take it without first talking to your healthcare provider.

The following dosage information was written using medical language for doctors and other healthcare professionals and is provided here for you to check your dosage. The dosage of this drug may differ for different patients. Therefore, always follow your doctor's instructions or the directions on the label. Contact your healthcare provider or pharmacist if you have any questions about the specific dosage of your medication after reviewing this information.

Adult Patients

Respiratory Tract Infections
Acute Bacterial Sinusitis

ORAL:
- 500 mg once every 24 hours for 10–14 days.
- Alternatively, 750 mg once every 24 hours for 5 days.

Acute Exacerbations of Chronic Bronchitis

ORAL:
- 500 mg once every 24 hours for 7 days.

Community-acquired Pneumonia (CAP)

ORAL:
- 500 mg once every 24 hours for 7–14 days.
- Alternatively, 750 mg once every 24 hours for 5 days can be used for treatment of CAP caused by *S. pneumoniae* (penicillin-susceptible strains), *H. influenzae*, *H. parainfluenzae*, *C. pneumoniae*, or *M. pneumoniae*.
- For empiric treatment of CAP, the IDSA and ATS recommend 750 mg once daily.

Nosocomial Pneumonia

ORAL:
- 750 mg once every 24 hours for 7–14 days.

Skin and Skin Structure Infections
Uncomplicated Infections

ORAL:
- 500 mg once every 24 hours for 7–10 days.

Complicated Infections

ORAL:
- 750 mg once every 24 hours for 7–14 days.

Urinary Tract Infections (UTIs) and Prostatitis
Uncomplicated UTIs

ORAL:
- 250 mg once every 24 hours for 3 days.

Complicated UTIs

ORAL:
- 250 mg once every 24 hours for 10 days.

Acute Pyelonephritis

ORAL:
- 250 mg once every 24 hours for 10 days.

Chronic Prostatitis

ORAL:
- 500 mg once every 24 hours for 28 days.

Anthrax
Postexposure Prophylaxis Following Inhalational Exposure

ORAL:
- 500 mg once daily. Initiate as soon as possible following suspected or confirmed exposure to aerosolized *B. anthracis*.
- Optimum duration of postexposure prophylaxis after an inhalation exposure to *B. anthracis* spores is unclear, but prolonged postexposure prophylaxis usually required. A duration of 60 days may be adequate for a low-dose exposure, but a duration >4 months may be necessary to reduce the risk following a high-dose exposure. CDC, US Working Group on Civilian Biodefense, and US Army Medical Research Institute of Infectious Diseases (USAMRIID) recommend that postexposure prophylaxis in unvaccinated individuals be continued for ≥60 days following a confirmed exposure (including in laboratory workers with confirmed exposures to *B. anthracis* cultures). The US Public Health Service Advisory Committee on Immunization Practices (ACIP) and USAMRIID recommend that individuals who are partially or fully vaccinated against anthrax receive postexposure prophylaxis for ≥30 days; if given in conjunction with anthrax vaccine, continue prophylaxis for at least 7–14 days after the third vaccine dose.
- Safety of levofloxacin given for >28 days has not been evaluated. Manufacturer states prolonged therapy should be used only when potential benefits outweigh risks.

Treatment of Inhalational Anthrax†

ORAL:
- 500 mg once daily for ≥60 days.
- Initial parenteral regimen preferred; use oral regimen for initial treatment only when a parenteral regimen is not available (e.g., supply or logistic problems because large numbers of individuals require treatment in a mass casualty setting). Continue for total duration of ≥60 days if inhalational anthrax occurred as the result of exposure to anthrax spores in the context of biologic warfare or bioterrorism.

Chlamydial Infections†
Urogenital Infections†

ORAL:
- 500 mg once daily for 7 days recommended by CDC and others.

Gonorrhea and Associated Infections†
Uncomplicated Urethral, Endocervical, or Rectal Gonorrhea†

ORAL:
- 250 mg as a single dose has been used for infections caused by susceptible *Neisseria gonorrhoeae*.
- Because of increased prevalence of quinolone-resistant *N. gonorrhoeae* (QRNG), CDC no longer recommends fluoroquinolones for treatment of gonorrhea or any associated infections involving *N. gonorrhoeae* (e.g., PID, epididymitis).
- Unless the presence of coexisting chlamydial infection has been excluded by appropriate testing, patients being treated for gonorrhea should also receive an anti-infective regimen effective for presumptive treatment of chlamydia (e.g., a single dose of oral azithromycin or a 7-day regimen of oral doxycycline).

Epididymitis†

ORAL:
- 500 mg once daily for 10 days recommended by CDC and others.
- Should be used *only* when epididymitis† most likely caused by sexually transmitted enteric bacteria (e.g., *Escherichia coli*) or when culture or nucleic acid amplification tests are negative for *N. gonorrhoeae*.

Mycobacterial Infections†
Active Tuberculosis†

ORAL:
- 0.5–1 g once daily. Must be used in conjunction with other antituberculosis agents.
- Multiple-drug regimen usually given for 12–18 months when rifampin-resistant *M. tuberculosis* are involved; for 18–24 months when isoniazid- and rifampin-resistant strains are involved; or for 24 months when the strain is resistant to isoniazid, rifampin, ethambutol, and/or pyrazinamide.

Nongonococcal Urethritis†

ORAL:
- 500 mg once daily for 7 days recommended by CDC.

Pelvic Inflammatory Disease†

ORAL:
- 500 mg once daily given for 14 days; used with or without oral metronidazole (500 mg twice daily for 14 days).
- Should be used for treatment of PID *only* when cephalosporins are not feasible, community prevalence and individual risk of gonorrhea is low, and in vitro susceptibility has been confirmed.

Travelers' Diarrhea†
Treatment of Travelers' Diarrhea†

ORAL:
- 500 mg once daily for 1–3 days.

Prevention of Travelers' Diarrhea†

ORAL:
- 500 mg once daily during the period of risk.
- Although anti-infective prophylaxis generally is discouraged, some clinicians state that it can be given during the period of risk (for ≤3 weeks) beginning the day of travel and continuing for 1 or 2 days after leaving the area of risk.

Prescribing Limits

Adult Patients

Do not exceed usual dosage or duration of therapy.

Special Populations

Hepatic Impairment
- Dosage adjustments not required.

Renal Impairment
- Dosage adjustment not needed for treatment of uncomplicated UTIs in adults with renal impairment.
- Dosage adjustment not needed for treatment of complicated UTIs or acute pyelonephritis in adults with $Cl_{cr} \geq 20$ mL/minute.
- For other indications, dosage adjustments required in adults with $Cl_{cr} < 50$ mL/minute.

Dosage for Treatment of Acute Bacterial Sinusitis, Acute Bacterial Exacerbations of Chronic Bronchitis, Community-acquired Pneumonia, Uncomplicated Skin and Skin Structure Infections, or Chronic Prostatitis in Adults with Renal Impairment

Cl_{cr} (mL/min)	Dosage
20–49	Initial 500-mg dose, then 250 mg once every 24 hours
10–19	Initial 500-mg dose, then 250 mg once every 48 hours
Hemodialysis or CAPD Patients	Initial 500-mg dose, then 250 mg once every 48 hours; supplemental doses not required after dialysis

Dosage for Treatment of Nosocomial Pneumonia or Complicated Skin and Skin Structure Infections in Adults with Renal Impairment

Cl_{cr} (mL/min)	Dosage
20–49	Initial 750-mg dose, then 750 mg once every 48 hours
10–19	Initial 750-mg dose, then 500 mg once every 48 hours
Hemodialysis or CAPD Patients	Initial 750-mg dose, then 500 mg once every 48 hours; supplemental doses not required after dialysis

Dosage for Treatment of Complicated UTIs or Acute Pyelonephritis in Adults with Renal Impairment	
Cl$_{cr}$ (mL/min)	Dosage
≥20	No dosage adjustment required
10–19	Initial 250-mg dose, then 250 mg once every 48 hours

Geriatric Patients
- No dosage adjustments except those related to renal impairment.

† *Use is not currently included in the labeling approved by the US Food and Drug Administration.*

Levorphanol Oral

(lee vor′ fa nole)

Brand Name: Levo-Dromoran®

Why is this medicine prescribed?

Levorphanol is used to relieve moderate to severe pain.

This medication is sometimes prescribed for other uses; ask your doctor or pharmacist for more information.

How should this medicine be used?

Levorphanol comes as a tablet to take by mouth. It usually is taken every 4 hours as needed. Follow the directions on your prescription label carefully, and ask your doctor or pharmacist to explain any part you do not understand. Take levorphanol exactly as directed.

Levorphanol can be habit-forming. Do not take a larger dose, take it more often, or for a longer period than your doctor tells you to.

What special precautions should I follow?

Before taking levorphanol,
- tell your doctor and pharmacist if you are allergic to codeine, levorphanol, or any other drugs.
- tell your doctor and pharmacist what prescription and nonprescription medications you are taking, especially other pain relievers; antidepressants; medications for cough, cold, or allergies; sedatives; sleeping pills; tranquilizers; and vitamins.
- tell your doctor if you have or have ever had liver or kidney disease, a history of alcoholism, lung or thyroid disease, heart disease, prostatic hypertrophy, or urinary problems.
- tell your doctor if you are pregnant, plan to become

pregnant, or are breast-feeding. If you become pregnant while taking levorphanol, call your doctor.
- if you are having surgery, including dental surgery, tell the doctor or dentist that you are taking levorphanol.
- you should know that this drug may make you drowsy. Do not drive a car or operate machinery until you know how this drug affects you.
- remember that alcohol can add to the drowsiness caused by this drug.

What should I do if I forget to take a dose?

Levorphanol usually is taken as needed. If your doctor has told you to take levorphanol regularly, take the missed dose as soon as you remember it. However, if it is almost time for the next dose, skip the missed dose and continue your regular dosing schedule. Do not take a double dose to make up for a missed one.

What side effects can this medicine cause?

Levorphanol may cause side effects. Tell your doctor if any of these symptoms are severe or do not go away:
- dizziness
- lightheadedness
- drowsiness
- upset stomach
- vomiting
- constipation
- stomach pain
- rash
- difficulty urinating

If you experience either of the following symptoms, call your doctor immediately:
- difficulty breathing
- fainting

If you experience a serious side effect, you or your doctor may send a report to the Food and Drug Administration's (FDA) MedWatch Adverse Event Reporting program online [at http://www.fda.gov/MedWatch/index.html] or by phone [1-800-332-1088].

What storage conditions are needed for this medicine?

Keep this medication in the container it came in, tightly closed, and out of reach of children. Store it at room temperature and away from excess heat and moisture (not in the bathroom). Throw away any medication that is outdated or no longer needed. Talk to your pharmacist about the proper disposal of your medication.

What should I do in case of overdose?

In case of overdose, call your local poison control center at 1-800-222-1222. If the victim has collapsed or is not breathing, call local emergency services at 911.

What other information should I know?

Keep all appointments with your doctor.

Do not let anyone else take your medication. Ask your

pharmacist any questions you have about refilling your prescription.

Talk to your doctor, pharmacist, or other healthcare professional if you have questions about dosing information for your medication.

Levothyroxine

(lee voe thye rox' een)

Brand Name: Levothroid®, Levoxyl®, Synthroid®, Unithroid®
Also available generically.

Important Warning

Thyroid hormone should not be used to treat obesity in patients with normal thyroid function. Levothyroxine is ineffective for weight reduction in normal thyroid patients and may cause serious or life-threatening toxicity, especially when taken with amphetamines. Talk to your doctor about the potential risks associated with this medication.

Why is this medicine prescribed?

Levothyroxine, a thyroid hormone, is used to treat hypothyroidism, a condition where the thyroid gland does not produce enough thyroid hormone. Without this hormone, the body cannot function properly, resulting in poor growth, slow speech, lack of energy, weight gain, hair loss, dry thick skin, and increased sensitivity to cold. When taken correctly, levothyroxine reverses these symptoms. Levothyroxine is also used to treat congenital hypothyroidism (cretinism) and goiter (enlarged thyroid gland).

This medication is sometimes prescribed for other uses; ask your doctor or pharmacist for more information.

How should this medicine be used?

Levothyroxine comes as a tablet to take by mouth. It usually is taken once a day on an empty stomach, 1/2 to 1 hour before breakfast. Follow the directions on your prescription label carefully, and ask your doctor or pharmacist to explain any part you do not understand. Take levothyroxine exactly as directed. Do not take more or less of it or take it more often than prescribed by your doctor.

The tablets may get stuck in your throat or cause choking or gagging; therefore, the tablet should be taken with a full glass of water.

If you are giving levothyroxine to an infant or child who cannot swallow the tablet, crush the tablet and mix it in 1 to 2 teaspoons of plain water. Give this mixture by spoon or dropper right away. Do not store this mixture. Only mix the crushed tablets with water. Do not mix with food or soybean infant formula.

Your doctor will probably start you on a low dose of levothyroxine and gradually increase your dose.

Levothyroxine controls hypothyroidism, but does not cure it. It may several weeks before you notice a change in your symptoms. Continue to take levothyroxine even if you feel well. Do not stop taking levothyroxine without talking to your doctor.

What special precautions should I follow?

Before taking levothyroxine,

- tell your doctor and pharmacist if you are allergic to levothyroxine, thyroid hormone, any other drugs, povidone iodine, tartrazine (a yellow dye in some processed foods and drugs), or foods such as lactose or corn starch. Levothroid and Eltroxin contain lactose, while Synthroid contains tartrazine and povidone. Eltroxin contains corn starch.
- tell your doctor and pharmacist what prescription and nonprescription medications you are taking, especially amphetamines; anticoagulants ('blood thinners') such as warfarin (Coumadin); antidepressants or anti-anxiety agents; arthritis medicine; aspirin; beta-blockers such as metoprolol (Lopressor, Toprol), propranolol (Inderal) or timolol (Blocadren, Timoptic); cancer chemotherapy agents; diabetes medications (insulin and tablets); digoxin (Lanoxin); estrogens; iron; methadone; oral contraceptives; phenytoin (Dilantin); steroids; theophylline (TheoDur); and vitamins.
- if you take an antacid, calcium carbonate (Tums), cholestyramine (Questran), colestipol (Colestid), iron, sodium polystrene sulfonate (Kayexalate), simethicone (Phazyme, Gas X), or sucralfate (Carafate), take it at least 4 hours before or 4 hours after you take levothyroxine.
- tell your doctor if you have or have ever had diabetes; hardening of the arteries (atherosclerosis); kidney disease; hepatitis; cardiovascular disease such as high blood pressure, chest pain (angina), arrhythmias, or heart attack; or an underactive adrenal or pituitary gland.
- tell your doctor if you are pregnant, plan to become pregnant or are breast-feeding. If you become pregnant while taking levothyroxine, call your doctor.
- if you have surgery, including dental surgery, tell the doctor or dentist that you are taking levothyroxine.

What special dietary instructions should I follow?

Unless your doctor tells you otherwise, continue your normal diet.

What should I do if I forget to take a dose?

Take the missed dose as soon as you remember it. However, if it is almost time for the next dose, skip the missed dose

---

and continue your regular dosing schedule. Do not take a double dose to make up for a missed one.

What side effects can this medicine cause?

Levothyroxine may cause side effects. Tell your doctor if any of these symptoms are severe or do not go away:
- weight loss
- tremor
- headache
- upset stomach
- vomiting
- diarrhea
- stomach cramps
- nervousness
- irritability
- insomnia
- excessive sweating
- increased appetite
- fever
- changes in menstrual cycle
- sensitivity to heat
- temporary hair loss, particularly in children during the first month of therapy

If you experience either of the following symptoms, call your doctor immediately:
- chest pain (angina)
- rapid or irregular heartbeat or pulse

If you experience a serious side effect, you or your doctor may send a report to the Food and Drug Administration's (FDA) MedWatch Adverse Event Reporting program online [at http://www.fda.gov/MedWatch/index.html] or by phone [1-800-332-1088].

What storage conditions are needed for this medicine?

Keep this medication in the container it came in, tightly closed, and out of reach of children. Store it at room temperature and away from excess heat and moisture (not in the bathroom). Throw away any medication that is outdated or no longer needed. Talk to your pharmacist about the proper disposal of your medication.

What should I do in case of overdose?

In case of overdose, call your local poison control center at 1-800-222-1222. If the victim has collapsed or is not breathing, call local emergency services at 911.

What other information should I know?

Keep all appointments with your doctor and the laboratory. Your doctor will order certain lab tests to check your response to levothyroxine.

Learn the brand name and generic name of your medication. Do not switch brands without talking to your doctor or pharmacist, as each brand of levothyroxine contains a slightly different amount of medication.

Do not let anyone else take your medication. Ask your pharmacist any questions you have about refilling your prescription.

Dosage Facts
For Informational Purposes

Caution: Do not change your dose, how often you take your medication, or the length of time you are to take it without first talking to your healthcare provider.

The following dosage information was written using medical language for doctors and other healthcare professionals and is provided here for you to check your dosage. The dosage of this drug may differ for different patients. Therefore, always follow your doctor's instructions or the directions on the label. Contact your healthcare provider or pharmacist if you have any questions about the specific dosage of your medication after reviewing this information.

General Dosage Information

Available as levothyroxine sodium; dosage is expressed in terms of the salt.

Adjust dosage carefully according to clinical and laboratory response to treatment. Avoid undertreatment or overtreatment.

Initiate dosage at a lower level in geriatric patients, in patients with functional or ECG evidence of cardiovascular disease, and in patients with severe, long-standing hypothyroidism.

Pediatric Patients

Hypothyroidism

ORAL:
- Initiate therapy at full replacement dosages as soon as possible after diagnosis of hypothyroidism to prevent deleterious effects on intellectual and physical growth and development; initiate dosage at a lower level in children with long-standing or severe hypothyroidism. The following dosages have been recommended:

Dosage for Management of Hypothyroidism in Pediatric Patients

Age	Daily Dose
0–3 months	10–15 mcg/kg
3–6 months	25–50 mcg or 8–10 mcg/kg
6–12 months	50–75 mcg or 6–8 mcg/kg
1–5 years	75–100 mcg or 5–6 mcg/kg
6–12 years	100–150 mcg or 4–5 mcg/kg
Older than 12 years (growth and puberty incomplete)	>150 mcg or 2–3 mcg/kg
Growth and puberty complete	1.6–1.7 mcg/kg

Alternatively, 25–50 mcg once daily has been recommended for otherwise healthy children <1 year of age; after 1 year of age, children may be given 3–5 mcg/kg daily until the adult dosage of about 150 mcg daily is reached in early or mid-adolescence.

In neonates at risk of cardiac failure, initiate at a lower dosage (e.g., 25 mcg daily); increase dosage at intervals of 4–6 weeks as needed based on clinical and laboratory response to treatment. In neonates with very low (<5 mcg/dL) or undetectable serum T_4 concentrations, usual initial dosage is 50 mcg daily.

When *transient* hypothyroidism is suspected, therapy may be temporarily discontinued when the child is older than 3 years of age to reassess the condition.

Hyperactivity in an older child may be minimized by initiating therapy at a dosage approximately one-fourth of the recommended full replacement dosage; increase dosage by an amount equal to one-fourth the full recommended replacement dosage at weekly intervals until the full recommended replacement dosage is reached.

For treatment of severe or long-standing hypothyroidism, usual initial dosage is 25 mcg daily. Increase dosage in increments of 25 mcg at intervals of 2–4 weeks until desired response is obtained.

Adult Patients

Hypothyroidism

ORAL:

- In otherwise healthy individuals <50 years of age and in those >50 years of age who have been recently treated for hyperthyroidism or who have been hypothyroid for only a short time (i.e., several months), usual initial oral dosage (full replacement dosage) is 1.7 mcg/kg daily (e.g., 100–125 mcg daily for a 70-kg adult) given as a single dose. Older patients may require <1 mcg/kg daily.
- Dosages >200 mcg daily seldom required; failure to respond adequately to oral dosages ≥ 300 mcg daily is rare and should prompt reevaluation of the diagnosis, or suggest presence of malabsorption, patient noncompliance, and/or drug interactions.
- For most patients >50 years of age, usual initial dosage is 25–50 mcg daily given as a single dose; increase dosage at intervals of 6–8 weeks.
- For management of severe or long-standing hypothyroidism, usual initial dosage is 12.5–25 mcg daily given as a single dose. Increase by increments of 25 mcg at intervals of 2–4 weeks until serum TSH concentrations return to normal; some clinicians suggest that dosage be adjusted at intervals of 4–8 weeks.
- For management of subclinical hypothyroidism (if considered necessary), initiate at lower dosages (e.g., 1 mcg/kg daily). If levothyroxine therapy is not initiated, monitor patients annually for changes in clinical status and thyroid laboratory parameters.

Pituitary TSH Suppression

Individualize dosage based on patient characteristics and nature of the disease. Target level for TSH suppression in management of well-differentiated thyroid cancer and thyroid nodules not established.

Thyroid Cancer

ORAL:

- Dosages >2 mcg/kg daily given as a single dose usually required to suppress TSH concentrations to <0.1 mU/L. In patients with high-risk tumors, target level for TSH suppression may be <0.01 mU/L.

Benign Nodules or Nontoxic Multinodular Goiter

ORAL:

- Suppress TSH concentrations to 0.1–0.5 mU/L for nodules and to 0.5–1 mU/L for multinodular goiter.

Special Populations

Patients with Cardiovascular Disease

Hypothyroidism

- Initiate therapy at lower doses than those recommended in patients without cardiovascular disease. For patients <50 years of age with underlying cardiovascular disease, usual initial dosage is 25–50 mcg daily given as a single dose; increase dosage at intervals of 6–8 weeks.
- If cardiac symptoms develop or worsen, reduce dosage or withhold therapy for 1 week and then cautiously restart therapy at a lower dose.

Geriatric Patients

Hypothyroidism

- Initiate therapy at lower doses than those recommended in younger patients.
- In geriatric patients with underlying cardiovascular disease, usual initial dosage is 12.5–25 mcg daily; increase dosage by increments of 12.5–25 mcg at intervals of 4–6 weeks until patient becomes euthyroid and serum TSH concentrations return to normal. If cardiac symptoms develop or worsen, reduce dosage or withhold therapy for 1 week and then cautiously restart therapy at a lower dose.

Lidocaine Transdermal

(lye′ doe kane)

Brand Name: Lidoderm®

Why is this medicine prescribed?

Lidocaine patches are used to relieve the pain of post-herpetic neuralgia (the burning, stabbing pains, or aches that may last for months or years after a shingles infection). Lidocaine is in a class of medications called local anesthetics. It works by stopping nerves from sending pain signals.

How should this medicine be used?

Lidocaine comes as a patch to apply to the skin. It is applied only once a day as needed for pain. Follow the directions on your prescription label carefully, and ask your doctor or pharmacist to explain any part you do not understand. Use lidocaine patches exactly as directed.

Your doctor will tell you how many lidocaine patches you may use at one time and the length of time you may wear the patches. Never apply more than three patches at one time, and never wear patches for more than 12 hours per day. Using too many patches or leaving patches on for too long may cause serious side effects.

To apply the patches, follow these steps:

1. Look at the skin that you plan to cover with a lidocaine patch. If the skin is broken or blistered, do not apply a patch to that area.
2. Use scissors to remove the outer seal from the package. Then pull apart the zipper seal.
3. Remove up to three patches from the package and press the zipper seal tightly together. The remaining patches may dry out if the zipper seal is not tightly closed.
4. Cut patch(es) to the size and shape that will cover your most painful area.
5. Peel the transparent liner off the back of the patch(es).
6. Press the patch(es) firmly onto your skin. If you are applying a patch to your face, be careful not to let it touch your eyes. If you do get lidocaine in your eye, wash it with plenty of water or saline solution.
7. Wash your hands after handling lidocaine patches.
8. Do not reuse lidocaine patches. After you are finished using a patch, remove it and dispose of it out of reach of children and pets. Used patches contain enough medication to seriously harm a child or pet.

Are there other uses for this medicine?

This medication may be prescribed for other uses; ask your doctor or pharmacist for more information.

What special precautions should I follow?

Before using lidocaine patches,

- tell your doctor and pharmacist if you are allergic to lidocaine; other local anesthetics such as bupivacaine (Marcaine), etidocaine (Duranest), mepivacaine (Carbocaine, Prolocaine), or prilocaine (Citanest); or any other medications.
- tell your doctor and pharmacist what prescription and nonprescription medications, vitamins, nutritional supplements, and herbal products you are taking. Be sure to mention any of the following: disopyramide (Norpace), flecainide (Tambocor), medications applied to the skin or mouth to treat pain, mexiletine (Mexitil), moricizine (Ethmozine), procainamide (Procanabid, Pronestyl), propafenone (Rhythmol), quinidine (Quinidex), and tocainide (Tonocard). Your doctor may need to change the doses of your medications or monitor you carefully for side effects.
- tell your doctor if you have or have ever had liver disease.
- tell your doctor if you are pregnant, plan to become pregnant, or are breast-feeding. If you become pregnant while using lidocaine patches, call your doctor.
- if you are having surgery, including dental surgery, tell the doctor or dentist that you are using lidocaine patches.

What special dietary instructions should I follow?

Unless your doctor tells you otherwise, continue your normal diet.

What should I do if I forget to take a dose?

This medication is usually taken as needed. If your doctor has told you to use lidocaine patches regularly, use the missed patch as soon as you remember it. However, if it is almost time for the next dose, skip the missed patch and continue your regular dosing schedule. Do not take a double dose to make up for a missed one.

What side effects can this medicine cause?

Lidocaine patches may cause side effects. If any of these symptoms occur, remove your patch and do not put it back on until the symptoms go away. Tell your doctor if any of these symptoms are severe or do not go away:

- burning or discomfort in the place you applied the patch
- redness or swelling of the skin under the patch

Some side effects can be serious. The following symptoms are uncommon, but if you experience any of them, call your doctor immediately:

- hives
- skin rash
- itching
- diffiiculty breathing or swallowing
- swelling of the face, throat, tongue, lips, eyes, hands, feet, ankles, or lower legs
- hoarseness
- cool, moist skin
- fast pulse or breathing
- unusual thirst
- upset stomach
- vomiting
- confusion
- weakness
- dizziness
- fainting

Lidocaine patches may cause other side effects. Call your doctor if you have any unusual problems while taking this medication.

If you experience a serious side effect, you or your doctor may send a report to the Food and Drug Administration's (FDA) MedWatch Adverse Event Reporting program online [at http://www.fda.gov/MedWatch/index.html] or by phone [1-800-332-1088].

What storage conditions are needed for this medicine?

Keep this medication in the container it came in, tightly closed, and out of reach of children. Store it at room tem-

perature and away from excess heat and moisture (not in the bathroom). Throw away any medication that is outdated or no longer needed. Talk to your pharmacist about the proper disposal of your medication.

What should I do in case of overdose?

If you wear too many patches or wear patches for too long, too much lidocaine may be absorbed into your blood. In that case, you may experience symptoms of an overdose.

In case of overdose, call your local poison control center at 1-800-222-1222. If the victim has collapsed or is not breathing, call local emergency services at 911.

Symptoms of overdose may include:
- lightheadedness
- nervousness
- inappropriate happiness
- confusion
- dizziness
- drowsiness
- ringing in the ears
- blurred or double vision
- vomiting
- feeling hot, cold, or numb
- twitching or shaking that you cannot control
- seizures
- loss of consciousness
- slow heartbeat

What other information should I know?

Keep all appointments with your doctor

Do not let anyone else take your medication. Ask your pharmacist any questions you have about refilling your prescription.

Talk to your doctor, pharmacist, or other healthcare professional if you have questions about dosing information for your medication.

Lidocaine Viscous

(lye' doe kane)

Brand Name: Xylocaine Viscous®

Why is this medicine prescribed?

Lidocaine viscous, a local anesthetic, is used to treat the pain of a sore or irritated mouth and throat often associated with cancer chemotherapy and certain medical procedures. Lidocaine viscous is not normally used for sore throats due to cold, flu, or infections such as strep throat.

This medication is sometimes prescribed for other uses; ask your doctor or pharmacist for more information.

How should this medicine be used?

Lidocaine viscous comes as a thick liquid and should be shaken well before using. Lidocaine viscous usually is used as needed but not more frequently than every 3 hours, with a maximum of eight doses in 24 hours. Follow the directions on your prescription label carefully, and ask your doctor or pharmacist to explain any part you do not understand. Use lidocaine exactly as directed. Do not use more or less of it or use it more often than prescribed by your doctor.

For a sore or irritated mouth, the dose should be placed in the mouth, swished around until the pain goes away, and spit out.

For a sore throat, the dose should be gargled and then may be swallowed. To avoid or decrease side effects, use the minimum amount of drug needed to relieve your pain.

Because lidocaine viscous decreases the feeling in your mouth and/or throat, it may affect your ability to swallow. Avoid eating for at least 1 hour after you have used this drug. You should also avoid chewing gum while using this medication.

What special precautions should I follow?

Before using lidocaine viscous,
- tell your doctor and pharmacist if you are allergic to lidocaine, anesthetics, or any other drugs.
- tell your doctor and pharmacist what prescription and nonprescription medications you are taking, including vitamins.
- tell your doctor if you are pregnant, plan to become pregnant, or are breast-feeding. If you become pregnant while taking lidocaine, call your doctor.

What should I do if I forget to take a dose?

Apply the missed dose as soon as you remember it. However, if it is almost time for the next dose, skip the missed dose and continue your regular dosing schedule. Do not use a double dose to make up for a missed one.

What side effects can this medicine cause?

Lidocaine viscous may cause side effects. If you experience any of the following symptoms, call your doctor immediately:
- drowsiness
- blurred or double vision
- shakiness
- irregular heartbeat
- vomiting
- seizures or convulsions
- ringing in the ears
- rash
- severe itching or burning

If you experience a serious side effect, you or your doctor may send a report to the Food and Drug Administration's (FDA) MedWatch Adverse Event Reporting program online [at http://www.fda.gov/MedWatch/index.html] or by phone [1-800-332-1088].

What storage conditions are needed for this medicine?

Keep this medication in the container it came in, tightly closed, and out of reach of children. Store it at room temperature and away from excess heat and moisture (not in the bathroom). Throw away any medication that is outdated or no longer needed. Talk to your pharmacist about the proper disposal of your medication.

What other information should I know?

Keep all appointments with your doctor.

Do not let anyone else take your medication. Ask your pharmacist any questions you have about refilling your prescription.

Talk to your doctor, pharmacist, or other healthcare professional if you have questions about dosing information for your medication.

Lindane

(lin′ dane)

Important Warning

Lindane cures lice and scabies, but it may cause serious side effects. Safer medications are available to treat these conditions. You should only use lindane if there is some reason you cannot use the other medications or if you have tried the other medications and they have not worked.

In rare cases, lindane has caused seizures and death. Most patients who experienced these severe side effects used too much lindane or used lindane too often or for too long, but a few patients experienced these problems even though they used lindane according to the directions. Babies; children; older people; people who weigh less than 110 lbs; and people who have skin conditions such as psoriasis, rashes, crusty scabby skin, or broken skin are more likely to experience the dangerous effects of lindane. These people should use lindane only if a doctor decides it is really needed.

Lindane should not be used to treat premature babies or people who have or have ever had seizures, especially if the seizures are hard to control.

Lindane is poisonous if too much is used or if it is used for too long or too often. Your doctor will tell you exactly how to use lindane. Follow these directions carefully. Do not use more lindane or leave the lindane on for a longer time than you are told. Do not use a second treatment of lindane even if you still have symptoms. You may be itchy for several weeks after your lice or scabies are killed.

Why is this medicine prescribed?

Lindane is used to cure infestations of scabies (small bugs that crawl under the skin and cause severe itching) and lice (small bugs that attach themselves to the skin on the head or pubic area ('crabs') and lay eggs called nits in the hair). Lindane is in a class of medications called scabicides and pediculicides. It works by killing the bugs and their eggs.

Lindane does not stop you from getting scabies or lice. You should only use lindane if you already have these conditions, not if you are afraid that you may become infested.

How should this medicine be used?

Lindane comes as a lotion to apply to the skin and a shampoo to apply to the hair and scalp. It should only be used once and then should not be used again. Follow the directions on the package or on your prescription label carefully, and ask your doctor or pharmacist to explain any part you do not understand. Use lindane exactly as directed. Do not use more or less of it or use it more often than directed by your doctor.

Before using lindane, ask your pharmacist or doctor for a copy of the manufacturer's information for the patient and read it carefully.

Lindane should only be used on the skin and hair. Never apply lindane to your mouth and never swallow it. Avoid getting lindane into your eyes.

When you apply lindane to yourself or someone else, wear gloves made of nitrile, sheer vinyl, or latex with neoprene. Do not wear gloves made of natural latex because they will not prevent lindane from reaching your skin. Throw away your gloves and wash your hands well when you are finished.

After using lindane, sanitize all the clothing, underwear, pajamas, sheets, pillowcases, and towels you have used recently. These items should be washed in very hot water or dry-cleaned.

Itching may still occur after successful treatment. Do not reapply lindane.

Lindane lotion is used only to treat scabies. Do not use it to treat lice. To use the lotion, follow these steps:
1. Your fingernails should be trimmed short and your skin should be clean, dry, and free of other oils, lotions, or creams. If you need to bathe or shower, wait 1 hour before applying lindane to allow your skin to cool.
2. Shake the lotion well.
3. Put some lotion on a toothbrush. Use the toothbrush to apply the lotion under your fingernails. Wrap the toothbrush in paper and throw it away. Do not use this toothbrush to brush your teeth because it may harm you.
4. Apply a thin layer of lotion all over your skin from your neck down to your toes (including the soles of your feet). You might not need all the lotion in the bottle.
5. Close the lindane bottle tightly and throw it away in a trashcan that is out of the reach of children. Do not save leftover lotion to use later.
6. You may dress in loose fitting clothing, but do not wear tight or plastic clothing or cover your skin with blankets.

Do not put plastic lined diapers on a baby who is being treated.

7. Leave the lotion on your skin for 8-12 hours, but no longer. If you leave the lotion on longer, it will not kill any more scabies, but it may cause seizures or other serious problems. Do not let anyone else touch your skin during this time. Other people may be harmed if their skin touches the lotion on your skin.

8. After 8-12 hours have passed, wash off all of the lotion with warm water. Do not use hot water.

Lindane shampoo is used only for pubic lice (crabs) and head lice. Do not use the shampoo if you have scabies. To use the shampoo, follow these steps:

1. Wash your hair with your regular shampoo at least 1 hour before applying lindane and dry it thoroughly. Do not use any creams, oils, or conditioners.

2. Shake the shampoo well. Apply just enough shampoo to make your hair, scalp, and the small hairs on the back of your neck wet. If you have pubic lice, apply the shampoo to the hair in your pubic area and the skin underneath. You might not need all of the shampoo in the bottle.

3. Close the lindane bottle tightly and throw it away in a trashcan that is out of the reach of children. Do not save leftover shampoo to use later.

4. Leave the lindane shampoo on your hair for exactly 4 minutes. Keep track of the time with a watch or clock. If you leave the lotion on for longer than 4 minutes, it will not kill any more lice, but it may cause seizures or other serious problems. Keep your hair uncovered during this time.

5. At the end of 4 minutes, use a small amount of warm water to lather the shampoo. Do not use hot water.

6. Wash all of the shampoo off of your hair and skin with warm water.

7. Dry your hair with a clean towel.

8. Comb your hair with a fine tooth comb (nit comb) or use tweezers to remove nits (lice eggs and larvae). You will probably need to ask someone to help you with this, especially if you have head lice.

Are there other uses for this medicine?

This medication should not be prescribed for other uses; ask your doctor or pharmacist for more information.

What special precautions should I follow?

Before using lindane,
- tell your doctor and pharmacist if you are allergic to lindane or any other medications.
- tell your doctor and pharmacist what prescription and nonprescription medications, vitamins, nutritional supplements, and herbal products you are taking. Be sure to mention any of the following: antidepressants (mood elevators); antibiotics such as cinoxacin (Cinobac), ciprofloxacin (Cipro), enoxacin (Penetrex), gatifloxacin (Tequin), imipenem/cilastin (Primaxin), levofloxacin (Levaquin), lomefloxacin (Maxequin), moxifloxacin (Avelox), nalidixic acid (NegGram), norfloxacin (Noroxin), ofloxacin (Floxin), penicillin, sparfloxacin (Zagam) and trovofloxacin and alatrofloxacin combination (Trovan); chloroquine sulfate; isoniazid (INH, Laniazid, Nydrazid); medications for mental illness; medications that suppress the immune system such as cyclosporine (Neoral, Sandimmune), mycophenolate mofetil (CellCept), and tacrolimus (Prograf); mepiridine (Demerol); methocarbamol (Robaxin); neostigmine (Prostigmin); pyridostigmine (Mestinon, Regonol); pyrimethamine (Daraprim), radiographic dyes; sedatives; sleeping pills; tacrine (Cognex); and theophylline (TheoDur, Theobid). Your doctor may need to change the doses of your medications or monitor you carefully for side effects.

- in addition to the conditions mentioned in the IMPORTANT WARNING section, tell your doctor if you have or have ever had human immunodeficiency virus (HIV) or acquired immunodeficiency syndrome (AIDS); seizures; a head injury; a tumor in your brain or spine; or liver disease. Also tell your doctor if you drink, used to drink, or have recently stopped drinking large amounts of alcohol and if you have recently stopped using sedatives (sleeping pills).

- tell your doctor if you are pregnant or are breast-feeding. If you are pregnant, wear gloves when applying lindane to another person to prevent its absorption through your skin. If you are breast-feeding, pump and discard your milk for 24 hours after you use lindane. Feed your baby stored breastmilk or formula during this time, and do not allow your baby's skin to touch the lindane on your skin.

- tell your doctor if you have recently used lindane.

- if you have scabies or pubic lice, tell your doctor if you have a sexual partner. This person should also be treated so he or she will not reinfect you. If you have head lice, all people who live in your household or who have been in close contact with you may need to be treated. Do not share your medication with other people because it may harm them.

What special dietary instructions should I follow?

Unless your doctor tells you otherwise, continue your normal diet.

What side effects can this medicine cause?

Lindane may cause side effects. Tell your doctor if any of these symptoms are severe or do not go away:
- skin rash
- itching or burning skin
- dry skin
- numbness or tingling of the skin
- hair loss

Some side effects can be serious. The following symptoms are uncommon, but if you experience any of them, call your doctor immediately:

- headache
- dizziness
- drowsiness
- shaking of your body that you cannot control
- seizures

Lindane may cause other side effects. Call your doctor if you have any unusual problems while taking this medication.

If you experience a serious side effect, you or your doctor may send a report to the Food and Drug Administration's (FDA) MedWatch Adverse Event Reporting program online [at http://www.fda.gov/MedWatch/index.html] or by phone [1-800-332-1088].

What storage conditions are needed for this medicine?

Keep this medication in the container it came in, tightly closed, and out of reach of children. Store it at room temperature and away from excess heat and moisture (not in the bathroom). Throw away any medication that is outdated or that remains after treatment. Talk to your pharmacist about the proper disposal of your medication.

What should I do in case of overdose?

In case of overdose, call your local poison control center at 1-800-222-1222. If the victim has collapsed or is not breathing, call local emergency services at 911.

If you accidentally get lindane in your mouth, call your local poison control center right away to find out how to get emergency help. If lindane gets into your eyes, wash them with water right away and get medical help if they are still irritated after washing.

What other information should I know?

Keep all appointments with your doctor.

Do not let anyone else use your medication. Your prescription is not refillable. See your doctor if you feel you need additional treatment.

Dosage Facts
For Informational Purposes

Caution: Do not change your dose, how often you take your medication, or the length of time you are to take it without first talking to your healthcare provider.

The following dosage information was written using medical language for doctors and other healthcare professionals and is provided here for you to check your dosage. The dosage of this drug may differ for different patients. Therefore, always follow your doctor's instructions or the directions on the label. Contact your healthcare provider or pharmacist if you have any questions

about the specific dosage of your medication after reviewing this information.

Pediatric Patients

Use with caution in children weighing <50 kg, especially infants.

Pediculosis

TOPICAL:
- Children ≥2 years of age: Apply about 30–60 mL of shampoo once to hair; amount of shampoo needed depends on the length of the hair (most patients require only 30 mL). After 4 minutes, add small quantities of water to the hair to form a good lather and then immediately and thoroughly rinse hair until all the lather is gone.
- Because of concerns about neurotoxicity, retreatment with lindane is not recommended.

Scabies

TOPICAL:
- Children ≥2 years of age: Apply lotion once into *all* skin surfaces (entire trunk and extremities) from the neck to the toes (including the soles of the feet).
- After 8–12 hours, lotion must be completely washed off the body using warm (not hot) water. Do *not* leave on the skin for >12 hours.
- Because of concerns about neurotoxicity, retreatment with lindane is not recommended.

Adult Patients

Pediculosis

TOPICAL:
- Apply about 30–60 mL of shampoo once to hair; amount of shampoo needed depends on the length of the hair (most patients require only 30 mL). After 4 minutes, add small quantities of water to the hair to form a good lather and then immediately and thoroughly rinse hair until all the lather is gone.
- Because of concerns about neurotoxicity, retreatment with lindane is not recommended.

Scabies

TOPICAL:
- Apply lotion once into *all* skin surfaces (entire trunk and extremities) from the neck to the toes (including the soles of the feet).
- Approximately 30 mL of the lotion is recommended for an average adult.
- After 8–12 hours, lotion must be completely washed off the body using warm (not hot) water. Do *not* leave on the skin for >12 hours.
- Because of concerns about neurotoxicity, retreatment with lindane is not recommended.

Prescribing Limits

Pediatric Patients

Pediculosis

TOPICAL:
- Children ≥2 years of age: Do *not* leave shampoo in the hair for >4 minutes and do not retreat.

Scabies

TOPICAL:
- Children ≥2 years of age: Do *not* leave lotion on the skin for >12 hours and do not retreat.

Adult Patients

Pediculosis

TOPICAL:
- Do *not* leave shampoo in the hair for >4 minutes and do not retreat.

Scabies

TOPICAL:
- Do *not* leave lotion on the skin for >12 hours and do not retreat.

Special Populations

Hepatic Impairment
- No specific dosage recommendations.

Renal Impairment
- No specific dosage recommendations.

Geriatric Patients
- No specific dosage recommendations.

Linezolid

(li ne′ zoh lid)

Brand Name: Zyvox®

Why is this medicine prescribed?

Linezolid is used to treat infections, including pneumonia, urinary tract infections, and infections of the skin and blood. Linezolid is in a class of antibacterials called oxazolidinones. It works by stopping the growth of bacteria.

How should this medicine be used?

Linezolid comes as a tablet and oral suspension (liquid) to take by mouth. It is usually taken with or without food twice a day (every 12 hours) for 10 to 28 days. Follow the directions on your prescription label carefully, and ask your doctor or pharmacist to explain any part you do not understand. Take linezolid exactly as directed. Do not take more or less of it or take it more often than prescribed by your doctor.

Before using the oral suspension, gently mix it by turning over the bottle three to five times. Do not shake.

Continue to take linezolid even if you feel well. Do not stop taking linezolid without talking to your doctor.

Are there other uses for this medicine?

This medication may be prescribed for other uses; ask your doctor or pharmacist for more information.

What special precautions should I follow?

Before taking linezolid,
- tell your doctor and pharmacist if you are allergic to linezolid or any other medications.
- tell your doctor and pharmacist what prescription and nonprescription medications, vitamins, nutritional supplements, and herbal products you are taking. Be sure to mention any of the following: antidepressants; cancer chemotherapy; cold remedies or decongestants containing pseudoephedrine or phenylpropanolamine; medications for migraine such as frovatriptan (Frova), naratriptan (Amerge), rizatriptan (Maxalt), sumatriptan (Imitrex), and zolmitriptan (Zomig); other antibiotics; and selective serotonin reuptake inhibitors (SSRIs) such as citalopram (Celexa), fluoxetine (Prozac, Sarafem), fluvoxamine (Luvox), paroxetine (Paxil), and sertraline (Zoloft). Your doctor may need to change the doses of your medications or monitor you carefully for side effects.
- tell your doctor if you have or have ever had high blood pressure, carcinoids, a tumor of the adrenal gland (pheochromocytoma), an overactive thyroid, or phenylketonuria.
- tell your doctor if you are pregnant, plan to become pregnant, or are breast-feeding. If you become pregnant while taking linezolid, call your doctor.

What special dietary instructions should I follow?

Avoid eating or drinking large amounts of foods and beverages containing tyramine while taking linezolid. These foods and beverages include alcoholic beverages, especially beer, Chianti, and other red wines; alcohol-free beer; cheeses (especially strong, aged, or processed varieties); sauerkraut; yogurt; raisins; bananas; sour cream; pickled herring; liver (especially chicken liver); dry sausage (including hard salami and pepperoni); canned figs; avocados; soy sauce; turkey; yeast extracts; papaya products (including certain meat tenderizers); fava beans; and broad bean pods.

What should I do if I forget to take a dose?

Take the missed dose as soon as you remember it. However, if it is almost time for the next dose, skip the missed dose and continue your regular dosing schedule. Do not take a double dose to make up for a missed one.

What side effects can this medicine cause?

Linezolid may cause side effects. Tell your doctor if any of these symptoms are severe or do not go away:
- diarrhea
- headache
- upset stomach
- vomiting
- difficulty falling asleep or staying asleep
- constipation

- rash
- dizziness
- fever

Some side effects can be serious. The following symptoms are uncommon, but if you experience any of them, call your doctor immediately:

- severe diarrhea
- fever, sore throat, and other signs of infection
- unusual bleeding or bruising
- pale skin
- lack of energy

Linezolid may cause other side effects. Call your doctor if you have any unusual problems while taking this medication.

If you experience a serious side effect, you or your doctor may send a report to the Food and Drug Administration's (FDA) MedWatch Adverse Event Reporting program online [at http://www.fda.gov/MedWatch/index.html] or by phone [1-800-332-1088].

What storage conditions are needed for this medicine?

Keep this medication in the container it came in, tightly closed, and out of reach of children. Store it at room temperature and away from excess heat and moisture (not in the bathroom). Throw away any medication that is outdated or no longer needed. The suspension should be used within 21 days. Talk to your pharmacist about the proper disposal of your medication.

What should I do in case of overdose?

In case of overdose, call your local poison control center at 1-800-222-1222. If the victim has collapsed or is not breathing, call local emergency services at 911.

What other information should I know?

Keep all appointments with your doctor and the laboratory. Your doctor will order certain blood tests to check your body's response to linezolid.

Do not let anyone else take your medication. Your prescription is probably not refillable. If you still have symptoms of infection after you finish the linezolid, call your doctor.

Dosage Facts
For Informational Purposes

Caution: Do not change your dose, how often you take your medication, or the length of time you are to take it without first talking to your healthcare provider.

The following dosage information was written using medical language for doctors and other healthcare professionals and is provided here for you to check your dosage. The dosage of this drug may differ for different patients. Therefore, always follow your doctor's instructions or the directions on the label. Contact your healthcare provider or pharmacist if you have any questions about the specific dosage of your medication after reviewing this information.

General Dosage Information

Safety and efficacy of >28 days of treatment have not been established.

Pediatric Patients

General Dosage for Neonates <7 Days of Age

ORAL:
- 10 mg/kg every 12 hours initially; consider 10 mg/kg every 8 hours in neonates with an inadequate response to the lower dosage. By 7 days of age, all neonates should receive 10 mg/kg every 8 hours.

Vancomycin-resistant Enterococcus faecium Infections

ORAL:
- Children 7 days through 11 years of age: 10 mg/kg every 8 hours for 14–28 days.
- Children ≥12 years of age: 600 mg every 12 hours for 14–28 days.

Respiratory Tract Infections
Nosocomial or Community-acquired Pneumonia

ORAL:
- Children 7 days through 11 years of age: 10 mg/kg every 8 hours for 10–14 days.
- Children ≥12 years of age: 600 mg every 12 hours for 10–14 days.

Skin and Skin Structure Infections
Uncomplicated Infections

ORAL:
- Children 7 days through 4 years of age: 10 mg/kg every 8 hours for 10–14 days.
- Children 5–11 years of age: 10 mg/kg every 12 hours for 10–14 days.
- Children ≥12 years of age: 600 mg every 12 hours for 10–14 days.

Complicated Infections

ORAL:
- Children 7 days through 11 years of age: 10 mg/kg every 8 hours for 10–14 days.
- Children ≥12 years of age: 600 mg every 12 hours for 10–14 days.

Adult Patients

Vancomycin-resistant Enterococcus faecium Infections

ORAL:
- 600 mg every 12 hours for 14–28 days.

Respiratory Tract Infections
Nosocomial or Community-acquired Pneumonia

ORAL:
- 600 mg every 12 hours for 10–14 days.

Skin and Skin Structure Infections
Uncomplicated Infections
ORAL:
- 400 mg every 12 hours for 10–14 days.

Complicated Infections
ORAL:
- 600 mg every 12 hours for 10–14 days.

Special Populations
Hepatic Impairment
- No dosage adjustments necessary in mild to moderate hepatic impairment; use with caution in severe impairment.

Renal Impairment
- No dosage adjustments recommended. Use with caution since metabolites may accumulate.
- For hemodialysis patients, administer after dialysis session.

Geriatric Patients
- Dosage adjustments not required.

Liothyronine

(lye oh thye′ roe neen)

Brand Name: Cytomel®
Also available generically.

> ## Important Warning
>
> Thyroid hormone should not be used to treat obesity in patients with normal thyroid function. Liothyronine is ineffective for weight reduction in normal thyroid patients and may cause serious or life-threatening toxicity, especially when taken with amphetamines. Talk to your doctor about the potential risks associated with this medication.

Why is this medicine prescribed?

Liothyronine, a thyroid hormone, is used to treat hypothyroidism, a condition where the thyroid gland does not produce enough thyroid hormone. Without this hormone, the body cannot function properly, resulting in poor growth, slow speech, lack of energy, weight gain, hair loss, dry thick skin, and increased sensitivity to cold. When taken correctly, liothyronine reverses these symptoms. Liothyronine is also used to treat goiter (enlarged thyroid gland) and to test for hyperthyroidism (a condition where the thyroid gland produces too much thyroid hormone).

How should this medicine be used?

Liothyronine comes as a tablet to take by mouth. It usually is taken as a single dose before breakfast every day. To con-
trol the symptoms of hypothyroidism you probably will need to take this medicine for the rest of your life. It may take about 2 weeks before you notice any change in your symptoms. Follow the directions on your prescription label carefully, and ask your doctor or pharmacist to explain any part you do not understand. Take liothyronine exactly as directed. Do not take more or less of it or take it more often than prescribed by your doctor.

Continue to take liothyronine even if you feel well. Do not stop taking liothyronine without talking to your doctor.

Are there other uses for this medicine?

This medication may be prescribed for other conditions; ask your doctor or pharmacist for more information.

What special precautions should I follow?

Before taking liothyronine,
- tell your doctor and pharmacist if you are allergic to liothyronine, thyroid hormone, or any other drugs.
- tell your doctor and pharmacist what prescription and nonprescription medications you are taking, especially amphetamines; antacids; anticancer medicines; anticoagulants ('blood thinners') such as warfarin (Coumadin); antidepressants or anti-anxiety agents; arthritis medications; aspirin; beta-blockers such as metoprolol (Lopressor, Toprol), propranolol (Inderal), or timolol (Blocadren, Timoptic); cholesterol-lowering resins such as cholestyramine (Questran) or colestipol (Colestid); diabetes medications (insulin and tablets); digoxin (Lanoxin); estrogens; iron; methadone; oral contraceptives; phenytoin (Dilantin); sodium polystyrene sulfonate (Kayexalate); steroids; sucralfate (Carafate); theophylline (TheoDur); and vitamins.
- if you take cholestyramine (Questran) or colestipol (Colestid), take it at least 4 hours before or 1 hour after taking liothyronine.
- tell your doctor if you have or have ever had diabetes; kidney disease; hepatitis; cardiovascular disease such as high blood pressure, hardening of the arteries (atherosclerosis), chest pain (angina), arrhythmias, or heart attack; or an underactive adrenal or pituitary gland.
- tell your doctor if you are pregnant, plan to become pregnant, or are breast-feeding. If you become pregnant while taking liothyronine, call your doctor.
- if you have surgery, including dental surgery, tell the doctor or dentist that you are taking liothyronine.

What special dietary instructions should I follow?

Unless your doctor tells you otherwise, continue your normal diet.

What should I do if I forget to take a dose?

Take the missed dose as soon as you remember it. However, if it is almost time for the next dose, skip the missed dose

and continue your regular dosing schedule. Do not take a double dose to make up for a missed one.

What side effects can this medicine cause?

Liothyronine may cause side effects. Tell your doctor if any of these symptoms are severe or do not go away:

- weight loss
- tremor
- headache
- upset stomach
- vomiting
- diarrhea
- stomach cramps
- nervousness
- irritability
- insomnia
- excessive sweating
- increased appetite
- fever
- changes in menstrual cycle
- sensitivity to heat
- temporary hair loss, particularly in children during the first month of therapy

If you experience either of the following symptoms, call your doctor immediately:

- chest pain (angina)
- rapid or irregular heartbeat or pulse

If you experience a serious side effect, you or your doctor may send a report to the Food and Drug Administration's (FDA) MedWatch Adverse Event Reporting program online [at http://www.fda.gov/MedWatch/index.html] or by phone [1-800-332-1088].

What storage conditions are needed for this medicine?

Keep this medication in the container it came in, tightly closed, and out of reach of children. Store it at room temperature and away from excess heat and moisture (not in the bathroom). Throw away any medication that is outdated or no longer needed. Talk to your pharmacist about the proper disposal of your medication.

What should I do in case of overdose?

In case of overdose, call your local poison control center at 1-800-222-1222. If the victim has collapsed or is not breathing, call local emergency services at 911.

What other information should I know?

Keep all appointments with your doctor and the laboratory. Your doctor will order certain lab tests to check your response to liothyronine.

Do not let anyone else take your medication. Ask your pharmacist any questions you have about refilling your prescription.

Dosage Facts

For Informational Purposes

Caution: Do not change your dose, how often you take your medication, or the length of time you are to take it without first talking to your healthcare provider.

The following dosage information was written using medical language for doctors and other healthcare professionals and is provided here for you to check your dosage. The dosage of this drug may differ for different patients. Therefore, always follow your doctor's instructions or the directions on the label. Contact your healthcare provider or pharmacist if you have any questions about the specific dosage of your medication after reviewing this information.

General Dosage Information

Available as liothyronine sodium; dosage expressed in terms of liothyronine.

Adjust dosage carefully according to clinical and laboratory response to treatment. Avoid undertreatment or overtreatment.

Initiate dosage at a lower level in geriatric patients, in patients with functional or ECG evidence of cardiovascular disease, and in patients with severe, long-standing hypothyroidism.

Pediatric Patients

Hypothyroidism

ORAL:

- Initiate therapy at full replacement dosages as soon as possible after diagnosis of hypothyroidism to prevent deleterious effects on intellectual and physical growth and development; initiate dosage at a lower level in children with long-standing or severe hypothyroidism.
- Initially, 5 mcg daily; increase by 5 mcg daily every 3–4 days until desired response is obtained.
- 20 mcg daily may be required for maintenance in infants, 50 mcg daily may be required for children ≥1 year of age, and full adult dosage may be required for children ≥3 years of age.
- When *transient* hypothyroidism is suspected, therapy may be temporarily discontinued when the child is >3 years of age to reassess the condition.

Adult Patients

Hypothyroidism
Mild Hypothyroidism

ORAL:

- Initially, 25 mcg daily. May increase by 12.5–25 mcg every 1–2 weeks until desired response is obtained. Usual maintenance dose is 25–75 mcg daily.

Severe Hypothyroidism

Initially, 5 mcg daily; may increase by 5–10 mcg every 1–2 weeks until desired response is obtained. Usual maintenance dose is 50–100 mcg daily.

Pituitary TSH Suppression
Nontoxic Goiter

ORAL:
- Initially, 5 mcg daily; may increase by 5–10 mcg daily every 1–2 weeks until a dosage of 25 mcg daily is reached. Thereafter, increase by 12.5–25 mcg every 1–2 weeks until desired response is obtained. Usual maintenance dose is 75 mcg daily.

T₃ Suppression Test

ORAL:
- 75–100 mcg daily for 7 days.

Special Populations

Hepatic Impairment
- No specific dosage recommendations at this time.

Renal Impairment
- No specific dosage recommendations at this time.

Patients with Cardiovascular Disease

Hypothyroidism

Oral
- Initiate at lower doses than those recommended in patients without cardiovascular disease. Initially 5 mcg daily; increase by ≤5mcg increments every 2 weeks. If cardiovascular symptoms develop or worsen, reduce dosage.

Geriatric Patients
- Select dosage with caution and at the lower end of usual range because of age-related decreases in hepatic, renal, and/or cardiac function and concomitant disease and drug therapy. In general, use lower doses.

Hypothyroidism

Oral
- Initially 5 mcg daily; may increase by 5 mcg daily every 1–2 weeks until desired response is obtained.

Lisdexamfetamine

(lis dex'' am fet a meen)

Brand Name: Vyvanse

Important Warning

Lisdexamfetamine can be habit-forming. Do not take a larger dose, take it more often, take it for a longer time, or take it in a different way than prescribed by your doctor. If you take too much lisdexamfetamine, you may find that the medication no longer controls your symptoms, you may feel a need to take large amounts of the medication, and you may experience symptoms such as rash, difficulty falling asleep or staying asleep, irritability, hyperactivity, and unusual changes in your personality or behavior. Tell your doctor if you drink or have ever drunk large amounts of alcohol, use or have ever used street drugs, or have overused prescription medications.

Do not stop taking lisdexamfetamine without talking to your doctor, especially if you have overused the medication. Your doctor will probably decrease your dose gradually and monitor you carefully during this time. You may develop severe depression and extreme tiredness if you suddenly stop taking lisdexamfetamine after overusing it.

Do not let anyone else take your medication. Store lisdexamfetamine in a safe place so that no one else can take it accidentally or on purpose. Keep track of how many tablets or capsules are left so you will know if any are missing.

Lisdexamfetamine may cause sudden death or serious heart problems, especially if the medication is misused.

Your doctor or pharmacist will give you the manufacturer's patient information sheet (Medication Guide) when you begin treatment with lisdexamfetamine and each time you refill your prescription. Read the information carefully and ask your doctor or pharmacist if you have any questions. You can also visit the Food and Drug Administration (FDA) website (http://www.fda.gov/cder) or the manufacturer's website to obtain the Medication Guide.

Why is this medicine prescribed?

Lisdexamfetamine is used as part of a treatment program for attention deficit hyperactivity disorder (ADHD; more difficulty focusing, controlling actions, and remaining still or quiet than other people who are the same age). Lisdexamfetamine is in a class of medications called central nervous system stimulants. It works by changing the amounts of certain natural substances in the brain.

How should this medicine be used?

Lisdexamfetamine comes as a capsule to be taken by mouth. The capsule is usually taken once a day in the morning with or without food. Take lisdexamfetamine at around the same time every day. Do not take lisdexamfetamine in the late afternoon or evening because it may cause difficulty falling asleep or staying asleep. Follow the directions on your prescription label carefully, and ask your doctor or pharmacist to explain any part you do not understand. Take lisdexamfetamine exactly as directed.

You may swallow the capsule whole, or you may open the capsule and sprinkle the entire contents into a glass of water. Drink the mixture right away. Do not store the water/capsule mixture for future use, and do not divide the contents of one capsule into more than one dose.

Your doctor will probably start you on a low dose of lisdexamfetamine and increase your dose gradually, not more often than once every week.

Your doctor may tell you to stop taking lisdexamfetamine from time to time to see if the medication is still needed. Follow these directions carefully.

Are there other uses for this medicine?

This medication may be prescribed for other uses; ask your doctor or pharmacist for more information.

What special precautions should I follow?

Before taking lisdexamfetamine,

- tell your doctor and pharmacist if you are allergic to amphetamine (in Adderall), benzphetamine (Didrex), dextroamphetamine (in Adderall, Dexedrine, Dextrostat), methamphetamine (Desoxyn) or any other medications.
- tell your doctor if you are taking monoamine oxidase (MAO) inhibitors, including isocarboxazid (Marplan), phenelzine (Nardil), selegiline (Eldepryl, Emsam, Zelapar), and tranylcypromine (Parnate), or if you have stopped taking them during the past 14 days. Your doctor will probably tell you not to take lisdexamfetamine until at least 14 days have passed since you last took an MAO inhibitor.
- tell your doctor and pharmacist what other prescription and nonprescription medications, vitamins, nutritional supplements, and herbal products you are taking. Be sure to mention any of the following: alpha blockers such as alfuzosin (Uroxatral), doxazosin (Cardura), prazosin (Minipress), tamsulosin (Flomax), and terazosin (Hytrin); antidepressants ('mood elevators'), antihistamines; beta blockers such as atenolol (Tenormin), labetalol (Normodyne), metoprolol (Lopressor, Toprol XL), nadolol (Corgard), and propranolol (Inderal); chlorpromazine (Thorazine); diuretics ('water pills') such as acetazolamide (Diamox); haloperidol (Haldol); lithium (Lithobid, Eskalith); narcotic medications for pain; medications for asthma, colds, and high blood pressure; certain medications for seizures such as ethosuximide (Zarontin), phenobarbital, and phenytoin (Dilantin); meperidine (Demerol); methenamine (Hiprex, Urex); propoxyphene (Darvon, Darvon-N); and sodium phosphate. Your doctor may need to change the doses of your medications or monitor you carefully for side effects.
- tell your doctor if you have glaucoma (an eye disease), hyperthyroidism (condition in which there is too much thyroid hormone in the body), or feelings of anxiety, tension, or agitation. Your doctor may tell you not to take lisdexamfetamine.
- tell your doctor if anyone in your family has or has ever had an irregular heartbeat or has died suddenly. Also tell your doctor if you have recently had a heart attack and if you have or have ever had a heart defect, high blood pressure, an irregular heartbeat, heart or blood vessel disease, or other heart problems. Your doctor will probably examine you to see if your heart and blood vessels are healthy before you start taking lisdexamfe-

tamine and will check your heart and blood pressure regularly during your treatment with lisdexamfetamine. Your doctor may tell you not to take lisdexamfetamine if you have a heart condition or if there is a high risk that you may develop a heart condition.
- tell your doctor if you or anyone in your family has or has ever had depression, bipolar disorder (mood that changes from depressed to abnormally excited), or mania (frenzied, abnormally excited mood), motor tics (repeated uncontrollable movements), verbal tics (repetition of sounds or words that is hard to control), or Tourette's syndrome (a condition characterized by the need to perform repeated motions or to repeat sounds or words), or has thought about or attempted suicide. Also tell your doctor if you have or have ever had mental illness, seizures, or an abnormal electroencephalogram (EEG; a test that measures electrical activity in the brain).
- tell your doctor if you are pregnant, plan to become pregnant, or are breast-feeding. If you become pregnant while taking lisdexamfetamine, call your doctor. You should not breastfeed while you are taking this medication.
- you should know that this medication may make it difficult for you to perform activities that require alertness or physical coordination. Do not drive a car or operate machinery until you know how this medication affects you.
- you should know that lisdexamfetamine should be used as part of a total treatment program for ADHD, which may include counseling and special education. Make sure to follow all of your doctor's and/or therapist's instructions.

What special dietary instructions should I follow?

Unless your doctor tells you otherwise, continue your normal diet.

What should I do if I forget to take a dose?

Take the missed dose as soon as you remember it. However, if it is almost time for the next dose, skip the missed dose and continue your regular dosing schedule. Do not take a double dose to make up for a missed one.

What side effects can this medicine cause?

Lisdexamfetamine may cause side effects. Tell your doctor if any of these symptoms are severe or do not go away:
- restlessness
- mood swings
- irritability
- difficulty falling asleep or staying asleep
- uncontrollable shaking of a part of the body
- dizziness
- headache
- dry mouth

- stomach pain
- nausea
- vomiting
- loss of appetite
- weight loss
- fever

Some side effects can be serious. If you experience any of these symptoms call your doctor immediately:

- fast or pounding heartbeat
- chest pain
- shortness of breath
- fainting
- seizures
- hallucinating (seeing things or hearing voices that do not exist)
- aggression
- frenzied, abnormally excited mood
- seizures
- tics
- blisters
- rash

Lisdexamfetamine may cause sudden death in children and teenagers who have heart defects or serious heart problems. This medication also may cause sudden death, heart attack or stroke in adults, especially adults with heart defects or serious heart problems. Talk to your doctor about the risks of taking this medication.

Lisdexamfetamine may slow children's growth or weight gain. Your child's doctor will watch his or her growth carefully. Talk to your child's doctor if you have concerns about your child's growth or weight gain while he or she is taking this medication. Talk to your child's doctor about the risks of giving lisdexamfetamine to your child.

Lisdexamfetamine may cause other side effects. Call your doctor if you have any unusual problems while taking this medication.

What storage conditions are needed for this medicine?

Keep this medication in the container it came in, tightly closed, and out of reach of children. Store it at room temperature and away from excess heat and moisture (not in the bathroom). Throw away any medication that is outdated or no longer needed. Talk to your pharmacist about the proper disposal of your medication.

What should I do in case of overdose?

In case of overdose, call your local poison control center at 1-800-222-1222. If the victim has collapsed or is not breathing, call local emergency services at 911.

Symptoms of overdose may include:

- restlessness
- confusion
- aggressive behavior
- feelings of panic

- hallucination (seeing things or hearing voices that do not exist)
- fast breathing
- uncontrollable shaking of a part of the body
- fever
- muscle weakness or aching
- tirednessor weakness
- depression
- fast or irregular heartbeat
- fainting
- dizziness
- blurred vision
- nausea
- vomiting
- diarrhea
- stomach cramps
- seizures
- coma (loss of consciousness for a period of time)

What other information should I know?

Keep all appointments with your doctor and the laboratory. Your doctor may order certain lab tests to check your body's response to lisdexamfetamine.

Before having any laboratory test, tell your doctor and the laboratory personnel that you are taking lisdexamfetamine.

This prescription is not refillable. Be sure to schedule appointments with your doctor on a regular basis so that you do not run out of medication.

Talk to your doctor, pharmacist, or other healthcare professional if you have questions about dosing information for your medication.

Lisinopril

(lyse in′ oh pril)

Brand Name: Prinivil®, Zestril®
Also available generically.

Important Warning
Do not take lisinopril if you are pregnant. If you become pregnant while taking lisinopril, call your doctor immediately. Lisinopril may harm the fetus.

Why is this medicine prescribed?

Lisinopril is used alone or in combination with other medications to treat high blood pressure. It is used in combination with other medications to treat heart failure. Lisinopril is also used to improve survival after a heart attack. Lisinopril is in a class of medications called angiotensin-converting enzyme (ACE) inhibitors. It works by decreasing certain chemicals that tighten the blood vessels, so blood flows more smoothly and the heart can pump blood more efficiently.

How should this medicine be used?

Lisinopril comes as a tablet to take by mouth. It is usually taken once a day. To help you remember to take lisinopril, take it around the same time every day. Follow the directions on your prescription label carefully, and ask your doctor or pharmacist to explain any part you do not understand. Take lisinopril exactly as directed. Do not take more or less of it or take it more often than prescribed by your doctor.

Your doctor will probably start you on a low dose of lisinopril and gradually increase your dose.

Lisinopril controls high blood pressure and heart failure but does not cure them. Continue to take lisinopril even if you feel well. Do not stop taking lisinopril without talking to your doctor.

Are there other uses for this medicine?

This medication may be prescribed for other uses; ask your doctor or pharmacist for more information.

What special precautions should I follow?

Before taking lisinopril,

- tell your doctor and pharmacist if you are allergic to lisinopril, enalapril (Vasotec), benazepril (Lotensin), captopril (Capoten), fosinopril (Monopril), moexipril (Univasc), perindopril (Aceon), quinapril (Accupril), ramipril (Altace), trandolapril (Mavik), or any other medications.
- tell your doctor and pharmacist what prescription and nonprescription medications, vitamins, nutritional supplements, and herbal products you are taking. Be sure to mention any of the following: aspirin and other non-steroidal anti-inflammatory medications (NSAIDs) such as indomethacin (Indocin); diuretics ('water pills'); lithium (Eskalith, Lithobid); and potassium supplements. Your doctor may need to change the doses of your medications or monitor you carefully for side effects.
- tell your doctor if you have or have ever had heart or kidney disease; diabetes; lupus; scleroderma; or angio-edema, a condition that causes difficulty swallowing or breathing and painful swelling of the the face, throat, tongue, lips, eyes, hands, feet, ankles, or lower legs.
- tell your doctor if you plan to become pregnant or are breast-feeding.
- if you are having surgery, including dental surgery, tell the doctor or dentist that you are taking lisinopril.
- you should know that diarrhea, vomiting, not drinking enough fluids, and sweating a lot can cause a drop in blood pressure, which may cause lightheadedness and fainting.

What special dietary instructions should I follow?

Talk to your doctor before using salt substitutes containing potassium. If your doctor prescribes a low-salt or low-sodium diet, follow these directions carefully.

What should I do if I forget to take a dose?

Take the missed dose as soon as you remember it. However, if it is almost time for the next dose, skip the missed dose and continue your regular regular dosing schedule. Do not take a double dose to make up for a missed one.

What side effects can this medicine cause?

Lisinopril may cause side effects. Tell your doctor if any of these symptoms are severe or do not go away:

- cough
- dizziness
- headache
- excessive tiredness
- upset stomach
- diarrhea
- weakness
- sneezing
- runny nose
- decrease in sexual ability
- rash

Some side effects can be serious. The following symptoms are uncommon, but if you experience any of them, call your doctor immediately:

- swelling of the face, throat, tongue, lips, eyes, hands, feet, ankles, or lower legs
- hoarseness
- difficulty breathing or swallowing
- fever, sore throat, chills, and other signs of infection
- yellowing of the skin or eyes
- lightheadedness
- fainting
- chest pain

Lisinopril may cause other side effects. Call your doctor if you have any unusual problems while taking this medication.

If you experience a serious side effect, you or your doctor may send a report to the Food and Drug Administration's (FDA) MedWatch Adverse Event Reporting program online [at http://www.fda.gov/MedWatch/index.html] or by phone [1-800-332-1088].

What storage conditions are needed for this medicine?

Keep this medication in the container it came in, tightly closed, and out of reach of children. Store it at room temperature and away from excess heat and moisture (not in the bathroom). Throw away any medication that is outdated or no longer needed. Talk to your pharmacist about the proper disposal of your medication.

What should I do in case of overdose?

In case of overdose, call your local poison control center at 1-800-222-1222. If the victim has collapsed or is not breathing, call local emergency services at 911.

Symptoms of overdose may include:

- lightheadedness
- fainting

What other information should I know?

Keep all appointments with your doctor and the laboratory. Your blood pressure should be checked regularly to determine your response to lisinopril. Your doctor may order certain lab tests to check your body's response to lisinopril.

Do not let anyone else take your medication. Ask your pharmacist any questions you have about refilling your prescription.

Dosage Facts
For Informational Purposes

Caution: Do not change your dose, how often you take your medication, or the length of time you are to take it without first talking to your healthcare provider.

The following dosage information was written using medical language for doctors and other healthcare professionals and is provided here for you to check your dosage. The dosage of this drug may differ for different patients. Therefore, always follow your doctor's instructions or the directions on the label. Contact your healthcare provider or pharmacist if you have any questions about the specific dosage of your medication after reviewing this information.

Pediatric Patients

Hypertension

ORAL:

- Children ≥6 years of age: Initially, 0.07 mg/kg (up to 5 mg) once daily. Adjust dosage until the desired BP goal is achieved (up to maximum dosage of 0.61 mg/kg or 40 mg daily).

Adult Patients

Hypertension

ORAL:

- Initially, 10 mg once daily as monotherapy. Adjust dosage to achieve BP control.
- In patients currently receiving diuretic therapy, discontinue diuretic, if possible, 2–3 days before initiating lisinopril. May cautiously resume diuretic therapy if BP not controlled adequately with lisinopril alone. If diuretic cannot be discontinued, increase sodium intake and initiate lisinopril at 5 mg daily under close medical supervision for at least 2 hours and until BP has stabilized for at least an additional hour.
- Usual dosage: 10–40 mg once daily.

- If effectiveness diminishes toward end of dosing interval in patients treated once daily (particularly likely with daily dosage of 10 mg), consider increasing dosage or administering drug in 2 divided doses.

Lisinopril/Hydrochlorothiazide Combination Therapy

ORAL:

- If BP is not adequately controlled by monotherapy with lisinopril or hydrochlorothiazide, can switch to the fixed-combination preparation containing lisinopril 10 mg and hydrochlorothiazide 12.5 mg or, alternatively, lisinopril 20 mg and hydrochlorothiazide 12.5 mg. Adjust dosage of either or both drugs according to patient's response; however, dosage of hydrochlorothiazide should not be increased for about 2–3 weeks after initiation of therapy.
- Can switch to the fixed-combination preparation if stable dosages of lisinopril or hydrochlorothiazide have been achieved.
- If BP is controlled by monotherapy with hydrochlorothiazide 25 mg daily but potassium loss is problematic, can switch to fixed-combination preparation containing lisinopril 10 mg and hydrochlorothiazide 12.5 mg.

CHF

ORAL:

- Initially, 2.5–5 mg daily. Monitor closely (especially patients with systolic BP <100 mg Hg) until BP has stabilized. To minimize risk of hypotension, reduce diuretic dosage, if possible.
- Usual dosage: 5–40 mg once daily.

AMI

ORAL:

- 5 mg within 24 hours post-MI, followed by 5 mg 24 hours after initial dose, 10 mg 48 hours after initial dose, and then 10 mg daily. Recommended maintenance dosage: 10 mg daily for 6 weeks.
- If low SBP (≤120 mm Hg) observed when lisinopril therapy is initiated or during the first 3 days post-MI, give lower dose (i.e., 2.5 mg).
- If hypotension (SBP <100 mm Hg) occurs, reduce maintenance dosage to 5 mg daily; may temporarily reduce further to 2.5 mg daily if needed.
- If prolonged hypotension (SBP <90 mm Hg lasting >1 hour) occurs, discontinue lisinopril.

Prescribing Limits

Pediatric Patients

Hypertension

ORAL:

- Children ≥6 years of age: Maximum 0.61 mg/kg or 40 mg daily.

Adult Patients

Hypertension

ORAL:

- Dosages up to 80 mg daily have been used, but no additional benefit observed.
- Dosage of lisinopril/hydrochlorothiazide fixed combination generally should not exceed lisinopril 80 mg and hydrochlorothiazide 50 mg daily.

Special Populations

Renal Impairment

Hypertension

- Initially, 5 mg once daily in adults with Cl_{cr} 10–30 mL/minute or 2.5 mg once daily in adults with Cl_{cr} <10 mL/minute (usually on hemodialysis). Titrate until BP is controlled or to maximum of 40 mg daily. Manufacturers do not recommend use in hypertensive pediatric patients with Cl_{cr} <30 mL/minute per 1.73 m².

- Lisinopril/hydrochlorothiazide fixed combinations are not recommended in patients with severe renal impairment.

CHF

- Initially, 2.5 mg once daily in CHF patients with moderate to severe renal impairment (Cl_{cr} ≤30 mL/minute or S_{cr} >3 mg/dL) under close medical supervision.

AMI

- Use with caution in AMI patients with S_{cr} >2 mg/dL. If renal impairment (S_{cr} >3 mg/dL or a doubling of baseline S_{cr}) occurs during lisinopril therapy, consider discontinuing therapy.

Volume- and/or Salt-depleted Patients

CHF

- Initially, 2.5 mg once daily in CHF patients with hyponatremia (serum sodium concentration <130 mEq/L) under close medical supervision.

Geriatric Patients

- Generally titrate dosage carefully, initiate therapy at the low end of the dosage range.

Lisinopril and Hydrochlorothiazide

(lyse in′ oh pril) (hye droe klor oh thye′ a zide)

Brand Name: Prinzide®, Zestoretic®

Important Warning

Do not take lisinopril and hydrochlorothiazide if you are pregnant. If you become pregnant while taking lisinopril and hydrochlorothiazide, call your doctor immediately. Lisinopril and hydrochlorothiazide may harm the fetus.

Why is this medicine prescribed?

The combination of lisinopril and hydrochlorothiazide is used to treat high blood pressure. Lisinopril is in a class of medications called angiotensin-converting enzyme (ACE) inhibitors. It works by decreasing certain chemicals that tighten the blood vessels, so blood flows more smoothly. Hydrochlorothiazide is in a class of medications called diuretics ('water pills'). It works by causing the kidneys to get rid of unneeded water and salt from the body into the urine.

How should this medicine be used?

The combination of lisinopril and hydrochlorothiazide comes as a tablet to take by mouth. It is usually taken once a day with or without food. To help you remember to take lisinopril and hydrochlorothiazide, take it around the same time every day. Follow the directions on your prescription label carefully, and ask your doctor or pharmacist to explain any part you do not understand. Take lisinopril and hydrochlorothiazide exactly as directed. Do not take more or less of it or take it more often than prescribed by your doctor.

Lisinopril and hydrochlorothiazide controls high blood pressure but does not cure it. Continue to take lisinopril and hydrochlorothiazide even if you feel well. Do not stop taking lisinopril and hydrochlorothiazide without talking to your doctor.

Are there other uses for this medicine?

This medication may be prescribed for other uses; ask your doctor or pharmacist for more information.

What special precautions should I follow?

Before taking lisinopril and hydrochlorothiazide,

- tell your doctor and pharmacist if you are allergic to lisinopril, hydrochlorothiazide, benazepril (Lotensin), captopril (Capoten), enalapril (Vasotec), fosinopril (Monopril), moexipril (Univasc), quinapril (Accupril), ramipril (Altace), trandolapril (Mavik), sulfa drugs, or any other medications.

- tell your doctor and pharmacist what prescription and nonprescription medications, vitamins, nutritional supplements, and herbal products you are taking. Be sure to mention any of the following: aspirin and other nonsteroidal anti-inflammatory medications (NSAIDs) such as ibuprofen (Advil, Motrin), indomethacin (Indocin), and naproxen (Aleve, Naprosyn); barbiturates such as phenobarbital (Luminal, Solfoton); cholestyramine (Questran); colestipol (Colestid); digoxin (Lanoxin); insulin or oral medications for diabetes; lithium (Eskalith, Lithobid); oral steroids such as dexamethasone (Decadron, Dexone), methylprednisolone (Medrol), and prednisone (Deltasone); other diuretics; other medications for high blood pressure; pain medications; and potassium supplements. Your doctor may need to change the doses of your medications or monitor you carefully for side effects.

- tell your doctor if you are on dialysis or are being treated with desensitization (a process to reduce your reaction to an allergen) and if you have or have ever had allergies; asthma; diabetes; gout; high cholesterol; collagen vascular disease such as lupus or scleroderma (a condition in which extra tissue grows on the skin and some organs); heart failure; any condition that causes you to urinate less than you normally do; a stroke or 'ministroke'; heart, kidney, or liver disease; or angioedema, a condition that causes difficulty swallowing or

breathing and painful swelling of the face, throat, tongue, lips, eyes, hands, feet, ankles, or lower legs.
- tell your doctor if you plan to become pregnant or are breast-feeding.
- if you are having surgery, including dental surgery, tell the doctor or dentist that you are taking lisinopril and hydrochlorothiazide.
- ask your doctor about the safe use of alcoholic beverages while you are taking lisinopril and hydrochlorothiazide. Alcohol can make the side effects from lisinopril and hydrochlorothiazide worse.
- you should know that diarrhea, vomiting, not drinking enough fluids, and sweating a lot can cause a drop in blood pressure, which may cause lightheadedness and fainting.
- you should know that lisinopril and hydrochlorothiazide may cause dizziness, lightheadedness, and fainting when you get up too quickly from a lying position. This is more common when you first start taking lisinopril and hydrochlorothiazide. To avoid this problem, get out of bed slowly, resting your feet on the floor for a few minutes before standing up.

What special dietary instructions should I follow?

Talk to your doctor before using salt substitutes containing potassium. If your doctor prescribes a low-salt or low-sodium diet, or an exercise program, follow these directions carefully.

What should I do if I forget to take a dose?

Take the missed dose as soon as you remember it. However, if it is almost time for the next dose, skip the missed dose and continue your regular dosing schedule. Do not take a double dose to make up for a missed one.

What side effects can this medicine cause?

Lisinopril and hydrochlorothiazide may cause side effects. Tell your doctor if any of these symptoms are severe or do not go away:
- dizziness
- headache
- cough
- excessive tiredness
- pain, burning, or tingling in the hands or feet
- decrease in sexual ability
- heartburn

Some side effects can be serious. The following symptoms are uncommon, but if you experience any of them, call your doctor immediately:
- swelling of the face, throat, tongue, lips, eyes, hands, feet, ankles, or lower legs
- hoarseness
- difficulty breathing or swallowing
- stomach pain
- upset stomach

- vomiting
- fever, sore throat, chills, and other signs of infection
- muscle pain, cramps, or weakness
- yellowing of the skin or eyes
- dry mouth
- thirst
- weakness
- restlessness
- confusion
- seizures
- decrease in urination
- lightheadedness
- fainting
- chest pain
- rapid, pounding, slow, or irregular heartbeat
- pain in big toe
- tingling in arms and legs
- loss of muscle tone
- weakness or heaviness in legs
- lack of energy
- cold, gray skin

Lisinopril and hydrochlorothiazide may cause other side effects. Call your doctor if you have any unusual problems while taking this medication.

If you experience a serious side effect, you or your doctor may send a report to the Food and Drug Administration's (FDA) MedWatch Adverse Event Reporting program online [at http://www.fda.gov/MedWatch/index.html] or by phone [1-800-332-1088].

What storage conditions are needed for this medicine?

Keep this medication in the container it came in, tightly closed, and out of reach of children. Store it at room temperature and away from excess heat and moisture (not in the bathroom). Throw away any medication that is outdated or no longer needed. Talk to your pharmacist about the proper disposal of your medication.

What should I do in case of overdose?

In case of overdose, call your local poison control center at 1-800-222-1222. If the victim has collapsed or is not breathing, call local emergency services at 911.

Symptoms of overdose may include:
- lightheadedness
- fainting
- blurred vision
- dry mouth
- thirst
- weakness
- drowsiness
- restlessness
- confusion
- seizures
- muscle pains or cramps
- infrequent urination

- upset stomach
- vomiting
- rapid or pounding heartbeat

What other information should I know?

Keep all appointments with your doctor and the laboratory. Your blood pressure should be checked regularly to determine your response to lisinopril and hydrochlorothiazide. Your doctor may order certain lab tests to check your body's response to lisinopril and hydrochlorothiazide.

Before having any laboratory test, tell your doctor and the laboratory personnel that you are taking lisinopril and hydrochlorothiazide.

Do not let anyone else take your medication. Ask your pharmacist any questions you have about refilling your prescription.

Dosage Facts
For Informational Purposes

Caution: Do not change your dose, how often you take your medication, or the length of time you are to take it without first talking to your healthcare provider.

The following dosage information was written using medical language for doctors and other healthcare professionals and is provided here for you to check your dosage. The dosage of this drug may differ for different patients. Therefore, always follow your doctor's instructions or the directions on the label. Contact your healthcare provider or pharmacist if you have any questions about the specific dosage of your medication after reviewing this information.

Adult Patients

Hypertension
Lisinopril/Hydrochlorothiazide Combination Therapy

ORAL:
- If BP is not adequately controlled by monotherapy with lisinopril or hydrochlorothiazide, can switch to the fixed-combination preparation containing lisinopril 10 mg and hydrochlorothiazide 12.5 mg or, alternatively, lisinopril 20 mg and hydrochlorothiazide 12.5 mg. Adjust dosage of either or both drugs according to patient's response; however, dosage of hydrochlorothiazide should not be increased for about 2–3 weeks after initiation of therapy.
- Can switch to the fixed-combination preparation if stable dosages of lisinopril or hydrochlorothiazide have been achieved.
- If BP is controlled by monotherapy with hydrochlorothiazide 25 mg daily but potassium loss is problematic, can switch to fixed-combination preparation containing lisinopril 10 mg and hydrochlorothiazide 12.5 mg.

Prescribing Limits
Adult Patients
Hypertension

ORAL:
- Dosage of lisinopril/hydrochlorothiazide fixed combination generally should not exceed lisinopril 80 mg and hydrochlorothiazide 50 mg daily.

Special Populations

Renal Impairment

Hypertension
- Lisinopril/hydrochlorothiazide fixed combinations are not recommended in patients with severe renal impairment.

Volume- and/or Salt-depleted Patients

CHF
- Initially, 2.5 mg once daily in CHF patients with hyponatremia (serum sodium concentration <130 mEq/L) under close medical supervision.

Lithium
(lith′ ee um)

Brand Name: Eskalith CR®, Eskalith®, Lithobid®
Also available generically.

Important Warning

Keep all appointments with your doctor and the laboratory. Your doctor will order certain lab tests to check your response to lithium.

Why is this medicine prescribed?

Lithium is used to treat and prevent episodes of mania (frenzied, abnormally excited mood) in people with bipolar disorder (manic depressive disorder; a disease that causes episodes of depression, episodes of mania, and other abnormal moods). Lithium is in a class of medications called antimanic agents. It works by decreasing abnormal activity in the brain.

How should this medicine be used?

Lithium comes as a tablet, capsule, extended-release (long-acting) tablet, and solution (liquid) to take by mouth. The tablets, capsules, and solution are usually taken three to four times a day. The extended-release tablets are usually taken two to three times a day. Take lithium at around the same times every day. Follow the directions on your prescription label carefully, and ask your doctor or pharmacist to explain any part you do not understand. Take lithium exactly as directed. Do not take more or less of it or take it more often than prescribed by your doctor.

Swallow the extended-release tablet whole; do not split, chew, or crush it.

Your doctor may increase or decrease the dose of your medication during your treatment. Follow these directions carefully.

Lithium may help to control your condition but will not cure it. It may take 1-3 weeks or longer for you to feel the full benefit of lithium. Continue to take lithium even if you feel well. Do not stop taking lithium without talking to your doctor.

Are there other uses for this medicine?

Lithium is also sometimes used to treat certain blood disorders, depression, schizophrenia (a mental illness that causes disturbed or unusual thinking, loss of interest in life, and strong or inappropriate emotions), disorders of impulse control (inability to resist the urge to perform a harmful action), and certain mental illnesses in children. Talk to your doctor about the risks of using this medication for your condition.

This medication may be prescribed for other uses; ask your doctor or pharmacist for more information.

What special precautions should I follow?

Before taking lithium,

- tell your doctor and pharmacist if you are allergic to lithium or any other medications.
- tell your doctor and pharmacist what prescription and nonprescription medications, vitamins, nutritional supplements, and herbal products you are taking or plan to take. Be sure to mention any of the following: acetazolamide (Diamox); aminophylline; angiotensin-converting enzyme (ACE) inhibitors such as benazepril (Lotensin), captopril (Capoten), enalapril (Vasotec), fosinopril (Monopril), lisinopril (Prinivil, Zestril), moexipril (Univasc), perindopril (Aceon), quinapril (Accupril), ramipril (Altace), and trandolapril (Mavik); angiotensin II receptor antagonists such as candesartan (Atacand), eprosartan (Teveten), irbesartan (Avapro), losartan (Cozaar), olmesartan (Benicar), telmisartan (Micardis), and valsartan (Diovan); antacids such as sodium bicarbonate; caffeine (found in certain medications to treat drowsiness and headaches); calcium channel blockers such as amlodipine (Norvasc), diltiazem (Cardizem, Dilacor, Tiazac, others), felodipine (Plendil), isradipine (DynaCirc), nicardipine (Cardene), nifedipine (Adalat, Procardia), nimodipine (Nimotop), nisoldipine (Sular), and verapamil (Calan, Covera, Isoptin, Verelan); carbamazepine (Tegretol); diuretics ('water pills'); medications for mental illness such as haloperidol (Haldol); methyldopa (Aldomet); metronidazole (Flagyl); nonsteroidal anti-inflammatory medications (NSAIDs) such as celecoxib (Celebrex), indomethacin (Indocin), and piroxicam (Feldene); potassium

iodide; phenytoin (Dilantin); selective serotonin reuptake inhibitors (SSRIs) such as citalopram (Celexa), duloxetine (Cymbalta), escitalopram (Lexapro), fluoxetine (Prozac, Sarafem), fluvoxamine (Luvox), paroxetine (Paxil), and sertraline (Zoloft); and theophylline (Theolair, Theochron). Your doctor may have to change the doses of your medication or monitor you more carefully for side effects.

- tell your doctor if you have or have ever had organic brain syndrome (any physical condition that affects the way your brain works); or thyroid, heart, or kidney disease. Also tell your doctor if you have severe diarrhea, excessive sweating, or fever. Call your doctor if you develop these symptoms during your treatment.
- tell your doctor if you are pregnant, plan to become pregnant, or are breast-feeding. If you become pregnant while taking lithium, call your doctor.
- if you are having surgery, including dental surgery, tell the doctor or dentist that you are taking lithium.
- you should know that this medication may make you drowsy. Do not drive a car or operate machinery until you know how this medication affects you.

What special dietary instructions should I follow?

It is important to follow a proper diet, including the right amounts of fluid and salt during your treatment. Your doctor will give you specific directions about the diet that is right for you. Follow these directions carefully.

Talk to your doctor about drinking drinks that contain caffeine, such as tea, coffee, cola, or chocolate milk.

What should I do if I forget to take a dose?

Take the missed dose as soon as you remember it. However, if it is almost time for the next dose, skip the missed dose and continue your regular dosing schedule. Do not take a double dose to make up for a missed one.

What side effects can this medicine cause?

Lithium may cause side effects. Tell your doctor if any of these symptoms are severe or do not go away:

- restlessness
- fine hand movements that are difficult to control
- loss of appetite
- stomach pain or bloating
- gas
- indigestion
- weight gain or loss
- dry mouth
- excessive saliva in the mouth
- tongue pain
- change in the ability to taste food
- swollen lips
- acne
- hair loss
- unusual discomfort in cold temperatures

- constipation
- depression
- joint or muscle pain
- thin, brittle fingernails or hair

Some side effects may be serious. If you experience any of the following symptoms, call your doctor immediately:

- tiredness
- shaking of a part of your body that you cannot control
- muscle weakness, stiffness, twitching, or tightness
- loss of coordination
- diarrhea
- vomiting
- excessive thirst
- frequent urination
- giddiness
- ringing in the ears
- slow, jerky movements
- movements that are unusual or difficult to control
- blackouts
- seizures
- slurred speech
- fast, slow, irregular, or pounding heartbeat
- chest tightness
- confusion
- hallucinations (seeing things or hearing voices that do not exist)
- crossed eyes
- painful, cold, or discolored fingers and toes
- headache
- pounding noises inside the head
- changes in vision
- paleness
- itching
- rash
- swelling of the eyes, face, lips, tongue, throat, hands, feet, ankles, or lower legs

Lithium may cause other side effects. Call your doctor if you experience any unusual symptoms while you are taking this medication.

If you experience a serious side effect, you or your doctor may send a report to the Food and Drug Administration's (FDA) MedWatch Adverse Event Reporting program online [at http://www.fda.gov/MedWatch/index.html] or by phone [1-800-332-1088].

What storage conditions are needed for this medicine?

Keep this medication in the container it came in, tightly closed, and out of reach of children. Store it at room temperature and away from excess heat and moisture (not in the bathroom). Throw away any medication that is outdated or no longer needed. Talk to your pharmacist about the proper disposal of your medication.

What should I do in case of overdose?

In case of overdose, call your local poison control center at 1-800-222-1222. If the victim has collapsed or is not breathing, call local emergency services at 911.

Symptoms of overdose may include:

- diarrhea
- vomiting
- upset stomach
- drowsiness
- muscle weakness
- loss of coordination

What other information should I know?

Do not let anyone else take your medication. Ask your pharmacist any questions you have about refilling your prescription.

Dosage Facts
For Informational Purposes

Caution: Do not change your dose, how often you take your medication, or the length of time you are to take it without first talking to your healthcare provider.

The following dosage information was written using medical language for doctors and other healthcare professionals and is provided here for you to check your dosage. The dosage of this drug may differ for different patients. Therefore, always follow your doctor's instructions or the directions on the label. Contact your healthcare provider or pharmacist if you have any questions about the specific dosage of your medication after reviewing this information.

General Dosage Information

Available as lithium carbonate and lithium citrate; dosages expressed in terms of the salts.

Pediatric Patients

Bipolar Disorder
Acute Episodes†

ORAL:
- Children ≤11 years of age: Usual dosages not established; lithium carbonate dosages of 15–20 mg/kg (about 0.4–0.5 mEq/kg) daily or equivalent lithium citrate dosages have been given in 2 or 3 divided doses. (Do not exceed usual adult dosages.)
- Children ≥12 years of age: Dosages usually are the same as those of adults.

Maintenance Dosages†

ORAL:
- Usual maintenance dosages have not been established; dosage should be adjusted according to serum lithium concentrations, patient tolerance, and clinical response.

Adult Patients

Bipolar Disorder
Acute Episodes

ORAL:

- Initially, 1.8 g daily as conventional lithium carbonate capsules or tablets, given in 3 or 4 divided doses, or 30 mL (about 48 mEq of lithium) of lithium citrate oral solution daily, given in 3 divided doses.
- Alternatively, 900 mg twice daily (morning and evening) or 600 mg 3 times daily as extended-release lithium carbonate tablets.

Maintenance Dosages

ORAL:

- 900 mg to 1.2 g daily as conventional lithium carbonate capsules or tablets, given in 3 or 4 divided doses, or 15–20 mL (about 24–32 mEq of lithium) of lithium citrate oral solution daily, given in 3 or 4 divided doses. This dosage generally provides serum lithium concentrations of 0.6–1.2 mEq/L.
- Alternatively, 900 mg to 1.2 g daily as extended-release lithium carbonate tablets, given in 2 or 3 divided doses.

Prescribing Limits

Pediatric Patients

Bipolar Disorder

ORAL:

- When calculating dosage based on weight, do not exceed usual adult dosage.

Adult Patients

Bipolar Disorder

ORAL:

- Maintenance dosage usually should not exceed 2.4 g of lithium carbonate (65 mEq) daily.

Special Populations

Geriatric Patients

- Select dosage with caution because of age-related decreases in hepatic, renal, and/or cardiac function and concomitant disease and drug therapy. Lower initial dosages (e.g., ≤900 mg of lithium carbonate daily) and more gradual dosage titration recommended.
- May have decreased renal function; monitor renal function and adjust dosage accordingly.
- Dosages that produce serum lithium concentrations at the lower end of therapeutic range may be sufficient for maintenance.

Pregnant Women

- Dosages generally need to be increased during pregnancy but should be reduced 1 week before parturition or when labor begins.

† Use is not currently included in the labeling approved by the US Food and Drug Administration.

Lodoxamide Ophthalmic

(loe dox' a mide)

Brand Name: Alomide®

Why is this medicine prescribed?

Lodoxamide is an antiallergy medication used to treat certain eye conditions.

This medication is sometimes prescribed for other uses; ask your doctor or pharmacist for more information.

How should this medicine be used?

Lodoxamide comes as eyedrops. It usually is applied up to four times a day. Therapy may be continued for 3 months. Follow the directions on your prescription label carefully, and ask your doctor or pharmacist to explain any part you do not understand. Use lodoxamide exactly as directed. Do not use more or less of it or use it more often than prescribed by your doctor.

To use the eyedrops, follow these instructions:

1. Wash your hands thoroughly with soap and water.
2. Use a mirror or have someone else put the drops in your eye.
3. Remove the protective cap. Make sure that the end of the dropper is not chipped or cracked.
4. Avoid touching the dropper tip against your eye or anything else.
5. Hold the dropper tip down at all times to prevent drops from flowing back into the bottle and contaminating the remaining contents.
6. Lie down or tilt your head back and gaze upward.
7. Holding the bottle between your thumb and index finger, place the dropper tip as near as possible to your eyelid without touching it.
8. Brace the remaining fingers of that hand against your cheek or nose.
9. With the index finger of your other hand, pull the lower lid of the eye down to form a pocket.
10. Drop the prescribed number of drops into the pocket made by the lower lid and the eye. Placing drops on the surface of the eyeball can cause stinging.
11. Close your eye and press lightly against the lower lid with your finger for 2-3 minutes to keep the medication in the eye. Do not blink.
12. Replace and tighten the cap right away. Do not wipe or rinse it off.
13. Wipe off any excess liquid from your cheek with a clean tissue. Wash your hands again.

What special precautions should I follow?

Before using lodoxamide eyedrops,

- tell your doctor and pharmacist if you are allergic to lodoxamide or any other drugs.
- tell your doctor and pharmacist what prescription and nonprescription medications you are taking, especially other eye medications and vitamins.
- tell your doctor if you are pregnant, plan to become pregnant, or are breast-feeding. If you become pregnant while using lodoxamide, call your doctor.
- tell your doctor if you wear soft contact lenses. Avoid wearing soft contact lenses while using lodoxamide because they may become damaged.

What should I do if I forget to take a dose?

Apply the missed dose as soon as you remember it. However, if it is almost time for the next dose, skip the missed dose and continue your regular dosing schedule. Do not apply a double dose to make up for a missed one.

What side effects can this medicine cause?

Lodoxamide may cause side effects. Tell your doctor if any of these symptoms are severe or do not go away:

- temporary stinging or burning in the eyes
- headache
- increased eye tearing
- dry eyes
- sneezing
- blurred or unstable vision

If you experience any of the following symptoms, stop using lodoxamide and call your doctor immediately:

- skin rash
- eye pain
- swelling in or around the eyes
- vision problems

If you experience a serious side effect, you or your doctor may send a report to the Food and Drug Administration's (FDA) MedWatch Adverse Event Reporting program online [at http://www.fda.gov/MedWatch/index.html] or by phone [1-800-332-1088].

What storage conditions are needed for this medicine?

Keep this medication in the container it came in, tightly closed, and out of reach of children. Store it at room temperature and away from excess heat and moisture (not in the bathroom). Do not use the eyedrops if the solution has changed color, is cloudy, or contains particles. Throw away any medication that is outdated or no longer needed. Talk to your pharmacist about the proper disposal of your medication.

What other information should I know?

Keep all appointments with your doctor. Your doctor will order certain eye tests to check your response to lodoxamide.

Do not let anyone else use your medication. Ask your pharmacist any questions you have about refilling your prescription.

Dosage Facts
For Informational Purposes

Caution: Do not change your dose, how often you take your medication, or the length of time you are to take it without first talking to your healthcare provider.

The following dosage information was written using medical language for doctors and other healthcare professionals and is provided here for you to check your dosage. The dosage of this drug may differ for different patients. Therefore, always follow your doctor's instructions or the directions on the label. Contact your healthcare provider or pharmacist if you have any questions about the specific dosage of your medication after reviewing this information.

General Dosage Information

Available as lodoxamide tromethamine; dosage expressed in terms of lodoxamide.

Pediatric Patients

Allergic Ocular Disorders

OPHTHALMIC:
- Children ≥2 years of age: 1 or 2 drops of a 0.1% solution in the affected eye(s) 4 times daily for up to 3 months.

Adult Patients

Allergic Ocular Disorders

OPHTHALMIC:
- 1 or 2 drops of a 0.1% solution in the affected eye(s) 4 times daily for up to 3 months.

Loperamide
(loe per′ a mide)

Brand Name: Anti-Diarrheal Formula®, Anti-Diarrheal Formula® Caplets®, Imodium® A-D, Imodium® A-D Caplets®, Imodium® Advanced Chewable Tablets as a combination product containing Loperamide Hydrochloride and Simethicone, Imodium®Advanced Caplets® as a combination product containing Loperamide Hydrochloride and Simethicone
Also available generically.

Why is this medicine prescribed?

Loperamide is used to control diarrhea. It is available with or without a prescription.

This medication is sometimes prescribed for other uses; ask your doctor or pharmacist for more information.

How should this medicine be used?

Loperamide comes as a tablet, capsule, and liquid to take by mouth. It usually is taken immediately after each loose bowel movement; it is sometimes taken on a schedule (one or more times a day) for chronic diarrhea. Follow the directions on the package or on your prescription label carefully, and ask your doctor or pharmacist to explain any part you do not understand. Take loperamide exactly as directed. Do not take more or less of it or take it more often than prescribed by your doctor.

If your symptoms do not improve within 2 days (10 days for chronic diarrhea) or if you develop a fever or bloody stools, call your doctor. Drink plenty of water or other beverages to replace fluids lost while having diarrhea.

What special precautions should I follow?

Before taking loperamide,
- tell your doctor and pharmacist if you are allergic to loperamide or any other drugs.
- tell your doctor and pharmacist what prescription and nonprescription medications you are taking.
- tell your doctor or pharmacist if you have a fever.
- tell your doctor and pharmacist if you are pregnant, plan to become pregnant, or are breast-feeding. If you become pregnant while taking loperamide, call your doctor.
- you should know that this drug may make you drowsy and dizzy. Do not drive a car or operate machinery until you know how this drug affects you.
- remember that alcohol can add to the drowsiness caused by this drug.

What should I do if I forget to take a dose?

If you are taking scheduled doses of loperamide, take the missed dose as soon as you remember it. However, if it is almost time for the next dose, skip the missed dose and continue your regular dosing schedule. Do not take a double dose to make up for a missed one.

What side effects can this medicine cause?

Loperamide may cause side effects. Tell your doctor if any of these symptoms are severe or do not go away:
- dry mouth
- dizziness
- drowsiness
- vomiting
- stomach pain, discomfort, or distention (enlargement)
- constipation
- fatigue

If you experience any of the following symptoms, call your doctor immediately:
- skin rash
- hives
- itching
- wheezing
- difficulty breathing

If you experience a serious side effect, you or your doctor may send a report to the Food and Drug Administration's (FDA) MedWatch Adverse Event Reporting program online [at http://www.fda.gov/MedWatch/index.html] or by phone [1-800-332-1088].

What storage conditions are needed for this medicine?

Keep this medication in the container it came in, tightly closed, and out of reach of children. Store it at room temperature and away from excess heat and moisture (not in the bathroom). Throw away any medication that is outdated or no longer needed. Talk to your pharmacist about the proper disposal of your medication.

What other information should I know?

Ask your pharmacist any questions you have about taking this medicine.

Dosage Facts
For Informational Purposes

Caution: Do not change your dose, how often you take your medication, or the length of time you are to take it without first talking to your healthcare provider.

The following dosage information was written using medical language for doctors and other healthcare professionals and is provided here for you to check your dosage. The dosage of this drug may differ for different patients. Therefore, always follow your doctor's instructions or the directions on the label. Contact your healthcare provider or pharmacist if you have any questions about the specific dosage of your medication after reviewing this information.

General Dosage Information

Available as loperamide hydrochloride; dosage expressed in terms of the salt.

Pediatric Patients

Acute Diarrhea

ORAL:
- Children 2–12 years of age: Dosage is based on age and body weight. The following pediatric dosages are recommended for the *first day* of therapy:

Initial Dosage for Children 2–12 Years of Age

Age (weight)	Dosage (initial 24 hours)
2–5 years (13–20 kg)	1 mg 3 times daily
6–8 years (20–30 kg)	2 mg twice daily
8–12 years (>30 kg)	2 mg 3 times daily

On the second and subsequent days of therapy, administer 0.1 mg/kg only after each unformed stool; do not exceed dosage appropriate for weight/age for the first day.

For *self-medication* (alone or combined with simethicone) of acute nonspecific diarrhea, determine dosage based on body weight if possible; otherwise use age. The following pediatric dosages are recommended:

Dosage for Self-Medication in Children 6–12 Years of Age

Age (weight)	Dosage
<6 years (≤21.4 kg)	Do not use unless directed by a clinician
6–8 years (21.8–26.8 kg)	2 mg after first unformed stool, followed by 1 mg after each subsequent unformed stool (not to exceed 4 mg in 24 hours)
9–11 years (27.3–43.2 kg)	2 mg after first unformed stool, followed by 1 mg after each subsequent unformed stool (not to exceed 6 mg in 24 hours)
≥12 years	4 mg after first unformed stool, followed by 2 mg after each subsequent unformed stool (not to exceed 8 mg in 24 hours)

Discontinue if there is no improvement after 48 hours of therapy.

Chronic Diarrhea

ORAL:
- Although a dosage of 0.08–0.24 mg/kg daily in 2 or 3 divided doses† has been used in a limited number of children for management of chronic diarrhea, therapeutic dosage for this age group not established.

Adult Patients

Acute Diarrhea

ORAL:
- Initially, 4 mg, followed by 2 mg after each unformed stool, up to a maximum of 16 mg daily.
- For *self-medication*, initial dosage (alone or combined with simethicone) is also 4 mg, followed by 2 mg after each subsequent unformed stool; however, do not exceed 8 mg in a 24-hour period unless directed by a clinician.

Chronic Diarrhea

ORAL:
- Initially, 4 mg, followed by 2 mg after each unformed stool until symptoms are controlled and then reduce for maintenance as required. When optimal dosage established, may administer as single or divided doses.
- In clinical trials, average maintenance dosage was 4–8 mg daily.
- If improvement after treatment with a maximum daily dosage of 16 mg is not observed within 10 days, symptoms are unlikely to be controlled by further administration. May continue therapy if diarrhea cannot be adequately controlled with diet or specific treatment.

Prescribing Limits

Pediatric Patients

Acute Diarrhea

ORAL:
- Children 2–5 years of age: Maximum 3 mg daily; not for *self-medication* unless directed by a clinician.
- Children 6–8 years of age: Maximum 4 mg daily. *Self-medication* should not exceed 2 days unless otherwise directed by a clinician.
- Children 9–11 years of age: Maximum 6 mg daily. *Self-medication* should not exceed 2 days unless otherwise directed by a clinician.
- Children ≥12 years of age: For *self-medication*, maximum 8 mg daily. *Self-medication* should not exceed 2 days unless otherwise directed by a clinician.

Adult Patients

Acute Diarrhea

ORAL:
- Maximum 16 mg daily.
- For *self-medication*, maximum 8 mg in a 24-hour period unless otherwise directed by a clinician.

Chronic Diarrhea

ORAL:
- 16 mg daily in divided doses.

† Use is not currently included in the labeling approved by the US Food and Drug Administration.

Lopinavir and Ritonavir

(loe pin′ a veer) (ri toe′ na veer)

Brand Name: Kaletra®

Why is this medicine prescribed?

The combination of lopinavir and ritonavir is used with other antiviral medications to treat human immunodeficiency virus (HIV) in patients with acquired immunodeficiency syndrome (AIDS). Lopinavir is in a class of medications called protease (pro' tee ace) inhibitors. It works by slowing the spread of HIV in the body. In this combination, ritonavir is used to increase the amount of lopinavir in the body so it can work better. Lopinavir and ritonavir is not a cure and may not decrease the number of HIV-related illnesses. Lopinavir and ritonavir does not prevent the spread of HIV to other people.

How should this medicine be used?

The combination of lopinavir and ritonavir comes as a capsule and a solution (liquid) to take by mouth. It is usually taken twice a day with food. Follow the directions on your prescription label carefully, and ask your doctor or pharmacist to explain any part you do not understand. Take lopinavir and ritonavir exactly as directed. Do not take more or less of it or take it more often than prescribed by your doctor.

Continue to take lopinavir and ritonavir even if you feel well. Do not stop taking lopinavir and ritonavir without talking to your doctor.

Are there other uses for this medicine?

This medication may be prescribed for other uses; ask your doctor or pharmacist for more information.

What special precautions should I follow?

Before taking lopinavir and ritonavir,
- tell your doctor and pharmacist if you are allergic to lopinavir, ritonavir (Norvir), or any other medications.
- do not take lopinavir and ritonavir if you are taking astemizole (Hismanal), cisapride (Propulsid), dihydroergotamine (D.H.E. 45, Migranal), ergonovine (Ergotrate Maleate), ergotamine (Cafatine, Cafergot, Cafetrate, others), flecainide (Tambocor), methylergonovine (Methergine), midazolam (Versed), pimozide (Orap), propafenone (Rythmol), terfenadine (Seldane), or triazolam (Halcion).
- tell your doctor and pharmacist what other prescription and nonprescription medications, vitamins, and nutritional supplements you are taking. Be sure to mention any of the following: anticoagulants ('blood thinners') such as warfarin (Coumadin); antifungals such as itra-

conazole (Sporanox) and ketoconazole (Nizoral); atovaquone (Mepron); calcium-channel blockers such as felodipine (Plendil), nicardipine (Cardene), and nifedipine (Adalat, Procardia); cholesterol-lowering medications such as atorvastatin (Lipitor), lovastatin (Mevacor), and simvastatin (Zocor); clarithromycin (Biaxin); disulfiram (Antabuse); medications for irregular heartbeats such as amiodarone (Cordarone, Pacerone), bepridil (Vascor), and quinidine (Quinidex); medications for seizures such as carbamazepine (Tegretol), phenobarbital (Luminal, Solfoton), and phenytoin (Dilantin); medications that suppress the immune system such as cyclosporine (Neoral, Sandimmune), Rapamune (sirolimus), and tacrolimus (Prograf); methadone (Dolophine); metronidazole (Flagyl); oral steroids such as dexamethasone (Decadron, Dexone); other antiviral medications such as amprenavir (Agenerase), delavirdine (Rescriptor), efavirenz (Sustiva), indinavir (Crixivan), nevirapine (Viramune), ritonavir (Norvir), and saquinavir (Fortovase, Invirase); rifabutin (Mycobutin); rifampin (Rifadin, Rimactane); and sildenafil (Viagra). Your doctor may need to change the doses of your medications or monitor you carefully for side effects.
- if you are taking didanosine, take it 1 hour before or 2 hours after lopinavir and ritonavir.
- tell your doctor what herbal products you are taking, especially products containing St. John's wort.
- tell your doctor if you have ever had pancreas disease and if you have or have ever had diabetes, liver disease, or hemophilia.
- you should know that lopinavir and ritonavir may decrease the effectiveness of oral contraceptives (birth control pills). Talk to your doctor about using another form of birth control.
- tell your doctor if you are pregnant, plan to become pregnant, or are breast-feeding. If you become pregnant while taking lopinavir and ritonavir, call your doctor. You should not breast-feed while taking lopinavir and ritonavir.
- you should know that lopinavir and ritonavir solution contains alcohol and may make you drowsy. Do not drive a car or operate machinery until you know how this medication affects you.
- remember that alcohol can add to the drowsiness caused by this medication.
- you should be aware that your body fat may increase or move to different areas of your body, such as your breasts and your upper back.

What special dietary instructions should I follow?

Unless your doctor tells you otherwise, continue your normal diet.

What should I do if I forget to take a dose?

Take the missed dose as soon as you remember it. However, if it is almost time for the next dose, skip the missed dose

and continue your regular dosing schedule. Do not take a double dose to make up for a missed one.

What side effects can this medicine cause?

Lopinavir and ritonavir may cause side effects. Tell your doctor if any of these symptoms are severe or do not go away:

- diarrhea
- weakness
- heartburn
- headache
- difficulty falling asleep or staying asleep
- rash

Some side effects can be serious. The following symptoms are uncommon, but if you experience any of them, call your doctor immediately:

- upset stomach
- vomiting
- stomach pain
- unusual bleeding or bruising
- extreme tiredness
- loss of appetite
- pain in the upper right part of the stomach
- yellowing of the skin or eyes
- flu-like symptoms

Lopinavir and ritonavir may cause high blood sugar. If you experience any of the following symptoms, call your doctor immediately:

- thirst
- dry mouth
- tiredness
- flushing
- dry skin
- frequent urination
- loss of appetite
- trouble breathing

Lopinavir and ritonavir may cause increases in levels of cholesterol and other fats (triglycerides) in the blood.

Lopinavir and ritonavir may cause other side effects. Call your doctor if you have any unusual problems while taking this medication.

If you experience a serious side effect, you or your doctor may send a report to the Food and Drug Administration's (FDA) MedWatch Adverse Event Reporting program online [at http://www.fda.gov/MedWatch/index.html] or by phone [1-800-332-1088].

What storage conditions are needed for this medicine?

Keep this medication in the container it came in, tightly closed, and out of reach of children. If you store lopinavir and ritonavir capsules or solution in the refrigerator, they can be used until the expiration date printed on the label. If you store them at room temperature, the capsules or solution should be used within 2 months. Throw away any medication that is outdated or no longer needed. Talk to your pharmacist about the proper disposal of your medication.

What should I do in case of overdose?

In case of overdose, call your local poison control center at 1-800-222-1222. If the victim has collapsed or is not breathing, call local emergency services at 911.

What other information should I know?

Keep all appointments with your doctor and the laboratory. Your doctor will order certain lab tests to check your body's response to lopinavir and ritonavir.

Do not let anyone else take your medication. Ask your pharmacist any questions you have about refilling your prescription.

Dosage Facts
For Informational Purposes

Caution: Do not change your dose, how often you take your medication, or the length of time you are to take it without first talking to your healthcare provider.

The following dosage information was written using medical language for doctors and other healthcare professionals and is provided here for you to check your dosage. The dosage of this drug may differ for different patients. Therefore, always follow your doctor's instructions or the directions on the label. Contact your healthcare provider or pharmacist if you have any questions about the specific dosage of your medication after reviewing this information.

General Dosage Information

Available as fixed combination containing lopinavir and ritonavir; dosage expressed in terms of both drugs.

Must be given in conjunction with other antiretrovirals. *If used with certain didanosine preparations, adjustment of treatment regimen recommended. If used with amprenavir, efavirenz, fosamprenavir, nelfinavir, or nevirapine, dosage adjustments recommended.*

Once-daily regimen may be used only in treatment-naive adults not receiving amprenavir, efavirenz, fosamprenavir, nelfinavir, or nevirapine. Once-daily regimen should *not* be used in treatment-experienced adults or patients receiving certain anticonvulsants (carbamazepine, phenobarbital, phenytoin).

Once-daily regimen should *not* be used in pediatric patients. Twice-daily regimen recommended for adolescents.

Pediatric Patients

Treatment of HIV Infection
Children ≤12 Years of Age Not Receiving
Amprenavir, Efavirenz, or Nevirapine

ORAL:
- Infants <6 months of age†: Lopinavir 300 mg/m² and ritonavir 75 mg/m² twice daily under investigation.

Dosage for Treatment of HIV Infection in Children 6 Months to 12 Years of Age Not Receiving Amprenavir, Efavirenz, or Nevirapine

Weight (kg)	Daily Dosage
7 to <15	lopinavir 12 mg/kg and ritonavir 3 mg/kg twice daily
15–40	lopinavir 10 mg/kg and ritonavir 2.5 mg/kg twice daily
>40	lopinavir 400 mg and ritonavir 100 mg (2 tablets or 5 mL of oral solution) twice daily

Alternatively, children 6 months to 12 years of age may receive lopinavir 230 mg/m^2 and ritonavir 57.5 mg/m^2 twice daily.

Children ≤12 Years of Age Receiving Amprenavir, Efavirenz, or Nevirapine

ORAL:

Dosage for Treatment of HIV Infection in Children 6 Months to 12 Years of Age Receiving Amprenavir, Efavirenz, or Nevirapine

Weight (kg)	Daily Dosage
7 to <15	lopinavir 13 mg/kg and ritonavir 3.25 mg/kg twice daily
15–45	lopinavir 11 mg/kg and ritonavir 2.75 mg/kg twice daily
>45	lopinavir 533 mg and ritonavir 133 mg (6.7 mL of oral solution) twice daily; alternatively, lopinavir 400 mg and ritonavir 100 mg (2 tablets) twice daily[1]

1. Some experts recommend that children weighing >50 kg receive lopinavir 600 mg and ritonavir 150 mg (3 tablets) twice daily.

Alternatively, children 6 months to 12 years of age may receive lopinavir 300 mg/m^2 and ritonavir 75 mg/m^2 twice daily.

Children >12 Years of Age

ORAL:
- Use adult dosage.
- Once-daily regimen not recommended.

Adult Patients

Treatment of HIV Infection

Treatment-naive Adults Not Receiving Amprenavir, Efavirenz, Fosamprenavir, Nelfinavir, or Nevirapine

ORAL:
- Lopinavir 400 mg and ritonavir 100 mg (2 tablets or 5 mL of oral solution) twice daily.
- Alternatively, lopinavir 800 mg and ritonavir 200 mg (4 tablets or 10 mL of oral solution) once daily.

Treatment-experienced Adults Not Receiving Amprenavir, Efavirenz, Fosamprenavir, Nelfinavir, or Nevirapine

ORAL:
- Lopinavir 400 mg and ritonavir 100 mg (2 tablets or 5 mL of oral solution) twice daily.
- Once-daily regimen not recommended.

Treatment-naive Adults Receiving Amprenavir, Efavirenz, Fosamprenavir, Nelfinavir, or Nevirapine

ORAL:
- Lopinavir 400 mg and ritonavir 100 mg (2 tablets) twice daily.
- Alternatively, lopinavir 533 mg and ritonavir 133 mg (6.7 mL of oral solution) twice daily.
- Once-daily regimen not recommended.

Treatment-experienced Adults Receiving Amprenavir, Efavirenz, Fosamprenavir, Nelfinavir, or Nevirapine

ORAL:
- Suspected reduced susceptibility to lopinavir (as determined by treatment history or laboratory studies): Consider lopinavir 600 mg and ritonavir 150 mg (3 tablets) twice daily. Use of this dosage with efavirenz associated with increased lopinavir and ritonavir concentrations.
- Alternatively, lopinavir 533 mg and ritonavir 133 mg (6.7 mL of oral solution) twice daily.
- Once-daily regimen not recommended.

Postexposure Prophylaxis of HIV†
Occupational Exposure†

ORAL:
- Lopinavir 400 mg and ritonavir 100 mg twice daily.
- Used in the preferred expanded regimen that includes lopinavir and ritonavir and 2 nucleoside reverse transcriptase inhibitors (NRTIs).
- Initiate postexposure prophylaxis as soon as possible following exposure (within hours rather than days) and continue for 4 weeks, if tolerated.

Nonoccupational Exposure†

ORAL:
- Lopinavir 400 mg and ritonavir 100 mg twice daily.
- Used in a PI-based regimen with 2 NRTIs. Fixed combination of lopinavir and ritonavir with (lamivudine or emtricitabine) and zidovudine is a preferred regimen; fixed combination of lopinavir and ritonavir with (lamivudine or emtricitabine) and (stavudine or abacavir or tenofovir or didanosine) is an alternative.
- Initiate postexposure prophylaxis as soon as possible following exposure (preferably ≤72 hours after exposure) and continue for 28 days.

Prescribing Limits
Pediatric Patients

Treatment of HIV Infection

ORAL:
- For those ≤12 years of age weighing >40 kg not receiving amprenavir, efavirenz, or nevirapine: Maximum dosage of lopinavir 400 mg and ritonavir 100 mg twice daily.
- For those ≤12 years of age weighing >45 kg receiving amprenavir, efavirenz, or nevirapine: Maximum dosage of lopinavir 533 mg and ritonavir 133 mg twice daily.

Loratadine

(lor at' a deen)

Brand Name: Alavert® Allergy & Sinus D-12 Hour (as a combination product containing Loratadine and Pseudoephedrine Sulfate), Alavert® Non-Drowsy Allergy Relief 24 Hour, Children's Claritin® Fruit Flavored Syrup 24 Hour, Claritin® 24 Hour, Claritin® Hives Relief, Claritin® RediTabs® 24 Hour, Claritin-D® 12 Hour (as a combination product containing Loratadine and Pseudoephedrine Sulfate), Claritin-D® 24 Hour (as a combination product containing Loratadine and Pseudoephedrine Sulfate)

Also available generically.

Why is this medicine prescribed?

Loratadine is used to temporarily relieve the symptoms of hay fever (allergy to pollen, dust, or other substances in the air) and other allergies. These symptoms include sneezing, runny nose, and itchy eyes, nose, or throat. Loratadine is also used to treat itching and redness caused by hives. However, loratadine does not prevent hives or other allergic skin reactions. Loratadine is in a class of medications called antihistamines. It works by blocking the action of histamine, a substance in the body that causes allergic symptoms.

Loratadine is also available in combination with pseudoephedrine (Sudafed, others). This monograph only includes information about the use of loratadine alone. If you are taking the loratadine and pseudoephedrine combination product, read the information on the package label or ask your doctor or pharmacist for more information.

How should this medicine be used?

Loratadine comes as a syrup (liquid), a tablet, and a rapidly disintegrating (dissolving) tablet to take by mouth. It is usually taken once a day with or without food. Follow the directions on the package label carefully, and ask your doctor or pharmacist to explain any part you do not understand. Take loratadine exactly as directed. Do not take more or less

of it or take it more often than directed on the package label or recommended by your doctor. If you take more loratadine than directed, you may experience drowsiness.

If you are taking the rapidly disintegrating tablet, follow the package directions to remove the tablet from the blister package without breaking the tablet. Do not try to push the tablet through the foil. After you remove the tablet from the blister package, immediately place it on your tongue and close your mouth. The tablet will quickly dissolve and can be swallowed with or without water.

Do not use loratadine to treat hives that are bruised or blistered, that are an unusual color, or that do not itch. Call your doctor if you have this type of hives.

Stop taking loratadine and call your doctor if your hives do not improve during the first 3 days of your treatment or if your hives last longer than 6 weeks. If you do not know the cause of your hives, call your doctor.

If you are taking loratadine to treat hives, and you develop any of the following symptoms, get emergency medical help right away: difficulty swallowing, speaking, or breathing; swelling in and around the mouth or swelling of the tongue; wheezing; drooling; dizziness; or loss of consciousness. These may be symptoms of a life-threatening allergic reaction called anaphylaxis. If your doctor suspects that you may experience anaphylaxis with your hives, he may prescribe an epinephrine injector (EpiPen). Do not use loratadine in place of the epinephrine injector.

Do not use this medication if the safety seal is open or torn.

Are there other uses for this medicine?

This medication may be recommended for other uses; ask your doctor or pharmacist for more information.

What special precautions should I follow?

Before taking loratadine,
- tell your doctor and pharmacist if you are allergic to loratadine, any other medications, or any of the ingredients in the type of loratadine you will be taking. Check the package label for a list of the ingredients.
- tell your doctor and pharmacist what prescription and nonprescription medications, vitamins, nutritional supplements and herbal products you are taking or plan to take. Be sure to mention medications for colds and allergies.
- tell your doctor if you have or have ever had asthma or kidney or liver disease.
- tell your doctor if you are pregnant, plan to become pregnant, or are breast-feeding. If you become pregnant while taking loratadine, call your doctor.
- if you have phenylketonuria (PKU, an inherited condition in which a special diet must be followed to prevent mental retardation), you should know that some brands of the orally disintegrating tablets may contain aspartame that forms phenylalanine.

What special dietary instructions should I follow?

Unless your doctor tells you otherwise, continue your normal diet.

What should I do if I forget to take a dose?

Take the missed dose as soon as you remember it. However, if it is almost time for the next dose, skip the missed dose and continue your regular dosing schedule. Do not take a double dose to make up for a missed one.

What side effects can this medicine cause?

Loratadine may cause side effects. Tell your doctor if any of these symptoms are severe or do not go away:

- headache
- dry mouth
- nosebleed
- sore throat
- mouth sores
- difficulty falling asleep or staying asleep
- nervousness
- weakness
- stomach pain
- diarrhea
- red or itchy eyes

Some side effects may be serious. If you experience any of the following symptoms, stop taking loratadine and call your doctor immediately:

- rash
- hives
- itching
- swelling of the eyes, face, lips, tongue, throat, hands, arms, feet, ankles, or lower legs
- hoarseness
- difficulty breathing or swallowing
- wheezing

What storage conditions are needed for this medicine?

Keep this medication in the container it came in, tightly closed, and out of reach of children. Store it at room temperature, away from excess heat and moisture (not in the bathroom) and away from light. Use the orally disintegrating tablets immediately after you remove them from the blister package, and within 6 months after you open the outer foil pouch. Write the date that you open the foil pouch on the product label so that you will know when 6 months have passed. Throw away any medication that is outdated or no longer needed. Talk to your pharmacist about the proper disposal of your medication.

What should I do in case of overdose?

In case of overdose, call your local poison control center at 1-800-222-1222. If the victim has collapsed or is not breathing, call local emergency services at 911.

Symptoms of overdose may include:

- fast or pounding heartbeat
- drowsiness
- headache
- unusual body movements

What other information should I know?

Keep all appointments with your doctor.

Ask your pharmacist any questions you have about loratadine.

Dosage Facts
For Informational Purposes

Caution: Do not change your dose, how often you take your medication, or the length of time you are to take it without first talking to your healthcare provider.

The following dosage information was written using medical language for doctors and other healthcare professionals and is provided here for you to check your dosage. The dosage of this drug may differ for different patients. Therefore, always follow your doctor's instructions or the directions on the label. Contact your healthcare provider or pharmacist if you have any questions about the specific dosage of your medication after reviewing this information.

General Dosage Information

Fixed-combination tablets formulated for 12-hour dosing contain 5 mg of loratadine and 60 mg of pseudoephedrine sulfate in an immediate-release outer shell and 60 mg of pseudoephedrine sulfate in an extended-release matrix core that slowly releases the drug.

Fixed-combination tablets formulated for 24-hour dosing contain 10 mg of loratadine in an immediate-release outer shell and 240 mg of pseudoephedrine sulfate in an extended-release matrix core that slowly releases the drug.

Pediatric Patients

Allergic Rhinitis

ORAL:

- *Self-medication* in children 2 to <6 years of age: 5 mg once daily (as oral solution).
- *Self-medication* in children ≥6 years of age: 10 mg once daily (as conventional or orally disintegrating tablets or oral solution).
- *Self-medication* in children ≥12 years of age: 5 mg every 12 hours (in fixed combination with 120 mg pseudoephedrine sulfate as the 12-hour formulation [e.g., Alavert® Allergy & Sinus, Claritin-D® 12 Hour]) or 10 mg once daily (in fixed combination with 240 mg pseudoephedrine sulfate as the 24-hour formulation [Claritin-D® 24 Hour]).

Chronic Idiopathic Urticaria

ORAL:

- Children 2–5 years of age: Not recommended for *self-medication*; a dosage of 5 mg once daily (as oral solution) has been recommended when clinicians *prescribe* the drug in children 2–5 years of age.
- *Self-medication* in children ≥6 years of age: 10 mg once daily.

Adult Patients

Allergic Rhinitis

ORAL:

- *Self-medication*: 10 mg once daily (as conventional or orally disintegrating tablets or oral solution).
- *Self-medication*: 5 mg every 12 hours (in fixed combination with 120 mg pseudoephedrine sulfate as the 12-hour formulation) or 10 mg once daily (in fixed combination with 240 mg pseudoephedrine sulfate as the 24-hour formulation).

Chronic Idiopathic Urticaria

ORAL:

- *Self-medication*: 10 mg once daily.

Prescribing Limits

Pediatric Patients

Allergic Rhinitis

Self-medication in children 2 to <6 years of age: Maximum 5 mg once daily (as oral solution).

Self-medication in children ≥6 years of age: Maximum 10 mg once daily (as conventional or orally disintegrating tablets or oral solution).

Self-medication in children ≥12 years of age: Maximum 10 mg daily (in fixed combination with pseudoephedrine sulfate as the 12-hour or 24-hour formulations).

Adult Patients

Allergic Rhinitis

Self-medication: Maximum 10 mg once daily (as conventional or orally disintegrating tablets or oral solution).

Self-medication: Maximum 10 mg daily (in fixed combination with pseudoephedrine sulfate as the 12-hour or 24-hour formulations).

Special Populations

Hepatic Impairment

- *Self-medication*: Consult a clinician.
- Children 2–5 years of age with hepatic failure: 5 mg *every other day* (as oral solution).
- Adults and children ≥6 years of age with hepatic failure: 10 mg *every other day* (as conventional or orally disintegrating tablets or oral solution).
- Fixed-combination loratadine/pseudoephedrine sulfate preparations generally should *not* be used in patients with hepatic impairment.

Renal Impairment

- *Self-medication*: Consult a clinician.
- Children 2–5 years of age with renal insufficiency (glomerular filtration rate <30 mL/minute): 5 mg *every other day* (as oral solution).
- Adults and children ≥6 years of age with renal insufficiency (glomerular filtration rate <30 mL/minute): 10 mg *every other day* (as conventional or orally disintegrating tablets or oral solution).
- Fixed-combination loratadine/pseudoephedrine sulfate preparations in adults and children ≥12 years of age with renal insufficiency (glomerular filtration rate <30 mL/minute): 5 mg of loratadine once daily (when the 12-hour formulation is used) or 10 mg of loratadine every other day (when the 24-hour formulation is used).

Lorazepam

(lor a′ ze pam)

Brand Name: Ativan®, Lorazepam Intensol®
Also available generically.

Why is this medicine prescribed?

Lorazepam is used to relieve anxiety.

This medication is sometimes prescribed for other uses; ask your doctor or pharmacist for more information.

How should this medicine be used?

Lorazepam comes as a tablet and concentrate (liquid) to take by mouth. It usually is taken two or three times a day and may be taken with or without food. Follow the directions on your prescription label carefully, and ask your doctor or pharmacist to explain any part you do not understand. Take lorazepam exactly as directed.

Lorazepam concentrate (liquid) comes with a specially marked dropper for measuring the dose. Ask your pharmacist to show you how to use the dropper. Dilute the concentrate in 1 ounce or more of water, juice, or carbonated beverages just before taking it. It also may be mixed with applesauce or pudding just before taking the dose.

Lorazepam can be habit-forming. Do not take a larger dose, take it more often, or for a longer time than your doctor tells you to. Tolerance may develop with long-term or excessive use, making the drug less effective. Do not take lorazepam for more than 4 months or stop taking this medication without talking to your doctor. Stopping the drug suddenly can worsen your condition and cause withdrawal symptoms (anxiousness, sleeplessness, and irritability). Your doctor probably will decrease your dose gradually.

Are there other uses for this medicine?

Lorazepam is also used to treat irritable bowel syndrome, epilepsy, insomnia, and nausea and vomiting from cancer treatment and to control agitation caused by alcohol withdrawal. Talk to your doctor about the possible risks of using this drug for your condition.

What special precautions should I follow?

Before taking lorazepam,

- tell your doctor and pharmacist if you are allergic to lorazepam, alprazolam (Xanax), chlordiazepoxide (Librium, Librax), clonazepam (Klonopin), clorazepate (Tranxene), diazepam (Valium), estazolam (ProSom), flurazepam (Dalmane), oxazepam (Serax), prazepam (Centrax), temazepam (Restoril), triazolam (Halcion), or any other drugs.
- tell your doctor and pharmacist what prescription and nonprescription medications you are taking, especially antihistamines; digoxin (Lanoxin); levodopa (Larodopa, Sinemet); medications for depression, seizures, pain, Parkinson's disease, asthma, colds, or allergies; muscle relaxants; oral contraceptives; probenecid (Benemid); rifampin (Rifadin); sedatives; sleeping pills; theophylline (Theo-Dur); tranquilizers; valproic acid (Depakene); and vitamins. These medications may add to the drowsiness caused by lorazepam.
- tell your doctor if you have or have ever had glaucoma; seizures; or lung, heart, or liver disease.
- tell your doctor if you are pregnant, plan to become pregnant, or are breast-feeding. If you become pregnant while taking lorazepam, call your doctor immediately.
- if you are having surgery, including dental surgery, tell the doctor or dentist that you are taking lorazepam.
- you should know that this drug may make you drowsy. Do not drive a car or operate machinery until you know how this drug affects you.
- remember that alcohol can add to the drowsiness caused by this drug.
- tell your doctor if you use tobacco products. Cigarette smoking may decrease the effectiveness of this drug.

What should I do if I forget to take a dose?

If you take several doses per day and miss a dose, skip the missed dose and continue your regular dosing schedule. Do not take a double dose to make up for a missed one.

What side effects can this medicine cause?

Side effects from lorazepam may occur and include:

- drowsiness
- dizziness
- tiredness
- weakness
- dry mouth
- diarrhea
- upset stomach
- changes in appetite

Tell your doctor if any of these symptoms are severe or do not go away:

- restlessness or excitement
- constipation
- difficulty urinating

- frequent urination
- blurred vision
- changes in sex drive or ability

If you experience any of the following symptoms, call your doctor immediately:

- shuffling walk
- persistent, fine tremor or inability to sit still
- fever
- difficulty breathing or swallowing
- severe skin rash
- yellowing of the skin or eyes
- irregular heartbeat

If you experience a serious side effect, you or your doctor may send a report to the Food and Drug Administration's (FDA) MedWatch Adverse Event Reporting program online [at http://www.fda.gov/MedWatch/index.html] or by phone [1-800-332-1088].

What storage conditions are needed for this medicine?

Keep this medication in the container it came in, tightly closed, and out of reach of children. Store it at room temperature and away from excess heat and moisture (not in the bathroom). Throw away any medication that is outdated or no longer needed. Talk to your pharmacist about the proper disposal of your medication.

What should I do in case of overdose?

In case of overdose, call your local poison control center at 1-800-222-1222. If the victim has collapsed or is not breathing, call local emergency services at 911.

What other information should I know?

Keep all appointments with your doctor and the laboratory. Your doctor will order certain lab tests to check your response to lorazepam.

Do not let anyone else take your medication. Ask your pharmacist any questions you have about refilling your prescription.

Dosage Facts
For Informational Purposes

Caution: Do not change your dose, how often you take your medication, or the length of time you are to take it without first talking to your healthcare provider.

The following dosage information was written using medical language for doctors and other healthcare professionals and is provided here for you to check your dosage. The dosage of this drug may differ for different patients. Therefore, always follow your doctor's instructions or the directions on the label. Contact your healthcare provider or pharmacist if you have any questions

about the specific dosage of your medication after reviewing this information.

Adult Patients

Anxiety

ORAL:

- Initially, 2–3 mg daily divided in 2 or 3 doses. Maintenance dosage of 1–10 mg daily (usually 2–6 mg) in divided doses, with the largest dose administered at bedtime. Increase dosage gradually if higher dosage is indicated; increase the evening dose before the daytime doses.
- For insomnia caused by anxiety, 2–4 mg as a single daily dose at bedtime.

Cancer Chemotherapy-induced Nausea and Vomiting†

ORAL:

- 2.5 mg the evening before and just after initiation of chemotherapy.

Special Populations

Hepatic Impairment

- Adjust oral dosage carefully in patients with severe hepatic insufficiency because oral therapy may exacerbate hepatic encephalopathy; lower than recommended dosages may be sufficient in these patients.

Geriatric Patients

- Cautious dosage selection recommended because of greater sensitivity and possible age-related decreases in hepatic or renal function; initiate therapy at the lower end of the usual range.

Anxiety Disorders

Oral

- Initially, 1–2 mg daily divided in 2 or 3 doses.

† Use is not currently included in the labeling approved by the US Food and Drug Administration.

Losartan

(loe sar′ tan)

Brand Name: Cozaar®

> ### Important Warning
>
> Do not take losartan if you are pregnant. If you become pregnant while taking losartan, call your doctor immediately. Losartan may harm the fetus.

Why is this medicine prescribed?

Losartan is used alone or in combination with other medications to treat high blood pressure. Losartan is in a class of medications called angiotensin II receptor antagonists. It works by blocking the action of certain chemicals that tighten the blood vessels so blood flows more smoothly.

How should this medicine be used?

Losartan comes as a tablet to take by mouth. It is usually taken once or twice a day with or without food. To help you remember to take losartan, take it around the same time every day. Follow the directions on your prescription label carefully, and ask your doctor or pharmacist to explain any part you do not understand. Take losartan exactly as directed. Do not take more or less of it or take it more often than prescribed by your doctor.

Losartan controls high blood pressure but does not cure it. Continue to take losartan even if you feel well. Do not stop taking losartan without talking to your doctor.

Are there other uses for this medicine?

Losartan is also used sometimes to treat congestive heart failure. Talk to your doctor about the possible risks of using this medication for your condition.

This medication may be prescribed for other uses; ask your doctor or pharmacist for more information.

What special precautions should I follow?

Before taking losartan,

- tell your doctor and pharmacist if you are allergic to losartan or any other medications.
- tell your doctor and pharmacist what prescription and nonprescription medications, vitamins, nutritional supplements, and herbal products you are taking. Be sure to mention any of the following: diuretics ('water pills'), indomethacin (Indocin), and potassium supplements. Your doctor may need to change the doses of your medications or monitor you carefully for side effects.
- tell your doctor if you have or have ever had heart failure or kidney or liver disease.
- tell your doctor if you plan to become pregnant or are breast-feeding.

What special dietary instructions should I follow?

Talk to your doctor before using salt substitutes containing potassium. If your doctor prescribes a low-salt or low-sodium diet, follow these directions carefully.

What should I do if I forget to take a dose?

Take the missed dose as soon as you remember it. However, if it is almost time for the next dose, skip the missed dose and continue your regular regular dosing schedule. Do not take a double dose to make up for a missed one.

What side effects can this medicine cause?

Losartan may cause side effects. Tell your doctor if any of these symptoms are severe or do not go away:

- dizziness
- runny nose
- sore throat

Some side effects can be serious. The following symptoms are uncommon, but if you experience any of them, call your doctor immediately:

- swelling of the face, throat, tongue, lips, eyes, hands, feet, ankles, or lower legs
- hoarseness
- difficulty breathing or swallowing
- fainting

Losartan may cause other side effects. Call your doctor if you have any unusual problems while taking this medication.

If you experience a serious side effect, you or your doctor may send a report to the Food and Drug Administration's (FDA) MedWatch Adverse Event Reporting program online [at http://www.fda.gov/MedWatch/index.html] or by phone [1-800-332-1088].

What storage conditions are needed for this medicine?

Keep this medication in the container it came in, tightly closed, and out of reach of children. Store it at room temperature and away from excess heat and moisture (not in the bathroom). Throw away any medication that is outdated or no longer needed. Talk to your pharmacist about the proper disposal of your medication.

What should I do in case of overdose?

In case of overdose, call your local poison control center at 1-800-222-1222. If the victim has collapsed or is not breathing, call local emergency services at 911.

Symptoms of overdose may include:

- dizziness
- fainting
- rapid or pounding heartbeat

What other information should I know?

Keep all appointments with your doctor. Your blood pressure should be checked regularly to determine your response to losartan.

Do not let anyone else take your medication. Ask your pharmacist any questions you have about refilling your prescription.

Dosage Facts
For Informational Purposes

Caution: Do not change your dose, how often you take your medication, or the length of time you are to take it without first talking to your healthcare provider.

The following dosage information was written using medical language for doctors and other healthcare pro-fessionals and is provided here for you to check your dosage. The dosage of this drug may differ for different patients. Therefore, always follow your doctor's instructions or the directions on the label. Contact your healthcare provider or pharmacist if you have any questions about the specific dosage of your medication after reviewing this information.

General Dosage Information

Available as losartan potassium; dosage expressed in terms of the salt.

Pediatric Patients

Hypertension

ORAL:

- Children ≥6 years of age: Initially, 0.7 mg/kg (up to 50 mg) once daily. Adjust dosage until the desired BP goal is achieved (up to maximum dosage of 1.4 mg/kg or 100 mg daily).

Adult Patients

Hypertension
Monotherapy

ORAL:

- Initially, 50 mg once daily in adults without intravascular volume depletion. Adjust dosage at approximately monthly intervals (more aggressively in high-risk patients) to achieve BP control.
- Usual dosage: 25–100 mg daily, given in 1 dose or 2 divided doses; no additional therapeutic benefit with higher dosages.
- If effectiveness diminishes toward end of dosing interval in patients treated once daily, consider increasing dosage or administering drug in 2 divided doses.

Combination Therapy

ORAL:

- If BP is not adequately controlled by monotherapy with losartan potassium or hydrochlorothiazide (25 mg daily), if BP is controlled but hypokalemia is problematic at this hydrochlorothiazide dosage, or in those with severe hypertension in whom the potential benefit of achieving prompt BP control outweighs the potential risk of initiating therapy with the commercially available fixed combination, can use the fixed-combination tablets once daily (losartan potassium 50 mg and hydrochlorothiazide 12.5 mg; then losartan potassium 100 mg and hydrochlorothiazide 25 mg, if BP remains uncontrolled after about 3 weeks of therapy [or after 2–4 weeks of therapy in those with severe hypertension]).
- If BP is not adequately controlled by monotherapy with losartan potassium 100 mg daily, can switch to fixed-combination tablets once daily (losartan potassium 100 mg and hydrochlorothiazide 12.5 mg; then losartan potassium 100 mg and hydrochlorothiazide 25 mg [administered as 2 tablets of the fixed combination containing 50 mg of losartan potassium and 12.5 mg of hydrochlorothiazide, or alternatively, as 1 tablet of the fixed combination containing 100 mg of losartan potassium and 25 mg of hydrochlorothiazide] if BP remains uncontrolled after about 3 weeks of therapy).

Prevention of Cardiovascular Morbidity and Mortality

ORAL:
- Initially, 50 mg once daily. Adjust dosage based on BP response. If indicated, add hydrochlorothiazide 12.5 mg daily and/or increase dosage of losartan to 100 mg once daily. Subsequently, may increase hydrochlorothiazide dosage to 25 mg once daily.

Diabetic Nephropathy

ORAL:
- Initially, 50 mg once daily. If BP is not adequately controlled, increase dosage to 100 mg once daily.

Prescribing Limits

Pediatric Patients

Hypertension

ORAL:
- Maximum 1.4 mg/kg or 100 mg daily.

Adult Patients

Hypertension
Combination Therapy

ORAL:
- Maximum 100 mg of losartan potassium and 25 mg of hydrochlorothiazide daily as the fixed combination.

Special Populations

Hepatic Impairment
- Manufacturer recommends initial dosage of 25 mg once daily in adults with a history of hepatic impairment.
- Losartan/hydrochlorothiazide fixed combination not recommended in patients with hepatic impairment.

Renal Impairment
- No initial dosage adjustments recommended by manufacturer for adults with renal impairment, including those undergoing hemodialysis. Use not recommended in pediatric patients with Cl_{cr} <30 mL/minute per 1.73 m^2.
- Losartan/hydrochlorothiazide fixed combination not recommended in patients with severe renal impairment.

Geriatric Patients
- No initial dosage adjustments necessary.

Volume- and/or Salt-depleted Patients
- Correct volume and/or salt depletion prior to initiation of therapy or initiate therapy under close medical supervision using lower initial dosage (25 mg once daily).
- Losartan/hydrochlorothiazide fixed combination not recommended in patients with intravascular volume depletion (e.g., patients receiving diuretics).

Losartan and Hydrochlorothiazide

(loe sar′ tan) (hye droe klor oh thye′ a zide)

Brand Name: Hyzaar®

Important Warning

Do not take losartan and hydrochlorothiazide if you are pregnant. If you become pregnant while taking losartan and hydrochlorothiazide, call your doctor immediately. Losartan and hydrochlorothiazide may harm the fetus.

Why is this medicine prescribed?

The combination of losartan and hydrochlorothiazide is used to treat high blood pressure. Losartan is in a class of medications called angiotensin II receptor antagonists. It works by blocking the action of certain chemicals that tighten the blood vessels, so blood flows more smoothly. Hydrochlorothiazide is in a class of medications called diuretics ('water pills'). It works by causing the kidneys to get rid of unneeded water and salt from the body into the urine.

How should this medicine be used?

The combination of losartan and hydrochlorothiazide comes as a tablet to take by mouth. It is usually taken once a day with or without food. To help you remember to take losartan and hydrochlorothiazide, take it around the same time every day. Follow the directions on your prescription label carefully, and ask your doctor or pharmacist to explain any part you do not understand. Take losartan and hydrochlorothiazide exactly as directed. Do not take more or less of it or take it more often than prescribed by your doctor.

Losartan and hydrochlorothiazide controls high blood pressure but does not cure it. Continue to take losartan and hydrochlorothiazide even if you feel well. Do not stop taking losartan and hydrochlorothiazide without talking to your doctor.

Are there other uses for this medicine?

This medication may be prescribed for other uses; ask your doctor or pharmacist for more information.

What special precautions should I follow?

Before taking losartan and hydrochlorothiazide,

- tell your doctor and pharmacist if you are allergic to losartan (Cozaar), hydrochlorothiazide (HCTZ, Hydrodiuril, Microzide), sulfa drugs, or any other medications.
- tell your doctor and pharmacist what prescription and nonprescription medications, vitamins, nutritional supplements, and herbal products you are taking. Be sure to mention any of the following: aspirin and other nonsteroidal anti-inflammatory medications (NSAIDs) such as indomethacin (Indocin); cholestyramine (Questran); colestipol (Colestid); insulin or oral medications for diabetes; lithium (Eskalith, Lithobid); narcotic pain medications; oral steroids such as dexamethasone (Decadron, Dexone), methylprednisolone (Medrol), and prednisone (Deltasone); other diuretics; other medications for high blood pressure; phenobarbital (Luminal, Solfoton); and potassium supplements. Your doctor may need to change the doses of your medications or monitor you carefully for side effects.
- tell your doctor if you have or have ever had gout; lupus; asthma; allergies; heart failure; diabetes; high blood levels of cholesterol or other fats (triglycerides); or liver or kidney disease.
- tell your doctor if you plan to become pregnant or are breast-feeding.
- if you are having surgery, including dental surgery, tell the doctor or dentist that you are taking losartan and hydrochlorothiazide.
- ask your doctor about the safe use of alcoholic beverages while you are taking losartan and hydrochlorothiazide. Alcohol can make the side effects from losartan and hydrochlorothiazide worse.
- you should know that diarrhea, vomiting, not drinking enough fluids, and sweating a lot can cause a drop in blood pressure, which may cause lightheadedness and fainting.

What special dietary instructions should I follow?

Talk to your doctor before using salt substitutes containing potassium. If your doctor prescribes a low-salt or low-sodium diet or an exercise program, follow these directions carefully.

What should I do if I forget to take a dose?

Take the missed dose as soon as you remember it. However, if it is almost time for the next dose, skip the missed dose and continue your regular dosing schedule. Do not take a double dose to make up for a missed one.

What side effects can this medicine cause?

Losartan and hydrochlorothiazide may cause side effects. Tell your doctor if any of these symptoms are severe or do not go away:

- dizziness
- runny nose
- sore throat
- back pain

Some side effects can be serious. The following symptoms are uncommon, but if you experience any of them, call your doctor immediately:

- swelling of the face, throat, tongue, lips, eyes, hands, feet, ankles, or lower legs
- hoarseness
- difficulty breathing or swallowing
- hives
- dry mouth
- thirst
- weakness
- drowsiness
- restlessness
- confusion
- seizures
- muscle pains or cramps
- infrequent urination
- upset stomach
- vomiting
- lightheadedness
- fainting
- rapid, pounding, or irregular heartbeat

Losartan and hydrochlorothiazide may cause other side effects. Call your doctor if you have any unusual problems while taking this medication.

If you experience a serious side effect, you or your doctor may send a report to the Food and Drug Administration's (FDA) MedWatch Adverse Event Reporting program online [at http://www.fda.gov/MedWatch/index.html] or by phone [1-800-332-1088].

What storage conditions are needed for this medicine?

Keep this medication in the container it came in, tightly closed, and out of reach of children. Store it at room temperature and away from excess heat and moisture (not in the bathroom). Throw away any medication that is outdated or no longer needed. Talk to your pharmacist about the proper disposal of your medication.

What should I do in case of overdose?

In case of overdose, call your local poison control center at 1-800-222-1222. If the victim has collapsed or is not breathing, call local emergency services at 911.

Symptoms of overdose may include:

- dizziness
- lightheadedness
- fainting
- rapid or pounding heartbeat

What other information should I know?

Keep all appointments with your doctor and the laboratory. Your blood pressure should be checked regularly to determine your response to losartan and hydrochlorothiazide. Your doctor may order certain blood tests to check your body's response to losartan and hydrochlorothiazide.

Before having any laboratory test, tell your doctor and the laboratory personnel that you are taking losartan and hydrochlorothiazide.

Do not let anyone else take your medication. Ask your pharmacist any questions you have about refilling your prescription.

Dosage Facts
For Informational Purposes

Caution: Do not change your dose, how often you take your medication, or the length of time you are to take it without first talking to your healthcare provider.

The following dosage information was written using medical language for doctors and other healthcare professionals and is provided here for you to check your dosage. The dosage of this drug may differ for different patients. Therefore, always follow your doctor's instructions or the directions on the label. Contact your healthcare provider or pharmacist if you have any questions about the specific dosage of your medication after reviewing this information.

General Dosage Information

Available as losartan potassium; dosage expressed in terms of the salt.

Adult Patients
Hypertension
Combination Therapy

ORAL:
- If BP is not adequately controlled by monotherapy with losartan potassium or hydrochlorothiazide (25 mg daily), if BP is controlled but hypokalemia is problematic at this hydrochlorothiazide dosage, or in those with severe hypertension in whom the potential benefit of achieving prompt BP control outweighs the potential risk of initiating therapy with the commercially available fixed combination, can use the fixed-combination tablets once daily (losartan potassium 50 mg and hydrochlorothiazide 12.5 mg; then losartan potassium 100 mg and hydrochlorothiazide 25 mg, if BP remains uncontrolled after about 3 weeks of therapy [or after 2–4 weeks of therapy in those with severe hypertension]).
- If BP is not adequately controlled by monotherapy with losartan potassium 100 mg daily, can switch to fixed-combination tablets once daily (losartan potassium 100 mg and hydrochlorothiazide 12.5 mg; then losartan potassium 100 mg and hydrochlorothiazide 25 mg [administered as 2 tablets of the fixed combination containing 50 mg of losar-

tan potassium and 12.5 mg of hydrochlorothiazide, or alternatively, as 1 tablet of the fixed combination containing 100 mg of losartan potassium and 25 mg of hydrochlorothiazide] if BP remains uncontrolled after about 3 weeks of therapy).

Prescribing Limits
Adult Patients
Hypertension
Combination Therapy

ORAL:
- Maximum 100 mg of losartan potassium and 25 mg of hydrochlorothiazide daily as the fixed combination.

Special Populations

Hepatic Impairment
- Losartan/hydrochlorothiazide fixed combination not recommended in patients with hepatic impairment.

Renal Impairment
- Losartan/hydrochlorothiazide fixed combination not recommended in patients with severe renal impairment.

Volume- and/or Salt-depleted Patients
- Losartan/hydrochlorothiazide fixed combination not recommended in patients with intravascular volume depletion (e.g., patients receiving diuretics).

Lovastatin

(loe′ va sta tin)

Brand Name: Advicor®, Altoprev®, Mevacor®
Also available generically.

Why is this medicine prescribed?

Lovastatin is used together with lifestyle changes (diet, weight-loss, exercise) to reduce the amount of cholesterol (a fat-like substance) and other fatty substances in the blood. Lovastatin is in a class of medications called HMG-CoA reductase inhibitors (statins). It works by slowing the production of cholesterol in the body.

Buildup of cholesterol and fats along the walls of the blood vessels (a process known as atherosclerosis) decreases blood flow and, therefore, the oxygen supply to the heart, brain, and other parts of the body. Lowering blood levels of cholesterol and fats may help to decrease your chances of getting heart disease, angina (chest pain), strokes, and heart attacks. In addition to taking a cholesterol-lowering medication, making certain changes in your daily habits can also lower your cholesterol blood levels. You should eat a diet that is low in saturated fat and cholesterol (see SPECIAL DIETARY), exercise 30 minutes on most, if not all days, and lose weight if you are overweight.

How should this medicine be used?

Lovastatin comes as a tablet and an extended-release (long-acting) tablet to take by mouth. The regular tablet is usually taken once or twice a day with meals. The extended-release tablet is usually taken once a day in the evening at bedtime. Take lovastatin at around the same time(s) every day. Follow the directions on your prescription label carefully, and ask your doctor or pharmacist to explain any part you do not understand. Take lovastatin exactly as directed. Do not take more or less of it or take it more often than prescribed by your doctor.

Swallow the extended-release tablets whole; do not split, chew, or crush them.

Your doctor may start you on a low dose of lovastatin and gradually increase your dose, not more than once every 4 weeks.

Continue to take lovastatin even if you feel well. Do not stop taking lovastatin without talking to your doctor.

Are there other uses for this medicine?

This medication may be prescribed for other uses; ask your doctor or pharmacist for more information.

What special precautions should I follow?

Before taking lovastatin,

- tell your doctor and pharmacist if you are allergic to lovastatin or any other medications.
- tell your doctor and pharmacist what prescription and nonprescription medications, vitamins, nutritional supplements, and herbal products you are taking or plan to take. Be sure to mention any of the following: amiodarone (Cordarone, Pacerone); anticoagulants ('blood thinners') such as warfarin (Coumadin); antifungal medications such as itraconazole (Sporanox) and ketoconazole (Nizoral); cimetidine (Tagamet); clarithromycin (Biaxin); cyclosporine (Neoral, Sandimmune); danazol (Danocrine); erythromycin (E.E.S., E-Mycin, Erythrocin); HIV protease inhibitors such as indinavir (Crixivan), ritonavir (Norvir) and saquinavir (Invirase, Fortovase); nefazodone (Serzone); other cholesterol-lowering medications such as fenofibrate (Tricor), gemfibrozil (Lopid), and niacin (nicotinic acid, Niacor, Niaspan); spironolactone (Aldactone); telithromycin (Ketek); and verapamil (Calan, Covera, Isoptin, Verelan). Your doctor may need to change the doses of your medications or monitor you carefully for side effects.
- tell your doctor if you have liver disease. Your doctor will probably tell you not to take lovastatin.
- tell your doctor if you drink large amounts of alcohol, if you have ever had liver disease or if you have or have ever had kidney disease.
- tell your doctor if you are pregnant, or plan to become pregnant. If you become pregnant while taking lovastatin, stop taking lovastatin and call your doctor immediately. Lovastatin may harm the fetus.
- do not breastfeed while you are taking this medication.
- if you are having surgery, including dental surgery, tell the doctor or dentist that you are taking lovastatin.
- ask your doctor about the safe use of alcoholic beverages while you are taking lovastatin. Alcohol can increase the risk of serious side effects.

What special dietary instructions should I follow?

Avoid drinking large amounts (more than 1 quart every day) of grapefruit juice while taking lovastatin.

Eat a low-cholesterol, low-fat diet. This kind of diet includes cottage cheese, fat-free milk, fish (not canned in oil), vegetables, poultry, egg whites, and polyunsaturated oils and margarines (corn, safflower, canola, and soybean oils). Avoid foods with excess fat in them such as meat (especially liver and fatty meat), egg yolks, whole milk, cream, butter, shortening, lard, pastries, cakes, cookies, gravy, peanut butter, chocolate, olives, potato chips, coconut, cheese (other than cottage cheese), coconut oil, palm oil, and fried foods.

What should I do if I forget to take a dose?

Take the missed dose as soon as you remember it. However, if it is almost time for the next dose, skip the missed dose and continue your regular dosing schedule. Do not take a double dose to make up for a missed one.

What side effects can this medicine cause?

Lovastatin may cause side effects. Tell your doctor if this symptom is severe or does not go away:

- constipation

Some side effects can be serious. The following symptoms are uncommon, but if you experience any of them, call your doctor immediately:

- muscle pain, tenderness, or weakness
- lack of energy
- fever
- yellowing of the skin or eyes
- pain in the upper right part of the stomach
- nausea
- extreme tiredness
- unusual bleeding or bruising
- loss of appetite
- flu-like symptoms
- rash
- hives
- itching
- difficulty breathing or swallowing
- swelling of the face, throat, tongue, lips, eyes, hands, feet, ankles, or lower legs
- hoarseness

Lovastatin may cause other side effects. Call your doctor if you have any unusual problems while taking this medication.

If you experience a serious side effect, you or your doctor may send a report to the Food and Drug Administration's (FDA) MedWatch Adverse Event Reporting program online [at http://www.fda.gov/MedWatch/index.html] or by phone [1-800-332-1088].

What storage conditions are needed for this medicine?

Keep this medication in the container it came in, tightly closed, and out of reach of children. Store it at room temperature and away from excess heat and moisture (not in the bathroom). Throw away any medication that is outdated or no longer needed. Talk to your pharmacist about the proper disposal of your medication.

What should I do in case of overdose?

In case of overdose, call your local poison control center at 1-800-222-1222. If the victim has collapsed or is not breathing, call local emergency services at 911.

What other information should I know?

Keep all appointments with your doctor and the laboratory. Your doctor will order certain lab tests before and during treatment to check your body's response to lovastatin.

Before having any laboratory test, tell your doctor and the laboratory personnel that you are taking lovastatin.

Do not let anyone else take your medication. Ask your pharmacist any questions you have about refilling your prescription.

Dosage Facts
For Informational Purposes

Caution: Do not change your dose, how often you take your medication, or the length of time you are to take it without first talking to your healthcare provider.

The following dosage information was written using medical language for doctors and other healthcare professionals and is provided here for you to check your dosage. The dosage of this drug may differ for different patients. Therefore, always follow your doctor's instructions or the directions on the label. Contact your healthcare provider or pharmacist if you have any questions about the specific dosage of your medication after reviewing this information.

Pediatric Patients

Dyslipidemias
Conventional Tablets

ORAL:
- Children 10-17 years of age: Initially, 10 mg once daily in patients who require small reductions in LDL-cholesterol. In patients who require reductions of ≥20%, initiate therapy at a dosage of 20 mg once daily.
- Adjust dosage at intervals of ≥ 4 weeks until the desired effect on lipoprotein concentrations is observed. Usual dosage range is 10–40 mg daily.

Adult Patients

Prevention of Cardiovascular Events or Dyslipidemias
Conventional Tablets

ORAL:
- Initially, 10 mg once daily in patients who require small reductions in LDL-cholesterol; in those who require reductions of ≥20%, 20 mg once daily.
- Adjust dosage at intervals of ≥ 4 weeks until the desired effect on lipoprotein concentrations is observed. Usual dosage range is 10–80 mg daily given in 1 or 2 divided doses.

Extended-release Tablets

ORAL:
- Initially, dosage is 20, 40, or 60 mg once daily. In patients who require small reductions in LDL-cholesterol, initiate therapy at a dosage of 10 mg once daily.
- Adjust dosage at intervals of ≥ 4 weeks until the desired effect on lipoprotein concentrations is observed. Usual dosage range is 10–60 mg once daily.

Lovastatin in Fixed Combination with Extended-release Niacin Tablets

ORAL:
- Determine dosage by identifying a stable dosage of extended-release niacin (Niaspan®). Patients receiving niacin preparations other than Niaspan® should be switched from their existing niacin therapy to Niaspan® and titrated to a stable dosage prior to switching to Advicor®. Once a stable dosage of Niaspan® is reached, switch patients directly to a niacin-equivalent dosage of Advicor®. In patients currently receiving a stable dosage of lovastatin, add Niaspan® and titrate slowly (using the recommended titration schedule) until a stable dosage of niacin has been reached, then switch patients to a niacin-equivalent dosage of Advicor®.
- Increase dosage by no more than 500 mg (of the niacin component) at 4-week intervals. Usual maintenance dosage ranges from 20 mg of lovastatin and 500 mg of extended-release niacin to 40 mg of lovastatin and 2 g of extended-release niacin once daily. In patients in whom therapy with Advicor® has been discontinued for an extended period (i.e., >7 days), reinstitute at the lowest available dosage. Because of differences in bioavailability, do *not* substitute 1 tablet of Advicor® 1 g/40 mg for 2 tablets of Advicor® 500 mg/20 mg, or vice versa.

Prescribing Limits

Pediatric Patients

Prevention of Cardiovascular Events or Dyslipidemias
Conventional Tablets

ORAL:
• Maximum 40 mg daily.

Adult Patients

Prevention of Cardiovascular Events or Dyslipidemias
Conventional Tablets

ORAL:
• Maximum 80 mg daily.

Lovastatin in Fixed-combination with Extended-release Niacin Tablets

ORAL:
• Maximum 40 mg of lovastatin and 2 g of extended-release niacin daily.

Special Populations

Hepatic Impairment
• Use with caution in patients who consume substantial amounts of alcohol and/or have a history of liver disease. Contraindicated in patients with active liver disease or unexplained, persistent increases in serum aminotransferase concentrations.

Renal Impairment
• Use with caution in patients with severe renal impairment (Cl_{cr} < 30 mL/min); dosage increases >20 mg daily should be carefully considered, and if deemed necessary, implemented with extreme caution.

Loxapine Oral

(lox′ a peen)

Brand Name: Loxitane®

Why is this medicine prescribed?

Loxapine is used to treat psychotic disorders and symptoms such as hallucinations, delusions, and hostility.

This medication is sometimes prescribed for other uses; ask your doctor or pharmacist for more information.

How should this medicine be used?

Loxapine comes as a capsule and liquid concentrate to take by mouth. It usually is taken two to four times a day. Follow the directions on your prescription label carefully, and ask your doctor or pharmacist to explain any part you do not understand. Take loxapine exactly as directed. Do not take more or less of it or take it more often than prescribed by your doctor.

Continue to take loxapine even if you feel well. Do not stop taking loxapine without talking to your doctor, especially if you have taken large doses for a long time. Your doctor probably will decrease your dose gradually. This drug must be taken regularly for a few weeks before its full effect is felt.

What special precautions should I follow?

Before taking loxapine,

• tell your doctor and pharmacist if you are allergic to loxapine or any other drugs.
• tell your doctor and pharmacist what prescription and nonprescription medications you are taking, especially antacids, antidepressants, antihistamines, appetite reducers (amphetamines), benztropine (Cogentin), bromocriptine (Parlodel), carbamazepine (Tegretol), dicyclomine (Bentyl), fluoxetine (Prozac), guanethidine (Ismelin), lithium, lorazepam (Ativan), medications for colds, meperidine (Demerol), methyldopa (Aldomet), phenytoin (Dilantin), propranolol (Inderal), sedatives, tetracycline, trihexyphenidyl (Artane), valproic acid (Depakane), and vitamins.
• tell your doctor if you have or have ever had depression; seizures; shock therapy; asthma; emphysema; chronic bronchitis; problems with your urinary system or prostate; glaucoma; history of alcohol abuse; thyroid problems; bad reaction to insulin; problems with your blood pressure; blood disorders; or heart, blood vessel, kidney, liver, or lung disease.
• tell your doctor if you are pregnant, plan to become pregnant, or are breast-feeding. If you become pregnant while taking loxapine, call your doctor.
• you should know that this drug may make you drowsy. Do not drive a car or operate machinery until you know how this drug affects you.
• remember that alcohol can add to the drowsiness caused by this drug.
• plan to avoid unnecessary or prolonged exposure to sunlight and to wear protective clothing, sunglasses, and sunscreen. Loxapine may make your skin sensitive to sunlight.

What special dietary instructions should I follow?

Loxapine may cause an upset stomach. Take loxapine with food or milk.

What should I do if I forget to take a dose?

Take the missed dose as soon as you remember it. However, if it is almost time for the next dose, skip the missed dose and continue your regular dosing schedule. Do not take a double dose to make up for a missed one.

What side effects can this medicine cause?

Loxapine may cause side effects. Your urine may turn pink or reddish-brown; this effect is not harmful. Tell your doctor if any of these symptoms are severe or do not go away:

- drowsiness
- dizziness
- blurred vision
- dry mouth
- upset stomach
- vomiting
- diarrhea
- constipation
- headache

If you experience any of the following symptoms, call your doctor immediately:

- tremor
- restlessness or pacing
- fine worm-like tongue movements
- unusual face, mouth, or jaw movements
- slow or difficult speech
- difficulty swallowing
- seizures
- fever
- yellowing of the skin or eyes

If you experience a serious side effect, you or your doctor may send a report to the Food and Drug Administration's (FDA) MedWatch Adverse Event Reporting program online [at http://www.fda.gov/MedWatch/index.html] or by phone [1-800-332-1088].

What storage conditions are needed for this medicine?

Keep this medication in the container it came in, tightly closed, and out of reach of children. Store it at room temperature and away from excess heat and moisture (not in the bathroom). Throw away any medication that is outdated or no longer needed. Talk to your pharmacist about the proper disposal of your medication.

What should I do in case of overdose?

In case of overdose, call your local poison control center at 1-800-222-1222. If the victim has collapsed or is not breathing, call local emergency services at 911.

What other information should I know?

Keep all appointments with your doctor and the laboratory. Your doctor will order certain lab tests to check your response to loxapine.

Do not let anyone else take your medication. Ask your pharmacist any questions you have about refilling your prescription.

Talk to your doctor, pharmacist, or other healthcare professional if you have questions about dosing information for your medication.

Lubiprostone

(loo bi pros' tone)

Brand Name: Amitiza®

Why is this medicine prescribed?

Lubiprostone is used to treat chronic idiopathic constipation (an ongoing condition that causes infrequent or difficult passing of stools) by relieving symptoms of abdominal pain, bloating, straining, and hard or lumpy stools. Lubiprostone is in a class of medications called laxatives. It works by increasing the amount of fluid that flows into the bowel and allowing the stool to pass more easily.

How should this medicine be used?

Lubiprostone comes as a capsule to take by mouth. It is usually taken with food twice a day. Take lubiprostone at around the same times every day. Follow the directions on your prescription label carefully, and ask your doctor or pharmacist to explain any part you do not understand. Take lubiprostone exactly as directed. Do not take more or less of it or take it more often than prescribed by your doctor.

Lubiprostone controls chronic idiopathic constipation but does not cure it. Continue to take lubiprostone even if you feel well. Do not stop taking lubiprostone without talking to your doctor. Your doctor will monitor your condition to see if you need to keep taking lubiprostone.

Are there other uses for this medicine?

This medication may be prescribed for other uses; ask your doctor or pharmacist for more information.

What special precautions should I follow?

Before taking lubiprostone,

- tell your doctor and pharmacist if you are allergic to lubiprostone or any other medications.
- tell your doctor and pharmacist what other prescription and nonprescription medications, vitamins, nutritional supplements, and herbal products you are taking or plan to take.
- tell your doctor if you have or have ever had a blockage in your stomach or bowels. Your doctor will probably tell you not to take lubiprostone.
- tell your doctor if you are pregnant, plan to become pregnant, or are breast-feeding. Your doctor will check to make sure that you are not pregant before you begin to take lubiprostone. You must use birth control while taking this medication. Talk to your doctor about the method of birth control that is best for you. If you become pregnant while taking lubiprostone, call your doctor right away.

What special dietary instructions should I follow?

Unless your doctor tells you otherwise, continue your normal diet.

What should I do if I forget to take a dose?

Take the missed dose as soon as you remember it. However, if it is almost time for the next dose, skip the missed dose and continue your regular dosing schedule. Do not take a double dose to make up for a missed one.

What side effects can this medicine cause?

Lubiprostone may cause side effects. Tell your doctor if any of these symptoms are severe or do not go away:

- nausea
- diarrhea
- bloating of stomach
- stomach pain
- gas
- vomiting
- heartburn
- dry mouth
- headache
- dizziness
- decreased feeling to touch
- swelling of the hands, feet, ankles, or lower legs
- discomfort in chest
- cough
- tiredness
- pain in joints, back, arms, or legs
- depression
- nervousness

Some side effects can be serious. If you experience the following symptom, call your doctor immediately:

- shortness of breath

Lubiprostone may cause other side effects. Call your doctor if you have any unusual problems while taking this medication.

What storage conditions are needed for this medicine?

Keep this medication in the container it came in, tightly closed, and out of reach of children. Store it at room temperature and away from excess heat and moisture (not in the bathroom). Throw away any medication that is outdated or no longer needed. Talk to your pharmacist about the proper disposal of your medication.

What should I do in case of overdose?

In case of overdose, call your local poison control center at 1-800-222-1222. If the victim has collapsed or is not breathing, call local emergency services at 911.

Symptoms of overdose may include:

- nausea
- vomiting
- diarrhea
- dizziness
- headache
- stomach pain
- flushing
- shortness of breath
- pale skin
- loss of consciousness
- loss of appetite
- weakness
- discomfort in chest
- dry mouth
- increased sweating
- skin irritation
- fainting

What other information should I know?

Keep all appointments with your doctor.

Do not let anyone else take your medication. Ask your pharmacist any questions you have about refilling your prescription.

Dosage Facts

For Informational Purposes

Caution: Do not change your dose, how often you take your medication, or the length of time you are to take it without first talking to your healthcare provider.

The following dosage information was written using medical language for doctors and other healthcare professionals and is provided here for you to check your dosage. The dosage of this drug may differ for different patients. Therefore, always follow your doctor's instructions or the directions on the label. Contact your healthcare provider or pharmacist if you have any questions about the specific dosage of your medication after reviewing this information.

Adult Patients

Chronic Idiopathic Constipation

ORAL:
- 24 mcg twice daily.

Magnesium Gluconate

(mag nee′ zhum gloo′ koe nate)

Brand Name: Almora®, Magtrate®, Magonate®

Why is this medicine prescribed?

Magnesium gluconate is used to treat low blood magnesium. Low blood magnesium is caused by gastrointestinal disorders, prolonged vomiting or diarrhea, kidney disease, or certain other conditions. Certain drugs lower magnesium levels as well.

This medication is sometimes prescribed for other uses; ask your doctor or pharmacist for more information.

How should this medicine be used?

Magnesium gluconate comes as a tablet and liquid to take by mouth. It usually is taken two to four times a day, depending on your condition. Follow the directions on your prescription label or package label carefully, and ask your doctor or pharmacist to explain any part you do not understand. Take magnesium gluconate exactly as directed. Do not take more or less of it or take it more often than prescribed by your doctor.

To prevent side effects, magnesium gluconate should be taken with meals. If you are taking an extended-release (long-acting) product, do not chew or crush the tablet. There are some tablets that can be crushed and mixed with food.

What special precautions should I follow?

Before taking magnesium gluconate,
- tell your doctor and pharmacist if you are allergic to magnesium gluconate or any other drugs.
- tell your doctor and pharmacist what prescription and nonprescription medications you are taking, especially other products with magnesium or tetracycline (Achromycin V, Panmycin, Sumycin), digoxin (Lanoxin), nitrofurantoin (Furadantin, Macrobid, Macrodantin), penicillamine (Cuprimine, Depen Titratable), and vitamins.
- tell your doctor if you have or have ever had kidney disease, stomach problems, or intestinal disease.
- tell your doctor if you are pregnant, plan to become pregnant, or are breast-feeding. If you become pregnant while taking magnesium gluconate, call your doctor.

What special dietary instructions should I follow?

A balanced diet usually provides enough magnesium. Sometimes supplements are necessary because of illness or medication use. Magnesium is found in a variety of foods, including green leafy vegetables, nuts, peas, beans, and cereal grains with the outer layers intact.

A high-fat diet may decrease the amount of magnesium you absorb from your diet. Over-cooking food also may decrease the amount of magnesium you absorb from your food. Follow the diet recommended by your doctor or dietitian. Ask if you are not sure you are getting enough vitamins and minerals.

What should I do if I forget to take a dose?

Take the missed dose as soon as you remember it. However, if it is almost time for the next dose, skip the missed dose and continue your regular dosing schedule. Do not take a double dose to make up for a missed one.

What side effects can this medicine cause?

Magnesium gluconate may cause side effects. Tell your doctor if either of these symptoms is severe or does not go away:
- diarrhea
- stomach upset

If you experience any of the following symptoms, call your doctor immediately:
- stomach cramps
- upset stomach
- vomiting
- flushing of skin
- dizziness

If you experience a serious side effect, you or your doctor may send a report to the Food and Drug Administration's (FDA) MedWatch Adverse Event Reporting program online [at http://www.fda.gov/MedWatch/index.html] or by phone [1-800-332-1088].

What storage conditions are needed for this medicine?

Keep this medication in the container it came in, tightly closed, and out of reach of children. Store it at room temperature and away from excess heat and moisture (not in the bathroom). Throw away any medication that is outdated or no longer needed. Talk to your pharmacist about the proper disposal of your medication.

What should I do in case of overdose?

In case of overdose, call your local poison control center at 1-800-222-1222. If the victim has collapsed or is not breathing, call local emergency services at 911.

What other information should I know?

Keep all appointments with your doctor and the laboratory. Your doctor will order certain lab tests to check your response to magnesium gluconate.

Do not let anyone else take your medication. Ask your pharmacist any questions you have about refilling your prescription.

Talk to your doctor, pharmacist, or other healthcare professional if you have questions about dosing information for your medication.

Magnesium Hydroxide

(mag nee′ zhum hye drox′ ide)

Brand Name: Milk of Magnesia®, Milk of Magnesia-Concentrated®, Phillips Milk of Magnesia®

Why is this medicine prescribed?

Magnesium hydroxide is used on a short-term basis to treat constipation.

This medication is sometimes prescribed for other uses; ask your doctor or pharmacist for more information.

How should this medicine be used?

Magnesium hydroxide come as a tablet and liquid to take by mouth. It usually is taken as needed for constipation. Follow the directions on the package or on your prescription label carefully, and ask your doctor or pharmacist to explain any part you do not understand. Take magnesium hydroxide exactly as directed. Do not take more or less of it or take it more often than prescribed by your doctor.

Shake the liquid well before each use.

What special precautions should I follow?

Before taking magnesium hydroxide,

- tell your doctor and pharmacist if you are allergic to magnesium hydroxide or any other drugs.
- tell your doctor and pharmacist what prescription and nonprescription medications you are taking, including vitamins.
- tell your doctor if you have or have ever had kidney disease.
- tell your doctor if you are pregnant, plan to become pregnant, or are breast-feeding. If you become pregnant while taking magnesium hydroxide, call your doctor.

What should I do if I forget to take a dose?

This medication usually is taken as needed. If your doctor has told you to take magnesium hydroxide regularly, take the missed dose as soon as you remember it. However, if it is almost time for the next dose, skip the missed dose and continue your regular dosing schedule. Do not take a double dose to make up for a missed one.

What side effects can this medicine cause?

Magnesium hydroxide may cause side effects. If you experience any of the following symptoms, call your doctor immediately:

- stomach cramps
- upset stomach
- vomiting
- diarrhea

If you experience a serious side effect, you or your doctor may send a report to the Food and Drug Administration's (FDA) MedWatch Adverse Event Reporting program online [at http://www.fda.gov/MedWatch/index.html] or by phone [1-800-332-1088].

What storage conditions are needed for this medicine?

Keep this medication in the container it came in, tightly closed, and out of reach of children. Store it at room temperature and away from excess heat and moisture (not in the bathroom). Throw away any medication that is outdated or no longer needed. Talk to your pharmacist about the proper disposal of your medication.

What other information should I know?

Ask your pharmacist any questions you have about taking this medicine.

Talk to your doctor, pharmacist, or other healthcare professional if you have questions about dosing information for your medication.

Magnesium Oxide

(mag nee′ zee um ox′ ide)

Brand Name: Mag-Ox®, Maox®, Uro-Mag®

Why is this medicine prescribed?

Magnesium is an element your body needs to function normally. Magnesium oxide may be used for different reasons. Some people use it as an antacid to relieve heartburn, sour stomach, or acid indigestion. Magnesium oxide also may be used as a laxative for short-term, rapid emptying of the bowel (before surgery, for example). It should not be used repeatedly. Magnesium oxide also is used as a dietary supplement when the amount of magnesium in the diet is not enough. Magnesium oxide is available without a prescription.

This medication is sometimes prescribed for other uses; ask your doctor or pharmacist for more information.

How should this medicine be used?

Magnesium oxide comes as a tablet and capsule to take by mouth. It usually is taken one to four times daily depending on which brand is used and what condition you have. Follow the directions on the package or on your prescription label carefully, and ask your doctor or pharmacist to explain any part you do not understand. Take magnesium oxide exactly as directed. Do not take more or less of it or take it more often than prescribed by your doctor.

Take any other medicine and magnesium oxide at least 2 hours apart.

If you are using magnesium oxide as a laxative, take it with a full glass (8 ounces) of cold water or fruit juice. Do not take a dose late in the day on an empty stomach.

Do not take magnesium oxide as an antacid for longer than 2 weeks unless your doctor tells you to. Do not take magnesium oxide as a laxative for more than 1 week unless your doctor tells you to.

What special precautions should I follow?

Before taking magnesium oxide,

- tell your doctor and pharmacist if you are allergic to magnesium oxide, other antacids or laxatives, or any other drugs.
- tell your doctor and pharmacist what prescription and nonprescription medications you are taking, especially other antacids or laxatives, anticoagulants ('blood thinners') such as warfarin (Coumadin), aspirin, diuretics ('water pills'), medicine for ulcers [cimetidine (Tagamet), ranitidine (Zantac)], and vitamins.
- tell your doctor if you have or have ever had heart, kidney, liver, or intestinal disease or high blood pressure.
- tell your doctor if you are pregnant, plan to become pregnant, or are breast-feeding. If you become pregnant while taking magnesium oxide, call your doctor immediately.
- tell your doctor if you are on a low-salt, low-sugar, or other special diet.

What should I do if I forget to take a dose?

If you are taking magnesium oxide on a regular schedule, take the missed dose as soon you remember it. However, if it is almost time for the next dose, skip the missed dose and continue your regular dosing schedule. Do not take a double dose to make up for a missed one.

What side effects can this medicine cause?

Magnesium oxide may cause side effects. To avoid unpleasant taste, take the tablet with citrus fruit juice or carbonated citrus drink. Tell your doctor if either of these symptoms are severe or do not go away:

- cramping
- diarrhea

If you experience any of the following symptoms, call your doctor immediately:

- rash or hives
- itching
- dizziness or lightheadedness
- mood or mental changes
- unusual tiredness
- weakness
- upset stomach
- vomiting

If you experience a serious side effect, you or your doctor may send a report to the Food and Drug Administration's (FDA) MedWatch Adverse Event Reporting program online [at http://www.fda.gov/MedWatch/index.html] or by phone [1-800-332-1088].

What storage conditions are needed for this medicine?

Keep this medication in the container it came in, tightly closed, and out of reach of children. Store it at room temperature and away from excess heat and moisture (not in the bathroom). Throw away any medication that is outdated or no longer needed. Talk to your pharmacist about the proper disposal of your medication.

What should I do in case of overdose?

In case of overdose, call your local poison control center at 1-800-222-1222. If the victim has collapsed or is not breathing, call local emergency services at 911.

What other information should I know?

If this medicine has been prescribed for you, keep all appointments with your doctor so that your response to magnesium can be checked.

Do not let anyone else take your medicine.

Talk to your doctor, pharmacist, or other healthcare professional if you have questions about dosing information for your medication.

Maprotiline

(ma proe′ ti leen)

Important Warning

A small number of children, teenagers, and young adults (up to 24 years of age) who took antidepressants ('mood elevators') such as maprotiline during clinical studies became suicidal (thinking about harming or killing oneself or planning or trying to do so). Children, teenagers, and young adults who take antidepressants to treat depression or other mental illnesses may be more likely to become suicidal than children, teenagers, and young adults who do not take antidepressants to treat these conditions. However, experts are not sure about how great this risk is and how much it should be considered in deciding whether a child or teenager should take an antidepressant. Children younger than 18 years of age should not normally take maprotiline, but in some cases, a doctor may decide that maprotiline is the best medication to treat a child's condition.

You should know that your mental health may change in unexpected ways when you take maprotiline or other antidepressants even if you are an adult over age 24. You may become suicidal, especially at the beginning of your treatment and any time that your dose is increased or decreased. You, your family, or your caregiver should call your doctor right away if you experience any of the following symptoms: new or worsening depression; thinking about harming or killing yourself, or planning or trying to do so; extreme worry; agitation; panic attacks; difficulty falling asleep or staying asleep; aggressive behavior; irritability; acting without thinking; severe restlessness; and frenzied abnormal excitement. Be sure that your family or caregiver knows which symptoms may be serious so they can call the doctor when you are unable to seek treatment on your own.

Your healthcare provider will want to see you often while you are taking maprotiline, especially at the beginning of your treatment. Be sure to keep all appointments for office visits with your doctor.

The doctor or pharmacist will give you the manufacturer's patient information sheet (medication guide) when you begin treatment with maprotiline. Read the information carefully and ask your doctor or pharmacist if you have any questions. You also can obtain the Medication Guide from the FDA website: http://www.fda.gov/cder/drug/antidepressants/antidepressants_MG_2007.pdf.

No matter what your age, before you take an antidepressant, you, your parent, or your caregiver should talk to your doctor about the risks and benefits of treating your condition with an antidepressant or with other treatments. You should also talk about the risks and benefits of not treating your condition. You should know that having depression or another mental illness greatly increases the risk that you will become suicidal. This risk is higher if you or anyone in your family has or has ever had bipolar disorder (mood that changes from depressed to abnormally excited) or mania (frenzied, abnormally excited mood) or has thought about or attempted suicide. Talk to your doctor about your condition, symptoms, and personal and family medical history. You and your doctor will decide what type of treatment is right for you.

Why is this medicine prescribed?

Maprotiline is used to treat depression, bipolar disorder (manic depressive disorder; a disease that causes episodes of depression, episodes of mania, and other abnormal moods), and anxiety. Maprotiline is in a class of medications called tetracyclic antidepressants. It works by increasing the amounts of certain natural substances in the brain that are needed to maintain mental balance.

How should this medicine be used?

Maprotiline comes as a tablet to take by mouth. It is usually taken one to three times a day and may be taken with or without food. Take maprotiline at around the same time(s) every day. Follow the directions on your prescription label carefully, and ask your doctor or pharmacist to explain any part you do not understand. Take maprotiline exactly as directed. Do not take more or less of it or take it more often than prescribed by your doctor.

It may take a few weeks or longer for you to feel the full benefit of maprotiline. Continue to take maprotiline even if you feel well. Do not stop taking maprotiline without talking to your doctor. Your doctor will probably want to decrease your dose gradually.

Are there other uses for this medicine?

This medication may be prescribed for other uses. Ask your doctor or pharmacist for more information.

What special precautions should I follow?

Before taking maprotiline,
- tell your doctor and pharmacist if you are allergic to maprotiline or any other medications.
- tell your doctor if you are taking a monoamine oxidase (MAO) inhibitor such as isocarboxazid (Marplan), phenelzine (Nardil), selegiline (Eldepryl, Emsam, Zelapar), and tranylcypromine (Parnate), or if you have taken an MAO inhibitor during the past 14 days. Your doctor will probably tell you that you should not take maprotiline.
- tell your doctor and pharmacist what prescription and nonprescription medications, vitamins, nutritional supplements and herbal products you are taking or plan to take. Be sure to mention any of the following: anticoagulants (blood thinners) such as warfarin (Coumadin); antihistamines; estrogens; fluoxetine (Prozac); levodopa (Sinemet, Larodopa); lithium (Eskalith, Lithobid); medication for high blood pressure, seizures, Parkinson's disease, asthma, colds, or allergies; methylphenidate (Ritalin); muscle relaxants; oral contraceptives; sedatives; sleeping pills; thyroid medication; and tranquilizers. Your doctor may need to change the doses of your medications or monitor you carefully for side effects.
- tell your doctor if you have or have ever had glaucoma (an eye condition), an enlarged prostate (a male reproductive gland), difficulty urinating, seizures, a brain tumor, a head injury, an overactive thyroid gland, or liver, kidney, or heart disease.
- tell your doctor if you are pregnant, plan to become pregnant, or are breast-feeding. If you become pregnant while taking maprotiline, call your doctor.
- if you are having surgery, including dental surgery, tell the doctor or dentist that you are taking maprotiline.
- you should know that this medication may make you drowsy. Do not drive a car or operate machinery until you know how this medication affects you.
- remember that alcohol can add to the drowsiness caused by this medication.
- tell your doctor if you use tobacco products. Cigarette smoking may decrease the effectiveness of this medication.

What special dietary instructions should I follow?

Unless your doctor tells you otherwise, continue your normal diet.

What should I do if I forget to take a dose?

Take the missed dose as soon as you remember it. However, if it is almost time for your next dose, skip the missed dose and continue your regular dosing schedule. Do not take a double dose to make up for a missed one.

What side effects can this medicine cause?

Maprotiline may cause side effects. Tell your doctor if any of these symptoms are severe or do not go away:

- nausea
- drowsiness
- weakness or tiredness
- nightmares
- dry mouth
- skin more sensitive to sunlight than usual
- changes in appetite or weight
- constipation
- difficulty urinating
- frequent urination
- blurred vision
- changes in sex drive or ability
- excessive sweating

Some side effects can be serious. If you experience any of the following symptoms or those listed in the IMPORTANT WARNING section, call your doctor immediately:

- jaw, neck, and back muscle spasms
- slow or difficult speech
- shuffling walk
- uncontrollable shaking of a part of the body
- fever, chills, sore throat, or flu-like symptoms
- difficulty breathing or swallowing
- rash
- yellowing of the skin or eyes
- irregular heartbeat

Maprotiline may cause other side effects. Call your doctor if you have any unusual problems while you are taking this medication.

If you experience a serious side effect, you or your doctor may send a report to the Food and Drug Administration's (FDA) MedWatch Adverse Event Reporting program online [at http://www.fda.gov/MedWatch/index.html] or by phone [1-800-332-1088].

What storage conditions are needed for this medicine?

Keep this medication in the container it came in, tightly closed, and out of reach of children. Store it at room temperature and away from excess heat and moisture (not in the bathroom). Throw away any medication that is outdated or no longer needed. Talk to your pharmacist about the proper disposal of your medication.

What should I do in case of overdose?

In case of overdose, call your local poison control center at 1-800-222-1222. If the victim has collapsed or is not breathing, call local emergency services at 911.

What other information should I know?

Keep all appointments with your doctor and the laboratory. Your doctor will order certain lab tests to check your response to maprotiline.

Do not let anyone else take your medication. Ask your pharmacist any questions you have about refilling your prescription.

Dosage Facts
For Informational Purposes

Caution: Do not change your dose, how often you take your medication, or the length of time you are to take it without first talking to your healthcare provider.

The following dosage information was written using medical language for doctors and other healthcare professionals and is provided here for you to check your dosage. The dosage of this drug may differ for different patients. Therefore, always follow your doctor's instructions or the directions on the label. Contact your healthcare provider or pharmacist if you have any questions about the specific dosage of your medication after reviewing this information.

General Dosage Information

Available as maprotiline hydrochloride; dosage expressed in terms of the salt.

Initiate therapy with low doses; slowly increase dosage as required.

Adult Patients

Major Depressive Disorder
Outpatients

ORAL:
- Initially, 75 mg daily for 2 weeks in patients with moderate to severe symptoms. After 2 weeks, gradually increase dosage in 25-mg increments, as tolerated. Usually, a maximum of 150 mg daily is effective in these patients.
- May increase dosage to 225 mg daily in patients with the most severe symptoms.
- After symptoms are controlled, gradually reduce dosage to the lowest level that will maintain relief of symptoms, generally 75–150 mg daily. Maintenance doses <200 mg daily may minimize the risk of seizures.

Hospitalized Patients

ORAL:
- Initially, 100–150 mg daily in patients with moderate to severe symptoms. If required, increase gradually as tolerated.

Usually, 150 mg daily is effective in most patients, but dosages as high as 225 mg daily may be necessary in some patients.

- After symptoms are controlled, gradually reduce dosage to the lowest level that will maintain relief of symptoms, generally 75–150 mg daily. Maintenance doses <200 mg daily may minimize the risk of seizures.

Prescribing Limits

Adult Patients

Major Depressive Disorder

ORAL:
- Maximum 225 mg daily.

Special Populations

Hepatic Impairment
- No specific dosage recommendations at this time.

Renal Impairment
- No specific dosage recommendations at this time

Geriatric Patients
- Initially, 25 mg daily. After 2 weeks, gradually increase dosage in 25-mg increments, as tolerated. Usually, 50–75 mg daily is effective in most patients.

Measles, Mumps, and Rubella Vaccines

Brand Name: Attenuvax®, M-M-R® II, Mumpsvax®, Meruvax® II, ProQuad®

Why get vaccinated?

Measles, mumps, and rubella are serious diseases.

Measles:
- Measles virus causes rash, cough, runny nose, eye irritation, and fever.
- It can lead to ear infection, pneumonia, seizures (jerking and staring), brain damage, and death.

Mumps:
- Mumps virus causes fever, headache, and swollen glands.
- It can lead to deafness, meningitis (infection of the brain and spinal cord covering), painful swelling of the testicles or ovaries, and, rarely, death.

Rubella (German Measles):
- Rubella virus causes rash, mild fever, and arthritis (mostly in women).
- If a woman gets rubella while she is pregnant, she could have a miscarriage or her baby could be born with serious birth defects.

You or your child could catch these diseases by being around someone who has them. They spread from person to person through the air. Measles, mumps, and rubella (MMR) vaccine can prevent these diseases. Most children who get their MMR shots will not get these diseases. Many more children would get them if we stopped vaccinating.

Who should get MMR vaccine and when?

Children should get **2 doses** of MMR vaccine:
- The first at 12-15 months of age
- and the second at 4-6 years of age.

These are the recommended ages. But children can get the second dose at any age, as long as it is at least 28 days after the first dose.

Some adults should also get MMR vaccine. Generally, anyone 18 years of age or older, who was born after 1956, should get at least one dose of MMR vaccine, unless they can show that they have had either the vaccines or the diseases. Ask your doctor or nurse for more information. MMR vaccine may be given at the same time as other vaccines.

Who should *not* get MMR vaccine or should wait?

- People should not get MMR vaccine who have ever had a life-threatening allergic reaction to gelatin, the antibiotic neomycin, or to a previous dose of MMR vaccine.
- People who are moderately or severely ill at the time the shot is scheduled should usually wait until they recover before getting MMR vaccine.
- Pregnant women should wait to get MMR vaccine until after they have given birth. Women should avoid getting pregnant for 4 weeks after getting MMR vaccine.

Some people should check with their doctor about whether they should get MMR vaccine, including anyone who:
- Has HIV/AIDS, or another disease that affects the immune system
- Is being treated with drugs that affect the immune system, such as steroids, for 2 weeks or longer
- Has any kind of cancer
- Is taking cancer treatment with x-rays or drugs
- Has ever had a low platelet count (a blood disorder)

People who recently had a transfusion or were given other blood products should ask their doctor when they may get MMR vaccine.

Ask your doctor or nurse for more information.

What are the risks from MMR vaccine?

A vaccine, like any medicine, is capable of causing serious problems, such as severe allergic reactions. The risk of MMR vaccine causing serious harm, or death, is extremely small. Getting MMR vaccine is much safer than getting any of these three diseases. Most people who get MMR vaccine do not have any problems with it.

Mild problems:
- Fever (up to 1 person out of 6)
- Mild rash (about 1 person out of 20)

- Swelling of glands in the cheeks or neck (rare)
- If these problems occur, it is usually within 7-12 days after the shot. They occur less often after the second dose.
  Moderate Problems:
- Seizure (jerking or staring) caused by fever (about 1 out of 3,000 doses)
- Temporary pain and stiffness in the joints, mostly in teenage or adult women (up to 1 out of 4)
- Temporary low platelet count, which can cause a bleeding disorder (about 1 out of 30,000 doses)
  Severe Problems (Very Rare):
- Serious allergic reaction (less than 1 out of a million doses)
- Several other severe problems have been known to occur after a child gets MMR vaccine. But this happens so rarely, experts cannot be sure whether they are caused by the vaccine or not. These include: deafness; long-term seizures, coma, or lowered consciousness; permanent brain damage.

What if there is a moderate or severe reaction?

What should I look for?

- Any unusual conditions, such as a serious allergic reaction, high fever or behavior changes. Signs of a serious allergic reaction include difficulty breathing, hoarseness or wheezing, hives, paleness, weakness, a fast heart beat or dizziness within a few minutes to a few hours after the shot. A high fever or seizure, if it occurs, would happen 1 or 2 weeks after the shot.

What should I do?

- Call a doctor, or get the person to a doctor right away.
- Tell your doctor what happened, the date and time it happened, and when the vaccination was given.
- Ask your health care provider to file a Vaccine Adverse Event Reporting System (VAERS) form if you have any reaction to the vaccine. Or call VAERS yourself at 1-800-822-7967, or visit their website at http://vaers.hhs.gov.

The National Vaccine Injury Compensation Program

In the rare event that you or your child has a serious reaction to a vaccine, a federal program has been created to help pay for the care of those who have been harmed.

For details about the National Vaccine Injury Compensation Program, call 1-800-338-2382 or visit the program's website at http://www.hrsa.gov/vaccinecompensation.

How can I learn more?

- Ask your doctor or other health care provider. They can give you the vaccine package insert or suggest other sources of information.
- Call your local or state health department's immunization program.

- Contact the Centers for Disease Control and Prevention (CDC): call 1-800-232-4636 (1-800-CDC-INFO) or visit the National Immunization Program's website at http://www.cdc.gov/nip.

MMR Vaccine Information Statement. U.S. Department of Health and Human Services/Centers for Disease Control and Prevention National Immunization Program. 1/15/2003.

Mebendazole

(me ben′ da zole)

Brand Name: Vermox®

Why is this medicine prescribed?

Mebendazole, an antiworm medication, kills parasites. It is used to treat roundworm, hookworm, pinworm, whipworm, and other worm infections.

This medication is sometimes prescribed for other uses; ask your doctor or pharmacist for more information.

How should this medicine be used?

Mebendazole comes as a chewable tablet. It usually is taken twice a day, in the morning and evening, for 3 days or as a single (one-time) dose. You may chew the tablets, swallow them whole, or crush and mix them with food. Treatment may have to be repeated in 2-3 weeks. Follow the directions on your prescription label carefully, and ask your doctor or pharmacist to explain any part you do not understand. Take mebendazole exactly as directed. Do not take more or less of it or take it more often than prescribed by your doctor.

What special precautions should I follow?

Before taking mebendazole,

- tell your doctor and pharmacist if you are allergic to mebendazole or any other drugs.
- tell your doctor and pharmacist what prescription and nonprescription medications you are taking, especially carbamazepine (Tegretol), phenytoin (Dilantin), and vitamins.
- tell your doctor if you have or have ever had stomach or liver disease.
- tell your doctor if you are pregnant, plan to become pregnant, or are breast-feeding. If you become pregnant while taking mebendazole, call your doctor.

What should I do if I forget to take a dose?

Take the missed dose as soon as you remember it. However, if it is almost time for the next dose, skip the missed dose and continue your regular dosing schedule. Do not take a double dose to make up for a missed one.

What side effects can this medicine cause?

Mebendazole may cause side effects. Tell your doctor if any of these symptoms are severe or do not go away:

- diarrhea
- stomach pain

What storage conditions are needed for this medicine?

Keep this medication in the container it came in, tightly closed, and out of reach of children. Store it at room temperature and away from excess heat and moisture (not in the bathroom). Throw away any medication that is outdated or no longer needed. Talk to your pharmacist about the proper disposal of your medication.

What should I do in case of overdose?

In case of overdose, call your local poison control center at 1-800-222-1222. If the victim has collapsed or is not breathing, call local emergency services at 911.

What other information should I know?

Keep all appointments with your doctor and the laboratory. Your doctor will order certain lab tests to check your response to mebendazole.

Do not let anyone else take your medication. Your prescription is probably not refillable. If you still have symptoms of infection after you finish the mebendazole, call your doctor.

Talk to your doctor, pharmacist, or other healthcare professional if you have questions about dosing information for your medication.

Meclizine

(mek′ li zeen)

Brand Name: Antivert®, Bonine®, Dramamine® Less Drowsy, Meni-D®
Also available generically.

Why is this medicine prescribed?

Meclizine is used to prevent and treat nausea, vomiting, and dizziness caused by motion sickness. It is most effective if taken before symptoms appear.

This medication is sometimes prescribed for other uses; ask your doctor or pharmacist for more information.

How should this medicine be used?

Meclizine comes as a regular and chewable tablet and a capsule. For motion sickness, meclizine should be taken 1 hour before you start to travel. Doses may be taken every 24 hours if needed. For dizziness caused by an ear condition, follow your doctor's directions. Follow the directions on your prescription label carefully, and ask your doctor or pharmacist to explain any part you do not understand. Take meclizine

exactly as directed. Do not take more or less of it or take it more often than prescribed by your doctor.

The chewable tablets may be chewed or swallowed whole.

What special precautions should I follow?

Before taking meclizine,

- tell your doctor and pharmacist if you are allergic to meclizine or any other drugs.
- tell your doctor and pharmacist what prescription and nonprescription medications you are taking, especially amobarbital (Amytal), medications for colds or allergies, pain medications, phenobarbital, sedatives, seizure medications, sleeping pills, tranquilizers, and vitamins. These drugs may increase the drowsiness caused by meclizine.
- tell your doctor if you have or have ever had glaucoma, an enlarged prostate, urinary tract blockage, or asthma.
- tell your doctor if you are pregnant, plan to become pregnant, or are breast-feeding. If you become pregnant while taking meclizine, call your doctor.

What should I do if I forget to take a dose?

Take the missed dose as soon as you remember it. However, if it is almost time for the next dose, skip the missed dose and continue your regular dosing schedule. Do not take a double dose to make up for a missed one.

What side effects can this medicine cause?

Meclizine may cause side effects. Tell your doctor if any of these symptoms are severe or do not go away:

- drowsiness or fatigue
- dry mouth

If you experience the following symptom, call your doctor immediately:

- blurred vision

If you experience a serious side effect, you or your doctor may send a report to the Food and Drug Administration's (FDA) MedWatch Adverse Event Reporting program online [at http://www.fda.gov/MedWatch/index.html] or by phone [1-800-332-1088].

What storage conditions are needed for this medicine?

Keep this medication in the container it came in, tightly closed, and out of reach of children. Store it at room temperature and away from excess heat and moisture (not in the bathroom). Throw away any medication that is outdated or no longer needed. Talk to your pharmacist about the proper disposal of your medication.

What should I do in case of overdose?

In case of overdose, call your local poison control center at 1-800-222-1222. If the victim has collapsed or is not breathing, call local emergency services at 911.

What other information should I know?

Keep all appointments with your doctor.

Do not let anyone else take your medication. Ask your pharmacist any questions you have about refilling your prescription.

Dosage Facts

For Informational Purposes

Caution: Do not change your dose, how often you take your medication, or the length of time you are to take it without first talking to your health-care provider.

The following dosage information was written using medical language for doctors and other healthcare professionals and is provided here for you to check your dosage. The dosage of this drug may differ for different patients. Therefore, always follow your doctor's instructions or the directions on the label. Contact your healthcare provider or pharmacist if you have any questions about the specific dosage of your medication after reviewing this information.

General Dosage Information

Available as meclizine hydrochloride; dosage expressed in terms of meclizine.

Pediatric Patients

Motion Sickness

ORAL:
- For *self-medication* in children ≥12 years of age, 25–50 mg once daily or as directed by clinician.

Adult Patients

Motion Sickness

ORAL:
- For *self-medication*, 25–50 mg once daily or as directed by clinician.

Vertigo

ORAL:
- 25–100 mg daily, administered in divided doses, depending on clinical response.

Meclofenamate

(me kloe fen am′ ate)

Important Warning

People who take nonsteroidal anti-inflammatory medications (NSAIDs) (other than aspirin) such as meclofenamate may have a higher risk of having a heart attack or a stroke than people who do not take these medications. These events may happen without warning and may cause death. This risk may be higher for people who take NSAIDs for a long time. Tell your doctor if you or anyone in your family has or has ever had heart disease, a heart attack, or a stroke, if you smoke, and if you have or have ever had high cholesterol, high blood pressure, or diabetes. Get emergency medical help right away if you experience any of the following symptoms: chest pain, shortness of breath, weakness in one part or side of the body, or slurred speech.

If you will be undergoing a coronary artery bypass graft (CABG; a type of heart surgery), you should not take meclofenamate right before or right after the surgery.

NSAIDs such as meclofenamate may cause ulcers, bleeding, or holes in the stomach or intestine. These problems may develop at any time during treatment, may happen without warning symptoms, and may cause death. The risk may be higher for people who take NSAIDs for a long time, are older in age, have poor health, or drink large amounts of alcohol while taking meclofenamate. Tell your doctor if you take any of the following medications: anticoagulants ('blood thinners') such as warfarin (Coumadin); aspirin; other NSAIDS such as ibuprofen (Advil, Motrin) and naproxen (Aleve, Naprosyn); or oral steroids such as dexamethasone (Decadron, Dexone), methylprednisolone (Medrol), and prednisone (Deltasone). Also tell your doctor if you have or have ever had ulcers, bleeding in your stomach or intestines, or other bleeding disorders. If you experience any of the following symptoms, stop taking meclofenamate and call your doctor: stomach pain, heartburn, vomiting a substance that is bloody or looks like coffee grounds, blood in the stool, or black and tarry stools.

Keep all appointments with your doctor and the laboratory. Your doctor will monitor your symptoms carefully and will probably order certain tests to check your body's response to meclofenamate. Be sure to tell your doctor how you are feeling so that your doctor can prescribe the right amount of medication to treat your condition with the lowest risk of serious side effects.

Your doctor or pharmacist will give you the manufacturer's patient information sheet (Medication Guide) when you begin treatment with meclofenamate and each time you refill your prescription. Read the information carefully and ask your doctor or pharmacist if you have any questions. You can also visit the Food and Drug Administration (FDA) website (http://www.fda.gov/cder) to obtain the Medication Guide.

Why is this medicine prescribed?

Meclofenamate is used to relieve pain, tenderness, swelling, and stiffness caused by osteoarthritis (arthritis caused by a breakdown of the lining of the joints) and rheumatoid arthritis (arthritis caused by swelling of the lining of the joints). It is also used to relieve other types of mild to moderate pain, including menstrual pain (pain that happens before or during a menstrual period). It also may be used to decrease bleeding in women who have abnormally heavy menstrual blood loss. Meclofenamate is in a class of medications called NSAIDs. It works by stopping the body's production of a substance that causes pain, fever, and inflammation.

How should this medicine be used?

Meclofenamate comes as a capsule to take by mouth. It is usually taken three or four times a day for arthritis, three times a day for heavy menstrual blood loss, or every 4-6 hours as needed for pain. Meclofenamate may be taken with food or milk to prevent upset stomach. If you take meclofenamate regularly, take it at the same times every day. Follow the directions on your prescription label carefully, and ask your doctor or pharmacist to explain any part you do not understand. Take meclofenamate exactly as directed. Do not take more or less of it or take it more often than prescribed by your doctor.

If you are taking meclofenamate to reduce heavy menstrual bleeding, your bleeding should decrease during your treatment. Call your doctor if your bleeding does not decrease or if you experience spotting or bleeding between menstrual periods.

If you are taking meclofenamate to relieve the symptoms of arthritis, your symptoms may begin to improve within a few days. It may take 2 to 3 weeks or longer for you to feel the full benefit of meclofenamate.

Are there other uses for this medicine?

Meclofenamate is also used to treat ankylosing spondylitis (arthritis that mainly affects the spine), gouty arthritis (joint pain caused by a build-up of certain substances in the joints), and psoriatic arthritis (arthritis that occurs with a long-lasting skin disease that causes scaling and swelling). Talk to your doctor about the risks of using this medication to treat your condition.

This medication is sometimes prescribed for other uses; ask your doctor or pharmacist for more information.

What special precautions should I follow?

Before taking meclofenamate,

- tell your doctor and pharmacist if you are allergic to meclofenamate, aspirin, or other NSAIDs such as ibuprofen (Advil, Motrin) and naproxen (Aleve, Naprosyn), any other medications, or any of the inactive ingredients in meclofenamate capsules. Ask your pharmacist for a list of the inactive ingredients.
- tell your doctor and pharmacist what prescription and nonprescription medications, vitamins, nutritional supplements, and herbal products you are taking or plan to take. Be sure to mention the medications listed in the IMPORTANT WARNING section and any of the following: angiotensin-converting enzyme (ACE) inhibitors such as benazepril (Lotensin), captopril (Capoten), enalapril (Vasotec), fosinopril (Monopril), lisinopril (Prinivil, Zestril), moexipril (Univasc), perindopril (Aceon), quinapril (Accupril), ramipril (Altace), and trandolapril (Mavik); diuretics ('water pills'); lithium (Eskalith, Lithobid); and methotrexate (Rheumatrex). Your doctor may need to change the doses of your medications or monitor you carefully for side effects.
- tell your doctor if you have or have ever had any of the conditions mentioned in the IMPORTANT WARNING section or asthma, especially if you also have frequent stuffed or runny nose or nasal polyps (swelling of the lining of the nose); swelling of the hands, feet, ankles, or lower legs; or liver or kidney disease.
- tell your doctor if you are pregnant, especially if you are in the last few months of your pregnancy, you plan to become pregnant, or you are breast-feeding. If you become pregnant while taking meclofenamate, call your doctor.
- if you are having surgery, including dental surgery, tell the doctor or dentist that you are taking meclofenamate.

What special dietary instructions should I follow?

Unless your doctor tells you otherwise, continue your normal diet.

What should I do if I forget to take a dose?

Take the missed dose as soon as you remember it. However, if it is almost time for the next dose, skip the missed dose and continue your regular dosing schedule. Do not take a double dose to make up for a missed one.

What side effects can this medicine cause?

Meclofenamate may cause side effects. Tell your doctor if any of these symptoms are severe or do not go away:

- diarrhea
- constipation
- gas
- sores in the mouth
- headache
- ringing in the ears

Some side effects can be serious. If you experience any of the following symptoms, or those mentioned in the IMPORTANT WARNING section, call your doctor immediately. Do not take any more meclofenamate until you speak to your doctor.

- blurred vision
- unexplained weight gain
- fever
- blisters
- rash
- itching
- hives
- swelling of the eyes, face, lips, tongue, throat, arms, hands, feet, ankles, or lower legs
- hoarseness
- difficulty breathing or swallowing
- yellowing of the skin or eyes
- excessive tiredness
- unusual bleeding or bruising
- lack of energy
- upset stomach
- loss of appetite
- pain in the upper right part of the stomach
- flu-like symptoms
- pale skin
- fast heartbeat
- cloudy, discolored, or bloody urine
- back pain
- difficult or painful urination

Meclofenamate may cause other side effects. Call your doctor if you have any unusual problems while taking this medication.

If you experience a serious side effect, you or your doctor may send a report to the Food and Drug Administration's (FDA) MedWatch Adverse Event Reporting program online [at http://www.fda.gov/MedWatch/index.html] or by phone [1-800-332-1088].

What storage conditions are needed for this medicine?

Keep this medication in the container it came in, tightly closed, and out of reach of children. Store it at room temperature and away from excess heat and moisture (not in the bathroom). Throw away any medication that is outdated or no longer needed. Talk to your pharmacist about the proper disposal of your medication.

What should I do in case of overdose?

In case of overdose, call your local poison control center at 1-800-222-1222. If the victim has collapsed or is not breathing, call local emergency services at 911.

Symptoms of overdoses may include:
- behavior that does not make sense
- agitation
- seizures
- decreased urination

What other information should I know?

Do not let anyone else take your medication. Ask your pharmacist any questions you have about refilling your prescription.

Dosage Facts
For Informational Purposes

Caution: Do not change your dose, how often you take your medication, or the length of time you are to take it without first talking to your health-care provider.

The following dosage information was written using medical language for doctors and other healthcare professionals and is provided here for you to check your dosage. The dosage of this drug may differ for different patients. Therefore, always follow your doctor's instructions or the directions on the label. Contact your healthcare provider or pharmacist if you have any questions about the specific dosage of your medication after reviewing this information.

General Dosage Information

Available as meclofenamate sodium; dosage expressed in terms of meclofenamic acid.

To minimize the potential risk of adverse cardiovascular and/or GI events, use lowest effective dosage and shortest duration of therapy consistent with the patient's treatment goals. Adjust dosage based on individual requirements and response; attempt to titrate to the lowest effective dosage.

Adult Patients

Inflammatory Diseases
Osteoarthritis or Rheumatoid Arthritis

ORAL:
- 200–400 mg daily in 3 or 4 equally divided doses. Initiate at lower dosage and adjust dose and frequency as necessary based on severity of symptoms and clinical response (maximum 400 mg daily).

Pain

ORAL:
- 50 mg every 4–6 hours. Some patients may require 100-mg doses for optimal pain relief (maximum 400 mg daily).

Dysmenorrhea or Menorrhagia

ORAL:
- 100 mg 3 times daily. Initiated at onset of menses and continue ≤ 6 days or until cessation of menses.

Prescribing Limits

Adult Patients

Inflammatory Diseases
Osteoarthritis or Rheumatoid Arthritis

ORAL:
- Maximum 400 mg daily.

Pain

ORAL:
- For mild to moderate pain, maximum 400 mg daily.

Dysmenorrhea or Menorrhagia

ORAL:
- Maximum 300 mg daily.

Special Populations

Renal Impairment
- Dosage reduction recommended in patients with renal impairment; monitor renal function.
- Use not recommended in patients with advanced renal disease.

Geriatric Patients
- Consider reduced initial dosage; monitor carefully.

Medroxyprogesterone

(me drox′ ee proe jes′ te rone)

Brand Name: Premphase® as a combination product containing Medroxyprogesterone Acetate, Conjugated Estrogens, and Conjugated Estrogens, Prempro® as a combination product containing Medroxyprogesterone Acetate and Conjugated Estrogens, Provera®

Also available generically.

Why is this medicine prescribed?

Medroxyprogesterone is used to treat abnormal menstruation (periods) or irregular vaginal bleeding. Medroxyprogesterone is also used to bring on a normal menstrual cycle in women who menstruated normally in the past but have not menstruated for at least 6 months and who are not pregnant or undergoing menopause (change of life). Medroxyprogesterone is also used to prevent overgrowth of the lining of the uterus (womb) and may decrease the risk of cancer of the uterus in patients who are taking estrogen. Medroxyprogesterone is in a class of medications called progestins. It works by stopping the growth of the lining of the uterus and by causing the uterus to produce certain hormones.

How should this medicine be used?

Medroxyprogesterone comes as a tablet to take by mouth. It is usually taken once a day on certain days of a regular monthly cycle. To help you remember to take medroxyprogesterone, take it at around the same time every day on the days you are scheduled to take it. Follow the directions on your prescription label carefully, and ask your doctor or pharmacist to explain any part you do not understand. Take medroxyprogesterone exactly as directed. Do not take more or less of it or take it more often than prescribed by your doctor.

Medroxyprogesterone may control your condition but will not cure it. Continue to take medroxyprogesterone according to your monthly schedule even if you feel well. Do not stop taking medroxyprogesterone without talking to your doctor.

Are there other uses for this medicine?

This medication may be prescribed for other uses; ask your doctor or pharmacist for more information.

What special precautions should I follow?

Before taking medroxyprogesterone,
- tell your doctor and pharmacist if you are allergic to medroxyprogesterone (Provera, Depo-Provera), any other medications, or corn.
- tell your doctor and pharmacist what prescription and nonprescription medications, vitamins, nutritional supplements, and herbal products you are taking. Be sure to mention aminoglutethimide (Cytadren). Your doctor may need to change the doses of your medications or monitor you carefully for side effects.
- tell your doctor if you have or have ever had cancer of the breasts or female organs; unexplained vaginal bleeding; a missed abortion (a pregnancy that ended when the unborn child died in the uterus but was not expelled from the body); blood clots in your legs, lungs, brain, or eyes; stroke or mini-stroke; seizures; migraine headaches; depression; asthma; diabetes; or heart, kidney, or liver disease.
- tell your doctor if you are pregnant, plan to become pregnant, or are breast-feeding. If you become pregnant while taking medroxyprogesterone, call your doctor immediately. Medroxyprogesterone should never be used to test for pregnancy or to prevent miscarriage during the first few months of pregnancy. Medroxyprogesterone has not been shown to prevent miscarriage and may harm the fetus.
- if you are having surgery, including dental surgery, tell the doctor or dentist that you are taking medroxyprogesterone.

What special dietary instructions should I follow?

Unless your doctor tells you otherwise, continue your normal diet.

What should I do if I forget to take a dose?

Take the missed dose as soon as you remember it. However, if it is almost time for the next dose, skip the missed dose and continue your regular dosing schedule. Do not take a double dose to make up for a missed one.

What side effects can this medicine cause?

Medroxyprogesterone may cause side effects. Tell your doctor if any of these symptoms are severe or do not go away:
- breasts that are tender or produce a liquid
- changes in menstrual flow
- irregular vaginal bleeding or spotting

- acne
- growth of hair on face
- loss of hair on scalp
- difficulty falling asleep or staying asleep
- drowsiness
- upset stomach
- weight gain or loss

Some side effects can be serious. The following symptoms are uncommon, but if you experience any of them, call your doctor immediately:

- pain, swelling, warmth, redness, or tenderness in one leg only
- slow or difficult speech
- dizziness or faintness
- weakness or numbness of an arm or leg
- shortness of breath
- coughing up blood
- sudden sharp or crushing chest pain
- fast or pounding heartbeat
- sudden vision changes or loss of vision
- double vision
- blurred vision
- bulging eyes
- missed periods
- depression
- yellowing of the skin or eyes
- fever
- hives
- skin rash
- itching
- difficulty breathing or swallowing
- swelling of the hands, feet, ankles, or lower legs

Some laboratory animals who were given medroxyprogesterone developed breast tumors. It is not known if medroxyprogesterone increases the risk of breast cancer in humans. Medroxyprogesterone may also increase the chance that you will develop a blood clot that moves to your lungs or brain. Talk to your doctor about the risks of taking this medication.

Medroxyprogesterone may cause other side effects. Call your doctor if you have any unusual problems while taking this medication.

If you experience a serious side effect, you or your doctor may send a report to the Food and Drug Administration's (FDA) MedWatch Adverse Event Reporting program online [at http://www.fda.gov/MedWatch/index.html] or by phone [1-800-332-1088].

What storage conditions are needed for this medicine?

Keep this medication in the container it came in, tightly closed, and out of reach of children. Store it at room temperature and away from excess heat and moisture (not in the bathroom). Throw away any medication that is outdated or no longer needed. Talk to your pharmacist about the proper disposal of your medication.

What should I do in case of overdose?

In case of overdose, call your local poison control center at 1-800-222-1222. If the victim has collapsed or is not breathing, call local emergency services at 911.

What other information should I know?

Keep all appointments with your doctor.

Before having any laboratory test, tell your doctor and the laboratory personnel that you are taking medroxyprogesterone.

Do not let anyone else take your medication. Ask your pharmacist any questions you have about refilling your prescription.

Dosage Facts
For Informational Purposes

Caution: Do not change your dose, how often you take your medication, or the length of time you are to take it without first talking to your health-care provider.

The following dosage information was written using medical language for doctors and other healthcare professionals and is provided here for you to check your dosage. The dosage of this drug may differ for different patients. Therefore, always follow your doctor's instructions or the directions on the label. Contact your healthcare provider or pharmacist if you have any questions about the specific dosage of your medication after reviewing this information.

General Dosage Information

Available as medroxyprogesterone acetate; dosage expressed in terms of the salt.

When used as a contraceptive or for the management of endometriosis, dosage does not need to be adjusted based on weight.

Adult Patients

Prevention of Endometrial Changes Associated with Estrogens

ORAL:
- 1.5–5 mg daily. Alternatively, 5–10 mg daily for 12–14 consecutive days per month.

Amenorrhea

ORAL:
- 5–10 mg daily for 5–10 days.
- To induce optimum secretory transformation of an endometrium that has been adequately primed with endogenous or exogenous estrogen, 10 mg daily for 10 days.

Uterine Bleeding

ORAL:
- 5–10 mg daily for 5–10 days beginning on the assumed or calculated 16th or 21st day of the menstrual cycle.
- To induce optimum secretory transformation of an endome-

trium that has been adequately primed with endogenous or exogenous estrogen, 10 mg daily for 10 days, beginning on the calculated 16th day of the menstrual cycle.

† Use is not currently included in the labeling approved by the US Food and Drug Administration.

Medroxyprogesterone Injection

(me drox′ ee proe jes′ te rone)

Brand Name: Depo-Provera, depo-subQ provera 104®

Also available generically.

Important Warning

Medroxyprogesterone injection may decrease the amount of calcium stored in your bones. The longer you use this medication, the more the amount of calcium in your bones may decrease. The amount of calcium in your bones may not return to normal even after you stop using medroxyprogesterone injection.

Loss of calcium from your bones may cause osteoporosis (a condition in which the bones become thin and weak) and may increase the risk that your bones might break at some time in your life, especially after menopause (change of life).

The amount of calcium in the bones usually increases during the teenage years. A decrease in bone calcium during this important time of bone strengthening may be especially serious. It is not known whether your risk of developing osteoporosis later in life is greater if you start to use medroxyprogesterone injection when you are a teenager or young adult. Tell your doctor if you or anyone in your family has osteoporosis; if you have or have ever had any other bone disease or anorexia nervosa (an eating disorder); or if you drink a lot of alcohol or smoke a great deal. Tell your doctor if you take any of the following medications: corticosteroids such as dexamethasone (Decadron, Dexone), methylprednisolone (Medrol), and prednisone (Deltasone); or medications for seizures such as carbamazepine (Tegretol), phenytoin (Dilantin), or phenobarbital (Luminal, Solfoton).

You should not use medroxyprogesterone injection for a long time (e.g., more than 2 years) unless no other method of birth control is right for you or no other medication will work to treat your condition. Your doctor may test your bones to be sure they are not becoming too thin before you continue to use medroxyprogesterone injection.

Keep all appointments with your doctor and the laboratory. Your doctor will monitor your health carefully to be sure you do not develop osteoporosis.

Talk to your doctor about the risks of using medroxyprogesterone injection.

Why is this medicine prescribed?

Medroxyprogesterone intramuscular (into a muscle) injection and medroxyprogesterone subcutaneous (under the skin) injection are used to prevent pregnancy. Medroxyprogesterone subcutaneous injection is also used to treat endometriosis [a condition in which the type of tissue that lines the uterus (womb) grows in other areas of the body and causes pain, heavy or irregular menstruation (periods), and other symptoms]. Medroxyprogesterone is in a class of medications called progestins. It works to prevent pregnancy by preventing ovulation (the release of eggs from the ovaries). Medroxyprogesterone also thins the lining of the uterus. This helps to prevent pregnancy in all women and slows the spread of tissue from the uterus to other parts of the body in women who have endometriosis. Medroxyprogesterone injection is a very effective method of birth control but does not prevent the spread of human immunodeficiency virus [HIV, the virus that causes acquired immunodeficiency syndrome (AIDS)] or other sexually transmitted diseases.

How should this medicine be used?

Medroxyprogesterone intramuscular injection comes as a suspension (liquid) to be injected into the buttocks or upper arm. It is usually given once every 3 months (13 weeks) by a health care provider in an office or clinic. Medroxyprogesterone subcutaneous injection comes as suspension to be injected just under the skin. It is usually injected once every 12-14 weeks by a health care provider in an office or clinic.

You must receive your first medroxyprogesterone subcutaneous or intramuscular injection only at a time when there is no possibility that you are pregnant. Therefore, you may only receive your first injection during the first 5 days of a normal menstrual period, during the first 5 days after you give birth if you are not planning to breastfeed your baby, or during the sixth week after giving birth if you are planning to breastfeed your baby. If you have been using a different method of birth control and are switching to medroxyprogesterone injection, your doctor will tell you when you should receive your first injection.

Are there other uses for this medicine?

This medication is sometimes prescribed for other uses; ask your doctor or pharmacist for more information.

What special precautions should I follow?

Before using medroxyprogesterone injection,
- tell your doctor and pharmacist if you are allergic to medroxyprogesterone (Depo-Provera, depo-subQ provera 104, Provera, in Prempro, in Premphase) or any other medications.

- tell your doctor and pharmacist what prescription and nonprescription medications, vitamins, nutritional supplements, and herbal products you are taking or plan to take. Be sure to mention the medications listed in the IMPORTANT WARNING section and aminogluteth-imide (Cytadren). Your doctor may need to change the doses of your medications or monitor you carefully for side effects.
- tell your doctor if you or anyone in your family has or has ever had breast cancer or diabetes. Also tell your doctor if you have or have ever had problems with your breasts such as lumps, bleeding from your nipples, an abnormal mammogram (breast x-ray), or fibrocystic breast disease (swollen, tender breasts and/or breast lumps that are not cancer); unexplained vaginal bleeding; irregular or very light menstrual periods; excessive weight gain or fluid retention before your period; blood clots in your legs, lungs, brain, or eyes; stroke or mini-stroke; migraine headaches; seizures; depression; high blood pressure; heart attack; asthma; or heart, liver, or kidney disease.
- tell your doctor if you think you might be pregnant, you are pregnant, or you plan to become pregnant. If you become pregnant while using medroxyprogesterone injection, call your doctor immediately. Medroxyproges-terone may harm the fetus.
- tell your doctor if you are breast-feeding. You may use medroxyprogesterone injection while you are breast-feeding as long as your baby is 6 weeks old when you receive your first injection. Some medroxyprogesterone may be passed to your baby in your breast milk but this has not been shown to be harmful. Studies of babies who were breastfed while their mothers were using medroxyprogesterone injection showed that the babies were not harmed by the medication.
- if you are having surgery, including dental surgery, tell the doctor or dentist that you are using medroxyproges-terone injection.
- you should know that your menstrual cycle will probably change while you are using medroxyprogesterone injection. At first, your periods will probably be irregular, and you may experience spotting between periods. If you continue to use this medication, your periods may stop completely. Your menstrual cycle will probably return to normal some time after you stop using this medication.

What special dietary instructions should I follow?

You should eat plenty of foods that are rich in calcium and vitamin D while you are taking medroxyprogesterone injection to help decrease the loss of calcium from your bones. Your doctor will tell you which foods are good sources of these nutrients and how many servings you need each day. Your doctor also may prescribe or recommend calcium or vitamin D supplements.

What should I do if I forget to take a dose?

If you miss an appointment to receive an injection of med-roxyprogesterone, call your doctor. You may not be protected from pregnancy if you do not receive your injections on schedule. If you do not receive an injection on schedule, your doctor will tell you when you should receive the missed injection. Your doctor will probably administer a pregnancy test to be sure that you are not pregnant before giving you the missed injection. You should use a different method of birth control, such as condoms until you receive the injection that you missed.

What side effects can this medicine cause?

Medroxyprogesterone may cause side effects. Tell your doctor if any of these symptoms are severe or do not go away:
- changes in menstrual periods (See SPECIAL PRECAU-TIONS)
- weight gain
- weakness
- tiredness
- nervousness
- irritability
- depression
- difficulty falling asleep or staying asleep
- hot flashes
- breast pain, swelling, or tenderness
- stomach cramps or bloating
- leg cramps
- back or joint pain
- acne
- loss of hair on scalp
- swelling, redness, irritation, burning, or itching of the vagina
- white vaginal discharge
- changes in sexual desire
- cold or flu symptoms
- pain, irritation, lumps, redness or scarring in the place where the medication was injected

Some side effects can be serious. The following side effects are uncommon, but if you experience any of them, call your doctor immediately:
- sudden shortness of breath
- sudden sharp or crushing chest pain
- coughing up blood
- severe headache
- upset stomach
- vomiting
- dizziness or faintness
- change or loss of vision
- double vision
- bulging eyes
- difficulty speaking
- weakness or numbness in an arm or leg
- seizure
- yellowing of the skin or eyes
- extreme tiredness

- pain, swelling, warmth, redness, or tenderness in one leg only
- menstrual bleeding that is heavier or lasts longer than normal
- severe pain or tenderness just below the waist
- rash
- hives
- itching
- difficulty breathing or swallowing
- swelling of the hands, feet, ankles, or lower legs
- difficult, painful, or frequent urination
- constant pain, pus, warmth, swelling, or bleeding in the place where the medication was injected

If you are younger than 35 years old and began to receive medroxyprogesterone injection in the last 4-5 years, you may have a slightly increased risk that you will develop breast cancer. Medroxyprogesterone injection may also increase the chance that you will develop a blood clot that moves to your lungs or brain. Talk to your doctor about the risks of using this medication.

Medroxyprogesterone injection is a long-acting birth control method. You might not become pregnant for some time after you receive your last injection. Talk to your doctor about the effects of using this medication if you plan to become pregnant in the near future.

Medroxyprogesterone injection may cause other side effects. Call your doctor if you have any unusual problems while taking this medication.

If you experience a serious side effect, you or your doctor may send a report to the Food and Drug Administration's (FDA) MedWatch Adverse Event Reporting program online [at http://www.fda.gov/MedWatch/index.html] or by phone [1-800-332-1088].

What storage conditions are needed for this medicine?

Your doctor will store the medication in his or her office.

What should I do in case of overdose?

In case of overdose, call your local poison control center at 1-800-222-1222. If the victim has collapsed or is not breathing, call local emergency services at 911.

What other information should I know?

You should have a complete physical exam, including blood pressure measurements, breast and pelvic exams, and a Pap test, at least yearly. Follow your doctor's directions for self-examining your breasts; report any lumps immediately.

Before you have any laboratory tests, tell the laboratory personnel that you are using medroxyprogesterone.

Dosage Facts
For Informational Purposes

Caution: Do not change your dose, how often you take your medication, or the length of time you

are to take it without first talking to your health-care provider.

The following dosage information was written using medical language for doctors and other healthcare professionals and is provided here for you to check your dosage. The dosage of this drug may differ for different patients. Therefore, always follow your doctor's instructions or the directions on the label. Contact your healthcare provider or pharmacist if you have any questions about the specific dosage of your medication after reviewing this information.

General Dosage Information

Available as medroxyprogesterone acetate; dosage expressed in terms of the salt.

When used as a contraceptive or for the management of endometriosis, dosage does not need to be adjusted based on weight.

Adult Patients

Contraception in Females
Medroxyprogesterone (Depo-Provera® Contraceptive, medroxyprogesterone acetate contraceptive)

IM:
- 150 mg every 3 months. Exclude possibility of pregnancy before administering the first dose and whenever ≥13 weeks have elapsed since the previous dose. Initiate during the first 5 days of a normal menstrual cycle, at 6 weeks postpartum in women who breast-feed, or within 5 days postpartum in those who do not breast-feed.

Medroxyprogesterone/Estradiol Fixed Combination (Lunelle®)

IM:
- Medroxyprogesterone acetate 25 mg and estradiol cypionate 5 mg (0.5 mL) monthly (every 28–30 days; not to exceed 33 days). Initiate during the first 5 days of a normal menstrual cycle, within 5 days of a complete first-trimester abortion, no earlier than 6 weeks postpartum in women who breast-feed, or no earlier than 4 weeks postpartum in those who do not breast-feed.
- If >33 days have elapsed since the previous injection, use an alternative (i.e., barrier) method of contraception and rule out pregnancy prior to continuing Lunelle®. Shortening the injection interval may alter menstrual pattern.
- When switching from other contraceptive methods, initiate Lunelle® in a manner that ensures continuous contraceptive coverage based on the mechanism of action of both methods (e.g., patients switching from oral contraceptives should be given an initial injection within 7 days after taking the last hormonally active tablet).

Medroxyprogesterone (depo-subQ provera 104®)

SUB-Q:
- 104 mg every 3 months (12–14 weeks). Exclude possibility of pregnancy before administering the first dose and whenever ≥14 weeks have elapsed since the previous dose. Initiate during the first 5 days of a normal menstrual cycle or ≥ 6 weeks postpartum in women who breast-feed.
- When switching from other contraceptive methods, initiate depo-subQ provera 104® in a manner that ensures continuous

contraceptive coverage based on the mechanism of action of both methods. Patients switching from combined contraceptives (estrogen plus progestin) should be given an initial injection within 7 days after taking the last hormonally active tablet or removing a transdermal patch or vaginal ring. Contraceptive coverage will be maintained when switching from medroxyprogesterone acetate contraceptive IM injection (e.g., Depo Provera® contraceptive injection) to depo-subQ provera 104® if the next injection is given within the dosing period recommended for the IM contraceptive injection.

Endometriosis

SUB-Q:
- depo-subQ provera 104®: 104 mg every 3 months (12–14 weeks). Exclude possibility of pregnancy before administering the first dose and whenever ≥14 weeks have elapsed since the previous dose. Initiate during the first 5 days of a normal menstrual cycle or ≥ 6 weeks postpartum in women who breast-feed.
- Benefit of therapy for >6 months not established; treatment for >2 years not recommended.

Endometrial Carcinoma

IM:
- Initially, 400–1000 mg once weekly. When improvement is noted and disease has stabilized (within weeks or months), maintain response with as little as 400 mg/month.

Renal Carcinoma

IM:
- Initially, 400–1000 mg once weekly. When improvement is noted and disease has stabilized (within weeks or months), maintain response with as little as 400 mg/month.

Paraphilia† in Males

IM:
- Initially, 200 mg 2 or 3 times daily. Alternatively, 500 mg once weekly.
- Adjust dose and/or frequency to an effective maintenance level according to patient response and tolerance and/or plasma testosterone concentration. Consult published protocols for more specific dosage information in these males.

† Use is not currently included in the labeling approved by the US Food and Drug Administration.

Mefloquine

(me′ floe kwin)

Brand Name: Lariam®

Why is this medicine prescribed?

Mefloquine is used to treat malaria (a serious infection that is spread by mosquitoes in certain parts of the world and can cause death) and to prevent malaria in travelers who visit areas where malaria is common. Mefloquine is in a class of medications called antimalarials. It works by killing the organisms that cause malaria.

How should this medicine be used?

Mefloquine comes as a tablet to take by mouth. If you are taking mefloquine to prevent malaria, you will probably take it once a week (on the same day each week). You will begin treatment 1-3 weeks before you travel to an area where malaria is common and should continue treatment for 4 weeks after you return from the area. If you are taking mefloquine to treat malaria, your doctor will tell you exactly how often you should take it. Always take mefloquine with food (preferably your main meal) and at least 8 ounces of water. Children may take smaller but more frequent doses of mefloquine. Follow the directions on your prescription label carefully, and ask your doctor or pharmacist to explain any part you do not understand. Take mefloquine exactly as directed. Do not take more or less of it or take it more often than prescribed by your doctor.

The tablets may be swallowed whole or crushed and mixed with a liquid such as water, milk, or sugar water.

If you are taking mefloquine to treat malaria, you may vomit soon after you take the medication. If you vomit less than 30 minutes after you take mefloquine, you should take another full dose of mefloquine. If you vomit 30-60 minutes after you take mefloquine, you should take another half dose of mefloquine. If you vomit again after taking the extra dose, call your doctor.

Are there other uses for this medicine?

This medication may be prescribed for other uses; ask your doctor or pharmacist for more information.

What special precautions should I follow?

Before taking mefloquine,
- tell your doctor and pharmacist if you are allergic to mefloquine, chloroquine (Aralen), hydroxychloroquine (Plaquenil), quinidine (Quinadex), quinine or any other medications.
- tell your doctor and pharmacist what prescription and nonprescription medications, vitamins, nutritional supplements, and herbal products you are taking. Be sure to mention any of the following: anticoagulants ('blood thinners'); antidepressants such as amitriptyline (Elavil), amoxapine (Asendin), clomipramine (Anafranil), desipramine (Norpramin), doxepin (Adapin, Sinequan), imipramine (Tofranil), nortriptyline (Aventyl, Pamelor), protriptyline (Vivactil), and trimipramine (Surmontil); antihistamines; calcium channel blockers such as amlodipine (Norvasc), diltiazem (Cardizem, Dilacor, Tiazac, others), felodipine (Plendil), isradipine (DynaCirc), nicardipine (Cardene), nifedipine (Adalat, Procardia), nimodipine (Nimotop), nisoldipine (Sular), and verapamil (Calan, Isoptin, Verelan); beta blockers such as atenolol (Tenormin), labetalol (Normodyne), metoprolol (Lopressor, Toprol XL), nadolol (Corgard), and propranolol (Inderal); chloroquine (Aralen); halofantrine (Halfan); hydroxychloroquine (Plaquenil); medication for diabetes, mental illness, seizures and up-

set stomach; medications for irregular heartbeat such as quinidine (Quinaglute, Quinidex); and quinine. Your doctor may need to change the doses of your medications or monitor you carefully for side effects.

- tell your doctor if you have or have ever had a mental illness such as depression, generalized anxiety disorder, psychosis (losing touch with reality), or schizophrenia (abnormal thoughts or feelings); seizures; or eye, liver or heart disease.
- tell your doctor if you are pregnant or plan to become pregnant. You should use birth control while you are visiting an area where malaria is common and while you are taking mefloquine and for 3 months after you stop taking it. If you become pregnant while taking mefloquine, call your doctor. You should not breastfeed while taking mefloquine.
- you should know that mefloquine may make you drowsy and dizzy. These symptoms may continue for a while after you stop taking mefloquine. Do not drive a car or operate machinery until you know how this medication affects you.
- you should know that mefloquine decreases your risk of becoming infected with malaria but does not guarantee that you will not become infected. You still need to protect yourself from mosquito bites by wearing long sleeves and long pants and using mosquito repellant and a bednet while you are in an area where malaria is common.
- you should know that the first symptoms of malaria are fever, chills, muscle pain, and headaches. If you are taking mefloquine to prevent malaria, call your doctor immediately if you develop any of these symptoms. Be sure to tell your doctor that you may have been exposed to malaria.
- you should plan what to do in case you experience serious side effects from mefloquine and have to stop taking the medication, especially if you are not near a doctor or pharmacy. You will have to get another medication to protect you from malaria. If no other medication is available, you will have to leave the area where malaria is common, and then get another medication to protect you from malaria.
- if you are taking mefloquine to treat malaria, your symptoms should improve within 48-72 hours after you finish your treatment. Call your doctor if your symptoms do not improve after this time.
- do not have any vaccinations (shots) without talking to your doctor. Your doctor may want you to finish all of your vaccinations 3 days before you start taking mefloquine.
- you should know that mefloquine may damage your liver or eyes if you take it for a long time. Your doctor will tell you if you should have your eyes and liver checked while taking mefloquine.

What special dietary instructions should I follow?

Unless your doctor tells you otherwise, continue your normal diet.

What should I do if I forget to take a dose?

Take the missed dose as soon as you remember it. However, if it is almost time for the next dose, skip the missed dose and continue your regular dosing schedule. Do not take a double dose to make up for a missed one.

What side effects can this medicine cause?

Mefloquine may cause side effects. Tell your doctor if any of these symptoms are severe or do not go away:

- upset stomach
- vomiting
- diarrhea
- stomach pain
- loss of appetite
- muscle pain
- dizziness
- loss of balance
- ringing in ears
- headache
- sleepiness
- difficulty falling or staying asleep
- unusual dreams

Some side effects can be serious. The following symptoms are uncommon, but if you experience any of them, call your doctor immediately:

- tingling in your fingers or toes
- difficulty walking
- seizures
- shaking of arms or legs that you cannot control
- nervousness or extreme worry
- depression
- changes in mood
- panic attack
- forgetfulness
- confusion
- hallucinations (seeing things or hearing voices that do not exist)
- violent behavior
- losing touch with reality
- feeling that others want to harm you
- thoughts of hurting or killing yourself
- rash

Mefloquine may cause other side effects. You may continue to experience side effects for some time after you take your last dose. Call your doctor if you have any unusual problems while taking this medication.

If you experience a serious side effect, you or your doctor may send a report to the Food and Drug Administration's (FDA) MedWatch Adverse Event Reporting program online [at http://www.fda.gov/MedWatch/index.html] or by phone [1-800-332-1088].

What storage conditions are needed for this medicine?

Keep this medication in the container it came in, tightly closed, and out of reach of children. Store it at room temperature and away from excess heat and moisture (not in the bathroom). Throw away any medication that is outdated or no longer needed. Talk to your pharmacist about the proper disposal of your medication.

What should I do in case of overdose?

In case of overdose, call your local poison control center at 1-800-222-1222. If the victim has collapsed or is not breathing, call local emergency services at 911.

Symptoms of overdose may include:
- upset stomach
- vomiting
- diarrhea
- stomach pain
- dizziness
- loss of balance
- headache
- sleepiness
- difficulty falling or staying asleep
- unusual dreams
- tingling in your fingers or toes
- difficulty walking
- seizures
- changes in mental health

What other information should I know?

Keep all appointments with your doctor and the laboratory. Your doctor may order certain lab tests and periodic eye examinations to check your body's response to mefloquine.

Do not let anyone else take your medication. Ask your pharmacist any questions you have about refilling your prescription.

Dosage Facts
For Informational Purposes

Caution: Do not change your dose, how often you take your medication, or the length of time you are to take it without first talking to your healthcare provider.

The following dosage information was written using medical language for doctors and other healthcare professionals and is provided here for you to check your dosage. The dosage of this drug may differ for different patients. Therefore, always follow your doctor's instructions or the directions on the label. Contact your healthcare provider or pharmacist if you have any questions about the specific dosage of your medication after reviewing this information.

General Dosage Information

Available as mefloquine hydrochloride; dosage usually expressed in terms of the salt. In the US, each 250 mg of mefloquine hydrochloride is equivalent to 228 mg of mefloquine base.

Dosage in children is based on body weight.

Pediatric Patients

Malaria
Prevention of P. vivax or P. falciparum Malaria

ORAL:
- Children weighing ≤45 kg: Approximately 5 mg/kg once weekly on the same day each week. (See Table.) Experience in infants <3 months of age or weighing <5 kg is limited.
- Children weighing >45 kg: 250 mg once weekly on the same day each week.

Dosage for Prevention of Malaria in Children Weighing ≤45 kg

Weight (kg)	Dosage Once Weekly
30–45	187.5 mg (¾ of a 250-mg tablet)
20–30	125 mg (½ of a 250-mg tablet)
10–20	62.5 mg (¼ of 250-mg tablet)
5–10	31.25 mg (⅛ of a 250-mg tablet)

Initiate prophylaxis 1–2 weeks prior to entering a malarious area and continue for 4 weeks after leaving the area. If there are concerns about tolerance or drug interactions, it may be advisable to initiate prophylaxis 2–4 weeks prior to travel in individuals receiving other drugs to ensure that the combination of drugs is well tolerated and to allow ample time if a switch to another antimalarial is required.

Terminal prophylaxis with primaquine may be indicated during the final 2 weeks of mefloquine prophylaxis if exposure occurred in areas where *P. ovale* or *P. vivax* are endemic.

Treatment of Uncomplicated P. vivax or P. falciparum Malaria

ORAL:
- Children ≥6 months of age: 20–25 mg/kg; dividing the dosage into 2 doses given 6–8 hours apart may reduce incidence and severity of adverse effects. Alternatively, CDC and some clinicians recommend that children weighing <45 kg may receive an initial dose of 15 mg/kg followed by a single dose of 10 mg/kg 6–12 hours later.
- If a response is not attained within 48–72 hours, an alternative antimalarial agent should be given; mefloquine should not be used for retreatment.
- For those with *P. vivax* malaria, a 14-day regimen of oral primaquine also may be indicated to provide a radical cure and prevent delayed attacks or relapse.

Presumptive Self-treatment of Malaria†

ORAL:
- An initial dose of 15 mg/kg followed by 10 mg/kg 12 hours later. Initiate presumptive self-treatment if malaria is sus-

pected (fever, chills, or other influenza-like illness) and professional medical care will not be available within 24 hours.
- *Not* recommended for presumptive self-treatment of malaria in those currently taking the drug for prophylaxis.

Adult Patients

Malaria
Prevention of P. vivax or P. falciparum Malaria
ORAL:
- 250 mg once weekly on the same day each week.
- Initiate prophylaxis 1–2 weeks prior to entering a malarious area and continue for 4 weeks after leaving the area. If there are concerns about tolerance or drug interactions, it may be advisable to initiate prophylaxis 3–4 weeks prior to travel in individuals receiving other drugs to ensure that the combination of drugs is well tolerated and to allow ample time if a switch to another antimalarial is required.
- Terminal prophylaxis with primaquine may be indicated during the final 2 weeks of mefloquine prophylaxis if exposure occurred in areas where *P. ovale* or *P. vivax* are endemic.

Treatment of Uncomplicated P. vivax or P. falciparum Malaria
ORAL:
- A single dose of 1250 mg. Alternatively, CDC and others recommend an initial dose of 750 mg followed by 500 mg given 6–12 hours later (total dose of 1250 mg).
- If a response is not attained within 48–72 hours, an alternative antimalarial agent should be given; mefloquine should not be used for retreatment.
- For those with *P. vivax* malaria, a 14-day regimen of oral primaquine also may be indicated to provide a radical cure and prevent delayed attacks or relapse.

Presumptive Self-treatment of Malaria†
ORAL:
- An initial dose of 750 mg followed by 500 mg given 12 hours later (total dose of 1250 mg). Initiate presumptive self-treatment if malaria is suspected (fever, chills, or other influenza-like illness) and professional medical care will not be available within 24 hours.
- *Not* recommended for presumptive self-treatment of malaria in individuals currently taking the drug for prophylaxis.

Prescribing Limits

Pediatric Patients

Malaria
Prevention of P. vivax or P. falciparum Malaria
ORAL:
- Maximum 1250 mg daily.

Special Populations
Hepatic Impairment
- No specific recommendations available regarding need for dosage adjustment in individuals with hepatic impairment. Increased mefloquine plasma concentrations may occur because of decreased elimination.

Renal Impairment
- No specific recommendations available regarding need for dosage adjustment in individuals with renal impairment.
- When used for prevention of malaria, limited data indicate

that dosage adjustment is not necessary in patients undergoing hemodialysis.

† Use is not currently included in the labeling approved by the US Food and Drug Administration.

Megestrol
(me jes′ trol)

Brand Name: Megace®, Megace® ES
Also available generically.

Why is this medicine prescribed?
Megestrol tablets are used to relieve the symptoms and reduce the suffering caused by advanced breast cancer and advanced endometrial cancer (cancer that begins in the lining of the uterus). Megestrol suspension is used to treat loss of appetite, malnutrition, and severe weight loss in patients with acquired immunodeficiency syndrome (AIDS). Megestrol should not be used to prevent loss of appetite and severe weight loss in patients who have not yet developed this condition. Megestrol is a man-made version of the human hormone progesterone. It treats breast cancer and endometrial cancer by affecting female hormones involved in cancer growth. It increases weight gain by increasing appetite.

How should this medicine be used?
Megestrol comes as a tablet, a suspension (liquid), and a concentrated suspension (Megace ES) to take by mouth. The tablets and suspension are usually taken several times a day. The concentrated suspension is usually taken once a day. Take megestrol at around the same time(s) every day. Follow the directions on your prescription label carefully, and ask your doctor or pharmacist to explain any part you do not understand. Take megestrol exactly as directed. Do not take more or less of it or take it more often than prescribed by your doctor.

Shake the liquid well before each use to mix the medication evenly.

The concentrated suspension is used in different dosages than the regular suspension. Do not switch from one to the other without talking to your doctor.

Do not stop taking megestrol without talking to your doctor.

Are there other uses for this medicine?
Megestrol is also sometimes used to treat malnutrition in patients with cancer, prostatic hypertrophy (enlargement of a male reproductive gland called the prostate), endometriosis (condition in which the type of tissue that lines the uterus grows in other areas of the body), and endometrial hyper-

plasia (overgrowth of the lining of the uterus). Talk to your doctor about the risks of using this medication for your condition.

What special precautions should I follow?

Before taking megestrol,

- tell your doctor and pharmacist if you are allergic to megestrol, any other medications, or any of the inactive ingredients in megestrol tablets, suspension, or concentrated suspension.. Ask your doctor or pharmacist for a list of the inactive ingredients.
- tell your doctor and pharmacist what prescription and nonprescription medications, vitamins, nutritional supplements, and herbal products you are taking or plan to take. Be sure to mention antibiotics and indinavir (Crixivan). Your doctor may need to adjust the doses of your medications or monitor you carefully for side effects.
- tell your doctor if you have or have ever had a blood clot anywhere in the body, a stroke, diabetes, or kidney or liver disease.
- tell your doctor if you are pregnant, plan to become pregnant, or are breast-feeding. If you become pregnant while taking megestrol, call your doctor immediately. Megestrol may harm the fetus. Do not breastfeed while you are taking megestrol.
- you should know that megestrol may interfere with the normal menstrual cycle (period) in women. However, you should not assume that you cannot become pregnant. Use a reliable method of birth control to prevent pregnancy.
- if you are having surgery, including dental surgery, during or shortly after your treatment, tell the doctor or dentist that you are taking megestrol.

What special dietary instructions should I follow?

Unless your doctor tells you otherwise, continue your normal diet.

What should I do if I forget to take a dose?

Take the missed dose as soon as you remember it. However, if it is almost time for the next dose, skip the missed dose and continue your regular dosing schedule. Do not take a double dose to make up for a missed one.

What side effects can this medicine cause?

Megestrol may cause side effects. Tell your doctor if any of these symptoms are severe or do not go away:

- impotence
- decreased sexual desire
- unexpected vaginal bleeding
- difficulty falling asleep or staying asleep
- gas
- rash

Some side effects can be serious. If you experience any of these symptoms, call your doctor immediately:

- nausea
- vomiting
- dizziness
- weakness
- blurred vision
- extreme thirst
- frequent urination
- extreme hunger
- leg pain
- difficulty breathing
- sharp, crushing chest pain or heaviness in chest
- slow or difficult speech
- weakness or numbness of an arm or leg

Megestrol may cause other side effects. Call your doctor if you have any unusual problems while taking this medication.

What storage conditions are needed for this medicine?

Keep this medication in the container it came in, tightly closed, and out of reach of children. Store it at room temperature and away from excess heat and moisture (not in the bathroom). Throw away any medication that is outdated or no longer needed. Talk to your pharmacist about the proper disposal of your medication.

What should I do in case of overdose?

In case of overdose, call your local poison control center at 1-800-222-1222. If the victim has collapsed or is not breathing, call local emergency services at 911.

What other information should I know?

Keep all appointments with your doctor and the laboratory. Your doctor may order certain lab tests to check your body's response to megestrol.

Do not let anyone else take your medication. Ask your pharmacist any questions you have about refilling your prescription.

Dosage Facts
For Informational Purposes

Caution: Do not change your dose, how often you take your medication, or the length of time you are to take it without first talking to your healthcare provider.

The following dosage information was written using medical language for doctors and other healthcare professionals and is provided here for you to check your dosage. The dosage of this drug may differ for different patients. Therefore, always follow your doctor's instructions or the directions on the label. Contact your healthcare provider or pharmacist if you have any questions about the specific dosage of your medication after reviewing this information.

General Dosage Information

Available as megestrol acetate; dosage expressed in terms of the salt.

Adult Patients

Breast Cancer

ORAL (TABLETS):
- 160 mg daily in 4 equally divided doses (40 mg 4 times daily); continue therapy for at least 2 months to determine antineoplastic effectiveness.
- Dosages of 480-1600 mg daily in divided doses have been used in clinical trials.

Endometrial Carcinoma

ORAL (TABLETS):
- 40–320 mg daily in divided doses; continue therapy for at least 2 months to determine antineoplastic effectiveness.

Cachexia

Treatment in HIV-infected Individuals

ORAL (ORAL SUSPENSION):
- Initially, 800 mg daily (20 mL per day).
- In clinical trials, 400 mg daily also has been used effectively.

ORAL (CONCENTRATED ORAL SUSPENSION [MEGACE® ES]):
- Initially, 625 mg daily.
- Clinically effective dosages are expected to range from 312.5–625 mg daily.

Treatment in Individuals with Neoplastic Disease†

ORAL:
- 480–600 mg daily generally have been used. However, some patients may exhibit weight gain with dosages as low as 160 mg daily.

Special Populations

Hepatic Impairment
- No specific dosage recommendations at this time.

Renal Impairment
- No specific dosage recommendations at this time.

Geriatric Patients
- Treatment of cachexia in HIV-infected individuals: Select dosage with caution because of age-related decreases in hepatic, renal, and/or cardiac function and concomitant disease and drug therapy.
- Treatment of breast cancer or endometrial cancer: No specific dosage recommendations at this time.

† Use is not currently included in the labeling approved by the US Food and Drug Administration.

Meloxicam

(mel ox′ i cam)

Brand Name: Mobic®

Important Warning

People who take nonsteroidal anti-inflammatory medications (NSAIDs) (other than aspirin) such as meloxicam may have a higher risk of having a heart attack or a stroke than people who do not take these medications. These events may happen without warning and may cause death. This risk may be higher for people who take NSAIDs for a long time. Tell your doctor if you or anyone in your family has or has ever had heart disease, a heart attack, or a stroke, if you smoke, and if you have or have ever had high cholesterol, high blood pressure, or diabetes. Get emergency medical help right away if you experience any of the following symptoms: chest pain, shortness of breath, weakness in one part or side of the body, or slurred speech.

If you will be undergoing a coronary artery bypass graft (CABG; a type of heart surgery), you should not take meloxicam right before or right after the surgery.

NSAIDs such as meloxicam may cause ulcers, bleeding, or holes in the stomach or intestine. These problems may develop at any time during treatment, may happen without warning symptoms, and may cause death. The risk may be higher for people who take NSAIDs for a long time, are older in age, have poor health, or drink large amounts of alcohol while you are taking meloxicam. Tell your doctor if you take any of the following medications: anticoagulants ('blood thinners') such as warfarin (Coumadin); aspirin; other NSAIDs such as ibuprofen (Advil, Motrin) or naproxen (Aleve, Naprosyn); or oral steroids such as dexamethasone (Decadron, Dexone), methylprednisolone (Medrol), and prednisone (Deltasone). Also tell your doctor if you have or have ever had ulcers or bleeding in your stomach or intestines, or other bleeding disorders. If you experience any of the following symptoms, stop taking meloxicam and call your doctor: stomach pain, heartburn, vomiting a substance that is bloody or looks like coffee grounds, blood in the stool, or black and tarry stools.

Keep all appointments with your doctor and the laboratory. Your doctor will monitor your symptoms carefully and will probably order certain tests to check your body's response to meloxicam. Be sure to tell your doctor how you are feeling so that your doctor can prescribe the right amount of medication

continued on next page

Important Warning (cont'd)

to treat your condition with the lowest risk of serious side effects.

Your doctor or pharmacist will give you the manufacturer's patient information sheet (Medication Guide) when you begin treatment with meloxicam and each time you refill your prescription. Read the information carefully and ask your doctor or pharmacist if you have any questions. You can also visit the Food and Drug Administration (FDA) website (http://www.fda.gov/cder) or the manufacturer's website to obtain the Medication Guide.

Why is this medicine prescribed?

Meloxicam is used to relieve pain, tenderness, swelling, and stiffness caused by osteoarthritis (arthritis caused by a breakdown of the lining of the joints) and rheumatoid arthritis (arthritis caused by swelling of the lining of the joints). Meloxicam is also used to relieve the pain, tenderness, swelling, and stiffness caused by juvenile rheumatoid arthritis (a type of arthritis that affects children) in children 2 years of age and older. Meloxicam is in a class of medications called nonsteroidal anti-inflammatory medications (NSAIDs). It works by stopping the body's production of a substance that causes pain, fever, and inflammation.

How should this medicine be used?

Meloxicam comes as a tablet and suspension (liquid) to take by mouth. It is usually taken once a day with or without food. Take meloxicam at the same time every day. Follow the directions on your prescription label carefully, and ask your doctor or pharmacist to explain any part you do not understand. Take meloxicam exactly as directed. Do not take more or less of it or take it more often than prescribed by your doctor.

Shake the suspension well before each use to mix the medication evenly.

Are there other uses for this medicine?

Meloxicam is also used sometimes to treat ankylosing spondylitis (arthritis that mainly affects the spine). Talk to your doctor about the possible risks of using this medication for your condition.

This medication may be prescribed for other uses; ask your doctor or pharmacist for more information.

What special precautions should I follow?

Before taking meloxicam,

- tell your doctor and pharmacist if you are allergic to meloxicam, aspirin or other NSAIDs such as ibuprofen (Advil, Motrin) and naproxen (Aleve, Naprosyn), or any other medications.
- tell your doctor and pharmacist what prescription and nonprescription medications, vitamins, nutritional supplements, and herbal products you are taking or plan to take. Be sure to mention the medications listed in the IMPORTANT WARNING section and any of the following: angiotensin-converting enzyme (ACE) inhibitors such as benazepril (Lotensin), captopril (Capoten), enalapril (Vasotec), fosinopril (Monopril), lisinopril (Prinivil, Zestril), and quinapril (Accupril); cholestyramine (Questran); diuretics ('water pills'); lithium (Eskalith, Lithobid, others); and methotrexate (Rheumatrex). Your doctor may need to change the doses of your medications or monitor you carefully for side effects.
- tell your doctor if you have or have ever had asthma, especially if you have frequent stuffed or runny nose or nasal polyps (swelling of the lining of the nose); swelling of the hands, feet, ankles, or lower legs; or kidney or liver disease.
- tell your doctor if you are pregnant, especially if you are in the last few months of your pregnancy, you plan to become pregnant, or you are breast-feeding. If you become pregnant while taking meloxicam, call your doctor.
- if you are having surgery, including dental surgery, tell the doctor or dentist that you are taking meloxicam.

What should I do if I forget to take a dose?

Take the missed dose as soon as you remember it. However, if it is almost time for the next dose, skip the missed dose and continue your regular dosing schedule. Do not take a double dose to make up for a missed one.

What side effects can this medicine cause?

Meloxicam may cause side effects. Tell your doctor if any of these symptoms are severe or do not go away:

- diarrhea
- constipation
- gas
- sore throat
- cough
- runny nose

Some side effects can be serious. If you experience any of the following symptoms, call your doctor immediately. Do not take any more meloxicam until you speak to your doctor:

- fever
- blisters
- rash
- hives
- itching
- swelling of the eyes, face, tongue, lips, throat, arms, hands, feet, ankles, or lower legs
- difficulty breathing or swallowing
- hoarseness
- pale skin
- fast heartbeat
- unexplained weight gain
- upset stomach
- excessive tiredness

- lack of energy
- yellowing of the skin or eyes
- pain in the right upper part of the stomach
- flu-like symptoms
- cloudy, discolored, or bloody urine
- back pain
- difficult or painful urination

Meloxicam may cause other side effects. Call your doctor if you have any unusual problems while taking this medication.

If you experience a serious side effect, you or your doctor may send a report to the Food and Drug Administration's (FDA) MedWatch Adverse Event Reporting program online [at http://www.fda.gov/MedWatch/index.html] or by phone [1-800-332-1088].

What storage conditions are needed for this medicine?

Keep this medication in the container it came in, tightly closed, and out of reach of children. Store it at room temperature and away from excess heat and moisture (not in the bathroom). Throw away any medication that is outdated or no longer needed. Talk to your pharmacist about the proper disposal of your medication.

What should I do in case of overdose?

In case of overdose, call your local poison control center at 1-800-222-1222. If the victim has collapsed or is not breathing, call local emergency services at 911.

Symptoms of overdose may include:
- lack of energy
- drowsiness
- upset stomach
- vomiting
- stomach pain
- bloody, black, or tarry stools
- vomiting a substance that is bloody or looks like coffee grounds
- difficulty breathing
- seizures
- coma

What other information should I know?

Do not let anyone else take your medication. Ask your pharmacist any questions you have about refilling your prescription.

Dosage Facts
For Informational Purposes

Caution: Do not change your dose, how often you take your medication, or the length of time you are to take it without first talking to your healthcare provider.

The following dosage information was written using medical language for doctors and other healthcare professionals and is provided here for you to check your dosage. The dosage of this drug may differ for different patients. Therefore, always follow your doctor's instructions or the directions on the label. Contact your healthcare provider or pharmacist if you have any questions about the specific dosage of your medication after reviewing this information.

General Dosage Information

To minimize the potential risk of adverse cardiovascular and/or GI events, use lowest effective dosage and shortest duration of therapy consistent with the patient's treatment goals. Adjust dosage based on individual requirements and response; attempt to titrate to the lowest effective dosage.

Pediatric Patients

Juvenile Arthritis

ORAL:
- Children ≥2 years of age: 0.125 mg/kg (maximum 7.5 mg) once daily. Higher dosages not associated with additional benefit.

Adult Patients

Osteoarthritis

ORAL:
- 7.5 mg once daily; may increase to 15 mg once daily.

Rheumatoid Arthritis

ORAL:
- 7.5 mg once daily; may increase to 15 mg once daily.

Prescribing Limits

Pediatric Patients

ORAL:
- Maximum 7.5 mg daily.

Adult Patients

ORAL:
- Maximum 15 mg daily.

Special Populations

Hepatic Impairment
- Dosage adjustment not necessary in patients with mild to moderate hepatic impairment; not studied in those with severe impairment.

Renal Impairment
- Dosage adjustment not necessary in patients with mild to moderate renal impairment (Cl_{cr} >15 mL/minute); not recommended in those with severe impairment.

Memantine

(mem′-an-teen)

Brand Name: Namenda®, Namenda® Titration Pak

Why is this medicine prescribed?

Memantine is used to treat the symptoms of Alzheimer's disease. Memantine is in a class of medications called NMDA receptor antagonists. It works by decreasing abnormal activity in the brain. Memantine can help people with Alzheimer's disease to think more clearly and perform daily activities more easily, but it is not a cure and does not stop the progression of the disease.

How should this medicine be used?

Memantine comes as a tablet to take by mouth. It is usually taken once or twice a day with or without food. Follow the directions on your prescription label carefully, and ask your doctor or pharmacist to explain any part you do not understand. To help you remember to take memantine, take it at around the same time(s) every day. Take memantine exactly as directed. Do not take more or less of it or take it more often than prescribed by your doctor.

Your doctor will probably start you on a low dose of memantine and gradually increase your dose, not more than once every week.

Memantine controls Alzheimer's disease but does not cure it. Continue to take memantine even if you feel well. Do not stop taking memantine without talking to your doctor.

Are there other uses for this medicine?

This medication may be prescribed for other uses; ask your doctor or pharmacist for more information.

What special precautions should I follow?

Before taking memantine,

- tell your doctor and pharmacist if you are allergic to memantine or any other medications.
- tell your doctor and pharmacist what prescription and nonprescription medications, vitamins, nutritional supplements, and herbal products you are taking. Be sure to mention any of the following: acetazolamide (Diamox); amantadine (Symmetrel); brinzolamide (Azopt); cimetidine (Tagamet); dextromethorphan (Robitussin, others); dichlorphenamide (Daranide); dorzolamide (Trusopt); methazolamide (GlaucTabs, Nepatazane); nicotine (Nicoderm, Nicorette, others); potassium citrate and citric acid (Cytra-K, Polycitra-K); ranitidine (Zantac); sodium bicarbonate (Soda Mint, baking soda); sodium citrate and citric acid (Bicitra, Oracit); and quinidine (Quinaglute, Quinidex). Your doctor may need to

change the doses of your medications or monitor you carefully for side effects.
- tell your doctor if you have or have ever had asthma, seizures, kidney disease, or repeated urinary tract infections.
- tell your doctor if you are pregnant, plan to become pregnant, or are breast-feeding. If you become pregnant while taking memantine, call your doctor.
- if you are having surgery, including dental surgery, tell the doctor or dentist that you are taking memantine.
- you should know that memantine may make you drowsy. Do not drive a car or operate machinery until you know how this medication affects you.
- tell your doctor if you use tobacco products. Cigarette smoking may decrease the effectiveness of this medication.

What special dietary instructions should I follow?

Tell your doctor if you are a vegetarian or if you usually eat large amounts of citrus fruits, vegetables, beans, or peas. Your doctor will tell you if you need to change your diet. If you do not regularly eat these foods, continue your normal diet.

What should I do if I forget to take a dose?

Take the missed dose as soon as you remember it. However, if it is almost time for the next dose, skip the missed dose and continue your regular dosing schedule. Do not take a double dose to make up for a missed one.

What side effects can this medicine cause?

Memantine may cause side effects. Tell your doctor if any of these symptoms are severe or do not go away:

- extreme tiredness
- dizziness
- confusion
- headache
- sleepiness
- constipation
- vomiting
- pain anywhere in your body, especially your back
- coughing

Some side effects can be serious. The following symptoms are uncommon, but if you experience any of them, call your doctor immediately:

- shortness of breath
- hallucination (seeing things or hearing voices that do not exist)

Memantine may cause other side effects. Call your doctor if you have any unusual problems while taking this medication.

If you experience a serious side effect, you or your doctor may send a report to the Food and Drug Administration's (FDA) MedWatch Adverse Event Reporting program online

[at http://www.fda.gov/MedWatch/index.html] or by phone [1-800-332-1088].

What storage conditions are needed for this medicine?

Keep this medication in the container it came in, tightly closed, and out of reach of children. Store it at room temperature and away from excess heat and moisture (not in the bathroom). Throw away any medication that is outdated or no longer needed. Talk to your pharmacist about the proper disposal of your medication.

What should I do in case of overdose?

In case of overdose, call your local poison control center at 1-800-222-1222. If the victim has collapsed or is not breathing, call local emergency services at 911.

Symptoms of overdose may include:

- restlessness
- hallucination (seeing things or hearing voices that do not exist)
- sleepiness
- loss of consciousness

What other information should I know?

Keep all appointments with your doctor.

Do not let anyone else take your medication. Ask your pharmacist any questions you have about refilling your prescription.

Dosage Facts
For Informational Purposes

Caution: Do not change your dose, how often you take your medication, or the length of time you are to take it without first talking to your healthcare provider.

The following dosage information was written using medical language for doctors and other healthcare professionals and is provided here for you to check your dosage. The dosage of this drug may differ for different patients. Therefore, always follow your doctor's instructions or the directions on the label. Contact your healthcare provider or pharmacist if you have any questions about the specific dosage of your medication after reviewing this information.

General Dosage Information

Available as memantine hydrochloride; dosage expressed in terms of memantine hydrochloride.

Tablets and oral solution are equivalent on a mg-per-mg basis.

Adult Patients

Alzheimer's Disease

ORAL:
- Initially, 5 mg once daily for 1 week.
- Subsequently, increase dosage to 10 mg daily (5 mg twice

daily) for ≥1 week, then 15 mg daily (administered as separate doses of 5 mg and 10 mg) for ≥1 week, and then to 20 mg daily (10 mg twice daily).
- Recommended target dosage: 20 mg daily given in 2 divided doses (10 mg twice daily).

Special Populations

Hepatic Impairment
- No specific dosage recommendations at this time.

Renal Impairment
- No dosage adjustment needed in patients with mild to moderate renal impairment. In patients with severe renal impairment (i.e., Cl_{cr} 5–29 mL/minute), a target dosage of 5 mg twice daily is recommended.

Geriatric Patients
- No specific dosage adjustments at this time.

Meningococcal Vaccine

Brand Name: Menactra®, Menomune®

What is meningococcal disease?

Meningococcal disease is a serious illness, caused by a bacteria. It is a leading cause of bacterial meningitis in children 2-18 years old in the United States.

Meningitis is an infection of fluid surrounding the brain and the spinal cord. Meningococcal disease also causes blood infections.

About 2,600 people get meningococcal disease each year in the U.S. 10-15% of these people die, in spite of treatment with antibiotics. Of those who live, another 11-19% lose their arms or legs, become deaf, have problems with their nervous systems, become mentally retarded, or suffer seizures or strokes.

Anyone can get meningococcal disease. But it is most common in infants less than one year of age and people with certain medical conditions, such as lack of a spleen. College freshmen who live in dormitories have an increased risk of getting meningococcal disease.

Meningococcal infections can be treated with drugs such as penicillin. Still, about 1 out of every ten people who get the disease dies from it, and many others are affected for life. This is why *preventing* the disease through use of meningococcal vaccine is important for people at highest risk.

Meningococcal vaccine

Two meningococcal vaccines are available in the U.S.:

- Meningococcal polysaccharide vaccine (MPSV4) has been available since the 1970s.
- Meningococcal conjugate vaccine (MCV4) was licensed in 2005.

Both vaccines can prevent 4 types of meningococcal disease, including 2 of the 3 types most common in the United States and a type that causes epidemics in Africa. Meningococcal vaccines cannot prevent all types of the disease. But they do protect many people who might become sick if they didn't get the vaccine.

Both vaccines work well, and protect about 90% of those who get it. MCV4 is expected to give better, longer-lasting protection.

MCV4 should also be better at preventing the disease from spreading from person to person.

Who should get meningococcal vaccine and when?

MCV4 is recommended for all children at their routine pre-adolescent visit (11-12 years of age). For those who have never gotten MCV4 previously, a dose is recommended at high school entry. Other adolescents who want to decrease their risk of meningococcal disease can also get the vaccine.

Meningococcal vaccine is also recommended for other people at increased risk for meningococcal disease:

- College freshmen living in dormitories.
- Microbiologists who are routinely exposed to meningococcal bacteria.
- U.S. military recruits.
- Anyone traveling to, or living in, a part of the world where meningococcal disease is common, such as parts of Africa.
- Anyone who has a damaged spleen, or whose spleen has been removed.
- Anyone who has terminal complement component deficiency (an immune system disorder).
- People who might have been exposed to meningitis during an outbreak.

MCV4 is the preferred vaccine for people 11-55 years of age in these risk groups, but MPSV4 can be used if MCV4 is not available. MPSV4 should be used for children 2-10 years old, and adults over 55, who are at risk.

People 2 years of age and older should get 1 dose. (Sometimes an additional dose is recommended for people who remain at high risk. Ask your provider.)

MPSV4 may be recommended for children 3 months to 2 years of age under special circumstances. These children should get 2 doses, 3 months apart.

Who should *not* get meningococcal vaccine or should wait?

- Anyone who has ever had a severe (life-threatening) allergic reaction to a previous dose of either meningococcal vaccine should not get another dose.
- Anyone who has a severe (life threatening) allergy to any vaccine component should not get the vaccine. Tell your doctor if you have any severe allergies.
- Anyone who is moderately or severely ill at the time the shot is scheduled should probably wait until they recover. Ask your doctor or nurse. People with a mild illness can usually get the vaccine.
- Anyone who has ever had Guillain-Barré Syndrome should talk with their doctor before getting MCV4.
- Meningococcal vaccines may be given to pregnant women. However, MCV4 is a new vaccine and has not been studied in pregnant women as much as MPSV4 has. It should be used only if clearly needed.
- Meningococcal vaccines may be given at the same time as other vaccines.

What are the risks from meningococcal vaccines?

A vaccine, like any medicine, could possibly cause serious problems, such as severe allergic reactions. The risk of meningococcal vaccine causing serious harm, or death, is extremely small.

Mild Problems:
- Up to about half of people who get meningococcal vaccines have mild side effects, such as redness or pain where the shot was given.
- If these problems occur, they usually last for 1 or 2 days. They are more common after MCV4 than after MPSV4.
- A small percentage of people who receive the vaccine develop a fever.

Severe Problems:
- Serious allergic reactions, within a few minutes to a few hours of the shot, are very rare.
- A serious nervous system disorder called Guillain-Barré Syndrome (or GBS) has been reported among some people who received MCV4. This happens so rarely that it is currently not possible to tell if the vaccine might be a factor. Even if it is, the risk is very small.

What if there is a moderate or severe reaction?

What should I look for?
- Any unusual condition, such as a high fever or behavior changes. Signs of a serious allergic reaction can include difficulty breathing, hoarseness or wheezing, hives, paleness, weakness, a fast heart beat or dizziness.

What should I do?
- Call a doctor, or get the person to a doctor right away.
- Tell your doctor what happened, the date and time it happened, and when the vaccination was given.
- Ask your health care provider to file a Vaccine Adverse Event Reporting System (VAERS) form if you have any reaction to the vaccine. Or call VAERS yourself at 1-800-822-7967, or visit their website at http://vaers.hhs.gov.

The National Vaccine Injury Compensation Program

In the rare event that you or your child has a serious reaction to a vaccine, a federal program has been created to help pay for the care of those who have been harmed.

For details about the National Vaccine Injury Compensation Program, call 1-800-338-2382 or visit the program's website at http://www.hrsa.gov/vaccinecompensation.

How can I learn more?

- Ask your doctor or other health care provider. They can give you the vaccine package insert or suggest other sources of information.
- Call your local or state health department's immunization program.
- Contact the Centers for Disease Control and Prevention (CDC): call 1-800-232-4636 (1-800-CDC-INFO) or visit the National Immunization Program's website at http://www.cdc.gov/nip.

Meningococcal Vaccine Information Statement. U.S. Department of Health and Human Services/Centers for Disease Control and Prevention National Immunization Program. 11/16/2006.

Meperidine

(me per' i deen)

Brand Name: Demerol® Hydrochloride, Demerol® Hydrochloride Syrup
Also available generically.

Why is this medicine prescribed?

Meperidine is used to relieve moderate to severe pain. Meperidine is in a class of medications called narcotic analgesics, a group of pain medications similar to morphine. It works by changing the way the body senses pain.

How should this medicine be used?

Meperidine comes as a tablet and a syrup (liquid) to take by mouth. It is usually taken with or without food every 3-4 hours as needed for pain. Follow the directions on your prescription label carefully, and ask your doctor or pharmacist to explain any part you do not understand. Take meperidine exactly as directed.

Swallow the tablets whole; do not split, chew, or crush them. People who are dependent on meperidine or who want to abuse the medication may consider crushing, chewing, snorting, or injecting it. Meperidine may cause serious side effects or death if it is taken in these ways.

If you are taking meperidine syrup, mix your dose with half a glass of water and swallow the mixture. Swallowing undiluted meperidine syrup may numb the mouth.

Your doctor will probably adjust your dose of meperidine during your treatment. Be sure to tell your doctor about any pain and side effects you experience while taking this medication. This will help your doctor find the dose that is best for you.

Meperidine can be habit forming. Do not take a larger dose, or take it more often or for a longer period of time than you were told by your doctor. If you have taken meperidine for longer than a few weeks, do not stop taking the medication without talking to your doctor. Your doctor will probably decrease your dose gradually. If you suddenly stop taking meperidine, you may experience withdrawal symptoms. Withdrawal symptoms may include: restlessness, watery eyes, stuffy nose, yawning, sweating, chills, muscle pain, irritability, nervousness, stomach pain, upset stomach, vomiting, loss of appetite, diarrhea, fast breathing, fast heartbeat, and back pain.

Are there other uses for this medicine?

This medication may be prescribed for other uses; ask your doctor or pharmacist for more information.

What special precautions should I follow?

Before taking meperidine,
- tell your doctor and pharmacist if you are allergic to meperidine or any other medications.
- tell your doctor and pharmacist what prescription and nonprescription medications, vitamins, nutritional supplements, and herbal products you are taking. Be sure to mention any of the following: acyclovir (Zovirax); antidepressants; butorphanol (Stadol NS); cimetidine (Tagamet); chlorpromazine (Thorazine); fluphenazine (Permitil, Prolixin); medications for anxiety, mental illness, pain, upset stomach, vomiting, and seizures; mesoridazine (Serentil); muscle relaxants such as baclofen (Lioresal), carisoprodol (Soma), cyclobenzaprine (Flexeril), methocarbamol (Robaxin), and tizanidine (Zanaflex); pentazocine (Talwin); perphenazine (Trilafon); phenytoin (Dilantin); prochlorperazine (Compazine); ritonavir (Norvir); sedatives; sleeping pills; thioridazine (Mellaril); trifluoperazine (Stelazine); triflupromazine (Vesprin); and tranquilizers. Also tell your doctor or pharmacist if you are taking the following medications or have stopped taking them within the past 2 weeks: monoamine oxidase (MAO) inhibitors including isocarboxazid (Marplan), phenelzine (Nardil), selegiline (Eldepryl), and tranylcypromine (Parnate). Your doctor may need to change the doses of your medications or monitor you carefully for side effects.
- tell your doctor if you use or have ever used street drugs, if you drink or have ever drunk large amounts of alcohol, and if you recently had surgery. Also tell your doctor if you have or have ever had Addison's disease (a

condition in which the body does not produce certain important chemicals); a head injury or a problem with pressure in your head or brain; mental illness; asthma, chronic obstructive pulmonary disease (COPD), or other conditions that affect your breathing; sickle cell anemia (a blood disease); pheochromocytoma (a type of tumor); an abnormally curved spine, especially if it causes breathing problems; enlarged prostate; urethral stricture (narrowing of the opening through which urine leaves the body); irregular heartbeat; seizures; stomach problems; or thyroid, liver, kidney, or lung disease.

- tell your doctor if you are pregnant, plan to become pregnant, or are breast-feeding. If you become pregnant while taking meperidine, call your doctor.
- if you are having surgery, including dental surgery, tell the doctor or dentist that you are taking meperidine.
- you should know that meperidine may make you drowsy. Do not drive a car or operate machinery until you know how this medication affects you.
- ask your doctor about the safe use of alcoholic beverages while you are taking meperidine. Alcohol and street drugs can make the side effects from meperidine worse and can cause serious harm or death.
- you should know that meperidine may cause dizziness, lightheadedness, and fainting when you get up too quickly from a lying position. This is more common when you first start taking meperidine. To avoid this problem, get out of bed slowly, resting your feet on the floor for a few minutes before standing up.

What special dietary instructions should I follow?

Unless your doctor tells you otherwise, continue your normal diet.

What should I do if I forget to take a dose?

This medication is usually taken as needed. If your doctor has told you to take meperidine regularly, take the missed dose as soon as you remember it. However, if it is almost time for the next dose, skip the missed dose and continue your regular dosing schedule. Do not take a double dose to make up for a missed one.

What side effects can this medicine cause?

Meperidine may cause side effects. Tell your doctor if any of these symptoms are severe or do not go away:
- lightheadedness
- dizziness
- weakness
- headache
- extreme calm
- mood changes
- confusion
- agitation

- upset stomach
- vomiting
- stomach pain or cramps
- constipation
- dry mouth
- flushing
- sweating
- changes in vision

Some side effects can be serious. The following symptoms are uncommon, but if you experience any of them or those listed in the IMPORTANT WARNING section, call your doctor immediately:
- slow or difficult breathing
- shaking hands that you cannot control
- muscle twitches or stiffening
- seizures
- hallucination (seeing things or hearing voices that do not exist)
- slow, fast, or pounding heartbeat
- difficulty urinating
- fainting
- rash
- hives

Meperidine may cause other side effects. Call your doctor if you have any unusual problems while taking this medication.

If you experience a serious side effect, you or your doctor may send a report to the Food and Drug Administration's (FDA) MedWatch Adverse Event Reporting program online [at http://www.fda.gov/MedWatch/index.html] or by phone [1-800-332-1088].

What storage conditions are needed for this medicine?

Keep this medication in the container it came in, tightly closed, and out of reach of children. Store it at room temperature and away from excess heat and moisture (not in the bathroom). Protect this medication from theft. Medication that is outdated or no longer needed should be flushed down the toilet, not thrown away. Talk to your pharmacist about the proper disposal of your medication.

What should I do in case of overdose?

In case of overdose, call your local poison control center at 1-800-222-1222. If the victim has collapsed or is not breathing, call local emergency services at 911.

Symptoms of overdose may include:
- slowed breathing
- extreme sleepiness
- coma
- loose, floppy muscles
- cold, clammy skin
- slow heartbeat
- upset stomach
- blurred vision

- dizziness
- fainting

What other information should I know?

Keep all appointments with your doctor.

Do not let anyone else take your medication. It is against the law to give this medication to anyone else. Ask your pharmacist any questions you have about refilling your prescription.

Dosage Facts
For Informational Purposes

Caution: Do not change your dose, how often you take your medication, or the length of time you are to take it without first talking to your healthcare provider.

The following dosage information was written using medical language for doctors and other healthcare professionals and is provided here for you to check your dosage. The dosage of this drug may differ for different patients. Therefore, always follow your doctor's instructions or the directions on the label. Contact your healthcare provider or pharmacist if you have any questions about the specific dosage of your medication after reviewing this information.

Pediatric Patients

Some experts discourage use in children.

Usual Dosage
ORAL:
- May receive 1.1–1.8 mg/kg (up to adult dose) orally, IM, or sub-Q every 3–4 hours as needed.
- Alternatively, 175 mg/m² daily in 6 divided doses orally, IM, or sub-Q.
- Single pediatric doses should not exceed 100 mg.

Adult Patients

Usual Dosage
ORAL:
- Usually, 50–150 mg every 3–4 hours as needed.

Prescribing Limits
Pediatric Patients

ORAL:
- Single pediatric doses should not exceed 100 mg.

Adult Patients

ORAL:
- Increased risk of toxicity from the active metabolite, normeperidine, when given for >48 hours or in total dosages exceeding 600 mg/24 hours.

Special Populations
Hepatic Impairment
- Adjustment in the dose, frequency, and/or duration of therapy may be necessary because accumulation of the drug and/or its toxic metabolite, normeperidine, can occur.

- Certain adverse effects secondary to CNS stimulation (e.g., seizures, agitation, irritability, nervousness, tremors, twitches, myoclonus) have been attributed to accumulation of normeperidine.
- Oral bioavailability may be increased substantially in these patients.

Renal Impairment
- Generally avoid in renal impairment, particularly repeated or high doses.
- If used, adjustment in the dose, frequency, and/or duration of meperidine therapy is likely to be necessary because accumulation of the drug and/or its toxic metabolite, normeperidine, can occur.
- Certain adverse effects secondary to CNS stimulation (e.g., seizures, agitation, irritability, nervousness, tremors, twitches, myoclonus) have been attributed to accumulation of normeperidine.

End-stage Renal Failure
- Avoid because of the risk of accumulation of the toxic metabolite, normeperidine.

Meperidine Hydrochloride Injection

(me per' i deen)

Brand Name: Demerol® Hydrochloride
Also available generically.

About Your Treatment

Your doctor has ordered meperidine, a strong analgesic (painkiller), to relieve your pain. The drug will be either injected into a large muscle (such as your buttock or hip) or added to an intravenous fluid that will drip through a needle or catheter placed in your vein or under your skin.

You may receive meperidine continuously for around-the-clock pain relief. Your doctor also may order other pain medications to make you more comfortable. This medication is sometimes prescribed for other uses; ask your doctor or pharmacist for more information.

Your health care provider (doctor, nurse, or pharmacist) may measure the effectiveness and side effects of your treatment using laboratory tests and physical examinations. It is important to keep all appointments with your doctor and the laboratory. The length of treatment depends on how you respond to the medication.

Precautions

Before administering meperidine,

- tell your doctor and pharmacist if you are allergic to meperidine or any other drugs.
- tell your doctor and pharmacist what prescription and nonprescription medications you are taking, especially other pain relievers; antidepressants; cough, cold, and allergy products; MAO inhibitors [phenelzine (Nardil) or tranylcypromine (Parnate)]; sedatives; sleeping pills; tranquilizers; and vitamins.
- tell your doctor if you have or have ever had liver or kidney disease, a history of alcoholism, lung or thyroid disease, heart disease, seizures, prostatic hypertrophy, or urinary problems.
- tell your doctor if you are pregnant, plan to become pregnant, or are breast-feeding. If you become pregnant while taking meperidine, call your doctor.
- you should know that this drug may make you drowsy. Do not drive a car or operate machinery until you know how this drug affects you.
- remember that alcohol can add to the drowsiness caused by this drug.

Administering Your Medication

Before you administer meperidine, look at the solution closely. It should be clear and free of floating material. Gently squeeze the bag or observe the solution container to make sure there are no leaks. Do not use the solution if it is discolored, if it contains particles, or if the bag or container leaks. Use a new solution, but show the damaged one to your health care provider.

It is important that you use your medication exactly as directed. Meperidine can be habit forming. Do not administer it more often or for a longer period than your doctor tells you. Do not change your dosing schedule without talking to your health care provider. Your health care provider may tell you to stop your infusion if you have a mechanical problem (such as a blockage in the tubing, needle, or catheter); if you have to stop an infusion, call your health care provider immediately so your therapy can continue.

Side Effects

Meperidine may cause side effects. Tell your health care provider if any of these symptoms are severe or do not go away:

- dizziness
- lightheadedness
- drowsiness
- mood changes
- upset stomach
- vomiting
- constipation
- sweating
- rash
- difficulty urinating

If you experience any of the following symptoms, call your health care provider immediately:

- difficulty breathing
- fainting
- muscle twitching
- seizures

If you experience a serious side effect, you or your doctor may send a report to the Food and Drug Administration's (FDA) MedWatch Adverse Event Reporting program online [at http://www.fda.gov/MedWatch/index.html] or by phone [1-800-332-1088].

Storage Conditions

- Your health care provider probably will give you a several-day supply of meperidine at a time. If you are receiving meperidine intravenously (in your vein), you probably will be told to store it in the refrigerator.
- Take your next dose from the refrigerator 1 hour before using it; place it in a clean, dry area to allow it to warm to room temperature.

If you are receiving meperidine intramuscularly (in your muscle), your health care provider will tell you how to store it properly.

Store your medication only as directed. Make sure you understand what you need to store your medication properly.

Keep your supplies in a clean, dry place when you are not using them, and keep all medications and supplies out of reach of children. Your health care provider will tell you how to throw away used needles, syringes, tubing, and containers to avoid accidental injury.

Overdose

In case of overdose, call your local poison control center at 1-800-222-1222. If the victim has collapsed or is not breathing, call local emergency services at 911.

Signs of Infection

If you are receiving meperidine in your vein or under your skin, you need to know the symptoms of a catheter-related infection (an infection where the needle enters your vein or skin). If you experience any of these effects near your intravenous catheter, tell your health care provider as soon as possible:

- tenderness
- warmth
- irritation
- drainage
- redness
- swelling
- pain

Dosage Facts
For Informational Purposes

Caution: Do not change your dose, how often you take your medication, or the length of time you are to take it without first talking to your health-care provider.

The following dosage information was written using medical language for doctors and other healthcare professionals and is provided here for you to check your dosage. The dosage of this drug may differ for different patients. Therefore, always follow your doctor's instructions or the directions on the label. Contact your healthcare provider or pharmacist if you have any questions about the specific dosage of your medication after reviewing this information.

Pediatric Patients

Some experts discourage use in children.

Usual Dosage

IM OR SUB-Q:
- May receive 1.1–1.8 mg/kg (up to adult dose) orally, IM, or sub-Q every 3–4 hours as needed.
- Alternatively, 175 mg/m² daily in 6 divided doses orally, IM, or sub-Q.
- Single pediatric doses should not exceed 100 mg.

IV:
- Do *not* use for PCA when analgesic consumption is expected to be high; risk of CNS excitatory toxicity from normeperidine.
- PCA (usually IV) via controlled-delivery device: Loading doses of 0.5–1.5 mg/kg, preferably titrated by clinician or nurse at bedside.
- PCA (usually IV) via controlled-delivery device: Maintenance doses (administered intermittently) of 0.1–0.2 mg/kg, self-administered usually no more frequently than every 6–12 minutes as a device-programmed lockout period.

Preoperative Dosage

IM OR SUB-Q:
- May receive 1–2.2 mg/kg (maximum up to the adult dose) IM or sub-Q 30–90 minutes before the beginning of anesthesia.

Adjunct to Anesthesia

IV INJECTION OR IV INFUSION:
- May be given by repeated slow IV injections of a dilute solution (e.g., containing 10 mg/mL) or by continuous IV infusion of a more dilute solution (e.g., containing 1 mg/mL).

Adult Patients

Usual Dosage

IM OR SUB-Q:
- Usually, 50–150 mg every 3–4 hours as needed.

IV INFUSION:
- Usually, 15–35 mg/hour.

IV:
- Do *not* use for PCA when analgesic consumption is expected to be high; risk of CNS excitatory toxicity from normeperidine.
- PCA (usually IV) via controlled-delivery device: Loading doses of 12.5–25 mg every 10 minutes, preferably titrated by clinician or nurse at bedside, up to 50–125 mg total.
- PCA (usually IV) via controlled-delivery device: Maintenance doses (self-administered intermittently) of 5–10 mg, self-administered usually no more frequently than every 6–12 minutes as a device-programmed lockout period.

Preoperative Dosage

IM OR SUB-Q:
- Usually, 50–100 mg IM or sub-Q 30–90 minutes before the beginning of anesthesia.

Adjunct to Anesthesia

IV INJECTION OR IV INFUSION:
- May be given by repeated slow IV injections of a dilute solution (e.g., containing 10 mg/mL) or by continuous IV infusion of a more dilute solution (e.g., containing 1 mg/mL).

Analgesia during Labor

IM OR SUB-Q:
- 50–100 mg when labor pains become regular; repeat at 1- to 3-hour intervals as needed.

Prescribing Limits

Pediatric Patients

IM OR SUB-Q:
- Single pediatric doses should not exceed 100 mg.

Adult Patients

IV, IM, OR SUB-Q:
- Increased risk of toxicity from the active metabolite, normeperidine, when given for >48 hours or in total dosages exceeding 600 mg/24 hours.

Special Populations

Hepatic Impairment
- Adjustment in the dose, frequency, and/or duration of therapy may be necessary because accumulation of the drug and/or its toxic metabolite, normeperidine, can occur.
- Certain adverse effects secondary to CNS stimulation (e.g., seizures, agitation, irritability, nervousness, tremors, twitches, myoclonus) have been attributed to accumulation of normeperidine.
- Oral bioavailability may be increased substantially in these patients.

Renal Impairment
- Generally avoid in renal impairment, particularly repeated or high doses.
- If used, adjustment in the dose, frequency, and/or duration of meperidine therapy is likely to be necessary because accumulation of the drug and/or its toxic metabolite, normeperidine, can occur.
- Certain adverse effects secondary to CNS stimulation (e.g., seizures, agitation, irritability, nervousness, tremors, twitches, myoclonus) have been attributed to accumulation of normeperidine.

End-stage Renal Failure

- Avoid because of the risk of accumulation of the toxic metabolite, normeperidine.

Meprobamate

(me proe ba′ mate)

Brand Name: Equagesic® as a combination product containing Meprobamate and Aspirin, Miltown®

Why is this medicine prescribed?

Meprobamate is used to treat anxiety disorders or for short-term relief of the symptoms of anxiety.

This medication is sometimes prescribed for other uses; ask your doctor or pharmacist for more information.

How should this medicine be used?

Meprobamate comes as a tablet and extended-release (long-acting) capsule to take by mouth. It usually is taken two to four times a day. Follow the directions on your prescription label carefully, and ask your doctor or pharmacist to explain any part you do not understand. Take meprobamate exactly as directed.

Do not open, chew, or crush tablets or extended-release capsules; swallow them whole.

Meprobamate can be habit-forming, do not take a larger dose, take it more often, or for a longer period than your doctor tells you to. Do not stop taking this drug without talking to your doctor, especially if you have been taking it for a long time. Your doctor probably will decrease your dose gradually.

What special precautions should I follow?

Before taking meprobamate,

- tell your doctor and pharmacist if you are allergic to meprobamate, carisoprodol, aspirin, tartrazine (a yellow dye in some processed foods and medications, including certain brands of meprobamate), or any other drugs.
- tell your doctor and pharmacist what prescription and nonprescription medications you are taking, especially medications for depression, cough, cold or asthma; sleep aids; and vitamins.
- tell your doctor if you have or have ever had kidney or liver disease, a history of alcohol or drug abuse, porphyria, or epilepsy.
- tell your doctor if you are pregnant, plan to become pregnant, or are breast-feeding. If you become pregnant while taking meprobamate, call your doctor.
- if you are having surgery, including dental surgery, tell the doctor or dentist that you are taking meprobamate.
- you should know that this drug may make you drowsy. Do not drive a car or operate machinery until you know how this drug affects you.
- remember that alcohol can add to the drowsiness caused by this drug.

What should I do if I forget to take a dose?

Do not take a missed dose when you remember it. Skip it completely; then take the next dose at the regularly scheduled time.

What side effects can this medicine cause?

Meprobamate may cause side effects. Tell your doctor if any of these symptoms are severe or do not go away:

- drowsiness
- upset stomach
- vomiting
- diarrhea
- headache
- difficulty coordinating movements
- excitement
- weakness

If you experience any of the following symptoms, call your doctor immediately:

- skin rash
- itching
- easy bruising
- bloody nose
- unusual bleeding
- tiny purple-colored skin spots
- sore throat
- fever
- difficulty breathing
- slurred speech
- staggering
- pounding or irregular heartbeat

If you experience a serious side effect, you or your doctor may send a report to the Food and Drug Administration's (FDA) MedWatch Adverse Event Reporting program online [at http://www.fda.gov/MedWatch/index.html] or by phone [1-800-332-1088].

What storage conditions are needed for this medicine?

Keep this medication in the container it came in, tightly closed, and out of reach of children. Store it at room temperature, away from excess heat and moisture (not in the bathroom). Throw away any medication that is outdated or no longer needed. Talk to your pharmacist about the proper disposal of your medication.

What should I do in case of overdose?

In case of overdose, call your local poison control center at 1-800-222-1222. If the victim has collapsed or is not breathing, call local emergency services at 911.

What other information should I know?

Keep all appointments with your doctor and the laboratory. Your doctor will order certain lab tests to check your response to meprobamate.

Call your doctor if you continue to have symptoms.

Do not let anyone else take your medication. Meprobamate is a controlled substance. Prescriptions may be refilled only a limited number of times; ask your pharmacist if you have any questions.

Talk to your doctor, pharmacist, or other healthcare professional if you have questions about dosing information for your medication.

Mesalamine

(me sal′ a meen)

Brand Name: Asacol®, Canasa®, Pentasa®, Rowasa®

Why is this medicine prescribed?

Mesalamine is used to treat ulcerative colitis (a condition in which part or all of the lining of the colon [large intestine] is swollen or worn away). Mesalamine delayed-release tablets and controlled-release capsules may be used to treat ulcerative colitis that affects any part of the colon. Mesalamine suppositories and enemas should only be used to treat inflammation of the lower part of the colon. Mesalamine is in a class of medications called anti-inflammatory agents. It works by stopping the body from producing a certain substance that may cause pain or inflammation.

How should this medicine be used?

Mesalamine comes as a delayed-release tablet and a controlled-release capsule to take by mouth and as a suppository and an enema to use in the rectum. The delayed-release tablet is usually taken three times a day, and the controlled-release capsule is usually taken four times a day. The suppository is usually used one to three times a day, and the enema is usually used once a day at bedtime. Follow the directions on your prescription label carefully, and ask your doctor or pharmacist to explain any part you do not understand. Take or use mesalamine exactly as directed. Do not take or use more or less of it or take or use it more often than prescribed by your doctor.

Swallow the tablets whole; do not split, chew, or crush them. Be careful not to break the protective coating on the tablets.

If you are unable to swallow the capsules, you may mix the contents of the capsules with water. Open a capsule and sprinkle all of the beads it contains in a small glass of water. Stir the beads into the water and drink the mixture right away. Do not store mixtures of beads and water for later use.

The enema and suppositories are for rectal use only.

You should begin to feel better during the first few days or weeks of your treatment with mesalamine. Continue to take or use mesalamine until you finish your prescription, even if you feel better at the beginning of your treatment.

Do not stop taking or using mesalamine without talking to your doctor.

Mesalamine suppositories and enemas may stain clothing, flooring, fabric and other surfaces. Take precautions to prevent staining when you use these medications.

If you are to use the enema, follow these steps:

1. Try to have a bowel movement. The medication will work best if your bowels are empty.
2. Use a scissors to cut the seal of the protective foil pouch that holds seven bottles of medication. Be careful not to squeeze or cut the bottles. Remove one bottle from the pouch.
3. Look at the liquid inside the bottle. It should be off-white or tan colored. The liquid may darken slightly if the bottles are left out of the foil pouch for a time. You may use liquid that has darkened a little bit, but do not use liquid that is dark brown.
4. Shake the bottle well to make sure the medication is mixed.
5. Remove the protective cover from the applicator tip. Be careful to hold the bottle by the neck so that the medication will not leak out of the bottle.
6. Lie on your left side with your lower (left) leg straight and your right leg bent toward your chest for balance. You can also kneel on a bed, resting your upper chest and one arm on the bed.
7. Gently insert the applicator tip into your rectum, pointing it slightly toward your navel (belly button). If this causes pain or irritation, try putting a small amount of personal lubricating jelly or petroleum jelly on the tip of the applicator before you insert it.
8. Hold the bottle firmly and tilt it slightly so that the nozzle is aimed toward your back. Squeeze the bottle slowly and steadily to release the medicine.
9. Withdraw the applicator. Remain in the same position for at least 30 minutes to allow the medicine to spread through your intestine. Try to keep the medicine inside of your body for about 8 hours (while you sleep).
10. Throw away the bottle in a trash can that is out of the reach of children and pets. Each bottle contains only one dose and should not be reused.

If you are to use the suppository, follow these steps:

1. Try to have a bowel movement just before using the suppository. The medication will work best if your bowels are empty.
2. Separate one suppository from the strip of suppositories. Hold the suppository upright and use your fingers to peel off the plastic wrapper. Try to handle the suppository as little as possible to avoid melting it with the heat of your hands.
3. You may put a small amount of personal lubricant jelly or Vaseline on the tip of the suppository so that it will be easier to insert.
4. Lie down on your left side and raise your right knee to your chest. (If you are left-handed, lie on your right side and raise your left knee.)
5. Using your finger, insert the suppository into the rectum,

pointed end first. Use gentle pressure to insert the suppository completely. Try to keep it in place for 1-3 hours or longer if possible.

6. Wash your hands thoroughly before you resume your normal activities.

If you will be using mesalamine enemas or suppositories, ask your pharmacist or doctor for a copy of the manufacturer's information for the patient that comes with the medication.

Are there other uses for this medicine?

This medication may be prescribed for other uses. Ask your doctor or pharmacist for more information.

What special precautions should I follow?

Before taking or using mesalamine,

- tell your doctor and pharmacist if you are allergic to mesalamine, balsalazide (Colazal); olsalazine (Dipentum); salicylate pain relievers such as aspirin, choline magnesium trisalicylate, choline salicylate (Arthropan), diflunisal (Dolobid), magnesium salicylate (Doan's, others), and salsalate; sulfasalazine (Azulfidine) or any other medications. If you will be using mesalamine enemas, tell your doctor if you are allergic to sulfites (substances used as food preservatives and found naturally in some foods) or any foods, dyes, or preservatives. Also tell your doctor if you are allergic to any of the ingredients in the type of mesalamine you will be using. Ask your pharmacist for a list of the ingredients.
- tell your doctor and pharmacist what prescription and nonprescription medications, vitamins, nutritional supplements, and herbal products you are taking or plan to take. Be sure to mention any of the following: aspirin or other nonsteroidal anti-inflammatory medications (NSAIDs) such as ibuprofen (Advil, Motrin) and naproxen (Aleve, Naprosyn); digoxin (Lanoxicaps, Lanoxin); or other medications for ulcerative colitis such as balsalazide (Colazal), olsalazine (Dipentum), or sulfasalazine (Azulfidine). Your doctor may need to change the doses of your medications or monitor you more carefully for side effects.
- tell your doctor if you have or have ever had pancreatitis (swelling of the pancreas), pericarditis (swelling of the sac around the heart), or liver or kidney disease. If you will be taking the delayed-release tablets, tell your doctor if you have or have ever had pyloric stenosis (condition in which the stomach does not empty normally). If you will be using the enemas, tell your doctor if you have asthma or allergies.
- tell your doctor if you are pregnant, plan to become pregnant, or are breast-feeding. If you become pregnant while taking mesalamine, call your doctor.
- you should know that mesalamine may cause a serious reaction. Many of the symptoms of this reaction are similar to the symptoms of ulcerative colitis, so it may be difficult to tell if you are experiencing a reaction to the

medication or a flare (episode of symptoms) of your disease. Call your doctor if you experience some or all of the following symptoms: stomach pain or cramping; bloody diarrhea; fever; headache; weakness; rash; or red, irritated eyes.

What special dietary instructions should I follow?

Unless your doctor tells you otherwise, continue your normal diet.

What should I do if I forget to take a dose?

Take or use the missed dose as soon as you remember it. However, if it is almost time for the next dose, skip the missed dose and continue your regular dosing schedule. Do not take or use a double dose to make up for a missed one.

What side effects can this medicine cause?

Mesalamine may cause side effects. Tell your doctor if any of these symptoms are severe or do not go away:

- headache
- muscle or joint pain, aching, tightness or stiffness
- back pain
- nausea
- vomiting
- heartburn
- burping
- constipation
- gas
- dry mouth
- sore throat
- cough
- flu-like symptoms
- stuffy head or runny nose
- ear pain
- anxiety
- sweating
- hemorrhoids
- pain in the rectum
- difficulty falling asleep or staying asleep
- acne
- slight hair loss

Some side effects can be serious. If you experience any of the following symptoms, call your doctor immediately:

- chest pain
- shortness of breath
- black or tarry stools
- bloody vomit
- vomiting material that looks like coffee grounds
- urinating more or less than usual
- blood in urine
- confusion
- swelling of any part of the body

Mesalamine may cause other side effects. Call your doctor if you have any unusual problems while you are taking or using this medication.

What storage conditions are needed for this medicine?

Keep this medication in the container it came in, tightly closed, and out of reach of children. Store it at room temperature and away from excess heat, light, and moisture (not in the bathroom). You may store mesalamine suppositories in the refrigerator but do not freeze them. Once you open the foil package of mesalamine enemas use all the bottles promptly, as directed by your doctor. Throw away any medication that is outdated or no longer needed. Talk to your pharmacist about the proper disposal of your medication.

What should I do in case of overdose?

In case of overdose, call your local poison control center at 1-800-222-1222. If the victim has collapsed or is not breathing, call local emergency services at 911.

What other information should I know?

If you are taking mesalamine delayed-release tablets, you may notice the tablet shell or part of the tablet shell in your stool. Tell your doctor if this happens several times.

Keep all appointments with your doctor and the laboratory. Your doctor may order certain lab tests before and during your treatment.

Do not let anyone else take or use your medicine. Ask your pharmacist any questions you have about refilling your prescription.

Dosage Facts
For Informational Purposes

Caution: Do not change your dose, how often you take your medication, or the length of time you are to take it without first talking to your healthcare provider.

The following dosage information was written using medical language for doctors and other healthcare professionals and is provided here for you to check your dosage. The dosage of this drug may differ for different patients. Therefore, always follow your doctor's instructions or the directions on the label. Contact your healthcare provider or pharmacist if you have any questions about the specific dosage of your medication after reviewing this information.

Pediatric Patients
Ulcerative Colitis† or Crohn's Disease†
ORAL:
- Delayed-release tablets have been given in an initial dosage of 20–30 mg/kg daily and then increased up to 60 mg/kg daily.

Adult Patients
Ulcerative Colitis
Management of Mildly to Moderately Active Ulcerative Colitis
ORAL:
- Delayed-release tablets: Usually, 2.4 g daily (given as two 400-mg delayed-release tablets 3 times daily) for 6 weeks.

Induction of Remission of Mildly to Moderately Active Ulcerative Colitis
ORAL:
- Extended-release capsules: Usually, 4 g daily in equally divided doses (given as four 250-mg extended-release capsules 4 times daily) for up to 8 weeks. Lower dosages (e.g., 2–4 g daily [in divided doses]) have been used†.

Maintenance of Remission
ORAL:
- Delayed-release tablets: Usually, 1.6 g daily in divided doses (given as four 400-mg delayed-release tablets) for 6 months. Dosages of 800 mg–4.8 g daily (in divided doses) also have been used.
- Extended-release capsules: Dosages of 1.5–3 g daily (in divided doses) have been used.
- Patients should be advised that ulcerative colitis rarely remits completely, and continued use of maintenance dosages of mesalamine may substantially decrease the risk of relapse.

Distal Ulcerative Colitis
RECTAL:
- Suppositories: Initially, 500 mg twice daily or 1 g (using 1-g suppositories) once daily at bedtime. If an inadequate response occurs after 2 weeks of therapy, dosage of the suppositories may be increased to 500 mg 3 times daily.
- Enema suspension: Usually, 4 g once daily (preferably at bedtime).
- Although clinical response may be apparent within 3–21 days, therapy with rectal mesalamine usually is continued for 3–6 weeks or until clinical and/or sigmoidoscopic remission is achieved.
- Efficacy of rectal therapy (in terms of modification of relapse rates) beyond 6 weeks has not been established, but mesalamine has been used rectally for prolonged periods (e.g., >1 year) in some patients.
- Lower dosages or less frequent administration of the rectal drug has been used in some patients†, particularly after initial remission is achieved.
- In some patients with distal ulcerative colitis in whom clinical remission occurred following daily administration of 4-g doses of the rectal suspension, dosage was reduced to 4 g every 2 or 3 nights or, occasionally, to less frequent administration. If clinical relapse occurred with such administration, dosage was increased to more frequent use. In some patients with distal ulcerative colitis or ulcerative proctosigmoiditis, the rectal suspension also has been used in dosages of 1–3 g daily.

Crohn's Disease†
Management of Mildly to Moderately Active Crohn's Disease†
ORAL:
- Adults have received dosages of 3.2–4.8 g daily (as delayed-release tablets) or 4 g daily (as extended-release capsules),

generally in divided doses. Lower dosages do not appear to be effective.

Prescribing Limits

Pediatric Patients

Ulcerative Colitis† or Crohn's Disease†

ORAL:
• Up to 60 mg/kg daily.

Adult Patients

Ulcerative Colitis
Management of Mildly to Moderately Active Ulcerative Colitis

ORAL:
• Delayed-release tablets: Up to 4.8 g daily in divided doses.
• Extended-release capsules: Up to 4 g daily in divided doses.

Induction of Remission of Mildly to Moderately Active Ulcerative Colitis

ORAL:
• Extended-release capsules: Up to 4 g daily in divided doses.

Maintenance of Remission

ORAL:
• Delayed-release tablets: Up to 4.8 g daily, in divided doses.
• Extended-release capsules†: Up to 3 g daily in divided doses.

Distal Ulcerative Colitis

RECTAL:
• Suppositories: Up to 500 mg 3 times daily.
• Enema suspension: Up to 4 g once daily.
• The drug has been used rectally for >1 year.

Crohn's Disease†
Management of Mildly to Moderately Active Crohn's Disease

ORAL:
• Delayed-release tablets: Up to 4.8 g daily in divided doses.
• Extended-release capsules: Up to 4 g daily in divided doses.

Maintenance of Remission

ORAL:
• Delayed-release tablets: Up to 4.8 g daily in divided doses.
• Extended-release capsules: Up to 3 g daily in divided doses.

Special Populations

Geriatric Patients
• Careful dosage selection recommended due to possible age-related decreases in hepatic, renal, and/or cardiac function and concomitant disease and drug therapy.

† Use is not currently included in the labeling approved by the US Food and Drug Administration.

Mesna

(mes′ na)

Brand Name: Mesnex®
Also available generically.

About Your Treatment

Your doctor has ordered the drug mesna to help treat your illness. Mesna can be injected into a vein or the liquid can be mixed in juice and taken by mouth. Depending on your treatment schedule, mesna will be given prior to and after each dose of chemotherapy or mixed in the same bag with your chemotherapy.

This medication is used to protect the bladder wall from the harmful effects of some cancer-fighting drugs.

Precautions

Before taking mesna,
• tell your doctor and pharmacist if you are allergic to mesna or any other drugs.
• tell your doctor and pharmacist what prescription and nonprescription medications you are taking, including vitamins.
• tell your doctor if you have or have ever had liver or kidney disease.
• tell your doctor if you are pregnant or breast-feeding. You should not plan to have children while receiving chemotherapy or for a while after treatments. (Talk to your doctor for further details.) Use a reliable method of birth control to prevent pregnancy.
• do not have any vaccinations (e.g., measles or flu shots) without talking to your doctor.

Side Effects

Side effects from mesna are common and include:
• bad taste in the mouth
• diarrhea or soft stools
• headache
• nausea
• vomiting

Tell your doctor if the following symptom is severe or lasts for several hours:
• fatigue

If you experience the following symptom, call your doctor immediately:
• blood in urine

If you experience a serious side effect, you or your doctor may send a report to the Food and Drug Administration's (FDA) MedWatch Adverse Event Reporting program online [at http://www.fda.gov/MedWatch/index.html] or by phone [1-800-332-1088].

Overdose

In case of overdose, call your local poison control center at 1-800-222-1222. If the victim has collapsed or is not breathing, call local emergency services at 911.

Dosage Facts
For Informational Purposes

Caution: Do not change your dose, how often you take your medication, or the length of time you are to take it without first talking to your healthcare provider.

The following dosage information was written using medical language for doctors and other healthcare professionals and is provided here for you to check your dosage. The dosage of this drug may differ for different patients. Therefore, always follow your doctor's instructions or the directions on the label. Contact your healthcare provider or pharmacist if you have any questions about the specific dosage of your medication after reviewing this information.

Adult Patients

Prophylaxis of Ifosfamide-induced Hemorrhagic Cystitis

If ifosfamide dosage is increased or decreased, maintain constant mesna-to-ifosfamide ratio.

IV:

- IV injection: For daily ifosfamide dosages <2.5 g/m², administer a mesna dosage equivalent to 20% weight/weight (w/w) of the daily ifosfamide dosage 15 minutes before or at the time of ifosfamide administration and then at 4 and 8 hours after the ifosfamide dose; total daily mesna dosage is equivalent to 60% w/w of the daily ifosfamide dosage. In patients receiving ifosfamide 1.2 g/m², administer mesna 240 mg/m² 15 minutes before or at the time of ifosfamide administration, followed by 240 mg/m² at 4 and 8 hours after the ifosfamide dose.
- Continuous IV infusion: For daily ifosfamide dosages <2.5 g/m², ASCO recommends administering a mesna loading dose equivalent to 20% w/w of the daily ifosfamide dosage by IV injection, followed by 40% w/w of the daily ifosfamide dosage by continuous IV infusion, continued for 12–24 hours after completion of the ifosfamide infusion.
- For daily ifosfamide dosages >2.5 g/m², there are insufficient data to recommend a mesna dosage; however, ASCO recommends more frequent and prolonged administration of mesna for maximum protection against urotoxicity.

IV, THEN ORAL:

- For daily ifosfamide dosages <2 g/m², administer a mesna dosage equivalent to 20% w/w of the daily ifosfamide dosage by IV injection at the time of ifosfamide administration, followed by 40% w/w of the daily ifosfamide dosage orally at 2 and 6 hours after the ifosfamide dose; total daily mesna dosage is equivalent to 100% w/w of the daily ifosfamide dosage.
- In patients receiving 1.2 g/m² of ifosfamide, administer mesna 240 mg/m² by IV injection at the time of ifosfamide administration, followed by 480 mg/m² orally at 2 and 6 hours after the ifosfamide dose.

- If patient vomits oral dose within 2 hours of administration, repeat dose or consider IV administration.

Prophylaxis of Cyclophosphamide-induced† Hemorrhagic Cystitis

IV:

- Mesna dosage equivalent to 60–160% w/w of the daily cyclophosphamide dosage, given by IV injection (in 3–5 divided doses daily) or by continuous IV infusion (continued for ≥24 hours after cyclophosphamide is discontinued).

Prescribing Limits

Adult Patients

Prophylaxis of Ifosfamide-induced Hemorrhagic Cystitis

IV:

- Maximum mesna dosage equivalent to 60% w/w of the daily ifosfamide dosage.
- Safety and efficacy of the recommended mesna-to-ifosfamide ratio not established for ifosfamide dosages >2.5 g/m² daily.

IV, THEN ORAL:

- Safety and efficacy of the recommended mesna-to-ifosfamide ratio not established for ifosfamide dosages >2 g/m² daily.

Special Populations

Geriatric Patients
- Cautious dosing recommended; always maintain constant mesna-to-ifosfamide ratio.

† Use is not currently included in the labeling approved by the US Food and Drug Administration.

Metaproterenol

(met a proe ter′ e nole)

Brand Name: Alupent®, Alupent® Inhalation Solution, Alupent® Syrup

Why is this medicine prescribed?

Metaproterenol is used to prevent and treat wheezing, shortness of breath, and troubled breathing caused by asthma, chronic bronchitis, emphysema, and other lung diseases. It relaxes and opens air passages in the lungs, making it easier to breathe.

This medication is sometimes prescribed for other uses; ask your doctor or pharmacist for more information.

How should this medicine be used?

Metaproterenol comes as tablets and syrup to take by mouth and as a solution and an aerosol to inhale by mouth. It usually is taken by oral inhalation as needed to relieve symptoms or every 3-4 hours to prevent symptoms or by mouth three or four times a day. Follow the directions on your prescription label carefully, and ask your doctor or pharmacist to explain any part you do not understand. Take metaproterenol exactly as directed. Do not take more or less of it or take it more often than prescribed by your doctor. If you are using metaproterenol as needed to relieve symptoms of asthma attacks, do not use more than 12 puffs per day.

Metaproterenol controls symptoms of asthma and other lung diseases but does not cure them. Continue to take metaproterenol even if you feel well. Do not stop taking metaproterenol without talking to your doctor.

Before you use the metaproterenol inhaler the first time, read the written instructions that come with it. Ask your doctor, pharmacist, or respiratory therapist to demonstrate the proper technique. Practice using the inhaler while in his or her presence.

To use the inhaler, follow these steps:

1. Shake the inhaler well.
2. Remove the protective cap.
3. Exhale (breathe out) as completely as possible through your nose while keeping your mouth shut.
4. *Open Mouth Technique:* Open your mouth wide, and place the open end of the mouthpiece about 1-2 inches from your mouth.
   Closed Mouth Technique: Place the open end of the mouthpiece well into your mouth, past your front teeth. Close your lips tightly around the mouthpiece.
5. Take a slow, deep breath through the mouthpiece and, at the same time, press down on the container to spray the medication into your mouth. Be sure that the mist goes into your throat and is not blocked by your teeth or tongue. Adults giving the treatment to young children may hold the child's nose closed to be sure that the medication goes into the child's throat.
6. Hold your breath for 5-10 seconds, remove the inhaler, and exhale slowly through your nose or mouth. If you take 2 puffs, wait 2 minutes and shake the inhaler well before taking the second puff.
7. Replace the protective cap on the inhaler.

If you have difficulty getting the medication into your lungs, a spacer (a special device that attaches to the inhaler) may help; ask your doctor, pharmacist, or respiratory therapist.

What special precautions should I follow?

Before taking metaproterenol,

- tell your doctor and pharmacist if you are allergic to metaproterenol or any other drugs.
- tell your doctor and pharmacist what prescription medications you are taking, especially atenolol (Tenormin); carteolol (Cartrol); labetalol (Normodyne, Trandate); metoprolol (Lopressor); nadolol (Corgard); phenelzine (Nardil); propranolol (Inderal); sotalol (Betapace); theophylline (Theo-Dur); timolol (Blocadren); tranylcypromine (Parnate); other medications for asthma, heart disease, or depression.
- tell your doctor and pharmacist what nonprescription medications and vitamins you are taking, including ephedrine, phenylephrine, phenylpropanolamine, or

pseudoephedrine. Many nonprescription products contain these drugs (e.g., diet pills and medications for colds and asthma), so check labels carefully. Do not take any of these medications without talking to your doctor (even if you never had a problem taking them before).

- tell your doctor if you have or have ever had irregular heartbeat, increased heart rate, glaucoma, heart disease, high blood pressure, an overactive thyroid gland, diabetes, or seizures.
- tell your doctor if you are pregnant, plan to become pregnant, or are breast-feeding. If you become pregnant while taking metaproterenol, call your doctor.
- if you are having surgery, including dental surgery, tell the doctor or dentist that you are taking metaproterenol.

What should I do if I forget to take a dose?

Take the missed dose as soon as you remember it. However, if it is almost time for the next dose, skip the missed dose and continue your regular dosing schedule. Do not take a double dose to make up for a missed one.

What side effects can this medicine cause?

Metaproterenol may cause side effects. Tell your doctor if any of these symptoms are severe or do not go away:

- tremor
- nervousness
- dizziness
- weakness
- headache
- upset stomach
- cough
- dry mouth
- throat irritation

If you experience any of the following symptoms, call your doctor immediately:

- increased difficulty breathing
- rapid or increased heart rate
- irregular heartbeat
- chest pain or discomfort

If you experience a serious side effect, you or your doctor may send a report to the Food and Drug Administration's (FDA) MedWatch Adverse Event Reporting program online [at http://www.fda.gov/MedWatch/index.html] or by phone [1-800-332-1088].

What storage conditions are needed for this medicine?

Keep this medication in the container it came in, tightly closed, and out of reach of children. Store it at room temperature and away from excess heat and moisture (not in the bathroom). Do not use the solution if it is pink, yellow, or darker than usual or if it has floating particles. Throw away any medication that is outdated or no longer needed. Talk to your pharmacist about the proper disposal of your medication. Avoid puncturing the container, and do not discard it in an incinerator or fire.

What should I do in case of overdose?

In case of overdose, call your local poison control center at 1-800-222-1222. If the victim has collapsed or is not breathing, call local emergency services at 911.

What other information should I know?

Keep all appointments with your doctor and the laboratory. Your doctor will order certain lab tests to check your response to metaproterenol.

To relieve dry mouth or throat irritation caused by metaproterenol inhalation, rinse your mouth with water, chew gum, or suck sugarless hard candy after using metaproterenol.

Inhalation devices require regular cleaning. Once a week, remove the drug container from the plastic mouthpiece, wash the mouthpiece with warm tap water, and dry it thoroughly.

Do not let anyone else take your medication. Ask your pharmacist any questions you have about refilling your prescription.

Talk to your doctor, pharmacist, or other healthcare professional if you have questions about dosing information for your medication.

Metaxalone

(me tax′ a lone)

Brand Name: Skelaxin®

Why is this medicine prescribed?

Metaxalone, a muscle relaxant, is used with rest, physical therapy, and other measures to relax muscles and relieve pain and discomfort caused by strains, sprains, and other muscle injuries.

This medication is sometimes prescribed for other uses; ask your doctor or pharmacist for more information.

How should this medicine be used?

Metaxalone comes as a tablet to take by mouth. It usually is taken three or four times a day. Follow the directions on your prescription label carefully, and ask your doctor or pharmacist to explain any part you do not understand. Take metaxalone exactly as directed. Do not take more or less of it or take it more often than prescribed by your doctor.

What special precautions should I follow?

Before taking metaxalone,
- tell your doctor and pharmacist if you are allergic to metaxalone or any other drugs.
- tell your doctor and pharmacist what prescription and nonprescription medications you are taking, especially medications for seizures, allergies, colds, or coughs; pain medications; sedatives; tranquilizers; and vitamins.
- tell your doctor if you have or have ever had kidney disease, liver disease, seizures, or a blood disorder.

- tell your doctor if you are pregnant, plan to become pregnant, or are breast-feeding. If you become pregnant while taking metaxalone, call your doctor immediately.
- you should know that this drug may make you drowsy. Do not drive a car or operate machinery until you know how metaxalone affects you.
- remember that alcohol can add to the drowsiness caused by this drug.

What should I do if I forget to take a dose?

Take the missed dose as soon as you remember it. However, if it is almost time for your next dose, skip the missed dose and continue your regular dosing schedule. Do not take a double dose to make up for a missed one.

What side effects can this medicine cause?

Metaxalone may cause side effects. Tell your doctor if any of these symptoms are severe or do not go away:
- drowsiness
- dizziness
- upset stomach
- vomiting
- headache
- nervousness

If you experience any of the following symptoms, call your doctor immediately:
- severe skin rash
- difficulty breathing
- yellowing of the skin or eyes
- unusual bruising or bleeding
- unusual tiredness or weakness
- seizures

If you experience a serious side effect, you or your doctor may send a report to the Food and Drug Administration's (FDA) MedWatch Adverse Event Reporting program online [at http://www.fda.gov/MedWatch/index.html] or by phone [1-800-332-1088].

What storage conditions are needed for this medicine?

Keep this medication in the container it came in, tightly closed, and out of reach of children. Store it at room temperature, away from excess heat and moisture (not in the bathroom). Throw away any medication that is outdated or no longer needed. Ask your pharmacist about the proper disposal of your medication.

What should I do in case of overdose?

In case of overdose, call your local poison control center at 1-800-222-1222. If the victim has collapsed or is not breathing, call local emergency services at 911.

What other information should I know?

Keep all appointments with your doctor.

Do not let anyone else take your medications. Ask your pharmacist any questions you have about refilling your prescription.

Dosage Facts
For Informational Purposes

Caution: Do not change your dose, how often you take your medication, or the length of time you are to take it without first talking to your healthcare provider.

The following dosage information was written using medical language for doctors and other healthcare professionals and is provided here for you to check your dosage. The dosage of this drug may differ for different patients. Therefore, always follow your doctor's instructions or the directions on the label. Contact your healthcare provider or pharmacist if you have any questions about the specific dosage of your medication after reviewing this information.

Pediatric Patients

Muscular Conditions

ORAL:
• Children >12 years of age: 800 mg 3 or 4 times daily.

Adult Patients

Muscular Conditions

ORAL:
• 800 mg 3 or 4 times daily.

Metformin

(met for' min)

Brand Name: Glucophage®, Glucophage ® XR, Fortamet®

Important Warning

Metformin may rarely cause a serious, life-threatening condition called lactic acidosis. Tell your doctor if you have or have ever had a heart attack; stroke; high blood pressure; diabetic ketoacidosis (blood sugar that is high enough to cause severe symptoms and requires emergency medical treatment) or coma; surgery to remove part of your small intestine; anemia (not enough red blood cells), or heart, kidney, lung, or liver disease.

Tell your doctor if you have recently had any of the following conditions, or if you develop them during treatment: serious infection; severe diarrhea, vomiting, or fever; or if you drink much less fluid than usual for any reason. You may have to stop taking metformin until you recover.

If you are having surgery, including dental surgery, any x-ray procedure in which dye is injected, or any major medical procedure, tell the doctor that you are taking metformin. You may need to stop taking metformin before the procedure and wait 48 hours to restart treatment. Your doctor will tell you exactly when you should stop taking metformin and when you should start taking it again.

Tell your doctor and pharmacist if you are taking or have taken the following medications: acyclovir (Zovirax); acetaminophen (Tylenol); aminoglycoside antibiotics such as amikacin (Amikin), gentamicin (Garamycin), Kanamycin (Kantrex), Neomycin (Neo-Fradin, Neo-Rx), netilmycin (netromycin), paramomycin (Humatin), streptomycin and tobramycin (Nebcin, Tobi); amphotericin B (Abelcet, Amphocin, others); angiotensin converting enzyme (ACE) inhibitors such as benazepril (Lotensin), captopril (Capoten), enalapril (Vasotec), fosinopril (Monopril), lisinopril (Prinvil, Zestril), moexipril (Univasc), perindopril (Aceon), quinapril (Accupril), ramipril (Altace), and trandolapril (Mavik); aspirin and other non-steroidal anti-inflammatory agents (NSAIDs) such as ibuprofen (Advil, Motrin) and naproxen (Aleve, Naprosyn); cancer chemotherapy medications; cyclosporine (Sandimmune, Neoral); dapsone (Avlosulfon); diuretics (water pills); foscarnet (Foscavir); gold compounds such as auranofin (Ridaura), aurothioglucose (Aurolate, Solganol), and gold sodium thiomalate (Myochrysine); hydralazine (Hydra-Zide); lithium (Eskalith, Lithobid); medications to treat human immunodeficiency virus (HIV) or acquired immunodeficiency syndrome (AIDS); methicillin (Staphcillin); nitrates; penicillin and sulfa antibiotics; penicillamine (Cuprimine, Depen); primaquine; propranolol (Inderal); rifampin (Rifadin, Rimactane); tacrolimus (Prograf); vancomycin (Vancocin); or if you have ever taken the Chinese weight-loss herb aristolochia.

If you experience any of the following symptoms, call your doctor immediately: extreme tiredness, weakness, or discomfort; upset stomach; vomiting; stomach pain; decreased appetite; deep and rapid breathing or shortness of breath; dizziness; light-headedness; fast or slow heartbeat; flushing of the skin; muscle pain; or feeling cold.

Tell your doctor if you regularly drink alcohol or sometimes drink large amounts of alcohol in a short time (binge drinking). Drinking alcohol increases your risk of developing lactic acidosis or may cause a decrease in blood sugar. Ask your doctor how much alcohol is safe to drink while you are taking metformin.

Keep all appointments with your doctor and the laboratory. Your doctor will order certain tests to check your body's response to metformin. Talk to your doctor about the risk(s) of taking metformin.

Why is this medicine prescribed?

Metformin is used alone or with other medications, including insulin, to treat type 2 diabetes (condition in which the body does not use insulin normally and therefore cannot control the amount of sugar in the blood). Metformin helps to control the amount of glucose (sugar) in your blood. It decreases the amount of glucose you absorb from your food and the amount of glucose made by your liver. Metformin also increases your body's response to insulin, a natural substance that controls the amount of glucose in the blood. Metformin is not used to treat type 1 diabetes (condition in which the body does not produce insulin and therefore cannot control the amount of sugar in the blood).

How should this medicine be used?

Metformin comes as a tablet and an extended-release (long-acting) tablet to take by mouth. The regular tablet is usually taken with meals two or three times a day. The extended-release tablet is usually taken once daily with the evening meal. To help you remember to take metformin, take it around the same time(s) every day. Follow the directions on your prescription label carefully, and ask your doctor or pharmacist to explain any part you do not understand. Take metformin exactly as directed. Do not take more or less of it or take it more often than prescribed by your doctor.

Swallow metformin extended-release tablets whole; do not split, chew, or crush them.

Your doctor may start you on a low dose of metformin and gradually increase your dose not more often than once every 1-2 weeks. You will need to monitor your blood sugar carefully so your doctor will be able to tell how well metformin is working.

Metformin controls diabetes but does not cure it. Continue to take metformin even if you feel well. Do not stop taking metformin without talking to your doctor.

Are there other uses for this medicine?

This medication may be prescribed for other uses; ask your doctor or pharmacist for more information.

What special precautions should I follow?

Before taking metformin,
- tell your doctor and pharmacist if you are allergic to metformin or any other medications.
- tell your doctor and pharmacist what other prescription and nonprescription medications, vitamins, nutritional supplements, and herbal products you are taking. Be sure to mention the medications listed in the IMPORTANT WARNING section and any of the following: amiloride (Midamor, Moduretic); antihistamines; beta-blockers such as atenolol (Tenormin), labetalol (Normodyne), metoprolol (Lopressor, Toprol XL), nadolol (Corgard), and propranolol (Inderal); calcium channel blockers such as amlodipine (Norvasc), diltiazem (Cardizem, Dilacor, Tiazac, others), felodipine (Lexxel, Plendil), isradipine (DynaCirc), nicardipine (Cardene), nifedipine (Adalat, Procardia), nimodipine (Nimotop), nisoldipine (Sular), and verapamil (Calan, Isoptin, Verelan); cimetidine (Tagamet); digoxin (Lanoxin, Lanoxicaps); furosemide (Lasix); hormone replacement therapy; insulin or other medications for diabetes; isoniazid (INH, Nydrazid); medications for asthma and colds; medications for mental illness and nausea such as fluphenazine (Prolixin), mesoridazine (Serentil), perphenazine (Trilafon), prochlorperazine (Compazine), promethazine (Phenergan), thioridazine (Mellaril), thiothixene (Navane), trifluoperazine (Stelazine), and triflupromazine (Vesprin); medications for thyroid disease; morphine (MS Contin, Roxanol, others); nicotinic acid; oral contraceptives (birth control pills); oral steroids such as dexamethasone (Decadron, Dexone), methylprednisolone (Medrol), and prednisone (Deltasone); phenytoin (Dilantin, Phenytek); procainamide (Procanbid); quinidine (Quinidex); quinine; ranitidine (Zantac); triamterene (Dyazide, Maxzide, others); or trimethoprim (Proloprim, Trimpex). Your doctor may need to change the doses of your medications or monitor you carefully for side effects.
- tell your doctor if you have or have ever had any medical condition, especially those mentioned in the IMPORTANT WARNING section.
- tell your doctor if you are pregnant, plan to become pregnant, or are breast-feeding. If you become pregnant while taking metformin, call your doctor.
- if you are using the extended release tablets, you should know that sometimes the tablet shell may appear in your stool. If this occurs, it is not harmful and will not affect the way the medication works.
- tell your doctor if you eat less or exercise more than usual. This can affect your blood sugar. Your doctor will give you instructions if this happens.

What special dietary instructions should I follow?

Be sure to follow all exercise and dietary recommendations made by your doctor or dietitian. It is important to eat a healthful diet.

What should I do if I forget to take a dose?

Take the missed dose as soon as you remember it. However, if it is almost time for the next dose, skip the missed dose and continue your regular dosing schedule. Do not take a double dose to make up for a missed one.

What side effects can this medicine cause?

This medication may cause changes in your blood sugar. You should know the symptoms of low and high blood sugar and what to do if you have these symptoms.

You may experience hypoglycemia (low blood sugar) while you are taking this medication. Your doctor will tell you what you should do if you develop hypoglycemia. He or she may tell you to check your blood sugar, eat or drink a food or beverage that contains sugar, such as hard candy or fruit juice, or get medical care. Follow these directions carefully if you have any of the following symptoms of hypoglycemia:

- shakiness
- dizziness or lightheadedness
- sweating
- nervousness or irritability
- sudden changes in behavior or mood
- headache
- numbness or tingling around the mouth
- weakness
- pale skin
- hunger
- clumsy or jerky movements

If hypoglycemia is not treated, severe symptoms may develop. Be sure that your family, friends, and other people who spend time with you know that if you have any of the following symptoms, they should get medical treatment for you immediately.

- confusion
- seizures
- loss of consciousness

Call your doctor immediately if you have any of the following symptoms of hyperglycemia (high blood sugar):

- extreme thirst
- frequent urination
- extreme hunger
- weakness
- blurred vision

If high blood sugar is not treated, a serious, life-threatening condition called diabetic ketoacidosis could develop. Call your doctor immediately if you have any of the these symptoms:

- dry mouth
- upset stomach and vomiting
- shortness of breath
- breath that smells fruity
- decreased consciousness

Metformin may cause side effects. Tell your doctor if any of these symptoms are severe, do not go away, go away and come back, or do not begin for some time after you begin taking metformin:

- diarrhea
- bloating
- stomach pain
- gas
- constipation
- unpleasant metallic taste in mouth
- heartburn
- headache
- sneezing
- cough
- runny nose
- flushing of the skin
- nail changes
- muscle pain

Some side effects can be serious. The following symptoms are uncommon, but if you experience any of them or those listed in the IMPORTANT WARNING section, call your doctor immediately:

- chest pain
- rash

Some female laboratory animals given high doses of metformin developed non-cancerous polyps (abnormal growths of tissue) in the uterus (womb). It is not known if metformin increases the risk of polyps in humans. Talk to your doctor about the risks of taking this medication.

Metformin may cause other side effects. Call your doctor if you have any unusual problems while taking this medication.

If you experience a serious side effect, you or your doctor may send a report to the Food and Drug Administration's (FDA) MedWatch Adverse Event Reporting program online [at http://www.fda.gov/MedWatch/index.html] or by phone [1-800-332-1088].

What storage conditions are needed for this medicine?

Keep this medication in the container it came in, tightly closed, and out of reach of children. Store it at room temperature and away from light excess heat and moisture (not in the bathroom). Throw away any medication that is outdated or no longer needed. Talk to your pharmacist about the proper disposal of your medication.

What should I do in case of overdose?

In case of overdose, call your local poison control center at 1-800-222-1222. If the victim has collapsed or is not breathing, call local emergency services at 911.

Symptoms of overdose may include:

- extreme tiredness
- weakness
- discomfort
- vomiting
- upset stomach
- stomach pain
- decreased appetite
- deep, rapid breathing
- shortness of breath
- dizziness
- light-headedness
- abnormally fast or slow heartbeat
- flushing of the skin
- muscle pain
- feeling cold

What other information should I know?

Keep all appointments with your doctor and the laboratory. Your blood sugar and glycosylated hemoglobin (HbA1c) should be checked regularly to determine your response to metformin. Your doctor may order other lab tests to check your response to metformin. Your doctor will also tell you how to check your response to this medication by measuring your blood or urine sugar levels at home. Follow these instructions carefully.

You should always wear a diabetic identification bracelet to be sure you get proper treatment in an emergency.

Do not let anyone else take your medication. Ask your pharmacist any questions you have about refilling your prescription.

Dosage Facts
For Informational Purposes

Caution: Do not change your dose, how often you take your medication, or the length of time you are to take it without first talking to your healthcare provider.

The following dosage information was written using medical language for doctors and other healthcare professionals and is provided here for you to check your dosage. The dosage of this drug may differ for different patients. Therefore, always follow your doctor's instructions or the directions on the label. Contact your healthcare provider or pharmacist if you have any questions about the specific dosage of your medication after reviewing this information.

General Dosage Information

Individualize dosage carefully based on patient's glycemic response and tolerance.

Pediatric Patients

Diabetes Mellitus

ORAL:

- Conventional tablets or oral solution in children 10–16 years of age: Initially, 500 mg twice daily with meals as monotherapy. Titrate dosage in increments of 500 mg daily at weekly intervals to a maximum of 2 g daily given in divided doses.

Adult Patients

Diabetes Mellitus
Initial Dosage in Previously Untreated Patients

ORAL:

- Conventional tablets or oral solution: Initially, 500 mg twice daily with the morning and evening meal. Titrate dosage by 500 mg daily at weekly intervals to a total of 2 g daily or to 850 mg twice daily after 2 weeks. Clinically important responses generally not observed at dosages <1.5 g daily. Usual maintenance dosage is 850 mg twice daily.
- Alternatively, give initial dosage of 500–850 mg once daily in the morning. If initial dosage is 850 mg daily, titrate dosage by 850 mg daily every *other* week to a total of 2 g daily.
- For additional glycemic control, administer up to a maximum daily dosage of 2.55 g given in divided doses.
- Extended-release tablets (Glucophage® XR) in patients ≥17 years of age: Initially, 500 mg once daily with the evening meal. Titrate dosage by 500 mg daily at weekly intervals to a maximum of 2 g daily. If glycemic control is not achieved with 2 g once daily, consider administering 1 g twice daily. If >2 g daily is required, switch to conventional tablet formulation and increase dosage up to 2.55 g daily in divided doses (preferably 3 doses for daily dosages >2 g).

- Extended-release tablets (Fortamet®) in patients ≥17 years of age: Initially, 1 g daily with the evening meal; 500 mg daily may be used when clinically appropriate. Titrate dosage by 500 mg daily at weekly intervals to a maximum of 2.5 g daily with the evening meal.

Initial Dosage of Metformin Hydrochloride in Fixed Combination with Glipizide (Metaglip®)

ORAL:

- Initially, 250 mg of metformin hydrochloride and 2.5 mg of glipizide once daily with a meal. For more severe hyperglycemia (fasting plasma glucose concentrations of 280–320 mg/dL), 500 mg of metformin hydrochloride and 2.5 mg of glipizide twice daily. Titrate in increments of one tablet (using the tablet strength at which therapy was initiated) daily at 2-week intervals until adequate blood glucose control is achieved or maximum daily dosage of 2 g of metformin hydrochloride and 10 mg of glipizide is reached.
- Efficacy of metformin hydrochloride and glipizide in fixed combination not established in patients with fasting plasma glucose concentrations >320 mg/dL. No experience with total initial daily dosages exceeding 2 g of metformin hydrochloride and 10 mg of glipizide.

Initial Dosage of Metformin Hydrochloride in Fixed Combination with Glyburide (Glucovance®)

ORAL:

- Initially, 250 mg of metformin hydrochloride and 1.25 mg of glyburide once daily with a meal. For more severe hyperglycemia (i.e., fasting plasma glucose concentrations >200 mg/dL or glycosylated hemoglobin >9%), 250 mg of metformin hydrochloride and 1.25 mg of glyburide twice daily with the morning and evening meal. Titrate dosage in increments of 250 mg of metformin hydrochloride and 1.25 mg of glyburide daily at 2-week intervals adequate control of blood glucose is achieved or a maximum daily dosage of 2 g of metformin hydrochloride and 10 mg of glyburide.
- The fixed combination of metformin hydrochloride 500 mg and glyburide 5 mg should not be used as initial therapy due to an increased risk of hypoglycemia.

Initial Dosage in Patients Transferred to Metformin Hydrochloride in Fixed Combination with Glipizide (Metaglip®)

ORAL:

- In previously treated patients, 500 mg of metformin hydrochloride and 2.5 or 5 mg of glipizide twice daily with the morning and evening meals. The initial dosage of glipizide and metformin hydrochloride in fixed combination should not exceed the daily dosage of metformin hydrochloride or glipizide (or the equivalent dosage of another sulfonylurea) previously received. Titrate dosage in increments not exceeding 500 mg of metformin hydrochloride and 5 mg of glipizide until adequate control of blood glucose is achieved or a maximum daily dosage of 2 g of metformin hydrochloride and 20 mg of glipizide is reached.
- For patients switching from combined therapy with separate preparations, the initial dosage of the fixed-combination preparation of glipizide and metformin hydrochloride should not exceed the daily dosages of glipizide (or equivalent dosage of another sulfonylurea antidiabetic agent) *and* metformin hydrochloride currently being taken. Use clinical judgment regarding whether to switch to the nearest equivalent dosage or to titrate dosage. Titrate dosage in increments of not more than 5 mg of glipizide and 500 mg of metformin hydrochlo-

ride until adequate control of blood glucose is achieved or maximum daily dosage of 20 mg of glipizide and 2 g of metformin hydrochloride is reached.

Initial Dosage in Patients Transferred to Metformin Hydrochloride in Fixed Combination with Glyburide (Glucovance®)

ORAL:

- Initially, 500 mg of metformin hydrochloride and 2.5 or 5 mg of glyburide twice daily with the morning and evening meal. For patients previously receiving metformin hydrochloride or glyburide (or another sulfonylurea agent), the initial dosage of metformin hydrochloride or glyburide should not exceed the dosage (or equivalent dosage) received previously. For patients previously receiving both metformin hydrochloride and glyburide (or another sulfonylurea agent) separately, the initial dosage should not exceed the previous dosage of metformin hydrochloride and glyburide (or the equivalent dosage of the other sulfonylurea) administered separately. Titrate dosage in increments not exceeding 500 mg of metformin hydrochloride and 5 mg of glyburide until adequate control of blood glucose is achieved or a maximum daily dosage of 2 g of metformin hydrochloride and 20 mg of glyburide is reached.
- For patients whose hyperglycemia is not adequately controlled on therapy with metformin hydrochloride in fixed combination with glyburide, a thiazolidinedione (e.g., pioglitazone, rosiglitazone) may be added at its recommended initial dosage and the dosage of the fixed combination may be continued unchanged. In patients requiring further glycemic control, titrate thiazolidinedione dosage upward as recommended.

Initial Dosage in Patients Transferred to Metformin Hydrochloride in Fixed Combination with Rosiglitazone (Avandamet®)

ORAL:

- In patients not adequately controlled on monotherapy with metformin hydrochloride or rosiglitazone, dosage of the fixed combination is based on the patient's current dosages of metformin hydrochloride and/or rosiglitazone. (See Table.) For replacement of concurrent therapy with the drugs given as separate tablets, dosage of the fixed combination is based on the patient's current dosages of metformin hydrochloride and/or rosiglitazone.

Initial Dosage of the Fixed Combination of Metformin Hydrochloride and Rosiglitazone (Avandamet®)

Prior Therapy Total Daily Dosage	Usual Initial Dosage of Avandamet®	
	Tablet strength	Number of tablets
Metformin Hydrochloride		
1 g	2 mg/500 mg	1 tablet twice daily
2 g	1 mg/500 mg	2 tablets twice daily
Rosiglitazone		
4 mg	2 mg/500 mg	1 tablet twice daily
8 mg	4 mg/500 mg	1 tablet twice daily

The tablet strength of the fixed combination that is selected should be the one that most closely provides the patient's existing dosage of metformin hydrochloride or rosiglitazone, respectively.

Individualize therapy in patients already receiving metformin hydrochloride at dosages not available in the fixed combination (i.e., dosages other than 1 or 2 g).

For patients switching from combined therapy with separate preparations, the initial dosage of the fixed-combination preparation of metformin hydrochloride and rosiglitazone should be the same as the daily dosage of metformin hydrochloride and rosiglitazone currently being taken.

If additional glycemic control is needed following transfer, titrate dosage upward in increments not exceeding 500 mg of metformin hydrochloride and/or 4 mg of rosiglitazone until adequate glycemic control is achieved or a maximum daily dosage of 2 g of metformin hydrochloride and 8 mg of rosiglitazone is reached.

Initial Metformin Hydrochloride Dosage in Patients Transferred from Insulin

ORAL:

- Initially, 500 mg once daily; increase dosage by 500 mg daily at weekly intervals adequate control of blood glucose is achieved or a maximum daily dosage of 2.5 g (conventional tablets) or 2 g (extended-release tablets) is reached. Concurrent insulin dosage initially remains unchanged. When fasting plasma glucose concentration decreases to <120 mg/dL, decrease insulin dosage by 10–25%.

Prescribing Limits

Pediatric Patients

ORAL:

- Children 10–16 years of age: Maximum 2 g daily as conventional tablets or oral solution.

Adult Patients

ORAL:

- Maximum 2.55 g daily (conventional tablets or oral solution; 2.5 g daily as Fortamet® extended-release tablets; or 2 g daily as certain other extended-release tablets (e.g., Glucophage®). Switch to conventional tablets for further dosage titration if required dosage exceeds 2 g daily while on extended-release tablets.
- For the fixed combination with glyburide, maximum daily dosage as second-line therapy is 2 g of metformin hydrochloride and 20 mg of glyburide. For the fixed combination with glipizide, maximum daily dosage is 2 g of metformin hydrochloride and 20 mg of glipizide. For the fixed combination with rosiglitazone, maximum daily dosage is 2 g of metformin hydrochloride and 8 mg of rosiglitazone.

Special Populations

Geriatric Patients

- Maintenance dosage generally should not be titrated to the maximum recommended for younger adults; limited data suggest reducing initial dosage by approximately 33% in geriatric patients.

Methadone

(meth′ a done)

Brand Name: Dolophine®, Methadose®, Methadose® Oral Concentrate
Also available generically.

Important Warning

Methadone may cause slowed breathing and irregular heartbeat which may be life-threatening. If you experience any of the following symptoms, call your doctor immediately: difficulty breathing; extreme drowsiness; slow, shallow breathing; fast, slow, pounding or irregular heartbeat; faintness; severe dizziness; or confusion.

The risk that you will experience serious or life-threatening side effects of methadone is greatest when you first start taking methadone, when you switch from another narcotic medication to methadone and when your doctor increases your dose of methadone. Your doctor may start you on a low dose of methadone and gradually increase your dose. Your doctor will monitor you closely during this time.

Follow the directions on your prescription label carefully and ask your doctor or pharmacist to explain any part you do not understand. Take methadone exactly as directed. Do not take more methadone or take methadone more often than prescribed by your doctor. If you are taking methadone to control pain, your pain may return before it is time for your next dose of methadone. If this happens, do not take an extra dose of methadone. You will still have methadone in your body after the pain relieving effect of the medication wears off. If you take extra doses, you may have too much methadone in your body and you may experience life-threatening side effects. Be aware that the pain relieving effects of methadone will last longer as your treatment continues for a longer time. Talk to your doctor if your pain is not controlled during your treatment with methadone.

Talk to your doctor about the risks of taking methadone for your condition.

Use of methadone to treat opiate addiction:

If you have been addicted to an opiate (narcotic drug such as heroin), and you are taking methadone to help you stop taking or continue not taking the drug, you must enroll in a treatment program. The treatment program must be approved by the state and federal governments and must treat patients according to specific federal laws. You may have to take your medication at the treatment program facility under the supervision of the program staff. Ask your doctor or the treatment program staff if you have any questions about enrolling in the program or taking or getting your medication.

Why is this medicine prescribed?

Methadone is used to relieve moderate to severe pain that has not been relieved by non-narcotic pain relievers. It also is used to prevent withdrawal symptoms in patients who were addicted to opiate drugs and are enrolled in treatment programs in order to stop taking or continue not taking the drugs. Methadone is in a class of medications called opiate (narcotic) analgesics. Methadone works to treat pain by changing the way the brain and nervous system respond to pain. It also works as a substitute for opiate drugs of abuse by producing similar effects and preventing withdrawal symptoms in people who have stopped using these drugs.

How should this medicine be used?

Methadone comes as a tablet, a dispersible tablet (can be dissolved in liquid), a solution (liquid), and a concentrated solution (liquid that must be diluted before use) to take by mouth. When methadone is used to relieve pain, it may be taken every 4 to 12 hours. If you take methadone as part of a treatment program, your doctor will prescribe the dosing schedule that is best for you.

Your doctor may change your dose of methadone during your treatment. Your doctor may decrease your dose or tell you to take methadone less often as your treatment continues. Ask your doctor or pharmacist if you have any questions about how much methadone you should take or how often you should take the medication.

Methadone can be habit-forming. Call your doctor if you find that you want to take extra medication or notice any other unusual changes in your behavior or mood.

Do not stop taking methadone without talking to your doctor. Your doctor will probably want to decrease your dose gradually. If you suddenly stop taking methadone, you may experience withdrawal symptoms such as restlessness, teary eyes, runny nose, yawning, sweating, chills, muscle pain, and widened pupils (black circles in the middle of the eyes).

If you are using the dispersible tablets, place one tablet in a liquid such as water or citrus fruit juice. Wait 1 minute to allow the tablet to dissolve and then drink the entire mixture.

If you are using methadone oral concentrate solution, you should mix your prescribed dose of medication in at least 1 ounce of liquid such as water, citrus fruit juice, Kool Aid®, Tang®, apple juice, or Crystal Light®.

Are there other uses for this medicine?

This medication may be prescribed for other uses; ask your doctor or pharmacist for more information.

What special precautions should I follow?

Before taking methadone,

- tell your doctor and pharmacist if you are allergic to methadone or any other medications.
- tell your doctor and pharmacist what prescription and nonprescription medications, vitamins, and nutritional supplements you are taking or plan to take. Be sure to mention any of the following: antidepressants such as amitriptyline (Elavil), amoxapine (Asendin), clomipramine (Anafranil), desipramine (Norpramin), doxepin (Adapin, Sinequan), imipramine (Tofranil), nortriptyline (Aventyl, Pamelor), protriptyline (Vivactil), and trimipramine (Surmontil); certain antifungals such as fluconazole (Diflucan), itraconazole (Sporanox), ketoconazole (Nizoral), and voriconazole (Vfend); antihistamines; buprenorphine (Subutex); butorphanol (Stadol NS); calcium channel blocking agents such as amlodipine (Norvasc), diltiazem (Cardizem, Dilacor, Tiazac, others), felodipine (Plendil), isradipine (DynaCirc), nicardipine (Cardene), nifedipine (Adalat, Procardia), nimodipine (Nimotop), nisoldipine (Sular), and verapamil (Calan, Covera, Isoptin, Verelan); diuretics ('water pills'); erythromycin (E.E.S., E-Mycin, Erythrocin); laxatives; medications for anxiety, mental illness, nausea, or pain; medications for HIV including abacavir (Ziagen), amprenavir (Agenerase), didanosine (Videx), efavirenz (Sustiva), lopinavir (in Kaletra), nelfinavir (Viracept), nevirapine (Viramune), ritonavir (Norvir, in Kaletra), stavudine (Zerit), and zidovudine (Retrovir); certain medications for irregular heartbeat such as disopyramide (Norpace), flecainide (Tambocor), mexiletine (Mexitil), moricizine (Ethmozine), procainamide (Procanbid, Pronestyl), propafenone (Rythmol), propranolol (Inderal), quinidine (Quinidex), and tocainide (Tonocard); certain medications for seizures such as carbamazepine (Carbatrol, Epitol, Tegretol), phenytoin (Dilantin, Phenytek); phenobarbital nalbuphine (Nubain); naloxone (Narcan); naltrexone (ReVia, Depade); pentazocine (Talwin); rifampin (Rifadin, Rimactane, in Rifamate); risperidone (Risperdal); sedatives; certain selective serotonin reuptake inhibitors (SSRIs) such as fluvoxamine (Luvox) and sertraline (Zoloft); sleeping pills; certain steroids such as cortisone, fludricortisone (Flurinef), and hydrocortisone (Cortef); and tranquilizers. Also tell your doctor or pharmacist if you are taking the following medications or have stopped taking them in the past 14 days: monoamine oxidase (MAO) inhibitors including isocarboxazid (Marplan), phenelzine (Nardil), selegiline (Eldepryl, Emsam, Zelpar), and tranylcypromine (Parnate). Many other medications may also interact with methadone, so be sure to tell your doctor about all the medications you are taking, even those that do not appear on this list. Your doctor may need to change the doses of your medications or monitor you carefully for side effects.
- tell your doctor what herbal products you are taking, especially St. John's wort.
- tell your doctor if you have or have ever had asthma or other breathing problems or a blockage in your intestine. Your doctor may tell you that you should not take methadone.
- tell your doctor if you have or have ever had a head injury, a brain tumor, a stroke, or any other condition that caused high pressure inside your skull; irregular heartbeat; urethral stricture (narrowing of the tube that carries urine out of the body), enlarged prostate (a male reproductive gland), or any other condition that causes difficulty urinating; Addison's disease (a condition in which the body does not make enough of certain natural substances); mental illness; chronic obstructive pulmonary disease (COPD; a group of lung diseases); kyphoscoliosis (condition in which the spine curves abnormally); sleep apnea (condition in which breathing stops for short periods during sleep); low levels of potassium or magnesium in your blood; or thyroid, heart, liver, or kidney disease. Also tell your doctor if you drink or have ever drunk large amounts of alcohol or if you use or have ever used street drugs or have overused prescription medications.
- tell your doctor if you are pregnant, plan to become pregnant, or are breast-feeding. If you become pregnant while taking methadone, call your doctor.
- if you are having surgery, including dental surgery, tell the doctor or dentist that you are taking methadone.
- you should know that this medication may make you drowsy. Do not drive a car or operate machinery until you know how this medication affects you.
- remember that alcohol can add to the drowsiness caused by this medication.
- tell your doctor if you use tobacco products. Cigarette smoking may decrease the effectiveness of this medication.
- you should know that methadone may cause dizziness when you get up too quickly from a lying position. This is more common when you first start taking methadone. To avoid this problem, get out of bed slowly, resting your feet on the floor for a few minutes before standing up.

What special dietary instructions should I follow?

Talk to your doctor about eating grapefruit and drinking grapefruit juice while taking this medicine.

What should I do if I forget to take a dose?

If your doctor has told you to take methadone regularly, take the missed dose as soon as you remember it. However, if it is almost time for the next dose, skip the missed dose and continue your regular dosing schedule. Do not take a double dose to make up for a missed one.

What side effects can this medicine cause?

Methadone may cause side effects. Tell your doctor if any of these symptoms are severe or do not go away:

- drowsiness
- weakness
- headache
- nausea
- vomiting
- constipation
- loss of appetite
- weight gain
- stomach pain
- dry mouth
- sweating
- flushing
- difficulty urinating
- swelling of the hands, arms, feet, and legs
- mood changes
- vision problems
- difficulty falling asleep or staying asleep
- decreased sexual desire or ability
- missed menstrual periods

Some side effects can be serious. If you experience any of the following symptoms or those mentioned in the IMPORTANT WARNING section, call your doctor immediately:

- seizures
- itching
- hives
- rash

Methadone may cause other side effects. Call your doctor if you have any unusual problems while you are taking this medication.

What storage conditions are needed for this medicine?

Keep this medication in the container it came in, tightly closed, and out of reach of children. Store it at room temperature and away from excess heat and moisture (not in the bathroom). Throw away any medication that is outdated or no longer needed. Talk to your pharmacist about the proper disposal of your medication.

Store methadone in a safe place so that no one else can take it accidentally or on purpose. Keep track of how many tablets or how much solution or concentrated solution is left so you will know if any is missing.

What should I do in case of overdose?

In case of overdose, call your local poison control center at 1-800-222-1222. If the victim has collapsed or is not breathing, call local emergency services at 911.

Symptoms of overdose may include:

- small, pinpoint pupils (black circles in the center of the eyes)
- slow or shallow breathing
- drowsiness
- cool, clammy, or blue skin
- loss of consciousness; coma
- limp muscles

What other information should I know?

Keep all appointments with your doctor, laboratory, and clinic. Your doctor will want to check your response to methadone.

This prescription is not refillable. If you continue to experience pain after you finish methadone, call your doctor. If you take this medication on a regular basis, be sure to schedule appointments with your doctor so that you do not run out of medication.

Dosage Facts
For Informational Purposes

Caution: Do not change your dose, how often you take your medication, or the length of time you are to take it without first talking to your healthcare provider.

The following dosage information was written using medical language for doctors and other healthcare professionals and is provided here for you to check your dosage. The dosage of this drug may differ for different patients. Therefore, always follow your doctor's instructions or the directions on the label. Contact your healthcare provider or pharmacist if you have any questions about the specific dosage of your medication after reviewing this information.

General Dosage Information

Available as methadone hydrochloride; dosage expressed in terms of the salt.

Pediatric Patients

Pain†

When selecting an initial dosage, consider the type, severity, and expected duration of the patient's pain; the age, general condition, and medical status of the patient; concurrent drug therapy; and the acceptable balance between pain relief and adverse effects.

Give the smallest effective dose in order to minimize development of tolerance and physical dependence.

ORAL:
- Dosage of 0.7 mg/kg daily in divided doses every 4–6 hours (maximum 10 mg per dose) has been suggested; carefully individualize dosage.

Adult Patients

Pain

When selecting an initial dosage, consider the type, severity, and expected duration of the patient's pain; the age, general condition, and medical status of the patient; concurrent drug therapy; and the acceptable balance between pain relief and adverse effects.

Give the smallest effective dose in order to minimize development of tolerance and physical dependence.

ORAL:
- 2.5–10 mg every 3–4 hours as necessary for the relief of severe pain. Titrate dosage to provide adequate analgesia; increase dosage slowly to avoid accumulation.

- Many clinicians suggest a dosage interval of 8–12 hours during chronic therapy to avoid accumulation and to minimize adverse effects.
- Dosage interval may range from 4–12 hours, since the duration of analgesia is relatively short during the first days of therapy but increases substantially with continued administration.
- Dose may need to be markedly reduced and/or the dosing interval increased after the first few doses based on assessments of pain relief, sedation, and other adverse effects.

Conversion from Other Opiate Therapy

For patients being transferred from therapy with other opiate agonists, dosage may be estimated based on comparisons with morphine sulfate. Select dosage carefully.

For patients being transferred from therapy with opiate agonists other than morphine, a comparative opiate agonist dosage table may be consulted to determine the equivalent morphine dosage.

ORAL:
- Dosage estimates obtained from must be individualized (e.g., based on prior opiate use, medical condition, concurrent drug therapy, anticipated use of analgesics for breakthrough pain).
- Administer the total daily dosage in divided doses (e.g., at 8-hour intervals) based on individual patient requirements.

Table 1. Conversion from Oral Morphine Sulfate to Oral Methadone Hydrochloride (for Chronic Administration)

Baseline Total Daily *Oral* Morphine Sulfate Dosage	Estimated Daily *Oral* Methadone Hydrochloride Dosage (as % of Total Daily Morphine Sulfate Dosage)
<100 mg	20–30%
100–300 mg	10–20%
300–600 mg	8–12%
600–1000 mg	5–10%
>1000 mg	<5%

Table 2. Conversion from Oral Morphine Sulfate to IV Methadone Hydrochloride (for Chronic Administration)

Baseline Total Daily *Oral* Morphine Sulfate Dosage	Estimated Daily *IV* Methadone Hydrochloride Dosage (as % of Total Daily Morphine Sulfate Dosage)
<100 mg	10–15%
100–300 mg	5–10%
300–600 mg	4–6%
600–1000 mg	3–5%
>1000 mg	<3%

Detoxification and Maintenance of Opiate Dependence

Detoxification

ORAL:
- Initiate when there are substantial opiate-agonist abstinence symptoms; determine initial dose based on the opiate tolerance of the patient.
- A single dose of 15–20 mg will often suppress withdrawal symptoms. Additional doses may be necessary if withdrawal symptoms are not suppressed or if they reappear. Usual dosage is 40 mg daily in single or divided doses, but higher dosage may be required.
- When the patient has been stabilized (i.e., substantial symptoms of withdrawal are absent) for 2 or 3 days, gradually decrease dosage daily or at 2-day intervals. Individualize and adjust dosage to keep withdrawal symptoms at a tolerable level. In hospitalized patients, reduce dosage by 20% daily; a more gradual reduction may be required in ambulatory patients.
- Adjust dosage to control abstinence symptoms without causing respiratory depression or marked sedation.

Maintenance

ORAL:
- Initially, up to 30 mg. Total dose on the first day should not exceed 40 mg unless it is documented that this total dose does not suppress withdrawal symptoms. Any substantial deviations from the manufacturer's labeling with regard to dose, frequency of administration, or conditions of use must be documented in the patient's record.
- Adjust initial dose based on opiate tolerance of the patient. Adjust subsequent dosage according to the requirements and response of the patient.
- Review maintenance dosage requirements regularly and reduce as indicated. All patients in a maintenance program should be given careful consideration for discontinuance of methadone therapy, especially after reaching a dosage of 10–20 mg daily.
- Once-daily dosing usually is adequate; there generally is no apparent advantage to divided doses. However, rapid metabolizers may not maintain adequate plasma concentrations with usual dosing regimens.

Prescribing Limits

Pediatric Patients

Pain†

ORAL:
- Single pediatric doses should not exceed 10 mg.

Special Populations

Hepatic Impairment
- Reduce initial dosage in patients with severe hepatic impairment.

Renal Impairment
- Reduce initial dosage in patients with severe renal impairment.

Geriatric and Debilitated Patients
- Reduce dosage in poor-risk and in very old patients.

† Use is not currently included in the labeling approved by the US Food and Drug Administration.

Methenamine

(meth en′ a meen)

Brand Name: Hiprex®, Mandelamine®, Urex®

Why is this medicine prescribed?

Methenamine, an antibiotic, eliminates bacteria that cause urinary tract infections. It usually is used on a long-term basis to treat chronic infections and to prevent recurrence of infections. Antibiotics will not work for colds, flu, or other viral infections.

This medication is sometimes prescribed for other uses; ask your doctor or pharmacist for more information.

How should this medicine be used?

Methenamine comes as a tablet and a liquid to take by mouth. It usually is taken either two times a day (every 12 hours) or four times a day (after meals and at bedtime). Follow the directions on your prescription label carefully, and ask your doctor or pharmacist to explain any part you do not understand. Take methenamine exactly as directed. Do not take more or less of it or take it more often than prescribed by your doctor.

Swallow the coated tablets whole. Do not crush or break them. Take the tablets with a full glass of water or with food. Shake the liquid well before each use to mix the drug evenly.

What special precautions should I follow?

Before taking methenamine,

- tell your doctor and pharmacist if you are allergic to methenamine, aspirin, tartrazine (a yellow dye in some processed foods and drugs), or any other drugs.
- tell your doctor and pharmacist what prescription and nonprescription medications you are taking, especially antacids, sulfamethizole, diuretics ('water pills'), and vitamins.
- tell your doctor if you have or have ever had kidney or liver disease.
- tell your doctor if you are pregnant, plan to become pregnant, or are breast-feeding. If you become pregnant while taking methenamine, call your doctor.

What special dietary instructions should I follow?

Methenamine may cause an upset stomach. Take methenamine with food or milk.

What should I do if I forget to take a dose?

Take the missed dose as soon as you remember it. However, if it is almost time for the next dose, skip the missed dose and continue your regular dosing schedule. Do not take a double dose to make up for a missed one.

What side effects can this medicine cause?

Methenamine may cause side effects. Tell your doctor if any of these symptoms are severe or do not go away:

- upset stomach
- vomiting
- diarrhea
- stomach cramps
- loss of appetite

If you experience any of the following symptoms, call your doctor immediately:

- skin rash
- hives
- itching (allergic reaction)

If you experience a serious side effect, you or your doctor may send a report to the Food and Drug Administration's (FDA) MedWatch Adverse Event Reporting program online [at http://www.fda.gov/MedWatch/index.html] or by phone [1-800-332-1088].

What storage conditions are needed for this medicine?

Keep this medication in the container it came in, tightly closed, and out of reach of children. Store it at room temperature and away from excess heat and moisture (not in the bathroom). Throw away any medication that is outdated or no longer needed. Talk to your pharmacist about the proper disposal of your medication.

What should I do in case of overdose?

In case of overdose, call your local poison control center at 1-800-222-1222. If the victim has collapsed or is not breathing, call local emergency services at 911.

What other information should I know?

Keep all appointments with your doctor and the laboratory. Your doctor will order certain lab tests to check your response to methenamine.

Do not let anyone else take your medication. Ask your pharmacist any questions you have about refilling your prescription.

Talk to your doctor, pharmacist, or other healthcare professional if you have questions about dosing information for your medication.

Methimazole

(meth im′ a zole)

Brand Name: Tapazole®

Why is this medicine prescribed?

Methimazole is used to treat hyperthyroidism, a condition that occurs when the thyroid gland produces too much thyroid hormone. It is also taken before thyroid surgery or radioactive iodine therapy.

This medication is sometimes prescribed for other uses; ask your doctor or pharmacist for more information.

How should this medicine be used?

Methimazole comes as a tablet and usually is taken three times a day, approximately every 8 hours, with food. Follow the directions on your prescription label carefully, and ask your doctor or pharmacist to explain any part you do not understand.

What special precautions should I follow?

Before taking methimazole,

- tell your doctor and pharmacist if you are allergic to methimazol, lactose, or any other drugs.
- tell your doctor and pharmacist what prescription and nonprescription medications you are taking, especially anticoagulants ('blood thinners') such as warfarin (Coumadin), beta blockers such as propranolol (Inderal), diabetes medications, digoxin (Lanoxin), theophylline (Theobid, Theo-Dur), and vitamins.
- tell your doctor if you have or have ever had any blood disease, such as decreased white blood cells (leukopenia), decreased platelets (thrombocytopenia), or aplastic anemia, or liver disease (hepatitis, jaundice).
- tell your doctor if you are pregnant, plan to become pregnant, or are breast-feeding. Methimazole should not be used during pregnancy or breast-feeding. If you become pregnant while taking methimazole, call your doctor immediately. Methimazole may harm the fetus.
- if you are having surgery, including dental surgery, tell the doctor or dentist that you are taking methimazole.

What special dietary instructions should I follow?

Methimazole may cause an upset stomach. Take methimazole with food or milk.

What should I do if I forget to take a dose?

Take the missed dose as soon as you remember it. However, if it is almost time for the next dose, skip the missed dose and continue your regular dosing schedule at evenly spaced, 8-hour intervals. Do not take a double dose to make up for a missed one.

What side effects can this medicine cause?

Methimazole may cause side effects. Tell your doctor if any of these symptoms are severe or do not go away:

- skin rash
- itching
- abnormal hair loss
- upset stomach
- vomiting
- loss of taste
- abnormal sensations (tingling, prickling, burning, tightness, and pulling)
- swelling
- joint and muscle pain
- drowsiness
- dizziness
- decreased white blood cells
- decreased platelets

If you experience any of the following symptoms, call your doctor immediately:

- sore throat
- fever
- headache
- chills
- unusual bleeding or bruising
- right-sided abdominal pain with decreased appetite
- yellowing of the skin or eyes
- skin eruptions

If you experience a serious side effect, you or your doctor may send a report to the Food and Drug Administration's (FDA) MedWatch Adverse Event Reporting program online [at http://www.fda.gov/MedWatch/index.html] or by phone [1-800-332-1088].

What storage conditions are needed for this medicine?

Keep this medication in the container it came in, tightly closed, and out of reach of children. Store it at room temperature and away from excess heat and moisture (not in the bathroom). Throw away any medication that is outdated or no longer needed. Talk to your pharmacist about the proper disposal of your medication.

What should I do in case of overdose?

In case of overdose, call your local poison control center at 1-800-222-1222. If the victim has collapsed or is not breathing, call local emergency services at 911.

What other information should I know?

Keep all appointments with your doctor and the laboratory.

Do not let anyone else take your medication. Ask your pharmacist any questions you have about refilling your prescription.

Talk to your doctor, pharmacist, or other healthcare professional if you have questions about dosing information for your medication.

Methocarbamol Oral

(meth oh kar′ ba mole)

Brand Name: Robaxin®
Also available generically.

Why is this medicine prescribed?

Methocarbamol, a muscle relaxant, is used with rest, physical therapy, and other measures to relax muscles and relieve pain and discomfort caused by strains, sprains, and other muscle injuries.

This medication is sometimes prescribed for other uses; ask your doctor or pharmacist for more information.

How should this medicine be used?

Methocarbamol comes as a tablet to take by mouth. It usually is taken four times a day at first, then it may be changed to three to six times a day. Follow the directions on your prescription label carefully, and ask your doctor or pharmacist to explain any part you do not understand. Take methocarbamol exactly as directed. Do not take more or less of it or take it more often than prescribed by your doctor.

What special precautions should I follow?

Before taking methocarbamol,
- tell your doctor and pharmacist if you are allergic to methocarbamol or any other drugs.
- tell your doctor and pharmacist what prescription and nonprescription medications you are taking, especially medications for seizures, depression, colds, or coughs; sedatives; tranquilizers; and vitamins
- tell your doctor if you are pregnant, plan to become pregnant, or are breast-feeding. If you become pregnant while taking methocarbamol, call your doctor.
- you should know that this drug may make you drowsy. Do not drive a car or operate machinery until you know how methocarbamol affects you.
- remember that alcohol can add to the drowsiness caused by this drug.

What should I do if I forget to take a dose?

Take the missed dose as soon as you remember it. However, if it is almost time for the next dose, skip the missed dose and continue your regular dosing schedule. Do not take a double dose to make up for a missed one.

What side effects can this medicine cause?

Methocarbamol may cause side effects. Methocarbamol may cause your urine to turn black, blue, or green. However, this effect is harmless. Tell your doctor if any of these symptoms are severe or do not go away:
- drowsiness
- dizziness
- upset stomach
- blurred vision
- fever

If you experience either of the following symptoms, call your doctor immediately:
- severe skin rash
- itching

If you experience a serious side effect, you or your doctor may send a report to the Food and Drug Administration's (FDA) MedWatch Adverse Event Reporting program online [at http://www.fda.gov/MedWatch/index.html] or by phone [1-800-332-1088].

What storage conditions are needed for this medicine?

Keep this medication in the container it came in, tightly closed, and out of reach of children. Store it at room temperature and away from excess heat and moisture (not in the bathroom). Throw away any medication that is outdated or no longer needed. Talk to your pharmacist about the proper disposal of your medication.

What should I do in case of overdose?

In case of overdose, call your local poison control center at 1-800-222-1222. If the victim has collapsed or is not breathing, call local emergency services at 911.

What other information should I know?

Keep all appointments with your doctor.

Do not let anyone else take your medication. Ask your pharmacist any questions you have about refilling your prescription.

Dosage Facts
For Informational Purposes

Caution: Do not change your dose, how often you take your medication, or the length of time you are to take it without first talking to your healthcare provider.

The following dosage information was written using medical language for doctors and other healthcare professionals and is provided here for you to check your dosage. The dosage of this drug may differ for different patients. Therefore, always follow your doctor's instructions or the directions on the label. Contact your healthcare provider or pharmacist if you have any questions about the specific dosage of your medication after reviewing this information.

Adult Patients
Muscular Conditions

ORAL:
- Usual initial dosage is 1.5 g 4 times daily for 2–3 days. For maintenance, decrease dosage to 4–4.5 g daily in 3–6 divided doses.

- A few patients may require initial dosage of 8 g daily in divided doses.

Methotrexate

(meth oh trex′ ate)

Brand Name: Rheumatrex®, Trexall®
Also available generically.

Important Warning

Methotrexate may cause very serious side effects. Some side effects of methotrexate may cause death. You should only use methotrexate to treat life-threatening cancer, or certain other conditions that are very severe and that cannot be treated with other medications. Talk to your doctor about the risks of taking methotrexate for your condition.

Tell your doctor if you have or have ever had excess fluid in your stomach area or in the space around your lungs and if you have or have ever had kidney disease. Also tell your doctor if you are taking aspirin or other nonsteroidal anti-inflammatory medications (NSAIDs) such as ibuprofen (Advil, Motrin) or naproxen (Aleve, Naprosyn) or are being treated with radiation therapy. These conditions and treatments may increase the risk that you will develop serious side effects of methotrexate. Your doctor will monitor you more carefully and may need to change the doses of your medications.

Methotrexate may cause liver damage. Tell your doctor if you are taking any of the following medications: acitretin (Soriatane), azathioprine (Imuran), isotretinoin (Accutane), sulfasalazine (Azulfidine), or tretinoin (Vesanoid). Tell your doctor if you drink or have ever drunk large amounts of alcohol and if you have or have ever had liver disease, Your doctor may tell you that you should not take methotrexate unless you have a life-threatening cancer. Also tell your doctor if you have diabetes. Do not drink alcohol while you are taking methotrexate. Call your doctor immediately if you experience any of the following symptoms: nausea, extreme tiredness, lack of energy, loss of appetite, pain in the upper right part of the stomach, yellowing of the skin or eyes, or flu-like symptoms.

Methotrexate may cause lung damage. Tell your doctor if you have or have ever had lung disease. Call your doctor immediately if you experience any of the following symptoms: dry cough, fever, or shortness of breath.

Methotrexate may cause kidney damage. Be sure to drink plenty of fluids during your treatment with methotrexate, especially if you exercise or are physically active. Call your doctor if you think you might be dehydrated (do not have enough fluid in your body). You may become dehydrated if you sweat excessively or if you vomit, have diarrhea, or have a fever.

Methotrexate may cause a decrease in the number of blood cells made by your bone marrow. Tell your doctor if you have or have ever had a low blood count (decrease in the number of blood cells in your body), anemia (red blood cells do not bring enough oxygen to all parts of the body), or any other problem with your blood cells. Your doctor may tell you not to take methotrexate unless you have a life-threatening cancer. Call your doctor immediately if you experience any of the following symptoms: sore throat, chills, fever, or other signs of infection; unusual bruising or bleeding; excessive tiredness; weakness; pale skin; dizziness; confusion; fast heartbeat; shortness of breath; or difficulty falling asleep or staying asleep.

Methotrexate may cause damage to your intestines. Tell your doctor if you have or have ever had stomach ulcers or ulcerative colitis (condition in which part or all of the lining of the intestine is swollen or worn away). If you develop sores in your mouth or diarrhea, stop taking methotrexate and call your doctor immediately.

Methotrexate may cause a severe rash that may be life-threatening. If you develop a rash, blisters, or a fever, call your doctor immediately.

Methotrexate may decrease the activity of your immune system, and you may develop serious infections. Tell your doctor if you have any type of infection and if you have or have ever had any condition that affects your immune system such as human immunodeficiency syndrome (HIV) or acquired immunodeficiency syndrome (AIDS). Your doctor may tell you that you should not take methotrexate unless you have a life-threatening cancer. If you experience signs of infection such as a sore throat, cough, fever, or chills, call your doctor immediately.

Taking methotrexate may increase the risk that you will develop lymphoma (cancer that begins in the cells of the immune system). If you do develop lymphoma, it might go away without treatment when you stop taking methotrexate, or it might need to be treated with chemotherapy.

If you are taking methotrexate to treat cancer, you may develop certain complications as methotrexate works to destroy the cancer cells. Your doctor will monitor you carefully and treat these complications if they occur.

Keep all appointments with your doctor and the laboratory. Your doctor will order lab tests before, during, and after your treatment to check your body's response to methotrexate and to treat side effects before they become severe.

Women who are taking methotrexate, or whose male partners are taking methotrexate are less likely to become pregnant than women who are not taking methotrexate or whose partners are not taking the medication. However, you should not assume that you or your partner cannot become pregnant while you are taking methotrexate. Tell your doctor if you or your partner is pregnant or plan to become pregnant. If you are female, you will need to take a pregnancy test before you begin taking methotrexate. Use a reliable method of birth control so that you or your partner will not become pregnant during or shortly after your treatment. If you are male, you and your female partner should continue to use birth control for 3 months after you stop taking methotrexate. If you are female, you should continue to use birth control until you have had one menstrual period that began after you stopped taking methotrexate. If you or your partner become pregnant, call your doctor immediately. Methotrexate may harm the fetus.

About Your Treatment

Your doctor has ordered methotrexate to help treat your illness. Methotrexate comes as a tablet to take by mouth. Your doctor will tell you how often you should take methotrexate. The schedule depends on the condition you have and on how your body responds to the medication.

You may take methotrexate on a rotating schedule that alternates several days when you take methotrexate with several days or weeks when you do not take the medication. Follow these directions carefully and ask your doctor or pharmacist if you do not know when to take your medication.

Follow the directions on your prescription label carefully and ask your doctor or pharmacist to explain anything you do not understand. Take methotrexate exactly as directed. Do not take more or less of it or take it more often than prescribed by your doctor. Do not stop taking methotrexate without talking to your doctor.

This medication is used to treat:
- severe psoriasis (a skin disease in which red, scaly patches form on some areas of the body) that cannot be controlled by other treatments.
- severe, active rheumatoid arthritis (a condition in which the body attacks its own joints, causing pain, swelling, and loss of function) that cannot be controlled by certain other medications.
- certain cancers that begin in the tissues that form around a fertilized egg in the uterus (womb)
- breast cancer
- certain cancers of the head and neck
- lung cancer
- certain types of lymphomas
- leukemia

Methotrexate is in a class of medications known as antimetabolites. Methotrexate treats cancer by slowing the growth of cancer cells. Methotrexate treats psoriasis by slowing the growth of skin cells. Methotrexate may treat rheumatoid arthritis by slowing the activity of the immune system.

If you are taking methotrexate to treat rheumatoid arthritis, it may take 3 to 6 weeks or longer for you to feel the full benefit of methotrexate. Continue to take methotrexate even if you feel well. Do not stop taking methotrexate without talking to your doctor.

If you are taking methotrexate once a week to treat rheumatoid arthritis and you forget a dose of your medication, take the missed dose as soon as you remember it. However, if more than 24 hours have passed, skip the missed dose and continue your regular dosing schedule. If you are taking methotrexate more often than once a week, ask your doctor what you should do if you miss a dose. Do not take a double dose to make up for a missed one.

Ask your pharmacist or doctor for a copy of the manufacturer's information for the patient.

Methotrexate is also sometimes used to treat Crohn's disease (a condition in which the immune system attacks the lining of the digestive tract, causing pain, diarrhea, weight loss, and fever). Talk to your doctor about the risks of using this medication for your condition.

This medication may be prescribed for other uses; ask your doctor or pharmacist for more information.

Precautions

Before taking methotrexate,
- tell your doctor and pharmacist if you are allergic to methotrexate, any other medications, or any of the inactive ingredients in methotrexate tablets. Ask your pharmacist for a list of the inactive ingredients.
- tell your doctor and pharmacist what prescription and nonprescription medications, vitamins, nutritional supplements, and herbal products you are taking or plan to take. Be sure to mention those listed in the IMPORTANT WARNING section and any of the following: certain antibiotics such as chloramphenicol (chloramycetin), penicillins, and tetracycline (Bristacycline, Sumycin); folic acid; other medications for rheumatoid arthritis; phenytoin (Dilantin); probenecid (Benemid); sulfonamides such as co-trimoxazole (Bactrim, Septra), sulfadiazine, sulfamethizole (Urobiotic), and sulfisoxazole (Gantrisin); and theopylline (Theochron, Theolair). Your doctor may need to change the doses of your medication or monitor you more carefully for side effects.
- in addition to the conditions listed in the IMPORTANT WARNING section, tell your doctor if you have or have ever had any other medical condition.
- tell your doctor if you are breast-feeding. You should not breastfeed during your treatment with methotrexate.
- before having surgery, including dental surgery, tell the doctor or dentist that you are taking methotrexate.
- plan to avoid unnecessary or prolonged exposure to sun-

light and to wear protective clothing, sunglasses, and sunscreen. Do not use sunlamps during your treatment with methotrexate. Methotrexate may make your skin sensitive to real or artificial sunlight. If you have psoriasis, your sores may get worse if you expose them to sunlight while you are taking methotrexate.

- do not have any vaccinations (injections to prevent disease) during your treatment with methotrexate without talking to your doctor.
- if you have rheumatoid arthritis, you should know that methotrexate will work best if you follow your doctor's instructions for resting and if you undergo physical therapy during your treatment.

Side Effects

Methotrexate may cause side effects. Tell your doctor if any of the following symptoms are severe or do not go away:

- swollen, tender gums
- headache
- hair loss
- acne
- changes in skin color
- irregular menstrual periods

Some side effects can be serious. If you experience any of the following symptoms or those listed in the IMPORTANT WARNING section, call your doctor immediately:

- chest pain
- fainting
- blurred vision
- sudden loss of vision
- difficulty speaking or slurred speech
- difficulty moving one or both sides of the body
- weakness or numbness of an arm or leg
- seizures
- pain or redness of one leg only
- urgent or frequent need to urinate
- blood in urine

Methotrexate may cause other side effects. Tell your doctor if you have any unusual problems while you are taking this medication.

Storage Conditions

Keep methotrexate in the container it came in, tightly closed, and out of reach of children. Store it at room temperature and away from excess heat and moisture (not in the bathroom). Throw away any medication that is outdated or no longer needed. Talk to your pharmacist about the proper disposal of your medication.

Overdose

In case of overdose, call your local poison control center at 1-800-222-1222. If the victim has collapsed or is not breathing, call local emergency services at 911.

It is important to get medical help right away when you realize that you have taken too much methotrexate. If you take an overdose of methotrexate, there is a medication that you can take to stop the overdose from causing serious harm. This medication works best when it is taken as soon as possible after the overdose.

Symptoms of overdose may include:

- sore throat, fever, chills, and other signs of infection
- unusual bruising or bleeding
- excessive tiredness
- weakness
- dizziness
- confusion
- fast heartbeat
- shortness of breath
- mouth sores
- nausea
- vomiting, especially vomit that is bloody or looks like coffee grounds
- bright red blood in stools
- black and tarry stools

Special Instructions

Do not let anyone else take your medication. Ask your pharmacist if you have any questions about refilling your prescription.

Dosage Facts
For Informational Purposes

Caution: Do not change your dose, how often you take your medication, or the length of time you are to take it without first talking to your healthcare provider.

The following dosage information was written using medical language for doctors and other healthcare professionals and is provided here for you to check your dosage. The dosage of this drug may differ for different patients. Therefore, always follow your doctor's instructions or the directions on the label. Contact your healthcare provider or pharmacist if you have any questions about the specific dosage of your medication after reviewing this information.

General Dosage Information

Available as methotrexate sodium; dosage is expressed in terms of methotrexate.

Various dosage schedules have been used; individualize dosage, route of administration, and duration of therapy according to disease being treated, other therapy employed, and condition, response, and tolerance of the patient. Consult published protocols for additional information on alternative regimens and dosages.

Pediatric Patients

Juvenile Rheumatoid Arthritis

ORAL:
- May administer an initial test dose prior to regular dosage schedule to detect possible sensitivity to adverse effects associated with the drug.

- Initially, 10 mg/m² once weekly. May adjust dosage gradually to achieve optimal response.
- Dosages up to 30 mg/m² weekly have been used in children, but published data are too limited to assess risk of serious toxicity at dosages >20 mg/m² weekly.
- Children receiving 20–30 mg/m² (0.65–1 mg/kg) weekly may have better absorption and fewer adverse GI effects if administered either IM or sub-Q.
- Optimum duration of therapy is unknown.

Adult Patients

Leukemia
ALL (Induction Therapy)

ORAL:
- Not generally a drug of choice, but 3.3 mg/m² daily in combination with prednisone 40–60 mg/m² daily for 4–6 weeks has been used.

ALL (Maintenance Therapy)

ORAL:
- After remission attained, 20–30 mg/m² total weekly dose, administered in divided doses twice weekly.

Lymphomas

ORAL:
- For Burkett's lymphoma (stage I or II), 10–25 mg daily for 4–8 days. In stage III Burkitt's lymphoma, commonly given with other antineoplastic agents. In all stages, several courses are usually administered, interposed with 7- to 10-day rest periods.
- Stage III lymphosarcomas may respond to combined drug therapy with methotrexate given in doses of 0.625–2.5 mg/kg daily.

Cutaneous T-cell Lymphoma; Mycosis Fungoides

ORAL:
- Usually, 5–50 mg weekly in early stages. Dose reduction or discontinuance is determined by hematologic monitoring and patient response.
- Also has been administered twice weekly in doses ranging from 15–37.5 mg in patients who have responded poorly to weekly therapy.

Psoriasis

ORAL:
- Administration of a single 5- to 10-mg dose 1 week prior to initiation of therapy has been recommended to detect idiosyncratic reactions.
- Divided oral dosage schedule: 2.5 mg at 12-hour intervals for 3 doses each week. May gradually adjust dosage by 2.5 mg/week to achieve optimal response; do not exceed 30 mg weekly ordinarily.
- Once optimal response obtained, reduce dosage schedule to lowest possible dose and longest possible rest period. Use may permit return to conventional topical therapy.

ORAL:
- Weekly single-dosage schedule: 10–25 mg as a single dose once weekly until adequate response achieved. May gradually adjust dosage to achieve optimal response; do not exceed 30 mg weekly ordinarily. Once optimal response obtained, reduce dosage schedule to lowest possible dose and longest possible rest period.

Rheumatoid Arthritis

ORAL:
- May administer an initial test dose prior to regular dosage schedule to detect possible sensitivity to adverse effects.
- Initially, 7.5 mg once weekly or a course once weekly of 2.5 mg administered at 12-hour intervals for 3 doses. May gradually adjust dosage to achieve an optimal response.
- At dosages >20 mg weekly, possible increased incidence and severity of serious toxic reactions, especially myelosuppression.
- Optimal duration of therapy is not known; limited data indicate that initial improvement is maintained for at least 2 years with continued therapy.

Trophoblastic Neoplasms

ORAL:
- Usually, 15–30 mg daily for 5 days. A repeat course may be given after a period of ≥1 week, provided all signs of residual toxicity have disappeared; 3–5 courses are usually employed. Clinical assessment before each course is essential.
- Therapy is usually evaluated by 24-hour quantitative analysis of urinary chorionic gonadotropin (hCG), which usually normalizes after third or fourth course; complete resolution of measurable lesions usually occurs 4–6 weeks later.
- 1 or 2 courses of therapy are usually given after normalization of urinary hCG concentrations is achieved.

Crohn's Disease†
Chronically Active Refractory Disease

ORAL:
- 12.5–22.5 mg once weekly has been administered for up to 1 year.

Prescribing Limits

Pediatric Patients

Juvenile Rheumatoid Arthritis

ORAL:
- Although there is experience with dosages up to 30 mg/m² weekly in children, published data are too limited to assess how dosages >20 mg/m² weekly might affect risk of serious toxicity.
- Children receiving 20–30 mg/m² (0.65–1 mg/kg) weekly may have better absorption and fewer GI effects if administered either IM or sub-Q.

Adult Patients

Psoriasis

ORAL:
- Do not ordinarily exceed 30 mg weekly.

Rheumatoid Arthritis

ORAL:
- Do not ordinarily exceed 20 mg weekly.
- Limited experience suggests substantial increase in incidence and severity of serious toxic reactions, especially bone marrow suppression, at dosages >20 mg weekly.

Special Populations

Renal Impairment
- Dose reduction and especially careful monitoring for toxicity required.

Geriatric Patients
- Select dosage with caution since hepatic and renal function and folate stores may be decreased; closely monitor for early signs of toxicity.

Patients with Ascites or Pleural Effusions
- Dose reduction and especially careful monitoring for toxicity required.

† Use is not currently included in the labeling approved by the US Food and Drug Administration.

Methsuximide Oral

(meth sux′ i mide)

Brand Name: Celontin® Kapseals®

Why is this medicine prescribed?

Methsuximide is used to treat a type of seizure called absence (petit mal) that cannot be treated with other medications. Methsuximide acts on the brain and nervous system in the treatment of epilepsy.

This medication is sometimes prescribed for other uses; ask your doctor or pharmacist for more information.

How should this medicine be used?

Methsuximide comes as a capsule to take by mouth. It is taken once a day at first, but the dosage may be increased gradually to two to four times a day. Follow the directions on your prescription label carefully, and ask your doctor or pharmacist to explain any part you do not understand. Take methsuximide exactly as directed. Do not take more or less of it or take it more often than prescribed by your doctor.

Continue to take methsuximide even if you feel well. Do not stop taking methsuximide without talking to your doctor, especially if you have taken large doses for a long time. Abruptly stopping the drug can cause seizures. Your doctor probably will decrease your dose gradually.

What special precautions should I follow?

Before taking methsuximide,
- tell your doctor and pharmacist if you are allergic to methsuximide or any other drugs.
- tell your doctor and pharmacist what prescription and nonprescription medications you are taking, especially other seizure medications, doxycycline (Vibramycin), isoniazid (INH), medications for colds or allergies such as chlorpheniramine (Chlor-Trimeton), medications for depression such as amitriptyline (Elavil), oral contraceptives, and vitamins. Methsuximide affects the action of other medications, and many medications can affect the action of methsuximide. Tell your doctor and pharmacist everything you are taking.
- tell your doctor if you have or have ever had kidney or liver disease or a blood disorder.
- tell your doctor if you are pregnant, plan to become pregnant, or are breast-feeding. If you become pregnant while taking methsuximide, call your doctor.
- if you are having surgery, including dental surgery, tell the doctor or dentist that you are taking methsuximide.
- you should know that this drug may make you drowsy. Do not drive a car or operate machinery until you know how this drug affects you.
- remember that alcohol can add to the drowsiness caused by this drug.
- plan to protect your eyes in the sun. Methsuximide may make your eyes more sensitive to light. Wear dark glasses in bright light.

What special dietary instructions should I follow?

Methsuximide may cause an upset stomach. Take methsuximide with food. Drink plenty of water.

What should I do if I forget to take a dose?

Take the missed dose as soon as you remember it. However, if it is within 4 hours of the next dose, skip the missed dose and continue your regular dosing schedule. Do not take a double dose to make up for a missed one.

What side effects can this medicine cause?

Methsuximide may cause side effects. Tell your doctor if any of these symptoms are severe or do not go away:
- drowsiness
- upset stomach
- vomiting
- constipation
- diarrhea
- stomach pain
- loss of taste and appetite
- weight loss
- irritability
- mental confusion
- depression
- insomnia
- nervousness
- headache

If you experience any of the following symptoms, call your doctor immediately:
- difficulty coordinating movements
- joint pain
- red, itchy skin rash
- easy bruising
- tiny purple-colored skin spots
- bloody nose
- unusual bleeding
- yellowing of the skin or eyes
- dark urine

- fever
- sore throat

If you experience a serious side effect, you or your doctor may send a report to the Food and Drug Administration's (FDA) MedWatch Adverse Event Reporting program online [at http://www.fda.gov/MedWatch/index.html] or by phone [1-800-332-1088].

What storage conditions are needed for this medicine?

Keep this medication in the container it came in, tightly closed, and out of reach of children. Store it at room temperature, away from light, excess heat, and moisture (not in the bathroom). Throw away any medication that is outdated or no longer needed. Talk to your pharmacist about the proper disposal of your medication.

What should I do in case of overdose?

In case of overdose, call your local poison control center at 1-800-222-1222. If the victim has collapsed or is not breathing, call local emergency services at 911.

What other information should I know?

Keep all appointments with your doctor and the laboratory. Your doctor will order certain lab tests to check your response to methsuximide.

Call your doctor if you continue to have seizures or convulsions while taking this medication.

If you give this drug to a child, observe and keep a record of the child's moods, behavior, attention span, hand-eye coordination, and ability to solve problems and perform tasks requiring thought. Ask the child's teacher to keep a similar record. This information can help the child's doctor determine whether to continue the drug or to change the dose or drug.

Wear identification (Medic Alert) indicating medication use and epilepsy.

Do not let anyone else take your medication. Ask your pharmacist any questions you have about refilling your prescription.

Talk to your doctor, pharmacist, or other healthcare professional if you have questions about dosing information for your medication.

Methyclothiazide

(meth i kloe thye′ a zide)

Brand Name: Aquatensen®, Enduron®

Why is this medicine prescribed?

Methyclothiazide, a 'water pill,' is used to treat high blood pressure and fluid retention caused by various conditions, including heart disease. It causes the kidneys to get rid of unneeded water and salt from the body into the urine.

This medicine is sometimes prescribed for other uses; ask your doctor or pharmacist for more information.

How should this medicine be used?

Methyclothiazide comes as a tablet to take by mouth. It usually is taken once a day in the morning. Follow the directions on your prescription label carefully, and ask your doctor or pharmacist to explain any part you do not understand. Take methyclothiazide exactly as directed. Do not take more or less of it or take it more often than prescribed by your doctor.

Methyclothiazide controls high blood pressure but does not cure it. Continue to take methyclothiazide even if you feel well. Do not stop taking methyclothiazide without talking to your doctor.

Are there other uses for this medicine?

Methyclothiazide may also be used to treat patients with diabetes insipidus and certain electrolyte disturbances and to prevent kidney stones in patients with high levels of calcium in their blood. Talk to your doctor about the possible risks of using this medicine for your condition.

What special precautions should I follow?

Before taking methyclothiazide,

- tell your doctor and pharmacist if you are allergic to methyclothiazide, sulfa drugs, or any other drugs.
- tell your doctor and pharmacist what prescription and nonprescription medications you are taking, especially other medications for high blood pressure, anti-inflammatory medications such as ibuprofen (Motrin, Nuprin) or naproxen (Aleve), corticosteroids (e.g., prednisone), lithium (Eskalith, Lithobid), medications for diabetes, probenecid (Benemid), and vitamins. If you also are taking cholestyramine or colestipol, take it at least 1 hour after methyclothiazide.
- tell your doctor if you have or have ever had diabetes, gout, or kidney, liver, thyroid, or parathyroid disease.
- tell your doctor if you are pregnant, plan to become pregnant, or are breast-feeding. If you become pregnant while taking methyclothiazide, call your doctor immediately.
- if you are having surgery, including dental surgery, tell the doctor or dentist that you are taking methyclothiazide.

- you should know that this drug may make you drowsy. Do not drive a car or operate machinery until you know how this drug affects you.
- remember that alcohol can add to the drowsiness caused by this drug.
- plan to avoid unnecessary or prolonged exposure to sunlight and to wear protective clothing, sunglasses, and sunscreen. Methyclothiazide may make your skin sensitive to sunlight.

What special dietary instructions should I follow?

Follow your doctor's directions. They may include following a daily exercise program or a low-salt or low-sodium diet, potassium supplements, and increased amounts of potassium-rich foods (e.g., bananas, prunes, raisins, and orange juice) in your diet.

What should I do if I forget to take a dose?

Take the missed dose as soon as you remember it. However, if it is almost time for your next dose, skip the missed dose and continue your regular dosing schedule. Do not take a double dose to make up for a missed one.

What side effects can this medicine cause?

Frequent urination should go away after you take methyclothiazide for a few weeks. Tell your doctor if any of these symptoms are severe or do not go away:
- muscle weakness
- dizziness
- cramps
- thirst
- stomach pain
- upset stomach
- vomiting
- diarrhea
- loss of appetite
- headache
- hair loss

If you experience any of the following symptoms, call your doctor immediately:
- sore throat with fever
- unusual bleeding or bruising
- severe skin rash with peeling skin
- difficulty breathing or swallowing

If you experience a serious side effect, you or your doctor may send a report to the Food and Drug Administration's (FDA) MedWatch Adverse Event Reporting program online [at http://www.fda.gov/MedWatch/index.html] or by phone [1-800-332-1088].

What storage conditions are needed for this medicine?

Keep this medicine in the container it came in, tightly closed, and out of reach of children. Store it at room temperature and away from excess heat and moisture (not in the bathroom). Throw away any medicine that is outdated or no longer needed. Talk to your pharmacist about the proper disposal of your medicine.

What should I do in case of overdose?

In case of overdose, call your local poison control center at 1-800-222-1222. If the victim has collapsed or is not breathing, call local emergency services at 911.

What other information should I know?

Keep all appointments with your doctor and the laboratory. Your blood pressure should be checked regularly, and blood tests should be done occasionally.

Do not let anyone else take your medicine. Ask your pharmacist any questions you have about refilling your prescription.

Talk to your doctor, pharmacist, or other healthcare professional if you have questions about dosing information for your medication.

Methyldopa
(meth ill doe′ pa)

Brand Name: Aldochlor® 250, Aldoril®
Also available generically.

Why is this medicine prescribed?

Methyldopa is used to treat high blood pressure. It works by relaxing the blood vessels so that blood can flow more easily through the body.

This medication is sometimes prescribed for other uses; ask your doctor or pharmacist for more information.

How should this medicine be used?

Methyldopa comes as a tablet and liquid to take by mouth. It usually is taken two to four times a day. Follow the directions on your prescription label carefully, and ask your doctor or pharmacist to explain any part you do not understand. Take methyldopa exactly as directed. Do not take more or less of it or take it more often than prescribed by your doctor.

The liquid should be shaken well before each dose.

Methyldopa controls high blood pressure but does not cure it. Continue to take methyldopa even if you feel well. Do not stop taking methyldopa without talking to your doctor.

Abruptly stopping methyldopa may increase blood pressure and cause unwanted side effects.

What special precautions should I follow?

Before taking methyldopa,
- tell your doctor and pharmacist if you are allergic to methyldopa, sulfites, or any other drugs.

- tell your doctor and pharmacist what prescription and nonprescription medications you are taking, especially haloperidol (Haldol), levodopa (Larodopa, Sinemet), lithium (Eskalith, Lithobid), other medications for high blood pressure, tolbutamide (Orinase), and vitamins.
- do not take with iron supplements or vitamins containing iron.
- tell you doctor if you have or have ever had kidney or liver disease, including hepatitis or cirrhosis.
- tell your doctor if you are pregnant, plan to become pregnant, or are breast-feeding. If you become pregnant while taking methyldopa, call your doctor.
- if you are having surgery, including dental surgery, tell the doctor or dentist that you are taking methyldopa.
- you should know that this drug may make you drowsy. Do not drive a car or operate machinery for 48-72 hours after you begin to take methyldopa or after your dose is increased.

What special dietary instructions should I follow?

Your doctor may prescribe a low-salt or low-sodium diet. Follow these directions carefully.

What should I do if I forget to take a dose?

Take the missed dose as soon as you remember it. However, if it is almost time for the next dose, skip the missed dose and continue your regular dosing schedule. Do not take a double dose to make up for a missed one.

What side effects can this medicine cause?

Methyldopa may cause side effects. Tell your doctor if any of these symptoms are severe or do not go away:
- drowsiness
- headache
- muscle weakness
- swollen ankles or feet
- upset stomach
- vomiting
- diarrhea
- gas
- dry mouth
- rash

If you experience any of the following symptoms, call your doctor immediately:
- unexplained fever
- extreme tiredness
- yellowing of the skin or eyes

If you experience a serious side effect, you or your doctor may send a report to the Food and Drug Administration's (FDA) MedWatch Adverse Event Reporting program online [at http://www.fda.gov/MedWatch/index.html] or by phone [1-800-332-1088].

What storage conditions are needed for this medicine?

Keep this medication in the container it came in, tightly closed, and out of reach of children. Store tablets at room temperature and away from excess heat and moisture (not in the bathroom). The liquid may be stored in the refrigerator or at room temperature. Throw away any medication that is outdated or no longer needed. Talk to your pharmacist about the proper disposal of your medication.

What should I do in case of overdose?

In case of overdose, call your local poison control center at 1-800-222-1222. If the victim has collapsed or is not breathing, call local emergency services at 911.

What other information should I know?

Keep all appointments with your doctor and the laboratory. Your blood pressure should be checked regularly to determine your response to methyldopa. Your doctor may order certain lab tests to monitor your red blood cell count and liver function.

Methyldopa may cause your urine to darken when it is exposed to air. This effect is harmless.

Do not let anyone else take your medication. Ask your pharmacist any questions you have about refilling your prescription.

Dosage Facts
For Informational Purposes

Caution: Do not change your dose, how often you take your medication, or the length of time you are to take it without first talking to your healthcare provider.

The following dosage information was written using medical language for doctors and other healthcare professionals and is provided here for you to check your dosage. The dosage of this drug may differ for different patients. Therefore, always follow your doctor's instructions or the directions on the label. Contact your healthcare provider or pharmacist if you have any questions about the specific dosage of your medication after reviewing this information.

General Dosage Information

Available as methyldopa or methyldopate hydrochloride; dosage expressed in terms of methyldopa or methyldopate hydrochloride, respectively.

Pediatric Patients

Hypertension
Monotherapy

ORAL:
- Initially, 10 mg/kg daily given in 2–4 divided doses.
- Adjust dosage until an adequate response is achieved. Max-

imum dosage is 65 mg/kg daily or 3 g daily, whichever is less.

Adult Patients

Hypertension
Monotherapy
ORAL:
- Initially, 250 mg 2 or 3 times daily for 2 days. Increase or decrease dosage every 2 days until an adequate response is achieved.
- For maintenance, manufacturers recommend 500–2000 mg daily given in 2–4 divided doses.
- JNC 7 recommends a lower usual dosage range of 125–500 mg twice daily; if needed, add another antihypertensive agent to the regimen rather than increasing maximum dosage >1 g daily because of poor patient tolerance.

Combination Therapy
ORAL:
- Methyldopa in fixed combination with hydrochlorothiazide: Initially, 250 mg of methyldopa and 15 mg of hydrochlorothiazide given 2–3 times daily, or 250 mg of methyldopa and 25 mg of hydrochlorothiazide given twice daily. Alternatively, 500 mg of methyldopa and either 30 or 50 mg of hydrochlorothiazide once daily.
- If tolerance occurs, add separate dosages of methyldopa or replace the fixed combination with each drug separately until the new effective dosage is reestablished by titration.
- Combination with hypotensive drugs other than thiazide diuretics: Initially, maximum recommended dosage is 500 mg daily in divided doses. Adjust dosage of other hypotensive drugs if necessary.

Prescribing Limits

Pediatric Patients

Hypertension
ORAL:
- Maximum 65 mg/kg daily or 3 g daily, whichever is less.

Adult Patients

Hypertension
ORAL:
- Maximum 3 g daily as maintenance therapy recommended by manufacturers. JNC 7 recommends maximum 1 g daily because of poor patient tolerance.
- Combination therapy with hypotensive drugs other than thiazide diuretics: Initially, maximum 500 mg daily in divided doses.

Special Populations
Renal Impairment
- Consider dosage reduction.

Geriatric Patients
- Consider dosage reduction to avoid syncope.

Methyldopa and Hydrochlorothiazide

(meth ill doe′ pa) (hye droe klor oh thye′ a zide)

Brand Name: Aldoril®

Why is this medicine prescribed?

The combination of methyldopa and hydrochlorothiazide is used to treat high blood pressure. Methyldopa works by relaxing the blood vessels so that blood can flow more easily through the body. Hydrochlorothiazide helps to lower blood pressure by eliminating unneeded water and salt from the body.

This medication is sometimes prescribed for other uses; ask your doctor or pharmacist for more information.

How should this medicine be used?

This medication comes as a tablet to take by mouth. It usually is taken two or three times a day. Follow the directions on your prescription label carefully, and ask your doctor or pharmacist to explain any part you do not understand. Take methyldopa and hydrochlorothiazide exactly as directed. Do not take more or less of it or take it more often than prescribed by your doctor.

This medication controls high blood pressure but does not cure it. Continue to take methyldopa and hydrochlorothiazide even if you feel well. Do not stop taking methyldopa and hydrochlorothiazide without talking to your doctor.

What special precautions should I follow?

Before taking methyldopa and hydrochlorothiazide,
- tell your doctor and pharmacist if you are allergic to methyldopa, hydrochlorothiazide, sulfa drugs, or any other drugs.
- tell your doctor and pharmacist what prescription and nonprescription medications you are taking, especially cholestyramine (Questran), digoxin (Lanoxin), haloperidol (Haldol), levodopa (Sinemet), lithium (Lithobid, Eskalith), MAO inhibitors [phenelzine (Nardil) and tranylcypromine (Parnate)], medications for diabetes, prednisone (Deltasone), probenecid (Benemid), tolbutamide (Orinase), and vitamins.
- do not take with iron supplements or vitamins containing iron.
- tell your doctor if you have or have ever had kidney or liver disease, diabetes, gout, or high blood cholesterol.
- tell your doctor if you are pregnant, plan to become pregnant, or are breast-feeding. If you become pregnant while taking methyldopa and hydrochlorothiazide, call your doctor.
- if you are having surgery, including dental surgery, tell the doctor or dentist that you are taking methyldopa and hydrochlorothiazide.

- you should know that this drug may make you drowsy. Do not drive a car or operate machinery for 48-72 hours after you begin to take this medication or after your dose is increased.
- ask your doctor about the safe use of alcohol while you are using methyldopa and hydrochlorothiazide. Alcohol can make the side effects from methyldopa and hydrochlorothiazide worse.

What special dietary instructions should I follow?

Your doctor may prescribe a low-salt or low-sodium diet. Follow these directions carefully.

What should I do if I forget to take a dose?

Take the missed dose as soon as you remember it. However, if it is almost time for the next dose, skip the missed dose and continue your regular dosing schedule. Do not take a double dose to make up for a missed one.

What side effects can this medicine cause?

Methyldopa and hydrochlorothiazide may cause side effects. Methyldopa and hydrochlorothiazide may cause your urine to darken when it is exposed to air; this effect is harmless. Tell your doctor if any of these symptoms are severe or do not go away:

- frequent urination
- dry mouth
- drowsiness
- headache
- upset stomach
- vomiting
- loss of appetite
- diarrhea
- gas
- rash

If you experience any of the following symptoms, call your doctor immediately:

- extreme tiredness
- muscle weakness or cramps
- unexplained fever
- yellowing of the skin or eyes
- trouble breathing
- swollen ankles or feet

If you experience a serious side effect, you or your doctor may send a report to the Food and Drug Administration's (FDA) MedWatch Adverse Event Reporting program online [at http://www.fda.gov/MedWatch/index.html] or by phone [1-800-332-1088].

What storage conditions are needed for this medicine?

Keep this medication in the container it came in, tightly closed, and out of reach of children. Store at room temperature and away from excess heat and moisture (not in the bathroom). Throw away any medication that is outdated or no longer needed. Talk to your pharmacist about the proper disposal of your medication.

What should I do in case of overdose?

In case of overdose, call your local poison control center at 1-800-222-1222. If the victim has collapsed or is not breathing, call local emergency services at 911.

What other information should I know?

Keep all appointments with your doctor and the laboratory. Your blood pressure should be checked regularly to determine your response to methyldopa and hydrochlorothiazide.

To relieve dry mouth caused by methyldopa and hydrochlorothiazide, chew gum or suck sugarless hard candy.

Do not let anyone else take your medication. Ask your pharmacist any questions you have about refilling your prescription.

Dosage Facts
For Informational Purposes

Caution: Do not change your dose, how often you take your medication, or the length of time you are to take it without first talking to your healthcare provider.

The following dosage information was written using medical language for doctors and other healthcare professionals and is provided here for you to check your dosage. The dosage of this drug may differ for different patients. Therefore, always follow your doctor's instructions or the directions on the label. Contact your healthcare provider or pharmacist if you have any questions about the specific dosage of your medication after reviewing this information.

General Dosage Information

Available as methyldopa or methyldopate hydrochloride; dosage expressed in terms of methyldopa or methyldopate hydrochloride, respectively.

Adult Patients

Hypertension
Combination Therapy

ORAL:
- Methyldopa in fixed combination with hydrochlorothiazide: Initially, 250 mg of methyldopa and 15 mg of hydrochlorothiazide given 2–3 times daily, or 250 mg of methyldopa and 25 mg of hydrochlorothiazide given twice daily. Alternatively, 500 mg of methyldopa and either 30 or 50 mg of hydrochlorothiazide once daily.
- If tolerance occurs, add separate dosages of methyldopa or replace the fixed combination with each drug separately until the new effective dosage is reestablished by titration.

Methylergonovine Oral

(meth il er goe noe' veen)

Brand Name: Methergine®, Methylergome-trine®

Why is this medicine prescribed?

Methylergonovine belongs to a class of drugs called ergot alkaloids. Methylergonovine is used to prevent or treat bleeding from the uterus that can happen after childbirth or an abortion.

This medication is sometimes prescribed for other uses; ask your doctor or pharmacist for more information.

How should this medicine be used?

Methylergonovine comes as a tablet to take by mouth three or four times a day. Follow the directions on your prescription label carefully, and ask your doctor or pharmacist to explain any part you do not understand. Take methylergonovine exactly as directed. Do not take more or less of it or take it more often than prescribed by your doctor.

What special precautions should I follow?

Before taking methylergonovine,

- tell your doctor and pharmacist if you are allergic to methylergonovine, other ergot alkaloids (Cafergot, Ergostat, Bellergal), or any other drugs.
- tell your doctor and pharmacist what prescription and nonprescription medications you are taking, especially other ergot alkaloids and vitamins.
- tell your doctor if you have or have ever had high blood pressure or blood vessel, heart, kidney, or liver disease.
- tell your doctor if you are pregnant, plan to become pregnant, or are breast-feeding. If you become pregnant while taking methylergonovine, call your doctor.

What should I do if I forget to take a dose?

Take the missed dose as soon as you remember it. However, if it is almost time for your next dose, skip the missed dose and continue your dosing schedule. Do not take a double dose to make up for a missed one.

What side effects can this medicine cause?

Methylergonovine may cause side effects. Tell your doctor if any of these symptoms are severe or do not go away:
- upset stomach
- vomiting
- diarrhea
- headache
- bad taste in mouth

If you experience any of the following symptoms, call your doctor immediately:

- seizures
- chest pain
- fast heartbeat
- difficulty breathing
- dizziness
- ringing in the ears
- leg cramps
- skin rash

If you experience a serious side effect, you or your doctor may send a report to the Food and Drug Administration's (FDA) MedWatch Adverse Event Reporting program online [at http://www.fda.gov/MedWatch/index.html] or by phone [1-800-332-1088].

What storage conditions are needed for this medicine?

Keep this medication in the container it came in, tightly closed, and out of reach of children. Store it at room temperature, away from light and excess heat and moisture (not in the bathroom). Throw away any medication that is outdated or no longer needed. Talk to your pharmacist about the proper disposal of your medication.

What should I do in case of overdose?

In case of overdose, call your local poison control center at 1-800-222-1222. If the victim has collapsed or is not breathing, call local emergency services at 911.

What other information should I know?

Keep all appointments with your doctor.

Do not let anyone else take your medication. Your prescription probably is not refillable. If you still have symptoms after you finish the methylergonovine, call your doctor.

Talk to your doctor, pharmacist, or other healthcare professional if you have questions about dosing information for your medication.

Methylphenidate

(meth il fen' i date)

Brand Name: Concerta®, Metadate®, Methylin®, Ritalin®
Also available generically.

Important Warning

Methylphenidate can be habit-forming. Do not take a larger dose, take it more often, take it for a longer time, or take it in a different way than prescribed by your doctor. If you take too much methylphenidate, you may find that the medication no longer controls your symptoms, you may feel a need to take large amounts of the medication, and you may experience unusual changes in your behavior. Tell your doctor if you drink or have ever drunk large amounts of alcohol, use or have ever used street drugs, or have overused prescription medications.

Do not stop taking methylphenidate without talking to your doctor, especially if you have overused the medication. Your doctor will probably decrease your dose gradually and monitor you carefully during this time. You may develop severe depression if you suddenly stop taking methylphenidate after overusing it.

Your doctor or pharmacist will give you the manufacturer's patient information sheet (Medication Guide) when you begin treatment with methylphenidate and each time you refill your prescription. Read the information carefully and ask your doctor or pharmacist if you have any questions. You can also visit the Food and Drug Administration (FDA) website (http://www.fda.gov/cder) or the manufacturer's website to obtain the Medication Guide.

Why is this medicine prescribed?

Methylphenidate is used as part of a treatment program for attention deficit hyperactivity disorder (ADHD; more difficulty focusing, controlling actions, and remaining still or quiet than other people who are the same age). Methylphenidate (Ritalin, Ritalin SR, Methylin, Methylin ER) is also used to treat narcolepsy (a sleep disorder that causes excessive daytime sleepiness and sudden attacks of sleep). Methylphenidate is in a class of medications called central nervous system (CNS) stimulants. It works by changing the amounts of certain natural substances in the brain.

How should this medicine be used?

Methylphenidate comes as an immediate-release tablet, a chewable tablet, a solution (liquid); an intermediate-acting (extended-release) tablet; a long-acting (extended-release) capsule, and a long-acting (extended release) tablet. The long-acting tablet and capsules supply some medication right away and release the remaining amount as a steady dose of medication over a long time. All of these forms of methylphenidate are taken by mouth. The regular tablets (Ritalin, Methylin), chewable tablets (Methylin), and solution (Methylin) are usually taken 2 to 3 times a day, preferably 35-40 minutes before meals. The last dose should be taken at least several hours before bedtime. The intermediate-acting extended release tablets (Ritalin SR, Metadate ER, Methylin ER) are usually taken once a day in the morning with or without food. The long-acting extended release capsule (Metadate CD) is usually taken once a day before breakfast; the long-acting extended-release tablet (Concerta) and capsule (Ritalin LA) are usually taken once a day in the morning with or without food.

Follow the directions on your prescription label carefully, and ask your doctor or pharmacist to explain any part you do not understand. Take methylphenidate exactly as directed.

You should thoroughly chew the chewable tablets and then drink a full glass (at least 8 ounces) of water or other liquid. If you take the chewable tablet without enough liquid, the tablet may swell and block your throat and may cause you to choke. If you have chest pain, vomiting, or trouble swallowing or breathing after taking the chewable tablet, you should call your doctor or get emergency medical treatment immediately.

Swallow the intermediate acting and long-acting extended-release tablets and capsules whole; do not split, chew, or crush them. However, if you cannot swallow the long-acting capsules (Metadate CD, Ritalin LA), you may carefully open the capsules and sprinkle the entire contents on a tablespoon of cool or room temperature applesauce. Swallow (without chewing) this mixture immediately after preparation and then drink a glass of water to make sure you have swallowed all of the medicine. Do not store the mixture for future use.

Your doctor may start you on a low dose of methylphenidate and gradually increase your dose, not more often than once every week.

Your condition should improve during your treatment. Call your doctor if your symptoms worsen at any time during your treatment or do not improve after one month.

Your doctor may tell you to stop taking methylphenidate from time to time to see if the medication is still needed. Follow these directions carefully.

Are there other uses for this medicine?

Methylphenidate should not be used to treat depression or excessive tiredness that is not caused by narcolepsy.

This medication is sometimes prescribed for other uses; ask your doctor or pharmacist for more information.

What special precautions should I follow?

Before taking methylphenidate,

- tell your doctor and pharmacist if you are allergic to methylphenidate or any other medications.
- tell your doctor if you are taking monoamine oxidase (MAO) inhibitors, including isocarboxazid (Marplan), phenelzine (Nardil), selegiline (Eldepryl), and tranylcypromine (Parnate), or have stopped taking them during the past 14 days. Your doctor will probably tell you not to take methylphenidate until at least 14 days have passed since you last took an MAO inhibitor.
- tell your doctor and pharmacist what prescription and nonprescription medications, vitamins, nutritional supplements, and herbal products you are taking. Be sure to mention any of the following: antidepressants ('mood elevators'); anticoagulants ('blood thinners') such as warfarin (Coumadin); clonidine (Catapres); guanabenz; medications for seizures such as phenobarbital, phenytoin (Dilantin), and primidone (Mysoline); and meth-

yldopa (Aldomet). If you are taking Ritalin LA, also tell your doctor if you take antacids.

- tell your doctor if you or anyone in your family has or has ever had Tourette's syndrome (a condition characterized by the need to perform repeated motions or to repeat sounds or words), facial or motor tics (repeated uncontrollable movements), or verbal tics (repetition of sounds or words that is hard to control), Also tell your doctor if you have glaucoma, or feelings of anxiety, tension, or agitation. Your doctor will probably tell you not to take methylphenidate.

- tell your doctor if anyone in your family has or has ever had an irregular heartbeat or has died suddenly. Also tell your doctor if you have recently had a heart attack and if you have or have ever had a heart defect, high blood pressure, an irregular heartbeat, heart or blood vessel disease, or other heart problems. Your doctor will probably examine you to see if your heart and blood vessels are healthy. Your doctor may tell you not to take methylphenidate if you have a heart condition or if there is a high risk that you may develop a heart condition.

- also tell your doctor if you have or ever have had seizures, or mental illness. If you are taking the chewable tablets, tell your doctor if you have trouble swallowing or if you have phenylketonuria (PKU, a disease in which you must avoid certain foods). If you are taking the long-acting extended-release tablet (Concerta), tell your doctor if you have a a narrowing or blockage of your digestive system.

- tell your doctor if you are pregnant, plan to become pregnant, or are breast-feeding. If you become pregnant while taking methylphenidate, call your doctor.

- if you are having surgery, including dental surgery, tell the doctor or dentist that you are taking methylphenidate.

- you should know that methylphenidate should be used as part of a total treatment program for ADHD, which may include counseling and special education. Make sure to follow all of your doctor's and/or therapist's instructions.

What should I do if I forget to take a dose?

Take the missed dose as soon as you remember it and take any remaining doses for that day at evenly spaced intervals, but do not take a dose at or near bedtime. However, if you remember a missed dose when it is almost time for your next scheduled dose, skip the missed dose. Do not take a double dose to make up for a missed one.

What side effects can this medicine cause?

Methylphenidate may cause side effects. Tell your doctor if any of these symptoms are severe or do not go away:

- nervousness
- difficulty falling asleep or staying asleep
- dizziness
- nausea

- vomiting
- loss of appetite
- stomach pain
- diarrhea
- headache
- painful menstruation

Some side effects can be serious. If you experience any of the following symptoms, call your doctor immediately:

- fast, pounding, or irregular heartbeat
- chest pain
- shortness of breath
- excessive tiredness
- slow or difficult speech
- dizziness or faintness
- weakness or numbness of an arm or leg
- seizures
- changes in vision or blurred vision
- agitation
- abnormal thoughts
- hallucinating (seeing things or hearing voices that do not exist)
- motor tics or verbal tics
- depression
- mood changes
- fever
- sore throat
- unusual bleeding or bruising
- muscle or joint pain
- hives
- rash
- itching
- difficulty breathing or swallowing

Methylphenidate may cause sudden death in children and teenagers with heart defects or serious heart problems. This medication also may cause sudden death, heart attack or stroke in adults, especially adults with heart defects or serious heart problems. Talk to your doctor about the risks of taking this medication.

Methylphenidate may slow children's growth or weight gain. Your child's doctor will watch his or her growth carefully. Talk to your child's doctor if you have concerns about your child's growth or weight gain while he or she is taking this medication. Talk to your child's doctor about the risks of giving methylphenidate to your child.

What storage conditions are needed for this medicine?

Keep this medication in the container it came in, tightly closed, and out of reach of children. Store it at room temperature, away from light and excess heat and moisture (not in the bathroom). Store methylphenidate in a safe place so that no one else can take it accidentally or on purpose. Keep track of how many tablets or capsules are left so you will know if any are missing. Throw away any medication that is outdated or no longer needed. Talk to your pharmacist about the proper disposal of your medication.

What should I do in case of overdose?

In case of overdose, call your local poison control center at 1-800-222-1222. If the victim has collapsed or is not breathing, call local emergency services at 911.

Symptoms of overdose may include:

- vomiting
- agitation
- shaking of hands that you cannot control
- muscle twitching
- seizures
- loss of consciousness
- inappropriate happiness
- confusion
- hallucinating (seeing things or hearing voices that do not exist)
- sweating
- flushing
- headache
- fever
- fast, pounding, or irregular heartbeat
- widening of pupils (black circles in the middle of the eyes)
- dry mouth

What other information should I know?

If you are taking methylphenidate long-acting tablets (Concerta), you may notice something that looks like a tablet in your stool. This is just the empty tablet shell, and this does not mean that you did not get your complete dose of medication.

Keep all appointments with your doctor and the laboratory. Your doctor may order certain lab tests to check your response to methylphenidate.

Do not let anyone else take your medication. This prescription is not refillable. Be sure to schedule appointments with your doctor on a regular basis so that you do not run out of medication.

Dosage Facts
For Informational Purposes

Caution: Do not change your dose, how often you take your medication, or the length of time you are to take it without first talking to your healthcare provider.

The following dosage information was written using medical language for doctors and other healthcare professionals and is provided here for you to check your dosage. The dosage of this drug may differ for different patients. Therefore, always follow your doctor's instructions or the directions on the label. Contact your healthcare provider or pharmacist if you have any questions about the specific dosage of your medication after reviewing this information.

General Dosage Information

Available as methylphenidate and methylphenidate hydrochloride; dosage of methylphenidate hydrochloride is expressed in terms of the salt.

Pediatric Patients

ADHD
Initial Therapy with Conventional Tablets or Oral Solution

ORAL:

- Initially, 5 mg twice daily, before breakfast and lunch. Increase dosage by 5–10 mg daily at weekly intervals based on response and tolerance, up to 60 mg daily; administer daily dosage in 2 or 3 divided doses.
- Some clinicians recommend an initial dosage of 0.25 mg/kg daily; if adverse effects are not observed, double daily dosage each week until 2 mg/kg daily is reached.
- Alternatively, dosage has been titrated over 28 days via daily-switch titration involving 5 randomly ordered repeats each of placebo and 5-, 10-, 15-, or 20-mg daily dosages (higher for children weighing >25 kg); each dose is repeated at breakfast and lunch, with a half dose given in the afternoon. The best dosage is selected based on clinical assessment of response.

Switching to Extended-release Tablets (Metadate® ER, Methylin® ER, Ritalin-SR®)

ORAL:

- Extended-release tablets can be substituted for conventional tablets at the nearest equivalent total daily dosage (e.g., patients receiving 10 mg as conventional tablets twice daily can be switched to 20 mg as extended-release tablets once daily).
- Usual dosage: 20–60 mg daily, given as 20–40 mg once daily or as 40 mg in the morning and 20 mg in the early afternoon.

Initial Therapy with Extended-release Capsules (Metadate® CD, Ritalin® LA)

ORAL:

- Metadate® CD: Initially, 20 mg once daily in the morning. Increase dosage by 10 or 20 mg daily at weekly intervals, up to 60 mg daily.
- Ritalin® LA: Initially, 20 mg once daily in the morning. Alternatively, initiate with 10 mg once daily when a lower initial dosage is appropriate. Increase dosage by 10 mg daily at weekly intervals, up to 60 mg daily.

Switching to Extended-release Capsules (Metadate® CD, Ritalin® LA)

ORAL:

Recommended Initial Dosages for Patients Being Switched from Conventional Tablets to Metadate® CD Extended-release Capsules

Previous Dosage (Conventional Tablets)	Initial Dosage (Metadate® CD Extended-release Capsules)
10 mg twice daily	20 mg once daily
20 mg twice daily	40 mg once daily

Adjust dosage of Metadate® CD by 10 or 20 mg daily at weekly intervals, up to 60 mg daily.

Recommended Initial Dosages for Patients Being Switched from Conventional or Extended-release Tablets to Ritalin® LA Extended-release Capsules

Previous Dosage	Initial Dosage (Ritalin® LA Extended-release Capsules)
Conventional Tablets	
5 mg twice daily	10 mg once daily
10 mg twice daily	20 mg once daily
15 mg twice daily	30 mg once daily
20 mg twice daily	40 mg once daily
30 mg twice daily	60 mg once daily
Extended-release Tablets	
20 mg daily	20 mg once daily
40 mg daily	40 mg once daily
60 mg daily	60 mg once daily

Adjust dosage of Ritalin® LA by 10 mg daily at weekly intervals, up to 60 mg daily.

For other conventional tablet regimens, substitute Ritalin® LA at the nearest daily dosage based on clinical judgment.

Initial Therapy with Extended-release Trilayer Core Tablets (Concerta®)

ORAL:
- Initially, 18 mg once daily in the morning. If adequate response does not occur, increase dosage at approximately weekly intervals up to 54 mg daily in children 6–12 years of age or 72 mg daily (maximum 2 mg/kg daily) in adolescents 13–17 years of age. Some clinicians state that dosage in children 6–12 years of age may be increased to 72 mg daily.

Switching to Extended-release Trilayer Core Tablets (Concerta®)

ORAL:
- For patients being switched from other drugs to methylphenidate (as extended-release trilayer core tablets), follow dosage recommendations for initial therapy with the extended-release trilayer core tablets.

Recommended Initial Dosages for Patients Being Switched from Conventional Tablets to Extended-release Trilayer Core Tablets

Previous Dosage (Conventional Tablets)	Initial Dosage (Concerta® Extended-release Trilayer Core Tablets)
5 mg given 2 or 3 times daily	18 mg once daily
10 mg given 2 or 3 times daily	36 mg once daily
15 mg given 2 or 3 times daily	54 mg once daily

Initial dosage as extended-release trilayer core tablets in patients being switched from conventional tablets should not exceed 54 mg daily. Adjust dosage at weekly intervals, up to 72 mg once daily. A 27-mg extended-release trilayer core tablet

also is available for patients who require a more gradual titration or who cannot tolerate a dosage of 36 mg daily.

Adult Patients

Narcolepsy

ORAL:
- Usual dosage of 10 mg (as conventional tablets or oral solution) 2 or 3 times daily; dosage range of 10–60 mg daily.

Prescribing Limits

Pediatric Patients

Conventional Tablets, Oral Solution, Extended-release Tablets, and Extended-release Capsules

Maximum 60 mg daily.

Extended-release Trilayer Core Tablets (Concerta®)

Initial therapy: Manufacturer recommends maximum dosage of 54 mg daily for children 6–12 years of age or 72 mg daily (maximum 2 mg/kg daily) for adolescents 13–17 years of age; however, some clinicians state that dosage for children 6–12 years of age may be increased to 72 mg daily.

Switched from other formulations: Maximum 72 mg daily.

Adult Patients

Maximum 60 mg daily.

Methylphenidate Transdermal

(meth il fen′ i date)

Brand Name: Daytrana®
Also available generically.

Important Warning

Methylphenidate can be habit-forming. Do not apply more patches, apply the patches more often, or leave the patches on for longer than prescribed by your doctor. If you use too much methylphenidate, you may find that the medication no longer controls your symptoms, you may feel a need to take large amounts of the medication, and you may experience unusual changes in your behavior. Tell your doctor if you drink or have ever drunk large amounts of alcohol, use or have ever used street drugs, or have overused prescription medications.

Do not stop using methylphenidate without talking to your doctor, especially if you have overused the medication. Your doctor will probably decrease your dose gradually and monitor you carefully during this time. You may develop severe depression if you suddenly stop using methylphenidate after over-using it.

Your doctor or pharmacist will give you the manufacturer's patient information sheet (Medication Guide) when you begin treatment with methylphenidate transdermal patches and each time you refill your prescription. Read the information carefully and ask your doctor or pharmacist if you have any questions. You can also visit the Food and Drug Administration (FDA) website (http://www.fda.gov/cder) or the manufacturer's website to obtain the Medication Guide.

Why is this medicine prescribed?

Methylphenidate transdermal patches are used to treat attention deficit hyperactivity disorder (ADHD; more difficulty focusing, controlling actions, and remaining still or quiet than other people who are the same age). Methylphenidate is in a class of medications called central nervous system stimulants. It works by changing the amounts of certain natural substances in the brain.

How should this medicine be used?

Transdermal methylphenidate comes as a patch to apply to the skin. It is usually applied once a day in the morning and left in place for up to 9 hours. Apply the methylphenidate patch at around the same time every day. Follow the directions on your prescription label carefully, and ask your doctor or pharmacist to explain any part you do not understand. Use methylphenidate patches exactly as directed.

Your doctor will probably start you on a low dose of methylphenidate and gradually increase your dose, not more often than once every week.

Your doctor may tell you to stop using methylphenidate patches from time to time to see if the medication is still needed. Follow these directions carefully.

Apply the patch to the hip area. Do not apply the patch to an open wound or cut, to skin that is irritated, red, or swollen, or to skin that is affected by a rash or other skin problem. Do not apply to the patch to the waistline because it may be rubbed off by tight clothing. Do not apply a patch to the same spot two days in a row; each morning apply the patch to the hip that did not have a patch the day before.

Methylphenidate patches should remain attached during normal daily activities, including swimming, showering, and bathing. If a patch does fall off, ask your child how and when this happened. When you notice that a patch has fallen off, you may apply a new patch to a different area of the same hip. However, you should remove the new patch at the time that you were scheduled to remove the original patch.

While you are wearing the patch, keep that hip away from direct sources of heat such as heating pads, electric blankets, and heated waterbeds.

To apply the patch, follow these steps:

1. Talk to your doctor about what time you should apply the patch. You should apply the patch 2 hours before the effects of the medication are needed.
2. Wash and dry the skin in the area where you plan to apply the patch. Be sure that the skin is free of powders, oils, and lotions.
3. Open the tray that contains the patches and throw away the drying agent that comes in the tray.
4. Remove one pouch from the tray and cut it open with scissors. Be careful not to cut the patch. Never use a patch that has been cut or damaged in any way.
5. Remove the patch from the pouch and hold it with the protective liner facing you.
6. Peel off half of the liner. Be careful not to touch the sticky side of the patch with your fingers.
7. Use the other half of the liner as a handle and apply the patch to the skin.
8. Press the patch firmly in place and smooth it down.
9. Hold the sticky half of the patch down with one hand. Use the other hand to pull back the other half of the patch and gently peel off the remaining piece of the protective liner.
10. Use the palm of your hand to press the entire patch firmly in place for about 30 seconds.
11. Go around the edges of the patch with your fingers to press them onto the skin. Be sure that the entire patch is firmly attached to the skin.
12. Throw away the empty pouch and the protective liner in a closed trash can that is out of reach of children and pets. Do not flush the pouch or liner down the toilet.
13. Wash your hands after you handle the patch.
14. Record the time that you applied the patch on the administration chart that comes with the patches. Use the timetable in the patient information that comes with the patches to find the time that the patch should be removed. Do not follow these times if your doctor has told you to use the patch for less than 9 hours. Follow your doctor's instructions carefully and ask your doctor if you do not know when you should remove the patch.
15. When it is time to remove the patch, use your fingers to peel it off slowly.
16. Fold the patch in half with the sticky sides together and press firmly to seal it shut. Flush the patch down the toilet or throw it away in a closed trash can that is out of the reach of children and pets.
17. If there is any adhesive left on the skin, gently rub the area with oil or lotion to remove it.
18. Wash your hands.
19. Record the time that you removed the patch and the way that you threw it away on the administration chart.

Ask your pharmacist or doctor for a copy of the manufacturer's information for the patient.

Are there other uses for this medicine?

Methylphenidate patches should not be used to treat depression or tiredness.

This medication may be prescribed for other uses; ask your doctor or pharmacist for more information.

What special precautions should I follow?

Before using methylphenidate,

- tell your doctor and pharmacist if you are allergic to methylphenidate, any other medications, any other skin patches, or any soaps, lotions, cosmetics, or adhesives that are applied to the skin.

- tell your doctor if you are taking a monoamine oxidase inhibitor (MAOI) such as isocarboxazid (Marplan), phenelzine (Nardil), tranylcypromine (Parnate), rasagiline (Azilect), or selegiline (Eldepryl), or if you have taken one of these medications during the past 14 days. Your doctor will probably tell you not to use methylphenidate patches until at least 14 days have passed since you last took an MAO inhibitor.

- tell your doctor and pharmacist what other prescription and nonprescription medications, vitamins, nutritional supplements, and herbal products you are taking or plan to take. Be sure to mention any of the following: anticoagulants ('blood thinners') such as warfarin (Coumadin); antidepressants such as clomipramine (Anafranil); desipramine (Norpramin) and imipramine (Tofranil); clonidine (Catapres); medications for high blood pressure; medications for seizures such as phenobarbital, phenytoin (Dilantin), and primidone (Mysoline); nonprescription medications used for colds, allergies, or nasal congestion; and selective serotonin reuptake inhibitors (SSRIs) such as citalopram (Celexa), escitalopram (Lexapro), fluoxetine (Prozac, Sarafem), fluvoxamine (Luvox), paroxetine (Paxil), and sertraline (Zoloft). Your doctor may need to change the doses of your medications or monitor you carefully for side effects.

- tell your doctor if you or anyone in your family has or has ever had Tourette's syndrome (a condition characterized by the need to perform repeated motions or to repeat sounds or words), motor tics (repeated uncontrollable movements), or verbal tics (repetition of sounds or words that is hard to control). Also tell your doctor if you have glaucoma, or feelings of anxiety, tension, or agitation. Your doctor will probably tell you not to use methylphenidate patches.

- tell your doctor if anyone in your family has or has ever had an irregular heartbeat or has died suddenly. Also tell your doctor if you have recently had a heart attack and if you have or have ever had a heart defect, high blood pressure, an irregular heartbeat, heart or blood vessel disease, or other heart problems. Your doctor will probably examine you to see if your heart and blood vessels are healthy. Your doctor may tell you not to use methylphenidate patches if you have a heart condition or if there is a high risk that you may develop a heart condition.

- tell your doctor if you or anyone in your family has or has ever had depression, bipolar disorder (mood that changes from depressed to abnormally excited), or mania (frenzied, abnormally excited mood), or has thought about or attempted suicide. Also tell your doctor if you have or have ever had seizures; an abnormal electroencephalogram (EEG; a test that measures electrical activity in the brain); mental illness; or a skin condition such as eczema (a condition that causes the skin to be dry, itchy, or scaly), psoriasis (a skin disease in which red scaly patches form on some areas of the body), or seborrheic dermatitis (condition in which flaky white or yellow scales form on the skin).

- tell your doctor if you are pregnant, plan to become pregnant, or are breast-feeding. If you become pregnant while using methylphenidate, call your doctor.

- if you are having surgery, including dental surgery, tell the doctor or dentist that you are using methylphenidate patches.

- you should know that methylphenidate should be used as part of a total treatment program for ADHD, which may include counseling and special education. Make sure to follow all of your doctor's and/or therapist's instructions.

What special dietary instructions should I follow?

Unless your doctor tells you otherwise, continue your normal diet.

What should I do if I forget to take a dose?

You may apply the missed patch as soon as you remember it. However, you should still remove the patch at your regular patch removal time. Do not apply extra patches to make up for a missed dose.

What side effects can this medicine cause?

Methylphenidate may cause side effects. Tell your doctor if any of these symptoms are severe or do not go away:

- nausea
- vomiting
- loss of appetite
- weight loss
- stuffed or runny nose
- swelling inside the nose
- redness or small bumps on the skin that was covered by the patch

Some side effects can be serious. If you experience any of these symptoms, call your doctor immediately:

- fast, pounding, or irregular heartbeat
- chest pain
- shortness of breath
- excessive tiredness
- slow or difficult speech
- dizziness or faintness
- weakness or numbness of an arm or leg
- blurred vision
- changes in vision
- rash
- swelling or blistering of the skin that was covered by the patch

- seizures
- motion tics or verbal tics
- abnormal thinking
- aggressive behavior
- changes in mood
- unusual sadness or crying
- depression
- hallucinations (seeing things or hearing voices that do not exist)

Methylphenidate patches may cause sudden death in children and teenagers with heart defects or serious heart problems. This medication also may cause heart attack or stroke in adults, especially adults with heart defects or serious heart problems. Talk to your doctor about the risks of using this medication.

Methylphenidate patches may slow children's growth or weight gain. Your child's doctor will watch his or her growth carefully. Talk to your child's doctor if you have concerns about your child's growth or weight gain while he or she is taking this medication. Talk to your child's doctor about the risks of giving methylphenidate patches to your child.

Methylphenidate patches may cause an allergic reaction. Some people who have an allergic reaction to methylphenidate patches may not be able to take methylphenidate by mouth in the future. Talk to your doctor about the risks of using methylphenidate patches.

Methylphenidate may cause other side effects. Call your doctor if you have any unusual problems while using this medication.

What storage conditions are needed for this medicine?

Keep this medication in the container it came in, tightly closed, and out of reach of children. Store it at room temperature and away from excess heat and moisture (not in the bathroom). Throw away any patches that are outdated or no longer needed by opening each pouch, folding each patch in half with the sticky sides together, and flushing the folded patches down the toilet or placing them in a closed trash can that is out of the reach of children and pets. Talk to your pharmacist about the proper disposal of your medication.

Store methylphenidate in a safe place so that no one else can take it accidentally or on purpose. Keep track of how many patches are left so you will know if any are missing.

What should I do in case of overdose?

If someone applies extra methylphenidate patches, remove the patches and clean the skin to remove any adhesive. Than call your local poison control center at 1-800-222-1222. If the victim has collapsed or is not breathing, call local emergency services at 911.

Symptoms of overdose may include:
- vomiting
- agitation
- uncontrollable shaking of a part of the body
- seizures

- coma (loss of consciousness for a period of time)
- extreme happiness
- confusion
- hallucinations (seeing things or hearing voices that do not exist)
- sweating
- flushing
- headache
- fever
- fast, pounding, or irregular heartbeat
- wide pupils (black circles in the middle of the eyes)
- dry mouth and nose

What other information should I know?

Keep all appointments with your doctor and the laboratory. Your doctor will order certain lab tests to check your body's response to methylphenidate.

Do not let anyone else take your medication. This prescription is not refillable. Be sure to schedule appointments with your doctor on a regular basis so that you do not run out of medication.

Dosage Facts
For Informational Purposes

Caution: Do not change your dose, how often you take your medication, or the length of time you are to take it without first talking to your healthcare provider.

The following dosage information was written using medical language for doctors and other healthcare professionals and is provided here for you to check your dosage. The dosage of this drug may differ for different patients. Therefore, always follow your doctor's instructions or the directions on the label. Contact your healthcare provider or pharmacist if you have any questions about the specific dosage of your medication after reviewing this information.

General Dosage Information

Available as methylphenidate and methylphenidate hydrochloride; dosage of methylphenidate hydrochloride is expressed in terms of the salt.

Pediatric Patients

ADHD
Initial Therapy with or Switching to Transdermal System

TRANSDERMAL:
- Individualize dosage titration, final dosage, and wear time according to patient's needs and response.
- Initially, apply one system delivering 10 mg/9 hours once daily (for initial therapy or for patients switching from other methylphenidate preparations). Increase dosage at weekly intervals, based on response and tolerance, by using the next larger dosage system (i.e., 1 system delivering 15 mg/9 hours, then 1 system delivering 20 mg/9 hours, and then 1 system delivering 30 mg/9 hours).

- If shorter duration of effect is desired or if late-day adverse effects appear, may remove system earlier than 9 hours. If aggravation of symptoms or other adverse events occur, reduce dosage or wear time or, if necessary, discontinue therapy.

Methylprednisolone Oral

(meth ill pred niss' oh lone)

Brand Name: Medrol®, Meprolone®
Also available generically.

Why is this medicine prescribed?

Methylprednisolone, a corticosteroid, is similar to a natural hormone produced by your adrenal glands. It is often used to replace this chemical when your body does not make enough of it. It relieves inflammation (swelling, heat, redness, and pain) and is used to treat certain forms of arthritis; skin, blood, kidney, eye, thyroid, and intestinal disorders (e.g., colitis); severe allergies; and asthma. Methylprednisolone is also used to treat certain types of cancer.

This medication is sometimes prescribed for other uses; ask your doctor or pharmacist for more information.

How should this medicine be used?

Methylprednisolone comes as a tablet to take by mouth. Your doctor will prescribe a dosing schedule that is best for you. Follow the directions on your prescription label carefully, and ask your doctor or pharmacist to explain any part you do not understand. Take methylprednisolone exactly as directed. Do not take more or less of it or take it more often than prescribed by your doctor.

Do not stop taking methylprednisolone without talking to your doctor. Stopping the drug abruptly can cause loss of appetite, upset stomach, vomiting, drowsiness, confusion, headache, fever, joint and muscle pain, peeling skin, and weight loss. If you take large doses for a long time, your doctor probably will decrease your dose gradually to allow your body to adjust before stopping the drug completely. Watch for these side effects if you are gradually decreasing your dose and after you stop taking the tablets. If these problems occur, call your doctor immediately. You may need to increase your dose of tablets temporarily or start taking them again.

What special precautions should I follow?

Before taking methylprednisolone,
- tell your doctor and pharmacist if you are allergic to methylprednisolone, aspirin, tartrazine (a yellow dye in some processed foods and drugs), or any other drugs.
- tell your doctor and pharmacist what prescription and nonprescription medications you are taking, especially anticoagulants ('blood thinners') such as warfarin (Coumadin), arthritis medications, aspirin, azithromycin (Zithromax), clarithromycin (Biaxin), cyclosporine (Neoral, Sandimmune), digoxin (Lanoxin), diuretics ('water pills'), erythromycin, estrogen (Premarin), ketoconazole (Nizoral), oral contraceptives, phenobarbital, phenytoin (Dilantin), rifampin (Rifadin), theophylline (Theo-Dur), and vitamins.
- if you have a fungal infection (other than on your skin), do not take methylprednisolone without talking to your doctor.
- tell your doctor if you have or have ever had liver, kidney, intestinal, or heart disease; diabetes; an underactive thyroid gland; high blood pressure; mental illness; myasthenia gravis; osteoporosis; herpes eye infection; seizures; tuberculosis (TB); or ulcers.
- tell your doctor if you are pregnant, plan to become pregnant, or are breast-feeding. If you become pregnant while taking methylprednisolone, call your doctor.
- if you are having surgery, including dental surgery, tell the doctor or dentist that you are taking methylprednisolone.
- if you have a history of ulcers or take large doses of aspirin or other arthritis medication, limit your consumption of alcoholic beverages while taking this drug. Methylprednisolone makes your stomach and intestines more susceptible to the irritating effects of alcohol, aspirin, and certain arthritis medications. This effect increases your risk of ulcers.

What special dietary instructions should I follow?

Your doctor may instruct you to follow a low-sodium, low-salt, potassium-rich, or high-protein diet. Follow these directions.

Methylprednisolone may cause an upset stomach. Take methylprednisolone with food or milk.

What should I do if I forget to take a dose?

When you start to take methylprednisolone, ask your doctor what to do if you forget a dose. Write down these instructions so that you can refer to them later.

If you take methylprednisolone once a day, take the missed dose as soon as you remember it. However, if it is almost time for the next dose, skip the missed dose and continue your regular dosing schedule. Do not take a double dose to make up for a missed one.

What side effects can this medicine cause?

Methylprednisolone may cause side effects. Tell your doctor if any of these symptoms are severe or do not go away:
- upset stomach
- stomach irritation
- vomiting
- headache
- dizziness
- insomnia

- restlessness
- depression
- anxiety
- acne
- increased hair growth
- easy bruising
- irregular or absent menstrual periods

If you experience any of the following symptoms, call your doctor immediately:

- skin rash
- swollen face, lower legs, or ankles
- vision problems
- cold or infection that lasts a long time
- muscle weakness
- black or tarry stool

If you experience a serious side effect, you or your doctor may send a report to the Food and Drug Administration's (FDA) MedWatch Adverse Event Reporting program online [at http://www.fda.gov/MedWatch/index.html] or by phone [1-800-332-1088].

What storage conditions are needed for this medicine?

Keep this medication in the container it came in, tightly closed, and out of reach of children. Store it at room temperature and away from excess heat and moisture (not in the bathroom). Throw away any medication that is outdated or no longer needed. Talk to your pharmacist about the proper disposal of your medication.

What should I do in case of overdose?

In case of overdose, call your local poison control center at 1-800-222-1222. If the victim has collapsed or is not breathing, call local emergency services at 911.

What other information should I know?

Keep all appointments with your doctor and the laboratory. Your doctor will order certain lab tests to check your response to methylprednisolone. Checkups are especially important for children because methylprednisolone can slow bone growth.

If your condition worsens, call your doctor. Your dose may need to be adjusted.

Carry an identification card that indicates that you may need to take supplementary doses (write down the full dose you took before gradually decreasing it) of methylprednisolone during periods of stress (injuries, infections, and severe asthma attacks). Ask your pharmacist or doctor how to obtain this card. List your name, medical problems, drugs and dosages, and doctor's name and telephone number on the card.

This drug makes you more susceptible to illnesses. If you are exposed to chicken pox, measles, or tuberculosis (TB) while taking methylprednisolone, call your doctor. Do not have a vaccination, other immunization, or any skin test while you are taking methylprednisolone unless your doctor tells you that you may.

Report any injuries or signs of infection (fever, sore throat, pain during urination, and muscle aches) that occur during treatment.

Your doctor may instruct you to weigh yourself every day. Report any unusual weight gain.

If your sputum (the matter you cough up during an asthma attack) thickens or changes color from clear white to yellow, green, or gray, call your doctor; these changes may be signs of an infection.

If you have diabetes, methylprednisolone may increase your blood sugar level. If you monitor your blood sugar (glucose) at home, test your blood or urine more frequently than usual. Call your doctor if your blood sugar is high or if sugar is present in your urine; your dose of diabetes medication and your diet may need to be changed.

Do not let anyone else take your medication. Ask your pharmacist any questions you have about refilling your prescription.

Dosage Facts
For Informational Purposes

Caution: Do not change your dose, how often you take your medication, or the length of time you are to take it without first talking to your healthcare provider.

The following dosage information was written using medical language for doctors and other healthcare professionals and is provided here for you to check your dosage. The dosage of this drug may differ for different patients. Therefore, always follow your doctor's instructions or the directions on the label. Contact your healthcare provider or pharmacist if you have any questions about the specific dosage of your medication after reviewing this information.

General Dosage Information

Available as methylprednisolone, methylprednisolone acetate, and methylprednisolone sodium succinate. Dosage of methylprednisolone sodium succinate or methylprednisolone acetate is expressed in terms of methylprednisolone or methylprednisolone acetate, respectively.

After a satisfactory response is obtained, decrease dosage in small decrements to the lowest level that maintains an adequate clinical response, and discontinue the drug as soon as possible.

Monitor patients continually for signs that indicate dosage adjustment is necessary, such as remissions or exacerbations of the disease and stress (surgery, infection, trauma).

High dosages may be required for acute situations of certain rheumatic disorders and collagen diseases; after a response has been obtained, drug often must be continued for long periods at low dosage.

High or massive dosages may be required in the treatment of pemphigus, exfoliative dermatitis, bullous dermatitis herpetiformis, severe erythema multiforme, or mycosis fungoides. Early initiation of systemic glucocorticoid therapy may be life-saving in pemphigus vulgaris. Reduce dosage gradually to the lowest effective level, but discontinuance may not be possible.

Massive dosages may be required for treatment of shock.

Pediatric Patients

Base pediatric dosage on severity of the disease and patient response rather than on strict adherence to dosage indicated by age, body weight, or body surface area.

Usual Dosage

ORAL:
- 0.117–1.66 mg/kg daily or 3.3–50 mg/m² daily, administered in 3 or 4 divided doses.

Adult Patients

Usual Dosage

ORAL:
- Initially, 2–60 mg daily, depending on disease being treated, and is usually divided into 4 doses.

Allergic Conditions

ORAL:
- For certain conditions (e.g., contact dermatitis, including poison ivy), 24 mg (6 tablets) for the first day, which is then tapered by 4 mg daily until 21 tablets have been administered.

Tapered Dosage Schedule

Day 1	Administer 24 mg (all 6 tablets on day 1 regardless of when the prescription is filled. For example, administer 24 mg (all 6 tablets) immediately as a single dose or divided in 2 or 3 doses and taken at intervals between the time the medicine is received and bedtime. Alternatively, administer 8 mg (2 tablets) twice daily (before breakfast and at bedtime) and 4 mg (1 tablet) twice daily (after lunch and dinner).
Day 2	Administer 4 mg (1 tablet) 3 times daily (before breakfast, after lunch, and after dinner) and 8 mg (2 tablets) at bedtime.
Day 3	Administer 4 mg (1 tablet) 4 times daily (before breakfast, after lunch, after dinner, and at bedtime).
Day 4	Administer 4 mg (1 tablet) 3 times daily (before breakfast, after lunch, and at bedtime).
Day 5	Administer 4 mg (1 tablet) twice daily (before breakfast and at bedtime).
Day 6	Administer 4 mg (1 tablet) before breakfast.

Some clinicians suggest tapering the dosage of the drug over 12 days may be associated with a lower incidence of flare-up of the dermatitis than that associated with 6-day therapy.

Acute Exacerbations of Multiple Sclerosis

ORAL:
- 160 mg daily for 1 week, followed by 64 mg every other day for a month.

† Use is not currently included in the labeling approved by the US Food and Drug Administration.

Methylprednisolone Sodium Succinate Injection

(meth il pred nis' oh lone)

Brand Name: A-methaPred®, Depo-Medrol®, Solu-Medrol®
Also available generically.

About Your Treatment

Your doctor has ordered methylprednisolone, a corticosteroid, to relieve inflammation (swelling, heat, redness, and pain). The drug will be added to an intravenous fluid that will drip through a needle or catheter placed in your vein for at least 1 hour per day.

Methylprednisolone is similar to a natural hormone produced by your adrenal glands. It is used to treat, but not cure, certain forms of arthritis; skin, blood, kidney, eye, thyroid, and intestinal disorders (e.g., colitis); and multiple sclerosis. This medication is sometimes prescribed for other uses; ask your doctor or pharmacist for more information.

Your health care provider (doctor, nurse, or pharmacist) may measure the effectiveness and side effects of your treatment using laboratory tests and physical examinations. It is important to keep all appointments with your doctor and the laboratory. The length of treatment depends on how you respond to the medication.

Precautions

Before administering methylprednisolone,
- tell your doctor and pharmacist if you are allergic to methylprednisolone, aspirin, or any other drugs.
- tell your doctor and pharmacist what prescription and nonprescription medications you are taking, especially anticoagulants ('blood thinners') such as warfarin (Coumadin), arthritis medications, aspirin, azithromycin (Zithromax), clarithromycin (Biaxin), cyclosporine (Neoral, Sandimmune), digoxin (Lanoxin), diuretics ('water pills'), erythromycin, estrogen (Premarin), ketoconazole (Nizoral), oral contraceptives, phenobarbital, phenytoin (Di-

lantin), rifampin (Rifadin), theophylline (Theo-Dur), and vitamins.

- tell your doctor if you have a fungal infection (other than on your skin); do not take methylprednisolone without talking to your doctor.
- tell your doctor if you have or have ever had liver, kidney, intestinal, or heart disease; diabetes; an underactive thyroid gland; high blood pressure; mental illness; myasthenia gravis; osteoporosis; herpes eye infection; seizures; tuberculosis (TB); or ulcers.
- tell your doctor if you are pregnant, plan to become pregnant, or are breast-feeding. If you become pregnant while taking methylprednisolone, call your doctor.
- if you are having surgery, including dental surgery, tell the doctor or dentist that you are taking methylprednisolone.

Administering Your Medication

Before you administer methylprednisolone, look at the solution closely. It should be clear and free of floating material. Gently squeeze the bag or observe the solution container to make sure there are no leaks. Do not use the solution if it is discolored, if it contains particles, or if the bag or container leaks. Use a new solution, but show the damaged one to your health care provider.

It is important that you use your medication exactly as directed. Do not change your dosing schedule without talking to your health care provider. Your health care provider may tell you to stop your infusion if you have a mechanical problem (such as a blockage in the tubing, needle, or catheter); if you have to stop an infusion, call your health care provider immediately so your therapy can continue.

Side Effects

Methylprednisolone may cause side effects. Tell your doctor if any of these symptoms are severe or do not go away:

- headache
- dizziness
- insomnia
- restlessness
- depression
- anxiety
- unusual moods
- increased sweating
- increased hair growth
- reddened face
- acne
- thinned skin
- easy bruising
- tiny purple skin spots
- irregular or absent menstrual periods

If you experience any of the following symptoms, call your doctor immediately:

- swollen feet, ankles, and lower legs
- muscle pain and weakness
- eye pain

- vision problems
- puffy skin (especially the face)
- a cold or infection that lasts a long time

Storage Conditions

- Your health care provider probably will give you a several-day supply of methylprednisolone at a time. You will be told how to prepare each dose.

Store your medication only as directed. Make sure you understand what you need to store your medication properly.

Keep your supplies in a clean, dry place when you are not using them, and keep all medications and supplies out of reach of children. Your health care provider will tell you how to throw away used needles, syringes, tubing, and containers to avoid accidental injury.

Overdose

In case of overdose, call your local poison control center at 1-800-222-1222. If the victim has collapsed or is not breathing, call local emergency services at 911.

Signs of Infection

If you are receiving methylprednisolone in your vein or under your skin, you need to know the symptoms of a catheter-related infection (an infection where the needle enters your vein or skin). If you experience any of these effects near your intravenous catheter, tell your health care provider as soon as possible:

- tenderness
- warmth
- irritation
- drainage
- redness
- swelling
- pain

Dosage Facts
For Informational Purposes

Caution: Do not change your dose, how often you take your medication, or the length of time you are to take it without first talking to your healthcare provider.

The following dosage information was written using medical language for doctors and other healthcare professionals and is provided here for you to check your dosage. The dosage of this drug may differ for different patients. Therefore, always follow your doctor's instructions or the directions on the label. Contact your healthcare provider or pharmacist if you have any questions about the specific dosage of your medication after reviewing this information.

General Dosage Information

Available as methylprednisolone, methylprednisolone acetate, and methylprednisolone sodium succinate. Dosage of methylprednisolone sodium succinate or methylprednisolone acetate is expressed in terms of methylprednisolone or methylprednisolone acetate, respectively.

After a satisfactory response is obtained, decrease dosage in small decrements to the lowest level that maintains an adequate clinical response, and discontinue the drug as soon as possible.

Monitor patients continually for signs that indicate dosage adjustment is necessary, such as remissions or exacerbations of the disease and stress (surgery, infection, trauma).

High dosages may be required for acute situations of certain rheumatic disorders and collagen diseases; after a response has been obtained, drug often must be continued for long periods at low dosage.

High or massive dosages may be required in the treatment of pemphigus, exfoliative dermatitis, bullous dermatitis herpetiformis, severe erythema multiforme, or mycosis fungoides. Early initiation of systemic glucocorticoid therapy may be lifesaving in pemphigus vulgaris. Reduce dosage gradually to the lowest effective level, but discontinuance may not be possible.

Massive dosages may be required for treatment of shock.

Pediatric Patients

Base pediatric dosage on severity of the disease and patient response rather than on strict adherence to dosage indicated by age, body weight, or body surface area.

Usual Dosage
Croup†

IV:
- Methylprednisolone sodium succinate: 1–2 mg/kg, followed by 0.5 mg/kg every 6–8 hours.

Pneumocystis jiroveci Pneumonia†

IV:
- Methylprednisolone sodium succinate in children >13 years of age with AIDS† and moderate to severe *Pneumocystis jiroveci* pneumonia: 30 mg twice daily for 5 days, followed by 30 mg once daily for 5 days, and then 15 mg once daily for 11 days (or until completion of the anti-infective regimen). Initiate within 24–72 hours of initial antipneumocystis therapy.

Acute Spinal Cord Injury†

IV:
- Methylprednisolone sodium succinate: 30 mg/kg IV (administered over 15 minutes), followed after 45 minutes by a continuous IV infusion of 5–6 mg/kg per hour for 23 hours.

Lupus Nephritis†

IV:
- Methylprednisolone sodium succinate: 30 mg/kg IV every other day for 6 doses.

Adult Patients

Usual Dosage

IV:
- Methylprednisolone sodium succinate: Usually, 10–250 mg; may repeat up to 6 times daily.

IV:
- Methylprednisolone sodium succinate: For high-dose therapy, administer 30 mg/kg over at least 30 minutes. May repeat every 4–6 hours for 48 hours. Continue high-dose therapy only until the condition stabilizes, usually ≤48–72 hours.

- For other conditions, 10–40 mg over several minutes. Administer subsequent doses IV depending on response and clinical condition.

Acute Exacerbations of Multiple Sclerosis

IV:
- For moderate to severe relapses, 1 g daily for 3–5 days, followed by 60 mg of oral prednisone daily, tapering the dosage over 12 days.
- Alternatively, 1 g or 15 mg/kg of IV methylprednisolone tapered over 15 days to 1 mg/kg, followed by oral prednisone or prednisolone in gradually decreasing dosages over several weeks to months.

Pneumocystis jiroveci Pneumonia

IV:
- In adults with AIDS† and moderate to severe *Pneumocystis jiroveci* pneumonia, 30 mg twice daily for 5 days, followed by 30 mg once daily for 5 days, and then 15 mg once daily for 11 days (or until completion of the anti-infective regimen). Initiate within 24–72 hours of initial antipneumocystis therapy.

Shock

IV:
- Life-threatening shock: massive doses of methylprednisolone as the sodium succinate such as 30 mg/kg by direct IV injection (over 3–15 minutes) initially and repeated every 4–6 hours if needed or 100–250 mg by direct IV injection (over 3–15 minutes) initially and repeated at 2- to 6-hour intervals as required.
- Alternatively, following the initial dose by direct IV injection, additional doses of 30 mg/kg may be administered by slow continuous IV infusion every 12 hours for 24–48 hours.
- Continue high-dose therapy only until the patient's condition has stabilized and usually not beyond 48–72 hours.

Acute Spinal Cord Injury†

IV:
- Methylprednisolone sodium succinate: Initially, 30 mg/kg of methylprednisolone by rapid IV injection over 15 minutes, followed in 45 minutes by IV infusion of 5.4 mg/kg per hour for 23 hours (total dose administered over 24 hours), has been recommended.

Lupus Nephritis†

IV:
- Methylprednisolone sodium succinate: 1 g IV (over a 1-hour period) daily for 3 consecutive days ("pulse" therapy).
- "Pulse" therapy has been followed by long-term oral prednisone or prednisolone therapy (0.5–1 mg/kg per day).

Optic Neuritis†

IV:
- 1 g daily for 3 days followed by oral prednisone 1 mg/kg daily for 11 days has been used.

† Use is not currently included in the labeling approved by the US Food and Drug Administration.

Metipranolol Ophthalmic

(met i pran' oh lol)

Brand Name: OptiPranolol®

Why is this medicine prescribed?

Metipranolol is used to treat glaucoma, a condition in which increased pressure in the eye can lead to gradual loss of vision. Metipranolol decreases the pressure in the eye.

This medication is sometimes prescribed for other uses; ask your doctor or pharmacist for more information.

How should this medicine be used?

Metipranolol comes as eyedrops. Metipranolol eyedrops usually are applied twice a day, at evenly spaced intervals. Follow the directions on your prescription label carefully, and ask your doctor or pharmacist to explain any part you do not understand. Do not use more or less of it or use it more often than prescribed by your doctor.

Metipranolol controls glaucoma but does not cure it. Continue to use metipranolol even if you feel well. Do not stop using metipranolol without talking to your doctor.

To use the eyedrops, follow these instructions:

1. Wash your hands thoroughly with soap and water.
2. Use a mirror or have someone else put the drops in your eye.
3. Remove the protective cap. Make sure that the end of the dropper is not chipped or cracked.
4. Avoid touching the dropper tip against your eye or anything else.
5. Hold the dropper tip down at all times to prevent drops from flowing back into the bottle and contaminating the remaining contents.
6. Lie down or tilt your head back.
7. Holding the bottle between your thumb and index finger, place the dropper tip as near as possible to your eyelid without touching it.
8. Brace the remaining fingers of that hand against your cheek or nose.
9. With the index finger of your other hand, pull the lower lid of the eye down to form a pocket.
10. Drop the prescribed number of drops into the pocket made by the lower lid and the eye. Placing drops on the surface of the eyeball can cause stinging.
11. Close your eye and press lightly against the lower lid with your finger for 2-3 minutes to keep the medication in the eye. Do not blink.
12. Replace and tighten the cap right away. Do not wipe or rinse it off.
13. Wipe off any excess liquid from your cheek with a clean tissue. Wash your hands again.

What special precautions should I follow?

Before using metipranolol eyedrops,

- tell your doctor and pharmacist if you are allergic to metipranolol, beta blockers, or any other drugs.
- tell your doctor and pharmacist what prescription and nonprescription medications you are taking, especially other eye medications; beta blockers such as atenolol (Tenormin), carteolol (Cartrol), labetalol (Normodyne, Trandate), metoprolol (Lopressor), nadolol (Corgard); propranolol (Inderal); sotalol (Betapace); or timolol (Blocadren); quinidine (Quinidex, Quinaglute Dura-Tabs); verapamil (Calan, Isoptin); and vitamins.
- tell your doctor if you have or have ever had thyroid, heart, or lung disease; congestive heart failure; or diabetes.
- tell your doctor if you are pregnant, plan to become pregnant, or are breast-feeding. If you become pregnant while using metipranolol, call your doctor immediately.
- if you are having surgery, including dental surgery, tell the doctor or dentist that you are using metipranolol.
- if you are using another eyedrop medication, use the eye medications at least 10 minutes apart.
- if you wear soft contact lenses, remove them before inserting metipranolol eyedrops, and wait 15 minutes before putting them back in.

What should I do if I forget to take a dose?

Apply the missed dose as soon as you remember it. However, if it is almost time for the next dose, skip the missed dose and continue your regular dosing schedule. Do not apply a double dose to make up for a missed one.

What side effects can this medicine cause?

Metipranolol may cause side effects. Tell your doctor if any of these symptoms are severe or do not go away:

- stinging or burning of the eye
- brow ache
- eye tearing
- sensitivity to light
- blurred vision after using the drops

If you experience any of the following symptoms, stop using metipranolol and call your doctor immediately:

- skin rash
- eye pain
- swelling in or around the eyes
- vision problems
- difficulty breathing
- rapid or strong heartbeat
- abnormal pulse
- headache
- dizziness
- depression
- fainting

If you experience a serious side effect, you or your doctor may send a report to the Food and Drug Administration's

(FDA) MedWatch Adverse Event Reporting program online [at http://www.fda.gov/MedWatch/index.html] or by phone [1-800-332-1088].

What storage conditions are needed for this medicine?

Keep this medication in the container it came in, tightly closed, and out of reach of children. Store it at room temperature and away from excess heat and moisture (not in the bathroom). Do not use the eyedrops if the solution has turned brown, is cloudy, or contains particles; obtain a fresh bottle. Throw away any medication that is outdated or no longer needed. Talk to your pharmacist about the proper disposal of your medication.

What other information should I know?

Keep all appointments with your doctor. Your doctor will order certain eye tests to check your response to metipranolol.

Do not let anyone else use your medication. Ask your pharmacist any questions you have about refilling your prescription.

Talk to your doctor, pharmacist, or other healthcare professional if you have questions about dosing information for your medication.

Metoclopramide Hydrochloride Injection

(met oh kloe pra' mide)

Brand Name: Reglan®
Also available generically.

About Your Treatment

Your doctor has ordered metoclopramide to relieve nausea and vomiting, stomach pain and bloating, loss of appetite, and a persistent feeling of fullness after meals. The drug will be added to an intravenous fluid that will drip through a needle or catheter placed in your vein for at least 15 minutes. This medication is sometimes prescribed for other uses; ask your doctor or pharmacist for more information.

Your health care provider (doctor, nurse, or pharmacist) may measure the effectiveness and side effects of your treatment using laboratory tests and physical examinations. It is important to keep all appointments with your doctor and the laboratory. The length of treatment depends on how you respond to the medication.

Precautions

Before administering metoclopramide,
- tell your doctor and pharmacist if you are allergic to metoclopramide or any other drugs.
- tell your doctor and pharmacist what prescription and nonprescription medications you are taking, especially barbiturates, insulin, narcotics, sedatives, tranquilizers, and vitamins.
- tell your doctor if you have or have ever had an adrenal tumor; seizures; Parkinson's disease; high blood pressure; heart, liver, or kidney disease; a history of mental illness or depression; or an intestinal blockage or bleeding.
- tell your doctor if you are pregnant, plan to become pregnant, or are breast-feeding. If you become pregnant while taking metoclopramide, call your doctor.
- you should know that this drug may make you drowsy. Do not drive a car or operate machinery until you know how this drug affects you.
- remember that alcohol can add to the drowsiness caused by this drug.

Administering Your Medication

Before you administer metoclopramide, look at the solution closely. It should be clear and free of floating material. Gently squeeze the bag or observe the solution container to make sure there are no leaks. Do not use the solution if it is discolored, if it contains particles, or if the bag or container leaks. Use a new solution, but show the damaged one to your health care provider.

It is important that you use your medication exactly as directed. Do not change your dosing schedule without talking to your health care provider. Your health care provider may tell you to stop your infusion if you have a mechanical problem (such as a blockage in the tubing, needle, or catheter); if you have to stop an infusion, call your health care provider immediately so your therapy can continue.

Side Effects

Metoclopramide may cause side effects. Tell your health care provider if any of these symptoms are severe or do not go away:
- drowsiness
- restlessness
- fatigue
- constipation
- diarrhea

If you experience any of the following symptoms, call your health care provider immediately:
- involuntary movements of the limbs or eyes
- spasm of the neck, face, and jaw muscles
- change in mood (depression)

If you experience a serious side effect, you or your doctor may send a report to the Food and Drug Administration's (FDA) MedWatch Adverse Event Reporting program online

[at http://www.fda.gov/MedWatch/index.html] or by phone [1-800-332-1088].

Storage Conditions

- Your health care provider probably will give you a several-day supply of metoclopramide at a time. If you are receiving metoclopramide intravenously (in your vein), you probably will be told to store it in the refrigerator or freezer.
- Take your next dose from the refrigerator 1 hour before using it; place it in a clean, dry area to allow it to warm to room temperature.
- If you are told to store additional metoclopramide in the freezer, always move a 24-hour supply to the refrigerator for the next day's use.
- Do not refreeze medications.

If you are receiving metoclopramide intramuscularly (in your muscle), your health care provider will tell you how to store it properly.

Store your medication only as directed. Make sure you understand what you need to store your medication properly.

Keep your supplies in a clean, dry place when you are not using them, and keep all medications and supplies out of reach of children. Your health care provider will tell you how to throw away used needles, syringes, tubing, and containers to avoid accidental injury.

Overdose

In case of overdose, call your local poison control center at 1-800-222-1222. If the victim has collapsed or is not breathing, call local emergency services at 911.

Signs of Infection

If you are receiving metoclopramide in your vein or under your skin, you need to know the symptoms of a catheter-related infection (an infection where the needle enters your vein or skin). If you experience any of these effects near your intravenous catheter, tell your health care provider as soon as possible:

- tenderness
- warmth
- irritation
- drainage
- redness
- swelling
- pain

Dosage Facts
For Informational Purposes

Caution: Do not change your dose, how often you take your medication, or the length of time you are to take it without first talking to your healthcare provider.

The following dosage information was written using medical language for doctors and other healthcare professionals and is provided here for you to check your dosage. The dosage of this drug may differ for different patients. Therefore, always follow your doctor's instructions or the directions on the label. Contact your healthcare provider or pharmacist if you have any questions about the specific dosage of your medication after reviewing this information.

General Dosage Information

Available as metoclopramide hydrochloride; dosage expressed in terms of metoclopramide.

Pediatric Patients

Intubation of the Small Intestine

IV:
- Children <6 years of age: Usually, one 0.1-mg/kg dose given by direct IV injection.
- Children 6–14 years of age: Usually, one 2.5- to 5-mg dose given by direct IV injection.
- Children >14 years of age: Usually, one 10-mg dose given by direct IV injection.

Radiographic Examination of the Upper GI Tract

IV:
- Children <6 years of age: Usually, one 0.1 mg/kg dose given by direct IV injection.
- Children 6–14 years of age: Usually, one 2.5- to 5-mg dose given by direct IV injection.

Adult Patients

Diabetic Gastric Stasis

IV:
- If symptoms are severe or oral use is not feasible, 10 mg 4 times daily, given by direct IV injection 30 minutes before meals and at bedtime. Continue until symptoms subside enough to allow oral administration.

IM:
- If symptoms are severe or oral use is not feasible, 10 mg 4 times daily, given 30 minutes before meals and at bedtime. Continue until symptoms subside enough to allow oral administration.

Prevention of Postoperative Nausea and Vomiting

IM:
- Usually, 10 mg administered near the end of the surgical procedure; 20 mg also may be used. Repeat every 4–6 hours as necessary.

Prevention of Cancer Chemotherapy-induced Emesis

IV:
- Initially, 2 mg/kg given by IV infusion 30 minutes before administration of highly emetogenic chemotherapy; repeat twice at 2-hour intervals. If vomiting is suppressed, may then decrease dosage to 1 mg/kg at 3-hour intervals for 3 additional doses. If vomiting is *not* suppressed after initial 3 doses, may continue 2-mg/kg doses at 3-hour intervals for 3 additional doses.

- For less emetogenic drugs or regimens, initial 1-mg/kg doses may be sufficient.
- Doses up to 2.75 mg/kg† have been used in patients receiving cisplatin alone or in combination with other antineoplastic agents when emesis was not adequately controlled with 2 mg/kg and substantial metoclopramide toxicity was *not* present.

Intubation of the Small Intestine

IV:
- Usually, one 10-mg dose given by direct IV injection.

Radiographic Examination of the Upper GI Tract

IV:
- Usually, one 10-mg dose given by direct IV injection.

Special Populations

Hepatic Impairment
- Dosage modification does not appear to be necessary.

Renal Impairment
- Modify dosage according to degree of renal impairment.
- In patients with Cl_{cr} <40 mL/minute, manufacturers recommend an initial dosage of approximately 50% of the usual dosage. Subsequently, increase or decrease dosage according to response and tolerance.

Geriatric Patients
- Administer lowest effective dosage. In geriatric patients with gastroesophageal reflux, initial 5-mg dose may be required due to possible sensitivity to therapeutic and/or adverse effects of metoclopramide.
- If parkinsonian symptoms occur, generally discontinue drug before initiating antiparkinsonian agents.

† *Use is not currently included in the labeling approved by the US Food and Drug Administration.*

Metoclopramide Oral

(met oh kloe pra′ mide)

Brand Name: Metoclopramide Hydrochloride Intensol®, Reglan®, Reglan® Syrup
Also available generically.

Why is this medicine prescribed?

Metoclopramide is used to relieve nausea and vomiting; heartburn, stomach pain, and bloating; and a persistent feeling of fullness after meals.

This medication is sometimes prescribed for other uses; ask your doctor or pharmacist for more information.

How should this medicine be used?

Metoclopramide comes as a tablet and liquid to take by mouth. Follow the directions on your prescription label carefully, and ask your doctor or pharmacist to explain any part you do not understand. Take metoclopramide exactly as directed. Do not take more or less of it or take it more often than prescribed by your doctor.

What special precautions should I follow?

Before taking metoclopramide,
- tell your doctor and pharmacist if you are allergic to metoclopramide or any other drugs.
- tell your doctor and pharmacist what prescription and nonprescription medications you are taking, especially amobarbital (Amytal), insulin, narcotics (pain medications), phenobarbital, sedatives, tranquilizers, and vitamins.
- tell your doctor if you have or have ever had an adrenal tumor; a seizure disorder; Parkinson's disease; high blood pressure; heart, liver, or kidney disease; a history of mental illness or depression; or an intestinal blockage or bleeding.
- tell your doctor if you are pregnant, plan to become pregnant, or are breast-feeding. If you become pregnant while taking metoclopramide, call your doctor.
- if you are having surgery, including dental surgery, tell the doctor or dentist that you are taking metoclopramide.
- you should know that this drug may make you drowsy. Do not drive a car or operate machinery until you know how this drug affects you.
- remember that alcohol can add to the drowsiness caused by this drug.

What should I do if I forget to take a dose?

Take the missed dose as soon as you remember it. However, if it is almost time for the next dose, skip the missed dose and continue your regular dosing schedule. Do not take a double dose to make up for a missed one.

What side effects can this medicine cause?

Metoclopramide may cause side effects. Tell your doctor if any of these symptoms are severe or do not go away:
- drowsiness
- restlessness
- fatigue
- constipation
- diarrhea

If you experience any of the following symptoms, call your doctor immediately:
- involuntary movements of the limbs or eyes
- spasm of the neck, face, and jaw muscles
- change in mood (depression)

If you experience a serious side effect, you or your doctor may send a report to the Food and Drug Administration's (FDA) MedWatch Adverse Event Reporting program online [at http://www.fda.gov/MedWatch/index.html] or by phone [1-800-332-1088].

What storage conditions are needed for this medicine?

Keep this medication in the container it came in, tightly closed, and out of reach of children. Store it at room temperature and away from excess heat and moisture (not in the bathroom). Throw away any medication that is outdated or no longer needed. Talk to your pharmacist about the proper disposal of your medication.

What should I do in case of overdose?

In case of overdose, call your local poison control center at 1-800-222-1222. If the victim has collapsed or is not breathing, call local emergency services at 911.

What other information should I know?

Keep all appointments with your doctor.

Do not let anyone else take your medication. Ask your pharmacist any questions you have about refilling your prescription.

Dosage Facts
For Informational Purposes

Caution: Do not change your dose, how often you take your medication, or the length of time you are to take it without first talking to your healthcare provider.

The following dosage information was written using medical language for doctors and other healthcare professionals and is provided here for you to check your dosage. The dosage of this drug may differ for different patients. Therefore, always follow your doctor's instructions or the directions on the label. Contact your healthcare provider or pharmacist if you have any questions about the specific dosage of your medication after reviewing this information.

General Dosage Information

Available as metoclopramide hydrochloride; dosage expressed in terms of metoclopramide.

Adult Patients

Diabetic Gastric Stasis

ORAL:
- 10 mg 4 times daily, given 30 minutes before meals and at bedtime. Continue for 2–8 weeks, depending on response and likelihood of continued well-being if drug is discontinued. Reinstitute at earliest symptom recurrence.

Prevention of Cancer Chemotherapy-induced Emesis

ORAL†:
- 2 mg/kg has been given 1 hour before administration of highly emetogenic chemotherapy and repeated 3 times at 2-hour intervals (i.e., at 1, 3, and 5 hours after initiation of chemotherapy); may give 2 additional doses at 3-hour inter-vals (i.e., at 8 and 11 hours after initiation of chemotherapy) for a total daily dose of 12 mg/kg.
- Total daily dose of 6 mg/kg has been used in patients who developed intolerable adverse effects with the higher daily dose.

Gastroesophageal Reflux

ORAL:
- Usually, 10–15 mg up to 4 times daily (30 minutes before each meal and at bedtime) for 4–12 weeks, depending on symptoms and response. Patients sensitive to therapeutic and/or adverse effects of metoclopramide may require initial dose of 5 mg.
- For intermittent symptoms or symptoms at specific times of the day, one 20-mg dose before the provoking situation may be preferred to daily administration of multiple doses.
- In patients with esophageal erosion and ulceration, 15 mg 4 times daily for 12 weeks has provided healing; monitor endoscopically because of the poor correlation between symptoms and healing.

Prescribing Limits

Adult Patients

Gastroesophageal Reflux

ORAL:
- Safety and efficacy beyond 12 weeks not established; use beyond 12 weeks is not recommended.

Special Populations

Hepatic Impairment
- Dosage modification does not appear to be necessary.

Renal Impairment
- Modify dosage according to degree of renal impairment.
- In patients with Cl_{cr} <40 mL/minute, manufacturers recommend an initial dosage of approximately 50% of the usual dosage. Subsequently, increase or decrease dosage according to response and tolerance.

Geriatric Patients
- Administer lowest effective dosage. In geriatric patients with gastroesophageal reflux, initial 5-mg dose may be required due to possible sensitivity to therapeutic and/or adverse effects of metoclopramide.
- If parkinsonian symptoms occur, generally discontinue drug before initiating antiparkinsonian agents.

† Use is not currently included in the labeling approved by the US Food and Drug Administration.

Metolazone

(me tole′ a zone)

Brand Name: Mykrox®, Zaroxolyn®

Why is this medicine prescribed?

Metolazone, a 'water pill,' is used to treat high blood pressure and fluid retention caused by various conditions, including heart disease. It causes the kidneys to get rid of unneeded water and salt from the body into the urine.

This medicine is sometimes prescribed for other uses; ask your doctor or pharmacist for more information.

How should this medicine be used?

Metolazone comes as a tablet to take by mouth. It usually is taken once a day in the morning. Follow the directions on your prescription label carefully, and ask your doctor or pharmacist to explain any part you do not understand. Take metolazone exactly as directed. Do not take more or less of it or take it more often than prescribed by your doctor.

Metolazone controls high blood pressure but does not cure it. Continue to take metolazone even if you feel well. Do not stop taking metolazone without talking to your doctor.

Are there other uses for this medicine?

Metolazone may also be used to treat patients with diabetes insipidus and certain electrolyte disturbances and to prevent kidney stones in patients with high levels of calcium in their blood. Talk to your doctor about the possible risks of using this medicine for your condition.

What special precautions should I follow?

Before taking metolazone,

- tell your doctor and pharmacist if you are allergic to metolazone, sulfa drugs, or any other drugs.
- tell your doctor and pharmacist what prescription and nonprescription medications you are taking, especially other medications for high blood pressure, anti-inflammatory medications such as ibuprofen (Motrin, Nuprin) or naproxen (Aleve), corticosteroids (e.g., prednisone), lithium (Eskalith, Lithobid), medications for diabetes, probenecid (Benemid), and vitamins. If you also are taking cholestyramine or colestipol, take it at least 1 hour after metolazone.
- tell your doctor if you have or have ever had diabetes, gout, or kidney, liver, thyroid, or parathyroid disease.
- tell your doctor if you are pregnant, plan to become pregnant, or are breast-feeding. If you become pregnant while taking metolazone, call your doctor immediately.
- if you are having surgery, including dental surgery, tell the doctor or dentist that you are taking metolazone.
- you should know that this drug may make you drowsy.

Do not drive a car or operate machinery until you know how this drug affects you.
- remember that alcohol can add to the drowsiness caused by this drug.
- plan to avoid unnecessary or prolonged exposure to sunlight and to wear protective clothing, sunglasses, and sunscreen. Metolazone may make your skin sensitive to sunlight.

What special dietary instructions should I follow?

Follow your doctor's directions. They may include following a daily exercise program or a low-salt or low-sodium diet, potassium supplements, and increased amounts of potassium-rich foods (e.g., bananas, prunes, raisins, and orange juice) in your diet.

What should I do if I forget to take a dose?

Take the missed dose as soon as you remember it. However, if it is almost time for your next dose, skip the missed dose and continue your regular dosing schedule. Do not take a double dose to make up for a missed one.

What side effects can this medicine cause?

Frequent urination should go away after you take metolazone for a few weeks. Tell your doctor if any of these symptoms are severe or do not go away:

- muscle weakness
- dizziness
- cramps
- thirst
- stomach pain
- upset stomach
- vomiting
- diarrhea
- headache
- hair loss

If you experience any of the following symptoms, call your doctor immediately:

- sore throat with fever
- unusual bleeding or bruising
- severe skin rash with peeling skin
- difficulty breathing or swallowing

If you experience a serious side effect, you or your doctor may send a report to the Food and Drug Administration's (FDA) MedWatch Adverse Event Reporting program online [at http://www.fda.gov/MedWatch/index.html] or by phone [1-800-332-1088].

What storage conditions are needed for this medicine?

Keep this medicine in the container it came in, tightly closed, and out of reach of children. Store it at room temperature and away from excess heat and moisture (not in the bathroom). Throw away any medicine that is outdated or no longer needed. Talk to your pharmacist about the proper disposal of your medicine.

What should I do in case of overdose?

In case of overdose, call your local poison control center at 1-800-222-1222. If the victim has collapsed or is not breathing, call local emergency services at 911.

What other information should I know?

Keep all appointments with your doctor and the laboratory. Your blood pressure should be checked regularly, and blood tests should be done occasionally.

Do not let anyone else take your medicine. Ask your pharmacist any questions you have about refilling your prescription.

Talk to your doctor, pharmacist, or other healthcare professional if you have questions about dosing information for your medication.

Metoprolol

(me toe′ proe lole)

Brand Name: Lopressor®, Lopressor® HCT, Toprol XL®

Also available generically.

Important Warning

Do not stop taking metoprolol without talking to your doctor. Suddenly stopping metoprolol may cause chest pain or heart attack. Your doctor will probably decrease your dose gradually.

Why is this medicine prescribed?

Metoprolol is used alone or in combination with other medications to treat high blood pressure. It also is used to prevent angina (chest pain) and to treat heart attacks. Extended-release (long-acting) metoprolol also is used in combination with other medications to treat heart failure. Metoprolol is in a class of medications called beta blockers. It works by slowing the heart rate and relaxing the blood vessels so the heart does not have to pump as hard.

How should this medicine be used?

Metoprolol comes as a tablet and an extended-release tablet to take by mouth. The regular tablet is usually taken once or twice a day with meals or immediately after meals. The extended-release tablet is usually taken once a day. To help you remember to take metoprolol, take it around the same time every day. Follow the directions on your prescription

label carefully, and ask your doctor or pharmacist to explain any part you do not understand. Take metoprolol exactly as directed. Do not take more or less of it or take it more often than prescribed by your doctor.

The long-acting tablet may be split. Swallow the whole or half tablets whole; do not chew or crush them.

Your doctor may start you on a low dose of metoprolol and gradually increase your dose.

Metoprolol controls high blood pressure and angina but does not cure them. Extended-release metoprolol controls heart failure but does not cure it. It may take a few weeks before you feel the full benefit of metoprolol. Continue to take metoprolol even if you feel well.

Are there other uses for this medicine?

Metoprolol is also used sometimes to prevent migraine headaches and to treat irregular heartbeat and movement disorders caused by medications for mental illness. Talk to your doctor about the possible risks of using this medication for your condition.

This medication may be prescribed for other uses; ask your doctor or pharmacist for more information.

What special precautions should I follow?

Before taking metoprolol,

- tell your doctor and pharmacist if you are allergic to metoprolol, acebutolol (Sectral), atenolol (Tenormin, in Tenoretic), betaxolol (Kerlone), bisoprolol (Zebeta, in Ziac), carvedilol (Coreg), Esmolol (Brevibloc), labetalol (Trandate), nadolol (Corgard, in Corzide), pindolol, propranolol (Inderal, Inderal LA, Innopran XL, in Inderide), sotalol (Betapace, Betapace AF, Sorine), timolol (Blocadren, in Timolide), any other medications, or any of the ingredients in metoprolol tablets. Ask your pharmacist for a list of the ingredients.
- tell your doctor and pharmacist what prescription and nonprescription medications, vitamins, nutritional supplements, and herbal products you are taking. Be sure to mention any of the following: bupropion (Wellbutrin), cimetidine (Tagamet), clonidine (Catapres), diphenhydramine (Benadryl), fluoxetine (Prozac, Sarafem), hydroxychloroquine, paroxetine (Paxil), propafenone (Rythmol), quinidine (Quinaglute, Quinidex), ranitidine (Zantac), reserpine (Serpalan, Serpasil, Serpatab), ritonavir (Norvir), terbinafine (Lamisil), and thioridazine (Mellaril), Your doctor may need to change the doses of your medications or monitor you carefully for side effects.
- tell your doctor if you have a slow heart rate, heart failure, problems with blood circulation, or pheochromocytoma (a tumor that develops on a gland near the kidneys and may cause high blood pressure and fast heartbeat). Your doctor may tell you not to take metoprolol.
- tell your doctor if you have or have ever had asthma or other lung disease; heart or liver disease; diabetes; se-

vere allergies; or an overactive thyroid gland (hyperthyroidism).

- tell your doctor if you are pregnant, plan to become pregnant, or are breast-feeding. If you become pregnant while taking metoprolol, call your doctor.
- if you are having surgery, including dental surgery, tell the doctor or dentist that you are taking metoprolol.
- you should know that metoprolol may make you drowsy. Do not drive a car or operate machinery until you know how this medication affects you.
- remember that alcohol can add to the drowsiness caused by this medication.
- you should know that if you have allergic reactions to different substances, your reactions may be worse while you are using metoprolol, and your allergic reactions may not respond to the usual doses of injectable epinephrine.

What special dietary instructions should I follow?

If your doctor prescribes a low-salt or low-sodium diet, follow these directions carefully.

What should I do if I forget to take a dose?

Take the missed dose as soon as you remember it. However, if it is almost time for the next dose, skip the missed dose and continue your regular dosing schedule. Do not take a double dose to make up for a missed one.

What side effects can this medicine cause?

Metoprolol may cause side effects. Tell your doctor if any of these symptoms are severe or do not go away:

- dizziness or lightheadedness
- tiredness
- depression
- upset stomach
- dry mouth
- stomach pain
- vomiting
- gas or bloating
- heartburn
- constipation
- rash or itching
- cold hands and feet
- runny nose

Some side effects can be serious. The following symptoms are uncommon, but if you experience any of them, call your doctor immediately:

- shortness of breath
- wheezing
- swelling of the hands, feet, ankles, or lower legs
- unusual weight gain
- fainting
- rapid, pounding, or irregular heartbeat

Metoprolol may cause other side effects. Call your doc-

tor if you have any unusual problems while taking this medication.

If you experience a serious side effect, you or your doctor may send a report to the Food and Drug Administration's (FDA) MedWatch Adverse Event Reporting program online [at http://www.fda.gov/MedWatch/index.html] or by phone [1-800-332-1088].

What storage conditions are needed for this medicine?

Keep this medication in the container it came in, tightly closed, and out of reach of children. Store it at room temperature and away from excess heat and moisture (not in the bathroom). Throw away any medication that is outdated or no longer needed. Talk to your pharmacist about the proper disposal of your medication.

What should I do in case of overdose?

In case of overdose, call your local poison control center at 1-800-222-1222. If the victim has collapsed or is not breathing, call local emergency services at 911.

Symptoms of overdose may include:

- dizziness
- fainting
- difficulty breathing or swallowing
- swelling of the hands, feet, ankles, or lower legs

What other information should I know?

Keep all appointments with your doctor. Your blood pressure should be checked regularly to determine your response to metoprolol. Your doctor may ask you to check your pulse (heart rate). Ask your pharmacist or doctor to teach you how to take your pulse. If your pulse is faster or slower than it should be, call your doctor.

Do not let anyone else take your medication. Ask your pharmacist any questions you have about refilling your prescription.

Dosage Facts
For Informational Purposes

Caution: Do not change your dose, how often you take your medication, or the length of time you are to take it without first talking to your healthcare provider.

The following dosage information was written using medical language for doctors and other healthcare professionals and is provided here for you to check your dosage. The dosage of this drug may differ for different patients. Therefore, always follow your doctor's instructions or the directions on the label. Contact your healthcare provider or pharmacist if you have any questions about the specific dosage of your medication after reviewing this information.

General Dosage Information

Available as metoprolol tartrate and metoprolol succinate; dosage expressed in terms of the tartrate.

Pediatric Patients

Hypertension†

ORAL:
- Some experts recommend an initial dosage of 1–2 mg/kg daily given in 2 divided doses. Increase dosage as necessary up to a maximum dosage of 6 mg/kg (up to 200 mg) daily given in 2 divided doses.

Adult Patients

Hypertension

ORAL:
- Initially, 50–100 mg given once daily (extended-release tablets) or in single or divided doses daily (conventional tablets). Increase dosage at weekly (or longer) intervals until optimum effect is achieved.
- If satisfactory BP response is not maintained throughout the day, larger doses, more frequent administration, or use of extended-release tablets may be required.

Angina
Long-term Management

ORAL:
- Initially, 100 mg given once daily (extended-release tablets) or in 2 divided doses daily (conventional tablets). Increase dosage at weekly intervals until optimum response is obtained or pronounced slowing of heart rate occurs.
- Usual maintenance dosage is 100–400 mg daily.

AMI

As soon as clinical condition allows, administer oral therapy (conventional tablets) to patients who have contraindications to or do not tolerate IV therapy during the early phase of definite or suspected AMI or to patients in whom therapy is delayed.

Late Treatment

ORAL:
- 100 mg twice daily for at least 3 months.

CHF

ORAL:
- Initially, 25 mg (extended-release tablets) once daily in adults with NYHA class II heart failure. In patients with more severe heart failure, use an initial dosage of 12.5 mg (extended-release tablets) once daily. Double the dosage every 2 weeks to a dosage of 200 mg or until highest tolerated dosage is reached.
- Some experts recommend initiation of therapy with 12.5 mg (extended-release tablets) daily or 6.25 mg (conventional tablets) twice daily for 2–4 weeks. If tolerated, increase to 25 mg daily for 2–4 weeks; subsequent dosages can be doubled every 2–4 weeks.
- If deterioration occurs during titration, increase dosage of concurrent diuretic and decrease dosage of metoprolol or temporarily discontinue metoprolol. Do not continue dosage titration until symptoms of worsening heart failure have stabilized. Initial difficulty in dosage titration should not preclude subsequent attempts to successfully titrate the dosage.

- Reduce dosage in patients with CHF who experience symptomatic bradycardia (e.g., dizziness) or 2nd or 3rd degree heart block.

Vascular Headache
Migraine†

ORAL:
- Dosages of 50–300 mg daily have been used in clinical studies; usual effective dosage was 200 mg daily.

Prescribing Limits

Pediatric Patients

Hypertension†

ORAL:
- Maximum 6 mg/kg (up to 200 mg) daily.

Adult Patients

Hypertension

ORAL:
- Dosages >400 mg (extended-release tablets) and 450 mg (conventional tablets) daily have not been studied.

Angina

ORAL:
- Dosages >400 mg daily have not been studied.

Supraventricular Tachyarrhythmias
Atrial Fibrillation†

ORAL:
- Maximum 100 mg twice daily.

CHF

ORAL:
- Up to 200 mg daily.

Special Populations

Hepatic Impairment
- Elimination occurs mainly in the liver; dosage reductions may be necessary.

Renal Impairment
- Dosage adjustments are not required.

Geriatric Patients
- Cautious dosage selection recommended; initiate therapy at the lower end of the dosage range.

† Use is not currently included in the labeling approved by the US Food and Drug Administration.

Metronidazole Injection

(me troe ni′ da zole)

Brand Name: Flagyl I.V.®, Flagyl®, Flagyl® I.V. RTU®, Metronidazole Injection RTU
Also available generically.

> ## Important Warning
>
> Metronidazole can cause cancer in laboratory animals. Talk to your doctor about the risks and benefits of using this medication.

About Your Treatment

Your doctor has ordered metronidazole, an antibiotic, to help treat your infection. The drug will be added to an intravenous fluid that will drip through a needle or catheter placed in your vein for 1 hour, three or four times a day.

Metronidazole eliminates bacteria that cause many infections, including meningitis; pneumonia; and stomach, skin, bone, joint, heart, and gynecological infections. This medication is sometimes prescribed for other uses; ask your doctor or pharmacist for more information.

Your health care provider (doctor, nurse, or pharmacist) may measure the effectiveness and side effects of your treatment using laboratory tests and physical examinations. It is important to keep all appointments with your doctor and the laboratory. The length of treatment depends on how your infection and symptoms respond to the medication.

Precautions

Before administering metronidazole,

- tell your doctor and pharmacist if you are allergic to metronidazole or any other drugs.
- tell your doctor and pharmacist what prescription and nonprescription medications you are taking, especially anticoagulants ('blood thinners') such as warfarin (Coumadin), astemizole (Hismanal), disulfiram (Antabuse), lithium (Lithobid), phenobarbital, phenytoin (Dilantin), and vitamins.
- tell your doctor if you have or have ever had blood, kidney, or liver disease or Crohn's disease.
- tell your doctor if you are pregnant, plan to become pregnant, or are breast-feeding. If you become pregnant while taking metronidazole, call your doctor.
- remember you should not drink alcoholic beverages while taking metronidazole. Alcohol may cause an upset stomach, vomiting, abdominal cramps, headache, sweating, and flushing (redness of the face).
- plan to avoid unnecessary or prolonged exposure to sunlight and to wear protective clothing, sunglasses, and sunscreen. Metronidazole may make your skin sensitive to sunlight.

Administering Your Medication

Before you administer metronidazole, look at the solution closely. It should be clear and free of floating material. Gently squeeze the bag or observe the solution container to make sure there are no leaks. Do not use the solution if it is discolored, if it contains particles, or if the bag or container leaks. Use a new solution, but show the damaged one to your health care provider.

It is important that you use your medication exactly as directed. Do not stop your therapy on your own for any reason because your infection could worsen and result in hospitalization. Do not change your dosing schedule without talking to your health care provider. Your health care provider may tell you to stop your infusion if you have a mechanical problem (such as a blockage in the tubing, needle, or catheter); if you have to stop an infusion, call your health care provider immediately so your therapy can continue.

Side Effects

Metronidazole may cause side effects. Tell your health care provider if any of these symptoms are severe or do not go away:

- vomiting
- upset stomach
- diarrhea
- loss of appetite
- dry mouth or sharp, unpleasant metallic taste
- dark or reddish-brown urine
- furry tongue or mouth or tongue irritation
- numbness or tingling of the hands or feet

If you experience any of the following symptoms, call your health care provider immediately:

- rash
- itching
- stuffy nose
- fever
- joint pain

If you experience a serious side effect, you or your doctor may send a report to the Food and Drug Administration's (FDA) MedWatch Adverse Event Reporting program online [at http://www.fda.gov/MedWatch/index.html] or by phone [1-800-332-1088].

Storage Conditions

- Your health care provider probably will give you a several-day supply of metronidazole at a time. You will be told to store it at room temperature and protect it from direct light.

Store your medication only as directed. Make sure you understand what you need to store your medication properly.

Keep your supplies in a clean, dry place when you are not using them, and keep all medications and supplies out of reach of children. Your health care provider will tell you how to throw away used needles, syringes, tubing, and containers to avoid accidental injury.

Overdose

In case of overdose, call your local poison control center at 1-800-222-1222. If the victim has collapsed or is not breathing, call local emergency services at 911.

Signs of Infection

If you are receiving metronidazole in your vein or under your skin, you need to know the symptoms of a catheter-related infection (an infection where the needle enters your vein or skin). If you experience any of these effects near your intravenous catheter, tell your health care provider as soon as possible:

- tenderness
- warmth
- irritation
- drainage
- redness
- swelling
- pain

Dosage Facts
For Informational Purposes

Caution: Do not change your dose, how often you take your medication, or the length of time you are to take it without first talking to your health-care provider.

The following dosage information was written using medical language for doctors and other healthcare professionals and is provided here for you to check your dosage. The dosage of this drug may differ for different patients. Therefore, always follow your doctor's instructions or the directions on the label. Contact your healthcare provider or pharmacist if you have any questions about the specific dosage of your medication after reviewing this information.

General Dosage Information

Available as metronidazole and metronidazole hydrochloride; dosage expressed in terms of metronidazole.

Pediatric Patients

General Dosage in Neonates†

IV:
- Neonates <1 week of age: AAP recommends 7.5 mg/kg every 24–48 hours in those weighing <1.2 g, 7.5 mg/kg every 24 hours in those weighing 1.2–2 kg, or 7.5 mg/kg every 12 hours in those weighing >2 kg.
- Neonates 1–4 weeks of age: AAP recommends 7.5 mg/kg every 24–48 hours in those weighing <1.2 kg, 7.5 mg/kg every 12 hours in those weighing 1.2–2 kg, and 15 mg/kg every 12 hours in those weighing >2 kg.

Tetanus†

IV:
- 30 mg/kg daily (up to 4 g daily) in 4 doses given for 10–14 days.

Adult Patients

IV, THEN ORAL:
- An initial IV loading dose of 15 mg/kg followed by IV maintenance doses of 7.5 mg/kg every 6 hours. After clinical improvement occurs, switch to oral metronidazole (7.5 mg/kg every 6 hours).
- Total duration of treatment usually is 7–10 days, but infections of bone and joints, lower respiratory tract, or endocardium may require longer treatment.

Amebiasis
Entamoeba histolytic Infections

IV:
- 500 mg every 6 hours for 10 days.

Clostridium difficile-associated Diarrhea and Colitis†

IV:
- 500–750 mg every 6–8 hours; use when oral therapy is not feasible.

Tetanus†

IV:
- 500 mg every 6 hours given for 7–10 days.

Perioperative Prophylaxis
Colorectal Surgery

IV:
- 0.5 g given at induction of anesthesia (within 0.5–1 hour prior to incision); used in conjunction with IV cefazolin (1–2 g).
- Manufacturer recommends 15 mg/kg by IV infusion over 30–60 minutes 1 hour prior to the procedure and, if necessary, 7.5 mg/kg by IV infusion over 30–60 minutes at 6 and 12 hours after the initial dose. The initial preoperative dose must be completely infused approximately 1 hour prior to surgery to ensure adequate serum and tissue concentrations of metronidazole at the time of incision. Prophylactic use of metronidazole should be limited to the day of surgery and should not be continued for more than 12 hours after surgery.

Special Populations

Hepatic Impairment
- Decrease dosage in patients with severe hepatic impairment and monitor plasma concentrations of the drug.

Geriatric Patients
- Select dosage with caution because of age-related decreases in hepatic function.

† Use is not currently included in the labeling approved by the US Food and Drug Administration.

Metronidazole Oral

(me troe ni′ da zole)

Brand Name: Flagyl®, Flagyl® 375, Flagyl® ER, Helidac® Therapy
Also available generically.

Important Warning

Metronidazole can cause cancer in laboratory animals. Talk to your doctor about the risks and benefits of using this medication.

Why is this medicine prescribed?

Metronidazole eliminates bacteria and other microorganisms that cause infections of the reproductive system, gastrointestinal tract, skin, vagina, and other areas of the body. Antibiotics will not work for colds, flu, or other viral infections.

This medication is sometimes prescribed for other uses; ask your doctor or pharmacist for more information.

How should this medicine be used?

Metronidazole comes as a tablet to take by mouth. It is usually taken two or three times a day for 5-10 days or longer. Follow the directions on your prescription label carefully, and ask your doctor or pharmacist to explain any part you do not understand. Take metronidazole exactly as directed. Do not take more or less of it or take it more often than prescribed by your doctor.

What special precautions should I follow?

Before taking metronidazole,

- tell your doctor and pharmacist if you are allergic to metronidazole or any other drugs.
- tell your doctor and pharmacist what prescription and nonprescription medications you are taking, especially anticoagulants ('blood thinners') such as warfarin (Coumadin), astemizole (Hismanal), disulfiram (Antabuse), lithium (Lithobid), phenobarbital, phenytoin (Dilantin), and vitamins.
- tell your doctor if you have or have ever had blood, kidney, or liver disease or Crohn's disease.
- tell your doctor if you are pregnant, plan to become pregnant, or are breast-feeding. If you become pregnant while taking metronidazole, call your doctor.
- know that you should not drink alcohol while taking this drug. Alcohol may cause an upset stomach, vomiting, stomach cramps, headaches, sweating, and flushing (redness of the face).
- plan to avoid unnecessary or prolonged exposure to sunlight and to wear protective clothing, sunglasses, and sunscreen. Metronidazole may make your skin sensitive to sunlight.

What should I do if I forget to take a dose?

Take the missed dose as soon as you remember it. However, if it is almost time for the next dose, skip the missed dose and continue your regular dosing schedule. Do not take a double dose to make up for a missed one.

What side effects can this medicine cause?

Metronidazole may cause side effects. Tell your doctor if any of these symptoms are severe or do not go away:

- vomiting
- diarrhea
- upset stomach
- loss of appetite
- dry mouth; sharp, unpleasant metallic taste
- dark or reddish-brown urine
- furry tongue; mouth or tongue irritation
- numbness or tingling of hands or feet

If you experience any of the following symptoms, call your doctor immediately:

- rash
- itching
- stuffy nose
- fever
- joint pain

If you experience a serious side effect, you or your doctor may send a report to the Food and Drug Administration's (FDA) MedWatch Adverse Event Reporting program online [at http://www.fda.gov/MedWatch/index.html] or by phone [1-800-332-1088].

What storage conditions are needed for this medicine?

Keep this medication in the container it came in, tightly closed, and out of reach of children. Store it at room temperature and away from excess heat and moisture (not in the bathroom). Throw away any medication that is outdated or no longer needed. Talk to your pharmacist about the proper disposal of your medication.

What should I do in case of overdose?

In case of overdose, call your local poison control center at 1-800-222-1222. If the victim has collapsed or is not breathing, call local emergency services at 911.

What other information should I know?

Keep all appointments with your doctor and the laboratory. Your doctor will order certain lab tests to check your response to metronidazole.

Do not let anyone else take your medication. Your prescription is probably not refillable. If you still have symptoms of infection after you finish the metronidazole, call your doctor.

Dosage Facts
For Informational Purposes

Caution: Do not change your dose, how often you take your medication, or the length of time you are to take it without first talking to your healthcare provider.

The following dosage information was written using medical language for doctors and other healthcare professionals and is provided here for you to check your dosage. The dosage of this drug may differ for different patients. Therefore, always follow your doctor's instructions or the directions on the label. Contact your healthcare provider or pharmacist if you have any questions about the specific dosage of your medication after reviewing this information.

General Dosage Information

Available as metronidazole and metronidazole hydrochloride; dosage expressed in terms of metronidazole.

Pediatric Patients

General Dosage in Neonates†

ORAL:
- Neonates <1 week of age: AAP recommends 7.5 mg/kg every 24–48 hours in those weighing <1.2 g, 7.5 mg/kg every 24 hours in those weighing 1.2–2 kg, or 7.5 mg/kg every 12 hours in those weighing >2 kg.
- Neonates 1–4 weeks of age: AAP recommends 7.5 mg/kg every 24–48 hours in those weighing <1.2 kg, 7.5 mg/kg every 12 hours in those weighing 1.2–2 kg, and 15 mg/kg every 12 hours in those weighing >2 kg.

General Dosage in Children ≥1 Month of Age†

ORAL:
- 15–35 mg/kg daily in 3 divided doses. AAP states oral route inappropriate for severe infections.

Amebiasis
Entamoeba histolytica Infections

ORAL:
- 35–50 mg/kg daily in 3 divided doses given for 7–10 (usually 10) days; follow-up with a luminal amebicide (e.g., iodoquinol, paromomycin).

Bacterial Vaginosis†

ORAL:
- Children weighing <45 kg: 15 mg/kg daily (up to 1 g) in 2 divided doses given for 7 days.
- Adolescents: 500 mg twice daily for 7 days.

Balantidiasis†

ORAL:
- 35–50 mg/kg daily in 3 divided doses given for 5 days.

Blastocystis hominis Infections†

ORAL:
- 20–35 mg/kg daily in 3 divided doses given for 10 days may improve symptoms in some patients.

Crohn's Disease†

ORAL:
- 10–20 mg/kg daily (up to 1 g daily) has been recommended for children with mild perianal Crohn's disease† or those intolerant to sulfasalazine or mesalamine.

Clostridium difficile-associated Diarrhea and Colitis†

ORAL:
- 30–50 mg/kg daily in 3 or 4 equally divided doses given for 7–10 days (not to exceed adult dosage).

Dientamoeba fragilis Infections†

ORAL:
- 20–40 mg/kg daily in 3 divided doses given for 10 days.

Dracunculiasis†

ORAL:
- 25 mg/kg daily (up to 750 mg) in 3 divided doses given for 10 days. Is not curative, but may decrease inflammation and facilitate worm removal.

Giardiasis†

ORAL:
- 15 mg/kg daily in 3 divided doses given for 5–7 days.

Nongonococcal Urethritis†

ORAL:
- Recurrent or persistent urethritis in adolescents: A single 2-g dose given in conjunction with a single 1-g dose of oral azithromycin (if azithromycin not used in the initial regimen).

Tetanus†

ORAL:
- 30 mg/kg daily (up to 4 g daily) in 4 doses given for 10–14 days.

Trichomoniasis†

ORAL:
- Prepubertal children weighing <45 kg: 15 mg/kg daily in 3 divided doses (up to 2 g daily) given for 7 days.
- Adolescents: A single 2-g dose or 500 mg twice daily for 7 days.

Prophylaxis in Sexual Assault Victims†

ORAL:
- Preadolescent children weighing <45 kg: 15 mg/kg daily given in 3 divided doses for 7 days given in conjunction with IM ceftriaxone and either oral azithromycin or oral erythromycin.
- Adolescents and preadolescent children weighing ≥45 kg: A single 2-g dose given in conjunction with IM ceftriaxone and either oral azithromycin or oral doxycycline.

Adult Patients

Anaerobic Bacterial Infections
Serious Infections

ORAL:
- 7.5 mg/kg every 6 hours (up to 4 g daily).

Gynecologic Infections
Pelvic Inflammatory Disease

ORAL:
- 500 mg twice daily given for 14 days; used in conjunction with a single IM dose of ceftriaxone (250 mg), cefoxitin (2

g with oral probenecid 1 g), or another parenteral cephalosporin (e.g., cefotaxime) and 14-day regimen of oral doxycycline (100 mg twice daily).

- Alternatively, 500 mg twice daily given for 14 days; used in conjunction with a 14-day regimen of oral ofloxacin (400 mg twice daily) or levofloxacin (500 mg once daily). Regimens containing a fluoroquinolone should only be considered when a parenteral cephalosporin is not feasible and the community prevalence and individual risk of gonorrhea is low.

Amebiasis
Entamoeba histolytic Infections

ORAL:

- 750 mg 3 times daily given for 5–10 (usually 10) days for intestinal amebiasis or 500–750 mg 3 times daily given for 5–10 (usually 10) days for amebic liver abscess. Alternatively, amebic liver abscess has been treated with 2.4 g once daily given for 1 or 2 days.
- Follow-up with a luminal amebicide (e.g., iodoquinol, paromomycin) after metronidazole.

Bacterial Vaginosis
Nonpregnant Women

ORAL:

- Conventional tablets: 500 mg twice daily given for 7 days. A single 2-g dose has been used (e.g., for patients who may be noncompliant with the multiple-dose regimen), but appears to be less effective than other regimens and is no longer recommended by CDC.
- Extended-release tablets: 750 mg once daily given for 7 days.

Pregnant Women

ORAL:

- Conventional tablets: 500 mg twice daily or 250 mg 3 times daily given for 7 days.
- Contraindicated during first trimester of pregnancy. In addition, single-dose regimens not recommended in pregnant women because of the slightly higher serum concentrations attained, which may reach fetal circulation.

Balantidiasis†

ORAL:

- 750 mg 3 times daily given for 5 days.

Blastocystis hominis Infections†

ORAL:

- 750 mg 3 times daily given for 10 days may improve symptoms in some patients.

Crohn's Disease†

ORAL:

- 400 mg twice daily or 1 g daily has been effective for treatment of active Crohn's disease†. For treatment of refractory perineal disease, 20 mg/kg (1–1.5 g) given in 3–5 divided doses daily has been employed.

Clostridium difficile-associated Diarrhea and Colitis†

ORAL:

- 750 mg to 2 g daily in 3 or 4 divided doses given for 7–14 days.
- Dose-ranging studies to determine comparative efficacy have not been performed; most commonly employed regimens are 250 mg 4 times daily or 500 mg 3 times daily given for 10 days.

Dientamoeba fragilis Infections†

ORAL:

- 500–750 mg 3 times daily given for 10 days.

Dracunculiasis†

ORAL:

- 250 mg 3 times daily given for 10 days. Is not curative, but may decrease inflammation and facilitate worm removal.

Giardiasis†

ORAL:

- 250 mg 3 times daily given for 5–7 days.

Helicobacter pylori Infection and Duodenal Ulcer Disease

ORAL:

- 250 mg in conjunction with tetracycline (500 mg) and bismuth subsalicylate (525 mg) 4 times daily (at meals and at bedtime) for 14 days; these drugs should be given concomitantly with an H_2-receptor antagonist in recommended dosage.

Nongonococcal Urethritis†

ORAL:

- Recurrent or persistent urethritis: A single 2-g dose given in conjunction with a single 1-g dose of oral azithromycin (if azithromycin not used in the initial regimen).

Trichomoniasis
Initial Treatment

ORAL:

- 2 g as a single dose or in 2 divided doses. Alternatively, 500 mg twice daily given for 7 days or 375 mg twice daily given for 7 days. Manufacturer also recommends 250 mg 3 times daily given for 7 days.

Retreatment

ORAL:

- 500 mg twice daily given for 7 days. If repeated failure occurs, CDC recommends 2 g once daily given for 5 days. Others recommend retreatment with 2–4 g daily for 7–14 days if metronidazole-resistant strains are involved.
- Do not administer repeat courses of treatment unless presence of *T. vaginalis* is confirmed by wet smear and/or culture and an interval of 4–6 weeks has passed since the initial course.
- If treatment of resistant infection is guided by in vitro susceptibility testing under aerobic conditions, some clinicians recommend that *T. vaginalis* strains exhibiting low-level resistance (minimum lethal concentration [MLC] <100 mcg/mL) be treated with 2 g daily for 3–5 days, those with moderate (intermediate) resistance (MLC 100–200 mcg/mL) be treated with 2–2.5 g daily for 7–10 days, and those with high-level resistance (MLC >200 mcg/mL) be treated with 3–3.5 g daily for 14–21 days. Because strains with high-level resistance are difficult to treat, CDC recommends that patients with culture-documented infection who do not respond to repeat regimens at dosages up to 2 g daily for 3–5 days and in whom the possibility of reinfection has been excluded should be managed in consultation with an expert (available through CDC).

Perioperative Prophylaxis
Colorectal Surgery

ORAL:
- 2 g with oral neomycin sulfate (2 g) given at 7 p.m. and 11 p.m. on day before surgery; used in conjunction with appropriate diet and catharsis.

Prophylaxis in Sexual Assault Victims†

ORAL:
- A single 2-g dose given in conjunction with IM ceftriaxone and either oral azithromycin or oral doxycycline.

Special Populations

Hepatic Impairment
- Decrease dosage in patients with severe hepatic impairment and monitor plasma concentrations of the drug.

Geriatric Patients
- Select dosage with caution because of age-related decreases in hepatic function.

† Use is not currently included in the labeling approved by the US Food and Drug Administration.

Metronidazole Topical

(me troe ni′ da zole)

Brand Name: MetroCream®, MetroGel®, MetroGel®-Vaginal, MetroLotion®, Noritate®
Also available generically.

Why is this medicine prescribed?

Metronidazole is used to treat acne rosacea (adult acne), a chronic condition in which the facial skin is inflamed and sores develop. Metronidazole decreases the redness and number of sores but may not be a cure. It is also used to treat some vaginal infections.

This medication is sometimes prescribed for other uses; ask your doctor or pharmacist for more information.

How should this medicine be used?

Metronidazole comes as a cream, lotion, or gel to be applied to your skin and as a gel to be used in the vagina. Metronidazole usually is used once or twice a day. It is used twice daily for 5 consecutive days to treat vaginal infections. Follow the directions on your prescription label carefully, and ask your doctor or pharmacist to explain any part you do not understand. Use metronidazole exactly as directed. Do not use more or less of it or use it more often than prescribed by your doctor.

If you are using metronidazole to treat acne, your symptoms probably will improve within 3 weeks and continue to improve over the following 6 weeks or more. Continue to use metronidazole. Do not stop using metronidazole without talking to your doctor. Your symptoms may worsen when you stop the drug.

For acne, wash the affected skin area with mild soap about 15-20 minutes before applying the medication. Apply a thin layer of cream, lotion, or gel and rub it gently into the affected area. Do not allow the gel to get into your eyes. You may then apply a moisturizer (if your skin is dry) and cosmetics. Ask your doctor for advice on what cosmetics to use.

Metronidazole gel for the vagina comes with a special applicator. Read the instructions provided with it and follow these steps:
1. Fill the special applicator that comes with the gel to the level indicated.
2. Lie on your back with your knees drawn upward and spread apart.
3. Gently insert the applicator into your vagina and push the plunger to release the medication.
4. Withdraw the applicator and wash it with soap and warm water.
5. Wash your hands promptly to avoid spreading the infection.

The dose should be applied when you lie down to go to bed. The drug works best if you do not get up again after applying the drug except to wash your hands and the applicator. You may wish to wear a sanitary napkin while using the vaginal gel to protect your clothing against stains. Do not use a tampon because it will absorb the drug. While using this drug, do not douche because it will wash the drug out of the vagina and decrease its effectiveness. Continue using this drug even if you get your period during the time of treatment.

What special precautions should I follow?

Before using metronidazole,
- tell your doctor and pharmacist if you are allergic to metronidazole or any other drugs.
- tell your doctor and pharmacist what prescription and nonprescription medications you are taking, especially anticoagulants ('blood thinners') such as warfarin (Coumadin) and vitamins.
- tell your doctor if you have or have ever had a central nervous system disease, liver or blood disease, or Crohn's disease.
- tell your doctor if you are pregnant, plan to become pregnant, or are breast-feeding. If you become pregnant while using metronidazole, call your doctor.
- plan to avoid unnecessary or prolonged exposure to sunlight and to wear protective clothing, sunglasses, and sunscreen. Metronidazole may make your skin sensitive to sunlight.

What special dietary instructions should I follow?

Do not drink alcohol while using the vaginal gel. Alcohol may cause an upset stomach, vomiting, stomach cramps, headaches, sweating, and flushing (redness of the face).

What should I do if I forget to take a dose?

Apply the acne cream, lotion, or gel as soon as you remember but do not apply a double dose to make up for a missed dose.

Apply the vaginal gel the next morning or night and continue with your usual dosing schedule.

What side effects can this medicine cause?

Metronidazole may cause side effects. Tell your doctor if any of these symptoms are severe or do not go away:

- increased skin redness, dryness, burning, irritation, or stinging

If you experience any of the following symptoms while using the vaginal gel, call your doctor immediately:

- stomach pain
- fever
- foul-smelling vaginal discharge

If you experience a serious side effect, you or your doctor may send a report to the Food and Drug Administration's (FDA) MedWatch Adverse Event Reporting program online [at http://www.fda.gov/MedWatch/index.html] or by phone [1-800-332-1088].

What storage conditions are needed for this medicine?

Keep this medication in the container it came in, tightly closed, and out of reach of children. Store it at room temperature and away from excess heat and moisture (not in the bathroom). Throw away any medication that is outdated or no longer needed. Talk to your pharmacist about the proper disposal of your medication.

What other information should I know?

Keep all appointments with your doctor. Metronidazole is for external use only. Do not let metronidazole get into your eyes, nose, or mouth, and do not swallow it. Do not apply dressings, bandages, cosmetics, lotions, or other skin medications to the area being treated unless your doctor tells you.

Do not have sexual intercourse during the 5 days that you use the vaginal gel.

Do not let anyone else use your medication. Ask your pharmacist any questions you have about refilling your prescription.

If you still have symptoms of infection after you finish the metronidazole, call your doctor.

Dosage Facts
For Informational Purposes

Caution: Do not change your dose, how often you take your medication, or the length of time you are to take it without first talking to your healthcare provider.

The following dosage information was written using medical language for doctors and other healthcare pro-

fessionals and is provided here for you to check your dosage. The dosage of this drug may differ for different patients. Therefore, always follow your doctor's instructions or the directions on the label. Contact your healthcare provider or pharmacist if you have any questions about the specific dosage of your medication after reviewing this information.

Pediatric Patients

Bacterial Vaginosis
Treatment in Nonpregnant Postmenarchal Females

INTRAVAGINAL:

- 0.75% gel: One applicatorful (approximately 37.5 g of metronidazole) once daily (at bedtime) or twice daily (in morning and evening) given for 5 consecutive days.

Adult Patients

Rosacea

TOPICAL:

- 0.75% cream or lotion: Apply thin film to cleansed, affected area twice daily (morning and evening) or as directed by clinician.
- 1% cream or gel: Apply thin film to cleansed, affected area once daily.
- Optimum treatment duration not established; has been continued for ≥21 weeks in clinical studies.
- Chronic therapy (usually intermittent) may be necessary, particularly for moderate to severe disease.
- Clinical improvement usually occurs within 3 weeks. Once adequate response occurs, adjust frequency and duration of treatment according to disease course.
- Although disease may remit during treatment, relapse occurs commonly following discontinuance.

Bacterial Vaginosis
Treatment in Nonpregnant Women

INTRAVAGINAL:

- 0.75% gel: One applicatorful (approximately 37.5 g of metronidazole) once daily (at bedtime) or twice daily (in morning and evening) given for 5 consecutive days.

Miconazole

(mi kon' a zole)

Brand Name: Desenex® Athlete's Foot Shake Powder, Desenex® Athlete's Foot Spray Powder, Desenex® Jock Itch Spray Powder, Desenex® Spray Liquid, Femizol-M®, Fungoid®, Lotrimin® AF Athlete's Foot Deodorant Spray Powder, Lotrimin® AF Athlete's Foot Powder, Lotrimin® AF Athlete's Foot Spray Liquid, Lotrimin® AF Athlete's Foot Spray Powder, Lotrimin® AF Jock Itch Spray Powder, Micatin® Athlete's Foot Cream, Micatin® Athlete's Foot Spray Liquid, Micatin® Athlete's Foot Spray Powder, Micatin® Jock Itch Cream, Micatin® Jock Itch Spray Powder, Monistat® 3, Monistat® 3 Combination Pack®, Monistat® 7, Monistat® 7 Combination Pack®, Monistat®1 Combination Pack Dual-Pak®, Monistat-Derm®, Ting® Antifungal Spray Powder, Ting® Spray Liquid, Zeasorb®-AF, Zeasorb®-AF Lotion

Why is this medicine prescribed?

Miconazole, an antifungal agent, is used for skin infections such as athlete's foot and jock itch and for vaginal yeast infections.

This medication is sometimes prescribed for other uses; ask your doctor or pharmacist for more information.

How should this medicine be used?

Miconazole comes as a cream, lotion, powder, spray liquid, and spray powder to be applied to the skin. It also comes as a cream and suppository to be inserted into the vagina. Miconazole is usually used once or twice a day for 1 month for athlete's foot or 2 weeks for other skin infections. For vaginal infections, it is used once a day at bedtime for 3 (Monistat-3) or 7 (Monistat-7) days. Follow the directions on the package or on your prescription label carefully, and ask your doctor or pharmacist to explain any part you do not understand. Use miconazole exactly as directed. Do not use more or less of it or use it more often than directed by your doctor.

It probably will take several days for improvement to be seen in skin infections.

Apply the topical forms of miconazole sparingly to the infected area after washing and drying the skin thoroughly. The cream and lotion should be rubbed gently into the skin. Wash your hands promptly.

If you are using miconazole vaginal cream or suppositories, read the instructions provided with the medication and follow these steps:

1. Fill the special applicator that comes with the cream to the level indicated, or unwrap a suppository and place it on the applicator as shown in the instructions.
2. Lie on your back with your knees drawn upward and spread apart.
3. Gently insert the applicator into the vagina, and push the plunger to release the medication.
4. Withdraw the applicator.
5. Discard the applicator if it is disposable. If the applicator is reusable, pull it apart and clean it with soap and warm water after each use.
6. Wash your hands promptly to avoid spreading the infection.

The dose should be applied when you lie down to go to bed. It works best if you do not get up after applying it except to wash your hands. You may wish to wear a sanitary napkin while using the suppositories or vaginal cream to protect your clothing against stains. Do not use a tampon because it will absorb the drug. Do not douche unless your doctor tells you to do so. Continue using miconazole vaginal cream or suppositories even if you get your period during treatment.

What special precautions should I follow?

Before using miconazole,
- tell your doctor and pharmacist if you are allergic to miconazole or any other drugs.
- tell your doctor and pharmacist what prescription and nonprescription medications you are taking, including vitamins.
- tell your doctor if you are pregnant, plan to become pregnant, or are breast-feeding. If you become pregnant while taking miconazole, call your doctor. Before using miconazole, tell your doctor if you are using a diaphragm or condom for birth control and are being treated for a vaginal infection. Miconazole vaginal cream and suppositories can interact with the latex in diaphragms and condoms, so use another method of birth control.

What should I do if I forget to take a dose?

Apply the missed dose as soon as you remember it. If you remember a missed dose at the time you are scheduled to apply the next one, omit the missed dose completely and use only the regularly scheduled dose. Do not use a double dose to make up for a missed one.

What side effects can this medicine cause?

Miconazole may cause side effects. If you experience any of the following symptoms, call your doctor immediately:
- increased burning, itching, or irritation of the skin or vagina
- stomach pain
- fever
- foul-smelling vaginal discharge

If you experience a serious side effect, you or your doctor may send a report to the Food and Drug Administration's (FDA) MedWatch Adverse Event Reporting program online [at http://www.fda.gov/MedWatch/index.html] or by phone [1-800-332-1088].

What storage conditions are needed for this medicine?

Keep this medication in the container it came in, tightly closed, and out of reach of children. Store it at room temperature and away from excess heat and moisture (not in the bathroom). Throw away any medication that is outdated or no longer needed. Talk to your pharmacist about the proper disposal of your medication.

What other information should I know?

Keep all appointments with your doctor. Miconazole is for external use only. Do not let miconazole get into your eyes, nose, or mouth, and do not swallow it. Do not apply dressings, bandages, cosmetics, lotions, or other skin medications to the area being treated unless your doctor tells you.

If you obtained the topical form of miconazole without a prescription and your symptoms do not improve within 4 weeks (2 weeks for jock itch), stop using it and talk to a pharmacist or doctor.

If this is the first time you have had vaginal itching and discomfort, talk to a doctor before using miconazole. If a doctor has told you before that you had a yeast infection and you have the same symptoms again, use the vaginal cream or suppositories as directed on the package.

Do not let anyone else use your medication. Ask your pharmacist any questions you have about refilling your prescription.

If you still have symptoms of infection after you finish the miconazole, call your doctor.

Talk to your doctor, pharmacist, or other healthcare professional if you have questions about dosing information for your medication.

Mifepristone

(mi fe′ pri stone)

Brand Name: Mifeprex®

> ## Important Warning
>
> Serious or life threatening vaginal bleeding may occur when a pregnancy is ended by miscarriage or by medical or surgical abortion. It is not known if taking mifepristone increases the risk that you will experience very heavy bleeding. Tell your doctor if you have or have ever had bleeding problems, an ectopic pregnancy ('tubal pregnancy' or pregnancy outside the uterus), anemia (less than normal number of red blood cells), or if you are taking anticoagulants ('blood thinners') such as warfarin (Coumadin), heparin, or aspirin. If you experience very heavy vaginal bleeding, such as soaking through two thick full-size sanitary pads every hour for two continuous hours, call your doctor immediately or seek emergency medical care.
>
> Serious or life threatening infections may occur when a pregnancy is ended by miscarriage or by medical or surgical abortion. A small number of patients died due to infections that they developed after they used mifepristone and misoprostol to end their pregnancies. Some of these patients had used misoprostol vaginally; vaginal use of oral misoprostol tablets has not been approved by the Food and Drug Administration (FDA). It is not known if mifepristone and/or misoprostol taken vaginally or by mouth caused these infections or deaths.
>
> If you develop a serious infection, you may not have many symptoms and your symptoms may not be very severe. You should call your doctor immediately if you experience any of the following symptoms: fever greater than 100.4 °F that lasts for more than 4 hours, severe pain or tenderness in the area below the waist, chills, fast heartbeat, or fainting.
>
> You should also call your doctor immediately if you have general symptoms of illness such as weakness, upset stomach, vomiting, diarrhea, or feeling sick more than 24 hours after taking mifepristone even if you do not have a fever or pain in the area below your waist.
>
> Your doctor will give you the manufacturer's patient information sheet (Medication Guide) to read before you begin treatment with mifepristone. You will also need to sign a patient agreement before taking mifepristone. Tell your doctor if you have questions about treatment with mifepristone or if you cannot follow the guidelines in the patient agreement.
>
> Talk to your doctor and decide whom to call and what to do in case of an emergency after taking mifepristone. Tell your doctor if you do not think that you will be able to follow this plan or to get medical treatment quickly in an emergency during the first two weeks after you take mifepristone. Take your medication guide with you if you visit an emergency room or seek emergency medical care so that the doctors who treat you will understand that you are undergoing a medical abortion.
>
> Keep all appointments with your doctor. These appointments are necessary to be sure that your pregnancy has ended and that you have not developed serious complications of medical abortion.
>
> Talk to your doctor about the risks of taking mifepristone.

Why is this medicine prescribed?

Mifepristone is used alone or in combination with misoprostol (Cytotec) to end an early pregnancy. Early pregnancy means it has been 49 days or less since your last menstrual period began. Mifepristone is in a class of medications called antiprogestational steroids. It works by blocking the activity of progesterone, a substance your body makes to help continue pregnancy.

How should this medicine be used?

Mifepristone comes as a tablet to take by mouth. It should be taken only in a clinic, medical office, or hospital under the supervision of a qualified doctor. You will take three tablets of mifepristone at one time on the first day. Two days later you must go back to your doctor. If your doctor is not certain that your pregnancy has ended, you will take two tablets of another medication called misoprostol. You may have vaginal bleeding for 9 to 30 days or longer. Fourteen days after taking mifepristone, you must go back to your doctor for an exam or ultrasound to make sure that the pregnancy has ended. Take mifepristone exactly as directed.

Are there other uses for this medicine?

Mifepristone is also sometimes used to end pregnancies when more than 49 days have passed since the woman's last menstrual period; as an emergency contraceptive after unprotected sexual intercourse ('morning-after pill'); to treat tumors of the brain, endometriosis (growth of uterus tissue outside the uterus), or fibroids (noncancerous tumors in the uterus); or to induce labor (to help start the birth process in a pregnant woman). Talk to your doctor about the possible risks of using this drug for your condition.

What special precautions should I follow?

Before taking mifepristone,

- tell your doctor if you are allergic to mifepristone; misoprostol (Arthrotec, Cytotec); other prostaglandins such as alprostadil, carboprost tromethamine (Hemabate), dinoprostone (Cervidil, Prepidil, Prostin E2), epoprostenol (Flolan), latanoprost (Xalatan), treprostinil (Remodulin); or any other medications.
- do not take mifepristone if you are taking any of the medications listed in the IMPORTANT WARNING section or corticosteroids such as beclomethasone (QVAR inhaler), betamethasone (Celestone), budesonide (Entocort, Pulmicort), cortisone (Cortone), dexamethasone (Decadron, Dexpak, Dexasone, others), fludrocortisone (Floriner), flunisolide (AeroBid); fluticasone (Advair, Flovent), hydrocortisone (Cortef, Cortenema, Hydrocortone), methylprednisolone (Medrol, Meprolone, others), prednisolone (Prelone, others), prednisone (Deltasone, Meticorten, Sterapred, others), and triamcinolone (Aristocort, Azmacort).
- tell your doctor what other prescription and nonprescription medications, vitamins, and nutritional supplements you are taking. Be sure to mention the medications listed in the IMPORTANT WARNING section and any of the following: amiodarone (Cordarone, Pacerone); astemizole; benzodiazepines such as alprazolam (Xanax), diazepam (Valium), midazolam (Versed), or triazolam (Halcion); buspirone (BuSpar); calcium

channel blockers such as amlodipine (Norvasc), diltiazem (Cardizem, Dilacor, Tiazac, others), felodipine (Lexxel, Plendil), nifedipine (Adalat, Procardia), nisoldipine (Sular), nitrendipine, or verapamil (Calan, Isoptin, Verelan); carbamazepine (Tegretol); chlorpheniramine (antihistamine in cough and cold products); cholesterol-lowering medications (statins) such as atorvastatin (Lipitor), cerivastatin, lovastatin (Mevacor), or simvastatin (Zocor); cimetidine (Tagamet); cisapride; clarithromycin (Biaxin, Prevpac); cyclosporine (Neoral, Sandimmune); dicloxacillin; erythromycin (E.E.S., EM-Mycin, Erythrocin); fluoxetine (Prozac, Sarafem); fluvoxamine (Luvox); haloperidol; furosemide; HIV protease inhibitors such as indinavir (Crixivan), nelfinavir (Viracept), ritonavir (Norvir), or saquinavir (Fortovase, Invirase); itraconazole (Sporanox); ketoconazole (Nizoral); methadone (Dolophine, Methadose); nefazodone (Serzone); phenobarbital (Luminal, Solfoton); phenytoin (Dilantin); pimozide (Orap); propranolol (Inderal); quinidine; quinine; rifampin (Rifadin, Rimactane); rifabutin (Mycobutin); tacrolimus (Prograf, Protopic); tamoxifen (Nolvadex); trazodone; troleandomycin (TAO); verapamil (Calan, Covera, Isoptin, Verelan, others); or vincristine (Vincasar). Your doctor may need to change the doses of your medications or monitor you carefully for side effects.
- tell your doctor what herbal products you are taking, especially St. John's wort.
- tell your doctor if you have or have ever had any of the conditions listed in the IMPORTANT WARNING section or any of the following: diabetes; high blood pressure; porphyria (an inherited blood disease that may cause skin or nervous system problems); adrenal failure (problems with your adrenal glands); or heart, kidney, liver, or lung disease
- tell your doctor if you have an intrauterine device (IUD) in place. It must be taken out before you take mifepristone.
- you should know that it is possible that mifepristone will not end your pregnancy. Your doctor will check to be sure that your pregnancy has ended when you return for your follow up appointments after you take mifepristone. If your pregnancy has not ended, you may choose to have surgery to end the pregnancy. If you do not have this surgery, your baby may be born with birth defects.
- tell your doctor if you are breast-feeding. You may need to stop breast-feeding for a few days after taking mifepristone.
- if you are having surgery, including dental surgery, tell the doctor or dentist that you have taken mifepristone.
- you should know that mifepristone may make you dizzy. Do not drive a car or operate machinery until you know how this medication affects you.
- tell your doctor if you smoke 10 or more cigarettes a day or if you have a history of heavy smoking.
- you should know that after ending a pregnancy with

mifepristone, you can become pregnant again right away, even before your period returns. If you do not want to become pregnant again, you should begin using birth control as soon as this pregnancy ends or before you start having sexual intercourse again.

What special dietary instructions should I follow?

Do not take mifepristone with grapefruit juice. Talk to your doctor about drinking grapefruit juice after taking this medication.

What should I do if I forget to take a dose?

You will only take mifepristone in your doctor's office or clinic, so you do not have to worry about forgetting to take a dose at home.

What side effects can this medicine cause?

Mifepristone may cause side effects. Tell your doctor if any of these symptoms are severe or do not go away:
- vaginal bleeding or spotting
- cramps
- pelvic pain
- vaginal burning, itching, or discharge
- headache
- tiredness
- difficulty falling asleep or staying asleep
- anxiety
- back or leg pain

Some side effects can be serious. If you experience any of the symptoms mentioned in the IMPORTANT WARNING section, call your doctor immediately.

Mifepristone may cause other side effects. Call your doctor if you have any unusual problems while taking this medication.

If you experience a serious side effect, you or your doctor may send a report to the Food and Drug Administration's (FDA) MedWatch Adverse Event Reporting program online [at http://www.fda.gov/MedWatch/index.html] or by phone [1-800-332-1088].

What storage conditions are needed for this medicine?

Your doctor will store the medication in his or her office.

What should I do in case of overdose?

In case of overdose, call your local poison control center at 1-800-222-1222. If the victim has collapsed or is not breathing, call local emergency services at 911.

Symptoms of overdose may include:
- dizziness
- fainting
- blurred vision
- upset stomach

- tiredness
- weakness
- shortness of breath
- fast heart beat

What other information should I know?

You should get mifepristone only from a doctor and use this medication only while under the care of a doctor. You should not buy mifepristone from other sources, such as the Internet, because you would bypass important safeguards to protect your health.

Do not let anyone else take your medication.

Dosage Facts
For Informational Purposes

Caution: Do not change your dose, how often you take your medication, or the length of time you are to take it without first talking to your healthcare provider.

The following dosage information was written using medical language for doctors and other healthcare professionals and is provided here for you to check your dosage. The dosage of this drug may differ for different patients. Therefore, always follow your doctor's instructions or the directions on the label. Contact your healthcare provider or pharmacist if you have any questions about the specific dosage of your medication after reviewing this information.

Adult Patients
Termination of Pregnancy

ORAL:
- 600 mg as a single dose. Two days later, administer misoprostol 400 mcg orally unless complete abortion confirmed.

Miglitol

(mig' li tol)

Brand Name: Glyset®

Why is this medicine prescribed?

Miglitol is used, alone or with other drugs, to treat type 2 diabetes (condition in which the body does not use insulin normally and, therefore, cannot control the amount of sugar in the blood), particularly in people whose diabetes cannot be controlled by diet alone. It slows the breakdown and absorption of table sugar and other complex sugars in the small intestine. This process results in decreased blood sugar (hypoglycemia) levels following meals.

This medication is sometimes prescribed for other uses; ask your doctor or pharmacist for more information.

How should this medicine be used?

Miglitol comes as a tablet to take by mouth. It is usually taken three times a day with the first bite of a meal. Follow the directions on your prescription label carefully, and ask your doctor or pharmacist to explain any part you do not understand. Take miglitol exactly as directed. Do not take more or less of it or take it more often than prescribed by your doctor.

What special precautions should I follow?

Before taking miglitol,
- tell your doctor and pharmacist if you are allergic to miglitol or any other drugs.
- tell your doctor and pharmacist what prescription and nonprescription medications you are taking, especially other medications for diabetes, digestive enzymes (Viokase, Pancrease, or Ultrase), digoxin (Lanoxin), propranolol (Inderal), ranitidine (Zantac), and vitamins.
- tell your doctor if you have or have ever had a chronic intestinal disease, inflammatory bowel disease, intestinal obstruction, or kidney disease.
- tell your doctor if you are pregnant, plan to become pregnant, or are breast-feeding. If you become pregnant while taking miglitol, call your doctor.

What special dietary instructions should I follow?

Miglitol is used in combination with proper diet and exercise to control blood sugar. Skipping or delaying meals or exercising more than usual may cause your blood sugar to fall too low (hypoglycemia). Maintaining the diet and exercise program suggested by your doctor will ensure that the drug works properly.

Alcohol may cause a decrease in blood sugar. Ask your doctor about the safe use of alcoholic beverages while you are taking miglitol.

What should I do if I forget to take a dose?

Take the missed dose as soon as you remember it. Remember that miglitol should only be taken with a meal. However, if it is almost time for the next dose, skip the missed dose and continue your regular dosing schedule. Do not take a double dose to make up for a missed one.

What side effects can this medicine cause?

When used in combination with insulin or other medications used to treat diabetes, miglitol may cause excessive lowering of blood sugar levels.

If you have any of the following symptoms, glucose products (Insta-Glucose or B-D Glucose tablets) should be used and you should call your doctor. Because miglitol blocks the breakdown of table sugar and other complex sugars, fruit juice or other products containing these sugars will not help to increase blood sugar. It is important that you and other members of your household understand this difference between miglitol and other medications used to treat diabetes.
- shakiness
- dizziness or lightheadedness
- sweating
- nervousness or irritability
- sudden changes in behavior or mood
- headache
- numbness or tingling around the mouth
- weakness
- pale skin
- hunger
- clumsy or jerky movements

If hypoglycemia is not treated, severe symptoms may develop. Be sure that your family, friends, and other people who spend time with you know that if you have any of the following symptoms, they should get medical treatment for you immediately.
- confusion
- seizures
- loss of consciousness

Call your doctor immediately if you have any of the following symptoms of hyperglycemia (high blood sugar):
- extreme thirst
- frequent urination
- extreme hunger
- weakness
- blurred vision

If high blood sugar is not treated, a serious, life-threatening condition called diabetic ketoacidosis could develop. Call your doctor immediately if you have any of these symptoms:
- dry mouth
- upset stomach and vomiting
- shortness of breath
- breath that smells fruity
- decreased consciousness

Miglitol may cause side effects. Tell your doctor if any of these symptoms are severe or do not go away:
- gas
- diarrhea
- stomach pain
- skin rash

What storage conditions are needed for this medicine?

Keep this medication in the container it came in, tightly closed, and out of reach of children. Store it at room temperature and away from excess heat and moisture (not in the bathroom). Throw away any medication that is outdated or no longer needed. Talk to your pharmacist about the proper disposal of your medication.

What should I do in case of overdose?

In case of overdose, call your local poison control center at 1-800-222-1222. If the victim has collapsed or is not breathing, call local emergency services at 911.

What other information should I know?

Keep all appointments with your doctor and the laboratory. Your blood sugar should be checked regularly to determine your response to miglitol. Your doctor will order certain lab tests to check your response to miglitol. Your doctor will also tell you how to check your response to this medication by measuring your blood or urine sugar levels at home. Follow these instructions carefully.

You should always wear a diabetic identification bracelet to be sure you get proper treatment in an emergency.

Do not let anyone else take your medication. Ask your pharmacist any questions you have about refilling your prescription.

Talk to your doctor, pharmacist, or other healthcare professional if you have questions about dosing information for your medication.

Minocycline Oral

(mi noe sye′ kleen)

Brand Name: Dynacin®, Minocin®, Myrac®
Also available generically.

Why is this medicine prescribed?

Minocycline is used to treat bacterial infections including pneumonia and other respiratory tract infections; acne; and infections of skin, genital, and urinary systems. It can also be used to eliminate bacteria from your nose and throat that may cause meningitis (swelling of tissues around the brain) in others, even though you may not have an infection. Minocycline is in a class of medications called tetracycline antibiotics. It works by preventing the growth and spread of bacteria. Antibiotics will not work for colds, flu, or other viral infections.

How should this medicine be used?

Minocycline comes as a regular capsule, a pellet-filled capsule, and a tablet, to take by mouth. It usually is taken twice a day (every 12 hours) but may be taken up to four times a day. Minocycline should be taken on an empty stomach, at least 1 hour before or 2 hours after meals. Drink a full glass of water with each dose. Follow the directions on your prescription label carefully, and ask your doctor or pharmacist to explain any part you do not understand. Take minocycline exactly as directed. Do not take more or less of it or take it more often than prescribed by your doctor.

Do not break, crush, or chew the regular or pellet-filled capsules; swallow them whole.

Are there other uses for this medicine?

This medication is sometimes prescribed for other uses; ask your doctor or pharmacist for more information.

What special precautions should I follow?

Before taking minocycline,

- tell your doctor and pharmacist if you are allergic to minocycline, tetracycline, doxycycline, or any other medications.
- tell your doctor and pharmacist what other prescription and nonprescription medications, vitamins, nutritional supplements, and herbal products you are taking or plan to take, especially acetaminophen (Tylenol, others), antacids, anticoagulants ('blood thinners') such as warfarin (Coumadin), cholesterol-lowering medications (statins), ergot-type medications such as bromocriptine (Parlodel), cabergoline (Dostinex), dihydroergotamine (D.H.E. 45, Migranal), ergoloid mesylates (Germinal, Hydergine), ergonovine (Ergotrate), ergotamine (Bellergal-S, Cafergot, Ergomar, Wigraine), methylergonovine (Methergine), methysergide (Sansert), and pergolide (Permax) iron products, isoniazid (INH, Nydrazid), methotrexate (Rheumatrex), niacin (nicotinic acid), penicillin, and rifampin (Rifadin, Rimactane). Also tell your doctor or pharmacist if you are taking isotretinoin (Accutane, Sotret, others) or have recently stopped taking it. Your doctor may need to change the doses of your medications or monitor you carefully for side effects. Minocycline decreases the effectiveness of some oral contraceptives; talk to your doctor about selecting another form of birth control to use while taking this medication.
- be aware that antacids, calcium supplements, iron products, and laxatives containing magnesium interfere with minocycline, making it less effective. Take minocycline 1 hour before or 2 hours after antacids (including sodium bicarbonate), calcium supplements, and laxatives containing magnesium. Take minocycline 2 hours before or 3 hours after iron preparations and vitamin products that contain iron.
- tell your doctor if you have or have ever had diabetes or kidney or liver disease.
- tell your doctor if you are pregnant, plan to become pregnant, or are breast-feeding. If you become pregnant while taking minocycline, call your doctor immediately. Minocycline can harm the fetus.
- if you are having surgery, including dental surgery, tell the doctor or dentist that you are taking minocycline.
- you should know that minocycline may make you lightheaded or dizzy. Do not drive a car or operate machinery until you know how this medication affects you. These effects may go away as you continue to take minocycline and usually go away quickly when you stop taking this medication.

- plan to avoid unnecessary or prolonged exposure to sunlight and to wear protective clothing, sunglasses, and sunscreen. Minocycline may make your skin sensitive to sunlight.
- you should know that when doxycycline is used during pregnancy or in babies or children up to age 8, it can cause the teeth to become permanently stained. Minocycline should not be used in children under age 8 except for inhalational anthrax or if your doctor decides it is needed.

What special dietary instructions should I follow?

Unless your doctor tells you otherwise, continue your normal diet.

What should I do if I forget to take a dose?

Take the missed dose as soon as you remember it. However, if it is almost time for the next dose, skip the missed dose and continue your regular dosing schedule. Do not take a double dose to make up for a missed one.

What side effects can this medicine cause?

Minocycline may cause side effects. Tell your doctor if any of these symptoms are severe or do not go away:
- itching of the rectum or vagina
- diarrhea
- dizziness or lightheadedness
- furry darkening or black discoloration of the tongue
- redness of the skin (sunburn)
- changes in skin color
- hearing loss or ringing in your ears

Some side effects can be serious. If you experience any of these symptoms, call your doctor immediately:
- severe headache
- blurred vision
- skin rash
- hives
- difficulty breathing or swallowing
- yellowing of the skin or eyes
- itching
- dark-colored urine
- light-colored bowel movements
- loss of appetite
- upset stomach
- vomiting
- stomach pain
- extreme tiredness or weakness
- confusion
- joint stiffness or swelling
- unusual bleeding or bruising
- decreased urination
- pain or discomfort in the mouth
- throat sores
- fever or chills

If you experience a serious side effect, you or your doctor may send a report to the Food and Drug Administration's (FDA) MedWatch Adverse Event Reporting program online [at http://www.fda.gov/MedWatch/index.html] or by phone [1-800-332-1088].

What storage conditions are needed for this medicine?

Keep this medication in the container it came in, tightly closed, and out of reach of children. Store it at room temperature and away from excess heat and moisture (not in the bathroom). Throw away any medication that is outdated or no longer needed. Talk to your pharmacist about the proper disposal of your medication.

What should I do in case of overdose?

In case of overdose, call your local poison control center at 1-800-222-1222. If the victim has collapsed or is not breathing, call local emergency services at 911.

Symptoms of overdose may include:
- dizziness
- upset stomach
- vomiting

What other information should I know?

Keep all appointments with your doctor and the laboratory. Your doctor will order certain lab tests to check your response to minocycline.

Before having any laboratory test, tell your doctor and the laboratory personnel that you are taking minocycline.

If you have diabetes, minocycline can cause false results in some tests for sugar in the urine. Check with your doctor before changing your diet or the dosage of your diabetes medicine.

Do not let anyone else take your medication. Your prescription is probably not refillable. If you still have symptoms of infection after you finish the minocycline, call your doctor.

Dosage Facts
For Informational Purposes

Caution: Do not change your dose, how often you take your medication, or the length of time you are to take it without first talking to your healthcare provider.

The following dosage information was written using medical language for doctors and other healthcare professionals and is provided here for you to check your dosage. The dosage of this drug may differ for different patients. Therefore, always follow your doctor's instructions or the directions on the label. Contact your healthcare provider or pharmacist if you have any questions about the specific dosage of your medication after reviewing this information.

General Dosage Information

Available as minocycline hydrochloride; dosage expressed in terms of minocycline.

Pediatric Patients

General Pediatric Dosage

ORAL:
- Children >8 years of age: 4 mg/kg initially followed by 2 mg/kg every 12 hours.

Mycobacterial Infections

Leprosy†

ORAL:
- Children 5–14 years of age: for treatment of single-lesion paucibacillary leprosy† in certain patient groups, WHO recommends a single-dose ROM regimen that includes a single 300-mg dose of rifampin, a single 200-mg dose of ofloxacin, and a single 50-mg dose of minocycline.
- Children <5 years of age: WHO recommends that an appropriately adjusted dose of each drug in the single-dose ROM regimen be used.

Adult Patients

General Adult Dosage

ORAL:
- 200 mg initially followed by 100 mg every 12 hours.
- Alternatively, if more frequent doses are preferred, 100–200 mg initially followed by 50 mg 4 times daily.

Acne

ORAL:
- 50 mg 1–3 times daily.

Chlamydial Infections

Uncomplicated Urethral, Endocervical, or Rectal Infections

ORAL:
- 100 mg every 12 hours given for ≥7 days.

Gonorrhea and Associated Infections

Uncomplicated Gonorrhea (except Urethritis or Anorectal in Men)

ORAL:
- 200 mg initially followed by 100 mg every 12 hours given for ≥ 4 days; follow-up cultures should be done within 2–3 days after completion of therapy.
- No longer recommended for gonorrhea by CDC or other experts.

Gonococcal Urethritis in Men

ORAL:
- 100 mg every 12 hours given for 5 days.
- No longer recommended for gonorrhea by CDC or other experts.

Mycobacterial Infections

Leprosy†

ORAL:
- For treatment of multibacillary leprosy† in those who cannot receive rifampin because of adverse effects, intercurrent disease (e.g., chronic hepatitis), or infection with rifampin-resistant *M. leprae*, WHO recommends supervised administration of a regimen of clofazimine (50 mg daily), ofloxacin (400 mg daily), and minocycline (100 mg daily) given for 6 months, followed by a regimen of clofazimine (50 mg daily) and mi-

nocycline (100 mg daily) given for at least an additional 18 months.
- For treatment of multibacillary leprosy in adults who will not accept or cannot tolerate clofazimine, WHO recommends supervised administration of a once-monthly ROM regimen that includes rifampin (600 mg once monthly), ofloxacin (400 mg once monthly), and minocycline (100 mg once monthly) given for 24 months.
- For treatment of single-lesion paucibacillary leprosy† in certain patient groups, WHO recommends a single-dose ROM regimen that includes a single 600-mg dose of rifampin, a single 400-mg dose of ofloxacin, and a single 100-mg dose of minocycline.

Mycobacterium marinum Infections

ORAL:
- Manufacturers state optimum dosage has not been established, but 100 mg every 12 hours for 6–8 weeks has been effective.
- 100 mg twice daily for ≥3 months recommended by ATS for treatment of cutaneous infections. A minimum of 4–6 weeks of treatment usually is necessary to determine whether the infection is responding.

Neisseria meningitidis Infections

N. meningitidis Carriers

ORAL:
- 100 mg every 12 hours given for 5 days.

Nocardiosis†

ORAL:
- 200 mg initially followed by 100 mg every 12 hours given for 12–18 months.

Nongonoccocal Urethritis

ORAL:
- 100 mg every 12 hours given for ≥ 7 days.

Rheumatoid Arthritis†

ORAL:
- 100 mg twice daily. A benefit may be evident within 1–3 months.

Syphilis

ORAL:
- 200 mg initially followed by 100 mg every 12 hours given for 10–15 days. Close follow-up and laboratory tests are recommended.

Vibrio Infections

Cholera

ORAL:
- 200 mg initially followed by 100 mg every 12 hours given for 2–3 days.

Prescribing Limits

Pediatric Patients

ORAL:
- Do not exceed usual adult dosage.

Minoxidil Oral

(mi nox′ i dill)

Brand Name: Loniten®
Also available generically.

Important Warning

Minoxidil may increase chest pain (angina) or cause other heart problems. It is important that you keep all appointments with your doctor so that you can be monitored for any symptoms or changes. If chest pain occurs or worsens while you are taking this medication, call your doctor immediately. Your doctor may prescribe other medicines as part of your minoxidil therapy. Do not stop taking these medications unless your doctor tells you to do so.

Why is this medicine prescribed?

Minoxidil is used with other drugs to treat high blood pressure. It works by relaxing the blood vessels so that blood can flow more easily through the body.

This medication is sometimes prescribed for other uses; ask your doctor or pharmacist for more information.

How should this medicine be used?

Minoxidil comes as a tablet to take by mouth. It usually is taken once or twice a day. Follow the directions on your prescription label carefully, and ask your doctor or pharmacist to explain any part you do not understand. Take minoxidil exactly as directed. Do not take more or less of it or take it more often than prescribed by your doctor.

Minoxidil controls high blood pressure but does not cure it. Continue to take minoxidil even if you feel well. Do not stop taking minoxidil without talking to your doctor.

What special precautions should I follow?

Before taking minoxidil,
- tell your doctor and pharmacist if you are allergic to minoxidil or any other drugs.
- tell your doctor and pharmacist what prescription and nonprescription medications you are taking, especially other medications for high blood pressure, diuretics ('water pills'), guanethidine, and vitamins.
- tell your doctor if you have or have ever had heart disease, a heart attack, pheochromocytoma, or kidney disease.
- tell your doctor if you are pregnant, plan to become pregnant, or are breast-feeding. If you become pregnant while taking minoxidil, call your doctor.
- if you are having surgery, including dental surgery, tell the doctor or dentist that you are taking minoxidil.
- you should know that this drug may make you drowsy. Do not drive a car or operate machinery until you know how it affects you.
- ask your doctor about the safe use of alcohol while you are taking minoxidil. Alcohol can make the side effects from minoxidil worse.

What special dietary instructions should I follow?

Your doctor may prescribe a low-salt or low-sodium diet. Follow these directions carefully.

What should I do if I forget to take a dose?

Take the missed dose as soon as you remember it. However, if it is almost time for the next dose, skip the missed dose and continue your regular dosing schedule. Do not take a double dose to make up for a missed one.

What side effects can this medicine cause?

Minoxidil may cause side effects. Tell your doctor if any of these symptoms are severe or do not go away:
- increase in size or darkness of fine body hair
- dizziness
- breast tenderness
- rash
- headache
- upset stomach
- vomiting

If you experience any of the following symptoms, or those listed in the IMPORTANT WARNING section, call your doctor immediately:
- fast heartbeat
- swollen ankles or feet
- unexplained weight gain
- difficulty breathing
- fainting

If you experience a serious side effect, you or your doctor may send a report to the Food and Drug Administration's (FDA) MedWatch Adverse Event Reporting program online [at http://www.fda.gov/MedWatch/index.html] or by phone [1-800-332-1088].

What storage conditions are needed for this medicine?

Keep this medication in the container it came in, tightly closed, and out of reach of children. Store at room temperature and away from excess heat and moisture (not in the bathroom). Throw away any medication that is outdated or no longer needed. Talk to your pharmacist about the proper disposal of your medication.

What should I do in case of overdose?

In case of overdose, call your local poison control center at 1-800-222-1222. If the victim has collapsed or is not breathing, call local emergency services at 911.

What other information should I know?

Keep all appointments with your doctor and the laboratory. Your blood pressure should be checked regularly to determine your response to minoxidil. Your doctor may order other tests such as EKG (electrocardiogram) to monitor your heart function.

Your doctor may ask you to check your pulse (heart rate) daily. Ask your doctor or pharmacist to teach you how. Call your doctor if your heart rate increases by more than 20 beats per minute while at rest.

Weigh yourself every day. Call your doctor if you experience rapid weight gain.

Do not let any one else take your medication. Ask your pharmacist any questions you have about refilling your prescription.

Dosage Facts
For Informational Purposes

Caution: Do not change your dose, how often you take your medication, or the length of time you are to take it without first talking to your healthcare provider.

The following dosage information was written using medical language for doctors and other healthcare professionals and is provided here for you to check your dosage. The dosage of this drug may differ for different patients. Therefore, always follow your doctor's instructions or the directions on the label. Contact your healthcare provider or pharmacist if you have any questions about the specific dosage of your medication after reviewing this information.

Pediatric Patients

Hypertension

ORAL:
- Children <12 years of age: Initially, 0.2 mg/kg (not to exceed 5 mg) once daily.
- Dosages may be increased at intervals of at least 3 days in increments of 50–100% until optimum BP response is achieved. If rapid control needed, adjust dosage every 6 hours; monitor BP closely.
- Usual effective dosage is 0.25–1 mg/kg daily in 1 or 2 doses up to a maximum dosage of 50 mg daily.
- Children >12 years of age: Initially, 2.5–5 mg once daily. Dosages may be increased at intervals of at least 3 days to 10 mg, 20 mg, and then 40 mg in 1 or 2 divided doses until optimum BP response is achieved. If rapid control needed, adjust dosage every 6 hours; monitor BP closely.
- Usual effective dosage is 10–40 mg daily in 1 or 2 doses up to maximum dosage of 100 mg daily.
- Some experts (JNC 7) recommend a usual dosage of 2.5–80 mg daily given in 1 or 2 divided doses daily.

Severe Hypertension†

Pediatric patients 1–17 years of age: For rapid reduction of blood pressure, 0.1–0.2 mg/kg may be used.

Adult Patients

Hypertension

ORAL:
- Initially, 2.5–5 mg once daily. Dosages may be increased at intervals of at least 3 days to 10 mg, 20 mg, and then 40 mg in 1 or 2 divided doses until optimum BP response is achieved. If rapid control needed, adjust dosage every 6 hours; monitor BP closely.
- Usual effective dosage is 10–40 mg daily in 1 or 2 doses up to maximum dosage of 100 mg daily.
- Some experts (JNC 7) recommend a usual dosage of 2.5–80 mg given in 1 or 2 divided doses daily.

Prescribing Limits

Pediatric Patients

Hypertension

ORAL:
- Children <12 years of age: maximum 50 mg daily.
- Children >12 years of age: maximum 100 mg daily.

Adult Patients

Hypertension

ORAL:
- Maximum 100 mg daily.

Special Populations

Renal Impairment
- Lower dosage may be required in renal failure or dialysis (about ⅓ less than in patients who are not receiving dialysis).
- Removed during dialysis. Some clinicians recommend administering minoxidil immediately after dialysis (if dialysis is at 9 am); if dialysis is after 3 p.m., the daily dose is given at 7 a.m. (i.e., 8 hours before dialysis).

Geriatric Patients
- Select dosage with caution because of age-related decreases in hepatic, renal, and/or cardiac function and concomitant disease and drug therapy.

† *Use is not currently included in the labeling approved by the US Food and Drug Administration.*

Minoxidil Topical

(mi nox′ i dill)

Brand Name: Rogaine®

Why is this medicine prescribed?

Minoxidil is used to stimulate hair growth and to slow balding. It is most effective for people under 40 years of age whose hair loss is recent. Minoxidil has no effect on receding hairlines. It does not cure baldness; most new hair is lost within a few months after the drug is stopped.

How should this medicine be used?

Minoxidil comes as a liquid to be applied to your scalp. Minoxidil usually is used twice a day.

Follow the directions on your package or prescription label carefully, and ask your doctor or pharmacist to explain any part you do not understand. Use minoxidil exactly as directed. Do not use more or less of it or use it more often than directed by your doctor.

Exceeding the recommended dosage does not produce greater or faster hair growth and may cause increased side effects. You must use minoxidil for at least 4 months, and possibly for up to 1 year, before you see any effect.

Three special applicators are provided: a metered-spray applicator for large scalp areas, an extender spray applicator (used with the metered-spray applicator) for small areas or under the hair, and a rub-on applicator.

Remove the outer and inner caps from the bottle, choose an applicator, and screw it tightly onto the bottle.

To use the extender spray applicator, first assemble the metered-spray applicator and then follow the instructions provided to attach the extender spray applicator. Pump the metered-spray or extender spray applicator six times for each dose. Try not to inhale the mist. Place the large cap on the metered-spray bottle or the small cap on the extender spray nozzle when not in use.

To use the rub-on applicator, hold the bottle upright and squeeze it until the upper chamber of the applicator is filled to the black line. Then turn the bottle upside down and rub on the medication. Place the large cap on the bottle when not in use. If you use your fingertips to apply the medication, wash them thoroughly afterwards.

Apply minoxidil to dry hair and scalp only. Do not apply it to other body areas, and keep it away from your eyes and sensitive skin. If it accidentally comes in contact with these areas, wash them with lots of cool water; call your doctor if they become irritated.

Do not apply minoxidil to a sunburned or irritated scalp.

What special precautions should I follow?

Before using minoxidil,
- tell your doctor and pharmacist if you are allergic to minoxidil or any other drugs.
- tell your doctor and pharmacist what prescription and nonprescription medications you are taking, especially guanethidine (Ismelin), other medications for high blood pressure, and vitamins.
- tell your doctor if you have or have ever had heart, kidney, liver, or scalp disease.
- tell your doctor if you are pregnant, plan to become pregnant, or are breast-feeding. If you become pregnant while using minoxidil, call your doctor.
- plan to avoid unnecessary or prolonged exposure to sunlight and to wear protective clothing, sunglasses, and sunscreen. Minoxidil may make your skin sensitive to sunlight.

What should I do if I forget to take a dose?

Skip the missed dose and continue your regular dosing schedule. Do not apply a double dose to make up for a missed one.

What side effects can this medicine cause?

Minoxidil may cause side effects. Tell your doctor if any of these symptoms are severe or do not go away:
- scalp itching, dryness, scaling, flaking, irritation, or burning

If you experience any of the following symptoms, call your doctor immediately:
- weight gain
- swelling of the face, ankles, hands, or stomach
- difficulty breathing (especially when lying down)
- rapid heartbeat
- chest pain
- lightheadedness

If you experience a serious side effect, you or your doctor may send a report to the Food and Drug Administration's (FDA) MedWatch Adverse Event Reporting program online [at http://www.fda.gov/MedWatch/index.html] or by phone [1-800-332-1088].

What storage conditions are needed for this medicine?

Keep this medication in the container it came in, tightly closed, and out of reach of children. Store it at room temperature and away from excess heat and moisture (not in the bathroom). Throw away any medication that is outdated or no longer needed. Talk to your pharmacist about the proper disposal of your medication.

What other information should I know?

Keep all appointments with your doctor. Minoxidil is for external use only. Do not let minoxidil get into your eyes, nose, or mouth, and do not swallow it. Do not apply dressings, bandages, cosmetics, lotions, or other skin medications to the area being treated unless your doctor tells you.

Do not let anyone else use your medication. Ask your pharmacist any questions you have about refilling your prescription.

Talk to your doctor, pharmacist, or other healthcare professional if you have questions about dosing information for your medication.

Mirtazapine

(mir taz′ a peen)

Brand Name: Remeron®, Remeron® SolTab®

Important Warning

A small number of children, teenagers, and young adults (up to 24 years of age) who took antidepressants ('mood elevators') such as mirtazapine during clinical studies became suicidal (thinking about harming or killing oneself or planning or trying to do so). Children, teenagers, and young adults who take antidepressants to treat depression or other mental illnesses may be more likely to become suicidal than children, teenagers, and young adults who do not take antidepressants to treat these conditions. However, experts are not sure about how great this risk is and how much it should be considered in deciding whether a child or teenager should take an antidepressant. Children younger than 18 years of age should not normally take mirtazapine, but in some cases, a doctor may decide that mirtazapine is the best medication to treat a child's condition.

You should know that your mental health may change in unexpected ways when you take mirtazapine or other antidepressants even if you are an adult over age 24. You may become suicidal, especially at the beginning of your treatment and any time that your dose is increased or decreased. You, your family, or your caregiver should call your doctor right away if you experience any of the following symptoms: new or worsening depression; thinking about harming or killing yourself, or planning or trying to do so; extreme worry; agitation; panic attacks; difficulty falling asleep or staying asleep; aggressive behavior; irritability; acting without thinking; severe restlessness; and frenzied abnormal excitement. Be sure that your family or caregiver knows which symptoms may be serious so they can call the doctor when you are unable to seek treatment on your own.

Your healthcare provider will want to see you often while you are taking mirtazapine, especially at the beginning of your treatment. Be sure to keep all appointments for office visits with your doctor.

The doctor or pharmacist will give you the manufacturer's patient information sheet (Medication Guide) when you begin treatment with mirtazapine. Read the information carefully and ask your doctor or pharmacist if you have any questions. You also can obtain the Medication Guide from the FDA website: http://www.fda.gov/cder/drug/antidepressants/antidepressants_MG_2007.pdf.

No matter what your age, before you take an antidepressant, you, your parent, or your caregiver should talk to your doctor about the risks and benefits of treating your condition with an antidepressant or with other treatments. You should also talk about the risks and benefits of not treating your condition. You should know that having depression or another mental illness greatly increases the risk that you will become suicidal. This risk is higher if you or anyone in your family has or has ever had bipolar disorder (mood that changes from depressed to abnormally excited) or mania (frenzied, abnormally excited mood) or has thought about or attempted suicide. Talk to your doctor about your condition, symptoms, and personal and family medical history. You and your doctor will decide what type of treatment is right for you.

Why is this medicine prescribed?

Mirtazapine is used to treat depression. Mirtazapine is in a class of medications called antidepressants. It works by increasing certain types of activity in the brain to maintain mental balance.

How should this medicine be used?

Mirtazapine comes as a tablet and as a disintegrating tablet to take by mouth. It usually is taken once a day at bedtime. It may be taken with or without food. Follow the directions on your prescription label carefully, and ask your doctor or pharmacist to explain any part you do not understand. Take mirtazapine exactly as directed. Do not take more or less of it or take it more often than prescribed by your doctor.

To take a mirtazapine disintegrating tablet, open the blister pack with dry hands and place the tablet on your tongue. The tablet will disintegrate on the tongue and can be swallowed with saliva. No water is needed to swallow disintegrating tablets. Once the tablet is removed from the blister pack, it cannot be stored. Do not split mirtazapine disintegrating tablets.

It may take several weeks or longer for you to feel the full benefit of mirtazapine. Continue to take mirtazapine even if you feel well. Do not stop taking mirtazapine without talking to your doctor. Your doctor probably will decrease your dose gradually.

Are there other uses for this medicine?

This medication is sometimes prescribed for other uses; ask your doctor or pharmacist for more information.

What special precautions should I follow?

Before taking mirtazapine,

- tell your doctor and pharmacist if you are allergic to mirtazapine or any other medications.
- tell your doctor and pharmacist what prescription and nonprescription medications, vitamins, nutritional supplements, and herbal products you are taking or plan to take. Be sure to tell the doctor if you are taking diazepam (Valium) and if you are taking an MAO inhibitor such as isocarboxazid (Marplan), phenelzine (Nardil), selegiline (Eldepryl, Emsam, Zelapar), and tranylcypromine (Parnate) or if you have stopped taking an MAO inhibitor within the past 14 days. Your doctor may tell you not to take mirtazapine.
- tell your doctor if you have or have ever had a heart attack, low blood pressure, heart or liver disease, or high cholesterol.
- tell your doctor if you are pregnant, plan to become pregnant, or are breast-feeding. If you become pregnant while taking mirtazapine, call your doctor.
- if you are having surgery, including dental surgery, tell the doctor or dentist that you are taking mirtazapine.
- you should know that this medication may make you drowsy. Do not drive a car or operate machinery until you know how this medication affects you.
- remember that alcohol can add to the drowsiness caused by this medication.
- if you have phenylketonuria (PKU, a inherited condition in which a special diet must be followed to prevent mental retardation), you should know that the orally disintegrating tablets contain aspartame that forms phenylalanine.

What special dietary instructions should I follow?

Unless your doctor tells you otherwise, continue your normal diet.

What should I do if I forget to take a dose?

Take the missed dose as soon as you remember it. However, if it is almost time for the next dose, skip the missed dose and continue your regular dosing schedule. Do not take a double dose to make up for a missed one.

What side effects can this medicine cause?

Mirtazapine may cause side effects. Tell your doctor if any of these symptoms are severe or do not go away:

- drowsiness
- dizziness
- anxiousness
- confusion
- increased weight and appetite
- dry mouth
- constipation
- nausea
- vomiting

Some side effects can be serious. If you experience any of the following symptoms or those listed in the IMPORTANT WARNING section, call your doctor immediately:

- flu-like symptoms, fever, chills, sore throat, mouth sores, or other signs of infection
- chest pain
- fast heartbeat
- seizures

Mirtazapine may cause other side effects. Call your doctor if you have any unusual problems while you are taking this medication.

If you experience a serious side effect, you or your doctor may send a report to the Food and Drug Administration's (FDA) MedWatch Adverse Event Reporting program online [at http://www.fda.gov/MedWatch/index.html] or by phone [1-800-332-1088].

What storage conditions are needed for this medicine?

Keep this medication in the container it came in, tightly closed, and out of reach of children. Store it at room temperature and away from excess heat and moisture (not in the bathroom). Throw away any medication that is outdated or no longer needed. Talk to your pharmacist about the proper disposal of your medication.

What should I do in case of overdose?

In case of overdose, call your local poison control center at 1-800-222-1222. If the victim has collapsed or is not breathing, call local emergency services at 911.

What other information should I know?

Keep all appointments with your doctor and the laboratory. Your doctor may order certain lab tests to check your response to mirtazapine.

Do not let anyone else take your medication. Ask your pharmacist any questions you have about refilling your prescription.

Dosage Facts
For Informational Purposes

Caution: Do not change your dose, how often you take your medication, or the length of time you are to take it without first talking to your healthcare provider.

The following dosage information was written using medical language for doctors and other healthcare professionals and is provided here for you to check your dosage. The dosage of this drug may differ for different patients. Therefore, always follow your doctor's instruc-

tions or the directions on the label. Contact your health-care provider or pharmacist if you have any questions about the specific dosage of your medication after reviewing this information.

Adult Patients
Major Depressive Disorder
ORAL:
- Initially, 15 mg daily. If no improvement, dosage may be increased up to a maximum of 45 mg daily at intervals of not less than 1–2 weeks.

Prescribing Limits
Adult Patients
Major Depressive Disorder
ORAL:
- Maximum 45 mg daily.

Special Populations
Hepatic Impairment
- Decreased clearance; however, no special population dosage recommendations at this time.

Renal Impairment
- Decreased clearance in patients with moderate to severe renal impairment; however, no special population dosage recommendations at this time.

Geriatric Patients
- Select dosage with caution because of age-related decreases in hepatic, renal, and/or cardiac function and concomitant disease and drug therapy.

Misoprostol
(mye soe prost′ ole)

Brand Name: Cytotec®
Also available generically.

Important Warning

Do not take misoprostol to prevent ulcers if you are pregnant or plan to become pregnant. Misoprostol may cause miscarriages, premature labor, or birth defects.

If you are a woman of childbearing age, you may take misoprostol to prevent ulcers only if you have had a negative pregnancy test in the past 2 weeks and if you use a reliable method of birth control while taking misoprostol. You must begin taking misoprostol on the second or third day of your menstrual period. If you become pregnant while taking misoprostol, stop taking it and call your doctor immediately.

Before taking misoprostol, ask your pharmacist or doctor for a copy of the manufacturer's information for the patient and read it carefully. Talk to your doctor about the risks of taking misoprostol.

Do not let anyone else take your medication, especially a woman who is or may become pregnant.

Why is this medicine prescribed?
Misoprostol is used to prevent ulcers in people who take certain arthritis or pain medicines, including aspirin, that can cause ulcers. It protects the stomach lining and decreases stomach acid secretion.

How should this medicine be used?
Misoprostol comes as a tablet to take by mouth. It is usually taken 4 times a day, after meals and at bedtime with food. Follow the directions on your prescription label carefully, and ask your doctor or pharmacist to explain any part you do not understand. Take misoprostol exactly as directed. Do not take more or less of it or take it more often than prescribed by your doctor.

Misoprostol must be taken regularly to be effective. Women should not take their first dose until the second or third day of their menstrual period (to be sure that they are not pregnant). Do not stop taking misoprostol without talking to your doctor.

Are there other uses for this medicine?
Misoprostol is also used sometimes to treat ulcers and to induce labor. Misoprostol is used in combination with mifepristone to end an early pregnancy. Talk to your doctor about the possible risks of using this drug for your condition.

This medication may be prescribed for other uses; ask your doctor or pharmacist for more information.

What special precautions should I follow?
Before taking misoprostol,
- tell your doctor and pharmacist if you are allergic to misoprostol or any other drugs.
- tell your doctor and pharmacist what prescription and nonprescription medications you are taking, especially antacids, aspirin, arthritis medications, and vitamins.
- tell your doctor if you are breast-feeding.

What should I do if I forget to take a dose?
Take the missed dose as soon as you remember it. However, if it is almost time for the next dose, skip the missed dose and continue your regular dosing schedule. Do not take a double dose to make up for a missed one.

What side effects can this medicine cause?

Misoprostol may cause side effects. Tell your doctor if any of these symptoms are severe or do not go away:

- diarrhea
- headache
- stomach pain
- upset stomach
- gas
- vomiting
- constipation
- indigestion

If you experience any of the following symptoms, call your doctor immediately:

- vomiting blood
- bloody or black, tarry stools

If you experience a serious side effect, you or your doctor may send a report to the Food and Drug Administration's (FDA) MedWatch Adverse Event Reporting program online [at http://www.fda.gov/MedWatch/index.html] or by phone [1-800-332-1088].

What storage conditions are needed for this medicine?

Keep this medication in the container it came in, tightly closed, and out of reach of children. Store it at room temperature and away from excess heat and moisture (not in the bathroom). Throw away any medication that is outdated or no longer needed. Talk to your pharmacist about the proper disposal of your medication.

What should I do in case of overdose?

In case of overdose, call your local poison control center at 1-800-222-1222. If the victim has collapsed or is not breathing, call local emergency services at 911.

What other information should I know?

Keep all appointments with your doctor.

Ask your pharmacist any questions you have about refilling your prescription.

Dosage Facts
For Informational Purposes

Caution: Do not change your dose, how often you take your medication, or the length of time you are to take it without first talking to your healthcare provider.

The following dosage information was written using medical language for doctors and other healthcare professionals and is provided here for you to check your dosage. The dosage of this drug may differ for different patients. Therefore, always follow your doctor's instructions or the directions on the label. Contact your health-

care provider or pharmacist if you have any questions about the specific dosage of your medication after reviewing this information.

General Dosage Information

Available as mifoprostol; dosage expressed in terms of mifoprostol.

Adult Patients

Prevention of NSAIA-Induced Ulcers

ORAL:

- 200 mcg 4 times daily. May reduce dosage to 100 mcg 4 times daily if higher dosage is not well tolerated; however, reduced dosage may be less effective. Alternatively, 200 mcg twice daily. Continue therapy for the duration of NSAIA therapy.

Gastric Ulcer†

ORAL:

- 100 or 200 mcg 4 times daily for 8 weeks.

Duodenal Ulcer†

ORAL:

- 100 or 200 mcg 4 times daily or 400 mcg twice daily for 4–8 weeks.

Termination of Pregnancy

ORAL:

- 400 mcg administered orally on day 3 (2 days after mifepristone administration) unless abortion has occurred and has been confirmed by clinical examination or ultrasonographic scan.

Special Populations

Renal Impairment

- Routine dosage reduction not required; however, dosage can be reduced if not tolerated.

Geriatric Patients

- Routine dosage reduction not required; however, dosage can be reduced if not tolerated.

† Use is not currently included in the labeling approved by the US Food and Drug Administration.

Modafinil

(moe daf′ i nil)

Brand Name: Provigil®

Why is this medicine prescribed?

Modafinil is used to treat excessive sleepiness caused by narcolepsy (a condition that causes excessive daytime sleepiness) or shift work sleep disorder (sleepiness during scheduled waking hours and difficulty falling asleep or staying asleep during scheduled sleeping hours in people who work at night or on rotating shifts). Modafinil is also used along with breathing devices or other treatments to prevent excessive sleepiness caused by obstructive sleep apnea/hypopnea syndrome (OSAHS; a sleep disorder in which the patient briefly stops breathing or breathes shallowly many times during sleep and therefore doesn't get enough restful sleep). Modafinil is in a class of medications called central nervous system (CNS) stimulants. It works by changing the amounts of certain natural substances in the area of the brain that controls sleep and wakefulness.

How should this medicine be used?

Modafinil comes as a tablet to take by mouth. It is usually taken once a day with or without food. If you are taking modafinil to treat narcolepsy or OSAHS, you will probably take it in the morning. If you are taking modafinil to treat shift work sleep disorder, you will probably take it 1 hour before the beginning of your work shift. Take modafinil at the same time every day. Do not change the time of day that you take modafinil without talking to your doctor. Follow the directions on your prescription label carefully, and ask your doctor or pharmacist to explain any part you do not understand. Take modafinil exactly as directed.

Modafinil may be habit forming. Do not take more or less of it or take it more often than prescribed by your doctor. If you take more than your prescribed dose, you may find it harder to fall asleep and stay asleep.

Modafinil may decrease your sleepiness, but it will not cure your sleep disorder. Continue to take modafinil even if you feel well. Do not stop taking modafinil without talking to your doctor.

Modafinil should not be used in place of getting enough sleep. Follow your doctor's advice about good sleep habits. Continue to use any breathing devices or other treatments that your doctor has prescribed to treat your condition, especially if you have OSAHS.

Are there other uses for this medicine?

This medication may be prescribed for other uses; ask your doctor or pharmacist for more information.

What special precautions should I follow?

Before taking modafinil,
- tell your doctor and pharmacist if you are allergic to modafinil or any other medications.
- tell your doctor and pharmacist what prescription and nonprescription medications, vitamins, nutritional supplements, and herbal products you are taking. Be sure to mention any of the following: anticoagulants ('blood thinners') such as warfarin (Coumadin); certain antidepressants such as clomipramine (Anafranil) and desipramine (Norpramin); certain antifungals such as itraconazole (Sporanox) and ketoconazole (Nizoral); cyclosporine (Neoral, Sandimmune); cyclophospha-

mide (Cytoxan, Neosar); diazepam (Valium); certain medications for seizures such as carbamazepine (Tegretol), phenobarbital (Luminal, Solfoton), and phenytoin (Dilantin); monoamine oxidase (MAO) inhibitors, including isocarboxazid (Marplan), phenelzine (Nardil), selegiline (Eldepryl), and tranylcypromine (Parnate); primidone (Mysoline); propranolol (Inderal); certain proton pump inhibitors such as lansoprazole (Prevacid), omeprazole (Prilosec), and pantoprazole (Protonix); selective serotonin reuptake inhibitors (SSRIs) such as as citalopram (Celexa), escitalopram (Lexapro), fluoxetine (Prozac, Sarafem), fluvoxamine (Luvox), paroxetine (Paxil), and sertraline (Zoloft); rifampin (Rifadin, Rimactane); and triazolam (Halcion). Many other medications may also interact with modafinil, so be sure to tell your doctor about all the medications you are taking, even those that do not appear on this list. Your doctor may need to change the doses of your medications or monitor you carefully for side effects.
- tell your doctor if you drink large amounts of alcohol, use or have ever used street drugs, or have overused prescription medications, especially stimulants. Also tell your doctor if you have ever had chest pain, an irregular heartbeat, or other heart problems after taking a stimulant, and if you have or have ever had high blood pressure, a heart attack, angina (chest pain), mental illness, or heart, liver, or kidney disease.
- you should know that modafinil may decrease the effectiveness of hormonal contraceptives (birth control pills, patches, rings, implants, injections, and intrauterine devices). Use another form of birth control while taking modafinil and for 1 month after you stop taking it. Talk to your doctor about types of birth control that will work for you while you are taking modafinil.
- tell your doctor if you are pregnant, plan to become pregnant, or are breast-feeding. If you become pregnant while taking modafinil, call your doctor.
- if you are having surgery, including dental surgery, tell the doctor or dentist that you are taking modafinil.
- you should know that modafinil may affect judgment or thinking and may not completely relieve the sleepiness caused by your disorder. Do not drive a car or operate machinery until you know how this medication affects you. If you avoided driving and other dangerous activities because of your sleep disorder, do not start performing these activities again without talking to your doctor even if you feel more alert.
- be aware that you should avoid drinking alcohol while taking modafinil.

What special dietary instructions should I follow?

Talk to your doctor about eating grapefruit or drinking grapefruit juice while you are taking this medication.

What should I do if I forget to take a dose?

You should skip the missed dose. Wait until the next time you are supposed to take modafinil, and then take your normal dose. If you take modafanil too late in your waking day, you may find it harder to go to sleep. Do not take a double dose to make up for a missed one.

What side effects can this medicine cause?

Modafinil may cause side effects. Tell your doctor if any of these symptoms are severe or do not go away:

- headache
- nervousness
- anxiety or restlessness
- dizziness
- difficulty falling asleep or staying asleep
- drowsiness
- depression
- mood swings
- upset stomach
- diarrhea
- constipation
- gas
- heartburn
- loss of appetite
- ulcers in the mouth
- unusual tastes
- sweating
- dry mouth
- excessive thirst
- runny nose
- nosebleed
- flushing
- tight muscles or difficulty moving
- back pain
- confusion
- shaking of a part of your body that you cannot control
- burning, tingling, or a numbness of the skin
- difficulty seeing or eye pain
- flu like symptoms

Some side effects can be serious. The following symptoms are uncommon, but if you experience any of them, call your doctor immediately:

- chest pain
- changes in mental health
- fast, pounding, or irregular heartbeat
- blood in the urine
- fever, sore throat, chills, and other signs of infection
- rash
- hives
- itching
- difficulty breathing or swallowing
- swelling of the face, throat, tongue, lips, eyes, hands, feet, ankles, or lower legs

Some children who took modafinil had a decrease in the number of their white blood cells (a type of blood cell that fights infection). Modafinil has not been shown to be safe for children under age 16. Talk to your child's doctor about the risks of giving modafinil to your child.

Modafinil may cause other side effects. Call your doctor if you have any unusual problems while taking this medication.

If you experience a serious side effect, you or your doctor may send a report to the Food and Drug Administration's (FDA) MedWatch Adverse Event Reporting program online [at http://www.fda.gov/MedWatch/index.html] or by phone [1-800-332-1088].

What storage conditions are needed for this medicine?

Keep this medication in the container it came in, tightly closed, and out of reach of children. Store it at room temperature and away from excess heat and moisture (not in the bathroom). Store modafinil in a safe place so that no one else can take it accidentally or on purpose. Keep track of how many tablets are left so you will know if any are missing.Throw away any medication that is outdated or no longer needed. Talk to your pharmacist about the proper disposal of your medication.

What should I do in case of overdose?

In case of overdose, call your local poison control center at 1-800-222-1222. If the victim has collapsed or is not breathing, call local emergency services at 911.

Symptoms of overdose may include:

- difficulty falling asleep or staying asleep
- agitation
- restlessness
- confusion
- hallucinations (seeing things or hearing voices that do not exist)
- nervousness
- shaking of a part of your body that you cannot control
- fast, slow or pounding heartbeat
- chest pain
- upset stomach
- diarrhea

What other information should I know?

Keep all appointments with your doctor.

Do not let anyone else take your medication. Ask your pharmacist any questions you have about refilling your prescription.

Dosage Facts
For Informational Purposes

Caution: Do not change your dose, how often you take your medication, or the length of time you are to take it without first talking to your healthcare provider.

The following dosage information was written using medical language for doctors and other healthcare pro-

fessionals and is provided here for you to check your dosage. The dosage of this drug may differ for different patients. Therefore, always follow your doctor's instructions or the directions on the label. Contact your healthcare provider or pharmacist if you have any questions about the specific dosage of your medication after reviewing this information.

Adult Patients

Narcolepsy

ORAL:
- 200 mg once daily.
- Dosages up to 400 mg daily have been well tolerated but may not be associated with increased therapeutic benefit.
- Long-term efficacy (>9 weeks) not systematically established. If clinician elects to prescribe for an extended time, periodically reevaluate long-term usefulness in the individual patient.

OSAHS

ORAL:
- 200 mg once daily.
- Dosages up to 400 mg daily have been well tolerated but may not be associated with increased therapeutic benefit.
- Long-term efficacy (>12 weeks) not systematically established. If clinician elects to prescribe for an extended time, periodically reevaluate long-term usefulness in the individual patient.

SWSD

ORAL:
- 200 mg once daily.
- Dosages up to 400 mg daily have been well tolerated but may not be associated with increased therapeutic benefit.
- Long-term efficacy (>12 weeks) not systematically established. If clinician elects to prescribe for an extended time, periodically reevaluate long-term usefulness in the individual patient.

Special Populations

Hepatic Impairment
- In patients with severe hepatic impairment (with or without cirrhosis), reduce dosage to 100 mg daily (i.e., one-half the usual recommended dosage).

Renal Impairment
- Current information inadequate to make specific dosage recommendations in patients with severe renal impairment.

Geriatric Patients
- Consider using lower than usual recommended dosage due to possible age-related decreases in renal and/or hepatic function.

Moexipril

(moe ex' i pril)

Brand Name: Uniretic® as a combination product containing Moexipril Hydrochloride and Hydrochlorothiazide, Univasc®

Also available generically.

Important Warning

Do not take moexipril if you are pregnant or breast-feeding. If you become pregnant while taking moexipril, call your doctor immediately.

Why is this medicine prescribed?

Moexipril is used to treat high blood pressure. It decreases certain chemicals that tighten the blood vessels, so blood flows more smoothly.

This medication is sometimes prescribed for other uses; ask your doctor or pharmacist for more information.

How should this medicine be used?

Moexipril comes as a tablet to take by mouth. It is usually taken once or twice a day and should be taken on an empty stomach 1 hour before or 2 hours after a meal. Follow the directions on your prescription label carefully, and ask your doctor or pharmacist to explain any part you do not understand. Take moexipril exactly as directed. Do not take more or less of it or take it more often than prescribed by your doctor.

Moexipril controls high blood pressure but does not cure it. Continue to take moexipril even if you feel well. Do not stop taking moexipril without talking to your doctor.

What special precautions should I follow?

Before taking moexipril,
- tell your doctor and pharmacist if you are allergic to moexipril or any other drugs.
- tell your doctor and pharmacist what prescription and nonprescription medications you are taking, especially diuretics ('water pills'), lithium (Eskalith, Lithobid), other medications for high blood pressure, potassium supplements, and vitamins.
- tell your doctor if you have or have ever had heart or kidney disease or diabetes.
- if you are having surgery, including dental surgery, tell the doctor or dentist that you are taking moexipril.

What special dietary instructions should I follow?

Talk to your doctor before using salt substitutes containing potassium. If your doctor prescribes a low-salt or low-sodium diet, follow these directions carefully.

What should I do if I forget to take a dose?

Take the missed dose as soon as you remember it. However, if it is almost time for the next dose, skip the missed dose and continue your regular regular dosing schedule. Do not take a double dose to make up for a missed one.

What side effects can this medicine cause?

Moexipril may cause side effects. Tell your doctor if any of these symptoms are severe or do not go away:

- cough
- dizziness or lightheadedness
- sore throat
- hoarseness
- excessive tiredness
- headache
- diarrhea
- vomiting
- fever
- muscle aches
- fast heartbeat

If you experience any of the following symptoms, call your doctor immediately:

- swelling of the face, eyes, lips, tongue, arms, or legs
- difficulty breathing or swallowing
- fainting
- rash

If you experience a serious side effect, you or your doctor may send a report to the Food and Drug Administration's (FDA) MedWatch Adverse Event Reporting program online [at http://www.fda.gov/MedWatch/index.html] or by phone [1-800-332-1088].

What storage conditions are needed for this medicine?

Keep this medication in the container it came in, tightly closed, and out of reach of children. Store it at room temperature and away from excess heat and moisture (not in the bathroom). Throw away any medication that is outdated or no longer needed. Talk to your pharmacist about the proper disposal of your medication.

What should I do in case of overdose?

In case of overdose, call your local poison control center at 1-800-222-1222. If the victim has collapsed or is not breathing, call local emergency services at 911.

What other information should I know?

Keep all appointments with your doctor and the laboratory. Your blood pressure should be checked regularly to determine your response to moexipril.

Do not let anyone else take your medication. Ask your pharmacist any questions you have about refilling your prescription.

Dosage Facts
For Informational Purposes

Caution: Do not change your dose, how often you take your medication, or the length of time you are to take it without first talking to your healthcare provider.

The following dosage information was written using medical language for doctors and other healthcare professionals and is provided here for you to check your dosage. The dosage of this drug may differ for different patients. Therefore, always follow your doctor's instructions or the directions on the label. Contact your healthcare provider or pharmacist if you have any questions about the specific dosage of your medication after reviewing this information.

General Dosage Information

Available as moexipril hydrochloride; dosage expressed in terms of the salt.

Adult Patients

Hypertension

ORAL:
- Initially, 7.5 mg once daily as monotherapy.
- In patients currently receiving diuretic therapy, discontinue diuretic, if possible, 2–3 days before initiating moexipril. May cautiously resume diuretic therapy if BP not controlled adequately with moexipril alone. If diuretic cannot be discontinued, increase sodium intake and give lower initial moexipril dose (3.75 mg) under close medical supervision.
- Usual dosage: 7.5–30 mg daily, given in 1 dose or 2 divided doses.
- If effectiveness diminishes toward end of dosing interval in patients treated once daily, consider increasing dosage or administering drug in 2 divided doses.

Moexipril/Hydrochlorothiazide Combination Therapy

ORAL:
- If BP is not adequately controlled by monotherapy with moexipril, can switch to the fixed-combination preparation containing moexipril hydrochloride 7.5 mg and hydrochlorothiazide 12.5 mg, moexipril hydrochloride 15 mg and hydrochlorothiazide 12.5 mg, or moexipril hydrochloride 15 mg and hydrochlorothiazide 25 mg. Adjust dosage of either or both drugs according to patient's response.

Prescribing Limits

Adult Patients

Hypertension

ORAL:
- Usually, maximum 30 mg daily. Dosages >60 mg daily have not been extensively evaluated in hypertensive patients.

Renal Impairment

Hypertension

ORAL:

- Initially, 3.75 mg once daily in patients with severe renal impairment (Cl_{cr} ≤40 mL/minute); titrate until BP is controlled or to maximum of 15 mg daily.
- Moexipril/hydrochlorothiazide fixed combination is not recommended in patients with severe renal impairment.

Volume- and/or Salt-depleted Patients

- Correct volume and/or salt depletion prior to initiation of therapy or initiate therapy under close medical supervision using lower initial dosage.

Molindone

(moe lin' done)

Brand Name: Moban®, Moban® Concentrate

Why is this medicine prescribed?

Molindone is used to treat schizophrenia and symptoms such as hallucinations, delusions, and hostility.

This medication is sometimes prescribed for other uses; ask your doctor or pharmacist for more information.

How should this medicine be used?

Molindone comes as a tablet and liquid concentrate to take by mouth. It usually is taken three or four times a day. Follow the directions on your prescription label carefully, and ask your doctor or pharmacist to explain any part you do not understand. Take molindone exactly as directed. Do not take more or less of it or take it more often than prescribed by your doctor.

The liquid concentrate must be diluted before use. It comes with a specially marked dropper for measuring the dose. Ask your pharmacist to show you how to use the dropper if you have difficulty. To dilute the liquid concentrate, add it to at least 2 ounces of water or fruit juice just before you take it. If any fruit juice gets on the dropper, rinse the dropper with tap water before replacing it in the bottle. Do not allow the liquid concentrate to touch your skin or clothing; it can irritate your skin. If you spill the liquid concentrate on your skin, wash it off immediately with soap and water.

Continue to take molindone even if you feel well. Do not stop taking molindone without talking to your doctor, especially if you have taken large doses for a long time. Your doctor probably will decrease your dose gradually. This drug must be taken regularly for a few weeks before its full effect is felt.

What special precautions should I follow?

Before taking molindone,

- tell your doctor and pharmacist if you are allergic to molindone, sulfites, or any other drugs.
- tell your doctor and pharmacist what prescription and nonprescription medications you are taking, especially antacids, antihistamines, appetite reducers (amphetamines), benztropine (Cogentin), bromocriptine (Parlodel), carbamazepine (Tegretol), dicyclomine (Bentyl), fluoxetine (Prozac), guanethidine (Ismelin), lithium, medications for colds, medications for depression, meperidine (Demerol), methyldopa (Aldomet), phenytoin (Dilantin), propranolol (Inderal), sedatives, tetracycline, trihexyphenidyl (Artane), valproic acid (Depakane), and vitamins.
- tell your doctor if you have or have ever had depression; seizures; shock therapy; asthma; emphysema; chronic bronchitis; problems with your urinary system or prostate; glaucoma; history of alcohol abuse; thyroid problems; bad reaction to insulin; angina; irregular heartbeat; problems with your blood pressure; blood disorders; or blood vessel, heart, kidney, liver, or lung disease.
- tell your doctor if you are pregnant, plan to become pregnant, or are breast-feeding. If you become pregnant while taking molindone, call your doctor.
- if you are having surgery, including dental surgery, tell the doctor or dentist that you are taking molindone.
- you should know that this drug may make you drowsy. Do not drive a car or operate machinery until you know how this drug affects you.
- remember that alcohol can add to the drowsiness caused by this drug.

What special dietary instructions should I follow?

Molindone may cause an upset stomach. Take molindone with food or milk.

What should I do if I forget to take a dose?

Take the missed dose as soon as you remember it and take any remaining doses for that day at evenly spaced intervals. However, if you remember a missed dose when it is almost time for your next scheduled dose, skip the missed dose. Do not take a double dose to make up for a missed one.

What side effects can this medicine cause?

Side effects from molindone are common. Your urine may turn pink or reddish-brown; this effect is not harmful. Tell your doctor if any of these symptoms are severe or do not go away:

- drowsiness
- dry mouth
- upset stomach
- vomiting
- diarrhea

- constipation
- restlessness
- headache

If you experience any of the following symptoms, call your doctor immediately:

- tremor
- restlessness or pacing
- fine worm-like tongue movements
- unusual face, mouth, or jaw movements
- shuffling walk
- slow, jerky movements
- seizures or convulsions
- fast, irregular, or pounding heartbeat
- difficulty urinating or loss of bladder control
- eye pain or discoloration
- difficulty breathing or fast breathing
- unusual tiredness or weakness
- unusual bleeding or bruising
- yellowing of the skin or eyes

If you experience a serious side effect, you or your doctor may send a report to the Food and Drug Administration's (FDA) MedWatch Adverse Event Reporting program online [at http://www.fda.gov/MedWatch/index.html] or by phone [1-800-332-1088].

What storage conditions are needed for this medicine?

Keep this medication in the container it came in, tightly closed, and out of reach of children. Store it at room temperature and away from excess heat and moisture (not in the bathroom). Protect the liquid from light. Throw away any medication that is outdated or no longer needed. Talk to your pharmacist about the proper disposal of your medication.

What should I do in case of overdose?

In case of overdose, call your local poison control center at 1-800-222-1222. If the victim has collapsed or is not breathing, call local emergency services at 911.

What other information should I know?

Keep all appointments with your doctor and the laboratory. Your doctor will order certain lab tests to check your response to molindone.

Do not let anyone else take your medication. Ask your pharmacist any questions you have about refilling your prescription.

Talk to your doctor, pharmacist, or other healthcare professional if you have questions about dosing information for your medication.

Mometasone Furoate

(moe met′ a sone)

Brand Name: Elocon®
Also available generically.

Why is this medicine prescribed?

Mometasone is used to relieve the itching and inflammation of numerous skin conditions.

This medication is sometimes prescribed for other uses; ask your doctor or pharmacist for more information.

How should this medicine be used?

Mometasone comes as a topical cream, ointment, and lotion. It usually is applied externally once a day. Follow the directions on your prescription label carefully, and ask your doctor or pharmacist to explain any part you do not understand. Use mometasone exactly as directed. Do not use more or less of it or use it more often than prescribed by your doctor.

To use mometasone cream or ointment, apply a thin film to the affected skin areas once daily.

To apply the lotion, place a few drops on the affected areas once daily and massage lightly until it disappears. To be most effective and economical, hold the nozzle of the bottle very close to the affected areas and gently squeeze.

What special precautions should I follow?

Before using mometasone,

- tell your doctor and pharmacist if you are allergic to mometasone or any other drugs.
- tell your doctor and pharmacist what prescription and nonprescription medications you are taking, including vitamins.
- tell your doctor if you have an infection or have ever had cataracts, glaucoma, or diabetes.
- tell your doctor if you are pregnant, plan to become pregnant, or are breast-feeding. If you become pregnant while using mometasone, call your doctor.

What should I do if I forget to take a dose?

Apply the missed dose as soon as you remember it and apply the remaining doses for that day at evenly spaced intervals if more than one dose a day is indicated by your doctor. Do not apply a double dose to make up for a missed dose.

What side effects can this medicine cause?

Mometasone may cause side effects. Tell your doctor if any of these symptoms are severe or do not go away:

- acne
- skin sores
- burning
- itching
- irritation

- dryness
- skin infection
- changes in skin color

If you experience any of the following symptoms, call your doctor immediately:

- treated area becomes infected (red, warm, or swollen)
- pus oozes from treated area
- if skin problem continues or worsens

If you experience a serious side effect, you or your doctor may send a report to the Food and Drug Administration's (FDA) MedWatch Adverse Event Reporting program online [at http://www.fda.gov/MedWatch/index.html] or by phone [1-800-332-1088].

What storage conditions are needed for this medicine?

Keep this medication in the container it came in, tightly closed, and out of reach of children. Store it at room temperature and away from excess heat and moisture (not in the bathroom). Throw away any medication that is outdated or no longer needed. Talk to your pharmacist about the proper disposal of your medication.

What other information should I know?

Keep all appointments with your doctor and the laboratory. Your skin condition should be checked to determine your response to mometasone.

Do not use mometasone on areas of your body other than as directed by your doctor, and do not use it for other skin problems. Do not wrap or bandage the treated area unless directed to do so by your doctor.

If you are using this medication on a child's diaper area, do not place tightly fitting diapers or plastic pants on the child. They can increase the absorption of mometasone through the skin, which can cause harmful effects.

Do not apply cosmetics, lotions, or other skin preparations to the treated area without talking to your doctor.

Do not let anyone else use your medication. Ask your pharmacist any questions you have about refilling your prescription.

Dosage Facts
For Informational Purposes

Caution: Do not change your dose, how often you take your medication, or the length of time you are to take it without first talking to your healthcare provider.

The following dosage information was written using medical language for doctors and other healthcare professionals and is provided here for you to check your dosage. The dosage of this drug may differ for different patients. Therefore, always follow your doctor's instructions or the directions on the label. Contact your healthcare provider or pharmacist if you have any questions

about the specific dosage of your medication after reviewing this information.

General Dosage Information

Available as mometasone furoate; dosage expressed in terms of the salt.

Pediatric Patients

Administer the least amount of topical preparations that provides effective therapy.

Corticosteroid-responsive Dermatoses
TOPICAL:
- Children ≥2 years of age: Apply 0.1% cream or ointment sparingly to affected area, usually once daily; safety and efficacy for >3 weeks not established. Cream and ointment also have been applied twice daily.
- Children ≥12 years of age: Apply a few drops of 0.1% lotion to affected area once daily.
- Discontinue when control is achieved; if improvement does not occur within 2 weeks, consider reassessment of the diagnosis.

Adult Patients
Corticosteroid-responsive Dermatoses
TOPICAL:
- Apply 0.1% cream or ointment sparingly to affected area, usually once daily. Cream and ointment also have been applied twice daily.
- Apply a few drops of 0.1% lotion to affected area once daily.
- Discontinue when control is achieved; if improvement does not occur within 2 weeks, consider reassessment of the diagnosis.

Prescribing Limits
Pediatric Patients
Corticosteroid-responsive Dermatoses
TOPICAL:
- Children ≥2 years of age: Safety and efficacy of therapy with 0.1% cream or ointment for >3 weeks have not been established.

Mometasone Nasal Inhalation

(moe met′ a sone)

Brand Name: Nasonex® Nasal Spray

Why is this medicine prescribed?

Mometasone nasal inhalation is used for the treatment and prevention of nasal symptoms of seasonal and year-round allergies, including runny nose, sneezing, and itchy nose. Mometasone nasal inhalation is in a class of medications called topical steroids. It works by reducing inflammation (swelling) in the nasal passages.

How should this medicine be used?

Mometasone comes as a spray to inhale through the nose. It is usually sprayed once a day in each nostril. To help you remember to use mometasone nasal inhalation, use it around the same time every day. Follow the directions on your prescription label carefully, and ask your doctor or pharmacist to explain any part you do not understand. Use mometasone nasal inhalation exactly as directed. Do not use more or less of it or use it more often than prescribed by your doctor.

Shake the pump well before each use.

Do not spray mometasone nasal inhalation into the eyes.

For the prevention of nasal symptoms of seasonal allergies, begin using mometasone nasal inhalation 2-4 weeks before the beginning of the pollen season.

Mometasone nasal inhalation controls the nasal symptoms of allergies but does not cure them. You should begin to feel an improvement in your nasal allergies within 1-2 days of the first dose of mometasone nasal inhalation. It may take 1-2 weeks until you feel the full benefit of mometasone nasal inhalation. Continue to use mometasone nasal inhalation even if you feel well.

Before you use mometasone nasal inhalation the first time, read the written instructions that come with it. Ask your doctor or pharmacist to show you how to use it. Practice using the inhaler while he or she watches.

To use the nasal inhalation, follow these steps:

1. Gently blow your nose to clear the nostrils.
2. Close one nostril. Tilt your head forward slightly and keep the bottle upright while inserting the nasal applicator into the other other nostril.
3. For each spray, press down firmly once on the shoulders of the white applicator using your forefinger and middle finger. Support the base of the bottle with your thumb. Breathe gently inward through the nostril.
4. Breathe out through the mouth.
5. Repeat in the other nostril.
6. Replace the plastic cap.

Before using a new pump of mometasone nasal inhalation for the first time, prime the pump by spraying ten times or until a fine spray appears. If you do not use the pump for more than 1 week, prime it again by spraying two times or until a fine spray appears.

Are there other uses for this medicine?

This medication may be prescribed for other uses; ask your doctor or pharmacist for more information.

What special precautions should I follow?

Before using mometasone nasal inhalation,

- tell your doctor and pharmacist if you are allergic to mometasone or any other medications.
- tell your doctor and pharmacist what prescription and nonprescription medications, vitamins, nutritional supplements, and herbal products you are taking.
- tell your doctor if you have a fungal, bacterial, or viral infection or a herpes infection of the eye and if you have or have ever had tuberculosis, glaucoma, or cataracts. Also tell your doctor if you have had a recent injury, surgery, or ulcer in the nose.
- tell your doctor if you are pregnant, plan to become pregnant, or are breast-feeding. If you become pregnant while using mometasone nasal inhalation, call your doctor.
- avoid exposure to measles and chicken pox. If you are exposed to one of these diseases while using mometasone nasal inhalation, call your doctor immediately.

What special dietary instructions should I follow?

Unless your doctor tells you otherwise, continue your normal diet.

What should I do if I forget to take a dose?

Take the missed dose as soon as you remember it. However, if it is almost time for the next dose, skip the missed dose and continue your regular dosing schedule. Do not take a double dose to make up for a missed one.

What side effects can this medicine cause?

Mometasone nasal inhalation may cause side effects. Tell your doctor if any of these symptoms are severe or do not go away:

- headache
- vomiting
- sore throat
- cough

Some side effects can be serious. The following symptoms are uncommon, but if you experience any of them, call your doctor immediately:

- wheezing
- vision changes
- yeast infection of the nose or throat

Mometasone nasal inhalation may cause children to grow more slowly. Talk to your doctor about the risks of taking this medication.

Mometasone nasal inhalation may cause other side effects. Call your doctor if you have any unusual problems while taking this medication.

If you experience a serious side effect, you or your doctor may send a report to the Food and Drug Administration's (FDA) MedWatch Adverse Event Reporting program online [at http://www.fda.gov/MedWatch/index.html] or by phone [1-800-332-1088].

What storage conditions are needed for this medicine?

Keep this medication in the container it came in, tightly closed, and out of reach of children. Store it at room temperature, away from light, and away from excess heat and moisture (not in the bathroom). Keep track of the number of sprays used from each bottle of mometasone nasal inhalation. Throw away the bottle after using 120 sprays. Throw away any medication that is outdated or no longer needed. Talk to your pharmacist about the proper disposal of your medication.

What other information should I know?

If your condition does not improve or becomes worse, call your doctor.

To clean the nasal applicator, remove the plastic cap and pull gently upward on the white nasal applicator so that it comes free. Wash the applicator and cap in cold water. Dry and replace the applicator, followed by the plastic cap.

Keep all appointments with your doctor.

Do not let anyone else take your medication. Ask your pharmacist any questions you have about refilling your prescription.

Dosage Facts
For Informational Purposes

Caution: Do not change your dose, how often you take your medication, or the length of time you are to take it without first talking to your healthcare provider.

The following dosage information was written using medical language for doctors and other healthcare professionals and is provided here for you to check your dosage. The dosage of this drug may differ for different patients. Therefore, always follow your doctor's instructions or the directions on the label. Contact your healthcare provider or pharmacist if you have any questions about the specific dosage of your medication after reviewing this information.

General Dosage Information

Available as mometasone furoate monohydrate; dosage expressed in terms of anhydrous mometasone furoate.

After priming, nasal spray pump delivers about 50 mcg of mometasone furoate per metered spray and about 120 metered doses per 17-g container.

Pediatric Patients

Titrate dosage to the lowest possible effective level.

Allergic Rhinitis
Treatment of Seasonal or Perennial Allergic Rhinitis

INTRANASAL INHALATION:
- Children 2–11 years of age: 50 mcg (1 spray) in each nostril once daily (100 mcg total daily dosage).
- Children ≥12 years of age: 100 mcg (2 sprays) in each nostril once daily (200 mcg total daily dosage).

Prophylaxis of Seasonal Allergic Rhinitis

INTRANASAL INHALATION:
- Children ≥12 years of age: 100 mcg (2 sprays) in each nostril once daily (200 mcg total daily dosage) starting 2–4 weeks prior to the anticipated start of the pollen season.

Adult Patients
Allergic Rhinitis
Treatment of Seasonal or Perennial Allergic Rhinitis

INTRANASAL INHALATION:
- 100 mcg (2 sprays) in each nostril once daily (200 mcg total daily dosage).

Prophylaxis of Seasonal Allergic Rhinitis

INTRANASAL INHALATION:
- 100 mcg (2 sprays) in each nostril once daily (200 mcg total daily dosage) starting 2–4 weeks prior to the anticipated start of the pollen season.

Montelukast

(mon te loo' kast)

Brand Name: Singulair®

Why is this medicine prescribed?

Montelukast is used to prevent difficulty breathing, chest tightness, wheezing and coughing caused by asthma. Montelukast is also used to prevent bronchospasm (breathing difficulties) during exercise. Montelukast is also used to treat the symptoms of seasonal (occurs only at certain times of the year), and perennial (occurs all year round) allergic rhinitis (a condition associated with sneezing and stuffy, runny or itchy nose). Montelukast is in a class of medications called leukotriene receptor antagonists (LTRAs). It works by blocking the action of substances in the body that cause the symptoms of asthma and allergic rhinitis.

How should this medicine be used?

Montelukast comes as a tablet, a chewable tablet, and granules to take by mouth. Montelukast is usually taken once a day with or without food. When montelukast is used to treat asthma, it should be taken in the evening. When montelukast is used to prevent breathing difficulties during exercise, it should be taken at least 2 hours before exercise. If you are taking montelukast once a day on a regular basis, you should not take an additional dose before exercising. When montelukast is used to treat allergic rhinitis, it may be taken at any time of day. Take montelukast at around the same time every day. Follow the directions on your prescription label carefully, and ask your doctor or pharmacist to explain any part you do not understand. Take montelukast exactly as directed. Do not take more or less of it or take it more often than prescribed by your doctor.

If you are giving the granules to your child, you should not open the foil pouch until your child is ready to take the medication. There are several ways that you can give the granules to your child, so choose the one that works best for you and your child. You may pour all of the granules directly from the packet into your child's mouth to be swallowed immediately. You may also pour the entire packet of granules onto a clean spoon and place the spoonful of medication in your child's mouth. If you prefer, you may mix the entire packet of granules in 1 teaspoon of cold or room temperature baby formula, breastmilk, applesauce, soft carrots, ice cream, or rice. You should not mix the granules with any other foods or liquids, but your child may drink any liquid right after he or she takes the granules. If you mix the granules with one of the allowed foods or drinks, use the mixtures within 15 minutes. Do not store unused mixtures of food, formula, or breast milk and the medication.

Do not use montelukast to treat a sudden attack of asthma symptoms. Your doctor will prescribe a short-acting inhaler to use during attacks. Talk to your doctor about how to treat symptoms of a sudden asthma attack. If your asthma symptoms get worse or if you have asthma attacks more often, be sure to call your doctor.

If you are taking montelukast to treat asthma, continue to take or use all other medications that your doctor has prescribed to treat your asthma. Do not stop taking any of your medications or change the doses of any of your medications unless your doctor tells you that you should. If your asthma is made worse by aspirin, do not take aspirin or other non-steroidal anti-inflammatory drugs (NSAIDs) during your treatment with montelukast.

Montelukast controls the symptoms of asthma and allergic rhinitis but does not cure these conditions. Continue to take montelukast even if you feel well. Do not stop taking montelukast without talking to your doctor.

Ask your pharmacist or doctor for a copy of the manufacturer's information for the patient.

Are there other uses for this medicine?

This medication may be prescribed for other uses; ask your doctor or pharmacist for more information.

What special precautions should I follow?

Before taking montelukast,
- tell your doctor and pharmacist if you are allergic to montelukast or any other medications.
- tell your doctor and pharmacist what prescription and nonprescription medications, vitamins, nutritional supplements, and herbal products you are taking or plan to take. Be sure to mention phenobarbital and rifampin (Rifadin, Rimactane). Your doctor may need to change the doses of your medications or monitor you more carefully for side effects.
- tell your doctor if you have or have ever had liver disease.
- tell your doctor if you are pregnant, plan to become pregnant, or are breast-feeding. If you become pregnant while taking montelukast, call your doctor.
- if you have phenylketonuria (PKU, a inherited condition in which a special diet must be followed to prevent mental retardation), you should know that the chewable tablets contain aspartame that forms phenylalanine.

What special dietary instructions should I follow?

Unless your doctor tells you otherwise, continue your normal diet.

What should I do if I forget to take a dose?

Skip the missed dose and continue your regular dosing schedule. Do not take a double dose to make up for a missed one. Do not take more than one dose of montelukast in a 24 hour period.

What side effects can this medicine cause?

Montelukast may cause side effects. Tell your doctor if any of these symptoms are severe or do not go away:
- headache
- dizziness
- heartburn
- stomach pain
- tiredness

Some side effects can be serious. If you experience any of the following symptoms, call your doctor immediately:
- difficulty breathing or swallowing
- swelling of the face, throat, tongue, lips, eyes, hands, feet, ankles, or lower legs
- hoarseness
- itching
- rash
- hives
- fever
- flu-like symptoms
- pins and needles or numbness in the arms or legs
- pain and swelling of the sinuses

Montelukast may cause other side effects. Call your doctor if you have any unusual problems while you are taking this medication.

If you experience a serious side effect, you or your doctor may send a report to the Food and Drug Administration's (FDA) MedWatch Adverse Event Reporting program online [at http://www.fda.gov/MedWatch/index.html] or by phone [1-800-332-1088].

What storage conditions are needed for this medicine?

Keep this medication in the container it came in, tightly closed, and out of reach of children. Store it at room temperature and away from excess heat and moisture (not in the bathroom). Throw away any medication that is outdated or no longer needed. Talk to your pharmacist about the proper disposal of your medication.

What should I do in case of overdose?

In case of overdose, call your local poison control center at 1-800-222-1222. If the victim has collapsed or is not breathing, call local emergency services at 911.

Symptoms of overdose may include:
- stomach pain
- sleepiness
- thirst
- headache
- vomiting
- restlessness or agitation

What other information should I know?

Keep all appointments with your doctor.

Do not let anyone else take your medication. Ask your pharmacist any questions you have about refilling your prescription.

Dosage Facts
For Informational Purposes

Caution: Do not change your dose, how often you take your medication, or the length of time you are to take it without first talking to your healthcare provider.

The following dosage information was written using medical language for doctors and other healthcare professionals and is provided here for you to check your dosage. The dosage of this drug may differ for different patients. Therefore, always follow your doctor's instructions or the directions on the label. Contact your healthcare provider or pharmacist if you have any questions about the specific dosage of your medication after reviewing this information.

General Dosage Information

Available as montelukast sodium; dosage expressed in terms of montelukast.

Pediatric Patients

Asthma

ORAL:
- Children 12 months to 5 years of age: 4 mg daily.
- Children 6–14 years of age: 5 mg daily.
- Adolescents ≥15 years of age: 10 mg daily.

Exercise-induced Bronchospasm

ORAL:
- Children 6–14 years of age: 5 mg daily.
- Adolescents ≥15 years of age: 10 mg daily.

Allergic Rhinitis

ORAL:
- Children 2–5 years of age: 4 mg daily.
- Children 6–14 years of age: 5 mg daily.
- Adolescents ≥15 years of age: 10 mg daily.

Adult Patients

Asthma

ORAL:
- 10 mg daily.

Exercise-induced Bronchospasm

ORAL:
- 10 mg daily.

Allergic Rhinitis

ORAL:
- 10 mg daily.

Urticaria†

ORAL:
- 5–20 mg daily.

Special Populations

Hepatic Impairment
- No dosage adjustment required in patients with mild to moderate hepatic impairment. Not evaluated in patients with severe hepatic impairment or hepatitis.

Renal Impairment
- No dosage adjustment required.

Geriatric Patients
- No dosage adjustment required.

† Use is not currently included in the labeling approved by the US Food and Drug Administration.

Morphine Oral

(mor′ feen)

Brand Name: Avinza®, Kadian®, MS Contin®, Oramorph® SR, Roxanol®, Roxanol®-T
Also available generically.

Important Warning

Morphine is available as long acting capsules or tablets. These capsules or tablets contain enough morphine to relieve pain for 12 or 24 hours and are designed to release the medication slowly over that period of time. It is very important not to split, chew, or crush these tablets or capsules and not to dissolve the beads contained in the capsules in any liquid before you swallow them. This would release all of the medication into your body at once and could cause serious health problems or death.

If you are taking Oramorph® SR or MS Contin® brand long-acting tablets or Avinza® or Kadian® brand long-acting capsules, you should swallow the tablets or capsules whole. If you are unable to swallow the capsules, you can carefully open a capsule, sprinkle all of the beads that it contains on a spoonful of cold or room temperature applesauce, and swallow the entire mixture immediately without chewing or crushing the beads. Then rinse your mouth with a little water and swallow the water to be sure that you have swallowed all the medication. Do not save mixtures of medication and applesauce for later.

If you are taking Avinza® brand long-acting capsules, you should not drink any drinks that contain alcohol or take any prescription or non-prescription medications that contain alcohol. Ask your doctor or pharmacist or check the list of ingredients if you do not know if a medication contains alcohol. Alcohol may cause the morphine in Avinza® brand long-acting capsules to be released in your body too quickly, causing serious health problems or death.

Why is this medicine prescribed?

Morphine is used to relieve moderate to severe pain. Morphine long-acting tablets and capsules are only used by patients who are expected to need medication to relieve moderate to severe pain around-the-clock for longer than a few days. Morphine is in a class of medications called opiate (narcotic) analgesics. It works by changing the way the body senses pain.

How should this medicine be used?

Morphine comes as a tablet, a solution (liquid), a controlled- or extended-release (long-acting) tablet, and a controlled- or sustained-release (long-acting) capsule all to take by mouth. The regular tablet and liquid usually are taken every 4 hours. The long acting tablet is usually taken every 8-12 hours. Kadian ®brand long-acting capsules are usually taken with or without food every 12 hours or every 24 hours. Avinza® brand long acting capsules are usually taken once a day. Follow the directions on your prescription label carefully, and ask your doctor or pharmacist to explain any part you do not understand.

If you are taking morphine solution, use the spoon or dropper that comes with the medication to measure your dose. Be sure that you know how many milliliters of the solution you should take. Ask your pharmacist if you have any questions about how much medication you should take or how to use the spoon or dropper.

If you are taking Kadian® brand long-acting capsules and you have a gastrostomy tube (surgically inserted feeding tube), ask your doctor or pharmacist how to administer the medication through your tube.

Your doctor may start you on a low dose of morphine and gradually increase your dose until your pain is controlled. Your doctor may adjust your dose at any time during your treatment if your pain is not controlled. If you feel that your pain is not controlled, call your doctor. Do not change the dose of your medication without talking to your doctor.

Morphine can be habit-forming. Take morphine exactly as directed. Do not take a larger dose, take it more often, or take it for a longer period of time or in a different way than prescribed by your doctor.

Do not stop taking morphine without talking to your doctor. Your doctor may decrease your dose gradually. If you suddenly stop taking morphine, you may experience withdrawal symptoms such as anxiety; sweating; difficulty falling asleep or staying asleep; chills; shaking of a part of your body that you cannot control; upset stomach; diarrhea; runny nose, sneezing or coughing; hair on your skin standing on end; or hallucinating (seeing things or hearing voices that do not exist).

Are there other uses for this medicine?

This medication is sometimes prescribed for other uses; ask your doctor or pharmacist for more information.

What special precautions should I follow?

Before taking morphine,
- tell your doctor and pharmacist if you are allergic to morphine, any other medications, or any of the inactive ingredients in the type of morphine tablets, capsules, or liquid you plan to take. Ask your pharmacist for a list of the inactive ingredients.
- tell your doctor and pharmacist what prescription and nonprescription medications, vitamins, nutritional supplements, and herbal products you are taking or plan to take. Be sure to mention any of the following: anticoagulants ('blood thinners') such as warfarin (Coumadin); antidepressants such as amitriptyline (Elavil), amoxapine (Asendin), clomipramine (Anafranil), desipramine (Norpramin), doxepin (Adapin, Sinequan), imipramine (Tofranil), nortriptyline (Aventyl, Pamelor), protriptyline (Vivactil), and trimipramine (Surmontil); antihistamines (found in cold and allergy medications); beta blockers such as atenolol (Tenormin), labetalol (Normodyne), metoprolol (Lopressor, Toprol XL), nadolol (Corgard), and propranolol (Inderal); buprenorphine (Subutex, in Suboxone); butorphanol (Stadol); cimetidine (Tagamet); diuretics ('water pills'); medications for anxiety, mental illness, pain, seizures, or upset stomach; muscle relaxants; nalbuphine (Nubain); pentazocine (Talwin, in Talacen); sedatives; sleeping pills; and tranquilizers. Also tell your doctor if you are taking any of the following medications or if you have stopped taking them within the past 2 weeks: monoamine oxidase (MAO) inhibitors, including isocarboxazid (Marplan), phenelzine (Nardil), procarbazine (Matulane), selegiline (Eldepryl), and tranylcypromine (Parnate). Your doctor may need to change the doses of your medications or monitor you more carefully for side effects.
- tell your doctor if you drink or have ever drunk large amounts of alcoholand if you have ever had major surgery. Also tell your doctor if you have or have ever had a head injury; a brain tumor; seizures; mental illness; difficulty swallowing; lung disease such as asthma, chronic obstructive pulmonary disease (COPD; a group of diseases that cause gradual loss of lung function), or other breathing problems; prostatic hypertrophy (en-

largement of a male reproductive gland); urinary problems; low blood pressure; irregular heartbeat; Addison's disease (condition in which the body does not make enough of certain natural substances); or liver, kidney, pancreatic, intestinal, or gallbladder disease.

- tell your doctor if you are pregnant, plan to become pregnant, or are breast-feeding. If you become pregnant while taking morphine, call your doctor.
- if you are having surgery, including dental surgery, tell the doctor or dentist that you are taking morphine.
- you should know that this medication may make you drowsy. Do not drive a car or operate machinery until you know how this medication affects you.
- talk to your doctor about the safe use of alcohol while you are taking this medication.
- you should know that morphine may cause dizziness, lightheadedness, and fainting when you get up too quickly from a lying position. To avoid this problem, get out of bed slowly, resting your feet on the floor for a few minutes before standing up.

What special dietary instructions should I follow?

Drink plenty of fluids while you are taking this medication.

What should I do if I forget to take a dose?

Take the missed dose as soon as you remember it. However, if it is almost time for the next dose, skip the missed dose and continue your regular dosing schedule. Do not take a double dose to make up for a missed one.

What side effects can this medicine cause?

Morphine may cause side effects. Tell your doctor if any of these symptoms are severe or do not go away:

- dizziness
- lightheadedness
- drowsiness
- upset stomach
- vomiting
- constipation
- diarrhea
- loss of appetite
- weight loss
- changes in ability to taste food
- dry mouth
- sweating
- weakness
- headache
- agitation
- nervousness
- mood changes
- confusion
- difficulty falling asleep or staying asleep
- stiff muscles
- shaking of a part of your body that you cannot control
- double vision

- red eyes
- small pupils (black circles in the middle of the eyes)
- eye movements that you cannot control
- chills
- flu symptoms
- decreased sexual desire or ability
- difficulty urinating or pain when urinating

Some side effects can be serious. If you experience any of the following symptoms, call your doctor immediately:

- slow, shallow, or irregular breathing
- blue or purple color to the skin
- fast or slow heartbeat
- seizures
- hallucinations (seeing things or hearing voices that do not exist)
- blurred vision
- fainting
- hives
- rash
- itching
- tightness in the throat
- difficulty swallowing
- swelling of the arms, hands, feet, ankles, or lower legs

Morphine may cause other side effects. Call your doctor if you have any unusual problems while taking this medication.

If you experience a serious side effect, you or your doctor may send a report to the Food and Drug Administration's (FDA) MedWatch Adverse Event Reporting program online [at http://www.fda.gov/MedWatch/index.html] or by phone [1-800-332-1088].

What storage conditions are needed for this medicine?

Keep this medication in the container it came in, tightly closed, and out of reach of children. Store it at room temperature and away from excess heat and moisture (not in the bathroom). Throw away any medication that is outdated or no longer needed. Talk to your pharmacist about the proper disposal of your medication.

Store morphine in a safe place so that no one else can take it accidentally or on purpose. Keep track of how many tablets or capsules or how much liquid is left so you will know if any medication is missing.

What should I do in case of overdose?

In case of overdose, call your local poison control center at 1-800-222-1222. If the victim has collapsed or is not breathing, call local emergency services at 911.

Symptoms of overdose may include:

- slow, shallow, or irregular breathing
- sleepiness
- loss of consciousness
- limp muscles
- cold, clammy skin
- small pupils

- slow heartbeat
- blurred vision
- upset stomach
- fainting

What other information should I know?

Keep all appointments with your doctor.

Do not let anyone else take your medication. This prescription is not refillable. If you are taking morphine to control your pain on a long term basis, be sure to schedule appointments with your doctor so that you do not run out of medication. If you are taking morphine on a short term basis, call your doctor if you continue to experience pain after you finish the medication.

Dosage Facts
For Informational Purposes

Caution: Do not change your dose, how often you take your medication, or the length of time you are to take it without first talking to your healthcare provider.

The following dosage information was written using medical language for doctors and other healthcare professionals and is provided here for you to check your dosage. The dosage of this drug may differ for different patients. Therefore, always follow your doctor's instructions or the directions on the label. Contact your healthcare provider or pharmacist if you have any questions about the specific dosage of your medication after reviewing this information.

General Dosage Information

Available as morphine sulfate; dosage usually expressed as the sulfate.

Should be given in the smallest effective dose and as infrequently as possible in order to minimize the development of tolerance and physical dependence.

In patients with severe, chronic pain, dosage should be adjusted according to the severity of the pain and the response and tolerance of the patient.

In patients with exceptionally severe, chronic pain or in those who have become tolerant to the analgesic effect of opiate agonists, it may be necessary to exceed the usual dosage.

Pediatric Patients

Pain
Moderate to Severe Pain
ORAL:
- Infants and children: 0.2–0.5 mg/kg every 4–6 hours (conventional tablets, oral solution).

Adult Patients

Pain (Oral Treatment)
Most manufacturers suggest that it is preferable to initiate and stabilize oral morphine sulfate therapy with a conventional (immediate-release) preparation and then switch the patient to an extended-release preparation (Avinza®, Kadian®, MS Contin®, Oramorph® SR) since titration of dosage may be more difficult with the latter preparations.

Dosing regimen must be individualized based on the patient's prior analgesic therapy.

Initial dosage of extended-release preparations should be based on the total daily dosage, potency, and specific characteristics of the current opiate agonist.

Other considerations should include the reliability of relative potency estimates used in calculating the equivalent morphine sulfate dosage, the degree of opiate experience and tolerance, the medical condition of the patient, concomitant drug therapy, and the nature and severity of the patient's pain.

It is preferable to underestimate the initial dosage of extended-release preparations than to inadvertently cause an overdosage of morphine sulfate.

Supplemental doses of a short-acting opiate agonist can be considered if breakthrough pain occurs with dosing regimens employing extended-release preparations.

When converting to another oral extended-release morphine sulfate preparation or to other oral or parenteral opiate analgesics, the manufacturer's labeling information should be consulted.

Oral Solutions or Conventional Tablets
ORAL:
- Usually, 10–30 mg every 4 hours as necessary or as directed by a physician.

Extended-release Capsules (Avinza®)
ORAL:
- Individualize dosage according to patient response and tolerance; do not exceed 1.6 g daily.
- Administer Avinza® no more frequently than once every 24 hours. The 60-, 90-, and 120-mg Avinza® capsules should be used only in opiate-tolerant patients.
- Switching from other oral morphine preparations to Avinza®: Use the prior total daily oral dosage and administer once every 24 hours. Supplemental doses of a short-acting opiate analgesic may be required for up to 4 days until the patient's response to Avinza® has stabilized.
- Switching from parenteral morphine or other non-morphine oral or parenteral opiate therapy to Avinza®: Calculate the opiate analgesic requirements during the previous 24 hours and convert to an equianalgesic dosage of Avinza®. Use conservative dosage conversion ratios to avoid toxicity.
- When used as the initial opiate in patients who do not have a proven tolerance to opiates: Usual initial dosage is 30 mg once daily; increase dosage by no more than 30 mg every 4 days. Dosage increases should be conservative in opiate-naive patients.

Extended-release Capsules (Kadian®)
ORAL:
- Individualize dosage according to patient response and tolerance; do not increase dosage more frequently than every other day.
- Administer Kadian® no more frequently than every 12 hours. Patients receiving once-daily Kadian® who experience excessive sedation or inadequate analgesia prior to the next dose should be switched to a twice-daily regimen. The 100-mg Kadian® capsules should be used only in opiate-tolerant patients.
- Switching from other oral morphine preparations to Kadian®:

Use the prior total daily oral dosage and give in 2 divided doses every 12 hours or once every 24 hours. First dose of Kadian® may be administered concurrently with the last dose of immediate-release opiate therapy because of the delayed peak plasma morphine concentrations produced by Kadian®.

- Switching from parenteral morphine or other non-morphine oral or parenteral opiate therapy to Kadian®: Calculate the opiate analgesic requirements during the previous 24 hours and convert to an equianalgesic dosage of Kadian®. Use conservative dosage conversion ratios to avoid toxicity.
- When used as the initial opiate in patients who do not have a proven tolerance to opiates: Initially 20 mg of Kadian®; increase by no more than 20 mg every other day.

Extended-release Tablets (MS Contin®)

ORAL:
- Individualize dosage according to patient response and tolerance.
- Interval between doses of MS Contin® should not exceed 12 hours in order to avoid administration of large single doses.
- Use 15-mg tablets when total daily dosage is expected to be <60 mg daily; use 30-mg tablets when total daily dosage is expected to be 60–120 mg daily. The 100- and 200-mg tablets of MS Contin® should be used only in patients who are opiate tolerant and require dosages of ≥200 mg daily.
- Switching from an immediate-release oral morphine preparation to MS Contin®: Use the prior total daily oral dosage and give in 2 divided doses every 12 hours or in 3 divided doses every 8 hours.
- Switching from parenteral morphine or other oral or parenteral non-morphine opiate to MS Contin®: Calculate the opiate analgesic requirements during the previous 24 hours and convert to an equianalgesic dosage of MS Contin®. Use conservative dosage conversion ratios to avoid toxicity.

Extended-release Tablets (Oramorph SR®)

ORAL:
- Individualize dosage according to patient response and tolerance.
- Dosing interval for Oramorph SR® should not exceed 12 hours because administration of large single doses may lead to acute overdosage. If pain is not controlled for the entire 12-hour interval, then the dosing interval may be decreased, but doses should be administered no more frequently than every 8 hours.
- Use 30-mg tablets if morphine sulfate requirement is ≤120 mg daily. Use 15-mg tablets if morphine sulfate requirement is low.
- Switching from other oral morphine preparations to Oramorph SR®: Use the prior total daily oral dosage and give in 2 divided doses every 12 hours.
- Switching from parenteral morphine or other oral or parenteral non-morphine opiate to Oramorph SR®: Calculate the opiate analgesic requirements during the previous 24 hours and convert to an equianalgesic dosage of Oramorph SR®. Use conservative dosage conversion ratios to avoid toxicity.

Prescribing Limits

Adult Patients

Analgesia

Avinza®

ORAL:
- Do not exceed 1.6 g daily.
- Administer no more frequently than every 24 hours. Increase dosage by no more than 30 mg every 4 days.

Kadian®

ORAL:
- Administer no more frequently than every 12 hours.

MS Contin®

ORAL:
- Interval between doses should not exceed 12 hours in order to avoid administration of large single doses.

Oramorph SR®

ORAL:
- Dosing interval should not exceed 12 hours because administration of large single doses may lead to acute overdosage.
- Administer no more frequently than every 8 hours.

Special Populations

Reduced dosage is indicated in poor-risk patients, in patients with substantial hepatic impairment, in very young or very old patients, and in patients receiving other CNS depressants.

Hepatic Impairment
- Reduce dosage in patients with severe hepatic impairment.

Renal Impairment
- Reduce dosage in patients with severe renal impairment, since the active metabolite morphine 6-glucuronide accumulates in such patients which can result in enhanced and prolonged opiate activity.

Geriatric and Debilitated Patients
- Reduce dosage in poor-risk patients and in very old patients.
- Administer epidurally or intrathecally with extreme caution and in reduced dosage in geriatric or debilitated patients.

Morphine Sulfate Injection

(mor′ feen)

Brand Name: Astramorph/PF®, Duramorph®, Infumorph®
Also available generically.

About Your Treatment

Your doctor has ordered morphine, a strong analgesic (painkiller), to relieve your pain. The drug will be either injected into a large muscle (such as your buttock or hip) or added to an intravenous fluid that will drip through a needle or catheter placed in your vein or under your skin.

You probably will receive morphine continuously for around-the-clock pain relief. Your doctor also may order other pain medications to make you more comfortable. This medication is sometimes prescribed for other uses; ask your doctor or pharmacist for more information.

Your health care provider (doctor, nurse, or pharmacist) may measure the effectiveness and side effects of your treatment using laboratory tests and physical examinations. It is important to keep all appointments with your doctor and the laboratory. The length of treatment depends on how you respond to the medication.

Precautions

Before administering morphine,

- tell your doctor and pharmacist if you are allergic to morphine, codeine (or medications that contain codeine such as Tylenol with Codeine), hydrocodone (e.g., Vicodin), hydromorphone (e.g., Dilaudid), oxycodone (e.g., Percocet), oxymorphone (Numorphan), or any other drugs.
- tell your doctor and pharmacist what prescription and nonprescription medications you are taking, especially other pain relievers; antidepressants; medications for cough, cold, or allergies; sedatives; sleeping pills; tranquilizers; and vitamins.
- tell your doctor if you have or have ever had liver or kidney disease, a history of alcoholism, lung or thyroid disease, heart disease, prostatic hypertrophy, or lung or urinary problems.
- tell your doctor if you are pregnant, plan to become pregnant, or are breast-feeding. If you become pregnant while taking morphine, call your doctor.
- you should know that this drug may make you drowsy. Do not drive a car or operate machinery until you know how this drug affects you.
- remember that alcohol can add to the drowsiness caused by this drug.
- tell your doctor if you use tobacco products. Cigarette smoking may decrease the effectiveness of this drug.

Administering Your Medication

Before you administer morphine, look at the solution closely. It should be clear and free of floating material. Gently squeeze the bag or observe the solution container to make sure there are no leaks. Do not use the solution if it is discolored, if it contains particles, or if the bag or container leaks. Use a new solution, but show the damaged one to your health care provider.

It is important that you use your medication exactly as directed. Morphine can be habit forming. Do not administer it more often or for a longer period than your doctor tells you. Do not change your dosing schedule without talking to your health care provider. Your health care provider may tell you to stop your infusion if you have a mechanical problem (such as a blockage in the tubing, needle, or catheter); if you have to stop an infusion, call your health care provider immediately so your therapy can continue.

Side Effects

Morphine may cause side effects. Tell your doctor if any of these symptoms are severe or do not go away:

- dizziness
- lightheadedness
- drowsiness
- upset stomach
- vomiting
- constipation
- stomach pain
- rash
- difficulty urinating

If you experience either of the following symptoms, call your doctor immediately:

- difficulty breathing
- fainting

If you experience a serious side effect, you or your doctor may send a report to the Food and Drug Administration's (FDA) MedWatch Adverse Event Reporting program online [at http://www.fda.gov/MedWatch/index.html] or by phone [1-800-332-1088].

Storage Conditions

- Your health care provider probably will give you several days supply of morphine at a time. If you are receiving morphine intravenously (in your vein), you probably will be told to store it in the refrigerator.
- Take your next dose from the refrigerator 1 hour before using it; place it in a clean, dry area to allow it to warm to room temperature.

If you are receiving morphine intramuscularly (in your muscle), your health care provider will tell you how to store it properly.

Store your medication only as directed. Make sure you understand what you need to store your medication properly.

Keep your supplies in a clean, dry place when you are not using them, and keep all medications and supplies out of reach of children. Your health care provider will tell you how to throw away used needles, syringes, tubing, and containers to avoid accidental injury.

Overdose

In case of overdose, call your local poison control center at 1-800-222-1222. If the victim has collapsed or is not breathing, call local emergency services at 911.

Signs of Infection

If you are receiving morphine in your vein or under your skin, you need to know the symptoms of a catheter-related infection (an infection where the needle enters your vein or skin). If you experience any of these effects near your intravenous catheter, tell your health care provider as soon as possible:

- tenderness
- warmth

- irritation
- drainage
- redness
- swelling
- pain

Dosage Facts
For Informational Purposes

Caution: Do not change your dose, how often you take your medication, or the length of time you are to take it without first talking to your healthcare provider.

The following dosage information was written using medical language for doctors and other healthcare professionals and is provided here for you to check your dosage. The dosage of this drug may differ for different patients. Therefore, always follow your doctor's instructions or the directions on the label. Contact your healthcare provider or pharmacist if you have any questions about the specific dosage of your medication after reviewing this information.

General Dosage Information

Available as morphine sulfate; dosage usually expressed as the sulfate.

Should be given in the smallest effective dose and as infrequently as possible in order to minimize the development of tolerance and physical dependence.

In patients with severe, chronic pain, dosage should be adjusted according to the severity of the pain and the response and tolerance of the patient.

In patients with exceptionally severe, chronic pain or in those who have become tolerant to the analgesic effect of opiate agonists, it may be necessary to exceed the usual dosage.

Pediatric Patients

Pain
Moderate to Severe Pain

IM OR SUB-Q:
- Neonates: 0.05–0.2 mg/kg every 2–4 hours as necessary.
- Infants and children: 0.1–0.2 mg/kg every 2–4 hours.
- Single pediatric doses should not exceed 10 mg.

IV:
- Neonates: 0.05–0.2 mg/kg every 2–4 hours as necessary. For continuous IV infusion, 0.025–0.05 mg/kg per hour.
- Infants and children: 0.1–0.2 mg/kg every 2–4 hours.
- Adolescents >12 years of age: 3–4 mg; may repeat in 5 minutes if needed.
- Single pediatric doses should not exceed 10 mg.
- PCA (usually IV) via controlled-delivery device: Loading doses of 0.05 mg/kg (preferably titrated by clinician or nurse at bedside, up to 0.05–0.2 mg/kg total) used. Maintenance doses (administered intermittently) of 10–20 mcg/kg, usually no more frequently than every 6–12 minutes as a device-programmed lockout period used for developmentally mature pediatric patients ≥7 years of age.

Cancer Pain (Severe, Chronic)

IV:
- Maintenance dosages of 0.025–2.6 mg/kg per hour (median: 0.04–0.07 mg/kg per hour) have been infused IV in children.

SUB-Q:
- Maintenance dosages of 0.025–1.79 mg/kg per hour (median: 0.06 mg/kg per hour) have been infused sub-Q in a limited number of children.

Sickle Cell Crisis (Severe Pain)

IV:
- Maintenance dosages of 0.03–0.15 mg/kg per hour have been infused IV in children.

Postoperative Analgesia

IV:
- Maintenance dosages of 0.01–0.04 mg/kg per hour have been infused.

Adult Patients

Pain (Other Routes)

IV:
- May administer 2.5–20 mg every 2–6 hours as needed or via continuous infusion at a rate of 0.8–10 mg per hour.
- Can be administered at a rate of 2–4 mg every 5 minutes, with some patients requiring as much as 25–30 mg before pain relief is adequate.

IM OR SUB-Q:
- May administer 2.5–20 mg every 2–6 hours as needed or via continuous infusion at a rate of 0.8–10 mg per hour.

Pain (MI)

To relieve pain and associated anxiety and provide potentially beneficial cardiovascular effects in adults with AMI, dosages of 2–15 mg have been administered parenterally.

IV:
- Preferred route since absorption following sub-Q or IM injection may be unpredictable, and repeated doses (up to every 5 minutes if necessary) in small increments (e.g., 1–4 mg) generally are preferred to larger and less frequent doses in order to minimize the risk of adverse effects (e.g., respiratory depression).
- Occasionally, patients may require relatively large cumulative doses (e.g., 2–3 mg/kg).
- Patients should be advised to notify their caretakers (e.g., nurse) immediately when discomfort occurs and describe its severity on a numeric scale (e.g., 1–10).

Cancer Pain

Individualize dosage according to the response and tolerance of the patient for sub-Q or continuous IV infusions.

CONTINUOUS IV:
- Initially 0.8–10 mg/hour and then increase to an effective dosage as necessary; an IV loading dose of ≥15 mg can be administered for initial relief of pain prior to initiating continuous IV infusion of the drug.
- Maintenance doses have ranged from 0.8–80 mg/hour infused IV, although higher (e.g., 150 mg/hour) maintenance dosages occasionally have been required.

Patient-controlled Analgesia (PCA)

IV:

- Adjust dosage according to the severity of the pain and response of the patient; consult the operator's manual for the patient-controlled infusion device for directions on administering the drug at the desired rate of infusion.
- Exercise care to avoid overdosage, which could result in respiratory depression, or abrupt cessation of therapy with the drug, which could precipitate opiate withdrawal.
- PCA via controlled-delivery device: Standard protocol uses loading dose of 1 mg, time between doses of 6 minutes (lockout period), and limit of 10 doses per hour. Loading doses of 2–4 mg every 10 minutes, preferably titrated by clinician or nurse at bedside, up to 6–16 mg total have been used for rapid control of pain. Maintenance doses (self-administered intermittently) of 0.5–2 mg, usually no more frequently than every 6–12 minutes as a device-programmed lockout period used.

Unstable Angina (Unresponsive to 3 Sublingual Doses of Nitroglycerin)

IV:

- 2–5 mg (repeated every 5–30 minutes as needed to relieve symptoms and maintain patient comfort) has been used.

Analgesia during Labor

SUB-Q OR IM:

- 10 mg.

Prescribing Limits

Pediatric Patients

Analgesia
Moderate to Severe Pain

IV, IM, OR SUB-Q:

- Single pediatric doses should not exceed 15 mg.

Special Populations

Reduced dosage is indicated in poor-risk patients, in patients with substantial hepatic impairment, in very young or very old patients, and in patients receiving other CNS depressants.

Hepatic Impairment

- Reduce dosage in patients with severe hepatic impairment.

Renal Impairment

- Reduce dosage in patients with severe renal impairment, since the active metabolite morphine 6-glucuronide accumulates in such patients which can result in enhanced and prolonged opiate activity.

Geriatric and Debilitated Patients

- Reduce dosage in poor-risk patients and in very old patients.
- Administer epidurally or intrathecally with extreme caution and in reduced dosage in geriatric or debilitated patients.

Moxifloxacin

Brand Name: Avelox®

Why is this medicine prescribed?

Moxifloxacin is in a class of drugs called fluoroquinolone antibiotics. It works by stopping the life cycle of bacteria. It is used to eliminate certain bacteria that cause infections in your lungs and sinuses. Antibiotics will not work for colds, flu, or other viral infections.

This medication is sometimes prescribed for other uses; ask your doctor or pharmacist for more information.

How should this medicine be used?

Moxifloxacin comes as tablet to take by mouth. It is usually taken once a day for 5 to 10 days. Moxifloxacin tablets should be swallowed whole with a full glass of water. It can be taken with or without food.

Follow the directions on your prescription label carefully, and ask your doctor or pharmacist to explain any part you do not understand. Use moxifloxacin exactly as directed. Do not use more or less of it or use it more often than prescribed by your doctor.

Continue to take moxifloxacin even if you feel well. Do not stop taking moxifloxacin without talking to your doctor.

Are there other uses for this medicine?

Moxifloxacin is used occasionally to treat prostatitis, osteomyelitis, traveler's diarrhea, gonorrheal cervicitis or urethritis, pelvic inflammatory disease, sinusitis, otitis media, septic arthritis, bacterial meningitis, bacteremia, and endocarditis, and to prevent infection in urological surgery. Talk to your doctor about the possible risks of using this drug for your condition.

What special precautions should I follow?

Before using moxifloxacin,

- tell your doctor and pharmacist if you are allergic to moxifloxacin, alatrofloxacin injection (Trovan), cinoxacin (Cinobac), ciprofloxacin (Cipro), enoxacin (Penetrex), gatifloxacin (Tequin), levofloxacin (Levaquin), lomefloxacin (Maxaquin), nalidixic acid (NegGram), norfloxacin (Noroxin), ofloxacin (Floxin), sparfloxacin (Zagam), trofloxacin tablets (Trovan), or any other drugs.
- tell your doctor and pharmacist what prescription and nonprescription medications you are taking, especially other antibiotics; amiodarone (Cordarone); cisapride (Propulsid); disopyramide (Norpace); diuretics ('water pills') such as furosemide (Lasix) and hydrochlorothiazide (Hydrodiuril); erythromycin (E-Mycin, Ery-Tab, PCE, others); medications for depression or other mental diseases; nonsteroidal anti-inflammatory agents; procainamide (Pronestyl); quinidine; sotalol (Betapace); and vitamins and herbal products.

- do not take with antacids containing magnesium or aluminum (Milk of Magnesia, Riopan, Maalox, Mylanta), sucralfate (Carafate), iron or zinc supplements, vitamins that contain iron or zinc, or didanosine (Videx) tablets or pediatric powder for oral solution. Take these medications at least 8 hours before or 4 hours after moxifloxacin.
- tell your doctor if you currently have diarrhea; have or have ever had liver disease, severe cerebral arteriosclerosis, or epilepsy; or if you have, have had, or have a family history of heart disease such as irregular rhythms, low potassium levels, bradycardia, or heart attacks.
- tell your doctor if you are pregnant or plan to become pregnant, or if you are breast-feeding. If you become pregnant while using moxifloxacin, call your doctor immediately.
- if you are having surgery, including dental surgery, tell the doctor or dentist that you are taking moxifloxacin.
- plan to avoid unnecessary or prolonged exposure to sunlight and to wear protective clothing, sunglasses, and sunscreen. Moxifloxacin may make your skin sensitive to sunlight.
- you should know that moxifloxacin may cause dizziness and lightheadedness. Do not drive a car or work on dangerous machinery until you know how moxifloxacin will affect you.

What special dietary instructions should I follow?

While taking moxifloxacin, you should drink at least eight full glasses of water or other liquid every day.

What should I do if I forget to take a dose?

Take the missed dose as soon as you remember it. However, if it is almost time for the next dose, skip the missed dose and continue your regular dosing schedule. Do not take a double dose to make up for a missed one.

What side effects can this medicine cause?

Side effects from moxifloxacin can occur. Tell your doctor if any of these symptoms are severe or do not go away:
- upset stomach
- diarrhea
- dizziness
- headache
- stomach pain
- vomiting
- change in taste

If you experience any of the following symptoms, call your doctor immediately:
- skin rash
- itching
- hives
- difficulty breathing or swallowing
- swelling of the face or throat

- fever
- yellowing of the skin or eyes
- dark urine
- pale or dark stools
- blood in urine
- sunburn or blistering
- confusion
- hallucinations
- depression
- suicidal thoughts
- fast or irregular heartbeat
- fainting
- pain, inflammation, or rupture of a tendon
- tremor
- extreme tiredness
- seizures or convulsions
- visual changes

If you experience a serious side effect, you or your doctor may send a report to the Food and Drug Administration's (FDA) MedWatch Adverse Event Reporting program online [at http://www.fda.gov/MedWatch/index.html] or by phone [1-800-332-1088].

What storage conditions are needed for this medicine?

Keep this medication in the container it came in, tightly closed, and out of reach of children. Store it at room temperature and away from excess heat and moisture (not in the bathroom). Throw away any medication that is outdated or no longer needed. Talk to your pharmacist about the proper disposal of your medication.

What should I do in case of overdose?

In case of overdose, call your local poison control center at 1-800-222-1222. If the victim has collapsed or is not breathing, call local emergency services at 911.

What other information should I know?

Moxifloxacin has not been tested in children younger than 18 years of age, so keep the medication out of reach of children.

Keep all appointments with your doctor and the laboratory. Your doctor may order certain lab tests to check your response to moxifloxacin.

Do not let anyone else take your medication. Your prescription is probably not refillable. If you still have symptoms of infection after you finish the moxifloxacin, call your doctor.

Dosage Facts
For Informational Purposes

Caution: Do not change your dose, how often you take your medication, or the length of time you are to take it without first talking to your healthcare provider.

The following dosage information was written using medical language for doctors and other healthcare professionals and is provided here for you to check your dosage. The dosage of this drug may differ for different patients. Therefore, always follow your doctor's instructions or the directions on the label. Contact your healthcare provider or pharmacist if you have any questions about the specific dosage of your medication after reviewing this information.

General Dosage Information

Available as moxifloxacin hydrochloride; dosage expressed in terms of moxifloxacin.

Dosage of oral and IV moxifloxacin is identical. Dosage adjustment not needed when switching from IV to oral administration, or vice versa.

Adult Patients

Respiratory Tract Infections
Acute Bacterial Sinusitis

ORAL:
• 400 mg once daily for 10 days.

Acute Bacterial Exacerbations of Chronic Bronchitis

ORAL:
• 400 mg once daily for 5 days.

Community-acquired Pneumonia (CAP)

ORAL:
• 400 mg once daily for 7–14 days.

Skin and Skin Structure Infections
Uncomplicated Infections

ORAL:
• 400 mg once daily for 7 days.

Complicated Infections

ORAL:
• 400 mg once daily for 7–21 days.

Anthrax†
Postexposure Prophylaxis Following Exposure in the Context of Biologic Warfare or Bioterrorism†

ORAL:
• 400 mg once daily for ≥60 days.
• Optimum duration of postexposure prophylaxis after an inhalation exposure to *B. anthracis* spores is unclear, but prolonged postexposure prophylaxis usually required. A duration of 60 days may be adequate for a low-dose exposure, but a duration >4 months may be necessary to reduce the risk following a high-dose exposure. CDC, US Working Group on Civilian Biodefense, and US Army Medical Research Institute of Infectious Diseases (USAMRIID) recommend that postexposure prophylaxis in unvaccinated individuals be continued for ≥60 days following a confirmed exposure (including in laboratory workers with confirmed exposures to *B. anthracis* cultures). The USPHS Advisory Committee on Immunization Practices (ACIP) and USAMRIID recommend that individuals who are partially or fully vaccinated against anthrax receive postexposure prophylaxis for ≥30 days; if given in conjunction with anthrax vaccine, continue prophylaxis for at least 7–14 days after the third vaccine dose.

Treatment of Inhalational Anthrax†

ORAL:
• 400 mg once daily for ≥60 days.
• Initial parenteral regimen preferred; use oral regimen for initial treatment only when a parenteral regimen is not available (e.g., supply or logistic problems because large numbers of individuals require treatment in a mass casualty setting). Continue for total duration of ≥60 days if inhalational anthrax occurred as the result of exposure to anthrax spores in the context of biologic warfare or bioterrorism.

Mycobacterial Infections†
Active Tuberculosis†

ORAL:
• 400 mg once daily. Must be used in conjunction with other antituberculosis agents.
• Multiple-drug regimen usually given for 12–18 months when rifampin-resistant *M. tuberculosis* are involved; for 18–24 months when isoniazid- and rifampin-resistant strains are involved; or for 24 months when the strain is resistant to isoniazid, rifampin, ethambutol, and/or pyrazinamide.

Prescribing Limits

Adult Patients

Do not exceed usual dosage or duration of therapy.

Special Populations

Hepatic Impairment
• Dosage adjustments not required in adults with mild or moderate hepatic impairment (Child-Pugh class A or B). Pharmacokinetics not evaluated in those with severe hepatic impairment (Child-Pugh class C).

Renal Impairment
• Dosage adjustments not required in adults with renal impairment, including those on hemodialysis or CAPD.

Geriatric Patients
• No dosage adjustments except those related to renal impairment.

† Use is not currently included in the labeling approved by the US Food and Drug Administration.

Moxifloxacin Ophthalmic

(mox ee flox′ a sin)

Brand Name: Vigamox®

Why is this medicine prescribed?

Moxifloxacin ophthalmic solution is used to treat bacterial conjunctivitis (pink eye; infection of the membrane that covers the outside of the eyeballs and the inside of the eyelids). Moxifloxacin ophthalmic solution is in a class of antibiotics called fluoroquinolones. It works by killing the bacteria that cause infection.

How should this medicine be used?

Moxifloxacin comes as an ophthalmic solution (eye drops) to place in the eyes. It is usually used three times a day for 7 days. To help you remember to use moxifloxacin ophthalmic solution, use it at around the same times every day. Follow the directions on your prescription label carefully, and ask your doctor or pharmacist to explain any part you do not understand. Use moxifloxacin ophthalmic solution exactly as directed. Do not use more or less of it or use it more often than prescribed by your doctor.

You should expect your symptoms to improve during your treatment. Call your doctor if your symptoms do not go away or get worse, or if you develop other problems with your eyes during your treatment.

Use moxifloxacin ophthalmic solution until you finish the prescription, even if you feel better. If you stop using moxifloxacin ophthalmic solution too soon, your infection may not be completely cured and the bacteria may become resistant to antibiotics.

When you use moxifloxacin ophthalmic solution, be careful not to let the tip of the bottle touch your eye, fingers, face, or any surface. If the tip does touch another surface, bacteria may get into the eye drops. Using eye drops that are contaminated with bacteria may cause serious damage to the eye or loss of vision. If you think your eye drops have become contaminated, call your doctor or pharmacist.

To use the eye drops, follow these steps:

1. Wash your hands thoroughly with soap and water.
2. Use a mirror or have someone else put the drops in your eye.
3. Remove the protective cap from the bottle. Make sure that the end of the dropper tip is not chipped or cracked.
4. Hold the bottle with the tip down at all times to prevent drops from flowing back into the bottle and contaminating the medication inside.
5. Lie down and gaze upward or tilt your head back.
6. Holding the bottle between your thumb and index finger, place the dropper tip as near as possible to your eyelid without touching it.
7. Brace the remaining fingers of that hand against your cheek or nose.
8. With the index finger of your other hand, pull the lower lid of the eye down to form a pocket.
9. Drop the prescribed number of drops into the pocket made by the lower lid and the eye. Placing drops on the surface of the eyeball can cause stinging.
10. Close your eye and press lightly against the lower lid with your finger for 2-3 minutes to keep the medication in the eye. Do not blink.
11. If your doctor told you to place moxifloxacin ophthalmic solution in both eyes, repeat steps 6-10 above for your other eye.
12. Replace the cap on the bottle and tighten it right away. Do not wipe or rinse off the tip.
13. Wipe off any excess liquid from your cheek with a clean tissue. Wash your hands again.

Are there other uses for this medicine?

This medication may be prescribed for other uses; ask your doctor or pharmacist for more information.

What special precautions should I follow?

Before using moxifloxacin ophthalmic solution,

- tell your doctor and pharmacist if you are allergic to moxifloxacin (Avelox, Vigamox), other quinolone antibiotics such as cinoxacin (Cinobac) (not available in the United States), ciprofloxacin (Cipro, Ciloxan), enoxacin (Penetrex) (not available in the United States), gatifloxacin (Tequin, Zymar), levofloxacin (Levaquin, Quixin, Iquix), lomefloxacin (Maxaquin), nalidixic acid (NegGram) (not available in the United States), norfloxacin (Noroxin), ofloxacin (Floxin, Ocuflox), sparfloxacin (Zagam), and trovafloxacin and alatrofloxacin combination (Trovan) (not available in the United States) or any other medications.
- tell your doctor and pharmacist what prescription and nonprescription medications, vitamins, nutritional supplements, and herbal products you are taking. Your doctor may need to change the doses of your medications or monitor you carefully for side effects.
- tell your doctor if you have or have ever had any medical condition.
- tell your doctor if you are pregnant, plan to become pregnant, or are breast-feeding. If you become pregnant while using moxifloxacin ophthalmic solution, call your doctor.
- tell your doctor if you wear contact lenses. You should not wear contact lenses while you have symptoms of bacterial conjunctivitis.
- you should know that bacterial conjunctivitis spreads easily. Wash your hands often, especially after you touch your eyes. When your infection goes away, you should wash or replace any eye makeup, contact lenses, or other objects that touched your infected eye(s).

What special dietary instructions should I follow?

Unless your doctor tells you otherwise, continue your normal diet.

What should I do if I forget to take a dose?

Place the missed dose in your eye(s) as soon as you remember it. However, if it is almost time for the next dose, skip the missed dose and continue your regular dosing schedule. Do not use a double dose to make up for a missed one.

What side effects can this medicine cause?

Moxifloxacin ophthalmic solution may cause side effects. Tell your doctor if any of these symptoms are severe or do not go away:

- red, irritated, itchy, or teary eyes
- blurred vision
- eye pain
- dry eyes
- broken blood vessels in the eyes
- runny nose
- cough

Some side effects can be serious. The following symptoms are uncommon, but if you experience any of them, call your doctor immediately:

- sore throat, fever, chills and other signs of infection
- ear pain or fullness
- rash
- hives
- itching
- difficulty breathing or swallowing
- swelling of the face, throat, tongue, lips, eyes, hands, feet, ankles, or lower legs

Moxifloxacin ophthalmic solution may cause other side effects. Call your doctor if you have any unusual problems while taking this medication.

If you experience a serious side effect, you or your doctor may send a report to the Food and Drug Administration's (FDA) MedWatch Adverse Event Reporting program online [at http://www.fda.gov/MedWatch/index.html] or by phone [1-800-332-1088].

What storage conditions are needed for this medicine?

Keep this medication in the container it came in, tightly closed, and out of reach of children. Store it at room temperature and away from excess heat and moisture (not in the bathroom). Throw away any medication that is outdated or no longer needed. Talk to your pharmacist about the proper disposal of your medication.

What other information should I know?

Keep all appointments with your doctor.

Do not let anyone else use your medication. Your prescription is probably not refillable. If you still have symptoms of infection after you finish the moxifloxacin ophthalmic solution, call your doctor.

Dosage Facts
For Informational Purposes

Caution: Do not change your dose, how often you take your medication, or the length of time you are to take it without first talking to your healthcare provider.

The following dosage information was written using medical language for doctors and other healthcare professionals and is provided here for you to check your dosage. The dosage of this drug may differ for different patients. Therefore, always follow your doctor's instructions or the directions on the label. Contact your health-

care provider or pharmacist if you have any questions about the specific dosage of your medication after reviewing this information.

General Dosage Information

Available as moxifloxacin hydrochloride; dosage expressed in terms of moxifloxacin.

Pediatric Patients

Bacterial Ophthalmic Infections
Conjunctivitis

OPHTHALMIC:

- Children ≥1 year of age: 1 drop of 0.5% solution in the affected eye(s) 3 times daily for 7 days.

Adult Patients

Bacterial Ophthalmic Infections
Conjunctivitis

OPHTHALMIC:

- 1 drop of 0.5% solution in the affected eye(s) 3 times daily for 7 days.

Mupirocin

(myoo peer' oh sin)

Brand Name: Bactroban®, Bactroban® Nasal
Also available generically.

Why is this medicine prescribed?

Mupirocin, an antibiotic, is used to treat impetigo as well as other skin infections caused by bacteria. It is not effective against fungal or viral infections.

This medication is sometimes prescribed for other uses; ask your doctor or pharmacist for more information.

How should this medicine be used?

Mupirocin comes in an ointment that is applied to the skin. Mupirocin usually is applied three times a day for 1-2 weeks. Follow the directions on your prescription label carefully, and ask your doctor or pharmacist to explain any part you do not understand. Use mupirocin exactly as directed. Do not use more or less of it or use it more often than prescribed by your doctor.

Wash the affected skin area thoroughly, and then gently apply a small amount (a thin film) of the ointment. You may cover the area with a sterile gauze dressing.

Do not apply mupirocin to your eyes.

Do not apply mupirocin to burns unless told to do so by your doctor.

What special precautions should I follow?

Before using mupirocin,

- tell your doctor and pharmacist if you are allergic to mupirocin or any other drugs.

- tell your doctor and pharmacist what prescription and nonprescription medications you are taking, especially chloramphenicol (Chloromycetin).
- tell your doctor if you are pregnant, plan to become pregnant, or are breast-feeding. If you become pregnant while taking mupirocin, call your doctor.

What should I do if I forget to take a dose?

Apply the missed dose as soon as you remember it. However, if it is almost time for the next dose, skip the missed dose and continue your regular dosing schedule. Do not apply a double dose to make up for a missed one.

What side effects can this medicine cause?

Mupirocin may cause side effects. Tell your doctor if any of these symptoms are severe or do not go away:
- burning, stinging, pain, itching, or rash

What storage conditions are needed for this medicine?

Keep this medication in the container it came in, tightly closed, and out of reach of children. Store it at room temperature and away from excess heat and moisture (not in the bathroom). Throw away any medication that is outdated or no longer needed. Talk to your pharmacist about the proper disposal of your medication.

What other information should I know?

Keep all appointments with your doctor. Mupirocin is for external use only. Do not let mupirocin ointment get into your eyes, nose, or mouth, and do not swallow it. Do not apply dressings, bandages, cosmetics, lotions, or other skin medications to the area being treated unless your doctor tells you.

Do not let anyone else use your medication. Ask your pharmacist any questions you have about refilling your prescription.

If you still have symptoms of infection after you finish the mupirocin, call your doctor.

Dosage Facts
For Informational Purposes

Caution: Do not change your dose, how often you take your medication, or the length of time you are to take it without first talking to your healthcare provider.

The following dosage information was written using medical language for doctors and other healthcare professionals and is provided here for you to check your dosage. The dosage of this drug may differ for different patients. Therefore, always follow your doctor's instructions or the directions on the label. Contact your healthcare provider or pharmacist if you have any questions

about the specific dosage of your medication after reviewing this information.

General Dosage Information

Available as mupirocin and mupirocin calcium; dosage expressed in terms of mupirocin.

Pediatric Patients

Skin Infections
Impetigo

TOPICAL:
- Children 2 months to 16 years of age: apply a small amount of mupirocin topical ointment to the affected area 3 times daily for 8–10 days.

Secondary Skin Infections (Lacerations, Sutured Wounds, Abrasions)

TOPICAL:
- Children 3 months to 16 years of age: apply a small amount of mupirocin calcium topical cream to the affected area 3 times daily for 10 days.

Nasal Carriage of Staphylococcus aureus

INTRANASAL:
- Children ≥12 years of age: apply one-half (approximately 0.25 g) of the ointment from a single-use tube of mupirocin calcium intranasal ointment into each nostril twice daily (morning and evening) for 5 days. Disperse the ointment throughout the nares, by closing nostrils and then pressing together and releasing the sides of the nose repetitively for 1 minute.

Adult Patients

Skin Infections
Impetigo

TOPICAL:
- Apply a small amount of mupirocin topical ointment to the affected area 3 times daily for 8–10 days.

Secondary Skin Infections (Lacerations, Sutured Wounds, Abrasions)

TOPICAL:
- Apply a small amount of mupirocin calcium topical cream to the affected area 3 times daily for 10 days.

Nasal Carriage of Staphylococcus aureus

INTRANASAL:
- Apply one-half (approximately 0.25 g) of the ointment from a single-use tube of mupirocin calcium 2% intranasal ointment into each nostril twice daily (morning and evening) for 5 days. Disperse the ointment throughout the nares, by closing nostrils and then pressing together and releasing the sides of the nose repetitively for 1 minute.

Mycophenolate

(mye koe fen′ oh late)

Brand Name: CellCept®

Important Warning

Mycophenolate may decrease your ability to fight infection. Wash your hands often and avoid people who are sick while you are taking this medication. If you experience any of the following symptoms, call your doctor immediately: sore throat; fever; chills; colds sores; blisters; swollen glands; extreme tiredness; loss of appetite; tingling or burning in one part of the body; general weak or sick feeling; and other signs of infection.

Mycophenolate may increase your risk of developing certain types of cancer, including lymphoma (a type of cancer that develops in the lymph system) and skin cancer. Plan to avoid unnecessary or prolonged exposure to real and artificial sunlight and light therapy and to wear protective clothing, sunglasses, and sunscreen. This will decrease your risk of developing skin cancer. Call your doctor if you experience any of the following symptoms: pain or swelling in the neck, groin, or armpits; a change in the appearance of a mole; skin changes; or sores that do not heal. Talk to your doctor about the risks of taking mycophenolate.

Why is this medicine prescribed?

Mycophenolate is used with other medications to prevent the body from rejecting kidney, heart, and liver transplants. Mycophenolate is in a class of medications called immunosuppressive agents. It works by weakening the body's immune system so it will not attack and reject the transplanted organ.

How should this medicine be used?

Mycophenolate comes as a capsule, a tablet, and a suspension (liquid) to take by mouth. It is usually taken twice a day on an empty stomach. Follow the directions on your prescription label carefully, and ask your doctor or pharmacist to explain any part you do not understand. Take mycophenolate exactly as directed. Do not take more or less of it or take it more often than prescribed by your doctor.

Swallow the tablets and capsules whole; do not split, chew, or crush them. Do not open the capsules.

Do not mix mycophenolate liquid with any other medication.

Be careful not to spill the liquid or to splash it onto your skin. If you do get the liquid on your skin, wash the area well with soap and water. If you get the liquid in your eyes, wash with plain water. Use wet paper towels to wipe up any spills.

Mycophenolate prevents transplant rejection only as long as you are taking the medication. Continue to take mycophenolate even if you feel well. Do not stop taking mycophenolate without talking to your doctor.

Are there other uses for this medicine?

Mycophenolate is also sometimes used to treat refractory uveitis (inflammation of the eyes that has not responded to other treatment), Churg-Strauss syndrome (a disease in which the body makes too many immune cells and they damage organs), and certain types of lupus nephritis (a disease in which the body attacks its own kidneys). Talk to your doctor about the possible risks of using this drug for your condition.

This medication may be prescribed for other uses; ask your doctor or pharmacist for more information.

What special precautions should I follow?

Before taking mycophenolate,

- tell your doctor and pharmacist if you are allergic to mycophenolate, mycophenolic acid, or any other medications.
- tell your doctor and pharmacist what other prescription and nonprescription medications, vitamins, nutritional supplements, and herbal products you are taking. Be sure to mention any of the following: acetazolamide (Diamox); acyclovir (Zovirax); antibiotics; azathioprine (Imuran); chlorothiazide (Diuril); cimetidine (Tagamet); cholestyramine (Questran); colestipol (Colestid); ethacrynic acid (Edecrin); furosemide (Lasix); ganciclovir (Cytovene); isoproterenol (Isuprel); meperidine (Demerol); morphine (MS Contin, MSIR, Oramorph); oral contraceptives (birth control pills); phenytoin (Dilantin); probenecid (Benemid); procainamide (Pronestyl); quinine; salicylate pain relievers such as aspirin, choline magnesium trisalicylate (Trisalate), choline salicylate (Arthropan), diflunisal (Dolobid), magnesium salicylate (Doan's, others) and salsalate (Argesic, Disalcid, Salgesic); and theophylline (TheoDur). Your doctor may need to change the doses of your medications or monitor you carefully for side effects.
- if you are taking antacids, take them 2 hours before or 4 hours after mycophenolate.
- tell your doctor if you have or have ever had Lesch-Nyhan or Keeley-Seegmiller syndrome (inherited diseases that cause high levels of a certain substance in the blood, joint pain, and problems with motion and behavior); any disease that affects your stomach, intestines, or digestive system; any type of cancer; phenylketonuria (an inherited diseases that requires patients to follow a special diet to prevent mental retardation); and liver or kidney disease.
- tell your doctor if you are pregnant, plan to become pregnant, or are breast-feeding. You must use two forms of birth control before beginning treatment with mycophenolate, during treatment, and for 6 weeks after treatment. Your doctor will not allow you to begin tak-

---

ing mycophenolate unless you have had a negative pregnancy test. If you become pregnant while you are taking mycophenolate, call your doctor immediately. Do not breastfeed while you are taking this medication.

- do not have any vaccinations (shots) without talking to your doctor.

What special dietary instructions should I follow?

Unless your doctor tells you otherwise, continue your normal diet.

What should I do if I forget to take a dose?

Take the missed dose as soon as you remember it. However, if it is almost time for the next dose, skip the missed dose and continue your regular dosing schedule. Do not take a double dose to make up for a missed one.

What side effects can this medicine cause?

Mycophenolate may cause side effects. Tell your doctor if any of these symptoms are severe or do not go away:

- diarrhea
- constipation
- stomach pain
- upset stomach
- vomiting
- difficulty falling asleep or staying asleep
- pain, especially in the back, muscles, or joints

Some side effects can be serious. The following symptoms are uncommon, but if you experience any of them or those listed in the IMPORTANT WARNING section, call your doctor immediately:

- swelling of the hands, feet, ankles, or lower legs
- difficulty breathing
- shaking hands that you cannot control
- unusual bruising or bleeding
- headache
- fast heartbeat
- excessive tiredness
- dizziness
- pale skin
- weakness
- black and tarry stools
- red blood in stools
- bloody vomit
- vomiting material that looks like coffee grounds
- loose, floppy muscles
- white patches in mouth or throat
- swelling of gums
- vision changes
- rash

Mycophenolate may cause other side effects. Call your doctor if you have any unusual problems while taking this medication.

If you experience a serious side effect, you or your doc-

tor may send a report to the Food and Drug Administration's (FDA) MedWatch Adverse Event Reporting program online [at http://www.fda.gov/MedWatch/index.html] or by phone [1-800-332-1088].

What storage conditions are needed for this medicine?

Keep this medication in the container it came in, tightly closed, and out of reach of children. Store it at room temperature and away from excess heat and moisture (not in the bathroom). Mycophenolate liquid may also be stored in a refrigerator, but should not be frozen. Throw away any unused mycophenolate liquid after 60 days and throw away any medication that is outdated or no longer needed. Talk to your pharmacist about the proper disposal of your medication.

What should I do in case of overdose?

In case of overdose, call your local poison control center at 1-800-222-1222. If the victim has collapsed or is not breathing, call local emergency services at 911.

Symptoms of overdose may include:

- upset stomach
- vomiting
- diarrhea
- fever, chills, and other signs of infection

What other information should I know?

Keep all appointments with your doctor and the laboratory. Your doctor will order certain lab tests to check your body's response to mycophenolate.

Do not let anyone else take your medication. Ask your pharmacist any questions you have about refilling your prescription.

Dosage Facts
For Informational Purposes

Caution: Do not change your dose, how often you take your medication, or the length of time you are to take it without first talking to your healthcare provider.

The following dosage information was written using medical language for doctors and other healthcare professionals and is provided here for you to check your dosage. The dosage of this drug may differ for different patients. Therefore, always follow your doctor's instructions or the directions on the label. Contact your healthcare provider or pharmacist if you have any questions about the specific dosage of your medication after reviewing this information.

General Dosage Information

Available as mycophenolate mofetil (oral capsules, tablets, for oral suspension) and mycophenolate mofetil hydrochloride (injection); dosage expressed in terms of mycophenolate mofetil.

Available as mycophenolate sodium (delayed-release tablets); dosage expressed in terms of mycophenolic acid.

Mycophenolate sodium delayed-release tablets should not be used interchangeably with mycophenolate mofetil tablets, capsules, or oral suspension without clinician supervision.

If neutropenia (ANC <1300/mm^3) develops, temporarily discontinue or reduce dosage.

Pediatric Patients

Renal Allotransplantation
Mycophenolate mofetil capsules, tablets, and oral suspension

ORAL:
- Children 3 months to 18 years of age: 600 mg/m^2 as the oral suspension twice daily (maximum 1 g twice daily).
- Children with a body surface area of 1.25–1.5 m^2: 750 mg as capsules twice daily.
- Children with a body surface area >1.5 m^2: 1 g as capsules or tablets twice daily.

Mycophenolate sodium delayed-release tablets

ORAL:
- Children 5–16 years of age: 400 mg/m^2 twice daily (maximum 720 mg twice daily).
- Children 5–16 years of age with a body surface area <1.19 m^2: accurate dosage cannot be administered using commercially available tablets.
- Children 5–16 years of age with a body surface area of 1.19–1.58 m^2: 1080 mg daily (given as three 180-mg tablets twice daily or as one 180-mg tablet and one 360-mg tablet twice daily).
- Children 5–16 years of age with a body surface >1.58 m^2: 1440 mg daily (given as four 180-mg tablets twice daily or two 360-mg tablets twice daily).

Adult Patients

Renal Allotransplantation
Mycophenolate mofetil capsules, tablets, and oral suspension

ORAL:
- 1 g twice daily. No efficacy advantage with dosage of 1.5 g twice daily; 2-g daily dosage associated with a superior safety profile compared with the 3-g daily dosage.

Mycophenolate sodium delayed-release tablets

ORAL:
- 720 mg twice daily.

Cardiac Allotransplantation
Mycophenolate mofetil capsules, tablets, and oral suspension

ORAL:
- 1.5 g twice daily.

Hepatic Allotransplantation
Mycophenolate mofetil capsules, tablets, and oral suspension

ORAL:
- 1.5 g twice daily.

Crohn's Disease†
Mycophenolate mofetil capsules, tablets, and oral suspension

ORAL:
- Dosages of 1–2 g daily have been used.

Prescribing Limits

Pediatric Patients

Renal Allotransplantation
Mycophenolate mofetil capsules, tablets, and oral suspension

ORAL:
- Children 3 months to 18 years of age: Maximum 1 g twice daily.

Mycophenolate sodium delayed-release tablets

ORAL:
- Children 5–16 years of age: Maximum 720 mg twice daily.

Special Populations

Hepatic Impairment

Renal Allotransplantation
- No dosage adjustment necessary in renal transplant recipients with severe hepatic parenchymal disease; not known whether dosage adjustment is needed for other hepatic diseases.

Cardiac Allotransplantation
- No data available for cardiac transplant recipients with severe hepatic parenchymal disease.

Renal Impairment

Renal Allotransplantation
- Dosage adjustment not necessary in renal transplant recipients experiencing postoperative delayed graft function.
- Mycophenolate mofetil capsules, tablets, or oral suspension or mycophenolate mofetil hydrochloride for injection: Avoid dosages >1 g twice daily in renal transplant recipients with severe chronic renal impairment (GFR <25 mL/minute per 1.73 m^2) beyond the immediate posttransplant period.

Cardiac Allotransplantation
- No data available for cardiac transplant recipients with severe chronic renal impairment.

Hepatic Allotransplantation
- No data available for hepatic transplant recipients with severe chronic renal impairment.

Geriatric Patients
- Mycophenolate mofetil capsules, tablets, or oral suspension: Select dosage carefully. Dosage adjustment based solely on age is not necessary in geriatric patients ≥65 years of age.
- Mycophenolate sodium delayed-release tablets: Maximum 720 mg twice daily.

† *Use is not currently included in the labeling approved by the US Food and Drug Administration.*

Nabilone

(nab′ i lone)

Brand Name: Cesamet®

Why is this medicine prescribed?

Nabilone is used to treat nausea and vomiting caused by cancer chemotherapy in people who have already taken other medications to treat this type of nausea and vomiting without good results. Nabilone is in a class of medications called cannabinoids. It works by affecting the area of the brain that controls nausea and vomiting.

How should this medicine be used?

Nabilone comes as a capsule to take by mouth. It is usually taken with or without food 2-3 times a day during a cycle of chemotherapy. Treatment with nabilone should begin 1-3 hours before the first dose of chemotherapy and may be continued for up to 48 hours after the end of the chemotherapy cycle. Take nabilone at around the same times every day. Follow the directions on your prescription label carefully, and ask your doctor or pharmacist to explain any part you do not understand. Take nabilone exactly as directed. Do not take more or less of it or take it more often than prescribed by your doctor.

Your doctor will probably start you on a low dose of nabilone and may gradually increase your dose if needed.

Nabilone helps control nausea and vomiting caused by cancer chemotherapy when taken as directed. Always take nabilone according to the schedule prescribed by your doctor even if you are not experiencing nausea or vomiting.

Nabilone may be habit forming. Do not take a larger dose, take it more often, or take it for a longer period of time than prescribed by your doctor. Call your doctor if you find that you want to take extra medication.

Are there other uses for this medicine?

This medication may be prescribed for other uses; ask your doctor or pharmacist for more information.

What special precautions should I follow?

Before taking nabilone,

- tell your doctor and pharmacist if you are allergic to nabilone, other cannabinoids such as dronabinol (Marinol) or marijuana (cannabis), any other medications, or any of the ingredients in nabilone capsules. Ask your pharmacist for a list of the ingredients.
- tell your doctor and pharmacist what prescription and nonprescription medications, vitamins, nutritional supplements, and herbal products you are taking or plan to take. Be sure to mention any of the following: antidepressants, including amitriptyline (in Limbitrol), amoxapine, desipramine (Norpramin) and fluoxetine (Prozac); antihistamines; amphetamines such as am-

phetamine (in Adderall), dextroamphetamine (Dexedrine, Dextrostat, in Adderall), and methamphetamine (Desoxyn); anticoagulants ('blood thinners') such as warfarin (Coumadin); atropine (Atropen, in Hycodan, in Lomotil, in Tussigon); codeine (in some cough syrups and pain relievers); barbiturates, including phenobarbital (Luminal) and secobarbital (Seconal, in Tuinal); buspirone (BuSpar); diazepam (Valium); digoxin (Lanoxicaps, Lanoxin); disulfiram (Antabuse); ipratropium (Atrovent); lithium (Eskalith, Lithobid); medications for anxiety, asthma, colds, irritable bowel disease, motion sickness, Parkinson's disease, seizures, ulcers, or urinary problems; muscle relaxants; naltrexone (Revia, Vivitrol); narcotic medications for pain; propranolol (Inderal); scopolamine (Transderm-Scop); sedatives; sleeping pills; tranquilizers; and theophylline (TheoDur, Theochron, Theolair). Your doctor may need to change the doses of your medications or monitor you carefully for side effects.

- tell your doctor if you or anyone in your family drinks or has ever drunk large amounts of alcohol or uses or has ever used street drugs such as marijuana. Also tell your doctor if you or anyone in your family has or has ever had a mental illness such as bipolar disorder (manic depressive disorder; a disease that causes episodes of depression, episodes of mania, and other abnormal moods), schizophrenia (a mental illness that causes disturbed or unusual thinking, loss of interest in life, and strong or inappropriate emotions) or depression. Also tell your doctor if you have or have ever had high blood pressure or heart, liver, or kidney disease.
- tell your doctor if you are pregnant, plan to become pregnant, or are breast-feeding. If you become pregnant while taking nabilone, call your doctor.
- if you are having surgery, including dental surgery, tell the doctor or dentist that you are taking nabilone.
- you should know that nabilone may make you drowsy and may cause changes in your mood, thinking, memory, judgment, or behavior. You may continue to have these symptoms for up to 72 hours after you finish your treatment with nabilone. You will need to be supervised by a responsible adult during and for several days after your treatment with nabilone. Do not drive a car operate machinery, or participate in dangerous activities while you are taking this medication and for several days after you finish your treatment.
- do not drink alcoholic beverages while you are taking nabilone. Alcohol can make the side effects from nabilone worse.
- you should know that nabilone may cause dizziness, lightheadedness, and fainting when you get up too quickly from a lying position. To avoid this problem, get out of bed slowly, resting your feet on the floor for a few minutes before standing up.

What special dietary instructions should I follow?

Unless your doctor tells you otherwise, continue your normal diet.

What should I do if I forget to take a dose?

Take the missed dose as soon as you remember it. However, if it is almost time for the next dose, skip the missed dose and continue your regular dosing schedule. Do not take a double dose to make up for a missed one.

What side effects can this medicine cause?

Nabilone may cause side effects. Tell your doctor if any of these symptoms are severe or do not go away:

- headache
- dizziness
- unsteady walking
- drowsiness
- sleep problems
- weakness
- dry mouth
- changes in appetite
- nausea
- "high", or elevated mood
- difficulty concentrating
- anxiety
- confusion
- depression

Some side effects can be serious. If you experience any of these symptoms, call your doctor immediately:

- fast heartbeat
- hallucinations (seeing things or hearing voices that do not exist)
- difficulty thinking clearly and understanding reality

Nabilone may cause other side effects. Call your doctor if you have any unusual problems while taking this medication.

What storage conditions are needed for this medicine?

Keep this medication in the container it came in, tightly closed, and out of reach of children. Store it at room temperature and away from excess heat and moisture (not in the bathroom). Throw away any medication that is outdated or no longer needed. Talk to your pharmacist about the proper disposal of your medication.

Store nabilone in a safe place so that no one else can take it accidentally or on purpose. Keep track of how many capsules are left so you will know if any are missing.

What should I do in case of overdose?

In case of overdose, call your local poison control center at 1-800-222-1222. If the victim has collapsed or is not breathing, call local emergency services at 911.

Symptoms of overdose may include:

- fast heartbeat
- dizziness
- lightheadedness
- fainting
- hallucinations
- anxiety
- changes in thinking, behavior, or mood
- confusion
- slowed breathing
- coma (loss of consciousness for a period of time)

What other information should I know?

Keep all appointments with your doctor.

Do not let anyone else take your medication. This prescription is not refillable. Be sure to see your doctor to get a new prescription before you begin each cycle of chemotherapy.

Talk to your doctor, pharmacist, or other healthcare professional if you have questions about dosing information for your medication.

Nabumetone

(na byoo′ me tone)

Brand Name: Relafen®
Also available generically.

Important Warning

People who take nonsteroidal anti-inflammatory medications (NSAIDs) (other than aspirin) such as nabumetone may have a higher risk of having a heart attack or a stroke than people who do not take these medications. These events may happen without warning and may cause death. This risk may be higher for people who take NSAIDs for a long time. Tell your doctor if you or anyone in your family has or has ever had heart disease, a heart attack, or a stroke, if you smoke, and if you have or have ever had high cholesterol, high blood pressure, or diabetes. Get emergency medical help right away if you experience any of the following symptoms: chest pain, shortness of breath, weakness in one part or side of the body, or slurred speech.

If you will be undergoing a coronary artery bypass graft (CABG; a type of heart surgery), you should not take nabumetone right before or right after the surgery.

NSAIDs such as nabumetone may cause ulcers, bleeding, or holes in the stomach or intestine. These

continued on next page

Important Warning (cont'd)

problems may develop at any time during treatment, may happen without warning symptoms, and may cause death. The risk may be higher for people who take NSAIDs for a long time, are older in age, have poor health, or who drink large amounts of alcohol while taking nabumetone. Tell your doctor if you take any of the following medications: anticoagulants ('blood thinners') such as warfarin (Coumadin); aspirin; other NSAIDs such as ibuprofen (Advil, Motrin) and naproxen (Aleve, Naprosyn); or oral steroids such as dexamethasone (Decadron, Dexone), methylprednisolone (Medrol), and prednisone (Deltasone). Also tell your doctor if you have or have ever had ulcers, bleeding in your stomach or intestines, or other bleeding disorders. If you experience any of the following symptoms, stop taking nabumetone and call your doctor: stomach pain, heartburn, vomiting a substance that is bloody or looks like coffee grounds, blood in the stool, or black and tarry stools.

Keep all appointments with your doctor and the laboratory. Your doctor will monitor your symptoms carefully and will probably order certain tests to check your body's response to nabumetone. Be sure to tell your doctor how you are feeling so that your doctor can prescribe the right amount of medication to treat your condition with the lowest risk of serious side effects.

Your doctor or pharmacist will give you the manufacturer's patient information sheet (Medication Guide) when you begin treatment with nabumetone and each time you refill your prescription. Read the information carefully and ask your doctor or pharmacist if you have any questions. You can also visit the Food and Drug Administration (FDA) website (http://www.fda.gov/cder) to obtain the Medication Guide.

Why is this medicine prescribed?

Nabumetone is used to relieve pain, tenderness, swelling, and stiffness caused by osteoarthritis (arthritis caused by a breakdown of the lining of the joints) and rheumatoid arthritis (arthritis caused by swelling of the lining of the joints). Nabumetone is in a class of medications called NSAIDs. It works by stopping the body's production of a substance that causes pain, fever, and inflammation.

How should this medicine be used?

Nabumetone comes as a tablet to take by mouth. It is usually taken once or twice a day with or without food. Take nabumetone at around the same time(s) every day. Follow the directions on your prescription label carefully, and ask your doctor or pharmacist to explain any part you do not understand. Take nabumetone exactly as directed. Do not take more or less of it or take it more often than prescribed by your doctor.

Your doctor may start you on a low dose of nabumetone and gradually increase your dose.

Are there other uses for this medicine?

This medication may be prescribed for other uses; ask your doctor or pharmacist for more information.

What special precautions should I follow?

Before taking nabumetone,

- tell your doctor and pharmacist if you are allergic to nabumetone, aspirin or other NSAIDs such as ibuprofen (Advil, Motrin) and naproxen (Aleve, Naprosyn), or any other medications.
- tell your doctor and pharmacist what prescription and nonprescription medications, vitamins, nutritional supplements, and herbal products you are taking or plan to take. Be sure to mention the medications listed in the IMPORTANT WARNING section and any of the following: angiotensin-converting enzyme (ACE) inhibitors such as benazepril (Lotensin), captopril (Capoten), enalapril (Vasotec), fosinopril (Monopril), lisinopril (Prinivil, Zestril), moexipril (Univasc), perindopril (Aceon), quinapril (Accupril), ramipril (Altace), and trandolapril (Mavik); diuretics ('water pills'); lithium (Eskalith, Lithobid); oral medications for diabetes; phenytoin (Dilantin, Phenytek); and methotrexate (Rheumatrex). Your doctor may need to change the doses of your medications or monitor you carefully for side effects.
- tell your doctor if you have or have ever had asthma, especially if you also have frequent stuffed or runny nose or nasal polyps (swelling of the lining of the nose); swelling of the hands, feet, ankles, or lower legs; or kidney or liver disease.
- tell your doctor if you are pregnant, especially if you are in the last few months of your pregnancy, you plan to become pregnant, or you are breast-feeding. If you become pregnant while taking nabumetone, call your doctor.
- if you are having surgery, including dental surgery, tell the doctor or dentist that you are taking nabumetone.
- plan to avoid unnecessary or prolonged exposure to sunlight and to wear protective clothing, sunglasses, and sunscreen. Nabumetone may make your skin sensitive to sunlight.

What special dietary instructions should I follow?

Unless your doctor tells you otherwise, continue your normal diet.

What should I do if I forget to take a dose?

Take the missed dose as soon as you remember it. However, if it is almost time for the next dose, skip the missed dose

and continue your regular dosing schedule. Do not take a double dose to make up for a missed one.

What side effects can this medicine cause?

Nabumetone may cause side effects. Tell your doctor if any of these symptoms are severe or do not go away:

- diarrhea
- constipation
- gas or bloating
- dizziness
- headache
- dry mouth
- sores in the mouth
- nervousness
- difficulty falling asleep or staying asleep
- increased sweating
- ringing in the ears

Some side effects can be serious. If you experience any of the following symptoms or those mentioned in the IMPORTANT WARNING section, call your doctor immediately. Do not take any more nabumetone until you speak to your doctor.

- unexpected weight gain
- yellowing of the skin or eyes
- lack of energy
- loss of appetite
- upset stomach
- pain in the upper right part of the stomach
- flu-like symptoms
- fever
- blisters
- rash
- itching
- hives
- swelling of the eyes, face, lips, tongue, throat, arms, hands, feet ankles, or lower legs
- difficulty breathing or swallowing
- hoarseness
- pale skin
- fast heartbeat
- cloudy, discolored, or bloody urine
- back pain
- difficult or painful urination

Nabumetone may cause other side effects. Call your doctor if you have any unusual problems while taking this medication.

If you experience a serious side effect, you or your doctor may send a report to the Food and Drug Administration's (FDA) MedWatch Adverse Event Reporting program online [at http://www.fda.gov/MedWatch/index.html] or by phone [1-800-332-1088].

What storage conditions are needed for this medicine?

Keep this medication in the container it came in, tightly closed, and out of reach of children. Store it at room tem-perature and away from excess heat and moisture (not in the bathroom). Throw away any medication that is outdated or no longer needed. Talk to your pharmacist about the proper disposal of your medication.

What should I do in case of overdose?

In case of overdose, call your local poison control center at 1-800-222-1222. If the victim has collapsed or is not breathing, call local emergency services at 911.

Symptoms of overdose may include:

- lack of energy
- drowsiness
- upset stomach
- vomiting
- stomach pain
- difficulty breathing
- seizures
- coma (loss of consciousness for a period of time)

What other information should I know?

Do not let anyone else take your medication. Ask your pharmacist any questions you have about refilling your prescription.

Dosage Facts
For Informational Purposes

Caution: Do not change your dose, how often you take your medication, or the length of time you are to take it without first talking to your healthcare provider.

The following dosage information was written using medical language for doctors and other healthcare professionals and is provided here for you to check your dosage. The dosage of this drug may differ for different patients. Therefore, always follow your doctor's instructions or the directions on the label. Contact your healthcare provider or pharmacist if you have any questions about the specific dosage of your medication after reviewing this information.

General Dosage Information

To minimize the potential risk of adverse cardiovascular and/or GI events, use lowest effective dosage and shortest duration of therapy consistent with the patient's treatment goals. Adjust dosage based on individual requirements and response; attempt to titrate to the lowest effective dosage.

Adult Patients

Inflammatory Diseases
Osteoarthritis or Rheumatoid Arthritis

ORAL:
- Initially, 1 g once daily. May increase dosage to 1.5–2 g daily, given as a single daily dose or 2 divided doses.
- Patients weighing <50 kg may be less likely to need dosages >1 g daily.

Prescribing Limits

Adult Patients

Inflammatory Diseases
Osteoarthritis or Rheumatoid Arthritis

ORAL:
- Maximum 2 g daily.

Special Populations

Renal Impairment
- Dosage adjustment not necessary in patients with mild renal impairment (Cl_{cr} >50 mL/minute).
- In patients with moderate renal impairment (Cl_{cr} 30–49 mL/minute), initiate at ≤750 mg daily (maximum initial dosage is 750 mg daily). Monitor renal function; may increase dosage to 1.5 g daily.
- In patients with severe renal impairment (Cl_{cr} <30 mL/minute), initiate at ≤500 mg daily (maximum inital dosage is 500 mg daily). Monitor renal function; may increase dosage to 1 g daily.

Nadolol

(nay doe′ lole)

Brand Name: Corgard®, Corzide® as a combination product containing Nadolol and Bendroflumethiazide

Also available generically.

Important Warning

Do not stop taking nadolol without talking to your doctor. Suddenly stopping nadolol may cause chest pain or heart attack. Your doctor will probably decrease your dose gradually.

Why is this medicine prescribed?

Nadolol is used alone or in combination with other medications to treat high blood pressure. It is also used to prevent angina (chest pain). Nadolol is in a class of medications called beta blockers. It works by slowing the heart rate and relaxing the blood vessels so the heart does not have to pump as hard.

How should this medicine be used?

Nadolol comes as a tablet to take by mouth. It is usually taken once a day with or without food. To help you remember to take nadolol, take it around the same time every day. Follow the directions on your prescription label carefully, and ask your doctor or pharmacist to explain any part you do not understand. Take nadolol exactly as directed. Do not take more or less of it or take it more often than prescribed by your doctor.

Your doctor may start you on a low dose of nadolol and gradually increase your dose.

Nadolol controls high blood pressure and angina but does not cure them. It may take a few weeks before you feel the full benefit of nadolol. Continue to take nadolol even if you feel well.

Are there other uses for this medicine?

Nadolol is also used sometimes to prevent migraine headaches, to treat irregular heartbeat, and to treat tremors caused by Parkinson's disease. Talk to your doctor about the possible risks of using this medication for your condition.

This medication may be prescribed for other uses; ask your doctor or pharmacist for more information.

What special precautions should I follow?

Before taking nadolol,
- tell your doctor and pharmacist if you are allergic to nadolol or any other medications.
- tell your doctor and pharmacist what prescription and nonprescription medications, vitamins, nutritional supplements, and herbal products you are taking. Be sure to mention any of the following: insulin and oral medications for diabetes; and reserpine. Your doctor may need to change the doses of your medications or monitor you carefully for side effects.
- tell your doctor if you have or have ever had asthma or other lung disease, a slow heart rate, heart or kidney disease, diabetes, severe allergies, or an overactive thyroid gland (hyperthyroidism).
- tell your doctor if you are pregnant, plan to become pregnant, or are breast-feeding. If you become pregnant while taking nadolol, call your doctor.
- if you are having surgery, including dental surgery, tell the doctor or dentist that you are taking nadolol.
- remember that alcohol can add to the drowsiness caused by this medication.
- you should know that if you have allergic reactions to different substances, your reactions may be worse while you are using nadolol, and your allergic reactions may not respond to the usual doses of injectable epinephrine.

What special dietary instructions should I follow?

If your doctor prescribes a low-salt or low-sodium diet, follow these directions carefully.

What should I do if I forget to take a dose?

Take the missed dose as soon as you remember it. However, if it is almost time for the next dose, skip the missed dose and continue your regular dosing schedule. Do not take a double dose to make up for a missed one.

What side effects can this medicine cause?

Nadolol may cause side effects. Tell your doctor if either of these symptoms is severe or does not go away:

- dizziness or lightheadedness
- excessive tiredness

Some side effects can be serious. The following symptoms are uncommon, but if you experience any of them, call your doctor immediately:

- shortness of breath
- swelling of the hands, feet, ankles, or lower legs
- unusual weight gain
- fainting

Nadolol may cause other side effects. Call your doctor if you have any unusual problems while taking this medication.

If you experience a serious side effect, you or your doctor may send a report to the Food and Drug Administration's (FDA) MedWatch Adverse Event Reporting program online [at http://www.fda.gov/MedWatch/index.html] or by phone [1-800-332-1088].

What storage conditions are needed for this medicine?

Keep this medication in the container it came in, tightly closed, and out of reach of children. Store it at room temperature and away from excess heat and moisture (not in the bathroom). Throw away any medication that is outdated or no longer needed. Talk to your pharmacist about the proper disposal of your medication.

What should I do in case of overdose?

In case of overdose, call your local poison control center at 1-800-222-1222. If the victim has collapsed or is not breathing, call local emergency services at 911.

Symptoms of overdose may include:

- dizziness
- fainting
- difficulty breathing or swallowing
- swelling of the hands, feet, ankles, or lower legs

What other information should I know?

Keep all appointments with your doctor. Your blood pressure should be checked regularly to determine your response to nadolol. Your doctor may ask you to check your pulse (heart rate). Ask your pharmacist or doctor to teach you how to take your pulse. If your pulse is faster or slower than it should be, call your doctor.

Do not let anyone else take your medication. Ask your pharmacist any questions you have about refilling your prescription.

Dosage Facts
For Informational Purposes

Caution: Do not change your dose, how often you take your medication, or the length of time you are to take it without first talking to your healthcare provider.

The following dosage information was written using medical language for doctors and other healthcare professionals and is provided here for you to check your dosage. The dosage of this drug may differ for different patients. Therefore, always follow your doctor's instructions or the directions on the label. Contact your healthcare provider or pharmacist if you have any questions about the specific dosage of your medication after reviewing this information.

Adult Patients

Hypertension
Monotherapy

ORAL:

- Initially, 20–40 mg daily.
- May gradually increase by 40–80 mg daily at 2- to 14-day intervals until optimum BP response is achieved.
- Manufacturers recommend usual maintenance dosage of 40–80 mg daily; dosages up to 240 or 320 mg daily may be needed.
- JNC 7 currently recommends 40–120 mg daily. It usually is preferable to add another antihypertensive agent to the regimen than to continue increasing nadolol dosage; continued increases may not be tolerated.

Combination Therapy

ORAL:

- Nadolol in fixed combination with bendroflumethiazide: Initially 40 mg of nadolol and 5 mg of bendroflumethiazide once daily. If needed, increase to 80 mg of nadolol and 5 mg of bendroflumethiazide once daily.
- If BP is not adequately controlled with the fixed combination alone, may gradually add another nondiuretic hypotensive agent, starting with 50% of the usual recommended starting dosage to avoid excessive reduction in BP.
- Use of fixed-combination preparations initially and for subsequent dosage adjustment generally is not recommended. Adjust by administering each drug separately, then use the fixed combination if the optimum maintenance dosage corresponds to the ratio in the combination preparation. Administer separately for subsequent dosage adjustment.

Angina
Chronic Stable Angina

ORAL:

- Initially, 40 mg daily. Gradually increase by 40–80 mg daily at 3- to 7-day intervals until optimum control of angina is obtained or there is pronounced slowing of the heart rate (i.e., <55 bpm).
- Usual maintenance dosage is 40 or 80 mg daily. Up to 160 or 240 mg daily may be needed.

Supraventricular Tachyarrhythmias†
Various Cardiac Arrhythmias†

ORAL:

- Maintenance dose: 60–160 mg daily in single or divided doses has been used.

Vascular Headache†
Prevention of Migraine†

ORAL:
- Usual effective dosage: 80–240 mg daily.

Prescribing Limits
Adult Patients
Angina

ORAL:
- Safety and efficacy of dosages >240 mg daily not established.

Special Populations

Renal Impairment
- Adjust intervals for usual dosage of nadolol alone or in fixed combination with bendroflumethiazide:

Cl$_{cr}$ (mL/minute per 1.73 m^2)	Dosage Interval
>50	24 h
31–50	24–36 h
10–30	24–48 h
<10	40–60 h

† *Use is not currently included in the labeling approved by the US Food and Drug Administration.*

Nafarelin

(naf a′ re lin)

Brand Name: Synarel®

Why is this medicine prescribed?

Nafarelin is a hormone used to treat symptoms of endometriosis such as pelvic pain, menstrual cramps, and painful intercourse. Nafarelin also is used to treat central precocious puberty (early puberty) in young boys and girls.

This medication is sometimes prescribed for other uses; ask your doctor or pharmacist for more information.

How should this medicine be used?

Nafarelin comes as a nasal spray. To use it, first clear your nasal passages by gently blowing your nose. Then insert the sprayer into a nostril. Sniff as you squeeze the sprayer once. To prevent mucus from entering the sprayer, release your grip after you remove the sprayer from your nose. Gently sniff two or three more times.

For treating endometriosis, initially nafarelin is used twice a day: one spray in one nostril in the morning and one spray in the other nostril in the evening. Nafarelin should be started between the second and fourth days of your menstrual period. Nafarelin should not be used for longer than 6 months to treat endometriosis.

For treating precocious puberty, initially nafarelin is used once a day as two sprays in each nostril each morning, for a total of four sprays each morning.

Follow the directions on your prescription label carefully, and ask your doctor or pharmacist to explain any part you do not understand. Nafarelin initially worsens symptoms before improving them. Use nafarelin exactly as directed. Do not use more or less of it or use it more often than prescribed by your doctor. Do not stop using nafarelin without talking to your doctor.

What special precautions should I follow?

Before using nafarelin,
- tell your doctor and pharmacist if you are allergic to nafarelin, gonadotropin-releasing hormones, or any other drugs.
- tell your doctor and pharmacist what prescription and nonprescription medications you are taking, especially anticonvulsants to treat seizures or epilepsy, nasal decongestants, steroids, and vitamins.
- tell your doctor if you have or have ever had osteoporosis or a family history of osteoporosis; ovarian cysts, ovarian tumors, or ovarian cancer; chronic rhinitis (runny nose); or a history of depression.
- tell your doctor if you are pregnant, plan to become pregnant, or are breast-feeding. It is important to use a non-hormonal means of contraception (birth control) while using nafarelin (e.g., condom or diaphragm). If you become pregnant while using nafarelin, call your doctor immediately.

What should I do if I forget to take a dose?

Use the missed dose as soon as you remember it. However, if it is almost time for the next dose, skip the missed dose and continue your regular dosing schedule. Do not use a double dose to make up for a missed one.

If doses are missed, you may experience breakthrough menstrual bleeding. Do not be alarmed, but inform your doctor.

What side effects can this medicine cause?

Nafarelin may cause side effects. Usually these symptoms are temporary, lasting only until your body adjusts to the medication. Tell your doctor if any of these symptoms are severe or do not go away:
- acne
- breast enlargement
- vaginal bleeding (menstruation should stop with this medication)
- mood swings
- increase in pubic hair
- body odor
- seborrhea (skin irritation)

- nasal irritation
- headache
- hot flashes
- insomnia
- change in weight
- vaginal dryness or vaginal discharge
- change in sex drive
- oily skin
- muscle aches
- rhinitis (runny nose)
- depression

If you experience any of the following symptoms, call your doctor immediately:

- stomach pain not related to menstruation
- shortness of breath or difficulty breathing
- chest pain
- rash
- severe itching

If you experience a serious side effect, you or your doctor may send a report to the Food and Drug Administration's (FDA) MedWatch Adverse Event Reporting program online [at http://www.fda.gov/MedWatch/index.html] or by phone [1-800-332-1088].

What storage conditions are needed for this medicine?

Keep this medication in the container it came in, tightly closed, and out of reach of children. Store it at room temperature and away from excess heat and moisture (not in the bathroom). Throw away any medication that is outdated or no longer needed. Talk to your pharmacist about the proper disposal of your medication.

What should I do in case of overdose?

In case of overdose, call your local poison control center at 1-800-222-1222. If the victim has collapsed or is not breathing, call local emergency services at 911.

What other information should I know?

If you must use a nasal decongestant, wait at least 2 hours after using the nafarelin spray.

Avoid sneezing or blowing your nose during or immediately after using nafarelin. This decreases nafarelin's effectiveness.

Keep all appointments with your doctor and the laboratory.

Do not let anyone else use your medication. Ask your pharmacist any questions you have about refilling your prescription.

Talk to your doctor, pharmacist, or other healthcare professional if you have questions about dosing information for your medication.

Nafcillin Sodium Injection

(naf sill′ in)

Brand Name: Unipen®
Also available generically.

About Your Treatment

Your doctor has ordered nafcillin, an antibiotic, to help treat your infection. The drug will be either injected into a large muscle (such as your buttock or hip) or added to an intravenous fluid that will drip through a needle or catheter placed in your vein for 30-60 minutes, four to six times a day.

Nafcillin eliminates bacteria that cause infections, including pneumonia; meningitis; and urinary tract, skin, bone, joint, blood, and heart valve infections. This medication is sometimes prescribed for other uses; ask your doctor or pharmacist for more information.

Your health care provider (doctor, nurse, or pharmacist) may measure the effectiveness and side effects of your treatment using laboratory tests and physical examinations. It is important to keep all appointments with your doctor and the laboratory. The length of treatment depends on how your infection and symptoms respond to the medication.

Precautions

Before administering nafcillin,

- tell your doctor and pharmacist if you are allergic to nafcillin, penicillin, cephalosporins [e.g., cefaclor (Ceclor), cefadroxil (Duricef), or cephalexin (Keflex)], or any other drugs.
- tell your doctor and pharmacist what prescription and nonprescription medications you are taking, especially antibiotics and vitamins.
- tell your doctor if you have or have ever had asthma; hay fever; or kidney, liver, or gastrointestinal disease (especially colitis).
- tell your doctor if you are pregnant, plan to become pregnant, or are breast-feeding. If you become pregnant while taking nafcillin, call your doctor.
- if you have diabetes and regularly check your urine for sugar, use Clinistix or TesTape. Do not use Clinitest tablets because nafcillin may cause false positive results.

Administering Your Medication

Before you administer nafcillin, look at the solution closely. It should be clear and free of floating material. Gently squeeze the bag or observe the solution container to make sure there are no leaks. Do not use the solution if it is discolored, if it contains particles, or if the bag or container leaks. Use a new solution, but show the damaged one to your health care provider.

It is important that you use your medication exactly as directed. Do not stop your therapy on your own for any reason because your infection could worsen and result in hospitalization. Do not change your dosing schedule without talking to your health care provider. Your health care provider may tell you to stop your infusion if you have a mechanical problem (such as a blockage in the tubing, needle, or catheter); if you have to stop an infusion, call your health care provider immediately so your therapy can continue.

Side Effects

Nafcillin may cause side effects. Tell your health care provider if either of these symptoms is severe or does not go away:

- upset stomach
- diarrhea

If you experience any of the following symptoms, call your health care provider immediately:

- rash
- itching
- fever
- chills
- facial swelling
- wheezing
- difficulty breathing
- unusual bleeding or bruising
- dizziness
- seizures
- sore mouth or throat

If you experience a serious side effect, you or your doctor may send a report to the Food and Drug Administration's (FDA) MedWatch Adverse Event Reporting program online [at http://www.fda.gov/MedWatch/index.html] or by phone [1-800-332-1088].

Storage Conditions

- Your health care provider probably will give you a several-day supply of nafcillin at a time. If you are receiving nafcillin intravenously (in your vein), you probably will be told to store it in the refrigerator or freezer.
- Take your next dose from the refrigerator 1 hour before using it; place it in a clean, dry area to allow it to warm to room temperature.
- If you are told to store additional nafcillin in the freezer, always move a 24-hour supply to the refrigerator for the next day's use.
- Do not refreeze medications.

If you are receiving nafcillin intramuscularly (in your muscle), your health care provider will tell you how to store it properly.

Store your medication only as directed. Make sure you understand what you need to store your medication properly.

Keep your supplies in a clean, dry place when you are not using them, and keep all medications and supplies out of reach of children. Your health care provider will tell you how to throw away used needles, syringes, tubing, and containers to avoid accidental injury.

Overdose

In case of overdose, call your local poison control center at 1-800-222-1222. If the victim has collapsed or is not breathing, call local emergency services at 911.

Signs of Infection

If you are receiving nafcillin in your vein or under your skin, you need to know the symptoms of a catheter-related infection (an infection where the needle enters your vein or skin). If you experience any of these effects near your intravenous catheter, tell your health care provider as soon as possible:

- tenderness
- warmth
- irritation
- drainage
- redness
- swelling
- pain

Dosage Facts
For Informational Purposes

Caution: Do not change your dose, how often you take your medication, or the length of time you are to take it without first talking to your healthcare provider.

The following dosage information was written using medical language for doctors and other healthcare professionals and is provided here for you to check your dosage. The dosage of this drug may differ for different patients. Therefore, always follow your doctor's instructions or the directions on the label. Contact your healthcare provider or pharmacist if you have any questions about the specific dosage of your medication after reviewing this information.

General Dosage Information

Available as nafcillin sodium; dosage expressed in terms of nafcillin.

Duration of treatment depends on type and severity of infection and should be determined by clinical and bacteriologic response of the patient. In severe staphylococcal infections, duration usually is ≥2 weeks; more prolonged therapy is necessary for treatment of osteomyelitis, endocarditis, or other metastatic infections.

Pediatric Patients

Staphylococcal Infections
General Dosage in Neonates

IV:
- Neonates <1 week of age: AAP and others recommend 25 mg/kg every 12 hours for those weighing ≤2 kg and 25 mg/kg every 8 hours for those weighing >2 kg. The higher dosages are recommended for meningitis.

- Neonates 1–4 weeks of age: AAP and others recommend 25 mg/kg every 12 hours for those weighing <1.2 kg; 25 mg/kg every 8 hours for those weighing 1.2–2 kg; and 25–35 mg/kg every 6 hours for those weighing >2 kg. The higher dosages are recommended for meningitis.

IM:

- 10 mg/kg twice daily recommended by manufacturer.
- Neonates <1 week of age: AAP and others recommend 25 mg/kg every 12 hours for those weighing ≦2 kg and 25 mg/kg every 8 hours for those weighing >2 kg. The higher dosages are recommended for meningitis.
- Neonates 1–4 weeks of age: AAP and others recommend 25 mg/kg every 12 hours for those weighing <1.2 kg; 25 mg/kg every 8 hours for those weighing 1.2 to 2 kg; and 25–35 mg/kg every 6 hours for those weighing >2 kg. The higher dosages are recommended for meningitis.

General Dosage in Infants and Children

IV:

- Children weighing ≥40 kg: manufacturer recommends 500 mg every 4 hours for mild to moderate infections and 1 g every 4 hours for severe infections.
- Children ≥1 month of age: AAP recommends 50–100 mg/kg daily in 4 divided doses for mild to moderate infections or 100–150 mg/kg daily in 4 divided doses for severe infections.

IM:

- Children weighing <40 kg: manufacturer recommends 25 mg/kg twice daily.
- Children weighing ≥40 kg: manufacturer recommends 500 mg every 4–6 hours for mild to moderate infections and 1 g every 4 hours for severe infections.
- Children ≥1 month of age: AAP recommends 50–100 mg/kg daily in 4 divided doses for mild to moderate infections or 100–150 mg/kg daily in 4 divided doses for severe infections.

Staphylococcal Native Valve Endocarditis

IV:

- AHA recommends 200 mg/kg daily given in divided doses every 4–6 hours for 6 weeks (maximum 12 g daily).
- In addition, during the first 3–5 days of nafcillin therapy, IM or IV gentamicin (3 mg/kg daily given in divided doses every 8 hours; dosage adjusted to achieve peak serum gentamicin concentrations approximately 3 mcg/mL and trough concentrations <1 mcg/mL) may be given concomitantly if the causative organism is susceptible to the drug.

Staphylococcal Prosthetic Valve Endocarditis

IV:

- AHA recommends 200 mg/kg daily given in divided doses every 4–6 hours for 6 weeks or longer (maximum 12 g daily).
- Used in conjunction with oral rifampin (20 mg/kg daily given in divided doses every 8 hours for 6 weeks or longer) and IM or IV gentamicin (3 mg/kg daily given in divided doses every 8 hours during the first 2 weeks of nafcillin therapy; dosage adjusted to achieve peak serum gentamicin concentrations approximately 3 mcg/mL and trough concentrations <1 mcg/mL).

Adult Patients

Staphylococcal Infections
General Adult Dosage

IV:

- 500 mg every 4 hours; severe infections may require 1 g every 4 hours.

IM:

- 500 mg every 4–6 hours; severe infections may require 1 g every 4 hours.

Acute or Chronic Staphylococcal Osteomyelitis

IV:

- 1–2 g every 4 hours.
- When used for treatment of acute or chronic osteomyelitis caused by susceptible penicillinase-producing staphylococci, parenteral therapy usually given for 3–8 weeks; follow-up with an oral penicillinase-resistant penicillin generally is recommended for treatment of chronic osteomyelitis.

Staphylococcal Native Valve Endocarditis

IV:

- AHA recommends 2 g every 4 hours for 4–6 weeks.
- Although benefits of concomitant aminoglycosides have not been clearly established, AHA states that IM or IV gentamicin (1 mg/kg every 8 hours) may be given concomitantly during the first 3–5 days of nafcillin therapy.

Staphylococcal Prosthetic Valve Endocarditis

IV:

- AHA recommends 2 g every 4 hours for ≥6 weeks in conjunction with oral rifampin (300 mg every 8 hours for 6 weeks or longer) and IM or IV gentamicin (1 mg/kg every 8 hours during the first 2 weeks of nafcillin therapy).

Staphylococcal Infections Related to Intravascular Catheters

IV:

- 2 g every 4 hours.

Special Populations

Hepatic Impairment

- Dosage adjustments not required unless renal function also impaired.

Renal Impairment

- Modification of dosage generally is unnecessary in patients with renal impairment alone; modification of dosage may be necessary in those with both severe renal impairment and hepatic impairment.

Naftifine Hydrochloride Topical

(naf' ti feen)

Brand Name: Naftin®

Why is this medicine prescribed?

Naftifine is used for skin infections such as athlete's foot, jock itch, and ringworm.

This medication is sometimes prescribed for other uses; ask your doctor or pharmacist for more information.

How should this medicine be used?

Naftifine comes as a cream and gel to apply to the skin. The cream is usually used once a day and the gel twice a day in the morning and evening for 2 to 4 weeks. Some infections require up to 6 weeks of treatment. Follow the directions on your prescription label carefully, and ask your doctor or pharmacist to explain any part you do not understand. Use naftifine exactly as directed. Do not use more or less of it or use it more often than prescribed by your doctor.

Thoroughly clean the infected area, allow it to dry, and then gently rub the medication in until most of it disappears. Use just enough medication to cover the affected area. You should wash your hands after applying the medication.

Continue to use naftifine even if you feel well. Do not stop using naftifine without talking to your doctor.

What special precautions should I follow?

Before using naftifine,
- tell your doctor and pharmacist if you are allergic to naftifine or any other drugs.
- tell your doctor and pharmacist what prescription and nonprescription drugs you are taking, including vitamins.
- tell your doctor if you are pregnant, plan to become pregnant, or are breast-feeding. If you become pregnant while using naftifine, call your doctor.

What should I do if I forget to take a dose?

Apply the missed dose as soon as you remember it. However, if it is almost time for the next dose, skip the missed dose and continue your regular dosing schedule. Do not apply a double dose to make up for a missed one.

What side effects can this medicine cause?

Naftifine may cause side effects. If you experience any of the following symptoms, call your doctor immediately:
- itching
- burning
- irritation or stinging
- redness
- dryness
- rash

If you experience a serious side effect, you or your doctor may send a report to the Food and Drug Administration's (FDA) MedWatch Adverse Event Reporting program online [at http://www.fda.gov/MedWatch/index.html] or by phone [1-800-332-1088].

What storage conditions are needed for this medicine?

Keep this medication in the container it came in, tightly closed, and out of reach of children. Store it at room temperature and away from excess heat and moisture (not in the bathroom). Throw away any medication that is outdated or no longer needed. Talk to your pharmacist about the proper disposal of your medication.

What other information should I know?

Keep all appointments with your doctor. Naftifine is for external use only. Do not let naftifine get into your eyes, nose or mouth, and do not swallow it. Do not apply dressings, bandages, cosmetics, lotions, or other skin medications to the area being treated unless your doctor tells you.

Do not let anyone else use your medication. Ask your pharmacist any questions you have about refilling your prescription. If you still have symptoms of infection after you finish the naftifine, call your doctor.

Talk to your doctor, pharmacist, or other healthcare professional if you have questions about dosing information for your medication.

Nalbuphine Injection

(nal' byoo feen)

Brand Name: Nubain®
Also available generically.

About Your Treatment

Your doctor has ordered nalbuphine, an analgesic (painkiller), to relieve your pain. The drug will be injected into a large muscle (such as your buttock or hip), under your skin, or into a vein.

You will probably receive nalbuphine every 3 to 6 hours as needed for pain. Your doctor may also order other pain medications to make you more comfortable. This medication is sometimes prescribed for other uses; ask your doctor or pharmacist for more information.

Your health care provider (doctor, nurse, or pharmacist) may measure the effectiveness and side effects of your treatment using laboratory tests and physical examinations. It is important to keep all appointments with your doctor and the laboratory. The length of treatment depends on how you respond to the medication.

Precautions

Before administering nalbuphine,

- tell your doctor and pharmacist if you are allergic to nalbuphine, medications containing sulfites, or any other drugs.
- tell your doctor and pharmacist what prescription and nonprescription medications you are taking, especially antidepressants; medications for cough, cold, or allergies; naloxone (Narcan); naltrexone (ReVia); other pain relievers; sedatives; sleeping pills; tranquilizers; and vitamins.
- tell your doctor if you have or have ever had breathing difficulties, including asthma and other respiratory diseases, liver or kidney disease, severe inflammatory bowel disease, or a history of drug dependence.
- tell your doctor if you are pregnant, plan to become pregnant, or are breast-feeding. If you become pregnant while taking nalbuphine, call your doctor.
- if you are having surgery, including dental surgery, tell the doctor or dentist that you are taking nalbuphine.
- you should know that this drug may make you drowsy. Do not drive a car or operate machinery until you know how nalbuphine will affect you.
- remember that alcohol can add to the drowsiness caused by this drug.

Administering Your Medication

Before you administer nalbuphine, look at the solution closely. It should be clear and free of floating material. Observe the solution container to make sure there are no leaks. Do not use the solution if it is discolored, if it contains particles, or if the container leaks. Use a new solution, but show the damaged one to your health care provider.

It is important that you use your medication exactly as directed. Nalbuphine can be habit forming. Do not administer it more often or for a longer period than your doctor tells you. Do not change your dosing schedule without talking to your health care provider.

Side Effects

Nalbuphine may cause side effects. Tell your doctor if any of these symptoms are severe or do not go away:

- dizziness
- lightheadedness
- drowsiness
- upset stomach
- vomiting
- dry mouth
- headache
- stomach cramps
- itchy skin
- bitter taste
- confusion or hallucinations

- feeling of heaviness
- unusual weakness

If you experience either of the following symptoms, call your doctor immediately:

- difficulty breathing
- fainting

If you experience a serious side effect, you or your doctor may send a report to the Food and Drug Administration's (FDA) MedWatch Adverse Event Reporting program online [at http://www.fda.gov/MedWatch/index.html] or by phone [1-800-332-1088].

Storage Conditions

- Your health care provider will probably give you a several-day supply of nalbuphine at a time and provide you with directions on how to prepare each dose. Store the vials at room temperature.

Store your medication only as directed. Make sure you understand what you need to store your medication properly.

Keep your supplies in a clean, dry place when you are not using them, and keep all medications and supplies out of the reach of children. Your health care provider will tell you how to throw away used needles, syringes, tubing, and containers to avoid accidental injury.

Signs of Infection

If you are receiving nalbuphine in your vein or under your skin, you need to know the symptoms of a catheter-related infection (an infection where the needle enters your vein or skin). If you experience any of these effects near your intravenous catheter, tell your health care provider as soon as possible:

- tenderness
- warmth
- irritation
- drainage
- redness
- swelling
- pain

Dosage Facts
For Informational Purposes

Caution: Do not change your dose, how often you take your medication, or the length of time you are to take it without first talking to your health-care provider.

The following dosage information was written using medical language for doctors and other healthcare professionals and is provided here for you to check your dosage. The dosage of this drug may differ for different patients. Therefore, always follow your doctor's instructions or the directions on the label. Contact your health-care provider or pharmacist if you have any questions about the specific dosage of your medication after reviewing this information.

General Dosage Information

Available as nalbuphine hydrochloride; dosage expressed in terms of the salt.

Adjust dosage according to the severity of pain, physical status of the patient, and other drugs that the patient is receiving.

Adult Patients

Pain

Patients Not Tolerant to Opiate Agonists

IV, IM, OR SUB-Q:
- 10 mg in a 70-kg patient (about 0.14 mg/kg). Repeat every 3–6 hours as necessary.

Patients Tolerant to Opiate Agonists

IV, IM, OR SUB-Q:
- Initially, administer 25% of the usual dose of nalbuphine in patients chronically receiving morphine, meperidine, codeine, or other opiate agonists with a similar duration of action.
- Observe the patient for signs or symptoms of withdrawal (e.g., abdominal cramps, nausea, vomiting, lacrimation, rhinorrhea, anxiety, restlessness, increased temperature, piloerection). If symptoms are troublesome, give IV morphine slowly in small increments until withdrawal symptoms are relieved. However, waiting until the abstinence syndrome abates is probably preferred. If withdrawal symptoms do not occur, increase dosage progressively until the desired level of analgesia is obtained.

Supplement to Balanced Anesthesia

IV:
- 0.3–3 mg/kg for induction of anesthesia. For maintenance, 0.25–0.5 mg/kg as necessary.

Prescribing Limits

Adult Patients

Pain

Patients Not Tolerant to Opiate Agonists

IV, IM, OR SUB-Q:
- Maximum 20 mg as a single dose; maximum 160 mg daily.

Special Populations

Hepatic Impairment
- Dosage reduction is recommended.

Renal Impairment
- Dosage reduction is recommended.

Naltrexone

(nal trex′ one)

Brand Name: Depade®, ReVia® (formerly Trexan®;

Also available generically.

Important Warning

Large doses of naltrexone may cause liver failure. Tell your doctor if you have liver or kidney disease. If you experience the following symptoms, stop taking naltrexone and call your doctor immediately: excessive tiredness, unusual bleeding or bruising, loss of appetite, pain in the upper right part of your stomach, dark urine, or yellowing of the skin or eyes.

Why is this medicine prescribed?

Naltrexone is used to help people who have a narcotic or alcohol addiction stay drug free. Naltrexone is used after the patient has stopped taking drugs or alcohol. It works by blocking the effects of narcotics or by decreasing the craving for alcohol.

This medication is sometimes prescribed for other uses; ask your doctor or pharmacist for more information.

How should this medicine be used?

Naltrexone comes as a tablet to take by mouth. It usually is taken once a day. Follow the directions on your prescription label carefully, and ask your doctor or pharmacist to explain any part you do not understand. Take naltrexone exactly as directed. Do not take more or less of it or take it more often than prescribed by your doctor.

Naltrexone helps decrease the craving for narcotics or alcohol but does not treat addiction. It is important that you attend all counseling, support group meetings, and other treatments prescribed by your doctor. Take naltrexone regularly. Do not stop taking it without talking to your doctor.

If, in the past 7-10 days, you have taken opioids (morphine, codeine, or others; ask your doctor or pharmacist for more information), tell your doctor before taking the first dose of naltrexone. Naltrexone will cause withdrawal if you have opioids in your blood.

Your doctor may perform a challenge test before you begin taking naltrexone. A small dose of naloxone (a drug similar to naltrexone) will be injected into your vein or under your skin, and you will be watched for symptoms of drug withdrawal. If you have symptoms, you will need to wait a few days before beginning naltrexone.

You should take naltrexone as directed by your physician. If you take heroin or any other opioid in small doses, you will not perceive any effect. Do not take large doses of heroin or any other narcotic; you may die or sustain serious injury, including coma.

What special precautions should I follow?

Before taking naltrexone,

- tell your doctor and pharmacist if you are allergic to naltrexone, other narcotics, or any other drugs.
- tell your doctor and pharmacist what prescription and nonprescription medications you are taking, especially anti-diarrhea drugs, medications for cough and colds, pain medication, and vitamins.
- tell your doctor if you have either of the conditions listed in the IMPORTANT WARNING section.
- tell your doctor if you are pregnant, plan to become pregnant, or are breast-feeding. If you become pregnant while taking naltrexone, call your doctor.
- if you are having surgery, including dental surgery, tell the doctor or dentist that you are taking naltrexone.
- you should know that this drug may make you drowsy. Do not drive a car or operate machinery until you know how this drug affects you.
- remember that alcohol can add to the drowsiness caused by this drug.
- you should know that if you take small doses of heroin or other narcotics while taking naltrexone, you will not feel any effects. If you take large doses of heroin or other narcotics while taking naltrexone, you may die, go into a coma, or have other serious injuries.

What should I do if I forget to take a dose?

If you miss your daily dose, take the missed dose as soon as you remember it. However, if you do not remember until the next day, skip the missed dose and continue your regular dosing schedule. Do not take a double dose to make up for a missed one.

If you are on a different dosing schedule, check with your pharmacist, nurse, or doctor.

What side effects can this medicine cause?

Naltrexone may cause side effects. Tell your doctor if any of these symptoms are severe or do not go away:

- upset stomach
- anxiety
- nervousness
- muscle or joint pain

If you experience any of the following symptoms or those listed in the IMPORTANT WARNING section, call your doctor immediately:

- confusion
- drowsiness
- hallucinations
- vomiting
- diarrhea
- bone and joint pain
- skin crawling
- stomach pain

- white bowel movements
- skin rash
- blurred vision

If you experience a serious side effect, you or your doctor may send a report to the Food and Drug Administration's (FDA) MedWatch Adverse Event Reporting program online [at http://www.fda.gov/MedWatch/index.html] or by phone [1-800-332-1088].

What storage conditions are needed for this medicine?

Keep this medication in the container it came in, tightly closed, and out of reach of children. Store it at room temperature and away from excess heat and moisture (not in the bathroom). Throw away any medication that is outdated or no longer needed. Talk to your pharmacist about the proper disposal of your medication.

What should I do in case of overdose?

In case of overdose, call your local poison control center at 1-800-222-1222. If the victim has collapsed or is not breathing, call local emergency services at 911.

What other information should I know?

Keep all appointments with your doctor and the laboratory. Your doctor will order certain lab tests to check your response to naltrexone.

Do not let anyone else take your medication. Ask your pharmacist any questions you have about refilling your prescription.

Dosage Facts
For Informational Purposes

Caution: Do not change your dose, how often you take your medication, or the length of time you are to take it without first talking to your healthcare provider.

The following dosage information was written using medical language for doctors and other healthcare professionals and is provided here for you to check your dosage. The dosage of this drug may differ for different patients. Therefore, always follow your doctor's instructions or the directions on the label. Contact your healthcare provider or pharmacist if you have any questions about the specific dosage of your medication after reviewing this information.

General Dosage Information

Available as naltrexone hydrochloride; dosage expressed in terms of the salt.

Adult Patients

Opiate Dependence
Induction of Therapy for Opiate Cessation
ORAL:
- Initiate induction regimen following completion of opiate detoxification and verification that the patient is free of opiates.
- Initially, 25 mg; if no evidence of withdrawal is present, begin 50 mg daily.
- Alternatively, some clinicians have administered 12.5 mg initially, followed by incremental increases of 12.5 mg daily until the usual dosage of 50 mg daily has been achieved.

Maintenance Therapy for Opiate Cessation
ORAL:
- 50 mg daily following induction of therapy.
- Alternatively, flexible dosing schedules (see table) have been suggested in an attempt to improve compliance. Administration of larger doses at longer intervals (e.g., 48–72 hours) may reduce opiate antagonist activity somewhat, but may improve compliance. Single doses >50 mg may increase risk of hepatic injury; weigh possible risks against probable benefits of flexible dosing.

Flexible Naltrexone Hydrochloride Dosing Schedules for Maintenance Therapy for Opiate Cessation

50 mg daily Monday through Friday and 100 mg on Saturday

100 mg every other day

150 mg every third day

100 mg on Monday and Wednesday and 150 mg on Friday

150 mg on Monday and 200 mg on Thursday

Ingestion of the naltrexone dose generally should be observed in a clinic setting or by a responsible family member to ensure compliance, in which case, regimens requiring less frequent visits may be more acceptable to the patient.

Monitor patient compliance by random testing of urine for naltrexone and 6-β-naltrexol or for the presence of opiates.

Optimum duration of maintenance therapy not established; base on individual requirements and response.

In patients who discontinue naltrexone prematurely and then desire to resume therapy following a relapse to opiate abuse, perform urinalysis for the presence of opiates and, if necessary, a naloxone challenge test prior to resuming therapy. If there is evidence of opiate dependence, conduct detoxification prior to reinitiation of naltrexone therapy.

Opiate Detoxification†
ORAL:
- Various dosage regimens have been used for rapid or ultra-rapid detoxification† of opiate dependence.
- The following regimen of naltrexone, given in conjunction with clonidine to attenuate withdrawal manifestations, has been studied.

Day of Detoxification Therapy	Clonidine Hydrochloride	Naltrexone Hydrochloride
Day 1	0.005 mg/kg initially; then titrated according to the severity of withdrawal and the adverse effects induced by clonidine	
Day 2	Administered every 4 hours to attenuate the withdrawal induced by naltrexone	Administered every 4 hours; 1 mg initially; then increased in 1-mg increments during the daytime on day 2
Day 3	Administered every 4 hours to attenuate the withdrawal induced by naltrexone; highest mean dosage was 2.3 mg daily on day 3	Administered every 4 hours; dosage increased in 2-mg increments during the daytime on day 3
Day 4	Administered only as needed to reduce signs and symptoms of withdrawal	10 mg 3 times daily
Day 5	Administered only as needed to reduce signs and symptoms of withdrawal	50 mg once daily

Alcohol Dependence
ORAL:
- 50 mg once daily, following verification that the patient is free of opiates.
- Optimum duration of therapy not established; safety and efficacy established only in short-term (up to 12 weeks) studies.

† Use is not currently included in the labeling approved by the US Food and Drug Administration.

Naproxen

(na prox′ en)

Brand Name: Aleve®, Anaprox®, Anaprox® DS, EC-Naprosyn®, Naprelan®, Naprosyn® Also available generically.

Important Warning

People who take nonsteroidal anti-inflammatory medications (NSAIDs) (other than aspirin) such as naproxen may have a higher risk of having a heart attack or a stroke than people who do not take these medications. These events may happen without warning and may cause death. This risk may be higher for people who take NSAIDs for a long time. Tell your doctor if you or anyone in your family has or has ever had heart disease, a heart attack, or a stroke, if you smoke, and if you have or have ever had high cholesterol, high blood pressure, or diabetes. Get emergency medical help right away if you experience any of the following symptoms: chest pain, shortness of breath, weakness in one part or side of the body, or slurred speech.

If you will be undergoing a coronary artery bypass graft (CABG; a type of heart surgery), you should not take naproxen right before or right after the surgery.

NSAIDs such as naproxen may cause ulcers, bleeding, or holes in the stomach or intestine. These problems may develop at any time during treatment, may happen without warning symptoms, and may cause death. The risk may be higher for people who take NSAIDs for a long time, are older in age, have poor health, or who drink three or more alcoholic drinks per day while taking naproxen. Tell your doctor if you take any of the following medications: anticoagulants ('blood thinners') such as warfarin (Coumadin); aspirin; other NSAIDs such as ibuprofen (Advil, Motrin) and ketoprofen (Orudis KT, Actron); or oral steroids such as dexamethasone (Decadron, Dexone), methylprednisolone (Medrol), and prednisone (Deltasone). Also tell your doctor if you have or have ever had ulcers, bleeding in your stomach or intestines, or other bleeding disorders. If you experience any of the following symptoms, stop taking naproxen and call your doctor: stomach pain, heartburn, vomiting a substance that is bloody or looks like coffee grounds, blood in the stool, or black and tarry stools.

Keep all appointments with your doctor and the laboratory. Your doctor will monitor your symptoms carefully and will probably order certain tests to check your body's response to naproxen. Be sure to tell your doctor how you are feeling so that your doctor can prescribe the right amount of medication to treat your condition with the lowest risk of serious side effects.

Your doctor or pharmacist will give you the manufacturer's patient information sheet (Medication Guide) when you begin treatment with prescription naproxen and each time you refill your prescription. Read the information carefully and ask your doctor or pharmacist if you have any questions. You can also visit the Food and Drug Administration (FDA) website (http://www.fda.gov/cder) or the manufacturer's website to obtain the Medication Guide.

Why is this medicine prescribed?

Prescription naproxen is used to relieve pain, tenderness, swelling, and stiffness caused by osteoarthritis (arthritis caused by a breakdown of the lining of the joints), rheumatoid arthritis (arthritis caused by swelling of the lining of the joints), juvenile arthritis (a form of joint disease in children), and ankylosing spondylitis (arthritis that mainly affects the spine). Prescription naproxen tablets, extended-release tablets, and suspension are also used to relieve shoulder pain caused by bursitis (inflammation of a fluid-filled sac in the shoulder joint), tendinitis (inflammation of the tissue that connects muscle to bone), gouty arthritis (attacks of joint pain caused by a build-up of certain substances in the joints), and pain from other causes, including menstrual pain (pain that happens before or during a menstrual period). Nonprescription naproxen is used to reduce fever and to relieve mild pain from headaches, muscle aches, arthritis, menstrual periods, the common cold, toothaches, and backaches. Naproxen is in a class of medications called NSAIDs. It works by stopping the body's production of a substance that causes pain, fever, and inflammation.

How should this medicine be used?

Prescription naproxen comes as a regular tablet, an enteric coated tablet (delayed-release tablet), an extended-release (long-acting) tablet, and a suspension (liquid) to take by mouth. The extended-release tablets are usually taken once a day. The tablets, enteric coated tablets, and suspension are usually taken twice a day for arthritis. The tablets and suspension are usually taken every 8 hours for gout, and every 6-8 hours as needed for pain. If you are taking naproxen on a regular basis, you should take it at the same time(s) every day.

Nonprescription naproxen comes as tablet and a gelatin coated tablet to take by mouth. It is usually taken with a full glass of water every 8-12 hours as needed. Nonprescription naproxen may be taken with food or milk to prevent stomach upset.

Follow the directions on the package or prescription label carefully, and ask your doctor or pharmacist to explain any part you do not understand. Take naproxen exactly as directed. Do not take more or less of it or take it more often than prescribed by your doctor or written on the package.

Shake the liquid well before each use to mix the medication evenly. Use the measuring cup provided to measure each dose of the liquid.

Swallow the enteric coated tablets and extended release tablets whole; do not split, chew, or crush them.

If you are taking naproxen to relieve the symptoms of arthritis, your symptoms may begin to improve within 1 week. It may take 2 weeks or longer for you to feel the full benefit of the medication.

Stop taking nonprescription naproxen and call your doctor if your symptoms get worse, you develop new or unexpected symptoms, the part of your body that was painful becomes red or swollen, your pain lasts for more than 10 days, or your fever lasts for more than 3 days.

Are there other uses for this medicine?

Naproxen is also sometimes used to treat Paget's disease of bone (a condition in which the bones become abnormally thick, fragile, and misshapen) and Bartter's syndrome (a condition in which the body does not absorb enough potassium, causing muscle cramping and weakness and other symptoms). Talk to your doctor about the risks of using this medication for your condition.

This medication is sometimes prescribed for other uses; ask your doctor or pharmacist for more information.

What special precautions should I follow?

Before taking naproxen,

- tell your doctor and pharmacist if you are allergic to naproxen, aspirin or other NSAIDs such as ibuprofen (Advil, Motrin) and ketoprofen (Orudis KT, Actron), any medications for pain or fever, or any other medications.
- tell your doctor and pharmacist what prescription and nonprescription medications, vitamins, nutritional supplements, and herbal products you are taking or plan to take. Be sure to mention the medications listed in the IMPORTANT WARNING section and any of the following: angiotensin-converting enzyme (ACE) inhibitors such as benazepril (Lotensin), captopril (Capoten), enalapril (Vasotec), fosinopril (Monopril), lisinopril (Prinivil, Zestril), moexipril (Univasc), perindopril (Aceon), quinapril (Accupril), ramipril (Altace), and trandolapril (Mavik); beta blockers such as atenolol (Tenormin), labetalol (Normodyne), metoprolol (Lopressor, Toprol XL), nadolol (Corgard), and propranolol (Inderal); diuretics ('water pills'); lithium (Eskalith, Lithobid), medications for diabetes, methotrexate (Rheumatrex); phenytoin (Dilantin); probenecid (Benemid); and sulfa antibiotics such as sulfisoxazole (Gantrisin) and sulfamethoxazole (in Bactrim, in Septra). If you are taking the enteric coated tablets, also tell your doctor if you are taking antacids or sucralfate (Carafate). Your doctor may need to change the doses of your medication or monitor you more carefully for side effects.

- do not take nonprescription naproxen with any other medication for pain unless your doctor tells you that you should.
- tell your doctor if you have been told to follow a low sodium diet and if you have or have ever had any of the conditions mentioned in the IMPORTANT WARNING section or asthma, especially if you also have frequent stuffed or runny nose or nasal polyps (swelling of the inside of the nose); swelling of the hands, arms, feet, ankles, or lower legs; anemia (red blood cells do not bring enough oxygen to all parts of the body); or liver or kidney disease.
- tell your doctor if you are pregnant, especially if you are in the last few months of your pregnancy, you plan to become pregnant, or you are breast-feeding. If you become pregnant while taking naproxen, call your doctor.
- if you are having surgery, including dental surgery, tell the doctor or dentist that you are taking naproxen.
- you should know that this medication may make you dizzy, drowsy, or depressed. Do not drive a car or operate machinery until you know how this drug affects you.
- remember that alcohol can add to the drowsiness caused by this medication.

What special dietary instructions should I follow?

Unless your doctor tells you otherwise, continue your normal diet.

What should I do if I forget to take a dose?

Take the missed dose as soon as you remember it. However, if it is almost time for the next dose, skip the missed dose and continue your regular dosing schedule. Do not take a double dose to make up for a missed one.

What side effects can this medicine cause?

Naproxen may cause side effects. Tell your doctor if any of these symptoms are severe or do not go away:

- constipation
- diarrhea
- gas
- sores in mouth
- excessive thirst
- headache
- dizziness
- lightheadedness
- drowsiness
- difficulty falling asleep or staying asleep
- burning or tingling in the arms or legs
- cold symptoms
- ringing in the ears
- hearing problems

Some side effects can be serious. If you experience any of the following symptoms, or those mentioned in the IM-

PORTANT WARNING section, call your doctor immediately. Do not take any more naproxen until you speak to your doctor:

- changes in vision
- feeling that the tablet is stuck in your throat
- unexplained weight gain
- sore throat, fever, chills, and other signs of infection
- blisters
- rash
- skin reddening
- itching
- hives
- swelling of the eyes, face, lips, tongue, throat, arms, hands, feet, ankles, or lower legs
- difficulty breathing or swallowing
- hoarseness
- excessive tiredness
- pain in the upper right part of the stomach
- upset stomach
- loss of appetite
- yellowing of the skin or eyes
- flu-like symptoms
- bruises or purple blotches under the skin
- pale skin
- fast heartbeat
- cloudy, discolored, or bloody urine
- back pain
- difficult or painful urination

Naproxen may cause other side effects. Call your doctor if you have any unusual problems while taking this medication.

If you experience a serious side effect, you or your doctor may send a report to the Food and Drug Administration's (FDA) MedWatch Adverse Event Reporting program online [at http://www.fda.gov/MedWatch/index.html] or by phone [1-800-332-1088].

What storage conditions are needed for this medicine?

Keep this medication in the container it came in, tightly closed, and out of reach of children. Store it at room temperature and away from excess heat and moisture (not in the bathroom). Throw away any medication that is outdated or no longer needed. Talk to your pharmacist about the proper disposal of your medication.

What should I do in case of overdose?

In case of overdose, call your local poison control center at 1-800-222-1222. If the victim has collapsed or is not breathing, call local emergency services at 911.

Symptoms of overdose may include:
- dizziness
- extreme tiredness
- confusion
- drowsiness
- stomach pain

- heartburn
- upset stomach
- vomiting
- slow or difficult breathing
- decreased urination

What other information should I know?

Before having any laboratory test, tell your doctor and the laboratory personnel that you are taking naproxen.

If you are taking prescription naproxen, do not let anyone else take your medication. Ask your pharmacist any questions you have about refilling your prescription.

Dosage Facts
For Informational Purposes

Caution: Do not change your dose, how often you take your medication, or the length of time you are to take it without first talking to your healthcare provider.

The following dosage information was written using medical language for doctors and other healthcare professionals and is provided here for you to check your dosage. The dosage of this drug may differ for different patients. Therefore, always follow your doctor's instructions or the directions on the label. Contact your healthcare provider or pharmacist if you have any questions about the specific dosage of your medication after reviewing this information.

General Dosage Information

Available as naproxen or naproxen sodium; *each 220, 275, 412.5, or 550 mg of naproxen sodium is approximately equivalent to 200, 250, 375, or 500 mg of naproxen, respectively.*

If changing from one strength to another or one dosage form to another, be aware that different dose strengths and formulations are not necessarily bioequivalent.

To minimize the potential risk of adverse cardiovascular and/or GI events, use lowest effective dosage and shortest duration of therapy consistent with the patient's treatment goals. Adjust dosage based on individual requirements and response; attempt to titrate to the lowest effective dosage.

Pediatric Patients

Inflammatory Diseases
Juvenile Rheumatoid Arthritis

ORAL:
- Naproxen 10 mg/kg daily in 2 divided doses.

Pain

ORAL:
- Naproxen sodium *self-medication* in children ≥12 years of age: Initially, 440 mg; usual dosage is 220 mg every 8–12 hours.

Fever

ORAL:
- Naproxen sodium *self-medication* in children ≥12 years of age: Initially, 440 mg; usual dosage is 220 mg every 8–12 hours.

Adult Patients

Inflammatory Diseases

Osteoarthritis, Rheumatoid Arthritis, or Ankylosing Spondylitis

ORAL:

Preparation	Dosage
Naproxen conventional tablets, delayed-release tablets, or suspension	250–500 mg twice daily; may increase dosage to 1.5 g daily for up to 6 months
Naproxen sodium conventional tablets	275–550 mg twice daily; may increase dosage to 1.65 g daily for up to 6 months
Naproxen sodium extended-release tablets	825 mg or 1.1 g once daily; may increase dosage to 1.65 g daily for up to 6 months

When naproxen conventional tablets are used in combination with lansoprazole (15 mg once daily), usual naproxen dosage is 375 or 500 mg twice daily.

Acute Tendinitis/Bursitis

ORAL:

Preparation	Dosage
Naproxen conventional tablets or suspension	500 mg initially, followed by 500 mg every 12 hours or 250 mg every 6–8 hours as needed
Naproxen sodium conventional tablets	550 mg initially, followed by 550 mg every 12 hours or 275 mg every 6–8 hours as needed
Naproxen sodium extended-release tablets	1.1 g once daily; may increase dosage to 1.65 g once daily for limited period

Gout

ORAL:

Preparation	Dosage
Naproxen conventional tablets or suspension	750 mg initially, followed by 250 mg every 8 hours until attack subsides
Naproxen sodium conventional tablets	825 mg initially, followed by 275 mg every 8 hours until attack subsides
Naproxen sodium extended-release tablets	1.1–1.65 g once on first day, followed by 1.1 g once daily until attack subsides

Pain

ORAL:

Preparation	Dosage
Naproxen conventional tablets or suspension	500 mg initially, followed by 500 mg every 12 hours or 250 mg every 6–8 hours as needed
Naproxen sodium conventional tablets	550 mg initially, followed by 550 mg every 12 hours or 275 mg every 6–8 hours as needed
Naproxen sodium extended-release tablets	1.1 g once daily; may increase dosage to 1.65 g once daily for limited period

Naproxen sodium for *self-medication* of minor aches and pain: Initially, 440 mg; usual dosage is 220 mg every 8–12 hours.

Dysmenorrhea

ORAL:

Preparation	Dosage
Naproxen conventional tablets or suspension	500 mg initially, followed by 500 mg every 12 hours or 250 mg every 6–8 hours as needed
Naproxen sodium conventional tablets	550 mg initially, followed by 550 mg every 12 hours or 275 mg every 6–8 hours as needed
Naproxen sodium extended-release tablets	1.1 g once daily; may increase dosage to 1.65 g once daily for limited period

Naproxen sodium *self-medication:* Initially, 440 mg; usual dosage is 220 mg every 8–12 hours.

Fever

ORAL:
- Naproxen sodium *self-medication*: Initially, 440 mg; usual dosage is 220 mg every 8–12 hours.

Prescribing Limits

Pediatric Patients

Pain

ORAL:
- Naproxen sodium *self-medication* in children ≥12 years of age: Maximum 440 mg in 8–12 hours; 660 mg in 24 hours. *Self-medication* should not exceed 10 days.

Fever

ORAL:
- Naproxen sodium *self-medication* in children ≥12 years of age: Maximum 440 mg in 8–12 hours; 660 mg in 24 hours. *Self-medication* should not exceed 3 days.

Adult Patients

Inflammatory Diseases
Osteoarthritis, Rheumatoid Arthritis, or Ankylosing Spondylitis

ORAL:
- As naproxen, maximum 1.5 g daily.
- As naproxen sodium, maximum 1.65 g daily.

Acute Tendinitis/Bursitis

ORAL:
- As naproxen, maximum 1.25 g on the first day; thereafter, 1 g daily. Maximum 1.5 g daily for limited period.
- As naproxen sodium, maximum 1.375 g on the first day; thereafter, 1.1 g daily. Maximum 1.65 g daily for limited period.

Pain

ORAL:
- As naproxen, maximum 1.25 g on the first day; thereafter, 1 g daily. Maximum 1.5 g daily for limited period.
- As naproxen sodium, maximum 1.375 g on the first day; thereafter, 1.1 g daily. Maximum 1.65 g daily for limited period.
- Naproxen sodium for *self-medication* of minor aches and pain: Maximum 440 mg in 8–12 hours; 660 mg in 24 hours. *Self-medication* should not exceed 10 days.

Dysmenorrhea

ORAL:
- As naproxen, maximum 1.25 g on the first day; thereafter, 1 g daily.
- As naproxen sodium, maximum 1.375 g on the first day; thereafter, 1.1 g daily.
- Naproxen sodium *self-medication*: Maximum 440 mg in 8–12 hours; 660 mg in 24 hours.

Fever

ORAL:
- Naproxen sodium *self-medication*: Maximum 440 mg in 8–12 hours; 660 mg in 24 hours. *Self-medication* should not exceed 3 days.

Special Populations

Hepatic Impairment
- Dosage adjustment may be needed if high doses required. Consider reduced initial dosage. Use lowest effective dosage.

Renal Impairment
- Consider reduced initial dosage.
- Not recommended for use in patients with moderate to severe renal impairment (Cl_{cr} <30 mL/minute).

Geriatric Patients
- Dosage adjustment may be needed if high doses required. Consider reduced initial dosage. Use lowest effective dosage.
- Maximum for *self-medication*, naproxen sodium 220 mg twice daily unless otherwise directed by a clinician.

Naratriptan

(nar' a trip tan)

Brand Name: Amerge

Why is this medicine prescribed?

Naratriptan is used to treat the symptoms of migraine headaches (severe, throbbing headaches that sometimes are accompanied by nausea and sensitivity to sound or light). Naratriptan is in a class of medications called selective serotonin receptor agonists. It works by narrowing blood vessels in the brain, stopping pain signals from being sent to the brain, and stopping the release of certain natural substances that cause pain, nausea, and other symptoms of migraine. Naratriptan does not prevent migraine attacks.

How should this medicine be used?

Naratriptan comes as a tablet to take by mouth. It should be taken at any time after a migraine headache starts. Usually only one tablet is needed. If you have no response to the first tablet, do not take a second tablet without consulting your doctor. If you have a partial response to the first tablet, or your headache returns, a second tablet may be taken 4 hours after the first tablet. Do not take more than two tablets of naratriptan in any 24-hour period. Follow the directions on your prescription label carefully, and ask your doctor or pharmacist to explain any part you do not understand. Take naratriptan exactly as directed. Do not take more or less of it or take it more often than prescribed by your doctor.

Naratriptan should be taken with plenty of water or other fluids.

Are there other uses for this medicine?

This medication is sometimes prescribed for other uses; ask your doctor or pharmacist for more information.

What special precautions should I follow?

Before taking naratriptan,
- tell your doctor and pharmacist if you are allergic to naratriptan, rizatriptan (Maxalt), sumatriptan (Imitrex), zolmitriptan (Zomig), or any other drugs.
- do not take naratriptan within 24 hours of another selective serotonin receptor agonist such as almotriptan (Axert), eletriptan (Relpax), frovatriptan (Frova), rizatriptan (Maxalt), sumatriptan (Imitrex), or zolmitriptan (Zomig); or ergot-type medications such as bromocriptine (Parlodel), cabergoline (Dostinex), dihydroergotamine (D.H.E. 45, Migranal), ergoloid mesylates (Germinal, Hydergine), ergonovine (Ergotrate), ergotamine (Bellergal-S, Cafergot, Ergomar, Wigraine), methylergonovine (Methergine), methysergide (Sansert), and pergolide (Permax).
- tell your doctor and pharmacist what prescription and nonprescription medications, vitamins, nutritional sup-

plements and herbal products you are taking or plan to take. Be sure to mention any of the following: oral contraceptives; selective serotonin reuptake inhibitors (SSRIs) such as citalopram (Celexa), escitalopram (Lexapro), fluoxetine (Prozac, Sarafem, in Symbyax), fluvoxamine, paroxetine (Paxil), and sertraline (Zoloft); and selective serotonin/norepinephrine reuptake inhibitors (SNRIs) such as duloxetine (Cymbalta) and venlafaxine (Effexor). Your doctor may need to change the doses of your medications or monitor you more carefully for side effects.

- tell your doctor if you have or have ever had high blood pressure; angina (recurring chest paint); a heart attack; diabetes; high cholesterol; obesity; coronary artery disease; menopause; or blood vessel, kidney, or liver disease.
- tell your doctor if you are pregnant, plan to become pregnant, or are breast-feeding. If you become pregnant while taking naratriptan, call your doctor.
- if you are having surgery, including dental surgery, tell your doctor or dentist that you are taking naratriptan.

What should I do if I forget to take a dose?

Naratriptan is not for routine use. Use it only to relieve your migraine headache as soon as migraine symptoms appear.

What side effects can this medicine cause?

Naratriptan may cause side effects. Tell your doctor if any of these symptoms are severe or do not go away:

- vision changes
- tingling sensations
- tiredness or weakness
- upset stomach
- dizziness
- warm or cold temperature sensations

If you experience any of the following symptoms, call your doctor immediately:

- pain or tightness in chest or throat
- rapid heartbeat
- difficulty breathing or shortness of breath
- redness, swelling, or itching of the eyelids, face, or lips
- sudden or severe stomach pain

What storage conditions are needed for this medicine?

Keep this medication in the container it came in, tightly closed, and out of reach of children. Store it at room temperature and away from excess heat and moisture (not in the bathroom). Throw away any medication that is outdated or no longer needed. Talk to your pharmacist about the proper disposal of your medication.

What should I do in case of overdose?

In case of overdose, call your local poison control center at 1-800-222-1222. If the victim has collapsed or is not breathing, call local emergency services at 911.

What other information should I know?

Keep all appointments with your doctor and the laboratory.

Call your doctor if you continue to have symptoms.

Do not let anyone else take your medication. Ask your pharmacist any questions you have about refilling your prescription.

Dosage Facts
For Informational Purposes

Caution: Do not change your dose, how often you take your medication, or the length of time you are to take it without first talking to your healthcare provider.

The following dosage information was written using medical language for doctors and other healthcare professionals and is provided here for you to check your dosage. The dosage of this drug may differ for different patients. Therefore, always follow your doctor's instructions or the directions on the label. Contact your healthcare provider or pharmacist if you have any questions about the specific dosage of your medication after reviewing this information.

General Dosage Information

Available as naratriptan hydrochloride; dosage is expressed in terms of naratriptan.

Adult Patients

Vascular Headaches
Migraine

ORAL:
- 1 or 2.5 mg as a single dose; individualize dosage selection, weighing the possible benefit (greater effectiveness) and risks (increased adverse effects) of the 2.5-mg dose.
- If headache recurs or only a partial response is achieved, may repeat dose once after 4 hours.
- Following failure to respond to the first dose, reconsider diagnosis of migraine prior to administration of a second dose.

Prescribing Limits

Adult Patients

Vascular Headaches
Migraine

ORAL:
- Maximum 5 mg in any 24-hour period.
- Safety of treating an average of >4 headaches per 30-day period not established.

Special Populations

Hepatic Impairment
- Contraindicated in patients with severe hepatic impairment. In patients with mild or moderate hepatic impairment, reduce initial dosage; maximum dosage of 2.5 mg per 24-hour period is recommended.

Renal Impairment
- Contraindicated in patients with severe renal impairment. In patients with mild or moderate renal impairment, reduce ini-

tial dosage; maximum dosage of 2.5 mg per 24-hour period is recommended.

Nateglinide Oral

(nuh tay′ gli nide)

Brand Name: Starlix®

Why is this medicine prescribed?

Nateglinide is used alone or in combination with other medications to treat type 2 diabetes (condition in which the body does not use insulin normally and therefore cannot control the amount of sugar in the blood) in people whose diabetes cannot be controlled by diet and exercise alone. Nateglinide belongs to a class of drugs called meglitinides. Nateglinide helps your body regulate the amount of glucose (sugar) in your blood. It decreases the amount of glucose by stimulating the pancreas to release insulin.

How should this medicine be used?

Nateglinide comes as a tablet to take by mouth. It is usually taken three times daily. Take nateglinide any time from 30 minutes before a meal to just before the meal. If you skip a meal, you need to skip the dose of nateglinide. If you add a meal, add a dose of nateglinide. Your doctor may gradually increase your dose, depending on your response to nateglinide. Monitor your blood glucose closely. Follow the directions on your prescription label carefully, and ask your doctor or pharmacist to explain any part you do not understand. Take nateglinide exactly as directed. Do not take more or less of it or take it more often than directed by the package label or prescribed by your doctor.

Nateglinide controls diabetes but does not cure it. Continue to take nateglinide even if you feel well. Do not stop taking nateglinide without talking with your doctor.

Are there other uses for this medicine?

This medication is sometimes prescribed for other uses; ask your doctor or pharmacist for more information.

What special precautions should I follow?

Before taking nateglinide,

- tell your doctor and pharmacist if you are allergic to nateglinide or any other drugs.
- tell your doctor and pharmacist what prescription and nonprescription medications you are taking, especially albuterol (Proventil, Ventolin); allergy or cold medications; aspirin and nonsteroidal anti-inflammatory drugs such as ibuprofen (Advil, Motrin) or naproxen (Aleve, Naprosyn); beta-blockers such as propranolol (Inderal); chloramphenicol (Chloromycetin); chlor-

promazine (Thorazine); corticosteroids such as dexamethasone (Decadron), methylprednisolone (Medrol), or prednisone (Deltasone, Orasone); diuretics ('water pills'); epinephrine; estrogens; fluphenazine (Prolixin); isoniazid (Rifamate); medications that contain alcohol or sugar; mesoridazine (Serentil); niacin; oral contraceptives (birth control pills); perphenazine (Trilafon); phenelzine (Nardil); probenecid (Benemid); prochlorperazine (Compazine); promazine (Sparine); promethazine (Phenergan); terbutaline (Brethine, Bricanyl); thioridazine (Mellaril); thyroid medication; tranylcypromine (Parnate); trifluoperazine (Stelazine); triflupromazine (Vesprin); trimeprazine (Temaril); and vitamins or herbal products.

- tell your doctor if you have or have ever had liver or pituitary disease, adrenal insufficiency, diabetic ketoacidosis, neuropathy (disease of the nervous system), or if you have been told you have type 1 diabetes mellitus (condition in which the body does not produce insulin and therefore cannot control the amount of sugar in the blood).
- tell your doctor if you are pregnant, plan to become pregnant, or are breast-feeding. If you become pregnant while taking nateglinide, call your doctor.
- if you are having surgery, including dental surgery, tell the doctor or dentist that you are taking nateglinide.
- tell your doctor if you have fever, infection, injury, or illness with vomiting or diarrhea. These may affect your blood sugar level.

What special dietary instructions should I follow?

Be sure to follow all exercise and dietary recommendations made by your doctor or dietitian. Calorie reduction, weight loss, and exercise will help control your diabetes and will also make nateglinide work better. It is important to eat a healthful diet. Alcohol may cause a decrease in blood sugar. Ask your doctor about the safe use of alcoholic beverages while you are taking nateglinide.

What should I do if I forget to take a dose?

Before you start taking nateglinide, ask your doctor what to do if you forget to take a dose. Write these directions down so you can refer to them later. As a general rule, if you have just begun to eat a meal, take the missed dose as soon as you remember it. However, if you have finished eating, or if it is almost time for the next dose, skip the missed dose and continue your regular dosing schedule. Do not take a double dose to make up for a missed one.

What side effects can this medicine cause?

This medication may cause changes in your blood sugar. You should know the symptoms of low and high blood sugar and what to do if you have these symptoms.

You may experience hypoglycemia (low blood sugar) while you are taking this medication. Your doctor will tell you what you should do if you develop hypoglycemia. He or she may tell you to check your blood sugar, eat or drink a food or beverage that contains sugar, such as hard candy or fruit juice, or get medical care. Follow these directions carefully if you have any of the following symptoms of hypoglycemia:

- shakiness
- dizziness or lightheadedness
- sweating
- nervousness or irritability
- sudden changes in behavior or mood
- headache
- numbness or tingling around the mouth
- weakness
- pale skin
- hunger
- clumsy or jerky movements

If hypoglycemia is not treated, severe symptoms may develop. Be sure that your family, friends, and other people who spend time with you know that if you have any of the following symptoms, they should get medical treatment for you immediately.

- confusion
- seizures
- loss of consciousness

Call your doctor immediately if you have any of the following symptoms of hyperglycemia (high blood sugar):

- extreme thirst
- frequent urination
- extreme hunger
- weakness
- blurred vision

If high blood sugar is not treated, a serious, life-threatening condition called diabetic ketoacidosis could develop. Call your doctor immediately if you have any of the these symptoms:

- dry mouth
- upset stomach and vomiting
- shortness of breath
- breath that smells fruity
- decreased consciousness

Nateglinide may cause side effects. Tell your doctor if any of these symptoms are severe or do not go away:

- headache
- nasal congestion
- runny nose
- joint aches
- back pain
- constipation
- cough
- flu-like symptoms

What storage conditions are needed for this medicine?

Keep this medication in the container it came in, tightly closed, and out of reach of children. Store it at room tem-perature and away from excess heat and moisture (not in the bathroom). Throw away any medication that is outdated or no longer needed. Talk to your pharmacist about the proper disposal of your medication.

What should I do in case of overdose?

In case of overdose, call your local poison control center at 1-800-222-1222. If the victim has collapsed or is not breathing, call local emergency services at 911.

What other information should I know?

Keep all appointments with your doctor and the laboratory. Your blood sugar and glycosylated hemoglobin (HbA1c) should be checked regularly to determine your response to nateglinide. Your doctor will also tell you how to check your response to this medication by measuring your blood or urine sugar levels at home. Follow these instructions carefully.

Keep yourself and your clothes clean. Wash cuts, scrapes, and other wounds quickly, and do not let them get infected.

You should always wear a diabetic identification bracelet to be sure you get proper treatment in an emergency.

Do not let anyone else take your medication. Ask your pharmacist any questions you have about refilling your prescription.

Dosage Facts
For Informational Purposes

Caution: Do not change your dose, how often you take your medication, or the length of time you are to take it without first talking to your healthcare provider.

The following dosage information was written using medical language for doctors and other healthcare professionals and is provided here for you to check your dosage. The dosage of this drug may differ for different patients. Therefore, always follow your doctor's instructions or the directions on the label. Contact your healthcare provider or pharmacist if you have any questions about the specific dosage of your medication after reviewing this information.

Adult Patients

Diabetes Mellitus

ORAL:
- 120 mg 3 times daily before meals. For patients who are near their goal glycosylated hemoglobin (HbA$_{1c}$) when nateglinide therapy is initiated, 60 mg 3 times daily before meals.

Special Populations

Hepatic Impairment
- No dosage adjustment necessary in patients with mild impairment. Use with caution in patients with moderate or severe impairment.

Renal Impairment
- No dosage adjustment necessary.

Geriatric Patients
- No dosage adjustment necessary.

Nedocromil Ophthalmic

(ne doe kroe′ mil)

Brand Name: Alocril®

Why is this medicine prescribed?

Nedocromil is used to treat itchy eyes caused by allergies. Symptoms of allergies occur when cells in your body called mast cells release substances after you come in contact with something to which you are allergic. Nedocromil is in a class of drugs called mast cell stabilizers. It works by stopping the release of these substances.

This medication is sometimes prescribed for other uses; ask your doctor or pharmacist for more information.

How should this medicine be used?

Nedocromil comes as eyedrops. One or two drops are usually applied to the affected eyes twice daily. Follow the directions on your prescription label carefully, and ask your doctor or pharmacist to explain any part you do not understand. Use nedocromil exactly as directed. Do not use more or less of it or use it more often than prescribed by your doctor.

Your allergy symptom (itchy eyes) should improve when you apply the eyedrops. If your symptoms do not improve or they worsen, call your doctor.

Continue to use nedocromil even if your eyes feel better. Continue to use it until you are no longer exposed to the substance that causes your symptoms, allergy season is over, or your doctor tells you to stop using it.

To use the eyedrops, follow these instructions:

1. Wash your hands thoroughly with soap and water.
2. Use a mirror or have someone else put the drops in your eye.
3. Remove the protective cap. Make sure the end of the dropper is not chipped or cracked.
4. Avoid touching the dropper tip against your eye or anything else.
5. Hold the dropper tip down at all times to prevent drops from flowing back into the bottle and contaminating the remaining contents.
6. Lie down or tilt your head back.
7. Holding the bottle between your thumb and index finger, place the dropper tip as near as possible to your eyelid without touching it.
8. Brace the remaining fingers of that hand against your cheek or nose.
9. With the index finger of your other hand, pull the lower lid of the eye down to form a pocket.
10. Drop the prescribed number of drops into the pocket made by the lower lid and the eye. Placing drops on the surface of the eyeball can cause stinging.
11. Close your eye and press lightly against the lower lid with your finger for 2-3 minutes to keep the medication in the eye. Do not blink.
12. Replace and tighten the cap right away. Do not wipe or rinse it off.
13. Wipe off any excess liquid from your cheek with a clean tissue. Wash your hands again.

What special precautions should I follow?

Before using nedocromil eyedrops,
- tell your doctor and pharmacist if you are allergic to nedocromil or any other drugs.
- tell your doctor and pharmacist what prescription and nonprescription medications you are taking, including vitamins or herbal products.
- tell you doctor if you wear contact lenses; you should not wear contact lenses while you have the allergy symptom of itchy eyes.

What should I do if I forget to take a dose?

Take the missed dose as soon as you remember it. However, if it is almost time for the next dose, skip the missed dose and continue your regular dosing schedule. Do not take a double dose to make up for a missed one.

What side effects can this medicine cause?

Nedocromil may cause side effects. Tell your doctor if any of these symptoms are severe or do not go away:
- stinging or burning of the eyes
- blurred vision
- increased eye redness or itching

What storage conditions are needed for this medicine?

Keep this medication in the container it came in, tightly closed, and out of reach of children. Store it at room temperature and away from excess heat and moisture (not in the bathroom). Throw away any medication that is outdated or no longer needed. Talk to your pharmacist about the proper disposal of your medication.

What other information should I know?

Keep all appointments with your doctor.

Do not let anyone else take your medication. Ask your pharmacist any questions you have about refilling your prescription.

Dosage Facts
For Informational Purposes

Caution: Do not change your dose, how often you take your medication, or the length of time you are to take it without first talking to your healthcare provider.

The following dosage information was written using medical language for doctors and other healthcare professionals and is provided here for you to check your dosage. The dosage of this drug may differ for different patients. Therefore, always follow your doctor's instructions or the directions on the label. Contact your healthcare provider or pharmacist if you have any questions about the specific dosage of your medication after reviewing this information.

General Dosage Information

Available as nedocromil sodium; dosage expressed in terms of the salt.

Pediatric Patients

Allergic Conjunctivitis

OPHTHALMIC:
- Children ≥3 years of age: 1 or 2 drops of a 2% solution in each eye twice daily.

Adult Patients

Allergic Conjunctivitis

OPHTHALMIC:
- 1 or 2 drops of a 2% solution in each eye twice daily.

Nedocromil Oral Inhalation

(ne doe kroe′ mil)

Brand Name: Tilade® Inhaler

Why is this medicine prescribed?

Nedocromil is used to prevent the wheezing, shortness of breath, and troubled breathing caused by asthma. It works by preventing the release of substances that cause inflammation (swelling) in the air passages of the lungs.

This medication is sometimes prescribed for other uses; ask your doctor or pharmacist for more information.

How should this medicine be used?

Nedocromil comes as an aerosol to inhale by mouth. It usually is inhaled four times a day to prevent asthma attacks. Follow the directions on your prescription label carefully, and ask your doctor or pharmacist to explain any part you do not understand. Use nedocromil exactly as directed. Do not use more or less of it or use it more often than prescribed by your doctor.

It may take up to 4 weeks for nedocromil to work. You should take it regularly for it to be effective. If your symptoms have not improved after 4 weeks, tell your doctor.

Nedocromil is used with a special inhaler. Before you use nedocromil inhalation for the first time, read the instructions for your device. Ask your doctor, pharmacist, or respiratory therapist to demonstrate the proper technique. Practice using the inhalation device while in his or her presence.

To use the inhaler, follow these steps:
1. Shake the inhaler well.
2. Remove the protective cap.
3. Exhale (breathe out) as completely as possible through your nose while keeping your mouth shut.
4. *Open Mouth Technique:* Open your mouth wide, and place the open end of the mouthpiece about 1-2 inches from your mouth.
   Closed Mouth Technique: Place the open end of the mouthpiece well into your mouth, past your front teeth. Close your lips tightly around the mouthpiece.
5. Take a slow, deep breath through the mouthpiece and, at the same time, press down on the container to spray the medication into your mouth. Be sure that the mist goes into your throat and is not blocked by your teeth or tongue. Adults giving the treatment to young children may hold the child's nose closed to be sure that the medication goes into the child's throat.
6. Hold your breath for 5-10 seconds, remove the inhaler, and exhale slowly through your nose or mouth. If you take 2 puffs, wait 2 minutes and shake the inhaler well before taking the second puff.
7. Replace the protective cap on the inhaler.

If you have difficulty getting the medication into your lungs, a spacer (a special device that attaches to the inhaler) may help; ask your doctor, pharmacist, or respiratory therapist.

What special precautions should I follow?

Before using nedocromil,
- tell your doctor and pharmacist if you are allergic to nedocromil or any other drugs.
- tell your doctor and pharmacist what prescription and nonprescription medications you are using, including vitamins.
- tell your doctor if you are pregnant, plan to become pregnant, or are breast-feeding. If you become pregnant while using nedocromil, call your doctor.

What should I do if I forget to take a dose?

Use the missed dose as soon as you remember it. However, if it is almost time for the next dose, skip the missed dose and continue your regular dosing schedule. Do not use a double dose to make up for a missed one.

What side effects can this medicine cause?

Nedocromil may cause side effects. Tell your doctor if any of these symptoms are severe or do not go away:

- sore throat
- bad taste in the mouth
- stomach pain
- cough
- stuffy nose
- itching or burning nasal passages
- sneezing
- headache

If you experience either of the following symptoms, call your doctor immediately:

- wheezing
- increased difficulty breathing

If you experience a serious side effect, you or your doctor may send a report to the Food and Drug Administration's (FDA) MedWatch Adverse Event Reporting program online [at http://www.fda.gov/MedWatch/index.html] or by phone [1-800-332-1088].

What storage conditions are needed for this medicine?

Keep this medication in the container it came in, tightly closed, and out of reach of children. Store it at room temperature and away from excess heat and moisture (not in the bathroom). Throw away any medication that is outdated or no longer needed. Talk to your pharmacist about the proper disposal of your medication. Avoid puncturing the aerosol container, and do not discard it in an incinerator or fire.

What other information should I know?

Keep all appointments with your doctor and the laboratory. Your doctor will order certain lab tests to check your response to nedocromil.

Do not use nedocromil to relieve an asthma attack that has already started; continue to use the medication prescribed for your acute attacks.

To relieve dry mouth or throat irritation caused by nedocromil inhalation, rinse your mouth with water, chew gum, or suck sugarless hard candy after each treatment.

Inhalation devices require regular cleaning. Once a week, remove the drug container from the plastic mouthpiece, wash the mouthpiece with warm tap water, and dry it thoroughly. Follow the written instructions for care of other inhalation devices.

Do not let anyone else use your medication. Ask your pharmacist any questions you have about refilling your prescription.

Dosage Facts

For Informational Purposes

Caution: Do not change your dose, how often you take your medication, or the length of time you are to take it without first talking to your healthcare provider.

The following dosage information was written using medical language for doctors and other healthcare professionals and is provided here for you to check your dosage. The dosage of this drug may differ for different patients. Therefore, always follow your doctor's instructions or the directions on the label. Contact your healthcare provider or pharmacist if you have any questions about the specific dosage of your medication after reviewing this information.

General Dosage Information

Available as nedocromil sodium, dosage expressed in terms of the salt.

The dose of nedocromil sodium is expressed as the amount delivered from the actuator of the inhaler per metered spray.

Oral inhalation aerosol delivers 2 mg from the valve and 1.75 mg from the actuator per metered spray. Each aerosol canister delivers ≥104 metered sprays.

Pediatric Patients

Asthma

ORAL INHALATION:

- Children ≥6 years of age: 3.5 mg (2 inhalations) 4 times daily at regular intervals (14 mg/day).
- Less frequent administration may be effective if asthma is well controlled at this dose (e.g., patients only need occasional β-agonist therapy and are not experiencing serious exacerbations).

Adult Patients

Asthma

ORAL INHALATION:

- 3.5 mg (2 inhalations) 4 times daily at regular intervals (14 mg/day).
- Less frequent administration may be effective if asthma is well controlled at this dose (e.g., patients only need occasional β-agonist therapy and are not experiencing serious exacerbations).

Prescribing Limits

Pediatric Patients

Asthma

ORAL INHALATION:

- Children ≥6 years of age: Maximum 3.5 mg (2 inhalations) 4 times daily (14 mg/day).

Adult Patients

Asthma

ORAL INHALATION:

- Maximum 3.5 mg (2 inhalations) 4 times daily (14 mg/day).

Special Populations

No special population dosage recommendations at this time.

Nefazodone

(nef ay′ zoe done)

Important Warning

A small number of children, teenagers, and young adults (up to 24 years of age) who took antidepressants ('mood elevators') such as nefazodone during clinical studies became suicidal (thinking about harming or killing oneself or planning or trying to do so). Children, teenagers, and young adults who take antidepressants to treat depression or other mental illnesses may be more likely to become suicidal than children, teenagers, and young adults who do not take antidepressants to treat these conditions. However, experts are not sure about how great this risk is and how much it should be considered in deciding whether a child or teenager should take an antidepressant. Children younger than 18 years of age should not normally take nefazodone, but in some cases, a doctor may decide that nefazodone is the best medication to treat a child's condition.

You should know that your mental health may change in unexpected ways when you take nefazodone or other antidepressants even if you are an adult over age 24. You may become suicidal, especially at the beginning of your treatment and any time that your dose is increased or decreased. You, your family, or your caregiver should call your doctor right away if you experience any of the following symptoms: new or worsening depression; thinking about harming or killing yourself, or planning or trying to do so; extreme worry; agitation; panic attacks; difficulty falling asleep or staying asleep; aggressive behavior; irritability; acting without thinking; severe restlessness; and frenzied abnormal excitement. Be sure that your family or caregiver knows which symptoms may be serious so they can call the doctor when you are unable to seek treatment on your own.

Your healthcare provider will want to see you often while you are taking nefazodone, especially at the beginning of your treatment. Be sure to keep all appointments for office visits with your doctor.

The doctor or pharmacist will give you the manufacturer's patient information sheet (Medication Guide) when you begin treatment with nefazodone. Read the information carefully and ask your doctor or pharmacist if you have any questions. You also can obtain the Medication Guide from the FDA website: http://www.fda.gov/cder/drug/antidepressants/antidepressants_MG_2007.pdf.

No matter what your age, before you take an antidepressant, you, your parent, or your caregiver should talk to your doctor about the risks and benefits of treating your condition with an antidepressant or with other treatments. You should also talk about the risks and benefits of not treating your condition. You should know that having depression or another mental illness greatly increases the risk that you will become suicidal. This risk is higher if you or anyone in your family has or has ever had bipolar disorder (mood that changes from depressed to abnormally excited) or mania (frenzied, abnormally excited mood) or has thought about or attempted suicide. Talk to your doctor about your condition, symptoms, and personal and family medical history. You and your doctor will decide what type of treatment is right for you.

Why is this medicine prescribed?

Nefazodone is used to treat depression. Nefazodone is in a class of medications called antidepressants. It works by increasing the amounts of certain natural substances in the brain that are needed to maintain mental balance.

How should this medicine be used?

Nefazodone comes as a tablet to take by mouth. It is usually taken two times a day and may be taken with or without food. Take nefazodone at around the same times every day. Follow the directions on your prescription label carefully, and ask your doctor or pharmacist to explain any part you do not understand. Take nefazodone exactly as directed. Do not take more or less of it or take it more often than prescribed by your doctor.

It may take a few weeks or longer for you to feel the full benefit of nefazodone. Continue to take nefazodone even if you feel well. Do not stop taking nefazodone without talking to your doctor. Your doctor will probably want to decrease your dose gradually.

Are there other uses for this medicine?

This medication may be prescribed for other uses; ask your doctor or pharmacist for more information.

What special precautions should I follow?

Before taking nefazodone,
- tell your doctor and pharmacist if you are allergic to nefazodone or any other medications.
- tell your doctor if you are taking alprazolam (Xanax), astemizole (Hismanal) (not available in the United States), cisapride (Propulsid) (not available in the United States), pimozide (Orap), or terfenadine (Seldane),(not available in the United States) if you are taking or have taken a monoamine oxidase (MAO) inhibitor such as isocarboxazid (Marplan), phenelzine (Nardil), selegiline (Eldepryl, Emsam, Zelapar) or tranylcypromine (Parnate), or if you have taken an MAO inhibitor in the past two weeks. Your doctor will probably tell you not to take nefazodone.

- tell your doctor and pharmacist what other prescription and nonprescription medications, vitamins, nutritional supplements, and herbal products you are taking or plan to take. Be sure to mention any of the following: anticoagulants ('blood thinners') such as warfarin (Coumadin); antihistamines; buspirone (Buspar); carbamazepine (Tegretol); cimetidine (Tagamet); cyclosporine (Neoral, Sandimmune); digoxin (Lanoxin); haloperidol (Haldol); levodopa (Sinemet, Larodopa); medication for high blood pressure, seizures, Parkinson's disease, asthma, colds, or allergies; methylphenidate (Ritalin); muscle relaxants; propranolol (Inderal); sedatives; sleeping pills; tacrolimus (Prograf); thyroid medications; tranquilizers; and triazolam (Halcion). If you have recently stopped taking fluoxetine (Prozac, Sarafem), you may have to wait several weeks before beginning to take nefazodone. Your doctor may need to change the doses of your medications or monitor you carefully for side effects.
- tell your doctor if you have or have ever had difficulty urinating; seizures; or kidney, liver, or heart disease.
- tell your doctor if you are pregnant, plan to become pregnant, or are breast-feeding. If you become pregnant while taking nefazodone, call your doctor.
- if you are having surgery, including dental surgery, tell the doctor or dentist that you are taking nefazodone.
- you should know that this medication may make you drowsy. Do not drive a car or operate machinery until you know how this medication affects you.
- remember that alcohol can add to the drowsiness caused by this medication. Avoid drinking alcohol while taking nefazodone.

What should I do if I forget to take a dose?

Take the missed dose as soon as you remember it. However, if it is almost time for your next dose, skip the missed dose and continue your regular dosing schedule. Do not take a double dose to make up for a missed one.

What side effects can this medicine cause?

Nefazodone may cause side effects. Call your doctor if any of these symptoms are severe or do not go away:
- nausea
- drowsiness
- weakness or tiredness
- nightmares
- dry mouth
- skin more sensitive to sunlight than usual
- changes in appetite or weight
- constipation
- difficulty urinating
- frequent urination
- blurred vision
- changes in sex drive or ability
- excessive sweating

Some side effects can be serious. If you experience any of the following symptoms or those listed in the IMPORTANT WARNINGS section, call your doctor immediately:
- jaw, neck, and back muscle spasms
- slow or difficult speech
- shuffling walk
- uncontrollable shaking of a part of the body
- fever
- difficulty breathing or swallowing
- rash
- irregular heartbeat
- seizures
- painful erections of the penis lasting more than 4 hours

Nefazodone may cause other side effects. Call your doctor if you have any unusual problems while you are taking this medication.

If you experience a serious side effect, you or your doctor may send a report to the Food and Drug Administration's (FDA) MedWatch Adverse Event Reporting program online [at http://www.fda.gov/MedWatch/index.html] or by phone [1-800-332-1088].

What storage conditions are needed for this medicine?

Keep this medication in the container it came in, tightly closed, and out of reach of children. Store it at room temperature and away from excess heat and moisture (not in the bathroom). Throw away any medication that is outdated or no longer needed. Talk to your pharmacist about the proper disposal of your medication.

What should I do in case of overdose?

In case of overdose, call your local poison control center at 1-800-222-1222. If the victim has collapsed or is not breathing, call local emergency services at 911.

What other information should I know?

Keep all appointments with your doctor and the laboratory. Your doctor may order certain lab tests to check your body's response to nefazodone.

Do not let anyone else take your medication. Ask your pharmacist any questions you have about refilling your prescription.

Dosage Facts
For Informational Purposes

Caution: Do not change your dose, how often you take your medication, or the length of time you are to take it without first talking to your health-care provider.

The following dosage information was written using medical language for doctors and other healthcare professionals and is provided here for you to check your dosage. The dosage of this drug may differ for different patients. Therefore, always follow your doctor's instruc-

tions or the directions on the label. Contact your health-care provider or pharmacist if you have any questions about the specific dosage of your medication after reviewing this information.

General Dosage Information

Available as nefazodone hydrochloride; dosage expressed in terms of the salt.

Adult Patients

Major Depressive Disorder

ORAL:
- Initially, 100 mg twice daily. Dosages may be increased by increments of 100–200 mg daily at intervals of not less than 1 week.
- Usual dosage: 300–600 mg daily.

Prescribing Limits

Adult Patients

Major Depressive Disorder

ORAL:
- Maximum dosage: 600 mg daily.

Special Populations

Geriatric or Debilitated Patients
- Initially, 50 mg twice daily. Subsequent dosage adjustments should be made in smaller increments and at longer intervals than in younger patients.
- Usual dosage in geriatric individuals: 200–400 mg daily.

Nelfinavir

(nel fin' a veer)

Brand Name: Viracept®, Viracept® Oral Powder

Important Warning

The effect of nelfinavir on the clinical progression of HIV infection, including the effect on the incidence of opportunistic infections or on overall survival, remains to be established.

Why is this medicine prescribed?

Nelfinavir is used in combination with other drugs, such as zidovudine (AZT), to treat human immunodeficiency virus (HIV) infections in patients with or without acquired immunodeficiency syndrome (AIDS). Nelfinavir is one of a class of drugs called protease (pro' tee ace) inhibitors, which slow the spread of HIV infection in the body.

This medication is sometimes prescribed for other uses; ask your doctor or pharmacist for more information.

How should this medicine be used?

Nelfinavir comes as a tablet and a powder to take by mouth. It usually is taken three times a day with a meal or light snack. Follow the directions on your prescription label carefully, and ask your doctor or pharmacist to explain any part you do not understand. Take nelfinavir exactly as directed. Do not take more or less of it or take it more often than prescribed by your doctor.

Nelfinavir powder may be added to water, milk, formula, soy milk, or dietary supplements. Your prescription label tells you how many scoops of powder to add to the liquid. Drink the entire mixture to get the full dose.

What special precautions should I follow?

Before taking nelfinavir,
- tell your doctor and pharmacist if you are allergic to nelfinavir or any other drugs.
- tell your doctor and pharmacist what prescription and nonprescription medications you are taking, especially amiodarone (Cordarone, Pacerone); astemizole (Hismanal); bromocriptine (Parlodel); cabergoline (Dostinex); carbamazepine (Tegretol); cisapride (Propulsid); cyclosporine (Neoral, Sandimmune); didanosine (Videx); ergot alkaloids such as dihydroergotamine (Migranal), ergoloid mesylates (Germinal, Hydergine) or ergotamine (Cafergot, Cafetrate, Wigraine, others); indinavir (Crixivan); ketoconazole (Nizoral); medications for high cholesterol, especially lovastatin (Mevacor) or simvastatin (Zocor); midazolam (Versed); pergolide (Permax); phenobarbital; phenytoin (Dilantin); quinidine (Quinaglute, Quinalan, Quinidex); rifabutin (Mycobutin); rifampin (Rifadin); ritonavir (Norvir); saquinavir (Invirase); sildenafil (Viagra); tacrolimus (Prograf); terfenadine (Seldane); triazolam (Halcion); and vitamins.
- tell your doctor and pharmacist what herbal products you are taking, especially St. John's wort.
- tell your doctor if you are taking birth control pills. Nelfinavir can decrease the effectiveness of oral contraceptives. You should use another method of birth control while taking this medication.
- tell your doctor if you have or have ever had liver disease.
- tell your doctor if you are pregnant, plan to become pregnant, or are breast-feeding. If you become pregnant while taking nelfinavir, call your doctor.
- if you are having surgery, including dental surgery, tell the doctor or dentist that you are taking nelfinavir.

What should I do if I forget to take a dose?

Take the missed dose as soon as you remember it. However, if it is almost time for the next dose, skip the missed dose and continue your regular dosing schedule. Do not take a double dose to make up for a missed one.

What side effects can this medicine cause?

Nelfinavir may cause side effects. Most symptoms are mild and improve with time. Tell your doctor if any of these symptoms are severe or do not go away:

- diarrhea
- upset stomach
- gas
- stomach pain
- shift in body fat

If you experience either of the following symptoms, call your doctor immediately:

- rash
- weakness

Nelfinavir may increase the sugar level in your blood. If you experience any of the following symptoms, call your doctor immediately:

- frequent urination
- increased thirst
- weakness
- dizziness
- headache

If you experience a serious side effect, you or your doctor may send a report to the Food and Drug Administration's (FDA) MedWatch Adverse Event Reporting program online [at http://www.fda.gov/MedWatch/index.html] or by phone [1-800-332-1088].

What storage conditions are needed for this medicine?

Keep this medication in the container it came in, tightly closed, and out of reach of children. Store it at room temperature and away from excess heat and moisture (not in the bathroom). After nelfinavir powder has been added to liquid, the mixture may be kept at room temperature for up to 6 hours. Throw away any medication that is outdated or no longer needed. Talk to your pharmacist about the proper disposal of your medication.

What should I do in case of overdose?

In case of overdose, call your local poison control center at 1-800-222-1222. If the victim has collapsed or is not breathing, call local emergency services at 911.

What other information should I know?

Nelfinavir is not a cure and does not prevent the spread of HIV infection to other people, so use precautions to avoid the spread of this infection.

Keep all appointments with your doctor and the laboratory. Your doctor will order certain lab tests to check your response to nelfinavir.

Do not let anyone else take your medication. Ask your pharmacist any questions you have about refilling your prescription.

Dosage Facts
For Informational Purposes

Caution: Do not change your dose, how often you take your medication, or the length of time you are to take it without first talking to your healthcare provider.

The following dosage information was written using medical language for doctors and other healthcare professionals and is provided here for you to check your dosage. The dosage of this drug may differ for different patients. Therefore, always follow your doctor's instructions or the directions on the label. Contact your healthcare provider or pharmacist if you have any questions about the specific dosage of your medication after reviewing this information.

General Dosage Information

Available as nelfinavir mesylate; dosage expressed as nelfinavir.

Must be given in conjunction with other antiretrovirals. *If used with didanosine, lopinavir, or indinavir, adjustment in the treatment regimen may be necessary.*

Pediatric Patients

Treatment of HIV Infection

ORAL:
- Neonates and children <2 years of age†: Reliably effective dosage not established. High interindividual variability in drug concentrations observed when 40 mg/kg every 12 hours was evaluated in neonates and infants up to 6 weeks of age; higher dosages are being investigated.
- Children 2–13 years of age: 45–55 mg/kg twice daily or 25–35 mg/kg 3 times daily.
- Children >13 years of age: 1.25 g (five 250-mg tablets or two 625-mg tablets) twice daily or 750 mg (three 250-mg tablets) 3 times daily.

Table 1. Pediatric Patients ≥2 Years of Age (Tablets)

Weight (kg)	No. of 250-mg Tablets 2 times daily (45–55 mg/kg 2 times daily)	No. of 250-mg Tablets 3 times daily (25–35 mg/kg 3 times daily)
10–12	2	1
13–18	3	2
19–20	4	2
≥21	4–5	3

Table 2. Pediatric Patients ≥2 years of Age (Oral Powder)

Weight (kg)	No. of Level 50-mg Scoops 2 times daily (45–55 mg/kg 2 times daily)	No. of Level 200-mg Teaspoons 2 times daily (45–55 mg/kg 2 times daily)	No. of Level 50-mg Scoops 3 times daily (25–35 mg/kg 3 times daily)	No. of Level 200-mg Teaspoons 3 times daily (25–35 mg/kg 3 times daily)
9 to <10.5	10	2½	6	1½
10.5 to <12	11	2¾	7	1¾
12 to <14	13	3¼	8	2
14 to <16	15	3¾	9	2¼
16 to <18	Use tablets	Use tablets	10	2½
18 to <23	Use tablets	Use tablets	12	3
≥23	Use tablets	Use tablets	15	3¾

Adult Patients

Treatment of HIV Infection

ORAL:
- 1.25 g (five 250-mg tablets or two 625-mg tablets) twice daily or 750 mg (three 250-mg tablets) 3 times daily.

Postexposure Prophylaxis of HIV†

Occupational Exposure†

ORAL:
- 1.25 g twice daily.
- Used in alternative expanded regimens that include nelfinavir and 2 NRTIs.
- Initiate postexposure prophylaxis as soon as possible following exposure (within hours rather than days) and continue for 4 weeks, if tolerated.

Nonoccupational Exposure†

ORAL:
- 1.25 g twice daily or 750 mg 3 times daily in conjunction with other antiretrovirals.
- Used in an alternative PI-based regimen that includes nelfinavir and (lamivudine or emtricitabine) and (zidovudine or stavudine or abacavir or tenofovir or didanosine).
- Initiate postexposure prophylaxis as soon as possible following exposure (preferably ≤72 hours after exposure) and continue for 28 days.

Prescribing Limits

Pediatric Patients

Treatment of HIV

ORAL:
- >2.5 g daily not studied in children.

Special Populations

Hepatic Impairment

Treatment of HIV Infection

ORAL:
- Dosage recommendations not available; use with caution.

Renal Impairment

Treatment of HIV Infection

ORAL:
- Dosage adjustments not necessary.

† Use is not currently included in the labeling approved by the US Food and Drug Administration.

Neomycin, Polymyxin, and Bacitracin Ophthalmic

(nee oh mye′ sin, pol i mix′ in, bass i tray′ sin)

Brand Name: AK-Trol®, Cortisporin® Ophthalmic Ointment, Cortisporin® Ophthalmic Suspension, Dexasporin®, Maxitrol®, Neosporin® Ophthalmic Ointment, Ocu-Spor-G®, Ocu-Trol®, Poly-Pred® Liquifilm®

Why is this medicine prescribed?

Neomycin, polymyxin, and bacitracin combination is used to treat eye and eyelid infections. Neomycin, polymyxin, and bacitracin are in a class of medications called antibiotics. Neomycin, polymyxin, and bacitracin combination works by stopping the growth of bacteria infecting a surface of the eye.

How should this medicine be used?

Neomycin, polymyxin, and bacitracin combination comes as an ophthalmic ointment to apply inside the lower lid of an infected eye. The ointment is usually applied to the eye every 3-4 hours for 7-10 days, as directed by your doctor. Follow the directions on your prescription label carefully, and ask your doctor or pharmacist to explain any part you do not understand. Use neomycin, polymyxin, and bacitracin ophthalmic ointment exactly as directed. Do not use more or less of it or use it more often than prescribed by your doctor.

Your eye or eyelid infection should begin getting better during the first few days of treatment with neomycin, polymyxin, and bacitracin combination. If your symptoms do not go away or get worse, call your doctor.

Continue to use neomycin, polymyxin, and bacitracin

combination as directed, even if your symptoms improve. Do not stop using neomycin, polymyxin, and bacitracin combination without talking to your doctor. If you stop using this medication too soon or skip doses, your infection may not be completely cured and bacteria may become resistant to antibiotics.

This medication is for use in the eye only. Do not let neomycin, polymyxin, and bacitracin combination get into your nose or mouth, and do not swallow it.

Never share your tube of ophthalmic ointment, even with someone who was also prescribed this medication. If more than one person uses the same tube, infection may spread.

To use the eye ointment, follow these steps:
1. Wash your hands well with soap and water.
2. Use a mirror or have someone else apply the ointment.
3. The ointment must be kept clean. Do not touch the tip of the tube against your eye, eyelid, fingers, or anything else.
4. Lie down and gaze upward or tilt your head back while standing.
5. Hold the tube between your thumb and index finger of the hand you usually use to hold a pencil. Place the tube as near to your eyelid as possible without touching it.
6. Brace the remaining fingers of your hand against your cheek or nose.
7. With the index finger of your other hand, pull the lower lid of your eye down to form a pocket.
8. Place the prescribed amount of ointment into the pocket made by your lower lid and eye.
9. Replace and tighten the cap right away.
10. Gently close your eyes and keep them closed for 1-2 minutes to allow the medication in the ointment to be absorbed.
11. Wipe off any excess ointment from outside or below your eye with a clean tissue. Wipe off any excess ointment from the outside of the tube with a clean tissue. Wash your hands again to remove any ointment.

Are there other uses for this medicine?

This medication may be prescribed for other uses; ask your doctor or pharmacist for more information.

What special precautions should I follow?

Before using neomycin, polymyxin, and bacitracin combination,
- tell your doctor and pharmacist if you are allergic to neomycin (Myciguent, others); polymyxin; bacitracin (Baciguent, others); aminoglycoside antibiotics such as amikacin (Amikin), gentamicin (Garamycin), kanamycin (Kantrex), paromycin (Humatin), streptomycin, and tobramycin (Nebcin, Tobi); zinc; or any other medications.
- tell your doctor and pharmacist what prescription and nonprescription medications, vitamins, nutritional supplements, and herbal products you are taking. Be sure to mention aminoglycoside antibiotics such as amikacin (Amikin), gentamicin (Garamycin), kanamycin (Kantrex), paromycin (Humatin), streptomycin, and tobramycin (Nebcin, Tobi). Your doctor may need to change the doses of your medications or monitor you carefully for side effects.
- tell your doctor if you have or have ever had hearing problems or kidney disease.
- tell your doctor if you are pregnant, plan to become pregnant, or are breast-feeding. If you become pregnant while taking neomycin, polymyxin, and bacitracin combination, call your doctor.

What special dietary instructions should I follow?

Unless your doctor tells you otherwise, continue your normal diet.

What should I do if I forget to take a dose?

Apply the missed dose as soon as you remember it. However, if it is almost time for the next dose, skip the missed dose and continue your regular dosing schedule. Do not apply a double dose to make up for a missed one.

What side effects can this medicine cause?

Neomycin, polymyxin, and bacitracin combination may cause side effects. If you experience any of the following symptoms, call your doctor immediately:
- eye pain
- irritation, burning, itching, swelling, or redness of the eye or eyelid
- worsening eye discharge
- red or scaly patches around eye or eyelid
- rash
- hives
- difficulty breathing or swallowing
- swelling of the face, throat, tongue, lips, eyes, hands, feet, ankles, or lower legs
- hoarseness
- chest tightness
- faintness
- dizziness

Neomycin, polymyxin, and bacitracin combination may cause other side effects. Call your doctor if you have any unusual problems while taking this medication.

If you experience a serious side effect, you or your doctor may send a report to the Food and Drug Administration's (FDA) MedWatch Adverse Event Reporting program online [at http://www.fda.gov/MedWatch/index.html] or by phone [1-800-332-1088].

What storage conditions are needed for this medicine?

Keep this medication in the container it came in, tightly closed, and out of reach of children. Store it at room temperature and away from excess heat and moisture (not in the bathroom). Throw away any medication that is outdated or no longer needed. Talk to your pharmacist about the proper disposal of your medication.

What other information should I know?

Keep all appointments with your doctor.

Ask your pharmacist any questions you have about refilling your prescription.

If you still have symptoms of infection after you finish the neomycin, polymyxin, and bacitracin combination prescription, call your doctor.

Talk to your doctor, pharmacist, or other healthcare professional if you have questions about dosing information for your medication.

Neomycin, Polymyxin, and Bacitracin Topical

(nee oh mye′ sin, pol i mix′ in, bass i tray′ sin)

Brand Name: Mycitracin®, Neosporin®, Triple Antibiotic Ointment®

Why is this medicine prescribed?

Neomycin, polymyxin, and bacitracin combination is used to prevent minor skin injuries such as cuts, scrapes, and burns from becoming infected. Neomycin, polymyxin, and bacitracin are in a class of medications called antibiotics. Neomycin, polymyxin, and bacitracin combination works by stopping the growth of bacteria.

How should this medicine be used?

Neomycin, polymyxin, and bacitracin combination comes as an ointment to apply to the skin. It is usually used one to three times a day. Neomycin, polymyxin, and bacitracin ointment is available without a prescription. However, your doctor may give you special directions on the proper use of this medication for your medical problem. Follow the directions on the package or those given to you by your doctor carefully, and ask your doctor or pharmacist to explain any part you do not understand. Use neomycin, polymyxin, and bacitracin combination exactly as directed. Do not use more or less of it or use it more often than prescribed by your doctor or written on the package.

This medication is for use only on the skin. Do not let neomycin, polymyxin, and bacitracin combination get into your eyes, nose, or mouth and do not swallow it.

You may use neomycin, polymyxin, and bacitracin combination to treat minor skin injuries. However, you should not use this medication to treat deep cuts, puncture wounds, animal bites, serious burns, or any injuries that affect large areas of your body. You should call your doctor or get emergency medical help if you have these types of injuries. A different treatment may be needed. You should also stop using this medication and call your doctor if you use this medication to treat a minor skin injury and your symptoms do not go away within 1 week.

Do not apply this medication to a child's diaper area, especially if the skin surface is broken or raw, unless told to do so by a doctor. If you are told to apply it to a child's diaper area, do not use tightly fitting diapers or plastic pants.

To use the ointment, follow these steps:

1. Wash your hands well with soap and water. Wash the injured area with soap and water and pat dry thoroughly with a clean towel.
2. Apply a small amount of the ointment (an amount equal to the size of your finger tip) to the injured skin. A thin layer is all that is needed. Do not touch the tip of the tube to your skin, hands, or anything else.
3. Replace and tighten the cap right away.
4. You may cover the affected area with a sterile bandage.
5. Wash your hands again.

Are there other uses for this medicine?

This medication may be prescribed for other uses; ask your doctor or pharmacist for more information.

What special precautions should I follow?

Before using neomycin, polymyxin, and bacitracin combination,

- tell your doctor and pharmacist if you are allergic to neomycin (Myciguent, others); polymyxin; bacitracin (Baciguent, others); aminoglycoside antibiotics such as amikacin (Amikin), gentamicin (Garamycin), kanamycin (Kantrex), paromycin (Humatin), and tobramycin (Nebcin, Tobi); zinc; or any other medications.
- tell your doctor and pharmacist what prescription and nonprescription medications, vitamins, nutritional supplements, and herbal products you are taking. Be sure to mention aminoglycoside antibiotics such as amikacin (Amikin), gentamicin (Garamycin), kanamycin (Kantrex), paromycin (Humatin), and tobramycin (Nebcin, Tobi). Your doctor may need to change the doses of your medications or monitor you carefully for side effects.
- tell your doctor if you have or have ever had hearing problems or kidney disease.
- tell your doctor if you are pregnant, plan to become pregnant, or are breast-feeding. If you become pregnant while using neomycin, polymyxin, and bacitracin combination, call your doctor.

What special dietary instructions should I follow?

Unless your doctor tells you otherwise, continue your normal diet.

What should I do if I forget to take a dose?

Apply the missed dose as soon as you remember it. However, if it is almost time for the next dose, skip the missed dose and continue your regular dosing schedule. Do not apply a double dose to make up for a missed one.

What side effects can this medicine cause?

Neomycin, polymyxin, and bacitracin combination may cause side effects. If you experience any of the following symptoms, call your doctor immediately:

- skin pain, irritation, burning, swelling, or redness
- itching
- rash
- hives
- red, scaly patches on skin
- difficulty breathing or swallowing
- swelling of the face, throat, tongue, lips, eyes, hands, feet, ankles, or lower legs
- hoarseness
- chest tightness
- faintness
- dizziness

Neomycin, polymyxin, and bacitracin combination may cause other side effects. Call your doctor if you have any unusual problems while taking this medication.

If you experience a serious side effect, you or your doctor may send a report to the Food and Drug Administration's (FDA) MedWatch Adverse Event Reporting program online [at http://www.fda.gov/MedWatch/index.html] or by phone [1-800-332-1088].

What storage conditions are needed for this medicine?

Keep this medication in the container it came in, tightly closed, and out of reach of children. Store it at room temperature and away from excess heat and moisture (not in the bathroom). Throw away any medication that is outdated or no longer needed. Talk to your pharmacist about the proper disposal of your medication.

What should I do in case of overdose?

You should not swallow neomycin, polymyxin, and bacitracin ointment. If someone does swallow this medication, call your local poison control center at 1-800-222-1222. If the victim has collapsed or is not breathing, call local emergency services at 911.

What other information should I know?

If your doctor has told you to use this medication, keep all appointments with your doctor. Call your doctor if you still have symptoms of infection after you finish using this medication as directed.

Ask your pharmacist any questions you have about neomycin, polymyxin, and bacitracin combination.

Talk to your doctor, pharmacist, or other healthcare professional if you have questions about dosing information for your medication.

Neomycin Topical

(nee oh mye′ sin)

Brand Name: Bactine® First Aid Antibiotic Plus Anesthetic as a combination product containing Neomycin Sulfate, Bacitracin Zinc, Lidocaine, and Polymyxin B Sulfate, Campho-Phenique® First Aid Antibiotic Plus Pain Reliever Maximum Strength as a combination product containing Neomycin Sulfate, Bacitracin Zinc, Lidocaine, and Polymyxin B Sulfate, Myciguent®, Mycitracin® Plus Pain Reliever as a combination product containing Neomycin Sulfate, Bacitracin Zinc, Lidocaine, and Polymyxin B Sulfate, Mycitracin® Triple Antibiotic First Aid Ointment Maximum Strength as a combination product containing Neomycin Sulfate, Bacitracin Zinc, and Polymyxin B Sulfate, Neo-Rx® Micronized Antibiotic Powder for Prescription Compounding, Neosporin® as a combination product containing Neomycin Sulfate, Bacitracin Zinc, and Polymyxin B Sulfate, Neosporin® G.U. Irrigant, Neosporin® Plus Maximum Strength First Aid Antibiotic/Pain Relieving Cream as a combination product containing Neomycin Sulfate, Polymyxin B Sulfate, and Pramoxine Hydrochloride, Neosporin® Plus Maximum Strength First Aid Antibiotic/Pain Relieving Ointment as a combination product containing Neomycin Sulfate, Bacitracin Zinc, Polymyxin B Sulfate, and Pramoxine Hydrochloride, Spectrocin® Plus as a combination product containing Neomycin Sulfate, Bacitracin Zinc, Lidocaine, and Polymyxin B Sulfate
Also available generically.

Why is this medicine prescribed?

Neomycin, an antibiotic, is used to prevent or treat skin infections caused by bacteria. It is not effective against fungal or viral infections.

This medication is sometimes prescribed for other uses; ask your doctor or pharmacist for more information.

How should this medicine be used?

Neomycin comes in cream and ointment that is applied to the skin. Neomycin usually is used one to three times a day.

Follow the directions on your prescription label carefully, and ask your doctor or pharmacist to explain any part you do not understand. Use neomycin exactly as directed. Do not use more or less of it or use it more often than prescribed by your doctor.

Thoroughly clean the infected area, allow it to dry, and then gently rub the medication in until most of it disappears. Use just enough medication to cover the affected area. You should wash your hands after applying the medication.

Do not apply neomycin to a child's diaper area, especially if the skin is raw, unless directed to do so by a doctor. If you are directed to apply neomycin to a child's diaper area, do not use tightly fitting diapers or plastic pants. They can increase the absorption of the drug, which can cause harmful effects.

Apply only small amounts of neomycin to scrapes, cuts, burns, sores, and wounds, and do not apply it more frequently than directed. Neomycin can be absorbed into the body through broken skin and cause kidney problems and hearing difficulty.

What special precautions should I follow?

Before using neomycin,
- tell your doctor and pharmacist if you are allergic to neomycin or any other drugs.
- tell your doctor and pharmacist what prescription and nonprescription medications you are taking, including vitamins.
- tell your doctor if you have or have ever had kidney disease.
- tell your doctor if you are pregnant, plan to become pregnant, or are breast-feeding. If you become pregnant while using neomycin, call your doctor.

What should I do if I forget to take a dose?

Apply the missed dose as soon as you remember it. However, if it is almost time for the next dose, skip the missed dose and continue your regular dosing schedule. Do not apply a double dose to make up for a missed one.

What side effects can this medicine cause?

Neomycin may cause side effects. If you experience any of the following symptoms, call your doctor immediately:
- irritation
- burning
- redness
- rash
- itching
- hearing difficulty
- decreased urination

If you experience a serious side effect, you or your doctor may send a report to the Food and Drug Administration's (FDA) MedWatch Adverse Event Reporting program online [at http://www.fda.gov/MedWatch/index.html] or by phone [1-800-332-1088].

What storage conditions are needed for this medicine?

Keep this medication in the container it came in, tightly closed, and out of reach of children. Store it at room temperature and away from excess heat and moisture (not in the bathroom). Neomycin may become discolored, but this change does not affect its action. Throw away any medication that is outdated or no longer needed. Talk to your pharmacist about the proper disposal of your medication.

What other information should I know?

Keep all appointments with your doctor. Neomycin is for external use only. Do not let neomycin get into your eyes, nose, or mouth, and do not swallow it. Do not apply dressings, bandages, cosmetics, lotions, or other skin medications to the area being treated unless your doctor tells you.

Do not let anyone else use your medication. Ask your pharmacist any questions you have about refilling your prescription.

If you still have symptoms of infection after you finish the neomycin, call your doctor.

Dosage Facts
For Informational Purposes

Caution: Do not change your dose, how often you take your medication, or the length of time you are to take it without first talking to your healthcare provider.

The following dosage information was written using medical language for doctors and other healthcare professionals and is provided here for you to check your dosage. The dosage of this drug may differ for different patients. Therefore, always follow your doctor's instructions or the directions on the label. Contact your healthcare provider or pharmacist if you have any questions about the specific dosage of your medication after reviewing this information.

General Dosage Information

Available as neomycin sulfate; dosage expressed in terms of the salt or the base.

Pediatric Patients

Superficial Skin Infections

TOPICAL:
- Children ≥2 years of age: Apply amount equal to the surface area of a fingertip to the affected area 1–3 times daily.

Adult Patients

Superficial Skin Infections

TOPICAL:
- Apply amount equal to the surface area of a fingertip to the affected area 1–3 times daily.

Nepafenac Ophthalmic

(ne-paf-fen'-ak)

Brand Name: Nevanac®

Why is this medicine prescribed?

Nepafenac ophthalmic is used to treat eye pain, redness, and swelling in patients who are recovering from cataract surgery (procedure to treat clouding of the lens in the eye). Nepafenac is in a class of medications called nonsteroidal anti-inflammatory medications (NSAIDs). It works by stopping the production of certain natural substances that cause pain and swelling.

How should this medicine be used?

Nepafenac ophthalmic comes as a suspension (liquid) to instill in the eyes. It is usually instilled three times a day beginning one day before cataract surgery, on the day of the surgery, and for 14 days after the surgery. Use nepafenac eye drops at around the same times every day. Follow the directions on your prescription label carefully, and ask your doctor or pharmacist to explain any part you do not understand. Use nepafenac eye drops exactly as directed. Do not use more or less of them or use them more often than prescribed by your doctor.

To use the eye drops, follow these steps:

1. Use a mirror or have someone else put the drops in your eye.
2. Wash your hands thoroughly with soap and water.
3. Shake the container well.
4. Remove the protective cap. Make sure that the end of the dropper is not chipped or cracked.
5. Avoid touching the dropper tip against your eye or anything else.
6. Lie down or tilt your head back and look upward.
7. Hold the bottle between your thumb and index finger and place the dropper tip as near as possible to your eyelid without touching it.
8. Brace the remaining fingers of that hand against your cheek or nose.
9. Use the index finger of your other hand to pull the lower lid of your eye down to form a pocket.
10. Drop the prescribed number of drops into the pocket made by the lower lid and the eye.
11. Close your eye and press lightly against the lower lid with your finger for 2-3 minutes to keep the medication in the eye. Do not blink.
12. Replace and tighten the cap right away. Do not rinse it off.
13. Wipe off any excess liquid from your cheek with a clean tissue. Wash your hands again.

Are there other uses for this medicine?

This medication may be prescribed for other uses; ask your doctor or pharmacist for more information.

What special precautions should I follow?

Before using nepafenac eye drops,
- tell your doctor and pharmacist if you are allergic to nepafenac; aspirin or other NSAIDs such as diclofenac (Voltaren), ibuprofen (Advil, Motrin), naproxen (Aleve, Naprosyn), or tolmetin (Tolectin); any other medications, or any of the ingredients in nepafenac eye drops. Ask your pharmacist for a list of the ingredients.
- tell your doctor and pharmacist what prescription and nonprescription medications, vitamins, nutritional supplements, and herbal products you are taking or plan to take. Be sure to mention any of the following: anticoagulants ('blood thinners') such as warfarin (Coumadin); aspirin and other NSAIDs such as ibuprofen (Advil, Motrin) and naproxen (Aleve, Naprosyn); and corticosteroid eye drops such as dexamethasone (Maxidex), fluorometholone (FML), hydrocortisone (in Cortisporin), loteprednol (Alrex, Lotemax), medrysone (HMS), prednisolone (Pred Mild), and rimexolone (Vexol). Your doctor may need to change the doses of your medications or monitor you carefully for side effects.
- tell your doctor if you have or have ever had diabetes, rheumatoid arthritis (arthritis caused by swelling of the lining of the joints), dry eye disease or any eye problem other than cataracts, or any condition that causes you to bleed easily.
- tell your doctor if you are pregnant, especially if you are in the last few months of your pregnancy, you plan to become pregnant, or you are breast-feeding. If you become pregnant while using nepafenac eye drops, call your doctor.
- if you wear contact lenses, remove them before you use nepafenac eye drops.

What special dietary instructions should I follow?

Unless your doctor tells you otherwise, continue your normal diet.

What should I do if I forget to take a dose?

Instill the missed dose as soon as you remember it. However, if it is almost time for the next dose, skip the missed dose and continue your regular dosing schedule. Do not instill extra eye drops to make up for a missed dose.

What side effects can this medicine cause?

Nepafenac eye drops may cause side effects. Tell your doctor if any of these symptoms are severe or do not go away:

- headache
- runny nose
- pain or pressure in the face
- upset stomach
- vomiting
- dry, itchy, or sticky eyes

Some side effects can be serious. If you experience any of these symptoms, call your doctor immediately:

- red or bloody eyes
- eye pain
- feeling that something is in the eye
- sensitivity to light
- blurred or decreased vision
- seeing specks or spots
- teary eyes
- eye discharge or crusting

Nepafenac eye drops may cause other side effects. Call your doctor if you have any unusual problems while using this medication.

If you experience a serious side effect, you or your doctor may send a report to the Food and Drug Administration's (FDA) MedWatch Adverse Event Reporting program online [at http://www.fda.gov/MedWatch/index.html] or by phone [1-800-332-1088].

What storage conditions are needed for this medicine?

Keep this medication in the container it came in, tightly closed, and out of reach of children. Store it at room temperature and away from excess heat and moisture (not in the bathroom). Throw away any medication that is outdated or no longer needed. Talk to your pharmacist about the proper disposal of your medication.

What other information should I know?

Keep all appointments with your doctor

Do not let anyone else use your medication. Ask your pharmacist any questions you have about refilling your prescription.

Dosage Facts
For Informational Purposes

Caution: Do not change your dose, how often you take your medication, or the length of time you are to take it without first talking to your healthcare provider.

The following dosage information was written using medical language for doctors and other healthcare professionals and is provided here for you to check your dosage. The dosage of this drug may differ for different patients. Therefore, always follow your doctor's instructions or the directions on the label. Contact your healthcare provider or pharmacist if you have any questions about the specific dosage of your medication after reviewing this information.

Pediatric Patients

Postoperative Ocular Inflammation and Pain

OPHTHALMIC:
- Patients ≥10 years of age: 1 drop of a 0.1% suspension in the affected eye(s) 3 times daily, beginning 1 day prior to cataract surgery and continuing on the day of the surgery and for 2 weeks after surgery.

Adult Patients

Postoperative Ocular Inflammation and Pain

OPHTHALMIC:
- 1 drop of a 0.1% suspension in the affected eye(s) 3 times daily, beginning 1 day prior to cataract surgery and continuing on the day of the surgery and for 2 weeks after surgery.

Nevirapine

(ne vye' ra peen)

Brand Name: Viramune®

Important Warning

Nevirapine can cause severe, life-threatening liver damage, skin reactions, and allergic reactions. Tell your doctor if you have or have ever had liver disease, especially hepatitis B or C. Tell your doctor if you have a rash or other skin condition before you start taking nevirapine. If you experience any of the following symptoms, stop taking nevirapine and call your doctor immediately: rash, especially if it is severe or comes along with any of the other symptoms on this list; excessive tiredness; lack of energy or general weakness; upset stomach; vomiting; loss of appetite; dark (tea colored) urine; pale stools; yellowing of the skin or eyes; pain in the upper right part of the stomach; fever; sore throat, chills, or other signs of infection; flu-like symptoms; muscle or joint aches; blisters; mouth sores; red or swollen eyes; hives; itching; swelling of the face, throat, tongue, lips, eyes, hands, feet, ankles, or lower legs; hoarseness; or difficulty breathing or swallowing.

If your doctor tells you to stop taking nevirapine because you had a serious skin or liver reaction, you should never take nevirapine again.

Your doctor will start you on a low dose of nevirapine and increase your dose after 14 days. This will decrease the risk that you will develop a serious skin reaction. If you develop any type of rash or any of the symptoms listed above while you are taking a low dose of nevirapine, call your doctor right away. Do not increase your dose until your rash or symptoms have gone away.

Keep all appointments with your doctor and the laboratory. Your doctor will order certain tests to check your body's response to nevirapine, especially during the first 18 weeks of your treatment.

Your doctor or pharmacist will give you the manufacturer's patient information sheet (Medication Guide) when you begin treatment with nevirapine and each time you refill your prescription. Read the information carefully and ask your doctor or pharmacist if you have any questions. You can also obtain the Medication Guide from the FDA website: http://www.fda.gov.

Talk to your doctor about the risks of taking nevirapine. There is a greater risk that you will develop serious liver damage during your treatment if you are a woman and if you have a high CD4 count (large number of a certain type of infection fighting cell in your blood).

Why is this medicine prescribed?

Nevirapine is used in combination with other medications to treat human immunodeficiency virus (HIV) infection in patients with or without acquired immunodeficiency syndrome (AIDS). Nevirapine is in a class of medications called non-nucleoside reverse transcriptase inhibitors (NNRTIs). It works by decreasing the amount of HIV in the blood. Nevirapine does not cure HIV and may not prevent you from developing HIV-related illnesses. Nevirapine does not prevent the spread of HIV to other people.

How should this medicine be used?

Nevirapine comes as a tablet and a suspension (liquid) to take by mouth. It is usually taken with or without food once a day for 2 weeks and twice a day after the first 2 weeks. Follow the directions on your prescription label carefully, and ask your doctor or pharmacist to explain any part you do not understand. Take nevirapine exactly as directed. Do not take more or less of it or take it more often than prescribed by your doctor.

Swallow nevirapine with liquids such as water, milk, or soda.

Shake the liquid gently before each use to mix the medication evenly. Use an oral dosing cup or dosing syringe to measure your dose. It is best to use a syringe, especially if your dose is less than 5 mL (1 teaspoon). If you use a dosing cup, first drink all of the medication that you measured in the dosing cup. Then fill the dosing cup with water and drink the water to be sure that you get your full dose.

Nevirapine may control HIV but will not cure it. Continue to take nevirapine even if you feel well. Do not stop taking nevirapine or any of the other medications that you are taking to treat HIV or AIDS without talking to your doctor. Your doctor will probably tell you to stop taking your medications in a certain order. If you miss doses or stop taking nevirapine, your condition may become more difficult to treat.

If you do not take nevirapine for 7 days or longer, do not start taking it again without talking to your doctor. Your doctor will start you on a low dose of nevirapine, and increase your dose after 2 weeks.

Are there other uses for this medicine?

Nevirapine is also sometimes used to prevent unborn babies whose mothers have HIV or AIDS from becoming infected with HIV during birth.

This medication may be prescribed for other uses; ask your doctor or pharmacist for more information.

What special precautions should I follow?

Before taking nevirapine,

- tell your doctor and pharmacist if you are allergic to nevirapine or any other medications.
- tell your doctor and pharmacist what prescription and nonprescription medications, vitamins, and nutritional supplements you are taking. Be sure to mention any of the following: anticoagulants ('blood thinners') such as warfarin (Coumadin); certain antifungals such as fluconazole (Diflucan), itraconazole (Sporanox), ketoconazole (Nizoral) and voriconazole (Vfend); calcium channel blockers such as diltiazem (Cardizem, Dilacor, Tiazac), nifedipine (Adalat, Procardia), and verapamil (Calan, Covera, Isoptin, Verelan); clarithromycin (Biaxin); certain cancer chemotherapy medications such as cyclophosphamide (Cytoxan); cisapride (Propulsid); cyclosporine (Neoral, Sandimmune); ergot alkaloids such as ergotamine (Cafergot, Ercaf, others); fentanyl (Duragesic, Actiq); medications for irregular heartbeat such as amiodarone (Cordarone) and disopyramide (Norpace); medications for seizures such as carbamazepine (Tegretol), clonazepam (Klonopin), and ethosuximide (Zarontin); methadone (Dolophine), other medications for HIV or AIDS such as amprenavir (Agenerase), atazanavir (Reyataz), efavirenz (Sustiva), indinavir (Crixivan); lopinavir and ritonavir combination (Kaletra), nelfinavir (Viracept) and saquinavir (Fortovase, Invirase); prednisone (Deltasone); rifabutin (Mycobutin), rifampin (Rifadin, Rimactane), sirolimus (Rapamune), and tacrolimus (Prograf). Many other medications may interact with nevirapine, so be sure to tell

your doctor about all the medications you are taking, even those that do not appear on this list. Your doctor may need to change the doses of your medications or monitor you more carefully for side effects.

- tell your doctor and pharmacist what herbal products you are taking, especially St. John's wort.
- tell your doctor if you have or have ever had kidney disease, especially if you are being treated with dialysis (treatment to clean the blood outside the body when the kidneys are not working well).
- tell your doctor if you are pregnant or plan to become pregnant. If you become pregnant while taking nevirapine, call your doctor. You should not breastfeed if you are infected with HIV or are taking nevirapine.
- tell your doctor if you are taking oral contraceptives ('birth control pills') to prevent pregnancy. Nevirapine may interfere with the action of oral contraceptives. Talk to your doctor about other methods of birth control that will work for you.
- you should know that your body fat may increase or move to other areas of your body such as your breasts, waist, or upper back.

What special dietary instructions should I follow?

Unless your doctor tells you otherwise, continue your normal diet.

What should I do if I forget to take a dose?

Take the missed dose as soon as you remember it. However, if it is almost time for the next dose, skip the missed dose and continue your regular dosing schedule. Do not take a double dose to make up for a missed one.

What side effects can this medicine cause?

Nevirapine may cause side effects. Tell your doctor if either of these symptoms is severe or does not go away:
- headache
- diarrhea

Some side effects can be serious. If you experience any of the symptoms listed in the IMPORTANT WARNING section, call your doctor immediately.

If you experience a serious side effect, you or your doctor may send a report to the Food and Drug Administration's (FDA) MedWatch Adverse Event Reporting program online [at http://www.fda.gov/MedWatch/index.html] or by phone [1-800-332-1088].

What storage conditions are needed for this medicine?

Keep this medication in the container it came in, tightly closed, and out of reach of children. Store it at room temperature and away from excess heat and moisture (not in the bathroom). Throw away any medication that is outdated or no longer needed. Talk to your pharmacist about the proper disposal of your medication.

What should I do in case of overdose?

In case of overdose, call your local poison control center at 1-800-222-1222. If the victim has collapsed or is not breathing, call local emergency services at 911.

Symptoms of overdose may include:
- swelling of the hands, feet, ankles, or lower legs
- painful red bumps on the skin
- excessive tiredness
- fever
- headache
- difficulty falling asleep or staying asleep
- upset stomach
- vomiting
- weight loss
- rash
- dizziness

What other information should I know?

Do not let anyone else take your medication. Ask your pharmacist any questions you have about refilling your prescription.

Dosage Facts
For Informational Purposes

Caution: Do not change your dose, how often you take your medication, or the length of time you are to take it without first talking to your healthcare provider.

The following dosage information was written using medical language for doctors and other healthcare professionals and is provided here for you to check your dosage. The dosage of this drug may differ for different patients. Therefore, always follow your doctor's instructions or the directions on the label. Contact your healthcare provider or pharmacist if you have any questions about the specific dosage of your medication after reviewing this information.

General Dosage Information

Available as nevirapine and nevirapine hemihydrate; dosage expressed in terms of nevirapine.

Must be given in conjunction with other antiretrovirals. *If used with indinavir, lopinavir, or saquinavir, adjustment in the treatment regimen necessary.*

Therapy should be initiated using a low dosage for the first 14 days since this appears to reduce frequency of rash. If rash occurs during this initial period, dosage should *not* be increased until the rash has resolved.

If nevirapine therapy has been interrupted for >7 days for any reason, therapy should be restarted using the recommended initial dosage.

Pediatric Patients

Treatment of HIV Infection

ORAL:
- Infants <2 months of age†: 5 mg/kg (or 120 mg/m²) once daily for the first 14 days of therapy, followed by 120 mg/m²

every 12 hours for the next 14 days, and then 200 mg/m² every 12 hours has been used.

- Children 2 months to 8 years of age: 4 mg/kg once daily for the first 14 days, followed by 7 mg/kg (maximum 200 mg) every 12 hours. Some experts recommend 120 mg/m² (maximum 200 mg) once daily for the first 14 days of therapy, followed by 120–200 mg/m² (maximum 200 mg) given every 12 hours. The higher dosage (i.e., 200 mg/m² twice daily) may be required.
- Children ≥8 years of age: 4 mg/kg daily for the first 14 days, followed by 4 mg/kg (maximum 200 mg) every 12 hours. Some experts recommend 120 mg/m² (maximum 200 mg) once daily for the first 14 days of therapy, followed by 120–200 mg/m² (maximum 200 mg) given every 12 hours.

Prevention of Maternal-fetal Transmission of HIV†

ORAL:

- Neonate: 2 mg/kg as a single dose given 48–72 hours after birth. Neonatal dose usually used in conjunction with a single intrapartum dose given to the mother at onset of labor.
- If mother received the intrapartum nevirapine dose <1 hour before delivery, some experts recommend the neonate receive 2 mg/kg as soon as possible after birth and an additional 2-mg/kg dose 48–72 hours after birth.

Adult Patients

Treatment of HIV Infection

ORAL:

- 200 mg once daily for the first 14 days, followed by 200 mg twice daily.

Prevention of Maternal-fetal Transmission of HIV†

ORAL:

- 200 mg given at the onset of labor. Maternal dose usually used in conjunction with a single dose given to the neonate after birth; if mother received the intrapartum nevirapine dose <1 hour before delivery, neonate may need 2 nevirapine doses.

Prescribing Limits

Pediatric Patients

Treatment of HIV Infection

ORAL:

- Children ≥2 months of age: 400 mg daily.

Special Populations

Hepatic Impairment

- Not clear whether dosage adjustment needed in patients with mild to moderate hepatic impairment. Not recommended in patients with moderate or severe hepatic impairment.

Renal Impairment

Treatment of HIV Infection

ORAL:

- Dosage adjustment not needed in patients with $Cl_{cr} \geq 20$ mL/minute.
- Administer 200 mg after each dialysis treatment.

Geriatric Patients

- Select dosage with caution because of age-related decreases in hepatic, renal, and/or cardiac function and concomitant disease and drug therapy.

† Use is not currently included in the labeling approved by the US Food and Drug Administration.

Niacin

(nye′ a sin)

Brand Name: Advicor®, Niacor®, Niaspan®
Also available generically.

Why is this medicine prescribed?

Niacin is used with diet changes (restriction of cholesterol and fat intake) to reduce the amount of cholesterol and certain fatty substances in your blood. Niacin is also used to prevent and treat pellagra (niacin deficiency), a disease caused by inadequate diet and other medical problems. Niacin is a B-complex vitamin.

How should this medicine be used?

Niacin comes as a tablet and an extended-release (long-acting) tablet to take by mouth. The regular tablet usually is taken two to three times a a day with meals, and the extended-release tablet is taken once a day, at bedtime, with food. Follow the directions on your prescription label or package label carefully, and ask your doctor or pharmacist to explain any part you do not understand. Take niacin exactly as directed. Do not take more or less of it or take it more often than prescribed by your doctor.

Swallow the extended-release tablets whole; do not split, chew, or crush them.

Your doctor will probably start you on a low dose of niacin and gradually increase your dose.

Continue to take niacin even if you feel well. Do not stop taking niacin without talking to your doctor.

Are there other uses for this medicine?

This medication is sometimes prescribed for other uses; ask your doctor or pharmacist for more information.

What special precautions should I follow?

Before taking niacin,

- tell your doctor and pharmacist if you are allergic to niacin, aspirin, tartrazine (a yellow dye in some processed foods and drugs), or any other drugs.
- tell your doctor and pharmacist what prescription and nonprescription medications you are taking, especially anticoagulants (blood thinners) such as warfarin (Cou-

madin), medications for high blood pressure or diabetes and other vitamins. If you take insulin or oral diabetes medication, your dose may need to be changed because niacin may increase the amount of sugar in your blood and urine.

- tell your doctor if you drink large amounts of alcohol and if you have or have ever had diabetes; gout; ulcers; allergies; jaundice (yellowing of the skin or eyes); or gallbladder, heart, or liver disease.
- tell your doctor if you are pregnant, plan to become pregnant, or are breast-feeding. If you become pregnant while taking niacin, call your doctor.
- if you are having surgery, including dental surgery, tell the doctor or dentist that you are taking niacin.
- you should know that this drug may make you drowsy. Do not drive a car or operate machinery until you know how this drug affects you.
- remember that alcohol can add to the drowsiness caused by this drug.
- you should know that niacin causes flushing (redness) of the face and neck. This side effect usually goes away after taking the medicine for a few weeks. Avoid drinking alcohol or hot drinks around the time you take niacin. Taking aspirin or another nonsteroidal anti-inflammatory medication such as ibuprofen (Advil, Motrin) or naproxen (Aleve, Naprosyn) 30 minutes before niacin may reduce the flushing. If you take extended-release niacin at bedtime, the flushing will probably happen while you are asleep. If you wake up and feel flushed, get up slowly, especially if you feel dizzy or faint.

What special dietary instructions should I follow?

If you take niacin to reduce the amount of cholesterol and fats in your blood, eat a low-cholesterol, low-fat diet. Follow the diet prescribed by your doctor.

What should I do if I forget to take a dose?

Take the missed dose as soon as you remember it. However, if it is almost time for the next dose, skip the missed dose and continue your regular dosing schedule. Do not take a double dose to make up for a missed one.

What side effects can this medicine cause?

Niacin may cause side effects. Tell your doctor if any of these symptoms are severe or do not go away:
- itching, stinging, tingling, or burning of the skin
- headache
- blurred vision
- upset stomach
- vomiting
- diarrhea
- heartburn
- bloating

If you experience any of the following symptoms, call your doctor immediately:

- dizziness
- faintness
- fast heartbeat
- yellowing of the skin or eyes

If you experience a serious side effect, you or your doctor may send a report to the Food and Drug Administration's (FDA) MedWatch Adverse Event Reporting program online [at http://www.fda.gov/MedWatch/index.html] or by phone [1-800-332-1088].

What storage conditions are needed for this medicine?

Keep this medication in the container it came in, tightly closed, and out of reach of children. Store it at room temperature and away from excess heat and moisture (not in the bathroom). Throw away any medication that is outdated or no longer needed. Talk to your pharmacist about the proper disposal of your medication.

What should I do in case of overdose?

In case of overdose, call your local poison control center at 1-800-222-1222. If the victim has collapsed or is not breathing, call local emergency services at 911.

What other information should I know?

Keep all appointments with your doctor and the laboratory. Your doctor will order certain lab tests to check your response to niacin.

Do not let anyone else take your medication. Ask your pharmacist any questions you have about refilling your prescription.

Dosage Facts
For Informational Purposes

Caution: Do not change your dose, how often you take your medication, or the length of time you are to take it without first talking to your healthcare provider.

The following dosage information was written using medical language for doctors and other healthcare professionals and is provided here for you to check your dosage. The dosage of this drug may differ for different patients. Therefore, always follow your doctor's instructions or the directions on the label. Contact your healthcare provider or pharmacist if you have any questions about the specific dosage of your medication after reviewing this information.

General Dosage Information

Commercially available as dietary supplements and as prescription-only preparations. Do not use these preparations interchangeably.

Pediatric Patients
Dietary Requirements

Recommended Daily Allowance (RDA) generally expressed in terms of niacin equivalents (NE). NE is calculated as follows: 1 mg of NE = 1 mg of niacin = 60 mg of tryptophan.

ORAL:

Age	RDA§	AI¶
0–6 months		2 mg of preformed niacin (0.3 mg/kg) daily
6–12 months		4 mg of NE (0.4 mg/kg) daily
1–3 years	6 mg of NE daily	
4–8 years	8 mg of NE daily	
9–13 years	12 mg of NE daily	
14–18 years	Boys: 16 mg of NE daily	
	Girls: 14 mg of NE daily	

§Recommended Dietary Allowance (RDA) is nutrient recommendation from National Academy of Sciences (NAS) for children and adults. The RDA for a given nutrient is the *goal* for dietary intake in individuals.
¶Adequate Intake (AI) is nutrient recommendation from NAS for infants ≤12 months of age; used when data are insufficient or too controversial to establish an RDA. AI set for infants ≤6 months of age is based on the observed mean niacin intake of infants fed principally human milk. AI set for infants 6–12 months of age is based on the AI for younger infants and data from adults.

Niacin Deficiency
Pellagra

ORAL:
- Niacin or niacinamide: 100–300 mg daily in divided doses.

Adult Patients
Prevention of Cardiovascular Events

ORAL:
- Extended-release niacin (Niaspan®): Initially, 500 mg once daily at bedtime. If response is inadequate, increase dosage by no more than 500 mg at 4-week intervals until desired effect is observed or maximum daily dosage of 2 g is reached.
- Usual maintenance dosage is 1–2 g once daily at bedtime.
- In patients previously treated with immediate-release preparations or in those who have discontinued extended-release niacin (Niaspan®) therapy for an extended period, titrate dosage as with initial therapy.

Dyslipidemias

ORAL:
- Immediate-release preparations: Initially, 100–500 mg 3 times daily. Increase dosage gradually (e.g., 300 mg daily at 4- to 7-day intervals) until desired effect is achieved. Usual maintenance dosage is 1.5–3 g daily given in 2 or 3 divided doses.
- Initial dosage of 250 mg daily following the evening meal recommended by manufacturer of Niacor® (immediate-release preparation). Increase dosage of Niacor® at 4- to 7-day intervals until desired effect is achieved or dosage of 1.5–2 g daily is reached. If adequate response is not achieved after 2 months, may then increase dosage at 2- to 4-week intervals to 3 g daily (1 g 3 times daily). Manufacturer of Niacor® states that higher doses (up to 6 g daily) occasionally may be required in patients with marked lipid abnormalities. Usual maintenance dosage recommended by manufacturer of Niacor® is 1–2 g daily given in 2 or 3 divided doses.
- Extended-release niacin (Niaspan®): Initially, 500 mg once daily at bedtime. If adequate response is not achieved after 4 weeks, increase dosage by no more than 500 mg at 4-week intervals until desired effect is observed. Usual maintenance dosage is 1–2 g once daily at bedtime. Titrate Niaspan® dosage as with initial therapy in patients previously treated with immediate-release niacin preparations or in those in whom therapy with extended-release niacin (Niaspan®) has been discontinued for a prolonged period.
- Extended-release niacin (Niaspan®) and lovastatin combination therapy: In patients already receiving a stable dosage of lovastatin, add Niaspan® (using recommended titration schedule). In patients already receiving a stable dosage of Niaspan®, add lovastatin (at initial dosage of 20 mg once daily). Adjust dosage at 4-week intervals.
- Fixed combination of extended-release niacin and lovastatin (Advicor®): Use only in patients already receiving a stable dosage of Niaspan®; in patients currently receiving niacin preparations other than Niaspan®, discontinue current niacin therapy and switch to Niaspan®. Once a stable Niaspan® dosage is reached, switch to Advicor® at the same niacin-equivalent dosage as Niaspan®. In patients currently receiving a stable dosage of lovastatin, add Niaspan® (using the recommended titration schedule) until a stable dosage has been reached, then switch to Advicor® at the same niacin-equivalent dosage as Niaspan®. Increase Advicor® dosage by no more than 500 mg (of the niacin component) at 4-week intervals. Usual maintenance dosage ranges from 500 mg of extended-release niacin and 20 mg of lovastatin to 2 g of extended-release niacin and 40 mg of lovastatin once daily. If Advicor® therapy has been discontinued for >7 days, reinstitute at the lowest available dosage. Because of differences in bioavailability, do *not* substitute 1 tablet of Advicor® 1 g/40 mg for 2 tablets of Advicor® 500 mg/20 mg, or vice versa.

Dietary Requirements

RDA generally expressed in terms of NE. NE is calculated as follows: 1 mg of NE = 1 mg of niacin = 60 mg of tryptophan.

ORAL:
- RDA for healthy men: 16 mg of NE daily.
- RDA for healthy women: 14 mg of NE daily.
- RDA for pregnant women: 18 mg of NE daily. Higher dosages required in women pregnant with >1 fetus.
- RDA for lactating women: 17 mg of NE daily. Higher dosages required in mothers nursing >1 infant.
- Higher dosages required in patients with Hartnup disease, liver cirrhosis, carcinoid syndrome, malabsorption syndrome, or in individuals receiving long-term isoniazid therapy or undergoing hemodialysis or peritoneal dialysis.

Niacin Deficiency
Pellagra

ORAL:
- Niacin or niacinamide: 300–500 mg daily in divided doses.

Hartnup Disease

ORAL:
- Niacin: 50–200 mg daily.

Prescribing Limits

Adult Patients

Prevention of Cardiovascular Events

ORAL:
- Extended-release niacin (Niaspan®): Maximum 2 g daily.

Dyslipidemias

ORAL:
- Immediate-release preparations: Maximum 4.5 g daily; manufacturer of Niacor® states that maximum of 6 g daily generally should not be exceeded.
- Extended-release niacin (Niaspan®): Maximum 2 g daily. When used in combination with lovastatin, maximum 2 g of Niaspan® and 40 mg of lovastatin daily.
- Fixed combination of extended-release niacin and lovastatin (Advicor®): Maximum 2 g of extended-release niacin and 40 mg of lovastatin daily.

Nicardipine

(nye kar′ de peen)

Brand Name: Cardene®, Cardene® SR
Also available generically.

Why is this medicine prescribed?

Nicardipine is used to treat high blood pressure. It relaxes your blood vessels so your heart does not have to pump as hard. It also increases the supply of blood and oxygen to the heart to control chest pain (angina). If taken regularly, nicardipine controls chest pain, but it does not stop chest pain once it starts. Your doctor may give you a different medication to take when you have chest pain.

This medication is sometimes prescribed for other uses; ask your doctor or pharmacist for more information.

How should this medicine be used?

Nicardipine comes as a regular capsule and as an extended-release (long-acting) capsule to take by mouth. The regular capsule is usually taken three times a day. The extended-release capsule is usually taken two times a day and is swallowed whole. Do not chew, divide, or crush the capsule. Follow the directions on your prescription label carefully, and ask your doctor or pharmacist to explain any part you do not understand. Take nicardipine exactly as directed. Do not take more or less of it or take it more often than prescribed by your doctor.

Nicardipine controls high blood pressure and chest pain (angina) but does not cure them. Continue to take nicardipine

even if you feel well. Do not stop taking nicardipine without talking to your doctor.

Are there other uses for this medicine?

Nicardipine is also used sometimes to treat congestive heart failure. Talk to your doctor about the possible risks of using this drug for your condition.

What special precautions should I follow?

Before taking nicardipine,
- tell your doctor and pharmacist if you are allergic to nicardipine or any other drugs.
- tell your doctor and pharmacist what prescription and nonprescription medications you are taking, especially carbamazepine (Tegretol); cimetidine (Tagamet); cyclosporine (Neoral, Sandimmune); fentanyl (Duragesic); heart and blood pressure medications such as beta-blockers, digoxin (Lanoxin), diuretics ('water pills'), and quinidine (Quinaglute, Quinidex); medications to treat glaucoma (increased pressure in the eye); phenytoin (Dilantin); ranitidine (Zantac); theophylline (Theo-Dur); and vitamins.
- tell your doctor if you have or have ever had heart, liver, or kidney disease.
- tell your doctor if you are pregnant, plan to become pregnant, or are breast-feeding. If you become pregnant while taking nicardipine, call your doctor.
- if you are having surgery, including dental surgery, tell your doctor or dentist that you are taking nicardipine.

What special dietary instructions should I follow?

Regular nicardipine capsules may be taken with or without food. The extended-release capsules should be taken with food, but avoid high-fat foods or high-fat meals.

Avoid drinking grapefruit juice or eating grapefruit 1 hour before or for 2 hours after taking nicardipine.

Talk to your doctor before using salt substitutes containing potassium. If your doctor prescribes a low-salt or low-sodium diet, follow these directions carefully.

What should I do if I forget to take a dose?

Take the missed dose as soon as you remember it. However, if it is almost time for the next dose, skip the missed dose and continue your regular dosing schedule. Do not take a double dose to make up for a missed one.

What side effects can this medicine cause?

Nicardipine may cause side effects. Tell your doctor if any of these symptoms are severe or do not go away:
- headache
- upset stomach
- dizziness or lightheadedness
- excessive tiredness
- flushing (feeling of warmth)

- numbness
- fast heartbeat
- muscle cramps
- constipation
- heartburn
- increased sweating
- dry mouth

If you experience any of the following symptoms, call your doctor immediately:

- swelling of the face, eyes, lips, tongue, arms, or legs
- difficulty breathing or swallowing
- fainting
- rash
- increase in frequency or severity of chest pain (angina)

If you experience a serious side effect, you or your doctor may send a report to the Food and Drug Administration's (FDA) MedWatch Adverse Event Reporting program online [at http://www.fda.gov/MedWatch/index.html] or by phone [1-800-332-1088].

What storage conditions are needed for this medicine?

Keep this medication in the container it came in, tightly closed, and out of reach of children. Store it at room temperature and away from excess heat and moisture (not in the bathroom). Throw away any medication that is outdated or no longer needed. Talk to your pharmacist about the proper disposal of your medication.

What should I do in case of overdose?

In case of overdose, call your local poison control center at 1-800-222-1222. If the victim has collapsed or is not breathing, call local emergency services at 911.

What other information should I know?

Keep all appointments with your doctor and the laboratory. Your blood pressure should be checked regularly to determine your response to nicardipine.

The extended-release capsule does not dissolve in the stomach after swallowing. It slowly releases medicine as it passes through your small intestines. It is not unusual to see the capsule shell in the stool.

Do not let anyone else take your medication. Ask your pharmacist any questions you have about refilling your prescription.

Dosage Facts
For Informational Purposes

Caution: Do not change your dose, how often you take your medication, or the length of time you are to take it without first talking to your healthcare provider.

The following dosage information was written using medical language for doctors and other healthcare professionals and is provided here for you to check your dosage. The dosage of this drug may differ for different patients. Therefore, always follow your doctor's instructions or the directions on the label. Contact your healthcare provider or pharmacist if you have any questions about the specific dosage of your medication after reviewing this information.

General Dosage Information

Available as nicardipine hydrochloride; dosage is expressed in terms of the salt.

Adult Patients

Hypertension
Conventional Capsules

ORAL:
- Initially, 20 mg 3 times daily.
- Adjust dosage according to patient's peak (approximately 1–2 hours after dosing, particularly during initiation of therapy) and trough (8 hours after dosing) BP responses, but generally no more frequently than at 3-day intervals.
- Usual dosage is 20–40 mg 3 times daily.

Extended-Release Capsules

ORAL:
- Initially, 30 mg twice daily.
- Adjust dosage according to BP response 2–4 hours after dosing as well as just prior to next dose.
- Usual dosage range is 30–60 mg twice daily.

Switching to Extended-Release Capsules

ORAL:
- Total daily dose of conventional tablets not a useful guide to judging effective dose of extended-release capsules. However, may administer the currently effective total daily dose of conventional capsules and adjust dosage according to BP response.

Angina
Conventional Capsules

ORAL:
- Initially, 20 mg 3 times daily. Adjust dosage according to patient tolerance and response at ≥3-day intervals.
- Usual dosage range is 20–40 mg 3 times daily.

Special Populations

Hepatic Impairment
- Conventional capsules: Initially, 20 mg twice daily in patients with severe hepatic impairment. Individualize dosage, but maintain a twice-daily dosing schedule.

Renal Impairment
- Conventional capsules: Initially, 20 mg 3 times daily. Titrate dosage carefully.
- Extended-release capsules: Initially, 30 mg twice daily. Titrate dosage carefully.

Geriatric Patients
- Cautious dosing recommended. For conventional and extended-release capsules, initiate therapy at low end of dosage range.

† Use is not currently included in the labeling approved by the US Food and Drug Administration.

Nicotine Gum

(nik' oh teen)

Brand Name: Nicorette®, Nicorette® DS
Also available generically.

Why is this medicine prescribed?

Nicotine chewing gum is used to help people stop smoking cigarettes. It acts as a substitute oral activity and provides a source of nicotine that reduces the withdrawal symptoms experienced when smoking is stopped.

How should this medicine be used?

Nicotine gum is used by mouth as a chewing gum and should not be swallowed. Follow the directions on the label, and ask your doctor or pharmacist to explain any part you do not understand. Use nicotine gum exactly as directed. Do not use more or less of it or use it more often unless prescribed by your doctor.

Usually treatment is started by using the 2-mg gum. Heavy smokers (those smoking more than 25 cigarettes per day) may start by using the 4-mg gum. Nicotine gum may be used regularly by chewing one piece of gum every 1-2 hours at first, or it may be used by chewing one piece of gum whenever you have the urge to smoke.

Nicotine gum should be chewed slowly until you can taste the nicotine or feel a slight tingling in your mouth. Then stop chewing and place (park) the chewing gum between your cheek and gum. When the tingling is almost gone (about 1 minute), start chewing again; repeat this procedure for about 30 minutes.

Do not chew nicotine gum too fast, do not chew more than one piece of gum at a time, and do not chew one piece too soon after another.

If you are using the 2-mg gum, do not chew more than 30 pieces a day if you are under the supervision of a doctor or 24 pieces a day if you are not under the supervision of a doctor. If you are using the 4-mg gum, do not chew more than 24 pieces a day.

Gradually begin reducing the amount of nicotine gum used after 2-3 months. This reduced use over time will help prevent nicotine-withdrawal symptoms.

Suggested tips to help reduce your use of nicotine gum gradually include:

1. Decrease the total number of pieces used per day by about 1 piece every 4-7 days.
2. Decrease the chewing time with each piece from the normal 30 minutes to 10-15 minutes for 4-7 days. Then gradually decrease the total number of pieces used per day.
3. Substitute one or more pieces of sugarless gum for an equal number of pieces of nicotine gum. Increase the number of pieces of sugarless gum substituted for nicotine gum every 4-7 days.
4. Replace 4-mg gum with 2-mg gum and apply any of the previous steps.

5. Consider stopping use of nicotine gum when your craving for nicotine is satisfied by one or two pieces of gum per day.

Use of nicotine gum for longer than 3 months is discouraged. Do not use nicotine gum longer than 6 months without talking with your doctor.

What special precautions should I follow?

Before using nicotine gum,

- tell your doctor and pharmacist what prescription and nonprescription medications you are taking, especially acetaminophen (Tylenol), caffeine, diuretics ('water pills'), imipramine (Tofranil), insulin, medications for high blood pressure, oxazepam (Serax), pentazocine (Talwin, Talwin NX, Talacen), propoxyphene (Darvon, E-Lor), propranolol (Inderal), theophylline (Theo-Dur), and vitamins.
- tell your doctor if you have or have ever had a heart attack, irregular heart rate, angina, ulcers, uncontrolled high blood pressure, overactive thyroid, pheochromocytoma, or a dental condition or disorder.
- tell your doctor if you are pregnant, plan to become pregnant, or are breast-feeding. If you become pregnant while using nicotine gum, stop using it and call your doctor immediately. Nicotine and nicotine gum may cause harm to the fetus.
- do not smoke cigarettes or use other nicotine products while using nicotine gum because nicotine overdose can occur.

What special dietary instructions should I follow?

Avoid eating and drinking (especially acidic beverages such as coffee or soft drinks) for 15 minutes before and during chewing of nicotine gum to prevent reduced absorption of nicotine.

What side effects can this medicine cause?

Nicotine may cause side effects. Tell your doctor if any of these symptoms are severe or do not go away:

- mouth ulcers
- jaw muscle aches
- dizziness
- headache
- upset stomach

If you experience any of the following symptoms, call your doctor immediately:

- seizures
- heart rhythm disturbances
- difficulty breathing

If you experience a serious side effect, you or your doctor may send a report to the Food and Drug Administration's (FDA) MedWatch Adverse Event Reporting program online [at http://www.fda.gov/MedWatch/index.html] or by phone [1-800-332-1088].

What storage conditions are needed for this medicine?

Keep this medication in the container it came in, tightly closed, and out of reach of children. Store it at room temperature and away from excess heat and moisture (not in the bathroom). Throw away any medication that is outdated or no longer needed. Talk to your pharmacist about the proper disposal of your medication.

What should I do in case of overdose?

In case of overdose, call your local poison control center at 1-800-222-1222. If the victim has collapsed or is not breathing, call local emergency services at 911.

What other information should I know?

Keep all appointments with your doctor.

Do not let anyone else take your medication. Ask your pharmacist any questions you have about refilling your prescription.

Dosage Facts
For Informational Purposes

Caution: Do not change your dose, how often you take your medication, or the length of time you are to take it without first talking to your healthcare provider.

The following dosage information was written using medical language for doctors and other healthcare professionals and is provided here for you to check your dosage. The dosage of this drug may differ for different patients. Therefore, always follow your doctor's instructions or the directions on the label. Contact your healthcare provider or pharmacist if you have any questions about the specific dosage of your medication after reviewing this information.

General Dosage Information

Available as nicotine polacrilex; dosage expressed in terms of nictoine.

Stop smoking completely before beginning buccal therapy.

Adult Patients
Smoking Cessation

ORAL:
- Patients who smoke < 25 cigarettes daily: Chew a 2-mg piece of gum every 2 hours during weeks 1–6; chew 1 piece every 2–4 hours during weeks 7–9; and chew 1 piece every 4–8 hours during weeks 10–12 of therapy. Alternatively, chew a 2-mg piece of gum whenever the urge to smoke occurs; do not exceed 2 pieces per hour.
- Patients who smoke ≥25 cigarettes daily: Chew a 4-mg piece of gum every 2 hours during weeks 1–6; chew 1 piece every 2–4 hours during weeks 7–9; and chew 1 piece every 4–8 hours during weeks 10–12 of therapy. Alternatively, chew 1 piece whenever the urge to smoke occurs; do not exceed 2 pieces per hour.
- Consult clinician if need for continued therapy at the end of regimen.

Prescribing Limits
Adult Patients

ORAL:
- Maximum 2 pieces of gum per hour (i.e., maximum 24 pieces daily).
- Maximum 12 weeks of therapy.

Special Populations

No specific dosage recommendations at this time.

Nicotine Lozenges

(nik′ oh teen)

Brand Name: Commit® lozenges
Also available generically.

Why is this medicine prescribed?

Nicotine lozenges are used to help people stop smoking. Nicotine lozenges are in a class of medications called smoking cessation aids. They work by providing nicotine to your body to decrease the withdrawal symptoms experienced when smoking is stopped and to reduce the urge to smoke.

How should this medicine be used?

Nicotine comes as a lozenge to slowly dissolve in the mouth. It is usually taken according to the directions on the package, at least 15 minutes after eating or drinking. Follow the directions on your medicine package carefully, and ask your doctor or pharmacist to explain any part you do not understand. Take nicotine lozenges exactly as directed. Do not take more or less of them or take them more often than prescribed by your doctor.

If you smoke your first cigarette within 30 minutes of waking up in the morning, you should use 4 mg nicotine lozenges. If you smoke your first cigarette more than 30 minutes after waking up in the morning, you should use 2 mg nicotine lozenges.

For Weeks 1 to 6 of treatment, you should use one lozenge every 1 to 2 hours. Using at least nine lozenges per day will increase your chance of quitting. For Weeks 7 to 9, you should use one lozenge every 2 to 4 hours. For Weeks 10 to 12, you should use one lozenge every 4 to 8 hours.

Do not use more than five lozenges in 6 hours or more than 20 lozenges per day. Do not use more than one lozenge at a time or use one lozenge right after another. Using too many lozenges at a time or one after another can cause side effects such as hiccups, heartburn, and nausea.

To take the lozenge, place it in your mouth and allow it to slowly dissolve. Do not chew or swallow lozenges. Once in a while, use your tongue to move the lozenge from one side of your mouth to the other. It should take 20 to 30 minutes to dissolve. Do not eat while the lozenge is in your mouth.

Stop using nicotine lozenges after 12 weeks. If you still feel the need to use nicotine lozenges, talk to your doctor.

Are there other uses for this medicine?

This medication may be used for other conditions; ask your doctor or pharmacist for more information.

What special precautions should I follow?

Before taking nicotine lozenges,

- tell your doctor and pharmacist if you are allergic to nicotine or any other medications.
- do not take nicotine lozenges if you are using any other nicotine smoking cessation aid, such as the nicotine patch, gum, inhaler, or nasal spray.
- tell your doctor and pharmacist what other prescription and nonprescription medications, vitamins, nutritional supplements, and herbal products you are taking or plan to take. Be sure to mention any of the following: non-nicotine smoking cessation aids, such as bupropion (Wellbutrin) or varenicline (Chantix), and medications for depression or asthma. Your doctor may need to change the doses of your medications once you stop smoking.
- tell your doctor if you have recently had a heart attack and if you have or have ever had heart disease, irregular heartbeat, high blood pressure, a stomach ulcer, diabetes, or phenylketonuria (PKU, a inherited condition in which a special diet must be followed to prevent mental retardation).
- tell your doctor if you are pregnant, plan to become pregnant, or are breast-feeding. If you become pregnant while taking nicotine lozenges, call your doctor.
- stop smoking completely. If you continue smoking while taking nicotine lozenges, you may have side effects.
- ask your doctor or pharmacist for advice and for written information to help you stop smoking. You are more likely to stop smoking during your treatment with nicotine lozenges if you get information and support from your doctor.

What special dietary instructions should I follow?

Unless your doctor tells you otherwise, continue your normal diet.

What side effects can this medicine cause?

Nicotine lozenges may cause side effects. Tell your doctor if either of these symptoms is severe or does not go away:

- heartburn
- sore throat

Some side effects can be serious. If you experience either of these symptoms, call your doctor immediately:

- mouth problems
- irregular or fast heartbeat

Nicotine lozenges may cause other side effects. Call your doctor if you have any unusual problems while taking this medication.

What storage conditions are needed for this medicine?

Keep this medication in the container it came in, tightly closed, and out of reach of children and pets. Store it at room temperature and away from excess heat and moisture (not in the bathroom). If you need to remove a lozenge, wrap it in paper and throw it away. Throw away any medication that is outdated or no longer needed. Talk to your pharmacist about the proper disposal of your medication.

What should I do in case of overdose?

In case of overdose, call your local poison control center at 1-800-222-1222. If the victim has collapsed or is not breathing, call local emergency services at 911.

Symptoms of overdose may include:

- nausea
- vomiting
- dizziness
- diarrhea
- weakness
- fast heartbeat

What other information should I know?

Keep all appointments with your doctor.

Ask your pharmacist any questions you have about nicotine lozenges.

Talk to your doctor, pharmacist, or other healthcare professional if you have questions about dosing information for your medication.

Nicotine Nasal Spray

(nik′ oh teen)

Brand Name: Nicotrol® NS
Also available generically.

Why is this medicine prescribed?

Nicotine nasal spray is used to help people stop smoking. Nicotine nasal spray should be used together with a smoking cessation program, which may include support groups, counseling, or specific behavior change techniques. Nicotine nasal spray is in a class of medications called smoking cessation aids. It works by providing nicotine to your body to decrease the withdrawal symptoms experienced when smoking is stopped and to reduce the urge to smoke.

How should this medicine be used?

Nicotine nasal spray comes as a liquid to spray into the nose. Follow the directions on your prescription label carefully, and ask your doctor or pharmacist to explain any part you do not understand. Use nicotine nasal spray exactly as directed. Do not use more or less of it or use it more often than prescribed by your doctor.

Follow your doctor's instructions about how many doses of nicotine spray you should use each day. Your doctor will probably tell you to start out using one or two doses per hour. Each dose is two sprays, one in each nostril. You should not use more than five doses per hour or 40 doses per day (24 hours). After you have used nicotine nasal spray for 8 weeks and your body adjusts to not smoking, your doctor may decrease your dose gradually over the next 4 to 6 weeks until you are not using nicotine inhalation any more. Follow your doctor's instructions for how to decrease your nicotine dose.

Nicotine nasal spray may be habit forming. Do not use a larger dose, use it more often, or use it for a longer period of time than prescribed by your doctor.

To use the nasal spray, follow these directions:

1. Wash your hands.
2. Gently blow your nose to clear your nasal passages.
3. Remove the cap of the nasal spray by pressing in the circles on the side of the bottle.
4. To prime the pump before the first use, hold the bottle in front of a tissue or paper towel. Pump the spray bottle six to eight times until a fine spray appears. Throw away the tissue or towel.
5. Tilt your head back slightly.
6. Insert the tip of the bottle as far as you comfortably can into one nostril, pointing the tip toward the back of your nose.
7. Breathe through your mouth.
8. Pump the spray firmly and quickly one time. Do not sniff, swallow, or inhale while spraying.
9. If your nose runs, gently sniff to keep the nasal spray in your nose. Wait 2 or 3 minutes before blowing your nose.
10. Repeat steps 6-8 for the second nostril.
11. Replace the cover on the spray bottle.
12. Any time you have not used the nasal spray for 24 hours, prime the pump in a tissue one or two times. However, do not prime too much as it will decrease the amount of medication in the container.

If you have not stopped smoking at the end of 4 weeks, talk to your doctor. Your doctor can try to help you understand why you were not able to stop smoking and make plans to try again.

Ask your pharmacist or doctor for a copy of the manufacturer's information for the patient.

Are there other uses for this medicine?

This medication may be prescribed for other uses; ask your doctor or pharmacist for more information.

What special precautions should I follow?

Before using nicotine nasal spray,

- tell your doctor and pharmacist if you are allergic to nicotine or any other medications.
- tell your doctor and pharmacist what prescription and nonprescription medications, vitamins, nutritional supplements, and herbal products you are taking or plan to take. Be sure to mention any of the following: acetaminophen (Tylenol); alpha blockers such as alfuzosin (Uroxatral), doxazosin (Cardura), prazosin (Minipress), tamsulosin (Flomax), and terazosin (Hytrin); beta blockers such as atenolol (Tenormin), labetalol (Normodyne), metoprolol (Lopressor, Toprol XL), nadolol (Corgard), and propranolol (Inderal); caffeine-containing medications (Esgic, Esgic Plus, Fioricet, NoDoz, Norgesic, others); cough and cold medications; imipramine (Tofranil); insulin; isoproterenol (Isuprel); oxazepam (Serax); pentazocine (Talacen, Talwin NX); and theophylline (TheoDur). Your doctor may need to change the doses of your medications once you stop smoking.
- tell your doctor if you have recently had a heart attack and if you have or have ever had nasal problems (allergies, sinus problems, or polyps), asthma, heart disease, angina, irregular heartbeat, problems with circulation such as Buerger's disease or Raynaud's phenomena, hyperthyroidism (an overactive thyroid), pheochromocytoma (a tumor on a small gland near the kidneys), insulin-dependent diabetes, ulcers, high blood pressure, and kidney or liver disease.
- tell your doctor if you are pregnant, plan to become pregnant, or are breast-feeding. If you become pregnant while using nicotine nasal spray, call your doctor. Nicotine may harm the fetus.
- stop smoking completely. If you continue smoking while using nicotine nasal spray, you may have side effects.
- you should know that even though you are using nicotine nasal spray, you may still have some smoking withdrawal symptoms. These include dizziness, anxiety, sleeping problems, depression, tiredness, and muscle pain. If you experience these symptoms, talk to your doctor about increasing your dose of nicotine inhalation.
- you may have some side effects when you first begin to use nicotine inhalation such as throat irritation, sneezing, coughing, watery eyes, or runny nose. Be sure to wait 5 minutes after using this medication before you drive a car or operate a motor vehicle.

What special dietary instructions should I follow?

Talk to your doctor about the safe use of caffeinated beverages while using this medication.

What side effects can this medicine cause?

Nicotine nasal spray may cause side effects. Tell your doctor if any of these symptoms are severe or do not go away:

- hot, peppery feeling in the back of the nose or throat
- runny nose
- throat irritation
- watering eyes
- sneezing
- coughing

Some side effects can be serious. If you experience any of these symptoms, call your doctor immediately:

- rapid heart rate

Nicotine nasal spray may cause other side effects. Call your doctor if you have any unusual problems while taking this medication.

What storage conditions are needed for this medicine?

Keep used and unused nicotine spray bottles out of the reach of children and pets. Store the bottles at room temperature and away from excess heat and moisture (not in the bathroom). Throw away used spray bottles with the child-resistant cover in place. Throw away any medication that is outdated or no longer needed. Talk to your pharmacist about the proper disposal of your medication.

What should I do in case of overdose?

If someone swallows nicotine nasal spray, call your local poison control center at 1-800-222-1222. If the victim has collapsed or is not breathing, call local emergency services at 911.

Symptoms of overdose may include:
- paleness
- cold sweat
- nausea
- drooling
- vomiting
- stomach pain
- diarrhea
- headache
- dizziness
- fainting
- problems with hearing and vision
- shaking of a part of your body that you cannot control
- confusion
- weakness
- seizures

What other information should I know?

Keep all appointments with your doctor.

Handle nicotine nasal spray carefully. If the bottle

drops, it may break. If this happens, wear rubber gloves and clean up the spill immediately with a cloth or paper towel. Avoid touching the liquid. Throw away the used cloth or paper towel in the trash. Pick up the broken glass carefully using a broom. Wash the area of the spill a few times. If even a small amount of nicotine solution comes in contact with the skin, lips, mouth, eyes, or ears, these areas should immediately be rinsed with plain water.

Do not let anyone else use your medication. Ask your pharmacist any questions you have about refilling your prescription.

Talk to your doctor, pharmacist, or other healthcare professional if you have questions about dosing information for your medication.

Nicotine Oral Inhalation

(nik′ oh teen)

Brand Name: Nicotrol® Inhaler
Also available generically.

Why is this medicine prescribed?

Nicotine oral inhalation is used to help people stop smoking. Nicotine oral inhalation should be used together with a smoking cessation program, which may include support groups, counseling, or specific behavioral change techniques. Nicotine inhalation is in a class of medications called smoking cessation aids. It works by providing nicotine to your body to decrease the withdrawal symptoms experienced when smoking is stopped and to reduce the urge to smoke.

How should this medicine be used?

Nicotine oral inhalation comes as a cartridge to inhale by mouth using a special inhaler. Follow the directions on your prescription label carefully, and ask your doctor or pharmacist to explain any part you do not understand. Use nicotine oral inhalation exactly as directed. Do not use more or less of it or use it more often than prescribed by your doctor.

Follow your doctor's instructions about how many nicotine cartridges you should use each day. Your doctor may increase or decrease your dose depending on your urge to smoke. After you have used nicotine inhalation for 12 weeks and your body adjusts to not smoking, your doctor may decrease your dose gradually over the next 6 to 12 weeks until you are not using nicotine inhalation any more. Follow your doctor's instructions for how to decrease your nicotine dose.

The nicotine in the cartridges is released by frequent puffing over 20 minutes. You may use up a cartridge all at once or puff on it for a few minutes at a time until the nicotine is finished. You may want to try different schedules to see what works best for you.

Ask your pharmacist or doctor for a copy of the manufacturer's information for the patient. Read the directions for how to use the inhaler and ask your doctor or pharmacist to show you the proper technique. Practice using the inhaler while in his or her presence.

If you have not stopped smoking at the end of 4 weeks, talk to your doctor. Your doctor can try to help you understand why you were not able to stop smoking and make plans to try again.

Are there other uses for this medicine?

This medication may be prescribed for other uses; ask your doctor or pharmacist for more information.

What special precautions should I follow?

Before using nicotine oral inhalation,
- tell your doctor and pharmacist if you are allergic to nicotine, menthol, or any other medications.
- tell your doctor and pharmacist what prescription and nonprescription medications, vitamins, nutritional supplements, and herbal products you are taking or plan to take. Be sure to mention any of the following: antidepressants such as amitriptyline (Elavil), amoxapine (Asendin), clomipramine (Anafranil), desipramine (Norpramin), doxepin (Adapin, Sinequan), imipramine (Tofranil), nortriptyline (Aventyl, Pamelor), protriptyline (Vivactil), and trimipramine (Surmontil); and theophylline (TheoDur). Your doctor may need to change the doses of your medications once you stop smoking.
- tell your doctor if you have recently had a heart attack and if you have or have ever had asthma, chronic obstructive pulmonary disease (COPD; emphysema or chronic bronchitis), heart disease, angina, irregular heartbeat, problems with circulation such as Buerger's disease or Raynaud's phenomena, hyperthyroidism (an overactive thyroid), pheochromocytoma (a tumor on a small gland near the kidneys), insulin-dependent diabetes, ulcers, high blood pressure, and kidney or liver disease.
- tell your doctor if you are pregnant, plan to become pregnant, or are breast-feeding. If you become pregnant while using nicotine inhalation, call your doctor. Nicotine may harm the fetus.
- stop smoking completely. If you continue smoking while using nicotine inhalation, you may have side effects.
- you should know that even though you are using nicotine inhalation, you may still have some smoking withdrawal symptoms. These include dizziness, anxiety, sleeping problems, depression, tiredness, and muscle pain. If you experience these symptoms, talk to your doctor about increasing your dose of nicotine inhalation.

What special dietary instructions should I follow?

Unless your doctor tells you otherwise, continue your normal diet.

What side effects can this medicine cause?

Nicotine oral inhalation may cause side effects. Tell your doctor if any of these symptoms are severe or do not go away:
- irritation in the mouth and throat
- cough
- runny nose
- taste changes
- pain of the jaw, neck, or back
- tooth problems
- sinus pressure and pain
- headache
- pain, burning, or tingling in the hands or feet
- gas

Some side effects can be serious. If you experience the following symptom, call your doctor immediately:
- rapid heart rate

Nicotine inhalation may cause other side effects. Call your doctor if you have any unusual problems while taking this medication.

What storage conditions are needed for this medicine?

Keep all the parts of the nicotine inhaler and used and unused nicotine cartridges out of the reach of children and pets. Store the mouthpiece in the plastic storage case. Store the cartridges at room temperature and away from excess heat and moisture (not in the bathroom). Throw away any medication that is outdated or no longer needed. Talk to your pharmacist about the proper disposal of your medication.

What should I do in case of overdose?

In case of overdose, call your local poison control center at 1-800-222-1222. If the victim has collapsed or is not breathing, call local emergency services at 911.

Symptoms of overdose may include:
- paleness
- cold sweat
- nausea
- drooling
- vomiting
- stomach pain
- diarrhea
- headache
- dizziness
- problems with hearing and vision
- shaking of a part of your body that you cannot control
- confusion
- weakness
- seizures

What other information should I know?

Keep all appointments with your doctor.

Do not let anyone else take your medication. Ask your pharmacist any questions you have about refilling your prescription.

Talk to your doctor, pharmacist, or other healthcare professional if you have questions about dosing information for your medication.

Nicotine Skin Patches

(nik' oh teen)

Brand Name: Nicoderm® CQ® Clear Step 3, NicoDerm® CQ® Step 1, NicoDerm® CQ® Step 2, NicoDerm® CQ® Step 3, Nicotrol® NS, Nicotrol® Step 1, Nicotrol® Step 2, Nicotrol® Step 3 Also available generically.

Why is this medicine prescribed?

Nicotine skin patches are used to help people stop smoking cigarettes. They provide a source of nicotine that reduces the withdrawal symptoms experienced when smoking is stopped.

How should this medicine be used?

Nicotine patches are applied directly to the skin. They are applied once a day, usually at the same time each day. Nicotine patches come in various strengths and may be used for various lengths of time. Follow the directions on your prescription label carefully, and ask your doctor or pharmacist to explain any part you do not understand. Use nicotine skin patches exactly as directed. Do not use more or less of them or use them more often than prescribed by your doctor.

Apply the patch to a clean, dry, hairless area of skin on the upper chest, upper arm, or hip as directed by the package directions. Avoid areas of irritated, oily, scarred, or broken skin.

Remove the patch from the package, peel off the protective strip, and immediately apply the patch to your skin. With the sticky side touching the skin, press the patch in place with the palm of your hand for about 10 seconds. Be sure the patch is held firmly in place, especially around the edges. Wash your hands with water alone after applying the patch. If the patch falls off or loosens, replace it with a new one.

You should wear the patch continuously for 16-24 hours, depending on the specific directions inside your nicotine patch package. The patch may be worn even while showering or bathing. Remove the patch carefully, and dispose of it by folding it in half with the sticky sides touching. After removing the used patch, apply the next patch to a different skin area to prevent skin irritation. Never wear two patches at once.

A switch to a lower strength patch may be considered after the first 2 weeks on the medication. A gradual reduction to lower strength patches is recommended to reduce nicotine- withdrawal symptoms. Nicotine patches may be used from 6 to 20 weeks depending on the specific instructions supplied with the patches.

What special precautions should I follow?

Before using nicotine skin patches,
- tell your doctor and pharmacist if you are allergic to adhesive tape or any drugs.
- tell your doctor and pharmacist what prescription and nonprescription medications you are taking, especially acetaminophen (Tylenol), caffeine, diuretics ('water pills'), imipramine (Tofranil), insulin, medications for high blood pressure, oxazepam (Serax), pentazocine (Talwin, Talwin NX, Talacen), propoxyphene (Darvon, E-Lor), propranolol (Inderal), theophylline (Theo-Dur), and vitamins.
- tell your doctor if you have or have ever had a heart attack, irregular heart rate, angina (chest pain), ulcers, uncontrolled high blood pressure, overactive thyroid, pheochromocytoma, or a skin condition or disorder.
- tell your doctor if you are pregnant, plan to become pregnant, or are breast-feeding. If you become pregnant while using nicotine skin patches, call your doctor immediately. Nicotine and nicotine skin patches may cause harm to the fetus.
- do not smoke cigarettes or use other nicotine products while using nicotine skin patches because nicotine overdose can result.

What should I do if I forget to take a dose?

Apply the missed dose as soon as you remember it. However, if it is almost time for the next dose, skip the missed dose and continue your regular dosing schedule. Do not apply a double dose to make up for a missed one.

What side effects can this medicine cause?

Nicotine skin patches may cause side effects. Tell your doctor if any of these symptoms are severe or do not go away:
- dizziness
- headache
- upset stomach
- vomiting
- diarrhea
- redness or swelling at the patch site

If you experience any of the following symptoms, call your doctor immediately:
- severe rash or swelling
- seizures
- abnormal heartbeat or rhythm
- difficulty breathing

If you experience a serious side effect, you or your doctor may send a report to the Food and Drug Administration's (FDA) MedWatch Adverse Event Reporting program online [at http://www.fda.gov/MedWatch/index.html] or by phone [1-800-332-1088].

What storage conditions are needed for this medicine?

Keep this medication in the container it came in, tightly closed, and out of reach of children. Store it at room temperature and away from excess heat and moisture (not in the bathroom). Throw away any medication that is outdated or no longer needed. Carefully throw away used patches by folding them with the sticky sides together and out of reach of children or pets.

What should I do in case of overdose?

In case of overdose, call your local poison control center at 1-800-222-1222. If the victim has collapsed or is not breathing, call local emergency services at 911.

What other information should I know?

Keep all appointments with your doctor.

Do not let anyone else use your medication. Ask your pharmacist any questions you have about refilling your prescription.

Dosage Facts
For Informational Purposes

Caution: Do not change your dose, how often you take your medication, or the length of time you are to take it without first talking to your health-care provider.

The following dosage information was written using medical language for doctors and other healthcare professionals and is provided here for you to check your dosage. The dosage of this drug may differ for different patients. Therefore, always follow your doctor's instructions or the directions on the label. Contact your healthcare provider or pharmacist if you have any questions about the specific dosage of your medication after reviewing this information.

General Dosage Information

Stop smoking completely before beginning transdermal nicotine therapy.

Adult Patients
Smoking Cessation

TRANSDERMAL:
- If cravings begin upon awakening, wear patch for 24 hours. If vivid dreams or sleep disruptions occur, wear patch for 16 hours; remove at bedtime and apply new patch upon awakening.

- *Self-medication* in patients who smoke ≤10 cigarettes daily: Initially, 14 mg daily for 6 weeks, then 7 mg daily for 2 weeks, then discontinue.
- *Self-medication* in patients who smoke >10 cigarettes daily: Initially, 21 mg daily for 4–6 weeks, then 14 mg daily for 2 weeks, then 7 mg daily for 2 weeks, then discontinue therapy.
- Consult clinician if need for continued therapy at the end of regimen.

Prescribing Limits
Adult Patients

TRANSDERMAL:
- *Self-medication* in patients who smoke ≤10 cigarettes: Maximum 8 weeks of therapy.
- *Self-medication* in patients who smoke >10 cigarettes daily: Maximum 10 weeks of therapy.
- Continued therapy for periods longer than usually recommended may be appropriate for certain patients to promote extended abstinence.

Special Populations

No specific dosage recommendations at this time.

Nifedipine
(nye fed′ i peen)

Brand Name: Adalat®, Adalat® CC, Nifedical® XL, Procardia XL®, Procardia®
Also available generically.

Why is this medicine prescribed?

Nifedipine is used to treat high blood pressure. It relaxes your blood vessels so your heart does not have to pump as hard. It also increases the supply of blood and oxygen to the heart to control chest pain (angina). If taken regularly, nifedipine controls chest pain, but it does not stop chest pain once it starts. Your doctor may give you a different medication to take when you have chest pain.

This medication is sometimes prescribed for other uses; ask your doctor or pharmacist for more information.

How should this medicine be used?

Nifedipine comes as a capsule and an extended-release tablet (long-acting) to take by mouth. It is usually taken one or three times a day. The extended-release tablet should be taken on an empty stomach, either 1 hour before or 2 hours after a meal, and should be swallowed whole. Do not chew, divide, or crush the tablet. Follow the directions on your prescription label carefully, and ask your doctor or pharmacist to explain any part you do not understand. Take nifedipine exactly as directed. Do not take more or less of it or take it more often than prescribed by your doctor.

Nifedipine controls high blood pressure and chest pain (angina) but does not cure them. Continue to take nifedipine even if you feel well. Do not stop taking nifedipine without talking to your doctor.

Are there other uses for this medicine?

Nifedipine is also used sometimes to treat migraine headaches, Raynaud's syndrome, congestive heart failure, and cardiomyopathy. Talk to your doctor about the possible risks of using this drug for your condition.

What special precautions should I follow?

Before taking nifedipine,
- tell your doctor and pharmacist if you are allergic to nifedipine or any other drugs.
- tell your doctor and pharmacist what prescription and nonprescription medications you are taking, especially cimetidine (Tagamet); fentanyl (Duragesic); heart and blood pressure medications like beta-blockers, digoxin (Lanoxin), warfarin (Coumadin), and quinidine (Quinaglute, Quinidex); phenytoin (Dilantin); ranitidine (Zantac); and vitamins.
- tell your doctor if you have or have ever had heart, liver, or kidney disease.
- tell your doctor if you are pregnant, plan to become pregnant, or are breast-feeding. If you become pregnant while taking nifedipine, call your doctor.
- if you are having surgery, including dental surgery, tell your doctor or dentist that you are taking nifedipine.

What special dietary instructions should I follow?

Nifedipine capsules may be taken with or without food, but the nifedipine extended-release tablets should be taken on an empty stomach, either 1 hour before or 2 hours after a meal.

Avoid drinking grapefruit juice or eating grapefruit while taking nifedipine.

Do not drink alcoholic beverages while taking this medication.

Talk to your doctor before using salt substitutes containing potassium. If your doctor prescribes a low-salt or low-sodium diet, follow these directions carefully.

What should I do if I forget to take a dose?

Take the missed dose as soon as you remember it. However, if it is almost time for the next dose, skip the missed dose and continue your regular dosing schedule. Do not take a double dose to make up for a missed one.

What side effects can this medicine cause?

Nifedipine may cause side effects. Tell your doctor if any of these symptoms are severe or do not go away:
- headache
- upset stomach
- dizziness or lightheadedness
- excessive tiredness
- flushing (feeling of warmth)
- heartburn
- fast heartbeat
- muscle cramps
- enlargement of gum tissue around teeth
- constipation
- nasal congestion
- cough
- decreased sexual ability

If you experience any of the following symptoms, call your doctor immediately:
- swelling of the face, eyes, lips, tongue, arms, or legs
- difficulty breathing or swallowing
- fainting
- rash
- yellowing of the skin or eyes
- increase in frequency or severity of chest pain (angina)

If you experience a serious side effect, you or your doctor may send a report to the Food and Drug Administration's (FDA) MedWatch Adverse Event Reporting program online [at http://www.fda.gov/MedWatch/index.html] or by phone [1-800-332-1088].

What storage conditions are needed for this medicine?

Keep this medication in the container it came in, tightly closed, and out of reach of children. Store it at room temperature and away from excess heat and moisture (not in the bathroom). Throw away any medication that is outdated or no longer needed. Talk to your pharmacist about the proper disposal of your medication.

What should I do in case of overdose?

In case of overdose, call your local poison control center at 1-800-222-1222. If the victim has collapsed or is not breathing, call local emergency services at 911.

What other information should I know?

Keep all appointments with your doctor and the laboratory. Your blood pressure should be checked regularly to determine your response to nifedipine.

Good dental hygiene decreases the chance and severity of gum swelling. Brush your teeth regularly and schedule dental cleanings every 6 months.

The extended-release tablet does not dissolve in the stomach after being swallowed. It slowly releases medicine as it passes through your small intestines. It is not unusual to see the tablet shell in the stool.

Do not let anyone else take your medication. Ask your pharmacist any questions you have about refilling your prescription.

Dosage Facts
For Informational Purposes

Caution: Do not change your dose, how often you take your medication, or the length of time you are to take it without first talking to your healthcare provider.

The following dosage information was written using medical language for doctors and other healthcare professionals and is provided here for you to check your dosage. The dosage of this drug may differ for different patients. Therefore, always follow your doctor's instructions or the directions on the label. Contact your healthcare provider or pharmacist if you have any questions about the specific dosage of your medication after reviewing this information.

General Dosage Information

Manufacturer states that two 30-mg Adalat® CC extended-release tablets may be interchanged with one 60-mg Adalat® CC extended-release tablet; however, three 30-mg Adalat® CC extended-release tablets should *not* be considered interchangeable with one 90-mg Adalat® CC extended-release tablet.

Pediatric Patients

Hypertension†
Extended-release Tablets

ORAL:
- Initially, 0.25–0.5 mg/kg daily given in 1 dose or 2 divided doses. Increase dosage as necessary up to a maximum dosage of 3 mg/kg (up to 120 mg) daily, given in 1 dose or 2 divided doses.

Adult Patients

Angina
Conventional Capsules

ORAL:
- Initially, 10 mg 3 times daily.
- Increase dosage gradually at 7- to 14-day intervals until optimum control of angina is obtained.
- May increase more rapidly to 90 mg daily in increments of 30 mg daily over a 3-day period if symptoms so warrant and patient's tolerance and response to therapy are frequently assessed.
- In hospitalized patients who are closely monitored, dosage may be increased in 10-mg increments at 4- to 6-hour intervals, as necessary to control pain and arrhythmias caused by ischemia. Single doses usually should not exceed 30 mg.
- Usual maintenance dosage is 10–20 mg 3 times daily. In some patients, especially those with evidence of coronary artery spasm, increased dosages of 20–30 mg 3 or 4 times daily and rarely, more than 120 mg daily may be necessary.

Extended-release Tablets

Initially, 30 or 60 mg once daily.

Increase dosage gradually at 7- to 14-day intervals until optimum control of angina is obtained.

Dosage may be increased more rapidly to 90 mg daily in increments of 30 mg daily after steady state is achieved (usually achieved on the second day of therapy with a given dose) if symptoms so warrant and patient's tolerance and response are frequently assessed.

In some patients, especially those with evidence of coronary artery spasm, higher dosages may be necessary. However, experience with antianginal dosages exceeding 90 mg once daily as extended-release tablets is limited and should be employed with caution and only when clinically necessary.

Extended-release tablets can be substituted for the conventional capsules at the nearest equivalent total daily dose.

Hypertension
Conventional Capsules

ORAL:
- *Not* recommended for use in the management of hypertension because of concerns about potential cardiovascular risks.

Extended-release Tablets

ORAL:
- Initially, 30 or 60 mg once daily.
- Increase dosage gradually at 7- to 14-day intervals until optimum control of BP is obtained.
- Dosage may be increased more rapidly, if symptoms so warrant and the patient's tolerance and response to therapy are frequently assessed.
- Usual maintenance dosage is 30–60 mg once daily.

Preeclampsia†

ORAL:
- Conventional capsules: 10 mg repeated at 20-minute intervals to a maximum total dosage of 30 mg. The drug should be used cautiously with magnesium sulfate since a precipitous drop in BP can occur.

Prescribing Limits

Pediatric Patients

Hypertension†

ORAL:
- Extended-release tablets: Maximum 3 mg/kg (up to 120 mg) daily.

Adult Patients

Angina

ORAL:
- Conventional liquid-filled capsules: Maximum 30 mg as a single dose. Maximum 180 mg daily.
- Extended-release tablets: Maximum 120 mg daily.

Hypertension

Extended-release tablets: Maximum 90 mg (Adalat® CC) or 120 mg (Procardia XL®) once daily. However, JNC currently recommends a lower maximum dosage of 60 mg daily.

† Use is not currently included in the labeling approved by the US Food and Drug Administration.

Nimodipine

(nye moe' di peen)

Brand Name: Nimotop®

Why is this medicine prescribed?

Nimodipine is used to treat symptoms resulting from a rup-
tured blood vessel in the brain (hemorrhage). It increases
blood flow to injured brain tissue.

This medication is sometimes prescribed for other uses;
ask your doctor or pharmacist for more information.

How should this medicine be used?

Nimodipine comes as a capsule to take by mouth. If a patient
cannot swallow the capsule, the medication can be given
through a feeding tube. It is usually taken every 4 hours for
21 days. Nimodipine should be taken on an empty stomach,
either 1 hour before a meal, or 2 hours after a meal. This
medication should be started within 4 days of the brain hemorrhage.

Follow the directions on your prescription label carefully, and ask your doctor or pharmacist to explain any part
you do not understand. Take nimodipine exactly as directed.
Do not take more or less of it or take it more often than
prescribed by your doctor.

Continue to take nimodipine even if you feel well. Do
not stop taking nimodipine without talking to your doctor.

Are there other uses for this medicine?

Nimodipine is also used sometimes to treat migraine headaches. Talk to your doctor about the possible risks of using
this drug for your condition.

What special precautions should I follow?

Before taking nimodipine,
- tell your doctor and pharmacist if you are allergic to
  nimodipine or any other drugs.
- tell your doctor and pharmacist what prescription and
  nonprescription medications you are taking, especially
  cimetidine (Tagamet), heart and blood pressure medicines, phenytoin (Dilantin), ranitidine (Zantac), and vitamins.
- tell your doctor if you have or have ever had heart, liver,
  or kidney disease.
- tell your doctor if you are pregnant, plan to become
  pregnant, or are breast-feeding. If you become pregnant
  while taking nimodipine, call your doctor.
- if you are having surgery, including dental surgery,
  tell your doctor or dentist that you are taking nimodipine.

What special dietary instructions should I follow?

Nimodipine should be taken on an empty stomach, either 1
hour before a meal or 2 hours after a meal.

Avoid drinking grapefruit juice or eating grapefruit
while taking nimodipine.

Talk to your doctor before using salt substitutes containing potassium. If your doctor prescribes a low-salt or
low-sodium diet, follow these directions carefully.

What should I do if I forget to take a dose?

Take the missed dose as soon as you remember it. However,
if it is almost time for the next dose, skip the missed dose
and continue your regular dosing schedule. Do not take a
double dose to make up for a missed one.

What side effects can this medicine cause?

Nimodipine may cause side effects. Tell your doctor if any
of these symptoms are severe or do not go away:
- headache
- dizziness or lightheadedness
- flushing (feeling of warmth)
- heartburn
- fast heartbeat
- slow heartbeat
- upset stomach
- stomach pain
- constipation
- depression, feeling low, or the 'blues'
- unusual bruising or bleeding

If you experience any of the following symptoms, call
your doctor immediately:
- swelling of the face, eyes, lips, tongue, arms, or legs
- difficulty breathing or swallowing
- fainting
- rash

If you experience a serious side effect, you or your doctor may send a report to the Food and Drug Administration's
(FDA) MedWatch Adverse Event Reporting program online
[at http://www.fda.gov/MedWatch/index.html] or by phone
[1-800-332-1088].

What storage conditions are needed for this medicine?

Keep this medication in the container it came in, tightly
closed, and out of reach of children. Store it at room temperature and away from excess heat and moisture (not in the
bathroom). Throw away any medication that is outdated or
no longer needed. Talk to your pharmacist about the proper
disposal of your medication.

What should I do in case of overdose?

In case of overdose, call your local poison control center at 1-800-222-1222. If the victim has collapsed or is not breathing, call local emergency services at 911.

What other information should I know?

Keep all appointments with your doctor and the laboratory.

Do not let anyone else take your medication. Ask your pharmacist any questions you have about refilling your prescription.

Dosage Facts

For Informational Purposes

Caution: Do not change your dose, how often you take your medication, or the length of time you are to take it without first talking to your healthcare provider.

The following dosage information was written using medical language for doctors and other healthcare professionals and is provided here for you to check your dosage. The dosage of this drug may differ for different patients. Therefore, always follow your doctor's instructions or the directions on the label. Contact your healthcare provider or pharmacist if you have any questions about the specific dosage of your medication after reviewing this information.

Adult Patients

Subarachnoid Hemorrhage

ORAL:
- 60 mg every 4 hours for 21 consecutive days. Initiate therapy as soon as possible after the occurrence of subarachnoid hemorrhage, preferably within 96 hours.
- It has been suggested that the drug may be discontinued after 14 consecutive days (but not earlier) in some uncomplicated cases in which early aneurysm surgery is performed.
- In patients in whom surgical repair of the aneurysm is performed relatively late (e.g., day 20), some clinicians suggest continuation of therapy for ≥5 days after surgery to minimize the possibility of postoperative vasospasm.
- It has been suggested that patients with unstable BP receive a lower dosage (e.g., 30 mg every 4 hours); however, the manufacturer states that the usual adult dosage should be used in such patients. (See Hypotension and Other Cardiovascular Effects under Cautions.)

Acute Ischemic Stroke†

ORAL:
- 120 mg daily given in divided doses for 21 or 28 days has been used.

Migraine†
Prophylaxis of Classic or Common Migraine†

ORAL:
- 120 mg daily given in divided doses has been used.

Special Populations

Hepatic Impairment

Subarachnoid Hemorrhage

ORAL:
- Initially, 30 mg every 4 hours.
- Monitor BP and heart rate closely. May use pharmacologic support of BP (e.g., vasopressors such as norepinephrine or dopamine), if necessary.

Renal Impairment
- No specific dosage recommendations.

Geriatric Patients
- Select dosage with caution because of age-related decreases in hepatic, renal, and/or cardiac function and concomitant disease and drug therapy.

† Use is not currently included in the labeling approved by the US Food and Drug Administration.

Nisoldipine

(nye′ sole di peen)

Brand Name: Sular®

Why is this medicine prescribed?

Nisoldipine is used to treat high blood pressure. It relaxes your blood vessels so your heart does not have to pump as hard.

This medication is sometimes prescribed for other uses; ask your doctor or pharmacist for more information.

How should this medicine be used?

Nisoldipine comes as an extended-release (long-acting) tablet to take by mouth. It is usually taken once a day. The tablet should be swallowed whole. Do not chew, divide, or crush the tablet. Follow the directions on your prescription label carefully, and ask your doctor or pharmacist to explain any part you do not understand. Take nisoldipine exactly as directed. Do not take more or less of it or take it more often than prescribed by your doctor.

Nisoldipine controls high blood pressure but does not cure it. Continue to take nisoldipine even if you feel well. Do not stop taking nisoldipine without talking to your doctor.

What special precautions should I follow?

Before taking nisoldipine,
- tell your doctor and pharmacist if you are allergic to nisoldipine or any other drugs.
- tell your doctor and pharmacist what prescription and nonprescription medications you are taking, especially cimetidine (Tagamet), fentanyl (Duragesic), heart and

blood pressure medications such as beta-blockers and diuretics ('water pills'), medications to treat glaucoma (increased pressure in the eye), phenytoin (Dilantin), rifampin (Rifadin, Rimactane), and vitamins.

- tell your doctor if you have or have ever had heart, liver, or kidney disease.
- tell your doctor if you are pregnant, plan to become pregnant, or are breast-feeding. If you become pregnant while taking nisoldipine, call your doctor.
- if you are having surgery, including dental surgery, tell your doctor or dentist that you are taking nisoldipine.

What special dietary instructions should I follow?

Nisoldipine tablets may be taken with or without food and should be swallowed whole. Do not chew, divide, or crush the tablet. Avoid taking nisoldipine with high-fat foods or high-fat meals.

Avoid drinking grapefruit juice or eating grapefruit while taking nisoldipine.

Talk to your doctor before using salt substitutes containing potassium. If your doctor prescribes a low-salt or low-sodium diet, follow these directions carefully.

What should I do if I forget to take a dose?

Take the missed dose as soon as you remember it. However, if it is almost time for the next dose, skip the missed dose and continue your regular dosing schedule. Do not take a double dose to make up for a missed one.

What side effects can this medicine cause?

Nisoldipine may cause side effects. Tell your doctor if any of these symptoms are severe or do not go away:

- headache
- upset stomach
- dizziness or lightheadedness
- flushing (feeling of warmth)
- fast heartbeat
- excessive tiredness
- nasal congestion
- sore throat

If you experience any of the following symptoms, call your doctor immediately:

- swelling of the face, eyes, lips, tongue, arms, or legs
- difficulty breathing or swallowing
- fainting
- rash

If you experience a serious side effect, you or your doctor may send a report to the Food and Drug Administration's (FDA) MedWatch Adverse Event Reporting program online [at http://www.fda.gov/MedWatch/index.html] or by phone [1-800-332-1088].

What storage conditions are needed for this medicine?

Keep this medication in the container it came in, tightly closed, and out of reach of children. Store it at room temperature and away from excess heat and moisture (not in the bathroom). Throw away any medication that is outdated or no longer needed. Talk to your pharmacist about the proper disposal of your medication.

What should I do in case of overdose?

In case of overdose, call your local poison control center at 1-800-222-1222. If the victim has collapsed or is not breathing, call local emergency services at 911.

What other information should I know?

Keep all appointments with your doctor and the laboratory. Your blood pressure should be checked regularly to determine your response to nisoldipine.

The extended-release tablet does not dissolve in the stomach after being swallowed. It slowly releases medicine as it passes through your small intestines. It is not unusual to see the tablet shell in the stool.

Do not let anyone else take your medication. Ask your pharmacist any questions you have about refilling your prescription.

Dosage Facts
For Informational Purposes

Caution: Do not change your dose, how often you take your medication, or the length of time you are to take it without first talking to your healthcare provider.

The following dosage information was written using medical language for doctors and other healthcare professionals and is provided here for you to check your dosage. The dosage of this drug may differ for different patients. Therefore, always follow your doctor's instructions or the directions on the label. Contact your healthcare provider or pharmacist if you have any questions about the specific dosage of your medication after reviewing this information.

Adult Patients

Hypertension
Extended-release Tablets

ORAL:
- Initially, 20 mg once daily.
- Increase as tolerated in increments of 10 mg daily at ≥ weekly intervals up to 60 mg once daily. Monitor BP carefully during initial titration or subsequent upward adjustment in dosage.
- Usual maintenance dosage is 20–40 mg once daily; however, JNC 7 recommends a usual dosage range of 10–40 mg daily.

Prescribing Limits

Adult Patients

Hypertension

ORAL:
- Maximum 60 mg daily.

Special Populations

Hepatic Impairment
- Initially, 10 mg daily; monitor BP response closely with each dosage adjustment.
- Reduce initial and maintenance dosages in patients with cirrhosis.

Renal Impairment
- Dosage modification not necessary in patients with mild to moderate renal impairment.

Geriatric Patients
- Initially, 10 mg daily; monitor BP response closely with each dosage adjustment.

Nitazoxanide

(nye ta zox′ a nide)

Brand Name: Alinia®

Why is this medicine prescribed?

Nitazoxanide is used to treat diarrhea in children and adults caused by the protozoa *Cryptosporidium* or *Giardia*. Protozoa are suspected as the cause when diarrhea lasts more than 7 days. Nitazoxanide is in a class of medications called antiprotozoal agents. It works by stopping the growth of certain protozoa that cause diarrhea.

How should this medicine be used?

Nitazoxanide comes as a tablet and a suspension (liquid) to take by mouth. It is usually taken with food every 12 hours for 3 days. Take nitazoxanide at around the same times every day. Follow the directions on your prescription label carefully, and ask your doctor or pharmacist to explain any part you do not understand. Take nitazoxanide exactly as directed. Do not take more or less of it or take it more often than prescribed by your doctor.

Shake the suspension well before each use to mix the medication evenly.

Are there other uses for this medicine?

This medication may be prescribed for other uses; ask your doctor or pharmacist for more information.

What special precautions should I follow?

Before taking nitazoxanide,
- tell your doctor and pharmacist if you are allergic to nitazoxanide or any other medications.
- tell your doctor and pharmacist what prescription and nonprescription medications, vitamins, nutritional supplements, and herbal products you are taking or plan to take. Be sure to mention any of the following: anticoagulants ('blood thinners') such as warfarin (Coumadin). Your doctor may need to change the doses of your medications or monitor you carefully for side effects.
- tell your doctor if you have or have ever had human immunodeficiency virus (HIV), problems with the immune system, or liver or kidney disease.
- tell your doctor if you are pregnant, plan to become pregnant, or are breast-feeding. If you become pregnant while taking nitazoxanide, call your doctor.

What special dietary instructions should I follow?

To prevent dehydration caused by diarrhea, make sure you or your child gets enough to drink. Take small, frequent sips of water, fruit juice, sports drinks, or broth.

What should I do if I forget to take a dose?

Take the missed dose as soon as you remember it. However, if it is almost time for the next dose, skip the missed dose and continue your regular dosing schedule. Do not take a double dose to make up for a missed one.

What side effects can this medicine cause?

Nitazoxanide may cause side effects. Tell your doctor if any of these symptoms are severe or do not go away:
- stomach pain
- headache
- upset stomach
- vomiting
- discolored urine

Some side effects can be serious. If you experience any of these symptoms, call your doctor immediately:
- skin rash
- itching

Nitazoxanide may cause other side effects. Call your doctor if you have any unusual problems while taking this medication.

If you experience a serious side effect, you or your doctor may send a report to the Food and Drug Administration's (FDA) MedWatch Adverse Event Reporting program online [at http://www.fda.gov/MedWatch/index.html] or by phone [1-800-332-1088].

What storage conditions are needed for this medicine?

Keep this medication in the container it came in, tightly closed, and out of reach of children. Store it at room temperature and away from excess heat and moisture (not in the bathroom). Throw away any medication that is outdated or no longer needed. Throw away any unused nitazoxanide suspension after 7 days. Talk to your pharmacist about the proper disposal of your medication.

What should I do in case of overdose?

In case of overdose, call your local poison control center at 1-800-222-1222. If the victim has collapsed or is not breathing, call local emergency services at 911.

What other information should I know?

Keep all appointments with your doctor.

Patients with diabetes should know that there are 1.48 grams of sucrose in each teaspoon of nitazoxanide suspension.

Do not let anyone else take your medication. Your prescription is probably not refillable. If you still have diarrhea after you finish the nitazoxanide, call your doctor.

Dosage Facts
For Informational Purposes

Caution: Do not change your dose, how often you take your medication, or the length of time you are to take it without first talking to your healthcare provider.

The following dosage information was written using medical language for doctors and other healthcare professionals and is provided here for you to check your dosage. The dosage of this drug may differ for different patients. Therefore, always follow your doctor's instructions or the directions on the label. Contact your healthcare provider or pharmacist if you have any questions about the specific dosage of your medication after reviewing this information.

General Dosage Information

Nitazoxanide tablets and oral suspension are not bioequivalent.

Pediatric Patients

Cryptosporidiosis

ORAL:
- Children 1–3 years of age: 100 mg every 12 hours for 3 days.
- Children 4–11 years of age: 200 mg every 12 hours for 3 days.
- Children ≥12 years of age: 500 mg every 12 hours for 3 days.

Giardiasis

ORAL:
- Children 1–3 years of age: 100 mg every 12 hours for 3 days.
- Children 4–11 years of age: 200 mg every 12 hours for 3 days.
- Children ≥12 years of age: 500 mg every 12 hours for 3 days.

Cestode (Tapeworm) Infections†
Hymenolepsis nana Infections†

ORAL:
- Children 1–3 years of age: 100 mg twice daily for 3 days.
- Children 4–11 years of age: 200 mg twice daily for 3 days.
- Children ≥12 years of age: 500 mg daily for 3 days.

Adult Patients

Cryptosporidiosis

ORAL:
- 500 mg every 12 hours for 3 days.

Giardiasis

ORAL:
- 500 mg every 12 hours for 3 days.

Cestode (Tapeworm) Infections†
Hymenolepsis nana Infections†

ORAL:
- 500 mg daily for 3 days.

† Use is not currently included in the labeling approved by the US Food and Drug Administration.

Nitrofurantoin

(nye troe fyoor an′ toyn)

Brand Name: Furadantin®, Macrobid®
Also available generically.

Why is this medicine prescribed?

Nitrofurantoin, an antibiotic, eliminates bacteria that cause urinary tract infections. Antibiotics will not work for colds, flu, or other viral infections.

This medication is sometimes prescribed for other uses; ask your doctor or pharmacist for more information.

How should this medicine be used?

Nitrofurantoin comes as a capsule and a liquid to take by mouth. Nitrofurantoin usually is taken two or four times a day for at least 7 days. Shake the oral liquid well before each use to mix the medication evenly. Take it with a full glass of water and with meals. Follow the directions on your prescription label carefully, and ask your doctor or pharmacist to explain any part you do not understand. Take nitrofurantoin exactly as directed. Do not take more or less of it or take it more often than prescribed by your doctor.

What special precautions should I follow?

Before taking nitrofurantoin,
- tell your doctor and pharmacist if you are allergic to nitrofurantoin or any other drugs.

- tell your doctor and pharmacist what prescription and nonprescription medications you are taking, especially antacids, antibiotics, benztropine (Cogentin), diphenhydramine (Benadryl), probenecid (Benemid), trihexyphenidyl (Artane), and vitamins.
- tell your doctor if you have anemia, kidney disease, lung disease, nerve damage, or glucose-6-phosphate dehydrogenase (G-6-PD) deficiency (an inherited blood disease).
- tell your doctor if you are pregnant, plan to become pregnant, or are breast-feeding. If you become pregnant while taking nitrofurantoin, call your doctor. Nitrofurantoin should not be taken by women in the last month of pregnancy.
- you should know that this drug may make you drowsy. Do not drive a car or operate machinery until you know how this drug affects you.
- remember that alcohol can add to the drowsiness caused by this drug.
- plan to avoid unnecessary or prolonged exposure to sunlight and to wear protective clothing, sunglasses, and sunscreen. Nitrofurantoin may make your skin sensitive to sunlight.

What should I do if I forget to take a dose?

Take the missed dose as soon as you remember it. However, if it is almost time for the next dose, skip the missed dose and take any remaining doses for that day at evenly spaced intervals. Do not take a double dose to make up for a missed one.

What side effects can this medicine cause?

Nitrofurantoin may cause side effects. Your urine may turn dark yellow or brown; this effect is harmless. Tell your doctor if any of these symptoms are severe or do not go away:
- upset stomach
- vomiting
- loss of appetite

If you experience any of the following symptoms, call your doctor immediately:
- difficulty breathing
- excessive tiredness
- fever or chills
- chest pain
- persistent cough
- numbness, tingling, or pinprick sensation in the fingers and toes
- muscle weakness
- swelling of the lips or tongue
- skin rash

If you experience a serious side effect, you or your doctor may send a report to the Food and Drug Administration's (FDA) MedWatch Adverse Event Reporting program online [at http://www.fda.gov/MedWatch/index.html] or by phone [1-800-332-1088].

What storage conditions are needed for this medicine?

Keep this medication in the container it came in, tightly closed, and out of reach of children. Store it at room temperature and away from excess heat and moisture (not in the bathroom). Throw away any medication that is outdated or no longer needed. Talk to your pharmacist about the proper disposal of your medication.

What should I do in case of overdose?

In case of overdose, call your local poison control center at 1-800-222-1222. If the victim has collapsed or is not breathing, call local emergency services at 911.

What other information should I know?

Keep all appointments with your doctor and the laboratory. Your doctor will order certain lab tests to check your response to nitrofurantoin.

If you have diabetes, use Clinistix or Tes-Tape instead of Clinitest to test your urine for sugar. Nitrofurantoin can cause Clinitest to show false results.

Do not let anyone else take your medication. Your prescription is probably not refillable. If you still have symptoms of infection after you finish the nitrofurantoin, call your doctor.

Dosage Facts
For Informational Purposes

Caution: Do not change your dose, how often you take your medication, or the length of time you are to take it without first talking to your healthcare provider.

The following dosage information was written using medical language for doctors and other healthcare professionals and is provided here for you to check your dosage. The dosage of this drug may differ for different patients. Therefore, always follow your doctor's instructions or the directions on the label. Contact your healthcare provider or pharmacist if you have any questions about the specific dosage of your medication after reviewing this information.

Pediatric Patients

Urinary Tract Infections (UTIs) in Children ≥1 Month of Age

ORAL:
- Capsules containing macrocrystals or suspension containing microcrystals: 5–7 mg/kg daily in 4 divided doses given for 7 days or for ≥3 days after urine becomes sterile.
- If used for long-term suppressive therapy, manufacturers states 1 mg/kg daily given as a single dose or in 2 equally divided doses may be adequate.

Urinary Tract Infections (UTIs) in Children >12 Years of Age

ORAL:
- Dual-release capsules: 100 mg every 12 hours for 7 days.

Adult Patients

Urinary Tract Infections (UTIs)

ORAL:
- Capsules containing macrocrystals or suspension containing microcrystals: 50–100 mg 4 times daily (50 mg 4 times daily for uncomplicated infections) given for 7 days or for ≥3 days after urine becomes sterile. If used for long-term suppressive therapy, manufacturer states 50–100 mg once daily at bedtime may be adequate.
- Dual-release capsules: 100 mg every 12 hours for 7 days.

Nitroglycerin Ointment

(nye troe gli ′ ser in)

Brand Name: Nitro-Bid®
Also available generically.

Why is this medicine prescribed?

Nitroglycerin ointment is used to prevent chest pain (angina). It works by relaxing the blood vessels to the heart, so the blood and oxygen supply to the heart is increased.

This medication is sometimes prescribed for other uses; ask your doctor or pharmacist for more information.

How should this medicine be used?

Nitroglycerin comes as an ointment to apply to the skin. It usually is applied three to six times a day. Your doctor may tell you to remove the ointment at a certain time each day. Follow the directions on your prescription label carefully, and ask your doctor or pharmacist to explain any part you do not understand. Use nitroglycerin ointment exactly as directed. Do not apply more or less of it or use it more often than prescribed by your doctor.

Nitroglycerin ointment controls chest pain but does not cure it. Continue to use nitroglycerin ointment even if you feel well. Do not stop using nitroglycerin ointment without talking to your doctor. Stopping the drug abruptly may cause chest pain.

Nitroglycerin ointment comes with paper with a ruled line for measuring the dose (in inches). Squeeze the ointment onto the paper, carefully measuring the amount specified on your prescription label. Use the paper to spread the ointment in a thin layer on a relatively hair-free area of skin (at least 2 inches by 3 inches) such as your chest. Do not rub in the ointment. Leave the paper on top of the ointment and hold it in place with an elastic bandage, hosiery, or tape. Wash your hands after applying the ointment; try not to get the ointment on your fingers.

Nitroglycerin can lose its effectiveness when used for a long time. This effect is called tolerance. If your angina attacks happen more often, last longer, or are more severe, call your doctor.

Are there other uses for this medicine?

Nitroglycerin is also used to improve circulation in patients with Raynaud's disease. Talk to your doctor about the possible risks of using this drug for your condition.

What special precautions should I follow?

Before using nitroglycerin ointment,
- tell your doctor and pharmacist if you are allergic to nitroglycerin ointment, tablets, or patches; isosorbide (Imdur, Isordil, Sorbitrate); or any other drugs.
- tell your doctor and pharmacist what prescription and nonprescription medications you are taking, especially aspirin; beta blockers such as atenolol (Tenormin), carteolol (Cartrol), labetalol (Normodyne, Trandate), metoprolol (Lopressor), nadolol (Corgard), propranolol (Inderal), sotalol (Betapace), and timolol (Blocadren); calcium channel blockers such as amlodipine (Norvasc), diltiazem (Cardizem), felodipine (Plendil), isradipine (DynaCirc), nifedipine (Procardia), and verapamil (Calan); dihydroergotamine (D.H.E. 45); sildenafil (Viagra); and vitamins.
- tell your doctor if you have or have ever had low red blood cell counts (anemia), glaucoma, or recent head trauma.
- tell your doctor if you are pregnant, plan to become pregnant, or are breast-feeding. If you become pregnant while using nitroglycerin ointment, call your doctor.
- if you are having surgery, including dental surgery, tell the doctor or dentist that you are using nitroglycerin ointment.
- you should know that this drug may make you drowsy and dizzy. Do not drive a car or operate machinery until you know how it affects you.
- ask your doctor about the safe use of alcoholic beverages while you are using nitroglycerin ointment. Alcohol can make the side effects from nitroglycerin ointment worse.

What should I do if I forget to take a dose?

Apply the missed dose as soon as you remember it. However, if it is almost time for the next dose, skip the missed dose and continue your regular dosing schedule. Do not apply a double dose to make up for a missed one.

What side effects can this medicine cause?

Side effects from nitroglycerin ointment are common. Tell your doctor if any of these symptoms are severe or do not go away:
- headache
- skin irritation or rash

- dizziness
- upset stomach
- headache
- flushing (feeling of warmth)

If you experience any of the following symptoms, call your doctor immediately:
- blurred vision
- dry mouth
- chest pain
- fainting

If you experience a serious side effect, you or your doctor may send a report to the Food and Drug Administration's (FDA) MedWatch Adverse Event Reporting program online [at http://www.fda.gov/MedWatch/index.html] or by phone [1-800-332-1088].

What storage conditions are needed for this medicine?

Keep this medication out of reach of children and away from toothpaste or other ointments and creams. Close the ointment tube tightly after each use. Store it at room temperature and away from excess heat and moisture (not in the bathroom). Throw away any medication that is outdated or no longer needed. Talk to your pharmacist about the proper disposal of your medication.

What should I do in case of overdose?

In case of overdose, call your local poison control center at 1-800-222-1222. If the victim has collapsed or is not breathing, call local emergency services at 911.

What other information should I know?

Keep all appointments with your doctor and the laboratory.

Nitroglycerin ointment should not be used for acute angina attacks. Continue to use nitroglycerin tablets or spray to relieve chest pain that has already started.

If headache continues, ask your doctor if you may take acetaminophen. Your nitroglycerin dose may need to be adjusted. Do not take aspirin or any other medication for headache while using nitroglycerin ointment unless you doctor tells you to.

If skin irritation continues, apply the ointment to a different area of skin.

Do not let anyone else use your medication. Ask your pharmacist any questions you have about refilling your prescription.

Dosage Facts
For Informational Purposes

Caution: Do not change your dose, how often you take your medication, or the length of time you are to take it without first talking to your healthcare provider.

The following dosage information was written using medical language for doctors and other healthcare professionals and is provided here for you to check your dosage. The dosage of this drug may differ for different patients. Therefore, always follow your doctor's instructions or the directions on the label. Contact your healthcare provider or pharmacist if you have any questions about the specific dosage of your medication after reviewing this information.

General Dosage Information

Carefully adjust dose according to the patient's requirements and response; use smallest effective dosage.

For IV administration, the type of IV administration set used (PVC or non-PVC) must be considered in dosage estimations. *IV dosages commonly used in early published studies were based on the use of PVC administration sets and are too high when non-PVC administration sets are used.*

Relative hemodynamic and antianginal tolerance may develop during prolonged infusions, contributing to the need for careful dosage titration.

Continuously monitor BP and heart rate, as well as other appropriate parameters (e.g., pulmonary capillary wedge pressure) in all patients. Adequate systemic BP and coronary perfusion pressure must be maintained.

Some patients with normal or low left ventricular filling pressures or pulmonary capillary wedge pressure may be extremely sensitive to the effects of IV nitroglycerin and may respond fully to dosages as low as 5 mcg/minute; these patients require particularly careful monitoring and dosage titration.

Adult Patients

Angina
Acute Symptomatic Relief and Acute Prophylactic Management

LINGUAL:
- Lingual solution using metered pump sprayer: 1 or 2 sprays (0.4 or 0.8 mg, respectively) onto or under the tongue; immediately close mouth.
- Additional single sprays may be given at intervals of approximately every 3–5 minutes as necessary if relief is not attained after the initial spray(s); maximum of 3 sprays (1.2 mg) should be given in a 15-minute period.
- If pain persists after a total of 3 doses within a 15-minute period, prompt medical attention is recommended.
- If used prophylactically, spray may be used 5–10 minutes before situations likely to provoke angina attacks.

SUBLINGUAL:
- Sublingual tablets: 0.3–0.6 mg is placed under the tongue or in the buccal pouch and allowed to dissolve.
- If relief is not attained after a single dose during an acute attack, additional doses may be given at 5-minute intervals.
- If pain persists after a total of 3 doses within a 15-minute period, prompt medical attention is recommended.
- If used prophylactically, place under the tongue or in the buccal pouch 5–10 minutes prior to engaging in activities likely to provoke angina attacks.

INTRABUCCAL:
- Extended-release buccal (transmucosal) tablets: place in buccal pouch and allow to dissolve undisturbed over a 3- to 5-hour period.

- If an angina attack occurs while a tablet is currently in place, another tablet may be administered on the opposite side from the one already in place.
- If an extended-release buccal tablet does not provide prompt relief of an acute attack, use of sublingual nitroglycerin is recommended.
- If a tablet is inadvertently swallowed, another tablet may be administered as a replacement.

Long-term Prophylactic Management of Angina

INTRABUCCAL:
- Extended-release buccal (transmucosal) tablets: initially 1 mg 3 times daily given every 5 hours during waking hours, with the patient's response assessed over a period of 4–5 days; titrate dosage upward incrementally until angina is effectively controlled or adverse effects preclude further increases.
- Maintenance: 2 mg 3 times daily with a dosing interval of 3– 5 hours.
- If angina occurs while a tablet is in place, the dose should be increased to the next tablet strength; if angina occurs after a tablet has dissolved, the dosing frequency should be increased.

ORAL:
- Extended-release capsules: 2.5–9 mg as an extended-release formulation has been administered orally every 8 or 12 hours.
- Do *not* use an extended-release formulation to treat acute attacks of angina because the onset of action of extended-release nitroglycerin formulations is not sufficiently rapid to abort acute attacks of angina.

TOPICAL (TRANSDERMAL SYSTEM):
- Usual initial dosage is 1 transdermal dosage system, delivering the smallest available dose of nitroglycerin in its dosage series, applied every 24 hours.
- To minimize the occurrence of tolerance to the effects of nitroglycerin, a nitrate-free interval of 10–12 hours has been recommended; however, the minimum nitrate-free interval necessary for restoration of full first-dose effects of nitrate therapy has not been determined.
- Dosage may be adjusted by changing to the next larger dosage system in the series or by a combination of dosage systems in the series.
- The transdermal systems should *not* be used to treat acute attacks of angina.

TOPICAL (OINTMENT):
- A suggested initial dosage is 0.5 inch, as squeezed from the tube, of the 2% ointment (i.e., approximately 7.5 mg) every 8 hours.
- Generally, spread over an area approximately equivalent to 3.5 by 2.25 inches or greater.
- Response to treatment is then assessed over the next several days.
- Dosage should be titrated upward until angina is effectively controlled or adverse effects preclude further increases.
- If angina occurs while the ointment is in place, the dose should be increased (e.g., in 0.5-inch increments).
- If angina occurs after the ointment has been in place for several hours, the frequency of dosing should be increased.
- Smallest effective dose should be administered 3 or 4 times daily, unless the patient's clinical response suggests a different regimen.
- When the dose to be applied is in multiples of whole inches,

unit-dose preparations that provide the equivalent of 1 inch of the 2% ointment may also be used.

Prescribing Limits

Adult Patients

Angina
Acute Symptomatic Relief and Acute Prophylactic Management
SUBLINGUAL:
- No more than 3 doses in a 15- to 30- minute period.

INTRABUCCAL:
- No more than 3 doses in a 15- to 30- minute period.

Special Populations

Hepatic Impairment
- No specific dosage recommendations for hepatic impairment.

Renal Impairment
- No dosage adjustments necessary for renal impairment.

Geriatric Patients
- Cautious dosage selection, usually starting at the low end of the dosing range, because of possible age-related decreases in hepatic, renal, and/or cardiac function and concomitant disease and drug therapy.

Nitroglycerin Skin Patches

(nye troe gli′ ser in)

Brand Name: Deponit®, Minitran®, Nitrek®, Nitro-Dur®

Also available generically.

Why is this medicine prescribed?

Nitroglycerin skin patches are used to prevent chest pain (angina). They work by relaxing the blood vessels to the heart, so the blood flow and oxygen supply to the heart is increased.

This medication is sometimes prescribed for other uses; ask your doctor or pharmacist for more information.

How should this medicine be used?

Nitroglycerin comes as a patch you apply to the skin. It is usually applied once a day. Your doctor may tell you to remove the patch at a certain time each day. Follow the directions on your prescription label carefully, and ask your doctor or pharmacist to explain any part you do not understand. Use the nitroglycerin skin patch exactly as directed. Do not apply it more or less often than prescribed by your doctor.

Nitroglycerin skin patches control chest pain but do not cure it. Continue to use the nitroglycerin skin patch even if you feel well. Do not stop using the nitroglycerin skin patch without talking to your doctor. Stopping the drug abruptly may cause chest pain.

Apply the patch to clean, dry skin that is relatively free of hair (above your knee) or upper arm (above your elbow). Avoid irritated, scarred, broken, and calloused skin. Select a different area each day to avoid skin irritation. Be sure to remove the patch before you apply another one.

If the patch loosens or falls off, replace it with a fresh one. Fold the used patch in half with the sticky sides together and dispose of it carefully. The patch still contains active medication that could be harmful to children or pets.

Nitroglycerin can lose its effectiveness when used for a long time. This effect is called tolerance. If your angina attacks happen more often, last longer, or are more severe, call your doctor.

What special precautions should I follow?

Before using a nitroglycerin skin patch,

- tell your doctor and pharmacist if you are allergic to nitroglycerin skin patches, tablets, capsules, or ointment; isosorbide (Imdur, Isordil, Sorbitrate); or any other drugs.
- tell your doctor and pharmacist what prescription and nonprescription medications you are taking, especially aspirin; beta blockers such as atenolol (Tenormin), carteolol (Cartrol), labetalol (Normodyne, Trandate), metoprolol (Lopressor), nadolol (Corgard), propranolol (Inderal), sotalol (Betapace), and timolol (Blocadren); calcium channel blockers such as amlodipine (Norvasc), diltiazem (Cardizem), felodipine (Plendil), isradipine (DynaCirc), nifedipine (Procardia), and verapamil (Calan, Isoptin); dihydroergotamine (D.H.E. 45); sildenafil (Viagra); and vitamins.
- tell your doctor if you have or have ever had low red blood cell counts (anemia), glaucoma, or recent head trauma.
- tell your doctor if you are pregnant, plan to become pregnant, or are breast-feeding. If you become pregnant while using a nitroglycerin skin patch, call your doctor.
- if you are having surgery, including dental surgery, tell the doctor or dentist that you are using a nitroglycerin skin patch.
- you should know that this drug may make you drowsy or dizzy. Do not drive a car or operate machinery until you know how this drug affects you.
- ask your doctor about the safe use of alcoholic beverages while you are using a nitroglycerin skin patch. Alcohol can make the side effects from the nitroglycerin skin patch worse.

What should I do if I forget to take a dose?

Apply the missed patch as soon as you remember it. Do not apply two patches to make up for a missed one.

What side effects can this medicine cause?

Side effects from nitroglycerin skin patches are common. Tell your doctor if any of these symptoms are severe or do not go away:

- headache
- skin irritation or rash
- dizziness
- upset stomach
- flushing (feeling of warmth)

If you experience any of the following symptoms, call your doctor immediately:

- blurred vision
- dry mouth
- chest pain
- fainting

If you experience a serious side effect, you or your doctor may send a report to the Food and Drug Administration's (FDA) MedWatch Adverse Event Reporting program online [at http://www.fda.gov/MedWatch/index.html] or by phone [1-800-332-1088].

What storage conditions are needed for this medicine?

Keep this medication out of reach of children. Store it at room temperature and away from excess heat and moisture (not in the bathroom). Throw away any medication that is outdated or no longer needed. Talk to your pharmacist about the proper disposal of your medication.

What should I do in case of overdose?

In case of overdose, call your local poison control center at 1-800-222-1222. If the victim has collapsed or is not breathing, call local emergency services at 911.

What other information should I know?

Keep all appointments with your doctor and the laboratory.

Nitroglycerin skin patches should not be used for acute angina attacks. Continue to use nitroglycerin tablets or spray to relieve chest pain that has already started.

If headache continues, ask your doctor if you may take acetaminophen. Your nitroglycerin dose may need to be adjusted. Do not take aspirin or any other medication for headache while using nitroglycerin skin patches unless you doctor tells you to.

Do not let anyone else use your medication. Ask your pharmacist any questions you have about refilling your prescription.

Please see the nitroglycerin ointment monograph to find dosing information for this medication.

Nitroglycerin Tablets, Capsules, and Sprays

(nye troe gli′ ser in)

Brand Name: Nitro-Bid®, Nitrogard®, Nitroglycerin Slocaps®, Nitrolingual® Pumpspray, NitroQuick®, Nitrostat®, Nitrotab®, Nitro-Time® Also available generically.

Why is this medicine prescribed?

Nitroglycerin is used to prevent chest pain (angina). It works by relaxing the blood vessels to the heart, so the blood flow and oxygen supply to the heart is increased.

This medication is sometimes prescribed for other uses; ask your doctor or pharmacist for more information.

How should this medicine be used?

Nitroglycerin comes as a sublingual tablet, buccal tablet, extended-release (long-acting) capsule, or spray to be used orally. The buccal extended-release tablets and the extended-release tablets and capsules are usually taken three to six times a day. Do not crush, chew, or divide the extended-release tablets or capsules. The sublingual tablet and spray are used as needed to relieve chest pain that has already started or to prevent pain before activities known to provoke attacks (e.g., climbing stairs, sexual activity, heavy exercise, or cold weather). The buccal extended-release tablets also may be used during an attack and just before situations known to provoke attacks. Follow the directions on your prescription label carefully, and ask your doctor or pharmacist to explain any part you do not understand. Take nitroglycerin exactly as directed. Do not take more or less of it or take it more often than prescribed by your doctor.

Nitroglycerin controls chest pain but does not cure it. Continue to use nitroglycerin even if you feel well. Do not stop taking nitroglycerin without talking to your doctor. Stopping the drug abruptly may cause chest pain.

Nitroglycerin can lose its effectiveness when used for a long time. This effect is called tolerance. If your angina attacks happen more often, last longer, or are more severe, call your doctor.

If you are using the buccal extended-release tablet, place the tablet between your cheek and gum and allow it to dissolve. Do not chew or swallow it. If you feel dizzy, sit down after placing the tablet in your mouth. Try not to swallow saliva until the tablet dissolves. Buccal extended-release tablets start to work within 2-3 minutes. To make the tablet dissolve faster, touch it with your tongue before placing it in your mouth or drink a hot liquid. If an attack occurs while you have a buccal extended-release tablet in place, place a second tablet on the opposite side of your mouth. If chest pain persists, use sublingual tablets, call for emergency as-

sistance, or go to a hospital emergency department immediately.

If you are taking nitroglycerin sublingual tablets or spray for acute chest pain, you should carry the tablets and spray with you at all times. Sit down when an acute attack occurs. The drug starts to work within 2 minutes and goes on working for up to 30 minutes. If you are taking nitroglycerin tablets and your chest pain is not relieved within 5 minutes, take another dose. If you are using nitroglycerin spray and your chest pain is not relieved in 3-5 minutes, repeat the process. Call for emergency assistance or go to a hospital emergency department if pain persists after you have taken three tablets (at 5-minute intervals) or have used three sprays (at 3-5 minute intervals) and 15 minutes have passed.

To use the tablets, place a tablet under your tongue or between your cheek and gum and allow it to dissolve. Do not swallow the tablet. Try not to swallow saliva too often until the tablet dissolves.

To use the spray, follow these steps:
1. Do not shake the drug container. Hold it upright with the opening of the spray mechanism as close as possible to your opened mouth.
2. Press the spray mechanism with your forefinger to release the spray. Spray the drug onto or under your tongue and close your mouth immediately. Do not inhale or swallow the spray.

Are there other uses for this medicine?

Nitroglycerin tablets also are used with other drugs to treat congestive heart failure and heart attacks. Talk to your doctor about the possible risks of using this drug for your condition.

What special precautions should I follow?

Before taking nitroglycerin,
- tell your doctor and pharmacist if you are allergic to nitroglycerin, isosorbide (Imdur, Isordil, Sorbitrate), or any other drugs.
- tell your doctor and pharmacist what prescription and nonprescription medications you are taking, especially aspirin; beta blockers such as atenolol (Tenormin), carteolol (Cartrol), labetalol (Normodyne, Trandate), metoprolol (Lopressor), nadolol (Corgard), propranolol (Inderal), sotalol (Betapace), and timolol (Blocadren); calcium channel blockers such as amlodipine (Norvasc), diltiazem (Cardizem), felodipine (Plendil), isradipine (DynaCirc), nifedipine (Procardia), and verapamil (Calan, Isoptin); dihydroergotamine (D.H.E. 45); sildenafil (Viagra); and vitamins.
- tell your doctor if you have low red blood cell counts (anemia), glaucoma, or recent head trauma.
- tell your doctor if you are pregnant, plan to become pregnant, or are breast-feeding. If you become pregnant while taking nitroglycerin, call your doctor.
- if you are having surgery, including dental surgery,

tell the doctor or dentist that you are taking nitroglycerin.

- you should know that this drug may make you drowsy or dizzy. Do not drive a car or operate machinery until you know how it affects you.
- ask your doctor about the safe use of alcoholic beverages while you are taking nitroglycerin. Alcohol can make the side effects from nitroglycerin worse.

What special dietary instructions should I follow?

Take nitroglycerin extended-release tablets and capsules on an empty stomach with a full glass of water.

What should I do if I forget to take a dose?

Take the missed dose as soon as you remember it. However, if it is almost time for the next dose, skip the missed dose and continue your regular dosing schedule. Do not take a double dose to make up for a missed one.

What side effects can this medicine cause?

Side effects from nitroglycerin are common. Tell your doctor if any of these symptoms are severe or do not go away:

- headache
- rash
- dizziness
- upset stomach
- flushing (feeling of warmth)

If you experience any of the following symptoms, call your doctor immediately:

- blurred vision
- dry mouth
- chest pain
- fainting

If you experience a serious side effect, you or your doctor may send a report to the Food and Drug Administration's (FDA) MedWatch Adverse Event Reporting program online [at http://www.fda.gov/MedWatch/index.html] or by phone [1-800-332-1088].

What storage conditions are needed for this medicine?

Keep this medication in the container it came in, tightly closed, and out of reach of children. Store it at room temperature and away from excess heat and moisture (not in the bathroom). Avoid puncturing the spray container and keep it away from excess heat. Do not open a container of sublingual nitroglycerin until you need a dose. Do not use tablets that are more than 12 months old. Throw away any medication that is outdated or no longer needed. Talk to your pharmacist about the proper disposal of your medication.

What should I do in case of overdose?

In case of overdose, call your local poison control center at 1-800-222-1222. If the victim has collapsed or is not breathing, call local emergency services at 911.

What other information should I know?

Keep all appointments with your doctor and the laboratory. Nitroglycerin extended-release capsules should not be used for acute angina attacks. Continue to use nitroglycerin tablets or spray to relieve chest pain that has already started.

If headache continues, ask your doctor if you may take acetaminophen. Your nitroglycerin dose may need to be adjusted. Do not take aspirin or any other medication for headache while taking nitroglycerin unless your doctor tells you to.

The tablets may cause a sweet, tingling sensation when placed under your tongue. This sensation is not an accurate indicator of drug strength; the absence of a tingling sensation does not mean that the drug is not working.

Do not let anyone else take your medication. Ask your pharmacist any questions you have about refilling your prescription.

Please see the nitroglycerin ointment monograph to find dosing information for this medication.

Nizatidine

(ni za' ti deen)

Brand Name: Axid®, Axid® AR Acid Reducer, Axid® Pulvules®

Why is this medicine prescribed?

Nizatidine is used to treat and prevent the recurrence of ulcers and to treat other conditions where the stomach makes too much acid. Nizatidine also is used to treat or prevent occasional heartburn, acid indigestion, or sour stomach. It decreases the amount of acid made in the stomach. Nizatidine is available with and without a prescription.

This medication is sometimes prescribed for other uses; ask your doctor or pharmacist for more information.

How should this medicine be used?

Nizatidine comes as a tablet and capsule to take by mouth. It usually is taken once daily at bedtime or twice a day with or without food. Follow the directions on the package or on your prescription label carefully, and ask your doctor or pharmacist to explain any part you do not understand. Take nizatidine exactly as directed. Do not take more or less of it or take it more often than prescribed by your doctor.

If symptoms of heartburn, acid indigestion, or sour stomach last for longer than 2 weeks while taking nizatidine, stop taking it and call your doctor.

What special precautions should I follow?

Before taking nizatidine,
- tell your doctor and pharmacist if you are allergic to nizatidine or any other drugs.
- tell your doctor and pharmacist what prescription and nonprescription medications you are taking, especially aspirin or antacids such as Maalox or Mylanta, and vitamins.
- tell your doctor if you have or have ever had kidney or liver disease.
- tell your doctor if you are pregnant, plan to become pregnant, or are breast-feeding. If you become pregnant while taking nizatidine, call your doctor.

What should I do if I forget to take a dose?

Take the missed dose as soon as you remember it. However, if it is almost time for the next dose, skip the missed dose and continue your regular dosing schedule. Do not take a double dose to make up for a missed one.

What side effects can this medicine cause?

Nizatidine may cause side effects. Tell your doctor if any of these symptoms are severe or do not go away:
- headache
- dizziness
- drowsiness
- constipation
- diarrhea
- stomach pain
- runny nose
- sneezing
- coughing
- sweating

If you have any of the following symptoms, call your doctor immediately:
- skin rash
- hives
- itching
- wheezing
- difficulty breathing

If you experience a serious side effect, you or your doctor may send a report to the Food and Drug Administration's (FDA) MedWatch Adverse Event Reporting program online [at http://www.fda.gov/MedWatch/index.html] or by phone [1-800-332-1088].

What storage conditions are needed for this medicine?

Keep this medication in the container it came in, tightly closed, and out of reach of children. Store it at room tem-perature and away from excess heat and moisture (not in the bathroom). Throw away any medication that is outdated or no longer needed. Talk to your pharmacist about the proper disposal of your medication.

What should I do in case of overdose?

In case of overdose, call your local poison control center at 1-800-222-1222. If the victim has collapsed or is not breathing, call local emergency services at 911.

What other information should I know?

Keep all appointments with your doctor.

Do not let anyone else take your medicine. Ask your pharmacist any questions you have about refilling your prescription.

Dosage Facts
For Informational Purposes

Caution: Do not change your dose, how often you take your medication, or the length of time you are to take it without first talking to your health-care provider.

The following dosage information was written using medical language for doctors and other healthcare professionals and is provided here for you to check your dosage. The dosage of this drug may differ for different patients. Therefore, always follow your doctor's instructions or the directions on the label. Contact your health-care provider or pharmacist if you have any questions about the specific dosage of your medication after reviewing this information.

Pediatric Patients

Erosive Esophagitis or GERD

ORAL:
- Children ≥12 years of age: 150 mg twice daily as oral solution for up to 8 weeks.

Gastroesophageal Reflux
Self-medication for Heartburn in Adolescents ≥12 years of Age

ORAL:
- 75 mg once or twice daily (maximum 150 mg in 24 hours continuously for 2 weeks) or as directed by clinician.

Self-medication for Prevention of Heartburn In Adolescents ≥12 Years of Age

ORAL:
- 75 mg once or twice daily (immediately or up to 1 hour before ingestion of causative food or beverage); maximum 150 mg in 24 hours continuously for 2 weeks or as directed by clinician.

Adult Patients

Gastroesophageal Reflux
Treatment of Esophagitis

ORAL:
- 150 mg twice daily for up to 12 weeks.
- 300 mg at bedtime also has been used, but is less effective and not considered appropriate therapy.

Self-medication for Heartburn

ORAL:
- 75 mg once or twice daily (maximum 150 mg in 24 hours continuously for 2 weeks) or as directed by clinician.

Self-medication for Prevention of Heartburn

ORAL:
- 75 mg once or twice daily (immediately or up to 1 hour before ingestion of causative food or beverage); maximum 150 mg in 24 hours continuously for 2 weeks or as directed by clinician.

Duodenal Ulcer
Treatment of Active Duodenal Ulcer

ORAL:
- 300 mg once daily at bedtime, or 150 mg twice daily.
- Healing may occur within 2 weeks in some, and within 4 weeks in most patients; some patients may benefit from an additional 4 weeks of therapy. Occasionally may be necessary to continue full-dose therapy for >6–8 weeks.
- Safety and efficacy of continuing full-dose therapy for > 8 weeks have not been established.

Maintenance of Healing of Duodenal Ulcer

ORAL:
- 150 mg once daily at bedtime.
- Some clinicians recommend continuing maintenance therapy for at least 1 year.
- Safety and efficacy of continuing maintenance therapy beyond 1 year have not been established.

Gastric Ulcer

ORAL:
- 150 mg twice daily or 300 mg once daily at bedtime for up to 8 weeks.
- Complete healing of gastric ulcers usually occurs within 8 weeks.
- Safety and efficacy for >8 weeks have not been established.

Prescribing Limits

Pediatric Patients

Erosive Esophagitis or GERD

ORAL:
- Maximum 300 mg daily for 8 weeks.

Gastroesophageal Reflux
Self-Medication For Heartburn in Adolescents ≥12 years of Age

ORAL:
- Maximum 150 mg in 24 hours continuously for 2 weeks.

Self-medication for Prevention of Heartburn in Adolescents ≥12 years of Age

ORAL:
- Maximum 150 mg in 24 hours continuously for 2 weeks.

Adult Patients

Gastroesophageal Reflux
Treatment of Esophagitis

ORAL:
- Safety and efficacy for >12 weeks not established.

Self-medication for Heartburn

ORAL:
- Maximum 150 mg in 24 hours continuously for 2 weeks.

Self-medication for Prevention of Heartburn

ORAL:
- Maximum 150 mg in 24 hours continuously for 2 weeks.

Duodenal Ulcer
Treatment of Active Duodenal Ulcer

ORAL:
- Safety and efficacy for >8 weeks not established.

Maintenance of Healing of Duodenal Ulcer

ORAL:
- Safety and efficacy for >1 year not established.

Gastric Ulcer
Short-term treatment of Active Benign Gastric Ulcer

ORAL:
- Safety and efficacy for >8 weeks not established.

Special Populations

Renal Impairment
- Modify doses and/or frequency of administration to the degree of renal impairment; clinical efficacy of recommended dosages have not been systematically evaluated.

Table 1. Nizatidine Dosage Based on Creatinine Clearance

Creatinine Clearance (mL/minute)	Dosage for Treatment of Esophagitis, Active Duodenal Ulcer, Active Benign Gastric Ulcer	Dosage for Maintenance of Healing of Duodenal Ulcer
20–50	150 mg once daily	150 mg once every other day
<20	150 mg once every other day	150 mg once every 3 days

Geriatric Patients
- Careful dosage selection recommended due to possible age-related decreases in renal function. Monitoring renal function may be useful.

Norelgestromin and Ethinyl Estradiol Transdermal System

(nor el jes' troe min) (eth' in il es tra dye' ole)

Brand Name: Ortho Evra®

Important Warning

Cigarette smoking increases the risk of serious side effects from the contraceptive patch, including heart attacks, blood clots, and strokes. This risk is higher for women over 35 years old and heavy smokers (15 or more cigarettes per day). If you use the contraceptive patch, you should not smoke.

Why is this medicine prescribed?

Norelgestromin and ethinyl estradiol transdermal system (patch) is used to prevent pregnancy. Norelgestromin is a progestin and ethinyl estradiol is an estrogen. Estrogen and progestin are two female sex hormones. Norelgestromin and ethinyl estradiol contraceptive patch works by preventing ovulation (the release of eggs from the ovaries) and by changing the cervical mucus and the lining of the uterus. The contraceptive patch is a very effective method of birth control, but it does not prevent the spread of human immunodeficiency virus [HIV; the virus that causes acquired immunodeficiency syndrome (AIDS)] and other sexually transmitted diseases.

How should this medicine be used?

Norelgestromin and ethinyl estradiol transdermal system comes as a patch to apply to the skin. One patch is applied once a week for 3 weeks, followed by a patch-free week. Follow the directions on your prescription label carefully, and ask your doctor or pharmacist to explain any part you do not understand. Use the contraceptive patch exactly as directed.

If you are just starting to use the contraceptive patch, you may apply your first patch on the first day of your menstrual period or the first Sunday after your period begins. If you apply your first patch after the first day of your menstrual period, you must use a backup method of birth control (such as a condom and/or a spermicide) for the first 7 days of the first cycle.

Always apply your new patch on the same day of the week (the Patch Change Day). Apply a new patch once a week for 3 weeks. During Week 4, remove the old patch but do not apply a new patch, and expect to begin your menstrual period. On the day after Week 4 ends, apply a new patch to start a new 4-week cycle even if your menstrual period has not started or has not ended. You should not go more than 7 days without a patch.

Apply the contraceptive patch to a clean, dry, intact, healthy area of skin on the buttock, abdomen, upper outer arm, or upper torso, in a place where it will not be rubbed by tight clothing. Do not place the contraceptive patch on the breasts or on skin that is red, irritated, or cut. Do not apply makeup, creams, lotions, powders, or other topical products to the skin area where the contraceptive patch is placed. Each new patch should be applied to a new spot on the skin to help avoid irritation.

Do not cut, decorate, or change the patch in any way. Do not use extra tape, glue, or wraps to hold the patch in place.

To use the contraceptive patch, follow these steps:
1. Open the foil pouch by tearing it along the edge.
2. Peel apart the foil pouch and open it flat.
3. Use your fingernail to lift one corner of the patch and peel the patch and its clear plastic liner off the foil liner. Sometimes patches can stick to the inside of the pouch; be careful not to remove the clear liner as you remove the patch.
4. Peel away half of the plastic liner. Avoid touching the sticky surface of the patch.
5. Apply the sticky surface of the patch to the skin and remove the other half of the plastic liner. Press down firmly on the patch with the palm of your hand for 10 seconds, making sure that the edges stick well.
6. After one week, remove the patch from your skin. Fold the used patch in half so that it sticks to itself and throw it away in a trash can that is out of the reach of children and pets. Do not flush the used patch down the toilet.

Check your patch every day to make sure it is sticking. If the patch has been partially or completely detached for less than one day, try to reapply it in the same place immediately. Do not try to reapply a patch that is no longer sticky, that has stuck to itself or another surface, that has any material stuck to its surface or that has loosened or fallen off before. Apply a new patch instead. Your Patch Change Day will stay the same. If the patch has been partially or completely detached for more than one day, or if you do not know how long the patch has been detached, you may not be protected from pregnancy. You must start a new cycle by applying a new patch immediately; the day that you apply the new patch becomes your new Patch Change Day. Use backup birth control for the first week of the new cycle.

If the skin under your patch becomes irritated, you may remove the patch and apply a new patch to a different spot on the skin. Leave the new patch in place until your regular Patch Change Day. Be sure to remove the old patch because you should never wear more than one patch at a time.

Ask your pharmacist or doctor for a copy of the manufacturer's information for the patient.

Are there other uses for this medicine?

This medication may be prescribed for other uses; ask your doctor or pharmacist for more information.

What special precautions should I follow?

Before using norelgestromin and ethinyl estradiol contraceptive patch,

- tell your doctor and pharmacist if you are allergic to estrogens, progestins, or any other medications.
- tell your doctor if you are using any other type of hormonal birth control, such as pills, rings, injections, or implants. Your doctor will tell you how and when you should stop using the other type of birth control and start using the contraceptive patch. Do not use any other type of hormonal birth control while you are using the contraceptive patch.
- tell your doctor and pharmacist what prescription and nonprescription medications, vitamins, and nutritional supplements you are taking. Be sure to mention any of the following: acetaminophen (APAP, Tylenol); antibiotics such as ampicillin; anticoagulants ('blood thinners') such as warfarin (Coumadin); antifungals such as itraconazole (Sporanox) and ketoconazole (Nizoral); ascorbic acid (vitamin C); atorvastatin (Lipitor); clofibrate; cyclosporine (Neoral, Sandimmune); griseofulvin (Fulvicin, Grifulvin, Grisactin); HIV protease inhibitors such as indinavir (Crixivan) and ritonavir (Norvir); medications for seizures such as carbamazepine (Tegretol), felbamate (Felbatol), phenobarbital (Luminal, Solfoton), oxcarbazepine (Trileptal), phenytoin (Dilantin), and topiramate (Topamax); morphine (Kadian, MS Contin, MSIR, others); oral steroids such as dexamethasone (Decadron, Dexone), methylprednisolone (Medrol), prednisone (Deltasone), and prednisolone (Prelone); rifampin (Rifadin, Rimactane); temazepam (Restoril); theophylline (Theobid, Theo-Dur); and thyroid medication such as levothyroxine (Levothroid, Levoxyl, Synthroid). Your doctor may need to change the doses of your medications or monitor you carefully for side effects.
- tell your doctor what herbal products you are taking, especially products containing St. John's wort.
- tell your doctor if you have recently had surgery or if you are on bedrest. Also tell your doctor if you have or have ever had a heart attack; a stroke; blood clots in your legs, lungs, or eyes; chest pain due to heart disease; cancer of the breasts, lining of the uterus, cervix, or vagina; vaginal bleeding between menstrual periods; hepatitis (swelling of the liver); yellowing of the skin or eyes, especially while you were pregnant or using hormonal contraceptives; a liver tumor; headaches that happen with other symptoms such as weakness or difficulty seeing or moving; high blood pressure; diabetes that has caused problems with your kidneys, eyes, nerves, or blood vessels; or heart valve disease. Your

doctor will probably tell you that you should not use the contraceptive patch.

- tell your doctor if you have recently given birth or had a miscarriage or abortion and if you weigh 198 lbs or more. Also tell your doctor if anyone in your family has ever had breast cancer and if you have or have ever had breast lumps, fibrocystic disease of the breast (condition in which lumps or masses that are not cancer form in the breasts) or an abnormal mammogram (x-ray of the breasts). Also tell your doctor if you have or have ever had high blood cholesterol and fats; diabetes; asthma; migraines or other types of headaches; depression; seizures; scanty or irregular menstrual periods; or liver, heart, gallbladder, or kidney disease.
- tell your doctor if you are pregnant, plan to become pregnant, or are breast-feeding. If you become pregnant while using norelgestromin and ethinyl estradiol contraceptive patch, call your doctor immediately. You should suspect that you are pregnant and call your doctor if you have used the contraceptive patch correctly and you have missed two periods in a row, or if you have not used the contraceptive patch correctly and you have missed one period.
- if you are having surgery, including dental surgery, tell the doctor or dentist that you are using norelgestromin and ethinyl estradiol contraceptive patch. Talk to your doctor about this as soon as your surgery is scheduled because your doctor may want you to stop using the contraceptive patch several weeks before your surgery.
- tell your doctor if you wear contact lenses. If you notice changes in your vision or ability to wear your lenses while using norelgestromin and ethinyl estradiol contraceptive patch, see an eye doctor.
- you should know that when you use the contraceptive patch, the average amount of estrogen in your blood will be higher than it would be if you used an oral contraceptive (birth control pill), and this may increase the risk of serious side effects such as blood clots in the legs or lungs. Two studies were done to learn more about this risk. One study found that women who used contraceptive patches were twice as likely to develop blood clots as women who used oral contraceptives. The other study found that women who used contraceptive patches were no more likely to develop blood clots than women who used oral contraceptives. Talk to your doctor about the birth control method that is best for you.

What special dietary instructions should I follow?

Unless your doctor tells you otherwise, continue your normal diet.

What should I do if I forget to take a dose?

If you forget to apply your patch at the start of any patch cycle (Week 1, Day 1), you may not be protected from pregnancy. Apply the first patch of the new cycle as soon as you remember. There is now a new Patch Change Day and a new Day 1. Use a backup method of birth control for one week.

If you forget to change your patch in the middle of the patch cycle (Week 2 or Week 3) for 1 or 2 days, apply a new patch immediately and apply the next patch on your usual Patch Change Day. If you forget to change your patch in the middle of the cycle for more than 2 days, you may not be protected from pregnancy. Stop the current cycle and start a new cycle immediately by applying a new patch. There is now a new Patch Change Day and a new Day 1. Use a backup method of birth control for 1 week.

If you forget to remove your patch at the end of the patch cycle (Week 4), take it off as soon as you remember. Start the next cycle on the usual Patch Change Day, the day after Day 28.

What side effects can this medicine cause?

Norelgestromin and ethinyl estradiol contraceptive patch may cause side effects. Tell your doctor if any of these symptoms are severe or do not go away:

- irritation, redness, or rash in the place where you applied the patch
- breast tenderness, enlargement, or discharge
- nausea
- vomiting
- stomach cramps or bloating
- weight gain or weight loss
- change in appetite
- brown or black skin patches
- acne
- swelling of the hands, feet, ankles, or lower legs
- hair loss
- bleeding or spotting between menstrual periods
- changes in menstrual flow
- painful or missed periods
- vaginal itching or irritation
- white vaginal discharge
- difficulty wearing contact lenses

Some side effects can be serious. If you experience any of the following symptoms, call your doctor immediately:

- sudden severe headache or vomiting
- speech problems
- dizziness or faintness
- weakness or numbness of an arm or leg
- sudden partial or complete loss of vision
- double vision
- bulging eyes
- sharp or crushing chest pain
- chest tightness
- coughing up blood
- shortness of breath
- calf pain
- severe stomach pain
- sleep problems, mood changes, and other signs of depression
- yellowing of the skin or eyes
- unusual bleeding

- loss of appetite
- extreme tiredness, weakness, or lack of energy
- fever
- dark-colored urine
- light-colored stool
- rash

Norelgestromin and ethinyl estradiol contraceptive patch may increase the risk of developing endometrial and breast cancer, gallbladder disease, liver tumors, heart attack, stroke, and blood clots. Talk to your doctor about the risks of using this medication.

Norelgestromin and ethinyl estradiol contraceptive patch may cause other side effects. Call your doctor if you have any unusual problems while taking this medication.

What storage conditions are needed for this medicine?

Keep this medication in the container it came in, tightly closed, and out of reach of children. Store it at room temperature and away from excess heat and moisture (not in the bathroom). Throw away any medication that is outdated or no longer needed. Talk to your pharmacist about the proper disposal of your medication.

What should I do in case of overdose?

In case of overdose, remove all the patches that were applied and call your local poison control center at 1-800-222-1222. If the victim has collapsed or is not breathing, call local emergency services at 911.

What other information should I know?

Keep all appointments with your doctor and the laboratory. You should have a complete physical examination every year, including blood pressure measurements, breast and pelvic exams, and a Pap test. Follow your doctor's directions for examining your breasts; report any lumps immediately.

Before you have any laboratory tests, tell the laboratory personnel that you use norelgestromin and ethinyl estradiol contraceptive patch, as this medication may interfere with some laboratory tests.

Do not let anyone else use your medication. Ask your pharmacist any questions you have about refilling your prescription.

Talk to your doctor, pharmacist, or other healthcare professional if you have questions about dosing information for your medication.

Norethindrone

(nor eth in′ drone)

Brand Name: Aygestin®

Why is this medicine prescribed?

Norethindrone is used to treat endometriosis, a condition in which the type of tissue that lines the uterus (womb) grows in other areas of the body and causes pain, heavy or irregular menstruation (periods), and other symptoms. Norethindrone is also used to treat abnormal periods or bleeding and to bring on a normal menstrual cycle in women who menstruated normally in the past but have not menstruated for at least 6 months and who are not pregnant or undergoing menopause (change of life). Norethindrone is also used as a test to see if the body is producing certain female hormones (natural substances that affect the uterus). Norethindrone is in a class of medications called progestins. It works by stopping the lining of the uterus from growing and by causing the uterus to produce certain hormones.

Norethindrone is also used to prevent pregnancy. Norethindrone is sold under different brand names and is taken in smaller amounts when it used to prevent pregnancy. This monograph does not include information on the use of norethindrone to prevent pregnancy. If you would like more information on that use of norethindrone, read the monograph called "Progestin Only Oral Contraceptives."

How should this medicine be used?

Norethindrone comes as a tablet to take by mouth. Norethindrone is taken on different schedules that depend on the condition that is being treated and on how well norethindrone works to treat the conditions. When norethindrone is used to treat endometriosis, it is usually taken once a day for 6 to 9 months or until breakthrough bleeding becomes bothersome. When norethindrone is used to bring on a normal cycle in women who have stopped menstruating, it is usually taken once a day for 5 to 10 days during the second half of the planned menstrual cycle. To help you remember to take norethindrone, take it at around the same time of day every day that you are scheduled to take it. Follow the directions on your prescription label carefully, and ask your doctor or pharmacist to explain any part you do not understand. Take norethindrone exactly as directed. Do not take more or less of it or take it more often than prescribed by your doctor.

If you are taking norethindrone for endometriosis, your doctor will probably start you on a low dose of norethindrone and gradually increase your dose, not more than once every 2 weeks.

Norethindrone may control your condition but will not cure it. Continue to take norethindrone even if you feel well. Do not stop taking norethindrone without talking to your doctor.

Are there other uses for this medicine?

This medication may be prescribed for other uses; ask your doctor or pharmacist for more information.

What special precautions should I follow?

Before taking norethindrone,

- tell your doctor and pharmacist if you are allergic to norethindrone, oral contraceptives ('birth control pills'), or any other medications.
- tell your doctor and pharmacist what prescription and nonprescription medications, vitamins, nutritional supplements, and herbal products you are taking. Be sure to mention medications for seizures such as carbamazepine (Tegretol), phenobarbital (Luminal, Solfoton), and phenytoin (Dilantin); and rifampin (Rifadin, Rimactane). Your doctor may need to change the doses of your medications or monitor you carefully for side effects.
- tell your doctor if you have recently had surgery or have been unable to move around for any reason and if you have or have ever had breast cancer; unexplained vaginal bleeding; a missed abortion (a pregnancy that ended when the unborn child died in the uterus but was not expelled from the body); blood clots in your legs, lungs, brain, or eyes; stroke or mini-stroke; coronary artery disease (clogged blood vessels leading to the heart); chest pain; a heart attack; thrombophilia (a condition in which the blood clots more easily); seizures; migraine headaches; depression; asthma; high cholesterol; diabetes; or heart, kidney, or liver disease.
- tell your doctor if you are pregnant, plan to become pregnant, or are breast-feeding. If you become pregnant while taking norethindrone, call your doctor immediately. Norethindrone should never be used to test for pregnancy.
- if you are having surgery, including dental surgery, tell the doctor or dentist that you are taking norethindrone.
- tell your doctor if you smoke cigarettes. Smoking may increase the risk that you will develop serious side effects of norethindrone.

What special dietary instructions should I follow?

Unless your doctor tells you otherwise, continue your normal diet.

What should I do if I forget to take a dose?

Take the missed dose as soon as you remember it. However, if it is almost time for the next dose, skip the missed dose and continue your regular dosing schedule. Do not take a double dose to make up for a missed one.

What side effects can this medicine cause?

Norethindrone may cause side effects. Tell your doctor if any of these symptoms are severe or do not go away:

- irregular vaginal bleeding or spotting
- changes in menstrual flow
- enlarged or tender breasts
- upset stomach
- weight changes
- difficulty falling asleep or staying asleep
- acne
- growth of hair on face

Some side effects can be serious. The following symptoms are uncommon, but if you experience any of them, call your doctor immediately:

- loss of vision
- blurred vision
- double vision
- bulging eyes
- migraine headache
- pain, warmth, or heaviness in the back of the lower leg
- shortness of breath
- coughing up blood
- sudden sharp or crushing chest pain
- heaviness in chest
- slow or difficult speech
- dizziness or faintness
- weakness or numbness of an arm or leg
- swelling of the arms, hands, feet, ankles, or lower legs
- yellowing of the skin or eyes
- depression
- mood swings
- brown patches on the face
- missed periods
- sudden, severe pain in the abdomen (area between the chest and waist)
- hives
- rash
- itching
- difficulty breathing or swallowing

Norethindrone may cause other side effects. Call your doctor if you have any unusual problems while taking this medication.

If you experience a serious side effect, you or your doctor may send a report to the Food and Drug Administration's (FDA) MedWatch Adverse Event Reporting program online [at http://www.fda.gov/MedWatch/index.html] or by phone [1-800-332-1088].

What storage conditions are needed for this medicine?

Keep this medication in the container it came in, tightly closed, and out of reach of children. Store it at room temperature and away from excess heat and moisture (not in the bathroom). Throw away any medication that is outdated or no longer needed. Talk to your pharmacist about the proper disposal of your medication.

What should I do in case of overdose?

In case of overdose, call your local poison control center at 1-800-222-1222. If the victim has collapsed or is not breathing, call local emergency services at 911.

What other information should I know?

Keep all appointments with your doctor and the laboratory. Your doctor may order certain lab tests to check your body's response to norethindrone.

Before having any laboratory test, tell your doctor and the laboratory personnel that you are taking norethindrone.

Do not let anyone else take your medication. Ask your pharmacist any questions you have about refilling your prescription.

Talk to your doctor, pharmacist, or other healthcare professional if you have questions about dosing information for your medication.

Norfloxacin

(nor flox′ a sin)

Brand Name: Noroxin®

Why is this medicine prescribed?

Norfloxacin is an antibiotic used to treat certain infections caused by bacteria, such as gonorrhea, prostate, and urinary tract infections. Antibiotics will not work for colds, flu, or other viral infections.

This medication is sometimes prescribed for other uses; ask your doctor or pharmacist for more information.

How should this medicine be used?

Norfloxacin comes as a tablet to take by mouth. It is usually taken every 12 hours (twice a day) for 7-28 days. To treat gonorrhea, a single dose is taken. Follow the directions on your prescription label carefully, and ask your doctor or pharmacist to explain any part you do not understand. Take norfloxacin exactly as directed. Do not take more or less of it or take it more often than prescribed by your doctor.

The tablets should be taken with a full glass of water.

Continue to take norfloxacin even if you feel well. Do not stop taking norfloxacin without talking to your doctor.

Are there other uses for this medicine?

Norfloxacin is also used sometimes to treat stomach infections. Talk to your doctor about the possible risks of using this drug for your condition.

What special precautions should I follow?

Before taking norfloxacin,

- tell your doctor and pharmacist if you are allergic to

norfloxacin, ciprofloxacin (Cipro), enoxacin (Penetrex), levofloxacin (Levaquin), lomefloxacin (Maxaquin), ofloxacin (Floxin), sparfloxacin (Zagam), cinoxacin (Cinobac), nalidixic acid (NegGram), or any other drugs.

- tell your doctor and pharmacist what prescription and nonprescription medications you are taking, especially other antibiotics, anticoagulants ('blood thinners') such as warfarin (Coumadin), cancer chemotherapy agents, cimetidine (Tagamet), cyclosporine (Neoral, Sandimmune), medications with caffeine (NoDoz, Vivarin), nitrofurantoin (Macrodantin), probenecid (Benemid), sucralfate (Carafate), theophylline (Theo-Dur), and vitamins.
- do not take with antacids (Mylanta, Maalox), didanosine (Videx) chewable/buffered tablets or oral solution, iron or zinc supplements, or vitamins that contain iron or zinc. Take them 2 hours before or after norfloxacin.
- tell your doctor if you have or have ever had kidney or liver disease, epilepsy, colitis, stomach problems, vision problems, heart disease, myasthenia gravis, or history of stroke.
- tell your doctor if you are pregnant, plan to become pregnant, or are breast-feeding. If you become pregnant while taking norfloxacin, call your doctor immediately.
- if you are having surgery, including dental surgery, tell the doctor or dentist that you are taking norfloxacin.
- you should know that this drug may cause dizziness, lightheadedness, and tiredness. Do not drive a car or work on dangerous machines until you know how norfloxacin will affect you.
- plan to avoid unnecessary or prolonged exposure to sunlight and to wear protective clothing, sunglasses, and sunscreen. Norfloxacin may make your skin sensitive to sunlight.

What special dietary instructions should I follow?

Take norfloxacin at least 1 hour before or 2 hours after meals or drinking or eating milk or dairy products. Take with a full glass of water. Drink at least eight full glasses of water or other liquid every day. Do not drink or eat a lot of caffeine-containing products as coffee, tea, cola, or chocolate. Norfloxacin increases nervousness, sleeplessness, heart pounding, and anxiety caused by caffeine.

What should I do if I forget to take a dose?

Take the missed dose as soon as you remember it. However, if it is almost time for the next dose, skip the missed dose and continue your regular dosing schedule. Do not take a double dose to make up for a missed one.

What side effects can this medicine cause?

Norfloxacin may cause side effects. Tell your doctor if any of these symptoms are severe or do not go away:
- upset stomach
- diarrhea

- vomiting
- stomach pain
- headache
- restlessness

If you experience any of the following symptoms, call your doctor immediately:
- skin rash
- itching
- hives
- difficulty breathing or swallowing
- swelling of the face or throat
- yellowing of the skin or eyes
- dark urine
- pale or dark stools
- blood in urine
- unusual tiredness
- sunburn or blistering
- seizures or convulsions
- vaginal infection
- vision changes
- pain, swelling, or rupture of a tendon in the shoulder, hand, or heel

If you experience a serious side effect, you or your doctor may send a report to the Food and Drug Administration's (FDA) MedWatch Adverse Event Reporting program online [at http://www.fda.gov/MedWatch/index.html] or by phone [1-800-332-1088].

What storage conditions are needed for this medicine?

Keep this medication in the container it came in, tightly closed, and out of reach of children. Store it at room temperature and away from excess heat and moisture (not in the bathroom). Keep away from light. Throw away any medication that is outdated or no longer needed. Talk to your pharmacist about the proper disposal of your medication.

What should I do in case of overdose?

In case of overdose, call your local poison control center at 1-800-222-1222. If the victim has collapsed or is not breathing, call local emergency services at 911.

What other information should I know?

Keep all appointments with your doctor and the laboratory. Your doctor will order certain lab tests to check your response to norfloxacin.

Do not let anyone else take your medication. Your prescription is probably not refillable. If you still have symptoms of infection after you finish the norfloxacin, call your doctor.

Dosage Facts
For Informational Purposes

Caution: Do not change your dose, how often you take your medication, or the length of time you

are to take it without first talking to your health-care provider.

The following dosage information was written using medical language for doctors and other healthcare professionals and is provided here for you to check your dosage. The dosage of this drug may differ for different patients. Therefore, always follow your doctor's instructions or the directions on the label. Contact your health-care provider or pharmacist if you have any questions about the specific dosage of your medication after reviewing this information.

Adult Patients

Urinary Tract Infections (UTIs) and Prostatitis
Uncomplicated UTIs

ORAL:
- 400 mg every 12 hours. Usual duration is 3 days for treatment of uncomplicated UTIs caused by susceptible *E. coli*, *K. pneumoniae*, or *P. mirabilis* or 7–10 days for treatment of uncomplicated UTIs caused by other susceptible bacteria.

Complicated UTIs

ORAL:
- 400 mg every 12 hours. Usual duration is ≥10–21 days.

Acute or Chronic Prostatitis Caused by E. coli

ORAL:
- 400 mg every 12 hours for 28 days.

GI Infections†
Gastroenteritis Caused by Susceptible Bacteria†

ORAL:
- 400 mg twice daily for 5 days. A duration of 3 days may be sufficient for some infections, including shigellosis or some *E. coli* infections.

Cholera†

ORAL:
- 400 mg twice daily for 3 days in conjunction with fluid and electrolyte replacement. A single 800-mg dose has been used in adults, but there is some evidence that a multiple-dose regimen is more effective than a single-dose regimen for treatment of severe cholera caused by *V. cholerae* 0139.

Treatment of Travelers' Diarrhea†

ORAL:
- 400 mg twice daily for 1–3 days.

Prevention of Travelers' Diarrhea†

ORAL:
- 400 mg once daily.
- Although anti-infective prophylaxis generally is discouraged, some clinicians state that it can be given during the period of risk (for ≤3 weeks) beginning the day of travel and continuing for 1 or 2 days after leaving the area of risk.

Gonorrhea
Uncomplicated Urethral, Endocervical, or Rectal Gonorrhea

ORAL:
- A single 800-mg dose.
- Because of increased prevalence of quinolone-resistant *Neis-seria gonorrhoeae* (QRNG), CDC no longer recommends fluoroquinolones for treatment of gonorrhea or any associated infections involving *N. gonorrhoeae* (e.g., PID, epididymitis).
- Unless the presence of coexisting chlamydial infection has been excluded by appropriate testing, patients being treated for gonorrhea should also receive an anti-infective regimen effective for presumptive treatment of chlamydia (e.g., a single dose of oral azithromycin or a 7-day regimen of oral doxycycline).

Prescribing Limits

Adult Patients

ORAL:
- Maximum 400 mg twice daily because of the risk of crystalluria.

Special Populations

Renal Impairment
- Dosage adjustments necessary in patients with severe renal impairment.
- Adults with Cl_{cr} ≤30 mL/minute per 1.73 m² should receive 400 mg once daily.

Geriatric Patients
- No dosage adjustments except those related to renal impairment.
- Select dosage with caution because of age-related decreases in renal impairment.

† Use is not currently included in the labeling approved by the US Food and Drug Administration.

Nortriptyline
(nor trip′ ti leen)

Brand Name: Aventyl®, Pamelor®
Also available generically.

Important Warning

A small number of children, teenagers, and young adults (up to 24 years of age) who took antidepressants ('mood elevators') such as nortriptyline during clinical studies became suicidal (thinking about harming or killing oneself or planning or trying to do so). Children, teenagers, and young adults who take antidepressants to treat depression or other mental illnesses may be more likely to become suicidal than children, teenagers, and young adults who do not take antidepressants to treat these conditions. However, experts are not sure about how great this risk is and how much it should be considered in deciding whether a child or teenager should take an antidepressant. Children younger than 18 years of age should not normally take nortriptyline, but in some cases, a doctor may decide that nortriptyline is the best medication to treat a child's condition.

You should know that your mental health may change in unexpected ways when you take nortriptyline or other antidepressants even if you are an adult over age 24. You may become suicidal, especially at the beginning of your treatment and any time that your dose is increased or decreased. You, your family, or your caregiver should call your doctor right away if you experience any of the following symptoms: new or worsening depression; thinking about harming or killing yourself, or planning or trying to do so; extreme worry; agitation; panic attacks; difficulty falling asleep or staying asleep; aggressive behavior; irritability; acting without thinking; severe restlessness; and frenzied abnormal excitement. Be sure that your family or caregiver knows which symptoms may be serious so they can call the doctor when you are unable to seek treatment on your own.

Your healthcare provider will want to see you often while you are taking nortriptyline, especially at the beginning of your treatment. Be sure to keep all appointments for office visits with your doctor.

The doctor or pharmacist will give you the manufacturer's patient information sheet (Medication Guide) when you begin treatment with nortriptyline. Read the information carefully and ask your doctor or pharmacist if you have any questions. You also can obtain the Medication Guide from the FDA website: http://www.fda.gov/cder/drug/antidepressants/antidepressants_MG_2007.pdf.

No matter what your age, before you take an antidepressant, you, your parent, or your caregiver should talk to your doctor about the risks and benefits of treating your condition with an antidepressant or with other treatments. You should also talk about the risks and benefits of not treating your condition. You should know that having depression or another mental illness greatly increases the risk that you will become suicidal. This risk is higher if you or anyone in your family has or has ever had bipolar disorder (mood that changes from depressed to abnormally excited) or mania (frenzied, abnormally excited mood) or has thought about or attempted suicide. Talk to your doctor about your condition, symptoms, and personal and family medical history. You and your doctor will decide what type of treatment is right for you.

Why is this medicine prescribed?

Nortriptyline is used to treat depression. Nortriptyline is in a group of medications called tricyclic antidepressants. It works by increasing the amounts of certain natural sub-

stances in the brain that are needed to maintain mental balance.

How should this medicine be used?

Nortriptyline comes as a capsule and an oral liquid to take by mouth. It is usually taken one to four times a day and may be taken with or without food. Take nortriptyline at around the same times every day. Follow the directions on your prescription label carefully, and ask your doctor or pharmacist to explain any part you do not understand. Take nortriptyline exactly as directed. Do not take more or less of it or take it more often than prescribed by your doctor.

Your doctor will probably start you on a low dose of nortriptyline and gradually increase your dose.

Continue to take nortriptyline even if you feel well. Do not stop taking nortriptyline without talking to your doctor. If you suddenly stop taking nortriptyline, you may experience withdrawal symptoms such as headache, nausea, and weakness. Your doctor will probably want to decrease your dose gradually.

Are there other uses for this medicine?

Nortriptyline is also sometimes used to treat panic disorders and post-herpetic neuralgia (the burning, stabbing pains, or aches that may last for months or years after a shingles infection). Nortriptyline is also sometimes used to help people stop smoking. Talk to your doctor about the possible risks of using this medication for your condition.

This medication may be prescribed for other uses. Ask your doctor or pharmacist for more information

What special precautions should I follow?

Before taking nortriptyline,

- tell your doctor and pharmacist if you are allergic to nortriptyline and other tricyclic antidepressants such as desipramine (Norpramin), clomipramine (Anafranil), imipramine (Tofranil), trimipramine (Surmontil), or any other medications.
- tell your doctor if you are taking a monoamine oxidase (MAO) inhibitor such as isocarboxazid (Marplan), phenelzine (Nardil), selegiline (Eldepryl, Emsam, Zelapar), and tranylcypromine (Parnate), or if you have stopped taking an MAO inhibitor within the past 14 days. Your doctor will probably tell you not to take nortriptyline.
- tell your doctor and pharmacist what prescription and nonprescription medications, vitamins, nutritional supplements and herbal products you are taking or plan to take. Be sure to mention any of the following: anticoagulants (blood thinners) such as warfarin (Coumadin); antihistamines; chlorpropamide (Diabinese); cimetidine (Tagamet); flecainide (Tambocor); guanethidine (Ismelin); lithium (Eskalith, Lithobid); medication for high blood pressure, seizures, Parkinson's disease, diabetes, asthma, nausea, mental illness, colds, or allergies; methylphenidate (Ritalin); muscle relaxants; propafenone

(Rhythmol); quinidine; sedatives; selective serotonin reuptake inhibitors such as selective serotonin reuptake inhibitors (SSRIs) such as citalopram (Celexa), escitalopram (Lexapro), fluoxetine (Prozac, Sarafem), fluvoxamine (Luvox), paroxetine (Paxil), and sertraline (Zoloft); sleeping pills; thyroid medication; and tranquilizers. Your doctor may need to change the doses of your medications or monitor you carefully for side effects.

- tell your doctor if you have recently had a heart attack. Your doctor may tell you not to take nortriptyline.
- tell your doctor if you have or have ever had glaucoma (an eye condition), an enlarged prostate (a male reproductive gland), difficulty urinating, diabetes, seizures, schizophrenia (a mental illness that causes disturbed or unusual thinking, loss of interest in life, and strong or inappropriate emotions), an overactive thyroid gland, or liver, kidney, or heart disease.
- tell your doctor if you are pregnant, plan to become pregnant, or are breast-feeding. If you become pregnant while taking nortriptyline, call your doctor.
- if you are having surgery, including dental surgery, tell the doctor or dentist that you are taking nortriptyline.
- you should know that this medication may make you drowsy. Do not drive a car or operate machinery until you know how this medication affects you.
- talk to your doctor about the safe use of alcohol while you are taking this medication.
- plan to avoid unnecessary or prolonged exposure to sunlight and to wear protective clothing, sunglasses, and sunscreen. Nortriptyline may make your skin sensitive to sunlight.

What special dietary instructions should I follow?

Unless your doctor tells you otherwise, continue your normal diet.

What should I do if I forget to take a dose?

Take the missed dose as soon as you remember it. However, if it is almost time for the next dose, skip the missed dose and continue your regular dosing schedule. Do not take a double dose to make up for a missed one.

What side effects can this medicine cause?

Nortriptyline may cause side effects. Tell your doctor if any of these symptoms are severe or do not go away:

- nausea
- drowsiness
- weakness or tiredness
- excitement or anxiety
- nightmares
- dry mouth
- changes in appetite or weight

- constipation
- difficulty urinating
- frequent urination
- blurred vision
- changes in sex drive or ability
- excessive sweating

Some side effects may be serious. If you experience any of the following symptoms or those listed in the IMPORTANT WARNING section, call your doctor immediately:

- jaw, neck, and back muscle spasms
- slow or difficult speech
- shuffling walk
- uncontrollable shaking of a part of the body
- fever
- difficulty breathing or swallowing
- rash
- yellowing of the skin or eyes
- irregular heartbeat

Nortriptyline may cause other side effects. Call your doctor if you have any unusual problems while you are taking this medication.

If you experience a serious side effect, you or your doctor may send a report to the Food and Drug Administration's (FDA) MedWatch Adverse Event Reporting program online [at http://www.fda.gov/MedWatch/index.html] or by phone [1-800-332-1088].

What storage conditions are needed for this medicine?

Keep this medication in the container it came in, tightly closed, and out of reach of children. Store it at room temperature and away from excess heat and moisture (not in the bathroom). Throw away any medication that is outdated or no longer needed. Talk to your pharmacist about the proper disposal of your medication.

What should I do in case of overdose?

In case of overdose, call your local poison control center at 1-800-222-1222. If the victim has collapsed or is not breathing, call local emergency services at 911.

Symptoms of overdose may include

- irregular heartbeat
- seizures
- coma (loss of consciousness for a period of time)
- confusion
- hallucination (seeing things that do not exist)
- widened pupils (dark circles in the middle of the eyes)
- drowsiness
- agitation
- fever
- low body temperature
- stiff muscles
- vomiting

What other information should I know?

Keep all appointments with your doctor and the laboratory. Your doctor may order certain lab tests to check your response to nortriptyline.

Do not let anyone else take your medication. Ask your pharmacist any questions you have about refilling your prescription.

Dosage Facts

For Informational Purposes

Caution: Do not change your dose, how often you take your medication, or the length of time you are to take it without first talking to your healthcare provider.

The following dosage information was written using medical language for doctors and other healthcare professionals and is provided here for you to check your dosage. The dosage of this drug may differ for different patients. Therefore, always follow your doctor's instructions or the directions on the label. Contact your healthcare provider or pharmacist if you have any questions about the specific dosage of your medication after reviewing this information.

General Dosage Information

Available as nortriptyline hydrochloride; dosage is expressed in terms of nortriptyline.

Adult Patients

Major Depressive Disorder

ORAL:
- Initially, 25 mg daily. Gradually adjust to level that produces maximal therapeutic effects (up to 200 mg daily).
- Usual dosage: Manufacturer recommends 75–100 mg daily, but some experts state usual dosage range is 50–200 mg daily. After symptoms are controlled, dosage should be gradually reduced to the lowest level that will maintain relief of symptoms.
- Hospitalized patients under close supervision may generally be given higher dosages than outpatients.

Smoking Cessation†

ORAL:
- 25 mg daily, and then gradually increase to a target dosage of 75–100 mg daily.
- Initiate nortriptyline therapy 10–28 days before date set for cessation of smoking.
- Nortriptyline was continued for approximately 12 weeks in clinical studies.

Prescribing Limits

Adult Patients

Major Depressive Disorder

ORAL:
- Manufacturer does not recommend dosages >150 mg daily, but higher dosages (e.g., 200 mg daily) have been used.

Special Populations

Geriatric Patients
- 30–50 mg daily.

† Use is not currently included in the labeling approved by the US Food and Drug Administration.

Nystatin

(nye stat′ in)

Brand Name: Mycostatin®, Mycostatin® Filmlok®, Mycostatin® Pastilles, Myco-Triacet® II as a combination product containing Nystatin and Triamcinolone Acetonide, Mytrex® as a combination product containing Nystatin and Triamcinolone Acetonide, Nystatin Ointment®, Nystat-Rx®, Nystop®, Pedi-Dri®

Why is this medicine prescribed?

Nystatin is used to treat fungal infections of the skin, mouth, vagina, and intestinal tract. Fungal medicines will not work for colds, flu, or other viral infections.

This medication is sometimes prescribed for other uses; ask your doctor or pharmacist for more information.

How should this medicine be used?

Nystatin comes as a tablet and a liquid to take by mouth; a soft lozenge (pastille) to be dissolved slowly in the mouth; a tablet and vaginal cream to be inserted into the vagina; and in powder, ointment, and cream to be applied to the skin.

Follow the directions on your prescription label carefully, and ask your doctor or pharmacist to explain any part you do not understand. Take nystatin exactly as directed. Do not take more or less of it or take it more often than prescribed by your doctor.

Allow the lozenges (pastilles) to dissolve slowly in your mouth. Do not chew or swallow lozenges whole. Continue to use nystatin lozenges (pastilles) for at least 48 hours after symptoms of your mouth infection disappear.

Nystatin liquid usually is used three to five times a day for mouth infections and three times a day for intestinal infections. Shake the bottle well before each use to mix the medication evenly. If you are using liquid nystatin for a mouth infection, place half of the dose in each side of the mouth and hold it there or swish it throughout the mouth for several minutes before swallowing. Good oral hygiene, including proper care of dentures, is important for the cure of mouth infections.

If you are using liquid nystatin for an intestinal infection, just swallow the liquid you measured from the dropper; there is no need to hold it or swish it in your mouth.

Nystatin skin ointment or cream usually is used several

times a day for skin infections. Wash the affected area thoroughly. Apply a small amount of cream or ointment and gently and thoroughly massage it into your skin. If you use this medication on your face, keep it out of your eyes.

If you are using powder for infected feet, dust the powder inside your shoes and stockings as well as on your feet.

Nystatin vaginal tablets and cream usually are used once or twice a day for vaginal infections. Nystatin vaginal tablets usually are used for 2 weeks in women who are not pregnant and for 3-6 weeks before delivery in pregnant women. Continue to use the vaginal tablets and cream even if symptoms improve after a few days. Insert the vaginal tablets or cream high into the vagina. They each come with a special applicator for inserting them and directions. Unwrap the vaginal tablets just before inserting them. Read the directions provided with the tablets or cream and follow these steps:

1. Fill the special applicator to the level indicated.
2. Lie on your back with your knees drawn upward and spread apart.
3. Gently insert the applicator into your vagina and push the plunger to release the medication.
4. Withdraw the applicator and wash it with soap and warm water.
5. Wash your hands promptly to avoid spreading the infection.

You may wish to wear a sanitary napkin while using the vaginal cream to protect your clothing against stains. Do not use a tampon because it will absorb the drug. Do not douche unless your doctor tells you to do so. Continue using nystatin vaginal cream or tablets even if you get your period during treatment.

What special precautions should I follow?

Before taking nystatin,

- tell your doctor and pharmacist if you are allergic to nystatin or any other drugs.
- tell your doctor and pharmacist what prescription and nonprescription medications you are taking, including vitamins.
- tell your doctor if you are pregnant, plan to become pregnant, or are breast-feeding. If you become pregnant while taking nystatin, call your doctor.

What should I do if I forget to take a dose?

Take the missed dose as soon as you remember it. However, if it is almost time for the next dose, skip the missed dose and continue your regular dosing schedule. Do not take a double dose to make up for a missed one.

What side effects can this medicine cause?

Nystatin may cause side effects. Tell your doctor if any of these symptoms from the vaginal tablets and cream or skin ointment or cream are severe or do not go away:

- itching
- irritation
- burning

If you experience any of the following symptoms from the oral tablets and liquid, call your doctor immediately:

- diarrhea
- upset stomach
- stomach pain
- skin rash

If you experience a serious side effect, you or your doctor may send a report to the Food and Drug Administration's (FDA) MedWatch Adverse Event Reporting program online [at http://www.fda.gov/MedWatch/index.html] or by phone [1-800-332-1088].

What storage conditions are needed for this medicine?

Keep this medication in the container it came in, tightly closed, and out of reach of children. Store the tablets and liquid at room temperature and away from excess heat and moisture (not in the bathroom). Store nystatin powder, lozenges (pastilles), and vaginal tablets and cream in the refrigerator. Do not allow nystatin to freeze. Throw away any medication that is outdated or no longer needed. Talk to your pharmacist about the proper disposal of your medication.

What other information should I know?

Keep all appointments with your doctor and the laboratory. Your doctor will order certain lab tests to check your response to nystatin.

Do not let anyone else take your medication. Your prescription is probably not refillable. If you still have symptoms of infection after you finish the nystatin, call your doctor.

Talk to your doctor, pharmacist, or other healthcare professional if you have questions about dosing information for your medication.

Nystatin and Triamcinolone

(nye stat′ in) (trye am sin′ oh lone)

Brand Name: Mycogen II®, Mycolog-II®, Myconel®, Myco-Triacet II®, Mytrex®, Tri-Statin®

Why is this medicine prescribed?

The combination of nystatin and triamcinolone is used to treat fungal skin infections. It relieves itching, inflammation, and pain.

This medication is sometimes prescribed for other uses; ask your doctor or pharmacist for more information.

How should this medicine be used?

The combination of nystatin and triamcinolone comes in ointment and cream to be applied to the skin. This medication usually is applied twice a day for no longer than 2 weeks. Follow the directions on your prescription label carefully, and ask your doctor or pharmacist to explain any part you do not understand. Use nystatin and triamcinolone exactly as directed. Do not use more or less of it or use it more often than prescribed by your doctor.

Wash the affected area thoroughly. Apply a small amount of cream or ointment and gently and thoroughly massage it into your skin.

If you use this medication on your face, keep it out of your eyes.

If you are using this medication on a child's diaper area, do not place tightly fitting diapers or plastic pants on the child. They can increase the absorption of triamcinolone, which can affect the child's growth.

What special precautions should I follow?

Before using nystatin and triamcinolone,

- tell your doctor and pharmacist if you are allergic to nystatin, triamcinolone, or any other drugs.
- tell your doctor and pharmacist what prescription and nonprescription medications you are taking, including vitamins.
- tell your doctor if you are pregnant, plan to become pregnant, or are breast-feeding. If you become pregnant while using nystatin and triamcinolone, call your doctor.

What should I do if I forget to take a dose?

Apply the missed dose as soon as you remember it. However, if it is almost time for the next dose, skip the missed dose and continue your regular dosing schedule. Do not apply a double dose to make up for a missed one.

What side effects can this medicine cause?

Nystatin and triamcinolone may cause side effects. If you experience any of the following symptoms, call your doctor immediately:

- acne
- skin sores
- itching
- irritation
- burning
- stinging

If you experience a serious side effect, you or your doctor may send a report to the Food and Drug Administration's (FDA) MedWatch Adverse Event Reporting program online [at http://www.fda.gov/MedWatch/index.html] or by phone [1-800-332-1088].

What storage conditions are needed for this medicine?

Keep this medication in the container it came in, tightly closed, and out of reach of children. Store it at room temperature and away from excess heat and moisture (not in the bathroom). Throw away any medication that is outdated or no longer needed. Talk to your pharmacist about the proper disposal of your medication.

What other information should I know?

Keep all appointments with your doctor. This medication is for external use only. Do not let nystatin and triamcinolone get into your eyes, nose, or mouth, and do not swallow it. Do not apply dressings, bandages, cosmetics, lotions, or other skin medications to the area being treated unless your doctor tells you.

Do not let anyone else use your medication. Ask your pharmacist any questions you have about refilling your prescription. If you still have symptoms of infection after you finish the nystatin and triamcinolone, call your doctor. Tell your doctor if your skin condition gets worse or does not go away.

Talk to your doctor, pharmacist, or other healthcare professional if you have questions about dosing information for your medication.

Octreotide Injection

(ok tree′ oh tide)

Brand Name: Sandostatin LAR® Depot, Sandostatin®

About Your Treatment

Your doctor has ordered octreotide to help control diarrhea and other symptoms of abdominal illness and other medical conditions such as intestinal tumors. Octreotide will be either injected subcutaneously (beneath the skin) or added to an intravenous fluid that will drip through a needle or catheter placed in your vein for 15-30 minutes, one to four times a day. This medication is sometimes prescribed for other uses; ask your doctor or pharmacist for more information.

Your health care provider (doctor, nurse, or pharmacist) may measure the effectiveness and side effects of your treatment using laboratory tests and physical examinations. It is important to keep all appointments with your doctor and the laboratory. The length of treatment depends on how you respond to the medication.

Precautions

Before administering octreotide,

- tell your doctor and pharmacist if you are allergic to octreotide or any other drugs.
- tell your doctor and pharmacist what prescription and nonprescription medications you are taking, especially antidiarrheals, cyclosporine (Neoral, Sandimmune), medications for diabetes or high blood pressure, and vitamins.
- tell your doctor if you have or have ever had diabetes or kidney or gallbladder disease.

- tell your doctor if you are pregnant, plan to become pregnant, or are breast-feeding. If you become pregnant while taking octreotide, call your doctor.
- you should know that this drug may make you drowsy. Do not drive a car or operate machinery until you know how this drug affects you.
- remember that alcohol can add to the drowsiness caused by this drug.

Administering Your Medication

Before you administer octreotide, look at the solution closely. It should be clear and free of floating material. Gently squeeze the bag or observe the solution container to make sure there are no leaks. Do not use the solution if it is discolored, if it contains particles, or if the bag or container leaks. Use a new solution, but show the damaged one to your health care provider.

It is important that you use your medication exactly as directed. Do not change your dosing schedule without talking to your health care provider. Your health care provider may tell you to stop your infusion if you have a mechanical problem (such as a blockage in the tubing, needle, or catheter); if you have to stop an infusion, call your health care provider immediately so your therapy can continue.

Side Effects

Octreotide may cause side effects. Pain or burning at the injection site may last for up to 15 minutes. Tell your health care provider if any of these symptoms are severe or do not go away:

- upset stomach
- vomiting
- diarrhea
- stomach pain
- bloating
- flatulence
- loose stools
- loss of appetite or increased hunger

If you experience any of the following symptoms, call your health care provider immediately:

- increased urination
- increased thirst
- difficulty breathing
- chills
- shakiness
- sweating
- weakness

If you experience a serious side effect, you or your doctor may send a report to the Food and Drug Administration's (FDA) MedWatch Adverse Event Reporting program online [at http://www.fda.gov/MedWatch/index.html] or by phone [1-800-332-1088].

Storage Conditions

- Your health care provider probably will give you a several-day supply of octreotide at a time. You will be told to store it in the refrigerator.

- Take your next dose from the refrigerator 1 hour before using it; place it in a clean, dry area to allow it to warm to room temperature.

Store your medication only as directed. Make sure you understand what you need to store your medication properly.

Keep your supplies in a clean, dry place when you are not using them, and keep all medications and supplies out of reach of children. Your health care provider will tell you how to throw away used needles, syringes, tubing, and containers to avoid accidental injury.

Overdose

In case of overdose, call your local poison control center at 1-800-222-1222. If the victim has collapsed or is not breathing, call local emergency services at 911.

Signs of Infection

If you are receiving octreotide in your vein or under your skin, you need to know the symptoms of a catheter-related infection (an infection where the needle enters your vein or skin). If you experience any of these effects near your intravenous catheter, tell your health care provider as soon as possible:

- tenderness
- warmth
- irritation
- drainage
- redness
- swelling
- pain

Dosage Facts
For Informational Purposes

Caution: Do not change your dose, how often you take your medication, or the length of time you are to take it without first talking to your healthcare provider.

The following dosage information was written using medical language for doctors and other healthcare professionals and is provided here for you to check your dosage. The dosage of this drug may differ for different patients. Therefore, always follow your doctor's instructions or the directions on the label. Contact your healthcare provider or pharmacist if you have any questions about the specific dosage of your medication after reviewing this information.

General Dosage Information

Available as octreotide acetate; dosage expressed in terms of octreotide.

Usual dosages are not well defined because of the wide variation in disease severity and response.

Individualize dosage according to patient response (symptomatic relief, biochemical response) and tolerance.

Initiate therapy with immediate-release injection administered sub-Q. If patient responds well after ≥2 weeks of sub-Q therapy, switch to long-acting suspension administered IM.

Maintain therapy with sub-Q injections of immediate-release injection for at least 2 weeks to establish tolerance before switching to long-acting suspension.

Pediatric Patients

Congenital Hyperinsulinism†

IV OR SUB-Q:

- Dosages of 3–40 mcg/kg (immediate-release injection) daily have been used in neonates and infants to stabilize plasma glucose levels prior to pancreatectomy, to treat recurrent postoperative hypoglycemia, and as an alternative medical treatment to diazoxide for control of hypoglycemia; however, experience in pediatric patients is limited.

Adult Patients

General

SUB-Q:

- Initially, 50–100 mcg (immediate-release injection) 1–3 times daily (usually 50 mcg once or twice daily). Subsequent dosage may be increased gradually according to patient response and tolerance and usually is given 2 or 3 times daily.

Carcinoid Tumors

SUB-Q:

- Initiate therapy with 100–600 mcg of immediate-release injection daily (average 300 mcg daily), given in 2–4 divided doses for at least 2 weeks.
- Median maintenance dosage (immediate-release injection) in clinical studies was approximately 450 mcg daily, clinical and biochemical benefits were obtained with as little as 50 mcg daily, dosages up to 1500 mcg daily sometimes were required; experience with dosages >750 mcg daily is limited.
- When switching to IM injection of long-acting suspension, continue sub-Q injections of immediate-release formulation at the previous dosage during at least the first 2 weeks of therapy with the long-acting suspension; sub-Q therapy (immediate-release injection) may be needed as long as 3–4 weeks to prevent exacerbation of disease symptoms.
- Temporary concomitant use of sub-Q therapy with immediate-release injection (at the dosage used prior to switching to the long-acting suspension) may be required to control exacerbation of symptoms that occur during IM therapy with long-acting suspension.

Carcinoid Crisis (Treatment)

Administer immediate-release injection by rapid IV injection or prolonged IV infusion.

IV:

- 50–500 mcg (immediate-release injection) administered by rapid IV injection and repeated as necessary.
- Alternatively, 50 mcg/hour (immediate-release injection) infused IV for 8–24 hours.

Carcinoid Crisis (Prophylaxis)

SUB-Q:

- 250–500 mcg (immediate-release injection) 1–2 hours prior to anesthetic induction has been used to prevent carcinoid crisis associated with surgery.
- 150–250 mcg (immediate-release injection) every 6–8 hours 24–48 hours prior to anesthetic induction or initiation of chemotherapy has been used.

Vasoactive Intestinal Peptide-secreting Tumors

SUB-Q:

- Initiate therapy with 200–300 mcg of immediate-release injection daily given in 2–4 divided doses for at least 2 weeks.
- Dosages range from 100–750 mcg (immediate-release injection) daily during this period; >450 mcg daily usually not required.
- When switching to IM injection of long-acting suspension, continue sub-Q injections of immediate-release injection at the previous dosage during at least the first 2 weeks of therapy with the long-acting suspension; sub-Q therapy (immediate-release injection) may be needed as long as 3–4 weeks to prevent exacerbation of disease symptoms.
- Temporary concomitant use of sub-Q therapy with immediate-release injection (at the dosage used prior to switching to the long-acting suspension) may be required to control exacerbation of symptoms that occur during IM therapy with long-acting suspension.

Acromegaly

Initiate therapy with low dosage immediate-release injection administered sub-Q to promote tolerance to adverse GI effects during titration.

Patients responding well to immediate-release injection (based on GH and IGF-I levels) and who tolerate the drug may be switched to the long-acting suspension administered IM.

SUB-Q:

- Initiate therapy with 150 mcg (immediate-release injection) daily given in 3 divided doses.
- Titrate dosage by tolerance, clinical effect, and evaluation of multiple GH levels. Adjust dosage based on GH levels measured at 1–4 hour intervals for 8–12 hours after sub-Q injection or alternatively, based on a single IGF-I level measured 2 weeks after initiation of therapy or a dosage change.
- 300–600 mcg (immediate-release injection) daily given in 3 divided doses generally results in maximum effect; up to 1500 mcg daily given in 3 divided doses may be needed in some cases.

Prescribing Limits

Adult Patients

General

Maximum recommended dosage has not been established; however, dosages ≥5 times usual (e.g., 1500–3000 mcg daily) have been used, and substantially higher single doses (e.g., up to 120 mg infused IV over 8 hours) reportedly have been administered without serious adverse effect.

Potential long-term effects (e.g., adverse GI and biliary effects) of relatively high dosages have not been fully elucidated. Possibility that clinical and/or biochemical response may diminish to some extent during prolonged therapy should be considered.

Carcinoid Tumors

SUB-Q:

- Limited experience with daily dosages exceeding 750 mcg (immediate-release injection); dosages up to 1500 mcg daily have been used.

Ofloxacin Ophthalmic

(oh flox′ a sin)

Brand Name: Ocuflox®
Also available generically.

Why is this medicine prescribed?

Ofloxacin ophthalmic is used to treat bacterial infections of the eye, including conjunctivitis (pink eye) and ulcers of the cornea. Ofloxacin is in a class of medications called quinolone antibiotics. It works by killing bacterial cells that cause infection.

How should this medicine be used?

Ofloxacin comes as an eyedrop to apply to the eye. It is usually applied to the affected eye(s) four or more times a day. Follow the directions on your prescription label carefully, and ask your doctor or pharmacist to explain any part you do not understand. Use ofloxacin exactly as directed. Do not use more or less of it or use it more often than prescribed by your doctor.

To apply the eyedrops, follow these steps:
1. Wash your hands thoroughly with soap and water.
2. Use a mirror or have someone else put the drops in your eye.
3. Make sure the end of the dropper is not chipped or cracked.
4. Avoid touching the dropper against your eye or anything else.
5. Hold the dropper tip down at all times to prevent drops from flowing back into the bottle and contaminating the remaining contents.
6. Lie down or tilt your head back.
7. Holding the bottle between your thumb and index finger, place the dropper as near as possible to your eyelid without touching it.
8. Brace the remaining fingers of that hand against your cheek or nose.
9. With the index finger of your other hand, pull the lower lid of the eye down to form a pocket.

10. Drop the prescribed number of drops into the pocket made by the lower lid and the eye. Placing the drops on the surface of the eyeball can cause stinging.
11. Close your eye and press lightly against the lower lid with your finger for 2-3 minutes to keep the medication in the eye. Do not blink.
12. Replace and tighten the cap right away. Do not wipe or rinse it off.
13. Wipe off any excess liquid from your cheek with a clean tissue. Wash your hands again.

Are there other uses for this medicine?

This medication may be prescribed for other uses; ask your doctor or pharmacist for more information.

What special precautions should I follow?

Before using ofloxacin ophthalmic,
- tell your doctor and pharmacist if you are allergic to ofloxacin, benzalkonium chloride, ciprofloxacin (Cipro), enoxacin (Penetrex), levofloxacin (Levaquin), lomefloxacin (Maxaquin), norfloxacin (Noroxin), sparfloxacin (Zagam), cinoxacin (Cinobac), nalidixic acid (NegGram), or any other medications.
- tell your doctor and pharmacist what prescription and nonprescription medications, vitamins, nutritional supplements, and herbal products you are taking. Be sure to mention any of the following: anticoagulants ('blood thinners') such as warfarin (Coumadin), cyclosporine (Neoral, Sandimmune), and theophylline (Theo-Dur). Your doctor may need to change the doses of your medications or monitor you carefully for side effects.
- tell your doctor if you are pregnant, plan to become pregnant, or are breast-feeding. If you become pregnant while using ofloxacin ophthalmic, call your doctor.
- you should know that ofloxacin solution contains benzalkonium chloride, which can be absorbed by soft contact lenses. Remove your contact lenses before applying ofloxacin and put them back in 10 minutes later.

What special dietary instructions should I follow?

Talk to your doctor about drinking coffee and other beverages containing caffeine while using this medicine.

What should I do if I forget to take a dose?

Apply the missed dose as soon as you remember it. However, if it is almost time for the next dose, skip the missed dose and continue your regular dosing schedule. Do not apply a double dose to make up for a missed one.

What side effects can this medicine cause?

Ofloxacin ophthalmic may cause side effects. Tell your doctor if any of these symptoms are severe or do not go away:
- eye burning or discomfort
- eye stinging or redness

- tearing eyes
- sensitivity to light
- blurred vision
- dry eyes

Some side effects can be serious. The following symptoms are uncommon, but if you experience any of them, call your doctor immediately:

- skin rash
- hives
- itching
- difficulty breathing or swallowing
- swelling of the face, throat, tongue, lips, eyes, hands, feet, ankles, or lower legs

Ofloxacin ophthalmic may cause other side effects. Call your doctor if you have any unusual problems while taking this medication.

If you experience a serious side effect, you or your doctor may send a report to the Food and Drug Administration's (FDA) MedWatch Adverse Event Reporting program online [at http://www.fda.gov/MedWatch/index.html] or by phone [1-800-332-1088].

What storage conditions are needed for this medicine?

Keep this medication in the container it came in, tightly closed, and out of reach of children. Store it at room temperature and away from excess heat and moisture (not in the bathroom). Throw away any medication that is outdated or no longer needed. Talk to your pharmacist about the proper disposal of your medication.

What other information should I know?

Keep all appointments with your doctor.

Do not let anyone else use your medication. Ask your pharmacist any questions you have about refilling your prescription.

Dosage Facts
For Informational Purposes

Caution: Do not change your dose, how often you take your medication, or the length of time you are to take it without first talking to your healthcare provider.

The following dosage information was written using medical language for doctors and other healthcare professionals and is provided here for you to check your dosage. The dosage of this drug may differ for different patients. Therefore, always follow your doctor's instructions or the directions on the label. Contact your healthcare provider or pharmacist if you have any questions about the specific dosage of your medication after reviewing this information.

Pediatric Patients

Bacterial Ophthalmic Infections
Conjunctivitis

OPHTHALMIC:

- Children≥1 year of age: 1 or 2 drops of 0.3% solution into affected eye(s) every 2–4 hours while awake for 2 days, then 1–2 drops 4 times daily for up to 5 more days.

Keratitis

OPHTHALMIC:

- Children≥1 year of age: 1 or 2 drops of 0.3% solution into affected eye(s) every 30 minutes while awake and then 4 and 6 hours after retiring, for 2 days. Beginning on the third day, instill 1 or 2 drops into affected eye(s) every hour while awake for up to an additional 4–6 days. Afterward, may instill 1 or 2 drops into affected eye(s) 4 times daily for additional 3 days or until clinical cure achieved.

Adult Patients

Bacterial Ophthalmic Infections
Conjunctivitis

OPHTHALMIC:

- 1 or 2 drops of 0.3% solution into affected eye(s) every 2–4 hours while awake for 2 days, then 1–2 drops 4 times daily for up to 5 more days.

Keratitis

OPHTHALMIC:

- 1 or 2 drops of a 0.3% solution into affected eye(s) every 30 minutes while awake and then 4 and 6 hours after retiring, for 2 days. Beginning on third day, instill 1 or 2 drops into affected eye(s) every hour while awake for up to an additional 4–6 days. Afterward, may instill 1 or 2 drops into affected eye(s) 4 times daily for additional 3 days or until clinical cure achieved.

Ofloxacin Oral

(oh floks' a sin)

Brand Name: Floxin®
Also available generically.

Why is this medicine prescribed?

Ofloxacin is an antibiotic used to treat certain infections caused by bacteria, such as pneumonia; bronchitis; venereal disease (VD); and prostate, skin, and urinary tract infections. Antibiotics will not work for colds, flu, or other viral infections.

How should this medicine be used?

Ofloxacin comes as a tablet to take by mouth. It is usually taken with or without food every 12 hours (twice a day) for 3-10 days. Some infections may take up to 6 weeks or longer. To treat VD, a single dose is taken. Follow the directions on your prescription label carefully, and ask your doctor or pharmacist to explain any part you do not understand. Take ofloxacin exactly as directed. Do not take more or less of it or take it more often than prescribed by your doctor.

The tablets should be taken with a full glass of water. Continue to take ofloxacin even if you feel well. Do not stop taking ofloxacin without talking to your doctor.

Are there other uses for this medicine?

This medication may be prescribed for other uses; ask your doctor or pharmacist for more information.

What special precautions should I follow?

Before taking ofloxacin,

- tell your doctor and pharmacist if you are allergic to ofloxacin, ciprofloxacin (Cipro), enoxacin (Penetrex), levofloxacin (Levaquin), lomefloxacin (Maxaquin), norfloxacin (Noroxin), sparfloxacin (Zagam), cinoxacin (Cinobac), nalidixic acid (NegGram), or any other medications.
- tell your doctor and pharmacist what prescription and nonprescription medications, vitamins, nutritional supplements, and herbal products you are taking or plan to take. Be sure to mention any of the following: other antibiotics, anticoagulants ('blood thinners') such as warfarin (Coumadin), cancer chemotherapy agents, cimetidine (Tagamet), cyclosporine (Neoral, Sandimmune), diabetes medication, probenecid (Benemid), sucralfate (Carafate), and theophylline (Theo-Dur). Your doctor may need to change the doses of your medications or monitor you carefully for side effects.
- if you are taking mineral supplements; antacids containing aluminum, calcium, or magnesium (Maalox, Mylanta, Tums); didanosine (Videx) chewable/buffered tablets or oral solution; sucralfate (Carafate); or vitamins containing iron or zinc, take ofloxacin two hours before or two hours after these medications.
- tell your doctor if you have or have ever had kidney or liver disease, diabetes, epilepsy, colitis, stomach problems, vision problems, heart disease, or history of stroke.
- tell your doctor if you are pregnant, plan to become pregnant, or are breast-feeding. If you become pregnant while taking ofloxacin, call your doctor.
- if you are having surgery, including dental surgery, tell the doctor or dentist that you are taking ofloxacin.
- you should know that this medication may cause dizziness, lightheadedness, and tiredness. Do not drive a car or work on dangerous machines until you know how ofloxacin will affect you.
- plan to avoid unnecessary or prolonged exposure to sunlight and to wear protective clothing, sunglasses, and sunscreen. Ofloxacin may make your skin sensitive to sunlight.

What special dietary instructions should I follow?

Drink at least eight full glasses of water or other liquid every day.

What should I do if I forget to take a dose?

Take the missed dose as soon as you remember it. However, if it is almost time for the next dose, skip the missed dose and continue your regular dosing schedule. Do not take a double dose to make up for a missed one.

What side effects can this medicine cause?

Ofloxacin may cause side effects. Tell your doctor if any of these symptoms are severe or do not go away:

- upset stomach
- diarrhea
- vomiting
- stomach pain
- headache
- restlessness
- difficulty falling asleep or staying asleep

Some side effects can be serious. If you experience any of these symptoms, call your doctor immediately:

- skin rash
- itching
- hives
- difficulty breathing or swallowing
- swelling of the face or throat
- yellowing of the skin or eyes
- dark urine
- pale or dark stools
- blood in urine
- unusual tiredness
- sunburn
- seizures or convulsions
- vaginal infection
- vision changes
- pain, inflammation, or rupture of a tendon

Ofloxacin may cause other side effects. Call your doctor if you have any unusual problems while taking this medication.

What storage conditions are needed for this medicine?

Keep this medication in the container it came in, tightly closed, and out of reach of children. Store it at room temperature and away from excess heat and moisture (not in the bathroom). Keep away from light. Throw away any medication that is outdated or no longer needed. Talk to your pharmacist about the proper disposal of your medication.

What should I do in case of overdose?

In case of overdose, call your local poison control center at 1-800-222-1222. If the victim has collapsed or is not breathing, call local emergency services at 911.

What other information should I know?

Keep all appointments with your doctor and the laboratory. Your doctor will order certain lab tests to check your response to ofloxacin.

Before having any laboratory test, tell your doctor and the laboratory personnel that you are taking ofloxacin.

Do not let anyone else take your medication. Your prescription is probably not refillable. If you still have symptoms of infection after you finish the ofloxacin, call your doctor.

Dosage Facts
For Informational Purposes

Caution: Do not change your dose, how often you take your medication, or the length of time you are to take it without first talking to your healthcare provider.

The following dosage information was written using medical language for doctors and other healthcare professionals and is provided here for you to check your dosage. The dosage of this drug may differ for different patients. Therefore, always follow your doctor's instructions or the directions on the label. Contact your healthcare provider or pharmacist if you have any questions about the specific dosage of your medication after reviewing this information.

Pediatric Patients

Mycobacterial Infections†
Single-lesion Paucibacillary Leprosy†

ORAL:
- Children 5–14 years of age: WHO recommends a single-dose ROM regimen that includes a single 300-mg dose of rifampin, a single 200-mg dose of ofloxacin, and a single 50-mg dose of minocycline.
- Children <5 years of age: WHO recommends that an appropriately adjusted dose of each drug in the above single-dose ROM regimen be used.

Adult Patients

General Adult Dosage

ORAL:
- 200–400 mg every 12 hours.
- Duration of treatment depends on the type and severity of infection and should be determined by clinical and bacteriologic response of the patient.

GI Infections
Treatment of Travelers' Diarrhea†

ORAL:
- 300 mg twice daily for 1–3 days.

Prevention of Travelers' Diarrhea†

ORAL:
- 300 mg once daily during the period of risk.
- Although anti-infective prophylaxis generally is discouraged, some clinicians state that it can be given during the period of risk (for ≤3 weeks) beginning the day of travel and continuing for 1 or 2 days after leaving the area of risk.

Respiratory Tract Infections
Acute Bacterial Exacerbations of Chronic Bronchitis

ORAL:
- 400 mg every 12 hours for 10 days.

Community-acquired Pneumonia

ORAL:
- 400 mg every 12 hours for 10 days.

Skin and Skin Structure Infections
Uncomplicated Infections

ORAL:
- 400 mg every 12 hours for 10 days.

Urinary Tract Infections (UTIs) and Prostatitis
Uncomplicated Cystitis Caused by E. coli or K. pneumoniae

ORAL:
- 200 mg every 12 hours for 3 days.

Uncomplicated Cystitis Caused by Other Susceptible Bacteria

ORAL:
- 200 mg every 12 hours for 7 days.

Complicated UTIs

ORAL:
- 200 mg every 12 hours for 10 days.

Prostatitis Caused by E. coli

ORAL:
- 300 mg every 12 hours for 6 weeks or longer.

Anthrax†
Postexposure Prophylaxis Following Exposure in the Context of Biologic Warfare or Bioterrorism†

ORAL:
- 400 mg twice daily for ≥60 days.
- Optimum duration of postexposure prophylaxis after an inhalation exposure to *B. anthracis* spores is unclear, but prolonged postexposure prophylaxis usually required. A duration of 60 days may be adequate for a low-dose exposure, but a duration >4 months may be necessary to reduce the risk following a high-dose exposure. CDC, US Working Group on Civilian Biodefense, and US Army Medical Research Institute of Infectious Diseases (USAMRIID) recommend that postexposure prophylaxis in unvaccinated individuals be continued for ≥60 days following a confirmed exposure (inlcuding in laboratory workers with confirmed exposures to *B. anthracis* cultures). The USPHS Advisory Committee on Immunization Practices (ACIP) and USAMRIID recommend that individuals who are partially or fully vaccinated against anthrax receive postexposure prophylaxis for ≥30 days; if given in conjunction with anthrax vaccine, continue prophylaxis for at least 7–14 days after the third vaccine dose.

Treatment of Inhalational Anthrax in a Mass Casualty Setting†

ORAL:
• 400 mg twice daily for ≥60 days.

Brucellosis†

ORAL:
• 400 mg once daily in conjunction with oral rifampin (600 mg once daily) given for 6 weeks was effective in some patients.

Chlamydial Infections
Urogenital Infections

ORAL:
• 300 mg every 12 hours for 7 days.

Gonorrhea and Associated Infections
Uncomplicated Urethral, Endocervical, or Rectal†
Gonorrhea

ORAL:
• 400 mg as a single dose has been used for infections caused by susceptible *Neisseria gonorrhea*.
• Because of increased prevalence of quinolone-resistant *Neisseria gonorrhoeae* (QRNG), CDC no longer recommends fluoroquinolones for treatment of gonorrhea or any associated infections involving *N. gonorrhoeae* (e.g., PID, epididymitis).
• Unless the presence of coexisting chlamydial infection has been excluded by appropriate testing, patients being treated for gonorrhea should also receive an anti-infective regimen effective for presumptive treatment of chlamydia (e.g., a single dose of oral azithromycin or a 7-day regimen of oral doxycycline).

Disseminated Gonococcal Infections†

ORAL:
• 400 twice daily recommended by CDC; given to complete ≥1 week of treatment after an initial parenteral regimen of ceftriaxone, cefotaxime, ceftizoxime (no longer commercially available in the US), or spectinomycin (not currently commercially available in the US).
• Because of increased prevalence of quinolone-resistant *Neisseria gonorrhoeae* (QRNG), CDC no longer recommends fluoroquinolones for treatment of gonorrhea or any associated infections involving *N. gonorrhoeae* (e.g., PID, epididymitis). Use as an alternative treatment option for disseminated infections *only* if in vitro susceptibility can be documented by culture.
• Unless the presence of coexisting chlamydial infection has been excluded by appropriate testing, patients being treated for gonorrhea should also receive an anti-infective regimen effective for presumptive treatment of chlamydia (e.g., a single dose of oral azithromycin or a 7-day regimen of oral doxycycline).

Epididymitis†

ORAL:
• 300 mg every 12 hours for 10 days recommended by CDC and others.
• Should be used *only* when epididymitis† most likely caused by sexually transmitted enteric bacteria (e.g., *E. coli*) or when culture or nucleic acid amplification tests are negative for *N. gonorrhoeae*.

Legionnaires' Disease†

ORAL:
• 400 mg every 12 hours for 2–3 weeks.

Mycobacterial Infections†
Leprosy†

ORAL:
• For treatment of multibacillary leprosy† in those who cannot receive rifampin because of adverse effects, intercurrent disease (e.g., chronic hepatitis), or infection with rifampin-resistant *Mycobacterium leprae*, WHO recommends supervised administration of a regimen of clofazimine (50 mg daily), ofloxacin (400 mg daily), and minocycline (100 mg daily) given for 6 months, followed by a regimen of clofazimine (50 mg daily) and minocycline (100 mg daily) given for at least an additional 18 months.
• For treatment of multibacillary leprosy† in adults who will not accept or cannot tolerate clofazimine, WHO recommends supervised administration of a once-monthly ROM regimen that includes rifampin (600 mg once monthly), ofloxacin (400 mg once monthly), and minocycline (100 mg once monthly) given for 24 months.
• For treatment of single-lesion paucibacillary leprosy† in certain patient groups, WHO recommends a single-dose ROM regimen that includes a single 600-mg dose of rifampin, a single 400-mg dose of ofloxacin, and a single 100-mg dose of minocycline.

M. fortuitum Infections†

ORAL:
• 300 or 600 mg once daily for 3–6 months.

Nongonococcal Urethritis and Cervicitis

ORAL:
• 300 mg every 12 hours for 7 days.

Pelvic Inflammatory Disease

ORAL:
• 400 mg every 12 hours for 10–14 days; used with or without oral metronidazole (500 mg twice daily for 14 days).
• Should be used for treatment of PID *only* when cephalosporins are not feasible, community prevalence and individual risk of gonorrhea is low, and in vitro susceptibility has been confirmed.

Rickettsial Infections†
Mediterranean Spotted Fever†

ORAL:
• 200 mg every 12 hours for 7 days was effective in some patients.

Q Fever†

ORAL:
• Acute Q fever† pneumonia caused by *Coxiella burnetii*: 600 mg daily for up to 16 days has been used.
• Q fever endocarditis†: 200 mg 3 times daily in conjunction with oral doxycycline (100 mg twice daily); long-term treatment (≥4 years) may be required.

Typhoid Fever and Other Salmonella Infections†
Mild to Moderate Typhoid Fever†

ORAL:
• 200–400 mg every 12 hours for 7–14 days.

Hepatic Impairment

- Maximum dosage of 400 mg daily in those with severe hepatic impairment (e.g., cirrhosis with or without ascites).

Renal Impairment

- Dosage adjustments required in adults with $Cl_{cr} \leq 50$ mL/minute.

Dosage in Adults with Renal Impairment

Cl_{cr} (mL/min)	Dosage
20–50	Usual initial dose, then usual dose once every 24 hours
<20	Usual initial dose, then 50% of usual dose once every 24 hours
Hemodialysis Patients	Initial 200-mg dose, then 100 mg once daily; supplemental doses not required after dialysis

Geriatric Patients

- No dosage adjustments except those related to renal impairment.

† *Use is not currently included in the labeling approved by the US Food and Drug Administration.*

Ofloxacin Otic

(oh floks′ a sin)

Brand Name: Floxin® Otic
Also available generically.

Why is this medicine prescribed?

Ofloxacin otic is used to treat outer ear infections in adults and children, chronic (long-lasting) middle ear infections in adults and children with a perforated eardrum (a condition where the eardrum has a hole in it), and acute (suddenly occurring) middle ear infections in children with ear tubes. Ofloxacin otic is in a class of medications called quinolone antibiotics. It works by killing the bacteria that cause infection.

How should this medicine be used?

Ofloxacin otic comes as a solution (liquid) to place into the ear. It is usually used once or twice a day for 7-14 days, depending on your condition. Use ofloxacin otic at around the same time(s) every day. Follow the directions on your prescription label carefully, and ask your doctor or pharmacist to explain any part you do not understand. Use of-loxacin otic exactly as directed. Do not use more or less of it or use it more often than prescribed by your doctor.

Ofloxacin otic is only for use in the ears. Do not use in the eyes.

You should begin to feel better during the first few days of treatment with ofloxacin otic. If your symptoms do not improve after one week or get worse, call your doctor.

Use ofloxacin otic until you finish the prescription, even if you feel better. If you stop using ofloxacin otic too soon or skip doses, your infection may not be completely treated and the bacteria may become resistant to antibiotics.

To use the eardrops, follow these steps:

1. Hold the bottle or single-dispensing container(s) in your hand for 1 or 2 minutes to warm the solution.
2. Lie down with the affected ear upward.
3. Place the prescribed number of drops or the contents of the prescribed number of single-dispensing containers into your ear.
4. If you are using a bottle of solution, be careful not to touch the tip to your ear, fingers, or any other surface.
5. For middle ear infections, push the tragus (small flap of cartilage just in front of the ear canal near the face) of the ear inward four times so that the drops will enter the middle ear.
6. Remain lying down with the affected ear upward for 5 minutes.
7. Repeat steps 1-6 for the opposite ear if necessary.

Are there other uses for this medicine?

This medication may be prescribed for other uses; ask your doctor or pharmacist for more information.

What special precautions should I follow?

Before using ofloxacin otic,

- tell your doctor and pharmacist if you are allergic to ofloxacin (Floxin), cinoxacin (Cinobac) (not available in the U.S.), ciprofloxacin (Cipro), enoxacin (Penetrex) (not available in the U.S.), gatifloxacin (Tequin) (not available in the U.S.), gemifloxacin (Factive), levofloxacin (Levaquin), lomefloxacin (Maxaquin), moxifloxacin (Avelox), nalidixic acid (NegGram), norfloxacin (Noroxin), sparfloxacin (Zagam) (not available in the U.S.), trovafloxacin and alatrofloxacin combination (Trovan) (not available in the U.S.), or any other medications.
- tell your doctor and pharmacist what prescription and nonprescription medications, vitamins, nutritional supplements, and herbal products you are taking or plan to take.
- tell your doctor if you are pregnant, plan to become pregnant, or are breast-feeding. If you become pregnant while using ofloxacin otic, call your doctor.
- you should know that you must keep your infected ear(s) clean and dry while using ofloxacin otic. Avoid getting the infected ear(s) wet while bathing, and avoid swimming unless your doctor has told you otherwise.

What special dietary instructions should I follow?

Unless your doctor tells you otherwise, continue your normal diet.

What should I do if I forget to take a dose?

Apply the missed dose as soon as you remember it. However, if it is almost time for the next dose, skip the missed dose and continue your regular dosing schedule. Do not use extra eardrops to make up for a missed dose.

What side effects can this medicine cause?

Ofloxacin otic may cause side effects. Tell your doctor if any of these symptoms are severe or do not go away:

- ear itching or pain
- change in taste
- dizziness

Some side effects can be serious. If you experience any of these symptoms, stop using ofloxacin otic call your doctor immediately:

- rash
- hives
- swelling of the face, throat, tongue, lips, eyes, hands, feet, ankles, or lower legs
- hoarseness
- difficulty swallowing or breathing

Ofloxacin otic may cause other side effects. Call your doctor if you have any unusual problems while using this medication.

What storage conditions are needed for this medicine?

Keep this medication in the container it came in, tightly closed, and out of reach of children. Store it at room temperature and away from excess heat and moisture (not in the bathroom). Protect from light. Throw away any medication that is outdated or no longer needed. Talk to your pharmacist about the proper disposal of your medication.

What should I do in case of overdose?

If someone swallows ofloxacin otic, call your local poison control center at 1-800-222-1222. If the victim has collapsed or is not breathing, call local emergency services at 911.

What other information should I know?

Keep all appointments with your doctor.

Do not let anyone else use your medication. Your prescription is probably not refillable. If you still have symptoms of infection after you finish the ofloxacin otic, call your doctor.

Dosage Facts
For Informational Purposes

Caution: Do not change your dose, how often you take your medication, or the length of time you are to take it without first talking to your healthcare provider.

The following dosage information was written using medical language for doctors and other healthcare professionals and is provided here for you to check your dosage. The dosage of this drug may differ for different patients. Therefore, always follow your doctor's instructions or the directions on the label. Contact your healthcare provider or pharmacist if you have any questions about the specific dosage of your medication after reviewing this information.

Pediatric Patients

Bacterial Otic Infections
Otitis Externa

OTIC:

- Children 6 months to 13 years of age: 5 drops of 0.3% solution into canal of affected ear(s) once daily for 7 days.
- Children ≥13 years of age: 10 drops of 0.3% solution into canal of affected ear(s) once daily for 7 days.

Acute Otitis Media

OTIC:

- Children 1–12 years of age with tympanostomy tubes: 5 drops of 0.3% solution into canal of affected ear(s) twice daily for 10 days.

Chronic Suppurative Otitis Media

OTIC:

- Children ≥12 years of age with perforated tympanic membranes: 10 drops of 0.3% solution into canal of affected ear(s) twice daily for 14 days.

Adult Patients

Bacterial Otic Infections
Otitis Externa

OTIC:

- 10 drops of 0.3% solution into canal of affected ear(s) once daily for 7 days.

Chronic Suppurative Otitis Media

OTIC:

- 10 drops of 0.3% solution into canal of affected ear(s) twice daily for 14 days in patients with perforated tympanic membranes.

Olanzapine

(oh lan′ za peen)

Brand Name: Symbyax® as a combination product containing Olanzapine and Fluoxetine Hydrochloride, Zyprexa®, Zydis®

Important Warning

Studies have shown that older adults with dementia (a brain disorder that affects the ability to remember, think clearly, communicate, and perform daily activities and that may cause changes in mood and personality) who take antipsychotics (medications for mental illness) such as olanzapine have an increased chance of death during treatment. Older adults with dementia may also have a greater chance of having a stroke or mini-stroke during treatment. If you experience any of the following symptoms, call your doctor immediately: slow or difficult speech, sudden dizziness or faintness, or weakness or numbness of an arm or leg.

Olanzapine is not approved by the Food and Drug Administration (FDA) for the treatment of behavior disorders in older adults with dementia. Talk to the doctor who prescribed this medication if you, a family member, or someone you care for has dementia and is taking olanzapine. For more information visit the FDA website: http://www.fda.gov/cder

Why is this medicine prescribed?

Olanzapine is used to treat the symptoms of schizophrenia (a mental illness that causes disturbed or unusual thinking, loss of interest in life, and strong or inappropriate emotions). It is also used to treat bipolar disorder (manic depressive disorder; a disease that causes episodes of depression, episodes of mania, and other abnormal moods). Olanzapine is in a class of medications called atypical antipsychotics. It works by changing the activity of certain natural substances in the brain.

How should this medicine be used?

Olanzapine comes as a tablet and an orally disintegrating tablet (tablet that dissolves quickly in the mouth) to take by mouth. It is usually taken once a day with or without food. Take olanzapine at around the same time every day. Follow the directions on your prescription label carefully, and ask your doctor or pharmacist to explain any part you do not understand. Take olanzapine exactly as directed. Do not take more or less of it or take it more often than prescribed by your doctor.

Do not try to push the orally disintegrating tablet through the foil. Instead, use dry hands to peel back the foil

packaging. Immediately take out the tablet and place it in your mouth. The tablet will quickly dissolve and can be swallowed with or without liquid.

Your doctor may start you on a low dose of olanzapine and gradually increase your dose.

Olanzapine may help control your symptoms, but it will not cure your condition. It may take several weeks or longer before you feel the full benefit of olanzapine. Continue to take olanzapine even if you feel well. Do not stop taking olanzapine without talking to your doctor. Your doctor will probably want to decrease your dose gradually.

Are there other uses for this medicine?

This medication may be prescribed for other uses; ask your doctor or pharmacist for more information.

What special precautions should I follow?

Before taking olanzapine,
- tell your doctor and pharmacist if you are allergic to olanzapine or any other medications.
- tell your doctor and pharmacist what prescription and nonprescription medications, vitamins, nutritional supplements, and herbal products you are taking or plan to take. Be sure to mention any of the following: antidepressants; antihistamines; carbamazepine (Tegretol); dopamine agonists such as bromocriptine (Parlodel), cabergoline (Dostinex), levodopa (Dopar, Larodopa), pergolide (Permax), and ropinirole (Requip); fluoroquinolone antibiotics including ciprofloxacin (Cipro), gatifloxacin (Tequin) (not available in the United States), levofloxacin (Levaquin), norfloxacin (Noroxin), ofloxacin (Floxin), others; fluvoxamine (Luvox); ipratropium (Atrovent); medications for anxiety, hypertension, irritable bowel disease, mental illness, motion sickness, Parkinson's disease, seizures, ulcers, or urinary problems; omeprazole (Prilosec); rifampin (Rifadin); sedatives; sleeping pills; ticlopidine (Ticlid); and tranquilizers. Your doctor may need to change the doses of your medications or monitor you carefully for side effects.
- tell your doctor if you use or have ever used street drugs or have overused prescription medications and if you have or have ever had a stroke, a mini-stroke, heart disease or a heart attack, an irregular heartbeat, seizures, breast cancer, any condition that makes it difficult for you to swallow, high or low blood pressure, liver or prostate disease, paralytic ileus (condition in which food cannot move through the intestine); or glaucoma (an eye condition), or if you or anyone in your family has or has ever had diabetes. Also tell your doctor if you have ever had to stop taking a medication for mental illness because of severe side effects.
- tell your doctor if you are pregnant or plan to become pregnant. If you become pregnant while taking olanzapine, call your doctor. Do not breast-feed if you are taking olanzapine.

- if you are having surgery, including dental surgery, tell the doctor or dentist that you are taking olanzapine.
- you should know that olanzapine may make you drowsy. Do not drive a car or operate machinery until you know how this medication affects you.
- you should know that alcohol can add to the drowsiness caused by this medication. Do not drink alcohol while taking olanzapine.
- tell your doctor if you use tobacco products. Cigarette smoking may decrease the effectiveness of this medication.
- you should know that you may experience hyperglycemia (increases in your blood sugar) while you are taking this medication, even if you do not already have diabetes. If you have schizophrenia, you are more likely to develop diabetes than people who do not have schizophrenia, and taking olanzapine or similar medications may increase this risk. Tell your doctor immediately if you have any of the following symptoms while you are taking olanzapine: extreme thirst, frequent urination, extreme hunger, blurred vision, or weakness. It is very important to call your doctor as soon as you have any of these symptoms, because high blood sugar can cause a serious condition called ketoacidosis. Ketoacidosis may become life-threatening if it is not treated at an early stage. Symptoms of ketoacidosis include: dry mouth, nausea and vomiting, shortness of breath, breath that smells fruity, and decreased consciousness.
- you should know that olanzapine may cause dizziness, lightheadedness, and fainting when you get up too quickly from a lying position. This is more common when you first start taking olanzapine. To avoid this problem, get out of bed slowly, resting your feet on the floor for a few minutes before standing up.
- you should know that olanzapine may make it harder for your body to cool down when it gets very hot. Tell your doctor if you plan to do vigorous exercise or be exposed to extreme heat.
- if you have phenylketonuria (PKU, an inherited condition in which a special diet must be followed to prevent mental retardation), you should know that the orally disintegrating tablets contain aspartame that forms phenylalanine.

What special dietary instructions should I follow?

Talk to your doctor about eating grapefruit and drinking grapefruit juice while taking this medicine.

Be sure to drink plenty of water every day while you are taking this medication.

What should I do if I forget to take a dose?

Take the missed dose as soon as you remember it. However, if it is almost time for the next dose, skip the missed dose and continue your regular dosing schedule. Do not take a double dose to make up for a missed one.

What side effects can this medicine cause?

Olanzapine may cause side effects. Tell your doctor if any of these symptoms are severe or do not go away:

- drowsiness
- dizziness
- restlessness
- unusual behavior
- depression
- difficulty falling asleep or staying asleep
- weakness
- difficulty walking
- constipation
- weight gain
- dry mouth
- pain in arms, legs, back, or joints

Some side effects can be serious. If you experience any of the following symptoms or those listed in the IMPORTANT WARNING section or the SPECIAL PRECAUTIONS section, call your doctor immediately:

- seizures
- changes in vision
- swelling of the arms, hands, feet, ankles, or lower legs
- unusual movements of your face or body that you cannot control
- fever
- very stiff muscles
- excess sweating
- fast or irregular heartbeat
- rash
- hives
- difficulty breathing or swallowing

Olanzapine may cause other side effects. Call your doctor if you have any unusual problems while taking this medication.

If you experience a serious side effect, you or your doctor may send a report to the Food and Drug Administration's (FDA) MedWatch Adverse Event Reporting program online [at http://www.fda.gov/MedWatch/index.html] or by phone [1-800-332-1088].

What storage conditions are needed for this medicine?

Keep this medication in the container it came in, tightly closed, and out of reach of children. Store it at room temperature and away from excess heat and moisture (not in the bathroom). Always store the orally disintegrating tablets in their sealed package, and use them immediately after opening the package. Throw away any medication that is outdated or no longer needed. Talk to your pharmacist about the proper disposal of your medication.

What should I do in case of overdose?

In case of overdose, call your local poison control center at 1-800-222-1222. If the victim has collapsed or is not breathing, call local emergency services at 911.

Symptoms of overdose may include:
- drowsiness
- slurred speech
- agitation
- fast heartbeat
- sudden movements that you cannot control
- coma (loss of consciousness for a period of time)

What other information should I know?

Keep all appointments with your doctor and the laboratory. Your doctor may order certain lab tests to check your body's response to olanzapine.

Do not let anyone else take your medication. Ask your pharmacist any questions you have about refilling your prescription.

Dosage Facts
For Informational Purposes

Caution: Do not change your dose, how often you take your medication, or the length of time you are to take it without first talking to your healthcare provider.

The following dosage information was written using medical language for doctors and other healthcare professionals and is provided here for you to check your dosage. The dosage of this drug may differ for different patients. Therefore, always follow your doctor's instructions or the directions on the label. Contact your healthcare provider or pharmacist if you have any questions about the specific dosage of your medication after reviewing this information.

Adult Patients

Schizophrenia

ORAL:
- Initially, 5–10 mg, usually as a single daily dose. Within several days, may increase by 5 mg daily, to a target dosage of 10 mg daily.
- Make subsequent dosage adjustments at intervals of not less than 7 days, usually in increments or decrements of 5 mg once daily.
- Increasing dosage beyond 10 mg daily usually does not result in greater efficacy; such increases generally should occur only after assessment of the patient's clinical status.
- Optimum duration of therapy currently is not known, but maintenance therapy with antipsychotic agents is well established. In responsive patients, continue as long as clinically necessary and tolerated, but at lowest possible effective dosage; reassess need for continued therapy periodically.

Bipolar Disorder
Acute Mania: Monotherapy

ORAL:
- Initially, 10–15 mg once daily. Make dosage adjustments in increments or decrements of 5 mg daily, at intervals of not less than 24 hours.
- Effective dosage in clinical studies generally ranged from 5–20 mg daily.

- If elect to use olanzapine for extended periods, periodically reevaluate the long-term usefulness for the individual patient.

Acute Mania: Combination Therapy

ORAL:
- Initially, 10 mg once daily when administered with lithium or divalproex sodium.
- Effective dosage of olanzapine in clinical studies generally ranged from 5–20 mg daily.
- No dosage adjustment for lithium or divalproex sodium is required when used in combination with olanzapine.

Acute Depression: Combination Therapy

ORAL:
- Initially, 6 mg in fixed combination with 25 mg of fluoxetine (Symbyax® 6/25) once daily in the evening.
- Increase dosage according to patient response and tolerance as indicated.
- In clinical trials, antidepressive efficacy was demonstrated at olanzapine dosages ranging from 6–12 mg daily and fluoxetine dosages ranging from 25–50 mg daily.
- If elect to use combined olanzapine and fluoxetine for extended periods, periodically reevaluate the long-term risks and benefits for the individual patient.

Prescribing Limits

Adult Patients

Schizophrenia

ORAL:
- Safety of dosages >20 mg daily not established.

Bipolar Disorder

ORAL:
- Safety of dosages >20 mg daily not established.
- Dosages >18 mg of olanzapine and 75 mg of fluoxetine in fixed-combination for acute depressive episodes not evaluated in clinical studies.

Special Populations

Initially, 5 mg orally daily in debilitated patients, in those predisposed to hypotension, in those who may be particularly sensitive to the effects of olanzapine, or in those who might metabolize olanzapine slowly (e.g., nonsmoking women ≥65 years of age); when indicated, adjust dosage with caution.

In fixed combination with fluoxetine for acute depressive episodes in bipolar disorder, an oral dosage of 6 mg of olanzapine and 25 mg of fluoxetine (Symbyax® 6/25) is recommended for initial and maintenance therapy in patients predisposed to hypotension, in those with hepatic impairment, or those who might metabolize the drugs(s) slowly (e.g., female gender, geriatric age, nonsmoking status); when indicated, adjust dosage with caution.

Geriatric Patients
- Careful dosage titration of oral olanzapine recommended in patients >65 years of age; initiate therapy at low end of dosage range.

Olmesartan

(all mi sar′ tan)

Brand Name: Benicar®, Benicar® HCT as a combination product containing Olmesartan Medoxomil and Hydrochlorothiazide

Important Warning

Do not take olmesartan if you are pregnant. If you become pregnant while taking olmesartan, call your doctor immediately. Olmesartan may harm the fetus.

Why is this medicine prescribed?

Olmesartan is used alone or in combination with other medications to treat high blood pressure. Olmesartan is in a class of medications called angiotensin II receptor antagonists. It works by blocking the action of certain chemicals that tighten the blood vessels, so blood flows more smoothly.

How should this medicine be used?

Olmesartan comes as a tablet to take by mouth. It is usually taken once a day with or without food. To help you remember to take olmesartan, take it around the same time every day. Follow the directions on your prescription label carefully, and ask your doctor or pharmacist to explain any part you do not understand. Take olmesartan exactly as directed. Do not take more or less of it or take it more often than prescribed by your doctor.

Your doctor may start you on a low dose of olmesartan and gradually increase your dose, not more than once every 2 weeks.

Olmesartan controls high blood pressure but does not cure it. It may take up to 2 weeks before you feel the full benefit of olmesartan. Continue to take olmesartan even if you feel well. Do not stop taking olmesartan without talking to your doctor.

Are there other uses for this medicine?

Olmesartan is sometimes also used to treat heart failure. Talk to your doctor about the possible risks of using this medication for your condition.

This medication may be prescribed for other uses; ask your doctor or pharmacist for more information.

What special precautions should I follow?

Before taking olmesartan,

- tell your doctor and pharmacist if you are allergic to olmesartan or any other medications.
- tell your doctor and pharmacist what prescription and nonprescription medications, vitamins, nutritional supplements, and herbal products you are taking. Be sure

to mention diuretics ('water pills'). Your doctor may need to change the doses of your medications or monitor you carefully for side effects.

- tell your doctor if you have or have ever had heart failure; kidney disease; or angioedema, a condition that causes difficulty swallowing or breathing and painful swelling of the the face, throat, tongue, lips, eyes, hands, feet, ankles, or lower legs.
- tell your doctor if you are planning to become pregnant or are breast-feeding.
- you should know that olmesartan may cause your blood pressure to drop too low, especially after your first dose. Your doctor may want you to take your first dose in his office so he can see how you react to this medication.

What special dietary instructions should I follow?

If your doctor prescribes a low-salt or low-sodium diet, follow these directions carefully.

What should I do if I forget to take a dose?

Take the missed dose as soon as you remember it. However, if it is almost time for the next dose, skip the missed dose and continue your regular dosing schedule. Do not take a double dose to make up for a missed one.

What side effects can this medicine cause?

Olmesartan may cause side effects. Tell your doctor if this symptom is severe or does not go away:

- dizziness

Some side effects can be serious. The following symptoms are uncommon, but if you experience any of them, call your doctor immediately:

- swelling of the face, throat, tongue, lips, eyes, hands, feet, ankles, or lower legs
- hoarseness
- difficulty swallowing or breathing

Olmesartan may cause other side effects. Call your doctor if you have any unusual problems while taking this medication.

If you experience a serious side effect, you or your doctor may send a report to the Food and Drug Administration's (FDA) MedWatch Adverse Event Reporting program online [at http://www.fda.gov/MedWatch/index.html] or by phone [1-800-332-1088].

What storage conditions are needed for this medicine?

Keep this medication in the container it came in, tightly closed, and out of reach of children. Store it at room temperature and away from excess heat and moisture (not in the bathroom). Throw away any medication that is outdated or no longer needed. Talk to your pharmacist about the proper disposal of your medication.

What should I do in case of overdose?

In case of overdose, call your local poison control center at 1-800-222-1222. If the victim has collapsed or is not breathing, call local emergency services at 911.

Symptoms of overdose may include:

- fainting
- dizziness
- blurred vision
- upset stomach
- fast or slow heartbeat

What other information should I know?

Keep all appointments with your doctor and the laboratory. Your blood pressure should be checked regularly to determine your response to olmesartan.

Do not let anyone else take your medication. Ask your pharmacist any questions you have about refilling your prescription.

Dosage Facts
For Informational Purposes

Caution: Do not change your dose, how often you take your medication, or the length of time you are to take it without first talking to your healthcare provider.

The following dosage information was written using medical language for doctors and other healthcare professionals and is provided here for you to check your dosage. The dosage of this drug may differ for different patients. Therefore, always follow your doctor's instructions or the directions on the label. Contact your healthcare provider or pharmacist if you have any questions about the specific dosage of your medication after reviewing this information.

General Dosage Information

Available as olmesartan medoxomil; dosage expressed in terms of the salt.

Adult Patients

Hypertension
Monotherapy

ORAL:

- Initially, 20 mg once daily in adults without intravascular volume depletion. Adjust dosage at approximately monthly intervals (more aggressively in high-risk patients) to achieve BP control.
- Usual dosage: 20–40 mg once daily; no additional therapeutic benefit with higher dosages or with twice-daily dosing.

Combination Therapy

ORAL:

- If BP is not adequately controlled by monotherapy with olmesartan or hydrochlorothiazide, can switch to fixed-combination olmesartan/hydrochlorothiazide tablets. In patients already receiving olmesartan medoxomil, initiate hydrochloro-thiazide at dosage of 12.5 mg once daily; in those receiving hydrochlororthiazide, consider reducing hydrochlo-rothiazide dosage to 12.5 mg and initiate olmesartan medoxomil at dosage of 20 mg once daily. Increase dosages to olmesartan medoxomil 40 mg and hydrochlorothiazide 25 mg once daily, if needed, to control BP.

Special Populations

Hepatic Impairment

- No initial dosage adjustments necessary in patients with moderate to severe hepatic impairment.

Renal Impairment

- Manufacturer states that no initial dosage adjustments necessary in patients with moderate to severe renal impairment (Cl_{cr} <40 mL/min). However, some clinicians recommend lower initial dose in patients with Cl_{cr} <20 mL/minute, with maximum dosage of 20 mg once daily in such patients.
- Dosage in patients with end-stage renal disease not determined.
- Olmesartan/hydrochlorothiazide fixed combination not recommended in patients with severe renal impairment.

Geriatric Patients

- No initial dosage adjustments necessary.

Volume- and/or Salt-depleted Patients

- Correct volume and/or salt depletion prior to initiation of therapy or initiate therapy under close medical supervision using lower initial dosage.

Olopatadine Ophthalmic

(oh loe pa ta' deen)

Brand Name: Patanol®

Why is this medicine prescribed?

Olopatadine is used to treat the symptoms of allergic pink eye. Olopatadine is in a class of medications called antihistamines. It works by blocking histamine, a substance in the body that causes allergic symptoms.

How should this medicine be used?

Olopatadine comes as an eyedrop to apply to the eye. It is usually applied to the affected eye(s) twice a day, around 6 to 8 hours apart. To help you remember to use olopatadine, use it around the same time every day. Follow the directions on your prescription label carefully, and ask your doctor or pharmacist to explain any part you do not understand. Use olopatadine exactly as directed. Do not use more or less of it or use it more often than prescribed by your doctor.

To apply the eyedrops, follow these steps:

1. Wash your hands thoroughly with soap and water.
2. Use a mirror or have someone else put the drops in your eye.

3. Make sure the end of the dropper is not chipped or cracked.
4. Avoid touching the dropper against your eye or anything else.
5. Hold the dropper tip down at all times to prevent drops from flowing back into the bottle and contaminating the remaining contents.
6. Lie down or tilt your head back.
7. Holding the bottle between your thumb and index finger, place the dropper as near as possible to your eyelid without touching it.
8. Brace the remaining fingers of that hand against your cheek or nose.
9. With the index finger of your other hand, pull the lower lid of the eye down to form a pocket.
10. Drop the prescribed number of drops into the pocket made by the lower lid and the eye. Placing the drops on the surface of the eyeball can cause stinging.
11. Close your eye and press lightly against the lower lid with your finger for 2-3 minutes to keep the medication in the eye. Do not blink.
12. Replace and tighten the cap right away. Do not wipe or rinse it off.
13. Wipe off any excess liquid from your cheek with a clean tissue. Wash your hands again.

Are there other uses for this medicine?

This medication may be prescribed for other uses; ask your doctor or pharmacist for more information.

What special precautions should I follow?

Before using olopatadine,

- tell your doctor and pharmacist if you are allergic to olopatadine, benzalkonium chloride, or any other medications.
- tell your doctor and pharmacist what prescription and nonprescription medications, vitamins, nutritional supplements, and herbal products you are taking.
- tell your doctor if you are pregnant, plan to become pregnant, or are breast-feeding. If you become pregnant while using olopatadine, call your doctor.
- you should know that you should not wear contact lenses if your eye(s) is/are red. If your eye is not red and you wear contact lenses, you should know that olopatadine solution contains benzalkonium chloride, which can be absorbed by soft contact lenses. Remove your contact lenses before applying olopatadine and put them back in 10 minutes later.

What special dietary instructions should I follow?

Unless your doctor tells you otherwise, continue your normal diet.

What should I do if I forget to take a dose?

Apply the missed dose as soon as you remember it. However, if it is almost time for the next dose, skip the missed dose and continue your regular dosing schedule. Do not apply a double dose to make up for a missed one.

What side effects can this medicine cause?

Olopatadine may cause side effects. Tell your doctor if any of these symptoms are severe or do not go away:

- headache
- blurred vision
- eye burning or stinging
- dry eyes
- sore throat
- taste changes

What storage conditions are needed for this medicine?

Keep this medication in the container it came in, tightly closed, and out of reach of children. Store it at room temperature and away from excess heat and moisture (not in the bathroom). Throw away any medication that is outdated or no longer needed. Talk to your pharmacist about the proper disposal of your medication.

What other information should I know?

Keep all appointments with your doctor.

Do not let anyone else use your medication. Ask your pharmacist any questions you have about refilling your prescription.

Dosage Facts
For Informational Purposes

Caution: Do not change your dose, how often you take your medication, or the length of time you are to take it without first talking to your healthcare provider.

The following dosage information was written using medical language for doctors and other healthcare professionals and is provided here for you to check your dosage. The dosage of this drug may differ for different patients. Therefore, always follow your doctor's instructions or the directions on the label. Contact your healthcare provider or pharmacist if you have any questions about the specific dosage of your medication after reviewing this information.

General Dosage Information

Available as olopatadine hydrochloride; dosage expressed in terms of olopatadine.

Pediatric Patients

Allergic Conjunctivitis

OPHTHALMIC:
- Children ≥3 years of age: 1 or 2 drops of a 0.1% solution in the affected eye(s) twice daily (at an interval of 6–8 hours).
- Once symptomatic improvement is established, continue therapy for as long as necessary to sustain improvement.

Adult Patients

Allergic Conjunctivitis

OPHTHALMIC:
- 1 or 2 drops of a 0.1% solution in the affected eye(s) twice daily (at an interval of 6–8 hours).
- Once symptomatic improvement is established, continue therapy for as long as necessary to sustain improvement.

Olsalazine

(ole sal′ a zeen)

Brand Name: Dipentum®

Why is this medicine prescribed?

Olsalazine, an anti-inflammatory medicine, is used to treat ulcerative colitis, a condition in which the bowel is inflamed. Olsalazine reduces the bowel inflammation, diarrhea (stool frequency), rectal bleeding, and abdominal pain.

This medication is sometimes prescribed for other uses; ask your doctor or pharmacist for more information.

How should this medicine be used?

Olsalazine comes as a capsule to take by mouth. It usually is taken twice a day after meals or with food to prevent stomach upset. Follow the directions on your prescription label carefully, and ask your doctor or pharmacist to explain any part you do not understand. Take olsalazine exactly as directed. Do not take more or less of it or take it more often than prescribed by your doctor.

What special precautions should I follow?

Before taking olsalazine,
- tell your doctor and pharmacist if you are allergic to olsalazine, aspirin or aspirin-like medicines, or any other drugs.
- tell your doctor and pharmacist what prescription and nonprescription medications you are taking, especially anticoagulants ('blood thinners') such as warfarin (Coumadin) and vitamins.
- tell your doctor if you are pregnant, plan to become pregnant, or are breast-feeding. If you become pregnant while taking osalazine, call your doctor.
- plan to avoid unnecessary or prolonged exposure to the sunlight and to wear protective clothing, sunglasses, and sunscreen. Olsalazine may make your skin sensitive to sunlight.

What should I do if I forget to take a dose?

Take the missed dose as soon as you remember it. However, if it is almost time for the next dose, skip the missed dose and continue your regular dosing schedule. Do not take a double dose to make up for a missed one.

What side effects can this medicine cause?

Olsalazine may cause side effects. Tell your doctor if any of these symptoms are severe or do not go away:
- stomach upset
- bloating
- loss of appetite
- blurred vision
- headache
- pain in joints
- dizziness

If you experience any of the following symptoms, call your doctor immediately:
- skin rash
- chest pain
- diarrhea
- unusual bleeding or bruising

If you experience a serious side effect, you or your doctor may send a report to the Food and Drug Administration's (FDA) MedWatch Adverse Event Reporting program online [at http://www.fda.gov/MedWatch/index.html] or by phone [1-800-332-1088].

What storage conditions are needed for this medicine?

Keep this medication in the container it came in, tightly closed, and out of reach of children. Store it at room temperature and away from excess heat and moisture (not in the bathroom). Throw away any medication that is outdated or no longer needed. Talk to your pharmacist about the proper disposal of your medication.

What other information should I know?

Keep all appointments with your doctor and the laboratory. Your doctor may order certain lab tests to check your response to olsalazine.

Do not let anyone else take your medicine. Ask your pharmacist any questions you have about refilling your prescription.

Dosage Facts
For Informational Purposes

Caution: Do not change your dose, how often you take your medication, or the length of time you are to take it without first talking to your healthcare provider.

The following dosage information was written using medical language for doctors and other healthcare professionals and is provided here for you to check your dosage. The dosage of this drug may differ for different patients. Therefore, always follow your doctor's instructions or the directions on the label. Contact your healthcare provider or pharmacist if you have any questions about the specific dosage of your medication after reviewing this information.

General Dosage Information

Dosage of olsalazine sodium, which is commercially available as the disodium salt, is expressed in terms of olsalazine sodium.

Daily dosage of 1g usually provides >0.9 g of mesalamine in the colon.

Adult Patients

Ulcerative Colitis

ORAL:
- 500 mg twice daily.

Omalizumab Injection

(oh mah lye zoo′ mab)

Brand Name: Xolair®

Why is this medicine prescribed?

Omalizumab injection is used to decrease the number of asthma attacks (wheezing, shortness of breath, and trouble breathing) in patients with allergic asthma whose symptoms are not controlled with inhaled steroids. Omalizumab is in a class of medications called monoclonal antibodies.It works by blocking the action of IgE cells (cells in the body that cause asthma symptoms) and stopping the release of substances in the body that cause an allergic response.

How should this medicine be used?

Omalizumab injection comes as a solution (liquid) to inject subcutaneously (under the skin). It is usually injected in a doctor's office once every 2 weeks or every 4 weeks.

Omalizumab may cause serious allergic reactions that are most likely to happen within 2 hours after you receive this medication, but may happen at any time during your treatment. You will have to stay at your doctor's office for at least 2 hours after you receive this medication.A doctor or nurse will watch you during this time to see if you are having a serious reaction to the medication. Tell your doctor or nurse right away if you experience any unusual symptoms, such as those listed in the SIDE EFFECTS section, after you receive omalizumab. Because an allergic reaction to omalizumab may happen after you leave your doctor's office, you may also be given another injectable medication for emergency use if you have certain side effects. Be sure that you know how to use this medication and to seek medical care immediately if these symptoms occur.

It may take some time before you feel the full benefit of omalizumab. Call your doctor if your asthma symptoms worsen. Talk to your doctor so that you know what to do if you have an asthma attack or breathing problems while receiving omalizumab. Do not decrease your dose or stop taking any other asthma medication that you may use to treat your condition, unless your doctor tells you to do so.

Are there other uses for this medicine?

This medication may be prescribed for other uses; ask your doctor or pharmacist for more information.

What special precautions should I follow?

Before using omalizumab injection,
- tell your doctor and pharmacist if you are allergic to omalizumab, or any other medications.
- tell your doctor and pharmacist what prescription and nonprescription medications, vitamins, nutritional supplements, and herbal products you are taking.
- tell your doctor if you are pregnant, plan to become pregnant, or are breast-feeding. If you become pregnant while using omalizumab, call your doctor.
- do not change the dose(s) of your other asthma medication(s) or stop taking them without talking to your doctor.

What special dietary instructions should I follow?

Unless your doctor tells you otherwise, continue your normal diet.

What should I do if I forget to take a dose?

If you miss an appointment to receive an injection of omalizumab you should call your health care doctor as soon as possible. The missed dose should be given as soon as it can be rescheduled.

What side effects can this medicine cause?

Omalizumab injection may cause side effects. Tell your doctor if any of these symptoms are severe or do not go away:
- pain, redness, swelling, warmth, burning, stinging, bruising, hardness (bump), or itching in the place omalizumab was injected
- pain, especially in joints, arms, or legs
- tiredness
- ear pain

Some side effects can be serious. The following symptoms are uncommon, but if you experience any of them, call your doctor or get medical care immediately:
- hives
- rash
- itching
- difficulty breathing or swallowing
- swelling of the face, throat, tongue, or lips
- tightness in chest
- flushing
- dizziness
- fainting
- fast heartbeat
- diarrhea
- vomiting
- stomach cramps

Omalizumab may increase the risk of developing cancer, including breast, skin, parotid (salivary gland, located near the mouth), and prostate cancer. Talk to your doctor about the risks of using this medication.

Omalizumab may cause other side effects. Call your doctor if you have any unusual problems while using this medication.

If you experience a serious side effect, you or your doctor may send a report to the Food and Drug Administration's (FDA) MedWatch Adverse Event Reporting program online [at http://www.fda.gov/MedWatch/index.html] or by phone [1-800-332-1088].

What storage conditions are needed for this medicine?

Your doctor will store this medication in his or her office.

What should I do in case of overdose?

In case of overdose, call your local poison control center at 1-800-222-1222. If the victim has collapsed or is not breathing, call local emergency services at 911.

What other information should I know?

Keep all appointments with your doctor.

Before having any laboratory test, tell your doctor and the laboratory personnel that you are taking or have taken omalizumab.

Dosage Facts
For Informational Purposes

Caution: Do not change your dose, how often you take your medication, or the length of time you are to take it without first talking to your healthcare provider.

The following dosage information was written using medical language for doctors and other healthcare professionals and is provided here for you to check your dosage. The dosage of this drug may differ for different patients. Therefore, always follow your doctor's instructions or the directions on the label. Contact your healthcare provider or pharmacist if you have any questions about the specific dosage of your medication after reviewing this information.

Pediatric Patients

Moderate to Severe Allergic Asthma

SUB-Q:
- Adolescents ≥12 years of age: 150–375 mg every 2 or 4 weeks. Base dosage and dosing frequency on total serum IgE concentrations, measured prior to therapy, and body weight (see Tables 1 and 2).

Adult Patients

Moderate to Severe Allergic Asthma

SUB-Q:
- 150–375 mg every 2 or 4 weeks. Base dosage and dosing frequency on total serum IgE concentrations, measured prior to therapy, and body weight (see Tables 1 and 2).

Table 1. Omalizumab Doses (mg) Administered Every 4 Weeks

Pre-treatment Serum IgE (IU/mL)	Body Weight (kg)			
	30–60	>60–70	>70–90	>90–150
≥30–100	150	150	150	300
>100–200	300	300	300	—a
>200–300	300	—a	—a	—a
>300–400	—a	—a	—a	—a
>400–500	—a	—a	—a	—a
>500–600	—a	—a	—a	—a

a see Table 2

Table 2. Omalizumab Doses (mg) Administered every 2 Weeks

Pre-treatment Serum IgE (IU/mL)	Body Weight (kg)			
	30–60	>60–70	>70–90	>90–150
>30–100	—a	—a	—a	—a
>100–200	—a	—a	—a	225
>200–300	—a	225	225	300
>300–400	225	225	300	—b
>400–500	300	300	375	—b
>500–600	300	375	—b	—b
>600–700	375	—b	—b	—b

a see Table 1
b Do not dose

Prescribing Limits

Pediatric Patients

Moderate to Severe Allergic Asthma

SUB-Q:
- Maximum 750 mg every 4 weeks.

Adult Patients

Moderate to Severe Allergic Asthma

SUB-Q:
- Maximum 750 mg every 4 weeks.

Special Populations

No special population (i.e., age, race, ethnicity, gender) dosage recommendations at this time.

Omeprazole

(oh me′ pray zol)

Brand Name: Prilosec®, Prilosec® OTC, Zegerid®

Also available generically.

Why is this medicine prescribed?

Prescription omeprazole is used alone or with other medications to treat ulcers (sores in the lining of the stomach or small intestine), gastroesophageal reflux disease (GERD), a condition in which backward flow of acid from the stomach causes heartburn and injury of the esophagus (tube that connects the mouth and stomach), and erosive esophagitis (swelling and wearing away of the lining of the esophagus). Omeprazole delayed-release capsules are also used to treat conditions in which the stomach produces too much acid. Omeprazole delayed-release capsules are also used in combination with other medications to eliminate *H. pylori* (a bacteria that causes ulcers) and possibly prevent new ulcers from developing in patients who have or have had ulcers of the small intestine. Omeprazole powder for suspension (to be mixed with water) is also used to prevent bleeding from the esophagus, stomach, or the top of the small intestine in people who have life-threatening illnesses. Nonprescription omeprazole is used to treat frequent heartburn (heartburn that occurs at least 2 days a week). Omeprazole is in a class of medications called proton-pump inhibitors. It works by decreasing the amount of acid made in the stomach.

How should this medicine be used?

Omeprazole comes as a delayed-release capsule, a nonprescription delayed-release tablet, a powder for suspension, and a regular capsule. The powder and regular capsule also contain sodium bicarbonate, a medication that decreases the amount of acid in the stomach and helps omeprazole to work quickly. The delayed-release capsules are usually taken once a day before a meal, but may be taken twice a day when used with other medications to eliminate *H. pylori* or up to three times a day when used to treat conditions in which the stomach produces too much acid. The capsules are usually taken once a day in the morning on an empty stomach one hour before a meal. The powder is usually taken once a day on an empty stomach one hour before a meal either in the morning or at bedtime. The nonprescription delayed-release tablets are usually taken once a day in the morning before eating. The nonprescription tablets should be taken for 14 days in a row, and additional 14-day treatments may be repeated once every 4 months if needed. To help you remember to take omeprazole, take it at around the same time(s) every day. Follow the directions on your prescription label or the package label carefully, and ask your doctor or pharmacist to explain any part you do not understand. Take omeprazole exactly as directed. Do not take more or less of it or

take it more often or for a longer period of time than prescribed by your doctor or stated on the package.

Swallow the regular omeprazole capsules with water. Do not swallow the capsules with any other liquid.

Swallow the delayed-release omeprazole capsules, the regular capsules, and the nonprescription delayed-release tablets whole; do not split, open, chew or crush them. Do not crush the nonprescription delayed-release tablets in food and do not open the regular capsules and mix the contents with food.

If you have difficulty swallowing the delayed-release capsules, you may add the contents of a delayed-release capsule to applesauce. Place one tablespoon of soft, cool applesauce in an empty bowl. Open the delayed-release capsule and carefully empty all the pellets inside the capsule onto the applesauce. Mix the pellets with the applesauce and swallow the mixture immediately with a glass of cool water. Do not chew or crush the pellets. Do not store the applesauce/pellet mixture for future use.

If you are taking the powder, you must mix it with water before use. Place 1-2 tablespoons of water into a small cup and add the contents of one powder packet. Mix well and drink the mixture immediately. Refill the cup with water and drink the water to be sure that you swallow all of the medication. Do not mix the medication with any other liquid or with food.

If you are taking the powder or the regular capsules, be sure that you are taking the strength and the number of capsules or powder packets that your doctor prescribed. If you were told to take one 40 mg capsule or powder packet, do not take two 20 mg capsules or powder packets instead. They do not contain the same amount of medication as one 40 mg capsule or packet. Ask your doctor or pharmacist if you have any questions about how many capsules or packets you should take.

Do not take nonprescription omeprazole for immediate relief of heartburn symptoms. It may take 1-4 days for you to feel the full benefit of the medication. Call your doctor if your symptoms get worse or do not improve after 14 days or if your symptoms return sooner than 4 months after you finish your treatment. Do not take nonprescription omeprazole for longer than 14 days or more often than once every 4 months without talking to your doctor.

Your doctor may prescribe omeprazole for 10-14 days to eliminate *H. pylori* or for 4-8 weeks or longer to treat other conditions. Continue to take omeprazole even if you feel well. Do not stop taking prescription omeprazole without talking to your doctor.

Are there other uses for this medicine?

This medication may be prescribed for other uses; ask your doctor or pharmacist for more information.

What special precautions should I follow?

Before taking omeprazole,

- tell your doctor and pharmacist if you are allergic

to omeprazole, esomeprazole (Nexium), lansoprazole (Prevacid), pantoprazole (Protonix), rabeprazole (Aciphex), any other medications, or any of the ingredients in the type of omeprazole you will be taking. Ask your pharmacist or check the package label for a list of the ingredients.

- tell your doctor and pharmacist what prescription and nonprescription medications, vitamins, nutritional supplements, and herbal products you are taking or plan to take. Be sure to mention any of the following: ampicillin (in Principen, in Unasyn); anticoagulants ('blood thinners') such as warfarin (Coumadin); atazanavir (Reyataz); cyclosporine (Neoral, Sandimmune); diazepam (Valium); digoxin (Lanoxicaps, Lanoxin) disulfiram (Antabuse); ketoconazole (Nizoral); medications for anxiety and seizures; phenytoin (Dilantin); sedatives; sleeping pills; tacrolimus (Prograf); tranquilizers; and vitamins or supplements containing iron. If you will be taking the regular capsules or powder, tell your doctor if you are taking any antacids or calcium supplements. Your doctor may need to change the doses of your medications or monitor you carefully for side effects.
- if you will be taking the regular capsules or the powder, tell your doctor if you have or have ever had low levels of calcium or potassium in your blood or excessive vomiting. Your doctor may tell you not to take omeprazole capsules or powder.
- if you plan to take nonprescription omeprazole, first tell your doctor if your heartburn has lasted 3 months or longer or if you have experienced any of the following symptoms: lightheadedness, sweating, or dizziness along with your heartburn; chest pain or shoulder pain; shortness of breath or wheezing; pain that spreads to your arms, neck, or shoulders; unexplained weight loss; nausea; vomiting, especially vomiting blood; stomach pain; difficulty swallowing or pain when you swallow; or black or bloody stools. You may have a more serious condition that cannot be treated with nonprescription medication.
- tell your doctor if you have or have ever had liver disease. If you will be taking the regular capsules or the powder, also tell your doctor if you have been told to limit the amount of sodium in your diet, if you have or have ever had low levels of potassium in your blood, or if you have or have ever had Bartter's syndrome (condition in which the kidneys cannot absorb potassium from the blood properly).
- tell your doctor if you are pregnant, plan to become pregnant, or are breast-feeding. If you become pregnant while taking omeprazole, call your doctor.

What special dietary instructions should I follow?

If you will be taking the regular capsules or the powder, your doctor may tell you to limit the amount of milk and other foods and drinks that are high in calcium that you eat and drink during your treatment. Follow these instructions carefully.

If you will be taking any other form of omeprazole, continue your normal diet unless your doctor tells you otherwise.

What should I do if I forget to take a dose?

Take the missed dose as soon as you remember it. However, if it is almost time for the next dose, skip the missed dose and continue your regular dosing schedule. Do not take a double dose to make up for a missed one.

What side effects can this medicine cause?

Omeprazole may cause side effects. Tell your doctor if any of these symptoms are severe or do not go away:
- stomach pain
- diarrhea
- constipation
- dizziness
- cough
- back pain

Some side effects can be serious. If you experience any of these symptoms, call your doctor immediately:
- rash
- hives
- itching
- swelling of the face, throat, tongue, lips, eyes, hands, feet, ankles, or lower legs
- difficulty breathing or swallowing
- hoarseness
- seizures
- muscle spasms, tightening, aching, or cramping
- burning or tingling of the lips, tongue, hands, or feet

Omeprazole may cause other side effects. Call your doctor if you have any unusual problems while taking this medication.

What storage conditions are needed for this medicine?

Keep this medication in the container it came in, tightly closed, and out of reach of children. Store it at room temperature and away from light, excess heat, and moisture (not in the bathroom). Throw away any medication that is outdated or no longer needed. Talk to your pharmacist about the proper disposal of your medication.

What should I do in case of overdose?

In case of overdose, call your local poison control center at 1-800-222-1222. If the victim has collapsed or is not breathing, call local emergency services at 911.

Symptoms of overdose may include:
- confusion
- drowsiness
- blurred vision
- fast or pounding heartbeat
- nausea

- vomiting
- sweating
- flushing (feeling of warmth)
- headache
- dry mouth

What other information should I know?

Keep all appointments with your doctor.

Do not let anyone else take your medication. If you are taking prescription omeprazole, ask your pharmacist any questions you have about refilling your prescription.

Dosage Facts
For Informational Purposes

Caution: Do not change your dose, how often you take your medication, or the length of time you are to take it without first talking to your healthcare provider.

The following dosage information was written using medical language for doctors and other healthcare professionals and is provided here for you to check your dosage. The dosage of this drug may differ for different patients. Therefore, always follow your doctor's instructions or the directions on the label. Contact your healthcare provider or pharmacist if you have any questions about the specific dosage of your medication after reviewing this information.

General Dosage Information

Available as omeprazole and omeprazole magnesium; dosage expressed in terms of omeprazole.

Pediatric Patients

Gastroesophageal Reflux
GERD.

ORAL (DELAYED-RELEASE CAPSULES):
- Children >2 years of age: Children weighing <20 kg: 10 mg once daily. Those weighing ≥20 kg: 20 mg once daily. Administered for 4 weeks in one study.

Treatment of Erosive Esophagitis.

ORAL (DELAYED-RELEASE CAPSULES):
- Children >2 years of age: Children weighing <20 kg: 10 mg daily. Those weighing ≥20 kg: 20 mg daily.
- On a mg/kg basis, dosage of omeprazole required to heal erosive esophagitis is greater in children than that required in adults. In an uncontrolled open-label study, dosages required for healing were 0.7–3.5 mg/kg daily (maximum 80 mg daily) for 3–6 months; about 90% of children healed in the first 3 months, and about 5% required a second course of treatment. Dosage of 0.7 mg/kg daily resulted in healing in 44% of children; an additional 28% of the children studied required a dosage of 1.4 mg/kg daily for healing to occur.

Maintenance of Healing of Erosive Esophagitis.

ORAL (DELAYED-RELEASE CAPSULES):
- Children >2 years of age: Children weighing <20 kg: 10 mg daily. Those weighing≥20 kg: 20 mg daily. Maintenance ther-

apy continued 2 years in one study. In an uncontrolled open-label study, maintenance dosages were half the dosages required for initial healing in 54% of children, while 46% required dosage increase (0.7–2.8 mg/kg daily) for all or part of the study.

Adult Patients

GERD
GERD without Erosive Esophagitis

ORAL (CAPSULES, DELAYED-RELEASE CAPSULES; POWDER FOR ORAL SUSPENSION):
- 20 mg once daily for up to 4 weeks.

Treatment of Erosive Esophagitis

ORAL (CAPSULES, DELAYED-RELEASE CAPSULES; POWDER FOR ORAL SUSPENSION):
- 20 mg once daily until healing occurs (usually within 4–8 weeks); 40 mg once daily may be required. May give an additional 4 weeks of therapy (up to 12 weeks for a single course). If recurs, consider additional 4–8 weeks of therapy.

Maintenance of Healing of Erosive Esophagitis

ORAL (CAPSULES, DELAYED-RELEASE CAPSULES; POWDER FOR ORAL SUSPENSION):
- 20 mg once daily. Chronic, lifelong therapy may be appropriate.

Self-medication for Frequent Heartburn

ORAL (DELAYED-RELEASE TABLETS):
- 20 mg daily in the morning for 14 days. Do not exceed recommended dosage or duration; do not administer more than one course every 4 months. May relieve symptoms within 24 hours, but 1–4 days may be required for complete relief.

Duodenal Ulcer
Treatment of Active Duodenal Ulcer

ORAL (CAPSULES, DELAYED-RELEASE CAPSULES; POWDER FOR SUSPENSION):
- 20 mg once daily until healing occurs (usually within 2–4 weeks); an additional 4 weeks of therapy may be beneficial. Patients who responded poorly to H_2-receptor antagonists may require up to 40 mg daily.

Treatment of Helicobacter pylori Infection and Duodenal Ulcer

ORAL (DELAYED-RELEASE CAPSULES):
- Triple therapy: 20 mg twice daily (morning and evening) for 10 days in conjunction with amoxicillin and clarithromycin; additional omeprazole therapy of 20 mg once daily for 18 days recommended if active ulcer present initially.
- Dual therapy: 40 mg once daily (in the morning) for 14 days in conjunction with clarithromycin; omeprazole 20 mg once daily for additional 14 days recommended if active ulcer present initially.

Gastric Ulcer
Treatment

ORAL (CAPSULES, DELAYED-RELEASE CAPSULES; POWDER FOR ORAL SUSPENSION):
- 40 mg once daily for 4–8 weeks.

Pathologic GI Hypersecretory Conditions
Zollinger-Ellison Syndrome

ORAL (DELAYED-RELEASE CAPSULES):
- 60 mg once daily initially. Adjust dosage according to patient response and tolerance; continue therapy as long as necessary.

Administer daily dosages >80 mg in divided doses. May require dosages of up to 360 mg daily (given in 3 divided doses).

Multiple Endocrine Adenomas

ORAL (DELAYED-RELEASE CAPSULES):

• 60 mg once daily initially. Adjust dosage according to patient response and tolerance; continue therapy as long as necessary. Administer daily dosages >80 mg in divided doses. May require dosages of up to 360 mg daily (given in 3 divided doses).

Systemic Mastocytosis

ORAL (DELAYED-RELEASE CAPSULES):

• 60 mg once daily initially. Adjust dosage according to patient response and tolerance; continue therapy as long as necessary. Administer daily dosages >80 mg in divided doses. May require dosages of up to 360 mg daily (given in 3 divided doses).

Upper GI Bleeding

Reduction of Risk of Upper GI Bleeding in Critically Ill Adults

ORAL (POWDER FOR ORAL SUSPENSION):

• Initially, 40 mg followed by 40 mg after 6–8 hours on the first day, then 40 mg once daily for up to 14 days. Safety and efficacy for >14 days not established.

Special Populations

Hepatic Impairment

• Consider dosage reduction, particularly in patients receiving long-term therapy for maintenance of healing of erosive esophagitis.

Asians

• Consider dosage reduction, especially in patients receiving long-term therapy for maintenance of healing of erosive esophagitis.

Ondansetron

(on dan′ se tron)

Brand Name: Zofran®, ZofranODT®

Why is this medicine prescribed?

Ondansetron is used to prevent nausea and vomiting caused by cancer chemotherapy, radiation therapy and surgery. Ondansetron is in a class of medications called 5-HT$_3$ receptor antagonists. It works by blocking the action of serotonin, a natural substance that may cause nausea and vomiting.

How should this medicine be used?

Ondansetron comes as a tablet, a rapidly disintegrating (dissolving) tablet, and an oral solution to take by mouth. The first dose of ondansetron is usually taken 30 minutes before the start of chemotherapy, 1 to 2 hours before the start of radiation therapy, or 1 hour before surgery. Additional doses are sometimes taken one to three times a day during chemotherapy or radiation therapy and for 1 to 2 days after the end of treatment. Follow the directions on your prescription label carefully, and ask your doctor or pharmacist to explain any part you do not understand. Take ondansetron exactly as directed. Do not take more or less of it or take it more often than prescribed by your doctor.

If you are taking the rapidly disintegrating tablet, remove the tablet from the package just before you take your dose. To open the package, do not try to push the tablet through the foil backing of the blister. Instead, use dry hands to peel back the foil backing. Gently remove the tablet and immediately place the tablet on the top of your tongue. The tablet will dissolve in a few seconds and can be swallowed with saliva.

Are there other uses for this medicine?

This medication may be prescribed for other uses. Ask your doctor or pharmacist for more information.

What special precautions should I follow?

Before taking ondansetron,

• tell your doctor and pharmacist if you are allergic to ondansetron, alosetron (Lotronex), dolasetron (Anzemet), granisetron (Kytril), palonosetron (Aloxi), any other medications, or any of the ingredients in ondansetron tablets or liquid. Ask your pharmacist for a list of the ingredients.

• tell your doctor and pharmacist what prescription and nonprescription medications, vitamins, nutritional supplements, and herbal products you are taking. Be sure to mention tramadol (Ultram, in Ultracet). Your doctor may need to change the doses of your medications or monitor you more carefully for side effects.

• tell your doctor if you have or have ever had liver disease.

• tell your doctor if you are pregnant, plan to become pregnant, or are breast-feeding. If you become pregnant while taking ondansetron, call your doctor.

• if you have phenylketonuria (PKU, an inherited condition in which a special diet must be followed to prevent mental retardation), you should know that the orally disintegrating tablets contain aspartame that forms phenylalanine.

What special dietary instructions should I follow?

Unless your doctor tells you otherwise, continue your usual diet.

What should I do if I forget to take a dose?

Take the missed dose as soon as you remember it. However, if it is almost time for the next dose, skip the missed dose and continue your regular dosing schedule. Do not take a double dose to make up for a missed one.

What side effects can this medicine cause?

Ondansetron may cause side effects. Tell your doctor if any of these symptoms are severe or do not go away:

- diarrhea
- headache
- constipation
- weakness
- tiredness
- dizziness

Some side effects can be serious. If you experience any of the following symptoms, call your doctor immediately:

- rash
- hives
- itching
- swelling of the eyes, face, lips, tongue, throat, hands, feet, ankles, or lower legs
- hoarseness
- difficulty breathing or swallowing
- shortness of breath
- noisy, high pitched breathing

Ondansetron may cause other side effects. Call your doctor if you have any unusual problems while you are taking this medication.

What storage conditions are needed for this medicine?

Keep this medication in the container it came in, tightly closed, and out of reach of children. Store the tablets and rapidly disintegrating tablets away from light, at room temperature or in the refrigerator. Store the solution at room temperature and away from light, excess heat, and moisture (not in the bathroom). Throw away any medication that is outdated or no longer needed. Talk to your pharmacist about the proper disposal of your medication.

What should I do in case of overdose?

In case of overdose, call your local poison control center at 1-800-222-1222. If the victim has collapsed or is not breathing, call local emergency services at 911.

Symptoms of overdose may include:

- sudden loss of vision for a short time
- dizziness or lightheadedness
- fainting
- constipation
- irregular heartbeat

What other information should I know?

Keep all appointments with your doctor.

Do not let anyone else take your medication. Ask your pharmacist any questions you have about refilling your prescription.

Dosage Facts
For Informational Purposes

Caution: Do not change your dose, how often you take your medication, or the length of time you are to take it without first talking to your healthcare provider.

The following dosage information was written using medical language for doctors and other healthcare professionals and is provided here for you to check your dosage. The dosage of this drug may differ for different patients. Therefore, always follow your doctor's instructions or the directions on the label. Contact your healthcare provider or pharmacist if you have any questions about the specific dosage of your medication after reviewing this information.

General Dosage Information

Available as ondansetron hydrochloride dihydrate (for oral or IV use) and as ondansetron base (orally disintegrating tablets); dosage expressed in terms of ondansetron.

Pediatric Patients

Cancer Chemotherapy-induced Nausea and Vomiting
Prevention

ORAL:

- Children 4–11 years of age: Initially, 4 mg given 30 minutes before administration of moderately emetogenic chemotherapy, followed by subsequent 4-mg doses given 4 and 8 hours after first dose. Continue with 4 mg every 8 hours for 1–2 days after completion of chemotherapy.
- Children ≥12 years of age: Initially, 8 mg given 30 minutes before administration of moderately emetogenic chemotherapy, followed by a subsequent 8-mg dose given 8 hours after first dose. Continue with 8 mg every 12 hours for 1–2 days after completion of chemotherapy.

Adult Patients

Cancer Chemotherapy-induced Nausea and Vomiting
Prevention

ORAL:

- Initially, 8 mg given 30 minutes before administration of moderately emetogenic chemotherapy, followed by a subsequent 8-mg dose given 8 hours after first dose. Continue with 8 mg every 12 hours for 1–2 days after completion of chemotherapy.
- 24 mg as a single dose given 30 minutes before administration of single-day highly emetogenic chemotherapy.

Postoperative Nausea and Vomiting
Prevention

ORAL:

- 16 mg as a single dose given 1 hour before induction of anesthesia.

Radiation-induced Nausea and Vomiting
Prevention, Usual Dosage

ORAL:

- Usually, 8 mg 3 times daily.

Prevention, for Total Body Irradiation

ORAL:
- 8 mg 1–2 hours before each fraction of radiotherapy administered each day.

Prevention, for Single High-dose Fraction Radiation to Abdomen

ORAL:
- 8 mg 1–2 hours before radiotherapy, with subsequent doses every 8 hours after the first dose for 1–2 days after completion of radiotherapy.

Prevention, for Daily Fractionated Radiation to Abdomen

ORAL:
- 8 mg 1–2 hours before radiotherapy, with subsequent doses every 8 hours after the first dose for each day radiotherapy is given.

Special Populations

Hepatic Impairment
- Do not exceed total daily dosage of 8 mg in patients with severe hepatic impairment (Child-Pugh score ≥10).

Renal Impairment
- No dosage adjustment required, but no experience to date with continuation beyond the first day of therapy.

Geriatric Patients
- No dosage adjustment required.

Ondansetron Injection

(on dan' se tron)

Brand Name: Zofran ®Injection

Why is this medicine prescribed?

Ondansetron injection is used to prevent nausea and vomiting caused by cancer chemotherapy and surgery. Ondansetron is in a class of medications called 5-HT$_3$ receptor antagonists. It works by blocking the action of serotonin, a natural substance that may cause nausea and vomiting.

How should this medicine be used?

Ondansetron comes as a solution (liquid) to be injected intravenously (into a vein) or into a muscle by a health care provider in a hospital or clinic. When ondansetron is used to prevent nausea and vomiting caused by chemotherapy, it is usually given 30 minutes before the start of chemotherapy. Additional doses may be given 4 hours after the first dose and 8 hours after the first dose. When ondansetron is used to prevent nausea and vomiting caused by surgery, it is usually given just before the surgery. Ondansetron is also sometimes given after surgery to patients who are experiencing nausea and vomiting and did not receive ondansetron before surgery.

Are there other uses for this medicine?

This medication may be prescribed for other uses. Ask your doctor or pharmacist for more information.

What special precautions should I follow?

Before taking ondansetron,
- tell your doctor and pharmacist if you are allergic to ondansetron, alosetron (Lotronex), dolasetron (Anzemet), granisetron (Kytril), palonosetron (Aloxi), or any other medications.
- tell your doctor and pharmacist what prescription and nonprescription medications, vitamins, nutritional supplements, and herbal products you are taking or plan to take. Be sure to mention tramadol (Ultram, in Ultracet). Your doctor may need to change the doses of your medications or monitor you more carefully for side effects.
- tell your doctor if you have or have ever had liver disease.
- tell your doctor if you are pregnant, plan to become pregnant, or are breast-feeding. If you become pregnant while taking ondansetron, call your doctor.

What special dietary instructions should I follow?

Unless your doctor tells you otherwise, continue your usual diet.

What side effects can this medicine cause?

Ondansetron may cause side effects. Tell your doctor if any of these symptoms are severe or do not go away:
- headache
- constipation
- drowsiness
- feeling cold
- numbness, burning, or tingling in the fingers or toes
- fever
- pain, redness, swelling, warmth, or burning in the place where ondansetron was injected

Some side effects can be serious. If you experience any of the following symptoms, call your doctor immediately:
- rash
- hives
- itching
- swelling of the eyes, face, lips, tongue, throat, hands, feet, ankles, or lower legs
- hoarseness
- difficulty breathing or swallowing
- shortness of breath
- noisy, high pitched breathing
- blurred vision or vision loss

Ondansetron may cause other side effects. Call your doctor if you have any unusual problems while you are taking this medication.

If you experience a serious side effect, you or your doctor may send a report to the Food and Drug Administration's

(FDA) MedWatch Adverse Event Reporting program online [at http://www.fda.gov/MedWatch/index.html] or by phone [1-800-332-1088].

What storage conditions are needed for this medicine?

This medication will be stored in the hospital or clinic.

What should I do in case of overdose?

In case of overdose, call your local poison control center at 1-800-222-1222. If the victim has collapsed or is not breathing, call local emergency services at 911.

Symptoms of overdose may include:

- sudden loss of vision for a short time
- dizziness or lightheadedness
- fainting
- constipation
- irregular heartbeat

What other information should I know?

Keep all appointments with your doctor.

Dosage Facts
For Informational Purposes

Caution: Do not change your dose, how often you take your medication, or the length of time you are to take it without first talking to your health-care provider.

The following dosage information was written using medical language for doctors and other healthcare professionals and is provided here for you to check your dosage. The dosage of this drug may differ for different patients. Therefore, always follow your doctor's instructions or the directions on the label. Contact your healthcare provider or pharmacist if you have any questions about the specific dosage of your medication after reviewing this information.

General Dosage Information

Available as ondansetron hydrochloride dihydrate (for oral or IV use) and as ondansetron base (orally disintegrating tablets); dosage expressed in terms of ondansetron.

Pediatric Patients

Cancer Chemotherapy-induced Nausea and Vomiting
Prevention

IV:
- Children 4–18 years of age: 0.15 mg/kg by IV infusion beginning 30 minutes before start of emetogenic chemotherapy, followed by subsequent 0.15-mg/kg doses given 4 and 8 hours after first dose.

Postoperative Nausea and Vomiting
Prevention

IV:
- Children 2–12 years of age weighing ≤40 kg: 0.1 mg/kg as a single dose by IV injection immediately before induction of anesthesia.
- Children 2–12 years of age weighing >40 kg: 4 mg as a single dose by IV injection immediately before induction of anesthesia.

Treatment

IV:
- Children 2–12 years of age weighing ≤40 kg: 0.1 mg/kg as a single dose by IV injection postoperatively, if nausea and/or vomiting occur shortly after surgery.
- Children 2–12 years of age weighing >40 kg: 4 mg as a single dose by IV injection postoperatively, if nausea and/or vomiting occur shortly after surgery.
- If adequate control of postoperative nausea and vomiting is not achieved after a single, prophylactic, preinduction IV dose, a second IV dose postoperatively does not provide additional control of nausea and vomiting.

Adult Patients

Cancer Chemotherapy-induced Nausea and Vomiting
Prevention

IV:
- 0.15 mg/kg by IV infusion beginning 30 minutes before administration of emetogenic chemotherapy, followed by 0.15 mg/kg infused 4 and 8 hours after first dose.
- Alternatively, 32 mg as a single dose by IV infusion beginning 30 minutes before administration of emetogenic chemotherapy.

Postoperative Nausea and Vomiting
Prevention

IV:
- 4 mg as a single dose by IV injection (undiluted) immediately before induction of anesthesia.
- Limited information available regarding dosage in patients weighing >80 kg.

IM:
- 4 mg as a single dose by IM injection (undiluted) as an alternative to IV administration.
- Limited information available regarding dosage in patients weighing >80 kg.

Treatment

IV:
- 4 mg as a single dose by IV injection (undiluted) postoperatively, if nausea and/or vomiting occur shortly after surgery.
- If adequate control of postoperative nausea and vomiting is not achieved after a single, prophylactic, preinduction IV dose, a second IV dose postoperatively does not provide additional control of nausea and vomiting.

Special Populations

Hepatic Impairment
- Do not exceed total daily dosage of 8 mg in patients with severe hepatic impairment (Child-Pugh score ≥10); no experience to date with continuation beyond the first day of IV therapy.

Renal Impairment
- No dosage adjustment required, but no experience to date with continuation beyond the first day of therapy.

Geriatric Patients
- No dosage adjustment required.

Orlistat

(or′ li stat)

Brand Name: alli®, Xenical®

Why is this medicine prescribed?

Orlistat (prescription and nonprescription) is used with an individualized low-calorie, low-fat diet and exercise program to help people lose weight. Prescription orlistat is used in overweight people who may also have high blood pressure, diabetes, high cholesterol, or heart disease. Orlistat is also used after weight-loss to help people keep from gaining back that weight. Orlistat is in a class of medications called lipase inhibitors. It works in the intestines by blocking absorption of some of the fat in foods eaten. This unabsorbed fat is then removed in stools from the body.

How should this medicine be used?

Orlistat comes as a capsule and a nonprescription capsule to take by mouth. It is usually taken three times a day with each main meal that contains fat. Take orlistat during a meal or up to 1 hour after a meal. If a meal is missed or does not have fat, you may skip your dose. Follow the directions on your prescription label or the package label carefully, and ask your doctor or pharmacist to explain any part you do not understand. Take orlistat exactly as directed. Do not take more or less of it or take it more often than prescribed by your doctor or stated on the package.

Ask your pharmacist or doctor for a copy of the manufacturer's information for the patient if orlistat is prescribed for you. For additional information about the nonprescription product, visit www.My Alli.com.

Are there other uses for this medicine?

This medication is sometimes prescribed for other uses; ask your doctor or pharmacist for more information.

What special precautions should I follow?

Before taking orlistat,
- tell your doctor and pharmacist if you are allergic to orlistat or any other medications.
- talk to your doctor if you are taking medications that suppress the immune system such as cyclosporine (Neoral, Sandimmune). If you are taking cyclosporine (Neoral, Sandimmune), take it 2 hours before or 2 hours after orlistat.

- tell your doctor and pharmacist what prescription and nonprescription, vitamins, nutritional supplements, and herbal products you are taking or plan to take. Be sure to mention any of the following: anticoagulants (''blood thinners'') such as warfarin (Coumadin); medications for diabetes, such as glipizide (Glucotrol), glyburide (DiaBeta, Dynase, Micronase), metformin (Glucophage), and insulin; medications to control blood pressure; medications for thyroid disease; and any other medications for weight loss.
- tell your doctor if you have if you have had an organ transplant or if you have cholestasis (condition in which the flow of bile from the liver is blocked) or malabsorption syndrome (problems absorbing food). Your doctor will probably tell you not to take orlistat.
- tell your doctor if you have or have ever had an eating disorder such as anorexia nervosa or bulimia, diabetes, kidney stones, pancreatitis (inflammation or swelling of the pancreas), or gallbladder or thyroid disease.
- tell your doctor if you are pregnant, plan to become pregnant, or are breast-feeding. Do not take orlistat if you are pregnant or breast-feeding.

What special dietary instructions should I follow?

Follow the diet program your doctor has given you. You should evenly divide the amount of daily fat, carbohydrates, and protein you eat over three main meals. If orlistat is taken with a diet high in fat (a diet with more than 30% of the total daily calories from fat), or with one meal very high in fat, it is more likely you will experience side effects from the medication.

Orlistat blocks your body's absorption of some fat-soluble vitamins and beta carotene. Therefore, when you use orlistat you should take a daily multivitamin that contains vitamins A, D, E, K, and beta-carotene. Read the label to find a multivitamin product that contains these vitamins. Take the multivitamin once a day, 2 hours before or 2 hours after taking orlistat, or take the multivitamin at bedtime. Ask your doctor or pharmacist any questions you might have about taking a multivitamin while you are taking orlistat.

While you are taking orlistat, you should avoid foods that have more than 30% fat. Read the labels on all the foods you buy. When eating meat, poultry (chicken) or fish, eat only 2 or 3 ounces (about the size of a deck of cards) for a serving. Choose lean cuts of meat and remove the skin from poultry. Fill up your meal plate with more grains, fruits, and vegetables. Replace whole-milk products with nonfat or 1% milk and reduced- or low-fat dairy items. Cook with less fat. Use vegetable oil spray when cooking. Salad dressings; many baked items; and prepackaged, processed, and fast foods are usually high in fat. Use the low- or nonfat versions of these foods and/or cut back on serving sizes. When dining out, ask how foods are prepared and request that they be prepared with little or no added fat.

What should I do if I forget to take a dose?

Take the missed dose as soon as you remember it unless it is more than 1 hour since you ate a main meal. If it is longer than 1 hour since you ate a main meal, skip the missed dose and continue on your regular dosing schedule. Do not take a double dose to make up for a missed one.

What side effects can this medicine cause?

Orlistat may cause side effects. The most common side effect of orlistat is changes in bowel movement (BM) habits. This generally occurs during the first weeks of treatment; however, it may continue throughout your use of orlistat. Tell your doctor if any of these symptoms are severe or do not go away:

- oily spotting on underwear or on clothing
- gas with oily spotting
- urgent need to have a bowel movement
- loose stools
- oily or fatty stools
- increased number of bowel movements
- difficulty controlling bowel movements
- pain or discomfort in the rectum (bottom)
- stomach pain
- irregular menstrual periods
- headache
- anxiety

Some side effects can be serious. If you experience any of these symptoms, call your doctor immediately:

- hives
- rash
- itching
- difficulty breathing or swallowing
- severe or continuous abdominal pain

If you experience a serious side effect, you or your doctor may send a report to the Food and Drug Administration's (FDA) MedWatch Adverse Event Reporting program online [at http://www.fda.gov/MedWatch/index.html] or by phone [1-800-332-1088].

What storage conditions are needed for this medicine?

Keep this medication in the container it came in, tightly closed, and out of reach of children. Store it at room temperature and away from excess heat, moisture (not in the bathroom), and light. Throw away any medication that is outdated or no longer needed. Talk to your pharmacist about the proper disposal of your medication.

What should I do in case of overdose?

In case of overdose, call your local poison control center at 1-800-222-1222. If the victim has collapsed or is not breathing, call local emergency services at 911.

What other information should I know?

Keep all appointments with your doctor.

You should also follow a program of regular physical activity or exercise while you are taking orlistat. However, before you start any new activity or exercise program, talk with your doctor or health care professional.

Do not let anyone else take your prescription medication. Ask your pharmacist any questions you have about refilling your prescription.

Dosage Facts
For Informational Purposes

Caution: Do not change your dose, how often you take your medication, or the length of time you are to take it without first talking to your healthcare provider.

The following dosage information was written using medical language for doctors and other healthcare professionals and is provided here for you to check your dosage. The dosage of this drug may differ for different patients. Therefore, always follow your doctor's instructions or the directions on the label. Contact your healthcare provider or pharmacist if you have any questions about the specific dosage of your medication after reviewing this information.

Adult Patients

Obesity

ORAL:
- 120 mg 3 times daily with each main meal containing fat. No additional benefit with dosages >120 mg 3 times daily.
- Reassess weight management and therapy periodically. Safety and efficacy beyond 2 years not established in clinical studies. However, if effective for weight loss or maintenance and no serious adverse effects occur, may continue orlistat as long as clinically indicated.

Orphenadrine

(or fen' a dreen)

Brand Name: Invagesic®, Norflex®, Norgesic® as a combination product containing Orphenadrine Citrate, Aspirin, and Caffeine, Norgesic® Forte as a combination product containing Orphenadrine Citrate, Aspirin, and Caffeine

Why is this medicine prescribed?

Orphenadrine is used with rest, physical therapy, and other measures to relieve pain and discomfort caused by strains, sprains, and other muscle injuries.

This medication is sometimes prescribed for other uses; ask your doctor or pharmacist for more information.

How should this medicine be used?

Orphenadrine comes as a tablet and an extended-release tablet to take by mouth. It is usually taken twice a day. Do not cut, crush, or chew the extended-release tablets; swallow them whole. Follow the directions on your prescription label carefully, and ask your doctor or pharmacist to explain any part you do not understand. Take orphenadrine exactly as directed. Do not take more or less of it or take it more often than prescribed by your doctor.

Are there other uses for this medicine?

Orphenadrine is also used occasionally to treat nighttime leg cramps. Talk to your doctor about the possible risks of using this drug for your condition.

What special precautions should I follow?

Before taking orphenadrine,

- tell your doctor and pharmacist if you are allergic to orphenadrine or any other drugs.
- tell your doctor and pharmacist what prescription and nonprescription medications you are taking, especially amantadine (Symadine, Symmetrel), fluphenazine (Prolixin), haloperidol (Haldol), medications for colds or allergies, medications for depression, perphenazine (Trilafon), prochlorperazine (Compazine), promethazine (Phenergan), sedatives, sleeping pills, trifluoperazine (Stelazine), and vitamins.
- tell your doctor if you have or have ever had glaucoma; myasthenia gravis; ulcers; a urinary tract or intestinal blockage; an enlarged prostate; an irregular heartbeat; or liver, kidney, or heart disease.
- tell your doctor if you are pregnant, plan to become pregnant, or are breast-feeding. If you become pregnant while taking orphenadrine, call your doctor.
- if you are having surgery, including dental surgery, tell the doctor or dentist that you are taking orphenadrine.
- you should know that this drug may make you drowsy. Do not drive a car or operate machinery until you know how orphenadrine will affect you.
- remember that alcohol can add to the drowsiness caused by this drug.

What should I do if I forget to take a dose?

Take the missed dose as soon as you remember it. However, if it is almost time for the next dose, skip the missed dose and continue your regular dosing schedule. Do not take a double dose to make up for a missed one.

What side effects can this medicine cause?

Orphenadrine may cause side effects. Tell your doctor if any of these symptoms are severe or do not go away:

- dry mouth
- drowsiness
- dizziness or lightheadedness
- upset stomach
- vomiting
- constipation
- difficulty urinating
- blurred vision
- headache

If you experience any of the following symptoms, call your doctor immediately:

- fast or irregular heartbeat
- fainting
- confusion
- hallucinations
- skin rash

If you experience a serious side effect, you or your doctor may send a report to the Food and Drug Administration's (FDA) MedWatch Adverse Event Reporting program online [at http://www.fda.gov/MedWatch/index.html] or by phone [1-800-332-1088].

What storage conditions are needed for this medicine?

Keep this medication in the container it came in, tightly closed, and out of reach of children. Store it at room temperature and away from excess heat and moisture (not in the bathroom). Throw away any medication that is outdated or no longer needed. Talk to your pharmacist about the proper disposal of your medication.

What should I do in case of overdose?

In case of overdose, call your local poison control center at 1-800-222-1222. If the victim has collapsed or is not breathing, call local emergency services at 911.

What other information should I know?

Keep all appointments with your doctor.

Do not let anyone else take your medication. Ask your pharmacist any questions you have about refilling your prescription.

Talk to your doctor, pharmacist, or other healthcare professional if you have questions about dosing information for your medication.

Oseltamivir

(os el tam′ i vir)

Brand Name: Tamiflu®

Why is this medicine prescribed?

Oseltamivir is used to treat some types of influenza infection ('flu') in adults and children (older than 1 year of age) who have had symptoms of the flu for no longer than 2 days. This medication is also used to prevent some types of flu in adults and children (older than 1 year of age) when they have spent time with someone who has the flu or when there is a flu outbreak. Oseltamivir is in a class of medications called neuraminidase inhibitors. It works by stopping the spread of the flu virus in the body. Oseltamivir helps shorten the time you have flu symptoms such as a stuffy or runny nose, sore throat, cough, muscle or joint aches, tiredness, headache, fever, and chills. Oseltamivir will not prevent bacterial infections which may occur as a complication of the flu.

How should this medicine be used?

Oseltamivir comes as a capsule and a suspension (liquid) to take by mouth. When oseltamivir is used to treat flu symptoms, it is usually taken twice daily (morning and evening) for 5 days. When oseltamivir is used to prevent flu, it is usually taken once a day for at least 10 days, or for up to 6 weeks during a community flu outbreak. Oseltamivir may be taken with or without food, but you can lessen the chance of getting an upset stomach by taking oseltamivir with food or milk. Follow the directions on your prescription label carefully, and ask your doctor or pharmacist to explain any part that you do not understand. Take oseltamivir exactly as directed. Do not take more or less of it or take it more often than prescribed by your doctor.

To prepare doses of oseltamivir liquid:

1. Shake the liquid well (for about 5 seconds) before each use to mix the medication evenly.
2. Open the bottle by pushing down on the cap and turning the cap at the same time.
3. Push the plunger of the measuring device completely down to the tip.
4. Insert the tip of the measuring device firmly into the opening on the top of the bottle.
5. Turn the bottle (with the measuring device attached) upside down.
6. Pull back on the plunger slowly until the amount of liquid prescribed by your doctor fills the measuring device to the appropriate marking. Some larger doses may need to be measured using the measuring device twice. If you are not sure how to correctly measure the dose your doctor has prescribed, ask your doctor or pharmacist.
7. Turn the bottle (with the measuring device attached) right side up and slowly remove the measuring device.
8. Take oseltamivir directly into your mouth from the measuring device; do not mix with any other liquids.
9. Replace the cap on the bottle and close tightly.
10. Remove the plunger from the rest of the measuring device and rinse both parts under running tap water. Allow the parts to air dry before putting back together for the next use.

Call your doctor or pharmacist to find out how you should measure your dose of oseltamivir solution if you do not have the measuring device.

Continue to take oseltamivir until you finish the prescription even if you start to feel better. Do not stop taking oseltamivir without talking to your doctor. If you stop taking oseltamivir too soon or skip doses, your infection may not be fully treated, or you may not be protected from the flu.

If you feel worse or develop new symptoms while taking oseltamivir, or if your flu symptoms do not start to get better, call your doctor.

Ask your pharmacist or doctor for a copy of the manufacturer's information for the patient.

Are there other uses for this medicine?

Oseltamivir may be used to treat and prevent infections from avian (bird) influenza (a virus that usually infects birds but can also cause serious illness in humans).

What special precautions should I follow?

Before taking oseltamivir,

- tell your doctor and pharmacist if you are allergic to oseltamivir or any other medications.
- tell your doctor what prescription and nonprescription medications, vitamins, nutritional supplements and herbal products you are taking or plan to take. Be sure to mention any of the following: medications that affect the immune system such as azathioprine (Imuran); cyclosporine (Neoral, Sandimmune); cancer chemotherapy medications; methotrexate (Rheumatrex); sirolimus (Rapamune); oral steroids such as dexamethasone (Decadron, Dexone), methylprednisolone (Medrol), and prednisone (Deltasone); or tacrolimus (Prograf). Your doctor may need to change the doses of your medications or monitor you carefully for side effects.
- tell your doctor if you have ever taken oseltamivir to treat or prevent the flu.
- tell your doctor if you have any disease or condition that affects your immune system such as human immunodeficiency virus (HIV) or acquired immunodeficiency syndrome (AIDS) or if you have heart, liver, lung, or kidney disease.
- tell your doctor if you are pregnant, plan to become pregnant, or are breast-feeding. If you become pregnant while taking oseltamivir, call your doctor.
- you should know that some people who took oseltamivir to treat flu became confused, behaved strangely, and in some cases harmed themselves. These symptoms were most common in children but were also experienced by

adults. If your child is taking oseltamivir, you should watch his or her behavior very carefully and call the doctor right away if he or she becomes confused or behaves abnormally. If you are taking oseltamivir, you, your family, or your caregiver should call the doctor right away if you become confused, behave abnormally, or think about harming yourself. Be sure that your family or caregiver knows which symptoms may be serious so they can call the doctor if you are unable to seek treatment on your own.

- ask your doctor if you should receive a flu vaccination each year. Oseltamivir does not take the place of a yearly flu vaccine. If you received or plan to receive the intranasal flu vaccine (FluMist; flu vaccine that is sprayed into the nose), you should tell your doctor before taking oseltamivir. Oseltamivir may interfere with the activity of the intranasal flu vaccine if it is taken up to 2 weeks after or up to 48 hours before the vaccine is administered.

What should I do if I forget to take a dose?

If you forget to take a dose, take it as soon as you remember it. If it is no longer than 2 hours before your next scheduled dose, skip the missed dose and continue your regular dosing schedule. If you miss several doses, call your doctor for directions. Do not take a double dose to make up for a missed one.

What side effects can this medicine cause?

Oseltamivir may cause side effects. Tell your doctor if any of these symptoms are severe or do not go away:

- nausea
- vomiting
- stomach pain
- diarrhea
- headache
- difficulty falling asleep or staying asleep
- cough
- dizziness

Some side effects can be serious. If you experience any of these symptoms or those mentioned in the SPECIAL PRECAUTIONS section, call your doctor immediately:

- rash, hives, or blisters on the skin
- itching
- swelling of the face or tongue
- difficulty breathing or swallowing
- hoarseness

What storage conditions are needed for this medicine?

Keep this medication in the container it came in and out of reach of children. Store the capsules at room temperature and away from excess heat and moisture (not in the bathroom). Keep the liquid in the refrigerator. Do not freeze oseltamivir liquid. Throw away any unused liquid medication after 10 days. Throw away any medication that is outdated or no longer needed. Talk to your pharmacist about the proper disposal of your medication.

What should I do in case of overdose?

In case of overdose, call your local poison control center at 1-800-222-1222. If the victim has collapsed or is not breathing, call local emergency services at 911.

Symptoms of overdose may include:

- nausea
- vomiting

What other information should I know?

Oseltamivir will not stop you from giving the flu to others. You should wash your hands frequently, and avoid practices such as sharing cups and utensils that can spread the virus to others.

Do not let anyone else take your medication. Your prescription is probably not refillable. If you still have symptoms of the flu after you finish taking oseltamivir, call your doctor.

Dosage Facts
For Informational Purposes

Caution: Do not change your dose, how often you take your medication, or the length of time you are to take it without first talking to your healthcare provider.

The following dosage information was written using medical language for doctors and other healthcare professionals and is provided here for you to check your dosage. The dosage of this drug may differ for different patients. Therefore, always follow your doctor's instructions or the directions on the label. Contact your healthcare provider or pharmacist if you have any questions about the specific dosage of your medication after reviewing this information.

General Dosage Information

Available as oseltamivir phosphate; dosage expressed in terms of oseltamivir.

Systemic availability of oseltamivir carboxylate from an extemporaneous oral preparation prepared from a bulk storage containers of the drug (not commercially available in the US) is expected to be the same as that from the commercially available preparations.

Pediatric Patients

Treatment of Influenza A and B Virus Infections

ORAL:

Dosage for Treatment of Influenza A and B in Children 1–12 Years of Age

Weight (kg)	Daily Dosage
≤15	30 mg twice daily for 5 days
>15 to 23	45 mg twice daily for 5 days
>23 to 40	60 mg twice daily for 5 days
>40	75 mg twice daily for 5 days

Children ≥13 years of age: 75 mg twice daily for 5 days.

Initiate oseltamivir treatment within 2 days after onset of symptoms; efficacy not established if treatment begins >40 hours after symptoms have been established.

Prevention of Influenza A and B Virus Infections

ORAL:

Dosage for Prevention of Influenza A and B in Children 1–12 Years of Age

Weight (kg)	Daily Dosage
≤15	30 mg once daily for 10 days
>15 to 23	45 mg once daily for 10 days
>23 to 40	60 mg once daily for 10 days
>40	75 mg once daily for 10 days

Children 1–12 years of age: Initiate oseltamivir prophylaxis within 2 days after exposure (e.g., close contact with infected individual). Usual duration is 10 days; duration >10 days not evaluated in this age group.

Children ≥13 years of age: 75 mg once daily for ≥10 days. Initiate oseltamivir prophylaxis within 2 days after exposure (e.g., close contact with infected individual). May be continued for up to 6 weeks during a community influenza outbreak.

Treatment of Avian Influenza A Virus Infections†

ORAL:

- Children: Dosage usually recommended for treatment of seasonal influenza A and B virus infections has been recommended. This dosage may be reasonable for early, mild cases of influenza A (H5N1) infection, but WHO and others state that severely ill patients may benefit from higher dosage and/or longer duration of therapy (i.e., 7–10 days).
- Initiate treatment as early as possible; the benefits of oseltamivir and optimal dosage for late-stage intervention in severe illness unknown.

Prevention of Avian Influenza A Virus Infections†

ORAL:

- Children: Dosage usually recommended for prophylaxis of seasonal influenza A and B virus infections has been rec-

ommended. No evidence to date that an increase in dosage or duration is necessary in individuals who have had a single exposure to influenza A (H5N1), but a longer duration of prophylaxis may be necessary in those with repeated or prolonged exposure.

- High-risk and moderate-risk exposure groups: Initiate as soon as possible and continue for 7–10 days after last known exposure.

Pandemic Influenza†

ORAL:

- Children: Dosage usually recommended for treatment or prophylaxis of seasonal influenza A and B virus infections is considered the *minimum* dosage required for treatment or prophylaxis of influenza in a pandemic situation. Clinical data on use of oseltamivir in pandemics not available.

Adult Patients

Treatment of Influenza A and B Virus Infections

ORAL:

- 75 mg twice daily for 5 days.
- Initiate oseltamivir treatment within 2 days after onset of symptoms; efficacy not established if treatment begins >40 hours after symptoms have been established.

Prevention of Influenza A and B Virus Infections

ORAL:

- 75 mg once daily given for at least 10 days. Initiate prophylaxis within 2 days after exposure (e.g., close contact with infected individual).
- 75 mg once daily has been given for up to 6 weeks during a community outbreak of influenza.

Treatment of Avian Influenza A Virus Infections†

ORAL:

- 75 mg twice daily for 5 days has been recommended. Dosage usually recommended for treatment of seasonal influenza A and B virus infections has been recommended. This dosage may be reasonable for early, mild cases of influenza A (H5N1) infection, but WHO and others state that severely ill patients may benefit from higher dosage (i.e., 150 mg twice daily in adults) and/or longer duration of therapy (i.e., 7–10 days).
- Initiate treatment as early as possible; benefits of oseltamivir and optimal dosage for late-stage intervention in severe illness unknown.

Prevention of Avian Influenza A Virus Infections†

ORAL:

- Dosage usually recommended for prophylaxis of seasonal influenza A and B virus infections has been recommended. No evidence to date that an increase in dosage or duration is necessary in individuals who have had a single exposure to influenza A (H5N1), but a longer duration of prophylaxis may be necessary in those with repeated or prolonged exposure.
- High-risk and moderate-risk exposure groups: Initiate as soon as possible and continue for 7–10 days after last known exposure.
- Preexposure prophylaxis or repeated or continuous postex-

posure prophylaxis may be necessary in individuals in high-risk situations (e.g., individuals directly involved in control and eradication of poultry outbreaks). Oseltamivir prophylaxis in a dosage of 75 mg daily generally well tolerated for up to 6 weeks.

- During avian influenza A (H7N7) outbreaks, 75 mg daily has been used for prophylaxis in exposed individuals.

Pandemic Influenza†

ORAL:

- Dosage recommended for treatment or prophylaxis of seasonal influenza A and B virus infections is considered the *minimum* dosage required for treatment or prophylaxis of influenza in a pandemic situation. Clinical data on use of oseltamivir in pandemics not available. Although 75-mg doses may provide adequate antiviral activity against a novel strain, preliminary data from animal studies suggest that higher doses and/or longer duration of treatment may be needed, especially if a pandemic is caused by a virulent strain (e.g., avian influenza A H5N1).
- Short-term prophylaxis (7–10 days) may be effective in reducing household transmission and long-term prophylaxis (4–8 weeks) presumably would provide protection during a pandemic wave of activity. Duration of prophylaxis needed for a ring prophylaxis strategy in an affected geographic area is uncertain, but would likely be 3–6 weeks if successful.

Special Populations

Hepatic Impairment

- Effect of hepatic dysfunction not fully determined. Manufacturer does not provide specific dosage recommendations; some clinicians suggest usual dosage can be used in those with mild to moderate hepatic impairment.

Renal Impairment

- Treatment of influenza A or B virus infections in patients with Cl$_{cr}$ 10–30 mL/min: 75 mg once daily for 5 days.
- Prevention of influenza A or B virus infections in patients with Cl$_{cr}$ 10–30 mL/min: 75 mg (as capsules) once every other day or 30 mg (as oral suspension) once daily.
- No dosage recommendations for patients with end-stage renal disease (Cl$_{cr}$ <10 mL/min) and those undergoing routine hemodialysis or CAPD.

Geriatric Patients

- No dosage adjustments except those related to renal impairment.

† *Use is not currently included in the labeling approved by the US Food and Drug Administration.*

Oxacillin Sodium Injection

(ox a sill′ in)

Brand Name: Bactocill®
Also available generically.

About Your Treatment

Your doctor has ordered oxacillin, an antibiotic, to help treat your infection. The drug will be either injected into a large muscle (such as your buttock or hip) or added to an intravenous fluid that will drip through a needle or catheter placed in your vein for about 30 minutes, four to six times a day.

Oxacillin eliminates bacteria that cause infections, including pneumonia; meningitis; and urinary tract, skin, bone, joint, blood, and heart valve infections. This medication is sometimes prescribed for other uses; ask your doctor or pharmacist for more information.

Your health care provider (doctor, nurse, or pharmacist) may measure the effectiveness and side effects of your treatment using laboratory tests and physical examinations. It is important to keep all appointments with your doctor and the laboratory. The length of treatment depends on how your infection and symptoms respond to the medication.

Precautions

Before administering oxacillin,

- tell your doctor and pharmacist if you are allergic to oxacillin, penicillin, cephalosporins [e.g., cefaclor (Ceclor), cefadroxil (Duricef), or cephalexin (Keflex)], or any other drugs.
- tell your doctor and pharmacist what prescription and nonprescription medications you are taking, especially antibiotics and vitamins.
- tell your doctor if you have or have ever had asthma; hay fever; or kidney, liver, or gastrointestinal disease (especially colitis).
- tell your doctor if you are pregnant, plan to become pregnant, or are breast-feeding. If you become pregnant while taking oxacillin, call your doctor.
- if you have diabetes and regularly check your urine for sugar, use Clinistix or TesTape. Do not use Clinitest tablets because oxacillin may cause false positive results.

Administering Your Medication

Before you administer oxacillin, look at the solution closely. It should be clear and free of floating material. Gently squeeze the bag or observe the solution container to make sure there are no leaks. Do not use the solution if it is discolored, if it contains particles, or if the bag or container leaks. Use a new solution, but show the damaged one to your health care provider.

It is important that you use your medication exactly as directed. Do not stop your therapy on your own for any reason because your infection could worsen and result in hospitalization. Do not change your dosing schedule without talking to your health care provider. Your health care provider may tell you to stop your infusion if you have a mechanical problem (such as a blockage in the tubing, needle, or catheter); if you have to stop an infusion, call your health care provider immediately so your therapy can continue.

Side Effects

Oxacillin may cause side effects. Tell your health care provider if either of these symptoms is severe or does not go away:

- upset stomach
- diarrhea

If you experience any of the following symptoms, call your health care provider immediately:

- rash
- itching
- fever
- chills
- facial swelling
- wheezing
- difficulty breathing
- unusual bleeding or bruising
- dizziness
- seizures
- sore mouth or throat

If you experience a serious side effect, you or your doctor may send a report to the Food and Drug Administration's (FDA) MedWatch Adverse Event Reporting program online [at http://www.fda.gov/MedWatch/index.html] or by phone [1-800-332-1088].

Storage Conditions

- Your health care provider probably will give you a several-day supply of oxacillin at a time. If you are receiving oxacillin intravenously (in your vein), you probably will be told to store it in the refrigerator or freezer.
- Take your next dose from the refrigerator 1 hour before using it; place it in a clean, dry area to allow it to warm to room temperature.
- If you are told to store additional oxacillin in the freezer, always move a 24-hour supply to the refrigerator for the next day's use.
- Do not refreeze medications.

If you are receiving oxacillin intramuscularly (in your muscle), your health care provider will tell you how to store it properly.

Store your medication only as directed. Make sure you understand what you need to store your medication properly.

Keep your supplies in a clean, dry place when you are not using them, and keep all medications and supplies out of reach of children. Your health care provider will tell you

how to throw away used needles, syringes, tubing, and containers to avoid accidental injury.

Overdose

In case of overdose, call your local poison control center at 1-800-222-1222. If the victim has collapsed or is not breathing, call local emergency services at 911.

Signs of Infection

If you are receiving oxacillin in your vein or under your skin, you need to know the symptoms of a catheter-related infection (an infection where the needle enters your vein or skin). If you experience any of these effects near your intravenous catheter, tell your health care provider as soon as possible:

- tenderness
- warmth
- irritation
- drainage
- redness
- swelling
- pain

Dosage Facts
For Informational Purposes

Caution: Do not change your dose, how often you take your medication, or the length of time you are to take it without first talking to your healthcare provider.

The following dosage information was written using medical language for doctors and other healthcare professionals and is provided here for you to check your dosage. The dosage of this drug may differ for different patients. Therefore, always follow your doctor's instructions or the directions on the label. Contact your healthcare provider or pharmacist if you have any questions about the specific dosage of your medication after reviewing this information.

General Dosage Information

Available as oxacillin sodium; dosage expressed in terms of oxacillin.

Duration of treatment depends on type and severity of infection and should be determined by clinical and bacteriologic response of the patient. For serious staphylococcal infections, duration usually is $\geq 1–2$ weeks; more prolonged therapy is necessary for treatment of osteomyelitis or endocarditis.

Pediatric Patients

Staphylococcal Infections
General Dosage in Neonates

IV OR IM:
- 25 mg/kg daily recommended by manufacturer.
- Neonates <1 week of age: AAP recommends 25 mg/kg every 12 hours for those weighing <1.2 kg; 25–50 mg/kg every 12

hours for those weighing 1.2 to 2 kg; and 25–50 mg/kg every 8 hours for those weighing >2 kg. The higher dosages are recommended for meningitis.
- Neonates 1–4 weeks of age: AAP recommends 25 mg/kg every 12 hours for those weighing <1.2 kg; 25–50 mg/kg every 8 hours for those weighing 1.2 to 2 kg; and 25–50 mg/kg every 6 hours for those weighing >2 kg. The higher dosages are recommended for meningitis.

Mild to Moderate Infections in Infants and Children

IV OR IM:
- Children weighing <40 kg: 50 mg/kg daily given in equally divided doses every 6 hours.
- Children weighing ≥40 kg: 250–500 mg every 4–6 hours.
- Children ≥1 month of age: AAP recommends 100–150 mg/kg daily in 4 divided doses.

Severe Infections in Infants and Children

IV OR IM:
- Children weighing <40 kg: 100–200 mg/kg daily given in equally divided doses every 4–6 hours.
- Children weighing ≥40 kg: 1 g every 4–6 hours.
- Children ≥1 month of age: AAP recommends 150–200 mg/kg daily in 4–6 divided doses.

Staphylococcal Native Valve Endocarditis

IV:
- AHA recommends 200 mg/kg daily given in divided doses every 4–6 hours for 6 weeks (maximum 12 g daily).
- In addition, during the first 3–5 days of oxacillin therapy, IM or IV gentamicin (3 mg/kg daily given in divided doses every 8 hours; dosage adjusted to achieve peak serum gentamicin concentrations approximately 3 mcg/mL and trough concentrations <1 mcg/mL) may be given concomitantly if the causative organism is susceptible to the drug.

Staphylococcal Prosthetic Valve Endocarditis

IV:
- AHA recommends 200 mg/kg daily given in divided doses every 4–6 hours for 6 weeks or longer (maximum 12 g daily).
- Used in conjunction with oral rifampin (20 mg/kg daily given in divided doses every 8 hours for 6 weeks or longer) and IM or IV gentamicin (3 mg/kg daily given in divided doses every 8 hours during the first 2 weeks of oxacillin therapy; dosage adjusted to achieve peak serum gentamicin concentrations approximately 3 mcg/mL and trough concentrations <1 mcg/mL).

Adult Patients

Staphylococcal Infections
Mild to Moderate Infections

IV OR IM:
- 250–500 mg every 4–6 hours.

Severe Infections

IV OR IM:
- 1 g every 4–6 hours.

Acute or Chronic Staphylococcal Osteomyelitis

IV:
- 1.5–2 g every 4 hours.
- When used for treatment of acute or chronic osteomyelitis caused by susceptible penicillinase-producing staphylococci, parenteral therapy generally continued for 3–8 weeks; follow-up with an oral penicillinase-resistant penicillin (e.g., di-

cloxacillin) generally recommended. In treatment of acute osteomyelitis, a shorter course of parenteral penicillinase-resistant therapy (5–28 days) followed by 3–6 weeks of oral penicillinase-resistant penicillin therapy also has been effective.

Staphylococcal Native Valve Endocarditis

IV:
- AHA recommends 2 g every 4 hours for 4–6 weeks.
- Although benefits of concomitant aminoglycosides have not been clearly established, AHA states that IM or IV gentamicin (1 mg/kg every 8 hours) may be given concomitantly during the first 3–5 days of oxacillin therapy.

Staphylococcal Prosthetic Valve Endocarditis

IV:
- AHA recommends 2 g every 4 hours for ≥6 weeks in conjunction with oral rifampin (300 mg every 8 hours for 6 weeks or longer) and IM or IV gentamicin (1 mg/kg every 8 hours during the first 2 weeks of oxacillin therapy).

Staphylococcal Infections Related to Intravascular Catheters

IV:
- 2 g every 4 hours.

Special Populations

Renal Impairment
- Modification of dosage generally is unnecessary in patients with renal impairment; some clinicians suggest that the lower range of the usual dosage (1 g IM or IV every 4–6 hours) be used in adults with Cl_{cr} <10 mL/minute.

Oxaliplatin Injection
(ox al″ i pla′ tin)

Brand Name: Eloxatin®

Important Warning

Oxaliplatin may cause severe allergic reactions. These allergic reactions may happen within a few minutes after you receive oxaliplatin and may cause death. Tell your doctor if you are allergic to oxaliplatin, carboplatin (Paraplatin), cisplatin (Platinol) or any other medications. If you experience any of the following symptoms, tell your doctor or other healthcare provider immediately: rash, hives, itching, reddening of the skin, difficulty breathing or swallowing, hoarseness, feeling as if your throat is closing, swelling of the lips and tongue, dizziness, lightheadness, or fainting.

Why is this medicine prescribed?

Oxaliplatin is used with other medications to treat advanced colon or rectal cancer (cancer that begins in the large intestine). Oxaliplatin is also used with other medications to prevent colon cancer from spreading in people who have had surgery to remove the tumor. Oxaliplatin is in a class of medications called platinum-containing antineoplastic agents. It works by killing cancer cells.

How should this medicine be used?

Oxaliplatin comes as a solution (liquid) to be injected into a vein. Oxaliplatin is administered by a doctor or nurse. It is usually given once every fourteen days.

Ask your pharmacist or doctor for a copy of the manufacturer's information for the patient.

Are there other uses for this medicine?

This medication may be prescribed for other uses; ask your doctor or pharmacist for more information.

What special precautions should I follow?

Before using oxaliplatin,
- tell your doctor and pharmacist what prescription and nonprescription medications, vitamins, nutritional supplements, and herbal products you are taking or plan to take. Be sure to mention oral anticoagulants ('blood thinners') such as warfarin (Coumadin). Your doctor may need to change the doses of your medications or monitor you carefully for side effects.
- tell your doctor if you have or have ever had kidney disease.
- tell your doctor if you are pregnant or plan to become pregnant. Oxaliplatin may harm the fetus. You should use birth control to prevent pregnancy during your treatment with oxaliplatin. Talk to your doctor about types of birth control that will work for you. If you become pregnant while taking oxaliplatin, call your doctor. Do not breast-feed during your treatment with oxaliplatin.
- if you are having surgery, including dental surgery, tell the doctor or dentist that you are using oxaliplatin.
- you should know that oxaliplatin may decrease your ability to fight infection. Stay away from people who are sick during your treatment with oxaliplatin.
- you should know that exposure to cold air or objects may make some of the side effects of oxaliplatin worse. You should not eat or drink anything colder than room temperature, touch any cold objects, go near air conditioners or freezers, wash your hands in cold water, or go outside in cold weather unless absolutely necessary for five days after you receive each dose of oxaliplatin. If you must go outside in cold weather, wear a hat, gloves, and a scarf, and cover your mouth and nose.

What special dietary instructions should I follow?

Unless your doctor tells you otherwise, continue your normal diet.

Do not eat or drink anything that is colder than room temperature for five days after you receive each dose of oxaliplatin.

What should I do if I forget to take a dose?

Call your doctor as soon as possible if you are unable to keep an appointment to receive oxaliplatin. It is very important that you receive your treatment on schedule.

What side effects can this medicine cause?

Oxaliplatin may cause side effects. Tell your doctor if any of these symptoms are severe or do not go away:
- numbness, burning, or tingling in the fingers, toes, hands, feet, mouth, or throat
- pain in the hands or feet
- increased sensitivity, especially to cold
- decreased sense of touch
- nausea
- vomiting
- diarrhea
- constipation
- gas
- stomach pain
- heartburn
- sores in the mouth
- loss of appetite
- change in the ability to taste food
- weight gain or loss
- hiccups
- dry mouth
- muscle, back, or joint pain
- tiredness
- anxiety
- depression
- difficulty falling asleep or staying asleep
- hair loss
- dry skin
- redness or peeling of the skin on the hands and feet
- sweating
- flushing

Some side effects can be serious. If you experience any of these symptoms or those listed in the IMPORTANT WARNING section, call your doctor immediately:
- stumbling or loss of balance when walking
- difficulty with everyday activities such as writing or fastening buttons
- difficulty speaking
- strange feeling in the tongue
- tightening of the jaw
- chest pain or pressure
- cough
- shortness of breath
- sore throat, fever, chills, and other signs of infection
- pain, redness, or swelling in the place where oxaliplatin was injected
- pain when urinating
- decreased urination

- unusual bruising or bleeding
- nosebleed
- blood in urine
- vomit that is bloody or looks like coffee grounds
- bright red blood in stool
- black and tarry stools
- pale skin
- weakness
- problems with vision
- swelling of the arms, hands, feet, ankles, or lower legs

Oxaliplatin may cause other side effects. Call your doctor if you have any unusual problems while taking this medication.

What should I do in case of overdose?

In case of overdose, call your local poison control center at 1-800-222-1222. If the victim has collapsed or is not breathing, call local emergency services at 911.

Symptoms of overdose may include:
- shortness of breath
- wheezing
- numbness or tingling in the fingers or toes
- vomiting
- chest pain
- slowed breathing
- slowed heartbeat
- tightening of the throat
- diarrhea

What other information should I know?

Keep all appointments with your doctor and the laboratory. Your doctor will order certain lab tests to check your body's response to oxaliplatin.

Dosage Facts
For Informational Purposes

Caution: Do not change your dose, how often you take your medication, or the length of time you are to take it without first talking to your healthcare provider.

The following dosage information was written using medical language for doctors and other healthcare professionals and is provided here for you to check your dosage. The dosage of this drug may differ for different patients. Therefore, always follow your doctor's instructions or the directions on the label. Contact your healthcare provider or pharmacist if you have any questions about the specific dosage of your medication after reviewing this information.

Adult Patients

Colorectal Cancer

IV:
- On day 1, administer oxaliplatin 85 mg/m^2 concurrently with leucovorin 200 mg/m^2 (in separate containers) by IV infusion

over 2 hours. Then administer fluorouracil 400 mg/m^2 by IV injection over 2–4 minutes, followed by fluorouracil 600 mg/m^2 by IV infusion over 22 hours.
- On day 2, administer leucovorin 200 mg/m^2 by IV infusion over 2 hours. Then administer fluorouracil 400 mg/m^2 by IV injection over 2–4 minutes, followed by fluorouracil 600 mg/m^2 by IV infusion over 22 hours.
- Repeat regimen at intervals of 2 weeks.

Dose Modification for Toxicity

To minimize acute toxicities, administer oxaliplatin over 6 hours; adjustment of infusion duration for fluorouracil or leucovorin not necessary.

If persistent grade 2 adverse neurosensory effects occur, reduce oxaliplatin dosage to 65 mg/m^2; dosage modification for fluorouracil or leucovorin not required. Discontinue therapy if persistent grade 3 neurosensory effects occur.

In patients who have recovered from grade 3 or 4 GI toxicity (that occurred despite prophylactic treatment), grade 4 neutropenia, or grade 3 or 4 thrombocytopenia, reduce oxaliplatin dosage to 65 mg/m^2 and reduce fluorouracil dosage by approximately 20% (i.e., to 300 mg/m^2 by IV injection over 2–4 minutes and 500 mg/m^2 by IV infusion over 22 hours). Do not administer next dose until neutrophil count >1500/mm^3 and platelet count $>75,000$/mm^3.

Special Populations

Renal Impairment
- Safety and efficacy not established; use with caution.

Oxandrolone

(ox an′ droe lone)

Brand Name: Oxandrin®

Important Warning

Medications similar to oxandrolone may have caused damage to the liver or spleen (a small organ just below the ribs) and tumors in the liver. Tell your doctor if you drink or have ever drunk large amounts of alcohol or used street drugs and if you have or have ever had liver disease. Tell your doctor and pharmacist if you are taking any of the following medications or herbal products: acetaminophen (Tylenol, others), cholesterol lowering medications (statins), comfrey tea, iron products, isoniazid (INH, Nydrazid), kava, methotrexate (Rheumatrex), niacin (nicotinic acid), or rifampin (Rifadin, Rimactane). If you experience any of the following symptoms, call your doctor immediately: upset stomach; extreme tiredness; unusual bruising or bleeding; lack of energy; loss of appetite; pain in the upper right part of the

continued on next page

Important Warning (cont'd)

stomach; yellowing of the skin or eyes; flu-like symptoms; pale, cool, or clammy skin; extreme thirst; fast but weak pulse; vomiting; or fast shallow breathing.

Oxandrolone may increase the amount of low density lipoprotein (LDL; 'bad cholesterol') and decrease the amount of high density lipoprotein (HDL; 'good cholesterol') in your blood. This may increase your risk of developing heart disease. Tell your doctor if you or anyone in your family has or has ever had high cholesterol, heart disease, a heart attack, chest pain, or a stroke. Also tell your doctor if you smoke or have ever smoked and if you have high blood pressure or diabetes.

Keep all appointments with your doctor and the laboratory. Your doctor will order certain tests to check your body's response to oxandrolone. Oxandrolone may damage the liver or increase LDL without causing symptoms. It is important to have regular laboratory tests to be sure that the liver is working properly and that LDL has not increased.

Talk to your doctor about the risks of taking oxandrolone.

Why is this medicine prescribed?

Oxandrolone is used with a diet and exercise program to cause weight gain in patients who have lost too much weight due to surgery, injury, or long lasting infections, or who are very underweight for unknown reasons. Oxandrolone is also used to treat bone pain in patients with osteoporosis (a condition in which the bones become thin and weak and break easily) and to prevent certain side effects in patients who take corticosteroids (a group of medications used to treat many conditions that involve inflammation or swelling of part of the body for a long time. Oxandrolone is in a class of medications called anabolic steroids. It works by increasing the amount of protein made by the body. This protein is used to build more muscle and increase body weight.

How should this medicine be used?

Oxandrolone comes as a tablet to take by mouth. It is usually taken two to four times a day. To help you remember to take oxandrolone, take it around the same times every day. Follow the directions on your prescription label carefully, and ask your doctor or pharmacist to explain any part you do not understand. Take oxandrolone exactly as directed. Do not take more or less of it or take it more often than prescribed by your doctor.

Your doctor will probably tell you to take oxandralone for 2-4 weeks. You may need to take oxandralone for additional 2-4 week periods if your weight decreases again.

Are there other uses for this medicine?

This medication may be prescribed for other uses; ask your doctor or pharmacist for more information.

What special precautions should I follow?

Before taking oxandrolone,

- tell your doctor and pharmacist if you are allergic to oxandrolone or any other medications.
- tell your doctor and pharmacist what other prescription and nonprescription medications, vitamins, nutritional supplements, and herbal products you are taking. Be sure to mention the medications listed in the IMPORTANT WARNING section and any of the following: anticoagulants ('blood thinners') such as warfarin (Coumadin); oral medications for diabetes; oral steroids such as dexamethasone (Decadron, Dexone), methylprednisolone (Medrol), and prednisone (Deltasone); and steroid creams, lotions, or ointments such as aclometasone (Aclovate), betamethasone (Diprolene, Diprosone, Valisone), clobetasol (temovate), desonide (DesOwen), desoximetasone (Topicort), diflorasone (Psorcon, Florone), fluoxinolone (Derma-Smoothe, Flurosyn, Synalar), fluocinonide (Lidex), flurandrenolide (Cordran), fluticasone (Cutivate), halcinonide (Halog), halobetasol (Ultravate), hydrocortisone (Cortizone, Westcort, others), mometasone (Elocon), and triamcinolone (Aristocort, Kenalog, others). Your doctor may need to change the doses of your medications or monitor you carefully for side effects.
- tell your doctor if you have or have ever had high levels of calcium in your blood, breast or prostate (a male reproductive organ) cancer, enlarged prostate, or kidney disease.
- tell your doctor if you are pregnant, plan to become pregnant, or are breast-feeding. If you become pregnant while taking oxandrolone, call your doctor immediately.

What special dietary instructions should I follow?

Unless your doctor tells you otherwise, continue your normal diet.

What should I do if I forget to take a dose?

Take the missed dose as soon as you remember it. However, if it is almost time for the next dose, skip the missed dose and continue your regular dosing schedule. Do not take a double dose to make up for a missed one.

What side effects can this medicine cause?

Oxandrolone may cause side effects. Tell your doctor if any of these symptoms are severe or do not go away:

- difficulty falling asleep or staying asleep
- depression
- nervousness or unusual excitement

- changes in sex drive or ability
- constipation

Some side effects can be serious. The following symptoms are uncommon, but if you experience any of them or those listed in the IMPORTANT WARNING section, call your doctor immediately. Some of these side effects may never go away if they are not treated immediately:

- swelling of the arms, hands, feet, ankles or lower legs
- new or worsening acne
- deepening of voice, increase in facial hair, baldness, and changes in genital structures in women
- abnormal menstrual periods
- enlarged penis or erections that come too often or do not go away
- pain, swelling, or decreased size of testes
- enlarged breasts
- frequent, difficult, or painful urination
- bone pain
- slowed heartbeat
- pain on your side (between your stomach and back)
- confusion
- extreme thirst
- muscle twitches or weakness
- tingling in arms or legs
- weakness or heaviness in legs
- changes in skin color

Oxandrolone may prevent normal growth in children. Children who take oxandrolone may be shorter as adults then they would have been if they had not taken the medication. Oxandrolone is more likely to interfere with the growth of younger children than older children. Your child's doctor will take x-rays regularly to be sure your child is growing normally. Talk to your child's doctor about the risks of giving this medication to your child.

Oxandrolone may decrease fertility in men. Talk to your doctor if your partner plans to become pregnant while you are taking oxandrolone.

Oxandrolone may cause other side effects. Call your doctor if you have any unusual problems while taking this medication.

If you experience a serious side effect, you or your doctor may send a report to the Food and Drug Administration's (FDA) MedWatch Adverse Event Reporting program online [at http://www.fda.gov/MedWatch/index.html] or by phone [1-800-332-1088].

What storage conditions are needed for this medicine?

Keep this medication in the container it came in, tightly closed, and out of reach of children. Store it at room temperature and away from excess heat and moisture (not in the bathroom). Throw away any medication that is outdated or no longer needed. Talk to your pharmacist about the proper disposal of your medication.

What should I do in case of overdose?

In case of overdose, call your local poison control center at 1-800-222-1222. If the victim has collapsed or is not breathing, call local emergency services at 911.

Symptoms of overdose may include:

- swelling of the arms, hands, feet, ankles, or lower legs

What other information should I know?

Before having any laboratory test, tell your doctor and the laboratory personnel that you are taking oxandrolone. Oxandrolone may affect the results of certain laboratory tests.

Do not let anyone else take your medication. Oxandrolone has not been shown to improve athletic ability. Ask your pharmacist any questions you have about refilling your prescription.

Talk to your doctor, pharmacist, or other healthcare professional if you have questions about dosing information for your medication.

Oxaprozin

(ox a proe′ zin)

Brand Name: Daypro®

Also available generically.

Important Warning

People who take nonsteroidal anti-inflammatory medications (NSAIDs) (other than aspirin) such as oxaprozin may have a higher risk of having a heart attack or a stroke than people who do not take these medications. These events may happen without warning and may cause death. This risk may be higher for people who take NSAIDs for a long time. Tell your doctor if you or anyone in your family has or has ever had heart disease, a heart attack, or a stroke, if you smoke, and if you have or have ever had high cholesterol, high blood pressure, or diabetes. Get emergency medical help right away if you experience any of the following symptoms: chest pain, shortness of breath, weakness in one part or side of the body, or slurred speech.

If you will be undergoing a coronary artery bypass graft (CABG; a type of heart surgery), you should not take oxaprozin right before or right after the surgery.

NSAIDs such as oxaprozin may cause ulcers, bleeding, or holes in the stomach or intestine. These problems may develop at any time during treatment, may happen without warning symptoms, and may

continued on next page

Important Warning (cont'd)

cause death. The risk may be higher for people who take NSAIDs for a long time, are older in age, have poor health. or drink large amounts of alcohol while you are taking oxaprozin. Tell your doctor if you take any of the following medications: anticoagulants ('blood thinners') such as warfarin (Coumadin); aspirin; other NSAIDs such as ibuprofen (Advil, Motrin) and naproxen (Aleve, Naprosyn); or oral steroids such as dexamethasone (Decadron, Dexone), methylprednisolone (Medrol), and prednisone (Deltasone). Also tell your doctor if you have or have ever had ulcers or bleeding in your stomach or intestines or other bleeding disorders. If you experience any of the following symptoms, stop taking oxaprozin and call your doctor: stomach pain, heartburn, vomiting a substance that is bloody or looks like coffee grounds, blood in the stool, or black and tarry stools.

Keep all appointments with your doctor and the laboratory. Your doctor will monitor your symptoms carefully and will probably order certain tests to check your body's response to oxaprozin. Be sure to tell your doctor how you are feeling so that your doctor can prescribe the right amount of medication to treat your condition with the lowest risk of serious side effects.

Your doctor or pharmacist will give you the manufacturer's patient information sheet (Medication Guide) when you begin treatment with oxaprozin and each time you refill your prescription. Read the information carefully and ask your doctor or pharmacist if you have any questions. You can also visit the Food and Drug Administration (FDA) website (http://www.fda.gov/cder) or the manufacturer's website to obtain the Medication Guide.

Why is this medicine prescribed?

Oxaprozin is used to relieve pain, tenderness, swelling, and stiffness caused by osteoarthritis (arthritis caused by a breakdown of the lining of the joints) and rheumatoid arthritis (arthritis caused by swelling of the lining of the joints). Oxaprozin is also used to relieve pain, tenderness, swelling, and stiffness caused by juvenile rheumatoid arthritis in children 6 years of age and older. Oxaprozin is in a class of medications called nonsteroidal anti-inflammatory medications (NSAIDs). It works by stopping the body's production of a substance that causes pain, fever, and inflammation.

How should this medicine be used?

Oxaprozin comes as a tablet to take by mouth. It is usually taken once or twice a day. Take oxaprozin at around the time(s) each day. Follow the directions on your prescription label carefully, and ask your doctor or pharmacist to explain any part you do not understand. Take oxaprozin exactly as directed. Do not take more or less of it or take it more often than prescribed by your doctor.

Are there other uses for this medicine?

This medication may be prescribed for other uses; ask your doctor or pharmacist for more information.

What special precautions should I follow?

Before taking oxaprozin,

- tell your doctor and pharmacist if you are allergic to oxaprozin, aspirin, or other NSAIDs such as ibuprofen (Advil, Motrin) and naproxen (Aleve, Naprosyn), or any other medications.
- tell your doctor and pharmacist what prescription and nonprescription medications, vitamins, nutritional supplements, and herbal products you are taking or plan to take. Be sure to mention the medications listed in the IMPORTANT WARNING section and any of the following: angiotensin-converting enzyme (ACE) inhibitors such as benazepril (Lotensin), captopril (Capoten), enalapril (Vasotec), fosinopril (Monopril), lisinopril (Prinivil, Zestril), moexipril (Univasc), perindopril (Aceon), quinapril (Accupril), ramipril (Altace), and trandolapril (Mavik); beta blockers such as atenolol (Tenormin), labetalol (Normodyne), metoprolol (Lopressor, Toprol XL), nadolol (Corgard), and propranolol (Inderal); diuretics ('water pills'); glyburide (DiBeta, Micronase); lithium (Eskalith, Lithobid); and methotrexate (Rheumatrex). Your doctor may need to change the doses of your medications or monitor you carefully for side effects.
- tell your doctor if you have or ever had asthma, especially if you also have frequent stuffed or runny nose or nasal polyps; swelling of the hands, feet, ankles, or lower legs; or kidney or liver disease.
- tell your doctor if you are pregnant, especially if you are in the last few months of your pregnancy, you plan to become pregnant, or you are breast-feeding. If you become pregnant while taking oxaprozin, call your doctor.
- if you are having surgery, including dental surgery, tell the doctor or dentist that you are taking oxaprozin.
- plan to avoid unnecessary or prolonged exposure to sunlight and to wear protective clothing, sunglasses, and sunscreen. Oxaprozin may make your skin sensitive to sunlight.

What special dietary instructions should I follow?

Unless your doctor tells you otherwise, continue your normal diet.

What should I do if I forget to take a dose?

Take the missed dose as soon as you remember it. However, if it is almost time for the next dose, skip the missed dose

and continue your regular dosing schedule. Do not take a double dose to make up for a missed one.

What side effects can this medicine cause?

Oxaprozin may cause side effects. Tell your doctor if any of these symptoms are severe or do not go away:

- diarrhea
- constipation
- vomiting
- gas or bloating
- drowsiness
- difficulty sleeping
- confusion
- depression
- dizziness
- headache
- ringing in the ears

Some side effects can be serious. If you experience any of the following symptoms or those mentioned in the IMPORTANT WARNING section, call your doctor immediately. Do not take any more oxaprozin until you speak to your doctor:

- unexplained weight gain
- fever
- blisters
- rash
- itching
- hives
- swelling of the eyes, face, lips, tongue, throat, hands, feet, ankles, or lower legs
- hoarseness
- difficulty breathing or swallowing
- yellowing of the skin or eyes
- lack of energy
- excessive tiredness
- upset stomach
- loss of appetite
- pain in the upper right part of the stomach
- flu-like symptoms
- pale skin
- fast heartbeat
- cloudy, discolored, or bloody urine
- back pain
- difficult or painful urination

Oxaprozin may cause other side effects. Call your doctor if you have any unusual problems while taking this medication.

If you experience a serious side effect, you or your doctor may send a report to the Food and Drug Administration's (FDA) MedWatch Adverse Event Reporting program online [at http://www.fda.gov/MedWatch/index.html] or by phone [1-800-332-1088].

What storage conditions are needed for this medicine?

Keep this medication in the container it came in, tightly closed, and out of reach of children. Store it at room temperature and away from excess heat and moisture (not in the bathroom). Throw away any medication that is outdated or no longer needed. Talk to your pharmacist about the proper disposal of your medication.

What should I do in case of overdose?

In case of overdose, call your local poison control center at 1-800-222-1222. If the victim has collapsed or is not breathing, call local emergency services at 911.

Symptoms of overdose may include:

- lack of energy
- drowsiness
- upset stomach
- vomiting
- stomach pain
- bloody, black, or tarry stools
- vomiting a substance that is bloody or looks like coffee grounds
- difficulty breathing
- seizures
- coma (loss of consciousness for a period of time)

What other information should I know?

Before having any laboratory test, tell your doctor and the laboratory personnel that you are taking oxaprozin.

Do not let anyone else take your medication. Ask your pharmacist any questions you have about refilling your prescription.

Dosage Facts
For Informational Purposes

Caution: Do not change your dose, how often you take your medication, or the length of time you are to take it without first talking to your healthcare provider.

The following dosage information was written using medical language for doctors and other healthcare professionals and is provided here for you to check your dosage. The dosage of this drug may differ for different patients. Therefore, always follow your doctor's instructions or the directions on the label. Contact your healthcare provider or pharmacist if you have any questions about the specific dosage of your medication after reviewing this information.

General Dosage Information

Available as oxaprozin and oxaprozin potassium; dosage expressed in terms of oxaprozin.

Attempt to titrate to the lowest effective dosage and shortest duration of therapy.

Pediatric Patients

Inflammatory Diseases
Juvenile Rheumatoid Arthritis

ORAL (OXAPROZIN):

Weight-based Dosage of Oxaprozin Tablets in Children 6–16 Years of Age

Weight (kg)	Dosage
22–31	600 mg daily
32–54	900 mg daily
≥55	1200 mg daily

Alternatively, 10–20 mg/kg daily was administered in one uncontrolled study.

Adult Patients

Inflammatory Diseases
Osteoarthritis or Rheumatoid Arthritis

ORAL (OXAPROZIN):
- Usual recommended dosage: 1200 mg once daily.
- Low-weight adults: 600 mg once daily. If response is inadequate, may increase with caution to 1200 mg daily.
- If rapid onset is required, a loading dose of 1200–1800 mg may be given; do not exceed 26 mg/kg.
- Reserve chronic doses >1200 mg for patients who weigh >50 kg, have normal hepatic and renal function, are at low risk for peptic ulcer, have severe symptoms, and have not experienced adverse GI, hepatic, renal, or dermatologic effects on lower dosages.

ORAL (OXAPROZIN POTASSIUM):
- Usual recommended dosage: 1200 mg once daily.
- Low-weight adults with mild osteoarthritis: 600 mg once daily.

Prescribing Limits

Pediatric Patients

ORAL:
- Oxaprozin: Maximum 1200 mg daily.

Adult Patients

ORAL:
- Oxaprozin: Maximum 1800 mg or 26 mg/kg daily, whichever is lower, in divided doses.
- Oxaprozin potassium: Maximum 1200 mg daily.

Special Populations

Hepatic Impairment
- No specific dosage recommendations at this time for well-compensated cirrhosis; use with caution in severe hepatic dysfunction.

Renal Impairment
- Oxaprozin: Initially, 600 mg daily in severe renal impairment or hemodialysis. Increase cautiously to 1200 mg daily if needed.
- Oxaprozin potassium: Not recommended in patients with advanced renal disease.

Geriatric Patients
- Consider dosage reduction; select dosage with caution because of age-related decreases in hepatic, renal, and/or cardiac function, and concomitant disease and drug therapy.

Oxazepam

(ox a′ ze pam)

Brand Name: Serax®

Why is this medicine prescribed?

Oxazepam is used to relieve anxiety. It also is used to control agitation caused by alcohol withdrawal.

This medication is sometimes prescribed for other uses; ask your doctor or pharmacist for more information.

How should this medicine be used?

Oxazepam comes as a tablet and capsule to take by mouth. It usually is taken three or four times a day and may be taken with or without food. Follow the directions on your prescription label carefully, and ask your doctor or pharmacist to explain any part you do not understand. Take oxazepam exactly as directed.

Oxazepam can be habit-forming. Do not take a larger dose, take it more often, or for a longer time than your doctor tells you to. Tolerance may develop with long-term or excessive use, making the drug less effective. This medication must be taken regularly to be effective. Do not skip doses even if you feel that you do not need them. Do not take oxazepam for more than 4 months or stop taking this medication without talking to your doctor. Stopping the drug suddenly can worsen your condition and cause withdrawal symptoms (anxiousness, sleeplessness, and irritability). Your doctor probably will decrease your dose gradually.

Are there other uses for this medicine?

Oxazepam is also used to treat irritable bowel syndrome. Talk to your doctor about the possible risks of using this drug for your condition.

What special precautions should I follow?

Before taking oxazepam,
- tell your doctor and pharmacist if you are allergic to oxazepam, alprazolam (Xanax); chlordiazepoxide (Librium, Librax), clonazepam (Klonopin), clorazepate (Tranxene), diazepam (Valium), estazolam (ProSom), flurazepam (Dalmane), lorazepam (Ativan), prazepam (Centrax), temazepam (Restoril), triazolam (Halcion), tartrazine (a yellow dye in some oxazepam tablets), aspirin, or any other drugs.

- tell your doctor and pharmacist what prescription and nonprescription medications you are taking, especially antihistamines; digoxin (Lanoxin); levodopa (Larodopa, Sinemet); medication for depression, seizures, Parkinson's disease, pain, asthma, colds, or allergies; muscle relaxants; oral contraceptives; phenytoin (Dilantin); probenecid (Benemid); rifampin (Rifadine); sedatives; sleeping pills; theophylline (Theo-Dur); tranquilizers; and vitamins. These medications may add to the drowsiness caused by oxazepam.
- tell your doctor if you have or have ever had glaucoma or seizures, or lung, heart, or liver disease.
- tell your doctor if you are pregnant, plan to become pregnant, or are breast-feeding. If you become pregnant while taking oxazepam, call your doctor immediately.
- if you are having surgery, including dental surgery, tell the doctor or dentist that you are taking oxazepam.
- you should know that this drug may make you drowsy. Do not drive a car or operate machinery until you know how this drug affects you.
- remember that alcohol can add to the drowsiness caused by this drug.
- tell your doctor if you use tobacco products. Cigarette smoking may decrease the effectiveness of this drug.

What should I do if I forget to take a dose?

If you take several doses per day and miss a dose, skip the missed dose and continue your regular dosing schedule. Do not take a double dose to make up for a missed one.

What side effects can this medicine cause?

Side effects from oxazepam may occur and include:
- drowsiness
- dizziness
- tiredness
- weakness
- dry mouth
- diarrhea
- upset stomach
- changes in appetite

Tell your doctor if any of these symptoms are severe or do not go away:
- restlessness or excitement
- constipation
- difficulty urinating
- frequent urination
- blurred vision
- changes in sex drive or ability

If you experience any of the following symptoms, call your doctor immediately:
- shuffling walk
- persistent, fine tremor or inability to sit still
- fever
- difficulty breathing or swallowing
- severe skin rash

- yellowing of the skin or eyes
- irregular heartbeat

If you experience a serious side effect, you or your doctor may send a report to the Food and Drug Administration's (FDA) MedWatch Adverse Event Reporting program online [at http://www.fda.gov/MedWatch/index.html] or by phone [1-800-332-1088].

What storage conditions are needed for this medicine?

Keep this medication in the container it came in, tightly closed, and out of reach of children. Store it at room temperature and away from excess heat and moisture (not in the bathroom). Throw away any medication that is outdated or no longer needed. Talk to your pharmacist about the proper disposal of your medication.

What should I do in case of overdose?

In case of overdose, call your local poison control center at 1-800-222-1222. If the victim has collapsed or is not breathing, call local emergency services at 911.

What other information should I know?

Keep all appointments with your doctor.

Do not let anyone else take your medication.

Talk to your doctor, pharmacist, or other healthcare professional if you have questions about dosing information for your medication.

Oxcarbazepine

(ox car baz' e peen)

Brand Name: Trileptal®

Why is this medicine prescribed?

Oxcarbazepine is used alone or in combination with other medications to treat certain types of seizures in people who have epilepsy. Oxcarbazepine is in a class of medications called anticonvulsants. It works by decreasing abnormal excitement in the brain.

How should this medicine be used?

Oxcarbazepine comes as a tablet and a suspension (liquid) to take by mouth. It is usually taken every 12 hours (twice a day)., with or without food. Take oxcarbazepine at around the same times every day. Follow the directions on your prescription label carefully, and ask your doctor or pharmacist to explain any part you do not understand. Take oxcarbazepine exactly as directed. Do not take more or less of it or take it more often than prescribed by your doctor.

Shake the suspension well right before each use to mix the medication evenly. Use the oral dosing syringe that came with the medication to withdraw the right amount of suspension from the bottle. You can swallow the suspension straight from the syringe, or you can mix it with a small glass of water and swallow the mixture. Wash the syringe with warm water and allow it to dry thoroughly after use.

Your doctor will probably start you on a low dose of oxcarbazepine and gradually increase your dose, not more often than once every three days. If you were taking another medication to treat your seizures and are switching to oxcarbazepine, your doctor may gradually decrease your dose of the other medication while increasing your dose of oxcarbazepine. Follow these directions carefully and ask your doctor if you are not sure how much medication you should take.

Oxcarbazepine may help control your seizures but will not cure your condition. Continue to take oxcarbazepine even if you feel well. Do not stop taking oxcarbazepine without talking to your doctor. If you suddenly stop taking oxcarbazepine, your seizures may get worse. Your doctor will probably decrease your dose gradually.

Are there other uses for this medicine?

Oxcarbazepine is also sometimes used to treat bipolar disorder (manic depressive disorder; a disease that causes episodes of depression, episodes of frenzied, abnormal excitement, and other abnormal moods). Talk to your doctor about the possible risks of using this medication for your condition.

This medication may be prescribed for other uses. Ask your doctor or pharmacist for more information.

What special precautions should I follow?

Before taking oxcarbazepine:

- tell your doctor and pharmacist if you are allergic to oxcarbazepine, carbamazepine (Carbatrol, Epitol, Equetro, Tegretol), any other medications, or any of the inactive ingredients in oxcarbazepine tablets or suspension. Ask your pharmacist for a list of the inactive ingredients in oxcarbazepine tablets or suspension.
- tell your doctor and pharmacist what prescription and nonprescription medications, vitamins, nutritional supplements, and herbal products you are taking or plan to take. Be sure to mention any of the following: amiodarone (Cordarone); amitriptyline (Elavil); calcium channel blockers such as amlodipine (Norvasc), diltiazem (Cardizem, Dilacor, Tiazac), felodipine (Plendil), isradipine (DynaCirc), nicardipine (Cardene), nifedipine (Procardia), nimodipine (Nimotop), nisoldipine (Sular), and verapamil (Calan, Covera, Isoptin, Verelan); chlorpromazine (Thorazine); clomipramine (Anafranil); cyclophosphamide (Cytoxan, Neosar); desmopressin (DDAVP, Minirin, Stimate); diazepam (Valium); diuretics ('water pills'); hormonal contraceptives (birth control pills, rings, patches, implants, injections, and intrauterine devices); indapamide (Natrilix); other medications for seizures such as carbamazepine (Carbatrol,

Epitol, Equetro, Tegretol), phenobarbital, phenytoin (Dilantin), and valproic acid (Depakene, Depakote); proton-pump inhibitors such as lansoprazole (Prevacid), omeprazole (Prilosec), and pantoprazole (Protonix); theophylline (Theo-Dur); and selective serotonin reuptake inhibitors (SSRIs) such as citalopram (Celexa), duloxetine (Cymbalta), escitalopram (Lexapro), fluoxetine (Prozac, Sarafem), fluvoxamine (Luvox), paroxetine (Paxil), and sertraline (Zoloft). Other medications may interact with oxcarbazepine, so be sure to tell your doctor and pharmacist about all the medications you are taking, even those that do not appear on this list. Your doctor may need to change the doses of your medications or monitor you carefully for side effects.

- tell your doctor if you have or have ever had kidney or liver disease.
- tell your doctor if you are pregnant, plan to become pregnant, or are breastfeeding. If you are using hormonal contraceptives, you should know that this type of birth control may not work well when taken with oxcarbazepine. Hormonal contraceptives should not be used as your only method of birth control while you are taking this medication. Talk to your doctor about birth control methods that will work for you. Call your doctor if you miss a period or think you may be pregnant while you are taking oxcarbazepine.
- you should know that this medication may make you drowsy or dizzy, or may cause vision changes. Do not drive a car or operate machinery until you know how this medication affects you.
- remember that alcohol can add to the drowsiness caused by this medication.

What should I do if I forget to take a dose?

Before you begin your treatment, talk to your doctor about what you should do if you accidentally miss a dose. Be sure to ask your doctor how long you should wait between taking a missed dose and taking your next scheduled dose of oxcarbazepine. Do not take a double dose to make up for a missed one.

What side effects can this medicine cause?

Oxcarbazepine may cause side effects. Tell your doctor if any of these symptoms are severe or do not go away:

- dizziness
- drowsiness
- vision changes
- double vision
- fast, repeating eye movements that you cannot control
- diarrhea
- constipation
- heartburn
- stomach pain
- loss of appetite
- changes in the way food tastes
- dry mouth

- weight gain
- shaking of a part of the body that you cannot control
- difficulty coordinating movements
- falling down
- slowed movements or thoughts
- speech problems
- forgetfulness
- difficulty concentrating
- nervousness
- mood swings
- back pain
- muscle weakness or sudden tightness
- acne
- toothache
- earache
- hot flushes
- increased sweating
- cold symptoms
- nosebleed
- swelling, redness, irritation, burning, or itching of the vagina
- white vaginal discharge

Some side effects can be serious. If you experience any of the following symptoms, call your doctor immediately:

- Swelling of the face, throat, tongue, lips, eyes, hands, feet, ankles, or lower legs
- seizures that last longer or happen more often than in the past
- headache
- unusual thirst
- upset stomach
- vomiting
- weakness
- confusion
- decreased alertness
- rash
- bumps or blisters in the mouth, on skin, or genitals
- red or purple-colored blotches or dots on skin
- red, irritated eyes
- itching
- fever
- swollen glands in the neck or under the arms
- yellowing of the skin or eyes
- unusual bruising or bleeding
- bleeding from the rectum or blood in stools
- sore throat, cough, chills, and other signs of infection
- increased, decreased, or painful urination
- joint pain
- chest pain

If you experience a serious side effect, you or your doctor may send a report to the Food and Drug Administration's (FDA) MedWatch Adverse Event Reporting program online [at http://www.fda.gov/MedWatch/index.html] or by phone [1-800-332-1088].

What storage conditions are needed for this medicine?

Keep this medication in the container it came in, tightly closed, and out of reach and sight of children. Store it at room temperature and away from excess heat and moisture (not in the bathroom). Throw away any unused suspension 7 weeks after the bottle is first opened and any medication that is outdated or no longer needed. Talk to your pharmacist about the proper disposal of your medication.

What should I do in case of overdose?

In case of overdose, call your local poison control center at 1-800-222-1222. If the victim has collapsed or is not breathing, call local emergency services at 911.

What other information should I know?

Keep all appointments with your doctor and the laboratory. Your doctor may order certain lab tests to check your response to oxcarbazepine.

Do not let anyone else take your medication. Ask your pharmacist any questions you have about refilling your prescription.

Dosage Facts
For Informational Purposes

Caution: Do not change your dose, how often you take your medication, or the length of time you are to take it without first talking to your healthcare provider.

The following dosage information was written using medical language for doctors and other healthcare professionals and is provided here for you to check your dosage. The dosage of this drug may differ for different patients. Therefore, always follow your doctor's instructions or the directions on the label. Contact your healthcare provider or pharmacist if you have any questions about the specific dosage of your medication after reviewing this information.

Pediatric Patients

Partial Seizures
Monotherapy

ORAL:
- Children 4–16 years of age: Initially, 8–10 mg/kg daily in 2 divided doses. Increase by 5 mg/kg every third day to recommended maintenance dosage.

Recommended Range of Maintenance Dosages during Monotherapy For Management of Partial Seizures in Pediatric Patients

Weight (kg)	Dosage Range (mg/day)
20	600–900
25	900–1200
30	900–1200
35	900–1500
40	900–1500
45	1200–1500
50	1200–1800
55	1200–1800
60	1200–2100
65	1200–2100
70	1500–2100

Combination Therapy

ORAL:

- Children 4–16 years of age: Initially, 8–10 mg/kg daily (≤600 mg daily) in 2 divided doses. Increase to the target maintenance dosage over 2 weeks.

Target Maintenance Dosage for Management of Partial Seizures in Combination with Other Anticonvulsant Agents in Pediatric Patients

Weight (kg)	Target Dosage (mg/day)
20–29	900
29.1–39	1200
>39	1800

Conversion to Monotherapy

ORAL:

- Children 4–16 years of age: Initially, 8–10 mg/kg daily in 2 divided doses. Increase dosage, based on patient response, by ≤10 mg/kg daily at weekly intervals to the recommended maintenance dosage for monotherapy. (See table under Monotherapy.) Observe patients closely during this transition phase.
- As oxcarbazepine replaces the existing anticonvulsant regimen, dosage of the other anticonvulsant(s) is simultaneously reduced and discontinued over 3–6 weeks. Observe patient closely during transition phase.

Adult Patients

Partial Seizures
Monotherapy

ORAL:

- Initially, 600 mg daily administered in 2 equally divided doses. Increase dosage by 300-mg daily increments every third day up to a dosage of 1200 mg daily.

Combination Therapy

ORAL:

- Initially, 600 mg daily in 2 equally divided doses. Increase dosage by 600-mg daily increments at approximately weekly intervals to recommended daily dosage of 1200 mg. Efficacy may be somewhat higher in patients receiving dosages >1200

mg daily, but most patients cannot tolerate daily dosages of 2400 mg, mainly because of adverse CNS effects.
- Observe patients closely and monitor plasma concentrations of concomitantly administered anticonvulsants during dosage titration of oxcarbazepine; plasma concentrations of these drugs may be altered when dosage of oxcarbazepine exceeds 1200 mg daily.

Conversion to Monotherapy

ORAL:

- Initially, 600 mg daily in 2 equally divided doses. Increase dosage by 600-mg daily increments at approximately weekly intervals to recommended daily dosage of 2400 mg, usually within 2–4 weeks.
- As oxcarbazepine replaces the existing anticonvulsant regimen, dosage of the other anticonvulsant(s) is simultaneously reduced and discontinued over 3–6 weeks. Observe patient closely during transition phase.

Special Populations

Hepatic Impairment

- No dosage adjustment required in patients with mild to moderate hepatic impairment.

Renal Impairment

- Initially, 300 mg daily in patients with CL_{cr} <30 mL/minute; increase dosage slowly based on patient response.

Geriatric Patients

- Manufacturer makes no specific dosage recommendations.

Oxiconazole

(ox i kon′ a zole)

Brand Name: Oxistat®

Why is this medicine prescribed?

Oxiconazole, an antifungal agent, is used to treat skin infections such as athlete's foot, jock itch, and ringworm.

This medication is sometimes prescribed for other uses; ask your doctor or pharmacist for more information.

How should this medicine be used?

Oxiconazole comes in a cream or lotion to be applied to your skin. Oxiconazole usually is applied once a day (in the evening) or twice a day (in the morning and evening). Follow the directions on your prescription label carefully, and ask your doctor or pharmacist to explain any part you do not understand. Use oxiconazole exactly as directed. Do not use more or less of it or use it more often than prescribed by your doctor.

Thoroughly clean the infected area, allow it to dry, and then gently rub the medication in until most of it disappears. Use just enough medication to cover the affected area. You should wash your hands after applying the medication.

What special precautions should I follow?

Before using oxiconazole,

- tell your doctor and pharmacist if you are allergic to oxiconazole or any other drugs.
- tell your doctor and pharmacist what prescription and nonprescription drugs you are taking, including vitamins.
- tell your doctor if you are pregnant, plan to become pregnant, or are breast-feeding. If you become pregnant while using oxiconazole, call your doctor.

What should I do if I forget to take a dose?

Apply the missed dose as soon as you remember it. However, if it is almost time for the next dose, skip the missed dose and continue your regular dosing schedule. Do not apply a double dose to make up for a missed one.

What side effects can this medicine cause?

Oxiconazole may cause side effects. Tell your doctor if any of these symptoms are severe or do not go away:

- itching
- burning
- redness
- dry or flaky skin
- tingling

If you experience any of the following symptoms, call your doctor immediately:

- pain
- swelling
- open sores
- skin rash

If you experience a serious side effect, you or your doctor may send a report to the Food and Drug Administration's (FDA) MedWatch Adverse Event Reporting program online [at http://www.fda.gov/MedWatch/index.html] or by phone [1-800-332-1088].

What storage conditions are needed for this medicine?

Keep this medication in the container it came in, tightly closed, and out of reach of children. Store it at room temperature and away from excess heat and moisture (not in the bathroom). Throw away any medication that is outdated or no longer needed. Talk to your pharmacist about the proper disposal of your medication.

What other information should I know?

Keep all appointments with your doctor. Oxiconazole is for external use only. Do not let oxiconazole get into your eyes, nose, or mouth, and do not swallow it. Do not apply dressings, bandages, cosmetics, lotions, or other skin medications to the area being treated unless your doctor tells you.

Do not let anyone else use your medication. Ask your pharmacist any questions you have about refilling your prescription.

If you still have symptoms of infection after you finish the oxiconazole, call your doctor.

Dosage Facts
For Informational Purposes

Caution: Do not change your dose, how often you take your medication, or the length of time you are to take it without first talking to your health-care provider.

The following dosage information was written using medical language for doctors and other healthcare professionals and is provided here for you to check your dosage. The dosage of this drug may differ for different patients. Therefore, always follow your doctor's instructions or the directions on the label. Contact your health-care provider or pharmacist if you have any questions about the specific dosage of your medication after reviewing this information.

General Dosage Information

Available as oxiconazole nitrate; dosage expressed in terms of oxiconazole.

Pediatric Patients

Dermatophytoses
Tinea Corporis or Tinea Cruris

TOPICAL:
- Apply 1% cream once or twice daily for 2 weeks.
- If clinical improvement does not occur after treatment, re-evaluate diagnosis.

Tinea Pedis

TOPICAL:
- Apply 1% cream once or twice daily for 1 month.
- If clinical improvement does not occur after treatment, re-evaluate diagnosis.

Pityriasis (Tinea) Versicolor

TOPICAL:
- Apply 1% cream once daily for 2 weeks.
- If clinical improvement does not occur after treatment, re-evaluate diagnosis.
- Normalization of hyper- or hypopigmented patches on trunk, neck, arms, and upper thighs is variable and may take months.

Adult Patients

Dermatophytoses
Tinea Corporis or Tinea Cruris

TOPICAL:
- Apply 1% cream or lotion once or twice daily for 2 weeks.
- If clinical improvement does not occur after treatment, re-evaluate diagnosis.

Tinea Pedis

TOPICAL:
- Apply 1% cream or lotion once or twice daily for 1 month.
- If clinical improvement does not occur after treatment, re-evaluate diagnosis.

Pityriasis (Tinea) Versicolor

TOPICAL:
- Apply 1% cream once daily for 2 weeks.
- If clinical improvement does not occur after treatment, re-evaluate diagnosis.
- Normalization of hyper- or hypopigmented patches on trunk, neck, arms, and upper thighs is variable and may take months.

Special Populations

No special population dosage recommendations at this time.

Oxybutynin

(ox i byoo′ ti nin)

Brand Name: Ditropan®, Ditropan XL®

Why is this medicine prescribed?

Oxybutynin is used to control urgent, frequent, or uncontrolled urination in people who have overactive bladder (a condition in which the bladder muscles have uncontrollable spasms), spina bifida (a disability that occurs when the spinal cord does not close properly before birth), or other conditions that affect the bladder muscles. Oxybutynin is in a class of medications called anticholinergics. It works by relaxing the bladder muscles to prevent urgent, frequent, or uncontrolled urination.

How should this medicine be used?

Oxybutynin comes as a tablet, a syrup, and an extended-release (long-acting) tablet to take by mouth. The tablets and syrup are usually taken two to four times a day. The extended-release tablet is usually taken once a day with or without food. Take oxybutynin at around the same time(s) every day. Follow the directions on your prescription label carefully, and ask your doctor or pharmacist to explain any part you do not understand. Take oxybutynin exactly as directed. Do not take more or less of it or take it more often than prescribed by your doctor.

Swallow the extended-release tablets whole with plenty of water or other liquid. Do not split, chew, or crush the extended-release tablets. Tell your doctor if you cannot swallow tablets.

Your doctor may start you on a low dose of oxybutynin and gradually increase your dose, not more than once every week.

Oxybutynin may control your symptoms, but will not cure your condition. Continue to take oxybutynin even if

you feel well. Do not stop taking oxybutynin without talking to your doctor.

You may notice some improvement in your symptoms within the first two weeks of your treatment. However, it may take six to eight weeks to experience the full benefit of oxybutynin. Talk to your doctor if your symptoms do not improve at all within eight weeks.

Are there other uses for this medicine?

This medication is sometimes prescribed for other uses; ask your doctor or pharmacist for more information.

What special precautions should I follow?

Before taking oxybutynin,
- tell your doctor and pharmacist if you are allergic to oxybutynin or any other medications.
- tell your doctor and pharmacist what prescription and nonprescription medications, vitamins, nutritional supplements, and herbal products you are taking or plan to take. Be sure to mention any of the following: amiodarone (Cordarone, Pacerone); certain antibiotics such as clarithromycin (Biaxin), erythromycin (E.E.S., E-Mycin, Erythrocin), and tetracycline (Bristamycin, Sumycin, Tetrex); certain antifungals such as itraconazole (Sporanox), miconazole (Monistat), and ketoconazole (Nizoral); antihistamines; aspirin and other nonsteroidal anti-inflammatory medications (NSAIDS) such as ibuprofen (Advil, Motrin) and naproxen (Aleve, Naprosyn); cimetidine (Tagamet); diltiazem (Cardizem, Dilacor, Tiazac); fluvoxamine; ipratropium (Atrovent); iron supplements; certain medications for human immunodeficiency virus (HIV) such as indinavir (Crixivan), nelfinavir (Viracept), and ritonavir (Norvir, in Kaletra); medications for irritable bowel disease, motion sickness, Parkinson's disease, ulcers, or urinary problems; medications for osteoporosis (a condition in which bones are weak, fragile, and can break easily) such as alendronate (Fosamax), ibandronate (Boniva), and risedronate (Actonel); nefazodone; potassium supplements; quinidine; and verapamil (Calan, Covera, Isoptin, Verelan). Your doctor may need to change the doses of your medications or monitor you carefully for side effects.
- tell your doctor if you have or have ever had benign prostatic hypertrophy (BPH; enlargement of the prostate, a male reproductive organ) or any other condition that makes it difficult for you to fully empty your bladder; any condition that prevents your stomach from emptying completely or slows the movement of food through your digestive system; or glaucoma (a serious eye condition that may cause loss of vision). Your doctor may tell you not to take oxybutynin.
- tell your doctor if you have or have ever had ulcerative colitis (sores in the intestine that cause stomach pain and diarrhea); gastroesophageal reflux disease (GERD; condition in which the contents of the stomach back up into the esophagus and cause pain and heartburn); hiatal

hernia (condition in which a portion of the wall of the stomach bulges outward, and may cause pain and heartburn); hyperthyroidism (condition in which there is too much thyroid hormone in the body); myasthenia gravis (a disorder of the nervous system that causes muscle weakness); fast or irregular heartbeat; high blood pressure; or heart, liver, or kidney disease.

- tell your doctor if you are pregnant, plan to become pregnant, or are breast-feeding. If you become pregnant while taking oxybutynin, call your doctor.
- if you are having surgery, including dental surgery, tell the doctor or dentist that you are taking oxybutynin.
- you should know that this medication may make you drowsy or cause blurred vision. Do not drive a car or operate machinery until you know how this medication affects you.
- talk to your doctor about the safe use of alcohol while you are taking this medication. Alcohol can make the side effects from oxybutynin worse.
- you should know that oxybutynin may make it harder for your body to cool down when it gets very hot. Avoid exposure to extreme heat, and call your doctor or get emergency medical treatment if you have fever or other signs of heat stroke such as dizziness, nausea, headache, confusion, and fast pulse after you are exposed to heat.

What special dietary instructions should I follow?

Talk to your doctor about eating grapefruit and drinking grapefruit juice while taking this medicine.

What should I do if I forget to take a dose?

If you are taking the tablet or syrup, take the missed dose as soon as you remember it. However, if it is almost time for the next dose, skip the missed dose and continue your regular dosing schedule. Do not take a double dose to make up for a missed one.

If you are taking the extended-release tablet and you remember more than eight hours before it is time for the next dose, take the missed dose right away. However, if your next dose is due in less than eight hours, skip the missed dose and continue your regular dosing schedule. Do not take a double dose to make up for the missed one.

What side effects can this medicine cause?

Oxybutynin may cause side effects. Tell your doctor if any of these symptoms are severe or do not go away:

- dry mouth
- blurred vision
- dry eyes, nose, or skin
- stomach pain
- constipation
- diarrhea
- nausea
- heartburn
- gas
- change in ability to taste food
- headache
- dizziness
- weakness
- confusion
- sleepiness
- difficulty falling asleep or staying asleep
- nervousness
- flushing
- swelling of the hands, arms, feet, ankles, or lower legs
- back or joint pain
- frequent, urgent, or painful urination
- rash

If you experience the following symptom, call your doctor immediately:

- fast, irregular, or pounding heartbeat

If you experience a serious side effect, you or your doctor may send a report to the Food and Drug Administration's (FDA) MedWatch Adverse Event Reporting program online [at http://www.fda.gov/MedWatch/index.html] or by phone [1-800-332-1088].

Oxybutynin may cause other side effects. Call your doctor if you have any unusual problems while you are taking this medication.

What storage conditions are needed for this medicine?

Keep this medication in the container it came in, tightly closed, and out of reach of children. Store it at room temperature and away from excess heat and moisture (not in the bathroom). Throw away any medication that is outdated or no longer needed. Talk to your pharmacist about the proper disposal of your medication.

What should I do in case of overdose?

In case of overdose, call your local poison control center at 1-800-222-1222. If the victim has collapsed or is not breathing, call local emergency services at 911.

Symptoms of overdose may include:
- restlessness
- uncontrollable shaking of a part of your body
- irritability
- seizures
- confusion
- hallucinations (seeing things or hearing voices that do not exist)
- flushing
- fever
- irregular heartbeat
- vomiting
- difficulty urinating
- slowed or difficult breathing
- inability to move

- coma (loss of consciousness for a period of time)
- memory loss
- agitation
- wide pupils (black circles in the centers of the eyes)
- dry skin

What other information should I know?

Keep all appointments with your doctor.

Do not let anyone else take your medication. Ask your pharmacist any questions you have about refilling your prescription.

If you are taking the extended-release tablet, you may notice something that looks like a tablet in your stool. This is just the empty tablet shell and does not mean that you did not get your complete dose of medication.

Dosage Facts
For Informational Purposes

Caution: Do not change your dose, how often you take your medication, or the length of time you are to take it without first talking to your healthcare provider.

The following dosage information was written using medical language for doctors and other healthcare professionals and is provided here for you to check your dosage. The dosage of this drug may differ for different patients. Therefore, always follow your doctor's instructions or the directions on the label. Contact your healthcare provider or pharmacist if you have any questions about the specific dosage of your medication after reviewing this information.

General Dosage Information

Conventional tablets, extended-release tablets, and oral solution available as oxybutynin chloride; dosage is expressed in terms of oxybutynin chloride.

Pediatric Patients

Overactive Bladder

ORAL:
- Conventional tablets or oral solution: 5 mg twice daily for children ≥5 years of age.
- Extended-release tablets: 5 mg once daily for children ≥6 years of age. Adjust dosage according to individual response and tolerance; increase dosage at 7-day intervals in increments of 5 mg up to maximum dosage of 20 mg once daily.

Adult Patients

Overactive Bladder

ORAL:
- Conventional tablets or oral solution: 5 mg 2–3 times daily.
- Extended-release tablets: 5 or 10 mg once daily. Adjust daily dosage according to individual response and tolerance; increase dosage at 7-day intervals in increments of 5 mg up to maximum dosage of 30 mg once daily.

Prescribing Limits
Pediatric Patients

Overactive Bladder

ORAL:
- Conventional tablets or oral solution: Maximum 5 mg 3 times daily.
- Extended-release tablets: Maximum 20 mg once daily.

Adult Patients

Overactive Bladder

ORAL:
- Conventional tablets or oral solution: Maximum 5 mg 4 times daily.
- Extended-release tablets: Maximum 30 mg once daily.

Special Populations

Geriatric Patients
- A lower initial dosage (2.5 mg 2 or 3 times daily) of conventional tablets or oral solution is recommended for frail geriatric patients.

Oxybutynin Transdermal
(ox i byoo′ ti nin)

Brand Name: Oxytrol®

Why is this medicine prescribed?

Oxybutynin transdermal patches are used to treat an overactive bladder (a condition in which the bladder muscles contract uncontrollably and cause frequent urination, urgent need to urinate, and inability to control urination). Oxybutynin is in a class of medications called anticholinergics. It works by relaxing the bladder muscles to prevent urgent, frequent, or uncontrolled urination.

How should this medicine be used?

Transdermal oxybutynin comes as a patch to apply to the skin. It is usually applied twice each week (every 3-4 days). You should apply transdermal oxybutynin on the same 2 days of the week every week. To help you remember to apply your patches on the right days, you should mark the calendar on the back of your package of medication. Follow the directions on your prescription label carefully, and ask your doctor or pharmacist to explain any part you do not understand. Use transdermal oxybutynin exactly as directed. Do not apply the patches more often than prescribed by your doctor.

You can apply oxybutynin patches anywhere on your stomach, hips, or buttocks except the area around your waistline. Choose an area where you think the patch will be comfortable for you, where it will not be rubbed by tight clothing, and where it will be protected from sunlight by clothing. After you apply a patch to a particular area, wait at least 1 week before applying another patch in that spot. Do not apply patches to skin that has wrinkles or folds; that you have recently treated with any lotion, oil, or powder; or that is oily, cut, scraped, or irritated. Before applying a patch, be sure the skin is clean and dry.

After you apply an oxybutynin patch, you should wear it all the time until you are ready to remove it and put on a fresh patch. If the patch loosens or falls off before it is time to replace it, try to press it back in place with your fingers. If the patch cannot be pressed back on, throw it away and apply a fresh patch to a different area. Replace the fresh patch on your next scheduled patch change day.

You may bathe, swim, shower, or exercise while you are wearing an oxybutynin patch. However, try not to rub on the patch during these activities, and do not soak in a hot tub for a long period of time while wearing a patch.

Transdermal oxybutynin controls the symptoms of overactive bladder but does not cure the condition. Continue to take transdermal oxybutynin even if you feel well. Do not stop taking transdermal oxybutynin without talking to your doctor.

To use the patches, follow these steps:

1. Open the protective pouch and remove the patch.
2. Peel the first piece of liner off the sticky side of the patch. A second strip of liner should remain stuck to the patch.
3. Press the patch firmly onto your skin with the sticky side down. Be careful not to touch the sticky side with your fingers.
4. Bend the patch in half and use your fingertips to roll the remaining part of the patch onto your skin. The second liner strip should fall off of the patch when you do this.
5. Press firmly on the surface of the patch to attach it tightly to your skin.
6. When you are ready to remove a patch, peel it off slowly and gently. Fold the patch in half with the sticky sides together and throw it away in a trash can that is out of reach of children and pets. Children and pets can be harmed if they chew on, play with, or wear used patches.
7. Wash the area that was under the patch with mild soap and warm water to remove any residue. If necessary, you can use baby oil or a medical adhesive removal pad to remove residue that will not come off with soap and water. Do not use alcohol, nail polish remover, or other solvents.
8. Apply a new patch to a different area immediately by following steps 1-5.

Are there other uses for this medicine?

This medication may be prescribed for other uses; ask your doctor or pharmacist for more information.

What special precautions should I follow?

Before using transdermal oxybutynin,

- tell your doctor and pharmacist if you are allergic to oxybutynin (Ditropan, Ditropan XL, Oxytrol), any other medications, medical tape products, or other skin patches.
- tell your doctor and pharmacist what prescription and nonprescription medications, vitamins, nutritional supplements and herbal products you are taking. Be sure to mention any of the following: antifungals such as fluconazole (Diflucan), itraconazole (Sporanox), ketoconazole (Nizoral), and miconazole (Micatin, Monistat); antihistamines; aspirin and other nonsteroidal anti-inflammatory medications (NSAIDs) such as ibuprofen (Advil, Motrin) and naproxen (Aleve, Naprosyn); chlorpromazine (Thorazine); cimetidine (Tagamet); clarithromycin (Biaxin); cyclosporine (Neoral, Sandimmune); danazol (Danocrine); delavirdine (Rescriptor); diltiazem (Cardizem, Dilacor, Tiazac); doxycycline (Doryx, Vibramycin); erythromycin (E.E.S., E-Mycin, Erythrocin); fluoxetine (Prozac, Sarafem); fluvoxamine (Luvox); HIV protease inhibitors such as indinavir (Crixivan) and ritonavir (Norvir); ipatropium (Atrovent); isoniazid (INH, Nydrazid); iron supplements; medications for osteoporosis or bone disease such as alendronate (Fosamax), etidronate (Didronel), ibandronate (Boniva), and risedronate (Actonel); medications for irritable bowel disease, motion sickness, Parkinson's disease, ulcers, or urinary problems; metronidazole (Flagyl); morphine (MSIR, Oramorph, others); nefazodone (Serzone); oral contraceptives (birth control pills); paroxetine (Paxil); potassium supplements (Slow-K, Klor-Con, others); qunidine (Quinaglute); tetracycline (Sumycin); troleandomycin (TAO); verapamil (Calan, Covera, Isoptin, Verelan); and zafirlukast (Accolate). Your doctor may need to change the doses of your medications or monitor you carefully for side effects.
- tell your doctor if you or any of your family members have or have ever had glaucoma (an eye disease that can cause vision loss) and if you have or have ever had any type of blockage in the bladder or digestive system; gastroesophageal reflux disease (GERD, a condition in which the contents of the stomach back up into the esophagus and cause pain and heartburn); myasthenia gravis (a disorder of the nervous system that causes muscle weakness); ulcerative colitis (sores in the intestine that cause stomach pain and diarrhea); benign prostatic hypertrophy (BPH, enlargement of the prostate, a male reproductive organ); or liver or kidney disease.
- tell your doctor if you are pregnant, plan to become pregnant, or are breast-feeding. If you become pregnant while using transdermal oxybutynin, call your doctor.
- if you are having surgery, including dental surgery, tell the doctor or dentist that you are using transdermal oxybutynin.

- you should know that transdermal oxybutynin may make you drowsy and may blur your vision. Do not drive a car or operate machinery until you know how this medication affects you.
- remember that alcohol can add to the drowsiness caused by this medication.
- you should know that transdermal oxybutynin may make it harder for your body to cool down when it gets very hot. Avoid exposure to extreme heat, and call your doctor or get emergency medical treatment if you have fever or other signs of heat stroke such as dizziness, upset stomach, headache, confusion, and fast pulse after you are exposed to heat.

What special dietary instructions should I follow?

Talk to your doctor about drinking grapefruit juice while taking this medicine.

What should I do if I forget to take a dose?

Remove the old patch and apply a new patch to a different spot as soon as you remember it. Replace the new patch on your next scheduled patch change day. Do not apply two patches to make up for a missed dose and never wear more than one patch at a time.

What side effects can this medicine cause?

Transdermal oxybutynin may cause side effects. Tell your doctor if any of these symptoms are severe or do not go away:

- redness, burning, or itching in the place where you applied a patch
- dry mouth
- constipation
- stomach pain
- gas
- upset stomach
- extreme tiredness
- drowsiness
- headache
- blurred vision
- flushing
- back pain

Some side effects can be serious. The following symptoms are uncommon, but if you experience any of them, call your doctor immediately:

- blisters, rash, or spots in the place where you applied a patch
- rash anywhere on the body
- painful urination

Transdermal oxybutynin may cause other side effects. Call your doctor if you have any unusual problems while using this medication.

If you experience a serious side effect, you or your doctor may send a report to the Food and Drug Administration's

(FDA) MedWatch Adverse Event Reporting program online [at http://www.fda.gov/MedWatch/index.html] or by phone [1-800-332-1088].

What storage conditions are needed for this medicine?

Keep this medication in the container it came in, tightly closed, and out of reach of children. Store the patches in their protective pouches and do not open a pouch until you are ready to apply the patch. Store this medication at room temperature and away from excess heat and moisture (not in the bathroom). Throw away any medication that is outdated or no longer needed. Talk to your pharmacist about the proper disposal of your medication.

What should I do in case of overdose?

In case of overdose, call your local poison control center at 1-800-222-1222. If the victim has collapsed or is not breathing, call local emergency services at 911.

Symptoms of overdose may include:

- flushing
- fever
- constipation
- dry skin
- sunken eyes
- extreme tiredness
- irregular heartbeat
- vomiting
- inability to urinate
- memory loss
- semi-awake state
- confusion
- wide pupils

What other information should I know?

Keep all appointments with your doctor

Do not let anyone else take your medication. Ask your pharmacist any questions you have about refilling your prescription.

Dosage Facts
For Informational Purposes

Caution: Do not change your dose, how often you take your medication, or the length of time you are to take it without first talking to your healthcare provider.

The following dosage information was written using medical language for doctors and other healthcare professionals and is provided here for you to check your dosage. The dosage of this drug may differ for different patients. Therefore, always follow your doctor's instructions or the directions on the label. Contact your healthcare provider or pharmacist if you have any questions about the specific dosage of your medication after reviewing this information.

General Dosage Information

Transdermal system available as oxybutynin; dosage is expressed in terms of oxybutynin.

Adult Patients

Overactive Bladder

TRANSDERMAL:
- 1 transdermal system (delivering 3.9 mg per day) twice weekly (every 3–4 days).

Oxycodone

(ox i koe′ done)

Brand Name: Endocodone®, OxyContin®, Oxydose®, OxyFast®, OxyIR®, Percolone®, Roxicodone®, Roxicodone® Intensol®
Also available generically.

Why is this medicine prescribed?

Oxycodone is used to relieve moderate to moderate-to-severe pain. It also is used to relieve postpartum, postoperative, and dental pain.

This medication is sometimes prescribed for other uses; ask your doctor or pharmacist for more information.

How should this medicine be used?

Oxycodone comes as a liquid and tablet to take by mouth. It usually is taken every 6 hours as needed; extended-release (long-acting) tablets usually are taken every 12 hours. Follow the directions on your prescription label carefully, and ask your doctor or pharmacist to explain any part you do not understand. Take oxycodone exactly as directed.

Swallow the extended-release tablet whole. Do not chew, break, or crush extended-release oxycodone tablets.

Oxycodone can be habit-forming. Do not take a larger dose, take it more often, or for a longer period than your doctor tells you to. If you have been taking oxycodone for more than a few weeks, do not stop taking oxycodone suddenly. Your doctor probably will decrease your dose gradually.

What special precautions should I follow?

Before taking oxycodone,
- tell your doctor and pharmacist if you are allergic to oxycodone, codeine, sulfites (some preparations of oxycodone contain sulfites and may cause allergic reactions), or any other drugs. If you are allergic to aspirin, tell your doctor and do not take any aspirin and oxycodone combination product (e.g., Percodan or Roxiprin).
- tell your doctor and pharmacist what prescription and nonprescription medications you are taking, especially other pain relievers; antidepressants; medications for cough, cold, allergies, dizziness, nausea, motion sickness; or schizophrenia; sedatives; sleeping pills; tranquilizers; and vitamins.
- tell your doctor if you have or have ever had hypothyroidism, Addison's disease, urethral stricture, prostatic hypertrophy, or lung or liver disease.
- tell your doctor if you are pregnant, plan to become pregnant, or are breast-feeding. If you become pregnant while taking oxycodone, call your doctor.
- if you are having surgery, including dental surgery, tell the doctor or dentist that you are taking oxycodone.
- you should know that this drug may make you drowsy. Do not drive a car or operate machinery until you know how this drug affects you.
- remember that alcohol can add to the drowsiness caused by this drug.

What should I do if I forget to take a dose?

Take the missed dose as soon as you remember it. However, if it is almost time for the next dose, skip the missed dose and continue your regular dosing schedule. Do not take a double dose to make up for a missed one.

What side effects can this medicine cause?

Oxycodone may cause side effects. Tell your doctor if any of these symptoms are severe or do not go away:
- upset stomach
- constipation
- dry mouth

If you experience any of the following symptoms, call your doctor immediately:
- rapid or slow heartbeat
- trouble breathing
- hives
- skin rash
- hallucinations
- yellowing of the skin or eyes
- headache
- vomiting
- dizziness

If you experience a serious side effect, you or your doctor may send a report to the Food and Drug Administration's (FDA) MedWatch Adverse Event Reporting program online [at http://www.fda.gov/MedWatch/index.html] or by phone [1-800-332-1088].

What storage conditions are needed for this medicine?

Keep this medication in the container it came in, tightly closed, and out of reach of children. Store it at room temperature and away from excess heat and moisture (not in the bathroom). Dispose of any medication that is outdated or no longer needed. Talk to your pharmacist about the proper disposal of your medication.

What should I do in case of overdose?

In case of overdose, call your local poison control center at 1-800-222-1222. If the victim has collapsed or is not breathing, call local emergency services at 911.

What other information should I know?

You may notice oxycodone tablets in your stool or colostomy bag. These tablets are empty, since the the medication has already been absorbed.

Keep all appointments with your doctor.

Do not let anyone else take your medication. Ask your pharmacist any questions you have about refilling your prescription.

Dosage Facts
For Informational Purposes

Caution: Do not change your dose, how often you take your medication, or the length of time you are to take it without first talking to your healthcare provider.

The following dosage information was written using medical language for doctors and other healthcare professionals and is provided here for you to check your dosage. The dosage of this drug may differ for different patients. Therefore, always follow your doctor's instructions or the directions on the label. Contact your healthcare provider or pharmacist if you have any questions about the specific dosage of your medication after reviewing this information.

General Dosage Information

Available as oxycodone hydrochloride and oxycodone terephthalate; dosage expressed in terms of the respective salt.

Pediatric Patients
Conventional Preparations

ORAL:
- Children <50 kg: Usually, initiate with 0.1–0.2 mg/kg every 3–4 hours as needed. Adjust according to response and tolerance.
- Children ≥50 kg: Usually, initiate with 5–10 mg every 3–4 hours as needed. Adjust according to response and tolerance.
- Children 6–12 Years of Age: 0.61 mg of the combined salts every 6 hours.
- Children ≥12 Years of Age: 1.22 mg of the combined salts every 6 hours.

Adult Patients
Conventional Preparations

ORAL:
- Usually, initiate with 5–10 mg every 3–4 hours as needed. Adjust according to response and tolerance.
- 4.88 mg every 6 hours as the combined salts.

Extended-release Tablets
Initial Therapy with Extended-release Tablets

ORAL:
- Initially, 10 mg every 12 hours. Patients previously receiving nonopiate analgesics may continue these drugs as dosage of the extended-release tablets is titrated to provide adequate analgesia.

Switching from Conventional Oxycodone Preparations to Extended-release Tablets

ORAL:
- Calculate the total daily dosage of the conventional preparation and give as extended-release tablets in 2 divided doses at 12-hour intervals.

Switching from Other Opiates to Extended-release Tablets

ORAL:
- The equivalent total daily dosage of oxycodone hydrochloride should be calculated based on standard conversion factors suggested by the manufacturer (table below) and administered as extended-release tablets in 2 divided doses at 12-hour intervals. Round *down* to the nearest whole tablet any calculated doses that do not correspond to an available tablet strength.

Converting Daily Opiate Dosages to Oxycodone (mg/day prior opiate × factor = mg/day oral oxycodone)

Prior Opiate	Factor Oral	Factor Parenteral
Oxycodone	1	—
Codeine	0.15	—
Hydrocodone	0.9	—
Hydromorphone	4	20
Levorphanol	7.5	15
Meperidine	0.1	0.4
Methadone	1.5	3
Morphine	0.5	3

Table to be used *only* for conversion to oral oxycodone.

More conservative conversion for patients receiving high-dose parenteral opiates (e.g., use 0.5 instead of 3 as multiplication factor for high-dose parenteral morphine).

Patients receiving fentanyl transdermal systems may receive extended-release tablets beginning 18 hours after removal of the transdermal system. Initially, dosage of approximately 10 mg every 12 hours as extended-release tablets can be substituted for each 25-mcg/hour increment in fentanyl transdermal system dosage. Monitor patient closely as clinical experience with this dosage conversion ratio is limited.

Switching from Extended-release Tablets

ORAL:

- When patients are switched from extended-release tablets to a parenteral opiate, conservative dose conversion ratios should be used to avoid toxicity.

Special Populations

Hepatic Impairment

Extended-release Tablets

- Initially, 33–50% of the usual dosage; titrate dosage carefully.

Renal Impairment

Extended-release Tablets

- Consider reduction of the initial dosage and adjust according to the clinical situation in impaired renal function ($Cl_{cr} < 60$ mL/minute).

Geriatric Patients

- Consider dosage reduction.

Oxycodone and Aspirin

(ox i koe′ done)

Brand Name: Endodan®, Percodan®, Roxiprin®

Why is this medicine prescribed?

The combination of oxycodone and aspirin is used to relieve moderate to moderately severe pain. Oxycodone is in a class of medications called narcotic analgesics. Aspirin is in a class of medications called nonsteroidal anti-inflammatory agents (NSAIDs). Oxycodone works by changing the way the brain and nervous system respond to pain. Aspirin works by decreasing pain messages received by the brain.

How should this medicine be used?

The combination of oxycodone and aspirin comes as a tablet to take by mouth. It is usually taken every 6 hours as needed. Follow the directions on your prescription label carefully, and ask your doctor or pharmacist to explain any part you do not understand. Take oxycodone and aspirin exactly as directed. Oxycodone can be habit-forming. Do not take more or less of this medication or take it more often or for a longer time than prescribed by your doctor.

Do not stop taking oxycodone and aspirin combination without talking to your doctor. Your doctor will probably decrease your dose gradually if you have been taking this medication for a long time.

Are there other uses for this medicine?

This medication may be prescribed for other uses; ask your doctor or pharmacist for more information.

What special precautions should I follow?

Before taking oxycodone and aspirin,

- tell your doctor and pharmacist if you are allergic to aspirin, oxycodone, or any other medications
- tell your doctor and pharmacist what other prescription and nonprescription medications, vitamins, nutritional supplements, and herbal products you are taking. Be sure to mention any of the following: acetazolamide (Diamox); angiotensin converting enzyme (ACE) inhibitors; antacids; anticoagulants ('blood thinners') such as warfarin (Coumadin); corticosteroids including cortisone (Cortone), dexamethasone (Decadron), hydrocortisone (Cortef), or prednisone (Deltasone); diuretics ('water pills'); medications for allergies, coughs or colds; other medications that contain aspirin; medications for anxiety, depression, or mental illness; medications for diabetes; medications for dizziness, nausea, or motion sickness; medications for gout, pain, or seizures; methotrexate; muscle relaxants; nizatidine (Axid); penicillins; phenybutazone; probenecid; sedatives; sleeping pills; sulfa antibiotics including sulfadiazine, sulfamethoxazole-trimethoprim (Bactrim, Septra), sulfamethizole (Urobiotic), sulfasalazine (Azulfidine), sulfisoxazole (Eryzole, Gantrisin, Pediazole); sulfinpyrazone (Anturane); or tranquilizers. Your doctor may need to change the doses of your medications or monitor you carefully for side effects.
- tell your doctor if you have recently had the flu, chickenpox, a head injury, or any sudden problem in your stomach or intestinal area; if you drink or have ever drunk large amounts of alcohol; or if you have or have ever had Addison's disease (condition where the adrenal gland does not produce enough hormones); anemia; asthma; gout; hemophilia or any other bleeding disorder; nasal polyps; prostatic hypertrophy (BPH, a condition where the prostate becomes large and can block urine flow); problems urinating; ulcers; or kidney, liver, thyroid or lung disease. Also tell your doctor if you have ever used street drugs or overused prescription drugs.
- tell your doctor if you are pregnant, plan to become pregnant, or are breast-feeding. If you become pregnant while taking oxycodone and aspirin combination, call your doctor.
- if you are having surgery, including dental surgery, tell the doctor or dentist that you are taking oxycodone and aspirin.
- you should know that oxycodone and aspirin may make you drowsy. Do not drive a car or operate machinery until you know how this medication affects you.
- remember that alcohol can add to the drowsiness caused by this medication.

What special dietary instructions should I follow?

Unless your doctor tells you otherwise, continue your normal diet.

What should I do if I forget to take a dose?

This medication usually is taken as needed. If your doctor has told you to take oxycodone and aspirin combination regularly, take the missed dose as soon as you remember it. However, if it is almost time for the next dose, skip the missed dose and continue your regular dosing schedule. Do not take a double dose to make up for a missed one.

What side effects can this medicine cause?

Oxycodone and aspirin combination may cause side effects. Lying down may help to relieve some of the following symptoms. Tell your doctor if any of these symptoms are severe or do not go away:

- dizziness
- lightheadedness
- drowsiness
- elevated or depressed mood
- upset stomach
- indigestion
- stomach pain
- vomiting
- constipation
- decreased appetite

Some side effects can be serious. The following symptoms are uncommon, but if you experience any of them, call your doctor immediately:

- hives
- skin rash
- itching
- difficulty breathing or swallowing
- swelling of the face, throat, tongue, lips, eyes, hands, feet, ankles, or lower legs
- hoarseness
- ringing in the ears
- decreased hearing
- abnormal bruising or bleeding
- bloody or black stools
- red blood in stools
- vomiting material that looks like coffee grounds
- bloody vomit
- extreme tiredness
- weakness
- confusion
- seizure
- yellowing of the skin or eyes

Oxycodone and aspirin combination may cause other side effects. Call your doctor if you have any unusual problems while taking this medication.

If you experience a serious side effect, you or your doctor may send a report to the Food and Drug Administration's (FDA) MedWatch Adverse Event Reporting program online [at http://www.fda.gov/MedWatch/index.html] or by phone [1-800-332-1088].

What storage conditions are needed for this medicine?

Keep this medication in the container it came in, tightly closed, and out of reach of children. Store it at room temperature and away from excess heat and moisture (not in the bathroom) and light. Throw away any medication that is outdated or no longer needed. Talk to your pharmacist about the proper disposal of your medication.

What should I do in case of overdose?

In case of overdose, call your local poison control center at 1-800-222-1222. If the victim has collapsed or is not breathing, call local emergency services at 911.

Symptoms of overdose may include:
- mild burning in throat or stomach
- vomiting
- dizziness
- extreme drowsiness
- mental confusion
- double vision
- abnormally elevated mood
- seeing things or hearing voices that do not exist (hallucinating)
- difficulty breathing
- bluish color around lips, fingernails, or toenails
- cold, clammy skin
- fever
- restlessness
- irritability
- incoherent speech
- shaking hands that you cannot control
- seizure
- loss of muscle tone
- decreased urination
- unresponsiveness
- coma
- decreased heart beat

What other information should I know?

Keep all appointments with your doctor.

Do not let anyone else take your medication. Ask your pharmacist any questions you have about refilling your prescription.

Talk to your doctor, pharmacist, or other healthcare professional if you have questions about dosing information for your medication.

Oxytocin Injection

(ox i toe′ sin)

Brand Name: Pitocin®, Syntocinon®

About Your Treatment

Your doctor has ordered oxytocin, a hormone, to stimulate contractions of the uterus and smooth muscle tissue. The drug will be either injected into a large muscle (such as your buttock or hip) or added to an intravenous fluid that will drip through a needle or catheter in your vein.

Oxytocin is a hormone produced by the hypothalamus and stored in the pituitary gland. It is used to help start or strengthen labor and to reduce bleeding after delivery. This medication is sometimes prescribed for other uses; ask your doctor or pharmacist for more information.

Your health care provider (doctor, nurse, or pharmacist) may measure the effectiveness and side effects of your treatment using laboratory tests and physical examinations. It is important to keep all appointments with your doctor and the laboratory. The length of treatment depends on how your symptoms respond to the medication.

Precautions

Before administering oxytocin,

- tell your doctor and pharmacist if you are allergic to oxytocin or any other drugs.
- tell your doctor and pharmacist what prescription and nonprescription medications you are taking, including vitamins.
- tell your doctor if you have or have ever had a premature delivery, herpes infection, eclampsia, cervical cancer, previous uterine surgery, prolapsed uterus, breech position, placenta previa, or other abnormal position of the fetus or umbilical cord.

Administering Your Medication

Before you administer oxytocin, look at the solution closely. It should be clear and free of floating material. Gently squeeze the bag or observe the solution container to make sure there are no leaks. Do not use the solution if it is discolored, if it contains particles, or if the bag or container leaks. Use a new solution, but show the damaged one to your health care provider.

It is important that you use your medication exactly as directed. Do not change your dosing schedule without talking to your health care provider. Your health care provider may tell you to stop your infusion if you have a mechanical problem (such as a blockage in the tubing, needle, or catheter); if you have to stop an infusion, call your health care provider immediately so your therapy can continue.

Side Effects

If you experience any of the following symptoms, call your health care provider immediately:

- chest pain or difficulty breathing
- confusion
- fast or irregular heartbeat
- severe headache
- irritation at the injection site

If you experience a serious side effect, you or your doctor may send a report to the Food and Drug Administration's (FDA) MedWatch Adverse Event Reporting program online [at http://www.fda.gov/MedWatch/index.html] or by phone [1-800-332-1088].

Storage Conditions

Store your medication only as directed. Make sure you understand what you need to store your medication properly.

Keep your supplies in a clean, dry place when you are not using them, and keep all medications and supplies out of reach of children. Your health care provider will tell you how to throw away used needles, syringes, tubing, and containers to avoid accidental injury.

Signs of Infection

If you are receiving oxytocin in your vein or under your skin, you need to know the symptoms of a catheter-related infection (an infection where the needle enters your vein or skin). If you experience any of these effects near your intravenous catheter, tell your health care provider as soon as possible:

- tenderness
- warmth
- irritation
- drainage
- redness
- swelling
- pain

Dosage Facts
For Informational Purposes

Caution: Do not change your dose, how often you take your medication, or the length of time you are to take it without first talking to your healthcare provider.

The following dosage information was written using medical language for doctors and other healthcare professionals and is provided here for you to check your dosage. The dosage of this drug may differ for different patients. Therefore, always follow your doctor's instructions or the directions on the label. Contact your healthcare provider or pharmacist if you have any questions about the specific dosage of your medication after reviewing this information.

Adult Patients

Dosage is determined by uterine response.

Labor Induction

CONTINUOUS IV INFUSION:

- Low-dose or high-dose regimens employed, depending on clinician preference.
- Maximum dosage not established; titrate according to response and tolerance.
- Monitor fetal heart rate and uterine contractions.
- Low-dose regimens and less frequent dose increases associated with decreased uterine hyperstimulation.
- High-dose regimens and more frequent dose increases associated with shorter labor, and less frequent cases of chorioamnionitis and cesarean delivery for dystocia but increased uterine hyperstimulation.
- Low-dose: Usually, initiate at 0.5–1 milliunit/minute.
- Generally, increase in low-dose regimen by 1- to 2-milliunits/minute at 30- to 60-minute intervals until a response is observed.
- Low-dose: Alternatively, initiate at 1–2 milliunits/minute.
- Generally, increase in alternative low-dose regimen by 2 milliunits/minute at 15-minute intervals.
- High-dose: Usually, initiate at about 6 milliunits/minute.
- Generally, increase in high-dose regimen by about 6 milliunits at 15-minute intervals.
- High-dose: Alternatively, initiate at 6 milliunits/minute.
- Generally, increase in alternative high-dose regimen by 6, 3, or 1 milliunits/minute at 20- to 40-minute intervals. If uterine hyperstimulation develops, do not exceed 3-milliunit/minute increases. If hyperstimulation recurs, do not exceed 1-milliunit/minute increases.
- May reduce infusion rate by similar amounts when the desired frequency of contractions is established (a uterine pattern comparable to spontaneous labor), without evidence of fetal distress, and labor has progressed to 5–6 cm dilation.
- At term, employ higher rates of infusion with caution; rates >9–10 milliunits/minute rarely are required.
- Before term, higher infusion rates may be necessary since uterine sensitivity to oxytocin is reduced secondary to decreased oxytocin receptors.

PULSATILE IV INFUSION:

- Infused via controlled-infusion device as periodic rapid pulse doses.
- Pulsatile dosing may better simulate spontaneous labor.
- Pulsatile dosing may reduce the total dose needed.
- Initiate at 1 milliunit/pulse (over 10 seconds) every 8 minutes for 3 doses per cycle, doubling the cycle dose as needed at 24-minute intervals (i.e., after each 3-dose cycle) until 32-milliunit pulse is achieved; thereafter, increase in 8-milliunit increments per cycle until adequate uterine activity is achieved.
- Alternatively, a computer-controlled, feedback-loop dosing is used where doses range from 0.67–20 milliunits/pulse (over 5 seconds), repeated no more frequently than every 5 minutes and no sooner than 30 seconds after a contraction reached baseline.
- Initiate the alternative regimen at 0.67 milliunits/pulse (over 5 seconds) every 5 minutes for 40 minutes; if inadequate labor, increase to 2 milliunits/pulse every 5 minutes for 40 minutes. Subsequent increase by 1-milliunit/pulse no more fre-

quently than after each 40-minute cycle. This regimen includes a computerized feedback loop measuring intrauterine waveform pressures to determine the timing of repeated doses.

Reduction of Postpartum Uterine Bleeding

Generally initiated after placental delivery and absence of additional fetuses is established.

IV:

- Infuse total of 10 units at 20–40 milliunits/minute; adjust rate to maintain uterine contraction and control uterine atony.

IM:

- 10 units.

Pregnancy Termination

IV:

- Infuse at 10–100 milliunits/minute.
- Maximum 30-unit cumulative dose within 12-hours because of water intoxication risk.

Evaluation of Fetal Respiratory Capability†

Oxytocin Challenge Test to Evaluate Fetal Distress in High-Risk Pregnancy†

IV:

- Initially, infuse at 0.5 milliunits/minute.
- May gradually increase at 15- to 30-minute intervals to a maximum of 20 milliunits/minute.
- Monitor fetal heart rate and uterine contractions immediately before and during oxytocin infusion.
- Discontinue infusion and compare baseline and oxytocin-induced fetal heart rates when 3 moderate uterine contractions occur within a 10-minute interval.
- Repeat in 1 week if no change in fetal heart rate occurs (negative response).
- Termination of pregnancy may be indicated if late deceleration of fetal heart rate occurs.

Prescribing Limits

Adult Patients

Labor Induction

No maximum dosage established.

Reduction of Postpartum Uterine Bleeding

IM:

- Total of 10 units.

IV:

- Usually, a total of 10 units.

Pregnancy Termination

IV:

- Maximum 30 units cumulative dose in 12-hours.

Oxytocin Challenge Test to Evaluate Fetal Distress†

IV:

- Maximum of 20 milliunits/minute.

† Use is not currently included in the labeling approved by the US Food and Drug Administration.

Palifermin

(pal ee fer′ min)

Brand Name: Kepivance®

About Your Treatment

Your doctor has ordered palifermin to help treat your illness. The drug is given by injection into a vein.

You will probably be given three doses of palifermin before you receive your cancer chemotherapy treatment and three doses of palifermin after you receive your cancer chemotherapy treatment. You will not be given palifermin on the same day that you are given your cancer chemotherapy treatment. Palifermin must be given at least 24 hours before and at least 24 hours after chemotherapy.

This medication is used to:

- prevent swelling, irritation and sores on the lining of the mouth and throat that may be caused by chemotherapy used to treat cancers of the blood or bone marrow (spongy tissue inside of bones where blood cells are formed).
- speed the healing of the lining of the mouth and throat if it is damaged by chemotherapy used to treat cancers of the blood or bone marrow.

Palifermin is in a class of drugs known as human keratinocyte growth factors. It stops sores from forming in the lining of the mouth and throat and helps the lining of the mouth and throat heal faster if it is damaged.

Palifermin may not be safe to use to prevent and treat mouth sores in patients who have other types of cancer. Palifermin may cause some tumors to grow faster.

This medication may be prescribed for other uses; ask your doctor or pharmacist for more information.

Precautions

Before taking palifermin,

- tell your doctor and pharmacist if you are allergic to palifermin, medications made from *E. coli* (a type of bacteria) proteins, or any other drugs. Ask your doctor if you are not sure if a medication you are allergic to is made from *E. coli* proteins.
- tell your doctor and pharmacist what prescription and nonprescription medications, vitamins, nutritional supplements, and herbal products you are taking. Your doctor may need to change the doses of your medications or monitor you carefully for side effects.
- tell your doctor if you have or have ever had any medical condition, especially liver or kidney disease.
- tell your doctor if you are pregnant or breast-feeding. If you become pregnant while taking palifermin, call your doctor.

Side Effects

Palifermin may cause side effects. Tell your doctor if any of these symptoms are severe or do not go away:

- thick tongue
- change in color of tongue
- change in ability to taste food
- increased or decreased sensitivity to touch, especially in and around the mouth
- burning or tingling, especially in and around the mouth
- joint pain

Some side effects can be serious. If you experience any of the following symptoms, call your doctor immediately:

- rash
- warm, red skin
- itching
- swelling of the hands, feet, ankles, or lower legs
- fever

Palifermin may cause other side effects. Call your doctor if you have any unusual problems while taking this drug.

If you experience a serious side effect, you or your doctor may send a report to the Food and Drug Administration's (FDA) MedWatch Adverse Event Reporting program online [at http://www.fda.gov/MedWatch/index.html] or by phone [1-800-332-1088].

Overdose

In case of overdose, call your local poison control center at 1-800-222-1222. If the victim has collapsed or is not breathing, call local emergency services at 911.

Symptoms of overdose may include:

- thick tongue
- change in color of tongue
- change in ability to taste food
- increased or decreased sensitivity to touch, especially in and around the mouth
- burning or tingling, especially in and around the mouth
- joint pain
- rash
- warm, red skin
- itching
- swelling of the hands, feet, ankles, or lower legs
- fever

Dosage Facts
For Informational Purposes

Caution: Do not change your dose, how often you take your medication, or the length of time you are to take it without first talking to your healthcare provider.

The following dosage information was written using medical language for doctors and other healthcare professionals and is provided here for you to check your dosage. The dosage of this drug may differ for different patients. Therefore, always follow your doctor's instructions or the directions on the label. Contact your healthcare provider or pharmacist if you have any questions about the specific dosage of your medication after reviewing this information.

Adult Patients

Chemotherapy-induced Oral Mucositis

IV:

- Initially, 60 mcg/kg daily, administered by direct IV injection on 3 consecutive days before and 3 consecutive days after myelotoxic chemotherapy (total of 6 doses).
- Administer the first 3 doses (doses 1–3) on the 3 consecutive days prior to myelotoxic chemotherapy, with the third dose administered *24–48 hours before* such chemotherapy. Administer the last 3 doses (doses 4–6) on the 3 consecutive days after myelotoxic chemotherapy, with the first of the 3 doses (i.e., dose 4) administered after, but on the same day as, hematopoietic stem cell infusion and at least 4 days after the previous dose (dose 3) of the drug.

Special Populations

No special population recommendations at this time.

Paliperidone

(pal ee per′ i done)

Brand Name: Invega®

Important Warning

Studies have shown that older adults with dementia (a brain disorder that affects the ability to remember, think clearly, communicate, and perform daily activities and may cause changes in mood and personality) who take antipsychotics (medications for mental illness) such as paliperidone have an increased risk of death during treatment. Older adults with dementia may also have a greater chance of having a stroke or ministroke during treatment. If you experience any of the following symptoms, call your doctor immediately: slow or difficult speech, dizziness, faintness, or weakness or numbness of an arm or leg.

Paliperidone is not approved by the Food and Drug Administration (FDA) for the treatment of behavior problems in older adults with dementia. Talk to the doctor who prescribed this medication, if you, a family member, or someone you care for has dementia and is taking paliperidone. For more information, visit the FDA website: http://www.fda.gov/cder

Why is this medicine prescribed?

Paliperidone is used to treat the symptoms of schizophrenia (a mental illness that causes disturbed or unusual thinking, loss of interest in life, and strong or inappropriate emotions). Paliperidone is in a class of medications called atypical antipsychotics. It works by changing the activity of certain natural substances in the brain.

How should this medicine be used?

Paliperidone comes as an extended-release (long-acting) tablet to take by mouth. It is usually taken once a day in the morning with or without food. Take paliperidone at around the same time every day. Follow the directions on your prescription label carefully, and ask your doctor or pharmacist to explain any part you do not understand. Take paliperidone exactly as directed. Do not take more or less of it or take it more often than prescribed by your doctor.

Swallow the tablets whole with plenty of water or other liquid. Do not split, chew, or crush the tablets. Tell your doctor if you cannot swallow tablets. Your doctor will probably prescribe another medication to treat your condition.

Talk to your doctor about how you are feeling during your treatment. If your symptoms are still bothersome, your doctor may gradually increase your dose, not more often than once every 5 days.

Paliperidone controls the symptoms of schizophrenia but does not cure the condition. Continue to take paliperidone even if you feel well. Do not stop taking paliperidone without talking to your doctor.

Are there other uses for this medicine?

This medication may be prescribed for other uses; ask your doctor or pharmacist for more information.

What special precautions should I follow?

Before taking paliperidone,

- tell your doctor and pharmacist if you are allergic to paliperidone, risperidone (Risperdal), or any other medications.
- tell your doctor and pharmacist what prescription and nonprescription medications, vitamins, nutritional supplements, and herbal products you are taking or plan to take. Be sure to mention any of the following: antidepressants; certain antibiotics such as erythromycin (E.E.S., E-Mycin, Erythrocin), gatifloxacin (Tequin) (not available in the United States), moxifloxacin (Avelox), and sparfloxacin (Zagam); certain antipsychotics such as chlorpromazine (Sonazine, Thorazine), pimozide (Orap), risperidone (Risperdal) and thioridazine; cisapride (Propulsid); levodopa (in Sinemet, in Stalevo); medications for anxiety, high blood pressure, or seizures; medications for irregular heartbeat such as amiodarone (Cordarone), disopyramide (Norpace), dofetilide (Tikosyn); procainamide (Procanbid, Pronestyl), quinidine (Quinidex), and sotalol (Betapace, Betapace AF); sedatives; sleeping pills; and tranquilizers. Your doctor may need to change the doses of your medications or monitor you carefully for side effects.
- tell your doctor if you have or have ever had a prolonged QT interval (a rare heart problem that may cause fainting or irregular heartbeat); slow or irregular heartbeat;

a heart attack; low levels of potassium or magnesium in your blood; seizures; a stroke; a head injury; a brain tumor; Parkinson's disease (a disorder of the nervous system that causes difficulties with movement, muscle control, and balance); diabetes; breast cancer; surgery involving the intestines; any condition that causes blockage or narrowing of the esophagus (tube that connects the mouth and stomach), stomach, or intestines such as cystic fibrosis (an inborn disease that causes problems with breathing, digestion, and reproduction), and inflammatory bowel disease (IBD; a group of conditions that cause swelling of the lining of the intestines); and kidney, heart, or liver disease. Also tell your doctor if you drink or have ever drunk large amounts of alcohol and if you use or have ever used street drugs or have overused prescription medications. Tell your doctor if you have ever had to stop taking a medication for mental illness because of severe side effects.

- tell your doctor if you are pregnant, or plan to become pregnant. If you become pregnant while taking paliperidone, call your doctor. Do not breast-feed while you are taking paliperidone.
- if you are having surgery, including dental surgery, tell the doctor or dentist that you are taking paliperidone.
- you should know that paliperidone may make you drowsy and may cause difficulty with thinking and movement. Do not drive a car or operate machinery until you know how this medication affects you.
- you should know that alcohol may add to the drowsiness caused by paliperidone. Do not drink alcoholic beverages while you are taking this medication.
- you should know that you may experience hyperglycemia (increases in your blood sugar) while you are taking this medication, even if you do not already have diabetes. If you have schizophrenia, you may be more likely to develop diabetes than people who do not have schizophrenia, and taking paliperidone or similar medications may increase this risk. Tell your doctor immediately if you have any of the following symptoms while you are taking paliperidone: extreme thirst, frequent urination, extreme hunger, blurred vision, or weakness. It is very important to call your doctor as soon as you have any of these symptoms, because high blood sugar can cause more serious symptoms, such as dry mouth, nausea and vomiting, shortness of breath, breath that smells fruity, or decreased consciousness, and may become life-threatening if it is not treated at an early stage.
- you should know that paliperidone may make it harder for your body to cool down when it gets very hot. Tell your doctor if you plan to exercise or be exposed to extreme heat.
- you should know that paliperidone may cause dizziness, lightheadedness, and fainting when you get up too quickly from a lying position. This is more common when you first start taking paliperidone or when your dose is increased. To avoid this problem, get out of bed slowly, resting your feet on the floor for a few minutes before standing up.

What special dietary instructions should I follow?

Unless your doctor tells you otherwise, continue your normal diet.

What should I do if I forget to take a dose?

Take the missed dose as soon as you remember it. However, if it is almost time for the next dose, skip the missed dose and continue your regular dosing schedule. Do not take a double dose to make up for a missed one.

What side effects can this medicine cause?

Paliperidone may cause side effects. Tell your doctor if any of these symptoms are severe or do not go away:

- dizziness
- extreme tiredness
- weakness
- headache
- dry mouth
- increased saliva
- weight gain
- stomach pain

Some side effects can be serious. If you experience any of these symptoms or those listed in the IMPORTANT WARNING section, call your doctor immediately:

- fever
- muscle pain or stiffness
- confusion
- fast, pounding, or irregular heartbeat
- sweating
- unusual movements of your face or body that you cannot control
- slow or stiff movements
- restlessness
- painful erection of the penis that lasts for hours

Paliperidone may cause other side effects. Call your doctor if you have any unusual problems while taking this medication.

What storage conditions are needed for this medicine?

Keep this medication in the container it came in, tightly closed, and out of reach of children. Store it at room temperature and away from excess heat and moisture (not in the bathroom). Throw away any medication that is outdated or no longer needed. Talk to your pharmacist about the proper disposal of your medication.

What should I do in case of overdose?

In case of overdose, call your local poison control center at 1-800-222-1222. If the victim has collapsed or is not breathing, call local emergency services at 911.

Symptoms of overdose may include:
- unusual movements of your face or body that you cannot control
- slow or stiff movements
- restlessness
- unsteadiness
- drowsiness
- fast heartbeat

What other information should I know?

Keep all appointments with your doctor.

Do not let anyone else take your medication. Ask your pharmacist any questions you have about refilling your prescription.

You may notice something that looks like a tablet in your stool. This is just the empty tablet shell and does not mean that you did not get your complete dose of medication.

Talk to your doctor, pharmacist, or other healthcare professional if you have questions about dosing information for your medication.

Palivizumab Injection

(pal i vi′ zu mab)

Brand Name: Synagis®

About Your Treatment

Your child's doctor has ordered palivizumab to help prevent a serious lower respiratory tract disease called respiratory syncytial virus (RSV). The drug will be injected into a large muscle (such as the thigh) once a month for several months.

It is important that your child receive this medicine each month during RSV season. Your health care provider will let you know when the monthly injections are no longer needed.

Your child's health care provider (doctor, nurse, or pharmacist) may measure the effectiveness and side effects of this treatment using laboratory tests and physical examinations. It is important to keep all appointments with your child's doctor and the laboratory. The length of treatment will be determined by your child's health care provider.

Precautions

Before administering palivizumab,
- tell your child's doctor and pharmacist if your child is allergic to palivizumab or has had a reaction to palivizumab or any other drugs.
- tell your doctor and pharmacist what prescription and nonprescription medications your child is taking, including vitamins.
- tell your child's doctor if your child has or has ever had bleeding problems or a low platelet count.

Administering Your Medication

Before you administer palivizumab to your child, you will need to mix it up. Your health care provider should show you how to mix and measure the first dose. You will need to use a needle and syringe to draw up 1 mL of sterile water into the syringe. Slowly add the sterile water to the palivizumab vial. Gently swirl the vial (do not shake it) for 30 seconds. You will then need to let the vial sit at room temperature for 20 minutes until the solution becomes clear. After 20 minutes, you are ready to give your child palivizumab. The solution should be clear and free of floating material. Do not use the solution if it is discolored or if it contains particles. Call your health care provider if you are unsure whether you should use the solution.

It is important to use this medicine exactly as directed. Do not stop giving this medicine to your child without talking to your child's health care provider. Do not change the dosing schedule without talking to your child's health care provider.

Side Effects

Palivizumab may cause side effects. Tell your child's health care provider if any of these symptoms are severe or do not go away:
- sore throat
- runny nose
- redness or irritation at injection site
- vomiting
- diarrhea

If your child experiences any of the following symptoms, call your child's health care provider immediately:
- severe skin rash
- itching
- hives
- difficulty breathing

If you experience a serious side effect, you or your doctor may send a report to the Food and Drug Administration's (FDA) MedWatch Adverse Event Reporting program online [at http://www.fda.gov/MedWatch/index.html] or by phone [1-800-332-1088].

Storage Conditions

- Your child's health care provider will probably give you a 1-month supply of palivizumab at a time. You will need to store it in the refrigerator.
- Do not allow palivizumab to freeze.
- Palivizumab must be used within 6 hours once you mix it. Your health care provider will give you directions on how to prepare each dose.

Store this medication only as directed. Make sure you understand what you need to store this medication properly.Keep your supplies in a clean, dry place when you are not using them, and keep all medications and supplies out of the reach of children. Your health care provider will tell you how to throw away used needles, syringes, and containers to avoid accidental injury.

Overdose

In case of overdose, call your local poison control center at 1-800-222-1222. If the victim has collapsed or is not breathing, call local emergency services at 911.

Signs of Infection

If you are receiving palivizumab under your skin, you need to know the symptoms of a catheter-related infection (an infection where the needle enters your skin). If you notice any of the following symptoms, tell your health care provider as soon as possible:

- fever
- unusual tiredness or weakness
- chills
- shaking
- loss of appetite
- redness around the injection site

Dosage Facts
For Informational Purposes

Caution: Do not change your dose, how often you take your medication, or the length of time you are to take it without first talking to your healthcare provider.

The following dosage information was written using medical language for doctors and other healthcare professionals and is provided here for you to check your dosage. The dosage of this drug may differ for different patients. Therefore, always follow your doctor's instructions or the directions on the label. Contact your healthcare provider or pharmacist if you have any questions about the specific dosage of your medication after reviewing this information.

Pediatric Patients

Respiratory Syncytial Virus (RSV) Infections
Prevention of RSV Lower Respiratory Tract Infections

IM:
- Infants at high risk for RSV disease: 15 mg/kg once monthly. Give first dose prior to beginning of RSV season and subsequent doses once monthly until end of season.
- Infants at high risk for RSV undergoing cardiopulmonary bypass: Give a supplemental 15-mg/kg dose as soon as possible after cardiopulmonary bypass (even if this is <1 month after the last dose). Thereafter, give usual doses once monthly.

Pamidronate Injection
(pa mi droe' nate)

Brand Name: Aredia®

About Your Treatment

Your doctor has ordered pamidronate to help treat your illness. The medication will be added to an intravenous fluid that will drip through a needle or catheter into your vein. You will receive your dose of pamidronate as an infusion (slow injection) that may last 2-24 hours. You may receive an infusion of pamidronate once every 3-4 weeks, once a day for 3 days in a row, or as a single dose that may be repeated after 1 week or longer. The treatment schedule depends on your condition.

Pamidronate is used to treat high levels of calcium in the blood that may be caused by certain types of cancer. Pamidronate is also used along with cancer chemotherapy to treat bone damage caused by multiple myeloma (cancer that begins in the plasma cells [white blood cells that produce substances needed to fight infection]) or by cancer that began in another part of the body but has spread to the bones. Pamidronate is also used to treat Paget's disease (a condition in which healthy bones are broken down and replaced by abnormally thick but weak bones). Pamidronate helps prevent bone breakdown and bone fractures. This medication is sometimes prescribed for other uses; ask your doctor or pharmacist for more information.

Your health care provider (doctor, nurse, or pharmacist) may measure the effectiveness and side effects of your treatment using laboratory tests and physical examinations. It is important to keep all appointments with your doctor. The length of treatment depends on your condition and on how you respond to the medication.

Precautions

Before administering pamidronate,
- tell your doctor and pharmacist if you are allergic to pamidronate, alendronate (Fosamax), etidronate (Didronel), risedronate (Actonel), tiludronate (Skelid), zoledronic acid (Zometa), any other medications, or any of the ingredients in pamidronate infusion. Ask your health care provider for a list of the ingredients.
- tell your doctor and pharmacist what prescription and nonprescription medications, vitamins, nutritional supplements and herbal products you are taking or plan to take. Be sure to mention any of the following: amphotericin B (Fungizone); antibiotics such as amikacin (Amikin), bacitracin; dapsone (Avlosulfon); foscarnet (Foscavir); ganciclovir (Cytovene); gentamicin (Garamycin), kanamaycin (Kantrex), methicillin (Staphcillin); neomycin (Neo-Rx, Neo-Fradin), netilmycin (Netromycin), paramomycin (Humatin), pentamidine (NebuPent); polymyxin (Aerosporin); rifampin (Rifadin, Rimactane); sulfonamides such as sulfamethoxazole and trimethoprim-

(Bactrim); streptomycin, tobramycin (Tobi, Nebcin), and valganciclovir (Valcyte); aspirin and other nonsteroidal anti-inflammatory medications such as ibuprofen (Advil, Motrin), and naproxen (Aleve, Naprosyn); aurothioglucose (Solganal); auranofin (Ridaura); cancer chemotherapy medications captopril (Capoten); cyclophosphamide (Cytoxan, Neosar); cyclosporine (Neoral, Sandimmune); gold sodium thiomalate (Myochrysine); lidocaine (Xylocaine, others); certain medications to treat or prevent malaria; nitrates; oral steroids such as dexamethasone (Decadron, Dexone), methylprednisolone (Medrol), and prednisone (Deltasone); penicillamine (Cuprimine, Depen); salicylate pain relievers; and tacrolimus (Prograf).

- tell your doctor if you have or have ever had an infection of the mouth or bones, gum disease or other problems with your teeth or mouth, or kidney or liver disease.
- tell your doctor if you are pregnant or are breast-feeding. Use a reliable method of birth control during your treatment with pamidronate. If you become pregnant while using pamidronate, call your doctor. Pamidronate may harm the fetus. Also talk to your doctor if you plan to become pregnant at any time in the future because pamidronate may remain in your body for years after you stop using it.
- if you are having surgery, tell the doctor that you are using pamidronate.
- you should know that pamidronate may cause serious problems with your jaw, especially if you have dental surgery or treatment while you are using the medication. A dentist should examine your teeth and perform any needed treatments before you start to use pamidronate. Be sure to brush your teeth and clean your mouth properly while you are using pamidronate. Talk to your doctor before having any dental treatments while you are using this medication. Call your doctor if you have any of the following symptoms: jaw pain; pain, swelling, or infection of the gums; sores or cuts on the gums that do not heal; loosening of teeth; numbness or a feeling of heaviness in the jaw; drainage of fluid from the gum or jaw; or seeing any exposed bone in your mouth.
- you should make sure your diet contains enough calcium and vitamins. You should discuss this with your health care provider.

Administering Your Medication

Before you administer pamidronate, look at the solution closely. It should be clear and free of floating material. Gently squeeze the bag or observe the solution container to make sure there are no leaks. Do not use the solution if it is discolored or if it contains particles. Use a new solution, but show the damaged one to your health care provider.

It is important that you use your medication exactly as directed. Do not stop your therapy on your own for any reason. Do not administer it more often or for longer periods than your doctor tells you. Do not change your dosing schedule without talking to your health care provider. Your health care provider may tell you to stop your infusion if you have a mechanical problem (such as blockage in the tubing, needle, or catheter); if you have to stop an infusion, call your health care provider immediately so your therapy can continue.

Side Effects

Pamidronate may cause side effects. Tell your doctor if any of these symptoms are severe or do not go away:

- bone, joint, or muscle pain
- slight fever
- loss of appetite
- upset stomach
- vomiting
- stomach pain
- constipation
- heartburn
- weakness
- dizziness
- headache
- increased sweating

If you experience any of the following symptoms, or those mentioned in the PRECAUTIONS section, call your health care provider immediately:

- seizures
- eye pain, swelling, itching, or redness
- blurred vision or changes in vision
- sensitivity to light
- fast or irregular heartbeat
- fainting
- sore throat, high fever, chills, cough, or other signs of infection
- unusual bruising or bleeding
- black and tarry stools
- red blood in stools
- bloody vomit
- vomiting material that looks like coffee grounds
- shortness of breath or fast breathing
- chest pain
- numbness or tingling in the arms, legs, lips, tongue, or the area around the mouth
- muscle cramps, spasms, or sudden muscle tightening
- depression
- personality changes
- difficult, frequent, or painful urination
- swelling of the face, throat, tongue, lips, eyes, hands, feet, ankles, or lower legs
- difficulty swallowing
- hoarseness
- hives
- rash
- itching

If you experience a serious side effect, you or your doctor may send a report to the Food and Drug Administration's (FDA) MedWatch Adverse Event Reporting program online [at http://www.fda.gov/MedWatch/index.html] or by phone [1-800-332-1088].

Storage Conditions

Store your medication only as directed. Make sure you understand how to store your medication properly. Do not use the solution after the expiration date and time written on the label of the medication. Keep your supplies in a clean, dry place when you are not using them, and keep all medications and supplies out of the reach of children. Your health care provider will tell you how to throw away used needles, syringes, tubing, and containers to avoid accidental injury.

Overdose

In case of overdose, call your local poison control center at 1-800-222-1222. If the victim has collapsed or is not breathing, call local emergency services at 911.

Symptoms of overdose may include:
- fever
- dizziness or lightheadedness
- blurred vision
- fainting
- changes in the way food tastes

Signs of Infection

If you are receiving pamidronate in your vein or under your skin, you need to know the symptoms of a catheter-related infection (an infection where the needle enters your vein or skin). If you experience any of these symptoms near your intravenous catheter, tell your health care provider as soon as possible:
- tenderness
- warmth
- irritation
- hardness or bump
- drainage
- redness
- swelling
- pain

Dosage Facts
For Informational Purposes

Caution: Do not change your dose, how often you take your medication, or the length of time you are to take it without first talking to your healthcare provider.

The following dosage information was written using medical language for doctors and other healthcare professionals and is provided here for you to check your dosage. The dosage of this drug may differ for different patients. Therefore, always follow your doctor's instructions or the directions on the label. Contact your healthcare provider or pharmacist if you have any questions about the specific dosage of your medication after reviewing this information.

General Dosage Information

Dosage of pamidronate disodium is expressed in terms of the salt.

Adult Patients

Hypercalcemia Associated with Malignancy
Moderate Hypercalcemia

IV:
- 60–90 mg as a single dose over at least 2–24 hours in those with albumin-corrected serum calcium concentration approximately 12–13.5 mg/dL.
- Consider retreatment if serum calcium concentrations do not return to normal or remain normal. Repeat the dose appropriate for the degree of hypercalcemia no sooner than 7 days after the initial dose in order to allow full response to the initial dose.

Severe Hypercalcemia

IV:
- 90-mg as a single dose over 2–24 hours in those with albumin-corrected serum calcium concentration >13.5 mg/dL.
- Consider retreatment if serum calcium concentrations do not return to normal or remain normal. Repeat the dose appropriate for the degree of hypercalcemia no sooner than 7 days after the initial dose in order to allow full response to the initial dose.

Paget's Disease of Bone

IV:
- Initially, 30 mg, administered as a 4-hour infusion, once daily on 3 consecutive days (total cumulative dose 90 mg for the course).
- Individualize the need for retreatment and base on patient response (e.g., increased serum alkaline phosphatase concentrations and urinary hydroxyproline). When clinically indicated, retreat with the same dosage that was required for initial treatment.

Osteolytic Bone Metastases of Breast Cancer

IV:
- Initially, 90 mg, administered as a 2-hour infusion, given once every 3–4 weeks. Optimum duration of such therapy is not known, but has been used at these intervals for 24 months.

Osteolytic Bone Lesions of Multiple Myeloma

IV:
- Initially, 90 mg, administered as a 4-hour infusion, given once monthly. Optimum duration of therapy currently is not known, but monthly doses have been administered for 21 months.

Prescribing Limits

Adult Patients

IV:
- Maximum 90 mg as a single dose. Duration of IV infusion should be no less than 2 hours.

Special Populations

Hepatic Impairment

- No dosage adjustment required in patients with mild to moderate hepatic impairment; not studied in patients with severe hepatic impairment.

Renal Impairment

- Withhold therapy in patients with bone metastases associated with solid tumors or with osteolytic lesions associated wtih multiple myeloma if renal function deteriorates (defined as an increase in serum creatinine concentration of at least 0.5 or 1 mg/dL in patients with normal [<1.4 mg/dL] or elevated [≥1.4 mg/dL] baseline serum creatinine concentrations, respectively) during therapy until serum creatinine concentrations return to within 10% of baseline levels.

Pancrelipase

(pan cre li′ pase)

Brand Name: Creon® 10 Minimicrospheres®, Creon® 20 Minimicrospheres®, Creon® 5 Minimicrospheres®, Ku-Zyme® HP, Lipram® 4500, Lipram®-CR10, Lipram®-CR20, Lipram®-CR5, Lipram®-PN10, Lipram®-PN16, Lipram®-PN20, Lipram®-UL12, Lipram®-UL18, Lipram®-UL20, Pancrease®, Pancrease® MT 10, Pancrease® MT 16, Pancrease® MT 20, Pancrease® MT 4, Pancrecarb® MS-16, Pancrecarb® MS-4, Pancrecarb® MS-8, Pangestyme®, Pangestyme® CN 10, Pangestyme® CN 20, Pangestyme® MT 16, Pangestyme® UL 12, Pangestyme® UL 18, Pangestyme® UL 20, Panokase®, Panokase® 16, Ultrase®, Ultrase® MT12, Ultrase® MT18, Ultrase® MT20, Viokase®, Viokase® 16, Viokase® 8

Why is this medicine prescribed?

Pancrelipase is used to improve digestion of foods and prevent frequent, fatty, foul-smelling bowel movements in people who have a condition that affects the pancreas (a gland that produces several substances that the body needs to function normally) such as cystic fibrosis (an inborn disease that causes problems with breathing, digestion, and reproduction), chronic pancreatitis (swelling of the pancreas that does not go away), or a blockage in the passages between the pancreas and the intestine, or who have had surgery to remove all or part of the pancreas or stomach. Pancrelipase is also sometimes used to test how well the pancreas is working. Pancrelipase is in a class of medications called enzymes. Pancrelipase acts in place of the natural substances normally made by the pancreas. It works by breaking down fats, proteins, and starches from food into smaller substances that can be absorbed from the intestine. This allows the body to use these substances for energy and prevents them from being passed as frequent, fatty bowel movements.

How should this medicine be used?

Pancrelipase comes as a powder, tablet, capsule that contains powder, delayed-release capsule that contains small coated beads, and delayed-release capsule that contains very small coated tablets to take by mouth. It is usually taken with food and plenty of water several times a day, often with every meal or snack. The number of times per day that you take pancrelipase depends on your condition and on how well you respond to treatment. Your doctor will tell you whether you should take pancrelipase before, during, or after meals and snacks. To help you remember to take pancrelipase, take it at around the same times every day. Follow the directions on your prescription label carefully, and ask your doctor or pharmacist to explain any part you do not understand. Take pancrelipase exactly as directed. Do not take more or less of it or take it more often than prescribed by your doctor.

You can mix pancrelipase powder or the contents of powder-filled pancrelipase capsules with liquids or soft foods, but be careful not to inhale any of the powder.

If you cannot swallow pancrelipase bead- or tablet-filled capsules whole, you can open the capsules and mix the beads or tablets with a small amount of a soft food such as pudding, applesauce, or gelatin. Certain foods such as dairy products may dissolve the protective coating of the beads or tablets, so ask your doctor or pharmacist before you mix the beads or tablets with any other soft food. Swallow the mixture right after you mix it without chewing or crushing the beads or tablets. After you swallow the mixture, drink a full glass of water or juice right away to wash down the medication.

Swallow pancrelipase powder, tablets, or the contents of opened capsules as soon as you put them in your mouth. Your mouth may become irritated if you suck on the tablets or hold them in your mouth.

Pancrelipase is sold under many brand names, and there are slight differences among the brand name products. Do not switch to a different brand of pancrelipase without talking to your doctor.

Your doctor will probably start you on a low dose of medication and gradually increase your dose depending on your response to treatment and the amount of fat in your diet. Be sure to tell your doctor how you are feeling and whether your bowel symptoms improve during your treatment. Do not change the dose of your medication unless your doctor tells you that you should.

Pancrelipase may control your symptoms but will not cure your condition. Continue to take pancrelipase even if you feel well. Do not stop taking pancrelipase without talking to your doctor.

Are there other uses for this medicine?

This medication may be prescribed for other uses; ask your doctor or pharmacist for more information.

What special precautions should I follow?

Before taking pancrelipase,

- tell your doctor and pharmacist if you are allergic to

pancrelipase, any other medications, or pork products. If you are taking Ultrase® brand capsules, tell your doctor if you are allergic to simethicone.

- tell your doctor and pharmacist what prescription and nonprescription medications, vitamins, nutritional supplements, and herbal products you are taking. Be sure to mention iron products. Your doctor may need to change the doses of your medications or monitor you carefully for side effects.
- tell your doctor if you have ever had surgery on your intestine and if you have or have ever had any disease of the pancreas that comes and goes, a blockage in your intestine at birth or later in life, short bowel syndrome (intestine shortened by surgery or infection), or inflammatory bowel disease (conditions such as Crohn's disease that cause swelling of the intestine and diarrhea or constipation).
- tell your doctor if you are pregnant, plan to become pregnant, or are breast-feeding. If you become pregnant while taking pancrelipase, call your doctor.

What special dietary instructions should I follow?

Your doctor or nutritionist will prescribe a diet specific for your nutritional needs. Follow these directions carefully.

Be sure to drink plenty of fluids throughout the day while you are taking this medication, especially if the weather is warm. Talk to your doctor about how much fluid you need to drink.

What should I do if I forget to take a dose?

Take the missed dose as soon as you remember it. However, if it is almost time for the next dose, skip the missed dose and continue your regular dosing schedule. Do not take a double dose to make up for a missed one.

What side effects can this medicine cause?

Pancrelipase may cause side effects. Tell your doctor if any of these symptoms are severe or do not go away:
- diarrhea
- constipation
- upset stomach
- vomiting
- stomach cramps
- bloating
- gas
- irritation around the anus

Some side effects can be serious. The following symptoms are uncommon, but if you experience any of them, call your doctor immediately:
- rash or other signs of allergic reaction
- diarrhea that is bloody or does not go away
- black, tarry stools
- stomach pain, cramps, or swelling
- pain or swelling in joints, especially the big toe

Pancrelipase may cause other side effects. Call your

doctor if you have any unusual problems while taking this medication.

If you experience a serious side effect, you or your doctor may send a report to the Food and Drug Administration's (FDA) MedWatch Adverse Event Reporting program online [at http://www.fda.gov/MedWatch/index.html] or by phone [1-800-332-1088].

What storage conditions are needed for this medicine?

Keep this medication in the container it came in, tightly closed, and out of reach of children. Store it at room temperature and away from excess heat and moisture (not in the bathroom). Do not refrigerate this medication. Throw away any medication that is outdated or no longer needed. Talk to your pharmacist about the proper disposal of your medication.

What should I do in case of overdose?

In case of overdose, call your local poison control center at 1-800-222-1222. If the victim has collapsed or is not breathing, call local emergency services at 911.

Symptoms of overdose may include:
- pain or swelling in joints, especially the big toe
- diarrhea

What other information should I know?

Keep all appointments with your doctor and the laboratory. Your doctor may order certain lab tests to check your body's response to pancrelipase.

Before having any laboratory test, tell your doctor and the laboratory personnel that you are taking pancrelipase.

Do not let anyone else take your medication. Ask your pharmacist any questions you have about refilling your prescription.

Talk to your doctor, pharmacist, or other healthcare professional if you have questions about dosing information for your medication.

Pantoprazole

(pan toe′ pra zole)

Brand Name: Protonix®

Why is this medicine prescribed?

Pantoprazole is used to treat gastroesophageal reflux disease (GERD), a condition in which backward flow of acid from the stomach causes heartburn and injury of the food pipe (esophagus). It is also used to treat conditions where the stomach produces too much acid, such as Zollinger-Ellison syndrome. Pantoprazole is in a class of medications called proton-pump inhibitors. It works by decreasing the amount of acid made in the stomach.

How should this medicine be used?

Pantoprazole comes as a delayed-release (long-acting) tablet to take by mouth. It is usually taken once or twice a day with or without food. To help you remember to take pantoprazole, take it around the same time every day. Follow the directions on your prescription label carefully, and ask your doctor or pharmacist to explain any part you do not understand. Take pantoprazole exactly as directed. Do not take more or less of it or take it more often than prescribed by your doctor.

Swallow the tablets whole; do not split, chew, or crush them.

Continue to take pantoprazole even if you feel well. Do not stop taking pantoprazole without talking to your doctor.

Are there other uses for this medicine?

This medicine may be prescribed for other uses; ask your doctor or pharmacist for more information.

What special precautions should I follow?

Before taking pantoprazole,
- tell your doctor and pharmacist if you are allergic to pantoprazole or any other medications.
- tell your doctor and pharmacist what prescription and nonprescription medications, vitamins, nutritional supplements, and herbal products you are taking. Be sure to mention any of the following: ampicillin (Omnipen, Polycillin, Totacillin); ketoconazole (Nizoral); and vitamins containing iron. Your doctor may need to change the doses of your medications or monitor you carefully for side effects.
- tell your doctor if you are pregnant, plan to become pregnant, or are breast-feeding. If you become pregnant while taking pantoprazole, call your doctor.

What special dietary instructions should I follow?

Unless your doctor tells you otherwise, continue your normal diet.

What should I do if I forget to take a dose?

Take the missed dose as soon as you remember it. However, if it is almost time for your next dose, skip the missed dose and continue your regular dosing schedule. Do not take a double dose to make up for a missed dose.

What side effects can this medicine cause?

Pantoprazole may cause side effects. Tell your doctor if any of these symptoms are severe or do not go away:
- diarrhea
- headache
- stomach pain
- gas or bloating

Pantoprazole may cause other side effects. Call your doctor if you have any unusual problems while taking this medication.

What storage conditions are needed for this medicine?

Keep this medication in the container it came in, tightly closed, and out of reach of children. Store it at room temperature and away from excess heat and moisture (not in the bathroom). Throw away any medication that is outdated or no longer needed. Talk to your pharmacist about the proper disposal of your medication.

What should I do in case of overdose?

In case of overdose, call your local poison control center at 1-800-222-1222. If the victim has collapsed or is not breathing, call local emergency services at 911.

What other information should I know?

Keep all appointments with your doctor.

Before having any laboratory test, tell your doctor and the laboratory personnel that you are taking pantoprazole.

Do not let anyone else take your medicine. Ask your pharmacist any questions you have about refilling your prescription.

Dosage Facts
For Informational Purposes

Caution: Do not change your dose, how often you take your medication, or the length of time you are to take it without first talking to your healthcare provider.

The following dosage information was written using medical language for doctors and other healthcare professionals and is provided here for you to check your dosage. The dosage of this drug may differ for different patients. Therefore, always follow your doctor's instructions or the directions on the label. Contact your healthcare provider or pharmacist if you have any questions about the specific dosage of your medication after reviewing this information.

General Dosage Information

Available as pantoprazole sodium; dosage expressed in terms of pantoprazole.

Adult Patients

GERD
Treatment of Erosive Esophagitis

ORAL:
- 40 mg once daily for up to 8 weeks. If not healed, consider additional 8 weeks of therapy.

Maintenance of Healing of Erosive Esophagitis

ORAL:
- 40 mg once daily. Not studied for >1 year of therapy. However, chronic, lifelong therapy with proton-pump inhibitor may be appropriate.

Pathologic GI Hypersecretory Conditions (e.g., Zollinger-Ellison Syndrome)

ORAL:
- 40 mg twice daily. Adjust dosage according to patient response and tolerance; continue therapy as long as necessary. May require dosages of up to 240 mg daily. Patients with Zollinger-Ellison syndrome have been treated for >2 years.

Special Populations

Hepatic Impairment
- No dosage adjustment necessary. Dosage exceeding 40 mg daily not studied in patients with hepatic impairment.

Papaverine

(pa pav′ er een)

Brand Name: Para-Time® SR

Why is this medicine prescribed?

Papaverine is used to improve blood flow in patients with circulation problems. It works by relaxing the blood vessels so that blood can flow more easily to the heart and through the body.

This medication is sometimes prescribed for other uses; ask your doctor or pharmacist for more information.

How should this medicine be used?

Papaverine comes as a tablet and extended-release (long-acting) capsule to take by mouth. The tablet usually is taken three to five times a day at evenly spaced intervals. The extended-release capsule usually is taken every 8-12 hours. Do not crush, chew, or divide the extended-release capsules. Follow the directions on your prescription label carefully, and ask your doctor or pharmacist to explain any part you do not understand. Take papaverine exactly as directed.

Papaverine may be habit-forming. Do not take larger doses, take it more often, or for a longer period than your doctor tells you to.

Papaverine controls high blood pressure but does not cure it. Continue to take papaverine even if you feel well. Do not stop taking papaverine without talking to your doctor.

Are there other uses for this medicine?

Papaverine is also used to treat impotence in men. Talk to your doctor about the possible risks of using this drug for your condition.

What special precautions should I follow?

Before taking papaverine,
- tell your doctor and pharmacist if you are allergic to papaverine or any other drugs.
- tell your doctor and pharmacist what prescription and nonprescription medications you are taking, especially levodopa (Larodopa, Sinemet) and vitamins.
- tell your doctor if you have or have ever had heart disease, an AV block (a heart rhythm disturbance), or glaucoma.
- tell your doctor if you are pregnant, plan to become pregnant, or are breast-feeding. If you become pregnant while taking papaverine, call your doctor.
- if you are having surgery, including dental surgery, tell the doctor or dentist that you are taking papaverine.
- you should know that this drug may make you drowsy or dizzy. Do not drive a car or operate machinery until you know how it affects you.
- ask your doctor about the safe use of alcohol while you are taking papaverine. Alcohol can make the side effects from papaverine worse.

What should I do if I forget to take a dose?

Take the missed dose as soon as you remember it. However, if it is almost time for the next dose, skip the missed dose and continue your regular dosing schedule. Do not take a double dose to make up for a missed one.

What side effects can this medicine cause?

Papaverine may cause side effects. Tell your doctor if any of these symptoms are severe or do not go away:
- flushing (feeling of warmth)
- sweating
- headache
- tiredness
- dizziness
- skin rash
- upset stomach
- loss of appetite
- diarrhea
- constipation
- stomach pain

If you experience either of the following symptoms, call your doctor immediately:
- yellowing of the skin or eyes
- irregular heartbeat

If you experience a serious side effect, you or your doctor may send a report to the Food and Drug Administration's (FDA) MedWatch Adverse Event Reporting program online [at http://www.fda.gov/MedWatch/index.html] or by phone [1-800-332-1088].

What storage conditions are needed for this medicine?

Keep this medication in the container it came in, tightly closed, and out of reach of children. Store at room temperature and away from excess heat and moisture (not in the bathroom). Throw away any medication that is outdated or no longer needed. Talk to your pharmacist about the proper disposal of your medication.

What should I do in case of overdose?

In case of overdose, call your local poison control center at 1-800-222-1222. If the victim has collapsed or is not breathing, call local emergency services at 911.

What other information should I know?

Keep all appointments with your doctor and the laboratory. Your doctor may order certain tests to monitor your liver function.

Do not let anyone else take your medication. Ask your pharmacist any questions you have about refilling your prescription.

Talk to your doctor, pharmacist, or other healthcare professional if you have questions about dosing information for your medication.

Paregoric

(par e gor′ ik)

Brand Name: Camphorated Tincture of Opium®

Why is this medicine prescribed?

Paregoric is used to relieve diarrhea. It decreases stomach and intestinal movement in the digestive system.

This medication is sometimes prescribed for other uses; ask your doctor or pharmacist for more information.

How should this medicine be used?

Paregoric comes as a liquid to take by mouth. It usually is taken one to four times a day or immediately after each loose bowel movement. Your prescription may be mixed with water before you take it; the water should turn cloudy white. Do not take more than six doses in 1 day. Follow the directions on your prescription label carefully, and ask your doctor or pharmacist to explain any part you do not understand. Take paregoric exactly as directed.

Paregoric can be habit-forming. Do not take a larger dose, take it more often, or for a longer period than your doctor tells you to.

If you have taken this medication for a long time, do not stop taking it suddenly. Your doctor probably will reduce your dose gradually.

What special precautions should I follow?

Before taking paregoric,
- tell your doctor and pharmacist if you are allergic to paregoric or any other drugs.

- tell your doctor and pharmacist what prescription and nonprescription medications you are taking, especially other pain relievers; antidepressants; medications for cough, cold, or allergies; sedatives; sleeping pills; tranquilizers; and vitamins.
- tell your doctor if you have or have ever had liver or kidney disease, a history of alcoholism or drug abuse, lung disease, or prostatic hypertrophy.
- tell your doctor if you are pregnant, plan to become pregnant, or are breast-feeding. If you become pregnant while taking paregoric, call your doctor.
- if you are having surgery, including dental surgery, tell the doctor or dentist that you are taking paregoric.
- you should know that this drug may make you drowsy. Do not drive a car or operate machinery until you know how this drug affects you.
- remember that alcohol can add to the drowsiness caused by this drug.

What should I do if I forget to take a dose?

Paregoric may be taken as needed. If your doctor has told you to take paregoric regularly, take the missed dose as soon as you remember it. However, if it is almost time for the next dose, skip the missed dose and continue your regular dosing schedule. Do not take a double dose to make up for a missed one.

What side effects can this medicine cause?

Paregoric may cause side effects. Tell your doctor if any of these symptoms are severe or do not go away:
- constipation
- upset stomach
- vomiting
- stomach pain
- drowsiness
- dizziness

If you experience the following symptom, call your doctor immediately:
- difficulty breathing

If you experience a serious side effect, you or your doctor may send a report to the Food and Drug Administration's (FDA) MedWatch Adverse Event Reporting program online [at http://www.fda.gov/MedWatch/index.html] or by phone [1-800-332-1088].

What storage conditions are needed for this medicine?

Keep this medication in the container it came in, tightly closed, and out of reach of children. Store it at room temperature and away from excess heat and moisture (not in the bathroom). Throw away any medication that is outdated or no longer needed. Talk to your pharmacist about the proper disposal of your medication.

What should I do in case of overdose?

In case of overdose, call your local poison control center at 1-800-222-1222. If the victim has collapsed or is not breathing, call local emergency services at 911.

What other information should I know?

Keep all appointments with your doctor and the laboratory. Your doctor may want to check your response to paregoric.

Do not let anyone else take your medication. Ask your pharmacist any questions you have about refilling your prescription.

Talk to your doctor, pharmacist, or other healthcare professional if you have questions about dosing information for your medication.

Paroxetine

(pa rox′ e teen)

Brand Name: Paxil®, Paxil® CR, Pexeva®
Also available generically.

Important Warning

A small number of children, teenagers, and young adults (up to 24 years of age) who took antidepressants ('mood elevators') such as paroxetine during clinical studies became suicidal (thinking about harming or killing oneself or planning or trying to do so). Children, teenagers, and young adults who take antidepressants to treat depression or other mental illnesses may be more likely to become suicidal than children, teenagers, and young adults who do not take antidepressants to treat these conditions. However, experts are not sure about how great this risk is and how much it should be considered in deciding whether a child or teenager should take an antidepressant. Children younger than 18 years of age should not normally take paroxetine, but in some cases, a doctor may decide that paroxetine is the best medication to treat a child's condition.

You should know that your mental health may change in unexpected ways when you take paroxetine or other antidepressants even if you are an adult over age 24. You may become suicidal, especially at the beginning of your treatment and any time that your dose is increased or decreased. You, your family, or your caregiver should call your doctor right away if you experience any of the following symptoms: new or worsening depression; thinking about harming or killing yourself, or planning or trying to do so; extreme worry; agitation; panic attacks; dif-

ficulty falling asleep or staying asleep; aggressive behavior; irritability; acting without thinking; severe restlessness; and frenzied abnormal excitement. Be sure that your family or caregiver knows which symptoms may be serious so they can call the doctor when you are unable to seek treatment on your own.

Your healthcare provider will want to see you often while you are taking paroxetine, especially at the beginning of your treatment. Be sure to keep all appointments for office visits with your doctor.

The doctor or pharmacist will give you the manufacturer's patient information sheet (Medication Guide) when you begin treatment with paroxetine. Read the information carefully and ask your doctor or pharmacist if you have any questions. You also can obtain the Medication Guide from the FDA website: http://www.fda.gov/cder/drug/antidepressants/antidepressants_MG_2007.pdf.

No matter what your age, before you take an antidepressant, you, your parent, or your caregiver should talk to your doctor about the risks and benefits of treating your condition with an antidepressant or with other treatments. You should also talk about the risks and benefits of not treating your condition. You should know that having depression or another mental illness greatly increases the risk that you will become suicidal. This risk is higher if you or anyone in your family has or has ever had bipolar disorder (mood that changes from depressed to abnormally excited) or mania (frenzied, abnormally excited mood) or has thought about or attempted suicide. Talk to your doctor about your condition, symptoms, and personal and family medical history. You and your doctor will decide what type of treatment is right for you.

Why is this medicine prescribed?

Paroxetine tablets, suspension (liquid), and extended-release (long-acting) tablets are used to treat depression, panic disorder (sudden, unexpected attacks of extreme fear and worry about these attacks), and social anxiety disorder (extreme fear of interacting with others or performing in front of others that interferes with normal life). Paroxetine tablets and oral solution are also used to treat obsessive compulsive disorder (bothersome thoughts that won't go away and the need to perform certain actions over and over), generalized anxiety disorder (excessive worrying that is difficult to control), and posttraumatic stress disorder (disturbing psychological symptoms that develop after a frightening experience). Paroxetine extended-release tablets are also used to treat premenstrual dysphoric disorder (PMDD, physical and psychological symptoms that occur before the onset of the menstrual period each month). Paroxetine is in a class of medications called selective serotonin reuptake inhibitors (SSRIs). It works by increasing the amount of serotonin, a natural substance in the brain that helps maintain mental balance.

How should this medicine be used?

Paroxetine comes as a tablet, a suspension (liquid), and a controlled-release (long-acting) tablet to take by mouth. It is usually taken once daily in the morning or evening, with or without food. You may want to take paroxetine with food to stop it from upsetting your stomach. Take paroxetine at around the same time every day. Follow the directions on your prescription label carefully, and ask your doctor or pharmacist to explain any part you do not understand. Take paroxetine exactly as directed. Do not take more or less of it or take it more often than prescribed by your doctor.

Shake the liquid well before each use to mix the medication evenly.

Swallow the extended-release and Pexeva® brand tablets whole; do not split, chew, or crush them.

Your doctor may start you on a low dose of paroxetine and gradually increase your dose, not more than once a week.

Paroxetine controls your condition but does not cure it. It may take several weeks or longer before you feel the full benefit of paroxetine. Continue to take paroxetine even if you feel well. Do not stop taking paroxetine without talking to your doctor. Your doctor will probably decrease your dose gradually. If you suddenly stop taking paroxetine, you may experience withdrawal symptoms such as depression; mood changes; frenzied or abnormally excited mood; irritability; anxiety; confusion; dizziness; headache; tiredness; numbness or tingling in the arms, legs, hands, or feet; unusual dreams; difficulty falling asleep or staying asleep; nausea; or sweating. Tell your doctor if you experience any of these symptoms when your dose of paroxetine is decreased.

Are there other uses for this medicine?

Paroxetine is also sometimes used to treat chronic headaches, tingling in the hands and feet caused by diabetes, and certain male sexual problems. Paroxetine is also used with other medications to treat bipolar disorder (mood that changes from depressed to abnormally excited). Talk to your doctor about the possible risks of using this drug for your condition.

This medication may be prescribed for other uses; ask your doctor or pharmacist for more information.

What special precautions should I follow?

Before taking paroxetine,

- tell your doctor and pharmacist if you are allergic to paroxetine or any other medications.
- tell your doctor if you are taking monoamine oxidase (MAO) inhibitors, including isocarboxazid (Marplan), phenelzine (Nardil), selegiline (Eldepryl, Emsam, Zelapar), and tranylcypromine (Parnate), or have stopped taking them within the past 2 weeks, or if you are taking thioridazine or pimozide (Orap). Your doctor will prob-

ably tell you not to take paroxetine. If you stop taking paroxetine, you should wait at least 2 weeks before you start to take an MAO inhibitor.

- tell your doctor and pharmacist what other prescription and nonprescription medications, and vitamins you are taking or plan to take. Be sure to mention any of the following: anticoagulants ('blood thinners') such as warfarin (Coumadin); antidepressants (mood elevators) such as amitriptyline (Elavil), amoxapine (Asendin), clomipramine (Anafranil), desipramine (Norpramin), doxepin (Adapin, Sinequan), imipramine (Tofranil), nortriptyline (Aventyl, Pamelor), protriptyline (Vivactil), and trimipramine (Surmontil); antihistamines; aspirin and other nonsteroidal anti-inflammatory medications (NSAIDs) such as ibuprofen (Advil, Motrin), and naproxen (Aleve, Naprosyn); atomoxetine (Straterra), atazanavir (Reyataz); bromocriptine (Parlodel); bupropion (Wellbutrin); buspirone (Buspar); celecoxib (Celebrex); chlorpromazine (Thorazine); cimetidine (Tagamet); clopidogrel (Plavix); codeine (found in many cough and pain medications); dexamethasone (Decadron); dextromethorphan (found in many cough medications); diazepam (Valium); dicloxacillin (Dynapen); digoxin (Lanoxin); dipyridamole (Persantine); diuretics ('water pills'); haloperidol (Haldol); isoniazid (INH, Nydrazid); lithium (Eskalith, Lithobid); medications for irregular heartbeat such as amiodarone (Cordarone, Pacerone), encainide (Enkaid), flecainide (Tambocor), mexiletine (Mexitil), moricizine (Ethmozine): propafenone (Rythmol), and quinidine (Quinidex); medications for mental illness and nausea; medications for migraine headaches such as almotriptan (Axert), eletriptan (Relpax), frovatriptan (Frova), naratriptan (Amerge), rizatriptan (Maxalt), sumatriptan (Imitrex), and zolmitriptan (Zomig); medications for seizures such as phenobarbital and phenytoin (Dilantin); meperidine (Demerol); methadone (Dolophine); metoclopramide (Reglan); metoprolol (Lopressor, Toprol XL); ondansetron (Zofran); other selective serotonin reuptake inhibitors such as citalopram (Celexa), fluoxetine (Prozac, Sarafem); fluvoxamine (Luvox); and sertraline (Zoloft); procyclidine (Kemadrin); propoxyphene (Darvon); propranolol (Inderal); ranitidine (Zantac); rifampin (Rifadin, Rimactane); risperidone (Risperdal); ritonavir (Norvir); tamoxifen (Nolvadex); terbinafine (Lamisil); theophylline (Theobid, Theo-Dur); ticlopidine (Ticlid); timolol (Blocadren); tramadol (Ultram); trazodone (Desyrel); and venlafaxine (Effexor). Your doctor may need to change the doses of your medications or monitor you carefully for side effects.
- tell your doctor what herbal products and nutritional supplements you are taking, especially St. John's wort and tryptophan.
- tell your doctor if you use or have ever used street drugs or have overused prescription medications, if you have recently had a heart attack, and if you have or have ever had glaucoma (an eye disease); seizures; bleeding from

your stomach or esophagus (tube that connects the mouth and stomach) or liver, kidney, or heart disease.

- tell your doctor if you are pregnant, plan to become pregnant, or are breast-feeding. If you become pregnant while taking paroxetine, call your doctor.
- you should know that paroxetine may make you drowsy and affect your judgment and thinking. Do not drive a car or operate machinery until you know how this medication affects you.
- ask your doctor about the safe use of alcoholic beverages while you are taking paroxetine.

What special dietary instructions should I follow?

Unless your doctor tells you otherwise, continue your normal diet.

What should I do if I forget to take a dose?

Take the missed dose as soon as you remember it. However, if it is almost time for the next dose, skip the missed dose and continue your regular dosing schedule. Do not take a double dose to make up for a missed one.

What side effects can this medicine cause?

Paroxetine may cause side effects. Tell your doctor if any of these symptoms are severe or do not go away:

- headache
- dizziness
- weakness
- difficulty concentrating
- nervousness
- forgetfulness
- confusion
- sleepiness or feeling "drugged"
- nausea
- vomiting
- diarrhea
- constipation
- gas
- stomach pain
- heartburn
- changes in ability to taste food
- decreased appetite
- weight loss or gain
- changes in sex drive or ability
- dry mouth
- sweating
- yawning
- sensitivity to light
- runny nose
- cough
- lump or tightness in throat
- pain in the back, muscles, joints, or anywhere in the body
- muscle weakness or tightness
- flushing

- problems with teeth
- unusual dreams
- painful or irregular menstruation

Some side effects can be serious. If you experience any of the following symptoms or those listed in the IMPORTANT WARNING section, call your doctor immediately:

- blurred vision
- rapid, pounding, or irregular heartbeat
- chest pain
- seizure
- abnormal bleeding or bruising
- sore throat, fever, chills, and other signs of infection
- uncontrollable shaking of a part of the body
- sudden muscle twitching or jerking that you cannot control
- numbness or tingling in your hands, feet, arms, or legs
- difficult, frequent, or painful urination
- swelling, itching, burning, or infection in the vagina
- painful erection that lasts for hours
- sudden upset stomach, vomiting, weakness, cramping, bloating, swelling, tightness in hands and feet, dizziness, headache and/or confusion
- hives
- skin rash
- itching
- swelling of the face, throat, tongue, lips, eyes, hands, feet, ankles, or lower legs
- hoarseness
- difficulty breathing or swallowing
- black and tarry stools
- red blood in stools
- bloody vomit
- vomiting material that looks like coffee grounds

Paroxetine may cause other side effects. Call your doctor if you have any unusual problems while taking this medication.

What storage conditions are needed for this medicine?

Keep this medication in the container it came in, tightly closed, and out of reach of children. Store it at room temperature and away from excess heat and moisture (not in the bathroom). Throw away any medication that is outdated or no longer needed. Talk to your pharmacist about the proper disposal of your medication.

What should I do in case of overdose?

In case of overdose, call your local poison control center at 1-800-222-1222. If the victim has collapsed or is not breathing, call local emergency services at 911.

Symptoms of overdose may include:

- drowsiness
- coma
- upset stomach
- uncontrollable shaking of a part of the body
- fast, pounding, irregular, or slow heartbeat
- confusion

- vomiting
- dizziness
- seizures
- fainting
- blurred vision
- extreme tiredness
- unusual bruising or bleeding
- lack of energy
- loss of appetite
- pain in the upper right part of the stomach
- flu-like symptoms
- yellowing of the skin and eyes
- aggressive behavior
- muscle pain, stiffness or weakness
- sudden muscle twitching or jerking that you cannot control
- dark red or brown urine
- difficulty urinating
- diarrhea
- frenzied, abnormally excited mood
- sweating
- fever
- difficulty walking

What other information should I know?

Keep all appointments with your doctor.

Do not let anyone else take your medication. Ask your pharmacist any questions you have about refilling your prescription.

Dosage Facts
For Informational Purposes

Caution: Do not change your dose, how often you take your medication, or the length of time you are to take it without first talking to your healthcare provider.

The following dosage information was written using medical language for doctors and other healthcare professionals and is provided here for you to check your dosage. The dosage of this drug may differ for different patients. Therefore, always follow your doctor's instructions or the directions on the label. Contact your healthcare provider or pharmacist if you have any questions about the specific dosage of your medication after reviewing this information.

General Dosage Information

Available as paroxetine hydrochloride; dosage expressed in terms of paroxetine.

Adult Patients

Major Depressive Disorder

ORAL:
- Conventional tablets or suspension: Initially, 20 mg once daily. If no improvement, dosage may be increased in 10-mg increments at weekly intervals.
- Extended-release tablets: Initially, 25 mg once daily. If no improvement, dosage may be increased in 12.5-mg increments at weekly intervals.
- Optimum duration not established; may require several months of therapy or longer. Antidepressant efficacy demonstrated for up to 1 year at mean dosage of 30 mg daily as conventional tablets or suspension, which corresponds to a 37.5 mg daily dosage as extended-release tablets.

Obsessive-Compulsive Disorder

ORAL:
- Conventional tablets or suspension: Initially, 20 mg once daily. If no improvement, dosage may be increased in 10-mg increments at weekly intervals, to 40 mg daily.
- Optimum duration not established; efficacy has been demonstrated in a 6-month relapse prevention trial. Obsessive-compulsive disorder is chronic and requires several months or longer of sustained therapy. May continue therapy in responding patients, but use lowest effective dosage and periodically reassess need for continued therapy.

Panic Disorder

ORAL:
- Conventional tablets or suspension: Initially, 10 mg once daily. If no improvement, dosage may be increased in 10-mg increments at weekly intervals, to 40 mg daily.
- Extended-release tablets: Initially, 12.5 mg once daily. If no improvement, dosage may be increased in 12.5-mg increments at weekly intervals.
- Optimum duration not established; efficacy demonstrated in a 3-month relapse prevention trial. May continue therapy in responding patients, but use lowest effective dosage and periodically reassess need for continued therapy.

Social Phobia

ORAL:
- Conventional tablets or suspension: 20 mg once daily; no additional clinical benefit was observed with higher dosages.
- Extended-release tablets: Initially, 12.5 mg once daily. If dosage is increased, use increments of 12.5-mg increments at weekly intervals.
- Long-term efficacy (>12 weeks) not demonstrated; may consider continuation in patient who responds, but use lowest effective dosage and periodically reassess need for continued therapy.

Anxiety Disorders

ORAL:
- Conventional tablets or suspension: Initially, 20 mg daily; no additional clinical benefit was observed with higher dosages. If needed, dosage may be increased in 10-mg increments at weekly intervals.
- Optimum duration not established; efficacy has been demonstrated in a 24-week relapse prevention trial. Generalized anxiety disorder is chronic. May continue therapy in responding patients. If used for extended periods, adjust dosage so that patients are maintained on lowest effective dosage and periodically reassess need for continued therapy.

Posttraumatic Stress Disorder

ORAL:
- Conventional tablets or suspension: 20 mg daily; insufficient evidence to suggest greater clinical benefit with higher dos-

ages. If needed, dosage may be increased in 10-mg increments at weekly intervals.
- Consider alternative therapy if patient fails to achieve ≥25% reduction in PTSD symptoms at week 8. If >75% reduction in PTSD symptoms and response maintained for ≥3 months, may consider up to 24 months of drug therapy. If used for extended periods, adjust dosage so that patients are maintained on lowest effective dosage and periodically reassess need for continued therapy.

Premenstrual Dysphoric Disorder

ORAL:
- Conventional tablets or suspension†: 5–30 mg daily.
- Extended-release tablets: Initially, 12.5 mg once daily; may be administered daily throughout menstrual cycle or only during luteal phase. Dosage may be increased in intervals of ≥1 week. Dosages of 12.5–25 mg were effective in clinical studies.

Premature Ejaculation†

ORAL:
- Conventional tablets or suspension: 10–40 mg once daily. Alternatively, 20 mg taken 3–4 hours before planned intercourse on an "as needed" basis.

Diabetic Neuropathy†

ORAL:
- Conventional tablets or suspension: 40 mg daily.

Chronic Headache†

ORAL:
- Conventional tablets or suspension: 10–50 mg daily for 3–9 months.

Prescribing Limits
Adult Patients
Major Depressive Disorder

ORAL:
- Conventional tablets or suspension: Maximum 50 mg daily.
- Extended-release tablets: 62.5 mg daily.

Obsessive-Compulsive Disorder

ORAL:
- Conventional tablets or suspension: Maximum 60 mg daily.

Panic Disorder

ORAL:
- Conventional tablets or suspension: Maximum 60 mg daily.
- Extended-release tablets: 75 mg daily.

Social Phobia

ORAL:
- Extended-release tablets: 37.5 mg daily.

Special Populations

Hepatic Impairment

ORAL:
- In patients with severe hepatic impairment, an initial dosage of 10 mg daily (as conventional tablets or suspension) or 12.5 mg daily (as extended-release tablets). If no clinical improvement is apparent, dosage may be titrated with caution up to a maximum of 40 mg daily (for conventional tablets or suspension) or 50 mg (for extended-release tablets).

Renal Impairment

ORAL:
- In patients with severe renal impairment, an initial dosage of 10 mg daily (as conventional tablets or suspension) or 12.5 mg daily (as extended-release tablets). If no clinical improvement is apparent, dosage may be titrated with caution up to a maximum of 40 mg daily (for conventional tablets or suspension) or 50 mg (for extended-release tablets).

Geriatric or Debilitated Patients
- Initially, 10 mg daily (as conventional tablets or suspension) or 12.5 mg daily (as extended-release tablets); if no clinical improvement is apparent, dosage may be titrated up to a maximum of 40 mg daily (as conventional tablets or suspension) or 50 mg daily (as extended-release tablets).

† Use is not currently included in the labeling approved by the US Food and Drug Administration.

Peginterferon alfa-2a

(peg in ter feer on)

Brand Name: Pegasys®

Important Warning

Peginterferon alfa-2a may cause or worsen the following conditions which may be serious or cause death: infections; mental illness including depression, mood and behavior problems, or thoughts of hurting or killing yourself; starting to use street drugs again if you used them in the past; ischemic disorders (conditions in which there is poor blood supply to an area of the body) such as angina (chest pain), heart attack, or colitis (inflammation of the bowels); and autoimmune disorders (conditions in which the immune system attacks one or more parts of the body) that may affect the blood, joints, kidneys, liver, lungs, muscles, skin, or thyroid gland. Tell your doctor if you have an infection; or if you have or have ever had an autoimmune disease; atherosclerosis (narrowing of the blood vessels from fatty deposits); cancer; chest pain; colitis; diabetes; heart attack; high blood pressure; high cholesterol; HIV (human immunodeficiency virus) or AIDS (acquired immunodeficiency syndrome); irregular heartbeat; mental illness including depression, anxiety, or thinking about or trying to kill yourself; liver disease other than hepatitis B or C; or heart, kidney, lung or thyroid disease. Also tell your doctor if you drink or have ever drunk large amounts of alcohol, or if you use or have ever used street drugs or have overused prescription medications. If you experience any of the following

continued on next page

Important Warning (cont'd)

symptoms, call your doctor immediately: bloody diarrhea or bowel movements; stomach pain, tenderness or swelling; chest pain; irregular heartbeat; changes in your mood or behavior; depression; irritability; anxiety; thoughts of killing or hurting yourself; hallucinating (seeing things or hearing voices that do not exist); frenzied or abnormally excited mood; loss of contact with reality; aggressive behavior; difficulty breathing; fever, chills, cough, sore throat, or other signs of infection; unusual bleeding or bruising; dark-colored urine; light colored bowel movements; extreme tiredness; yellowing of the skin or eyes; severe muscle or joint pain; or worsening of an autoimmune disease.

Keep all appointments with your doctor and the laboratory. Your doctor will order certain tests to check your body's response to peginterferon alfa-2a.

Your doctor and pharmacist will give you the manufacturer's patient information sheet (Medication Guide) when you begin treatment with peginterferon alfa-2a and each time you refill your prescription. Read the information carefully and ask your doctor or pharmacist if you have any questions. You can also visit the Food and Drug Administration (FDA) website (www.fda.gov/cder) or the manufacturer's website to obtain the Medication Guide.

Talk to your doctor about the risks of using peginterferon alfa-2a.

Use with ribavirin (Copegus, Rebetol):

You may take peginterferon with another medication called ribavirin (Copegus, Rebetol). Ribavirin may help peginterferon work better to treat your condition, but it may also cause serious side effects. The rest of this section tells about the risks of taking ribavirin. Your doctor and pharmacist will give you the manufacturer's patient information sheet (Medication Guide) when you begin treatment with ribavirin and each time you refill your prescription. Read the information carefully and ask your doctor or pharmacist if you have any questions. You can also visit the Food and Drug Administration (FDA) website (www.fda.gov/cder) or the manufacturer's website to obtain the Medication Guide

Ribavirin may cause anemia (condition in which there is a decrease in the number of red blood cells). Tell your doctor if you have ever had a heart attack and if you have or have ever had high blood pressure, breathing problems, any condition that affects your blood such as sickle cell anemia (inherited condition in which the red blood cells are abnormally shaped and cannot bring oxygen to all parts of the body) or thalassemia (Mediterranean anemia; a condition in which the red blood cells do not contain enough of the substance needed to carry oxygen), or heart disease. If you experience any of the following symptoms, call your doctor immediately: excessive tiredness, pale skin, headache, dizziness, confusion, fast heartbeat, weakness, shortness of breath, or chest pain.

For female patients who are taking ribavirin:

Do not take ribavirin if you are pregnant or plan to become pregnant. You should not start taking ribavirin until a pregnancy test has shown that you are not pregnant. You must use two forms of birth control and be tested for pregnancy every month during your treatment and for 6 months afterward. Call your doctor immediately if you become pregnant during this time. Ribavirin may cause harm or death to the fetus.

For male patients who are taking ribavirin:

Do not take ribavirin if your partner is pregnant or plans to become pregnant. If you have a partner who can become pregnant, you should not start taking ribavirin until a pregnancy test shows that she is not pregnant. You must use two forms of birth control, including a condom with spermicide during your treatment and for 6 months afterward. Your partner must be tested for pregnancy every month during this time. Call your doctor immediately if your partner becomes pregnant. Ribavirin may cause harm or death to the fetus.

Why is this medicine prescribed?

Peginterferon alfa-2a is used alone or in combination with ribavirin (a medication) to treat chronic (long-term) hepatitis C infection (swelling of the liver caused by a virus) in people who show signs of liver damage and who have not been treated with interferon alpha (medication similar to peginterferon alfa-2a) in the past. Peginterferon alfa-2a is also used to treat chronic hepatitis B infection (swelling of the liver caused by a virus) in people who show signs of liver damage. Peginterferon alfa-2a is in a class of medications called interferons. Peginterferon is a combination of interferon and polyethylene glycol, which helps the interferon stay active in your body for a longer period of time. Peginterferon works by decreasing the amount of hepatitis C virus (HCV) or hepatitis B virus (HBV) in the body. Peginterferon alfa-2a may not cure hepatitis C or hepatitis B or prevent you from developing complications of hepatitis C or hepatitis B such as cirrhosis (scarring) of the liver, liver failure, or liver cancer. Peginterferon alfa-2a may not prevent the spread of hepatitis C or hepatitis B to other people.

How should this medicine be used?

Peginterferon alfa-2a comes as a solution (liquid) in a vial and a prefilled syringe to inject subcutaneously (into the fatty layer just under the skin). It is usually injected once a week, on the same day of the week, and at around the same time of day. Follow the directions on your prescription label carefully, and ask your doctor or pharmacist to explain any part you do not understand. Use peginterferon alfa-2a exactly as directed. Do not use more or less of this medication or use it more often than prescribed by your doctor.

Your doctor will probably start you on an average dose of peginterferon alfa-2a. Your doctor may decrease your dose if you experience serious side effects of the medication. Be sure to tell your doctor how you are feeling during your treatment and ask your doctor or pharmacist if you have questions about the amount of medication you should take.

Continue to use peginterferon alfa-2a even if you feel well. Do not stop using peginterferon alfa-2a without talking to your doctor.

Only use the brand and type of interferon that your doctor prescribed. Do not use another brand of interferon or switch between peginterferon alfa-2a in vials and prefilled syringes without talking to your doctor. If you switch to a different brand or type of interferon, your dose may need to be changed.

You can inject peg-interferon alfa-2a yourself or have a friend or relative give you the injections. Before you use peg-interferon alfa-2a for the first time, read the written instructions that come with it. Ask your doctor or pharmacist to show you or the person who will be injecting the medication how to inject it. If another person will be injecting the medication for you, be sure that he or she knows how to avoid accidental needlesticks to prevent the spread of hepatitis.

You can inject peginterferon alfa-2a anywhere on your stomach or thighs, except your navel (belly button) and waistline. Use a different spot for each injection. Do not use the same injection spot two times in a row. Do not inject peginterferon alfa-2a into an area where the skin is sore, red, bruised, scarred, infected, or abnormal in any way.

Never reuse syringes, needles, or vials of peginterferon alfa-2a. Throw away used needles and syringes in a puncture resistant container, and throw away used vials of medication in the trash. Talk to your doctor or pharmacist about how to dispose of the puncture resistant container.

Before you use peginterferon alfa-2a, look at the solution in the vial or the prefilled syringe closely. It should be clear and free of floating particles. Check the vial or syringe to make sure there are no leaks and check the expiration date. Do not use the solution if it is expired, discolored, cloudy, contains particles, or is in a leaky vial or syringe. Use a new solution, and show the damaged or expired one to your doctor or pharmacist.

To prepare peginterferon alfa-2a in vials for injection, follow these steps:

1. Find a clean, comfortable area and collect the supplies you will need: unused syringe, unused needle, and several alcohol pads.
2. Remove a vial of peginterferon alfa-2a from the refrigerator.
3. Warm the vial of peginterferon alfa-2a by rolling it gently in the palms of your hands for about 1 minute. Do not shake the vial.
4. Wash your hands with soap and warm water. Dry your

hands with a paper towel and use the towel to turn off the faucet.

5. Flip off the plastic top covering the vial opening and clean the rubber stopper with an alcohol pad.
6. Remove the needle and syringe from their packaging. If the needle and syringe were packaged separately, attach the needle to the end of the syringe. Remove the clear protective needle cap from the end of the needle. If there is an orange cap attached to the end of the syringe above the needle, do not remove it. This is to protect you from accidental needle sticks.
7. Pull the syringe plunger back so that the end of it is lined up with the mark on the syringe barrel that matches your prescribed dose. If you are not sure which mark on the syringe matches your dose, stop and call your doctor or pharmacist before you inject any medication.
8. Hold the syringe straight up and down and push the needle down through the center of the medication vial stopper.
9. Be sure that the tip of the needle is in the empty space above the liquid in the vial. Push down slowly on the plunger to inject all the air from the syringe into the vial.
10. Keep the needle inside the vial and turn both the vial and the needle upside down. Hold the vial and syringe straight up. Make sure the needle tip is in the medication liquid, not in the space above it, to prevent bubbles from forming in the syringe.
11. Slowly pull back on the plunger to fill the syringe with medication up to the mark that matches your dose.
12. Pull the syringe straight out of the vial. Do not touch the needle to anything.
13. Remove air bubbles from the syringe by holding the syringe with the needle pointing up to the ceiling. Use your thumb and finger to gently tap the syringe to bring air bubbles to the top. Push the plunger slightly to push air bubbles out of the syringe without squirting out any liquid.
14. Keep the syringe pointing up until you are ready to give your dose. See below for injection instructions.

To prepare a prefilled syringe of peginterferon alfa-2a, follow these steps:

1. Find a clean comfortable area and collect the supplies you will need: prefilled syringe, needle with needle guard, and several alcohol pads.
2. Remove a prefilled syringe from the refrigerator and warm it by gently rolling it in your hands for 1 minute. Be careful not to shake the syringe.
3. Wash your hands with soap and warm water. Dry your hands with a paper towel and use the towel to turn off the faucet.
4. Remove the needle from the package, but keep the plastic cap on the needle until you are ready to inject the medication.
5. Remove the rubber cap on the tip of the syringe and throw it away.

6. Put the needle on the end of the syringe barrel so that it fits tightly. Keep the syringe in a horizontal position until you are ready to use it. If you need to set the syringe down, make sure the plastic needle cap (shield) is covering the needle. Do not touch the needle to anything.

7. Remove the plastic cap from the needle shield, but do not remove the orange needle guard attached to the syringe above the needle.

8. Hold the syringe with the needle pointing toward the ceiling. Using your thumb and finger, tap the syringe to bring any air bubbles to the top. Press the plunger in slightly to push any air bubbles out of the syringe.

9. Slowly and carefully push down on the plunger rod until the edge of the plunger is lined up with the mark on the syringe barrel that matches your dose. If you are not sure which mark on the syringe matches your dose, stop and call your doctor or pharmacist before you inject any medication. Do not save or reuse any medication that you squirt out of the syringe.

10. Do not let the needle touch any surface. See below for injection instructions.

To inject a dose of peginterferon alfa-2a, follow these steps:

1. Gently tap the skin in the place where you plan to inject peginterferon alfa-2a. Use an alcohol pad to clean the skin in the injection spot and allow it to air dry for 10 seconds.

2. Hold the needle with the point facing up. Use your thumb and forefinger to pinch up a fold of skin at the injection spot.

3. Hold the syringe like a pencil at a 45 or 90 degree angle to your skin. In one quick motion, insert the needle as far as it will go into the pinched area of skin. Pull back slightly on the syringe plunger. If blood comes into the syringe, the needle has entered a blood vessel. Do not inject. Pull out the needle and throw away the syringe and needle in a puncture proof container. Choose a different spot to inject your medication and start the injection process over using new supplies. If no blood appears, let go of the pinched skin and slowly push the plunger all the way down so that all of the medication is injected.

4. Pull the needle out at the same angle you put it into your skin. Wipe the injection spot with an alcohol pad.

5. If you used a syringe with an orange needle-stick protection device, put the free end of the orange needle guard on a flat surface and push down on it until it clicks and covers the needle.

6. Throw away your syringe and needle in a puncture-proof container right away. If you used a vial of peginterferon alfa-2a, throw it away. Each vial can only be used once.

Are there other uses for this medicine?

This medication may be prescribed for other uses; ask your doctor or pharmacist for more information.

What special precautions should I follow?

Before using peginterferon alfa-2a,

- tell your doctor and pharmacist if you are allergic to peginterferon alfa-2a, other alpha interferons, any other medications, benzyl alcohol, or polyethylene glycol (PEG). Ask your doctor if you are not sure if a medication you are allergic to is an alpha interferon.

- tell your doctor and pharmacist what other prescription and nonprescription medications, vitamins, nutritional supplements, and herbal products you are taking or plan to take. Be sure to mention any of the following: clozapine (Clozaril); cyclobenzaprine (Flexeril); imipramine (Tofranil); certain medications for HIV or AIDS such as abacavir (Ziagen, in Epzicom, in Trizivir), didanosine (ddI or Videx), emtricitabine (Emtriva, in Truvada), lamivudine (Epivir, in Combivir, in Epzicom, in Trizivir), stavudine (Zerit), tenofovir (Viread, in Truvada), zalcitabine (HIVID), and zidovudine (Retrovir, in Combivir, in Trizivir); methadone (Dolophine, Methadose); mexilitene (Mexitil); naproxen (Aleve, Anaprox, Naprosyn, others); riluzole (Rilutek); tacrine (Cognex); and theophyilline (TheoDur, others). Your doctor may need to change the doses of your medications or monitor you carefully for side effects.

- tell your doctor or pharmacist if you have ever had an organ transplant (surgery to replace an organ in the body). Also tell your doctor if you have or have ever had any of the conditions mentioned in the IMPORTANT WARNING section or any of the following: anemia (red blood cells do not bring enough oxygen to other parts of the body), or problems with your eyes or pancreas.

- tell your doctor if you are pregnant, plan to become pregnant or are breast-feeding. Peginterferon alfa-2a may harm the fetus or cause you to miscarry (lose your baby). Talk to your doctor about using birth control while you are taking this medication. You should not breastfeed while you are taking this medication.

- if you are having surgery, including dental surgery, tell the doctor or dentist that you are taking peginterferon alfa-2a.

- you should know that peginterferon alfa-2a may make you dizzy, confused, or drowsy. Do not drive a car or operate machinery until you know how this medication affects you.

- you should know that you may experience flu-like symptoms such as headache, fever, chills, tiredness, muscle aches, and joint pain during your treatment with peginterferon alfa-2a. If these symptoms are bothersome, ask your doctor if you should take an over-the-counter pain and fever reducer before you inject each dose of peginterferon alfa-2a. You may want to inject peginterferon alfa-2a at bedtime so that you can sleep through the symptoms.

What special dietary instructions should I follow?

Drink plenty of fluids while you are taking this medication.

What should I do if I forget to take a dose?

If you remember the missed dose no longer than 2 days after you were scheduled to inject it, inject the missed dose as soon as you remember it. Then inject your next dose on your regularly scheduled day the following week. If more than 2 days have passed since the day you were scheduled to inject the medication, ask your doctor or pharmacist what you should do. Do not use a double dose or use more than one dose in 1 week to make up for a missed dose.

What side effects can this medicine cause?

Peginterferon alfa-2a may cause side effects. Tell your doctor if any of these symptoms are severe or do not go away:

- bruising, pain, redness, swelling, or irritation in the place you injected peginterferon alfa-2a
- upset stomach
- vomiting
- heartburn
- change in the way things taste
- dry mouth
- loss of appetite
- weight loss
- diarrhea
- dry or itchy skin
- hair loss
- difficulty falling asleep or staying asleep
- difficulty concentrating or remembering
- sweating
- dizziness

Some side effects can be serious. The following symptoms are uncommon, but if you experience any of them, or those listed in the IMPORTANT WARNING section, call your doctor immediately:

- blurred vision, vision changes, or loss of vision
- pale skin
- fast heartbeat
- lower back pain
- rash
- hives
- swelling of the face, throat, tongue, lips, eyes, hands, feet, ankles, or lower legs
- difficulty swallowing
- hoarseness

Peginterferon alfa-2a may cause other side effects. Call your doctor if you have any unusual problems while taking this medication.

If you experience a serious side effect, you or your doctor may send a report to the Food and Drug Administration's (FDA) MedWatch Adverse Event Reporting program online [at http://www.fda.gov/MedWatch/index.html] or by phone [1-800-332-1088].

What storage conditions are needed for this medicine?

Keep this medication in the container it came in, tightly closed, and out of reach of children. Store it in the refrigerator, but do not freeze it. Do not leave peginterferon alfa-2a outside of the refrigerator for more than 24 hours (1 day). Keep peginterferon alfa-2a away from light. Throw away any medication that is outdated or no longer needed. Talk to your pharmacist about the proper disposal of your medication.

What should I do in case of overdose?

In case of overdose, call your local poison control center at 1-800-222-1222. If the victim has collapsed or is not breathing, call local emergency services at 911.

If the victim has not collapsed, call the doctor who prescribed this medication. The doctor may want to order lab tests.

Symptoms of overdose may include

- tiredness
- unusual bleeding or bruising
- fever, sore throat, chills, cough, or other signs of infection

What other information should I know?

Do not let anyone else use your medication. Ask your pharmacist any questions you have about refilling your prescription.

Dosage Facts
For Informational Purposes

Caution: Do not change your dose, how often you take your medication, or the length of time you are to take it without first talking to your healthcare provider.

The following dosage information was written using medical language for doctors and other healthcare professionals and is provided here for you to check your dosage. The dosage of this drug may differ for different patients. Therefore, always follow your doctor's instructions or the directions on the label. Contact your healthcare provider or pharmacist if you have any questions about the specific dosage of your medication after reviewing this information.

General Dosage Information

Because there are differences in the potencies and in recommended dosages between the commercially available peginterferon alfa preparations, it is recommended that the peginterferon alfa preparation selected for the patient be used throughout the treatment regimen. Patients should be cautioned *not* to change brands of peginterferon alfa without consulting their clinician.

Dosage of peginterferon alfa and/or ribavirin should be adjusted in patients who develop adverse neuropsychiatric (i.e., depression) or hematologic effects. If serious adverse effects or laboratory abnormalities occur during concomitant peginterferon alfa and oral ribavirin therapy, the dosage of one or both drugs should be modified or therapy discontinued, if appropriate, until the adverse reactions abate. If intolerance persists after dosage adjustments, both peginterferon alfa and oral ribavirin should be discontinued.

Adult Patients

Treatment of Chronic Hepatitis C Virus (HCV) Infection
Comcomitant Therapy with Peginterferon Alfa-2a (Pegasys®) and Ribavirin

SUB-Q:
- Adults with HCV monoinfection (without coexisting HIV infection): 180 mcg once weekly in conjunction with oral ribavirin (800 mg–1.2 g daily, depending on HCV genotype). (See Table.)

Adult Dosage of Pegasys® and Ribavirin for Patients with HCV Monoinfection

HCV Genotype	Pegasys® Dosage	Ribavirin Dosage	Duration
1,4	180 mcg	500 mg twice daily in those weighing <75 kg or 600 mg twice daily in those weighing ≥75 kg	48 weeks
2,3	180 mcg	400 mg twice daily	24 weeks
5,6	Data insufficient to make dosage recommendations	Data insufficient to make dosage recommendations	

Adults with HCV and HIV coinfection: 180 mcg once weekly in conjunction with oral ribavirin (800 mg daily in 2 doses) for 48 weeks, regardless of HCV genotype.

Monotherapy with Peginterferon Alfa-2a (Pegasys®)

SUB-Q:
- Adults with monoinfection (without coexisting HIV infection): 180 mcg once weekly for 48 weeks.
- Adults with HIV coinfection: 180 mcg once weekly for 48 weeks.

Special Populations

Hepatic Impairment

Treatment of Chronic Hepatitis C Virus (HCV) Infection
Peginterferon Alfa-2a (Pegasys®)

SUB-Q:
- In patients with progressive ALT increases above baseline values, decrease Pegasys® dosage to 135 mcg once weekly. If increases in ALT concentrations progress despite dosage reduction or are accompanied by increased bilirubin or evidence of hepatic decompensation, immediately discontinue the drug.

Renal Impairment

Treatment of Chronic Hepatitis C Virus (HCV) Infection
Peginterferon Alfa-2a (Pegasys®)

SUB-Q:
- Patients with end-stage renal disease requiring hemodialysis: Reduce dosage to 135 mcg once weekly. Monitor closely for signs and symptoms of interferon toxicity.

Geriatric Patients
- Cautious dosage selection because of age-related decreases in renal function. Use peginterferon alfa with caution in those with Cl_{cr} <50 mL/minute; concomitant oral ribavirin should not be used in those with Cl_{cr} <50 mL/minute.

Patients Who Develop Depression during Treatment
- In patients who develop mild mental depression, usual dosage of Pegasys® may be continued if the patient is evaluated once weekly (by office visit and/or phone).
- If a patient develops moderate depression, dosage should be reduced and the patient evaluated once weekly (office visit at least every other week). If a patient develops moderate depression while receiving Pegasys®, reduce dosage to 135 mcg daily (a reduction to 90 mcg daily may be needed in some cases). If symptoms improve with the reduced dosage and remain stable for 4 weeks, reduced dosage can be continued or dosage can be increased to the usual dosage.
- If a patient develops severe depression, permanently discontinue Pegasys® and provide immediate psychiatric consultation.

Patients Who Develop Hematologic Effects during Therapy
- Dosage of Pegasys® should be decreased to 135 mcg once weekly in patients with ANC <750/mm³; withhold the drug in those with ANC <500/mm³. If ANC increases to >1000/mm³, Pegasys® may be resumed at a dosage of 90 mcg once weekly with close monitoring. If platelet counts decrease to <50,000/mm³, reduce Pegasys® dosage to 90 mcg once weekly; discontinue the drug in those with platelet counts <25,000/mm³.
- Although usual dosage of Pegasys® can be continued in patients with abnormal decreases in hemoglobin concentrations, concomitant oral ribavirin dosage should be decreased to 600 mg daily (200 mg every morning and 400 every evening) if hemoglobin concentrations decrease to <10 g/dL in patients with no preexisting cardiovascular disease or if hemoglobin concentrations decrease by ≥2 g/dL during any 4-week period in patients with a history of stable cardiovascular disease. Concomitant oral ribavirin should be permanently discontinued if hemoglobin concentrations decrease to <8.5 g/dL in patients with no preexisting cardiovascular disease or if hemoglobin concentrations fall to <12 g/dL after 4 weeks of reduced ribavirin dosage in patients with a history of stable cardiovascular disease.

Peginterferon alfa-2b

(peg in ter feer on)

Brand Name: PEG-Intron®

Important Warning

Peginterferon alfa-2b may cause or worsen the following conditions that may be serious or cause death: infections; mental illness including depression, mood and behavior problems, or thoughts of hurting or killing yourself or others; starting to use street drugs again if you used them in the past; ischemic disorders (conditions in which there is poor blood supply to an area of the body) such as angina (chest pain), heart attack, or colitis (inflammation of the bowels); and autoimmune disorders (conditions in which the immune system attacks one or more parts of the body) that may affect the blood, joints, kidneys, liver, lungs, muscles, skin, or thyroid gland. Tell your doctor if you have an infection; or if you have or have ever had an autoimmune disease; atherosclerosis (narrowing of the blood vessels from fatty deposits); cancer; chest pain; colitis; diabetes; heart attack; high blood pressure; high cholesterol; HIV (human immunodeficiency virus) or AIDS (acquired immunodeficiency syndrome); irregular heartbeat; mental illness including depression, anxiety, or thinking about or trying to kill yourself; liver disease other than hepatitis C; or heart, kidney, lung or thyroid disease. Also tell your doctor if you drink or have ever drunk large amounts of alcohol, or if you use or have ever used street drugs or have overused prescription medications. If you experience any of the following symptoms, call your doctor immediately: bloody diarrhea or bowel movements; stomach pain, tenderness or swelling; chest pain; irregular heartbeat; changes in your mood or behavior; depression; irritability; anxiety; thoughts of killing or hurting yourself; hallucinating (seeing things or hearing voices that do not exist); frenzied or abnormally excited mood; loss of contact with reality; aggressive behavior; difficulty breathing; fever, chills, cough, sore throat, or other signs of infection; unusual bleeding or bruising; dark-colored urine; light colored bowel movements; extreme tiredness; yellowing of the skin or eyes; severe muscle or joint pain; or worsening of an autoimmune disease.

Keep all appointments with your doctor and the laboratory. Your doctor will order certain tests to check your body's response to peginterferon alfa-2b.

Your doctor and pharmacist will give you the manufacturer's patient information sheet (Medication Guide) when you begin treatment with peginterferon alfa-2b and each time you refill your prescription. Read the information carefully and ask your doctor or pharmacist if you have any questions. You can also visit the Food and Drug Administration (FDA) website (www.fda.gov/cder) or the manufacturer's website to obtain the Medication Guide.

Talk to your doctor about the risks of using peginterferon alfa-2b.

Use with ribavirin (Copegus, Rebetol):

You may take peginterferon alpha-2b with another medication called ribavirin (Copegus, Rebetol). Ribavirin may help peginterferon alpha-2b work better to treat your condition, but it may also cause serious side effects. The rest of this section presents the risks of taking ribavirin. If you are taking ribavirin, you should read this information carefully. Your doctor and pharmacist will give you the manufacturer's patient information sheet (Medication Guide) when you begin treatment with ribavirin and each time you refill your prescription. Read the information carefully and ask your doctor or pharmacist if you have any questions. You can also visit the Food and Drug Administration (FDA) website (www.fda.gov/cder) or the manufacturer's website to obtain the Medication Guide.

Ribavirin may cause anemia (condition in which there is a decrease in the number of red blood cells). Tell your doctor if you have ever had a heart attack and if you have or have ever had high blood pressure, breathing problems, any condition that affects your blood such as sickle cell anemia (inherited condition in which the red blood cells are abnormally shaped and cannot bring oxygen to all parts of the body) or thalassemia (Mediterranean anemia; a condition in which the red blood cells do not contain enough of the substance needed to carry oxygen), or heart disease. If you experience any of the following symptoms, call your doctor immediately: excessive tiredness, pale skin, headache, dizziness, confusion, fast heartbeat, weakness, shortness of breath, or chest pain.

For female patients who are taking ribavirin:

Do not take ribavirin if you are pregnant or plan to become pregnant. You should not start taking ribavirin until a pregnancy test has shown that you are not pregnant. You must use two forms of birth control and be tested for pregnancy every month during your treatment and for 6 months afterward. Call your doctor immediately if you become pregnant during this time. Ribavirin may cause harm or death to the fetus.

For male patients who are taking ribavirin:

Do not take ribavirin if your partner is pregnant or plans to become pregnant. If you have a partner who can become pregnant, you should not start taking ribavirin until a pregnancy test shows that she is **continued on next page**

Why is this medicine prescribed?

Peginterferon alfa-2b is used alone or in combination with ribavirin (a medication) to treat chronic (long-term) hepatitis C infection (swelling of the liver caused by a virus) in people who show signs of liver damage and who have not been treated with interferon alpha (medication similar to peginterferon alfa-2b) in the past. Peginterferon alfa-2b is in a class of medications called interferons. Peginterferon alpha-2b is a combination of interferon and polyethylene glycol, which helps the interferon stay active in your body for a longer period of time. Peginterferon alpha-2b works by decreasing the amount of hepatitis C virus (HCV) in the body. Peginterferon alfa-2b may not cure hepatitis C or prevent you from developing complications of hepatitis C such as cirrhosis (scarring) of the liver, liver failure, or liver cancer. Peginterferon alfa-2b may not prevent the spread of hepatitis C to other people.

How should this medicine be used?

Peginterferon alfa-2b comes as a powder in a vial and in a single dose injection pen to mix with liquid and inject subcutaneously (in the fatty layer just under the skin). It is usually injected once a week on the same day of the week, at or around the same time of day. Follow the directions on your prescription label carefully, and ask your doctor or pharmacist to explain any part you do not understand. Use peginterferon alfa-2b exactly as directed. Do not use more or less of this medication or use it more often or for a longer period of time than prescribed by your doctor.

Peginterferon alfa-2b controls hepatitis C but may not cure it. Continue to use peginterferon alfa-2b even if you feel well. Do not stop using peginterferon alfa-2b without talking to your doctor.

Only use the brand and type of interferon that your doctor prescribed. Do not use another brand of interferon or switch between peginterferon alfa-2b in vials and injection pens without talking to your doctor. If you switch to a different brand or type of interferon, your dose may need to be changed.

You can inject peginterferon alfa-2b yourself or have a friend or relative give you the injections. Before you use peginterferon alfa-2b for the first time, read the written instructions that come with it. Ask your doctor or pharmacist to show you or the person who will be injecting the medication how to inject it. If another person will be injecting the medication for you, be sure that he or she knows how to avoid accidental needle sticks to prevent the spread of HCV.

You can inject peginterferon alfa-2b anywhere on the outer part of your upper arms, your thighs, or your stomach except your navel (belly button) and waist. Do not inject into your stomach if you are very thin. Use a different spot for each injection. Do not inject peginterferon alfa-2b into an area where the skin is sore, red, bruised, scarred, irritated, or infected; has stretch marks or lumps; or is abnormal in any way.

Never reuse or share syringes, needles, injection pens, or vials of medication. Throw away used needles, syringes, and injection pens in a puncture-resistant container and throw away used vials of medication in the trash. Talk to your doctor or pharmacist about how to dispose of the puncture-resistant container.

To use peginterferon alfa-2b injection pen, follow these steps:

1. Take the carton containing the injection pen out of the refrigerator and allow time for it to reach room temperature. Check the expiration date printed on the carton, and do not use the carton if the expiration date has passed. Check to be sure the carton contains the following supplies: injection pen, disposable needle, and alcohol swabs. You may also need an adhesive bandage and a piece of sterile gauze to use after your injection.
2. Look in the window of the injection pen and make sure that the cartridge holder chamber contains a white to off-white tablet that is whole or in pieces, or a powder.
3. Wash your hands thoroughly with soap and water, rinse, and towel dry. It is important to keep your work area, your hands, and the injection site clean to prevent infection.
4. Hold the injection pen upright (dose button down). You can use the bottom of the carton as a dosing tray to hold the pen in place. Press the two halves of the pen together firmly until you hear a click.
5. Wait several seconds for the powder to completely dissolve.
6. Gently turn the injection pen upside down twice to mix the solution. Do not shake the injection pen.
7. Turn the injection pen right side up and look through the window to see if the mixed solution is completely dissolved. If there is still foam, wait until it settles. It is normal to see some small bubbles near the top of the solution. If the solution is not clear or if you see particles, do not use it, and call your doctor or pharmacist.
8. Place the injection pen into the dose tray, with the dosing button on the bottom. Wipe the rubber cover of the injection pen with an alcohol pad.
9. Remove the protective paper tab from the injection needle. Keep the injection pen upright in the dose tray and gently push the injection needle straight onto the injection pen. Screw the needle securely in place. You may see some liquid trickle out from under the cap for a few seconds. Wait until this stops before going to the next step.
10. Remove the injection pen from the dose tray. Hold the pen firmly and pull the dosing button out as far as it

will go, until you see the dark bands (lines) below the dosing button. Be careful not to push the dosing button in until you are ready to inject the medication.

11. Turn the dosing button until the number that matches your prescribed dose is lined up with the dosing tab. If you are not sure which number matches your dose, stop, and call your doctor or pharmacist before you inject any medication.

12. Choose your injection spot and clean the skin in the area with an alcohol pad. Wait for the area to dry.

13. Remove the outer cap from the injection pen needle. There may be liquid around the inner needle cap. This is normal. Once the skin at the injection spot is dry, pull off the inner needle cap. Be careful not to touch the needle to anything.

14. Hold the injection pen with your fingers wrapped around the pen body barrel and your thumb on the dosing button.

15. With your other hand, pinch up the skin in the area you have cleaned for the injection. Insert the needle into the pinched skin at an angle of 45 to 90 degrees.

16. Inject the medication by pressing the dosing button down slowly and firmly until you can't push it any further. Keep your thumb pressed down on the dosing button for an additional 5 seconds to make sure you get the complete dose.

17. Pull the injection pen needle out of your skin at the same angle you put it into your skin.

18. Gently press the injection spot with a small bandage or sterile gauze if necessary for a few seconds, but do not massage or rub the injection site.

19. If there is bleeding, cover the injection spot with an adhesive bandage.

20. Throw away the injection pen with the needle still attached in a puncture-proof container. Do not recap the needle.

21. Two hours after the injection, check the injection spot for redness, swelling, or tenderness. If you have a skin reaction and it doesn't clear up in a few days or it worsens, call your doctor or nurse.

To use peginterferon alfa-2b in vials, follow these steps:

1. Wash your hands thoroughly with soap and water, rinse, and towel dry.

2. Check the expiration date printed on the carton of peginterferon alfa-2b and do not use the carton if the expiration date has passed. Take the following supplies out of the carton and place them on a clean work area: a vial of peginterferon alfa-2b, a vial of sterile water for injection (diluent), two syringes with needles attached, and alcohol pads.

3. Remove the protective wrapper from one of the syringes.

4. Flip off the protective caps from the tops of the peginterferon alfa-2b vial and the diluent vial. Clean the rubber stoppers on the tops of both vials with an alcohol pad.

5. Remove the protective needle cap and fill the syringe with air by pulling the plunger back to the 0.7 mL mark on the barrel.

6. Hold the sterile water vial upright without touching the cleaned top with your hands.

7. Insert the syringe needle through the rubber stopper and press down on the plunger to inject the air from the syringe into the vial.

8. Turn the vial upside down with the syringe still attached, and make sure the tip of the needle is in the liquid. Withdraw 0.7 mL of sterile water by pulling the syringe plunger back to exactly the 0.7 mL mark.

9. Remove the needle from the diluent vial by pulling it straight up out of the rubber stopper. Do not touch the needle to anything.

10. Insert the needle through the rubber stopper of the peginterferon alfa-2b vial, and place the needle tip against the glass wall of the vial.

11. Slowly inject the 0.7 mL of sterile water so that it runs down the glass inside the vial. Do not aim the stream of sterile water at the white powder in the bottom of the vial.

12. Remove the needle from the vial by pulling the syringe straight out of the rubber stopper. Hold the safety sleeve tightly and pull it over the needle until you hear a click and the green stripe on the sleeve covers the red stripe on the needle. Throw away the syringe in a puncture-proof container.

13. Gently swirl the vial in a circular motion until the powder is completely dissolved. If the solution is cold, roll the vial gently in your hands to warm it.

14. If air bubbles have formed, wait until the solution has settled and all the bubbles have risen to the top of the solution and disappeared before going on to the next step.

15. Look carefully at the liquid in the bottle. Do not inject the liquid unless it is clear, colorless, and does not contain particles.

16. Clean the rubber stopper on the vial of peginterferon alfa-2b again with another alcohol pad.

17. Remove the protective packaging from the second syringe. Remove the protective cap from the needle of the syringe.

18. Fill the syringe with air by pulling the plunger back to the mL mark that matches your prescribed dose. If you are not sure which mark on the syringe matches your dose, stop and call your doctor or pharmacist before you inject the medication.

19. Hold the vial of peginterferon alfa-2b upright without touching the cleaned top of the vial with your hands.

20. Insert the syringe needle into the peginterferon alfa-2b solution vial, and press down on the plunger to inject the air into the vial.

21. Hold the vial and syringe and slowly turn the vial upside down with the needle still inside the vial. Keep the tip of the needle in the solution.

22. Slowly pull the syringe plunger back to the correct mark

to withdraw the amount of peginterferon alfa-2b that your doctor prescribed.

23. Pull the syringe straight out of the vial. Do not touch the needle to anything.

24. Check for air bubbles in the syringe. If you see any bubbles, hold the syringe with the needle pointing up and gently tap the syringe until the bubbles rise. Then, carefully push the syringe plunger in slowly until the bubbles disappear, without pushing any of the solution out of the syringe.

25. Choose an injection spot and clean the skin in the area with an alcohol pad. Wait for the area to dry.

26. Remove the protective cap from the needle. Make sure the safety sleeve of the syringe is pushed firmly against the rim of the syringe so that the needle is fully exposed.

27. Pinch up a 2-inch fold of loose skin at the injection spot. With your other hand, pick up the syringe and hold it like a pencil with the point (bevel) of the needle facing up. Push the needle approximately 1/4 inch into the pinched skin at a 45- to 90-degree angle, using a quick, dart-like thrust.

28. Let the pinched skin loose and use that hand to help hold the syringe barrel.

29. Pull the plunger of the syringe back very slightly. If blood comes into the syringe, the needle has entered a blood vessel. Do not inject. Pull the needle out at the same angle you put it into the skin, and throw the syringe away in a puncture-proof container. Repeat the steps above to prepare a new dose using a new syringe and a new vial. If no blood comes into the syringe, inject the medication by gently pressing the plunger all the way down the syringe barrel.

30. Hold an alcohol pad near the needle and pull the needle straight out of the skin. Press the alcohol pad over the injection site for several seconds. Do not rub or massage the injection site. If there is bleeding, cover it with a bandage.

31. Cover the syringe with the safety sleeve the same way that you covered the first syringe. (See Step 12 above.) Throw away the syringe and the needle in a puncture-proof container.

32. Two hours after the injection, check the injection spot for redness, swelling, or tenderness. If you have a skin reaction and it doesn't clear up in a few days or it worsens, call your doctor or nurse.

Are there other uses for this medicine?

This medication may be prescribed for other uses; ask your doctor or pharmacist for more information.

What special precautions should I follow?

Before taking peginterferon alfa-2b,

- tell your doctor and pharmacist if you are allergic to peginterferon alfa-2b, other alpha interferons, any other medications, or polyethylene glycol (PEG). Ask your doctor if you are not sure if a medication you are allergic to is an alpha interfereon.

- tell your doctor and pharmacist what other prescription and nonprescription medications, vitamins, nutritional supplements, and herbal products you are taking or plan to take. Be sure to mention the medications listed in the IMPORTANT WARNING section and methadone (Dolophine, Methadose). Your doctor may need to change the doses of your medications or monitor you carefully for side effects.

- tell your doctor or pharmacist if you have ever had an organ transplant (surgery to replace a part of the body) or if you have or have ever had any of the conditions mentioned in the IMPORTANT WARNING section or any of the following: sleep problems, or problems with your eyes or pancreas.

- tell your doctor if you are pregnant, plan to become pregnant, or are breast-feeding. Peginterferon alfa-2b may harm the fetus or cause you to miscarry (lose your baby). Talk to your doctor about using birth control while you are taking this medication. You should not breastfeed while you are taking this medication.

- if you are having surgery, including dental surgery, tell the doctor or dentist that you are taking peginterferon alfa-2b.

- you should know that peginterferon alfa-2b may make you drowsy, dizzy, or confused. Do not drive a car or operate machinery until you know how this medication affects you.

- you should know that you may experience flu-like symptoms such as fever, chills, muscle aches, and joint pain during your treatment with peginterferon alfa-2b. If these symptoms are bothersome, ask your doctor if you should take an over-the-counter pain and fever reducer before you inject each dose of peginterferon alfa-2b. You may want to inject peginterferon alfa-2b at bedtime so that you can sleep through the symptoms.

- plan to get plenty of rest and regular light exercise during your treatment. Talk to your doctor about safe ways to exercise during your treatment.

What special dietary instructions should I follow?

Drink at least 10 full glasses of water or clear juices without caffeine or alcohol every day during your treatment with peginterferon alfa-2b. Be especially careful to drink enough fluid during the first weeks of your treatment.

Be sure to eat well during your treatment. If you have an upset stomach or don't have an appetite, eat healthy snacks or several smaller meals throughout the day.

What should I do if I forget to take a dose?

If you remember the missed dose no later than the day after you were scheduled to inject it, inject the missed dose as soon as you remember it. Then inject your next dose on your regularly scheduled day the following week. If you do not remember the missed dose until several days have passed, check with your doctor about what to do. Do not double the next dose or take more than one dose a week without talking to your doctor.

What side effects can this medicine cause?

Peginterferon alfa-2b may cause side effects. Tell your doctor if any of these symptoms are severe or do not go away:

- bruising, pain, redness, swelling, itching, or irritation in a place where you injected peginterferon alfa-2b
- upset stomach
- vomiting
- loss of appetite
- change in the way things taste
- diarrhea
- constipation
- heartburn
- weight loss
- headache
- dizziness
- confusion
- hair loss or thinning
- itching
- difficulty concentrating
- feeling cold or hot all the time
- changes to your skin
- dry mouth
- sweating
- flushing
- runny nose
- difficulty falling asleep or staying asleep

Some side effects can be serious. The following symptoms are uncommon, but if you experience any of them, or those listed in the IMPORTANT WARNING section, call your doctor immediately:

- rash
- hives
- difficulty swallowing
- swelling of the face, throat, tongue, lips, eyes, hands, feet, ankles, or lower legs
- hoarseness
- fast heartbeat
- pale skin
- lower back pain

Peginterferon alfa-2b may cause other side effects. Call your doctor if you have any unusual problems while taking this medication.

If you experience a serious side effect, you or your doctor may send a report to the Food and Drug Administration's (FDA) MedWatch Adverse Event Reporting program online [at http://www.fda.gov/MedWatch/index.html] or by phone [1-800-332-1088].

What storage conditions are needed for this medicine?

Keep this medication in the container it came in, tightly closed, and out of reach of children. Store peginterferon alfa-2b injection pens in the refrigerator, and do not expose them to heat. Store vials of peginterferon alfa-2b powder at room temperature and away from excess heat and moisture (not in the bathroom). It is best to inject peginterferon alfa-2b solution in vials or injection pens immediately after mixing. If necessary, vials or injection pens containing prepared peginterferon alfa-2b solution may be stored in the refrigerator for up to 24 hours. Do not freeze peginterferon alfa-2b. Throw away any medication that is outdated or no longer needed. Talk to your pharmacist about the proper disposal of your medication.

What should I do in case of overdose?

In case of overdose, call your local poison control center at 1-800-222-1222. If the victim has collapsed or is not breathing, call local emergency services at 911.

If the victim has not collapsed, call the doctor who prescribed this medication. The doctor may want to examine the victim more closely and perform laboratory tests.

What other information should I know?

Do not let anyone else use your medication or any of your injection supplies. Ask your pharmacist any questions you have about refilling your prescription.

Dosage Facts
For Informational Purposes

Caution: Do not change your dose, how often you take your medication, or the length of time you are to take it without first talking to your healthcare provider.

The following dosage information was written using medical language for doctors and other healthcare professionals and is provided here for you to check your dosage. The dosage of this drug may differ for different patients. Therefore, always follow your doctor's instructions or the directions on the label. Contact your healthcare provider or pharmacist if you have any questions about the specific dosage of your medication after reviewing this information.

General Dosage Information

Because there are differences in the potencies and in recommended dosages between the commercially available peginterferon alfa preparations, it is recommended that the peginterferon alfa preparation selected for the patient be used throughout the treatment regimen. Patients should be cautioned *not* to change brands of peginterferon alfa without consulting their clinician.

Dosage of peginterferon alfa and/or ribavirin should be adjusted in patients who develop adverse neuropsychiatric (i.e., depression) or hematologic effects. If serious adverse effects or laboratory abnormalities occur during concomitant peginterferon alfa and oral ribavirin therapy, the dosage of one or both drugs should be modified or therapy discontinued, if appropriate, until the adverse reactions abate. If intolerance persists after dosage adjustments, both peginterferon alfa and oral ribavirin should be discontinued.

Adult Patients

Treatment of Chronic Hepatitis C Virus (HCV) Infection
Comcomitant Therapy with Peginterferon Alfa-2b (PEG-Intron®) and Ribavirin

SUB-Q:
- 1.5 mcg/kg once weekly in conjunction with oral ribavirin (400 mg twice daily).
- The appropriate volume of reconstituted PEG-Intron® to be administered in conjunction with oral ribavirin is based on the solution strength used and the patient's weight as suggested in the following table, and may be adjusted according to the patient's response and tolerance.

Adult Dosage of PEG-Intron® for Concomitant Therapy

Redipen® or Vial Strength (mcg per 0.5 mL)	Weight (kg)	Once Weekly Dose (mcg)	Volume of PEG-Intron® to Administer (mL)
50	<40	50	0.5
80	40–50	64	0.4
80	51–60	80	0.5
120	61–75	96	0.4
120	76–85	120	0.5
150	>85	150	0.5

Monotherapy with Peginterferon Alfa-2b (PEG-Intron®)

SUB-Q:
- 1 mcg/kg once weekly for 1 year. The appropriate volume of reconstituted peginterferon alfa-2b is based on the solution strength used and the patient's weight as suggested in the following table, and may be adjusted according to the patient's response and tolerance.

Adult Dosage of PEG-Intron® for Monotherapy

Redipen® or Vial Strength (mcg per 0.5 mL)	Weight (kg)	Once Weekly Dose (mcg)	Volume of PEG-Intron® to Administer (mL)
50	≤45	40	0.4
50	46–56	50	0.5
80	57–72	64	0.4
80	73–88	80	0.5
120	89–106	96	0.4
120	107–136	120	0.5
150	137–160	150	0.5

Special Populations

Renal Impairment

Treatment of Chronic Hepatitis C Virus (HCV) Infection
Peginterferon Alfa-2b (PEG-Intron®)

SUB-Q:
- Patients with moderate renal impairment (Cl_{cr} 30–50 mL/minute): Reduce dosage by 25%.
- Patients with severe renal impairment (Cl_{cr} 10–29 mL/minute): Reduce dosage by 50%.
- Discontinue if renal function decreases during treatment.

Geriatric Patients
- Cautious dosage selection because of age-related decreases in renal function. Use peginterferon alfa with caution in those with Cl_{cr} <50 mL/minute; concomitant oral ribavirin should not be used in those with Cl_{cr} <50 mL/minute.

Patients Who Develop Depression during Treatment
- In patients who develop mild mental depression, usual dosage of PEG-Intron® may be continued if the patient is evaluated once weekly (by office visit and/or phone).
- If a patient develops moderate depression, dosage should be reduced and the patient evaluated once weekly (office visit at least every other week).
- If the patient develops moderate depression while receiving PEG-Intron®, reduce dosage by 50% for at least 4–8 weeks. If symptoms improve with the reduced dosage and remain stable for 4 weeks, reduced dosage can be continued or dosage can be increased to the usual dosage.
- If a patient develops severe depression, permanently discontinue PEG-Intron® and provide immediate psychiatric consultation.

Patients Who Develop Hematologic Effects during Therapy
- Dosage of PEG-Intron® should be decreased by 50% in patients who have leukocyte counts <1500/mm³, neutrophil counts <750/mm³, or platelet counts <80,000/mm³; usual dosage of oral ribavirin can be continued in these patients. In those with hemoglobin concentrations <10 g/dL, usual dosage of PEG-Intron® can be continued but oral ribavirin dosage should be decreased by 200 mg daily. Both peginterferon alfa-2b and oral ribavirin should be permanently discontinued in patients who have hemoglobin concentrations <8.5 g/dL, leukocyte counts <1000/mm³, neutrophil counts <500/mm³, or platelet counts <50,000/mm³. For patients with preexisting stable cardiovascular disease, PEG-Intron® dosage should be decreased by 50% and ribavirin dosage decreased by 200 mg daily if hemoglobin concentrations decrease more than 2 g/dL during any 4-week period; both drugs should be permanently discontinued if hemoglobin concentrations fall to <12 g/dL after 4 weeks of such reduced dosages.

Pemetrexed Injection

(pem″ e trex′ ed)

Brand Name: Alimta®

Why is this medicine prescribed?

Pemetrexed is used with another chemotherapy (anti-cancer) medication to treat malignant pleural mesothelioma (a type of cancer that affects the inside lining of the chest cavity). Pemetrexed is also used to treat non-small cell lung cancer. Pemetrexed is in a class of medications called antifolate antineoplastic agents. It works by blocking the action of a certain substance in the body that may help cancer cells multiply.

How should this medicine be used?

Pemetrexed comes as a solution (liquid) to be injected into a vein. Pemetrexed is administered by a doctor or nurse in a medical office or infusion center. It is usually given once every 21 days.

Your doctor will probably tell you to take other medications, such as folic acid (a vitamin), vitamin B$_{12}$, and a corticosteroid such as dexamethasone (Decadron) to decrease some of the side effects of this medication. Your doctor will give you directions for taking these medications. Follow your doctor's directions carefully. Ask your doctor or pharmacist to explain any part you do not understand. If you miss a dose of one of these medications, call your doctor.

Your doctor will ask you to have regular blood tests before and during treatment with pemetrexed. Your doctor may change your dose of pemetrexed or delay treatment based on the results of the blood tests.

Ask your pharmacist or doctor for a copy of the manufacturer's information for the patient.

Are there other uses for this medicine?

This medication may be prescribed for other uses; ask your doctor or pharmacist for more information.

What special precautions should I follow?

Before taking pemetrexed,

- tell your doctor and pharmacist if you are allergic to pemetrexed, mannitol, or any other medications.
- tell your doctor and pharmacist what other prescription and nonprescription medications, vitamins, nutritional supplements, and herbal products you are taking or plan to take. Be sure to mention any of the following: aspirin and other nonsteroidal anti-inflammatory medications (NSAIDs) such as ibuprofen (Advil, Motrin) and naproxen (Aleve, Naprosyn), or probenecid. Your doctor may need to change the doses of your medications or monitor you carefully for side effects.
- tell your doctor if you have a pleural effusion (excess

fluid between the linings around the lung), ascites (excess fluid in the abdomen); or have or have ever had kidney or liver disease.

- tell your doctor if you are pregnant or plan to become pregnant. You should use birth control to prevent pregnancy during your treatment with pemetrexed. If you become pregnant while using this medication, call your doctor. Pemetrexed may harm the fetus.
- tell your doctor if you are breast-feeding. You should not breast-feed during your treatment with pemetrexed.

What special dietary instructions should I follow?

Unless your doctor tells you otherwise, continue your normal diet.

What should I do if I forget to take a dose?

If you miss an appointment to receive a dose of pemetrexed, call your doctor as soon as possible.

What side effects can this medicine cause?

Pemetrexed may cause side effects. Tell your doctor if any of these symptoms are severe or do not go away:

- nausea
- vomiting
- constipation
- loss of appetite
- weight loss
- tiredness
- weakness
- pale skin
- headache
- dizziness
- confusion
- fast heartbeat
- difficulty falling asleep or staying asleep
- changes in mood
- depression
- joint or muscle pain

Some side effects can be serious. If you experience any of these symptoms, call your doctor immediately:

- diarrhea
- sores and/or redness in the mouth or throat or on the lips
- unusual bleeding or bruising
- sore throat, fever, chills, cough or other signs of infection
- chest pain
- difficulty breathing or swallowing
- slow or difficult speech
- dizziness or faintness
- weakness or numbness of an arm or leg
- pain, burning, numbness, or tingling in the hands or feet
- hives
- rash
- itching
- decreased urination

Pemetrexed may cause other side effects. Call your doctor if you have any unusual problems while taking this medication.

What should I do in case of overdose?

In case of overdose, call your local poison control center at 1-800-222-1222. If the victim has collapsed or is not breathing, call local emergency services at 911.

Symptoms of overdose may include:

- rash
- sores and/or redness in the mouth or throat or on the lips
- unusual bleeding or bruising
- sore throat, fever, chills, cough or other signs of infection
- extreme tiredness
- weakness
- pale skin
- headache
- dizziness
- confusion
- fast heartbeat
- difficulty falling asleep or staying asleep

What other information should I know?

Keep all appointments with your doctor and the laboratory. Your doctor will order certain lab tests to check your body's response to pemetrexed.

Dosage Facts
For Informational Purposes

Caution: Do not change your dose, how often you take your medication, or the length of time you are to take it without first talking to your healthcare provider.

The following dosage information was written using medical language for doctors and other healthcare professionals and is provided here for you to check your dosage. The dosage of this drug may differ for different patients. Therefore, always follow your doctor's instructions or the directions on the label. Contact your healthcare provider or pharmacist if you have any questions about the specific dosage of your medication after reviewing this information.

General Dosage Information

Available as pemetrexed disodium heptahydrate; dosage expressed in terms of anhydrous pemetrexed.

Adult Patients

Malignant Pleural Mesothelioma

IV:

- 500 mg/m^2 on day 1 of a 21-day cycle. Used in conjunction with cisplatin 75 mg/m^2 on day 1 of a 21-day cycle; initiate cisplatin infusion 30 minutes after completion of pemetrexed infusion.
- Consult published protocols for information on administration of cisplatin.
- Adjust subsequent dosages of pemetrexed and cisplatin based on nadir blood counts (i.e., ANCs, platelet counts) and maximum nonhematologic toxicity from preceding dose.
- Do not administer repeat course until ANCs $\geq$1500/mm^3, platelet count $\geq$100,000/mm^3, and Cl$_{cr}$ $\geq$45 mL/minute.

Non-small Cell Lung Cancer

IV:

- 500 mg/m^2 on day 1 of a 21-day cycle.
- Adjust subsequent dosages based on nadir blood counts (i.e., ANCs, platelet counts) and maximum nonhematologic toxicity from preceding dose.
- Do not administer repeat course until ANCs $\geq$1500/mm^3, platelet count $\geq$100,000/mm^3, and Cl$_{cr}$ $\geq$45 mL/minute.

Dosage Modification for Toxicity

Delay treatment to allow time for recovery from toxicity.

Hematologic Toxicity

Reduce dose according to nadir ANC and platelet count. (See Table 1.)

Discontinue therapy if patient experiences grade 3 or 4 hematologic toxicity after 2 dose reductions.

Table 1. Recommended Dosage Modification for Hematologic Toxicity of Pemetrexed Monotherapy or Pemetrexed and Cisplatin Combination Therapy

Toxicity	Dose of Pemetrexed	Dose of Cisplatin
Nadir ANC <500/mm^3 and nadir platelets $\geq$50,000/mm^3	75% of previous dose	75% of previous dose
Nadir platelets <50,000/mm^3, regardless of nadir ANC	50% of previous dose	50% of previous dose

Nonhematologic Toxicity (Except Neurotoxicity)

Reduce dose based on toxicity type and severity. (See Table 2.)

Interrupt therapy for grade 3 (except grade 3 elevation in serum transaminase values) or 4 nonhematologic toxicity until resolution to at least pretreatment values.

Dosage modification not required for grade 3 elevation in serum transaminase values.

Discontinue if patient experiences grade 3 or 4 nonhematologic toxicity (except grade 3 elevation in serum transaminase values) after 2 dose reductions.

Table 2. Recommended Dosage Modification for Nonhematologic Toxicity (Except Neurotoxicity) of Pemetrexed Monotherapy or Pemetrexed and Cisplatin Combination Therapy

Toxicity and National Cancer Institute (NCI) Common Toxicity Criteria Grade	Dose of Pemetrexed	Dose of Cisplatin
Any grade 3 or 4 nonhematologic toxicity (except neurotoxicity), excluding grade 3 or 4 mucositis or grade 3 elevation in serum transaminase values	75% of previous dose	75% of previous dose
Any diarrhea requiring hospitalization (regardless of grade) or grade 3 or 4 diarrhea	75% of previous dose	75% of previous dose
Grade 3 or 4 mucositis	50% of previous dose	100% of previous dose

Neurotoxicity

Reduce cisplatin dose for grade 2 neurotoxicity; no change in pemetrexed dose needed. (See Table 3.)

Discontinue immediately for grade 3 or 4 neurotoxicity.

Table 3. Recommended Dosage Modifications for Neurotoxicity of Pemetrexed Monotherapy or Pemetrexed and Cisplatin Combination Therapy

NCI Common Toxicity Criteria Grade	Dose of Pemetrexed	Dose of Cisplatin
0–1	100% of previous dose	100% of previous dose
2	100% of previous dose	50% of previous dose

Special Populations

Renal Impairment

- $Cl_{cr} \geq 45$ mL/minute: Routine dosage adjustment not required.
- $Cl_{cr} < 45$ mL/minute: Insufficient information to make dosage recommendation; use *not* recommended.

Geriatric Patients

- No dosage adjustments except those recommended for all patients.

Penbutolol

(pen byoo' toe lole)

Brand Name: Levatol®

Why is this medicine prescribed?

Penbutolol is used to treat high blood pressure. This medication is sometimes prescribed for other uses; ask your doctor or pharmacist for more information.

How should this medicine be used?

Penbutolol comes as a tablet to take by mouth. It is usually taken once a day. Follow the directions on your prescription label carefully and ask your doctor or pharmacist to explain any part you do not understand. Take penbutolol exactly as directed. Do not take more or less of it or take it more often than prescribed by your doctor.

Penbutolol helps control your condition but will not cure it. Continue to take penbutolol even if you feel well. Do not stop taking penbutolol without talking to your doctor.

What special precautions should I follow?

Before taking penbutolol,

- tell your doctor and pharmacist if you are allergic to penbutolol or any other drugs.
- tell your doctor and pharmacist what prescription and nonprescription medications you are taking, especially medications for migraine headaches, asthma, allergies, colds, or pain; other medications for heart disease or high blood pressure; reserpine (Serpasil); and vitamins.
- tell your doctor if you have or have ever had asthma; diabetes; heart block; an overactive thyroid; or heart, lung, liver, or kidney disease.
- tell your doctor if you are pregnant, plan to become pregnant, or are breast-feeding. If you become pregnant while taking penbutolol, call your doctor.
- if you are having surgery, including dental surgery, tell your doctor or dentist that you take penbutolol.

What should I do if I forget to take a dose?

Take the missed dose as soon as you remember it. However, if it is almost time for the next dose, skip the missed dose and continue your regular dosing schedule. Do not take a double dose to make up for a missed one.

What side effects can this medicine cause?

Penbutolol may cause side effects. Tell your doctor if any of these symptoms are severe or do not go away:

- upset stomach
- diarrhea
- cough
- dizziness or lightheadedness
- excessive tiredness

- headache
- difficulty sleeping
- sweating
- decreased sexual ability
- memory loss

If you experience any of the following symptoms, call your doctor immediately:

- chest pain
- difficulty breathing or swallowing
- fainting
- slow or irregular heartbeat
- depression
- easy bruising or bleeding

If you experience a serious side effect, you or your doctor may send a report to the Food and Drug Administration's (FDA) MedWatch Adverse Event Reporting program online [at http://www.fda.gov/MedWatch/index.html] or by phone [1-800-332-1088].

What storage conditions are needed for this medicine?

Keep this medication in the container it came in, tightly closed, and out of reach of children. Store it at room temperature and away from excess heat and moisture (not in the bathroom). Throw away any medication that is outdated or no longer needed. Talk to your pharmacist about the proper disposal of your medication.

What should I do in case of overdose?

In case of overdose, call your local poison control center at 1-800-222-1222. If the victim has collapsed or is not breathing, call local emergency services at 911.

What other information should I know?

Keep all appointments with your doctor and the laboratory.

Your blood pressure should be checked regularly to determine your response to penbutolol. Your doctor may ask you to check your pulse (heart rate). Ask your pharmacist or doctor to teach you how to take your pulse. If your pulse is faster or slower than it should be, call your doctor.

Do not let anyone else take your medication. Ask your pharmacist any questions you have about refilling your prescription.

Talk to your doctor, pharmacist, or other healthcare professional if you have questions about dosing information for your medication.

Penciclovir Cream

(pen sye′ kloe veer)

Brand Name: Denavir®

Why is this medicine prescribed?

Penciclovir is used on the lips and faces of adults to treat cold sores caused by herpes simplex virus. Penciclovir does not cure herpes infections but decreases pain and itching if applied when the earliest symptoms first appear.

This medication is sometimes prescribed for other uses; ask your doctor or pharmacist for more information.

How should this medicine be used?

Penciclovir comes as a cream. It is usually used externally every 2 hours while you are awake for 4 days. Follow the directions on your prescription label carefully, and ask your doctor or pharmacist or doctor to explain any part you do not understand. Use penciclovir exactly as directed. Do not use more or less of it or use it more often than prescribed by your doctor. Use this medication as soon as possible after symptoms appear.

Clean and dry the area before applying the cream to avoid spreading the infection. Rub the cream in gently, using enough cream to cover all sores completely.

Continue to use penciclovir even if you feel well. Do not stop using penciclovir without talking to your doctor.

What special precautions should I follow?

Before using penciclovir,

- tell your doctor and pharmacist if you are allergic to penciclovir, acyclovir (Zovirax), or any other drugs.
- tell your doctor and pharmacist what prescription and nonprescription medications you are taking, including vitamins.
- tell your doctor if you are pregnant, plan to become pregnant, or are breast-feeding. If you become pregnant while taking penciclovir, call your doctor.

What should I do if I forget to take a dose?

Apply the missed dose as soon as you remember it and apply any remaining doses for that day at evenly spaced intervals. However, if it is almost time for the next dose, skip the missed dose and continue your regular dosing schedule. Do not apply a double dose to make up for a missed one.

What side effects can this medicine cause?

Penciclovir may cause side effects. Tell your doctor if any of these symptoms are severe or do not go away:

- headache
- irritation at the site of application

What storage conditions are needed for this medicine?

Keep this medication in the container it came in, tightly closed, and out of reach of children. Store it at room temperature and away from excess heat and moisture (not in the bathroom). Throw away any medication that is outdated or no longer needed. Talk to your pharmacist about the proper disposal of your medication.

What other information should I know?

Keep all appointments with your doctor. Penciclovir should only be used on the lips and face. Avoid getting it in your eyes. Keep the infected area clean and dry.

Do not let anyone else use your medication. Ask your pharmacist any questions you have about refilling your prescription. If you still have symptoms of infection after you finish the penciclovir, call your doctor.

Dosage Facts

For Informational Purposes

Caution: Do not change your dose, how often you take your medication, or the length of time you are to take it without first talking to your healthcare provider.

The following dosage information was written using medical language for doctors and other healthcare professionals and is provided here for you to check your dosage. The dosage of this drug may differ for different patients. Therefore, always follow your doctor's instructions or the directions on the label. Contact your healthcare provider or pharmacist if you have any questions about the specific dosage of your medication after reviewing this information.

Adult Patients

Herpes Labialis

TOPICAL:
- Rub 1% cream gently into the affected area every 2 hours while awake (about 9, but at least 6, times daily) for 4 days. Use sufficient quantity to adequately cover all lesions of the lips and surrounding skin.
- Initiate at the earliest sign or symptom (i.e., within 1 hour of the prodrome or appearance of the first lesion) of herpes labialis.

Penicillin G Potassium or Sodium Injection

(pen i sill' in)

Brand Name: Pfizerpen®
Also available generically.

About Your Treatment

Your doctor has ordered penicillin, an antibiotic, to help treat your infection. The drug will be either injected into a large muscle (such as your buttock or hip) or added to an intravenous fluid that will drip through a needle or catheter placed in your vein for 30 minutes or more, four to six times a day.

Penicillin eliminates bacteria that cause many kinds of infections, including pneumonia; meningitis; and skin, bone, joint, stomach, blood, and heart valve infections. This medication is sometimes prescribed for other uses; ask your doctor or pharmacist for more information.

Your health care provider (doctor, nurse, or pharmacist) may measure the effectiveness and side effects of your treatment using laboratory tests and physical examinations. It is important to keep all appointments with your doctor and the laboratory. The length of treatment depends on how your infection and symptoms respond to the medication.

Precautions

Before administering penicillin,
- tell your doctor and pharmacist if you are allergic to penicillin, cephalosporins [e.g., cefaclor (Ceclor), cefadroxil (Duricef), or cephalexin (Keflex)], or any other drugs.
- tell your doctor and pharmacist what prescription and nonprescription medications you are taking, especially other antibiotics, anticoagulants ('blood thinners') such as warfarin (Coumadin), aspirin or other nonsteroidal anti-inflammatory medications such as naproxen (Anaprox) or ibuprofen (Motrin), atenolol (Tenormin), diuretics ('water pills'), oral contraceptives, probenecid (Benemid), and vitamins.
- tell your doctor if you have or have ever had kidney or liver disease, allergies, asthma, blood disease, colitis, stomach problems, or hay fever.
- tell your doctor if you are pregnant, plan to become pregnant, or are breast-feeding. If you become pregnant while taking penicillin, call your doctor.
- if you have diabetes and regularly check your urine for sugar, use Clinistix or TesTape. Do not use Clinitest tablets because penicillin may cause false positive results.

Administering Your Medication

Before you administer penicillin, look at the solution closely. It should be clear and free of floating material. Gently squeeze the bag or observe the solution container to make sure there are no leaks. Do not use the solution if it is discolored, if it contains particles, or if the bag or container leaks. Use a new solution, but show the damaged one to your health care provider.

It is important that you use your medication exactly as directed. Do not stop your therapy on your own for any reason because your infection could worsen and result in hospitalization. Do not change your dosing schedule without talking to your health care provider. Your health care provider may tell you to stop your infusion if you have a mechanical problem (such as a blockage in the tubing, needle, or catheter); if you have to stop an infusion, call your health care provider immediately so your therapy can continue.

Side Effects

Penicillin may cause side effects. Tell your health care provider if either of these symptoms is severe or does not go away:

- upset stomach
- diarrhea

If you experience any of the following symptoms, call your health care provider immediately:

- rash
- itching
- fever
- chills
- facial swelling
- wheezing
- difficulty breathing
- unusual bleeding or bruising
- dizziness
- seizures
- sore mouth or throat

If you experience a serious side effect, you or your doctor may send a report to the Food and Drug Administration's (FDA) MedWatch Adverse Event Reporting program online [at http://www.fda.gov/MedWatch/index.html] or by phone [1-800-332-1088].

Storage Conditions

- Your health care provider probably will give you a several-day supply of penicillin at a time. If you are receiving penicillin intravenously (in your vein), you probably will be told to store it in the refrigerator or freezer.
- Take your next dose from the refrigerator 1 hour before using it; place it in a clean, dry area to allow it to warm to room temperature.
- If you are told to store additional penicillin in the freezer, always move a 24-hour supply to the refrigerator for the next day's use.
- Do not refreeze medications.

If you are receiving penicillin intramuscularly (in your muscle), your health care provider will tell you how to store it properly.

Store your medication only as directed. Make sure you understand what you need to store your medication properly.

Keep your supplies in a clean, dry place when you are not using them, and keep all medications and supplies out of reach of children. Your health care provider will tell you how to throw away used needles, syringes, tubing, and containers to avoid accidental injury.

Overdose

In case of overdose, call your local poison control center at 1-800-222-1222. If the victim has collapsed or is not breathing, call local emergency services at 911.

Signs of Infection

If you are receiving penicillin in your vein or under your skin, you need to know the symptoms of a catheter-related infection (an infection where the needle enters your vein or skin). If you experience any of these effects near your intravenous catheter, tell your health care provider as soon as possible:

- tenderness
- warmth
- irritation
- drainage
- redness
- swelling
- pain

Dosage Facts
For Informational Purposes

Caution: Do not change your dose, how often you take your medication, or the length of time you are to take it without first talking to your healthcare provider.

The following dosage information was written using medical language for doctors and other healthcare professionals and is provided here for you to check your dosage. The dosage of this drug may differ for different patients. Therefore, always follow your doctor's instructions or the directions on the label. Contact your healthcare provider or pharmacist if you have any questions about the specific dosage of your medication after reviewing this information.

General Dosage Information

Dosage of penicillin G potassium, penicillin G sodium, penicillin G benzathine, penicillin G procaine, and fixed combination of penicillin G benzathine and penicillin G procaine is expressed in terms of USP penicillin G units.

Pediatric Patients

General Dosage for Neonates
Penicillin G Potassium or Penicillin G Sodium

IV OR IM:

- Neonates <1 week of age: AAP recommends 25,000–50,000 units/kg every 12 hours in those weighing ≤2 kg and 25,000–50,000 units/kg every 8 hours for those weighing >2 kg.

- Neonates 1–4 weeks of age: AAP recommends 25,000–50,000 units/kg every 12 hours in those weighing <1.2 kg, 25,000–50,000 units every 8 hours for those weighing 1.2–2 kg, and 25,000–50,000 units every 6 hours for those weighing >2 kg.

Penicillin G Procaine

IM:

- Neonates <1 week of age: AAP recommends 50,000 units/kg every 24 hours in those weighing ≥1.2 kg.
- Neonates 1–4 weeks of age: AAP recommends 50,000 units/kg every 24 hours in those weighing ≥1.2 kg.

General Pediatric Dosage
Penicillin G Benzathine

IM:

- Children ≥1 month of age: AAP recommends 600,000 units/kg daily in children weighing <27.3 kg or 1.2 million units/kg daily for those weighing ≥27.3 kg for treatment of mild to moderate infections. Inappropriate for severe infections according to AAP.

Penicillin G Potassium or Penicillin G Sodium

IV OR IM:

- Children ≥1 month of age: AAP recommends 25,000–50,000 units/kg daily given in 4 divided doses for treatment of mild to moderate infections and 250,000–400,000 units/kg daily given in 4–6 divided doses for treatment of severe infections.

Penicillin G Procaine

IM:

- Children ≥1 month of age: AAP recommends 25,000–50,000 units/kg daily given in 1 or 2 divided doses for treatment of mild to moderate infections. Inappropriate for severe infections according to AAP.

Fixed Combination of Penicillin G Benzathine and Penicillin G Procaine

IM:

- Treatment of S. pyogenes infections (upper respiratory tract, skin and soft-tissue, scarlet fever, erysipelas): A single dose containing 1.2 million units (2 mL of Bicillin® C-R 900/300) usually sufficient. Alternatively, if Bicillin® C-R is used, children weighing <13.6 kg may receive 600,000 units, those weighing 13.6–27.2 kg may receive 0.9–1.2 million units, and those weighing >27.2 kg may receive 2.4 million units. When Bicillin® C-R is used, the dose usually is given at a single session using multiple IM sites; alternatively, if compliance regarding the return visit is assured, the total dose can be divided and half given on day 1 and half on day 3.
- Treatment of S. pneumoniae infections (except meningitis): 1.2 units (2 mL of Bicillin® C-R 900/300) as a single dose repeated every 2 or 3 days until temperature is normal for 48 hours. Alternatively, if Bicillin® C-R is used, 600,000 units as a single dose repeated every 2 or 3 days until temperature is normal for 48 hours. Other penicillin formulations (penicillin G potassium or penicillin G sodium) may be necessary for severe infections.

Endocarditis
Treatment of Native Valve Endocarditis Caused by Viridans Streptococci or S. bovis

IV:

- Penicillin G potassium or penicillin G sodium (for penicillin-susceptible strains; MIC≤0.1 mcg/mL): 200,000 units daily given in 4–6 equally divided doses for 4 weeks. Alternatively, 200,000 units daily given in 4–6 divided doses for 2 weeks in conjunction with IM or IV gentamicin (3 mg/kg daily in 3 divided doses for 2 weeks; dosage adjusted to achieve peak serum gentamicin concentrations approximately 3 mcg/mL and trough concentrations <1 mcg/mL).
- Penicillin G potassium or penicillin G sodium (for relatively resistant strains; MIC >0.1–0.5 mcg/mL): 300,000 units daily given in 4–6 equally divided doses for 4 weeks; used in conjunction with IM or IV gentamicin (3 mg/kg daily in 3 divided doses for 4 weeks; dosage adjusted to achieve peak serum gentamicin concentrations approximately 3 mcg/mL and trough concentrations <1 mcg/mL).
- Penicillin G potassium or penicillin G sodium (for nutritionally variant or strains with high-level resistance; MIC >0.5 mcg/mL): 300,000 units daily given in 4–6 equally divided doses for 4–6 weeks; used in conjunction with IM or IV gentamicin (3 mg/kg daily in 3 divided doses for 4–6 weeks; dosage adjusted to achieve peak serum gentamicin concentrations approximately 3 mcg/mL and trough concentrations <1 mcg/mL).

Treatment of Enterococcal Endocarditis

IV:

- Penicillin G potassium or penicillin G sodium: 300,000 units daily given in 4–6 equally divided doses for 4–6 weeks; used in conjunction with IM or IV gentamicin (3 mg/kg daily in 3 divided doses for 4–6 weeks; dosage adjusted to achieve peak serum gentamicin concentrations approximately 3 mcg/mL and trough concentrations <1 mcg/mL).

Meningitis
Meningitis Caused by S. pneumoniae

IV:

- Penicillin G potassium or penicillin G sodium: AAP recommends 250,000–400,000 units/kg daily given in 4–6 divided doses in those ≥1 month of age. A dosage of 250,000 units/kg daily given in 6 divided doses generally results in mean CSF concentrations of 0.8 mcg/mL sustained throughout the 4 hours between infusions.

Meningitis Caused by S. agalactiae (Group B Streptococci)

IV:

- Penicillin G potassium or penicillin G sodium: AAP recommends 250,000–450,000 units/kg daily IV in 3 divided doses in neonates ≤7 days of age or 450,000 units/kg daily IV in 4 divided doses in neonates >7 days of age.
- Penicillin G potassium or penicillin G sodium: AAP recommends 250,000–400,000 units/kg daily given IV in 4–6 divided doses in those ≥1 month of age. A dosage of 250,000 units/kg daily given in 6 divided doses generally results in mean CSF concentrations of 0.8 mcg/mL sustained throughout the 4 hours between infusions.

Pharyngitis and Tonsillitis

IM:

- Penicillin G benzathine: AAP, AHA, and IDSA recommend a single dose of 600,000 units for those weighing ≤27 kg and a single dose of 1.2 million units for those weighing >27 kg.
- Penicillin G benzathine: Manufacturer recommends a single dose of 300,000–600,000 units in those weighing <27 kg and a single dose of 900,000 units in older children.

Anthrax
Treatment of Naturally Occurring or Endemic Anthrax

IV:
- Penicillin G potassium or penicillin G sodium: 100,000–150,000 units/kg daily given in divided doses every 4–6 hours.
- Continue for ≥14 days after symptoms abate.

Treatment of Inhalational, GI, or Oropharyngeal Anthrax

IV:
- Penicillin G potassium or penicillin G sodium: 50,000 units/kg IV every 6 hours in children <12 years of age.

Postexposure Prophylaxis Following Exposure in the Context of Biologic Warfare or Bioterrorism

IM:
- Penicillin G procaine: 25,000 units/kg (maximum 1.2 million units) every 12 hours; use only if penicillin susceptibility is confirmed.
- Total duration of postexposure prophylaxis usually is 60 days. Safety data for penicillin G procaine administered at the dosage recommended for prophylaxis of anthrax supports a duration of therapy of ≤2 weeks, and clinicians must consider the risks versus benefits of administering penicillin G procaine for >2 weeks or switching to an appropriate alternative anti-infective (e.g., oral amoxicillin or penicillin V).

Diphtheria
Treatment of Diphtheria

IV:
- Penicillin G potassium or penicillin G sodium: 100,000–150,000 units/kg daily given IV in 4 divided doses daily for 14 days; used as an adjunct to diphtheria antitoxin.

IM:
- Penicillin G procaine: CDC recommends 300,000 units daily in those weighing ≤10 kg or 600,000 units daily in those weighing >10 kg as an adjunct to diphtheria antitoxin. AAP recommends 25,000–50,000 units/kg daily (maximum 1.2 million units daily) given in 2 divided doses for 14 days.

Prevention of Diphtheria in Close Contacts

IM:
- Penicillin G benzathine: A single dose of 600,000 units in children <6 years of age or weighing <30 kg or 1.2 million units in those ≥6 years of age or weighing ≥30 kg.
- Provide prophylaxis regardless of immunization status and closely monitor for symptoms of diphtheria for 7 days.
- In addition, contacts who are inadequately immunized against diphtheria (i.e., have previously received <3 doses of diphtheria toxoid) or whose immunization status is unknown should receive an immediate dose of an age-appropriate diphtheria toxoid preparation and the primary series should be completed according to the recommended schedule.
- Contacts who are fully immunized should receive an immediate booster dose of an age-appropriate diphtheria toxoid preparation if it has been ≥5 years since their last booster dose.

Elimination of Diphtheria Carrier State

IM:
- Penicillin G potassium or penicillin G sodium: 300,000–400,000 units daily given in divided doses for 10–12 days.
- Penicillin G benzathine: A single dose of 600,000 units in children <6 years of age or weighing <30 kg or 1.2 million units in those ≥6 years of age or weighing ≥30 kg.
- Obtain follow-up cultures ≥2 weeks after treatment of diphtheria carriers; if cultures are positive, a 10-day course of oral erythromycin should be given and additional follow-up cultures obtained.

Listeria Infections
Serious Listeria Infections in Neonates

IV:
- Penicillin G potassium or penicillin G sodium: 500,000 to 1 million units daily.

Lyme Disease†
Early or Late Lyme Disease with Serious Neurologic, Cardiac, and/or Arthritic Manifestations†

IV:
- Penicillin G potassium or penicillin G sodium: 200,000–400,000 units/kg daily (maximum 18–24 million units daily) given in 4 or 6 divided doses (every 4 or 6 hours) for 14–28 days.

Severe Lyme Carditis†

IV:
- Penicillin G potassium or penicillin G sodium: 200,000–400,000 units/kg daily (maximum 18–24 million units daily) given in 4 or 6 divided doses (every 4–6 hours) for 14–21 days.

Syphilis

Fixed combination of penicillin G benzathine and penicillin G procaine (Bicillin® C-R, Bicillin® C-R 900/300) should *not* be used for treatment of any form of syphilis.

Neonates with Proven or Presumed Congenital Syphilis

IV:
- Penicillin G potassium or penicillin G sodium: CDC and AAP recommend 100,000–150,000 units/kg daily (administered as 50,000 units/kg IV every 12 hours during the first 7 days of life and every 8 hours thereafter) for a total duration of 10 days. CDC and AAP state that if >1 day of therapy is missed, the entire course of therapy should be readministered.

IM:
- Penicillin G benzathine: Manufacturer recommends a single dose of 50,000 units/kg. CDC and AAP state that penicillin G benzathine is not recommended for treatment of known congenital syphilis; these experts recommend IV penicillin G potassium or sodium or IM penicillin G procaine for neonates with proven or highly probable congenital syphilis.
- Penicillin G procaine: CDC and AAP recommend 50,000 units/kg once daily for 10 days; if >1 day of therapy is missed, the entire course should be readministered.

Children ≥1 Month of Age with Suspected Congenital Syphilis or Late and Previously Untreated Congenital Syphilis

IV:
- Penicillin G potassium or penicillin G sodium: 200,000–300,000 units/kg daily (given as 50,000 units/kg every 4–6 hours) for 10 days. Some clinicians recommend that this regimen be followed by a regimen of IM penicillin G benzathine (50,000 units/kg once weekly for 1–3 weeks).

IM:
- Penicillin G benzathine: 50,000 units/kg once weekly for 3 weeks.

Primary or Secondary Syphilis in Children ≥1 Month of Age

IM:
- Penicillin G benzathine: A single dose of 50,000 units/kg (up to 2.4 million units).

Primary or Secondary Syphilis in Adolescents

IM:
- Penicillin G benzathine: A single dose of 2.4 million units. For HIV-infected adolescents, some clinicians suggest that additional doses of 2.4 million units be given once weekly for a total of 3 weeks of therapy.
- Penicillin G procaine: Manufacturer recommends 600,000 units daily for 8 days. CDC recommends use of penicillin G benzathine for primary or secondary syphilis.

Latent Syphilis or Tertiary Syphilis in Children ≥1 Month of Age

IM:
- Penicillin G benzathine: CDC and AAP recommend that early latent syphilis be treated with a single dose of 50,000 units/kg (up to 2.4 million units) and that those with late latent syphilis or latent syphilis of unknown duration receive 50,000 units/kg (up to 2.4 million units) once weekly for 3 successive weeks (up to a maximum total dosage of 7.2 million units).

Latent Syphilis or Tertiary Syphilis in Adolescents

IM:
- Penicillin G benzathine: For early latent syphilis (syphilis of <1-year duration), CDC recommends a single dose of 2.4 million units. For late latent syphilis, latent syphilis of unknown duration, and tertiary syphilis, CDC recommends 2.4 million units once weekly for 3 successive weeks (7.2 million units total). These regimens also can be used to treat early latent syphilis, late latent syphilis, or syphilis of unknown duration in HIV-infected adolescents, provided they have a normal CSF examination.
- Penicillin G procaine: Manufacturer recommends 600,000 units daily for 10–15 days. CDC recommends use of penicillin G benzathine for latent or tertiary syphilis.

Neurosyphilis in Children

IV:
- Penicillin G potassium or penicillin G sodium: AAP recommends 200,000–300,000 units/kg daily for 10–14 days; some clinicians recommend that this regimen be followed by a single IM dose of 50,000 units/kg of penicillin G benzathine (up to 2.4 million units).

IM:
- Penicillin G benzathine: Manufacturer recommends 2.4 million units once weekly for 3 weeks. CDC recommends use of penicillin G potassium or sodium or penicillin G procaine for treatment of neurosyphilis.

Neurosyphilis in Adolescents

IV:
- Penicillin G potassium or penicillin G sodium: 18–24 million units daily (given as 3–4 million units every 4 hours or by continuous IV infusion) for 10–14 days; some clinicians recommend that this regimen be followed by a regimen of IM penicillin G benzathine (2.4 million units once weekly for up to 3 weeks).

IM:
- Penicillin G benzathine: Manufacturer recommends 2.4 million units once weekly for 3 weeks. CDC recommends use of penicillin G potassium or sodium or penicillin G procaine for treatment of neurosyphilis.
- Penicillin G procaine: CDC states that 2.4 million units may be given once daily for 10–14 days in conjunction with oral probenecid (500 mg every 6 hours) if compliance can be ensured; some clinicians recommend that this regimen be followed by a regimen of IM penicillin G benzathine (2.4 million units once weekly for up to 3 weeks).

Yaws, Pinta, and Bejel

IM:
- Penicillin G benzathine: A single dose of 300,000 units in children <6 years of age or a single dose of 1.2 million units in children 6–15 years of age.

Prevention of Rheumatic Fever Recurrence

IM:
- Penicillin G benzathine: 1.2 million units once every 3–4 weeks. The 4-week regimen recommended for most patients in the US.
- Long-term, continuous prophylaxis for 5 years or into adulthood required.

Adult Patients

General Adult Dosage
Penicillin G Potassium or Penicillin G Sodium

IV OR IM:
- Treatment of severe streptococcal or staphylococcal infections: Minimum 5 million units daily. Some clinicians suggest that adults with meningitis caused by susceptible organisms receive 15 million units daily given IV in divided doses every 4 hours.

Fixed Combination of Penicillin G Benzathine and Penicillin G Procaine

IM:
- Treatment of S. pyogenes infections (upper respiratory tract, skin and soft-tissue, scarlet fever, erysipelas): 2.4 million units. The dose usually is given at a single session using multiple IM sites; alternatively, if compliance regarding the return visit is assured, the total dose can be divided and 1.2 million units given on day 1 and 1.2 million units given on day 3.
- Treatment of S. pneumoniae infections (except meningitis): 1.2 units as a single dose repeated every 2 or 3 days until temperature is normal for 48 hours. Other penicillin formulations (penicillin G potassium or penicillin G sodium) may be necessary for severe infections.

Endocarditis
Treatment of Endocarditis Caused by S. pyogenes (Group A Streptococci)

IM:
- Penicillin G procaine: Manufacturer recommends 600,000 to 1 million units daily. AHA states that penicillin G potassium or sodium usually preferred.

Native Valve Endocarditis Caused by Penicillin-susceptible Staphylococci

IV:
- Penicillin G potassium or penicillin G sodium: 12–18 million units daily (by continuous IV infusion or in 6 equally divided doses) given for 4–6 weeks.

Treatment of Endocarditis Caused by Viridans Streptococci or S. bovis

IV:
- Penicillin G potassium or penicillin G sodium (penicillin susceptible strains; MIC ≤0.1 mcg/mL): 12–18 million units daily (by continuous IV infusion or in 6 equally divided doses) given for 4 weeks for native valve endocarditis. Alternatively, 12–18 million units daily (by continuous IV infusion or in 6 equally divided doses) given for 2 weeks in conjunction with IM or IV gentamicin (1 mg/kg every 8 hours given for 2 weeks). The 2-week regimen is not recommended for patients with complications such as extracardiac foci of infection or intracardiac abscesses.
- Penicillin G potassium or penicillin G sodium (nutritionally variant or relatively resistant strains; MIC >0.1 and <0.5 mcg/mL): 18 million units daily (by continuous IV infusion or in 6 equally divided IV doses) for 4 weeks in conjunction with IM or IV gentamicin (1 mg/kg every 8 hours during the first 2 weeks).
- Penicillin G potassium or penicillin G sodium (high level penicillin resistance; MIC >5 mcg/mL): 18–30 million units daily (by continuous IV infusion or in 6 equally divided IV doses) for 4–6 weeks in conjunction with IM or IV gentamicin (1 mg/kg every 8 hours for 4–6 weeks).

Treatment of Enterococcal Endocarditis

IV:
- Penicillin G potassium or penicillin G sodium: 18–30 million units daily (by continuous IV infusion or in 6 equally divided IV doses) given for 4–6 weeks in conjunction with IM or IV gentamicin (1 mg/kg every 8 hours given for 4–6 weeks). Treatment with both drugs generally should be continued for 4–6 weeks, but patients who had symptoms of infection for >3 months before treatment was initiated and patients with prosthetic heart valves require ≥6 weeks of therapy with both drugs.

Pharyngitis and Tonsillitis

IM:
- Penicillin G benzathine: A single dose of 1.2 million units.

Respiratory Tract Infections

IM:
- Penicillin G procaine: 600,000 to 1 million units daily for ≥10 days.

Septicemia

IV:
- Penicillin G potassium or penicillin G sodium: 20–80 million units daily.

Skin and Skin Structure Infections

IM:
- Penicillin G procaine: 600,000 to 1 million units daily for ≥10 days.

Actinomycosis

IV:
- Penicillin G potassium or penicillin G sodium: 1–6 million units daily for cervicofacial infections or 10–20 million units daily for pulmonary or abdominal infections.
- Prolonged therapy (1.5–18 months or longer) may be necessary. Many clinicians recommend that patients with pulmonary actinomycosis or other severe infections receive 4–6 weeks of IV therapy followed by 6–12 additional months of oral therapy (e.g., penicillin V, a tetracycline).

Anthrax
Treatment of Naturally Occurring or Endemic Anthrax

IV:
- Penicillin G potassium or penicillin G sodium: Minimum parenteral dosage is 5 million units daily given in divided doses; IV dosages up to 20 million units daily have been used in the treatment of anthrax septicemia and intestinal, pulmonary, and meningeal anthrax. Some clinicians recommend that adults receive IV penicillin G in a dosage of 8–12 million units daily given in divided doses every 4–6 hours.

Treatment of Inhalational, GI, or Oropharyngeal Anthrax

IV:
- Penicillin G potassium or penicillin G sodium: 4 million units IV every 4 hours suggested if used for treatment of anthrax in the context of biologic warfare or bioterrorism when the organism has been shown to be susceptible to penicillin.
- Oral anti-infective therapy may be substituted for IV therapy as soon as the patient's clinical condition improves.
- Because of the possible persistence of anthrax spores in lung tissue following an aerosol exposure in the context of biologic warfare or bioterrorism, the CDC and other experts recommend that anti-infective therapy should be continued for 60 days.

Treatment of Cutaneous Anthrax

IM:
- Penicillin G procaine: 600,000 to 1 million units daily.
- Although 5–10 days of treatment may be adequate for mild, uncomplicated cutaneous anthrax that occurs as the result of naturally occurring or endemic exposures to anthrax, 60 days of treatment necessary it occurs as the result of exposure to aerosolized *B. anthracis* spores (e.g., in context of biologic warfare or bioterrorism).

Postexposure Prophylaxis Following Exposure in the Context of Biologic Warfare or Bioterrorism

IM:
- Penicillin G procaine: 1.2 million units every 12 hours; use only if penicillin susceptibility is confirmed.
- Total duration of postexposure prophylaxis usually is 60 days. Safety data for penicillin G procaine administered at the dosage recommended for prophylaxis of anthrax supports a duration of therapy of ≤2 weeks, and clinicians must consider the risks versus benefits of administering penicillin G procaine for >2 weeks or switching to an appropriate alternative anti-infective (e.g., oral amoxicillin or penicillin V).

Clostridium Infections
Tetanus

IV OR IM:

- Penicillin G potassium or penicillin G sodium: 20 million units daily; used as an adjunct to antitoxin.

Botulism

IV:

- Penicillin G potassium or penicillin G sodium: When used in the management of wound botulism as an adjunct to botulinum antitoxin (available from the CDC), 2 million units every 4 hours in conjunction with IV metronidazole (250 mg every 6 hours). Anti-infectives have no known direct effects on botulinum toxin but may be indicated to eradicate *C. botulinum* at the wound site.

Diphtheria
Treatment of Diphtheria

IV:

- Penicillin G potassium or penicillin G sodium: 100,000–150,000 units/kg daily given IV in 4 divided doses daily for 14 days; used as an adjunct to diphtheria antitoxin.

Prevention of Diphtheria in Close Contacts

IM:

- Penicillin G benzathine: A single dose of 1.2 million units.
- Penicillin G procaine: 300,000–600,000 units daily for 14 days as an adjunct to diphtheria antitoxin.
- Provide prophylaxis regardless of immunization status and closely monitor for symptoms of diphtheria for 7 days.
- In addition, contacts who are inadequately immunized against diphtheria (i.e., have previously received <3 doses of diphtheria toxoid) or whose immunization status is unknown should receive an immediate dose of an age-appropriate diphtheria toxoid preparation and the primary series should be completed according to the recommended schedule.
- Contacts who are fully immunized should receive an immediate booster dose of an age-appropriate diphtheria toxoid preparation if it has been ≥5 years since their last booster dose.

Elimination of Diphtheria Carrier State

IM:

- Penicillin G benzathine: A single dose of 1.2 million units.
- Penicillin G procaine: 300,000 units daily for 10 days.
- Obtain follow-up cultures ≥2 weeks after treatment of diphtheria carriers; if cultures are positive, a 10-day course of oral erythromycin should be given and additional follow-up cultures obtained.

Erysipelothrix rhusiopathiae Infections
Endocarditis Caused by Erysipelothrix rhusiopathiae

IV:

- Penicillin G potassium or penicillin G sodium: 2–20 million units daily for 4–6 weeks.

Uncomplicated Infections (e.g., Erysipeloid) Caused by Erysipelothrix rhusiopathiae

IM:

- Penicillin G procaine: 600,000 to 1 million units daily.

Fusobacterium Infections
Oropharyngeal, Lower Respiratory Tract, and Genital Infections

IV OR IM:

- Penicillin G potassium or penicillin G sodium: 5–10 million units daily.

Necrotizing Ulcerative Gingivitis

IM:

- Penicillin G procaine: 600,000 to 1 million units daily.

Listeria Infections
Endocarditis or Meningitis Caused by Listeria

IV:

- Penicillin G potassium or penicillin G sodium: 15–20 million units daily given for 4 weeks for endocarditis or for 2 weeks for meningitis.

Lyme Disease†
Early or Late Lyme Disease with Serious Neurologic, Cardiac, and/or Arthritic Manifestations†

IV:

- Penicillin G potassium or penicillin G sodium: 18–24 million units daily given in 6 divided doses (every 4 hours) for 14–28 days.

Severe Lyme Carditis

IV:

- Penicillin G potassium or penicillin G sodium: 18–24 million units daily given in 4 or 6 divided doses (every 4 or 6 hours) for 14–21 days.

Neisseria meningitidis Infections
Meningitis

IV:

- Penicillin G potassium or penicillin G sodium: 20–30 million units daily given by continuous IV infusion for ≥10–14 days.

Pasteurella multocida Infections
Bacteremia or Meningitis Caused by P. multocida

IV OR IM:

- Penicillin G potassium or penicillin G sodium: 4–6 million units daily for 2 weeks.

Rat-bite Fever

IV:

- Penicillin G potassium or penicillin G sodium: 12–15 million units daily for ≥3–4 weeks.

IM:

- Penicillin G procaine: 600,000 to 1 million units daily.

Syphilis

Fixed combination of penicillin G benzathine and penicillin G procaine (Bicillin® C-R, Bicillin® C-R 900/300) should *not* be used for treatment of any form of syphilis.

Primary or Secondary Syphilis

IM:

- Penicillin G benzathine: A single dose of 2.4 million units. For HIV-infected adults, some clinicians suggest that additional doses of 2.4 million units be given once weekly for a total of 3 weeks of therapy. For pregnant women, some clinicians recommend that a second penicillin G benzathine dose of 2.4 million units be administered 1 week after the initial dose.

- Penicillin G procaine: Manufacturer recommends 600,000 units daily for 8 days. CDC recommends use of penicillin G benzathine (not penicillin G procaine) for primary or secondary syphilis.

Latent Syphilis or Tertiary Syphilis

IM:

- Penicillin G benzathine: For early latent syphilis (syphilis of <1-year duration), CDC recommends a single dose of 2.4 million units. For late latent syphilis, latent syphilis of unknown duration, and tertiary syphilis, CDC recommends 2.4 million units once weekly for 3 successive weeks (7.2 million units total). These regimens also can be used to treat early latent syphilis, late latent syphilis, or syphilis of unknown duration in HIV-infected adults, provided they have a normal CSF examination.
- Penicillin G procaine: Manufacturer recommends 600,000 units daily for 10–15 days. CDC recommends use of penicillin G benzathine (not penicillin G procaine) for latent or tertiary syphilis.

Neurosyphilis

IV:

- Penicillin G potassium or penicillin G sodium: 18–24 million units daily (given as 3–4 million units every 4 hours or by continuous IV infusion) for 10–14 days; some clinicians recommend that this regimen be followed by a regimen of IM penicillin G benzathine (2.4 million units once weekly for up to 3 weeks).

IM:

- Penicillin G benzathine: Manufacturer recommends 2.4 million units once weekly for 3 weeks. CDC recommends use of penicillin G potassium or sodium or penicillin G procaine (with probenecid) for treatment of neurosyphilis.
- Penicillin G procaine: CDC states that 2.4 million units may be given once daily for 10–14 days in conjunction with oral probenecid (500 mg every 6 hours) if compliance can be ensured; some clinicians recommend that this regimen be followed by a regimen of IM penicillin G benzathine (2.4 million units once weekly for up to 3 weeks).

Yaws, Pinta, and Bejel

IM:

- Penicillin G benzathine: A single dose of 1.2 million units.
- Penicillin G procaine: Manufacturer states dosage is the same as that recommended for the corresponding stage of syphilis.

Prevention of Perinatal Group B Streptococcal (GBS) Disease†

IV:

- Penicillin G potassium or penicillin G sodium: A single dose of 5 million units of IV penicillin G be given at onset of labor or after membrane rupture followed by 2.5 million units IV every 4 hours until delivery.

Prevention of Rheumatic Fever Recurrence

IM:

- Penicillin G benzathine: 1.2 million units once every 3–4 weeks. The 4-week regimen recommended for most patients in the US.
- Long-term, continuous prophylaxis required.

Recommended Duration of Prophylaxis for Prevention of Rheumatic Fever Recurrence

Patient Category	Duration
Rheumatic fever without carditis	5 years or until 21 years of age, whichever is longer
Rheumatic fever with carditis but no residual heart disease (no valvular disease)	10 years or well into adulthood, whichever is longer
Rheumatic fever with carditis and residual heart disease (persistent valvular disease)	At least 10 years since last episode and at least until 40 years of age; sometimes for life

Special Populations

Renal Impairment

- In patients with impaired renal function, doses and/or frequency of administration of penicillin G must be modified in response to the degree of impairment, severity of the infection, and susceptibility of the causative organism.
- Some clinicians suggest that patients who are uremic but have a Cl_{cr} >10 mL/minute receive a full loading dose of IM or IV penicillin G potassium or sodium followed by one-half the usual dose every 4–5 hours and that patients with Cl_{cr} <10 mL/minute receive a full loading dose followed by one-half the usual dose every 8–10 hours.
- Alternatively, some clinicians suggest that if the usual dosing interval for penicillin G potassium or sodium in patients with normal renal function (Cl_{cr} >50 mL/minute) is every 6 or 8 hours, then the usual dose should be given at 8- to 12-hour intervals or 12- to 18-hour intervals in patients with Cl_{cr} <10–50 or less than 10 mL/minute, respectively.
- Some clinicians suggest that a maximum dosage of 4–10 million units of penicillin G potassium or sodium daily be used in adults with severe renal failure.
- In patients with impaired hepatic function in addition to impaired renal function, further dosage reductions may be advisable.

† *Use is not currently included in the labeling approved by the US Food and Drug Administration.*

Penicillin V Potassium Oral

(pen i sil′ in)

Brand Name: Beepen-VK®, Betapen-VK®, Ledercillin VK®, Pen-Vee K®, Robicillin VK®, V-Cillin K®, Veetids®
Also available generically.

Why is this medicine prescribed?

Penicillin V potassium is an antibiotic used to treat certain infections caused by bacteria such as pneumonia, scarlet fever, and ear, skin, and throat infections. It also is used to prevent recurrent rheumatic fever and chorea. Antibiotics will not work for colds, flu, or other viral infections.

This medication is sometimes prescribed for other uses; ask your doctor or pharmacist for more information.

How should this medicine be used?

Penicillin V potassium comes as a tablet and liquid to take by mouth. It is usually taken every 6 hours (four times a day) or every 8 hours (three times a day). Follow the directions on your prescription label carefully, and ask your doctor or pharmacist to explain any part you do not understand. Take penicillin V potassium exactly as directed. Do not take more or less of it or take it more often than prescribed by your doctor.

Shake the liquid well before each use to mix the medication evenly.

The tablets should be swallowed whole and taken with a full glass of water.

Continue to take penicillin V potassium even if you feel well. Do not stop taking penicillin V potassium without talking to your doctor.

What special precautions should I follow?

Before taking penicillin V potassium,
- tell your doctor and pharmacist if you are allergic to penicillin V potassium, tartrazine (a yellow dye in some processed foods and drugs), or any other drugs.
- tell your doctor and pharmacist what prescription and nonprescription medications you are taking, especially other antibiotics, anticoagulants ('blood thinners') such as warfarin (Coumadin), atenolol (Tenormin), aspirin or other nonsteroidal anti-inflammatory medicine such as naproxen (Anaprox) or ibuprofen (Motrin), oral contraceptives, probenecid (Benemid), and vitamins.
- tell your doctor if you have or have ever had kidney or liver disease, allergies, asthma, blood disease, colitis, stomach problems, or hay fever.
- tell your doctor if you are pregnant, plan to become pregnant, or are breast-feeding. If you become pregnant while taking penicillin V potassium, call your doctor.
- if you are having surgery, including dental surgery, tell the doctor or dentist that you are taking penicillin V potassium.

What special dietary instructions should I follow?

Take penicillin V potassium at least 1 hour before or 2 hours after meals.

What should I do if I forget to take a dose?

Take the missed dose as soon as you remember it. However, if it is almost time for the next dose, skip the missed dose and continue your regular dosing schedule. Do not take a double dose to make up for a missed one.

What side effects can this medicine cause?

Penicillin V potassium may cause side effects. Tell your doctor if any of these symptoms are severe or do not go away:
- upset stomach
- diarrhea
- vomiting
- mild skin rash

If you experience any of the following symptoms, call your doctor immediately:
- severe skin rash
- itching
- hives
- difficulty breathing or swallowing
- wheezing
- vaginal infection

If you experience a serious side effect, you or your doctor may send a report to the Food and Drug Administration's (FDA) MedWatch Adverse Event Reporting program online [at http://www.fda.gov/MedWatch/index.html] or by phone [1-800-332-1088].

What storage conditions are needed for this medicine?

Keep this medication in the container it came in, tightly closed, and out of reach of children. Store the tablets at room temperature and away from excess heat and moisture (not in the bathroom). Throw away any medication that is outdated or no longer needed. Keep liquid medicine in the refrigerator, tightly closed, and throw away any unused medication after 14 days. Do not freeze. The liquid is good for 7 days at room temperature. Talk to your pharmacist about the proper disposal of your medication.

What should I do in case of overdose?

In case of overdose, call your local poison control center at 1-800-222-1222. If the victim has collapsed or is not breathing, call local emergency services at 911.

What other information should I know?

Keep all appointments with your doctor and the laboratory. Your doctor will order certain lab tests to check your response to penicillin V potassium.

If you are diabetic, use Clinistix or TesTape (not Clinitest) to test your urine for sugar while taking this drug.

Do not let anyone else take your medication. Your prescription is probably not refillable. If you still have symptoms of infection after you finish the penicillin V potassium, call your doctor.

Dosage Facts
For Informational Purposes

Caution: Do not change your dose, how often you take your medication, or the length of time you are to take it without first talking to your healthcare provider.

The following dosage information was written using medical language for doctors and other healthcare professionals and is provided here for you to check your dosage. The dosage of this drug may differ for different patients. Therefore, always follow your doctor's instructions or the directions on the label. Contact your healthcare provider or pharmacist if you have any questions about the specific dosage of your medication after reviewing this information.

General Dosage Information

Available as the potassium salt. Dosage usually expressed as mg of penicillin V, but may be expressed in terms of USP penicillin V units.

Potency of penicillin V potassium preparations containing 125, 250, or 500 mg of penicillin V is approximately equivalent to 200,000, 400,000, or 800,000 USP penicillin V units, respectively.

Pediatric Patients

Pharyngitis and Tonsillitis

ORAL:
- Children: 250 mg 2 or 3 times daily for 10 days.
- Adolescents ≥12 years of age: 500 mg 2 or 3 times daily for 10 days or 250 mg 3 or 4 times daily for 10 days.
- Follow-up throat cultures not indicated in asymptomatic patients, but recommended 2–7 days after treatment in those who remain symptomatic, develop recurring symptoms, or have a history of rheumatic fever and are at unusually high risk for recurrence.

Other Streptococcal Infections

ORAL:
- Adolescents ≥12 years of age: 125–250 mg every 6 to 8 hours for 10 days for mild to moderate infections.
- Adolescents ≥12 years of age: 250–500 mg every 6 hours for mild to moderate infections caused by susceptible *S. pneumoniae*; continue until afebrile for at least 2 days.

Skin and Skin Structure Infections

ORAL:
- Adolescents ≥12 years of age: 250–500 mg every 6–8 hours.

Prevention of Rheumatic Fever Recurrence

ORAL:
- 125–250 mg twice daily. AHA recommends 250 mg twice daily.
- Long-term, continuous prophylaxis for ≥ 5 years or into adulthood required.

Prevention of Bacterial Endocarditis
Patients Undergoing Certain Dental or Upper Respiratory Tract Procedures

ORAL:
- Children weighing <27 kg: 1 g given 1 hour prior to the procedure and 500 mg 6 hours later.
- Children weighing ≥27 kg: 2 g given 1 hour prior to the procedure and 1 g 6 hours later.

Prevention of S. pneumonia Infections in Asplenic Individuals

ORAL:
- Children <5 years of age: 125 mg twice daily.
- Children ≥5 years of age: 250 mg twice daily.
- In infants with sickle cell anemia, initiate penicillin V prophylaxis as soon as diagnosis is established (preferably by 2 months of age); continue until approximately 5 years of age. Appropriate duration in children with asplenia from other causes unknown; some experts recommend that asplenic children at high risk receive prophylaxis throughout childhood and into adulthood.

Necrotizing Ulcerative Gingivitis

ORAL:
- Adolescents ≥12 years of age: 250–500 mg every 6–8 hours for mild to moderate infections.

Anthrax
Postexposure Prophylaxis

ORAL:
- 50 mg/kg daily given in 4 divided doses for 60 days for postexposure prophylaxis following exposure to *B. anthracis* spores (inhalational anthrax)†; use only if penicillin susceptibility confirmed.

Cutaneous Anthrax

ORAL:
- 25–50 mg/kg daily given in 2 or 4 divided doses for treatment of uncomplicated cutaneous anthrax† resulting from naturally occurring or endemic exposure to anthrax.
- 7–10 days of treatment may be adequate if cutaneous anthrax occurred as the result of natural or endemic exposures; 60 days of treatment necessary if it occurred as the result of exposure to aerosolized anthrax spores (e.g., in context of biologic warfare or bioterrorism).

Adult Patients

Pharyngitis and Tonsillitis

ORAL:
- 500 mg 2 or 3 times daily for 10 days or 250 mg 3 or 4 times daily for 10 days.

Other Streptococcal Infections

ORAL:
- 125–250 mg every 6 to 8 hours for 10 days for mild to moderate infections.

- 250–500 mg every 6 hours for mild to moderate infections caused by susceptible *S. pneumoniae*; continue until afebrile for at least 2 days.

Skin and Skin Structure Infections

ORAL:
- 250–500 mg every 6–8 hours.

Prevention of Rheumatic Fever Recurrence

ORAL:
- 125–250 mg twice daily. AHA recommends 250 mg twice daily.
- Long-term, continuous prophylaxis required.

Recommended Duration of Prophylaxis for Prevention of Rheumatic Fever Recurrence

Patient Category	Duration
Rheumatic fever without carditis	5 years or until 21 years of age, whichever is longer
Rheumatic fever with carditis but no residual heart disease (no valvular disease)	10 years or well into adulthood, whichever is longer
Rheumatic fever with carditis and residual heart disease (persistent valvular disease)	At least 10 years since last episode and at least until 40 years of age; sometimes for life

Prevention of Bacterial Endocarditis

Patients Undergoing Certain Dental or Upper Respiratory Tract Procedures

ORAL:
- 2 g given 1 hour prior to the procedure and 1 g 6 hours later.

Necrotizing Ulcerative Gingivitis

ORAL:
- 250–500 mg every 6–8 hours for mild to moderate infections.

Anthrax

Postexposure Prophylaxis

ORAL:
- 7.5 mg/kg 4 times daily for 60 days for postexposure prophylaxis following suspected or confirmed exposure to *B. anthracis* spores (inhalational anthrax)†; use only if penicillin susceptibility confirmed.

Cutaneous Anthrax

ORAL:
- 200–500 mg 4 times daily for treatment of uncomplicated cutaneous anthrax† resulting from naturally occurring or endemic exposure to anthrax.
- 7–10 days of treatment may be adequate if cutaneous anthrax occurred as the result of natural or endemic exposures; 60 days of treatment necessary if it occurred as the result of exposure to aerosolized anthrax spores (e.g., in context of biologic warfare or bioterrorism).

Actinomycosis

ORAL:
- 2–4 g daily given in divided doses every 6 hours for 6–12 months for follow-up treatment of actinomycosis† after initial 4–6 weeks of parenteral treatment.
- For mild cervicofacial actinomycosis, use a 2-month regimen of penicillin V.

Whipple' Disease

ORAL:
- 1–1.5 g daily.

† Use is not currently included in the labeling approved by the US Food and Drug Administration.

Pentamidine Inhalation

(pen tam′ i deen)

Brand Name: NebuPent®, Pentacarinat®, Pentam® 300

Also available generically.

Why is this medicine prescribed?

Pentamidine is an anti-infective agent that helps to treat or prevent pneumonia caused by the organism Pneumocystis carinii.

This medication is sometimes prescribed for other uses; ask your doctor or pharmacist for more information.

How should this medicine be used?

Pentamidine comes as a solution to be inhaled using a nebulizer. It usually is used once every 4 weeks. Inhalation of pentamidine delivers the drug directly to your lungs. Your doctor, nurse, or pharmacist will show you how to use the nebulizer. Follow the directions on your prescription label carefully, and ask your doctor or pharmacist to explain any part you do not understand. Take pentamidine exactly as directed. Do not take more or less of it or take it more often than prescribed by your doctor.

What special precautions should I follow?

Before taking pentamidine,
- tell your doctor and pharmacist if you are allergic to pentamidine or any other drugs.
- tell your doctor and pharmacist what prescription and nonprescription medications you are taking or have recently taken, especially antibiotics, amphotericin B (Fungizone), cisplatin (Platinol), foscarnet (Foscavir), and vitamins.
- tell your doctor if you have or have ever had asthma;

hay fever; high or low blood pressure; diabetes; high or low blood sugar; anemia; severe skin allergic reaction; or heart, kidney, liver, or pancreatic disease.

- tell your doctor if you are pregnant, plan to become pregnant, or are breast-feeding. If you become pregnant while taking pentamidine, call your doctor.

What should I do if I forget to take a dose?

Take the missed dose as soon as you remember it. However, if it is almost time for the next dose, skip the missed dose and continue your regular dosing schedule. Do not take a double dose to make up for a missed one.

What side effects can this medicine cause?

Pentamidine may cause side effects. Tell your doctor if any of these symptoms are severe or do not go away:

- fatigue
- metallic taste
- cough
- dizziness
- burning sensation in your throat
- decreased appetite
- lightheadedness or faintness
- itching
- upset stomach
- vomiting
- night sweats or chills

If you experience any of the following symptoms, call your doctor immediately:

- chest pain
- abnormal heartbeat
- shortness of breath or difficulty breathing
- skin rash
- confusion
- slurred speech

If you experience a serious side effect, you or your doctor may send a report to the Food and Drug Administration's (FDA) MedWatch Adverse Event Reporting program online [at http://www.fda.gov/MedWatch/index.html] or by phone [1-800-332-1088].

What storage conditions are needed for this medicine?

Keep this medication in the container it came in, tightly closed, and out of reach of children. Store it at room temperature and away from excess heat and moisture (not in the bathroom). Throw away any medication that is outdated or no longer needed. Talk to your pharmacist about the proper disposal of your medication.

What should I do in case of overdose?

In case of overdose, call your local poison control center at 1-800-222-1222. If the victim has collapsed or is not breathing, call local emergency services at 911.

What other information should I know?

Keep all appointments with your doctor and the laboratory. Your doctor will order certain lab tests to check your response to pentamidine.

You may develop a cough while using aerosol pentamidine. The cough may be more severe if you smoke or have a history of asthma. If you experience cough or difficulty breathing, call your doctor. Your doctor may suggest slowing the aerosol stream or may prescribe a bronchodilator (medication that opens the airways) to use before your pentamidine inhalation.

Do not let anyone else take your medication. Ask your pharmacist any questions you have about refilling your prescription.

Dosage Facts
For Informational Purposes

Caution: Do not change your dose, how often you take your medication, or the length of time you are to take it without first talking to your healthcare provider.

The following dosage information was written using medical language for doctors and other healthcare professionals and is provided here for you to check your dosage. The dosage of this drug may differ for different patients. Therefore, always follow your doctor's instructions or the directions on the label. Contact your healthcare provider or pharmacist if you have any questions about the specific dosage of your medication after reviewing this information.

General Dosage Information

Available as pentamidine isethionate in the US; dosage expressed as pentamidine isethionate.

May be available outside the US as the mesylate salt; dosage of the mesylate salt is expressed as the base. Consider that dosages used in some published references may be unclear since the salt employed may not be specified.

Pediatric Patients

Pneumocystis jiroveci (Pneumocystis carinii) Pneumonia
Primary Prophylaxis

INHALATION:

- Children ≥5 years of age†: 300 mg every 4 weeks (once monthly). The child must be capable of effectively using a nebulizer; other appropriate agents (co-trimoxazole, dapsone, atovaquone) recommended for younger children.
- In HIV-infected children 1–5 years of age, primary prophylaxis should be initiated if CD4+ T-cell counts are <500/mm³ or CD4+ percentage is <15%. In HIV-infected children 6–12 years of age, primary prophylaxis should be initiated if CD4+ T-cell counts are <200/mm³ or CD4+ percentage is <15%.
- Adolescents†: Dosage and criteria for initiation or discontinuance of primary prophylaxis in this age group are the same as those recommended for adults.

Prevention of Recurrence (Secondary Prophylaxis)

INHALATION:

- Children ≥5 years of age†: 300 mg every 4 weeks (once monthly). The child must be capable of effectively using a nebulizer; other appropriate agents (co-trimoxazole, dapsone, atovaquone) recommended for younger children.
- The safety of discontinuing secondary prophylaxis in HIV-infected children receiving potent antiretroviral therapy has not been extensively studied. Children who have a history pneumocystis pneumonia should receive life-long suppressive therapy to prevent recurrence.
- Adolescents†: Dosage and criteria for initiation or discontinuance of secondary prophylaxis in this age group are the same as those recommended for adults.

Adult Patients

Pneumocystis jiroveci (Pneumocystis carinii) Pneumonia
Primary Prophylaxis

INHALATION:

- 300 mg every 4 weeks (once monthly).
- Initiate primary prophylaxis in patients with CD4+ T-cell counts <200/mm³ or a history of oropharyngeal candidiasis. Also consider primary prophylaxis if CD4+ T-cell percentage is <14% or there is a history of an AIDS-defining illness.
- Primary prophylaxis can be discontinued in adults and adolescents responding to potent antiretroviral therapy who have a sustained (≥3 months) increase in CD4+ T-cell counts from <200/mm³ to >200/mm³. However, it should be restarted if CD4+ T-cell count decreases to <200/mm³.

Prevention of Recurrence (Secondary Prophylaxis)

INHALATION:

- 300 mg every 4 weeks (once monthly).
- Initiate long-term suppressive therapy or chronic maintenance therapy (secondary prophylaxis) in those with a history of *P. jiroveci* pneumonia to prevent recurrence.
- Discontinuance of secondary prophylaxis is recommended in those who have a sustained (≥3 months) increase in CD4+ T-cell counts to >200/mm³ since such prophylaxis appears to add little benefit in terms of disease prevention and discontinuance reduces the medication burden, the potential for toxicity, drug interactions, selection of drug-resistant pathogens, and cost.
- Reinitiate secondary prophylaxis if CD4+ T-cell count decreases to <200/mm³ or if *P. jiroveci* pneumonia recurs at a CD4+ T-cell count >200/mm³. It probably is prudent to continue secondary prophylaxis for life in those who had *P. jiroveci* episodes when they had CD4+ T-cell counts >200/mm³.

Special Populations

Renal Impairment

- Some clinicians suggest that dosage adjustment may be needed if parenteral pentamidine is used in patients with severe renal impairment. Manufacturer states that parenteral pentamidine should be used with caution in patients with renal impairment and that safety and efficacy of alternative dosage regimens have not been established in these patients.

† Use is not currently included in the labeling approved by the US Food and Drug Administration.

Pentamidine Isethionate Injection

(pen tam′ i deen)

Brand Name: Pentam®
Also available generically.

About Your Treatment

Your doctor has ordered pentamidine, an anti-infective agent, to help treat pneumonia caused by the organism Pneumocystis carinii. The drug will be either injected into a large muscle (such as your buttock or hip) or added to an intravenous fluid that will drip through a needle or catheter placed in your vein for 60 to 120 minutes, once a day. This medication is sometimes prescribed for other uses; ask your doctor or pharmacist for more information.

Your health care provider (doctor, nurse, or pharmacist) may measure the effectiveness and side effects of your treatment using laboratory tests and physical examinations. It is important to keep all appointments with your doctor and the laboratory. The length of treatment depends on how your infection and symptoms respond to the medication.

Precautions

Before administering pentamidine,

- tell your doctor and pharmacist if you are allergic to pentamidine or any other drugs.
- tell your doctor and pharmacist what prescription and nonprescription medications you are taking, especially antibiotics, amphotericin B (Fungizone), cisplatin (Platinol), foscarnet (Foscavir), and vitamins.
- tell your doctor if you have or have ever had asthma; hay fever; high or low blood pressure; diabetes; high or low blood sugar; anemia; severe skin allergic reaction; or heart, kidney, liver, or pancreatic disease.
- tell your doctor if you are pregnant, plan to become pregnant, or are breast-feeding. If you become pregnant while taking pentamidine, call your doctor.

Administering Your Medication

Before you administer pentamidine, look at the solution closely. It should be clear and free of floating material. Gently squeeze the bag or observe the solution container to make sure there are no leaks. Do not use the solution if it is discolored, if it contains particles, or if the bag or container leaks. Use a new solution, but show the damaged one to your health care provider.

It is important that you use your medication exactly as directed. Do not stop your therapy on your own for any reason because your infection could worsen and result in hospitalization. Do not change your dosing schedule without talking to your health care provider. Your health care provider may tell you to stop your infusion if you have a mechanical problem (such as a blockage in the tubing, needle, or catheter); if you have to stop an infusion, call your health care provider immediately so your therapy can continue.

Side Effects

Pentamidine may cause side effects. These side effects include kidney damage, but it is usually mild or moderate and reversible when the drug is stopped. Drink plenty of fluids while receiving pentamidine to minimize the risk. You also may experience lightheadedness and faintness after a dose of pentamidine. To minimize this risk, lie down while receiving this medication and do not administer it more quickly than directed.

Pentamidine also may cause low blood sugar (hypoglycemia). Symptoms include cold sweats, clammy feeling, dizziness, weakness, nervousness, unusual hunger, abnormal heartbeat, blurred vision, confusion, slurred speech, and unconsciousness. These effects may be severe and can occur even after pentamidine is discontinued. Pentamidine also may cause high blood sugar (hyperglycemia). Symptoms include frequent urination, increased thirst, weakness, dizziness, and headache. Your health care provider will advise you what to do if you develop low or high blood sugar; write down these directions so that you can refer to them later.

Tell your health care provider if any of these symptoms are severe or do not go away:
- upset stomach
- vomiting
- stomach pain
- diarrhea
- decreased appetite
- metallic taste

If you experience any of the following symptoms, call your health care provider immediately:
- rash
- itching
- unusual bleeding or bruising
- flushed, dry skin
- fruity breath odor
- increased thirst
- increased urination
- hallucinations
- difficulty breathing
- seizures
- drowsiness
- sore mouth or throat

If you experience a serious side effect, you or your doctor may send a report to the Food and Drug Administration's (FDA) MedWatch Adverse Event Reporting program online [at http://www.fda.gov/MedWatch/index.html] or by phone [1-800-332-1088].

Storage Conditions

- Your health care provider will probably give you a 1- or 2-day supply of pentamidine at a time. If you are receiving pentamidine intravenously (in your vein),

your health care provider will tell you to store it at room temperature in a clean, dry place.

If you are receiving pentamidine intramuscularly (in your muscle), your health care provider will tell you how to store it properly.

Store your medication only as directed. Make sure you understand what you need to store your medication properly.

Keep your supplies in a clean, dry place when you are not using them, and keep all medications and supplies out of reach of children. Your health care provider will tell you how to throw away used needles, syringes, tubing, and containers to avoid accidental injury.

Overdose

In case of overdose, call your local poison control center at 1-800-222-1222. If the victim has collapsed or is not breathing, call local emergency services at 911.

Signs of Infection

If you are receiving pentamidine in your vein or under your skin, you need to know the symptoms of a catheter-related infection (an infection where the needle enters your vein or skin). If you experience any of these effects near your intravenous catheter, tell your health care provider as soon as possible:
- tenderness
- warmth
- irritation
- drainage
- redness
- swelling
- pain

Dosage Facts
For Informational Purposes

Caution: Do not change your dose, how often you take your medication, or the length of time you are to take it without first talking to your healthcare provider.

The following dosage information was written using medical language for doctors and other healthcare professionals and is provided here for you to check your dosage. The dosage of this drug may differ for different patients. Therefore, always follow your doctor's instructions or the directions on the label. Contact your healthcare provider or pharmacist if you have any questions about the specific dosage of your medication after reviewing this information.

General Dosage Information

Available as pentamidine isethionate in the US; dosage expressed as pentamidine isethionate.

May be available outside the US as the mesylate salt; dosage of the mesylate salt is expressed as the base. Consider that dosages used in some published references may be unclear since the salt employed may not be specified.

Pediatric Patients

Pneumocystis jiroveci (Pneumocystis carinii) Pneumonia
Treatment

IV OR IM:

- Children >4 months of age: 3–4 mg/kg once daily for 14–21 days.
- Adolescents: 3–4 mg/kg once daily for 14–21 days.
- Some patients may require more prolonged treatment; manufacturer cautions that therapy for >21 days may be associated with increased toxicity.

African Trypanosomiasis†
Treatment of Trypanosoma brucei gambiense Infections†

IM:

- 4 mg/kg once daily for 10 days recommended by CDC and others.

Leishmaniasis†
Treatment of Cutaneous Leishmaniasis†

IV OR IM:

- 2–3 mg/kg once daily or every other day for 4–7 doses.

Treatment of Visceral Leishmaniasis Caused by Leishmania donovani (Kala-azar)†

IV OR IM:

- 2–4 mg/kg once daily or every other day for 15–30 doses recommended by CDC and others. Some clinicians recommend 4 mg 3 times weekly for 15–25 doses.

Adult Patients

Pneumocystis jiroveci (Pneumocystis carinii) Pneumonia
Treatment

IV OR IM:

- 3–4 mg/kg once daily for 14–21 days.
- Some patients may require more prolonged treatment; manufacturer cautions that therapy for >21 days may be associated with increased toxicity.

African Trypanosomiasis†
Treatment of Trypanosoma brucei gambiense Infections†

IM:

- 4 mg/kg once daily for 10 days recommended by CDC and others.

Leishmaniasis†
Treatment of Cutaneous Leishmaniasis†

IV OR IM:

- 2–3 mg/kg once daily or every other day for 4–7 doses.

Treatment of Visceral Leishmaniasis Caused by Leishmania donovani (Kala-azar)†

IV OR IM:

- 2–4 mg/kg once daily or every other day for 15–30 doses recommended by CDC and others. Some clinicians recommend 4 mg 3 times weekly for 15–25 doses.

Special Populations

Renal Impairment

- Some clinicians suggest that dosage adjustment may be needed if parenteral pentamidine is used in patients with severe renal impairment. Manufacturer states that parenteral pentamidine should be used with caution in patients with renal impairment and that safety and efficacy of alternative dosage regimens have not been established in these patients.

† Use is not currently included in the labeling approved by the US Food and Drug Administration.

Pentazocine and Naloxone

(pen taz' oh seen) (nal ox' one)

Brand Name: Talwin Nx®

Why is this medicine prescribed?

The combination of pentazocine and naloxone is used to relieve moderate to severe pain.

This medication is sometimes prescribed for other uses; ask your doctor or pharmacist for more information.

How should this medicine be used?

The combination of pentazocine and naloxone comes as a tablet to take by mouth. It usually is taken every 3-4 hours as needed. Do not crush or chew the tablets. Follow the directions on your prescription label carefully, and ask your doctor or pharmacist to explain any part you do not understand. Take pentazocine and naloxone exactly as directed.

Pentazocine can be habit-forming. Do not take a larger dose, take it more often, or for a longer period than your doctor tells you to.

What special precautions should I follow?

Before taking pentazocine and naloxone,

- tell your doctor and pharmacist if you are allergic to pentazocine, naloxone, sulfites, or any other drugs.
- tell your doctor and pharmacist what prescription and nonprescription medications you are taking, other pain relievers; antidepressants [especially fluoxetine (Prozac)]; medications for cough, cold, or allergies; sedatives; sleeping pills; tranquilizers; and vitamins.
- tell your doctor if you have or have ever had liver or kidney disease; a history of alcoholism or seizure disorders; lung or thyroid disease; heart disease; prostatic hypertrophy; or biliary or urinary problems.
- tell your doctor if you are pregnant, plan to become pregnant, or are breast-feeding. If you become pregnant

while taking pentazocine and naloxone, call your doctor.

- if you are having surgery, including dental surgery, tell the doctor or dentist that you are taking pentazocine and naloxone.
- you should know that this drug may make you drowsy. Do not drive a car or operate machinery until you know how this drug affects you.
- remember that alcohol can add to the drowsiness caused by this drug.

What should I do if I forget to take a dose?

This medication usually is taken as needed. If your doctor has told you to take pentazocine and naloxone regularly, take the missed dose as soon as you remember it. However, if it is almost time for the next dose, skip the missed dose and continue your regular dosing schedule. Do not take a double dose to make up for a missed one.

What side effects can this medicine cause?

Pentazocine and naloxone may cause side effects. Tell your doctor if any of these symptoms are severe or do not go away:

- confusion
- feeling very tired
- dizziness
- lightheadedness
- drowsiness
- mood changes
- headache
- upset stomach
- vomiting
- constipation
- stomach pain
- rash
- difficulty urinating

If you experience any of the following symptoms, call your doctor immediately:

- difficulty breathing
- fast heartbeat
- fainting
- hallucinations

If you experience a serious side effect, you or your doctor may send a report to the Food and Drug Administration's (FDA) MedWatch Adverse Event Reporting program online [at http://www.fda.gov/MedWatch/index.html] or by phone [1-800-332-1088].

What storage conditions are needed for this medicine?

Keep this medication in the container it came in, tightly closed, and out of reach of children. Store it at room temperature and away from excess heat and moisture (not in the bathroom). Throw away any medication that is outdated or no longer needed. Talk to your pharmacist about the proper disposal of your medication.

What should I do in case of overdose?

In case of overdose, call your local poison control center at 1-800-222-1222. If the victim has collapsed or is not breathing, call local emergency services at 911.

What other information should I know?

Keep all appointments with your doctor.

Do not let anyone else take your medication. Ask your pharmacist any questions you have about refilling your prescription.

Dosage Facts
For Informational Purposes

Caution: Do not change your dose, how often you take your medication, or the length of time you are to take it without first talking to your healthcare provider.

The following dosage information was written using medical language for doctors and other healthcare professionals and is provided here for you to check your dosage. The dosage of this drug may differ for different patients. Therefore, always follow your doctor's instructions or the directions on the label. Contact your healthcare provider or pharmacist if you have any questions about the specific dosage of your medication after reviewing this information.

General Dosage Information

Available as pentazocine and naloxone hydrochlorides; dosage expressed in terms of the bases.

Adjust dosage according to severity of pain, physical status of the patient, and other drugs that the patient is receiving.

Adult Patients

Pain

ORAL:
- Initially, 50 mg every 3–4 hours. Increase dosage to 100 mg when needed (maximum 600 mg daily).

Prescribing Limits

Adult Patients

Pain

ORAL:
- Maximum 600 mg daily.

Special Populations

Hepatic Impairment
- Doses and/or frequency of administration may need to be decreased, particularly when administered orally, in patients with hepatic impairment (e.g., cirrhosis).

Geriatric Patients
- Cautious dosage selection recommended; initiate therapy at the lower end of the usual range.

Pentobarbital Oral and Rectal

(pen toe bar′ bi tal)

Brand Name: Nembutal®, Nembutal® Sodium, Nembutal® Sodium Solution

Why is this medicine prescribed?

Pentobarbital, a barbiturate, is used in the short-term treatment of insomnia (to help you fall asleep and stay asleep for a proper rest). It is also used as a sedative to relieve anxiety and induce sleep before surgery.

This medication is sometimes prescribed for other uses; ask your doctor or pharmacist for more information.

How should this medicine be used?

Pentobarbital comes as a capsule and liquid to take by mouth and as a suppository to be used rectally. The capsule or liquid is taken at bedtime as needed for insomnia or two to four times a day for anxiety. Take pentobarbital on an empty stomach, at least 1 hour before or 2 hours after meals. The suppositories are inserted at bedtime as needed for insomnia or two to four times a day for anxiety. Follow the directions on your prescription label carefully, and ask your doctor or pharmacist to explain any part you do not understand. Take pentobarbital exactly as directed.

Pentobarbital can be habit-forming; do not take a larger dose, take it more often, or for a longer time than your doctor tells you to. Do not stop taking pentobarbital without talking to your doctor, especially if you have taken large doses for a long time. Your doctor probably will decrease your dose gradually.

To insert a pentobarbital suppository, follow these steps:

1. Remove the wrapper.
2. Dip the tip of the suppository in water.
3. Lie down on your left side and raise your right knee to your chest. (A left-handed person should lie on the right side and raise the left knee.)
4. Using your finger, insert the suppository into the rectum, about 1/2 to 1 inch in infants and children and 1 inch in adults. Hold it in place for a few moments.
5. Stand up after about 15 minutes. Wash your hands thoroughly and resume your normal activities.

What special precautions should I follow?

Before taking pentobarbital,
- tell your doctor and pharmacist if you are allergic to pentobarbital, aspirin, tartrazine (a yellow dye in some processed foods and drugs), or any other drugs.
- tell your doctor and pharmacist what prescription and nonprescription medications you are taking, especially acetaminophen (Tylenol), antihistamines, chloramphen-

icol (Chloromycetin), digitoxin (Crystodigin), diuretics ('water pills'), doxycycline (Vibramycin), griseofulvin (Grisactin), medications for depression or seizures, metronidazole (Flagyl), oral contraceptives, propranolol (Inderal), quinidine, rifampin, sedatives, sleeping pills, steroids (for asthma), theophylline (Theo-Dur), tranquilizers, and vitamins.
- tell your doctor if you have a fever or pain or if you have or have ever had liver or kidney disease, asthma, hyperthyroidism, diabetes, anemia, a history of alcoholism or drug abuse, or heart or lung problems.
- tell your doctor if you are pregnant, plan to become pregnant, or are breast-feeding. If you become pregnant while taking pentobarbital, call your doctor.
- if you are having surgery, including dental surgery, tell the doctor or dentist that you are taking pentobarbital.
- you should know that this drug may make you drowsy. Do not drive a car or operate machinery until you know how this drug affects you.
- remember that alcohol can add to the drowsiness caused by this drug.

What should I do if I forget to take a dose?

Do not take a missed dose when you remember it. Skip the missed dose and continue your regular dosing schedule. Do not take a double dose to make up for a missed one.

What side effects can this medicine cause?

Pentobarbital may cause side effects. Tell your doctor if any of these symptoms are severe or do not go away:
- drowsiness
- headache
- depression
- excitement
- joint or muscle pain
- upset stomach
- diarrhea
- constipation

If you experience any of the following symptoms, call your doctor immediately:
- skin rash
- itching
- sore throat
- fever
- easy bruising
- bloody nose
- unusual bleeding

If you experience a serious side effect, you or your doctor may send a report to the Food and Drug Administration's (FDA) MedWatch Adverse Event Reporting program online [at http://www.fda.gov/MedWatch/index.html] or by phone [1-800-332-1088].

What storage conditions are needed for this medicine?

Keep this medication in the container it came in, tightly closed, and out of reach of children. Store it at room tem-

perature and away from excess heat and moisture (not in the bathroom). Throw away any medication that is outdated or no longer needed. Talk to your pharmacist about the proper disposal of your medication.

What should I do in case of overdose?

In case of overdose, call your local poison control center at 1-800-222-1222. If the victim has collapsed or is not breathing, call local emergency services at 911.

What other information should I know?

Keep all appointments with your doctor.

Do not let anyone else take your medication. Ask your pharmacist any questions you have about refilling your prescription.

Talk to your doctor, pharmacist, or other healthcare professional if you have questions about dosing information for your medication.

Pentosan Polysulfate

(pen′ toe san pol i sul′ fate)

Brand Name: Elmiron®

Why is this medicine prescribed?

Pentosan polysulfate is used to relieve bladder pain and discomfort related to interstitial cystitis, a disease that causes swelling and scarring of the bladder wall. Pentosan polysulfate is similar to a class of medications called low molecular weight heparins. It works by preventing irritation of the bladder walls.

How should this medicine be used?

Pentosan polysulfate comes as a capsule to take by mouth. It is usually taken with water three times a day, 1 hour before or 2 hours after meals. Follow the directions on your prescription label carefully, and ask your doctor or pharmacist to explain any part you do not understand. Take pentosan polysulfate exactly as directed. Do not take more or less of it or take it more often than prescribed by your doctor.

Are there other uses for this medicine?

This medication may be prescribed for other uses; ask your doctor or pharmacist for more information.

What special precautions should I follow?

Before taking pentosan polysulfate,
- tell your doctor and pharmacist if you are allergic to pentosan polysulfate, danaparoid (Orgaran), heparin, or any other medications.
- tell your doctor and pharmacist what prescription and

nonprescription medications, vitamins, nutritional supplements, and herbal products you are taking. Be sure to mention any of the following: anticoagulants ('blood thinners') such as warfarin (Coumadin) and aspirin. Your doctor may need to change the doses of your medications or monitor you carefully for side effects.
- tell your doctor if you have or have ever had an aneurysm, hemophilia, ulcers, low platelet count, an intestinal blockage, or liver or spleen disease.
- tell your doctor if you are pregnant, plan to become pregnant, or are breast-feeding. If you become pregnant while taking pentosan polysulfate, call your doctor.
- if you are having surgery, including dental surgery, tell the doctor or dentist that you are taking pentosan polysulfate.
- you should know that pentosan polysulfate has a blood-thinning effect and may cause increased bleeding.

What special dietary instructions should I follow?

Unless your doctor tells you otherwise, continue your normal diet.

What should I do if I forget to take a dose?

Take the missed dose as soon as you remember it. However, if it is almost time for the next dose, skip the missed dose and continue your regular dosing schedule. Do not take a double dose to make up for a missed one.

What side effects can this medicine cause?

Pentosan polysulfate may cause side effects. Tell your doctor if any of these symptoms are severe or do not go away:
- hair loss
- diarrhea
- upset stomach
- heartburn
- headache
- rash
- stomach pain
- difficulty falling asleep or staying asleep
- moodiness
- dizziness

Some side effects can be serious. The following symptoms are uncommon, but if you experience any of them, call your doctor immediately:
- unusual bruising or bleeding
- nosebleed
- heavy gum bleeding
- black and tarry stools
- red blood in stools
- bloody vomit
- vomiting material that looks like coffee grounds

Pentosan polysulfate may cause other side effects. Call your doctor if you have any unusual problems while taking this medication.

If you experience a serious side effect, you or your doctor may send a report to the Food and Drug Administration's (FDA) MedWatch Adverse Event Reporting program online [at http://www.fda.gov/MedWatch/index.html] or by phone [1-800-332-1088].

What storage conditions are needed for this medicine?

Keep this medication in the container it came in, tightly closed, and out of reach of children. Store it at room temperature and away from excess heat and moisture (not in the bathroom). Throw away any medication that is outdated or no longer needed. Talk to your pharmacist about the proper disposal of your medication.

What should I do in case of overdose?

In case of overdose, call your local poison control center at 1-800-222-1222. If the victim has collapsed or is not breathing, call local emergency services at 911.

What other information should I know?

Keep all appointments with your doctor. Your doctor will examine you after 3 months to see if your symptoms have improved.

Do not let anyone else take your medication. Ask your pharmacist any questions you have about refilling your prescription.

Talk to your doctor, pharmacist, or other healthcare professional if you have questions about dosing information for your medication.

Pentoxifylline

(pen tox i′ fi leen)

Brand Name: Pentoxil®, Trental®
Also available generically.

Why is this medicine prescribed?

Pentoxifylline is used to improve blood flow in patients with circulation problems to reduce aching, cramping, and tiredness in the hands and feet. It works by decreasing the thickness (viscosity) of blood. This change allows your blood to flow more easily, especially in the small blood vessels of the hands and feet.

This medication is sometimes prescribed for other uses; ask your doctor or pharmacist for more information.

How should this medicine be used?

Pentoxifylline comes as an extended-release (long-acting) tablet to take by mouth. It usually is taken three times a day. Do not break, crush, or chew the tablets; swallow them whole. Follow the directions on your prescription label carefully, and ask your doctor or pharmacist to explain any part you do not understand. Take pentoxifylline exactly as directed. Do not take more or less of it or take it more often than prescribed by your doctor.

Although you may feel the effects of this medication in 2-4 weeks, you may need to take it for up to 8 weeks before you feel the full effect of pentoxifylline.

Pentoxifylline controls the symptoms of circulation problems, but does not cure them. Continue to take pentoxifylline even if you feel well. Do not stop taking pentoxifylline without talking to your doctor.

Are there other uses for this medicine?

Pentoxifylline also is used for leg ulcers, strokes, high-altitude sickness, eye and ear disorders, and sickle cell disease and to treat pain from diabetic neuropathy. Talk to your doctor about the possible risks of using this drug for your condition.

What special precautions should I follow?

Before taking pentoxifylline,

- tell your doctor and pharmacist if you are allergic to caffeine-containing products (coffee, tea, colas), pentoxifylline, theobromine, theophylline (Theo-Dur), or any other drugs.
- tell your doctor and pharmacist what prescription and nonprescription medications you are taking, especially anticoagulants ('blood thinners') such as warfarin (Coumadin) and vitamins.
- tell your doctor if you have or have ever had kidney disease.
- tell your doctor if you are pregnant, plan to become pregnant, or are breast-feeding. If you become pregnant while taking pentoxifylline, call your doctor.
- if you are having surgery, including dental surgery, tell the doctor or dentist that you are taking pentoxifylline.
- you should know that this drug may make you drowsy or dizzy. Do not drive a car or operate machinery until you know how it affects you.

What special dietary instructions should I follow?

Take pentoxifylline with meals to prevent upset stomach. If symptoms continue, tell your doctor. Your dose may need to be decreased.

What should I do if I forget to take a dose?

Take the missed dose as soon as you remember it. However, if it is almost time for the next dose, skip the missed dose and continue your regular dosing schedule. Do not take a double dose to make up for a missed one.

What side effects can this medicine cause?

Pentoxifylline may cause side effects. Tell your doctor if any of these symptoms are severe or do not go away:

- upset stomach
- vomiting
- gas
- dizziness
- headache

If you experience either of the following symptoms, call your doctor immediately:

- chest pain
- fast heartbeat

If you experience a serious side effect, you or your doctor may send a report to the Food and Drug Administration's (FDA) MedWatch Adverse Event Reporting program online [at http://www.fda.gov/MedWatch/index.html] or by phone [1-800-332-1088].

What storage conditions are needed for this medicine?

Keep this medication in the container it came in, tightly closed, and out of reach of children. Store it at room temperature and away from excess heat and moisture (not in the bathroom). Throw away any medication that is outdated or no longer needed. Talk to your pharmacist about the proper disposal of your medication.

What should I do in case of overdose?

In case of overdose, call your local poison control center at 1-800-222-1222. If the victim has collapsed or is not breathing, call local emergency services at 911.

What other information should I know?

Keep all appointments with your doctor and the laboratory. Your blood pressure may need to be checked regularly, especially if you are taking other heart medications.

Do not let anyone else take your medication. Ask your pharmacist any questions you have about refilling your prescription.

Dosage Facts
For Informational Purposes

Caution: Do not change your dose, how often you take your medication, or the length of time you are to take it without first talking to your healthcare provider.

The following dosage information was written using medical language for doctors and other healthcare professionals and is provided here for you to check your dosage. The dosage of this drug may differ for different patients. Therefore, always follow your doctor's instructions or the directions on the label. Contact your healthcare provider or pharmacist if you have any questions about the specific dosage of your medication after reviewing this information.

Adult Patients

Peripheral Vascular Disease

ORAL:
- 400 mg 3 times daily. Continue for at least 8 weeks to determine efficacy. Reduce dosage to 400 mg twice daily if adverse GI and/or CNS effects develop. Discontinue if adverse effects persist at this lower dosage. Efficacy was demonstrated in clinical studies of 6-months duration.

Perindopril

(per in′ doe pril)

Brand Name: Aceon®

Important Warning

Do not take perindopril if you are pregnant. If you become pregnant while taking perindopril, call your doctor immediately. Perindopril may harm the fetus.

Why is this medicine prescribed?

Perindopril is used alone or in combination with other medications to treat high blood pressure. Perindopril is in a class of medications called angiotensin-converting enzyme (ACE) inhibitors. It makes blood flow more smoothly by preventing the production of certain natural chemicals that tighten the blood vessels.

How should this medicine be used?

Perindopril comes as a tablet to take by mouth. It is usually taken once or twice a day. Follow the directions on your prescription label carefully, and ask your doctor or pharmacist to explain any part you do not understand. Take perindopril exactly as directed. Do not take more or less of it or take it more often than prescribed by your doctor.

Your doctor may start you on a low dose of perindopril and gradually increase your dose.

Perindopril controls high blood pressure but does not cure it. Continue to take perindopril even if you feel well. Do not stop taking perindopril without talking to your doctor.

Are there other uses for this medicine?

This medication may be prescribed for other uses; ask your doctor or pharmacist for more information.

What special precautions should I follow?

Before taking perindopril,

- tell your doctor and pharmacist if you are allergic to perindopril, benazepril (Lotensin), captopril (Capoten), enalapril (Vasotec), fosinopril (Monopril), lisinopril

(Prinivil, Zestril), moexipril (Univasc), quinapril (Accupril), ramipril (Altace), trandolapril (Mavik), or any other medications.

- tell your doctor and pharmacist what prescription and nonprescription medications, vitamins, nutritional supplements, and herbal products you are taking. Be sure to mention any of the following: cyclosporine (Neoral, Sandimmune), diuretics ('water pills'), heparin, indomethacin (Indocin), lithium (Eskalith, Lithobid), and potassium supplements (K-Dur, Klor-Con, others). Your doctor may need to change the doses of your medications or monitor you carefully for side effects.
- tell your doctor if you are on dialysis and if have or have ever had heart failure; lupus (SLE); scleroderma; diabetes; swelling of the face, throat, tongue, lips, eyes, hands, feet, ankles, and/or lower legs (angioedema); or kidney or liver disease.
- tell your doctor if you plan to become pregnant or are breast-feeding.
- you should know that diarrhea, vomiting, not drinking enough fluids, and sweating a lot can cause a drop in blood pressure, which may cause lightheadedness and fainting.

What special dietary instructions should I follow?

Talk to your doctor before using salt substitutes containing potassium. If your doctor prescribes a low-salt or low-sodium diet, follow these directions carefully.

What should I do if I forget to take a dose?

Take the missed dose as soon as you remember it. However, if it is almost time for the next dose, skip the missed dose and continue your regular dosing schedule. Do not take a double dose to make up for a missed one.

What side effects can this medicine cause?

Perindopril may cause side effects. Tell your doctor if any of these symptoms are severe or do not go away:

- cough
- headache
- weakness
- dizziness
- diarrhea
- stomach pain
- upset stomach

Some side effects can be serious. The following symptoms are uncommon, but if you experience any of them, call your doctor immediately:

- swelling of the face, throat, tongue, lips, eyes, hands, feet, ankles, or lower legs
- hoarseness
- difficulty swallowing or breathing
- lightheadedness
- fainting

- fever, sore throat, chills, and other signs of infection
- irregular or rapid heartbeats

Perindopril may cause other side effects. Call your doctor if you have any unusual problems while taking this medication.

If you experience a serious side effect, you or your doctor may send a report to the Food and Drug Administration's (FDA) MedWatch Adverse Event Reporting program online [at http://www.fda.gov/MedWatch/index.html] or by phone [1-800-332-1088].

What storage conditions are needed for this medicine?

Keep this medication in the container it came in, tightly closed, and out of reach of children. Store it at room temperature and away from excess heat and moisture (not in the bathroom). Throw away any medication that is outdated or no longer needed. Talk to your pharmacist about the proper disposal of your medication.

What should I do in case of overdose?

In case of overdose, call your local poison control center at 1-800-222-1222. If the victim has collapsed or is not breathing, call local emergency services at 911.

What other information should I know?

Keep all appointments with your doctor.

Do not let anyone else take your medication. Ask your pharmacist any questions you have about refilling your prescription.

Dosage Facts
For Informational Purposes

Caution: Do not change your dose, how often you take your medication, or the length of time you are to take it without first talking to your healthcare provider.

The following dosage information was written using medical language for doctors and other healthcare professionals and is provided here for you to check your dosage. The dosage of this drug may differ for different patients. Therefore, always follow your doctor's instructions or the directions on the label. Contact your healthcare provider or pharmacist if you have any questions about the specific dosage of your medication after reviewing this information.

General Dosage Information

Available as perindopril erbumine; dosage expressed in terms of perindopril erbumine.

Adult Patients

Hypertension

ORAL:
- Initially, 4 mg once daily as monotherapy. Adjust dosage at approximately monthly intervals (more aggressively in high-risk patients) to achieve BP control.
- In patients currently receiving diuretic therapy, discontinue diuretic, if possible, 2–3 days before initiating perindopril. May cautiously resume diuretic therapy if BP not controlled adequately with perindopril alone. If diuretic cannot be discontinued, initiate therapy at 2–4 mg daily (given in 1 dose or 2 divided doses) under close medical supervision for several hours until BP has stabilized.
- Usual dosage: 4–8 mg once daily.

Prescribing Limits

Adult Patients

Hypertension

ORAL:
- Maximum 16 mg daily.

Special Populations

Renal Impairment

Hypertension
- Initially, 2 mg daily in patients with renal impairment (Cl$_{cr}$ >30 mL/minute); titrate until BP is controlled or to maximum of 8 mg daily.

Geriatric Patients

Hypertension
- Initially, 4 mg daily, given in 1 dose or 2 divided doses. Adjust dosage to achieve BP control. Administer dosages >8 mg daily with caution and under close medical supervision.

Permethrin

(per meth′ rin)

Brand Name: Elimite®, Nix® Creme Rinse
Also available generically.

Why is this medicine prescribed?

Permethrin kills parasites and their eggs. It is used to treat scabies (a skin infestation) and lice infestations of the head, body, and pubic area ('crabs'). Permethrin does not prevent these infestations.

How should this medicine be used?

Permethrin comes in a cream and liquid (cream rinse) to use externally. Usually, one application of permethrin completely eliminates the parasites. However, the treatment may need to be repeated after 1 week; call your doctor if signs of infestation (live parasites) reappear. Follow the directions on the package or on your prescription label carefully, and ask your doctor or pharmacist to explain any part you do not understand. Use permethrin exactly as directed. Do not use more or less of it or use it more often than directed by your doctor.

Wear rubber gloves when applying it if you have open cuts or scratches on your hands. If this medication accidentally gets in your eyes, rinse them thoroughly with water for at least 5 minutes.

If you are to use the liquid, follow these steps:
1. Shampoo your hair using your regular shampoo.
2. Thoroughly rinse and towel dry your hair and scalp.
3. Allow your hair to air dry for a few minutes.
4. Do not stand (or sit) in a shower or bathtub; lean over a sink to apply permethrin to your head.
5. Shake the bottle of liquid well.
6. Thoroughly wet the hair and scalp with the liquid. Cover the areas behind your ears and the back of your neck.
7. Keep permethrin on your hair for 10 minutes before rinsing it off thoroughly with water.
8. Dry your hair with a clean towel.
9. Comb your hair with a fine tooth comb to remove nits (lice eggs and larvae).
10. Wash your hands to remove the medication.

If you are to use the cream, follow these steps:
1. Wash your entire body or take a shower.
2. Thoroughly massage the cream into your skin over your entire body, from your head to your toes.
3. Leave the cream on for 8-14 hours.
4. Wash the cream off after 8-14 hours by taking another shower.

If you have head lice, wash combs and brushes with permethrin liquid and rinse them thoroughly with water to remove the drug.

What special precautions should I follow?

Before using permethrin,
- tell your doctor and pharmacist if you are allergic to permethrin or any other drugs.
- tell your doctor and pharmacist what prescription and nonprescription medications you are taking, including vitamins.
- tell your doctor if you are pregnant or are breast-feeding. If you are pregnant, wear gloves when applying permethrin to another person to prevent its absorption through your skin.

What side effects can this medicine cause?

Permethrin may cause side effects. Tell your doctor if any of these symptoms are severe or do not go away:
- skin irritation
- rash
- redness
- swelling

What storage conditions are needed for this medicine?

Keep this medication in the container it came in, tightly closed, and out of reach of children. Store it at room temperature and away from excess heat and moisture (not in the bathroom). Throw away any medication that is outdated or no longer needed. Talk to your pharmacist about the proper disposal of your medication.

What other information should I know?

Keep all appointments with your doctor. Permethrin is for external use only. Do not let permethrin get into your eyes, nose, or mouth, and do not swallow it. Do not apply dressings, bandages, cosmetics, lotions, or other skin medications to the area being treated unless your doctor tells you.

After using permethrin, machine-wash (or dry clean) all clothing, bed linen, and towels that you have used in the last 2 days. Use hot water. Dry everything in a hot dryer for at least 20 minutes. Thoroughly clean all bathtubs, showers, and toilets in your home with rubbing alcohol.

You may have transmitted the parasites to family members and close contacts (including sexual contacts); advise them to see a doctor if they develop symptoms of infestation.

If you have scabies and your skin has become sensitive to the parasite, itching may persist for several weeks after the treatment. However, this itching does not mean that the treatment was a failure. Call your doctor if you have questions.

Do not let anyone else use your medication. Ask your pharmacist any questions you have about permethrin.

Dosage Facts
For Informational Purposes

Caution: Do not change your dose, how often you take your medication, or the length of time you are to take it without first talking to your healthcare provider.

The following dosage information was written using medical language for doctors and other healthcare professionals and is provided here for you to check your dosage. The dosage of this drug may differ for different patients. Therefore, always follow your doctor's instructions or the directions on the label. Contact your healthcare provider or pharmacist if you have any questions about the specific dosage of your medication after reviewing this information.

Pediatric Patients

Pediculosis
Pediculosis Capitis

TOPICAL:
- Lotion (cream rinse): apply a sufficient amount (30–60 mL) to washed and towel-dried hair to thoroughly saturate the hair and the scalp (including the areas behind the ears and the nape of the neck). After 10 minutes, rinse with water.

- One treatment usually is successful; treatment may be repeated with 1% permethrin cream rinse or an alternative pediculicide after 7–10 days if lice or nits are detected at the hair-skin junction. Some clinicians recommend a second treatment routinely 1 week later to achieve maximum results.
- In resistant cases of pediculosis capitis, some clinicians recommend leaving the cream rinse on for a longer period of time (e.g., 30–60 minutes)† or as an alternative, application of 5% cream† to the hair, covering it with a shower cap, and leaving it on overnight to overcome the ectoparasite's resistance to lower concentrations of the drug.

Scabies

TOPICAL:
- Cream: apply a thin, uniform layer and massage gently and thoroughly into *all* skin surfaces (entire trunk and extremities) from the neck to the toes (including the soles of the feet). Wash off (by showering or bathing) after 8–14 hours.
- One application of 5% cream usually is successful in eradicating scabies.
- No consensus on the need for retreatment; some experts recommend retreatment if symptoms persist after 1 week, while others recommend retreatment only if live mites are observed. Still others recommend routine retreatment (i.e., 2 courses), particularly in severe cases with diffuse cutaneous findings.
- CDC recommends retreating patients who do not respond to permethrin with an alternative regimen.
- Many clinicians recommend follow-up examinations of patients 2 and 4 weeks after treatment. If the patient is not clear of new lesions at either examination, it should be considered a treatment failure; such treatment failures may be secondary to failure to treat all exposed individuals or failure to apply the drug properly. If the patient is clear of new lesions when examined at 2 weeks, but has new lesions at 4 weeks, it should be considered a reinfestation rather than a treatment failure.

Demodicidosis†
D. folliculorum or D. brevis Infestations†

TOPICAL:
- Permethrin 1% and permethrin 5% have been used; effective dosage regimen not established.

Adult Patients

Pediculosis
Pediculosis Capitis

TOPICAL:
- Lotion (cream rinse): apply a sufficient amount (30–60 mL) to washed and towel-dried hair to thoroughly saturate the hair and the scalp (including the areas behind the ears and the nape of the neck). After 10 minutes, rinse with water.
- One treatment usually is successful; treatment may be repeated with 1% permethrin cream or an alternative pediculicide after 7–10 days if lice or nits are detected at the hair-skin junction. Some clinicians recommend a second treatment routinely 1 week later to achieve maximum results.
- In resistant cases of pediculosis capitis, some clinicians recommend leaving the cream rinse on for a longer period of time (e.g., 30–60 minutes)† or as an alternative, application of 5% cream† to the hair, covering it with a shower cap, and leaving it on overnight to overcome the ectoparasite's resistance to lower concentrations of the drug.

Pediculosis Pubis

TOPICAL:

- Lotion (cream rinse) or cream: thoroughly saturate the pubic and other affected areas; allow to remain for 10 minutes and then rinse off with water.
- CDC recommends reevaluating the patient 1 week after treatment if symptoms persist; retreatment may be necessary if lice are found or eggs are observed. If retreatment in necessary, CDC recommends use of an alternative regimen.
- Routine retreatment 7–10 days after initial treatment is recommended by some clinicians, but if used correctly, one treatment with 1% cream rinse usually is effective.

Scabies

TOPICAL:

- Cream: apply a thin layer uniformly and massage gently and thoroughly into *all* skin surfaces (entire trunk and extremities) from the neck to the toes (including the soles of the feet). Usual dosage to treat an average adult is 30 g of 5% cream. Wash off (by showering or bathing) after 8–14 hours.
- One application of 5% cream usually is successful in eradicating scabies.
- No consensus on the need for retreatment; some experts recommend retreatment if symptoms persist after 1 week, while others recommend retreatment only if live mites are observed. Still others recommend routine retreatment (i.e., 2 courses), particularly in severe cases with diffuse cutaneous findings.
- CDC recommends retreating patients who do not respond to permethrin with an alternative regimen.
- Many clinicians recommend follow-up examinations of patients 2 and 4 weeks after treatment. If the patient is not clear of new lesions at either examination, it should be considered a treatment failure; such treatment failures may be secondary to failure to treat all exposed individuals or failure to apply the drug properly. If the patient is clear of new lesions when examined at 2 weeks, but has new lesions at 4 weeks, it should be considered a reinfestation rather than a treatment failure.

Demodicidosis†
D. folliculorum or D. brevis Infestations†

TOPICAL:

- Permethrin 1% and permethrin 5% have been used; effective dosage regimen not established.

† Use is not currently included in the labeling approved by the US Food and Drug Administration.

Perphenazine Oral

(per fen′ a zeen)

Brand Name: Trilafon®

Why is this medicine prescribed?

Perphenazine is used to treat schizophrenia and symptoms such as hallucinations, delusions, and hostility.

This medication is sometimes prescribed for other uses; ask your doctor or pharmacist for more information.

How should this medicine be used?

Perphenazine comes as a tablet and liquid concentrate to take by mouth. It usually is taken three times a day. Follow the directions on your prescription label carefully, and ask your doctor or pharmacist to explain any part you do not understand. Take perphenazine exactly as directed. Do not take more or less of it or take it more often than prescribed by your doctor.

The liquid concentrate must be diluted before use. It comes with a specially marked dropper for measuring the dose. Ask your pharmacist to show you how to use the dropper if you have difficulty. To dilute the liquid concentrate, add it to at least 2 ounces of milk, water, or orange soda or pineapple, apricot, prune, orange, tomato, or grapefruit juice just before you take it. Do not add it to drinks with caffeine (cola, coffee), tannics (tea), or pectinates (apple juice). If any of the drink gets on the dropper, rinse the dropper with tap water before replacing it in the bottle. Do not allow the liquid concentrate to touch your skin or clothing; it can irritate your skin. If you spill the liquid concentrate on your skin, wash it off immediately with soap and water.

Continue to take perphenazine even if you feel well. Do not stop taking perphenazine without talking to your doctor, especially if you have taken large doses for a long time. Your doctor probably will decrease your dose gradually. This drug must be taken regularly for a few weeks before its full effect is felt.

What special precautions should I follow?

Before taking perphenazine,

- tell your doctor and pharmacist if you are allergic to perphenazine, sulfites, or any other drugs.
- tell your doctor and pharmacist what prescription and nonprescription medications you are taking, especially antacids, antihistamines, appetite reducers (amphetamines), benztropine (Cogentin), bromocriptine (Parlodel), carbamazepine (Tegretol), dicyclomine (Bentyl), fluoxetine (Prozac), guanethidine (Ismelin), lithium, medications for colds, medications for depression, meperidine (Demerol), methyldopa (Aldomet), phenytoin (Dilantin), propranolol (Inderal), sedatives, trihexyphenidyl (Artane), valproic acid (Depakene), and vitamins.

- tell your doctor if you have or have ever had depression; seizures; shock therapy; asthma; emphysema; chronic bronchitis; problems with your urinary system or prostate; glaucoma; history of alcohol abuse; thyroid problems; bad reaction to insulin; angina; irregular heartbeat; problems with your blood pressure; blood disorders; blood vessel, heart, kidney, liver, or lung disease.
- tell your doctor if you are pregnant, plan to become pregnant, or are breast-feeding. If you become pregnant while taking perphenazine, call your doctor.
- if you are having surgery, including dental surgery, tell the doctor or dentist that you are taking perphenazine.
- you should know that this drug may make you drowsy. Do not drive a car or operate machinery until you know how this drug affects you.
- remember that alcohol can add to the drowsiness caused by this drug.
- plan to avoid unnecessary or prolonged exposure to sunlight and to wear protective clothing, sunglasses, and sunscreen. Perphenazine may make your skin sensitive to sunlight.

What special dietary instructions should I follow?

Perphenazine may cause an upset stomach. Take perphenazine with food or milk.

What should I do if I forget to take a dose?

Take the missed dose as soon as you remember it and take any remaining doses for that day at evenly spaced intervals. However, if you remember a missed dose when it is almost time for your next scheduled dose, skip the missed dose. Do not take a double dose to make up for a missed one.

What side effects can this medicine cause?

Side effects from perphenazine may occur. Your urine may turn pink or reddish-brown; this effect is not harmful. Tell your doctor if any of these symptoms are severe or do not go away:

- drowsiness
- dizziness
- blurred vision
- dry mouth
- upset stomach
- vomiting
- diarrhea
- constipation
- restlessness
- headache
- weight gain

If you experience any of the following symptoms, call your doctor immediately:

- tremor
- restlessness or pacing
- fine worm-like tongue movements
- unusual face, mouth, or jaw movements
- shuffling walk
- seizures or convulsions
- fast, irregular, or pounding heartbeat
- difficulty urinating
- yellowing of the skin or eyes

If you experience a serious side effect, you or your doctor may send a report to the Food and Drug Administration's (FDA) MedWatch Adverse Event Reporting program online [at http://www.fda.gov/MedWatch/index.html] or by phone [1-800-332-1088].

What storage conditions are needed for this medicine?

Keep this medication in the container it came in, tightly closed, and out of reach of children. Store it at room temperature and away from excess heat and moisture (not in the bathroom). Protect the liquid from light. Throw away any medication that is outdated or no longer needed. Talk to your pharmacist about the proper disposal of your medication.

What should I do in case of overdose?

In case of overdose, call your local poison control center at 1-800-222-1222. If the victim has collapsed or is not breathing, call local emergency services at 911.

What other information should I know?

Keep all appointments with your doctor and the laboratory. Your doctor will order certain lab tests to check your response to perphenazine.

Do not let anyone else take your medication. Ask your pharmacist any questions you have about refilling your prescription.

Talk to your doctor, pharmacist, or other healthcare professional if you have questions about dosing information for your medication.

Phenazopyridine

(fen az oh peer' i deen)

Brand Name: Azo-Dine®, Azo-Gesic®, Azo-Natural®, Azo-Standard®, Baridium®, Prodium®, Pyridium®, Pyridium® Plus as a combination product containing Phenazopyridine Hydrochloride, Butabarbital, and Hyoscyamine Hydrobromide, Re-Azo®, UTI Relief®

Also available generically.

Why is this medicine prescribed?

Phenazopyridine relieves urinary tract pain, burning, irritation, and discomfort, as well as urgent and frequent urination caused by urinary tract infections, surgery, injury, or examination procedures. However, phenazopyridine is not an antibiotic; it does not cure infections.

This medication is sometimes prescribed for other uses; ask your doctor or pharmacist for more information.

How should this medicine be used?

Phenazopyridine comes as a tablet to take by mouth. It usually is taken three times a day after meals. Do not chew or crush the tablets; swallow them whole with a full glass of water. You may stop taking this drug when pain and discomfort completely disappear. Follow the directions on your prescription label carefully, and ask your doctor or pharmacist to explain any part you do not understand. Take phenazopyridine exactly as directed. Do not take more or less of it or take it more often than prescribed by your doctor.

What special precautions should I follow?

Before taking phenazopyridine,
- tell your doctor and pharmacist if you are allergic to phenazopyridine or any other drugs.
- tell your doctor and pharmacist what prescription and nonprescription medications you are taking, including vitamins.
- tell your doctor if you have or have ever had kidney disease or glucose-6-phosphate dehydrogenase (G-6-PD) deficiency (an inherited blood disease).
- tell your doctor if you are pregnant, plan to become pregnant, or are breast-feeding. If you become pregnant while taking phenazopyridine, call your doctor.

What should I do if I forget to take a dose?

Take the missed dose as soon as you remember it. However, if it is almost time for the next dose, skip the missed dose and continue your regular dosing schedule. Do not take a double dose to make up for a missed one.

What side effects can this medicine cause?

Phenazopyridine may cause side effects. Your urine may turn a red-orange or brown; this effect is harmless. Tell your doctor if any of these symptoms are severe or do not go away:
- headache
- dizziness
- upset stomach

If you experience any of the following symptoms, call your doctor immediately:
- yellowing of the skin or eyes
- fever
- confusion
- skin discoloration (blue to bluish-purple)
- shortness of breath
- skin rash
- sudden decrease in the amount of urine
- swelling of the face, fingers, feet, or legs

If you experience a serious side effect, you or your doctor may send a report to the Food and Drug Administration's (FDA) MedWatch Adverse Event Reporting program online [at http://www.fda.gov/MedWatch/index.html] or by phone [1-800-332-1088].

What storage conditions are needed for this medicine?

Keep this medication in the container it came in, tightly closed, and out of reach of children. Store it at room temperature and away from excess heat and moisture (not in the bathroom). Throw away any medication that is outdated or no longer needed. Talk to your pharmacist about the proper disposal of your medication.

What should I do in case of overdose?

In case of overdose, call your local poison control center at 1-800-222-1222. If the victim has collapsed or is not breathing, call local emergency services at 911.

What other information should I know?

Keep all appointments with your doctor and the laboratory. Your doctor will order certain lab tests to check your response to phenazopyridine.

Phenazopyridine can interfere with laboratory tests, including urine tests for glucose (sugar) and ketones. If you have diabetes, you should use Clinitest rather than Tes-Tape or Clinistix to test your urine for sugar. Urine tests for ketones (Acetest and Ketostix) may give false results. Before you have any tests, tell the laboratory personnel and doctor that you take this medication.

Phenazopyridine stains clothing and contact lenses. Avoid wearing contact lenses while taking this medicine.

Do not let anyone else take your medication. Your prescription is probably not refillable.

If you still have symptoms after you finish the phenazopyridine, call your doctor.

Dosage Facts
For Informational Purposes

Caution: Do not change your dose, how often you take your medication, or the length of time you are to take it without first talking to your healthcare provider.

The following dosage information was written using medical language for doctors and other healthcare professionals and is provided here for you to check your dosage. The dosage of this drug may differ for different patients. Therefore, always follow your doctor's instructions or the directions on the label. Contact your healthcare provider or pharmacist if you have any questions about the specific dosage of your medication after reviewing this information.

General Dosage Information

Available as phenazopyridine hydrochloride; dosage expressed in terms of the salt.

Pediatric Patients

Urinary Tract Mucosal Anesthesia or Analgesia

Relief of Irritation Due to Trauma, Surgery, Endoscopic Procedures, or the Passage of Sounds or Catheters

ORAL:
- 12 mg/kg daily, in 3 divided doses.
- Discontinue when pain and discomfort are relieved, usually after 3–15 days.

Relief of Irritation Due to Infection

ORAL:
- 12 mg/kg daily, in 3 divided doses, for no more than 2 days; use in combination with an anti-infective agent and then continue therapy with anti-infective agent alone.

Adult Patients

Urinary Tract Mucosal Anesthesia or Analgesia

Relief of Irritation Due to Trauma, Surgery, Endoscopic Procedures, or the Passage of Sounds or Catheters

ORAL:
- Usually, 200 mg 3 times daily.
- Discontinue when pain and discomfort are relieved, usually after 3–15 days.

Relief of Irritation Due to Infection

ORAL:
- Usually, 200 mg 3 times daily for no more than 2 days; use in combination with an anti-infective agent and then continue therapy with anti-infective agent alone.

Self-Medication

ORAL:
- 190 mg 3 times daily for up to 2 days.
- Consult clinician if symptoms persist for >2 days.

Prescribing Limits

Pediatric Patients

Urinary Tract Anesthesia or Analgesia
Relief of Irritation Due to Infection

ORAL:
- Maximum 12 mg/kg daily, in 3 divided doses, for no more than 2 days.

Adult Patients

Urinary Tract Anesthesia or Analgesia
Relief of Irritation Due to Infection

ORAL:
- Maximum 200 mg 3 times daily for no more than 2 days.

Self-Medication

ORAL:
- Maximum 190 mg 3 times daily for no more than 2 days.

Phenelzine
(fen′ el zeen)

Brand Name: Nardil®
Also available generically.

Important Warning

A small number of children, teenagers, and young adults (up to 24 years of age) who took antidepressants ('mood elevators') such as phenelzine during clinical studies became suicidal (thinking about harming or killing oneself or planning or trying to do so). Children, teenagers, and young adults who take antidepressants to treat depression or other mental illnesses may be more likely to become suicidal than children, teenagers, and young adults who do not take antidepressants to treat these conditions. However, experts are not sure about how great this risk is and how much it should be considered in deciding whether a child or teenager should take an antidepressant. Children younger than 18 years of age should not normally take phenelzine, but in some cases, a doctor may decide that phenelzine is the best medication to treat a child's condition.

You should know that your mental health may change in unexpected ways when you take phenelzine or other antidepressants even if you are an adult over age 24. You may become suicidal, especially at the beginning of your treatment and any time that your dose is increased or decreased. You, your family, or your caregiver should call your doctor right away if you experience any of the following symptoms: new or worsening depression; thinking about harming or killing yourself, or planning or trying to do so; extreme worry; agitation; panic attacks; difficulty falling asleep or staying asleep; aggressive behavior; irritability; acting without thinking; severe restlessness; and frenzied abnormal excitement. Be sure that your family or caregiver knows which symptoms may be serious so they can call the doctor when you are unable to seek treatment on your own.

Your healthcare provider will want to see you often while you are taking phenelzine, especially at the beginning of your treatment. Be sure to keep all appointments for office visits with your doctor.

The doctor or pharmacist will give you the manufacturer's patient information sheet (Medication Guide) when you begin treatment with phenelzine. Read the information carefully and ask your doctor or pharmacist if you have any questions. You also can obtain the Medication Guide from the FDA web-

continued on next page

Important Warning (cont'd)

site: http://www.fda.gov/cder/drug/antidepressants/antidepressants_MG_2007.pdf.

No matter what your age, before you take an antidepressant, you, your parent, or your caregiver should talk to your doctor about the risks and benefits of treating your condition with an antidepressant or with other treatments. You should also talk about the risks and benefits of not treating your condition. You should know that having depression or another mental illness greatly increases the risk that you will become suicidal. This risk is higher if you or anyone in your family has or has ever had bipolar disorder (mood that changes from depressed to abnormally excited) or mania (frenzied, abnormally excited mood) or has thought about or attempted suicide. Talk to your doctor about your condition, symptoms, and personal and family medical history. You and your doctor will decide what type of treatment is right for you.

Why is this medicine prescribed?

Phenelzine is used to treat depression in people who have not been helped by other medications. Phenelzine is in a class of medications called monoamine oxidase inhibitors (MAOIs). It works by increasing the amounts of certain natural substances that are needed to maintain mental balance.

How should this medicine be used?

Phenelzine comes as a tablet to take by mouth. It is usually taken three times a day. Follow the directions on your prescription label carefully, and ask your doctor or pharmacist to explain any part you do not understand. Take phenelzine exactly as directed. Do not take more or less of it or take it more often than prescribed by your doctor.

Your doctor will probably start you on a low dose of phenelzine and gradually increase your dose. After your symptoms have improved, your doctor will probably gradually decrease your dose. Follow these directions carefully.

Phenelzine controls the symptoms of depression but does not cure the condition. It may take 4 weeks or longer for you to feel the full benefit of phenelzine. Continue to take phenelzine even if you feel well. Do not stop taking phenelzine without talking to your doctor. Your doctor probably will want to decrease your dose gradually. If you suddenly stop taking phenelzine, you may experience withdrawal symptoms such as nightmares, agitation, loss of contact with reality, nausea, vomiting, and weakness.

Are there other uses for this medicine?

This medication may be prescribed for other uses; ask your doctor or pharmacist for more information.

What special precautions should I follow?

Before taking phenelzine,

- tell your doctor and pharmacist if you are allergic to phenelzine or any other medications.
- tell your doctor if you are taking, have recently taken, or plan to take any of the following prescription and non-prescription medications: certain other antidepressants including amitriptyline (Elavil), amoxapine, clomipramine (Anafranil), desipramine (Norpramin), doxepin (Sinequan), imipramine (Tofranil), maprotiline, mirtazapine (Remeron), nortriptyline (Pamelor), protriptyline (Vivactil), and trimipramine (Surmontil); amphetamines such as amphetamine (in Adderall), benzphetamine (Didrex), dextroamphetamine (Dexedrine, Dextrostat, in Adderall), and methamphetamine (Desoxyn); bupropion (Wellbutrin, Zyban); buspirone (BuSpar); caffeine (No-Doz, Quick-Pep, Vivarin); cyclobenzaprine (Flexeril); dexfenfluramine (Redux) (not available in the U.S.); dextromethorphan (Robitussin, others); duloxetine (Cymbalta); epinephrine (Epipen, Primatene Mist); guanethidine (Ismelin) (not available in the U.S.); levodopa (Larodopa, in Sinemet); medications for allergies, cough and cold symptoms, hay fever; anxiety, sinus problems, or weight loss (diet pills, appetite suppressants); medications for seizures such as carbamazepine (Tegretol); narcotic medications for pain; nasal decongestants, including nose drops and sprays; other MAOIs such as isocarboxazid (Marplan); pargyline (not available in the U.S.), procarbazine (Matulane), tranylcypromine (Parnate), and selegiline (Eldepryl, Emsam, Zelapar); meperidine (Demerol); methyldopa (Aldomet); 'pep pills'; sedatives; selective serotonin reuptake inhibitors such as citalopram (Celexa), escitalopram (Lexapro), fluoxetine (Prozac), fluvoxamine (Luvox), paroxetine (Paxil), and sertraline (Zoloft); sleeping pills; tranquilizers; venlafaxine (Effexor); and medications containing alcohol (Nyquil, elixirs, others). Your doctor may tell you not to take tranylcypromine if you are taking or have recently stopped taking one or more of these medications.
- tell your doctor and pharmacist what other prescription and nonprescription medications, vitamins, and herbal products you are taking or plan to take. Be sure to mention any of the following: barbiturates such as pentobarbital (Nembutal), phenobarbital (Luminal), and secobarbital (Seconal); beta blockers such as atenolol (Tenormin), labetalol (Normodyne), metoprolol (Lopressor, Toprol XL), nadolol (Corgard), and propranolol (Inderal); doxepin cream (Zonelon), insulin and oral medications for diabetes; and medication for high blood pressure including diuretics ('water pills'), and reserpine (Serpalan). Your doctor may need to change the doses of your medications and monitor you carefully for side effects.
- you should know that phenelzine may remain in your body for several weeks after you stop taking the medi-

cation. During the first few weeks after your treatment ends, tell your doctor and pharmacist that you have recently stopped taking phenelzine before you start taking any new medications.

- tell your doctor if you are taking any nutritional supplements, especially phenylalanine (DLPA)(contained in aspartame sweetened products such as diet sodas and foods, over-the-counter medications, and some prescription medications), rauwolfia, tyrosine, or tryptophan.
- tell your doctor if you have or have ever had pheochromocytoma (a tumor on a small gland near the kidneys) or heart or liver disease. Your doctor may tell you not to take phenelzine.
- tell your doctor if you use street drugs. Also tell your doctor if you have or have ever had high blood pressure; diabetes; seizures; schizophrenia (a mental illness that causes disturbed thinking, loss of interest in life, and strong or unusual emotions); agitation; or hyperactivity or other movement disorders.
- tell your doctor if you are pregnant, plan to become pregnant, or are breast-feeding. If you become pregnant while taking phenelzine, call your doctor.
- if you are having surgery, including dental surgery, tell the doctor or dentist that you are taking phenelzine.
- you should know that this medication may make you drowsy. Do not drive a car or operate machinery until you know how this medication affects you.
- do not drink alcohol while you are taking phenelzine. Alcohol can make the side effects of phenelzine worse.
- you should know that phenelzine may cause dizziness, lightheadedness, and fainting when you get up too quickly from a lying position. This is more common when you first start taking phenelzine. To avoid this problem, get out of bed slowly, resting your feet on the floor for a few minutes before standing up.

What special dietary instructions should I follow?

You may experience a serious reaction if you eat foods that are high in tyramine during your treatment with phenelzine. Tyramine is found in many foods, including meat, poultry, fish, or cheese that has been smoked, aged, improperly stored, or spoiled; certain fruits, vegetables, and beans; alcoholic beverages; and yeast products that have fermented. Your doctor or dietitian will tell you which foods you must avoid completely, and which foods you may eat in small amounts. You should also avoid foods and drinks that contain caffeine during your treatment with phenelzine. Follow these directions carefully. Ask your doctor or dietitian if you have any questions about what you may eat and drink during your treatment.

What should I do if I forget to take a dose?

Take the missed dose as soon as you remember it. However, if it is almost time for your next dose, skip the missed dose and continue your regular dosing schedule. Do not take a double dose to make up for a missed one.

What side effects can this medicine cause?

Phenelzine may cause side effects. Tell your doctor if any of the following symptoms are severe or do not go away:

- drowsiness
- weakness
- dizziness
- dry mouth
- constipation
- weight gain
- decreased sexual ability
- uncontrollable shaking of any part of the body
- muscle twitching or jerking

Some side effects can be serious. If you experience any of the following symptoms or those listed in the IMPORTANT WARNING section, call your doctor immediately:

- headache
- slow, fast, or pounding heartbeat
- neck stiffness or soreness
- chest pain
- nausea
- vomiting
- sweating
- wide pupils (black circles in the middle of the eyes)
- eyes more sensitive to light than usual
- swelling of face, throat, arms, hands, feet, ankles, or lower legs
- difficulty breathing or swallowing
- yellowing of the skin or eyes

Phenelzine may cause other side effects. Call your doctor if you experience any unusual problems while you are taking this medication.

What storage conditions are needed for this medicine?

Keep this medication in the container it came in, tightly closed, and out of reach of children. Store it at room temperature and away from excess heat and moisture (not in the bathroom). Throw away any medication that is outdated or no longer needed. Talk to your pharmacist about the proper disposal of your medication.

What should I do in case of overdose?

In case of overdose, call your local poison control center at 1-800-222-1222. If the victim has collapsed or is not breathing, call local emergency services at 911.

Symptoms of overdose may include:

- drowsiness
- dizziness
- faintness
- irritability
- hyperactivity
- agitation
- headache

- hallucinations (seeing things or hearing voices that do not exist)
- tightening of the jaw
- stiffly arched back
- seizures
- coma (loss of consciousness for a period of time)
- fast, irregular pulse
- chest pain
- slowed breathing
- fever
- sweating
- cool, clammy skin

What other information should I know?

Keep all appointments with your doctor and the laboratory. Your doctor will check your blood pressure regularly during your treatment with phenelzine.

Do not let anyone else take your medication. Ask your pharmacist any questions you have about refilling your prescription.

Dosage Facts
For Informational Purposes

Caution: Do not change your dose, how often you take your medication, or the length of time you are to take it without first talking to your healthcare provider.

The following dosage information was written using medical language for doctors and other healthcare professionals and is provided here for you to check your dosage. The dosage of this drug may differ for different patients. Therefore, always follow your doctor's instructions or the directions on the label. Contact your healthcare provider or pharmacist if you have any questions about the specific dosage of your medication after reviewing this information.

General Dosage Information

Available as phenelzine sulfate; dosage expressed in terms of phenelzine.

Adult Patients

Major Depressive Disorder

ORAL:
- Initially, 15 mg 3 times daily. Increase fairly rapidly to at least 60 mg, as tolerated. 90 mg daily may be required.
- After maximum benefit obtained (usually in 2–6 weeks), gradually reduce dosage to the lowest level that will maintain relief of symptoms.
- Maintenance doses may be as low as 15 mg daily or every other day.

Special Populations

Hepatic Impairment
- No specific dosage recommendations at this time; however, should not be used in patients with a history of liver disease or abnormal liver function tests.

Renal Impairment
- No specific dosage recommendations at this time; however, should not be used in patients with severe renal function impairment.

Geriatric Patients
- Select dosage with caution, usually starting at a lower dose and increasing more gradually, because of age-related decreases in hepatic, renal, and/or cardiac function and concomitant disease and drug therapy.

Phenobarbital

(fee noe bar′ bi tal)

Brand Name: Luminal® Sodium
Also available generically.

Why is this medicine prescribed?

Phenobarbital, a barbiturate, is used to control epilepsy (seizures) and as a sedative to relieve anxiety. It is also used for short-term treatment of insomnia to help you fall asleep.

This medication is sometimes prescribed for other uses; ask your doctor or pharmacist for more information.

How should this medicine be used?

Phenobarbital comes as a tablet, capsule, and elixir (liquid) to take by mouth. You may obtain a specially marked measuring spoon from your pharmacist to be sure of an accurate dose of the liquid. It usually is taken one to three times a day and may be taken with or without food. If you take phenobarbital once a day, take it at bedtime. Follow the directions on your prescription label carefully, and ask your doctor or pharmacist to explain any part you do not understand. Take phenobarbital exactly as directed. If you are taking phenobarbital to control convulsions or seizures, follow the exact schedule prescribed by your doctor.

Phenobarbital can be habit-forming. Do not use phenobarbital for more than 2 weeks if it is being used to help you sleep. Do not take a larger dose, take it more often, or for a longer time than your doctor tells you to. Tolerance may develop with long-term or excessive use, making the drug less effective. This medication must be taken regularly to be effective. Do not skip doses even if you feel that you do not need them. Call your doctor if you have convulsions or seizures while taking phenobarbital. Do not stop taking this drug without talking to your doctor, especially if you have been taking it for a long time. Stopping the drug suddenly can cause withdrawal symptoms (anxiousness, sleeplessness, and irritability). Your doctor probably will decrease your dose gradually.

What special precautions should I follow?

Before taking phenobarbital,
- tell your doctor and pharmacist if you are allergic to phenobarbital or any other drugs.

- tell your doctor and pharmacist what prescription and nonprescription medications you are taking, especially acetaminophen (Tylenol); anticoagulants such as warfarin (Coumadin); carbamazepine (Tegretol); chloramphenicol (Chloromycetin); clonazepam (Klonopin); disulfiram (Antabuse); doxycycline (Vibramycin); felodipine (Plendil); fenoprofen (Nalfon); griseofulvin (Fulvicin); MAO inhibitors [phenelzine (Nardil) or tranylcypromine (Parnate)]; medications for depression, seizures, pain, asthma, colds, or allergies; metoprolol (Lopressor); metronidazole (Flagyl); muscle relaxants; phenylbutazone (Azolid, Butazolidin); propranolol (Inderal); quinidine; rifampin (Rifadin); sedatives; sleeping pills; steroids; theophylline (Theo-Dur); tranquilizers; valproic acid (Depakene); verapamil (Calan); and vitamins. These medications may add to the drowsiness caused by phenobarbital.
- tell your doctor if you have or have ever had anemia or seizures, or lung, heart, or liver disease.
- use a method of birth control other than oral contraceptives while taking this medication. Phenobarbital can decrease the effectiveness of oral contraceptives.
- tell your doctor if you are pregnant, plan to become pregnant, or are breast-feeding. If you become pregnant while taking phenobarbital, call your doctor immediately.
- if you are having surgery, including dental surgery, tell the doctor or dentist that you are taking phenobarbital.
- you should know that this drug may make you drowsy. Do not drive a car or operate machinery until you know how this drug affects you.
- remember that alcohol can add to the drowsiness caused by this drug.

What should I do if I forget to take a dose?

If you take several doses per day, take the missed dose as soon as you remember it and take any remaining doses for that day at evenly spaced intervals. However, if it is almost time for the next dose, skip the missed dose and continue your regular dosing schedule. Do not take a double dose to make up for a missed one.

What side effects can this medicine cause?

Side effects from phenobarbital may occur and include:
- drowsiness
- headache
- dizziness
- depression
- excitement (especially in children)
- upset stomach
- vomiting

Tell your doctor if any of these symptoms are severe or do not go away:
- nightmares
- increased dreaming
- constipation
- joint or muscle pain

If you experience any of the following symptoms, call your doctor immediately:
- seizures
- mouth sores
- sore throat
- easy bruising
- bloody nose
- unusual bleeding
- fever
- difficulty breathing or swallowing
- severe skin rash

If you experience a serious side effect, you or your doctor may send a report to the Food and Drug Administration's (FDA) MedWatch Adverse Event Reporting program online [at http://www.fda.gov/MedWatch/index.html] or by phone [1-800-332-1088].

What storage conditions are needed for this medicine?

Keep this medication in the container it came in, tightly closed, and out of reach of children. Store it at room temperature and away from excess heat and moisture (not in the bathroom). Throw away any medication that is outdated or no longer needed. Talk to your pharmacist about the proper disposal of your medication.

What should I do in case of overdose?

In case of overdose, call your local poison control center at 1-800-222-1222. If the victim has collapsed or is not breathing, call local emergency services at 911.

What other information should I know?

Keep all appointments with your doctor and the laboratory. Your doctor will order certain lab tests to check your response to phenobarbital.

If you are taking phenobarbital to control seizures and have an increase in their frequency or severity, call your doctor. Your dose may need to be adjusted. If you use phenobarbital for seizures, carry identification (Medic Alert) stating that you have epilepsy and that you are taking phenobarbital.

Do not let anyone else take your medication. Ask your pharmacist any questions you have about refilling your prescription.

Dosage Facts
For Informational Purposes

Caution: Do not change your dose, how often you take your medication, or the length of time you are to take it without first talking to your healthcare provider.

The following dosage information was written using medical language for doctors and other healthcare professionals and is provided here for you to check your

dosage. The dosage of this drug may differ for different patients. Therefore, always follow your doctor's instructions or the directions on the label. Contact your healthcare provider or pharmacist if you have any questions about the specific dosage of your medication after reviewing this information.

General Dosage Information

Available as phenobarbital sodium; dosage expressed in terms of the salt.

Pediatric Patients

Anxiety

ORAL:
- 6 mg/kg daily or 180 mg/m² daily, in 3 equally divided doses.

Surgery

ORAL:
- 1–3 mg/kg preoperatively.

Drug Withdrawal

ORAL:
- Infants: 3–10 mg/kg daily. After symptoms are relieved, decrease dosage gradually and withdraw drug completely over a 2-week period.

Seizure Disorders

ORAL:
- 15–50 mg 2 or 3 times daily. Alternatively, 3–5 mg/kg or 125 mg/m² daily.

Prevention of Febrile Seizures

ORAL:
- 3–4 mg/kg daily.

Status Epilepticus

Hyperbilirubinemia in Neonates†

ORAL:
- 7 mg/kg per day from the first to fifth day of life.

Cholestasis†

ORAL:
- Children <12 years of age: Dosages of 3–12 mg/kg daily in 2 or 3 divided doses have been used.

Adult Patients

Insomnia and Anxiety

Anxiety

ORAL:
- 30–120 mg daily.

Insomnia

ORAL:
- 100–320 mg.

Drug Withdrawal

ORAL:
- 30-mg dose for each 100- to 200-mg dose of the barbiturate or nonbarbiturate hypnotic that the patient has been taking daily, administered in 3 or 4 divided doses. If the patient shows signs of withdrawal on the first day, a loading dose of 100–200 mg of phenobarbital sodium may be administered IM in addition to the oral dose.
- After stabilization on phenobarbital sodium, decrease the to-

tal daily dose of phenobarbital sodium by 30 mg per day. After withdrawal symptoms are relieved, gradually decrease dosage and withdraw completely over a 2-week period.

Seizure Disorders

ORAL:
- 100–300 mg daily, usually at bedtime.

Cholestasis†

ORAL:
- Dosages of 90–180 mg daily in 2 or 3 divided doses have been used.

Special Populations

Hepatic Impairment
- Dosage reduction recommended in patients with hepatic impairment; avoid use in patients with marked hepatic impairment.

Renal Impairment
- Dosage reduction recommended.

Geriatric Patients
- Dosage reduction recommended.

† Use is not currently included in the labeling approved by the US Food and Drug Administration.

Phenoxybenzamine

(fen ox ee ben′ za meen)

Brand Name: Dibenzyline®

Why is this medicine prescribed?

Phenoxybenzamine is used to treat episodes of high blood pressure and sweating related to pheochromocytoma.

This medication is sometimes prescribed for other uses; ask your doctor or pharmacist for more information.

How should this medicine be used?

Phenoxybenzamine comes as a capsule to take by mouth. It usually is taken two or three times a day. Follow the directions on your prescription label carefully, and ask your doctor or pharmacist to explain any part you do not understand. Take phenoxybenzamine exactly as directed. Do not take more or less of it or take it more often than prescribed by your doctor.

Phenoxybenzamine controls symptoms related to pheochromocytoma and controls bladder symptoms but does not cure them. Continue to take phenoxybenzamine even if you feel well. Do not stop taking phenoxybenzamine without talking to your doctor.

Are there other uses for this medicine?

Phenoxybenzamine is also used to control bladder problems such as urgency, frequency, and inability to control urination in patients with neurogenic bladder, functional outlet obstruction, and partial prostatic obstruction. Talk to your doctor about the possible risks of using this drug for your condition.

What special precautions should I follow?

Before taking phenoxybenzamine,

- tell your doctor and pharmacist if you are allergic to phenoxybenzamine or any other drugs.
- tell your doctor and pharmacist what prescription and nonprescription medications you are taking, especially medications for diet control, high blood pressure, asthma, cough, colds, allergies, and glaucoma; and vitamins.
- tell your doctor if you have or have ever had heart or kidney disease, a stroke, or transient ischemic attacks (TIA).
- tell your doctor if you are pregnant, plan to become pregnant, or are breast-feeding. If you become pregnant while taking phenoxybenzamine, call your doctor immediately.
- if you are having surgery, including dental surgery, tell the doctor or dentist that you are taking phenoxybenzamine.
- you should know that this drug may make you drowsy. Do not drive a car or operate machinery until you know how this drug affects you.
- remember that alcohol can add to the drowsiness caused by this drug.

What should I do if I forget to take a dose?

Take the missed dose as soon as you remember it. However, if it is almost time for the next dose, skip the missed dose and continue your regular dosing schedule. Do not take a double dose to make up for a missed one.

What side effects can this medicine cause?

Phenoxybenzamine may cause side effects. Tell your doctor if any of these symptoms are severe or do not go away:

- nasal congestion
- dizziness
- upset stomach
- sexual dysfunction (difficulty ejaculating)
- dizziness

If you experience any of the following symptoms, call your doctor immediately:

- fainting
- fast heartbeat
- vomiting

If you experience a serious side effect, you or your doctor may send a report to the Food and Drug Administration's (FDA) MedWatch Adverse Event Reporting program online [at http://www.fda.gov/MedWatch/index.html] or by phone [1-800-332-1088].

What storage conditions are needed for this medicine?

Keep this medication in the container it came in, tightly closed, and out of reach of children. Store it at room temperature and away from excess heat and moisture (not in the bathroom). Throw away any medication that is outdated or no longer needed. Talk to your pharmacist about the proper disposal of your medication.

What should I do in case of overdose?

In case of overdose, call your local poison control center at 1-800-222-1222. If the victim has collapsed or is not breathing, call local emergency services at 911.

What other information should I know?

Keep all appointments with your doctor and the laboratory. Your blood pressure should be checked regularly to determine your response to phenoxybenzamine.

Do not let anyone else take your medication. Ask your pharmacist any questions you have about refilling your prescription.

Talk to your doctor, pharmacist, or other healthcare professional if you have questions about dosing information for your medication.

Phentermine

(fen′ ter meen)

Brand Name: Adipex-P®, Ionamin®
Also available generically.

Why is this medicine prescribed?

Phentermine is used, in combination with diet and exercise, to help you lose weight. It works by decreasing your appetite.

This medication is sometimes prescribed for other uses; ask your doctor or pharmacist for more information.

How should this medicine be used?

Phentermine comes in tablets and extended-release capsules. It usually is taken as a single daily dose in the morning or three times a day 30 minutes before meals. Follow the directions on your prescription label carefully, and ask your doctor or pharmacist to explain any part you do not understand. Take phentermine exactly as directed.

Most people take the drug for 3-6 weeks; the length of treatment depends on how you respond to the medication. Phentermine can be habit-forming. Do not take a larger dose, take it more often, or for a longer period than your doctor tells you to.

To prevent side effects, phentermine should be taken with meals. If you are taking an extended-release (long-acting) product, do not chew or crush the tablet. There are some tablets that can be crushed and mixed with food.

What special precautions should I follow?

Before taking phentermine,

- tell your doctor and pharmacist if you are allergic to phentermine or any other drugs.
- tell your doctor and pharmacist what prescription and nonprescription medications you are taking, especially fluoxetine (Prozac), fluvoxamine (Luvox), guanethidine, insulin, MAO inhibitors [phenelzine (Nardil) and tranylcypromine (Parnate)] even if you stopped taking them within the past 2 weeks, medications for weight loss and depression, paroxetine (Paxil), sertraline (Zoloft), and vitamins.
- tell your doctor if you have or have ever had heart disease, high blood pressure, arteriosclerosis (narrowing of the arteries), hyperthyroidism (overactive thyroid gland), diabetes, glaucoma, or a history of drug abuse.
- tell your doctor if you are pregnant, plan to become pregnant, or are breast-feeding. If you become pregnant while taking phentermine, call your doctor.
- you should know that this drug may make you drowsy. Do not drive a car or operate machinery until you know how this drug affects you.
- remember that alcohol can add to the drowsiness caused by this drug.
- if you have diabetes, you may need a larger dose of insulin while taking phentermine. Call your doctor if you have questions or problems.

What special dietary instructions should I follow?

Follow the diet and exercise program your doctor has given you. Phentermine works best in combination with a diet program.

What should I do if I forget to take a dose?

Take the missed dose as soon as you remember it. However, if it is almost time for the next dose, skip the missed dose and continue your regular dosing schedule. Do not take a double dose to make up for a missed one.

What side effects can this medicine cause?

Phentermine may cause side effects. Tell your doctor if any of these symptoms are severe or do not go away:

- dry mouth
- unpleasant taste
- diarrhea
- constipation
- vomiting

If you experience any of the following symptoms, call your doctor immediately:

- increased blood pressure
- heart palpitations
- restlessness
- dizziness
- tremor
- insomnia
- shortness of breath
- chest pain
- dizziness
- swelling of the legs and ankles
- difficulty doing exercise that you have been able to do

If you experience a serious side effect, you or your doctor may send a report to the Food and Drug Administration's (FDA) MedWatch Adverse Event Reporting program online [at http://www.fda.gov/MedWatch/index.html] or by phone [1-800-332-1088].

What storage conditions are needed for this medicine?

Keep this medication in the container it came in, tightly closed, and out of reach of children. Store it at room temperature and away from excess heat and moisture (not in the bathroom). Throw away any medication that is outdated or no longer needed. Talk to your pharmacist about the proper disposal of your medication.

What should I do in case of overdose?

In case of overdose, call your local poison control center at 1-800-222-1222. If the victim has collapsed or is not breathing, call local emergency services at 911.

What other information should I know?

Keep all appointments with your doctor and the laboratory. Your doctor will order certain lab tests to check your response to phentermine.

Do not let anyone else take your medication. Ask your pharmacist any questions you have about refilling your prescription.

Dosage Facts
For Informational Purposes

Caution: Do not change your dose, how often you take your medication, or the length of time you are to take it without first talking to your healthcare provider.

The following dosage information was written using medical language for doctors and other healthcare professionals and is provided here for you to check your dosage. The dosage of this drug may differ for different patients. Therefore, always follow your doctor's instructions or the directions on the label. Contact your healthcare provider or pharmacist if you have any questions

about the specific dosage of your medication after reviewing this information.

General Dosage Information

Available as phentermine resin complex; dosage expressed in terms of phentermine. Also available as phentermine hydrochloride; dosage expressed in terms of phentermine hydrochloride.

Adjust dosage according to individual response and tolerance; use the smallest dosage required to produce the desired response.

Adult Patients

Exogenous Obesity

ORAL:
- Phentermine (as resin complex): Usual dosage is 15 or 30 mg once daily.
- Phentermine hydrochloride: Usual dosage is 8 mg 3 times daily (given 30 minutes before meals) or 15–37.5 mg once daily (in the morning). Alternatively, 18.75 mg twice daily.

Special Populations

Geriatric Patients
- Select dosage with caution, starting at lower end of dosage range.

Phenylephrine

(fen il ef′ rin)

Brand Name: Sudafed PE®
Also available generically.

Why is this medicine prescribed?

Phenylephrine is used to relieve nasal discomfort caused by colds, allergies, and hay fever. It is also used to relieve sinus congestion and pressure. Phenylephrine is in a class of medications called nasal decongestants. It works by reducing swelling of the nasal passages.

How should this medicine be used?

Phenylephrine comes as a tablet to take by mouth. It is usually taken every 4 hours as needed. Do not take more than 6 doses in a 24-hour period. Follow the directions on the package label carefully, and ask your doctor or pharmacist to explain any part you do not understand. Take phenylephrine exactly as directed. Do not take more or less of it or take it more often than prescribed by your doctor.

Your symptoms should improve during your treatment. If your symptoms do not get better within 7 days or if you have a fever, stop taking phenylephrine and call your doctor.

Are there other uses for this medicine?

This medication may be prescribed for other uses; ask your doctor or pharmacist for more information.

What special precautions should I follow?

Before taking phenylephrine,
- tell your doctor and pharmacist if you are allergic to phenylephrine or any other medications.
- do not take phenylephrine if you are taking monoamine oxidase (MAO) inhibitors, including isocarboxazid (Marplan), phenelzine (Nardil), selegiline (Eldepryl), and tranylcypromine (Parnate), or have stopped taking them within the past 2 weeks.
- tell your doctor and pharmacist what other prescription and nonprescription medications, vitamins, nutritional supplements, and herbal products you are taking or plan to take. You should know that phenylephrine may in used in combination with other medications to treat colds, allergies, and sinus headaches. Be sure to read the information provided for the patient when taking combination products to be sure that you are not taking additional medications that contain the same ingredient.
- tell your doctor if you have or have ever had high blood pressure, diabetes, trouble urinating because of an enlarged prostate gland, or thyroid or heart disease.
- tell your doctor if you are pregnant, plan to become pregnant, or are breast-feeding. If you become pregnant while taking phenylephrine, call your doctor.
- if you are having surgery, including dental surgery, tell the doctor or dentist that you are taking phenylephrine.

What special dietary instructions should I follow?

Unless your doctor tells you otherwise, continue your normal diet.

What should I do if I forget to take a dose?

This medication is usually taken as needed. If your doctor has told you to take phenylephrine regularly, take the missed dose as soon as you remember it. However, if it is almost time for the next dose, skip the missed dose and continue your regular dosing schedule. Do not take a double dose to make up for a missed one.

What side effects can this medicine cause?

Phenylephrine may cause side effects. Some side effects can be serious. If you experience any of these symptoms, stop using phenylephrine and call your doctor immediately:
- nervousness
- dizziness
- sleeplessness

Phenylephrine may cause other side effects. Call your doctor if you have any unusual problems while taking this medication.

If you experience a serious side effect, you or your doctor may send a report to the Food and Drug Administration's (FDA) MedWatch Adverse Event Reporting program online [at http://www.fda.gov/MedWatch/index.html] or by phone [1-800-332-1088].

What storage conditions are needed for this medicine?

Keep this medication in the container it came in, tightly closed, and out of reach of children. Store it at room temperature and away from excess heat and moisture (not in the bathroom). Throw away any medication that is outdated or no longer needed. Talk to your pharmacist about the proper disposal of your medication.

What should I do in case of overdose?

In case of overdose, call your local poison control center at 1-800-222-1222. If the victim has collapsed or is not breathing, call local emergency services at 911.

What other information should I know?

Ask your pharmacist any questions you have about phenylephrine.

Dosage Facts
For Informational Purposes

Caution: Do not change your dose, how often you take your medication, or the length of time you are to take it without first talking to your healthcare provider.

The following dosage information was written using medical language for doctors and other healthcare professionals and is provided here for you to check your dosage. The dosage of this drug may differ for different patients. Therefore, always follow your doctor's instructions or the directions on the label. Contact your healthcare provider or pharmacist if you have any questions about the specific dosage of your medication after reviewing this information.

Pediatric Patients
Nasal Congestion

ORAL:
- *Self-medication* in children 2–5 years of age: 2.5 mg every 4 hours.
- *Self-medication* in children 6–11 years of age: 5 mg every 4 hours.
- *Self-medication* in children ≥12 years of age: Usually, 10 mg every 4 hours.
- May be administered in fixed combination with other drugs.
- Discontinue therapy if symptoms persist for >7 days or are accompanied by fever or if nervousness, dizziness, or insomnia occurs.

Adult Patients
Nasal Congestion

ORAL:
- *Self-medication*: Usually, 10 mg every 4 hours. May be administered in fixed combination with other drugs.
- Discontinue therapy if symptoms persist for >7 days or are accompanied by fever or if nervousness, dizziness, or insomnia occurs.

Prescribing Limits
Pediatric Patients
Nasal Congestion

ORAL:
- *Self-medication* in children 2–5 years of age: Maximum 15 mg in any 24-hour period.
- *Self-medication* in children 6–11 years of age: Maximum 30 mg in any 24-hour period.
- *Self-medication* in children ≥12 years of age: Maximum 60 mg in any 24-hour period.

Adult Patients
Hypotension
Nasal Congestion

ORAL:
- *Self-medication*: Maximum 60 mg in any 24-hour period.

Phenytoin Oral
(fen′ i toyn)

Brand Name: Dilantin®, Dilantin® Infatabs®, Dilantin® Kapseals®, Dilantin-125®, Phenytek® Also available generically.

Why is this medicine prescribed?

Phenytoin is used to treat various types of convulsions and seizures. Phenytoin acts on the brain and nervous system in the treatment of epilepsy.

This medication is sometimes prescribed for other uses; ask your doctor or pharmacist for more information.

How should this medicine be used?

Phenytoin comes as a capsule, extended-release (long-acting) capsule, chewable tablet, and liquid to take by mouth. It usually is taken two or three times a day. However, the extended-release capsules may be taken only once a day, usually at bedtime. Follow the directions on your prescription label carefully, and ask your doctor or pharmacist to explain any part you do not understand. Take phenytoin exactly as directed. Do not take more or less of it or take it more often than prescribed by your doctor.

Shake the liquid well before each use.

Do not open, crush, or chew the extended-release capsules; swallow them whole.

Continue to take phenytoin even if you feel well. Do not stop taking phenytoin without talking to your doctor, especially if you have taken large doses for a long time. Abruptly stopping the drug can cause seizures. Your doctor probably will decrease your dose gradually.

Are there other uses for this medicine?

Phenytoin is also used to control arrhythmias (irregular heartbeat) and to treat migraine headaches and facial nerve pain.

Talk to your doctor about the possible risks of using this drug for your condition.

What special precautions should I follow?

Before taking phenytoin,

- tell your doctor and pharmacist if you are allergic to phenytoin or any other drugs.
- tell your doctor and pharmacist what prescription and nonprescription medications you are taking, especially other seizure medications, acetaminophen (Tylenol), antacids such as Mylanta or Maalox, anticoagulants ('blood thinners') such as warfarin (Coumadin), chloramphenicol (Chloromycetin), cimetidine (Tagamet), disopyramide (Norpace), doxycycline (Vibramycin), fluconazole (Diflucan), heart medications such as digoxin, ibuprofen (Advil), isoniazid (INH), lithium, medications for anxiety such as diazepam (Valium), medications for colds or allergies such as chlorpheniramine (Chlor-Trimeton), medications for depression such as amitriptyline (Elavil), meperidine (Demerol), omeprazole (Prilosec), oral contraceptives, pyridoxine (vitamin B6), quinidine, rifampin, sedatives such as phenobarbital, sucralfate (Carafate), theophylline (Theo-Dur), tranquilizers such as chlorpromazine (Thorazine), and other vitamins. Phenytoin affects the action of other medications, and many medications can affect the action of phenytoin. Tell your doctor and pharmacist everything you are taking.
- tell your doctor if you have or have ever had irregular heartbeat; low blood pressure; problems with your blood sugar; a blood disorder; or heart, kidney, or liver disease.
- tell your doctor if you are pregnant, plan to become pregnant, or are breast-feeding. If you become pregnant while taking phenytoin, call your doctor.
- if you are having surgery, including dental surgery, tell the doctor or dentist that you are taking phenytoin.
- you should know that this drug may make you drowsy. Do not drive a car or operate machinery until you know how this drug affects you.
- remember that alcohol can add to the drowsiness caused by this drug.

What special dietary instructions should I follow?

Phenytoin may cause an upset stomach. Take phenytoin with food. If you are on enteral feeding, it is best to take phenytoin 2 hours before or after the enteral feeding. Drink plenty of water when taking this medicine.

What should I do if I forget to take a dose?

Take the missed dose as soon as you remember it. However, if it is almost time for the next dose, skip the missed dose and continue your regular dosing schedule. Do not take a double dose to make up for a missed one.

What side effects can this medicine cause?

Side effects from phenytoin may occur. Tell your doctor if any of these symptoms are severe or do not go away:

- drowsiness
- redness, irritation, bleeding, and swelling of the gums
- upset stomach
- vomiting
- constipation
- stomach pain
- loss of taste and appetite
- weight loss
- difficulty swallowing
- mental confusion
- blurred or double vision
- insomnia
- nervousness
- muscle twitching
- headache
- increased hair growth

If you experience any of the following symptoms, call your doctor immediately:

- difficulty coordinating movements
- skin rash
- easy bruising
- tiny purple-colored skin spots
- bloody nose
- slurred speech
- unusual bleeding
- yellowing of the skin or eyes
- dark urine
- swollen glands
- fever
- sore throat

If you experience a serious side effect, you or your doctor may send a report to the Food and Drug Administration's (FDA) MedWatch Adverse Event Reporting program online [at http://www.fda.gov/MedWatch/index.html] or by phone [1-800-332-1088].

What storage conditions are needed for this medicine?

Keep this medication in the container it came in, tightly closed, and out of reach of children. Store it at room temperature, away from excess heat and moisture (not in the bathroom). Protect the extended-release capsules and liquid from light. Do not freeze the liquid. Throw away any medication that is outdated or no longer needed. Talk to your pharmacist about the proper disposal of your medication.

What should I do in case of overdose?

In case of overdose, call your local poison control center at 1-800-222-1222. If the victim has collapsed or is not breathing, call local emergency services at 911.

What other information should I know?

Keep all appointments with your doctor and the laboratory. Your doctor will order certain lab tests to check your response to phenytoin.

Phenytoin capsules and tablets (and different brands of phenytoin) have different effects. Do not change brands of phenytoin without talking to your doctor.

Call your doctor if you continue to have seizures or convulsions while taking this medication.

If you give this drug to a child, observe and keep a record of the child's moods, behavior, attention span, hand-eye coordination, and ability to solve problems and perform tasks requiring thought. Ask the child's teacher to keep a similar record. This information can help the child's doctor determine whether to continue the drug or to change the dose or drug.

Wear identification (Medic Alert) indicating medication use and epilepsy.

Do not let anyone else take your medication. Ask your pharmacist any questions you have about refilling your prescription.

Dosage Facts

For Informational Purposes

Caution: Do not change your dose, how often you take your medication, or the length of time you are to take it without first talking to your healthcare provider.

The following dosage information was written using medical language for doctors and other healthcare professionals and is provided here for you to check your dosage. The dosage of this drug may differ for different patients. Therefore, always follow your doctor's instructions or the directions on the label. Contact your healthcare provider or pharmacist if you have any questions about the specific dosage of your medication after reviewing this information.

General Dosage Information

Each 100 mg of phenytoin sodium contains approximately 92 mg of phenytoin; consider the difference when switching from the base to its sodium salt or vice versa.

Pediatric Patients

Seizure Disorders

ORAL:
- Usual dosage: Initially, 5 mg/kg or 250 mg/m² daily in 2 or 3 equally divided doses; total dosage ≤300 mg daily.
- Therapeutic serum concentrations achieved more rapidly with a 500- to 600-mg oral loading dose, in divided doses, fol-

lowed by usual maintenance dosage 24 hours after initiating loading dose.
- Adjust subsequent dosage carefully and slowly according to the patient's requirements.
- Neonates, maintenance dosage: Usually, 3–5 mg/kg daily.
- Infants 1–12 months of age, maintenance dosage: Usually, 4–8 mg/kg daily.
- Children 1–11 years of age, maintenance dosage: 4–10 mg/kg daily.
- Adolescents, 12–17 years of age, maintenance dosage: 4–8 mg/kg daily.

Adult Patients

Seizure Disorders
Prompt-Release preparations

ORAL:
- Usual dosage: Initially, 100 mg 3 times daily.
- A period of 5–10 days may be required to achieve anticonvulsant effects.
- Increases to >300 mg daily may lead to markedly increased serum phenytoin concentrations; therefore, adjust dosage above this level carefully and slowly.
- Therapeutic serum concentrations achieved more rapidly with a 1-g oral loading dose given as 400, 300, and 300 mg at 2-hour intervals, followed by usual maintenance dosage 24 hours after initiating loading dose.
- Increase daily dosage gradually, if necessary, in increments of 100 mg every 2–4 weeks until desired response is achieved.
- Dosing at 100 mg 4 times daily may benefit some patients, and others may require dosages up to 200 mg 3 times daily.
- Optimum daily dose: Varies considerably but usually in the range of 4–7 mg/kg (300–600 mg daily for most adults).

Extended-Release Preparations

ORAL:
- For patients stabilized on a dosage of 100 mg 3 times daily, once-daily dosing with 300 mg as extended phenytoin sodium capsules may be considered.
- Do *not* use prompt phenytoin sodium capsules *nor* oral phenytoin base suspensions or chewable tablets for once-daily dosing.

Cardiac Arrhythmias
Ventricular Tachycardia

ORAL:
- 100 mg 2–4 times daily.

Paroxysmal Atrial Tachycardia

ORAL:
- 100 mg 2–4 times daily.

Cardiac Glycoside Intoxication

ORAL:
- 100 mg 2–4 times daily.

Prescribing Limits

Pediatric Patients

Seizure Disorders

ORAL:
- Total dosage should not exceed 300 mg daily.

Adult Patients

Seizure Disorders
Prompt-Release Preparations

ORAL:
- Increases in dosage to >300 mg daily may lead to markedly increased serum phenytoin concentrations; therefore, adjust dosage above this level carefully and slowly.

Special Populations

Hepatic Impairment
- Consider reduced maintenance dosage in hepatic cirrhosis. Do *not* use oral loading-dose regimens.

Renal Impairment
- Do *not* use oral loading-dose regimens.
- End-stage renal impairment generally can receive usual loading and maintenance dosages initially, adjusting as necessary.

Geriatric Patients
- May show early signs of toxicity.
- Geriatric patients with heart disease: It has been recommended that the drug be given at a rate of 50 mg over 2–3 minutes.

Obese Patients
- Ideal or nonobese weight probably correlates best with maintenance dosages. Loading doses may require adjustment for increased volume of distribution.

Pregnancy
- Monitor phenytoin therapy closely (phenytoin concentrations may decline) to ensure optimum seizure control.

Phytonadione

(fye toe na dye' one)

Brand Name: Mephyton®

Why is this medicine prescribed?

Phytonadione (vitamin K) is used to prevent bleeding in people with blood clotting problems or too little vitamin K in the body. Phytonadione is in a class of medications called vitamins. It works by providing vitamin K that is needed for blood to clot normally in the body.

How should this medicine be used?

Phytonadione comes as a tablet to take by mouth. It should be taken as directed by your doctor. Your doctor may sometimes prescribe another medication (bile salts) to take with phytonadione. Follow the directions on your prescription label carefully, and ask your doctor or pharmacist to explain any part you do not understand. Do not stop taking phytonadione without talking to your doctor. Take phytonadione exactly as directed. Do not take more or less of it or take it more often than prescribed by your doctor.

Are there other uses for this medicine?

This medication is sometimes prescribed for other uses; ask your doctor or pharmacist for more information.

What special precautions should I follow?

Before taking phytonadione,
- tell your doctor and pharmacist if you are allergic to phytonadione, any other medications, or any of the ingredients in phytonadione tablets. Ask your pharmacist for a list of the ingredients.
- Do not take anticoagulants ('blood thinners') such as warfarin (Coumadin) while you are taking phytonadione unless told to do so by your doctor.
- tell your doctor and pharmacist what prescription and nonprescription medications, vitamins, nutritional supplements, and herbal products you are taking or plan to take. Be sure to mention any of the following: antibiotics; salicylate pain relievers such as aspirin or aspirin-containing products, choline magnesium trisalicylate, choline salicylate (Arthropan), diflunisal (Dolobid), magnesium salicylate (Doan's, others), and salsalate (Argesic, Disalcid, Salgesic). Your doctor may need to change the doses of your medications or monitor you carefully for side effects.
- if you are taking orlistat (Xenical), take it 2 hours before or 2 hours after phytonadione.
- tell your doctor if you have or have ever had liver disease.
- tell your doctor if you are pregnant, plan to become pregnant, or are breast-feeding. If you become pregnant while taking phytonadione, call your doctor.

What special dietary instructions should I follow?

Talk to your doctor about the amount of vitamin K-rich foods to include in your diet while taking phytonadione. Do not increase or decrease your normal intake of foods such as green leafy vegetables, liver, broccoli, and cauliflower without checking with your doctor.

What should I do if I forget to take a dose?

Take the missed dose as soon as you remember it. However, if it is almost time for the next dose, skip the missed dose and continue your regular dosing schedule. Tell your doctor if you miss any doses. Do not take a double dose to make up for a missed one.

What side effects can this medicine cause?

Phytonadione may cause side effects. If you experience the following symptom, call your doctor immediately:
- unusual bruising or bleeding

What storage conditions are needed for this medicine?

Keep this medication in the container it came in, tightly closed, and out of reach of children. You should always protect phytonadione from light. Store it at room temperature and away from excess heat and moisture (not in the bathroom). Throw away any medication that is outdated or no longer needed. Talk to your pharmacist about the proper disposal of your medication.

What other information should I know?

Keep all appointments with your doctor and the laboratory. Your doctor will order certain lab tests to check your response to phytonadione.

Do not let anyone else take your medication. Ask your pharmacist any questions you have about refilling your prescription.

Dosage Facts
For Informational Purposes

Caution: Do not change your dose, how often you take your medication, or the length of time you are to take it without first talking to your healthcare provider.

The following dosage information was written using medical language for doctors and other healthcare professionals and is provided here for you to check your dosage. The dosage of this drug may differ for different patients. Therefore, always follow your doctor's instructions or the directions on the label. Contact your healthcare provider or pharmacist if you have any questions about the specific dosage of your medication after reviewing this information.

General Dosage Information

Dose, frequency of administration, and duration of treatment depend on the severity of the prothrombin deficiency and the response of the patient.

Pediatric Patients

Hemorrhagic Disease of the Newborn
Prophylaxis

ORAL:
- Alternatively, 1–2 mg orally† (can use injection formulation) immediately after delivery. Several oral doses, administered over a period of up to 3 months, may be required (e.g., at 1–2 weeks and 4 weeks of age in breast-fed infants, repeatedly if diarrhea occurs in breast-fed infants).

Treatment

- Empiric administration should not replace proper laboratory evaluation of the coagulation mechanism.
- A prompt response (shortening of the prothrombin time in 2–4 hours) following phytonadione usually is diagnostic of hemorrhagic disease of the newborn, and failure to respond indicates another diagnosis or coagulation disorder.

Dietary and Replacement Requirements
Healthy Infants ≤6 Months of Age

ORAL:
- 2 mcg daily.

Healthy Infants 7–12 Months of Age

ORAL:
- 2.5 mcg daily.

Healthy Children 1–3 Years of Age

ORAL:
- 30 mcg daily.

Healthy Children 4–8 Years of Age

ORAL:
- 55 mcg daily.

Healthy Children 9–13 Years of Age

ORAL:
- 60 mcg daily.

Healthy Children 14–18 Years of Age

ORAL:
- 75 mcg daily.

Adult Patients

Anticoagulant-induced Hypoprothrombinemia

ORAL:
- Usual initial dosage: 2.5–10 mg. Initial doses up to 25 mg have been used.
- Subsequent frequency and dosage should be determined by prothrombin time response and/or clinical condition.
- Dose may be repeated in 12–48 hours.
- *Rarely*, larger doses (e.g., 50 mg) may be required; however, administer lowest effective dosage so that refractoriness to further anticoagulant therapy is minimized and prothrombin time is not decreased below the effective anticoagulant level.

Hypoprothrombinemia from Other Causes

ORAL:
- Usual initial dosage: 2.5–25 mg, depending on deficiency, severity, and response. *Rarely*, larger doses (e.g., 50 mg) may be required.
- Determine subsequent frequency and dosage by prothrombin time response and/or clinical condition in addition to reduction or discontinuance of drug (if drug therapy causing hypoprothrombinemia).

Dietary and Replacement Requirements
Healthy Men ≥ 19 Years of Age

ORAL:
- 120 mcg daily.

Healthy Women ≥19 Years of Age

ORAL:
- 90 mcg daily.
- Limited data suggest that the vitamin K status in pregnant women does not differ from that in nonpregnant women. Therefore, NAS states that the AI of vitamin K does not need to be increased during pregnancy (i.e., pregnant women can receive the usual AI appropriate for their age).
- Available evidence indicates that the vitamin K status of lactating women is comparable to that of nonlactating women. Vitamin K is not distributed in clinically important amounts into milk, and the AI for lactating women does not differ from that for nonlactating women.

Pilocarpine Ophthalmic

(pye loe kar′ peen)

Brand Name: Isopto® Carpine, Pilopine HS®
Also available generically.

Why is this medicine prescribed?

Pilocarpine is used to treat glaucoma, a condition in which increased pressure in the eye can lead to gradual loss of vision. Pilocarpine relieves the symptoms of glaucoma.

This medication is sometimes prescribed for other uses; ask your doctor or pharmacist for more information.

How should this medicine be used?

Pilocarpine comes in eyedrops, eye gel, and a controlled-release system (Ocusert Pilo). The eyedrops usually are applied two to four times daily. The gel usually is applied once daily and at bedtime. The controlled-release system is used once a week and should be applied at bedtime. Follow the directions on your prescription label carefully, and ask your doctor or pharmacist to explain any part you do not understand. Use pilocarpine exactly as directed. Do not use more or less of it or use it more often than prescribed by your doctor.

Pilocarpine controls glaucoma, but does not cure it. Continue to use pilocarpine even if you feel well. Do not stop using pilocarpine without talking to your doctor.

To use the eyedrops, follow these steps:
1. Wash your hands thoroughly with soap and water.
2. Use a mirror or have someone else put the drops in your eye.
3. Remove the protective cap. Make sure that the end of the dropper is not chipped or cracked.
4. Avoid touching the dropper tip against your eye or anything else.
5. Hold the dropper tip down at all times to prevent drops from flowing back into the bottle and contaminating the remaining contents.
6. Lie down or tilt your head back.
7. Holding the bottle between your thumb and index finger, place the dropper tip as near as possible to your eyelid without touching it.
8. Brace the remaining fingers of that hand against your cheek or nose.
9. With the index finger of your other hand, pull the lower lid of the eye down to form a pocket.
10. Drop the prescribed number of drops into the pocket made by the lower lid and the eye. Placing drops on the surface of the eyeball can cause stinging.
11. Close your eye and press lightly against the lower lid with your finger for 2-3 minutes to keep the medication in the eye. Do not blink.
12. Replace and tighten the cap right away. Do not wipe or rinse it off.
13. Wipe off any excess liquid from your cheek with a clean tissue. Wash your hands again.

To use the eye gel, follow these instructions:
1. Wash your hands thoroughly with soap and water.
2. Use a mirror or have someone else apply the gel.
3. Remove the protective cap. Avoid touching the tip of the tube against your eye or anything else. The gel must be kept clean.
4. Tilt your head forward slightly.
5. Holding the tube between your thumb and index finger, place the tube as near as possible to your eyelid without touching it.
6. Brace the remaining fingers of that hand against your cheek or nose.
7. With the index finger of your other hand, pull the lower lid of your eye down to form a pocket.
8. Place a small amount of gel into the pocket made by the lower lid and the eye. A 1/2-inch strip of gel usually is enough unless otherwise directed by your doctor.
9. Gently close your eyes and keep them closed for 1-2 minutes to allow the medication to be absorbed.
10. Replace and tighten the cap right away.
11. Wipe off any excess gel from your eyelids and lashes with a clean tissue. Wash your hands again.

To use the controlled-release system,
1. Wash your hands thoroughly with soap and water before handling it.
2. Follow the written patient instructions, and place the system in your eye at bedtime.
3. Place the system either in the pocket formed at the lower part of the eye by the lower eyelid and eyeball or, preferably, at the upper part of the eye under the upper eyelid. (It is less likely to come out when placed at the upper part of the eye.)
4. The system is to stay in your eye for 7 days. If it comes out, rinse it with cool tap water and replace it in your eye. Discard the system if it is damaged or contaminated, and insert a new one.

5. To prevent the system from coming out at night, work the system from the lower part of your eye to the upper part (under the upper eyelid) by gently pressing it (with a clean finger) through your closed eyelid at bedtime.

6. Check to be sure that the system is in place each night when you go to bed and when you wake up. If one becomes lost, you can either replace it or replace the systems in both eyes so that both eyes are on the same replacement schedule.

What special precautions should I follow?

Before using pilocarpine eyedrops,

- tell your doctor and pharmacist if you are allergic to pilocarpine or any other drugs.
- tell your doctor and pharmacist what prescription and nonprescription medications you are taking, including vitamins.
- tell your doctor if you have or have ever had asthma, intestinal disease, ulcers, high blood pressure, heart disease, an overactive thyroid gland, seizures, Parkinson's disease, or an obstruction in the urinary tract.
- tell your doctor if you are pregnant, plan to become pregnant, or are breast-feeding. If you become pregnant while using pilocarpine, call your doctor immediately.
- if you are having surgery, including dental surgery, tell the doctor or dentist that you are using pilocarpine.
- if you are using another eyedrop medication, use the eye medications at least 10 minutes apart.

What should I do if I forget to take a dose?

Apply the missed drops or gel as soon as you remember it. However, if it is almost time for the next dose, skip the missed dose and continue your regular dosing schedule.

Do not apply a double dose to make up for a missed one.

What side effects can this medicine cause?

Pilocarpine may cause side effects. Tell your doctor if any of these symptoms are severe or do not go away:

- blurred or dim vision
- stinging, burning, or discomfort in the eye
- itching or redness of the eye
- tearing or swelling of the eye
- redness of the eyelids
- headache

If you experience any of the following symptoms, call your doctor immediately:

- sweating
- muscle tremors
- upset stomach
- vomiting

- diarrhea
- difficulty breathing
- watering of the mouth
- dizziness
- weakness

If you experience a serious side effect, you or your doctor may send a report to the Food and Drug Administration's (FDA) MedWatch Adverse Event Reporting program online [at http://www.fda.gov/MedWatch/index.html] or by phone [1-800-332-1088].

What storage conditions are needed for this medicine?

Keep the drops and gel in the container they came in, tightly closed, and out of reach of children. Store them at room temperature and away from excess heat and moisture (not in the bathroom). Store the controlled-release system in the refrigerator. Throw away any medication that is outdated or no longer needed. Talk to your pharmacist about the proper disposal of your medication.

What other information should I know?

Keep all appointments with your doctor. Your doctor will order certain eye tests to check your response to pilocarpine.

Do not let anyone else use your medication. Ask your pharmacist any questions you have about refilling your prescription.

Dosage Facts
For Informational Purposes

Caution: Do not change your dose, how often you take your medication, or the length of time you are to take it without first talking to your healthcare provider.

The following dosage information was written using medical language for doctors and other healthcare professionals and is provided here for you to check your dosage. The dosage of this drug may differ for different patients. Therefore, always follow your doctor's instructions or the directions on the label. Contact your healthcare provider or pharmacist if you have any questions about the specific dosage of your medication after reviewing this information.

General Dosage Information

Available as pilocarpine hydrochloride; dosage expressed in terms of the salt.

Adjust concentration and frequency of solution instillation according to patient requirements and response, as determined by tonometric readings.

In patients with heavily pigmented irides, higher solution concentrations may be required.

Adjust dosage of ophthalmic gel based on periodic tonometric readings.

Adult Patients

Open-Angle Glaucoma

OPHTHALMIC:

- 1–2 drops of a 1–4% solution in the eye(s) every 4–12 hours. Solution concentrations >4% are only occasionally more effective than lower concentrations.
- Apply a 1.3-cm (0.5-inch) ribbon of a 4% gel into lower conjunctival sac once daily at bedtime.

Acute Angle-Closure Glaucoma

OPHTHALMIC:

- 1 drop of a 2% solution in the affected eye every 5–10 minutes for 3–6 doses, followed by 1 drop every 1–3 hours until pressure is controlled. To prevent a bilateral attack, 1 drop of a 1–2% solution in the unaffected eye every 6–8 hours.

Ocular Surgery

Iridectomy

OPHTHALMIC:

- 1 drop of a 2% solution 4 times immediately prior to iridectomy has been used.

Congenital Glaucoma (Goniotomy)

OPHTHALMIC:

- 1 drop of a 2% solution every 6 hours prior to surgery has been used.
- May use a 2% solution to fill the gonioscopic lens prior to goniotomy, or may administer 1 drop of a 2% solution every 6 hours plus 3 times in the 30 minutes immediately preceding goniotomy, with or without concomitant administration of acetazolamide.

Ophthalmologic Examinations

OPHTHALMIC:

- 1 drop of a 1% solution in the affected eye(s).

Pimecrolimus Topical

(pim e krow′ li mus)

Brand Name: Elidel®

Important Warning

A small number of patients who used pimecrolimus cream or another similar medication developed skin cancer or lymphoma (cancer in a part of the immune system). There is not enough information available to tell whether pimecrolimus cream caused these pa-

tients to develop cancer. Studies of transplant patients and laboratory animals and an understanding of the way pimecrolimus works suggest that there is possibility that people who use pimecrolimus cream have a greater risk of developing cancer. More study is needed to understand this risk.

Follow these directions carefully to decrease the possible risk that you will develop cancer during your treatment with pimecrolimus cream:

- Use pimecrolimus cream only when you have symptoms of eczema. Stop using pimecrolimus cream when your symptoms go away or when your doctor tells you that you should stop. Do not use pimecrolimus cream continuously for a long time.
- Call your doctor if you have used pimecrolimus cream for 6 weeks and your eczema symptoms have not improved. A different medication may be needed.
- Call your doctor if your eczema symptoms come back after your treatment with pimecrolimus cream.
- Apply pimecrolimus cream only to skin that is affected by eczema. Use the smallest amount of cream that is needed to control your symptoms.
- Do not use pimecrolimus cream to treat eczema in children who are younger than 2 years old.
- Tell your doctor if you have or have ever had cancer, especially skin cancer, or any condition that affects your immune system. Ask your doctor if you are not sure if a condition that you have has affected your immune system. Pimecrolimus may not be right for you.
- Protect your skin from real and artificial sunlight during your treatment with pimecrolimus cream. Do not use sun lamps or tanning beds, and do not undergo ultraviolet light therapy. Stay out of the sunlight as much as possible during your treatment, even when the medication is not on your skin. If you need to be outside in the sun, wear loose fitting clothing to protect the treated skin, and ask your doctor about other ways to protect your skin from the sun.

Your doctor or pharmacist will give you the manufacturer's patient information sheet (Medication Guide) when you begin treatment with pimecrolimus and each time you refill your prescription. Read the information carefully and ask your doctor or pharmacist if you have any questions. You can also visit the Food and Drug Administration (FDA) website (http://www.fda.gov/cder) or the manufacturer's website to obtain the Medication Guide.

Talk to your doctor about the risks of using pimecrolimus.

Why is this medicine prescribed?

Pimecrolimus is used to control the symptoms of eczema (atopic dermatitis; a skin disease that causes the skin to be dry and itchy and to sometimes develop red, scaly rashes). Pimecrolimus is only used to treat patients who cannot use other medications for eczema, or whose symptoms were not controlled by other medications. Pimecrolimus is in a class of medications called topical calcineurin inhibitors. It works by stopping the immune system from producing substances that may cause eczema.

How should this medicine be used?

Pimecrolimus comes as a cream to apply to the skin. It is usually applied twice a day for up to 6 weeks at a time. Follow the directions on your prescription label carefully, and ask your doctor or pharmacist to explain any part you do not understand. Apply pimecrolimus cream exactly as directed. Do not apply more or less of it or apply it more often than prescribed by your doctor.

Pimecrolimus cream is only for use on the skin. Be careful not to get pimecrolimus cream in your eyes or mouth. If you get pimecrolimus cream in your eyes, rinse them with cold water. If you swallow pimecrolimus cream, call your doctor.

To use the cream, follow these steps:

1. Wash your hands with soap and water.
2. Be sure that the skin in the affected area is dry.
3. Apply a thin layer of pimecrolimus cream to all affected areas of your skin. You can apply pimecrolimus to all affected skin surfaces including your head, face, and neck.
4. Rub the cream into your skin gently and completely.
5. Wash your hands with soap and water to remove any leftover pimecrolimus cream. Do not wash your hands if you are treating them with pimecrolimus cream.
6. You may cover the treated areas with normal clothing, but do not use any bandages, dressings, or wraps.
7. Be careful not to wash the cream from affected areas of your skin. Do not swim, shower, or bathe immediately after applying pimecrolimus cream. Ask your doctor if you should apply more pimecrolimus cream after you swim, shower, or bathe.
8. After you apply pimecrolimus cream and allow time for it be completely absorbed into your skin, you may apply moisturizers, sunscreen, or makeup to the affected area. Ask your doctor about the specific products you plan to use.

Are there other uses for this medicine?

This medication may be prescribed for other uses; ask your doctor or pharmacist for more information.

What special precautions should I follow?

Before using pimecrolimus cream,

- tell your doctor and pharmacist if you are allergic to pimecrolimus or any other medications.

- tell your doctor and pharmacist what prescription and nonprescription medications, vitamins, nutritional supplements, and herbal products you are taking. Be sure to mention any of the following: antifungals such as fluconazole (Diflucan), itraconazole (Sporanox), and ketoconazole (Nizoral); calcium channel blockers such as diltiazem (Cardizem, Dilacor, Tiazac, others), and verapamil (Calan, Isoptin, Verelan); cimetidine (Tagamet); clarithromycin (Biaxin); cyclosporine (Neoral, Sandimmune); danazol (Danocrine); delavirdine (Rescriptor); erythromycin (E.E.S., E-Mycin, Erythrocin); fluoxetine (Prozac, Sarafem); fluvoxamine (Luvox); HIV protease inhibitors such as indinavir (Crixivan), and ritonavir (Norvir); isoniazid (INH, Nydrazid); metronidazole (Flagyl); nefazodone; oral contraceptives (birth control pills); other ointments, creams, or lotions; troleandomycin (TAO); and zafirlukast (Accolate). Your doctor may need to change the doses of your medications or monitor you carefully for side effects.
- tell your doctor if you have or have ever had Netherton's syndrome (an inherited condition that causes the skin to be red, itchy, and scaly), redness and peeling of most of your skin, any other skin disease, or any type of skin infection, especially chicken pox, shingles (a skin infection in people who have had chicken pox in the past), herpes (cold sores), or eczema herpeticum (viral infection that causes fluid filled blisters to form on the skin of people who have eczema). Also tell your doctor if your eczema rash has turned crusty or blistered or if you think that your eczema rash is infected.
- tell your doctor if you are pregnant, plan to become pregnant, or are breast-feeding. If you become pregnant while taking pimecrolimus, call your doctor.
- ask your doctor about the safe use of alcohol during your treatment with pimecrolimus cream. Your face may become flushed or red or feel hot if you drink alcohol during your treatment.
- avoid exposure to chicken pox, shingles and other viruses. If you are exposed to one of these viruses while using pimecrolimus, call your doctor immediately.
- you should know that good skin care and moisturizers may help relieve the dry skin caused by eczema. Talk to your doctor about the moisturizers you should use, and always apply them after applying pimecrolimus cream.

What special dietary instructions should I follow?

Talk to your doctor about eating grapefruit and drinking grapefruit juice while taking this medicine.

What should I do if I forget to take a dose?

Apply the missed dose as soon as you remember it. However, if it is almost time for the next dose, skip the missed dose and continue your regular dosing schedule. Do not apply extra cream to make up for a missed dose.

What side effects can this medicine cause?

Pimecrolimus may cause side effects. Tell your doctor if any of these symptoms are severe or do not go away:

- burning, warmth, stinging, soreness, or redness in the areas where you applied pimecrolimus (call your doctor if this lasts more than 1 week)
- warts, bumps, or other growths on skin
- eye irritation
- headache
- cough
- red, stuffy or runny nose
- nosebleed
- diarrhea
- painful menstrual periods

Some side effects can be serious. If you experience any of the following symptoms, call your doctor immediately:

- sore or red throat
- fever
- flu-like symptoms
- ear pain, discharge, and other signs of infection
- hives
- new or worsening rash
- itching
- swelling of the face, throat, tongue, lips, eyes, hands, feet, ankles, or lower legs
- difficulty breathing or swallowing
- crusting, oozing, blistering or other signs of skin infection
- cold sores
- chicken pox or other blisters
- swollen glands in the neck

Pimecrolimus may cause other side effects. Call your doctor if you have any unusual problems while taking this medication.

If you experience a serious side effect, you or your doctor may send a report to the Food and Drug Administration's (FDA) MedWatch Adverse Event Reporting program online [at http://www.fda.gov/MedWatch/index.html] or by phone [1-800-332-1088].

What storage conditions are needed for this medicine?

Keep this medication in the container it came in, tightly closed, and out of reach of children. Store it at room temperature and away from excess heat and moisture (not in the bathroom). Throw away any medication that is outdated or no longer needed. Talk to your pharmacist about the proper disposal of your medication.

What other information should I know?

Keep all appointments with your doctor.

Do not let anyone else take your medication. Ask your pharmacist any questions you have about refilling your prescription.

Dosage Facts
For Informational Purposes

Caution: Do not change your dose, how often you take your medication, or the length of time you are to take it without first talking to your health-care provider.

The following dosage information was written using medical language for doctors and other healthcare professionals and is provided here for you to check your dosage. The dosage of this drug may differ for different patients. Therefore, always follow your doctor's instructions or the directions on the label. Contact your healthcare provider or pharmacist if you have any questions about the specific dosage of your medication after reviewing this information.

Pediatric Patients

Atopic Dermatitis

TOPICAL:
- Children ≥2 years of age: Apply to affected areas twice daily.
- Treatment effects usually evident within 15 days; erythema and infiltration or papulation generally reduced within 8 days. Discontinue treatment following resolution of signs and symptoms (e.g., pruritus, rash, erythema). If manifestations persist beyond 6 weeks, reexamine patient and confirm diagnosis.

Adult Patients

Atopic Dermatitis

TOPICAL:
- Apply to affected areas twice daily.
- Treatment effects usually evident within 15 days; erythema and infiltration or papulation generally reduced within 8 days. Discontinue treatment following resolution of signs and symptoms (e.g., pruritus, rash, erythema). If manifestations persist beyond 6 weeks, reexamine patient and confirm diagnosis.

Prescribing Limits

Pediatric Patients

Atopic Dermatitis

TOPICAL:
- For short-term and intermittent use only; avoid continuous long-term use. Safety of noncontinuous use for >1 year not established.

Adult Patients

Atopic Dermatitis

TOPICAL:
- For short-term and intermittent use only; avoid continuous long-term use. Safety of noncontinuous use for >1 year not established.

Pimozide

(pi′ moe zide)

Brand Name: Orap®

Why is this medicine prescribed?

Pimozide is used to control tics (unusual movements or sounds that the patient may be able to hold back for a short time but cannot really control) caused by Tourette's disorder. Pimozide should only be used in patients who cannot take other medications or who have taken other medications without good results. Pimozide should only be used to treat severe tics that stop the patient from learning, working, or performing normal activities. Pimozide is in a class of medications called antipsychotics. It works by decreasing abnormal excitement in the brain.

How should this medicine be used?

Pimozide comes as a tablet to take by mouth. It is usually taken with or without food once a day at bedtime or twice a day. To help you remember to take pimozide, take it around the same time every day. Follow the directions on your prescription label carefully, and ask your doctor or pharmacist to explain any part you do not understand. Take pimozide exactly as directed. Do not take more or less of it or take it more often than prescribed by your doctor.

Your doctor will probably start you on a low dose of pimozide and gradually increase your dose, not more than once every 2 or 3 days.

Pimozide controls Tourette's disorder but does not cure it. It may take some time before you feel the full benefit of pimozide. Continue to take pimozide even if you feel well. Do not stop taking pimozide without talking to your doctor. You may experience a serious reaction if you suddenly stop taking pimozide. Your doctor will probably decrease your dose gradually.

Are there other uses for this medicine?

Pimozide is also used sometimes to treat schizophrenia, and certain behavior, personality, movement, and psychiatric disorders in adults. Pimozide should not be prescribed for other uses in children. Talk to your doctor about the possible risks of using this medication for your condition.

What special precautions should I follow?

Before taking pimozide,

- tell your doctor and pharmacist if you are allergic to pimozide, other medications for mental illness, or any other medications.
- do not take antibiotics such as azithromycin (Zithromax, Z-Pak), clarithromycin (Biaxin), dirithromycin (Dynabac), erythromycin (E.E.S., E-Mycin, Erythrocin), and

troleandomycin (TAO); antifungals such as fluconazole (Diflucan), itraconazole (Sporanox), and ketoconazole (Nizoral); dofetilide (Tikosyn); chlorpromazine (Ormazine, Thorazine); cyclosporine (Neoral, Sandimmune); danazol (Danocrine); delavirdine (Rescriptor); diltiazem (Cardizem, Dilacor, Tiazac); dolasetron (Anzemet); fluoxetine (Prozac, Sarafem); fluvoxamine (Luvox); gatifloxacin (Tequin); HIV protease inhibitors such as indinavir (Crixivan), nelfinavir (Viracept), saquinavir (Fortovase, Invirase), and ritonavir (Norvir); medication for irregular heartbeat such as amiodarone (Cordarone), disopyramide (Norpace), procainamide (Procanabid, Pronestyl), quinidine (Cardioquin, Quinaglute, Quinidex), and sotalol (Betapace); mefloquine (Lariam); mesoridazine (Serentil); metronidazole (Flagyl); moxifloxacin (Avelox); nefazadone (Serzone); oral contraceptives (birth control pills); pentamidine (Nebu-Pent); sertraline (Zoloft); sparfloxacin (Zagam); tacrolimus (Prograf); thioridazine (Mellaril); verapamil (Calan, Covera, Isoptin, Verelan); zafirlukast (Accolate); zileuton (Zyflo); and ziprasidone (Geodon) while taking pimozide.
- tell your doctor if you are taking medications that may cause tics, including amphetamines such as amphetamine (Adderall) and dextroamphetamine (Dexadrine, Dextrostat); pemoline (Cylert); and methyphenidate (Concerta, Ritalin). Your doctor may tell you to stop taking your medication for a while before you start taking pimozide. This will let your doctor see if your tics were caused by the other medication and can be treated by stopping it.
- tell your doctor and pharmacist what other prescription and nonprescription medications, vitamins, nutritional supplements, and herbal products you are taking. Be sure to mention any of the following: antidepressants (mood elevators); diuretics ('water pills'); medications for anxiety, mental illness, pain, and seizures; sedatives; sleeping pills; and tranquilizers. Your doctor may need to change the doses of your medications or monitor you carefully for side effects.
- tell your doctor if you have or have ever had breast cancer; an irregular heartbeat; Parkinson's disease; glaucoma; problems with urination; seizures; low levels of potassium or magnesium in your blood; and heart, prostate, liver, or kidney disease.
- tell your doctor if you are pregnant, plan to become pregnant, or are breast-feeding. If you become pregnant while taking pimozide, call your doctor.
- if you are having surgery, including dental surgery, tell the doctor or dentist that you are taking pimozide.
- you should know that pimozide may make you drowsy. Do not drive a car or operate machinery until you know how this medication affects you.
- remember that alcohol can add to the drowsiness caused by this medication.
- you should know that pimozide may make it harder for your body to cool down when it gets very hot. Tell your

doctor if you plan to do vigorous exercise or be exposed to extreme heat.

What special dietary instructions should I follow?

Talk to your doctor about drinking grapefruit juice while taking this medicine.

What should I do if I forget to take a dose?

Take the missed dose as soon as you remember it. However, if it is almost time for the next dose, skip the missed dose and continue your regular dosing schedule. Do not take a double dose to make up for a missed one.

What side effects can this medicine cause?

Pimozide may cause side effects. Tell your doctor if any of these symptoms are severe or do not go away:

- sleepiness
- headache
- weakness
- dry mouth
- diarrhea
- constipation
- unusual hunger or thirst
- muscle tightness
- changes in posture
- difficulty falling or staying asleep
- nervousness
- changes in behavior
- changes in taste
- eyes sensitive to light
- changes in vision
- decreased sexual ability
- rash

Some side effects can be serious. The following symptoms are uncommon, but if you experience any of them, call your doctor immediately:

- unusual movements of your body or face that you cannot control
- high fever
- muscle stiffness
- confusion
- sweating
- fast heartbeat
- shuffling walk
- restlessness
- difficulty moving any part of your body
- difficulty speaking

At high doses, pimozide has caused tumors in mice. This does not necessarily mean that pimozide will also cause tumors in humans. Pimozide may also cause other serious side effects. Talk to your doctor about the risks of taking this medication.

Pimozide may cause other side effects. Call your doctor if you have any unusual problems while taking this medication.

If you experience a serious side effect, you or your doctor may send a report to the Food and Drug Administration's (FDA) MedWatch Adverse Event Reporting program online [at http://www.fda.gov/MedWatch/index.html] or by phone [1-800-332-1088].

What storage conditions are needed for this medicine?

Keep this medication in the container it came in, tightly closed, and out of reach of children. Store it at room temperature and away from excess heat and moisture (not in the bathroom). Throw away any medication that is outdated or no longer needed. Talk to your pharmacist about the proper disposal of your medication.

What should I do in case of overdose?

In case of overdose, call your local poison control center at 1-800-222-1222. If the victim has collapsed or is not breathing, call local emergency services at 911.

Symptoms of overdose may include:

- difficulty moving body
- shuffling walk
- dizziness
- headache
- fainting
- blurred vision
- upset stomach
- coma
- difficulty breathing

What other information should I know?

Keep all appointments with your doctor and the laboratory. Your doctor will order certain lab tests to check your body's response to pimozide.

Do not let anyone else take your medication. Ask your pharmacist any questions you have about refilling your prescription.

Dosage Facts
For Informational Purposes

Caution: Do not change your dose, how often you take your medication, or the length of time you are to take it without first talking to your healthcare provider.

The following dosage information was written using medical language for doctors and other healthcare professionals and is provided here for you to check your dosage. The dosage of this drug may differ for different patients. Therefore, always follow your doctor's instructions or the directions on the label. Contact your healthcare provider or pharmacist if you have any questions about the specific dosage of your medication after reviewing this information.

General Dosage Information

Initiate therapy with low dosage and adjust dosage gradually.

Pediatric Patients

Tourette's Syndrome

ORAL:

- Children <12 years of age†: Reliable dose-response data for drug effects on tic manifestations not available.
- Children ≥12 years of age: Initially, 0.05 mg/kg daily, preferably at bedtime. May increase dosage every third day to a maximum of 0.2 mg/kg daily, not to exceed 10 mg daily.
- During prolonged maintenance therapy, use lowest possible effective dosage. Once adequate response is achieved, make periodic attempts (e.g., every 6–12 months) to reduce dosage to determine whether initial intensity and frequency of tics persist.
- In attempts to reduce dosage, consider possibility that observed increases of tic intensity and frequency may represent a transient, withdrawal-related phenomenon rather than return of the syndrome's symptoms. Allow 1–2 weeks to elapse before concluding that an increase in tic manifestations is a function of the underlying disorder rather than a response to drug withdrawal.
- If therapy is to be discontinued, gradually reduce dosage.

Adult Patients

Tourette's Syndrome

ORAL:

- Initially, 1–2 mg daily in divided doses. May increase dosage every other day according to patient's tolerance and therapeutic response. Some clinicians suggest that dosage be increased at longer intervals (e.g., every 5–7 days), until manifestations decrease by ≥70%, adverse effects occur without symptomatic benefit, or symptomatic benefit and adverse effects occur simultaneously.
- If minimal adverse effects occur (e.g., not interfering with functioning) before adequate response is achieved, hold further dosage increase until adverse effects resolve. If adverse effects interfere with functioning but are not severe, can reduce dosage by 1-mg increments at weekly intervals until such effects resolve.
- If severe adverse effects occur, immediately reduce dosage by 50% or withhold drug. Once serious adverse effects resolve, can reinstitute with more gradual titration, increasing dosage at intervals ranging from 7–30 days.
- Most patients are adequately treated with dosages <0.2 mg/kg daily or 10 mg daily, whichever is less; higher dosages not recommended.
- During prolonged maintenance therapy, use lowest possible effective dosage. Once adequate response is achieved, make periodic attempts (e.g., every 6–12 months) to reduce dosage to determine whether initial intensity and frequency of tics persist.
- In attempts to reduce dosage, consider possibility that observed increases of tic intensity and frequency may represent a transient, withdrawal-related phenomenon rather than return of the syndrome's symptoms. Allow 1–2 weeks to elapse before concluding that an increase in tic manifestations is a function of the underlying disorder rather than a response to drug withdrawal.
- If therapy is to be discontinued, gradually reduce dosage.

Prescribing Limits

Pediatric Patients

Tourette's Syndrome

ORAL:

- Children ≥12 years of age: Maximum 0.2 mg/kg, not exceeding 10 mg daily.

Adult Patients

Tourette's Syndrome

ORAL:

- Dosages >0.2 mg/kg or 10 mg daily not recommended.

† Use is not currently included in the labeling approved by the US Food and Drug Administration.

Pindolol

(pin′ doe lole)

Brand Name: Visken®
Also available generically.

Important Warning
Do not stop taking pindolol without talking to your doctor first. If pindolol is stopped suddenly, it may cause chest pain or heart attack in some people.

Why is this medicine prescribed?

Pindolol is used to treat high blood pressure. It works by relaxing your blood vessels so your heart doesn't have to pump as hard.

This medication is sometimes prescribed for other uses; ask your doctor or pharmacist for more information.

How should this medicine be used?

Pindolol comes as a tablet to take by mouth. It usually is taken two times a day. Follow the directions on your prescription label carefully, and ask your doctor or pharmacist to explain any part you do not understand. Take pindolol exactly as directed. Do not take more or less of it or take it more often than prescribed by your doctor.

Pindolol helps control your condition but will not cure it. Continue to take pindolol even if you feel well. Do not stop taking pindolol without talking to your doctor.

Are there other uses for this medicine?

Pindolol is also used sometimes to prevent angina (chest pain) and heart attacks. Talk to your doctor about the possible risks of using this drug for your condition.

What special precautions should I follow?

Before taking pindolol,

- tell your doctor and pharmacist if you are allergic to pindolol or any other drugs.
- tell your doctor and pharmacist what prescription and nonprescription medications you are taking, especially other medications for heart disease or high blood pressure, reserpine, thioridazine (Mellaril), and vitamins.
- tell your doctor if you have or have ever had asthma or other lung disease; diabetes; severe allergies; thyroid problems; or heart, liver, or kidney disease.
- tell your doctor if you are pregnant, plan to become pregnant, or are breast-feeding. If you become pregnant while taking pindolol, call your doctor.
- if you are having surgery, including dental surgery, tell the doctor or dentist that you are taking pindolol.
- you should know that this drug may make you drowsy. Do not drive a car or operate machinery until you know how this drug affects you.
- remember that alcohol can add to the drowsiness caused by this drug.

What special dietary instructions should I follow?

Talk to your doctor before using salt substitutes containing potassium. If your doctor prescribes a low-salt or low-sodium diet, follow these directions carefully.

What should I do if I forget to take a dose?

Take the missed dose as soon as you remember it. However, if it is almost time for the next dose, skip the missed dose and continue your regular dosing schedule. Do not take a double dose to make up for a missed one.

What side effects can this medicine cause?

Pindolol may cause side effects. Tell your doctor if any of these symptoms are severe or do not go away:

- dizziness or lightheadedness
- excessive tiredness
- difficulty sleeping
- unusual dreams
- upset stomach
- heartburn
- cold hands or feet
- muscle or joint pain

If you experience any of the following symptoms, call your doctor immediately:

- difficulty breathing
- sore throat and fever
- unusual bleeding
- swelling of the feet or hands
- unusual weight gain
- chest pain
- slow, irregular heartbeat

If you experience a serious side effect, you or your doctor may send a report to the Food and Drug Administration's (FDA) MedWatch Adverse Event Reporting program online [at http://www.fda.gov/MedWatch/index.html] or by phone [1-800-332-1088].

What storage conditions are needed for this medicine?

Keep this medication in the container it came in, tightly closed, and out of reach of children. Store it at room temperature and away from excess heat and moisture (not in the bathroom). Throw away any medication that is outdated or no longer needed. Talk to your pharmacist about the proper disposal of your medication.

What should I do in case of overdose?

In case of overdose, call your local poison control center at 1-800-222-1222. If the victim has collapsed or is not breathing, call local emergency services at 911.

What other information should I know?

Keep all appointments with your doctor and the laboratory. Your doctor will need to determine your response to pindolol. Your doctor may ask you to check your pulse (heart rate). Ask your pharmacist or doctor to teach you how to take your pulse. If your pulse is faster or slower than it should be, call your doctor.

Do not let anyone else take your medication. Ask your pharmacist any questions you have about refilling your prescription.

Dosage Facts
For Informational Purposes

Caution: Do not change your dose, how often you take your medication, or the length of time you are to take it without first talking to your healthcare provider.

The following dosage information was written using medical language for doctors and other healthcare professionals and is provided here for you to check your dosage. The dosage of this drug may differ for different patients. Therefore, always follow your doctor's instructions or the directions on the label. Contact your healthcare provider or pharmacist if you have any questions about the specific dosage of your medication after reviewing this information.

Adult Patients
Hypertension

ORAL:

- Initially, 5 mg twice daily. Increase dosage gradually by 10 mg daily at 3- to 4-week intervals as necessary up to 60 mg daily. The usual maintenance dosage range is 10–40 mg daily, given in 2 divided doses.

Angina†

ORAL:
• 15–40 mg daily, given in 3 or 4 divided doses.

Prescribing Limits

Adult Patients

Hypertension

ORAL:
• Maximum 60 mg daily.

Special Populations

Hepatic Impairment
• Dosage must be modified in response to the degree of hepatic impairment.

† Use is not currently included in the labeling approved by the US Food and Drug Administration.

Pioglitazone

(pye oh gli′ ta zone)

Brand Name: Actos®, ActoPLUSMet® (as a combination product containing pioglitazone and metformin), Duetact® (as a combination product containing pioglitazone and glimepiride)

Important Warning

Pioglitazone and other similar medications for diabetes may cause or worsen congestive heart failure (condition in which the heart is unable to pump enough blood to the other parts of the body). Before you start to take pioglitazone, tell your doctor if you have or have ever had congestive heart failure, especially if your heart failure is so severe that you must limit your activity and are only comfortable when you are at rest or you must remain in a chair or bed. Also tell your doctor if you were born with a heart defect, and if you have or have ever had swelling of the arms, hands, feet, ankles, or lower legs; heart disease; high cholesterol or fats in the blood; high blood pressure; coronary artery disease (narrowing of the blood vessels that lead to the heart); a heart attack; or an irregular heartbeat. Your doctor may tell you not to take pioglitazone or may monitor you carefully during your treatment.

If you develop congestive heart failure, you may experience certain symptoms. Tell your doctor immediately if you have any of the following symptoms, especially when you first start taking pioglitazone or after your dose is increased: large weight gain in a short period of time; shortness of breath;

swelling of the arms, hands, feet, ankles, or lower legs; swelling or pain in the stomach; waking up short of breath during the night; needing to sleep with extra pillows in order to breathe while lying down; frequent dry cough; or increased tiredness.

Talk to your doctor about the risks of taking pioglitazone.

Why is this medicine prescribed?

Pioglitazone is used with a diet and exercise program and sometimes with other medications, to treat type 2 diabetes (condition in which the body does not use insulin normally and, therefore, cannot control the amount of sugar in the blood). Pioglitazone is in a class of medications called thiazolidinediones. It works by increasing the body's sensitivity to insulin, a natural substance that helps control blood sugar levels. Pioglitazone is not used to treat type 1 diabetes (condition in which the body does not produce insulin and therefore cannot control the amount of sugar in the blood) or diabetic ketoacidosis (a serious condition that may develop if high blood sugar is not treated).

How should this medicine be used?

Pioglitazone comes as a tablet to take by mouth. It is usually taken once daily with or without meals. Take pioglitazone at around the same time every day. Follow the directions on your prescription label carefully, and ask your doctor or pharmacist to explain any part you do not understand. Take pioglitazone exactly as directed. Do not take more or less of it or take it more often than prescribed by your doctor.

Your doctor may start you on a low dose of pioglitazone and gradually increase your dose.

Pioglitazone controls type 2 diabetes but does not cure it. It may take 2 weeks for your blood sugar to decrease and several weeks longer for you to feel the full effect of pioglitazone. Continue to take pioglitazone even if you feel well. Do not stop taking pioglitazone without talking to your doctor.

Are there other uses for this medicine?

This medication may be prescribed for other uses; ask your doctor or pharmacist for more information.

What special precautions should I follow?

Before taking pioglitazone,
• tell your doctor and pharmacist if you are allergic to pioglitazone or any other medications.
• tell your doctor and pharmacist what prescription and nonprescription medications, vitamins, nutritional supplements and herbal products you are taking or plan to take. Be sure to mention any of the following: atorvastatin (Lipitor), gemfibrozil (Lopid), hormonal contraceptives (birth control pills, patches, rings, implants, and injections), ketoconazole (Nizoral), midazolam, montelukast (Singulair), nifedipine (Procardia), and rif-

ampin (Rifadin, Rifater, in Rifamate). Your doctor may need to change the doses of your medications or monitor you carefully for side effects.

- tell your doctor if you have or have ever had any of the conditions mentioned in the IMPORTANT WARNING section or liver disease.
- tell your doctor if you are pregnant, plan to become pregnant, or are breast-feeding. If you become pregnant while taking pioglitazone, call your doctor. Do not breastfeed while you are taking pioglitazone.
- if you have not yet experienced menopause (change of life; end of monthly periods) you should know that pioglitazone may increase the chance that you will become pregnant even if you do not have regular monthly periods or you have a condition that prevents you from ovulating (releasing an egg from the ovaries). Talk to your doctor about methods of birth control that will work for you.
- if you will be having surgery, including dental surgery, tell the doctor or dentist that you are taking pioglitazone.
- ask your doctor what to do if you get sick, develop an infection or fever, experience unusual stress, or are injured. These conditions can affect your blood sugar and the amount of pioglitazone you may need.

What special dietary instructions should I follow?

Be sure to follow all exercise and dietary recommendations made by your doctor or dietitian. It is important to eat a healthy diet, exercise regularly, and lose weight if necessary. This will help to control your diabetes and help pioglitazone work more effectively.

Alcohol may cause a decrease in blood sugar. Ask your doctor about the safe use of alcoholic beverages while you are taking pioglitazone.

What should I do if I forget to take a dose?

If you remember that same day, take the missed dose as soon as your remember it. However, if you do not remember until the next day, skip the missed dose and continue your regular dosing schedule. Do not take more than one dose in one day and do not take a double dose to make up for a missed one.

What side effects can this medicine cause?

This medication may cause changes in your blood sugar. You should know the symptoms of low and high blood sugar and what to do if you have these symptoms.

You may experience hypoglycemia (low blood sugar) if you are taking this medication in combination with other medications used to treat diabetes. Your doctor will tell you what you should do if you develop hypoglycemia. He or she may tell you to check your blood sugar, eat or drink a food or beverage that contains sugar, such as hard candy or fruit juice, or get medical care. Follow these directions carefully if you have any of the following symptoms of hypoglycemia:

- shakiness

- dizziness or lightheadedness
- sweating
- nervousness or irritability
- sudden changes in behavior or mood
- headache
- numbness or tingling around the mouth
- weakness
- pale skin
- hunger
- clumsy or jerky movements

If hypoglycemia is not treated, severe symptoms may develop. Be sure that your family, friends, and other people who spend time with you know that if you have any of the following symptoms, they should get medical treatment for you immediately.

- confusion
- seizures
- loss of consciousness

Call your doctor immediately if you have any of the following symptoms of hyperglycemia (high blood sugar):

- extreme thirst
- frequent urination
- extreme hunger
- weakness
- blurred vision

If high blood sugar is not treated, a serious, life-threatening condition called diabetic ketoacidosis could develop. Call your doctor immediately if you have any of these symptoms:

- dry mouth
- upset stomach and vomiting
- shortness of breath
- breath that smells fruity
- decreased consciousness

Pioglitazone may cause side effects. Tell your doctor if any of these symptoms are severe or do not go away:

- runny nose and other cold symptoms
- headache
- muscle pain
- tooth or mouth pain
- sore throat

Some side effects can be serious. If you experience any of the following symptoms or those mentioned in the IMPORTANT WARNING section, call your doctor immediately:

- nausea
- vomiting
- loss of appetite
- excessive tiredness
- dark urine
- yellowing of the skin or whites of the eyes
- blurred vision
- vision loss

In clinical studies, more people who took pioglitazone developed bladder cancer than people who did not take pioglitazone. Talk to your doctor about the risk of taking this medication.

In clinical studies, more women who took pioglitazone developed fractures, especially of the hands, arms, feet, ankles, and lower legs than women who did not take pioglitazone. Men who took pioglitazone did not have a greater risk of developing fractures than men who did not take the medication. If you are a woman, talk to your doctor about the risk of taking this medication.

Pioglitazone may cause other side effects. Call your doctor if you have any unusual problems while you are taking this medication.

What storage conditions are needed for this medicine?

Keep this medication in the container it came in, tightly closed, and out of reach of children. Store it at room temperature and away from excess heat and moisture (not in the bathroom). Throw away any medication that is outdated or no longer needed. Talk to your pharmacist about the proper disposal of your medication.

What should I do in case of overdose?

In case of overdose, call your local poison control center at 1-800-222-1222. If the victim has collapsed or is not breathing, call local emergency services at 911.

What other information should I know?

Keep all appointments with your doctor, your eye doctor, and the laboratory. Your doctor will probably order regular eye examinations and certain laboratory tests to check your body's response to rosiglitazone. Your blood sugar and glycosolated hemoglobin should be checked regularly to determine your response to pioglitazone. Your doctor will also tell you how to check your response to pioglitazone by measuring your blood or urine sugar levels at home. Follow these directions carefully.

You should always wear a diabetic identification bracelet to be sure you get proper treatment in an emergency.

Do not let anyone else take your medication. Ask your pharmacist any questions you have about refilling your prescription.

Dosage Facts
For Informational Purposes

Caution: Do not change your dose, how often you take your medication, or the length of time you are to take it without first talking to your healthcare provider.

The following dosage information was written using medical language for doctors and other healthcare professionals and is provided here for you to check your dosage. The dosage of this drug may differ for different patients. Therefore, always follow your doctor's instructions or the directions on the label. Contact your healthcare provider or pharmacist if you have any questions about the specific dosage of your medication after reviewing this information.

General Dosage Information

Available as pioglitazone hydrochloride; dosage expressed in terms of pioglitazone.

Adult Patients

Diabetes Mellitus
Monotherapy

ORAL:
- Initially, 15 or 30 mg once daily. If response is inadequate, increase dosage in increments, up to a maximum dosage of 45 mg daily. If response is inadequate with monotherapy, consider combination therapy.

Combination with Other Antidiabetic Agents

ORAL:
- May continue current dosage of the sulfonylurea, metformin, or insulin upon initiation of pioglitazone.
- Combination therapy with a sulfonylurea: Initially, 15 or 30 mg once daily. If hypoglycemia occurs, reduce sulfonylurea dosage.
- Combination therapy with metformin: Initially, 15 or 30 mg once daily. Adjustment of metformin dosage unlikely.
- Combination therapy with insulin: Initially, 15 or 30 mg once daily. If hypoglycemia occurs or if fasting plasma glucose (FPG) concentrations decrease to <100 mg/dL, decrease insulin dosage by 10–25%. Further adjustments should be individualized based on therapeutic response.

Prescribing Limits

Adult Patients

Maximum 45 mg daily (as monotherapy or in combination with a sulfonylurea, metformin, or insulin).

Special Populations

Renal Impairment
- No dosage adjustment necessary.

Geriatric Patients
- No dosage adjustment necessary.

CHF
- Should be initiated at the lowest approved dosage in patients with type 2 diabetes and systolic CHF (NYHA class II). If subsequent dosage escalation is necessary, increase dosage gradually only after several months of treatment. Monitor carefully for weight gain, edema, or other manifestations of CHF exacerbation. Use not recommended in patients with more severe CHF (NYHA class III or IV).

Pirbuterol Acetate Oral Inhalation

(peer byoo' ter ole)

Brand Name: Maxair Autohaler®

Why is this medicine prescribed?

Pirbuterol is used to prevent and treat wheezing, shortness of breath, and troubled breathing caused by asthma, chronic bronchitis, emphysema, and other lung diseases. Pirbuterol is in a class of medications called beta-agonist bronchodilators. It works by relaxing and opening air passages in the lungs, making it easier to breathe.

How should this medicine be used?

Pirbuterol comes as an aerosol to inhale by mouth. It is usually taken as 1-2 puffs every 4-6 hours as needed to relieve symptoms or every 4-6 hours to prevent symptoms. Follow the directions on your prescription label carefully, and ask your doctor or pharmacist to explain any part you do not understand. Use pirbuterol exactly as directed. Do not use more or less of it or use it more often than prescribed by your doctor. Do not use more than 12 puffs in 24 hours.

Pirbuterol controls symptoms of asthma and other lung diseases but does not cure them. Do not stop using pirbuterol without talking to your doctor.

Before you use the pirbuterol inhaler the first time, read the written instructions that come with it. Ask your doctor, pharmacist, or respiratory therapist to demonstrate the proper technique. Practice using the inhaler while in his or her presence.

The pirbuterol inhaler should be primed (tested) before you use it the first time and any time it has not been used for 48 hours. To prime the inhaler, follow these steps:

1. Remove the mouthpiece cover by pulling down the lip on the back of the cover.
2. Point the mouthpiece away from yourself and other people so that the priming sprays will go into the air.
3. Push the lever up so it stays up.
4. Push the white test fire slide on the bottom of the mouthpiece in the direction indicated by the arrow on the test fire slide. A priming spray will be released.
5. To release a second priming spray, return the lever to its down position and repeat steps 2-4.
6. After the second priming spray is released, return the lever to its down position.

To use the inhaler, follow these steps:

1. Remove the mouthpiece cover by pulling down the lip on the back of the cover. Make sure there are no foreign objects in the mouthpiece.
2. Hold the inhaler upright so that the arrows point up. Then raise the lever so that it snaps into place and stays up.
3. Hold the inhaler around the middle and shake gently several times.
4. Continue to hold the inhaler upright and exhale (breathe out) normally.
5. Seal your lips tightly around the mouthpiece and inhale (breathe in) deeply through the mouthpiece with steady force. You will hear a click and feel a soft puff when the medicine is released. Do not stop when you hear and feel the puff; continue to take a full, deep breath.
6. Take the inhaler away from you mouth, hold your breath for 10 seconds, then exhale slowly.
7. Continue to hold the inhaler upright while lowering the lever. Lower the lever after each inhalation.
8. If your doctor has told you to take more than one inhalation, wait 1 minute and then repeat steps 2-7.
9. When you have finished using the inhaler, make sure the lever is down and replace the mouthpiece cover.

Are there other uses for this medicine?

This medication may be prescribed for other uses; ask your doctor or pharmacist for more information.

What special precautions should I follow?

Before using pirbuterol,

- tell your doctor and pharmacist if you are allergic to pirbuterol or any other drugs.
- tell your doctor and pharmacist what prescription medications you are taking, especially atenolol (Tenormin); carteolol (Cartrol); labetalol (Normodyne, Trandate); metoprolol (Lopressor); nadolol (Corgard); phenelzine (Nardil); propranolol (Inderal); sotalol (Betapace); theophylline (Theo-Dur); timolol (Blocadren); tranylcypromine (Parnate); other medications for asthma, heart disease, or depression.
- tell your doctor and pharmacist what nonprescription medications and vitamins you are taking, including ephedrine, phenylephrine, phenylpropanolamine, or pseudoephedrine. Many nonprescription products contain these drugs (e.g., diet pills and medications for colds and asthma), so check labels carefully. Do not take any of these medications without talking to your doctor (even if you never had a problem taking them before).
- tell your doctor if you have or have ever had an irregular heartbeat, increased heart rate, glaucoma, heart disease, high blood pressure, an overactive thyroid gland, diabetes, or seizures.
- tell your doctor if you are pregnant, plan to become pregnant, or are breast-feeding. If you become pregnant while using pirbuterol, call your doctor.
- if you are having surgery, including dental surgery, tell the doctor or dentist that you are using pirbuterol.

What should I do if I forget to take a dose?

Use the missed dose as soon as you remember it. However, if it is almost time for the next dose, skip the missed dose and continue your regular dosing schedule. Do not take a double dose to make up for a missed one.

What side effects can this medicine cause?

Pirbuterol may cause side effects. Tell your doctor if any of these symptoms are severe or do not go away:

- tremor
- nervousness
- dizziness
- weakness
- headache
- upset stomach
- diarrhea
- cough
- dry mouth
- throat irritation

If you experience any of the following symptoms, call your doctor immediately:

- increased difficulty breathing
- rapid or increased heartbeat
- irregular heartbeat
- chest pain or discomfort

If you experience a serious side effect, you or your doctor may send a report to the Food and Drug Administration's (FDA) MedWatch Adverse Event Reporting program online [at http://www.fda.gov/MedWatch/index.html] or by phone [1-800-332-1088].

What storage conditions are needed for this medicine?

Keep this medication in the container it came in, tightly closed, and out of reach of children. Store it at room temperature and away from excess heat and moisture (not in the bathroom). Throw away any medication that is outdated or no longer needed. Talk to your pharmacist about the proper disposal of your medication. Avoid puncturing the container, and do not discard it in an incinerator or fire.

What other information should I know?

Keep all appointments with your doctor and the laboratory. Your doctor will order certain lab tests to check your response to pirbuterol.

To relieve dry mouth or throat irritation, rinse your mouth with water, chew gum, or suck sugarless hard candy after using pirbuterol.

Inhalation devices require regular cleaning. Once a week, remove the mouthpiece cover, turn the inhaler upside down and wipe the mouthpiece with a clean dry cloth. Gently tap the back of the inhaler so the flap comes down and the spray hole can be seen. Clean the surface of the flap with a dry cotton swab.

Do not let anyone else use your medication. Ask your pharmacist any questions you have about refilling your prescription.

Talk to your doctor, pharmacist, or other healthcare professional if you have questions about dosing information for your medication.

Piroxicam

(peer ox' i kam)

Brand Name: Feldene®
Also available generically.

Important Warning

People who take nonsteroidal anti-inflammatory medications (NSAIDs) (other than aspirin) such as piroxicam may have a higher risk of having a heart attack or a stroke than people who do not take these medications. These events may happen without warning and may cause death. This risk may be higher for people who take NSAIDs for a long time. Tell your doctor if you or anyone in your family has or has ever had heart disease, a heart attack, or a stroke, if you smoke, and if you have or have ever had high cholesterol, high blood pressure, or diabetes. Get emergency medical help right away if you experience any of the following symptoms: chest pain, shortness of breath, weakness in one part or side of the body, or slurred speech.

If you will be undergoing a coronary artery bypass graft (CABG; a type of heart surgery), you should not take piroxicam right before or right after the surgery.

NSAIDs such as piroxicam may cause ulcers, bleeding, or holes in the stomach or intestine. These problems may develop at any time during treatment, may happen without warning symptoms, and may cause death. The risk may be higher for people who take NSAIDs for a long time, are older in age, have poor health, or drink large amounts of alcohol while you are taking piroxicam. Tell your doctor if you take any of the following medications: anticoagulants ('blood thinners') such as warfarin (Coumadin); aspirin; other NSAIDs such as ibuprofen (Advil, Motrin) and naproxen (Aleve, Naprosyn); or oral steroids such as dexamethasone (Decadron, Dexone), methylprednisolone (Medrol), and prednisone (Deltasone). Also tell your doctor if you have or have ever had ulcers or bleeding in your stomach or intestines or other bleeding disorders. If you experience any of the following symptoms, stop taking piroxicam and call your doctor: stomach pain, heartburn, vomiting a substance that is bloody or looks like coffee grounds, blood in the stool, or black and tarry stools.

Keep all appointments with your doctor and the laboratory. Your doctor will monitor your symptoms carefully and will probably order certain tests to check your body's response to piroxicam. Be sure to tell your doctor how you are feeling so that your doctor can prescribe the right amount of medication to treat your condition with the lowest risk of serious side effects.

Your doctor or pharmacist will give you the manufacturer's patient information sheet (Medication Guide) when you begin treatment with piroxicam and each time you refill your prescription. Read the information carefully and ask your doctor or pharmacist if you have any questions. You can also visit the Food and Drug Administration (FDA) website (http://www.fda.gov/cder) or the manufacturer's website to obtain the Medication Guide.

Why is this medicine prescribed?

Piroxicam is used to relieve pain, tenderness, swelling, and stiffness caused by osteoarthritis (arthritis caused by a breakdown of the lining of the joints) and rheumatoid arthritis (arthritis caused by swelling of the lining of the joints). Piroxicam is in a class of medications called NSAIDs. It works by stopping the body's production of a substance that causes pain, fever, and inflammation.

How should this medicine be used?

Piroxicam comes as a capsule to take by mouth. It is usually taken once or twice a day. Take piroxicam at around the same time(s) every day. Follow the directions on your prescription label carefully, and ask your doctor or pharmacist to explain any part you do not understand. Take piroxicam exactly as directed. Do not take more or less of it or take it more often than prescribed by your doctor.

Piroxicam will help control your symptoms but will not cure your condition. It may take 8-12 weeks or longer before you feel the full benefit of piroxicam.

Are there other uses for this medicine?

Piroxicam is also sometimes used to treat gouty arthritis (attacks of severe joint pain and swelling caused by a build-up of certain substances in the joints) and ankylosing spondylitis (arthritis that mainly affects the spine). It is also sometimes used to relieve muscle pain and swelling, menstrual pain, and pain after surgery or childbirth. Talk to your doctor about the risks of using this medication for your condition.

What special precautions should I follow?

Before taking piroxicam,
- tell your doctor and pharmacist if you are allergic to piroxicam, aspirin, or other NSAIDs such as ibuprofen (Advil, Motrin) and naproxen (Aleve, Naprosyn), or any other medications.
- tell your doctor and pharmacist what prescription and nonprescription medications, vitamins, nutritional supplements, and herbal products you are taking or plan to take. Be sure to mention the medications listed in the IMPORTANT WARNING section and any of the following: angiotensin-converting enzyme (ACE) inhibi-

tors such as benazepril (Lotensin), captopril (Capoten), enalapril (Vasotec), fosinopril (Monopril), lisinopril (Prinivil, Zestril), moexipril (Univasc), perindopril (Aceon), quinapril (Accupril), ramipril (Altace), and trandolapril (Mavik); diuretics ('water pills'); lithium (Eskalith, Lithobid); medications for diabetes; methotrexate (Rheumatrex); and phenytoin (Dilantin).
- tell your doctor if you have or have ever had asthma, especially if you also have frequent stuffy or runny nose or nasal polyps (swelling of the lining of the nose); swelling of the hands, feet, ankles, or lower legs; or liver, or kidney disease.
- tell your doctor if you are pregnant, especially if you are in the last few months of your pregnancy, you plan to become pregnant, or you are breast-feeding. If you become pregnant while taking piroxicam, call your doctor.
- if you are having surgery, including dental surgery, tell the doctor or dentist that you are taking piroxicam.

What special dietary instructions should I follow?

Unless your doctor tells you otherwise, continue your normal diet.

What should I do if I forget to take a dose?

Take the missed dose as soon as you remember it. However, if it is almost time for the next dose, skip the missed dose and continue your regular dosing schedule. Do not take a double dose to make up for a missed one.

What side effects can this medicine cause?

Piroxicam may cause side effects. Tell your doctor if any of these symptoms are severe or do not go away:
- diarrhea
- constipation
- gas
- headache
- dizziness
- ringing in the ears

Some side effects can be serious. If you experience any of the following symptoms or those mentioned in the IMPORTANT WARNING section, call your doctor immediately. Do not take any more piroxicam until you speak to your doctor.
- vision problems
- unexplained weight gain
- fever
- blisters
- joint pain
- rash
- itching
- hives
- swelling of the eyes, face, lips, tongue, throat, arms, hands, feet, ankles, or lower legs
- difficulty breathing or swallowing

- hoarseness
- pale skin
- fast hearbeat
- excessive tiredness
- unusual bleeding or bruising
- lack of energy
- upset stomach
- loss of appetite
- pain in the upper right part of the stomach
- flu-like symptoms
- yellowing of the skin or eyes
- cloudy, discolored, or bloody urine
- back pain
- difficult or painful urination

Piroxicam may cause other side effects. Call your doctor if you have any unusual problems while taking this medication.

If you experience a serious side effect, you or your doctor may send a report to the Food and Drug Administration's (FDA) MedWatch Adverse Event Reporting program online [at http://www.fda.gov/MedWatch/index.html] or by phone [1-800-332-1088].

What storage conditions are needed for this medicine?

Keep this medication in the container it came in, tightly closed, and out of reach of children. Store it at room temperature and away from excess heat and moisture (not in the bathroom). Throw away any medication that is outdated or no longer needed. Talk to your pharmacist about the proper disposal of your medication.

What should I do in case of overdose?

In case of overdose, call your local poison control center at 1-800-222-1222. If the victim has collapsed or is not breathing, call local emergency services at 911.

Symptoms of overdose may include:
- lack of energy
- drowsiness
- upset stomach
- vomiting
- stomach pain
- bloody, black, or tarry stools
- vomiting a substance that is bloody or looks like coffee grounds
- difficulty breathing
- coma (loss of consciousness for a period of time)

What other information should I know?

Do not let anyone else take your medication. Ask your pharmacist any questions you have about refilling your prescription.

Dosage Facts
For Informational Purposes

Caution: Do not change your dose, how often you take your medication, or the length of time you are to take it without first talking to your healthcare provider.

The following dosage information was written using medical language for doctors and other healthcare professionals and is provided here for you to check your dosage. The dosage of this drug may differ for different patients. Therefore, always follow your doctor's instructions or the directions on the label. Contact your healthcare provider or pharmacist if you have any questions about the specific dosage of your medication after reviewing this information.

General Dosage Information

To minimize the potential risk of adverse cardiovascular and/or GI events, use lowest effective dosage and shortest duration of therapy consistent with patient's treatment goals. Adjust dosage based on individual requirements and response; attempt to titrate to lowest effective dosage.

Adult Patients

Inflammatory Diseases
Osteoarthritis or Rheumatoid Arthritis

ORAL:
- Initially, 20 mg daily.Adjust dosage based on response and tolerance; 30 or 40 mg daily may be required for maintenance therapy, although 20 mg daily is usually adequate.

Prescribing Limits

Adult Patients

Inflammatory Diseases

ORAL:
- Dosages >20 mg daily associated with increased frequency of adverse GI effects.

Special Populations

Hepatic Impairment

Inflammatory Diseases
- Dosage reduction may be required.

Pneumococcal Conjugate Vaccine

Brand Name: Prevnar®

Why get vaccinated?

Infection with *Streptococcus pneumoniae* bacteria can cause serious illness and death. Invasive pneumococcal disease is responsible for about 200 deaths each year among children under 5 years old. It is the leading cause of bacterial meningitis in the United States. (Meningitis is an infection of the covering of the brain).

Pneumococcal infection causes severe disease in children under five years old. Before a vaccine was available, each year pneumococcal infection caused: over 700 cases of meningitis, 13,000 blood infections, and about 5 million ear infections.

It can also lead to other health problems, including: pneumonia, deafness, brain damage.

Children under 2 years old are at highest risk for serious disease.

Pneumococcus bacteria are spread from person to person through close contact.

Pneumococcal infections can be hard to treat because the bacteria have become resistant to some of the drugs that have been used to treat them. This makes prevention of pneumococcal infections even more important.

Pneumococcal conjugate vaccine can help prevent serious pneumococcal disease, such as meningitis and blood infections. It can also prevent some ear infections. But ear infections have many causes, and pneumococcal vaccine is effective against only some of them.

Pneumococcal conjugate vaccine

Pneumococcal conjugate vaccine is approved for infants and toddlers. Children who are vaccinated when they are infants will be protected when they are at greatest risk for serious disease.

Some older children and adults may get a different vaccine called pneumococcal polysaccharide vaccine. There is a separate Vaccine Information Statement for people getting this vaccine.

Who should get the vaccine and when?

- **Children Under 2 Years of Age**

    The routine schedule for pneumococcal conjugate vaccine is 4 doses, one dose at each of these ages: 2 months, 6 months, 4 months, 12-15 months.

    Children who weren't vaccinated at these ages can still get the vaccine. The number of doses needed depends on the child's age. Ask your health care provider for details.

- **Children Between 2 and 5 Years of Age**

    Pneumococcal conjugate vaccine is also recommended for children between 2 and 5 years old who have not already gotten the vaccine and are at high risk of serious pneumococcal disease. This includes children who: have sickle cell disease; have a damaged spleen or no spleen; have HIV/AIDS; have other diseases that affect the immune system, such as diabetes, cancer, or liver disease, or who take medications that affect the immune system, such as chemotherapy or steroids; or have chronic heart or lung disease.

    The vaccine should be considered for all other children under 5 years, especially those at higher risk of serious pneumococcal disease. This includes children who: are under 3 years of age; are of Alaska Native, American Indian or African American descent; or attend group day care.

    The number of doses needed depends on the child's age. Ask your health care provider for more details.

    Pneumococcal conjugate vaccine may be given at the same time as other vaccines.

Which children should not get pneumococcal conjugate vaccine or should wait?

Children should not get pneumococcal conjugate vaccine if they had a serious (life-threatening) allergic reaction to a previous dose of this vaccine, or have a severe allergy to a vaccine component. Tell your health-care provider if your child has ever had a severe reaction to any vaccine, or has any severe allergies.

Children with minor illnesses, such as a cold, may be vaccinated. But children who are moderately or severely ill should usually wait until they recover before getting the vaccine.

What are the risks from pneumococcal conjugate vaccine?

In studies (nearly 60,000 doses), pneumococcal conjugate vaccine was associated with only mild reactions:

- Up to about 1 infant out of 4 had redness, tenderness, or swelling where the shot was given.
- Up to about 1 out of 3 had a fever of over 100.4°F, and up to about 1 in 50 had a higher fever (over 102.2°F).
- Some children also became fussy or drowsy, or had a loss of appetite.

So far, no serious reactions have been associated with this vaccine. However, a vaccine, like any medicine, could cause serious problems, such as a severe allergic reaction. The risk of this vaccine causing serious harm, or death, is extremely small.

What if there is a moderate or severe reaction?

What should I look for?

- Look for any unusual condition, such as a serious allergic reaction, high fever, or unusual behavior.

- Serious allergic reactions are extremely rare with any vaccine. If one were to occur, it would most likely be within a few minutes to a few hours after the shot. Signs can include: difficulty breathing, weakness, hives, hoarseness or wheezing, fast heart beat, paleness, swelling of the throat, dizziness.

What should I do?

- Call a doctor, or get the person to a doctor right away.
- Tell your doctor what happened, the date and time it happened, and when the vaccination was given.
- Ask your health care provider to file a Vaccine Adverse Event Reporting System (VAERS) form if you have any reaction to the vaccine. Or call VAERS yourself at 1-800-822-7967, or visit their website at http://vaers.hhs.gov.

The National Vaccine Injury Compensation Program

In the rare event that you or your child has a serious reaction to a vaccine, a federal program has been created to help pay for the care of those who have been harmed.

For details about the National Vaccine Injury Compensation Program, call 1-800-338-2382 or visit the program's website at http://www.hrsa.gov/vaccinecompensation.

How can I learn more?

- Ask your doctor or other health care provider. They can give you the vaccine package insert or suggest other sources of information.
- Call your local or state health department's immunization program.
- Contact the Centers for Disease Control and Prevention (CDC): call 1-800-232-4636 (1-800-CDC-INFO) or visit the National Immunization Program's website at http://www.cdc.gov/nip.

Pneumococcal Conjugate Vaccine Information Statement. U.S. Department of Health and Human Services/Centers for Disease Control and Prevention National Immunization Program. 9/30/2002.

Pneumococcal Polysaccharide Vaccine

Brand Name: Pneumovax® 23

Why get vaccinated?

Pneumococcal disease is a serious disease that causes much sickness and death. In fact, pneumococcal disease kills more people in the United States each year than all other vaccine preventable diseases combined. Anyone can get pneumococcal disease. However, some people are at greater

risk from the disease. These include people 65 and older, the very young, and people with special health problems such as alcoholism, heart or lung disease, kidney failure, diabetes, HIV infection, or certain types of cancer.

Pneumococcal disease can lead to serious infections of the lungs (pneumonia), the blood (bacteremia), and the covering of the brain (meningitis). About 1 out of every 20 people who get pneumococcal pneumonia dies from it, as do about 2 people out of 10 who get bacteremia and 3 people out of 10 who get meningitis. People with the special health problems mentioned above are even more likely to die from the diease.

Drugs such as penicillin were once effective in treating these infections; but the disease has become more resistant to these drugs, making treatment of pneumococcal infections more difficult. This makes prevention of the disease through vaccination even more important.

Pneumococcal polysaccharide vaccine (PPV)

The pneumococcal polysaccharide vaccine (PPV) protects against 23 types of pneumococcal bacteria. Most healthy adults who get the vaccine develop protection to most or all of these types within 2 to 3 weeks of getting the shot. Very old people, children under 2 years of age, and people with some long-term illnesses might not respond as well or at all.

Who should get PPV?

- All adults 65 years of age or older.
- Anyone over 2 years of age who has a long term health problem such as: heart disease, lung disease, sickle cell disease, diabetes, alcoholism, cirrhosis, leaks of cerebrospinal fluid.
- Anyone over 2 years of age who has a disease or condition that lowers the body's resistance to infection, such as: Hodgkin's disease; lymphoma, leukemia; kidney failure; multiple myeloma; nephrotic syndrome; HIV infection or AIDS; damaged spleen, or no spleen; organ transplant.
- Anyone over 2 years of age who is taking any drug or treatment that lowers the body's resistance to infection, such as: long-term steroids, certain cancer drugs, radiation therapy.
- Alaskan Natives and certain Native American populations.

How many doses of PPV are needed?

Usually one dose of PPV is all that is needed. However, under some circumstances a second dose may be given.

A second dose is also recommended for people who:
- have a damaged spleen or no spleen
- have sickle-cell disease
- have HIV infection or AIDS
- have cancer, leukemia, lymphoma, multiple myeloma
- have kidney failure

- have nephrotic syndrome
- have had an organ or bone marrow transplant
- are taking medication that lowers immunity (such as chemotherapy or long-term steroids)

Children 10 years old and younger may get this second dose 3 years after the first dose. Those older than 10 should get it 5 years after the first dose.

Other facts about getting the vaccine

Otherwise healthy children who often get ear infections, sinus infections, or other upper respiratory diseases do not need to get PPV because of these conditions.

PPV may be less effective in some people, especially those with lower resistance to infection. But these people should still be vaccinated, because they are more likely to get seriously ill from pneumococcal disease.

Pregnancy: The safety of PPV for pregnant women has not yet been studied. There is no evidence that the vaccine is harmful to either the mother or the fetus, but pregnant women should consult with their doctor before being vaccinated. Women who are at high risk of pneumococcal disease should be vaccinated before becoming pregnant, if possible.

What are the risks from PPV?

PPV is a very safe vaccine.

About half of those who get the vaccine have very mild side effects, such as redness or pain where the shot is given. Less than 1% develop a fever, muscle aches, or more severe local reactions.

Severe allergic reactions have been reported very rarely. As with any medicine, there is a very small risk that serious problems, even death, could occur after getting a vaccine.

Getting the disease is much more likely to cause serious problems than getting the vaccine.

What if there is a moderate or severe reaction?

What should I look for?

- Severe allergic reaction (hives, difficulty breathing, shock).

 What should I do?

- Call a doctor, or get the person to a doctor right away.
- Tell your doctor what happened, the date and time it happened, and when the vaccination was given.
- Ask your health care provider to file a Vaccine Adverse Event Reporting System (VAERS) form if you have any reaction to the vaccine. Or call VAERS yourself at 1-800-822-7967, or visit their website at http://vaers.hhs.gov.

The National Vaccine Injury Compensation Program

In the rare event that you or your child has a serious reaction to a vaccine, a federal program has been created to help pay for the care of those who have been harmed.

For details about the National Vaccine Injury Compensation Program, call 1-800-338-2382 or visit the program's website at http://www.hrsa.gov/vaccinecompensation.

How can I learn more?

- Ask your doctor or other health care provider. They can give you the vaccine package insert or suggest other sources of information.
- Call your local or state health department's immunization program.
- Contact the Centers for Disease Control and Prevention (CDC): call 1-800-232-4636 (1-800-CDC-INFO) or visit the National Immunization Program's website at http://www.cdc.gov/nip.

Pneumococcal Polysaccharide Vaccine Information Statement. U.S. Department of Health and Human Services/ Centers for Disease Control and Prevention National Immunization Program. 7/29/1997.

Polio Vaccine

Brand Name: IPOL®, Orimune® Trivalent

What is polio?

Polio is a disease caused by a virus. It enters a child's (or adult's) body through the mouth. Sometimes it does not cause serious illness. But sometimes it causes paralysis (can't move arm or leg). It can kill people who get it, usually by paralyzing the muscles that help them breathe.

Polio used to be very common in the United States. It paralyzed and killed thousands of people a year before we had a vaccine for it.

Why get vaccinated?

Inactivated Polio Vaccine (IPV) can prevent polio.

History: A 1916 polio epidemic in the United States killed 6,000 people and paralyzed 27,000 more. In the early 1950's there were more than 20,000 cases of polio each year. Polio vaccination was begun in 1955. By 1960 the number of cases had dropped to about 3,000, and by 1979 there were only about 10. The success of polio vaccination in the U.S. and other countries sparked a world-wide effort to eliminate polio.

Today: No wild polio has been reported in the United States for over 20 years. But the disease is still common in some parts of the world. It would only take one case of polio from another country to bring the disease back if we were not protected by vaccine. If the effort to eliminate the disease from the world is successful, some day we won't need polio vaccine. Until then, we need to keep getting our children vaccinated.

Why is Oral Polio Vaccine no longer recommended?

There are two kinds of polio vaccine: IPV, which is the shot recommended in the United States today, and a live, oral polio vaccine (OPV), which is drops that are swallowed.

Until recently OPV was recommended for most children in the United States. OPV helped us rid the country of polio, and it is still used in many parts of the world.

Both vaccines give immunity to polio, but OPV is better at keeping the disease from spreading to other people. However, for a few people (about one in 2.4 million), OPV actually causes polio. Since the risk of getting polio in the United States is now extremely low, experts believe that using oral polio vaccine is no longer worth the slight risk, except in limited circumstances which your doctor can describe. The polio shot (IPV) does not cause polio.

Who should get polio vaccine and when?

IPV is a shot, given in the leg or arm, depending on age. Polio vaccine may be given at the same time as other vaccines.

Children: Most people should get polio vaccine when they are children. Children get 4 doses of IPV, at these ages: 2 months, 6-18 months, 4 months, 4-6 years.

Adults: Most adults do not need polio vaccine because they were already vaccinated as children. But three groups of adults are at higher risk and should consider polio vaccination: (1) people traveling to areas of the world where polio is common, (2) laboratory workers who might handle polio virus, and (3) health care workers treating patients who could have polio.

Adults in these three groups who have never been vaccinated against polio should get 3 doses of IPV: the first dose at any time, the second dose 1 to 2 months later, the third dose 6 to 12 months after the second.

Adults in these three groups who have had 1 or 2 doses of polio vaccine in the past should get the remaining 1 or 2 doses. It doesn't matter how long it has been since the earlier dose(s).

Adults in these three groups who have had 3 or more doses of polio vaccine (either IPV or OPV) in the past may get a booster dose of IPV.

Ask your health care provider for more information.

Who should *not* get IPV or should wait?

These people should not get IPV:

- Anyone who has ever had a life-threatening allergic reaction to the antibiotics neomycin, streptomycin or polymyxin B should not get the polio shot.
- Anyone who has a severe allergic reaction to a polio shot should not get another one.

These people should wait:

- Anyone who is moderately or severely ill at the time the shot is scheduled should usually wait until they recover before getting polio vaccine. People with minor illnesses, such as a cold, *may* be vaccinated.

What are the risks from IPV?

Some people who get IPV get a sore spot where the shot was given. The vaccine used today has never been known to cause any serious problems, and most people don't have any problems at all with it.

However, a vaccine, like any medicine, could cause serious problems, such as a severe allergic reaction. The risk of a polio shot causing serious harm, or death, is extremely small.

What if there is a serious reaction?

What should I look for?

- Look for any unusual condition, such as a serious allergic reaction, high fever, or unusual behavior.
- If a serious allergic reaction occurred, it would happen within a few minutes to a few hours after the shot. Signs of a serious allergic reaction can include difficulty breathing, weakness, hoarseness or wheezing, a fast heart beat, hives, dizziness, paleness, or swelling of the throat.

What should I do?

- Call a doctor, or get the person to a doctor right away.
- Tell your doctor what happened, the date and time it happened, and when the vaccination was given.
- Ask your health care provider to file a Vaccine Adverse Event Reporting System (VAERS) form if you have any reaction to the vaccine. Or call VAERS yourself at 1-800-822-7967, or visit their website at http://vaers.hhs.gov.

The National Vaccine Injury Compensation Program

In the rare event that you or your child has a serious reaction to a vaccine, a federal program has been created to help pay for the care of those who have been harmed.

For details about the National Vaccine Injury Compensation Program, call 1-800-338-2382 or visit the program's website at http://www.hrsa.gov/vaccinecompensation.

How can I learn more?

- Ask your doctor or other health care provider. They can give you the vaccine package insert or suggest other sources of information.
- Call your local or state health department's immunization program.
- Contact the Centers for Disease Control and Prevention (CDC): call 1-800-232-4636 (1-800-CDC-INFO) or visit the National Immunization Program's website at http://www.cdc.gov/nip.

Polio Vaccine Information Statement. U.S. Department of Health and Human Services/Centers for Disease Control and Prevention National Immunization Program. 1/1/2000.

Polyethylene Glycol 3350

(pol ee eth′ i leen glye′ col)

Brand Name: MiraLax®

Why is this medicine prescribed?

Polyethylene glycol 3350 is used to treat occasional constipation. Polyethylene glycol 3350 is in a class of medications called osmotic laxatives. It works by causing water to be retained with the stool. This increases the number of bowel movements and softens the stool so it is easier to pass.

How should this medicine be used?

Polyethylene glycol 3350 comes as a powder to be mixed with a liquid and taken by mouth. It is usually taken once a day as needed for up to 2 weeks. Follow the directions on your prescription label carefully, and ask your doctor or pharmacist to explain any part you do not understand. Take polyethylene glycol 3350 exactly as directed.

Polyethylene glycol 3350 may be habit-forming. Do not take a larger dose, take it more often, or take it for a longer period of time than your doctor tells you to.

It may take 2 to 4 days for polyethylene glycol 3350 to produce a bowel movement.

To use the powder, follow these steps:

1. If you are using polyethylene glycol 3350 from a bottle, use the measuring line on the bottle cap to measure a single dose (about 1 heaping tablespoon). If you are using polyethylene glycol 3350 packets, each packet contains a single dose.
2. Pour the powder into a cup containing 8 ounces of water, juice, soda, coffee, or tea.
3. Stir to dissolve the powder.
4. Drink immediately.

Are there other uses for this medicine?

This medication may be prescribed for other uses; ask your doctor or pharmacist for more information.

What special precautions should I follow?

Before taking polyethylene glycol 3350,

- tell your doctor and pharmacist if you are allergic to polyethylene glycol or any other medications.
- tell your doctor and pharmacist what prescription and nonprescription medications, vitamins, nutritional supplements, and herbal products you are taking.
- tell your doctor if you have or have ever had a bowel obstruction (blockage in the intestine) and if you have symptoms of bowel obstruction (upset stomach, vomiting, and stomach pain or bloating).
- tell your doctor if you are pregnant, plan to become

pregnant, or are breast-feeding. If you become pregnant while taking polyethylene glycol 3350, call your doctor.

What special dietary instructions should I follow?

Eat a well-balanced diet that includes fiber-rich foods, such as unprocessed bran, whole-grain bread, and fresh fruits and vegetables. Drink plenty of fluids and exercise regularly.

What should I do if I forget to take a dose?

This medication is usually taken as needed.

What side effects can this medicine cause?

Polyethylene glycol 3350 may cause side effects. Tell your doctor if any of these symptoms are severe or do not go away:

- upset stomach
- bloating
- cramping
- gas

Some side effects can be serious. The following symptoms are uncommon, but if you experience either of them, call your doctor immediately:

- diarrhea
- hives

Polyethylene glycol 3350 may cause other side effects. Call your doctor if you have any unusual problems while taking this medication.

If you experience a serious side effect, you or your doctor may send a report to the Food and Drug Administration's (FDA) MedWatch Adverse Event Reporting program online [at http://www.fda.gov/MedWatch/index.html] or by phone [1-800-332-1088].

What storage conditions are needed for this medicine?

Keep this medication in the container it came in, tightly closed, and out of reach of children. Store it at room temperature and away from excess heat and moisture (not in the bathroom). Throw away any medication that is outdated or no longer needed. Talk to your pharmacist about the proper disposal of your medication.

What should I do in case of overdose?

In case of overdose, call your local poison control center at 1-800-222-1222. If the victim has collapsed or is not breathing, call local emergency services at 911.

Symptoms of overdose may include:

- diarrhea
- thirst
- confusion
- seizure

What other information should I know?

Keep all appointments with your doctor.

Do not let anyone else take your medication. Ask your

pharmacist any questions you have about refilling your prescription.

Talk to your doctor, pharmacist, or other healthcare professional if you have questions about dosing information for your medication.

Polyethylene glycol-electrolyte solution (PEG-ES)

(pol ee eth′ i leen glye′ col)

Brand Name: CoLyte®, GoLYTELY®

Why is this medicine prescribed?

Polyethylene glycol-electrolyte solution (PEG-ES) is used to cleanse the bowel before a gastrointestinal examination or surgery. It works by causing diarrhea.

This medication is sometimes prescribed for other uses; ask your doctor or pharmacist for more information.

How should this medicine be used?

Polyethylene glycol-electrolyte solution (PEG-ES) comes as a powder to take by mouth. You should prepare the solution in the container; follow the instructions on the label carefully. An 8-ounce glass of solution should be rapidly swallowed every 10 minutes until the prescribed amount of liquid has been taken or your stool is watery, clear, and free of solid matter. Your doctor will tell you at what time you should begin drinking PEG-ES. You should not eat for at least 3-4 hours before you are told to begin drinking PEG-ES. You should not take any oral medications within 1 hour of starting PEG-ES. You should begin having bowel movements within 1 hour of beginning PEG-ES. Follow the directions on your prescription label carefully, and ask your doctor or pharmacist to explain any part you do not understand. Take PEG-ES exactly as directed. Do not take more or less of it or take it more often than prescribed by your doctor.

What special precautions should I follow?

Before taking PEG-ES,
- tell your doctor and pharmacist if you are allergic to PEG-ES or any other drugs.
- tell your doctor and pharmacist what prescription and nonprescription medications you are taking, including vitamins or herbal products.
- tell your doctor if you have or have ever had a gastrointestinal disease or obstruction.
- tell your doctor if you are pregnant, plan to become pregnant, or are breastfeeding.

What side effects can this medicine cause?

PEG-ES may cause side effects. Tell your doctor if any of these symptoms are severe or do not go away:
- upset stomach
- stomach pain
- bloating
- vomiting
- rectal irritation

If you experience any of the following symptoms, call your doctor immediately:
- rash
- hives
- skin irritation

If you experience a serious side effect, you or your doctor may send a report to the Food and Drug Administration's (FDA) MedWatch Adverse Event Reporting program online [at http://www.fda.gov/MedWatch/index.html] or by phone [1-800-332-1088].

What storage conditions are needed for this medicine?

Keep this medication in the container it came in, tightly closed, and out of reach of children. Store the mixed solution in the refrigerator and use it within 48 hours. Throw away any medication that is outdated or no longer needed. Talk to your pharmacist about the proper disposal of your medication.

What other information should I know?

Keep all appointments with your doctor and the laboratory.

Do not let anyone else take your medication. Ask your pharmacist any questions you have about refilling your prescription.

Talk to your doctor, pharmacist, or other healthcare professional if you have questions about dosing information for your medication.

Posaconazole

(poe″ sa kon′ a zole)

Brand Name: Noxafil®

Why is this medicine prescribed?

Posaconazole is used to prevent serious fungal infections in people with a weakened ability to fight infection. Posaconazole is also used to treat yeast infections of the mouth and throat including yeast infections that could not be treated successfully with other medications. Posaconazole is in a class of antifungals called triazoles. It works by slowing the growth of fungi that cause infection.

How should this medicine be used?

Posaconazole comes as a suspension (liquid) to take by mouth. Each dose should be taken with a full meal or liquid nutritional supplement. When posaconazole is used to prevent fungal infections, it is usually taken three times a day. When posaconazole is used to treat yeast infections of the mouth and throat, it is usually taken once or twice a day. The length of your treatment depends on your general health, the type of infection you have, and how well you respond to this medication. Take posaconazole at around the same times every day. Follow the directions on your prescription label carefully, and ask your doctor or pharmacist to explain any part you do not understand. Take posaconazole exactly as directed. Do not take more or less of it or take it more often than prescribed by your doctor.

Shake the liquid well before each use to mix the medication evenly.

Posaconazole comes with a dosing spoon to measure your dose. The spoon should be rinsed thoroughly with water after each use and before storing.

Continue to take posaconazole until your doctor tells you that you should stop, even if you feel better. Do not stop taking posaconazole without talking to your doctor. If you stop taking posaconazole too soon, your infection may not be completely treated.

Are there other uses for this medicine?

This medication may be prescribed for other uses; ask your doctor or pharmacist for more information.

What special precautions should I follow?

Before taking posaconazole,

- tell your doctor and pharmacist if you are allergic to posaconazole; other antifungal medications such as fluconazole (Diflucan), itraconazole (Sporanox), ketoconazole (Nizoral), or voriconazole (Vfend); simethicone; any other medications; or any of the ingredients in posaconazole. Ask your pharmacist for a list of the ingredients.
- do not take posaconazole if you are taking any of the following medications: astemizole (Hismanal) (not available in the U.S.); cisapride (Propulsid); ergot-type medications such as bromocriptine (Parlodel), cabergoline (Dostinex), dihydroergotamine (D.H.E. 45, Migranal), ergoloid mesylates (Germinal, Hydergine), ergonovine (Ergotrate), ergotamine (Bellergal-S, Cafergot, Ergomar, Wigraine), methylergonovine (Methergine), and pergolide (Permax); halofantrine (Halfan) (not available in the U.S.); pimozide (Orap); quinidine; or terfenadine (Seldane) (not available in the U.S.).
- tell your doctor and pharmacist what other prescription and nonprescription medications, vitamins, nutritional supplements, and herbal products you are taking or plan to take. Be sure to mention any of the following: benzodiazepines such as alprazolam (Xanax), diazepam (Valium), midazolam (Versed), and triazolam (Hal-

cion); calcium channel blockers such as amlodipine (Norvasc), diltiazem (Cardizem, Dilacor, Tiazac, others), felodipine (Plendil), nifedipine (Adalat, Procardia), nisoldipine (Sular), and verapamil (Calan, Isoptin, Verelan); cholesterol-lowering medications (statins) such as atorvastatin (Lipitor), lovastatin (Mevacor), and simvastatin (Zocor); cimetidine (Tagamet); cyclosporine (Gengraf, Neoral, Sandimmune); erythromycin (E.E.S., E-Mycin, Erythrocin), glipizide (Glucotrol); phenytoin (Dilantin, Phenytek); rifabutin (Mycobutin); sirolimus (Rapamune); tacrolimus (Prograf); vinblastine; and vincristine. Many other medications may also interact with posaconazole, so be sure to tell your doctor about all the medications you are taking, even those that do not appear on this list. Your doctor may need to change the doses of your medications or monitor you carefully for side effects.

- tell your doctor if you cannot eat a full meal or liquid nutritional supplement and if you have or have ever had an irregular heartbeat; kidney or liver disease; or low levels of calcium, magnesium, or potassium in your blood. Also tell your doctor if you develop severe diarrhea or vomiting at any time during your treatment.
- tell your doctor if you are pregnant, plan to become pregnant, or are breast-feeding. If you become pregnant while taking posaconazole, call your doctor.

What special dietary instructions should I follow?

Unless your doctor tells you otherwise, continue your normal diet.

What should I do if I forget to take a dose?

Take the missed dose as soon as you remember it. However, if it is almost time for the next dose, skip the missed dose and continue your regular dosing schedule. Do not take a double dose to make up for a missed one.

What side effects can this medicine cause?

Posaconazole may cause side effects. Tell your doctor if any of these symptoms are severe or do not go away;

- fever
- headache
- chills or shaking
- dizziness
- weakness
- swelling of the hands, feet, ankles, or lower legs
- diarrhea
- vomiting
- stomach pain
- constipation
- heartburn
- weight loss
- rash
- itching
- back or muscle pain

- sores on the lips, mouth, or throat
- difficulty falling asleep or staying asleep
- anxiety
- increased sweating
- nosebleeds
- coughing

Some side effects can be serious. If you experience any of these symptoms, call your doctor immediately:

- unusual bruising or bleeding
- extreme tiredness
- lack of energy
- loss of appetite
- nausea
- pain in the upper right part of the stomach
- yellowing of the skin or eyes
- flu-like symptoms
- dark urine
- pale stools
- fast, pounding, or irregular heartbeat
- sudden loss of consciousness
- shortness of breath
- decreased urination

Posaconazole may cause other side effects. Call your doctor if you have any unusual problems while taking this medication.

What storage conditions are needed for this medicine?

Keep this medication in the container it came in, tightly closed, and out of reach of children. Store it at room temperature and away from excess heat and moisture (not in the bathroom). Do not freeze this medication. Throw away any medication that is outdated or no longer needed. Talk to your pharmacist about the proper disposal of your medication.

What should I do in case of overdose?

In case of overdose, call your local poison control center at 1-800-222-1222. If the victim has collapsed or is not breathing, call local emergency services at 911.

What other information should I know?

Keep all appointments with your doctor and the laboratory. Your doctor will order certain lab tests to check your body's response to posaconazole.

Do not let anyone else take your medication. Ask your pharmacist any questions you have about refilling your prescription. If you still have symptoms of infection after you finish taking posaconazole, call your doctor.

Talk to your doctor, pharmacist, or other healthcare professional if you have questions about dosing information for your medication.

Potassium

(poe tass' i um)

Brand Name: Glu-K®, K⁺ 10®, K⁺ 8®, K⁺ Care®, K⁺ Care® Effervescent Tablets, Kaochlor® 10%, Kaon® Elixir, Kaon-Cl® 20% Elixir, Kaon-Cl-10®, Kay Ciel®, K-Dur® 10, K-Dur® 20, K-Lor®, Klor-Con® 10, Klor-Con® 8, Klor-Con® Powder, Klor-Con®/25 Powder, Klor-Con®/EF, Klotrix®, K-Lyte/CL® 50 Effervescent Tablets, K-Lyte/CL® Effervescent Tablets, K-Lyte® DS Effervescent Tablets, K-Lyte® Effervescent Tablets, K-Tab® Filmtab®, Micro-K®, Quic-K®, Rum-K®, Slow-K®, Tri-K®, Twin-K®

Why is this medicine prescribed?

Potassium is essential for the proper functioning of the heart, kidneys, muscles, nerves, and digestive system. Usually the food you eat supplies all of the potassium you need. However, certain diseases (e.g., kidney disease and gastrointestinal disease with vomiting and diarrhea) and drugs, especially diuretics ('water pills'), remove potassium from the body. Potassium supplements are taken to replace potassium losses and prevent potassium deficiency.

This medication is sometimes prescribed for other uses; ask your doctor or pharmacist for more information.

How should this medicine be used?

Potassium comes in oral liquid, powder, granules, effervescent tablets, regular tablets, extended-release (long-acting) tablets, and extended-release capsules. It usually is taken two to four times a day, with or immediately after meals. Follow the directions on your prescription label carefully, and ask your doctor or pharmacist to explain any part you do not understand. Take potassium exactly as directed. Do not take more or less of it or take it more often than prescribed by your doctor.

Take all forms of potassium with a full glass of water or fruit juice.

Add the liquid to water. Dissolve the powder, granules, or effervescent tablets in cold water or fruit juice according to the manufacturer's directions or the directions on your prescription label; mix the drug well just before you take it. Cold liquids help mask the unpleasant taste.

Swallow extended-release tablets and capsules whole. Do not chew them or dissolve them in your mouth.

What special precautions should I follow?

Before taking potassium,

- tell your doctor and pharmacist if you are allergic to potassium or any other drugs.
- tell your doctor and pharmacist what prescription and nonprescription medications you are taking, especially angiotensin converting enzyme (ACE) inhibitors such

as captopril (Capoten), enalapril (Vasotec), and lisinopril (Prinivil, Zestril); diuretics ('water pills'); and vitamins. Do not take potassium if you are taking amiloride (Midamor), spironolactone (Aldactone), or triamterene (Dyrenium).

- tell your doctor if you have or have ever had heart, kidney, or Addison's (adrenal gland) disease.
- tell your doctor if you are pregnant, plan to become pregnant, or are breast-feeding. If you become pregnant while taking potassium, call your doctor.
- if you are having surgery, including dental surgery, tell the doctor or dentist that you are taking potassium.

What special dietary instructions should I follow?

If you are using a salt substitute, tell your doctor. Many salt substitutes contain potassium. Your doctor will consider this source in determining your dose of potassium supplement. Your doctor may advise you to use a potassium-containing salt substitute and to eat potassium-rich foods (e.g., bananas, prunes, raisins, and milk).

What should I do if I forget to take a dose?

Take the missed dose as soon as you remember it and take any remaining doses for that day at evenly spaced intervals. Do not take a double dose to make up for a missed one.

What side effects can this medicine cause?

Potassium may cause side effects. Tell your doctor if any of these symptoms are severe or do not go away:
- upset stomach
- vomiting
- diarrhea

If you experience any of the following symptoms, call your doctor immediately:
- mental confusion
- listlessness
- tingling, prickling, burning, tight, or pulling sensation of arms, hands, legs, or feet
- heaviness or weakness of legs
- cold, pale, gray skin
- stomach pain
- unusual stomach bulging
- black stools

If you experience a serious side effect, you or your doctor may send a report to the Food and Drug Administration's (FDA) MedWatch Adverse Event Reporting program online [at http://www.fda.gov/MedWatch/index.html] or by phone [1-800-332-1088].

What storage conditions are needed for this medicine?

Keep this medication in the container it came in, tightly closed, and out of reach of children. Store it at room temperature and away from excess heat and moisture (not in the bathroom). Throw away any medication that is outdated or no longer needed. Talk to your pharmacist about the proper disposal of your medication.

What should I do in case of overdose?

In case of overdose, call your local poison control center at 1-800-222-1222. If the victim has collapsed or is not breathing, call local emergency services at 911.

What other information should I know?

Keep all appointments with your doctor and the laboratory. Your doctor will order certain lab tests to check your response to potassium. You may have electrocardiograms (EKGs) and blood tests to see if your dose needs to be changed.

Do not let anyone else take your medication. Ask your pharmacist any questions you have about refilling your prescription.

Dosage Facts
For Informational Purposes

Caution: Do not change your dose, how often you take your medication, or the length of time you are to take it without first talking to your healthcare provider.

The following dosage information was written using medical language for doctors and other healthcare professionals and is provided here for you to check your dosage. The dosage of this drug may differ for different patients. Therefore, always follow your doctor's instructions or the directions on the label. Contact your healthcare provider or pharmacist if you have any questions about the specific dosage of your medication after reviewing this information.

General Dosage Information

Dosage of potassium supplements usually expressed as mEq of potassium.

Normal adult daily potassium requirement and usual dietary intake of potassium is 40–80 mEq; infants may require 2–3 mEq/kg or 40 mEq/m^2 daily.

Dosage must be carefully individualized according to the patient's requirements and response.

To avoid serious hyperkalemia, replacement of potassium deficits must be undertaken gradually, usually over a 3- to 7-day period depending on the severity of the deficit.

Potassium replacement requirements can be estimated only by clinical condition and response, ECG monitoring, and/or plasma potassium determinations.

Dosage Equivalents of Oral Potassium Salts

40 mEq of potassium is provided by approximately:

3.9 g of potassium acetate

4.0 g of potassium bicarbonate

3.0 g of potassium chloride

4.3 g of potassium citrate

9.4 g of potassium gluconate

5.4 g of monobasic potassium phosphate

3.5 g of dibasic potassium phosphate

Pediatric Patients

Hypokalemia
Prevention or Treatment

ORAL:

- If used in pediatric patients†, do not exceed 3 mEq/kg daily in young children.

Adult Patients

Hypokalemia
Prevention

ORAL:

- Average dosage approximately 20 mEq daily. Usually should not exceed 150 mEq daily.

Treatment

ORAL:

- Usual dosage is 40–100 mEq or more daily. Usually should not exceed 150 mEq daily.

Prescribing Limits

Pediatric Patients

Hypokalemia†
Prevention or Treatment†

ORAL:

- 3 mEq/kg daily for young children.

Adult Patients

Hypokalemia
Prevention or Treatment

ORAL:

- Usually should not exceed 150 mEq daily.

Special Populations

Renal Impairment

- Cautious dosage selection and careful monitoring recommended in patients with renal impairment.

Geriatric Patients

- Select dosage with caution, starting at low end of dosage range, because of age-related decreases in hepatic, renal, and/or cardiac function and concomitant disease and drug therapy.

† *Use is not currently included in the labeling approved by the US Food and Drug Administration.*

Pramipexole

(pra mi pex′ ole)

Brand Name: Mirapex®

Why is this medicine prescribed?

Pramipexole is used alone or with other medications to treat the symptoms of Parkinson's disease (PD; a disorder of the nervous system that causes difficulties with movement, muscle control, and balance), including shaking of parts of the body, stiffness, slowed movements, and problems with balance. Pramipexole is also used to treat restless legs syndrome (RLS; a condition that causes discomfort in the legs and a strong urge to move the legs, especially at night and when sitting or lying down). Pramipexole is in a class of medications called dopamine agonists. It works by acting in place of dopamine, a natural substance in the brain that is needed to control movement.

How should this medicine be used?

Pramipexole comes as a tablet to take by mouth. When pramiprexole is used to treat Parkinson's disease, it is usually taken three times a day. When pramiprexole is used to treat restless legs syndrome, it is usually taken once a day, 2 to 3 hours before bedtime. Pramipexole may be taken with or without food, but taking pramipexole with food may help to prevent nausea that may be caused by the medication. Follow the directions on your prescription label carefully and ask your doctor or pharmacist to explain any part you do not understand. Take pramipexole exactly as directed. Do not take more or less of it or take it more often than prescribed by your doctor.

Your doctor will start you on a low dose of pramipexole and gradually increase your dose. Your doctor will probably not increase your dose more often than once every 4 to 7 days. It may take several weeks before you reach a dose that works for you.

If you are taking pramipexole to treat restless legs syndrome, you should know that as your treatment continues, your symptoms may worsen, may begin earlier in the evening or afternoon, or may occur in the early morning. Call your doctor if your symptoms worsen or if they begin to occur at different times than in the past.

Pramipexole controls the symptoms of Parkinson's disease and restless legs syndrome but does not cure these conditions. Continue to take pramipexole even if you feel well. Do not stop taking pramipexole without talking to your doctor. If you are taking pramipexole to treat Parkinson's disease and you suddenly stop taking the medication, you may experience, fever, muscle stiffness, changes in consciousness, and other symptoms. Your doctor will probably decrease your dose gradually over 7 days.

If you stop taking pramipexole for any reason, do not start to take the medication again without talking to your doctor. Your doctor will probably want to increase your dose again gradually.

Are there other uses for this medicine?

This medication is sometimes prescribed for other uses; ask your doctor or pharmacist for more information.

What special precautions should I follow?

Before taking pramipexole,

- tell your doctor and pharmacist if you are allergic to pramipexole or any other medications, or any of the ingredients in pramipexole tablets. Ask your doctor or pharmacist for a list of the inactive ingredients.
- tell your doctor and pharmacist what prescription and nonprescription medications vitamins, nutritional supplements and herbal products you are taking or plan to take. Be sure to mention any of the following: amantadine (Symadine, Symmetrel); antidepressants; antihistamines; cimetidine (Tagamet); diltiazem (Cardiazem, Dilacor XR); levodopa (Larodopa, Dopar, in Sinemet); medications for allergies, anxiety, mental illness, nausea, and seizures; metoclopramide (Reglan); quinidine; quinine; ranitidine (Zantac, Zantac 75); sedatives; sleeping pills; tranquilizers; triamterene (Dyrenium, in Dyazide, in Maxzide); and verapamil (Isoptin, Calan, Verelan, and others). Your doctor may need to change the doses of your medications or monitor you carefully for side effects.
- tell your doctor if you have or have ever had an urge to gamble that was difficult to control, trouble controlling movement of your muscles, a sleep disorder other than restless legs syndrome, dizziness, fainting, low blood pressure, or heart or kidney disease.
- tell your doctor if you are pregnant or plan to become pregnant. If you become pregnant while taking pramipexole, call your doctor. Do not breast-feed while you are taking pramipexole.
- if you are having surgery, including dental surgery, tell your doctor or dentist that you are taking pramipexole.
- you should know that pramipexole may make you drowsy or may cause you to suddenly fall asleep during your regular daily activities. You might not feel drowsy before you suddenly fall asleep. Do not drive a car or operate machinery at the beginning of your treatment until you know how pramipexole will affect you. If you suddenly fall asleep while you are doing something such as watching television or riding in a car, or if you become very drowsy, call your doctor. Do not drive or operate machinery until you talk to your doctor.
- remember that alcohol can add to the drowsiness caused by this medication. Tell your doctor if you regularly drink alcoholic beverages.
- you should know that pramipexole may cause dizziness, lightheadedness, nausea, fainting, or sweating when you get up too quickly from a sitting or lying position. This is more common when you first start taking pramipexole, or when your dose is increased. To avoid this problem, get out of the chair or bed slowly, resting your feet on the floor for a few minutes before standing up.

What special dietary instructions should I follow?

Unless your doctor tells you otherwise, continue your normal diet.

What should I do if I forget to take a dose?

If you are taking pramipexole to treat Parkinson's disease, take the missed dose as soon as you remember it. However, if it is almost time for the next dose, skip the missed dose and continue your regular dosing schedule. Do not take a double dose to make up for a missed one.

If you are taking pramipexole to treat restless legs syndrome, skip the missed dose. Take your regular dose 2 to 3 hours before your next bedtime. Do not double the next dose to make up for the missed dose.

What side effects can this medicine cause?

Pramipexole may cause side effects. Tell your doctor if any of these symptoms are severe or do not go away:

- nausea
- abnormal body movements and motions
- weakness
- dizziness
- drowsiness
- difficulty falling asleep or staying asleep
- difficulty remembering or thinking
- confusion
- abnormal thoughts or dreams
- heartburn
- constipation
- diarrhea
- loss of appetite
- weight loss
- dry mouth
- joint pain
- frequent urination or urgent need to urinate
- difficulty urinating or pain when urinating
- decreased sexual interest or ability
- swelling of the arms, hands, feet, ankles, or lower legs

Some side effects can be serious. If you experience any of the following symptoms, call your doctor immediately:

- hallucinations (seeing things or hearing voices that do not exist)
- changes in vision
- chest pain
- shortness of breath
- dark, red, or cola-colored urine
- muscle tenderness
- muscle stiffness or aching
- muscle weakness

Some people who took medications such as pramipexole to treat Parkinson's disease or restless legs syndrome developed gambling problems, an increased interest in sex, or overeating problems. There is not enough information to tell whether the people developed these problems because they took the medication or for other reasons. Call your doctor if you have difficulty controlling any of these behaviors. Tell your family members about these risks so that they can call the doctor even if you do not realize that your behavior has become a problem.

People who have Parkinson's disease may have a greater risk of developing melanoma (a type of skin cancer) than people who do not have Parkinson's disease. There is not enough information to tell whether medications used to treat Parkinson's disease such as pramipexole increase the risk of developing skin cancer. You should have regular skin examinations to check for melanoma while you are taking pramipexole even if you do not have Parkinson's disease. Talk to your doctor about the risk of taking pramipexole.

Pramipexole may cause other side effects. Call your doctor if you have any unusual problems while you are taking this medication.

If you experience a serious side effect, you or your doctor may send a report to the Food and Drug Administration's (FDA) MedWatch Adverse Event Reporting program online [at http://www.fda.gov/MedWatch/index.html] or by phone [1-800-332-1088].

What storage conditions are needed for this medicine?

Keep this medication in the container it came in, tightly closed, and out of reach of children. Store it at room temperature and away from excess heat and moisture (not in the bathroom). Throw away any medication that is outdated or no longer needed. Talk to your pharmacist about the proper disposal of your medication.

What should I do in case of overdose?

In case of overdose, call your local poison control center at 1-800-222-1222. If the victim has collapsed or is not breathing, call local emergency services at 911.

What other information should I know?

Keep all appointments with your doctor.

Do not let anyone else take your medication. Ask your pharmacist any questions you have about refilling your prescription.

Dosage Facts
For Informational Purposes

Caution: Do not change your dose, how often you take your medication, or the length of time you are to take it without first talking to your healthcare provider.

The following dosage information was written using medical language for doctors and other healthcare professionals and is provided here for you to check your dosage. The dosage of this drug may differ for different patients. Therefore, always follow your doctor's instructions or the directions on the label. Contact your healthcare provider or pharmacist if you have any questions about the specific dosage of your medication after reviewing this information.

General Dosage Information

Available as pramipexole dihydrochloride; dosage expressed in terms of the monohydrated form of this salt.

Adult Patients

Parkinsonian Syndrome

ORAL:
- Initiate at a low dosage and increase slowly (at intervals of $\geq 5-7$ days) until the maximum therapeutic response is achieved.

Usual Initial Dosage of Pramipexole Dihydrochloride for the Treatment of Parkinsonian Syndrome

Week of Therapy	Daily Dosage Schedule	Total Daily Dose
1	0.125 mg 3 times daily	0.375 mg daily
2	0.25 mg 3 times daily	0.75 mg daily
3	0.5 mg 3 times daily	1.5 mg daily
4	0.75 mg 3 times daily	2.25 mg daily
5	1 mg 3 times daily	3 mg daily
6	1.25 mg 3 times daily	3.75 mg daily
7	1.5 mg 3 times daily	4.5 mg daily

Continually reevaluate and adjust the dosage according to the needs of the patient in an effort to find a dosage schedule that provides maximum relief of symptoms with minimum adverse effects.

In a fixed-dose study in patients with early parkinsonian syndrome, dosages >1.5 mg daily (i.e., 3, 4.5, or 6 mg daily) were not associated with additional therapeutic benefit. As the dosage increased over the range from 1.5 mg to 6 mg daily, the incidence of postural hypotension, nausea, constipation, somnolence, and amnesia increased.

When pramipexole is used as an adjunct to levodopa, consider reducing the levodopa dosage.

Discontinue pramipexole therapy gradually over a period of 1 week.

Special Populations

Renal Impairment

Parkinsonian Syndrome

ORAL:
- Modify dosage and/or frequency of administration in response to the degree of renal impairment.

Recommended Dosage of Pramipexole Dihydrochloride for Patients with Renal Impairment

Cl$_{cr}$	Initial Dosage	Maximum Dosage
≥60 mL/minute	0.125 mg 3 times daily	1.5 mg 3 times daily
35–59 mL/minute	0.125 mg twice daily	1.5 mg twice daily
15–34 mL/minute	0.125 mg once daily	1.5 mg once daily
<15 mL/minute	Not adequately studied; no specific recommendation	
Hemodialysis	Not adequately studied; no specific recommendation	

Geriatric Patients
• No dosage adjustments necessary, since therapy is initiated at a low dosage and titrated according to clinical response.

Pramlintide Injection

(pram′ lin tide)

Brand Name: Symlin®

Important Warning

You will use pramlintide with mealtime insulin to control your blood sugar levels. When you use insulin, there is a chance that you will experience hypoglycemia (low blood sugar). This risk may be greater during the first 3 hours after you inject pramlintide, especially if you have Type 1 diabetes (condition in which the body does not produce insulin and therefore cannot control the amount of sugar in the blood). You may harm yourself or others if your blood sugar drops while you are involved in an activity that requires you to be alert or to think clearly. Do not drive a car or use heavy machinery until you know how pramlintide affects your blood sugar. Talk to your doctor about what other activities you should avoid while you are using pramlintide.

Tell your doctor if you have had diabetes for a long time, if you have diabetic nerve disease, if you cannot tell when your blood sugar is low, and if you needed medical treatment for hypoglycemia several times in the past 6 months. Also tell your doctor if you are taking any of the following medications: angiotensin converting enzyme (ACE) inhibitors used

to treat high blood pressure, heart disease, or diabetic kidney disease; beta blockers such as atenolol (Tenormin), labetalol (Normodyne), metoprolol (Lopressor, Toprol XL), nadolol (Corgard), and propranolol (Inderal); clonidine (Catapres); disopyramide (Norpace); fenofibrate (Lofibra, Tricor); fluoxetine (Prozac, Sarafem); gemfibrozil (Lopid); guanethidine (Ismelin); other medications for diabetes; monoamine oxidase (MAO) inhibitors such as isocarboxazid (Marplan), phenelzine (Nardil), selegiline (Eldepryl), and tranylcypromine (Parnate); pentoxifylline (Trental); propoxyphene (Darvon); reserpine (Serpalan, Serpasil); salicylate pain relievers such as aspirin; and sulfonamide antibiotics such as trimethoprim/sulfamethoxazole (Bactrim, Septra).

While you are using pramlintide, you must measure your blood sugar before and after every meal and at bedtime. You also will need to see or talk to your doctor often, and frequently change your doses of pramlintide and insulin according to your doctor's directions. Tell your doctor if you think that it will be difficult for you to do these things, if you have had difficulty checking your blood sugar or using your insulin correctly in the past, or if you find it difficult to manage your treatment after you start using pramlintide.

Your doctor will decrease your dose of insulin when you start using pramlintide. Your doctor will start you on a low dose of pramlintide and will gradually increase your dose. Call your doctor right away if you have an upset stomach during this time; your dose may need to be changed or you may have to stop using pramlintide. Your doctor will probably change your dose of insulin once you are using a dose of pramlintide that is right for you. Follow all of these directions carefully and ask your doctor or pharmacist right away if you are not sure how much insulin or pramlintide you should use.

The risk of hypoglycemia may be greater in certain situations. Call your doctor if you plan to be more active than usual. If you have any of the following conditions you should not use pramlintide and should call your doctor to find out what to do:
• you plan to skip a meal.
• you plan to eat a meal with less than 250 calories or 30 grams of carbohydrates.
• you cannot eat because you are sick.
• you cannot eat because you are scheduled for surgery or a medical test.
• your blood sugar is very low before a meal.

Alcohol may cause a decrease in blood sugar. Ask your doctor about the safe use of alcoholic beverages while you are using pramlintide.

Call your doctor right away if your blood sugar is lower than normal or if you have any of the following symptoms of low blood sugar: hunger, headache, sweating, shaking of a part of your body that

continued on next page

Important Warning (cont'd)

you cannot control, irritability, difficulty concentrating, loss of consciousness, coma, or a seizure. Be sure that you always have a fast acting source of sugar such as hard candy, juice, glucose tablets, or glucagon available to treat hypoglycemia.

Your doctor or pharmacist will give you the manufacturer's patient information sheet (Medication Guide) when you begin treatment with pramlintide and each time you refill your prescription. Read the information carefully and ask your doctor or pharmacist if you have any questions. You can also obtain the Medication Guide from the FDA website: http://www.fda.gov.

Why is this medicine prescribed?

Pramlintide is used with mealtime insulin to control blood sugar levels in people who have diabetes. Pramlintide is only used to treat patients whose blood sugar could not be controlled by insulin or insulin and an oral medication for diabetes. Pramlintide is in a class of medications called antihyperglycemics. It works by slowing the movement of food through the stomach. This prevents blood sugar from rising too high after a meal, and may decrease appetite and cause weight loss.

How should this medicine be used?

Pramlintide comes as a solution (liquid) to inject subcutaneously (just under the skin). It is usually injected several times a day, before each meal that includes at least 250 calories or 30 grams of carbohydrate. Follow the directions on your prescription label carefully, and ask your doctor or pharmacist to explain any part you do not understand. Use pramlintide exactly as directed. Do not use more or less of it or use it more often than prescribed by your doctor.

Pramlintide controls diabetes but does not cure it. Continue to use pramlintide even if you feel well. Do not stop using pramlintide without talking to your doctor. If you do stop using pramlintide for any reason, do not start using it again without talking to your doctor.

Use a U-100 insulin syringe to inject pramlintide. It is best to use the 0.3-mL size. Use the table in the medication guide to find the number of insulin syringe units that matches your prescribed dose (in micrograms [mcg]) of pramlintide. Ask your doctor or pharmacist if you are not sure how many syringe units of medication you will need to inject.

Use a new syringe and needle for each injection. Do not mix pramlintide and insulin in the same syringe, and do not use the same syringe or needle to inject pramlintide and insulin one after another. Throw away your needle and syringe in a puncture-resistant container that is out of the reach of children. Talk to your doctor or pharmacist about how to throw away the puncture-resistant container.

You can inject pramlintide anywhere on your stomach or thigh. Do not inject pramlintide into your arm. Choose a different spot to inject pramlintide every day. Be sure that the spot you choose is more than 2 inches away from the spot where you will inject insulin.

You should inject pramlintide under the skin the same way that you inject insulin. Allow the vial of pramlintide to warm to room temperature before you inject the medication. Look at the liquid in the vial before you inject it, and do not use it if it is cloudy. If you have questions about injecting pramlintide, ask your doctor or pharmacist.

Are there other uses for this medicine?

This medication may be prescribed for other uses; ask your doctor or pharmacist for more information.

What special precautions should I follow?

Before using pramlintide,

- tell your doctor and pharmacist if you are allergic to pramlintide, any other medications, or metacresol.
- tell your doctor and pharmacist what prescription and nonprescription medications, vitamins, nutritional supplements, and herbal products you are taking. Be sure to mention the medications listed in the IMPORTANT WARNING section and any of the following: antihistamines; certain antidepressants ('mood elevators') called tricyclic antidepressants; certain medications to treat asthma, diarrhea, lung disease, mental illness, motion sickness, overactive bladder, pain, Parkinson's disease, stomach or intestinal cramps, ulcers, and upset stomach; cisapride (Propulsid); laxatives; metoclopramide (Reglan); and stool softeners. Your doctor may need to change the doses of your medications or monitor you carefully for side effects.
- if you are taking a medication for pain such as acetaminophen (Tylenol), take it at least 1 hour before or 2 hours after you use pramlintide.
- tell your doctor if you have or have ever had gastroparesis (slowed movement of food from the stomach to the small intestine) and if you are being treated with dialysis (treatment to clean the blood outside the body when the kidneys are not working well).
- tell your doctor if you are pregnant, plan to become pregnant, or are breast-feeding. If you become pregnant while using pramlintide, call your doctor.
- if you are having surgery, including dental surgery, tell the doctor or dentist that you are using pramlintide.

What special dietary instructions should I follow?

Your doctor, dietitian, or diabetes educator will help you create a meal plan that works for you. Follow the meal plan carefully.

What should I do if I forget to take a dose?

Skip the missed dose and use your usual dose of pramlintide before your next major meal. Do not use a double dose to make up for a missed one.

What side effects can this medicine cause?

Pramlintide may cause side effects. Tell your doctor if any of these symptoms are severe or do not go away:

- redness, swelling, bruising, or itching in the place where you injected pramlintide
- loss of appetite
- stomach pain
- indigestion
- upset stomach
- excessive tiredness
- dizziness
- coughing
- sore throat
- joint pain

Some side effects can be serious. If you experience any of the symptoms listed in the IMPORTANT WARNING section, call your doctor immediately.

Pramlintide may cause other side effects. Call your doctor if you have any unusual problems while using this medication.

If you experience a serious side effect, you or your doctor may send a report to the Food and Drug Administration's (FDA) MedWatch Adverse Event Reporting program online [at http://www.fda.gov/MedWatch/index.html] or by phone [1-800-332-1088].

What storage conditions are needed for this medicine?

Keep this medication in the container it came in, tightly closed, and out of reach of children. Keep unopened vials of pramlintide in the refrigerator, but do not freeze them. Throw away any vials that were frozen or exposed to heat. You may store opened vials of pramlintide in the refrigerator or at room temperature, and you must use them within 28 days. Throw away any medication left in an opened vial after 28 days and any medication that is outdated or no longer needed. Talk to your pharmacist about the proper disposal of your medication.

What should I do in case of overdose?

In case of overdose, call your local poison control center at 1-800-222-1222. If the victim has collapsed or is not breathing, call local emergency services at 911.

Symptoms of overdose may include:

- upset stomach
- vomiting
- diarrhea
- dizziness
- flushing

What other information should I know?

Do not let anyone else use your medication. Ask your pharmacist any questions you have about refilling your prescription.

Dosage Facts
For Informational Purposes

Caution: Do not change your dose, how often you take your medication, or the length of time you are to take it without first talking to your healthcare provider.

The following dosage information was written using medical language for doctors and other healthcare professionals and is provided here for you to check your dosage. The dosage of this drug may differ for different patients. Therefore, always follow your doctor's instructions or the directions on the label. Contact your healthcare provider or pharmacist if you have any questions about the specific dosage of your medication after reviewing this information.

General Dosage Information

Available as pramlintide acetate; dosage expressed in terms of pramlintide.

Dosage expressed in mcg; dosage must be converted to insulin unit equivalents if administered using a U-100 insulin syringe.

Prior to initiating therapy, reduce preprandial, rapid-acting, short-acting, or fixed-mix insulin dosages by 50%.

Once maintenance dosage of pramlintide is attained and nausea (if experienced) has subsided, adjust dosage of preprandial insulin to achieve optimal glycemic control.

Adult Patients

Diabetes Mellitus
Type 1 Diabetes Mellitus

SUB-Q:

- Initially, 15 mcg immediately before each major meal, up to 4 times daily.
- Increase dosage in increments of 15 mcg to 30, 45, or 60 mcg, as tolerated, before each major meal, when no clinically important nausea has occurred for ≥3 days at the current dosage level.
- If nausea persists at the 45- or 60-mcg dosage level, reduce dosage to 30 mcg before each major meal.
- If the 30-mcg dosage is not tolerated, consider discontinuance of therapy.
- If pramlintide is reinitiated following a discontinuance for any reason, use initial dosage and dosage titration schedule.

Type 2 Diabetes Mellitus

SUB-Q:

- Initially, 60 mcg immediately before each major meal, up to 3 times daily.
- Increase dosage to 120 mcg before each major meal, when no clinically important nausea has occurred for 3–7 days.
- If nausea persists at dosage of 120 mcg, reduce dosage to 60 mcg before each major meal.
- If pramlintide is reinitiated following a discontinuance for any reason, use initial dosage and dosage titration schedule.

Prescribing Limits

Adult Patients

Diabetes Mellitus

Type 1 Diabetes Mellitus

SUB-Q:
- Maximum daily dosage not established; however, in clinical studies, has been administered up to 4 times daily before each major meal.

Type 2 Diabetes Mellitus

SUB-Q:
- Maximum daily dosage not established; however, in clinical studies, has been administered up to 3 times daily before each major meal.

Special Populations

Hepatic Impairment
- No dosage adjustment required.

Renal Impairment
- No dosage adjustment required.

Geriatric Patients
- Careful dosage selection recommended due to possible age-related increased sensitivity to hypoglycemia; careful patient selection for full understanding of insulin adjustments and glucose monitoring is recommended.

Pramoxine

(pra mox′ een)

Brand Name: Fleet® Pain-Relief, Itch-X®, PrameGel®, Prax®, Proctofoam®, Tronolane®

Why is this medicine prescribed?

Pramoxine is used to temporarily relieve pain and itching from insect bites; poison ivy, poison oak, or poison sumac; minor cuts, scrapes, or burns; minor skin irritation or rashes; or dry, itchy skin. Pramoxine also may be used to treat soreness, burning, itching, and pain from hemorrhoids ("piles") and other minor rectal irritations or itching. Pramoxine is in a class of medications called topical anesthetics. It works by stopping nerves from sending pain signals.

How should this medicine be used?

Pramoxine comes as a gel or spray to apply to the skin. Pramoxine also comes as a cream, foam, lotion, or solution (liquid) to apply to the rectal area. The solution comes as individual pledgets (medicated wipes for one time use). Pramoxine is usually applied to the affected area several times a day. Pramoxine cream or pledgets may be used up to five times a day; the spray or gel may be used 3 or 4 times daily. Pramoxine hemorrhoidal cream, lotion, and foam may be applied after bowel movements as needed or directed. Fol-

low the directions on the package or on your prescription label carefully, and ask your doctor or pharmacist to explain any part you do not understand. Use pramoxine exactly as directed. Do not use more or less of it or use it more often or for a longer time than described on the package or prescribed by your doctor.

If your symptoms continue for longer than seven days, your condition worsens, or your condition clears up for a few days and then comes back, stop using pramoxine and call your doctor.

Be careful not to get pramoxine into your eyes or nose. If pramoxine gets into your eyes, flush them with water and call your doctor.

You should not apply pramoxine to open wounds, areas of skin that are damaged or blistered, deep wounds, or large areas. Unless directed by your doctor, do not use bandages or wraps after pramoxine is applied.

Do not put moistened medication pads, cream, gel, or foam into your rectum with your fingers or any device.

To use pramoxine cream, gel, or spray, or lotion, follow these steps:
1. Wash your hands.
2. Clean the affected area with mild soap and warm water. Rinse thoroughly.
3. Pat affected area dry with a clean, soft cloth or tissue.
4. Apply small amount of pramoxine to affected area.
5. Wash hands thoroughly.

To use pramoxine pledgets, follow these steps:
1. Wash your hands.
2. Clean affected rectal area with mild soap and warm water. Rinse thoroughly.
3. Gently dry by patting or blotting with a clean, soft cloth or tissue.
4. Open sealed pouch and remove pledget.
5. Apply medication from pledget to affected rectal area by patting. If needed, fold pledget and leave in place for up to 15 minutes.
6. Remove pledget, and throw away, out of reach of children.
7. Wash your hands thoroughly.

To use pramoxine hemorrhoidal foam, follow these steps:
1. Wash your hands.
2. Clean affected area with mild soap and warm water. Rinse thoroughly.
3. Gently dry by patting or blotting with a clean, soft cloth or tissue.
4. Shake the foam container.
5. Squirt a small amount of foam onto a clean tissue and apply to affected rectal area.
6. Wash your hands thoroughly.

Are there other uses for this medicine?

This medication may be prescribed for other uses; ask your doctor or pharmacist for more information.

What special precautions should I follow?

Before using pramoxine,

- tell your doctor and pharmacist if you are allergic to pramoxine, other topical anesthetics, or any other medication.
- tell your doctor and pharmacist what other prescription and nonprescription medications, vitamins, nutritional supplements, and herbal products you are using.
- tell your doctor if you are pregnant, plan to become pregnant, or are breast-feeding. If you become pregnant while taking pramoxine, call your doctor.

What special dietary instructions should I follow?

Unless your doctor tells you otherwise, continue your normal diet.

What should I do if I forget to take a dose?

Apply the missed dose as soon as you remember it. However, if it is almost time for the next dose, skip the missed dose and continue your regular dosing schedule. Do not apply a double dose to make up for a missed one.

What side effects can this medicine cause?

Pramoxine may cause side effects. Tell your doctor if any of these symptoms are severe or do not go away:

- redness, irritation, swelling, burning, stinging, or pain at affected area
- dryness at affected area

Some side effects can be serious. The following symptoms are uncommon, but if you experience any of them, call your doctor immediately:

- bleeding at affected area
- hives
- skin rash
- severe itching
- difficulty breathing or swallowing
- swelling of the face, throat, tongue, lips, eyes, hands, feet, ankles, or lower legs
- hoarseness

Pramoxine may cause other side effects. Call your doctor if you have any unusual problems while taking this medication.

If you experience a serious side effect, you or your doctor may send a report to the Food and Drug Administration's (FDA) MedWatch Adverse Event Reporting program online [at http://www.fda.gov/MedWatch/index.html] or by phone [1-800-332-1088].

What storage conditions are needed for this medicine?

Keep this medication in the container it came in, tightly closed, and out of reach of children. Store it at room temperature and away from excess heat and moisture (not in the bathroom). Keep pramoxine aerosol container, spray or lotion away from fire, flame, or extreme heat. Throw away any medication that is outdated or no longer needed. Do not throw pramoxine aerosol containers away in an incinerator. Talk to your pharmacist about the proper disposal of your medication.

What should I do in case of overdose?

In case of overdose, call your local poison control center at 1-800-222-1222. If the victim has collapsed or is not breathing, call local emergency services at 911.

What other information should I know?

Keep all appointments with your doctor.

Ask your pharmacist or doctor any questions you have about pramoxine.

Talk to your doctor, pharmacist, or other healthcare professional if you have questions about dosing information for your medication.

Pravastatin

(pra′ va stat in)

Brand Name: Pravachol®, Pravigard® PAC

Why is this medicine prescribed?

Pravastatin is used together with lifestyle changes (diet, weight-loss, exercise) to reduce the amount of cholesterol (a fat-like substance) and other fatty substances in the blood. Pravastatin is in a class of medications called HMG-CoA reductase inhibitors (statins). It works by slowing the production of cholesterol in the body.

Buildup of cholesterol and other fats along the walls of the blood vessels (a process known as atherosclerosis) decreases blood flow and, therefore, the oxygen supply to the heart, brain, and other parts of the body. Lowering blood levels of cholesterol and other fats may help to decrease your chances of getting heart disease, angina (chest pain), strokes, and heart attacks. In addition to taking a cholesterol-lowering medication, making certain changes in your daily habits can also lower your cholesterol blood levels. You should eat a diet that is low in saturated fat and cholesterol (see SPECIAL DIETARY), exercise 30 minutes on most, if not all days, and lose weight if you are overweight.

How should this medicine be used?

Pravastatin comes as a tablet to take by mouth. It is usually taken once a day with or without food. Take pravastatin at around the same time every day. Follow the directions on your prescription label carefully, and ask your doctor or pharmacist to explain any part you do not understand. Take pravastatin exactly as directed. Do not take more or less of it or take it more often than prescribed by your doctor.

Your doctor may start you on a low dose of pravastatin and gradually increase your dose, not more than once every 4 weeks.

Continue to take pravastatin even if you feel well. Do not stop taking pravastatin without talking to your doctor.

Are there other uses for this medicine?

This medication may be prescribed for other uses; ask your doctor or pharmacist for more information.

What special precautions should I follow?

Before taking pravastatin,
- tell your doctor and pharmacist if you are allergic to pravastatin or any other medications.
- tell your doctor and pharmacist what prescription and nonprescription medications, vitamins, nutritional supplements, and herbal products you are taking or plan to take. Be sure to mention any of the following: cimetidine (Tagamet); cyclosporine (Neoral, Sandimmune); ketoconazole (Nizoral); other cholesterol-lowering medications such as fenofibrate (Tricor), gemfibrozil (Lopid), and niacin (nicotinic acid, Niacor, Niaspan); and spironolactone (Aldactone). Your doctor may need to change the doses of your medications or monitor you carefully for side effects.
- if you are taking cholestyramine (Questran) or colestipol (Cholestid), take them 4 hours before or 1 hour after pravastatin. If you are taking antacids, take them 1 hour before pravastatin.
- tell your doctor if you have liver disease. Your doctor will probably tell you not to take pravastatin.
- tell your doctor if you drink large amounts of alcohol, if you have ever had liver disease or if you have or have ever had kidney disease.
- tell your doctor if you are pregnant or plan to become pregnant. If you become pregnant while taking pravastatin, stop taking pravastatin and call your doctor immediately. Pravastatin may harm the fetus.
- do not breast-feed while you are taking this medication.
- if you are having surgery, including dental surgery, tell the doctor or dentist that you are taking pravastatin.
- ask your doctor about the safe use of alcoholic beverages while you are taking pravastatin. Alcohol can increase the risk of serious side effects.

What special dietary instructions should I follow?

Eat a low-cholesterol, low-fat diet. This kind of diet includes cottage cheese, fat-free milk, fish (not canned in oil), vegetables, poultry, egg whites, and polyunsaturated oils and margarines (corn, safflower, canola, and soybean oils). Avoid foods with excess fat in them such as meat (especially liver and fatty meat), egg yolks, whole milk, cream, butter, shortening, lard, pastries, cakes, cookies, gravy, peanut butter, chocolate, olives, potato chips, coconut, cheese (other than cottage cheese), coconut oil, palm oil, and fried foods.

What should I do if I forget to take a dose?

Take the missed dose as soon as you remember it. However, if it is almost time for the next dose, skip the missed dose and continue the regular dosing schedule. Do not take a double dose to make up for a missed one.

What side effects can this medicine cause?

Pravastatin may cause side effects. Tell your doctor if either of these symptoms is severe or does not go away:
- heartburn
- headache

Some side effects can be serious. The following symptoms are uncommon, but if you experience any of them, call your doctor immediately:
- muscle pain, tenderness, or weakness
- lack of energy
- fever
- yellowing of the skin or eyes
- pain in the upper right part of the stomach
- nausea
- extreme tiredness
- unusual bleeding or bruising
- loss of appetite
- flu-like symptoms
- rash
- hives
- itching
- difficulty breathing or swallowing
- swelling of the face, throat, tongue, lips, eyes, hands, feet, ankles, or lower legs
- hoarseness

Pravastatin may cause other side effects. Call your doctor if you have any unusual problems while taking this medication.

If you experience a serious side effect, you or your doctor may send a report to the Food and Drug Administration's (FDA) MedWatch Adverse Event Reporting program online [at http://www.fda.gov/MedWatch/index.html] or by phone [1-800-332-1088].

What storage conditions are needed for this medicine?

Keep this medication in the container it came in, tightly closed, and out of reach of children. Store it at room temperature and away from excess heat and moisture (not in the bathroom). Throw away any medication that is outdated or no longer needed. Talk to your pharmacist about the proper disposal of your medication.

What should I do in case of overdose?

In case of overdose, call your local poison control center at 1-800-222-1222. If the victim has collapsed or is not breathing, call local emergency services at 911.

What other information should I know?

Keep all appointments with your doctor and the laboratory. Your doctor will order certain lab tests before and during treatment to check your body's response to pravastatin.

Before having any laboratory test, tell your doctor and the laboratory personnel that you are taking pravastatin.

Do not let anyone else take your medication. Ask your pharmacist any questions you have about refilling your prescription.

Dosage Facts

For Informational Purposes

Caution: Do not change your dose, how often you take your medication, or the length of time you are to take it without first talking to your healthcare provider.

The following dosage information was written using medical language for doctors and other healthcare professionals and is provided here for you to check your dosage. The dosage of this drug may differ for different patients. Therefore, always follow your doctor's instructions or the directions on the label. Contact your healthcare provider or pharmacist if you have any questions about the specific dosage of your medication after reviewing this information.

General Dosage Information

Available as pravastatin sodium; dosage expressed in terms of pravastatin.

Pediatric Patients

Dyslipidemias

ORAL:
- Children 8–13 years of age: 20 mg once daily. Dosages exceeding 20 mg daily have not been evaluated.
- Adolescents 14–18 years of age: 40 mg once daily. Dosages exceeding 40 mg daily have not been evaluated.
- Re-evaluate in adulthood and modify therapy appropriately to achieve adult target LDL-cholesterol goals.

Adult Patients

Dyslipidemias and Prevention of Cardiovascular Events

ORAL:
- Initially, 40 mg once daily. If antilipemic response is inadequate, increase dosage to 80 mg daily. Adjust dosage at intervals of ≥4 weeks until the desired effect on lipoprotein concentrations is observed.

Special Populations

Hepatic Impairment
- Initially, 10 mg once daily in patients with a history of substantial hepatic impairment.
- Use with caution in patients who consume substantial amounts of alcohol, in patients who have a history of liver disease, or in those with manifestations of liver disease (e.g., jaundice); monitor such patients closely. Contraindicated in patients with active liver disease or unexplained, persistent increases in serum aminotransferase concentrations.

Renal Impairment
- Initially, 10 mg once daily in patients with a history of substantial renal impairment.

Prazosin

(pra′ zoe sin)

Brand Name: Minipress®
Also available generically.

Why is this medicine prescribed?

Prazosin is used alone or in combination with other medications to treat high blood pressure. Prazosin is in a class of medications called alpha-blockers. It works by relaxing the blood vessels so that blood can flow more easily through the body.

How should this medicine be used?

Prazosin comes as a capsule to take by mouth. It usually is taken two or three times a day at evenly spaced intervals. The first time taking prazosin, you should take it before you go to bed. Follow the directions on your prescription label carefully, and ask your doctor or pharmacist to explain any part you do not understand. Take prazosin exactly as directed. Do not take more or less of it or take it more often than prescribed by your doctor.

Your doctor will probably start you on a low dose of prazosin and gradually increase your dose.

Prazosin controls high blood pressure but does not cure it. Continue to take prazosin even if you feel well. Do not stop taking prazosin without talking to your doctor.

Are there other uses for this medicine?

Prazosin is also used to treat benign prostatic hyperplasia (BPH, noncancerous enlargement of the prostate), congestive heart failure, pheochromocytoma (adrenal gland tumor), and Raynaud's disease (condition where the fingers and toes change skin color from white to blue to red when exposed to hot or cold temperatures). Talk to your doctor about the possible risks of using this medication for your condition.

This medication may be prescribed for other uses; ask your doctor or pharmacist for more information.

What special precautions should I follow?

Before taking prazosin,
- tell your doctor and pharmacist if you are allergic to prazosin, alfuzosin (Uroxatral), doxazosin (Cardura), terazosin (Hytrin), or any other medications.
- tell your doctor and pharmacist what other prescription

and nonprescription medications, vitamins, nutritional supplements, and herbal products you are taking or plan to take. Be sure to mention: beta-blockers such as propranolol (Inderal); medications for erectile dysfunction (ED) such as sildenafil (Viagra), tadalafil (Cialis), or vardenafil (Levitra); and other medications for high blood pressure.

- tell your doctor if you have narcolepsy (a sleep disorder that may cause extreme sleepiness, sudden uncontrollable urge to sleep during daily activities) or if you have or have ever had prostate cancer or liver disease.
- tell your doctor if you are pregnant, plan to become pregnant, or are breast-feeding. If you become pregnant while taking prazosin, call your doctor.
- if you are having surgery, including dental surgery, tell the doctor or dentist that you are taking prazosin. If you need to have eye surgery at any time during or after your treatment, be sure to tell your doctor that you are taking or have taken prazosin.
- you should know that this drug may make you drowsy or dizzy. Do not drive a car, operate machinery, or perform dangerous tasks for 24 hours after the first time you take prazosin or after your dose is increased.
- ask your doctor about the safe use of alcoholic beverages while you are taking prazosin. Alcohol can make the side effects from prazosin worse.
- you should know that prazosin may cause dizziness, lightheadedness, and fainting when you get up too quickly from a lying position. This is more common when you first start taking prazosin, when your dose is increased, or when another blood pressure medication is added to your treatment. To help avoid this problem, get out of bed slowly, resting your feet on the floor for a few minutes before standing up. If you experience these symptoms, sit or lie down. These symptoms may also occur if you drink alcohol, stand for long periods of time, exercise, or if the weather is hot. If these symptoms do not improve, call your doctor.

What special dietary instructions should I follow?

Follow your doctor's directions for your meals, including advice for a reduced salt (sodium) diet.

What should I do if I forget to take a dose?

Take the missed dose as soon as you remember it. However, if it is almost time for the next dose, skip the missed dose and continue your regular dosing schedule. Do not take a double dose to make up for a missed one. Check with your doctor if you have missed two or more doses.

What side effects can this medicine cause?

Prazosin may cause side effects. Tell your doctor if any of these symptoms or those listed in the SPECIAL PRECAUTIONS section are severe or do not go away:
- weakness

- tiredness
- headache
- nausea

Some side effects can be serious. If you experience any of the following symptoms, call your doctor immediately:
- hives
- rash
- itching
- difficulty breathing
- fast, pounding, or irregular heartbeat
- chest pain
- painful erection of the penis that lasts for hours

What storage conditions are needed for this medicine?

Keep this medication in the container it came in, tightly closed, and out of reach of children. Store it at room temperature and away from excess heat and moisture (not in the bathroom). Throw away any medication that is outdated or no longer needed. Talk to your pharmacist about the proper disposal of your medication.

What should I do in case of overdose?

In case of overdose, call your local poison control center at 1-800-222-1222. If the victim has collapsed or is not breathing, call local emergency services at 911.

Symptoms of overdose may include:
- drowsiness
- decreased reflexes
- dizziness
- lightheadedness
- fainting

What other information should I know?

Keep all appointments with your doctor and the laboratory. Your blood pressure should be checked regularly to determine your response to prazosin.

Before having any laboratory test, tell your doctor and the laboratory personnel that you are taking prazosin.

Do not let anyone else take your medication. Ask your pharmacist any questions you have about refilling your prescription.

Dosage Facts
For Informational Purposes

Caution: Do not change your dose, how often you take your medication, or the length of time you are to take it without first talking to your healthcare provider.

The following dosage information was written using medical language for doctors and other healthcare professionals and is provided here for you to check your dosage. The dosage of this drug may differ for different patients. Therefore, always follow your doctor's instruc-

tions or the directions on the label. Contact your healthcare provider or pharmacist if you have any questions about the specific dosage of your medication after reviewing this information.

General Dosage Information

Available as prazosin hydrochloride; dosage expressed in terms of prazosin.

Individualize dosage according to patient response and tolerance. Initiate at low dosage to minimize frequency of postural hypotension and syncope.

Postural effects are most likely to occur 2–6 hours after a dose; monitor BP during this period after first dose and with any dosage increases.

If therapy is interrupted for a few days, restart using initial dosage regimen.

Pediatric Patients

Hypertension†

ORAL:
- Initially, 0.05–0.1 mg/kg daily given in 3 divided doses. Increase dosage as necessary up to a maximum of 0.5 mg/kg daily given in 3 divided doses.

Adult Patients

Hypertension
Monotherapy

ORAL:
- Initially, 1 mg 2 or 3 times daily. Do *not* initiate with higher dosages. May increase dosage gradually to 20 mg daily given in divided doses.
- Usual maintenance dosage: 6–15 mg daily given in divided doses.
- Careful monitoring of BP is recommended during initial titration or subsequent upward dosage adjustment; avoid large or abrupt reductions in BP.
- For the acute management of severe hypertension, initially, 1–2 mg; dosage may be repeated after 1 hour, if necessary.

Combination Therapy

ORAL:
- When other hypotensive agents or diuretics are added to existing prazosin therapy, reduce dosage to 1 or 2 mg 3 times daily; gradually increase according to patient's response and tolerance.
- Initial use of fixed combination with polythiazide is not recommended; adjust by administering each drug separately, then use the fixed combination if the optimum maintenance dosage corresponds to the ratio of drugs in the combination preparation. Administer separately for subsequent dosage adjustment.

Prescribing Limits

Pediatric Patients

Hypertension†

ORAL:
- Maximum 0.5 mg/kg daily.

Adult Patients

Hypertension

ORAL:
- Maximum 20 mg daily.

Special Populations

Hepatic Impairment
- No specific dosage recommendations at this time.

Renal Impairment
- Initially, 1 mg twice daily. Patients with chronic renal failure may require only small doses.

Geriatric Patients
- No specific dosage recommendations at this time; generally increase dosage more slowly in geriatric hypertensive patients than in younger adults.

† *Use is not currently included in the labeling approved by the US Food and Drug Administration.*

Prazosin and Polythiazide

(pra′ zoe sin) (pol i thye′ a zide)

Brand Name: Minizide®

Important Warning

Prazosin and polythiazide should not be the first medicine you use for high blood pressure. Your medications must be carefully adjusted to treat high blood pressure. If you have not been on any medication for high blood pressure before prazosin and polythiazide, check with your doctor again before taking it.

Why is this medicine prescribed?

The combination of prazosin and polythiazide is used to treat high blood pressure. It is a combination of two medicines. Prazosin, an alpha-block antihypertensive, works by relaxing blood vessels so that blood can flow more easily through the body. Polythiazide, a thiazide diuretic ('water pill'), causes the kidneys to get rid of unneeded water and salt from the body into the urine.

This medication is sometimes prescribed for other uses; ask your doctor or pharmacist for more information.

How should this medicine be used?

The combination of prazosin and polythiazide comes as a capsule to take by mouth. It is usually taken two to three times a day. Follow the directions on your prescription label carefully, and ask your doctor or pharmacist to explain any part you do not understand. Take prazosin and polythiazide exactly as directed. Do not take more or less of it or take it more often than prescribed by your doctor.

The combination of prazosin and polythiazide controls

high blood pressure but does not cure it. Continue to take prazosin and polythiazide even if you feel well. Do not stop taking prazosin and polythiazide without talking to your doctor.

What special precautions should I follow?

Before taking prazosin and polythiazide,

- tell your doctor and pharmacist if you are allergic to prazosin, polythiazide, other thiazide drugs, chlorothiazide, sulfa drugs, doxazosin, terazosin, or any other drugs.
- tell your doctor and pharmacist what prescription and nonprescription medications you are taking, especially anti-inflammatory medications such as ibuprofen (Motrin, Nuprin) or Naproxen (Aleve); beta-adrenergic blockers such as atenolol (Tenormin), carteolol (Cartrol), labetalol (Normodyne, Trandate), metoprolol (Lopressor), nadolol (Corgard), propranolol (Inderal), sotalol (Betapace), and timolol (Blocadren); clonidine (Catapres); corticosteroids (such as prednisone [Deltasone, Orasone, others], betamethasone [Celestone], cortisone [Cortone], dexamethasone [Decadron, others], hydrocortisone, or methylprednisolone [Medrol, Solu-Medrol, others]); guanadrel (Hylorel); guanethidine (Ismelin); indomethacin (Indocin); lithium (Eskalith, Lithobid), medications for diabetes; other medications for high blood pressure; probenecid (Benemid); reserpine (Serpalan, Serpasil); verapamil (Calan); and vitamins and herbal products.
- tell your doctor if you have or have ever had asthma; liver, thyroid, or kidney disease; high cholesterol; diabetes; gout; difficulty urinating; or systemic lupus erythematosus (SLE).
- tell your doctor if you are pregnant, plan to become pregnant, or are breast-feeding. If you become pregnant while taking prazosin and polythiazide, call your doctor immediately.
- if you are having surgery, including dental surgery, tell the doctor or dentist that you are taking prazosin and polythiazide.
- you should know that this drug may make you drowsy or dizzy. Do not drive a car or operate machinery for 24 hours after the first time you take prazosin and polythiazide or after your dose is increased.
- remember that alcohol can add to the drowsiness caused by this drug.
- plan to avoid unnecessary or prolonged exposure to sunlight and to wear protective clothing, sunglasses, and sunscreen. Prazosin and polythiazide may make your skin sensitive to sunlight.
- you should know that this drug may make you dizzy when you get up from sitting or laying down. Be sure you get up slowly.

What special dietary instructions should I follow?

Follow your doctor's directions. They may include following a daily exercise program or a low-salt or low-sodium diet, potassium supplements, and increased amounts of potassium-rich foods (e.g., bananas, prunes, raisins, and orange juice) in your diet.

What should I do if I forget to take a dose?

Take the missed dose as soon as you remember it. However, if it is almost time for the next dose, skip the missed dose and continue your regular dosing schedule. Do not take a double dose to make up for a missed one. Check with your doctor if you have missed two or more doses.

What side effects can this medicine cause?

Prazosin and polythiazide may cause side effects. Tell your doctor if any of these symptoms are severe or do not go away:

- dizziness
- drowsiness
- weakness
- tiredness
- blurred vision
- ringing in the ears
- stuffy nose
- bloody nose
- headache
- upset stomach
- vomiting
- diarrhea
- muscle weakness
- thirst or dry mouth
- abdominal pain
- constipation
- joint pain
- cramps or muscle pain
- decreased or increased urination
- hair loss
- loss of appetite
- decreased sexual ability or interest

If you experience any of the following symptoms, call your doctor immediately:

- difficulty breathing
- difficulty swallowing
- fast heartbeat
- irregular heartbeat
- chest pain
- sore throat with fever
- fainting
- unusual bleeding or bruising
- severe skin rash with peeling skin
- yellowing of the skin or whites of the eyes
- infection

If you experience a serious side effect, you or your doctor may send a report to the Food and Drug Administration's (FDA) MedWatch Adverse Event Reporting program online [at http://www.fda.gov/MedWatch/index.html] or by phone [1-800-332-1088].

What storage conditions are needed for this medicine?

Keep this medication in the container it came in, tightly closed, and out of reach of children. Store it at room temperature and away from excess heat and moisture (not in the bathroom). Throw away any medication that is outdated or no longer needed. Talk to your pharmacist about the proper disposal of your medication.

What should I do in case of overdose?

In case of overdose, call your local poison control center at 1-800-222-1222. If the victim has collapsed or is not breathing, call local emergency services at 911.

What other information should I know?

Keep all appointments with your doctor and the laboratory. Your blood pressure should be checked regularly to determine your response to prazosin and polythiazide.

Before having laboratory tests, tell your doctor and the laboratory personnel that you are taking prazosin and polythiazide. This drug interferes with some laboratory tests.

Do not let anyone else take your medication. Ask your pharmacist any questions you have about refilling your prescription.

Talk to your doctor, pharmacist, or other healthcare professional if you have questions about dosing information for your medication.

Prednisolone Ophthalmic

(pred niss' oh lone)

Brand Name: AK-Pred®, Blephamide®, Blephamide® Liquifilm®, Econopred® Plus, Inflamase® Forte, Inflamase® Mild, Poly-Pred® Liquifilm®, Pred Forte®, Pred Mild®, Pred-G®, Pred-G® Liquifilm®, Vasocidin® as a combination product containing Prednisolone Sodium Phosphate and Sulfacetamide Sodium

Why is this medicine prescribed?

Prednisolone reduces the irritation, redness, burning, and swelling of eye inflammation caused by chemicals, heat, radiation, infection, allergy, or foreign bodies in the eye. It sometimes is used after eye surgery.

This medication is sometimes prescribed for other uses; ask your doctor or pharmacist for more information.

How should this medicine be used?

Prednisolone comes as eyedrops and eye ointment. Follow the directions on your prescription label carefully, and ask your doctor or pharmacist to explain any part you do not understand. Use prednisolone exactly as directed. Do not use more or less of it or use it more often than prescribed by your doctor.

If you are using the suspension form of prednisolone eyedrops (Pred Forte, Pred Mild, Econopred, Econopred Plus), shake the bottle well before each dose. It is not necessary to shake prednisolone eyedrop solution (AK-Pred, Inflamase Mild, Inflamase Forte).

Continue to use prednisolone even if you feel well. Do not stop using prednisolone without talking to your doctor.

To use the eyedrops, follow these instructions:
1. Wash your hands thoroughly with soap and water.
2. Use a mirror or have someone else put the drops in your eye.
3. If using prednisolone suspension eyedrops, shake the bottle well for 10 seconds.
4. Remove the protective cap. Make sure that the end of the dropper is not chipped or cracked.
5. Avoid touching the dropper tip against your eye or anything else.
6. Hold the dropper tip down at all times to prevent drops from flowing back into the bottle and contaminating the remaining contents.
7. Lie down or tilt your head back.
8. Holding the bottle between your thumb and index finger, place the dropper tip as near as possible to your eyelid without touching it.
9. Brace the remaining fingers of that hand against your cheek or nose.
10. With the index finger of your other hand, pull the lower lid of the eye down to form a pocket.
11. Drop the prescribed number of drops into the pocket made by the lower lid and the eye. Placing drops on the surface of the eyeball can cause stinging.
12. Close your eye and press lightly against the lower lid with your finger for 2-3 minutes to keep the medication in the eye. Do not blink.
13. Replace and tighten the cap right away. Do not wipe or rinse it off.
14. Wipe off any excess liquid from your cheek with a clean tissue. Wash your hands again.

To use the eye ointment, follow these instructions:
1. Wash your hands thoroughly with soap and water.
2. Use a mirror or have someone else apply the ointment.
3. Avoid touching the tip of the tube against your eye or anything else. The ointment must be kept clean.
4. Tilt your head forward slightly.
5. Holding the tube between your thumb and index finger, place the tube as near as possible to your eyelid without touching it.
6. Brace the remaining fingers of that hand against your cheek or nose.
7. With the index finger of your other hand, pull the lower lid of your eye down to form a pocket.
8. Place a small amount of ointment into the pocket made by the lower lid and the eye. A 1/2-inch strip of oint-

ment usually is enough unless otherwise directed by your doctor.

9. Gently close your eyes and keep them closed for 1-2 minutes to allow the medication to be absorbed.
10. Replace and tighten the cap right away.
11. Wipe off any excess ointment from your eyelids and lashes with a clean tissue. Wash your hands again.

What special precautions should I follow?

Before using prednisolone eyedrops or eye ointment,

- tell your doctor and pharmacist if you are allergic to prednisolone or any other drugs.
- tell your doctor and pharmacist what prescription and nonprescription medications you are taking, including vitamins.
- tell your doctor if you have or have ever had glaucoma or diabetes.
- tell your doctor if you are pregnant, plan to become pregnant, or are breast-feeding. If you become pregnant while using prednisolone, call your doctor immediately.

What should I do if I forget to take a dose?

Apply the missed dose as soon as you remember it. Use any remaining doses for that day at evenly spaced intervals. However, if you remember a missed dose at the time the next one is due, use only the regularly scheduled dose. Do not apply a double dose to make up for a missed one.

What side effects can this medicine cause?

Prednisolone may cause side effects. Tell your doctor if any of these symptoms are severe or do not go away:

- temporary eye burning or stinging
- temporary blurred vision

If you experience the following symptom, call your doctor immediately:

- eye pain

If you experience a serious side effect, you or your doctor may send a report to the Food and Drug Administration's (FDA) MedWatch Adverse Event Reporting program online [at http://www.fda.gov/MedWatch/index.html] or by phone [1-800-332-1088].

What storage conditions are needed for this medicine?

Keep this medication in the container it came in, tightly closed, and out of reach of children. Store it at room temperature and away from excess heat and moisture (not in the bathroom). Throw away any medication that is outdated or no longer needed. Talk to your pharmacist about the proper disposal of your medication.

What other information should I know?

Keep all appointments with your doctor.

Do not let anyone else use your medication. Ask your pharmacist any questions you have about refilling your prescription.

If you still have symptoms of eye irritation after you finish the prednisolone, call your doctor.

Talk to your doctor, pharmacist, or other healthcare professional if you have questions about dosing information for your medication.

Prednisone
(pred′ ni sone)

Brand Name: Prednisone Intensol®, Sterapred®, Sterapred® DS
Also available generically.

Why is this medicine prescribed?

Prednisone is used alone or with other medications to treat the symptoms of low corticosteroid levels (lack of certain substances that are usually produced by the body and are needed for normal body functioning). Prednisone is also used to treat other conditions in patients with normal corticosteroid levels. These conditions include certain types of arthritis; severe allergic reactions; multiple sclerosis (a disease in which the nerves do not function properly); lupus (a disease in which the body attacks many of its own organs); and certain conditions that affect the lungs, skin, eyes, kidneys blood, thyroid, stomach, and intestines. Prednisone is also sometimes used to treat the symptoms of certain types of cancer. Prednisone is in a class of medications called corticosteroids. It works to treat patients with low levels of corticosteroids by replacing steroids that are normally produced naturally by the body. It works to treat other conditions by reducing swelling and redness and by changing the way the immune system works.

How should this medicine be used?

Prednisone comes as a tablet, a solution (liquid), and a concentrated solution to take by mouth. Prednisone is usually taken with food one to four times a day or once every other day. Your doctor will probably tell you to take your dose(s) of prednisone at certain time(s) of day every day. Your personal dosing schedule will depend on your condition and on how you respond to treatment. Follow the directions on your prescription label carefully, and ask your doctor or pharmacist to explain any part you do not understand. Take prednisone exactly as directed. Do not take more or less of it or take it more often or for a longer period of time than prescribed by your doctor.

If you are taking the concentrated solution, use the specially marked dropper that comes with the medication to measure your dose. You may mix the concentrated solution with juice, other flavored liquids, or soft foods such as applesauce.

Your doctor may change your dose of prednisone often during your treatment to be sure that you are always taking the lowest dose that works for you. Your doctor may also need to change your dose if you experience unusual stress on your body such as surgery, illness, infection, or a severe asthma attack. Tell your doctor if your symptoms improve or get worse or if you get sick or have any changes in your health during your treatment.

If you are taking prednisone to treat a long-lasting disease, the medication may help control your condition but will not cure it. Continue to take prednisone even if you feel well. Do not stop taking prednisone without talking to your doctor. If you suddenly stop taking prednisone, your body may not have enough natural steroids to function normally. This may cause symptoms such as extreme tiredness, weakness, slowed movements, upset stomach, weight loss, changes in skin color, sores in the mouth, and craving for salt. Call your doctor if you experience these or other unusual symptoms while you are taking decreasing doses of prednisone or after you stop taking the medication.

Are there other uses for this medicine?

Prednisone is also sometimes used with antibiotics to treat a certain type of pneumonia in patients with acquired immunodeficiency syndrome (AIDS). Talk to your doctor about the risks of using this drug for your condition.

This medication may be prescribed for other uses; ask your doctor or pharmacist for more information.

What special precautions should I follow?

Before taking prednisone,
- tell your doctor and pharmacist if you are allergic to prednisone, any other medications, or any of the inactive ingredients in prednisone tablets or solutions. Ask your doctor or pharmacist for a list of the inactive ingredients.
- tell your doctor and pharmacist what prescription and nonprescription medications, vitamins, and nutritional supplements you are taking or plan to take. Be sure to mention any of the following: amiodarone (Cordarone, Pacerone); anticoagulants ('blood thinners') such as warfarin (Coumadin); certain antifungals such as fluconazole (Diflucan), itraconazole (Sporanox), ketoconazole (Nizoral) and voriconazole (Vfend); aprepitant (Emend); aspirin; carbamazepine (Carbatrol, Epitol, Tegretol); cimetidine (Tagamet); clarithromycin (Biaxin, in Prevpak); cyclosporine (Neoral, Sandimmune); delavirdine (Rescriptor); diltiazem (Cardizem, Dilacor, Tiazac, others); dexamethasone (Decadron, Dexpak); diuretics ('water pills'); efavirenz (Sustiva); fluoxetine (Prozac, Sarafem); fluvoxamine (Luvox); griseofulvin (Fulvicin, Grifulvin, Gris-PEG); HIV protease inhibitors including atazanavir (Reyataz), indinavir (Crixivan), lopinavir (in Kaletra), nelfinavir (Viracept), ritonavir (Norvir, in Kaletra), and saquinavir (Fortovase, Invirase); hormonal contraceptives (birth control pills, patches, rings, implants, and injections); lovastatin (Altocor, Mevacor); medications for diabetes; nefazodone; nevirapine (Viramune); phenobarbital; phenytoin (Dilantin, Phenytek); rifabutin (Mycobutin), rifampin (Rifadin, Rimactane, in Rifamate); sertraline (Zoloft); troleandomycin (TAO); verapamil (Calan, Covera, Isoptin, Verelan); and zafirlukast (Accolate). Your doctor may need to change the doses of your medications or monitor you carefully for side effects.
- tell your doctor what herbal products you are taking or plan to take, especially St. John's wort.
- tell your doctor if you have an eye infection now or have ever had eye infections that come and go and if you have or have ever had threadworms (a type of worm that can live inside the body); diabetes; high blood pressure; emotional problems; mental illness; myasthenia gravis (a condition in which the muscles become weak); osteoporosis (condition in which the bones become weak and fragile and can break easily); seizures; tuberculosis (TB); ulcers; or liver, kidney, intestinal, heart, or thyroid disease.
- tell your doctor if you are pregnant, plan to become pregnant, or are breast-feeding. If you become pregnant while taking prednisone, call your doctor.
- if you are having surgery, including dental surgery, or need emergency medical treatment, tell the doctor, dentist, or medical staff that you are taking or have recently stopped taking prednisone. You should carry a card or wear a bracelet with this information in case you are unable to speak in a medical emergency.
- do not have any vaccinations (shots to prevent diseases) without talking to your doctor.
- you should know that prednisone may decrease your ability to fight infection and may prevent you from developing symptoms if you get an infection. Stay away from people who are sick and wash your hands often while you are taking this medication. Be sure to avoid people who have chicken pox or measles. Call your doctor immediately if you think you may have been around someone who had chicken pox or measles.

What special dietary instructions should I follow?

Your doctor may instruct you to follow a low-salt, high potassium, or high calcium diet. Your doctor may also prescribe or recommend a calcium or potassium supplement. Follow these directions carefully.

Talk to your doctor about eating grapefruit and drinking grapefruit juice while you are taking this medication.

What should I do if I forget to take a dose?

When you start to take prednisone, ask your doctor what to do if you forget to take a dose. Write down these instructions so that you can refer to them later. Call your doctor or pharmacist if you miss a dose and do not know what to do. Do not take a double dose to make up for a missed dose.

What side effects can this medicine cause?

Prednisone may cause side effects. Tell your doctor if any of these symptoms are severe or do not go away:

- headache
- dizziness
- difficulty falling asleep or staying asleep
- inappropriate happiness
- extreme changes in mood
- changes in personality
- bulging eyes
- acne
- thin, fragile skin
- red or purple blotches or lines under the skin
- slowed healing of cuts and bruises
- increased hair growth
- changes in the way fat is spread around the body
- extreme tiredness
- weak muscles
- irregular or absent menstrual periods
- decreased sexual desire
- heartburn
- increased sweating

Some side effects can be serious. If you experience any of the following symptoms, call your doctor immediately:

- vision problems
- eye pain, redness, or tearing
- sore throat, fever, chills, cough, or other signs of infection
- seizures
- depression
- loss of contact with reality
- confusion
- muscle twitching or tightening
- shaking of the hands that you cannot control
- numbness, burning, or tingling in the face, arms, legs, feet, or hands
- upset stomach
- vomiting
- lightheadedness
- irregular heartbeat
- sudden weight gain
- shortness of breath, especially during the night
- dry, hacking cough
- swelling or pain in the stomach
- swelling of the eyes, face, lips, tongue, throat, arms, hands, feet, ankles, or lower legs
- difficulty breathing or swallowing
- rash
- hives
- itching

Prednisone may slow growth and development in children. Your child's doctor will watch his or her growth carefully. Talk to your child's doctor about the risks of giving prednisone to your child.

Prednisone may increase the risk that you will develop osteoporosis. Talk to your doctor about the risks of taking prednisone and about things that you can do to decrease the chance that you will develop osteoporosis.

Some patients who took prednisone or similar medications developed a type of cancer called Kaposi's sarcoma. Talk to your doctor about the risks of taking prednisone.

Prednisone may cause other side effects. Call your doctor if you have any unusual problems while you are taking this medication.

If you experience a serious side effect, you or your doctor may send a report to the Food and Drug Administration's (FDA) MedWatch Adverse Event Reporting program online [at http://www.fda.gov/MedWatch/index.html] or by phone [1-800-332-1088].

What storage conditions are needed for this medicine?

Keep this medication in the container it came in, tightly closed, and out of reach of children. Store it at room temperature and away from excess heat and moisture (not in the bathroom). Throw away any medication that is outdated or no longer needed. Talk to your pharmacist about the proper disposal of your medication.

What should I do in case of overdose?

In case of overdose, call your local poison control center at 1-800-222-1222. If the victim has collapsed or is not breathing, call local emergency services at 911.

What other information should I know?

Keep all appointments with your doctor and the laboratory. Your doctor will order certain lab tests to check your body's response to prednisone.

If you are having any skin tests such as allergy tests or tuberculosis tests, tell the doctor or technician that you are taking prednisone.

Do not let anyone else take your medication. Ask your pharmacist any questions you have about refilling your prescription.

Dosage Facts
For Informational Purposes

Caution: Do not change your dose, how often you take your medication, or the length of time you are to take it without first talking to your healthcare provider.

The following dosage information was written using medical language for doctors and other healthcare professionals and is provided here for you to check your dosage. The dosage of this drug may differ for different patients. Therefore, always follow your doctor's instructions or the directions on the label. Contact your healthcare provider or pharmacist if you have any questions about the specific dosage of your medication after reviewing this information.

General Dosage Information

After a satisfactory response is obtained, decrease dosage in small decrements to the lowest level that maintains an adequate clinical response, and discontinue the drug as soon as possible.

Monitor patients continually for signs that indicate dosage adjustment is necessary, such as remissions or exacerbations of the disease and stress (surgery, infection, trauma).

High dosages may be required for acute situations of certain rheumatic disorders and collagen diseases. After a response has been obtained, drug often must be continued for long periods at low dosage.

High or massive dosages may be required in the treatment of pemphigus, exfoliative dermatitis, bullous dermatitis herpetiformis, severe erythema multiforme, or mycosis fungoides. Early initiation of systemic glucocorticoid therapy may be lifesaving in pemphigus vulgaris. Reduce dosage gradually to the lowest effective level, but discontinuance may not be possible.

Pediatric Patients

Base pediatric dosage on severity of the disease and patient response rather than on strict adherence to dosage indicated by age, body weight, or body surface area.

Usual Dosage

ORAL:
- 0.14–2 mg/kg daily or 4–60 mg/m² daily in 4 divided doses.

Pneumocystis jiroveci (Pneumocystis carinii) Pneumonia

ORAL:
- Adolescents >13 years of age with moderate to severe *Pneumocystis jiroveci* (formerly *Pneumocystis carinii*) pneumonia and acquired immunodeficiency syndrome† (AIDS): 40 mg twice daily for 5 days, followed by 40 mg once daily for 5 days, and then 20 mg once daily for 11 days (or until completion of the anti-infective regimen) currently is recommended. Initiate glucocorticoid therapy within 24–72 hours of initial antipneumocystis therapy. Consult published protocols and the most current clinical guidelines.

Allergic Conditions

ORAL:
- For certain conditions (e.g., contact dermatitis, including poison ivy), 30 mg (6 tablets) for the first day, which is then tapered by 5 mg daily until 21 tablets have been administered (see Tapered Dosage Schedule table).

Tapered Dosage Schedule

Day 1	Administer 10 mg twice daily (before breakfast and at bedtime) and 5 mg twice daily (after lunch and dinner).
Day 2	Administer 5 mg 3 times daily (before breakfast, after lunch, and after dinner) and 10 mg at bedtime.
Day 3	Administer 5 mg 4 times daily (before breakfast, after lunch, after dinner, and at bedtime).
Day 4	Administer 5 mg 3 times daily (before breakfast, after lunch, and at bedtime).
Day 5	Administer 5 mg twice daily (before breakfast and at bedtime).
Day 6	Administer 5 mg before breakfast.

Adult Patients

Usual Dosage

ORAL:
- Initially, 5–60 mg daily, depending on the disease being treated, usually in 2–4 divided doses.

Pneumocystis jiroveci (Pneumocystis carinii) Pneumonia

ORAL:
- Adults with moderate to severe *Pneumocystis jiroveci* (formerly *Pneumocystis carinii*) pneumonia and acquired immunodeficiency syndrome† (AIDS): 40 mg twice daily for 5 days, followed by 40 mg once daily for 5 days, and then 20 mg once daily for 11 days (or until completion of the anti-infective regimen) currently is recommended. Initiate within 24–72 hours of initial antipneumocystis therapy. Consult published protocols and the most current clinical guidelines.

Allergic Conditions

ORAL:
- For certain conditions (e.g., contact dermatitis, including poison ivy), 30 mg (6 tablets) for the first day, which is then tapered by 5 mg daily until 21 tablets have been administered (see Tapered Dosage Schedule table).

Tapered Dosage Schedule

Day 1	Administer 10 mg twice daily (before breakfast and at bedtime) and 5 mg twice daily (after lunch and dinner)
Day 2	Administer 5 mg 3 times daily (before breakfast, after lunch, and after dinner) and 10 mg at bedtime
Day 3	Administer 5 mg 4 times daily (before breakfast, after lunch, after dinner, and at bedtime)
Day 4	Administer 5 mg 3 times daily (before breakfast, after lunch, and at bedtime)
Day 5	Administer 5 mg twice daily (before breakfast and at bedtime)
Day 6	Administer 5 mg before breakfast

Advanced Pulmonary or Extrapulmonary Tuberculosis

ORAL:
- For severe systemic and respiratory complications of advanced pulmonary tuberculosis: 40–60 mg daily, tapered over 4–8 weeks.
- Tuberculous meningitis: 1 mg/kg daily for 30 days, followed by gradual tapering of the dosage over a period of weeks, has been suggested.
- Tuberculous pericarditis: 60 mg daily tapered over 6–12 weeks.
- Tuberculous pleurisy: 20–40 mg daily tapered over 4–8 weeks.
- Mediastinal lymphadenopathy associated with primary intrathoracic tuberculosis: 2–5 mg/kg per day (or equivalent), with dosage reduction to 1 mg/kg per day over the first week and tapered over the next 5 weeks.

Multiple Sclerosis

ORAL:

• For acute exacerbations, the manufacturer recommends 200 mg daily for 1 week followed by 80 mg every other day for 1 month. Alternatively, 60 mg daily tapering over 12 days following IV methylprednisolone (1 g daily for 3–5 days) has been used.

Optic Neuritis

ORAL:

• 1 mg/kg daily for 11 days following IV methylprednisolone therapy (1 g daily for 3 days).

† Use is not currently included in the labeling approved by the US Food and Drug Administration.

Pregabalin

(pre gab′ a lin)

Brand Name: Lyrica®

Why is this medicine prescribed?

Pregabalin is used to relieve neuropathic pain (pain from damaged nerves) that can occur in your arms, hands fingers, legs, feet, or toes if you have diabetes or in the area of your rash if you have shingles (a painful rash that occurs after infection with herpes zoster). It is also used in combination with other medications to treat certain types of seizures in patients with epilepsy. Pregabalin is in a class of medications called anticonvulsants. It works by changing the amounts of certain natural substances in the brain.

How should this medicine be used?

Pregabalin comes as a capsule to take by mouth. It is usually taken with or without food two or three times a day. Take pregabalin at around the same times every day. Follow the directions on your prescription label carefully, and ask your doctor or pharmacist to explain any part you do not understand. Take pregabalin exactly as directed. Do not take more or less of it or take it more often than prescribed by your doctor.

Your doctor will probably start you on a low dose of pregabalin and gradually increase your dose over the first week of treatment.

Pregabalin may be habit forming. Do not take a larger dose, take it more often, or take it for a longer period of time than prescribed by your doctor.

Pregabalin controls your pain or seizures but does not cure them. It may take several weeks or longer before you feel the full benefit of pregabalin. Continue to take pregabalin even if you feel well.

Do not stop taking pregabalin without talking to your doctor. If you suddenly stop taking pregabalin, your seizures may become worse or you may experience withdrawal symptoms (e.g., trouble falling asleep or staying asleep, upset stomach, diarrhea, or headache). Your doctor will decrease your dose gradually over at least a week.

Ask your pharmacist or doctor for a copy of the manufacturer's information for the patient.

Are there other uses for this medicine?

This medication may be prescribed for other uses; ask your doctor or pharmacist for more information.

What special precautions should I follow?

Before taking pregabalin,

• tell your doctor and pharmacist if you are allergic to pregabalin, any other medications, or any of the ingredients in pregabalin capsules.

• tell your doctor and pharmacist what other prescription and nonprescription medications, vitamins, nutritional supplements, and herbal products you are taking or plan to take. Be sure to mention any of the following: antidepressants, antihistamines, medications for anxiety, mental illness, or seizures pioglitazone (Actos), rosiglitazone (Avandia), sedatives, sleeping pills, and tranquilizers. Your doctor may need to change the doses of your medications or monitor you carefully for side effects.

• tell your doctor if you have or have ever had problems with your vision, bleeding problems or blood disorders (low platelets), or heart or kidney problems.

• tell your doctor if you are pregnant, plan to become pregnant, or are breast-feeding. If you become pregnant while taking pregabalin, call your doctor. If you are male, tell your doctor if you plan to father a child. In studies in animals, pregabalin was associated with sperm problems in males and birth defects (physical problems that are present at birth). It is not known if similar effects would be found in humans.

• if you are having surgery, including dental surgery, tell the doctor or dentist that you are taking pregabalin.

• you should know that pregabalin may make you dizzy or drowsy. Do not drive a car or operate machinery until you know how this medication affects you.

• remember that alcohol can add to the drowsiness caused by this medication.

What special dietary instructions should I follow?

Unless your doctor tells you otherwise, continue your normal diet.

What should I do if I forget to take a dose?

If you forget to take a dose and remember a few hours later, take the missed dose as soon as you remember it. However, if it is almost time for the next dose, skip the missed dose and continue your regular dosing schedule. Do not take a double dose to make up for a missed one.

What side effects can this medicine cause?

Pregabalin may cause side effects. Tell your doctor if any of these symptoms are severe or do not go away:

- dry mouth
- constipation
- gas
- tiredness
- dizziness
- difficulty concentrating or paying attention
- confusion
- lack of coordination
- shaking hands that you cannot control
- unsteady walking
- shortness of breath
- weight gain
- pain, including back pain

Some side effects can be serious. If you experience any of these symptoms, call your doctor immediately:

- blurred vision or changes in eyesight
- swelling of the of the face, hands, feet, ankles, or lower legs
- muscle pain, tenderness, or weakness
- fever
- redness or sores on your skin (if you have diabetes)
- bleeding or bruising
- chest pain

Pregabalin has caused tumors in the blood vessels of laboratory animals (mice) in some studies. It is not known if pregablin causes this effect in humans. Talk to your doctor about the risks of taking this medication.

Pregabalin may cause other side effects. Call your doctor if you have any unusual problems while taking this medication.

If you experience a serious side effect, you or your doctor may send a report to the Food and Drug Administration's (FDA) MedWatch Adverse Event Reporting program online [at http://www.fda.gov/MedWatch/index.html] or by phone [1-800-332-1088].

What storage conditions are needed for this medicine?

Keep this medication in the container it came in, tightly closed, and out of reach of children. Store it at room temperature and away from excess heat and moisture (not in the bathroom). Throw away any medication that is outdated or no longer needed. Talk to your pharmacist about the proper disposal of your medication.

What should I do in case of overdose?

In case of overdose, call your local poison control center at 1-800-222-1222. If the victim has collapsed or is not breathing, call local emergency services at 911.

What other information should I know?

Keep all appointments with your doctor and the laboratory. Your doctor may order certain lab tests to check your body's response to pregabalin.

Do not let anyone else take your medication. Ask your pharmacist any questions you have about refilling your prescription.

Dosage Facts
For Informational Purposes

Caution: Do not change your dose, how often you take your medication, or the length of time you are to take it without first talking to your healthcare provider.

The following dosage information was written using medical language for doctors and other healthcare professionals and is provided here for you to check your dosage. The dosage of this drug may differ for different patients. Therefore, always follow your doctor's instructions or the directions on the label. Contact your healthcare provider or pharmacist if you have any questions about the specific dosage of your medication after reviewing this information.

General Dosage Information

Efficacy and adverse effects dose related, although effect of dosage escalation rate on tolerability not studied.

Adult Patients

Seizure Disorders
Partial Seizures

ORAL:

- Initially, 75 mg twice daily or 50 mg 3 times daily (initial dosage not to exceed 150 mg daily). Increase dosage up to a maximum of 600 mg daily, based on individual patient response and tolerability.
- Effective maintenance dosage is 150–600 mg daily, administered in 2 or 3 divided doses.
- Dosage recommendations for use of pregabalin in conjunction with gabapentin not available, since such regimens not evaluated in controlled clinical studies.

Neuropathic Pain
Postherpetic Neuralgia

ORAL:

- Initially, 150 mg daily (75 mg twice daily or 50 mg 3 times daily). Increase dosage to 300 mg daily within 1 week based on efficacy and tolerability.
- Recommended maintenance dosage is 150–300 mg daily in 2 or 3 divided doses.
- May increase dosage up to 600 mg daily (administered in 2 or 3 divided doses) in those who tolerate the drug but do not experience adequate pain relief following 2–4 weeks of treatment with pregabalin 300 mg daily.
- Because of risk for dose-dependent adverse effects and higher rates of treatment discontinuance secondary to adverse effects, reserve dosages exceeding 300 mg daily for those who

have continuing pain and are tolerating the 300-mg daily dosage.

Diabetic Neuropathy

ORAL:

- Initially, 150 mg daily in 3 divided doses (50 mg 3 times daily); increase dosage within 1 week up to a maximum of 300 mg daily (administered in 3 divided doses), based on efficacy and tolerability.
- Higher pregabalin dosages (i.e., dosages exceeding 600 mg daily) provide no additional benefit, but may increase risk of adverse effects.

Prescribing Limits

Adult Patients

Seizure Disorders and Neuropathic Pain

ORAL:

- Maximum 600 mg daily.

Special Populations

Renal Impairment

- Modify dosage of pregabalin in adults with renal impairment (Cl_{cr} <60 mL/minute) based on Cl_{cr}.

Table 1. Pregabalin Dosage Adjustment in Patients with Renal Impairment

Usual Dosage Regimen (for Patients with Creatinine Clearances of ≥60 mL/min)	Creatinine Clearance (mL/min)	Adjusted Dosage Regimen
150 mg daily given in 2 or 3 divided doses	30–60	75 mg daily given in 2 or 3 divided doses
	15–30	25–50 mg daily given as a single dose or in 2 divided doses
	<15	25 mg once daily
300 mg daily given in 2 or 3 divided doses	30–60	150 mg daily given in 2 or 3 divided doses
	15–30	75 mg daily given as a single dose or in 2 divided doses
	<15	25–50 mg once daily
600 mg daily given in 2 or 3 divided doses	30–60	300 mg daily given in 2 or 3 divided doses
	15–30	150 mg daily given as a single dose or in 2 divided doses
	<15	75 mg once daily

Patients undergoing hemodialysis should receive a supplemental dose immediately following each 4-hour dialysis session. Individuals receiving the 25-mg once-daily dosage regimen should receive a supplemental dose of 25 or 50 mg, those receiving the 25- to 50-mg once-daily dosage regimen should receive a supplemental dose of 50 or 75 mg, and those receiving the 75-mg once-daily dosage regimen should receive a supplemental dose of 100 or 150 mg.

Geriatric Patients

- Adjust dosage for geriatric patients with renal impairment.

Primaquine

(prim′ a kwin)

Why is this medicine prescribed?

Primaquine is used alone or with another medication to treat malaria (a serious infection that is spread by mosquitoes in certain parts of the world and can cause death) and to prevent the disease from coming back in people that are infected with malaria. Primaquine is in a class of medications called antimalarials. It works by killing the organisms that cause malaria.

How should this medicine be used?

Primaquine comes as a tablet to take by mouth. It is usually taken once a day for 14 days. Take primaquine at around the same time every day. Follow the directions on your prescription label carefully, and ask your doctor or pharmacist to explain any part you do not understand. Take primaquine exactly as directed. Do not take more or less of it or take it more often or for a longer period of time than prescribed by your doctor.

Take primaquine until you finish the prescription, even if you feel better. If you stop taking primaquine too soon or skip doses, your infection may not be completely treated.

Are there other uses for this medicine?

Primaquine is also sometimes used to treat Pneumocystis jiroveci pneumonia (lung disease caused by fungus). Talk to your doctor about the risks of using this drug for your condition.

This medication may be prescribed for other uses; ask your doctor or pharmacist for more information.

What special precautions should I follow?

Before taking primaquine,

- tell your doctor and pharmacist if you are allergic to primaquine, any other medications, or any of the ingredients in primaquine tablets. Ask your pharmacist for a list of the ingredients.
- tell your doctor if you are taking penicillin; cephalosporins such as cephalexin (Keflex), cefaclor, cefuroxime (Ceftin), cefdinir (Omnicef), or cefpodoxime (Vantin); levodopa (in Sinemet); medications to treat cancer; methyldopa (Aldomet); or quinidine. Your doctor will probably tell you not to take primaquine. Also do not

take primaquine if you are taking or have recently taken quinacrine (not available in the US).

- tell your doctor and pharmacist what other prescription and nonprescription medications, vitamins, nutritional supplements, and herbal products you are taking or plan to take.
- tell your doctor if you have or have ever had rheumatoid arthritis, hemolytic anemia (a condition with an abnormally low number of red blood cells), lupus erythematosus (a disease that occurs when the body's tissues are attacked by antibodies from its own immune system), methemoglobinemia (a condition with defective red blood cells that are unable to carry oxygen to the tissues in the body), nicotinamide adenine dinucleotide (NADH) deficiency (a genetic condition), glucose-6-phosphate dehydrogenase (G6PD) deficiency (a genetic condition), or if you or someone in your family has had a reaction after eating fava beans.
- tell your doctor if you are pregnant, plan to become pregnant, or are breast-feeding. If you become pregnant while taking primaquine, call your doctor.

What special dietary instructions should I follow?

Unless your doctor tells you otherwise, continue your normal diet.

What should I do if I forget to take a dose?

Take the missed dose as soon as you remember it. However, if it is almost time for the next dose, skip the missed dose and continue your regular dosing schedule. Do not take a double dose to make up for a missed one.

What side effects can this medicine cause?

Primaquine may cause side effects. Tell your doctor if any of these symptoms are severe or do not go away:

- nausea
- vomiting
- heartburn
- abdominal cramps

Some side effects can be serious. If you experience any of these symptoms, call your doctor immediately:

- tiredness
- pale skin
- shortness of breath
- fast heartbeat
- yellowing of the skin or eyes
- dark colored urine
- headache
- lack of energy
- grey-bluish color of lips and/or skin
- nervousness
- seizure
- weak pulse
- confusion
- sore throat, fever, cough, or other signs of infection

- fainting
- dizziness
- blurred vision

Primaquine may cause other side effects. Call your doctor if you have any unusual problems while taking this medication.

What storage conditions are needed for this medicine?

Keep this medication in the container it came in, tightly closed, and out of reach of children. Store it at room temperature and away from excess heat and moisture (not in the bathroom). Throw away any medication that is outdated or no longer needed. Talk to your pharmacist about the proper disposal of your medication.

What should I do in case of overdose?

In case of overdose, call your local poison control center at 1-800-222-1222. If the victim has collapsed or is not breathing, call local emergency services at 911.

Symptoms of overdose may include:

- abdominal cramps
- vomiting
- heartburn
- grey-bluish color of lips and/or skin
- headache
- lack of energy
- nervousness
- seizure
- weak pulse
- confusion
- fainting
- dizziness
- blurred vision

What other information should I know?

Keep all appointments with your doctor and the laboratory. Your doctor may order certain lab tests to check your body's response to primaquine.

Before having any laboratory test, tell your doctor and the laboratory personnel that you are taking primaquine.

Do not let anyone else take your medication. Ask your pharmacist any questions you have about refilling your prescription.

Dosage Facts
For Informational Purposes

Caution: Do not change your dose, how often you take your medication, or the length of time you are to take it without first talking to your healthcare provider.

The following dosage information was written using medical language for doctors and other healthcare professionals and is provided here for you to check your

dosage. The dosage of this drug may differ for different patients. Therefore, always follow your doctor's instructions or the directions on the label. Contact your healthcare provider or pharmacist if you have any questions about the specific dosage of your medication after reviewing this information.

General Dosage Information

Available as primaquine phosphate; dosage usually expressed in terms of primaquine. Each 26.3 mg of primaquine phosphate is equivalent to 15 mg of primaquine.

Pediatric Patients

Malaria

Radical Cure and Prevention of Delayed Attacks or Relapse of P. ovale or P. vivax Malaria

ORAL:
- 0.6 mg/kg (1 mg/kg of primaquine phosphate) once daily for 14 days.

Terminal Prophylaxis to Prevent Delayed Primary Attacks or Relapse of P. ovale or P. vivax Malaria

ORAL:
- 0.6 mg/kg (1 mg/kg of primaquine phosphate) once daily for 14 days.
- When used in individuals who have left areas where *P. ovale* or *P. vivax* are endemic, administer primaquine during the last 2 weeks of, or immediately following, primary prophylaxis with chloroquine, doxycycline, or mefloquine. If fixed-combination of atovaquone and proguanil is used for primary prophylaxis, administer primaquine either during the last 7 days of atovaquone and proguanil prophylaxis and then for an additional 7 days, or alternatively, for 14 days after atovaquone and proguanil prophylaxis is discontinued.

Primary Prophylaxis of Malaria (Including Chloroquine-resistant P. falciparum Malaria)†

ORAL:
- 0.6 mg/kg (1 mg/kg of primaquine phosphate) once daily. Initiate prophylaxis 1–2 days prior to entering a malarious area and continue for 3–7 days after leaving the area.

Adult Patients

Malaria

Radical Cure and Prevention of Delayed Attacks or Relapse of P. ovale or P. vivax Malaria

ORAL:
- 30 mg of primaquine (52.6 mg of primaquine phosphate) once daily for 14 days recommended by CDC and others. Manufacturer recommends 15 mg of primaquine (26.3 mg of primaquine phosphate) once daily for 14 days.
- As an alternative to the daily regimen or in patients with borderline G-6-PD deficiency, CDC recommends 45 mg of primaquine (79 mg of primaquine phosphate) once weekly for 8 weeks. Consultation with an expert in infectious disease and/or tropical medicine is recommended if this alternative regimen is considered for individuals with borderline G-6-PD deficiency.

Terminal Prophylaxis to Prevent Delayed Primary Attacks or Relapse of P. ovale or P. vivax Malaria

ORAL:
- 30 mg of primaquine (52.6 mg of primaquine phosphate) once daily for 14 days recommended by CDC and others. Manu-

facturer recommends 15 mg of primaquine (26.3 mg of primaquine phosphate) once daily for 14 days.
- When used in individuals who have left areas where *P. ovale* or *P. vivax* are endemic, administer primaquine during the last 2 weeks of, or immediately following, prophylaxis with chloroquine, doxycycline, or mefloquine. If the fixed-combination atovaquone and proguanil is used for primary prophylaxis, administer primaquine either during the last 7 days of atovaquone and proguanil prophylaxis and then for an additional 7 days, or alternatively, for 14 days after atovaquone and proguanil prophylaxis is discontinued.

Primary Prophylaxis of Malaria (Including Chloroquine-resistant P. falciparum Malaria)†

ORAL:
- 30 mg of primaquine once daily. Initiate prophylaxis 1–2 days prior to entering a malarious area and continue for 3–7 days after leaving the area.

Pneumocystis jiroveci (Pneumocystis carinii) Pneumonia†

Treatment of Mild to Moderate Infections

ORAL:
- 15–30 mg of primaquine once daily for 21 days; used in conjunction with IV clindamycin (600–900 mg every 6–8 hours) or oral clindamycin (300–450 mg orally every 6–8 hours) given for 21 days.

Prescribing Limits

Pediatric Patients

Pediatric dosage should not exceed usual adult dosage.

† Use is not currently included in the labeling approved by the US Food and Drug Administration.

Primidone

(pri′ mi done)

Brand Name: Mysoline®

Why is this medicine prescribed?

Primidone is used to control seizures.

This medication is sometimes prescribed for other uses; ask your doctor or pharmacist for more information.

How should this medicine be used?

Primidone comes as a tablet and suspension (liquid) to take by mouth. It usually is taken once a day at bedtime when you first use it, and then the dosage is gradually increased to three or four times a day. It may be taken with food. Shake the suspension well before each use. Follow the directions on your prescription label carefully, and ask your doctor or pharmacist to explain any part you do not understand. Take primidone exactly as directed. Do not take more or less of it or take it more often than your doctor tells you to.

This medication must be taken regularly to be effective. Do not skip doses even if you feel that you do not need them. Do not stop taking this drug until your doctor specifically tells you to do so. Stopping the drug abruptly can cause seizures. Your doctor probably will decrease your dose gradually.

Are there other uses for this medicine?

Primidone is also used to treat tremors. Talk to your doctor about the possible risks of using this drug for your condition.

What special precautions should I follow?

Before taking primidone,

- tell your doctor and pharmacist if you are allergic to primidone or any other drugs. Also, tell your doctor if you ever had a bad reaction to amobarbital (Amytal), butabarbital (Butisol), pentobarbital (Nembutal), phenobarbital, or secobarbital (Seconal).
- tell your doctor and pharmacist what prescription and nonprescription medications you are taking, especially acetazolamide (Diamox); anticoagulants ('blood thinners') such as warfarin (Coumadin); antihistamines; carbamazepine (Tegretol); disulfiram (Antabuse); doxycycline (Vibramycin); griseofulvin (Fulvicin); isoniazid (INH, Laniazid, Nydrazid); MAO inhibitors [phenelzine (Nardil) or tranylcypromine (Parnate)]; medications for depression, seizures, pain, asthma, colds, or allergies; muscle relaxants; nicotinamide; oral contraceptives; phenytoin (Dilantin); sedatives; sleeping pills; steroids; tranquilizers; valproic acid (Depakene); and vitamins.
- tell your doctor if you have or have ever had anemia or lung, kidney, or liver disease.
- use a method of birth control other than oral contraceptives while taking this medication. Primidone can decrease the effectiveness of oral contraceptives.
- tell your doctor if you are pregnant, plan to become pregnant, or are breast-feeding. If you become pregnant while taking primidone, call your doctor immediately.
- if you are having surgery, including dental surgery, tell the doctor or dentist that you are taking primidone.
- you should know that this drug may make you drowsy. Do not drive a car or operate machinery until you know how this drug affects you.
- remember that alcohol can add to the drowsiness caused by this drug.

What should I do if I forget to take a dose?

Take the missed dose as soon as you remember it and take any remaining doses for that day at evenly spaced intervals. However, if you remember a missed dose at the time you are scheduled to take the next one, skip the missed dose completely. Do not take a double dose to make up for the missed one.

What side effects can this medicine cause?

Side effects from primidone may occur and include:
- drowsiness
- incoordination
- irritability
- excitement (in children)
- upset stomach
- tiredness
- headache
- changes in appetite

Tell your doctor if any of these symptoms are severe or do not go away:
- restlessness or excitement
- hair loss
- swollen eyelids or legs
- double vision
- blurred vision
- changes in sex drive or ability

If you experience any of the following symptoms, call your doctor immediately:
- seizures
- sore throat
- fever
- severe skin rash
- yellowing of the skin or eyes
- dark urine
- bloody nose
- unusual bleeding
- tiny purple skin spots
- easy bruising

If you experience a serious side effect, you or your doctor may send a report to the Food and Drug Administration's (FDA) MedWatch Adverse Event Reporting program online [at http://www.fda.gov/MedWatch/index.html] or by phone [1-800-332-1088].

What storage conditions are needed for this medicine?

Keep this medication in the container it came in, tightly closed, and out of reach of children. Store it at room temperature and away from excess heat and moisture (not in the bathroom). Do not freeze the suspension. Throw away any medication that is outdated or no longer needed. Talk to your pharmacist about the proper disposal of your medication.

What should I do in case of overdose?

In case of overdose, call your local poison control center at 1-800-222-1222. If the victim has collapsed or is not breathing, call local emergency services at 911.

What other information should I know?

Keep all appointments with your doctor and the laboratory. Your doctor will order certain lab tests to check your response to primidone. Your dose may need to be adjusted frequently, especially when you first take primidone.

Differences in effectiveness may be seen with different brands of this medication. Switching brands is not recommended without the advice of your pharmacist. Call your doctor if you continue to have seizures. Carry identification (Medic Alert) stating that you have epilepsy and that you are taking primidone.

Do not let anyone else take your medication. Ask your pharmacist any questions you have about refilling your prescription.

Talk to your doctor, pharmacist, or other healthcare professional if you have questions about dosing information for your medication.

Probenecid

(proe ben' e sid)

Brand Name: Col-Probenecid® (as a combination product containing Probenecid and Colchicine)

Why is this medicine prescribed?

Probenecid is used to treat chronic gout and gouty arthritis. It is used to prevent attacks related to gout, not treat them once they occur. It acts on the kidneys to help the body eliminate uric acid. Probenecid is also used to make certain antibiotics more effective by preventing the body from passing them in the urine.

This medication is sometimes prescribed for other uses; ask your doctor or pharmacist for more information.

How should this medicine be used?

Probenecid comes in a tablet to take by mouth. It usually is taken two times a day when prescribed for chronic gout or gouty arthritis and four times a day when prescribed with antibiotics to make them more effective. Follow the directions on your prescription label carefully, and ask your doctor or pharmacist to explain any part you do not understand. Take probenecid exactly as directed. Do not take more or less of it or take it more often than prescribed by your doctor.

Probenecid may increase the frequency of gout attacks during the first 6-12 months that you take it, although it will eventually prevent them. Another drug, such as colchicine, may be prescribed to decrease this effect.

What special precautions should I follow?

Before taking probenecid,
- tell your doctor and pharmacist if you are allergic to probenecid or any other drugs.
- tell your doctor and pharmacist what prescription and nonprescription medications you are taking, especially aminosalicylic acid, antibiotics, aspirin, cancer chemotherapy agents (methotrexate), clofibrate (Atromid-S), dapsone, diflunisal (Dolobid), diuretics ('water pills'), heparin, indomethacin (Indocin), medication for anxiety, nitrofurantoin (Macrodantin, Macrobid), oral diabetes medications, pyrazinamide, salsalate (Disalcid),

and vitamins. Because aspirin products may affect the way your body responds to probenecid, you should avoid them while taking probenecid. If you need something to relieve minor pain or fever, ask your doctor or pharmacist to recommend an aspirin substitute, such as acetaminophen (Tylenol).
- tell your doctor if you have or have ever had ulcers, kidney stones, a kidney disorder, or a blood disorder.
- tell your doctor if you are pregnant, plan to become pregnant, or are breast-feeding. If you become pregnant while taking probenecid, call your doctor immediately.
- tell your doctor if you plan to have surgery involving a general anesthetic.
- if you are having any urine tests done, tell your doctor and the laboratory personnel that you are taking probenecid because it may affect the results of the test.

What special dietary instructions should I follow?

Drink at least six to eight full glasses of water a day while taking probenecid to prevent kidney stones, unless directed to do otherwise by your doctor.

Probenecid may cause an upset stomach. Take with food or antacids.

What should I do if I forget to take a dose?

Take the missed dose as soon as you remember it. However, if it is almost time for the next dose, skip the missed dose and continue your regular dosing schedule. Do not take a double dose to make up for a missed one.

What side effects can this medicine cause?

Probenecid may cause side effects. Tell your doctor if any of these symptoms are severe or do not go away:
- headache
- upset stomach
- vomiting
- loss of appetite
- dizziness

If you experience any of the following symptoms, call your doctor immediately:
- severe skin rash
- difficulty breathing or swallowing
- unusual bleeding or bruising

If you experience a serious side effect, you or your doctor may send a report to the Food and Drug Administration's (FDA) MedWatch Adverse Event Reporting program online [at http://www.fda.gov/MedWatch/index.html] or by phone [1-800-332-1088].

What storage conditions are needed for this medicine?

Keep this medication in the container it came in, tightly closed, and out of reach of children. Store it at room temperature and away from excess heat and moisture (not in the

---

bathroom). Throw away any medication that is outdated or no longer needed. Talk to your pharmacist about the proper disposal of your medication.

What should I do in case of overdose?

In case of overdose, call your local poison control center at 1-800-222-1222. If the victim has collapsed or is not breathing, call local emergency services at 911.

What other information should I know?

Keep all appointments with your doctor and the laboratory. Your doctor will order certain lab tests to check your response to probenecid.

Do not let anyone else take your medication. Ask your pharmacist any questions you have about refilling your prescription.

Talk to your doctor, pharmacist, or other healthcare professional if you have questions about dosing information for your medication.

Procainamide Oral

(proe kane a′ mide)

Brand Name: Procanbid®
Also available generically.

Important Warning

Antiarrhythmic drugs, including procainamide, may increase the risk of death. Tell your doctor if you have had a heart attack within the past two years. Procainamide should be used only to treat life-threatening arrhythmias (irregular heartbeats).

Procainamide may cause a decrease in the number of cells in your bone marrow. Procainamide may also cause symptoms of lupus.

Keep all appointments with your doctor and the laboratory. Your doctor will order certain lab tests to check your response to procainamide.

If you experience any of the following symptoms, call your doctor immediately: fever, chills, sore throat, bruising, bleeding, muscle aches or weakness, stomach or chest pain, skin rash, or blisters on the cheek, tongue and lips.

Talk to your doctor about the risks of taking procainamide.

Why is this medicine prescribed?

Procainamide is used to treat abnormal heart rhythms. It works by making your heart more resistant to abnormal activity.

How should this medicine be used?

Procainamide comes as a capsule and tablet to take by mouth. Immediate-acting procainamide usually is taken every 3 or 4 hours. The long-acting product is usually taken every 6 or 12 hours. Do not cut, crush, or chew extended-release (long-acting) tablets; swallow them whole. You may see a waxy core in your stool if you are taking the extended-release product; this is normal.

Follow the directions on your prescription label carefully, and ask your doctor or pharmacist to explain any part you do not understand. Take procainamide exactly as directed. Do not take more or less of it or take it more often than prescribed by your doctor.

Procainamide helps control your condition but will not cure it. Continue to take procainamide even if you feel well. Do not stop taking procainamide without talking to your doctor.

Are there other uses for this medicine?

This medication should not be prescribed for other uses; ask your doctor or pharmacist for more information.

What special precautions should I follow?

Before taking procainamide,

- tell your doctor and pharmacist if you are allergic to procainamide, anesthetics, aspirin, or any other drugs.
- tell your doctor and pharmacist what prescription and nonprescription medications you are taking, especially digoxin (Lanoxin) or drugs for high blood pressure, and vitamins.
- in addition to the condition listed in the IMPORTANT WARNING section, tell your doctor if you have or have ever had lupus, heart disease, high blood pressure, kidney or liver disease, or myasthenia gravis.
- tell your doctor if you are pregnant, plan to become pregnant, or are breast-feeding. If you become pregnant while taking procainamide, call your doctor.
- if you are having surgery, including dental surgery, tell the doctor or dentist that you are taking procainamide.
- you should know that this drug may make you dizzy. Do not drive a car or operate machinery until you know how this drug affects you.
- remember that alcohol can add to the dizziness caused by this drug.
- talk to your doctor about the use of cigarettes and caffeine-containing beverages. These products may increase the irritability of your heart and interfere with the action of procainamide.

What should I do if I forget to take a dose?

Take the missed dose as soon as you remember it. However, if it is almost time for the next dose, skip the missed dose and continue your regular dosing schedule. Do not take a double dose to make up for a missed one.

What side effects can this medicine cause?

Procainamide may cause side effects. Tell your doctor if any of these symptoms are severe or do not go away:

- dizziness or lightheadedness
- loss of appetite
- upset stomach
- vomiting
- bitter taste

If you experience the following symptom or any of those listed in the IMPORTANT WARNING section, call your doctor immediately:

- irregular heartbeat

If you experience a serious side effect, you or your doctor may send a report to the Food and Drug Administration's (FDA) MedWatch Adverse Event Reporting program online [at http://www.fda.gov/MedWatch/index.html] or by phone [1-800-332-1088].

What storage conditions are needed for this medicine?

Keep this medication in the container it came in, tightly closed, and out of reach of children. Store it at room temperature and away from excess heat and moisture (not in the bathroom). Throw away any medication that is outdated or no longer needed. Talk to your pharmacist about the proper disposal of your medication.

What should I do in case of overdose?

In case of overdose, call your local poison control center at 1-800-222-1222. If the victim has collapsed or is not breathing, call local emergency services at 911.

What other information should I know?

Keep all appointments with your doctor and the laboratory. Your doctor will need to determine your response to procainamide.

Take procainamide at the same time each day in regularly spaced intervals. Changing the time of your doses prevents procainamide from working effectively.

Do not let anyone else take your medication. Ask your pharmacist any questions you have about refilling your prescription.

Dosage Facts
For Informational Purposes

Caution: Do not change your dose, how often you take your medication, or the length of time you are to take it without first talking to your healthcare provider.

The following dosage information was written using medical language for doctors and other healthcare professionals and is provided here for you to check your dosage. The dosage of this drug may differ for different patients. Therefore, always follow your doctor's instructions or the directions on the label. Contact your healthcare provider or pharmacist if you have any questions about the specific dosage of your medication after reviewing this information.

General Dosage Information

Available as procainamide hydrochloride; dosage expressed in terms of the salt.

Adjust dosage carefully according to individual requirements and response, age, renal function, and the general condition and cardiovascular status of the patient.

Monitor BP, cardiac function (via ECG) and also renal function (i.e. Cl_{cr}), especially when given IV or when given orally for prolonged periods and in patients with increased risk of adverse reactions to procainamide, such as patients >50 years of age or those with severe heart disease, hypotension, or hepatic or renal disease.

Reduce dosage in renal insufficiencyand/or CHF and in critically ill patients; determine plasma concentrations of procainamide and its major metabolite (N-acetyl procainamide) and adjust dosage to maintain desired concentrations.

Pediatric Patients

Ventricular and Supraventricular Arrhythmias

ORAL (CONVENTIONAL TABLETS OR CAPSULES):
- 15–50 mg/kg *daily* (not to exceed 4 g in 24 hours), given in divided doses (every 3–6 hours).

Adult Patients

Ventricular Arrhythmias

ORAL (CONVENTIONAL TABLETS OR CAPSULES):
- Usual dosage: Initially, up to 50 mg/kg daily (to achieve therapeutic plasma procainamide concentrations), given in divided doses every 3 hours.
- 6.25 mg/kg has been administered every 3 hours for VPCs.

ORAL (EXTENDED-RELEASE TABLETS DESIGNED FOR ADMINISTRATION EVERY 6 HOURS):
- Usual dosage: Up to 50 mg/kg daily given in equally divided doses at 6-hour intervals.
- Maintenance: One-fourth of the total required daily dose may be given every 6 hours.

ORAL (EXTENDED-RELEASE TABLETS DESIGNED FOR ADMINISTRATION EVERY 12 HOURS [PROCANBID®]):
- Usual dosage: Up to 50 mg/kg (2–5 g, depending on weight) daily, given in equally divided doses at 12-hour intervals.
- Maintenance: One-half of the total required daily dose may be given every 12 hours.
- Patients receiving other formulations of procainamide may be switched to Procanbid® extended-release tablets at the nearest equivalent total daily dosage; however, retitration with Procanbid® is recommended.

Supraventricular Tachyarrhythmias
Conversion of Atrial Fibrillation and Paroxysmal Atrial Tachycardia

ORAL (CONVENTIONAL TABLETS OR CAPSULES):
- Initially, 1.25 g; if no change in ECG, give 750 mg 1 hour later.

- Give additional doses of 0.5–1 g every 2 hours until normal sinus rhythm is restored or until toxic effects appear.

Conversion of Atrial Flutter

ORAL (CONVENTIONAL TABLETS OR CAPSULES):
- Individualize dosage according to the therapeutic response.

Maintainance of Normal Sinus Rhythm after Conversion

ORAL (CONVENTIONAL TABLETS OR CAPSULES):
- Usual dosage: 0.5–1 g every 4–6 hours.

Maintenance Therapy of Atrial Fibrillation and Paroxysmal Atrial Tachycardia

ORAL (EXTENDED-RELEASE TABLETS DESIGNED FOR ADMINISTRATION EVERY 6 HOURS):
- One-fourth of the total required daily dose given every 6 hours; usual dosage is 1 g every 6 hours.

Prescribing Limits

Pediatric Patients

Ventricular and Supraventricular Arrhythmias

ORAL (CONVENTIONAL TABLETS OR CAPSULES):
- Maximum daily dosage is 4 g.

Special Populations

Hepatic Impairment
- No specific dosage recommendations.

Renal Impairment
- Adjust dosage because of risk of drug accumulation and toxicity secondary to decreased clearance and increased elimination half-life.

Geriatric Patients
- Monitor ECG and renal function and dose cautiously, especially prolonged therapy. Maintenance dosage generally lower than that in younger adults; base dosage on response, tolerance, and serum concentrations.

† Use is not currently included in the labeling approved by the US Food and Drug Administration.

Prochlorperazine

(proe klor per′ a zeen)

Brand Name: Compazine®, Compazine® Spansule®, Compazine® Syrup, Compro®
Also available generically.

Why is this medicine prescribed?

Prochlorperazine is used to treat the nausea and vomiting caused by radiation therapy, cancer chemotherapy, surgery, and other conditions. It is also used to treat psychotic symptoms such as hallucinations and hostility.

This medication is sometimes prescribed for other uses; ask your doctor or pharmacist for more information.

How should this medicine be used?

Prochlorperazine comes as a tablet, extended-release (long-acting) capsule, oral liquid, and rectal suppository. Prochlorperazine usually is taken three or four times a day (tablets), or once or twice a day (extended-release capsules). Follow the directions on your prescription label carefully, and ask your doctor or pharmacist to explain any part you do not understand. Take prochlorperazine exactly as directed. Do not take more or less of it or take it more often than prescribed by your doctor.

Although prochlorperazine is not habit-forming, do not stop taking it abruptly, especially if you have been taking it for a long time. Your doctor probably will decrease your dose gradually.

Do not open extended-release capsules; swallow them whole.

Do not allow the liquid to touch your skin; it can cause irritation.

If you are to insert a rectal suppository, follow these steps:
1. If the suppository feels soft, hold it under cold, running water for 1 minute. Then remove the wrapper.
2. Dip the tip of the suppository in water.
3. Lie down on your left side and raise your right knee to your chest. (A left-handed person should lie on the right side and raise the left knee.)
4. Using your finger, insert the suppository into the rectum, about 1/2 to 1 inch in children and 1 inch in adults. Hold the suppository in place for a few moments.
5. Stand up after about 15 minutes. Wash your hands thoroughly and resume your normal activities.

What special precautions should I follow?

Before taking prochlorperazine,
- tell your doctor and pharmacist if you are allergic to prochlorperazine, any tranquilizer, or any other drugs.
- tell your doctor and pharmacist what prescription and nonprescription medications you are taking, especially antihistamines, lithium (Eskalith, Lithobid), medications for depression and Parkinson's disease, muscle relaxants, narcotics (pain medication), sedatives, seizure medication, sleeping pills, and vitamins.
- be sure a child younger than 16 years of age does not have symptoms of Reye's syndrome (sudden, severe, and persistent vomiting; unusual behavior; fever; and seizures). Call your child's doctor immediately if your child experiences any of these symptoms. Do not give prochlorperazine or aspirin to the child.
- tell your doctor if you have or have ever had heart, liver, or kidney disease; a bad reaction to insulin; shock therapy; glaucoma; an enlarged prostate; difficulty urinating; asthma, emphysema, chronic bronchitis, or lung disease; Parkinson's disease; or seizures.

- tell your doctor if you are pregnant, plan to become pregnant, or are breast-feeding. If you become pregnant while taking prochlorperazine, call your doctor.
- if you are having surgery, including dental surgery, tell the doctor or dentist that you are taking prochlorperazine.
- you should know that this drug may make you drowsy. Do not drive a car or operate machinery until you know how this drug affects you.
- remember that alcohol can add to the drowsiness caused by this drug.
- plan to avoid unnecessary or prolonged exposure to sunlight and to wear protective clothing, sunglasses, and sunscreen. Prochlorperazine may make your skin sensitive to sunlight.

What should I do if I forget to take a dose?

Take the missed dose as soon as you remember it. However, if it is almost time for the next dose, skip the missed dose and continue your regular dosing schedule. Do not take a double dose to make up for a missed one.

What side effects can this medicine cause?

Prochlorperazine may cause side effects. Tell your doctor if this symptom is severe or does not go away:

- drowsiness

If you experience any of the following symptoms, call your doctor immediately:

- jaw, neck, and back muscle spasms
- fine worm-like tongue movements
- rhythmic face, mouth, or jaw movements
- slow or difficult speech
- difficulty swallowing
- restlessness and pacing
- tremors
- shuffling walk
- skin rash
- yellowing of the skin or eyes

If you experience a serious side effect, you or your doctor may send a report to the Food and Drug Administration's (FDA) MedWatch Adverse Event Reporting program online [at http://www.fda.gov/MedWatch/index.html] or by phone [1-800-332-1088].

What storage conditions are needed for this medicine?

Keep this medication in the container it came in, tightly closed, and out of reach of children. Store it at room temperature and away from excess heat and moisture (not in the bathroom). Throw away any medication that is outdated or no longer needed. Talk to your pharmacist about the proper disposal of your medication.

What should I do in case of overdose?

In case of overdose, call your local poison control center at 1-800-222-1222. If the victim has collapsed or is not breathing, call local emergency services at 911.

What other information should I know?

Keep all appointments with your doctor.

Do not let anyone else take your medication. Ask your pharmacist any questions you have about refilling your prescription.

Dosage Facts
For Informational Purposes

Caution: Do not change your dose, how often you take your medication, or the length of time you are to take it without first talking to your healthcare provider.

The following dosage information was written using medical language for doctors and other healthcare professionals and is provided here for you to check your dosage. The dosage of this drug may differ for different patients. Therefore, always follow your doctor's instructions or the directions on the label. Contact your healthcare provider or pharmacist if you have any questions about the specific dosage of your medication after reviewing this information.

General Dosage Information

Available as prochlorperazine, prochlorperazine edisylate, or prochlorperazine maleate; dosage expressed in terms of prochlorperazine.

Pediatric Patients

Children should receive the lowest possible effective dosage, and parents should be instructed not to exceed the prescribed dosage.

Use not recommended in children <2 years of age or those weighing <9 kg.

Prescriptions for 2.5-mg pediatric suppositories should be written as "2 ½ mg" to avoid confusion with 25-mg adult suppositories.

Psychotic Disorders
ORAL OR RECTAL:
- Children 2–12 years of age: Initially, 2.5 mg 2 or 3 times daily. Dosage may be increased according to patient's therapeutic response and tolerance, but usually should not exceed 20 and 25 mg daily for children 2–5 and 6–12 years of age, respectively.
- Dosage for children <2 years of age or those weighing <9 kg not established.

Nausea and Vomiting

ORAL OR RECTAL:

Dosage for Treatment of Severe Nausea and Vomiting in Children ≥2 Years of Age

Weight (kg)	Daily Dosage
≤9	Use not recommended
9.1–13.2	2.5 mg once or twice daily
13.6–17.7	2.5 mg 2 or 3 times daily
18.2–38.6	2.5 mg 3 times daily or 5 mg twice daily

　　　Alternatively, in children ≥2 years of age and weighing >9 kg: 0.4 mg/kg or 10 mg/m² daily given in 3 or 4 divided doses.

　　　Generally, it is not necessary to continue therapy for >24 hours.

Adult Patients

Psychotic Disorders

ORAL:
- 5 or 10 mg (as conventional tablets or oral solution) 3 or 4 times daily in office patients and outpatients with relatively mild symptomatology.
- Initially, 10 mg (as conventional tablets or oral solution) 3 or 4 times daily for hospitalized or well-supervised patients with moderate to severe symptomatology. Gradually increase dosage every 2 or 3 days until symptoms are controlled or adverse effects become troublesome. Although some patients exhibit optimum response with 50–75 mg daily, dosages up to 150 mg daily may be required in severely disturbed patients.

Nonpsychotic Anxiety

ORAL:
- 5 mg (as conventional tablets or oral solution) 3 or 4 times daily for ≤12 weeks.
- Alternatively, a dosage of 15 mg (as extended-release capsules) once daily upon arising or 10 mg (as extended-release capsules) every 12 hours may be used.

Nausea and Vomiting

ORAL:
- Usually, 5 or 10 mg (as conventional tablets or oral solution) 3 or 4 times daily.
- Alternatively, 15 mg (as extended-release capsules) once daily upon arising or 10 mg (as extended-release capsules) every 12 hours may be used; some patients subsequently may require a dosage of 30 mg (using the appropriate number of 10- or 15-mg extended-release capsules) once daily in the morning.
- Dosages >40 mg daily should be used only in resistant cases.

RECTAL:
- 25 mg twice daily.

Prescribing Limits

Pediatric Patients

Psychotic Disorders

ORAL OR RECTAL:
- Maximum 10 mg daily for the first day.
- Subsequently, maximum 20 and 25 mg daily for children 2–5 and 6–12 years of age, respectively.

Nausea and Vomiting

ORAL OR RECTAL:

Maximum Dosage for Treatment of Severe Nausea and Vomiting in Children ≥2 Years of Age

Weight (kg)	Maximum Daily Dosage
≤9	Use not recommended
9.1–13.2	Maximum 7.5 mg daily
13.6–17.7	Maximum 10 mg daily
18.2–38.6	Maximum 15 mg daily

Adult Patients

Nonpsychotic Anxiety

ORAL:
- Maximum 20 mg daily; do not administer for >12 weeks.

Nausea and Vomiting

ORAL:
- Dosages >40 mg daily should be used only in resistant cases.

Special Populations

Geriatric Patients
- Generally, select dose at lower end of recommended range; increase dosage gradually and monitor closely.

Debilitated or Emaciated Patients
- Increase dosage gradually.

Procyclidine

(proe sye′ kli deen)

Brand Name: Kemadrin®

Why is this medicine prescribed?

Procyclidine is used to treat parkinsonism (slowed movements, stiffness of the body, uncontrollable body movements, weakness, tiredness, soft voice, and other symptoms caused by damaged nerves in the brain). Procyclidine is also used to treat problems with moving and drooling that may be caused by certain medications for mental illness. Procyclidine is in a class of medications called antispasmodics or antimuscarinics. It works by preventing sudden tightening of the muscles.

How should this medicine be used?

Procyclidine comes as a tablet to take by mouth. It is usually taken 3 times a day during or after meals and is sometimes also taken at bedtime. Take procyclidine at around the same times every day. Follow the directions on your prescription label carefully, and ask your doctor or pharmacist to explain any part you do not understand. Take procyclidine exactly as directed. Do not take more or less of it or take it more often than prescribed by your doctor.

Your doctor will probably start you on a low dose of procyclidine and gradually increase your dose.

Procyclidine may help control your symptoms but will not cure your condition. Continue to take procyclidine even if you feel well. Do not stop taking procyclidine without talking to your doctor.

Are there other uses for this medicine?

This medication may be prescribed for other uses; ask your doctor or pharmacist for more information.

What special precautions should I follow?

Before taking procyclidine,

- tell your doctor and pharmacist if you are allergic to procyclidine, any other medications, or any of the ingredients in procyclidine tablets. Ask your pharmacist for a list of the ingredients in procyclidine tablets.
- tell your doctor and pharmacist what prescription and nonprescription medications, vitamins, nutritional supplements, and herbal products you are taking or plan to take. Your doctor may need to change the doses of your medications or monitor you carefully for side effects.
- tell your doctor if you have or have ever had glaucoma (an eye disease), enlargement of the prostate (a male reproductive gland), low blood pressure, mental illness, fast or irregular heartbeat, ulcers, colitis (swelling of the intestine), difficulty urinating, or heart, kidney, liver, lung, nervous system, or thyroid disease.
- tell your doctor if you are pregnant, plan to become pregnant, or are breast-feeding. If you become pregnant while taking procyclidine, call your doctor.
- you should know that procyclidine may make you drowsy or dizzy or cause blurred vision. Do not drive a car or operate machinery until you know how this medication affects you.
- you should know that procyclidine may make it harder for your body to cool down when it gets very hot. Drink plenty of fluids and be careful while exercising or participating in outside activities, especially in warm weather.

What special dietary instructions should I follow?

Unless your doctor tells you otherwise, continue your normal diet.

What should I do if I forget to take a dose?

Take the missed dose as soon as you remember it. However, if it is almost time for the next dose, skip the missed dose and continue your regular dosing schedule. Do not take a double dose to make up for a missed one.

What side effects can this medicine cause?

Procyclidine may cause side effects. Tell your doctor if any of these symptoms are severe or do not go away:

- dry mouth
- widening of the pupils (black circle in the middle of the eye)
- blurred vision
- upset stomach
- vomiting
- stomach pain
- constipation
- giddiness
- lightheadedness
- muscle weakness
- rash

Some side effects can be serious. The following symptoms are uncommon, but if you experience any of them, call your doctor immediately:

- confusion
- disorientation
- agitation
- hallucinations (seeing things or hearing voices that do not exist)
- fever
- pain, swelling, redness, or hardness of the cheek
- drainage of pus in the mouth

Procyclidine may cause other side effects. Call your doctor if you have any unusual problems while taking this medication.

If you experience a serious side effect, you or your doctor may send a report to the Food and Drug Administration's (FDA) MedWatch Adverse Event Reporting program online [at http://www.fda.gov/MedWatch/index.html] or by phone [1-800-332-1088].

What storage conditions are needed for this medicine?

Keep this medication in the container it came in, tightly closed, and out of reach of children. Store it at room temperature and away from excess heat and moisture (not in the bathroom). Throw away any medication that is outdated or no longer needed. Talk to your pharmacist about the proper disposal of your medication.

What should I do in case of overdose?

In case of overdose, call your local poison control center at 1-800-222-1222. If the victim has collapsed or is not breathing, call local emergency services at 911.

What other information should I know?

Keep all appointments with your doctor.

Do not let anyone else take your medication. Ask your pharmacist any questions you have about refilling your prescription.

Dosage Facts
For Informational Purposes

Caution: Do not change your dose, how often you take your medication, or the length of time you are to take it without first talking to your healthcare provider.

The following dosage information was written using medical language for doctors and other healthcare professionals and is provided here for you to check your dosage. The dosage of this drug may differ for different patients. Therefore, always follow your doctor's instructions or the directions on the label. Contact your healthcare provider or pharmacist if you have any questions about the specific dosage of your medication after reviewing this information.

General Dosage Information

Available as procyclidine hydrochloride; dosage expressed in terms of the salt.

Adjust dosage carefully according to individual requirements and response.

Adult Patients

Parkinsonian Syndrome

Younger and postencephalitic patients require and tolerate a higher dosage than geriatric patients or those with arteriosclerosis.

Therapy-Naive Patients

ORAL:
- Initially, 2.5 mg 3 times daily after meals. As tolerated, gradually increase to 5 mg 3 times daily or the minimum dosage needed to control symptoms. If needed, administer an additional 5-mg dose at bedtime.
- If bedtime dosage is not tolerated, total daily dosage may be administered in 3 divided doses.

Patients Transferring from Other Antiparkinsonian Therapy

ORAL:
- Gradually substitute 2.5 mg 3 times daily for all or part of original drug. Increase procyclidine dose as needed while decreasing other drug until complete replacement achieved.

Drug-Induced Extrapyramidal Reactions

ORAL:
- Initially, 2.5 mg 3 times daily; increase by 2.5-mg increments until symptoms controlled.
- Usual dosage: 10–20 mg daily.

Special Populations

No special population dosage recommendations at this time.

Progesterone
(proe jes' ter one)

Brand Name: Prometrium®

Why is this medicine prescribed?

Progesterone is used as a part of hormone replacement therapy in women who have passed menopause (the change of life) and have not had a hysterectomy (surgery to remove the uterus). Hormone replacement therapy usually includes estrogen, which is used to treat symptoms of menopause and reduce the risk of developing certain diseases. However, estrogen can also cause abnormal thickening of the lining of the uterus and increase the risk of developing uterine cancer. Progesterone helps to prevent this thickening and decreases the risk of developing uterine cancer. Progesterone is also used to bring on menstruation (period) in women of childbearing age who have had normal periods and then stopped menstruating. Progesterone is in a class of medications called progestins (female hormones). It works as part of hormone replacement therapy by decreasing the amount of estrogen in the uterus. It works to bring on menstruation by replacing the natural progesterone that some women are missing.

How should this medicine be used?

Progesterone comes as a capsule to take by mouth. It is usually taken once a day in the evening or at bedtime. You will probably take progesterone on a rotating schedule that alternates 10-12 days when you take progesterone with 16-18 days when you do not take the medication. Your doctor will tell you exactly when to take progesterone. To help you remember to take progesterone, take it around the same time in the evening. Follow the directions on your prescription label carefully, and ask your doctor or pharmacist to explain any part you do not understand. Take progesterone exactly as directed. Do not take more or less of it or take it more often than prescribed by your doctor.

Continue to take progesterone as directed even if you feel well. Do not stop taking progesterone without talking to your doctor.

Are there other uses for this medicine?

This medication may be prescribed for other uses; ask your doctor or pharmacist for more information.

What special precautions should I follow?

Before taking progesterone,
- tell your doctor and pharmacist if you are allergic to progesterone, oral contraceptives (birth control pills), hormone replacement therapy, any other medications, or peanuts.
- tell your doctor and pharmacist what other prescription and nonprescription medications, vitamins, and nutri

tional supplements you are taking. Be sure to mention any of the following: amiodarone (Cordarone, Pacerone); antifungals such as fluconazole (Diflucan), itraconazole (Sporanox), and ketoconazole (Nizoral); cimetidine (Tagamet); clarithromycin (Biaxin); cyclosporine (Neoral, Samdimmune); danazol (Danocrine); delaviridine (Rescriptor); diltiazem (Cardizem, Dilacor, Tiazac); erythromycin (E.E.S, E-Mycin, Erythrocin); fluoxetine (Prozac, Sarafem); fluvoxamine (Luvox); HIV protease inhibitors such as indinavir (Crixivan), ritonavir (Norvir), and saquinavir (Fortovase); isoniazid (INH, Nydrazid); lansoprazole (Prevacid, Prevpac); metronidazole (Flagyl); nefazodone (Serzone); omeprazole (Prilosec); oral contraceptives (birth control pills); ticlopidine (Ticlid); troleandomycin (TAO); verapamil (Calan, Covera, Isoptin, Verelan); and zafirlukast (Accolate). Your doctor may need to change the doses of your medications or monitor you carefully for side effects.

- tell your doctor what herbal products you are taking, especially St. John's wort.
- tell your doctor if you have or have ever had unexplained vaginal bleeding between periods; a miscarriage in which some tissue was left in the uterus; cancer of the breasts or female organs; seizures; migraine headaches; asthma; diabetes; depression; blood clots in the legs, lungs, eyes, brain, or anywhere in the body; stroke or ministroke; vision problems; or liver, kidney, heart, or gallbladder disease.
- tell your doctor if you are pregnant, plan to become pregnant, or are breast-feeding. If you become pregnant while taking progesterone, call your doctor.
- if you are having surgery, including dental surgery, tell the doctor or dentist that you are taking progesterone.
- you should know that progesterone may make you dizzy or drowsy. Do not drive a car or operate machinery until you know how this medication affects you. If progesterone does make you dizzy or drowsy, take your daily dose at bedtime.
- you should know that progesterone may cause dizziness, lightheadedness, and fainting when you get up too quickly from a lying position. This is more common when you first start taking progesterone. To avoid this problem, get out of bed slowly, resting your feet on the floor for a few minutes before standing up.

What special dietary instructions should I follow?

Talk to your doctor about drinking grapefruit juice while taking this medication.

What should I do if I forget to take a dose?

Take the missed dose as soon as you remember it. However, if it is almost time for the next dose, skip the missed dose and continue your regular dosing schedule. Do not take a double dose to make up for a missed one.

What side effects can this medicine cause?

Progesterone may cause side effects. Tell your doctor if any of these symptoms are severe or do not go away:
- headache
- breast tenderness or pain
- upset stomach
- vomiting
- diarrhea
- constipation
- tiredness
- muscle, joint, or bone pain
- mood swings
- irritability
- excessive worrying
- runny nose
- sneezing
- cough
- vaginal discharge
- problems urinating

Some side effects can be serious. The following symptoms are uncommon, but if you experience any of them, call your doctor immediately:
- breast lumps
- migraine headache
- severe dizziness or faintness
- slow or difficult speech
- weakness or numbness of an arm or leg
- lack of coordination or loss of balance
- shortness of breath
- fast heartbeat
- sharp chest pain
- coughing up blood
- leg swelling or pain
- loss of vision or blurred vision
- bulging eyes
- double vision
- unexpected vaginal bleeding
- shaking hands that you cannot control
- seizures
- stomach pain or swelling
- depression
- hives
- skin rash
- itching
- difficulty breathing or swallowing
- swelling of the face, throat, tongue, lips, eyes, hands, feet, ankles, or lower legs
- hoarseness

Laboratory animals who were given progesterone developed tumors. It is not known if progesterone increases the risk of tumors in humans. Talk to your doctor about the risks of taking this medication.

Medications like progesterone may cause abnormal blood clotting. This may cut off the blood supply to the brain, heart, lungs, or eyes and cause serious problems. Call your doctor if you experience any of the symptoms listed above as serious side effects. Talk to your doctor about the risks of taking this medication.

Progesterone may cause other side effects. Call your doctor if you have any unusual problems while taking this medication.

If you experience a serious side effect, you or your doctor may send a report to the Food and Drug Administration's (FDA) MedWatch Adverse Event Reporting program online [at http://www.fda.gov/MedWatch/index.html] or by phone [1-800-332-1088].

What storage conditions are needed for this medicine?

Keep this medication in the container it came in, tightly closed, and out of reach of children. Store it at room temperature and away from excess heat and moisture (not in the bathroom). Throw away any medication that is outdated or no longer needed. Talk to your pharmacist about the proper disposal of your medication.

What should I do in case of overdose?

In case of overdose, call your local poison control center at 1-800-222-1222. If the victim has collapsed or is not breathing, call local emergency services at 911.

What other information should I know?

Keep all appointments with your doctor.

Before having any laboratory test or biopsy (removal of tissue for testing), tell your doctor and the laboratory personnel that you are taking progesterone.

Do not let anyone else take your medication. Ask your pharmacist any questions you have about refilling your prescription.

Talk to your doctor, pharmacist, or other healthcare professional if you have questions about dosing information for your medication.

Progestin-Only Oral Contraceptives

(pro jes' tin)

Brand Name: Micronor®, Nor-Q.D.®, Ovrette®

Why is this medicine prescribed?

Progestin-only oral contraceptives are used to prevent pregnancy. Progestin is a female hormone. It works by preventing the release of eggs from the ovaries (ovulation) and changing the cervical mucus and the lining of the uterus. Progestin-only oral contraceptives are a very effective

method of birth control, but they do not prevent the spread of AIDS and other sexually transmitted diseases.

How should this medicine be used?

Progestin-only oral contraceptives come as tablets to take by mouth. They are taken once a day, every day at the same time. Follow the directions on your prescription label carefully, and ask your doctor or pharmacist to explain any part you do not understand. Take progestin-only oral contraceptives exactly as directed. Do not take more or less of it or take it more often than prescribed by your doctor.

Progestin-only oral contraceptives come in packs of 28 pills. Begin the next pack the day after the last pack is finished.

It is best to start taking progestin-only oral contraceptives on the first day of your menstrual period. If you start taking progestin-only oral contraceptives on another day, use a backup method of birth control (such as a condom and/or a spermicide) for the next 48 hours. If you have had a miscarriage or an abortion, you can start taking progestin-only oral contraceptives the next day.

Progestin-only oral contraceptives are safe for use by breast-feeding mothers. If you are fully breastfeeding (not giving your baby any food or formula), you may start taking this medication 6 weeks after delivery. If you are partially breast-feeding (giving your baby some food or formula), you should start taking this medication by 3 weeks after delivery.

Before taking progestin-only oral contraceptives, ask your pharmacist or doctor for a copy of the manufacturer's information for the patient and read it carefully.

Are there other uses for this medicine?

This medication may be prescribed for other uses; ask your doctor or pharmacist for more information.

What special precautions should I follow?

Before taking progestin-only oral contraceptives,
- tell your doctor and pharmacist if you are allergic to progestins, aspirin, tartrazine (a yellow food coloring), or any other medications.
- tell your doctor and pharmacist what prescription and nonprescription medications, vitamins, nutritional supplements, and herbal products you are taking. Be sure to mention any of the following: carbamazepine (Tegretol), phenobarbital (Luminal, Solfoton), phenytoin (Dilantin), and rifampin (Rifadin). Your doctor may need to change the doses of your medications or monitor you carefully for side effects.
- tell your doctor if you have or have ever had breast lumps or breast cancer, vaginal bleeding between menstrual periods, liver tumors, liver disease, or diabetes.
- tell your doctor if you are pregnant or plan to become pregnant. If you become pregnant while taking progestin-only contraceptives, call your doctor.
- tell your doctor if you use tobacco products. Cigarette smoking may increase the risk of heart attacks and

strokes. You should not smoke while taking this medication.

What special dietary instructions should I follow?

Unless your doctor tells you otherwise, continue your normal diet.

What should I do if I forget to take a dose?

Take the missed dose as soon as you remember it, and go back to taking progestin-only contraceptives at your regular time. If you take a dose more than 3 hours late, be sure to use a backup method of birth control for the next 48 hours. If you are not sure what to do about the pills you have missed, keep taking progestin-only contraceptives and use a backup method of birth control until you speak to your doctor.

What side effects can this medicine cause?

Progestin-only oral contraceptives may cause side effects. Tell your doctor if any of these symptoms are severe or do not go away:

- irregular menstrual periods
- headache
- breast pain
- upset stomach
- dizziness
- acne
- increased hair growth

Some side effects can be serious. The following symptoms are uncommon, but if you experience any of them, call your doctor immediately:

- bleeding that lasts a long time
- lack of menstrual periods
- severe stomach pain

Combined estrogen and progestin oral contraceptives may increase the risk of getting breast cancer, endometrial cancer, and liver tumors. It is not known whether progestin-only oral contraceptives also increase the risks of these conditions. Talk to your doctor about the risks of taking this medication.

Progestin-only oral ontraceptives may cause other side effects. Call your doctor if you have any unusual problems while taking this medication.

If you experience a serious side effect, you or your doctor may send a report to the Food and Drug Administration's (FDA) MedWatch Adverse Event Reporting program online [at http://www.fda.gov/MedWatch/index.html] or by phone [1-800-332-1088].

What storage conditions are needed for this medicine?

Keep this medication in the container it came in, tightly closed, and out of reach of children. Store it at room temperature and away from excess heat and moisture (not in the bathroom). Throw away any medication that is outdated or no longer needed. Talk to your pharmacist about the proper disposal of your medication.

What should I do in case of overdose?

In case of overdose, call your local poison control center at 1-800-222-1222. If the victim has collapsed or is not breathing, call local emergency services at 911.

What other information should I know?

Keep all appointments with your doctor.

Before you have any laboratory tests, tell the laboratory personnel that you take progestin-only oral contraceptives, as this medication may interfere with some laboratory tests.

Rarely, women can become pregnant even if they are taking oral contraceptives. You should get a pregnancy test if it has been more than 45 days since your last period or if your period is late and you missed one or more doses or took them late and had sex without a backup method of birth control.

If you want to become pregnant, stop taking progestin-only contraceptives. Progestin-only contraceptives should not delay your ability to get pregnant.

Do not let anyone else take your medication. Ask your pharmacist any questions you have about refilling your prescription.

Talk to your doctor, pharmacist, or other healthcare professional if you have questions about dosing information for your medication.

Promethazine

(proe meth' a zeen)

Brand Name: Phenadoz®, Phenergan®, Promethegan®, Prometh® VC syrup

Important Warning

Promethazine may cause breathing to slow or stop, and may cause death in children. Promethazine should not be given to babies or children who are younger than 2 years old and should be given with caution to children who are 2 years of age or older. Promethazine should not routinely be used to treat vomiting in children; it should only be used in specific cases when a doctor decides that it is needed. Tell your child's doctor if your child has any condition that affects his/her breathing such as lung disease, asthma, sleep apnea (stops breathing for short periods of time during sleep). Tell your doctor or pharmacist about all the medications your child is taking, especially barbiturates such as phenobarbital

(Luminal), medications for anxiety, narcotic medications for pain, sedatives, sleeping pills, and tranquilizers. Call your child's doctor immediately and get emergency medical treatment if your child has difficulty breathing, wheezes, slows or pauses in breathing, or stops breathing.

Talk to your doctor about the risks of giving promethazine to your child.

Why is this medicine prescribed?

Promethazine is used to relieve the symptoms of allergic reactions such as allergic rhinitis (runny nose and watery eyes caused by allergy to pollen, mold or dust), allergic conjunctivitis (red, watery eyes caused by allergies), allergic skin reactions, and allergic reactions to blood or plasma products. Promethazine is used with other medications to treat anaphylaxis (sudden, severe allergic reactions). Promethazine is also used to relax and sedate patients before and after surgery, during labor, and at other times. Promethazine is also used to prevent and control upset stomach and vomiting that may occur after surgery, and to help relieve pain after surgery. Promethazine is also used to prevent and treat motion sickness. Promethazine is in a class of medications called phenothiazines. It works by blocking the action of a certain natural substance in the body.

How should this medicine be used?

Promethazine comes as a tablet and syrup (liquid) to take by mouth and as a suppository to use rectally.When promethazine is used to treat allergies, it is usually taken one to four times daily, before meals and/or at bedtime. When promethazine is used to treat motion sickness, it is taken 30-60 minutes before travel and again after 8-12 hours if needed. On longer trips, promethazine is usually taken in the morning and before the evening meal on each day of travel. When promethazine is used to treat or prevent upset stomach and vomiting it is usually taken every 4-6 hours as needed. Promethazine may also be taken at bedtime the night before surgery to relieve anxiety and produce quiet sleep. Follow the directions on your prescription label carefully, and ask your doctor or pharmacist to explain any part you do not understand. Take promethazine exactly as directed. Do not take more or less of it or take it more often than prescribed by your doctor.

Promethazine suppositories are for rectal use only. Do not try to swallow the suppositories or insert in any other part of your body.

To insert a promethazine suppository, follow these steps:
1. If the suppository feels soft, hold it under cold, running water for 1 minute. Remove the wrapper.
2. Dip the tip of the suppository in water.
3. Lie down on your left side and raise your right knee to your chest. (A left-handed person should lie on the right side and raise the left knee.)
4. Using your finger, insert the suppository into the rectum,

about 1/2 to 1 inch in children who are 2 years of age older and 1 inch in adults. Hold it in place for a few moments.
5. Stand up after about 15 minutes. Wash your hands thoroughly and resume your normal activities.

Are there other uses for this medicine?

This medication may be prescribed for other uses; ask your doctor or pharmacist for more information.

What special precautions should I follow?

Before taking promethazine,
- tell your doctor and pharmacist if you are allergic to promethazine, other phenothiazines (certain medications used to treat mental illness, upset stomach, vomiting, severe hiccups, and other conditions) or any other medications. Also tell your doctor and pharmacist if you have ever had an unusual or unexpected reaction when you took promethazine, another phenothiazine, or any other medication. Ask your doctor or pharmacist if you do not know if a medication you are allergic to is a phenothiazine.
- tell your doctor and pharmacist what prescription and nonprescription medications, vitamins, nutritional supplements and herbal products you are taking or plan to take. Be sure to mention any of the following: antidepressants ('mood elevators') such as amitriptyline (Elavil), amoxapine (Asendin), clomipramine (Anafranil), desipramine (Norpramin), doxepin (Adapin, Sinequan), imipramine (Tofranil), nortriptyline (Aventyl, Pamelor), protriptyline (Vivactil), and trimipramine (Surmontil); antihistamines; azathioprine (Imuran); barbiturates such as phenobarbital (Luminal); cancer chemotherapy; epinephrine (Epipen); ipratropium (Atrovent) medications for anxiety, irritable bowel disease, mental illness, motion sickness, Parkinson's disease, seizures, ulcers, or urinary problems; monoamine oxidase inhibitors (MAOIs) such as isocarboxazid (Marplan), phenelzine (Nardil), tranylcypromine (Parnate), and selegiline (Eldepryl); narcotics and other pain medication; sedatives; sleeping pills; and tranquilizers.
- tell your doctor if you have or have ever had an enlarged prostate (a male reproductive gland); glaucoma (an eye disease); seizures; ulcers, blockage in the passage between the stomach and intestine; blockage in the bladder; asthma or other lung disease; sleep apnea; cancer; or heart, kidney, or liver disease. If you will be giving promethazine to a child, also tell the child's doctor if the child has any of the following symptoms before he or she receives the medication: vomiting, listlessness, drowsiness, confusion, aggression, seizures, yellowing of the skin or eyes, weakness, or flu-like symptoms. Also tell the child's doctor if the child has not been drinking normally, has had excessive vomiting or diarrhea, or appears dehydrated.
- tell your doctor if you are pregnant or plan to become

pregnant. If you become pregnant while taking promethazine, call your doctor. Do not breastfeed while you are taking promethazine.

- if you are having surgery, including dental surgery, tell the doctor or dentist that you are taking promethazine.
- you should know that this drug may make you drowsy. Do not drive a car or operate machinery until you know how this drug affects you. If you are giving promethazine to a child, watch the child to be sure he or she does not get hurt while riding a bike or participating in other activities that could be dangerous.
- remember that alcohol can add to the drowsiness caused by this medication.
- plan to avoid unnecessary or prolonged exposure to sunlight and to wear protective clothing, sunglasses, and sunscreen. Promethazine may make your skin sensitive to sunlight.

What should I do if I forget to take a dose?

Take the missed dose as soon as you remember it. However, if it is almost time for the next dose, skip the missed dose and continue your regular dosing schedule. Do not take a double dose to make up for a missed one.

What side effects can this medicine cause?

Promethazine can cause side effects. Tell your doctor if any of these symptoms are severe or do not go away:

- dry mouth
- drowsiness
- listlessness
- difficulty falling asleep or staying asleep
- nightmares
- dizziness
- ringing in ears
- blurred or double vision
- loss of coordination
- upset stomach
- vomiting
- nervousness
- restlessness
- hyperactivity
- abnormally happy mood
- stuffy nose
- itching

Some side effects can be serious. If you experience any of the following symptoms, call your doctor immediately:

- wheezing
- slowed breathing
- breathing stops for a short time
- fever
- sweating
- stiff muscles
- decreased alertness
- fast or irregular pulse or heartbeat
- faintness
- abnormal or uncontrollable movements

- hallucinations (seeing things or hearing voices that do not exist)
- confusion
- overwhelming or unmanageable fear or emotion
- seizures
- shaking of a part of the body that you cannot control
- unusual bruising or bleeding
- sore throat, fever, chills, and other signs of infection
- uncontrolled eye movements
- tongue sticking out
- abnormal neck position
- inability to respond to people around you
- yellowing of the skin or eyes
- rash
- hives
- swelling of the face, eyes, lips, tongue, throat, arms, hands, feet, ankles, or lower legs
- hoarseness
- difficulty breathing or swallowing

If you experience a serious side effect, you or your doctor may send a report to the Food and Drug Administration's (FDA) MedWatch Adverse Event Reporting program online [at http://www.fda.gov/MedWatch/index.html] or by phone [1-800-332-1088].

What storage conditions are needed for this medicine?

Keep this medication in the carton or container it came in, tightly closed, and out of reach of children. Store promethazine tablets and liquid at room temperature and away from excess heat and moisture (not in the bathroom). Store promethazine suppositories in the refrigerator. Protect the medication from light. Throw away any medication that is outdated or no longer needed. Talk to your pharmacist about the proper disposal of your medication.

What should I do in case of overdose?

In case of overdose, call your local poison control center at 1-800-222-1222. If the victim has collapsed or is not breathing, call local emergency services at 911.

Symptoms of overdose may include:

- difficulty breathing
- slowed or stopped breathing
- dizziness
- lightheadedness
- fainting
- loss of consciousness
- fast heartbeat
- tight muscles that are difficult to move
- loss of coordination
- continuous twisting movements of the hands and feet
- dry mouth
- wide pupils (black circles in the middle of the eyes)
- flushing
- upset stomach
- constipation

- abnormal excitement or agitation
- nightmares

What other information should I know?

Keep all appointments with your doctor.

Promethazine can interfere with the results of home pregnancy tests. Talk to your doctor if you think you might be pregnant while you are taking promethazine. Do not try to test for pregnancy at home.

Before having any laboratory test, tell your doctor and the laboratory personnel that you are taking promethazine.

Do not let anyone else take your medication. Ask your pharmacist any questions you have about refilling your prescription.

Talk to your doctor, pharmacist, or other healthcare professional if you have questions about dosing information for your medication.

Propafenone

(proe pa feen' one)

Brand Name: Rythmol®
Also available generically.

Important Warning

Antiarrhythmic drugs, including propafenone, may increase the risk of death. Tell your doctor if you have had a heart attack within the past two years.

Propafenone should be used only to treat life-threatening arrhythmias (irregular heartbeats). Talk to your doctor about the risk of taking propafenone.

Why is this medicine prescribed?

Propafenone is used to treat arrhythmias and to maintain a normal heart rate. It acts on the heart muscle to improve the heart's rhythm.

How should this medicine be used?

Propafenone comes as a tablet to take by mouth. It usually is taken every 8 hours. This medication is sometimes started in the hospital where your response can be monitored. Follow the directions on your prescription label carefully, and ask your doctor or pharmacist to explain any part you do not understand. Take propafenone exactly as directed. Do not take more or less of it or take it more often than prescribed by your doctor.

Propafenone controls irregular heartbeats, but does not cure them. Continue to take propafenone even if you feel well. Do not stop taking propafenone without talking to your doctor. Your heartbeat may become irregular if you suddenly stop taking propafenone.

Are there other uses for this medicine?

This medication should not be prescribed for other uses; ask your doctor or pharmacist for more information.

What special precautions should I follow?

Before taking propafenone,

- tell your doctor and pharmacist if you are allergic to propafenone or any other drugs.
- tell your doctor and pharmacist what prescription and nonprescription medications you are taking, especially anticoagulants ('blood thinners') such as warfarin (Coumadin), beta blockers such as atenolol (Tenormin), carteolol (Cartrol), labetalol (Normodyne, Trandate), metoprolol (Lopressor), nadolol (Corgard), propranolol (Inderal), sotalol (Betapace), and timolol (Blocadren); cimetidine (Tagamet); cyclosporine (Neoral, Sandimmune); digoxin (Lanoxin); quinidine (Quinaglute); rifampin (Rifadin); and vitamins.
- in addition to the condition listed in the IMPORTANT WARNING section, tell your doctor if you have or have ever had liver or kidney disease, congestive heart failure, a pacemaker, chronic bronchitis, asthma, or emphysema.
- tell your doctor if you are pregnant, plan to become pregnant, or are breast-feeding. If you become pregnant while taking propafenone, call your doctor.
- if you are having surgery, including dental surgery, tell the doctor or dentist that you are taking propafenone.
- you should know that this drug may make you drowsy or dizzy. Do not drive a car or operate machinery until you know how it affects you.

What special dietary instructions should I follow?

Talk to your doctor about your diet. Foods and salt substitutes containing potassium can affect the action of propafenone.

What should I do if I forget to take a dose?

Take the missed dose if you remember it within 4 hours. If you do not remember it until 4 or more hours after the scheduled time, skip the missed dose and continue your regular dosing schedule. Do not take a double dose to make up for a missed one.

What side effects can this medicine cause?

Propafenone may cause side effects. Tell your doctor if any of these symptoms are severe or do not go away:

- dizziness
- drowsiness
- dry mouth
- headache

- upset stomach
- diarrhea
- constipation
- vomiting
- loss of appetite
- taste changes
- gas
- blurred vision

If you experience any of the following symptoms, call your doctor immediately:

- difficulty breathing
- chest pain
- irregular heartbeat
- increased or decreased heartbeat
- fainting
- skin rash
- unexplained fever, chills, or sore throat
- unusual bleeding or bruising

If you experience a serious side effect, you or your doctor may send a report to the Food and Drug Administration's (FDA) MedWatch Adverse Event Reporting program online [at http://www.fda.gov/MedWatch/index.html] or by phone [1-800-332-1088].

What storage conditions are needed for this medicine?

Keep this medication in the container it came in, tightly closed, and out of reach of children. Store it at room temperature and away from excess heat and moisture (not in the bathroom). Throw away any medication that is outdated or no longer needed. Talk to your pharmacist about the proper disposal of your medication.

What should I do in case of overdose?

In case of overdose, call your local poison control center at 1-800-222-1222. If the victim has collapsed or is not breathing, call local emergency services at 911.

What other information should I know?

Keep all appointments with your doctor and the laboratory. Your doctor may want to evaluate the effectiveness of propafenone with physical examinations, EKG (electrocardiogram) tests, and blood tests.

Do not let anyone else take your medication. Ask your pharmacist any questions you have about refilling your prescription.

Dosage Facts
For Informational Purposes

Caution: Do not change your dose, how often you take your medication, or the length of time you are to take it without first talking to your healthcare provider.

The following dosage information was written using medical language for doctors and other healthcare professionals and is provided here for you to check your dosage. The dosage of this drug may differ for different patients. Therefore, always follow your doctor's instructions or the directions on the label. Contact your healthcare provider or pharmacist if you have any questions about the specific dosage of your medication after reviewing this information.

General Dosage Information

Adjust dosage carefully according to individual requirements and response, patient tolerance, and the general condition and cardiovascular status of the patient.

Consider dosage reduction in patients who develop excessive prolongation of the PR interval, excessive QRS widening, or second- or third-degree AV block.

Usually do not use oral loading doses (conventional [immediate-release] tablets) since acute toxicity may occur. However, oral loading doses (e.g., 450–750 mg as conventional [immediate-release] tablets) have been used with apparent safety for conversion of recent-onset atrial fibrillation to normal sinus rhythm† in individuals without heart failure.

Pediatric Patients

Supraventricular Arrhythmias

ORAL (CONVENTIONAL [IMMEDIATE-RELEASE] TABLETS):
- Maximum daily dosage 600 mg/m².

Adult Patients

Paroxysmal Atrial Fibrillation/Flutter and Paroxysmal Supraventricular Tachyarrhythmias

ORAL (CONVENTIONAL [IMMEDIATE-RELEASE] TABLETS):
- Initially, 150 mg every 8 hours.
- Increase dosage after 3–4 days to 225 mg 3 times daily (every 8 hours) if necessary.
- If desired therapeutic response is not attained after an additional 3–4 days, increase dosage to 300 mg 3 times daily (every 8 hours).

ORAL (EXTENDED-RELEASE CAPSULES):
- Initially, 225 mg every 12 hours.
- Increase dosage after ≥5 days to 325 mg every 12 hours if necessary.
- If desired therapeutic response is not attained after an additional 5 days, increase dosage to 425 mg every 12 hours.
- If a dose is missed, only administer the next scheduled dose; do *not* double next dose.
- When switching from conventional (immediate-release) tablets to extended-release capsules, the dosage conversion ratio is *not* a 1:1 substitution (e.g., a patient who currently is receiving 150 mg every 8 hours of conventional (immediate-release) tablets may be switched to 325 mg of extended-release capsules every 12 hours).

Conversion of Atrial Fibrillation to Normal Sinus Rhythm†

ORAL (CONVENTIONAL [IMMEDIATE-RELEASE] TABLETS):
- 150–600 mg, as a single dose.

Self-administration for Conversion of PAF†

ORAL (CONVENTIONAL [IMMEDIATE-RELEASE] TABLETS):

- Adults weighing 70 kg or more: May use a single oral loading dose of 600 mg 5 minutes after noting the onset of palpitations.
- Adults weighing < 70 kg: May use a single oral loading dose of 450 mg 5 minutes after noting the onset of palpitations.
- Do not take more than a single oral dose during a 24-hour period.

Ventricular Arrhythmias

ORAL (CONVENTIONAL [IMMEDIATE-RELEASE] TABLETS):

- Initially, 150 mg every 8 hours.
- Increase dosage after 3–4 days to 225 mg 3 times daily if necessary.
- If desired therapeutic response is not attained after an additional 3–4 days, increase dosage to 300 mg 3 times daily.

Prescribing Limits

Pediatric Patients

Supraventricular Arrhythmias

ORAL (CONVENTIONAL [IMMEDIATE-RELEASE] TABLETS):

- Maximum daily dosage is 600 mg/m².

Adult Patients

Supraventricular Arrhythmias

ORAL (CONVENTIONAL [IMMEDIATE-RELEASE] TABLETS):

- Maximum daily dosage is 900 mg.

Life-threatening Ventricular Arrhythmias

ORAL (CONVENTIONAL [IMMEDIATE-RELEASE] TABLETS):

- Maximum daily dosage is 900 mg.

Special Populations

Hepatic Impairment

- When conventional (immediate-release) tablets are used, reduce dosage by approximately 70–80%; monitor patients for signs of toxicity, including hypotension, somnolence, bradycardia, conduction disturbances, seizures, and/or ventricular arrhythmias.

Geriatric Patients and Those with Myocardial Damage

- During initiation of therapy (conventional [immediate-release] tablets), gradual dosage escalation should be performed in geriatric patients and those with marked previous myocardial ischemia.

† Use is not currently included in the labeling approved by the US Food and Drug Administration.

Propantheline

(proe pan′ the leen)

Brand Name: Pro-Banthine®

Why is this medicine prescribed?

Propantheline is used with other medication to treat ulcers.

This medication is sometimes prescribed for other uses; ask your doctor or pharmacist for more information.

How should this medicine be used?

Propantheline comes as a tablet. Propantheline usually is taken four times a day, 30 minutes before meals and at bedtime. Follow the directions on your prescription label carefully, and ask your doctor or pharmacist to explain any part you do not understand. Take propantheline exactly as directed. Do not take more or less of it or take it more often than prescribed by your doctor.

What special precautions should I follow?

Before taking propantheline,

- tell your doctor and pharmacist if you are allergic to propantheline or any other drugs.
- tell your doctor and pharmacist what prescription and nonprescription medications you are taking, especially amantadine (Symmetrel), antihistamines, digoxin (Lanoxin), disopyramide (Norpace), glutethimide (Doriden), levodopa (Larodopa, Sinemet), meperidine (Demerol), extended-release potassium chloride tablets, quinidine (Quinaglute), tranquilizers, medications for depression and Parkinson's disease, and vitamins. Take propantheline at least 1 hour before taking antacids and at least 2 hours after ketoconazole (Nizoral) tablets.
- tell your doctor if you have or have ever had colitis; glaucoma; an enlarged prostate gland; high blood pressure; an overactive thyroid gland; liver, heart, blood vessel, or kidney disease; myasthenia gravis; difficulty urinating; or asthma, bronchitis, emphysema, or lung disease.
- tell your doctor if you are pregnant, plan to become pregnant, or are breast-feeding. If you become pregnant while taking propantheline, call your doctor.
- if you are having surgery, including dental surgery, tell the doctor or dentist that you are taking propantheline.
- you should know that this drug may make you drowsy. Do not drive a car or operate machinery until you know how this drug affects you.
- remember that alcohol can add to the drowsiness caused by this drug.

What should I do if I forget to take a dose?

Take the missed dose as soon as you remember it. However, if it is almost time for the next dose, skip the missed dose

and continue your regular dosing schedule. Do not take a double dose to make up for a missed one.

What side effects can this medicine cause?

Propantheline may cause side effects. Tell your doctor if any of these symptoms are severe or do not go away:

- dry mouth
- increased sensitivity of your eyes to light
- dizziness
- nervousness
- difficulty sleeping
- headache
- loss of sense of taste
- upset stomach
- vomiting
- bloating
- confusion (especially in the elderly)
- blurred vision
- constipation

If you experience any of the following symptoms, call your doctor immediately:

- fast heartbeat
- heart palpitations
- eye pain
- difficulty urinating
- skin rash
- itching

If you experience a serious side effect, you or your doctor may send a report to the Food and Drug Administration's (FDA) MedWatch Adverse Event Reporting program online [at http://www.fda.gov/MedWatch/index.html] or by phone [1-800-332-1088].

What storage conditions are needed for this medicine?

Keep this medication in the container it came in, tightly closed, and out of reach of children. Store it at room temperature and away from excess heat and moisture (not in the bathroom). Throw away any medication that is outdated or no longer needed. Talk to your pharmacist about the proper disposal of your medication.

What should I do in case of overdose?

In case of overdose, call your local poison control center at 1-800-222-1222. If the victim has collapsed or is not breathing, call local emergency services at 911.

What other information should I know?

Keep all appointments with your doctor.

Do not let anyone else take your medication. Ask your pharmacist any questions you have about refilling your prescription.

Talk to your doctor, pharmacist, or other healthcare professional if you have questions about dosing information for your medication.

Propoxyphene

(proe pox′ i feen)

Brand Name: Darvocet A500® as a combination product containing Propoxyphene Napsylate and Acetaminophen, Darvocet-N® 100 as a combination product containing Propoxyphene Napsylate and Acetaminophen, Darvocet-N® 50 as a combination product containing Propoxyphene Napsylate and Acetaminophen, Darvon® Compound-65 Pulvules®, Darvon® Pulvules®, Darvon-N®, E-Lor®, PC-CAP®, Propocet® 100 as a combination product containing Propoxyphene Napsylate and Acetaminophen, Wygesic®

Also available generically.

Important Warning

Propoxyphene in high doses, taken by itself or in combination with other drugs, has been associated with drug-related deaths. Do not take propoxyphene in combination with other drugs that cause drowsiness: alcohol, tranquilizers, sleep aids, antidepressant drugs, or antihistamines. Do not take a larger dose, take it more often, or for a longer period than your doctor tells you to.

Why is this medicine prescribed?

Propoxyphene is used to relieve mild to moderate pain.

This medication is sometimes prescribed for other uses; ask your doctor or pharmacist for more information.

How should this medicine be used?

Propoxyphene comes as a tablet, capsule, and liquid to take by mouth. It usually is taken every 4 hours as needed. Follow the directions on your prescription label carefully, and ask your doctor or pharmacist to explain any part you do not understand. Take propoxyphene exactly as directed.

Propoxyphene can be habit-forming.

Shake the liquid well before each use.

What special precautions should I follow?

Before taking propoxyphene,

- tell your doctor and pharmacist if you are allergic to propoxyphene or any other drugs.
- tell your doctor and pharmacist what prescription and nonprescription medications you are taking, especially other pain relievers; anticoagulants ('blood-thinners') such as warfarin (Coumadin); antidepressants; antihistamines; medications for cough, cold, or allergies; muscle relaxants; sedatives; seizure medications; sleeping pills; tranquilizers; and vitamins.

- tell your doctor if you have or have ever had liver or kidney disease, or a history of alcoholism.
- tell your doctor if you are pregnant, plan to become pregnant, or are breast-feeding. If you become pregnant while taking propoxyphene, call your doctor.
- if you are having surgery, including dental surgery, tell the doctor or dentist that you are taking propoxyphene.
- you should know that this drug may make you drowsy. Do not drive a car or operate machinery until you know how this drug affects you.
- remember that alcohol can add to the drowsiness caused by this drug.

What should I do if I forget to take a dose?

Propoxyphene usually is taken as needed. If your doctor has told you to take propoxyphene regularly, take the missed dose as soon as you remember it. However, if it is almost time for the next dose, skip the missed dose and continue your regular dosing schedule. Do not take a double dose to make up for a missed one.

What side effects can this medicine cause?

Propoxyphene may cause side effects. Tell your doctor if any of these symptoms are severe or do not go away:

- dizziness
- lightheadedness
- drowsiness
- upset stomach
- vomiting
- constipation
- stomach pain
- skin rash
- mood changes
- headache

If you experience the following symptom, call your doctor immediately:

- difficulty breathing

If you experience a serious side effect, you or your doctor may send a report to the Food and Drug Administration's (FDA) MedWatch Adverse Event Reporting program online [at http://www.fda.gov/MedWatch/index.html] or by phone [1-800-332-1088].

What storage conditions are needed for this medicine?

Keep this medication in the container it came in, tightly closed, and out of reach of children. Store it at room temperature and away from excess heat and moisture (not in the bathroom). Throw away any medication that is outdated or no longer needed. Talk to your pharmacist about the proper disposal of your medication.

What should I do in case of overdose?

In case of overdose, call your local poison control center at 1-800-222-1222. If the victim has collapsed or is not breathing, call local emergency services at 911.

What other information should I know?

Keep all appointments with your doctor.

Do not let anyone else take your medication. Ask your pharmacist any questions you have about refilling your prescription.

Dosage Facts
For Informational Purposes

Caution: Do not change your dose, how often you take your medication, or the length of time you are to take it without first talking to your healthcare provider.

The following dosage information was written using medical language for doctors and other healthcare professionals and is provided here for you to check your dosage. The dosage of this drug may differ for different patients. Therefore, always follow your doctor's instructions or the directions on the label. Contact your healthcare provider or pharmacist if you have any questions about the specific dosage of your medication after reviewing this information.

General Dosage Information

Available as propoxyphene hydrochloride and propoxyphene napsylate; dosage expressed in terms of the salt.

Propoxyphene napsylate 100 mg is equivalent to propoxyphene hydrochloride 65 mg.

Adult Patients

Pain

ORAL:
- Propoxyphene hydrochloride: Usual dosage is 65 mg every 4 hours as needed. Doses <65 mg have questionable efficacy.
- Propoxyphene napsylate: Usual dosage is 100 mg every 4 hours as needed.

Prescribing Limits
Adult Patients
Pain

ORAL:
- Propoxyphene hydrochloride: Maximum 390 mg daily.
- Propoxyphene napsylate: Maximum 600 mg daily.

Special Populations

Hepatic Impairment
- Consider dosage reduction.

Renal Impairment
- Consider dosage reduction.

Geriatric Patients
- Consider increase in dosing interval.

Propranolol Oral

(proe pran' oh lole)

Brand Name: Inderal®, Inderal® LA, Inderide®, Innopran® XL, Propranolol Hydrochloride Intensol®

Also available generically.

Important Warning

Do not stop taking propranolol without talking to your doctor first. If propranolol is stopped suddenly, it may cause chest pain or heart attack in some people.

Why is this medicine prescribed?

Propranolol is used to treat high blood pressure. It is also used to prevent angina (chest pain) and heart attacks. It works by relaxing your blood vessels so your heart doesn't have to pump as hard. Propranolol is also used to treat abnormal heart rhythms.

Propranolol is also used to prevent migraine headaches and tremors.

This medication is sometimes prescribed for other uses; ask your doctor or pharmacist for more information.

How should this medicine be used?

Propranolol comes as a tablet or capsule to take by mouth. It also comes as a solution or concentrate. The extended-release (long-acting) product usually is taken once a day. Immediate-acting propranolol may be taken two, three, or four times a day. The number of doses depends on why it is being taken.

Do not cut, crush, or chew extended-release tablets; swallow them whole. Dilute the concentrated oral liquid with water, juice, or soft drinks, or mix it with applesauce or pudding just before taking it.

Follow the directions on your prescription label carefully, and ask your doctor or pharmacist to explain any part you do not understand. Take propranolol exactly as directed. Do not take more or less of it or take it more often than prescribed by your doctor.

Propranolol helps control your condition but will not cure it. Continue to take propranolol even if you feel well. Do not stop taking propranolol without talking to your doctor.

What special precautions should I follow?

Before taking propranolol,
- tell your doctor and pharmacist if you are allergic to propranolol or any other drugs.
- tell your doctor and pharmacist what prescription and nonprescription medications you are taking, especially cimetidine (Tagamet); medications for migraine headaches, asthma, allergies, colds, or pain; other medications for heart disease or high blood pressure; reserpine; and vitamins.
- tell your doctor if you have or have ever had asthma or other lung disease; heart, liver, or kidney disease; diabetes; severe allergies; or thyroid problems.
- tell your doctor if you are pregnant, plan to become pregnant, or are breast-feeding. If you become pregnant while taking propranolol, call your doctor.
- if you are having surgery, including dental surgery, tell the doctor or dentist that you are taking propranolol.
- you should know that this drug may make you drowsy. Do not drive a car or operate machinery until you know how this drug affects you.
- remember that alcohol can add to the drowsiness caused by this drug.

What special dietary instructions should I follow?

Talk to your doctor before using salt substitutes containing potassium. If your doctor prescribes a low-salt or low-sodium diet, follow these directions carefully.

What should I do if I forget to take a dose?

Take the missed dose as soon as you remember it. However, if it is almost time for the next dose, skip the missed dose and continue your regular dosing schedule. Do not take a double dose to make up for a missed one.

What side effects can this medicine cause?

Propranolol may cause side effects. Tell your doctor if any of these symptoms are severe or do not go away:
- dizziness or lightheadedness
- difficulty sleeping
- excessive tiredness
- upset stomach
- vomiting
- rash
- diarrhea
- constipation

If you experience any of the following symptoms, call your doctor immediately:
- difficulty breathing
- sore throat
- unusual bleeding
- swelling of the feet or hands
- unusual weight gain
- chest pain
- slow, irregular heartbeat

If you experience a serious side effect, you or your doctor may send a report to the Food and Drug Administration's (FDA) MedWatch Adverse Event Reporting program online [at http://www.fda.gov/MedWatch/index.html] or by phone [1-800-332-1088].

What storage conditions are needed for this medicine?

Keep this medication in the container it came in, tightly closed, and out of reach of children. Store it at room temperature and away from excess heat and moisture (not in the bathroom). Throw away any medication that is outdated or no longer needed. Talk to your pharmacist about the proper disposal of your medication.

What should I do in case of overdose?

In case of overdose, call your local poison control center at 1-800-222-1222. If the victim has collapsed or is not breathing, call local emergency services at 911.

What other information should I know?

Keep all appointments with your doctor and the laboratory. Your doctor will need to determine your response to propranolol. Your doctor may ask you to check your pulse (heart rate). Ask your pharmacist or doctor to teach you how to take your pulse. If your pulse is faster or slower than it should be, call your doctor.

Do not let anyone else take your medication. Ask your pharmacist any questions you have about refilling your prescription.

Dosage Facts
For Informational Purposes

Caution: Do not change your dose, how often you take your medication, or the length of time you are to take it without first talking to your healthcare provider.

The following dosage information was written using medical language for doctors and other healthcare professionals and is provided here for you to check your dosage. The dosage of this drug may differ for different patients. Therefore, always follow your doctor's instructions or the directions on the label. Contact your healthcare provider or pharmacist if you have any questions about the specific dosage of your medication after reviewing this information.

Pediatric Patients

Usual Dosage

ORAL:
- Conventional tablets: 2–4 mg/kg daily in 2 equally divided doses. Weight-adjusted initial dosage is approximate; adjust dosage according to response, up to 16 mg/kg daily.
- Do not calculate dosage based on body surface area; may result in excessive plasma concentrations.
- If propranolol is to be discontinued, decrease dosage gradually over 7–14 days.

Hypertension

ORAL:
- Conventional tablets: initially, 1 mg/kg daily in 2 equally divided doses. Adjust according to response and tolerance.
- Usual maintenance dosage is 2–4 mg/kg daily in 2 equally divided doses, up to 16 mg/kg daily.
- Alternatively, some experts recommend a usual initial dosage of 1–2 mg/kg daily given in 2 or 3 divided doses. Increase dosage as necessary up to a maximum dosage of 4 mg/kg (up to 640 mg) daily given in 2 or 3 divided doses.

Cardiac Arrhythmias

ORAL:
- Initially, 1.5–2 mg/kg daily; titrate upward as necessary to 16 mg/kg daily in 4 divided doses to control the arrhythmia.
- Dosages >4 mg/kg daily may be necessary for the management of supraventricular tachyarrhythmias.

Thyrotoxicosis
Treatment of Tachyarrhythmias in Neonates with Thyrotoxicosis

ORAL:
- 2 mg/kg daily in 2–4 divided doses has been used. Higher dosages occasionally may be needed.

Adult Patients

Hypertension
Monotherapy

ORAL:
- Conventional tablets or oral solution: initially, 40 mg twice daily. Usual effective dosage is 120–240 mg daily.
- Extended-release capsules: initially, 80 mg once daily. Usual effective dosage is 120–160 mg once daily.
- Increase dosage gradually at 3- to 7-day intervals until optimum affect is achieved; some patients may require doses of 640 mg daily.

Fixed Combination Therapy

ORAL:
- Propranolol in fixed combination with hydrochlorothiazide: administer in 2 divided doses daily (up to 160 mg of propranolol and 50 mg of hydrochlorothiazide total daily dosage).
- Combination preparation is inappropriate with propranolol dosages >160 mg daily due to excessive dosage of the thiazide component. May gradually add another antihypertensive agent when necessary using half of the usual initial dosage to avoid an excessive decrease in BP.
- Initial use of fixed-combination preparations is not recommended; adjust by administering each drug separately, then use the fixed combination if the optimum maintenance dosage corresponds to the drug dosages in the combination preparation. Administer separately for subsequent dosage adjustment.

Angina
Chronic Stable Angina

ORAL:
- Conventional tablets or oral solution: usual dosage is 80–320 mg daily in 2–4 divided doses. More than 320 mg daily has been recommended when there is only a partial response to usual dosage.
- Extended-release capsules: initially, 80 mg daily. Gradually increase dosage at 3- to 7-day intervals as needed to control symptoms. Optimum response usually occurs at 160 mg daily, but there is wide variation in response.

Unstable Angina or Non-ST-Segment Elevation/Non-Q-Wave MI

ORAL:

- Conventional tablets or oral solution: initially, 40–80 mg every 6–8 hours; thereafter, maintain on 20–80 mg twice daily. Titrate to target heart rate of 50–60 bpm in patients with unstable angina in the absence of dose-limiting adverse effects.

Cardiac Arrhythmias

ORAL:

- Conventional tablets or oral solution: usually 10–30 mg 3 or 4 times daily.

Ventricular Fibrillation after MI

ORAL:

- Maintenance dose: 180–320 mg daily in divided doses has been recommended.

Slowing of Ventricular Response during Acute Atrial Fibrillation

ORAL:

- Maintenance dosage for persistent atrial fibrillation: 80–240 mg daily in divided doses.

Hypertrophic Subaortic Stenosis

ORAL:

- Conventional tablets or oral solution: 20–40 mg 3 or 4 times daily.
- Extended-release capsules: 80–160 mg once daily.

Pheochromocytoma
Prior to Surgery

ORAL:

- Conventional tablets or oral solution: 60 mg daily in divided doses (in conjunction with an α-adrenergic blocking agent) for 3 days prior to surgery.

Adjunctive Treatment for Inoperable Pheochromocytoma.

ORAL:

- 30 mg daily in divided doses (in conjunction with an α-adrenergic blocker).

Vascular Headache
Prevention of Common Migraine

ORAL:

- Conventional tablets or oral solution: initially, 80 mg daily in divided doses.
- Extended-release capsules: 80 mg once daily.
- Gradually increase dosage to achieve optimum response; usual effective dosage is 80–240 mg daily.
- Discontinue if response is inadequate after 4–6 weeks; gradual withdrawal over several weeks may be advisable.

AMI
Mortality Reduction after AMI

ORAL:

- Conventional tablets or oral solution: 180–240 mg daily in divided doses, beginning 5–21 days after infarction. Higher dosage may be necessary for patients with coexisting conditions (e.g., angina, hypertension).
- Administered in 3–4 divided doses daily in clinical studies, but twice-daily dosing also may be adequate.
- Optimum benefit may be achieved when oral therapy with β-adrenergic blocking agent is continued for at least 1–3 years after infarction (when not contraindicated); some experts recommend continuing therapy *indefinitely* unless contraindicated.

Essential Tremor
Routine Therapy

ORAL:

- Conventional tablets: initially, 40 mg twice daily.
- Response is variable and dosage must be individualized; optimal suppression of tremor usually occurs with 120–320 mg daily in 3 divided doses.
- Complete suppression of tremor rarely is achieved; dosages exceeding 320 mg daily may not provide substantial added benefit but are associated with an increased risk of adverse effects.
- Extended-release capsules: usual dosages administered once daily each morning appear to be at least as effective as equivalent dosages of conventional tablets administered in divided doses daily.

Intermittent Therapy

ORAL:

- Conventional tablets: 80–120 mg as a single dose 1–3 hours before planned activity or anticipated stress associated with tremor.

Prescribing Limits

Pediatric Patients

Hypertension

ORAL:

- Maximum 16 mg/kg daily; however, some experts recommend a maximum dosage of 4 mg/kg (up to 640 mg) daily.

Adult Patients

Angina

ORAL:

- 320 mg daily; some clinicians recommend higher dosage if there is only a partial response to usual dosage.

AMI

ORAL:

- 240 mg daily.

Essential Tremor

ORAL:

- 320 mg daily; higher dosages do not provide substantial added benefit and are associated with an increased risk of adverse effects.

Special Populations

Hepatic Impairment
- Use with caution.

Renal Impairment
- Dosage adjustments not required. Use with caution.

Geriatric Patients
- Use caution in dosage selection; initiate therapy at low end of dosage range.

Propylthiouracil

(proe pill thye oh yoor′ a sill)

Why is this medicine prescribed?

Propylthiouracil is used to treat hyperthyroidism, a condition that occurs when the thyroid gland produces too much thyroid hormone. It also is taken before thyroid surgery or radioactive iodine therapy.

How should this medicine be used?

Propylthiouracil comes as a tablet and is usually taken three times a day, approximately every 8 hours, with food. Follow the directions on your prescription label carefully, and ask your doctor or pharmacist to explain any part you do not understand. Take propylthiouracil exactly as directed. Do not take more or less of it or take it more often than prescribed by your doctor.

Are there other uses for this medicine?

This medication may be prescribed for other uses; ask your doctor or pharmacist for more information.

What special precautions should I follow?

Before taking propylthiouracil,

- tell your doctor and pharmacist if you are allergic to propylthiouracil or any other drugs.
- tell your doctor and pharmacist what prescription and nonprescription medications you are taking, especially anticoagulants ('blood thinners') such as warfarin (Coumadin), diabetes medications, digoxin (Lanoxin), and vitamins.
- tell your doctor if you have or have ever had any blood disease, such as decreased white blood cells (leukopenia), decreased platelets (thrombocytopenia), or aplastic anemia, or liver disease (hepatitis, jaundice).
- tell your doctor if you are pregnant, plan to become pregnant, or are breast-feeding. If you become pregnant while taking propylthiouracil, call your doctor immediately.
- if you are having surgery, including dental surgery, tell the doctor or dentist that you are taking propylthiouracil.

What special dietary instructions should I follow?

Unless your doctor tells you otherwise, continue your normal diet.

What should I do if I forget to take a dose?

Take the missed dose as soon as you remember it. However, if it is almost time for the next dose, skip the missed dose and continue your regular dosing schedule at evenly spaced, 8-hour intervals. Do not take a double dose to make up for a missed one.

What side effects can this medicine cause?

Propylthiouracil may cause side effects. Tell your doctor if any of these symptoms are severe or do not go away:

- skin rash
- itching
- abnormal hair loss
- upset stomach
- vomiting
- loss of taste
- abnormal sensations (tingling, prickling, burning, tightness, and pulling)
- swelling
- joint and muscle pain
- drowsiness
- dizziness
- decreased white blood cells
- decreased platelets

Some side effects can be serious. The following symptoms are uncommon, but if you experience any of them, call your doctor immediately:

- sore throat
- fever
- headache
- chills
- unusual bleeding or bruising
- right-sided abdominal pain with decreased appetite
- yellowing of the skin or eyes
- skin eruptions

Propylthiouracil may cause other side effects. Call your doctor if you have any unusual problems while taking this medication.

If you experience a serious side effect, you or your doctor may send a report to the Food and Drug Administration's (FDA) MedWatch Adverse Event Reporting program online [at http://www.fda.gov/MedWatch/index.html] or by phone [1-800-332-1088].

What storage conditions are needed for this medicine?

Keep this medication in the container it came in, tightly closed, and out of reach of children. Store it at room temperature and away from excess heat and moisture (not in the bathroom). Throw away any medication that is outdated or no longer needed. Talk to your pharmacist about the proper disposal of your medication.

What should I do in case of overdose?

In case of overdose, call your local poison control center at 1-800-222-1222. If the victim has collapsed or is not breathing, call local emergency services at 911.

What other information should I know?

Keep all appointments with your doctor and the laboratory.

Do not let anyone else take your medication. Ask your pharmacist any questions you have about refilling your prescription.

Talk to your doctor, pharmacist, or other healthcare professional if you have questions about dosing information for your medication.

Protriptyline

(proe trip′ ti leen)

Brand Name: Vivactil®
Also available generically.

Important Warning

A small number of children, teenagers, and young adults (up to 24 years of age) who took antidepressants ('mood elevators') such as protriptyline during clinical studies became suicidal (thinking about harming or killing oneself or planning or trying to do so). Children, teenagers, and young adults who take antidepressants to treat depression or other mental illnesses may be more likely to become suicidal than children, teenagers, and young adults who do not take antidepressants to treat these conditions. However, experts are not sure about how great this risk is and how much it should be considered in deciding whether a child or teenager should take an antidepressant. Children younger than 18 years of age should not normally take protriptyline, but in some cases, a doctor may decide that protriptyline is the best medication to treat a child's condition.

You should know that your mental health may change in unexpected ways when you take protriptyline or other antidepressants even if you are an adult over age 24. You may become suicidal, especially at the beginning of your treatment and any time that your dose is increased or decreased. You, your family, or your caregiver should call your doctor right away if you experience any of the following symptoms: new or worsening depression; thinking about harming or killing yourself, or planning or trying to do so; extreme worry; agitation; panic attacks; difficulty falling asleep or staying asleep; aggressive behavior; irritability; acting without thinking; severe restlessness; and frenzied abnormal excitement. Be sure that your family or caregiver knows which symptoms may be serious so they can call the doctor when you are unable to seek treatment on your own.

Your healthcare provider will want to see you often while you are taking protriptyline, especially at the beginning of your treatment. Be sure to keep all appointments for office visits with your doctor.

The doctor or pharmacist will give you the manufacturer's patient information sheet (Medication Guide) when you begin treatment with protriptyline.

Read the information carefully and ask your doctor or pharmacist if you have any questions. You also can obtain the Medication Guide from the FDA website: http://www.fda.gov/cder/drug/antidepressants/ antidepressants_MG_2007.pdf.

No matter what your age, before you take an antidepressant, you, your parent, or your caregiver should talk to your doctor about the risks and benefits of treating your condition with an antidepressant or with other treatments. You should also talk about the risks and benefits of not treating your condition. You should know that having depression or another mental illness greatly increases the risk that you will become suicidal. This risk is higher if you or anyone in your family has or has ever had bipolar disorder (mood that changes from depressed to abnormally excited) or mania (frenzied, abnormally excited mood) or has thought about or attempted suicide. Talk to your doctor about your condition, symptoms, and personal and family medical history. You and your doctor will decide what type of treatment is right for you.

Why is this medicine prescribed?

Protriptyline is used to treat depression. Protriptyline is in a class of medications called tricyclic antidepressants. It works by increasing the amounts of certain natural substances in the brain that help maintain mental balance.

How should this medicine be used?

Protriptyline comes as a tablet to take by mouth. It is usually taken three or four times a day. Take protriptyline at around the same times every day. Follow the directions on your prescription label carefully, and ask your doctor or pharmacist to explain any part you do not understand. Take protriptyline exactly as directed. Do not take more or less of it or take it more often than prescribed by your doctor.

Your doctor will probably start you on a low dose of protriptyline and gradually increase your dose. Your doctor may decrease your dose after your condition is controlled.

Protriptyline controls depression but does not cure it. Continue to take protriptyline even if you feel well. Do not stop taking protriptyline without talking to your doctor. If you suddenly stop taking protriptyline, you may experience withdrawal symptoms such as nausea, headache, and lack of energy.

Are there other uses for this medicine?

This medication may be prescribed for other uses; ask your doctor or pharmacist for more information.

What special precautions should I follow?

Before taking protriptyline,
- tell your doctor and pharmacist if you are allergic to protriptyline or any other medications.

- tell your doctor if you are taking cisapride (Propulsid) (not available in the U.S.) or monoamine oxidase (MAO) inhibitors such as isocarboxazid (Marplan); phenelzine (Nardil), selegiline (Eldepryl, Emsam, Zelapar), and tranylcypromine (Parnate), or if you have taken an MAO inhibitor during the past 14 days. Your doctor will probably tell you that you should not take protriptyline.
- tell your doctor and pharmacist what other prescription and nonprescription medications, vitamins, nutritional supplements, and herbal products you are taking or plan to take. Be sure to mention any of the following: amiodarone (Cordarone, Pacerone); antihistamines; bupropion (Wellbutrin); celecoxib (Celebrex); cimetidine (Tagamet); doxorubicin (Adriamycin); guanethidine (Ismelin); ipratropium (Atrovent); medications for anxiety, asthma, colds, diabetes, irritable bowel disease, mental illness, motion sickness, Parkinson's disease, seizures, ulcers, or urinary problems; medications for irregular heartbeat such as flecainide (Tambocor), moricizine (Ethmozine), and propafenone (Rythmol); methadone (Dolophine); metoclopramide (Reglan); other antidepressants; quinidine; ranitidine (Zantac); reserpine (Serpasil); ritonavir (Norvir); selective serotonin reuptake inhibitors (SSRIs) such as citalopram (Celexa), fluoxetine (Prozac, Sarafem), fluvoxamine (Luvox), paroxetine (Paxil), and sertraline (Zoloft); sedatives; sleeping pills; terbinafine (Lamisil); thyroid medications; tramadol (Ultram); and tranquilizers. Tell your doctor or pharmacist if you have stopped taking fluoxetine (Prozac, Sarafem) in the past 5 weeks. Your doctor may need to change the doses of your medications or monitor you carefully for side effects.
- tell your doctor if you have recently had a heart attack. Your doctor will probably tell you not to take protriptyline.
- tell your doctor if you drink large amounts of alcohol; if you are undergoing electroshock therapy (procedure in which small electric shocks are administered to the brain to treat certain mental illnesses); or if you have or have ever had glaucoma (an eye disease), an enlarged prostate (a male reproductive organ), difficulty urinating, mental illness, seizures, hyperthyroidism (an overactive thyroid gland), or diabetes.
- tell your doctor if you are pregnant, plan to become pregnant, or are breast-feeding. If you become pregnant while taking protriptyline, call your doctor.
- if you are having surgery, including dental surgery, tell the doctor or dentist that you are taking protriptyline.
- you should know that protriptyline may make you drowsy. Do not drive a car or operate machinery until you know how this medication affects you.
- remember that alcohol can add to the drowsiness caused by this medication.
- plan to avoid unnecessary or prolonged exposure to sunlight and to wear protective clothing, sunglasses, and sunscreen. Protriptyline may make your skin sensitive to sunlight.
- you should know that protriptyline may cause dizziness, lightheadedness, and fainting when you get up too quickly from a lying position. This is more common when you first start taking protriptyline. To avoid this problem, get out of bed slowly, resting your feet on the floor for a few minutes before standing up.

What special dietary instructions should I follow?

Unless your doctor tells you otherwise, continue your normal diet.

What should I do if I forget to take a dose?

Take the missed dose as soon as you remember it. However, if it is almost time for the next dose, skip the missed dose and continue your regular dosing schedule. Do not take a double dose to make up for a missed one.

What side effects can this medicine cause?

Protriptyline may cause side effects. Tell your doctor if any of these symptoms are severe or do not go away:

- nausea
- vomiting
- diarrhea
- loss of appetite
- weight changes
- unusual taste in the mouth
- stomach pain or cramps
- heartburn
- dry mouth
- constipation
- drowsiness
- dizziness
- nightmares
- headaches
- frequent urination, especially at night
- difficulty urinating
- wide pupils
- changes in sex drive or ability
- breast enlargement in men and women
- unsteadiness
- ringing in ears
- hair loss
- flushing
- sweating
- black tongue

Some side effects can be serious. If you experience any of the following symptoms or those listed in the IMPORTANT WARNING section, call your doctor immediately:

- slow or difficult speech
- weakness or numbness of an arm or a leg
- crushing chest pain
- rapid, pounding, or irregular heartbeat
- rash or hives

- itching
- swelling of the face or tongue
- yellowing of the skin or eyes
- jaw, neck, and back muscle spasms
- uncontrollable shaking of a part of the body
- fainting
- blurred vision
- difficulty walking
- unusual bleeding or bruising
- seizures
- confusion
- hallucination (seeing things or hearing voices that do not exist)
- believing things that are not true
- fever
- pain, burning, or tingling in the hands or feet

Protriptyline may cause other side effects. Call your doctor if you have any unusual problems while taking this medication.

If you experience a serious side effect, you or your doctor may send a report to the Food and Drug Administration's (FDA) MedWatch Adverse Event Reporting program online [at http://www.fda.gov/MedWatch/index.html] or by phone [1-800-332-1088].

What storage conditions are needed for this medicine?

Keep this medication in the container it came in, tightly closed, and out of reach of children. Store it at room temperature and away from excess heat and moisture (not in the bathroom). Throw away any medication that is outdated or no longer needed. Talk to your pharmacist about the proper disposal of your medication.

What should I do in case of overdose?

In case of overdose, call your local poison control center at 1-800-222-1222. If the victim has collapsed or is not breathing, call local emergency services at 911.

Symptoms of overdose may include:

- irregular heartbeat
- loss of consciousness
- fainting
- seizures
- confusion
- problems concentrating
- hallucination (seeing things or hearing voices that do not exist)
- agitation
- drowsiness
- stiff muscles
- vomiting
- fever
- cold body temperature

What other information should I know?

Keep all appointments with your doctor.

Do not let anyone else take your medication. Ask your pharmacist any questions you have about refilling your prescription.

Dosage Facts
For Informational Purposes

Caution: Do not change your dose, how often you take your medication, or the length of time you are to take it without first talking to your healthcare provider.

The following dosage information was written using medical language for doctors and other healthcare professionals and is provided here for you to check your dosage. The dosage of this drug may differ for different patients. Therefore, always follow your doctor's instructions or the directions on the label. Contact your healthcare provider or pharmacist if you have any questions about the specific dosage of your medication after reviewing this information.

General Dosage Information

Available as protriptyline hydrochloride; dosage expressed in terms of the salt.

Adult Patients

Major Depressive Disorder

ORAL:

- Initially, 15–40 mg daily, depending on the severity of the condition being treated. Adjust dosage gradually until maximal therapeutic effect with minimal toxicity is achieved. May increase up to 60 mg daily if needed.
- After symptoms are controlled, gradually reduce dosage to the lowest level that will maintain relief of symptoms.

Prescribing Limits

Adult Patients

Major Depressive Disorder

ORAL:

- Maximum 60 mg daily.

Special Populations

Hepatic Impairment

ORAL:

- No specific dosage recommendations at this time.

Renal Impairment

ORAL:

- No specific dosage recommendations at this time.

Geriatric Patients

- Initially, 5 mg 3 times daily. May increase gradually if necessary; however, monitor for cardiac abnormalities at doses >20 mg daily.
- After symptoms are controlled, gradually reduce dosage to the lowest level that will maintain relief of symptoms.

Pseudoephedrine

(soo doe e fed′ rin)

Brand Name: Decofed®, Dimetapp® Decongestant Infant Drops, Drixoral® Nasal Decongestant, Efidac 24® Pseudoephedrine, Genaphed®, Kidkare® Decongestant Drops, Pedia Relief®, PediaCare® Infants' Oral Decongestant Drops, Simply Stuffy®, Sudafed® 12 Hour Caplets®, Sudafed® 24 Hour, Sudafed® Children's Nasal Decongestant, Sudafed® Nasal Decongestant, Suphedrin®, Su-Phedrin®, Suphedrin® Children's, Triaminic® AM Decongestant Syrup, Triaminic® Infant Oral Decongestant Drops
Also available generically.

Why is this medicine prescribed?

Pseudoephedrine is used to relieve nasal discomfort caused by colds, allergies, and hay fever. It is also used to relieve sinus congestion and pressure. Pseudoephedrine is in a class of medications called sympathomimetic agents that are used as nasal decongestants. It works by causing narrowing of the blood vessels of swollen nasal mucous membranes to reduce nasal congestion and allow drainage of sinus passages.

How should this medicine be used?

Pseudoephedrine comes as a regular tablet, a chewable tablet, a 12-hour extended-release (long-acting) tablet, a 24-hour extended-release tablet, a solution (liquid), and a concentrated solution (drops). The regular tablets, chewable tablets, liquid, or drops usually are taken every 4-6 hours, but you should not take more than 4 doses in a 24-hour period. The 12-hour extended-release tablets usually are taken every 12 hours, and you should not take more than 2 doses in a 24-hour period. The 24-hour extended-release tablets usually are taken once a day, and you should not take more than one dose in a 24-hour period. To help prevent trouble sleeping, take the last dose of the day several hours before bedtime. Follow the directions on the package label or on your prescription label carefully, and ask your doctor or pharmacist to explain any part you do not understand. Take pseudoephedrine exactly as directed. Do not take more or less of it or take it more often than prescribed by your doctor.

Your symptoms should improve during your treatment. If your symptoms do not get better within 7 days or if you have a fever, stop taking pseudoephedrine and call your doctor.

Do not break, crush, or chew extended-release tablets; swallow them whole.

Do not give extended-release tablets to children younger than 12 years of age.

Are there other uses for this medicine?

This medication is sometimes prescribed for other uses; ask your doctor or pharmacist for more information.

What special precautions should I follow?

Before taking pseudoephedrine,

- tell your doctor and pharmacist if you are allergic to pseudoephedrine or any other medications.
- do not take pseudoephedrine if you are taking monoamine oxidase (MAO) inhibitors, including isocarboxazid (Marplan), phenelzine (Nardil), selegiline (Eldepryl), and tranylcypromine (Parnate), or have stopped taking them within the past 2 weeks. If you stop taking pseudoephedrine you should wait at least 2 weeks before you start to take an MAO inhibitor.
- tell your doctor and pharmacist what prescription and nonprescription medications, vitamins, nutritional supplements, and herbal products you are taking or plan to take, especially medications for diet or appetite control, asthma, or high blood pressure.
- tell your doctor if you have or have ever had high blood pressure, glaucoma, diabetes, difficulty urinating (due to an enlarged prostate gland), or thyroid, heart, or kidney disease. If you are taking pseudoephedrine 24-hour extended-release tablets, tell your doctor if you have had a narrowing or blockage of your digestive system.
- tell your doctor if you are pregnant, plan to become pregnant, or are breast-feeding. If you become pregnant while taking pseudoephedrine, call your doctor.
- if you are having surgery, including dental surgery, tell the doctor or dentist that you are taking pseudoephedrine.

What special dietary instructions should I follow?

Caffeine-containing beverages (coffee, tea, and cola) may increase the restlessness and insomnia caused by pseudoephedrine in sensitive individuals, so you may wish to reduce your consumption of these beverages.

What should I do if I forget to take a dose?

Take the missed dose as soon as you remember it. However, if it is almost time for the next dose, skip the missed dose and continue your regular dosing schedule. Do not take a double dose to make up for a missed one.

What side effects can this medicine cause?

Pseudoephedrine may cause side effects. Tell your doctor if any of these symptoms are severe or do not go away:

- restlessness
- upset stomach

Some side effects can be serious. If you experience any of the following symptoms, call your doctor immediately:

- nervousness

- dizziness
- difficulty sleeping
- stomach pain
- vomiting
- difficulty breathing
- fast or irregular heartbeat
- weakness
- palpitations
- shaking of a part of the body that you cannot control
- seeing things or hearing voices that do not exist (hallucinating)

If you experience a serious side effect, you or your doctor may send a report to the Food and Drug Administration's (FDA) MedWatch Adverse Event Reporting program online [at http://www.fda.gov/MedWatch/index.html] or by phone [1-800-332-1088].

What storage conditions are needed for this medicine?

Keep this medication in the container it came in, tightly closed, and out of reach of children. Store it at room temperature and away from excess heat and moisture (not in the bathroom). The chewable tablets and concentrated solution (drops) should be protected from light; store in the outer carton until the medication is used. Throw away any medication that is outdated or no longer needed. Talk to your pharmacist about the proper disposal of your medication.

What should I do in case of overdose?

In case of overdose, call your local poison control center at 1-800-222-1222. If the victim has collapsed or is not breathing, call local emergency services at 911.

What other information should I know?

If you are taking pseudoephedrine 24-hour extended-release tablets, you may notice something that looks like a tablet in your stool. This is just the empty tablet shell, and this does not mean that you did not get your complete dose of medication.

You should know that pseudoephedrine may used in combination with other medications to treat colds, allergies, and sinus headaches. Be sure to read the information provided for the patient when taking combination products to be sure that you are not taking additional medications that contain the same ingredient.

Ask your pharmacist any questions you have about pseudoephedrine.

Dosage Facts
For Informational Purposes

Caution: Do not change your dose, how often you take your medication, or the length of time you are to take it without first talking to your healthcare provider.

The following dosage information was written using medical language for doctors and other healthcare professionals and is provided here for you to check your dosage. The dosage of this drug may differ for different patients. Therefore, always follow your doctor's instructions or the directions on the label. Contact your healthcare provider or pharmacist if you have any questions about the specific dosage of your medication after reviewing this information.

General Dosage Information

Single-entity preparation: Available as pseudoephedrine hydrochloride; dosage expressed in terms of the salt.

Fixed-combination preparation: available as pseudoephedrine hydrochloride or pseudoephedrine sulfate.

Pediatric Patients

Nasal Congestion, Sinus Congestion, and Other Respiratory Conditions

ORAL:
- *Self-medication* in children <2 years of age: Consult a pediatrician.
- *Self-medication* in children 2–5 years of age: 15 mg every 4–6 hours. Alternatively, some pediatricians recommend 4 mg/kg or 125 mg/m² daily, given in 4 divided doses.
- *Self-medication* in children 6–11 years of age: 30 mg every 4–6 hours.
- *Self-medication* in children ≥12 years of age: 60 mg (as conventional tablets) every 4–6 hours, 120 mg (as extended-release tablets) every 12 hours, or 240 mg (as extended-release core tablets) once daily.
- Discontinue therapy if symptoms persist for >7 days or are accompanied by fever.

Adult Patients

Nasal Congestion, Sinus Congestion, and Other Respiratory Conditions

ORAL:
- *Self-medication*: 60 mg (as conventional tablets) every 4–6 hours, 120 mg (as extended-release tablets) every 12 hours, or 240 mg (as extended-release core tablets) once daily.
- Discontinue therapy if symptoms persist for >7 days or are accompanied by fever.

Otitic Barotrauma†

ORAL:
- Air travelers: 120 mg (as extended-release tablets) 30 minutes before flight departure.
- Underwater divers: 60 mg 30 minutes before diving.

Prescribing Limits

Pediatric Patients

Nasal Congestion, Sinus Congestion, and Other Respiratory Conditions

ORAL:
- *Self-medication* in children 2–5 years of age: Maximum 60 mg in any 24-hour period.
- *Self-medication* in children 6–11 years of age: Maximum 120 mg in any 24-hour period.
- *Self-medication* in children ≥12 years of age: Maximum 240

mg in any 24-hour period (as conventional tablets, 120-mg extended-release tablets, or 240-mg extended-release core tablets).

Adult Patients

Nasal Congestion, Sinus Congestion, and Other Respiratory Conditions

ORAL:

- *Self-medication*: Maximum 240 mg in any 24-hour period (as conventional tablets, 120-mg extended-release tablets, or 240-mg extended-release core tablets).

† Use is not currently included in the labeling approved by the US Food and Drug Administration.

Pseudoephedrine and Triprolidine

(soo doe e fed′ rin) (trye proe′ li deen)

Brand Name: Actifed®, Allerfrim®, Triafed®

Why is this medicine prescribed?

The combination of pseudoephedrine (a decongestant) and triprolidine (an antihistamine) relieves itchy, watery eyes; sneezing; and runny or stuffy nose caused by hay fever, allergies, and the common cold.

This medication is sometimes prescribed for other uses; ask your doctor or pharmacist for more information.

How should this medicine be used?

The combination of pseudoephedrine and triprolidine comes in capsules, tablets, extended-release (long-acting) capsules, and liquid to take by mouth. It usually is taken every 4-6 hours or every 12 hours (extended-release capsules) as needed. Follow the directions on your prescription label carefully, and ask your doctor or pharmacist to explain any part you do not understand. Take pseudoephedrine and triprolidine exactly as directed. Do not take more or less of it or take it more often than prescribed by your doctor.

Do not open extended-release capsules; swallow them whole.

Do not give this medication to children less than 12 years of age unless a doctor directs you to do so.

What special precautions should I follow?

Before taking pseudoephedrine and triprolidine,

- tell your doctor and pharmacist if you are allergic to pseudoephedrine, triprolidine, or any other drugs.
- tell your doctor and pharmacist what prescription and nonprescription medications you are taking, especially medications for asthma, high blood pressure, or sei-

zures; muscle relaxants; narcotics (pain medications); sedatives; sleeping pills; tranquilizers; and vitamins. Do not take this drug if you have taken an MAO inhibitor [phenelzine (Nardil) or tranylcypromine (Parnate)] in the last 2 weeks.

- tell your doctor if you have or have ever had heart disease, high blood pressure, difficulty urinating (due to an enlarged prostate gland), glaucoma, asthma, an overactive thyroid gland, ulcers, seizures, or diabetes.
- tell your doctor if you are pregnant, plan to become pregnant, or are breast-feeding. If you become pregnant while taking pseudoephedrine and triprolidine, call your doctor.
- if you are having surgery, including dental surgery, tell the doctor or dentist that you are taking pseudoephedrine and triprolidine.
- you should know that this drug may make you drowsy. Do not drive a car or operate machinery until you know how this drug affects you.
- remember that alcohol can add to the drowsiness caused by this drug.

What special dietary instructions should I follow?

Pseudoephedrine and triprolidine may cause an upset stomach. Take pseudoephedrine and triprolidine with food or milk.

What should I do if I forget to take a dose?

Take the missed dose as soon as you remember it. However, if it is almost time for the next dose, skip the missed dose and continue your regular dosing schedule. Do not take a double dose to make up for a missed one.

What side effects can this medicine cause?

Pseudoephedrine and triprolidine may cause side effects. Tell your doctor if any of these symptoms are severe or do not go away:

- dry mouth, nose, and throat
- upset stomach
- difficulty sleeping
- chest congestion
- headache
- diarrhea
- drowsiness

If you experience any of the following symptoms, call your doctor immediately:

- muscle weakness
- vision problems
- skin rash
- excitement
- difficulty breathing
- fast heartbeat
- tremors
- difficult or painful urination
- hallucinations

If you experience a serious side effect, you or your doctor may send a report to the Food and Drug Administration's (FDA) MedWatch Adverse Event Reporting program online [at http://www.fda.gov/MedWatch/index.html] or by phone [1-800-332-1088].

What storage conditions are needed for this medicine?

Keep this medication in the container it came in, tightly closed, and out of reach of children. Store it at room temperature and away from excess heat and moisture (not in the bathroom). Throw away any medication that is outdated or no longer needed. Talk to your pharmacist about the proper disposal of your medication.

What should I do in case of overdose?

In case of overdose, call your local poison control center at 1-800-222-1222. If the victim has collapsed or is not breathing, call local emergency services at 911.

What other information should I know?

Keep all appointments with your doctor.

Do not let anyone else take your medication. Ask your pharmacist any questions you have about refilling your prescription.

Talk to your doctor, pharmacist, or other healthcare professional if you have questions about dosing information for your medication.

Psyllium

(sil′ i yum)

Brand Name: Fiberall®, Hydrocil Instant®, Konsyl®, Metamucil®, Modane Bulk Powder®, Perdiem Fiber®, Serutan®, Siblan®

Why is this medicine prescribed?

Psyllium, a bulk-forming laxative, is used to treat constipation. It absorbs liquid in the intestines, swells, and forms a bulky stool, which is easy to pass.

This medication is sometimes prescribed for other uses; ask your doctor or pharmacist for more information.

How should this medicine be used?

Psyllium comes as a powder, granules, and wafer to take by mouth. It usually is taken one to three times daily. Follow the directions on the package or on your prescription label carefully, and ask your doctor or pharmacist to explain any part you do not understand. Take psyllium exactly as directed. Do not take more or less of it or take it more often than prescribed by your doctor.

The powder and granules must be mixed with 8 ounces of a pleasant tasting liquid, such as fruit juice, right before use. Chew wafers thoroughly. For psyllium to work properly and to prevent side effects, you must drink at least 8 ounces of liquid when you take it.

Do not take psyllium for longer than 1 week unless your doctor tells you to.

Are there other uses for this medicine?

Your doctor also may prescribe psyllium to treat diarrhea or high cholesterol. Talk to your doctor about the possible risks of using this drug for your condition.

What special precautions should I follow?

Before taking psyllium,

- tell your doctor and pharmacist if you are allergic to psyllium or any other drugs.
- tell your doctor and pharmacist what prescription and nonprescription medications you are taking, including vitamins. Do not take digoxin (Lanoxin), salicylates (aspirin), or nitrofurantoin (Macrodantin, Furadantin, Macrobid) within 3 hours of taking psyllium.
- tell your doctor if you have or have ever had diabetes mellitus, heart disease, high blood pressure, kidney disease, rectal bleeding, intestinal blockage, or difficulty swallowing.
- tell your doctor if you are pregnant, plan to become pregnant, or are breast-feeding. If you become pregnant while taking psyllium, call your doctor.
- tell your pharmacist or doctor if you are on a low-sugar or low-sodium diet.
- be careful not to breathe in psyllium powder when mixing a dose. It can cause allergic reactions when accidentally inhaled.

What special dietary instructions should I follow?

To prevent constipation, drink plenty of fluids, exercise regularly, and eat a high-fiber diet, including whole-grain (e.g., bran) cereals, fruits, and vegetables.

What should I do if I forget to take a dose?

If you are taking scheduled doses of psyllium, take the missed dose as soon as you remember it. However, if it is almost time for the next dose, skip the missed dose and continue your dosing schedule. Do not take a double dose to make up for a missed one.

What side effects can this medicine cause?

Psyllium may cause side effects. If you have any of the following symptoms, call your doctor immediately:

- difficulty breathing
- stomach pain
- difficulty swallowing
- skin rash

- itching
- upset stomach
- vomiting

If you experience a serious side effect, you or your doctor may send a report to the Food and Drug Administration's (FDA) MedWatch Adverse Event Reporting program online [at http://www.fda.gov/MedWatch/index.html] or by phone [1-800-332-1088].

What storage conditions are needed for this medicine?

Keep this medication in the container it came in, tightly closed, and out of reach of children. Store it at room temperature and away from excess heat and moisture (not in the bathroom). Throw away any medication that is outdated or no longer needed. Talk to your pharmacist about the proper disposal of your medication.

What other information should I know?

Ask your doctor or pharmacist any questions you have about taking this medicine.

Talk to your doctor, pharmacist, or other healthcare professional if you have questions about dosing information for your medication.

Pyrantel

(pi ran' tel)

Brand Name: Ascarel®, Pin-X®, Reese's® Pinworm Medicine, Reese's® Pinworm Medicine Caplets®

Why is this medicine prescribed?

Pyrantel, an antiworm medication, is used to treat roundworm, hookworm, pinworm, and other worm infections.

This medication is sometimes prescribed for other uses; ask your doctor or pharmacist for more information.

How should this medicine be used?

Pyrantel comes as a capsule and a liquid to take by mouth. It usually is taken as a single dose for pinworm and roundworm infections. The dose usually is repeated after 2 weeks for pinworm infections. For hookworm infections, pyrantel usually is taken once a day for 3 days. Pyrantel may be taken with food, juice, or milk or on an empty stomach.

Shake the liquid well to mix the medication evenly. Pyrantel may be mixed with milk or fruit juice. Follow the directions on your prescription label carefully, and ask your doctor or pharmacist to explain any part you do not understand. Take pyrantel exactly as directed. Do not take more or less of it or take it more often than prescribed by your doctor.

What special precautions should I follow?

Before taking pyrantel,

- tell your doctor and pharmacist if you are allergic to pyrantel or any other drugs.
- tell your doctor and pharmacist what prescription and nonprescription medications you are taking, especially piperazine (another antiworm medication), and vitamins.
- tell your doctor if you have or have ever had anemia or liver disease.
- tell your doctor if you are pregnant, plan to become pregnant, or are breast-feeding. If you become pregnant while taking pyrantel, call your doctor.

What should I do if I forget to take a dose?

Take the missed dose as soon as you remember it. However, if it is almost time for the next dose, skip the missed dose and continue your regular dosing schedule. Do not take a double dose to make up for a missed one.

What side effects can this medicine cause?

Pyrantel may cause side effects. Tell your doctor if any of these symptoms are severe or do not go away:

- upset stomach
- vomiting
- diarrhea
- loss of appetite
- stomach cramps
- stomach pain
- straining and pain during bowel movements

What storage conditions are needed for this medicine?

Keep this medication in the container it came in, tightly closed, and out of reach of children. Store it at room temperature and away from excess heat and moisture (not in the bathroom). Throw away any medication that is outdated or no longer needed. Talk to your pharmacist about the proper disposal of your medication.

What other information should I know?

Keep all appointments with your doctor and the laboratory. Your doctor will order certain lab tests to check your response to pyrantel.

Do not let anyone else take your medication. Your prescription is probably not refillable. If you still have symptoms of infection after you finish the pyrantel, call your doctor.

Talk to your doctor, pharmacist, or other healthcare professional if you have questions about dosing information for your medication.

Pyrazinamide

(peer a zin′ a mide)

Why is this medicine prescribed?

Pyrazinamide kills or stops the growth of certain bacteria that cause tuberculosis (TB). It is used with other drugs to treat tuberculosis.

This medication is sometimes prescribed for other uses; ask your doctor or pharmacist for more information.

How should this medicine be used?

Pyrazinamide comes as a tablet to take by mouth. It usually is taken once a day (at the same time each day) or in larger doses twice a week. Pyrazinamide may be taken with or without food. Follow the directions on your prescription label carefully, and ask your pharmacist or doctor to explain any part you do not understand. Take pyrazinamide exactly as directed. Do not take more or less of it or take it more often than prescribed by your doctor.

What special precautions should I follow?

Before taking pyrazinamide,

- tell your doctor and pharmacist if you are allergic to pyrazinamide, niacin, ethionamide (Trecator-SC), or any other drugs.
- tell your doctor and pharmacist what prescription and nonprescription medications you are taking, especially allopurinol (Zyloprim), colchicine and/or probenecid (Col-Probenecid, Benemid), ethionamide (Trecator-SC), and vitamins.
- tell your doctor if you have or have ever had gout, liver or kidney disease, or diabetes.
- tell your doctor if you are pregnant, plan to become pregnant, or are breast-feeding. If you become pregnant while taking pyrazinamide, call your doctor.
- plan to avoid unnecessary or prolonged exposure to sunlight and to wear protective clothing, sunglasses, and sunscreen. Pyrazinamide may make your skin sensitive to sunlight.

What should I do if I forget to take a dose?

Take the missed dose as soon as you remember it. However, if it is almost time for the next dose, skip the missed dose and take only your regularly scheduled dose. Do not take a double dose to make up for a missed one.

What side effects can this medicine cause?

Pyrazinamide may cause side effects. Tell your doctor if any of these symptoms are severe or do not go away:

- upset stomach
- fatigue

If you experience any of the following symptoms, call your doctor immediately:

- skin rash
- fever
- vomiting
- loss of appetite
- yellowing of the skin or eyes
- darkened urine
- pain and swelling in the joints
- unusual bleeding or bruising
- difficult urination

If you experience a serious side effect, you or your doctor may send a report to the Food and Drug Administration's (FDA) MedWatch Adverse Event Reporting program online [at http://www.fda.gov/MedWatch/index.html] or by phone [1-800-332-1088].

What storage conditions are needed for this medicine?

Keep this medication in the container it came in, tightly closed, and out of reach of children. Store it at room temperature and away from excess heat and moisture (not in the bathroom). Throw away any medication that is outdated or no longer needed. Talk to your pharmacist about the proper disposal of your medication.

What should I do in case of overdose?

In case of overdose, call your local poison control center at 1-800-222-1222. If the victim has collapsed or is not breathing, call local emergency services at 911.

What other information should I know?

Keep all appointments with your doctor and the laboratory. Your doctor will order certain lab tests to check your response to pyrazinamide.

If you have diabetes, pyrazinamide may interfere with urine ketone tests. If you use urine ketone tests, check with your doctor about using other types of tests while taking pyrazinamide.

Do not let anyone else take your medication. Ask your pharmacist any questions you have about refilling your prescription.

Talk to your doctor, pharmacist, or other healthcare professional if you have questions about dosing information for your medication.

Pyrethrin and Piperonyl Butoxide

(pi reth′ rin) (pi′ per on il)

Brand Name: A-200® Lice Killing Shampoo, Lice Treatment® Maximum Strength Shampoo, Licide®, Pronto® Lice-Killing Shampoo Kit, Pyrinyl® Plus Liquid, RID® Maximum Strength Lice Killing Shampoo, RID® Mousse, Tisit® Blue Gel, Tisit® Liquid, Tisit® Shampoo

Why is this medicine prescribed?

Pyrethrin with piperonyl butoxide kills parasites and their eggs. It is used to treat scabies (a skin infestation) and lice infestations of the head, body, and pubic area ('crabs'). Pyrethrin with piperonyl butoxide does not prevent these infestations.

How should this medicine be used?

The pyrethrin and piperonyl butoxide combination comes in liquid, gel, and shampoo form. Usually, one application of pyrethrin with piperonyl butoxide is effective. However, the treatment may need to be repeated after 1 week; call your doctor if signs of infestation (live parasites) reappear. Follow the directions on the package or on your prescription label carefully, and ask your doctor or pharmacist to explain any part you do not understand. Use pyrethrin and piperonyl butoxide exactly as directed. Do not use more or less of it or use it more often than directed by your doctor.

Wear rubber gloves when applying it if you have open cuts or scratches on your hands. If this medication accidentally gets in your eyes, rinse them thoroughly with water for at least 5 minutes.

To use the liquid or gel, follow these steps:
1. Use enough medication to cover the affected hairy area and adjacent areas. Ask your pharmacist or doctor any questions you have about where to apply the medication.
2. Leave the medication on for exactly 10 minutes.
3. Thoroughly wash the area with warm water and soap or regular shampoo.
4. Dry with a clean towel.
5. Wash your hands to remove the medication.
6. Dress in clean clothes.

To use the shampoo, follow these steps:
1. Shake the shampoo before using it. Then thoroughly cover your dry hair and scalp or skin with shampoo.
2. Use a small amount of water to work the shampoo into your hair until a lather forms.
3. Leave the shampoo on for exactly 10 minutes.
4. Rinse your hair thoroughly with water.
5. Dry your hair with a clean towel.
6. Comb your hair with a fine tooth comb to remove nits (lice eggs and larvae).
7. Wash your hands to remove the medication.

If you have head lice, wash combs and brushes with the liquid, gel, or shampoo and rinse them thoroughly with water to remove the drug.

What special precautions should I follow?

Before using pyrethrin and piperonyl butoxide,
- tell your doctor and pharmacist if you are allergic to pyrethrin, piperonyl butoxide, ragweed, petroleum products, or any other drugs.
- tell your doctor and pharmacist what prescription and nonprescription medications you are taking, including vitamins.
- tell your doctor if you are pregnant or are breast-feeding. If you are pregnant, wear gloves when applying this medication to another person to prevent its absorption through your skin.

What side effects can this medicine cause?

Pyrethrin and piperonyl butoxide may cause side effects. Tell your doctor if any of these symptoms are severe or do not go away:
- skin irritation
- rash
- redness
- swelling

What storage conditions are needed for this medicine?

Keep this medication in the container it came in, tightly closed, and out of reach of children. Store it at room temperature and away from excess heat and moisture (not in the bathroom). Throw away any medication that is outdated or no longer needed. Talk to your pharmacist about the proper disposal of your medication.

What other information should I know?

Keep all appointments with your doctor. Pyrethrin and piperonyl butoxide is for external use only. Do not let pyrethrin and piperonyl butoxide get into your eyes, nose, or mouth, and do not swallow it. Do not apply dressings, bandages, cosmetics, lotions, or other skin medications to the area being treated unless your doctor tells you.

After using pyrethrin and piperonyl butoxide, machine-wash (or dry clean) all clothing, bed linen, and towels that you have used in the last 2 days. Use hot water. Dry everything in a hot dryer for at least 20 minutes. Thoroughly clean all bathtubs, showers, and toilets in your home with rubbing alcohol.

You may have transmitted the parasites to family members and close contacts (including sexual contacts); advise them to see a doctor if they develop symptoms of infestation.

If you have scabies and your skin has become sensitive to the parasite, itching may persist for several weeks after the treatment. However, this itching does not mean that the treatment was a failure. Call your doctor if you have questions.

Do not let anyone else use your medication. Ask your pharmacist any questions you have about pyrethrin and piperonyl butoxide.

Talk to your doctor, pharmacist, or other healthcare professional if you have questions about dosing information for your medication.

Pyridostigmine

(peer id oh stig′ meen)

Brand Name: Mestinon®, Mestinon® Syrup, Mestinon® Timespan®

Why is this medicine prescribed?

Pyridostigmine is used to decrease muscle weakness resulting from myasthenia gravis.

This medication is sometimes prescribed for other uses; ask your doctor or pharmacist for more information.

How should this medicine be used?

Pyridostigmine comes as a regular tablet, an extended-release (long-acting) tablet, and a syrup to take by mouth. It usually is taken once, twice, or several times a day, depending on the type of tablet. Your doctor may change your dose, depending on how you respond to the drug. When you first start taking pyridostigmine, your doctor may want you to keep a daily record of the time you take each dose, how long you feel better after taking each dose, and if you have side effects. This record will help the doctor decide how much drug is best for you.

Follow the directions on your prescription label carefully, and ask your doctor or pharmacist to explain any part you do not understand. Take pyridostigmine exactly as directed. Do not take more or less of it or take it more often than prescribed by your doctor.

Continue to take pyridostigmine even if you feel well. Do not stop taking pyridostigmine without talking to your doctor.

Pyridostigmine overdose can cause severe illness, including muscle weakness. It is very hard to tell the difference between too little and too much pyridostigmine. Call your doctor immediately if your symptoms become worse.

What special precautions should I follow?

Before taking pyridostigmine,
- tell your doctor and pharmacist if you are allergic to pyridostigmine, bromides, or any other drugs.
- tell your doctor and pharmacist what prescription and nonprescription medications you are taking, especially allergy or cold medications, dexamethasone (Decadron), hydrocortisone (Hydrocortone), magnesium-containing products, medications for heart arrhythmias, sleeping pills, and vitamins.
- tell your doctor if you have or have ever had intestinal or bladder blockage, asthma, seizures, heart or kidney disease, thyroid problems, or stomach ulcers.
- tell your doctor if you are pregnant, plan to become pregnant, or are breast-feeding. If you become pregnant while taking pyridostigmine, call your doctor.
- you should know that this drug may make you drowsy. Do not drive a car or operate machinery until you know how this drug affects you.
- remember that alcohol can add to the drowsiness caused by this drug.

What special dietary instructions should I follow?

Pyridostigmine may cause an upset stomach. Take pyridostigmine with food or milk.

What should I do if I forget to take a dose?

Take the missed dose as soon as you remember it. However, if you remember a missed dose near the time you are supposed to take the next dose, take only the regularly scheduled dose. Do not take a double dose to make up for a missed one.

What side effects can this medicine cause?

Pyridostigmine may cause side effects. Tell your doctor if any of these symptoms are severe or do not go away:
- upset stomach
- diarrhea
- vomiting
- drooling
- pale skin
- cold sweats
- blurred vision
- watery eyes
- increased urge to urinate
- anxiousness and feelings of panic
- muscle weakness

If you experience any of the following symptoms, call your doctor immediately:
- severe itching, skin rash, or hives
- slurred speech
- confusion
- seizures
- difficulty breathing

If you experience a serious side effect, you or your doctor may send a report to the Food and Drug Administration's (FDA) MedWatch Adverse Event Reporting program online [at http://www.fda.gov/MedWatch/index.html] or by phone [1-800-332-1088].

What storage conditions are needed for this medicine?

Keep this medication in the container it came in, tightly closed, and out of reach of children. Store it at room tem-

perature and away from excess heat and moisture (not in the bathroom). Throw away any medication that is outdated or no longer needed. Talk to your pharmacist about the proper disposal of your medication.

What should I do in case of overdose?

In case of overdose, call your local poison control center at 1-800-222-1222. If the victim has collapsed or is not breathing, call local emergency services at 911.

What other information should I know?

Keep all appointments with your doctor and the laboratory. Your doctor will order certain lab tests to check your response to pyridostigmine.

Do not let anyone else take your medication. Ask your pharmacist any questions you have about refilling your prescription.

Talk to your doctor, pharmacist, or other healthcare professional if you have questions about dosing information for your medication.

Pyridoxine

(peer i dox' een)

Available generically.

Why is this medicine prescribed?

Pyridoxine, vitamin B_6, is required by your body for utilization of energy in the foods you eat, production of red blood cells, and proper functioning of nerves. It is used to treat and prevent vitamin B_6 deficiency resulting from poor diet, certain medications, and some medical conditions.

This medication is sometimes prescribed for other uses; ask your doctor or pharmacist for more information.

How should this medicine be used?

Pyridoxine comes in regular and extended-release (long-acting) tablets. It usually is taken once a day. Follow the directions on your prescription label or package label carefully, and ask your doctor or pharmacist to explain any part you do not understand. Take pyridoxine exactly as directed. Do not take more or less of it or take it more often than prescribed by your doctor.

Do not chew, crush, or cut extended-release tablets; swallow them whole.

What special precautions should I follow?

Before taking pyridoxine,

- tell your doctor and pharmacist if you are allergic to pyridoxine or any other drugs.
- tell your doctor and pharmacist what prescription and nonprescription medications you are taking, especially

levodopa (Larodopa, Sinemet), phenobarbital, phenytoin (Dilantin), and other vitamins.
- tell your doctor if you are pregnant, plan to become pregnant, or are breast-feeding. If you become pregnant while taking pyridoxine, call your doctor.

What special dietary instructions should I follow?

Your doctor may tell you to eat more foods containing vitamin B_6, especially whole-grain cereals, fish, vegetables, beans, and liver and other organ meat.

What should I do if I forget to take a dose?

Take the missed dose as soon as you remember it. However, if it is almost time for the next dose, skip the missed dose and continue your regular dosing schedule. Do not take a double dose to make up for a missed one.

What side effects can this medicine cause?

Pyridoxine may cause side effects. Tell your doctor if any of these symptoms are severe or do not go away:
- upset stomach
- headache
- sleepiness
- tingling, prickling, burning, or sensation of tightness of the hands and feet

What storage conditions are needed for this medicine?

Keep this medication in the container it came in, tightly closed, and out of reach of children. Store it at room temperature and away from excess heat and moisture (not in the bathroom). Throw away any medication that is outdated or no longer needed. Talk to your pharmacist about the proper disposal of your medication.

What should I do in case of overdose?

In case of overdose, call your local poison control center at 1-800-222-1222. If the victim has collapsed or is not breathing, call local emergency services at 911.

What other information should I know?

Keep all appointments with your doctor and the laboratory. Your doctor will order certain lab tests to check your response to pyridoxine.

Do not let anyone else take your medication. Ask your pharmacist any questions you have about refilling your prescription.

Talk to your doctor, pharmacist, or other healthcare professional if you have questions about dosing information for your medication.

Quetiapine

(kwe tye′ a peen)

Brand Name: Seroquel®

Important Warning

Use in Older Adults:

Studies have shown that older adults with dementia (a brain disorder that affects the ability to remember, think clearly, communicate, and perform daily activities and that may cause changes in mood and personality) who take antipsychotics (medications for mental illness) such as quetiapine have an increased risk of death during treatment. If you experience any of the following symptoms, call your doctor immediately: slow or difficult speech, sudden dizziness or faintness, or weakness or numbness of an arm or leg.

Quetiapine is not approved by the Food and Drug Administration (FDA) for the treatment of behavioral problems in older adults with dementia. Talk to the doctor who prescribed this medication if you, a family member, or someone you care for has dementia and is taking quetiapine. For more information visit the FDA website: http://www.fda.gov/cder

Risk of Suicidality:

A small number of children, teenagers, and young adults (up to 24 years of age) who took antidepressants ('mood elevators') such as quetiapine during clinical studies became suicidal (thinking about harming or killing oneself or planning or trying to do so). Children, teenagers, and young adults who take antidepressants to treat depression or other mental illnesses may be more likely to become suicidal than children, teenagers, and young adults who do not take antidepressants to treat these conditions. However, experts are not sure about how great this risk is and how much it should be considered in deciding whether a child or teenager should take an antidepressant. Children younger than 18 years of age should not normally take quetiapine, but in some cases, a doctor may decide that quetiapine is the best medication to treat a child's condition.

You should know that your mental health may change in unexpected ways when you take quetiapine or other antidepressants even if you are an adult over age 24. You may become suicidal, especially at the beginning of your treatment and any time that your dose is increased or decreased. You, your family, or your caregiver should call your doctor right away if you experience any of the following symptoms: new or worsening depression; thinking about harming or killing yourself, or planning or trying to do so; extreme worry; agitation; panic attacks; difficulty falling asleep or staying asleep; aggressive behavior; irritability; acting without thinking; severe restlessness; and frenzied abnormal excitement. Be sure that your family or caregiver knows which symptoms may be serious so they can call the doctor when you are unable to seek treatment on your own.

Your healthcare provider will want to see you often while you are taking quetiapine, especially at the beginning of your treatment. Be sure to keep all appointments for office visits with your doctor.

The doctor or pharmacist will give you the manufacturer's patient information sheet (Medication Guide) when you begin treatment with quetiapine. Read the information carefully and ask your doctor or pharmacist if you have any questions. You also can obtain the Medication Guide from the FDA website: http://www.fda.gov/cder/drug/antidepressants/antidepressants_MG_2007.pdf.

No matter what your age, before you take an antidepressant, you, your parent, or your caregiver should talk to your doctor about the risks and benefits of treating your condition with an antidepressant or with other treatments. You should also talk about the risks and benefits of not treating your condition. You should know that having depression or another mental illness greatly increases the risk that you will become suicidal. This risk is higher if you or anyone in your family has or has ever had bipolar disorder (mood that changes from depressed to abnormally excited) or mania (frenzied, abnormally excited mood) or has thought about or attempted suicide. Talk to your doctor about your condition, symptoms, and personal and family medical history. You and your doctor will decide what type of treatment is right for you.

Why is this medicine prescribed?

Quetiapine is used to treat the symptoms of schizophrenia (a mental illness that causes disturbed or unusual thinking, loss of interest in life, and strong or inappropriate emotions). It is also used to treat episodes of mania (frenzied, abnormally excited or irritated mood) or depression in patients with bipolar disorder (manic depressive disorder; a disease that causes episodes of depression, episodes of mania, and other abnormal moods). Quetiapine is in a class of medications called atypical antipsychotics. It works by changing the activity of certain natural substances in the brain.

How should this medicine be used?

Quetiapine comes as a tablet to take by mouth. It is usually taken one to three times a day. Take quetiapine at around the same time(s) every day. Follow the directions on your prescription label carefully, and ask your doctor or pharmacist to explain any part you do not understand. Take quetiapine exactly as directed. Do not take more or less of it or take it more often than prescribed by your doctor.

Your doctor will probably start you on a low dose of quetiapine and gradually increase your dose during the first week of your treatment. Ask your doctor or pharmacist if you have any questions about the amount of medication you should take each day at the beginning of your treatment

Quetiapine may help control your symptoms but will not cure your condition. Continue to take quetiapine even if you feel well. Do not stop taking quetiapine without talking to your doctor. If you suddenly stop taking quetiapine, you may experience withdrawal symptoms such as nausea, vomiting, and difficulty falling asleep or staying asleep. Your doctor will probably want to decrease your dose gradually.

Are there other uses for this medicine?

This medication may be prescribed for other uses; ask your doctor or pharmacist for more information.

What special precautions should I follow?

Before taking quetiapine,

- tell your doctor and pharmacist if you are allergic to quetiapine or any other medications.
- tell your doctor and pharmacist what prescription and nonprescription medications, vitamins, nutritional supplements and herbal products you are taking or plan to take. Be sure to mention any of the following: antidepressants; certain antifungals such as fluconazole (Diflucan), itraconazole (Sporanox), ketoconazole (Nizoral), and voriconazole (Vfend); antihistamines; barbiturates; carbamazepine (Tegretol); divalproex (Depakote); dopamine agonists such as bromocriptine (Parlodel), cabergoline (Dostinex), levodopa (Dopar, Larodopa), pergolide (Permax), and ropinirole (Requip); erythromycin (E.E.S., E-Mycin, Erythrocin); lorazepam (Ativan); medications for anxiety, high blood pressure, irritable bowel disease, mental illness, motion sickness, Parkinson's disease, ulcers, or urinary problems; phenobarbital (Luminal); phenytoin (Dilantin); rifampin (Rifadin, Rimactane); sedatives; oral steroids such as dexamethasone (Decadron, Dexone), methylprednisolone (Medrol), and prednisone (Deltasone); sleeping pills; thioridazine (Mellaril); and tranquilizers. Your doctor may need to change the doses of your medications or monitor you carefully for side effects.
- tell your doctor if you or anyone in your family has or has ever had diabetes. Also tell your doctor if you have ever used street drugs or overused prescription medications and if you have or have ever had any condition that makes it difficult for you to swallow, or seizures, high cholesterol, high or low blood pressure, a heart attack, a stroke, breast cancer or thyroid, heart or liver disease. If you have ever had to stop taking a medication for mental illness because of severe side effects, be sure to tell your doctor.
- tell your doctor if you are pregnant or plan to become pregnant. If you become pregnant while taking quetiapine, call your doctor. Do not breastfeed while taking quetiapine.
- if you are having surgery, including dental surgery, tell your doctor or dentist that you are taking quetiapine.
- you should know that quetiapine may make you drowsy. Do not drive a car or operate machinery until you know how this medication affects you.
- you should know that alcohol can add to the drowsiness caused by this medication. Do not drink alcohol while taking quetiapine.
- you should know that you may experience hyperglycemia (increases in your blood sugar) while you are taking this medication, even if you do not already have diabetes. If you have schizophrenia, you are more likely to develop diabetes than people who do not have schizophrenia, and taking quetiapine or similar medications may increase this risk. Tell your doctor immediately if you have any of the following symptoms while you are taking quetiapine: extreme thirst, frequent urination, extreme hunger, blurred vision, or weakness. It is very important to call your doctor as soon as you have any of these symptoms, because high blood sugar can cause a serious condition called ketoacidosis. Ketoacidosis may become life-threatening if it is not treated at an early stage. Symptoms of ketoacidosis include: dry mouth, nausea and vomiting, shortness of breath, breath that smells fruity, and decreased consciousness.
- you should know that quetiapine may make it harder for your body to cool down when it gets very hot. Tell your doctor if you plan to do vigorous exercise or be exposed to extreme heat.
- you should know that quetiapine may cause dizziness, lightheadedness, and fainting when you get up too quickly from a lying position. This is more common when you first start taking quetiapine and when your dose is increased. To avoid this problem, get out of bed slowly, resting your feet on the floor for a few minutes before standing up.

What special dietary instructions should I follow?

Talk to your doctor about eating grapefruit and drinking grapefruit juice while taking this medicine.

Be sure to drink plenty of water every day while you are taking this medication.

What should I do if I forget to take a dose?

Take the missed dose as soon as you remember it. However, if it is almost time for the next dose, skip the missed dose and continue your regular dosing schedule. Do not take a double dose to make up for a missed one.

What side effects can this medicine cause?

Quetiapine may cause side effects. Tell your doctor if any of these symptoms are severe or do not go away:

- drowsiness
- dizziness
- pain
- weakness
- dry mouth
- indigestion
- constipation
- stomach pain
- headache
- excessive weight gain
- sore throat

Some side effects can be serious. If you experience any of the following symptoms or those listed in the IMPORTANT WARNING or SPECIAL PRECAUTIONS section, call your doctor immediately:

- fainting
- seizures
- changes in vision
- uncontrollable movements of your arms, legs, tongue, face, or lips
- painful erection of the penis that lasts for hours
- fever
- muscle stiffness, pain, or weakness
- excess sweating
- fast or irregular heartbeat
- confusion
- unusual bleeding or bruising
- hives
- rash
- blisters
- difficulty breathing or swallowing

Quetiapine may cause other side effects. Call your doctor if you have any unusual problems while taking this medication.

Quetiapine has caused cataracts in laboratory animals. It is not known if quetiapine may cause cataracts in humans. You will need to have eye exams to check for cataracts at the beginning of your treatment and every six months during your treatment. Talk to your doctor about the risks of taking quetiapine.

If you experience a serious side effect, you or your doctor may send a report to the Food and Drug Administration's (FDA) MedWatch Adverse Event Reporting program online [at http://www.fda.gov/MedWatch/index.html] or by phone [1-800-332-1088].

What storage conditions are needed for this medicine?

Keep this medication in the container it came in, tightly closed, and out of reach of children. Store it at room temperature and away from excess heat and moisture (not in the bathroom). Throw away any medication that is outdated or no longer needed. Talk to your pharmacist about the proper disposal of your medication.

What should I do in case of overdose?

In case of overdose, call your local poison control center at 1-800-222-1222. If the victim has collapsed or is not breathing, call local emergency services at 911.

Symptoms of overdose may include:

- drowsiness
- dizziness
- fainting
- fast heartbeat

What other information should I know?

Keep all appointments with your doctor.

Do not let anyone else take your medication. Ask your pharmacist any questions you have about refilling your prescription.

Dosage Facts
For Informational Purposes

Caution: Do not change your dose, how often you take your medication, or the length of time you are to take it without first talking to your healthcare provider.

The following dosage information was written using medical language for doctors and other healthcare professionals and is provided here for you to check your dosage. The dosage of this drug may differ for different patients. Therefore, always follow your doctor's instructions or the directions on the label. Contact your healthcare provider or pharmacist if you have any questions about the specific dosage of your medication after reviewing this information.

General Dosage Information

Available as quetiapine fumarate; dosage is expressed in terms of quetiapine.

Reinitiating therapy: In patients previously treated with quetiapine, dosage titration is not necessary if reinitiated after a drug-free period <1 week; if reinitiated after a drug-free period >1 week, generally titrate dosage as with initial therapy.

Adult Patients

Schizophrenia

ORAL:
- Initially, 25 mg twice daily.
- Increase dosage in increments of 25–50 mg 2 or 3 times daily on the second or third day, as tolerated, to a target dosage of 300–400 mg daily in 2 or 3 divided doses by the fourth day.
- Make subsequent dosage adjustments at intervals of not less than 2 days, usually in increments or decrements of 25–50 mg twice daily.
- Dosages ranging from 150–750 mg daily were effective in clinical trials. Dosages >300 mg daily usually do not result

in greater efficacy, but dosages of 400–500 mg daily have been required in some patients.

- Optimum duration of therapy currently not known, but efficacy of maintenance therapy with antipsychotics is well established. Continue therapy in responsive patients as long as clinically necessary and tolerated but at lowest possible effective dosage; reassess need for continued therapy and optimal dosage periodically (e.g., at least annually).
- If discontinuance is considered, precautions include slow, gradual dose reduction over many months, more frequent clinician visits, and use of early intervention strategies.

Bipolar Disorder
Acute Mania
ORAL:
- Initially, 100 mg daily in 2 divided doses. Increase dosage (in increments of ≤100 mg daily in 2 divided doses) to 400 mg daily on the fourth day of therapy. Make subsequent adjustments in increments of ≤200 mg daily to reach a dosage of up to 800 mg daily by the sixth day of therapy.
- Majority of patients respond to 400–800 mg daily.
- Optimum duration not established; efficacy has been demonstrated in two 12-week monotherapy trials and one 3-week adjunct therapy trial. If used for extended periods, periodically reevaluate long-term risks and benefits for the individual patient.

Prescribing Limits
Adult Patients
Schizophrenia
ORAL:
- Safety of dosages >800 mg daily not established.

Bipolar Disorder
Acute Mania
ORAL:
- Safety of dosages >800 mg daily not established.

Special Populations
Hepatic Impairment
- Initially, 25 mg daily; increase dosage by 25–50 mg daily according to clinical response and tolerability until an effective dosage is reached.

Renal Impairment
- No dosage adjustment necessary.

Patients at Risk of Orthostatic Hypotension
- Consider a slower rate of dosage titration and a lower target dosage in geriatric patients and in patients who are debilitated or have a predisposition to hypotensive reactions. Adjust dosage with caution.
- Initially, 25 mg twice daily to minimize risk of orthostatic hypotension and associated syncope. If hypotension occurs during dosage titration, return to previous dosage in titration schedule.

Quinapril
(kwin′ a pril)

Brand Name: Accupril®, Accuretic® as a combination product containing Quinapril Hydrochloride and Hydrochlorothiazide

Important Warning

Do not take quinapril if you are pregnant. If you become pregnant while taking quinapril, call your doctor immediately. Quinapril may harm the fetus.

Why is this medicine prescribed?

Quinapril is used alone or in combination with other medications to treat high blood pressure. It is used in combination with other medications to treat heart failure. Quinapril is in a class of medications called angiotensin-converting enzyme (ACE) inhibitors. It works by decreasing certain chemicals that tighten the blood vessels, so blood flows more smoothly and the heart can pump blood more efficiently.

How should this medicine be used?

Quinapril comes as a tablet to take by mouth. It is usually taken once or twice a day. To help you remember to take quinapril, take it around the same time every day. Follow the directions on your prescription label carefully, and ask your doctor or pharmacist to explain any part you do not understand. Take quinapril exactly as directed. Do not take more or less of it or take it more often than prescribed by your doctor.

Your doctor will probably start you on a low dose of quinapril and gradually increase your dose, not more than once every one or two weeks.

Quinapril controls high blood pressure and heart failure but does not cure them. Continue to take quinapril even if you feel well. Do not stop taking quinapril without talking to your doctor.

Are there other uses for this medicine?

This medication may be prescribed for other uses; ask your doctor or pharmacist for more information.

What special precautions should I follow?

Before taking quinapril,
- tell your doctor and pharmacist if you are allergic to quinapril, benazepril (Lotensin), captopril (Capoten), enalapril (Vasotec), fosinopril (Monopril), lisinopril (Prinivil, Zestril), moexipril (Univasc), perindopril (Aceon), ramipril (Altace), trandolapril (Mavik), or any other medications.
- tell your doctor and pharmacist what prescription and nonprescription medications, vitamins, nutritional sup-

plements, and herbal products you are taking. Be sure to mention any of the following: diuretics ('water pills'); lithium (Eskalith, Lithobid); potassium supplements; and tetracycline (Sumycin). Your doctor may need to change the doses of your medications or monitor you carefully for side effects.

- tell your doctor if you have or have ever had heart, liver, or kidney disease; lupus; scleroderma; diabetes; or angioedema, a condition that causes difficulty swallowing or breathing and painful swelling of the the face, throat, tongue, lips, eyes, hands, feet, ankles, or lower legs.
- tell your doctor if you plan to become pregnant or are breast-feeding.
- if you are having surgery, including dental surgery, tell the doctor or dentist that you are taking quinapril.
- you should know that diarrhea, vomiting, not drinking enough fluids, and sweating a lot can cause a drop in blood pressure, which may cause lightheadedness and fainting.

What special dietary instructions should I follow?

Talk to your doctor before using salt substitutes containing potassium. If your doctor prescribes a low-salt or low-sodium diet, follow these directions carefully.

What should I do if I forget to take a dose?

Take the missed dose as soon as you remember it. However, if it is almost time for the next dose, skip the missed dose and continue your regular dosing schedule. Do not take a double dose to make up for a missed one.

What side effects can this medicine cause?

Quinapril may cause side effects. Tell your doctor if any of these symptoms are severe or do not go away:
- dizziness
- excessive tiredness
- cough
- upset stomach
- vomiting

Some side effects can be serious. The following symptoms are uncommon, but if you experience any of them, call your doctor immediately:
- swelling of the face, throat, tongue, lips, eyes, hands, feet, ankles, or lower legs
- hoarseness
- difficulty breathing or swallowing
- yellowing of the skin or eyes
- fever, sore throat, chills, and other signs of infection
- chest pain
- lightheadedness
- fainting

Quinapril may cause other side effects. Call your doctor if you have any unusual problems while taking this medication.

If you experience a serious side effect, you or your doctor may send a report to the Food and Drug Administration's (FDA) MedWatch Adverse Event Reporting program online [at http://www.fda.gov/MedWatch/index.html] or by phone [1-800-332-1088].

What storage conditions are needed for this medicine?

Keep this medication in the container it came in, tightly closed, and out of reach of children. Store it at room temperature and away from excess heat and moisture (not in the bathroom). Throw away any medication that is outdated or no longer needed. Talk to your pharmacist about the proper disposal of your medication.

What should I do in case of overdose?

In case of overdose, call your local poison control center at 1-800-222-1222. If the victim has collapsed or is not breathing, call local emergency services at 911.

Symptoms of overdose may include:
- lightheadedness
- fainting

What other information should I know?

Keep all appointments with your doctor and the laboratory. Your blood pressure should be checked regularly to determine your response to quinapril. Your doctor may order certain lab tests to check your body's response to quinapril.

Do not let anyone else take your medication. Ask your pharmacist any questions you have about refilling your prescription.

Dosage Facts
For Informational Purposes

Caution: Do not change your dose, how often you take your medication, or the length of time you are to take it without first talking to your healthcare provider.

The following dosage information was written using medical language for doctors and other healthcare professionals and is provided here for you to check your dosage. The dosage of this drug may differ for different patients. Therefore, always follow your doctor's instructions or the directions on the label. Contact your healthcare provider or pharmacist if you have any questions about the specific dosage of your medication after reviewing this information.

General Dosage Information

Available as quinapril hydrochloride; dosage expressed in terms of quinapril.

Pediatric Patients

Hypertension†

ORAL:

- Some experts recommend an initial dosage of 5–10 mg once daily. Increase dosage as necessary to a maximum dosage of 80 mg once daily.

Adult Patients

Hypertension

ORAL:

- Initially, 10 or 20 mg once daily as monotherapy. Adjust dosage at ≥2-week intervals to achieve BP control.
- In patients currently receiving diuretic therapy, discontinue diuretic, if possible, 2–3 days before initiating quinapril. May cautiously resume diuretic therapy if BP not controlled adequately with quinapril alone. If diuretic cannot be discontinued, increase sodium intake and initiate quinapril at 5 mg daily under close medical supervision for several hours and until BP has stabilized.
- Usual dosage: 20–80 mg daily, given in 1 dose or 2 divided doses.
- If effectiveness diminishes toward end of dosing interval in patients treated once daily, consider increasing dosage or administering drug in 2 divided doses.

Quinapril/Hydrochlorothiazide Combination Therapy

ORAL:

- If BP is not adequately controlled by monotherapy with quinapril or hydrochlorothiazide, can switch to the fixed-combination preparation containing quinapril 10 mg and hydrochlorothiazide 12.5 mg or, alternatively, quinapril 20 mg and hydrochlorothiazide 12.5 mg. Adjust dosage of either or both drugs according to patient's response.
- If BP is controlled by monotherapy with hydrochlorothiazide 25 mg daily but potassium loss is problematic, can switch to fixed-combination preparation containing quinapril 10 mg and hydrochlorothiazide 12.5 mg or, alternatively, quinapril 20 mg and hydrochlorothiazide 12.5 mg.
- If BP is controlled with quinapril 20 mg and hydrochlorothiazide 25 mg (administered separately) and if no clinically important electrolyte disturbance is observed, can switch to the fixed-combination preparation containing these corresponding doses for convenience.

CHF

ORAL:

- Initially, 5 mg twice daily. Monitor closely for ≥2 hours until BP has stabilized. To minimize risk of hypotension, reduce diuretic dosage, if possible.
- Adjust dosage at weekly intervals to reach usual dosage.
- Usual dosage: 20–40 mg daily, given in 2 equally divided doses.

Prescribing Limits

Pediatric Patients

Hypertension†

ORAL:

- Maximum 80 mg daily.

Special Populations

Renal Impairment

Hypertension

ORAL:

- Initially, 10 mg once daily in adults with Cl_{cr} >60 mL/minute; 5 mg once daily in those with Cl_{cr} 30–60 mL/minute; or 2.5 mg once daily in those with Cl_{cr} 10–30 mL/minute. Titrate at 2-week intervals until BP is controlled.
- Quinapril/hydrochlorothiazide fixed combinations are not recommended in patients with severe renal impairment (Cl_{cr} ≤30 mL/minute or S_{cr} >3 mg/dL).

CHF

ORAL:

- Initially (first day), 5 mg in patients with moderate renal impairment (Cl_{cr} >30 mL/minute) or 2.5 mg in patients with severe renal impairment (Cl_{cr} 10–30 mL/minute) under close medical supervision. If well tolerated, administer as twice-daily regimen on subsequent days. Titrate at weekly intervals based on clinical and hemodynamic response.

Geriatric Patients

Hypertension

Oral

- Initially, 10 mg once daily as monotherapy. Adjust dosage at ≥2-week intervals to achieve BP control.

† Use is not currently included in the labeling approved by the US Food and Drug Administration.

Quinidine Oral

(kwin′ i deen)

Available generically.

Important Warning

Studies have shown that some antiarrhythmic drugs may increase the risk of death, especially if you have had a previous heart attack. This information also may apply to quinidine. Quinidine usually is used only to treat life-threatening arrhythmias.

Why is this medicine prescribed?

Quinidine is used to treat abnormal heart rhythms. It works by making your heart more resistant to abnormal activity. Quinidine is also used to treat malaria.

This medication is sometimes prescribed for other uses; ask your doctor or pharmacist for more information.

How should this medicine be used?

Quinidine comes as a tablet to take by mouth. Immediate-acting quinidine usually is taken three or four times a day. The extended-release (long-acting) product usually is taken two or three times a day. Do not cut, crush, or chew extended-release tablets; swallow them whole.

Follow the directions on your prescription label carefully, and ask your doctor or pharmacist to explain any part you do not understand. Take quinidine exactly as directed. Do not take more or less of it or take it more often than prescribed by your doctor.

Quinidine helps control your condition but will not cure it. Continue to take quinidine even if you feel well. Do not stop taking quinidine without talking to your doctor.

What special precautions should I follow?

Before taking quinidine,
- tell your doctor and pharmacist if you are allergic to quinidine, quinine, or any other drugs.
- tell your doctor and pharmacist what prescription and nonprescription medications you are taking, especially anticoagulants ('blood thinners') such as warfarin (Coumadin); antidepressants; cimetidine (Tagamet); codeine products; diltiazem (Cardizem, Dilacor, Tiazac); medication for heart disease or high blood pressure; medications for seizures, sleep, or an infection; and vitamins.
- tell your doctor if you have an infection or have or have ever had myasthenia gravis; heart, kidney, or liver disease; or muscle weakness.
- tell your doctor if you are pregnant, plan to become pregnant, or are breast-feeding. If you become pregnant while taking quinidine, call your doctor.
- if you are having surgery, including dental surgery, tell the doctor or dentist that you are taking quinidine.
- you should know that this drug may make you dizzy. Do not drive a car or operate machinery until you know how this drug affects you.
- remember that alcohol can add to the dizziness caused by this drug.
- talk to your doctor about the use of cigarettes and caffeine-containing beverages. These products may increase the irritability of your heart and interfere with the action of quinidine.
- do not change brands of medication without talking to your doctor.

What special dietary instructions should I follow?

Avoid drinking grapefruit juice while taking quinidine. Do not change the amount of salt in your diet without talking to your doctor.

What should I do if I forget to take a dose?

Take the missed dose as soon as you remember it. However, if it is almost time for the next dose, skip the missed dose and continue your regular dosing schedule. Do not take a double dose to make up for a missed one.

What side effects can this medicine cause?

Quinidine may cause side effects. Tell your doctor if any of these symptoms are severe or do not go away:
- diarrhea
- stomach pain and cramps
- dizziness or lightheadedness
- headache
- fatigue
- weakness
- rash
- vision changes
- difficulty sleeping
- tremor

If you experience any of the following symptoms, call your doctor immediately:
- irregular heartbeat
- chest pain
- skin rash
- hearing changes (ringing or loss of hearing)
- vision changes (blurred or light sensitivity)
- unusual bleeding or bruising

If you experience a serious side effect, you or your doctor may send a report to the Food and Drug Administration's (FDA) MedWatch Adverse Event Reporting program online [at http://www.fda.gov/MedWatch/index.html] or by phone [1-800-332-1088].

What storage conditions are needed for this medicine?

Keep this medication in the container it came in, tightly closed, and out of reach of children. Store it at room temperature and away from excess heat and moisture (not in the bathroom). Throw away any medication that is outdated or no longer needed. Talk to your pharmacist about the proper disposal of your medication.

What should I do in case of overdose?

In case of overdose, call your local poison control center at 1-800-222-1222. If the victim has collapsed or is not breathing, call local emergency services at 911.

What other information should I know?

Keep all appointments with your doctor and the laboratory. Your doctor will need to determine your response to quinidine.

Take quinidine at the same time each day in regularly spaced intervals. Changing the time of your doses prevents quinidine from working effectively.

Do not let anyone else take your medication. Ask your pharmacist any questions you have about refilling your prescription.

Dosage Facts
For Informational Purposes

Caution: Do not change your dose, how often you take your medication, or the length of time you are to take it without first talking to your healthcare provider.

The following dosage information was written using medical language for doctors and other healthcare professionals and is provided here for you to check your dosage. The dosage of this drug may differ for different patients. Therefore, always follow your doctor's instructions or the directions on the label. Contact your healthcare provider or pharmacist if you have any questions about the specific dosage of your medication after reviewing this information.

General Dosage Information

Available as quinidine sulfate and quinidine gluconate. Dosage for treatment of arrhythmias usually expressed in terms of the salt; dosage for treatment of malaria expressed in terms of the base or salt.

On a molar basis, approximately 267 mg of quinidine gluconate is equivalent to 200 mg of quinidine sulfate.

Each 100 mg of quinidine gluconate contains 62.5 mg of quinidine.

Pediatric Patients

Quinidine Sulfate
Arrhythmias†

ORAL:
- 20–50 mg/kg (usually 30 mg/kg) daily or 900 mg/m^2 daily, given in 4 or 5 divided doses.

Adult Patients

Quinidine Sulfate
Arrhythmias

ORAL:
- Conversion of atrial fibrillation: 200 mg every 2 or 3 hours for 5–8 doses in adults. Increase the individual dose each day until normal sinus rhythm is restored or toxic effects occur.
- Alternatively, 300–400 mg every 6 hours.
- If successful conversion of atrial fibrillation does not occur with plasma concentrations of 9 mcg/mL, further increases in dosage generally are unsuccessful and increase the possibility of toxicity.
- Treatment of paroxysmal supraventricular tachycardias (including paroxysmal atrial tachycardia and paroxysmal AV junctional rhythm): 400–600 mg every 2–3 hours until the paroxysm is terminated.
- Treatment of paroxysmal VT: 400–600 mg every 2–3 hours; however, dosages up to 600 mg every hour for 10 hours have been given.
- Treatment of atrial and ventricular premature contractions: 200–300 mg 3 or 4 times daily in adults.
- To maintain normal sinus rhythm after conversion: 200–400 mg 3 or 4 times daily.
- Alternatively, 600 mg as an extended-release formulation may be given every 8–12 hours.

- Some patients may require larger doses or more frequent administration, but dosage should be increased only after careful evaluation of the patient, including ECG monitoring and determination of plasma quinidine concentration.

Uncomplicated P. falciparum Malaria†

ORAL:
- 300–600 mg or 10 mg/kg of quinidine sulfate every 8 hours for 5–7 days.

Quinidine Gluconate
Arrhythmias

ORAL:
- Suppression and prevention of atrial, AV junctional, and VPCs: 324–660 mg as an extended-release preparation every 8–12 hours.
- Maintenance of normal sinus rhythm following conversion: 648 mg every 12 hours or 324–660 mg every 8 hours as an extended-release preparation. Some may be maintained in normal sinus rhythm on 324–330 mg of an extended-release preparation every 8–12 hours, while others may require larger doses or more frequent administration (e.g., every 6 hours).

Prescribing Limits

Adult Patients

Arrhythmias
Quinidine Sulfate

ORAL:
- 3–4 g daily.

Special Populations

Hepatic Impairment
- Consider dosage reduction to avoid toxicity.

Renal Impairment
- Consider dosage reduction to avoid toxicity.
- In patients with severe malaria receiving IV quinidine gluconate, initial loading doses and maintenance IV infusion rates generally do not need to be reduced in those with renal failure. If renal failure persists or clinical improvement does not occur in such patients, CDC recommends reducing maintenance IV infusion rate by one-third to one-half on the third day of treatment.

CHF
- Consider dosage reduction to avoid toxicity.

Geriatric Patients
- Select dosage with caution because of age-related decreases in hepatic, renal, and/or cardiac function and concomitant disease and drug therapy.

† Use is not currently included in the labeling approved by the US Food and Drug Administration.

Quinine

(kwye′ nine)

Available generically.

Why is this medicine prescribed?

Quinine is used to prevent and treat malaria.

This medication is sometimes prescribed for other uses; ask your doctor or pharmacist for more information.

How should this medicine be used?

Quinine comes in capsules and tablets to take by mouth. It usually is taken three times a day (every 8 hours) for 3 days for malaria attacks, twice a day for 6 weeks to prevent or suppress malaria, and at bedtime for leg cramps. Follow the directions on your prescription label carefully, and ask your doctor or pharmacist to explain any part you do not understand. Take quinine exactly as directed. Do not take more or less of it or take it more often than prescribed by your doctor.

Since quinine is very bitter, do not chew tablets before swallowing them.

Are there other uses for this medicine?

Quinine is also used to treat nighttime leg muscle cramps. Talk to your doctor about the possible risks of using this drug for your condition.

What special precautions should I follow?

Before taking quinine,
- tell your doctor and pharmacist if you are allergic to quinine, quinidine, or any other drugs.
- tell your doctor and pharmacist what prescription and nonprescription medications you are taking, especially acetazolamide, antacids, anticoagulants ('blood thinners') such as warfarin (Coumadin), cimetidine (Tagamet), digitoxin, digoxin (Lanoxin), quinidine, and vitamins. Do not take antacids that contain aluminum (e.g., aluminum hydroxide) or sodium bicarbonate without talking to your doctor. Also, avoid tonic water and nonprescription cold preparations that contain quinine.
- tell your doctor if you have or have ever had G-6-PD deficiency (an inherited blood disease), ringing ears, eye problems, or blackwater fever.
- tell your doctor if you are pregnant, plan to become pregnant, or are breast-feeding. If you become pregnant while taking quinine, call your doctor immediately.
- if you are having surgery, including dental surgery, tell the doctor or dentist that you are taking quinine.

What should I do if I forget to take a dose?

Take the missed dose as soon as you remember it, and take any remaining doses for that day at evenly spaced intervals.

However, if you take only one dose per day at bedtime, skip the missed dose completely. Do not take a double dose to make up for a missed one.

What side effects can this medicine cause?

Quinine may cause side effects. Tell your doctor if any of these symptoms are severe or do not go away:
- stomach pain
- vomiting
- stomach upset
- dizziness
- headache
- sweating
- restlessness
- confusion
- apprehension

If you experience any of the following symptoms, call your doctor immediately:
- skin rash
- difficulty breathing
- swelling of the face
- fever
- vision problems or changes
- difficulty hearing or ringing in the ears
- faintness
- easy bruising
- unusual bleeding
- sore throat
- fast heartbeat
- chest pain

If you experience a serious side effect, you or your doctor may send a report to the Food and Drug Administration's (FDA) MedWatch Adverse Event Reporting program online [at http://www.fda.gov/MedWatch/index.html] or by phone [1-800-332-1088].

What storage conditions are needed for this medicine?

Keep this medication in the container it came in, tightly closed, and out of reach of children. Store it at room temperature and away from excess heat and moisture (not in the bathroom). Throw away any medication that is outdated or no longer needed. Talk to your pharmacist about the proper disposal of your medication.

What should I do in case of overdose?

In case of overdose, call your local poison control center at 1-800-222-1222. If the victim has collapsed or is not breathing, call local emergency services at 911.

What other information should I know?

Keep all appointments with your doctor.

Do not let anyone else take your medication. Ask your pharmacist any questions you have about refilling your prescription.

Dosage Facts

For Informational Purposes

Caution: Do not change your dose, how often you take your medication, or the length of time you are to take it without first talking to your healthcare provider.

The following dosage information was written using medical language for doctors and other healthcare professionals and is provided here for you to check your dosage. The dosage of this drug may differ for different patients. Therefore, always follow your doctor's instructions or the directions on the label. Contact your healthcare provider or pharmacist if you have any questions about the specific dosage of your medication after reviewing this information.

General Dosage Information

Available as quinine sulfate; dosage expressed in terms of the salt.

Pediatric Patients

Malaria

Treatment of Uncomplicated Chloroquine-resistant P. falciparum or P. vivax Malaria

ORAL:

- 10 mg/kg 3 times daily for 3 or 7 days as determined by the geographic origin of the infecting parasite (3 days if malaria was acquired in Africa or South America or 7 days if acquired in Southeast Asia). Used in conjunction with doxycycline, tetracycline, or clindamycin for treatment of *P. falciparum* malaria or in conjunction with doxycycline for treatment of *P. vivax* malaria.
- Children <8 years of age who should not receive tetracyclines: 10 mg/kg 3 times daily for 3–7 days if used in conjunction with clindamycin for *P. falciparum* malaria or for 7 days if used alone for *P. falciparum* or *P. vivax* malaria.
- For those with *P. vivax* malaria, a 14-day regimen of oral primaquine also may be indicated to provide a radical cure and prevent delayed attacks or relapse.

Treatment of Severe P. falciparum Malaria

ORAL:

- 10 mg/kg 3 times daily to complete 3 or 7 days of total IV quinidine gluconate and oral quinine sulfate therapy as determined by the geographic origin of the infecting parasite (3 days if malaria was acquired in Africa or South America or 7 days if acquired in Southeast Asia).
- IV quinidine gluconate used initially; after ≥24 hours and after parasitemia is reduced to <1% and oral therapy is tolerated, oral quinine is substituted. The drugs are used in conjunction with a 7-day regimen of another antimalarial agent (e.g., doxycycline, tetracycline, or clindamycin) administered IV or orally as tolerated.

Presumptive Self-treatment of Malaria†

ORAL:

- 10 mg/kg 3 times daily for 3 or 7 days as determined by the geographic origin of the infecting parasite (3 days if malaria was acquired in Africa or South America or 7 days if acquired

in Southeast Asia) in conjunction with a 7-day regimen of doxycycline.
- Initiate presumptive self-treatment if malaria is suspected (fever, chills, or other influenza-like illness) and professional medical care will not be available within 24 hours.
- *Not* recommended for presumptive self-treatment of malaria in those currently taking the drug for prophylaxis.

Babesiosis†

ORAL:

- 25 mg/kg daily in 3 divided doses given for 7–10 days; used in conjunction with oral clindamycin (20–40 mg/kg daily in 3 divided doses for 7–10 days).

Adult Patients

Malaria

Treatment of Uncomplicated Chloroquine-resistant P. falciparum or P. vivax Malaria

ORAL:

- 650 mg every 8 hours for 3 or 7 days as determined by the geographic origin of the infecting parasite (3 days if malaria was acquired in Africa or South America or 7 days if acquired in Southeast Asia.) Used in conjunction with doxycycline, tetracycline, or clindamycin for treatment of *P. falciparum* malaria or in conjunction with doxycycline for treatment of *P. vivax* malaria.
- For those with *P. vivax* malaria, a 14-day regimen of oral primaquine also may be indicated to provide a radical cure and prevent delayed attacks or relapse.

Treatment of Severe P. falciparum Malaria

ORAL:

- 650 mg every 8 hours to complete 3 or 7 days of total quinidine and quinine therapy as determined by the geographic origin of the infecting parasite (3 days if malaria was acquired in Africa or South America or 7 days if acquired in Southeast Asia).
- IV quinidine gluconate used initially; after ≥24 hours and after parasitemia is reduced to <1% and oral therapy is tolerated, oral quinine is substituted. The drugs are used in conjunction with a 7-day regimen of another antimalarial agent (e.g., doxycycline, tetracycline, or clindamycin) administered IV or orally as tolerated.

Presumptive Self-treatment of Malaria†

ORAL:

- 650 mg every 8 hours given for 3 or 7 days (3 days if malaria was acquired in Africa or South America or 7 days if acquired in Southeast Asia) in conjunction with a 7-day regimen of doxycycline.
- Initiate presumptive self-treatment if malaria is suspected (fever, chills, or other influenza-like illness) and professional medical care will not be available within 24 hours.
- *Not* recommended for self-treatment of malaria in individuals currently taking the drug for prophylaxis.

Prevention of Malaria†

ORAL:

- 325 mg every 12 hours; continue prophylaxis for 6 weeks after leaving the malarious area.
- Terminal prophylaxis with primaquine may also be indicated if exposure occurred in areas where *P. ovale* or *P. vivax* are endemic. Primaquine terminal prophylaxis generally is ad-

ministered during the final 14 days of, or immediately following, quinine sulfate prophylaxis.

Nocturnal Recumbency Leg Muscle Cramps†

ORAL:
- 200–300 mg at bedtime. If necessary, 1 dose after the evening meal and 1 dose at bedtime. When leg cramps do not occur after several consecutive nights, discontinue quinine to determine if continued therapy is necessary.

Babesiosis†

ORAL:
- 650 mg 3 times daily for 7–10 days; used in conjunction with oral clindamycin (600 mg 3 times daily for 7–10 days).

Prescribing Limits

Pediatric Patients

Malaria
Treatment of Uncomplicated or Severe Malaria

ORAL:
- Do not exceed usual adult dosage.

Special Populations

Pregnant Women

Treatment of Uncomplicated Chloroquine-resistant P. falciparum Malaria
- Oral: 650 mg every 8 hours for 3 days if malaria was acquired in Africa or South America or 7 days if acquired in Southeast Asia where relative resistance to quinine has been reported; used in conjunction with a 7-day regimen of clindamycin.

Treatment of Uncomplicated Chloroquine-resistant P. vivax Malaria
- Oral: 650 mg every 8 hours for 7 days (regardless of where infection was acquired); used without clindamycin. Then, give chloroquine (300 mg once weekly) as prophylaxis for duration of the pregnancy until primaquine can be given after delivery to provide a radical cure.

† Use is not currently included in the labeling approved by the US Food and Drug Administration.

Rabeprazole

(ra be' pray zole)

Brand Name: AcipHex®

Why is this medicine prescribed?

Rabeprazole is used to treat conditions where the stomach produces too much acid, including ulcers, gastroesophageal reflux disease (GERD), and Zollinger-Ellison syndrome. Rabeprazole is used in combination with other medications to eliminate *H. pylori*, a bacteria that causes ulcers. Rabeprazole is in a class of medications called proton-pump inhibitors. It works by decreasing the amount of acid made in the stomach.

How should this medicine be used?

Rabeprazole comes as a delayed-release (long-acting) tablet to take by mouth. It is usually taken once a day for 4 to 8 weeks, but it is sometimes taken for a longer time. When taken for ulcers, rabeprazole should be taken after the morning meal. When taken in combination with other medications to eliminate *H. pylori*, rabeprazole is taken twice a day, with the morning and evening meals, for 7 days. Follow the directions on your prescription label carefully, and ask your doctor or pharmacist to explain any part you do not understand. Take rabeprazole exactly as directed. Do not take more or less of it or take it more often than prescribed by your doctor.

Swallow the tablets whole; do not split, chew, or crush them.

Are there other uses for this medicine?

This medication may be prescribed for other uses; ask your doctor or pharmacist for more information.

What special precautions should I follow?

Before taking rabeprazole,
- tell your doctor and pharmacist if you are allergic to rabeprazole, lansoprazole (Prevacid), omeprazole (Prilosec), pantoprazole (Protonix), or any other medications.
- tell your doctor and pharmacist what prescription and nonprescription medications, vitamins, nutritional supplements, and herbal products you are taking. Be sure to mention any of the following: cyclosporine (Neoral, Sandimmune), digoxin (Lanoxin), and ketoconazole (Nizoral). Your doctor may need to change the doses of your medications or monitor you carefully for side effects.
- tell your doctor if you have or have ever had liver disease.
- tell your doctor if you are pregnant, plan to become pregnant, or are breast-feeding. If you become pregnant while taking rabeprazole, call your doctor.

What special dietary instructions should I follow?

Unless your doctor tells you otherwise, continue your normal diet.

What should I do if I forget to take a dose?

Take the missed dose as soon as you remember it. However, if it is almost time for the next dose, skip the missed dose and continue your regular dosing schedule. Do not take a double dose to make up for a missed one.

What side effects can this medicine cause?

Rabeprazole may cause side effects. Tell your doctor if these symptoms are severe or do not go away:

- headache
- upset stomach
- diarrhea
- stomach pain
- vomiting
- constipation
- dry mouth
- increased or decreased appetite
- muscle or bone pain
- drowsiness
- dizziness
- difficulty falling asleep or staying asleep

There may be other side effects from rabeprazole. Call your doctor if you have any unusual problems while taking this medication.

What storage conditions are needed for this medicine?

Keep this medication in the container it came in, tightly closed, and out of reach of children. Store it at room temperature and away from excess heat and moisture (not in the bathroom). Throw away any medication that is outdated or no longer needed. Talk to your pharmacist about the proper disposal of your medication.

What should I do in case of overdose?

In case of overdose, call your local poison control center at 1-800-222-1222. If the victim has collapsed or is not breathing, call local emergency services at 911.

What other information should I know?

Keep all appointments with your doctor and the laboratory.

Do not let anyone else take your medication. Ask your pharmacist any questions you have about refilling your prescription.

Dosage Facts
For Informational Purposes

Caution: Do not change your dose, how often you take your medication, or the length of time you are to take it without first talking to your healthcare provider.

The following dosage information was written using medical language for doctors and other healthcare professionals and is provided here for you to check your dosage. The dosage of this drug may differ for different patients. Therefore, always follow your doctor's instructions or the directions on the label. Contact your healthcare provider or pharmacist if you have any questions about the specific dosage of your medication after reviewing this information.

General Dosage Information

Available as rabeprazole sodium; dosage expressed in terms of the salt.

Adult Patients

GERD
GERD without Erosive Esophagitis

ORAL:
- 20 mg once daily for 4 weeks; may give additional 4 weeks if symptoms are not completely resolved.

Treatment of Erosive Esophagitis

ORAL:
- 20 mg once daily for 4–8 weeks. If not healed after 8 weeks, consider additional 8 weeks of therapy (up to 16 weeks for a single course).

Maintenance of Healing of Erosive Esophagitis

ORAL:
- 20 mg once daily. Chronic, lifelong therapy may be appropriate.

Duodenal Ulcer
Treatment of Active Duodenal Ulcer

ORAL:
- 20 mg once daily for up to 4 weeks; some patients may require additional therapy.

Helicobacter pylori Infection and Duodenal Ulcer Disease

ORAL:
- Triple therapy: 20 mg twice daily for 7 days in conjunction with amoxicillin and clarithromycin.

Pathologic GI Hypersecretory Conditions (e.g., Zollinger-Ellison Syndrome)

ORAL:
- 60 mg once daily. Dosages up to 100 mg once daily or 60 mg twice daily have been used. Divided doses may be required. Adjust dosage as needed, continue treatment as long as necessary. Has been used continuously for up to 1 year.

Rabies Vaccine

Brand Name: Imovax®, RabAvert®

What is rabies?

Rabies is a serious disease. It is caused by a virus. Rabies is mainly a disease of animals. Humans get rabies when they are bitten by infected animals.

At first there might not be any symptoms. But weeks, or even years after a bite, rabies can cause pain, fatigue, headaches, fever, and irritability. These are followed by seizures, hallucinations, and paralysis. Rabies is almost always fatal.

Wild animals—especially bats—are the most common source of human rabies infection in the United States.

Skunks, raccoons, dogs, and cats can also transmit the disease.

Human rabies is rare in the United States. There have been only 39 cases diagnosed since 1990. However, between 16,000 and 39,000 people are treated each year for possible exposure to rabies after animal bites. Also, rabies is far more common in other parts of the world, with about 40,000–70,000 rabies-related deaths each year. Bites from unvaccinated dogs cause most of these cases. Rabies vaccine can prevent rabies.

Rabies vaccine

Rabies vaccine is given to people at high risk of rabies to protect them if they are exposed. It can also prevent the disease if it is given to a person *after* they have been exposed.

Rabies vaccine is made from killed rabies virus. It cannot cause rabies.

Who should get rabies vaccine and when?

Preventive Vaccination (No Exposure):

- People at high risk of exposure to rabies, such as veterinarians, animal handlers, rabies laboratory workers, spelunkers, and rabies biologics production workers should be offered rabies vaccine.
- The vaccine should also be considered for: (1) people whose activities bring them into frequent contact with rabies virus or with possibly rabid animals, and (2) international travelers who are likely to come in contact with animals in parts of the world where rabies is common.
- The pre-exposure schedule for rabies vaccination is 3 doses, given at the following times: (1) Dose 1: As appropriate, (2) Dose 2: 7 days after Dose 1, and (3) Dose 3: 21 days or 28 days after Dose 1.
- For laboratory workers and others who may be repeatedly exposed to rabies virus, periodic testing for immunity is recommended, and booster doses should be given as needed. (Testing or booster doses are not recommended for travelers.) Ask your doctor for details.

Vaccination After an Exposure:

- Anyone who has been bitten by an animal, or who otherwise may have been exposed to rabies, should see a doctor immediately.
- A person who is exposed and has never been vaccinated against rabies should get 5 doses of rabies vaccine — one dose right away, and additional doses on the 3rd, 7th, 14th, and 28th days. They should also get a shot of Rabies Immune Globulin at the same time as the first dose. This gives immediate protection.
- A person who has been previously vaccinated should get 2 doses of rabies vaccine — one right away and another on the 3rd day. Rabies Immune Globulin is not needed.

Tell your doctor if...

Talk with a doctor before getting rabies vaccine if you:

- ever had a serious (life-threatening) allergic reaction to a previous dose of rabies vaccine, or to any component of the vaccine,
- have a weakened immune system because of: HIV/AIDS or another disease that affects the immune system; treatment with drugs that affect the immune system, such as steroids; cancer, or cancer treatment with radiation or drugs.

If you have a minor illness, such as a cold, you can be vaccinated. If you are moderately or severely ill, you should probably wait until you recover before getting a routine (non-exposure) dose of rabies vaccine. **If you have been exposed to rabies virus, you should get the vaccine regardless of any other illnesses you may have.**

What are the risks from rabies vaccine?

A vaccine, like any medicine, is capable of causing serious problems, such as severe allergic reactions. The risk of a vaccine causing serious harm, or death, is extremely small. Serious problems from rabies vaccine are very rare.

Mild Problems:

- soreness, redness, swelling, or itching where the shot was given (30% - 74%)
- headache, nausea, abdominal pain, muscle aches, dizziness (5% - 40%)

Moderate Problems:

- hives, pain in the joints, fever (about 6% of booster doses)
- illness resembling Guillain-Barré Syndrome (GBS), with complete recovery (very rare)

Other nervous system disorders have been reported after rabies vaccine, but this happens so rarely that it is not known whether they are related to the vaccine.

NOTE: Several brands of rabies vaccine are available in the United States, and reactions may vary between brands. Your provider can give you more information about a particular brand.

What if there is a moderate or severe reaction?

What should I look for?

- Any unusual condition, such as a high fever or behavior changes. Signs of a serious allergic reaction can include difficulty breathing, hoarseness or wheezing, hives, paleness, weakness, a fast heart beat or dizziness.

What should I do?

- Call a doctor, or get the person to a doctor right away.
- Tell your doctor what happened, the date and time it happened, and when the vaccination was given.
- Ask your health care provider to file a Vaccine Adverse Event Reporting System (VAERS) form if you have any reaction to the vaccine. Or call VAERS yourself

at 1-800-822-7967, or visit their website at http://vaers.hhs.gov.

The National Vaccine Injury Compensation Program

In the rare event that you or your child has a serious reaction to a vaccine, a federal program has been created to help pay for the care of those who have been harmed.

For details about the National Vaccine Injury Compensation Program, call 1-800-338-2382 or visit the program's website at http://www.hrsa.gov/vaccinecompensation.

How can I learn more?

- Ask your doctor or other health care provider. They can give you the vaccine package insert or suggest other sources of information.
- Call your local or state health department's immunization program.
- Contact the Centers for Disease Control and Prevention (CDC): call 1-800-232-4636 (1-800-CDC-INFO) or visit the National Immunization Program's website at http://www.cdc.gov/nip

Rabies Vaccine Information Statement. U.S. Department of Health and Human Services/Centers for Disease Control and Prevention National Immunization Program. 1/12/2006.

Raloxifene

(ral ox′ i feen)

Brand Name: Evista®

Why is this medicine prescribed?

Raloxifene is used to prevent and treat osteoporosis, a disease common in women past menopause, which results in bones that break easily. Raloxifene is in a class of medications called selective estrogen receptor modulators (SERMs). It works by acting similar to estrogen, a female hormone produced by the body. Like estrogen, raloxifene increases the density of bone.

How should this medicine be used?

Raloxifene comes as a tablet to take by mouth. It is usually taken once a day at any time, with or without food. To help you remember to take raloxifene, take it around the same time every day. Follow the directions on your prescription label carefully, and ask your doctor or pharmacist to explain any part you do not understand. Take raloxifene exactly as directed. Do not take more or less of it or take it more often than prescribed by your doctor.

Continue to take raloxifene even if you feel well. Do not stop taking raloxifene without talking to your doctor.

Ask your pharmacist or doctor for a copy of the manufacturer's information for the patient.

Are there other uses for this medicine?

This medication may be prescribed for other uses; ask your doctor or pharmacist for more information. There is interest in possible beneficial effects of raloxifene on breast cancer risk in women.

What special precautions should I follow?

Before taking raloxifene,

- tell your doctor and pharmacist if you are allergic to raloxifene or any other drugs.
- tell your doctor and pharmacist what prescription and nonprescription medications, vitamins, nutritional supplements, and herbal products you are taking. Be sure to mention any of the following: anticoagulants ('blood thinners') such as warfarin (Coumadin), cholestyramine (Questran) or colestipol (Colestid), diazepam (Valium, Valrelease, Zetran), diazoxide (Proglycem), and estrogen or hormone replacement therapy (ERT or HRT). Your doctor may need to change the doses of your medications or monitor you carefully for side effects.
- tell your doctor if you have cancer and if you have or have ever had breast lumps or cancer, high blood cholesterol or triglycerides, blood clots (e.g., in the legs, lung, or eye), phlebitis in the leg, heart failure, or liver disease.
- tell your doctor if you are pregnant, plan to become pregnant, or are breast-feeding. If you become pregnant while taking raloxifene, call your doctor immediately. Raloxifene may harm the fetus.
- if you are having surgery, including dental surgery, tell the doctor or dentist that you are taking raloxifene.
- you should know that raloxifene increases the risk of blood clots. Because being inactive also increases the risk of blood clots, you should stop taking raloxifene 72 hours before a long period of lying down (for example, when recovering from surgery or when on bedrest). Resume taking raloxifene once you become active again. During long trips, make sure to get up and walk around every once in a while.
- you should know that raloxifene has not been found to cause spotting or menstrual-like bleeding nor to increase the risk of cancer of the uterine lining. However, tell your doctor if you develop unexplained vaginal bleeding or spotting.
- you should know that raloxifene has not been found to cause breast tenderness or swelling nor to increase the risk of breast cancer. However, tell your doctor if you notice any changes in your breasts.

What special dietary instructions should I follow?

Follow all dietary and exercise recommendations, including those regarding calcium and vitamin D supplements.

What should I do if I forget to take a dose?

Take the missed dose as soon as you remember it. However, if it is almost time for your next dose, skip the missed dose and continue your regular dosing schedule. Do not take a double dose to make up for a missed one.

What side effects can this medicine cause?

Raloxifene may cause side effects. Tell your doctor if any of these symptoms are severe or do not go away:

- hot flashes (more common in the first 6 months of raloxifene therapy)
- leg cramps
- swelling of the hands, feet, ankles, or lower legs

Some side effects can be serious. The following symptoms are uncommon, but if you experience any of them, call your doctor immediately:

- sudden chest pain or chest heaviness
- difficulty breathing or coughing up blood
- pain, swelling, or warmth in the calves, legs, hands, or feet
- sudden change in your vision such as vision loss or blurring

If you experience a serious side effect, you or your doctor may send a report to the Food and Drug Administration's (FDA) MedWatch Adverse Event Reporting program online [at http://www.fda.gov/MedWatch/index.html] or by phone [1-800-332-1088].

What storage conditions are needed for this medicine?

Keep this medication in the container it came in, tightly closed, and out of reach of children. Store it at room temperature and away from excess heat and moisture (not in the bathroom). Throw away any medication that is outdated or no longer needed. Talk to your pharmacist about the proper disposal of your medication.

What should I do in case of overdose?

In case of overdose, call your local poison control center at 1-800-222-1222. If the victim has collapsed or is not breathing, call local emergency services at 911.

What other information should I know?

Keep all appointments with your doctor and the laboratory. You should have a complete physical examination, including blood pressure measurements, breast and pelvic exams, and a Pap test at least yearly. Follow your doctor's directions for examining your breasts; report any lumps immediately. Your doctor may order certain lab tests to check your body's response to raloxifene.

Before you have any laboratory tests, tell the person doing the test that you take raloxifene, as this medication may interfere with some lab tests.

Do not let anyone else take your medication. Ask your pharmacist any questions you have about refilling your prescription.

Dosage Facts
For Informational Purposes

Caution: Do not change your dose, how often you take your medication, or the length of time you are to take it without first talking to your healthcare provider.

The following dosage information was written using medical language for doctors and other healthcare professionals and is provided here for you to check your dosage. The dosage of this drug may differ for different patients. Therefore, always follow your doctor's instructions or the directions on the label. Contact your healthcare provider or pharmacist if you have any questions about the specific dosage of your medication after reviewing this information.

General Dosage Information

Available as raloxifene hydrochloride; dosage expressed in terms of the salt.

Adult Patients

Osteoporosis
Prevention in Postmenopausal Women

ORAL:
- Usual dosage: 60 mg daily.
- No additional benefit observed with higher dosages (e.g., 150 mg daily).

Treatment in Postmenopausal Women

ORAL:
- Usual dosage: 60 mg daily.
- Higher dosages (e.g., 120 mg daily) associated with lower incidence of vertebral fracture in women with ≥1 baseline fracture; no additional benefit in women without baseline vertebral fractures.

Breast Cancer
Reduction in the Incidence of Invasive Breast Cancer in Postmenopausal Women at High Risk†

ORAL:
- 60 mg daily; duration of STAR trial was 5 years.

† Use is not currently included in the labeling approved by the US Food and Drug Administration.

Ramelteon

(ram el' tee on)

Brand Name: Rozerem®

Why is this medicine prescribed?

Ramelteon is used to help patients who have sleep-onset insomnia (difficulty falling asleep) fall asleep more quickly. Ramelteon is in a class of medications called melatonin receptor agonists. It works similarly to melatonin, a natural substance in the brain that is needed for sleep.

How should this medicine be used?

Ramelteon comes as a tablet to take by mouth. It is usually taken once a day, no earlier than 30 minutes before bedtime. Do not take ramelteon with or shortly after a high fat meal. Follow the directions on your prescription label carefully, and ask your doctor or pharmacist to explain any part you do not understand. Take ramelteon exactly as directed. Do not take more or less of it or take it more often than prescribed by your doctor.

You may become sleepy soon after you take ramelteon. After you take ramelteon, you should complete any necessary bedtime preparations and go to bed. Do not plan any other activities for this time.

Your insomnia should improve after you begin treatment with ramelteon. Call your doctor if your insomnia does not improve at the beginning of your treatment. Also call your doctor if your insomnia gets worse or you notice unusual changes in your behavior at any time during your treatment.

Are there other uses for this medicine?

This medication may be prescribed for other uses; ask your doctor or pharmacist for more information.

What special precautions should I follow?

Before taking ramelteon,

- tell your doctor and pharmacist if you are allergic to ramelteon or any other medications.
- tell your doctor and pharmacist what prescription and nonprescription medications, vitamins, nutritional supplements, and herbal products you are taking or plan to take. Be sure to mention any of the following: amiodarone (Cordarone, Pacerone); certain antifungals such as fluconazole (Diflucan), itraconazole (Sporanox), ketoconazole (Nizoral), and voriconazole (Vfend); aprepitant (Emend); cimetidine (Tagamet); clarithromycin (Biaxin, in Prevpac); clopidogrel (Plavix); efavirenz (Sustiva); HIV protease inhibitors including atazanavir (Reyataz), indinavir (Crixivan), lopinavir (in Kaletra), nelfinavir (Viracept), ritonavir (Norvir, in Kaletra), and saquinavir (Fortovase, Invirase); fluoroquinolone antibiotics including ciprofloxacin (Cipro), gatifloxacin (Tequin), levofloxacin (Levaquin), norfloxacin (Noroxin), ofloxacin (Floxin), others; fluvastatin (Lescol) fluvoxamine (Luvox); metronidazole (Flagyl); nefazodone; rifampin (Rifadin, Rimactane); sulfamethoxazole (Bactrim, Septra); sulfinpyrazone (Anturane); ticlopidine (Ticlid); and zarfirlukast (Accolate). Your doctor may need to change the doses of your medications or monitor you carefully for side effects.
- tell your doctor if you have or have ever had chronic obstructive pulmonary disease (COPD, damage to the lungs that makes breathing difficult), sleep apnea (breathing stops for a short time during sleep), depression, or liver disease.
- tell your doctor if you are pregnant, plan to become pregnant, or are breast-feeding. If you become pregnant while taking ramelteon, call your doctor.
- you should know that ramelteon may make you drowsy during the daytime. Do not drive a car or operate machinery until you know how this medication affects you.
- ask your doctor about the safe use of alcoholic beverages while you are taking ramelteon. Alcohol can add to the drowsiness caused by ramelteon.

What special dietary instructions should I follow?

Talk to your doctor about eating grapefruit and drinking grapefruit juice while taking this medicine.

What should I do if I forget to take a dose?

Do not take a double dose to make up for a missed one.

What side effects can this medicine cause?

Ramelteon may cause side effects. Tell your doctor if any of these symptoms are severe or do not go away:

- drowsiness or tiredness
- dizziness
- upset stomach
- changes in the way food tastes
- muscle or joint pain
- stuffy or runny nose, cough, or other cold symptoms
- flu-like symptoms

Some side effects can be serious. If you experience any of these symptoms, call your doctor:

- stopping of menstrual periods
- milky discharge from the nipples
- decreased sexual desire
- fertility problems
- depression

Ramelteon may cause other side effects. Call your doctor if you have any unusual problems while taking this medication.

If you experience a serious side effect, you or your doctor may send a report to the Food and Drug Administration's (FDA) MedWatch Adverse Event Reporting program online [at http://www.fda.gov/MedWatch/index.html] or by phone [1-800-332-1088].

What storage conditions are needed for this medicine?

Keep this medication in the container it came in, tightly closed, and out of reach of children. Store it at room temperature and away from excess heat and moisture (not in the bathroom). Throw away any medication that is outdated or no longer needed. Talk to your pharmacist about the proper disposal of your medication.

What should I do in case of overdose?

In case of overdose, call your local poison control center at 1-800-222-1222. If the victim has collapsed or is not breathing, call local emergency services at 911.

What other information should I know?

Keep all appointments with your doctor.

Do not let anyone else take your medication. Ask your pharmacist any questions you have about refilling your prescription.

Dosage Facts
For Informational Purposes

Caution: Do not change your dose, how often you take your medication, or the length of time you are to take it without first talking to your healthcare provider.

The following dosage information was written using medical language for doctors and other healthcare professionals and is provided here for you to check your dosage. The dosage of this drug may differ for different patients. Therefore, always follow your doctor's instructions or the directions on the label. Contact your healthcare provider or pharmacist if you have any questions about the specific dosage of your medication after reviewing this information.

Adult Patients
Insomnia

ORAL:
• 8 mg.

Special Populations

Hepatic Impairment
• Increased exposure to drug and active metabolite. No specific dosage recommendations at this time. However, use with caution in patients with moderate hepatic impairment; avoid use in patients with severe hepatic impairment.

Renal Impairment
• No dosage adjustment necessary in patients with mild, moderate, or severe renal impairment or in those requiring chronic hemodialysis.

Ramipril
(ra mi′ pril)

Brand Name: Altace®
Also available generically.

Important Warning

Do not take ramipril if you are pregnant. If you become pregnant while taking ramipril, call your doctor immediately. Ramipril may harm the fetus.

Why is this medicine prescribed?

Ramipril is used alone or in combination with other medications to treat high blood pressure. It is also used to reduce the risk of heart attack and stroke in patients at risk for these problems and to improve survival in patients with heart failure after a heart attack. Ramipril is in a class of medications called angiotensin-converting enzyme (ACE) inhibitors. It works by decreasing certain chemicals that tighten the blood vessels, so blood flows more smoothly and the heart can pump blood more efficiently.

How should this medicine be used?

Ramipril comes as a capsule to take by mouth. It is usually taken once or twice a day with or without food. To help you remember to take ramipril, take it around the same time every day. Follow the directions on your prescription label carefully, and ask your doctor or pharmacist to explain any part you do not understand. Take ramipril exactly as directed. Do not take more or less of it or take it more often than prescribed by your doctor.

Swallow the capsule whole, or open the capsule and sprinkle the contents on a small amount of applesauce (about 4 oz.) or in 4 oz. of water or apple juice. Eat or drink the entire mixture. This mixture can be prepared in advance and stored for 24 hours at room temperature or 48 hours in the refrigerator.

Your doctor will probably start you on a low dose of ramipril and gradually increase your dose.

Ramipril controls high blood pressure and heart failure but does not cure them. Continue to take ramipril even if you feel well. Do not stop taking ramipril without talking to your doctor.

Are there other uses for this medicine?

This medication may be prescribed for other uses; ask your doctor or pharmacist for more information.

What special precautions should I follow?

Before taking ramipril,
• tell your doctor and pharmacist if you are allergic to ramipril, benazepril (Lotensin), captopril (Capoten),

enalapril (Vasotec), fosinopril (Monopril), lisinopril (Prinivil, Zestril), moexipril (Univasc), perindopril (Aceon), quinapril (Accupril), trandolapril (Mavik), or any other medications.

- tell your doctor and pharmacist what prescription and nonprescription medications, vitamins, nutritional supplements, and herbal products you are taking. Be sure to mention any of the following: aspirin and other non-steroidal anti-inflammatory medications (NSAIDs) such as indomethacin (Indocin); diuretics ('water pills'); lithium (Eskalith, Lithobid); and potassium supplements. Your doctor may need to change the doses of your medications or monitor you carefully for side effects.
- tell your doctor if you have or have ever had heart, liver, or kidney disease; lupus; scleroderma; diabetes; or angioedema, a condition that causes difficulty swallowing or breathing and painful swelling of the the face, throat, tongue, lips, eyes, hands, feet, ankles, or lower legs.
- tell your doctor if you plan to become pregnant or are breast-feeding.
- if you are having surgery, including dental surgery, tell the doctor or dentist that you are taking ramipril.
- you should know that diarrhea, vomiting, not drinking enough fluids, and sweating a lot can cause a drop in blood pressure, which may cause lightheadedness and fainting.

What special dietary instructions should I follow?

Talk to your doctor before using salt substitutes containing potassium. If your doctor prescribes a low-salt or low-sodium diet, follow these directions carefully.

What should I do if I forget to take a dose?

Take the missed dose as soon as you remember it. However, if it is almost time for the next dose, skip the missed dose and continue your regular regular dosing schedule. Do not take a double dose to make up for a missed one.

What side effects can this medicine cause?

Ramipril may cause side effects. Tell your doctor if any of these symptoms are severe or do not go away:
- headache
- dizziness
- cough
- upset stomach
- vomiting
- excessive tiredness
- weakness

Some side effects can be serious. The following symptoms are uncommon, but if you experience any of them, call your doctor immediately:
- swelling of the face, throat, tongue, lips, eyes, hands, feet, ankles, or lower legs
- hoarseness
- difficulty breathing or swallowing

- yellowing of the skin or eyes
- fever, sore throat, chills, and other signs of infection
- lightheadedness
- fainting

Ramipril may cause other side effects. Call your doctor if you have any unusual problems while taking this medication.

If you experience a serious side effect, you or your doctor may send a report to the Food and Drug Administration's (FDA) MedWatch Adverse Event Reporting program online [at http://www.fda.gov/MedWatch/index.html] or by phone [1-800-332-1088].

What storage conditions are needed for this medicine?

Keep this medication in the container it came in, tightly closed, and out of reach of children. Store it at room temperature and away from excess heat and moisture (not in the bathroom). Throw away any medication that is outdated or no longer needed. Talk to your pharmacist about the proper disposal of your medication.

What should I do in case of overdose?

In case of overdose, call your local poison control center at 1-800-222-1222. If the victim has collapsed or is not breathing, call local emergency services at 911.

Symptoms of overdose may include:
- lightheadedness
- fainting

What other information should I know?

Keep all appointments with your doctor and the laboratory. Your blood pressure should be checked regularly to determine your response to ramipril. Your doctor may order certain lab tests to check your body's response to ramipril.

Do not let anyone else take your medication. Ask your pharmacist any questions you have about refilling your prescription.

Dosage Facts
For Informational Purposes

Caution: Do not change your dose, how often you take your medication, or the length of time you are to take it without first talking to your healthcare provider.

The following dosage information was written using medical language for doctors and other healthcare professionals and is provided here for you to check your dosage. The dosage of this drug may differ for different patients. Therefore, always follow your doctor's instructions or the directions on the label. Contact your healthcare provider or pharmacist if you have any questions about the specific dosage of your medication after reviewing this information.

Adult Patients

Hypertension

ORAL:
- Initially, 1.25–2.5 mg once daily in patients not receiving diuretic therapy. Adjust dosage at approximately monthly intervals (more aggressively in high-risk patients) to achieve BP control.
- In patients currently receiving diuretic therapy, discontinue diuretic, if possible, 2–3 days before initiating ramipril. May cautiously resume diuretic therapy if BP not controlled adequately with ramipril alone. If diuretic cannot be discontinued, increase sodium intake or initiate ramipril at 1.25 mg daily under close medical supervision.
- Usual dosage: 2.5–20 mg daily, given in 1 dose or 2 divided doses.
- If effectiveness diminishes toward end of dosing interval in patients treated once daily, consider increasing dosage or administering drug in 2 divided doses.

CHF after MI

ORAL:
- Initially, 2.5 mg twice daily, beginning as early as 2 days after MI. If hypotension occurs, reduce dosage to 1.25 mg twice daily. After 1 week at initial dosage, adjust dosage as tolerated at 3-week intervals to target dosage of 5 mg twice daily.
- Following initial dose, monitor closely for ≥ 2 hours and until BP has stabilized for at least an additional hour. To minimize risk of hypotension, reduce diuretic dosage, if possible.

Prevention of Cardiovascular Events

ORAL:
- Initially, 2.5 mg once daily for 1 week, followed by 5 mg once daily for 3 weeks; subsequently increase dosage as tolerated to maintenance dosage of 10 mg once daily. In patients with hypertension or those with recent MI, may administer total daily dosage in divided doses.

Special Populations

Renal Impairment
- Initial dosage of 1.25 mg once daily recommended in patients with renal artery stenosis.
- In patients with $Cl_{cr} < 40$ mL/minute per 1.73 m², 25% of the usual doses are expected to induce full therapeutic concentrations of ramiprilat.

Hypertension

ORAL:
- Initially, 1.25 mg once daily in patients with $Cl_{cr} < 40$ mL/minute per 1.73 m². Titrate until BP is controlled or to maximum dosage of 5 mg daily.

CHF after MI

ORAL:
- Initially, 1.25 mg once daily in patients with $Cl_{cr} < 40$ mL/minute per 1.73 m². May increase dosage to 1.25 mg twice daily; subsequently titrate according to clinical response and tolerance up to maximum dosage of 2.5 mg twice daily.

Volume-and/or Salt-Depleted Patients
- Correct volume and/or salt depletion prior to initiation of therapy or initiate therapy at dosage of 1.25 mg once daily.

Ranibizumab Injection

(ra'' ni biz' oo mab)

Brand Name: Lucentis®

Why is this medicine prescribed?

Ranibizumab is used to treat wet age-related macular degeneration (AMD; an ongoing disease of the eye that causes loss of the ability to see straight ahead and may make it more difficult to read, drive, or perform other daily activities). Ranibizumab is in a class of medications called vascular endothelial growth factor A (VEGF-A) antagonists. It works by blocking abnormal blood vessel growth and leakage in the eye(s) that may cause vision loss in people with wet AMD.

How should this medicine be used?

Ranibizumab comes as a solution (liquid) to be injected into the eye by a doctor. It is usually given in a doctor's office every month. Your doctor may give you injections on a different schedule if that is best for you.

Before you receive a ranibizumab injection, your doctor will clean your eye to prevent infection and numb your eye to reduce discomfort during the injection. You may feel pressure in your eye when the medication is injected. After your injection, your doctor will need to examine your eyes before you leave the office.

Ranibizumab controls wet AMD, but does not cure it. Your doctor will watch you carefully to see how well ranibizumab works for you. Talk to your doctor about how long you should continue treatment with ranibizumab.

Are there other uses for this medicine?

This medication may be prescribed for other uses; ask your doctor or pharmacist for more information.

What special precautions should I follow?

Before receiving ranibizumab injection,
- tell your doctor and pharmacist if you are allergic to ranibizumab or any other medications.
- tell your doctor and pharmacist what other prescription and nonprescription medications, vitamins, nutritional supplements, and herbal products you are taking or plan to take. Be sure to mention if you have received verteporfin (Visudyne) recently.
- tell your doctor if you have or have ever had glaucoma (an eye disease) or an infection in or around your eyes.
- tell your doctor if you are pregnant, plan to become pregnant, or are breast-feeding. If you become pregnant while taking ranibizumab, call your doctor.
- your doctor may prescribe antibiotic eye drops for you to use for a few days after you receive each injection. Talk to your doctor about how to use these eye drops.

- ask your doctor if there are any activities you should avoid during your treatment with ranibizumab injection.
- you should know that your eyes will be dilated (treated with eye drops that widen the pupils) before you receive each ranibizumab injection. This may make your eyes sensitive to bright light and may make it difficult for you to drive. Bring a hat or sunglasses to your appointment and plan to have someone drive you home after your treatment.
- talk to your doctor about testing your vision at home during your treatment. Check your vision in both eyes as directed by your doctor, and call your doctor if there are any changes in your vision.

What special dietary instructions should I follow?

Unless your doctor tells you otherwise, continue your normal diet.

What should I do if I forget to take a dose?

If you miss an appointment to receive ranibizumab, call your doctor as soon as possible.

What side effects can this medicine cause?

Ranibizumab may cause side effects. Tell your doctor if any of these symptoms are severe or do not go away:
- headache
- dry or itchy eyes
- teary eyes
- feeling that something is in your eye
- nausea
- back pain

Some side effects can be serious. If you experience any of these symptoms, call your doctor immediately:
- reddening of eye
- eye sensitivity to light
- eye pain
- decrease or changes in vision
- bleeding in or around the eye
- swelling of the eye or eyelid
- seeing "floaters" or small specks
- seeing flashing lights
- chest pain
- shortness of breath
- sweating
- slow or difficult speech
- dizziness or faintness
- weakness or numbness of an arm or leg

Ranibizumab may cause other side effects. Call your doctor if you have any unusual problems while receiving this medication.

What should I do in case of overdose?

In case of overdose, call your local poison control center at 1-800-222-1222. If the victim has collapsed or is not breathing, call local emergency services at 911.

What other information should I know?

Keep all appointments with your doctor. Your doctor will need to examine your eyes to see if you are developing serious side effects within 2 to 7 days after you receive each ranibizumab injection.

Talk to your doctor, pharmacist, or other healthcare professional if you have questions about dosing information for your medication.

Ranitidine
(ra nye′ te deen)

Brand Name: Tritec®, Zantac®, Zantac® 75, Zantac® EFFERdose®, Zantac® Syrup
Also available generically.

Why is this medicine prescribed?

Ranitidine is used to treat ulcers; gastroesophageal reflux disease (GERD), a condition in which backward flow of acid from the stomach causes heartburn and injury of the food pipe (esophagus); and conditions where the stomach produces too much acid, such as Zollinger-Ellison syndrome. Over-the-counter ranitidine is used to prevent and treat symptoms of heartburn associated with acid indigestion and sour stomach. Ranitidine is in a class of medications called H_2 blockers. It decreases the amount of acid made in the stomach.

How should this medicine be used?

Ranitidine comes as a tablet, an effervescent tablet, effervescent granules, and a syrup to take by mouth. It is usually taken once a day at bedtime or two to four times a day. Over-the-counter ranitidine comes as a tablet to take by mouth. It is usually taken once or twice a day. To prevent symptoms, it is taken 30-60 minutes before eating or drinking foods that cause heartburn. Follow the directions on your prescription or the package label carefully, and ask your doctor or pharmacist to explain any part you do not understand. Take ranitidine exactly as directed. Do not take more or less of it or take it more often than prescribed by your doctor.

Dissolve ranitidine effervescent tablets and granules in a full glass (6-8 ounces) of water before drinking.

Do not take over-the-counter ranitidine for longer than 2 weeks unless your doctor tells you to. If symptoms of heartburn, acid indigestion, or sour stomach last longer than 2 weeks, stop taking ranitidine and call your doctor.

Are there other uses for this medicine?

Ranitidine is also used sometimes to treat upper gastrointestinal bleeding and to prevent stress ulcers, stomach damage from use of nonsteroidal anti-inflammatory medications

(NSAIDs), and aspiration of stomach acid during anesthesia. Talk to your doctor about the risks of using this medication for your condition.

This medication may be prescribed for other uses; ask your doctor or pharmacist for more information.

What special precautions should I follow?

Before taking ranitidine,

- tell your doctor and pharmacist if you are allergic to ranitidine or any other medications.
- tell your doctor and pharmacist what prescription and nonprescription medications, vitamins, nutritional supplements, and herbal products you are taking. Be sure to mention either of the following: anticoagulants ('blood thinners') such as warfarin (Coumadin); and triazolam (Halcion). Your doctor may need to change the doses of your medications or monitor you carefully for side effects.
- tell your doctor if you have or have ever had porphyria, phenylketonuria, or kidney or liver disease.
- tell your doctor if you are pregnant, plan to become pregnant, or are breast-feeding. If you become pregnant while taking ranitidine, call your doctor.

What special dietary instructions should I follow?

Unless your doctor tells you otherwise, continue your normal diet.

What should I do if I forget to take a dose?

Take the missed dose as soon as you remember it. However, if it is almost time for the next dose, skip the missed dose and continue your regular dosing schedule. Do not take a double dose to make up for a missed one.

What side effects can this medicine cause?

Ranitidine may cause side effects. Tell your doctor if any of these symptoms are severe or do not go away:

- headache
- constipation
- diarrhea
- upset stomach
- vomiting
- stomach pain

Ranitidine may cause other side effects. Call your doctor if you have any unusual problems while taking this medication.

What storage conditions are needed for this medicine?

Keep this medication in the container it came in, tightly closed, and out of reach of children. Store it at room temperature and away from excess heat and moisture (not in the bathroom). Throw away any medication that is outdated or

no longer needed. Talk to your pharmacist about the proper disposal of your medication.

What should I do in case of overdose?

In case of overdose, call your local poison control center at 1-800-222-1222. If the victim has collapsed or is not breathing, call local emergency services at 911.

What other information should I know?

Keep all appointments with your doctor.

Before having any laboratory test, tell your doctor and the laboratory personnel that you are taking ranitidine.

Do not let anyone else take your medicine. Ask your pharmacist any questions you have about refilling your prescription.

Dosage Facts
For Informational Purposes

Caution: Do not change your dose, how often you take your medication, or the length of time you are to take it without first talking to your healthcare provider.

The following dosage information was written using medical language for doctors and other healthcare professionals and is provided here for you to check your dosage. The dosage of this drug may differ for different patients. Therefore, always follow your doctor's instructions or the directions on the label. Contact your healthcare provider or pharmacist if you have any questions about the specific dosage of your medication after reviewing this information.

General Dosage Information

Available as ranitidine hydrochloride; dosage expressed in terms of ranitidine.

Pediatric Patients

Duodenal Ulcer
Treatment of Active Duodenal Ulcer

ORAL:
- Children 1 month to 16 years of age: 2–4 mg/kg daily given as 2 equally divided doses.
- Maximum 300 mg daily.

Maintenance of Healing of Duodenal Ulcer

ORAL:
- Children 1 month to 16 years of age: 2–4 mg/kg once daily.
- Maximum 150 mg daily.

Gastric Ulcer
Treatment

ORAL:
- Children 1 month to 16 years of age: 2–4 mg/kg daily given as 2 equally divided doses.
- Maximum 300 mg daily.

Maintenance of Healing of Gastric Ulcer

ORAL:
- Children 1 month to 16 years of age: 2–4 mg/kg once daily.
- Maximum 150 mg daily.

Gastroesophageal Reflux
Treatment of GERD

ORAL:
- Children 1 month to 16 years of age: 5–10 mg/kg daily, usually administered as 2 equally divided doses.

Treatment of Erosive Esophagitis

ORAL:
- Children 1 month to 16 years of age: 5–10 mg/kg daily, usually administered as 2 equally divided doses.

Self-medication for Heartburn

ORAL:
- Children ≥12 years of age: 75 or 150 mg once or twice daily for up to 2 weeks.
- Maximum 150 mg (as 75-mg tablets) or 300 mg (as 150-mg tablets) in 24 hours continuously for 2 weeks.

Self-medication for Prevention of Heartburn

ORAL:
- Children ≥12 years of age: 75 mg or 150 mg once or twice daily continuously for up to 2 weeks; administer 30–60 minutes before ingestion of causative food or beverage.
- Maximum 150 mg (as 75-mg tablets) or 300 mg (as 150-mg tablets) in 24 hours continuously for 2 weeks.

Adult Patients

Duodenal Ulcer
Treatment of Active Duodenal Ulcer

ORAL:
- Usual dosage: 150 mg twice daily.
- Alternative: 300 mg daily after evening meal or at bedtime for optimum convenience and compliance.
- 100 mg twice daily reported to be as effective in healing ulcers as 150 mg twice daily.
- Healing usually within 4 weeks; may occur in 2 weeks.
- Additional 4 weeks of therapy may be beneficial.

Maintenance of Healing of Duodenal Ulcer

ORAL:
- 150 mg daily at bedtime.

Gastric Ulcer

ORAL:
- 150 mg twice daily.
- Healing usually within 6 weeks.

Maintenance of Gastric Ulcer Healing

ORAL:
- 150 mg daily at bedtime.

Gastroesophageal Reflux
Treatment of GERD

ORAL:
- 150 mg twice daily.

Treatment of Erosive Esophagitis

ORAL:
- 150 mg 4 times daily.

Maintenance of Healing of Erosive Esophagitis

ORAL:
- 150 mg twice daily.

Self-medication for Heartburn

ORAL:
- 75 mg or 150 mg once or twice daily.
- Maximum 150 mg (as 75-mg tablets) or 300 mg (as 150-mg tablets) in 24 hours continuously for 2 weeks.

Self-medication for Prevention of Heartburn

ORAL:
- 75 or 150 mg once or twice daily; administer 30–60 minutes before ingestion of causative food or beverage.
- Maximum 150 mg (as 75-mg tablets) or 300 mg (as 150-mg tablets) in 24 hours continuously for 2 weeks.

Pathologic GI Hypersecretory Conditions

ORAL:
- 150 mg twice daily; may administer more frequently, if needed.
- Adjust dosage according to patient response.
- Dosages up to 6 g daily have been used for severe disease.
- Continue as long as necessary.

Prescribing Limits

Pediatric Patients

Gastroesophageal Reflux
Self-medication for Heartburn

ORAL:
- Adolescents ≥12 years of age: Maximum 150 mg (as 75-mg tablets) or 300 mg (as 150-mg tablets) in 24 hours continuously for 2 weeks.

Self-medication for Prevention of Heartburn

ORAL:
- Adolescents ≥12 years of age: Maximum 150 mg (as 75-mg tablets) or 300 mg (as 150-mg tablets) in 24 hours continuously for 2 weeks.

Duodenal Ulcer
Treatment of Active Duodenal Ulcer

ORAL:
- Children 1 month to 16 years of age: Maximum 300 mg daily.

Maintenance of Healing of Duodenal Ulcer:

ORAL:
- Children 1 month to 16 years of age: Maximum 150 mg daily.

Gastric Ulcer
Treatment of Gastric Ulcer

ORAL:
- Children 1 month to 16 years of age: Maximum 300 mg daily.

Maintenance of Healing of Gastric Ulcer

ORAL:
- Children 1 month to 16 years of age: Maximum 150 mg daily.

Adult Patients

Gastroesophageal Reflux
Self-Medication for Heartburn

ORAL:
- Maximum 150 mg (as 75-mg tablets) or 300 mg (as 150-mg tablets) in 24 hours continuously for 2 weeks.

Self-medication for Prevention of Heartburn

ORAL:
- Maximum 150 mg (as 75-mg tablets) or 300 mg (as 150-mg tablets) in 24 hours continuously for 2 weeks.

Duodenal Ulcer
Treatment of Active Duodenal Ulcer

ORAL:
- Safety and efficacy for >8 weeks have not been established.

Gastric Ulcer
Treatment of Active Benign Gastric Ulcer

ORAL:
- Safety and efficacy for >6 weeks have not been established.

Special Populations

Renal Impairment

Cl_{cr} <50 mL/minute

ORAL:
- 150 mg once every 24 hours. If necessary, may cautiously increase dosage frequency to every 12 hours or more frequently.

Hemodialysis

Decreases blood levels; administer at the end of hemodialysis.

Geriatric Patients
- Careful dosage selection recommended because of possible age-related decrease in renal function.

Ranitidine Hydrochloride Injection

(ra ni′ ti deen)

Brand Name: Zantac®, Zantac® Premixed
Also available generically.

About Your Treatment

Your doctor has ordered ranitidine hydrochloride to decrease the acid produced by your stomach.

Ranitidine may be added to an intravenous fluid that will drip through a needle or catheter placed in your vein for 15-20 minutes, one to four times a day. It also may be added to your total parenteral nutrition (TPN) solution.

Ranitidine decreases acid in your stomach to help treat an ulcer or prevent one from developing. Ranitidine helps to decrease the stomach pain, diarrhea, and loss of appetite that ulcers can cause. This medication is sometimes prescribed for other uses; ask your doctor or pharmacist for more information.

Your health care provider (doctor, nurse, or pharmacist)

may measure the effectiveness and side effects of your treatment using laboratory tests and physical examinations. It is important to keep all appointments with your doctor and the laboratory. The length of treatment depends on how you respond to the medication.

Precautions

Before administering ranitidine,
- tell your doctor and pharmacist if you are allergic to ranitidine or any other drugs.
- tell your doctor and pharmacist what prescription and nonprescription medications you are taking, especially acetaminophen (Tylenol), anticoagulants ('blood thinners') such as warfarin (Coumadin), propantheline, and vitamins.
- tell your doctor if you have or have ever had kidney or liver disease or acute porphyria.
- tell your doctor if you are pregnant, plan to become pregnant, or are breast-feeding. If you become pregnant while taking ranitidine, call your doctor.

Administering Your Medication

Before you administer ranitidine, look at the solution closely. It should be clear and free of floating material. Gently squeeze the bag or observe the solution container to make sure there are no leaks. Do not use the solution if it is discolored, if it contains particles, or if the bag or container leaks. Use a new solution, but show the damaged one to your health care provider.

It is important that you use your medication exactly as directed. Do not change your dosing schedule without talking to your health care provider. Your health care provider may tell you to stop your infusion if you have a mechanical problem (such as a blockage in the tubing, needle, or catheter); if you have to stop an infusion, call your health care provider immediately so your therapy can continue.

Side Effects

Ranitidine may cause side effects. Tell your health care provider if any of these symptoms are severe or do not go away:
- headache
- dizziness
- constipation
- diarrhea
- stomach pain
- upset stomach

Storage Conditions

- Your health care provider probably will give you a several-day supply of ranitidine at a time. If you are receiving ranitidine intravenously (in your vein), you probably will be told to store it in the refrigerator or freezer.
- Take your next dose from the refrigerator 1 hour before using it; place it in a clean, dry area to allow it to warm to room temperature.

- If you are told to store additional ranitidine in the freezer, always move a 24-hour supply to the refrigerator for the next day's use.
- Do not refreeze medications.

If you are receiving ranitidine mixed with TPN, you may be directed to keep it in a clean, dry area away from heat.

Store your medication only as directed. Make sure you understand what you need to store your medication properly.

Keep your supplies in a clean, dry place when you are not using them, and keep all medications and supplies out of reach of children. Your health care provider will tell you how to throw away used needles, syringes, tubing, and containers to avoid accidental injury.

Overdose

In case of overdose, call your local poison control center at 1-800-222-1222. If the victim has collapsed or is not breathing, call local emergency services at 911.

Signs of Infection

If you are receiving ranitidine in your vein or under your skin, you need to know the symptoms of a catheter-related infection (an infection where the needle enters your vein or skin). If you experience any of these effects near your intravenous catheter, tell your health care provider as soon as possible:

- tenderness
- warmth
- irritation
- drainage
- redness
- swelling
- pain

Dosage Facts
For Informational Purposes

Caution: Do not change your dose, how often you take your medication, or the length of time you are to take it without first talking to your healthcare provider.

The following dosage information was written using medical language for doctors and other healthcare professionals and is provided here for you to check your dosage. The dosage of this drug may differ for different patients. Therefore, always follow your doctor's instructions or the directions on the label. Contact your healthcare provider or pharmacist if you have any questions about the specific dosage of your medication after reviewing this information.

General Dosage Information

Available as ranitidine hydrochloride; dosage expressed in terms of ranitidine.

Pediatric Patients

Duodenal Ulcer
Treatment of Active Duodenal Ulcer

IV:
- Children 1 month to 16 years of age: 2–4 mg/kg daily given as divided doses every 6–8 hours.
- Maximum 50 mg every 6–8 hours.

Maintenance of Healing of Duodenal Ulcer

Increase Gastric pH in Neonates Undergoing ECMO

IV:
- Neonates (<1 month of age) at risk for GI hemorrhage: Consider 2 mg/kg every 12–24 hours (or as continuous infusion).
- A dose of 2 mg/kg usually is sufficient to increase gastric pH to >4 for at least 15 hours.

Adult Patients

General parenteral dosage (in hospitalized patients with pathologic hypersecretory conditions or intractable duodenal ulcer, or short-term use when oral therapy is not feasible):

INTERMITTENT DIRECT IV INJECTION:
- 50 mg every 6–8 hours.
- Increase dosage when necessary by administering 50 mg more frequently.
- Maximum 400 mg daily.

INTERMITTENT IV INFUSION:
- 50 mg every 6–8 hours.
- Increase dosage when necessary by administering 50 mg more frequently.
- Maximum 400 mg daily.

CONTINUOUS IV INFUSION:
- 150 mg/24 hours (6.25 mg/hour). Also see Pathologic GI Hypersecretory Conditions under Dosage.

Pathologic GI Hypersecretory Conditions
CONTINUOUS IV INFUSION:
- Initiate at 1 mg/kg per hour.
- Titrate upward in 0.5 mg/kg per hour increments and redetermine gastric acid secretion if symptoms occur or gastric acid output is >10 mEq per hour after 4 hours.
- Dosages up to 2.5 mg/kg per hour and infusion rates up to 220 mg/hour have been used.

Prescribing Limits

Adult Patients

General parenteral dosage (hospitalized patients with pathologic hypersecretory conditions or intractable duodenal ulcer, or short-term use when oral therapy is not feasible):

INTERMITTENT DIRECT IV:
- Maximum 400 mg daily.
- Maximum 50 mg per dose.
- Maximum concentration 2.5 mg/mL (50 mg/20 mL).
- Maximum injection rate: 4 mL/minute (i.e., over 5 minutes).

INTERMITTENT IV INFUSION:
- Maximum 400 mg daily.
- Maximum 50 mg per dose.
- Maximum concentration 0.5 mg/mL (50 mg/100 mL).
- Maximum infusion rate: 5–7 mL/minute (100 mL over 15–20 minutes).

- Commercially available infusion solution (50 mg in 50 mL of 0.45% sodium chloride): over 15–20 minutes.

Pathologic GI Hypersecretory Conditions

CONTINUOUS IV INFUSION:
- Zollinger-Ellison Syndrome: Maximum concentration 2.5 mg/mL.
- Up to 2.5 mg/kg per hour or 220 mg/hour has been used.

Special Populations

Renal Impairment

Cl_{cr} <50 mL/minute

INTERMITTENT DIRECT IV:
- 50 mg every 18–24 hours. If necessary, may cautiously increase dosage frequency to every 12 hours or more frequently.

INTERMITTENT IV INFUSION:
- 50 mg every 18–24 hours. If necessary, may cautiously increase dosage frequency to every 12 hours or more frequently.

CONTINUOUS IV INFUSION:
- Not evaluated.

Hemodialysis

Decreases blood levels; administer at the end of hemodialysis.

Geriatric Patients
- Careful dosage selection recommended because of possible age-related decrease in renal function.

Ranolazine

(ra noe′ la zeen)

Brand Name: Ranexa®

Why is this medicine prescribed?

Ranolazine is used with other medications to treat angina (chest pain or pressure that is felt when the heart does not get enough oxygen) that is a symptom of an ongoing condition. Ranolazine is used to treat people who still experience angina even when they take other medications to treat the condition. Ranolazine may prevent episodes of angina, but it cannot be used to relieve an episode of angina that has already begun. Ranolazine is in a class of medications called anti-ischemics. The exact way that ranolazine works is not known at this time.

How should this medicine be used?

Ranolazine comes as an extended-release (long-acting) tablet to take by mouth. It is usually taken with or without food two times a day. Take ranolazine at around the same times every day. Follow the directions on your prescription label carefully, and ask your doctor or pharmacist to explain any part you do not understand. Take ranolazine exactly as directed. Do not take more or less of it or take it more often than prescribed by your doctor.

Swallow the tablets whole; do not break, chew, or crush them.

Your doctor will probably start you on a low dose of ranolazine and gradually increase your dose.

Do not take ranolazine to treat a sudden attack of angina. Your doctor will tell you what you should do if you experience an attack of angina. Make sure that you understand these directions.

Ranolazine may help to control your condition but will not cure it. Continue to take ranolazine even if you feel well. Do not stop taking ranolazine without talking to your doctor.

Are there other uses for this medicine?

This medication may be prescribed for other uses; ask your doctor or pharmacist for more information.

What special precautions should I follow?

Before taking ranolazine,
- tell your doctor and pharmacist if you are allergic to ranolazine, any other medications, or any of the ingredients in ranolazine tablets. Ask your pharmacist for a list of the ingredients.
- tell your doctor if you are taking any of the following medications: certain antibiotics such as clarithromycin (Biaxin, in Prevpac), erythromycin (E.E.S., E-Mycin, Erythrocin), moxifloxacin (Avelox), sparfloxacin (Zagam) (not available in the United States) and troleandomycin (TAO); certain antifungals such as fluconazole (Diflucan), itraconazole (Sporanox), ketoconazole (Nizoral), and voriconazole (Vfend); certain antipsychotics (medications to treat mental illness) including thioridazine (Mellaril) and ziprasidone (Geodon); cisapride (Propulsid) (not available in the United States); diltiazem (Cardizem, Tiazac, Dilacor); certain medications to treat human immunodeficiency virus (HIV) or acquired immunodeficiency syndrome (AIDS) such as atazanavir (Reyataz), delavirdine (Rescriptor), efavirenz (Sustiva), indinavir (Crixivan), lopinavir (in Kaletra), nelfinavir (Viracept), ritonavir (Norvir, in Kaletra), and saquinavir (Invirase); medications for irregular heartbeat such as amiodarone (Cordarone, Pacerone), disopyramide (Norpace), dofetilide (Tikosyn), procainamide (Procanbid, Pronestyl), quinidine (Quinidex), and sotalol (Betapace); pimozide (Orap); and verapamil (Calan, Covera, Isoptin, Verelan). Your doctor may tell you not to take ranolazine if you are taking one or more of these medications.
- tell your doctor and pharmacist what other prescription and nonprescription medications, vitamins, nutritional supplements, and herbal products you are taking or plan to take. Be sure to mention any of the following: certain antidepressants such as amitriptyline (Elavil), amoxapine (Asendin), clomipramine (Anafranil), desipramine (Norpramin), doxepin (Adapin, Sinequan), imipramine (Tofranil), nortriptyline (Aventyl, Pamelor), protriptyline (Vivactil), and trimipramine (Surmontil); cyclo-

sporine (Neoral, Sandimmune); digoxin (Lanoxicaps, Lanoxin); and simvastatin (in Vytorin, Zocor). Your doctor may need to change the doses of your medications or monitor you carefully for side effects. Many other medications may also interact with ranolazine, so be sure to tell your doctor about all the medications you are taking, even those that do not appear on this list or the list above.

- tell your doctor if you have or have ever had a prolonged QT interval (a rare heart problem that may cause fainting or irregular heartbeat) or liver disease. Your doctor may tell you that you should not take ranolazine.
- tell your doctor if anyone in your family has or has ever had a prolonged QT interval and if you or anyone in your family has or has ever had a fast, slow, or irregular heartbeat; an abnormal electrocardiogram (EKG, ECG, heart rhythm test), or low levels of potassium in the blood. Also tell your doctor if you have or have ever had kidney disease.
- tell your doctor if you are pregnant, plan to become pregnant, or are breast-feeding. If you become pregnant while taking ranolazine, call your doctor. You should not breast-feed while taking ranolazine.
- you should know that ranolazine may make you dizzy and lightheaded. Do not drive a car, operate machinery, or participate in activities requiring mental alertness and coordination until you know how this medication affects you.

What special dietary instructions should I follow?

Do not drink grapefruit juice or eat grapefruit products while taking this medication.

What should I do if I forget to take a dose?

Skip the missed dose and continue your regular dosing schedule. Do not take a double dose to make up for a missed one.

What side effects can this medicine cause?

Ranolazine may cause side effects. Tell your doctor if any of these symptoms are severe or do not go away:
- nausea
- constipation
- headache
- dizziness

Some side effects can be serious. If you experience either of these symptoms, call your doctor immediately:
- fast, pounding, or irregular heartbeat
- fainting

Ranolazine may cause prolonged QT interval, a serious or life-threatening condition. Talk to your doctor about the risks of taking this medication.

Ranolazine may cause other side effects. Call your doctor if you have any unusual problems while taking this medication.

What storage conditions are needed for this medicine?

Keep this medication in the container it came in, tightly closed, and out of reach of children. Store it at room temperature and away from excess heat and moisture (not in the bathroom). Throw away any medication that is outdated or no longer needed. Talk to your pharmacist about the proper disposal of your medication.

What should I do in case of overdose?

In case of overdose, call your local poison control center at 1-800-222-1222. If the victim has collapsed or is not breathing, call local emergency services at 911.
    Symptoms of overdose may include:
- nausea
- vomiting
- dizziness
- confusion
- double vision
- pain, burning, numbness, or tingling in any part of the body
- fainting
- loss of consciousness

What other information should I know?

Keep all appointments with your doctor.
    Do not let anyone else take your medication. Ask your pharmacist any questions you have about refilling your prescription.

Talk to your doctor, pharmacist, or other healthcare professional if you have questions about dosing information for your medication.

Rasagiline

(ra sa′ ji leen)

Brand Name: Azilect®

Why is this medicine prescribed?

Rasagiline is used alone or in combination with another medication to treat the symptoms of Parkinson's disease (a slowly progressing disease of the nervous system causing a fixed face without expression, tremor at rest, slowing of movements, walking with shuffling steps, stooped posture and muscle weakness). Rasagiline is in a class of medications called monoamine oxidase (MAO) type B inhibitors. It works by increasing the amounts of certain natural substances in the brain.

How should this medicine be used?

Rasagiline comes as a tablet to take by mouth. It is usually taken once a day with or without food. Take rasagiline at around the same time every day. Follow the directions on your prescription label carefully, and ask your doctor or pharmacist to explain any part you do not understand. Take rasagiline exactly as directed. Do not take more or less of it or take it more often than prescribed by your doctor.

Are there other uses for this medicine?

This medication may be prescribed for other uses; ask your doctor or pharmacist for more information.

What special precautions should I follow?

Before taking rasagiline,

- tell your doctor and pharmacist if you are allergic to rasagiline or any other medications.
- tell your doctor if you are taking amphetamines (Adderall, Dexedrine, DextroStat); antidepressants such as amitriptyline (Elavil), amoxapine (Asendin), clomipramine (Anafranil), desipramine (Norpramin), doxepin (Adapin, Sinequan), imipramine (Tofranil), mirtazapine (Remeron), nortriptyline (Aventyl, Pamelor), protriptyline (Vivactil), and trimipramine (Surmontil); ephedrine; cough and cold products containing dextromethorphan (DM; in Robitussin Cough Calmers, Sucrets Cough Control, Suppress, others), phenylephrine (Sudafed PE, others), phenylpropanolamine (not available in the U.S.), or pseudoephedrine (Pediacare, Sudafed, Suphedrine, others); cyclobenzaprine (Flexeril); diet or weight-control products containing ephedrine; meperidine (Demerol); methadone (Dolophine, Methadose); other MAO inhibitors such as phenelzine (Nardil), selegiline (Eldepryl), or tranylcypromine (Parnate); nasal and oral decongestants; propoxyphene (Darvon, in Darvocet-N, others); serotonin-norepinephrine reuptake inhibitors such as duloxetine (Cymbalta) and venlafaxine (Effexor); selective serotonin reuptake inhibitors (SSRIs) such as citalopram (Celexa), escitalopram (Lexapro), fluoxetine (Prozac, Sarafem), fluvoxamine (Luvox), paroxetine (Paxil), and sertraline (Zoloft); St. John's wort; or tramadol (Ultram, in Ultracet). Your doctor will probably tell you not to take these medications while taking rasagiline and for at least 14 days after stopping rasagiline.
- tell your doctor and pharmacist what other prescription and nonprescription medications, vitamins, nutritional supplements, and herbal products you are taking or plan to take. Be sure to mention any of the following: atazanavir (Reyataz); cimetidine (Tagamet); fluoroquinolone antibiotics including ciprofloxacin (Cipro), gatifloxacin (Tequin), levofloxacin (Levaquin), norfloxacin (Noroxin), ofloxacin (Floxin), others; and ticlopidine (Ticlid). Your doctor may need to change the doses of your medications or monitor you carefully for side effects.
- tell your doctor if you have pheochromocytoma (a tumor on a small gland near the kidneys). Your doctor will probably tell you not to take rasagiline.

- tell your doctor if you have or have ever had kidney or liver disease.
- tell your doctor if you are pregnant, plan to become pregnant, or are breast-feeding. If you become pregnant while taking rasagiline, call your doctor.
- if you are having surgery, including dental surgery, tell the doctor or dentist that you are taking rasagiline. Your doctor will probably tell you to stop taking rasagiline at least 14 days before elective surgery.
- you should know that rasagiline may cause dizziness, lightheadedness, and fainting when you get up too quickly from a lying position. This is more common during the first 2 months of taking rasagiline. To avoid this problem, get out of bed slowly, resting your feet on the floor for a few minutes before standing up.
- you should know that rasagiline may cause serious, life-threatening high blood pressure when taken with certain medications or foods. Carefully follow your doctor's instructions about medications and foods to be avoided. Call your doctor right away if you have a severe headache, blurred vision, or any of the other symptoms listed below as serious side effects.
- you should know that patients who took rasagiline had a higher risk of melanoma (a type of skin cancer) than people in the general population. It is not known whether this increased risk is caused by Parkinson's disease or rasagiline. You should have regular visits with a dermatologist to examine your skin for melanoma.

What special dietary instructions should I follow?

Do NOT eat the following foods, which contain tyramine, while taking rasagiline and for 2 weeks after you stop taking it: pickled herring; dried sausage; hard salami; spoiled or improperly stored meat, poultry, fish, and liver; fava bean pods; aged cheeses; tap beer and unpasteurized beers; red wine; concentrated yeast extract; sauerkraut; and most soybean products, including soy sauce and tofu.

You MAY eat the following foods, which contain little or no tyramine, while taking rasagiline: fresh meat, poultry, and fish; fresh processed meats such as lunch meats, hot dogs, breakfast sausage, and cooked sliced ham; processed cheeses; mozzarella cheese; ricotta cheese; cottage cheese; yogurt; bottled and canned beers; white wine; Brewer's yeast; baker's yeast; and soy milk.

Talk to your doctor about eating grapefruit and drinking grapefruit juice while taking this medicine.

What should I do if I forget to take a dose?

Do not take a double dose to make up for a missed one. Skip the missed dose and take your next dose at the usual time the next day.

What side effects can this medicine cause?

Rasagiline may cause side effects. Tell your doctor if any of these symptoms are severe or do not go away:

- mild headache
- joint or neck pain
- heartburn
- stomach pain
- constipation
- diarrhea
- loss of appetite
- weight loss
- flu-like symptoms
- fever
- sweating
- runny nose
- red, swollen, and/or itchy eyes
- dry mouth
- unsteadiness, wobbliness, or lack of coordination
- lack of energy
- sleepiness
- depression
- pain, burning, numbness, or tingling in the hands or feet
- rash
- black and blue marks

Some side effects can be serious. If you experience any of these symptoms, call your doctor immediately:

- severe headache
- blurred vision
- difficulty thinking
- seizures
- chest pain
- nausea
- vomiting
- shortness of breath or difficulty breathing
- unconsciousness
- slow or difficult speech
- dizziness or faintness
- weakness or numbness of an arm or leg
- hallucinating (seeing things or hearing voices that do not exist)

Rasagiline may cause other side effects. Call your doctor if you have any unusual problems while taking this medication.

What storage conditions are needed for this medicine?

Keep this medication in the container it came in, tightly closed, and out of reach of children. Store it at room temperature and away from excess heat and moisture (not in the bathroom). Throw away any medication that is outdated or no longer needed. Talk to your pharmacist about the proper disposal of your medication.

What should I do in case of overdose?

In case of overdose, call your local poison control center at 1-800-222-1222. If the victim has collapsed or is not breathing, call local emergency services at 911.

Symptoms of rasagiline overdose may occur as late as 1 to 2 days after the overdose. Symptoms of overdose may include:

- drowsiness
- dizziness
- faintness
- irritability
- seizures
- hyperactivity
- agitation
- severe headache
- hallucinating
- difficulty opening the mouth
- rigid body spasm that may include an arched back
- seizures
- unconsciousness
- fast or irregular heart beat
- pain in the area between the stomach and chest
- difficulty breathing
- fever
- sweating
- cool, clammy skin

What other information should I know?

Keep all appointments with your doctor.

Do not let anyone else take your medication. Ask your pharmacist any questions you have about refilling your prescription.

Talk to your doctor, pharmacist, or other healthcare professional if you have questions about dosing information for your medication.

Repaglinide

(re pag′ lin ide)

Brand Name: Prandin®

Why is this medicine prescribed?

Repaglinide is used to treat type 2 diabetes (condition in which the body does not use insulin normally and, therefore, cannot control the amount of sugar in the blood). Repaglinide helps your body regulate the amount of glucose (sugar) in your blood. It decreases the amount of glucose by stimulating the pancreas to release insulin.

This medication is sometimes prescribed for other uses; ask your doctor or pharmacist for more information.

How should this medicine be used?

Repaglinide comes as a tablet to take by mouth. The tablets are taken before meals, any time from 30 minutes before a meal to just before the meal. If you skip a meal, you need to skip the dose of repaglinide. If you add an extra meal, you need to take an extra dose of repaglinide. Your doctor may gradually increase your dose, depending on your response to repaglinide. Follow the directions on your prescription label carefully, and ask your doctor or pharmacist to explain any part you do not understand. Take repaglinide exactly as directed. Do not take more or less of it or take it more often than directed by the package label or prescribed by your doctor.

Continue to take repaglinide even if you feel well. Do not stop taking repaglinide without talking to your doctor.

What special precautions should I follow?

Before taking repaglinide,

- tell your doctor and pharmacist if you are allergic to repaglinide or any other drugs.
- tell your doctor and pharmacist what prescription and nonprescription medications you are taking, especially acetophenazine (Tindal), aspirin, blood pressure medicines, carbamazepine (Tegretol), chloramphenicol (Chloromycetin), chlorpromazine (Thorazine), corticosteroids, diuretics ('water pills'), drugs for arthritis, erythromycin, troglitazone (Rezulin), estrogens, fluphenazine (Prolixin), isoniazid (Rifamate), ketoconazole (Nizoral), mesoridazine (Serentil), oral contraceptives, perphenazine (Trilafon), phenelzine (Nardil), phenobarbital (Luminal), phenytoin (Dilantin), probenecid (Benemid), prochlorperazine (Compazine), promazine (Sparine), promethazine (Phenergan), rifampin (Rifadin, Rimactane), thioridazine (Mellaril), tranylcypromine (Parnate), trifluoperazine (Stelazine), triflupromazine (Vesprin), trimeprazine (Temaril), vitamins, or warfarin (Coumadin).
- tell your doctor if you have or have ever had liver or kidney disease or if you have been told you have type I diabetes mellitus.
- tell your doctor if you are pregnant, plan to become pregnant, or are breast-feeding. If you become pregnant while taking repaglinide, call your doctor.
- if you are having surgery, including dental surgery, tell the doctor or dentist that you are taking repaglinide.

What special dietary instructions should I follow?

Be sure to follow all exercise and dietary recommendations made by your doctor or dietitian. It is important to eat a healthful diet.

Alcohol may cause a decrease in blood sugar. Ask your doctor about the use of alcoholic beverages while you are taking repaglinide.

What should I do if I forget to take a dose?

If you have just begun to eat a meal, take the missed dose as soon as you remember it. However, if you have finished eating, skip the missed dose and continue your regular dosing schedule. Do not take a double dose to make up for a missed one.

What side effects can this medicine cause?

This medication may cause changes in your blood sugar. You should know the symptoms of low and high blood sugar and what to do if you have these symptoms.

You may experience hypoglycemia (low blood sugar) while you are taking this medication. Your doctor will tell you what you should do if you develop hypoglycemia. He or she may tell you to check your blood sugar, eat or drink a food or beverage that contains sugar, such as hard candy or fruit juice, or get medical care. Follow these directions carefully if you have any of the following symptoms of hypoglycemia:

- shakiness
- dizziness or lightheadedness
- sweating
- nervousness or irritability
- sudden changes in behavior or mood
- headache
- numbness or tingling around the mouth
- weakness
- pale skin
- hunger
- clumsy or jerky movements

If hypoglycemia is not treated, severe symptoms may develop. Be sure that your family, friends, and other people who spend time with you know that if you have any of the following symptoms, they should get medical treatment for you immediately.

- confusion
- seizures
- loss of consciousness

Call your doctor immediately if you have any of the following symptoms of hyperglycemia (high blood sugar):

- extreme thirst
- frequent urination
- extreme hunger
- weakness
- blurred vision

If high blood sugar is not treated, a serious, life-threatening condition called diabetic ketoacidosis could develop. Call your doctor immediately if you have any of these symptoms:

- dry mouth
- upset stomach and vomiting
- shortness of breath
- breath that smells fruity
- decreased consciousness

Repaglinide may cause side effects. Tell your doctor if any of these symptoms are severe or do not go away:

- headache
- nasal congestion
- joint aches
- back pain

- constipation
- diarrhea

What storage conditions are needed for this medicine?

Keep this medication in the container it came in, tightly closed and out of reach of children. Store it at room temperature and away from excess heat and moisture (not in the bathroom). Throw away any medication that is outdated or no longer needed. Talk to your pharmacist about the proper disposal of your medication.

What should I do in case of overdose?

In case of overdose, call your local poison control center at 1-800-222-1222. If the victim has collapsed or is not breathing, call local emergency services at 911.

What other information should I know?

Keep all appointments with your doctor and the laboratory. Your blood sugar and glycosylated hemoglobin (HbA1c) should be checked regularly to determine your response to repaglinide. Your doctor will also tell you how to check your response to this medication by measuring your blood or urine sugar levels at home. Follow these instructions carefully.

You should always wear a diabetic identification bracelet to be sure you get proper treatment in an emergency.

Do not let anyone else take your medication. Ask your pharmacist any questions you have about refilling your prescription.

Dosage Facts
For Informational Purposes

Caution: Do not change your dose, how often you take your medication, or the length of time you are to take it without first talking to your healthcare provider.

The following dosage information was written using medical language for doctors and other healthcare professionals and is provided here for you to check your dosage. The dosage of this drug may differ for different patients. Therefore, always follow your doctor's instructions or the directions on the label. Contact your healthcare provider or pharmacist if you have any questions about the specific dosage of your medication after reviewing this information.

Adult Patients
Diabetes Mellitus

ORAL:
- Initially, 0.5 mg (the minimum effective dosage) preprandially 2–4 times daily (depending on meal patterns) in patients not previously treated with oral antidiabetic agents or in those who have relatively good glycemic control (i.e., glycosylated hemoglobin <8%).

- Patients with glycosylated hemoglobin ≥8% despite treatment with other oral antidiabetic agents: initially, 1 or 2 mg with or preceding each meal.
- Approximately 90% of maximal glucose-lowering effect is achieved with dosage of 1 mg 3 times daily.
- May double dosage at no less than weekly intervals until desired fasting blood glucose concentration (e.g., 80–140 mg/dL with infrequent hypoglycemic episodes) is achieved or maximum daily dosage of 16 mg (e.g., 4 mg four times daily depending on meal patterns) is attained.
- Safety and efficacy of higher dosages (8–20 mg 3–4 times daily before meals) not established.

Prescribing Limits
Adult Patients
Diabetes Mellitus

ORAL:
- Maximum daily dosage of 16 mg (e.g., 4 mg four times daily depending on meal patterns) recommended by manufacturer; higher dosages have been used.

Special Populations

Renal Impairment
- Mild to moderate renal dysfunction: No adjustment in initial dosage necessary. May administer usual initial dosage but use caution with subsequent dosage increases.
- Severe renal impairment (e.g., Cl_{cr} 20–40 mL/minute): Initiate dosage of 0.5 mg daily and titrate carefully.
- Use not established in patients with Cl_{cr} <20 mL/minute or those with renal failure requiring hemodialysis.

Hepatic Impairment
- Use with caution. Manufacturer recommends same initial dosage used in patients with normal hepatic function, but should make subsequent dosage adjustments at longer than usual intervals (e.g., 3 months) to allow full assessment of response. Some clinicians suggest lower initial dosage in patients with hepatic impairment.

Reserpine

(re ser' peen)

Brand Name: Serpalan®, Serpasil®

Why is this medicine prescribed?

Reserpine is used to treat high blood pressure. It works by decreasing your heart rate and relaxing the blood vessels so that blood can flow more easily through the body. It also is used to treat severe agitation in patients with mental disorders.

This medication is sometimes prescribed for other uses; ask your doctor or pharmacist for more information.

How should this medicine be used?

Reserpine comes as a tablet to take by mouth. It usually is taken once daily. Follow the directions on your prescription label carefully, and ask your doctor or pharmacist to explain any part you do not understand. Take reserpine exactly as directed. Do not take more or less of it or take it more often than prescribed by your doctor.

Reserpine controls high blood pressure or symptoms of agitation, but does not cure them. Continue to take reserpine even if you feel well. Do not stop taking reserpine without talking to your doctor. Abruptly stopping reserpine may increase blood pressure and cause unwanted side effects.

What special precautions should I follow?

Before taking reserpine,

- tell your doctor and pharmacist if you are allergic to reserpine, aspirin, tartrazine (a yellow dye in some processed foods and medications), or any other drugs.
- tell your doctor and pharmacist what prescription and nonprescription medications you are taking, especially amitriptyline (Elavil), clomipramine (Anafranil), desipramine (Norpramin), digoxin (Lanoxin), doxepin (Adepin, Sinequan), ephedrine, epinephrine, imipramine (Tofranil), MAO inhibitors [phenelzine (Nardil) and tranylcypromine (Parnate)], methylphenidate (Ritalin), nortriptyline (Aventyl, Pamelor), phenylephrine, protriptyline (Vivactil), quinidine (Quinaglute), trimipramine (Surmontil), and vitamins.
- tell your doctor if you have or have ever had kidney disease, gallstones, ulcers, ulcerative colitis, a history of depression, or electric shock therapy.
- tell your doctor if you are pregnant, plan to become pregnant, or are breast-feeding. If you become pregnant while taking reserpine, call your doctor.
- if you are having surgery, including dental surgery, tell the doctor or dentist that you are taking reserpine.
- you should know that this drug may make you drowsy or dizzy. Do not drive a car or operate machinery until you know how it affects you.
- ask your doctor about the safe use of alcohol while you are taking reserpine. Alcohol can make the side effects from reserpine worse.

What special dietary instructions should I follow?

Your doctor may prescribe a low-salt or low-sodium diet. Follow these directions carefully.

What should I do if I forget to take a dose?

Do not take the missed dose when you remember it; skip the missed dose and continue your regular dosing schedule. Do not take a double dose to make up for a missed one.

What side effects can this medicine cause?

Reserpine may cause side effects. Tell your doctor if any of these symptoms are severe or do not go away:

- dizziness
- loss of appetite
- diarrhea
- upset stomach
- vomiting
- stuffy nose
- headache
- dry mouth
- decreased sexual ability

If you experience any of the following symptoms, call your doctor immediately:

- depression
- nightmares
- fainting
- slow heartbeat
- chest pain
- swollen ankles or feet

If you experience a serious side effect, you or your doctor may send a report to the Food and Drug Administration's (FDA) MedWatch Adverse Event Reporting program online [at http://www.fda.gov/MedWatch/index.html] or by phone [1-800-332-1088].

What storage conditions are needed for this medicine?

Keep this medication in the container it came in, tightly closed, and out of reach of children. Store at room temperature and away from excess heat and moisture (not in the bathroom). Throw away any medication that is outdated or no longer needed. Talk to your pharmacist about the proper disposal of your medication.

What should I do in case of overdose?

In case of overdose, call your local poison control center at 1-800-222-1222. If the victim has collapsed or is not breathing, call local emergency services at 911.

What other information should I know?

Keep all appointments with your doctor and the laboratory. Your blood pressure should be checked regularly to determine your response to reserpine.

Your doctor may ask you to check your pulse (heart rate) daily and will tell you how rapid it should be. Ask your doctor or pharmacist to teach you how to take your pulse. If your pulse is slower than it should be, call your doctor before taking reserpine that day.

Weigh yourself every day. Call your doctor if you experience rapid weight gain.

Do not let anyone else take your medication. Ask your pharmacist any questions you have about refilling your prescription.

Talk to your doctor, pharmacist, or other healthcare professional if you have questions about dosing information for your medication.

Retapamulin

(re′ te pam′ ue lin)

Brand Name: Altabax®

Why is this medicine prescribed?

Retapamulin is used to treat impetigo (a skin infection caused by bacteria) in children and adults. Retapamulin is in a class of medications called antibacterials. It works by killing and stopping the growth of bacteria on the skin.

How should this medicine be used?

Retapamulin comes as an ointment to be applied in a thin layer to the skin. It is usually used two times a day for 5 days. Apply retapamulin at around the same times every day. Follow the directions on your prescription label carefully, and ask your doctor or pharmacist to explain any part you do not understand. Use retapamulin exactly as directed. Do not use more or less of it or use it more often than prescribed by your doctor.

The infected area of the skin should begin to look better during the first few days of treatment with retapamulin. If your symptoms do not improve after using this medication for 3 to 4 days or get worse, call your doctor.

Retapamulin is for use only on the infected area of the skin. Do not let retapamulin ointment get into your eyes, or inside your mouth, or nose, or inside the female genital area. Do not swallow this medication.

Use retapamulin until you finish the prescription, even if the infection looks better. If you stop using retapamulin too soon or skip doses, the infection may not be completely gone and the bacteria could become difficult to treat with another antibiotic.

To use the ointment, follow these steps:

1. Use a clean cotton swab to spread a thin layer of retapamulin on the skin that is infected.
2. Cover the treated area with a bandage or clean gauze to protect the area and prevent accidental spread of the ointment to the eyes or other areas, especially in young children.
3. Wash your hands after applying retapamulin if the hands are not to be treated.

Ask your pharmacist or doctor for a copy of the manufacturer's information for the patient.

What special precautions should I follow?

Before taking retapamulin,

- tell your doctor and pharmacist if you are allergic to retapamulin, or any other medications. Ask your pharmacist for a list of the ingredients.
- tell your doctor and pharmacist what other prescription and nonprescription medications, vitamins, nutritional supplements, and herbal products you are taking or plan to take.
- tell your doctor if you are pregnant, plan to become pregnant, or are breast-feeding.

What special dietary instructions should I follow?

Unless your doctor tells you otherwise, continue your normal diet.

What should I do if I forget to take a dose?

Apply the missed dose as soon as you remember it. However, if it is almost time for the next dose, skip the missed dose and continue your regular dosing schedule. Do not apply extra ointment to make up for a missed dose.

What side effects can this medicine cause?

Retapamulin may cause side effects. Tell your doctor if any of these symptoms are severe or do not go away:

- irritation at the in the place where you applied the ointment
- blisters
- burning
- redness
- swelling
- oozing from the place where you applied the ointment
- itching
- diarrhea
- headache

Retapamulin may cause other side effects. Call your doctor if you have any unusual problems while taking this medication.

What storage conditions are needed for this medicine?

Keep this medication in the container it came in, tightly closed, and out of reach of children. Store it at room temperature and away from excess heat and moisture (not in the bathroom). Throw away any medication that is outdated or no longer needed. Talk to your pharmacist about the proper disposal of your medication.

What should I do in case of overdose?

In case of overdose, call your local poison control center at 1-800-222-1222. If the victim has collapsed or is not breathing, call local emergency services at 911.

What other information should I know?

Keep all appointments with your doctor.

Do not let anyone else take your medication. Your prescription is probably not refillable. If you still have symptoms of infection after you finish retapamulin, call your doctor.

Talk to your doctor, pharmacist, or other healthcare professional if you have questions about dosing information for your medication.

Ribavirin

(rye ba vye′ rin)

Brand Name: Copegus®, Rebetol®

Also available generically.

Important Warning

Ribavirin will not treat hepatitis C (a virus that infects the liver and may cause severe liver damage or liver cancer) unless it is taken with another medication. If you have hepatitis C, your doctor will prescribe another medication to take with ribavirin. Take both medications exactly as directed.

Ribavirin may cause anemia (condition in which there is a decrease in the number of red blood cells). Tell your doctor if you have ever had a heart attack and if you have or have ever had high blood pressure, breathing problems, any condition that affects your blood such as sickle cell anemia (inherited condition in which the red blood cells are abnormally shaped and cannot bring oxygen to all parts of the body) or thalassemia (Mediterranean anemia; a condition in which the red blood cells do not contain enough of the substance needed to carry oxygen), or heart disease. If you experience any of the following symptoms, call your doctor immediately: excessive tiredness, pale skin, headache, dizziness, confusion, fast heartbeat, weakness, shortness of breath, or chest pain.

Keep all appointments with your doctor and the laboratory. Your doctor will order blood tests before you start taking ribavirin and often during the first 4 weeks of your treatment.

Your doctor or pharmacist will give you the manufacturer's patient information sheet (Medication Guide) when you begin treatment with ribavirin and each time you refill your prescription. Read the information carefully and ask your doctor or pharmacist if you have any questions. You also can obtain the Medication Guide from the FDA website: http://www.fda.gov/cder/foi/label/2002/21511_Copegus_lbl.pdf.

Talk to your doctor about the risks of taking ribavirin.

For female patients:

Do not take ribavirin if you are pregnant or plan to become pregnant. You should not start taking ribavirin until a pregnancy test has shown that you are not pregnant. You must use two forms of birth control and be tested for pregnancy every month during your treatment and for 6 months afterward. Call your doctor immediately if you become pregnant during this time. Ribavirin may cause harm or death to the fetus.

For male patients:

Do not take ribavirin if your partner is pregnant or plans to become pregnant. If you have a partner who can become pregnant, you should not start taking ribavirin until a pregnancy test shows that she is not pregnant. You must use two forms of birth control, including a condom with spermicide during your treatment and for 6 months afterward. Your partner must be tested for pregnancy every month during this time. Call your doctor immediately if your partner becomes pregnant. Ribavirin may cause harm or death to the fetus.

Why is this medicine prescribed?

Ribavirin is used with another medication called an interferon to treat hepatitis C. Ribavirin is in a class of antiviral medications called nucleoside analogues. It works by stopping the virus that causes hepatitis C from spreading inside the body. It is not known if treatment that includes ribavirin and another medication cures hepatitis C infection, prevents liver damage that may be caused by hepatitis C, or prevents the spread of hepatitis C to other people.

How should this medicine be used?

Ribavirin comes as a tablet, a capsule and an oral solution (liquid) to take by mouth. It is usually taken twice a day, in the morning and the evening, for 24-48 weeks or longer. Take ribavirin tablets with food. Take ribavirin capsules and oral solution with food, unless your doctor tells you that you may take ribavirin with or without food. In that case, be sure to take the medication the same way every day. It is best to take ribavirin at around the same times every day. Follow the directions on your prescription label carefully, and ask your doctor or pharmacist to explain any part you do not understand. Take ribavirin exactly as directed. Do not take more or less of it or take it more often than prescribed by your doctor.

Shake the liquid well before each use to mix the medication evenly. Be sure to wash the measuring spoon or cup after use each time you measure the liquid.

Your doctor may decrease your dose or tell you to stop taking ribavirin for a short time if you develop side effects of the medication. Call your doctor if you are bothered by side effects of ribavirin. Do not decrease your dose or stop taking ribavirin unless your doctor tells you that you should.

Are there other uses for this medicine?

Ribavirin is also sometimes used to treat viral hemorrhagic fevers (viruses that can cause bleeding inside and outside of the body, problems with many organs, and death). In the event of biological warfare, ribavirin may be used to treat viral hemorrhagic fever that has been spread deliberately. Ribavirin is also sometimes used to treat severe acute respiratory syndrome (SARS; a virus that may cause breathing problems, pneumonia, and death). Talk to your doctor about the possible risks of using this drug for your condition.

This medication may be prescribed for other uses; ask your doctor or pharmacist for more information.

What special precautions should I follow?

Before taking ribavirin,

- tell your doctor and pharmacist if you are allergic to ribavirin or any other medications. If you are taking ribavirin tablets, tell your doctor if you are allergic to corn.
- tell your doctor and pharmacist what other prescription and nonprescription medications, vitamins, nutritional supplements, and herbal products you are taking. Be sure to mention the medications listed in the IMPORTANT WARNING section and any of the following: medications for anxiety, depression, or any other mental illness; medications for human immunodeficiency virus (HIV) or acquired immunodeficiency syndrome (AIDS) such as didanosine (Videx), stavudine (Zerit), and zidovudine (Retrovir); and medications that supress the immune system such as cancer chemotherapy, cyclosporine (Neoral, Sandimmune), sirolimus (Rapamune), and tacrolimus (Prograf). If you are taking ribavirin capsules, tell your doctor if you are taking antacids. Your doctor may need to change the doses of your medications or monitor you carefully for side effects.
- tell your doctor if you drink or have ever drunk large amounts of alcohol, if you use or have ever used street drugs, if you have ever thought about killing yourself or planned or tried to do so, and if you have ever had an organ transplant. Also tell your doctor if you have or have ever had a mental illness such as depression, anxiety, or psychosis (loss of contact with reality); cancer; psoriasis (an inherited skin condition); HIV or AIDS; diabetes; sarcoidosis (a condition in which abnormal tissue grows in parts of the body such as the lungs); Gilbert's syndrome (a mild liver condition that may cause yellowing of the skin or eyes); gout (a type of arthritis caused by crystals deposited in the joints); any type of liver disease other than hepatitis C; or thyroid, kidney, pancreas, eye, or lung disease.
- tell your doctor if you have ever taken any medication to treat hepatitis C. Be sure that your doctor has your complete medical records and knows how well you responded to other treatments for hepatitis C.
- tell your doctor if you are breast-feeding. You should not breastfeed while you are taking ribavirin.
- you should know that ribavirin may make you drowsy, dizzy, or confused. Do not drive a car or operate machinery until you know how this medication affects you.
- do not drink alcoholic beverages while you are taking ribavirin. Alcohol can make your liver disease worse.

What special dietary instructions should I follow?

Be sure to drink plenty of fluids while you are taking ribavirin.

What should I do if I forget to take a dose?

If you remember the missed dose that same day, take the medication right away. However, if you do not remember the missed dose until the next day, call your doctor to find out what to do. Do not take a double dose to make up for a missed one.

What side effects can this medicine cause?

Ribavirin may cause side effects. Tell your doctor if any of these symptoms are severe or do not go away:

- cough
- upset stomach
- vomiting
- diarrhea
- constipation
- heartburn
- loss of appetite
- weight loss
- changes in ability to taste food
- dry mouth
- difficulty concentrating
- difficulty falling asleep or staying asleep
- memory loss
- rash
- dry, irritated, or itchy skin
- sweating
- painful or irregular menstruation (period)
- muscle or bone pain
- hair loss

Some side effects can be serious. The following symptoms are uncommon, but if you experience any of them, or those listed in the IMPORTANT WARNING section, call your doctor immediately:

- hives
- swelling of the face, throat, tongue, lips, eyes, hands, feet, ankles, or lower legs
- hoarseness
- difficulty swallowing or breathing
- pain in the stomach or lower back
- bloody diarrhea
- bright red blood in stools
- black, tarry stools
- unusual bleeding or bruising
- vision changes
- fever, chills, and other signs of infection
- depression
- thinking about hurting or killing yourself
- mood changes
- excessive worry
- irritability
- starting to use street drugs or alcohol again if you used these substances in the past
- worsening of psoriasis that you had before you started to take ribavirin
- intolerance to cold

Ribavirin may slow growth and weight gain in children. Talk to your child's doctor about the risks of giving this medication to your child.

Ribavirin may cause other side effects. Call your doctor if you have any unusual problems while taking this medication.

If you experience a serious side effect, you or your doctor may send a report to the Food and Drug Administration's (FDA) MedWatch Adverse Event Reporting program online [at http://www.fda.gov/MedWatch/index.html] or by phone [1-800-332-1088].

What storage conditions are needed for this medicine?

Keep this medication in the container it came in, tightly closed, and out of reach of children. Store ribavirin tablets and capsules at room temperature and away from excess heat and moisture (not in the bathroom). Store ribavirin oral solution in the refrigerator or at room temperature. Throw away any medication that is outdated or no longer needed. Talk to your pharmacist about the proper disposal of your medication.

What should I do in case of overdose?

In case of overdose, call your local poison control center at 1-800-222-1222. If the victim has collapsed or is not breathing, call local emergency services at 911.

What other information should I know?

Do not let anyone else take your medication. Ask your pharmacist any questions you have about refilling your prescription.

Dosage Facts
For Informational Purposes

Caution: Do not change your dose, how often you take your medication, or the length of time you are to take it without first talking to your healthcare provider.

The following dosage information was written using medical language for doctors and other healthcare professionals and is provided here for you to check your dosage. The dosage of this drug may differ for different patients. Therefore, always follow your doctor's instructions or the directions on the label. Contact your healthcare provider or pharmacist if you have any questions about the specific dosage of your medication after reviewing this information.

Pediatric Patients

Treatment of Chronic Hepatitis C Virus (HCV) Infection
Concomitant Therapy with Ribavirin and Interferon Alfa-2b (Rebetol® and Intron® A)

ORAL:
- Capsules or oral solution: 15 mg/kg daily in 2 divided doses in conjunction with sub-Q interferon alfa. Use oral solution in those weighing ≤25 kg and in those who cannot swallow capsules.
- HCV genotype 1: Recommended duration is 48 weeks. Assess virologic response after 24 weeks of treatment; consider discontinuing if HCV RNA is not below the limits of detection.
- HCV genotype 2,3: Recommended duration is 24 weeks.
- Safety and efficacy of >48 weeks of treatment not established in pediatric patients.

Pediatric Dosage of Rebetol® and Intron® A for Concomitant Therapy

Weight (kg)	Rebetol® Dosage (Capsules)	Intron® A Dosage
25–36	200 mg in morning and 200 mg in evening	3 million units/m² sub-Q 3 times weekly
37–49	200 mg in morning and 400 mg in evening	3 million units/m² sub-Q 3 times weekly
50–61	400 mg in morning and 400 mg in evening	3 million units/m² sub-Q 3 times weekly
>61	400 mg in morning and 600 mg in evening in those weighing <75 kg or 600 mg in morning and 600 mg in evening in those weighing ≥75 kg	Use usual adult dosage

Dosage modification may be necessary if adverse hematologic effects occur.

Viral Hemorrhagic Fevers†
Treatment of Viral Hemorrhagic Fevers in Context of Biologic Warfare or Bioterrorism†

ORAL:
- US Army Medical Research Institute of Infectious Diseases (USAMRIID) and US Working Group on Civilian Biodefense recommend initial loading dose of 30 mg/kg, followed by 15 mg/kg daily given in 2 divided doses. Duration of treatment is 10 days.
- IV regimen usually preferred. Oral regimen may be used when parenteral preparation cannot be obtained or would be impractical (e.g., when large numbers of individuals require treatment in a mass casualty setting).

Adult Patients

Treatment of Chronic Hepatitis C Virus (HCV) Infection

Concomitant Therapy with Ribavirin Tablets and Peginterferon Alfa-2a (Pegasys®)

ORAL:

- Adults with HCV and HIV coinfection: 800 mg daily in 2 divided doses (regardless of HCV genotype) in conjunction with sub-Q peginterferon alfa-2a (180 mcg once weekly) for 48 weeks.
- Adults with HCV monoinfection (without coexisting HIV infection): 800 mg–1.2 g daily in 2 divided doses (depending on HCV genotype) in conjunction with sub-Q peginterferon alfa-2a (180 mcg once weekly). (See Table.)

Adult Dosage of Ribavirin Tablets and Pegasys® for Patients with HCV Monoinfection

HCV Genotype	Ribavirin Tablets Dosage	Pegasys® Dosage	Duration
1,4	500 mg twice daily in those weighing <75 kg or 600 mg twice daily in those weighing ≥75 kg	180 mcg sub-Q once weekly	48 weeks
2,3	400 mg twice daily	180 mcg sub-Q once weekly	24 weeks
5,6	Data insufficient to make dosage recommendations	Data insufficient to make dosage recommendations	

Dosage modification may be necessary if adverse hematologic effects occur.

Concomitant Therapy with Ribavirin Capsules and Peginterferon Alfa-2b (PEG-Intron®)

ORAL:

- 800 mg daily (400 mg twice daily) in conjunction with sub-Q PEG-Intron®. Continue regimen for 24–48 weeks in treatment-naive patients, depending on baseline disease characteristics, virologic response, and/or tolerability.
- Dosage modification may be necessary if adverse hematologic effects occur.

Concomitant Therapy with Ribavirin Capsules and Interferon Alfa-2b (Intron® A)

ORAL:

- Adults weighing ≤75 kg: 1 g daily (400 mg every morning and 600 mg every evening) in conjunction with sub-Q Intron® A.
- Adults weighing >75 kg: 1.2 g daily (600 mg twice daily) in conjunction with sub-Q Intron® A.

- Continue regimen for 24–48 weeks in treatment-naive patients, depending on baseline disease characteristics, virologic response, and/or tolerability.
- Dosage modification may be necessary if adverse hematologic effects occur.

Viral Hemorrhagic Fevers

Treatment of Crimean-Congo Hemorrhagic Fever†

ORAL:

- Initial loading dose of 30 mg/kg, followed by 15 mg/kg every 6 hours for 4 days and then 7.5 mg/kg every 8 hours for 6 days has been used.

Treatment of Viral Hemorrhagic Fevers in Context of Biologic Warfare or Bioterrorism†

ORAL:

- USAMRIID and US Working Group on Civilian Biodefense recommend initial loading dose of 2 g, followed by 1.2 daily given in 2 divided doses for those weighing >75 kg or 1 g daily (400 mg in the morning and 600 mg in the evening) for those weighing ≤75 kg. Duration of treatment is 10 days.
- IV regimen usually preferred. Oral regimen may be used when parenteral preparation cannot be obtained or would be impractical (e.g., when large numbers of individuals require treatment in a mass casualty setting).

Special Populations

Geriatric Patients

- Cautious dosage selection because of age-related decreases in renal, hepatic, and/or cardiac function. Initiate therapy at the lower end of the dosing range.

Patients Who Develop Hematologic Effects during Therapy

Treatment of Chronic Hepatitis C Virus (HCV) Infection

- In pediatric patients with no cardiovascular disease, decrease Rebetol® dosage to 7.5 mg/kg daily in 2 divided doses if hemoglobin concentration decreases to <10 g/dL; permanently discontinue the drug if concentration decreases to <8.5 g/dL. In those with history of cardiovascular disease, decrease Rebetol® dosage to 7.5 mg/kg daily in 2 divided doses if hemoglobin decreases by ≥2 g/dL during any 4-week period; permanently discontinue the drug if hemoglobin is <12 g/dL after 4 weeks of a reduced ribavirin dosage.

- In adults with no cardiovascular disease, decrease dosage of ribavirin capsules or tablets to 600 mg daily (200 mg in morning and 400 mg in evening) if hemoglobin concentration decreases to <10 g/dL; permanently discontinue the drug if concentration decreases to <8.5 g/dL. In those with history of stable cardiovascular disease, decrease dosage of ribavirin capsules or tablets to 600 mg daily (200 mg in morning and 400 mg in evening) if hemoglobin decreases by ≥2 g/dL during any 4-week period; permanently discontinue the drug if hemoglobin is <12 g/dL after 4 weeks of a reduced ribavirin dosage.

† *Use is not currently included in the labeling approved by the US Food and Drug Administration.*

Rifabutin

(rif' a byoo tin)

Brand Name: Mycobutin®

Why is this medicine prescribed?

Rifabutin helps to prevent or slow the spread of Mycobacterium avium complex (MAC) disease in patients with human immunodeficiency virus (HIV) infection.

This medication is sometimes prescribed for other uses; ask your doctor or pharmacist for more information.

How should this medicine be used?

Rifabutin comes as a capsule to take by mouth. Rifabutin usually is taken once or twice a day. Take it on an empty stomach, 1 hour before or 2 hours after meals. If you have difficulty swallowing the capsule, you may empty its contents into applesauce. Follow the directions on your prescription label carefully, and ask your doctor or pharmacist to explain any part you do not understand. Take rifabutin exactly as directed. Do not take more or less of it or take it more often than prescribed by your doctor.

What special precautions should I follow?

Before taking rifabutin,

- tell your doctor and pharmacist if you are allergic to rifabutin, niacin, ethionamide (Trecator-SC), or any other drugs.
- tell your doctor and pharmacist what prescription and nonprescription medications you are taking, especially anticoagulants ('blood thinners') such as warfarin (Coumadin), blood pressure or heart disease medication, diabetes medications, digoxin (Lanoxin), methadone, oral contraceptives, zidovudine (Retrovir), and vitamins. Rifabutin decreases the effectiveness of some oral contraceptives; another form of birth control should be used while taking this drug.
- tell your doctor if you have or have ever had blood disorders or active tuberculosis.
- tell your doctor if you are pregnant, plan to become pregnant, or are breast-feeding. If you become pregnant while taking rifabutin, call your doctor.

What should I do if I forget to take a dose?

Take the missed dose as soon as you remember it. However, if it is almost time for the next dose, skip the missed dose and continue your regular dosing schedule. Do not take a double dose to make up for a missed one.

What side effects can this medicine cause?

Rifabutin may cause side effects. Skin, tears, saliva, sweat, urine, and stools may turn orange-brown; this side effect is normal and will stop when you finish taking this medication.

Tell your doctor if any of these symptoms are severe or do not go away:

- upset stomach or cramps
- vomiting
- headache
- altered sense of taste

If you experience any of the following symptoms, call your doctor immediately:

- chest pain
- skin rash
- muscle aches
- severe headache
- fatigue
- sore throat
- flu-like symptoms
- vision changes
- unusual bruising or bleeding
- yellowing of the skin or eyes

If you experience a serious side effect, you or your doctor may send a report to the Food and Drug Administration's (FDA) MedWatch Adverse Event Reporting program online [at http://www.fda.gov/MedWatch/index.html] or by phone [1-800-332-1088].

What storage conditions are needed for this medicine?

Keep this medication in the container it came in, tightly closed, and out of reach of children. Store it at room temperature and away from excess heat and moisture (not in the bathroom). Throw away any medication that is outdated or no longer needed. Talk to your pharmacist about the proper disposal of your medication.

What should I do in case of overdose?

In case of overdose, call your local poison control center at 1-800-222-1222. If the victim has collapsed or is not breathing, call local emergency services at 911.

What other information should I know?

Keep all appointments with your doctor and the laboratory. Your doctor will order certain lab tests to check your response to rifabutin.

Do not let anyone else take your medication. Ask your pharmacist any questions you have about refilling your prescription.

Talk to your doctor, pharmacist, or other healthcare professional if you have questions about dosing information for your medication.

Rifampin

(rif′ am pin)

Brand Name: Rifadin®, Rifamate® as a combination product containing Rifampin and Isoniazid, Rifater® as a combination product containing Rifampin, Isoniazid, and Pyrazinamide, Rimactane®

Why is this medicine prescribed?

Rifampin eliminates bacteria that cause tuberculosis (TB). It is generally used with other drugs to treat tuberculosis or to eliminate Neisseria meningitidis (a bacteria) and to prevent you from giving these infections to others. However, rifampin is not used to treat Neisseria meningitidis infection.

This medication is sometimes prescribed for other uses; ask your doctor or pharmacist for more information.

How should this medicine be used?

Rifampin comes as a capsule to take by mouth. It usually is taken once a day. You will probably be taking it for at least 3 months and possibly for up to 2 years. Rifampin works best on an empty stomach; take it 1 hour before or at least 2 hours after a meal. If you have difficulty swallowing the capsule, you may empty its contents into applesauce or jelly. Follow the directions on your prescription label carefully, and ask your doctor or pharmacist to explain any part you do not understand. Take rifampin exactly as directed. Do not take more or less of it or take it more often than prescribed by your doctor.

What special precautions should I follow?

Before taking rifampin,

- tell your doctor and pharmacist if you are allergic to rifampin or any other drugs.
- tell your doctor and pharmacist what prescription and nonprescription medications you are taking, especially anticoagulants ('blood thinners') such as warfarin (Coumadin), cyclosporine (Neoral, Sandimmune), estrogen, hydrocortisone (Hydrocortone), medications for heart disease or diabetes, methadone, prednisone (Deltasone), theophylline (Theo-Dur), verapamil (Calan, Isoptin), and vitamins. Rifampin alters the effectiveness of oral contraceptives; use another method of birth control while taking this medication. Ask your doctor or pharmacist for advice.
- tell your doctor if you have or have ever had liver disease.
- tell your doctor if you are pregnant, plan to become pregnant, or are breast-feeding. If you become pregnant while taking rifampin, call your doctor.
- you should know that this drug may make you drowsy. Do not drive a car or operate machinery until you know how this drug affects you.
- remember that alcohol can add to the drowsiness caused by this drug.

What should I do if I forget to take a dose?

Take the missed dose as soon as you remember it. However, if it is almost time for the next dose, skip the missed dose and continue your regular dosing schedule. Do not take a double dose to make up for a missed one.

What side effects can this medicine cause?

Rifampin may cause side effects. Your urine, stools, saliva, sputum, sweat, and tears may turn red-orange; this effect is harmless. Tell your doctor if any of these symptoms are severe or do not go away:

- headache
- muscle pain
- bone pain
- heartburn
- upset stomach
- vomiting
- stomach cramps
- chills
- diarrhea

If you experience any of the following symptoms, call your doctor immediately:

- skin rash (hives)
- sores on skin or in the mouth
- fever
- yellowing of the skin or eyes

If you experience a serious side effect, you or your doctor may send a report to the Food and Drug Administration's (FDA) MedWatch Adverse Event Reporting program online [at http://www.fda.gov/MedWatch/index.html] or by phone [1-800-332-1088].

What storage conditions are needed for this medicine?

Keep this medication in the container it came in, tightly closed, and out of reach of children. Store it at room temperature and away from excess heat and moisture (not in the bathroom). Throw away any medication that is outdated or no longer needed. Talk to your pharmacist about the proper disposal of your medication.

What should I do in case of overdose?

In case of overdose, call your local poison control center at 1-800-222-1222. If the victim has collapsed or is not breathing, call local emergency services at 911.

What other information should I know?

Keep all appointments with your doctor and the laboratory. Your doctor will order certain lab tests to check your response to rifampin.

Do not let anyone else take your medication. Ask your

pharmacist any questions you have about refilling your prescription.

Talk to your doctor, pharmacist, or other healthcare professional if you have questions about dosing information for your medication.

Rifaximin

(ri fax′ i men)

Brand Name: Xifaxan®

Why is this medicine prescribed?

Rifaximin is used to treat traveler's diarrhea caused by certain bacteria. Rifaximin is in a class of medications called antibiotics. It works by preventing the bacteria from growing inside the intestine (gut). Rifaximin will not work to treat bloody diarrhea or diarrhea with fever.

How should this medicine be used?

Rifaximin comes as a tablet to take by mouth. It is usually taken with or without food three times a day for 3 days. To help you remember to take rifaximin, take it around the same times every day. Follow the directions on your prescription label carefully, and ask your doctor or pharmacist to explain any part you do not understand. Take rifaximin exactly as directed. Do not take more or less of it or take it more often than prescribed by your doctor.

Your symptoms should improve within 24 to 48 hours after you start taking rifaximin. If your symptoms do not go away or they get worse, or you develop a fever or bloody diarrhea, call your doctor.

Take rifaximin until you finish the prescription, even if you feel better. If you stop taking rifaximin too soon your infection may not be completely cured and bacteria may become resistant to antibiotics.

Are there other uses for this medicine?

This medication may be prescribed for other uses; ask your doctor or pharmacist for more information.

What special precautions should I follow?

Before taking rifaximin,
- tell your doctor and pharmacist if you are allergic to rifaximin, rifabutin (Mycobutin), rifampin (Rifadin, Rifamate, Rifater, Rimactane), rifapentine (Priftin), or any other medications.
- tell your doctor and pharmacist what other prescription and nonprescription medications, vitamins, nutritional supplements, and herbal products you are taking or have recently taken. Be sure to mention antibiotics. Your doctor may have to change the doses of your medica-

tions, monitor you carefully for side effects or treat your diarrhea differently.
- tell your doctor if you have or have ever had any medical condition.
- tell your doctor if you are pregnant, plan to become pregnant, or are breast-feeding. If you become pregnant while taking rifaximin, call your doctor.

What special dietary instructions should I follow?

Unless your doctor tells you otherwise, continue your normal diet.

What should I do if I forget to take a dose?

Take the missed dose as soon as you remember it. However, if it is almost time for the next dose, skip the missed dose and continue your regular dosing schedule. Do not take a double dose to make up for a missed one.

What side effects can this medicine cause?

Rifaximin may cause side effects. Tell your doctor if this symptom is severe or does not go away:
- vomiting

Some side effects can be serious. The following symptoms are uncommon, but if you experience any of them, call your doctor immediately:
- hives
- skin rash
- itching
- difficulty breathing or swallowing
- swelling of the face, throat, tongue, lips, eyes, hands, feet, ankles, or lower legs
- hoarseness
- fever, chills, sore throat, and other signs of infection

Rifaximin may cause other side effects. Call your doctor if you have any unusual problems while taking this medication.

If you experience a serious side effect, you or your doctor may send a report to the Food and Drug Administration's (FDA) MedWatch Adverse Event Reporting program online [at http://www.fda.gov/MedWatch/index.html] or by phone [1-800-332-1088].

What storage conditions are needed for this medicine?

Keep this medication in the container it came in, tightly closed, and out of reach of children. Store it at room temperature and away from excess heat and moisture (not in the bathroom). Throw away any medication that is outdated or no longer needed. Talk to your pharmacist about the proper disposal of your medication.

What should I do in case of overdose?

In case of overdose, call your local poison control center at 1-800-222-1222. If the victim has collapsed or is not breathing, call local emergency services at 911.

What other information should I know?

Keep all appointments with your doctor.

Do not let anyone else take your medication. Your prescription is probably not refillable. If you still have symptoms of infection after you finish the rifaximin, call your doctor.

Dosage Facts
For Informational Purposes

Caution: Do not change your dose, how often you take your medication, or the length of time you are to take it without first talking to your healthcare provider.

The following dosage information was written using medical language for doctors and other healthcare professionals and is provided here for you to check your dosage. The dosage of this drug may differ for different patients. Therefore, always follow your doctor's instructions or the directions on the label. Contact your healthcare provider or pharmacist if you have any questions about the specific dosage of your medication after reviewing this information.

Pediatric Patients

Travelers' Diarrhea Caused by Noninvasive Strains of E. coli
Treatment

ORAL:
- Adolescents ≥12 years of age: 200 mg 3 times daily for 3 days.

Adult Patients

Travelers' Diarrhea Caused by Noninvasive Strains of E. coli
Treatment

ORAL:
- 200 mg 3 times daily for 3 days.

Hepatic Encephalopathy†
Treatment

ORAL:
- 600–1200 mg daily (usually in 3 divided doses) for 7–21 days has been used.

Special Populations

Hepatic Impairment
- No specific dosage adjustments recommended.

Renal Impairment
- Not specifically studied in renal impairment, but clinically important differences in elimination not expected.

Geriatric Patients
- Not specifically studied in patients ≥65 years of age.

† Use is not currently included in the labeling approved by the US Food and Drug Administration.

Riluzole
(ril′ yoo zole)

Brand Name: Rilutek®

Why is this medicine prescribed?

Riluzole is used to slow the progress of amyotrophic lateral sclerosis (ALS or Lou Gehrig's disease). The drug also may delay the need for a tracheostomy (breathing tube), but it is not a cure for ALS.

This medication is sometimes prescribed for other uses; ask your doctor or pharmacist for more information.

How should this medicine be used?

Riluzole comes as a tablet to take by mouth. It usually is taken twice a day, every 12 hours. You should take it at the same time each day (usually in the morning and in the evening). Follow the directions on your prescription label carefully, and ask your doctor or pharmacist to explain any part you do not understand. Take riluzole exactly as directed. Do not take more or less of it or take it more often than prescribed by your doctor.

Riluzole slows progression of ALS but does not cure it. Continue to take riluzole even if you feel well. Do not stop taking riluzole without talking to your doctor.

What special precautions should I follow?

Before taking riluzole,
- tell your doctor and pharmacist if you are allergic to riluzole or any other drugs.
- tell your doctor and pharmacist what prescription and nonprescription medications you are taking, especially amitriptyline (Elavil), caffeine-containing products, ciprofloxacin (Cipro), ofloxacin (Floxin), omeprazole (Prilosec), rifampin (Rifadin), theophylline (Theo-Dur), and vitamins.
- tell your doctor if you have or have ever had blood disorders or anemia or kidney or liver disease.
- tell your doctor if you are pregnant, plan to become pregnant, or are breast-feeding. If you become pregnant while taking riluzole, call your doctor.
- if you are having surgery, including dental surgery, tell the doctor or dentist that you are taking riluzole.
- you should know that this drug may make you drowsy. Do not drive a car or operate machinery until you know how this drug affects you.
- remember that alcohol can add to the drowsiness caused by this drug.
- tell your doctor if you use tobacco products. Cigarette smoking may decrease the effectiveness of this drug.

What special dietary instructions should I follow?

Take riluzole on an empty stomach (1 hour before or 2 hours after meals). Do not drink or eat a lot of caffeine-containing products, such as coffee, tea, cola, or chocolate. Avoid eating charcoal-broiled foods.

What should I do if I forget to take a dose?

Take the missed dose as soon as you remember it. However, if it is almost time for the next dose, skip the missed dose and continue your regular dosing schedule. Do not take a double dose to make up for a missed one.

What side effects can this medicine cause?

Riluzole may cause side effects. Tell your doctor if any of these symptoms are severe or do not go away:

- dizziness
- tiredness
- upset stomach
- stomach pain
- diarrhea
- muscle weakness or aches
- loss of appetite
- headache

If you experience any of the following symptoms, call your doctor immediately:

- difficulty breathing
- fever
- depression

If you experience a serious side effect, you or your doctor may send a report to the Food and Drug Administration's (FDA) MedWatch Adverse Event Reporting program online [at http://www.fda.gov/MedWatch/index.html] or by phone [1-800-332-1088].

What storage conditions are needed for this medicine?

Keep this medication in the container it came in, tightly closed, and out of reach of children. Store it at room temperature, away from light and excess heat and moisture (not in the bathroom). Throw away any medication that is outdated or no longer needed. Talk to your pharmacist about the proper disposal of your medication.

What should I do in case of overdose?

In case of overdose, call your local poison control center at 1-800-222-1222. If the victim has collapsed or is not breathing, call local emergency services at 911.

What other information should I know?

Keep all appointments with your doctor and the laboratory. Your doctor will order certain lab tests to check your response to riluzole.

Riluzole can affect your body's ability to fight infection. If you have any illness, especially one with a fever, call your doctor.

Do not let anyone else take your medication. Ask your pharmacist any questions you have about refilling your prescription.

Dosage Facts
For Informational Purposes

Caution: Do not change your dose, how often you take your medication, or the length of time you are to take it without first talking to your healthcare provider.

The following dosage information was written using medical language for doctors and other healthcare professionals and is provided here for you to check your dosage. The dosage of this drug may differ for different patients. Therefore, always follow your doctor's instructions or the directions on the label. Contact your healthcare provider or pharmacist if you have any questions about the specific dosage of your medication after reviewing this information.

Adult Patients

Amyotrophic Lateral Sclerosis

ORAL:
- 50 mg every 12 hours.

Prescribing Limits

Adult Patients

Amyotrophic Lateral Sclerosis

ORAL:
- Maximum 50 mg every 12 hours; higher daily dosages provide no additional benefit but may increase the risk of adverse effects.

Special Populations

Hepatic Impairment
- Use with caution; however, no specific dosage recommendations.
- Discontinue therapy if ALT is >10 times ULN or if jaundice develops.
- Manufacturer states that there is no experience with reinitiating therapy in patients whose therapy was discontinued for ALT >5 times ULN.

Renal Impairment
- Use with caution; however, no specific dosage recommendations.

Geriatric Patients
- Use with caution; however, no specific dosage recommendations.

Rimantadine

(ri man' ta deen)

Brand Name: Flumadine®, Flumadine® Syrup
Also available generically.

Why is this medicine prescribed?

Rimantadine is used to prevent and treat infections caused by influenza A virus.

This medication is sometimes prescribed for other uses; ask your doctor or pharmacist for more information.

How should this medicine be used?

Rimantadine comes as a tablet and a liquid to take by mouth. It usually is taken once or twice a day for 2-12 weeks. A flu vaccine also will be given. Follow the directions on your prescription label carefully, and ask your doctor or pharmacist to explain any part you do not understand. Take rimantadine exactly as directed. Do not take more or less of it or take it more often than prescribed by your doctor.

What special precautions should I follow?

Before taking rimantadine,

- tell your doctor and pharmacist if you are allergic to rimantadine or any other drugs.
- tell your doctor and pharmacist what prescription and nonprescription medications you are taking, especially acetaminophen, aspirin, cimetidine (Tagamet), and vitamins.
- tell your doctor if you have or have ever had liver disease, seizures, or blood disorders.
- tell your doctor if you are pregnant, plan to become pregnant, or are breast-feeding. If you become pregnant while taking rimantadine, call your doctor.

What special dietary instructions should I follow?

Rimantadine may cause an upset stomach. Take rimantadine with food or milk.

What should I do if I forget to take a dose?

Take the missed dose as soon as you remember it. However, if it is almost time for the next dose, skip the missed dose and continue your regular dosing schedule. Do not take a double dose to make up for a missed one.

What side effects can this medicine cause?

Rimantadine may cause side effects. Tell your doctor if any of these symptoms are severe or do not go away:

- upset stomach
- nervousness
- tiredness
- difficulty sleeping and concentrating
- lightheadedness

If you experience any of the following symptoms, call your doctor immediately:

- skin rash
- yellowing of the skin or eyes
- mood changes
- mental confusion
- vision changes

If you experience a serious side effect, you or your doctor may send a report to the Food and Drug Administration's (FDA) MedWatch Adverse Event Reporting program online [at http://www.fda.gov/MedWatch/index.html] or by phone [1-800-332-1088].

What storage conditions are needed for this medicine?

Keep this medication in the container it came in, tightly closed, and out of reach of children. Store it at room temperature and away from excess heat and moisture (not in the bathroom). Throw away any medication that is outdated or no longer needed. Talk to your pharmacist about the proper disposal of your medication.

What should I do in case of overdose?

In case of overdose, call your local poison control center at 1-800-222-1222. If the victim has collapsed or is not breathing, call local emergency services at 911.

What other information should I know?

Keep all appointments with your doctor and the laboratory. Your doctor will order certain lab tests to check your response to rimantadine.

Do not let anyone else take your medication. Your prescription is probably not refillable. If you still have symptoms of infection after you finish the rimantadine, call your doctor.

Dosage Facts
For Informational Purposes

Caution: Do not change your dose, how often you take your medication, or the length of time you are to take it without first talking to your healthcare provider.

The following dosage information was written using medical language for doctors and other healthcare professionals and is provided here for you to check your dosage. The dosage of this drug may differ for different patients. Therefore, always follow your doctor's instructions or the directions on the label. Contact your healthcare provider or pharmacist if you have any questions about the specific dosage of your medication after reviewing this information.

General Dosage Information

Available as rimantadine hydrochloride; dosage expressed in terms of rimantadine hydrochloride.

Pediatric Patients

Treatment of Influenza A Virus Infections

ORAL:
- Children ≥13 years of age†: 100 mg twice daily.
- Initiate rimantadine treatment as soon as possible, preferably within 24–48 hours after onset of symptoms and continue for up to 5 days or 24–48 hours after symptoms disappear.

Prevention of Influenza A Virus Infections

ORAL:
- Children 1–9 years of age: 5 mg/kg (maximum 150 mg) once daily.
- Children ≥10 years of age: 100 mg twice daily. AAP recommends 5 mg/kg daily in 2 divided doses in those weighing <40 kg or 100 mg twice daily in those weighing ≥40 kg.
- For prophylaxis of influenza A when influenza virus vaccine is contraindicated or unavailable or when a poor antibody response to the vaccine is expected (e.g., severe immunodeficiency, HIV infection), rimantadine can be started in anticipation of an influenza A outbreak and before or after contact with individuals with influenza A virus infection. Can be given for the duration of an influenza A outbreak in the community, which may be as long as 6–12 weeks. Manufacturer states that safety and efficacy for >6 weeks not established.
- For prophylaxis in conjunction with influenza virus vaccine, rimantadine should be administered for 2 weeks after vaccine administration. Children <9 years of age receiving influenza virus vaccine for the first time may require rimantadine prophylaxis for up to 6 weeks following vaccination or until 2 weeks after the second dose of vaccine.

Adult Patients

Treatment of Influenza A Virus Infections

ORAL:
- 100 mg twice daily.
- Initiate rimantadine treatment as soon as possible, preferably within 24–48 hours after onset of symptoms and continue for up to 5 days or 24–48 hours after symptoms disappear.

Prevention of Influenza A Virus Infections

ORAL:
- 100 mg twice daily.
- For prophylaxis of influenza A when influenza virus vaccine is contraindicated or unavailable or when a poor antibody response to the vaccine is expected (e.g., severe immunodeficiency, HIV infection), rimantadine can be started in anticipation of an influenza A outbreak and before or after contact with individuals with influenza A virus infection. Can be given for the duration of an influenza A outbreak in the community, which may be as long as 6–12 weeks. Manufacturer states that safety and efficacy for >6 weeks not established.
- For prophylaxis in conjunction with influenza virus vaccine, rimantadine should be administered for 2 weeks after vaccine administration.

Prescribing Limits

Pediatric Patients

Prevention of Influenza A Virus Infections

ORAL:
- Children 1–9 years of age: Maximum 150 mg daily.

Special Populations

Hepatic Impairment

Treatment or Prevention of Influenza A Virus Infections

- 100 mg daily in patients with severe hepatic impairment.

Renal Impairment

Treatment or Prevention of Influenza A Virus Infections

- 100 mg daily in patients with severe renal impairment (Cl_{cr} ≤10 mL/minute). Further dosage adjustments may be needed.

Geriatric Patients
- ≥65 years of age: 100 mg daily recommended by the manufacturer; ACIP and others recommend 100 mg daily in those who experienced adverse effects with the usual adult dosage.
- Geriatric individuals residing in nursing homes: 100 mg daily.

† Use is not currently included in the labeling approved by the US Food and Drug Administration.

Risedronate

(ris ed' roe nate)

Brand Name: Actonel®, Actonel® with Calcium

Why is this medicine prescribed?

Risedronate is used to prevent and treat osteoporosis (a condition in which the bones become thin and weak and break easily) in women who have undergone menopause (change of life; end of menstrual periods) and in men and women who are taking glucocorticoids (corticosteroids; a type of medication that may cause osteoporosis). Risedronate is also used to treat osteoporosis in men. Risedronate is also used to treat Paget's disease of bone (a condition in which the bones are soft and weak and may be deformed, painful, or easily broken). Risedronate is in a class of medications called bisphosphonates. It works by preventing bone breakdown and increasing bone density (thickness).

How should this medicine be used?

Risedronate comes as a tablet to take by mouth. It is usually taken on an empty stomach once a day in the morning or once a week in the morning. If you are taking risedronate once a week, take it on the same day every week. Follow the directions on your prescription label carefully, and ask your doctor or pharmacist to explain any part you do not understand. Take risedronate exactly as directed. Do not take more or less of it or take it more often or for a longer period of time than prescribed by your doctor.

Risedronate may not work properly and may damage the esophagus (tube between the mouth and stomach) or cause sores in the mouth if it is not taken according to the following instructions. Tell your doctor if you do not understand, you do not think you will remember, or you are unable to follow these instructions:

- You must take risedronate immediately after you get out of bed in the morning and before you eat or drink anything. Never take risedronate at bedtime or before you wake up and get out of bed for the day.
- Swallow the tablets with a full glass (6 to 8 ounces) of plain water while you are sitting or standing. Never take risedronate with tea, coffee, juice, mineral water, milk, other dairy drinks, or any liquid other than plain water.
- Swallow the tablets whole. Do not split, chew, or crush them. Do not suck on the tablets or hold them in your mouth for any length of time.
- After you take risedronate, do not eat, drink, or take any other medications for at least 30 minutes. Do not lie down for at least 30 minutes after you take risedronate. Sit upright or stand upright until at least 30 minutes have passed.

Risedronate controls osteoporosis and Paget's disease of bone but does not cure these conditions. Risedronate helps to treat and prevent osteoporosis only as long as it is taken regularly. Continue to take risedronate even if you feel well. Do not stop taking risedronate without talking to your doctor.

Ask your pharmacist or doctor for a copy of the manufacturer's information for the patient.

Are there other uses for this medicine?

This medication may be prescribed for other uses; ask your doctor or pharmacist for more information.

What special precautions should I follow?

Before taking risedronate,

- tell your doctor and pharmacist if you are allergic to risedronate or any other medications.
- tell your doctor and pharmacist what prescription and nonprescription medications, vitamins, nutritional supplements, and herbal products you are taking or plan to take. Be sure to mention any of the following: aspirin and other nonsteroidal anti-inflammatory medications (NSAIDs) such as ibuprofen (Advil, Motrin) and naproxen (Aleve, Naprosyn); cancer chemotherapy; and oral steroids such as dexamethasone (Decadron, Dexone), methylprednisolone (Medrol), and prednisone (Deltasone). Your doctor may need to change the doses of your medications or monitor you carefully for side effects.

- if you are taking any other oral medications including vitamins, supplements, or antacids, take them at least 30 minutes after you take risedronate.
- tell your doctor if you have or have ever had a low level of calcium in your blood and if you are unable to sit upright or stand upright for at least 30 minutes. Your doctor may tell you that you should not take risedronate.
- tell your doctor if you are undergoing radiation therapy; if you have or have ever had difficulty swallowing; heartburn, ulcers, or other problems with your stomach or esophagus; anemia (condition in which the red blood cells do not bring enough oxygen to all the parts of the body); cancer; any type of infection, especially in your mouth; problems with your mouth, teeth, or gums; any condition that stops your blood from clotting normally; dental or kidney disease.
- tell your doctor if you are pregnant or are breast-feeding. Also tell your doctor if you plan to become pregnant at any time in the future, because risedronate may remain in your body for years after you stop taking it. Call your doctor if you become pregnant during or after your treatment with risedronate.
- you should know that risedronate may cause serious problems with your jaw, especially if you have dental surgery or treatment while you are taking the medication. A dentist should examine your teeth and perform any needed treatments before you start to take risedronate. Be sure to brush your teeth and clean your mouth properly while you are taking risedronate. Talk to your doctor before having any dental treatments while you are taking this medication.
- talk to your doctor about other things you can do to prevent osteoporosis from developing or worsening. Your doctor will probably tell you to avoid smoking and drinking large amounts of alcohol and to follow a regular program of weight-bearing exercise.

What special dietary instructions should I follow?

You should eat plenty of foods that are rich in calcium and vitamin D while you are taking risedronate. Your doctor will tell you which foods are good sources of these nutrients and how many servings you need each day. If you find it difficult to eat enough of these foods, tell your doctor. In that case, your doctor can prescribe or recommend a supplement.

What should I do if I forget to take a dose?

If you miss a dose of once-daily risedronate, do not take it later in the day. Skip the missed dose and take one dose the next morning as usual. If you miss a dose of once-weekly risedronate, do not take it later in the day. Take one dose the morning after you remember. Then return to taking one dose once each week on your regularly scheduled day. Never take a double dose to make up for a missed one, and never take more than one dose in one day.

What side effects can this medicine cause?

Risedronate may cause side effects. Tell your doctor if any of these symptoms are severe or do not go away:

- nausea
- burping
- dry mouth
- stomach pain
- diarrhea
- constipation
- gas
- headache
- dizziness
- depression
- anxiety
- weakness
- leg cramps
- bone, joint, and/or muscle pain
- back pain
- flu-like symptoms
- fever, chills, sore throat, cough, and other signs of infection
- frequent or urgent need to urinate
- painful urination
- runny nose
- dry eyes
- ringing in the ears

Some side effects can be serious. If you experience any of the following side effects, call your doctor immediately before you take any more risedronate:

- difficulty swallowing or pain when swallowing
- new or worsening heartburn
- chest pain
- bloody vomit
- vomiting material that looks like coffee grounds
- black, tarry, or bloody stools
- itching
- rash
- hives
- blisters on skin
- swelling of the face, throat, tongue, lips, eyes, hands, feet, ankles, or lower legs
- difficulty breathing
- hoarseness
- swollen, red, or painful eyes
- sensitivity to light

Risedronate may cause other side effects. Call your doctor if you have any unusual problems while taking this medication.

What storage conditions are needed for this medicine?

Keep this medication in the container it came in, tightly closed, and out of reach of children. Store it at room temperature and away from excess heat and moisture (not in the bathroom). Throw away any medication that is outdated or no longer needed. Talk to your pharmacist about the proper disposal of your medication.

What should I do in case of overdose?

In case of overdose, give the victim a full glass of milk and call your local poison control center at 1-800-222-1222. If the victim has collapsed or is not breathing, call local emergency services at 911.

Symptoms of overdose may include:

- numbness or tingling around mouth or in hands or feet
- muscle spasms, cramps, or twitches
- seizures

What other information should I know?

Keep all appointments with your doctor and the laboratory.

Before having any laboratory test or bone imaging study, tell your doctor and the laboratory personnel that you are taking risedronate.

Do not let anyone else take your medication. Ask your pharmacist any questions you have about refilling your prescription.

Dosage Facts
For Informational Purposes

Caution: Do not change your dose, how often you take your medication, or the length of time you are to take it without first talking to your healthcare provider.

The following dosage information was written using medical language for doctors and other healthcare professionals and is provided here for you to check your dosage. The dosage of this drug may differ for different patients. Therefore, always follow your doctor's instructions or the directions on the label. Contact your healthcare provider or pharmacist if you have any questions about the specific dosage of your medication after reviewing this information.

General Dosage Information

Available as risedronate sodium; dosage expressed in terms of the salt.

Adult Patients

Osteoporosis
Prevention of Postmenopausal Osteoporosis

ORAL:
- 5 mg once *daily* or 35 mg once *weekly*.

Treatment of Postmenopausal Osteoporosis

ORAL:
- 5 mg once *daily* or 35mg once *weekly*.

Corticosteroid-induced Osteoporosis
Prevention of Corticosteroid-induced Osteoporosis

ORAL:
- 5 mg once *daily*.
- Continue risedronate as long as patient continues to receive corticosteroid therapy.

Treatment of Corticosteroid-induced Osteoporosis

ORAL:
- 5 mg once *daily*.
- Continue risedronate as long as patient continues to receive corticosteroid therapy.

Paget's Disease of Bone

ORAL:
- 30 mg once daily for 2 months.
- Consider retreatment (same dosage and duration) after a 2-month posttreatment evaluation period if relapse occurs or if initial treatment failed to normalize serum alkaline phosphatase concentrations.

Prescribing Limits

Adult Patients

Paget's Disease of Bone

ORAL:
- Safety and efficacy not established for >1 course of retreatment.

Special Populations

Hepatic Impairment
- Dosage adjustments are not necessary.

Renal Impairment
- Dosage adjustments are not necessary in patients with mild to moderate impairment ($Cl_{cr} \geq 30$ mL/minute). Use is not recommended in patients with severe impairment ($Cl_{cr} < 30$ mL/minute).

Risperidone

(ris per′ i done)

Brand Name: Risperdal®, Risperdal® M-TAB®

Important Warning

Studies have shown that older adults with dementia (a brain disorder that affects the ability to remember, think clearly, communicate, and perform daily activities and that may cause changes in mood and personality) who take antipsychotics (medications for mental illness) such as risperidone have an increased risk of death during treatment. Older adults with dementia may also have a greater chance of having a stroke or mini-stroke during treatment. Tell your doctor and pharmacist if you are taking furosemide (Lasix). If you experience any of the following symptoms, call your doctor immediately: slow or difficult speech, sudden dizziness or faintness, or weakness or numbness of an arm or leg.

Risperidone is not approved by the Food and Drug Administration (FDA) for the treatment of behavior problems in older adults with dementia. Talk to the doctor who prescribed this medication if you, a family member, or someone you care for has dementia and is taking risperidone. For more information visit the FDA website: http://www.fda.gov/cder

Why is this medicine prescribed?

Risperidone is used to treat the symptoms of schizophrenia (a mental illness that causes disturbed or unusual thinking, loss of interest in life, and strong or inappropriate emotions). It is also used to treat episodes of mania (frenzied, abnormally excited, or irritated mood) or mixed episodes (symptoms of mania and depression that happen together) in patients with bipolar disorder (manic depressive disorder; a disease that causes episodes of depression, episodes of mania, and other abnormal moods). Risperidone is also used to treat behavior problems such as aggression and self-injury and sudden mood changes in teenagers and children 5-16 years of age who have autism (a condition that causes repetitive behavior, difficulty interacting with others, and problems with communication). Risperidone is in a class of medications called atypical antipsychotics. It works by changing the activity of certain natural substances in the brain.

How should this medicine be used?

Risperidone comes as a tablet, a solution (liquid), and an orally disintegrating tablet (tablet that dissolves quickly in the mouth) to take by mouth. It is usually taken once or twice a day with or without food. Take risperidone at around the same time(s) every day. Follow the directions on your prescription label carefully, and ask your doctor or pharmacist to explain any part you do not understand. Take risperidone exactly as directed. Do not take more or less of it or take it more often than prescribed by your doctor.

Use the dropper provided to measure your dose of risperidone oral solution. You can take the oral solution with water, orange juice, coffee, or low-fat milk. Do not take the solution with tea or cola.

Do not try to push the orally disintegrating tablet through the foil. Instead, use dry hands to peel back the foil packaging. Immediately take out the tablet and place it on your tongue. The tablet will quickly dissolve and can be swallowed with or without liquid. Do not chew or crush the tablet.

Your doctor will probably start you on a low dose of risperidone and gradually increase your dose to allow your body to adjust to the medication.

Risperidone may help control your symptoms but will

not cure your condition. It may take several weeks or longer before you feel the full benefit of risperidone. Continue to take risperidone even if you feel well. Do not stop taking risperidone without talking to your doctor. If you suddenly stop taking risperidone, your symptoms may return and your illness may become harder to treat.

Are there other uses for this medicine?

This medication may be prescribed for other uses; ask your doctor or pharmacist for more information.

What special precautions should I follow?

Before taking risperidone,

- tell your doctor and pharmacist if you are allergic to risperidone or any other medications.
- tell your doctor and pharmacist what prescription and nonprescription medications, vitamins, nutritional supplements and herbal products you are taking or plan to take. Be sure to mention any of the following: antidepressants; carbamazepine (Tegretol); cimetidine (Tagamet); clozapine (Clozaril); dopamine agonists such as bromocriptine (Parlodel), cabergoline (Dostinex), levodopa (Dopar, Larodopa), pergolide (Permax), and ropinirole (Requip); levodopa (Dopar, Sinemet); medications for anxiety, high blood pressure, or seizures; other medications for mental illness; paroxetine (Paxil); phenobarbital (Luminal, Solfoton); phenytoin (Dilantin); quinidine (Quinaglute, Quinidex); ranitidine (Zantac); rifampin (Rifadin, Rimactane); sedatives; sleeping pills; tranquilizers; and valproic acid (Depakote, Depakene). Your doctor may need to change the doses of your medications or monitor you carefully for side effects.
- tell your doctor if you use or have ever used street drugs or large amounts of alcohol or if you have ever overused prescription medications and if you have or have ever had Parkinson's disease (PD; a disorder of the nervous system that causes difficulties with movement, muscle control, and balance); difficulty swallowing; breast cancer; angina (chest pain); irregular heartbeat; high or low blood pressure; heart failure; a heart attack; a stroke; seizures; or heart, kidney or liver disease; or if you or anyone in your family has or has ever had diabetes. Also tell your doctor if you have ever had to stop taking a medication for mental illness because of severe side effects.
- tell your doctor if you are pregnant or plan to become pregnant. If you become pregnant while taking risperidone, call your doctor. Do not breastfeed while taking risperidone.
- if you are having surgery, including dental surgery, tell the doctor or dentist that you are taking risperidone.
- you should know that risperidone may make you drowsy. Do not drive a car or operate machinery until you know how this medication affects you.
- you should know that alcohol can add to the drowsiness caused by this medication. Do not drink alcohol while taking risperidone.

- you should know that you may experience hyperglycemia (increases in your blood sugar) while you are taking this medication, even if you do not already have diabetes. If you have schizophrenia, you are more likely to develop diabetes than people who do not have schizophrenia, and taking risperidone or similar medications may increase this risk. Tell your doctor immediately if you have any of the following symptoms while you are taking risperidone: extreme thirst, frequent urination, extreme hunger, blurred vision, or weakness. It is very important to call your doctor as soon as you have any of these symptoms, because high blood sugar that is not treated can cause a serious condition called ketoacidosis. Ketoacidosis may become life-threatening if it is not treated at an early stage. Symptoms of ketoacidosis include: dry mouth, upset stomach and vomiting, shortness of breath, breath that smells fruity, and decreased consciousness.
- you should know that risperidone may make it harder for your body to cool down when it gets very hot or warm up when it gets very cold. Tell your doctor if you plan to do vigorous exercise or be exposed to extremely high or low temperatures.
- you should know that risperidone may cause dizziness, lightheadedness, and fainting when you get up too quickly from a lying position. This is more common when you first start taking risperidone. To avoid this problem, get out of bed slowly, resting your feet on the floor for a few minutes before standing up.
- if you have phenylketonuria (PKU, an inherited condition in which a special diet must be followed to prevent mental retardation), you should know that the orally disintegrating tablets contain aspartame which forms phenylalanine.

What special dietary instructions should I follow?

Unless your doctor tells you otherwise, continue your normal diet.

What should I do if I forget to take a dose?

Take the missed dose as soon as you remember it. However, if it is almost time for the next dose, skip the missed dose and continue your regular dosing schedule. Do not take a double dose to make up for a missed one.

What side effects can this medicine cause?

Risperidone may cause side effects. Tell your doctor if any of these symptoms are severe or do not go away:

- drowsiness
- dizziness
- diarrhea
- constipation
- heartburn
- dry mouth
- increased appetite
- weight gain

- stomach pain
- anxiety
- agitation
- restlessness
- dreaming more than usual
- difficulty falling asleep or staying asleep
- decreased sexual interest or ability
- runny nose
- cough
- sore throat
- muscle or joint pain
- dry or discolored skin
- difficulty urinating

Some side effects can be serious. If you experience any of the following symptoms or those listed in the IMPORTANT WARNING section or the SPECIAL PRECAUTIONS section, call your doctor immediately:

- fever
- muscle stiffness
- confusion
- fast or irregular pulse
- sweating
- unusual movements of your face or body that you cannot control
- faintness
- seizures
- slow movements or shuffling walk
- rash
- hives
- itching
- difficulty breathing or swallowing
- painful erection of the penis that lasts for hours

Risperidone may cause children to gain more weight than expected and for boys and male adolescents to have an increase in the size of their breasts. Talk to your doctor about the risks of giving this medication to your child.

Risperidone may cause other side effects. Call your doctor if you have any unusual problems while taking this medication.

If you experience a serious side effect, you or your doctor may send a report to the Food and Drug Administration's (FDA) MedWatch Adverse Event Reporting program online [at http://www.fda.gov/MedWatch/index.html] or by phone [1-800-332-1088].

What storage conditions are needed for this medicine?

Keep this medication in the container it came in, tightly closed, and out of reach of children. Store it at room temperature and away from excess heat and moisture (not in the bathroom). Always store the orally disintegrating tablets in their sealed package, and use them immediately after opening the package. Throw away any medication that is outdated or no longer needed. Talk to your pharmacist about the proper disposal of your medication.

What should I do in case of overdose?

In case of overdose, call your local poison control center at 1-800-222-1222. If the victim has collapsed or is not breathing, call local emergency services at 911.

Symptoms of overdose may include:

- drowsiness
- fast, pounding, or irregular heartbeat
- upset stomach
- blurred vision
- fainting
- dizziness
- seizures

What other information should I know?

Keep all appointments with your doctor and the laboratory. Your doctor may order certain lab tests to check your body's response to risperidone.

Do not let anyone else take your medication. Ask your pharmacist any questions you have about refilling your prescription.

Dosage Facts
For Informational Purposes

Caution: Do not change your dose, how often you take your medication, or the length of time you are to take it without first talking to your healthcare provider.

The following dosage information was written using medical language for doctors and other healthcare professionals and is provided here for you to check your dosage. The dosage of this drug may differ for different patients. Therefore, always follow your doctor's instructions or the directions on the label. Contact your healthcare provider or pharmacist if you have any questions about the specific dosage of your medication after reviewing this information.

General Dosage Information

If reinitiated after a drug-free period, titrate oral dosage as with initial therapy.

Adult Patients

Schizophrenia

ORAL:
- Initially, 1 mg twice daily, with increases in increments of 1 mg twice daily on second and third day, as tolerated, to target dosage of 6–8 mg daily (once daily or in 2 equally divided doses) recommended by manufacturer. Make subsequent dosage adjustments at intervals of ≥7 days.
- Alternatively, an initial dosage of 1–2 mg daily, with increases in increments of 0.5–1 mg daily titrated over 6–7 days, as tolerated, to target dosage of 4 mg daily may be more appropriate in most otherwise healthy adult patients.
- Lower initial dosages (e.g., 1 mg daily) and slower dosage titrations to an initial target dosage of 2 mg daily may be

appropriate for younger patients and those being treated for their first psychotic episode. Titrate dosage up to 4 mg daily depending on clinical response and adverse neurologic effects; 1–3 mg may be optimal.
- Maximal efficacy generally observed in dosage range of 4–8 mg daily; dosages >6 mg daily did not result in greater efficacy, but were associated with more adverse effects (e.g., extrapyramidal symptoms).
- Efficacy maintained for up to 2 years, but optimum duration of therapy currently is not known. In responsive patients, continue as long as clinically necessary and tolerated, but at lowest possible effective dosage; periodically reassess need for continued therapy.

Bipolar Disorder
Acute Manic or Mixed Episodes

ORAL:
- Initially 2–3 mg once daily.
- Adjust dosage, if indicated, in increments or decrements of 1 mg daily at intervals of not less than 24 hours.
- Antimanic efficacy demonstrated in dosage range of 1–6 mg daily; dosages >6 mg daily not studied.
- Not studied >3 weeks. If elect to use risperidone for extended periods, periodically reevaluate long-term risks and benefits for the individual patient.

Prescribing Limits
Adult Patients

Schizophrenia

ORAL:
- Dosages >6 mg (in 2 divided doses) generally not recommended; safety of dosages >16 mg daily not established.

Bipolar Disorder
Acute Manic or Mixed Episodes

ORAL:
- Safety and efficacy of dosages >6 mg not established.

Special Populations

Hepatic Impairment
- Oral: Initially, 0.5 mg twice daily in patients with severe hepatic impairment; increase dosage in increments of ≤0.5 mg twice daily. If increase in dosage beyond 1.5 mg twice daily is planned, adjust at intervals of at least 1 week; slower titration may be appropriate in some patients.

Renal Impairment
- Oral: Initially, 0.5 mg twice daily in patients with severe renal impairment; increase dosage in increments of ≤0.5 mg twice daily. If increase in dosage beyond 1.5 mg twice daily is planned, adjust at intervals of at least 1 week; slower titration may be appropriate in some patients.

Geriatric, Debilitated, or Hypotensive Patients
- Oral: Initially, 0.5 mg twice daily in geriatric or debilitated patients and patients either predisposed to hypotension or for whom hypotension would pose a risk; increase dosage in increments of ≤0.5 mg twice daily. If increase in dosage beyond 1.5 mg twice daily is planned, adjust at intervals of at least 1 week; slower titration may be appropriate in some patients. If a once-daily dosage regimen is considered, titrate on a twice-daily regimen for 2–3 days at the target dosage before switching to a once-daily regimen.

- Alternatively, in geriatric patients, initially give 0.25 mg daily; gradually increase dosage as tolerated.

Ritonavir
(ri toe′ na veer)

Brand Name: Norvir®, Norvir® Softgel

Important Warning

Serious or potentially life-threatening reactions can occur when ritonavir is taken along with certain drugs. Therefore, do not take ritonavir with alprazolam (Xanax); amiodarone (Cordarone); astemizole (Hismanal); belladonna, phenobarbital, and ergotamine tartrate (Bellergal-S, Bel-Phen-Ergot S, Phenerbel-S); bepridil (Vascor); bromocriptine (Parlodel); bupropion (Wellbutrin); cabergoline (Dostinex); cisapride (Propulsid); clorazepate (Tranxene); clozapine (Clozaril); diazepam (Valium); dihydroergotamine (D.H.E. 45, Migranal); disopyramide (Norpace); encainide (Enkaid); ergoloid mesylates (Germinal, Hydergine); ergonovine (Ergotrate Maleate); ergotamine (Cafatine, Cafergot, Cafetrate, others); estazolam (ProSom); flecainide (Tambocor); fluoxetine (Prozac, Sarafem); flurazepam (Dalmane); meperidine (Demerol); methylergonovine (Methergine); methysergide (Sansert); mexiletine (Mexitil); midazolam (Versed); nefazadone (Serzone); pergolide (Permax); pimozide (Orap); piroxicam (Feldene); propafenone (Rythmol); propoxyphene (Darvon); quinidine; rifabutin (Mycobutin); terfenadine (Seldane); triazolam (Halcion); or zolpidem (Ambien).

Why is this medicine prescribed?

Ritonavir is used to treat human immunodeficiency virus (HIV) infection. It belongs to a class of drugs called protease (pro' tee ace) inhibitors, which slow the spread of HIV infection in the body. It is usually taken with other antiviral medications. Ritonavir is not a cure and may not decrease the number of HIV-related illnesses. Ritonavir does not prevent the spread of HIV to other people.

This medication is sometimes prescribed for other uses; ask your doctor or pharmacist for more information.

How should this medicine be used?

Ritonavir comes as a capsule and liquid to take by mouth. It is usually taken every 12 hours (twice a day). Follow the directions on your prescription label carefully, and ask your doctor or pharmacist to explain any part you do not understand. Take ritonavir exactly as directed. Do not take more or less of it or take it more often than prescribed by your doctor.

Mix just one dose at a time and take the whole dose within 1 hour of mixing. Rinse the cup after each dose.

Continue to take ritonavir even if you feel well. Do not stop taking ritonavir without talking to your doctor.

What special precautions should I follow?

Before taking ritonavir,
- tell your doctor and pharmacist if you are allergic to ritonavir or any other drugs.
- in addition to the drugs listed in the IMPORTANT WARNING section, also tell your doctor and pharmacist what other prescription and nonprescription medications you are taking, especially anticoagulants ('blood thinners') such as warfarin (Coumadin), cholesterol-lowering medications such as lovastatin (Mevacor) and simvastatin (Zocor), clarithromycin (Biaxin), desipramine (Norpramin), didanosine (Videx), disulfiram (Antabuse), heart medications, indinavir (Crixivan), ketoconazole (Nizoral), medications for depression and seizures, medications that suppress the immune system such as cyclosporine (Neoral, Sandimmune) and tacrolimus (Prograf), meperidine (Demerol), Methadone (Dolobid), metronidazole (Flagyl), oral contraceptives (birth control pills), pain relievers, rifabutin (Mycobutin), rifampin (Rifadin, Rimactane), saquinavir (Invirase), sildenafil (Viagra), theophylline (Theo-Dur), vitamins, and nutritional supplements.
- tell your doctor and pharmacist what herbal products you are taking, especially St. John's wort and products containing St. John's wort.
- tell your doctor if you have or have ever had liver disease, diabetes, hemophilia, or a history of alcohol abuse.
- tell your doctor if you are pregnant, plan to become pregnant, or are breast-feeding. If you become pregnant while taking ritonavir, call your doctor immediately.
- tell your doctor if you drink alcohol.

What special dietary instructions should I follow?

Take ritonavir with food. Ritonavir liquid may be taken alone or mixed with chocolate milk or the food supplements Ensure or Advera. Do not mix it with any other fluids.

What should I do if I forget to take a dose?

Take the missed dose as soon as you remember it. However, if it is almost time for the next dose, skip the missed dose and continue your regular dosing schedule. Do not take a double dose to make up for a missed one.

What side effects can this medicine cause?

Side effects from ritonavir may occur. Tell your doctor if any of these symptoms are severe or do not go away:
- loss of strength or weakness
- upset stomach
- vomiting
- diarrhea or loose stools
- headache
- dizziness
- shift in body fat

If you experience any of the following symptoms, call your doctor immediately:
- rash
- hives
- difficulty breathing
- swelling of the tongue or lips
- tingling sensation or numbness in the hands, feet, or around the lips
- excessive tiredness
- lack of energy
- loss of appetite
- pain in the upper right part of the stomach
- yellowing of the skin or eyes

Ritonavir may increase the sugar level in your blood. If you experience any of the following symptoms, call your doctor immediately:
- frequent urination
- increased thirst
- weakness
- dizziness
- headache

If you experience a serious side effect, you or your doctor may send a report to the Food and Drug Administration's (FDA) MedWatch Adverse Event Reporting program online [at http://www.fda.gov/MedWatch/index.html] or by phone [1-800-332-1088].

What storage conditions are needed for this medicine?

Keep this medication in the container it came in, tightly closed, and out of reach of children. Keep retonavir capsules and liquid in the refrigerator; do not freeze. The liquid bottle in use can be stored in a cool area for up to 30 days. Throw away any medication that is outdated or no longer needed. Talk to your pharmacist about the proper disposal of your medication.

What should I do in case of overdose?

In case of overdose, call your local poison control center at 1-800-222-1222. If the victim has collapsed or is not breathing, call local emergency services at 911.

What other information should I know?

Keep all appointments with your doctor and the laboratory. Your doctor will order certain lab tests to check your response to ritonavir.

Do not let anyone else take your medication. Ask your pharmacist any questions you have about refilling your prescription.

Dosage Facts
For Informational Purposes

Caution: Do not change your dose, how often you take your medication, or the length of time you are to take it without first talking to your healthcare provider.

The following dosage information was written using medical language for doctors and other healthcare professionals and is provided here for you to check your dosage. The dosage of this drug may differ for different patients. Therefore, always follow your doctor's instructions or the directions on the label. Contact your healthcare provider or pharmacist if you have any questions about the specific dosage of your medication after reviewing this information.

General Dosage Information

Must be given in conjunction with other antiretrovirals. *Low-dose ritonavir used with amprenavir, atazanavir, darunavir, fosamprenavir, indinavir, saquinavir, or tipranavir in ritonavir-boosted regimens. If used with didanosine, adjustment in the treatment regimen recommended.*

To minimize nausea associated with initiation of standard-dosage ritonavir therapy, initiate therapy using a dose escalation schedule.

Pediatric Patients
Treatment of HIV Infection

ORAL:
- >1 month of age: Initially, 250 mg/m² twice daily, increase in increments of 50 mg/m² every 12 hours (i.e., by 100 mg/m² daily) at intervals of 2–3 days as tolerated up to 350–400 mg/m² twice daily (not >600 mg twice daily).
- If a dosage of 400 mg/m² twice daily is not tolerated (due to adverse effects), use highest dosage that is tolerated or consider use of an alternative PI.

Pediatric Dosage Using Oral Solution

Body Surface Area (m²)	Twice daily dose of 250 mg/ m²	Twice daily dose of 300 mg/ m²	Twice daily dose of 350 mg/ m²	Twice daily dose of 400 mg/ m²
0.2	0.6 mL (50 mg)	0.75 mL (60 mg)	0.9 mL (70 mg)	1 mL (80 mg)
0.25	0.8 mL (62.5 mg)	0.9 mL (75 mg)	1.1 mL (87.5 mg)	1.25 mL (100 mg)
0.5	1.6 mL (125 mg)	1.9 mL (150 mg)	2.2 mL (175 mg)	2.5 mL (200 mg)
0.75	2.3 mL (187.5 mg)	2.8 mL (225 mg)	3.3 mL (262.5 mg)	3.75 mL (300 mg)
1	3.1 mL (250 mg)	3.75 mL (300 mg)	4.4 mL (350 mg)	5 mL (400 mg)
1.25	3.9 mL (312.5 mg)	4.7 mL (375 mg)	5.5 mL (437.5 mg)	6.25 mL (500 mg)
1.5	4.7 mL (375 mg)	5.6 mL (450 mg)	6.6 mL (525 mg)	7.5 ml (600 mg)

Adult Patients
Treatment of HIV Infection

ORAL:
- Initially 300 mg twice daily, increase dosage every 2–3 days by 100 mg twice daily up to a dosage of 600 mg twice daily. Alternatively, some experts recommend 300 mg twice daily initially, then increase over 5 days to 600 mg twice daily; others recommend 300 mg twice daily on days 1 and 2, 400 mg twice daily on days 3–5, 500 mg twice daily on days 6–13, and 600 mg twice daily thereafter.

Low-dose Ritonavir for Ritonavir-boosted Regimens

ORAL:
- 100 or 200 mg once daily or 100–400 mg twice daily depending on the other PI.

Prescribing Limits
Pediatric Patients
Treatment of HIV Infection

ORAL:
- 600 mg twice daily.

Special Populations

Hepatic Impairment
- Dosage adjustment not necessary in patients with mild to moderate hepatic impairment; data not available for severe hepatic impairment.

Renal Impairment
- Dosage adjustments not necessary.

Geriatric Patients
- Select dosage carefully; initiate therapy at the low end of the dosing range.

Rituximab Injection

(ri tux' i mab)

Brand Name: Rituxan®

Important Warning

Some people who received rituximab experienced severe reactions to the medication. Some of these people died within 24 hours after they received a dose of rituximab. Most of these deaths happened after the first dose of rituximab. Tell your doctor if you have or have ever had chronic lymphocytic leukemia (CLL; a type of cancer that begins in the white blood cells), mantle cell lymphoma (a fast-growing cancer that begins in the cells of the immune system), an irregular heartbeat, or heart or lung disease. If you have any of these conditions, or if you are female, there is a greater chance that you will experience a serious reaction to rituximab. If you experience any of the following symptoms, tell your doctor or other health care provider immediately: hives; swelling of the lips, tongue, or throat; difficulty breathing or swallowing; dizziness; fainting; shortness of breath; wheezing; blurred vision; headache; pounding or irregular heartbeat; fast or weak pulse; loss of consciousness, fast breathing; pale or bluish skin; pain in the chest that may spread to other parts of the upper body; weakness; excessive tiredness; sweating; or anxiety.

When rituximab is used to treat non-Hodgkin's lymphoma (NHL; a type of cancer that begins in a type of white blood cells that normally fight infection) it may cause a condition called tumor lysis syndrome (TLS; a group of symptoms caused by the fast breakdown of cancer cells). TLS may cause kidney failure and the need for dialysis treatment. Tell your doctor if you are also receiving cisplatin (Platinol). If you notice that you need to urinate less often than usual or that you produce less urine than usual, tell your doctor immediately.

Rituximab has caused severe skin reactions. These reactions have caused death. If you experience any of the following symptoms, tell your doctor immediately: painful sores, ulcers, blisters, rash, or peeling skin.

Some people who received rituximab developed progressive multifocal leukoencephalopathy (PML; a rare infection of the brain that cannot be treated, prevented, or cured and that usually causes death or severe disability) during or after their treatment. If you experience any of the following symptoms, call your doctor immediately: difficulty thinking clearly or walking, loss of strength, vision problems, or any other unusual symptoms that develop suddenly.

Talk to your doctor about the risks of using rituximab.

Why is this medicine prescribed?

Rituximab is used alone or with other medications to treat certain types of non-Hodgkin's lymphoma (NHL; a type of cancer that begins in a type of white blood cells that normally fights infection). Rituximab is also used with another medication to treat the symptoms of rheumatoid arthritis (RA; a condition in which the body attacks its own joints, causing pain, swelling, and loss of function) in people who have already been treated with a certain type of medication called a tumor necrosis factor (TNF) inhibitor. Rituximab is in a class of medications called biologic antineoplastic agents. It treats NHL by causing the death of blood cells that have multiplied abnormally. It treats rheumatoid arthritis by causing the death of certain blood cells that may cause the immune system to attack the joints.

How should this medicine be used?

Rituximab comes as a solution (liquid) to be injected into a vein. Rituximab is administered by a doctor or nurse in a medical office or infusion center. When rituximab is used to treat rheumatoid arthritis, it is usually given as 2 doses spaced 2 weeks apart. When rituximab is used to treat NHL it is either given once a week for 4-8 weeks or on the first day of each chemotherapy cycle. Your dosing schedule will depend on the condition that you have, the other medications you are using, and how well your body responds to treatment.

Rituximab must be given slowly. It may take several hours or longer to receive your first dose of rituximab, so you should plan to spend most of the day at the medical office or infusion center. After the first dose, you may receive your medication more quickly, depending on how you respond to treatment.

You may experience symptoms such as fever, shaking chills, tiredness, headache, or nausea while you are receiving a dose of rituximab, especially the first dose. Tell your doctor or other healthcare provider if you experience these symptoms while you are receiving your medication. Your doctor may prescribe other medications to help prevent or relieve these symptoms. Your doctor may tell you to take these medications before you receive each dose of rituximab.

Ask your pharmacist or doctor for a copy of the manufacturer's information for the patient.

Are there other uses for this medicine?

This medication may be prescribed for other uses; ask your doctor or pharmacist for more information.

What special precautions should I follow?

Before using rituximab,

- tell your doctor and pharmacist if you are allergic to rituximab or any other medications.
- tell your doctor and pharmacist what prescription and nonprescription medications, vitamins, nutritional supplements, and herbal products you are taking or plan to take. Be sure to mention the medication in the IMPORTANT WARNING section and either of the following: medications for high blood pressure and other medications for rheumatoid arthritis. Your doctor may need to change the doses of your medications or monitor you carefully for side effects.
- tell your doctor if you have any of the conditions mentioned in the IMPORTANT WARNING section and if you have or have ever had hepatitis B or other viruses such as chicken pox, herpes (a virus that may cause cold sores or outbreaks of blisters in the genital area), West Nile virus (a virus that is spread through mosquito bites and may cause serious symptoms), or cytomegalovirus (a common virus that usually only causes serious symptoms in people who have weakend immune systems or who are infected at birth). Also tell your doctor if you have any type of infection now or if you have or have ever had an infection that would not go away or an infection that comes and goes.
- tell your doctor if you are pregnant or plan to become pregnant. Rituximab may harm the fetus. You should use birth control to prevent pregnancy during your treatment with rituximab and for up to 12 months after your treatment. Talk to your doctor about types of birth control that will work for you. If you become pregnant while using rituximab, call your doctor.
- tell your doctor if you are breast-feeding. You should not breast-feed during your treatment with rituximab or for some time after your treatment
- if you are having surgery, including dental surgery, tell the doctor or dentist that you are using rituximab.
- you should know that you may be drowsy or dizzy after you receive a dose of rituximab. Do not drive a car or operate machinery until you know how this medication affects you. Plan to have someone else drive you home from the medical office or infusion center after you receive your treatment.
- ask your doctor whether you should receive any vaccinations before you begin your treatment with rituximab. Do not have any vaccinations during your treatment without talking to your doctor.

What special dietary instructions should I follow?

Unless your doctor tells you otherwise, continue your normal diet.

What should I do if I forget to take a dose?

If you miss an appointment to receive rituximab, call your doctor right away.

What side effects can this medicine cause?

Rituximab may cause side effects. Tell your doctor if any of these symptoms are severe or do not go away:

- nausea
- vomiting
- diarrhea
- heartburn
- weight gain
- muscle or back pain
- flushing
- night sweats
- tiredness
- weakness
- numbness, burning or tingling in the hands or feet
- runny nose

Some side effects can be serious. If you experience any of these symptoms or those listed in the IMPORTANT WARNING section, call your doctor immediately:

- stomach area pain
- unusual bruising or bleeding
- sore throat, fever, chills, or other signs of infection
- chest tightness
- joint pain or soreness

Rituximab may cause other side effects. Call your doctor if you have any unusual problems while using this medication.

What should I do in case of overdose?

In case of overdose, call your local poison control center at 1-800-222-1222. If the victim has collapsed or is not breathing, call local emergency services at 911.

What other information should I know?

Keep all appointments with your doctor and the laboratory. Your doctor will order certain lab tests to check your body's response to rituximab.

Dosage Facts
For Informational Purposes

Caution: Do not change your dose, how often you take your medication, or the length of time you are to take it without first talking to your healthcare provider.

The following dosage information was written using medical language for doctors and other healthcare professionals and is provided here for you to check your dosage. The dosage of this drug may differ for different patients. Therefore, always follow your doctor's instructions or the directions on the label. Contact your health-

care provider or pharmacist if you have any questions about the specific dosage of your medication after reviewing this information.

Adult Patients

Non-Hodgkin's Lymphoma
Relapsed or Refractory Low-grade or Follicular, Antigen CD20-positive, B-cell Non-Hodgkin's Lymphoma

IV:
- 375 mg/m² administered by IV infusion once weekly for 4 weeks or 8 weeks.
- If disease subsequently progresses, administer an additional course of 375 mg/m² once weekly for 4 weeks.

Previously Untreated Follicular, Antigen CD20-Positive, B-Cell Non-Hodgkin's Lymphoma

IV:
- 375 mg/m² administered by IV infusion on day 1 of each cycle of CVP chemotherapy for up to 8 infusions.

Previously Untreated Low-Grade, Antigen CD20-Positive, B-Cell Non-Hodgkin's Lymphoma

IV:
- For patients with stable disease or a partial or complete response following 6–8 cycles of CVP chemotherapy, 375 mg/m² administered by IV infusion once weekly for 4 infusions; repeat every 6 months for up to 16 infusions.

Diffuse Large B-cell, Antigen CD20-positive, Non-Hodgkin's Lymphoma

IV:
- 375 mg/m² administered by IV infusion on day 1 of each chemotherapy cycle for up to 8 infusions.

Radioimmunotherapy with Rituximab and Ibritumomab

IV:
- Administer rituximab 250 mg/m² within 4 hours prior to an imaging dose of indium In 111 ibritumomab tiuxetan (coupled with 1 or more whole body scans to assess distribution); 7–9 days later, administer rituximab 250 mg/m² within 4 hours prior to a therapeutic dose of yttrium Y 90 ibritumomab tiuxetan.

Rheumatoid Arthritis

IV:
- Two doses of 1 g each given by IV infusion 2 weeks apart.

Therapy Interruptions or Discontinuance for Toxicity

Depending on the nature and severity of rituximab-related toxicities, slowing of the infusion rate, interruption of the infusion, or discontinuance of the drug may be required; provide appropriate treatment as indicated.

Prescribing Limits

Adult Patients

Non-Hodgkin's Lymphoma
Relapsed or Refractory Low-grade or Follicular, Antigen CD20-positive, B-cell Non-Hodgkin's Lymphoma

IV:
- Safety and efficacy of >2 courses of therapy not established.

Previously Untreated Follicular, Antigen CD20-Positive, B-Cell Non-Hodgkin's Lymphoma

IV:
- Maximum 8 infusions.

Previously Untreated Low-Grade, Antigen CD20-Positive, B-Cell Non-Hodgkin's Lymphoma

IV:
- Maximum 16 infusions.

Diffuse Large B-cell, Antigen CD20-positive, Non-Hodgkin's Lymphoma

IV:
- Maximum 8 cycles of therapy (i.e., 8 rituximab infusions recommended.

Rheumatoid Arthritis

IV:
- Safety and efficacy of >2 doses (i.e., 1 course of therapy) not established in controlled clinical trials. Limited experience in uncontrolled setting with 2–5 courses (2 doses per course; subsequent courses generally administered 24 weeks, but no sooner than 16 weeks, after previous course).

Special Populations

No special population dosage recommendations at this time.

Rivastigmine
(ri va stig' meen)

Brand Name: Exelon®

Why is this medicine prescribed?

Rivastigmine is used to treat dementia (a brain disorder that affects the ability to remember, think clearly, communicate, and perform daily activities and may cause changes in mood and personality) in people with Alzheimer's disease (a brain disease that slowly destroys the memory and ability to think, learn, communicate and handle daily activities). Rivastigmine is also used to treat dementia in people with Parkinson's disease (a brain and nervous system disease with symptoms of slowing of movement, muscle weakness, shuffling walk, and loss of memory). Rivastigmine is in a class of medications called cholinesterase inhibitors. It improves mental function (such as memory and thinking) by increasing the amount of a certain natural substance in the brain.

How should this medicine be used?

Rivastigmine comes as a capsule and solution (liquid) to take by mouth. It is usually taken twice a day with meals in the morning and evening. Follow the directions on your prescription label carefully, and ask your doctor or pharmacist to explain any part you do not understand. Take rivastigmine exactly as directed. Do not take more or less of it or take it more often than prescribed by your doctor.

Your doctor will start you on a low dose of rivastigmine and slowly increase your dose, not more than once every 2 weeks.

Rivastigmine may improve the ability to think and remember or slow the loss of these abilities, but does not cure Alzheimer's disease or dementia in people with Parkinson's disease. Continue to take rivastigmine even if you feel well. Do not stop taking rivastigmine without talking to your doctor.

If you are taking rivastigmine oral solution, ask your pharmacist or doctor for a copy of the manufacturer's instructions for use. Carefully read these instructions. Always use the oral dosing syringe that comes with rivastigmine solution to measure your dose. Talk to your doctor or pharmacist if you have questions about how to measure your dose of rivastigmine solution.

Rivastigmine oral solution may be swallowed directly from the syringe or mixed with a liquid before use. Mix it with a small glass of water, cold fruit juice, or soda. Be sure to stir the mixture completely. Do not mix this medication with any liquid other than the ones listed. If the medication is mixed with water, juice, or soda, it must be taken within 4 hours.

To take a dose of rivastigmine solution, follow these steps:

1. Remove the oral dosing syringe that came with this medication from its protective case.
2. Push down and twist off the child-resistant cap to open the bottle of rivastigmine solution.
3. Put the tip of the oral syringe into the white stopper opening on top of the bottle.
4. While holding the syringe straight up, pull up on the plunger to the mark on the syringe that equals your dose.
5. Check the liquid in the syringe for air bubbles. If there are large air bubbles, gently move the syringe plunger up and down a few times. Do not worry about a few tiny air bubbles.
6. Make sure the plunger is on the mark on the syringe that equals your dose.
7. Remove the oral syringe from the bottle by pulling up on it.
8. Swallow your dose from the syringe directly, or mix it with the liquid you have chosen. Drink or swallow all of the solution.
9. Wipe off the outside of the oral syringe with a clean tissue, and put the syringe back into its case.
10. Close the child-resistant cap on the bottle of medication.

Are there other uses for this medicine?

Rivastigmine is also used sometimes to treat Lewy body dementia (a condition in which the brain develops abnormal protein structures, and the brain and nervous system are destroyed over time). Talk to your doctor about the possible risks of using this medication for your condition.

What special precautions should I follow?

Before taking rivastigmine,

- tell your doctor and pharmacist if you are allergic to rivastigmine, neostigmine (Prostigmin), physostigmine (Antilirium, Isopto Eserine), pyridostigmine (Mestinon, Regonol), any other medications, or any of the ingredients in rivastigmine solution. Ask your pharmacist for a list of the ingredients..
- tell your doctor and pharmacist what prescription and nonprescription medications, vitamins, nutritional supplements, and herbal products you are taking or plan to take. Be sure to mention any of the following: antihistamines; aspirin and other nonsteroidal anti-inflammatory medications (NSAIDs) such as ibuprofen (Advil, Motrin) and naproxen (Aleve, Naprosyn); bethanechol (Duvoid, Urabeth, Urecholine); ipratropium (Atrovent); and medications for Alzheimer's disease, glaucoma, irritable bowel disease, motion sickness, myasthenia gravis, Parkinson's disease, ulcers, or urinary problems. Your doctor may need to change the doses of your medications or monitor you carefully for side effects.
- tell your doctor if you have or have ever had asthma, an enlarged prostate or other condition that blocks the flow of urine, ulcers, abnormal heart beats, or other heart or lung disease.
- tell your doctor if you are pregnant, plan to become pregnant, or are breast-feeding. If you become pregnant while taking rivastigmine, call your doctor.
- if you are having surgery, including dental surgery, tell the doctor or dentist that you are taking rivastigmine.

What special dietary instructions should I follow?

Unless your doctor tells you otherwise, continue your normal diet.

What should I do if I forget to take a dose?

Take the missed dose as soon as you remember it. However, if it is almost time for the next dose, skip the missed dose and continue your regular dosing schedule. Do not take a double dose to make up for a missed one.

If you miss taking rivastigmine for more than a few days, talk to your doctor before starting to take it again. You will probably have to restart taking it at a lower dose.

What side effects can this medicine cause?

Rivastigmine may cause side effects. Tell your doctor if any of these symptoms are severe or do not go away:

- nausea
- vomiting
- loss of appetite
- heartburn or indigestion
- stomach pain
- weight loss
- diarrhea

- constipation
- gas
- weakness
- dizziness
- headache
- extreme tiredness
- lack of energy
- tremor or worsening of tremor
- increased sweating
- difficulty falling asleep or staying asleep
- confusion

Some side effects can be serious. The following symptoms are uncommon, but if you experience any of them, call your doctor immediately:
- fainting
- black and tarry stools
- red blood in stools
- bloody vomit
- vomiting material that looks like coffee grounds
- difficulty urinating
- painful urination
- seizures
- depression
- anxiety
- aggressive behavior
- hearing voices or seeing things that do not exist)
- uncontrollable movements and muscle contractions

Rivastigmine may cause other side effects. Call your doctor if you have any unusual problems while taking this medication.

If you experience a serious side effect, you or your doctor may send a report to the Food and Drug Administration's (FDA) MedWatch Adverse Event Reporting program online [at http://www.fda.gov/MedWatch/index.html] or by phone [1-800-332-1088].

What storage conditions are needed for this medicine?

Keep this medication in the container it came in, tightly closed, and out of reach of children. Store it at room temperature and away from excess heat and moisture (not in the bathroom). Store rivastigmine solution in an upright position. Do not place rivastigmine solution in the freezer or allow rivastigmine solution to freeze. Throw away any medication that is outdated or no longer needed. Talk to your pharmacist about the proper disposal of your medication.

What should I do in case of overdose?

In case of overdose, call your local poison control center at 1-800-222-1222. If the victim has collapsed or is not breathing, call local emergency services at 911.

Symptoms of overdose may include:
- nausea
- vomiting
- increased saliva
- sweating

- slow heart beat
- inability to hold urine
- slowed thinking and movement
- dizziness
- fainting
- blurred vision
- difficulty breathing
- loss of consciousness
- seizure

What other information should I know?

Keep all appointments with your doctor.

Do not let anyone else take your medication. Ask your pharmacist any questions you have about refilling your prescription.

Dosage Facts
For Informational Purposes

Caution: Do not change your dose, how often you take your medication, or the length of time you are to take it without first talking to your healthcare provider.

The following dosage information was written using medical language for doctors and other healthcare professionals and is provided here for you to check your dosage. The dosage of this drug may differ for different patients. Therefore, always follow your doctor's instructions or the directions on the label. Contact your healthcare provider or pharmacist if you have any questions about the specific dosage of your medication after reviewing this information.

General Dosage Information

Available as rivastigmine tartrate; dosage is expressed in terms of rivastigmine.

Adult Patients

Alzheimer's Disease

ORAL:
- Initially, 1.5 mg twice daily.
- If well tolerated, increase dosage after ≥2 weeks to 3 mg twice daily; attempt to increase dosage to 4.5 mg twice daily and 6 mg twice daily after ≥2 weeks of treatment at the previous dosage.
- If adverse effects intolerable, discontinue for several doses and then resume at the same or the immediately preceding (lower) dosage in the titration regimen. However, if therapy is interrupted for more than several days, restart drug using the recommended initial dosage (i.e., 1.5 mg twice daily) and titration schedule until the previous maintenance dosage is reached (to decrease the risk of severe vomiting and related sequelae [e.g., spontaneous esophageal rupture].)

Prescribing Limits

Adult Patients

Alzheimer's Disease

ORAL:
- Maximum 6 mg twice daily.

Special Populations

Hepatic Impairment
- Decreased clearance; however, dosage adjustment may not be necessary since dosage is titrated to adverse effect tolerability.

Renal Impairment
- Clearance decreased with moderate impairment and *increased* with severe impairment; however, dosage adjustment may not be necessary since dosage is titrated to adverse effect tolerability.

Rizatriptan

(rye za trip′ tan)

Brand Name: Maxalt®, Maxalt-MLT®

Why is this medicine prescribed?

Rizatriptan is used to treat the symptoms of migraine headaches (severe, throbbing headaches that sometimes are accompanied by nausea and sensitivity to sound and light). Rizatriptan is in a class of medications called selective serotonin receptor agonists. It works by narrowing blood vessels in the brain, stopping pain signals from being sent to the brain, and stopping the release of certain natural substances that cause pain, nausea, and other symptoms of migraine. Rizatriptan does not prevent migraine attacks.

How should this medicine be used?

Rizatriptan comes as a tablet and an orally disintegrating tablet to take by mouth. It should be taken at the first sign of a migraine headache. If you are at risk for heart disease and you have never taken rizatriptan before, you may need to take the first dose in your doctor's office. Usually only one dose is needed. If pain is not relieved with the first dose, your doctor may prescribe a second dose to be taken 2 hours after the first dose. Do not take more than 30 mg of rizatriptan in any 24-hour period. If you are also taking propranolol (Inderal), you should not take more than 15 mg of rizatriptan in any 24-hour period. Follow the directions on the package or prescription label carefully, and ask your doctor or pharmacist to explain any part you do not understand. Take rizatriptan exactly as directed. Do not take more or less of it or take it more often than directed by the package label or prescribed by your doctor.

The orally disintegrating tablet should not be removed from the package until just before it is taken. The packet should be opened with dry hands, and the orally disintegrating tablet should be placed on the tongue, where it will dissolve and be swallowed with saliva.

Are there other uses for this medicine?

This medication is sometimes prescribed for other uses; ask your doctor or pharmacist for more information.

What special precautions should I follow?

Before taking rizatriptan
- tell your doctor and pharmacist if you are allergic to rizatriptan, naratriptan (Amerge), sumatriptan (Imitrex), zolmitriptan (Zomig), or any other drugs.
- do not take rizatriptan if you have taken a monoamine oxidase inhibitor (MAOI) such as isocarboxazid (Marplan), phenelzine (Nardil), selegiline (Emsam, Eldepryl), and tranylcypromine (Parnate) during the last two weeks or if you have taken another medication for migraine headaches such as dihydroergotamine (D.H.E. 45, Migranal), methysergide (Sansert), almotriptan (Axert), eletriptan (Relpax), frovatriptan (Frova), naratriptan (Amerge), sumatriptan (Imitrex), or zolmitriptan (Zomig) during the past 24 hours.
- tell your doctor and pharmacist what prescription and nonprescription medications, vitamins, nutritional supplements, or herbal products you are taking or plan to take. Be sure to mention any of the following: selective serotonin reuptake inhibitors such as citalopram (Celexa), escitalopram (Lexapro), fluoxetine (Prozac, Sarafem, in Symbyax), fluvoxamine, paroxetine (Paxil), and sertraline (Zoloft); and selective serotonin/norepinephrine reuptake inhibitors (SNRIs) such as duloxetine (Cymbalta) and venlafaxine (Effexor). Your doctor may need to change the doses of your medications or monitor you more carefully for side effects..
- tell your doctor if you smoke, if you have a strong family history of heart disease, if you are postmenopausal, or if you are a man over 40. Also tell your doctor if you have or have ever had high blood pressure; phenylketonuria; angina (recurring chest pain); a heart attack; diabetes; high cholesterol; obesity; stroke; transient ischemic attack (mini-stroke); ischemic bowel disease; coronary artery disease; seizures; or blood vessel, kidney, or liver disease.
- tell your doctor if you are pregnant, plan to become pregnant, or are breast-feeding. If you become pregnant while taking rizatriptan, call your doctor.
- you should know that this drug may make you drowsy. Do not drive a car or operate machinery until you know how rizatriptan will affect you.
- remember that alcohol can add to the drowsiness caused by this drug. Do not drink alcohol while taking this medication.
- tell your doctor if you use or have ever used tobacco products. A history of tobacco use or cigarette smoking while taking rizatriptan may increase the risk associated with taking rizatriptan.
- plan to avoid unnecessary or prolonged exposure to sunlight and sun lamps and to wear protective clothing, sunglasses, and sunscreen. Rizatriptan may make your skin sensitive to sunlight.

What should I do if I forget to take a dose?

Rizatriptan is not for routine use. Use it only to relieve a migraine headache as soon as symptoms appear.

What side effects can this medicine cause?

Rizatriptan may cause side effects. Tell your doctor if any of these symptoms are severe or do not go away:

- drowsiness
- dizziness
- fatigue
- tingling or numb feeling
- upset stomach
- stomach pain
- vomiting
- diarrhea
- muscle pain or cramps
- tremors
- chills
- flushing (feeling of warmth)
- dry mouth

If you experience any of the following symptoms, call your doctor immediately:

- chest pain, tightness, or heaviness
- fast or irregular heartbeats
- throat pain or tightness
- difficulty breathing
- redness, swelling, or itching of the eyelids, face, or lips
- rash
- changes in vision

What storage conditions are needed for this medicine?

Keep this medication in the container it came in, tightly closed, and out of reach of children. Do not remove tablets from the blister pack until just before use. Store the medication at room temperature and away from excess heat and moisture (not in the bathroom). Throw away any medication that is outdated or no longer needed. Talk to your pharmacist about the proper disposal of your medication.

What should I do in case of overdose?

In case of overdose, call your local poison control center at 1-800-222-1222. If the victim has collapsed or is not breathing, call local emergency services at 911.

What other information should I know?

Keep all appointments with your doctor and the laboratory.

Read the patient information that comes with your prescription before you begin to take rizatriptan, and read it again every time you have your prescription filled in case the patient information changes.

Call your doctor if you continue to have migraine headache symptoms after the first dose.

Do not let anyone else take your medication. Ask your pharmacist any questions you have about refilling your prescription.

Dosage Facts
For Informational Purposes

Caution: Do not change your dose, how often you take your medication, or the length of time you are to take it without first talking to your healthcare provider.

The following dosage information was written using medical language for doctors and other healthcare professionals and is provided here for you to check your dosage. The dosage of this drug may differ for different patients. Therefore, always follow your doctor's instructions or the directions on the label. Contact your healthcare provider or pharmacist if you have any questions about the specific dosage of your medication after reviewing this information.

General Dosage Information

Available as rizatriptan benzoate; dosage is expressed in terms of rizatriptan.

Adult Patients

Vascular Headaches
Migraine

ORAL:
- 5 or 10 mg as a single dose; individualize dosage selection, weighing the possible benefit (greater effectiveness) and risks (increased adverse effects) of the 10-mg dose.
- Additional doses may be administered at intervals of ≥2 hours, up to a maximum dosage of 30 mg in any 24-hour period.
- Following failure to respond to first dose, reconsider diagnosis of migraine prior to administration of a second dose.

Prescribing Limits

Adult Patients

Vascular Headaches
Migraine

ORAL:
- Maximum 30 mg in any 24-hour period.
- Safety of treating an average of >4 headaches per 30-day period has not been established.

Ropinirole

(roe pin′ i role)

Brand Name: Requip®

Why is this medicine prescribed?

Ropinirole is used alone or with other medications to treat the symptoms of Parkinson's disease (PD; a disorder of the nervous system that causes difficulties with movement, muscle control, and balance), including shaking of parts of the body, stiffness, slowed movements, and problems with balance. Ropinirole is also used to treat restless legs syndrome (RLS; a condition that causes discomfort in the legs and a strong urge to move the legs, especially at night and when sitting or lying down). Ropinirole is in a class of medications called dopamine agonists. It works by acting in place of dopamine, a natural substance in the brain that is needed to control movement.

How should this medicine be used?

Ropinirole comes as a tablet to take by mouth. When ropinirole is used to treat Parkinson's disease, it is usually taken three times a day. When ropinirole is used to treat restless legs syndrome, it is usually taken once a day, 1 to 3 hours before bedtime. Ropinirole may be taken with or without food, but taking ropinirole with food may help to prevent nausea that may be caused by the medication. Follow the directions on your prescription label carefully and ask your doctor or pharmacist to explain any part you do not understand. Take ropinirole exactly as directed. Do not take more or less of it or take it more often than prescribed by your doctor.

Your doctor will start you on a low dose of ropinirole and gradually increase your dose. If you are taking ropinirole to treat Parkinson's disease, your doctor will probably not increase your dose more often than once a week. If you are taking ropinirole to treat restless legs syndrome, your doctor will probably increase your dose after 2 days, again at the end of the first week, and then not more often than once a week. It may take several weeks before you reach a dose that works for you. If you are taking ropinirole to treat restless legs syndrome, you may receive a starter kit that contains tablets of increasing strength to be taken during the first 2 weeks of your treatment. The dose of medication you will need depends on how well the medication works for you and may be different than the doses contained in the kit. Your doctor will tell you how to use the kit and whether you should take all the tablets it contains. Follow these directions carefully.

Ropinirole controls the symptoms of Parkinson's disease and restless legs syndrome but does not cure these conditions. Continue to take ropinirole even if you feel well. Do not stop taking ropinirole without talking to your doctor. If you are taking ropinirole to treat Parkinson's disease and you suddenly stop taking the medication, you may experience fever, fast heartbeat, muscle stiffness, sweating, and other symptoms. Your doctor will probably decrease your dose gradually.

If you stop taking ropinirole for any reason, do not start to take the medication again without talking to your doctor. Your doctor will probably want to increase your dose again gradually.

What special precautions should I follow?

Before taking ropinirole,

- tell your doctor and pharmacist if you are allergic to ropinirole, any other medications, or any of the ingredients in ropinirole tablets. Ask your doctor or pharmacist for a list of the inactive ingredients.
- tell your doctor and pharmacist what prescription and nonprescription medications, vitamins, nutritional supplements and herbal products you are taking or plan to take. Be sure to mention any of the following: antidepressants ('mood elevators'); antipsychotics (medications for mental illness); cimetidine (Tagamet, Tagamet HB); fluoroquinolone antibiotics such as ciprofloxacin (Cipro), and norfloxacin (Noroxin); fluvoxamine (Luvox); levodopa (in Sinemet, in Stalevo); medications for anxiety and seizures; medications that contain estrogen such as hormone replacement therapy and hormonal contraceptives (birth control pill, patches, rings, or injections); medications that cause drowsiness; metoclopramide (Reglan); mexiletine (Mexitil); sedatives; sleeping pills; and tranquilizers. Your doctor may need to change the doses of your medications or monitor you carefully for side effects.
- tell your doctor if you have ever had an urge to gamble that was difficult to control and if you have or have ever had a sleep disorder other than restless legs syndrome; or heart, liver, or kidney disease.
- tell your doctor if you are pregnant, plan to become pregnant, or are breast-feeding. If you become pregnant while taking ropinirole, call your doctor.
- you should know that ropinirole may make you drowsy or may cause you to suddenly fall asleep during your regular daily activities. You might not feel drowsy before you suddenly fall asleep. Do not drive a car or operate machinery at the beginning of your treatment until you know how the medication affects you. If you suddenly fall asleep while you are doing something such as watching television or riding in a car, or if you become very drowsy, call your doctor. Do not drive or operate machinery until you talk to your doctor.
- remember that alcohol can add to the drowsiness caused by this medication. Tell your doctor if you regularly drink alcoholic drinks.
- tell your doctor if you use tobacco products. Call your doctor if you start or stop smoking during your treatment with ropinirole. Smoking may decrease the effectiveness of this medication.
- you should know that ropinirole may cause dizziness, lightheadedness, nausea, or sweating when you get up

too quickly from a sitting or lying position. This is more common when you first start taking ropinirole. To avoid this problem, get out of the chair or bed slowly, resting your feet on the floor for a few minutes before standing up.

What special dietary instructions should I follow?

Unless your doctor tells you otherwise, continue your normal diet.

What should I do if I forget to take a dose?

If you are taking ropinirole to treat Parkinson's disease, take the missed dose as soon as you remember it. However, if it is almost time for the next dose, skip the missed dose and continue your regular dosing schedule. Do not take a double dose to make up for a missed one.

If you are taking ropinirole to treat restless legs syndrome, skip the missed dose. Take your regular dose 1 to 3 hours before your next bedtime. Do not double the next dose to make up for the missed dose.

What side effects can this medicine cause?

Ropinirole may cause side effects. Tell your doctor if any of these symptoms are severe or do not go away:

- nausea
- vomiting
- dizziness
- drowsiness
- weakness
- headache
- heartburn
- stomach pain
- constipation
- sweating
- confusion
- anxiety
- abnormal body movements
- slowed or decreased movements
- numbness, burning, or tingling in the hands, arms, feet, or legs
- frequent or urgent need to urinate
- difficulty urinating or pain when urinating
- runny nose, sore throat, and other cold symptoms
- joint pain
- swelling of the hands, arms, feet, ankles, or lower legs
- dry mouth

Some side effects can be serious. If you experience any of the following symptoms, call your doctor immediately:

- hallucinations (seeing things or hearing voices that do not exist)
- fainting
- slow or irregular heartbeat
- shortness of breath
- double vision or other problems with vision

Some people who took medications such as ropinirole to treat Parkinson's disease developed gambling problems. There is not enough information to tell whether the people developed these problems because they took the medication or for other reasons. Call your doctor if you have an urge to gamble that is difficult to control. Tell your family members about this risk so that they can call the doctor even if you do not realize that your gambling has become a problem.

People who have Parkinson's disease may have a greater risk of developing melanoma (a type of skin cancer) than people who do not have Parkinson's disease. There is not enough information to tell whether medications used to treat Parkinson's disease such as ropinirole increase the risk of developing skin cancer. You should have regular skin examinations to check for melanoma while you are taking ropinirole even if you do not have Parkinson's disease. Talk to your doctor about the risk of taking ropinirole.

Ropinirole may cause other side effects. Call your doctor if you have any unusual problems while you are taking this medication.

What storage conditions are needed for this medicine?

Keep this medication in the container it came in, tightly closed, and out of reach of children. Store it at room temperature and away from direct sunlight, excess heat, and moisture (not in the bathroom). Throw away any medication that is outdated or no longer needed. Talk to your pharmacist about the proper disposal of your medication.

What should I do in case of overdose?

In case of overdose, call your local poison control center at 1-800-222-1222. If the victim has collapsed or is not breathing, call local emergency services at 911.

Symptoms of overdose may include:

- nausea
- vomiting
- dizziness
- hallucinations
- sweating
- fear when in small or closed space
- body movements that are difficult to control
- pounding heartbeat
- weakness
- nightmares
- coughing
- fainting
- chest pain
- confusion

What other information should I know?

Keep all appointments with your doctor.

Do not let anyone else take your medication. Ask your pharmacist any questions you have about refilling your prescription.

Dosage Facts
For Informational Purposes

Caution: Do not change your dose, how often you take your medication, or the length of time you are to take it without first talking to your health-care provider.

The following dosage information was written using medical language for doctors and other healthcare professionals and is provided here for you to check your dosage. The dosage of this drug may differ for different patients. Therefore, always follow your doctor's instructions or the directions on the label. Contact your healthcare provider or pharmacist if you have any questions about the specific dosage of your medication after reviewing this information.

General Dosage Information

Available as ropinirole hydrochloride; dosage expressed in terms of ropinirole.

Adult Patients

Parkinsonian Syndrome

ORAL:
- Initiate at a low dosage and increase slowly until the maximum therapeutic response is achieved.

Table 1. Usual Initial Dosage of Ropinirole for the Treatment of Parkinsonian Syndrome

Week of Therapy	Daily Dosage Schedule	Total Daily Dose
1	0.25 mg 3 times daily	0.75 mg daily
2	0.5 mg 3 times daily	1.5 mg daily
3	0.75 mg 3 times daily	2.25 mg daily
4	1 mg 3 times daily	3 mg daily
After week 4		Daily dosage may be increased by 1.5 mg daily each week up to 9 mg daily, and then by up to 3 mg daily each week to a total daily dosage of 24 mg

Continually reevaluate and adjust the dosage according to the needs of the patient in an effort to find a dosage schedule that provides maximum relief of symptoms with minimum adverse effects.

When ropinirole is used as an adjunct to levodopa, the levodopa dosage may be decreased gradually as tolerated.

Discontinue ropinirole therapy gradually over a period of 1 week. Reduce the frequency of administration from 3 times daily to twice daily for 4 days and then to once daily for 3 days before complete discontinuance of the drug.

If therapy is interrupted for a substantial period of time, reinitiation at initial recommended dosage (see Table 1) may be warranted.

Restless Legs Syndrome

ORAL:
- Initiate at a low dosage and increase slowly based on clinical response and tolerability.

Table 2. Usual Initial Dosage of Ropinirole for the Treatment of Restless Legs Syndrome

Day/Week of Therapy	Daily Dosage
Days 1 and 2	0.25 mg once daily
Days 3–7	0.5 mg once daily
Week 2	1 mg once daily
Week 3	1.5 mg once daily
Week 4	2 mg once daily
Week 5	2.5 mg once daily
Week 6	3 mg once daily
Week 7	4 mg once daily

Has been discontinued without gradually reducing the dosage in patients receiving up to 4 mg once daily.

If therapy is interrupted for a substantial period of time, reinitiation at initial recommended dosage (see Table 2) may be warranted.

Prescribing Limits

Adult Patients

Parkinsonian Syndrome

ORAL:
- Dosages >24 mg daily have not been evaluated in clinical trials.

Restless Legs Syndrome

ORAL:
- Safety and efficacy not established for dosages >4 mg once daily.

Special Populations

Hepatic Impairment
- Titrate dosage carefully. Manufacturer makes no specific recommendations for dosage adjustment.

Renal Impairment
- No dosage adjustments necessary in patients with Cl_{cr} of 30–50 mL/minute. Manufacturer makes no specific recommendations for dosage adjustment in patients with severe renal impairment.

Geriatric Patients
- No dosage adjustments necessary in patients >65 years of age, since therapy is initiated at a low dosage and titrated according to clinical response.

Rosiglitazone

(roe si gli′ ta zone)

Brand Name: Avandia®, Avandaryl® (as a combination product containing rosiglitazone and glimepiride), Avandamet® (as a combination product containing rosiglitazone and metformin)

Important Warning

Rosiglitazone and other similar medications for diabetes may cause or worsen congestive heart failure (condition in which the heart is unable to pump enough blood to the other parts of the body). Some studies have shown that people who take rosiglitazone and insulin are more likely to have a heart attack or to die of heart problems than people who take insulin alone. Before you start to take rosiglitazone, tell your doctor if you have or have ever had congestive heart failure, especially if your heart failure is so severe that you must limit your activity and are only comfortable when you are at rest or you must remain in a chair or bed. Also tell your doctor if you were born with a heart defect, and if you have or have ever had swelling of the arms, hands, feet, ankles, or lower legs; heart disease; high blood pressure; coronary artery disease (narrowing of the blood vessels that lead to the heart); a heart attack; an irregular heartbeat; or high cholesterol or fats in the blood. Your doctor may tell you not to take rosiglitazone or may monitor you carefully during your treatment.

If you develop congestive heart failure or other heart problems, you may experience certain symptoms. Tell your doctor immediately if you have any of the following symptoms, especially when you first start taking rosiglitazone or after your dose is increased: large weight gain in a short period of time; shortness of breath; swelling of the arms, hands, feet, ankles, or lower legs; chest pain; swelling or pain in the stomach; waking up short of breath during the night; needing to sleep with extra pillows in order to breathe while lying down; frequent dry cough; or increased tiredness.

Talk to your doctor about the risks of taking rosiglitazone.

Why is this medicine prescribed?

Rosiglitazone is used along with a diet and exercise program and sometimes with one or more other medications to treat type 2 diabetes (condition in which the body does not use insulin normally and therefore cannot control the amount of sugar in the blood). Rosiglitazone is in a class of medications called thiazolidinediones. It works by increasing the body's sensitivity to insulin, a natural substance that helps control blood sugar levels. Rosiglitazone is not used to treat type 1 diabetes (condition in which the body does not produce insulin and therefore cannot control the amount of sugar in the blood) or diabetic ketoacidosis (a serious condition that may occur if high blood sugar is not treated).

How should this medicine be used?

Rosiglitazone comes as a tablet to take by mouth. It is usually taken once or twice daily with or without meals. Take rosiglitazone at about the same time(s) every day. Follow the directions on your prescription label carefully, and ask your doctor or pharmacist to explain any part you do not understand. Take rosiglitazone exactly as directed. Do not take more or less of it or take it more often than prescribed by your doctor.

Your doctor may increase your dose of rosiglitazone after 8-12 weeks, based on your body's response to the medication.

Rosiglitazone helps control type 2 diabetes but does not cure it. It may take 2 weeks for your blood sugar to decrease, and 2-3 months or longer for you to feel the full benefit of rosiglitazone. Continue to take rosiglitazone even if you feel well. Do not stop taking rosiglitazone without talking to your doctor.

Are there other uses for this medicine?

This medication may be prescribed for other uses; ask your doctor or pharmacist for more information.

What special precautions should I follow?

Before taking rosiglitazone,

- tell your doctor and pharmacist if you are allergic to rosiglitazone or any other medications.
- tell your doctor and pharmacist what prescription and nonprescription medications, vitamins, nutritional supplements, and herbal products you are taking or plan to take. Be sure to mention any of the following: gemfibrozil (Lopid), insulin and other medications for diabetes, montelukast (Singulair), and rifampin (Rifadin, Rimactane, in Rifamate). Your doctor may need to change the doses of your medications or monitor you carefully for side effects.
- tell your doctor if you have or have ever had any of the conditions mentioned in the IMPORTANT WARNING section or diabetic eye disease such as macular edema (swelling of the back of the eye); or liver disease. Also tell your doctor if you have ever taken troglitazone (Rezulin, no longer available in the United States), especially if you stopped taking it because you experienced side effects.
- tell your doctor if you are pregnant or plan to become pregnant. If you become pregnant while taking rosiglitazone, call your doctor. Do not breastfeed while you are taking rosiglitazone.
- if you have not yet experienced menopause (change of

life; end of monthly menstrual periods) you should know that rosiglitazone may increase the chance that you will become pregnant even if you do not have regular monthly periods or you have a condition that prevents you from ovulating (releasing an egg from the ovaries). Talk to your doctor about methods of birth control that will work for you.

- if you will be having surgery, including dental surgery, tell the doctor or dentist that you are taking rosiglitazone.
- ask your doctor what to do if you get sick, develop an infection or fever, experience unusual stress, or are injured. These conditions can affect your blood sugar and the amount of rosiglitazone you may need.

What special dietary instructions should I follow?

Be sure to follow all exercise and dietary recommendations made by your doctor or dietitian. It is important to eat a healthy diet, exercise regularly, and lose weight if necessary. This will help to control your diabetes and help rosiglitazone work more effectively

What should I do if I forget to take a dose?

Take the missed dose as soon as you remember it. However, if it is time for the next dose, skip the missed dose and continue your regular dosing schedule. Do not take a double dose to make up for a missed one.

What side effects can this medicine cause?

This medication may cause changes in your blood sugar. You should know the symptoms of low and high blood sugar and what to do if you have these symptoms.

You may experience hypoglycemia (low blood sugar) if you are taking this medication in combination with other medications used to treat diabetes. Your doctor will tell you what you should do if you develop hypoglycemia. He or she may tell you to check your blood sugar, eat or drink a food or beverage that contains sugar, such as hard candy or fruit juice, or get medical care. Follow these directions carefully if you have any of the following symptoms of hypoglycemia:

- shakiness
- dizziness or lightheadedness
- sweating
- nervousness or irritability
- sudden changes in behavior or mood
- headache
- numbness or tingling around the mouth
- weakness
- pale skin
- hunger
- clumsy or jerky movements

If hypoglycemia is not treated, severe symptoms may develop. Be sure that your family, friends, and other people who spend time with you know that if you have any of the

following symptoms, they should get medical treatment for you immediately.

- confusion
- seizures
- loss of consciousness

Call your doctor immediately if you have any of the following symptoms of hyperglycemia (high blood sugar):

- extreme thirst
- frequent urination
- extreme hunger
- weakness
- blurred vision

If high blood sugar is not treated, a serious, life-threatening condition called diabetic ketoacidosis could develop. Call your doctor immediately if you have any of these symptoms:

- dry mouth
- upset stomach and vomiting
- shortness of breath
- breath that smells fruity
- decreased consciousness

Rosiglitazone may cause side effects. Tell your doctor if any of these symptoms are severe or do not go away:

- headache
- runny nose and other cold symptoms
- sore throat
- back pain
- painful or irregular menstrual periods

Some side effects can be serious. If you experience any of the following symptoms, or those listed in the IMPORTANT WARNING section, call your doctor immediately:

- loss of appetite
- nausea
- vomiting
- dark urine
- yellowing of the skin or eyes
- blurred vision
- vision loss
- difficulty seeing colors
- difficulty seeing in the dark
- pale skin
- dizziness
- swelling of the eyes, face, lips, tongue, or throat
- hoarseness
- difficulty swallowing or breathing
- hives
- itching
- fever
- blisters

Rosiglitazone may cause other side effects. Call your doctor if you experience any unusual problems while you are taking this medication.

In clinical studies, more women who took rosiglitazone experienced fractures, especially of the hands, arms, feet, ankles, and lower legs than women who did not take rosiglitazone. Men who took rosiglitazone did not have a greater risk of experiencing fractures than men who did not take the medication. If you are a woman, talk to your doctor about the risk of taking this medication.

What storage conditions are needed for this medicine?

Keep this medication in the container it came in, tightly closed, and out of reach of children. Store it at room temperature and away from light, excess heat, and moisture (not in the bathroom). Throw away any medication that is outdated or no longer needed. Talk to your pharmacist about the proper disposal of your medication.

What should I do in case of overdose?

In case of overdose, call your local poison control center at 1-800-222-1222. If the victim has collapsed or is not breathing, call local emergency services at 911.

What other information should I know?

Keep all appointments with your doctor, your eye doctor, and the laboratory. Your doctor will probably order regular eye examinations and certain laboratory tests to check your body's response to rosiglitazone. Your blood sugar and glycosylated hemoglobin should be checked regularly to determine your response to rosiglitazone. Your doctor may also tell you how to check your response to rosiglitazone by measuring your blood or urine sugar levels at home. Follow these directions carefully.

You should always wear a diabetic identification bracelet to be sure you get proper treatment in an emergency.

Do not let anyone else take your medication. Ask your pharmacist any questions you have about refilling your prescription.

Dosage Facts
For Informational Purposes

Caution: Do not change your dose, how often you take your medication, or the length of time you are to take it without first talking to your healthcare provider.

The following dosage information was written using medical language for doctors and other healthcare professionals and is provided here for you to check your dosage. The dosage of this drug may differ for different patients. Therefore, always follow your doctor's instructions or the directions on the label. Contact your healthcare provider or pharmacist if you have any questions about the specific dosage of your medication after reviewing this information.

General Dosage Information

Available as rosiglitazone maleate; dosage expressed in terms of rosiglitazone.

Adult Patients

Diabetes Mellitus
Monotherapy

ORAL:
- Initially, 4 mg daily in 1 or 2 divided doses (morning and evening). If response is inadequate after 8–12 weeks, increase dosage to 8 mg daily. In clinical studies, a dosage of 4 mg twice daily resulted in the greatest reduction in fasting plasma glucose (FPG) concentrations and glycosylated hemoglobin (HbA_{1c}).

Combination Therapy with Other Antidiabetic Agents

ORAL:
- May continue current dosage of the sulfonylurea, metformin, or insulin upon initiation of rosiglitazone.
- Combination therapy with a sulfonylurea: 4 mg daily in 1 or 2 divided doses. If hypoglycemia occurs, reduce sulfonylurea dosage.
- Combination therapy with metformin: Initially, 4 mg daily in 1 or 2 divided doses. Need for adjustment of metformin dosage unlikely.
- Combination therapy with insulin: 4 mg daily in 1 or 2 divided doses. If hypoglycemia occurs or if FPG concentrations decrease to <100 mg/dL, decrease insulin dosage by 10–25%. Further adjustments should be individualized based on therapeutic response. Discontinue combination therapy in patients who do not respond (i.e., reduction in HbA_{1c} or insulin dosage) after 4–5 months of therapy or in patients with substantial adverse effects.

Rosiglitazone/Metformin Fixed-combination Therapy

ORAL:
- In patients inadequately controlled on metformin monotherapy, the usual initial dosage of rosiglitazone (in fixed combination with metformin hydrochloride) is 4 mg daily, given in 2 divided doses with meals.
- In patients inadequately controlled on rosiglitazone monotherapy, the usual initial dosage of metformin hydrochloride (in fixed combination with rosiglitazone) is 1 g daily, given in 2 divided doses with meals.
- Tablet strength of fixed-combination preparation should most closely match patient's existing dosage of rosiglitazone or metformin hydrochloride. (See Table.)

Initial Dosage of the Fixed Combination of Rosiglitazone and Metformin Hydrochloride (Avandamet[*])

Prior Therapy Total Daily Dosage	Usual Initial Dosage of Avandamet®	
	Tablet strength	Number of tablets
Metformin Hydrochloride[a]		
1 g	2 mg/500 mg	1 tablet twice daily
2 g	2 mg/1 g	1 tablet twice daily
Rosiglitazone		
4 mg	2 mg/500 mg	1 tablet twice daily
8 mg	4 mg/500 mg	1 tablet twice daily

[a]For patients on dosages of metformin hydrochloride between 1 and 2 g daily, initiation of fixed-combination preparation requires individualization of therapy.

For patients switching from combined therapy with separate preparations, the initial dosage of the fixed-combination preparation should be the same as the daily dosage of metformin hydrochloride and rosiglitazone currently being taken.

If additional glycemic control is needed, may increase dosage in increments of 4 mg of rosiglitazone and/or 500 mg of metformin hydrochloride until adequate glycemic control is achieved or a maximum dosage of 8 mg of rosiglitazone and 2 g of metformin hydrochloride is reached.

Prescribing Limits

Adult Patients

Conventional tablets: Maximum 8 mg daily (as monotherapy); no additional benefit from 12-mg daily dosages. Dosages >4 mg daily in combination with a sulfonylurea or insulin not studied or recommended.

Fixed-combination preparation: Maximum 8 mg of rosiglitazone and 2 g of metformin hydrochloride.

Special Populations

Renal Impairment
- Conventional tablets: No dosage adjustment necessary.
- Fixed-combination preparation: Contraindicated

Geriatric Patients
- Conventional tablets: No dosage adjustment necessary.
- Fixed-combination preparation: Cautious dosing recommended. Carefully assess renal function with each dosage adjustment to minimize risk of lactic acidosis. Do not titrate to maximum recommended dosage.

Other Populations
- Fixed-combination preparation: Do not titrate to maximum recommended dosage in debilitated or malnourished patients.

Rosuvastatin

(roe soo′ va sta tin)

Brand Name: Crestor®

Why is this medicine prescribed?

Rosuvastatin is used together with lifestyle changes (diet, weight-loss, exercise) to reduce the amount of cholesterol (a fat-like substance) and other fatty substances in your blood. Rosuvastatin is in a class of medications called HMG-CoA reductase inhibitors (statins). It works by slowing the production of cholesterol in the body.

Buildup of cholesterol and other fats along the walls of the blood vessels (a process known as atherosclerosis) decreases blood flow and, therefore, the oxygen supply to the heart, brain, and other parts of the body. Lowering blood levels of cholesterol and fats may help to decrease your chances of getting heart disease, angina (chest pain), strokes, and heart attacks. In addition to taking a cholesterol-lowering medication, making certain changes in your daily habits can also lower your cholesterol blood levels. You should eat a diet that is low in saturated fat and cholesterol (see SPECIAL DIETARY), exercise 30 minutes on most, if not all days, and lose weight if you are overweight.

How should this medicine be used?

Rosuvastatin comes as a tablet to take by mouth. It is usually taken once a day with or without food. Take rosuvastatin at around the same time every day. Follow the directions on your prescription label carefully, and ask your doctor or pharmacist to explain any part you do not understand. Take rosuvastatin exactly as directed. Do not take more or less of it or take it more often than prescribed by your doctor.

Your doctor will probably start you on a low dose of rosuvastatin and gradually increase your dose, not more than once every 2-4 weeks.

Continue to take rosuvastatin even if you feel well. Do not stop taking rosuvastatin without talking to your doctor.

Are there other uses for this medicine?

This medication may be prescribed for other uses; ask your doctor or pharmacist for more information.

What special precautions should I follow?

Before taking rosuvastatin,
- tell your doctor and pharmacist if you are allergic to rosuvastatin or any other medications.
- tell your doctor and pharmacist what prescription and nonprescription medications, vitamins, nutritional supplements, and herbal products you are taking or plan to take. Be sure to mention any of the following: anticoagulants ('blood thinners') such as warfarin (Coumadin); cimetidine (Tagamet); cyclosporine (Neoral, Sandimmune); ketoconazole (Nizoral); other medications for high cholesterol such as clofibrate (Atromid-S), fenofibrate (Tricor), gemfibrozil (Lopid), and niacin (Niaspan, Niacor); and spironolactone (Aldactone). Your doctor may need to change the doses of your medications or monitor you carefully for side effects.
- if you are taking aluminum and magnesium hydroxide antacids (Mylanta, Maalox), take them at least 2 hours after rosuvastatin.
- tell your doctor if you have liver disease. Your doctor will probably tell you not to take rosuvastatin.
- tell your doctor if you drink large amounts of alcohol and if you have ever had liver disease or if you have or have ever had kidney or thyroid disease.
- tell your doctor if you are pregnant or plan to become pregnant. If you become pregnant while taking rosuvastatin, call your doctor immediately. Rosuvastatin may harm the fetus.
- do not breastfeed while taking rosuvastatin.
- if you are having surgery, including dental surgery, tell the doctor or dentist that you are taking rosuvastatin.
- ask your doctor about the safe use of alcoholic beverages while you are taking rosuvastatin. Alcohol can increase the risk of serious side effects.

What special dietary instructions should I follow?

Eat a low-cholesterol, low-fat diet. This kind of diet includes cottage cheese, fat-free milk, fish (not canned in oil), vegetables, poultry, egg whites, and polyunsaturated oils and margarines (corn, safflower, canola, and soybean oils). Avoid foods with excess fat in them such as meat (especially liver and fatty meat), egg yolks, whole milk, cream, butter, shortening, lard, pastries, cakes, cookies, gravy, peanut butter, chocolate, olives, potato chips, coconut, cheese (other than cottage cheese), coconut oil, palm oil, and fried foods.

What should I do if I forget to take a dose?

Take the missed dose as soon as you remember it. However, if it is almost time for the next dose, skip the missed dose and continue your regular dosing schedule. Do not take a double dose to make up for a missed one.

What side effects can this medicine cause?

Rosuvastatin may cause side effects. Tell your doctor if any of these symptoms are severe or do not go away:

- constipation
- heartburn
- dizziness
- difficulty falling asleep or staying asleep
- depression
- joint pain
- cough

Some side effects can be serious. The following symptoms are uncommon, but if you experience any of them, call your doctor immediately:

- muscle pain, tenderness, or weakness
- lack of energy
- fever
- chest pain
- yellowing of the skin or eyes
- pain in the upper right part of the abdomen
- nausea
- extreme tiredness
- unusual bleeding or bruising
- loss of appetite
- flu-like symptoms
- sore throat, chills, or other signs of infection
- rash
- hives
- itching
- difficulty breathing or swallowing
- swelling of the face, throat, tongue, lips, eyes, hands, feet, ankles, or lower legs
- hoarseness
- numbness or tingling in fingers or toes

Rosuvastatin may cause other side effects. Call your doctor if you have any unusual problems while taking this medication.

If you experience a serious side effect, you or your doctor may send a report to the Food and Drug Administration's (FDA) MedWatch Adverse Event Reporting program online [at http://www.fda.gov/MedWatch/index.html] or by phone [1-800-332-1088].

What storage conditions are needed for this medicine?

Keep this medication in the container it came in, tightly closed, and out of reach of children. Store it at room temperature and away from excess heat and moisture (not in the bathroom). Throw away any medication that is outdated or no longer needed. Talk to your pharmacist about the proper disposal of your medication.

What should I do in case of overdose?

In case of overdose, call your local poison control center at 1-800-222-1222. If the victim has collapsed or is not breathing, call local emergency services at 911.

What other information should I know?

Keep all appointments with your doctor and the laboratory. Your doctor will order certain lab tests to check your body's response to rosuvastatin.

Before having any laboratory test, tell your doctor and the laboratory personnel that you are taking rosuvastatin.

Do not let anyone else take your medication. Ask your pharmacist any questions you have about refilling your prescription.

Dosage Facts
For Informational Purposes

Caution: Do not change your dose, how often you take your medication, or the length of time you are to take it without first talking to your healthcare provider.

The following dosage information was written using medical language for doctors and other healthcare professionals and is provided here for you to check your dosage. The dosage of this drug may differ for different patients. Therefore, always follow your doctor's instructions or the directions on the label. Contact your healthcare provider or pharmacist if you have any questions about the specific dosage of your medication after reviewing this information.

General Dosage Information

Available as rosuvastatin calcium; dosage expressed in terms of rosuvastatin.

When initiating statin therapy or switching from another statin, select appropriate initial dosage, then carefully adjust dosage according to individual requirements and response.

Adult Patients

Dyslipidemias
Primary Hypercholesterolemia and Mixed Dyslipidemia

ORAL:

- Usual initial dosage is 10 mg once daily. Initiate at 5 mg once daily in patients requiring less aggressive LDL-cholesterol reductions, patients with predisposing factors for myopathy, or patients at risk of increased exposure to rosuvastatin (e.g., Asian patients, patients receiving concomitant cyclosporine therapy, patients with severe renal impairment). Initiate at 20 mg once daily in patients with marked hypercholesterolemia (LDL-cholesterol >190 mg/dL) and aggressive lipid targets.
- Determine serum lipoprotein concentrations within 2–4 weeks after initiating and/or titrating therapy and adjust dosage accordingly. Usual maintenance dosage is 5–40 mg once daily.
- Reserve 40-mg daily dosage for patients who have not achieved their LDL-cholesterol goal with the 20-mg daily dosage.

Homozygous Familial Hypercholesterolemia

ORAL:

- Initially, 20 mg once daily. Dosage can be increased up to 40 mg once daily.

Hypertriglyceridemia

ORAL:

- Initially, 10 mg once daily. Usual maintenance dosage is 5–40 mg once daily.

Prescribing Limits

Adult Patients

Dyslipidemias

ORAL:

- Maximum 40 mg once daily.

Special Populations

Asian Patients
- Initially, 5 mg once daily. When contemplating dosage escalation in patients experiencing inadequate response with 5, 10, or 20 mg daily, consider potential for increased systemic exposure in Asian patients relative to Caucasian patients.

Renal Impairment
- Dosage modification not necessary in patients with mild to moderate renal impairment.
- Patients with severe renal impairment (Cl_{cr} <30 mL/minute) not undergoing hemodialysis: Initially, 5 mg once daily; dosage can be increased up to 10 mg once daily.

Rotavirus Vaccine

Brand Name: RotaTeq®

What is rotavirus?

Rotavirus is a virus that causes severe diarrhea, mostly in babies and young children. It is often accompanied by vomiting and fever. Rotavirus is not the only cause of severe diarrhea, but it is one of the most serious. Each year in the United States rotavirus is responsible for:

- more than 400,000 doctor visits
- more than 200,000 emergency room visits
- 55,000 to 70,000 hospitalizations
- 20-60 deaths

Almost all children in the U.S. are infected with rotavirus before their 5th birthday. Children are most likely to get rotavirus disease between November and May, depending on the part of the country. Your child can get rotavirus infection by being around other children who are already infected.

Rotavirus vaccine

Better hygiene and sanitation have not been very good at reducing rotavirus disease. Rotavirus vaccine is the best way to protect children against rotavirus disease.

Rotavirus vaccine is an oral (swallowed) vaccine; it is not given by injection.

Rotavirus vaccine will not prevent diarrhea or vomiting caused by other germs, but it is very good at preventing diarrhea and vomiting caused by rotavirus. About 98% of children who get the vaccine are protected from *severe* rotavirus diarrhea, and about 74% do not get rotavirus diarrhea at all.

Children who get the vaccine are also much less likely to be hospitalized or to see a doctor because of rotavirus infection.

Who should get rotavirus vaccine and when?

- Children should get 3 doses of rotavirus vaccine. They are recommended at these ages: 2 months of age, 4 months of age, and 6 months of age.
- The first dose should be given between 6 and 12 weeks of age. The vaccine has not been studied when started among children outside that age range.
- Children should have gotten all 3 doses by 32 weeks of age.
- Rotavirus vaccine may be given at the same time as other childhood vaccines. Children who get the vaccine may be fed normally afterward.

Who should *not* get rotavirus vaccine or should wait?

- A child who has had a severe (life-threatening) allergic reaction to a dose of rotavirus vaccine should not get another dose. A child who has a severe (life threatening) allergy to any component of rotavirus vaccine should not get the vaccine. Tell your doctor if your child has any severe allergies that you know of.
- Children who are moderately or severely ill at the time the vaccination is scheduled should probably wait until they recover. This includes children who have diarrhea or vomiting. Ask your doctor or nurse. Children with mild illnesses should usually get the vaccine.
- Check with your doctor if your child has any ongoing digestive problems.
- Check with your doctor if your child's immune system is weakened because of: HIV/AIDS, or any other disease that affects the immune system; treatment with drugs such as long-term steroids; cancer, or cancer treatment with x-rays or drugs.
- Check with your doctor if your child recently had a blood transfusion or received any other blood product (such as immune globulin).
- In the late 1990s a different type of rotavirus vaccine was used. This vaccine was found to be associated with an uncommon type of bowel obstruction called "intussusception," and was taken off the market. The new rotavirus vaccine has been tested with more than 70,000 children and has not been associated with intussusception. However, once a person has had intussusception, from any cause, they are at higher risk for getting it again. **So as a precaution, it is suggested that if a child has had intussusception they should not get rotavirus vaccine.**

What are the risks from rotavirus vaccine?

A vaccine, like any medicine, could possibly cause serious problems, such as severe allergic reactions. The risk of rotavirus vaccine causing serious harm, or death, is extremely small. Getting rotavirus vaccine is much safer than getting the disease.

Mild Problems:

- Children are slightly (1-3%) more likely to have mild, temporary diarrhea or vomiting within 7 days after getting a dose of rotavirus vaccine than children who have not gotten the vaccine.

Moderate or Severe Problems:

- Moderate or severe problems have not been associated with this vaccine.
- If rare reactions occur with any new product, they may not be identified until thousands, or millions, of people have used it. Like all vaccines, rotavirus vaccine will continue to be monitored for unusual or severe problems.

What if there is a moderate or severe reaction?

What should I look for?

- Any unusual condition, such as a high fever or behavior changes. Signs of a serious allergic reaction can include difficulty breathing, hoarseness or wheezing, hives, paleness, weakness, a fast heart beat or dizziness.

What should I do?

- Call a doctor, or get the person to a doctor right away.
- Tell your doctor what happened, the date and time it happened, and when the vaccination was given.
- Ask your health care provider to file a Vaccine Adverse Event Reporting System (VAERS) form if you have any reaction to the vaccine. Or call VAERS yourself at 1-800-822-7967, or visit their website at http://vaers.hhs.gov.

The National Vaccine Injury Compensation Program

In the rare event that you or your child has a serious reaction to a vaccine, a federal program has been created to help pay for the care of those who have been harmed.

For details about the National Vaccine Injury Compensation Program, call 1-800-338-2382 or visit the program's website at http://www.hrsa.gov/vaccinecompensation.

How can I learn more?

- Ask your doctor or other health care provider. They can give you the vaccine package insert or suggest other sources of information.
- Call your local or state health department's immunization program.
- Contact the Centers for Disease Control and Prevention (CDC): call 1-800-232-4636 (1-800-CDC-INFO) or visit the National Immunization Program's website at http://www.cdc.gov/nip

Rotavirus Vaccine Information Statement. U.S. Department of Health and Human Services/Centers for Disease Control and Prevention National Immunization Program. 4/12/2006.

Salmeterol Oral Inhalation

(sal me′ te role)

Brand Name: Serevent®

Important Warning

In a large clinical study, more patients with asthma who used salmeterol died of asthma problems than patients with asthma who did not use salmeterol. If you have asthma, use of salmeterol may increase the chance that you will experience serious or fatal asthma problems. Your doctor will only prescribe salmeterol if other medications have not controlled your asthma or if your asthma is so severe that two medications are needed to control it. Salmeterol should not be the first or the only medication that you use to treat your asthma.

Do not use salmeterol if you have asthma that is quickly getting worse. Tell your doctor if you have had many severe asthma attacks or if you have ever been hospitalized because of asthma symptoms. If you have any of the following signs of worsening asthma, call your doctor immediately:

- your short-acting inhaler [inhaled medication such as albuterol (Proventil, Ventolin) that is used to treat sudden attacks of asthma symptoms] does not work as well as it did in the past
- you need to use more puffs than usual of your short-acting inhaler or use it more often
- you need to use four or more puffs per day of your short-acting inhaler for two or more days in a row
- you use more than one canister (200 inhalations) of your short-acting inhaler during an 8-week period
- your peak-flow meter (home device used to test breathing) results show your breathing problems are worsening
- you need to go to the emergency room for asthma treatment.
- your symptoms do not improve after you use salmeterol regularly for one week or your symptoms get worse at any time during your treatment

Talk to your doctor about the risks of using this medication.

Your doctor or pharmacist will give you the manufacturer's patient information sheet (Medication Guide) when you begin treatment with salmeterol and each time you refill your prescription. Read the information carefully and ask your doctor or pharmacist if you have any questions. You can also visit the Food and Drug Administration (FDA) website (http://www.fda.gov/cder) or the manufacturer's website to obtain the Medication Guide.

Why is this medicine prescribed?

Salmeterol is used to treat wheezing, shortness of breath, and breathing difficulties caused by asthma and chronic obstructive pulmonary disease (COPD; a group of lung diseases that includes chronic bronchitis and emphysema). It also is used to prevent bronchospasm (breathing difficulties) during exercise. Salmeterol is in a class of medications called long-acting beta agonists (LABAs). It works by relaxing and opening air passages in the lungs, making it easier to breathe.

How should this medicine be used?

Salmeterol comes as a dry powder to inhale by mouth using a specially designed inhaler. When salmeterol is used to treat asthma or COPD, it is usually used twice a day, in the morning and evening, about 12 hours apart. Use salmeterol at around the same times every day. When salmeterol is used to prevent breathing difficulties during exercise, it is usually used at least 30 minutes before exercise, but not more often than once every 12 hours. If you are using salmeterol twice a day on a regular basis, do not use another dose before exercising. Follow the directions on your prescription label carefully, and ask your doctor or pharmacist to explain any part you do not understand. Use salmeterol exactly as directed. Do not use more or less of it or use it more often than prescribed by your doctor.

Talk to your doctor about how you should take your other oral or inhaled medications for asthma during your treatment with salmeterol. If you were taking a corticosteroid (a type of medication used to prevent airway swelling in patients with asthma), you doctor will probably tell you to continue taking it just as you did before you began using salmeterol. If you were using a short acting beta agonist inhaler such as albuterol (Proventil, Ventolin) on a regular basis, your doctor will probably tell you to stop using it regularly, but to continue to use it to treat sudden attacks of asthma symptoms. Follow these directions carefully. Do not change the way you use any of your medications without talking to your doctor.

Do not use salmeterol during an attack of asthma or COPD. Your doctor will prescribe a short-acting inhaler to use during attacks.

Salmeterol controls the symptoms of asthma and other lung diseases but does not cure these conditions. Do not stop using salmeterol without talking to your doctor. If you suddenly stop using salmeterol, your symptoms may worsen.

Before you use the salmeterol inhaler the first time, ask your doctor, pharmacist, or respiratory therapist to show you how to use it. Practice using the inhaler while he or she watches.

To use the inhaler, follow these steps:

1. If you will be using a new inhaler for the first time, remove it from the box and the foil wrapper. Fill in the blanks on the inhaler label with the date that you opened the pouch and the date 6 weeks later when you must replace the inhaler.
2. Hold the inhaler in one hand, and put the thumb of your other hand on the thumbgrip. Push your thumb away from you as far as it will go until the mouthpiece appears and snaps into position.
3. Hold the inhaler in a level, horizontal position with the mouthpiece toward you. Slide the lever away from you as far as it will go until it clicks.
4. Every time the lever is pushed back, a dose is ready to inhale. You will see the number in the dose counter go down. Do not waste doses by closing or tilting the inhaler, playing with the lever, or advancing the lever more than once.
5. Hold the inhaler level and away from your mouth, and breathe out as far as you comfortably can.
6. Keep the inhaler in a level, flat position. Put the mouthpiece to your lips. Breathe in quickly and deeply though the inhaler, not through your nose.
7. Remove the inhaler from your mouth, and hold your breath for 10 seconds or as long as you comfortably can. Breathe out slowly.
8. You will probably taste or feel the salmeterol powder released by the inhaler. Even if you do not, do not inhale another dose. If you are not sure you are getting your dose of salmeterol, call your doctor or pharmacist.
9. Put your thumb on the thumbgrip and slide it back toward you as far as it will go. The device will click shut.

Never exhale into the inhaler, take the inhaler apart, or wash the mouthpiece or any part of the inhaler. Keep the inhaler dry. Do not use the inhaler with a spacer.

Are there other uses for this medicine?

This medication may be prescribed for other uses; ask your doctor or pharmacist for more information.

What special precautions should I follow?

Before using salmeterol,
- tell your doctor and pharmacist if you are allergic to salmeterol, any other medications, milk protein, or any foods.
- tell your doctor if you use another LABA such as fluticasone and salmeterol combination (Advair) or formoterol (Foradil). These medications should not be used with salmeterol. Your doctor will tell you which medication you should use and which medication you should stop using.
- tell your doctor and pharmacist what prescription and nonprescription medications, vitamins, nutritional supplements, and herbal products you are taking. Be sure to mention any of the following: beta blockers such as atenolol (Tenormin), labetalol (Normodyne), metopro-

lol (Lopressor, Toprol XL), nadolol (Corgard), and propranolol (Inderal); diuretics ('water pills'); and other medications for asthma or COPD. Also tell your doctor or pharmacist if you are taking the following medications or have stopped taking them within the past 2 weeks: antidepressants such as amitriptyline (Elavil), amoxapine (Asendin), clomipramine (Anafranil), desipramine (Norpramin), doxepin (Adapin, Sinequan), imipramine (Tofranil), nortriptyline (Aventyl, Pamelor), protriptyline (Vivactil), and trimipramine (Surmontil); and monoamine oxidase (MAO) inhibitors including isocarboxazid (Marplan), phenelzine (Nardil), selegiline (Eldepryl), and tranylcypromine (Parnate). Your doctor may need to change the doses of your medications or monitor you carefully for side effects.
- tell your doctor if you have or have ever had irregular heartbeat, high blood pressure, hyperthyroidism (overactive thyroid), diabetes, seizures, or liver or heart disease.
- tell your doctor if you are pregnant, plan to become pregnant, or are breast-feeding. If you become pregnant while using salmeterol, call your doctor.

What special dietary instructions should I follow?

Unless your doctor tells you otherwise, continue your normal diet.

What should I do if I forget to take a dose?

Skip the missed dose and continue your regular dosing schedule. Do not inhale a double dose to make up for a missed one.

What side effects can this medicine cause?

Salmeterol may cause side effects. Tell your doctor if any of these symptoms are severe or do not go away:
- shaking of a part of your body that you cannot control
- headache
- nervousness
- dizziness
- cough
- stuffed nose
- runny nose
- ear pain
- pale skin
- muscle pain, stiffness, or cramps
- sore throat
- throat irritation
- flu-like symptoms
- nausea
- heartburn
- tooth pain
- dry mouth
- sores or white patches in the mouth
- red or irritated eyes

- difficulty falling asleep or staying asleep
- burning or tingling of the hands or feet

Some side effects can be serious. If you experience any of the following symptoms, call your doctor immediately:

- coughing, wheezing, or chest tightness that begins soon after you inhale salmeterol
- fast or pounding heartbeat
- chest pain
- rash
- hives
- swelling of the face, throat, tongue, lips, eyes, hands, feet, ankles, or lower legs
- hoarseness
- choking or difficulty swallowing
- loud, high-pitched breathing

Salmeterol may cause other side effects. Call your doctor if you have any unusual problems while you are taking this medication.

If you experience a serious side effect, you or your doctor may send a report to the Food and Drug Administration's (FDA) MedWatch Adverse Event Reporting program online [at http://www.fda.gov/MedWatch/index.html] or by phone [1-800-332-1088].

What storage conditions are needed for this medicine?

Keep this medication in the container it came in, tightly closed, and out of reach of children. Store it at room temperature and away from excess heat and moisture (not in the bathroom). Throw away the inhaler 6 weeks after you remove it from the foil overwrap or after every blister has been used (when the dose indicator reads 0), whichever comes first. Talk to your pharmacist about the proper disposal of your medication.

What should I do in case of overdose?

In case of overdose, call your local poison control center at 1-800-222-1222. If the victim has collapsed or is not breathing, call local emergency services at 911.

Symptoms of overdose may include:

- seizures
- chest pain
- dizziness
- fainting
- blurred vision
- fast, pounding, or irregular heartbeat
- nervousness
- headache
- shaking of a part of your body that you cannot control
- muscle cramps or weakness
- dry mouth
- nausea
- dizziness
- excessive tiredness
- lack of energy
- difficulty falling asleep or staying asleep

What other information should I know?

Keep all appointments with your doctor.

Do not let anyone else use your medication. Ask your pharmacist any questions you have about refilling your prescription.

Dosage Facts
For Informational Purposes

Caution: Do not change your dose, how often you take your medication, or the length of time you are to take it without first talking to your healthcare provider.

The following dosage information was written using medical language for doctors and other healthcare professionals and is provided here for you to check your dosage. The dosage of this drug may differ for different patients. Therefore, always follow your doctor's instructions or the directions on the label. Contact your healthcare provider or pharmacist if you have any questions about the specific dosage of your medication after reviewing this information.

General Dosage Information

Available as salmeterol xinafoate; dosage expressed in terms of salmeterol.

Each blister in the Serevent® device contains 50 mcg of salmeterol as salmeterol xinafoate inhalation powder. However, the precise amount of drug delivered to the lungs depends on factors such as the patient's inspiratory flow.

Pediatric Patients

Asthma

ORAL INHALATION:
- Serevent® Diskus®: 50 mcg (1 inhalation) twice daily in children ≥4 years of age.

Exercise-induced Bronchospasm

ORAL INHALATION:
- 50 mcg (1 inhalation) administered via the Serevent® Diskus® device at least 30 minutes before exercise for children ≥4 years of age.

Adult Patients

Asthma

ORAL INHALATION:
- Serevent® Diskus®: 50 mcg (1 inhalation) twice daily.

Exercise-induced Bronchospasm

ORAL INHALATION:
- Serevent® Diskus®: 50 mcg (1 inhalation) administered at least 30 minutes before exercise.

COPD

ORAL INHALATION:
- Serevent® Diskus®: 50 mcg (1 inhalation) twice daily.

Pediatric Patients

Asthma

ORAL:

- Children ≥4 years of age receiving Serevent® Diskus®: Maximum 50 mcg (1 inhalation) twice daily.

Exercise-induced Bronchospasm

ORAL INHALATION:

- Serevent® Diskus®: 50 mcg (1 inhalation) twice daily (every 12 hours) in children ≥4 years of age.

Adult Patients

Asthma

ORAL INHALATION:

- Serevent® Diskus®: Maximum 50 mcg (1 inhalation) twice daily.

Exercise-induced Bronchospasm

ORAL INHALATION:

- Serevent® Diskus®: 50 mcg (1 inhalation) twice daily (every 12 hours).

COPD

ORAL INHALATION:

- Serevent® Diskus®: 50 mcg (1 inhalation) twice daily.

Special Populations

Hepatic Impairment

- Decreased clearance.
- Monitor patients closely; however, dosage adjustments not required.

Renal Impairment

- Pharmacokinetics have not been studied; dosage adjustments not required.

Saquinavir

(sa kwin' a veer)

Brand Name: Invirase®, Fortovase®

Important Warning

Roche Pharmaceuticals has announced that Fortovase® brand saquinavir capsules will no longer be available in the United States by February 15, 2006. This action is not based on any known safety problems with Fortovase, but is being taken because Fortovase is not widely used. If you are taking Fortovase, talk to your doctor about switching to another treatment.

Invirase® brand hard gelatin capsules and tablets and Fortovase® brand soft gelatin capsules all contain saquinavir, but can not be substituted for one another. Invirase must be taken with another medication called ritonavir (Norvir), which is called "boosted" therapy. Fortovase may be taken without ritonavir, but it must be taken more often and at a different dose than Invirase. Do not take Fortovase and Invirase at the same time. Take only the brand of saquinavir that was prescribed by your doctor and do not switch to the other brand of saquinavir unless your doctor tells you that you should. Each time you have your prescription filled, look at the brand name printed on your prescription label and at the tablets or capsules inside your bottle to be sure that you have received the right medication. Ask your doctor if you have not yet started taking saquinavir and don't know how your tablets or capsules should look.

Why is this medicine prescribed?

Saquinavir is used in combination with other medications to treat human immunodeficiency virus (HIV) infection in patients with or without acquired immunodeficiency syndrome (AIDS). Saquinavir is in a class of antiviral medications called protease inhibitors. It works by slowing the spread of HIV in the body. Saquinavir does not cure HIV and may not prevent you from developing HIV-related illnesses. Saquinavir does not prevent the spread of HIV to other people.

How should this medicine be used?

Saquinavir comes as a hard gelatin capsule (Invirase), a tablet (Invirase), and a soft gelatin capsule (Fortovase) to take by mouth. The hard gelatin capsule and tablet are usually taken with ritonavir (Norvir) two times a day with a meal or up to 2 hours after a full meal. The soft gelatin capsule is usually taken three times a day with a meal or up to 2 hours after a meal. Take saquinavir at around the same times every day. It may be easier to remember to take saquinavir if you take it with meals. Follow the directions on your prescription label carefully, and ask your doctor or pharmacist to explain any part you do not understand. Take saquinavir exactly as directed. Do not take more or less of it or take it more often than prescribed by your doctor.

Continue to take saquinavir even if you feel well. Do not stop taking saquinavir without talking to your doctor. If you miss doses, take less than the prescribed dose or stop taking saquinavir, your condition may become more difficult to treat.

Are there other uses for this medicine?

Saquinavir soft gelatin capsules are also used to help prevent infection in health care workers or other people who were accidentally exposed to HIV. Talk to your doctor about the possible risks of using this medication for your condition.

This medication may be prescribed for other uses; ask your doctor or pharmacist for more information.

What special precautions should I follow?

Before taking saquinavir,

- tell your doctor and pharmacist if you are allergic to saquinavir, any other medications, or any of the ingredients in saquinavir. Ask your pharmacist for a list of the ingredients.
- do not take astemizole (Hismanal) (no longer available in the United States); cisapride (Propulsid) (no longer available in the United States); ergot medications such as dihydroergotamine (Migranal), ergoloid mesylates (Germinal, Hydergine), ergonovine (Ergotrate), ergotamine (Cafergot, Wigraine), methylergonovine (Methergine), and methysergide (Sansert); medications for irregular heartbeat such as amiodarone (Cordarone, Pacerone), bepridil (not available in the United States), flecainide (Tambocor), propafenone (Rhythmol), or quinidine (Quinidex); midazolam (Versed); pimozide (Orap); rifampin (Rifadin, Rimactane, in Rifamate); terfenadine (Seldane) (no longer available in the United States); or triazolam (Halcion) while taking saquinavir.
- tell your doctor and pharmacist what other prescription and nonprescription medications, vitamins, and nutritional supplements you are taking or plan to take. Be sure to mention any of the following: anticoagulants ('blood thinners') such as warfarin (Coumadin); antifungals such as fluconazole (Diflucan), itraconazole (Sporanox), ketoconazole (Nizoral), and voriconazole (Vfend); aprepitant (Emend); benzodiazepines such as alprazolam (Xanax), clorazepate (ClorazeCaps, Tranxene, others), diazepam (Valium), and flurazepam (Dalmane); buspirone (BuSpar); calcium channel blockers such as amlodipine (Norvasc), diltiazem (Cardizem, Dilacor, Tiazac, others), felodipine (Plendil), isradipine (DynaCirc), nicardipine (Cardene), nifedipine (Adalat, Procardia), nimodipine (Nimotop), nisoldipine (Sular), and verapamil (Calan, Covera, Isoptin, Verelan); cholesterol-lowering medications (statins) such as atorvastatin (Lipitor), lovastatin (Advicor, Altocor, Mevacor), and simvastatin (Zocor); chlorpheniramine (antihistamine in over-the-counter cough and cold medications); cimetidine (Tagamet); clarithromycin (Biaxin, in Prevpac); clindamycin (Cleocin); dapsone (Avlosulfon); dexamethasone (Decadron, Dexone); disopyramide (Norpace); erythromycin (E.E.S., E-Mycin, Erythrocin); fentanyl (Duragesic); fluoxetine (Prozac, Sarafem); fluvoxamine (Luvox); griseofulvin (Fulvicin, Grifulvin, Gris-PEG); haloperidol (Haldol); hormonal contraceptives (birth control pills, rings, and patches); immunosuppressants such as cyclosporine (Neoral, Sandimmune), tacrolimus (Protopic), or rapamycin (sirolimus, Rapamune); insulin or oral medications for diabetes; isoniazid (INH, Nydrazid); medications to treat erectile dysfunction such as sildenafil (Viagra), tadalafil (Cialis), and vardenafil (Levitra); medications to treat HIV or AIDS including atazanavir (Reyataz), delavir-

dine (Rescriptor), efavirenz (Sustiva), indinavir (Crixivan), lopinavir (in Kaletra), nelfinavir (Viracept), nevirapine (Viramune), or ritonavir (Norvir, in Kaletra); medications to treat seizures such as carbamazepine (Carbatrol, Epitol, Tegretol), phenytoin (Dilantin, Phenytek), and phenobarbital (Luminal, Solfoton); methadone (Dolophine, Methadose); nefazodone; phenylbutazone (Azolid, Butazolidin, others) (no longer available in the United States); propranolol (Inderal, in Inderide); quinine; ranitidine (Zantac); rifabutin (Mycobutin); sertraline (Zoloft); tamoxifen (Nolvadex); trazodone; tricyclic antidepressants including amitriptyline (in Limbitrol), clomipramine (Anafranil), desipramine (Norpramin), doxepin (Sinequan), imipramine (Tofranil), others; troleandomycin (TAO); vincristine; and zafirlukast (Accolate). Other medications may interact with saquinavir, so be sure to tell your doctor and pharmacist about all the medications you are taking, even those that do not appear on this list. Your doctor may need to change the doses of your medications or monitor you carefully for side effects.
- tell your doctor what herbal products you are taking or plan to take, especially St. John's wort and garlic capsules.
- tell your doctor if you drink or have ever drunk large amounts of alcohol, if you have ever taken any form of saquinavir in the past, and if you or anyone in your family has or has ever had diabetes. Also tell your doctor if you have or have ever had high cholesterol or triglycerides (fats in the blood); hemophilia (a bleeding disorder); or heart, kidney, or liver disease.
- tell your doctor if you are pregnant or plan to become pregnant. If you become pregnant while taking saquinavir, call your doctor. You should not breastfeed if you are infected with HIV or are taking saquinavir.
- if you are having surgery, including dental surgery, tell the doctor or dentist that you are taking saquinavir.
- you should be aware that your body fat may increase or move to different areas of your body, such as your upper back, neck ("buffalo hump"), breasts, and around your stomach. You may notice a loss of body fat from your face, legs, and arms.

What special dietary instructions should I follow?

Talk to your doctor about eating grapefruit and drinking grapefruit juice while taking this medication.

What should I do if I forget to take a dose?

Take the missed dose as soon as you remember it. However, if it is almost time for the next dose, skip the missed dose and continue your regular dosing schedule. Do not take a double dose to make up for a missed one.

What side effects can this medicine cause?

Saquinavir may cause side effects. Tell your doctor if any of these symptoms are severe or do not go away:

- diarrhea
- stomach pain
- upset stomach
- vomiting
- heartburn
- gas or bloating
- constipation
- change in the way food tastes
- increased appetite
- sores in mouth
- headache
- weakness
- tiredness
- dizziness
- anxiety
- depression
- difficulty falling asleep or staying asleep
- runny nose
- pain, burning, numbness, or tingling in the hands or feet
- warts
- muscle or back pain
- changes in sex drive

Some side effects can be serious. If you experience any of these symptoms, call your doctor immediately:

- rash
- itching
- chest pain
- shortness of breath
- flu-like symptoms
- fever
- yellowing of the skin or eyes
- extreme tiredness
- lack of energy
- loss of appetite
- pain in the upper right part of the stomach
- cough

Saquinavir may increase the sugar level in your blood. If you experience any of the following symptoms, call your doctor immediately:

- thirst
- dry mouth
- tiredness
- flushing
- dry lips or skin
- frequent urination
- loss of appetite
- trouble breathing or fast breathing
- upset stomach
- vomiting
- fruity breath
- loss of consciousness

Saquinavir may cause other side effects. Call your doctor if you have any unusual problems while taking this medication.

If you experience a serious side effect, you or your doctor may send a report to the Food and Drug Administration's (FDA) MedWatch Adverse Event Reporting program online [at http://www.fda.gov/MedWatch/index.html] or by phone [1-800-332-1088].

What storage conditions are needed for this medicine?

Keep this medication in the container it came in, tightly closed, and out of reach of children. Store it at room temperature and away from excess heat and moisture (not in the bathroom). Throw away any medication that is outdated or no longer needed. Talk to your pharmacist about the proper disposal of your medication.

What should I do in case of overdose?

In case of overdose, call your local poison control center at 1-800-222-1222. If the victim has collapsed or is not breathing, call local emergency services at 911.

Symptoms of overdose may include:

- throat pain

What other information should I know?

Keep all appointments with your doctor and the laboratory. Your doctor will order certain lab tests before and during treatment to check your body's response to saquinavir.

Do not let anyone else take your medication. Ask your pharmacist any questions you have about refilling your prescription.

Dosage Facts
For Informational Purposes

Caution: Do not change your dose, how often you take your medication, or the length of time you are to take it without first talking to your healthcare provider.

The following dosage information was written using medical language for doctors and other healthcare professionals and is provided here for you to check your dosage. The dosage of this drug may differ for different patients. Therefore, always follow your doctor's instructions or the directions on the label. Contact your healthcare provider or pharmacist if you have any questions about the specific dosage of your medication after reviewing this information.

General Dosage Information

Available as saquinavir mesylate; dosage expressed as saquinavir.

Must be given in conjunction with other antiretrovirals. *If used with efavirenz or nelfinavir, dosage adjustment recommended.*

Pediatric Patients

Treatment of HIV Infection

ORAL:

- Adolescents ≥16 years of age: 1 g twice daily in conjunction with low-dose ritonavir (100 mg twice daily). Alternatively, 1 g twice daily in conjunction with usual dosage of lopinavir/ritonavir twice daily.

Adult Patients

Treatment of HIV Infection

ORAL:

- 1 g twice daily in conjunction with low-dose ritonavir (100 mg twice daily). Alternatively, 1 g twice daily in conjunction with usual dosage of lopinavir/ritonavir twice daily.

Postexposure Prophylaxis of HIV†

Occupational Exposure†

ORAL:

- 1 g twice daily with low-dose ritonavir (100 mg twice daily).
- Used in alternative expanded regimens that include saquinavir with low-dose ritonavir and 2 NRTIs.
- Initiate postexposure prophylaxis as soon as possible following exposure (within hours rather than days) and continue for 4 weeks, if tolerated.

Nonoccupational Exposure†

ORAL:

- 1 g twice daily in conjunction with low-dose ritonavir (100 mg twice daily) or, alternatively, 400 mg twice daily in conjunction with low-dose ritonavir (400 mg twice daily).
- Used in alternative PI-based regimens that include ritonavir-boosted saquinavir and (lamivudine or emtricitabine) and (zidovudine or stavudine or abacavir or tenofovir or didanosine).
- Initiate postexposure prophylaxis as soon as possible following exposure (preferably ≤72 hours after exposure) and continue for 28 days.

Special Populations

Hepatic Impairment

Treatment of HIV Infection

- Dosage recommendations not available; use with caution in mild to moderate hepatic impairment. Contraindicated in severe hepatic impairment.

Renal Impairment

Treatment of HIV Infection

- No initial dosage adjustment needed. Use with caution in severe renal impairment.

Geriatric Patients

- Select dosage with caution because of age-related decreases in hepatic, renal, and/or cardiac function and concomitant disease and drug therapy.

† Use is not currently included in the labeling approved by the US Food and Drug Administration.

Sargramostim Injection

(sar gram′ oh stim)

Brand Name: Leukine®

About Your Treatment

Your doctor has ordered sargramostim to help your bone marrow make new white blood cells. The drug will be either given subcutaneously (beneath your skin) or added to an intravenous fluid that will drip through a needle or catheter placed in your vein for 2 hours once a day for 14-21 days.

Sargramostim is a synthetic version of substances naturally produced by your body. It helps you to fight infections so you can receive your next chemotherapy cycle as scheduled.

Your health care provider (doctor, nurse, or pharmacist) may measure the effectiveness and side effects of your treatment using laboratory tests and physical examinations. It is important to keep all appointments with your doctor and the laboratory. The length of treatment depends on how you respond to the medication.

Precautions

Before administering sargramostim,

- tell your doctor and pharmacist if you are allergic to any drugs.
- tell your doctor and pharmacist what prescription and nonprescription medications you are taking, especially cancer chemotherapy medications, dexamethasone (Decadron), lithium (Lithobid), prednisone, zidovudine (AZT, Retrovir), and vitamins.
- tell your doctor if you are pregnant, plan to become pregnant, or are breast-feeding. If you become pregnant while taking sargramostim, call your doctor.

Administering Your Medication

Before you administer sargramostim, look at the solution closely. It should be clear and free of floating material. Observe the solution container to make sure there are no leaks. Do not use the solution if it is discolored, if it contains particles, or if the container leaks. Use a new solution, but show the damaged one to your health care provider.

It is important that you use your medication exactly as directed. Do not change your dosing schedule without talking to your health care provider. Patients with severe anemia often feel very tired and weak. Most patients start to feel better about 6 weeks after starting sargramostim. Do not stop your therapy on your own for any reason because your ability to avoid blood transfusions could be hampered.

Side Effects

The most common side effect during sargramostim therapy is mild bone pain, usually in the lower back or pelvis and lasting only a few days. Another common side effect is a flu-like syndrome with fever, fatigue, chills, and muscle aches. Your doctor may recommend that you take acetaminophen or other painkillers.

Tell your health care provider if any of these symptoms are severe or do not go away:

- headache
- diarrhea
- skin rash or itching
- weakness
- dizziness or faintness
- flushing of the face

If you experience any of the following symptoms, call your health care provider immediately:

- fever
- shortness of breath
- sudden weight gain
- swelling of the lower legs or feet

If you experience a serious side effect, you or your doctor may send a report to the Food and Drug Administration's (FDA) MedWatch Adverse Event Reporting program online [at http://www.fda.gov/MedWatch/index.html] or by phone [1-800-332-1088].

Storage Conditions

- Your health care provider probably will give you a several-day supply of sargramostim at a time. Your health care provider may give you directions on how to prepare each dose. Store the vials in the refrigerator.
- Take your next dose from the refrigerator 1 hour before using it; place it in a clean, dry area to allow it to warm to room temperature.
- Avoid shaking the vial. Use a vial only once, and do not reenter a needle into a vial. Discard unused portions and outdated medication.
- Do not allow sargramostim to freeze.

Store your medication only as directed. Make sure you understand what you need to store your medication properly.

Keep your supplies in a clean, dry place when you are not using them, and keep all medications and supplies out of reach of children. Your health care provider will tell you how to throw away used needles, syringes, tubing, and containers to avoid accidental injury.

Overdose

In case of overdose, call your local poison control center at 1-800-222-1222. If the victim has collapsed or is not breathing, call local emergency services at 911.

Signs of Infection

If you are receiving sargramostim in your vein or under your skin, you need to know the symptoms of a catheter-related infection (an infection where the needle enters your vein or skin). If you experience any of these effects near your intravenous catheter, tell your health care provider as soon as possible:

- tenderness
- warmth
- irritation
- drainage
- redness
- swelling
- pain

Dosage Facts
For Informational Purposes

Caution: Do not change your dose, how often you take your medication, or the length of time you are to take it without first talking to your healthcare provider.

The following dosage information was written using medical language for doctors and other healthcare professionals and is provided here for you to check your dosage. The dosage of this drug may differ for different patients. Therefore, always follow your doctor's instructions or the directions on the label. Contact your healthcare provider or pharmacist if you have any questions about the specific dosage of your medication after reviewing this information.

General Dosage Information

If a severe adverse reaction occurs, reduce dosage by 50% or temporarily discontinue therapy until the reaction abates.

Discontinue therapy if blast cells appear on the leukocyte differential or if disease progression occurs.

Temporarily discontinue therapy or reduce dosage by 50% if the ANC is >20,000/mm³ or if the platelet count is >500,000/mm³. Base decision to interrupt therapy or reduce dosage on the clinical condition of the patient.

Pediatric Patients

Neutropenia Associated with HIV Infection and Antiretroviral Therapy†

IV OR SUB-Q:
- Adolescents: Dosage of 250 mcg/m² administered by IV infusion or sub-Q injection once daily for 2–4 weeks has been used.

Adult Patients

Autologous or Allogeneic Bone Marrow Transplantation

IV:
- 250 mcg/m² once daily, administered by IV infusion over 2 hours. Initiate therapy 2–4 hours after infusion of bone marrow (but no sooner than 24 hours after the last course of radiation therapy or the last dose of chemotherapy). Do not initiate therapy until the posttransplantation ANC is <500/mm³. Continue until the ANC is >1500/mm³ for 3 consecutive days.

Peripheral Blood Progenitor Cell Transplantation
Mobilization of Hematopoietic Progenitor Cells

IV OR SUB-Q:

- 250 mcg/m² daily, administered by continuous IV infusion over 24 hours or by sub-Q injection once daily. Continue therapy throughout the period of PBPC collection. Usually, initiate PBPC collection by day 5 of therapy and perform daily until protocol-specified targets are achieved.
- Reduce dosage by 50% if the leukocyte count increases to >50,000/mm³.

Administration Following Reinfusion of PBPC Collection

IV OR SUB-Q:

- To accelerate myeloid engraftment following autologous PBPC transplantation, 250 mcg/m² daily, administered by continuous IV infusion over 24 hours or by sub-Q injection once daily. Initiate immediately following infusion of PBPC and continue until the ANC is >1500/mm³ for 3 consecutive days.

Bone Marrow Transplantation Failure or Engraftment Delay

IV:

- Initially, 250 mcg/m² administered by IV infusion over 2 hours once daily for 14 consecutive days. Discontinue for 7 consecutive days.
- If engraftment has not occurred after this 7-day interval, administer a second course of therapy. For the second course of therapy, administer 250 mcg/m² by IV infusion over 2 hours once daily for 14 consecutive days. Discontinue for 7 consecutive days.
- If engraftment has not occurred after this 7-day interval, administer a third course of therapy. For the third course of therapy, administer 500 mcg/m² by IV infusion over 2 hours once daily for 14 consecutive days.

Leukemias
Acute Myelogenous Leukemia

IV:

- Initially, 250 mcg/m² administered by IV infusion over 4 hours once daily. Initiate therapy on approximately day 11 or 4 days following completion of induction therapy; use only if the bone marrow is hypoplastic with <5% blast cells on day 10. If a second cycle of induction chemotherapy is necessary, administer sargramostim therapy approximately 4 days after completion of chemotherapy; use only if the bone marrow is hypoplastic with <5% blast cells. Continue sargramostim until the ANC is >1500/mm³ for 3 consecutive days or for a maximum of 42 days.
- Temporarily discontinue therapy or reduce dosage by 50% if the ANC is >20,000/mm³.
- Discontinue therapy immediately if leukemia regrowth occurs.

Myelodysplastic Syndromes† and Aplastic Anemia†
Myelodysplastic Syndromes†

IV:

- Dosages of 15–500 mcg/m² once daily, administered by IV infusion over 1–12 hours, have been used. Alternatively, dosages of 30–500 mcg/m² daily, administered by continuous IV infusion over 24 hours, have been used.

Aplastic Anemia†

IV:

- Dosages of 15–480 mcg/m² once daily, administered by IV infusion over 1–12 hours, have been used. Alternatively, dosages of 120–500 mcg/m² daily, administered by continuous IV infusion over 24 hours, have been used.

Neutropenia Associated with HIV Infection and Antiretroviral Therapy†

IV OR SUB-Q:

- Dosage of 250 mcg/m² administered by IV infusion or sub-Q injection once daily for 2–4 weeks has been used.

Prescribing Limits
Adult Patients

Bone Marrow Transplantation Failure or Engraftment Delay

IV:

- Maximum 3 courses of therapy (500 mcg/m² daily during the third course) recommended.

Leukemias
Acute Myelogenous Leukemia

IV:

- Maximum 250 mcg/m² once daily for 42 days.

† Use is not currently included in the labeling approved by the US Food and Drug Administration.

Scopolamine Patch

(skoe pol′ a meen)

Brand Name: Scopace®, Transderm Scōp®

Why is this medicine prescribed?

Scopolamine is used to prevent nausea and vomiting caused by motion sickness.

This medication is sometimes prescribed for other uses; ask your doctor or pharmacist for more information.

How should this medicine be used?

Scopolamine comes as a patch to be placed on the skin behind your ear. Apply one patch to a clean, dry, hairless area behind the ear. The patch should be applied at least 4 hours before its effects will be needed. Each patch is good for 3 days. Follow the directions on your prescription label carefully, and ask your doctor or pharmacist to explain any part you do not understand. Use the scopolamine patch exactly as directed.

To apply the patch, follow the directions provided by the manufacturer and these steps:

1. After washing the area behind the ear, wipe the area with a clean, dry tissue to ensure that the area is dry.
2. Remove the patch from its protective pouch. To expose

the adhesive surface of the patch, the clear plastic protective strip should be peeled off and discarded. Contact with the exposed adhesive layer should be avoided to prevent contamination of fingers with scopolamine. Temporary blurred vision and dilation of the pupils may result if scopolamine comes into contact with your eyes.

3. Place the adhesive side against the skin.
4. Press the patch firmly for 10-20 seconds. Be sure that the edges adhere to your skin.
5. After you have placed the patch behind your ear, wash your hands thoroughly.

At the end of 3 days, or when the scopolamine patch is no longer needed, remove the patch and throw it away. Wrap the patch in tissue or paper to avoid exposing anyone else to the remaining medication. Wash your hands and the area behind your ear thoroughly to remove any traces of scopolamine from the area. If a new patch needs to be applied, place a fresh patch on the hairless area behind your other ear.

What special precautions should I follow?

Before using scopolamine patches,

- tell your doctor and pharmacist if you are allergic to scopolamine or any other drugs.
- tell your doctor and pharmacist what prescription and nonprescription medications you are taking, especially medications that decrease mental alertness; cough, cold, and allergy products; and vitamins.
- tell your doctor if you have or have ever had glaucoma; heart, liver, or kidney disease; stomach or intestinal obstruction; or difficulty urinating.
- tell your doctor if you are pregnant, plan to become pregnant, or are breast-feeding. If you become pregnant while using scopolamine patches, call your doctor immediately.
- if you are having surgery, including dental surgery, tell the doctor or dentist that you are using scopolamine patches.
- you should know that this drug may make you drowsy. Do not drive a car or operate machinery until you know how scopolamine patches will affect you. This is especially important during the first 3-5 days of therapy and when your dose is increased.
- talk to your doctor about the safe use of alcohol while taking this drug. Alcohol increases the side effects caused by scopolamine patches.

What should I do if I forget to take a dose?

Apply the missed patch as soon as you remember it. Do not apply more than one patch at a time.

What side effects can this medicine cause?

Scopolamine patches may cause side effects. Tell your doctor if any of these symptoms are severe or do not go away:

- drowsiness
- disorientation
- dry mouth
- blurred vision
- dilated pupils
- confusion
- hallucinations
- difficulty urinating
- rash

If you experience any of the following symptoms, remove the patch and call your doctor immediately:

- eye pain
- dizziness
- rapid pulse

If you experience a serious side effect, you or your doctor may send a report to the Food and Drug Administration's (FDA) MedWatch Adverse Event Reporting program online [at http://www.fda.gov/MedWatch/index.html] or by phone [1-800-332-1088].

What storage conditions are needed for this medicine?

Keep this medication in the container it came in, tightly closed, and out of reach of children. Store it at room temperature and away from excess heat and moisture (not in the bathroom). Throw away any medication that is outdated or no longer needed. Talk to your pharmacist about the proper disposal of your medication.

What should I do in case of overdose?

In case of overdose, call your local poison control center at 1-800-222-1222. If the victim has collapsed or is not breathing, call local emergency services at 911.

What other information should I know?

Keep all appointments with your doctor and the laboratory.

The patch is not affected by limited exposure to water during bathing or swimming.

Do not let anyone else use your medication. Ask your pharmacist any questions you have about refilling your prescription.

Dosage Facts
For Informational Purposes

Caution: Do not change your dose, how often you take your medication, or the length of time you are to take it without first talking to your healthcare provider.

The following dosage information was written using medical language for doctors and other healthcare professionals and is provided here for you to check your dosage. The dosage of this drug may differ for different patients. Therefore, always follow your doctor's instructions or the directions on the label. Contact your healthcare provider or pharmacist if you have any questions

about the specific dosage of your medication after reviewing this information.

General Dosage Information

Tablets and injection: Available as scopolamine hydrobromide; dosage expressed in terms of the salt.

Adult Patients

Motion Sickness

TRANSDERMAL:
- Usually, one scopolamine system applied ≥4 hours prior to anticipated exposure to motion.
- May use for up to 72 hours if necessary or may remove during the 72-hour period when an antiemetic effect is no longer required.
- When necessary to continue beyond 72 hours, remove the initially applied system and place another system behind the ear at a different site.

Postoperative Nausea and Vomiting

TRANSDERMAL:
- Apply one transdermal system the evening before scheduled surgery.
- For cesarean section, apply 1 hour prior to surgery to minimize exposure of the infant to the drug.
- Allow patch to remain in place for 24 hours following surgery, then remove and discard.

Secobarbital

(see koe bar′ bi tal)

Brand Name: Seconal® Sodium Pulvules®

Why is this medicine prescribed?

Secobarbital, a barbiturate, is used in the short-term treatment of insomnia to help you fall asleep and stay asleep through the night. It is also used as a sedative to relieve anxiety before surgery.

This medication is sometimes prescribed for other uses; ask your doctor or pharmacist for more information.

How should this medicine be used?

Secobarbital comes as a capsule to take by mouth. It usually is taken at bedtime as needed for sleep. Follow the directions on your prescription label carefully, and ask your doctor or pharmacist to explain any part you do not understand. Your prescription is not refillable. Take secobarbital exactly as directed.

Secobarbital can be habit-forming. Do not use secobarbital for more than 2 weeks. Do not take a larger dose, take it more often, or for a longer time than your doctor tells you to. Tolerance may develop with long-term or excessive use, making the drug less effective. If your sleep problems con-

tinue, talk to your doctor, who will determine whether this drug is right for you.

What special precautions should I follow?

Before taking secobarbital,
- tell your doctor and pharmacist if you are allergic to secobarbital or any other drugs.
- tell your doctor and pharmacist what prescription and nonprescription medications you are taking, especially acetaminophen (Tylenol); anticoagulants ('blood thinners') such as warfarin (Coumadin); antihistamines; carbamazepine (Tegretol); clonazepam (Klonopin); disulfiram (Antabuse); felodipine (Plendil); fenoprofen (Nalfon); MAO inhibitors [phenelzine (Nardil) or tranylcypromine (Parnate)]; medications for depression, seizures, pain, asthma, colds, or allergies; metoprolol (Lopressor); metronidazole (Flagyl); muscle relaxants; propranolol (Inderal); rifampin (Rifadin); sedatives; sleeping pills; steroids; theophylline (Theo-Dur); tranquilizers; valproic acid (Depakene); verapamil (Calan); and vitamins. These medications may add to the drowsiness caused by secobarbital.
- tell your doctor if you have or have ever had anemia; asthma; seizures; or lung, heart, or liver disease.
- use a method of birth control other than oral contraceptives while taking this medication. Secobarbital can decrease the effectiveness of oral contraceptives.
- tell your doctor if you are pregnant, plan to become pregnant, or are breast-feeding. If you become pregnant while taking secobarbital, call your doctor immediately.
- if you are having surgery, including dental surgery, tell the doctor or dentist that you are taking secobarbital.
- you should know that this drug may make you drowsy. Do not drive a car or operate machinery until you know how this drug affects you.
- remember that alcohol can add to the drowsiness caused by this drug.

What should I do if I forget to take a dose?

Do not take the missed dose when you remember it. Skip it completely; then take the next dose at the regularly scheduled time. Do not take a double dose to make up for a missed one.

What side effects can this medicine cause?

Side effects from secobarbital may occur and include:
- drowsiness
- headache
- dizziness
- depression
- excitement (especially in children)
- upset stomach

Tell your doctor if any of these symptoms are severe or do not go away:
- vomiting
- nightmares

- increased dreaming
- constipation
- joint or muscle pain

If you experience any of the following symptoms, call your doctor immediately:

- mouth sores
- sore throat
- easy bruising
- bloody nose
- unusual bleeding
- fever
- difficulty breathing or swallowing
- severe skin rash

If you experience a serious side effect, you or your doctor may send a report to the Food and Drug Administration's (FDA) MedWatch Adverse Event Reporting program online [at http://www.fda.gov/MedWatch/index.html] or by phone [1-800-332-1088].

What storage conditions are needed for this medicine?

Keep this medication in the container it came in, tightly closed, and out of reach of children. Store it at room temperature and away from excess heat and moisture (not in the bathroom). Throw away any medication that is outdated or no longer needed. Talk to your pharmacist about the proper disposal of your medication.

What should I do in case of overdose?

In case of overdose, call your local poison control center at 1-800-222-1222. If the victim has collapsed or is not breathing, call local emergency services at 911.

What other information should I know?

Keep all appointments with your doctor and the laboratory. Your doctor will order certain lab tests to check your response to secobarbital.

Do not let anyone else take your medication.

Talk to your doctor, pharmacist, or other healthcare professional if you have questions about dosing information for your medication.

Selegiline

(se le′ ji leen)

Brand Name: Eldepryl®, Zelapar®
Also available generically.

Why is this medicine prescribed?

Selegiline is used to help control the symptoms of Parkinson's disease (PD; a disorder of the nervous system that causes difficulties with movement, muscle control, and balance) in people who are taking levodopa and carbidopa combination (Sinemet). Selegiline may help people with Parkinson's disease by decreasing the dose of levodopa/carbidopa needed to control symptoms, stopping the effects of levodopa/carbidopa from wearing off between doses, and increasing the length of time that levodopa/carbidopa will continue to control symptoms. Selegiline is in a group of medications called monoamine oxidase type B (MAO-B) inhibitors. It works by increasing the amount of dopamine (a natural substance that is needed to control movement) in the brain.

How should this medicine be used?

Selegiline comes as a capsule and an orally disintegrating (dissolving) tablet to take by mouth. The capsule is usually taken twice a day with breakfast and with lunch. The orally disintegrating tablet is usually taken once a day before breakfast without food, water, or other liquids. Follow the directions on your prescription label carefully, and ask your doctor or pharmacist to explain any part you do not understand. Take selegiline exactly as directed. Do not take more or less of it or take it more often than prescribed by your doctor. If you take too much selegiline, you may experience a sudden and dangerous increase in your blood pressure.

If you are taking the orally disintegrating tablet, do not remove the blister that contains the tablets from the outer pouch until you are ready to take a dose. When it is time for your dose, remove the blister card from the outer pouch and use dry hands to peel open one blister. Do not try to push the tablet through the foil. Place the tablet on your tongue and wait for it to dissolve. Do not swallow the tablet. Do not eat or drink anything for 5 minutes before you take the tablet and for 5 minutes after you take the tablet.

If you are taking the orally disintegrating tablet, your doctor may start you on a low dose of selegiline and increase your dose after six weeks.

Tell your doctor if you experience nausea, stomach pain, or dizziness. Your doctor may decrease your dose of levodopa/carbidopa during your treatment with selegiline, especially if you experience these symptoms or other unusual symptoms. Follow these directions carefully and ask your doctor or pharmacist if you do not know how much medication you should take. Do not change the doses of any of your medications unless your doctor tells you that you should.

Selegiline may help to control the symptoms of PD, but it will not cure the condition. Do not stop taking selegiline without talking with your doctor. If you suddenly stop taking medications for Parkinson's disease such as selegiline, you may experience fever, sweating, stiff muscles, and loss of consciousness. Call your doctor if you experience these or other unusual symptoms after you stop taking selegiline.

Are there other uses for this medicine?

This medication may be prescribed for other uses; ask your doctor or pharmacist for more information.

What special precautions should I follow?

Before taking selegiline,
- tell your doctor and pharmacist if you are allergic to selegiline, or any other medications.
- tell your doctor if you are taking, have recently taken, or plan to take any of the following prescription and nonprescription medications: dextromethorphan (Robitussin); meperidine (Demerol); methadone (Dolophine); propoxyphene (Darvon); tramadol (Ultram, in Ultracet); and other medications that contain selegiline (Eldepryl, Emsam, Zelapar). Your doctor may tell you not to take selegiline if you are taking or have recently taken any of these medications. If you stop taking selegiline, your doctor may tell you not to take these medications until at least 14 days have passed since you last took selegiline.
- tell your doctor and pharmacist what prescription and nonprescription medications, vitamins, nutritional supplements, and herbal products you are taking. Be sure to mention any of the following: antidepressants such as amitriptyline (Elavil) and imipramine (Tofranil); carbamazepine (Carbatrol, Equetro); medications for cough and cold symptoms or for weight loss; nafcillin; phenobarbital; phenytoin (Dilantin); selective serotonin reuptake inhibitors such as citalopram (Celexa), escitalopram (Lexapro), fluoxetine (Prozac), fluvoxamine (Luvox), paroxetine (Paxil), and sertraline (Zoloft); and rifampin (Rifadin, Rimactane). Your doctor may need to change the doses of your medications or monitor you more carefully for side effects.
- tell your doctor if you have or have ever had liver or kidney disease.
- if you have phenylketonuria (PKU; an inherited condition in which a special diet must be followed to prevent mental retardation), you should know that the orally disintegrating tablets contain aspartame that forms phenylalanine.
- tell your doctor if you are pregnant, plan to become pregnant, or are breast-feeding. If you become pregnant while taking selegiline, call your doctor.
- you should know that selegiline may cause dizziness, lightheadedness, and fainting when you get up too quickly from a lying position. This is more common when you first start taking selegiline. To avoid this problem, get out of bed slowly, resting your feet on the floor for a few minutes before standing up.

What special dietary instructions should I follow?

Ask your doctor if you need to avoid any foods during your treatment with selegiline. Your doctor will probably tell you that you may continue your normal diet as long as you take selegiline exactly as directed.

What should I do if I forget to take a dose?

Take the missed dose as soon as you remember it. However, if it is almost time for your next dose, skip the missed dose and continue your regular dosing schedule. Do not take a double dose to make up for a missed one.

What side effects can this medicine cause?

Selegiline may cause side effects. Tell your doctor if any of these symptoms are severe or do not go away:
- dizziness
- lightheadedness
- fainting
- dry mouth
- nausea
- vomiting
- stomach pain
- difficulty swallowing
- heartburn
- diarrhea
- gas
- constipation
- difficulty falling asleep or staying asleep
- unusual dreams
- sleepiness
- depression
- pain, especially in the legs or back
- muscle pain or weakness
- purple blotches on the skin
- rash
- redness, irritation, or sores in the mouth (if you are taking the orally disintegrating tablets)

Some side effects can be serious. If you experience any of the following symptoms, call your doctor immediately:
- severe headache
- chest pain
- fast, irregular, or pounding heartbeat
- sweating
- sudden, severe nausea and vomiting
- confusion
- stiff or sore neck
- uncontrollable shaking of a part of your body
- unusual movements that are difficult to control
- hallucinations (seeing thing or hearing voices that do not exist)
- difficulty breathing

People who have PD may have an increased risk of developing melanoma (a type of skin cancer). There is not enough information to tell whether selegiline or other medications for PD increase the risk of melanoma. Talk to your doctor about the risks of taking selegiline and about whether you should have your skin examined during your treatment.

Selegiline may cause other side effects. Call your doctor if you have any unusual problems while you are taking this medication.

What storage conditions are needed for this medicine?

Keep this medication in the container it came in, tightly closed, and out of reach of children. Store it at room temperature and away from excess heat and moisture (not in the bathroom). Throw away any medication that is outdated or no longer needed. Throw away any unused orally disintegrating tablets three months after you open the protective pouch. Talk to your pharmacist about the proper disposal of your medication.

What should I do in case of overdose?

In case of overdose, call your local poison control center at 1-800-222-1222. If the victim has collapsed or is not breathing, call local emergency services at 911.

Symptoms of overdose may include:
- drowsiness
- dizziness
- faintness
- irritability
- hyperactivity
- agitation
- severe headache
- hallucinations (seeing things or hearing voices that do not exist)
- jaw tightness
- stiffness and arching of the back
- seizures
- coma (loss of consciousness for a period of time)
- fast and irregular pulse
- chest pain
- slowed breathing
- sweating
- fever
- cold, clammy skin

What other information should I know?

Keep all appointments with your doctor.

Do not let anyone else take your medication. Ask your pharmacist any questions you have about refilling your prescription.

Dosage Facts
For Informational Purposes

Caution: Do not change your dose, how often you take your medication, or the length of time you are to take it without first talking to your healthcare provider.

The following dosage information was written using medical language for doctors and other healthcare professionals and is provided here for you to check your dosage. The dosage of this drug may differ for different patients. Therefore, always follow your doctor's instructions or the directions on the label. Contact your healthcare provider or pharmacist if you have any questions about the specific dosage of your medication after reviewing this information.

General Dosage Information

Available as selegiline hydrochloride; dosage expressed in terms of the salt.

Adult Patients
Parkinsonian Syndrome

ORAL:
- Usual dosage: 5 mg twice daily.
- Some clinicians suggest an initial dosage of 2.5 mg daily in patients receiving concomitant levodopa/carbidopa; may increase dosage gradually up to 5 mg twice daily.

Prescribing Limits
Adult Patients
Parkinsonian Syndrome

ORAL:
- Maximum 10 mg daily.

Special Populations

No special population dosage recommendations.

Selegiline Transdermal
(se le′ ji leen)

Brand Name: Emsam®

Important Warning

A small number of children, teenagers, and young adults (up to 24 years of age) who took antidepressants ('mood elevators') such as transdermal selegiline during clinical studies became suicidal (thinking about harming or killing oneself or planning or trying to do so). Children, teenagers, and young adults who take antidepressants to treat depression or other mental illnesses may be more likely to become suicidal than children, teenagers, and young adults who do not take antidepressants to treat these conditions. However, experts are not sure about how great this risk is and how much it should be considered in deciding whether a child or teenager should take an antidepressant. Children younger than 18 years of

continued on next page

Important Warning (cont'd)

age should not normally take transdermal selegiline, but in some cases, a doctor may decide that transdermal selegiline is the best medication to treat a child's condition.

You should know that your mental health may change in unexpected ways when you take transdermal selegiline or other antidepressants even if you are an adult over age 24. You may become suicidal, especially at the beginning of your treatment and any time that your dose is increased or decreased. You, your family, or your caregiver should call your doctor right away if you experience any of the following symptoms: new or worsening depression; thinking about harming or killing yourself, or planning or trying to do so; extreme worry; agitation; panic attacks; difficulty falling asleep or staying asleep; aggressive behavior; irritability; acting without thinking; severe restlessness; and frenzied abnormal excitement. Be sure that your family or caregiver knows which symptoms may be serious so they can call the doctor when you are unable to seek treatment on your own.

Your healthcare provider will want to see you often while you are taking transdermal selegiline, especially at the beginning of your treatment. Be sure to keep all appointments for office visits with your doctor.

The doctor or pharmacist will give you the manufacturer's patient information sheet (Medication Guide) when you begin treatment with transdermal selegiline. Read the information carefully and ask your doctor or pharmacist if you have any questions. You also can obtain the Medication Guide from the FDA website: http://www.fda.gov/cder/drug/antidepressants/antidepressants_MG_2007.pdf.

No matter what your age, before you take an antidepressant, you, your parent, or your caregiver should talk to your doctor about the risks and benefits of treating your condition with an antidepressant or with other treatments. You should also talk about the risks and benefits of not treating your condition. You should know that having depression or another mental illness greatly increases the risk that you will become suicidal. This risk is higher if you or anyone in your family has or has ever had bipolar disorder (mood that changes from depressed to abnormally excited) or mania (frenzied, abnormally excited mood) or has thought about or attempted suicide. Talk to your doctor about your condition, symptoms, and personal and family medical history. You and your doctor will decide what type of treatment is right for you.

Why is this medicine prescribed?

Transdermal selegiline is used to treat depression. Selegiline is in a class of medications called monoamine oxidase (MAO) inhibitors. It works by increasing the amounts of certain natural substances that are needed to maintain mental balance.

How should this medicine be used?

Transdermal selegiline comes as a patch to apply to the skin. It is usually applied once a day and left in place for 24 hours. Remove your old selegiline patch and apply a new patch at around the same time every day. Follow the directions on your prescription label carefully, and ask your doctor or pharmacist to explain any part you do not understand. Use transdermal selegiline exactly as directed. Do not apply more patches or apply patches more often than prescribed by your doctor.

Your doctor may start you on a low dose of transdermal selegiline and gradually increase your dose, not more often than once every 2 weeks.

Transdermal selegiline controls depression but does not cure it. Your condition may begin to improve after you have used transdermal selegiline for one week or longer. However, you should continue to use transdermal selegiline even if you feel well. Do not stop using transdermal selegiline without talking to your doctor.

Apply selegiline patches to dry, smooth skin anywhere on your upper chest, your back (between your neck and your waist), your upper thigh, or the outer surface of your upper arm. Choose an area where the patch will not be rubbed by tight clothing. Do not apply selegiline patches to skin that is hairy, oily, irritated, broken, scarred, or calloused.

After you apply a selegiline patch, you should wear it all the time until you are ready to remove it and put on a fresh patch. If the patch loosens or falls off before it is time to replace it, try to press it back in place with your fingers. If the patch cannot be pressed back on, throw it away and apply a fresh patch to a different area. Replace the fresh patch at your regularly scheduled patch change time.

Do not cut selegiline patches.

While you are wearing a selegiline patch, protect the patch from direct heat such as heating pads, electric blankets, heat lamps, saunas, hot tubs, and heated water beds. Do not expose the patch to direct sunlight for very long.

To use the patches, follow these steps:

1. Choose the area where you will apply the patch. Wash the area with soap and warm water. Rinse off all of the soap and dry the area with a clean towel.
2. Open the protective pouch and remove the patch.
3. Peel the first piece of liner off the sticky side of the patch. A second strip of liner should remain stuck to the patch.
4. Press the patch firmly onto your skin with the sticky side down. Be careful not to touch the sticky side with your fingers.
5. Remove the second strip of protective liner and press the rest of the sticky side of the patch firmly against your skin. Be sure that the patch is pressed flat against the skin with no bumps or folds and that it is firmly attached.
6. Wash your hands with soap and water to remove any medicine that may have gotten on them. Do not touch your eyes until you have washed your hands.

7. After 24 hours, peel the patch off slowly and gently. Fold the patch in half with the sticky sides together and throw it away in a trash can that is out of reach of children and pets. Children and pets can be harmed if they chew on, play with, or wear used patches.

8. Wash the area that was under the patch with mild soap and warm water to remove any residue. If necessary, you can use baby oil or a medical adhesive removal pad to remove residue that will not come off with soap and water. Do not use alcohol, nail polish remover, or other solvents.

9. Apply a new patch to a different area immediately by following steps 1 to 6.

Are there other uses for this medicine?

This medication may be prescribed for other uses; ask your doctor or pharmacist for more information.

What special precautions should I follow?

Before using transdermal selegiline,

- tell your doctor and pharmacist if you are allergic to selegiline or any other medications.
- tell your doctor if you are taking, have recently taken, or plan to take any of the following prescription and non-prescription medications, herbal products, or nutritional supplements: amphetamines (stimulants, 'uppers') such as amphetamine (in Adderall), benzphetamine (Didrex), dextroamphetamine (Dexedrine, Dextrostat, in Adderall), and methamphetamine (Desoxyn); antidepressants such as amitriptyline (Elavil) and imipramine (Tofranil); bupropion (Wellbutrin, Zyban); buspirone (BuSpar); carbamazepine (Tegretol); cyclobenzaprine (Flexeril); dextromethorphan (Robitussin); medications for cough and cold symptoms or for weight loss; meperidine (Demerol); methadone (Dolophine); mirtazapine (Remeron); other monoamine oxidase inhibitors such as isocarboxazid (Marplan), phenelzine (Nardil), oral selegiline (Eldepryl, Zelapar), and tranylcypromine (Parnate); oxcarbazepine (Trileptal); pentazocine (Talwin); propoxyphene (Darvon); selective serotonin reuptake inhibitors such as citalopram (Celexa), escitalopram (Lexapro), fluoxetine (Prozac), fluvoxamine (Luvox), paroxetine (Paxil), and sertraline (Zoloft); selective serotonin and norepinephrine reuptake inhibitors (SSNRIs) such as duloxetine (Cymbalta) and venlafaxine (Effexor); St. John's wort; tramadol (Ultram, in Ultracet); and tyramine supplements. Your doctor may tell you not to use transdermal selegiline until 1 or more weeks have passed since you last took one of these medications. If you stop using transdermal selegiline, your doctor will probably tell you not to take any of these medications until at least two weeks have passed since you stopped using transdermal selegiline.
- tell your doctor and pharmacist what other prescription and nonprescription medications and vitamins you are taking or plan to take. Your doctor may need to change

the doses of your medications or monitor you carefully for side effects.

- you should know that selegiline may remain in your body for several weeks after you stop using the medication. During the first few weeks after your treatment ends, tell your doctor and pharmacist that you have recently stopped using selegiline before you start taking any new medications.
- tell your doctor if you have or have ever had pheochromocytoma (a tumor on a small gland near the kidneys). Your doctor may tell you that you should not use transdermal selegiline.
- tell your doctor if you tend to get dizzy or faint and if you have or have ever had seizures, a heart attack, or heart disease.
- tell your doctor if you are pregnant, plan to become pregnant, or are breast-feeding. If you become pregnant while using transdermal selegiline, call your doctor.
- if you are having surgery, including dental surgery, tell the doctor or dentist that you are using transdermal selegiline
- you should know that transdermal selegiline may make you drowsy. Do not drive a car or operate machinery until you know how this medication affects you.
- talk to your doctor about the safe use of alcoholic beverages while you are using transdermal selegiline.
- you should know that transdermal selegiline may cause dizziness, lightheadedness, and fainting when you get up too quickly from a lying position. This is more common when you first start using transdermal selegiline. To avoid this problem, get out of bed slowly, resting your feet on the floor for a few minutes before standing up.

What special dietary instructions should I follow?

You may need to follow a special diet during your treatment with transdermal selegiline. This depends on the strength of the patches you are using. If you are using the 6 mg/24 hour patch, you may continue your normal diet.

If you are using the 9 mg/24 hour patch or the 12 mg/24 hour patch, you may experience a serious reaction if you eat foods that are high in tyramine during your treatment. Tyramine is found in many foods, including meat, poultry, fish, or cheese that has been smoked, aged, improperly stored, or spoiled; certain fruits, vegetables, and beans; alcoholic beverages; and yeast products that have fermented. Your doctor or dietitian will tell you which foods you must avoid completely, and which foods you may eat in small amounts. Follow these directions carefully. Ask your doctor or dietitian if you have any questions about what you may eat and drink during your treatment.

What should I do if I forget to take a dose?

If you forget to change your patch after 24 hours, remove the old patch, apply a new patch as soon as you remember and continue your regular dosing schedule. Do not apply an extra patch to make up for a missed dose.

What side effects can this medicine cause?

Transdermal selegiline may cause side effects. Tell your doctor if any of these symptoms are severe or do not go away:

- redness of the area where you applied the patch
- diarrhea
- heartburn
- dry mouth
- weight loss
- rash

Some side effects can be serious. If you experience any of these symptoms or those listed in the IMPORTANT WARNING section, call your doctor immediately:

- severe headache
- fast, slow, or pounding heartbeat
- chest pain
- stiff or sore neck
- nausea
- vomiting
- sweating
- confusion
- widened pupils (black circles in the middle of the eyes)
- sensitivity of the eyes to light

Transdermal selegiline may cause other side effects. Call your doctor if you have any unusual problems while taking this medication.

What storage conditions are needed for this medicine?

Keep this medication in the container it came in, tightly closed, and out of reach of children. Store it at room temperature and away from excess heat and moisture (not in the bathroom). Store the patches in their protective pouches and do not open a pouch until you are ready to apply the patch. Throw away any medication that is outdated or no longer needed. Talk to your pharmacist about the proper disposal of your medication.

What should I do in case of overdose?

In case of overdose, call your local poison control center at 1-800-222-1222. If the victim has collapsed or is not breathing, call local emergency services at 911.

Symptoms of overdose may include:

- drowsiness
- dizziness
- faintness
- irritability
- hyperactivity
- agitation
- severe headache
- hallucinations (seeing things or hearing voices that do not exist)
- jaw tightness
- stiffness and arching of the back
- seizures
- coma (loss of consciousness for a period of time)
- fast and irregular pulse
- chest pain
- slowed breathing
- sweating
- fever
- cold, clammy skin

What other information should I know?

Keep all appointments with your doctor.

Do not let anyone else take your medication. Ask your pharmacist any questions you have about refilling your prescription.

Talk to your doctor, pharmacist, or other healthcare professional if you have questions about dosing information for your medication.

Selenium Sulfide

(se lee' nee um)

Brand Name: Exsel®, Head and Shoulders Intensive Treatment Dandruff Shampoo®, Selsun®, Selsun Blue®

Why is this medicine prescribed?

Selenium sulfide, an anti-infective agent, relieves itching and flaking of the scalp and removes the dry, scaly particles that are commonly referred to as dandruff or seborrhea. It is also used to treat tinea versicolor, a fungal infection of the skin.

This medication is sometimes prescribed for other uses; ask your doctor or pharmacist for more information.

How should this medicine be used?

Selenium sulfide comes in a lotion and is usually applied as a shampoo. As a shampoo, selenium sulfide usually is used twice a week for the first 2 weeks and then once a week for 2, 3, or 4 weeks, depending on your response. For skin infections, selenium sulfide usually is applied once a day for 7 days. Follow the directions on the package or on your prescription label carefully, and ask your doctor or pharmacist to explain any part you do not understand. Use selenium sulfide exactly as directed. Do not use more or less of it or use it more often than directed by your doctor.

Do not use this medication if your scalp or the skin area to be treated is cut or scratched.

Avoid getting selenium sulfide in your eyes. If the medication gets into your eyes accidentally, rinse them with clear water for several minutes.

Do not leave selenium sulfide on your hair, scalp, or skin for long periods (e.g., overnight) because it is irritating. Rinse off all of the lotion.

Do not use this medication on children younger than 2 years of age without a doctor's permission.

To use the lotion as a shampoo, follow these steps:

1. Remove all jewelry; selenium sulfide may damage it.
2. Wash your hair with ordinary shampoo and rinse it well.
3. Shake the lotion well.
4. Massage 1-2 teaspoonsful of the lotion into your wet scalp.
5. Leave the lotion on your scalp for 2-3 minutes.
6. Rinse your scalp three or four times with clean water.
7. Repeat Steps 4, 5, and 6.
8. If you are using selenium sulfide before or after bleaching, tinting, or permanent waving your hair, rinse your hair with cool water for at least 5 minutes after applying selenium sulfide to prevent discolored hair.
9. Wash your hands well and clean under your nails to remove any lotion.

If your doctor tells you to use the lotion on your skin, apply a small amount of water with the lotion to the affected area and massage it to form a lather. Leave the lotion on your skin for 10 minutes; then rinse it thoroughly.

What special precautions should I follow?

Before using selenium sulfide,

- tell your doctor and pharmacist if you are allergic to selenium sulfide or any other drugs.
- tell your doctor and pharmacist what prescription and non-prescription medications you are taking, including vitamins.
- tell your doctor if you are pregnant, plan to become pregnant, or are breast-feeding. If you become pregnant while using selenium sulfide, call your doctor.

What should I do if I forget to take a dose?

Apply the missed dose as soon as you remember it. However, if it is almost time for the next dose, skip the missed dose and continue your regular dosing schedule. Do not apply a double dose to make up for a missed one.

What side effects can this medicine cause?

Selenium sulfide may cause side effects. Tell your doctor if any of these symptoms are severe or do not go away:

- oiliness or dryness of hair and scalp
- hair loss
- hair discoloration

If you experience either of the following symptoms, call your doctor immediately:

- scalp irritation
- skin irritation

If you experience a serious side effect, you or your doctor may send a report to the Food and Drug Administration's (FDA) MedWatch Adverse Event Reporting program online [at http://www.fda.gov/MedWatch/index.html] or by phone [1-800-332-1088].

What storage conditions are needed for this medicine?

Keep this medication in the container it came in, tightly closed, and out of reach of children. Store it at room temperature and away from excess heat and moisture (not in the bathroom). Throw away any medication that is outdated or no longer needed. Talk to your pharmacist about the proper disposal of your medication.

What other information should I know?

Keep all appointments with your doctor. Selenium sulfide is for external use only. Do not let selenium sulfide get into your eyes, nose, or mouth, and do not swallow it. Do not apply dressings, bandages, cosmetics, lotions, or other skin medications to the area being treated unless your doctor tells you.

Do not let anyone else use your medication. Ask your pharmacist any questions you have about refilling your prescription.

Tell your doctor if your skin condition gets worse or does not go away.

Talk to your doctor, pharmacist, or other healthcare professional if you have questions about dosing information for your medication.

Sertraline

(ser′ tra leen)

Brand Name: Zoloft®

Important Warning

A small number of children, teenagers, and young adults (up to 24 years of age) who took antidepressants ('mood elevators') such as sertraline during clinical studies became suicidal (thinking about harming or killing oneself or planning or trying to do so). Children, teenagers, and young adults who take antidepressants to treat depression or other mental illnesses may be more likely to become suicidal than children, teenagers, and young adults who do not take antidepressants to treat these conditions. However, experts are not sure about how great this risk is and how much it should be considered in deciding whether a child or teenager should take an antidepressant.

You should know that your mental health may change in unexpected ways when you take sertraline or other antidepressants even if you are an adult over age 24. You may become suicidal, especially at the beginning of your treatment and any time that your dose is increased or decreased. You, your family, or your caregiver should call your doctor right away if you experience any of the following symptoms: new or worsening depression; thinking about harming or killing yourself, or planning or trying to do so; ex-

continued on next page

Important Warning (cont'd)

treme worry; agitation; panic attacks; difficulty falling asleep or staying asleep; aggressive behavior; irritability; acting without thinking; severe restlessness; and frenzied abnormal excitement. Be sure that your family or caregiver knows which symptoms may be serious so they can call the doctor when you are unable to seek treatment on your own.

Your healthcare provider will want to see you often while you are taking sertraline, especially at the beginning of your treatment. Be sure to keep all appointments for office visits with your doctor.

The doctor or pharmacist will give you the manufacturer's patient information sheet (Medication Guide) when you begin treatment with sertraline. Read the information carefully and ask your doctor or pharmacist if you have any questions. You also can obtain the Medication Guide from the FDA website: http://www.fda.gov/cder/drug/antidepressants/antidepressants_MG_2007.pdf.

No matter what your age, before you take an antidepressant, you, your parent, or your caregiver should talk to your doctor about the risks and benefits of treating your condition with an antidepressant or with other treatments. You should also talk about the risks and benefits of not treating your condition. You should know that having depression or another mental illness greatly increases the risk that you will become suicidal. This risk is higher if you or anyone in your family has or has ever had bipolar disorder (mood that changes from depressed to abnormally excited) or mania (frenzied, abnormally excited mood) or has thought about or attempted suicide. Talk to your doctor about your condition, symptoms, and personal and family medical history. You and your doctor will decide what type of treatment is right for you.

Why is this medicine prescribed?

Sertraline is used to treat depression, obsessive-compulsive disorder (bothersome thoughts that won't go away and the need to perform certain actions over and over), panic attacks (sudden, unexpected attacks of extreme fear and worry about these attacks), posttraumatic stress disorder (disturbing psychological symptoms that develop after a frightening experience), and social anxiety disorder (extreme fear of interacting with others or performing in front of others that interferes with normal life). It is also used to relieve the symptoms of premenstrual dysphoric disorder, including mood swings, irritability, bloating, and breast tenderness. Sertraline is in a class of antidepressants called selective serotonin reuptake inhibitors (SSRIs). It works by increasing the amounts of serotonin, a natural substance in the brain that helps maintain mental balance.

How should this medicine be used?

Sertraline comes as a tablet and a concentrate (liquid) to take by mouth. It is usually taken once daily in the morning or evening. To treat premenstrual dysphoric disorder, sertraline is taken once a day, either every day of the month or on certain days of the month. Take sertraline at around the same time every day. Follow the directions on your prescription label carefully, and ask your doctor or pharmacist to explain any part you do not understand. Take sertraline exactly as directed. Do not take more or less of it or take it more often than prescribed by your doctor.

Sertraline concentrate must be diluted before use. Immediately before taking it, use the provided dropper to remove the amount of concentrate your doctor has told you to take. Mix the concentrate with 4 ounces (1/2 cup) of water, ginger ale, lemon or lime soda, lemonade, or orange juice. Do not mix the concentrate with any liquids other than the ones listed. Drink immediately.

Your doctor may start you on a low dose of sertraline and gradually increase your dose, not more than once a week.

It may take a few weeks or longer before you feel the full benefit of sertraline. Continue to take sertraline even if you feel well. Do not stop taking sertraline without talking to your doctor.

Are there other uses for this medicine?

Sertraline is also used sometimes to treat headaches and sexual problems. Talk to your doctor about the possible risks of using this medication for your condition.

This medication may be prescribed for other uses; ask your doctor or pharmacist for more information.

What special precautions should I follow?

Before taking sertraline,

- tell your doctor and pharmacist if you are allergic to sertraline or any other medications. Before taking sertraline liquid concentrate, tell your doctor if you are allergic to latex.
- tell your doctor if you are taking monoamine oxidase (MAO) inhibitors, including isocarboxazid (Marplan), phenelzine (Nardil), selegiline (Eldepryl, Emsam, Zelapar), and tranylcypromine (Parnate), or have stopped taking them within the past two weeks, or if you are taking pimozide (Orap). Your doctor will probably tell you not to take sertraline. If you stop taking sertraline, you should wait at least 2 weeks before you start to take an MAO inhibitor.
- do not take disulfiram (Antabuse) while taking sertraline concentrate.
- tell your doctor and pharmacist what other prescription and nonprescription medications, vitamins, nutritional supplements, and herbal products you are taking or plan to take. Be sure to mention any of the following: anticoagulants ('blood thinners') such as warfarin (Coumadin); antidepressants (mood elevators) such as amitriptyline (Elavil), amoxapine (Asendin), clomipramine (Anafranil), desipra-

mine (Norpramin), doxepin (Adapin, Sinequan), imipramine (Tofranil), nortriptyline (Aventyl, Pamelor), protriptyline (Vivactil), and trimipramine (Surmontil); aspirin and other nonsteroidal anti-inflammatory medications (NSAIDs) such as ibuprofen (Advil, Motrin) and naproxen (Aleve, Naprosyn); cimetidine (Tagamet); diazepam (Valium); digoxin (Lanoxin); lithium (Eskalith, Lithobid); medications for anxiety, mental illness, Parkinson's disease, and seizures; medications for irregular heartbeat such as flecainide (Tambocor) and propafenone (Rythmol); oral medications for diabetes such as tolbutamide (Orinase); medications for migraine headaches such as almotriptan (Axert), eletriptan (Relpax), frovatriptan (Frova), naratriptan (Amerge), rizatriptan (Maxalt), sumatriptan (Imitrex), and zolmitriptan (Zomig); sedatives; sleeping pills; and tranquilizers. Your doctor may need to change the doses of your medications or monitor you carefully for side effects.

- tell your doctor if you have recently had a heart attack and if you have or have ever had seizures or liver or heart disease.
- tell your doctor if you are pregnant, plan to become pregnant, or are breast-feeding. If you become pregnant while taking sertraline, call your doctor.
- you should know that sertraline may make you drowsy. Do not drive a car or operate machinery until you know how this medication affects you.
- ask your doctor about the safe use of alcoholic beverages while you are taking sertraline.

What special dietary instructions should I follow?

Unless your doctor tells you otherwise, continue your normal diet.

What should I do if I forget to take a dose?

Take the missed dose as soon as you remember it. However, if it is almost time for the next dose, skip the missed dose and continue your regular dosing schedule. Do not take a double dose to make up for a missed one.

What side effects can this medicine cause?

Sertraline may cause side effects. Tell your doctor if any of these symptoms are severe or do not go away:
- nausea
- diarrhea
- constipation
- vomiting
- dry mouth
- gas or bloating
- loss of appetite
- weight changes
- drowsiness
- dizziness
- excessive tiredness
- headache

- pain, burning, or tingling in the hands or feet
- nervousness
- uncontrollable shaking of a part of the body
- sore throat
- changes in sex drive or ability
- excessive sweating

Some side effects can be serious. If you experience any of the following symptoms or those listed in the IMPORTANT WARNING section, call your doctor immediately:
- blurred vision
- seizures
- abnormal bleeding or bruising
- hallucinating (seeing things or hearing voices that do not exist)

Sertraline may cause other side effects. Call your doctor if you have any unusual problems while taking this medication.

What storage conditions are needed for this medicine?

Keep this medication in the container it came in, tightly closed, and out of reach of children. Store it at room temperature and away from excess heat and moisture (not in the bathroom). Throw away any medication that is outdated or no longer needed. Talk to your pharmacist about the proper disposal of your medication.

What should I do in case of overdose?

In case of overdose, call your local poison control center at 1-800-222-1222. If the victim has collapsed or is not breathing, call local emergency services at 911.

Symptoms of overdose may include:
- hair loss
- changes in sex drive or ability
- drowsiness
- excessive tiredness
- difficulty falling asleep or staying asleep
- diarrhea
- vomiting
- rapid, pounding or irregular heartbeat
- nausea
- dizziness
- excitement
- uncontrollable shaking of a part of the body
- seizures
- hallucinating (hearing voices or seeing things that do not exist)
- unconsciousness
- fainting

What other information should I know?

Keep all appointments with your doctor.

Do not let anyone else take your medication. Ask your pharmacist any questions you have about refilling your prescription.

Dosage Facts
For Informational Purposes

Caution: Do not change your dose, how often you take your medication, or the length of time you are to take it without first talking to your healthcare provider.

The following dosage information was written using medical language for doctors and other healthcare professionals and is provided here for you to check your dosage. The dosage of this drug may differ for different patients. Therefore, always follow your doctor's instructions or the directions on the label. Contact your healthcare provider or pharmacist if you have any questions about the specific dosage of your medication after reviewing this information.

General Dosage Information

Available as sertraline hydrochloride; dosage is expressed in terms of sertraline.

Pediatric Patients

OCD

ORAL:
- Children 6–12 years of age: Initially, 25 mg once daily.
- Adolescents 13–17 years of age: Initially, 50 mg once daily.
- Dosage may be increased at weekly intervals according to clinical response.
- Avoid excessive dosages in children.
- Optimum duration not established; may require several months of therapy or longer.

Adult Patients

Major Depressive Disorder

ORAL:
- Initially, 50–100 mg once daily. Dosage may be increased at weekly intervals according to clinical response.
- Optimum duration not established; may require several months of therapy or longer.

OCD

ORAL:
- Initially, 50 mg once daily. Dosage may be increased at weekly intervals according to clinical response.
- Optimum duration not established; may require several months of therapy or longer.

Panic Disorder

ORAL:
- Initially, 25 mg once daily. After 1 week, increase to 50 mg once daily. Dosage may be increased at weekly intervals according to clinical response.
- Optimum duration not established; may require several months of therapy or longer.

PTSD

ORAL:
- Initially, 25 mg once daily. After 1 week, increase to 50 mg once daily. Dosage may then be increased at weekly intervals according to clinical response.
- Optimum duration not established; may require several months of therapy or longer.

PMDD

ORAL:
- Initially, 50 mg once daily given continuously throughout the menstrual cycle or just during the luteal phase (i.e., starting 2 weeks prior to the anticipated onset of menstruation and continuing through the first full day of menses).
- Dosage may be increased in 50-mg increments at the onset of each new menstrual cycle.
- If a dosage of 100 mg daily has been established with luteal phase dosing, titrate dosage using a 50 mg daily dosage for the first 3 days of each luteal phase dosing period.
- Optimum duration not established; periodically assess need for dosage adjustment and continued therapy.

Social Phobia

ORAL:
- Initially, 25 mg once daily. After 1 week, increase to 50 mg once daily. Dosage may be increased at weekly intervals according to clinical response.
- Optimum duration not established; may require several months of therapy or longer.

Premature Ejaculation†

ORAL:
- 25–50 mg daily. Alternatively, 25–50 mg daily on an "as needed" basis.

Prescribing Limits

Pediatric Patients

OCD

ORAL:
- Maximum 200 mg daily.

Adult Patients

Major Depressive Disorder

ORAL:
- Maximum 200 mg daily.

OCD

ORAL:
- Maximum 200 mg daily.

Panic Disorder

ORAL:
- Maximum 200 mg daily.

PTSD

ORAL:
- Maximum 200 mg daily.

PMDD

ORAL:
- Maximum 150 mg daily when administered continuously or 100 mg daily when administered during the luteal phase only.

Social Phobia

ORAL:
- Maximum 200 mg daily.

Special Populations

Hepatic Impairment

- Decreased clearance; lower dosages or less frequent administration recommended.

Renal Impairment

- No dosage adjustments needed. Not substantially removed by dialysis; supplemental doses may be unnecessary after dialysis.

† *Use is not currently included in the labeling approved by the US Food and Drug Administration.*

Shingles (Zoster) Vaccine

Brand Name: Zostavax®

What is shingles?

Shingles is a painful skin rash, often with blisters. It is also called herpes zoster. A shingles rash usually appears on one side of the face or body and lasts from 2 to 4 weeks. Its main symptom is pain, which can be quite severe. Other symptoms of shingles can include fever, headache, chills and upset stomach. Very rarely, a shingles infection can lead to pneumonia, hearing problems, blindness, brain inflammation (encephalitis) or death.

For about 1 person in 5, severe pain can continue even after the rash clears up. This is called post-herpetic neuralgia.

Shingles is caused by the varicella zoster virus, the same virus that causes chickenpox. Only someone who has had a case of chickenpox, or gotten chickenpox vaccine, can get shingles. The virus stays in your body. It can reappear many years later to cause a case of shingles.

You can't catch shingles from another person with shingles. However, a person who has never had chickenpox (or chickenpox vaccine) could get chickenpox from someone with shingles. This is not very common.

Shingles is far more common in people 50 and older than in younger people. It is also more common in people whose immune systems are weakened because of a disease such as cancer, or drugs such as steroids or chemotherapy. At least 1 million people a year in the United States get shingles.

Shingles vaccine

A vaccine for shingles was licensed in 2006. In clinical trials, the vaccine prevented shingles in about half of people 60 years of age and older. It can also reduce the pain associated with shingles.

A single dose of shingles vaccine is indicated for adults 60 years of age and older.

Which people should not get shingles vaccine or should wait?

A person should not get shingles vaccine who:

- has ever had a life-threatening allergic reaction to gelatin, the antibiotic neomycin, or any other component of shingles vaccine. Tell your doctor if you have any severe allergies.
- has a weakened immune system because of HIV/AIDS or another disease that affects the immune system; treatment with drugs that affect the immune system, such as steroids; cancer treatment such as radiation or chemotherapy; a history of cancer affecting the bone marrow or lymphatic system, such as leukemia or lymphoma.
- has active, untreated tuberculosis.
- is pregnant, or might be pregnant. Women should not become pregnant until at least three months after getting shingles vaccine.

Someone with a minor illness, such as a cold, may be vaccinated. But anyone who is moderately or severely ill should usually wait until they recover before getting the vaccine. This includes anyone with a temperature of 101.3°F or higher.

What are the risks from shingles vaccine?

A vaccine, like any medicine, could possibly cause serious problems, such as severe allergic reactions. However, the risk of a vaccine causing serious harm, or death, is extremely small. No serious problems have been identified with shingles vaccine. Like all vaccines, shingles vaccine is being closely monitored for unusual or severe problems.

Mild Problems:

- Redness, soreness, swelling, or itching at the site of the injection (about 1 person in 3).
- Headache (about 1 person in 70).

What if there is a moderate or severe reaction?

What should I look for?

- Any unusual condition, such as a high fever or behavior changes. Signs of a serious allergic reaction can include difficulty breathing, hoarseness or wheezing, hives, paleness, weakness, a fast heart beat or dizziness. These usually occur within the first few hours after vaccination.

What should I do?

- Call a doctor, or get the person to a doctor right away.
- Tell your doctor what happened, the date and time it happened, and when the vaccination was given.
- Ask your health care provider to file a Vaccine Adverse Event Reporting System (VAERS) form if you have any reaction to the vaccine. Or call VAERS yourself at 1-800-822-7967, or visit their website at http://vaers.hhs.gov.

The National Vaccine Injury Compensation Program

In the rare event that you or your child has a serious reaction to a vaccine, a federal program has been created to help pay for the care of those who have been harmed.

For details about the National Vaccine Injury Compensation Program, call 1-800-338-2382 or visit the program's website at http://www.hrsa.gov/vaccinecompensation.

How can I learn more?

- Ask your doctor or other health care provider. They can give you the vaccine package insert or suggest other sources of information.
- Call your local or state health department's immunization program.
- Contact the Centers for Disease Control and Prevention (CDC): call 1-800-232-4636 (1-800-CDC-INFO) or visit the National Immunization Program's website at http://www.cdc.gov/nip

Shingles (Zoster) Vaccine Information Statement. U.S. Department of Health and Human Services/Centers for Disease Control and Prevention National Immunization Program. 9/11/2006.

Sibutramine

(si byoo' tra meen)

Brand Name: Meridia®

Why is this medicine prescribed?

Sibutramine is used in combination with a reduced calorie diet and exercise to help people who are overweight lose weight and maintain their weight loss. Sibutramine is in a class of medications called appetite suppressants. It works by acting on appetite control centers in the brain to decrease appetite.

How should this medicine be used?

Sibutramine comes as a capsule to take by mouth. It is usually taken with or without food once a day. To help you remember to take sibutramine, take it around the same time every day. Follow the directions on your prescription label carefully, and ask your doctor or pharmacist to explain any part you do not understand. Take sibutramine exactly as directed. Sibutramine can be habit forming. Do not take more or less of it or take it more often or for a longer time than prescribed by your doctor.

Your doctor may start you on a low dose of sibutramine and increase your dose, after you have been taking sibutramine for at least 4 weeks. Your doctor may decrease your dose if you experience certain side effects while you are taking your starting dose.

You will probably lose weight soon after you begin taking sibutramine and following your diet and exercise program. Be sure to monitor your weight, and call your doctor if you do not lose at least 4 pounds during your first 4 weeks of therapy. Your doctor may wish to change your dose of sibutramine.

You may not continue to lose weight after your first 6 months of treatment. However, you should continue to take sibutramine even if you have stopped losing weight. If you stop taking sibutramine, you may gain weight. Do not stop taking sibutramine without talking to your doctor.

Are there other uses for this medicine?

This medication may be prescribed for other uses; ask your doctor or pharmacist for more information.

What special precautions should I follow?

Before taking sibutramine,

- tell your doctor and pharmacist if you are allergic to sibutramine or any other medications.
- do not take sibutramine if you are taking monoamine oxidase (MAO) inhibitors, including isocarboxazid (Marplan), phenelzine (Nardil), selegiline (Eldepryl), and tranylcypromine (Parnate), or have stopped taking them within the past 2 weeks. Do not start taking these drugs for at least 2 weeks after you stop taking sibutramine.
- do not take other prescription or non-prescription medications, herbal products or nutritional supplements to help you lose weight such as benzphetamine (Didrex), methamphetamine (Desoxyn), phendimetrazine (Adipost, Bontril, others), and phentermine (Adipex-P, Phentride, others) while you are taking sibutramine.
- tell your doctor and pharmacist what other prescription and nonprescription medications, vitamins, nutritional supplements, and herbal products you are taking. Be sure to mention any of the following: amiodarone (Cordarone); anticoagulants ('blood thinners') such as warfarin (Coumadin); antifungals such as fluconazole (Diflucan), itraconazole (Sporanox), and ketoconazole (Nizoral); caffeine-containing products including NoDoz, and Vivarin; cancer chemotherapy medications; clarithromycin (Biaxin, Prevpac); clopidogrel (Plavix); cyclosporine (Neoral, Sandimmune); danazol (Danocrine); delavirdine (Rescriptor); diltiazem (Cardizem, Dilacor, Tiazac); erythromycin (E.E.S., E-Mycin, Erythrocin); fentanyl (Actiq, Duragesic); gold salts such as auranofin (Ridaura) and aurothioglucose (Solganal); heparin; HIV protease inhibitors such as indinavir (Crixivin), nelfinavir (Viracept), ritonavir (Norvir), and saquinavir (Fortovase, Invirase); isoniazid (INH, Nydrazid); lithium (Eskalith, Lithobid); medications for allergies, coughs, and colds; medications for depression; medications for high blood pressure; medications for migraine headaches such as dihydroergotamine mesylate (Migranal), ergoloid mesylates (Gerimal, Hydergine), ergonovine (Ergotrate, Meth-

ergine); ergotamine (Bellamine, Cafergot, others), frovatriptan (Frova), methysergide (Sansert), naratriptan (Amerge), rizatriptan (Maxalt), sumatriptan (Imitrex), and zolmitriptan (Zomig); medications for nausea such as alosetron (Lotronex), dolasetron (Anzemet), granisetron (Kytril), ondansetron (Zofran) and palonosetron (Aloxi); medications for anxiety, mental illness, seizures, and pain; meperidine (Demerol, Mepergan); metronidazole (Flagyl); muscle relaxants; pentazocine (Talcen, Talwin); quinine; quinidine (Quinidex); salicylate pain relievers such as aspirin, choline magnesium trisalicylate, choline salicylate (Arthropan), diflunisal (Dolobid), magnesium salicylate (Doan's, others), and salsalate (Argesic, Disalcid, Salgesic); sedatives; sleeping pills; sulfa antibiotics such as sulfadiazine, sulfamethizole (Urobiotic), sulfamethoxazole and trimethoprim (Bactrim, Septra), sulfasalazine (Azulfidine), sulfisoxazole (Gatrisin, Pediazole); ticlopidine (Ticlid); tranquilizers; troleandomycin (TAO); tryptophan; verapamil (Calan, Covera, Isoptin, Verelan); or zafirlukast (Accolate). Your doctor may need to change the doses of your medications or monitor you carefully for side effects.

- tell your doctor if you have or have ever had an eating disorder such as anorexia nervosa (abnormal focus on being thin that causes patient to eat very little and exercise excessively) or bulimia nervosa (eating large amounts of food and then removing the food from the body using diuretics (water pills), laxatives, or vomiting); cancer; chest pain; congestive heart failure (heart is unable to pump blood well enough); depression; gallstones (clumps of hardened material that can block the passages from the liver to intestine); glaucoma (an eye disease); a heart attack; hemophilia or other bleeding problems; high blood pressure; irregular heart beat; migraine headaches; osteoporosis (thinning and weakening of the bones); Parkinson's disease (a disorder of the nervous system that causes difficulties with movement, muscle control, and balance); seizures; a stroke or ministroke; pulmonary hypertension (high pressure in the vessel that moves blood from the heart to the lungs); or kidney, liver, or thyroid disease. Also tell your doctor if you have ever used street drugs or overused prescription medications.
- tell your doctor if you are pregnant or are breast-feeding. You should use effective birth control to be sure you do not become pregnant while you are taking sibutramine. Ask your doctor if you need help choosing a method of birth control.
- if you are having surgery, including dental surgery, tell the doctor or dentist that you are taking sibutramine.
- you should know that sibutramine may make you drowsy and may affect your judgment, your ability to think, and your coordination. Do not drive a car or operate machinery until you know how this medication affects you.
- remember that alcohol can add to the drowsiness caused by this medication. Ask your doctor about the safe use of alcoholic beverages while you are taking sibutramine.
- ask your doctor about drinking coffee, tea, or caffeinated beverages while taking sibutramine. Caffeine may make the side effects from sibutramine worse.

What special dietary instructions should I follow?

Follow the diet and exercise program your doctor has given you.

Talk to your doctor about drinking grapefruit juice while taking this medicine.

What should I do if I forget to take a dose?

Take the missed dose as soon as you remember it. However, if it is almost time for the next dose, skip the missed dose and continue your regular dosing schedule. Do not take a double dose to make up for a missed one.

What side effects can this medicine cause?

Sibutramine may cause side effects. Tell your doctor if any of these symptoms are severe or do not go away:
- headache
- change in appetite
- constipation
- heartburn
- dry mouth
- weakness
- back pain
- nervousness
- difficulty falling asleep or staying asleep
- runny nose
- flu-like symptoms
- flushing
- painful menstrual periods

Some side effects can be serious. The following symptoms are uncommon, but if you experience any of them, call your doctor immediately:
- fast or pounding heart beat
- chest pain
- shortness of breath
- upset stomach
- stomach pain
- vomiting
- extreme excitement
- restlessness
- anxiety
- depression
- dizziness
- lightheadedness
- fainting
- confusion
- uncoordinated or abnormal movement
- muscle stiffness
- shaking hands that you cannot control
- seizures

- shivering
- excessive sweating
- fever
- sore throat
- large pupils (black area in center of eyes)
- change in vision
- eye pain
- hives
- skin rash
- itching
- difficulty speaking, breathing, or swallowing
- hoarseness
- swelling of the face, throat, tongue, lips, eyes, hands, feet, ankles, or lower legs
- unusual bleeding or bruising

Sibutramine may cause other side effects. Call your doctor if you have any unusual problems while taking this medication.

If you experience a serious side effect, you or your doctor may send a report to the Food and Drug Administration's (FDA) MedWatch Adverse Event Reporting program online [at http://www.fda.gov/MedWatch/index.html] or by phone [1-800-332-1088].

What storage conditions are needed for this medicine?

Keep this medication in the container it came in, tightly closed, and out of reach of children. Store it at room temperature and away from excess heat and moisture (not in the bathroom) and light. Throw away any medication that is outdated or no longer needed. Talk to your pharmacist about the proper disposal of your medication.

What should I do in case of overdose?

In case of overdose, call your local poison control center at 1-800-222-1222. If the victim has collapsed or is not breathing, call local emergency services at 911.

Symptoms of overdose may include:
- fast heart beat

What other information should I know?

Keep all appointments with your doctor. Your doctor will monitor your blood pressure and heart rate (pulse) frequently while you are taking sibutramine.

Do not let anyone else take your medication. Ask your pharmacist any questions you have about refilling your prescription.

Dosage Facts
For Informational Purposes

Caution: Do not change your dose, how often you take your medication, or the length of time you are to take it without first talking to your healthcare provider.

The following dosage information was written using medical language for doctors and other healthcare professionals and is provided here for you to check your dosage. The dosage of this drug may differ for different patients. Therefore, always follow your doctor's instructions or the directions on the label. Contact your healthcare provider or pharmacist if you have any questions about the specific dosage of your medication after reviewing this information.

General Dosage Information

Available as sibutramine hydrochloride monohydrate; dosage expressed in terms of the monohydrate.

Adult Patients

Obesity

ORAL:
- Initially, 10 mg once daily.
- If weight loss is inadequate (e.g., <1.8 kg of weight loss) after 4 weeks of treatment, consider increasing dosage to 15 mg daily or discontinuance; take BP and heart rate into account.
- Reserve 5-mg daily dose for patients who do not tolerate 10 mg daily.
- Safety and efficacy >2 years not established in clinical studies.

Prescribing Limits

Adult Patients

Obesity

ORAL:
- Maximum 15 mg daily.

Special Populations

Hepatic Impairment
- Mild or moderate hepatic impairment: Dosage adjustment not needed.

Geriatric Patients
- Select dosage with caution.

Sildenafil

(sil den' a fil)

Brand Name: Viagra®

Why is this medicine prescribed?

Sildenafil is used to treat erectile dysfunction (impotence; inability to get or keep an erection) in men. Sildenafil is in a class of medications called phosphodiesterase (PDE) inhibitors. It works by increasing blood flow to the penis during sexual stimulation. This increased blood flow can cause an erection. Sildenafil does not cure erectile dysfunction or increase sexual desire. Sildenafil does not prevent pregnancy or the spread of sexually transmitted diseases such as human immunodeficiency virus (HIV).

How should this medicine be used?

Sildenafil comes as a tablet to take by mouth. It should be taken as needed about 1 hour before sexual activity. However, sildenafil can be taken anytime from 4 hours to 30 minutes before sexual activity. Sildenafil usually should not be taken more than once every 24 hours. If you have certain health conditions or are taking certain medications, your doctor may tell you to take sildenafil less often. Follow the directions on your prescription label carefully, and ask your doctor or pharmacist to explain any part you do not understand. Take sildenafil exactly as directed. Do not take more or less of it or take it more often than prescribed by your doctor.

You can take sildenafil with or without food. However, if you take sildenafil with a high-fat meal, it will take longer for the medication to start to work.

Your doctor will probably start you on an average dose of sildenafil and increase or decrease your dose depending on your response to the medication. Tell your doctor if sildenafil is not working well or if you are experiencing side effects.

Are there other uses for this medicine?

This medication is sometimes prescribed for other uses; ask your doctor or pharmacist for more information.

What special precautions should I follow?

Before taking sildenafil,

- tell your doctor and pharmacist if you are allergic to sildenafil or any other medications.
- do not take sildenafil if you are taking taking or have recently taken nitrates such as isosorbide dinitrate (Isordil), isosorbide mononitrate (Imdur, ISMO), and nitroglycerin (Nitro-BID, Nitro-Dur, Nitroquick, Nitrostat, others). Nitrates come as tablets, sublingual (under the tongue) tablets, sprays, patches, pastes, and ointments. Ask your doctor if you are not sure whether any of your medications contain nitrates.
- do not take street drugs containing nitrates such as amyl nitrate and butyl nitrate ('poppers') while taking sildenafil.
- tell your doctor and pharmacist what prescription and nonprescription medications, vitamins, and nutritional supplements you are taking or plan to take, especially alpha blockers such as alfuzosin (Uroxatral), doxazosin (Cardura), prazosin (Minipress), tamsulosin (Flomax), and terazosin (Hytrin); amiodarone (Cordarone, Pacerone); amlodipine (Norvasc); certain antifungals such as fluconazole (Diflucan), griseofulvin (Fulvicin, Grifulvin, Gris-PEG), itraconazole (Sporanox), ketoconazole (Nizoral), and voriconazole (Vfend); aprepitant (Emend); carbamazepine (Carbatrol, Epitol, Tegretol); cimetidine (Tagamet, Tagamet HB); clarithromycin (Biaxin, in Prevpac); cyclosporine (Neoral, Sandimmune); delaviridine (Rescriptor); dexamethasone (Decadron, Dexpak); diltiazem (Cardizem, Dilacor, Tiazac, others); efavirenz (Sus-

tiva); erythromycin (E.E.S., E-Mycin, Erythrocin); fluoxetine (Prozac, Sarafem); fluvoxamine (Luvox); HIV protease inhibitors including atazanavir (Reyataz), indinavir (Crixivan), lopinavir (in Kaletra), nelfinavir (Viracept), ritonavir (Norvir, in Kaletra), and saquinavir (Fortovase, Invirase); lovastatin (Advicor, Altocor, Mevacor); nefazodone; nevirapine (Viramune); other medications or devices to treat erectile dysfunction; phenobarbital; phenytoin (Dilantin, Phenytek); rifabutin (Mycobutin); rifampin (Rifadin, Rimactane); sertraline (Zoloft); troleandomycin (TAO); verapamil (Calan, Covera, Isoptin, Verelan); and zafirlukast (Accolate).
- tell your doctor what herbal products you are taking or plan to take, especially St. John's wort.
- tell your doctor if you smoke and if you have ever had an erection that lasted for several hours. Also tell your doctor if you have or have ever had a bleeding disorder, a stomach ulcer; heart, kidney, or liver disease; a heart attack; an irregular heartbeat; chest pain; a stroke; high or low blood pressure; high cholesterol; blood cell problems such as sickle cell anemia (a disease of the red blood cells), multiple myeloma (cancer of the plasma cells), or leukemia (cancer of the white blood cells); conditions affecting the shape of the penis (e.g., angulation, cavernosal fibrosis, or Peyronie's disease); or diabetes. Also tell your doctor if you or any of your family members have or have ever had an eye disease such as retinitis pigmentosa or if you have ever had severe vision loss, especially if you were told that the vision loss was caused by a blockage of blood flow to the nerves that help you see. Tell your doctor if you have ever been advised by a health care professional to avoid sexual activity for medical reasons or if you have ever experienced chest pain during sexual activity.
- you should know that sildenafil is only for use in males. Women should not take sildenafil, especially if they are or could become pregnant or are breast-feeding. If a pregnant woman takes sildenafil, she should call her doctor.
- if you are having surgery, including dental surgery, tell your doctor or dentist that you take sildenafil.
- you should know that sexual activity may be a strain on your heart, especially if you have heart disease. If you have chest pain during sexual activity, call your doctor immediately and avoid sexual activity until your doctor tells you otherwise.
- tell all your health care providers that you are taking sildenafil. If you ever need emergency medical treatment for a heart problem, the health care providers who treat you will need to know when you last took sildenafil.

What special dietary instructions should I follow?

Talk to your doctor about eating grapefruit and drinking grapefruit juice while taking this medicine.

What side effects can this medicine cause?

Sildenafil may cause side effects. Tell your doctor if any of these symptoms are severe or do not go away:

- headache
- upset stomach
- diarrhea
- dizziness or lightheadedness
- flushing (feeling of warmth)
- stuffy nose

Some side effects can be serious. If you experience any of the following symptoms, call your doctor immediately:

- sudden severe loss of vision (see below for more information)
- blurred vision
- changes in color vision (seeing a blue tinge on objects or having difficulty telling the difference between blue and green)
- painful erection
- prolonged erection (longer than 4 hours)
- fainting
- chest pain
- itching or burning during urination
- rash

Some patients experienced a sudden loss of some or all of their vision after they took sildenafil or other medications that are similar to sildenafil. The vision loss was permanent in some cases. It is not known if the vision loss was caused by the medication. If you experience a sudden loss of vision while you are taking sildenafil, call your doctor immediately. Do not take any more doses of sildenafil or similar medications such as tadalafil (Cialis) or vardenafil (Levitra) until you talk to your doctor.

Sildenafil may cause other side effects. Call your doctor if you have any unusual problems while you are taking this medication.

If you experience a serious side effect, you or your doctor may send a report to the Food and Drug Administration's (FDA) MedWatch Adverse Event Reporting program online [at http://www.fda.gov/MedWatch/index.html] or by phone [1-800-332-1088].

What storage conditions are needed for this medicine?

Keep this medication in the container it came in, tightly closed, and out of reach of children. Store it at room temperature and away from excess heat and moisture (not in the bathroom). Throw away any medication that is outdated or no longer needed. Talk to your pharmacist about the proper disposal of your medication.

What should I do in case of overdose?

In case of overdose, call your local poison control center at 1-800-222-1222. If the victim has collapsed or is not breathing, call local emergency services at 911.

What other information should I know?

Keep all appointments with your doctor.

Do not let anyone else take your medication. Ask your pharmacist any questions you have about refilling your prescription.

Dosage Facts
For Informational Purposes

Caution: Do not change your dose, how often you take your medication, or the length of time you are to take it without first talking to your healthcare provider.

The following dosage information was written using medical language for doctors and other healthcare professionals and is provided here for you to check your dosage. The dosage of this drug may differ for different patients. Therefore, always follow your doctor's instructions or the directions on the label. Contact your healthcare provider or pharmacist if you have any questions about the specific dosage of your medication after reviewing this information.

General Dosage Information

Available as sildenafil citrate; dosage expressed in terms of sildenafil.

Adult Patients

Erectile Dysfunction

ORAL:
- Initially, 50 mg. Depending on effectiveness and tolerance, increase dosage to a maximum of 100 mg or decrease to 25 mg.

PAH

ORAL:
- 20 mg 3 times daily. Efficacy of lower dosages not established.

Prescribing Limits

Adult Patients

Erectile Dysfunction

ORAL:
- Maximum 100 mg daily.

PAH

ORAL:
- Dosages up to 80 mg 3 times daily have been studied but have not been more effective than recommended dosage of 20 mg 3 times daily.

Special Populations

Hepatic Impairment

Erectile Dysfunction

ORAL:
- Reduce initial dose to 25 mg.

PAH

ORAL:
- No dosage adjustments necessary for mild to moderate hepatic impairment (Child-Pugh class A and B). Not studied in severe hepatic impairment (Child-Pugh class C).

Renal Impairment

Erectile Dysfunction

ORAL:
• If Cl_{cr} is <30 mL/minute, reduce initial dose to 25 mg.

PAH

ORAL:
• No dosage adjustment needed, even in severe impairment (Cl_{cr} <30 mL/minute).

Geriatric Patients

Erectile Dysfunction

Oral
• Reduce initial dose to 25 mg in men ≥65 years of age.

PAH

Oral
• Select dosage with caution because of age-related decreases in hepatic, renal, and/or cardiac function and concomitant disease and drug therapy.

Silver Sulfadiazine

(sil' ver sul fa dye' a zeen)

Brand Name: Silvadene®, SSD Cream®, Thermazene®

Why is this medicine prescribed?

Silver sulfadiazine, a sulfa drug, is used to prevent and treat infections of second- and third-degree burns. It kills a wide variety of bacteria.

This medication is sometimes prescribed for other uses; ask your doctor or pharmacist for more information.

How should this medicine be used?

Silver sulfadiazine comes in a cream. Silver sulfadiazine usually is applied once or twice a day. Follow the directions on your prescription label carefully, and ask your doctor or pharmacist to explain any part you do not understand. Use silver sulfadiazine exactly as directed. Do not use more or less of it or use it more often than prescribed by your doctor.

Do not apply this drug to infants less than 2 months of age.

Do not stop using silver sulfadiazine until your doctor tells you to do so. Your burn must be healed so that infection is no longer a problem. Gently wash the burned skin area daily to help remove dead skin. If your burn becomes infected or if your infection worsens, call your doctor.

Before applying the medication, clean the burned area and remove any dead or burned skin. Always wear a sterile, disposable glove when you apply silver sulfadiazine. Cover the cleaned burned area with a 1/16-inch thickness of cream. Keep the burned area covered with cream at all times; reapply the cream to any area that becomes uncovered.

What special precautions should I follow?

Before using silver sulfadiazine,
• tell your doctor and pharmacist if you are allergic to silver sulfadiazine, sulfa drugs, or any other drugs.
• tell your doctor and pharmacist what prescription and nonprescription medications you are taking, including vitamins.
• tell your doctor if you have or have ever had liver or kidney disease.
• tell your doctor if you are pregnant, plan to become pregnant, or are breast-feeding. If you become pregnant while using silver sulfadiazine, call your doctor.

What should I do if I forget to take a dose?

Apply the missed dose as soon as you remember it. However, if it is almost time for the next dose, skip the missed dose and continue your regular dosing schedule. Do not apply a double dose to make up for a missed one.

What side effects can this medicine cause?

Silver sulfadiazine may cause side effects. Tell your doctor if any of these symptoms are severe or do not go away:
• pain
• burning
• itching

If you experience any of the following symptoms, call your doctor immediately:
• unusual bleeding or bruising
• fever
• sore throat
• yellowing of the skin or eyes
• blood in urine
• aching joints
• unusual weakness or tiredness
• skin rash

If you experience a serious side effect, you or your doctor may send a report to the Food and Drug Administration's (FDA) MedWatch Adverse Event Reporting program online [at http://www.fda.gov/MedWatch/index.html] or by phone [1-800-332-1088].

What storage conditions are needed for this medicine?

Keep this medication in the container it came in, tightly closed, and out of reach of children. Store it at room temperature and away from excess heat and moisture (not in the bathroom). Throw away any medication that is outdated or no longer needed. Talk to your pharmacist about the proper disposal of your medication.

What other information should I know?

Keep all appointments with your doctor.

Silver sulfadiazine is for external use only. Do not let silver sulfadiazine get into your eyes, nose, or mouth, and do not swallow it. Do not apply dressings, bandages, cosmetics, lotions, or other skin medications to the area being treated unless your doctor tells you.

Do not let anyone else use your medication. Ask your pharmacist any questions you have about refilling your prescription.

Tell your doctor if your skin condition gets worse or does not go away.

Talk to your doctor, pharmacist, or other healthcare professional if you have questions about dosing information for your medication.

Simethicone

(sye meth' i kone)

Brand Name: Alka-Seltzer® Gas Relief Maximum Strength Softgels®, Flatulex® Drops, GasAid® Maximum Strength Softgels®, Gas-X®, Gas-X® Extra Strength, Gas-X® Extra Strength Liquid, Gas-X® Extra Strength Softgels®, Genasyme®, Genasyme® Drops, Maalox® Anti-Gas Extra Strength, Maalox® Anti-Gas Regular Strength, Mylanta® Gas Relief, Mylanta® Gas Relief Gelcaps®, Mylanta® Gas Relief Maximum Strength, Mylicon® Infant's Drops, Phazyme® Infant Drops, Phazyme®-125 Softgels®, Phazyme®-166 Maximum Strength, Phazyme®-166 Maximum Strength Softgels®

Also available generically.

Why is this medicine prescribed?

Simethicone is used to treat the symptoms of gas such as uncomfortable or painful pressure, fullness, and bloating.

This medication is sometimes prescribed for other uses; ask your doctor or pharmacist for more information.

How should this medicine be used?

Simethicone comes as regular tablets, chewable tablets, capsules, and liquid to take by mouth. It usually is taken four times a day, after meals and at bedtime. Follow the directions on the package or on your prescription label carefully, and ask your doctor or pharmacist to explain any part you do not understand. Take simethicone exactly as directed. Do not take more or less of it or take it more often than prescribed by your doctor.

Swallow the regular tablets and capsules whole. Chewable tablets should be chewed thoroughly before being swallowed; do not swallow them whole. Do not take more than six simethicone tablets or eight simethicone capsules each day unless your doctor tells you to. The liquid may be mixed with 1 ounce of cool water or infant formula.

What special precautions should I follow?

Before taking simethicone,
- tell your doctor and pharmacist if you are allergic to simethicone or any other drugs.
- tell your doctor and pharmacist what prescription and nonprescription medications you are taking, including vitamins.
- tell your doctor if you are pregnant, plan to become pregnant, or are breast-feeding. If you become pregnant while taking simethicone, call your doctor.

What should I do if I forget to take a dose?

If you are taking simethicone on a regular schedule, take the missed dose as soon you remember it. However, if it is almost time for the next dose, skip the missed dose and continue your regular dosing schedule. Do not take a double dose to make up for a missed one.

What side effects can this medicine cause?

When taken as directed, simethicone usually has no side effects.

What storage conditions are needed for this medicine?

Keep this medication in the container it came in, tightly closed, and out of reach of children. Store it at room temperature and away from excess heat and moisture (not in the bathroom). Throw away any medication that is outdated or no longer needed. Talk to your pharmacist about the proper disposal of your medication.

What other information should I know?

Ask your doctor or pharmacist any questions you have about taking this medicine.

Dosage Facts
For Informational Purposes

Caution: Do not change your dose, how often you take your medication, or the length of time you are to take it without first talking to your healthcare provider.

The following dosage information was written using medical language for doctors and other healthcare professionals and is provided here for you to check your dosage. The dosage of this drug may differ for different patients. Therefore, always follow your doctor's instructions or the directions on the label. Contact your healthcare provider or pharmacist if you have any questions about the specific dosage of your medication after reviewing this information.

Pediatric Patients

Flatulence, Functional Gastric Bloating, and Postoperative Gas Pain

ORAL:

- Usual dosage in children >12 years of age: 40–125 mg 4 times daily as needed after meals and at bedtime.
- *Self-medication* in children <2 years of age (<10.9 kg): 20 mg (0.3 mL) as needed after meals and at bedtime as oral drops; do not exceed 12 doses (i.e., 240 mg) daily.
- *Self-medication* in children 2–12 years of age (>10.9 kg): 40 mg as needed after meals and at bedtime; do not exceed 12 doses (i.e., 480 mg) daily.
- *Self-medication* in children >12 years of age: 40–125 mg as needed after meals and at bedtime; do not exceed 500 mg daily.

Adult Patients

Flatulence, Functional Gastric Bloating, and Postoperative Gas Pain

ORAL:

- Usual dosage: 40–125 mg 4 times daily as needed after meals and at bedtime.
- *Self-medication*: 40–250 mg as needed after meals and at bedtime; do not exceed 500 mg daily.

Diagnostic Aid Prior to Gastroscopy or Radiography of the Intestine

ORAL:

- 67 mg as a single dose of oral suspension, in 2.5 mL of water.

Prescribing Limits

Pediatric Patients

Flatulence, Functional Gastric Bloating, and Postoperative Gas Pain

ORAL:

- *Self-medication* in children <2 years of age (weight <10.9 kg): Maximum 12 doses (i.e., 240 mg) daily.
- *Self-medication* in children 2–12 years of age (weight >10.9 kg): Maximum 12 doses (i.e., 480 mg) daily.
- *Self-medication* in children >12 years of age: Maximum 500 mg daily.

Adult Patients

Flatulence, Functional Gastric Bloating, and Postoperative Gas Pain

ORAL:

- *Self-medication*: Maximum 500 mg daily.

Special Populations

No special population dosage recommendations at this time.

Simvastatin

(sim′ va stat in)

Brand Name: Vytorin®, Zocor®

Why is this medicine prescribed?

Simvastatin is used together with lifestyle changes (diet, weight-loss, exercise) to reduce the amount of cholesterol (a fat-like substance) and certain other fatty substances in your blood. Simvastatin is in a class of medications called HMG-CoA reductase inhibitors (statins). It works by slowing the production of cholesterol in the body.

Buildup of cholesterol and fats along the walls of your arteries (a process known as atherosclerosis) decreases blood flow and, therefore, the oxygen supply to your heart, brain, and other parts of your body. Lowering your blood level of cholesterol and fats may help to decrease your chances of getting heart disease, angina (chest pain), strokes, and heart attacks. In addition to taking a cholesterol-lowering medication, making certain changes in your daily habits can also lower your cholesterol blood levels. You should eat a diet that is low in saturated fat and cholesterol (see SPECIAL DIETARY), exercise 30 minutes on most, if not all days, and lose weight if you are overweight.

How should this medicine be used?

Simvastatin comes as a tablet to take by mouth. It usually is taken one to three times a day. Take simvastatin at around the same time(s) every day. Follow the directions on your prescription label carefully, and ask your doctor or pharmacist to explain any part you do not understand. Take simvastatin exactly as directed. Do not take more or less of it or take it more often than prescribed by your doctor.

Your doctor may start you on a low dose of simvastatin and gradually increase your dose, not more than once every 4 weeks.

Continue to take simvastatin even if you feel well. Do not stop taking simvastatin without talking to your doctor.

Are there other uses for this medicine?

This medication may be prescribed for other uses; ask your doctor or pharmacist for more information.

What special precautions should I follow?

Before taking simvastatin,

- tell your doctor and pharmacist if you are allergic to simvastatin or any other medications.
- tell your doctor and pharmacist what prescription and nonprescription medications, vitamins, nutritional supplements, and herbal products you are taking or plan to take. Be sure to mention any of the following: amiodarone (Cordarone, Pacerone); antifungal medications such as itraconazole (Sporanox) and ketoconazole (Nizoral); anticoagulants ('blood thinners') such as warfa-

rin (Coumadin); cholestyramine (Questran), clarithromycin (Biaxin), clofibrate (Atromid-S), cyclosporine (Sandimmune, Neoral), danazol; digoxin (Lanoxin), erythromycin (E.E.S., E-Mycin, Erythrocin); HIV protease inhibitors such as indinavir (Crixivan), ritonavir (Norvir) and saquinavir (Invirase, Fortovase); nefazodone (Serzone); other cholesterol-lowering medications such as fenofibrate (Tricor), gemfibrozil (Lopid), and niacin (nicotinic acid, Niacor, Niaspan); nefazodone (Serzone), and telithromycin (Ketek); and verapamil (Calan, Covera, Isoptin, Verelan). Your doctor may need to change the doses of your medications or monitor you carefully for side effects.

- tell your doctor if you have liver disease. Your doctor will probably tell you not to take simvastatin.
- tell your doctor if you drink large amounts of alcohol, if you have ever had liver disease or if you have or have ever had kidney disease.
- tell your doctor if you are pregnant or plan to become pregnant. If you become pregnant while taking simvastatin, stop taking simvastatin and call your doctor immediately. Simvastatin can harm the fetus.
- Do not breast-feed while you are taking this medication.
- if you are having surgery, including dental surgery, tell the doctor or dentist that you are taking simvastatin.
- ask your doctor about the safe use of alcoholic beverages while you are taking simvastatin. Alcohol can increase the risk of serious side effects.

What special dietary instructions should I follow?

Avoid drinking large quantities (more than 1 quart a day) of grapefruit juice while taking simvastatin.

Eat a low-cholesterol, low-fat diet. This kind of diet includes cottage cheese, fat-free milk, fish (not canned in oil), vegetables, poultry, egg whites, and polyunsaturated oils and margarines (corn, safflower, canola, and soybean oils). Avoid foods with excess fat in them such as meat (especially liver and fatty meat), egg yolks, whole milk, cream, butter, shortening, lard, pastries, cakes, cookies, gravy, peanut butter, chocolate, olives, potato chips, coconut, cheese (other than cottage cheese), coconut oil, palm oil, and fried foods.

What should I do if I forget to take a dose?

Take the missed dose as soon as you remember it. However, if it is almost time for the next dose, skip the missed dose and continue the regular dosing schedule. Do not take a double dose to make up for a missed one.

What side effects can this medicine cause?

Simvastatin may cause side effects. Tell your doctor if any of these symptoms are severe or do not go away:
- constipation

If you experience the following symptoms, call your doctor immediately:
- muscle pain, tenderness, or weakness
- lack of energy
- fever
- yellowing of the skin or eyes
- pain in the upper right part of the stomach
- nausea
- extreme tiredness
- unusual bleeding or bruising
- loss of appetite
- flu-like symptoms
- rash
- hives
- itching
- difficulty breathing or swallowing
- swelling of the face, throat, tongue, lips, eyes, hands, feet, ankles, or lower legs
- hoarseness

If you experience a serious side effect, you or your doctor may send a report to the Food and Drug Administration's (FDA) MedWatch Adverse Event Reporting program online [at http://www.fda.gov/MedWatch/index.html] or by phone [1-800-332-1088].

What storage conditions are needed for this medicine?

Keep this medication in the container it came in, tightly closed, and out of reach of children. Store it at room temperature and away from excess heat and moisture (not in the bathroom). Throw away any medication that is outdated or no longer needed. Talk to your pharmacist about the proper disposal of your medication.

What should I do in case of overdose?

In case of overdose, call your local poison control center at 1-800-222-1222. If the victim has collapsed or is not breathing, call local emergency services at 911.

What other information should I know?

Keep all appointments with your doctor and the laboratory. Your doctor will order certain lab tests before and during treatment to check your response to simvastatin.

Before having any laboratory test, tell your doctor and the laboratory personnel that you are taking simvastatin.

Do not let anyone else take your medication. Ask your pharmacist any questions you have about refilling your prescription.

Dosage Facts
For Informational Purposes

Caution: Do not change your dose, how often you take your medication, or the length of time you

are to take it without first talking to your health-care provider.

The following dosage information was written using medical language for doctors and other healthcare professionals and is provided here for you to check your dosage. The dosage of this drug may differ for different patients. Therefore, always follow your doctor's instructions or the directions on the label. Contact your healthcare provider or pharmacist if you have any questions about the specific dosage of your medication after reviewing this information.

Pediatric Patients

Dyslipidemias

ORAL:
- Children ≥10 years of age: 10 mg once daily.
- Adjust dosage at intervals of ≥4 weeks until the desired effect on lipoprotein concentrations is observed. Usual dosage range is 10–40 mg daily.

Adult Patients

Dyslipidemias and Prevention of Cardiovascular Events

ORAL:
- Initially, 20–40 mg once daily.
- Patients with CHD or CHD risk equivalents: Initially, 40 mg once daily.
- Adjust dosage at intervals of no less than 4 weeks until the desired effect on lipoprotein concentrations is observed. Usual dosage range is 5–80 mg daily.
- Simvastatin-ezetimibe fixed combination (Vytorin®): Initially, simvastatin 20 mg and ezetimibe 10 mg once daily in the evening. In patients requiring less aggressive LDL-cholesterol lowering, consider lower dosage (simvastatin 10 mg and ezetimibe 10 mg once daily). In patients requiring LDL-cholesterol reductions >55%, give simvastatin 40 mg and ezetimibe 10 mg once daily. Determine serum lipoprotein concentrations 2 weeks after initiation of therapy and adjust dosage as needed. Usual maintenance dosage is simvastatin 10–80 mg and ezetimibe 10 mg once daily.

Homozygous Familial Hypercholesterolemia

ORAL:
- 40 mg once daily in the evening or 80 mg daily in 3 divided doses of 20 mg, 20 mg, and an evening dose of 40 mg.
- Simvastatin-ezetimibe fixed combination (Vytorin®): Initially, simvastatin 40 or 80 mg and ezetimibe 10 mg once daily in the evening.

Prescribing Limits

Pediatric Patients

ORAL:
- Children ≥10 years of age: Maximum 40 mg once daily.

Special Populations

Hepatic Impairment
- Use with caution in patients who consume substantial amounts of alcohol and/or have a history of liver disease. Contraindicated in patients with active liver disease or unexplained, persistent increases in serum aminotransferase concentrations.

Renal Impairment
- Dosage modification is not necessary in patients with mild to moderate impairment. In patients with severe renal impairment, initially, 5 mg once daily. Use with caution; monitor closely.
- Simvastatin-ezetimibe fixed combination (Vytorin®): Dosage modification is not necessary in patients with mild to moderate impairment. In patients with severe renal impairment, do not use unless patient already has tolerated treatment with simvastatin at dosage of ≥5 mg daily; in such patients, exercise caution and monitor closely.

Sirolimus

(sir oh′ li mus)

Brand Name: Rapamune®

Important Warning

Sirolimus may increase the risk of infection and lymphoma. If you experience any of the following symptoms, call your doctor immediately: fever, sore throat, chills, frequent or painful urination, or other signs of infection.

Keep all appointments with your doctor and the laboratory. Your doctor will order certain tests to check your body's response to sirolimus.

Talk to your doctor about the risks of taking sirolimus.

Why is this medicine prescribed?

Sirolimus is used in combination with other medications to prevent rejection of kidney transplants. Sirolimus is in a class of medications called immunosuppressants. It works by suppressing the body's immune system.

How should this medicine be used?

Sirolimus comes as a tablet and a solution (liquid) to take by mouth. It is usually taken once a day, either always with food or always without food. To help you remember to take sirolimus, take it around the same time every day. Follow the directions on your prescription label carefully, and ask your doctor or pharmacist to explain any part you do not understand. Take sirolimus exactly as directed. Do not take more or less of it or take it more often than prescribed by your doctor.

Continue to take sirolimus even if you feel well. Do not stop taking sirolimus without talking to your doctor.

To use the bottles of solution, follow these steps:
1. Open the solution bottle. On first use, insert the plastic tube with stopper tightly into the bottle until it is even with the top of the bottle. Do not remove from the bottle.

2. For each use, tightly insert one of the amber syringes with the plunger fully pushed in into the opening in the plastic tube.

3. Draw up the amount of solution your doctor has prescribed by gently pulling out the plunger of the syringe until the bottom of the black line of the plunger is even with the correct mark on the syringe. Keep the bottle upright. If bubbles form in the syringe, empty the syringe into the bottle and repeat this step.

4. Empty the syringe into a glass or plastic cup containing at least 2 ounces (1/4 cup) of water or orange juice. Do not use apple juice, grapefruit juice, or other liquids. Stir vigorously for 1 minute and drink immediately.

5. Refill the cup with at least 4 ounces (1/2 cup) of water or orange juice. Stir vigorously and drink the rinse solution.

6. Throw away the used syringe.

If you need to carry a filled syringe with you, snap a cap onto the syringe and put the syringe in the carrying case. Use the medication in the syringe within 24 hours.

To use the pouches of solution, follow these steps:

1. Before opening the pouch, squeeze the pouch from the neck area to push the contents into the lower part of the pouch.

2. Fold the marked area on the pouch and carefully cut with scissors.

3. Squeeze the entire contents of the pouch into a glass or plastic cup containing at least 2 ounces (1/4 cup) of water or orange juice. Do not use apple juice, grapefruit juice, or other liquids. Stir vigorously for 1 minute and drink immediately.

4. Refill the cup with at least 4 ounces (1/2 cup) of water or orange juice. Stir vigorously and drink the rinse solution.

Are there other uses for this medicine?

Sirolimus also is used sometimes to treat psoriasis. Talk to your doctor about the possible risks of using this medication for your condition.

This medication may be prescribed for other uses; ask your doctor or pharmacist for more information.

What special precautions should I follow?

Before taking sirolimus,

- tell your doctor and pharmacist if you are allergic to sirolimus or any other medications.
- tell your doctor and pharmacist what prescription and nonprescription medications, vitamins, and nutritional supplements you are taking. Be sure to mention any of the following: amphotericin B (Abelcet, AmBisome, Amphocin, Fungizone); antifungals such as clotrimazole (Lotrimin), fluconazole (Diflucan), itraconazole (Sporanox), and ketoconazole (Nizoral); bromocriptine (Parlodel); cimetidine (Tagamet); cisapride (Propulsid); clarithromycin (Biaxin); danazol (Danocrine); diltiazem (Cardizem, Dilacor, Tiazac); erythromycin (E.E.S., E-

Mycin, Erythrocin); HIV protease inhibitors such as indinavir (Crixivan) and ritonavir (Norvir); medications for seizures such as carbamazepine (Tegretol), phenobarbital (Luminal, Solfoton), and phenytoin (Dilantin); metoclopramide (Reglan); nicardipine (Cardene); rifabutin (Mycobutin); rifampin (Rifadin, Rimactane); rifapentine (Priftin); troleandomycin (TAO); and verapamil (Calan, Covera, Isoptin, Verelan). Your doctor may need to change the doses of your medications or monitor you carefully for side effects.

- if you are taking cyclosporine (Neoral) soft gelatin capsules or solution, take them 4 hours before sirolimus.
- tell your doctor what herbal products you are taking, especially St. John's wort.
- tell your doctor if you have or have ever had high cholesterol or triglycerides or liver disease.
- tell your doctor if you are pregnant, plan to become pregnant, or are breast-feeding. You should use an effective method of birth control before starting to take sirolimus, while taking sirolimus, and for 12 weeks after stopping sirolimus. If you become pregnant while taking sirolimus, call your doctor.
- if you are having surgery, including dental surgery, tell the doctor or dentist that you are taking sirolimus.
- plan to avoid unnecessary or prolonged exposure to sunlight and to wear protective clothing, sunglasses, and sunscreen. Sirolimus may increase your risk for skin cancer.
- do not have any vaccinations (e.g., measles or flu shots) without talking to your doctor.

What special dietary instructions should I follow?

Avoid drinking large amounts of grapefruit juice while taking this medicine.

What should I do if I forget to take a dose?

Take the missed dose as soon as you remember it. However, if it is almost time for the next dose, skip the missed dose and continue your regular dosing schedule. Do not take a double dose to make up for a missed one.

What side effects can this medicine cause?

Sirolimus may cause side effects. Tell your doctor if any of these symptoms are severe or do not go away:

- stomach pain
- weakness
- back pain
- headache
- constipation
- diarrhea
- upset stomach
- vomiting
- swelling of the hands, feet, ankles, or lower legs
- weight gain
- joint pain

- difficulty falling asleep or staying asleep
- tremor
- rash
- fever

Some side effects can be serious. The following symptoms are uncommon, but if you experience any of them or those listed in the IMPORTANT WARNING section, call your doctor immediately:

- pale skin
- unusual bleeding or bruising
- cough
- shortness of breath

Sirolimus may cause other side effects. Call your doctor if you have any unusual problems while taking this medication.

If you experience a serious side effect, you or your doctor may send a report to the Food and Drug Administration's (FDA) MedWatch Adverse Event Reporting program online [at http://www.fda.gov/MedWatch/index.html] or by phone [1-800-332-1088].

What storage conditions are needed for this medicine?

Keep this medication in the container it came in, tightly closed, and out of reach of children. Store tablets at room temperature and away from excess heat and moisture (not in the bathroom). Keep liquid medication in the refrigerator, closed tightly, and throw away any unused medication one month after the bottle is opened. Do not freeze. If needed, you may store the pouches for up to 24 hours and the bottles for up to 15 days at room temperature. Throw away any medication that is outdated or no longer needed. Talk to your pharmacist about the proper disposal of your medication.

What should I do in case of overdose?

In case of overdose, call your local poison control center at 1-800-222-1222. If the victim has collapsed or is not breathing, call local emergency services at 911.

What other information should I know?

Keep all appointments with your doctor and the laboratory. Your doctor may order certain lab tests to check your body's response to sirolimus.

Do not let anyone else take your medication. Ask your pharmacist any questions you have about refilling your prescription.

Dosage Facts
For Informational Purposes

Caution: Do not change your dose, how often you take your medication, or the length of time you are to take it without first talking to your healthcare provider.

The following dosage information was written using medical language for doctors and other healthcare professionals and is provided here for you to check your dosage. The dosage of this drug may differ for different patients. Therefore, always follow your doctor's instructions or the directions on the label. Contact your healthcare provider or pharmacist if you have any questions about the specific dosage of your medication after reviewing this information.

Pediatric Patients

Renal Allotransplantion
Concomitant Sirolimus and Cyclosporine Therapy

ORAL:

- Children ≥13 years of age who weigh ≥40 kg: Initially, 6 mg as a loading dose in *de novo* renal transplant recipients. Maintenance dosage of 2 mg daily.
- Children ≥13 years of age who weigh <40 kg: Initially, 3 mg/m² as a loading dose in *de novo* renal transplant recipients. Maintenance dosage of 1 mg/m² daily.

Sirolimus Therapy following Cyclosporine Withdrawal

ORAL:

- Children ≥13 years of age: As cyclosporine is gradually discontinued over 4- to 8-week period, increase sirolimus dosage (by approximately 4-fold) to maintain trough whole blood concentrations 12–24 ng/mL (chromatographic method). If subsequent dosage adjustment is required, manufacturer states that new dosage can be estimated based on the following equation:

New sirolimus dosage = current sirolimus dosage
× (target concentration / current concentration)

- Loading dose may be necessary if a considerable increase in trough sirolimus concentrations is required. Estimate loading dose based on the following equation:

Sirolimus loading dose = 3 × (new maintenance dosage
− current maintenance dosage)

Adult Patients

Renal Allotransplantion
Concomitant Sirolimus and Cyclosporine Therapy

ORAL:

- Initially, 6 mg as a loading dose in *de novo* renal transplant recipients. Maintenance dosage of 2 mg daily.

Sirolimus Therapy following Cyclosporine Withdrawal

ORAL:

- As cyclosporine is gradually discontinued over 4- to 8-week period, increase sirolimus dosage (by approximately 4-fold) to maintain trough whole blood concentrations of 12–24 ng/mL (chromatographic method). If subsequent dosage adjustment is required, manufacturer states that new dosage can be estimated based on the following equation:

New sirolimus dosage = current sirolimus dosage
× (target concentration / current concentration)

- Loading dose may be necessary if a considerable increase in trough sirolimus concentrations is required. Estimate loading dose based on the following equation:

Sirolimus loading dose = 3 × (new maintenance dosage
− current maintenance dosage)

Prescribing Limits

Pediatric Patients

Renal Allotransplantation

ORAL:
- Children ≥13 years of age who weigh ≥40 kg: Maximum 40 mg within 1-day period.

Adult Patients

Renal Allotransplantation

ORAL:
- Maximum 40 mg within 1-day period.

Special Populations

Hepatic Impairment
- Reduce maintenance dose by one-third in patients with hepatic impairment; loading dose does not require modification.

Renal Impairment
- Dosage reduction is not necessary.

Geriatric Patients
- Dosage adjustments based solely on advanced age do not appear to be necessary.

Black Patients
- Limited data suggest that 5 mg daily may be more effective than 2 mg daily; however, manufacturer states that potential benefit of higher dose must be weighed against an increased risk of dose-dependent adverse effects.

Sitagliptin

(sit a glip′ tin)

Brand Name: Januvia®

Why is this medicine prescribed?

Sitagliptin is used along with diet and exercise and sometimes with other medications to lower blood sugar levels in patients with type 2 diabetes (condition in which blood sugar is too high because the body does not produce or use insulin normally). Sitagliptin is in a class of medications called dipeptidyl peptidase-4 (DPP-4) inhibitors. It works by increasing the amounts of certain natural substances that lower blood sugar when it is high.

How should this medicine be used?

Sitagliptin comes as a tablet to take by mouth. It is usually taken once a day with or without food. Take sitagliptin at around the same time every day. Follow the directions on your prescription label carefully, and ask your doctor or pharmacist to explain any part you do not understand. Take sitagliptin exactly as directed. Do not take more or less of it or take it more often than prescribed by your doctor.

Sitagliptin helps to control high blood sugar but does not cure diabetes. Continue to take sitagliptin even if you feel well. Do not stop taking sitagliptin without talking to your doctor.

Ask your pharmacist or doctor for a copy of the manufacturer's information for the patient.

Are there other uses for this medicine?

This medication may be prescribed for other uses; ask your doctor or pharmacist for more information.

What special precautions should I follow?

Before taking sitagliptin,
- tell your doctor and pharmacist if you are allergic to sitagliptin or any other medications.
- tell your doctor and pharmacist what prescription and nonprescription medications, vitamins, nutritional supplements, and herbal products you are taking or plan to take. Be sure to mention any of the following: digoxin (Lanoxicaps, Lanoxin); insulin; and certain oral medications for diabetes including acetohexamide, chlorpropamide (Diabinese), glimepiride (Amaryl), glipizide (Glucotrol, in Metaglip), glyburide (Diabeta, Glycron, Micronase), tolazamide (Tolinase), and tolbutamide. Your doctor may need to change the doses of your medications or monitor you carefully for side effects.
- tell your doctor if you have or have ever had type 1 diabetes (condition in which the body does not make insulin and therefore can not control the amount of sugar in the blood), diabetic ketoacidosis (a serious condition that may occur when blood sugar is too high), or kidney disease.
- tell your doctor if you are pregnant, plan to become pregnant, or are breast-feeding. If you become pregnant while taking sitagliptin, call your doctor.
- if you are having surgery, including dental surgery, tell the doctor or dentist that you are taking sitagliptin.
- talk to your doctor about what you should do if you get hurt or if you develop a fever or infection. These conditions may affect your blood sugar.
- talk to your doctor about the symptoms of high and low blood sugar and other complications of diabetes, what to do if you develop these symptoms, and how to prevent these conditions.

What special dietary instructions should I follow?

Be sure to follow all diet and exercise recommendations made by your doctor or dietician.

What should I do if I forget to take a dose?

Take the missed dose as soon as you remember it. However, if it is almost time for the next dose, skip the missed dose and continue your regular dosing schedule. Do not take a double dose to make up for a missed one.

What side effects can this medicine cause?

Sitagliptin may cause side effects. Tell your doctor if any of these symptoms are severe or do not go away:

- stuffed or runny nose
- sore throat
- headache
- stomach pain
- diarrhea

Sitagliptin may cause other side effects. Call your doctor if you have any unusual problems while taking this medication.

What storage conditions are needed for this medicine?

Keep this medication in the container it came in, tightly closed, and out of reach of children. Store it at room temperature and away from excess heat and moisture (not in the bathroom). Throw away any medication that is outdated or no longer needed. Talk to your pharmacist about the proper disposal of your medication.

What should I do in case of overdose?

In case of overdose, call your local poison control center at 1-800-222-1222. If the victim has collapsed or is not breathing, call local emergency services at 911.

What other information should I know?

Keep all appointments with your doctor and the laboratory. Your blood sugar and glycosylated hemoglobin (HbA1c) should be checked regularly to determine your response to sitagliptin. Your doctor will also tell you how to check your response to sitagliptin by measuring your blood or urine sugar levels at home. Follow these instructions carefully.

Do not let anyone else take your medication. Ask your pharmacist any questions you have about refilling your prescription.

Talk to your doctor, pharmacist, or other healthcare professional if you have questions about dosing information for your medication.

Sodium Bicarbonate

(soe′ dee um bye kar′ bon ate)

Why is this medicine prescribed?

Sodium bicarbonate is an antacid used to relieve heartburn and acid indigestion. Your doctor also may prescribe sodium bicarbonate to make your blood or urine less acidic in certain conditions.

This medication is sometimes prescribed for other uses; ask your doctor or pharmacist for more information.

How should this medicine be used?

Sodium bicarbonate comes as a tablet and powder to take by mouth. Sodium bicarbonate is taken one to four times a day, depending on the reason you take it. Follow the directions on your prescription label carefully, and ask your doctor or pharmacist to explain any part you do not understand. Take sodium bicarbonate exactly as directed. Do not take more or less of it or take it more often than prescribed by your doctor.

If you are using sodium bicarbonate as an antacid, it should be taken 1-2 hours after meals, with a full glass of water. If you are using sodium bicarbonate for another reason, it may be taken with or without food. Do not take sodium bicarbonate on an overly full stomach.

Dissolve sodium bicarbonate powder in at least 4 ounces of water. Measure powdered doses carefully using a measuring spoon.

Do not use sodium bicarbonate for longer than 2 weeks unless your doctor tells you to. If sodium bicarbonate does not improve your symptoms, call your doctor.

Do not give sodium bicarbonate to children under 12 years of age unless your doctor tells you to.

What special precautions should I follow?

Before taking sodium bicarbonate,

- tell your doctor and pharmacist what prescription and nonprescription medications you are taking, especially other antacids, aspirin or aspirin-like medicines, benzodiazepines, flecainide (Tambocor), iron, ketoconazole (Nizoral), lithium (Eskalith, Lithobid), methenamine (Hiprex, Urex), methotrexate, quinidine, sulfa-containing antibiotics, tetracycline (Sumycin), or vitamins. Take sodium bicarbonate at least 2 hours apart from other medicines.
- tell your doctor if you have or have ever had high blood pressure, congestive heart failure, or kidney disease or if you have recently had bleeding in your stomach or intestine.
- tell your doctor if you are pregnant, plan to become pregnant, or are breast-feeding. If you become pregnant while taking sodium bicarbonate, call your doctor.

What special dietary instructions should I follow?

This medicine increases the amount of sodium in your body. If you are on a sodium-restricted diet, check with your doctor before taking sodium bicarbonate.

What should I do if I forget to take a dose?

If your doctor has told you to take sodium bicarbonate on a certain schedule, take the missed dose as soon as you remember it. However, if it is almost time for the next dose, skip the missed dose and continue your regular dosing schedule. Do not take a double dose to make up for a missed one.

What side effects can this medicine cause?

Sodium bicarbonate may cause side effects. Tell your doctor if any of these symptoms are severe or do not go away:

- increased thirst
- stomach cramps
- gas

If you have any of the following symptoms, stop taking sodium bicarbonate and call your doctor immediately:

- severe headache
- upset stomach
- vomit that resembles coffee grounds
- loss of appetite
- irritability
- weakness
- frequent urge to urinate
- slow breathing
- swelling of feet or lower legs
- bloody, black, or tarry stools
- blood in your urine

If you experience a serious side effect, you or your doctor may send a report to the Food and Drug Administration's (FDA) MedWatch Adverse Event Reporting program online [at http://www.fda.gov/MedWatch/index.html] or by phone [1-800-332-1088].

What storage conditions are needed for this medicine?

Keep this medication in the container it came in, tightly closed, and out of reach of children. Store it at room temperature and away from excess heat and moisture (not in the bathroom). Throw away any medication that is outdated or no longer needed. Talk to your pharmacist about the proper disposal of your medication.

What should I do in case of overdose?

In case of overdose, call your local poison control center at 1-800-222-1222. If the victim has collapsed or is not breathing, call local emergency services at 911.

What other information should I know?

If your doctor has prescribed sodium bicarbonate, keep all scheduled appointments so that your response to the medicine can be checked.

Dosage Facts
For Informational Purposes

Caution: Do not change your dose, how often you take your medication, or the length of time you are to take it without first talking to your healthcare provider.

The following dosage information was written using medical language for doctors and other healthcare professionals and is provided here for you to check your dosage. The dosage of this drug may differ for different patients. Therefore, always follow your doctor's instructions or the directions on the label. Contact your healthcare provider or pharmacist if you have any questions about the specific dosage of your medication after reviewing this information.

General Dosage Information

Each 84 mg or 1 g of sodium bicarbonate contains 1 or about 12 mEq, respectively, each of sodium and bicarbonate ions.

Pediatric Patients

Alkalinization of Urine

ORAL:
- 1–10 mEq (84–840 mg) per kg daily, adjusted according to response.

Adult Patients

Acidosis Associated with Chronic Renal Failure

ORAL:
- Initially, 20–36 mEq daily, given in divided doses when plasma bicarbonate concentration is less than 15 mEq/L. Titrate dosage to provide a plasma bicarbonate concentration of about 18–20 mEq/L. To relieve symptoms and prevent or stabilize renal failure and osteomalacia in patients with renal tubular acidosis, higher dosages of sodium bicarbonate are necessary.
- Distal (type 1) renal tubular acidosis: Initially, 0.5–2 mEq/kg daily, given in 4 or 5 divided doses. Titrate dosage until hypercalciuria and acidosis are controlled, and according to the response and tolerance of the patient. Alternatively, 48–72 mEq (about 4–6 g) daily.
- Proximal (type 2) renal tubular acidosis: 4–10 mEq/kg daily, given in divided doses.

Alkalinization of Urine

ORAL:
- Initially, 48 mEq (4 g), followed by 12–24 mEq (1–2 g) every 4 hours. Dosages of 30–48 mEq (2.5–4 g) every 4 hours, up to 192 mEq (16 g) daily, may be required in some patients. Titrate dosage to maintain the desired urinary pH.

† Use is not currently included in the labeling approved by the US Food and Drug Administration.

Sodium Oxybate

(ox′ i bate)

Brand Name: Xyrem®

Important Warning

Sodium oxybate is another name for GHB, a substance that is often illegally sold and abused, especially by young adults in social settings such as nightclubs. Sodium oxybate may be harmful when taken by people other than the person for whom it was prescribed. Do not sell or give your sodium oxybate to anyone else; selling or sharing it is against the law. Store sodium oxybate in a safe place, such as a locked cabinet or box, so that no one else can take it accidentally or on purpose. Keep track of how much liquid is left in your bottle so you will know if any is missing.

Take sodium oxybate exactly as directed. Do not take more of it or take it more often than prescribed by your doctor. If you take too much sodium oxybate, you may experience life-threatening symptoms including seizures, slowed or stopped breathing, loss of consciousness, and coma. You may also develop a craving for sodium oxybate, feel a need to take larger and larger doses, or want to continue taking sodium oxybate even though it causes unpleasant symptoms. If you have taken sodium oxybate in amounts larger than prescribed by your doctor, and you suddenly stop taking it, you may experience withdrawal symptoms such as difficulty falling asleep or staying asleep, restlessness, anxiety, abnormal thinking, loss of contact with reality, sleepiness, upset stomach, shaking of a part of your body that you cannot control, sweating, muscle cramps, and fast heartbeat.

Sodium oxybate may cause serious side effects even if it is taken as directed. Do not take antidepressants; medications for anxiety, mental illness, or seizures; sedatives; sleeping pills; or tranquilizers while you are taking sodium oxybate. Do not drink alcohol while you are taking sodium oxybate. Tell your doctor if you snore and if you have or have ever had lung disease, difficulty breathing, sleep apnea (a sleep disorder that causes breathing to stop for short periods during sleep), seizures, or depression. Also tell your doctor if you have ever thought about harming or killing yourself or planned or tried to do so, if you use or have ever used street drugs, or if you have overused prescription medications. If you experience any of the following symptoms, call your doctor immediately: depression, confusion, abnormal thoughts, thoughts of harming or killing yourself, anxiety, feeling that others want to harm you, hallucinations (seeing things or hearing voices that do not exist), loss of contact with reality, agitation, memory problems, breathing problems, snoring, sleep apnea, slowed or stopped breathing, or excessive drowsiness during the day.

Sodium oxybate is not available at retail pharmacies. A special program is in place to distribute the medication and provide information about the medication. You will receive written information and an instructional video about the safe use of sodium oxybate. Your medication will be mailed to you from a central pharmacy after you have read the information and talked to a pharmacist. Ask your doctor if you have any questions about how you will receive your medication.

Your doctor or pharmacist will give you the manufacturer's patient information sheet (Medication Guide) when you begin treatment with sodium oxybate and each time you refill your prescription. Read the information carefully and ask your doctor or pharmacist if you have any questions. You can also obtain the Medication Guide from the FDA website: http://www.fda.gov/cder/drug/infopage/xyrem/medicationguide.htm.

Keep all appointments with your doctor. You should see your doctor at least every 3 months.

Talk to your doctor about the risks of taking sodium oxybate.

Why is this medicine prescribed?

Sodium oxybate is used to prevent attacks of cataplexy (episodes of muscle weakness that begin suddenly and last for a short time) in patients who have narcolepsy (a sleep disorder that may cause extreme sleepiness, sudden uncontrollable urge to sleep during daily activities, and cataplexy). Sodium oxybate is in a class of medications called central nervous system depressants. The way that sodium oxybate works to treat cataplexy is not known.

How should this medicine be used?

Sodium oxybate comes as a solution (liquid) to mix with water and take by mouth. It is usually taken twice each night because sodium oxybate wears off after a short time and the effects of one dose will not last for the entire night. The first dose is taken at bedtime, and a second dose is taken 2 1/2 to 4 hours after the first dose. Sodium oxybate must be taken on an empty stomach, so the first dose should be taken several hours after the evening meal. Try to allow the same amount of time between your evening meal and your first dose of sodium oxybate every night. Follow the directions on your prescription label carefully, and ask your doctor or pharmacist to explain any part you do not understand.

Do not take your bedtime dose of sodium oxybate until you are in bed and are ready to go to sleep for the night.

Sodium oxybate begins to work very quickly and you may have an upset stomach or feel dizzy or lightheaded if you take the medication before you go to bed for the night.

Place your second dose of sodium oxybate in a safe place near your bed before you go to sleep. Use an alarm clock to be sure that you will wake up in time to take the second dose. If you wake up before the alarm goes off and it has been at least 2 1/2 hours since you took your first dose, take your second dose, turn off the alarm, and go back to sleep.

Your doctor will probably start you on a low dose of sodium oxybate and gradually increase your dose, not more often than once every 2 weeks.

Sodium oxybate may help to control your symptoms but will not cure your condition. Continue to take sodium oxybate even if you feel well. Do not stop taking sodium oxybate without talking to your doctor. Your doctor will probably want to decrease your dose gradually. If you suddenly stop taking sodium oxybate, you may have more attacks of cataplexy and you may experience anxiety and difficulty falling asleep or staying asleep.

To prepare doses of sodium oxybate, follow these steps:

1. Open the carton that your medicine came in and remove the bottle of medication and the measuring device.
2. Remove the measuring device from its wrapper.
3. Open the bottle by pushing down on the cap and turning the cap counterclockwise (to the left) at the same time.
4. Place the open bottle upright on a table.
5. Hold the bottle upright with one hand. Use your other hand to place the tip of the measuring device in the center opening on the top of the bottle. Press the tip firmly into the opening.
6. Hold the bottle and measuring device with one hand. Use your other hand to pull back on the plunger until it is even with the marking that matches the dose your doctor prescribed. Be sure to keep the bottle upright to allow the medication to flow into the measuring device.
7. Remove the measuring device from the top of the bottle. Place the tip of the measuring device in one of the dosing cups provided with the medication.
8. Press down on the plunger to empty the medication into the dosing cup.
9. Add 2 ounces (60 mL, 1/4 cup, or about 4 tablespoons) of tap water to the dosing cup. The medication will taste best if you mix it with cold water. Do *not* mix the medication with fruit juice, soft drinks, or any other liquid.
10. Repeat steps 5-9 to prepare a dose of sodium oxybate in the second dosing cup.
11. Place the caps on both dosing cups. Turn each cap clockwise (to the right) until it clicks and locks in place.
12. Rinse the measuring device with water.
13. Replace the cap on the bottle of sodium oxybate and return the bottle and measuring device to the safe place where they are stored. Place both prepared dosing cups of medication in a safe place near your bed.
14. When it is time for you to take the first dose of sodium oxybate, press down on the cap and turn it counterclock-

wise (to the left). Drink all of the liquid while you are sitting on your bed. Put the cap back on the cup, turn it clockwise (to the right) to lock it in place, and lie down right away.
15. When you wake up 2 1/2 - 4 hours later to take the second dose, repeat step 14.

Are there other uses for this medicine?

This medication may be prescribed for other uses; ask your doctor or pharmacist for more information.

What special precautions should I follow?

Before taking sodium oxybate,

- tell your doctor and pharmacist if you are allergic to sodium oxybate or any other medications.
- tell your doctor and pharmacist what other prescription and nonprescription medications, vitamins, nutritional supplements, and herbal products you are taking. Be sure to mention the medications listed in the IMPORTANT WARNING section and levodopa (Larodopa, in Sinemet). Your doctor may need to change the doses of your medications or monitor you carefully for side effects.
- tell your doctor if you are following a low salt diet for medical reasons and if you have or have ever had succinic semialdehyde dehydrogenase deficiency (an inherited condition in which certain substances build up in the body and cause retardation and developmental delays), heart failure, high blood pressure, or liver or kidney disease.
- tell your doctor if you are pregnant, plan to become pregnant, or are breast-feeding. If you become pregnant while taking sodium oxybate, call your doctor.
- if you are having surgery, including dental surgery, tell the doctor or dentist that you are taking sodium oxybate.
- you should know that you will be very sleepy for at least 6 hours after you take sodium oxybate, and you may also be drowsy during the daytime. Do not drive a car, operate machinery, or perform any other dangerous activities for at least 6 hours after you take your medication. Avoid dangerous activities at all times until you know how sodium oxybate affects you.

What special dietary instructions should I follow?

Unless your doctor tells you otherwise, continue your normal diet.

What should I do if I forget to take a dose?

If you miss the first dose of sodium oxybate, you may take a dose when the second dose is scheduled; do not take a second dose of sodium oxybate that night. If you miss the second dose, skip the missed dose and continue your regular dosing schedule on the next night. Do not take a double dose to make up for a missed one. Always allow at least 2 1/2 hours between doses of sodium oxybate.

What side effects can this medicine cause?

Sodium oxybate may cause side effects. Tell your doctor if any of these symptoms are severe or do not go away:
- bedwetting
- headache
- dizziness
- upset stomach
- vomiting
- diarrhea
- heartburn
- stomach pain
- back pain
- weakness
- difficulty falling asleep or staying asleep
- sweating
- flu-like symptoms
- ringing in the ears
- problems with vision
- painful or irregular menstrual periods
- abnormal sensitivity to touch or sound

Some side effects can be serious. The following symptoms are uncommon, but if you experience any of them or those listed in the IMPORTANT WARNING section, call your doctor immediately:
- sleepwalking
- abnormal dreams
- sore throat, fever, chills, and other signs of infection

Sodium oxybate may cause other side effects. Call your doctor if you have any unusual problems while taking this medication.

If you experience a serious side effect, you or your doctor may send a report to the Food and Drug Administration's (FDA) MedWatch Adverse Event Reporting program online [at http://www.fda.gov/MedWatch/index.html] or by phone [1-800-332-1088].

What storage conditions are needed for this medicine?

Keep this medication in the container it came in, tightly closed, and out of reach of children and pets. Store it at room temperature and away from excess heat and moisture (not in the bathroom). Throw away any medication that is outdated or no longer needed. Throw away unused mixtures of sodium oxybate and water 24 hours after you prepare them. When you are ready to throw away a bottle of sodium oxybate, pour any remaining medication down the drain, use a marker to destroy the bottle label, and throw away the bottle with your household trash. Ask your doctor or call the central pharmacy if you have questions about the proper disposal of your medication.

What should I do in case of overdose?

In case of overdose, call your local poison control center at 1-800-222-1222. If the victim has collapsed or is not breathing, call local emergency services at 911.

Symptoms of overdose may include:
- confusion
- problems with coordination
- agitation
- loss of consciousness
- coma
- slow, shallow, or interrupted breathing
- loss of bladder control
- loss of bowel control
- vomiting
- sweating
- headache
- blurred vision
- muscle jerks or twitches
- seizure
- slow heartbeat
- low body temperature
- weak muscles

What other information should I know?

Ask your doctor or call the central pharmacy if you have any questions about refilling your prescription.

Dosage Facts
For Informational Purposes

Caution: Do not change your dose, how often you take your medication, or the length of time you are to take it without first talking to your healthcare provider.

The following dosage information was written using medical language for doctors and other healthcare professionals and is provided here for you to check your dosage. The dosage of this drug may differ for different patients. Therefore, always follow your doctor's instructions or the directions on the label. Contact your healthcare provider or pharmacist if you have any questions about the specific dosage of your medication after reviewing this information.

Pediatric Patients
Narcolepsy

ORAL:
- Adolescents ≥16 years of age: Initially, 4.5 g nightly in 2 doses of 2.25 g each. Increase dosage in increments of 1.5 g daily (0.75 g per dose) at 1- to 2-week intervals to a maximum dosage of 9 g daily.

Adult Patients

Narcolepsy

ORAL:
- Initially, 4.5 g nightly in 2 doses of 2.25 g each. Increase dosage in increments of 1.5 g daily (0.75 g per dose) at 1- to 2-week intervals to a maximum dosage of 9 g daily.

Prescribing Limits

Pediatric Patients

Narcolepsy

ORAL:
- Adolescents ≥16 years of age: Maximum 9 g daily.

Adult Patients

Narcolepsy

ORAL:
- Maximum 9 g daily.

Special Populations

Hepatic Impairment
- Initially, 2.25 g nightly in 2 doses of 1.125 g each; adjust subsequent dosages to achieve desired effect. Closely monitor for potential adverse effects.

Renal Impairment
- Dosage adjustment not expected to be necessary.

Sodium Polystyrene Sulfonate

(pol ee stye′ reen)

Brand Name: Kayexalate®, Kionex®, SPS®
Also available generically.

Why is this medicine prescribed?

Sodium polystyrene sulfonate is used to treat increased amounts of potassium in the body.

How should this medicine be used?

Sodium polystyrene sulfonate comes as a powder and suspension to take by mouth. It may also be used as a rectal enema. It is usually taken one to four times a day. The powder should be mixed with water or syrup as directed by your doctor. Shake the liquid (suspension) well before each use. Follow the directions on your prescription label carefully, and ask your doctor or pharmacist to explain any part you do not understand. Take sodium polystyrene sulfonate exactly as directed. Do not take more or less of it or take it more often than prescribed by your doctor.

Sodium polystyrene sulfonate controls high potassium when taken as directed by your doctor. Do not stop taking sodium polystyrene sulfonate without talking to your doctor.

What special precautions should I follow?

Before taking sodium polystyrene sulfonate,
- tell your doctor and pharmacist if you are allergic to sodium polystyrene sulfonate or any other drugs.
- tell your doctor and pharmacist what prescription and nonprescription medications you are taking, especially antacids, digoxin, diuretics ('water pills'), laxatives, and vitamins or herbal products.
- tell your doctor if you have or have ever had heart or kidney disease, hypertension, or constipation.
- tell your doctor if you are pregnant, plan to become pregnant, or are breast-feeding. If you become pregnant while taking sodium polystyrene sulfonate, call your doctor.
- tell your doctor if you are on a sodium-restricted diet.

What special dietary instructions should I follow?

Talk to your doctor before using salt substitutes containing potassium. If your doctor prescribes a low-salt or low-sodium diet, follow these directions carefully.

What should I do if I forget to take a dose?

Take the missed dose as soon as you remember it. However, if it is almost time for the next dose, skip the missed dose and continue your regular dosing schedule. Do not take a double dose to make up for a missed one.

What side effects can this medicine cause?

Sodium polystyrene sulfonate may cause side effects. Tell your doctor if any of these symptoms are severe or do not go away:
- constipation
- diarrhea
- upset stomach
- nausea
- vomiting

If you experience any of the following symptoms, call your doctor immediately:
- confusion
- muscle weakness
- unusual swelling
- irregular heartbeat
- rectal or lower stomach pain
- increased thirst

If you experience a serious side effect, you or your doctor may send a report to the Food and Drug Administration's (FDA) MedWatch Adverse Event Reporting program online [at http://www.fda.gov/MedWatch/index.html] or by phone [1-800-332-1088].

What storage conditions are needed for this medicine?

Keep this medication in the container it came in, tightly closed, and out of reach of children. Store it at room temperature (unless told otherwise by your pharmacist) and away from excess heat and moisture (not in the bathroom). Throw away any medication that is outdated or no longer needed. Talk to your pharmacist about the proper disposal of your medication. If you prepare sodium polystyrene sulfonate from a powder, refrigerate the mixed suspension. Do not use a suspension more than 24 hours after you have prepared it.

What other information should I know?

Keep all appointments with your doctor and the laboratory.

Do not let anyone else take your medication. Ask your pharmacist any questions you have about refilling your prescription.

Dosage Facts
For Informational Purposes

Caution: Do not change your dose, how often you take your medication, or the length of time you are to take it without first talking to your healthcare provider.

The following dosage information was written using medical language for doctors and other healthcare professionals and is provided here for you to check your dosage. The dosage of this drug may differ for different patients. Therefore, always follow your doctor's instructions or the directions on the label. Contact your healthcare provider or pharmacist if you have any questions about the specific dosage of your medication after reviewing this information.

Pediatric Patients
Hyperkalemia

ORAL:
- Infants and small children: Reduced dosage recommended. Calculate dosage based on the fact that 1 g of the resin binds approximately 1 mEq of potassium.
- Oral administration not recommended in neonates.

RECTAL:
- Reduced dosage recommended. Calculate dosage based on the fact that 1 g of the resin binds approximately 1 mEq of potassium.
- Use with caution.

Adult Patients
Hyperkalemia

ORAL:
- 15 g (approximately 4 level teaspoonfuls of the powder or 60 mL of the commercially available suspension) 1–4 times daily (average 15–60 g daily).

RECTAL:
- 30–50 g (120–200 mL of the commercially available suspension) every 6 hours or as necessary.

Prescribing Limits
Adult Patients
Hyperkalemia

ORAL:
- 15 g 4 times daily (60 g daily).

RECTAL:
- 50 g every 6 hours.

Solifenacin

(sol i fen' a cin)

Brand Name: VESIcare®

Why is this medicine prescribed?

Solifenacin is used to treat overactive bladder (a condition in which the bladder muscles contract uncontrollably and cause frequent urination, urgent need to urinate, and inability to control urination). Solifenacin is in a class of medications called anticholinergics. It works by relaxing the bladder muscles to prevent urgent, frequent, or uncontrolled urination.

How should this medicine be used?

Solifenacin comes as a tablet to take by mouth. It is usually taken once a day with or without food. To help you remember to take solifenacin, take it at around the same time every day. Follow the directions on your prescription label carefully, and ask your doctor or pharmacist to explain any part you do not understand. Take solifenacin exactly as directed. Do not take more or less of it or take it more often than prescribed by your doctor.

Swallow the tablets whole; do not split, chew, or crush them. Swallow the tablets with water or another liquid.

Your doctor will probably start you on a low dose of solifenacin and increase your dose later in your treatment.

Solifenacin may help to control your symptoms but will not cure your condition. Continue to take solifenacin even if you feel well. Do not stop taking solifenacin without talking to your doctor.

Are there other uses for this medicine?

This medication may be prescribed for other uses; ask your doctor or pharmacist for more information.

What special precautions should I follow?

Before taking solifenacin,

- tell your doctor and pharmacist if you are allergic to solifenacin, any other medications, or corn.
- tell your doctor and pharmacist what prescription and nonprescription medications, vitamins, and nutritional supplements you are taking. Be sure to mention any of the following: amiodarone (Cordarone, Pacerone); antifungals such as fluconazole (Diflucan), itraconazole (Sporanox), and ketoconazole (Nizoral); carbamazepine (Tegretol); cimetidine (Tagamet); cisapride (Propulsid); clarithromycin (Biaxin); cyclosporine (Neoral, Sandimmune); danazol (Danocrine); delavirdine (Rescriptor); dexamethasone (Decadron); diltiazem (Cardizem, Dilacor, Tiazac); disopyramide (Norpace); dofetilide (Tikosyn); erythromycin (E.E.S., E-Mycin, Erythrocin); ethosuximide (Zarontin); fluoxetine (Prozac, Sarafem); fluvoxamine (Luvox); HIV protease inhibitors such as indinavir (Crixivan) and ritonavir (Norvir); isoniazid (INH, Nydrazid); metronidazole (Flagyl); moxifloxacin (Avelox); nefazodone; phenobarbital (Luminal, Solfoton); phenytoin (Dilantin); pimozide (Orap); procainamide (Procanbid, Pronestyl); quinidine (Quinaglute, Quinidex); rifabutin (Mycobutin); rifampin (Rifadin, Rimactane); sotalol (Betapace); sparfloxacin (Zagam); thioridazine (Mellaril); troglitazone (Rezulin); troleandomycin (TAO); verapamil (Calan, Covera, Isoptin, Verelan); and zafirlukast (Accolate). Your doctor may need to change the doses of your medications or monitor you carefully for side effects.
- tell your doctor what herbal products you are taking, especially St. John's wort.
- tell your doctor if you or any of your family members have or have ever had prolonged QT interval (a problem with the way electricity is conducted in the heart that may cause fainting) or unexplained fainting; and if you have or have ever had glaucoma (an eye disease that can cause vision loss); any type of blockage in the bladder or digestive system; difficulty emptying your bladder or a weak urine stream; myasthenia gravis (a disorder of the nervous system that causes muscle weakness); ulcerative colitis (sores in the intestine that cause stomach pain and diarrhea); benign prostatic hypertrophy (BPH, enlargement of the prostate, a male reproductive organ); constipation; or liver or kidney disease.
- tell your doctor if you are pregnant or plan to become pregnant. If you become pregnant while taking solifenacin, call your doctor. Do not take solifenacin while you are breastfeeding.
- if you are having surgery, including dental surgery, tell the doctor or dentist that you are taking solifenacin.
- you should know that solifenacin may cause blurred vision. Do not drive a car or operate machinery until you know how this medication affects you.
- you should know that solifenacin may make it harder for your body to cool down when it gets very hot. Avoid exposure to extreme heat, and call your doctor or get emergency medical treatment if you have fever or other signs of heat stroke such as dizziness, upset stomach, headache, confusion, and fast pulse after you are exposed to heat.

What special dietary instructions should I follow?

Talk to your doctor about drinking grapefruit juice while taking this medicine.

What should I do if I forget to take a dose?

Skip the missed dose and take your next dose at the regular time the next day. Do not take two doses of solifenacin in the same day.

What side effects can this medicine cause?

Solifenacin may cause side effects. Tell your doctor if any of these symptoms are severe or do not go away:

- dry mouth
- constipation
- stomach pain
- upset stomach
- vomiting
- heartburn
- dry eyes
- blurred vision
- extreme tiredness

Some side effects can be serious. The following symptoms are uncommon, but if you experience any of them, call your doctor immediately:

- severe stomach pain
- constipation that lasts longer than 3 days
- painful or frequent urination
- bloody or cloudy urine
- back pain
- swelling of the face, throat, tongue, lips, eyes, hands, feet, ankles, or lower legs
- hoarseness
- difficulty breathing or swallowing

Solifenacin may cause other side effects. Call your doctor if you have any unusual problems while taking this medication.

If you experience a serious side effect, you or your doctor may send a report to the Food and Drug Administration's (FDA) MedWatch Adverse Event Reporting program online [at http://www.fda.gov/MedWatch/index.html] or by phone [1-800-332-1088].

What storage conditions are needed for this medicine?

Keep this medication in the container it came in, tightly closed, and out of reach of children. Store it at room temperature and away from excess heat and moisture (not in the bathroom). Throw away any medication that is outdated or no longer needed. Talk to your pharmacist about the proper disposal of your medication.

What should I do in case of overdose?

In case of overdose, call your local poison control center at 1-800-222-1222. If the victim has collapsed or is not breathing, call local emergency services at 911.

Symptoms of overdose may include:

- flushing
- dry mouth
- dry eyes
- blurred vision
- enlarged pupils (black circle in the middle of the eye)
- confusion
- fever
- fast heartbeat
- shaking hands that you cannot control
- difficulty walking
- hallucinations (seeing things or hearing voices that do not exist)
- coma
- collapse

What other information should I know?

Keep all appointments with your doctor.

Do not let anyone else take your medication. Ask your pharmacist any questions you have about refilling your prescription.

Dosage Facts

For Informational Purposes

Caution: Do not change your dose, how often you take your medication, or the length of time you are to take it without first talking to your healthcare provider.

The following dosage information was written using medical language for doctors and other healthcare professionals and is provided here for you to check your dosage. The dosage of this drug may differ for different patients. Therefore, always follow your doctor's instructions or the directions on the label. Contact your healthcare provider or pharmacist if you have any questions about the specific dosage of your medication after reviewing this information.

General Dosage Information

Available as solifenacin succinate; dosage expressed in terms of the salt.

Adult Patients

Overactive Bladder

ORAL:
- Initially, 5 mg once daily. If well tolerated, may increase to 10 mg once daily.

Prescribing Limits

Adult Patients

Overactive Bladder

ORAL:
- Maximum 10 mg daily.

Special Populations

Hepatic Impairment
- Maximum 5 mg daily in patients with moderate hepatic impairment (Child-Pugh class B).
- Use *not* recommended in patients with severe hepatic impairment (Child-Pugh class C).

Renal Impairment
- Maximum 5 mg daily in patients with severe renal impairment (Cl$_{cr}$ <30 mL/minute).

Sotalol

(soe′ ta lole)

Brand Name: Betapace AF®, Betapace®, Sorine®

Also available generically.

Important Warning

Sotalol can cause irregular heartbeats. For the first three days you take sotalol, you will have to be in a facility where your heart can be monitored. Tell your doctor if you have or have ever had kidney disease.

Betapace and Betapace AF are used for different types of irregular heartbeats and should not be used interchangeably. Make sure your doctor knows which product you have been taking.

Why is this medicine prescribed?

Sotalol is used to treat irregular heartbeats. Sotalol is in a class of medications called antiarrhythmics. It works by acting on the heart muscle to improve the heart's rhythm.

How should this medicine be used?

Sotalol comes as a tablet to take by mouth. Sotalol (Betapace) is usually taken twice a day and sotalol (Betapace AF) is usually taken once or twice a day on an empty stomach, at least 2 hours after or 1 hour before breakfast and your evening meal. Follow the directions on your prescription label carefully, and ask your doctor or pharmacist to explain any part you do not understand. Take sotalol exactly as directed. Do not take more or less of it or take it more often than prescribed by your doctor.

Sotalol controls your condition but does not cure it. Continue to take sotalol even if you feel well. Do not stop taking sotalol without talking to your doctor. If sotalol is stopped suddenly, it may cause chest pain or heart attack.

Are there other uses for this medicine?

This medication may be prescribed for other uses; ask your doctor or pharmacist for more information.

What special precautions should I follow?

Before taking sotalol,

- tell your doctor and pharmacist if you are allergic to sotalol or any other drugs.
- tell your doctor and pharmacist what prescription and nonprescription medications you are taking, especially medications for migraine headaches, diabetes, asthma, allergies, colds, or pain; other medications for high blood pressure or heart disease; reserpine; and vitamins.
- if you are taking aluminum- or magnesium-containing antacids (Maalox, Mylanta), take them at least 2 hours before or after sotalol.
- in addition to the condition listed in the IMPORTANT WARNING section, tell your doctor if you have or have ever had heart or liver disease; asthma or other lung disease; disease of the blood vessels; severe allergies; diabetes; or an overactive thyroid gland.
- tell your doctor if you are pregnant, plan to become pregnant, or are breast-feeding. If you become pregnant while taking sotalol, call your doctor.
- if you are having surgery, including dental surgery, tell the doctor or dentist that you are taking sotalol.
- you should know that this drug may make you drowsy. Do not drive a car or operate machinery until you know how this drug affects you.
- remember that alcohol can add to the drowsiness caused by this drug.

What special dietary instructions should I follow?

Talk to your doctor before using salt substitutes containing potassium. If your doctor prescribes a low-salt or low-sodium diet, follow these directions carefully.

What should I do if I forget to take a dose?

Take the missed dose as soon as you remember it. However, if it is almost time for the next dose, skip the missed dose and continue your regular dosing schedule. Do not take a double dose to make up for a missed one.

What side effects can this medicine cause?

Sotalol may cause side effects. Tell your doctor if any of these symptoms are severe or do not go away:

- dizziness
- lightheadedness
- excessive tiredness
- headache
- constipation
- diarrhea
- upset stomach
- muscle aches

If you experience any of the following symptoms, call your doctor immediately:

- shortness of breath or wheezing
- swelling of the feet and lower legs
- chest pain

If you experience a serious side effect, you or your doctor may send a report to the Food and Drug Administration's (FDA) MedWatch Adverse Event Reporting program online [at http://www.fda.gov/MedWatch/index.html] or by phone [1-800-332-1088].

What storage conditions are needed for this medicine?

Keep this medication in the container it came in, tightly closed, and out of reach of children. Store it at room temperature and away from excess heat and moisture (not in the bathroom). Throw away any medication that is outdated or no longer needed. Talk to your pharmacist about the proper disposal of your medication.

What should I do in case of overdose?

In case of overdose, call your local poison control center at 1-800-222-1222. If the victim has collapsed or is not breathing, call local emergency services at 911.

What other information should I know?

Keep all appointments with your doctor and the laboratory. Your blood pressure should be checked regularly to determine your response to sotalol. Your doctor may ask you to check your pulse (heart rate). Ask your pharmacist or doctor to teach you how to take your pulse. If your pulse is faster or slower than it should be, call your doctor.

Do not let anyone else take your medication. Ask your pharmacist any questions you have about refilling your prescription.

Dosage Facts
For Informational Purposes

Caution: Do not change your dose, how often you take your medication, or the length of time you are to take it without first talking to your healthcare provider.

The following dosage information was written using medical language for doctors and other healthcare professionals and is provided here for you to check your dosage. The dosage of this drug may differ for different patients. Therefore, always follow your doctor's instructions or the directions on the label. Contact your healthcare provider or pharmacist if you have any questions about the specific dosage of your medication after reviewing this information.

General Dosage Information

Prior to dose escalation, monitor for efficacy (e.g., PES, Holter) and safety (e.g., QT interval, heart rate, electrolytes) to reduce the risk of precipitating arrhythmias.

Pediatric Patients

Dosage for children ≤2 years of age must be calculated by multiplying the recommended initial dosage for children ≥2 years of age (i.e., 30 mg/m² 3 times daily) by an age-dependent factor obtained from the age and factor graph in the manufacturer prescribing information. (See Table 1.)

For children ≥2 years of age, normalize initial and incremental dosage based on body surface area.

The manufacturer states that reaching plasma concentrations occurring within the therapeutic adult range is an appropriate guide.

ORAL:

Table 1. Initial Pediatric Dosages (age-adjusted)

Age*	Initial dosage calculation (dosage for children ≥2 years of age [30 mg/m²] multiplied by an age-dependent factor)**	Total Initial Daily Dosage
Neonates about 1 week of age	30 mg/m² X 0.3 (9 mg/m²) three times daily	27 mg/m² daily
Infants 1 month of age	30 mg/m² X 0.68 (20 mg/m²) three times daily	60 mg/m² daily
Infants 20 months of age	30 mg/m² X 0.97 (29.1 mg/m²) three times daily	87.3 mg/m² daily
Children ≥2 years of age	30 mg/m² X 1 (30 mg/m²) three times daily	90 mg/m² daily (equivalent to initial 160 mg daily adult dosage)

*To obtain dosages for ages not mentioned in this table, see age/factor graph in manufacturer prescribing information
**See age/factor graph in manufacturer prescribing information for age-dependent factor

Children ≤2 years of age: dosage may be increased using similar calculations (e.g., multiply dose by age-dependent factor). (See age and factor graph in manufacturer prescribing information).

Children ≥2 years of age: dosage may be increased gradually up to 60 mg/m² three times daily (equivalent to 360 mg daily adult dosage).

Allow at least 36 hours between dose increments to attain steady state plasma concentrations.

Time to reach steady-state plasma concentration is longer in neonates and infants, and decreases with increasing age up to about 2 years of age; in neonates, time to steady-state may be a week or longer.

Adult Patients

Life-threatening Ventricular Arrhythmias

ORAL:
- Initially, 80 mg twice daily. If necessary, dosage may be increased gradually after appropriate evaluation to 240–320 mg daily given in divided doses; allow 3 days between dosing increments.
- Usual maintenance dosage: 160–320 mg daily in divided doses.
- May increase to 480–640 mg daily in divided doses, but risk of potentially serious toxicity increases with such doses; use only when potential benefits outweigh the possible risks.

Supraventricular Arrhythmias

Individualize dosage carefully according to renal function and QT interval. Use not recommended if baseline QT interval is >450 msec.

If a dose is missed, take only the next scheduled dose; do not double a dose.

Initiation and Dosage Titration

Initially, 80 mg twice daily in adults with normal renal function (Cl$_{cr}$ > 60 mL/minute) and a near normal QT interval (≤450 msec). If arrhythmia is well controlled (e.g., no recurrences of atrial fibrillation or flutter) during first 3 days of inpatient monitoring and QT interval is <500 msec, may discharge patient on current treatment with an adequate supply to allow uninterrupted therapy until the outpatient prescription is filled.

Discontinue or reduce dosage if QT interval is ≥500 msec during inpatient dosage-titration phase.

If atrial fibrillation or flutter recur during initiation, may increase dosage gradually to 120 or 160 mg twice daily (the maximum recommended dosage), allowing 3 days of inpatient monitoring between dosing increments.

For recurrences after completion of inpatient monitoring despite therapy at lower than maximum recommended dosage, readmit to an institutional setting and increase dosage gradually after appropriate evaluation to maximum of 160 mg twice daily, allowing inpatient monitoring for an additional 3 days for each increase in dosage.

In a large dose-ranging study, 120 mg twice daily was most effective in delaying the time to a recurrence of atrial fibrillation or flutter.

Maintenance Dosage

If QT interval is ≥520 msec or if JT interval is ≥430 msec in patients with a QRS interval >100 msec, reduce dosage and monitor until the QT or JT interval returns to <520 or 430 msec, respectively.

Discontinue therapy if QT interval is ≥520 msec at the lowest maintenance dosage of 80 mg twice daily.

Prescribing Limits

Adult Patients

Life-threatening Ventricular Arrhythmias

ORAL:
- Maximum 480–640 mg daily in divided doses.

Supraventricular Arrhythmias

ORAL:
- Maximum 320 mg daily (160 mg twice daily); increased incidence of torsades de pointes with higher dosages.

Special Populations

Renal Impairment
- Adjust dosage if Cl_{cr} is <60 mL/minute.
- Dosage in children with renal impairment has not been established. However, decreased dosage or increased dosage intervals are recommended for all age groups with renal impairment.

Ventricular Arrhythmias

ORAL:
- Initially, in adults, 80 mg; modify frequency according to the following table:

Cl_{cr} (mL/minute)	Dosing Interval (hours)
>60	12
30–59	24
10–29	36–48
<10	individualize

Increase dosage only after a given dose has been repeated at least 5 or 6 times at the dosing interval appropriate for the degree of renal impairment.

Administer with extreme caution in patients with renal failure undergoing hemodialysis; possible increased elimination half-life in anuric patients.

Supraventricular Arrhythmias

Contraindicated if Cl_{cr} <40 mL/minute.

If a dose is missed, take only the next scheduled dose; do not double a dose (may increase risk of sotalol-induced arrhythmias).

Initiate therapy in a setting that can provide dosage adjustments based on Cl_{cr} and continuous ECG monitoring (e.g., QT interval) for at least 5–6 days (when steady-state plasma concentrations are reached) after initiation.

Initiation and Dosage Titration

Initially, 80 mg once daily for Cl_{cr} of 40–60 mL/minute. If arrhythmia is well controlled (e.g., no recurrences of atrial fibrillation or flutter) during inpatient monitoring of the first 5–6 doses and the QT interval is <500 msec, may discharge patient on current treatment.

Reduce dosage or discontinue if QT_c interval is prolonged to ≥500 msec after first or subsequent daily dosage.

If recurrences of atrial fibrillation or flutter occur during initiation of therapy at a daily dosage of 80 mg, may increase dosage gradually after appropriate evaluation to 120 or 160 mg once daily, allowing inpatient monitoring for 5–6 doses between dosing increments.

For recurrences after completion of inpatient monitoring despite therapy at lower than maximum recommended dosage, readmit to an institutional setting and increase dosage gradually after appropriate evaluation to a maximum of 160 mg once daily, allowing inpatient monitoring for 5–6 doses between dosing increments.

>160 mg once daily is not recommended (increased incidence of torsades de pointes).

Geriatric Patients
- Modification of dosage based on age alone is not necessary.
- Because geriatric patients may have decreased renal function and because patients with renal impairment may be at increased risk of sotalol-induced toxicity, monitor closely and adjust dosage accordingly.

Spironolactone

(speer on oh lak′ tone)

Brand Name: Aldactone®
Also available generically.

Important Warning

Spironolactone has caused tumors in laboratory animals. Talk to your doctor about the risks and benefits of using this medication for your condition.

Why is this medicine prescribed?

Spironolactone is used to treat certain patients with hyperaldosteronism (the body produces too much aldosterone, a naturally occurring hormone); low potassium levels; and in patients with edema (fluid retention) caused by various conditions, including heart, liver, or kidney disease. Spironolactone is also used alone or with other medications to treat high blood pressure. Spironolactone is in a class of medications called aldosterone receptor antagonists. It causes the kidneys to eliminate unneeded water and sodium from the body into the urine, but reduces the loss of potassium from the body.

How should this medicine be used?

Spironolactone comes as a tablet to take by mouth. It usually is taken once a day in the morning or sometimes twice a day. Take spironolactone at around the same time(s) every day. Follow the directions on your prescription label carefully, and ask your doctor or pharmacist to explain any part you do not understand. Take spironolactone exactly as directed. Do not take more or less of it or take it more often than prescribed by your doctor.

Your doctor may start you on a low dose of spironolactone and gradually increase your dose.

Spironolactone controls high blood pressure and hyperaldosteronism, but does not cure these conditions. It may take about 2 weeks or longer before the full effect of spironolactone occurs. Continue to take spironolactone even if you feel well. Do not stop taking spironolactone without talking to your doctor.

Are there other uses for this medicine?

Spironolactone also is used in combination with other medicines to treat precocious puberty (a condition causing children to enter puberty too soon, resulting in the development of sexual characteristics in girls usually younger than 8 years of age and in boys usually younger than 9 years of age) or myasthenia gravis (MG, a disease in which the nerves do not function properly and patients may experience weakness; numbness; loss of muscle coordination; and problems with vision, speech, and bladder control). Spironolactone also may be used to treat certain female patients with abnormal facial hair. Talk to your doctor about the possible risks of using this medication for your condition.

This medication is sometimes prescribed for other uses; ask your doctor or pharmacist for more information.

What special precautions should I follow?

Before taking spironolactone,

- tell your doctor and pharmacist if you are allergic to spironolactone; any other medications; or the ingredients in spironolactone tablets. Ask your pharmacist for a list of the ingredients.
- tell your doctor if you are taking amiloride (Midamor), potassium supplements, triamterene (Dyrenium). Your doctor may tell you not to take spironolactone if you are taking one or more of these medications.
- tell your doctor and pharmacist what prescription and nonprescription medications, vitamins, nutritional supplements, and herbal products you are taking or plan to take. Be sure to mention angiotensin-converting enzyme (ACE) inhibitors such as benazepril (Lotensin), captopril (Capoten), enalapril (Vasotec), fosinopril (Monopril), lisinopril (Prinivil, Zestril), moexipril (Univasc), perindopril, (Aceon), quinapril (Accupril), ramipril (Altace), and trandolapril (Mavik); aspirin and other non-steroidal anti-inflammatory medications (NSAIDS) such as ibuprofen (Advil, Motrin), indomethacin (Indocin), and naproxen (Aleve, Naprosyn); barbiturates such as phenobarbital; digoxin (Digitek, Lanoxicaps, Lanoxin); diuretics ('water pills'); lithium (Eskalith, Lithobid); medications to treat high blood pressure; narcotic medications for pain; and oral steroids such as dexamethasone (Decadron, Dexone), methylprednisolone (Medrol), and prednisone (Deltasone).

- tell your doctor if you have kidney disease. Your doctor may tell you not to take spironolactone.
- tell your doctor if you have or have ever had liver disease.
- tell your doctor if you are pregnant, or plan to become pregnant. If you become pregnant while taking spironolactone, call your doctor. Do not breastfeed if you are taking spironolactone.
- if you are having surgery, including dental surgery, tell the doctor or dentist that you are taking spironolactone.
- you should know that drinking alcohol with this medication may cause dizziness, lightheadedness, and fainting when you get up too quickly from a lying position. Talk to your doctor about drinking alcohol while you are taking spironolactone.

What special dietary instructions should I follow?

Follow your doctor's directions for your meals, including advice for a reduced-salt (sodium) diet and daily exercise program. Avoid potassium-containing salt substitutes while you are taking this medication. Talk with your doctor about the amount of potassium-rich foods (e.g., bananas, prunes, raisins, and orange juice) that you may have in your diet.

What should I do if I forget to take a dose?

Take the missed dose as soon as you remember it. However, if it is almost time for your next dose, skip the missed dose and continue your regular dosing schedule. Do not take a double dose to make up for a missed one.

What side effects can this medicine cause?

Spironolactone may cause side effects. Tell your doctor if any of these symptoms are severe or do not go away:

- vomiting
- diarrhea
- stomach pain or cramps
- dry mouth
- thirst
- dizziness
- unsteadiness
- headache
- enlarged or painful breasts in men or women
- irregular menstrual periods
- vaginal bleeding in post-menopausal ('after the change of life', the end of monthly menstrual periods) women
- difficulty maintaining or achieving an erection
- deepening of voice
- increased hair growth on parts of the body
- drowsiness
- tiredness
- restlessness

If you experience any of the following symptoms, call your doctor immediately:

- muscle weakness, pain, or cramps

- pain, burning, numbness, or tingling in the hands or feet
- inability to move arms or legs
- changes in heartbeat
- confusion
- nausea
- extreme tiredness
- unusual bleeding or bruising
- lack of energy
- loss of appetite
- pain in the upper right part of the stomach
- yellowing of the skin or eyes
- fever, sore throat, cough, chills, and other signs of infection
- flu-like symptoms
- cold, gray skin
- rash
- hives
- itching
- difficulty breathing or swallowing
- vomiting blood
- blood in stools
- decreased urination
- blurred vision
- fainting

If you experience a serious side effect, you or your doctor may send a report to the Food and Drug Administration's (FDA) MedWatch Adverse Event Reporting program online [at http://www.fda.gov/MedWatch/index.html] or by phone [1-800-332-1088].

What storage conditions are needed for this medicine?

Keep this medicine in the container it came in, tightly closed, and out of reach of children. Store it at room temperature and away from excess heat and moisture (not in the bathroom). Throw away any medicine that is outdated or no longer needed. Talk to your pharmacist about the proper disposal of your medicine.

What should I do in case of overdose?

In case of overdose, call your local poison control center at 1-800-222-1222. If the victim has collapsed or is not breathing, call local emergency services at 911.

Symptoms of overdose may include:

- drowsiness
- confusion
- rash
- nausea
- vomiting
- dizziness
- diarrhea
- tingling in arms and legs
- loss of muscle tone
- weakness or heaviness in legs
- confusion
- lack of energy

- cold, gray skin
- irregular or slow heartbeat

What other information should I know?

Keep all appointments with your doctor and the laboratory. Your doctor will order certain lab tests to check your body's response to spironolactone.

Before having any laboratory test, tell your doctor and the laboratory personnel that you are taking spironolactone.

Do not let anyone else take your medicine. Ask your pharmacist any questions you have about refilling your prescription.

Dosage Facts
For Informational Purposes

Caution: Do not change your dose, how often you take your medication, or the length of time you are to take it without first talking to your healthcare provider.

The following dosage information was written using medical language for doctors and other healthcare professionals and is provided here for you to check your dosage. The dosage of this drug may differ for different patients. Therefore, always follow your doctor's instructions or the directions on the label. Contact your healthcare provider or pharmacist if you have any questions about the specific dosage of your medication after reviewing this information.

Pediatric Patients

Edema†

ORAL:
- 3.3 mg/kg (up to 100 mg) daily as a single dose or in divided doses.
- Alternatively, initial dosage of 60 mg/m² daily in divided doses.

Hypertension†

ORAL:
- Initially, 1 mg/kg daily as a single dose or in 2 divided doses. Increase dosage as necessary up to a maximum of 3.3 mg/kg (up to 100 mg) daily as a single dose or in 2 divided doses.

Primary Aldosteronism†
Diagnosis

ORAL:
- 125–375 mg/m² in divided doses over 24 hours.
- If serum potassium concentration increases during therapy but decreases when the drug is discontinued, a presumptive diagnosis of primary aldosteronism should be considered.

Adult Patients

Edema

ORAL:
- Initially, 100 mg daily. Range: 25–200 mg daily.
- As monotherapy, administer usual initial dosage for ≥5 days; if response is satisfactory, titrate dosage to optimal dosage.

- If response is not satisfactory after initial 5 days of therapy, add a thiazide or loop diuretic. Do *not* adjust spironolactone dosage during combined diuretic therapy.
- Spironolactone in combination with hydrochlorothiazide: spironolactone 100 mg daily and hydrochlorothiazide 100 mg daily as a single dose or in divided doses. Range: spironolactone 25–200 mg daily and hydrochlorothiazide 25–200 mg daily as a single dose or in divided doses.
- Initial use of fixed-combination preparations is not recommended; adjust by administering each drug separately, then use the fixed combination if the optimum maintenance dosage corresponds to the ratio of drugs in the combination preparation. Administer separately for subsequent dosage adjustment.

Hypertension

Lower dosage and combination therapy recommended by JNC 7; higher spironolactone dosage may result in intolerable adverse effects.

Carefully monitor BP during initial titration or subsequent upward adjustment in dosage.

Adjust dosage at approximately monthly intervals.

Monotherapy

ORAL:
- Usual initial dosage: 50–100 mg daily as a single dose or in divided doses. Full hypotensive response may require 2 weeks.
- Usual dosage recommended by JNC 7: 25–50 mg daily.

Spironolactone/Hydrochlorothiazide Combination Therapy

ORAL:
- Spironolactone 50–100 mg daily and hydrochlorothiazide 50–100 mg daily as a single dose or in divided doses.
- Initial use of fixed-combination spironolactone/hydrochlorothiazide preparations is not recommended; adjust by administering each drug separately, then use the fixed combination if the optimum maintenance dosage corresponds to the ratio of drugs in the combination preparation. Administer separately for subsequent dosage adjustment.

CHF

ORAL:
- Initially, 12.5–25 mg daily used in patients receiving an ACE inhibitor and a loop diuretic with or without a cardiac glycoside.
- Increase to 50 mg daily after 8 weeks in patients who exhibit signs and symptoms of progressive heart failure and have serum potassium concentrations <5.5 mEq/L.
- Decrease to 25 mg every other day if hyperkalemia occurs.

Primary Aldosteronism
Diagnosis

ORAL:
- 400 mg daily for 3–4 weeks. Correction of hypokalemia and hypertension provides presumptive evidence for the diagnosis of primary aldosteronism.
- Alternatively, 400 mg daily for 4 days. If serum potassium concentration increases during spironolactone therapy but decreases when the drug is discontinued, consider presumptive diagnosis of primary aldosteronism.

Medical Therapy Prior to Adrenalectomy

ORAL:
- Patients with a definitive diagnosis: 100–400 mg daily before surgery.

Treatment Of Primary Aldosteronism

ORAL:
- Initially, 400 mg daily.
- Maintenance dosage: 100–300 mg daily. Use lowest effective dosage for long-term maintenance therapy.

Hypokalemia

ORAL:
- 25–100 mg daily.

Hirsutism†

ORAL:
- 50–200 mg daily. Regression of hirsutism evident within 2 months, maximal within 6 months, and has been maintained for ≥16 months with continued therapy.

Prescribing Limits

Pediatric Patients

Hypertension†

ORAL:
- Maximum 3.3 mg/kg (up to 100 mg) daily.

† Use is not currently included in the labeling approved by the US Food and Drug Administration.

Spironolactone and Hydrochlorothiazide

(speer on oh lak′ tone) (hye droe klor oh thye′ a zide)

Brand Name: Aldactazide®, Spironazide®, Spirozide®

Important Warning

Spironolactone has caused tumors in laboratory animals. Talk to your doctor about the risks and benefits of using this medicine for your condition.

Why is this medicine prescribed?

The combination of spironolactone and hydrochlorothiazide, a 'water pill,' is used to treat high blood pressure and fluid retention caused by various conditions, including heart disease. It causes the kidneys to eliminate unneeded water and salt from the body into the urine.

This medicine is sometimes prescribed for other uses; ask your doctor or pharmacist for more information.

How should this medicine be used?

The combination of spironolactone and hydrochlorothiazide comes as a tablet to take by mouth. It usually is taken once a day in the morning with food. Follow the directions on your prescription label carefully, and ask your doctor or pharmacist to explain any part you do not understand. Take spironolactone and hydrochlorothiazide exactly as directed. Do not take more or less of it or take it more often than prescribed by your doctor.

This medication controls high blood pressure but does not cure it. Continue to take spironolactone and hydrochlorothiazide even if you feel well. Do not stop taking spironolactone and hydrochlorothiazide without talking to your doctor.

What special precautions should I follow?

Before taking spironolactone and hydrochlorothiazide,

- tell your doctor and pharmacist if you are allergic to spironolactone, hydrochlorothiazide, sulfa drugs, or any other drugs.
- tell your doctor and pharmacist what prescription and nonprescription medications you are taking, especially aspirin; captopril (Capoten); digoxin (Lanoxin); enalapril (Vasotec); lisinopril (Prinivil, Zestril); lithium (Eskalith, Lithobid); medications for arthritis, diabetes, or high blood pressure; potassium supplements; and vitamins. Do not take this medicine if you are taking amiloride or triamterene.
- tell your doctor if you have or have ever had diabetes, gout, or kidney or liver disease.
- tell your doctor if you are pregnant, plan to become pregnant, or are breast-feeding. If you become pregnant while taking spironolactone and hydrochlorothiazide, call your doctor.
- if you are having surgery, including dental surgery, tell the doctor or dentist that you are taking spironolactone and hydrochlorothiazide.
- you should know that this drug may make you drowsy. Do not drive a car or operate machinery until you know how this drug affects you.
- remember that alcohol can add to the drowsiness caused by this drug.

What special dietary instructions should I follow?

Follow your doctor's directions for a low-salt or low-sodium diet and daily exercise program. Avoid potassium-containing salt substitutes. Limit your intake of potassium-rich foods (e.g., bananas, prunes, raisins, and orange juice). Ask your doctor for advice on how much of these foods you may have.

What should I do if I forget to take a dose?

Take the missed dose as soon as you remember it. However, if it is almost time for the next dose, skip the missed dose and continue your regular dosing schedule. Do not take a double dose to make up for a missed one.

What side effects can this medicine cause?

Spironolactone and hydrochlorothiazide may cause side effects. Tell your doctor if any of these symptoms are severe or do not go away:

- upset stomach
- vomiting
- diarrhea
- loss of appetite
- stomach pain
- gas
- frequent urination
- dizziness
- headache
- enlarged or painful breasts
- irregular menstrual periods
- drowsiness

If you experience any of the following symptoms, call your doctor immediately:

- muscle weakness or cramps
- rapid, excessive weight loss
- fatigue
- slow or irregular heartbeat
- sore throat
- unusual bruising or bleeding
- yellowing of the skin or eyes
- skin rash
- vomiting blood
- fever
- confusion

If you experience a serious side effect, you or your doctor may send a report to the Food and Drug Administration's (FDA) MedWatch Adverse Event Reporting program online [at http://www.fda.gov/MedWatch/index.html] or by phone [1-800-332-1088].

What storage conditions are needed for this medicine?

Keep this medicine in the container it came in, tightly closed, and out of reach of children. Store it at room temperature and away from excess heat and moisture (not in the bathroom). Throw away any medicine that is outdated or no longer needed. Talk to your pharmacist about the proper disposal of your medicine.

What should I do in case of overdose?

In case of overdose, call your local poison control center at 1-800-222-1222. If the victim has collapsed or is not breathing, call local emergency services at 911.

What other information should I know?

Keep all appointments with your doctor and the laboratory. Your blood pressure should be checked regularly, and blood tests should be done occasionally.

Do not let anyone else take your medicine. Ask your pharmacist any questions you have about refilling your prescription.

Dosage Facts
For Informational Purposes

Caution: Do not change your dose, how often you take your medication, or the length of time you are to take it without first talking to your healthcare provider.

The following dosage information was written using medical language for doctors and other healthcare professionals and is provided here for you to check your dosage. The dosage of this drug may differ for different patients. Therefore, always follow your doctor's instructions or the directions on the label. Contact your healthcare provider or pharmacist if you have any questions about the specific dosage of your medication after reviewing this information.

Adult Patients

Edema

ORAL:
- As monotherapy, administer usual initial dosage for ≥5 days; if response is satisfactory, titrate dosage to optimal dosage.
- If response is not satisfactory after initial 5 days of therapy, add a thiazide or loop diuretic. Do *not* adjust spironolactone dosage during combined diuretic therapy.
- Spironolactone in combination with hydrochlorothiazide: spironolactone 100 mg daily and hydrochlorothiazide 100 mg daily as a single dose or in divided doses. Range: spironolactone 25–200 mg daily and hydrochlorothiazide 25–200 mg daily as a single dose or in divided doses.
- Initial use of fixed-combination preparations is not recommended; adjust by administering each drug separately, then use the fixed combination if the optimum maintenance dosage corresponds to the ratio of drugs in the combination preparation. Administer separately for subsequent dosage adjustment.

Hypertension

Lower dosage and combination therapy recommended by JNC 7; higher spironolactone dosage may result in intolerable adverse effects.

Carefully monitor BP during initial titration or subsequent upward adjustment in dosage.

Adjust dosage at approximately monthly intervals.

Spironolactone/Hydrochlorothiazide Combination Therapy

ORAL:
- Spironolactone 50–100 mg daily and hydrochlorothiazide 50–100 mg daily as a single dose or in divided doses.
- Initial use of fixed-combination sprionolactone/hydrochlorothiazide preparations is not recommended; adjust by administering each drug separately, then use the fixed combination if the optimum maintenance dosage corresponds to the ratio of drugs in the combination preparation. Administer separately for subsequent dosage adjustment.

Hypokalemia

ORAL:
- 25–100 mg daily.

Hirsutism†

ORAL:
- 50–200 mg daily. Regression of hirsutism evident within 2 months, maximal within 6 months, and has been maintained for ≥16 months with continued therapy.

† Use is not currently included in the labeling approved by the US Food and Drug Administration.

Stavudine
(stav′ yoo deen)

Brand Name: Zerit®

Important Warning

Stavudine, when used alone or in combination with other antiviral medications, may cause serious and possibly deadly damage to the liver and pancreas and a life-threatening condition called lactic acidosis. Tell your doctor if you have or have ever had liver or pancreas disease or gallstones, and if you have taken medication to treat HIV for a long time. Also tell your doctor if you drink or have ever drunk large quantities of alcohol and if you are taking didanosine (Videx) or hydroxyurea (Droxia, Hydrea). Tell your doctor if you are pregnant or plan to become pregnant. If you become pregnant while taking stavudine, call your doctor.

If you experience any of the following symptoms, call your doctor immediately: upset stomach, vomiting, unusual or unexpected stomach pain, sudden weight loss, extreme weakness or tiredness, shortness of breath, fast breathing, weakness in arms or legs, and any sudden change in your general health. Keep all appointments with your doctor and the laboratory. Your doctor will order certain lab tests to check your response to stavudine.

Why is this medicine prescribed?

Stavudine is used in combination with other antiviral medications to treat human immunodeficiency virus (HIV) infection in patients with or without acquired immunodeficiency syndrome (AIDS). Stavudine is in a class of antiviral medications called nucleoside analogue reverse transcriptase inhibitors (NRTIs). It works by slowing the spread of HIV in the body. Stavudine does not cure HIV and may not prevent you from developing HIV-related illnesses. Stavudine does not prevent the spread of HIV to other people.

How should this medicine be used?

Stavudine comes as a capsule and a solution (liquid) to take by mouth. It is usually taken twice a day (every 12 hours), with or without food and with plenty of water. To help you remember to take stavudine, take it at around the same time each day. Follow the directions on your prescription label carefully, and ask your doctor or pharmacist to explain any part you do not understand. Take stavudine exactly as directed. Do not take more or less of it or take it more often than prescribed by your doctor.

If you are giving the oral solution to a child, shake the bottle well before each use to mix the medication evenly. Use the measuring cup provided to measure the child's dose.

Stavudine controls HIV infection but does not cure it. Continue to take stavudine even if you feel well. Do not stop taking stavudine without talking to your doctor. If you miss doses or suddenly stop taking stavudine, your condition may become more difficult to treat.

Are there other uses for this medicine?

Stavudine is also sometimes used in combination with other medications to prevent HIV infection in health care workers or other people who were accidentally exposed to HIV. Talk to your doctor about the possible risks of using this medication for your condition.

This medication may be prescribed for other uses; ask your doctor or pharmacist for more information.

What special precautions should I follow?

Before taking stavudine,
- tell your doctor and pharmacist if you are allergic to stavudine or any other medications.
- tell your doctor and pharmacist what prescription and nonprescription medications, vitamins, nutritional supplements and herbal products you are taking. Be sure to mention those listed in the IMPORTANT WARNING section and zidovudine (Retrovir, also an ingredient in the combination products Combivir and Trizivir). Your doctor may need to change the doses of your medications or monitor you more carefully for side effects.
- tell your doctor if you have or have ever had kidney disease, diabetes (if you are taking stavudine solution), or peripheral neuropathy (a type of nerve damage that causes tingling, numbness, and pain in the hands and feet).
- tell your doctor if you are breast-feeding. You should not breastfeed if you are infected with HIV or if you are taking stavudine.
- you should know that stavudine may cause side effects that must be treated right away before they become serious. Children who are taking stavudine may not be able to tell you about the side effects they are feeling.

If you are giving stavudine to a child, ask the child's doctor how you can tell if the child is having these serious side effects.
- you should know that your body fat may increase or move to different areas of your body such as your breasts and your upper back.

What special dietary instructions should I follow?

Unless your doctor tells you otherwise, continue your normal diet.

What should I do if I forget to take a dose?

Take the missed dose as soon as you remember it. However, if it is almost time for the next dose, skip the missed dose and continue your regular dosing schedule. Do not take a double dose to make up for a missed one.

What side effects can this medicine cause?

Stavudine may cause side effects. Tell your doctor if either of these symptoms is severe or does not go away:
- headache
- diarrhea

Some side effects can be serious. If you experience the following symptoms or any of those listed in the IMPORTANT WARNING section, call your doctor immediately:
- numbness, tingling, burning or pain in the hands or feet
- difficulty moving your hands and feet
- rash

If you experience a serious side effect, you or your doctor may send a report to the Food and Drug Administration's (FDA) MedWatch Adverse Event Reporting program online [at http://www.fda.gov/MedWatch/index.html] or by phone [1-800-332-1088].

What storage conditions are needed for this medicine?

Keep this medication in the container it came in, tightly closed, and out of reach of children. Store the capsules at room temperature and away from excess heat and moisture (not in the bathroom). Store the solution in the refrigerator and throw away the unused portion after 30 days. Throw away any medication that is outdated or no longer needed. Talk to your pharmacist about the proper disposal of your medication.

What should I do in case of overdose?

In case of overdose, call your local poison control center at 1-800-222-1222. If the victim has collapsed or is not breathing, call local emergency services at 911.

Symptoms of overdose may include:
- numbness, tingling, or pain in the hands or feet
- difficulty moving hands or feet
- upset stomach

- vomiting
- unusual or unexpected stomach pain
- weakness or tiredness
- shortness of breath
- weakness in arms and legs

What other information should I know?

Do not let anyone else take your medication. Ask your pharmacist any questions you have about refilling your prescription.

Dosage Facts
For Informational Purposes

Caution: Do not change your dose, how often you take your medication, or the length of time you are to take it without first talking to your healthcare provider.

The following dosage information was written using medical language for doctors and other healthcare professionals and is provided here for you to check your dosage. The dosage of this drug may differ for different patients. Therefore, always follow your doctor's instructions or the directions on the label. Contact your healthcare provider or pharmacist if you have any questions about the specific dosage of your medication after reviewing this information.

General Dosage Information

Must be given in conjunction with other antiretrovirals.

Pediatric Patients

Treatment of HIV Infection

ORAL:
- Birth to 13 days of age: 0.5 mg/kg every 12 hours.
- ≥14 days of age weighing <30 kg: 1 mg/kg every 12 hours.
- ≥30 kg to <60 kg: 30 mg twice daily.
- ≥60 kg: 40 mg twice daily.
- Temporarily interrupt stavudine if peripheral neuropathy occurs. If peripheral neuropathy resolves completely, reinitiate using doses 50% of the usually recommended pediatric dose.

Adult Patients

Treatment of HIV

ORAL:
- <60 kg: 30 mg twice daily.
- ≥60 kg: 40 mg twice daily.
- Temporarily interrupt stavudine if peripheral neuropathy occurs. If peripheral neuropathy resolves, reinitiate with 15 mg twice daily in those weighing <60 kg and 20 mg twice daily in those weighing ≥60 kg.

Postexposure Prophylaxis of HIV†
Occupational Exposure†

ORAL:
- <60 kg: 30 mg twice daily.
- ≥60 kg: 40 mg twice daily; if toxicity develops, use 20–30 mg twice daily.

- Used in alternative basic regimens with lamivudine or emtricitabine.
- Initiate postexposure prophylaxis as soon as possible following exposure (within hours rather than days) and continue for 4 weeks, if tolerated.

Nonoccupational Exposure†

ORAL:
- <60 kg: 30 mg twice daily.
- ≥60 kg: 40 mg twice daily.
- Used in an alternative nonnucleoside reverse transcriptase inhibitor-based (NNRTI-based) regimen that includes efavirenz and (lamivudine or emtricitabine) and stavudine and in various alternative HIV protease inhibitor-based (PI-based) regimens that include a PI (with or without low-dose ritonavir) and (lamivudine or emtricitabine) and stavudine.
- Initiate postexposure prophylaxis as soon as possible following exposure (preferably ≤72 hours after exposure) and continue for 28 days.

Special Populations

Renal Impairment

Treatment of HIV Infection

- Consider a reduction in the dose and/or an increase in the dosing interval in pediatric patients with renal impairment; data insufficient to recommend a specific dose adjustment.

Table 1. Dosage in Adults with Renal Impairment

Cl_{cr} (mL/minute)	Weighing <60 kg	Weighing ≥60 kg
≥50	30 mg every 12 hours	40 mg every 12 hours
26–50	15 mg every 12 hours	20 mg every 12 hours
10–25	15 mg every 24 hours	20 mg every 24 hours
Hemodialysis Patients	15 mg every 24 hours given after completion of dialysis and at the same time of day on days that patient does not undergo hemodialysis	20 mg every 24 hours given after completion of dialysis and at the same time of day on days that patient does not undergo hemodialysis

† *Use is not currently included in the labeling approved by the US Food and Drug Administration.*

Stimulant Laxatives

Brand Name: Bisacodyl®, Cascara Sagrada®, Castor Oil®, Dulcolax®, Ex-Lax Gentle Nature®, Fleet Laxative®, Gentlax®, Senna®, Senokot®

Why is this medicine prescribed?

Stimulant laxatives are used to treat constipation or before rectal or bowel examinations or surgery. They work by increasing the movement in your bowel. They also are used to treat certain conditions of the intestinal tract.

This medication is sometimes prescribed for other uses; ask your doctor or pharmacist for more information.

How should this medicine be used?

Stimulant laxatives come in many different forms, including liquids, powders, granules, tablets, and suppositories. Follow the directions on your package or prescription label carefully, and ask your doctor or pharmacist to explain any part you do not understand. Take stimulant laxatives exactly as directed. Do not take more or less of it or take it more often than prescribed by your doctor.

Take stimulant laxatives on an empty stomach with a full 8-ounce glass of water. Results occur more slowly if the medicine is taken with food. Most stimulant laxatives are taken at bedtime, with results by morning; however, some products may take up to 24 hours to produce a bowel movement.

Castor oil acts more quickly than the other laxatives, so do not take castor oil at bedtime. To avoid the bad taste of castor oil, chill it in the refrigerator and mix it with cold orange juice just before drinking. Castor oil should not be used routinely to treat constipation.

Do not crush or chew bisacodyl tablets. Do not take them within 1 hour of drinking milk or taking antacids.

If you are to insert a suppository, follow these steps:

1. Remove the wrapper.
2. Dip the tip of the suppository in lukewarm water.
3. Lie down on your left side and raise your right knee to your chest. (A left-handed person should lie on the right side and raise the left knee.)
4. Using your finger, insert the suppository high into your rectum. Hold it in place for a few moments. Try to keep it there for as long as possible.
5. Wash your hands thoroughly.

Do not use stimulant laxatives for longer than 1 week, unless your doctor tells you to. Do not take more than the recommended dose; overuse of stimulant laxatives may cause serious side effects. Call your doctor if you do not have a bowel movement after taking a stimulant laxative.

Use of stimulant laxatives over a long period may lead to dependence. Overuse results in permanent damage to your intestine and colon. If your symptoms do not improve while using a stimulant laxative, call your doctor. Do not give a stimulant laxative to a child less than 10 years old, unless your doctor tells you to.

What special precautions should I follow?

Before taking stimulant laxatives,

- tell your doctor and pharmacist if you are allergic to any other drugs.
- tell your doctor and pharmacist what prescription and nonprescription medications you are taking, especially antacids; antibiotics; pain or seizure medicines; medicines for depression, heart disease, or blood pressure; and vitamins.
- tell your doctor if you have or have ever had diabetes, heart disease, high blood pressure, or intestinal disease.
- tell your doctor if you are pregnant, plan to become pregnant, or are breast-feeding. If you become pregnant while taking stimulant laxatives, call your doctor.

What special dietary instructions should I follow?

A regular diet and exercise program is important for regular bowel function. Eat a high-fiber diet and drink plenty of liquids (six to eight glasses) each day. Avoid food that causes constipation, such as processed cheese. If you are on a low-sugar, low-calorie, or low-sodium diet, check with your doctor or pharmacist before taking a stimulant laxative.

What should I do if I forget to take a dose?

If you are taking scheduled doses of stimulant laxatives, take the missed dose as soon as you remember it. However, if it is almost time for the next dose, skip the missed dose and continue your regular dosing schedule. Do not take a double dose to make up for the missed one.

What side effects can this medicine cause?

Stimulant laxatives may cause side effects. Cascara and senna commonly cause yellow-brown urine; this is harmless. Tell your doctor if any of these symptoms are severe or do not go away:

- diarrhea
- upset stomach
- vomiting
- irritation
- stomach cramping

If you have any of the following symptoms, stop taking stimulant laxatives and call your doctor immediately:

- bloody stools
- severe cramping
- pain
- weakness
- dizziness
- unusual tiredness
- rectal bleeding

If you experience a serious side effect, you or your doctor may send a report to the Food and Drug Administration's

(FDA) MedWatch Adverse Event Reporting program online [at http://www.fda.gov/MedWatch/index.html] or by phone [1-800-332-1088].

What storage conditions are needed for this medicine?

Keep this medication in the container it came in, tightly closed, and out of reach of children. Store it at room temperature and away from excess heat and moisture (not in the bathroom). Throw away any medication that is outdated or no longer needed. Talk to your pharmacist about the proper disposal of your medication.

What other information should I know?

Ask your pharmacist any questions you have about taking this medicine.

Talk to your doctor, pharmacist, or other healthcare professional if you have questions about dosing information for your medication.

Stool Softeners

Brand Name: Colace®, Dialose®, Docusate®, DOS®, Doxinate®, Fleet Sof-Lax®, Hemaspan®, Modane Soft®, Surfak®
Also available generically.

Why is this medicine prescribed?

Stool softeners are used on a short-term basis to relieve constipation by people who should avoid straining during bowel movements because of heart conditions, hemorrhoids, and other problems. They soften stools, making them easier to pass.

This medication is sometimes prescribed for other uses; ask your doctor or pharmacist for more information.

How should this medicine be used?

Stool softeners come as a capsule, tablet, liquid, and syrup to take by mouth. A stool softener usually is taken at bedtime. Follow the directions on the package or your prescription label carefully, and ask your doctor or pharmacist to explain any part you do not understand. Take stool softeners exactly as directed. Do not take more or less of it or take it more often than prescribed by your doctor.

Take capsules and tablets with a full glass of water. The liquid comes with a specially marked dropper for measuring the dose. Ask your pharmacist to show you how to use it if you have difficulty. Mix the liquid (not the syrup) with 4 ounces of milk, fruit juice, or formula to mask its bitter taste.

One to three days of regular use usually are needed for this medicine to take effect. Do not take stool softeners for more than 1 week unless your doctor directs you to. If sudden changes in bowel habits last longer than 2 weeks or if your stools are still hard after you have taken this medicine for 1 week, call your doctor.

What special precautions should I follow?

Before taking stool softeners,

- tell your doctor and pharmacist if you are allergic to any drugs.
- tell your doctor and pharmacist what prescription and nonprescription medications you are taking, especially aspirin and vitamins. Do not take mineral oil while taking stool softeners.
- tell your doctor if you are pregnant, plan to become pregnant, or are breast-feeding. If you become pregnant while taking stool softeners, call your doctor.

What should I do if I forget to take a dose?

This medication usually is taken as needed. If your doctor has told you to take stool softeners regularly, take the missed dose as soon as you remember it. However, if it is almost time for the next dose, skip the missed dose and continue your regular dosing schedule. Do not take a double dose to make up for a missed one.

What side effects can this medicine cause?

Stool softeners may cause side effects. Tell your doctor if any of these symptoms are severe or do not go away:

- stomach or intestinal cramps
- upset stomach
- throat irritation (from oral liquid)

If you experience any of the following symptoms, call your doctor immediately:

- skin rash (hives)
- difficulty breathing or swallowing
- fever
- vomiting
- stomach pain

If you experience a serious side effect, you or your doctor may send a report to the Food and Drug Administration's (FDA) MedWatch Adverse Event Reporting program online [at http://www.fda.gov/MedWatch/index.html] or by phone [1-800-332-1088].

What storage conditions are needed for this medicine?

Keep this medication in the container it came in, tightly closed, and out of reach of children. Store it at room temperature and away from excess heat and moisture (not in the bathroom). Throw away any medication that is outdated or no longer needed. Talk to your pharmacist about the proper disposal of your medication.

What other information should I know?

Ask your pharmacist any questions you have about taking this medicine.

Dosage Facts
For Informational Purposes

Caution: Do not change your dose, how often you take your medication, or the length of time you are to take it without first talking to your healthcare provider.

The following dosage information was written using medical language for doctors and other healthcare professionals and is provided here for you to check your dosage. The dosage of this drug may differ for different patients. Therefore, always follow your doctor's instructions or the directions on the label. Contact your healthcare provider or pharmacist if you have any questions about the specific dosage of your medication after reviewing this information.

General Dosage Information

Administered in doses only large enough to produce softening of the stools.

Oral dosage varies widely according to the severity of the condition and the response of the patient and should be adjusted to individual response.

Pediatric Patients
Constipation

May be administered in divided doses, but usually one bedtime dose is sufficient.

Initially, doses at the higher end of the dosage ranges may be required.

ORAL:
- Children <2 years of age: Usually, 25 mg (range: 20–50 mg) daily.
- Children 2–12 years of age: Usually, 50–150 mg daily.
- Children >12 years of age: Usually, 50–360 mg daily.

ORAL, ALTERNATIVE DOSING (E.G., LIQUID FORMULATIONS):
- Children <3 years of age: 10–40 mg daily.
- Children 3–6 years of age: 20–60 mg daily.
- Children 6–12 years of age: 40–150 mg daily.

Adult Patients
Constipation

ORAL:
- Usually, 50–360 mg daily.

ORAL, ALTERNATIVE DOSING (E.G., LIQUID FORMULATIONS):
- 50–500 mg daily.

Special Populations

Hepatic Impairment
- No specific dosage recommendations for hepatic impairment.

Renal Impairment
- No specific dosage recommendations for renal impairment.

Geriatric Patients
- No specific geriatric dosage recommendations.

Sucralfate

(soo' kral fate)

Brand Name: Carafate®

Why is this medicine prescribed?

Sucralfate is used to treat ulcers. It adheres to damaged ulcer tissue and protects against acid and enzymes so healing can occur.

This medication is sometimes prescribed for other uses; ask your doctor or pharmacist for more information.

How should this medicine be used?

Sucralfate comes as a tablet and liquid to take by mouth. It usually is taken four times a day, 1 hour before meals and at bedtime. Take sucralfate on an empty stomach, 2 hours after or 1 hour before meals. Follow the directions on your prescription label carefully, and ask your doctor or pharmacist to explain any part you do not understand. Take sucralfate exactly as directed. Do not take more or less of it or take it more often than prescribed by your doctor.

Shake liquid sucralfate well before measuring doses.

This medicine must be taken regularly to be effective. It may take up to 8 weeks for ulcers to heal.

Are there other uses for this medicine?

Sucralfate is also used to protect the stomach lining when taking aspirin and for mouth sores that occur with cancer chemotherapy. Talk to your doctor about the possible risks of using this drug for your condition.

What special precautions should I follow?

Before taking sucralfate,
- tell your doctor and pharmacist if you are allergic to sucralfate or any other drugs.
- tell your doctor and pharmacist what prescription and nonprescription medications you are taking, especially antacids (Mylanta, Maalox), anticoagulants ('blood thinners') such as warfarin (Coumadin), cinoxacin (Cinobac), ciprofloxacin (Cipro), digoxin (Lanoxin), enoxacin (Penetrex), ketoconazole (Nizoral), levofloxacin (Levaquin), lomefloxacin (Maxaquin), nalidixic acid (NegGram), norfloxacin (Noroxin), ofloxacin (Floxin), phenytoin (Dilantin), quinidine, sparfloxacin (Zagam), tetracycline (Sumycin), and vitamins. If you are taking any of these medicines, do not take them within 2 hours of taking sucralfate.

- tell your doctor if you have or have ever had heart or kidney disease or diabetes.
- tell your doctor if you are pregnant, plan to become pregnant, or are breast-feeding. If you become pregnant while taking sucralfate, call your doctor.

What should I do if I forget to take a dose?

Take the missed dose as soon as you remember it. However, if it is almost time for the next dose, skip the missed dose and continue your regular dosing schedule. Do not take a double dose to make up for a missed one.

What side effects can this medicine cause?

Sucralfate may cause side effects. To avoid constipation, abdominal pain, and gas, eat a high-fiber diet (extra fruits, vegetables, salads, and bran) and drink plenty of fluids.

If you experience any of the following symptoms, call your doctor immediately:

- passing red or black stools
- coughing up or vomiting material that is bright red or looks like coffee grounds

If you experience a serious side effect, you or your doctor may send a report to the Food and Drug Administration's (FDA) MedWatch Adverse Event Reporting program online [at http://www.fda.gov/MedWatch/index.html] or by phone [1-800-332-1088].

What storage conditions are needed for this medicine?

Keep this medication in the container it came in, tightly closed, and out of reach of children. Store it at room temperature and away from excess heat and moisture (not in the bathroom). Throw away any medication that is outdated or no longer needed. Talk to your pharmacist about the proper disposal of your medication.

What other information should I know?

Keep all appointments with your doctor and the laboratory. Your doctor will order certain lab tests to check your response to sucralfate.

Do not let anyone else take your medication. Ask your pharmacist any questions you have about refilling your prescription.

Talk to your doctor, pharmacist, or other healthcare professional if you have questions about dosing information for your medication.

Sulfacetamide Ophthalmic

(sul fa see′ ta mide)

Brand Name: AK-Sulf, Bleph-10, Blephamide®, FML-S®, Sulf-10
Also available generically.

Why is this medicine prescribed?

Sulfacetamide stops the growth of bacteria that cause certain eye infections. It is used to treat eye infections and to prevent them after injuries.

This medication is sometimes prescribed for other uses; ask your doctor or pharmacist for more information.

How should this medicine be used?

Sulfacetamide comes as eyedrops and eye ointment. The eyedrops usually are applied every 2-3 hours during the day and less frequently at night; the ointment usually is applied four times a day and at bedtime. Follow the directions on your prescription label carefully, and ask your doctor or pharmacist to explain any part you do not understand. Use sulfacetamide exactly as directed. Do not use more or less of it or use it more often than prescribed by your doctor.

To use the eyedrops, follow these instructions:

1. Wash your hands thoroughly with soap and water.
2. Use a mirror or have someone else put the drops in your eye.
3. Remove the protective cap. Make sure that the end of the dropper is not chipped or cracked and that the eyedrops are clear (not cloudy).
4. Avoid touching the dropper tip against your eye or anything else.
5. Hold the dropper tip down at all times to prevent drops from flowing back into the bottle and contaminating the remaining contents.
6. Lie down or tilt your head back.
7. Holding the bottle between your thumb and index finger, place the dropper tip as near as possible to your eyelid without touching it.
8. Brace the remaining fingers of that hand against your cheek or nose.
9. With the index finger of your other hand, pull the lower lid of the eye down to form a pocket.
10. Drop the prescribed number of drops into the pocket made by the lower lid and the eye. Placing drops on the surface of the eyeball can cause stinging.
11. Close your eye and press lightly against the lower lid with your finger for 2-3 minutes to keep the medication in the eye. Do not blink.
12. Replace and tighten the cap right away. Do not wipe or rinse it off.

13. Wipe off any excess liquid from your cheek with a clean tissue. Wash your hands again.

To use the eye ointment, follow these instructions:

1. Wash your hands thoroughly with soap and water.
2. Use a mirror or have someone else apply the ointment.
3. Avoid touching the tip of the tube against your eye or anything else. The ointment must be kept clean.
4. Tilt your head forward slightly.
5. Holding the tube between your thumb and index finger, place the tube as near as possible to your eyelid without touching it.
6. Brace the remaining fingers of that hand against your cheek or nose.
7. With the index finger of your other hand, pull the lower lid of your eye down to form a pocket.
8. Place a small amount of ointment into the pocket made by the lower lid and the eye. A 1/2-inch strip of ointment usually is enough unless otherwise directed by your doctor.
9. Gently close your eyes and keep them closed for 1-2 minutes to allow the medication to be absorbed.
10. Replace and tighten the cap right away.
11. Wipe off any excess ointment from your eyelids and lashes with a clean tissue. Wash your hands again.

What special precautions should I follow?

Before using sulfacetamide eyedrops or eye ointment,

- tell your doctor and pharmacist if you are allergic to sulfacetamide, sulfa drugs, sulfites, or any other drugs.
- tell your doctor and pharmacist what prescription and nonprescription medications you are taking, especially other eye medications and vitamins.
- tell your doctor if you are pregnant, plan to become pregnant, or are breast-feeding. If you become pregnant while using sulfacetamide, call your doctor immediately.
- tell your doctor if you wear soft contact lenses. If the brand of sulfacetamide you are using contains benzalkonium chloride, wait at least 15 minutes after using the medicine to put in soft contact lenses.

What should I do if I forget to take a dose?

Apply the missed dose as soon as you remember it. However, if it is almost time for the next dose, skip the missed dose and continue your regular dosing schedule. Do not apply a double dose to make up for a missed one.

What side effects can this medicine cause?

Sulfacetamide may cause side effects. Tell your doctor if any of these symptoms are severe or do not go away:

- temporary stinging or burning of the eye
- increased redness, itching, or swelling of the eye that continues for more than 48 hours

What storage conditions are needed for this medicine?

Keep this medication in the container it came in, tightly closed, and out of the reach of children. Store it at room temperature and away from excess heat and moisture (not in the bathroom). Do not let it freeze and do not use discolored eyedrops (yellowish brown to deep reddish brown). Throw away any unused part of your prescription. Do not save it to use for another infection. Talk to your pharmacist about the proper disposal of your medication.

What other information should I know?

Keep all appointments with your doctor.

Do not let anyone else use your medication. Ask your pharmacist any questions you have about refilling your prescription.

If you still have symptoms of infection after you finish the sulfacetamide, call your doctor.

Dosage Facts
For Informational Purposes

Caution: Do not change your dose, how often you take your medication, or the length of time you are to take it without first talking to your healthcare provider.

The following dosage information was written using medical language for doctors and other healthcare professionals and is provided here for you to check your dosage. The dosage of this drug may differ for different patients. Therefore, always follow your doctor's instructions or the directions on the label. Contact your healthcare provider or pharmacist if you have any questions about the specific dosage of your medication after reviewing this information.

Pediatric Patients

Bacterial Ophthalmic Infections

OPHTHALMIC:

- Ointment: apply ribbon of ointment (approximately 1.25–2.5 cm in length) in the conjunctival sac every 3–4 hours and at bedtime. Alternatively, the ointment may be applied at night in conjunction with daytime use of the ophthalmic solution.
- Solution: 1 or 2 drops of solution into the lower conjunctival sac every 2–3 hours initially and less frequently at night. Usual duration of treatment is 7–10 days.

Chlamydial Ophthalmic Infections
Trachoma

OPHTHALMIC:

- Ointment†: apply ribbon of ointment to the affected eye(s) twice daily for 2 months or twice daily for the first 5 days of each month for 6 months in conjunction with systemic anti-infectives.
- Solution: 2 drops in the conjunctival sac of the affected eye(s) every 2 hours in conjunction with systemic anti-infectives.

Adult Patients

Bacterial Ophthalmic Infections

OPHTHALMIC:

- Ointment: apply ribbon of ointment (approximately 1.25–2.5 cm in length) in the conjunctival sac every 3–4 hours and at bedtime. Alternatively, the ointment may be applied at night in conjunction with daytime use of the ophthalmic solution.
- Solution: 1 or 2 drops of solution into the lower conjunctival sac every 2–3 hours initially and less frequently at night. Usual duration of treatment is 7–10 days.

Chlamydial Ophthalmic Infections
Trachoma

OPHTHALMIC:

- Ointment†: apply ribbon of ointment to the affected eye(s) twice daily for 2 months or twice daily for the first 5 days of each month for 6 months in conjunction with systemic anti-infectives.
- Solution: 2 drops in the conjunctival sac of the affected eye(s) every 2 hours in conjunction with systemic anti-infectives.

† Use is not currently included in the labeling approved by the US Food and Drug Administration.

Sulfadiazine

(sul fa dye′ a zeen)

Brand Name: Microsulfon®

Why is this medicine prescribed?

Sulfadiazine, a sulfa drug, eliminates bacteria that cause infections, especially urinary tract infections. Antibiotics will not work for colds, flu, or other viral infections.

This medication is sometimes prescribed for other uses; ask your doctor or pharmacist for more information.

How should this medicine be used?

Sulfadiazine comes as a tablet to take by mouth. It is usually taken three to six times a day. Follow the directions on your prescription label carefully, and ask your doctor or pharmacist to explain any part you do not understand. Take sulfadiazine exactly as directed. Do not take more or less of it or take it more often than prescribed by your doctor.

The tablets should be taken with a full glass of water.

Continue to take sulfadiazine even if you feel well. Do not stop taking sulfadiazine without talking to your doctor.

What special precautions should I follow?

Before taking sulfadiazine,

- tell your doctor and pharmacist if you are allergic to sulfadiazine, any other sulfa drugs, diuretic ('water pills'), oral diabetes medications, or any other drugs.
- tell your doctor and pharmacist what prescription and nonprescription medications you are taking, especially anticoagulants ('blood thinners') such as warfarin (Coumadin), diabetes medications, diuretics ('water pills'), and vitamins.
- tell your doctor if you have or have ever had liver or kidney disease, asthma, severe allergies, or glucose-6-phosphate dehydrogenase (G-6PD) deficiency (an inherited blood disease).
- tell your doctor if you are pregnant, plan to become pregnant, or are breast-feeding. If you become pregnant while taking sulfadiazine, call your doctor.
- plan to avoid unnecessary or prolonged exposure to sunlight and to wear protective clothing, sunglasses, and sunscreen. Sulfadiazine may make your skin sensitive to sunlight.

What special dietary instructions should I follow?

You should drink plenty of fluids and take sulfadiazine on an empty stomach.

What should I do if I forget to take a dose?

Take the missed dose as soon as you remember it. However, if it is almost time for the next dose, skip the missed dose and continue your regular dosing schedule. Do not take a double dose to make up for a missed one.

What side effects can this medicine cause?

Sulfadiazine may cause side effects. Tell your doctor if any of these symptoms are severe or do not go away:

- diarrhea
- upset stomach
- loss of appetite
- dizziness

If you experience any of the following symptoms, call your doctor immediately:

- rash or skin changes
- sore throat
- fever
- headache
- joint or muscle aches
- yellowing of the skin or eyes
- swelling of the lips or tongue
- swallowing problems
- tiredness
- weakness
- blood in urine
- difficulty breathing
- unusual bleeding or bruising
- ringing in ears

If you experience a serious side effect, you or your doctor may send a report to the Food and Drug Administration's (FDA) MedWatch Adverse Event Reporting program online [at http://www.fda.gov/MedWatch/index.html] or by phone [1-800-332-1088].

What storage conditions are needed for this medicine?

Keep this medication in the container it came in, tightly closed and out of reach of children. Store it at room temperature and away from excess heat and moisture (not in the bathroom). Throw away any medication that is outdated or no longer needed. Talk to your pharmacist about the proper disposal of your medication.

What should I do in case of overdose?

In case of overdose, call your local poison control center at 1-800-222-1222. If the victim has collapsed or is not breathing, call local emergency services at 911.

What other information should I know?

Keep all appointments with your doctor.

Do not let anyone else take your medication. Your prescription is probably not refillable.

If you still have symptoms of an infection after you finish sulfadiazine, call your doctor.

Talk to your doctor, pharmacist, or other healthcare professional if you have questions about dosing information for your medication.

Sulfasalazine

(sul fa sal′ a zeen)

Brand Name: Azulfidine®, Azulfidine® EN-tabs®

Also available generically.

Why is this medicine prescribed?

Sulfasalazine is used to treat bowel inflammation, diarrhea (stool frequency), rectal bleeding, and abdominal pain in patients with ulcerative colitis, a condition in which the bowel is inflamed. Sulfasalazine delayed-release (Azulfidine EN-tabs) is also used to treat rheumatoid arthritis in adults and children whose disease has not responded well to other medications. Sulfasalazine is in a class of medications called anti-inflammatory drugs. It works by reducing inflammation (swelling) inside the body.

How should this medicine be used?

Sulfasalazine comes as regular and delayed-release (enteric-coated) tablets. It usually is taken four times a day in evenly spaced doses throughout the day so that no more than 8 hours separates any two doses, if possible. Take sulfasalazine after a meal or with a light snack, then drink a full glass of water. Follow the directions on your prescription label carefully, and ask your doctor or pharmacist to explain any part you do not understand. Take sulfasalazine exactly as directed.

Do not take more or less of it or take it more often than prescribed by your doctor.

Swallow tablets whole; do not crush or chew them.

Drink plenty of fluids (at least six to eight glasses of water or other beverage per day) while taking sulfasalazine.

Continue to take sulfasalazine even if you feel well. Do not stop taking sulfasalazine without talking to your doctor.

Are there other uses for this medicine?

Sulfasalazine is also used to treat bowel inflammation, diarrhea (stool frequency), rectal bleeding, and abdominal pain in Crohn's disease. Talk to your doctor about the possible risks of using this drug for your condition.

What special precautions should I follow?

Before taking sulfasalazine,

- tell your doctor if you are allergic to sulfasalazine, sulfapyridine, aspirin, choline magnesium trisalicylate (Triosal, Trilisate), choline salicylate (Arthropan), mesalamine (Asacol, Pentasa, Rowasa), salsalate (Argesic-SA, Disalcid, Salgesic, others), sulfa drugs, trisalicylate (Tricosal, Trilisate), or any other drugs.
- tell your doctor and pharmacist what prescription and nonprescription medications you are taking, especially digoxin (Lanoxin), folic acid, and vitamins.
- tell your doctor if you have or have ever had asthma, kidney or liver disease, porphyria, blood problems, or blockage in your intestine or urinary tract.
- tell your doctor if you are pregnant, plan to become pregnant, or are breast-feeding. If you become pregnant while taking sulfasalazine, call your doctor.
- plan to avoid unnecessary or prolonged exposure to sunlight and to wear protective clothing, sunglasses, and sunscreen. Sulfasalazine may make your skin sensitive to sunlight.

What should I do if I forget to take a dose?

Take the missed dose as soon as you remember it. However, if it is almost time for your next dose, skip the missed dose and continue your regular dosing schedule. Do not take a double dose to make up for a missed one.

What side effects can this medicine cause?

Sulfasalazine may cause side effects. Sulfasalazine causes temporary infertility in males. Fertility returns when the medicine is stopped. It can also cause your urine or skin to turn yellowish-orange; this effect is harmless.

Tell your doctor if any of these symptoms are severe or do not go away:

- diarrhea
- headache
- loss of appetite
- upset stomach
- vomiting
- stomach pain

If you have any of the following symptoms, stop taking sulfasalazine and call your doctor immediately:

- skin rash
- itching
- hives
- swelling
- sore throat
- fever
- joint or muscle aches
- pale or yellow skin
- difficulty swallowing
- tiredness
- unusual bleeding or bruising
- weakness

If you experience a serious side effect, you or your doctor may send a report to the Food and Drug Administration's (FDA) MedWatch Adverse Event Reporting program online [at http://www.fda.gov/MedWatch/index.html] or by phone [1-800-332-1088].

What storage conditions are needed for this medicine?

Keep this medication in the container it came in, tightly closed, and out of reach of children. Store it at room temperature and away from excess heat and moisture (not in the bathroom). Throw away any medication that is outdated or no longer needed. Talk to your pharmacist about the proper disposal of your medication.

What should I do in case of overdose?

In case of overdose, call your local poison control center at 1-800-222-1222. If the victim has collapsed or is not breathing, call local emergency services at 911.

What other information should I know?

Keep all appointments with your doctor and the laboratory. Your doctor may order certain lab tests to check your response to sulfasalazine.

Do not let anyone else take your medicine. Ask your pharmacist any questions you have about refilling your prescription.

Dosage Facts
For Informational Purposes

Caution: Do not change your dose, how often you take your medication, or the length of time you are to take it without first talking to your healthcare provider.

The following dosage information was written using medical language for doctors and other healthcare professionals and is provided here for you to check your dosage. The dosage of this drug may differ for different patients. Therefore, always follow your doctor's instructions or the directions on the label. Contact your health-care provider or pharmacist if you have any questions about the specific dosage of your medication after reviewing this information.

Pediatric Patients

Ulcerative Colitis

ORAL:
- Conventional tablets in children $\geq$ 2 years of age: initial dosage is 40–60 mg/kg daily in 3–6 divided doses and usual maintenance dosage is 30 mg/kg daily in 4 divided doses. Interval between doses should not exceed 8 hours.
- Delayed-release tablets in children $\geq$6 years of age: initial dosage is 40–60 mg/kg daily in 3–6 divided doses and usual maintenance dosage is 30 mg/kg daily in 4 divided doses. Interval between doses should not exceed 8 hours.

Crohn's Disease†

ORAL:
- Initiate therapy with 25–40 mg/kg daily and increase to 50–75 mg/kg daily (maximum daily dosage 4 g).

Juvenile Arthritis
Polyarticular Course

ORAL:
- Delayed-release tablets in children $\geq$6 years of age: 30–50 mg/kg daily in 2 equally divided doses; the maximum dosage usually is 2 g daily.
- To reduce GI intolerance, the manufacturers recommend that therapy be initiated with ¼ to ⅓ of the planned maintenance dosage, and that dosage be increased at weekly intervals until the planned maintenance dosage is achieved (usually at week 4).

Adult Patients

Ulcerative Colitis

ORAL:
- Conventional or delayed-release tablets: initial dosage is 3–4 g daily given in equally divided doses; interval between doses should not exceed 8 hours. In some patients, it may be advantageous to initiate therapy with a dosage of 1–2 g daily to lessen adverse GI effects. Usual maintenance dosage is 2 g daily in 4 divided doses, although some clinicians advocate a lower maintenance dosage of 1–1.5 g daily if necessary to prevent adverse effects.
- Dosage as high as 12 g daily has been used for initial therapy, but dosage >4 g daily is accompanied by increased incidence of adverse effects. Generally avoid dosage >4 g daily unless serum concentrations of total sulfapyridine and the phenotype of the patient are known.
- Efficacy of maintenance therapy appears to be dose related, but potential benefits of dosages >2 g daily must be weighed against the risks of increased adverse effects and the necessity for more careful patient monitoring.

Crohn's Disease†

ORAL:
- Mildly to moderately active disease: 3–6 g daily (as conventional or delayed-release tablets) has been used.
- Maintenance: 1.5–3 g daily (as conventional or delayed-release tablets) has been used, although such dosages do not appear to be more effective than placebo when used in patients with medically induced remission.

Rheumatoid Arthritis

ORAL:

- Delayed-release tablets: 2–3 g daily given in equally divided doses every 12 hours.
- It may be advantageous to initiate therapy with a dosage of 0.5–1 g daily to lessen adverse GI effects. The manufacturers recommend that patients receive 0.5 g every evening the first week of therapy, 0.5 g twice daily (morning and evening) the second week, 0.5 g every morning and 1 g every evening the third week, and 1 g twice daily (morning and evening) thereafter.
- A response to sulfasalazine (manifested by improvement in the number and extent of actively inflamed joints) may not occur until after 4–12 weeks of therapy.
- Patients receiving sulfasalazine dosages >2 g daily should be carefully monitored.

Prescribing Limits

Pediatric Patients

Juvenile Arthritis

ORAL:

- Maximum of 2 g daily.

Crohn's Disease†

ORAL:

- Maximum of 4 g daily.

† Use is not currently included in the labeling approved by the US Food and Drug Administration.

Sulfinpyrazone

(sul fin peer′ a zone)

Brand Name: Anturane®

Why is this medicine prescribed?

Sulfinpyrazone is used to treat gouty arthritis. It works by lowering the amount of uric acid in your blood, preventing gout attacks. The drug helps prevent attacks but will not treat an attack once it has started.

This medication is sometimes prescribed for other uses; ask your doctor or pharmacist for more information.

How should this medicine be used?

Sulfinpyrazone comes as a tablet and capsule to take by mouth. Sulfinpyrazone usually is taken twice a day. Take with food or milk. Follow the directions on your prescription label carefully, and ask your doctor or pharmacist to explain any part you do not understand. Take sulfinpyrazone exactly as directed. Do not take more or less of it or take it more often than prescribed by your doctor.

Sulfinpyrazone helps control gout but does not cure it. Continue to take sulfinpyrazone even if you feel well. Do not stop taking sulfinpyrazone without talking to your doctor.

Are there other uses for this medicine?

Sulfinpyrazone may be used after a heart attack. Talk to your doctor about the possible risks of using this drug for your condition.

What special precautions should I follow?

Before taking sulfinpyrazone,

- tell your doctor and pharmacist if you are allergic to sulfinpyrazone or any other drugs.
- tell your doctor and pharmacist what prescription and nonprescription medications you are taking, especially anticoagulants ('blood thinners') such as warfarin (Coumadin), acetaminophen (Tylenol), aspirin or products that contain aspirin, cholestyramine (Questran), diuretics ('water pills'), niacin (Nicobid, Slo-Niacin), theophylline (Theo-Dur), tolbutamide (Orinase), verapamil (Calan, Isoptin), and vitamins.
- tell your doctor if you have or have ever had peptic ulcer disease, kidney disease, or any blood disease.
- tell your doctor if you are pregnant, plan to become pregnant, or are breast-feeding. If you become pregnant while taking sulfinpyrazone, call your doctor.
- if you are having surgery, including dental surgery, tell the doctor or dentist that you are taking sulfinpyrazone.
- you should know that this drug may make you drowsy. Do not drive a car or operate machinery until you know how this drug affects you.
- remember that alcohol can add to the drowsiness caused by this drug. Also, alcohol may increase the amount of uric acid in your blood. Do not drink alcohol while taking sulfinpyrazone before checking with your doctor.

What special dietary instructions should I follow?

Sulfinpyrazone helps your body get rid of uric acid through your urine. This process may cause kidney stones. To help prevent kidney stones, be sure to drink 10-12 glasses (8 ounces each) of fluid each day or drink enough water to keep your urine a light yellow color.

What should I do if I forget to take a dose?

Take the missed dose as soon as you remember it. However, if it is almost time for the next dose, skip the missed dose and continue your regular dosing schedule. Do not take a double dose to make up for a missed one.

What side effects can this medicine cause?

Sulfinpyrazone may cause side effects. Tell your doctor if any of these symptoms are severe or do not go away:

- upset stomach
- vomiting
- loss of appetite

- joint pain, redness, or swelling

If you experience any of the following symptoms, call your doctor immediately:

- difficulty breathing
- tightness in the chest
- skin rash
- unusual bruising or bleeding
- fever
- sore throat
- mouth sores
- swollen or painful glands
- painful urination
- change in the amount of urine
- lower back or side pain
- blood in urine or stool

If you experience a serious side effect, you or your doctor may send a report to the Food and Drug Administration's (FDA) MedWatch Adverse Event Reporting program online [at http://www.fda.gov/MedWatch/index.html] or by phone [1-800-332-1088].

What storage conditions are needed for this medicine?

Keep this medication in the container it came in, tightly closed, and out of reach of children. Store it at room temperature and away from excess heat and moisture (not in the bathroom). Throw away any medication that is outdated or no longer needed. Talk to your pharmacist about the proper disposal of your medication.

What should I do in case of overdose?

In case of overdose, call your local poison control center at 1-800-222-1222. If the victim has collapsed or is not breathing, call local emergency services at 911.

What other information should I know?

Keep all appointments with your doctor and the laboratory. Your doctor will order certain lab tests to check your response to sulfinpyrazone.

Do not let anyone else take your medication. Ask your pharmacist any questions you have about refilling your prescription.

Talk to your doctor, pharmacist, or other healthcare professional if you have questions about dosing information for your medication.

Sulindac

(sul in' dak)

Brand Name: Clinoril®
Also available generically.

Important Warning

People who take nonsteroidal anti-inflammatory medications (NSAIDs) (other than aspirin) such as sulindac may have a higher risk of having a heart attack or a stroke than people who do not take these medications. These events may happen without warning and may cause death. This risk may be higher for people who take NSAIDs for a long time. Tell your doctor if you or anyone in your family has or has ever had heart disease, a heart attack, or a stroke, if you smoke, and if you have or have ever had high cholesterol, high blood pressure, or diabetes. Get emergency medical help right away if you experience any of the following symptoms: chest pain, shortness of breath, weakness in one part or side of the body, or slurred speech.

If you will be undergoing a coronary artery bypass graft (CABG; a type of heart surgery), you should not take sulindac right before or right after the surgery.

NSAIDs such as sulindac may cause ulcers, bleeding, or holes in the stomach or intestine. These problems may develop at any time during treatment, may happen without warning symptoms, and may cause death. The risk may be higher for people who take NSAIDs for a long time, are older in age, have poor health, or drink large amounts of alcohol while you are taking sulindac. Tell your doctor if you take any of the following medications: anticoagulants ('blood thinners') such as warfarin (Coumadin); aspirin; other NSAIDs such as diflunisal (Dolobid), ibuprofen (Advil, Motrin) or naproxen (Aleve, Naprosyn), or oral steroids such as dexamethasone (Decadron, Dexone), methylprednisolone (Medrol), and prednisone (Deltasone). Also tell your doctor if you have or have ever had ulcers or bleeding in your stomach or intestines, or other bleeding disorders. If you experience any of the following symptoms, stop taking sulindac and call your doctor: stomach pain, heartburn, vomiting a substance that is bloody or looks like coffee grounds, blood in the stool, or black and tarry stools.

Keep all appointments with your doctor and the laboratory. Your doctor will monitor your symptoms carefully and will probably order certain tests to check your body's response to sulindac. Be sure to

continued on next page

Important Warning (cont'd)

tell your doctor how you are feeling so that your doctor can prescribe the right amount of medication to treat your condition with the lowest risk of serious side effects.

Your doctor or pharmacist will give you the manufacturer's patient information sheet (Medication Guide) when you begin treatment with sulindac and each time you refill your prescription. Read the information carefully and ask your doctor or pharmacist if you have any questions. You can also visit the Food and Drug Administration (FDA) website (http://www.fda.gov/cder) or the manufacturer's website to obtain the Medication Guide.

Why is this medicine prescribed?

Sulindac is used to relieve pain, tenderness, swelling, and stiffness caused by osteoarthritis (arthritis caused by a breakdown of the lining of the joints), rheumatoid arthritis (arthritis caused by swelling of the lining of the joints), and ankylosing spondylitis (arthritis that mainly affects the spine). Sulindac also is used to treat pain in the shoulder caused by bursitis (inflammation of a fluid-filled sac in the shoulder joint) and tendinitis (inflammation of the tissue that connects muscle to bone). It is also used to relieve gouty arthritis (attacks of severe joint pain and swelling caused by a build-up of certain substances in the joints). Sulindac is in a class of medications called NSAIDs. It works by stopping the body's production of a substance that causes pain, fever, and inflammation.

How should this medicine be used?

Sulindac comes as a tablet to take by mouth. It is usually taken with food twice a day. Take sulindac at around the same times each day. Follow the directions on your prescription label carefully, and ask your doctor or pharmacist to explain any part you do not understand. Take sulindac exactly as directed. Do not take more or less of it or take it more often than prescribed by your doctor.

Sulindac helps control arthritis pain but does not cure arthritis. If you are taking sulindac to treat arthritis pain, it may take 1 week or longer before you feel the full benefit of sulindac.

Are there other uses for this medicine?

Sulindac is also sometimes used to reduce the number of polyps (abnormal growths) in the colon (large intestine) and rectum in patients with familial adenomatous polyposis (a condition in which hundreds or thousands of polyps form in the colon and cancer may develop). Talk to your doctor about the risks of using this medication for your condition.

This medication is sometimes prescribed for other uses; ask your doctor or pharmacist for more information.

What special precautions should I follow?

Before taking sulindac,

- tell your doctor and pharmacist if you are allergic to sulindac, aspirin or or other NSAIDs such as ibuprofen (Advil, Motrin) and naproxen (Aleve, Naprosyn), or any other medications.
- tell your doctor and pharmacist what prescription and nonprescription medications, vitamins, nutritional supplements, and herbal products you are taking or plan to take. Be sure to mention the medications listed in the IMPORTANT WARNING section and any of the following: angiotensin-converting enzyme (ACE) inhibitors such as benazepril (Lotensin), captopril (Capoten), enalapril (Vasotec), fosinopril (Monopril), lisinopril (Prinivil, Zestril), moexipril (Univasc), perindopril (Aceon), quinapril (Accupril), ramipril (Altace), and trandolapril (Mavik); angiotensin II receptor antagonists such as candesartan (Atacand), eprosartan (Teveten), irbesartan (Avapro), losartan (Cozaar), olmesartan (Benicar), telmisartan (Micardis), valsartan (Diovan); cyclosporine (Neoral, Sandimmune); diuretics ('water pills'); lithium (Eskalith, Lithobid); oral medications for diabetes; methotrexate (Rheumatrex); and probenecid (Benemid).
- tell your doctor if you have or have ever had any of the conditions mentioned in the IMPORTANT WARNING section or asthma, especially if you also have frequent stuffed or runny nose or nasal polyps (swelling of the lining of the nose); kidney stones; swelling of the hands, arms, feet, ankles, or lower legs; or liver or kidney disease.
- tell your doctor if you are pregnant, especially if you are in the last few months of your pregnancy, you plan to become pregnant, or you are breast-feeding. If you become pregnant while taking sulindac, call your doctor.
- if you are having surgery, including dental surgery, tell the doctor or dentist that you are taking sulindac.

What special dietary instructions should I follow?

Unless your doctor tells you otherwise, continue your normal diet.

What should I do if I forget to take a dose?

Take the missed dose as soon as you remember it. However, if it is almost time for the next dose, skip the missed dose and continue your regular dosing schedule. Do not take a double dose to make up for a missed one.

What side effects can this medicine cause?

Sulindac may cause side effects. Tell your doctor if any of these symptoms are severe or do not go away:

- headache
- dizziness

- nervousness
- diarrhea
- constipation
- gas
- ringing in the ears

Some side effects can be serious. If you experience any of the following symptoms, or those mentioned in the IMPORTANT WARNING section, call your doctor immediately. Do not take any more sulindac until you speak to your doctor:

- unexplained weight gain
- fever
- chills
- cough
- sweating
- flushing
- muscle or joint pain
- chest pain
- blisters
- rash
- itching
- hives
- swelling of the eyes, face, lips, tongue, throat, arms, hands, feet, ankles, or lower legs
- difficulty breathing or swallowing
- hoarseness
- pale skin
- fast hearbeat
- excessive tiredness
- unusual bleeding or bruising
- lack of energy
- upset stomach
- loss of appetite
- pain in the upper right part of the stomach
- flu-like symptoms
- yellowing of the skin or eyes
- cloudy, discolored, or bloody urine
- back pain
- difficult or painful urination
- blurred vision or other problems with sight

Sulindac may cause other side effects. Call your doctor if you have any unusual problems while taking this medication.

If you experience a serious side effect, you or your doctor may send a report to the Food and Drug Administration's (FDA) MedWatch Adverse Event Reporting program online [at http://www.fda.gov/MedWatch/index.html] or by phone [1-800-332-1088].

What storage conditions are needed for this medicine?

Keep this medication in the container it came in, tightly closed, and out of reach of children. Store it at room temperature and away from excess heat and moisture (not in the bathroom). Throw away any medication that is outdated or no longer needed. Talk to your pharmacist about the proper disposal of your medication.

What should I do in case of overdose?

In case of overdose, call your local poison control center at 1-800-222-1222. If the victim has collapsed or is not breathing, call local emergency services at 911.

Symptoms of overdose may include:

- loss of consciousness
- fainting
- dizziness
- blurred vision
- upset stomach
- decreased urination

What other information should I know?

Do not let anyone else take your medication. Ask your pharmacist any questions you have about refilling your prescription.

Dosage Facts
For Informational Purposes

Caution: Do not change your dose, how often you take your medication, or the length of time you are to take it without first talking to your healthcare provider.

The following dosage information was written using medical language for doctors and other healthcare professionals and is provided here for you to check your dosage. The dosage of this drug may differ for different patients. Therefore, always follow your doctor's instructions or the directions on the label. Contact your healthcare provider or pharmacist if you have any questions about the specific dosage of your medication after reviewing this information.

General Dosage Information

To minimize the potential risk of adverse cardiovascular and/or GI events, use lowest effective dosage and shortest duration of therapy consistent with the patient's treatment goals. Adjust dosage based on individual requirements and response; attempt to titrate to the lowest effective dosage.

Adult Patients

Inflammatory Diseases
Osteoarthritis, Rheumatoid Arthritis, or Ankylosing Spondylitis

ORAL:
- Initially, 150 mg twice daily. Adjust dosage based on response.

Acute Painful Shoulder

ORAL:
- 200 mg twice daily; reduce dosage based on response. 7–14 days of therapy usually adequate.

Gout

ORAL:
- 200 mg twice daily; reduce dosage based on response. 7 days of therapy usually adequate.

Colorectal Polyps†

ORAL:
- 150 mg twice daily.

Prescribing Limits

Adult Patients

Inflammatory Diseases

ORAL:
- Maximum 400 mg daily.

Special Populations

Hepatic Impairment
- Dosage reduction may be required.

Renal Impairment
- Dosage reduction may be required.

† *Use is not currently included in the labeling approved by the US Food and Drug Administration.*

Sumatriptan Injection

(soo ma trip′ tan)

Brand Name: Imitrex Injection®

Why is this medicine prescribed?

Sumatriptan is used to treat the symptoms of migraine headaches (severe, throbbing headaches that sometimes are accompanied by nausea and sensitivity to sound and light). Sumatriptan is in a class of medications called selective serotonin receptor agonists. It works by narrowing blood vessels in the brain and by stopping pain signals from being sent to the brain. Sumatriptan does not prevent migraine attacks.

How should this medicine be used?

Sumatriptan is taken by injection, just under your skin, as soon as your migraine symptoms appear. You should feel relief of your symptoms within 1 hour (maybe within 10 minutes). If your symptoms then return after the first injection, you may take a second injection after 1 hour. But do not use more than two injections in a 24-hour period. Follow the directions on your prescription label carefully, and ask your doctor or pharmacist to explain any part you do not understand. Take sumatriptan exactly as directed. Do not take more or less of it or take it more often than prescribed by your doctor.

Sumatriptan comes in an autoinjection device so that you can self-inject this medication into your thigh or deltoid area (shoulder joint). Your doctor or pharmacist should show you how to load the injector and administer the medication. Also read the instruction pamphlet and be sure that you understand the correct injection technique before you use the autoinjector.

Try the autoinjector for the first time in your doctor's office so that he/she can be sure that you are using it correctly and can monitor any side effects.

Are there other uses for this medicine?

This medication is sometimes prescribed for other uses; ask your doctor or pharmacist for more information.

What special precautions should I follow?

Before using sumatriptan,
- tell your doctor and pharmacist if you are allergic to sumatriptan or any other drugs.
- do not use sumatriptan if you have taken a monoamine oxidase inhibitor (MAOI) such as isocarboxazid (Marplan), phenelzine (Nardil), selegiline (Eldepryl, Emsam) or tranylcypromine (Parnate) during the past 2 weeks or if you have taken another medication for migraine headaches such as dihydroergotamine (D.H.E. 45, Migranal), methysergide (Sansert), almotriptan (Axert), eletriptan (Relpax), frovatriptan (Frova), naratriptan (Amerge), rizatriptan (Maxalt, Maxalt-MLT), or zolmitriptan (Zomig) during the past 24 hours.
- tell your doctor and pharmacist what prescription and nonprescription medications, vitamins, herbal products and nutritional supplements you are taking or plan to take. Be sure to mention any of the following: selective serotonin reuptake inhibitors (SSRIs) such as citalopram (Celexa), escitalopram (Lexapro), fluoxetine (Prozac, Sarafem, in Symbyax), fluvoxamine, paroxetine (Paxil), and sertraline (Zoloft), and selective serotonin/norepinephrine reuptake inhibitors (SNRIs) such as duloxetine (Cymbalta) and venlafaxine (Effexor). Your doctor may need to change the doses of your medications or monitor you carefully for side effects.
- tell your doctor if you smoke, if you have a strong family history of heart disease, if you are postmenopausal, or if you are a man over 40. Also tell your doctor if you have or have ever had high blood pressure; angina (recurring chest pain); a heart attack; diabetes; high cholesterol; obesity; stroke; transient ischemic attack (mini-stroke); ischemic bowel disease; coronary artery disease; seizures; or blood vessel, kidney, or liver disease.
- tell your doctor if you are pregnant, plan to become pregnant, or are breast-feeding. If you become pregnant while taking sumatriptan, call your doctor.

What should I do if I forget to take a dose?

Sumatriptan is not for routine use. Use it only to relieve your migraine headache as soon as symptoms of the migraine appear.

What side effects can this medicine cause?

Sumatriptan may cause side effects. Tell your doctor if any of these symptoms are severe or do not go away:

- pain or redness at the site of injection
- flushing
- tingling feeling
- feeling of warmth or heaviness
- drowsiness
- upset stomach
- vomiting
- muscle cramps

If you experience any of the following symptoms, call your doctor immediately:

- pain or tightness in chest or throat
- fast heartbeat
- difficulty breathing
- wheezing
- redness, swelling, or itching of the eyelids, face, or lips
- skin rash, lumps, or hives
- changes in vision

What storage conditions are needed for this medicine?

Keep this medication in the container it came in, tightly closed, and out of reach of children. Store it at room temperature, away from light, excess heat, and moisture (not in the bathroom). Throw away any medication that is outdated or no longer needed. Talk to your pharmacist about the proper disposal of needles, syringes, and the medication.

What should I do in case of overdose?

In case of overdose, call your local poison control center at 1-800-222-1222. If the victim has collapsed or is not breathing, call local emergency services at 911.

What other information should I know?

Keep all appointments with your doctor.

Never inject this medication any place except under the skin of your thigh or shoulder.

Call your doctor if you continue to have symptoms.

Do not let anyone else take your medication. Ask your pharmacist any questions you have about refilling your prescription.

Dosage Facts
For Informational Purposes

Caution: Do not change your dose, how often you take your medication, or the length of time you are to take it without first talking to your healthcare provider.

The following dosage information was written using medical language for doctors and other healthcare professionals and is provided here for you to check your dosage. The dosage of this drug may differ for different patients. Therefore, always follow your doctor's instructions or the directions on the label. Contact your healthcare provider or pharmacist if you have any questions about the specific dosage of your medication after reviewing this information.

General Dosage Information

Available as sumatriptan (nasal solution) and sumatriptan succinate (tablets and injection); dosage expressed in terms of sumatriptan.

Following failure to respond to first dose, reconsider diagnosis of migraine prior to administration of a second dose.

Adult Patients

Vascular Headaches
Migraine

SUB-Q:

- ≤6 mg as a single dose. If dose-limiting adverse effects occur with 6-mg dose, lower doses (e.g., 4 mg) may be given. In patients receiving doses other than 4 or 6 mg, only the single-dose vials containing 6 mg/0.5 mL should be used to provide the desired dose.
- If headache recurs, a 6-mg *sub-Q* dose may be repeated once after ≥1 hour or additional *oral* doses may be administered at intervals ≥2 hours, up to a maximum *oral* dosage of 100 mg daily.
- If patient does not respond to first 6-mg dose, additional doses are unlikely to provide benefit.

Cluster Headache

SUB-Q:

- ≤6 mg as a single dose. If dose-limiting adverse effects occur with 6-mg dose, lower doses may be administered using only single-dose vials; use autoinjection device only with prefilled, unit-of-use syringes containing 6 mg.
- If headache recurs, 6-mg dose may be repeated once after ≥1 hour, up to a maximum dosage of 12 mg in any 24-hour period.
- If patient does not respond to first 6-mg dose, additional doses are unlikely to provide benefit.

Prescribing Limits

Adult Patients

Vascular Headaches

Migraine

SUB-Q:
- Maximum 6 mg as a single dose; do not exceed 12 mg (i.e., two 6-mg doses given ≥1 hour apart) in any 24-hour period.

Cluster Headache

SUB-Q:
- Maximum 6 mg as a single dose; do not exceed 12 mg (i.e., two 6-mg doses given ≥1 hour apart) in any 24-hour period.

Special Populations

Hepatic Impairment
- Contraindicated in patients with severe hepatic impairment.

Patients Receiving MAO-A Inhibitors
- Concurrent or recent (within 2 weeks) use of MAO-A inhibitor and *oral* or *intranasal* sumatriptan is contraindicated; *sub-Q* sumatriptan is not generally recommended, but if concomitant use is clinically warranted, decrease sumatriptan *sub-Q* dosage and administer under careful medical supervision.

Sumatriptan Oral and Nasal

(soo ma trip′ tan)

Brand Name: Imitrex®

Why is this medicine prescribed?

Sumatriptan is used to treat the symptoms of migraine headaches (severe, throbbing headaches that sometimes is accompanied by nausea or sensitivity to sound and light). Sumatriptan is in a class of medications called selective serotonin receptor agonists. It works by narrowing blood vessels in the head and stopping pain signals from being sent to the brain. Sumatriptan does not prevent migraine attacks.

How should this medicine be used?

Sumatriptan comes as a tablet to take by mouth and a nasal spray. It should be used at the first sign of a migraine headache. If you are at risk for heart disease and you have never taken sumatriptan before, you may need to take the first dose in your doctor's office. Usually only one dose is needed. If pain is not relieved with the first dose, your doctor may prescribe a second dose to be taken after at least 2 hours. Do not take more than 200mg of the tablets or 40

mg of the nasal spray in any 24-hour period. Follow the directions on your prescription label carefully, and ask your doctor or pharmacist to explain any part you do not understand. Take sumatriptan exactly as directed. Do not take more or less of it or take it more often than prescribed by your doctor.

Take the tablet with plenty of water or other fluids.

To use the nasal spray, follow the package directions or ask or your doctor or pharmacist to explain any part you do not understand.

Are there other uses for this medicine?

This medication is sometimes prescribed for other uses; ask your doctor or pharmacist for more information.

What special precautions should I follow?

Before taking sumatriptan,
- tell your doctor and pharmacist if you are allergic to sumatriptan or any other drugs.
- do not take sumatriptan if you have taken a monoamine oxidase inhibitor (MAOI) such as isocarboxazid (Marplan), phenelzine (Nardil), selegiline (Emsam, Eldepryl), or tranylcypromine (Parnate) during the past 2 weeks or if you have taken another medication for migraine headaches such as dihydroergotamine (D.H.E. 45, Migranal), methysergide (Sansert), almotriptan (Axert), eletriptan (Relpax), frovatriptan (Frova), naratriptan (Amerge), rizatriptan (Maxalt, Maxalt-MLT), or zolmitriptan (Zomig) during the past 24 hours.
- tell your doctor and pharmacist what prescription and nonprescription medications, vitamins, nutritional supplements, and herbal products you are taking or plan to take. Be sure to mention any of the following: selective serotonin reuptake inhibitors (SSRIs) such as citalopram (Celexa), escitalopram (Lexapro), fluoxetine (Prozac, Sarafem, in Symbyax), fluvoxamine, paroxetine (Paxil), and sertraline (Zoloft); and selective serotonin/norepinephrine reuptake inhibitors (SNRIs) such as duloxetine (Cymbalta) and venlafaxine (Effexor). Your doctor may need to change the doses of your medications or monitor you more carefully for side effects.
- tell your doctor if you smoke, if you have a strong family history of heart disease, if you are postmenopausal, or if you are a man over 40. Also tell your doctor if you have or have ever had high blood pressure; angina (recurring chest pain); a heart attack; diabetes; high cholesterol; obesity; stroke; transient ischemic attack (mini-stroke); ischemic bowel disease; coronary artery disease; seizures; or blood vessel, kidney, or liver disease.
- tell your doctor if you are pregnant, plan to become pregnant, or are breast-feeding. If you become pregnant while taking sumatriptan, call your doctor.
- you should know that this drug may make you drowsy. Do not drive a car or operate machinery until you know how this drug affects you.

- remember that alcohol can add to the drowsiness caused by this drug.

What should I do if I forget to take a dose?

Sumatriptan is not for routine use. Use it only to relieve your migraine headache as soon as symptoms of the migraine appear.

What side effects can this medicine cause?

Sumatriptan may cause side effects. Tell your doctor if any of these symptoms are severe or do not go away:
- flushing
- tingling feeling
- feeling of warmth or heaviness
- drowsiness
- dizziness
- upset stomach
- diarrhea
- vomiting
- irritation of the nose
- muscle cramps

If you experience any of the following symptoms, call your doctor immediately:
- pain or tightness in chest or throat
- sudden or severe stomach pain
- fast heartbeat
- difficulty breathing
- wheezing
- redness, swelling, or itching of the eyelids, face, or lips
- skin rash, lumps, or hives
- change in vision

What storage conditions are needed for this medicine?

Keep this medication in the container it came in, tightly closed, and out of reach of children. Store it at room temperature, away from excess heat and moisture (not in the bathroom). Throw away any medication that is outdated or no longer needed. Talk to your pharmacist about the proper disposal of your medication.

What should I do in case of overdose?

In case of overdose, call your local poison control center at 1-800-222-1222. If the victim has collapsed or is not breathing, call local emergency services at 911.

What other information should I know?

Keep all appointments with your doctor.

Call your doctor if you continue to have symptoms.

Do not let anyone else take your medication. Ask your pharmacist any questions you have about refilling your prescription.

Dosage Facts
For Informational Purposes

Caution: Do not change your dose, how often you take your medication, or the length of time you are to take it without first talking to your health-care provider.

The following dosage information was written using medical language for doctors and other healthcare professionals and is provided here for you to check your dosage. The dosage of this drug may differ for different patients. Therefore, always follow your doctor's instructions or the directions on the label. Contact your health-care provider or pharmacist if you have any questions about the specific dosage of your medication after reviewing this information.

General Dosage Information

Available as sumatriptan (nasal solution) and sumatriptan succinate (tablets and injection); dosage expressed in terms of sumatriptan.

Following failure to respond to first dose, reconsider diagnosis of migraine prior to administration of a second dose.

Adult Patients

Vascular Headaches
Migraine

ORAL:
- 25, 50, or 100 mg as a single dose. Individualize dosage selection, weighing the possible benefit (greater effectiveness) and risks (increased adverse effects) of the 50- or 100-mg dose; 100-mg dose may not provide substantially greater effect than 50-mg dose.
- If headache recurs or partial response occurs after initial dose, additional oral doses may be administered at intervals of ≥2 hours, up to a maximum oral dosage of 200 mg daily.
- If headache recurs after an initial *sub-Q* dose, additional *oral* doses may be administered at intervals ≥2 hours, up to a maximum *oral* dosage of 100 mg daily.

INTRANASAL:
- 5, 10, or 20 mg as a single dose; individualize dosage selection, weighing the possible benefit (greater effectiveness) and risks (increased adverse effects) of the 20-mg dose. Doses >20 mg provide no additional benefit.
- To achieve a 10-mg dose, administer a single 5-mg dose into each nostril.
- If headache recurs, dose may be repeated once after 2 hours, up to a maximum dosage of 40 mg daily.

Prescribing Limits

Adult Patients

Vascular Headaches
Migraine

ORAL:
- Maximum 200 mg daily; do not exceed 100 mg daily if following an initial *sub-Q* dose.
- Safety of treating an average of >4 headaches per 30-day period has not been established.

INTRANASAL:
- Maximum 40 mg daily.
- Safety of treating an average of >4 headaches per 30-day period has not been established.

Special Populations

Hepatic Impairment
- Contraindicated in patients with severe hepatic impairment. Unpredictable increases in bioavailability following *oral* administration in patients with hepatic impairment. If *oral* therapy is deemed advisable in these patients, do not exceed 50 mg as a single dose.

Patients Receiving MAO-A Inhibitors
- Concurrent or recent (within 2 weeks) use of MAO-A inhibitor and *oral* or *intranasal* sumatriptan is contraindicated.

Sunscreens

Brand Name: Bullfrog®, Coppertone®, Hawaiian Tropic®, PreSun®, Sundown®

Why is this medicine prescribed?

Sunscreens help to prevent sunburn and reduce the harmful effects of the sun such as premature skin aging and skin cancer.

How should this medicine be used?

Sunscreens come in cream, lotion, gel, stick, spray, and lip balm. They are for external use only; do not swallow them. Sunscreens should be applied between 30 minutes and 2 hours before sun exposure. In general, they should be reapplied after every 80 minutes spent in the water or perspiring heavily or every 2 hours spent out of the water. Follow the directions on the label carefully, and ask your pharmacist to explain any part you do not understand.

Ask your pharmacist or doctor about which sunscreen product to use. The choice depends on your sunburn and tanning history, skin type, use of other medications, and reasons for using a sunscreen. You want a product with the appropriate sun protection factor (SPF) for you. In most cases, an SPF of greater than 30 is not necessary and is not recommended.

If you are using a sunscreen to prevent drug-induced photosensitivity reactions or to prevent ultraviolet-induced disorders, choose a broad-spectrum product. Ask your pharmacist for advice.

If you will be swimming or sweating heavily, choose a sunscreen that is labeled waterproof or very water resistant.

Talk to your doctor before using a sunscreen on an infant less than 6 months old. Use a sunscreen with a high SPF (e.g., 30) in children older than 6 months.

Sunscreens should be applied liberally to all exposed areas. The average adult in a bathing suit should apply 9 half-teaspoon size portions as follows:
- **Face and neck:** 1 half-teaspoon portion
- **Arms and shoulders:** 1 half-teaspoon portion to each arm
- **Torso:** 1 half-teaspoon portion each to front and back
- **Legs and top of feet:** 2 half-teaspoon portions to each leg

What special precautions should I follow?

Before using sunscreens,
- tell your doctor and pharmacist if you are allergic to sunscreens, diuretics ('water pills'), sulfonamides, oral diabetic drugs, acetazolamide (Diamox), or any other drugs.
- tell your doctor and pharmacists what topical medications you are taking.

What should I do if I forget to take a dose?

If you forget to apply sunscreen and remember while you are being exposed to the sun, apply it as soon as possible.

What side effects can this medicine cause?

Sunscreens may cause side effects. Tell your doctor if either of these symptoms are severe or do not go away:
- skin rash
- irritation

What storage conditions are needed for this medicine?

Keep this medication in the container it came in, tightly closed, and out of reach of children.

What other information should I know?

Ask your pharmacist any questions you have about sunscreens.

Talk to your doctor, pharmacist, or other healthcare professional if you have questions about dosing information for your medication.

Tacrine

(tak′ reen)

Brand Name: Cognex®

Why is this medicine prescribed?

Tacrine is used to treat the symptoms of Alzheimer's disease, but it does not cure the disease.

This medication is sometimes prescribed for other uses; ask your doctor or pharmacist for more information.

How should this medicine be used?

Tacrine comes as a capsule to take by mouth. It usually is taken four times a day. Take tacrine on an empty stomach (1 hour before or 2 hours after meals). Follow the directions on your prescription label carefully, and ask your doctor or pharmacist to explain any part you do not understand. Take tacrine exactly as directed. Do not take more or less of it or take it more often than prescribed by your doctor.

Continue to take tacrine even if you feel well. Do not stop taking tacrine without talking to your doctor, especially if you have taken large doses for a long time. Your doctor probably will decrease your dose gradually. This drug must be taken regularly for a few weeks before its full effect is felt.

What special precautions should I follow?

Before taking tacrine,

- tell your doctor and pharmacist if you are allergic to tacrine or any other drugs.
- tell your doctor and pharmacist what prescription and nonprescription medications you are taking, especially atropine-like drugs (belladonna, dicyclomine, and scopolamine); bethanechol; cimetidine (Tagamet); cold, sinus, and allergy medications; fluvoxamine (Luvox); neostigmine; nonsteroidal anti-inflammatory medicine such as aspirin, ibuprofen (Advil, Motrin, or Nuprin), indomethacin (Indocin), and naproxen (Naprosyn); theophylline (Theo-Dur); ulcer medications; and vitamins.
- tell your doctor if you have or have ever had ulcers; seizures; problems with your urinary system; asthma; or blood vessel, heart, kidney, liver, lung, or stomach disease. Also tell your doctor if you have experienced yellowing of the skin or eyes when you took tacrine in the past.
- tell your doctor if you are pregnant, plan to become pregnant, or are breast-feeding. If you become pregnant while taking tacrine, call your doctor.
- if you are having surgery, including dental surgery, tell the doctor or dentist that you are taking tacrine.
- you should know that this drug may make you drowsy. Do not drive a car or operate machinery until you know how this drug affects you.
- remember that alcohol can add to the drowsiness caused by this drug.

What should I do if I forget to take a dose?

Take the missed dose as soon as you remember it and take any remaining doses for that day at evenly spaced intervals. However, if you remember a missed dose when it is almost time for your next scheduled dose, skip the missed dose. Do not take a double dose to make up for a missed one.

What side effects can this medicine cause?

Tacrine may cause side effects. Tell your doctor if any of these symptoms are severe or do not go away:

- upset stomach
- vomiting
- diarrhea
- loss of balance
- heartburn
- muscle aches
- headache
- loss of appetite

If you experience any of the following symptoms, call your doctor immediately:

- rash
- yellowing of the skin or eyes
- changes in stool color
- stomach pain
- difficulty urinating

If you experience a serious side effect, you or your doctor may send a report to the Food and Drug Administration's (FDA) MedWatch Adverse Event Reporting program online [at http://www.fda.gov/MedWatch/index.html] or by phone [1-800-332-1088].

What storage conditions are needed for this medicine?

Keep this medication in the container it came in, tightly closed, and out of reach of children. Store it at room temperature and away from excess heat and moisture (not in the bathroom). Throw away any medication that is outdated or no longer needed. Talk to your pharmacist about the proper disposal of your medication.

What should I do in case of overdose?

In case of overdose, call your local poison control center at 1-800-222-1222. If the victim has collapsed or is not breathing, call local emergency services at 911.

What other information should I know?

Keep all appointments with your doctor and the laboratory. Your doctor will order certain lab tests to check your response to tacrine.

Do not let anyone else take your medication. Ask your pharmacist any questions you have about refilling your prescription.

Dosage Facts
For Informational Purposes

Caution: Do not change your dose, how often you take your medication, or the length of time you are to take it without first talking to your health-care provider.

The following dosage information was written using medical language for doctors and other healthcare professionals and is provided here for you to check your dosage. The dosage of this drug may differ for different patients. Therefore, always follow your doctor's instructions or the directions on the label. Contact your health-care provider or pharmacist if you have any questions about the specific dosage of your medication after reviewing this information.

General Dosage Information

Available as tacrine hydrochloride; dosage expressed in terms of tacrine.

Adjust dosage or discontinue therapy in patients with serum ALT elevations as required.

Adult Patients

Alzheimer's Disease
Initiation and Titration

ORAL:
- Initially, 10 mg 4 times daily for at least 4 weeks.
- If well tolerated and increased serum ALT concentrations have not occurred, increase dosage to 20 mg 4 times daily; if tolerated, increase dosage in 40-mg daily increments (divided into 4 doses daily) at 4-week intervals up to a maximum of 160 mg daily (40 mg 4 times daily).

Dosage Adjustment for ALT Elevations

ORAL:
- If serum ALT concentrations are ≤3 times the ULN, continue usual dosages.
- If serum ALT concentrations are >3 times to ≤5 times the ULN, reduce dosage by 40 mg daily. Resume usual dosages when ALT concentrations have returned to within normal limits.
- If serum ALT concentrations are >5 times the ULN, withhold tacrine. Consider rechallenge when ALT concentrations have returned to within normal limits.

Rechallenge

ORAL:
- Initially, 10 mg 4 times daily for at least 6 weeks. If tolerated with no unacceptable changes in serum ALT concentrations, resume recommended dosage titration schedule.

Prescribing Limits

Adult Patients

Alzheimer's Disease

ORAL:
- Maximum 160 mg daily (40 mg 4 times daily).

Special Populations
Hepatic Impairment
- Reduced clearance is likely; dosage adjustments should be considered.

Tacrolimus
(ta kroe' li mus)

Brand Name: Prograf®

Important Warning

Tacrolimus increases your risk of getting infections. Avoid people with contagious diseases, such as the flu and colds. Keep cuts and scratches clean. Use good personal hygiene, especially for your mouth, teeth, skin, hair, and hands. Tacrolimus also may increase your risk of getting certain types of cancer. Talk to your doctor about this risk.

Why is this medicine prescribed?

Tacrolimus is used to prevent rejection of liver transplants. Sometimes it is used to prevent rejection of other types of transplants.

This medication is sometimes prescribed for other uses; ask your doctor or pharmacist for more information.

How should this medicine be used?

Tacrolimus comes as a capsule to take by mouth and in an injectable form. It usually is taken twice a day. Follow the directions on your prescription label carefully, and ask your doctor or pharmacist to explain any part you do not understand. Take tacrolimus exactly as directed. Do not take more or less of it or take it more often than prescribed by your doctor.

Continue to take tacrolimus even if you feel well. Do not stop taking tacrolimus without talking to your doctor. You will probably take tacrolimus for a long time.

What special precautions should I follow?

Before taking tacrolimus,
- tell your doctor and pharmacist if you are allergic to tacrolimus or any other drugs.
- tell your doctor and pharmacist what prescription and nonprescription medications you are taking, especially amiloride (Midamor, Moduretic), bromocriptine (Parlodel), carbamazepine (Tegretol), cimetidine (Tagamet), cisapride (Propulsid), clarithromycin (Biaxin), clotrimazole (Mycelex, Lotrimin), cyclosporine (Neoral, Sandimmune), danazol (Danocrine), diltiazem (Cardi-

zem), erythromycin (E-Mycin), fluconazole (Diflucan), ganciclovir (Cytovene), HIV protease inhibitors such as indinavir (Crixivan) and ritonavir (Norvir), itraconazole (Sporanox), ketoconazole (Nizoral), methylprednisolone (Medrol), metoclopramide (Reglan), nefazodone (Serzone), nicardipine (Cardene), nifedipine (Adalat, Procardia), omeprazole (Prilosec), oral contraceptives (birth control pills), phenobarbital, phenytoin (Dilantin), rifabutin (Mycobutin), rifampin (Rifadin, Rimactane), spironolactone (Aldactone), triamterene-containing drugs (Dyazide, Dyrenium, Maxzide), troleandomycin (Tao), verapamil (Calan, Isoptin), and vitamins. Do not take antacids within 2 hours of taking tacrolimus.

- tell your doctor and pharmacist what herbal products you are taking, especially St. John's wort and products containing St. John's Wort.
- tell your doctor if you have or have ever had heart or kidney disease or diabetes.
- tell your doctor if you are pregnant, plan to become pregnant, or are breast-feeding. If you become pregnant while taking tacrolimus, call your doctor.
- if you are having surgery, including dental surgery, tell the doctor or dentist that you are taking tacrolimus.

What special dietary instructions should I follow?

Avoid eating grapefruit or drinking grapefruit juice while taking tacrolimus.

What should I do if I forget to take a dose?

Take the missed dose as soon as you remember it. However, if it is almost time for the next dose, skip the missed dose and continue your regular dosing schedule. Do not take a double dose to make up for a missed one.

What side effects can this medicine cause?

Tacrolimus may cause side effects. Tell your doctor if any of these symptoms are severe or do not go away:

- diarrhea
- upset stomach
- vomiting
- stomach pain
- loss of appetite
- insomnia

If you experience any of the following symptoms, call your doctor immediately:

- fever
- sore throat
- chills
- frequent or painful urination
- decreased urination
- severe or continued headaches
- swelling of the feet, ankles, lower legs, and hands
- weight gain
- tremor
- weakness
- unusual bleeding or bruising

- skin rash
- itching
- hives
- difficulty breathing
- wheezing
- yellowing of the skin or eyes
- seizures

If you experience a serious side effect, you or your doctor may send a report to the Food and Drug Administration's (FDA) MedWatch Adverse Event Reporting program online [at http://www.fda.gov/MedWatch/index.html] or by phone [1-800-332-1088].

What storage conditions are needed for this medicine?

Keep this medication in the container it came in, tightly closed, and out of reach of children. Store it at room temperature and away from excess heat and moisture (not in the bathroom). Throw away any medication that is outdated or no longer needed. Talk to your pharmacist about the proper disposal of your medication.

What should I do in case of overdose?

In case of overdose, call your local poison control center at 1-800-222-1222. If the victim has collapsed or is not breathing, call local emergency services at 911.

What other information should I know?

Keep all appointments with your doctor and the laboratory. Your doctor will order certain lab tests to check your response to tacrolimus and do blood tests to see how your liver and kidneys are working.

Tacrolimus can raise your blood pressure. Talk to your doctor about checking your blood pressure regularly.

Before receiving any vaccinations, tell your doctor that you are taking tacrolimus.

Do not let anyone else take your medication. Ask your pharmacist any questions you have about refilling your prescription.

Dosage Facts
For Informational Purposes

Caution: Do not change your dose, how often you take your medication, or the length of time you are to take it without first talking to your healthcare provider.

The following dosage information was written using medical language for doctors and other healthcare professionals and is provided here for you to check your dosage. The dosage of this drug may differ for different patients. Therefore, always follow your doctor's instructions or the directions on the label. Contact your healthcare provider or pharmacist if you have any questions about the specific dosage of your medication after reviewing this information.

General Dosage Information

Available as anhydrous tacrolimus; dosage expressed in terms of anhydrous drug.

Individualize dosage based on clinical assessments of organ rejection and patient tolerability.

Dosage requirements generally decline with continued therapy; long-term administration is necessary to prevent rejection.

Pediatric Patients

Hepatic Allotransplantation

Children generally appear to require higher dosages than adults on a weight basis to achieve comparable blood concentrations.

ORAL:
- Initially, 150–200 mcg/kg (0.15–0.2 mg/kg) daily, administered in 2 divided doses every 12 hours; initiate therapy no earlier than 6 hours after liver transplantation.

IV:
- Initially, 30–50 mcg/kg (0.03–0.05 mg/kg) daily commencing after revascularization of the graft.
- Continue IV therapy only until the patient can tolerate oral therapy. In most cases, therapy can be switched to the oral route within 2–4 days. Initiate oral tacrolimus 8–12 hours after IV infusion is discontinued.

Adult Patients

Hepatic Allotransplantation

ORAL:
- Initially, 100–150 mcg/kg (0.1–0.15 mg/kg) daily, administered in 2 divided doses every 12 hours; initiate therapy no earlier than 6 hours after liver transplantation.

IV:
- Initially, 30–50 mcg/kg (0.03–0.05 mg/kg) daily commencing after revascularization of the graft. Adults should receive a dosage at the lower end of this range.
- Continue IV therapy only until the patient can tolerate oral therapy. In most cases, therapy can be switched to the oral route within 2–4 days. Initiate oral tacrolimus 8–12 hours after IV infusion is discontinued.

Renal Allotransplantation

Black renal transplant patients may require higher doses than patients of other races to maintain comparable whole blood trough drug concentrations.

ORAL:
- Usual initial dosage: 200 mcg/kg (0.2 mg/kg) daily, administered in 2 divided doses every 12 hours. Therapy may be administered within 24 hours of kidney transplantation, but should be delayed until renal function has recovered (e.g., S_{cr} ≤4 mg/dL).

IV:
- Initially, 30–50 mcg/kg (0.03–0.05 mg/kg) daily commencing after revascularization of the graft. Adults should receive a dosage at the lower end of this range.
- Continue IV therapy only until the patient can tolerate oral therapy.

Special Populations

Hepatic Impairment
- Initiate therapy with the lowest dosage in the recommended range.

- Further dosage reduction may be required (e.g., in patients with severe hepatic impairment [Child-Pugh score ≥10]).

Renal Impairment
- Initiate therapy with the lowest dosage in the recommended range. Further dosage reduction may be required.
- Delay initiation of therapy for ≥48 hours in patients who develop postoperative oliguria.

Tacrolimus Topical

(ta kroe′ li mus)

Brand Name: Protopic®

Important Warning

A small number of patients who used tacrolimus ointment or another similar medication developed skin cancer or lymphoma (cancer in a part of the immune system). There is not enough information available to tell whether tacrolimus ointment caused these patients to develop cancer. Studies of transplant patients and laboratory animals and an understanding of the way tacrolimus works suggest that there is a possibility that people who use tacrolimus ointment have a greater risk of developing cancer. More study is needed to understand this risk.

Follow these directions carefully to decrease the possible risk that you will develop cancer during your treatment with tacrolimus ointment:

- Use tacrolimus ointment only when you have symptoms of eczema. Stop using tacrolimus ointment when your symptoms go away or when your doctor tells you that you should stop. Do not use tacrolimus ointment continuously for a long time.
- Call your doctor if you have used tacrolimus ointment for 6 weeks and your eczema symptoms have not improved, or if your symptoms get worse at any time during your treatment. A different medication may be needed.
- Call your doctor if your eczema symptoms come back after your treatment with tacrolimus ointment.
- Apply tacrolimus ointment only to skin that is affected by eczema. Use the smallest amount of ointment that is needed to control your symptoms.
- Do not use tacrolimus ointment to treat eczema in children who are younger than 2 years old. Do not use tacrolimus ointment 0.1% to treat eczema in children who are between 2 and 15 years old. Only tacrolimus ointment 0.03% may be used to treat children in this age group.

- Tell your doctor if you have or have ever had cancer, especially skin cancer, or any condition that affects your immune system. Ask your doctor if you are not sure if a condition that you have has affected your immune system. Tacrolimus may not be right for you.
- Protect your skin from real and artificial sunlight during your treatment with tacrolimus ointment. Do not use sun lamps or tanning beds, and do not undergo ultraviolet light therapy. Stay out of the sunlight as much as possible during your treatment, even when the medication is not on your skin. If you need to be outside in the sun, wear loose fitting clothing to protect the treated skin, and ask your doctor about other ways to protect your skin from the sun.

    Your doctor or pharmacist will give you the manufacturer's patient information sheet (Medication Guide) when you begin treatment with tacrolimus and each time you refill your prescription. Read the information carefully and ask your doctor or pharmacist if you have any questions. You can also visit the Food and Drug Administration (FDA) website (http://www.fda.gov/cder) or the manufacturer's website to obtain the Medication Guide.

    Talk to your doctor about the risks of using tacrolimus ointment.

Why is this medicine prescribed?

Tacrolimus ointment is used to treat the symptoms of eczema (atopic dermatitis; a skin disease that causes the skin to be dry and itchy and to sometimes develop red, scaly rashes) in patients who cannot use other medications for their condition or whose eczema has not responded to another medication. Tacrolimus is in a class of medications called topical calcineurin inhibitors. It works by stopping the immune system from producing substances that may cause eczema.

How should this medicine be used?

Tacrolimus comes as an ointment to apply to the skin. It is usually applied twice a day to the affected area. To help you remember to apply tacrolimus ointment, apply it at around the same times every day. Follow the directions on your prescription label carefully, and ask your doctor or pharmacist to explain any part you do not understand. Use tacrolimus exactly as directed. Do not use more or less of it or use it more often than prescribed by your doctor.

To use the ointment, follow these steps:
1. Wash your hands with soap and water.
2. Be sure that the skin in the affected area is dry.
3. Apply a thin layer of tacrolimus ointment to all affected areas of your skin.
4. Rub the ointment into your skin gently and completely.
5. Wash your hands with soap and water to remove any leftover tacrolimus ointment. Do not wash your hands if you are treating them with tacrolimus.
6. You may cover the treated areas with normal clothing, but do not use any bandages, dressings, or wraps.
7. Be careful not to wash the ointment off of affected areas of your skin. Do not swim, shower, or bathe immediately after applying tacrolimus ointment.

Are there other uses for this medicine?

This medication may be prescribed for other uses; ask your doctor or pharmacist for more information.

What special precautions should I follow?

Before using tacrolimus ointment,
- tell your doctor and pharmacist if you are allergic to tacrolimus ointment, injection, or capsules (Prograf), or any other medications.
- tell your doctor and pharmacist what prescription and nonprescription medications, vitamins, nutritional supplements, and herbal products you are taking. Be sure to mention any of the following: antifungals such as fluconazole (Diflucan), itraconazole (Sporanox), and ketoconazole (Nizoral); calcium channel blockers such as diltiazem (Cardizem, Dilacor, Tiazac) and verapamil (Calan, Covera, Isoptin, Verelan); cimetidine (Tagamet); erythromycin (E.E.S., E-Mycin, Erythrocin); and other ointments, creams, or lotions. Your doctor may need to change the doses of your medications or monitor you carefully for side effects.
- tell your doctor if you have a skin infection and if you have or have ever had kidney disease, Netherton's syndrome (an inherited condition that causes the skin to be red, itchy, and scaly), redness and peeling of most of your skin, any other skin disease, or any type of skin infection, especially chicken pox, shingles (a skin infection in people who have had chicken pox in the past), herpes (cold sores), or eczema herpeticum (viral infection that causes fluid filled blisters to form on the skin of people who have eczema). Also tell your doctor if your eczema rash has turned crusty or blistered or you think your eczema rash is infected.
- tell your doctor if you are pregnant, plan to become pregnant, or are breast-feeding. If you become pregnant while using tacrolimus ointment, call your doctor.
- if you are having surgery, including dental surgery, tell the doctor or dentist that you are using tacrolimus ointment.
- ask your doctor about the safe use of alcoholic beverages while you are using tacrolimus ointment. Your skin or face may become flushed or red and feel hot if you drink alcohol during your treatment.
- avoid exposure to chicken pox, shingles, and other viruses. If you are exposed to one of these viruses while using tacrolimus ointment, call your doctor immediately.
- you should know that good skin care and moisturizers

may help relieve the dry skin caused by eczema. Talk to your doctor about the moisturizers you should use, and always apply them after applying tacrolimus ointment.

What special dietary instructions should I follow?

Talk to your doctor about eating grapefruit and drinking grapefruit juice while you are taking this medicine.

What should I do if I forget to take a dose?

Apply the missed dose as soon as you remember it. However, if it is almost time for the next dose, skip the missed dose and continue your regular dosing schedule. Do not apply extra ointment to make up for a missed dose.

What side effects can this medicine cause?

Tacrolimus ointment may cause side effects. Tell your doctor if any of these symptoms are severe or do not go away:
- skin burning, stinging, redness or soreness
- tingling skin
- increased sensitivity of the skin to hot or cold temperatures
- itching
- acne
- swollen or infected hair follicles
- headache
- muscle or back pain
- flu-like symptoms
- stuffy or runny nose
- nausea

Some side effects can be serious. If you experience any of the following symptoms, call your doctor immediately:
- swollen glands
- rash
- crusting, oozing, blistering or other signs of skin infection
- cold sores
- chicken pox or other blisters
- swelling of the hands, arms, feet, ankles, or lower legs

Tacrolimus ointment may cause other side effects. Call your doctor if you have any unusual problems while taking this medication.

If you experience a serious side effect, you or your doctor may send a report to the Food and Drug Administration's (FDA) MedWatch Adverse Event Reporting program online [at http://www.fda.gov/MedWatch/index.html] or by phone [1-800-332-1088].

What storage conditions are needed for this medicine?

Keep this medication in the container it came in, tightly closed, and out of reach of children. Store it at room temperature and away from excess heat and moisture (not in the bathroom). Throw away any medication that is outdated or no longer needed. Talk to your pharmacist about the proper disposal of your medication.

What should I do in case of overdose?

In case of overdose, call your local poison control center at 1-800-222-1222. If the victim has collapsed or is not breathing, call local emergency services at 911.

What other information should I know?

Keep all appointments with your doctor.

Do not let anyone else use your medication. Ask your pharmacist any questions you have about refilling your prescription.

Dosage Facts
For Informational Purposes

Caution: Do not change your dose, how often you take your medication, or the length of time you are to take it without first talking to your healthcare provider.

The following dosage information was written using medical language for doctors and other healthcare professionals and is provided here for you to check your dosage. The dosage of this drug may differ for different patients. Therefore, always follow your doctor's instructions or the directions on the label. Contact your healthcare provider or pharmacist if you have any questions about the specific dosage of your medication after reviewing this information.

Pediatric Patients

Atopic Dermatitis

TOPICAL:
- Children 2–15 years of age: Apply 0.03% ointment to affected areas twice daily, approximately 12 hours apart.
- Adolescents ≥16 years of age: Apply 0.03 or 0.1% ointment to affected areas twice daily, approximately 12 hours apart.
- Discontinue treatment following resolution of signs and symptoms (e.g., pruritus, rash, erythema). If manifestations persist beyond 6 weeks, reexamine patient and confirm diagnosis.

Adult Patients

Atopic Dermatitis

TOPICAL:
- Apply 0.03 or 0.1% ointment to affected areas twice daily, approximately 12 hours apart.
- Discontinue treatment following resolution of signs and symptoms (e.g., pruritus, rash, erythema). If manifestations persist beyond 6 weeks, reexamine patient and confirm diagnosis.

Prescribing Limits

Pediatric Patients

Atopic Dermatitis

TOPICAL:

- For short-term and intermittent use only; avoid continuous long-term use. Safety of noncontinuous use for >1 year not established.

Adult Patients

Atopic Dermatitis

TOPICAL:

- For short-term and intermittent use only; avoid continuous long-term use. Safety of noncontinuous use for >1 year not established.

Special Populations

Hepatic Impairment

- No dosage adjustment appears necessary; effect of hepatic impairment on the pharmacokinetics of topical tacrolimus has not been evaluated.

Renal Impairment

- No dosage adjustment appears necessary. Effect of renal impairment on the pharmacokinetics of topical tacrolimus has not been evaluated; following IV administration of tacrolimus, elimination in patients with renal dysfunction is similar to that in healthy individuals.

Tadalafil

(tah da′ la fil)

Brand Name: Cialis®

Why is this medicine prescribed?

Tadalafil is used to treat erectile dysfunction (impotence; inability to get or keep an erection) in men. Tadalafil is in a class of medications called phosphodiesterase (PDE) inhibitors. It works by increasing blood flow to the penis during sexual stimulation. This increased blood flow can cause an erection. Tadalafil does not cure erectile dysfunction or increase sexual desire. Tadalafil does not prevent pregnancy or the spread of sexually transmitted diseases such as human immunodeficiency virus (HIV).

How should this medicine be used?

Tadalafil comes as a tablet to take by mouth. It is usually taken with or without food before sexual activity. Your doctor will help you decide the best time for you to take tadalafil before sexual activity. Tadalafil should not be taken more often than once every 24 hours. If you have certain health conditions or are taking certain medications, your doctor may tell you to take tadalafil less often. Follow the directions on your prescription label carefully, and ask your doctor or pharmacist to explain any part you do not understand. Take tadalafil exactly as directed. Do not take more or less of it or take it more often than prescribed by your doctor.

Your doctor will probably start you on an average dose of tadalafil and increase or decrease your dose depending on your response to the medication. Tell your doctor if tadalafil is not working well or if you are experiencing side effects.

Are there other uses for this medicine?

This medication may be prescribed for other uses; ask your doctor or pharmacist for more information.

What special precautions should I follow?

Before taking tadalafil,

- tell your doctor and pharmacist if you are allergic to tadalafil or any other medications.
- do not take tadalafil if you are taking or have recently taken nitrates such as isosorbide dinitrate (Isordil), isosorbide mononitrate (Imdur, ISMO), and nitroglycerin (Nitro-BID, Nitro-Dur, Nitroquick, Nitrostat, others). Nitrates come as tablets, sublingual (under the tongue) tablets, sprays, patches, pastes, and ointments. Ask your doctor if you are not sure whether any of your medications contain nitrates.
- do not take street drugs containing nitrates such as amyl nitrate and butyl nitrate ('poppers') while taking tadalafil.
- tell your doctor and pharmacist what other prescription and nonprescription medications, vitamins, and nutritional supplements you are taking or plan to take. Be sure to mention any of the following: alpha blockers such as alfuzosin (Uroxatral), doxazosin (Cardura), prazosin (Minipress), tamsulosin (Flomax), and terazosin (Hytrin); amiodarone (Cordarone, Pacerone); certain antifungals such as fluconazole (Diflucan), griseofulvin (Fulvicin, Grifulvin, Gris-PEG), itraconazole (Sporanox), ketoconazole (Nizoral), voriconazole (Vfend); aprepitant (Emend); carbamazepine (Tegretol); cimetidine (Tagamet); clarithromycin (Biaxin); cyclosporine (Neoral, Sandimmune); danazol (Danocrine); delavirdine (Rescriptor); dexamethasone (Decadron); diltiazem (Cardizem, Dilacor, Tiazac); efavirenz (Sustiva); erythromycin (E.E.S., E-Mycin, Erythrocin); ethosuximide (Zarontin); fluoxetine (Prozac, Sarafem); fluvoxamine (Luvox); HIV protease inhibitors including atazanavir (Reyataz), indinavir (Crixivan), lopinavir (in Kaletra), nelfinavir (Viracept), ritonavir (Norvir, in Kaletra), and saquinavir (Fortovase, Invirase); isoniazid (INH, Nydrazid); lovastatin (Altocor, Mevacor); medications for high blood pressure; metronidazole (Flagyl); nefazodone (Serzone); nevirapine (Viramune); other medications or treatments for erectile dysfunction; phenobarbital; phenytoin (Dilantin); rifabutin (Mycobutin); rifampin (Rifadin, Rimactane); sertraline (Zoloft); troleandomycin (TAO); verapamil (Calan, Covera, Isoptin,

Verelan); and zafirlukast (Accolate). Your doctor may need to change the doses of your medications or monitor you carefully for side effects.

- tell your doctor what herbal products you are taking, especially St. John's wort.
- tell your doctor if you smoke and if you have ever had an erection that lasted more than 4 hours. Also tell your doctor if you have or have ever had a condition that affects the shape of the penis, such as angulation, cavernosal fibrosis, or Peyronie's disease; diabetes; high cholesterol; high or low blood pressure; irregular heartbeat; a heart attack; angina (chest pain); a stroke; ulcers in the stomach or intestine; a bleeding disorder; blood cell problems such as sickle cell anemia (a disease of the red blood cells), multiple myeloma (cancer of the plasma cells), or leukemia (cancer of the white blood cells); and liver, kidney, or heart disease. Also tell your doctor if you or any of your family members have or have ever had an eye disease such as retinitis pigmentosa or if you have ever had severe vision loss, especially if you were told that the vision loss was caused by a blockage of blood flow to the nerves that help you see. Tell your doctor if you have ever been advised by a health care professional to avoid sexual activity for medical reasons or if you have ever experienced chest pain during sexual activity.
- you should know that tadalafil is only for use in males. Women should not take tadalafil, especially if they are or could become pregnant or are breast-feeding. If a pregnant woman takes tadalafil, she should call her doctor.
- if you are having surgery, including dental surgery, tell the doctor or dentist that you are taking tadalafil.
- ask your doctor about the safe use of alcoholic beverages while you are taking tadalafil. Alcohol can make the side effects from tadalafil worse. Your doctor will tell you how much alcohol you may drink while you are taking this medication.
- you should know that sexual activity may be a strain on your heart, especially if you have heart disease. If you have chest pain during sexual activity, call your doctor immediately and avoid sexual activity until your doctor tells you otherwise.
- tell all your health care providers that you are taking tadalafil. If you ever need emergency medical treatment for a heart problem, the health care providers who treat you will need to know when you last took tadalafil.

What special dietary instructions should I follow?

Talk to your doctor about eating grapefruit and drinking grapefruit juice while taking this medicine.

What side effects can this medicine cause?

Tadalafil may cause side effects. Tell your doctor if any of these symptoms are severe or do not go away:

- headache
- indigestion or heartburn
- flushing
- pain in the back, muscles, or any limb
- stuffy or runny nose

If you experience any of the following symptoms, call your doctor immediately:

- sudden severe loss of vision (see below for more information)
- blurred vision
- changes in color vision (seeing a blue tinge on objects or having difficulty telling the difference between blue and green)
- erection that lasts longer than 4 hours
- chest pain
- hives
- rash

Tadalafil may cause other side effects. Call your doctor if you have any unusual problems while taking this medication.

Some patients experienced a sudden loss of some or all of their vision after they took tadalafil or other medications that are similar to tadalafil. The vision loss was permanent in some cases. It is not known if the vision loss was caused by the medication. If you experience a sudden loss of vision while you are taking tadalafil, call your doctor immediately. Do not take any more doses of tadalafil or similar medications such as sildenafil (Viagra) or vardenafil (Levitra) until you talk to your doctor.

If you experience a serious side effect, you or your doctor may send a report to the Food and Drug Administration's (FDA) MedWatch Adverse Event Reporting program online [at http://www.fda.gov/MedWatch/index.html] or by phone [1-800-332-1088].

What storage conditions are needed for this medicine?

Keep this medication in the container it came in, tightly closed, and out of reach of children. Store it at room temperature and away from excess heat and moisture (not in the bathroom). Throw away any medication that is outdated or no longer needed. Talk to your pharmacist about the proper disposal of your medication.

What should I do in case of overdose?

In case of overdose, call your local poison control center at 1-800-222-1222. If the victim has collapsed or is not breathing, call local emergency services at 911.

Symptoms of overdose may include:

- headache
- indigestion or heartburn
- flushing
- pain in the back, muscles, or any limb
- stuffy or runny nose
- erection that lasts longer than 4 hours

What other information should I know?

Keep all appointments with your doctor.

Do not let anyone else take your medication. Ask your pharmacist any questions you have about refilling your prescription.

Dosage Facts

For Informational Purposes

Caution: Do not change your dose, how often you take your medication, or the length of time you are to take it without first talking to your healthcare provider.

The following dosage information was written using medical language for doctors and other healthcare professionals and is provided here for you to check your dosage. The dosage of this drug may differ for different patients. Therefore, always follow your doctor's instructions or the directions on the label. Contact your healthcare provider or pharmacist if you have any questions about the specific dosage of your medication after reviewing this information.

Adult Patients

Erectile Dysfunction

ORAL:
- Initially, 10 mg. Depending on effectiveness and tolerance, increase dosage to a maximum of 20 mg or decrease to 5 mg.

Prescribing Limits

Adult Patients

Erectile Dysfunction

ORAL:
- Maximum 20 mg daily.

Special Populations

Hepatic Impairment
- In patients with mild to moderate hepatic impairment (Child-Pugh class A or B), maximum dosage is 10 mg once daily. Use not recommended in patients with severe hepatic impairment (Child-Pugh class C).

Renal Impairment
- If Cl_{cr} is 31–50 mL/minute, reduce initial dosage to 5 mg once daily; maximum dosage is 10 mg administered no more frequently than once every 48 hours. If Cl_{cr} is <30 mL/minute), including patients undergoing hemodialysis, maximum dosage is 5 mg administered no more frequently than once daily.

Geriatric Patients
- No dosage adjustments necessary based solely on age.

Tamoxifen

(ta mox′ i fen)

Brand Name: Nolvadex®
Also available generically.

Important Warning

Tamoxifen may cause cancer of the uterus (womb), strokes, and blood clots in the lungs. These conditions may be serious or fatal. Tell your doctor if you have ever had a blood clot in the lungs or legs, a stroke, or a heart attack. Also tell your doctor if you smoke, if you have high blood pressure or diabetes, if your ability to move around during your waking hours is limited, or if you are taking anticoagulants ('blood thinners') such as warfarin (Coumadin). If you experience any of the following symptoms during or after your treatment, call your doctor immediately: abnormal vaginal bleeding; irregular menstrual periods; changes in vaginal discharge, especially if the discharge becomes bloody, brown, or rusty; pain or pressure in the pelvis (the stomach area below the belly button); leg swelling or tenderness; chest pain; shortness of breath; coughing up blood; sudden weakness, tingling, or numbness in your face, arm, or leg, especially on one side of your body; sudden confusion; difficulty speaking or understanding; sudden difficulty seeing in one or both eyes; sudden difficulty walking; dizziness; loss of balance or coordination; or sudden severe headache.

Keep all appointments with your doctor. You will need to have gynecological examinations (examinations of the female organs) regularly to find early signs of cancer of the uterus.

If you are thinking about taking tamoxifen to reduce the chance that you will develop breast cancer, you should talk to your doctor about the risks and benefits of this treatment. You and your doctor will decide whether the possible benefit of tamoxifen treatment is worth the risks of taking the medication. If you need to take tamoxifen to treat breast cancer, the benefits of tamoxifen outweigh the risks.

Your doctor or pharmacist will give you the manufacturer's patient information sheet (Medication Guide) when you begin treatment with tamoxifen and each time you refill your prescription. Read the information carefully and ask your doctor or pharmacist if you have any questions. You can also visit the Food and Drug Administration (FDA) website (http://www.fda.gov/cder) or the manufacturer's website to obtain the Medication Guide.

About Your Treatment

Your doctor has prescribed tamoxifen for you. Tamoxifen comes as a tablet to take by mouth.

This medication is used to:

- treat breast cancer that has spread to other parts of the body in men and women.
- treat early breast cancer in women who have already been treated with surgery, radiation, and/or chemotherapy.
- reduce the risk of developing a more serious type of breast cancer in women who have had ductal carcinoma in situ (DCIS; a type of breast cancer that does not spread outside of the milk duct where it forms) and who have been treated with surgery and radiation.
- reduce the risk of breast cancer in women who are at high risk for the disease due to their age, personal medical history, and family medical history.

Tamoxifen is in a class of medications known as antiestrogens. It blocks the activity of estrogen (a female hormone) in the breast. This may stop the growth of some breast tumors that need estrogen to grow.

Tamoxifen is usually taken once or twice a day with or without food. Take tamoxifen at around the same time(s) every day. Follow the directions on your prescription label carefully, and ask your doctor or pharmacist to explain anything you do not understand. Take tamoxifen exactly as directed. Do not take more or less of it or take it more often than prescribed by your doctor.

Swallow tamoxifen tablets whole; do not split, chew, or crush them. Swallow the tablets with water or any other nonalcoholic drink.

If you are taking tamoxifen to prevent breast cancer, you will probably take it for five years. If you are taking tamoxifen to treat breast cancer, your doctor will decide how long your treatment will last. Do not stop taking tamoxifen without talking to your doctor.

If you forget to take a dose of tamoxifen, take the missed dose as soon as you remember it, and take your next dose as usual. However, if it is almost time for your next dose, skip the missed dose and continue your regular dosing schedule. Do not take a double dose to make up for a missed one.

Tamoxifen is also used sometimes to induce ovulation (egg production) in women who do not produce eggs but wish to become pregnant. Tamoxifen is also sometimes used to treat McCune-Albright syndrome (a condition that may cause bone disease, early sexual development, and dark colored spots on the skin in children). Talk to your doctor about the possible risks of using this drug for your condition.

This medication may be prescribed for other uses; ask your doctor or pharmacist for more information.

Precautions

Before taking tamoxifen,

- tell your doctor and pharmacist if you are allergic to tamoxifen or any other medications.

- tell your doctor and pharmacist what prescription and nonprescription medications, vitamins, nutritional supplements, and herbal products you are taking or plan to take. Be sure to mention any of the following: aminoglutethimide (Cytadren); anastrazole (Arimidex), bromocriptine (Parlodel); cancer chemotherapy medication such as cyclophosphamide (Cytoxan, Neosar) letrozole (Femara); medroxyprogesterone (Depo-Provera, Provera, in Prempro); phenobarbital; and rifampin (Rifadin, Rimactane). Your doctor may need to change the doses of your medications or monitor you carefully for side effects.
- in addition to the conditions listed in the IMPORTANT WARNING section, tell your doctor if you have or have ever had high blood levels of cholesterol.
- tell your doctor if you are pregnant or plan to become pregnant. You should not plan to become pregnant while taking tamoxifen or for 2 months after your treatment. Your doctor may perform a pregnancy test or tell you to begin your treatment during your menstrual period to be sure that you are not pregnant when you begin taking tamoxifen. You will need to use a reliable nonhormonal method of birth control to prevent pregnancy while you are taking tamoxifen and for 2 months after your treatment. Talk to your doctor about the types of birth control that are right for you, and continue to use birth control even if you do not have regular menstrual periods during your treatment. Stop taking tamoxifen and call your doctor right away if you think you have become pregnant during your treatment. Tamoxifen may harm the fetus.
- tell your doctor if you are breast-feeding. You should not breastfeed during your treatment with tamoxifen.
- tell all of your doctors and other health care providers that you are taking tamoxifen.
- you will still need to look for early signs of breast cancer since it is possible to develop breast cancer even during treatment with tamoxifen. Talk to your doctor about how often you should examine your breasts yourself, have a doctor examine your breasts, and have mammograms (x-ray examinations of the breasts). Call your doctor right away if you find a new lump in your breast.

Side Effects

Tamoxifen may cause side effects. Tell your doctor if any of these symptoms are severe or do not go away:

- increased bone or tumor pain
- pain or reddening around the tumor site
- hot flashes
- nausea
- excessive tiredness
- dizziness
- depression
- headache
- thinning of hair
- weight loss
- stomach cramps

- constipation
- loss of sexual desire or ability (in men)

Some side effects can be serious. If you experience any of the following symptoms or those listed in the IMPORTANT WARNING section, call your doctor immediately:

- vision problems
- loss of appetite
- yellowing of the skin or eyes
- unusual bruising or bleeding
- fever
- blisters
- rash
- swelling of the eyes, face, lips, tongue, throat, hands, arms, feet, ankles, or lower legs
- thirst
- muscle weakness
- restlessness

Tamoxifen may increase the risk that you will develop other cancers, including liver cancer. Talk to your doctor about this risk.

Tamoxifen may increase the risk that you will develop cataracts (clouding of the lens in the eye) that may need to be treated with surgery. Talk to your doctor about this risk.

Tamoxifen may cause other side effects. Call your doctor if you have any unusual problems while taking this medication.

Storage Conditions

Keep tamoxifen in the container it came in, tightly closed, and out of reach of children. Store it at room temperature and away from excess heat and moisture (not in the bathroom). Throw away any medication that is outdated or no longer needed. Talk to your pharmacist about the proper disposal of your medication.

Overdose

In case of overdose, call your local poison control center at 1-800-222-1222. If the victim has collapsed or is not breathing, call local emergency services at 911.

Symptoms of overdose may include:

- uncontrollable shaking of a part of the body
- unsteadiness
- dizziness

Special Instructions

- Keep all appointments with your doctor and the laboratory. Your doctor will order certain lab tests to check your body's response to tamoxifen.
- Before having any laboratory test, tell your doctor and the laboratory personnel that you are taking tamoxifen.
- Do not let anyone else take your medication. Talk to your pharmacist if you have any questions about refilling your prescription.

Dosage Facts
For Informational Purposes

Caution: Do not change your dose, how often you take your medication, or the length of time you are to take it without first talking to your healthcare provider.

The following dosage information was written using medical language for doctors and other healthcare professionals and is provided here for you to check your dosage. The dosage of this drug may differ for different patients. Therefore, always follow your doctor's instructions or the directions on the label. Contact your healthcare provider or pharmacist if you have any questions about the specific dosage of your medication after reviewing this information.

General Dosage Information

Available as tamoxifen citrate; dosage expressed in terms of tamoxifen.

Adult Patients

Breast Cancer
Adjuvant Therapy

ORAL:
- 20–40 mg daily. Current data from clinical studies support 5 years of adjuvant therapy.

Ductal Carcinoma in Situ

ORAL:
- 20 mg daily for 5 years.

Metastatic Breast Cancer

ORAL:
- 20–40 mg daily.

Reduction in the Incidence of Breast Cancer in Women at High Risk

ORAL:
- 20 mg daily for 5 years.

Prescribing Limits

Adult Patients

Breast Cancer
Adjuvant Therapy

ORAL:
- No evidence that dosages >20 mg daily are more effective.

Tamsulosin

(tam soo′ loe sin)

Brand Name: Flomax®

Why is this medicine prescribed?

Tamsulosin is used in men to treat the symptoms of an enlarged prostate (benign prostatic hyperplasia or BPH) which include difficulty urinating (hesitation, dribbling, weak stream, and incomplete bladder emptying), painful urination, and urinary frequency and urgency. Tamsulosin is in a class of medications called alpha blockers. It works by relaxing the muscles in the prostate and bladder so that urine can flow easily.

How should this medicine be used?

Tamsulosin comes as a capsule to take by mouth. It is usually taken once a day. Take tamsulosin 30 minutes after the same meal each day. Follow the directions on your prescription label carefully, and ask your doctor or pharmacist to explain any part you do not understand. Take tamsulosin exactly as directed. Do not take more or less of it or take it more often than prescribed by your doctor.

Swallow tamsulosin capsules whole; do not split, chew, crush, or open them.

Your doctor will probably start you on a low dose of tamsulosin and may increase your dose after 2 to 4 weeks.

Tamsulosin may help control your condition, but it will not cure it. Continue to take tamsulosin even if you feel well. Do not stop taking tamsulosin without talking to your doctor.

Are there other uses for this medicine?

This medication may be prescribed for other uses; ask your doctor or pharmacist for more information.

What special precautions should I follow?

Before taking tamsulosin,

- tell your doctor and pharmacist if you are allergic to tamsulosin, sulfa medications, or any other medications.
- tell your doctor and pharmacist what prescription and nonprescription medications, vitamins, nutritional supplements and herbal products you are taking or plan to take. Be sure to mention any of the following: other alpha blocker medications such as alfuzosin (Uroxatral), doxazosin (Cardura), prazosin (Minipress), and terazosin (Hytrin); anticoagulants ('blood thinners') such as warfarin (Coumadin); cimetidine (Tagamet); and medications for erectile dysfunction (ED) such as sildenafil (Viagra), tadalafil (Cialis), or vardenafil (Levitra); Your doctor may need to change the doses of your medications or monitor you more carefully for side effects.
- tell your doctor if you have or have ever had prostate cancer or liver or kidney disease.
- you should know that tamsulosin is only for use in men.

Women should not take tamsulosin, especially if they are pregnant or could become pregnant or are breastfeeding. If a pregnant woman takes tamsulosin, she should call her doctor.

- if you are having surgery, including dental surgery, tell the doctor or dentist that you are taking tamsulosin. If you need to have eye surgery at any time during or after your treatment, be sure to tell your doctor that you are taking or have taken tamsulosin.
- you should know that this medication may make you drowsy or dizzy. Do not drive a car, operate machinery, or perform dangerous tasks until you know how this medication affects you.
- you should know that tamsulosin may cause dizziness, lightheadedness, a spinning sensation, and fainting, especially when you get up too quickly from a lying position. This is more common when you first start taking tamsulosin or after your dose is increased. To help avoid this problem, get out of bed slowly, resting your feet on the floor for a few minutes before standing up. Call your doctor if these symptoms are severe or do not go away.

What should I do if I forget to take a dose?

Take the missed dose as soon as you remember it. However, if it is almost time for the next dose, skip the missed dose and continue your regular dosing schedule. Do not take a double dose to make up for a missed one. If you interrupt your treatment for several days or longer, call your doctor before restarting the medication, especially if you take more than one capsule of tamsulosin a day.

What side effects can this medicine cause?

Tamsulosin may cause side effects. Tell your doctor if any of these symptoms or those in the SPECIAL PRECAUTIONS section are severe or do not go away:

- sleepiness
- difficulty falling asleep or staying asleep
- weakness
- back pain
- diarrhea
- runny or stuffy nose
- pain or pressure in the face
- sore throat, cough, fever, chills, or other signs of infection
- blurred vision
- difficulty ejaculating

Some side effects can be serious. If you experience any of the following symptoms, call your doctor immediately:

- painful erection of the penis that lasts for hours
- rash
- itching
- hives
- swelling of the eyes, face, tongue, lips, throat, arms, hands, feet, ankles, or lower legs

What storage conditions are needed for this medicine?

Keep this medication in the container it came in, tightly closed, and out of reach of children. Store it at room temperature and away from excess heat and moisture (not in the bathroom). Throw away any medication that is outdated or no longer needed. Talk to your pharmacist about the proper disposal of your medication.

What should I do in case of overdose?

In case of overdose, call your local poison control center at 1-800-222-1222. If the victim has collapsed or is not breathing, call local emergency services at 911.

Symptoms of overdose may include:

- dizziness
- fainting
- blurred vision
- upset stomach
- headache

What other information should I know?

Keep all appointments with your doctor.

Do not let anyone else take your medication. Ask your pharmacist any questions you have about refilling your prescription.

Dosage Facts
For Informational Purposes

Caution: Do not change your dose, how often you take your medication, or the length of time you are to take it without first talking to your healthcare provider.

The following dosage information was written using medical language for doctors and other healthcare professionals and is provided here for you to check your dosage. The dosage of this drug may differ for different patients. Therefore, always follow your doctor's instructions or the directions on the label. Contact your healthcare provider or pharmacist if you have any questions about the specific dosage of your medication after reviewing this information.

General Dosage Information

Available as tamsulosin hydrochloride; dosage is expressed in terms of the salt.

Adult Patients

BPH

ORAL:

- Initially, 0.4 mg once daily. Allow 2–4 weeks to assess response at initial dosage. May increase dosage to 0.8 mg once daily, if necessary, to improve urinary flow rates and reduce symptoms.
- If administration is interrupted for several days at either dos-

age (i.e., 0.4 or 0.8 mg daily), reinitiate therapy at dosage of 0.4 mg once daily.

Special Populations

Hepatic Impairment

- Dosage adjustment not necessary in patients with moderate hepatic impairment.

Renal Impairment

- Dosage adjustment not necessary in patients with mild to severe renal impairment (Cl_{cr} 10–70 mL/minute per 1.73 m²).
- Not studied in patients with end-stage renal disease (Cl_{cr} <10 mL/minute per 1.73 m²).

Telbivudine

(tel biv′ ue deen)

Brand Name: Tyzeka®

Important Warning

Telbivudine can cause serious or life-threatening damage to the liver and a condition called lactic acidosis (a build-up of an acid in the blood). Tell your doctor if you drink or have ever drunk large amounts of alcohol, if you use or have ever used injectable street drugs, and if you have or have ever had cirrhosis (scarring) of the liver or any liver disease other than hepatitis B. Tell your doctor and pharmacist if you are taking or have taken the following medications: acetaminophen (Tylenol, others); cholesterol-lowering medications (statins); iron products; isoniazid (INH, Nydrazid); medications to treat human immunodeficiency virus (HIV) or acquired immunodeficiency syndrome (AIDS); methotrexate (Rheumatrex); niacin (nicotinic acid); or rifampin (Rifadin, Rimactane). If you experience any of the following symptoms, call your doctor immediately: yellowing of the skin or eyes; dark-colored urine; light-colored bowel movements; difficulty breathing; stomach pain; or swelling; nausea; vomiting; unusual muscle pain; loss of appetite for at least several days; lack of energy; extreme weakness or tiredness; feeling cold, especially in the arms or legs; dizziness or lightheadedness; or fast or irregular heartbeat.

Do not stop taking telbivudine without talking to your doctor. When you stop taking telbivudine your hepatitis may get worse. This is most likely to happen during the first several months after you stop taking telbivudine. Be careful not to miss doses or run out of telbivudine. Refill your prescription at least 5 days before you expect that you will need the new supply of medication. If you experience any of the following symptoms after you stop taking telbi-

continued on next page

Important Warning (cont'd)

vudine, call your doctor immediately: extreme tiredness, weakness, nausea, vomiting, loss of appetite, yellowing of the skin or eyes, dark-colored urine, or light-colored bowel movements.

Keep all appointments with your doctor and the laboratory before, during, and after your treatment with telbivudine. Your doctor will order certain tests to check your body's response to telbivudine during this time.

Talk to your doctor about the risks of taking telbivudine.

Why is this medicine prescribed?

Telbivudine is used for chronic (long term) hepatitis B infection (swelling of the liver caused by a virus) in people who may also show signs of liver damage. Telbivudine is in a class of medications called nucleoside analogues. It works by decreasing the amount of hepatitis B virus (HBV) in the body. Telbivudine does not cure hepatitis B and may not prevent complications of chronic hepatitis B, such as cirrhosis of the liver or liver cancer. Telbivudine does not prevent the spread of hepatitis B to other people through sexual contact, sharing needles, or contact with blood.

How should this medicine be used?

Telbivudine comes as a tablet to take by mouth. It is usually taken once a day with or without food. Take telbivudine at around the same time every day. Follow the directions on your prescription label carefully, and ask your doctor or pharmacist to explain any part you do not understand. Take telbivudine exactly as directed. Do not take more or less of it or take it more often than prescribed by your doctor.

Ask your pharmacist or doctor for a copy of the manufacturer's information for the patient.

Are there other uses for this medicine?

This medication may be prescribed for other uses; ask your doctor or pharmacist for more information.

What special precautions should I follow?

Before taking telbivudine,

- tell your doctor and pharmacist if you are allergic to telbivudine or any other medications.
- tell your doctor and pharmacist what other prescription and nonprescription medications, vitamins, nutritional supplements, and herbal products you are taking or plan to take. Be sure to mention the medications listed in the IMPORTANT WARNING section and any of the following: chloroquine (Aralen); erythromycin (E.E.S., E-Mycin, Erythrocin); fenofibrate (Antara, Lofibra, Triglide); gemfibrozil (Lopid); hydroxychloroquine (Plaquenil); medications to prevent rejection of a transplanted organ, such as cyclosporine (Neoral, Sandimmune) or tacrolimus (Prograf); medications to treat fungal infec-

tions such as fluconazole (Diflucan), itraconazole (Sporanox), ketoconazole (Nizoral), posaconazole (Noxafil), or voriconazole (Vfend); oral steroids such as dexamethasone (Decadron, Dexone), methylprednisolone (Medrol), and prednisone; (Deltasone), penicillamine (Cuprimine); probenecid; or zidovudine (AZT, Retrovir, in Combivir, in Trizivir). Your doctor may need to change the doses of your medications or monitor you carefully for side effects.

- Tell your doctor if you have or have ever had a liver transplant (surgery to replace a diseased liver), or kidney disease.
- Tell your doctor if you are pregnant, plan to become pregnant, or are breast-feeding. If you become pregnant while taking telbivudine, call your doctor. Do not breastfeed while you are taking telbivudine.
- If you are having surgery, including dental surgery, tell the doctor or dentist that you are taking telbivudine.

What special dietary instructions should I follow?

Unless your doctor tells you otherwise, continue your normal diet.

What should I do if I forget to take a dose?

Take the missed dose as soon as you remember it. However, if it is almost time for the next dose, skip the missed dose and continue your regular dosing schedule. Do not take a double dose to make up for a missed one.

What side effects can this medicine cause?

Telbivudine may cause side effects. Tell your doctor if any of these symptoms are severe or do not go away:

- headache
- diarrhea
- back or joint pain
- difficulty falling asleep or staying asleep
- itching
- rash

Some side effects can be serious. If you experience any of these symptoms, or those listed in the IMPORTANT WARNING section, call your doctor immediately:

- muscle aches, pain, weakness, or tenderness

Telbivudine may cause other side effects. Call your doctor if you have any unusual problems while taking this medication.

What storage conditions are needed for this medicine?

Keep this medication in the container it came in, tightly closed, and out of reach of children and pets. Store it at room temperature and away from excess heat and moisture (not in the bathroom). Throw away any medication that is outdated or no longer needed. Talk to your pharmacist about proper disposal of your medication.

What should I do in case of overdose?

In case of overdose, call your local poison control center at 1-800-222-1222. If the victim has collapsed or is not breathing, call local emergency services at 911.

What other information should I know?

Keep all appointments with your doctor and the laboratory.

Do not let anyone else take your medication. Ask your pharmacist any questions you have about refilling your prescription.

Talk to your doctor, pharmacist, or other healthcare professional if you have questions about dosing information for your medication.

Telithromycin

(tel ith roe mye′ sin)

Brand Name: Ketek®

Important Warning

Telithromycin may cause worsening of symptoms, including breathing problems, when taken by people with myasthenia gravis (a disease that causes muscle weakness). These breathing problems may be severe or life-threatening and may cause death. Tell your doctor if you have myasthenia gravis. You should not take telithromycin if you have this condition.

Your doctor or pharmacist will give you the manufacturer's patient information sheet (Medication Guide) when you begin treatment with telithromycin and each time you refill your prescription. Read the information carefully and ask your doctor or pharmacist if you have any questions. You can also visit the Food and Drug Administration (FDA) website (http://www.fda.gov/cder) or the manufacturer's website to obtain the Medication Guide.

Why is this medicine prescribed?

Telithromycin is used to treat certain types of pneumonia (an infection of the lungs) that is caused by bacteria. Telithromycin is in a class of medications called ketolide antibiotics. It works by killing bacteria. Antibiotics will not kill viruses that can cause colds, flu, or other infections.

How should this medicine be used?

Telithromycin comes as a tablet to take by mouth. It is usually taken with or without food once a day for 7-10 days. To help you remember to take telithromycin, take it around the same time every day. Follow the directions on your pre-scription label carefully, and ask your doctor or pharmacist to explain any part you do not understand. Take telithromycin exactly as directed. Do not take more or less of it or take it more often than prescribed by your doctor.

Swallow the tablets whole; do not split, chew, or crush them.

You should start to feel better early in your treatment. Call your doctor if your condition does not improve while you are taking telithromycin. Take telithromycin until you finish the prescription, even if you feel better. If you stop taking telithromycin too soon or if you skip doses of telithromycin, your infection may not be cured and the bacteria may become resistant to antibiotics.

Are there other uses for this medicine?

This medication may be prescribed for other uses; ask your doctor or pharmacist for more information.

What special precautions should I follow?

Before taking telithromycin,

- tell your doctor and pharmacist if you are allergic to telithromycin, azithromycin (Zithromax), clarithromycin (Biaxin), dirithromycin (Dynabac, no longer available in the U.S.), erythromycin (E.E.S., E-Mycin, Erythrocin), troleandomycin (TAO, no longer available in the U.S.), or any other medications.
- do not take telithromycin if you are taking cisapride (Propulsid, no longer available in the U.S.) or pimozide (Orap).
- tell your doctor if you have had hepatitis (swelling of the liver) or jaundice (yellowing of the skin or eyes) while taking telithromycin or azithromycin (Zithromax), clarithromycin (Biaxin), dirithromycin (Dynabac, no longer available in the U.S.), erythromycin (E.E.S., E-Mycin, Erythrocin), or troleandomycin (TAO, no longer available in the U.S.). Your doctor will tell you not to take telithromycin.
- tell your doctor and pharmacist what other prescription and nonprescription medications, vitamins, nutritional supplements, and herbal products you are taking or plan to take. Be sure to mention any of the following: anticoagulants ('blood thinners') such as warfarin (Coumadin); antifungals such as itraconazole (Sporanox) and ketoconazole (Nizoral); carbamazepine (Tegretol); cholesterol-lowering medications such as atorvastatin (Lipitor, in Caduet), lovastatin (Altoprev, Mevacor, in Advicor), and simvastatin (Zocor, in Vytorin); cyclosporine (Neoral, Sandimmune); digoxin (Lanoxin); diuretics ('water pills'); ergot-type medications such as bromocriptine (Parlodel), cabergoline (Dostinex), dihydroergotamine (D.H.E. 45, Migranal), ergoloid mesylates (Germinal, Hydergine), ergonovine (Ergotrate), ergotamine (Bellergal-S, Cafergot, Ergomar, Wigraine), methylergonovine (Methergine), methysergide (Sansert), and pergolide (Permax); medications for irregular heartbeat, including amiodarone (Cordarone, Pacerone),

dofetilide (Tikosyn), disopyramide (Norpace), procain-amide (Procanbid), quinidine, or sotalol (Betapace); metoprolol (Lopressor, Toprol XL); midazolam (Versed); phenobarbital (Luminal, Solfoton); phenytoin (Dilantin); repaglinide (Prandin); rifabutin (Mycobutin); rifampin (Rifadin, Rimactane); sirolimus (Rapamune); tacrolimus (Prograf); and triazolam (Halcion). Your doctor may need to change the doses of your medications or monitor you carefully for side effects.

- if you are taking theophylline (Theo-24, Theobid, Theo-Dur, others), take it 1 hour before or after telithromycin.
- tell your doctor if you or anyone in your family has or has had a heart problem that may cause fainting and a slow or irregular heartbeat, or heart disease; or if you have low blood levels of potassium or magnesium; or kidney or liver disease.
- tell your doctor if you are pregnant, plan to become pregnant, or are breast-feeding. If you become pregnant while taking telithromycin, call your doctor.
- if you are having surgery, including dental surgery, tell the doctor or dentist that you are taking telithromycin.
- you should know that telithromycin may cause dizziness or fainting. If you feel lightheaded and have severe nausea or vomiting, do not drive a car, operate machinery or participate in dangerous activities. If you faint, call your doctor before taking another dose of telithromycin.
- you should know that antibiotics, including telithromycin, may cause an infection in the intestines with symptoms of watery diarrhea, diarrhea that does not go away, or bloody stools; stomach cramps; or fever. Call your doctor if you have these symptoms. These symptoms can occur up to two months after finishing treatment.
- you should know that telithromycin may cause liver damage, which may be severe or life-threatening. This reaction may happen at any time while you are taking telithromycin or right after you finish taking this medication. Stop taking telithromycin and call your doctor right away if you have any of the following symptoms: tiredness, lack of energy, unusual bleeding or bruising, loss of appetite, nausea, itchy skin, dark urine, light-colored stools, yellowing of your skin or eyes, pain or tenderness in the upper right part of your stomach, swelling of the abdomen, or flu-like symptoms.
- you should know that telithromycin may cause vision problems, including blurred vision, difficulty focusing, and seeing double. These problems usually happen after the first or second dose and last for a few hours. To avoid these problems, avoid quick changes in looking from things far away to things close by. Do not drive a car, operate machinery, or participate in dangerous activities until you know how this medication affects you. If you have vision problems while taking telithromycin, call your doctor before taking another dose.

What special dietary instructions should I follow?

Unless your doctor tells you otherwise, continue your normal diet.

What should I do if I forget to take a dose?

Take the missed dose as soon as you remember it. However, if it is almost time for the next dose, skip the missed dose and continue your regular dosing schedule. Never take more than one dose of telithromycin in 24 hours. Do not take a double dose to make up for a missed one.

What side effects can this medicine cause?

Telithromycin may cause side effects. Tell your doctor if any of these symptoms are severe or do not go away:

- diarrhea
- nausea
- vomiting
- headache
- dizziness

Some side effects can be serious. If you experience any of these symptoms, or those listed in the SPECIAL PRECAUTIONS section, call your doctor immediately:

- fainting
- rapid, irregular, or pounding heartbeat
- hives
- rash
- itching
- difficulty breathing or swallowing
- swelling of the face, throat, tongue, lips, eyes, hands, feet, ankles, or lower legs
- hoarseness

Telithromycin may cause other side effects. Call your doctor if you have any unusual problems while taking this medication.

What storage conditions are needed for this medicine?

Keep this medication in the container it came in, tightly closed, and out of reach of children. Store it at room temperature and away from excess heat and moisture (not in the bathroom). Throw away any medication that is outdated or no longer needed. Talk to your pharmacist about the proper disposal of your medication.

What should I do in case of overdose?

In case of overdose, call your local poison control center at 1-800-222-1222. If the victim has collapsed or is not breathing, call local emergency services at 911.

What other information should I know?

Keep all appointments with your doctor.

Do not let anyone else take your medication. Your prescription is probably not refillable. If you still have symptoms of infection after you finish the telithromycin, call your doctor.

Dosage Facts
For Informational Purposes

Caution: Do not change your dose, how often you take your medication, or the length of time you are to take it without first talking to your healthcare provider.

The following dosage information was written using medical language for doctors and other healthcare professionals and is provided here for you to check your dosage. The dosage of this drug may differ for different patients. Therefore, always follow your doctor's instructions or the directions on the label. Contact your healthcare provider or pharmacist if you have any questions about the specific dosage of your medication after reviewing this information.

Adult Patients

Respiratory Tract Infections
Community-acquired Pneumonia

ORAL:
- 800 mg once daily for 7–10 days.

Special Populations

Hepatic Impairment
- Hepatic impairment: Dosage adjustment not required.
- Hepatic impairment with coexisting severe renal impairment (Cl_{cr} <30 mL/minute or undergoing hemodialysis): Use reduced dosage of 400 mg once daily.

Renal Impairment
- Mild to moderate renal impairment: Dosage adjustment not required.
- Severe renal impairment (Cl_{cr} <30 mL/minute or undergoing hemodialysis): Use reduced dosage of 600 mg once daily. On dialysis days, administer daily dose after dialysis session.
- Severe renal impairment (Cl_{cr} <30 mL/minute or undergoing hemodialysis) with coexisting hepatic impairment: Use reduced dosage of 400 mg once daily.

Geriatric Patients
- Routine dosage adjustment based on age not required.

Telmisartan
(tel mi sar′ tan)

Brand Name: Micardis®, Micardis® HCT as a combination product containing Telmisartan and Hydrochlorothiazide

Important Warning

Do not take telmisartan if you are pregnant. If you become pregnant while taking telmisartan, call your doctor immediately. Telmisartan may harm the fetus.

Why is this medicine prescribed?

Telmisartan is used alone or in combination with other medications to treat high blood pressure. Telmisartan is in a class of medications called angiotensin II receptor antagonists. It works by blocking the action of certain chemicals that tighten the blood vessels, so blood flows more smoothly.

How should this medicine be used?

Telmisartan comes as a tablet to take by mouth. It is usually taken once a day with or without food. To help you remember to take telmisartan, take it around the same time every day. Follow the directions on your prescription label carefully, and ask your doctor or pharmacist to explain any part you do not understand. Take telmisartan exactly as directed. Do not take more or less of it or take it more often than prescribed by your doctor.

Your doctor may start you on a low dose of telmisartan and gradually increase your dose.

Telmisartan controls high blood pressure but does not cure it. Continue to take telmisartan even if you feel well. Do not stop taking telmisartan without talking to your doctor.

Are there other uses for this medicine?

Telmisartan is also used sometimes to treat congestive heart failure. Talk to your doctor about the possible risks of using this medication for your condition.

This medication may be prescribed for other uses; ask your doctor or pharmacist for more information.

What special precautions should I follow?

Before taking telmisartan,
- tell your doctor and pharmacist if you are allergic to telmisartan or any other medications.
- tell your doctor and pharmacist what prescription and nonprescription medications, vitamins, nutritional supplements, and herbal products you are taking. Be sure to mention any of the following: anticoagulants ('blood thinners') such as warfarin (Coumadin); digoxin (Lan-

oxin); and diuretics ('water pills'). Your doctor may need to change the doses of your medications or monitor you carefully for side effects.

- tell your doctor if you have or have ever had heart failure or kidney or liver disease.
- tell your doctor if you plan to become pregnant or are breast-feeding.

What special dietary instructions should I follow?

If your doctor prescribes a low-salt or low-sodium diet, follow these directions carefully.

What should I do if I forget to take a dose?

Take the missed dose as soon as you remember it. However, if it is almost time for the next dose, skip the missed dose and continue your regular dosing schedule. Do not take a double dose to make up for a missed one.

What side effects can this medicine cause?

Telmisartan may cause side effects. Tell your doctor if any of these symptoms are severe or do not go away:

- runny nose
- sore throat
- back pain
- sinus pain
- diarrhea

Some side effects can be serious. The following symptoms are uncommon, but if you experience any of them, call your doctor immediately:

- swelling of the face, throat, tongue, lips, eyes, hands, feet, ankles, or lower legs
- hoarseness
- difficulty breathing or swallowing
- fainting

Telmisartan may cause other side effects. Call your doctor if you have any unusual problems while taking this medication.

If you experience a serious side effect, you or your doctor may send a report to the Food and Drug Administration's (FDA) MedWatch Adverse Event Reporting program online [at http://www.fda.gov/MedWatch/index.html] or by phone [1-800-332-1088].

What storage conditions are needed for this medicine?

Keep this medication in the container it came in, tightly closed, and out of reach of children. Store it at room temperature and away from excess heat and moisture (not in the bathroom). Throw away any medication that is outdated or no longer needed. Talk to your pharmacist about the proper disposal of your medication.

What should I do in case of overdose?

In case of overdose, call your local poison control center at 1-800-222-1222. If the victim has collapsed or is not breathing, call local emergency services at 911.

Symptoms of overdose may include:

- dizziness
- fainting
- rapid or pounding heartbeat

What other information should I know?

Keep all appointments with your doctor. Your blood pressure should be checked regularly to determine your response to telmisartan.

Do not let anyone else take your medication. Ask your pharmacist any questions you have about refilling your prescription.

Dosage Facts
For Informational Purposes

Caution: Do not change your dose, how often you take your medication, or the length of time you are to take it without first talking to your healthcare provider.

The following dosage information was written using medical language for doctors and other healthcare professionals and is provided here for you to check your dosage. The dosage of this drug may differ for different patients. Therefore, always follow your doctor's instructions or the directions on the label. Contact your healthcare provider or pharmacist if you have any questions about the specific dosage of your medication after reviewing this information.

Adult Patients

Hypertension
Monotherapy

ORAL:

- Initially, 40 mg once daily in adults without intravascular volume depletion. Adjust dosage at approximately monthly intervals (more aggressively in high-risk patients) to achieve BP control.
- Usual dosage: 20–80 mg once daily; no additional therapeutic benefit with higher dosages.

Combination Therapy

ORAL:

- If BP is not adequately controlled by monotherapy with telmisartan 80 mg daily, can switch to fixed-combination tablets (telmisartan 80 mg and hydrochlorothiazide 12.5 mg; then telmisartan 160 mg and hydrochlorothiazide 25 mg), administered once daily.
- If BP is not adequately controlled by monotherapy with hydrochlorothiazide 25 mg or if BP is controlled but hypokalemia is problematic at this dosage, can use fixed-combination tablets containing telmisartan 80 mg and hydrochlorothiazide 12.5 mg, administered once daily. Can increase dosage

to telmisartan 160 mg and hydrochlorothiazide 25 mg, if needed, to control BP.

Special Populations

Hepatic Impairment

- Initiate therapy under close medical supervision in patients with obstructive biliary disease or hepatic impairment.
- If fixed-combination tablets are used in patients with obstructive biliary disease or hepatic impairment, recommended initial dosage is telmisartan 40 mg and hydrochlorothiazide 12.5 mg daily. Use of fixed combination not recommended in those with severe hepatic impairment.

Renal Impairment

- No initial dosage adjustments necessary in patients with Cl_{cr} >30 mL/minute. Manufacturer makes no specific recommendations regarding telmisartan monotherapy in those with Cl_{cr} ≤30 mL/minute.
- Telmisartan/hydrochlorothiazide fixed combination not recommended in patients with Cl_{cr} <30 mL/minute.

Geriatric Patients

- No initial dosage adjustments necessary.

Volume- and/or Salt-Depleted Patients

- Correct volume and/or salt depletion prior to initiation of therapy or initiate therapy under close medical supervision using lower initial dosage.

Temazepam

(te maz' e pam)

Brand Name: Restoril®
Also available generically.

Why is this medicine prescribed?

Temazepam is used on a short-term basis to help you fall asleep and stay asleep through the night.

This medication is sometimes prescribed for other uses; ask your doctor or pharmacist for more information.

How should this medicine be used?

Temazepam comes as a capsule to take by mouth and may be taken with or without food. It usually is taken before bedtime when needed. Follow the directions on your prescription label carefully, and ask your doctor or pharmacist to explain any part you do not understand. Take temazepam exactly as directed.

Temazepam can be habit-forming. Do not take a larger dose, take it more often, or for a longer period than your doctor tells you to. Tolerance may develop with long-term or excessive use, making the drug less effective. Do not take temazepam for more than 5 weeks or stop taking this medication without talking to your doctor. Stopping the drug suddenly can cause withdrawal symptoms (anxiousness, sleeplessness, and irritability). Your doctor probably will de-

crease your dose gradually. You may experience sleeping difficulties the first one or two nights after stopping this medication. If your sleep problems continue, talk to your doctor, who will determine whether this drug is right for you.

What special precautions should I follow?

Before taking temazepam,

- tell your doctor and pharmacist if you are allergic to temazepam, alprazolam (Xanax), chlordiazepoxide (Librium, Librax), clonazepam (Klonopin), clorazepate (Tranxene), diazepam (Valium), estazolam (ProSom), flurazepam (Dalmane), lorazepam (Ativan), oxazepam (Serax), prazepam (Centrax), triazolam (Halcion), or any other drugs.
- tell your doctor and pharmacist what prescription and nonprescription medications you are taking, especially antihistamines; cimetidine (Tagamet); digoxin (Lanoxin); disulfiram (Antabuse); isoniazid (INH, Laniazid, Nydrazid); medications for depression, seizures, Parkinson's disease, pain, asthma, colds, or allergies; muscle relaxants; oral contraceptives; probenecid (Benemid); rifampin (Rifadin); sedatives; sleeping pills; theophylline (Theo-Dur); tranquilizers; and vitamins. These medications may add to the drowsiness caused by temazepam.
- tell your doctor if you have or have ever had glaucoma; seizures; or lung, heart, or liver disease.
- tell your doctor if you are pregnant, plan to become pregnant, or are breast-feeding. If you become pregnant while taking temazepam, call your doctor immediately.
- if you are having surgery, including dental surgery, tell the doctor or dentist that you are taking temazepam.
- you should know that this drug may make you drowsy. Do not drive a car or operate machinery until you know how this drug affects you.
- remember that alcohol can add to the drowsiness caused by this drug.
- tell your doctor if you use tobacco products. Cigarette smoking may decrease the effectiveness of this drug.

What should I do if I forget to take a dose?

If you miss a dose, skip the missed dose and continue your regular dosing schedule. Do not take a double dose to make up for a missed one.

What side effects can this medicine cause?

Side effects from temazepam may occur and include:

- headache
- heartburn
- diarrhea
- hangover effect (grogginess)
- drowsiness
- dizziness or lightheadedness
- weakness
- dry mouth

Tell your doctor if any of these symptoms are severe or do not go away:

- constipation
- difficulty urinating
- frequent urination
- blurred vision

If you experience any of the following symptoms, call your doctor immediately:

- jaw, neck, and back muscle spasms
- slow or difficult speech
- persistent, fine tremor or inability to sit still
- fever
- difficulty breathing or swallowing
- severe skin rash
- yellowing of the skin or eyes
- irregular heartbeat

If you experience a serious side effect, you or your doctor may send a report to the Food and Drug Administration's (FDA) MedWatch Adverse Event Reporting program online [at http://www.fda.gov/MedWatch/index.html] or by phone [1-800-332-1088].

What storage conditions are needed for this medicine?

Keep this medication in the container it came in, tightly closed, and out of reach of children. Store it at room temperature and away from excess heat and moisture (not in the bathroom). Throw away any medication that is outdated or no longer needed. Talk to your pharmacist about the proper disposal of your medication.

What should I do in case of overdose?

In case of overdose, call your local poison control center at 1-800-222-1222. If the victim has collapsed or is not breathing, call local emergency services at 911.

What other information should I know?

Keep all appointments with your doctor and the laboratory.

Do not let anyone else take your medication.

Dosage Facts
For Informational Purposes

Caution: Do not change your dose, how often you take your medication, or the length of time you are to take it without first talking to your healthcare provider.

The following dosage information was written using medical language for doctors and other healthcare professionals and is provided here for you to check your dosage. The dosage of this drug may differ for different patients. Therefore, always follow your doctor's instructions or the directions on the label. Contact your healthcare provider or pharmacist if you have any questions

about the specific dosage of your medication after reviewing this information.

Adult Patients

Insomnia

ORAL:
- 7.5–30 mg; 15 mg is the usual recommended dose. In patients with transient insomnia, 7.5 mg may be sufficient.

Special Populations

Geriatric or Debilitated Patients
- Possible increased sensitivity to benzodiazepines. Initially, 7.5 mg.

Tenofovir
(te noe′ fo veer)

Brand Name: Atripla ® as a combination product containing Efavirenz, Emtricitabine, and Tenofovir, Truvada® as a combination product containing Tenofovir and Emtricitabine, Viread®

Important Warning

Tenofovir, when used alone or in combination with other antiviral medications, may cause serious damage to the liver and a condition called lactic acidosis. Tell your doctor if you drink large amounts of alcohol and if you have or have ever had liver disease.

If you experience any of the following symptoms, call your doctor immediately: upset stomach, loss of appetite, excessive tiredness, weakness, dark yellow or brown urine, unusual bleeding or bruising, flu-like symptoms, yellowing of the skin or eyes, and pain in the upper right part of your stomach.

Keep all appointments with your doctor and the laboratory. Your doctor will order certain lab tests to check your body's response to tenofovir.

Why is this medicine prescribed?

Tenofovir is used in combination with other antiviral medications to treat human immunodeficiency virus (HIV) in patients with acquired immunodeficiency syndrome (AIDS). Tenofovir is in a class of antiviral medications called reverse transcriptase inhibitors. It works by slowing the spread of HIV in the body. Tenofovir is not a cure and may not decrease the number of HIV-related illnesses. Tenofovir does not prevent the spread of HIV to other people.

How should this medicine be used?

Tenofovir comes as a tablet to take by mouth. It is usually taken once a day with a meal. Follow the directions on your prescription label carefully, and ask your doctor or pharmacist to explain any part you do not understand. Take tenofovir exactly as directed. Do not take more or less of it or take it more often than prescribed by your doctor.

Continue to take tenofovir even if you feel well. Do not stop taking tenofovir without talking to your doctor.

Are there other uses for this medicine?

This medication may be prescribed for other uses; ask your doctor or pharmacist for more information.

What special precautions should I follow?

Before taking tenofovir,

- tell your doctor and pharmacist if you are allergic to tenofovir or any other medications.
- tell your doctor and pharmacist what prescription and nonprescription medications, vitamins, nutritional supplements, and herbal products you are taking. Be sure to mention any of the following: antiviral medications such as acyclovir (Zovirax), cidofovir (Vistide), ganciclovir (Cytovene, Vitasert), valacyclovir (Valtrex), and valganciclovir (Valcyte); aspirin and other nonsteroidal antiinflammatory medications (NSAIDs) such as indomethacin (Indocin); didanosine (Videx); diuretics ('water pills'); penicillin (Pen Vee K, Veetids, others); and probenecid (Benemid). Your doctor may need to change the doses of your medications or monitor you carefully for side effects.
- if you are taking didanosine (Videx), take it 1 hour before or 2 hours after tenofovir.
- in addition to the condition listed in the IMPORTANT WARNING section, tell your doctor if you have or have ever had kidney disease.
- tell your doctor if you are pregnant, plan to become pregnant, or are breast-feeding. If you become pregnant while taking tenofovir, call your doctor. You should not breastfeed while taking tenofovir.
- you should be aware that your body fat may increase or move to different areas of your body, such as your breasts and your upper back.

What special dietary instructions should I follow?

Unless your doctor tells you otherwise, continue your normal diet.

What should I do if I forget to take a dose?

Take the missed dose as soon as you remember it. However, if it is almost time for the next dose, skip the missed dose and continue your regular dosing schedule. Do not take a double dose to make up for a missed one.

What side effects can this medicine cause?

Tenofovir may cause side effects. Tell your doctor if any of these symptoms are severe or do not go away:

- upset stomach
- diarrhea
- vomiting
- gas
- loss of appetite

Some side effects can be serious. If you experience any of those listed in the IMPORTANT WARNING section, call your doctor immediately.

Tenofovir may cause other side effects. Call your doctor if you have any unusual problems while taking this medication.

If you experience a serious side effect, you or your doctor may send a report to the Food and Drug Administration's (FDA) MedWatch Adverse Event Reporting program online [at http://www.fda.gov/MedWatch/index.html] or by phone [1-800-332-1088].

What storage conditions are needed for this medicine?

Keep this medication in the container it came in, tightly closed, and out of reach of children. Store it at room temperature and away from excess heat and moisture (not in the bathroom). Throw away any medication that is outdated or no longer needed. Talk to your pharmacist about the proper disposal of your medication.

What should I do in case of overdose?

In case of overdose, call your local poison control center at 1-800-222-1222. If the victim has collapsed or is not breathing, call local emergency services at 911.

What other information should I know?

Do not let anyone else take your medication. Ask your pharmacist any questions you have about refilling your prescription.

Dosage Facts
For Informational Purposes

Caution: Do not change your dose, how often you take your medication, or the length of time you are to take it without first talking to your healthcare provider.

The following dosage information was written using medical language for doctors and other healthcare professionals and is provided here for you to check your dosage. The dosage of this drug may differ for different patients. Therefore, always follow your doctor's instructions or the directions on the label. Contact your healthcare provider or pharmacist if you have any questions about the specific dosage of your medication after reviewing this information.

General Dosage Information

Available as tenofovir disodium fumarate; dosage expressed in terms of tenofovir disodium fumarate.

Dosage of Truvada® and Atripla® expressed as number of tablets.

Viread® and Truvada® must be given in conjunction with other antiretrovirals. Atripla® may be used alone or in conjunction with other antiretrovirals.

If used with atazanavir, adjustment in treatment regimen necessary. If used with didanosine, adjustment of didanosine dosage necessary.

Pediatric Patients

Treatment of HIV Infection†

ORAL:
- Children 2–8 years of age: 8 mg/kg once daily under investigation.
- Children >8 years of age: Median dose 210 mg/m² (maximum 300 mg) once daily under investigation.

Adult Patients

Treatment of HIV Infection

ORAL:
- 300 mg once daily.
- Truvada®: 1 tablet once daily.
- Atripla®: 1 tablet once daily.

Postexposure Prophylaxis of HIV†

Occupational Exposure†

ORAL:
- 300 mg once daily.
- Used in basic regimens with lamivudine or emtricitabine.
- Initiate postexposure prophylaxis as soon as possible following exposure (within hours rather than days) and continue for 4 weeks, if tolerated.

Nonoccupational Exposure†

ORAL:
- 300 mg once daily.
- Used in preferred nonnucleoside reverse transcriptase-based (NNRTI-based) regimens that includes efavirenz and (lamivudine or emtricitabine) and (zidovudine or tenofovir); also used in various alternative HIV protease inhibitor-based (PI-based) regimens that include a PI (with or without low-dose ritonavir) and (lamivudine or emtricitabine) and tenofovir.
- Initiate postexposure prophylaxis as soon as possible following exposure (preferably ≤72 hours after exposure) and continue for 28 days.

Special Populations

Hepatic Impairment

Treatment of HIV Infection

ORAL:
- Dosage adjustment not needed.

Renal Impairment

Treatment of HIV Infection

- Adjust dosage if Cl_{cr} <50 mL/minute.

Viread® Dosage in Adults with Renal Impairment

Cl_{cr} (mL/min)	Dosage
30–49	300 mg once every 48 hours
10–29	300 mg twice weekly
Hemodialysis patients	300 mg once every 7 days or after a total of approximately 12 hours of hemodialysis (assuming 3 hemodialysis sessions/week each lasting approximately 4 hours)

Manufacturer states dosage recommendations not available for patients with Cl_{cr} <10 mL/minute who are not undergoing hemodialysis. Some clinicians recommend 300 mg once every 7 days in those with end-stage renal disease.

Truvada® Dosage in Adults with Renal Impairment

Cl_{cr} (mL/minute)	Dose and Dosing Interval
≥50	One tablet every 24 hours
30–49	One tablet every 48 hours (monitor clinical response and renal function since dosage has not been evaluated clinically)
<30 (including hemodialysis patients)	Not recommended

Atripla®: Dosage adjustment not necessary in patients with Cl_{cr} ≥50 mL/minute. Not recommended in patients with Cl_{cr} < 50 mL/minute.

Geriatric Patients
- Select dosage with caution because of age-related decreases in hepatic, renal, and/or cardiac function and concomitant disease and drug therapy.

† Use is not currently included in the labeling approved by the US Food and Drug Administration.

Terazosin

(ter ay′ zoe sin)

Brand Name: Hytrin®
Also available generically.

Why is this medicine prescribed?

Terazosin is used in men to treat the symptoms of an enlarged prostate (benign prostatic hyperplasia or BPH), which include difficulty urinating (hesitation, dribbling, weak stream, and incomplete bladder emptying), painful urination, and urinary frequency and urgency. It also is used alone or in combination with other medications to treat high blood pressure. Terazosin is in a class of medications called alpha-blockers. It relieves the symptoms of BPH by relaxing the muscles of the bladder and prostate. It lowers blood pressure by relaxing the blood vessels so that blood can flow more easily through the body.

How should this medicine be used?

Terazosin comes as a capsule to take by mouth. It is usually taken with or without food once a day at bedtime or twice a day. Follow the directions on your prescription label carefully, and ask your doctor or pharmacist to explain any part you do not understand. Take terazosin exactly as directed. Do not take more or less of it or take it more often than prescribed by your doctor.

Your doctor will start you on a low dose of terazosin and gradually increase your dose. If you stop taking terazosin for a few days or longer, call your doctor. Your doctor usually will start you again on the lowest dose of terazosin and gradually increase your dose.

Terazosin controls high blood pressure and the symptoms of BPH but does not cure them. It may take 4 to 6 weeks or longer before you feel the full benefit of terazosin for BPH. Continue to take terazosin even if you feel well. Do not stop taking terazosin without talking to your doctor.

Are there other uses for this medicine?

This medication may be prescribed for other uses; ask your doctor or pharmacist for more information.

What special precautions should I follow?

Before taking terazosin,

- tell your doctor and pharmacist if you are allergic to terazosin, doxazosin (Cardura, Cardura XL), prazosin (Minipress, in Minizide), or any other medications.
- tell your doctor and pharmacist what prescription and nonprescription medications, vitamins, nutritional supplements, and herbal products you are taking or plan to take. Be sure to mention any of the following: medications for erectile dysfunction (ED) such as sildenafil (Viagra), tadalafil (Cialis), or vardenafil (Levitra); and other medications for high blood pressure, especially verapamil (Calan, Covera, Isoptin, Verelan). Your doctor may need to change the doses of your medications or monitor you carefully for side effects.
- tell your doctor if you have or have ever had prostate cancer.
- tell your doctor if you are pregnant, plan to become pregnant, or are breast-feeding. If you become pregnant while taking terazosin, call your doctor.
- if you are having surgery, including dental surgery, tell the doctor or dentist that you are taking terazosin. If you need to have eye surgery at any time during or after your treatment, be sure to tell your doctor that you are taking or have taken terazosin.
- you should know that terazosin may make you drowsy or dizzy. Do not drive a car, operate machinery or perform dangerous tasks for 12 hours after the first time you take terazosin or after your dose is increased, and until you know how this medication affects you.
- you should know that terazosin may cause dizziness, lightheadedness, and fainting when you get up too quickly from a lying position. This is more common when you first start taking terazosin, when your dose is increased, or when treatment with terazosin is stopped for several days and then restarted. To avoid this problem, get out of bed slowly, resting your feet on the floor for a few minutes before standing up. If you experience these symptoms, sit or lie down. If these symptoms do not improve, call your doctor.

What special dietary instructions should I follow?

Follow your doctor's directions for your meals, including advice for a reduced salt (sodium) diet.

What should I do if I forget to take a dose?

Take the missed dose as soon as you remember it. However, if it is almost time for the next dose, skip the missed dose and continue your regular dosing schedule. Do not take a double dose to make up for a missed one. Check with your doctor if you have missed two or more doses.

What side effects can this medicine cause?

Terazosin may cause side effects. Tell your doctor if any of these symptoms or those listed in the SPECIAL PRECAUTIONS section are severe or do not go away:

- weakness
- tiredness
- stuffy or runny nose
- back pain
- nausea
- weight gain
- decreased sexual ability
- blurred vision
- swelling of the hands, feet, ankles, or lower legs
- pain, burning, numbness, or tingling in the hands or feet

Some side effects can be serious. If you experience any of these symptoms, call your doctor immediately:

- hives
- rash
- itching
- shortness of breath
- rapid, pounding, or irregular heartbeat
- painful erection of the penis that lasts for hours

Terazosin may cause other side effects. Call your doctor if you have any unusual problems while taking this medication.

What storage conditions are needed for this medicine?

Keep this medication in the container it came in, tightly closed, and out of reach of children. Store it at room temperature and away from light and excess heat and moisture (not in the bathroom). Throw away any medication that is outdated or no longer needed. Talk to your pharmacist about the proper disposal of your medication.

What should I do in case of overdose?

In case of overdose, call your local poison control center at 1-800-222-1222. If the victim has collapsed or is not breathing, call local emergency services at 911.

Symptoms of overdose may include:

- dizziness
- lightheadedness
- fainting
- blurred vision

What other information should I know?

Keep all appointments with your doctor. Your blood pressure should be checked regularly to determine your response to terazosin.

Do not let anyone else take your medication. Ask your pharmacist any questions you have about refilling your prescription.

Dosage Facts
For Informational Purposes

Caution: Do not change your dose, how often you take your medication, or the length of time you are to take it without first talking to your healthcare provider.

The following dosage information was written using medical language for doctors and other healthcare professionals and is provided here for you to check your dosage. The dosage of this drug may differ for different patients. Therefore, always follow your doctor's instructions or the directions on the label. Contact your healthcare provider or pharmacist if you have any questions about the specific dosage of your medication after reviewing this information.

General Dosage Information

Available as terazosin hydrochloride; dosage expressed in terms of terazosin.

Individualize dosage according to patient response and tolerance. Initiate at low dosage to minimize frequency of postural hypotension and syncope.

Monitor BP 2–3 hours after dosing and at end of dosing interval to determine whether peak and trough responses are similar and to assess potential manifestations (e.g., dizziness, palpitations) of an excessive response.

If therapy is interrupted for several days or longer, restart using initial dosage regimen.

Pediatric Patients

Hypertension†

ORAL:
- Initially, 1 mg once daily. Increase dosage as necessary up to a maximum of 20 mg once daily.

Adult Patients

Hypertension

ORAL:
- Initially, 1 mg daily at bedtime. May increase dosage gradually to 5 mg daily, with further titration up to 20 mg daily if BP is not controlled.
- Each increase should be delayed until BP has stabilized at a given dosage.

BPH

ORAL:
- Initially, 1 mg daily at bedtime. May increase daily dosage to 2 mg and thereafter to 5 mg and 10 mg, if necessary, to reduce symptoms and/or improve urinary flow rates.

Prescribing Limits

Pediatric Patients

Hypertension†

ORAL:
- Maximum 20 mg daily.

Adult Patients

Hypertension

ORAL:
- Maximum 40 mg daily.

BPH

ORAL:
- Maximum 20 mg daily.

Special Populations

Hepatic Impairment
- Manufacturer makes no specific dosage recommendations; effects on the pharmacokinetics of terazosin have not been elucidated.

Renal Impairment
- Clinically important alterations in the pharmacokinetics of terazosin not observed to date; dosage adjustment not necessary.
- Administration of supplemental doses of the drug following hemodialysis does not appear to be necessary.

Geriatric Patients
- Use with caution; generally, increase dosage more slowly in geriatric patients than in younger adults.

† Use is not currently included in the labeling approved by the US Food and Drug Administration.

Terbinafine

(ter′ bin a feen)

Brand Name: Lamisil®, Lamisil® AT

Why is this medicine prescribed?

Terbinafine is used to treat fungal infections of the toenail and fingernail. Terbinafine is in a class of medications called antifungals. It works by stopping the growth of fungi.

How should this medicine be used?

Terbinafine comes as a tablet to take by mouth. It is usually taken once a day for 6 weeks for fingernail fungus and once a day for 12 weeks for toenail fungus. Follow the directions on your prescription label carefully, and ask your doctor or pharmacist to explain any part you do not understand. Take terbinafine exactly as directed. Do not take more or less of it or take it more often than prescribed by your doctor.

Your fungus may not be completely cured until a few months after you finish taking terbinafine. This is because it takes time for a healthy nail to grow in.

Are there other uses for this medicine?

This medication may be prescribed for other uses; ask your doctor or pharmacist for more information.

What special precautions should I follow?

Before taking terbinafine,
- tell your doctor and pharmacist if you are allergic to terbinafine or any other medications.
- tell your doctor and pharmacist what prescription and nonprescription medications, vitamins, nutritional supplements, and herbal products you are taking. Be sure to mention any of the following: anticoagulants (blood thinners) such as warfarin (Coumadin); antidepressants such as amitriptyline (Elavil), amoxapine (Asendin), clomipramine (Anafranil), desipramine (Norpramin), doxepin (Adapin, Sinequan), imipramine (Tofranil), nortriptyline (Aventyl, Pamelor), protriptyline (Vivactil), and trimipramine (Surmontil); beta-blockers such as atenolol (Tenormin), labetalol (Normodyne), metoprolol (Lopressor, Toprol XL), nadolol (Corgard), and propranolol (Inderal); cimetidine (Tagamet); medications that suppress the immune system such as azathioprine (Imuran), cyclosporine (Neoral, Sandimmune), methotrexate (Rheumatrex), sirolimus (Rapamune), and tacrolimus (Prograf); rifampin (Rifadin, Rimactane); and selegiline (Eldepryl). Your doctor may need to change the doses of your medications or monitor you carefully for side effects.
- tell your doctor if you have or have ever had kidney or liver disease, human immunodeficiency virus (HIV), or acquired immunodeficiency syndrome (AIDS).
- tell your doctor if you are pregnant, plan to become pregnant, or are breast-feeding. If you become pregnant while taking terbinafine, call your doctor. You should not take terbinafine while breast-feeding.

What special dietary instructions should I follow?

Unless your doctor tells you otherwise, continue your normal diet.

What should I do if I forget to take a dose?

Take the missed dose as soon as you remember it. However, if it is almost time for the next dose, skip the missed dose and continue your regular dosing schedule. Do not take a double dose to make up for a missed one.

What side effects can this medicine cause?

Terbinafine may cause side effects. Tell your doctor if any of these symptoms are severe or do not go away:
- diarrhea
- upset stomach
- stomach pain
- rash
- itching
- hives
- changes in taste or loss of taste

Some side effects can be serious. The following symptoms are uncommon, but if you experience any of them, call your doctor immediately:
- upset stomach that does not go away
- loss of appetite
- extreme tiredness
- vomiting
- pain in the right upper part of the stomach
- dark urine
- pale stools
- severe skin rash that keeps getting worse
- fever, sore throat, and other signs of infection

Terbinafine may cause other side effects. Call your doctor if you have any unusual problems while taking this medication.

If you experience a serious side effect, you or your doctor may send a report to the Food and Drug Administration's (FDA) MedWatch Adverse Event Reporting program online [at http://www.fda.gov/MedWatch/index.html] or by phone [1-800-332-1088].

What storage conditions are needed for this medicine?

Keep this medication in the container it came in, tightly closed, and out of reach of children. Store it at room temperature and away from excess heat and moisture (not in the bathroom). Throw away any medication that is outdated or no longer needed. Talk to your pharmacist about the proper disposal of your medication.

What should I do in case of overdose?

In case of overdose, call your local poison control center at 1-800-222-1222. If the victim has collapsed or is not breathing, call local emergency services at 911.

What other information should I know?

Keep all appointments with your doctor and the laboratory. Your doctor may order certain lab tests to check your body's response to terbinafine.

Do not let anyone else take your medication. Ask your pharmacist any questions you have about refilling your prescription.

Dosage Facts
For Informational Purposes

Caution: Do not change your dose, how often you take your medication, or the length of time you are to take it without first talking to your healthcare provider.

The following dosage information was written using medical language for doctors and other healthcare professionals and is provided here for you to check your dosage. The dosage of this drug may differ for different patients. Therefore, always follow your doctor's instructions or the directions on the label. Contact your healthcare provider or pharmacist if you have any questions about the specific dosage of your medication after reviewing this information.

General Dosage Information

Available as terbinafine hydrochloride; dosage expressed in terms of terbinafine.

Adult Patients

Onychomycosis
Fingernails

ORAL:
- 250 mg daily given for 6 weeks. More prolonged treatment generally has not been more effective, although some patients may benefit from extended and/or repeated courses of terbinafine.
- Fingernail infections usually are reevaluated ≥18 weeks after completion of treatment.

Toenails

ORAL:
- 250 mg daily given for 12 weeks. Some patients who do not respond to the initial 12-week regimen may respond to a second course.
- Toenail infections usually are reevaluated 6–9 months after completion of therapy.

Terbutaline
(ter byoo′ ta leen)

Brand Name: Brethine®

Why is this medicine prescribed?

Terbutaline is used to prevent and treat wheezing, shortness of breath, and troubled breathing caused by asthma, chronic bronchitis, emphysema, and other lung diseases. It relaxes and opens air passages in the lungs, making it easier to breathe.

This medication is sometimes prescribed for other uses; ask your doctor or pharmacist for more information.

How should this medicine be used?

Terbutaline comes as tablets to take by mouth and as an aerosol to inhale by mouth. The tablets usually are taken three times a day. The aerosol is used as needed to relieve symptoms or every 4-6 hours to prevent symptoms. Follow the directions on your prescription label carefully, and ask your doctor or pharmacist to explain any part you do not understand. Take terbutaline exactly as directed. Do not take more or less of it or take it more often than prescribed by your doctor.

Terbutaline controls symptoms of asthma and other lung diseases but does not cure them. Continue to use terbutaline even if you feel well. Do not stop using terbutaline without talking to your doctor.

Before you use the terbutaline inhaler the first time, read the written instructions that come with it. Ask your doctor, pharmacist, or respiratory therapist to demonstrate the proper technique. Practice using the inhaler while in his or her presence.

To use the inhaler, follow these steps:
1. Shake the inhaler well.
2. Remove the protective cap.
3. Exhale (breathe out) as completely as possible through your nose while keeping your mouth shut.
4. *Open Mouth Technique:* Open your mouth wide, and place the open end of the mouthpiece about 1-2 inches from your mouth.
   Closed Mouth Technique: Place the open end of the mouthpiece well into your mouth, past your front teeth. Close your lips tightly around the mouthpiece.
5. Take a slow, deep breath through the mouthpiece and, at the same time, press down on the container to spray the medication into your mouth. Be sure that the mist goes into your throat and is not blocked by your teeth or tongue. Adults giving the treatment to young children may hold the child's nose closed to be sure that the medication goes into the child's throat.
6. Hold your breath for 5-10 seconds, remove the inhaler, and exhale slowly through your nose or mouth. If you take 2 puffs, wait 2 minutes and shake the inhaler well before taking the second puff.
7. Replace the protective cap on the inhaler.

If you have difficulty getting the medication into your lungs, a spacer (a special device that attaches to the inhaler) may help; ask your doctor, pharmacist, or respiratory therapist.

Are there other uses for this medicine?

Terbutaline tablets are also used to prevent premature labor in pregnancy. The tablets usually are taken every 4-6 hours until the baby is delivered. Talk to your doctor about the possible risks of using this drug for your condition.

What special precautions should I follow?

Before using terbutaline,
- tell your doctor and pharmacist if you are allergic to terbutaline or any other drugs.
- tell your doctor and pharmacist what prescription medications you are taking, especially atenolol (Tenormin), carteolol (Cartrol), labetalol (Normodyne, Trandate), metoprolol (Lopressor), nadolol (Corgard), phenelzine (Nardil), propranolol (Inderal), sotalol (Betapace), theophylline (Theo-Dur), timolol (Blocadren), tranylcypromine (Parnate), other medications for asthma, heart disease, or depression.
- tell your doctor and pharmacist what nonprescription medications and vitamins you are taking, including ephedrine, phenylephrine, phenylpropanolamine, or pseudoephedrine. Many nonprescription products contain these drugs (e.g., diet pills and medications for colds and asthma), so check labels carefully. Do not take any of these medications without talking to your doctor (even if you never had a problem taking them before).
- tell your doctor if you have or have ever had an irregular heartbeat, increased heart rate, glaucoma, heart disease, high blood pressure, an overactive thyroid gland, diabetes, or seizures.
- tell your doctor if you are pregnant, plan to become pregnant, or are breast-feeding. If you become pregnant while using terbutaline, call your doctor.
- if you are having surgery, including dental surgery, tell the doctor or dentist that you are using terbutaline.

What should I do if I forget to take a dose?

Use the missed dose as soon as you remember it. However, if it is almost time for the next dose, skip the missed dose and continue your regular dosing schedule. Do not use a double dose to make up for a missed one.

What side effects can this medicine cause?

Terbutaline may cause side effects. Tell your doctor if any of these symptoms are severe or do not go away:
- tremor
- nervousness
- dizziness
- drowsiness
- weakness
- headache
- upset stomach
- flushing
- sweating
- dry mouth
- throat irritation

If you experience any of the following symptoms, call your doctor immediately:
- increased difficulty breathing
- rapid or increased heart rate
- irregular heartbeat
- chest pain or discomfort

If you experience a serious side effect, you or your doctor may send a report to the Food and Drug Administration's (FDA) MedWatch Adverse Event Reporting program online [at http://www.fda.gov/MedWatch/index.html] or by phone [1-800-332-1088].

What storage conditions are needed for this medicine?

Keep this medication in the container it came in, tightly closed, and out of reach of children. Store it at room temperature and away from excess heat and moisture (not in the bathroom). Throw away any medication that is outdated or no longer needed. Talk to your pharmacist about the proper disposal of your medication. Avoid puncturing the container, and do not discard it in an incinerator or fire.

What should I do in case of overdose?

In case of overdose, call your local poison control center at 1-800-222-1222. If the victim has collapsed or is not breathing, call local emergency services at 911.

What other information should I know?

Keep all appointments with your doctor and the laboratory. Your doctor will order certain lab tests to check your response to terbutaline.

To relieve dry mouth or throat irritation caused by terbutaline inhalation, rinse your mouth with water, chew gum, or suck sugarless hard candy after using terbutaline.

Inhalation devices require regular cleaning. Once a week, remove the drug container from the plastic mouthpiece, wash the mouthpiece with warm tap water, and dry it thoroughly.

Do not let any one else use your medication. Ask your pharmacist any questions you have about refilling your prescription.

Talk to your doctor, pharmacist, or other healthcare professional if you have questions about dosing information for your medication.

Terconazole Vaginal Cream, Vaginal Suppositories

(ter kon′ a zole)

Brand Name: Terazol® 3, Terazol® 7
Also available generically.

Why is this medicine prescribed?

Terconazole is used to treat fungal and yeast infections of the vagina.

This medication is sometimes prescribed for other uses; ask your doctor or pharmacist for more information.

How should this medicine be used?

Terconazole comes as a cream and suppository to insert into the vagina. It is usually used daily at bedtime for either 3 or 7 days. Follow the directions on your prescription label carefully, and ask your doctor or pharmacist to explain any part you do not understand. Use terconazole exactly as directed. Do not use more or less of it or use it more often than prescribed by your doctor.

To use the vaginal cream or vaginal suppositories, read the instructions provided with the medication and follow these steps:

1. To use the cream, fill the special applicator that comes with the cream to the level indicated. To use the suppository, unwrap it, wet it with lukewarm water, and place it on the applicator as shown in the accompanying instructions.
2. Lie on your back with your knees drawn upward and spread apart.
3. Insert the applicator high into your vagina (unless you are pregnant), and then push the plunger to release the medication. If you are pregnant, insert the applicator gently. If you feel resistance (hard to insert), do not try to insert it further; call your doctor.
4. Withdraw the applicator.
5. Pull the applicator apart and clean it with soap and warm water after each use.
6. Wash your hands promptly to avoid spreading the infection.

The dose should be applied when you lie down to go to bed. The drug works best if you do not get up again after applying it except to wash your hands. You may wish to wear a sanitary napkin to protect your clothing against stains. Do not use a tampon because it will absorb the drug. Do not douche unless your doctor tells you to do so.

Continue to use terconazole even if you feel well. Do not stop using terconazole without talking to your doctor. Continue using this medication during your menstrual period.

What special precautions should I follow?

Before using terconazole,
- tell your doctor and pharmacist if you are allergic to terconazole or any other drugs.
- tell your doctor and pharmacist what prescription and nonprescription drugs you are taking, especially antibiotic medications and vitamins.
- tell your doctor if you have or have ever had problems with your immune system, human immunodeficiency virus infection (HIV), acquired immunodeficiency syndrome (AIDS), or diabetes.
- tell your doctor if you are pregnant, plan to become pregnant, or are breast-feeding. If you become pregnant while using terconazole, call your doctor immediately. Terconazole may harm the fetus.

What should I do if I forget to take a dose?

Insert the missed dose as soon as you remember it. However, if it is almost time for the next dose, skip the missed dose and continue your regular dosing schedule. Do not insert a double dose to make up for a missed one.

What side effects can this medicine cause?

Terconazole may cause side effects. Tell your doctor if any of these symptoms are severe or do not go away:
- headache
- missed menstrual periods

If you experience any of the following symptoms, call your doctor immediately:
- burning in vagina when cream or suppository is inserted
- irritation in vagina when cream or suppository is inserted
- stomach pain
- fever
- foul-smelling vaginal discharge

If you experience a serious side effect, you or your doctor may send a report to the Food and Drug Administration's (FDA) MedWatch Adverse Event Reporting program online [at http://www.fda.gov/MedWatch/index.html] or by phone [1-800-332-1088].

What storage conditions are needed for this medicine?

Keep this medication tightly closed, in the container it came in, and out of reach of children. Store it at room temperature and away from excess heat and moisture (not in the bathroom). Throw away any medication that is outdated or no longer needed. Talk to your pharmacist about the proper disposal of your medication.

What other information should I know?

Keep all appointments with your doctor. Terconazole is for external use only. Do not let cream get into your eyes or mouth, and do not swallow it. Do not swallow the suppositories.

Refrain from sexual intercourse. An ingredient in the cream may weaken certain latex products like condoms or diaphragms; do not use such products within 72 hours of using this medication. Wear clean cotton panties (or panties with cotton crotches), not panties made of nylon, rayon, or other synthetic fabrics.

Do not let anyone else use your medication. Ask your pharmacist any questions you have about refilling your prescription. If you still have symptoms of infection after you finish the terconazole, call your doctor.

Dosage Facts
For Informational Purposes

Caution: Do not change your dose, how often you take your medication, or the length of time you are to take it without first talking to your healthcare provider.

The following dosage information was written using medical language for doctors and other healthcare professionals and is provided here for you to check your dosage. The dosage of this drug may differ for different patients. Therefore, always follow your doctor's instructions or the directions on the label. Contact your healthcare provider or pharmacist if you have any questions about the specific dosage of your medication after reviewing this information.

Adult Patients
Uncomplicated Vulvovaginal Candidiasis

INTRAVAGINAL:
- Cream: one applicatorful of 0.4% cream once daily at bedtime for 7 consecutive days or one applicatorful of 0.8% cream once daily at bedtime for 3 consecutive days.
- Suppository: one 80-mg vaginal suppository once daily at bedtime for 3 consecutive days.

Complicated Vulvovaginal Candidiasis
Recurrent Vulvovaginal Infections Caused by Candida albicans

INTRAVAGINAL:
- CDC and others recommend an initial intensive regimen (7–14 days of an intravaginal azole or 3-dose regimen of oral fluconazole) to achieve mycologic remission, followed by an appropriate maintenance regimen (6-month regimen of once-weekly oral fluconazole or, alternatively, an intravaginal azole given intermittently).

Other Complicated Vulvovaginal Infections

INTRAVAGINAL:
- CDC and others recommend 7–14 days of an intravaginal azole for vulvovaginal candidiasis that is severe, caused by Candida other than C. albicans, or occurring in women with underlying medical conditions.
- HIV-infected patients: Use same regimen recommended for other patients. Some experts recommend a duration of 3–7 days. Maintenance regimen of an intravaginal azole can be considered for those with recurrent episodes; routine primary or secondary prophylaxis (long-term suppressive or chronic maintenance therapy) not recommended.

Special Populations

Hepatic Impairment
- No specific dosage recommendations at this time.

Renal Impairment
- No specific dosage recommendations at this time.

Geriatric Patients
- No specific dosage recommendations at this time.

Teriparatide (rDNA origin) Injection

(terr ih par′ a tyd)

Brand Name: Forteo®

Important Warning

Teriparatide causes osteosarcoma (cancer of the bones) in laboratory rats. It is possible that teriparatide may also increase the chances that humans will develop this rare but serious cancer. Because of this risk, teriparatide should not be used to prevent osteoporosis, to treat mild osteoporosis, or by people who can take other medications for osteoporosis. You should not use teriparatide unless you have osteoporosis and at least one of the following conditions is met: you have already had at least one bone fracture; your doctor has determined that you are at high risk of fractures; or you cannot take or do not respond to other medications for osteoporosis. Tell your doctor if you have or have ever had a bone disease such as Paget's disease, bone cancer or a cancer that has spread to the bone, or radiation therapy of the bones. Your doctor will order certain tests to see if teriparatide is right for you.

Talk to your doctor about the risks of taking teriparatide.

Why is this medicine prescribed?

Teriparatide is used to treat osteoporosis in men and postmenopausal women who are at high risk of fractures (broken bones). Osteoporosis is a disease that causes bones to weaken and break more easily. Teriparatide contains a synthetic form of natural human hormone called parathyroid hormone (PTH). It reduces the risk of fractures by causing the body to build new bone and by increasing bone strength and density (thickness).

How should this medicine be used?

Teriparatide comes as a solution to inject in the fatty layer just under the skin (subcutaneously). It is usually injected once a day. To help you remember to take teriparatide, take it around the same time every day. Follow the directions on your prescription label carefully, and ask your doctor or pharmacist to explain any part you do not understand. Use teriparatide exactly as directed. Do not use more or less of it or use it more often than prescribed by your doctor.

You can inject teriparatide yourself or have a friend or relative perform the injections. Before you use teriparatide yourself the first time, read the written instructions that come with it. Ask your doctor or pharmacist to show you or the person who will be injecting the medication how to inject it. The instructions for use include solutions to problems you may have when you try to use teriparatide. Check the instructions if you have difficulty following the directions below.

Teriparatide comes in a pen that contains enough medication for 28 doses. Use a new needle for each injection. Needles are sold separately. Ask your doctor or pharmacist if you have questions about the type of needles to use. Dispose of used needles in a puncture-resistant container. Talk to your doctor or pharmacist about how to dispose of the puncture-resistant container.

To inject teriparatide, follow these steps:

1. Remove your teriparatide pen from the refrigerator and check to be sure it is safe to use. It should be labeled with the correct name of the medication and an expiration date that has not passed and should contain a clear colorless solution. Do not use the syringe if it is expired, is cloudy, or contains flakes. Do not remove the pen from the refrigerator until you are ready to begin the injection process. There is no need to allow the medication to warm up before use.
2. Wash your hands with soap and water.
3. Pull off the pen cap and wipe the rubber seal on the end of the pen with an alcohol swab.
4. Get a fresh needle to attach to the pen. Remove the paper tab from the outer needle shield but do not remove the cap. Place the needle over the end of the pen and turn it to the right until it is tight.
5. Hold the pen with the needle pointing up and remove both needle shields. You may throw away the inner shield, but save the outer shield to use when you remove the needle.
6. Turn the dose knob to the right until an arrow appears in the dose window. The raised notches on the pen and dose knob will be in line.
7. Pull the dose knob out until you see a zero in the dose window.
8. Turn the knob to the right until the number 1 appears in the dose window.
9. Hold the pen with the needle pointing up and gently tap the clear cartridge holder with your finger so that air bubbles collect near the top.
10. Push the injection button all the way up with your thumb. A small amount of liquid will come out of the needle. Keep pressing until the liquid stops coming out. A diamond will appear in the dose window. If no liquid

comes out of the needle when you push the button, repeat steps 6-10.
11. Turn the knob to the right until an arrow appears in the dose window. The raised notches on the dose knob and pen will be in line.
12. Pull the dose knob out until you see a zero in the dose window.
13. Turn the knob to the right until the number 2 appears in the dose window. The pen is now ready to inject.
14. Choose an injection site on either of your thighs or your stomach, and clean it as directed by your doctor. Be sure a chair or bed is nearby so you can sit or lie down if you are dizzy after the injection.
15. Gently pinch up a fold of skin, and push the needle straight in. Look at the dose window to be sure it still shows the number 2.
16. Use your thumb to push the injection button all the way in. Hold the button down while counting slowly to 5.
17. Remove the needle from your skin. You should see a diamond in the dose window. If you do not see a diamond, you did not receive the full dose, and you should call your doctor for directions.
18. Carefully replace the outer needle shield. Your doctor will show you how to do this. Remove the capped needle by turning it to the left; throw it away.
19. Put the cap back onto the pen and check the markings on the cartridge holder. These markings tell how much medication is left in the pen. Be sure your next pen is ready when the bottom of the plunger reaches the 60 mark.
20. Put the pen back in the refrigerator right away.

Teriparatide controls osteoporosis but does not cure it. Continue to take teriparatide even if you feel well. Do not stop taking teriparatide without talking to your doctor.

Are there other uses for this medicine?

This medication may be prescribed for other uses; ask your doctor or pharmacist for more information.

What special precautions should I follow?

Before taking teriparatide,

- tell your doctor and pharmacist if you are allergic to teriparatide, mannitol, or any other medications.
- tell your doctor and pharmacist what prescription and nonprescription medications, vitamins, nutritional supplements, and herbal products you are taking. Be sure to mention either of the following: digoxin (Digitek, Lanoxin) and hydrochlorothiazide (HCTZ, Hydrodiuril, Microzide). Your doctor may need to change the doses of your medications or monitor you carefully for side effects.
- in addition to the conditions listed in the IMPORTANT WARNING section, tell your doctor if you have or have ever had any condition that causes you to have too much calcium in your blood, such as disease of the parathyroid gland; kidney or urinary tract stones; and liver, kidney, or heart disease.

- you should know that teriparatide should only be used by women once they have passed menopause and, therefore, cannot become pregnant or breastfeed. Teriparatide should not be used during pregnancy or while breast-feeding.
- you should know that teriparatide may cause fast heartbeat, dizziness, lightheadedness, and fainting when you get up too quickly from a lying position. This is more common when you first start taking teriparatide. To avoid this problem, get out of bed slowly, resting your feet on the floor for a few minutes before standing up. Be sure a chair is nearby when you inject teriparatide so you can sit down if you get dizzy.

What special dietary instructions should I follow?

It is important that you get enough calcium and vitamin D while you are taking teriparatide. Your doctor may prescribe supplements if your dietary intake is not enough. Talk to your doctor about doing weight-bearing exercise. Also talk to your doctor about avoiding cigarette smoking and avoiding drinking large amounts of alcohol.

What should I do if I forget to take a dose?

Take the missed dose as soon as you remember it that day. However, if the day has already passed, skip the missed dose and continue your regular dosing schedule. Never inject more than one dose per day.

What side effects can this medicine cause?

Teriparatide may cause side effects. Tell your doctor if any of these symptoms or those listed in the SPECIAL PRECAUTIONS section are severe or do not go away:

- pain
- headache
- weakness
- diarrhea
- heartburn or sour stomach
- leg cramps
- dizziness
- depression

Some side effects can be serious. The following symptoms are uncommon, but if you experience any of them call your doctor immediately:

- chest pain
- fainting
- difficulty breathing
- fever, sore throat, chills, and other signs of infection
- upset stomach
- vomiting
- constipation
- lack of energy
- muscle weakness

Teriparatide may cause other side effects. Call your doctor if you have any unusual problems while taking this medication.

If you experience a serious side effect, you or your doctor may send a report to the Food and Drug Administration's (FDA) MedWatch Adverse Event Reporting program online [at http://www.fda.gov/MedWatch/index.html] or by phone [1-800-332-1088].

What storage conditions are needed for this medicine?

Keep this medication in the pen it came in with the cap on and without a needle attached, tightly closed, and out of reach of children. Store it in the refrigerator but do not freeze it. Protect it from light. Throw away any medication that is outdated or no longer needed. Throw away the pen 28 days after you first use it, even if it is not empty. Talk to your pharmacist about the proper disposal of your medication.

What should I do in case of overdose?

In case of overdose, call your local poison control center at 1-800-222-1222. If the victim has collapsed or is not breathing, call local emergency services at 911.

Symptoms of overdose may include:

- upset stomach
- vomiting
- dizziness
- headache
- lightheadedness and fainting on standing
- constipation
- lack of energy
- muscle weakness

What other information should I know?

Keep all appointments with your doctor and the laboratory. Your doctor will order certain lab tests to check your body's response to teriparatide.

Do not let anyone else take your medication. Never share a teriparatide pen. Ask your pharmacist any questions you have about refilling your prescription.

Dosage Facts
For Informational Purposes

Caution: Do not change your dose, how often you take your medication, or the length of time you are to take it without first talking to your healthcare provider.

The following dosage information was written using medical language for doctors and other healthcare professionals and is provided here for you to check your dosage. The dosage of this drug may differ for different patients. Therefore, always follow your doctor's instructions or the directions on the label. Contact your healthcare provider or pharmacist if you have any questions about the specific dosage of your medication after reviewing this information.

Adult Patients

Osteoporosis in Postmenopausal Women

SUB-Q:
- 20 mcg once daily.

Osteoporosis in Men

SUB-Q:
- 20 mcg once daily.

Testosterone Buccal

(tes tos' ter one)

Brand Name: Striant®
Also available generically.

Why is this medicine prescribed?

Testosterone buccal systems are used to treat the symptoms of low testosterone in men who do not produce enough natural testosterone. Testosterone is a hormone that is usually produced by the body that contributes to the growth, development, and functioning of the male sexual organs and typical male characteristics. Symptoms of low testosterone include decreased sexual desire and ability, extreme tiredness, low energy, depression, and loss of certain male characteristics such as muscular build and deep voice. Testosterone buccal systems work by supplying synthetic testosterone to replace the testosterone that is normally produced naturally.

How should this medicine be used?

Buccal testosterone comes as a system (tablet shaped patch) to apply to the upper gum. It is usually applied twice a day around every 12 hours. To help you remember to apply testosterone buccal systems, apply them at about the same times each day. It may be convenient to apply the systems after you eat breakfast and brush your teeth, and after dinner. Follow the directions on your prescription label carefully, and ask your doctor or pharmacist to explain any part you do not understand. Apply testosterone buccal systems exactly as directed. Do not apply more or fewer systems or apply the systems more often than prescribed by your doctor.

You should apply testosterone buccal systems to the areas of your upper gum that are above the left and right incisors (the teeth just to the left and right of the two front teeth). Alternate sides at every dose so that you never apply a system to the same side 2 doses in a row.

Testosterone buccal systems only work when applied to the upper gum. Although the systems look like tablets, you should not chew or swallow them.

Testosterone buccal systems will soften and mold to the shape of your gum and will gradually release medication. However, they will not dissolve completely in your mouth and must be removed after 12 hours.

You may brush your teeth; use mouthwash; use tobacco products; chew gum; eat; and drink alcoholic or nonalcoholic beverages while you are wearing a testosterone buccal system. However, these activities may cause the system to fall off your gum. After you are finished the activity, check to be sure the system is still in place.

If your testosterone buccal system does not stick or falls off within 8 hours after you apply it, replace it with a new system immediately and apply your next dose at the regularly scheduled time. If your system falls off more than 8 hours after you apply it, apply a new system immediately and do not apply a new system at the regularly scheduled time. The replacement system will take the place of your next dose.

Testosterone buccal systems may control your condition but will not cure it. Continue to use testosterone even if you feel well. Do not stop using testosterone without talking to your doctor. If you stop using testosterone, your symptoms may return.

To apply testosterone buccal systems, follow these steps:
1. Push one system out through the back of the blister card. Notice that one side of the system is flat and is marked with the company logo and the other side is curved.
2. Place the system on your fingertip with the flat side against your finger.
3. Gently press the curved side of the system against the proper area of your upper gum. Push the system as high up on your gum as possible.
4. Place your finger on the outside of your upper lip over the spot where you applied the testosterone buccal system. Press down on the spot for 30 seconds to help the system stick to your gum.
5. The testosterone buccal system should now be stuck to your gum. If it is stuck to your cheek, you may leave it in place. The system will still release medication properly when stuck to your cheek

To remove testosterone buccal systems, follow these steps:
1. Gently slide the system to the front or back of your mouth to loosen it.
2. Slide the system down from your gum to a tooth. Be careful not to scratch your gum.
3. Remove the system from your mouth and thow it away in a trash can that is out of the reach of children and pets. Children and pets can be harmed if they chew on or play with used systems.
4. Apply a new system following the directions above.

Are there other uses for this medicine?

This medication may be prescribed for other uses; ask your doctor or pharmacist for more information.

What special precautions should I follow?

Before using testosterone buccal systems,
- tell your doctor and pharmacist if you are allergic to testosterone, soy, or any other medications.

- tell your doctor and pharmacist what prescription and nonprescription medications, vitamins, nutritional supplements, and herbal products you are taking. Be sure to mention any of the following: insulin (Humulin, Humalog, Novolin, others) or oral steroids such as dexamethasone, (Decadron, Dexone), methylprednisolone (Medrol), and prednisone (Deltasone). Your doctor may need to change the doses of your medications or monitor you carefully for side effects.
- tell your doctor if you have a family history of prostate cancer, if you smoke or work with heavy metals such as cadmium, and if you have or have ever had breast or prostate cancer; enlarged prostate; diabetes; or heart, kidney, liver, or lung disease.
- you should know that testosterone buccal systems are only for use in men. Women should not use this medication, especially if they are or may become pregnant or are breast-feeding. Testosterone may harm the fetus.
- you should check your gums regularly while you are using this medication. Call your doctor if you notice any changes in your gums.

What special dietary instructions should I follow?

Unless your doctor tells you otherwise, continue your normal diet.

What should I do if I forget to take a dose?

Remove the old system and apply a new one as soon as you remember it. If you remember within 8 hours after the usual application time, keep the new system in place until your next scheduled application time. If you remember more than 8 hours after the usual application time, do not remove the new system at the next scheduled application time.

What side effects can this medicine cause?

Testosterone buccal systems may cause side effects. Tell your doctor if any of these symptoms are severe or do not go away:
- irritation, redness, pain, tenderness, swelling, toughening, or blistering of gums
- stinging of lips
- toothache
- unpleasant or bitter taste in mouth
- difficulty tasting food
- headache
- stomach pain or cramps
- acne
- nervousness
- swelling of nose

Some side effects can be serious. The following symptoms are uncommon, but if you experience any of them, call your doctor immediately:
- swelling of the hands, feet, ankles, and lower legs
- sudden unexplained weight gain
- difficulty breathing, especially at night

- erections of the penis that happen too often or do not go away
- upset stomach
- vomiting
- stomach pain or cramping
- loss of appetite
- extreme tiredness
- yellowing of the skin or eyes
- dark urine
- light colored stool
- difficulty urinating
- breast pain or enlargement
- depression or other mood changes

Medications similar to testosterone that are taken by mouth for a long time may cause serious damage to the liver or liver cancer. Testosterone buccal systems have not been shown to cause this damage. Testosterone may increase the risk of developing prostate cancer. Talk to your doctor about the risks of taking this medication.

Testosterone buccal systems may cause other side effects. Call your doctor if you have any unusual problems while using this medication.

If you experience a serious side effect, you or your doctor may send a report to the Food and Drug Administration's (FDA) MedWatch Adverse Event Reporting program online [at http://www.fda.gov/MedWatch/index.html] or by phone [1-800-332-1088].

What storage conditions are needed for this medicine?

Keep this medication in the container it came in, tightly closed, and out of reach of children. Store it at room temperature and away from excess heat and moisture (not in the bathroom). Protect this medication from theft. Throw away any medication that is outdated or no longer needed. Talk to your pharmacist about the proper disposal of your medication.

What should I do in case of overdose?

In case of overdose, call your local poison control center at 1-800-222-1222. If the victim has collapsed or is not breathing, call local emergency services at 911.

Symptoms of overdose may include:
- slow or difficult speech
- faintness
- weakness or numbness of an arm or leg

What other information should I know?

Keep all appointments with your doctor and the laboratory. Your doctor may order certain lab tests to check your body's response to testosterone buccal systems.

Before having any laboratory tests, tell your doctor and the laboratory personnel that you are using testosterone buccal systems. This medication may affect the results of certain laboratory tests.

Do not let anyone else take your medication. Ask your

pharmacist any questions you have about refilling your prescription.

Dosage Facts
For Informational Purposes

Caution: Do not change your dose, how often you take your medication, or the length of time you are to take it without first talking to your healthcare provider.

The following dosage information was written using medical language for doctors and other healthcare professionals and is provided here for you to check your dosage. The dosage of this drug may differ for different patients. Therefore, always follow your doctor's instructions or the directions on the label. Contact your healthcare provider or pharmacist if you have any questions about the specific dosage of your medication after reviewing this information.

General Dosage Information

Available as testosterone; dosage expressed in terms of testosterone.

Adult Patients

Male Hypogonadism

INTRABUCCAL:
- 30 mg (1 extended-release transmucosal tablet) twice daily (morning and evening) about 12 hours apart. Serum testosterone concentration may be determined just prior to the morning dose at 4–12 weeks after initiation of intrabuccal therapy; if total serum testosterone concentration is excessive, discontinue intrabuccal therapy and consider alternative treatments.

Testosterone Topical

(tes tos' ter one)

Brand Name: Androgel®, Testim®
Also available generically.

Why is this medicine prescribed?

Testosterone topical gel is used to treat the symptoms of low testosterone in men who do not produce enough natural testosterone. Testosterone is a hormone that is usually produced by the body that is needed for the growth and functioning of the male sexual organs and for the development of typical male characteristics. Symptoms of low testosterone include decreased sexual desire and ability, extreme tiredness, low energy, depression, brittle bones that may break easily, and loss of certain male characteristics such as muscular build and deep voice. Testosterone gel works by supplying testosterone to replace the testosterone that is normally produced in the body.

How should this medicine be used?

Topical testosterone comes as a gel to apply to the skin. It is usually applied once a day. It is best to apply testosterone gel in the morning. To help you remember to use testosterone gel, use it at around the same time every day. Follow the directions on your prescription label carefully, and ask your doctor or pharmacist to explain any part you do not understand. Use testosterone gel exactly as directed. Do not apply more or less of it or apply it more often than prescribed by your doctor.

AndroGel® and Testim® brand gels both contain testosterone, but they are manufactured differently and are used in slightly different ways. Be sure that you know which brand of gel you are using and how and where you should apply it. Read the manufacturer's patient information that came with your gel carefully.

You can apply AndroGel® anywhere on your shoulders, upper arms, or abdomen (area between your chest and your waist). You can apply Testim® anywhere on your shoulders or upper arms, but you should *not* apply it to your abdomen. You should *not* apply either gel to your penis or scrotum or to skin that has sores, cuts, or irritation.

Be careful not to get testosterone gel in your eyes. If you do get testosterone gel in your eyes, wash them right away with warm, clean water. Call a doctor if your eyes become irritated.

You should not shower, bathe, swim, or wash the place where you applied the medication for at least 2 hours after you apply Testim® gel or at least 5-6 hours after you apply AndroGel®. Once in while, you may shower, bathe or swim as soon as 1 hour after you apply AndroGel®, but you should usually wait the full 5-6 hours. If you usually take a bath or shower in the morning, be sure to take your bath or shower before you apply either brand of testosterone gel.

Testosterone gel comes in single use tubes and packets and a multiple use pump. The pump releases a specific amount of testosterone gel each time the top is pressed. You will probably need to press the top of the pump four to eight times to get your full dose of testosterone gel. Your doctor or pharmacist will tell you how many times to press the pump for each dose, and how many doses your pump contains. Throw away the pump after you have used that number of doses even if it is not empty.

Testosterone gel may catch fire. Stay away from open flames and do not smoke while you are applying testosterone gel and until the gel has dried completely.

Your doctor may start you on a low dose of testosterone gel and gradually increase your dose, not more than once every two weeks.

Testosterone gel may control your condition but will not cure it. Continue to use testosterone gel even if you feel well. Do not stop using testosterone gel without talking to your doctor. If you stop using testosterone gel, your symptoms may return.

To use testosterone gel, follow these steps:

1. Be sure that the skin in the place where you plan to apply testosterone gel is completely dry.
2. Open your container of testosterone gel. If you are using a packet, fold the top edge at the perforation and tear across the packet along the perforation. If you are using a tube, unscrew the cap. If you are using a pump for the first time, press down on the top of the pump three times and discard the medication that comes out down a drain or in a trash can that is safe from children and pets.
3. Squeeze the packet or tube or press down on the top of the pump the right number of times to place the medication on the palm of your hand. It may be easier to apply testosterone gel if you squeeze the medication onto your palm and apply it to your skin in small portions.
4. Apply the medication to the area you have chosen.
5. Throw away the empty packet or tube in a trash can that is safe from children and pets.
6. Wash your hands with soap and water right away.
7. Allow the medication to dry for a few minutes before you cover the area with clothing.

Are there other uses for this medicine?

This medication may be prescribed for other uses; ask your doctor or pharmacist for more information.

What special precautions should I follow?

Before using testosterone gel,

- tell your doctor and pharmacist if you are allergic to testosterone, any other medications, or soy.
- tell your doctor and pharmacist what prescription and nonprescription medications, vitamins, nutritional supplements, and herbal products you are taking. Be sure to mention any of the following: inhaled steroids such as beclomethasone (QVAR), budesonide (Pulmicort), flunisolide (AeroBid), fluticasone (Flovent), and triamcinolone (Azmacort); insulin (Humalin, Humalog, Novolin, others); oral steroids such as dexamethasone (Decadron, Dexone), methylprednisolone (Medrol), and prednisone (Deltasone); propranolol (Inderal); and steroid creams, lotions, or ointments such as alclometasone (Aclovate), betamethasone (Diprolene, Diprosone, Valisone), clobetasol (Temovate), desonide (DesOwen), desoximetasone (Topicort), diflorasone (Psorcon, Florone), fluocinolone (Derma-Smoothe, Flurosyn, Synalar), fluocinonide (Lidex), flurandrenolide (Cordran), fluticasone (Cutivate), halcinonide (Halog), halobetasol (Ultravate), hydrocortisone (Cortizone, Westcort, others), mometasone (Elocon), and triamcinolone (Aristocort). Your doctor may need to change the doses of your medications or monitor you carefully for side effects.
- tell your doctor if you or anyone in your family has or has ever had prostate cancer or if a doctor has told you that you might have prostate cancer if you smoke or work with heavy metals such as cadmium and if you have or have ever had breast cancer, diabetes, or heart, kidney, liver, or lung disease.

- you should know that testosterone gel is only for use in men. Women should not use this medication, especially if they are or may become pregnant or are breastfeeding. Testosterone may harm the fetus.
- you should know that testosterone gel can harm people who touch the skin where you applied it. It is most harmful to women, especially if they are pregnant, and children. Cover the place where you applied testosterone gel with a shirt to prevent others from touching it. If you expect direct skin contact with someone else, you should wash the place where you applied testosterone gel with soap and water first. However, it is best to wait several hours after you apply the medication before you wash the area. If someone else touches the testosterone gel in your container or the place where you applied testosterone gel, that person should wash the area with soap and water as soon as possible. Tell your doctor if your female partner or anyone who has touched testosterone gel develops acne or grows hair in new places on his or her body.

What special dietary instructions should I follow?

Unless your doctor tells you otherwise, continue your normal diet.

What should I do if I forget to take a dose?

If your next scheduled dose is not due for 12 hours or longer, apply the missed dose as soon as you remember it. However, if your next dose is due in less than 12 hours, skip the missed dose and continue your regular dosing schedule. Do not apply a double dose to make up for a missed one.

What side effects can this medicine cause?

Testosterone gel may cause side effects. Tell your doctor if any of these symptoms are severe or do not go away:

- breast enlargement and/or pain
- decreased sexual desire
- acne
- hair loss
- hot flushes
- depression
- mood changes
- nervousness
- headache
- difficulty falling asleep or staying asleep
- teary eyes
- changes in ability to smell or taste

Some side effects can be serious. The following symptoms are uncommon, but if you experience any of them, call your doctor immediately:

- swelling of the hands, feet, ankles, or lower legs
- breathing problems, especially during sleep
- erections that happen too often or that last too long
- difficulty urinating
- frequent urination, especially at night

- upset stomach
- vomiting
- yellow or darkened skin

Medications similar to testosterone that are taken by mouth for a long time may cause serious damage to the liver or liver cancer. Testosterone gel has not been shown to cause this damage. Testosterone may increase the risk of developing prostate cancer. Talk to your doctor about the risks of taking this medication.

Testosterone gel may cause other side effects. Call your doctor if you have any unusual problems while taking this medication.

If you experience a serious side effect, you or your doctor may send a report to the Food and Drug Administration's (FDA) MedWatch Adverse Event Reporting program online [at http://www.fda.gov/MedWatch/index.html] or by phone [1-800-332-1088].

What storage conditions are needed for this medicine?

Keep this medication in the container it came in, tightly closed, and out of reach of children. Store it at room temperature and away from excess heat and moisture (not in the bathroom). Throw away any medication that is outdated or no longer needed. Talk to your pharmacist about the proper disposal of your medication.

What should I do in case of overdose?

In case of overdose, call your local poison control center at 1-800-222-1222. If the victim has collapsed or is not breathing, call local emergency services at 911.

Symptoms of overdose may include:

- slow or difficult speech
- faintness
- weakness or numbness of an arm or leg

What other information should I know?

Keep all appointments with your doctor and the laboratory. Your doctor will order certain lab tests to check your body's response to testosterone gel.

Before having any laboratory test, tell your doctor and the laboratory personnel that you are using testosterone gel.

Do not let anyone else use your medication. Ask your pharmacist any questions you have about refilling your prescription.

Dosage Facts
For Informational Purposes

Caution: Do not change your dose, how often you take your medication, or the length of time you are to take it without first talking to your health-care provider.

The following dosage information was written using medical language for doctors and other healthcare pro-

fessionals and is provided here for you to check your dosage. The dosage of this drug may differ for different patients. Therefore, always follow your doctor's instructions or the directions on the label. Contact your healthcare provider or pharmacist if you have any questions about the specific dosage of your medication after reviewing this information.

General Dosage Information

Available as testosterone; dosage expressed in terms of testosterone. Also available as testosterone enanthante or testosterone cypionate; dosage expressed in terms of the salts.

AndroGel® unit-dose packets contain 2.5 or 5 g of gel (25 or 50 mg of testosterone). Each depression of the metered-dose pump delivers 1.25 g of gel (12.5 mg of testosterone) after priming.

Testim® unit-dose tubes contain 5 g of gel (50 mg of testosterone).

Adult Patients
Male Hypogonadism

TOPICAL (GEL):

- AndroGel® and Testim®: Apply 50 mg of testosterone (5 g of 1% gel) once daily, preferably in the morning; this dose delivers about 5 mg of testosterone systemically. Adjust dosage according to serum testosterone concentrations obtained approximately 14 days after initiating daily application of the gel.
- AndroGel®: If serum testosterone concentrations are below the normal range or the clinical response is inadequate, the dosage can be increased initially to 75 mg of testosterone (7.5 g of 1% gel) and, if necessary, subsequently to 100 mg of testosterone (10 g of 1% gel).
- Testim®: If serum testosterone concentrations are below the normal range or the clinical response is inadequate, the dosage can be increased to 100 mg of testosterone (10 g of 1% gel).

Testosterone Transdermal

(tes tos' ter one)

Brand Name: Androderm®, Testoderm®, Testoderm® TTS

Also available generically.

Why is this medicine prescribed?

Testosterone transdermal patches are used to treat the symptoms of low testosterone in men who do not produce enough natural testosterone. Testosterone is a hormone that is usually produced by the body that contributes to the growth, development, and functioning of the male sexual organs and typical male characteristics. Symptoms of low testosterone include decreased sexual desire and ability, extreme tiredness, low energy, depression, and loss of certain male characteristics such as muscular build and deep voice. Testosterone patches work by supplying synthetic testosterone to replace testosterone that is normally produced naturally.

How should this medicine be used?

Transdermal testosterone comes as a patch to apply to the skin. It is usually applied once daily, and the schedule depends on the type of patch. Androderm patches are applied each night between 8 pm and midnight and left on for 24 hours. Testoderm patches are applied at the same time every morning (or any other regular time of day or night if the morning is inconvenient) and left on for 22-24 hours. Follow the directions on your prescription label carefully, and ask your doctor or pharmacist to explain any part you do not understand. Use testosterone patches exactly as directed. Do not apply more or fewer patches or apply the patches more often than prescribed by your doctor.

Androderm and Testoderm brand patches both contain testosterone, but they are manufactured differently and are intended for use on different parts of the body. Be sure you know which type of patch you are using and where, when, and how you are to apply your patches. Carefully read the manufacturer's patient information that comes with your patches.

If you are using Androderm patches, you should choose a spot on your back, stomach, thighs, or upper arms to apply your patch(es). Be sure that the spot you have chosen is not oily, hairy, likely to perspire heavily, over a bone such as a shoulder or hip, or likely to be under pressure from sitting or sleeping. Do not apply to the scrotum or a skin area with open sores or irritation. Also be sure that the patch will stay flat against the skin and will not be pulled or stretched during normal activity. Choose a different spot each night and wait at least 7 days before applying another patch to a spot you have used.

If you are using Testoderm patches, you should apply them to your scrotum. Before you begin treatment, you should shave the hair from the area. Stretch your scrotal skin and shave with short gentle strokes of a disposable razor. Do not use soap, water, lotions, creams, or chemical hair removers. You should shave the area whenever hair has grown back, usually once or twice a week.

Androderm patches may be worn while swimming, bathing, or showering. However, Testoderm patches should be removed before water activities and placed on a clean, dry surface with the shiny side facing up. After water activities, dry your body and reapply the patch using the regular procedure.

If a patch becomes loose, smooth it down with your fingers. If it falls off, try to reapply the same patch. If the patch cannot be reapplied, apply a new one. However, if an Androderm patch falls off after twelve noon or if a Testoderm patch falls off after you have worn it for 12 hours, do not apply a new patch until your next scheduled application time.

Testosterone patches may control your condition but will not cure it. It may take up to 8 weeks before you feel the full benefit of testosterone. Continue to use testosterone patches even if you feel well. Do not stop using testosterone patches without talking to your doctor. If you stop using testosterone, your symptoms may return.

To use Androderm patches, follow these steps:

1. Clean and dry the spot where you will apply the patch.
2. Tear the foil pouch along the edge and remove the patch.
3. Peel the protective liner and silver disc off the patch and throw them away.
4. Place the patch on your skin with the sticky side down and press down firmly with your palm for 10 seconds. Be sure it is completely stuck to your skin, especially around the edges.
5. When you are ready to remove the patch, pull it off the skin and throw it away in a trash can that is out of the reach of children and pets. Children and pets can be harmed if they chew on or play with used patches.
6. Apply a new patch immediately by following steps 1-4.

To use Testoderm patches, follow these steps:

1. Be sure that your scrotum and your hands are warm and dry.
2. Tear the pouch along the top edge and remove the patch.
3. Peel the clear plastic liner off the patch and throw it away.
4. Warm the patch by holding it a few inches away from a mild heat source such as a light bulb or blowdryer.
5. Sit or stand in a comfortable position. Stretch the skin of your scrotum to smooth out the folds.
6. Press the shiny side of the patch onto your scrotum. Cup your hand over the patch and hold it in place for 10 seconds.
7. Be sure that the edges of the patch are pressed firmly against your skin. If the patch falls off, repeat steps 4-6. Be sure to warm the patch again and try holding it in place for longer than 10 seconds.
8. Put on close fitting underwear to hold the patch in place. If the patch still falls off, wearing an athletic supporter may help.
9. When you are ready to remove the patch, gently peel it off the skin and throw it away in a trash can that is out of the reach of children and pets. Children and pets can be harmed if they chew on or play with used patches.

Are there other uses for this medicine?

This medication may be prescribed for other uses; ask your doctor or pharmacist for more information.

What special precautions should I follow?

Before using testosterone patches,

- tell your doctor and pharmacist if you are allergic to testosterone, ethanol, or any other medications.
- tell your doctor and pharmacist what prescription and nonprescription medications, vitamins, nutritional supplements, and herbal products you are taking. Be sure

to mention any of the following: anticoagulants ('blood thinners') such as warfarin (Coumadin); insulin (Humalin, Humalog, Novolin, others); oral steroids such as dexamethasone (Decadron, Dexone), methylprednisolone (Medrol), and prednisone (Deltasone); and propranolol (Inderal). Your doctor may need to change the doses of your medications or monitor you carefully for side effects.

- tell your doctor if you have a family history of prostate cancer, if you smoke or work with heavy metals such as cadmium and if you have or have ever had a blood disorder, breast or prostate cancer, diabetes, or heart, kidney, liver, or lung disease.
- you should know that transdermal testosterone is only for use in men. Women should not use this medication, especially if they are or may become pregnant or are breastfeeding. Testosterone may harm the fetus.
- you should know that Androderm and Testoderm patches may be worn during sexual activity. It is very unlikely that your partner will be exposed to more than slight amounts of testosterone. However, there is a slight possiblity that the patch may be transferred to the partner's skin. If this happens, remove the patch and wash the area well. Call a doctor immediately if your female partner develops bad acne or grows hair in new places on her body.
- if you are using Androderm patches, your skin may become irritated in the place where you apply the patch(es). If this happens, you may apply a small amount of hydrocortisone cream to the area after removing your patch(es). Only use hydrocortisone cream; do not use an ointment. If your skin remains irritated after this treatment, call your doctor.

What special dietary instructions should I follow?

Unless your doctor tells you otherwise, continue your normal diet.

What should I do if I forget to take a dose?

Apply the missed patch(es) as soon as you remember. However, if it is almost time for the next dose, skip the missed dose and continue your regular dosing schedule. Do not apply extra patches to make up for a missed dose.

What side effects can this medicine cause?

Transdermal testosterone may cause side effects. Tell your doctor if any of these symptoms are severe or do not go away:

- itching, pain, or irritation of scrotum if you are using Testoderm patches
- burn-like blisters, pain, redness, hardness, or itching in the place you applied Androderm patches
- enlarged or tender breasts
- acne
- depression

- headache
- dizziness
- pain anywhere in the body, especially the back

Some side effects can be serious. The following symptoms are uncommon, but if you experience any of them, call your doctor immediately:

- erections that happen too often or that do not go away
- upset stomach
- vomiting
- yellowing of skin or eyes
- ankle swelling
- changes in skin color
- difficulty breathing while awake or asleep
- pain in pelvis (area between hips)
- difficult, frequent, or painful urination
- painful ejaculation
- fever or chills
- black and tarry stools
- red blood in stools
- bloody vomit
- vomiting material that looks like coffee grounds
- slow or difficult speech
- faintness
- weakness or numbness of an arm or leg
- rash

Medications similar to testosterone that are taken by mouth for a long time may cause serious damage to the liver or liver cancer. Transdermal testosterone has not been shown to cause this damage. Testosterone may increase the risk of developing prostate cancer. Talk to your doctor about the risks of taking this medication.

Testosterone may cause other side effects. Call your doctor if you have any unusual problems while taking this medication.

If you experience a serious side effect, you or your doctor may send a report to the Food and Drug Administration's (FDA) MedWatch Adverse Event Reporting program online [at http://www.fda.gov/MedWatch/index.html] or by phone [1-800-332-1088].

What storage conditions are needed for this medicine?

Keep this medication in the container it came in, tightly closed, and out of reach of children. Store it at room temperature and away from excess heat and moisture (not in the bathroom). Use patches immediately after opening the protective pouch. Androderm patches may burst if exposed to extreme heat or pressure. Do not use damaged patches. Throw away any medication that is outdated or no longer needed. Talk to your pharmacist about the proper disposal of your medication.

What should I do in case of overdose?

If you wear too many patches, or wear patches for too long, too much testosterone may be absorbed into your bloodstream. In that case, you may experience symptoms of an overdose.

In case of overdose, call your local poison control center at 1-800-222-1222. If the victim has collapsed or is not breathing, call local emergency services at 911.

Symptoms of overdose may include:
- slow or difficult speech
- faintness
- weakness or numbness of an arm or leg

What other information should I know?

Keep all appointments with your doctor and the laboratory. Your doctor will order certain lab tests to check your body's response to testosterone.

Testosterone can interfere with the results of certain laboratory tests. Before having any tests, tell your doctor and the laboratory personnel that you are taking testosterone.

Do not let anyone else take your medication. Ask your pharmacist any questions you have about refilling your prescription.

Dosage Facts

For Informational Purposes

Caution: Do not change your dose, how often you take your medication, or the length of time you are to take it without first talking to your healthcare provider.

The following dosage information was written using medical language for doctors and other healthcare professionals and is provided here for you to check your dosage. The dosage of this drug may differ for different patients. Therefore, always follow your doctor's instructions or the directions on the label. Contact your healthcare provider or pharmacist if you have any questions about the specific dosage of your medication after reviewing this information.

General Dosage Information

Available as testosterone; dosage expressed in terms of testosterone. Also available as testosterone enanthante or testosterone cypionate; dosage expressed in terms of the salts.

Adult Patients

Male Hypogonadism

TOPICAL (TRANSDERMAL SYSTEM):
- Usual initial dosage is 1 system delivering 5 mg/24 hours or 2 systems delivering 2.5 mg/24 hours applied to the skin nightly.
- Adjust dosage according to morning serum testosterone concentrations. Depending on requirements, increase dosage to 7.5 mg once daily (administered nightly as 1 system delivering 5 mg/24 hours plus 1 system delivering 2.5 mg/24 hours or as 3 systems delivering 2.5 mg/24 hours) or decrease dosage to 2.5 mg once daily (administered nightly as 1 system delivering 2.5 mg/24 hours).

Tetanus and Diphtheria Vaccine

Brand Name: Decavac®

About the Diseases

Tetanus and diphtheria are serious diseases. Tetanus is caused by a germ that enters the body through a cut or wound. Diphtheria spreads when germs pass from an infected person to the nose or throat of others.

TETANUS (Lockjaw) causes painful tightening of the muscles, usually all over the body. It can lead to "locking" of the jaw so the victim cannot open his mouth or swallow. Tetanus leads to death in about 1 out of 10 cases.

DIPHTHERIA causes a thick covering in the back of the throat. It can lead to breathing problems, paralysis, heart failure, and even death.

Benefits of the vaccines

Vaccination is the best way to protect against tetanus and diphtheria. Because of vaccination, there are many fewer cases of these diseases. Cases are rare in children because most get DTaP (Diphtheria, Tetanus, and acellular Pertussis) or DT (Diphtheria and Tetanus) vaccines. There would be many more cases if we stopped vaccinating people.

When should you get Td vaccine?

Td is made for people 7 years of age and older.

People who have not gotten at least 3 doses of any tetanus and diphtheria vaccine (DTP, DTaP or DT) during their lifetime should do so using Td. After a person gets the third dose, a Td dose is needed every 10 years all through life.

Other vaccines may be given at the same time as Td.

Tell your doctor or nurse if the person getting the vaccine:
- ever had a serious allergic reaction or other problem with Td, or any other tetanus and diphtheria vaccine (DTP, DTaP or DT)
- now has a moderate or severe illness
- is pregnant

What are the risks from Td vaccine?

As with any medicine, there are very small risks that serious problems, even death, could occur after getting a vaccine. The risks from the vaccine are much smaller than the risks from the diseases if people stopped using vaccine. Almost all people who get Td have no problems from it.

Mild Problems:
- Soreness, redness, or swelling where the shot was given.
- If these problems occur, they usually start within hours to a day or two after vaccination. They may last 1-2 days.

- These problems can be worse in adults who get Td vaccine very often. Acetaminophen or ibuprofen (non-aspirin pain relievers) may be used to reduce soreness.
  Severe Problems (Rare):
- Serious allergic reaction
- Deep, aching pain and muscle wasting in upper arm(s), This starts 2 days to 4 weeks after the shot, and may last many months.

What if there is a serious reaction?

What should I do?
- Call a doctor, or get the person to a doctor right away.
- Tell your doctor what happened, the date and time it happened, and when the vaccination was given.
- Ask your health care provider to file a Vaccine Adverse Event Reporting System (VAERS) form if you have any reaction to the vaccine. Or call VAERS yourself at 1-800-822-7967, or visit their website at http://vaers.hhs.gov.

The National Vaccine Injury Compensation Program

In the rare event that you or your child has a serious reaction to a vaccine, a federal program has been created to help pay for the care of those who have been harmed.

For details about the National Vaccine Injury Compensation Program, call 1-800-338-2382 or visit the program's website at http://www.hrsa.gov/vaccinecompensation.

How can I learn more?

- Ask your doctor or other health care provider. They can give you the vaccine package insert or suggest other sources of information.
- Call your local or state health department's immunization program.
- Contact the Centers for Disease Control and Prevention (CDC): call 1-800-232-4636 (1-800-CDC-INFO) or visit the National Immunization Program's website at http://www.cdc.gov/nip

Td Vaccine Information Statement. U.S. Department of Health and Human Services/Centers for Disease Control and Prevention National Immunization Program. 6/10/1994.

Tetanus, Diphtheria, and Pertussis (Tdap) Vaccine

Brand Name: Adacel®, Boostrix®

Why get vaccinated?

Tdap (Tetanus, Diphtheria, Pertussis) vaccine can protect adolescents and adults against three serious diseases. Tetanus, diphtheria, and pertussis are all caused by bacteria. Diphtheria and pertussis are spread from person to person. Tetanus enters the body through cuts, scratches, or wounds.

TETANUS (Lockjaw) causes painful tightening of the muscles, usually all over the body. It can lead to "locking" of the jaw so the victim cannot open his mouth or swallow. Tetanus leads to death in about 2 out of 10 cases.

DIPHTHERIA causes a thick covering in the back of the throat. It can lead to breathing problems, paralysis, heart failure, and even death.

PERTUSSIS (Whooping Cough) causes severe coughing spells, vomiting, and disturbed sleep. It can lead to weight loss, incontinence, rib fractures and passing out from violent coughing, pneumonia, and hospitalization due to complications. In 2004 there were more than 25,000 cases of pertussis in the U.S. More than 8,000 of these cases were among adolescents and more than 7,000 were among adults. Up to 2 in 100 adolescents and 5 in 100 adults with pertussis are hospitalized or have complications.

Tdap and related vaccines

Vaccines for Adolescents and Adults:
- **Tdap** was licensed in 2005. It is the first vaccine for adolescents and adults that protects against all three diseases.
- **Td** (tetanus and diphtheria) vaccine has been used for many years as booster doses for adolescents and adults. It does not contain pertussis vaccine.

Vaccines for Children Younger than 7 Years:
- **DTaP** vaccine is given to children to protect them from these three diseases. Immunity can fade over time, and periodic "booster" doses are needed by adolescents and adults to keep immunity strong. (DTP is an older version of DTaP. It is no longer used in the United States.)
- **DT** contains diphtheria and tetanus vaccines. It is used for children younger than 7 who should not get pertussis vaccine.

Who should get Tdap vaccine and when?

Adolescents 11 through 18 years of age should get one booster dose of Tdap.
- A dose of Tdap is recommended for adolescents who

got DTaP or DTP as children but have not yet gotten a dose of Td. The preferred age is 11-12.

- Adolescents who have already gotten a booster dose of Td are encouraged to get a dose of Tdap as well, for protection against pertussis. Waiting at least 5 years between Td and Tdap is encouraged, but not required.
- Adolescents who did not get all their scheduled doses of DTaP or DTP as children should complete the series using a combination of Td and Tdap.

Adults 19 through 64 years of age should substitute Tdap for one booster dose of Td. Td should be used for later booster doses.

- Adults who expect to have close contact with an infant younger than 12 months of age should get a dose of Tdap. Waiting at least 2 years since the last dose of Td is suggested, but not required.
- Healthcare workers who have direct patient contact in hospitals or clinics should get a dose of Tdap. A 2-year interval since the last Td is suggested, but not required.

An adolescent or adult who gets a severe cut or burn might need protection against tetanus infection. Tdap may be used if the person has not had a previous dose. Td should be used rather than Tdap if Tdap is not available, and for: anybody who has already gotten Tdap; adults 65 years of age and older; children 7 through 9 years of age.

If vaccination is needed during pregnancy, Td usually is preferred over Tdap. Ask your doctor. New mothers who have never received a dose of Tdap should get a dose as soon as possible after delivery. Tdap may be given at the same time as other vaccines.

Who should *not* get Tdap vaccine or should wait?

- Anyone who has had a life-threatening allergic reaction after a dose of DTP, DTaP, DT, or Td vaccine should not get Tdap.
- Anyone who has a severe allergy to any component of the vaccine should not get Tdap. Tell your health care provider if the person getting the vaccine has any known severe allergies.
- Talk with your doctor if the person getting the vaccine has a severe allergy to latex. Some Tdap vaccines should not be given to people with a severe latex allergy.
- Anyone who went into a coma or had a long seizure within 7 days after a dose of DTP or DTaP should not get Tdap, unless a cause other than the vaccine was found.
- Talk to your doctor if the person getting the vaccine: has epilepsy or another nervous system problem; had severe swelling or severe pain after a previous dose of any vaccine containing tetanus, diphtheria or pertussis; or has had Guillain Barré Syndrome (GBS).
- Anyone who has a moderate or severe illness on the day the shot is scheduled should usually wait until they recover before getting the vaccine. Those with a mild illness or low fever can usually be vaccinated.

What are the risks from Tdap vaccine?

A vaccine, like any medicine, could possibly cause serious problems, such as severe allergic reactions. However, the risk of a vaccine causing serious harm, or death, is extremely small. If rare reactions occur with any new product, they may not be identified until many thousands, or even millions, of people have used the product. Like all vaccines, Tdap is being closely monitored for unusual or severe problems.

Clinical trials (testing before the vaccine was licensed) involved about 4,200 adolescents and about 1,800 adults. The following problems were reported. These are similar to problems reported after Td vaccine.

Mild Problems (Noticeable, but did not interfere with activities):

- Pain (about 3 in 4 adolescents and 2 in 3 adults)
- Redness or swelling (about 1 in 5)
- Mild fever of at least 100.4°F (up to about 1 in 25 adolescents and 1 in 100 adults)
- Headache (about 4 in 10 adolescents and 3 in 10 adults)
- Tiredness (about 1 in 3 adolescents and 1 in 4 adults)
- Nausea, vomiting, diarrhea, stomach ache (up to 1 in 4 adolescents and 1 in 10 adults)
- Other mild problems reported include chills, body aches, sore joints, rash, and swollen lymph glands.

Moderate Problems (Interfered with activities, but did not require medical attention):

- Pain at the injection site (about 1 in 20 adolescents and 1 in 100 adults)
- Redness or swelling (up to about 1 in 16 adolescents and 1 in 25 adults)
- Fever over 102°F (about 1 in 100 adolescents and 1 in 250 adults)
- Nausea, vomiting, diarrhea, stomach ache (up to 3 in 100 adolescents and 1 in 100 adults)
- Headache (1 in 300)

Severe Problems (Unable to perform usual activities; required medical attention):

- None were seen among adolescents.
- In the adult clinical trial, two adults had nervous system problems after getting the vaccine. These may or may not have been caused by the vaccine. They went away on their own and did not cause any permanent harm.
- A severe allergic reaction could occur after any vaccine.They are estimated to occur less than once in a million doses.

A person who gets these diseases is much more likely to have severe complications than a person who gets Tdap vaccine.

What if there is a severe reaction?

What should I look for?

- Any unusual condition, such as a high fever or behavior changes. Signs of a serious allergic reaction can include difficulty breathing, hoarseness or wheezing, hives, paleness, weakness, a fast heart beat or dizziness.

What should I do?

- Call a doctor, or get the person to a doctor right away.
- Tell your doctor what happened, the date and time it happened, and when the vaccination was given.
- Ask your health care provider to file a Vaccine Adverse Event Reporting System (VAERS) form if you have any reaction to the vaccine. Or call VAERS yourself at 1-800-822-7967, or visit their website at http://vaers.hhs.gov.

The National Vaccine Injury Compensation Program

In the rare event that you or your child has a serious reaction to a vaccine, a federal program has been created to help pay for the care of those who have been harmed.

For details about the National Vaccine Injury Compensation Program, call 1-800-338-2382 or visit the program's website at http://www.hrsa.gov/vaccinecompensation.

How can I learn more?

- Ask your doctor or other health care provider. They can give you the vaccine package insert or suggest other sources of information.
- Call your local or state health department's immunization program.
- Contact the Centers for Disease Control and Prevention (CDC): call 1-800-232-4636 (1-800-CDC-INFO) or visit the National Immunization Program's website at http://www.cdc.gov/nip

Tdap Vaccine Information Statement. U.S. Department of Health and Human Services/Centers for Disease Control and Prevention National Immunization Program. 7/12/2006.

Tetracycline

(tet ra sye′ kleen)

Brand Name: Helidac Therapy® as a combination product containing Tetracycline, Metronidazole, and Bismuth subsalicylate, Sumycin®, Sumycin® Syrup
Also available generically.

Why is this medicine prescribed?

Tetracycline, is used to treat bacterial infections, including pneumonia and other respiratory tract infections; acne; infections of skin, genital and urinary systems; and the infection that causes stomach ulcers (Helicobacter pylori). It also may be used as an alternative to other medications for the treatment of Lyme disease and for the treatment and prevention of anthrax (after inhalational exposure). Tetracycline is in a class of medications called tetracycline antibiotics. It works by preventing the growth and spread of bacteria. Antibiotics will not work for colds, flu, or other viral infections.

How should this medicine be used?

Tetracycline comes as a capsule and suspension (liquid) to take by mouth. It is usually taken two to four times daily. Tetracycline should be taken on an empty stomach, at least 1 hour before or 2 hours after meals or snacks. Drink a full glass of water with each dose of tetracycline. Do not take tetracycline with food, especially dairy products such as milk, yogurt, cheese, and ice cream. Follow the directions on your prescription label carefully, and ask your doctor or pharmacist to explain any part you do not understand. Take tetracycline exactly as directed. Do not take more or less of it or take it more often than prescribed by your doctor.

Shake the liquid well before each use to mix the medication evenly.

Are there other uses for this medicine?

This medication is sometimes prescribed for other uses; ask your doctor or pharmacist for more information.

What special precautions should I follow?

Before taking tetracycline,

- tell your doctor and pharmacist if you are allergic to tetracycline, minocycline, doxycycline, sulfites, or any other medications.
- tell your doctor and pharmacist what prescription and nonprescription medicines, vitamins, nutritional supplements, and herbal products you are taking or plan to take, especially antacids, anticoagulants ('blood thinners') such as warfarin (Coumadin), and penicillin. Tetracycline may decrease the effectiveness of some oral contraceptives; another method of birth control should be used while taking this drug.
- be aware that antacids, calcium supplements, iron products, and laxatives containing magnesium interfere with tetracycline, making it less effective. Take tetracycline 1 hour before or 2 hours after antacids (including sodium bicarbonate), calcium supplements, and laxatives containing magnesium. Take tetracycline 2 hours before or 3 hours after iron preparations and vitamin products that contain iron.
- tell your doctor if you have or have ever had diabetes, allergies, asthma, hay fever, hives, or kidney or liver disease.
- tell your doctor if you are pregnant, plan to become pregnant, or are breast-feeding. If you become pregnant while taking tetracycline, call your doctor immediately. Tetracycline can harm the fetus.
- if you are having surgery, including dental surgery, tell the doctor or dentist that you are taking tetracycline.
- plan to avoid unnecessary or prolonged exposure to sunlight and to wear protective clothing, sunglasses, and sunscreen. Tetracycline may make your skin sensitive to sunlight.
- you should know that when tetracycline is used during pregnancy or in babies or children up to age 8, it can cause the teeth to become permanently stained. Tetra-

cycline should not be used in children under age 8 unless your doctor decides it is needed.

What special dietary instructions should I follow?

Unless your doctor tells you otherwise, continue your normal diet.

What should I do if I forget to take a dose?

Take the missed dose as soon as you remember it. However, if it is almost time for the next dose, skip the missed dose and continue your regular dosing schedule. Do not take a double dose to make up for a missed one.

What side effects can this medicine cause?

Tetracycline may cause side effects. Tell your doctor if any of these symptoms are severe or do not go away:

- upset stomach
- diarrhea
- itching of the rectum or vagina
- sore mouth
- redness of the skin (sunburn)
- changes in skin color

Some side effects can be serious. If you experience any of these symptoms, call your doctor immediately:

- severe headache
- blurred vision
- skin rash
- hives
- difficulty breathing or swallowing
- yellowing of the skin or eyes
- itching
- dark-colored urine
- light-colored bowel movements
- loss of appetite
- upset stomach
- vomiting
- stomach pain
- extreme tiredness or weakness
- confusion
- joint stiffness or swelling
- unusual bleeding or bruising
- decreased urination
- pain or discomfort in the mouth
- throat sores
- fever or chills

If you experience a serious side effect, you or your doctor may send a report to the Food and Drug Administration's (FDA) MedWatch Adverse Event Reporting program online [at http://www.fda.gov/MedWatch/index.html] or by phone [1-800-332-1088].

What storage conditions are needed for this medicine?

Keep this medication in the container it came in, tightly closed, and out of reach of children. Store it at room temperature and away from excess heat and moisture (not in the bathroom). Throw away any medication that is outdated or no longer needed. Talk to your pharmacist about the proper disposal of your medication.

What should I do in case of overdose?

In case of overdose, call your local poison control center at 1-800-222-1222. If the victim has collapsed or is not breathing, call local emergency services at 911.

What other information should I know?

Keep all appointments with your doctor and the laboratory. Your doctor will order certain lab tests to check your response to tetracycline.

Before having any laboratory test, tell your doctor and the laboratory personnel that you are taking tetracycline.

If you have diabetes, tetracycline causes false results in some tests for sugar in the urine. Check with your doctor before changing your diet or the dosage of your diabetes medicine.

Do not let anyone else take your medication. Your prescription is probably not refillable. If you still have symptoms of infection after you finish the tetracycline, call your doctor.

Dosage Facts
For Informational Purposes

Caution: Do not change your dose, how often you take your medication, or the length of time you are to take it without first talking to your healthcare provider.

The following dosage information was written using medical language for doctors and other healthcare professionals and is provided here for you to check your dosage. The dosage of this drug may differ for different patients. Therefore, always follow your doctor's instructions or the directions on the label. Contact your healthcare provider or pharmacist if you have any questions about the specific dosage of your medication after reviewing this information.

General Dosage Information

Available as tetracycline and tetracycline hydrochloride; dosage expressed in terms of tetracycline hydrochloride.

Pediatric Patients

General Pediatric Dosage

ORAL:
- Children >8 years of age: 25–50 mg/kg daily in 4 divided doses.

Balantidiasis†

ORAL:
- Children ≥8 years of age: 40 mg/kg daily (up to 2 g) in 4 divided doses given for 10 days.

Brucellosis

ORAL:

- Children ≥8 years of age: 30–40 mg/kg daily (up to 2 g) in 4 divided doses. Duration of treatment usually is 4–6 weeks; more prolonged treatment may be necessary for severe infections or when there are complications.
- If infection is severe or if endocarditis, meningitis, or osteomyelitis are present, administer IM streptomycin or gentamicin during the first 7–14 days of tetracycline therapy. Rifampin can be administered concomitantly (with or without an aminoglycoside) to decrease the risk of relapse.

Dientamoeba fragilis Infection†

ORAL:

- Children ≥8 years of age: 40 mg/kg daily (up to 2 g) in 4 divided doses given for 10 days.

Malaria†

Treatment of Uncomplicated Chloroquine-resistant P. falciparum Malaria†

ORAL:

- Children ≥8 years of age: 6.25 mg/kg 4 times daily given for 7 days; used in conjunction with oral quinine sulfate (10 mg/kg 3 times daily given for 3 days if infection was acquired in Africa or South America or for 7 days if acquired in Southeast Asia).

Treatment of Uncomplicated P. vivax Malaria†

ORAL:

- Children ≥8 years of age: 6.25 mg/kg 4 times daily given for 7 days; used in conjunction with oral quinine sulfate (10 mg/kg 3 times daily given for 3 days if infection was acquired in Africa or South America or for 7 days if acquired in Southeast Asia).
- In addition, a 14-day regimen of oral primaquine (0.6 mg/kg once daily) also may be indicated to provide a radical cure and prevent delayed attacks or relapse of P. vivax malaria.

Treatment of Severe P. falciparum Malaria†

ORAL:

- Children ≥8 years of age: 6.25 mg/kg 4 times daily given for 7 days; used in conjunction with IV quinidine gluconate (followed by oral quinine sulfate) given for a total duration of 3–7 days. If an IV tetracycline is necessary initially, use IV doxycycline until oral therapy can be tolerated.

Plague

Treatment of Pneumonic Plague

ORAL:

- Children >8 years of age: 25–50 mg/kg daily in 4 divided doses given for ≥10–14 days.
- Prompt initiation of treatment (within 18–24 hours of symptom onset) is essential. A parenteral regimen (e.g., IM streptomycin, IM or IV gentamicin, IV doxycycline) is preferred for initial treatment; an oral regimen may be substituted when the patient's condition improves or if a parenteral regimen is unavailable.

Postexposure Prophylaxis following High-risk Exposure†

ORAL:

- Children >8 years of age: 25–50 mg/kg daily in 2 or 4 equally divided doses.
- Duration of prophylaxis following exposure to plague aerosol

or a patient with suspected pneumonic plague is 7 days or the duration of exposure risk plus 7 days.

Syphilis

Primary or Secondary Syphilis

ORAL:

- Children >8 years of age: 500 mg 4 times daily given for 14 days.

Latent Syphilis or Tertiary Syphilis (Except Neurosyphilis)

ORAL:

- Children >8 years of age: 500 mg 4 times daily given for 14 days for early latent syphilis (duration <1 year) or 500 mg 4 times daily given for 28 days for late latent syphilis (duration ≥1 year), latent syphilis of unknown duration, or tertiary syphilis.

Vibrio Infections

Cholera

ORAL:

- Children >8 years of age: 50 mg/kg daily in 4 divided doses given for 3 days.

Adult Patients

General Adult Dosage

ORAL:

- 1–2 g daily in 2–4 divided doses.
- 500 mg twice daily or 250 mg 4 times daily may be adequate for mild to moderate infections; severe infections may required 500 mg 4 times daily.

Respiratory Tract Infections

Mycoplasma pneumoniae Infections

ORAL:

- 1–2 g daily in 2–4 equally divided doses. Duration of treatment usually is 1–4 weeks.

Acne

ORAL:

- 1 g daily given in divided doses; when improvement occurs in 1–2 weeks, decrease slowly to a maintenance dosage of 125–500 mg daily. Continue maintenance dosage until clinical improvement allows discontinuation of the drug.

Actinomycosis

ORAL:

- 1–2 g daily for 6–12 months as follow-up to penicillin G.

Anthrax

Postexposure Prophylaxis following Exposure in the Context of Biologic Warfare or Bioterrorism

ORAL:

- 500 mg every 6 hours given for ≥60 days.
- Optimum duration of postexposure prophylaxis after an inhalation exposure to B. anthracis spores is unclear, but prolonged postexposure prophylaxis usually required. A duration of 60 days may be adequate for a low-dose exposure, but a duration >4 months may be necessary to reduce the risk following a high-dose exposure. CDC recommends that postexposure prophylaxis following a confirmed exposure (including in laboratory workers with confirmed exposures to B. anthracis cultures) be continued for 60 days. The US Working Group on Civilian Biodefense and the US Army Medical Research Institute of Infectious Diseases (USAMRIID) rec-

ommends that postexposure prophylaxis be continued for *at least* 60 days in individuals who are not fully immunized against anthrax and when anthrax vaccine is unavailable or cannot be used for postexposure vaccination.

Treatment of Inhalational Anthrax

ORAL:
- 500 mg every 6 hours.
- Initial parenteral regimen preferred; use oral regimen for initial treatment only when a parenteral regimen is not available (e.g., supply or logistic problems because large numbers of individuals require treatment in a mass casualty setting). Continue for total duration of ≥60 days if inhalational anthrax occurred as the result of exposure to anthrax spores in the context of biologic warfare or bioterrorism.

Balantidiasis†

ORAL:
- 500 mg 4 times daily given for 10 days.

Brucellosis

ORAL:
- 500 mg 4 times daily given for 3 weeks.
- If infection is severe or if endocarditis, meningitis, or osteomyelitis are present, administer IM streptomycin or gentamicin during the first 7–14 days of tetracycline therapy. Rifampin can be administered concomitantly to decrease the risk of relapse (with or without an aminoglycoside).

Burkholderia Infections†
Melioidosis†

ORAL:
- 2–3 g daily given for 1–3 months. In severe cases, some clinicians recommend concomitant chloramphenicol during the first month. In patients with extrapulmonary suppurative lesions, continue tetracycline therapy for 6–12 months.

Campylobacter Infections
Campylobacter fetus Infections

ORAL:
- 1–2 g daily given for 10 days.

Chancroid

ORAL:
- 1–2 g daily given for 2–4 weeks.

Chlamydial Infections
Uncomplicated Urethral, Endocervical, or Rectal Infections

ORAL:
- 500 mg 4 times daily given for ≥7 days.

Psittacosis (Ornithosis)

ORAL:
- 500 mg 4 times daily given for ≥10–14 days after defervescence.

Dientamoeba fragilis Infection†

ORAL:
- 500 mg 4 times daily for 10 days.

Gonorrhea and Associated Infections
Uncomplicated Gonorrhea

ORAL:
- 500 mg 4 times daily given for 7 days. No longer recommended for gonorrhea by CDC or other experts.

Empiric Treatment of Epididymitis†

ORAL:
- 500 mg 4 times daily given for 10 days; as follow-up to a single dose of IM ceftriaxone.

Granuloma Inguinale (Donovanosis)

ORAL:
- 1–2 g daily given for 2–4 weeks.

Helicobacter pylori Infection and Duodenal Ulcer Disease

ORAL:
- 500 mg in conjunction with metronidazole (250 mg) and bismuth subsalicylate (525 mg) 4 times daily (at meals and at bedtime) for 14 days; these drugs should be given concomitantly with usual dosage of an H_2-receptor antagonist.

Leptospirosis†

ORAL:
- 1–2 g daily given for 5–7 days.

Malaria†
Treatment of Uncomplicated Chloroquine-resistant P. falciparum Malaria†

ORAL:
- 250 mg 4 times daily given for 7 days; used in conjunction with quinine sulfate (650 mg 3 times daily given for 3 days if malaria was acquired in Africa or South America or for 7 days if acquired in Southeast Asia).

Treatment of Uncomplicated P. vivax Malaria†

ORAL:
- 250 mg 4 times daily given for 7 days; used in conjunction with oral quinine sulfate (650 mg 3 times daily given for 3 days if malaria was acquired in Africa or South America or for 7 days if acquired in Southeast Asia).
- In addition, a 14-day regimen of oral primaquine (30 mg once daily) also may be indicated to provide a radical cure and prevent delayed attacks or relapse of *P. vivax* malaria.

Treatment of Severe *P. falciparum* Malaria†

ORAL:
- 250 mg 4 times daily for 7 days; used in conjunction with IV quinidine gluconate (followed by oral quinine sulfate) given for a total duration of 3–7 days. If an IV tetracycline is necessary initially, use IV doxycycline until oral therapy can be tolerated.

Plague
Treatment

ORAL:
- 2–4 g daily in 4 divided doses given for ≥10–14 days.
- Prompt initiation of treatment (within 18–24 hours of symptom onset) is essential. A parenteral regimen (e.g., IM streptomycin, IM or IV gentamicin, IV doxycycline) is preferred for initial treatment; an oral regimen may be substituted when the patient's condition improves or if a parenteral regimen is unavailable.

Postexposure Prophylaxis following High-risk Exposure†

ORAL:
- 1–2 g daily in 2 or 4 divided doses.
- Duration of prophylaxis following exposure to plague aerosol or a patient with suspected pneumonic plague is 7 days or the duration of exposure risk plus 7 days.

Relapsing Fever

ORAL:
- 1–2 g daily until afebrile for 7 days. A single 500-mg dose may be effective in some patients.

Rickettsial Infections

ORAL:
- 1–2 g daily in 2–4 divided doses. Duration of treatment usually is ≥3–7 days or until patients has been afebrile for approximately 2–3 days.

Q Fever

ORAL:
- 500 mg every 6 hours given for ≥14 days for treatment of acute Q fever.
- For prophylaxis against Q fever†, 500 mg every 6 hours given for ≥5–7 days may prevent clinical disease if initiated 8–12 days after exposure; such prophylaxis is not effective and may only prolong the onset of disease if given immediately (1–7 days) after exposure.

Syphilis
Primary or Secondary Syphilis

ORAL:
- 500 mg 4 times daily given for 14 days recommended by CDC and others. Manufacturer recommends a total dosage of 30–40 g in equally divided doses given over 10–15 days.

Latent Syphilis or Tertiary Syphilis (Except Neurosyphilis)

ORAL:
- 500 mg 4 times daily given for 14 days for early latent syphilis (duration <1 year) or 500 mg 4 times daily given for 28 days for late latent syphilis (duration≥1 year), latent syphilis of unknown duration, or tertiary syphilis.

Tularemia
Treatment

ORAL:
- 500 mg 4 times daily given for ≥14–21 days. Relapse may occur as long as 6 months after treatment with tetracycline; however, retreatment with the same dosage usually is curative.

Postexposure Prophylaxis following High-risk Exposure†

ORAL:
- 500 mg 4 times daily.
- Initiate postexposure prophylaxis within 24 hours of exposure and continue for ≥14 days.

Vibrio Infections
Cholera

ORAL:
- 1–2 g daily given for 2–3 days. 500 mg 4 times daily for 3 days also has been recommended.

Yaws

ORAL:
- 1–2 g daily given for 10–14 days.

Prescribing Limits
Pediatric Patients

Malaria
Treatment of Severe P. falciparum Malaria†

ORAL:
- Children ≥8 years of age: Maximum 1g daily.

Special Populations

Renal Impairment
- Adjust dosage by decreasing doses or increasing dosing interval.

† *Use is not currently included in the labeling approved by the US Food and Drug Administration.*

Tetrahydrozoline Ophthalmic

(tet ra hye droz' a leen)

Brand Name: A.R.® Eye Drops as a combination product containing Tetrahydrozoline Hydrochloride and Zinc Sulfate, Collyrium Fresh®, Murine® Plus, Optigene® 3, Tyzine®, Visine®, Visine® A.C. as a combination product containing Tetrahydrozoline Hydrochloride and Zinc Sulfate, Visine® Moisturizing

Why is this medicine prescribed?

Tetrahydrozoline is used to relieve minor eye irritation and redness caused by colds, pollen, and swimming.

This medication is sometimes prescribed for other uses; ask your doctor or pharmacist for more information.

How should this medicine be used?

Tetrahydrozoline comes as eyedrops. The eyedrops usually are applied to the affected eyes three or four times a day. Follow the directions on the package label or your prescription label carefully, and ask your doctor or pharmacist to explain any part you do not understand. Use tetrahydrozoline exactly as directed. Do not use more or less of it or use it more often than directed by your doctor.

To use the eyedrops, follow these instructions:
1. Wash your hands thoroughly with soap and water.
2. Use a mirror or have someone else put the drops in your eye.
3. Remove the protective cap. Make sure that the end of the dropper is not chipped or cracked.
4. Avoid touching the dropper tip against your eye or anything else.
5. Hold the dropper tip down at all times to prevent drops

from flowing back into the bottle and contaminating the remaining contents.

6. Lie down or tilt your head back.

7. Holding the bottle between your thumb and index finger, place the dropper tip as near as possible to your eyelid without touching it.

8. Brace the remaining fingers of that hand against your cheek or nose.

9. With the index finger of your other hand, pull the lower lid of the eye down to form a pocket.

10. Drop the prescribed number of drops into the pocket made by the lower lid and the eye. Placing drops on the surface of the eyeball can cause stinging.

11. Close your eye and press lightly against the lower lid with your finger for 2-3 minutes to keep the medication in the eye. Do not blink.

12. Replace and tighten the cap right away. Do not wipe or rinse it off.

13. Wipe off any excess liquid from your cheek with a clean tissue. Wash your hands again.

What special precautions should I follow?

Before using tetrahydrozoline eyedrops,

- tell your doctor and pharmacist if you are allergic to tetrahydrozoline or any other drugs.
- tell your doctor and pharmacist what prescription and nonprescription medications you are taking, especially eye medications, medications for high blood pressure, MAO inhibitors [phenelzine (Nardil) and tranylcypromine (Parnate)], and vitamins.
- tell your doctor if you have any eye disease or infection, heart disease, high blood pressure, or an overactive thyroid gland.
- tell your doctor if you are pregnant, plan to become pregnant, or are breast-feeding. If you become pregnant while using tetrahydrozoline, call your doctor immediately.
- if you are having surgery, including dental surgery, tell your doctor or dentist that you are using tetrahydrozoline. You may have to stop using tetrahydrozoline for a short time.
- tell your doctor if you wear soft contact lenses. If the brand of tetrahydrozoline you are taking contains benzalkonium chloride, wait at least 15 minutes after using the medicine to put in soft contact lenses.

What should I do if I forget to take a dose?

Apply the missed dose as soon as you remember it. However, if it is almost time for the next dose, skip the missed dose and continue your regular dosing schedule. Do not apply a double dose to make up for a missed one.

What side effects can this medicine cause?

Tetrahydrozoline may cause side effects. Tell your doctor if any of these symptoms are severe or do not go away:

- stinging or burning of the eye

- blurred vision
- increased eye redness or irritation

If you experience any of the following symptoms, stop using tetrahydrozoline and call your doctor immediately:

- headache
- sweating
- fast or irregular heartbeat
- nervousness

If you experience a serious side effect, you or your doctor may send a report to the Food and Drug Administration's (FDA) MedWatch Adverse Event Reporting program online [at http://www.fda.gov/MedWatch/index.html] or by phone [1-800-332-1088].

What storage conditions are needed for this medicine?

Keep this medication in the container it came in, tightly closed, and out of reach of children. Store it at room temperature and away from excess heat and moisture (not in the bathroom). If the medication becomes discolored, do not use it; obtain a fresh bottle. Throw away any medication that is outdated or no longer needed. Talk to your pharmacist about the proper disposal of your medication.

What other information should I know?

Keep all appointments with your doctor.

Do not let anyone else use your medication. Ask your pharmacist any questions you have about tetrahydrozoline or your prescription.

If you still have symptoms of eye irritation after using tetrahydrozoline as directed, call your doctor.

Talk to your doctor, pharmacist, or other healthcare professional if you have questions about dosing information for your medication.

Thalidomide

(tha li' doe mide)

Brand Name: Thalomid®

Important Warning

Tell your doctor if you are pregnant, plan to become pregnant, or are breast-feeding. If you become pregnant while taking thalidomide, stop taking thalidomide and call your doctor immediately. Thalidomide can cause pregnancy loss or severe birth defects.

Before starting treatment, women of childbearing age should have a pregnancy test. Your doctor will not give you a prescription for thalidomide until a negative pregnancy test has been obtained. Your

continued on next page

Important Warning (cont'd)

doctor will order pregnancy tests often during your treatment; it is important that you keep these appointments. Women of childbearing age who are taking thalidomide should not have sexual intercourse or should use two forms of birth control for at least 1 month before beginning thalidomide therapy, during thalidomide therapy, and for 1 month after stopping thalidomide therapy. If your period is irregular, late, or you miss a period during treatment with thalidomide, call your doctor immediately.

If you are a sexually active male, you will need to use barrier contraception, such as condoms, while taking thalidomide.

Why is this medicine prescribed?

Thalidomide is used to treat and prevent skin conditions caused by erythema nodosum leprosum (ENL).

This medication is sometimes prescribed for other uses; ask your doctor or pharmacist for more information.

How should this medicine be used?

Thalidomide comes as a capsule to take by mouth. Thalidomide is usually taken once a day at bedtime, but at least 1 hour after the evening meal. Take thalidomide with a glass of water. Follow the directions on your prescription label carefully, and ask your doctor or pharmacist to explain any part you do not understand. Take thalidomide exactly as directed. Do not take more or less of it or take it more often than prescribed by your doctor.

Are there other uses for this medicine?

Thalidomide is also used sometimes to treat Kaposi's sarcoma, primary brain malignancies, chronic graft versus host disease, Behcet's disease, aphthous ulcers, systemic lupus erythematosus (SLE), adult Langerhans cell histiocytosis, rheumatoid arthritis, and Jessner's lymphocytic infiltration of the skin. Talk to your doctor about the possible risks of using this drug for your condition.

What special precautions should I follow?

Before taking thalidomide,
- tell your doctor and pharmacist if you are allergic to thalidomide or any other drugs.
- tell your doctor and pharmacist if you are taking any other medications, including amprenavir (Agenerase), barbiturates, carbamazepine (Carbatrol, Epitol, Tegretol), chlorpromazine (Ormazine, Thorazine), griseofulvin (Fulvicin, Grifulvin, Grisactin, others), indinavir (Crixivan), nelfinavir (Viracept), phenytoin (Dilantin), reserpine (Serpalan, Serpasil, others), rifabutin (Mycobutin), rifampin (Rifadin, Rimactane), ritonavir (Norvir), saquinavir (Fortovase, Invirase), and vitamins. If you are using oral contraceptives to prevent pregnancy while taking thalidomide, you should be aware of med-

ications that may affect the effectiveness of oral contraceptives. Ask your pharmacist for more information.
- tell your doctor if you have or have ever had human immunodeficiency virus (HIV), acquired immunodeficiency syndrome (AIDS), or neutropenia.
- you should know that this drug may make you drowsy. Do not drive a car or operate machinery until you know how thalidomide will affect you.
- remember that alcohol can add to the drowsiness caused by this drug.
- plan to avoid unnecessary or prolonged exposure to sunlight and sun lamps and to wear protective clothing, sunglasses, and sunscreen. Thalidomide may make your skin sensitive to sunlight.
- be aware that you should not give blood or donate sperm during treatment with thalidomide.
- thalidomide may cause dizziness and decreases in blood pressure that could result in falls. After lying down, you should sit upright for a few minutes before standing up.

What should I do if I forget to take a dose?

Take the missed dose as soon as you remember it. However, if it is almost time for the next dose, skip the missed dose and continue your regular dosing schedule. Do not take a double dose to make up for a missed one.

What side effects can this medicine cause?

Thalidomide may cause side effects. Tell your doctor if any of these symptoms are severe or do not go away:
- drowsiness
- dizziness
- slow heartbeats

If you experience any of the following symptoms, call your doctor immediately:
- rash
- numbness, tingling, pain, or a burning sensation in the hands or feet
- fever

If you experience a serious side effect, you or your doctor may send a report to the Food and Drug Administration's (FDA) MedWatch Adverse Event Reporting program online [at http://www.fda.gov/MedWatch/index.html] or by phone [1-800-332-1088].

What storage conditions are needed for this medicine?

Keep this medication in the container it came in, tightly closed, and out of reach of children. Store it at room temperature and away from excess heat and moisture (not in the bathroom). Throw away any medication that is outdated or no longer needed. Talk to your pharmacist about the proper disposal of your medication.

What should I do in case of overdose?

In case of overdose, call your local poison control center at 1-800-222-1222. If the victim has collapsed or is not breathing, call local emergency services at 911.

What other information should I know?

Keep all appointments with your doctor and the laboratory. Your doctor will order laboratory tests to monitor your response to thalidomide.

Do not let anyone else take your medication. Ask your pharmacist any questions you have about refilling your prescription. Tell your doctor if your skin condition gets worse or does not go away.

Talk to your doctor, pharmacist, or other healthcare professional if you have questions about dosing information for your medication.

Thiamine

(thye′ a min)

Available generically.

Why is this medicine prescribed?

Thiamine is a vitamin used by the body to break down sugars in the diet. The medication helps correct nerve and heart problems that occur when a person's diet does not contain enough thiamine.

This medication is sometimes prescribed for other uses; ask your doctor or pharmacist for more information.

How should this medicine be used?

Thiamine comes in tablets to take by mouth. It is usually taken three times a day with meals. If you have a thiamine deficiency, your doctor may prescribe thiamine for 1 month or more. Follow the directions on your prescription label or package label carefully, and ask your doctor or pharmacist to explain any part you do not understand. Take thiamine exactly as directed. Do not take more or less of it or take it more often than prescribed by your doctor.

Thiamine should be taken with meals. If you are taking an extended-release (long-acting) product, do not chew or crush the tablet. There are some tablets that can be crushed and mixed with food.

What special precautions should I follow?

Before taking thiamine,

- tell your doctor and pharmacist if you are allergic to thiamine or any other drugs.
- tell your doctor and pharmacist what prescription and nonprescription medications you are taking, including other vitamins.
- tell your doctor if you are pregnant, plan to become pregnant, or are breast-feeding. If you become pregnant while taking thiamine, call your doctor.
- if you are having surgery, including dental surgery, tell the doctor or dentist that you are taking thiamine.

What special dietary instructions should I follow?

Your doctor may suggest that you eat more potatoes, whole-grain cereals and breads, meats (especially pork and liver), peas, beans, and nuts to increase the thiamine in your diet.

What should I do if I forget to take a dose?

Take the missed dose as soon as you remember it. However, if it is almost time for the next dose, skip the missed dose and continue your regular dosing schedule. Do not take a double dose to make up for a missed one.

What side effects can this medicine cause?

Thiamine tablets usually do not cause any side effects.

What storage conditions are needed for this medicine?

Keep this medication in the container it came in, tightly closed, and out of reach of children. Store it at room temperature and away from excess heat and moisture (not in the bathroom). Throw away any medication that is outdated or no longer needed. Talk to your pharmacist about the proper disposal of your medication.

What should I do in case of overdose?

In case of overdose, call your local poison control center at 1-800-222-1222. If the victim has collapsed or is not breathing, call local emergency services at 911.

What other information should I know?

Keep all appointments with your doctor and the laboratory. Your doctor will order certain lab tests to check your response to thiamine.

Do not let anyone else take your medication. Ask your pharmacist any questions you have about refilling your prescription.

Talk to your doctor, pharmacist, or other healthcare professional if you have questions about dosing information for your medication.

Thioridazine

(thye oh rid' a zeen)

Available generically.

Important Warning

Thioridazine can cause life-threatening irregular heartbeat. You should only take thioridazine if your schizophrenia has not responded to other medications.

If you experience any of the following symptoms, call your doctor immediately: fast, irregular, or pounding heartbeat, dizziness, lightheadedness, fainting or seizures. Talk to your doctor about the risks of taking thioridazine.

Why is this medicine prescribed?

Thioridazine is used to treat schizophrenia and symptoms such as hallucinations, delusions, and hostility.

How should this medicine be used?

Thioridazine comes as a tablet, liquid suspension, and liquid concentrate to take by mouth. It is usually taken two to four times a day. Follow the directions on your prescription label carefully, and ask your doctor or pharmacist to explain any part you do not understand. Take thioridazine exactly as directed. Do not take more or less of it or take it more often than prescribed by your doctor.

Shake the liquid suspension well before each use to mix the medication evenly. You may obtain a specially marked measuring spoon from your pharmacist to be sure of an accurate dose.

The liquid concentrate must be diluted before use. It comes with a specially marked dropper for measuring the dose. Ask your pharmacist to show you how to use the dropper if you have difficulty. To dilute the liquid concentrate, add it to at least 2 ounces of water, orange juice, or grape juice before taking it. If any of the juice gets on the dropper, rinse the dropper with tap water before replacing it in the bottle. Do not allow the liquid concentrate to touch your skin or clothing; it can irritate your skin. If you spill the liquid concentrate on your skin, wash it off immediately with soap and water.

Continue to take thioridazine even if you feel well. Do not stop taking thioridazine without talking to your doctor, especially if you have taken large doses for a long time. Your doctor probably will decrease your dose gradually. This drug must be taken regularly for a few weeks before its full effect is felt.

Are there other uses for this medicine?

This medication should not be prescribed for other uses; ask your doctor or pharmacist for more information.

What special precautions should I follow?

Before taking thioridazine,

- tell your doctor and pharmacist if you are allergic to thioridazine or any other drugs.
- tell your doctor and pharmacist what prescription and nonprescription medications you are taking, especially antacids, antidepressant medications, antihistamines, appetite reducers (amphetamines), benztropine (Cogentin), bromocriptine (Parlodel), carbamazepine (Tegretol), dicyclomine (Bentyl), fluoxetine (Prozac), fluvoxamine (Luvox), guanethidine (Ismelin), lithium, medication for colds, meperidine (Demerol), methyldopa (Aldomet), paroxetine (Paxil), phenytoin (Dilantin), pindolol (Visken), propranolol (Inderal), sedatives, trihexyphenidyl (Artane), valproic acid (Depakane), and vitamins.
- tell your doctor if you have or have ever had depression; seizures; shock therapy; asthma; emphysema; chronic bronchitis; problems with your urinary system or prostate; glaucoma; history of alcohol abuse; thyroid problems; bad reaction to insulin; angina; irregular heartbeat; problems with your blood pressure; blood disorders; or blood vessel, heart, kidney, liver, or lung disease.
- tell your doctor if you are pregnant, plan to become pregnant, or are breast-feeding. If you become pregnant while taking thioridazine, call your doctor.
- if you are having surgery, including dental surgery, tell the doctor or dentist that you are taking thioridazine.
- you should know that this drug may make you drowsy. Do not drive a car or operate machinery until you know how this drug affects you.
- remember that alcohol can add to the drowsiness caused by this drug.
- plan to avoid unnecessary or prolonged exposure to sunlight and to wear protective clothing, sunglasses, and sunscreen. Thioridazine may make your skin sensitive to sunlight.

What special dietary instructions should I follow?

Thioridazine may cause an upset stomach. Take thioridazine with food or milk.

What should I do if I forget to take a dose?

Take the missed dose as soon as you remember it and take any remaining doses for that day at evenly spaced intervals. However, if you remember a missed dose when it is almost time for your next scheduled dose, skip the missed dose. Do not take a double dose to make up for a missed one.

If you take thioridazine once a day at bedtime and do not remember it until the next morning, omit the missed dose. Do not take a double dose to make up for a missed one.

What side effects can this medicine cause?

Side effects from thioridazine may occur. Your urine may turn pink or reddish-brown; this effect is not harmful. Tell your doctor if any of these symptoms are severe or do not go away:

- drowsiness
- dizziness
- blurred vision
- dry mouth
- upset stomach
- vomiting
- diarrhea
- constipation
- restlessness
- headache
- weight gain

If you experience any of the following symptoms or the one listed in the IMPORTANT WARNING section, call your doctor immediately:

- tremor
- restlessness or pacing
- fine worm-like tongue movements
- unusual face, mouth, or jaw movements
- difficulty swallowing
- shuffling walk
- seizures or convulsions
- difficulty urinating or loss of bladder control
- yellowing of the skin or eyes

If you experience a serious side effect, you or your doctor may send a report to the Food and Drug Administration's (FDA) MedWatch Adverse Event Reporting program online [at http://www.fda.gov/MedWatch/index.html] or by phone [1-800-332-1088].

What storage conditions are needed for this medicine?

Keep this medication in the container it came in, tightly closed, and out of reach of children. Store it at room temperature and away from excess heat and moisture (not in the bathroom). Protect the liquid from light. Throw away any medication that is outdated or no longer needed. Talk to your pharmacist about the proper disposal of your medication.

What should I do in case of overdose?

In case of overdose, call your local poison control center at 1-800-222-1222. If the victim has collapsed or is not breathing, call local emergency services at 911.

What other information should I know?

Keep all appointments with your doctor and the laboratory. Your doctor will order certain lab tests to check your response to thioridazine.

Do not let anyone else take your medication. Ask your pharmacist any questions you have about refilling your prescription.

Talk to your doctor, pharmacist, or other healthcare professional if you have questions about dosing information for your medication.

Thiothixene Oral

(thye oh thix' een)

Brand Name: Navane®

Why is this medicine prescribed?

Thiothixene is used to treat schizophrenia and symptoms such as hallucinations, delusions, and hostility.

This medication is sometimes prescribed for other uses; ask your doctor or pharmacist for more information.

How should this medicine be used?

Thiothixene comes as a capsule and liquid concentrate to take by mouth. It usually is taken two or three times a day. Follow the directions on your prescription label carefully, and ask your doctor or pharmacist to explain any part you do not understand. Take thiothixene exactly as directed. Do not take more or less of it or take it more often than prescribed by your doctor.

The liquid concentrate must be diluted before use. It comes with a specially marked dropper for measuring the dose. Ask your pharmacist to show you how to use the dropper if you have difficulty. To dilute the liquid concentrate, add it to at least 2 ounces of milk, water, soft drink, tomato or fruit juice, or soup just before you take it. If any beverage or soup gets on the dropper, rinse the dropper with tap water before replacing it in the bottle. Do not allow the liquid concentrate to touch your skin or clothing; it can irritate your skin. If you spill the liquid concentrate on your skin, wash it off immediately with soap and water.

Continue to take thiothixene even if you feel well. Do not stop taking thiothixene without talking to your doctor, especially if you have taken large doses for a long time. Your doctor probably will decrease your dose gradually. This drug must be taken regularly for a few weeks before its full effect is felt.

What special precautions should I follow?

Before taking thiothixene,

- tell your doctor and pharmacist if you are allergic to thiothixene or any other drugs.
- tell your doctor and pharmacist what prescription and nonprescription medications you are taking, especially antacids, antihistamines, appetite reducers (amphetamines), benztropine (Cogentin), bromocriptine (Parlodel), carbamazepine (Tegretol), fluoxetine (Prozac), guanethidine (Ismelin), lithium, medications for colds, medication for depression, meperidine (Demerol), methyldopa (Aldomet), phenytoin (Dilantin), propran-

olol (Inderal), sedatives such as secobarbital (Seconal), trihexyphenidyl (Artane), valproic acid (Depakane), and vitamins.

- tell your doctor if you have or have ever had depression; seizures; shock therapy; asthma; emphysema; chronic bronchitis; problems with your urinary system or prostate; glaucoma; history of alcohol abuse; thyroid problems; bad reaction to insulin; angina; irregular heartbeat; problems with your blood pressure; blood disorders; blood vessel, heart, kidney, liver, or lung disease.
- tell your doctor if you are pregnant, plan to become pregnant, or are breast-feeding. If you become pregnant while taking thiothixene, call your doctor.
- if you are having surgery, including dental surgery, tell the doctor or dentist that you are taking thiothixene.
- you should know that this drug may make you drowsy. Do not drive a car or operate machinery until you know how this drug affects you.
- remember that alcohol can add to the drowsiness caused by this drug.
- plan to avoid unnecessary or prolonged exposure to sunlight and to wear protective clothing, sunglasses, and sunscreen. Thiothixene may make your skin sensitive to sunlight.

What special dietary instructions should I follow?

Thiothixene may cause an upset stomach. Take thiothixene with food or milk.

What should I do if I forget to take a dose?

Take the missed dose as soon as you remember it and take any remaining doses for that day at evenly spaced intervals. However, if you remember a missed dose when it is almost time for your next scheduled dose, skip the missed dose. Do not take a double dose to make up for a missed one.

What side effects can this medicine cause?

Side effects from thiothixene may occur. Your urine may turn pink or reddish-brown; this effect is not harmful. Tell your doctor if any of these symptoms are severe or do not go away:

- drowsiness
- dizziness or blurred vision
- dry mouth
- upset stomach
- vomiting
- diarrhea
- constipation
- restlessness
- headache
- weight gain

If you experience any of the following symptoms, call your doctor immediately:

- tremor
- restlessness or pacing
- fine worm-like tongue movements
- unusual face, mouth, or jaw movements
- shuffling walk
- seizures or convulsions
- fast, irregular, or pounding heartbeat
- difficulty urinating or loss of bladder control
- yellowing of the skin or eyes

If you experience a serious side effect, you or your doctor may send a report to the Food and Drug Administration's (FDA) MedWatch Adverse Event Reporting program online [at http://www.fda.gov/MedWatch/index.html] or by phone [1-800-332-1088].

What storage conditions are needed for this medicine?

Keep this medication in the container it came in, tightly closed, and out of reach of children. Store it at room temperature and away from excess heat and moisture (not in the bathroom). Protect the liquid from light. Throw away any medication that is outdated or no longer needed. Talk to your pharmacist about the proper disposal of your medication.

What should I do in case of overdose?

In case of overdose, call your local poison control center at 1-800-222-1222. If the victim has collapsed or is not breathing, call local emergency services at 911.

What other information should I know?

Keep all appointments with your doctor and the laboratory. Your doctor will order certain lab tests to check your response to thiothixene.

Do not let anyone else take your medication. Ask your pharmacist any questions you have about refilling your prescription.

Talk to your doctor, pharmacist, or other healthcare professional if you have questions about dosing information for your medication.

Thyroid

(thye′ roid)

Brand Name: Armour® Thyroid
Also available generically.

Important Warning

Thyroid hormone should not be used to treat obesity in patients with normal thyroid function. Thyroid medication is ineffective for weight reduction in normal thyroid patients and may cause serious or life-threatening toxicity, especially when taken with amphetamines (benzphetamine [Didrex], dextroamphetamine [Dexedrine, in Adderall], methamphetamine [Desoxyn]). Talk to your doctor about the potential risks associated with this medication.

Why is this medicine prescribed?

Thyroid is a hormone produced by the body. When taken correctly, thyroid is used to treat the symptoms of hypothyroidism (a condition where the thyroid gland does not produce enough thyroid hormone). Symptoms of hypothyroidism include lack of energy, depression, constipation, weight gain, hair loss, dry skin, dry coarse hair, muscle cramps, decreased concentration, aches and pains, swelling of the legs, and increased sensitivity to cold. Thyroid is also used to treat goiter (enlarged thyroid gland). Thyroid is in a class of medications called thyroid agents. It works by supplying the thyroid hormone normally produced by the body.

How should this medicine be used?

Thyroid comes as a tablet to take by mouth. It usually is taken once a day before breakfast. Take thyroid at around the same time every day. Follow the directions on your prescription label carefully, and ask your doctor or pharmacist to explain any part you do not understand. Take thyroid exactly as directed. Do not take more or less of it or take it more often than prescribed by your doctor.

Your doctor will probably start you on a low dose of thyroid and gradually increase your dose.

Thyroid helps control the symptoms of hypothyroidism, but does not cure this condition. It may take up to several weeks before you notice any change in your symptoms. To control the symptoms of hypothyroidism, you probably will need to take thyroid for the rest of your life. Continue to take thyroid even if you feel well. Do not stop taking thyroid without talking to your doctor.

Are there other uses for this medicine?

This medication is sometimes prescribed for other uses; ask your doctor or pharmacist for more information.

What special precautions should I follow?

Before taking thyroid,

- tell your doctor and pharmacist if you are allergic to thyroid, any other medications, pork, or any of the ingredients in thyroid tablets. Ask your pharmacist for a list of the ingredients.
- tell your doctor and pharmacist what other prescription and nonprescription medications, vitamins, and nutritional supplements you are taking or plan to take. Be sure to mention any of the following: androgens such as danazol or testosterone; anticoagulants ('blood thinners') such as warfarin (Coumadin); antidepressants; aprepitant (Emend); carbamazepine (Carbatrol, Epitol, Tegretol); diabetes medications that you take by mouth; digoxin (Lanoxin); efavirenz (Sustiva); estrogen (hor-

mone replacement therapy) griseofulvin (Fulvicin, Grifulvin, Gris-PEG); human growth hormone (Genotropin); insulin; lovastatin (Altocor, Mevacor); nevirapine (Viramune); oral contraceptives containing estrogen; oral steroids such as dexamethasone (Decadron, Dexone, Dexpak), methylprednisolone (Medrol), and prednisone (Deltasone); phenobarbital (Luminal, Solfoton); phenytoin (Dilantin, Phenytek); potassium iodide (contained in Elixophyllin-Kl, Pediacof, KIE); rifabutin (Mycobutin); rifampin (Rifadin, Rimactane, in Rifamate); ritonavir (Norvir, in Kaletra); salicylate pain relievers such as aspirin and aspirin-containing products, choline magnesium trisalicylate, choline salicylate (Arthropan), diflunisal (Dolobid), magnesium salicylate (Doan's, others), and salsalate (Argesic, Disalcid, Salgesic); strong iodine solution (Lugol's Solution); and theophylline (Elixophyllin, Theolair, Theo-24, Quibron, others).

- if you take cholestyramine (Questran) or colestipol (Colestid), take it at least 4 hours before taking your thyroid medication. If you take antacids, ironcontaining medications or nutritional supplements, simethicone, or sucralfate (Carafate), take them at least 4 hours before or 4 hours after taking your thyroid medication.
- tell your doctor what herbal products you are taking, especially St John's wort.
- tell your doctor if you have or have ever had diabetes; osteoporosis; hardening or narrowing of the arteries (atherosclerosis); cardiovascular disease such as high blood pressure, high blood cholesterol and fats, angina (chest pain), arrhythmias, or heart attack; malabsorption diseases (conditions that cause a decrease in absorption from the intestine); an underactive adrenal or pituitary gland; or kidney or liver disease.
- tell your doctor if you are pregnant, plan to become pregnant, or are breast-feeding. If you become pregnant while taking thyroid, call your doctor.
- if you are having surgery, including dental surgery, tell the doctor or dentist that you are taking thyroid.

What special dietary instructions should I follow?

Unless your doctor tells you otherwise, continue your normal diet.

What should I do if I forget to take a dose?

Take the missed dose as soon as you remember it. However, if it is almost time for the next dose, skip the missed dose and continue your regular dosing schedule. Do not take a double dose to make up for a missed one. Tell your doctor if you miss two or more doses of thyroid in a row.

What side effects can this medicine cause?

Thyroid may cause side effects. Tell your doctor if any of these symptoms are severe or do not go away:

- weight loss
- shaking of a part of your body that you cannot control

- headache
- nausea
- vomiting
- diarrhea
- stomach cramps
- hyperactivity
- anxiety
- irritability or rapid changes in mood
- difficulty falling asleep or staying asleep
- flushing
- increased appetite
- fever
- changes in menstrual cycle
- muscle weakness
- temporary hair loss, particularly in children during the first month of therapy

Some side effects can be serious. If you experience any of the following symptoms, call your doctor immediately:

- rash
- difficulty breathing or swallowing
- chest pain
- rapid or irregular heartbeat
- swelling of the hands, feet, ankles, or lower legs
- excessive sweating
- sensitivity or intolerance to heat
- nervousness
- seizure

Thyroid may cause other side effects. Call your doctor if you have any unusual problems while taking this medication.

If you experience a serious side effect, you or your doctor may send a report to the Food and Drug Administration's (FDA) MedWatch Adverse Event Reporting program online [at http://www.fda.gov/MedWatch/index.html] or by phone [1-800-332-1088].

What storage conditions are needed for this medicine?

Keep this medication in the container it came in, tightly closed, and out of reach of children. Store it at room temperature and away from excess heat and moisture (not in the bathroom). Throw away any medication that is outdated or no longer needed. Talk to your pharmacist about the proper disposal of your medication.

What should I do in case of overdose?

In case of overdose, call your local poison control center at 1-800-222-1222. If the victim has collapsed or is not breathing, call local emergency services at 911.

What other information should I know?

Keep all appointments with your doctor and the laboratory. Your doctor will order certain lab tests to check your response to thyroid.

Before having any laboratory test, tell your doctor and the laboratory personnel that you are taking thyroid.

Thyroid tablets may have a strong odor. This does not mean that the medication is spoiled or unable to be used.

Learn the brand name and generic name of your medication. Check your medication each time you have your prescription refilled or receive a new prescription. Do not switch brands without talking to your doctor or pharmacist, as each brand of thyroid contains a slightly different amount of medication.

Do not let anyone else take your medication. Ask your pharmacist any questions you have about refilling your prescription.

Dosage Facts
For Informational Purposes

Caution: Do not change your dose, how often you take your medication, or the length of time you are to take it without first talking to your healthcare provider.

The following dosage information was written using medical language for doctors and other healthcare professionals and is provided here for you to check your dosage. The dosage of this drug may differ for different patients. Therefore, always follow your doctor's instructions or the directions on the label. Contact your healthcare provider or pharmacist if you have any questions about the specific dosage of your medication after reviewing this information.

General Dosage Information

Adjust dosage carefully according to clinical and laboratory response to treatment. Avoid undertreatment or overtreatment.

Initiate dosage at a lower level in geriatric patients, in patients with functional or ECG evidence of cardiovascular disease, and in patients with severe, long-standing hypothyroidism.

Pediatric Patients

Hypothyroidism

ORAL:
- Initiate therapy at full replacement dosages as soon as possible after diagnosis of hypothyroidism to prevent deleterious effects on intellectual and physical growth and development.

Dosage for Management of Hypothyroidism in Children

Age	Daily Dose	Daily Dose by Weight
0–6 months	15–30 mg	4.8–6 mg/kg
6–12 months	30–45 mg	3.6–4.8 mg/kg
1–5 years	45–60 mg	3–3.6 mg/kg
6–12 years	60–90 mg	2.4–3 mg/kg
>12 years	>90 mg	1.2–1.8 mg/kg

When *transient* hypothyroidism is suspected, therapy may be temporarily discontinued for 2–8 weeks when the child is older than 3 years of age to reassess the condition.

Adult Patients

Hypothyroidism

ORAL:
- Initially, 30 mg daily given as a single dose. Increase dosage by increments of 15 mg daily every 2–3 weeks as needed.
- For management of long-standing hypothyroidism, usual initial dosage is 15 mg daily given as a single dose.
- Usual maintenance dosage: 60–120 mg daily given as a single dose.
- Failure to respond to 180 mg daily suggests lack of compliance or malabsorption.

Pituitary TSH Suppression

Individualize dosage based on patient characteristics and nature of the disease.

Thyroid Cancer

ORAL:
- Suppress TSH to low or undetectable levels. Larger doses than those used for replacement therapy are required.

Special Populations

Hepatic Impairment
- No specific dosage recommendations at this time.

Renal Impairment
- No specific dosage recommendations at this time.

Patients with Cardiovascular Disease

Hypothyroidism
- Initiate therapy at lower doses than those recommended in patients without cardiovascular disease. Usual initial dosage is 15–30 mg daily given as a single dose. If cardiovascular symptoms develop or worsen, reduce dosage.

Geriatric Patients

Hypothyroidism
- Initiate therapy at lower doses than those recommended in younger patients. Usual initial dosage is 15–30 mg daily given as a single dose.

Tiagabine

(ty ag′ a been)

Brand Name: Gabitril®

Why is this medicine prescribed?

Tiagabine is used in combination with other medications to treat partial seizures (a type of epilepsy). Tiagabine is in a class of medications called anticonvulsants. It is not known exactly how tiagabine works, but it increases the amount of natural chemicals in the brain which prevent seizure activity.

How should this medicine be used?

Tiagabine comes as a tablet to take by mouth. It usually is taken with food two to four times a day. However, for the first week of treatment will only take tiagabine once a day. Your doctor will slowly increase your dose (not more often than once each week) until you reach the dose of tiagabine you are to take regularly. To help you remember to take tiagabine, take it around the same time(s) every day. Follow the directions on your prescription label carefully, and ask your doctor or pharmacist to explain any part you do not understand. Take tiagabine exactly as directed. Do not take more or less of it or take it more often than prescribed by your doctor.

Continue to take tiagabine even if you feel well. Do not stop taking tiagabine without talking to your doctor. Abruptly stopping this medication can cause seizures. Your doctor will probably decrease your dose gradually.

Are there other uses for this medicine?

Tiagabine should not be prescribed for other uses. Ask your doctor or pharmacist for more information.

What special precautions should I follow?

Before taking tiagabine,
- tell your doctor and pharmacist if you are allergic to tiagabine or any other medications.
- tell your doctor and pharmacist what other prescription and nonprescription medications, vitamins, and nutritional supplements you are taking. Be sure to mention any of the following: amiodarone (Cordarone, Pacerone); anticonvulsants such as carbamazepine (Tegretol), ethosuximide (Zarontin), gabapentin (Neurontin), lamotrigine (Lamictal), phenobarbital (Luminal, Solfoton), phenytoin (Dilantin, Phenytek), primidone (Mysoline), and valproic acid (Depakene, Depakote); anticholinesterases such as physostigmine (Antilirium), pyridostigmine (Mestinon, Regonol), and neostigmine (Prostigmin); antidepressants; antifungals such as fluconazole (Diflucan), itraconazole (Sporanox), and ketoconazole (Nizoral); chloroquine sulfate (Aralen); clarithromycin (Biaxin, in Prevpac); contrast dyes used during radiology procedures (CAT scans, X-rays); cyclosporine (Neoral, Sandimmune); dexamethasone (Decadron, Dexpak); diazepam (Valium); dicloxacillin; diltiazem (Cardizem, Dilacor, Tiazac, others; erythromycin (E.E.S., E-Mycin, Erythrocin); furosemide (Lasix); griseofulvin (Fulvicin-U/F, Grifulvin V, Gris-PEG); isoniazid (INH, Laniazid, Nydrazid); imipenem-cilastatin (Primaxin); lovastatin (Altocor, Mevacor, in Advicor); medications to treat HIV infection including delavirdine (Rescriptor); efavirenz (Sustiva); nevirapine (Viramune); and ritonavir (Norvir, in Kaletra); medications that may make you drowsy, such as cough, cold, and allergy products, medications for anxiety, muscle relaxants, pain medications, sedatives, sleeping pills, or tranquilizers; medications for mental illness; methocarbamol (Robaxin); mycophenolate mofetil (CellCept);

penicillins; phenylbutazone (no longer available in the US); propranolol (Inderal, Inderide); quinidine (Quinidex); quinolones such as cinoxacin (Cinobac) (no longer available in the US), ciprofloxacin (Cipro), enoxacin (Penetrex) (no longer available in the US), gatifloxacin (Tequin), levofloxacin (Levaquin), lomefloxacin (Maxequin), nalidixic acid (NegGram)(no longer available in the US), norfloxacin (Noroxin), ofloxacin (Floxin), sparfloxacin (Zagam) and trovafloxacin/alatrofloxacin combination (Trovan) (no longer available in the US); rifabutin (Mycobutin); rifampin (Rifadin, Rifamate, Rimactane, others); stimulants such as caffeine-containing products and decongestants; tacrolimus (Prograf); triazolam (Halcion); troleandomycin (TAO); verapamil (Calan, Covera, Isoptin, Verelan); warfarin (Coumadin); or zafirlukast (Accolate).

- tell your doctor what herbal products you are taking, especially St. John's wort
- tell your doctor if you have or have ever had a severe rash caused by taking a medication; status epilepticus (seizures following one another without a break); eye, or liver disease.
- tell your doctor if you are pregnant, plan to become pregnant, or are breast-feeding. If you become pregnant while taking tiagabine, call your doctor immediately.
- if you are having surgery, including dental surgery, tell the doctor or dentist that you are taking tiagabine.
- you should know that tiagabine may make you drowsy and may affect your ability to think clearly. Do not drive a car or operate machinery until you know how this drug will affect you.
- remember that alcohol may add to the drowsiness caused by this medication. Ask your doctor about the safe use of alcoholic beverages while you are taking tiagabine.
- you should know that seizures, including status epilepticus, have occurred in people without epilepsy who take tiagabine. These seizures usually occurred soon after beginning treatment with tiagabine or near the time of a dose increase, but also have also occurred at other times during treatment.

What special dietary instructions should I follow?

Talk to your doctor about drinking grapefruit juice while taking this medication.

What should I do if I forget to take a dose?

Take the missed dose as soon as you remember it. However, if it is almost time for the next dose, skip the missed dose and continue your regular dosing schedule. Do not take a double dose to make up for a missed one. If you have missed more than one dose, call your doctor for instructions about re-starting your medication.

What side effects can this medicine cause?

Tiagabine may cause side effects. Tell your doctor if any of these symptoms are severe or do not go away:

- dizziness
- drowsiness
- lack of energyor weakness
- wobbliness, unsteadiness, or incoordination causing difficulty walking
- depression
- hostility or anger
- irritability
- confusion
- difficulty concentrating or paying attention
- abnormal thinking
- speech or language problems
- increased appetite
- upset stomach
- stomach pain
- nervousness
- difficulty falling asleep or staying asleep
- itching
- bruising
- painful or frequent urination

Some side effects can be serious. The following symptoms are uncommon, but if you experience any of them, call your doctor immediately:

- rash
- sores on the inside of your mouth, nose, eyes or throat
- flu-like symptoms
- changes in vision
- severe weakness
- shaking hands you cannot control
- numbness, pain, burning, or tingling in the hands or feet
- seizures, including status epilepticus

If you experience a serious side effect, you or your doctor may send a report to the Food and Drug Administration's (FDA) MedWatch Adverse Event Reporting program online [at http://www.fda.gov/MedWatch/index.html] or by phone [1-800-332-1088].

What storage conditions are needed for this medicine?

Keep this medication in the container it came in, tightly closed, and out of reach of children. Store it at room temperature and away from excess heat and moisture (not in the bathroom). Throw away any medication that is outdated or no longer needed. Talk to your pharmacist about the proper disposal of your medication.

What should I do in case of overdose?

In case of overdose, call your local poison control center at 1-800-222-1222. If the victim has collapsed or is not breathing, call local emergency services at 911.

Symptoms of overdose may include:

- tiredness
- weakness
- wobbliness, unsteadiness, or incoordination causing difficulty walking
- shaking hands you cannot control

- confusion
- speech or language problems
- agitation
- anger or hostility
- depression
- vomiting
- loss of consciousness
- abnormal, uncontrollable muscle contractions
- temporary inability to move (paralysis)
- seizures, including status epilepticus

What other information should I know?

Keep all appointments with your doctor and the laboratory.

Do not let anyone else take your medication. Ask your pharmacist any questions you have about refilling your prescription.

Dosage Facts

For Informational Purposes

Caution: Do not change your dose, how often you take your medication, or the length of time you are to take it without first talking to your healthcare provider.

The following dosage information was written using medical language for doctors and other healthcare professionals and is provided here for you to check your dosage. The dosage of this drug may differ for different patients. Therefore, always follow your doctor's instructions or the directions on the label. Contact your healthcare provider or pharmacist if you have any questions about the specific dosage of your medication after reviewing this information.

General Dosage Information

Available as tiagabine hydrochloride; dosage expressed in terms of the salt.

Dosage is based on whether a hepatic enzyme-inducing anticonvulsant drug (e.g., carbamazepine, phenobarbital, phenytoin, primidone) is administered concomitantly.

Patients receiving a combination of enzyme-inducing and non-enzyme-inducing anticonvulsants (e.g., carbamazepine and valproate) should be considered to have induced hepatic microsomal enzymes.

Modification of tiagabine dosage may be required with the addition of a hepatic enzyme-inducing anticonvulsant, dosage change of these drugs, or their discontinuance from the regimen.

Unless clinically indicated, modification of concomitant anticonvulsant therapy is not necessary when tiagabine is added to an anticonvulsant regimen.

Administration of a loading dose is not recommended. Increase dosage slowly; avoid rapid increases in dosage and/or large dosage increments.

Consider dosage retitration if a patient misses multiple doses.

Pediatric Patients

Partial Seizures
Patients Receiving Hepatic Enzyme-inducing Anticonvulsants

ORAL:
- Adolescents 12–18 years of age: Initially, 4 mg once daily for the first week. Daily dosage may be increased to 4 mg twice daily beginning with the second week; thereafter, the total daily dosage (administered in 2–4 divided doses) may be increased by 4–8 mg at weekly intervals until a clinical response is achieved or a total daily dosage of 32 mg is reached.
- See manufacturer's prescribing information for typical dosing titration regimen.

Patients Not Receiving Hepatic Enzyme-inducing Anticonvulsants

ORAL:
- Adolescents 12–18 years of age: Use lower dosage and a slower dosage titration schedule than that used in those receiving an enzyme-inducing anticonvulsant.
- Systemic exposure following administration of a 12-mg dose in a patient not receiving a hepatic enzyme-inducing drug is expected to be comparable to that of a 32-mg dose in a patient receiving a hepatic enzyme-inducing drug.

Adult Patients

Partial Seizures
Patients Receiving Hepatic Enzyme-inducing Anticonvulsants

ORAL:
- Initially, 4 mg once daily for the first week. Beginning with the second week, the total daily dosage (administered as 2–4 divided doses) may be increased by 4–8 mg at weekly intervals until a clinical response is achieved or a total daily dosage of 56 mg is reached.
- Usual maintenance dosage: 32–56 mg daily administered as 2–4 divided doses.
- See manufacturer's prescribing information for typical dosing titration regimen.

Patients Not Receiving Hepatic Enzyme-inducing Anticonvulsants

ORAL:
- Use lower dosage and a slower dosage titration schedule than that used in those receiving an enzyme-inducing anticonvulsant.
- Systemic exposure following administration of a 12- or 22-mg dose in a patient not receiving a hepatic enzyme-inducing drug is expected to be comparable to that of a 32- or 56-mg dose in a patient receiving a hepatic enzyme-inducing drug.

Prescribing Limits

Pediatric Patients

Partial Seizures

ORAL:
- Daily dosages >32 mg have been tolerated in a limited number of adolescents for a relatively short duration.

Adult Patients

Partial Seizures

ORAL:
- Dosages >56 mg daily have not been systemically evaluated.

Ticlopidine

(tye kloe′ pi deen)

Brand Name: Ticlid®

Important Warning

Ticlopidine may cause a decrease in white blood cells, which fight infection in the body. If you have fever, chills, sore throat, or other signs of an infection, call your doctor immediately.

Ticlopidine may also cause a potentially life-threatening decrease in platelets, which may occur as part of a syndrome that includes injury to red blood cells, causing anemia, kidney abnormalities, neurologic changes, and fever. This condition is called thrombotic thrombocytopenic purpura (TTP).

Call your doctor immediately if you have yellowing of the skin or eyes, pinpoint dots (rash) on the skin, pale color, fever, difficulty speaking, seizures, weakness on a side of the body, or dark urine.

Keep all appointments with your doctor and the laboratory. Your doctor will order lab tests, especially during the first 3 months of treatment, to check your response to ticlopidine.

Why is this medicine prescribed?

Ticlopidine is used to reduce the risk of stroke. It works by preventing excessive blood clotting.

This medication is sometimes prescribed for other uses; ask your doctor or pharmacist for more information.

How should this medicine be used?

Ticlopidine comes as a tablet to take by mouth. It usually is taken twice a day. Follow the directions on your prescription label carefully, and ask your doctor or pharmacist to explain any part you do not understand. Take ticlopidine exactly as directed. Do not take more or less of it or take it more often than prescribed by your doctor.

Continue to take ticlopidine even if you feel well. Do not stop taking ticlopidine without talking to your doctor.

Are there other uses for this medicine?

Ticlopidine also is used before open heart surgery and in the treatment of sickle cell disease, certain types of kidney disease (primary glomerulonephritis), and blocked arteries in the legs. Talk to your doctor about the possible risks of using this drug for your condition.

What special precautions should I follow?

Before taking ticlopidine,
- tell your doctor and pharmacist if you are allergic to ticlopidine or any other drugs.
- tell your doctor and pharmacist what prescription and nonprescription medications you are taking, especially antacids, anticoagulants ('blood thinners') such as warfarin (Coumadin), aspirin, cimetidine (Tagamet), digoxin (Lanoxin), theophylline (Theo-Dur), and vitamins.
- if you also take antacids (Maalox, Mylanta) take them 1 hour before or 2 hours after taking ticlopidine.
- tell your doctor if you have or have ever had liver disease, bleeding disorders, bleeding ulcers, low blood cell counts (neutropenia, thrombocytopenia, anemia, TTP), kidney disease, high blood cholesterol, or high blood fats (triglycerides).
- tell your doctor if you are pregnant, plan to become pregnant, or are breast-feeding. If you become pregnant while taking ticlopidine, call your doctor.
- if you are having surgery, including dental surgery, tell the doctor or dentist that you are taking ticlopidine. Your doctor may tell you to stop taking ticlopidine 10-14 days before your procedure. Follow these directions.

What special dietary instructions should I follow?

Take ticlopidine with meals or just after eating to prevent upset stomach.

What should I do if I forget to take a dose?

Take the missed dose as soon as you remember it. However, if it is almost time for the next dose, skip the missed dose and continue your regular dosing schedule. Do not take a double dose to make up for a missed one.

What side effects can this medicine cause?

Ticlopidine may cause side effects. Tell your doctor if any of these symptoms are severe or do not go away:
- upset stomach
- diarrhea
- vomiting
- stomach pain
- loss of appetite
- gas
- headache
- itching

If you experience any of the following symptoms, or

those listed in the IMPORTANT WARNING section, call your doctor immediately:

- fever, sore throat, or other signs of infection
- unusual bleeding or bruising
- light-colored stools
- skin rash

If you experience a serious side effect, you or your doctor may send a report to the Food and Drug Administration's (FDA) MedWatch Adverse Event Reporting program online [at http://www.fda.gov/MedWatch/index.html] or by phone [1-800-332-1088].

What storage conditions are needed for this medicine?

Keep this medication in the container it came in, tightly closed, and out of reach of children. Store it at room temperature and away from excess heat and moisture (not in the bathroom). Throw away any medication that is outdated or no longer needed. Talk to your pharmacist about the proper disposal of your medication.

What should I do in case of overdose?

In case of overdose, call your local poison control center at 1-800-222-1222. If the victim has collapsed or is not breathing, call local emergency services at 911.

What other information should I know?

Ticlopidine prevents blood from clotting so it may take longer than usual for you to stop bleeding if you are cut or injured. Avoid activities that have a high risk of causing injury. Call your doctor if bleeding is unusual.

Do not let anyone else take your medication. Ask your pharmacist any questions you have about refilling your prescription.

Dosage Facts
For Informational Purposes

Caution: Do not change your dose, how often you take your medication, or the length of time you are to take it without first talking to your healthcare provider.

The following dosage information was written using medical language for doctors and other healthcare professionals and is provided here for you to check your dosage. The dosage of this drug may differ for different patients. Therefore, always follow your doctor's instructions or the directions on the label. Contact your healthcare provider or pharmacist if you have any questions about the specific dosage of your medication after reviewing this information.

General Dosage Information

Available as ticlopidine hydrochloride; dosage expressed in terms of the salt.

Adult Patients

Thrombotic Stroke

ORAL:
- 250 mg twice daily.

Prevention of Coronary Artery Stent Thrombosis

ORAL:
- Manufacturer recommends 250 mg twice daily for up to 30 days in conjunction with antiplatelet dosages of aspirin.
- Alternatively, some clinicians suggest a ticlopidine loading dose† of 500 mg at least 6 hours prior to stent implantation, followed by 250 mg twice daily for 2 weeks in patients receiving bare-metal stents.
- For aspirin-intolerant patients, some clinicians recommend a ticlopidine loading dose† of 500 mg at least 24 hours prior to stent implantation.

Prescribing Limits

Adult Patients

Thrombotic Stroke

ORAL:
- Therapy has been continued for 5.8 years or longer in some patients.

Special Populations

Renal Impairment
- Reduce dosage or discontinue therapy if hemorrhagic or hematopoietic complications occur.

† Use is not currently included in the labeling approved by the US Food and Drug Administration.

Tiludronate

(tye loo′ droe nate)

Brand Name: Skelid®

Why is this medicine prescribed?

Tiludronate, a bisphosphonate, is used to treat Paget's disease. It slows the weakening of bone by decreasing the breakdown of bone.

This medication is sometimes prescribed for other uses; ask your doctor or pharmacist for more information.

How should this medicine be used?

Tiludronate comes as a tablet to take by mouth. It should be taken once a day on an empty stomach. Do not remove tablets from the foil strip until you are ready to take them. Tiludronate should be taken with a full glass (6-8 ounces) of plain water. Wait at least 2 hours before eating, drinking, or taking other medications. Do not take tiludronate with mineral water, coffee, orange juice, grapefruit juice, milk, or other dairy products.

Follow the directions on your prescription label carefully, and ask your doctor or pharmacist to explain any part you do not understand. Take tiludronate exactly as directed. Do not take more or less of it or take it more often than prescribed by your doctor. Your doctor will probably prescribe tiludronate for 3 months. Do not stop taking tiludronate without talking to your doctor.

What special precautions should I follow?

Before taking tiludronate,
- tell your doctor and pharmacist if you are allergic to tiludronate, alendronate, clodrinate, etidronate, risendronate, pamidronate, or any other drugs.
- tell your doctor and pharmacist what prescription and nonprescription medications you are taking, especially antacids (such as aluminum hydroxide [Amphogel], magnesium oxide [Mag-Ox], or aluminum magnesium [Riopan]); aspirin products (such as aspirin or diflunisal [Dolobid]); calcium products; indomethacin (Indocin); mineral or vitamin supplements containing calcium, iron, magnesium, or aluminum; and other vitamins or herbal products.
- tell your doctor if you have or have ever had abnormalities of your esophagus; an overactive parathyroid gland; upper gastrointestinal disease such as ulcers, gastritis, heartburn, chronic stomach problems, or duodenitis; kidney disease; a history of neuroleptic malignant syndrome (high temperature with rigid muscles and abnormal consciousness); below-normal calcium levels in your blood; or low levels of vitamin D.
- tell your doctor if you are pregnant, plan to become pregnant, or are breast-feeding. If you become pregnant while taking tiludronate, call your doctor immediately.
- if you are having surgery, including dental surgery, tell the doctor or dentist that you are taking tiludronate.

What special dietary instructions should I follow?

It is important that you get enough calcium and vitamin D while you are taking tiludronate. Your doctor may prescribe supplements if your dietary intake is not enough.

Remember that tiludronate should be taken on an empty stomach, at least 2 hours after eating or taking medications. It should be taken with at least 6-8 ounces of water. Food, drinks, and other drugs (including vitamins, calcium, and vitamin D) should not be taken for at least 2 hours after taking tiludronate.

What should I do if I forget to take a dose?

Take the missed dose as soon as you remember it. However, if it is almost time for the next dose, skip the missed dose and continue your regular dosing schedule. Do not take a double dose to make up for a missed one.

What side effects can this medicine cause?

Tiludronate may cause side effects. Tell your doctor if any of these symptoms are severe or do not go away:
- upset stomach
- diarrhea
- stomach irritation or pain
- gas
- constipation
- vomiting
- decreased appetite
- swelling of the feet or legs
- headache
- dizziness
- nasal congestion
- muscle, joint, or bone pain
- red or irritated eyes
- throat pain
- difficulty sleeping
- tingling in extremities
- nervousness
- muscle contractions

If you experience any of the following symptoms, call your doctor immediately:
- rash
- blurred or decreased vision
- chest pain
- difficulty swallowing
- coughing
- fever
- sinus or respiratory infection

If you experience a serious side effect, you or your doctor may send a report to the Food and Drug Administration's (FDA) MedWatch Adverse Event Reporting program online [at http://www.fda.gov/MedWatch/index.html] or by phone [1-800-332-1088].

What storage conditions are needed for this medicine?

Keep this medication in the container it came in, tightly closed, and out of reach of children. Do not remove tablets from foil strip until you are ready to take them. Store this medication at room temperature and away from excess heat and moisture (not in the bathroom). Talk to your pharmacist about the proper disposal of your medication.

What should I do in case of overdose?

In case of overdose, call your local poison control center at 1-800-222-1222. If the victim has collapsed or is not breathing, call local emergency services at 911.

What other information should I know?

Keep all appointments with your doctor and the laboratory. Your doctor may order certain laboratory tests to check your response to tiludronate.

Do not let anyone else take your medication. Ask your pharmacist any questions you have about refilling your prescription.

Talk to your doctor, pharmacist, or other healthcare professional if you have questions about dosing information for your medication.

Timolol Ophthalmic

(tye′ moe lole)

Brand Name: Timoptic®, Timoptic-XE®
Also available generically.

Why is this medicine prescribed?

Timolol is used to treat glaucoma, a condition in which increased pressure in the eye can lead to gradual loss of vision. Timolol decreases the pressure in the eye.

This medication is sometimes prescribed for other uses; ask your doctor or pharmacist for more information.

How should this medicine be used?

Timolol comes as eyedrops and eye gel. Timolol eyedrops usually are applied once or twice a day, at evenly spaced intervals, until pressure in your eyeball is controlled (about 4 weeks). Then you may be able to use it once a day. Timolol gel usually is applied once a day. Follow the directions on your prescription label carefully, and ask doctor or pharmacist to explain any part you do not understand. Use timolol exactly as directed. Do not use more or less of it or use it more often than prescribed by your doctor.

Timolol controls glaucoma but does not cure it. Continue to use timolol even if you feel well. Do not stop using timolol without talking to your doctor.

To use the eyedrops or eye gel, follow these instructions:

1. Wash your hands thoroughly with soap and water.
2. Use a mirror or have someone else put the drops in your eye.
3. If you are using the eye gel, invert the container and shake it once. (There is no need to shake the solution.) Make sure that the end of the dropper is not chipped or cracked.
4. Avoid touching the dropper tip against your eye or anything else. If the tip touches anything, it can become contaminated with bacteria that can cause serious eye infections.
5. Hold the dropper tip down at all times to prevent drops from flowing back into the bottle and contaminating the remaining contents.
6. Lie down or tilt your head back.
7. Holding the bottle between your thumb and index finger, place the dropper tip as near as possible to your eyelid without touching it.
8. Brace the remaining fingers of that hand against your cheek or nose.
9. With the index finger of your other hand, pull the lower lid of the eye down to form a pocket.
10. Drop the prescribed number of drops into the pocket made by the lower lid and the eye. Placing drops on the surface of the eyeball can cause stinging.
11. Close your eye and press lightly against the lower lid with your finger for 2-3 minutes to keep the medication in the eye. Do not blink.
12. Replace and tighten the cap right away. Do not wipe or rinse it off.
13. Wipe off any excess liquid from your cheek with a clean tissue. Wash your hands again.

What special precautions should I follow?

Before using timolol eyedrops or eye gel,

- tell your doctor and pharmacist if you are allergic to timolol, beta blockers, or any other drugs.
- tell your doctor and pharmacist what prescription and nonprescription medications you are taking, especially other eye medications; beta blockers such as atenolol (Tenormin), carteolol (Cartrol), esmolol (Breviblic), labetalol (Normodyne, Trandate), metoprolol (Lopressor), nadolol (Corgard), propranolol (Inderal), sotalol (Betapace), and timolol (Blocadren); quinidine (Quinidex, Quinaglute Dura-Tabs); verapamil (Calan, Isoptin); and vitamins.
- tell your doctor if you have or have ever had thyroid, heart, or lung disease; congestive heart failure; myasthenia gravis; or diabetes.
- tell your doctor if you are pregnant, plan to become pregnant, or are breast-feeding. If you become pregnant while using timolol, call your doctor immediately.
- if you are having surgery, including dental surgery, tell the doctor or dentist that you are using timolol.
- if you are using another eyedrop medication, use the eye medications at least 10 minutes apart.
- if you have eye surgery, an eye injury, or develop an eye infection while taking timolol eyedrops or eye gel, ask your doctor if you can continue using the same container of timolol.
- if you wear soft contact lenses, remove them before using timolol, and wait until 15 minutes after using timolol to put them back in.

What should I do if I forget to take a dose?

Apply the missed dose as soon as you remember it. However, if it is almost time for the next dose, skip the missed dose and continue your regular dosing schedule. Do not apply a double dose to make up for a missed one.

What side effects can this medicine cause?

Timolol may cause side effects. Tell your doctor if any of these symptoms are severe or do not go away:

- eye irritation

- double vision
- headache
- depression
- dizziness
- upset stomach

If you experience any of the following symptoms, stop using timolol and call your doctor immediately:

- slow or irregular heartbeat
- difficulty breathing
- sudden weight gain
- swelling of the feet or lower legs
- fainting

If you experience a serious side effect, you or your doctor may send a report to the Food and Drug Administration's (FDA) MedWatch Adverse Event Reporting program online [at http://www.fda.gov/MedWatch/index.html] or by phone [1-800-332-1088].

What storage conditions are needed for this medicine?

Keep this medication in the container it came in, tightly closed, and out of reach of children. Store it at room temperature and away from excess heat and moisture (not in the bathroom). If it becomes discolored or cloudy, obtain a fresh bottle. Throw away any medication that is outdated or no longer needed. Talk to your pharmacist about the proper disposal of your medication.

What other information should I know?

Keep all appointments with your doctor. Your doctor will order certain eye tests to check your response to timolol.

Do not let anyone else use your medication. Ask your pharmacist any questions you have about refilling your prescription.

Dosage Facts
For Informational Purposes

Caution: Do not change your dose, how often you take your medication, or the length of time you are to take it without first talking to your healthcare provider.

The following dosage information was written using medical language for doctors and other healthcare professionals and is provided here for you to check your dosage. The dosage of this drug may differ for different patients. Therefore, always follow your doctor's instructions or the directions on the label. Contact your healthcare provider or pharmacist if you have any questions about the specific dosage of your medication after reviewing this information.

General Dosage Information

Available as timolol maleate or timolol (as the hemihydrate); dosage is expressed in terms of timolol.

Adult Patients
Ocular Hypertension and Glaucoma

OCULAR ADMINISTRATION:
- Timolol ophthalmic solution: initially, 1 drop of a 0.25% solution in the affected eye(s) twice daily. May increase dosage to 1 drop of a 0.5% solution in the affected eye(s) twice daily if necessary. May then reduce dosage to 1 drop of the effective strength in the affected eye(s) once daily if satisfactory IOP is maintained.
- Timolol ophthalmic gel-forming solution: 1 drop of a 0.25 or 0.5% solution in the affected eye(s) once daily.
- Fixed-combination timolol/dorzolamide solution: 1 drop in the affected eye(s) twice daily.

Prescribing Limits
Adult Patients
Ocular Hypertension and Glaucoma

OCULAR ADMINISTRATION:
- Timolol ophthalmic solution: Dosages >1 drop of a 0.5% solution in the affected eye(s) twice daily generally do not produce further reduction in IOP.
- Timolol ophthalmic gel-forming solution: Dosages >1 drop of a 0.5% solution in the affected eye(s) once daily not studied.

Timolol Oral

(tye′ moe lole)

Brand Name: Blocadren®, Timolide®
Also available generically.

Important Warning

Do not stop taking timolol without talking to your doctor first. If timolol is stopped suddenly, it may cause chest pain or heart attack in some people.

Why is this medicine prescribed?

Timolol is used to treat high blood pressure. It also is used to prevent angina (chest pain) and heart attacks. It works by relaxing your blood vessels so your heart doesn't have to pump as hard. Timolol also is used to prevent migraine headaches.

This medication is sometimes prescribed for other uses; ask your doctor or pharmacist for more information.

How should this medicine be used?

Timolol comes as a tablet to take by mouth. It usually is taken one or two times a day. Follow the directions on your prescription label carefully, and ask your doctor or pharmacist to explain any part you do not understand. Take timolol exactly as directed. Do not take more or less of it or take it more often than prescribed by your doctor.

Timolol helps control your condition but will not cure it. Continue to take timolol even if you feel well. Do not stop taking timolol without talking to your doctor.

What special precautions should I follow?

Before taking timolol,
- tell your doctor and pharmacist if you are allergic to timolol or any other drugs.
- tell your doctor and pharmacist what prescription and nonprescription medications you are taking, especially aspirin and other nonsteroidal anti-inflammatory drugs (NSAIDs) such as ibuprofen (Advil, Motrin) and naproxen (Aleve, Naprosyn), clonidine (Catapres), digoxin (Lanoxin), diltiazem (Cardizem, Dilacor, Tiazac), medications for glaucoma, nifedipine (Adalat, Procardia), other medications for heart disease or high blood pressure, quinidine (Quinidex, Quinaglute Dura-Tabs), reserpine (Serpalan, Serpasil), verapamil (Calan, Covera, Verelan), and vitamins.
- tell your doctor if you have or have ever had asthma or other lung disease; heart, liver, or kidney disease; diabetes; severe allergies; muscle disease; or thyroid problems.
- tell your doctor if you are pregnant, plan to become pregnant, or are breast-feeding. If you become pregnant while taking timolol, call your doctor.
- if you are having surgery, including dental surgery, tell the doctor or dentist that you are taking timolol.
- you should know that this drug may make you drowsy. Do not drive a car or operate machinery until you know how this drug affects you.
- remember that alcohol can add to the drowsiness caused by this drug.

What special dietary instructions should I follow?

Talk to your doctor before using salt substitutes containing potassium. If your doctor prescribes a low-salt or low-sodium diet, follow these directions carefully.

What should I do if I forget to take a dose?

Take the missed dose as soon as you remember it. However, if it is almost time for the next dose, skip the missed dose and continue your regular dosing schedule. Do not take a double dose to make up for a missed one.

What side effects can this medicine cause?

Timolol may cause side effects. Tell your doctor if any of these symptoms are severe or do not go away:
- dizziness or lightheadedness
- excessive tiredness
- heartburn
- headache
- cold hands and feet

If you experience any of the following symptoms, call your doctor immediately:
- difficulty breathing
- swelling of the feet or hands
- unusual weight gain
- chest pain
- slow, irregular heartbeat

If you experience a serious side effect, you or your doctor may send a report to the Food and Drug Administration's (FDA) MedWatch Adverse Event Reporting program online [at http://www.fda.gov/MedWatch/index.html] or by phone [1-800-332-1088].

What storage conditions are needed for this medicine?

Keep this medication in the container it came in, tightly closed, and out of reach of children. Store it at room temperature and away from excess heat and moisture (not in the bathroom). Throw away any medication that is outdated or no longer needed. Talk to your pharmacist about the proper disposal of your medication.

What should I do in case of overdose?

In case of overdose, call your local poison control center at 1-800-222-1222. If the victim has collapsed or is not breathing, call local emergency services at 911.

What other information should I know?

Keep all appointments with your doctor and the laboratory. Your doctor will need to determine your response to timolol. Your doctor may ask you to check your pulse (heart rate). Ask your pharmacist or doctor to teach you how to take your pulse. If your pulse is faster or slower than it should be, call your doctor.

Do not let anyone else take your medication. Ask your pharmacist any questions you have about refilling your prescription.

Dosage Facts
For Informational Purposes

Caution: Do not change your dose, how often you take your medication, or the length of time you are to take it without first talking to your healthcare provider.

The following dosage information was written using medical language for doctors and other healthcare professionals and is provided here for you to check your dosage. The dosage of this drug may differ for different patients. Therefore, always follow your doctor's instructions or the directions on the label. Contact your healthcare provider or pharmacist if you have any questions about the specific dosage of your medication after reviewing this information.

General Dosage Information

Available as timolol maleate; dosage expressed in terms of the salt.

Adult Patients

Hypertension
Monotherapy

ORAL:

- Initially, 10 mg twice daily.
- Increase dosage gradually at weekly (or longer) intervals until optimum effect is obtained.
- Usual maintenance dosage is 20–40 mg daily, given in 2 divided doses; once daily dosing may be possible in some patients. Increases up to a maximum of 60 mg daily (given in 2 divided doses) may be necessary.

Timolol/Hydrochlorothiazide Combination Therapy

ORAL:

- Timolol/hydrochlorothiazide fixed combination is not recommended for initial therapy; adjust initial and subsequent dosages by administering each drug separately. May use if optimum maintenance dosage corresponds to ratio in the commercial combination preparation.

AMI

ORAL:

- Usual dosage is 10 mg twice daily.
- Initiation within 7–28 days following AMI reduces cardio-vascular mortality and nonfatal reinfarction. Some experts recommend initiation within a few days after AMI (if not already initiated acutely).
- Optimum benefit may be achieved when oral β-adrenergic blocking agent is continued for at least 1–3 years after infarction (if not contraindicated). Some experts recommend continuing *indefinitely* unless contraindicated.

Angina
Chronic Stable Angina Pectorist†

ORAL:

- 15–45 mg daily, given in 3 or 4 divided doses. Adjust dosage according to clinical response and to maintain a resting heart rate of 55–60 bpm.

Unstable Angina or Non-ST-segment Elevation MI†

In patients at high risk for ischemic events, ACC and AHA suggest initiation with IV loading dose of a β-blocker (in patients who tolerate IV therapy) followed by oral therapy; oral therapy is recommended for lower risk patients.

ORAL:

- 10 mg twice daily.
- The target resting heart rate is 50–60 bpm in the absence of dose-limiting adverse effects.

Vascular Headaches
Migraine

ORAL:

- Initially, 10 mg twice daily. Adjust dosage according to clinical response and patient tolerance; do not exceed 30 mg daily, given in divided doses (e.g., 10 mg in the morning and 20 mg in the evening).
- During maintenance therapy, can administer 20-mg daily dosage as a single rather than divided dose; some patients may respond adequately to 10 mg once daily.

- If an adequate response is not achieved after 6–8 weeks at the maximum recommended dosage, discontinue therapy.

Prescribing Limits

Adult Patients

Hypertension

ORAL:

- Maximum 60 mg daily.

Vascular Headaches (Migraine)

ORAL:

- Maximum 30 mg daily.

Special Populations

Hepatic Impairment

- Must modify doses and/or frequency of administration in response to degree of hepatic impairment.

Renal Impairment

- Must modify doses and/or frequency of administration in response to degree of renal impairment.

Geriatric Patients

- Select dosage with caution because of age-related decreases in hepatic, renal, and/or cardiac function and concomitant disease and drug therapy. Initiate at low end of dosing range.

† Use is not currently included in the labeling approved by the US Food and Drug Administration.

Tinidazole

(tye ni′ da zole)

Brand Name: Tindamax®

Important Warning

Another medication that is similar to tinidazole has caused cancer in laboratory animals. It is not known whether tinidazole increases the risk of developing cancer in laboratory animals or in humans. Talk to your doctor about the risks and benefits of using this medication.

Why is this medicine prescribed?

Tinidazole is used to treat trichomoniasis (a sexually transmitted disease that can affect men and women), giardiasis (an infection of the intestine that can cause diarrhea, gas, and stomach cramps), and amebiasis (an infection of the intestine that can cause diarrhea, gas, and stomach cramps and can spread to other organs such as the liver). Tinidazole is in a class of medications called antiprotozoal agents. It works by killing the organisms that can cause infection.

How should this medicine be used?

Tinidazole comes as a suspension (liquid) prepared by the pharmacist and a tablet to take by mouth. It is usually taken with food as a single dose or once a day for 3 to 5 days. To help you remember to take tinidazole (if you are to take it for more than one day), take it around the same time every day. Follow the directions on your prescription label carefully, and ask your doctor or pharmacist to explain any part you do not understand. Take tinidazole exactly as directed. Do not take more or less of it or take it more often than prescribed by your doctor.

Shake the liquid well before each use to mix the medication evenly.

Take tinidazole until you finish the prescription, even if you feel better. If you stop taking tinidazole too soon or skip doses, your infection may not be completely cured and bacteria may become resistant to antibiotics

Are there other uses for this medicine?

This medication may be prescribed for other uses; ask your doctor or pharmacist for more information.

What special precautions should I follow?

Before taking tinidazole,
- tell your doctor and pharmacist if you are allergic to tinidazole, metronidazole (Flagyl), or any other medications.
- tell your doctor and pharmacist what prescription and nonprescription medications, vitamins, nutritional supplements, and herbal products you are taking. Be sure to mention any of the following: anticoagulants ('blood thinners') such as warfarin (Coumadin); antifungals such as fluconazole (Diflucan), itraconazole (Sporanox), and ketoconazole (Nizoral); carbamazepine (Tegretol); cimetidine (Tagamet); clarithromycin (Biaxin); cyclosporine (Neoral, Sandimmune); danazol (Danocrine); delavirdine (Rescriptor); dexamethasone (Decadron); diltiazem (Cardizem, Dilacor; Tiazac); erythromycin (E.E.S., E-Mycin, Erythrocin); ethosuximide (Zarontin); fluorouracil (Adrucil); fluoxetine (Prozac, Sarafem); fluvoxamine (Luvox); fosphenytoin (Cerebyx); HIV protease inhibitors such as indinavir (Crixivan) and ritonavir (Norvir); isoniazid (INH, Nydrazid); lithium (Lithobid); metronidazole (Flagyl); nefazodone (Serzone); oral contraceptives (birth control pills); oxytetracycline (Terramycin); phenobarbital (Luminal, Solfoton); phenytoin (Dilantin); rifabutin (Mycobutin); rifampin (Rifadin, Rimactane); tacrolimus (Prograf); troglitazone (Rezulin); troleandomycin (TAO); verapamil (Calan, Covera, Isoptin, Verelan); and zafirlukast (Accolate). Also tell your doctor if you are taking disulfiram (Antabuse) or have stopped taking it within the past 2 weeks. Your doctor may need to change the doses of your medications or monitor you carefully for side effects.
- if you are taking cholestyramine (Questran), you should not take it at the same time that you take tinidazole. Ask your doctor or pharmacist how to space doses of these medications.
- tell your doctor if you have a yeast infection now; if you are being treated with dialysis (mechanical removal of waste in patients with kidney failure); or if you have or have ever had seizures or nervous system, blood, or liver disease.
- tell your doctor if you are pregnant or plan to become pregnant. If you become pregnant while taking tinidazole, call your doctor. Do not breastfeed while you are taking tinidazole and for 3 days after you finish your treatment.
- know that you should not drink alcohol while you are taking this medication and for 3 days afterwards. Alcohol may cause an upset stomach, vomiting, stomach cramps, headaches, sweating, and flushing (redness of the face).

What special dietary instructions should I follow?

Talk to your doctor about drinking grapefruit juice while taking this medication.

What should I do if I forget to take a dose?

Take the missed dose as soon as you remember it. However, if it is almost time for the next dose, skip the missed dose and continue your regular dosing schedule. Do not take a double dose to make up for a missed one.

What side effects can this medicine cause?

Tinidazole may cause side effects. Tell your doctor if any of these symptoms are severe or do not go away:
- sharp, unpleasant metallic taste
- upset stomach
- vomiting
- loss of appetite
- constipation
- stomach pain or cramps
- headache
- tiredness or weakness
- dizziness

Some side effects can be serious. The following symptoms are uncommon, but if you experience any of them, call your doctor immediately:
- seizures
- numbness or tingling of hands or feet
- rash
- hives
- swelling of the face, throat, tongue, lips, eyes, hands, feet, ankles, or lower legs
- hoarseness
- difficulty swallowing or breathing

If you experience a serious side effect, you or your doctor may send a report to the Food and Drug Administration's

(FDA) MedWatch Adverse Event Reporting program online [at http://www.fda.gov/MedWatch/index.html] or by phone [1-800-332-1088].

What storage conditions are needed for this medicine?

Keep this medication in the container it came in, tightly closed, and out of reach of children. Store it at room temperature and away from excess heat and moisture (not in the bathroom). Protect the medication from light. Throw away any medication that is outdated or no longer needed. Throw away any remaining liquid after 7 days. Talk to your pharmacist about the proper disposal of your medication.

What should I do in case of overdose?

In case of overdose, call your local poison control center at 1-800-222-1222. If the victim has collapsed or is not breathing, call local emergency services at 911.

What other information should I know?

Keep all appointments with your doctor and the laboratory. Your doctor may order certain lab tests to check your body's response to tinidazole. Before having any laboratory test, tell your doctor and the laboratory personnel that you are taking tinidazole.

Do not let anyone else take your medication. Your prescription is probably not refillable. If you still have symptoms of infection after you finish the tinidazole, call your doctor.

Dosage Facts
For Informational Purposes

Caution: Do not change your dose, how often you take your medication, or the length of time you are to take it without first talking to your healthcare provider.

The following dosage information was written using medical language for doctors and other healthcare professionals and is provided here for you to check your dosage. The dosage of this drug may differ for different patients. Therefore, always follow your doctor's instructions or the directions on the label. Contact your healthcare provider or pharmacist if you have any questions about the specific dosage of your medication after reviewing this information.

Pediatric Patients

Amebiasis
Entamoeba Histolytic Infections
ORAL:
- Children >3 years of age (intestinal amebiasis): 50 mg/kg (up to 2 g) once daily given for 3 days; follow-up with an oral luminal amebicide (e.g., iodoquinol, paromomycin).
- Children >3 years of age (amebic liver abscess): 50 mg/kg (up to 2 g) once daily given for 3–5 days; follow-up with an oral luminal amebicide (e.g., iodoquinol, paromomycin).

Giardiasis
ORAL:
- Children >3 years of age: 50 mg/kg (up to 2 g) given as a single dose.

Trichomoniasis†
ORAL:
- Children >3 years of age†: 50 mg/kg (up to 2 g) given as a single dose.

Adult Patients

Amebiasis
Entamoeba Histolytic Infections
ORAL:
- Intestinal amebiasis: 2 g once daily given for 3 days; follow-up with an oral luminal amebicide (e.g., iodoquinol, paromomycin).
- Amebic liver abscess: 2 g once daily for 3–5 days; follow-up with an oral luminal amebicide (e.g., iodoquinol, paromomycin).

Giardiasis
ORAL:
- 2 g given as a single dose.

Trichomoniasis
ORAL:
- 2 g given as a single dose.
- Treat sexual partners of the patient simultaneously using the same dosage.
- For treatment failure following a metronidazole regimen (e.g., single 2-g dose of metronidazole), CDC recommends retreatment with a single 2-g dose of tinidazole; if retreatment fails, CDC recommends tinidazole 2 g once daily for 5 days. If multiple-dose regimen fails, consult a specialist.

Nongonococcal Urethritis†
ORAL:
- CDC recommends a single 2-g dose of tinidazole in conjunction with a single1-g dose of oral azithromycin (if azithromycin not used in the initial regimen) for treatment of recurrent and persistent urethritis in patients who previously received a recommended regimen.

Prescribing Limits

Pediatric Patients

ORAL:
- Children >3 years of age: Maximum 50 mg/kg (up to 2 g) daily or as a single dose.

Special Populations

Hepatic Impairment
- Data insufficient to make specific dosage recommendations. Use usual dosage with caution.

Renal Impairment
- Dosage adjustments not needed, unless patient is undergoing hemodialysis.
- If given on a day that hemodialysis is performed, administer an additional dose (equivalent to 50% of the recommended dose) after the dialysis session.

Geriatric Patients
- Select dosage with caution because of age-related decreases in hepatic, renal, and/or cardiac function and concomitant disease and drug therapy.

† Use is not currently included in the labeling approved by the US Food and Drug Administration.

Tiotropium Oral Inhalation

(tee oh tro′ pee um)

Brand Name: Spiriva® HandiHaler®

Why is this medicine prescribed?

Tiotropium is used to prevent wheezing, shortness of breath, and difficulty breathing in patients with chronic obstructive pulmonary disease (COPD, a group of diseases that affect the lungs and airways) such as chronic bronchitis (swelling of the air passages that lead to the lungs) and emphysema (damage to air sacs in the lungs). Tiotropium is in a class of medications called bronchodilators. It works by relaxing and opening the air passages to the lungs to make breathing easier.

How should this medicine be used?

Tiotropium comes as a capsule to use with a specially designed inhaler. You will use the inhaler to breathe in the dry powder contained in the capsules. Tiotropium is usually inhaled once a day in the morning or evening. To help you remember to inhale tiotropium, inhale it around the same time every day. Follow the directions on your prescription label carefully, and ask your doctor or pharmacist to explain any part you do not understand. Use tiotropium exactly as directed. Do not inhale more or less of it or inhale it more often than prescribed by your doctor.

Tiotropium will only work if you use the inhaler it comes with to inhale the powder in the capsules. Never swallow tiotropium capsules and never try to inhale them using any other inhaler. Never use your tiotropium inhaler to take any other medication.

Do not use tiotropium to treat a sudden attack of wheezing or shortness of breath. Your doctor will probably prescribe a different medication to use when you have great difficulty breathing.

Tiotropium controls COPD but does not cure it. It may take a few weeks before you feel the full benefits of tiotropium. Continue to take tiotropium even if you feel well. Do not stop taking tiotropium without talking to your doctor.

Be careful not to get tiotropium powder in your eyes. If tiotropium powder gets into your eyes, your vision may become blurred and you may be sensitive to light. Call your doctor if this happens.

To use the inhaler, follow these steps:

1. Use the diagram in the patient information that came with your medication to help you learn the names of the parts of your inhaler. You should be able to find the dust cap, mouthpiece, base, piercing button, and center chamber.
2. Pick up one blister card of tiotropium capsules and tear it along the perforation. You should now have two strips that each contain three capsules.
3. Put away one of the strips for later. Use the tab to carefully peel back the foil on the other blister strip until the STOP line. This should fully uncover one capsule. The other two capsules on the strip should still be sealed in their packaging. Plan to use those capsules on the next 2 days.
4. Pull upward on the dust cap of your inhaler to open it.
5. Open the mouthpiece of the inhaler. Remove the tiotropium capsule from the package and place it in the center chamber of the inhaler.
6. Close the mouthpiece firmly until it clicks, but do not close the dust cap.
7. Hold the inhaler so that the mouthpiece is on top. Press the green piercing button once, then let it go.
8. Breathe out completely without putting any part of the inhaler in or near your mouth.
9. Bring the inhaler up to your mouth and close your lips tightly around the mouthpiece.
10. Hold your head upright and breathe in slowly and deeply. You should breathe just fast enough to hear the capsule vibrate. Continue to breathe in until your lungs are full.
11. Hold your breath for as long as you can comfortably do so. Take the inhaler out of your mouth while you are holding your breath.
12. Breathe normally for a short time.
13. Repeat steps 8-11 to inhale any medication that may be left in your inhaler.
14. Open the mouthpiece and tilt the inhaler to spill out the used capsule. Throw the used capsule away out of the reach of children and pets. You may see a small amount of powder remaining in the capsule. This is normal and does not mean that you did not get your full dose.
15. Close the mouthpiece and dust cap and store the inhaler in a safe place.

Are there other uses for this medicine?

This medication may be prescribed for other uses; ask your doctor or pharmacist for more information.

What special precautions should I follow?

Before using tiotropium,
- tell your doctor and pharmacist if you are allergic to tiotropium, atropine (Atropen, Sal-Tropine, Ocu-Tropine), ipratropium (Atrovent), or any other medications.

- tell your doctor and pharmacist what prescription and nonprescription medications, vitamins, nutritional supplements, and herbal products you are taking. Be sure to mention any of the following: amiodarone (Cordarone); antihistamines; atropine (Atropen, Sal-Tropine, Ocu-Tropine); cisapride (Propulsid); disopyramide (Norpace); dofetilide (Tikosyn); erythromycin (E.E.S, E-Mycin, Erythrocin); eye drops; ipratropium (Atrovent); medications for irritable bowel disease, motion sickness, Parkinson's disease, ulcers, or urinary problems; moxifloxacin (Avelox); pimozide (Orap); procainamide (Procanbid, Pronestyl); quinidine (Quinidex); sotalol (Betapace); sparfloxacin (Zagam); and thioridazine (Mellaril). Your doctor may need to change the doses of your medications or monitor you carefully for side effects.
- tell your doctor if you have or have ever had glaucoma (an eye disease that can cause vision loss), urinary problems, irregular heart beat, or prostate (a male reproductive organ) or kidney disease.
- tell your doctor if you are pregnant, plan to become pregnant, or are breast-feeding. If you become pregnant while taking tiotropium, call your doctor.
- if you are having surgery, including dental surgery, tell the doctor or dentist that you are taking tiotropium.

What special dietary instructions should I follow?

Unless your doctor tells you otherwise, continue your normal diet.

What should I do if I forget to take a dose?

Inhale the missed dose as soon as you remember it. However, if it is almost time for the next dose, skip the missed dose and continue your regular dosing schedule. Do not inhale a double dose to make up for a missed one.

What side effects can this medicine cause?

Tiotropium may cause side effects. Tell your doctor if any of these symptoms are severe or do not go away:
- dry mouth
- constipation
- stomach pain
- vomiting
- indigestion
- muscle pain
- nosebleed
- runny nose
- sneezing
- painful white patches in mouth

Some side effects can be serious. The following symptoms are uncommon, but if you experience any of them, call your doctor immediately:
- hives
- skin rash
- itching

- difficulty breathing or swallowing
- swellling of the face, throat, tongue, lips, eyes, hands, feet, ankles, or lower legs
- hoarseness
- chest pain
- sore throat, fever, chills, and other signs of infection
- headaches or other signs of a sinus infection
- painful or difficult urination
- fast heart beat
- eye pain
- blurred vision
- seeing halos around lights or seeing colored images
- red eyes

Tiotropium may cause other side effects. Call your doctor if you have any unusual problems while using this medication.

If you experience a serious side effect, you or your doctor may send a report to the Food and Drug Administration's (FDA) MedWatch Adverse Event Reporting program online [at http://www.fda.gov/MedWatch/index.html] or by phone [1-800-332-1088].

What storage conditions are needed for this medicine?

Keep this medication in the container it came in, tightly closed, and out of reach of children. Store it at room temperature and away from excess heat and moisture (not in the bathroom). Do not open the blister package surrounding a capsule until just before you are ready to use it. If you accidentally open the package of a capsule that you cannot use immediately, throw away that capsule. Never store capsules inside the inhaler. Throw away any medication that is outdated or no longer needed. Talk to your pharmacist about the proper disposal of your medication.

What should I do in case of overdose?

In case of overdose, call your local poison control center at 1-800-222-1222. If the victim has collapsed or is not breathing, call local emergency services at 911.

Symptoms of overdose may include:
- dry mouth
- stomach pain
- constipation
- shaking hands that you cannot control
- changes in thinking
- blurred vision
- red eyes
- fast heartbeat
- difficulty urinating

What other information should I know?

Keep all appointments with your doctor.

You will receive a new inhaler with each 30 day supply of medication. Normally, you will not need to clean your inhaler during the 30 days you use it. However, if you do need to clean your inhaler, you should open the dust cap and mouthpiece and then press the piercing button to open the base. Then rinse the entire inhaler with warm water but without any soaps or detergents. Tip out excess water and leave the inhaler to air dry for 24 hours with the dust cap, mouthpiece, and base open. Do not wash your inhaler in the dishwasher and do not use it after you wash it until it has been allowed to dry for 24 hours. You may also clean the outside of the mouthpiece with a moist (not wet) tissue.

Do not let anyone else take your medication. Ask your pharmacist any questions you have about refilling your prescription.

Dosage Facts
For Informational Purposes

Caution: Do not change your dose, how often you take your medication, or the length of time you are to take it without first talking to your healthcare provider.

The following dosage information was written using medical language for doctors and other healthcare professionals and is provided here for you to check your dosage. The dosage of this drug may differ for different patients. Therefore, always follow your doctor's instructions or the directions on the label. Contact your healthcare provider or pharmacist if you have any questions about the specific dosage of your medication after reviewing this information.

General Dosage Information

Available as tiotropium bromide monohydrate; dosage expressed in terms of anhydrous tiotropium.

Each capsule contains 18 mcg of tiotropium as an inhalation powder. However, the precise amount of drug delivered to the lungs depends on factors such as the patient's inspiratory flow.

Adult Patients

COPD

ORAL INHALATION:
- 18 mcg (contents of one capsule) once daily.

Special Populations

Hepatic Impairment
- No dosage adjustments required.

Renal Impairment
- No dosage adjustments required.

Geriatric Patients
- No dosage adjustments required.

Tipranavir
(tip ra′ na veer)

Brand Name: Aptivus®

Important Warning

Tipranavir taken with ritonavir (Norvir) may cause bleeding in the brain. This condition may be life-threatening. Tell your doctor if you have recently had surgery or if you have recently been injured in any way. Also tell your doctor if you have a bleeding disorder such as hemophilia (condition in which the blood does not clot normally). Tell your doctor and pharmacist if you are taking any of the following medications: anticoagulants ('blood thinners') such as warfarin (Coumadin), aspirin, cilostazol (Pletal), clopidogrel (Plavix), or ticlopidine (Ticlid). If you need to get emergency medical treatment for any reason, be sure to tell all of the doctors who treat you that you are taking tipranavir. Call your doctor immediately if you experience unusual bruising or bleeding during your treatment with tipranavir.

Tipranavir taken with ritonavir (Norvir) may cause liver damage that may be life-threatening. Tell your doctor if you have or have ever had hepatitis (swelling of the liver caused by a virus) or any other liver disease. Tell your doctor and pharmacist if you are taking acetaminophen (Tylenol, others); cholesterol lowering medications (statins) such as atorvastatin (Lipitor), lovastatin (Mevacor) and simvastatin (Zocor); iron products; isoniazid (INH, Nydrazid); methotrexate (Rheumatrex); niacin (nicotinic acid); rifampin (Rifadin, Rimactane); and salicylate pain relievers (aspirin, others). If you experience any of the following symptoms, stop taking tipranavir and call your doctor immediately: tiredness; flu-like symptoms; loss of appetite; upset stomach; pain, ache, swelling, or sensitivity on your right side below your ribs; yellowing of the skin or eyes; dark (tea-colored) urine; or pale bowel movements.

Keep all appointments with your doctor and the laboratory. Your doctor will order certain tests to check your body's response to tipranavir.

Talk to your doctor about the risks of taking tipranavir.

Why is this medicine prescribed?

Tipranavir is used with ritonavir (Norvir) and at least two other medications to treat human immunodeficiency virus (HIV). Tipranavir is in a class of medications called protease inhibitors. It works by slowing the spread of HIV in the body. Tipranavir does not cure HIV infection and may not prevent you from developing HIV-related illnesses. Tipranavir does not prevent you from spreading HIV to other people.

How should this medicine be used?

Tipranavir comes as a capsule to take by mouth. It is usually taken with food and with ritonavir twice a day. Take tipranavir and ritonavir at around the same times every day. Follow the directions on your prescription label carefully, and ask your doctor or pharmacist to explain any part you do not understand. Take tipranavir exactly as directed. Do not take more or less of it or take it more often than prescribed by your doctor.

Do not take tipranavir without ritonavir.

Swallow the capsules whole; do not chew them.

Tipranavir controls HIV but does not cure it. Continue to take tipranavir even if you feel well. Do not stop taking tipranavir without talking to your doctor. If you stop taking tipranavir or skip doses, your condition may become more difficult to treat. When your supply of tipranavir starts to run low, get more from your doctor or pharmacist.

Ask your doctor or pharmacist for a copy of the manufacturer's information for the patient. Read this information carefully and ask your doctor or pharmacist if you have any questions.

Are there other uses for this medicine?

This medication may be prescribed for other uses; ask your doctor or pharmacist for more information.

What special precautions should I follow?

Before taking tipranavir,

- tell your doctor and pharmacist if you are allergic to tipranavir, ritonavir (Norvir), sulfa medications, any other medications, or any of the ingredients in tipranavir. Ask your pharmacist if you are unsure if a medication you are allergic to is a sulfa medication.
- do not take tipranavir if you are taking astemizole (Hismanal) (no longer available in the United States); cisapride (Propulsid) (no longer available in the United States); ergot medications for migraines such as dihydroergotamine (D.H.E. 45, Migranal), ergoloid mesylate (Hydergine), ergotamine (Bellamine, Cafergot, Ergomar, others), or methylergonovine (Methergine); certain medications for irregular heartbeat including amiodarone (Pacerone), bepridil (Vascor) (no longer available in the United States), flecainide (Tambocor), propafenone (Rythmol), or quinidine (Quinaglute); midazolam (Versed); pimozide (Orap); terfenadine (Seldane) (no longer available in the United States); and triazolam (Halcion).
- tell your doctor and pharmacist what other prescription and nonprescription medications, vitamins, and nutritional supplements you are taking or plan to take. Be sure to mention the medications listed in the IMPORTANT WARNING section and any of the following: antifungal medications such as fluconazole (Diflucan),

itraconazole (Sporanox), ketoconazole (Nizoral), or voriconazole (Vfend); calcium-channel blockers such as diltiazem (Cardizem, Dilacor, Tiazac, others), felodipine (Lexxel, Plendil), nicardipine (Cardene), nisoldipine (Sular), or verapamil (Calan, Covera, Isoptin, Verelan, others); clarithromycin (Biaxin, in Prevpac); desipramine (Norpramin); disulfiram (Antabuse); immunosuppressants such as cyclosporine (Neoral, Sandimmune), sirolimus (Rapamune), or tacrolimus (Prograf); medications for diabetes such as glimepiride (Amaryl), glipizide (Glucotrol, in Metaglip), glyburide (Diabeta, Glycron, Glynase, Micronase, others), pioglitazone (Actos, in Actoplus), repaglinide (Prandin), or tolbutamide; certain medications for erectile dysfunction including sildenafil (Viagra), tadalafil (Cialis), or vardenafil (Levitra); other medications for HIV including amprenavir (Agenerase), lopinavir (in Kaletra), and saquinavir (Invirase); meperidine (Demerol, in Mepergan); methadone (Dolophine, Methadose); metronidazole (Flagyl); rifabutin (Mycobutin); and selective-serotonin reuptake inhibitors (SSRIs) such as fluoxetine (Prozac, Sarafem, in Symbyax), paroxetine (Paxil), or sertraline (Zoloft). Many other medications may also interact with tipranavir, so be sure to tell your doctor about all the medications you are taking, even those that do not appear on this list. Be sure to talk to your doctor or pharmacist before you begin taking any new medications during your treatment with tipranavir. Your doctor may need to change the doses of your medications or monitor you carefully for side effects.

- if you are taking didanosine, take it 2 hours before or 2 hours after you take tipranavir.
- if you are taking antacids, take them 2 hours before or 4 hours after you take tipranavir.
- tell your doctor what herbal products you are taking, especially St. John's wort.
- tell your doctor if you have or have ever had diabetes or high blood sugar; high blood cholesterol or triglycerides (blood fats); or an infection that comes and goes such as tuberculosis (TB), cytomegalovirus (CMV), herpes, shingles, or pneumonia.
- tell your doctor if you are pregnant, plan to become pregnant, or are breast-feeding. If you become pregnant while taking tipranavir, call your doctor. Do not breast-feed if you are infected with HIV or are taking tipranavir.
- you should know that tipranavir may decrease the effectiveness of hormonal contraceptives (birth control pills, rings, patches, and injections). Talk to your doctor about other ways to prevent pregnancy while you are taking this medication.
- if you are having surgery, including dental surgery, tell the doctor or dentist that you are taking tipranavir.
- plan to avoid unnecessary or prolonged exposure to sunlight and to wear protective clothing, sunglasses, and sunscreen. Tipranavir may make your skin sensitive to sunlight.

- you should know that your body fat may increase or move to different areas of your body such as your breasts and upper back.

What special dietary instructions should I follow?

Talk to your doctor about eating grapefruit and drinking grapefruit juice while taking this medicine.

What should I do if I forget to take a dose?

Take the missed dose as soon as you remember it. However, if it is almost time for the next dose, skip the missed dose and continue your regular dosing schedule. Do not take a double dose to make up for a missed one.

What side effects can this medicine cause?

Tipranavir may cause hyperglycemia (high blood sugar). Call your doctor if you have any of the following symptoms of hyperglycemia:

- extreme thirst
- frequent urination
- extreme hunger
- weakness
- blurred vision

If high blood sugar is not treated, a serious, life-threatening condition called diabetic ketoacidosis could develop. Call your doctor immediately if you have any of the these symptoms:

- dry mouth
- upset stomach and vomiting
- shortness of breath
- breath that smells fruity
- decreased consciousness

Tipranavir may cause side effects. Tell your doctor if any of these symptoms are severe or do not go away:

- diarrhea
- vomiting
- headache
- difficulty falling asleep or staying asleep
- depression

Some side effects can be serious. If you experience any of these symptoms or those listed in the IMPORTANT WARNING section, call your doctor immediately:

- fever, chills, cough, or other signs of infection
- rash
- itching
- throat tightness
- difficulty breathing or swallowing
- joint pain or stiffness

Tipranavir may cause other side effects. Call your doctor if you have any unusual problems while taking this medication.

What storage conditions are needed for this medicine?

Keep this medication in the container it came in, tightly closed, and out of reach of children. Store unopened bottles of tipranavir capsules in the refrigerator. Store opened bottles of tipranavir at room temperature, and away from excess heat and moisture (not in the bathroom). Throw away any unused tipranavir capsules 60 days after you open the bottle Mark the date you open the bottle of tipranavir on the label so you will know when it is time to throw the remaining medication away. Throw away any medication that is outdated or no longer needed. Talk to your pharmacist about the proper disposal of your medication.

What should I do in case of overdose?

In case of overdose, call your local poison control center at 1-800-222-1222. If the victim has collapsed or is not breathing, call local emergency services at 911.

What other information should I know?

Do not let anyone else take your medication. Ask your pharmacist any questions you have about refilling your prescription.

Dosage Facts
For Informational Purposes

Caution: Do not change your dose, how often you take your medication, or the length of time you are to take it without first talking to your healthcare provider.

The following dosage information was written using medical language for doctors and other healthcare professionals and is provided here for you to check your dosage. The dosage of this drug may differ for different patients. Therefore, always follow your doctor's instructions or the directions on the label. Contact your healthcare provider or pharmacist if you have any questions about the specific dosage of your medication after reviewing this information.

Adult Patients

Treatment of HIV Infection

ORAL:
- 500 mg twice daily *boosted* with low-dose ritonavir (200 mg twice daily).

Special Populations

Hepatic Impairment
- Dosage adjustment not needed in mild hepatic impairment (Child-Pugh class A). Contraindicated in moderate or severe hepatic impairment (Child-Pugh class B or C).

Renal Impairment
- Renal clearance of tipranavir negligible; decreased total body clearance not expected in renal impairment. Some experts state dosage adjustment not necessary.

Geriatric Patients
- Select dosage with caution because of age-related decreases in hepatic, renal, and/or cardiac function and concomitant disease and drug therapy.

Tizanidine

(tye zan′ i deen)

Brand Name: Zanaflex®
Also available generically.

Why is this medicine prescribed?

Tizanidine, a muscle relaxant, is used to help relax certain muscles in your body. It relieves the spasms and increased muscle tone caused by medical problems such as multiple sclerosis or spinal injury.

This medication is sometimes prescribed for other uses; ask your doctor or pharmacist for more information.

How should this medicine be used?

Tizanidine comes as a tablet to take by mouth. It usually is taken two or three times a day. Follow the directions on your prescription label carefully, and ask your doctor or pharmacist to explain any part you do not understand. Take tizanidine exactly as directed. Do not take more or less of it or take it more often than prescribed by your doctor.

What special precautions should I follow?

Before taking tizanidine,
- tell your doctor and pharmacist if you are allergic to tizanidine or any other drugs.
- tell your doctor and pharmacist what prescription and nonprescription medications you are taking, including other medications that cause drowsiness, medications for high blood pressure, oral contraceptives, and vitamins.
- tell your doctor if you have or have ever had kidney or liver disease.
- tell your doctor if you are pregnant, plan to become pregnant, or are breast-feeding. If you become pregnant while taking tizanidine, call your doctor immediately.
- if you are having surgery, including dental surgery, tell the doctor or dentist that you are taking tizanidine.
- you should know that this drug may make you drowsy. Do not drive a car or operate machinery until you know how this drug affects you.
- remember that alcohol can add to the drowsiness caused by this drug.

What should I do if I forget to take a dose?

If you take several doses per day, take the missed dose as soon as you remember it and take any remaining doses for that day at evenly spaced intervals. However, if you remember a missed dose when it is almost time for your next scheduled dose, skip the missed dose. Do not take a double dose to make up for a missed one.

What side effects can this medicine cause?

Side effects from tizanidine can occur. Tell your doctor if any of these symptoms are severe or do not go away:
- dizziness
- upset stomach
- vomiting
- tingling sensation in the arms, legs, hands, and feet
- dry mouth
- increased muscle spasms

If you experience either of the following symptoms, call your doctor immediately:
- yellowing of the skin or eyes
- unexplained flu-like symptoms

If you experience a serious side effect, you or your doctor may send a report to the Food and Drug Administration's (FDA) MedWatch Adverse Event Reporting program online [at http://www.fda.gov/MedWatch/index.html] or by phone [1-800-332-1088].

What storage conditions are needed for this medicine?

Keep this medication in the container it came in, tightly closed, and out of reach of children. Store it at room temperature and away from excess heat and moisture (not in the bathroom). Throw away any medication that is outdated or no longer needed. Talk to your pharmacist about the proper disposal of your medication.

What should I do in case of overdose?

In case of overdose, call your local poison control center at 1-800-222-1222. If the victim has collapsed or is not breathing, call local emergency services at 911.

What other information should I know?

Keep all appointments with your doctor and the laboratory. Your doctor will order certain lab tests to check your response to tizanidine.

Do not let anyone else take your medication. Ask your pharmacist any questions you have about refilling your prescription.

Dosage Facts
For Informational Purposes

Caution: Do not change your dose, how often you take your medication, or the length of time you

are to take it without first talking to your health-care provider.

The following dosage information was written using medical language for doctors and other healthcare professionals and is provided here for you to check your dosage. The dosage of this drug may differ for different patients. Therefore, always follow your doctor's instructions or the directions on the label. Contact your health-care provider or pharmacist if you have any questions about the specific dosage of your medication after reviewing this information.

General Dosage Information

Available as tizanidine hydrochloride; dosage expressed in terms of tizanidine.

Adult Patients

Spasticity

ORAL:
- Initially, 4 mg; single doses <8 mg not effective in clinical trials, but 4-mg dose used to minimize the incidence of common dose-related adverse effects (e.g., orthostatic hypotension).
- Repeat 4-mg dose every 6–8 hours as needed for a maximum of 3 doses in 24 hours.
- Increase dosage gradually in increments of 2–4 mg daily over a period of 2–4 weeks until optimum therapeutic effects are obtained with tolerable adverse effects.

Prescribing Limits

Adult Patients

Spasticity

ORAL:
- Maximum 36 mg in a 24-hour period.

Special Populations

Renal Impairment
- Initiate with caution in patients with renal impairment (Cl_{cr} <25 mL/minute). In these patients, use smaller individual doses during dosage titration; if higher doses are needed, increase the amount of each individual dose rather than increasing the frequency of dosing.

Tobramycin Ophthalmic

(toe bra mye′ sin)

Brand Name: AK-Tob®, TobraDex®, Tobrex® Also available generically.

Why is this medicine prescribed?

Tobramycin kills bacteria that cause certain eye infections.

This medication is sometimes prescribed for other uses; ask your doctor or pharmacist for more information.

How should this medicine be used?

Tobramycin comes as eyedrops and eye ointment. The eye drops usually are applied every 4-8 hours; the ointment usually is applied two to four times a day. Follow the directions on your prescription label carefully, and ask your doctor or pharmacist to explain any part you do not understand. Use tobramycin exactly as directed. Do not use more or less of it or use it more often than prescribed by your doctor.

To use the eyedrops, follow these instructions:
1. Wash your hands thoroughly with soap and water.
2. Use a mirror or have someone else put the drops in your eye.
3. Remove the protective cap. Make sure that the end of the dropper is not chipped cracked.
4. Avoid touching the dropper tip against your eye or anything else.
5. Hold the dropper tip down at all times to prevent drops from flowing back into the bottle and contaminating the remaining contents.
6. Lie down or tilt your head back.
7. Holding the bottle between your thumb and index finger, place the dropper tip as near as possible to your eyelid without touching it.
8. Brace the remaining fingers of that hand against your cheek or nose.
9. With the index finger of your other hand, pull the lower lid of the eye down to form a pocket.
10. Drop the prescribed number of drops into the pocket made by the lower lid and the eye. Placing drops on the surface of the eyeball can cause stinging.
11. Close your eye and press lightly against the lower lid with your finger for 2-3 minutes to keep the medication in the eye. Do not blink.
12. Replace and tighten the cap right away. Do not wipe or rinse it off.
13. Wipe off any excess liquid from your cheek with a clean tissue. Wash your hands again.

To use the eye ointment, follow these instructions:
1. Wash your hands thoroughly with soap and water.
2. Use a mirror or have someone else apply the ointment.
3. Remove the protective cap. Avoid touching the tip of the tube against your eye or anything else. The ointment must be kept clean.
4. Tilt your head forward slightly.
5. Holding the tube between your thumb and index finger, place the tube as near as possible to your eyelid without touching it.
6. Brace the remaining fingers of that hand against your cheek or nose.
7. With the index finger of your other hand, pull the lower lid of your eye down to form a pocket.
8. Place a small amount of ointment into the pocket made by the lower lid and the eye. A 1/2-inch strip of oint-

ment usually is enough unless otherwise directed by your doctor.

9. Gently close your eyes and keep them closed for 1-2 minutes to allow the medication to be absorbed.
10. Replace and tighten the cap right away.
11. Wipe off any excess ointment from your eyelids and lashes with a clean tissue. Wash your hands again.

What special precautions should I follow?

Before using tobramycin eyedrops or eye ointment,

- tell your doctor and pharmacist if you are allergic to tobramycin, other antibiotics, or any other drugs.
- tell your doctor and pharmacist what prescription and nonprescription medications you are taking, especially other eye medications and vitamins.
- tell your doctor if you are pregnant, plan to become pregnant, or are breast-feeding. If you become pregnant while using tobramycin, call your doctor immediately.
- tell your doctor if you wear soft contact lenses. If the brand of tobramycin you are using contains benzalkonium chloride, wait at least 15 minutes after using the medicine to put in soft contact lenses.

What should I do if I forget to take a dose?

Apply the missed dose as soon as you remember it. However, if it is almost time for the next dose, skip the missed dose and continue your regular dosing schedule. Do not apply a double dose to make up for a missed one.

What side effects can this medicine cause?

Tobramycin may cause side effects. Tell your doctor if any of these symptoms are severe or do not go away:

- eye tearing
- itching, stinging, or burning of the eye
- swelling of the eye
- temporary blurred vision (from the ointment)

What storage conditions are needed for this medicine?

Keep this medication in the container it came in, tightly closed, and out of reach of children. Store it at room temperature and away from excess heat and moisture (not in the bathroom). Throw away any medication that is outdated or no longer needed. Talk to your pharmacist about the proper disposal of your medication.

What other information should I know?

Keep all appointments with your doctor.

Do not let anyone else use your medication. Ask your pharmacist any questions you have about refilling your prescription.

If you still have symptoms of infection after you finish the tobramycin, call your doctor.

Dosage Facts
For Informational Purposes

Caution: Do not change your dose, how often you take your medication, or the length of time you are to take it without first talking to your healthcare provider.

The following dosage information was written using medical language for doctors and other healthcare professionals and is provided here for you to check your dosage. The dosage of this drug may differ for different patients. Therefore, always follow your doctor's instructions or the directions on the label. Contact your healthcare provider or pharmacist if you have any questions about the specific dosage of your medication after reviewing this information.

Pediatric Patients

Bacterial Ophthalmic Infections

OPHTHALMIC:

- Tobramycin ophthalmic ointment: Apply a ribbon of ointment (approximately 1.25 cm [0.5 inch]) to the affected eye(s) 2–3 times daily for mild to moderate infections. For severe infections, apply every 3–4 hours; when improvement occurs, decrease frequency of application.
- Tobramycin and dexamethasone ophthalmic ointment: Apply a ribbon of ointment (approximately 1.25 cm [0.5 inch]) into the conjunctival sac of affected eye(s) up to 3 or 4 times daily.
- Tobramycin ophthalmic solution: 1–2 drops of 0.3% solution in the affected eye(s) every 4 hours for mild to moderate infections. For severe infections, 2 drops of a 0.3% solution in the affected eye(s) every hour; when improvement occurs, decrease frequency of application.
- Tobramycin and dexamethasone ophthalmic suspension: 1–2 drops in the affected eye(s) every 4–6 hours. During the initial 24–48 hours, dosing may be increased to every 2 hours. When improvement occurs, decrease frequency of application. Do not discontinue prematurely.

Adult Patients

Bacterial Ophthalmic Infections

OPHTHALMIC:

- Tobramycin ophthalmic ointment: Apply a ribbon of ointment (approximately 1.25 cm [0.5 inch]) to the affected eye(s) 2–3 times daily for mild to moderate infections. For severe infections, apply every 3–4 hours; when improvement occurs, decrease frequency of application.
- Tobramycin and dexamethasone ophthalmic ointment: Apply a ribbon of ointment (approximately 1.25 cm [0.5 inch]) into the conjunctival sac of affected eye(s) up to 3 or 4 times daily.
- Tobramycin ophthalmic solution: 1–2 drops of 0.3% solution in the affected eye(s) every 4 hours for mild to moderate infections. For severe infections, 2 drops of a 0.3% solution in the affected eye(s) every hour; when improvement occurs, decrease frequency of application.
- Tobramycin and dexamethasone ophthalmic suspension: 1–2 drops into the conjunctival sac of affected eye(s) every 4–6 hours. During the initial 24–48 hours, dosing may be increased

to every 2 hours. When improvement occurs, decrease frequency of application. Do not discontinue prematurely.

- Loteprednol etabonate and tobramycin ophthalmic suspension: 1–2 drops into the conjunctival sac of affected eye(s) every 4–6 hours. During the initial 24–48 hours, dosing may be increased to every 1–2 hours. When improvement occurs, decrease frequency of application. Do not discontinue prematurely.

Tolazamide

(tole az′ a mide)

Brand Name: Tolinase®

Important Warning

Oral hypoglycemic drugs, including tolazamide, have been associated with increased cardiovascular mortality. Talk to your doctor about the possible risks, benefits, and alternatives of using this drug for your condition.

Why is this medicine prescribed?

Tolazamide is used to treat type 2 diabetes (condition in which the body does not use insulin normally and therefore cannot control the amount of sugar in the blood), particularly in people whose diabetes cannot be controlled by diet alone. Tolazamide lowers blood sugar by stimulating the pancreas to secrete insulin and helping the body use insulin efficiently. The pancreas must produce insulin for this medication to work. Tolazamide is not used to treat type 1 diabetes (condition in which the body does not produce insulin and therefore cannot control the amount of sugar in the blood).

This medication is sometimes prescribed for other uses; ask your doctor or pharmacist for more information.

How should this medicine be used?

Tolazamide comes in tablets to take by mouth. It is usually taken once a day with breakfast. Follow the directions on your prescription label carefully, and ask your doctor or pharmacist to explain any part you do not understand. Take tolazamide exactly as directed. Do not take more or less of it or take it more often than prescribed by your doctor.

Continue to take tolazamide even if you feel well. Do not stop taking tolazamide without talking to your doctor.

What special precautions should I follow?

Before taking tolazamide,
- tell your doctor and pharmacist if you are allergic to tolazamide or any other drugs.

- tell your doctor and pharmacist what prescription and nonprescription medications you are taking, especially antibiotics, anticoagulants ('blood thinners') such as warfarin (Coumadin), dexamethasone (Decadron), diuretics ('water pills'), estrogens, isoniazid (INH), MAO inhibitors [phenelzine (Nardil) and tranylcypromine (Parnate)], medications for high blood pressure and heart disease, niacin, oral contraceptives, phenytoin (Dilantin), prednisone, probenecid (Benemid), and vitamins.
- tell your doctor if you have or have ever had liver, kidney, thyroid, adrenal, heart, or pituitary disease.
- tell your doctor if you are pregnant, plan to become pregnant, or are breast-feeding. If you become pregnant while taking tolazamide, call your doctor.
- if you are having surgery, including dental surgery, tell the doctor or dentist that you are taking tolazamide.
- plan to avoid unnecessary or prolonged exposure to sunlight and to wear protective clothing, sunglasses, and sunscreen. Tolazamide may make your skin sensitive to sunlight.

What special dietary instructions should I follow?

Be sure to follow all exercise and dietary recommendations made by your doctor or dietitian. It is important to eat a healthful diet.

Alcohol may cause a decrease in blood sugar. Ask your doctor about the safe use of alcoholic beverages while you are taking tolazamide.

What should I do if I forget to take a dose?

Before you start to take tolazamide, ask your doctor what you should do if you forget to take a dose. Write down these directions so you can refer to them later.

As a general rule, take the missed dose as soon as you remember it unless it is almost time for the next dose. Do not take a double dose to make up for a missed one.

What side effects can this medicine cause?

This medication may cause changes in your blood sugar. You should know the symptoms of low and high blood sugar and what to do if you have these symptoms.

You may experience hypoglycemia (low blood sugar) while you are taking this medication. Your doctor will tell you what you should do if you develop hypoglycemia. He or she may tell you to check your blood sugar, eat or drink a food or beverage that contains sugar, such as hard candy or fruit juice, or get medical care. Follow these directions carefully if you have any of the following symptoms of hypoglycemia:
- shakiness
- dizziness or lightheadedness
- sweating
- nervousness or irritability
- sudden changes in behavior or mood
- headache

- numbness or tingling around the mouth
- weakness
- pale skin
- hunger
- clumsy or jerky movements

If hypoglycemia is not treated, severe symptoms may develop. Be sure that your family, friends, and other people who spend time with you know that if you have any of the following symptoms, they should get medical treatment for you immediately.

- confusion
- seizures
- loss of consciousness

Call your doctor immediately if you have any of the following symptoms of hyperglycemia (high blood sugar):

- extreme thirst
- frequent urination
- extreme hunger
- weakness
- blurred vision

If high blood sugar is not treated, a serious, life-threatening condition called diabetic ketoacidosis could develop. Call your doctor immediately if you have any of these symptoms:

- dry mouth
- upset stomach and vomiting
- shortness of breath
- breath that smells fruity
- decreased consciousness

Tolazamide may cause side effects. If you experience any of the following symptoms, call your doctor immediately:

- skin rash
- itching or redness
- exaggerated sunburn
- yellowing of the skin or eyes
- light-colored stools
- dark urine
- unusual bleeding or bruising
- fever
- sore throat

If you experience a serious side effect, you or your doctor may send a report to the Food and Drug Administration's (FDA) MedWatch Adverse Event Reporting program online [at http://www.fda.gov/MedWatch/index.html] or by phone [1-800-332-1088].

What storage conditions are needed for this medicine?

Keep this medication in the container it came in, tightly closed, and out of reach of children. Store it at room temperature and away from excess heat and moisture (not in the bathroom). Throw away any medication that is outdated or no longer needed. Talk to your pharmacist about the proper disposal of your medication.

What should I do in case of overdose?

In case of overdose, call your local poison control center at 1-800-222-1222. If the victim has collapsed or is not breathing, call local emergency services at 911.

What other information should I know?

Keep all appointments with your doctor and the laboratory. Your doctor will order certain lab tests to check your response to tolazamide. Your doctor will also tell you how to check your response to this medication by measuring your blood or urine sugar levels at home. Follow these instructions carefully.

You should always wear a diabetic identification bracelet to be sure you get proper treatment in an emergency.

Do not let anyone else take your medication. Ask your pharmacist any questions you have about refilling your prescription.

Talk to your doctor, pharmacist, or other healthcare professional if you have questions about dosing information for your medication.

Tolbutamide

(tole byoo′ ta mide)

Brand Name: Orinase®
Also available generically.

> ## Important Warning
>
> Oral hypoglycemic drugs, including tolbutamide, have been associated with increased cardiovascular mortality. Talk to your doctor about the possible risks, benefits, and alternatives of using this drug for your condition.

Why is this medicine prescribed?

Tolbutamide is used to treat type 2 diabetes (condition in which the body does not use insulin normally and therefore cannot control the amount of sugar in the blood), particularly in people whose diabetes cannot be controlled by diet alone. Tolbutamide lowers blood sugar by stimulating the pancreas to secrete insulin and helping the body use insulin efficiently. The pancreas must produce insulin for this drug to work. Tolbutamide is not used to treat type 1 diabetes (condition in which the body does not produce insulin and therefore cannot control the amount of sugar in the blood).

This medication is sometimes prescribed for other uses; ask your doctor or pharmacist for more information.

How should this medicine be used?

Tolbutamide comes in tablets to take by mouth. It is usually taken several times a day. Follow the directions on your prescription label carefully, and ask your doctor or pharmacist to explain any part you do not understand. Take tolbutamide exactly as directed. Do not take more or less of it or take it more often than prescribed by your doctor.

Continue to take tolbutamide even if you feel well. Do not stop taking tolbutamide without talking to your doctor.

What special precautions should I follow?

Before taking tolbutamide,
- tell your doctor and pharmacist if you are allergic to tolbutamide or any other drugs.
- tell your doctor and pharmacist what prescription and nonprescription medications you are taking, especially antibiotics, anticoagulants ('blood thinners') such as warfarin (Coumadin), dexamethasone (Decadron), diuretics ('water pills'), estrogens, isoniazid (INH), MAO inhibitors [phenelzine (Nardil) and tranylcypromine (Parnate)], medications for high blood pressure or heart disease, niacin, oral contraceptives, phenytoin (Dilantin), prednisone, probenecid (Benemid), and vitamins.
- tell your doctor if you have or have ever had heart or kidney disease.
- tell your doctor if you are pregnant, plan to become pregnant, or are breast-feeding. If you become pregnant while taking tolbutamide, call your doctor immediately.
- if you are having surgery, including dental surgery, tell the doctor or dentist that you are taking tolbutamide.
- plan to avoid unnecessary or prolonged exposure to sunlight and to wear protective clothing, sunglasses, and sunscreen. Tolbutamide may make your skin sensitive to sunlight.

What special dietary instructions should I follow?

Be sure to follow all exercise and dietary recommendations made by your doctor or dietitian. It is important to eat a healthful diet.

Alcohol may cause a decrease in blood sugar. Ask your doctor about the safe use of alcoholic beverages while you are taking tolbutamide.

What should I do if I forget to take a dose?

Before you start to take tolbutamide, ask your doctor what you should do if you forget to take a dose. Write these directions down so that you can refer to them later.

As a general rule, take the missed dose as soon as you remember it unless it is almost time for the next dose. Do not take a double dose to make up for a missed one.

What side effects can this medicine cause?

This medication may cause changes in your blood sugar. You should know the symptoms of low and high blood sugar and what to do if you have these symptoms.

You may experience hypoglycemia (low blood sugar) while you are taking this medication. Your doctor will tell you what you should do if you develop hypoglycemia. He or she may tell you to check your blood sugar, eat or drink a food or beverage that contains sugar, such as hard candy or fruit juice, or get medical care. Follow these directions carefully if you have any of the following symptoms of hypoglycemia:
- shakiness
- dizziness or lightheadedness
- sweating
- nervousness or irritability
- sudden changes in behavior or mood
- headache
- numbness or tingling around the mouth
- weakness
- pale skin
- hunger
- clumsy or jerky movements

If hypoglycemia is not treated, severe symptoms may develop. Be sure that your family, friends, and other people who spend time with you know that if you have any of the following symptoms, they should get medical treatment for you immediately.
- confusion
- seizures
- loss of consciousness

Call your doctor immediately if you have any of the following symptoms of hyperglycemia (high blood sugar):
- extreme thirst
- frequent urination
- extreme hunger
- weakness
- blurred vision

If high blood sugar is not treated, a serious, life-threatening condition called diabetic ketoacidosis could develop. Call your doctor immediately if you have any of these symptoms:
- dry mouth
- upset stomach and vomiting
- shortness of breath
- breath that smells fruity
- decreased consciousness

Tolbutamide may cause side effects. If you experience any of the following symptoms, call your doctor immediately:
- skin rash
- itching or redness
- exaggerated sunburn
- yellowing of the skin or eyes
- light-colored stools
- dark urine

- unusual bleeding or bruising
- fever
- sore throat

If you experience a serious side effect, you or your doctor may send a report to the Food and Drug Administration's (FDA) MedWatch Adverse Event Reporting program online [at http://www.fda.gov/MedWatch/index.html] or by phone [1-800-332-1088].

What storage conditions are needed for this medicine?

Keep this medication in the container it came in, tightly closed, and out of reach of children. Store it at room temperature and away from excess heat and moisture (not in the bathroom). Throw away any medication that is outdated or no longer needed. Talk to your pharmacist about the proper disposal of your medication.

What should I do in case of overdose?

In case of overdose, call your local poison control center at 1-800-222-1222. If the victim has collapsed or is not breathing, call local emergency services at 911.

What other information should I know?

Keep all appointments with your doctor and the laboratory. Your doctor will order certain lab tests to check your response to tolbutamide. Your doctor will also tell you how to check your response to this medication by measuring your blood or urine sugar levels at home. Follow these instructions carefully.

You should always wear a diabetic identification bracelet to be sure you get proper treatment in an emergency.

Do not let anyone else take your medication. Ask your pharmacist any questions you have about refilling your prescription.

Dosage Facts
For Informational Purposes

Caution: Do not change your dose, how often you take your medication, or the length of time you are to take it without first talking to your healthcare provider.

The following dosage information was written using medical language for doctors and other healthcare professionals and is provided here for you to check your dosage. The dosage of this drug may differ for different patients. Therefore, always follow your doctor's instructions or the directions on the label. Contact your healthcare provider or pharmacist if you have any questions about the specific dosage of your medication after reviewing this information.

Adult Patients
Diabetes Mellitus
Initial Dosage in Previously Untreated Patients

ORAL:
- Initially, 1–2 g daily. Subsequently, increase or decrease dosage based on patient response.

Initial Dosage in Patients Transferred from Other Oral Antidiabetic Agents

ORAL:
- Conservative dosing recommended. May discontinue other oral antidiabetic agent immediately; a transition period or loading doses are not required. During transfer from chlorpropamide (a sulfonylurea with a longer elimination half-life), use cautious dosing for 2 weeks to prevent hypoglycemia.

Initial Dosage in Patients Transferred from Insulin

ORAL:
- Initially, 1–2 g daily if insulin requirements were ≤20 units daily. Abruptly discontinue insulin.
- Initially, 1–2 g daily if insulin requirements were 20–40 units daily, and concurrently reduce insulin dosage by 30–50%. Subsequently, adjust insulin dosage according to therapeutic response.
- Initially, 1–2 g daily if insulin requirements were >40 units daily, and concurrently reduce insulin dosage by 20%. Subsequently, adjust insulin dosage according to therapeutic response.

Maintenance Dosage

ORAL:
- Usual maintenance dosage: 250 mg–3 g daily. Patients who do not respond to 2 g daily will not respond to a higher dosage; however, temporary increases to >2 g may be required to maintain control in some patients. Maintenance dosages >2 g daily are seldom required.
- If inadequate glycemic control occurs in patients previously controlled on tolbutamide, temporary small dosage increases may restore adequate control.

Prescribing Limits
Adult Patients
Diabetes Mellitus

ORAL:
- Maximum 3 g daily.

Special Populations

Hepatic Impairment
- Conservative initial and maintenance dosages recommended.

Renal Impairment
- Conservative initial and maintenance dosages recommended.

Geriatric Patients
- Conservative initial and maintenance dosages recommended.

Debilitated or Malnourished Patients
- Conservative initial and maintenance dosages recommended.

Tolcapone

(tole′ ka pone)

Brand Name: Tasmar®

Important Warning

Tolcapone may cause life threatening liver damage. Tell your doctor if you have or have ever had liver disease. Keep all appointments with your doctor and the laboratory. Your doctor will order certain laboratory tests before and during treatment to check your response to tolcapone.

If you experience any of the following symptoms, call your doctor immediately: upset stomach that does not go away, extreme tiredness, lack of energy, yellowing of the skin or whites of eyes, tenderness on the right upper side of the stomach, itching, loss of appetite, pale stools, or dark urine.

Why is this medicine prescribed?

Tolcapone is used in combination with levodopa and carbidopa to treat the signs and symptoms of Parkinson's disease.

This medication is sometimes prescribed for other uses; ask your doctor or pharmacist for more information.

How should this medicine be used?

Tolcapone comes as a tablet to take by mouth. It is usually taken three times a day. Your doctor will most likely prescribe this in addition to levodopa and carbidopa (Sinemet). Follow the directions on your prescription label carefully, and ask your doctor or pharmacist to explain any part you do not understand. Take tolcapone exactly as directed. Do not take more or less of it or take it more often than prescribed by your doctor.

Tolcapone controls symptoms of Parkinson's disease but does not cure it. Continue to take tolcapone even if you feel well. Do not stop taking tolcapone without talking to your doctor. Abrupt discontinuation of tolcapone may cause high fever and confusion.

What special precautions should I follow?

Before taking tolcapone,
- tell your doctor and pharmacist if you are allergic to tolcapone or any other drugs.
- tell your doctor and pharmacist what prescription and nonprescription medications you are taking, especially anticoagulants (''blood thinners'') such as warfarin (Coumadin), desipramine (Norpramin), dobutamine (Dobutrex), drugs that cause drowsiness (sedatives, tranquilizers, and sleeping pills), isoproterenol (Isuprel),

MAO inhibitors [phenelzine (Nardil) or tranylcypromine (Parnate)], methyldopa (Aldomet), and vitamins.
- in addition to the condition listed in the IMPORTANT WARNING section, tell your doctor if you have or have ever had heart or kidney disease or rhabdomyolysis (skeletal muscle disease).
- tell your doctor if you are pregnant, plan to become pregnant, or are breast-feeding. If you become pregnant while taking tolcapone, call your doctor.
- if you are having surgery, including dental surgery, tell your doctor or dentist that you are taking tolcapone.
- you should know that this drug may make you drowsy. Do not drive a car or operate machinery until you know how tolcapone will affect you.
- remember that alcohol can add to the drowsiness caused by this drug.

What special dietary instructions should I follow?

Tolcapone may cause an upset stomach. Tolcapone may be taken with food to reduce nausea.

What should I do if I forget to take a dose?

Take the missed dose as soon as you remember it. However, if it is almost time for the next dose, skip the missed dose and continue your regular dosing schedule. Do not take a double dose to make up for a missed one.

What side effects can this medicine cause?

Tolcapone may cause side effects. Tell your doctor if any of these symptoms are severe or do not go away:
- sleep disturbances
- excessive dreaming
- diarrhea
- dizziness
- vomiting
- increased sweating

If you experience any of the following symptoms, or any of those listed in the IMPORTANT WARNING section, call your doctor immediately:
- hallucinations
- confusion
- irregular heartbeat

If you experience a serious side effect, you or your doctor may send a report to the Food and Drug Administration's (FDA) MedWatch Adverse Event Reporting program online [at http://www.fda.gov/MedWatch/index.html] or by phone [1-800-332-1088].

What storage conditions are needed for this medicine?

Keep this medication in the container it came in, tightly closed, and out of reach of children. Store it at room temperature and away from excess heat and moisture (not in the bathroom). Throw away any medication that is outdated or

---

no longer needed. Talk to your pharmacist about the proper disposal of your medication.

What should I do in case of overdose?

In case of overdose, call your local poison control center at 1-800-222-1222. If the victim has collapsed or is not breathing, call local emergency services at 911.

What other information should I know?

Do not let anyone else take your medication. Ask your pharmacist any questions you have about refilling your prescription.

Dosage Facts
For Informational Purposes

Caution: Do not change your dose, how often you take your medication, or the length of time you are to take it without first talking to your healthcare provider.

The following dosage information was written using medical language for doctors and other healthcare professionals and is provided here for you to check your dosage. The dosage of this drug may differ for different patients. Therefore, always follow your doctor's instructions or the directions on the label. Contact your healthcare provider or pharmacist if you have any questions about the specific dosage of your medication after reviewing this information.

Adult Patients
Parkinsonian Syndrome

ORAL:
- Usual dosage: 100 mg 3 times daily.
- Reserve higher dosage (200 mg 3 times daily) for situations when the anticipated incremental benefit is justified. If the patient fails to show the expected clinical benefit while receiving 200 mg 3 times daily for 3 weeks, discontinue the drug.

Special Populations

Renal Impairment
- Dosage adjustment not required in patients with mild to moderate renal impairment (Cl_{cr} >30 mL/minute). Safety not evaluated in patients with Cl_{cr} <25 mL/minute.

Tolmetin
(tole′ met in)

Brand Name: Tolectin®, Tolectin® DS
Also available generically.

Important Warning

People who take nonsteroidal anti-inflammatory medications (NSAIDs) (other than aspirin) such as tolmetin may have a higher risk of having a heart attack or a stroke than people who do not take these medications. These events may happen without warning and may cause death. This risk may be higher for people who take NSAIDs for a long time. Tell your doctor if you or anyone in your family has or has ever had heart disease, a heart attack, or a stroke, if you smoke, and if you have or have ever had high cholesterol, high blood pressure, or diabetes. Get emergency medical help right away if you experience any of the following symptoms: chest pain, shortness of breath, weakness in one part or side of the body, or slurred speech.

If you will be undergoing a coronary artery bypass graft (CABG; a type of heart surgery), you should not take tolmetin right before or right after the surgery.

NSAIDs such as tolmetin may cause ulcers, bleeding, or holes in the stomach or intestine. These problems may develop at any time during treatment, may happen without warning symptoms, and may cause death. The risk may be higher for people who take NSAIDs for a long time, are older in age, have poor health, or drink large amounts of alcohol while taking tolmetin. Tell your doctor if you take any of the following medications: anticoagulants ('blood thinners') such as warfarin (Coumadin); aspirin; other NSAIDs such as ibuprofen (Advil, Motrin) and naproxen (Aleve, Naprosyn); or oral steroids such as dexamethasone (Decadron, Dexone), methylprednisolone (Medrol), and prednisone (Deltasone). Also tell your doctor if you have or have ever had ulcers, bleeding in your stomach or intestines, or other bleeding disorders. If you experience any of the following symptoms, stop taking tolmetin and call your doctor: stomach pain, heartburn, vomiting a substance that is bloody or looks like coffee grounds, blood in the stool, or black and tarry stools.

Keep all appointments with your doctor and the laboratory. Your doctor will monitor your symptoms carefully and will probably order certain tests to check your body's response to tolmetin. Be sure to tell your doctor how you are feeling so that your doctor can prescribe the right amount of medication to treat your condition with the lowest risk of serious side effects.

Your doctor or pharmacist will give you the manufacturer's patient information sheet (Medication Guide) when you begin treatment with tolmetin and each time you refill your prescription. Read the information carefully and ask your doctor or pharmacist if you have any questions. You can also visit the Food and Drug Administration (FDA) website (http://www.fda.gov/cder) to obtain the Medication Guide.

Why is this medicine prescribed?

Tolmetin is used to relieve pain, tenderness, swelling, and stiffness caused by osteoarthritis (arthritis caused by a breakdown of the lining of the joints) and rheumatoid arthritis (arthritis caused by swelling of the lining of the joints). Tolmetin is also used to relieve pain, tenderness, swelling, and stiffness caused by juvenile rheumatoid arthritis in children 2 years of age and older. Tolmetin is in a class of medications called NSAIDs. It works by stopping the body's production of a substance that causes pain, fever, and inflammation.

How should this medicine be used?

Tolmetin comes as a tablet and a capsule to take by mouth. Adults usually take tolmetin three times a day on an empty stomach, and children older than 2 years of age usually take tolmetin three or four times a day on an empty stomach. Take tolmetin at around the same times every day. It is best to take the first dose of the day just after waking in the morning and to take the last dose of the day at bedtime. Follow the directions on your prescription label carefully, and ask your doctor or pharmacist to explain any part you do not understand. Take tolmetin exactly as directed. Do not take more or less of it or take it more often than prescribed by your doctor.

Tell your doctor if tolmetin upsets your stomach. Your doctor may tell you to take tolmetin with an antacid to prevent stomach upset. Your doctor will tell you which antacids are safe to take with tolmetin.

Tolmetin may help to control your symptoms but will not cure your condition. Your symptoms may improve within one week after you start to take tolmetin, but it may take several weeks or longer for you to feel the full benefit of the medication. Talk to your doctor about how tolmetin is working for you.

Are there other uses for this medicine?

Tolmetin is also used to treat ankylosing spondylitis (arthritis that mainly affects the spine). It is also sometimes used to treat certain conditions that cause muscle strain or swelling in the shoulder or elbow and injuries such as recent sprains.

This medication is sometimes prescribed for other uses; ask your doctor or pharmacist for more information.

What special precautions should I follow?

Before taking tolmetin,
- tell your doctor and pharmacist if you are allergic to tolmetin, aspirin, or other NSAIDs such as ibuprofen (Advil, Motrin) and naproxen (Aleve, Naprosyn), any other medications, or any of the inactive ingredients in tolmetin tablets or capsules. Ask your pharmacist for a list of the inactive ingeredients.
- tell your doctor and pharmacist what prescription and nonprescription medications, vitamins, nutritional supplements, and herbal products you are taking or plan to take. Be sure to mention the medications listed in the IMPORTANT WARNING section and any of the following: angiotensin-converting enzyme (ACE) inhibitors such as benazepril (Lotensin), captopril (Capoten), enalapril (Vasotec), fosinopril (Monopril), lisinopril (Prinivil, Zestril), moexipril (Univasc), perindopril (Aceon), quinapril (Accupril), ramipril (Altace), and trandolapril (Mavik); diuretics ('water pills'); lithium (Eskalith, Lithobid); and methotrexate (Rheumatrex). Your doctor may need to change the doses of your medications or monitor you carefully for side effects.
- tell your doctor if you have or have ever had any of the conditions mentioned in the IMPORTANT WARNING section or asthma, especially if you also have frequent stuffed or runny nose or nasal polyps (swelling of the lining of the nose); swelling of the hands, feet, ankles, or lower legs; or liver or kidney disease.
- tell your doctor if you are pregnant, especially if you are in the last few months of your pregnancy, you plan to become pregnant, or you are breast-feeding. If you become pregnant while taking tolmetin, call your doctor.
- if you are having surgery, including dental surgery, tell the doctor or dentist that you are taking tolmetin.
- you should know that this drug may make you dizzy. Do not drive a car or operate machinery until you know how this drug affects you.

What special dietary instructions should I follow?

Unless your doctor tells you otherwise, continue your normal diet.

What should I do if I forget to take a dose?

Take the missed dose as soon as you remember it. However, if it is almost time for the next dose, skip the missed dose and continue your regular dosing schedule. Do not take a double dose to make up for a missed one.

What side effects can this medicine cause?

Tolmetin may cause side effects. Tell your doctor if any of these symptoms are severe or do not go away:

- diarrhea
- constipation
- gas
- weight gain or loss
- headache
- depression
- skin irritation
- ringing in the ears

Some side effects can be serious. If you experience any of the following symptoms, or those mentioned in the IMPORTANT WARNING section, call your doctor immediately. Do not take any more tolmetin until you speak to your doctor:

- changes in vision
- unexplained weight gain
- fever
- blisters
- rash
- itching
- hives
- swelling of the eyes, face, lips, tongue, throat, arms, hands, feet, ankles, or lower legs
- difficulty breathing or swallowing
- hoarseness
- yellowing of the skin or eyes
- excessive tiredness
- unusual bleeding or bruising
- lack of energy
- upset stomach
- loss of appetite
- pain in the upper right part of the stomach
- flu-like symptoms
- pale skin
- fast heartbeat
- cloudy, discolored, or bloody urine
- back pain
- difficult or painful urination

Tolmetin may cause other side effects. Call your doctor if you have any unusual problems while taking this medication.

If you experience a serious side effect, you or your doctor may send a report to the Food and Drug Administration's (FDA) MedWatch Adverse Event Reporting program online [at http://www.fda.gov/MedWatch/index.html] or by phone [1-800-332-1088].

What storage conditions are needed for this medicine?

Keep this medication in the container it came in, tightly closed, and out of reach of children. Store it at room temperature and away from excess heat and moisture (not in the bathroom). Throw away any medication that is outdated or no longer needed. Talk to your pharmacist about the proper disposal of your medication.

What should I do in case of overdose?

In case of overdose, call your local poison control center at 1-800-222-1222. If the victim has collapsed or is not breathing, call local emergency services at 911.

What other information should I know?

Before having any laboratory test, tell your doctor and the laboratory personnel that you are taking tolmetin.

Do not let anyone else take your medication. Ask your pharmacist any questions you have about refilling your prescription.

Dosage Facts
For Informational Purposes

Caution: Do not change your dose, how often you take your medication, or the length of time you are to take it without first talking to your healthcare provider.

The following dosage information was written using medical language for doctors and other healthcare professionals and is provided here for you to check your dosage. The dosage of this drug may differ for different patients. Therefore, always follow your doctor's instructions or the directions on the label. Contact your healthcare provider or pharmacist if you have any questions about the specific dosage of your medication after reviewing this information.

General Dosage Information

Available as tolmetin sodium; dosage expressed in terms of tolmetin.

Adjust dosage according to the patient's response and tolerance. Attempt to titrate to the lowest effective dosage and shortest duration of therapy.

Pediatric Patients

Inflammatory Diseases
Juvenile Rheumatoid Arthritis

ORAL:
- Children ≥2 years of age: Initially, 20 mg/kg daily in 3–4 divided doses. After 1–2 weeks, may adjust dosage until a satisfactory response is achieved, to a maximum 30 mg/kg daily in divided doses. Usual effective dosage 15–30 mg/kg daily.

Adult Patients

Inflammatory Diseases
Rheumatoid Arthritis and Osteoarthritis

ORAL:
- Initially, 400 mg 3 times daily. After 1–2 weeks, may adjust dosage until a satisfactory response is achieved, to a maximum 1800 mg daily in divided doses. Usual effective dosage is 600–1800 mg daily in 3 divided doses.

Ankylosing Spondylitis†

ORAL:
- 600–1600 mg daily in divided doses.

Adhesive Capsulitis Shoulder†

ORAL:
- 600 or 1200 mg daily in divided doses.

Radiohumeral Bursitis†

ORAL:
- 600 or 1200 mg daily in divided doses.

Local Trauma†

ORAL:
- 600 or 1200 mg daily in divided doses.

Prescribing Limits

Pediatric Patients

Inflammatory Diseases
Juvenile Rheumatoid Arthritis

ORAL:
- Children ≥2 years of age: Maximum 30 mg/kg daily.

Adult Patients

Inflammatory Diseases
Rheumatoid Arthritis and Osteoarthritis

ORAL:
- Maximum 1800 mg daily.

Special Populations

Hepatic Impairment
- No specific dosage recommendations at this time.

Renal Impairment
- No specific dosage recommendations at this time; not recommended in advanced renal disease.

Geriatric Patients
- No specific dosage recommendations at this time.

† Use is not currently included in the labeling approved by the US Food and Drug Administration.

Tolnaftate
(tole naf' tate)

Brand Name: Aftate® for Athlete's Foot Aerosol Spray Liquid, Aftate® for Athlete's Foot Aerosol Spray Powder, Aftate® for Jock Itch Aerosol Spray Powder, Breezee® Mist Antifungal Foot Powder, Tinactin®, Tinactin® Jock Itch Cream, Tinactin® Jock Itch Spray Powder, Tinactin® Liquid Aerosol, Tinactin® Powder Aerosol, Ting® Antifungal Cream, Ting® Antifungal Spray
Also available generically.

Why is this medicine prescribed?

Tolnaftate stops the growth of fungi that cause skin infections, including athlete's foot, jock itch, and ringworm.

This medication is sometimes prescribed for other uses; ask your doctor or pharmacist for more information.

How should this medicine be used?

Tolnaftate comes as a cream, liquid, powder, gel, spray powder, and spray liquid for application to the skin. Tolnaftate usually is applied twice a day. Follow the directions on the package or on your prescription label carefully, and ask your doctor or pharmacist to explain any part you do not understand. Use tolnaftate exactly as directed. Do not use more or less of it or use it more often than directed by your doctor.

The burning and soreness of athlete's foot or the itching of jock itch should decrease within 2-3 days. Continue treatment for at least 2 weeks after symptoms disappear. A total of 4-6 weeks of treatment may be necessary.

Thoroughly clean the infected area, allow it to dry, and then gently rub the medication in until most of it disappears. Use just enough medication to cover the affected area. You should wash your hands after applying the medication.

Spray and powder forms should be applied between the toes; socks and shoes should be treated lightly. Sprays should be shaken well before each use to mix the medication and then sprayed from a distance of at least 6 inches.

What special precautions should I follow?

Before using tolnaftate,
- tell your doctor and pharmacist if you are allergic to tolnaftate or any other drugs.
- tell your doctor and pharmacist what prescription and nonprescription medications you are taking, including vitamins.
- tell your doctor if you are pregnant, plan to become pregnant, or are breast-feeding. If you become pregnant while using tolnaftate, call your doctor.

What should I do if I forget to take a dose?

Apply the missed dose as soon as you remember it. However, if it is almost time for the next dose, skip the missed dose and continue your regular dosing schedule. Do not apply a double dose to make up for a missed one.

What side effects can this medicine cause?

Tolnaftate may cause side effects. If you experience the following symptom, call your doctor:

- skin irritation

If you experience a serious side effect, you or your doctor may send a report to the Food and Drug Administration's (FDA) MedWatch Adverse Event Reporting program online [at http://www.fda.gov/MedWatch/index.html] or by phone [1-800-332-1088].

What storage conditions are needed for this medicine?

Keep this medication in the container it came in, tightly closed, and out of reach of children. Store it at room temperature and away from excess heat and moisture (not in the bathroom). Do not puncture spray cans or throw them into a fire. Throw away any medication that is outdated or no longer needed. Talk to your pharmacist about the proper disposal of your medication.

What other information should I know?

Keep all appointments with your doctor. Tolnaftate is for external use only. Do not let tolnaftate get into your eyes, nose, or mouth, and do not swallow it. Do not apply dressings, bandages, cosmetics, lotions, or other skin medications to the area being treated unless your doctor tells you.

Do not let anyone else use your medication. Ask your pharmacist any questions you have about refilling your prescription. If you still have symptoms of infection after you finish the tolnaftate, call your doctor.

Dosage Facts
For Informational Purposes

Caution: Do not change your dose, how often you take your medication, or the length of time you are to take it without first talking to your healthcare provider.

The following dosage information was written using medical language for doctors and other healthcare professionals and is provided here for you to check your dosage. The dosage of this drug may differ for different patients. Therefore, always follow your doctor's instructions or the directions on the label. Contact your healthcare provider or pharmacist if you have any questions about the specific dosage of your medication after reviewing this information.

Pediatric Patients

Dermatophytoses
Tinea Corporis or Tinea Cruris

TOPICAL:
- Children ≥2 years of age: Apply to affected area twice daily (morning and night) for 4 weeks for tinea corporis or 2 weeks for tinea cruris.
- If improvement does not occur after 4 weeks of treatment, diagnosis and therapy should be reevaluated.

Tinea Pedis

TOPICAL:
- Children ≥2 years of age: Apply to affected area twice daily (morning and night) for 4 weeks.
- If improvement does not occur after 4 weeks of treatment, diagnosis and therapy should be reevaluated.
- Daily use after treatment may help prevent reinfection.

Pityriasis (Tinea) Versicolor†

TOPICAL:
- Children ≥2 years of age: Apply to affected area twice daily (morning and night).
- If improvement does not occur after 4 weeks of treatment, diagnosis and therapy should be reevaluated.

Adult Patients

Dermatophytoses
Tinea Corporis or Tinea Cruris

TOPICAL:
- Apply to affected area twice daily (morning and night) for 4 weeks for tinea corporis or 2 weeks for tinea cruris.
- If improvement does not occur after 4 weeks of treatment, diagnosis and therapy should be reevaluated.

Tinea Pedis

TOPICAL:
- Apply to affected area twice daily (morning and night) for 4 weeks.
- If improvement does not occur after 4 weeks of treatment, diagnosis and therapy should be reevaluated.
- Daily use after treatment may help prevent reinfection.

Pityriasis (Tinea) Versicolor†

TOPICAL:
- Apply to affected area twice daily (morning and night).
- If improvement does not occur after 4 weeks of treatment, diagnosis and therapy should be reevaluated.

† Use is not currently included in the labeling approved by the US Food and Drug Administration.

Tolterodine

(tole ter′ a deen)

Brand Name: Detrol®, Detrol® LA

Why is this medicine prescribed?

Tolterodine is used to relieve urinary difficulties, including frequent urination and inability to control urination. Tolterodine is in a class of medications called antimuscarinics. It works by preventing bladder contraction.

How should this medicine be used?

Tolterodine comes as a tablet and an extended-release (long-acting) capsule to take by mouth. The tablet is usually taken twice a day. The extended-release capsule is usually taken once a day with liquids. Follow the directions on your prescription label carefully, and ask your doctor or pharmacist to explain any part you do not understand. Take tolterodine exactly as directed. Do not take more or less of it or take it more often than prescribed by your doctor.

Swallow the extended-release capsules whole; do not split, chew, or crush them.

Are there other uses for this medicine?

This medication is sometimes prescribed for other uses; ask your doctor or pharmacist for more information.

What special precautions should I follow?

Before taking tolterodine,

- tell your doctor and pharmacist if you are allergic to tolterodine or any other drugs.
- tell your doctor and pharmacist what prescription and nonprescription medications you are taking, especially clarithromycin (Biaxin), erythromycin (E-mycin, Ery-Tab, others), fluconazole (Diflucan), itraconazole (Sporanox), ketoconazole (Nizoral), medications for glaucoma, and vitamins.
- tell your doctor if you have or have ever had kidney or liver disease, glaucoma, or an obstructive gastrointestinal disease, such as pyloric stenosis.
- tell your doctor if you are pregnant, plan to become pregnant, or are breast-feeding. If you become pregnant while taking tolterodine, call your doctor.

What should I do if I forget to take a dose?

Take the missed dose as soon as you remember it. However, if it is almost time for the next dose, skip the missed dose and continue your regular dosing schedule. Do not take a double dose to make up for a missed one.

What side effects can this medicine cause?

Tolterodine may cause side effects. Tell your doctor if any of these symptoms are severe or do not go away:

- dry mouth
- blurred vision
- upset stomach
- headache
- constipation
- dry eyes
- dizziness

If you experience any of the following symptoms, call your doctor immediately:

- difficulty urinating
- rash
- chest pain

If you experience a serious side effect, you or your doctor may send a report to the Food and Drug Administration's (FDA) MedWatch Adverse Event Reporting program online [at http://www.fda.gov/MedWatch/index.html] or by phone [1-800-332-1088].

What storage conditions are needed for this medicine?

Keep this medication in the container it came in, tightly closed, and out of reach of children. Store it at room temperature and away from excess heat and moisture (not in the bathroom). Throw away any medication that is outdated or no longer needed. Talk to your pharmacist about the proper disposal of your medication.

What should I do in case of overdose?

In case of overdose, call your local poison control center at 1-800-222-1222. If the victim has collapsed or is not breathing, call local emergency services at 911.

What other information should I know?

Keep all appointments with your doctor.

Do not let anyone else take your medication. Ask your pharmacist any questions you have about refilling your prescription.

Dosage Facts
For Informational Purposes

Caution: Do not change your dose, how often you take your medication, or the length of time you are to take it without first talking to your healthcare provider.

The following dosage information was written using medical language for doctors and other healthcare professionals and is provided here for you to check your dosage. The dosage of this drug may differ for different patients. Therefore, always follow your doctor's instructions or the directions on the label. Contact your healthcare provider or pharmacist if you have any questions about the specific dosage of your medication after reviewing this information.

General Dosage Information

Available as tolterodine tartrate; dosage expressed in terms of the salt.

Adult Patients

Overactive Bladder

ORAL:
- Conventional tablets: Initially, 2 mg twice daily. May reduce dosage to 1 mg twice daily according to individual response and tolerance.
- Extended-release capsules: Initially, 4 mg once daily. May reduce dosage to 2 mg once daily according to individual response and tolerance; however, efficacy data for this lower dosage are limited.

Special Populations

Renal Impairment
- 1 mg twice daily (as conventional tablets) or 2 mg once daily (as extended-release capsules) in patients with substantially reduced renal function.

Hepatic Impairment
- 1 mg twice daily (as conventional tablets) or 2 mg once daily (as extended-release capsules) in patients with substantially reduced hepatic function.

Geriatric Patients
- No dosage adjustments required for otherwise healthy geriatric patients.

Topiramate

(toe pyre′ a mate)

Brand Name: Topamax®

Why is this medicine prescribed?

Topiramate is used with other medications to treat certain types of seizures in patients with epilepsy or Lennox-Gastaut syndrome (a disorder that causes seizures and developmental delays). Topiramate is used to treat patients who continue to have seizures even when they take other anti-seizure medications. Topiramate is in a class of medications called anticonvulsants. It works by decreasing abnormal excitement in the brain.

How should this medicine be used?

Topiramate comes as a tablet and a sprinkle capsule to take by mouth. It is usually taken with or without food twice a day in the morning and evening. Take topiramate at around the same times every day. Follow the directions on your prescription label carefully, and ask your doctor or pharmacist to explain any part you do not understand. Take topiramate exactly as directed. Do not take more or less of it or take it more often than prescribed by your doctor.

Topiramate tablets have a bitter taste and lose their effectiveness quickly when broken, so you should swallow them whole. Do not split, chew, or crush them.

Your doctor will probably start you on a low dose of topiramate and gradually increase your dose, not more than once every week.

Topiramate may control your seizures but will not cure your condition. Continue to take topiramate even if you feel well. Do not stop taking topiramate without talking to your doctor. If you suddenly stop taking topiramate, you may have severe seizures. Your doctor will probably decrease your dose gradually.

The sprinkle capsules may be swallowed whole or opened and poured over food. To take the sprinkle capsule with food, follow these steps:
1. Prepare a teaspoonful of soft food such as applesauce, custard, ice cream, oatmeal, pudding, or yogurt.
2. Hold the capsule upright over the food. You should be able to read the word 'TOP' on the capsule.
3. Twist off the clear part of the capsule and pour the entire contents onto the spoonful of food.
4. Swallow the entire mixture immediately without chewing.
5. Have a drink to wash down the mixture and to be sure that you swallow all of it.

Are there other uses for this medicine?

Topiramate is also sometimes used to treat cluster headaches and infantile spasms (a condition that causes uncontrolled stiffening of the body in babies). Talk to your doctor about the risks of using this medication for your condition.

This medication may be prescribed for other uses; ask your doctor or pharmacist for more information.

What special precautions should I follow?

Before taking topiramate,
- tell your doctor and pharmacist if you are allergic to topiramate or any other medications.
- tell your doctor and pharmacist what prescription and nonprescription medications, vitamins, nutritional supplements, and herbal products you are taking. Be sure to mention any of the following: acetazolamide (Diamox); antidepressants; antihistamines; cholestyramine (Questran); dichlorphenamide (Daranide); digoxin (Lanoxin, Digitek); ipratropium (Atrovent); iron; isoniazid (INH, Nydrazid); medications for irritable bowel disease, mental illness, motion sickness, Parkinson's disease, ulcers, or urinary problems; metformin (Glucophage); methazolamide; oral contraceptives (birth control pills); other medications for seizures such as carbamazepine (Tegretol), and phenytoin (Dilantin, Phenytek); salicylate pain relievers such as aspirin, choline magnesium trisalicylate (Trisalate), choline salicylate (Arthropan), diflunisal (Dolobid), magnesium salicylate (Doan's, others), and salsalate (Argesic, Disalcid, Salgesic); sedatives; sleeping pills; tranquilizers; valproic acid (Depakene, Depakote); and zonisamide (Zonegran). Your doctor may need to change the doses of your medications or monitor you carefully for side effects.

- tell your doctor if you or any family members have or have ever had kidney stones, if you drink or have ever drunk large amounts of alchohol, and if you have or have ever had diabetes; glaucoma (a type of eye disease); nearsightedness; any disease that affects your breathing such as asthma or chronic obstructive pulmonary disease (COPD); or liver or kidney disease.
- tell your doctor if you are pregnant, plan to become pregnant, or are breast-feeding. If you become pregnant while taking topiramate, call your doctor.
- if you are having surgery, including dental surgery, tell the doctor or dentist that you are taking topiramate.
- you should know that topiramate may make you drowsy, dizzy, confused, or unable to concentrate. Do not drive a car or operate machinery until you know how this medication affects you.
- ask your doctor about the safe use of alcoholic beverages while you are taking topiramate. Alcohol can cause seizures or make seizures worse.
- if you are taking oral contraceptives (birth control pills), tell your doctor if unexpected bleeding or spotting occurs. Topiramate can decrease the effectiveness of oral contraceptives.
- you should know that topiramate can prevent you from sweating and make it harder for your body to cool down when it gets very hot. This happens most often in warm weather and to children who take topiramate. Avoid exposure to heat, drink plenty of fluids and tell your doctor if you have a fever, headache, muscle cramps, an upset stomach, or are not sweating as usual.
- you should know that you may be more likely to develop a kidney stone while you are taking topiramate. Drink 6-8 glasses of water every day to prevent kidney stones from forming.

What special dietary instructions should I follow?

Talk to your doctor about increasing the amount of food you eat if you lose weight while you are taking topiramate.

Talk to your doctor before changing your diet or beginning any type of weight loss program. Do not follow a ketogenic diet (a high-fat, low-carbohydrate diet used to control seizures) or any other high-fat, low-carbohydrate diet, such as the Atkin's diet, while taking this medication.

What should I do if I forget to take a dose?

Take the missed dose as soon as you remember it. However, if it is almost time for the next dose, skip the missed dose and continue your regular dosing schedule. Do not take a double dose to make up for a missed one. You may have seizures if you miss doses of topiramate.

What side effects can this medicine cause?

You may experience hypoglycemia (low blood sugar) while you are taking this medication. Your doctor will tell you what you should do if you develop hypoglycemia. He or she may tell you to check your blood sugar, eat or drink a food or beverage that contains sugar, such as hard candy or fruit juice, or get medical care. Follow these directions carefully if you have any of the following symptoms of hypoglycemia:

- shakiness
- dizziness or lightheadedness
- sweating
- nervousness or irritability
- sudden changes in behavior or mood
- headache
- numbness or tingling around the mouth
- weakness
- pale skin
- hunger
- clumsy or jerky movements

If hypoglycemia is not treated, severe symptoms may develop. Be sure that your family, friends, and other people who spend time with you know that if you have any of the following symptoms, they should get medical treatment for you immediately.

- confusion
- seizures
- loss of consciousness

Topiramate may cause other side effects. Tell your doctor if any of these symptoms are severe or do not go away:

- slow thinking or movements
- difficulty concentrating
- speech problems, especially difficulty thinking of specific words
- memory problems
- lack of coordination
- trouble walking
- confusion
- nervousness
- aggressive behavior
- irritability
- mood swings
- depression
- headache
- extreme tiredness
- drowsiness
- weakness
- extreme thirst
- weight loss
- constipation
- diarrhea
- gas
- heartburn
- change in ability to taste food
- swelling of the tongue
- overgrowth of the gums
- dry mouth
- increased saliva
- trouble swallowing
- nosebleed
- teary or dry eyes
- back, muscle, or bone pain

- missed menstrual periods
- excessive menstrual bleeding
- skin problems or changes in skin color
- dandruff
- hair loss
- growth of hair in unusual places
- runny nose
- difficulty falling or staying asleep

Some side effects can be serious. The following symptoms are uncommon, but if you experience any of them, call your doctor immediately:

- blurred vision
- eye pain
- double vision
- tingling in fingers or toes
- shaking hands that you cannot control
- restlessness, inability to sit still
- crossed eyes
- worsening of seizures
- slow heart rate
- pounding or irregular heartbeat
- chest pain
- trouble breathing
- fast, shallow breathing
- inability to respond to things around you
- upset stomach
- vomiting
- stomach pain
- loss of appetite
- excessive hunger
- unintentional loss of urine
- difficult or painful urination
- unusual bruising or bleeding
- sore throat, fever, chills, and other signs of infection
- muscle weakness
- bone pain

Topiramate may cause osteoporosis (a condition in which bones can break more easily) in adults and rickets (abnormal, curved bone growth) in children. Topiramate may also slow the growth of children. These conditions can be caught early and prevented through regular laboratory tests. Talk to your doctor about the risks of taking topiramate.

Topiramate may cause other side effects. Call your doctor if you have any unusual problems while taking this medication.

If you experience a serious side effect, you or your doctor may send a report to the Food and Drug Administration's (FDA) MedWatch Adverse Event Reporting program online [at http://www.fda.gov/MedWatch/index.html] or by phone [1-800-332-1088].

What storage conditions are needed for this medicine?

Keep this medication in the container it came in, tightly closed, and out of reach of children. Tablets should be stored at room temperature and away from excess heat and mois-

ture (not in the bathroom). Sprinkle capsules should be stored at or below 77° F. Never store broken tablets or mixtures of sprinkles and soft food. These should be used right away or thrown away. Throw away any medication that is outdated or no longer needed. Talk to your pharmacist about the proper disposal of your medication.

What should I do in case of overdose?

In case of overdose, call your local poison control center at 1-800-222-1222. If the victim has collapsed or is not breathing, call local emergency services at 911.

Symptoms of overdose may include:

- seizures
- drowsiness
- speech problems
- blurred vision
- double vision
- trouble thinking
- tiredness
- loss of coordination
- loss of consciousness
- coma
- fainting
- dizziness
- stomach pain
- upset stomach
- vomiting
- excessive hunger
- agitation
- depression
- shortness of breath
- confusion
- loss of appetite
- pounding or irregular heartbeat
- fast, shallow breathing
- inability to respond to things around you
- muscle weakness
- bone pain

What other information should I know?

Keep all appointments with your doctor and the laboratory. Your doctor will order certain lab tests to check your body's response to topiramate.

Do not let anyone else take your medication. Ask your pharmacist any questions you have about refilling your prescription.

Dosage Facts
For Informational Purposes

Caution: Do not change your dose, how often you take your medication, or the length of time you are to take it without first talking to your healthcare provider.

The following dosage information was written using medical language for doctors and other healthcare pro-

fessionals and is provided here for you to check your dosage. The dosage of this drug may differ for different patients. Therefore, always follow your doctor's instructions or the directions on the label. Contact your healthcare provider or pharmacist if you have any questions about the specific dosage of your medication after reviewing this information.

Pediatric Patients

Seizure Disorders

Partial Seizures, Primary Generalized Tonic-Clonic Seizures, or Seizures Associated with Lennox-Gastaut Syndrome

ORAL:
- Initially, 25 mg (or less based on a range of 1–3 mg/kg daily) given nightly for the first week in children 2–16 years of age. Increase dosage at 1- or 2-week intervals in increments of 1–3 mg/kg daily, administered in 2 divided doses, to achieve optimal clinical response.
- Maintenance, 5–9 mg/kg daily in 2 divided doses.
- Alternatively, some clinicians recommend an initial dosage of 0.5–1 mg/kg daily, with slow titration (in increments of 1–3 mg/kg every other week or in increments of 0.5–1 mg/kg per week) to obtain optimal efficacy with minimal adverse effects.

Adult Patients

Seizure Disorders
Partial Seizures

ORAL:
- Initially, 25–50 mg daily. Increase dosage at weekly intervals in increments of 25–50 mg to achieve optimal clinical response.
- Recommended maintenance dosage is 200–400 mg daily, administered in 2 equally divided doses (morning and evening).
- Titration in increments of 25 mg/week is associated with a lower incidence of cognitive and psychiatric adverse effects and lower discontinuance rates but may delay the time to reach an effective dosage.
- Dosages >400 mg daily generally have not produced substantial additional improvement, but may improve seizure control in some patients, if tolerated.

Primary Generalized Tonic-Clonic Seizures

ORAL:
- Initially, 25–50 mg daily. Increase dosage at weekly intervals in increments of 25–50 mg to achieve optimal clinical response.
- Recommended maintenance dosage is 400 mg daily, administered in 2 equally divided doses (morning and evening).
- Titration in increments of 25 mg/week is associated with a lower incidence of cognitive and psychiatric adverse effects and lower discontinuance rates but may delay the time to reach an effective dosage.

Seizures Associated with Lennox-Gastaut Syndrome

ORAL:
- Manufacturer makes no specific dosage recommendations; in 1 controlled trial, topiramate was initiated at dosage of 1 mg/kg and titrated over 2 weeks to target dosage of approximately 6 mg/kg daily.

Migraine Prophylaxis

ORAL:
- Recommended total daily dosage is 100 mg, administered in 2 divided doses. Titrate therapy using the following schedule:

Table 1. Topiramate Dosage Titration Schedule for Migraine Prophylaxis in Adults

	Morning Dose	Evening Dose
Week 1	None	25 mg
Week 2	25 mg	25 mg
Week 3	25 mg	50 mg
Week 4	50 mg	50 mg

Titrate dosage based on clinical outcome. Use longer intervals between dose adjustments if required.

Prescribing Limits

Adult Patients

Seizure Disorders

ORAL:
- Dosages >1.6 g daily in patients with seizure disorders have not been studied.

Special Populations

Hepatic Impairment
- Clearance may be decreased; however, manufacturer makes no specific recommendations regarding dosage adjustment.

Renal Impairment
- If Cl_{cr} is <70 mL/minute per 1.73 m², decrease daily adult dosage by 50%. Patients with renal impairment will require a longer time to reach steady state at each dosage level.
- Patients undergoing hemodialysis may require a supplemental dose following dialysis session; base amount on duration of dialysis, clearance rate of dialysis system, and the patient's effective renal clearance of topiramate.

Geriatric Patients
- If Cl_{cr} <70 mL/minute per 1.73 m², dosage adjustment may be necessary.

Torsemide Oral

(tore′ se mide)

Brand Name: Demadex Oral®

Why is this medicine prescribed?

Torsemide, a 'water pill,' is used to reduce the swelling and fluid retention caused by various medical problems, including heart or liver disease. It also is used to treat high blood pressure. It causes the kidneys to get rid of unneeded water and salt from the body into the urine.

This medicine is sometimes prescribed for other uses; ask your doctor or pharmacist for more information.

How should this medicine be used?

Torsemide comes as a tablet to take by mouth. It usually is taken once a day in the morning. Follow the directions on your prescription label carefully, and ask your doctor or pharmacist to explain any part you do not understand. Take torsemide exactly as directed. Do not take more or less of it or take it more often than prescribed by your doctor.

Torsemide controls high blood pressure but does not cure it. Continue to take torsemide even if you feel well. Do not stop taking torsemide without talking to your doctor.

What special precautions should I follow?

Before taking torsemide,

- tell your doctor and pharmacist if you are allergic to torsemide, sulfa drugs, or any other drugs.
- tell your doctor and pharmacist what prescription and nonprescription medications you are taking, especially other medications for high blood pressure, corticosteroids (e.g., prednisone), digoxin (Lanoxin), indomethacin (Indocin), lithium (Eskalith, Lithobid), probenecid (Benemid), and vitamins.
- tell your doctor if you have or have ever had diabetes, gout, or kidney or liver disease.
- tell your doctor if you are pregnant, plan to become pregnant, or are breast-feeding. Do not breast-feed while taking this medicine. If you become pregnant while taking torsemide, call your doctor.
- if you are having surgery, including dental surgery, tell the doctor or dentist that you are taking torsemide.

What special dietary instructions should I follow?

Follow your doctor's directions. They may include a daily exercise program and a low-sodium or low-salt diet, potassium supplements, and increased amounts of potassium-rich foods (e.g., bananas, prunes, raisins, and orange juice) in your diet.

What should I do if I forget to take a dose?

Take the missed dose as soon as you remember it. However, if it is almost time for your next dose, skip the missed dose and continue your regular dosing schedule. Do not take a double dose to make up for a missed one.

What side effects can this medicine cause?

Frequent urination may last for up to 6 hours after a dose and should decrease after you take torsemide for a few weeks. Tell your doctor if any of these symptoms are severe or do not go away:

- muscle cramps
- weakness
- dizziness
- faintness
- fatigue
- headache
- confusion
- thirst
- upset stomach
- vomiting

If you have either of the following symptoms, call your doctor immediately:

- rapid, excessive weight loss
- vomiting blood

If you experience a serious side effect, you or your doctor may send a report to the Food and Drug Administration's (FDA) MedWatch Adverse Event Reporting program online [at http://www.fda.gov/MedWatch/index.html] or by phone [1-800-332-1088].

What storage conditions are needed for this medicine?

Keep this medicine in the container it came in, tightly closed, and out of reach of children. Store it at room temperature and away from excess heat and moisture (not in the bathroom). Throw away any medicine that is outdated or no longer needed. Talk to your pharmacist about the proper disposal of your medicine.

What should I do in case of overdose?

In case of overdose, call your local poison control center at 1-800-222-1222. If the victim has collapsed or is not breathing, call local emergency services at 911.

What other information should I know?

Keep all appointments with your doctor and the laboratory. Your blood pressure should be checked regularly, and blood tests should be done occasionally.

Do not let anyone else take your medicine. Ask your pharmacist any questions you have about refilling your prescription.

Talk to your doctor, pharmacist, or other healthcare professional if you have questions about dosing information for your medication.

Tramadol

(tra′ ma dole)

Brand Name: Ultram®, Ultram® ER, Ultracet® (combination with acetaminophen)
Also available generically.

Why is this medicine prescribed?

Tramadol is used to relieve moderate to moderately severe pain. Tramadol extended-release tablets are only used by people who are expected to need medication to relieve pain around-the-clock for a long time. Tramadol is in a class of medications called opiate agonists. It works by changing the way the body senses pain.

How should this medicine be used?

Tramadol comes as a tablet and an extended-release (long-acting) tablet to take by mouth. The regular tablet is usually taken with or without food every 4-6 hours as needed. The extended-release tablet should be taken once a day. Take the extended-release tablet at about the same time of day every day, and either always take it with food or always take it without food. Take tramadol exactly as directed. Do not take more medication as a single dose or take more doses per day than prescribed by your doctor. Taking more tramadol than prescribed by your doctor may cause serious side effects or death.

Your doctor may start you on a low dose of tramadol and gradually increase the amount of medication you take, not more often than every 3 days if you are taking the regular tablets or every 5 days if you are taking the extended-release tablets.

Swallow the extended-release tablets whole; do not split, chew, or crush them. Do not snort (inhale powder from crushed tablet) or inject the dissolved extended-release tablets. Taking this medication in a way that is not recommended may cause serious side effects or death.

Tramadol can be habit-forming. Do not take a larger dose, take it more often, or take it for a longer period of time than prescribed by your doctor. Call your doctor if you find that you want to take extra medication or if you notice any other unusual changes in your behavior or mood.

Do not stop taking tramadol without talking to your doctor. Your doctor will probably decrease your dose gradually. If you suddenly stop taking tramadol you may experience withdrawal symptoms such as nervousness; panic; sweating; difficulty falling asleep or staying asleep; runny nose, sneezing, or cough; numbness, pain, burning, or tingling in your hands or feet; hair standing on end; chills; nausea; uncontrollable shaking of a part of your body; diarrhea; or rarely, hallucinations (seeing things or hearing voices that do not exist).

Are there other uses for this medicine?

This medication is sometimes prescribed for other uses; ask your doctor or pharmacist for more information.

What special precautions should I follow?

Before taking tramadol,
- tell your doctor and pharmacist if you are allergic to tramadol or other opiate pain or cough medications such as meperidine (Demerol), morphine (Avinza, Kadian, MS Contin), codeine (in some pain medications and cough syrups), hydrocodone (in Vicodin), hydromorphone (Dilaudid), oxycodone (OxyContin, in Percocet), propoxyphene (Darvon, Darvon N, in Darvocet), any other medications, or any of the ingredients in tramadol tablets or extended-release tablets. Ask your pharmacist for a list of ingredients in tramadol tablets or extended release tablets.
- tell your doctor and pharmacist what other prescription and nonprescription medications, vitamins, and nutritional supplements you are taking. Be sure to mention any of the following: antifungal medications such as ketoconazole (Nizoral); digoxin (Lanoxin); erythromycin (E.E.S., E-Mycin, Erythrocin); monoamine oxidase (MAO) inhibitors, including isocarboxazid (Marplan), phenelzine (Nardil), selegiline (Eldepryl, Emsam, Zelapar), and tranylcypromine (Parnate); medications for anxiety, mental illness, nausea, and pain; medications for seizures, such as carbamazepine (Tegretol); muscle relaxants such as cyclobenzaprine (Flexeril); promethazine (Phenergan); quinidine; rifampin (Rifadin, Rifamate, Rimactane, others); sedatives; sleeping pills; selective serotonin reuptake inhibitors (SSRIs) such as citalopram (Celexa), fluoxetine (Prozac, Sarafem), fluvoxamine (Luvox), paroxetine (Paxil), and sertraline (Zoloft); tranquilizers; tricyclic antidepressants such as amitriptyline (Elavil), amoxapine (Asendin), clomipramine (Anafranil), desipramine (Norpramin), doxepin (Adapin, Sinequan), imipramine (Tofranil), nortriptyline (Aventyl, Pamelor), protriptyline (Vivactil), and trimipramine (Surmontil); and warfarin (Coumadin). Many other medications may also interact with tramadol, so be sure to tell your doctor about all the medications you are taking, even those that do not appear on this list. Your doctor may need to change the doses of your medications or monitor you carefully for side effects.
- tell your doctor what herbal products you are taking, especially St. John's wort.
- tell your doctor if you have or have ever had seizures; an infection in your brain or spine; a head injury, a brain tumor, a stroke, or any other condition that caused high pressure inside your skull; depression or thoughts about harming or killing yourself or planning or trying to do so; diabetes; breathing problems or lung disease; or kidney or liver disease. Also tell your doctor if you drink or have ever drunk large amounts of alcohol, use or have ever used street drugs, or have overused prescription medications.
- tell your doctor if you are pregnant, plan to become pregnant, or are breast-feeding. If you become pregnant while taking tramadol, call your doctor.
- if you are having surgery, including dental surgery, tell the doctor or dentist that you are taking tramadol.
- you should know that this medication may make you drowsy and may affect your coordination. Do not drive a car or operate machinery until you know how this medication affects you.
- talk to your doctor about the safe use of alcohol while you are taking this medication. Alcohol can make the side effects from tramadol worse.
- you should know that tramadol may cause dizziness, lightheadedness, and fainting when you get up from a lying position. To avoid this, get out of bed slowly,

resting your feet on the floor for a few minutes before standing up.

What special dietary instructions should I follow?

Talk to your doctor about drinking grapefruit juice while you are taking this medication.

What should I do if I forget to take a dose?

If your doctor has told you to take tramadol regularly, take the missed dose as soon as you remember it. However, if it is almost time for the next dose, skip the missed dose and continue your regular dosing schedule. Do not take a double dose to make up for a missed one.

What side effects can this medicine cause?

Tramadol may cause side effects. Tell your doctor if any of these symptoms are severe or do not go away:

- dizziness
- weakness
- sleepiness
- difficulty falling asleep or staying asleep
- headache
- nervousness
- agitation
- uncontrollable shaking of a part of the body
- muscle tightness
- changes in mood
- drowsiness
- heartburn or indigestion
- nausea
- vomiting
- diarrhea
- constipation
- itching
- sweating
- chills
- dry mouth

Some side effects can be serious. If you experience any of these symptoms or those listed in the SPECIAL PRE-CAUTIONS section, call your doctor immediately:

- seizures
- sores on the inside of your mouth, nose, eyes, or throat
- flu-like symptoms
- hives
- rash
- difficulty swallowing or breathing
- swelling of the face, throat, tongue, lips, eyes, hands, feet, ankles, or lower legs
- hoarseness
- hallucinations (seeing things or hearing voices that do not exist)

If you experience a serious side effect, you or your doctor may send a report to the Food and Drug Administration's (FDA) MedWatch Adverse Event Reporting program online

[at http://www.fda.gov/MedWatch/index.html] or by phone [1-800-332-1088].

Tramadol may cause other side effects. Tell your doctor if you have any unusual problems while you are taking this medication.

What storage conditions are needed for this medicine?

Keep this medication in the container it came in, tightly closed, and out of reach of children. Store it at room temperature and away from excess heat and moisture (not in the bathroom). Throw away any medication that is outdated or no longer needed. Talk to your pharmacist about the proper disposal of your medication.

What should I do in case of overdose?

In case of overdose, call your local poison control center at 1-800-222-1222. If the victim has collapsed or is not breathing, call local emergency services at 911.

Symptoms of overdose may include:

- decreased size of the pupil (the black circle in the center of the eye)
- difficulty breathing
- extreme drowsiness
- unconsciousness
- coma
- seizure
- heart attack

What other information should I know?

Keep all appointments with your doctor.

Do not let anyone else take your medication. Ask your pharmacist any questions you have about refilling your prescription.

Dosage Facts
For Informational Purposes

Caution: Do not change your dose, how often you take your medication, or the length of time you are to take it without first talking to your healthcare provider.

The following dosage information was written using medical language for doctors and other healthcare professionals and is provided here for you to check your dosage. The dosage of this drug may differ for different patients. Therefore, always follow your doctor's instructions or the directions on the label. Contact your healthcare provider or pharmacist if you have any questions about the specific dosage of your medication after reviewing this information.

General Dosage Information

Available as tramadol hydrochloride; dosage expressed in terms of the salt.

Adult Patients

Pain

Conventional Tablets

ORAL:

- Initially, 25 mg daily in the morning; titrate dosage slowly to reduce risk of adverse effects. Increase dosage in 25-mg increments as separate doses every 3 days to a dosage of 100 mg daily (25 mg 4 times daily); then may increase total daily dosage by 50 mg every 3 days as tolerated, up to 200 mg daily (50 mg 4 times daily.) After titration, 50–100 mg can be given every 4–6 hours, up to 400 mg daily.
- If more rapid onset of analgesia is required, may initiate therapy at 50–100 mg every 4–6 hours (up to 400 mg daily), but risk of adverse events may be increased.

Extended-release Tablets

ORAL:

- Initially, 100 mg once daily; increase dosage in 100-mg increments every 5 days, as needed and tolerated, up to 300 mg daily.

Fixed Combination with Acetaminophen

ORAL:

- 75 mg of tramadol hydrochloride every 4–6 hours as needed (up to 300 mg daily).

Prescribing Limits

Adult Patients

Pain

Conventional Tablets

ORAL:

- Maximum 400 mg daily.

Extended-release Tablets

ORAL:

- Maximum 300 mg daily.

Fixed Combination with Acetaminophen

ORAL:

- Maximum 300 mg daily.

Special Populations

Hepatic Impairment

- In patients with cirrhosis, 50 mg (as conventional tablets) every 12 hours.
- Extended-release tablets not recommended for use in patients with severe (Child-Pugh class C) hepatic impairment. Available tablet strengths do not provide sufficient dosing flexibility for safe use in these patients.
- Tramadol in fixed combination with acetaminophen not recommended in patients with hepatic impairment.

Renal Impairment

- Reduced dosage recommended in patients with severe renal impairment (Cl_{cr} <30 mL/minute).

Severe Renal Impairment

- Conventional tablets: 50–100 mg of tramadol every 12 hours (maximum 200 mg daily). In hemodialysis patients, administer the patient's regular dose on dialysis days (not substantially removed by dialysis).
- Fixed combination with acetaminophen: Maximum of 75 mg of tramadol hydrochloride (in combination with acetaminophen) every 12 hours.

- Extended-release tablets not recommended. Available tablet strengths do not provide sufficient dosing flexibility for safe use.

Geriatric Patients

- Cautious dosage selection; initiate therapy at the lower end of the dosage range.
- In patients >75 years of age, maximum 300 mg daily.

Trandolapril

(tran dole′ a pril)

Brand Name: Mavik®, Tarka® as a combination product containing Trandolapril and Verapamil Hydrochloride

---

Important Warning

Do not take trandolapril if you are pregnant. If you become pregnant while taking trandolapril, call your doctor immediately. Trandolapril may harm the fetus.

Why is this medicine prescribed?

Trandolapril is used alone or in combination with other medications to treat high blood pressure. It is also used to improve survival in patients with heart failure after a heart attack. Trandolapril is in a class of medications called angiotensin-converting enzyme (ACE) inhibitors. It works by decreasing certain chemicals that tighten the blood vessels, so blood flows more smoothly and the heart can pump blood more efficiently.

How should this medicine be used?

Trandolapril comes as a tablet to take by mouth. It is usually taken once or twice a day with or without food. To help you remember to take trandolapril, take it around the same time every day. Follow the directions on your prescription label carefully, and ask your doctor or pharmacist to explain any part you do not understand. Take trandolapril exactly as directed. Do not take more or less of it or take it more often than prescribed by your doctor.

Your doctor will probably start you on a low dose of trandolapril and gradually increase your dose, not more than once a week.

Trandolapril controls high blood pressure but does not cure it. Continue to take trandolapril even if you feel well. Do not stop taking trandolapril without talking to your doctor.

Are there other uses for this medicine?

This medication may be prescribed for other uses; ask you doctor or pharmacist for more information.

What special precautions should I follow?

Before taking trandolapril,

- tell your doctor and pharmacist if you are allergic to trandolapril, benazepril (Lotensin), captopril (Capoten), enalapril (Vasotec), fosinopril (Monopril), lisinopril (Prinivil, Zestril), moexipril (Univasc), perindopril (Aceon), quinapril (Accupril), ramipril (Altace), or any other medications.
- tell your doctor and pharmacist what prescription and nonprescription medications, vitamins, nutritional supplements, and herbal products you are taking. Be sure to mention any of the following: diuretics ('water pills'); lithium (Eskalith, Lithobid); and potassium supplements. Your doctor may need to change the doses of your medications or monitor you carefully for side effects.
- tell your doctor if you have recently had severe vomiting or diarrhea and if you have or have ever had heart, liver, or kidney disease; lupus; scleroderma; or diabetes.
- tell your doctor if you plan to become pregnant or are breast-feeding.
- if you are having surgery, including dental surgery, tell the doctor or dentist that you are taking trandolapril.
- you should know that diarrhea, vomiting, not drinking enough fluids, and sweating a lot can cause a drop in blood pressure, which may cause lightheadedness and fainting.

What special dietary instructions should I follow?

Talk to your doctor before using salt substitutes containing potassium. If your doctor prescribes a low-salt or low-sodium diet, follow these directions carefully.

What should I do if I forget to take a dose?

Take the missed dose as soon as you remember it. However, if it is almost time for the next dose, skip the missed dose and continue your regular dosing schedule. Do not take a double dose to make up for a missed one.

What side effects can this medicine cause?

Trandolapril may cause side effects. Tell your doctor if any of these symptoms are severe or do not go away:

- cough
- dizziness
- muscle pain

Some side effects can be serious. The following symptoms are uncommon, but if you experience any of them, call your doctor immediately:

- swelling of the face, throat, tongue, lips, eyes, hands, feet, ankles, or lower legs
- hoarseness
- difficulty breathing or swallowing
- yellowing of the skin or eyes
- fever, sore throat, chills, and other signs of infection

- lightheadedness
- fainting

Trandolapril may cause other side effects. Call your doctor if you have any unusual problems while taking this medication.

If you experience a serious side effect, you or your doctor may send a report to the Food and Drug Administration's (FDA) MedWatch Adverse Event Reporting program online [at http://www.fda.gov/MedWatch/index.html] or by phone [1-800-332-1088].

What storage conditions are needed for this medicine?

Keep this medication in the container it came in, tightly closed, and out of reach of children. Store it at room temperature and away from excess heat and moisture (not in the bathroom). Throw away any medication that is outdated or no longer needed. Talk to your pharmacist about the proper disposal of your medication.

What should I do in case of overdose?

In case of overdose, call your local poison control center at 1-800-222-1222. If the victim has collapsed or is not breathing, call local emergency services at 911.

Symptoms of overdose may include:

- lightheadedness
- fainting

What other information should I know?

Keep all appointments with your doctor and the laboratory. Your blood pressure should be checked regularly to determine your response to trandolapril. Your doctor may order certain lab tests to check your body's response to trandolapril.

Do not let anyone else take your medication. Ask your pharmacist any questions you have about refilling your prescription.

Dosage Facts
For Informational Purposes

Caution: Do not change your dose, how often you take your medication, or the length of time you are to take it without first talking to your healthcare provider.

The following dosage information was written using medical language for doctors and other healthcare professionals and is provided here for you to check your dosage. The dosage of this drug may differ for different patients. Therefore, always follow your doctor's instructions or the directions on the label. Contact your healthcare provider or pharmacist if you have any questions about the specific dosage of your medication after reviewing this information.

Adult Patients

Hypertension

ORAL:

- Initially, 2 mg once daily in black patients and 1 mg once daily in patients of other races as monotherapy. Adjust dosage at intervals of ≥1 week.
- In patients currently receiving diuretic therapy, discontinue diuretic, if possible, 2–3 days before initiating trandolapril. May cautiously resume diuretic therapy if BP not controlled adequately with trandolapril alone. If diuretic cannot be discontinued, initiate therapy at 0.5 mg daily under close medical supervision for several hours until BP has stabilized.
- Usual dosage: 2–4 mg once daily.
- If 4 mg once daily does not adequately control BP, consider administering drug in 2 divided doses. If trandolapril monotherapy does not adequately control BP, consider adding a diuretic.
- Limited clinical experience with dosages >8 mg daily.

Trandolapril/Verapamil Combination Therapy

ORAL:

- Adjust dosage by first administering each drug separately. For patients receiving verapamil (up to 240 mg) and trandolapril (up to 8 mg) in separate tablets once daily, replacement with the fixed combination can be attempted using tablets containing the same component doses.

Heart Failure or Left Ventricular Dysfunction after AMI

ORAL:

- Initially, 1 mg once daily; therapy may be initiated about 3–5 days after AMI.
- Titrate dosage as tolerated to a target dosage of 4 mg once daily; if 4 mg daily is not tolerated, may continue therapy at the highest tolerated dosage.

Prescribing Limits

Adult Patients

Hypertension

ORAL:

- Limited clinical experience with dosages >8 mg daily.

Special Populations

Hepatic Impairment

Hypertension

ORAL:

- Reduced initial dosage (0.5 mg once daily) recommended in patients with hepatic cirrhosis; titrate subsequent dosage according to BP response.

Heart Failure or Left Ventricular Dysfunction after AMI

ORAL:

- Reduced initial dosage (0.5 mg once daily) recommended in patients with hepatic cirrhosis; titrate subsequent dosage as tolerated according to response.

Renal Impairment

Hypertension

ORAL:

- Reduced initial dosage (0.5 mg once daily) recommended in patients with severe renal impairment (Cl_{cr} <30 mL/minute); titrate subsequent dosage according to BP response.

Heart Failure or Left Ventricular Dysfunction after AMI

ORAL:

- Reduced initial dosage (0.5 mg once daily) recommended in patients with severe renal impairment (Cl_{cr} <30 mL/minute); titrate subsequent dosage as tolerated according to response.

Tranylcypromine

(tran il sip′ roe meen)

Brand Name: Parnate®
Also available generically.

Important Warning

A small number of children, teenagers, and young adults (up to 24 years of age) who took antidepressants ('mood elevators') such as tranylcypromine during clinical studies became suicidal (thinking about harming or killing oneself or planning or trying to do so). Children, teenagers, and young adults who take antidepressants to treat depression or other mental illnesses may be more likely to become suicidal than children, teenagers, and young adults who do not take antidepressants to treat these conditions. However, experts are not sure about how great this risk is and how much it should be considered in deciding whether a child or teenager should take an antidepressant. Children younger than 18 years of age should not normally take tranylcypromine, but in some cases, a doctor may decide that tranylcypromine is the best medication to treat a child's condition.

You should know that your mental health may change in unexpected ways when you take tranylcypromine or other antidepressants even if you are an adult over age 24. You may become suicidal, especially at the beginning of your treatment and any time that your dose is increased or decreased. You, your family, or your caregiver should call your doctor right away if you experience any of the following symptoms: new or worsening depression; thinking about harming or killing yourself, or planning or trying to do so; extreme worry; agitation; panic attacks; difficulty falling asleep or staying asleep; aggressive behavior; irritability; acting without thinking; severe restlessness; and frenzied abnormal excitement. Be sure that your family or caregiver knows which symptoms may be serious so they can call the doctor when you are unable to seek treatment on your own.

Your healthcare provider will want to see you often while you are taking tranylcypromine, especially at the beginning of your treatment. Be sure to keep all appointments for office visits with your doctor.

The doctor or pharmacist will give you the manufacturer's patient information sheet (Medication Guide) when you begin treatment with tranylcypromine. Read the information carefully and ask your doctor or pharmacist if you have any questions. You also can obtain the Medication Guide from the FDA website: http://www.fda.gov/cder/drug/antidepressants/antidepressants_MG_2007.pdf.

No matter what your age, before you take an antidepressant, you, your parent, or your caregiver should talk to your doctor about the risks and benefits of treating your condition with an antidepressant or with other treatments. You should also talk about the risks and benefits of not treating your condition. You should know that having depression or another mental illness greatly increases the risk that you will become suicidal. This risk is higher if you or anyone in your family has or has ever had bipolar disorder (mood that changes from depressed to abnormally excited) or mania (frenzied, abnormally excited mood) or has thought about or attempted suicide. Talk to your doctor about your condition, symptoms, and personal and family medical history. You and your doctor will decide what type of treatment is right for you.

Why is this medicine prescribed?

Tranylcypromine is used to treat depression in people who have not been helped by other medications. Tranylcypromine is in a class of medications called monoamine oxidase inhibitors (MAOIs). It works by increasing the amounts of certain natural substances that are needed to maintain mental balance.

How should this medicine be used?

Tranylcypromine comes as a tablet to take by mouth. It is usually taken twice a day. Take tranylcypromine at around the same times every day. Follow the directions on your prescription label carefully, and ask your doctor or pharmacist to explain any part you do not understand. Take tranylcypromine exactly as directed.

Tranylcypromine may be habit-forming. Do not take a larger dose, take it more often, or take it for a longer period of time than prescribed by your doctor. Call your doctor if you find that you want to take extra medication or you notice any other unusual changes in your behavior or mood.

Your doctor will probably start you on a low dose of tranylcypromine and gradually increase your dose, not more often than once every 1-3 weeks. After your symptoms improve, your doctor will probably gradually decrease your dose of tranylcypromine.

Tranylcypromine controls the symptoms of depression but does not cure the condition. It may take 3 weeks or longer for you to feel the full benefit of tranylcypromine. Continue to take tranylcypromine even if you feel well. Do not stop taking tranylcypromine without talking to your doctor. Your doctor will probably want to decrease your dose gradually.

Are there other uses for this medicine?

This medication is sometimes prescribed for other uses; ask your doctor or pharmacist for more information.

What special precautions should I follow?

Before taking tranylcypromine,
- tell your doctor and pharmacist if you are allergic to tranylcypromine or any other medications.
- tell your doctor if you are taking, you have recently taken, or you plan to take any of the following prescription or non-prescription medications: certain other antidepressants including amitriptyline (Elavil), amoxapine, clomipramine (Anafranil), desipramine (Norpramin), doxepin (Sinequan), imipramine (Tofranil), maprotiline, nortriptyline (Pamelor), protriptyline (Vivactil), and trimipramine (Surmontil); amphetamines such as amphetamine (in Adderall), benzphetamine (Didrex), dextroamphetamine (Dexedrine, Dextrostat, in Adderall), and methamphetamine (Desoxyn); bupropion (Wellbutrin, Zyban); buspirone (BuSpar); caffeine (No-Doz, Quick-Pep, Vivarin); cyclobenzaprine (Flexeril); dexfenfluramine (Redux) (not available in the U.S.); dextromethorphan (Robitussin, others); diuretics ('water pills'); levodopa (Larodopa, in Sinemet); medications for allergies, cough and cold symptoms, and hay fever; medications for high blood pressure such as guanethidine (Ismelin) (not available in the U.S.), methyldopa (Aldomet), and reserpine (Serpalan); medications for Parkinson's disease, anxiety, or weight loss (diet pills); medications for seizures such as carbamazepine (Tegretol); narcotic medications for pain; other MAOIs such as isocarboxazid (Marplan); pargyline (not available in the U.S.), phenelzine (Nardil), procarbazine (Matulane), and selegiline (Eldepryl); meperidine (Demerol); sedatives; selective serotonin reuptake inhibitors such as citalopram (Celexa), duloxetine (Cymbalta), escitalopram (Lexapro), fluoxetine (Prozac), fluvoxamine (Luvox), paroxetine (Paxil), and sertraline (Zoloft); sleeping pills; tranquilizers; and medications containing alcohol (Nyquil, elixirs, others). Your doctor may tell you not to take tranylcypromine if you are taking or have recently stopped taking one or more of these medications.
- tell your doctor and pharmacist what other prescription and nonprescription medications, vitamins, and herbal products you are taking or plan to take. Be sure to mention any of the following: disulfiram (Antabuse), doxepin cream (Zonalon), insulin and oral medications for diabetes, and medications for nausea or mental illness. Your doctor may need to change the doses of your medications or monitor you carefully for side effects.
- you should know that tranylcypromine may remain in your body for several weeks after you stop taking the medication. During the first few weeks after your treatment ends, tell your doctor and pharmacist that you have recently stopped taking tranylcypromine before you start taking any new medications.

- tell your doctor if you are taking any nutritional supplements, especially tryptophan.
- tell your doctor if you have or have ever had high blood pressure; frequent or severe headaches; pheochromocytoma (a tumor on a small gland near the kidneys); a stroke or mini-stroke; or heart, blood vessel, or liver disease. Your doctor may tell you not to take tranylcypromine.
- tell your doctor if you use or have ever used street drugs or have overused prescription medications. Tell your doctor if you have or have ever had anxiety, agitation, diabetes, seizures, or kidney or thyroid disease.
- tell your doctor if you are pregnant, plan to become pregnant, or are breast-feeding. If you become pregnant while taking tranylcypromine, call your doctor.
- if you are having surgery, including dental surgery, or any x-ray procedure, tell the doctor or dentist that you are taking tranylcypromine.
- you should know that this medication may make you drowsy. Do not drive a car or operate machinery until you know how this medication affects you.
- remember that alcohol can add to the drowsiness caused by this medication. Do not drink alcohol while you are taking tranylcypromine.
- you should know that tranylcypromine may cause dizziness, lightheadedness, and fainting when you get up too quickly from a lying position. This is more common when you first start taking tranylcypromine. To avoid this problem, get out of bed slowly, resting your feet on the floor for a few minutes before standing up.

What special dietary instructions should I follow?

You may experience a serious reaction if you eat foods that are high in tyramine during your treatment with tranylcypromine. Tyramine is found in many foods, including meat, poultry, fish, or cheese that has been smoked, aged, improperly stored, or spoiled; certain fruits, vegetables, and beans; alcoholic beverages; and yeast products that have fermented. Your doctor or dietitian will tell you which foods you must avoid completely, and which foods you may eat in small amounts. You should also avoid foods and drinks that contain caffeine during your treatment with tranylcypromine. Follow these directions carefully. Ask your doctor or dietitian if you have any questions about what you may eat and drink during your treatment.

What should I do if I forget to take a dose?

Take the missed dose as soon as you remember it. However, if it is almost time for your next dose, skip the missed dose and continue your regular dosing schedule. Do not take a double dose to make up for a missed one.

What side effects can this medicine cause?

Tranylcypromine may cause side effects. Tell your doctor if any of these symptoms are severe or do not go away:

- drowsiness
- weakness
- dry mouth
- loss of appetite
- diarrhea
- constipation
- stomach pain
- blurred vision
- chills
- ringing in the ears
- muscle tightening or jerking
- uncontrollable shaking of any part of the body
- numbness, burning, or tingling in the arms or legs
- difficulty urinating
- decreased sexual ability
- hair loss
- rash

Some side effects can be serious. If you experience any of the following symptoms or those listed in the IMPORTANT WARNING section, call your doctor immediately:

- headache
- slow, fast, or pounding heartbeat
- chest pain or tightness
- tightening of the throat
- nausea
- sweating
- fever
- cold, clammy skin
- dizziness
- neck stiffness or soreness
- sensitivity to light
- widened pupils (black circles in the middle of the eyes)
- swelling of arms, hands, feet, ankles, or lower legs
- unusual bleeding or bruising
- pain in the upper right part of the stomach
- flu-like symptoms
- yellowing of the skin or eyes

Tranylcypromine may cause other side effects. Call your doctor if you have any unusual problems while you are taking this medication.

If you experience a serious side effect, you or your doctor may send a report to the Food and Drug Administration's (FDA) MedWatch Adverse Event Reporting program online [at http://www.fda.gov/MedWatch/index.html] or by phone [1-800-332-1088].

What storage conditions are needed for this medicine?

Keep this medication in the container it came in, tightly closed, and out of reach of children. Store it at room temperature and away from excess heat and moisture (not in the bathroom). Throw away any medication that is outdated or no longer needed. Talk to your pharmacist about the proper disposal of your medication.

What should I do in case of overdose?

In case of overdose, call your local poison control center at 1-800-222-1222. If the victim has collapsed or is not breathing, call local emergency services at 911.

Symptoms of overdose may include:

- difficulty falling asleep or staying asleep
- restlessness
- anxiety
- agitation
- confusion
- unclear speech
- dizziness
- weakness
- drowsiness
- headache
- muscle twitching
- fever
- stiffness
- coma (loss of consciousness for a period of time)

What other information should I know?

Keep all appointments with your doctor. Your doctor will check your blood pressure often during your treatment with tranylcypromine.

Do not let anyone else take your medication. Ask your pharmacist any questions you have about refilling your prescription.

Dosage Facts

For Informational Purposes

Caution: Do not change your dose, how often you take your medication, or the length of time you are to take it without first talking to your healthcare provider.

The following dosage information was written using medical language for doctors and other healthcare professionals and is provided here for you to check your dosage. The dosage of this drug may differ for different patients. Therefore, always follow your doctor's instructions or the directions on the label. Contact your healthcare provider or pharmacist if you have any questions about the specific dosage of your medication after reviewing this information.

General Dosage Information

Available as tranylcypromine sulfate; dosage expressed in terms of tranylcypromine.

Adult Patients

Major Depressive Disorder

ORAL:
- 30 mg daily in 2 divided doses. If no improvement after 2–3 weeks, dosage may be increased in increments of 10 mg daily at 1- to 3-week intervals to a maximum 60 mg daily.
- Transferring from another MAO inhibitor: Initially, 15 mg daily in 2 divided doses for at least 7 days.

- After maximum benefit obtained, gradually reduce dosage to the lowest level that will maintain relief of symptoms.

Prescribing Limits

Adult Patients

Major Depressive Disorder

ORAL:
- Maximum 60 mg daily.

Special Populations

Hepatic Impairment
- No specific dosage recommendations at this time; however, should not be used in patients with a history of liver disease or abnormal liver function tests.

Renal Impairment
- No specific dosage recommendations at this time; however, should not be used in patients with severe renal function impairment.

Geriatric Patients
- Select dosage with caution, usually starting at a lower dose, because of age-related decreases in hepatic, renal, and/or cardiac function and concomitant disease and drug therapy.

Travoprost Ophthalmic

(tra′ voe prost)

Brand Name: Travatan®

Why is this medicine prescribed?

Travoprost is used to treat eye conditions, including glaucoma and ocular hypertension, in which increased pressure can lead to a gradual loss of vision. Travoprost is used for patients who cannot use other eye medications for their condition or whose eye condition has not responded to another medication. Travoprost is in a class of medications called prostanoid agonists. It lowers pressure in the eye by increasing the flow of natural eye fluids out of the eye.

How should this medicine be used?

Travoprost comes as an eyedrop to apply to the eye. It is usually applied to the affected eye(s) once a day in the evening. To help you remember to use travoprost, use it around the same time every day. Follow the directions on your prescription label carefully, and ask your doctor or pharmacist to explain any part you do not understand. Use travoprost exactly as directed. Do not use more or less of it or use it more often than prescribed by your doctor.

Travoprost controls glaucoma and ocular hypertension but does not cure them. Continue to use travoprost even if you feel well. Do not stop using travoprost without talking to your doctor.

To apply the eyedrops, follow these steps:

1. Wash your hands thoroughly with soap and water.

2. Use a mirror or have someone else put the drops in your eye.
3. Make sure the end of the dropper is not chipped or cracked.
4. Avoid touching the dropper against your eye or anything else.
5. Hold the dropper tip down at all times to prevent drops from flowing back into the bottle and contaminating the remaining contents.
6. Lie down or tilt your head back.
7. Holding the bottle between your thumb and index finger, place the dropper as near as possible to your eyelid without touching it.
8. Brace the remaining fingers of that hand against your cheek or nose.
9. With the index finger of your other hand, pull the lower lid of the eye down to form a pocket.
10. Drop the prescribed number of drops into the pocket made by the lower lid and the eye. Placing the drops on the surface of the eyeball can cause stinging.
11. Close your eye and press lightly against the lower lid with your finger for 2-3 minutes to keep the medication in the eye. Do not blink.
12. Replace and tighten the cap right away. Do not wipe or rinse it off.
13. Wipe off any excess liquid from your cheek with a clean tissue. Wash your hands again.

Are there other uses for this medicine?

This medication may be prescribed for other uses; ask your doctor or pharmacist for more information.

What special precautions should I follow?

Before using travoprost,

- tell your doctor and pharmacist if you are allergic to travoprost, benzalkonium chloride, or any other medications.
- tell your doctor and pharmacist what prescription and nonprescription medications, vitamins, nutritional supplements, and herbal products you are taking.
- if you are using another topical eye medication, apply it at least 5 minutes before or after travoprost.
- tell your doctor if you have inflammation (swelling) of the eye or a torn or missing lens and if you have or have ever had liver or kidney disease.
- tell your doctor if you are pregnant, plan to become pregnant, or are breast-feeding. If you become pregnant while using travoprost, call your doctor immediately.
- you should know that pregnant women should avoid touching travoprost solution. If a pregnant woman comes into contact with the contents of the travoprost bottle, she should immediately wash the exposed area with soap and water.
- you should know that travoprost solution contains benzalkonium chloride, which can be absorbed by soft contact lenses. If you wear contact lenses, remove them before applying travoprost and put them back in 15 minutes later.

- if you have an eye injury, infection, or surgery while using travoprost, ask your doctor if you should continue using the same eyedrops container.

What special dietary instructions should I follow?

Unless your doctor tells you otherwise, continue your normal diet.

What should I do if I forget to take a dose?

Apply the missed dose as soon as you remember it. However, if it is almost time for the next dose, skip the missed dose and continue your regular dosing schedule. Do not apply a double dose to make up for a missed one.

What side effects can this medicine cause?

Travoprost may cause side effects. Tell your doctor if any of these symptoms are severe or do not go away:

- eye pain or irritation
- blurred vision
- dry eyes
- eye tearing
- headache

Some side effects can be serious. The following symptoms are uncommon, but if you experience any of them, call your doctor immediately:

- sensitivity to light
- abnormal vision
- pink eye
- redness or swelling of the eyelid

Travoprost may change the color of your eye (to brown) and darken the skin around the eye. It may also cause your eyelashes to grow longer and thicker and darken in color. These changes usually occur slowly, but they may be permanent. If you use travoprost in only one eye, you should know that there may be a difference between your eyes after taking travoprost. Call your doctor if you notice these changes.

Travoprost may cause other side effects. Call your doctor if you have any unusual problems while taking this medication.

If you experience a serious side effect, you or your doctor may send a report to the Food and Drug Administration's (FDA) MedWatch Adverse Event Reporting program online [at http://www.fda.gov/MedWatch/index.html] or by phone [1-800-332-1088].

What storage conditions are needed for this medicine?

Keep this medication in the container it came in, tightly closed, and out of reach of children. Store it at room temperature and away from excess heat and moisture (not in the bathroom). Throw away any medication that is outdated or no longer needed. Talk to your pharmacist about the proper disposal of your medication.

What other information should I know?

Keep all appointments with your doctor.

Do not let anyone else use your medication. Ask your pharmacist any questions you have about refilling your prescription.

Dosage Facts
For Informational Purposes

Caution: Do not change your dose, how often you take your medication, or the length of time you are to take it without first talking to your healthcare provider.

The following dosage information was written using medical language for doctors and other healthcare professionals and is provided here for you to check your dosage. The dosage of this drug may differ for different patients. Therefore, always follow your doctor's instructions or the directions on the label. Contact your healthcare provider or pharmacist if you have any questions about the specific dosage of your medication after reviewing this information.

Adult Patients
Ocular Hypertension and Glaucoma

OPHTHALMIC:
- One drop of a 0.004% solution in the affected eye(s) once daily in the evening.
- More frequent dosing may paradoxically diminish the IOP-lowering effect of the drug.

Trazodone

(traz' oh done)

Important Warning

A small number of children, teenagers, and young adults (up to 24 years of age) who took antidepressants ('mood elevators') such as trazodone during clinical studies became suicidal (thinking about harming or killing oneself or planning or trying to do so). Children, teenagers, and young adults who take antidepressants to treat depression or other mental illnesses may be more likely to become suicidal than children, teenagers, and young adults who do not take antidepressants to treat these conditions. However, experts are not sure about how great this risk is and how much it should be considered in deciding whether a child or teenager should take an antidepressant. Children younger than 18 years of age should not normally take trazodone, but in some cases, a doctor may decide that trazodone is the best medication to treat a child's condition.

You should know that your mental health may change in unexpected ways when you take trazodone or other antidepressants even if you are an adult over age 24. You may become suicidal, especially at the beginning of your treatment and any time that your dose is increased or decreased. You, your family, or your caregiver should call your doctor right away if you experience any of the following symptoms: new or worsening depression; thinking about harming or killing yourself, or planning or trying to do so; extreme worry; agitation; panic attacks; difficulty falling asleep or staying asleep; aggressive behavior; irritability; acting without thinking; severe restlessness; and frenzied abnormal excitement. Be sure that your family or caregiver knows which symptoms may be serious so they can call the doctor when you are unable to seek treatment on your own.

Your healthcare provider will want to see you often while you are taking trazodone, especially at the beginning of your treatment. Be sure to keep all appointments for office visits with your doctor.

The doctor or pharmacist will give you the manufacturer's patient information sheet (Medication Guide) when you begin treatment with trazodone. Read the information carefully and ask your doctor or pharmacist if you have any questions. You also can obtain the Medication Guide from the FDA website: http://www.fda.gov/cder/drug/antidepressants/antidepressants_MG_2007.pdf.

No matter your age, before you take an antidepressant, you, your parent, or your caregiver should talk to your doctor about the risks and benefits of treating your condition with an antidepressant or with other treatments. You should also talk about the risks and benefits of not treating your condition. You should know that having depression or another mental illness greatly increases the risk that you will become suicidal. This risk is higher if you or anyone in your family has or has ever had bipolar disorder (mood that changes from depressed to abnormally excited) or mania (frenzied, abnormally excited mood) or has thought about or attempted suicide. Talk to your doctor about your condition, symptoms, and personal and family medical history. You and your doctor will decide what type of treatment is right for you.

Why is this medicine prescribed?

Trazodone is used to treat depression. Trazodone is in a class of medications called serotonin modulators. It works by increasing the amount of serotonin, a natural substance in the brain that helps maintain mental balance.

How should this medicine be used?

Trazodone comes as a tablet to take by mouth. It is usually taken with a meal or light snack two or more times a day. To help you remember to take trazodone, take it around the same times every day. Follow the directions on your prescription label carefully, and ask your doctor or pharmacist to explain any part you do not understand. Take trazodone exactly as directed. Do not take more or less of it, take it more often, or take it for a longer time than prescribed by your doctor.

Your doctor may start you on a low dose of trazodone and gradually increase your dose, not more than once every 3 to 4 days. Your doctor may decrease your dose once your condition is controlled.

Trazodone controls depression, but does not cure it. It may take 2 weeks or longer before you feel the full benefit of trazodone. Continue to take trazodone even if you feel well. Do not stop taking trazodone without talking to your doctor. Your doctor will probably decrease your dose gradually.

Are there other uses for this medicine?

Trazodone is also sometimes used to treat schizophrenia (a mental illness that causes disturbed or unusual thinking, loss of interest in life, and strong or inappropriate emotions); anxiety (excessive worry); and alcohol abuse. Trazodone is also sometimes used to control abnormal, uncontrollable movements that may be experienced as side effects of other medications. Talk to your doctor about the possible risks of using this medication for your condition.

This medication may be prescribed for other uses. Ask your doctor or pharmacist for more information.

What special precautions should I follow?

Before taking trazodone,
- tell your doctor and pharmacist if you are allergic to trazodone or any other medications.
- tell your doctor and pharmacist what other prescription and nonprescription medications, vitamins, and nutritional supplements you are taking or plan to take. Be sure to mention any of the following: anticoagulants ('blood thinners') such as warfarin (Coumadin); antidepressants, antifungal medications such as fluconazole (Diflucan), itraconazole (Sporanox), and ketoconazole (Nizoral); cimetidine (Tagamet); clarithromycin (Biaxin, Prevpac); cyclosporine (Neoral, Sandimmune); danazol (Danocrine); delaviridine (Rescriptor); dexamethasone (Decadron); digoxin (Digitek, Lanoxin, Lanoxicaps); diltiazem (Cardizem, Dilacor, Tiazac); erythromycin (E.E.S., E-Mycin, Erythrocin); HIV protease inhibitors such as indinavir (Crixivan), nelfinavir (Viracept), ritonavir (Norvir), and saquinavir (Fortovase, Invirase); isoniazid (INH, Nydrazid); medications for allergies, cough or colds; medications for anxiety, high blood pressure, irregular heartbeat, mental illness or pain; medication for seizures such as carbamazepine (Tegretol), ethosuximide (Zarontin), phenobarbital (Lu-

minal, Solfoton), and phenytoin (Dilantin); metronidazole (Flagyl); muscle relaxants; nefazodone; oral contraceptives (birth control pills); rifabutin (Mycobutin); rifampin (Rifadin, Rimactane); sedatives; selective serotonin reuptake inhibitors (SSRIs) such as fluoxetine (Prozac, Sarafem) and fluvoxamine (Luvox); sleeping pills; tranquilizers; troleandomycin (TAO); verapamil (Calan, Isoptin, Verelan); or zafirlukast (Accolate). Also, tell your doctor or pharmacist if you are taking the following medications, called MAO inhibitors, or if you have stopped taking them within the past 2 weeks: isocarboxazid (Marplan), phenelzine (Nardil), selegiline (Eldepryl, Emsam, Zelapar), or tranylcypromine (Parnate). Your doctor may need to change the doses of your medications or monitor you carefully for side effects.
- tell your doctor what herbal products you are taking, especially St. John's wort.
- tell your doctor if you are being treated with electroshock therapy (procedure in which small electric shocks are administered to the brain to treat certain mental illnesses) and if you have or have ever had cancer; a heart attack, irregular heart beat; high blood pressure; human immunodeficiency virus (HIV) or acquired immunodeficiency syndrome (AIDS); low white blood cell count; or heart disease.
- tell your doctor if you are pregnant, plan to become pregnant, or are breast-feeding. If you become pregnant while taking trazodone, call your doctor.
- if you are having surgery, including dental surgery, tell the doctor or dentist that you are taking trazodone.
- you should know that trazodone may make you drowsy and affect your judgment. Do not drive a car or operate machinery until you know how this medication affects you. If drowsiness is a problem, ask your doctor about taking part of your dose at bedtime.
- ask your doctor about the safe use of alcoholic beverages while you are taking trazodone. Alcohol can make the side effects from trazodone worse.
- you should know that trazodone may cause dizziness, lightheadedness, and fainting when you get up too quickly from a lying position. To avoid this problem, get out of bed slowly, resting your feet on the floor for a few minutes before standing up.

What special dietary instructions should I follow?

Talk to your doctor about eating grapefruit and drinking grapefruit juice while taking this medicine.

What should I do if I forget to take a dose?

Take the missed dose as soon as you remember it. However, if it is almost time for the next dose, skip the missed dose and continue your regular dosing schedule. Do not take a double dose to make up for a missed one.

What side effects can this medicine cause?

Trazodone may cause side effects. Tell your doctor if any of these symptoms are severe or do not go away:

- headache or heaviness in head
- nausea
- vomiting
- bad taste in mouth
- stomach pain
- diarrhea
- constipation
- changes in appetite or weight
- weakness or tiredness
- nervousness
- decreased ability to concentrate or remember things
- confusion
- nightmares
- muscle pain
- dry mouth
- sweating
- blurred vision
- tired, red, or itchy eyes
- ringing in ears

Some side effects can be serious. If you experience any of the following symptoms or those listed in the IMPORTANT WARNING section, call your doctor immediately:

- chest pain
- fast, pounding, or irregular heartbeat
- shortness of breath
- fever, sore throat, chills, or other signs of infection
- hives
- skin rash
- itching
- difficulty breathing or swallowing
- swelling of the face, throat, tongue, lips, eyes, hands, feet, ankles, or lower legs
- hoarseness
- decreased coordination
- uncontrollable shaking of a part of the body
- numbness, burning, or tingling in the arms, legs, hands, or feet
- dizziness or lightheadedness
- fainting
- painful erection that lasts longer than normal

Trazodone may cause painful, long lasting erections in males. In some cases emergency and/or surgical treatment has been required and, in some of these cases, permanent damage has occurred. Talk to your doctor about the risk of taking trazodone.

Trazodone may cause other side effects. Call your doctor if you have any unusual problems while taking this medication.

If you experience a serious side effect, you or your doctor may send a report to the Food and Drug Administration's (FDA) MedWatch Adverse Event Reporting program online [at http://www.fda.gov/MedWatch/index.html] or by phone [1-800-332-1088].

What storage conditions are needed for this medicine?

Keep this medication in the container it came in, tightly closed, and out of reach of children. Store it at room temperature and away from excess heat and moisture (not in the bathroom). Throw away any medication that is outdated or no longer needed. Talk to your pharmacist about the proper disposal of your medication.

What should I do in case of overdose?

In case of overdose, call your local poison control center at 1-800-222-1222. If the victim has collapsed or is not breathing, call local emergency services at 911.

Symptoms of overdose may include:

- vomiting
- drowsiness
- changes in heartbeat
- seizures
- difficulty breathing
- painful erection that does not go away

What other information should I know?

Keep all appointments with your doctor.

Do not let anyone else take your medication. Ask your pharmacist any questions you have about refilling your prescription.

Dosage Facts
For Informational Purposes

Caution: Do not change your dose, how often you take your medication, or the length of time you are to take it without first talking to your healthcare provider.

The following dosage information was written using medical language for doctors and other healthcare professionals and is provided here for you to check your dosage. The dosage of this drug may differ for different patients. Therefore, always follow your doctor's instructions or the directions on the label. Contact your healthcare provider or pharmacist if you have any questions about the specific dosage of your medication after reviewing this information.

General Dosage Information

Available as trazodone hydrochloride; dosage is expressed in terms of the salt.

Adult Patients

Major Depressive Disorder

ORAL:
- Initially, 150 mg daily, given in divided doses. Daily dosage may be increased in 50-mg increments every 3 or 4 days based on patient's response and tolerance.

Tretinoin

(tret′ i noyn)

Brand Name: Avita®, Renova® Emollient, Retin-A®, Retin-A® Micro®
Also available generically.

Why is this medicine prescribed?

Tretinoin is used to treat acne. It promotes peeling of affected skin areas and unclogs pores. Tretinoin controls acne but does not cure it.

This medication is sometimes prescribed for other uses; ask your doctor or pharmacist for more information.

How should this medicine be used?

Tretinoin comes in topical liquid, cream, and gel. Tretinoin usually is used daily at bedtime or once every 2 or 3 days. Follow the directions on your prescription label carefully, and ask your doctor or pharmacist to explain any part you do not understand. Use tretinoin exactly as directed. Do not use more or less of it or use it more often than prescribed by your doctor.

Your acne probably will get worse (red, scaling skin and an increase in acne sores) during the first 7-10 days that you use this medication. Nevertheless, continue to use it; the acne sores should disappear. Usually 2-3 weeks (and sometimes more than 6 weeks) of regular use of tretinoin is required before improvement is seen.

Use only nonmedicated cosmetics on cleansed skin. Do not use topical preparations with a lot of alcohol, menthol, spices, or lime (e.g., shaving lotions, astringents, and perfumes); they can sting your skin, especially when you first use tretinoin.

Do not use any other topical medications, especially benzoyl peroxide, salicylic acid (wart remover), and dandruff shampoos containing sulfur or resorcinol unless your doctor directs you to do so. If you have used any of these topical medications recently, ask your doctor if you should wait before using tretinoin.

If you are to apply any form of tretinoin, follow these steps:

1. Wash your hands and affected skin area thoroughly with mild, bland soap (not medicated or abrasive soap or soap that dries the skin) and water. To be sure that your skin is thoroughly dry, wait 20-30 minutes before applying tretinoin.
2. Use clean fingertips, a gauze pad, or a cotton swab to apply the medication.
3. Use enough medication to cover the affected area lightly. Do not oversaturate the gauze pad or cotton swab.

Apply the medication to the affected skin area only (e.g., skin with acne sores).

What special precautions should I follow?

Before using tretinoin,

• tell your doctor and pharmacist if you are allergic to tretinoin or any other drugs.
• tell your doctor and pharmacist what prescription and nonprescription medications you are taking, including vitamins.
• tell your doctor if you are pregnant, plan to become pregnant, or are breast-feeding. If you become pregnant while using tretinoin, call your doctor.
• plan to avoid unnecessary or prolonged exposure to sunlight and to wear protective clothing, sunglasses, and sunscreen. Tretinoin may make your skin sensitive to sunlight.

What should I do if I forget to take a dose?

If you use tretinoin once a day, skip the missed dose completely. Do not use this medication more often than once a day. If you use tretinoin every 2 or 3 days and remember a missed dose within 12 hours of the time when you should have applied it, apply the missed dose immediately. Otherwise, skip the missed dose; do not apply a double dose.

What side effects can this medicine cause?

Tretinoin may cause side effects. Tell your doctor if any of these symptoms are severe or do not go away:
• warmth or slight stinging of the skin
• lightening or darkening of the skin
• red, scaling skin
• increase in acne sores
• swelling, blistering, or crusting of the skin

What storage conditions are needed for this medicine?

Keep this medication in the container it came in, tightly closed, and out of reach of children. Store it at room temperature and away from excess heat and moisture (not in the bathroom). Throw away any medication that is outdated or no longer needed. Talk to your pharmacist about the proper disposal of your medication.

What other information should I know?

Keep all appointments with your doctor. Tretinoin is for external use only. Do not let tretinoin get into your eyes, the corner of your nose, or mouth, or any broken skin, and do not swallow it. Do not apply dressings, bandages, cosmetics, lotions, or other skin medications to the area being treated unless your doctor tells you.

Do not let anyone else use your medication. Ask your pharmacist any questions you have about refilling your prescription.

Tell your doctor if your skin condition gets worse or does not go away.

Dosage Facts
For Informational Purposes

Caution: Do not change your dose, how often you take your medication, or the length of time you are to take it without first talking to your healthcare provider.

The following dosage information was written using medical language for doctors and other healthcare professionals and is provided here for you to check your dosage. The dosage of this drug may differ for different patients. Therefore, always follow your doctor's instructions or the directions on the label. Contact your healthcare provider or pharmacist if you have any questions about the specific dosage of your medication after reviewing this information.

Pediatric Patients

Acne

TOPICAL:
- Adolescents ≥12 years of age: Apply once daily at bedtime.
- Because of potential to cause severe irritation and peeling, therapy can be initiated using a lower concentration cream or gel applied every 2 or 3 days at bedtime; if tolerated, solution or higher concentration cream or gel can be used.
- Initial response (redness, scaling, and possibly more pronounced comedones) occurs within 7–10 days. Therapeutic effects usually are apparent after 2–3 weeks; optimal effects may require >6 weeks of therapy.
- Relapses generally occur within 3–6 weeks after therapy is discontinued.

Adult Patients

Acne

TOPICAL:
- Apply once daily at bedtime.
- Because of potential to cause severe irritation and peeling, therapy can be initiated using a lower concentration cream or gel applied every 2 or 3 days at bedtime; if tolerated, solution or higher concentration cream or gel can be used.
- Initial response (redness, scaling, and possibly more pronounced comedones) occurs within 7–10 days. Therapeutic effects usually are apparent after 2–3 weeks; optimal effects may require >6 weeks of therapy.
- Relapses generally occur within 3–6 weeks after therapy is discontinued.

Photoaging

TOPICAL:
- Apply a pea-sized amount of the 0.02 or 0.05% cream once daily at bedtime.

- Individualize dosage according to patient response and tolerance, depending on skin type, degree of photoaging present, race, and/or age of the patient. Mild scaling can be used as a guide in determining tolerance level.
- If therapy is not well tolerated, may reduce frequency to every other night or every third night.
- Maintenance regimen of 2–4 applications weekly suggested for some patients once maximum response has been achieved.
- Therapeutic response occurs gradually over 6 months; clinically important decreases in fine wrinkles may not be apparent for 8 weeks.
- Therapeutic effects may be lost when therapy and accompanying comprehensive skin care and sun avoidance are discontinued.

Prescribing Limits

Adult Patients

Photoaging

TOPICAL:
- Safety and efficacy of therapy with 0.02% cream for >52 weeks or with 0.05% cream for >48 weeks not established.

Triamcinolone Nasal Inhalation

(trye am sin' oh lone)

Brand Name: Nasacort® AQ Nasal Spray, Nasacort® HFA Nasal Inhaler

Why is this medicine prescribed?

Triamcinolone, a corticosteroid, is used to prevent allergy symptoms including sneezing, itching, and runny or stuffed nose.

This medication is sometimes prescribed for other uses; ask your doctor or pharmacist for more information.

How should this medicine be used?

Triamcinolone comes as a solution to inhale through the nose. It usually is inhaled one to four times a day at evenly spaced intervals. Follow the directions on your prescription label carefully, and ask your doctor or pharmacist to explain any part you do not understand. Use triamcinolone exactly as directed. Do not use more or less of it or use it more often than prescribed by your doctor.

Triamcinolone controls allergy symptoms but does not cure them. Continue to use triamcinolone even if you feel well. Do not stop using triamcinolone without talking to your doctor.

Before you use triamcinolone the first time, read the written instructions that come with it. Ask your doctor, pharmacist, or respiratory therapist to demonstrate the proper technique. Practice using the inhaler while in his or her presence.

Before using triamcinolone, gently blow your nose to clear your nasal passages. Avoid blowing your nose for 15 minutes after inhaling the prescribed dose.

What special precautions should I follow?

Before using triamcinolone,

- tell your doctor and pharmacist if you are allergic to triamcinolone or any other drugs.
- tell your doctor and pharmacist what prescription and nonprescription medications you are taking, especially anticoagulants ('blood thinners') such as warfarin (Coumadin), arthritis medication, aspirin, cyclosporine (Neoral, Sandimmune), digoxin (Lanoxin), diuretics ('water pills'), estrogen (Premarin), ketoconazole (Nizoral), oral contraceptives, phenobarbital, phenytoin (Dilantin), rifampin (Rifadin), theophylline (Theo-Dur), and vitamins.
- if you have a nose infection or a fungal infection (other than on your skin), do not use triamcinolone without talking to your doctor.
- tell your doctor if you have or have ever had tuberculosis (TB); liver, kidney, intestinal, or heart disease; diabetes; an underactive thyroid gland; high blood pressure; mental illness; myasthenia gravis; osteoporosis; herpes eye infection; seizures; or ulcers.
- tell your doctor if you are pregnant, plan to become pregnant, or are breast-feeding. If you become pregnant while using triamcinolone, call your doctor.

What should I do if I forget to take a dose?

Use the missed dose as soon as you remember it. However, if it is almost time for the next dose, skip the missed dose and continue your regular dosing schedule. Do not use a double dose to make up for a missed one.

What side effects can this medicine cause?

Triamcinolone may cause side effects. Tell your doctor if any of these symptoms are severe or do not go away:

- headache
- nasal irritation or dryness
- sore throat
- sneezing
- nosebleed

If you experience any of the following symptoms, call your doctor immediately:

- increased difficulty breathing
- swollen face, lower legs, or ankles
- vision problems
- cold or infection that lasts a long time
- muscle weakness

If you experience a serious side effect, you or your doctor may send a report to the Food and Drug Administration's (FDA) MedWatch Adverse Event Reporting program online [at http://www.fda.gov/MedWatch/index.html] or by phone [1-800-332-1088].

What storage conditions are needed for this medicine?

Keep this medication in the container it came in, tightly closed, and out of reach of children. Store it at room temperature and away from excess heat and moisture (not in the bathroom). Throw away any medication that is outdated or no longer needed. Talk to your pharmacist about the proper disposal of your medication. Avoid puncturing the aerosol container, and do not discard it in an incinerator or fire.

What other information should I know?

Keep all appointments with your doctor. Your symptoms may improve after just a few days. If they do not improve within 3 weeks, call your doctor.

Avoid exposure to chicken pox and measles. This drug makes you more susceptible to these illnesses. If you are exposed to them while using triamcinolone, call your doctor. Do not have a vaccination or other immunization unless your doctor tells you that you may.

Report any injuries or signs of infection (fever, sore throat, pain during urination, and muscle aches) that occur during treatment.

If your sputum (the matter that you cough up during an asthma attack) thickens or changes color from clear white to yellow, green, or gray, call your doctor; these changes may be signs of an infection.

Inhalation devices require regular cleaning, and some require periodic replacement. Follow the directions that come with your inhaler.

Do not let anyone else use your medication. Ask your pharmacist any questions you have about refilling your prescription.

Dosage Facts
For Informational Purposes

Caution: Do not change your dose, how often you take your medication, or the length of time you are to take it without first talking to your healthcare provider.

The following dosage information was written using medical language for doctors and other healthcare professionals and is provided here for you to check your dosage. The dosage of this drug may differ for different patients. Therefore, always follow your doctor's instructions or the directions on the label. Contact your healthcare provider or pharmacist if you have any questions about the specific dosage of your medication after reviewing this information.

General Dosage Information

After priming, nasal spray pump delivers about 55 mcg of triamcinolone acetonide per metered spray and about 30 or 120 metered doses per 6.5-g or 16.5-g container, respectively.

Once optimal symptomatic relief is achieved, reduce dosage gradually to the lowest effective level.

Intranasal triamcinolone acetonide should not be continued beyond 3 weeks in the absence of adequate symptomatic improvement.

Pediatric Patients

Seasonal Allergic Rhinitis

INTRANASAL INHALATION:
- Children 6–11 years of age: Initially 55 mcg (1 spray) in each nostril once daily (110 mcg total). May be increased to 110 mcg (2 sprays) in each nostril once daily (220 mcg total).
- Children ≥12 years of age: 110 mcg (2 sprays) in each nostril once daily (220 mcg total).

Perennial Allergic Rhinitis

INTRANASAL INHALATION:
- Children 6–12 years of age: Initially 55 mcg (1 spray) in each nostril once daily (110 mcg total). Maximum, 110 mcg (2 sprays) in each nostril once daily (220 mcg total).
- Children ≥12 years of age: Initially 110 mcg (2 sprays) in each nostril once daily (220 mcg total).

Adult Patients

Seasonal Allergic Rhinitis

INTRANASAL INHALATION:
- 110 mcg (2 sprays) in each nostril once daily (220 mcg total).

Perennial Allergic Rhinitis

INTRANASAL INHALATION:
- 110 mcg (2 sprays) in each nostril once daily (220 mcg total).

Prescribing Limits

Pediatric Patients

Seasonal or Perennial Allergic Rhinitis

INTRANASAL INHALATION:
- Children 6–12 years of age: Maximum 220 mcg (2 sprays in each nostril) daily.

Adult Patients

Seasonal or Perennial Allergic Rhinitis

INTRANASAL INHALATION:
- Maximum 220 mcg (2 sprays in each nostril) daily.

Perennial Allergic Rhinitis

INTRANASAL INHALATION:
- Maximum 220 mcg (2 sprays in each nostril) daily.

Special Populations

Hepatic Impairment
- No specific dosage recommendations at this time.

Renal Impairment
- No specific dosage recommendations at this time.

Geriatric Patients
- No specific dosage recommendations at this time.

Triamcinolone Oral

(trye am sin′ oh lone)

Brand Name: Aristocort®

Why is this medicine prescribed?

Triamcinolone, a corticosteroid, is similar to a natural hormone produced by your adrenal glands. It often is used to replace this chemical when your body does not make enough of it. It relieves inflammation (swelling, heat, redness, and pain) and is used to treat certain forms of arthritis; skin, blood, kidney, eye, thyroid, and intestinal disorders (e.g., colitis); severe allergies; and asthma. Triamcinolone is also used to treat certain types of cancer.

This medication is sometimes prescribed for other uses; ask your doctor or pharmacist for more information.

How should this medicine be used?

Triamcinolone comes as a tablet and syrup to be taken by mouth. Your doctor will prescribe a dosing schedule that is best for you. Follow the directions on your prescription label carefully, and ask your doctor or pharmacist to explain any part you do not understand.

Do not stop taking triamcinolone without talking to your doctor. Stopping the drug abruptly can cause loss of appetite, upset stomach, vomiting, drowsiness, confusion, headache, fever, joint and muscle pain, peeling skin, and weight loss. If you take large doses for a long time, your doctor probably will decrease your dose gradually to allow your body to adjust before stopping the drug completely. Watch for these side effects if you are gradually decreasing your dose and after you stop taking the tablets or oral liquid, even if you switch to an inhalation. If these problems occur, call your doctor immediately. You may need to increase your dose of tablets or liquid temporarily or start taking them again.

Take triamcinolone exactly as directed. Do not take more or less of it or take it more often than prescribed by your doctor.

What special precautions should I follow?

Before taking triamcinolone,
- tell your doctor and pharmacist if you are allergic to triamcinolone, aspirin, tartrazine (a yellow dye in some processed foods and drugs), or any other drugs.
- tell your doctor and pharmacist what prescription and nonprescription medications you are taking, especially anticoagulants ('blood thinners') such as warfarin (Coumadin), arthritis medications, aspirin, cyclosporine (Neoral, Sandimmune), digoxin (Lanoxin), diuretics ('water pills'), estrogen (Premarin), ketoconazole (Nizoral), oral contraceptives, phenobarbital, phenytoin (Dilantin), rifampin (Rifadin), theophylline (Theo-Dur), and vitamins.
- if you have a fungal infection (other than on your skin), do not take triamcinolone without talking to your doctor.

- tell your doctor if you have or have ever had liver, kidney, intestinal, or heart disease; diabetes; an underactive thyroid gland; high blood pressure; mental illness; myasthenia gravis; osteoporosis; herpes eye infection; seizures; tuberculosis (TB); or ulcers.
- tell your doctor if you are pregnant, plan to become pregnant, or are breast-feeding. If you become pregnant while taking triamcinolone, call your doctor.
- if you are having surgery, including dental surgery, tell the doctor or dentist that you are taking triamcinolone.
- if you have a history of ulcers or take large doses of aspirin or other arthritis medication, limit your consumption of alcoholic beverages while taking this drug. Triamcinolone makes your stomach and intestines more susceptible to the irritating effects of alcohol, aspirin, and certain arthritis medications. This effect increases your risk of ulcers.

What special dietary instructions should I follow?

Your doctor may instruct you to follow a low-sodium, low-salt, potassium-rich, or high-protein diet. Follow these directions.

Triamcinolone may cause an upset stomach. Take triamcinolone with food or milk.

What should I do if I forget to take a dose?

When you start to take triamcinolone, ask your doctor what to do if you forget a dose. Write down these instructions so that you can refer to them later.

If you take triamcinolone once a day, take the missed dose as soon as you remember it. However, if it is almost time for the next dose, skip the missed dose and continue your regular dosing schedule. Do not take a double dose to make up for a missed one.

What side effects can this medicine cause?

Triamcinolone may cause side effects. Tell your doctor if any of these symptoms are severe or do not go away:
- upset stomach
- stomach irritation
- vomiting
- headache
- dizziness
- insomnia
- restlessness
- depression
- anxiety
- acne
- increased hair growth
- easy bruising
- irregular or absent menstrual periods

If you experience any of the following symptoms, call your doctor immediately:
- skin rash
- swollen face, lower legs, or ankles
- vision problems

- cold or infection that lasts a long time
- muscle weakness
- black or tarry stool

If you experience a serious side effect, you or your doctor may send a report to the Food and Drug Administration's (FDA) MedWatch Adverse Event Reporting program online [at http://www.fda.gov/MedWatch/index.html] or by phone [1-800-332-1088].

What storage conditions are needed for this medicine?

Keep this medication in the container it came in, tightly closed, and out of reach of children. Store it at room temperature and away from excess heat and moisture (not in the bathroom). Throw away any medication that is outdated or no longer needed. Talk to your pharmacist about the proper disposal of your medication.

What should I do in case of overdose?

In case of overdose, call your local poison control center at 1-800-222-1222. If the victim has collapsed or is not breathing, call local emergency services at 911.

What other information should I know?

Keep all appointments with your doctor and the laboratory. Your doctor will order certain lab tests to check your response to triamcinolone. Checkups are especially important for children because triamcinolone can slow bone growth.

Carry an identification card that indicates that you may need to take supplementary doses (write down the full dose you took before gradually decreasing it) of triamcinolone during periods of stress (injuries, infections, and severe asthma attacks). Ask your pharmacist or doctor how to obtain this card. List your name, medical problems, drugs and dosages, and doctor's name and telephone number on the card.

This drug makes you more susceptible to illnesses. If you are exposed to chicken pox, measles, or tuberculosis (TB) while taking triamcinolone, call your doctor. Do not have a vaccination, other immunization, or any skin test while you are taking triamcinolone unless your doctor tells you that you may.

Report any injuries or signs of infection (fever, sore throat, pain during urination, and muscle aches) that occur during treatment.

Your doctor may instruct you to weigh yourself every day. Report any unusual weight gain.

If your sputum (the matter you cough up during an asthma attack) thickens or changes color from clear white to yellow, green, or gray, call your doctor; these changes may be signs of an infection.

If you have diabetes, triamcinolone may increase your blood sugar level. If you monitor your blood sugar (glucose) at home, test your blood or urine more frequently than usual. Call your doctor if your blood sugar is high or if sugar is present in your urine; your dose of diabetes medication and your diet may need to be changed.

Do not let anyone else take your medication. Ask your pharmacist any questions you have about refilling your prescription.

Dosage Facts
For Informational Purposes

Caution: Do not change your dose, how often you take your medication, or the length of time you are to take it without first talking to your healthcare provider.

The following dosage information was written using medical language for doctors and other healthcare professionals and is provided here for you to check your dosage. The dosage of this drug may differ for different patients. Therefore, always follow your doctor's instructions or the directions on the label. Contact your healthcare provider or pharmacist if you have any questions about the specific dosage of your medication after reviewing this information.

General Dosage Information

Available as triamcinolone, triamcinolone acetonide, and triamcinolone hexacetonide. Dosage of triamcinolone acetonide or hexacetonide is expressed in terms of the respective salt.

After a satisfactory response is obtained, decrease dosage in small decrements to the lowest level that maintains an adequate clinical response, and discontinue the drug as soon as possible.

Monitor patients continually for signs that indicate dosage adjustment is necessary, such as remissions or exacerbations of the disease and stress (surgery, infection, trauma).

High dosages may be required for acute situations of certain rheumatic disorders and collagen diseases; after a response has been obtained, drug often must be continued for long periods at low dosage.

High or massive dosages may be required in the treatment of pemphigus, exfoliative dermatitis, bullous dermatitis herpetiformis, severe erythema multiforme, or mycosis fungoides. Early initiation of systemic glucocorticoid therapy may be life-saving in pemphigus vulgaris. Reduce dosage gradually to the lowest effective level, but discontinuance may not be possible.

Pediatric Patients

Base pediatric dosage on severity of the disease and patient response rather than on strict adherence to dosage indicated by age, body weight, or body surface area.

Usual Dosage

ORAL:
- Some clinicians recommend 0.117–1.66 mg/kg daily or 3.3–50 mg/m² daily, administered in 4 divided doses.

Neoplastic Diseases

ORAL:
- In children with acute leukemia, usually 1 mg/kg daily, but up to 2 mg/kg may be necessary. Initial response usually observed within 6–21 days and therapy continued for 4–6 weeks.

Adult Patients

Usual Dosage

ORAL:
- Initially, 4–48 mg daily, usually administered in 1–4 doses, depending on disease being treated.

Asthma

ORAL:
- For severe or incapacitating asthma, 8–16 mg daily.

Adrenocortical Insufficiency

ORAL:
- Usually, 4–12 mg daily in addition to mineralocorticoid therapy.

Rheumatic Disorders and Collagen Diseases

ORAL:
- In patients with rheumatoid arthritis, acute gouty arthritis, ankylosing spondylitis, select cases of psoriatic arthritis, acute and subacute bursitis, or acute nonspecific tenosynovitis, initially, 8–16 mg once daily (morning) or on alternate days. Occasionally, more effective relief achieved with administration 2–4 times daily.
- In patients with systemic lupus erythematosus, initially, 20–32 mg daily until desired response is achieved, then reduce to maintenance dosage. In patients with more severe symptoms, ≥48 mg daily initially and higher maintenance dosages may be required.
- In patients with acute rheumatic carditis, initially, 20–60 mg daily until desired clinical response achieved. Reduce dosage and continue maintenance therapy for ≥6–8 weeks (seldom required for >3 months).

Dermatologic Diseases

ORAL:
- In patients with pemphigus, bullous dermatitis herpetiformis, severe erythema multiforme, exfoliative dermatitis, or mycosis fungoides, initially, 8–16 mg daily. Alternatitvely, alternative-day therapy is well tolerated and may be assiocated with fewer adverse effects.
- In patients with severe psoriasis, 8–16 mg daily. Maintenance period depends on clinical response.

Allergic Conditions

ORAL:
- In patients with acute seasonal or perennial allergic rhinitis, 8–12 mg daily to alleviate acute distress; intractable cases may require high initial and maintenance dosages.
- In patients with contact dermatitis or atopic dermatitis, short-courses of 8–16 mg daily to supplement topical therapy.

Ocular Disorders

ORAL:
- In patients with allergic conjunctivitis, keratitis, iridocyclitis, chorioretinitis, anterior segment inflammation, diffuse posterior uveitis and choroiditis, optic neuritis, or sympathetic ophthalmia, initially, 12–40 mg daily for short duration, depending on severity of condition.

Hematologic Disorders

ORAL:
- 16–60 mg daily, with dosage reduction after adequate clinical response.

Neoplastic Diseases

ORAL:

- In patients with acute leukemia and lymphoma, usually, 16–40 mg daily; dosages as high as 100 mg daily may be necessary for treatment of leukemia.

Nephrotic Syndrome and Lupus Nephritis

ORAL:

- Average 16–20 mg (up to 48 mg) daily, until diuresis occurs. After diuresis begins, continue treatment until maximal or complete remission occurs, then reduce dosage gradually and discontinue. In less severe disease, maintenance dosage as low as 4 mg may be adequate.

Tuberculous Meningitis

ORAL:

- Average 32–48 mg daily in single or divided doses.

Triamcinolone Oral Inhalation

(trye am sin′ oh lone)

Brand Name: Azmacort® Oral Inhaler

Important Warning

If you are switching (or have recently switched) from oral triamcinolone (or another oral corticosteroid such as betamethasone, dexamethasone, methylprednisolone, prednisolone, or prednisone) to triamcinolone inhalation and have an injury, infection, or severe asthma attack, take a full dose (even if you have been gradually decreasing your dose) of oral triamcinolone (or the other oral corticosteroid) and call your doctor for additional instructions.

Carry an identification card that indicates that you may need to take supplementary doses (write down the full dose you took before gradually decreasing it) of the corticosteroid during periods of stress (injuries, infections, and severe asthma attacks). Ask your pharmacist or doctor how to obtain this card. List your name, medical problems, drugs and dosages, and doctor's name and telephone number on the card.

Why is this medicine prescribed?

Triamcinolone, a corticosteroid, is used to prevent wheezing, shortness of breath, and troubled breathing caused by severe asthma and other lung diseases.

This medication is sometimes prescribed for other uses; ask your doctor or pharmacist for more information.

How should this medicine be used?

Triamcinolone comes as an aerosol to use by oral inhalation. It usually is inhaled three or four times a day at evenly spaced intervals. Follow the directions on your prescription label carefully, and ask your doctor or pharmacist to explain any part you do not understand. Use triamcinolone exactly as directed. Do not use more or less of it or use it more often than prescribed by your doctor.

Triamcinolone controls symptoms of asthma and other lung diseases but does not cure them. Continue to use triamcinolone even if you feel well. Do not stop using triamcinolone without talking to your doctor.

Before you use the triamcinolone inhaler the first time, read the written instructions that come with it. Ask your doctor, pharmacist, or respiratory therapist to demonstrate the proper technique. Practice using the inhaler while in his or her presence.

To use the inhaler, follow these steps:

1. Shake the inhaler well.
2. Remove the protective cap.
3. Exhale (breathe out) as completely as possible through your nose while keeping your mouth shut.
4. *Open Mouth Technique:* Open your mouth wide, and place the open end of the mouthpiece about 1-2 inches from your mouth.
   Closed Mouth Technique: Place the open end of the mouthpiece well into your mouth, past your front teeth. Close your lips tightly around themouthpiece.
5. Take a slow, deep breath through the mouthpiece and, at the same time, press down on the container to spray the medication into your mouth. Be sure that the mist goes into your throat and is not blocked by your teeth or tongue. Adults giving the treatment to young children may hold the child's nose closed to be sure that the medication goes into the child's throat.
6. Hold your breath for 5-10 seconds, remove the inhaler, and exhale slowly through your nose or mouth. If you take 2 puffs, wait 2 minutes and shake the inhaler well before taking the second puff.
7. Replace the protective cap on the inhaler.

After each treatment, rinse your mouth with water or mouthwash.

If you have difficulty getting the medication into your lungs, a spacer (a special device that attaches to the inhaler) may help; ask your doctor, pharmacist, or respiratory therapist.

What special precautions should I follow?

Before using triamcinolone,

- tell your doctor and pharmacist if you are allergic to triamcinolone or any other drugs.
- tell your doctor and pharmacist what prescription and nonprescription medications you are taking, especially arthritis medications, aspirin, digoxin (Lanoxin), diuretics ('water pills'), estrogen (Premarin), ketoconazole (Nizoral), oral contraceptives, phenobarbital, phenytoin (Dilantin), rifampin (Rifadin), theophylline (Theo-Dur), and vitamins.

- if you have a fungal infection (other than on your skin), do not take triamcinolone without talking to your doctor.
- tell your doctor if you have or have ever had liver, kidney, intestinal, or heart disease; diabetes; an underactive thyroid gland; high blood pressure; mental illness; myasthenia gravis; osteoporosis; herpes eye infection; seizures; or ulcers.
- tell your doctor if you are pregnant, plan to become pregnant, or are breast-feeding. If you become pregnant while using triamcinolone, call your doctor.
- if you have a history of ulcers or take large doses of aspirin or other arthritis medication, limit your consumption of alcoholic beverages while taking this drug. Triamcinolone makes your stomach and intestines more susceptible to the irritating effects of alcohol, aspirin, and certain arthritis medications. This effect increases your risk of ulcers.

What special dietary instructions should I follow?

Your doctor may instruct you to follow a low-sodium, low-salt, potassium-rich, or high-protein diet. Follow these directions.

What should I do if I forget to take a dose?

Use the missed dose as soon as you remember it. However, if it is almost time for the next dose, skip the missed dose and continue your regular dosing schedule. Do not use a double dose to make up for a missed one.

What side effects can this medicine cause?

Triamcinolone may cause side effects. Tell your doctor if any of these symptoms are severe or do not go away:
- dry or irritated throat and mouth
- cough
- difficult or painful speech

If you experience any of the following symptoms, call your doctor immediately:
- skin rash
- increased difficulty breathing
- white spots or sores in your mouth
- swollen face, lower legs, or ankles
- vision problems
- cold or infection that lasts a long time
- muscle weakness

If you experience a serious side effect, you or your doctor may send a report to the Food and Drug Administration's (FDA) MedWatch Adverse Event Reporting program online [at http://www.fda.gov/MedWatch/index.html] or by phone [1-800-332-1088].

What storage conditions are needed for this medicine?

Keep this medication in the container it came in, tightly closed, and out of reach of children. Store it at room temperature and away from excess heat and moisture (not in the bathroom). Throw away any medication that is outdated or no longer needed. Talk to your pharmacist about the proper disposal of your medication. Avoid puncturing the aerosol container, and do not discard it in an incinerator or fire.

What other information should I know?

Keep all appointments with your doctor and the laboratory. Your doctor will order certain lab tests to check your response to triamcinolone.

Triamcinolone is not used for rapid relief of breathing problems. If you do not have another inhaler for prompt relief of breathing difficulty, ask your doctor to prescribe one.

If your doctor has prescribed a bronchodilator (a drug to be inhaled for rapid relief of difficult breathing), use it several minutes before you use your triamcinolone inhaler so that triamcinolone can reach deep into your lungs.

Avoid exposure to chicken pox and measles. This drug can make you more susceptible to these illnesses. If you are exposed to them while using triamcinolone, call your doctor. Do not have a vaccination or other immunization unless your doctor tells you that you may.

Report any injuries or signs of infection (fever, sore throat, pain during urination, and muscle aches) that occur during treatment.

If your sputum (the matter you cough up during an asthma attack) thickens or changes color from clear white to yellow, green, or gray, call your doctor; these changes may be signs of an infection.

Inhalation devices require regular cleaning. Once a week, remove the drug container from the plastic mouthpiece, wash the mouthpiece with warm tap water, and dry it thoroughly.

Do not let anyone else use your medication. Ask your pharmacist any questions you have about refilling your prescription.

Dosage Facts
For Informational Purposes

Caution: Do not change your dose, how often you take your medication, or the length of time you are to take it without first talking to your healthcare provider.

The following dosage information was written using medical language for doctors and other healthcare professionals and is provided here for you to check your dosage. The dosage of this drug may differ for different patients. Therefore, always follow your doctor's instructions or the directions on the label. Contact your healthcare provider or pharmacist if you have any questions about the specific dosage of your medication after reviewing this information.

General Dosage Information

Available as triamcinolone acetonide. Dosage of triamcinolone acetonide is expressed in terms of the respective salt.

Triamcinolone acetonide oral aerosol inhaler delivers

about 100 mcg of drug per metered spray. Commercially available aerosol delivers at least 240 metered sprays; do not use after 240 actuations.

Pediatric Patients

Asthma

ORAL INHALATION:

- Triamcinolone acetonide in children <6 years of age: manufacturer does not recommended use in this age group.
- Triamcinolone acetonide in children 6–12 years of age: Initially, 100 or 200 mcg (1 or 2 sprays) 3 or 4 times daily (300–800 mcg total) or 200–400 mcg (2–4 sprays) twice daily (400–800 mcg total); adjust dosage according to patient response. Maximum dosage recommended by manufacturer is 1200 mcg (12 sprays) daily; some experts state that higher dosages may be used in children with severe persistent asthma.
- Continually monitor patients for signs that indicate dosage adjustment is necessary (e.g., remissions or exacerbations of disease and stress [surgery, infection, trauma]).

Adult Patients

Asthma

ORAL INHALATION:

- Triamcinolone acetonide: Initially, 200 mcg (2 sprays) 3 or 4 times daily (600 or 800 mcg total) or 400 mcg (4 sprays) twice daily. In adults with severe asthma, it may be advisable to start with 12–16 sprays daily (1200–1600 mcg total), and then reduce dosage to the lowest effective level. Maximum 1600 mcg (16 sprays) daily recommended by manufacturer, but some experts state that higher dosages may be used.

Prescribing Limits

Pediatric Patients

Asthma

ORAL INHALATION:

- Triamcinolone acetonide in children 6–12 years of age: Manufacturer recommends that dosage not exceed 1200 mcg (12 sprays) daily.

Adult Patients

Asthma

ORAL INHALATION:

- Triamcinolone acetonide: Manufacturer recommends that dosage not exceed 1600 mcg (16 sprays) daily.

Special Populations

Geriatric Patients

- Generally, initiate oral inhalation therapy at low end of dosage range, reflecting greater frequency of decreased hepatic, renal, or cardiac function, and of concomitant disease or other drug therapy.

Triamcinolone Topical

(trye am sin' oh lone)

Brand Name: Aristocort®, Aristocort® A, Flutex®, Kenalog®, Kenalog® in Orabase®, Kenalog® Spray, Myco® II as a combination product containing Triamcinolone Acetonide and Nystatin, Mycogen® II as a combination product containing Triamcinolone Acetonide and Nystatin, Mycolog® II as a combination product containing Triamcinolone Acetonide and Nystatin, Mycolog®-II as a combination product containing Triamcinolone Acetonide and Nystatin, Myco-Triacet® II as a combination product containing Triamcinolone Acetonide and Nystatin, Mytrex® as a combination product containing Triamcinolone Acetonide and Nystatin, N.T.A.® Cream as a combination product containing Triamcinolone Acetonide and Nystatin, N.T.A.® Ointment as a combination product containing Triamcinolone Acetonide and Nystatin, NGT® as a combination product containing Triamcinolone Acetonide and Nystatin, Triacet®, Tri-Statin® II as a combination product containing Triamcinolone Acetonide and Nystatin

Also available generically.

Why is this medicine prescribed?

Triamcinolone is used to treat the itching, redness, dryness, crusting, scaling, inflammation, and discomfort of various skin conditions. It is also used to relieve the discomfort of mouth sores.

This medication is sometimes prescribed for other uses; ask your doctor or pharmacist for more information.

How should this medicine be used?

Triamcinolone comes in ointment, cream, lotion, liquid, and aerosol (spray) in various strengths for use on the skin and as a paste for use in the mouth. It usually is applied two to four times a day. For mouth sores, it is applied at bedtime and, if necessary, two or three times daily, preferably after meals. Follow the directions on your prescription label carefully, and ask your doctor or pharmacist to explain any part you do not understand. Use triamcinolone exactly as directed. Do not use more or less of it or use it more often than prescribed by your doctor. Do not apply it to other areas of your body or wrap or bandage the treated area unless directed to do so by your doctor.

Wash or soak the affected area thoroughly before applying the medicine, unless it irritates your skin. Apply the ointment, cream, liquid, or lotion sparingly in a thin film and rub it in gently.

To use the lotion or liquid on your scalp, part your hair, apply a small amount of the medicine on the affected area, and rub it in gently. Protect the area from washing and rubbing until the lotion or liquid dries. You may wash your hair as usual but not right after applying the medicine.

To apply an aerosol, shake well and spray on the affected area holding the container about 3 to 6 inches away. Spray for about 2 seconds to cover an area the size of your hand. Take care not to inhale the vapors. If you are spraying near your face, cover your eyes.

To apply the paste, press a small amount on the mouth sore without rubbing until a thin film develops. You may need to use more paste if the mouth sore is large. If the mouth sore does not begin to heal within 7 days, call your doctor.

Avoid prolonged use on the face, in the genital or rectal areas, and in skin creases and armpits unless directed to do so by your doctor.

If you are using triamcinolone on your face, keep it out of your eyes.

Do not apply cosmetics or other skin preparations on the treated area without talking with your doctor.

If you are using triamcinolone on a child's diaper area, do not use tight-fitting diapers or plastic pants. Such use may increase side effects.

If your doctor tells you to wrap or bandage the treated area, follow these instructions:
1. Soak the area in water or wash it well.
2. While the skin is moist, gently rub the medication into the affected areas.
3. Cover the area with plastic wrap (such as Saran Wrap or Handi-Wrap). The plastic may be held in place with a gauze or elastic bandage or adhesive tape on the normal skin beside the treated area. (Instead of using plastic wrap, plastic gloves may be used for the hands, plastic bags for the feet, or a shower cap for the scalp.)
4. Carefully seal the edges of the plastic to make sure the wrap adheres closely to the skin. If the affected area is moist, you can leave the edges of the plastic wrap partly unsealed or puncture the wrap to allow excess moisture to escape.
5. Leave the plastic wrap in place as long as directed by your doctor. Usually plastic wraps are left in place no more than 12 hours each day.
6. Cleanse the skin and reapply the medication each time a new plastic wrapping is applied. Do not discontinue treatment abruptly without talking to your doctor.

What special precautions should I follow?

Before using triamcinolone,
- tell your doctor and pharmacist if you are allergic to triamcinolone or any other drugs.
- tell your doctor and pharmacist what prescription and nonprescription medications you are taking, especially cancer chemotherapy agents, other topical medications, and vitamins.
- tell your doctor if you have an infection or if you have ever had diabetes, glaucoma, cataracts, a circulation disorder, or an immune disorder.
- tell your doctor if you are pregnant, plan to become pregnant, or are breast-feeding. If you become pregnant while using triamcinolone, call your doctor immediately.

What should I do if I forget to take a dose?

Apply the missed dose as soon as you remember it. However, if it is almost time for the next dose, skip the missed dose and continue your regular dosing schedule. Do not apply a double dose to make up for a missed one.

What side effects can this medicine cause?

Side effects from triamcinolone can occur. Tell your doctor if any of these symptoms are severe or do not go away:
- drying or cracking of the skin
- acne
- itching
- burning
- change in skin color

If you experience any of the following symptoms, call your doctor immediately:
- severe skin rash
- difficulty breathing or swallowing
- wheezing
- skin infection (redness, swelling, or oozing of pus)

If you experience a serious side effect, you or your doctor may send a report to the Food and Drug Administration's (FDA) MedWatch Adverse Event Reporting program online [at http://www.fda.gov/MedWatch/index.html] or by phone [1-800-332-1088].

What storage conditions are needed for this medicine?

Keep this medication in the container it came in, tightly closed, and out of reach of children. Store it according to the package instructions. Throw away any medication that is outdated or no longer needed. Do not use it to treat other skin conditions. Talk to your pharmacist about the proper disposal of your medications.

What other information should I know?

Keep all appointments with your doctor.

Do not let anyone else use your medication. Ask your pharmacist any questions you have about refilling your prescription.

Dosage Facts
For Informational Purposes

Caution: Do not change your dose, how often you take your medication, or the length of time you are to take it without first talking to your healthcare provider.

The following dosage information was written using medical language for doctors and other healthcare professionals and is provided here for you to check your

dosage. The dosage of this drug may differ for different patients. Therefore, always follow your doctor's instructions or the directions on the label. Contact your healthcare provider or pharmacist if you have any questions about the specific dosage of your medication after reviewing this information.

General Dosage Information

Available as triamcinolone acetonide; dosage expressed in terms of the salt.

Pediatric Patients

Administer the least amount of topical preparations that provides effective therapy.

Corticosteroid-responsive Dermatoses

TOPICAL:
- Apply appropriate preparations of triamcinolone acetonide sparingly 2–4 times daily.
- Apply 0.1 and 0.5% creams 2–3 times daily according to severity of the condition.
- Apply aerosol 3–4 times daily.

Adult Patients

Corticosteroid-responsive Dermatoses

TOPICAL:
- Apply appropriate preparations of triamcinolone acetonide sparingly 2–4 times daily.
- Apply 0.1 and 0.5% creams 2–3 times daily according to severity of the condition.
- Apply aerosol 3–4 times daily.
- Apply paste at bedtime and, if necessary, 2 or 3 times daily, preferably after meals. If substantial regeneration or repair of oral tissues does not occur after 7 days, further investigate the etiology of the lesions.

Triamterene

(trye am′ ter een)

Brand Name: Dyrenium®
Also available generically.

Why is this medicine prescribed?

Triamterene is used alone or with other medications to treat edema (fluid retention; excess fluid held in body tissues) caused by various conditions, including liver and heart disease. Triamterene is in a class of medications called diuretics ('water pills'). It causes the kidneys to eliminate unneeded water and sodium from the body into the urine, but reduces the loss of potassium.

How should this medicine be used?

Triamterene comes as a capsule to take by mouth. It usually is taken once a day in the morning after breakfast or twice a day after breakfast and lunch. It is best to take triamterene earlier in the day so that frequent trips to the bathroom do not interfere with nighttime sleep. Take triamterene at around the same time(s) every day. Follow the directions on your prescription label carefully, and ask your doctor or pharmacist to explain any part you do not understand. Take triamterene exactly as directed. Do not take more or less of it or take it more often than prescribed by your doctor.

Are there other uses for this medicine?

Triamterene is used in combination with other diuretics to treat high blood pressure.

This medicine may be prescribed for other uses; ask your doctor or pharmacist for more information.

What special precautions should I follow?

Before taking triamterene,
- tell your doctor and pharmacist if you are allergic to triamterene or any other medications (Dyazide, Maxzide).
- do not take triamterene if you are taking amiloride (Midamor), spironolactone (Aldactone), or other medications containing triamterene.
- tell your doctor and pharmacist what prescription and nonprescription medications, vitamins, nutritional supplements, and herbal products you are taking or plan to take. Be sure to mention angiotensin-converting enzyme (ACE) inhibitors such as benazepril (Lotensin), captopril (Capoten), enalapril (Vasotec), fosinopril (Monopril), lisinopril (Prinivil, Zestril), moexipril (Univasc), perindopril, (Aceon), quinapril (Accupril), ramipril (Altace), and trandolapril (Mavik); lithium (Eskalith, Lithobid); non-steroidal anti-inflammatory medications (NSAIDS) such as ibuprofen (Advil, Motrin) and naproxen (Aleve, Naprosyn); medications for diabetes, or high blood pressure; other diuretics; and potassium supplements. Your doctor may need to change the doses of your medications or monitor you carefully for side effects.
- tell your doctor if you have or have ever had diabetes, gout, kidney stones, or heart, kidney, or liver disease.
- tell your doctor if you are pregnant or plan to become pregnant. If you become pregnant while taking triamterene, call your doctor. Do not breastfeed if you are taking triamterene.
- if you are having surgery, including dental surgery, tell the doctor or dentist that you are taking triamterene.
- plan to avoid unnecessary or prolonged exposure to sunlight and to wear protective clothing, sunglasses, and sunscreen. Triamterene may make your skin sensitive to sunlight.

What special dietary instructions should I follow?

Follow your doctor's directions for your meals, including advice for a reduced salt (sodium) diet and daily exercise program. Avoid potassium-containing salt substitutes while you are taking this medication. Talk with your doctor about the amount of potassium-rich foods (e.g., bananas, prunes, raisins, and orange juice) that you may have in your diet.

What should I do if I forget to take a dose?

Take the missed dose as soon as you remember it. However, if it is almost time for your next dose, skip the missed dose and continue your regular dosing schedule. Do not take a double dose to make up for a missed one.

What side effects can this medicine cause?

Triamterene may cause side effects. Tell your doctor if any of these symptoms are severe or do not go away:

- vomiting
- dizziness
- headache

Some side effects can be serious. If you experience any of the following symptoms, call your doctor immediately:

- muscle weakness or cramps
- slow or irregular heartbeat
- diarrhea
- rash
- difficulty breathing or swallowing
- upset stomach
- extreme tiredness
- unusual bleeding or bruising
- lack of energy
- loss of appetite
- pain in the upper right part of the stomach
- yellowing of the skin or eyes
- flu-like symptoms
- sore throat
- severe dry mouth
- unusual bruising or bleeding

If you experience a serious side effect, you or your doctor may send a report to the Food and Drug Administration's (FDA) MedWatch Adverse Event Reporting program online [at http://www.fda.gov/MedWatch/index.html] or by phone [1-800-332-1088].

What storage conditions are needed for this medicine?

Keep this medicine in the container it came in, tightly closed, and out of reach of children. Store it at room temperature and away from excess heat and moisture (not in the bathroom). Throw away any medicine that is outdated or no longer needed. Talk to your pharmacist about the proper disposal of your medicine.

What should I do in case of overdose?

In case of overdose, call your local poison control center at 1-800-222-1222. If the victim has collapsed or is not breathing, call local emergency services at 911.

Symptoms of overdose may include:

- upset stomach
- vomiting
- weakness or tiredness
- dizziness

What other information should I know?

Keep all appointments with your doctor and the laboratory. Your doctor will order certain lab tests to check your body's response to triamterene.

Do not let anyone else take your medicine. Ask your pharmacist any questions you have about refilling your prescription.

Dosage Facts
For Informational Purposes

Caution: Do not change your dose, how often you take your medication, or the length of time you are to take it without first talking to your healthcare provider.

The following dosage information was written using medical language for doctors and other healthcare professionals and is provided here for you to check your dosage. The dosage of this drug may differ for different patients. Therefore, always follow your doctor's instructions or the directions on the label. Contact your healthcare provider or pharmacist if you have any questions about the specific dosage of your medication after reviewing this information.

General Dosage Information

Individualize dosage according to patient's requirements and response.

If added to an existing antihypertensive regimen, initially reduce dosage of each antihypertensive agent and then individualize dosage according to patient's requirements and response.

Abrupt discontinuance may result in rebound kaliuresis; taper dosage gradually.

Different commercially available fixed-combination triamterene/hydrochlorothiazide preparations may *not* be therapeutic equivalents. The oral bioavailabilities of the individual drugs and the amounts and ratios of these drugs in various commercially available fixed-combination preparations may differ.

Pediatric Patients

Usual Dosage†

ORAL:
- Initially, 2–4 mg/kg daily or 115 mg/m² daily, given in a single dose or 2 divided doses after meals.
- If necessary, increase dosage to 6 mg/kg daily. Do not exceed 300 mg daily.

Hypertension†

ORAL:
- Initially, 1–2 mg/kg daily given in 2 divided doses after meals. Increase dosage as necessary up to 3–4 mg/kg daily given in 2 divided doses. Do not exceed 300 mg daily.

Adult Patients

Edema
Monotherapy

ORAL:
- Initially, 100 mg twice daily after meals. After edema is controlled, usual maintenance dosage is 100 mg daily or every other day. Do not exceed 300 mg daily.

Combination Therapy

ORAL:

- When Dyazide®, Maxzide® or Maxzide®-25 mg, or therapeutically equivalent formulations of these combinations are used, the usual dosage in terms of triamterene is 37.5–75 mg once daily.
- Patients receiving 25 mg of hydrochlorothiazide who become hypokalemic may be switched to Maxzide®-25 mg (37.5 mg triamterene/25 mg hydrochlorothiazide).
- Patients receiving 50 mg of hydrochlorothiazide who become hypokalemic may be switched to Maxzide® (75 mg triamterene/50 mg hydrochlorothiazide).

Hypertension

Monotherapy

ORAL:

- Usual dosage recommended by JNC 7 as monotherapy: 50–100 mg daily. Some patients may benefit from dividing the daily dosage into 2 doses.

Combination Therapy

ORAL:

- Usually combined with a kaliuretic diuretic.
- In conjunction with a kaliuretic diuretic, an initial triamterene dosage of 25 mg once daily has been recommended. Titrate dosage upward as needed and tolerated to a suggested maximum triamterene dosage of 100 mg daily.
- Initially, administer each drug separately to adjust dosage.
- May use in fixed combination with hydrochlorothiazide if optimum maintenance dosage corresponds to drug ratio in combination preparation.
- Administer each drug separately whenever dosage adjustment is necessary.
- When Dyazide®, Maxzide® or Maxzide®-25 mg, or therapeutically equivalent formulations of these combinations are used, the usual dosage in terms of triamterene is 37.5–75 mg once daily.
- Patients receiving 25 mg of hydrochlorothiazide who become hypokalemic may be switched to Maxzide®-25 mg (37.5 mg triamterene/25 mg hydrochlorothiazide).
- Patients receiving 50 mg of hydrochlorothiazide who become hypokalemic may be switched to Maxzide® (75 mg triamterene/50 mg hydrochlorothiazide).
- If BP is not adequately controlled by use of 75 mg once daily (of triamterene in the fixed combination of triamterene/hydrochlorothiazide), another antihypertensive agent may be added.

Prescribing Limits

Pediatric Patients

ORAL:

- Maximum 300 mg daily.

Adult Patients

ORAL:

- Maximum 300 mg daily.
- The manufacturer states there is no clinical experience to date with dosages of fixed-combination Maxzide® or Maxzide®-25 mg exceeding 75 mg of triamterene and 50 mg of hydrochlorothiazide daily.

Special Populations

Hepatic Impairment

- No specific dosage recommendations for hepatic impairment; caution if using fixed combination with hydrochlorothiazide because of risk of precipitating hepatic coma.

Renal Impairment

- No specific dosage recommendations for renal impairment; do not use in patients with renal impairment and elevated serum potassium; discontinue in patients who develop hyperkalemia while on the drug.

† Use is not currently included in the labeling approved by the US Food and Drug Administration.

Triamterene and Hydrochlorothiazide

(trye am′ ter een) (hye droe klor oh thye′ a zide)

Brand Name: Dyazide®, Maxzide®

Why is this medicine prescribed?

The combination of triamterene and hydrochlorothiazide is used to treat high blood pressure and edema (fluid retention; excess fluid held in body tissues) in patients who have lower amounts of potassium in their bodies or for whom low potassium levels in the body could be dangerous. The combination of triamterene and hydrochlorothiazide is in a class of medications called diuretics ('water pills'). It causes the kidneys to get rid of unneeded water and sodium from the body into the urine, but reduces the loss of potassium.

How should this medicine be used?

The combination of triamterene and hydrochlorothiazide comes as a capsule and tablet to take by mouth. It usually is taken once a day. It is best to take this medication earlier in the day so that frequent trips to the bathroom do not interfere with nighttime sleep. Take triamterene and hydrochlorothiazide at around the same time every day. Follow the directions on your prescription label carefully, and ask your doctor or pharmacist to explain any part you do not understand. Take triamterene and hydrochlorothiazide exactly as directed. Do not take more or less of it or take it more often than prescribed by your doctor.

This medication controls high blood pressure but does not cure it. Continue to take triamterene and hydrochlorothiazide even if you feel well. Do not stop taking triamterene and hydrochlorothiazide without talking to your doctor.

Are there other uses for this medicine?

This medicine may be prescribed for other uses; ask your doctor or pharmacist for more information.

What special precautions should I follow?

Before taking triamterene and hydrochlorothiazide,

- tell your doctor and pharmacist if you are allergic to triamterene, hydrochlorothiazide, sulfonamide-derived medications ('sulfa drugs'), or any other medications.

- do not take triamterene and hydrochlorothiazide if you are taking amiloride (Midamor), spironolactone (Aldactone), or other medications containing triamterene.
- tell your doctor and pharmacist what prescription and nonprescription medications, vitamins, nutritional supplements, and herbal products you are taking or plan to take. Be sure to mention amphotericin B (Amphocin, Fungizone); angiotensin-converting enzyme (ACE) inhibitors such as benazepril (Lotensin), captopril (Capoten), enalapril (Vasotec), fosinopril (Monopril), lisinopril (Prinivil, Zestril), moexipril (Univasc), perindopril, (Aceon), quinapril (Accupril), ramipril (Altace), and trandolapril (Mavik); anticoagulants ('blood thinners') such as warfarin (Coumadin); barbiturates (phenobarbital); digoxin (Lanoxin); laxatives; lithium (Eskalith, Lithobid); medications for diabetes, gout, or high blood pressure; methenamine (Hiprex, Urex); narcotic pain relievers; nonsteroidal anti-inflammatory medications (NSAIDs) such as ibuprofen (Advil, Motrin) and naproxen (Aleve, Naprosyn); oral steroids such as dexamethasone (Decadron, Dexone), methylprednisolone (Medrol), and prednisone (Deltasone); and potassium supplements. Your doctor may need to change the doses of your medications or monitor you carefully for side effects.
- tell your doctor if you have or have ever had kidney stones, systemic lupus erythematosus (SLE, a chronic inflammatory condition), diabetes, gout, or thyroid, heart, kidney, or liver disease.
- tell your doctor if you are pregnant or plan to become pregnant. Do not breastfeed if you are taking triamterene and hydrochlorothiazide. If you become pregnant while taking triamterene and hydrochlorothiazide, call your doctor.
- if you are having surgery, including dental surgery, tell the doctor or dentist that you are taking triamterene and hydrochlorothiazide.
- plan to avoid unnecessary or prolonged exposure to sunlight and to wear protective clothing, sunglasses, and sunscreen. Triamterene and hydrochlorothiazide may make your skin sensitive to sunlight.
- you should know that triamterene and hydrochlorothiazide may cause dizziness, lightheadedness, and fainting when you get up too quickly from a lying position. This is more common when you first start taking triamterene and hydrochlorothiazide and may be made worse by drinking alcohol. To avoid this problem, get out of bed slowly, resting your feet on the floor for a few minutes before standing up.

What special dietary instructions should I follow?

Follow your doctor's directions for your meals, including advice for a reduced salt (sodium) diet. Avoid potassium-containing salt substitutes while you are taking this medication. Talk with your doctor about the amount of potassium-rich foods (e.g., bananas, prunes, raisins, and orange juice) that you may have in your diet.

What should I do if I forget to take a dose?

Take the missed dose as soon as you remember it. However, if it is almost time for the next dose, skip the missed dose and continue your regular dosing schedule. Do not take a double dose to make up for a missed one.

What side effects can this medicine cause?

Triamterene and hydrochlorothiazide may cause side effects. Tell your doctor if any of these symptoms are severe or do not go away:

- gas
- frequent urination
- dizziness
- headache

Some side effects can be serious. If you experience any of the following symptoms, call your doctor immediately:

- rash or hives
- difficulty breathing or swallowing
- pain in the upper stomach area
- swelling or tenderness of stomach area
- upset stomach
- vomiting
- fever
- rapid pulse
- extreme tiredness
- unusual bruising or bleeding
- loss of appetite
- yellowing of skin or eyes
- flu-like symptoms
- muscle weakness or cramps
- feelings of numbness, tingling, pricking, burning, or creeping on the skin
- inability to move arms and legs
- slow or irregular heartbeat
- severe dry mouth
- severe thirst
- muscle pain or fatigue
- decreased urination

If you experience a serious side effect, you or your doctor may send a report to the Food and Drug Administration's (FDA) MedWatch Adverse Event Reporting program online [at http://www.fda.gov/MedWatch/index.html] or by phone [1-800-332-1088].

What storage conditions are needed for this medicine?

Keep this medicine in the container it came in, tightly closed, and out of reach of children. Store it at room temperature and away from excess heat and moisture (not in the bathroom). Throw away any medicine that is outdated or no longer needed. Talk to your pharmacist about the proper disposal of your medicine.

What should I do in case of overdose?

In case of overdose, call your local poison control center at 1-800-222-1222. If the victim has collapsed or is not breathing, call local emergency services at 911.

Symptoms of overdose may include:
- increased urination
- upset stomach
- vomiting
- weakness or tiredness
- fever

What other information should I know?

Keep all appointments with your doctor and the laboratory. Your doctor will order certain lab tests to check your body's response to triamterene.

Before having any laboratory test, tell your doctor and the laboratory personnel that you are taking triamterene and hydrochlorothiazide.

Do not let anyone else take your medicine. Ask your pharmacist any questions you have about refilling your prescription.

Talk to your doctor, pharmacist, or other healthcare professional if you have questions about dosing information for your medication.

Triazolam

(trye ay′ zoe lam)

Brand Name: Halcion®
Also available generically.

Why is this medicine prescribed?

Triazolam is used on a short-term basis to help you fall asleep and stay asleep through the night.

This medication is sometimes prescribed for other uses; ask your doctor or pharmacist for more information.

How should this medicine be used?

Triazolam comes as a tablet to take by mouth and may be taken with or without food. It usually is taken before bedtime when needed. Follow the directions on your prescription label carefully, and ask your doctor or pharmacist to explain any part you do not understand. Take triazolam exactly as directed.

Triazolam can be habit-forming. Do not take a larger dose, take it more often, or for a longer period than your doctor tells you to. Tolerance may develop with long-term or excessive use, making the medications less effective. Triazolam should be used only for short periods, such as a few days and generally no longer than 1-2 weeks. If your sleep problems continue, talk to your doctor, who will determine whether this drug is right for you.

What special precautions should I follow?

Before taking triazolam,
- tell your doctor and pharmacist if you are allergic to triazolam, alprazolam (Xanax), chlordiazepoxide (Librium, Librax), clonazepam (Klonopin), clorazepate (Tranxene), diazepam (Valium), estazolam (ProSom), flurazepam (Dalmane), lorazepam (Ativan), oxazepam (Serax), prazepam (Centrax), temazepam (Restoril), or any other drugs.
- tell your doctor and pharmacist what prescription and nonprescription medications you are taking, especially amiodarone (Cordarone, Pacerone); antihistamines; azithromycin (Zithromax); cimetidine (Tagamet); clarithromycin (Biaxin); cyclosporine (Neoral, Sandimmune); digoxin (Lanoxin); diltiazem (Cardizem, Dilacor, Tiazac); disulfiram (Antabuse); ergotamine (Cafatine, Cafergot, Wigraine, others); erythromycin (Erythrocin); isoniazid (INH, Laniazid, Nydrazid); itraconazole (Sporanox); ketoconazole (Nizoral); medications for depression, seizures, Parkinson's disease, pain, asthma, colds, or allergies; muscle relaxants; nefazodone (Serzone); nicardipine (Cardene); nifedipine (Adalat, Procardia); oral contraceptives; probenecid (Benemid); ranitidine (Zantac); rifampin (Rifadin); sedatives; sleeping pills; theophylline (Theo-Dur); tranquilizers; verapamil (Calan, Covera-HS, Verelan); and vitamins. These medications may add to the drowsiness caused by triazolam.
- tell your doctor if you have or have ever had glaucoma; seizures; or lung, heart, or liver disease.
- tell your doctor if you are pregnant, plan to become pregnant, or are breast-feeding. If you become pregnant while taking triazolam, call your doctor immediately.
- if you are having surgery, including dental surgery, tell the doctor or dentist that you are taking triazolam.
- you should know that this drug may make you drowsy. Do not drive a car or operate machinery until you know how this drug affects you.
- remember that alcohol can add to the drowsiness caused by this drug.
- tell your doctor if you use tobacco products. Cigarette smoking may decrease the effectiveness of this drug.

What special dietary instructions should I follow?

Do not eat grapefruit or drink grapefruit juice while taking triazolam; it may change the effectiveness of this medication.

What should I do if I forget to take a dose?

If you miss a dose, skip the missed dose and continue your regular dosing schedule. Do not take a double dose to make up for a missed one.

What side effects can this medicine cause?

Triazolam may cause side effects such as:
- headache
- heartburn

- diarrhea
- hangover effect (grogginess)
- drowsiness
- dizziness or lightheadedness
- weakness
- dry mouth

Tell your doctor if any of these symptoms are severe or do not go away:

- constipation
- difficulty urinating
- frequent urination
- blurred vision

If you experience any of the following symptoms, call your doctor immediately:

- jaw, neck, and back muscle spasms
- slow or difficult speech
- persistent, fine tremor or inability to sit still
- fever
- difficulty breathing or swallowing
- severe skin rash
- yellowing of the skin or eyes
- irregular heartbeat

If you experience a serious side effect, you or your doctor may send a report to the Food and Drug Administration's (FDA) MedWatch Adverse Event Reporting program online [at http://www.fda.gov/MedWatch/index.html] or by phone [1-800-332-1088].

What storage conditions are needed for this medicine?

Keep this medication in the container it came in, tightly closed, and out of reach of children. Store it at room temperature and away from excess heat and moisture (not in the bathroom). Throw away any medication that is outdated or no longer needed. Talk to your pharmacist about the proper disposal of your medication.

What should I do in case of overdose?

In case of overdose, call your local poison control center at 1-800-222-1222. If the victim has collapsed or is not breathing, call local emergency services at 911.

What other information should I know?

Keep all appointments with your doctor and the laboratory.
Do not let anyone else take your medication.

Dosage Facts
For Informational Purposes

Caution: Do not change your dose, how often you take your medication, or the length of time you are to take it without first talking to your healthcare provider.

The following dosage information was written using medical language for doctors and other healthcare pro-fessionals and is provided here for you to check your dosage. The dosage of this drug may differ for different patients. Therefore, always follow your doctor's instructions or the directions on the label. Contact your healthcare provider or pharmacist if you have any questions about the specific dosage of your medication after reviewing this information.

General Dosage Information

Individualize dosage; use the smallest effective dose.

Some adverse effects (e.g., amnesia, dizziness, drowsiness, lightheadedness) appear to be dose related. Inconclusive whether other effects (e.g., confusion, bizarre or abnormal behavior, agitation, hallucinations) are dose related.

Adult Patients

Insomnia

ORAL:
- Usual dose is 0.25 mg.
- In some patients (e.g., those with low body weight), 0.125 mg may be adequate.
- Reserve 0.5-mg dose for exceptional cases in which the patient does not respond adequately to a lower dose.

Prescribing Limits

Adult Patients

Insomnia

ORAL:
- Maximum 0.5 mg daily.

Special Populations

Hepatic Impairment
- No specific dosage recommendations.

Renal Impairment
- No specific dosage recommendations.

Geriatric or Debilitated Patients
- Usual dosages in healthy geriatric patients should be approximately half those in younger adults.
- Initially, 0.125 mg daily. Increased risk of adverse (e.g., behavioral) effects if therapy is initiated at doses >0.125 mg.
- Reserve 0.25-mg dose for exceptional cases in which the patient does not respond adequately to a lower dose.

Trifluoperazine Oral

(trye floo oh per′ a zeen)

Brand Name: Stelazine®

Why is this medicine prescribed?

Trifluoperazine is used to treat schizophrenia and symptoms such as hallucinations, delusions, and hostility. It is also used short-term to treat anxiety in some patients.

This medication is sometimes prescribed for other uses; ask your doctor or pharmacist for more information.

How should this medicine be used?

Trifluoperazine comes as a tablet and liquid concentrate to take by mouth. It usually is taken one or two times a day. Follow the directions on your prescription label carefully, and ask your doctor or pharmacist to explain any part you do not understand. Take trifluoperazine exactly as directed. Do not take more or less of it or take it more often than prescribed by your doctor.

The liquid concentrate must be diluted before use. It comes with a specially marked dropper for measuring the dose. Ask your pharmacist to show you how to use the dropper if you have difficulty. To dilute the liquid concentrate, add it to at least 2 ounces of milk, water, soft drink, coffee, tea, tomato or fruit juice, soup, or pudding just before you take it. If any beverage, soup, or pudding gets on the dropper, rinse the dropper with tap water before replacing it in the bottle. Do not allow the liquid concentrate to touch your skin or clothing; it can irritate your skin. If you spill the liquid concentrate on your skin, wash it off immediately with soap and water.

Continue to take trifluoperazine even if you feel well. Do not stop taking trifluoperazine without talking to your doctor, especially if you have taken large doses for a long time. Your doctor probably will decrease your dose gradually. This drug must be taken regularly for a few weeks before its full effect is felt.

What special precautions should I follow?

Before taking trifluoperazine,

- tell your doctor and pharmacist if you are allergic to trifluoperazine, sulfites, or any other drugs.
- tell your doctor and pharmacist what prescription and nonprescription medications you are taking, especially antacids, antihistamines, appetite reducers (amphetamines), benztropine (Cogentin), bromocriptine (Parlodel), carbamazepine (Tegretol), fluoxetine (Prozac), guanethidine (Ismelin), lithium, medication for colds, medication for depression, meperidine (Demerol), methyldopa (Aldomet), phenytoin (Dilantin), propranolol (Inderal), sedatives, trihexyphenidyl (Artane), valproic acid (Depakane), and vitamins.
- tell your doctor if you have or have ever had depression; seizures; shock therapy; asthma; emphysema; chronic bronchitis; problems with your urinary system or prostate; glaucoma; a history of alcohol abuse; thyroid problems; bad reaction to insulin; angina; irregular heartbeat; problems with your blood pressure; blood disorders; blood vessel, heart, kidney, liver, or lung disease.
- tell your doctor if you are pregnant, plan to become pregnant, or are breast-feeding. If you become pregnant while taking trifluoperazine, call your doctor.
- if you are having surgery, including dental surgery, tell the doctor or dentist that you are taking trifluoperazine.
- you should know that this drug may make you drowsy. Do not drive a car or operate machinery until you know how this drug affects you.
- remember that alcohol can add to the drowsiness caused by this drug.
- plan to avoid unnecessary or prolonged exposure to sunlight and to wear protective clothing, sunglasses, and sunscreen. Trifluoperazine may make your skin sensitive to sunlight.

What special dietary instructions should I follow?

Trifluoperazine may cause an upset stomach. Take trifluoperazine with food or milk.

What should I do if I forget to take a dose?

Take the missed dose as soon as you remember it and take any remaining doses for that day at evenly spaced intervals. However, if you remember a missed dose when it is almost time for your next scheduled dose, skip the missed dose. Do not take a double dose to make up for a missed one.

If you take trifluoperazine once a day at bedtime and do not remember it until the next morning, omit the missed dose. Do not take a double dose to make up for a missed one.

What side effects can this medicine cause?

Trifluoperazine may cause side effects. Your urine may turn pink or reddish-brown; this effect is not harmful. Tell your doctor if any of these symptoms are severe or do not go away:

- drowsiness
- dizziness or blurred vision
- dry mouth
- upset stomach
- vomiting
- diarrhea
- constipation
- restlessness
- headache
- weight gain

If you experience any of the following symptoms, call your doctor immediately:

- tremor
- restlessness or pacing
- fine worm-like tongue movements
- unusual face, mouth, or jaw movements
- shuffling walk
- seizures or convulsions
- fast, irregular, or pounding heartbeat
- difficulty urinating or loss of bladder control
- yellowing of the skin or eyes

If you experience a serious side effect, you or your doctor may send a report to the Food and Drug Administration's (FDA) MedWatch Adverse Event Reporting program online [at http://www.fda.gov/MedWatch/index.html] or by phone [1-800-332-1088].

What storage conditions are needed for this medicine?

Keep this medication in the container it came in, tightly closed, and out of reach of children. Store it at room temperature and away from excess heat and moisture (not in the bathroom). Protect the liquid from light. Throw away any medication that is outdated or no longer needed. Talk to your pharmacist about the proper disposal of your medication.

What should I do in case of overdose?

In case of overdose, call your local poison control center at 1-800-222-1222. If the victim has collapsed or is not breathing, call local emergency services at 911.

What other information should I know?

Keep all appointments with your doctor and the laboratory. Your doctor will order certain lab tests to check your response to trifluoperazine.

Do not let anyone else take your medication. Ask your pharmacist any questions you have about refilling your prescription.

Talk to your doctor, pharmacist, or other healthcare professional if you have questions about dosing information for your medication.

Trihexyphenidyl

(trye hex ee fen' i dil)

Brand Name: Artane®, Artane Sequels®, Trihexane®, Trihexy-2®, Trihexy-5®
Also available generically.

Why is this medicine prescribed?

Trihexyphenidyl is used to treat the symptoms of Parkinson's disease and tremors caused by other medical problems or drugs.

This medication is sometimes prescribed for other uses; ask your doctor or pharmacist for more information.

How should this medicine be used?

Trihexyphenidyl comes as a tablet, liquid, and extended-release (long-acting) capsule to take by mouth. It usually is taken three or four times a day (with meals and at bedtime). The controlled-release capsules are taken once a day (after breakfast) or twice a day, every 12 hours. You may have to take trihexyphenidyl for a long time to treat Parkinson's disease. However, trihexyphenidyl may only be needed for a short period to treat other conditions. Follow the directions on your prescription label carefully, and ask your doctor or pharmacist to explain any part you do not understand. Take trihexyphenidyl exactly as directed. Do not take more or less of it or take it more often than prescribed by your doctor.

Do not stop taking trihexyphenidyl suddenly without talking with your doctor, especially if you are also taking other medications. Sudden stoppage can cause symptoms of Parkinson's disease to return.

Do not open the extended-release capsules and do not chew the tablets. Swallow them whole.

What special precautions should I follow?

Before taking trihexyphenidyl,

- tell your doctor and pharmacist if you are allergic to trihexyphenidyl or any other drugs.
- tell your doctor and pharmacist what prescription and nonprescription medications you are taking, especially amantadine (Symmetrel), digoxin, haloperidol (Haldol), levodopa (Larodopa, Sinemet), tranquilizers, and vitamins.
- tell your doctor if you have or have ever had kidney or liver disease, myasthenia gravis, heart or blood pressure problems, problems with your urinary system or prostate, or stomach problems.
- tell your doctor if you are pregnant, plan to become pregnant, or are breast-feeding. If you become pregnant while taking trihexyphenidyl, call your doctor.
- if you are having surgery, including dental surgery, tell the doctor or dentist that you are taking trihexyphenidyl.
- you should know that this drug may make you drowsy. Do not drive a car or operate machinery until you know how this drug affects you.
- remember that alcohol can add to the drowsiness caused by this drug.

What special dietary instructions should I follow?

Trihexyphenidyl may cause an upset stomach. Take trihexyphenidyl with food or milk.

What should I do if I forget to take a dose?

Take the missed dose as soon as you remember it. However, if it is almost time for the next dose, skip the missed dose and continue your regular dosing schedule. Do not take a double dose to make up for a missed one.

What side effects can this medicine cause?

Trihexyphenidyl may cause side effects. Tell your doctor if any of these symptoms are severe or do not go away:

- drowsiness
- dizziness or blurred vision
- dry mouth
- upset stomach
- vomiting
- diarrhea
- constipation
- increased eye sensitivity to light
- difficulty urinating

If you experience any of the following symptoms, call your doctor immediately:

- skin rash
- fast, irregular, or pounding heartbeat
- fever
- confusion
- depression
- delusions or hallucinations
- eye pain

If you experience a serious side effect, you or your doctor may send a report to the Food and Drug Administration's (FDA) MedWatch Adverse Event Reporting program online [at http://www.fda.gov/MedWatch/index.html] or by phone [1-800-332-1088].

What storage conditions are needed for this medicine?

Keep this medication in the container it came in, tightly closed, and out of reach of children. Store it at room temperature and away from excess heat and moisture (not in the bathroom). Throw away any medication that is outdated or no longer needed. Talk to your pharmacist about the proper disposal of your medication.

What should I do in case of overdose?

In case of overdose, call your local poison control center at 1-800-222-1222. If the victim has collapsed or is not breathing, call local emergency services at 911.

What other information should I know?

Keep all appointments with your doctor and the laboratory. Your doctor will order certain lab tests to check your response to trihexyphenidyl.

Do not let anyone else take your medication. Ask your pharmacist any questions you have about refilling your prescription.

Dosage Facts
For Informational Purposes

Caution: Do not change your dose, how often you take your medication, or the length of time you are to take it without first talking to your healthcare provider.

The following dosage information was written using medical language for doctors and other healthcare professionals and is provided here for you to check your dosage. The dosage of this drug may differ for different patients. Therefore, always follow your doctor's instructions or the directions on the label. Contact your healthcare provider or pharmacist if you have any questions about the specific dosage of your medication after reviewing this information.

General Dosage Information

Available as trihexyphenidyl hydrochloride; dosage expressed in terms of the salt.

Adjust dosage carefully according to individual requirements and response.

Adult Patients
Parkinsonian Syndrome

ORAL:
- Initially, 1 mg on first day. Dosages may be increased in 2-mg increments at 3- to 5-day intervals up to a maximum of 6–10 mg daily.
- Postencephalitic patients: 12–15 mg daily may be required.
- When trihexylphenidyl is used as an adjunct to levodopa, consider reducing levodopa and trihexyphenidyl dosages. Generally, 3–6 mg daily of trihexyphenidyl hydrochloride is adequate.
- If trihexyphenidyl is replacing another antiparkisonian agent, increase trihexyphenidyl dose as needed while decreasing other drug dose until complete replacement is achieved.

Drug-Induced Extrapyramidal Reactions

ORAL:
- Usual dosage: 5–15 mg total daily dosage.
- Initially, 1 mg; if extrapyramidal reactions are not controlled within a few hours, progressively increase dosage until control is achieved.
- Alternatively, to achieve a more rapid control, reduce dosage of the drug causing the reaction, then adjust the dosage of both drugs to attain the desired drug effect without extrapyramidal symptoms. Once control of extrapyramidal reactions has been maintained for several days, dosage of trihexyphenidyl may be reduced or discontinued.

Prescribing Limits
Adult Patients
Parkinsonian Syndrome

ORAL:
- Maximum of 6–10 mg daily in most patients; postencephalitic patients may require 12–15 mg daily.

Special Populations

Hepatic Impairment
- No specific dosage recommendations at this time.

Renal Impairment
- No specific dosage recommendations at this time.

Geriatric Patients
- Patients ≥60 years of age: Initiate with low dosage; titrate dosage gradually.

Trimethobenzamide

(trye meth oh ben′ za mide)

Brand Name: Tigan®

Important Warning

In April 2007, the Food and Drug Administration (FDA) announced that suppositories containing trimethobenzamide may no longer be marketed in the United States. The FDA made this decision because **continued on next page**

```
Important Warning (cont'd)
```
trimethobenzamide suppositories have not been shown to work to treat nausea and vomiting. If you are currently using trimethobenzamide suppositories, you should call your doctor or other healthcare professional to talk about switching to another treatment.

Why is this medicine prescribed?

Trimethobenzamide is used to treat nausea and vomiting that may occur after surgery. It is also used to control nausea caused by gastroenteritis ('stomach flu'; a virus that may cause nausea, vomiting, and diarrhea). Trimethobenzamide is in a class of medications called antihistamines. Trimethobenzamide may work by decreasing activity in the area of the brain that causes nausea and vomiting.

How should this medicine be used?

Trimethobenzamide comes as a capsule to take by mouth. Trimethobenzamide usually is taken three or four times a day. Take trimethobenzamide at around the same times every day. Follow the directions on your prescription label carefully, and ask your doctor or pharmacist to explain any part you do not understand. Take trimethobenzamide exactly as directed. Do not take more or less of it or take it more often than prescribed by your doctor.

Are there other uses for this medicine?

This medication is sometimes prescribed for other uses; ask your doctor or pharmacist for more information.

What special precautions should I follow?

Before taking trimethobenzamide,
- tell your doctor and pharmacist if you are allergic to trimethobenzamide or any other medications.
- tell your doctor and pharmacist what prescription and nonprescription medications, vitamins, nutritional supplements and herbal products you are taking or plan to take. Be sure to mention any of the following: antidepressants; antihistamines; barbiturates such as phenobarbital (Luminal); belladonna alkaloids (Donnatal); medications for anxiety, mental illness, pain and seizures; other medications for nausea and vomiting; sedatives; sleeping pills; and tranquilizers. Your doctor may need to change the doses of your medications or monitor you more carefully for side effects.
- tell your doctor if you have Reye's Syndrome (a condition affecting the brain and liver that can happen after a viral illness), encephalitis (inflammation of the brain), or a high fever, or if you have or have ever had liver disease. If you will be giving trimethobenzamide to a child, also tell the child's doctor if the child has any of the following symptoms before he or she receives the medication: vomiting, listlessness, drowsiness, confusion, aggression, seizures, yellowing of the skin or eyes, weakness, or flu-like symptoms. Also tell the child's doctor if the child has not been drinking normally, has had excessive vomiting or diarrhea, or appears dehydrated.
- tell your doctor if you are pregnant, plan to become pregnant, or are breast-feeding. If you become pregnant while taking trimethobenzamide, call your doctor.
- if you are having surgery, including dental surgery, tell the doctor or dentist that you are taking trimethobenzamide.
- you should know that this medication may make you drowsy. Do not drive a car or operate machinery until you know how this medication affects you.
- ask your doctor about the safe use of alcoholic beverages while you are taking trimethobenzamide. Alcohol can make the side effects from trimethobenzamide worse.

What special dietary instructions should I follow?

Unless your doctor tells you otherwise, continue your normal diet.

What should I do if I forget to take a dose?

Take the missed dose as soon as you remember it. However, if it is almost time for the next dose, skip the missed dose and continue your regular dosing schedule. Do not take a double dose to make up for a missed one.

What side effects can this medicine cause?

Trimethobenzamide may cause side effects. Tell your doctor if any of these symptoms are severe or do not go away:
- drowsiness
- dizziness
- headache
- depression
- diarrhea

Some side effects can be serious. If you experience any of the following symptoms, call your doctor immediately:
- rash
- backward arching of the head, neck, and back
- muscle cramps
- uncontrollable shaking of a part of the body
- slow, jerking movements
- shuffling walk
- slow speech
- confusion
- blurred vision
- yellowing of the skin or eyes
- seizures
- coma (loss of consciousness for a period of time)

Trimethobenzamide may cause other side effects. Call your doctor if you have any unusual problems while you are taking this medication.

If you experience a serious side effect, you or your doctor may send a report to the Food and Drug Administration's (FDA) MedWatch Adverse Event Reporting program online [at http://www.fda.gov/MedWatch/index.html] or by phone [1-800-332-1088].

What storage conditions are needed for this medicine?

Keep this medication in the container it came in, tightly closed, and out of reach of children. Store it at room temperature and away from excess heat and moisture (not in the bathroom). Throw away any medication that is outdated or no longer needed. Talk to your pharmacist about the proper disposal of your medication.

What other information should I know?

Keep all appointments with your doctor.

Do not let anyone else take your medication. Ask your pharmacist any questions you have about refilling your prescription.

Talk to your doctor, pharmacist, or other healthcare professional if you have questions about dosing information for your medication.

Trimethoprim

(trye meth′ oh prim)

Brand Name: Proloprim®
Also available generically.

Why is this medicine prescribed?

Trimethoprim eliminates bacteria that cause urinary tract infections. It is used in combination with other drugs to treat certain types of pneumonia. It also is used to treat 'travelers' diarrhea.' Antibiotics will not work for colds, flu, or other viral infections.

This medication is sometimes prescribed for other uses; ask your doctor or pharmacist for more information.

How should this medicine be used?

Trimethoprim comes as a tablet to take by mouth. It usually is taken one or two times a day. Trimethoprim may be taken with or without food. Follow the directions on your prescription label carefully, and ask your pharmacist or doctor to explain any part you do not understand. Take trimethoprim exactly as directed. Do not take more or less of it or take it more often than prescribed by your doctor.

What special precautions should I follow?

Before taking trimethoprim,
- tell your doctor and pharmacist if you are allergic to trimethoprim, sulfa drugs, diuretics ('water pills', oral diabetes medications, or any other drugs.
- tell your doctor and pharmacist what prescription and nonprescription medications you are taking, especially phenytoin (Dilantin) and vitamins.

- tell your doctor if you have or have ever had anemia or liver or kidney disease.
- tell your doctor if you are pregnant, plan to become pregnant, or are breast-feeding. If you become pregnant while taking trimethoprim, call your doctor immediately.

What special dietary instructions should I follow?

Take trimethoprim on an empty stomach, 1 hour before or 2 hours after meals. However, if you experience nausea, you may take trimethoprim with food.

Drink at least eight glasses of liquid (water, tea, coffee, soft drinks, milk, and fruit juice) every day.

What should I do if I forget to take a dose?

Take the missed dose as soon as you remember it. However, if it is almost time for your next dose, skip the missed dose and continue your dosing schedule. Do not take a double dose to make up for a missed one.

What side effects can this medicine cause?

Trimethoprim may cause side effects. Tell your doctor if any of these symptoms are severe or do not go away:
- upset stomach
- vomiting
- diarrhea

If you experience any of the following symptoms, call your doctor immediately:
- rash (hives)
- itching
- difficulty breathing or swallowing
- sore throat
- fever or chills
- mouth sores
- unusual bruising or bleeding
- yellowing of the skin or eyes
- paleness
- joint aches
- bluish-colored fingernails, lips, or skin

If you experience a serious side effect, you or your doctor may send a report to the Food and Drug Administration's (FDA) MedWatch Adverse Event Reporting program online [at http://www.fda.gov/MedWatch/index.html] or by phone [1-800-332-1088].

What storage conditions are needed for this medicine?

Keep this medication in the container it came in, tightly closed, and out of reach of children. Store it at room temperature and away from excess heat and moisture (not in the bathroom). Throw away any medication that is outdated or no longer needed. Talk to your pharmacist about the proper disposal of your medication.

What should I do in case of overdose?

In case of overdose, call your local poison control center at 1-800-222-1222. If the victim has collapsed or is not breathing, call local emergency services at 911.

What other information should I know?

Keep all appointments with your doctor and the laboratory. Your doctor will order certain lab tests to check your response to trimethoprim.

Do not let anyone else take your medication. Your prescription is probably not refillable. If you still have symptoms of infection after you finish the trimethoprim, call your doctor.

Dosage Facts
For Informational Purposes

Caution: Do not change your dose, how often you take your medication, or the length of time you are to take it without first talking to your healthcare provider.

The following dosage information was written using medical language for doctors and other healthcare professionals and is provided here for you to check your dosage. The dosage of this drug may differ for different patients. Therefore, always follow your doctor's instructions or the directions on the label. Contact your healthcare provider or pharmacist if you have any questions about the specific dosage of your medication after reviewing this information.

Pediatric Patients

Acute Otitis Media (AOM)

ORAL:
- Children ≥6 months of age: 10 mg/kg daily in 2 divided doses every 12 hours given for 10 days.

Adult Patients

Urinary Tract Infections (UTIs)
Acute, Uncomplicated UTIs

ORAL:
- 100 mg every 12 hours or 200 mg once daily for 10–14 days.

Pneumocystis jiroveci (Pneumocystis carinii) Pneumonia†
Treatment of PCP†

ORAL:
- 5 mg/kg 3 times daily for 21 days; used in conjunction with dapsone (100 mg once daily for 21 days).

Special Populations

Renal Impairment

Urinary Tract Infections (UTIs)
Acute, Uncomplicated UTIs

ORAL:
- Doses and/or frequency of administration must be modified in response to the degree of renal impairment.

- 50 mg every 12 hours in adults with Cl_{cr} 15–30 mL/minute.
- Manufacturers recommend the drug not be used in patients with Cl_{cr} <15 mL/minute; some clinicians suggest the drug can be used in reduced dosages in these patients.

Geriatric Patients
- Cautious dosage selection because of age-related decreases in renal, hepatic, and/or cardiac function. Initiate therapy at the lower end of the dosing range.

† Use is not currently included in the labeling approved by the US Food and Drug Administration.

Trimetrexate Glucuronate

(tri me trex′ ate)

Brand Name: Neutrexin®

Important Warning

It is important to remember to take trimetrexate with leucovorin as directed by your doctor. If you miss a dose, take it as soon as you remember. If it is almost time for the next dose, skip the missed dose and continue with your regular dosing schedule. Call your doctor if you miss a dose.

About Your Treatment

Your doctor has ordered the drug trimetrexate to help treat your illness. The drug can be given by injection into a vein.

This medication is used to treat:
- infections caused by the bacteria *Pneumocystis carinii* in patients that do not have a fully functioning immune system

This medication is sometimes prescribed for other uses; ask your doctor or pharmacist for more information.

Trimetrexate resembles a normal nutrient needed for cell growth. The *Pneumocystis* bacteria and cancer cells take in trimetrexate, which then interferes with their growth. You also will be given the drug leucovorin with each trimetrexate treatment. Leucovorin replaces the same needed nutrient in normal cells. *Pneumocystis* bacteria and cancer cells cannot use leucovorin. Take leucovorin exactly as prescribed by your doctor.

Precautions

Before taking trimetrexate,
- tell your doctor and pharmacist if you are allergic to trimetrexate or any other drugs.
- tell your doctor and pharmacist what prescription and

nonprescription medications you are taking, especially acetaminophen (Tylenol), aspirin, clotrimazole (Mycelex), erythromycin, fluconazole (Diflucan), ketoconazole (Nizoral), miconazole (Monistat), rifabutin (Mycobutin), rifampin (Rifadin), zidovudine (AZT, Retrovir), and vitamins.

- tell your doctor if you have or have ever had kidney or liver disease, stomach ulcers, or intestinal disease.
- you should know that trimetrexate may interfere with the normal menstrual cycle (period) in women and may stop sperm production in men. However, you should not assume that you cannot get pregnant or that you cannot get someone else pregnant. Women who are pregnant or breast-feeding should tell their doctors before they begin taking this drug. You should not plan to have children while receiving chemotherapy or for a while after treatments. (Talk to your doctor for further details.) Use a reliable method of birth control to prevent pregnancy. Trimetrexate may harm the fetus.
- do not have any vaccinations (e.g., measles or flu shots) without talking to your doctor.

Side Effects

Side effects from trimetrexate may occur and include:

- nausea
- loss of appetite or weight

Tell your doctor if either of these symptoms is severe or lasts for several hours:

- mouth blistering
- fatigue

If you experience any of the following symptoms, call your doctor immediately:

- painful urination or red urine
- black, tarry stools
- diarrhea
- unusual bruising or bleeding
- fever
- cough
- difficulty swallowing
- dizziness
- chills
- shortness of breath
- severe vomiting
- rash
- yellowing of the skin or eyes

If you experience a serious side effect, you or your doctor may send a report to the Food and Drug Administration's (FDA) MedWatch Adverse Event Reporting program online [at http://www.fda.gov/MedWatch/index.html] or by phone [1-800-332-1088].

Overdose

In case of overdose, call your local poison control center at 1-800-222-1222. If the victim has collapsed or is not breathing, call local emergency services at 911.

Special Instructions

- The most common side effect of trimetrexate is a decrease in the number of blood cells. Your doctor may order tests before, during, and after your treatment to see if your blood cells are affected by the drug.

Talk to your doctor, pharmacist, or other healthcare professional if you have questions about dosing information for your medication.

Trimipramine

(trye mi′ pra meen)

Brand Name: Surmontil®
Also available generically.

Important Warning

A small number of children, teenagers, and young adults (up to 24 years of age) who took antidepressants ('mood elevators') such as trimipramine during clinical studies became suicidal (thinking about harming or killing oneself or planning or trying to do so). Children, teenagers, and young adults who take antidepressants to treat depression or other mental illnesses may be more likely to become suicidal than children, teenagers, and young adults who do not take antidepressants to treat these conditions. However, experts are not sure about how great this risk is and how much it should be considered in deciding whether a child or teenager should take an antidepressant. Children younger than 18 years of age should not normally take trimipramine, but in some cases, a doctor may decide that trimipramine is the best medication to treat a child's condition.

You should know that your mental health may change in unexpected ways when you take trimipramine or other antidepressants even if you are an adult over age 24. You may become suicidal, especially at the beginning of your treatment and any time that your dose is increased or decreased. You, your family, or your caregiver should call your doctor right away if you experience any of the following symptoms: new or worsening depression; thinking about harming or killing yourself, or planning or trying to do so; extreme worry; agitation; panic attacks; difficulty falling asleep or staying asleep; aggressive behavior; irritability; acting without thinking; severe restlessness; and frenzied abnormal excitement. Be sure that your family or caregiver knows which symptoms may be serious so they can call the doctor when you are unable to seek treatment on your own.

continued on next page

Important Warning (cont'd)

Your healthcare provider will want to see you often while you are taking trimipramine, especially at the beginning of your treatment. Be sure to keep all appointments for office visits with your doctor.

The doctor or pharmacist will give you the manufacturer's patient information sheet (Medication Guide) when you begin treatment with trimipramine. Read the information carefully and ask your doctor or pharmacist if you have any questions. You also can obtain the Medication Guide from the FDA website: http://www.fda.gov/cder/drug/antidepressants/antidepressants_MG_2007.pdf.

No matter your age, before you take an antidepressant, you, your parent, or your caregiver should talk to your doctor about the risks and benefits of treating your condition with an antidepressant or with other treatments. You should also talk about the risks and benefits of not treating your condition. You should know that having depression or another mental illness greatly increases the risk that you will become suicidal. This risk is higher if you or anyone in your family has or has ever had bipolar disorder (mood that changes from depressed to abnormally excited) or mania (frenzied, abnormally excited mood) or has thought about or attempted suicide. Talk to your doctor about your condition, symptoms, and personal and family medical history. You and your doctor will decide what type of treatment is right for you.

Why is this medicine prescribed?

Trimipramine is used to treat depression. Trimipramine is in a class of medications called tricyclic antidepressants. It works by increasing the amount of certain natural substances in the brain that are needed to maintain mental balance.

How should this medicine be used?

Trimipramine comes as a capsule to take by mouth. It is usually taken one to three times a day. Take trimipramine at around the same time(s) every day. Follow the directions on your prescription label carefully, and ask your doctor or pharmacist to explain any part you do not understand. Take trimipramine exactly as directed. Do not take more or less of it or take it more often than prescribed by your doctor.

Your doctor will start you on a low dose of trimipramine and gradually increase your dose.

It may take up to 4 weeks before you feel the benefit of trimipramine. Continue to take trimipramine even if you feel well. Do not stop taking trimipramine without talking to your doctor.

Are there other uses for this medicine?

This medication may be prescribed for other uses; ask your doctor or pharmacist for more information.

What special precautions should I follow?

Before taking trimipramine,

- tell your doctor and pharmacist if you are allergic to trimipramine, clomipramine (Anafranil), desipramine (Norpramin), imipramine (Tofranil), or any other medications.
- tell your doctor if you are taking monoamine oxidase (MAO) inhibitors, including isocarboxazid (Marplan), phenelzine (Nardil) selegiline (Eldepryl, Emsam, Zelapar) and tranylcypromine (Parnate) or if you have taken an MAO inhibitor during the past 14 days. Your doctor will probably tell you not to take trimipramine.
- tell your doctor and pharmacist what prescription and nonprescription medications, vitamins, nutritional supplements, and herbal products you are taking or plan to take. Be sure to mention any of the following: cimetidine (Tagamet); decongestants; guanethidine (Ismelin); ipratropium (Atrovent); medications for irritable bowel disease, motion sickness, Parkinson's disease, ulcers, or urinary problems; medications for irregular heartbeats such as quinidine (Quinidex), flecainide (Tambocor), and propafenone (Rythmol); other antidepressants; and selective serotonin reuptake inhibitors (SSRIs) such as fluoxetine (Prozac, Sarafem), paroxetine (Paxil), and sertraline (Zoloft). Tell your doctor or pharmacist if you have stopped taking fluoxetine (Prozac, Sarafem) in the past 5 weeks. Your doctor may need to change the doses of your medications or monitor you carefully for side effects.
- tell your doctor if you have recently had a heart attack. Your doctor will probably tell you not to take trimipramine.
- tell your doctor if you have or have ever had glaucoma (an eye condition), enlargement of the prostate (a male reproductive gland), difficulty urinating, thyroid disease, seizures, or heart, kidney, or liver disease.
- tell your doctor if you are pregnant, plan to become pregnant, or are breast-feeding. If you become pregnant while taking trimipramine, call your doctor.
- if you are having surgery, including dental surgery, tell the doctor or dentist that you are taking trimipramine.
- you should know that trimipramine may make you drowsy. Do not drive a car or operate machinery until you know how this medication affects you.
- remember that alcohol can add to the drowsiness caused by this medication.
- plan to avoid unnecessary or prolonged exposure to sunlight and to wear protective clothing, sunglasses, and sunscreen. Trimipramine may make your skin sensitive to sunlight.

What special dietary instructions should I follow?

Unless your doctor tells you otherwise, continue your normal diet.

What should I do if I forget to take a dose?

Take the missed dose as soon as you remember it. However, if it is almost time for the next dose, skip the missed dose and continue your regular dosing schedule. Do not take a double dose to make up for a missed one.

What side effects can this medicine cause?

Trimipramine may cause side effects. Tell your doctor if any of these symptoms are severe or do not go away:
- nausea
- vomiting
- diarrhea
- stomach pain
- drowsiness
- weakness or tiredness
- excitement or anxiety
- confusion
- dizziness
- headache
- nightmares
- dry mouth
- changes in appetite or weight
- constipation
- difficulty urinating
- frequent urination
- blurred vision
- changes in sex drive or ability
- excessive sweating
- ringing in the ears
- pain, burning, or tingling in the hands or feet

Some side effects can be serious. If you experience any of the following symptoms or those listed in the IMPORTANT WARNING section, call your doctor immediately:
- jaw, neck, and back muscle spasms
- slow or difficult speech
- shuffling walk
- uncontrollable shaking of a part of the body
- fever and sore throat
- difficulty breathing or swallowing
- rash
- yellowing of the skin or eyes
- seizures
- seeing things or hearing voices that do not exist (hallucinating)
- chest pain
- pounding or irregular heartbeat

Trimipramine may cause other side effects. Call your doctor if you have any unusual problems while taking this medication.

If you experience a serious side effect, you or your doctor may send a report to the Food and Drug Administration's (FDA) MedWatch Adverse Event Reporting program online [at http://www.fda.gov/MedWatch/index.html] or by phone [1-800-332-1088].

What storage conditions are needed for this medicine?

Keep this medication in the container it came in, tightly closed, and out of reach of children. Store it at room temperature and away from excess heat and moisture (not in the bathroom). Throw away any medication that is outdated or no longer needed. Talk to your pharmacist about the proper disposal of your medication.

What should I do in case of overdose?

In case of overdose, call your local poison control center at 1-800-222-1222. If the victim has collapsed or is not breathing, call local emergency services at 911.

What other information should I know?

Keep all appointments with your doctor.

Do not let anyone else take your medication. Ask your pharmacist any questions you have about refilling your prescription.

Dosage Facts
For Informational Purposes

Caution: Do not change your dose, how often you take your medication, or the length of time you are to take it without first talking to your healthcare provider.

The following dosage information was written using medical language for doctors and other healthcare professionals and is provided here for you to check your dosage. The dosage of this drug may differ for different patients. Therefore, always follow your doctor's instructions or the directions on the label. Contact your healthcare provider or pharmacist if you have any questions about the specific dosage of your medication after reviewing this information.

General Dosage Information

Available as trimipramine maleate; dosage expressed in terms of trimipramine.

Pediatric Patients

Major Depressive Disorder

ORAL:
- Adolescents: Initially, 50 mg daily; may increase gradually to 100 mg daily, as tolerated.

Adult Patients

Major Depressive Disorder
Outpatients

ORAL:
- Initially, 75 mg daily; may increase gradually to 150 mg daily.
- After symptoms are controlled, gradually reduce dosage to the lowest level that will maintain relief of symptoms, usually 50–150 mg daily. Continue therapy for at least 3 months to prevent relapse.

Hospitalized Patients

ORAL:
- Initially, 100 mg daily; dosage may be increased gradually to 200 mg daily after a few days. If there is no improvement after 2–3 weeks at 200 mg daily, dosage may be increased to a maximum of 250–300 mg daily (administered in divided doses).
- After symptoms are controlled, dosage should be gradually reduced to the lowest level that will maintain relief of symptoms. Continue therapy for at least 3 months to prevent relapse.

Prescribing Limits

Pediatric Patients

Major Depressive Disorder

ORAL:
- Adolescents: Maximum 100 mg daily.

Adult Patients

Major Depressive Disorder

Outpatients

ORAL:
- Maximum 200 mg daily.

Hospitalized Patients

ORAL:
- Maximum 300 mg daily.

Special Populations

Hepatic Impairment
- No specific dosage recommendations at this time.

Renal Impairment
- No specific dosage recommendations at this time.

Geriatric Patients
- Initially, 50 mg daily; may gradually increase to a maximum of 100 mg daily, as tolerated.

Trospium

(trose′ pee um)

Brand Name: Sanctura®

Why is this medicine prescribed?

Trospium is used to treat an overactive bladder (a condition in which the bladder muscles contract uncontrollably and cause frequent urination, urgent need to urinate, and inability to control urination). Trospium is in a class of medications called anticholinergics. It works by relaxing the bladder muscles to prevent urgent, frequent, or uncontrolled urination.

How should this medicine be used?

Trospium comes as a tablet to take by mouth. It is usually taken twice a day on an empty stomach or one hour before meals. Trospium is sometimes taken once a day at bedtime. To help you remember to take trospium, take it around the same time every day. Follow the directions on your prescription label carefully, and ask your doctor or pharmacist to explain any part you do not understand. Take trospium exactly as directed. Do not take more or less of it or take it more often than prescribed by your doctor.

Are there other uses for this medicine?

This medication may be prescribed for other uses; ask your doctor or pharmacist for more information.

What special precautions should I follow?

Before taking trospium,
- tell your doctor and pharmacist if you are allergic to trospium, any other medications, or wheat.
- tell your doctor and pharmacist what other prescription and nonprescription medications, vitamins, nutritional supplements, and herbal products you are taking. Be sure to mention any of the following: antihistamines; digoxin (Lanoxin); ipratropium (Atrovent); medications for irritable bowel disease, motion sickness, Parkinson's disease, ulcers, or urinary problems; metformin (Glucophage); morphine (MSIR, Oramorph, others); procainamide; tenofovir (Viread); and vancomycin (Vancocin). Your doctor may need to change the doses of your medications or monitor you carefully for side effects.
- tell your doctor if you have or have ever had glaucoma (an eye disease that can cause vision loss); any type of blockage in the bladder or digestive system; myasthenia gravis (a disorder of the nervous system that causes muscle weakness); ulcerative colitis (sores in the intestine that cause stomach pain and diarrhea); benign prostatic hypertrophy (BPH, enlargement of the prostate, a male reproductive organ); or liver or kidney disease.
- tell your doctor if you are pregnant, plan to become pregnant, or are breast-feeding. If you become pregnant while taking trospium, call your doctor.
- if you are having surgery, including dental surgery, tell the doctor or dentist that you are taking trospium.
- you should know that trospium may make you drowsy or dizzy and may cause blurred vision. Do not drive a car or operate machinery until you know how this medication affects you.
- remember that alcohol can add to the drowsiness caused by this medication.
- you should know that trospium may make it harder for your body to cool down when it gets very hot. Avoid exposure to extreme heat, and call your doctor or get emergency medical treatment if you have fever or other signs of heat stroke such as dizziness, upset stomach, headache, confusion, and fast pulse after you are exposed to heat.

What special dietary instructions should I follow?

Unless your doctor tells you otherwise, continue your normal diet.

What should I do if I forget to take a dose?

Take the missed dose 1 hour before your next meal. However, if you are due to take your next dose at that time, skip the missed dose and continue your normal dosing schedule. Do not take a double dose to make up for a missed one.

What side effects can this medicine cause?

Trospium may cause side effects. Tell your doctor if any of these symptoms are severe or do not go away:

- dry mouth
- constipation
- headache

Some side effects can be serious. The following symptoms are uncommon, but if you experience any of them, call your doctor immediately:

- difficulty urinating
- rash
- hives
- itching
- difficulty breathing or swallowing

If you experience a serious side effect, you or your doctor may send a report to the Food and Drug Administration's (FDA) MedWatch Adverse Event Reporting program online [at http://www.fda.gov/MedWatch/index.html] or by phone [1-800-332-1088].

What storage conditions are needed for this medicine?

Keep this medication in the container it came in, tightly closed, and out of reach of children. Store it at room temperature and away from excess heat and moisture (not in the bathroom). Throw away any medication that is outdated or no longer needed. Talk to your pharmacist about the proper disposal of your medication.

What should I do in case of overdose?

In case of overdose, call your local poison control center at 1-800-222-1222. If the victim has collapsed or is not breathing, call local emergency services at 911.

Symptoms of overdose may include:

- fast heartbeat
- widened pupils (black circle in the middle of the eye)
- sensitivity to light

What other information should I know?

Keep all appointments with your doctor.

Do not let anyone else take your medication. Ask your pharmacist any questions you have about refilling your prescription.

Dosage Facts
For Informational Purposes

Caution: Do not change your dose, how often you take your medication, or the length of time you are to take it without first talking to your healthcare provider.

The following dosage information was written using medical language for doctors and other healthcare professionals and is provided here for you to check your dosage. The dosage of this drug may differ for different patients. Therefore, always follow your doctor's instructions or the directions on the label. Contact your healthcare provider or pharmacist if you have any questions about the specific dosage of your medication after reviewing this information.

General Dosage Information

Available as trospium chloride; dosage expressed in terms of the salt.

Adult Patients

Overactive Bladder

ORAL:
- 20 mg twice daily.

Special Populations

Hepatic Impairment
- Use caution in patients with moderate or severe hepatic impairment.

Renal Impairment
- In patients with severe renal impairment (Cl_{cr} <30 mL/minute), decrease dosage to 20 mg once daily at bedtime.

Geriatric Patients
- In geriatric patients ≥75 years of age, may decrease dosage to 20 mg once daily based on patient tolerance.

Ursodiol

(er′ soe dye ol)

Brand Name: Actigall®

Why is this medicine prescribed?

Ursodiol is used to dissolve gallstones in patients who do not want surgery or cannot have surgery to remove gallstones. Ursodiol is also used to prevent the formation of gallstones in overweight patients who are losing weight very quickly. Ursodiol is a bile acid, a substance naturally produced by the body that is stored in the gallbladder. It works by decreasing the production of cholesterol and by dissolving the cholesterol in bile so that it cannot form stones.

This medication is sometimes prescribed for other uses; ask your doctor or pharmacist for more information.

How should this medicine be used?

Ursodiol comes as a capsule to take by mouth. It is usually taken two or three times a day to treat gallstones and two times a day to prevent gallstones in patients who are losing weight quickly. Follow the directions on your prescription label carefully, and ask your doctor or pharmacist to explain any part you do not understand. Take ursodiol exactly as directed. Do not take more or less of it or take it more often than prescribed by your doctor.

This drug must be taken for months to have an effect. You may need to take ursodiol for up to 2 years. Your gallstones may not completely dissolve, and even if your gallstones do dissolve you may have gallstones again within 5 years after successful treatment with ursodiol. Continue to take ursodiol even if you feel well. Do not stop taking ursodiol without talking to your doctor.

What special precautions should I follow?

Before taking ursodiol,

- tell your doctor and pharmacist if you are allergic to ursodiol, bile acids, or any other drugs.
- tell your doctor and pharmacist what prescription and nonprescription medications you are taking, especially antacids that contain aluminum (Amphojel, Gaviscon, Maalox, Mylanta, others), cholestyramine (LoCHOLEST, Prevalite, Questran), clofibrate (Atromid-S), colestipol (Colestid), medications that lower lipid or cholesterol levels, medications that contain estrogen (including birth control pills), and vitamins and herbal products.
- tell your doctor if you have or have ever had disease of the liver, gallbladder, pancreas, or bile duct.
- tell your doctor if you are pregnant, plan to become pregnant, or are breast-feeding. If you become pregnant while taking ursodiol, call your doctor.

What should I do if I forget to take a dose?

Take the missed dose as soon as you remember it. However, if it is almost time for the next dose, skip the missed dose and continue your regular dosing schedule. Do not take a double dose to make up for a missed one.

What side effects can this medicine cause?

Side effects from ursodiol can occur. Tell your doctor if any of these symptoms are severe or do not go away:

- diarrhea
- constipation
- upset stomach
- indigestion
- dizziness
- vomiting
- cough

- sore throat
- runny nose
- back pain
- muscle and joint pain
- hair loss

If you experience any of the following symptoms, call your doctor immediately:

- frequent urination or pain when you urinate
- cough with fever

If you experience a serious side effect, you or your doctor may send a report to the Food and Drug Administration's (FDA) MedWatch Adverse Event Reporting program online [at http://www.fda.gov/MedWatch/index.html] or by phone [1-800-332-1088].

What storage conditions are needed for this medicine?

Keep this medication in the container it came in, tightly closed, and out of reach of children. Store it at room temperature and away from excess heat and moisture (not in the bathroom). Throw away any medication that is outdated or no longer needed. Talk to your pharmacist about the proper disposal of your medication.

What should I do in case of overdose?

In case of overdose, call your local poison control center at 1-800-222-1222. If the victim has collapsed or is not breathing, call local emergency services at 911.

What other information should I know?

Keep all appointments with your doctor and the laboratory. Your doctor will order blood tests to check your liver function every few months while you take ursodiol. You will also have a type of x-ray called ultrasound imaging to see how your gallstones are responding to ursodiol.

Do not let anyone else take your medication. Ask your pharmacist any questions you have about refilling your prescription.

Talk to your doctor, pharmacist, or other healthcare professional if you have questions about dosing information for your medication.

Valacyclovir

(val ay sye′ kloe veer)

Brand Name: Valtrex® Caplets

Why is this medicine prescribed?

Valacyclovir is used to treat herpes zoster (shingles) and genital herpes. It does not cure herpes infections but decreases pain and itching, helps sores to heal, and prevents new ones from forming.

This medication is sometimes prescribed for other uses; ask your doctor or pharmacist for more information.

How should this medicine be used?

Valacyclovir comes as a tablet to take by mouth. It is usually taken every 8 hours (three times a day) for 7 days to treat shingles. To treat genital herpes it is usually taken twice a day for 5 days. Follow the directions on your prescription label carefully, and ask your doctor or pharmacist to explain any part you do not understand. Take valacyclovir exactly as directed. Do not take more or less of it or take it more often than prescribed by your doctor. Use this medication as soon as possible after symptoms appear.

Continue to take valacyclovir even if you feel well. Do not stop taking valacyclovir without talking to your doctor.

What special precautions should I follow?

Before taking valacyclovir,

- tell your doctor and pharmacist if you are allergic to acyclovir (Zovirax), valacyclovir, or any other drugs.
- tell your doctor and pharmacist what prescription and nonprescription medications you are taking, especially cimetidine (Tagamet), probenecid (Benemid), and vitamins.
- tell your doctor if you have or have ever had kidney or liver disease, problems with your immune system, human immunodeficiency virus infection (HIV), or acquired immunodeficiency syndrome (AIDS).
- tell your doctor if you are pregnant, plan to become pregnant, or are breast-feeding. If you become pregnant while taking valacyclovir, call your doctor.

What should I do if I forget to take a dose?

Take the missed dose as soon as you remember it, and take any remaining doses for that day at evenly spaced intervals. However, if it is almost time for the next dose, skip the missed dose and continue your regular dosing schedule. Do not take a double dose to make up for a missed one.

What side effects can this medicine cause?

Valacyclovir may cause side effects. Tell your doctor if any of these symptoms are severe or do not go away:

- headache
- upset stomach
- vomiting
- diarrhea or loose stools
- constipation

If you experience any of the following side effects, call your doctor immediately:

- rash
- itching
- confusion
- yellowness of the skin or eyes
- fever
- blood in the urine

If you experience a serious side effect, you or your doctor may send a report to the Food and Drug Administration's (FDA) MedWatch Adverse Event Reporting program online [at http://www.fda.gov/MedWatch/index.html] or by phone [1-800-332-1088].

What storage conditions are needed for this medicine?

Keep this medication in the container it came in, tightly closed, and out of reach of children. Store it at room temperature and away from excess heat and moisture (not in the bathroom). Throw away any medication that is outdated or no longer needed. Talk to your pharmacist about the proper disposal of your medication.

What should I do in case of overdose?

In case of overdose, call your local poison control center at 1-800-222-1222. If the victim has collapsed or is not breathing, call local emergency services at 911.

What other information should I know?

Keep all appointments with your doctor and the laboratory. Your doctor will order certain lab tests to check your response to valacyclovir.

Do not have sexual intercourse when you can see the genital herpes lesions. However, genital herpes can be spread even when there are no symptoms.

Do not let anyone else take your medication. Ask your pharmacist any questions you have about refilling your prescription. If you still have symptoms of infection after you finish the valacyclovir, call your doctor.

Dosage Facts
For Informational Purposes

Caution: Do not change your dose, how often you take your medication, or the length of time you are to take it without first talking to your healthcare provider.

The following dosage information was written using medical language for doctors and other healthcare professionals and is provided here for you to check your dosage. The dosage of this drug may differ for different patients. Therefore, always follow your doctor's instructions or the directions on the label. Contact your healthcare provider or pharmacist if you have any questions about the specific dosage of your medication after reviewing this information.

General Dosage Information

Available as valacyclovir hydrochloride; dosage expressed in terms of valacyclovir.

Pediatric Patients

Genital Herpes, Herpes Labialis, Mucocutaneous Herpes Simplex Virus (HSV) Infections, and Herpes Zoster

ORAL:
- Adolescents should receive dosage recommended for adults.

Adult Patients

Genital Herpes
Treatment of First Episodes

ORAL:
- Immunocompetent adults: 1 g twice daily for 7–10 days. CDC suggests duration of treatment may be extended if healing is incomplete after 10 days.
- HIV-infected adults: 1 g twice daily for 7–14 days recommended by CDC and others.
- Initiate therapy within 48 hours of onset of signs and symptoms; efficacy not established if initiated >72 hours after onset of signs or symptoms.

Episodic Treatment of Recurrent Episodes

ORAL:
- Immunocompetent adults: 500 mg twice daily for 3 days. Alternatively, CDC recommends 1 g once daily for 5 days†.
- HIV-infected adults: CDC recommends 1 g twice daily for 5–10 days; may be continued for 7–14 days.
- Initiate therapy at first sign or symptom of an episode; efficacy not established if initiated >24 hours after onset of signs or symptoms.

Suppressive Therapy of Recurrent Episodes

ORAL:
- Immunocompetent adults: 1g once daily. Alternatively, 500 mg once daily for those with a history of ≤9 recurrences per year.
- HIV-infected adults: 500 mg twice daily.
- Manufacturer states safety and efficacy not established beyond a duration of 1 year in immunocompetent or 6 months in HIV-infected individuals.
- Because frequency of recurrent episodes diminishes over time in many patients, CDC and others recommend suppressive antiviral therapy be discontinued periodically (e.g., once yearly) to assess the need for continued therapy.

Reduction of Transmission

ORAL:
- 500 mg once daily in source partner with a history of ≤9 recurrences per year.
- Efficacy for reducing transmission not established beyond a duration of 8 months in discordant couples.

Herpes Labialis

ORAL:
- Immunocompetent adults: 2 g every 12 hours for 1 day; treatment for cold sores should not exceed 1 day.
- Initiate treatment at earliest symptom of cold sore (e.g., tingling, itching, burning); efficacy not established if initiated after development of clinical signs of cold sore (e.g., papule, vesicle, ulcer).

Mucocutaneous Herpes Simplex Virus (HSV) Infections
Chronic Suppression of Recurrent Episodes

ORAL:
- HIV-infected adults: 500 mg twice daily for chronic suppressive or maintenance therapy (secondary prophylaxis) of HSV infections in those who have frequent or severe recurrences.

Herpes Zoster

ORAL:
- Immunocompetent adults: 1 g 3 times daily for 7 days.
- Local dermatomal herpes zoster in HIV-infected adults or adolescents†: 1 g 3 times daily for 7–10 days recommended by CDC and others.
- Initiate therapy at earliest sign or symptom (preferably within 48 hours of rash onset); efficacy not established if initiated >72 hours after rash onset.

Special Populations

Hepatic Impairment
- Dosage adjustments not recommended for patients with cirrhosis.

Renal Impairment

Genital Herpes

ORAL:

Dosage for Treatment of Genital Herpes in Renal Impairment

Cl_{cr} (mL/min)	Daily Dosage
First Episodes	
≥50	1 g every 12 hours
30–49	1 g every 12 hours
10–29	1 g once every 24 hours
<10	500 mg once every 24 hours
Episodic Treatment of Recurrent Episodes	
≥50	500 mg every 12 hours
30–49	500 mg every 12 hours
10–29	500 mg once every 24 hours
<10	500 mg once every 24 hours
Suppressive Therapy of Recurrent Episodes (Immunocompetent with >9 Episodes/Year)	
≥50	1 g once every 24 hours
30–49	1 g once every 24 hours
10–29	500 mg once every 24 hours
<10	500 mg once every 24 hours
Suppressive Therapy of Recurrent Episodes (Immunocompetent with <9 Episodes/Year)	
≥50	500 mg once every 24 hours
30–49	500 mg once every 24 hours
10–29	500 mg once every 48 hours
<10	500 mg once every 48 hours
Suppressive Therapy of Recurrent Episodes (HIV-infected Individuals)	
≥50	500 mg every 12 hours
30–49	500 mg every 12 hours
10–29	500 mg once every 24 hours
<10	500 mg once every 24 hours

Herpes Labialis

ORAL:

Dosage for Treatment of Herpes Labialis in Renal Impairment

Cl_{cr} (mL/min)	Daily Dosage
≥50	2 g every 12 hours for 1 day
30–49	1 g every 12 hours for 1 day
10–29	500 mg every 12 hours for 1 day
<10	A single dose of 500 mg

Herpes Zoster

ORAL:

Dosage for Treatment of Herpes Zoster in Renal Impairment

Cl_{cr} (mL/min)	Daily Dosage
≥50	1 g every 8 hours
30–49	1 g every 12 hours
10–29	1 g once every 24 hours
<10	500 mg once every 24 hours

Hemodialysis

Usual dose should be administered after hemodialysis.

Peritoneal Dialysis

Supplemental doses unnecessary following CAPD or CAVHD.

Geriatric Patients
- No dosage adjustments except those related to renal impairment.

† Use is not currently included in the labeling approved by the US Food and Drug Administration.

Valganciclovir

(val gan sye′ kloh veer)

Brand Name: Valcyte®

Important Warning

Valganciclovir may lower the number of all types of cells in your blood, causing serious and life-threatening problems. Tell your doctor if you have or have ever had anemia (red blood cells do not bring enough oxygen to all parts of the body); neutropenia (less than normal number of white blood cells); thrombocytopenia (less than normal number of platelets); or other blood or bleeding problems. Tell your doctor if you have ever developed blood problems as a side effect of any medication. Tell your doctor and phar-

macist if you are taking or have taken any of the following medications: anticoagulants ('blood thinners') such as warfarin (Coumadin); cancer chemotherapy medications; dapsone; flucytosine, (Ancobon); heparin; immunosuppressants such as azathioprine (Azasan, Imuran), cyclosporine (Neoral, Sandimmune), methotrexate (Rheumatrex), sirolimus (Rapamune), and tacrolimus (Prograf); interferons (Infergen, Intron A, PEGASYS, PEG-Intron, Roferon-A); medications to treat human immunodeficiency virus (HIV) and acquired immunodeficiency syndrome (AIDS) including didanosine (Videx), zalcitabine (HIVID), or zidovudine (Retrovir, AZT); nonsteroidal anti-inflammatory medications to treat pain and swelling such as aspirin, ibuprofen (Advil, Motrin), naproxen (Aleve, Naprosyn), and others; pentamidine (NebuPent, Pentam); pyrimethamine (Daraprim, in Fansidar); steroids such as dexamethasone (Decadron), prednisone (Deltasone), or others; trimethoprim/sufamethoxazole (cotrimoxazole, Bactrim, Septra); or if you have received or are receiving radiation (X-ray) therapy. If you experience any of the following symptoms, call your doctor immediately: excessive tiredness; pale skin; headache; dizziness; confusion; fast heartbeat; difficulty falling asleep or staying asleep; weakness; shortness of breath; unusual bleeding or bruising; or sore throat, fever, chills, cough, or other signs of infection.

Keep all appointments with your doctor and the laboratory. Your doctor will order certain tests to check your body's response to valganciclovir.

Laboratory animals who were given valganciclovir developed birth defects. It is not known if valganciclovir causes birth defects in people. If you can become pregnant, you should use effective birth control while taking valganciclovir. If you are a man and your partner can become pregnant, you should use a condom while taking valganciclovir and for 90 days after your treatment. Talk to your doctor if you have questions about birth control. Do not take valganciclovir if you are pregnant or plan to become pregnant. If you become pregnant while taking valganciclovir, call your doctor immediately.

Laboratory animals who were given valganciclovir developed a lower sperm count (fewer male reproductive cells) and fertility problems. It is not known if valganciclovir causes lower sperm counts in men or problems with fertility in women.

Laboratory animals who were given valganciclovir developed cancer. It is not known if valganciclovir increases the risk of cancer in humans.

Talk to your doctor about the risks of taking valganciclovir.

Ask your pharmacist or doctor for a copy of the manufacturer's information for the patient and read it carefully before you start taking this medication and each time you get a refill.

Why is this medicine prescribed?

Valganciclovir is used to treat cytomegalovirus (CMV) retinitis (eye infection that can cause blindness) in people who have acquired immunodeficiency syndrome (AIDS). Valganciclovir is also used to prevent cytomegalovirus (CMV) disease in people who have received a heart, kidney, or kidney-pancreas transplant and who have a chance of getting CMV disease. Valganciclovir is in a class of medications called antivirals. It works by preventing the spread of CMV disease or slowing the growth of CMV.

How should this medicine be used?

Valganciclovir comes as a tablet to take by mouth. It is usually taken with food once or twice a day. To help you remember to take valganciclovir, take it around the same time(s) every day. Follow the directions on your prescription label carefully, and ask your doctor or pharmacist to explain any part you do not understand. Take valganciclovir exactly as directed. Do not take more or less of it or take it more often than prescribed by your doctor.

If you used to take ganciclovir (Cytovene), your doctor may have prescribed valganciclovir for you to take instead. Valganciclovir changes into ganciclovir in your body. However, valganciclovir tablets contain a different amount of medication and are taken differently than ganciclovir capsules. Do not take the same number of valganciclovir tablets at the same times that you used to take ganciclovir capsules Take valganciclovir according to the directions you were given by your doctor. Talk to your doctor or pharmacist if you have questions about taking valganciclovir.

Swallow the tablets whole; do not split, chew, break or crush them.

Be careful when handling valganciclovir tablets. Do not allow your skin, eyes, mouth, or nose to come into contact with broken or crushed valganciclovir tablets. If such contact occurs, wash your skin well with soap and water or rinse your eyes well with plain water.

Your doctor may start you on a high dose of valganciclovir and decrease your dose after several weeks. Valganciclovir does not cure CMV retinitis. You may develop CMV retinitis or your symptoms may get worse while you are taking valganciclovir. However, valganciclovir may prevent blindness caused by CMV retinitis. It is important that you see your doctor regularly and continue to take valganciclovir for as long as your doctor tells you that you should. Do not stop taking valganciclovir without talking to your doctor and try not to miss any doses. If you stop taking valganciclovir even for a short time, your condition may become worse and may be more difficult to treat.

Are there other uses for this medicine?

This medication may be prescribed for other uses; ask your doctor or pharmacist for more information.

What special precautions should I follow?

Before taking valganciclovir,
- tell your doctor and pharmacist if you are allergic to valganciclovir, acyclovir (Zovirax), ganciclovir (Cytovene or Cytovene-IV), or any other medications.
- do not take ganciclovir (Cytovene, Cytovene-IV) while you are taking valganciclovir.
- tell your doctor and pharmacist what other prescription and nonprescription medications, vitamins, nutritional supplements, and herbal products you are taking. Be sure to mention the medications listed in the IMPORTANT WARNING section and any of the following: aminoglycoside antibiotics such as amikacin (Amikin), gentamicin (Garamycin), neomycin (Neo-Rx, Neo-Fradin), netilmycin (Netromycin), streptomycin, tobramycin (Nebcin, Tobi), and others; amphotericin B (Fungizone); captopril (Capoten, in Capozide); diuretics ('water pills'); foscarnet (Foscavir); gold compounds such as auranofin (Ridaura) or aurothioglucose (Solganal); imipenem-cilastatin (Primaxin); immune globulin (gamma globulin, IGIV, BayGam, Carimmune, Gammagard, others): methicillin (Staphcillin); muromonab-CD3 (OKT3); mycophenolate mofetil (CellCept); nitrates such as isosorbide dinitrate (Isordil, Sorbitrate) or nitroglycerin products; penicillamine (Cuprimine, Depen); primaquine; probenecid; rifampin (Rifadin, Rimactane); or other nucleoside analogues such as acyclovir (Zovirax), famciclovir (Famvir), and ribavirin (Copegus, Rebetol, Virazole, in Rebetron). Your doctor may need to change the doses of your medications or monitor you carefully for side effects.
- tell your doctor if you have or have ever had the conditions mentioned in the IMPORTANT WARNING section or any of the following conditions: seizures; an eye problem other than CMV retinitis; high blood pressure; higher than normal calcium in your blood; kidney, or liver disease; or if you are being treated with hemodialysis (a special machine that removes waste products from blood).
- tell your doctor if you are breast-feeding. You should not breastfeed while taking valganciclovir. Talk to your doctor about when you may safely begin breastfeeding after you stop taking valganciclovir.
- if you are having surgery, including dental surgery, tell the doctor or dentist that you are taking valganciclovir.
- you should know that valganciclovir may make you drowsy, dizzy, unsteady, confused, less alert, or cause seizures. Do not drive a car or operate machinery until you know how this medication affects you.

What special dietary instructions should I follow?

Unless your doctor tells you otherwise, continue your normal diet.

What should I do if I forget to take a dose?

Take the missed dose as soon as you remember it. Then take the next dose at the usual scheduled time. However, if it is almost time for the next dose, skip the missed dose and continue your regular dosing schedule. Do not take a double dose to make up for a missed one.

What side effects can this medicine cause?

Valganciclovir may cause side effects. Tell your doctor if any of these symptoms are severe or do not go away:

- diarrhea
- upset stomach
- vomiting
- stomach pain
- loss of appetite
- thirst
- constipation
- headache
- back pain
- leg swelling
- trouble walking

Some side effects can be serious. The following symptoms are uncommon, but if you experience any of them or those listed in the IMPORTANT WARNING section, call your doctor immediately:

- seeing specks, flashes of light, or a dark curtain over everything
- decreased urination
- swelling of the hands, arms, feet, ankles, or lower legs
- hives
- rash
- itching
- yellowing of the skin or eyes
- shaking hands that you cannot control
- numbness, pain, burning, or tingling in the hands or feet
- seizures

Valganciclovir may cause other side effects. Call your doctor if you have any unusual problems while taking this medication.

If you experience a serious side effect, you or your doctor may send a report to the Food and Drug Administration's (FDA) MedWatch Adverse Event Reporting program online [at http://www.fda.gov/MedWatch/index.html] or by phone [1-800-332-1088].

What storage conditions are needed for this medicine?

Keep this medication in the container it came in, tightly closed, and out of reach of children. Store it at room temperature and away from excess heat and moisture (not in the bathroom). Throw away any medication that is outdated or no longer needed. Talk to your pharmacist about the proper disposal of your medication.

What should I do in case of overdose?

In case of overdose, call your local poison control center at 1-800-222-1222. If the victim has collapsed or is not breathing, call local emergency services at 911.

Symptoms of overdose may include:

- upset stomach
- vomiting
- stomach pain
- diarrhea

- shaking hands that you cannot control
- seizures
- decreased urination
- bloody urine
- sore throat, fever, chills, cough, or other signs of infection
- excessive tiredness
- pale skin
- yellowing of the skin or eyes
- headache
- dizziness
- confusion
- fast heartbeat
- difficulty falling asleep or staying asleep
- weakness
- shortness of breath
- unusual bleeding or bruising

What other information should I know?

Your doctor may order regular eye exams while you are taking this medication. Keep all appointments with the ophthalmologist (appointments for eye exams).

Before having any laboratory test, tell your doctor and the laboratory personnel that you are taking valganciclovir.

Do not let anyone else take your medication. Do not let your valganciclovir supply run out. Ask your pharmacist any questions you have about refilling your prescription.

Dosage Facts
For Informational Purposes

Caution: Do not change your dose, how often you take your medication, or the length of time you are to take it without first talking to your healthcare provider.

The following dosage information was written using medical language for doctors and other healthcare professionals and is provided here for you to check your dosage. The dosage of this drug may differ for different patients. Therefore, always follow your doctor's instructions or the directions on the label. Contact your healthcare provider or pharmacist if you have any questions about the specific dosage of your medication after reviewing this information.

General Dosage Information

Available as valganciclovir hydrochloride; dosage expressed in terms of valganciclovir.

Valganciclovir tablets and ganciclovir capsules are not bioequivalent; valganciclovir tablets cannot be substituted for ganciclovir capsules on a one-to-one basis.

Adult Patients
CMV Retinitis

ORAL:
- Initial (induction) therapy: 900 mg twice daily for 21 days.
- After completion of induction therapy or in patients with in-

active CMV retinitis, use a maintenance dosage of 900 mg once daily.

Prevention of CMV Disease in Transplant Recipients

ORAL:
- Kidney, heart, and kidney-pancreas transplant patients at high risk: 900 mg once daily starting within 10 days of transplantation and continued until 100 days posttransplantation.

Special Populations

Renal Impairment
- Adjust dosage if Cl_{cr} <60 mL/minute.

Dosage for Treatment of CMV Retinitis in Renal Impairment

Cl_{cr} (mL/min)	Induction Dosage	Maintenance Dosage
40–59	450 mg twice daily	450 mg once daily
25–39	450 mg once daily	450 mg every 2 days
10–24	450 mg every 2 days	450 mg twice weekly

No dosage recommendations for hemodialysis patients; do not use in patients undergoing hemodialysis (Cl_{cr} <10 mL/minute).

Valproic Acid

(val proe′ ik)

Brand Name: Depakene®, Depakote®, Depakote® ER, Depakote® Sprinkle
Also available generically.

Important Warning

Valproic acid may cause serious or life threatening damage to the liver. The risk of developing liver damage is greatest in children who are younger than 2 years old and in people who are taking more than one medication to prevent seizures, or who have any of the following conditions: a severe seizure disorder and mental retardation; certain inherited diseases that prevent the body from changing food to energy normally; any condition that affects the ability to think, learn, and understand; or liver disease. Tell your doctor or your child's doctor if you or your child have any of these conditions. Your child should not take any other medications to control seizures while he or she is taking valproic acid. If you notice that your seizures are more severe or happen more often or if you experience any of the following symptoms, call your doctor immediately: excessive tiredness, lack of

energy, weakness, stomach pain, loss of appetite, nausea, vomiting, or swelling of the face.

Valproic acid may cause serious or life-threatening damage to the pancreas. This may occur at any time during your treatment. If you experience any of the following symptoms, call your doctor immediately: stomach pain, nausea, vomiting, or loss of appetite.

Keep all appointments with your doctor and the laboratory. Your doctor will order certain lab tests to check your response to valproic acid.

Talk to your doctor about the risks of taking valproic acid or of giving valproic acid to your child.

Before you start to take valproic acid, tell your doctor if you are pregnant or plan to become pregnant. If you become pregnant while taking valproic acid, call your doctor immediately. Valproic acid can cause birth defects. Be sure to read the manufacturer's information for women who could become pregnant. Talk to your doctor about the risk of taking valproic acid during pregnancy.

Why is this medicine prescribed?

Valproic acid is used alone or with other medications to treat certain types of seizures. Valproic acid is also used to treat mania (episodes of frenzied, abnormally excited mood) in people with bipolar disorder (manic-depressive disorder; a disease that causes episodes of depression, episodes of mania, and other abnormal moods). It is also used to prevent migraine headaches, but not to relieve headaches that have already begun. Valproic acid is in a class of medications called anticonvulsants. It works by increasing the amount of a certain natural substance in the brain.

How should this medicine be used?

Valproic acid comes as a capsule, an extended-release (long-acting) tablet, a delayed-release (slow to begin working) tablet, a sprinkle capsule (capsule that contains small beads of medication that can be sprinkled on food), and a syrup (liquid) to take by mouth. The syrup, capsules, delayed-release tablets, and sprinkle capsules are usually taken two or more times daily. The extended-release tablets are usually taken once a day. Take valproic acid at around the same time(s) every day. Take valproic acid with food to help prevent the medication from upsetting your stomach. Follow the directions on your prescription label carefully, and ask your doctor or pharmacist to explain any part you do not understand. Take valproic acid exactly as directed. Do not take more or less of it or take it more often than prescribed by your doctor.

Swallow the regular capsules and extended-release tablets whole; do not split, chew, or crush them.

You can swallow the sprinkle capsules whole, or you can open the capsules and sprinkle the beads they contain on a teaspoonful of soft food, such as applesauce or pudding. Swallow the mixture of food and medication beads right after you prepare it. Be careful not to chew the beads. Do not store unused mixtures of food and medication.

Do not mix the syrup into any carbonated drink.

Your doctor may start you on a low dose of valproic acid and gradually increase your dose, not more often than once a week.

Valproic acid may help to control your condition but will not cure it. Continue to take valproic acid even if you feel well. Do not stop taking valproic acid without talking to your doctor. If you suddenly stop taking valproic acid, you may experience a severe, long-lasting and possibly life-threatening seizure. Your doctor will probably decrease your dose gradually.

Are there other uses for this medicine?

Valproic acid is also sometimes used to treat outbursts of aggression in children with attention deficit hyperactivity disorder (ADHD; more difficulty focusing or remaining still or quiet than other people who are the same age), chorea (a group of conditions that affect the ability to control body movements), and certain conditions that affect thinking, learning, and understanding. Talk to your doctor about the possible risks of using this medication for your condition.

This medication is sometimes prescribed for other uses. Ask your doctor or pharmacist for more information.

What special precautions should I follow?

Before taking valproic acid,

- tell your doctor and pharmacist if you are allergic to valproic acid any other medications, or any of the ingredients in the type of valproic acid that has been prescribed for you. Ask your pharmacist for a list of the ingredients.
- tell your doctor and pharmacist what prescription and nonprescription medications, vitamins, nutritional supplements, and herbal products you are taking or plan to take. Be sure to mention any of the following: acyclovir (Zovirax); antidepressants ('mood elevators') such as amitriptyline (Elavil) and nortriptyline (Pamelor); anticoagulants ('blood thinners') such as warfarin (Coumadin); aspirin; clonazepam (Klonopin); diazepam (Valium); medications for anxiety or mental illness; other medications for seizures such as carbamazepine (Tegretol), ethosuximide (Zarontin), felbamate (Felbatol), phenobarbital, phenytoin (Dilantin), primidone (Mysoline), lamotrigine (Lamictal), mephobarbital (Mebaral), and topiramate (Topamax); meropenem (Merrem IV); rifampin (Rifadin); sedatives; sleeping pills; tolbutamide; tranquilizers; and zidovudine (Retrovir). Your doctor may need to change the doses of your medications or monitor you carefully for side effects.
- tell your doctor if you have or have ever had a urea cycle disorder (one of a group of conditions that affect the ability to change protein from food into energy). Your doctor will probably tell you not to take valproic acid.
- tell your doctor if anyone in your family has ever had a urea cycle disorder or has died of unknown causes in the first months of life. Also tell your doctor if you have or have ever had episodes of vomiting, extreme tiredness and/or irritability; episodes of confusion and loss of ability to think and understand, especially during pregnancy or after childbirth; coma (loss of consciousness for a period of time); mental retardation; difficulty coordinating your movements; human immunodeficiency virus (HIV); cytomegalovirus (CMV; a virus that can cause symptoms in people who have weak immune systems); hyperlipidemia (higher than normal amount of fats in the blood); or kidney disease.

- tell your doctor if you are breast-feeding.
- if you are having surgery, including dental surgery, tell the doctor or dentist that you are taking valproic acid.
- you should know that valproic acid may make you drowsy. Do not drive a car or operate machinery until you know how this medication affects you.
- remember that alcohol can add to the drowsiness caused by this medication.

What special dietary instructions should I follow?

Unless your doctor tells you otherwise, continue your normal diet. Be sure to drink plenty of water or other liquids while you are taking valproic acid.

What should I do if I forget to take a dose?

Take the missed dose as soon as you remember it. However, if it is almost time for your next dose, skip the missed dose and continue your regular dosing schedule. Do not take a double dose to make up for a missed one.

What side effects can this medicine cause?

Valproic acid may cause side effects. Tell your doctor if any of these symptoms are severe or do not go away:

- drowsiness
- dizziness
- headache
- diarrhea
- constipation
- heartburn
- changes in appetite
- weight changes
- back pain
- agitation
- mood swings
- abnormal thinking
- memory loss
- uncontrollable shaking of a part of the body
- loss of coordination
- uncontrollable movements of the eyes
- blurred or double vision
- ringing in the ears
- stuffed or runny nose
- sore throat
- hair loss

Some side effects can be serious. If you experience any of the following symptoms or those listed in the IMPORTANT WARNING section, call your doctor immediately:

- unusual bruising or bleeding
- tiny purple spots on the skin
- fever
- blisters or rash
- itching
- hives
- confusion
- difficulty breathing or swallowing
- swollen glands
- weakness in the joints
- depression
- thinking about killing yourself or planning or trying to do so

Valproic acid may cause other side effects. Call your doctor if you have any unusual problems while taking this medication.

What storage conditions are needed for this medicine?

Keep this medication in the container it came in, tightly closed, and out of reach of children. Store it at room temperature, away from excess heat and moisture (not in the bathroom). Throw away any medication that is outdated or no longer needed. Talk to your pharmacist about the proper disposal of your medication.

What should I do in case of overdose?

In case of overdose, call your local poison control center at 1-800-222-1222. If the victim has collapsed or is not breathing, call local emergency services at 911.

Symptoms of overdose may include:

- sleepiness
- irregular heartbeat
- coma (loss of consciousness for a period of time)

What other information should I know?

If you are taking the sprinkle capsules, you may notice the medication beads in your stool. This is normal and does not mean that you did not get the full dose of medication.

If you have diabetes and your doctor has told you to test your urine for ketones, tell the doctor that you are taking valproic acid. Valproic acid can cause false results on urine tests for ketones.

Before having any laboratory test, tell your doctor and the laboratory personnel that you are taking valproic acid.

Do not let anyone else take your medication. Ask your pharmacist any questions you have about refilling your prescription.

Dosage Facts
For Informational Purposes

Caution: Do not change your dose, how often you take your medication, or the length of time you are to take it without first talking to your healthcare provider.

The following dosage information was written using medical language for doctors and other healthcare professionals and is provided here for you to check your dosage. The dosage of this drug may differ for different patients. Therefore, always follow your doctor's instructions or the directions on the label. Contact your healthcare provider or pharmacist if you have any questions about the specific dosage of your medication after reviewing this information.

General Dosage Information

Dosage of valproate sodium and divalproex sodium is expressed in terms of valproic acid.

Must adjust dosage carefully and slowly according to individual requirements and response.

An anticonvulsant therapeutic range of 50–100 mcg/mL has been suggested; seizure control occasionally may occur with lower or higher concentrations, but >150 mcg/mL usually is toxic.

For acute manic or mixed episodes in bipolar disorder, usually dosed to clinical response with trough plasma concentrations of 50–125 mcg/mL.

To minimize adverse GI effects, give dosages >250 mg daily in 2 or more divided doses.

When delayed-release tablets are administered, a twice-daily dosing regimen is suggested whenever feasible and appears to adequately maintain plasma valproic acid concentrations in most patients.

When extended-release tablets are administered, a once-daily dosing regimen is used.

If a patient misses a dose of extended-release tablets, take the dose as soon as possible, unless it is almost time for the next dose. If the patient skips a dose, do *not* take a double dose of extended-release tablets to make up for the missed dose.

When switching to divalproex sodium delayed-release tablets in patients receiving valproic acid, the same daily dose and schedule should be used.

After stabilization with divalproex sodium therapy, the daily dose may be divided and administered 2 or 3 times daily, in selected patients.

Frequency of adverse effects (particularly hepatic effects) may be dose related; weigh carefully the benefit of improved seizure control that may accompany higher dosages against the risk of adverse effects.

Pediatric Patients

Consider risk of increased fatal hepatotoxicity in children <2 years of age.

Neonates: Ability to eliminate valproic acid is markedly reduced.

Children 3 months to 10 years of age: Consider the possibility that the 50% increased clearance (on a proportionate weight basis) relative to older children and adults may affect dosage.

Children >10 years of age and adolescents: Pharmacokinetic parameters approximate those of adults.

Seizure Disorders
Complex Partial Seizures (Monotherapy and Adjunctive Therapy)

Dosages titrated up to 100 mg/kg daily in 3 or 4 divided doses may be needed in some patients, especially with concurrent enzyme inducers (e.g., phenytoin, carbamazepine).

ORAL (CONVENTIONAL AND DELAYED-RELEASE PREPARATIONS):

- Dosages apply to conventional (capsules and solution) and delayed-release (tablets) dosage forms of valproic acid (active moiety), valproate sodium, and disodium valproate.
- Initial dosage: 10–15 mg/kg daily.
- Increase valproic acid therapy by 5- to 10-mg/kg daily at weekly intervals, usually up to 60 mg/kg daily according to response.
- When used adjunctively, may continue concurrent anticonvulsant therapy, adjusting dosages according to response and tolerance.
- Alternatively, may attempt to decrease dosage of the current anticonvulsant by 25% every 2 weeks, either starting concomitantly with initiation of valproic acid therapy or delayed by 1–2 weeks if there is a concern that seizures are likely to occur with a reduction.
- Speed and duration of withdrawal of the current anticonvulsant can be highly variable; monitor patients closely during this period for increased seizure frequency.
- When converting a patient from a current anticonvulsant to valproic acid therapy for the treatment of complex partial seizures, valproic acid therapy should be initiated at usual starting doses.

Simple or Complex Absence Seizures

Dosages titrated up to 100 mg/kg daily in 3 or 4 divided doses may be needed in some patients, especially with concurrent enzyme inducers (e.g., phenytoin, carbamazepine).

ORAL (CONVENTIONAL AND DELAYED-RELEASE PREPARATIONS):

- Dosages apply to conventional (capsules and solution) and delayed-release (tablets) dosage forms of valproic acid (active moiety), valproate sodium, and disodium valproate.
- Initial dosage: 10–15 mg/kg daily.
- Increase by 5- to 10-mg/kg daily at weekly intervals, usually up to 60 mg/kg daily according to response.

Other Seizure Disorders†

Dosages titrated up to 100 mg/kg daily in 3 or 4 divided doses may be needed in some patients, especially with concurrent enzyme inducers (e.g., phenytoin, carbamazepine).

ORAL (CONVENTIONAL AND DELAYED-RELEASE PREPARATIONS):

- Dosages apply to conventional (capsules and solution) and delayed-release (tablets) dosage forms of valproic acid (active moiety), valproate sodium, and disodium valproate.
- Initial dosage: 10–15 mg/kg daily.
- Increase by 5- to 10-mg/kg daily at weekly intervals, usually up to 60 mg/kg daily according to response.

Adult Patients

Seizure Disorders
Complex Partial Seizures

Dosages titrated up to 100 mg/kg daily in 3 or 4 divided doses may be needed in some patients, especially with concurrent enzyme inducers (e.g., phenytoin, carbamazepine).

ORAL (CONVENTIONAL, DELAYED-, AND EXTENDED-RELEASE PREPARATIONS):

- Dosages apply to conventional (capsules and solution), delayed-release (tablets), and extended-release (tablets) dosage forms of valproic acid (active moiety), valproate sodium, and disodium valproate.
- Initial dosage: 10–15 mg/kg daily.

- Increase by 5- to 10-mg/kg daily at weekly intervals, usually up to 60 mg/kg daily according to response.
- When used adjunctively, may continue concurrent anticonvulsant therapy, adjusting dosages according to response and tolerance.
- Alternatively, may attempt to decrease dosage of the current anticonvulsant by 25% every 2 weeks, either starting concomitantly with initiation of valproic acid therapy or delayed by 1–2 weeks if there is a concern that seizures are likely to occur with a reduction.
- Speed and duration of withdrawal of the current anticonvulsant can be highly variable; monitor patients closely during this period for increased seizure frequency.

Simple or Complex Absence Seizures

Dosages titrated up to 100 mg/kg daily in 3 or 4 divided doses may be needed in some patients, especially with concurrent enzyme inducers (e.g., phenytoin, carbamazepine).

ORAL (CONVENTIONAL, DELAYED-, AND EXTENDED-RELEASE PREPARATIONS):

- Dosages apply to conventional (capsules and solution), delayed-release (tablets), and extended-release (tablets) dosage forms of valproic acid (active moiety), valproate sodium, and disodium valproate.
- Initial dosage: 15 mg/kg daily.
- Increase by 5- to 10-mg/kg daily at weekly intervals, usually up to 60 mg/kg daily according to response.

Seizure Disorders
Conversion from Delayed-release (Depakote®) to Extended-release (Depakote® ER) Tablets

ORAL:

- When converting a patient whose seizure disorder is controlled with delayed-release tablets (Depakote®) to the extended-release tablets (Depakote® ER), give the drug once daily using a total daily dose that is 8–20% higher than the corresponding delayed-release dosage that the patient was receiving.
- For patients whose delayed-release daily dosage cannot be directly converted to a corresponding commercially available extended-release dosage, consider increasing the delayed-release total daily dosage to the next higher dosage before converting to the appropriate extended-release dosage.

Other Seizure Disorders†

Dosages titrated up to 100 mg/kg daily in 3 or 4 divided doses may be needed in some patients, especially with concurrent enzyme inducers (e.g., phenytoin, carbamazepine).

ORAL (CONVENTIONAL, DELAYED-, AND EXTENDED-RELEASE PREPARATIONS):

- Dosages apply to conventional (capsules and solution), delayed-release (tablets), and extended-release (tablets) dosage forms of valproic acid (active moiety), valproate sodium, and disodium valproate.
- Initial dosage: 10–15 mg/kg daily.
- Increase by 5- to 10-mg/kg daily at weekly intervals, usually up to 60 mg/kg daily according to response.

Bipolar Disorder
Manic or Mixed Episodes

ORAL:

- Initially, 750 mg daily in divided doses as delayed-release tablets or 25 mg/kg once daily as extended-release tablets for acute episodes.

- For acute episodes, increase dosage as quickly as possible to achieve the lowest therapeutic dose producing the desired clinical effect or desired serum concentration; however, the manufacturer recommends that the dose not exceed 60 mg/kg daily.
- Usually dosed to clinical response with trough plasma concentrations of 50–125 mcg/mL.
- Efficacy beyond 3 weeks not systematically evaluated; if continued, periodically reevaluate long-term usefulness and risk for the individual patient.
- Safety for longer-term antimanic therapy is supported by data from record reviews involving approximately 360 patients treated for >3 months.
- Dosing guidelines for maintenance therapy† are less evidence-based than those for acute therapy, and dosages lower than those employed for acute therapy occasionally have been used.

Migraine Prophylaxis
With or without Aura
ORAL:
- Initially, 250 mg *twice* daily as delayed-release tablets (Depakote®) or 500 mg *once* daily as extended-release tablets (Depakote® ER).
- Maintenance: After 1 week at the initial dosage, may titrate according to response up to 1 g daily; no evidence of additional benefit with higher dosages.
- If a patient requires smaller dosage adjustment than that available using the extended-release tablets, use the delayed-release tablets instead.

Schizophrenia†
ORAL:
- In general, for adjunctive therapy, administer in the same dosages, and with the same resulting therapeutic plasma concentrations, as those for the management of seizure disorders.

Prescribing Limits
Pediatric Patients
Seizure Disorders
ORAL:
- Usual maximum recommended dosage is 60 mg/kg daily; up to 100 mg/kg daily may be necessary in some patients, but monitor plasma concentrations.

Adult Patients
Seizure Disorders
ORAL:
- Usual maximum recommended dosage is 60 mg/kg daily; up to 100 mg/kg daily may be necessary in some patients, but monitor plasma concentrations.

Bipolar Disorder
Manic or Mixed Episodes
ORAL:
- Maximum recommended dosage is 60 mg/kg daily.

Migraine Prophylaxis
With or without Aura
ORAL:
- Maximum recommended dosage is 1 g daily.

Special Populations
Hepatic Impairment
- Decreased clearance.

- Because of decreased protein binding, monitoring *total* (bound + unbound) drug concentrations may be misleading.

Renal Impairment
- Decreased (by 27%) clearance of unbound (active) drug.
- Dosage adjustment does not appear necessary.
- Because of decreased protein binding, monitoring *total* (bound + unbound) drug concentrations may be misleading.

Neonates
- Markedly decreased ability to eliminate the drug in patients ≤2 months of age.
- Refractory seizures: Oral loading dose of 20 mg/kg, followed by 10 mg/kg every 12 hours.
- Consider risk of increased fatal hepatotoxicity in children <2 years of age.

Geriatric Patients
- Starting dosage should be reduced because of a decrease in clearance of unbound valproic acid; subsequent dosage should be increased more slowly in geriatric patients.
- Consider dosage reduction or discontinuance in geriatric patients with decreased food or fluid intake and in those with excessive somnolence.
- Determine ultimate therapeutic dosage on the basis of tolerability and clinical response.

Gender
- No dosage adjustment based solely on gender.

Race
- Potential effects not studied.

† Use is not currently included in the labeling approved by the US Food and Drug Administration.

Valsartan
(val sar′ tan)

Brand Name: Diovan®, Diovan® HCT as a combination product containing Valsartan and Hydrochlorothiazide

> ## Important Warning
>
> Do not take valsartan if you are pregnant. If you become pregnant while taking valsartan, call your doctor immediately. Valsartan may harm the fetus.

Why is this medicine prescribed?
Valsartan is used alone or in combination with other medications to treat high blood pressure. It is also used to treat heart failure in people who cannot take angiotensin-converting enzyme (ACE) inhibitors. Valsartan is in a class of medications called angiotensin II receptor antagonists. It works by blocking the action of certain chemicals that tighten the blood vessels, so blood flows more smoothly.

How should this medicine be used?

Valsartan comes as a tablet to take by mouth. For the treatment of high blood pressure, it is usually taken once a day with or without food. For the treatment of heart failure, it is usually taken twice a day with or without food. To help you remember to take valsartan, take it around the same time every day. Follow the directions on your prescription label carefully, and ask your doctor or pharmacist to explain any part you do not understand. Take valsartan exactly as directed. Do not take more or less of it or take it more often than prescribed by your doctor.

Your doctor may start you on a low dose of valsartan and gradually increase your dose.

Valsartan controls high blood pressure and heart failure but does not cure them. Continue to take valsartan even if you feel well. Do not stop taking valsartan without talking to your doctor.

Are there other uses for this medicine?

This medication may be prescribed for other uses; ask your doctor or pharmacist for more information.

What special precautions should I follow?

Before taking valsartan,

- tell your doctor and pharmacist if you are allergic to valsartan or any other medications.
- tell your doctor and pharmacist what prescription and nonprescription medications, vitamins, nutritional supplements, and herbal products you are taking. Be sure to mention the following: angiotensin-converting enzyme (ACE) inhibitors such as benazepril (Lotensin), captopril (Capoten), enalapril (Vasotec), fosinopril (Monopril), lisinopril (Prinivil, Zestril), moexipril (Univasc), perindopril (Aceon), quinapril (Accupril), ramipril (Altace), and trandolapril (Mavik); beta blockers such as atenolol (Tenormin), labetalol (Normodyne), metoprolol (Lopressor, Toprol XL), nadolol (Corgard), and propranolol (Inderal); and diuretics ('water pills'). Your doctor may need to change the doses of your medications or monitor you carefully for side effects.
- tell your doctor if you have or have ever had kidney or liver disease.
- tell your doctor if you plan to become pregnant or are breast-feeding.

What special dietary instructions should I follow?

If your doctor prescribes a low-salt or low-sodium diet, follow these directions carefully.

What should I do if I forget to take a dose?

Take the missed dose as soon as you remember it. However, if it is almost time for the next dose, skip the missed dose and continue your regular dosing schedule. Do not take a double dose to make up for a missed one.

What side effects can this medicine cause?

Valsartan may cause side effects. Tell your doctor if any of these symptoms are severe or do not go away:

- dizziness
- headache
- excessive tiredness
- diarrhea
- stomach pain
- back pain
- joint pain

Some side effects can be serious. The following symptoms are uncommon, but if you experience any of them, call your doctor immediately:

- swelling of the face, throat, tongue, lips, eyes, hands, feet, ankles, or lower legs
- hoarseness
- difficulty breathing or swallowing
- fainting

Valsartan may cause other side effects. Call your doctor if you have any unusual problems while taking this medication.

If you experience a serious side effect, you or your doctor may send a report to the Food and Drug Administration's (FDA) MedWatch Adverse Event Reporting program online [at http://www.fda.gov/MedWatch/index.html] or by phone [1-800-332-1088].

What storage conditions are needed for this medicine?

Keep this medication in the container it came in, tightly closed, and out of reach of children. Store it at room temperature and away from excess heat and moisture (not in the bathroom). Throw away any medication that is outdated or no longer needed. Talk to your pharmacist about the proper disposal of your medication.

What should I do in case of overdose?

In case of overdose, call your local poison control center at 1-800-222-1222. If the victim has collapsed or is not breathing, call local emergency services at 911.

Symptoms of overdose may include:

- dizziness
- fainting
- rapid or pounding heartbeat

What other information should I know?

Keep all appointments with your doctor and the laboratory. Your blood pressure should be checked regularly to determine your response to valsartan.

Do not let anyone else take your medication. Ask your pharmacist any questions you have about refilling your prescription.

Dosage Facts
For Informational Purposes

Caution: Do not change your dose, how often you take your medication, or the length of time you are to take it without first talking to your health-care provider.

The following dosage information was written using medical language for doctors and other healthcare professionals and is provided here for you to check your dosage. The dosage of this drug may differ for different patients. Therefore, always follow your doctor's instructions or the directions on the label. Contact your healthcare provider or pharmacist if you have any questions about the specific dosage of your medication after reviewing this information.

Adult Patients

Hypertension
Monotherapy

ORAL:
- Initially, 80 or 160 mg once daily in adults without intravascular volume depletion. Adjust dosage at approximately monthly intervals (more aggressively in high-risk patients) to achieve BP control.
- Usual dosage: 80–320 mg given once daily. However, at dosages >80 mg daily, addition of diuretic produces greater BP reduction than increases in valsartan dosage.

Combination Therapy

ORAL:
- If BP is not adequately controlled by monotherapy with valsartan, can switch to fixed-combination tablets once daily (valsartan 80 or 160 mg and hydrochlorothiazide 12.5 mg; then valsartan 160 mg and hydrochlorothiazide 12.5 mg or valsartan 160 mg and hydrochlorothiazide 25 mg, if BP remains uncontrolled after about 3–4 weeks of therapy).
- If BP is not adequately controlled by monotherapy with hydrochlorothiazide 25 mg or if BP is controlled but hypokalemia is problematic at this dosage, can switch to the fixed-combination tablets once daily (valsartan 80 or 160 mg and hydrochlorothiazide 12.5 mg; then valsartan 160 mg and hydrochlorothiazide 25 mg, if BP remains uncontrolled after about 3–4 weeks of therapy).

CHF

ORAL:
- Initially, 40 mg twice daily. Increase dosage to 160 mg twice daily (maximum dosage used in clinical trials) or highest tolerated dosage.

Special Populations

Hepatic Impairment
- No initial dosage adjustments necessary in patients with mild to moderate hepatic impairment. Cautious dosing recommended in those with severe impairment.

Renal Impairment
- No initial dosage adjustments necessary in patients with mild to moderate renal impairment. Cautious dosing recommended in those with severe impairment.

Geriatric Patients
- No initial dosage adjustments necessary.

Volume- and/or Salt-Depleted Patients
- Correct volume and/or salt depletion prior to initiation of therapy or initiate therapy under close medical supervision.

Vancomycin
(van koe mye' sin)

Brand Name: Vancocin®
Also available generically.

Why is this medicine prescribed?

Vancomycin is used to treat colitis (inflammation of the intestine caused by certain bacteria) that may occur after antibiotic treatment. Vancomycin is in a class of medications called glycopeptide antibiotics. It works by killling bacteria in the intestines. Vancomycin will not kill bacteria or treat infections in any other part of the body when taken by mouth. Antibiotics will not work for colds, flu, or other viral infections.

How should this medicine be used?

Vancomycin comes as a capsule to take by mouth. It is usually taken 3-4 times a day for 7-10 days. To help you remember to take vancomycin, take it around the same times every day. Follow the directions on your prescription label carefully, and ask your doctor or pharmacist to explain any part you do not understand. Take vancomycin exactly as directed. Do not take more or less of it or take it more often than prescribed by your doctor.

Take vancomycin until you finish the prescription, even if you feel better. If you stop taking vancomycin too soon or miss doses, your infection may not be completely cured and bacteria may become resistant to antibiotics.

Are there other uses for this medicine?

This medication should not be prescribed for other uses; ask your doctor or pharmacist for more information.

What special precautions should I follow?

Before taking vancomycin,
- tell your doctor and pharmacist if you are allergic to vancomycin, or any other medications.
- tell your doctor and pharmacist what prescription and nonprescription medications, vitamins, nutritional supplements, and herbal products you are taking. Be sure to mention amikacin (Amikin), amphotericin B (Fungizone), bacitracin, cisplatin (Platinol), colistin, gentamicin (Garamycin), kanamycin (Kantrex), polymyxin B, streptomycin, and tobramycin (Nebcin).
- tell your doctor if you have or have ever had inflammatory bowel disease (swelling of the intestine that can

cause painful cramps or diarrhea), including Crohn's disease and ulcerative colitis; hearing loss; or kidney disease.

- tell your doctor if you are pregnant, plan to become pregnant, or are breast-feeding. If you become pregnant while taking Vancomycin, call your doctor.

What special dietary instructions should I follow?

Unless your doctor tells you otherwise, continue your normal diet.

What should I do if I forget to take a dose?

Take the missed dose as soon as you remember it. However, if it is almost time for the next dose, skip the missed dose and continue your regular dosing schedule. Do not take a double dose to make up for a missed one.

What side effects can this medicine cause?

Vancomycin may cause side effects. Tell your doctor if this symptom is severe or does not go away:

- upset stomach

Some side effects can be serious. The following symptoms are uncommon, but if you experience any of them, call your doctor immediately:

- sore throat, fever, chills, and other signs of infection
- hives
- skin rash
- itching
- difficulty breathing or swallowing
- redness of the skin above the waist
- pain and muscle tightness of the chest and back
- unusual bleeding or bruising
- fainting
- dizziness
- blurred vision
- ringing in the ears

If you experience a serious side effect, you or your doctor may send a report to the Food and Drug Administration's (FDA) MedWatch Adverse Event Reporting program online [at http://www.fda.gov/MedWatch/index.html] or by phone [1-800-332-1088].

What storage conditions are needed for this medicine?

Keep this medication in the container it came in, tightly closed, and out of reach of children. Store it at room temperature and away from excess heat and moisture (not in the bathroom). Throw away any medication that is outdated or no longer needed. Talk to your pharmacist about the proper disposal of your medication.

What should I do in case of overdose?

In case of overdose, call your local poison control center at 1-800-222-1222. If the victim has collapsed or is not breathing, call local emergency services at 911.

What other information should I know?

Keep all appointments with your doctor.

Do not let anyone else take your medication. Your prescription is probably not refillable. If you still have symptoms of infection after you finish the vancomycin, call your doctor.

Dosage Facts
For Informational Purposes

Caution: Do not change your dose, how often you take your medication, or the length of time you are to take it without first talking to your healthcare provider.

The following dosage information was written using medical language for doctors and other healthcare professionals and is provided here for you to check your dosage. The dosage of this drug may differ for different patients. Therefore, always follow your doctor's instructions or the directions on the label. Contact your healthcare provider or pharmacist if you have any questions about the specific dosage of your medication after reviewing this information.

General Dosage Information

Available as vancomycin hydrochloride; dosage expressed in terms of vancomycin.

Pediatric Patients

Clostridium difficile-associated Diarrhea and Colitis

ORAL:
- 40 mg/kg given in 3 or 4 divided doses for 7–10 days.

Staphylococcal Enterocolitis

ORAL:
- 40 mg/kg given in 3 or 4 divided doses for 7–10 days.

Prescribing Limits
Pediatric Patients

Maximum 2 g daily.

For treatment of endocarditis, AHA and IDSA state pediatric dosage should not exceed recommended adult dosage.

Adult Patients

Maximum 2 g daily.

For treatment of endocarditis, AHA and IDSA recommend maximum 2 g daily unless serum concentrations are inappropriately low. These experts recommend dosage be adjusted to obtain peak serum concentrations (1 hour after completion of IV infusion) of 30–45 mcg/mL and trough concentrations of 10–15 mcg/mL.

Special Populations

Hepatic Impairment
- Limited data suggest dosage adjustments not necessary.

Geriatric Patients
• Cautious dosage selection (usually starting at the low end of the dosing range) because of age-related decreases in renal function.

† Use is not currently included in the labeling approved by the US Food and Drug Administration.

Vardenafil
(var den′ a fil)

Brand Name: Levitra®

Why is this medicine prescribed?

Vardenafil is used to treat erectile dysfunction (impotence; inability to get or keep an erection) in men. Vardenafil is in a class of medications called phosphodiesterase (PDE) inhibitors. It works by increasing blood flow to the penis during sexual stimulation. This increased blood flow can cause an erection. Vardenafil does not cure erectile dysfunction or increase sexual desire. Vardenafil does not prevent pregnancy or the spread of sexually transmitted diseases such as human immunodeficiency virus (HIV).

How should this medicine be used?

Vardenafil comes as a tablet to take by mouth. It is usually taken as needed, with or without food, 60 minutes before sexual activity. Vardenafil usually should not be taken more often than once every 24 hours. If you have certain health conditions or are taking certain medications, your doctor may tell you to take vardenafil less often. Follow the directions on your prescription label carefully, and ask your doctor or pharmacist to explain any part you do not understand. Take vardenafil exactly as directed. Do not take more or less of it or take it more often than prescribed by your doctor.

Your doctor will probably start you on an average dose of vardenafil and increase or decrease your dose depending on your response to the medication. Tell your doctor if vardenafil is not working well or if you are experiencing side effects.

Are there other uses for this medicine?

This medication may be prescribed for other uses; ask your doctor or pharmacist for more information.

What special precautions should I follow?

Before taking vardenafil,
• tell your doctor and pharmacist if you are allergic to vardenafil or any other medications.
• do not take vardenafil if you are taking or have recently taken nitrates such as isosorbide dinitrate (Isordil), isosorbide mononitrate (Imdur, ISMO), and nitroglycerin (Nitro-BID, Nitro-Dur, Nitroquick, Nitrostat, others). Nitrates come as tablets, sublingual (under the tongue)

tablets, sprays, patches, pastes, and ointments. Ask your doctor if you are not sure if any of your medications contain nitrates.
• do not take street drugs containing nitrates such as amyl-nitrate and butyl nitrate ('poppers') while taking vardenafil.
• tell your doctor and pharmacist what other prescription and nonprescription medications, vitamins, and nutritional supplements you are taking or plan to take. Be sure to mention any of the following: alpha blockers such as alfuzosin (Uroxatral), doxazosin (Cardura), prazosin (Minipress), tamsulosin (Flomax), and terazosin (Hytrin); amiodarone (Cordarone); antifungals such as fluconazole (Diflucan), griseofulvin (Fulvicin, Grifulvin, Gris-PEG), itraconazole (Sporanox), and ketoconazole (Nizoral); aprepitant (Emend); carbamazepine (Carbatrol, Epitol, Tegretol); clarithromycin (Biaxin); cyclosporine (Neoral, Sandimmune); danazol (Danocrine); delavirdine (Rescriptor); dexamethasone (Decadron, Dexpak); diltiazem (Cardizem, Dilacor, Tiazac); disopyramide (Norpace); efavirenz (Sustiva); erythromycin (E.E.S., E-Mycin, Erythrocin); fluoxetine (Prozac, Sarafem); fluvoxamine (Luvox); HIV protease inhibitors including atazanavir (Reyataz), indinavir (Crixivan), lopinavir (in Kaletra), nelfinavir (Viracept), ritonavir (Norvir, in Kaletra), and saquinavir (Fortovase, Invirase); isoniazid (INH, Nydrazid); lovastatin (Altocor, Mevacor); medications for high blood pressure or irregular heartbeat; metronidazole (Flagyl); nevirapine (Viramune); other medications or treatments for erectile dysfunction; nefazodone (Serzone); paroxetine (Paxil); phenobarbital; phenytoin (Dilantin, Phenytek); procainamide (Procanbid, Pronestyl); quinidine (Quinidex); rifabutin (Mycobutin); rifampin (Rifadin, Rimactane, in Rifamate); sertraline (Zoloft); sotalol (Betapace); troleandomycin (TAO); verapamil (Calan, Covera, Isoptin, Verelan); and zafirlukast (Accolate). Your doctor may need to change the doses of your medications or monitor you carefully for side effects.
• tell your doctor what herbal products you are taking, especially St. John's wort.
• tell your doctor if you smoke and if you have ever had an erection that lasted more than 4 hours. Also tell your doctor if you have or have ever had a condition that affects the shape of the penis, such as angulation, cavernosal fibrosis, or Peyronie's disease; diabetes; high cholesterol; high or low blood pressure; irregular heartbeat; a heart attack; angina (chest pain); a stroke; ulcers in the stomach or intestine; a bleeding disorder; blood cell problems such as sickle cell anemia (a disease of the red blood cells), multiple myeloma (cancer of the plasma cells), or leukemia (cancer of the white blood cells); and liver, kidney, or heart disease. Also tell your doctor if you or any of your family members have or have ever had long QT syndrome (a heart condition) or retinitis pigmentosus (an eye disease) or if you have ever had severe vision loss, especially if you were told

that the vision loss was caused by a blockage of blood flow to the nerves that help you see. Tell your doctor if you have ever been advised by a health care professional to avoid sexual activity for medical reasons.

- you should know that vardenafil is only for use in males. Women should not take vardenafil, especially if they are or could become pregnant or are breast-feeding. If a pregnant woman takes vardenafil, she should call her doctor.
- if you are having surgery, including dental surgery or any dental procedure, tell the doctor or dentist that you are taking vardenafil.
- you should know that sexual activity may be a strain on your heart, especially if you have heart disease. If you have chest pain during sexual activity, call your doctor immediately and avoid sexual activity until your doctor tells you otherwise.
- tell all your health care providers that you are taking vardenafil. If you ever need emergency medical treatment for a heart problem, the health care providers who treat you will need to know when you last took vardenafil.

What special dietary instructions should I follow?

Talk to your doctor about eating grapefruit or drinking grapefruit juice while taking this medicine.

What side effects can this medicine cause?

Vardenafil may cause side effects. Tell your doctor if any of these symptoms are severe or do not go away:
- headache
- upset stomach
- heartburn
- dizziness
- flushing
- stuffy or runny nose
- flu-like symptoms

Some side effects can be serious. If you experience any of the following symptoms, call your doctor immediately:
- erection that lasts longer than 4 hours
- sudden severe loss of vision (see below for more information)
- blurred vision
- changes in color vision (seeing blue tinge on objects, difficulty telling the difference between blue and green, or difficulty seeing at night)
- swelling of the face, throat, tongue, lips, eyes, hands, feet, ankles, or lower legs
- hoarseness
- difficulty breathing or swallowing
- fainting
- hives
- rash

Vardenafil may cause other side effects. Call your doctor if you have any unusual problems while taking this medication.

Some patients experienced a sudden loss of some or all of their vision after they took vardenafil or other medications that are similar to vardenafil. The vision loss was permanent in some cases. It is not known if the vision loss was caused by the medication. If you experience a sudden loss of vision while you are taking vardenafil, call your doctor immediately. Do not take any more doses of vardenafil or similar medications such as sildenafil (Viagra) or tadalafil until you talk to your doctor.

If you experience a serious side effect, you or your doctor may send a report to the Food and Drug Administration's (FDA) MedWatch Adverse Event Reporting program online [at http://www.fda.gov/MedWatch/index.html] or by phone [1-800-332-1088].

What storage conditions are needed for this medicine?

Keep this medication in the container it came in, tightly closed, and out of reach of children. Store it at room temperature and away from excess heat and moisture (not in the bathroom). Throw away any medication that is outdated or no longer needed. Talk to your pharmacist about the proper disposal of your medication.

What should I do in case of overdose?

In case of overdose, call your local poison control center at 1-800-222-1222. If the victim has collapsed or is not breathing, call local emergency services at 911.

Symptoms of overdose may include:
- back or muscle pain
- blurred vision

What other information should I know?

Keep all appointments with your doctor.

Do not let anyone else take your medication. Ask your pharmacist any questions you have about refilling your prescription.

Dosage Facts
For Informational Purposes

Caution: Do not change your dose, how often you take your medication, or the length of time you are to take it without first talking to your healthcare provider.

The following dosage information was written using medical language for doctors and other healthcare professionals and is provided here for you to check your dosage. The dosage of this drug may differ for different patients. Therefore, always follow your doctor's instructions or the directions on the label. Contact your healthcare provider or pharmacist if you have any questions about the specific dosage of your medication after reviewing this information.

General Dosage Information

Available as vardenafil hydrochloride; dosage expressed in terms of vardenafil.

Adult Patients

Erectile Dysfunction

ORAL:
- Initially, 10 mg. Depending on effectiveness and tolerance, increase dosage to a maximum of 20 mg or decrease to 5 mg. Administer no more frequently than once daily.

Prescribing Limits

Adult Patients

Erectile Dysfunction

ORAL:
- Maximum 20 mg daily.

Special Populations

Hepatic Impairment
- In patients with moderate hepatic impairment (Child-Pugh class B), decrease initial dosage to 5 mg; maximum dosage is 10 mg once daily. Not studied in patients with severe hepatic impairment (Child-Pugh class C).

Renal Impairment
- Dosage adjustments not required in patients with patients with mild (Cl_{cr} of 50–80 mL/minute) to severe (Cl_{cr} <30 mL/minute) renal impairment. Not studied in patients requiring renal dialysis.

Geriatric Patients
- Reduce initial dose to 5 mg given no more frequently than once daily in men ≥65 years of age.

Varenicline

(var en′ i kleen)

Brand Name: Chantix®

Why is this medicine prescribed?

Varenicline is used to help people stop smoking. Varenicline is in a class of medications called smoking cessation aids. It works by blocking the pleasant effects of nicotine (from smoking) on the brain.

How should this medicine be used?

Varenicline comes as a tablet to take by mouth. It is usually taken once or twice a day with a full glass of water after eating. Take varenicline at around the same time(s) every day. If you are taking varenicline twice a day, take one dose in the morning and one dose in the evening. Follow the directions on your prescription label carefully, and ask your doctor or pharmacist to explain any part you do not understand. Take varenicline exactly as directed. Do not take more or less of it or take it more often than prescribed by your doctor.

Your doctor will probably start you on a low dose of varenicline and gradually increase your dose over the first week of treatment.

Set a quit date to stop smoking, and start taking var-

enicline 1 week before that date. You may continue to smoke during this first week, but make sure to try to stop smoking on the date you have chosen.

It may take several weeks for you to feel the full benefit of varenicline. You may slip and smoke during your treatment. If this happens, you may still be able to stop smoking. Continue to take varenicline and to try not to smoke.

You will probably take varenicline for 12 weeks. If you have completely stopped smoking at the end of 12 weeks, your doctor may tell you to take varenicline for another 12 weeks. This may help keep you from starting to smoke again.

If you have not stopped smoking at the end of 12 weeks, talk to your doctor. Your doctor can try to help you understand why you were not able to stop smoking and make plans to try to quit again.

Are there other uses for this medicine?

This medication may be prescribed for other uses; ask your doctor or pharmacist for more information.

What special precautions should I follow?

Before taking varenicline,
- tell your doctor and pharmacist if you are allergic to varenicline or any other medications.
- tell your doctor and pharmacist what prescription and nonprescription medications, vitamins, nutritional supplements, and herbal products you are taking or plan to take. Be sure to mention any of the following: anticoagulants ('blood thinners') such as warfarin (Coumadin); insulin; other medications to help you stop smoking such as bupropion (Wellbutrin, Zyban) and nicotine gum, inhaler, lozenges, nasal spray, or skin patches; and theophylline (TheoDur). Your doctor may need to change the doses of some of your medications once you stop smoking.
- tell your doctor if you have or have ever had kidney disease.
- tell your doctor if you are pregnant, plan to become pregnant, or are breast-feeding. If you become pregnant while taking varenicline, call your doctor.
- ask your doctor for advice and for written information to help you stop smoking. You are more likely to stop smoking during your treatment with varenicline if you get information and support from your doctor.

What special dietary instructions should I follow?

Unless your doctor tells you otherwise, continue your normal diet.

What should I do if I forget to take a dose?

Take the missed dose as soon as you remember it. However, if it is almost time for the next dose, skip the missed dose and continue your regular dosing schedule. Do not take a double dose to make up for a missed one.

What side effects can this medicine cause?

Varenicline may cause side effects. Tell your doctor if any of these symptoms are severe or do not go away:

- nausea
- constipation
- gas
- vomiting
- heartburn
- bad taste in the mouth
- increased or decreased appetite
- trouble falling asleep or staying asleep
- abnormal dreams or nightmares
- drowsiness
- headache
- rash

Varenicline may cause other side effects. Call your doctor if you have any unusual problems while taking this medication.

What storage conditions are needed for this medicine?

Keep this medication in the container it came in, tightly closed, and out of reach of children. Store it at room temperature and away from excess heat and moisture (not in the bathroom). Throw away any medication that is outdated or no longer needed. Talk to your pharmacist about the proper disposal of your medication.

What should I do in case of overdose?

In case of overdose, call your local poison control center at 1-800-222-1222. If the victim has collapsed or is not breathing, call local emergency services at 911.

What other information should I know?

Keep all appointments with your doctor.

Do not let anyone else take your medication. Ask your pharmacist any questions you have about refilling your prescription.

Dosage Facts
For Informational Purposes

Caution: Do not change your dose, how often you take your medication, or the length of time you are to take it without first talking to your healthcare provider.

The following dosage information was written using medical language for doctors and other healthcare professionals and is provided here for you to check your dosage. The dosage of this drug may differ for different patients. Therefore, always follow your doctor's instructions or the directions on the label. Contact your healthcare provider or pharmacist if you have any questions about the specific dosage of your medication after reviewing this information.

General Dosage Information

Available as varenicline tartrate; dosage expressed in terms of varenicline.

Adult Patients

Smoking Cessation

ORAL:

- 0.5 mg once daily on days 1–3, followed by 0.5 mg twice daily on days 4–7, and then 1 mg twice daily from day 8 through the end of 12 weeks of treatment. Initiate 1 week before the target smoking cessation date.
- Titrate dosage during the initial week of treatment to reduce the incidence of drug-related nausea. Dosage may be reduced temporarily or permanently in patients who experience intolerable adverse effects.
- In patients who have successfully stopped smoking by the end of 12 weeks of initial treatment, consider an additional 12 weeks of therapy to increase the likelihood of long-term abstinence.
- Patients unable to quit smoking during 12 weeks of treatment or those who have relapsed after varenicline therapy should make another attempt to quit smoking once factors responsible for such failure have been identified and addressed.

Prescribing Limits

Adult Patients

ORAL:
- 1 mg twice daily.

Special Populations

Hepatic Impairment
- No dosage adjustment is needed in patients with hepatic impairment.

Renal Impairment
- No dosage adjustment needed in patients with mild to moderate renal impairment.
- If Cl_{cr} is <30 mL/minute, initially administer 0.5 mg once daily; titrate dosage as needed to a maximum of 0.5 mg twice daily.
- In patients with end-stage renal disease undergoing hemodialysis, maximum dosage is 0.5 mg once daily.

Geriatric Patients
- Select dosage carefully and monitor renal function.

Varicella (Chickenpox) Vaccine

Brand Name: Varivax®, ProQuad®

Why get vaccinated?

Chickenpox (also called varicella) is a common childhood disease. It is usually mild, but it can be serious, especially in young infants and adults.

- It causes a rash, itching, fever, and tiredness.

- It can lead to severe skin infection, scars, pneumonia, brain damage, or death.
- The chickenpox virus can be spread from person to person through the air, or by contact with fluid from chickenpox blisters.
- A person who has had chickenpox can get a painful rash called shingles years later.
- Before the vaccine, about 11,000 people were hospitalized for chickenpox each year in the United States.
- Before the vaccine, about 100 people died each year as a result of chickenpox in the United States.

Chickenpox vaccine can prevent chickenpox. Most people who get chickenpox vaccine will not get chickenpox. But if someone who has been vaccinated does get chickenpox, it is usually very mild. They will have fewer blisters, are less likely to have a fever, and will recover faster.

Who should get chickenpox vaccine and when?

Routine
- Children who have never had chickenpox should get 2 doses of chickenpox vaccine at these ages: 12-15 months of age, and 4-6 years of age (may be given earlier, if at least 3 months after the 1st dose)
- People 13 years of age and older (who have never had chickenpox or received chickenpox vaccine) should get two doses at least 28 days apart.

Catch-Up
- Children or adolescents who are not fully vaccinated should receive one or two doses of chickenpox vaccine. The timing of these doses depends on the person's age. Ask your provider. Chickenpox vaccine may be given at the same time as other vaccines.

Note: Chickenpox vaccine may be given along with measles-mumps-rubella (MMR) vaccine in a combination vaccine called MMRV.

Who should *not* get chickenpox vaccine or should wait?

- People should not get chickenpox vaccine if they have ever had a life-threatening allergic reaction to gelatin, the antibiotic neomycin, or a previous dose of chickenpox vaccine.
- People who are moderately or severely ill at the time the shot is scheduled should usually wait until they recover before getting chickenpox vaccine.
- Pregnant women should wait to get chickenpox vaccine until after they have given birth. Women should not get pregnant for 1 month after getting chickenpox vaccine.
- Some people should check with their doctor about whether they should get chickenpox vaccine, including anyone who: has HIV/AIDS or another disease that affects the immune system; is being treated with drugs that affect the immune system, such as steroids, for 2 weeks or longer; has any kind of cancer; is getting cancer treatment with radiation or drugs.

- People who recently had a transfusion or were given other blood products should ask their doctor when they may get chickenpox vaccine.

What are the risks from chickenpox vaccine?

Getting chickenpox vaccine is much safer than getting chickenpox disease. Most people who get chickenpox vaccine do not have any problems with it. However, a vaccine, like any medicine, is capable of causing serious problems, such as severe allergic reactions. The risk of chickenpox vaccine causing serious harm, or death, is extremely small.

Mild Problems:
- Soreness or swelling where the shot was given (about 1 out of 5 children and up to 1 out of 3 adolescents and adults)
- Fever (1 person out of 10, or less)
- Mild rash, up to a month after vaccination (1 person out of 20, or less). It is possible for these people to infect other members of their household, but this is extremely rare.
- Note: MMRV vaccine has been associated with higher rates of fever (up to about 1 person in 5) and measles-like rash (about 1 person in 20) than MMR and varicella vaccines given separately.

Moderate Problems:
- Seizure (jerking or staring) caused by fever (less than 1 person out of 1,000).

Severe Problems:
- Pneumonia (very rare)
- Other serious problems, including severe brain reactions and low blood count, have been reported after chickenpox vaccination. These happen so rarely experts cannot tell whether they are caused by the vaccine or not. If they are, it is extremely rare.

What if there is a moderate or severe reaction?

What should I look for?
- Any unusual condition, such as a high fever or behavior changes. Signs of a serious allergic reaction can include difficulty breathing, hoarse ness or wheezing, hives, paleness, weakness, a fast heart beat or dizziness.

What should I do?
- Call a doctor, or get the person to a doctor right away.
- Tell your doctor what happened, the date and time it happened, and when the vaccination was given.
- Ask your health care provider to file a Vaccine Adverse Event Reporting System (VAERS) form if you have any reaction to the vaccine. Or call VAERS yourself at 1-800-822-7967, or visit their website at http://vaers.hhs.gov.

The National Vaccine Injury Compensation Program

In the rare event that you or your child has a serious reaction to a vaccine, a federal program has been created to help pay for the care of those who have been harmed.

For details about the National Vaccine Injury Compensation Program, call 1-800-338-2382 or visit the program's website at http://www.hrsa.gov/vaccinecompensation.

How can I learn more?

- Ask your doctor or other health care provider. They can give you the vaccine package insert or suggest other sources of information.
- Call your local or state health department's immunization program.
- Contact the Centers for Disease Control and Prevention (CDC): call 1-800-232-4636 (1-800-CDC-INFO) or visit the National Immunization Program's website at http://www.cdc.gov/nip.

Varicella Vaccine Information Statement. U.S. Department of Health and Human Services/Centers for Disease Control and Prevention National Immunization Program. 1/10/2007.

Venlafaxine

(ven′ la fax een)

Brand Name: Effexor®, Effexor® XR
Also available generically.

Important Warning

A small number of children, teenagers, and young adults (up to 24 years of age) who took antidepressants ('mood elevators') such as venlafaxine during clinical studies became suicidal (thinking about harming or killing oneself or planning or trying to do so). Children, teenagers, and young adults who take antidepressants to treat depression or other mental illnesses may be more likely to become suicidal than children, teenagers, and young adults who do not take antidepressants to treat these conditions. However, experts are not sure about how great this risk is and how much it should be considered in deciding whether a child or teenager should take an antidepressant. Children younger than 18 years of age should not normally take venlafaxine, but in some cases, a doctor may decide that venlafaxine is the best medication to treat a child's condition.

You should know that your mental health may change in unexpected ways when you take venlafaxine or other antidepressants even if you are an adult over age 24. You may become suicidal, especially at the beginning of your treatment and any time that your dose is increased or decreased. You, your family, or your caregiver should call your doctor right away if you experience any of the following symptoms: new or worsening depression; thinking about harming or killing yourself, or planning or trying to do so; extreme worry; agitation; panic attacks; difficulty falling asleep or staying asleep; aggressive behavior; irritability; acting without thinking; severe restlessness; and frenzied abnormal excitement. Be sure that your family or caregiver knows which symptoms may be serious so they can call the doctor when you are unable to seek treatment on your own.

Your healthcare provider will want to see you often while you are taking venlafaxine, especially at the beginning of your treatment. Be sure to keep all appointments for office visits with your doctor.

The doctor or pharmacist will give you the manufacturer's patient information sheet (Medication Guide) when you begin treatment with venlafaxine. Read the information carefully and ask your doctor or pharmacist if you have any questions. You also can obtain the Medication Guide from the FDA website: http://www.fda.gov/cder/drug/antidepressants/antidepressants_MG_2007.pdf.

No matter your age, before you take an antidepressant, you, your parent, or your caregiver should talk to your doctor about the risks and benefits of treating your condition with an antidepressant or with other treatments. You should also talk about the risks and benefits of not treating your condition. You should know that having depression or another mental illness greatly increases the risk that you will become suicidal. This risk is higher if you or anyone in your family has or has ever had bipolar disorder (mood that changes from depressed to abnormally excited) or mania (frenzied, abnormally excited mood) or has thought about or attempted suicide. Talk to your doctor about your condition, symptoms, and personal and family medical history. You and your doctor will decide what type of treatment is right for you.

Why is this medicine prescribed?

Venlafaxine is used to treat depression. Venlafaxine extended-release (long-acting) capsules are also used to treat generalized anxiety disorder (excessive worrying that is difficult to control), social anxiety disorder (extreme fear of interacting with others or performing in front of others that interferes with normal life), and panic disorder (sudden, unexpected attacks of extreme fear and worry about these attacks). Venlafaxine is in a class of medications called selective serotonin and norepinephrine reuptake inhibitors (SNRIs). It works by increasing the amounts of serotonin and norepinephrine, natural substances in the brain that help maintain mental balance.

How should this medicine be used?

Venlafaxine comes as a tablet or extended-release capsule to take by mouth. The tablet is usually taken two or three times a day with food. The extended-release capsule is usually taken once daily in the morning or evening with food. Take venlafaxine at around the same time(s) every day. Follow the directions on your prescription label carefully, and ask your doctor or pharmacist to explain any part you do not understand. Take venlafaxine exactly as directed. Do not take more or less of it or take it more often or for a longer period of time than prescribed by your doctor.

Swallow the extended-release capsule whole; do not split, chew or crush it, or place it in water. If you cannot swallow the extended-release capsule, you may carefully open the capsule and sprinkle the entire contents on a spoonful of applesauce. Swallow (without chewing) this mixture immediately after preparation and then drink a glass of water to make sure that you have swallowed all of the medication.

Your doctor will probably start you on a low dose of venlafaxine and gradually increase your dose, not more often than once every 4 to 7 days. Tell your doctor how you are feeling during your treatment so that your doctor can adjust your dose properly.

Venlafaxine controls depression but does not cure it. It may take 6 to 8 weeks or longer for you to feel the full benefit of this medication. Continue to take venlafaxine even if you feel well. Do not stop taking venlafaxine without talking to your doctor. Your doctor will probably decrease your dose gradually. If you suddenly stop taking venlafaxine, you may experience withdrawal symptoms such as agitation; anxiety; confusion; sad mood; irritability; frenzied or abnormal excitement; lack of coordination; trouble falling asleep or staying asleep; nightmares; nausea; vomiting; loss of appetite; diarrhea; dry mouth; sweating; ringing in the ears; seizures; or burning, tingling, numbness, or electric shock-like feelings in any part of the body. Tell your doctor if you experience any of these symptoms while you are decreasing your dose of venlafaxine or soon after you stop taking venlafaxine.

Are there other uses for this medicine?

Venlafaxine is also sometimes used to treat hot flashes (hot flushes; sudden strong feelings of heat and sweating) in women who have experienced menopause ('change of life'; the end of monthly menstrual periods) or who are taking medication to treat breast cancer. Talk to your doctor or pharmacist about the risks of using venlafaxine to treat your condition.

This medication is sometimes prescribed for other uses; ask your doctor or pharmacist for more information.

What special precautions should I follow?

Before taking venlafaxine,
- tell your doctor and pharmacist if you are allergic to venlafaxine, any other medications, or any of the ingredients in venlafaxine tablets or extended-release capsules. Ask your pharmacist for a list of the ingredients.
- tell your doctor if you are taking a monoamine oxidase (MAO) inhibitor, such as isocarboxazid (Marplan), phenelzine (Nardil), selegiline (Eldepryl, Emsam, Zelapar), and tranylcypromine (Parnate), or if you have stopped taking one of these medications within the past 14 days.

Your doctor will probably tell you that you should not take venlafaxine. If you stop taking venlafaxine, your doctor will tell you that you should wait at least 7 days before you start to take an MAO inhibitor.
- tell your doctor and pharmacist what other prescription and nonprescription medications, vitamins, or nutritional supplements you are taking or plan to take. Be sure to mention any of the following: anticoagulants ('blood thinners') such as warfarin (Coumadin); amiodarone (Cordarone, Pacerone); other antidepressants; cimetidine (Tagamet); clozapine (Clozaril); diuretics ('water pills'); duloxetine (Cymbalta); haloperidol (Haldol); imipramine (Tofranil); indinavir (Crixivan); ketoconazole (Nizoral); linezolid (Zyvox); lithium; medications for anxiety, mental illness, pain, seizures, or weight loss; medications for migraine such as almotriptan (Axert), eletriptan (Relpax), frovatriptan (Frova), naratriptan (Amerge), rizatriptan (Maxalt), sumatriptan (Imitrex), and zolmitriptan (Zomig); methadone (Dolophine); phentermine (Adipex P, Ionamin); ritonavir (Norvir); sedatives; selective serotonin reuptake inhibitors (SSRIs) such as citalopram (Celexa), fluoxetine (Prozac, Sarafem), fluvoxamine (Luvox), paroxetine (Paxil), and sertraline (Zoloft); sleeping pills; tramadol (Ultram); and tranquilizers. Your doctor may need to change the doses of your medications or monitor you carefully for side effects.
- tell your doctor what nutritional supplements and herbal products you are taking, especially St. John's wort and tryptophan.
- tell your doctor if you have ever used illegal drugs or overused prescription medications. Also tell your doctor if you have recently had a heart attack and if you have or have ever had high blood pressure, high blood cholesterol glaucoma (an eye disease), high pressure in the eyes (a condition that can lead to glaucoma), seizures, or heart, kidney, liver, or thyroid disease.
- tell your doctor if you are pregnant, plan to become pregnant, or are breast-feeding. If you become pregnant while taking venlafaxine, call your doctor.
- if you are having surgery, including dental surgery, tell the doctor or dentist that you are taking venlafaxine.
- you should know that this medication may make you drowsy. Do not drive a car or operate machinery until you know how this medication affects you.
- remember that alcohol can add to the drowsiness caused by this medication.

What special dietary instructions should I follow?

Unless your doctor tells you otherwise, continue your normal diet.

What should I do if I forget to take a dose?

Take the missed dose as soon as you remember it. However, if it is almost time for your next dose, skip the missed dose and continue your regular dosing schedule. Do not take a double dose to make up for a missed one. If you are taking the extended-release capsules, do not take more than one dose per day.

What side effects can this medicine cause?

Venlafaxine may cause side effects. Call your doctor if any of the following symptoms are severe or do not go away:

- drowsiness
- weakness or tiredness
- dizziness
- headache
- nightmares
- nausea
- vomiting
- stomach pain
- constipation
- diarrhea
- gas
- heartburn
- burping
- dry mouth
- change in ability to taste food
- loss of appetite
- weight loss
- uncontrollable shaking of a part of the body
- pain, burning, numbness, or tingling in part of the body
- muscle tightness
- twitching
- yawning
- sweating
- hot flashes or flushing
- frequent urination
- difficulty urinating
- sore throat, chills, or other signs of infection
- ringing in the ears
- changes in sexual desire or ability
- enlarged pupils (black circles in the middle of the eyes)

Some side effects can be serious. If you experience any of the following symptoms or those listed in the IMPORTANT WARNING section, call your doctor immediately:

- rash
- hives
- itching
- difficulty breathing or swallowing
- chest pain
- fast, pounding, or irregular heartbeat
- seizures
- unusual bruising or bleeding
- small purple spots on the skin
- eye pain or redness
- changes in vision
- fever
- problems with coordination
- hallucinations (seeing things or hearing voices that do not exist)
- coma (loss of consciousness for a period of time)

Venlafaxine may slow growth and weight gain in chil-

dren. If your child is taking venlafaxine, your child's doctor will watch your child's growth carefully. Talk to your child's doctor about the risks of giving venlafaxine to your child.

Venlafaxine may cause other side effects. Call your doctor if you have any unusual problems while you are taking this medication.

What storage conditions are needed for this medicine?

Keep this medication in the container it came in, tightly closed, and out of reach of children. Store it at room temperature and away from excess heat and moisture (not in the bathroom). Throw away any medication that is outdated or no longer needed. Talk to your pharmacist about the proper disposal of your medication.

What should I do in case of overdose?

In case of overdose, call your local poison control center at 1-800-222-1222. If the victim has collapsed or is not breathing, call local emergency services at 911.

Symptoms of overdose may include:

- dizziness
- nausea
- vomiting
- burning, tingling, or numbness of the hands and feet
- increased size of the pupil (black center of the eye)
- muscle pain
- hot and cold spells
- sleepiness
- seizures
- fast, slow, or irregular heartbeat
- coma (loss of consciousness for a period of time)

What other information should I know?

Keep all appointments with your doctor and the laboratory. Your doctor will check your blood pressure often and order certain lab tests to check your response to venlafaxine.

Do not let anyone else take your medication. Ask your pharmacist any questions you have about refilling your prescription.

Dosage Facts
For Informational Purposes

Caution: Do not change your dose, how often you take your medication, or the length of time you are to take it without first talking to your healthcare provider.

The following dosage information was written using medical language for doctors and other healthcare professionals and is provided here for you to check your dosage. The dosage of this drug may differ for different patients. Therefore, always follow your doctor's instructions or the directions on the label. Contact your healthcare provider or pharmacist if you have any questions about the specific dosage of your medication after reviewing this information.

General Dosage Information

Available as venlafaxine hydrochloride; dosage expressed in terms of venlafaxine.

Adult Patients

Major Depressive Disorder

ORAL:
- Initially, 75 mg daily administered in 2 or 3 divided doses as conventional tablets or as a single daily dose when using the extended-release capsules. Alternatively, an initial dosage of 37.5 mg daily as extended-release capsules for the first 4–7 days (followed by an increase to 75 mg daily) may be considered for some patients. If no improvement, dosage may be increased by increments of up to 75 mg daily at intervals of not less than 4 days up to a maximum dosage of 375 mg daily (usually administered in 3 divided doses) as conventional tablets or 225 mg daily as extended-release capsules..
- No additional benefit demonstrated from dosages >225 mg daily as conventional tablets in clinical studies in moderately depressed outpatients, but patients with more severe depression responded to higher dosages (mean dosage of 350 mg daily).
- If desired, conventional tablets may be switched to the extended-release capsules at the nearest equivalent daily venlafaxine dosage (e.g., change 37.5 mg administered twice daily as conventional tablets to 75-mg extended-release capsule administered once daily). Individualize dosage adjustments as necessary.
- Optimum duration not established; may require several months of therapy or longer. Antidepressant efficacy demonstrated for up to 6 months with venlafaxine extended-release capsules and for up to 1 year with conventional tablets.
- Periodically reassess need for continued therapy and appropriateness of dosage.

Generalized Anxiety Disorder

ORAL:
- Initially, 75 mg once daily as extended-release capsules. In some patients, it may be desirable to initiate therapy with a dosage of 37.5 mg daily given for the first 4–7 days, followed by an increase to 75 mg daily. If no improvement, dosage may be increased in increments of up to 75 mg daily (up to a maximum dosage of 225 mg daily as extended-release capsules) at intervals of not less than 4 days.
- Optimum duration not established; efficacy demonstrated in a 6-month clinical trial. Periodically reassess need for continued therapy.

Social Phobia

ORAL:
- Initially, 75 mg once daily as extended-release capsules. In some patients, it may be desirable to initiate therapy with a dosage of 37.5 mg daily given for the first 4–7 days, followed by an increase to 75 mg daily. If no improvement, dosage may be increased in increments of up to 75 mg daily (up to a maximum dosage of 225 mg daily as extended-release capsules) at intervals of not less than 4 days.
- Optimum duration not established; long-term efficacy (>12 weeks) not demonstrated. Periodically reassess need for continued therapy.

Panic Disorder

ORAL:
- Initially, 37.5 mg once daily as extended-release capsules for 7 days. If no improvement, increase dosage may be increased

in increments of up to 75 mg daily at intervals of not less than 7 days. In clinical trials, 37.5 mg once daily was given initially for 7 days, then 75 mg once daily for 7 days; thereafter, dosage was increased in increments of 75 mg daily every 7 days if necessary. Certain patients not responding to 75 mg once daily may benefit from dosage increases up to a maximum of approximately 225 mg daily.
- Optimum duration not established; longer-term efficacy (>12 weeks) in prolonging time to relapse in responding patients demonstrated in a controlled trial. Periodically reassess need for continued therapy.

Vasomotor Symptoms†

Optimum dosage for vasomotor symptoms† in women with breast cancer and in postmenopausal women not established. Initially, some clinicians recommend 37.5 mg once daily as extended-release capsules; may increase as necessary to 75 mg once daily. 75 mg once daily as extended-release capsules appeared optimal in one study. Further dosage increases may not provide additional benefit but are potentially more toxic.

Prescribing Limits

Adult Patients

Major Depression

ORAL:
- Maximum 375 mg daily (generally in 3 equally divided doses) as conventional tablets or 225 mg daily as extended-release capsules.

Generalized Anxiety Disorder

ORAL:
- Maximum 225 mg daily as extended-release capsules.

Social Phobia

ORAL:
- Maximum 225 mg daily as extended-release capsules.

Panic Disorder

ORAL:
- Maximum 225 mg daily as extended-release capsules.

Special Populations

Hepatic Impairment

ORAL:
- Extended-release capsules: Reduce initial dosage by 50% in patients with moderate hepatic impairment.
- Conventional tablets: Reduce total daily dosage by 50% in patients with moderate hepatic impairment.
- In patients with cirrhosis, may be desirable to individualize dosages. May be necessary to reduce dosage of conventional tablets by >50%.

Renal Impairment

ORAL:
- When using conventional tablets or extended-release capsules, reduce total daily dosage by 25–50% in patients with mild-to-moderate renal impairment and by 50% in those undergoing hemodialysis. Withhold dosages until the dialysis period is complete (4 hours).

† *Use is not currently included in the labeling approved by the US Food and Drug Administration.*

Verapamil

(ver ap′ a mil)

Brand Name: Calan®, Calan® SR Caplets®, Covera-HS®, Isoptin® SR, Verelan®, Verelan® PM

Also available generically.

Why is this medicine prescribed?

Verapamil is used to treat irregular heartbeats (arrhythmias) and high blood pressure. It relaxes your blood vessels so your heart does not have to pump as hard. It also increases the supply of blood and oxygen to the heart to control chest pain (angina). If taken regularly, verapamil controls chest pain, but it does not stop chest pain once it starts. Your doctor may give you a different medication to take when you have chest pain.

This medication is sometimes prescribed for other uses; ask your doctor or pharmacist for more information.

How should this medicine be used?

Verapamil comes as a regular tablet and as an extended-release (long-acting) tablet and capsule to take by mouth. The regular tablet is usually taken three times a day. The extended-release tablet and capsule are usually taken one or two times a day and should be swallowed whole. Do not chew, divide, or crush the extended-release tablet or capsule. Follow the directions on your prescription label carefully, and ask your doctor or pharmacist to explain any part you do not understand. Take verapamil exactly as directed. Do not take more or less of it or take it more often than prescribed by your doctor.

Verapamil controls arrhythmias, high blood pressure, and chest pain (angina) but does not cure them. Continue to take verapamil even if you feel well. Do not stop taking verapamil without talking to your doctor.

Are there other uses for this medicine?

Verapamil is also used sometimes to treat migraine headaches and cardiomyopathy. Talk to your doctor about the possible risks of using this drug for your condition.

What special precautions should I follow?

Before taking verapamil,

- tell your doctor and pharmacist if you are allergic to verapamil or any other drugs.
- tell your doctor and pharmacist what prescription and nonprescription medications you are taking, especially aspirin, carbamazepine (Tegretol); cyclosporine (Neoral, Sandimmune); fentanyl (Duragesic); heart and blood pressure medications such as beta-blockers, digoxin (Lanoxin), disopyramide (Norpace), flecainide (Tambocor), quinidine (Quinaglute, Quinidex), diuretics ('water pills'), or any other blood pressure lowering medication; lithium (Eskalith, Lithobid); medications to treat depression; medications to treat glaucoma (increased pressure in the eye); phenobarbital; rifampin (Rifadin, Rimactane); theophylline (Theo-Dur); and vitamins.
- tell your doctor if you have or have ever had heart, liver, or kidney disease, muscular dystrophy, or gastrointestinal obstruction (strictures).
- tell your doctor if you are pregnant, plan to become pregnant, or are breast-feeding. If you become pregnant while taking verapamil, call your doctor.
- if you are having surgery, including dental surgery, tell your doctor or dentist that you are taking verapamil.
- you should know that verapamil may increase the effects of alcohol and make them last longer.

What special dietary instructions should I follow?

Verapamil may cause an upset stomach. Take verapamil with food or milk.

Talk to your doctor before using salt substitutes containing potassium. If your doctor prescribes a low-salt or low-sodium diet, follow these directions carefully.

What should I do if I forget to take a dose?

Take the missed dose as soon as you remember it. However, if it is almost time for the next dose, skip the missed dose and continue your regular dosing schedule. Do not take a double dose to make up for a missed one.

What side effects can this medicine cause?

Verapamil may cause side effects. Tell your doctor if any of these symptoms are severe or do not go away:

- constipation
- dizziness or lightheadedness
- headache
- upset stomach
- heartburn
- excessive tiredness
- flushing (feeling of warmth)
- slow heartbeat
- vivid, unusual dreams

If you experience any of the following symptoms, call your doctor immediately:

- swelling of the face, eyes, lips, tongue, arms, or legs
- difficulty breathing or swallowing
- fainting
- rash
- yellowing of the skin or eyes
- fever
- increase in frequency or severity of chest pain (angina)

If you experience a serious side effect, you or your doctor may send a report to the Food and Drug Administration's (FDA) MedWatch Adverse Event Reporting program online [at http://www.fda.gov/MedWatch/index.html] or by phone [1-800-332-1088].

What storage conditions are needed for this medicine?

Keep this medication in the container it came in, tightly closed, and out of reach of children. Store it at room temperature and away from excess heat and moisture (not in the bathroom). Throw away any medication that is outdated or no longer needed. Talk to your pharmacist about the proper disposal of your medication.

What should I do in case of overdose?

In case of overdose, call your local poison control center at 1-800-222-1222. If the victim has collapsed or is not breathing, call local emergency services at 911.

What other information should I know?

Keep all appointments with your doctor and the laboratory. Your blood pressure should be checked regularly to determine your response to verapamil.

Your doctor may ask you to check your pulse (heart rate) daily and will tell you how fast it should be. If your pulse is slower than it should be, call your doctor for directions on taking verapamil that day. Ask your doctor or pharmacist to teach you how to check your pulse.

The extended-release tablet (Covera) does not dissolve in the stomach after being swallowed. It slowly releases medicine as it passes through the small intestines. It is not unusual to see the tablet shell eliminated in the stool.

Do not let anyone else take your medication. Ask your pharmacist any questions you have about refilling your prescription.

Dosage Facts
For Informational Purposes

Caution: Do not change your dose, how often you take your medication, or the length of time you are to take it without first talking to your healthcare provider.

The following dosage information was written using medical language for doctors and other healthcare professionals and is provided here for you to check your dosage. The dosage of this drug may differ for different patients. Therefore, always follow your doctor's instructions or the directions on the label. Contact your healthcare provider or pharmacist if you have any questions about the specific dosage of your medication after reviewing this information.

General Dosage Information

Available as verapamil hydrochloride; dosage expressed in terms of the salt.

Adult Patients

Supraventricular Tachyarrhythmias
PSVT Prophylaxis

ORAL:
- Usual dosage: 240–480 mg daily given in 3 or 4 divided doses as conventional tablets (Calan®).

Ventricular Rate Control in Atrial Fibrillation or Flutter

ORAL:
- Usual dosage: 240–320 mg daily given in 3 or 4 divided doses as conventional tablets (Calan®).

Angina

ORAL:
- Usual initial dosage: 80 mg 3 or 4 times daily as conventional tablets (Calan®). Gradually increase dosage by 80-mg increments at weekly intervals or, in patients with unstable angina, at daily intervals until optimum control of angina is obtained.
- Alternatively, usual initial dosage of 180 mg at bedtime as extended-release core tablets (Covera-HS®). If adequate response does not occur, may increase dosage to 240 mg daily, and subsequently by 120-mg increments to 480 mg daily at bedtime.

Hypertension
Monotherapy

ORAL:
- Recommended dosages vary by formulation. Adjust dosage at approximately monthly intervals (more aggressively in high-risk patients) to achieve BP control.
- When switching from conventional tablets (Calan®) to extended-release capsules (Verelan®) or tablets (Calan® SR, Isoptin® SR), can use same total daily dosage.

Table 1. Recommended Dosages for Management of Hypertension

Formulation	Initial Dosage	Dosage Titration Regimen	Usual Dosages
Controlled extended-release capsules (Verelan PM®)	200 mg once daily at bedtime	Manufacturer states that dosage may be increased to 300 mg once daily and then to 400 mg once daily, if required	JNC 7 recommends usual range of 120–360 mg once daily
Extended-release capsules (Verelan®)	120 mg once daily in the morning	Manufacturer states that dosage may be increased to 180 mg once daily and then to 240 mg once daily, with subsequent increases in 120-mg increments to 480 mg once daily, if required	120–240 mg once daily

Conventional tablets (Calan®)	80 mg 3 times daily		JNC 7 recommends usual range of 80–320 mg daily, given in 2 divided doses
Extended-release tablets (Calan®SR, Isoptin® SR)	180 mg once daily in the morning	Increase dosage to 240 mg each morning Subsequently, increase dosage to 360 mg daily, given in 2 divided doses (either 180 mg in the morning + 180 mg in the evening or 240 mg in the morning + 120 mg in the evening) Manufacturer states that dosage may be increased to 240 mg every 12 hours, if required	JNC 7 recommends usual range of 120–360 mg daily, given in 1 or 2 divided doses
Extended-release core tablets (Covera-HS®)	180 mg once daily at bedtime	Manufacturer states that dosage may be increased to 240 mg once daily, with subsequent increases to 360 mg once daily and then to 480 mg once daily, if required	JNC 7 recommends usual range of 120–360 mg once daily

Combination Therapy

ORAL:

- If BP is not adequately controlled by monotherapy with verapamil (up to 240 mg daily) or trandolapril (up to 8 mg daily), can switch to fixed-combination tablets using tablets containing the same component doses.

Special Populations

Hepatic Impairment

- Reduce usual daily doses by up to 60–70% in patients with severe hepatic dysfunction.

Angina

ORAL:

- Usual dosage in patients with decreased hepatic function: 40 mg (as conventional tablets) 3 times daily.

Hypertension

ORAL:

- Controlled extended-release capsules (Verelan®PM): Manufacturer states that initial dosage of 100 mg daily at bedtime rarely may be necessary in patients with impaired hepatic function.

Renal Impairment

- Supplemental doses not necessary in patients undergoing hemodialysis.

Hypertension

ORAL:

- Controlled extended-release capsules (Verelan®PM): Manufacturer states that initial dosage of 100 mg daily at bedtime rarely may be necessary in patients with impaired renal function.

Geriatric Patients

Supraventricular Tachyarrhythmias

- Use slower infusion rates (over ≥3 minutes) in geriatric patients in order to minimize risk of adverse effects.

Angina

- Usual dosage: 40 mg (as conventional tablets) 3 times daily.

Hypertension

- Lower initial dosage recommended for treatment of hypertension in geriatric patients.

Table 2. Recommended Initial Dosages for Management of Hypertension in Geriatric Patients

Formulation	Initial Dosage
Extended-release capsules (Verelan®)	120 mg once daily in the morning
Controlled extended-release capsules (Verelan PM®)	100 mg daily at bedtime may rarely be necessary
Conventional tablets (Calan®)	40 mg 3 times daily
Extended-release tablets (Calan®SR, Isoptin®)	120 mg once daily in the morning

Small-stature Patients

Hypertension

- Lower initial dosage recommended for treatment of hypertension in patients with small stature.

Table 3. Recommended Initial Dosages for Management of Hypertension in Small-stature Patients

Formulation	Initial Dosage
Extended-release capsules (Verelan®)	120 mg once daily in the morning
Controlled extended-release capsules (Verelan PM®)	100 mg daily at bedtime may rarely be necessary
Conventional tablets (Calan®)	40 mg 3 times daily
Extended-release tablets (Calan®SR, Isoptin®)	120 mg once daily in the morning

Verapamil and Trandolapril

(ver ap' a mil) (tran dole' a pril)

Brand Name: Tarka®

Important Warning

Do not take verapamil and trandolapril if you are pregnant or breast-feeding. If you become pregnant while taking verapamil and trandolapril, call your doctor immediately.

Why is this medicine prescribed?

The combination of verapamil and trandolapril is used to treat high blood pressure. It is a combination of two medications. It decreases certain chemicals that tighten the blood vessels, so blood flows more smoothly. It also relaxes your blood vessels so your heart does not have to pump as hard.

This medication is sometimes prescribed for other uses; ask your doctor or pharmacist for more information.

How should this medicine be used?

The combination of verapamil and trandolapril comes as a tablet to take by mouth. It is usually taken once a day. The tablet should be swallowed whole. Do not chew, divide, or crush the tablets. Follow the directions on your prescription label carefully, and ask your doctor or pharmacist to explain any part you do not understand. Take verapamil and trandolapril exactly as directed. Do not take more or less of it or take it more often than prescribed by your doctor.

The combination of verapamil and trandolapril controls high blood pressure but does not cure it. Continue to take verapamil and trandolapril even if you feel well. Do not stop taking verapamil and trandolapril without talking to your doctor.

What special precautions should I follow?

Before taking verapamil and trandolapril,

- tell your doctor and pharmacist if you are allergic to trandolapril, verapamil, benazepril, captopril, enalapril, fosinopril, lisinopril, moexipril, quinapril, ramipril, or any other drugs.
- tell your doctor and pharmacist what prescription and nonprescription medications you are taking, especially albuterol (Volmax, Proventil [tablets and syrup only], Ventolin [tablets and syrup only]); allopurinol (Zyloprim); antacids; betamethasone (Celestone); carbamazepine (Tegretol); chemotherapy medications; cimetidine (Tagamet); cortisone (Cortone); cyclosporine (Neoral, Sandimmune); dantrolene (Dantrium); dexamethasone (Decadron, Dexone); diuretics ('water pills'); fentanyl (Duragesic); fludrocortisone (Florinef); heart and blood pressure medications such as beta-adrenergic blockers, digoxin (Lanoxin), disopyramide (Norpace), flecainide (Tambocor), procainamide (Procan), and quinidine (Quinaglute, Quinadex); hydrocortisone (Cortef, Hydrocortone); lithium (Eskalith, Lithobid); medications that suppress your immune system; medications to treat depression or psychiatric conditions; medications to treat glaucoma (increased pressure in the eye); medications to treat pain; muscle relaxants; methylprednisolone (Medrol); nonsteroidal anti-inflammatory drugs; other medications for high blood pressure or diabetes; phenobarbital; phenytoin (Dilantin); potassium supplements; prednisolone (Prelone); prednisone (Deltasone, Orasone); rifampin (Rifadin, Rimactane); theophylline; tranquilizers; triamcinolone (Aristocort); and vitamins or herbal products.
- tell your doctor if you have or have ever had heart, liver, or kidney disease; a recent heart attack; an irregular heartbeat; muscular dystrophy; gastrointestinal obstruction (strictures); or diabetes.
- if you are having surgery, including dental surgery, tell the doctor or dentist that you are taking verapamil and trandolapril.
- you should know that this drug may make you drowsy. Do not drive a car or operate machinery until you know how verapamil and trandolapril will affect you.
- remember that alcohol can add to the drowsiness caused by this drug. Do not drink alcohol while taking this medication.

What special dietary instructions should I follow?

Verapamil and trandolapril may cause an upset stomach. Take verapamil and trandolapril with food or milk. Talk to your doctor before using salt substitutes containing potassium. If your doctor prescribes a low-salt or low-sodium diet, follow these directions carefully.

What should I do if I forget to take a dose?

Take the missed dose as soon as you remember it. However, if it is almost time for the next dose, skip the missed dose and continue your regular dosing schedule. Do not take a double dose to make up for a missed one.

What side effects can this medicine cause?

Verapamil and trandolapril may cause side effects. Tell your doctor if any of these symptoms are severe or do not go away:

- cough
- dizziness or lightheadedness
- sore throat
- hoarseness
- excessive tiredness
- headache
- diarrhea
- constipation
- upset stomach

- heartburn
- flushing (feeling of warmth)
- slow heartbeat
- vivid, unusual dreams

If you experience any of the following symptoms, call your doctor immediately:

- swelling of the face, eyes, lips, tongue, arms, or legs
- difficulty breathing or swallowing
- fainting
- rash
- yellowing of the skin or eyes
- fever
- increase in frequency or severity of chest pain (angina)

If you experience a serious side effect, you or your doctor may send a report to the Food and Drug Administration's (FDA) MedWatch Adverse Event Reporting program online [at http://www.fda.gov/MedWatch/index.html] or by phone [1-800-332-1088].

What storage conditions are needed for this medicine?

Keep this medication in the container it came in, tightly closed, and out of reach of children. Store it at room temperature and away from excess heat and moisture (not in the bathroom). Throw away any medication that is outdated or no longer needed. Talk to your pharmacist about the proper disposal of your medication.

What should I do in case of overdose?

In case of overdose, call your local poison control center at 1-800-222-1222. If the victim has collapsed or is not breathing, call local emergency services at 911.

What other information should I know?

Keep all appointments with your doctor and the laboratory. Your blood pressure should be checked regularly to determine your response to verapamil and trandolapril.

Your doctor may ask you to check your pulse (heart rate) daily and will tell you how fast it should be. If your pulse is slower than it should be, call your doctor for directions on taking verapamil and trandolapril that day. Ask your doctor or pharmacist to teach you how to check your pulse.

Do not let anyone else take your medication. Ask your pharmacist any questions you have about refilling your prescription.

Dosage Facts
For Informational Purposes

Caution: Do not change your dose, how often you take your medication, or the length of time you are to take it without first talking to your health-care provider.

The following dosage information was written using medical language for doctors and other healthcare professionals and is provided here for you to check your dosage. The dosage of this drug may differ for different patients. Therefore, always follow your doctor's instructions or the directions on the label. Contact your healthcare provider or pharmacist if you have any questions about the specific dosage of your medication after reviewing this information.

Adult Patients

Hypertension
Trandolapril/Verapamil Combination Therapy

ORAL:
- Adjust dosage by first administering each drug separately. For patients receiving verapamil (up to 240 mg) and trandolapril (up to 8 mg) in separate tablets once daily, replacement with the fixed combination can be attempted using tablets containing the same component doses.

Voriconazole

(vohr ih kon′ uh zohl)

Brand Name: Vfend®

Why is this medicine prescribed?

Voriconazole is used to treat serious fungal infections such as invasive aspergillosis (a fungal infection that begins in the lungs and spreads through the bloodstream to other organs) and esophageal candidiasis (infection by a yeast-like fungus that may cause white patching in the mouth and throat). Voriconazole is in a class of antifungal medications called triazoles. It works by slowing the growth of the fungi that cause infection.

How should this medicine be used?

Voriconazole comes as a tablet and a suspension (liquid) to take by mouth. It is usually taken every 12 hours on an empty stomach, at least 1 hour before or 1 hour after a meal. To help you remember to take voriconazole, take it at around the same times every day. Follow the directions on your prescription label carefully, and ask your doctor or pharmacist to explain any part you do not understand. Take voriconazole exactly as directed. Do not take more or less of it or take it more often than prescribed by your doctor.

If you are taking voriconazole suspension, shake the closed bottle for about 10 seconds before each use to mix the medication evenly. Do not mix the suspension with any other medications, water, or any other liquid. Always use the measuring device that comes with your medication. You may not get the right amount of medication if you use a household spoon to measure your dose.

At the beginning of your treatment, you may receive voriconazole by intravenous (into a vein) injection. When you begin taking voriconazole by mouth, your doctor may start you on a low dose and increase your dose if your condition does not improve. Your doctor also may decrease your dose if you experience side effects from voriconazole.

The length of your treatment depends on your general health, the type of infection you have, and how well you respond to the medication. If you are taking voriconazole for esophageal candidiasis, you will take it for at least 14 days. If you are taking voriconazole for aspergillosis, you may take it for several months or longer. Continue to take voriconazole even if you feel well. Do not stop taking voriconazole without talking to your doctor.

Are there other uses for this medicine?

This medication may be prescribed for other uses; ask your doctor or pharmacist for more information.

What special precautions should I follow?

Before taking voriconazole,
- tell your doctor and pharmacist if you are allergic to voriconazole; other antifungal medications such as fluconazole (Diflucan), itraconazole (Sporonox), or ketoconazole (Nizoral); or any other medications.
- do not take voriconazole if you are taking any of the following medications: astemizole (Hismanal) (not available in the United States); carbamazepine (Tegretol); cisapride (Propulsid); efavirenz (Sustiva); ergot-type medications such as dihydroergotamine (D.H.E. 45, Migranal), ergoloid mesylates (Germinal, Hydergine), ergonovine (Ergotrate), ergotamine (Bellergal-S, Cafergot, Ergomar, Wigraine), methylergonovine (Methergine), and methysergide (Sansert); phenobarbital (Luminal, Solfoton); pimozide (Orap); quinidine (Quinadex, Quinaglute); mephobarbital (Mebaral); rifabutin (Mycobutin); rifampin (Rifadin, Rimactane); ritonavir (Norvir, in Kaletra); sirolimus (Rapamune); and terfenadine (Seldane) (not available in the United States).
- tell your doctor and pharmacist what other prescription and nonprescription medications, vitamins, and nutritional supplements you are taking. Be sure to mention any of the following: amiodarone (Cordarone); anticoagulants ('blood thinners') such as warfarin (Coumadin); benzodiazepines such as alprazolam (Xanax), diazepam (Valium), midazolam (Versed), and triazolam (Halcion); calcium channel blockers such as amlodipine (Norvasc), felodipine (Plendil), isradipine (DynaCirc), nicardipine (Cardene), nifedipine (Adalat, Procardia), nimodipine (Nimotop), and nisoldipine (Sular); cholesterol-lowering medications (statins) such as atorvastatin (Lipitor), fluvastatin (Lescol), lovastatin (Mevacor), pravastatin (Pravachol), and simvastatin (Zocor); cyclosporine (Neoral, Sandimmune); disopyramide (Norpace); dofetilide (Tikosyn); erythromycin (E.E.S., E-Mycin, Erythrocin); medications for diabetes such as glipizide (Glucotrol), glyburide (Diabeta, Micronase, Glycron, others), and tolbutamide (Orinase); medications for HIV

such as amprenavir (Agenerase), atazanavir (Reyataz), delavirdine (Rescriptor), fosamprenavir (Lexiva), nelfinavir (Viracept), nevirapine (Viramune), and saquinavir (Fortovase, Invirase); methadone (Dolophine); moxifloxacin (Avelox); phenytoin (Dilantin); procainamide (Procanbid, Pronestyl); proton-pump inhibitors such as esomeprazole (Nexium), lansoprazole (Prevacid), omeprazole (Prilosec), pantoprazole (Protonix), and rabeprazole (AcipHex); sotalol (Betapace); sparfloxacin (Zagam); tacrolimus (Prograf); thioridazine (Mellaril); vinblastine; and vincristine (Vincasar). Many other medications may also interact with voriconazole, so be sure to tell your doctor about all the medications you are taking, even those that do not appear on this list. Your doctor may need to change the doses of your medications or monitor you carefully for side effects.
- tell your doctor what herbal products you are taking, especially St. John's wort.
- tell your doctor if you have ever been treated with chemotherapy medications for cancer and if you have or have ever had cardiomyopathy (enlarged or thickened heart muscle that stops the heart from pumping blood normally), cancer of the blood cells, any condition that makes it difficult for you to digest sucrose or lactose, or liver or kidney disease.
- tell your doctor if you are pregnant, plan to become pregnant, or are breast-feeding. If you become pregnant while taking voriconazole, call your doctor.
- you should know that voriconazole may cause blurred vision or other problems with your eyesight and may make your eyes sensitive to bright light. Do not drive a car at night while taking voriconazole. Do not drive a car during the day or operate machinery if you have any problems with your vision while you are taking this medication.
- plan to avoid unnecessary or prolonged exposure to sunlight and to wear protective clothing, sunglasses, and sunscreen. Voriconazole may make your skin sensitive to sunlight.

What special dietary instructions should I follow?

Talk to your doctor about eating grapefruit and drinking grapefruit juice while taking this medicine.

What should I do if I forget to take a dose?

Take the missed dose as soon as you remember it. However, if it is almost time for the next dose, skip the missed dose and continue your regular dosing schedule. Do not take a double dose to make up for a missed one.

What side effects can this medicine cause?

Voriconazole may cause side effects. Tell your doctor if any of these symptoms are severe or do not go away:
- blurred or abnormal vision
- difficulty seeing colors

- sensitivity to bright light
- diarrhea
- vomiting
- headache
- dizziness
- dry mouth
- flushing

Some side effects can be serious. The following symptoms are uncommon, but if you experience any of them, call your doctor immediately:

- fever
- chills or shaking
- fast heartbeat
- fast breathing
- confusion
- upset stomach
- extreme tiredness
- unusual bruising or bleeding
- lack of energy
- loss of appetite
- pain in the upper right part of the stomach
- yellowing of the skin or eyes
- flu-like symptoms
- hallucinations (seeing things or hearing voices that do not exist)
- chest pain
- rash
- hives
- itching
- difficulty breathing or swallowing
- swelling of the hands, feet, ankles, or lower legs

Voriconazole may cause other side effects. Call your doctor if you have any unusual problems while taking this medication.

If you experience a serious side effect, you or your doctor may send a report to the Food and Drug Administration's (FDA) MedWatch Adverse Event Reporting program online [at http://www.fda.gov/MedWatch/index.html] or by phone [1-800-332-1088].

What storage conditions are needed for this medicine?

Keep this medication in the container it came in, tightly closed, and out of reach of children. Store it at room temperature and away from excess heat and moisture (not in the bathroom). Do not refrigerate or freeze the medication. Throw away any medication that is outdated or no longer needed. Throw away any unused suspension after 14 days. Talk to your pharmacist about the proper disposal of your medication.

What should I do in case of overdose?

In case of overdose, call your local poison control center at 1-800-222-1222. If the victim has collapsed or is not breathing, call local emergency services at 911.

Symptoms of overdose may include:

- sensitivity to light
- widened pupils (black circles in the middle of the eyes)
- closed eyes
- drooling
- loss of balance while moving
- depression
- shortness of breath
- seizures
- swollen stomach
- extreme tiredness

What other information should I know?

Keep all appointments with your doctor and the laboratory. Your doctor will order certain lab tests to check your body's response to voriconazole.

Do not let anyone else take your medication. Ask your pharmacist any questions you have about refilling your prescription. If you still have symptoms of infection after you finish the voriconazole, call your doctor.

Dosage Facts
For Informational Purposes

Caution: Do not change your dose, how often you take your medication, or the length of time you are to take it without first talking to your healthcare provider.

The following dosage information was written using medical language for doctors and other healthcare professionals and is provided here for you to check your dosage. The dosage of this drug may differ for different patients. Therefore, always follow your doctor's instructions or the directions on the label. Contact your healthcare provider or pharmacist if you have any questions about the specific dosage of your medication after reviewing this information.

General Dosage Information

Duration of therapy should be based on the severity of the patient's underlying disease, recovery from immunosuppression, and response to the drug.

Pediatric Patients

Treatment of Aspergillosis and Other Fungal Infections

ORAL:
- Children 9 months to 15 years of age†: After initial IV regimen, maintenance dosage of 100 mg twice daily in those weighing <40 kg or 200 mg twice daily in those weighing ≥40 kg.

Adult Patients

Treatment of Aspergillosis

ORAL:
- Adults weighing <40 kg: After initial IV regimen, maintenance dosage of 100 mg every 12 hours; if response is inadequate, increase to 150 mg every 12 hours. If not tolerated,

decrease dosage by increments of 50 mg to a minimum of 100 mg every 12 hours.
- Adults weighing ≥40 kg: After initial IV regimen, maintenance dosage of 200 mg every 12 hours; if response is inadequate, increase to 300 mg every 12 hours. If not tolerated, decrease dosage by increments of 50 mg to a minimum of 200 mg every 12 hours.

Candida Infection
Treatment of Candidemia and Disseminated Infections
ORAL:
- Adults weighing <40 kg: After initial IV regimen, maintenance dosage of 100 mg every 12 hours; if response is inadequate, increase to 150 mg every 12 hours. If not tolerated, decrease dosage by increments of 50 mg to a minimum of 100 mg every 12 hours.
- Adults weighing ≥40 kg: After initial IV regimen, maintenance dosage of 200 mg every 12 hours; if response is inadequate, increase to 300 mg every 12 hours. If not tolerated, decrease dosage by increments of 50 mg to a minimum of 200 mg every 12 hours.
- Continue for at least 14 days after symptoms have resolved or after the last positive culture, whichever is longer.

Treatment of Esophageal Candidiasis
ORAL:
- Adults weighing <40 kg: 100 mg every 12 hours.
- Adults weighing ≥40 kg: 200 mg every 12 hours.
- Continue for ≥14 days and for ≥7 days after resolution of symptoms.

Treatment of Fusarium and Scedosporium Infections
ORAL:
- Adults weighing <40 kg: After initial IV regimen, maintenance dosage of 100 mg every 12 hours; if response is inadequate, increase to 150 mg every 12 hours. If not tolerated, decrease dosage by increments of 50 mg to a minimum of 100 mg every 12 hours.
- Adults weighing ≥40 kg: After initial IV regimen, maintenance dosage of 200 mg every 12 hours; if response is inadequate, increase to 300 mg every 12 hours. If not tolerated, decrease dosage by increments of 50 mg to a minimum of 200 mg every 12 hours.

Special Populations
Hepatic Impairment
- Use usual loading dose regimen in patients with mild-to-moderate hepatic cirrhosis (Child-Pugh class A or B); decrease maintenance dosages by 50%.
- Not studied in patients with severe cirrhosis (Child-Pugh class C) or in those with chronic hepatitis B (HBV) or hepatitis C virus (HCV) infection.

Renal Impairment
- Dosage adjustment of oral voriconazole not needed.

Geriatric Patients
- No dosage adjustments required.

Concomitant Phenytoin Therapy
- If used with phenytoin, voriconazole dosage adjustment recommended.

† Use is not currently included in the labeling approved by the US Food and Drug Administration.

Vorinostat
(vor in′ oh stat)

Brand Name: Zolinza®

Why is this medicine prescribed?
Vorinostat is used to treat cutaneous T-cell lymphoma (CTCL, a type of cancer) in people whose disease has not improved, has gotten worse, or has come back after taking other medications. Vorinostat is in a class of medications called histone deacetylase (HDAC) inhibitors. It works by killing or stopping the growth of cancer cells.

How should this medicine be used?
Vorinostat comes as a capsule to take by mouth. It is usually taken once a day with food. Your doctor will tell you whether to take vorinostat every day or only on some days of the week. Take vorinostat at around the same time every day. Follow the directions on your prescription label carefully, and ask your doctor or pharmacist to explain any part you do not understand. Take vorinostat exactly as directed. Do not take more or less of it or take it more often than prescribed by your doctor.

Swallow the capsules whole; do not open, chew, or crush them. If you are not able to swallow the capsules whole, call your doctor. If vorinostat capsules are accidentally opened or crushed, do not touch the capsules or the powder. If the powder from an open or crushed capsule gets on your skin or in your eyes or nose, wash the area well with plenty of water and call your doctor.

Ask your pharmacist or doctor for a copy of the manufacturer's information for the patient.

Are there other uses for this medicine?
This medication may be prescribed for other uses; ask your doctor or pharmacist for more information.

What special precautions should I follow?
Before taking vorinostat,
- tell your doctor and pharmacist if you are allergic to vorinostat or any other medications.
- tell your doctor and pharmacist what prescription and nonprescription medications, vitamins, nutritional supplements, and herbal products you are taking or plan to

take. Be sure to mention any of the following: amiodarone (Cordarone), anticoagulants ('blood thinners') such as warfarin (Coumadin), cisapride (Propulsid) (no longer available in the US), disopyramide (Norpace), dofetilide (Tikosyn), erythromycin (E.E.S., E-Mycin, Erythrocin), medications to treat heart arrhythmias; moxifloxacin (Avelox), pimozide (Orap), procainamide (Procanbid, Pronestyl), quinidine (Quinidex), sotalol (Betapace, Betapace AF), sparfloxacin (Zagam), thioridazine (Mellaril), and valproic acid (Depakene). Your doctor may need to change the doses of your medications or monitor you carefully for side effects.

- tell your doctor if you have nausea, vomiting, or diarrhea; and if you have or have ever had a blood clot in the lungs or a vein (blood vessel); high blood sugar or diabetes; arrhythmias (abnormal heart beat or heart rhythm problems); and heart, kidney, or liver disease.
- tell your doctor if you are pregnant, plan to become pregnant, or are breast-feeding. Vorinostat may cause harm to the fetus. If you become pregnant while taking vorinostat, call your doctor immediately.
- you should know that vorinostat may make you drowsy. Do not drive a car or operate machinery until you know how this medication affects you.
- you should know that vorinostat may cause an increase in blood glucose. If you have diabetes or high blood sugar, check your blood sugar as often as directed by your doctor. If your blood sugar is higher than usual, call your doctor. Tell your doctor immediately if you have any of the following symptoms while you are taking vorinostat: extreme thirst, frequent urination, extreme hunger, blurred vision, or weakness. It is very important to call your doctor as soon as you have any of these symptoms, because high blood sugar that is not treated can cause a serious condition called ketoacidosis. Ketoacidosis may become life-threatening if it is not treated at an early stage. Symptoms of ketoacidosis include: dry mouth, upset stomach and vomiting, shortness of breath, breath that smells fruity, and decreased consciousness. Call your doctor if you are unable to eat or drink normally due to nausea, vomiting, or diarrhea while you are taking vorinostat. Your doctor may need to change your diet or medication to help control your blood sugar while you are taking vorinostat.

What special dietary instructions should I follow?

Make sure to drink at least eight 8-ounce cups of water or other liquids every day while taking vorinostat so you do not become dehydrated.

Unless your doctor tells you otherwise, continue your normal diet.

What should I do if I forget to take a dose?

Take the missed dose as soon as you remember it. However, if it is almost time for the next dose, skip the missed dose and continue your regular dosing schedule. Do not take a double dose to make up for a missed one.

What side effects can this medicine cause?

Vorinostat may cause side effects. Tell your doctor if any of these symptoms are severe or do not go away:
- diarrhea
- nausea
- loss of appetite
- weight loss
- vomiting
- constipation
- extreme tiredness
- chills
- change in the way things taste
- dry mouth
- hair loss
- dizziness
- swelling of the legs, feet, or ankles
- itching
- cough
- fever
- headache
- muscle aches

Some side effects can be serious. If you experience any of these symptoms, call your doctor immediately:
- unusual bleeding or bruising
- pale skin
- sudden swelling, redness, warmth, pain, and/or tenderness in a leg
- skin redness or change in skin color
- sudden sharp chest pain
- shortness of breath
- coughing up blood
- sweating
- fast heartbeat
- fainting
- feeling anxious

Vorinostat may cause other side effects. Call your doctor if you have any unusual problems while taking this medication.

What storage conditions are needed for this medicine?

Keep this medication in the container it came in, tightly closed, and out of reach of children. Store it at room temperature and away from excess heat and moisture (not in the bathroom). Throw away any medication that is outdated or no longer needed. Talk to your pharmacist about the proper disposal of your medication.

What should I do in case of overdose?

In case of overdose, call your local poison control center at 1-800-222-1222. If the victim has collapsed or is not breathing, call local emergency services at 911.

What other information should I know?

Keep all appointments with your doctor and the laboratory. Your doctor will order certain lab tests to check your body's response to vorinostat.

Before having any laboratory test, tell your doctor and the laboratory personnel that you are taking vorinostat.

Do not let anyone else take your medication. Ask your pharmacist any questions you have about refilling your prescription.

Talk to your doctor, pharmacist, or other healthcare professional if you have questions about dosing information for your medication.

Warfarin

(war′ far in)

Brand Name: Coumadin®
Also available generically.

Important Warning

Warfarin may cause severe bleeding that can be life-threatening and even cause death. Tell your doctor if you have or have ever had a blood or bleeding disorder; bleeding problems, especially in your stomach or your esophagus (tube from the throat to the stomach), intestines, urinary tract or bladder, or lungs; high blood pressure; heart attack; angina (chest pain or pressure); heart disease; pericarditis (swelling of the lining (sac) around the heart); endocarditis (infection of one or more heart valves); a stroke or ministroke; aneurysm (weakening or tearing of an artery or vein); anemia (low number of red blood cells in the blood); cancer; chronic diarrhea; or kidney, or liver disease. Also tell your doctor if you fall often or have had a recent serious injury or surgery. Bleeding is more likely during warfarin treatment for people over 65 years of age, and it is also more likely during the first few weeks of warfarin treatment. It is also more likely for people who take high doses of warfarin, or take this medication for a long time. The risk for bleeding while taking warfarin is also higher for people participating in an activity or sport that may result in serious injury. Tell your doctor and pharmacist if you are taking or plan to take any prescription or nonprescription medications, vitamins, nutritional supplements, and herbal or botanical products (See SPECIAL PRECAUTIONS), as some of these products may increase the risk for bleeding while you are taking warfarin. If you experience any of the following symptoms, call your doctor immediately: pain, swelling, or discomfort, bleeding from

a cut that does not stop in the usual amount of time, nosebleeds or bleeding from your gums, coughing up or vomiting blood or material that looks like coffee grounds, unusual bleeding or bruising, increased menstrual flow or vaginal bleeding, pink, red, or dark brown urine, red or tarry black bowel movements, headache, dizziness, or weakness.

Keep all appointments with your doctor and the laboratory. Your doctor will order certain tests to check your body's response to warfarin.

Your doctor or pharmacist will give you the manufacturer's patient information sheet (Medication Guide) when you begin treatment with warfarin and each time you refill your prescription. Read the information carefully and ask your doctor or pharmacist if you have any questions. You can also visit the Food and Drug Administration (FDA) website (http://www.fda.gov/cder) or the manufacturer's website to obtain the Medication Guide.

Talk to your doctor about the risk(s) of taking warfarin.

Why is this medicine prescribed?

Warfarin is used to prevent blood clots from forming or growing larger in your blood and blood vessels. Warfarin is in a class of medications called anticoagulants ('blood thinners'). It is prescribed for people with certain types of irregular heartbeat, people with prosthetic (replacement or mechanical) heart valves, and people who have suffered a heart attack. Warfarin is also used to treat or prevent venous thrombosis (swelling and blood clot in a vein) and pulmonary embolism (a blood clot in the lung). It works by decreasing the clotting ability of the blood.

How should this medicine be used?

Warfarin comes as a tablet to take by mouth. It usually is taken once a day with or without food. Take warfarin at around the same time every day. Follow the directions on your prescription label carefully, and ask your doctor or pharmacist to explain any part you do not understand. Take warfarin exactly as directed. Do not take more or less of it or take it more often than prescribed by your doctor. Call your doctor immediately if you take more than your prescribed dose of warfarin.

Your doctor will probably start you on a low dose of warfarin and gradually increase or decrease your dose based on the results of your blood tests. Make sure you understand any new dosing instructions from your doctor.

Continue to take warfarin even if you feel well. Do not stop taking warfarin without talking to your doctor.

Are there other uses for this medicine?

This medication may be prescribed for other uses; ask your doctor or pharmacist for more information.

What special precautions should I follow?

Before taking warfarin,

- tell your doctor and pharmacist if you are allergic to warfarin or any other medications.
- do not take more two or more medications that contain warfarin at the same time. Be sure to check with your doctor or pharmacist if you are uncertain that a medication may contain warfarin or warfarin sodium.
- tell your doctor and pharmacist what prescription and nonprescription medications, vitamins, and nutritional supplements you are taking or plan to take, especially antibiotics; aspirin or aspirin-containing products and other nonsteroidal anti-inflammatory drugs such as ibuprofen (Advil, Motrin) and naproxen (Aleve, Naprosyn); heparin; medications for cancer, cholesterol, colds and allergies, depression, diabetes, digestive problems (including ulcers and heartburn), gout, heart disease, mental illness, pain, seizures thyroid problems, and tuberculosis; streptokinase; ticlopidine; or urokinase. Many other medications may also interact with warfarin, so be sure to tell your doctor about all the medications you are taking, even those that do not appear on this list. Do not take any new medications or stop taking any medication without talking to your doctor.
- tell your doctor and pharmacist what herbal or botanical products you are taking, especially bromelains, coenzyme Q10 (ubidecarenone), cranberry products, danshen, dong quai, garlic, Ginkgo biloba, ginseng, and St. John's wort. There are many other herbal or botanical products which might affect your body's response to warfarin. Do not start or stop taking any herbal products without talking to your doctor.
- tell your doctor if you have or have ever had a thyroid condition or diabetes. Also tell your doctor if you have an infection, a gastrointestinal illness such as diarrhea, or sprue (an allergic reaction to protein found in grains that causes diarrhea), or an indwelling catheter (a flexible plastic tube that is placed into the bladder to allow the urine to drain out).
- tell your doctor if you are pregnant, think you might be pregnant, plan to become pregnant, or become pregnant while taking warfarin. You should not take warfarin if you are pregnant. Talk to your doctor about the use of effective birth control while taking warfarin. If you become pregnant while taking warfarin, call your doctor immediately. Warfarin may harm the fetus.
- tell your doctor if you are breast-feeding.
- if you are having surgery, including dental surgery or a procedure, tell the doctor or dentist that you are taking warfarin. Your doctor may tell you to stop taking warfarin before the surgery or procedure or change your dosage of warfarin before the surgery or procedure. Follow your doctor's directions carefully and keep all appointments with the laboratory if your doctor requests blood tests to determine the appropriate dosage of warfarin.
- tell your doctor if you drink or have ever drunk large amounts of alcohol. Your doctor will probably tell you not to take warfarin. Avoid drinking alcohol while you are taking this medication.
- if you are going to receive an immunization, such as a flu shot, or any other injection into a muscle, tell the health care professional that you are taking warfarin.

What special dietary instructions should I follow?

Eat a normal, healthy diet with the same amount of foods that contain vitamin K; ask your doctor or pharmacist for a list of foods that contain vitamin K. Be sure to talk to your doctor before you make any changes in your diet or try to gain or lose weight. Do not eat large amounts of leafy, green vegetables or certain vegetable oils, such as soybean or canola, that contain large amounts of vitamin K. Avoid juice or products that contain cranberries. Ask your doctor about eating licorice while taking warfarin.

What should I do if I forget to take a dose?

Take the missed dose as soon as you remember it, if it is the same day that you were to take the dose. Do not take a double dose the next day to make up for a missed one. Talk to your doctor if you miss a dose of warfarin.

What side effects can this medicine cause?

Warfarin may cause side effects. Tell your doctor if any of these symptoms are severe or do not go away:

- gas
- tiredness
- pale skin

If you experience any of the following symptoms, or those listed in the IMPORTANT WARNING section, call your doctor immediately:

- hives,
- rash,
- itching,
- difficulty breathing or swallowing,
- diarrhea,
- fever,
- infection,
- nausea,
- loss of appetite,
- pain in the upper right part of the stomach,
- yellowing of the skin or eyes,
- flu-like symptoms,
- chest, stomach, joint, or muscle pain,
- difficultly in moving any part of your body,
- feelings of numbness, tingling, pricking, burning, or creeping on the skin.

You should know that warfarin may cause necrosis or gangrene (death of skin or other body tissues). Call your doctor immediately if you notice a purplish or darkened color, skin changes, ulcers, or an unusual problem in any area of your skin or body, or if you have a severe pain that occurs suddenly, or color or temperature change in any area of your body. Call your doctor immediately if your toes become painful or become purple or dark in color. You may need medical care right away to prevent amputation (removal) of your affected body part.

Warfarin may cause other side effects. Call your doctor if you have any unusual problems while taking this medication.

What storage conditions are needed for this medicine?

Keep this medication in the container it came in, tightly closed, and out of reach of children. Store it at room temperature and away from excess heat, moisture (not in the bathroom), and light. Throw away any medication that is outdated or no longer needed. Talk to your pharmacist about the proper disposal of your medication.

What should I do in case of overdose?

In case of overdose, call your local poison control center at 1-800-222-1222. If the victim has collapsed or is not breathing, call local emergency services at 911.

Symptoms of overdose may include:

- blood or darkened blood in bowel movements,
- spitting or coughing up blood,
- heavy bleeding with your period,
- blood in urine or vomit,
- small, flat, round red spots under the skin,
- unusual bruising,
- continued oozing or bleeding from minor cuts.

What other information should I know?

Warfarin prevents blood from clotting so it may take longer than usual for you to stop bleeding if you are cut or injured. Avoid activities that have a high risk of causing injury. Call your doctor if bleeding is unusual or if you fall and get hurt, especially if you hit your head.

Carry an identification card or wear a bracelet that indicates that you take warfarin. Ask your pharmacist or doctor how to obtain this card or bracelet. List your name, medical problems, drugs and dosages, and doctor's name and telephone number on the card.

Tell all your healthcare providers that you take warfarin.

Do not let anyone else take your medication. Ask your pharmacist any questions you have about refilling your prescription.

Dosage Facts
For Informational Purposes

Caution: Do not change your dose, how often you take your medication, or the length of time you are to take it without first talking to your healthcare provider.

The following dosage information was written using medical language for doctors and other healthcare professionals and is provided here for you to check your dosage. The dosage of this drug may differ for different patients. Therefore, always follow your doctor's instructions or the directions on the label. Contact your healthcare provider or pharmacist if you have any questions about the specific dosage of your medication after reviewing this information.

General Dosage Information

Available as warfarin sodium; dosage expressed in terms of the salt.

Pediatric Patients

Venous Thrombosis and Pulmonary Embolism
Treatment or Secondary Prevention

ORAL:

- Neonates with homozygous protein C deficiency and associated purpura fulminans: Maintenance of an INR of 2.5–4.5 long-term suggested.
- Children >2 months of age with first episode idiopathic thromboembolic event: Follow-up anticoagulation after heparin or an LMW heparin with dosage adjusted to maintain a target INR of 2.5 (range 2–3) for at least 6 months.
- Children >2 months of age with first episode thromboembolic event secondary to precipitating factors: Maintenance of a target INR of 2.5 (range 2–3) is suggested for 3 months or until resolution of such factors. Such factors include cancer, trauma/surgery, congenital heart disease, or systemic lupus erythematosus.
- Children >2 months of age with recurrent thromboembolic events secondary to precipitating factors after previous 3 months of oral anticoagulation: Continued maintenance of a target INR of 2.5 (range 2–3) is suggested for another 3 months or until resolution of such factors.
- Children with recurrent idiopathic thromboembolic events: Indefinite oral anticoagulation at low (INR of 1.3–1.8) to moderate intensity (INR of 2–3) suggested.
- Children >2 months of age with central venous catheter-associated venous thromboembolic events: Adjust dosage to maintain target INR of 2.5 (range 2–3) for 3 months.
- Children >2 months of age with first DVT associated with a central venous catheter after previous 3 months of oral anticoagulation for catheter-related thrombosis: Continue anticoagulation at a lower intensity (INR 1.5–1.8) until the central venous catheter is removed.
- Children >2 months of age with recurrent thrombosis associated with a central venous catheter after previous 3 months of oral anticoagulation: Continue anticoagulation at a lower intensity (INR 1.5–1.8) until the central venous catheter is removed.
- Children >2 months of age with breakthrough thrombosis associated with central venous catheters despite low-intensity oral anticoagulation: Increase of the anticoagulation to an INR of 2–3 until the catheter is removed or for a minimum of 3 months.
- Children >2 months of age receiving long-term total parenteral nutrition via a central venous catheter: Continuous dos-

age at INR 2–2.5 suggested or alternatively, for the first 3 months after each central venous catheter is inserted.

Cardiovascular Conditions†

ORAL:

- Giant coronary aneurysms following Kawasaki disease†: Adjustment of dosage to maintain an INR of 2–3 with aspirin (3–5 mg/kg daily) is suggested to reduce subsequent thrombosis and infarction.
- Neonates and children with dilated cardiomyopathy†: Primary prophylaxis at INR of 2–3 suggested while the child is awaiting a cardiac transplant.
- Fontan surgery for congenital univentricular heart lesions†: Maintenance of an INR of 2–3 following full-dose heparin suggested for primary prevention of thromboembolic events; the optimal duration of therapy unknown.

Cerebral Thromboembolism

Acute Cerebral Venous Sinus Thrombosis†

ORAL:

- Secondary prevention†: Follow-up oral anticoagulation at a target INR of 2.5 (range 2–3) for 3–6 months after therapy with unfractionated heparin or an LMW heparin.

Adult Patients

Venous Thrombosis and Pulmonary Embolism

Treatment or Secondary Prevention

ORAL:

- As follow-up to therapy with heparin or an LMW heparin, initial dose is 5–10 mg daily. Adjust subsequent daily dosage to achieve and maintain a target INR of 2.5 (range 2–3) for ≥3 months.
- Individualize length of treatment of DVT or pulmonary embolism based on age, comorbid conditions, and the likelihood of recurrence.
- DVT or pulmonary embolism with reversible or time-limited risk factors for venous thromboembolism: Adjust dosage to maintain a target INR of 2.5 (range 2–3) for at least 3 months.
- First episode of idiopathic DVT: Adjust dosage to maintain a target INR of 2.5 (range 2–3) for at least 6–12 months.
- First episode of DVT or pulmonary embolism and continuing risk factors: Adjust dosage to maintain a target INR of 2.5 (range 2–3) for at least 6–12 months. Such factors include cancer, antithrombin III or protein C or S deficiencies, antiphospholipid antibody syndrome, factor V Leiden or prothrombin 20210A gene mutations, homocysteinemia, and high levels of factor VII.
- First episode of DVT or pulmonary embolism with antiphospholipid antibodies or ≥2 thrombophilic conditions: Adjust dosage to maintain a target INR of 2.5 (range 2–3) for 12 months. Indefinite anticoagulation suggested in these patients.
- Consider long-term therapy in patients with risk factors for recurrent thromboembolism, including venous insufficiency, idiopathic venous thromboembolism, and history of thrombotic events (≥2 episodes).

Prophylaxis in Hip-replacement Surgery

ORAL:

- Initially, 5–10 mg daily with dosage adjusted to achieve a target INR of 2.5 (range 2–3) for ≥10 days.
- Initiate prophylaxis for venous thromboembolism perioperatively (the evening before or after surgery).

- Extended prophylaxis for ≤28–35 days with warfarin, fondaparinux, or LMW heparin recommended.

Prophylaxis in Hip-fracture Surgery

ORAL:

- Initially, 5–10 mg daily with dosage adjusted to achieve a target INR of 2.5 (range 2–3) for ≥10 days.
- Initiate prophylaxis for venous thromboembolism preoperatively with heparin or a LMW heparin if surgery is delayed or after surgery once hemostasis has been demonstrated. Continue prophylactic anticoagulant therapy with warfarin, a LMW heparin, or fondaparinux following surgery for 28–35 days.

Prophylaxis in Knee-replacement Surgery

ORAL:

- Initially, 5–10 mg daily with dosage adjusted to achieve a target INR of 2.5 (range 2–3) for 10 days.
- Initiate prophylaxis for venous thromboembolism perioperatively (the evening before or after surgery).

Prophylaxis in Trauma

ORAL:

- Acute spinal cord injury: Following initial therapy with an LMW heparin, adjust warfarin sodium dosage to a target INR of 2.5 (range 2–3) in the rehabilitation phase. Continue prophylactic anticoagulant therapy following trauma for a minimum of 3 months or until completion of the inpatient phase of rehabilitation.
- Trauma patients with impaired mobility: Adjust dosage to a target INR of 2.5 (range 2–3) after hospital discharge.

Embolism Associated with Atrial Fibrillation/Flutter

ORAL:

- Adjust dosage for long-term oral anticoagulation to a target INR of 2.5 (range 2–3) in patients who are at high risk for stroke.
- For atrial fibrillation persisting for >48 hours after open-heart surgery: Maintain a target INR of 2.5 (range 2–3) in patients at high risk for stroke for several weeks following reversion to normal sinus rhythm.
- Atrial flutter and mitral stenosis: Adjust dosage to maintain a target INR of 2.5 (range 2–3).

Thromboprophylaxis during Cardioversion of Atrial Fibrillation/ Flutter

ORAL:

- Initiate at least 3–4 weeks prior to cardioversion (target INR of 2.5, range 2–3) and continue after the procedure until normal sinus rhythm has been maintained for 3–4 weeks. For emergency cardioversion, administer for ≥4 weeks as follow-up anticoagulation after initiating periprocedural IV heparin.

Embolism Associated with Valvular Heart Disease

ORAL:

- Mitral valve disease associated with rheumatic fever or mitral valve regurgitation: Adjust dosage to prolong the INR to a target of 2.5 (range 2–3) in patients who have either concurrent paroxysmal or chronic persistent atrial fibrillation or a history of systemic embolism (e.g., stroke). Add aspirin (75–100 mg daily) to therapy in patients who have a breakthrough embolic event.

- Rheumatic mitral valve disease with left atrial hypertrophy (left atrial diameter exceeding 5.5 cm) and normal sinus rhythm: Long-term anticoagulation at a target INR of 2.5 (range 2–3).
- Mitral valve prolapse and a history of systemic embolism (e.g., stroke), or recurrent TIAs despite aspirin therapy: Maintain a target INR of 2.5 (range 2–3).
- Mitral annular calcification complicated by systemic embolism (noncalcific systemic embolism): Long-term prophylaxis at a target INR of 2.5 (range 2–3) suggested.
- Patients undergoing percutaneous mitral valvuloplasty: Maintain a target INR of 2.5 (range 2–3) for 3 weeks prior to the procedure and for 4 weeks after the procedure.

Thromboembolism Associated with Prosthetic Heart Valves
Prophylaxis

ORAL:

- Bioprosthetic valve in the aortic position: Adjust dosage to maintain a target INR of 2.5 (range 2–3) during the first 3 months.
- Bioprosthetic valve in the mitral position: Adjust dosage to maintain a target INR of 2.5 (range 2–3) for the first 3 months.
- Mitral bioprosthetic heart valve and additional risk factors (atrial fibrillation, left ventricular dysfunction, prior thromboembolism, hypercoagulable states): Maintenance of a target INR of 3 (range 2.5–3.5) for ≥3 months recommended by ACC and AHA.
- Bioprosthetic valves with evidence of a left atrial thrombus at valve replacement surgery: Adjust dosage to maintain a target INR of 2.5 (range 2–3) for the first 3 months.
- Patients with bioprosthetic valves who have a history of systemic embolism: Maintenance of a target INR of 2.5 (range 2–3) for 3–12 months recommended by ACCP.
- Patients with newer (e.g., bileaflet, Medtronic disk) mechanical heart valves in the aortic position with no additional risk factors: Adjust dosage to a target INR of 2.5 (range 2–3) long-term.
- Tilting disk valves and bileaflet mechanical heart valves in the mitral position: Adjust dosage to maintain a target INR of 3 (range 2.5–3.5) long-term.
- Mechanical valves and additional risk factors (atrial fibrillation, left atrial enlargement, endocardial damage, low ejection fraction): Long-term oral anticoagulation at a target INR of 3 (range 2.5–3.5) and low-dose aspirin (75–100 mg daily).
- First-generation mechanical valve (e.g., caged ball, caged disk): Combination therapy with warfarin (dosage adjusted to a target INR of 3 [range 2.5–3.5]) and aspirin (75–100 mg daily) is recommended long-term.

Treatment

ORAL:

- Breakthrough embolic event despite dosage adjusted to maintain a target INR of 2.5 (range 2–3): Increase dosage to achieve and maintain a target INR of 3 (range 2.5–3.5) and add aspirin (75–100 mg daily).
- Breakthrough embolic event despite target INR of 3 (range 2.5–3.5): Increase dosage to a target INR of 4 (range 3.5–4.5).
- Breakthrough embolic event in patients receiving a combination of low-dose aspirin (80–100 mg daily) and warfarin: ACC and AHA suggest increasing the dosage of warfarin

first. Increase the aspirin dosage (to 325 mg daily) if the higher warfarin dosage does not prevent embolic events.
- Breakthrough embolic event on aspirin therapy alone: Increase the aspirin dosage to 325 mg daily or initiate warfarin to achieve and maintain a target INR of 2.5 (range 2–3).
- Patients with large valve thrombosis in whom surgical intervention is not feasible and thrombolytic therapy is successful: Follow-up anticoagulation to IV unfractionated heparin and overlap agents until attainment of a target INR of 3.5 (range 3–4) or 4 (range 3.5–4.5) in patients with aortic or mitral prosthetic valves, respectively.
- Patients with some residual valve thrombosis after partially successful thrombolytic therapy: Adjust dosage to achieve a target INR of 3 (range 2.5–3.5) and institute adjusted-dose sub-Q unfractionated heparin twice daily for 3 months.
- Patients with small valve thrombus who are in NYHA class I or II heart failure and who are hemodynamically stable with IV unfractionated heparin: May be transferred from IV unfractionated heparin therapy to the combination of sub-Q adjusted-dose unfractionated heparin (to achieve an aPTT of 55–80 seconds) and adjusted-dose warfarin therapy (adjusted to maintain a target INR of 3 [range 2.5–3.5]) for 1–3 months as an alternative to thrombolytic therapy or reoperation. Upon resolution of the small valve thrombus, increase dosage to maintain a target INR of 3.5 (range 3–4) for prosthetic aortic valves or a target INR of 4 (range 3.5–4.5) for prosthetic mitral valves; institute concomitant low-dose aspirin therapy.

ST-Segment Elevation MI
Treatment or Secondary Prevention

ORAL:

- As follow-up after heparin or LMW heparin therapy, initiate warfarin therapy after the initial 2 days of hospitalization to maintain a target INR of 2.5 (range 2–3) for 3 months in patients at increased risk of systemic or pulmonary embolism (e.g., history of previous systemic embolism, ventricular mural thrombus or severe left ventricular dysfunction, venous thromboembolism, or severe heart failure).
- Hospitalized patients with DVT or pulmonary embolism: Initiate concurrently with full-dose LMW heparin and continue for a minimum of 5 days until a target INR of 2.5 (range 2–3) is obtained.
- Manufacturer recommends initiation of therapy in patients at 2–4 weeks postinfarction with dosage adjusted to maintain a target INR of 3 (range 2.5–3.5). Where meticulous INR monitoring is standard and routinely accessible, ACCP recommends long-term (up to 4 years) anticoagulation with high-intensity warfarin (target INR of 3 [range 2.5–3.5]) or moderate-intensity (target INR of 2.5 [range 2–3]) warfarin and low-dose aspirin in both high- and low-risk patients following MI.
- In patients with AMI who are at increased risk for bleeding complications or who are receiving concomitant aspirin therapy, maintain the INR at the lower end of this suggested range.
- ACCP recommends oral anticoagulation (target INR 2.5, range 2–3) in addition to low-dose (≤100 mg daily) aspirin for 3 months following MI in high-risk patients (e.g., large anterior MI, substantial heart failure, intracardiac thrombus visible on echocardiography, history of thromboembolism).
- ACC and AHA recommend initiation at hospital discharge in patients with documented left ventricular thrombus or extensive wall motion abnormality. Adjust dosage to maintain a

target INR of 2.5 (range 2–3) for 3 months or indefinitely in patients without an increased risk for bleeding.

- ACC and AHA recommend long-term prophylaxis, initiated at hospital discharge in patients without stent implantation who have other coexisting conditions that warrant anticoagulation (i.e., left ventricular thrombus, cerebral emboli, wall motion abnormality). Adjust dosage to maintain a target INR of 3 (range 2.5–3.5) or a target INR of 2.5 (range 2–3) with concomitant aspirin (75–162 mg daily).
- Patients unable to take aspirin who do not undergo stent implantation, as an alternative to clopidogrel: Adjust dosage to maintain a target INR of 3 (range 2.5-3.5).
- Recent MI and persistent atrial fibrillation: Adjust dosage to maintain a target INR of 2.5 (range 2–3) indefinitely.

Primary Prevention

ORAL:
- Patients at high risk for CAD, as an alternative to aspirin therapy alone: Adjust dosage to maintain a target INR of 1.5.

Cerebral Thromboembolism
Secondary Prevention

ORAL:
- TIAs or mild ischemic stroke and concurrent atrial fibrillation: Adjust dosage to maintain a target INR of 2.5 (range 2–3) long-term, provided no contraindications to therapy exist.
- Patients at high risk for recurrent stroke from other cardiac sources: Maintenance of a target INR of 2.5 (range 2–3) with concomitant aspirin (75–162 mg daily) recommended by ACC and AHA. Cardiac sources of embolism include mechanical prosthetic heart valves, recent MI, left ventricular thrombus, dilated cardiomyopathies, marantic endocarditis, and extensive wall-motion abnormalities.
- Recent MI complicated by ischemic stroke and left ventricular thrombus or akinetic segment: Adjust dosage to maintain a target INR of 2.5 (range 2–3) with aspirin (75–162 mg daily) therapy for ≥3 months.
- Acute phase of cerebral venous sinus thrombosis†: Follow-up oral anticoagulation (target INR of 2.5 [range 2–3]) for 3–6 months after unfractionated heparin or an LMW heparin.

Treatment/Secondary Prevention in Arterial Vascular Surgery†

ORAL:
- Pulmonary thromboendarterectomy: Indefinite oral anticoagulation a target INR of 2.5 (range 2–3).
- Patients who are ineligible for pulmonary endarterectomy: Indefinite oral anticoagulation at a target INR of 2.5 (range 2–3).

Special Populations

Hepatic Impairment
- Possible increased anticoagulant effect. May require lower initial and maintenance dosages.

Renal Impairment
- Possible increased anticoagulant effect in moderate to severe renal impairment. No dosage adjustments required.

Geriatric Patients
- Possible increased anticoagulant effect. Lower initial (≤5 mg) and maintenance dosages recommended. Adjust dosage to maintain INR at the lower end of the range of 2–3.
- In patients >75 years of age who are considered at high risk

for bleeding complications but do not have frank contraindications, use a lower target INR of 2 (range: 1.6–2.5) for primary prevention of stroke and systemic embolism.

Asian Patients
- Possible increased anticoagulant effect. May require lower initial and maintenance dosages.

† Use is not currently included in the labeling approved by the US Food and Drug Administration.

Zafirlukast

(za fir′ loo kast)

Brand Name: Accolate®
Also available generically.

Why is this medicine prescribed?

Zafirlukast is used to prevent asthma symptoms. Zafirlukast is in a class of medications called leukotriene receptor antagonists (LTRAs). It works by blocking the action of certain natural substances that cause swelling and tightening of the airways.

How should this medicine be used?

Zafirlukast comes as a tablet to take by mouth. It is usually taken two times a day, 1 hour before or 2 hours after meals. Try to take zafirlukast at around the same times every day. Follow the directions on your prescription label carefully, and ask your doctor or pharmacist to explain any part you do not understand. Take zafirlukast exactly as directed. Do not take more or less of it or take it more often than prescribed by your doctor.

Do not use zafirlukast to treat a sudden attack of asthma symptoms. Your doctor will prescribe a short-acting inhaler to use during attacks. Talk to your doctor about how to treat symptoms of a sudden asthma attack.

Continue to take or use all other medications that your doctor has prescribed to treat your asthma. Do not stop taking any of your medications or change the doses of any of your medications unless your doctor tells you that you should.

Zafirlukast may help control asthma symptoms, but it does not cure asthma. Continue to take zafirlukast even if you feel well. Do not stop taking zafirlukast without talking to your doctor.

Are there other uses for this medicine?

Zafirlukast is also sometimes used to treat allergic rhinitis (hay fever; runny nose, watery eyes, and other symptoms caused by an allergic reaction to pollen or other substances in the air). Zafirlukast is also sometimes used to prevent breathing difficulties during exercise in people who have asthma.

What special precautions should I follow?

Before taking zafirlukast,

- tell your doctor and pharmacist if you are allergic to zafirlukast or any other medications.
- tell your doctor and pharmacist what prescription and nonprescription medications, vitamins, nutritional supplements, and herbal products you are taking or plan to take. Be sure to mention any of the following: anticoagulants ('blood thinners') such as warfarin (Coumadin); aspirin or aspirin-containing products; calcium channel blockers such as amlodipine (Norvasc, in Caduet), diltiazem (Cardizem, Tiazac), felodipine (Plendil), isradipine (Dynacirc), nicardipine (Cardene), nifedipine (Adalat, Procardia, others), nimodipine (Nimotop), nisoldipine (Sular), or verapamil (Calan, Covera, Isoptin, Verelan); carbamazepine (Equetro, Tegretol); cisapride (Propulsid) (not available in the U.S.); cyclosporine (Neoral, Sandimmune); erythromycin (E.E.S, Erythrocin); phenytoin (Dilantin); theophylline (Theo-Dur, others); and tolbutamide. Other medications may also interact with zafirlukast, so be sure to tell your doctor about all the medications you are taking, even those that do not appear on this list. Your doctor may need to change the doses of your medications or monitor you more carefully for side effects.
- tell your doctor if you have or have ever had liver disease.
- tell your doctor if you are pregnant or plan to become pregnant. If you become pregnant while taking zafirlukast, call your doctor.
- do not breastfeed while you are taking zafirlukast.

What special dietary instructions should I follow?

Unless your doctor tells you otherwise, continue your normal diet.

What should I do if I forget to take a dose?

Take the missed dose as soon as you remember it. However, if it is almost time for the next dose, skip the missed dose and continue your regular dosing schedule. Do not take a double dose to make up for a missed one.

What side effects can this medicine cause?

Zafirlukast may cause side effects. Tell your doctor if this symptom is severe or does not go away.

- headache

Some side effects can be serious. If you experience any of the following symptoms, call your doctor immediately.

- nausea
- loss of appetite
- pain in the right upper part of your stomach

- excessive tiredness
- lack of energy
- itching
- yellowing of the skin or eyes
- flu-like symptoms
- rash
- swelling of the eyes, face, lips, tongue, or throat
- difficulty breathing or swallowing
- hoarseness
- pain, burning, numbness, or tingling in the hands or feet

Zafirlukast may cause other side effects. Call your doctor if you have any unusual problems while you are taking this medication.

What storage conditions are needed for this medicine?

Keep this medication in the container it came in, tightly closed, and out of reach of children. Store it at room temperature and away from light, excess heat, and moisture (not in the bathroom). Throw away any medication that is outdated or no longer needed. Talk to your pharmacist about the proper disposal of your medication.

What should I do in case of overdose?

In case of overdose, call your local poison control center at 1-800-222-1222. If the victim has collapsed or is not breathing, call local emergency services at 911.

Symptoms of overdose may include:

- nausea
- rash

What other information should I know?

Keep all appointments with your doctor and the laboratory. Your doctor may order certain lab tests to check your response to zafirlukast.

Do not let anyone else take your medication. Ask your pharmacist any questions you have about refilling your prescription.

Dosage Facts
For Informational Purposes

Caution: Do not change your dose, how often you take your medication, or the length of time you are to take it without first talking to your healthcare provider.

The following dosage information was written using medical language for doctors and other healthcare professionals and is provided here for you to check your dosage. The dosage of this drug may differ for different patients. Therefore, always follow your doctor's instructions or the directions on the label. Contact your healthcare provider or pharmacist if you have any questions about the specific dosage of your medication after reviewing this information.

Pediatric Patients

Asthma

ORAL:
- Children 5–11 years of age: 10 mg twice daily.
- Children ≥12 years of age: 20 mg twice daily.

Adult Patients

Asthma

ORAL:
- 20 mg twice daily.

Allergic Rhinitis†

ORAL:
- 20 or 40 mg as a single dose prior to environmental exposure to ragweed pollen.

Special Populations

Hepatic Impairment
- Manufacturer does not make specific dosage recommendations for patients with hepatic impairment. However, consider dosage reduction; decreased clearance reported in patients with stable alcoholic cirrhosis. Not evaluated in patients with hepatitis or in long-term studies of patients with cirrhosis.

Renal Impairment
- Dosage adjustment not required.

Geriatric Patients
- Dosage adjustment not required.

† Use is not currently included in the labeling approved by the US Food and Drug Administration.

Zaleplon

(zal′ e plon)

Brand Name: Sonata®

Why is this medicine prescribed?

Zaleplon is used for short-term treatment of insomnia to help you fall asleep.

This medication is sometimes prescribed for other uses; ask your doctor or pharmacist for more information.

How should this medicine be used?

Zaleplon comes as a capsule to take by mouth. It is usually taken once a day at bedtime or after going to bed if you cannot fall asleep. This medication is usually taken for 7-10 days. Follow the directions on your prescription label carefully, and ask your doctor or pharmacist to explain any part you do not understand. Take zaleplon exactly as directed. Do not take zaleplon unless you will be able to sleep for at least 4 hours after taking the dose.

Zaleplon can be habit-forming; do not take a larger dose, take it more often, or take it for a longer period than your doctor tells you to. Do not stop taking zaleplon without talking to your doctor.

Zaleplon can lose its effectiveness if used for long periods of time. If you experience difficulty falling asleep, call your doctor.

What special precautions should I follow?

Before taking zaleplon,
- tell your doctor and pharmacist if you are allergic to zaleplon, aspirin, tartarzine (a yellow dye in some processed foods and drugs), or any other drugs.
- tell your doctor and pharmacist what prescription and nonprescription medications you are taking, especially allergy medications; antihistamines; barbiturates; cimetidine (Tagamet); cold medicines; imipramine (Tofranil); medications for depression; medications for seizures such as phenytoin (Dilantin), carbamazepine (Eptitol, Tegretol, others), and phenobarbital (Solfoton); pain relievers; rifampin (Rifadin, Rimactane); thioridazine (Mellaril); tranquilizers; and vitamins and herbal products.
- tell your doctor if you have or have ever had kidney or liver disease, a history of alcohol or drug abuse or depression, asthma, breathing problems, or allergies.
- tell your doctor if you are pregnant, plan to become pregnant, or are breast-feeding. If you become pregnant while taking zaleplon, call your doctor.
- if you are having surgery, including dental surgery, tell the doctor or dentist that you are taking zaleplon.
- you should know that this drug may make you drowsy. Do not drive a car or operate machinery until you know how zaleplon will affect you.
- remember that alcohol can add to the drowsiness caused by this drug.

What special dietary instructions should I follow?

Do not take zaleplon with or right after a high-fat or heavy meal.

What should I do if I forget to take a dose?

Do not take a missed dose when you remember it. Skip the missed dose and take the next dose at the regularly scheduled time.

What side effects can this medicine cause?

Zaleplon may cause side effects. Tell your doctor if any of these symptoms are severe or do not go away:
- drowsiness
- dizziness
- lightheadedness
- lack of coordination
- headache
- constipation
- dry mouth
- muscle aches

If you experience any of the following symptoms, call your doctor immediately:

- skin rash
- itching
- fast or irregular heartbeat
- chest pain
- difficulty breathing
- fever
- behavior changes or acting differently
- mental confusion
- abnormal thinking or dreams
- hallucinations
- depression
- worsening of insomnia
- problems with memory

If you experience a serious side effect, you or your doctor may send a report to the Food and Drug Administration's (FDA) MedWatch Adverse Event Reporting program online [at http://www.fda.gov/MedWatch/index.html] or by phone [1-800-332-1088].

What storage conditions are needed for this medicine?

Keep this medication in the container it came in, tightly closed, and out of reach of children. Store it at room temperature and away from excess heat and moisture (not in the bathroom). Throw away any medication that is outdated or no longer needed. Talk to your pharmacist about the proper disposal of your medication.

What should I do in case of overdose?

In case of overdose, call your local poison control center at 1-800-222-1222. If the victim has collapsed or is not breathing, call local emergency services at 911.

What other information should I know?

Keep all appointments with your doctor.

Do not let anyone else take your medication. Zaleplon is a controlled substance. Prescriptions may be refilled only a limited number of times; ask your pharmacist if you have any questions.

Dosage Facts

For Informational Purposes

Caution: Do not change your dose, how often you take your medication, or the length of time you are to take it without first talking to your healthcare provider.

The following dosage information was written using medical language for doctors and other healthcare professionals and is provided here for you to check your dosage. The dosage of this drug may differ for different patients. Therefore, always follow your doctor's instructions or the directions on the label. Contact your healthcare provider or pharmacist if you have any questions about the specific dosage of your medication after reviewing this information.

Adult Patients

Insomnia

ORAL:
- Individualize dosage.
- Adults <65 years of age: 10 mg. Although risk of certain adverse effects appears to be dose dependent, 20-mg doses have been adequately tolerated; may consider if unresponsive to a trial of lower dosage.
- Generally, limit use to 7–10 days; reevaluate patient if plan to use >2–3 weeks.

Prescribing Limits

Adult Patients

Insomnia

Doses >20 mg not adequately studied; not recommended by manufacturer.

Special Populations

Hepatic Impairment
- In patients with mild to moderate hepatic impairment, 5 mg; doses >10 mg not recommended. Not recommended in patients with severe hepatic impairment.

Renal Impairment
- No dosage adjustment necessary in patients with mild to moderate renal impairment. Not adequately studied in patients with severe renal impairment.

Geriatric Patients
- In adults ≥65 years of age, 5 mg may be sufficient; doses >10 mg not recommended.

Debilitated or Low-weight Patients
- In debilitated patients or low-weight patients <65 years of age, 5 mg may be sufficient; doses >10 mg not recommended.

Patients Receiving Cimetidine
- In patients receiving cimetidine concomitantly, initial dose of 5 mg recommended.

Zanamivir Inhalation

(za na′ mi veer)

Brand Name: Relenza®

Why is this medicine prescribed?

Zanamivir is used in adults and children to treat some types of influenza ('flu') in people who have had symptoms of the flu for less than 2 days. This medication is also used to prevent some types of flu in adults and children when they have spent time with someone who has the flu or when there is a flu outbreak. Zanamivir is in a class of medications called neuraminidase inhibitors. It works by stopping the growth and spread of the flu virus in your body. Zanamivir helps shorten the time you have flu symptoms such as nasal congestion, sore throat, cough, muscle aches, tiredness, weakness, headache, fever, and chills.

How should this medicine be used?

Zanamivir comes as a powder to inhale (breathe in) by mouth. To treat influenza, two inhalations of zanamivir are used twice daily for 5 days. You should inhale the doses about 12 hours apart and at the same time each day. However, on the first day of treatment, your doctor may tell you to inhale the doses closer together. To help prevent the spread of influenza in people living in the same household, two inhalations of zanamivir are used once a day for 10 days. To help prevent the spread of influenza in a community, two inhalations of zanamivir are used once a day for 28 days. When using zanamivir to prevent influenza it should be inhaled at around the same time every day. Follow the directions on your prescription label carefully, and ask your doctor or pharmacist to explain any part you do not understand. Use zanamivir exactly as directed. Do not use more or less of it or use it more often than prescribed by your doctor.

Zanamivir comes with a plastic inhaler called a Diskhaler (device for inhaling powder) and five Rotadisks (circular foil blister packs containing four doses of medication). Do not put a hole in or open any medication blister pack until inhaling a dose with the Diskhaler. Carefully read the manufacturer's instructions that describe how to prepare and inhale a dose of zanamivir using the Diskhaler. Be sure to ask your pharmacist or doctor if you have any questions about how to prepare or inhale this medication.

Follow the directions on your prescription label carefully, and ask your doctor or pharmacist to explain any part that you do not understand. Use zanamivir exactly as directed. Do not use more or less of it or use it more often than prescribed by your doctor.

The use of the inhaler for a child should be supervised by an adult who understands how to use zanamivir and has been instructed in its use by a healthcare provider.

Continue to take zanamivir even if you start to feel better. Do not stop taking zanamivir without talking to your doctor.

If you feel worse or develop new symptoms during or after treatment, or if your flu symptoms do not start to get better, call your doctor.

Ask your pharmacist or doctor for a copy of the manufacturer's information for the patient.

Are there other uses for this medicine?

This medication may be prescribed for other uses; ask your doctor or pharmacist for more information.

What special precautions should I follow?

Before using zanamivir,
- tell your doctor and pharmacist if you are allergic to

zanamivir, any other medications, any food products, or lactose (milk proteins).
- tell your doctor and pharmacist what prescription and nonprescription medications, vitamins, nutritional supplements, and herbal products you are taking or plan to take. Your doctor may need to change the doses of your medications or monitor you carefully for side effects.
- tell your doctor if you have or have ever had asthma or other breathing problems, bronchitis (swelling of the air passages that lead to the lungs), emphysema (damage to air sacs in the lungs); or heart, kidney, liver, or other lung disease.
- if you use an inhaled medication to treat asthma, emphysema, or other breathing problems and you are scheduled to take that medication at the same time as zanamivir, you should take your regular medication before taking zanamivir.
- tell your doctor if you are pregnant, plan to become pregnant, or are breast-feeding. If you become pregnant while taking zanamivir, call your doctor.
- you should know that zanamivir may cause serious or life-threatening breathing problems, more commonly in patients with asthma or emphysema. If you have trouble breathing or have wheezing after your dose of zanamivir, stop using zanamivir and get medical attention. If you have difficulty breathing, and have been prescribed a rescue medication, use your rescue medication immediately and then call for medical attention. Do not take any more zanamivir without first talking to your doctor.

What special dietary instructions should I follow?

Unless your doctor tells you otherwise, continue your normal diet.

What should I do if I forget to take a dose?

If you forget to inhale a dose, inhale it as soon as you remember it. If it is 2 hours or less until the next dose, skip the missed dose and continue your regular dosing schedule. Do not inhale a double dose to make up for a missed one.

What side effects can this medicine cause?

Zanamivir may cause side effects. Tell your doctor if any of these symptoms are severe or do not go away:
- headache
- dizziness
- nausea
- vomiting
- diarrhea
- cough
- irritation of the nose
- infection of the ear, nose, sinuses, throat, or bronchi (breathing tubes of the lung)

If you experience any of the following symptoms, call your doctor immediately:

- difficulty breathing
- wheezing
- shortness of breath
- hives
- rash
- itching
- difficulty swallowing
- swelling of the face, throat, tongue, lips, eyes, hands, feet, ankles, or lower legs
- hoarseness

If you experience a serious side effect, you or your doctor may send a report to the Food and Drug Administration's (FDA) MedWatch Adverse Event Reporting program online [at http://www.fda.gov/MedWatch/index.html] or by phone [1-800-332-1088].

What storage conditions are needed for this medicine?

Keep this medication in the container it came in and out of reach of children. Store it at room temperature and away from excess heat and moisture (not in the bathroom). Throw away any medication that is outdated or no longer needed. Talk to your pharmacist about the proper disposal of your medication.

What should I do in case of overdose?

In case of overdose, call your local poison control center at 1-800-222-1222. If the victim has collapsed or is not breathing, call local emergency services at 911.

What other information should I know?

You should maintain proper hygiene, wash your hands frequently, and avoid situations such as sharing cups and utensils that can spread the influenza virus to others.

Ask your doctor if you should receive a flu vaccination each year. Zanamivir does not take the place of a yearly flu vaccine.

The Diskhaler should only be used for zanamivir. Do not use the Diskhaler to take other medications that you inhale.

Do not let anyone else use your medication. Your prescription is probably not refillable.

Dosage Facts
For Informational Purposes

Caution: Do not change your dose, how often you take your medication, or the length of time you are to take it without first talking to your healthcare provider.

The following dosage information was written using medical language for doctors and other healthcare professionals and is provided here for you to check your dosage. The dosage of this drug may differ for different patients. Therefore, always follow your doctor's instruc-

tions or the directions on the label. Contact your healthcare provider or pharmacist if you have any questions about the specific dosage of your medication after reviewing this information.

Pediatric Patients

Treatment of Influenza A and B Virus Infections

ORAL INHALATION:
- Children ≥7 years of age: 2 inhalations (one 5-mg blister per inhalation for a total dose of 10 mg) twice daily (approximately 12 hours apart) for 5 days. Initiate zanamivir treatment within 2 days after onset of symptoms; efficacy not established if treatment begins >2 days after onset of symptoms.
- Whenever possible, the first day of treatment should include 2 doses provided there is at least 2 hours between doses; on subsequent days, doses should be given about 12 hours apart (morning and evening) at approximately the same time each day.

Prevention of Influenza A and B Virus Infections
Household Setting

ORAL INHALATION:
- Adolescents and children ≥5 years of age: 2 inhalations (one 5-mg blister per inhalation for a total dose of 10 mg) once daily for 10 days. Administer at approximately the same time each day. Efficacy in household settings not established if zanamivir prophylaxis initiated >1.5 days after onset of symptoms in the index case.

Community Outbreak

ORAL INHALATION:
- Adolescents: 2 inhalations (one 5-mg blister per inhalation for a total dose of 10 mg) once daily for 28 days. Administer at approximately the same time each day. Efficacy in community outbreaks not established if zanamivir prophylaxis initiated >5 days after the outbreak is identified in the community. Safety and efficacy of prophylaxis given for >28 days not evaluated.

Adult Patients

Treatment of Influenza A and B Virus Infections

ORAL INHALATION:
- 2 inhalations (one 5-mg blister per inhalation for a total dose of 10 mg) twice daily (approximately 12 hours apart) for 5 days. Initiate zanamivir treatment within 2 days after onset of symptoms; efficacy not established if treatment begins after 48 hours of symptoms.
- Whenever possible, the first day of treatment should include 2 doses provided there is at least 2 hours between doses; on subsequent days, doses should be given about 12 hours apart (morning and evening) at approximately the same time each day.

Prevention of Influenza A and B Virus Infections
Household Setting

ORAL INHALATION:
- 2 inhalations (one 5-mg blister per inhalation for a total dose of 10 mg) once daily for 10 days. Administer at approximately the same time each day. Efficacy in household settings

not established if zanamivir prophylaxis initiated >1.5 days after onset of symptoms in the index case.

Community Outbreak

ORAL INHALATION:

- 2 inhalations (one 5-mg blister per inhalation for a total dose of 10 mg) once daily for 28 days. Administer at approximately the same time each day. Efficacy in community outbreaks not established if zanamivir prophylaxis initiated >5 days after the outbreak is identified in the community. Safety and efficacy of prophylaxis given for >28 days not evaluated.

Zidovudine Oral

(zye doe′ vue deen)

Brand Name: Combivir® as a combination product containing Zidovudine and Lamivudine, Retrovir®, Retrovir® Syrup, Trizivir® as a combination product containing Zidovudine, Abacavir Sulfate, and Lamivudine
Also available generically.

Important Warning

Zidovudine may decrease the number of a certain type of white blood cell in the blood and cause anemia and muscle disorders. When used alone or in combination with other antiviral medications, zidovudine can also cause serious damage to the liver and a blood condition called lactic acidosis.

Call your doctor immediately if you experience any of the following symptoms: upset stomach, loss of appetite, dark yellow or brown urine, unusual bleeding or bruising, flu-like symptoms, yellowing of the skin or eyes, and pain in the upper right part of your stomach, muscle weakness, lack of strength, muscle pain, shortness of breath, unusual tiredness or weakness, and pale skin.

It is extremely important to keep all appointments with your doctor and the laboratory. Your doctor will order certain lab tests to check your response to zidovudine.

Why is this medicine prescribed?

Zidovudine is used alone or with other medications to treat human immunodeficiency virus (HIV) infection in patients with or without acquired immunodeficiency syndrome (AIDS). It will slow the spread of HIV infection in the body. Zidovudine is not a cure and may not decrease the number of HIV-related illnesses. Zidovudine does not prevent the spread of HIV to other people except when given to HIV-positive pregnant women. Zidovudine is given to HIV-pos-

itive pregnant women to prevent the infection from going to the baby. However, HIV infection may still occur in the infant despite this treatment.

This medication is sometimes prescribed for other uses; ask your doctor or pharmacist for more information.

How should this medicine be used?

Zidovudine comes as a capsule, tablet, and syrup to take by mouth. It is usually taken three to four times a day. In some cases it may be taken five times a day. Follow the directions on your prescription label carefully, and ask your doctor or pharmacist to explain any part you do not understand. Take zidovudine exactly as directed. Do not take more or less of it or take it more often than prescribed by your doctor.

Continue to take zidovudine even if you feel well. Do not stop taking zidovudine without talking to your doctor.

Are there other uses for this medicine?

Zidovudine is also used sometimes to treat health care workers and other individuals exposed to HIV infection after accidental contact with HIV-contaminated blood, tissues, or other body fluids. Talk to your doctor about the possible risks of using this drug for your condition.

What special precautions should I follow?

Before taking zidovudine,

- tell your doctor and pharmacist if you are allergic to zidovudine or any other drugs.
- tell your doctor and pharmacist what prescription and nonprescription medications you are taking, especially acetaminophen, acyclovir (Zovirax), aspirin, cimetidine (Tagamet), fluconazole (Diflucan), foscarnet (Foscavir), ganciclovir (Cytovene), indomethacin (Indocin), interferon, lorazepam (Ativan), oxazepam (Serax), probenecid (Benemid), valproic acid (Depakene, Depakote), and vitamins.
- tell your doctor if you have or have ever had liver or kidney disease, any disease or swelling of the muscle, anemia, a history of alcohol abuse, or bleeding or other blood problems.
- tell your doctor if you are pregnant, plan to become pregnant, or are breast-feeding. If you become pregnant while taking zidovudine, call your doctor.
- tell your doctor if you drink alcohol.

What special dietary instructions should I follow?

Zidovudine should be taken at least 30 minutes before or 1 hour after a meal. You should take it sitting up with plenty of water.

What should I do if I forget to take a dose?

Take the missed dose as soon as you remember it. However, if it is almost time for the next dose, skip the missed dose

and continue your regular dosing schedule. Do not take a double dose to make up for a missed one.

What side effects can this medicine cause?

Zidovudine may cause side effects. Tell your doctor if any of these symptoms are severe or do not go away:

- stomach pain
- diarrhea or loose stools
- constipation
- headache
- dizziness
- difficulty sleeping

If you experience the following symptom, or any of those listed in the IMPORTANT WARNING section, call your doctor immediately:

- rash

If you experience a serious side effect, you or your doctor may send a report to the Food and Drug Administration's (FDA) MedWatch Adverse Event Reporting program online [at http://www.fda.gov/MedWatch/index.html] or by phone [1-800-332-1088].

What storage conditions are needed for this medicine?

Keep this medication in the container it came in, tightly closed, and out of reach of children. Store it at room temperature and away from excess heat and moisture (not in the bathroom). Throw away any medication that is outdated or no longer needed. Talk to your pharmacist about the proper disposal of your medication.

What should I do in case of overdose?

In case of overdose, call your local poison control center at 1-800-222-1222. If the victim has collapsed or is not breathing, call local emergency services at 911.

What other information should I know?

Do not let anyone else take your medication. Ask your pharmacist any questions you have about refilling your prescription.

Dosage Facts
For Informational Purposes

Caution: Do not change your dose, how often you take your medication, or the length of time you are to take it without first talking to your healthcare provider.

The following dosage information was written using medical language for doctors and other healthcare professionals and is provided here for you to check your dosage. The dosage of this drug may differ for different patients. Therefore, always follow your doctor's instructions or the directions on the label. Contact your health-care provider or pharmacist if you have any questions about the specific dosage of your medication after reviewing this information.

General Dosage Information

Used in conjunction with other antiretrovirals for treatment of HIV infection or for postexposure prophylaxis of HIV; may be used alone or in conjunction with other antiretrovirals for prevention of maternal-fetal transmission of HIV. The fixed-combination preparation containing zidovudine, abacavir, and lamivudine may be used alone or in conjunction with other antiretrovirals.

Dosage of Combivir® and Trizivir® expressed as number of tablets.

IV dosing regimen of 1 mg/kg every 4 hours is equivalent to an oral regimen of 100 mg every 4 hours.

Modification of zidovudine dosage is necessary in adults or pediatric patients who develop anemia and/or neutropenia. Substantial anemia (hemoglobin <7.5 g/dL or a reduction >25% from baseline) and/or neutropenia (granulocyte count <750/mm³ or a reduction >50% from baseline) may require dose interruption until evidence of bone marrow recovery occurs. If bone marrow recovery occurs following interruption of therapy, reinitiation of zidovudine therapy may be appropriate.

Pediatric Patients
Treatment of HIV Infection

ORAL:

- Premature neonates: 2 mg/kg every 12 hours; frequency of administration may be increased to every 8 hours at 2 weeks of age in neonates with ≥30 weeks gestation at birth or at 4 weeks of age in those with <30 weeks gestation at birth.
- Neonates and infants <6 weeks of age: 2 mg/kg every 6 hours.
- Infants and children 6 weeks to 12 years of age: 160 mg/m² (maximum 200 mg) every 8 hours. 180–240 mg/m² every 12 hours has been used by some investigators to improve compliance.
- Adolescents ≥12 years of age: 200 mg 3 times daily or 300 mg twice daily.
- Combivir®: 1 tablet twice daily in adolescents ≥12 years of age.
- Trizivir®: 1 tablet twice daily in adolescents weighing ≥40 kg.

Prevention of Maternal-fetal Transmission of HIV
3-Part Zidovudine Regimen

ORAL:

- Premature neonates: Initiate therapy with 2 mg/kg every 12 hours; frequency of administration may be increased to every 8 hours at 2 weeks of age in neonates with >30 weeks gestation at birth or at 4 weeks of age in those with <30 weeks gestation at birth.
- Neonates: 2 mg/kg every 6 hours starting within 12 hours after birth and continued through 6 weeks of age.
- Used in conjunction with antepartum and intrapartum zidovudine in the mother.

Zidovudine and Lamivudine Regimen

ORAL:

- Neonates born to women who received no antiretroviral therapy prior to labor: 4 mg/kg every 12 hours given for 7 days

in conjunction with a 7-day regimen of oral lamivudine (2 mg/kg every 12 hours).
- Used in conjunction with intrapartum regimen of oral zidovudine and lamivudine in the mother.

Adult Patients

Treatment of HIV Infection

ORAL:
- 600 mg daily in divided doses. Usually given in a dosage of 200 mg 3 times daily or 300 mg twice daily.
- Combivir®: 1 tablet twice daily.
- Trizivir®: 1 tablet twice daily. Patient should weigh ≥40 kg.

Prevention of Maternal-fetal Transmission of HIV
3-Part Zidovudine Regimen

ORAL:
- 100 mg 5 times daily or 200 mg 3 times daily or 300 mg twice daily initiated at 14–34 weeks of pregnancy and continued until the start of labor. At start of labor, switch to IV zidovudine.
- Used in conjunction with a 6-week zidovudine regimen in the neonate.

Zidovudine and Lamivudine Regimen

ORAL:
- Women in labor who have received no prior antiretroviral therapy: 600 mg at onset of labor, then 300 mg every 3 hours during labor. Given in conjunction with oral lamivudine (150 mg at onset of labor, then 150 mg every 12 hours during labor).
- Used in conjunction with a 7-day regimen of oral zidovudine and lamivudine in the neonate.

Postexposure Prophylaxis of HIV†
Occupational Exposure†

ORAL:
- 200 mg 3 times daily or 300 mg twice daily.
- Used in basic regimens with lamivudine or emtricitabine.
- Initiate postexposure prophylaxis as soon as possible following exposure (within hours rather than days) and continue for 4 weeks, if tolerated.

Nonoccupational Exposure†

ORAL:
- 200 mg 3 times daily or 300 mg twice daily.
- Used in preferred nonnucleoside reverse transcriptase inhibitor-based (NNRTI-based) regimens that include efavirenz and (lamivudine or emtricitabine) and (zidovudine or tenofovir) or preferred HIV protease inhibitor-based (PI-based) regimens that include fixed combination of lopinavir and ritonavir and (lamivudine or emtricitabine) and zidovudine. Also used in various alternative PI-based regimens that include a PI (with or without low-dose ritonavir) and (lamivudine or emtricitabine) and zidovudine.
- Initiate postexposure prophylaxis as soon as possible following exposure (preferably ≤72 hours after exposure) and continue for 28 days.

Prescribing Limits
Pediatric Patients
Treatment of HIV Infection

ORAL:
- Children 6 weeks to 12 years of age: Maximum 200 mg every 8 hours.

Special Populations

Hepatic Impairment

Treatment of HIV Infection
- Insufficient clinical experience to recommend dosage adjustment for patients with mild to moderate hepatic impairment or liver cirrhosis; a reduction in dosage may be necessary in these patients and frequent monitoring for hematologic toxicities advised.

Renal Impairment

Treatment of HIV Infection

ORAL:
- 100 mg every 6 to 8 hours for patients with end-stage renal disease maintained on hemodialysis or peritoneal dialysis.

Geriatric Patients
- Select dosage with caution because of age-related decreases in hepatic, renal, and/or cardiac function and concomitant disease and drug therapy.

† Use is not currently included in the labeling approved by the US Food and Drug Administration.

Zileuton

(zye loo′ ton)

Brand Name: Zyflo® Filmtab®
Also available generically.

Why is this medicine prescribed?

Zileuton is used to prevent asthma symptoms. It works by blocking the formation of substances that cause inflammation, fluid retention, mucous secretion, and constriction in your lungs.

This medication is sometimes prescribed for other uses; ask your doctor or pharmacist for more information.

How should this medicine be used?

Zileuton comes as a tablet to take by mouth. It usually is taken four times a day. Follow the directions on your prescription label carefully, and ask your doctor or pharmacist to explain any part you do not understand. Take zileuton exactly as directed. Do not take more or less of it or take it more often than prescribed by your doctor.

Zileuton controls asthma symptoms but does not cure them. Continue to take zileuton even if you feel well. Do not stop taking zileuton without talking to your doctor.

What special precautions should I follow?

Before taking zileuton,

- tell your doctor and pharmacist if you are allergic to zileuton or any other drugs.
- tell your doctor and pharmacist what prescription and nonprescription medications you are taking, especially anticoagulants ('blood thinners') such as warfarin (Coumadin), propranolol (Inderal), terfenadine (Seldane), theophylline (Theo-Dur), and vitamins.
- tell your doctor if you have or have ever had liver disease or if you consume alcohol regularly.
- tell your doctor if you are pregnant, plan to become pregnant, or are breast-feeding. If you become pregnant while taking zileuton, call your doctor.

What special dietary instructions should I follow?

Ask your doctor for advice on how much alcohol is safe to drink while you are taking this medicine.

What should I do if I forget to take a dose?

Take the missed dose as soon as you remember it. However, if it is almost time for the next dose, skip the missed dose and continue your regular dosing schedule. Do not take a double dose to make up for a missed one.

What side effects can this medicine cause?

Zileuton may cause side effects. Tell your doctor if any of these symptoms are severe or do not go away.

- headache
- upset stomach
- heartburn
- vomiting
- constipation
- nervousness
- dizziness
- insomnia
- gas

If you experience any of the following symptoms, call your doctor immediately.

- stomach pain
- fatigue
- itching
- yellowing of the skin or eyes
- flu-like symptoms

If you experience a serious side effect, you or your doctor may send a report to the Food and Drug Administration's (FDA) MedWatch Adverse Event Reporting program online [at http://www.fda.gov/MedWatch/index.html] or by phone [1-800-332-1088].

What storage conditions are needed for this medicine?

Keep this medication in the container it came in, tightly closed, and out of reach of children. Store it at room temperature and away from excess heat and moisture (not in the bathroom). Throw away any medication that is outdated or no longer needed. Talk to your pharmacist about the proper disposal of your medication.

What should I do in case of overdose?

In case of overdose, call your local poison control center at 1-800-222-1222. If the victim has collapsed or is not breathing, call local emergency services at 911.

What other information should I know?

Keep all appointments with your doctor and the laboratory. Your doctor will order certain lab tests to monitor your liver function while you are taking zileuton.

Call your doctor if your asthma symptoms do not improve or worsen.

Zileuton will not stop an acute attack that has already started. Continue to use the medication prescribed for your acute attacks.

Do not let anyone else take your medication. Ask your pharmacist any questions you have about refilling your prescription.

Dosage Facts
For Informational Purposes

Caution: Do not change your dose, how often you take your medication, or the length of time you are to take it without first talking to your healthcare provider.

The following dosage information was written using medical language for doctors and other healthcare professionals and is provided here for you to check your dosage. The dosage of this drug may differ for different patients. Therefore, always follow your doctor's instructions or the directions on the label. Contact your healthcare provider or pharmacist if you have any questions about the specific dosage of your medication after reviewing this information.

Pediatric Patients

Asthma

ORAL:
- Children $\geq$12 years of age: 600 mg 4 times daily.

Adult Patients

Asthma

ORAL:
- 600 mg 4 times daily.

Prescribing Limits
Pediatric Patients

Asthma

ORAL:
- Children $\geq$12 years of age: Maximum 2.4 g daily.

Adult Patients

Asthma

ORAL:
- Maximum 2.4 g daily.

Special Populations

Hepatic Impairment
- No specific dosage recommendations at this time. Do not use in patients with active liver disease or transaminases ≥3 times the ULN.

Renal Impairment
- Dosage adjustment not required.

Geriatric Patients
- Dosage adjustment not required.

Ziprasidone

(zi pray′ si done)

Brand Name: Geodon®

Important Warning

Studies have shown that older adults with dementia (a brain disorder that affects the ability to remember, think clearly, communicate, and perform daily activities and that may cause changes in mood and personality) who take antipsychotics (medications for mental illness) such as ziprasidone have an increased risk of death during treatment. Older adults with dementia may also have a greater chance of having a stroke or mini-stroke during treatment. If you experience any of the following symptoms, call your doctor immediately: slow or difficult speech, sudden dizziness or faintness, or weakness or numbness of an arm or leg.

Ziprasidone is not approved by the Food and Drug Administration (FDA) for the treatment of behavior problems in older adults with dementia. Talk to the doctor who prescribed this medication if you, a family member, or someone you care for has dementia and is taking ziprasidone. For more information visit the FDA website: http://www.fda.gov/cder

Why is this medicine prescribed?

Ziprasidone is used to treat the symptoms of schizophrenia (a mental illness that causes disturbed or unusual thinking, loss of interest in life, and strong or inappropriate emotions). It is also used to treat episodes of mania (frenzied, abnor-mally excited or irritated mood) or mixed episodes (symptoms of mania and depression that happen together) in patients with bipolar disorder (manic depressive disorder; a disease that causes episodes of depression, episodes of mania, and other abnormal moods). Ziprasidone is in a class of medications called atypical antipsychotics. It works by changing the activity of certain natural substances in the brain.

How should this medicine be used?

Ziprasidone comes as a capsule to take by mouth. It is usually taken twice a day with food. Take ziprasidone at around the same times every day. Follow the directions on your prescription label carefully, and ask your doctor or pharmacist to explain any part you do not understand. Take ziprasidone exactly as directed. Do not take more or less of it or take it more often than prescribed by your doctor.

Your doctor may start you on a low dose of ziprasidone and gradually increase your dose.

Ziprasidone may help control your symptoms but will not cure your condition. Continue to take ziprasidone even if you feel well. Do not stop taking ziprasidone without talking to your doctor.

Are there other uses for this medicine?

This medication may be prescribed for other uses; ask your doctor or pharmacist for more information.

What special precautions should I follow?

Before taking ziprasidone,
- tell your doctor and pharmacist if you are allergic to ziprasidone or any other medications.
- tell your doctor if you are taking amiodarone (Cordarone, Pacerone), chlorpromazine (Thorazine), cisapride (Propulsid) (no longer available in the U.S.), disopyramide (Norpace), dofetilide (Tikosyn), dolasetron (Anzemet), droperidol (Inapsine), erythromycin (E.E.S., E-Mycin, Erythrocin), gatifloxacin (Tequin)(no longer available in the U.S.), halofantrine (Halfan)(no longer available in the U.S.), levomethadyl (ORLAAM) (no longer available in the U.S.), mefloquine (Lariam), mesoridazine (Serentil)(no longer available in the U.S..), moxifloxacin (Avelox), pentamidine (NebuPent, Pentam 300), pimozide (Orap), procainamide (Procanbid, Promine, Pronestyl), quinidine (Quinidex), sotalol (Betapace), sparfloxacin (Zagam), tacrolimus (Prograf), or thioridazine (Mellaril). Your doctor may tell you not to take ziprasidone if you are taking one or more of these medications.
- tell your doctor and pharmacist what other prescription and nonprescription medications, vitamins, nutritional supplements, and herbal products you are taking or plan to take. Be sure to mention any of the following: antidepressants; certain antifungals such as fluconazole (Diflucan), itraconazole (Sporanox), ketoconazole (Nizoral), and voriconazole (Vfend); aprepitant (Emend);

carbamazepine (Tegretol); clarithromycin (Biaxin, in Prevpac); cyclosporine (Neoral, Sandimmune); delavirdine (Rescriptor); diltiazem (Cardizem, Dilacor, Tiazac, others); diuretics ('water pills'); dopamine agonists such as bromocriptine (Parlodel), cabergoline (Dostinex), levodopa (Dopar, Larodopa), pergolide (Permax), and ropinirole (Requip); efavirenz (Sustiva); fluoxetine (Prozac, Sarafem); fluvoxamine (Luvox); HIV protease inhibitors including atazanavir (Reyataz), indinavir (Crixivan), lopinavir (in Kaletra), nelfinavir (Viracept), ritonavir (Norvir, in Kaletra), and saquinavir (Fortovase, Invirase); hormonal contraceptives (birth control pills, rings, patches, implants, and injections); lovastatin (Mevacor, in Advicor); medications for anxiety, high blood pressure or seizures; nefazodone; sertraline (Zoloft); sleeping pills; tranquilizers; troleandomycin (TAO)(no longer available in the U.S..); verapamil (Calan, Covera, Isoptin, Verelan); and zafirlukast (Accolate). Your doctor may need to change the doses of your medications or monitor you carefully for side effects.

- tell your doctor if you use or have ever used street drugs or have overused prescription medications or if you have recently had a heart attack or have trouble swallowing. Also tell your doctor if you have or have ever had heart or liver disease, breast cancer, heart failure, an irregular heartbeat, a stroke or mini-stroke, or seizures, or if you or anyone in your family has or has ever had diabetes. Also tell your doctor if you have ever had to stop taking a medication for mental illness because of severe side effects.
- tell your doctor if you are pregnant or plan to become pregnant. If you become pregnant while taking ziprasidone, call your doctor. Do not breast-feed while taking ziprasidone.
- you should know that ziprasidone may make you drowsy. Do not drive a car or operate machinery until you know how this medication affects you.
- you should know that alcohol can add to the drowsiness caused by this medication. Do not drink alcohol while taking ziprasidone.
- you should know that you may experience hyperglycemia (increases in your blood sugar) while you are taking this medication, even if you do not already have diabetes. If you have schizophrenia, you are more likely to develop diabetes than people who do not have schizophrenia, and taking ziprasidone or similar medications may increase this risk. Tell your doctor immediately if you have any of the following symptoms while you are taking ziprasidone: extreme thirst, frequent urination, extreme hunger, blurred vision, or weakness. It is very important to call your doctor as soon as you have any of these symptoms, because high blood sugar that is not treated can cause a serious condition called ketoacidosis. Ketoacidosis may become life-threatening if it is not treated at an early stage. Symptoms of ketoacidosis include: dry mouth, nausea and vomiting, shortness of breath, breath that smells fruity, and decreased consciousness.
- you should know that ziprasidone may cause dizziness, lightheadedness, and fainting when you get up too quickly from a lying position. This is more common when you first start taking ziprasidone. To avoid this problem, get out of bed slowly, resting your feet on the floor for a few minutes before standing up.
- you should know that ziprasidone may make it harder for your body to cool down when it gets very hot. Tell your doctor if you plan to do vigorous exercise or be exposed to extreme heat.

What special dietary instructions should I follow?

Talk to your doctor about eating grapefruit and drinking grapefruit juice while taking this medicine.

Be sure to drink plenty of water every day while you are taking this medication.

What should I do if I forget to take a dose?

Take the missed dose as soon as you remember it. However, if it is almost time for the next dose, skip the missed dose and continue your regular dosing schedule. Do not take a double dose to make up for a missed one.

What side effects can this medicine cause?

Ziprasidone may cause side effects. Tell your doctor if any of these symptoms are severe or do not go away:

- drowsiness
- headache
- restlessness
- anxiety
- constipation
- diarrhea
- loss of appetite
- muscle pain
- runny nose, sneezing
- cough
- weight gain

Some side effects can be serious. If you experience any of the following symptoms or those listed in the IMPORTANT WARNING section or the SPECIAL PRECAUTIONS section, call your doctor immediately:

- unusual movements of your face or body that you cannot control
- fast, irregular, or pounding heartbeat
- rash or hives
- fever
- muscle stiffness
- confusion
- sweating
- painful erection of the penis that lasts for hours

Ziprasidone may cause other side effects. Call your doctor if you have any unusual problems while taking this medication.

If you experience a serious side effect, you or your doctor may send a report to the Food and Drug Administration's (FDA) MedWatch Adverse Event Reporting program online [at http://www.fda.gov/MedWatch/index.html] or by phone [1-800-332-1088].

What storage conditions are needed for this medicine?

Keep this medication in the container it came in, tightly closed, and out of reach of children. Store it at room temperature and away from excess heat and moisture (not in the bathroom). Throw away any medication that is outdated or no longer needed. Talk to your pharmacist about the proper disposal of your medication.

What should I do in case of overdose?

In case of overdose, call your local poison control center at 1-800-222-1222. If the victim has collapsed or is not breathing, call local emergency services at 911.

Symptoms of overdose may include:
- drowsiness
- slurred speech
- sudden movements that you cannot control
- uncontrollable shaking of a part of the body
- anxiety

What other information should I know?

Keep all appointments with your doctor and the laboratory. Your doctor may order certain lab tests to check your body's response to ziprasidone.

Do not let anyone else take your medication. Ask your pharmacist any questions you have about refilling your prescription.

Dosage Facts
For Informational Purposes

Caution: Do not change your dose, how often you take your medication, or the length of time you are to take it without first talking to your healthcare provider.

The following dosage information was written using medical language for doctors and other healthcare professionals and is provided here for you to check your dosage. The dosage of this drug may differ for different patients. Therefore, always follow your doctor's instructions or the directions on the label. Contact your healthcare provider or pharmacist if you have any questions about the specific dosage of your medication after reviewing this information.

General Dosage Information

Available as ziprasidone hydrochloride or ziprasidone mesylate; oral dosage expressed in terms of hydrochloride monohydrate.

Adult Patients
Schizophrenia

ORAL:
- Initially, 20 mg twice daily.
- Dosage may be increased after a minimum of 2 days. Observe patients for several weeks prior to upward titrations of dosage to ensure use of the lowest effective dosage.
- In patients responding to ziprasidone therapy, continue the drug as long as clinically necessary and tolerated, but at lowest possible effective dosage; periodically reassess need for continued therapy. Efficacy maintained for up to 52 weeks in clinical trials, but optimum duration of therapy currently is not known.

Bipolar Disorder

ORAL:
- Initially, 40 mg twice daily on day 1. Increase dosage to 60 or 80 mg twice daily on the second day.
- Subsequent dosage adjustments based on efficacy and tolerability may be made within a dosage range of 40–80 mg twice daily.
- Efficacy for long-term use (i.e., >3 weeks) or for prophylactic use in patients with bipolar disorder not systematically evaluated. If used for extended periods, periodically reevaluate the long-term risks and benefits for the individual patient.

Prescribing Limits
Adult Patients
Schizophrenia

ORAL:
- Maximum 80 mg twice daily.

Bipolar Disorder

ORAL:
- Maximum 80 mg twice daily.

Zoledronic Acid Injection

(zoe′ le dron ik)

Brand Name: Zometa®

Why is this medicine prescribed?

Zoledronic acid is used to treat high levels of calcium in the blood that may be caused by certain types of cancer. Zoledronic acid is also used along with cancer chemotherapy to treat bone damage caused by multiple myeloma [cancer that begins in the plasma cells (white blood cells that produce substances needed to fight infection)] or by cancer that began in another part of the body but has spread to the bones. Zoledronic acid is not cancer chemotherapy, and it will not slow or stop the spread of cancer. However, it can be used to treat bone disease in patients who have cancer. Zoledronic acid is in a class of medications called bisphosphonates. It works by slowing bone breakdown and decreasing the amount of calcium released from the bones into the blood.

How should this medicine be used?

Zoledronic acid comes as a solution (liquid) to infuse (inject slowly) intravenously (into a vein) over at least 15 minutes. It is usually injected by a health care provider in a doctor's office, hospital, or clinic. When zoledronic acid is used to treat high blood levels of calcium caused by cancer it is usually given as a single dose. A second dose may be given at least 7 days after the first dose if blood calcium does not drop to normal levels or remain at normal levels. When zoledronic acid is used to treat bone damage caused by multiple myeloma or cancer that has spread to the bones, it is usually given once every 3-4 weeks.

Your doctor will prescribe a calcium supplement and a multivitamin containing vitamin D to take during your treatment. You should take these supplements every day.

Are there other uses for this medicine?

This medication may be prescribed for other uses; ask your doctor or pharmacist for more information.

What special precautions should I follow?

Before taking zoledronic acid,
- tell your doctor and pharmacist if you are allergic to zoledronic acid; other bisphosphonates such as alendronate (Fosamax), etidronate (Didronel), pamidronate (Aredia), risedronate (Actonel), or tiludronate (Skelid); or any other medications.
- tell your doctor and pharmacist what prescription and nonprescription medications, vitamins, nutritional supplements, and herbal products you are taking. Be sure to mention any of the following: acetaminophen (Tylenol); amphotericin B (Fungizone); aminoglycoside antibiotics such as amikacin (Amikin), gentamycin (Garamycin), kanamaycin (Kantrex), neomycin (Neo-Rx, Neo-Fradin), netilmycin (Netromycin), paramomycin (Humatin), streptomycin, and tobramycin (Tobi, Nebcin); aspirin and other nonsteroidal anti-inflammatory medications such as ibuprofen (Advil, Motrin), and naproxen (Aleve, Naprosyn); aurothioglucose (Solganal), auranofin (Ridaura); bacitracin; cancer chemotherapy drugs such as carmustine (BCNU), cisplatin (Platinol AQ), cyclophosphamide (Cytoxan, Neosar); daunorubicin (DaunoXome, Cerubidine), doxorubicin (Adriamycin, Rubex), ifosfamide (Ifex), lomustine (CeeNU), and streptozocin (Zanosar); captopril (Capoten); cyclosporine (Neoral, Sandimmune); dapsone (Avlosulfon); foscarnet (Foscavir); gold sodium thiomalate (Myochrysine); loop diuretics ('water pills') such as bumetanide (Bumex), ethacrynic acid (Edecrin), and furosemide (Lasix); methicillin (Staphcillin); nitrates; oral steroids such as dexamethasone (Decadron, Dexone), methylprednisolone (Medrol), and prednisone (Delta-

sone); penicillamine (Cuprimine, Depen); pentamidine (NebuPent); primaquine; rifampin (Rifadin, Rimactane); salicylate pain relievers; sulfonamides such as sulfamethoxazole and trimethoprim (Bactrim); thalidomide (Thalomid); and tacrolimus (Prograf). Your doctor may need to change the doses of your medications or monitor you carefully for side effects.
- tell your doctor if you are being treated wtih radiation therapy and if you have or have ever had heart failure (condition in which the heart cannot pump enough blood to other parts of the body); anemia (condition in which red blood cells cannot bring enought oxygen to the other parts of the body); any condition that stops your blood from clotting normally; problems with your mouth, teeth, or gums; an infection, especially in your mouth; asthma, especially if it is made worse by aspirin; or kidney or liver disease.
- tell your doctor if you are pregnant. You should use a reliable method of birth control to prevent pregnancy while you are taking zoledronic acid. If you become pregnant while taking zoledronic acid, call your doctor. Talk to your doctor if you plan to become pregnant at any time in the future because zoledronic acid may remain in your body for years after you stop taking it. Do not breastfeed while you are taking zoledronic acid.
- you should know that zoledronic acid may cause serious problems with your jaws, especially if you have dental surgery or treatment while you are taking the medication. A dentist should examine your teeth and perform any needed treatments before you start to take zoledronic acid. Be sure to brush your teeth and clean your mouth properly while you are taking zoledronic acid. Talk to your doctor before having any dental treatments while you are taking this medication.

What special dietary instructions should I follow?

Unless your doctor tells you otherwise, continue your normal diet.

What should I do if I forget to take a dose?

If you miss an appointment to receive a zoledronic acid infusion, call your doctor as soon as possible.

What side effects can this medicine cause?

Zoledronic acid may cause side effects. Tell your doctor if any of these symptoms are severe or do not go away:
- redness or swelling in the place where you received your injection
- red, swollen, or teary eyes
- constipation
- upset stomach
- vomiting
- diarrhea
- stomach pain
- loss of appetite

- weight loss
- heartburn
- difficulty swallowing
- mouth sores
- pain anywhere in the body
- excessive worry
- agitation
- difficulty falling asleep or staying asleep
- white patches in the mouth
- swelling, redness, irritation, burning, or itching of the vagina
- white vaginal discharge
- hair loss

Some side effects can be serious. The following symptoms are uncommon, but if you experience any of them, call your doctor immediately:

- fever, chills, and other signs of infection
- bone, joint, or muscle pain, and other flu-like symptoms
- rash
- itching
- chest pain
- coughing
- weakness
- muscle cramps
- fast, pounding, or irregular heartbeat
- dizziness
- depression
- difficulty walking
- seizures
- confusion
- leg swelling
- shortness of breath
- sudden tightening of muscles
- numbness, burning, or tingling in fingers or toes
- dry mouth
- decreased urination
- sunken eyes
- sluggishness
- headache
- pale skin
- unusual bruising or bleeding
- frequent urination, especially at night
- excessive thirst
- hallucinations (seeing things or hearing voices that do not exist)
- muscle weakness
- double vision
- difficulty speaking
- jaw or mouth pain

Zoledronic acid may cause other side effects. Call your doctor if you have any unusual problems while taking this medication.

If you experience a serious side effect, you or your doctor may send a report to the Food and Drug Administration's (FDA) MedWatch Adverse Event Reporting program online [at http://www.fda.gov/MedWatch/index.html] or by phone [1-800-332-1088].

What storage conditions are needed for this medicine?

Your doctor will store this medication in his or her office and give it to you as needed.

What should I do in case of overdose?

In case of overdose, call your local poison control center at 1-800-222-1222. If the victim has collapsed or is not breathing, call local emergency services at 911.

Symptoms of overdose may include:

- fever
- tingling in hands or feet
- weakness
- muscle cramps
- fast, pounding, or irregular heartbeat
- dizziness
- depression
- difficulty walking
- seizures
- confusion
- shortness of breath
- sudden tightening of muscles
- numbness, burning, or tingling in fingers or toes
- muscle weakness
- double vision
- difficulty speaking

What other information should I know?

Keep all appointments with your doctor and the laboratory. Your doctor will order certain lab tests to check your body's response to zoledronic acid.

Dosage Facts
For Informational Purposes

Caution: Do not change your dose, how often you take your medication, or the length of time you are to take it without first talking to your healthcare provider.

The following dosage information was written using medical language for doctors and other healthcare professionals and is provided here for you to check your dosage. The dosage of this drug may differ for different patients. Therefore, always follow your doctor's instructions or the directions on the label. Contact your healthcare provider or pharmacist if you have any questions about the specific dosage of your medication after reviewing this information.

General Dosage Information

Available as zoledronic acid (as the monohydrate); dosage expressed in terms of the anhydrous drug.

Adult Patients

Hypercalcemia Associated with Malignancy

IV:

- 4 mg as a single dose in patients with an albumin-corrected serum calcium concentration of ≥12 mg/dL.
- Consider retreatment if serum calcium concentrations do not return to normal or do not remain normal. Initial dose can be repeated ≥7 days after treament initiation to allow full response to initial dose.

Bone Metastases of Solid Tumors and Osteolytic Lesions of Multiple Myeloma

IV:

- 4 mg once every 3–4 weeks in patients with baseline Cl_{cr} >60 mL/minute. Optimum duration of such therapy is not known, but has been used at the recommended interval for 4–12 months.
- If renal function deteriorates (defined as an increase in S_{cr} of ≥0.5 mg/dL) in patients with a baseline S_{cr} of <1.4 mg/dL, withhold therapy until S_{cr} returns to within 10% of baseline levels. Reinitiate therapy at the same dosage used prior to treatment interruption.

Prescribing Limits

Adult Patients

Hypercalcemia Associated with Malignancy

IV:

- Maximum 4 mg as a single dose. Safety and efficacy of >1 course of retreatment not established.

Bone Metastases of Solid Tumors and Osteolytic Lesions of Multiple Myeloma

IV:

- Maximum 4 mg as a single dose.

Special Populations

Hepatic Impairment

- No dosage recommendations at this time.

Renal Impairment

Hypercalcemia Associated with Malignancy

IV:

- Dosage adjustments are not necessary in patients with mild to moderate renal impairment (S_{cr} <4.5 mg/dL).

Bone Metastases of Solid Tumors and Osteolytic Lesions of Multiple Myeloma

IV:

- In patients with mild to moderate renal impairment (baseline Cl_{cr} of 30–60 mL/minute), lower initial dosages of zoledronic acid are recommended.

Table 2. Initial Dosage in Adults with Bone Metastases of Solid Tumors and Osteolytic Lesions of Multiple Myeloma Based on Renal Function

Calculated Cl_{cr} (mL/minute)	IV Dosage
>60	4 mg every 3–4 weeks
50–60	3.5 mg every 3–4 weeks
40–49	3.3 mg every 3–4 weeks
30–39	3 mg every 3–4 weeks

If renal function deteriorates (defined as an increase in S_{cr} of ≥1 mg/dL) in patients with a baseline S_{cr} of ≥1.4 mg/dL, withhold therapy until S_{cr} returns to within 10% of baseline levels. Reinitiate therapy at the same dosage that was used prior to the treatment interruption. Studies in this patient population included individuals with S_{cr} <3 mg/dL.

Geriatric Patients

- No dosage recommendations at this time.

Zolmitriptan Nasal

(zohl mi trip′ tan)

Brand Name: Zomig®

Why is this medicine prescribed?

Zolmitriptan is used to treat the symptoms of migraine headaches (severe, throbbing headaches that sometimes are accompanied by other symptoms such as nausea and sensitivity to sound and light). Zolmitriptan is in a class of medications called selective serotonin (5-HT) receptor agonists. It works by narrowing blood vessels around the brain and stopping the release of certain natural substances that cause pain, nausea, and other symptoms of migraine. Zolmitriptan does not prevent migraine attacks.

How should this medicine be used?

Zolmitriptan comes as a spray to inhale through the nose. It is usually used during a migraine attack. If your symptoms improve after you use zolmitriptan but return after 2 hours or longer, you may use a second dose of zolmitriptan. However, if your symptoms do not improve after you use zolmitriptan, do not use a second dose without talking to your doctor. Do not use more than two sprays of zolmitriptan in a 24-hour period. Call your doctor if you need to use zolmitriptan nasal spray to treat more than four headaches in 1 month. Follow the directions on your prescription label carefully, and ask your doctor or pharmacist to explain any part you do not understand. Use zolmitriptan exactly as directed. Do not use more or less of it or use it more often than prescribed by your doctor.

Do not use zolmitriptan to treat a headache that feels

different than your usual migraine attacks. Call your doctor to find out what you should do.

If you have certain risk factors for heart disease, your doctor may ask you to use your first dose of zolmitriptan in the doctor's office or other medical facility where you can be monitored for serious reactions.

Ask your pharmacist or doctor for a copy of the manufacturer's information for the patient.

To use the nasal spray, follow these steps:

1. Read all of the manufacturer's instructions for using the nasal spray before you use your first dose.
2. Blow your nose gently.
3. Remove the protective cap from the sprayer.
4. Hold the sprayer between your fingers and thumb, but be careful not to press the plunger.
5. Use your other hand to block one nostril by pressing firmly on the side of your nose.
6. Put the tip of the sprayer into your other nostril as far as feels comfortable and tilt your head back slightly. Be careful not to press the plunger or spray the medication in your eyes.
7. Breathe in gently through your nose. At the same time, press the plunger firmly with your thumb. The plunger may feel stiff and you may hear a click.
8. Keep your head slightly tilted back and remove the tip from your nose.
9. Breathe gently through your mouth for 5-10 seconds. It is normal to feel liquid in your nose or the back of your throat.
10. The sprayer only contains one dose of medication. After you have used it, throw it away in a trash can that is out of the reach of children and pets.

Are there other uses for this medicine?

This medication may be prescribed for other uses; ask your doctor or pharmacist for more information.

What special precautions should I follow?

Before using zolmitriptan,

- tell your doctor and pharmacist if you are allergic to zolmitriptan or any other medications.
- do not use zolmitriptan if you have taken any of the following medications in the past 24 hours: other selective serotonin receptor agonists such as almotriptan (Axert), eletriptan (Relpax), frovatriptan (Frova), naratriptan (Amerge), rizatriptan (Maxalt), or sumatriptan (Imitrex); or ergot-type medications such as bromocriptine (Parlodel), cabergoline (Dostinex), dihydroergotamine (D.H.E. 45, Migranal), ergoloid mesylates (Germinal, Hydergine), ergonovine (Ergotrate), ergotamine (Bellergal-S, Cafergot, Ergomar, Wigraine), methylergonovine (Methergine), methysergide (Sansert), and pergolide (Permax).
- do not use zolmitriptan if you are taking a monoamine oxidase A (MAO-A) inhibitor such as isocarboxazid (Marplan), phenelzine (Parnate), or tranylcypromine

(Nardil) or if you have taken one of these medications in the past 2 weeks.

- tell your doctor and pharmacist what other prescription and nonprescription medications, vitamins, nutritional supplements, and herbal products you are taking or plan to take. Be sure to mention any of the following: acetaminophen (Tylenol); cimetidine (Tagamet); oral contraceptives ('birth control pills'); propranolol (Inderal); selective serotonin reuptake inhibitors (SSRIs) such as citalopram (Celexa), escitalopram (Lexapro), fluoxetine (Prozac, Sarafem, in Symbyax), fluvoxamine, paroxetine (Paxil), and sertraline (Zoloft); and selective serotonin/norepinephrine reuptake inhibitors (SNRIs) such as duloxetine (Cymbalta) and venlafaxine (Effexor). Your doctor may need to change the doses of your medications or monitor you carefully for side effects.
- tell your doctor if you smoke, if you or any family members have or have ever had heart disease, if you have gone through menopause (change of life), and if you have or have ever had a heart attack; angina (chest pain); pounding or irregular heartbeat; shortness of breath; a stroke or 'mini-stroke'; high blood pressure; high cholesterol; diabetes; seizures; circulation problems such as varicose veins, blood clots in the legs, Raynaud's disease (problems with blood flow to the fingers, toes, ears, and nose) or ischemic bowel disease (bloody diarrhea and stomach pain caused by decreased blood flow to the intestines); or liver or kidney disease.
- tell your doctor if you are pregnant, plan to become pregnant, or are breast-feeding. If you plan to be sexually active while you are using this medication, talk to your doctor about effective methods of birth control. If you become pregnant while taking zolmitriptan, call your doctor.
- you should know that zolmitriptan may make you drowsy. Do not drive a car or operate machinery until you know how this medication affects you.
- talk to your doctor about your headache symptoms. Zolmitriptan should not be used to treat certain types of migraine headaches (hemiplegic or basilar) or other types of headaches (such as cluster headaches).

What special dietary instructions should I follow?

Unless your doctor tells you otherwise, continue your normal diet.

What side effects can this medicine cause?

Zolmitriptan may cause side effects. Tell your doctor if any of these symptoms are severe or do not go away:

- sore or irritated nose
- sensitive skin, especially around the nose
- dry mouth
- unusual taste in the mouth
- upset stomach
- dizziness

- weakness
- burning or tingling feeling

Some side effects can be serious. If you experience any of these symptoms, call your doctor immediately:

- pain, tightness, pressure, or heaviness in the chest, throat, or jaw
- slow or difficult speech
- dizziness or faintness
- problems with vision
- weakness or numbness of an arm or leg
- fast, pounding, or irregular heartbeat
- bloody diarrhea
- stomach pain
- paleness or blue color of the fingers and toes
- shortness of breath
- swelling of the eyes, face, lips, tongue, or throat
- difficulty swallowing
- hoarseness

Zolmitriptan may cause other side effects. Call your doctor if you have any unusual problems while taking this medication.

What storage conditions are needed for this medicine?

Keep this medication in the container it came in, tightly closed, and out of reach of children. Store it at room temperature and away from excess heat and moisture (not in the bathroom). Throw away any medication that is outdated or no longer needed. Talk to your pharmacist about the proper disposal of your medication.

What should I do in case of overdose?

In case of overdose, call your local poison control center at 1-800-222-1222. If the victim has collapsed or is not breathing, call local emergency services at 911.

Symptoms of overdose may include:

- sleepy, quiet state

What other information should I know?

Keep all appointments with your doctor.

Do not let anyone else take your medication. Ask your pharmacist any questions you have about refilling your prescription.

Dosage Facts
For Informational Purposes

Caution: Do not change your dose, how often you take your medication, or the length of time you are to take it without first talking to your healthcare provider.

The following dosage information was written using medical language for doctors and other healthcare professionals and is provided here for you to check your dosage. The dosage of this drug may differ for different

patients. Therefore, always follow your doctor's instructions or the directions on the label. Contact your healthcare provider or pharmacist if you have any questions about the specific dosage of your medication after reviewing this information.

General Dosage Information

Due to similarity in systemic exposure, dosage adjustments with oral and intranasal formulations should be similar; doses <5 mg can be achieved only through use of oral formulations.

Adult Patients

Vascular Headaches
Migraine

INTRANASAL:

- 5 mg (1 spray) as a single dose; individualize selection of dosage and administration route.
- If headache recurs, dose may be repeated after 2 hours.
- Following failure to respond to first dose, reconsider diagnosis of migraine prior to administration of a second dose.

Prescribing Limits

Adult Patients

Vascular Headaches
Migraine

INTRANASAL:

- Maximum 10 mg in any 24-hour period.
- Safety of treating an average of >4 headaches per 30-day period has not been established.

Special Populations

Hepatic Impairment

- Generally use <2.5 mg as a single oral dose in patients with moderate to severe hepatic impairment; concurrent BP monitoring recommended.
- Recommended doses can be achieved only with oral formulations; use of intranasal formulation not recommended.

Zolmitriptan Oral

(zohl mi trip′ tan)

Brand Name: Zomig®, Zomig-ZMT®

Why is this medicine prescribed?

Zolmitriptan is used to treat the symptoms of migraine headache (severe throbbing headache that sometimes is experienced with other symptoms such as upset stomach and sensitivity to sound and light). Zolmitriptan is in a class of medications called selective serotonin (5-HT) receptor agonists. It works by reducing swelling of blood vessels around the brain and blocking the release of certain natural substances that cause pain, upset stomach, and other symptoms of migraine. Zolmitriptan does not prevent migraine attacks.

How should this medicine be used?

Zolmitriptan comes as a tablet and an orally disintegrating tablet (tablet that dissolves quickly in the mouth) to take by mouth. It is usually taken during a migraine attack. If your symptoms improve after you take zolmitriptan but return after 2 hours or longer, you may take a second dose. However, if your symptoms do not improve after you take zolmitriptan, do not take a second dose without calling your doctor. Your doctor will tell you the maximum number of tablets or orally disintegrating tablets you may take in a 24 hour period. Call your doctor if you need to take zolmitriptan to treat more than 3 headaches in one month. Follow the directions on your prescription label carefully, and ask your doctor or pharmacist to explain any part you do not understand. Take zolmitriptan exactly as directed. Do not take more or less of it or take it more often than prescribed by your doctor.

Do not take zolmitriptan to treat a headache that feels different than your usual migraine attacks. Call your doctor to find out what you should do.

If you have certain risk factors for heart disease, your doctor may ask you to take your first dose of zolmitriptan in the doctor's office or other medical facility where you can be monitored for serious reactions.

If your doctor has prescribed a dose lower than 2.5 mg, you may use your fingers to break the 2.5 mg tablet on the line that divides it in half. However, you should not break or split the orally disintegrating tablet.

To take the orally disintegrating tablet, use dry hands to peel back the foil packaging. Immediately take out the tablet and place it on your tongue. The tablet will quickly dissolve and can be swallowed with saliva. No water is needed to swallow disintegrating tablets. Do not open the foil packaging or remove the orally disintegrating tablet until just before you are ready to take it.

Ask your pharmacist or doctor for a copy of the manufacturer's information for the patient.

Are there other uses for this medicine?

This medication may be prescribed for other uses; ask your doctor or pharmacist for more information.

What special precautions should I follow?

Before taking zolmitriptan,
- tell your doctor and pharmacist if you are allergic to zolmitriptan or any other medications.
- do not take zolmitriptan if you have taken any of the following medications in the past 24 hours: other selective serotonin receptor (5-HT) agonists such as almotriptan (Axert), eletriptan (Relpax), frovatriptan (Frova), naratriptan (Amerge), rizatriptan (Maxalt), or sumatriptan (Imitrex); or ergot-type medications such as bromocriptine (Parlodel), cabergoline (Dostinex), dihydroergotamine (D.H.E. 45, Migranal), ergoloid mesylates (Germinal, Hydergine), ergonovine (Ergotrate), ergotamine (Bellergal-S, Cafergot, Ergomar, Wigraine),

methylergonovine (Methergine), methysergide (Sansert), and pergolide (Permax).
- do not take zolmitriptan if you are taking a monoamine oxidase A (MAO-A) inhibitor such as isocarboxazid (Marplan), phenelzine (Parnate), or tranylcypromine (Nardil) or if you have taken one of these medications in the past 2 weeks.
- tell your doctor and pharmacist what other prescription and nonprescription medications, vitamins, nutritional supplements, or herbal products you are taking or plan to take. Be sure to mention any of the following: acetaminophen (Tylenol), cimetidine (Tagamet), oral contraceptives ('birth control pills'), propranolol (Inderal), and selective serotonin reuptake inhibitors (SSRIs) such as citalopram (Celexa), duloxetine (Cymbalta), escitalopram (Lexapro), fluoxetine (Prozac, Sarafem), fluvoxamine (Luvox), paroxetine (Paxil), and sertraline (Zoloft). Your doctor may need to change the doses of your medications or monitor you carefully for side effects.
- tell your doctor if you smoke, if you or any family members have or have ever had heart disease, if you have gone through menopause (change of life), and if you have or have ever had a heart attack; angina (chest pain); pounding or irregular heartbeat; shortness of breath; a stroke or 'mini-stroke'; high blood pressure; high cholesterol; diabetes; seizures; circulation problems such as varicose veins, blood clots in the legs, Raynaud's disease (problems with blood flow to the fingers, toes, ears, and nose), or ischemic bowel disease (bloody diarrhea and stomach pain caused by decreased blood flow to the intestines); or liver or kidney disease.
- tell your doctor if you are pregnant, plan to become pregnant, or are breast-feeding. If you plan to be sexually active while you are taking this medication, talk to your doctor about effective methods of birth control. If you become pregnant while taking zolmitriptan, call your doctor.
- you should know that this medication may cause drowsiness and dizziness. Do not drive a car or operate machinery until you know how zolmitriptan affects you.
- talk to your doctor about your headache symptoms. Zolmitriptan should not be used to treat certain types of migraine headaches (hemiplegic or basilar) or other types of headaches (such as cluster headaches).
- if you have phenylketonuria (PKU, a inherited condition in which a special diet must be followed to prevent mental retardation), you should know that the orally disintegrating tablets contain aspartame which forms phenylalanine.

What special dietary instructions should I follow?

Unless your doctor tells you otherwise, continue your normal diet.

What side effects can this medicine cause?

Zolmitriptan may cause side effects. Tell your doctor if any of these symptoms are severe or do not go away:

- burning or tingling feeling
- feeling warm or cold
- drowsiness
- dry mouth
- upset stomach
- heartburn
- sweating
- weakness

Some side effects can be serious. If you experience any of the following symptoms, call your doctor immediately:

- pain, tightness, pressure, or heaviness in the chest, throat, or jaw
- muscle aches
- slow or difficult speech
- dizziness or faintness
- weakness or numbness of an arm or leg
- fast, pounding, or irregular heartbeat
- bloody diarrhea
- stomach pain
- paleness or blue color of the fingers and toes
- shortness of breath
- swelling of the eyes, face, lips, tongue, or throat,
- difficulty swallowing
- hoarseness
- rash or lumps on the skin

If you experience a serious side effect, you or your doctor may send a report to the Food and Drug Administration's (FDA) MedWatch Adverse Event Reporting program online [at http://www.fda.gov/MedWatch/index.html] or by phone [1-800-332-1088].

What storage conditions are needed for this medicine?

Keep this medication in the container it came in, tightly closed, and out of reach of children. Store it at room temperature and away from excess heat and moisture (not in the bathroom). Throw away any medication that is outdated or no longer needed and any orally disintegrating tablets that you removed from the blister pack but did not use immediately. Talk to your pharmacist about the proper disposal of your medication.

What should I do in case of overdose?

In case of overdose, call your local poison control center at 1-800-222-1222. If the victim has collapsed or is not breathing, call local emergency services at 911.

Symptoms of overdose may include:
- sleepy, quiet state.

What other information should I know?

Keep all appointments with your doctor and the laboratory.

Do not let anyone else take your medication. Ask your pharmacist any questions you have about refilling your prescription.

Dosage Facts
For Informational Purposes

Caution: Do not change your dose, how often you take your medication, or the length of time you are to take it without first talking to your health-care provider.

The following dosage information was written using medical language for doctors and other healthcare professionals and is provided here for you to check your dosage. The dosage of this drug may differ for different patients. Therefore, always follow your doctor's instructions or the directions on the label. Contact your healthcare provider or pharmacist if you have any questions about the specific dosage of your medication after reviewing this information.

General Dosage Information

Due to similarity in systemic exposure, dosage adjustments with oral and intranasal formulations should be similar; doses <5 mg can be achieved only through use of oral formulations.

Adult Patients

Vascular Headaches
Migraine

ORAL:
- Initially, ≤ 2.5 mg. In clinical studies, single oral doses of 1 (not commercially available in US), 2.5, or 5 mg were effective, but the 2.5- and 5-mg doses were effective in a greater proportion of patients. The 5-mg dose appears to offer little additional benefit and is associated with increased risk of adverse effects.
- If headache recurs, dose may be repeated after ≥ 2 hours.
- Following failure to respond to first dose, reconsider diagnosis of migraine prior to administration of a second dose.

Prescribing Limits

Adult Patients

Vascular Headaches
Migraine

ORAL:
- Maximum 10 mg in any 24-hour period.
- Safety of treating an average of >3 headaches per 30-day period has not been established.

Special Populations

Hepatic Impairment
- Generally use <2.5 mg as a single oral dose in patients with moderate to severe hepatic impairment; concurrent BP monitoring recommended.
- Recommended doses can be achieved only with oral formulations; use of intranasal formulation not recommended.

Zolpidem

(zole pi′ dem)

Brand Name: Ambien®, Ambien CR®

Why is this medicine prescribed?

Zolpidem is used to treat insomnia (difficulty falling asleep or staying asleep). Zolpidem belongs to a class of medications called sedative-hypnotics. It works by slowing activity in the brain to allow sleep.

How should this medicine be used?

Zolpidem comes as a tablet and an extended-release (long acting) tablet to take by mouth. It is usually taken as needed at bedtime. Zolpidem will work faster if it is not taken with a meal or immediately after a meal. Follow the directions on your prescription label carefully, and ask your doctor or pharmacist to explain any part you do not understand. Take zolpidem exactly as directed.

You will probably become very sleepy soon after you take zolpidem and will remain sleepy for some time after you take the medication. Plan to go to bed right after you take zolpidem, and to stay in bed for 7-8 hours. Do not take zolpidem if you will be unable to remain asleep for 7-8 hours after taking the medication. If you get up too soon after taking zolpidem, you may experience memory problems.

Swallow the extended release tablets whole; do not split, chew, or crush them.

Your sleep problems should improve within 7-10 days after you start taking zolpidem. Call your doctor if your sleep problems do not improve during this time or if they get worse at any time during your treatment.

Zolpidem should normally be taken for short periods of time. If you take zolpidem for 2 weeks or longer, zolpidem may not help you sleep as well as it did when you first began to take the medication. If you take zolpidem for a long time, you also may develop dependence ('addiction'; a need to continue taking the medication) on zolpidem. Talk to your doctor about the risks of taking zolpidem for 2 weeks or longer. Do not take a larger dose of zolpidem, take it more often, or take it for a longer time than prescribed by your doctor.

Do not stop taking zolpidem without talking to your doctor, especially if you have taken it for longer than 2 weeks. If you suddenly stop taking zolpidem, you may develop unpleasant feelings or you may experience more severe withdrawal symptoms such as seizures, shakiness, stomach and muscle cramps, vomiting, sweating, and rarely, seizures.

You may have more difficulty falling asleep or staying asleep on the first night after you stop taking zolpidem than you did before you started taking the medication. This is normal and usually gets better without treatment after one or two nights.

Ask your doctor or pharmacist for a copy of the manufacturer's information for the patient.

Are there other uses for this medicine?

This medication may be prescribed for other uses; ask your doctor or pharmacist for more information.

What special precautions should I follow?

Before taking zolpidem,

- tell your doctor and pharmacist if you are allergic to zolpidem or any other medications.
- tell your doctor and pharmacist what prescription and nonprescription medications, vitamins, nutritional supplements, and herbal products you are taking or plan to take. Be sure to mention any of the following: antidepressants ('mood elevators') such as imipramine (Tofranil); itraconazole (Sporanox); medications for anxiety, colds or allergies, mental illness, pain, or seizures; rifampin (Rifadin, Rimactane); sedatives; sertraline (Zoloft); sleeping pills; and tranquilizers. Your doctor may need to change the doses of your medications or monitor you carefully for side effects.
- tell your doctor if you drink or have ever drunk large amounts of alcohol, use or have ever used street drugs, or have overused prescription medications. Also tell your doctor if you have or have ever had depression; a problem with heavy snoring; sleep apnea (condition in which the patient briefly stops breathing many times during the night); other breathing problems such as asthma, bronchitis, and emphysema; myasthenia gravis (condition that causes weakness of certain muscles); or liver or kidney disease.
- tell your doctor if you are pregnant or plan to become pregnant. If you become pregnant while taking zolpidem, call your doctor. Do not breastfeed while you are taking zolpidem.
- if you are having surgery, including dental surgery, tell the doctor or dentist that you are taking zolpidem.
- you should know that zolpidem may make you drowsy during the day, and may increase the risk that you will fall. Take extra care not to fall and do not drive a car or operate machinery until you know how this medication affects you.
- do not drink alcohol during your treatment with zolpidem. Alcohol can make the side effects of zolpidem worse.
- you should know that some people who took zolpidem got out of bed and drove their cars, prepared and ate food, had sex, made phone calls, or were involved in other activities while partially asleep. After they woke up, these people were usually unable to remember what they had done. Call your doctor right away if you find out that you have been driving or doing anything else while you were sleeping.
- you should know that your mental health may change in unexpected ways while you are taking this medica-

tion. It is hard to tell if these changes are caused by zolpidem or if they are caused by physical or mental illnesses that you already have or suddenly develop. Tell your doctor right away if you experience any of the following symptoms: aggressiveness, strange or unusually outgoing behavior, hallucinations (seeing things or hearing voices that do not exist), feeling as if you are outside of your body, memory problems, difficulty concentrating, slowed speech or movements; new or worsening depression, thinking about killing yourself, confusion, and any other changes in your usual thoughts, mood, or behavior. Be sure that your family knows which symptoms may be serious so that they can call the doctor if you are unable to seek treatment on your own.

What special dietary instructions should I follow?

Unless your doctor tells you otherwise, continue your normal diet.

What should I do if I forget to take a dose?

Zolpidem should only be taken at bedtime. If you did not take zolpidem at bedtime and you are unable to fall asleep, you may take zolpidem if you will be able to remain in bed for 7-8 hours afterward. Do not take zolpidem if you are not ready to go to sleep right away and stay asleep for at least 7-8 hours.

What side effects can this medicine cause?

Zolpidem may cause side effects. Tell your doctor if any of these symptoms are severe or do not go away:
- drowsiness
- weakness
- headache
- dizziness
- 'drugged feeling'
- unsteady walking
- difficulty keeping balance
- constipation
- diarrhea
- gas
- heartburn
- stomach pain or tenderness
- changes in appetite
- uncontrollable shaking of a part of the body
- burning or tingling in the hands, arms, feet, or legs
- unusual dreams
- dry mouth or throat
- ringing, pain, or itching in the ears
- eye redness
- muscle aches or cramps
- joint, back, or neck pain
- heavy menstrual bleeding

Some side effects can be serious. If you experience any of the following symptoms, call your doctor immediately:

- rash
- hives
- itching
- swelling of the eyes, face, lips, tongue, or throat
- feeling that the throat is closing
- difficulty breathing or swallowing
- hoarseness
- shortness of breath
- nausea
- vomiting
- pounding heartbeat
- chest pain
- blurred vision or other vision problems

Zolpidem may cause other side effects. Call your doctor if you have any unusual problems while you are taking this medication.

If you experience a serious side effect, you or your doctor may send a report to the Food and Drug Administration's (FDA) MedWatch Adverse Event Reporting program online [at http://www.fda.gov/MedWatch/index.html] or by phone [1-800-332-1088].

What storage conditions are needed for this medicine?

Keep this medication in the container it came in, tightly closed, and out of reach of children. Store it at room temperature, away from excess heat and moisture (not in the bathroom). Throw away any medication that is outdated or no longer needed. Talk to your pharmacist about the proper disposal of your medication.

What should I do in case of overdose?

In case of overdose, call your local poison control center at 1-800-222-1222. If the victim has collapsed or is not breathing, call local emergency services at 911.

Symptoms of overdose may include:
- drowsiness
- coma (loss of consciousness for a period of time)
- slowed breathing or heartbeat

What other information should I know?

Keep all appointments with your doctor.

Do not let anyone else take your medication. Ask your pharmacist if you have any questions about refilling your prescription.

Dosage Facts
For Informational Purposes

Caution: Do not change your dose, how often you take your medication, or the length of time you are to take it without first talking to your healthcare provider.

The following dosage information was written using medical language for doctors and other healthcare pro-

fessionals and is provided here for you to check your dosage. The dosage of this drug may differ for different patients. Therefore, always follow your doctor's instructions or the directions on the label. Contact your healthcare provider or pharmacist if you have any questions about the specific dosage of your medication after reviewing this information.

General Dosage Information

Available as zolpidem tartrate; dosage is expressed in terms of the salt.

Individualize dosage; use smallest effective dose.

Adult Patients

Insomnia

ORAL:
- 10 mg (as conventional tablets) or 12.5 mg (as extended-release tablets).

Prescribing Limits

Adult Patients

Insomnia

ORAL:
- Maximum 10 mg daily as conventional tablets. Higher doses (e.g., 15 or 20 mg) occasionally have been used but may be associated with increased risk of adverse effects, including abuse potential.

Special Populations

Hepatic Impairment
- Prolonged elimination. Initially, 5 mg (as conventional tablets) or 6.25 mg (as extended-release tablets).

Renal Impairment
- Possible pharmacokinetic alterations. Manufacturer recommends close monitoring but states that dosage reduction is not necessary; some clinicians recommend that dosage reduction be considered.

Geriatric or Debilitated Patients
- Possible increased sensitivity to sedatives and hypnotics. Initially, 5 mg (as conventional tablets) or 6.25 mg (as extended-release tablets).

Zonisamide

(zoe nis' a mide)

Brand Name: Zonegran®
Also available generically.

Why is this medicine prescribed?

Zonisamide is used in combination with other medications to treat seizures in adults with epilepsy. Zonisamide is in a class of medications called anticonvulsants. It works by decreasing abnormal excitement in the brain.

How should this medicine be used?

Zonisamide comes as a capsule to take by mouth. It is usually taken once or twice a day with or without food. To help you remember to take zonisamide, take it around the same time every day. Follow the directions on your prescription label carefully, and ask your doctor or pharmacist to explain any part you do not understand. Take zonisamide exactly as directed. Do not take more or less of it or take it more often than prescribed by your doctor.

Swallow the capsules whole; do not split, chew, or crush them.

Your doctor will probably start you on a low dose of zonisamide and gradually increase your dose, not more than once every 2 weeks.

Zonisamide controls epilepsy but does not cure it. It may take 2 weeks or longer before you feel the full benefit of zonisamide. Continue to take zonisamide even if you feel well. Do not stop taking zonisamide without talking to your doctor. If you suddenly stop taking zonisamide, your seizures may become worse. Your doctor will probably decrease your dose gradually.

Are there other uses for this medicine?

This medication may be prescribed for other uses; ask your doctor or pharmacist for more information.

What special precautions should I follow?

Before taking zonisamide,
- tell your doctor and pharmacist if you are allergic to zonisamide, celecoxib (Celebrex), diuretics ('water pills'), oral medications for diabetes, sulfa drugs, or any other medications.
- tell your doctor and pharmacist what prescription and nonprescription medications, vitamins, nutritional supplements, and herbal products you are taking. Be sure to mention any of the following: antifungals such as fluconazole (Diflucan), itraconazole (Sporanox), and ketoconazole (Nizoral); antihistamines; carbamazepine (Carbatrol, Tegretol), cimetidine (Tagamet); clarithromycin (Biaxin); cyclosporine (Neoral, Sandimmune); danazol (Danocrine); delavirdine (Rescriptor); dexamethasone (Decadron, Dexpak), diltiazem (Cardizem, Dilacor, Tiazac); ethosuximide (Zarontin), erythromycin (E.E.S., E-Mycin, Erythrocin); fluoxetine (Prozac, Sarafem); fluvoxamine (Luvox); HIV protease inhibitors such as indinavir (Crixivan) and ritonavir (Norvir); ipratropium (Atrovent); isoniazid (INH, Nydrazid); medications for irritable bowel disease, motion sickness, Parkinson's disease, ulcers, or urinary problems; metronidazole (Flagyl); nefazodone (Serzone); oral contraceptives (birth control pills); oral medications for glaucoma such as acetazolamide (Diamox); phenobarbital (Luminal, Solfoton); phenytoin (Dilantin); primidone (Mysoline); rifabutin (Mycobutin), rifampin (Rifadin, Rimactane); troglitazone (Rezulin); troleandomycin (TAO); valproic acid (Depak-

ene, Depakote); verapamil (Calan, Covera, Isoptin, Verelan); and zafirlukast (Accolate). Your doctor may need to change the doses of your medications or monitor you carefully for side effects.

- tell your doctor if you have or have ever had liver or kidney disease.
- tell your doctor if you are pregnant, plan to become pregnant, or are breast-feeding. If you become pregnant while taking zonisamide, call your doctor. Zonisamide may harm the fetus.
- if you are having surgery, including dental surgery, tell the doctor or dentist that you are taking zonisamide.
- you should know that zonisamide may make you drowsy. Do not drive a car or operate machinery until you know how this medication affects you.
- remember that alcohol can add to the drowsiness caused by this medication.
- you should know that you may be more likely to develop kidney stones while taking zonisamide. You should drink 6-8 glasses of water daily to help prevent kidney stones from forming.
- you should know that zonisamide can prevent you from sweating and make it harder for your body to cool down when it gets very hot. This happens most often in warm weather and to children who take zonisamide. (Children should not normally take zonisamide, but in some cases, a doctor will decide whether it is the best choice.) You should avoid exposure to heat and notify your doctor if you have a fever and/or are not sweating as usual.

What special dietary instructions should I follow?

Talk to your doctor about eating grapefruit and drinking grapefruit juice while taking this medicine.

What should I do if I forget to take a dose?

Take the missed dose as soon as you remember it. However, if it is almost time for the next dose, skip the missed dose and continue your regular dosing schedule. Do not take a double dose to make up for a missed one.

What side effects can this medicine cause?

Zonisamide may cause side effects. Tell your doctor if any of these symptoms are severe or do not go away:
- drowsiness
- loss of appetite
- upset stomach
- vomiting
- weight loss
- changes in taste
- dizziness
- constipation
- dry mouth
- headache
- confusion
- irritability

- difficulty falling asleep or staying asleep
- difficulty with memory
- pain, burning, or tingling in the hands or feet
- difficulty focusing eyes
- double vision
- sneezing
- runny nose

Some side effects can be serious. The following symptoms are uncommon, but if you experience any of them, call your doctor immediately:
- rash
- worsening or longer lasting seizures
- sudden back pain
- stomach pain
- pain when urinating
- bloody or dark urine
- fever
- sore throat
- sores in mouth
- easy bruising
- depression
- unusual thoughts
- difficulty thinking of words or trouble speaking
- difficulty thinking or concentrating
- lack of coordination
- difficulty walking

Zonisamide may cause other side effects. Call your doctor if you have any unusual problems while taking this medication.

If you experience a serious side effect, you or your doctor may send a report to the Food and Drug Administration's (FDA) MedWatch Adverse Event Reporting program online [at http://www.fda.gov/MedWatch/index.html] or by phone [1-800-332-1088].

What storage conditions are needed for this medicine?

Keep this medication in the container it came in, tightly closed, and out of reach of children. Store it at room temperature and away from excess heat and moisture (not in the bathroom). Throw away any medication that is outdated or no longer needed. Talk to your pharmacist about the proper disposal of your medication.

What should I do in case of overdose?

In case of overdose, call your local poison control center at 1-800-222-1222. If the victim has collapsed or is not breathing, call local emergency services at 911.

Symptoms of overdose may include:
- slow heartbeat
- difficulty breathing
- dizziness
- fainting
- loss of consciousness

What other information should I know?

Keep all appointments with your doctor and the laboratory. Your doctor may order certain lab tests to check your body's response to zonisamide.

Do not let anyone else take your medication. Ask your pharmacist any questions you have about refilling your prescription.

Dosage Facts
For Informational Purposes

Caution: Do not change your dose, how often you take your medication, or the length of time you are to take it without first talking to your healthcare provider.

The following dosage information was written using medical language for doctors and other healthcare professionals and is provided here for you to check your dosage. The dosage of this drug may differ for different patients. Therefore, always follow your doctor's instructions or the directions on the label. Contact your healthcare provider or pharmacist if you have any questions about the specific dosage of your medication after reviewing this information.

Adult Patients

Seizure Disorders
Partial Seizures

ORAL:
- Initially, 100 mg daily.
- Dosage may be increased to 200 mg daily, with further increases to 300 and 400 mg daily; allow ≥2 weeks between dosage changes (to achieve steady state at each dosage level). Some clinicians may prefer to administer lower dosages for longer periods (in order to fully assess safety at steady state).
- Dosages >400 mg daily may not be associated with increased therapeutic benefit.
- Adverse effects occur more frequently at dosages ≥300 mg daily.

Prescribing Limits
Adult Patients

Seizure Disorders
Partial Seizures

ORAL:
- Limited experience with dosages >600 mg daily.

Special Populations

Hepatic Impairment
- Titrate dosage slowly.

Renal Impairment
- Titrate dosage slowly.

Canadian Trade Name Index

Selected brand-names of Canadian medications are listed below. When a Canadian brand-name drug is listed in this index, the US generic name of the equivalent drug will be shown as "see (US generic name)." The listing of selected brand names in this index is intended only for ease of reference. There are other brand name products that have not been included in the book. Because a brand name is listed in this index does not mean that the authors or organizations represented have any particular knowledge that the brand listed has properties different from other brands of the same drug, nor is it intended as a recommendation of the drugs listed. Additionally, if a brand name product is not listed it does not indicate that the product has been evaluated to be unsatisfactory of substandard.

A

Abelcet, *see* Amphotericin B Injection
Abenol, *see* Acetaminophen
Absorbine JR Antifungal Liquid, *see* Tolnaftate
Accolate, *see* Zafirlukast
Accupril, *see* Quinapril
Accuretic, *see* Hydrochlorothiazide and Quinapril
Accutane, *see* Isotretinoin
Acet, *see* Acetaminophen
Acet Codeine, *see* Acetaminophen and Codeine
Acetazolam, *see* Acetazolamide Oral
Acetazone Forte, *see* Chlorzoxazone and Acetaminophen
Achieve, *see* Folic Acid and Potassium
Acid Control, *see* Famotidine Oral
Acid Reducer, *see* Ranitidine Oral
Acide Folique, *see* Folic Acid
Acidhalt, *see* Famotidine Oral
ACN, *see* Sodium Chloride (Catheter Flush) Injection
Actifed, *see* Pseudoephedrine
Actifed Plus, *see* Pseudoephedrine and Acetaminophen
Activa Balance, *see* Folic Acid
Actonel, *see* Risedronate
Actos, *see* Pioglitazone
Acular, *see* Ketorolac Ophthalmic and Ketorolac Oral
AD HP, *see* Hyoscyamine
Adalat XL, *see* Nifedipine
Adaptagen, *see* Epinephrine Injection
Addipak Sodium Chloride, *see* Sodium Chloride (Catheter Flush) Injection
Adeks - DPS, *see* Pyridoxine and Phytonadione Oral
Adeks, *see* Folic Acid and Phytonadione Oral
ADR II, *see* Potassium
Adrenalin, *see* Epinephrine Injection
Adrenalinum, *see* Epinephrine Injection
Adriamycin, *see* Doxorubicin
Adrien Gagnon Multi-vitamines et Mineraux, *see* Folic Acid and Potassium
Adrisin, *see* Sodium Chloride (Catheter Flush) Injection
Advair, *see* Fluticasone and Salmeterol
Advicor, *see* Lovastatin
Advil, *see* Ibuprofen
Advil Cold and Sinus, *see* Ibuprofen and Pseudoephedrine
Advil Cold and Sinus Plus, *see* Chlorpheniramine, Ibuprofen, and Pseudoephedrine
Aerius, *see* Desloratadine
Agenerase, *see* Amprenavir
Aggrenox, *see* Dipyridamole
A-hydrocort Inj, *see* Hydrocortisone Injection
AK Mycin, *see* Erythromycin
AK Spor, *see* Neomycin Topical
AK Trol, *see* Dexamethasone Oral and Dexamethasone Ophthalmic
Akarpine, *see* Pilocarpine Ophthalmic
Alcabase, *see* Potassium
Alcomicin, *see* Gentamicin Ophthalmic
Aldactazide, *see* Hydrochlorothiazide and Spironolactone
Aldactone, *see* Spironolactone
Aldara, *see* Imiquimod
Alertec, *see* Modafinil
Alertonic, *see* Thiamine and Pyridoxine
Alka-Seltzer, *see* Sodium Bicarbonate
Alkeran, *see* Melphalan
Allegra, *see* Fexofenadine
Allegra-D, *see* Pseudoephedrine and Fexofenadine
Aller-aide, *see* Diphenhydramine Oral
Allerdryl, *see* Diphenhydramine Oral
Allergy + Sinus Relief Extra Strength, *see* Acetaminophen, Chlorpheniramine, and Pseudoephedrine

Allergy Eye Drops, *see* Tetrahydrozoline Ophthalmic
Allergy Sinus Headache Caplets, *see* Acetaminophen, Pseudoephedrine, Diphenhydramine Oral
Allergy-Relief, *see* Cetirizine Hydrochloride
Allernix, *see* Diphenhydramine Oral
Aller-Relief, *see* Cetirizine Hydrochloride
Allertin, *see* Loratadine
Alloprin, *see* Allopurinol
Alocril, *see* Nedocromil Ophthalmic and Nedocromil Oral Inhalation
Alomide, *see* Lodoxamide Ophthalmic
Alphagan, *see* Brimonidine Ophthalmic
Altace, *see* Ramipril
Amaryl, *see* Glimepiride
Ambisome, *see* Amphotericin B Injection
Amerge, *see* Naratriptan
Amevive, *see* Alefacept Injection
Amikin, *see* Amikacin Sulfate Injection
Amox, *see* Amoxicillin
Amphotec, *see* Amphotericin B Injection
Anafranil, *see* Clomipramine
Anandron, *see* Nilutamide
Ansaid, *see* Flurbiprofen Oral
Anti-diarrheal Caplets, *see* Loperamide
Anugesic-HC, *see* Pramoxine
Anusol Plus, *see* Pramoxine
Anzemet, *see* Dolasetron and Abacavir
APAP, *see* Acetaminophen
Apresoline, *see* Hydralazine
Arava, *see* Leflunomide
Aredia, *see* Pamidronate Injection
Aribosan B31, *see* Nitroglycerin Ointment and Colchicine Oral
Aricept, *see* Donepezil
Arimidex, *see* Anastrozole
Aristocort, *see* Triamcinolone Topical and Triamcinolone Nasal Inhalation
Arnix HP, *see* Colchicine Oral
Art HP, *see* Colchicine Oral
Arthrotec, *see* Misoprostol
Artritol, *see* Acetaminophen
Artrol, *see* Sodium Bicarbonate
Atacand, *see* Candesartan
Atacand Plus, *see* Candesartan and Hydrochlorothiazide
Atarax, *see* Hydroxyzine
Atasol, *see* Acetaminophen
Ativan, *see* Lorazepam
Atridox, *see* Doxycycline
Atropinum, *see* Atropine Ophthalmic
Atrovent, *see* Ipratropium Bromide Oral Inhalation and Albuterol
Avalide, *see* Hydrochlorothiazide and Irbesartan
Avandamet, *see* Rosiglitazone and Metformin
Avandia, *see* Rosiglitazone
Avapro, *see* Irbesartan
Avaxim, *see* Hepatitis A Vaccine
Aveeno Anti-itch, *see* Pramoxine
Avelox, *see* Moxifloxacin
Aventyl, *see* Nortriptyline
Avodart, *see* Dutasteride
Avonex, *see* Interferon Beta-1b Injection
Axid, *see* Nizatidine
Azopt, *see* Brinzolamide Ophthalmic

B

Bactroban, *see* Mupirocin
Balminil, *see* Guaifenesin, Pseudoephedrine and Diphenhydramine Oral
Barriere HC, *see* Hydrocortisone Topical

Bellergal Spacetabs, *see* Phenobarbital
Beminal, *see* Pyridoxine
Benadryl, *see* Diphenhydramine Oral
Bentylol, *see* Dicyclomine
Benylin, *see* Guaifenesin, Pseudoephedrine, and Acetaminophen
Benzaclin, *see* Clindamycin
Benzamycin, *see* Erythromycin
Betacaine Gel, *see* Lidocaine Viscous
Betaderm, *see* Betamethasone Topical
Betagan, *see* Levobunolol Ophthalmic
Betaloc, *see* Metoprolol Oral
Betaxin, *see* Thiamine
Betnesol Retention Enema, *see* Betamethasone Topical
Betoptic S, *see* Betaxolol Ophthalmic
Bevifer, *see* Thiamine and Pyridoxine
Bextra, *see* Valdecoxib
Biaxin, *see* Clarithromycin Oral
Bicnu, *see* Carmustine
Bismutal, *see* Guaifenesin
Bonamine, *see* Meclizine
Bricanyl, *see* Terbutaline
Bronchophan, *see* Guaifenesin
Burinex, *see* Bumetanide
Buspar, *see* Buspirone
Bustab, *see* Buspirone
Busulfex, *see* Busulfan

C

Caduet, *see* Atorvastatin and Amlodipine
Caelyx, *see* Doxorubicin
Caladryl lotion, *see* Pramoxine
Calcijex, *see* Calcitriol
Calcimar, *see* Calcitonin Salmon Injection
Calmex, *see* Diphenhydramine Oral
Calmylin, *see* Diphenhydramine Oral, Guaifenesin, and Pseudoephedrine
Caltine, *see* Calcitonin Salmon Injection
Candistatin, *see* Nystatin
Canesten, *see* Clotrimazole
Capex, *see* Fluocinolone Topical
Capoten, *see* Captopril
Carbolith, *see* Lithium
Cardizem, *see* Diltiazem
Cardura, *see* Doxazosin
Carthamex cap, *see* Pyridoxine
Casodex, *see* Bicalutamide
Catapres, *see* Clonidine Tablets and Skin Patches
Caverject, *see* Alprostadil
Ceclor, *see* Cefaclor
Ceenu, *see* Lomustine
Cefotan, *see* Cefotetan Disodium Injection
Ceftin, *see* Cefuroxime Oral
Cefzil, *see* Cefprozil
Celebrex, *see* Celecoxib
Celestone, *see* Betamethasone
Celexa, *see* Citalopram
Cellcept, *see* Mycophenolate Oral
Celontin, *see* Methsuximide Oral
Cephanol, *see* Acetaminophen
Ceporacin, *see* Cephalothin Sodium Injection
Cerezyme, *see* Imiglucerase Injection
Cerubidine, *see* Daunorubicin
Cervidil, *see* Dinoprostone
Chlorinum, *see* Chloral Hydrate
Chlor-tripolon, *see* Chlorpheniramine and Loratadine
Chlorum, *see* Chloral Hydrate
Ciloxan, *see* Ciprofloxacin Oral

Cimicifuga Plex, *see* Thyroid
Cipralex, *see* Escitalopram
Cipro, *see* Ciprofloxacin Oral
Ciprodex, *see* Ciprofloxacin and Dexamethasone
Claforan, *see* Cefotaxime Sodium Injection
Claritin, *see* Loratadine
Clarus, *see* Isotretinoin
Clavulin, *see* Amoxicillin
Climara, *see* Estradiol Transdermal System
Clindasol, *see* Clindamycin
Clindets, *see* Clindamycin
Clindoxyl Gel, *see* Clindamycin
Clobex, *see* Clobetasol
Clomid, *see* Clomiphene
Clonapam, *see* Clonazepam
Clotrimaderm, *see* Clotrimazole
Clozaril, *see* Clozapine
Colestid, *see* Colestipol
Coltalin Cold & Allergy, *see* Acetaminophen and Chlorpheniramine
Combantrin, *see* Pyrantel
Combigan, *see* Timolol Ophthalmic and Brimonidine Ophthalmic
Combivent, *see* Ipratropium Bromide Oral Inhalation and Albuterol
Combivir, *see* Zidovudine Oral and Lamivudine
Comtan, *see* Entacapone
Concerta, *see* Methylphenidate
Copaxone, *see* Glatiramer Injection
Coptin, *see* Sulfadiazine and Trimethoprim
Cordarone, *see* Amiodarone Oral
Coreg, *see* Carvedilol
Corgard, *see* Nadolol
Coricidin II, *see* Chlorpheniramine and Acetaminophen
Cort Sym, *see* Chloral Hydrate
Cortate, *see* Hydrocortisone Topical
Cortef, *see* Hydrocortisone Oral
Cortenema, *see* Hydrocortisone Topical
Cortisporin, *see* Hydrocortisone Topical and Neomycin Topical
Cortoderm, *see* Hydrocortisone Topical
Corytab, *see* Acetaminophen
Cosopt, *see* Timolol Ophthalmic and Dorzolamide Ophthalmic
Coumadin, *see* Warfarin
Covera-HS, *see* Verapamil
Coversyl, *see* Perindopril
Coversyl Plus, *see* Indapamide and Perindopril
Cozaar, *see* Losartan Potassium
Cresophene, *see* Dexamethasone Oral
Crixivan, *see* Indinavir
Cyclomen, *see* Danazol
Cytogam, *see* Cytomegalovirus Immune Globulin Intravenous Injection
Cytomel, *see* Liothyronine
Cytosar, *see* Cytarabine
Cytovene, *see* Ganciclovir Sodium Injection
Cytoxan, *see* Cyclophosphamide

D

Dalacin C, *see* Clindamycin
Dalmacol, *see* Doxylamine
Dalmane, *see* Flurazepam
Damylin, *see* Diphenhydramine Oral
Dantrium, *see* Dantrolene Oral
Daypro, *see* Oxaprozin
DDAVP, *see* Desmopressin
Declomycin, *see* Demeclocycline
Depakene, *see* Valproic Acid
Depocyt, *see* Cytarabine
Depo-Provera, *see* Medroxyprogesterone
Dermazin, *see* Silver Sulfadiazine
Dermovate, *see* Clobetasol
Detrol, *see* Tolterodine
Dexasone, *see* Dexamethasone Ophthalmic
Diabeta, *see* Glyburide
Diacomp, *see* Pyridoxine
Diahalt, *see* Loperamide
Diamel, *see* Folic Acid
Diamine, *see* Folic Acid
Diamox Sequels, *see* Acetazolamide Oral
Diarr-eze, *see* Loperamide
Diastat Rectal Delivery System, *see* Diazepam

Diazemuls, *see* Diazepam
Diclectin, *see* Doxylamine and Pyridoxine
Diclophen, *see* Dicyclomine and Phenobarbital
Didrocal, *see* Etidronate
Didronel, *see* Etidronate
Diflucan, *see* Fluconazole Oral
Dilantin, *see* Phenytoin Oral
Dilaudid, *see* Hydromorphone Hydrochloride
Dilotab II, *see* Acetaminophen
Dimetane, *see* Brompheniramine and Guaifenesin
Dimetapp, *see* Brompheniramine
Diocarpine, *see* Pilocarpine Ophthalmic
Diogent, *see* Gentamicin Ophthalmic
Diomycin, *see* Erythromycin
Dioptrol, *see* Dexamethasone Ophthalmic
Diosporin, *see* Neomycin Topical
Diovan, *see* Valsartan
Diovan-HCT, *see* Hydrochlorothiazide and Valsartan
Diovol Plus, *see* Simethicone
Dipentum, *see* Olsalazine
Diphenist, *see* Diphenhydramine Oral
Diprolene, *see* Betamethasone Topical
Ditropan, *see* Oxybutynin
Divalproex, *see* Valproic Acid
Dixarit, *see* Clonidine Tablets and Skin Patches
Dobutrex, *see* Dobutamine Hydrochloride Injection
Dormex, *see* Diphenhydramine Oral
Dormiphen, *see* Diphenhydramine Oral
Doxazosin, *see* Doxazosin
Doxepine, *see* Doxepin
Doxycin, *see* Doxycycline
Duo Trav, *see* Travoprost Ophthalmic and Timolol Ophthalmic
Duovent UDV, *see* Ipratropium Bromide Oral Inhalation and Albuterol
Duragesic, *see* Fentanyl Citrate Injection
Duralith, *see* Lithium
Duraphat, *see* Fluoride
Duricef, *see* Cefadroxil
Duvoid, *see* Bethanechol

E

Ecostatin, *see* Econazole Topical
Edecrin, *see* Ethacrynic Acid
Edemnix hp, *see* Colchicine Oral
EES, *see* Erythromycin
Effexor, *see* Venlafaxine
Efudex, *see* Fluorouracil
Elavil, *see* Amitriptyline
Eligard, *see* Leuprolide
Elocom, *see* Mometasone
Elo-vate, *see* Pyridoxine
Eltroxin, *see* Levothyroxine
Enbrel, *see* Etanercept
Enca, *see* Minocycline Oral
Endantadine, *see* Amantadine
Endocet, *see* Acetaminophen
Endomethasone, *see* Dexamethasone Oral
Entex LA, *see* Guaifenesin and Pseudoephedrine
Entocort, *see* Budesonide
Epaxal, *see* Hepatitis A Vaccine
Epival ECT, *see* Valproic Acid
Eprex, *see* Epoetin Alfa Injection
Ergodryl, *see* Diphenhydramine Oral
Erybid, *see* Erythromycin
EryC, *see* Erythromycin
Erysol Gel, *see* Erythromycin
Erythromid, *see* Erythromycin
Estalis, *see* Estradiol Transdermal System
Estrace, *see* Estradiol Transdermal System
Estracomb, *see* Estradiol Transdermal System
Estraderm, *see* Estradiol Transdermal System
Estradot, *see* Estradiol Transdermal System
Estring, *see* Estradiol Transdermal System
Estrogel, *see* Estradiol Transdermal System
Estroven, *see* Folic Acid
Ethyol, *see* Amifostine
Etibi, *see* Ethambutol
Etrafon, *see* Amitriptyline and Perphenazine Oral
Euflex, *see* Flutamide
Euglucon, *see* Glyburide
Euthyrox, *see* Levothyroxine
Evista, *see* Raloxifene

Exdol, *see* Acetaminophen
Exelon, *see* Rivastigmine
Ezetrol, *see* Ezetimibe

F

Famvir, *see* Famciclovir
Fibroplex, *see* Pyridoxine
Flagyl, *see* Metronidazole Topical
Flagystatin, *see* Metronidazole Topical and Nystatin
Flamazine, *see* Silver Sulfadiazine
Flomax, *see* Tamsulosin
Flonase, *see* Fluticasone Nasal Inhalation
Floradix, *see* Folic Acid
Florazole, *see* Metronidazole Topical
Florinef, *see* Fludrocortisone Acetate
Flovent, *see* Fluticasone Oral Inhalation
Floxin, *see* Ofloxacin Injection
Fludara, *see* Fludarabine Phosphate
Fluoderm, *see* Fluocinolone Topical
Fluoron, *see* Fluoride
Fluoroplex, *see* Fluorouracil
Folacal, *see* Folic Acid
Formulex, *see* Dicyclomine
Fortaplex, *see* Pyridoxine and Thiamine
Fortaz, *see* Ceftazidime Injection
Forteo, *see* Teriparatide (rDNA origin) Injection
Fortolin, *see* Acetaminophen
Fortovase, *see* Saquinavir
Forza-10, *see* Folic Acid
Fosamax, *see* Alendronate
Fragmin, *see* Dalteparin Sodium Injection
Froben, *see* Flurbiprofen Oral
Fungicure, *see* Tolnaftate
Fungizone, *see* Amphotericin B Injection

G

Gamastan S/D, *see* Immune Globulin Intravenous Injection
Gamimune N, *see* Immune Globulin Intravenous Injection
Gammagard S/D, *see* Immune Globulin Intravenous Injection
Gamunex, *see* Immune Globulin Intravenous Injection
Garamycin, *see* Gentamicin Sulfate Injection and Gentamicin Ophthalmic
Garasone, *see* Betamethasone Topical and Gentamicin Ophthalmic
Gemzar, *see* Gemcitabine Hydrochloride
Gentak, *see* Gentamicin Ophthalmic
Gliadel, *see* Carmustine
Glucobay, *see* Acarbose
Gluconorm, *see* Repaglinide
Glucophage, *see* Metformin
Glumetza, *see* Metformin
Glycon, *see* Metformin
Gynazole, *see* Butoconazole Vaginal Cream

H

Halcion, *see* Triazolam
Haldol, *see* Haloperidol Oral
Halog, *see* Halcinonide Topical
Halotestin, *see* Fluoxymesterone
Havrix, *see* Hepatitis A Vaccine
Heptovir, *see* Lamivudine
Herceptin, *see* Trastuzumab
Hexit, *see* Lindane
Histenol, *see* Pseudoephedrine and Acetaminophen
Hivid, *see* Zalcitabine
Humalog, *see* Insulin Lispro
Humate-P, *see* Antihemophilic Factor (Human)
Humira, *see* Adalimumab Injection
Hycamtin, *see* Topotecan Hydrochloride
Hycort Retention Enema, *see* Hydrocortisone Topical
Hydergine, *see* Ergoloid Mesylates
Hydrea, *see* Hydroxyurea
Hydrosone, *see* Hydrocortisone Topical
Hytrin, *see* Terazosin
Hyzaar, *see* Hydrochlorothiazide and Losartan Potassium

I

Idamycin, *see* Idarubicin
Ifex, *see* Ifosfamide
Imitrex, *see* Sumatriptan Oral and Nasal
Imodium, *see* Loperamide
Impril, *see* Imipramine

Imuran, *see* Azathioprine
Inderal, *see* Propranolol Oral
Indocid, *see* Indomethacin
Intal, *see* Cromolyn Sodium Nasal Solution
Invirase, *see* Saquinavir
Ionamin, *see* Phentermine
Isoptin, *see* Verapamil
Isopto Carpine, *see* Pilocarpine Ophthalmic
Isotamine, *see* Isoniazid
Isotamine B, *see* Isoniazid and Pyridoxine

K

Kaletra, *see* Ritonavir
Kayexalate, *see* Sodium Polystyrene Sulfonate
Keflex, *see* Cephalexin
Kenalog, *see* Triamcinolone Topical
Keppra, *see* Levetiracetam
Kidrolase, *see* Asparaginase
Kineret, *see* Anakinra
Kivexa, *see* Abacavir and Lamivudine
Kogenate FS, *see* Antihemophilic Factor (Recombinant)
Kwellada-P, *see* Permethrin
Kytril, *see* Granisetron

L

Lamictal, *see* Lamotrigine
Lamisil, *see* Terbinafine
Lanoxin, *see* Digoxin Oral
Lantus, *see* Insulin Glargine
Lanvis, *see* Thioguanine
Largactil, *see* Chlorpromazine
Lasix, *see* Furosemide
Lescol, *see* Fluvastatin
Leukeran, *see* Chlorambucil
Leustatin, *see* Cladribine
Levaquin, *see* Levofloxacin Injection
Levate, *see* Amitriptyline
Levo-T, *see* Levothyroxine
Liberator, *see* Loratadine
Librax, *see* Chlordiazepoxide
Lidodan, *see* Lidocaine Viscous
Lioresal, *see* Baclofen Oral
Lipidil, *see* Fenofibrate
Lipitor, *see* Atorvastatin
Lithane, *see* Lithium
Locacorten Vioform, *see* Clioquinol Topical
Lomine, *see* Dicyclomine
Loniten, *see* Minoxidil Oral
Loperacap, *see* Loperamide
Lopid, *see* Gemfibrozil
Lopresor, *see* Metoprolol Oral
Losec, *see* Omeprazole
Lotensin, *see* Benazepril
Lotriderm, *see* Betamethasone Topical and Clotrimazole
Lovenox, *see* Enoxaparin Injection
Lozide, *see* Indapamide
Lumigan, *see* Bimatoprost Ophthalmic
Lupron, *see* Leuprolide
Luvox, *see* Fluvoxamine

M

Maalox, *see* Simethicone
Macrobid, *see* Nitrofurantoin
Macrodantin, *see* Nitrofurantoin
Malarone, *see* Atovaquone
Matulane, *see* Procarbazine
Mavik, *see* Trandolapril
Maxalt, *see* Rizatriptan
Maxidex, *see* Dexamethasone Ophthalmic
Maxilene, *see* Lidocaine Viscous
Maxipime, *see* Cefepime Injection
Maxitrol, *see* Dexamethasone Ophthalmic and Neomycin Topical
Mazepine, *see* Carbamazepine
Medrol, *see* Methylprednisolone Sodium Succinate Injection
Medroxy, *see* Medroxyprogesterone
Mefenamic, *see* Mefenamic Acid
Megace, *see* Megestrol
Mepron, *see* Atovaquone
Meridia, *see* Sibutramine
Merrem, *see* Meropenem Injection
Mersyndol, *see* Doxylamine and Acetaminophen
Mestinon, *see* Pyridostigmine
Metadol, *see* Methadone Oral

Methoxacet, *see* Acetaminophen and Methocarbamol Oral
Methoxisal, *see* Methocarbamol Oral
Metreton, *see* Chlorpheniramine and Prednisone Oral
Metrogel, *see* Metronidazole Topical
Mevacor, *see* Lovastatin
Miacalcin, *see* Calcitonin Salmon Injection
Micardis, *see* Telmisartan
Micardis Plus, *see* Telmisartan and Hydrochlorothiazide
Micatin, *see* Miconazole Injection
Micozole, *see* Miconazole Injection
Mielocol, *see* Guaifenesin
Minipress, *see* Prazosin
Minirin, *see* Desmopressin
Minitran, *see* Nitroglycerin Ointment
Minocin, *see* Minocycline Oral
Minox, *see* Minoxidil Topical
Mirapex, *see* Pramipexole
Mobicox, *see* Meloxicam
Moduret, *see* Hydrochlorothiazide
Monistat, *see* Miconazole Injection
Monitan, *see* Acebutolol
Monoclate-P, *see* Antihemophilic Factor (Human)
Monocor, *see* Bisoprolol
Monopril, *see* Fosinopril
Monurol, *see* Fosfomycin
Motrin, *see* Ibuprofen
Muse, *see* Alprostadil
Mustargen, *see* Mechlorethamine
Mutamycin, *see* Mitomycin
Mycobutin, *see* Rifabutin
Mycostatin, *see* Nystatin
Myleran, *see* Busulfan
Myocet, *see* Doxorubicin
Myotonachol, *see* Bethanechol

N

Nadryl, *see* Diphenhydramine Oral
Naftin, *see* Naftifine Hydrochloride Topical
Nalcrom, *see* Cromolyn Sodium Nasal Solution
Naprosyn, *see* Naproxen
Nardil, *see* Phenelzine
Nasacort, *see* Triamcinolone Nasal Inhalation
Nasonex, *see* Mometasone Nasal Inhalation
Navane, *see* Thiothixene Oral
Navelbine, *see* Vinorelbine Tartrate
Neggram, *see* Nalidixic Acid
Nembutal, *see* Pentobarbital Oral and Rectal
Neoral, *see* Cyclosporine Injection
Neosporin, *see* Neomycin Topical
Neupogen, *see* Filgrastim
Neurontin, *see* Gabapentin
Neutragel, *see* Fluoride
Neutrexin, *see* Trimetrexate Glucuronate
Nexium, *see* Esomeprazole
Nidagel, *see* Metronidazole Topical
Nimotop, *see* Nimodipine
Nitro-Dur, *see* Nitroglycerin Ointment
Nitrol, *see* Nitroglycerin Ointment
Nix, *see* Permethrin
Nizoral, *see* Ketoconazole
Nolvadex, *see* Tamoxifen
Norflex, *see* Orphenadrine
Norgesic, *see* Orphenadrine
Noritate, *see* Metronidazole Topical
Norvasc, *see* Amlodipine
Norventyl, *see* Nortriptyline
Norvir, *see* Ritonavir
Novamilor, *see* Hydrochlorothiazide
Novamoxin, *see* Amoxicillin
Novoxapam, *see* Oxazepam
Nubain, *see* Nalbuphine Injection
Nyaderm, *see* Nystatin
Nytol, *see* Diphenhydramine Oral

O

Octostim, *see* Desmopressin
Ocuflox, *see* Ofloxacin Oral
Oesclim, *see* Estradiol Transdermal System
Opticrom, *see* Cromolyn Sodium Nasal Solution
Optimyxin, *see* Neomycin Topical
Oracort, *see* Triamcinolone Nasal Inhalation
Orap, *see* Pimozide
Orfenace, *see* Orphenadrine
Ovol, *see* Simethicone

Oxeze, *see* Formoterol Oral Inhalation
Oxizole, *see* Oxiconazole
Oxpam, *see* Oxazepam
Oxycontin, *see* Oxycodone

P

Palafer CF, *see* Folic Acid
Panadol, *see* Acetaminophen
Pantoloc, *see* Pantoprazole
Parafon Forte, *see* Chlorzoxazone and Acetaminophen
Paraplatin-AQ, *see* Carboplatin
Pariet, *see* Rabeprazole
Parlodel, *see* Bromocriptine
Parnate, *see* Tranylcypromine
Patanol, *see* Olopatadine Ophthalmic
Paxil, *see* Paroxetine
PCE, *see* Erythromycin
Pediacol, *see* Simethicone
Pediaphen, *see* Acetaminophen
Pediapred, *see* Prednisolone Ophthalmic
Pediazole, *see* Erythromycin
Pen-Vee, *see* Penicillin V Potassium Oral
Pepcid, *see* Famotidine Oral
Pepsotol, *see* Sodium Bicarbonate
Percocet, *see* Acetaminophen and Oxycodone
Permax, *see* Pergolide
Persantine, *see* Dipyridamole
Pertudoron, *see* Quinine
Pharmorubicin, *see* Epirubicin Injection
Phazyme, *see* Simethicone
Phenazo, *see* Phenazopyridine
Phenergan, *see* Promethazine
Phen-Oris, *see* Clioquinol Topical
Pilopine, *see* Pilocarpine Ophthalmic
Pitrex, *see* Tolnaftate
Plaquenil, *see* Hydroxychloroquine
Plavix, *see* Clopidogrel
Plendil, *see* Felodipine
Polytrim, *see* Trimethoprim
Pramegel, *see* Pramoxine
Pramox HC, *see* Hydrocortisone Topical and Pramoxine
Prandase, *see* Acarbose
Pravachol, *see* Pravastatin
Pravasa, *see* Pravastatin
Prepidil, *see* Dinoprostone
Preterax, *see* Indapamide and Perindopril
Prevacid, *see* Lansoprazole
Prevex HC, *see* Hydrocortisone Topical
Prinivil, *see* Lisinopril
Prinzide, *see* Hydrochlorothiazide and Lisinopril
Probeta, *see* Levobunolol Ophthalmic
Procan SR, *see* Procainamide Oral
Proclearz Antifungal, *see* Tolnaftate
Proctodan-HC, *see* Pramoxine
Proctofoam HC, *see* Pramoxine
Proctol Ointment, *see* Hydrocortisone Topical
Proctosedyl Ointment, *see* Hydrocortisone Topical
Procytox, *see* Cyclophosphamide
Prograf, *see* Tacrolimus
Proleukin, *see* Aldesleukin
Prolopa, *see* Levodopa
Propecia, *see* Finasteride
Propine, *see* Dipivefrin Ophthalmic
Proscar, *see* Finasteride
Prostin E2, *see* Dinoprostone
Prostin VR, *see* Alprostadil
Protopic, *see* Tacrolimus
Protrin, *see* Sulfamethoxazole and Trimethoprim
Protylol, *see* Dicyclomine
Provera, *see* Medroxyprogesterone
Prozac, *see* Fluoxetine
Pulmicort, *see* Budesonide
Pulmicort Turbuhaler, *see* Budesonide Inhalation Powder
Pulmophylline Elx, *see* Theophylline
Pulmozyme, *see* Dornase Alfa
Purinethol, *see* Mercaptopurine
PVF-K, *see* Penicillin V Potassium Oral

Q

Qvar, *see* Beclomethasone Oral Inhalation

R

R & C Shampoo, *see* Pyrethrin and Piperonyl Butoxide
Rapamune, *see* Sirolimus

Pregnancy Precaution Listing

The following medicines, selected from those included in this publication, have specific precautions in regard to use during pregnancy. For specific information, consult the individual drug information monograph; look in the index for the page number.

The use of any medicine during pregnancy must be carefully considered. The physician and the patient must balance the expected benefits against the possible risks.

Absence of a drug from the list is not meant to imply that it is safe for use in pregnant patients. For many drugs, it is not known whether a problem exists; experimentation on pregnant women is generally not done. Knowledge is usually gained only from the accumulated experience over many years in giving a drug to pregnant women who needed its benefits. Also, well-planned studies in pregnant animals may reveal problems, although the relation of such findings to pregnant humans and their babies may not be known. Problems suggested by animal studies are often included in the warnings in this book.

Readers are reminded that the information in this text is selected and not considered to be complete.

Risk factors (A, B, C, D, X) have been assigned to all drugs, based on the level of risk the drug poses to the fetus. Risk factors are designed to help the reader quickly classify a drug for use during pregnancy. They do not refer to breast-feeding risk. Because they tend to oversimplify a complex topic, they should always be used in conjunction with the accompanying text. The definitions for the factors are those used by the Food and Drug Administration (Federal Register 1980;44:37434-67). In some cases, more than one risk factor is listed with a short explanation.

Category	Description
A	Studies in pregnant women have not shown an increased risk of birth defects.
B	Animal studies have shown no evidence of harm to the fetus; however, there are no good-quality studies in pregnant women **or** Animal studies have shown an adverse effect, but studies in pregnant women have failed to show a risk to the fetus.
C	Animal studies have shown an adverse effect, and there are no good-quality studies in pregnant women **or** No animal studies have been conducted, and there are no good-quality studies in pregnant women.
D	Studies in pregnant women have found a risk to the fetus. However, the benefits of taking this drug may outweigh the potential risk.
X	Studies in animals or pregnant women have found proof of birth defects. The drug should not be used in women who are or may become pregnant.

A

α_1-Proteinase Inhibitor - **C**
Abacavir - **C**
Abarelix - **X**
Abatacept - **C**
Abciximab - **C**
Acamprosate - **C**
Acarbose - **B**
Acebutolol - **B**
Acetaminophen - **B**
Acetylcysteine - **B**
Acyclovir (Systemic) - **B**
Acyclovir (Topical) - **B**
Adalimumab - **B**
Adapalene - **C**
Adefovir - **C**
Adenosine - **C**
Agalsidase Beta - **B**
Albumin Human - **C**
Albuterol - **C**
Aldesleukin - **C**
Alefacept - **B**
Alemtuzumab - **C**
Alendronate - **C**
Alfuzosin - **B**
Alitretinoin - **D**
Allopurinol - **C**
Almotriptan - **C**
Alosetron - **B**
Alprazolam - **D**
Alteplase - **C**
Amantadine - **C**
Amifostine - **C**
Amikacin - **D**
Aminocaproic Acid - **C**
Aminolevulinic Acid - **C**
Amiodarone - **D**
Amitriptyline - **C**
Amlodipine - **C**
Amoxicillin - **B**
Amoxicillin/Clavulanate - **B**
Amphetamine - **C**
Amphotericin B - **B**

Ampicillin - **B**
Ampicillin/Sulbactam - **B**
Amprenavir - **C**
Anakinra - **B**
Anastrozole - **D**
Anthrax Vaccine - **D**
Apomorphine - **C**
Apraclonidine - **C**
Aprepitant - **B**
Aprotinin - **B**
Argatroban - **B**
Aripiprazole - **C**
Arsenic Trioxide - **D**
Articaine - **C**
Asparaginase - **C**
Aspirin - **C**; **D** (3rd trimester)
Atazanavir - **B**
Atenolol - **D**
Atomoxetine - **C**
Atorvastatin - **X**
Atovaquone/Proguanil - **C**
Atracurium - **C**
Atropine - **C**
Azacitidine - **D**
Azathioprine - **D**
Azelaic Acid - **B**
Azelastine - **C**
Azithromycin - **B**
Aztreonam - **B**

B

Bacitracin - **C**
Bacitracin (EENT) - **C**
Baclofen - **C**
Balsalazide - **B**
Basiliximab - **B**
Beclomethasone (EENT) - **C**
Beclomethasone (Systemic) - **C**
Benazepril - **C** (1st trimester); **D** (2nd and 3rd trimesters)
Benzocaine - **C**
Benzonatate - **C**
Benztropine - **C**
Betamethasone - **C**

Betamethasone - **C**
Betaxolol - **C**
Betaxolol - **C**
Bevacizumab - **C**
Bexarotene (Systemic) - **X**
Bexarotene (Topical) - **X**
Bicalutamide - **X**
Bimatoprost - **C**
Biperiden - **C**
Bisacodyl - **B** (base); safety not established for bisacodyl tannex
Bisoprolol - **C**
Bivalirudin - **B**
Bleomycin - **D**
Bortezomib - **D**
Bosentan - **X**
Botulinum Toxin Type A - **C**
Botulinum Toxin Type B - **C**
Brimonidine - **B**
Brinzolamide - **C**
Bromfenac - **C**
Budesonide (EENT) - **B**
Budesonide (Systemic) - **B** (orally inhaled powder and inhalation suspension); **C** (oral capsules)
Bumetanide - **C**
Bupivacaine - **C**
Buprenorphine - **C**
Bupropion - **B**
Buspirone - **B**
Busulfan - **D**
Butenafine - **B**
Butoconazole - **C**
Butorphanol - **C**

C

Calcipotriene - **C**
Calcitonin - **C**
Calcitriol - **C**
Calcium Salts - **C**
Candesartan - **C** (1st trimester); **D** (2nd and 3rd trimesters)
Capecitabine - **D**
Captopril - **C** (1st trimester); **D** (2nd and 3rd trimesters)
Carbamazepine - **D**

Carbenicillin - **B**
Carboplatin - **D**
Carisoprodol - **C**
Carmustine - **D**
Carvedilol - **C**
Caspofungin - **C**
Castor Oil - **X**
Cefaclor - **B**
Cefadroxil - **B**
Cefazolin - **B**
Cefdinir - **B**
Cefditoren - **B**
Cefepime - **B**
Cefixime - **B**
Cefotaxime - **B**
Cefotetan - **B**
Cefoxitin - **B**
Cefpodoxime - **B**
Cefprozil - **B**
Ceftazidime - **B**
Ceftibuten - **B**
Ceftizoxime - **B**
Ceftriaxone - **B**
Cefuroxime - **B**
Celecoxib - **C** (Avoid use in 3rd trimester)
Cephalexin - **B**
Cetirizine - **B**
Cetrorelix - **X**
Cetuximab - **C**
Cevimeline - **C**
Chlorambucil - **D**
Chloramphenicol - **C**
Chlorhexidine (EENT) - **B** (oral solution); **C** (subgingival pellets)
Chlorhexidine (Topical) - **B**
Chloroquine - **C** (Avoid use during pregnancy)
Chlorothiazide - **C**
Chlorpheniramine - **B** (Not recommended during the 3rd trimester)
Chlorthalidone - **B**
Chlorzoxazone - **C**
Cholestyramine - **C**
Ciclesonide - **C**
Ciclopirox - **B**
Cidofovir - **C**
Cilostazol - **C**
Cimetidine - **B**
Cinacalcet - **C**
Ciprofloxacin - **C**
Ciprofloxacin (EENT) - **C**
Cisplatin - **D**
Citalopram - **C**
Clarithromycin - **C**
Clindamycin - **B**
Clindamycin (Topical) - **B**
Clobetasol - **C**
Clofarabine - **D**
Clomipramine - **C**
Clonazepam - **D**
Clonidine - **C**
Clopidogrel - **B**
Clotrimazole (Topical) - **B**
Clozapine - **B**
Codeine - **C**
Colchicine - **C** (oral)
Colesevelam - **B**
Colestipol - **B**
Co-trimoxazole - **C**
Cromolyn - **C**
Cromolyn - **B**
Cyclobenzaprine - **B**
Cyclophosphamide - **D**
Cyclosporine - **C**
Cyclosporine (EENT) - **C**
Cyproheptadine - **B**
Cytarabine - **D**

D

Dacarbazine - **C**
Daclizumab - **C**
Dactinomycin - **D**
Dalteparin - **B** (Multiple-dose vials containing benzyl alcohol should not be used in pregnant women)

Danazol - **X**
Dantrolene - **C**
Daptomycin - **B**
Darbepoetin Alfa - **C**
Darifenacin - **C**
Daunorubicin - **D**
Decitabine - **D**
Deferasirox - **C**
Delavirdine - **C**
Demeclocycline - **D**
Denileukin - **C**
Desipramine - **C**
Desloratadine - **C**
Dexamethasone - **C**
Dexamethasone (EENT) - **C**
Dexmedetomidine - **C** (Use during labor and delivery is not recommended)
Dexmethylphenidate - **C**
Dexrazoxane - **C**
Dextroamphetamine - **C**
Dextromethorphan - **C**
Diazepam - **D**
Diazoxide - **C**
Diclofenac - **C** (Avoid use in 3rd trimester)
Diclofenac (Topical) - **B** (Avoid use in 3rd trimester)
Dicloxacillin - **B**
Dicyclomine - **B**
Didanosine - **B**
Diflunisal - **C** (Avoid use in 3rd trimester)
Digoxin - **C**
Dihydroergotamine - **X**
Diltiazem - **C**
Dimenhydrinate - **C**
Diphenhydramine - **B**
Diphenoxylate - **C**
Dipivefrin - **B**
Dipyridamole - **B**
Disopyramide - **C**
Disulfiram - **C**
Dobutamine - **B**
Docetaxel - **D**
Dofetilide - **C**
Dolasetron - **B**
Donepezil - **C**
Dopamine - **C**
Dornase Alfa - **B**
Dorzolamide - **C**
Doxazosin - **C**
Doxorubicin - **D**
Doxycycline - **D**
Doxycycline (EENT) - **D**
Dronabinol - **C**
Droperidol - **C**
Drotrecogin Alfa - **C**
Duloxetine - **C**
Dutasteride - **X**

E

Econazole - **C**
Efalizumab - **C**
Efavirenz - **D**
Eflornithine - **C**
Eletriptan - **C**
Emedastine - **B**
Emtricitabine - **B**
Enalapril - **C** (1st trimester); **D** (2nd and 3rd trimesters)
Enfuvirtide - **B**
Enoxaparin - **B**
Entacapone - **C**
Entecavir - **C**
Ephedrine - **C**
Epinastine - **C**
Epinephrine - **C**
Epinephrine (EENT) - **C**
Epirubicin - **D**
Eplerenone - **B**
Epoetin Alfa - **C**
Epoprostenol - **B**
Eprosartan - **C** (1st trimester); **D** (2nd and 3rd trimesters)
Eptifibatide - **B**
Ergotamine - **X**
Erlotinib - **D**

Ertapenem - **B**
Erythromycin (EENT) - **B**
Erythromycin (Systemic) - **B**
Erythromycin (Topical) - **B**
Escitalopram - **C**
Esmolol - **C**
Esomeprazole - **B**
Estradiol - **X**
Estramustine - **X**
Estrogen-Progestin Combinations - **X**
Estrogens, Conjugated - **X**
Estropipate, Esterified Estrogens - **X**
Eszopiclone - **C**
Etanercept - **B**
Etidronate - **C**
Etodolac - **C** (Avoid use in 3rd trimester)
Etoposide - **D**
Exemestane - **D**
Exenatide - **C**
Ezetimibe - **C**

F

Famciclovir - **B**
Famotidine - **B**
Felbamate - **C**
Felodipine - **C**
Fenofibrate - **C**
Fentanyl - **C**
Fexofenadine - **C**
Filgrastim - **C**
Finasteride - **X**
Flecainide - **C**
Floxuridine - **D**
Fluconazole - **C**
Flucytosine - **C**
Fludarabine - **D**
Fludrocortisone - **C**
Flumazenil - **C**
Flunisolide (EENT) - **C**
Fluocinolone - **C**
Fluocinolone (Topical) - **C**
Fluorouracil - **D**
Fluoxetine - **C**
Fluphenazine - **C**
Flurbiprofen - **C**
Flutamide - **D**
Fluticasone - **C**
Fluticasone (EENT) - **C**
Fluvastatin - **X**
Fluvoxamine - **C**
Folic Acid - **A**
Fondaparinux - **B**
Formoterol - **C**
Fosamprenavir - **C**
Foscarnet - **C**
Fosinopril - **C** (1st trimester); **D** (2nd and 3rd trimesters)
Fosphenytoin - **D**
Frovatriptan - **C**
Fulvestrant - **D**
Furosemide - **C**

G

Gabapentin - **C**
Galantamine - **B**
Gallium Nitrate - **C**
Ganciclovir - **C**
Ganirelix - **X**
Gatifloxacin (EENT) - **C**
Gatifloxacin (Systemic) - **C**
Gefitinib - **D**
Gemcitabine - **D**
Gemfibrozil - **C**
Gemifloxacin - **C**
Gemtuzumab - **D**
Gentamicin (EENT) - **C**
Gentamicin (Systemic) - **D**
Glatiramer - **B**
Glimepiride - **C**
Glipizide - **C**
Glyburide - **B**
Glycopyrrolate - **B**
Goserelin - **D** (advanced breast cancer); **X** (endometriosis, endometrial-thinning agent)

Granisetron - **B**
Griseofulvin - **C**
Guaifenesin - **C**

H

Haemophilus influenzae type b Vaccine - **C**
Haloperidol - **C**
Heparin - **C**
Hepatitis B Vaccine - **C**
Hetastarch - **C**
Histrelin - **X**
Human Papillomavirus (HPV) Vaccine - **B**
Hydralazine - **C**
Hydrochlorothiazide - **B**
Hydrocodone - **C**
Hydrocortisone (Systemic) - **C**
Hydrocortisone (Topical) - **C**
Hydromorphone - **C**
Hydroxychloroquine - **C**
Hydroxyurea - **D**
Hydroxyzine - **C** (Contraindicated in early pregnancy)

I

Ibandronate - **C**
Ibritumomab - **D**
Ibuprofen - **C** (Avoid use in 3rd trimester)
Ibutilide - **C**
Idarubicin - **D**
Ifosfamide - **D**
Iloprost - **C**
Imatinib - **D**
Imiglucerase - **C**
Imipenem/Cilastatin - **C**
Imipramine - **D**
Imiquimod - **C**
Inamrinone - **C**
Indapamide - **B**
Indinavir - **C**
Indomethacin - **C** (Avoid use in 3rd trimester)
Infliximab - **B**
Influenza Vaccine - **C**
Insulin - **B**
Insulin Aspart - **C**
Insulin Detemir - **C**
Insulin Glargine - **C**
Insuline Glulisine - **C**
Insulin Human - **B**
Insulin Lispro - **B**
Interferon Beta - **C**
Interferon Gamma - **C**
Ipratropium (EENT) - **B**
Ipratropium (Systemic) - **B**
Irbesartan - **C** (1st trimester); **D** (2nd and 3rd trimesters)
Irinotecan - **D**
Iron Dextran - **C**
Iron Sucrose - **B**
Isoproterenol - **C**
Isosorbide - **C**
Isotretinoin - **X**
Isradipine - **C**
Itraconazole - **C**
Ivermectin - **C**

J

Japanese Encephalitis Vaccine - **C**

K

Ketoconazole (Systemic) - **C**
Ketoconazole (Topical) - **C**
Ketoprofen - **C** (Avoid use in 3rd trimester)
Ketorolac - **C** (Avoid use in 3rd trimester)
Ketotifen - **C**

L

Labetalol - **C**
Lactulose - **B**
Lamivudine - **C**
Lamotrigine - **C**
Lansoprazole - **B**
Lanthanum - **C**
Laronidase - **B**

Latanoprost - **C**
Leflunomide - **X**
Lepirudin - **B**
Letrozole - **D**
Leucovorin - **C**
Leuprolide - **X**
Levalbuterol - **C**
Levetiracetam - **C**
Levodopa/Carbidopa - **C**
Levofloxacin (EENT) - **C**
Levofloxacin (Systemic) - **C**
Levothyroxine - **A**
Lidocaine (Local) - **B**
Lidocaine (Systemic) - **B**
Lindane - **C**
Linezolid - **C**
Lisinopril - **C** (1st trimester); **D** (2nd and 3rd trimesters)
Lithium - **D**
Lodoxamide - **B**
Lomustine - **D**
Loperamide - **B**
Lopinavir and Ritonavir - **C**
Loracarbef - **B**
Loratadine - **B**
Lorazepam - **D**
Losartan - **C** (1st trimester); **D** (2nd and 3rd trimesters)
Loteprednol - **C**
Lovastatin - **X**
Lubiprostone - **C**
Lutropin Alfa - **X**

M

Magnesium Sulfate - **A or B**
Mannitol - **C**
Meclizine - **B**
Medroxyprogesterone - **X**
Mefloquine - **C**
Megestrol - **X** (Oral Suspensions); **D** (Tablets)
Meloxicam - **C** (Avoid use in 3rd trimester)
Memantine - **B**
Meningococcal Vaccine - **C**
Meperidine - **C**
Meropenem - **B**
Mesalamine - **B**
Mesna - **B**
Metaxalone - **B**
Metformin - **B**
Methadone - **C**
Methocarbamol - **C**
Methotrexate - **X**
Methyldopa - **C** (IV injection); **B** (tablets)
Methylphenidate - **C**
Methylprednisolone - **C**
Methyltestosterone - **X**
Metoclopramide - **B**
Metoprolol - **C**
Metronidazole - **B** (Contraindicated during the first trimester of pregnancy)
Metronidazole - **B**
Mexiletine - **C**
Micafungin - **C**
Miconazole - **C**
Midazolam - **D**
Midodrine - **C**
Mifepristone - **X**
Miglustat - **X**
Milrinone - **C**
Mineral Oil - **C**
Minocycline - **D**
Minocycline (EENT) - **D**
Minoxidil - **C**
Mirtazapine - **C**
Misoprostol - **X**
Mitomycin - **C**
Mitotane - **C**
Mitoxantrone - **D**
Modafinil - **C**
Moexipril - **C** (1st trimester); **D** (2nd and 3rd trimesters)
Mometasone (EENT) - **C**
Mometasone (Topical) - **C**
Montelukast - **B**
Morphine - **C**

Moxifloxacin (EENT) - **C**
Moxifloxacin (Systemic) - **C**
Mupirocin - **B**
Mycophenolate - **C**

N

Nabumetone - **C** (Avoid use in 3rd trimester)
Nadolol - **C**
Nafcillin - **B**
Nalbuphine - **B**
Naloxone - **B/C**
Naltrexone - **C**
Naphazoline - **C**
Naproxen - **C** (Avoid use in 3rd trimester)
Naratriptan - **C**
Natalizumab - **C**
Nateglinide - **C**
Nedocromil - **B**
Nedocromil - **B**
Nefazodone - **C**
Nelarabine - **D**
Nelfinavir - **B**
Nepafenac - **C**
Neomycin - **C**
Neomycin - **C**
Nepafenac - **C**
Nesiritide - **C**
Nevirapine - **C**
Niacin - **C**
Nicardipine - **C**
Nicotine - **D**
Nifedipine - **C**
Nilutamide - **C**
Nimodipine - **C**
Nisoldipine - **C**
Nitazoxanide - **B**
Nitric Oxide - **C**
Nitrofurantoin - **B**
Nitroglycerin - **C**
Nizatidine - **B**
Norepinephrine - **C**
Norfloxacin - **C**
Nortriptyline - **D**
Nystatin - **A** (vaginal tablets)

O

Octreotide - **B**
Ofloxacin - **C**
Ofloxacin (EENT) - **C**
Olmesartan - **C** (1st trimester); **D** (2nd and 3rd trimesters)
Olopatadine - **C**
Olsalazine - **C**
Omalizumab - **B**
Omega-3-acid Ethyl Esters - **C**
Omeprazole - **C**
Ondansetron - **B**
Orlistat - **B** (use not recommended)
Oseltamivir - **C**
Oxacillin - **B**
Oxaliplatin - **D**
Oxcarbazepine - **C**
Oxiconazole - **B**
Oxybutynin - **B**
Oxycodone - **B/C**
Oxymetazoline - **C**

P

Paclitaxel - **D**
Palifermin - **C**
Paliperidone - **C**
Palivizumab - **C** (Not indicated for use in adults)
Palonosetron - **B**
Pamidronate - **D**
Pancuronium - **C**
Pantoprazole - **B**
Paroxetine - **C**
Pegaptanib - **B**
Pegaspargase - **C**
Pegfilgrastim - **C**
Peginterferon Alfa - **C** (when used alone); **X** (when used with ribavirin)

gvisomant - **B**
Pemetrexed - **D**
Pemirolast - **C**
Penciclovir - **B**
Penicillin G - **B**
Penicillin V - **B**
Pentamidine - **C**
Pentazocine - **C**
Pentoxifylline - **C**
Pergolide - **B**
Perindopril - **C** (1st trimester); **D** (2nd and 3rd trimesters)
Permethrin - **B**
Phenazopyridine - **B**
Phenobarbital - **B** (oral); **D** (IV)
Phentermine - **C**
Phentolamine - **C**
Phenylephrine - **C**
Phenytoin - **D**
Physostigmine - **C**
Phytonadione - **C**
Pilocarpine - **C**
Pimecrolimus - **C**
Pimozide - **C**
Pindolol - **B**
Pioglitazone - **C**
Piperacillin/Tazobactam - **B**
Piroxicam - **C**
Pneumococcal Conjugate Vaccine - **C**
Pneumococcal Polysaccharide Vaccine - **C**
Podofilox - **C**
Polymyxin B - **C**
Posaconazole - **C**
Potassium Supplements - **C**
Pramipexole - **C**
Pramlintide - **C**
Pravastatin - **X**
Prazosin - **C**
Prednisolone - **C**
Prednisone - **C**
Pregabalin - **C**
Primaquine - **C**
Procainamide - **C**
Procarbazine - **D**
Prochlorperazine - **C**
Procyclidine - **C**
Promethazine - **C**
Propafenone - **C**
Propofol - **B**
Propoxyphene - **C**; **D** (if used for prolonged periods)
Propranolol - **C**
Prussian Blue - **C**
Pseudoephedrine - **C**

Q
Quetiapine - **C**
Quinapril - **C** (1st trimester); **D** (2nd and 3rd trimesters)
Quinidine - **C**
Quinine - **X**
Quinupristin/Dalfopristin - **B**

R
Rabeprazole - **B**
Rabies Vaccine - **C**
Raloxifene - **X**
Ramelteon - **C**
Ramipril - **C** (1st trimester); **D** (2nd and 3rd trimesters)
Ranitidine - **B**
Ranolazine - **C**
Rasagiline - **C**
Rasburicase - **C**
Repaglinide - **C**
Reteplase - **C**
Ribavirin - **X**
Rifaximin - **C**
Riluzole - **C**
Rimantadine - **C**
Risedronate - **C**

Risperidone - **C**
Ritonavir - **B**
Rituximab - **C**
Rivastigmine - **B**
Rizatriptan - **C**
Rocuronium - **C**
Ropinirole - **C**
Rosiglitazone - **C**
Rosuvastatin - **X**

S
Salmeterol - **C**
Saquinavir - **B**
Sargramostim - **C**
Scopolamine - **C**
Selegiline - **C**
Sertaconazole - **C**
Sevelamer - **C**
Shingles (Zoster) Vaccine - **C**
Sibutramine - **C**
Sildenafil - **B**
Simethicone - **C**
Simvastatin - **X**
Sirolimus - **C**
Sitagliptin - **B**
Sodium Bicarbonate - **C**
Sodium Ferric Gluconate - **B**
Sodium Nitroprusside - **C**
Sodium Oxybate - **B**
Sodium Polystyrene Sulfonate - **C**
Solifenacin - **C**
Sotalol - **B**
Spectinomycin - **B**
Spironolactone - **C**
Stavudine - **C**
Succinylcholine - **C**
Sufentanil - **C**
Sulconazole - **C**
Sulfacetamide - **C**
Sulfasalazine - **B**
Sulindac - **C** (avoid use in 3rd trimester)
Sumatriptan - **C**
Sunitinib - **D**

T
Tacrine - **C**
Tacrolimus (Systemic) - **C**
Tacrolimus (Topical) - **C**
Tadalafil - **B**
Talc - **B**
Tamoxifen - **D**
Tamsulosin - **B**
Tazarotene - **X**
Tegaserod - **B**
Telithromycin - **C**
Telmisartan - **C** (1st trimester); **D** (2nd and 3rd trimesters)
Temazepam - **X**
Temozolomide - **D**
Tenecteplase - **C**
Teniposide - **D**
Tenofovir - **B**
Terazosin - **C**
Terbinafine (Systemic) - **B**
Terbinafine (Topical) - **B**
Terconazole (Topical) - **C**
Teriparatide - **C**
Testosterone - **X**
Tetanus and Diphtheria Vaccine - **C**
Tetanus, Diphtheria, and Pertussis (Tdap) Vaccine - **C**
Tetracycline - **D**
Thioguanine - **D**
Thiopental - **C**
Thrombin - **C**
Tiagabine - **C**
Ticarcillin/Clavulanate - **B**
Ticlopidine - **B**
Tigecycline - **D**

Timolol (EENT) - **C**
Timolol (Systemic) - **C**
Tinidazole - **B**
Tinzaparin - **B**
Tioconazole - **B**
Tiotropium - **C**
Tipranavir - **C**
Tirofiban - **B**
Tizanidine - **C**
Tobramycin (EENT) - **B**
Tobramycin (Systemic) - **D**
Tolcapone - **C**
Tolnaftate - **C**
Tolterodine - **C**
Topiramate - **C**
Topotecan - **D**
Toremifene - **D**
Torsemide - **B**
Tositumomab - **X**
Tramadol - **C**
Trandolapril - **C** (1st trimester); **D** (2nd and 3rd trimesters)
Trastuzumab - **B**
Travoprost - **C**
Trazodone - **C**
Treprostinil - **B**
Tretinoin - **C**
Tretinoin - **D**
Triamcinolone (EENT) - **C**
Triamcinolone (Systemic) - **C**
Triamcinolone (Topical) - **C**
Triamterene - **C**
Triazolam - **X**
Trifluridine - **C**
Trihexyphenidyl - **C**
Trimethoprim - **C**
Triptorelin - **X**
Tromethamine - **C**
Trospium - **C**
Typhoid Vaccine - **C**

V
Valacyclovir - **B**
Valganciclovir - **C**
Valproate/Divalproex - **D**
Valsartan - **C** (1st trimester); **D** (2nd and 3rd trimesters)
Vancomycin - **B** (oral); **C** (IV)
Vardenafil - **B**
Varenicline - **C**
Varicella (Chickenpox) Vaccine - **C**
Vasopressin - **C**
Vecuronium - **C**
Venlafaxine - **C**
Verapamil - **C**
Verteporfin - **C**
Vinblastine - **D**
Vincristine - **D**
Voriconazole - **D**

W
Warfarin - **X**

Y
Yellow Fever Vaccine - **C**

Z
Zalcitabine - **C**
Zaleplon - **C**
Zanamivir - **C**
Ziconotide - **C**
Zidovudine - **C**
Zileuton - **C**
Ziprasidone - **C**
Zoledronic Acid - **D**
Zolmitriptan - **C**
Zolpidem - **C**
Zonisamide - **C**

Immunization Schedules, US

Recommended Immunization Schedule for Persons Aged 0–6 Years

UNITED STATES • 2007

Vasine▼ Age►	Birth	1 month	2 months	4 months	6 months	12 months	15 months	18 months	19–23 months	2–3 years	4–6 years
Hepatitis B[1]	HepB	HepB		see footnote 1		HepB			HepB Series		
Rotavirus			Rota	Rota	Rota						
Diphtheria, Tetanus, Pertussis			DTaP	DTaP	DTaP		DTaP				DTaP
Haemophilus influenzae type b			Hib	Hib	*Hib*	Hib		Hib			
Pneumococcal[2]			PCV	PCV	PCV	PCV				PCV / PPV	
Inactivated Poliovirus			IPV	IPV		IPV					IPV
Influenza[3]						Influenza (Yearly)					
Measles, Mumps, Rubella						MMR					MMR
Varicella						Varicella					Varicella
Hepatitis A						HepA (2 doses)				HepA Series	
Meningococcal										MPSV4	

☐ Range of recommended ages   ☐ Catch-up immunization   ☐ Certain high-risk groups

This schedule gives the recommended ages for routine administration of currently licensed childhood vaccines for children aged 0–6 years. The information is based on the 2007 recommendations by the Advisory Committee on Immunization Practices, the American Academy of Pediatrics, and the American Academy of Family Physicians. Additional information is available at www.cdc.gov/vaccines/recs/schedules/default.htm#child. Because these recommendations may change or new vaccines may become available, always check with your child's doctor for the most current immunization information.

Footnotes to table 1

1) Hepatitis B vaccine (4-month dose): When hepatitis B vaccine is given as a shot in combination with other vaccines, a dose at 4 months may be given. If hepatitis B vaccine is given alone, then a dose at 4 months is not needed.

2) Pneumococcal vaccine: Two types of pneumococcal vaccine are available. Pneumococcal conjugate vaccine (PCV) can be given to certain high-risk patients at ages 24-59 months and pneumococcal polysaccharide vaccine (PPV) can be given to children 2 years or older in certain high risk groups.

3) Influenza vaccine: Two doses of influenza vaccine (as a shot or nasal spray) are recommended for children 9 years and younger who are receiving the vaccine for the first time.

Source: Adapted from Centers for Disease Control and Prevention. Recommended childhood immunization schedule – United States, 2007. Pediatrics. 2007; 119.

Recommended Immunization Schedule for Persons Aged 7–18 Years

UNITED STATES • 2007

Vaccine ▼ Age ▶	7–10 years	11–12 YEARS	13–14 years 15 years 16–18 years
Tetanus, Diphtheria, Pertussis[1]	see footnote 1	Tdap	Tdap
Human Papillomavirus[2]	see footnote 2	HPV (3 doses)	HPV Series
Meningococcal[3]		MCV4	MCV4[3] / MCV4
Pneumococcal		PPV	
Influenza[4]		Influenza (Yearly)	
Hepatitis A		HepA Series	
Hepatitis B		HepB Series	
Inactivated Poliovirus		IPV Series	
Measles, Mumps, Rubella		MMR Series	
Varicella		Varicella Series	

Range of recommended ages

Catch-up immunization

Certain high-risk groups

This schedule gives the recommended ages for routine administration of currently licensed childhood vaccines for children aged 7–18 years. The information is based on the 2007 recommendations by the Advisory Committee on Immunization Practices, the American Academy of Pediatrics, and the American Academy of Family Physicians. Additional information is available at www.cdc.gov/vaccines/recs/schedules/default.htm#child. Because these recommendations may change or new vaccines may become available, always check with your child's doctor for the most current immunization information.

Footnotes to table 2

1) Tetanus and diphtheria toxoids and pertussis vaccine (Tdap): Give a dose at age 11–12 years for those who have completed the recommended childhood DTP/DTaP vaccination series and have not received a tetanus and diphtheria toxoids vaccine (Td) booster dose. Adolescents aged 13–18 years who missed the 11–12 year Td/Tdap booster dose should also receive a single dose of Tdap if they have completed the recommended childhood DTP/DTaP vaccination series.

2) Human papillomavirus vaccine (HPV): Give the first dose of the HPV vaccine series to females at age 11–12 years. Then give the second dose 2 months after the first dose and the third dose 6 months after the first dose. The HPV vaccine series may be given to females at age 13–18 years if not previously vaccinated.

3) Meningococcal vaccine: Two types of vaccine are available - MPSV4 for children aged 2–10 years and MCV4 (or MPSV4) for older children. The MCV4 may be given at age 11–12 years and to previously unvaccinated adolescents at high school entry (at approximately age 15 years). MCV4 (or MPSV4 is an acceptable alternative) is recommended for previously unvaccinated college freshmen living in dormitories.

4) Influenza vaccine: Two doses of influenza vaccine (as a shot or nasal spray) are recommended for children 9 years and younger who are receiving the vaccine for the first time.

Source: Adapted from Centers for Disease Control and Prevention. Recommended childhood immunization schedule – United States, 2007. Pediatrics. 2007; 119.

Recommended Adult Immunization Schedule
United States, October 2006–September 2007

Age group (yrs) ▶ Vaccine ▼	19–49 years	50–64 years	≥65 years
Tetanus, diphtheria, pertussis (Td/Tdap)[1]	1-dose Td booster every 10 yrs Substitute 1 dose of Tdap for Td		
Human papillomavirus (HPV)[2]	3 doses (females)		
Measles, mumps, rubella (MMR)	1 or 2 doses	1 dose	
Varicella[3,6]	2 doses (0, 4–8 wks)	2 doses (0, 4–8 wks)	
Influenza[4]	1 dose annually	1 dose annually	
Pneumococcal (polysaccharide)[5]	1–2 doses		1 dose
Hepatitis A	2 doses (0, 6–12 mos, or 0, 6–18 mos)		
Hepatitis B	3 doses (0, 1–2, 4–6 mos)		
Meningococcal			

For all persons in this category who meet the age requirements and who lack evidence of immunity (e.g., lack documentation of vaccination or have no evidence of prior infection)

Recommended if some other risk factor is present (e.g., on the basis of medical, occupational, lifestyle, or other indications)

This schedule provides the recommended US immunization schedule for adults. The information is based on recommendations by the Advisory Committee on Immunization Practices, the American Academy of Family Physicians, and the American College of Obstetricians and Gynecologists. Additional information is available at www.cdc.gov/vaccines/recs/schedules/adult-schedule.htm. Because these recommendations may change or new vaccines may become available, always check with your doctor for the most current immunization information.

Footnotes to table 3

1) Tetanus, diphtheria, and acellular pertussis (Td/Tdap): Tdap or tetanus and diphtheria (Td) vaccine may be used; Tdap should replace a single dose of Td for adults aged <65 years who have not previously received a dose of Tdap (either in the primary series, as a booster, or for wound management).

2) Human papillomavirus (HPV) vaccination: HPV vaccination is recommended for all females aged <26 years who have not completed the vaccine series. Ideally, vaccine should be administered before potential exposure to HPV through sexual activity; however, women who are sexually active should still be vaccinated.

3) Varicella vaccination: All adults without evidence of immunity to varicella should receive 2 doses of varicella vaccine.

4) Influenza vaccination: Healthy, nonpregnant persons aged 5–49 years without high-risk medical conditions who do not come into contact with severely immunocompromised persons in special care units can receive either intranasally administered influenza vaccine (FluMist®) or inactivated vaccine. Other persons should receive the inactivated vaccine.

5) Revaccination with pneumococcal polysaccharide vaccine: For persons aged >65 years, one-time revaccination if they were vaccinated >5 years previously and were aged <65 years at the time of primary vaccination.

6) Shingles (Zoster) vaccine: After the adult immunization schedule for 2006-07 was finalized, the Advisory Committee on Immunization Practices (ACIP) provided an additional recommendation that one dose of shingles vaccine be given to adults 60 years of age and older even if they have already had an episode of shingles (herpes zoster).

Source: Adapted from Centers for Disease Control and Prevention. Recommended adult immunization schedule – United States, October 2006 – September 2007. MMWR. 2006; 55Q1-4.

M⁓y Medication Record

It is important for you to keep a record of all of the prescription and nonprescription (over-the-counter) drugs you are taking, as well as any products such as vitamins, minerals, or other dietary supplements. This record is the most important contribution that you can make to medication safety and good medication management. You should bring this list with you each time you visit a doctor or other healthcare professional or if you are admitted to a hospital. It is also an important resource to carry with you in case of emergencies.

Please see the sample version of "My Medication Record" as an example of how to fill out this form. A tear-out version is provided for your use, as well as a permanent copy on the inside back cover of this book. Additional forms may be accessed online at www.consumerdrugreference.com.

My Medication Record

Name: John Smith   **Birth Date:** 5 / 29 / 50

Allergies: Penicillin

Medication Name	What is it For?	Dose	How Often?	Prescribed by: (phone #)	Start/Stop Dates
Zoloft (sertraline)	Depression	100 mg	Once per day in the morning	Dr. John Doe, 123-456-7890	Start 2/5/06

SAMPLE

This handy form can help you use medicine safely. Keep it up-to-date, and bring it with you to each hospital or doctor's visit.

My Medication Record

Name: _____

Birth Date: ___ / ___ / ___

Allergies: _____

Medication Name	What is it For?	Dose	How Often?	Prescribed by: (phone #)	Start/Stop Dates